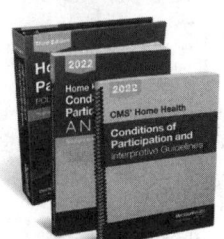

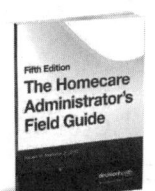

Complete Home Health

ICD-10-CM

Diagnosis Coding Manual

Ensure diagnosis coding and billing compliance

International Classification of Diseases,
10th Revision, Clinical Modification (ICD-10-CM)

2022 EDITION

Published by:

decisionhealth
an hcpro brand

AHCC
Home of BMSC & Caring Professionals

All the codes, indexes and other material in the International Classification of Diseases, 10th Revision, Clinical Modification (ICD-10-CM) are taken from official ICD-10-CM data tables and instructions from the National Center for Health Statistics (NCHS) and authorized for use by Medicare providers by the Centers for Medicare and Medicaid Services (CMS). NCHS serves as the World Health Organization (WHO) Collaborating Center for the Family of International Classifications for North America, and in this capacity is responsible for coordination of all official disease classification activities in the United States relating to the ICD and its use, interpretation, and periodic revision.

The tips and related content found in this coding manual are derived from CMS guidance, the official coding guidelines and Coding Clinic guidance. Additional proprietary information contained herein is compiled from DecisionHealth products ***Home Health Line***, ***Home Health Coding Center*** and ***Diagnosis Coding Pro for Home Health***.

Every reasonable effort has been made to ensure the accuracy of the information contained herein. However, the ultimate responsibility for correct coding lies with the provider of services. DecisionHealth, its employees, agents and staff make no representation, warranty or guarantee that use of the content herein ensures payment or will prevent disputes with Medicare or other third-party payers, and will not bear responsibility or liability for the results or consequences resulting from the use of this book.

Product Code: DHPABHHICD22
ISBN: 978-1-64535-127-6

decisionhealth
an hcpro brand

Subject Matter Expert Contributors

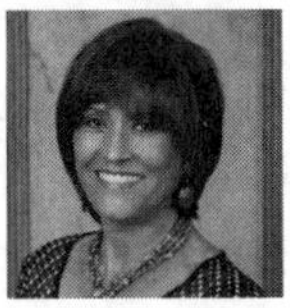

Lisa Selman-Holman, JD, BSN, RN, HCS-D, HCS-O, COS-C, is a 30-year veteran of home care as a registered nurse and attorney. She is the founder of Selman-Holman & Associates, a home care management and consulting company based in Denton, Texas, and the coding service CoDR – Coding Done Right. She is the Chair of the Board of Medical Specialty Coding and Compliance (BMSC) and one of the developers of the HCS-D examinations. Lisa is an AHIMA Approved ICD-10-CM/PCS Trainer.

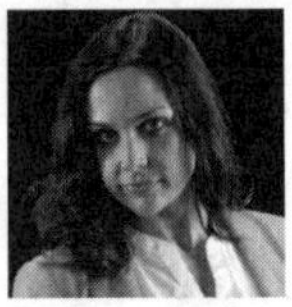

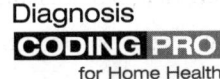

Brandi Whitemyer, RN, CDIP, COS-C, HCS-D, HCS-O, is a consultant and home health and hospice coding expert. She has more than 18 years of experience in post-acute healthcare as the previous owner of a full-service coding and consulting company, along with experience in the development of coding, billing/revenue cycle and clinical education resources for post-acute care. For the past 11 years, Brandi has worked with agencies on survey compliance, medical reviews and appeals of Medicare denials, writing corrective action plans and developing policy, managing revenue cycle and billing compliance, coding and quality assurance processes, and coding and OASIS education.

Also contributing subject matter expertise to the Coding Manual:

J'non Griffin, RN, MHA, WCC, HCS-D, HCS-H, COS-C, AHIMA-Approved ICD-10-CM Trainer/Ambassador, is the president of Home Health Solutions – A Simione Coding Company. Griffin offers home health consulting on many topics including quality assurance and performance improvement, program development, coding and OASIS review, staff education and plan of care compilation. Griffin has experience as a field nurse, director and executive with home health and hospice agencies.

DecisionHealth's 2022 Complete Home Health ICD-10-CM Diagnosis Coding Manual Team

Maria Tsigas, Product Director, Information
Susana Lambert, Production Editor & Coordinator
Dmitriy Bonin, Database Developer
Diana Chi, .NET Web Developer
AnnMarie Lemoine, Team Lead, Creative Layout
Nicole Grande, Senior Layout Artist

DecisionHealth
100 Winners Circle, Suite 300
Brentwood, TN 37027
store.decisionhealth.com

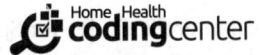

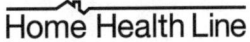

Table of Contents

Understanding this Manual

Before you can code a patient's diagnosis, it's important to understand how to use the ICD-10-CM manual. ICD-10-CM code(s) establish medical necessity for services rendered, and can impact the episodic payment a home health agency (HHA) receives under the Patient Driven Groupings Model (PDGM) payment system.

DecisionHealth's *Complete Home Health ICD-10-CM Diagnosis Coding Manual* contains many icons and highlights that call attention to key indicators and serve as triggers to alert you to instances when you may need additional information to accurately assign a specific code.

Here are the icons used in this Manual, and what they are calling attention to:

- $P This icon indicates the code is an acceptable primary diagnosis in PDGM and depending on its clinical group, will generate case-mix points and determine payment amount. **IMPORTANT:** This list is current as of the 1/1/21 PDGM grouper update. To view a list of all PDGM acceptable primary diagnoses along with their assigned clinical group, visit **decisionhealth.com/pdf/pdgm.zip.** If CMS updates the list after the Manual has published, we will upload the new list to this folder.
- !Q This icon indicates "questionable encounter" and appears on those codes that are NOT acceptable as primary diagnoses in PDGM. Under PDGM, failure to use a primary diagnosis code that fits into one of the clinical groups could result in claims getting kicked back to providers. **IMPORTANT:** This list is current as of the 1/1/21 PDGM grouper update. To view a list of all questionable encounter codes, visit **decisionhealth.com/pdf/pdgm.zip.** If CMS updates the list after the Manual has published, we will upload the new list to this folder.
- $H $L These icons are placed on those codes that can generate either a High or Low comorbidity adjustment in PDGM. In addition to assigning one principal diagnosis, you can assign up to 24 secondary diagnoses, and receive a comorbidity adjustment. **Only one adjustment is applied per episode.** Comorbidity adjustments fall into one of three categories: no, low or high. The adjustments are designed to account for the additional resource use required for patients with complex needs. To qualify for a **low** comorbidity adjustment, the claim must include **one secondary diagnosis** found within one of 12 comorbidity subgroups associated with higher resource use. To qualify for a **high** comorbidity adjustment, the claim must include **two or more secondary diagnoses** that fall within 34 comorbidity subgroup interactions that account for 18 distinct comorbidity subgroups. **IMPORTANT:** This list is current as of the 1/1/21 PDGM grouper update. To view a list of of those codes eligible for the low and high adjustment along with their subgroups, visit **decisionhealth.com/pdf/pdgm.zip.** If CMS updates the list after the Manual has published, we will upload the new list to this folder.
- $P !Q When both these icons appear on a code, it indicates that one or more of the 7th character codes are acceptable primary diagnoses and one or more are not acceptable. Note, you will find most of these instances in Chapter 19. To view a list of all PDGM acceptable primary diagnoses, visit **decisionhealth.com/pdf/pdgm.zip.**
- 4 5 6 7 These icons indicate that an additional character is required to make the code valid. When a 7th character is required, there is a box indicating what the 7th character means. Also, all codes requiring a 7th character will have a dash at the end of them indicating they are not valid until a 7th character is added. The 7th character is used in certain chapters to provide information about the characteristic of the encounter. For example in Chapter 19 (Injury, poisoning and certain other consequences of external causes), the 7th character indicates one of the following:
  - A = Initial encounter
  - D = Subsequent encounter
  - S = Sequela

  Additional examples of 7th character use can be found in Chapters 13 (musculoskeletal), 15 – 16 (obstetrics) and 20 (external causes).
- x7 This icon appears on codes that require a 7th character but are less than six characters. ICD-10-CM utilizes a placeholder character "X" for these codes. The placeholder "X" should be assigned for all characters less than six, and the 7th character must always be the 7th character of the code. Where a placeholder exists, the X must be used in order for the code to be considered a valid code. For these codes, we've already placed the X placeholders in the code for you; however, you will still need to choose the appropriate 7th character. An example of the x7 is at category T36 (Poisoning by, adverse effect of and underdosing of systemic antibiotics).
- Unspecified This indicator appears on codes that are described as 'unspecified'. Codes titled "unspecified" are for use when the information in

the medical record is insufficient to assign a more specific code. For those categories for which an unspecified code is not provided, the "other specified" code may represent both other and unspecified. Diagnoses codes that are too vague — meaning the code does not provide adequate information to support the need for home health services — won't fit into any of the groupings under PDGM; therefore it is imperative for home health coders to be as specific as possible when coding a condition.

- ✚ This indicator appears on codes with the instruction to "use additional code when documentation is present." Also, when a code contains instructions to "use additional code," "code first," and/or "code also," these instructions are highlighted in red to alert you that an additional code is required when assigning that particular code.
- M This icon indicates a manifestation code. Be alerted to these codes because they can never be coded alone and are never allowed to be listed as the primary diagnosis. Icons and educational notes help coders spot manifestation codes and sequence them properly – the etiology, or underlying condition, is sequenced first followed by the manifestation. In addition to the icon, these codes are highlighted in yellow with italic font in the Tabular to emphasize their importance. For example, see category F02 (Dementia in other diseases classified elsewhere) in the Tabular. In the Alphabetic Index, the etiology and manifestation conditions are listed together with the etiology code listed first followed by the manifestation code in brackets. For example, when you look up "dementia, with Parkinsonism" in the Index, code G31.83 (Parkinsonism) is listed first, followed by the manifestation code *[F02.80]*.
- ⊟ Be alerted to codes that require you to identify the specific side of the body, or both sides. Note, for bilateral sites, the final character of the codes indicates laterality. Example: L89.012 (Pressure ulcer of **right** elbow, stage 2).
- **Px** Z codes (found in Chapter 21) may be used as either a first-listed or secondary code, depending on the circumstances of the encounter. Certain Z codes may only be used as first-listed or principal diagnosis – these are indicated with a **Px** icon in the Tabular. The Z codes that may only be reported as the principal/first-listed diagnosis also are listed in the ICD-10 guidelines.
- H Look for this icon in the Tabular List to help identify acceptable hospice non-cancer diagnoses. ***Note:*** This is not an exhaustive list; it is just a starting point. Because of the expansion in coding diagnoses that contribute to the prognosis of 6 months or less, there are hundreds of codes that can be coded by hospice. The ones marked in the Manual with the hospice icon are those listed in the PGBA hospice LCD as well as those categories that are common hospice non-cancer diagnoses, such as I69 and I50. For more information on coding hospice diagnoses, see the Hospice section in the back of the Manual.
- ▲★ These icons in the Tabular alert you to codes that were newly added ★ or revised ▲ for the upcoming code year.

Tips, guidelines, alerts and definitions

This Manual provides our exclusive *DecisionHealth* content in the form of tips, guidelines, alerts and definitions in the Tabular that guide you on how to use a specific code to avoid common mistakes. Keep an eye out for the following indicators in the Tabular:

- CODING TIPS✓ Tips specific to home health ICD-10 coding that guide you, raise red flags and will help you code correctly.
- GUIDELINES ICD-10 guidelines embedded in the Tabular at the code level to alert you to the specific home health rules you need to be aware of to code accurately.
- ALERTS Specific "Alerts" on codes that are being denied with information on how to properly assign them to avoid having the claim denied.
- DEFINITION Definitions appear throughout to help you identify diseases and conditions to enhance coding and critical thinking skills.

Additional features

Other features of the Manual that help coders make the right choices and improve coding skills include:

- Home health **scenarios:** More than 100 home health scenarios and code assignment answers can be used to teach and learn proper coding. Look for these at the back of each Tabular chapter. Note that some disease chapters that are uncommon in home health, do not have scenarios. **Important:** Chapter 18 contains examples of scenarios in which it would be common to assign a symptom code in the primary position. However, these scenarios have been updated to demonstrate the importance of securing a more definitive diagnosis. Remember, the majority of symptom codes do not fit into any of the groupings under PDGM, and assigning one in the primary position could result in a claim denial.

- Narrative **chapter introductions** quickly give a sense of the codes you'll find in that specific disease chapter. The introductory comments before each chapter highlight the basics of what is covered in the section, including sequencing issues and guidance for assigning the top home care diagnoses. All introductions are written in plain English to help home health staff understand what is in the chapter.
- **Hospice coding primer:** In the back of the book you'll find hospice coding guidance based on the Hospice Wage Index rule and expert analysis to ensure accurate coding of hospice claims.
- **Official coding guidelines:** The FY2022 official coding guidelines are in a separate packet, delivered with your Coding Manual.

Defining ICD-10-CM & its conventions

Background on ICD-10

The National Center for Health Statistics (NCHS), the federal agency responsible for use of the International Statistical Classification of Diseases and Related Health Problems, 10th revision (ICD-10) in the United States, has developed a clinical modification for morbidity purposes. The ICD-10 was initially used to code and classify mortality data from death certificates, having replaced ICD-9 for this purpose as of Jan. 1, 1999. ICD-10-CM then replaced ICD-9-CM, volumes 1 and 2 as of Oct. 1, 2015.

The World Health Organization (WHO) owns and publishes the ICD-10 classification, and authorized the development of an adaptation of ICD-10 for use in the United States.

ICD-10-CM was developed following a thorough evaluation by a technical advisory panel and additional consultation with physician groups, clinical coders, and others to assure clinical accuracy and utility.

The American Hospital Association (AHA) and the American Health Information Management Association (AHIMA) conducted a field test for ICD-10-CM in summer 2003.

The clinical modification represents a significant improvement over ICD-9-CM. Specific improvements include: the addition of information relevant to ambulatory and managed care encounters; expanded injury codes; the creation of combination diagnosis/symptom codes to reduce the number of codes needed to fully describe a condition; the addition of sixth and seventh characters; laterality; and greater specificity in code assignment. The new structure allows further expansion than was possible with ICD-9-CM.

On Jan. 16, 2009, the Department of Health and Human Services (HHS) published a final rule adopting ICD-10-CM (and ICD-10-PCS) to replace ICD-9-CM in HIPAA-covered transactions, effective Oct. 1, 2013. However, that effective date was postponed twice and the implementation finally occurred on Oct. 1, 2015. *[www.cdc.gov/nchs/icd/icd10cm.htm#10update.]*

What is ICD-10-CM?

ICD-10-CM, or the International Classification of Diseases, 10th Edition, Clinical Modification, applies to all covered entities. A number of other countries have also moved to ICD-10, including:

- United Kingdom (1995);
- France (1997);
- Australia (1998);
- Germany (2000); and
- Canada (2001).

The ICD-10-CM system is an improvement in that it provides a higher level of detail and the ability to expand to capture new technologies and advancements in clinical medicine. ICD-10-CM will lead to more accurate payment for services rendered, and facilitate evaluation of medical processes and outcomes, according to CMS.

ICD-10-CM/PCS consists of two parts:

- **ICD-10-CM for diagnosis coding:** This is the diagnosis classification system developed by the Centers for Disease Control and Prevention for use in all U.S. health care treatment settings. It consists of the Alphabetic Index an the Tabular List, and uses 3–7 alpha and numeric digits and full code titles;
- **ICD-10-PCS for inpatient procedure coding:** This is the procedure classification system developed by the Centers for Medicare & Medicaid Services (CMS) for use in the U.S. for inpatient hospital settings **ONLY. Home health does *not* use ICD-10 procedure codes.**

Breakdown of ICD-10-CM

To select a code that corresponds to a diagnosis or reason for the visit documented in the medical record, first locate the term in the Alphabetic Index, and then verify the code in the Tabular List. Make sure to read and adhere to all instructional notations that appear in both the Alphabetic Index and the Tabular List.

You must use both the Alphabetic Index and Tabular List when locating and assigning a code. The Alphabetic Index does not always provide the full code. Selection of the full code, including laterality and any applicable 7th character, can only be done in the Tabular List. A dash (-) at the end of an Alphabetic Index entry or Tabular code indicates that additional characters are required. Even when a dash is not included at the Alphabetic Index, you must refer to the Tabular List to verify that no 7th character is required.

Tabular List

The Tabular List is a numerical listing of the ICD-10 codes and their descriptors classified to etiology of conditions or to conditions that affect a specific body system. The Tabular List explains the details of how coding a particular condition must be done. Includes and Excludes 1 and 2 notes give more guidance, and can help validate code selection or steer you to another area.

ICD-10-CM diagnosis codes are composed of codes with 3, 4, 5, 6 or 7 characters. Codes with three characters are included as the heading of a category that may be further subdivided by the use of fourth and/or fifth characters and/or sixth characters, which provide greater detail.

A three-character code is to be used only if it is not further subdivided. A code is invalid if it has not been coded to the full number of characters required for that code, including the 7th character, if applicable.

The tabular code list contains categories, subcategories and codes. Characters for categories, subcategories and codes may be either a letter or a number. All categories are three characters. Subcategories are either 4 or 5 characters. Codes may be 3, 4, 5, 6 or 7 characters.

Here's an example:

M1a: Chronic Gout

M1a.3: Chronic gout due to renal impairment

M1a.33: Chronic gout due to renal impairment, wrist

M1a.332: Chronic gout due to renal impairment, left wrist

The appropriate code or codes from A00.0 through T88.9-, Z00.-- Z99.89 must be used to identify diagnoses, symptoms, conditions, problems, complaints or other reason(s) for the encounter/visit.

Codes that describe symptoms and signs, as opposed to diagnoses, are acceptable for reporting purposes when a related definitive diagnosis has not been established (confirmed) by the provider. ICD-10 Chapter 18, Symptoms, Signs, and Abnormal Clinical and Laboratory Findings, Not Elsewhere Classified (codes R00.0 - R99), contains many, but not all codes for symptoms.

Alphabetic Index

You should not code directly from the Alphabetic Index. First, review the medical record to extract the pertinent written descriptions of the disease or symptoms. Then, look up the condition, injury, or sign/symptom in the Index, and then verify the code(s) in the Tabular Listing.

The Alphabetic Index is an index of diseases, injuries, symptoms and other reasons for a patient encounter. The main terms are in boldface type and should never be referenced by anatomical site. When using the Index, you would reference the "condition," or other key words to locate potential diagnosis assignment.

When consulting the Alphabetic Index, several codes listed may seem applicable at first. To determine which one is correct, consult the Tabular List. In reviewing the Tabular List, pay attention to the chapter and subsection in which the code appears. This can help in the selection of the correct code when several alternatives may appear suitable. Follow all instructional notes at the category and specific code areas.

Subterms are indented under the main term and indicate the site, type, or etiology for conditions or injuries. More specificity in the condition will be further indented to the right, as needed. Connecting words such as "with," "due to," "in," or "associated with" indicate a relationship between the main term and the subterm.

The word "with" or "in" should be interpreted to mean "associated with" or "due to" when it appears in a code title, the Alphabetic Index, or an instructional note in the Tabular List. The classification presumes a causal relationship between the two conditions linked by these terms. These conditions should be coded as related even in the absence of provider documentation explicitly linking them, unless the documentation clearly states the conditions are unrelated or when another guideline exists that specifically requires a documented linkage between two conditions (e.g., sepsis guideline for "acute organ dysfunction that is not clearly associated with the sepsis"), according to the official coding guidelines conventions.

Another important coding convention is the etiology/manifestation convention. When two codes are required to indicate etiology and manifestation, the manifestation code will appear italicized and in [brackets] following the etiology code. The conditions are to be assigned as listed: the etiology code precedes the *[manifestation code]* in sequencing.

Neoplasm Table

In the Alphabetic Index also contains the Neoplasm Table. The Neoplasm Table appears at the end of the Alphabetic Index.

In the Neoplasm Table, codes listed with a dash (–) following the code have a required 5th character for laterality. The tabular list must be reviewed for the complete code.

Table of Drugs and Chemicals

After the Neoplasm Table is the Table of Drugs and Chemicals. This table contains a classification of drugs and other chemical substances associated with poisonings and external causes of adverse effects. The table's rows identify the substance and the columns define the intent: poisoning, accidental (unintentional); poisoning, intentional self-harm; poisoning, assault; poisoning, undetermined; adverse effect; and underdosing.

There often is confusion as to when coding a poisoning is appropriate versus when coding an adverse effect is appropriate. In ICD-10, when the drug was correctly prescribed and properly administered and the patient experienced a problem, it is an adverse effect. Assign the code for the nature of the adverse effect followed by the code for the adverse effect of the drug (T36-T50).

Unlike an adverse effect, a poisoning involves a scenario in which the drug was *not* taken correctly. Poisoning codes have an associated intent: accidental, intentional self-harm, assault and undetermined. List the poisoning code first, followed by the symptoms (effects).

Index to External Cause of Injuries

The final section of the Alphabetic Index is the Index to External Cause of Injuries. This section classifies environmental events, circumstances, and conditions as the *cause of* injury, poisoning and other adverse effects. The Index to External Cause of Injuries is organized by main terms that describe the accident, circumstance, event, or specific agent causing the injury or other adverse effect.

ICD-10-CM Guidelines

All necessary coding guidance can be found in the ICD-10-CM Coding Guidelines and the instructional notes embedded within the Tabular.

ICD-10-CM Conventions

The conventions for ICD-10-CM are the general rules for use independent of the guidelines. These conventions are incorporated within the Alphabetic Index and Tabular List as instructional notes. You should take note of the following key conventions:

Abbreviations

- NEC – Not elsewhere classifiable: This abbreviation represents "other specified." When a specific code is not available for a condition, the Alphabetic Index directs the coder to the "other specified" code in the Tabular List.
- NOS – Not otherwise specified: This abbreviation is the equivalent of unspecified.

Punctuation

- [ ] Brackets are used in the Tabular List to enclose synonyms, alternative wording or explanatory phrases. Brackets are used in the Alphabetic Index to identify manifestation codes.
- () Parentheses are used in both the Alphabetic Index and Tabular List to enclose supplementary words that may be present or absent in the statement of a disease or procedure without affecting the code number to which it is assigned. The terms within the parentheses are referred to as nonessential modifiers.

  The nonessential modifiers in the Alphabetic Index to Diseases apply to subterms following a main term except when a nonessential modifier and a subentry are mutually exclusive, the subentry takes precedence. For example, in the ICD-10-CM Alphabetic Index under the main term Enteritis, "acute" is a nonessential modifier and "chronic" is a subentry. In this case, the nonessential modifier "acute" does not apply to the subentry "chronic."
- **:** Colons are used in the Tabular List after an incomplete term, which needs one or more of the modifiers following the colon to make it assignable to a given category.

Instructional Notations

- INCLUDES This note appears immediately under a three character code title to further define, or give examples of, the content of the category.
- **Excludes Notes:** ICD-10 has two types of excludes notes. Each type of note has a different definition.
  - EXCLUDES 1 Excludes 1 means "not coded here." An Excludes 1 note indicates that the code excluded should ***never*** be used at the same time as the code above the Excludes 1 note. An Excludes 1 is used when two conditions cannot occur together, such as a congenital form versus an acquired form of the same condition. ***Note:*** You may code two conditions together, even if one or both of them is listed in an Excludes 1 note, as long as they are ***not related***.
  - EXCLUDES 2 Excludes 2 means "not included here." An Excludes 2 note indicates that the condition excluded is not part of the condition represented by the code, but a patient may have both conditions at the same time. When an Excludes 2 note appears under a code, it is acceptable to use both the code and the excluded code together, when appropriate.

Laterality

Some ICD-10-CM codes indicate laterality, specifying whether the condition occurs on the left, right or is bilateral. If no bilateral code is provided and the condition is bilateral, assign separate codes for both the left and right side. If the side is not identified in the medical record, assign the code for the unspecified side.

Deep dive into ICD-10 conventions & guidelines

The coding conventions always take precedence over the coding guidelines.

A keen understanding of how coding conventions and guidelines interact will help you navigate through thorny scenarios where guidance sometimes is contradictory, and where getting it wrong can lead to claim rejections and cash-flow interruptions.

Section I of the *Official Coding Guidelines* encases the coding conventions, general coding guidelines and chapter-specific coding guidelines. While conventions always supersede both sets of guidelines, general and chapter-specific guidelines carry the same weight.

Build your foundation with ICD-10 conventions

The following are a few of the ***ICD-10 coding conventions***, along with specific examples that will apply to home health. Master these before moving on to studying ICD-10 coding guidelines, as these instructions will always take precedence:

Etiology-manifestation sequencing *[I.A.13]*: A manifestation code must be sequenced directly after its etiology, and it can never be coded primary. As a convention, this sequencing instruction will trump other instructions in the guidelines, such as the rule to sequence a residual code before its related sequela code *[I.B.10]*.

The 7th character *[I.A.5]*: Certain ICD-10 codes require the use of a 7th character, such as fracture codes, which are coded on home health claims instead of an aftercare code. The code will be considered invalid if the 7th character is not included, or isn't assigned in the 7th position. ***Example:*** Consider the code for a fracture of the shaft of the right fibula in ICD-10, S82.401. By itself, S82.401 is invalid; it needs a 7th character, such as "D" for subsequent encounter for closed fracture with routine healing. "D" will be the 7th character most commonly used for the care of fractures in home health.

The placeholder character *[I.A.4]*: A placeholder character "x" is used to fill in unused spaces with certain ICD-10 codes that require a 7th character designation, but the most subdivided form of the code doesn't contain at least six characters. ***Example:*** Home health will often use these placeholder characters with external cause codes found in Chapter 20. Many of these codes are made up of only four characters, but require a 7th character to describe the type of encounter, whether initial (A), subsequent (D) or sequela (S). Consider X10.2 for Contact with fats and cooking oils, which is only four digits, but needs the 7th character to be valid. This code requires two placeholder x's to result in X10.2xxD (Contact with fat and cooking oils, subsequent encounter). Note that when placeholders are required, the x's must be used in order for the code to be valid. ***Note:*** Invalid codes due to missing 7th characters or placeholder x's were among the top reasons for claims being returned for provider (RTP'd) in the first several months following the ICD-10 implementation.

Excludes 1 and Excludes 2 notes *[I.A.12.a/b]*: ICD-10 employs two types of Excludes notes.

An **Excludes 1** note means that two conditions can ***never*** be coded together. ***Example***: An Excludes 1 note at the E10.- category level (Type 1 diabetes mellitus) lists E11.- which is the category that contains codes for Type 2 diabetes mellitus. This means you can never assign a code from the E10.- category along with a code from the E11.- category. ***Note:*** You may code two conditions together, even if one or both of them is listed in an Excludes 1 note, as long as they are ***not related***.

An **Excludes 2** note implies that two conditions ***could be coded*** on the same claim if appropriate. ***Example***: A home health patient could have both an acute bronchitis infection on top of chronic obstructive bronchitis, a form of COPD. The ICD-10 code for acute obstructive bronchitis is J20.9, and it carries an Excludes 2 note that lists codes from the J44.- category (Other chronic obstructive pulmonary disease). The Excludes 2 note communicates that the acute bronchitis is not the same as chronic obstructive bronchitis, but they can be assigned together if both are diagnosed.

The **word "with" or "in" should be interpreted** to mean "associated with" or "due to" when it appears in a code title, the Alphabetic Index (either under a main term or subterm), or an instructional note in the Tabular List. The classification presumes a causal relationship between the two conditions linked by these terms. These conditions should be coded as related even in the absence of provider documentation explicitly linking them, unless the documentation clearly states the conditions are unrelated or when another guideline exists that specifically requires a documented linkage between two conditions (e.g., sepsis guideline for "acute organ dysfunction that is not clearly associated with the sepsis"). The word "with" in the Alphabetic Index is sequenced immediately following the main term or subterm, not in alphabetical order.

Take note of key ICD-10 guidelines

Further your grasp of ICD-10 by developing a thorough understanding of ***ICD-10 coding guidelines***, once you'd laid a firm foundation on the coding conventions. These ICD-10 guidelines will have a direct impact on home health coding:

Laterality *[I.B.13]*: The ICD-10 code set provides a way to capture laterality — that is, a right or left side, or bilateral, designation. ***Example***: Consider the M17.- category for Osteoarthritis of knee. A fourth character of "0" indicates that the condition is primary and bilateral (on both sides). If that patient's osteoarthritis is primary and confined to his right knee, for example, the correct code would be M17.11 (Unilateral primary osteoarthritis, right knee).

Coders can assign a unilateral code in the case of a patient who had a condition on both sides of the body, but for whom treatment resolved the condition on one side and it still exists on the other. An example of this would be a patient whose cataract in one eye is resolved through surgery but who still has a cataract in the other eye. However, if the treatment on the first side didn't resolve the condition completely, the bilateral code should still be used, according to coding guidelines.

Sequelae *[I.B.10]*: What were known as late effects in ICD-9 are ***sequela*** in ICD-10, and are governed by the rules in this guideline. The condition currently at hand, that resulted from the past illness or injury, i.e. the residual, is to be coded ***before*** the sequela form of the code for the now-resolved illness or injury. ***Example:*** Consider a woman being treated in home health for a contracture of her right hand that resulted from a third-degree burn suffered several years ago. The contracture is the residual and is coded with M24.541 (Contracture, right hand). It is immediately followed by the sequela form of the code for the injury that caused it, the burn, T23.301S (Burn of third degree of right hand, unspecified site, sequela). Notice the 7th character "S" on the code, which designates it as a sequela, as opposed to an active condition.

Steps to Accurate Coding

Recording diagnoses is the responsibility of the attending physician. As of Jan. 1, 1998, physicians are required by law to provide the diagnosis information for Medicare and Medicaid patients (*Balanced Budget Act, HR 2015 Sec 4317*). Failure to do so can result in prosecution. The physician must supply the diagnosis code for all services and testing performed or ordered, including home health care. Although the law provides for the physician to provide the diagnosis codes, home health providers do not always find this to be true. OASIS assessment strategies allow diagnosis information to be obtained through assessment with verification from the physician. The plan of care lists the conditions that require or may impact home health care; these conditions are listed in following forms: plan of care, OASIS and the claim form (UB-04).

Warning: The hospital discharge diagnosis is not always the reason home care is provided. There should be close scrutiny of the primary diagnosis assigned. The home health PPS rule states that the only clinicians who can determine the primary and secondary or other diagnoses are the assessing clinicians, including the registered nurse, and physical, occupational, or speech therapists. The assigned codes on the OASIS comprehensive assessment must match the home health plan of care, as well as those on the home health claim submitted.

Basic Coding Steps

Review the plan of care and assessment to find the reason(s) for home health services. The need for medically necessary skilled services is used in judging the relevancy of a diagnosis to the plan of care (POC) and to the OASIS. A review of qualifications for various skilled services under the home health benefit can be found in Chapter 7 of the Medicare Benefit Policy Manual.

To select a code in the classification that corresponds to a diagnosis or reason for visit documented in a medical record, first locate the term in the Alphabetic Index, and then verify the code in the Tabular List. You should read and be guided by instructional notations that appear in both the Alphabetic Index and Tabular list. It is essential to use both the Alphabetic Index and Tabular List when locating and assigning a code. The format of the Alphabetic Index and the Tabular list are dictionary style: Main terms in the Alphabetic Index are set flush with the left- hand margin and printed in bold type.

The Alphabetic Index does not always provide the full code. Selection of the full code, including laterality and 7th character, can only be completed in the Tabular. A dash (-) at the end of a code at the Alphabetic Index will indicate that additional characters are required. Even if a dash is not included at the Alphabetic Index entry, it is necessary to refer to the Tabular List to verify that no 7th character is required.

Follow any instructions that direct you to "see" another code. This is a crucial step that must be completed.

Identify any manifestation code (these codes will have two selections with a code in brackets following the main code). This pair is to be assigned with the etiology preceding the manifestation. For example: Dementia with Lewy Bodies: G31.83 first listed, *[F02.80]* follows etiology.

General Coding Guidelines

The ICD-10-CM coding guidelines are revised and approved by the American Hospital Association, the American Health Information Management Association, the Centers for Medicare and Medicaid Services and the National Center for Health Statistics. They state:

1. The appropriate code or codes from A00.0 through T88.9, Z00.0-Z99.8 are used to identify diagnoses, symptoms, conditions, problems, complaints, or other reason(s) for encounter/visit.
2. For accurate reporting of ICD-10-CM diagnosis codes, the documentation should describe the patient's condition using terminology that includes specific diagnoses as well as symptoms, problems, or reasons for the encounter. There are ICD-10-CM codes to describe all of these.
3. Codes that describe symptoms and signs, as opposed to diagnoses, are acceptable for reporting purposes when a diagnosis has not been established (confirmed) by the physician. Chapter 18, Symptoms, Signs and Abnormal Clinical and Laboratory Findings, Note Elsewhere Classified (codes R00.0-R99), contains many, but not all, codes for symptoms.
4. ICD-10-CM is composed of codes with three, four, five, six or seven characters. Codes with three characters are included in ICD-10-CM as the headings for categories of codes that may be further subdivided by the use of fourth and/ or fifth characters and/or sixth characters, which provide greater specificity.

A three-character code is to be used only if it is not further subdivided. A code is invalid if it has not been coded to the full number of characters required for that code, including the seventh character, if applicable.

Rules for selecting the primary and secondary diagnoses codes come from OASIS requirements and ICD-10-CM guidelines. OASIS instructions state to follow the official guidelines for coding.

In the Alphabetic Index, reference the entire "indented" series of codes following a main term. These indented terms underneath the main bold term are called "sub entries." Their purpose is to add specificity to the code.

These "sub entries" change the code term and increase the specificity of a code. The first code at the main bold term is usually an unspecified code, also known as 'not otherwise specified' (NOS). Only use NOS codes if you do not have access to more specific information.

The word "with" in the Alphabetic Index is sequenced immediately following the main term or subterm, not in alphabetical order.

The word "with" or "in" should be interpreted to mean "associated with" or "due to" when it appears in a code title, the Alphabetic Index, or an instructional note in the Tabular List. The classification presumes a causal relationship between the two conditions linked by these terms in the Alphabetic Index or Tabular List, according to the official coding guidelines.

These conditions should be coded as related even in the absence of provider documentation explicitly linking them, unless the documentation clearly states the conditions are unrelated. For conditions not specifically linked by these relational terms in the classification, provider documentation must link the conditions in order to code them as related.

An example is diabetes and the manifestations listed underneath the word 'with' in the alphabetical index, but the convention also applies to other instances where the word 'with' is a sub entry under a main term in the alpha listing. However, if there is ever uncertainty as to the relationship between two conditions, query the physician.

Write down the code possibilities and verify in the Tabular List the accurate code assignment. Be sure to read the notes at the Tabular List for the accurate code assignment and sequencing. The patient's primary focus of care for the home health episode will be the principal code choice, unless official coding guidelines otherwise apply.

Assign the code(s) selected in proper sequence. List first the ICD-10-CM code for the diagnosis, condition, problem, or other reason for the home health visit documented in the medical record as chiefly responsible for the services provided. List additional codes that describe any coexisting conditions managed during the episode of care.

If more than one diagnosis is treated concurrently, the diagnosis that represents the most acute condition and requires the most intensive services should be entered first. The primary diagnosis is the diagnosis most related to the POC; most acute diagnosis; and the chief reason for providing home care. The secondary or other diagnoses must be relevant to the care rendered. Include conditions actively addressed and any comorbid conditions affecting the patient's responsiveness to treatment and rehabilitative prognosis, even if the condition is not the focus of any home health treatment itself. A diagnosis, once listed, must be supported by documentation in the comprehensive assessment (OASIS) and in the plan of care.

Do not assign a diagnosis documented as "probable," "suspected," "questionable," "rule-out," or "working." Rather, code the condition(s) to the highest degree of certainty for the visit, such as symptoms, signs, or other reasons.

Chronic conditions treated on an ongoing basis may be coded and reported as many times as the patient receives treatment and care for the condition. A chronic condition, even if not the focus of care, will always impact the care and should be coded as a pertinent diagnosis. These diagnoses also should be addressed in the plan of care. Do not code conditions that are resolved, i.e. no longer exist, or do not impact the home health plan of care.

As a home care provider, you should try to select an ICD-10 code from Chapters 1 – 19 that best describes the patient's current, active condition under treatment. However, be aware that there also are additional codes (supplemental classification) that are important to coding. Z codes identify conditions other than illness that result in the use of health care services. For example, Z47.1 describes aftercare following joint replacement surgery. In addition, V, W, X, and Y codes classify external causes of morbidity, such as X11.0- (Contact with hot water in a bath or tub), and include codes for adverse effects and poisonings.

Code to the highest level of specificity

The diagnosis codes are made up of three, four, five, six, or seven characters. When coding the patient's condition, the ICD-10-CM code must be taken to the highest level of specificity.

If a three-character category further subdivides into 4th, 5th, 6th, or 7th characters, the completed code must include the appropriate 4th, 5th, 6th, and 7th characters, as indicated. A three-character code category is to be used only if it is not further subdivided into 4th, 5th, 6th, or 7th character requirements. For example, Unspecified viral encephalitis (A86), Unspecified mood disorder (F39), Microencephalopathy (Q02), Unspecified urinary incontinence (R32), Nondiabetic hypoglycemic coma (E15), are all examples where three characters represent the highest specificity.

Where 4th, 5th, 6th and/or 7th character subclassifications are provided, they must be assigned or the result will be an invalid Medicare claim. Assigning the highest degree of specificity will enable Medicare to properly classify the severity of the patient's condition. Additionally, you will avoid having your Medicare claim rejected.

Using combination codes

ICD-10-CM includes a number of codes referred to as "combination codes." A combination code is a single code used to classify two diagnoses, or a diagnosis with an associated secondary process (manifestation), or a diagnosis with an associated complication. Not all conditions may be captured by the use of combination codes, but some may, and in those cases, the combination code should be assigned. Assign only the combination code when that code fully identifies the diagnostic conditions involved or when the Alphabetic Index so directs. Multiple coding should not be used when the classification provides a combination code that clearly identifies all of the elements documented in the diagnosis.

For example, many diabetes codes in the ICD-10-CM code set utilize combination codes to capture both the diabetes and a manifestation of the diabetes within one ICD-10 code. Type 2 diabetes mellitus with unspecified diabetic retinopathy with macular edema is coded to E11.311. This is an example of using a combination code that classifies a diagnosis with an associated secondary process (manifestation) within the combination code. No second code is assigned for the retinopathy or macular edema, as the single combination code includes these conditions.

Only when the combination code lacks specificity in describing the manifestation or complication, an additional code should be used. In such a case, sequencing guidelines for the specific combination code will indicate to "use an additional code." For example, when assigning the combination code E11.22, Type 2 diabetes with diabetic chronic kidney disease, an additional code is required to identify the stage of chronic kidney disease. Instructions at the code level will indicate to use an additional code to identify the stage of chronic kidney disease (N18.1 – N18.6), which should be sequenced following the E11.22 code.

Manifestation coding steps

In certain cases, ICD-10-CM requires that more than one code be assigned to report a condition. This requirement, termed "etiology/manifestation coding" often involves both a disease (etiology) and one of its manifestations. The ICD-10-CM manual clearly shows the instances where manifestation coding is required. You'll notice that these codes are listed in the Alphabetic Index with the etiology code listed first, followed by the manifestation code italicized in brackets. The code appearing in brackets is always to be sequenced second. Additionally, these codes appear in the Tabular List with a "code first" note at the manifestation code and a "use additional code" note at the etiology code. Coding conventions require that these sequencing guidelines be followed and failure to follow correct sequencing for a manifestation/etiology code pair may result in return of the claim to the provider.

To help you identify them, manifestation codes in the Tabular List are italicized and highlighted in yellow with an 'M' to the left of the code. Manifestation codes may never appear in the principal diagnosis field, and must be preceded by the code for the underlying condition (etiology). Every manifestation code in the Tabular List is accompanied by instructions to report the etiology first.

The sequencing instructions in the ICD-10-CM Coding Guidelines for manifestation coding for a single condition are only intended to apply to diagnoses that are required to be sequenced a certain way by the coding guidelines, e.g., manifestations, sequelae, complications.

Therefore, unless an agency encounters such a situation when consulting the Alphabetic Index or Tabular List, it should continue to list the primary reason for home care in the principal diagnosis field as it has always done. ICD-10-CM guidelines, except in the case of manifestation coding and other specific sequencing guidelines, do not direct users to report the root cause of a patient's health problems when a more proximate diagnosis is available. For example, consider neurogenic bladder in a stable MS patient or radiculitis in a stable MS patient. In these cases, when the proximate diagnosis (neurogenic bladder or radiculitis) is the main reason for home care, it is reported as the primary diagnosis, and the underlying condition (MS) is a secondary diagnosis. Always consult the Official Coding Guidelines and instructions for guidance on sequencing.

Sequela coding steps

A "sequela" is the residual effect (condition produced) after the acute phase of an injury or illness has terminated. The residual effect may be apparent early, such as after an acute phase of illness (e.g., CVA), or it may occur much later, a year or more, as with a previous injury. Examples of sequelae include: scar formation due to a healed burn, deviated septum due to a nasal fracture, and infertility due to tubal occlusion from old tuberculosis. Coding of sequelae generally requires two codes sequenced in the following order: the condition or nature of the sequela is sequenced first. The sequela code is sequenced second.

An exception to this general sequencing guideline includes instances where the code for the sequela is followed by a manifestation code identified in the Tabular List, or the sequela code has been expanded (at the 4th, 5th or 6th character levels) to include the manifestation(s) (for example, I69.391, Dysphagia following cerebral infarction, should be sequenced prior to the code for the type of dysphagia).

To identify the sequela code, reference the word "sequela" in the Alphabetic Index.

Coding from the Table of Drugs and Chemicals

Knowing when to use a code to indicate a poisoning or an adverse event can be tricky. Consider the following ICD-10-CM rules when coding poisonings and adverse events.

A substance used incorrectly is poisoning in ICD-10 terms. However, it's also considered a poisoning if the patient's condition is caused by the interaction between a therapeutic drug used correctly and a nonprescription drug or alcohol. For example, a patient may present with acute liver failure because he correctly took Valium, but he also consumed ethyl alcohol. This would be considered a poisoning.

When a patient presents with a poisoning, list the combination code for the drug or substance causing the poisoning code first (and the circumstance), then follow with a code for the effect of the poisoning.

In the Valium and alcohol example above, you would first code T51.0X1D (accidental poisoning by alcohol, subsequent encounter), followed by T42.4X1D (accidental poisoning due to Valium, subsequent episode) followed by K72.00 (Acute hepatic failure without coma).

Check the documentation for the following clues that the condition is considered a poisoning: wrong medication given or taken, wrong dosage given or taken, medication given to or taken by the wrong person, intoxication (other than cumulative, see "adverse effect"), or the term "overdose."

ICD-10-CM also includes codes for underdosing of a medication. Underdosing refers to taking less than is prescribed by a provider or manufacturer's instruction. Do not assign codes for underdosing as a primary diagnosis under any condition. Rather, the medical condition for which the underdosed medication was prescribed should be assigned, if this condition relapsed or exacerbated. A code for non-compliance (Z91.12-, Z91.13-) should be assigned with a code for underdosing when appropriate.

A substance used correctly, but with an unintended reaction, is considered an adverse effect for ICD-10 purposes. This includes a bad interaction between two or more therapeutic drugs that have been used correctly.

When coding an adverse effect, sequence the nature of the adverse effect first, then follow with the appropriate combination code from T36 – T50 for the adverse effect of the drug.

Terms you might see in your physician's documentation that signal an adverse effect include: "allergic reaction," "cumulative effect" of a drug (toxicity), "hypersensitivity" to a drug, "idiosyncratic reaction," "paradoxical reaction," or "synergistic reaction."

Remember to always check the Tabular List when coding from the Table of Drugs and Chemicals.

What happens if you choose the wrong code?

If a diagnosis is listed on the billing form and no supporting documentation is found in the medical record, there may be financial consequences for the home health entity, and the discrepancy is an audit liability.

Conditions for which there is no supporting documentation should not be reported. Query the physician if there are questions on documentation.

CMS has software programs that scan forms (OASIS, UB-04) for discrepancies (i.e., final diagnosis code submitted not matching the codes on the UB-04, OASIS, etc.). This could suspend payment and require additional document review by the MAC and other government contractors.

Prospective audits should be conducted by the home health agency to ensure accurate capture of the appropriate ICD-10-CM codes as well as consistency across forms (plan of care, OASIS and UB-04). Careful attention must be paid to the differences in the coding rules between home health agencies and hospitals/physicians.

Also consider that correct coding is a requirement of HIPAA compliance.

FY2022 Code Change Summary

Starting Oct. 1, 2021, coders will be able to assign **U09.9** (Post COVID-19 condition, unspecified) to capture post COVID-19 conditions — or cases when a patient continues to have lingering symptoms after the infection is gone.

This code is not to be used in cases that are still presenting with active COVID-19. However, an exception is made in cases of re-infection with COVID-19, occurring with a condition related to prior COVID-19, according to the FY2022 Tabular addenda.

Coders should list U09.9 secondary to specific codes for lingering conditions such as chronic respiratory failure (J96.1-), loss of smell (R43.8), loss of taste (R43.8), multisystem inflammatory syndrome (M35.81), pulmonary embolism (I26.-) and pulmonary fibrosis (J84.10), according to new tabular instructions for the code

Overall, the FY2022 update includes159 new codes, an additional 130 revisions to Tabular instructions and code descriptions, and 32 codes deemed invalid.

Other notable updates

- A new code to capture depression — **F32.A** (Depression, unspecified). The addition of a code for depression NOS is more clinically accurate versus assigning these patients a 'major depressive disorder' code, say coding experts. Major depressive disorder has specific clinical criteria and an unspecified depression may not meet those criteria
- The Tabular instruction at category **I20-I25** (Ischemic heart diseases) has changed. The note stating "Use Additional code to identify presence of hypertension (I10-I16)" has been deleted, and replaced with: "**Code also** the presence of hypertension (I10-I16)".
- New code **I5A** to capture non-ischemic myocardial injury (non-traumatic).
- 8 new codes to further capture irritant contact dermatitis. More specifically, irritant contact dermatitis due to friction or contact with body fluids (**L24.A-**) and irritant contact dermatitis related to stoma or fistula (**L24.B-**).
- Chapter 13 accounts for 20 code changes, including an expansion of the category for Sjogren syndrome (**M35.0-**) and a new series of codes for non-radiographic axial spondyloarthritis (**M45.A-**). The diagnosis code for low back pain (M54.5) has been expanded to distinguish vertebrogenic low back pain (**M54.51**) from other types.
- Six new codes to add specificity to coughs (R05), including acute (**R05.1**), subacute (**R05.2**), chronic (**R05.3**), cough syncope (**R05.4**), other specified (**R05.8**), and unspecified (**R05.9**).
- 12 new codes that describe poisonings, adverse effects and underdosing for synthetic cannabinoids (**T40.71-, T40.72-**). For example, **T40.721A** (Poisoning by synthetic cannabinoids, accidental (unintentional), initial encounter) and **T40.725A** (Adverse effect of synthetic cannabinoids, initial encounter). These codes **replace the T40.7X-** codes (Poisoning by, adverse effect of and underdosing of cannabis (derivatives)), which are deemed invalid in the FY2022 update.
- 11 new codes to capture various social determinants of health including **Z55.5** (Less than a high school diploma), **Z58.6** (Inadequate drinking-water supply) and **Z59.00** (Homelessness unspecified). Home health industry experts noted that the addition of social determinants of health codes are beneficial as they will be important items in OASIS-E.

Quick Reference Guide to Alphabetic Index Search Terms

Use this tool to help you more efficiently locate correct codes in the alphabetic index

Diagnosis	Term to search for in the index
Pressure ulcer	Search "ulcer, pressure" and then to body site affected
Pseudogout	Search under "chondrocalcinosis"
Chronic nephritis due to systemic lupus erythematosus	Search under "lupus, nephritis"
Hip fracture	Search under "fracture, femur, upper end, neck"
Alzheimer's disease	Search under "disease, Alzheimer's"
Crohn's disease	Search under "Enteritis, regional"
Status of replaced joint	Ankle: Search under "presence, ankle joint implant" Elbow: Search under "presence, elbow joint implant" Finger: Search under "presence, finger joint implant" Hip: Search under "presence, hip joint implant" Knee: Search under "presence, knee joint implant" Shoulder: Search under "presence, shoulder joint implant" Wrist: Search under "presence, wrist joint implant" Specified NEC: Search under "presence, joint implant, specified joint NEC"
Heart failure	Search under "failure, heart"
COPD (Chronic obstructive pulmonary disease)	Search under "disease, pulmonary, chronic obstructive"
PVD (peripheral vascular disease)	Search under "disease, vascular, peripheral"
Diabetic ulcer	Search under "diabetes, with, foot ulcer" OR Search under "diabetes, with, skin ulcer NEC"
Amputation stump infection	Search under "complication, amputation stump NEC, infection or inflammation"
Coronary artery disease	Search under "disease, heart, ischemic, atherosclerotic"
Coronary artery disease with angina	Of native vessel: Search under "arteriosclerosis, coronary, native vessel, with angina pectoris" Of bypass graft: Search under "arteriosclerosis, coronary, bypass graft, with angina pectoris"
Toe ulcer	Search under "ulcer, lower limb, toe"
Gastric ulcer	Search under "ulcer, stomach"
Lower limb amputation status	Above knee: Search under "absence, extremity, lower" Below knee: Search under "absence, extremity, below knee"
Upper limb amputation status	Above elbow: Search under "absence, arm, above elbow" Below elbow: Search under "absence, arm, below elbow"
Osteomyelitis in the foot	Acute: Search under "osteomyelitis, acute, metatarsus" Chronic: Search under "osteomyelitis, chronic, metatarsus"
Parkinson's disease	Search under "Parkinsonism"
Major recurrent depression	Search under "disorder, depressive, recurrent"

Quick Reference Guide to Alphabetic Index Search Terms (cont.)

Diagnosis	Term to search for in the index
Surgical wound infection	Search under "Complication, surgical procedure, wound infection"
Cerebral autosomal dominant, with subcortical infarcts and leukoencephalopathy (CADASIL)	Search under "Arteriopathy, cerebral autosomal dominant, with subcortical infarcts and leukoencephalopathy (CADASIL)" or "CADASIL (cerebral autosomal dominant arteriopathy with subcortical infarcts andleukoencephalopathy)"
Elevated blood pressure reading, no diagnosis of hypertension	Search under "Hypertension, transient"
Lacunar infarction or stroke	Search under "Infarct, lacunar"
Paraplegia due to current injury	Code to injury with seventh character A
Paraplegia as sequela of previous injury	Code to injury with seventh character S
Postprocedural sepsis	Search under "Sepsis, postprocedural"

Abnormal, abnormality, abnormalities - *continued*
- fluid - *continued*
  - thorax (bronchial washings) (pleural fluid) — *see* Abnormal, specimen, respiratory organs
  - vaginal — *see* Abnormal, specimen, female genital organs
- form
  - teeth K00.2
  - uterus — *see* Anomaly, uterus
- function studies
  - auditory R94.120
  - bladder R94.8
  - brain R94.09
  - cardiovascular R94.30
  - ear R94.128
  - endocrine NEC R94.7
  - eye NEC R94.118
  - kidney R94.4
  - liver R94.5
  - nervous system
    - central NEC R94.09
    - peripheral NEC R94.138
  - pancreas R94.8
  - placenta R94.8
  - pulmonary R94.2
  - special senses NEC R94.128
  - spleen R94.8
  - thyroid R94.6
  - vestibular R94.121
- gait — *see* Gait
  - hysterical F44.4
- gastrin secretion E16.4
- globulin R77.1
  - cortisol-binding E27.8
  - thyroid-binding E07.89
- glomerular, minor — *see also* N00-N07 with fourth character .0 N05.0
- glucagon secretion E16.3
- glucose tolerance (test) (non-fasting) R73.09
- gravitational (G) forces or states (effect of) T75.81
- hair (color) (shaft) L67.9
  - specified NEC L67.8
- hard tissue formation in pulp (dental) K04.3
- head movement R25.0
- heart
  - rate R00.9
    - specified NEC R00.8
  - shadow R93.1
  - sounds NEC R01.2
- hemoglobin (disease) — *see also* Disease, hemoglobin D58.2
  - trait — *see* Trait, hemoglobin, abnormal
- histology NEC R89.7
- immunological findings R89.4
  - in serum R76.9
    - specified NEC R76.8
- increase in appetite R63.2
- involuntary movement — *see* Abnormal, movement, involuntary
- jaw closure M26.51
- karyotype R89.8
- kidney function test R94.4
- knee jerk R29.2
- leukocyte (cell) (differential) NEC D72.9
- liver function test — *see also* Elevated, liver function, test R79.89
- loss of
  - height R29.890
  - weight R63.4
- mammogram NEC R92.8
  - calcification (calculus) R92.1
  - microcalcification R92.0
- Mantoux test R76.11
- movement (disorder) — *see also* Disorder, movement
  - head R25.0
  - involuntary R25.9
    - fasciculation R25.3
    - of head R25.0
    - spasm R25.2
    - specified type NEC R25.8
    - tremor R25.1

Abnormal, abnormality, abnormalities - *continued*
- myoglobin (Aberdeen) (Annapolis) R89.7
- neonatal screening P09.9
  - for
    - congenital adrenal hyperplasia P09.2
    - congenital endocrine disease P09.2
    - congenital hematologic disorders P09.3
    - critical congenital heart disease P09.5
    - cystic fibrosis P09.4
    - hemoglobinothies P09.3
    - hypothyroidism P09.2
    - inborn errors of metabolism P09.1
    - neonatal hearing loss P09.6
    - red cell membrane defects P09.3
    - sickle cell P09.3
    - specified NEC P09.8
- oculomotor study R94.113
- palmar creases Q82.8
- Papanicolaou (smear)
  - anus R85.619
    - atypical squamous cells cannot exclude high grade squamous intraepithelial lesion (ASC-H) R85.611
    - atypical squamous cells of undetermined significance (ASC-US) R85.610
    - cytologic evidence of malignancy R85.614
    - high grade squamous intraepithelial lesion (HGSIL) R85.613
    - human papillomavirus (HPV) DNA test
      - high risk positive R85.81
      - low risk postive R85.82
    - inadequate smear R85.615
    - low grade squamous intraepithelial lesion (LGSIL) R85.612
    - satisfactory anal smear but lacking transformation zone R85.616
    - specified NEC R85.618
    - unsatisfactory smear R85.615
  - bronchial washings R84.6
  - cerebrospinal fluid R83.6
  - cervix R87.619
    - atypical squamous cells cannot exclude high grade squamous intraepithelial lesion (ASC-H) R87.611
    - atypical squamous cells of undetermined significance (ASC-US) R87.610
    - cytologic evidence of malignancy R87.614
    - high grade squamous intraepithelial lesion (HGSIL) R87.613
    - inadequate smear R87.615
    - low grade squamous intraepithelial lesion (LGSIL) R87.612
    - non-atypical endometrial cells R87.618
    - satisfactory cervical smear but lacking transformation zone R87.616
    - specified NEC R87.618
    - thin preparaton R87.619
    - unsatisfactory smear R87.615
  - nasal secretions R84.6
  - nipple discharge R89.6
  - peritoneal fluid R85.69
  - pleural fluid R84.6
  - prostatic secretions R86.6
  - saliva R85.69
  - seminal fluid R86.6
  - sites NEC R89.6
  - sputum R84.6
  - synovial fluid R89.6
  - throat scrapings R84.6
  - vagina R87.629
    - atypical squamous cells cannot exclude high grade squamous intraepithelial lesion (ASC-H) R87.621
    - atypical squamous cells of undetermined significance (ASC-US) R87.620
    - cytologic evidence of malignancy R87.624
    - high grade squamous intraepithelial lesion (HGSIL) R87.623
    - inadequate smear R87.625
    - low grade squamous intraepithelial lesion (LGSIL) R87.622

Abnormal, abnormality, abnormalities - *continued*
- Papanicolaou (smear) - *continued*
  - vagina - *continued*
    - specified NEC R87.628
    - thin preparation R87.629
    - unsatisfactory smear R87.625
  - vulva R87.69
  - wound secretions R89.6
- partial thromboplastin time (PTT) R79.1
- pelvis (bony) — *see* Deformity, pelvis
- percussion, chest (tympany) R09.89
- periods (grossly) — *see* Menstruation
- phonocardiogram R94.39
- plantar reflex R29.2
- plasma
  - protein R77.9
    - specified NEC R77.8
  - viscosity R70.1
- pleural (folds) Q34.0
- posture R29.3
- product of conception O02.9
  - specified type NEC O02.89
- prothrombin time (PT) R79.1
- pulmonary
  - artery, congenital Q25.79
  - function, newborn P28.89
  - test results R94.2
- pulsations in neck R00.2
- pupillary H21.56-
  - function (reaction) (reflex) — *see* Anomaly, pupil, function
- radiological examination — *see* Abnormal, diagnostic imaging
- red blood cell (s) (morphology) (volume) R71.8
- reflex — *see* Reflex
- renal function test R94.4
- response to nerve stimulation R94.130
- retinal correspondence H53.31
- retinal function study R94.111
- rhythm, heart — *see also* Arrhythmia
- saliva — *see* Abnormal, specimen, digestive organs
- scan
  - kidney R94.4
  - liver R93.2
  - thyroid R94.6
- secretion
  - gastrin E16.4
  - glucagon E16.3
- semen, seminal fluid — *see* Abnormal, specimen, male genital organs
- serum level (of)
  - acid phosphatase R74.8
  - alkaline phosphatase R74.8
  - amylase R74.8
  - enzymes R74.9
    - specified NEC R74.8
  - lipase R74.8
  - triacylglycerol lipase R74.8
- shape
  - gravid uterus — *see* Anomaly, uterus
- sinus venosus Q21.1
- size, tooth, teeth K00.2
- spacing, tooth, teeth, fully erupted M26.30
- specimen
  - digestive organs (peritoneal fluid) (saliva) R85.9
    - cytology R85.69
    - drug level R85.2
    - enzyme level R85.0
    - histology R85.7
    - hormones R85.1
    - immunology R85.4
    - microbiology R85.5
    - nonmedicinal level R85.3
    - specified type NEC R85.89
  - female genital organs (secretions) (smears) R87.9
    - cytology R87.69
      - cervix R87.619
        - human papillomavirus (HPV) DNA test
          - high risk positive R87.810

Abnormal, abnormality, abnormalities - *continued*
- specimen - *continued*
  - female genital organs (secretions) (smears) - *continued*
    - cytology - *continued*
      - cervix - *continued*
        - human papillomavirus (HPV) DNA test - *continued*
          - low risk positive R87.820
        - inadequate (unsatisfactory) smear R87.615
        - non-atypical endometrial cells R87.618
        - specified NEC R87.618
      - vagina R87.629
        - human papillomavirus (HPV) DNA test
          - high risk positive R87.811
          - low risk positive R87.821
        - inadequate (unsatisfactory) smear R87.625
      - vulva R87.69
    - drug level R87.2
    - enzyme level R87.0
    - histological R87.7
    - hormones R87.1
    - immunology R87.4
    - microbiology R87.5
    - nonmedicinal level R87.3
    - specified type NEC R87.89
  - male genital organs (prostatic secretions) (semen) R86.9
    - cytology R86.6
    - drug level R86.2
    - enzyme level R86.0
    - histological R86.7
    - hormones R86.1
    - immunology R86.4
    - microbiology R86.5
    - nonmedicinal level R86.3
    - specified type NEC R86.8
  - nipple discharge — *see* Abnormal, specimen, specified
  - respiratory organs (bronchial washings) (nasal secretions) (pleural fluid) (sputum) R84.9
    - cytology R84.6
    - drug level R84.2
    - enzyme level R84.0
    - histology R84.7
    - hormones R84.1
    - immunology R84.4
    - microbiology R84.5
    - nonmedicinal level R84.3
    - specified type NEC R84.8
  - specified organ, system and tissue NOS R89.9
    - cytology R89.6
    - drug level R89.2
    - enzyme level R89.0
    - histology R89.7
    - hormones R89.1
    - immunology R89.4
    - microbiology R89.5
    - nonmedicinal level R89.3
    - specified type NEC R89.8
  - synovial fluid — *see* Abnormal, specimen, specified
  - thorax (bronchial washings) (pleural fluids) — *see* Abnormal, specimen, respiratory organs
  - vagina (secretion) (smear) R87.629
  - vulva (secretion) (smear) R87.69
  - wound secretion — *see* Abnormal, specimen, specified
- spermatozoa — *see* Abnormal, specimen, male genital organs
- sputum (amount) (color) (odor) R09.3
- stool (color) (contents) (mucus) R19.5
  - bloody K92.1
  - guaiac positive R19.5
- synchondrosis Q78.8
- thermography — *see also* Abnormal, diagnostic imaging R93.89
- thyroid-binding globulin E07.89
- tooth, teeth (form) (size) K00.2
- toxicology (findings) R78.9
- transport protein E88.09
- tumor marker NEC R97.8
- ultrasound results — *see* Abnormal, diagnostic imaging
- umbilical cord complicating delivery O69.9
- urination NEC R39.198
- urine (constituents) R82.90
  - bile R82.2
  - cytological examination R82.89
  - drugs R82.5
  - fat R82.0
  - glucose R81
  - heavy metals R82.6
  - hemoglobin R82.3
  - histological examination R82.89
  - ketones R82.4
  - microbiological examination (culture) R82.79
  - myoglobin R82.1
  - positive culture R82.79
  - protein — *see* Proteinuria
  - specified substance NEC R82.998
    - chromoabnormality NEC R82.91
  - substances nonmedical R82.6
- uterine hemorrhage — *see* Hemorrhage, uterus
- vectorcardiogram R94.39
- visually evoked potential (VEP) R94.112
- white blood cells D72.9
  - specified NEC D72.89
- X-ray examination — *see* Abnormal, diagnostic imaging

Abnormity (any organ or part) — *see* Anomaly

Abocclusion M26.29
- hemolytic disease (newborn) P55.1
- incompatibility reaction ABO — *see* Complication(s), transfusion, incompatibility reaction, ABO

Abolition, language R48.8

Aborter, habitual or recurrent — *see* Loss (of), pregnancy, recurrent

Abortion (complete) (spontaneous) O03.9
- with
  - retained products of conception — *see* Abortion, incomplete
- attempted (elective) (failed) O07.4
  - complicated by O07.30
    - afibrinogenemia O07.1
    - cardiac arrest O07.36
    - chemical damage of pelvic organ (s) O07.34
    - circulatory collapse O07.31
    - cystitis O07.38
    - defibrination syndrome O07.1
    - electrolyte imbalance O07.33
    - embolism (air) (amniotic fluid) (blood clot) (fat) (pulmonary) (septic) (soap) O07.2
    - endometritis O07.0
    - genital tract and pelvic infection O07.0
    - hemolysis O07.1
    - hemorrhage (delayed) (excessive) O07.1
    - infection
      - genital tract or pelvic O07.0
      - urinary tract O07.38
    - intravascular coagulation O07.1
    - laceration of pelvic organ (s) O07.34
    - metabolic disorder O07.33
    - oliguria O07.32
    - oophoritis O07.0
    - parametritis O07.0
    - pelvic peritonitis O07.0
    - perforation of pelvic organ (s) O07.34
    - renal failure or shutdown O07.32
    - salpingitis or salpingo-oophoritis O07.0
    - sepsis O07.37
    - shock O07.31
    - specified condition NEC O07.39
    - tubular necrosis (renal) O07.32

Abortion (complete) (spontaneous) - *continued*
- attempted (elective) (failed) - *continued*
  - complicated by - *continued*
    - uremia O07.32
    - urinary tract infection O07.38
    - venous complication NEC O07.35
      - embolism (air) (amniotic fluid) (blood clot) (fat) (pulmonary) (septic) (soap) O07.2
- complicated (by) (following) O03.80
  - afibrinogenemia O03.6
  - cardiac arrest O03.86
  - chemical damage of pelvic organ (s) O03.84
  - circulatory collapse O03.81
  - cystitis O03.88
  - defibrination syndrome O03.6
  - electrolyte imbalance O03.83
  - embolism (air) (amniotic fluid) (blood clot) (fat) (pulmonary) (septic) (soap) O03.7
  - endometritis O03.5
  - genital tract and pelvic infection O03.5
  - hemolysis O03.6
  - hemorrhage (delayed) (excessive) O03.6
  - infection
    - genital tract or pelvic O03.5
    - urinary tract O03.88
  - intravascular coagulation O03.6
  - laceration of pelvic organ (s) O03.84
  - metabolic disorder O03.83
  - oliguria O03.82
  - oophoritis O03.5
  - parametritis O03.5
  - pelvic peritonitis O03.5
  - perforation of pelvic organ (s) O03.84
  - renal failure or shutdown O03.82
  - salpingitis or salpingo-oophoritis O03.5
  - sepsis O03.87
  - shock O03.81
  - specified condition NEC O03.89
  - tubular necrosis (renal) O03.82
  - uremia O03.82
  - urinary tract infection O03.88
  - venous complication NEC O03.85
    - embolism (air) (amniotic fluid) (blood clot) (fat) (pulmonary) (septic) (soap) O03.7
- failed — *see* Abortion, attempted
- habitual or recurrent N96
  - with current abortion — *see* categories O03-O04
  - without current pregnancy N96
  - care in current pregnancy O26.2-
- incomplete (spontaneous) O03.4
  - complicated (by) (following) O03.30
    - afibrinogenemia O03.1
    - cardiac arrest O03.36
    - chemical damage of pelvic organ (s) O03.34
    - circulatory collapse O03.31
    - cystitis O03.38
    - defibrination syndrome O03.1
    - electrolyte imbalance O03.33
    - embolism (air) (amniotic fluid) (blood clot) (fat) (pulmonary) (septic) (soap) O03.2
    - endometritis O03.0
    - genital tract and pelvic infection O03.0
    - hemolysis O03.1
    - hemorrhage (delayed) (excessive) O03.1
    - infection
      - genital tract or pelvic O03.0
      - urinary tract O03.38
    - intravascular coagulation O03.1
    - laceration of pelvic organ (s) O03.34
    - metabolic disorder O03.33
    - oliguria O03.32
    - oophoritis O03.0
    - parametritis O03.0
    - pelvic peritonitis O03.0
    - perforation of pelvic organ (s) O03.34
    - renal failure or shutdown O03.32
    - salpingitis or salpingo-oophoritis O03.0

Abortion (complete) (spontaneous) - *continued*
incomplete (spontaneous) - *continued*
complicated (by) (following) - *continued*
sepsis O03.37
shock O03.31
specified condition NEC O03.39
tubular necrosis (renal) O03.32
uremia O03.32
urinary infection O03.38
venous complication NEC O03.35
embolism (air) (amniotic fluid) (blood clot) (fat) (pulmonary) (septic) (soap) O03.2
induced (encounter for) Z33.2
complicated by O04.80
afibrinogenemia O04.6
cardiac arrest O04.86
chemical damage of pelvic organ (s) O04.84
circulatory collapse O04.81
cystitis O04.88
defibrination syndrome O04.6
electrolyte imbalance O04.83
embolism (air) (amniotic fluid) (blood clot) (fat) (pulmonary) (septic) (soap) O04.7
endometritis O04.5
genital tract and pelvic infection O04.5
hemolysis O04.6
hemorrhage (delayed) (excessive) O04.6
infection
genital tract or pelvic O04.5
urinary tract O04.88
intravascular coagulation O04.6
laceration of pelvic organ (s) O04.84
metabolic disorder O04.83
oliguria O04.82
oophoritis O04.5
parametritis O04.5
pelvic peritonitis O04.5
perforation of pelvic organ (s) O04.84
renal failure or shutdown O04.82
salpingitis or salpingo-oophoritis O04.5
sepsis O04.87
shock O04.81
specified condition NEC O04.89
tubular necrosis (renal) O04.82
uremia O04.82
urinary tract infection O04.88
venous complication NEC O04.85
embolism (air) (amniotic fluid) (blood clot) (fat) (pulmonary) (septic) (soap) O04.7
inevitable O03.4
missed O02.1
spontaneous — *see* Abortion (complete) (spontaneous)
threatened O20.0
threatened (spontaneous) O20.0
tubal O00.10-
with intrauterine pregnancy O00.11-
Abortus fever A23.1
Aboulomania F60.7
Abrami's disease D59.8
Abramov-Fiedler myocarditis (acute isolated myocarditis) I40.1
Abrasion T14.8
abdomen, abdominal (wall) S30.811
alveolar process S00.512
ankle S90.51-
antecubital space — *see* Abrasion, elbow
anus S30.817
arm (upper) S40.81-
auditory canal — *see* Abrasion, ear
auricle — *see* Abrasion, ear
axilla — *see* Abrasion, arm
back, lower S30.810
breast S20.11-
brow S00.81
buttock S30.810
calf — *see* Abrasion, leg
canthus — *see* Abrasion, eyelid
cheek S00.81
internal S00.512

Abrasion - *continued*
chest wall — *see* Abrasion, thorax
chin S00.81
clitoris S30.814
cornea S05.0-
costal region — *see* Abrasion, thorax
dental K03.1
digit (s)
foot — *see* Abrasion, toe
hand — *see* Abrasion, finger
ear S00.41-
elbow S50.31-
epididymis S30.813
epigastric region S30.811
epiglottis S10.11
esophagus (thoracic) S27.818
cervical S10.11
eyebrow — *see* Abrasion, eyelid
eyelid S00.21-
face S00.81
finger (s) S60.41-
index S60.41-
little S60.41-
middle S60.41-
ring S60.41-
flank S30.811
foot (except toe (s) alone) S90.81-
toe — *see* Abrasion, toe
forearm S50.81-
elbow only — *see* Abrasion, elbow
forehead S00.81
genital organs, external
female S30.816
male S30.815
groin S30.811
gum S00.512
hand S60.51-
head S00.91
ear — *see* Abrasion, ear
eyelid — *see* Abrasion, eyelid
lip S00.511
nose S00.31
oral cavity S00.512
scalp S00.01
specified site NEC S00.81
heel — *see* Abrasion, foot
hip S70.21-
inguinal region S30.811
interscapular region S20.419
jaw S00.81
knee S80.21-
labium (majus) (minus) S30.814
larynx S10.11
leg (lower) S80.81-
knee — *see* Abrasion, knee
upper — *see* Abrasion, thigh
lip S00.511
lower back S30.810
lumbar region S30.810
malar region S00.81
mammary — *see* Abrasion, breast
mastoid region S00.81
mouth S00.512
nail
finger — *see* Abrasion, finger
toe — *see* Abrasion, toe
nape S10.81
nasal S00.31
neck S10.91
specified site NEC S10.81
throat S10.11
nose S00.31
occipital region S00.01
oral cavity S00.512
orbital region — *see* Abrasion, eyelid
palate S00.512
palm — *see* Abrasion, hand
parietal region S00.01
pelvis S30.810
penis S30.812
perineum
female S30.814
male S30.810
periocular area — *see* Abrasion, eyelid
phalanges

Abrasion - *continued*
phalanges - *continued*
finger — *see* Abrasion, finger
toe — *see* Abrasion, toe
pharynx S10.11
pinna — *see* Abrasion, ear
popliteal space — *see* Abrasion, knee
prepuce S30.812
pubic region S30.810
pudendum
female S30.816
male S30.815
sacral region S30.810
scalp S00.01
scapular region — *see* Abrasion, shoulder
scrotum S30.813
shin — *see* Abrasion, leg
shoulder S40.21-
skin NEC T14.8
sternal region S20.319
submaxillary region S00.81
submental region S00.81
subungual
finger (s) — *see* Abrasion, finger
toe (s) — *see* Abrasion, toe
supraclavicular fossa S10.81
supraorbital S00.81
temple S00.81
temporal region S00.81
testis S30.813
thigh S70.31-
thorax, thoracic (wall) S20.91
back S20.41-
front S20.31-
throat S10.11
thumb S60.31-
toe (s) (lesser) S90.416
great S90.41-
tongue S00.512
tooth, teeth (dentifrice) (habitual) (hard tissues) (occupational) (ritual) (traditional) K03.1
trachea S10.11
tunica vaginalis S30.813
tympanum, tympanic membrane — *see* Abrasion, ear
uvula S00.512
vagina S30.814
vocal cords S10.11
vulva S30.814
wrist S60.81-
Abrism — *see* Poisoning, food, noxious, plant
Abruptio placentae O45.9-
with
afibrinogenemia O45.01-
coagulation defect O45.00-
specified NEC O45.09-
disseminated intravascular coagulation O45.02-
hypofibrinogenemia O45.01-
specified NEC O45.8-
Abruption, placenta — *see* Abruptio placentae
Abscess (connective tissue) (embolic) (fistulous) (infective) (metastatic) (multiple) (pernicious) (pyogenic) (septic) L02.91
with
diverticular disease (intestine) K57.80
with bleeding K57.81
large intestine K57.20
with
bleeding K57.21
small intestine K57.40
with bleeding K57.41
small intestine K57.00
with
bleeding K57.01
large intestine K57.40
with bleeding K57.41
lymphangitis - code by site under Abscess
abdomen, abdominal
cavity K65.1
wall L02.211
abdominopelvic K65.1

Abscess (connective tissue) (embolic) (fistulous) (infective) (metastatic) (multiple) (pernicious) (pyogenic) (septic) - *continued*
accessory sinus — *see* Sinusitis
adrenal (capsule) (gland) E27.8
alveolar K04.7
  with sinus K04.6
amebic A06.4
  brain (and liver or lung abscess) A06.6
  genitourinary tract A06.82
  liver (without mention of brain or lung abscess) A06.4
  lung (and liver) (without mention of brain abscess) A06.5
  specified site NEC A06.89
  spleen A06.89
anerobic A48.0
ankle — *see* Abscess, lower limb
anorectal K61.2
antecubital space — *see* Abscess, upper limb
antrum (chronic) (Highmore) — *see* Sinusitis, maxillary
anus K61.0
apical (tooth) K04.7
  with sinus (alveolar) K04.6
appendix K35.33
areola (acute) (chronic) (nonpuerperal) N61.1
  puerperal, postpartum or gestational — *see* Infection, nipple
arm (any part) — *see* Abscess, upper limb
artery (wall) I77.89
atheromatous I77.2
auricle, ear — *see* Abscess, ear, external
axilla (region) L02.41-
  lymph gland or node L04.2
back (any part, except buttock) L02.212
Bartholin's gland N75.1
  with
    abortion — *see* Abortion, by type complicated by, sepsis
    ectopic or molar pregnancy O08.0
  following ectopic or molar pregnancy O08.0
Bezold's — *see* Mastoiditis, acute
bilharziasis B65.1
bladder (wall) — *see* Cystitis, specified type NEC
bone (subperiosteal) — *see also* Osteomyelitis, specified type NEC
  accessory sinus (chronic) — *see* Sinusitis
  chronic or old — *see* Osteomyelitis, chronic
  jaw (lower) (upper) M27.2
  mastoid — *see* Mastoiditis, acute, subperiosteal
  petrous — *see* Petrositis
  spinal (tuberculous) A18.01
    nontuberculous — *see* Osteomyelitis, vertebra
bowel K63.0
brain (any part) (cystic) (otogenic) G06.0
  amebic (with abscess of any other site) A06.6
  gonococcal A54.82
  pheomycotic (chromomycotic) B43.1
  tuberculous A17.81
breast (acute) (chronic) (nonpuerperal) N61.1
  newborn P39.0
  puerperal, postpartum, gestational — *see* Mastitis, obstetric, purulent
broad ligament N73.2
  acute N73.0
  chronic N73.1
Brodie's (localized) (chronic) M86.8X-
bronchi J98.09
buccal cavity K12.2
bulbourethral gland N34.0
bursa M71.00
  ankle M71.07-
  elbow M71.02-
  foot M71.07-
  hand M71.04-
  hip M71.05-
  knee M71.06-

Abscess (connective tissue) (embolic) (fistulous) (infective) (metastatic) (multiple) (pernicious) (pyogenic) (septic) - *continued*
bursa - *continued*
  multiple sites M71.09
  pharyngeal J39.1
  shoulder M71.01-
  specified site NEC M71.08
  wrist M71.03-
buttock L02.31
canthus — *see* Blepharoconjunctivitis
cartilage — *see* Disorder, cartilage, specified type NEC
cecum K35.33
cerebellum, cerebellar G06.0
  sequelae G09
cerebral (embolic) G06.0
  sequelae G09
cervical (meaning neck) L02.11
  lymph gland or node L04.0
cervix (stump) (uteri) — *see* Cervicitis
cheek (external) L02.01
  inner K12.2
chest J86.9
  with fistula J86.0
  wall L02.213
chin L02.01
choroid — *see* Inflammation, chorioretinal
circumtonsillar J36
cold (lung) (tuberculous) — *see also* Tuberculosis, abscess, lung
  articular — *see* Tuberculosis, joint
colon (wall) K63.0
colostomy K94.02
conjunctiva — *see* Conjunctivitis, acute
cornea H16.31-
corpus
  cavernosum N48.21
  luteum — *see* Oophoritis
Cowper's gland N34.0
cranium G06.0
cul-de-sac (Douglas') (posterior) — *see* Peritonitis, pelvic, female
cutaneous — *see* Abscess, by site
dental K04.7
  with sinus (alveolar) K04.6
dentoalveolar K04.7
  with sinus K04.6
diaphragm, diaphragmatic K65.1
Douglas' cul-de-sac or pouch — *see* Peritonitis, pelvic, female
Dubois A50.59
ear (middle) — *see also* Otitis, media, suppurative
  acute — *see* Otitis, media, suppurative, acute
  external H60.0-
entamebic — *see* Abscess, amebic
enterostomy K94.12
epididymis N45.4
epidural G06.2
  brain G06.0
  spinal cord G06.1
epiglottis J38.7
epiploon, epiploic K65.1
erysipelatous — *see* Erysipelas
esophagus K20.80
ethmoid (bone) (chronic) (sinus) J32.2
external auditory canal — *see* Abscess, ear, external
extradural G06.2
  brain G06.0
    sequelae G09
  spinal cord G06.1
extraperitoneal K68.19
eye — *see* Endophthalmitis, purulent
eyelid H00.03-
face (any part, except ear, eye and nose) L02.01
fallopian tube — *see* Salpingitis
fascia M72.8
fauces J39.1
fecal K63.0
femoral (region) — *see* Abscess, lower limb
filaria, filarial — *see* Infestation, filarial

Abscess (connective tissue) (embolic) (fistulous) (infective) (metastatic) (multiple) (pernicious) (pyogenic) (septic) - *continued*
finger (any) — *see also* Abscess, hand
  nail — *see* Cellulitis, finger
foot L02.61-
forehead L02.01
frontal sinus (chronic) J32.1
gallbladder K81.0
genital organ or tract
  female (external) N76.4
  male N49.9
    multiple sites N49.8
    specified NEC N49.8
gestational mammary O91.11-
gestational subareolar O91.11-
gingival — *see* Periodontitis, localized
gland, glandular (lymph) (acute) — *see* Lymphadenitis, acute
gluteal (region) L02.31
gonorrheal — *see* Gonococcus
groin L02.214
gum — *see* Periodontitis, localized
hand L02.51-
head NEC L02.811
  face (any part, except ear, eye and nose) L02.01
heart — *see* Carditis
heel — *see* Abscess, foot
helminthic — *see* Infestation, helminth
hepatic (cholangitic) (hematogenic) (lymphogenic) (pylephlebitic) K75.0
  amebic A06.4
hip (region) — *see* Abscess, lower limb
horseshoe K61.31
ileocecal K35.33
ileostomy (bud) K94.12
iliac (region) L02.214
  fossa K35.33
infraclavicular (fossa) — *see* Abscess, upper limb
inguinal (region) L02.214
  lymph gland or node L04.1
intersphincteric K61.4
intestine, intestinal NEC K63.0
  rectal K61.1
intra-abdominal — *see also* Abscess, peritoneum K65.1
  following procedure T81.43
    obstetrical O86.03
  postprocedural T81.43
    retroperitoneal K68.11
intracranial G06.0
intramammary — *see* Abscess, breast
intramuscular, following procedure T81.42
  obstetrical O86.02
intraorbital — *see* Abscess, orbit
intraperitoneal K65.1
intrasphincteric (anus) K61.4
intraspinal G06.1
intratonsillar J36
ischiorectal (fossa) (specified NEC) K61.39
jaw (bone) (lower) (upper) M27.2
joint — *see* Arthritis, pyogenic or pyemic
  spine (tuberculous) A18.01
    nontuberculous — *see* Spondylopathy, infective
kidney N15.1
  with calculus N20.0
    with hydronephrosis N13.6
  puerperal (postpartum) O86.21
knee — *see also* Abscess, lower limb
  joint M00.9
labium (majus) (minus) N76.4
lacrimal
  caruncle — *see* Inflammation, lacrimal, passages, acute
  gland — *see* Dacryoadenitis
  passages (duct) (sac) — *see* Inflammation, lacrimal, passages, acute
lacunar N34.0
larynx J38.7
lateral (alveolar) K04.7
  with sinus K04.6
leg (any part) — *see* Abscess, lower limb

Abscess (connective tissue) (embolic) (fistulous) (infective) (metastatic) (multiple) (pernicious) (pyogenic) (septic) - *continued*
lens H27.8
lingual K14.0
tonsil J36
lip K13.0
Littre's gland N34.0
liver (cholangitic) (hematogenic) (lymphogenic) (pylephlebitic) (pyogenic) K75.0
amebic (due to Entamoeba histolytica) (dysenteric) (tropical) A06.4
with
brain abscess (and liver or lung abscess) A06.6
lung abscess A06.5
loin (region) L02.211
lower limb L02.41-
lumbar (tuberculous) A18.01
nontuberculous L02.212
lung (miliary) (putrid) J85.2
with pneumonia J85.1
due to specified organism (see Pneumonia, in (due to))
amebic (with liver abscess) A06.5
with
brain abscess A06.6
pneumonia A06.5
lymph, lymphatic, gland or node (acute) — *see also* Lymphadenitis, acute
mesentery I88.0
malar M27.2
mammary gland — *see* Abscess, breast
marginal, anus K61.0
mastoid — *see* Mastoiditis, acute
maxilla, maxillary M27.2
molar (tooth) K04.7
with sinus K04.6
premolar K04.7
sinus (chronic) J32.0
mediastinum J85.3
meibomian gland — *see* Hordeolum
meninges G06.2
mesentery, mesenteric K65.1
mesosalpinx — *see* Salpingitis
mons pubis L02.215
mouth (floor) K12.2
muscle — *see* Myositis, infective
myocardium I40.0
nabothian (follicle) — *see* Cervicitis
nasal J32.9
nasopharyngeal J39.1
navel L02.216
newborn P38.9
with mild hemorrhage P38.1
without hemorrhage P38.9
neck (region) L02.11
lymph gland or node L04.0
nephritic — *see* Abscess, kidney
nipple N61.1
associated with
lactation — *see* Pregnancy, complicated by
pregnancy — *see* Pregnancy, complicated by
nose (external) (fossa) (septum) J34.0
sinus (chronic) — *see* Sinusitis
omentum K65.1
operative wound T81.49
orbit, orbital — *see* Cellulitis, orbit
otogenic G06.0
ovary, ovarian (corpus luteum) — *see* Oophoritis
oviduct — *see* Oophoritis
palate (soft) K12.2
hard M27.2
palmar (space) — *see* Abscess, hand
pancreas (duct) — *see* Pancreatitis, acute
parafrenal N48.21
parametric, parametrium N73.2
acute N73.0
chronic N73.1
paranephric N15.1
parapancreatic — *see* Pancreatitis, acute

Abscess (connective tissue) (embolic) (fistulous) (infective) (metastatic) (multiple) (pernicious) (pyogenic) (septic) - *continued*
parapharyngeal J39.0
pararectal K61.1
parasinus — *see* Sinusitis
parauterine — *see also* Disease, pelvis, inflammatory N73.2
paravaginal — *see* Vaginitis
parietal region (scalp) L02.811
parodontal — *see* Periodontitis, aggressive, localized
parotid (duct) (gland) K11.3
region K12.2
pectoral (region) L02.213
pelvis, pelvic
female — *see* Disease, pelvis, inflammatory
male, peritoneal K65.1
penis N48.21
gonococcal (accessory gland) (periurethral) A54.1
perianal K61.0
periapical K04.7
with sinus (alveolar) K04.6
periappendicular K35.33
pericardial I30.1
pericecal K35.33
pericemental — *see* Periodontitis, aggressive, localized
pericholecystic — *see* Cholecystitis, acute
pericoronal — *see* Periodontitis, aggressive, localized
peridental — *see* Periodontitis, aggressive, localized
perimetric — *see also* Disease, pelvis, inflammatory N73.2
perinephric, perinephritic — *see* Abscess, kidney
perineum, perineal (superficial) L02.215
urethra N34.0
periodontal (parietal) — *see* Periodontitis, aggressive, localized
apical K04.7
periosteum, periosteal — *see also* Osteomyelitis, specified type NEC
with osteomyelitis — *see also* Osteomyelitis, specified type NEC
acute — *see* Osteomyelitis, acute
chronic — *see* Osteomyelitis, chronic
peripharyngeal J39.0
peripleuritic J86.9
with fistula J86.0
periprostatic N41.2
perirectal K61.1
perirenal (tissue) — *see* Abscess, kidney
perisinuous (nose) — *see* Sinusitis
peritoneum, peritoneal (perforated) (ruptured) K65.1
with appendicitis — *see also* Appendicitis K35.33
pelvic
female — *see* Peritonitis, pelvic, female
male K65.1
postoperative T81.49
puerperal, postpartum, childbirth O85
tuberculous A18.31
peritonsillar J36
perityphlic K35.33
periureteral N28.89
periurethral N34.0
gonococcal (accessory gland) (periurethral) A54.1
periuterine — *see also* Disease, pelvis, inflammatory N73.2
perivesical — *see* Cystitis, specified type NEC
petrous bone — *see* Petrositis
phagedenic NOS L02.91
chancroid A57
pharynx, pharyngeal (lateral) J39.1
pilonidal L05.01
pituitary (gland) E23.6
pleura J86.9
with fistula J86.0

Abscess (connective tissue) (embolic) (fistulous) (infective) (metastatic) (multiple) (pernicious) (pyogenic) (septic) - *continued*
popliteal — *see* Abscess, lower limb
postcecal K35.33
postlaryngeal J38.7
postnasal J34.0
postoperative (any site) — *see also* Infection, postoperative wound T81.49
retroperitoneal K68.11
postpharyngeal J39.0
posttonsillar J36
post-typhoid A01.09
pouch of Douglas — *see* Peritonitis, pelvic, female
premammary — *see* Abscess, breast
prepatellar — *see* Abscess, lower limb
presacral K68.19
prostate N41.2
gonococcal (acute) (chronic) A54.22
psoas muscle K68.12
puerperal - code by site under Puerperal, abscess
pulmonary — *see* Abscess, lung
pulp, pulpal (dental) K04.01
irreversible K04.02
reversible K04.01
rectovaginal septum K63.0
rectovesical — *see* Cystitis, specified type NEC
rectum K61.1
renal — *see* Abscess, kidney
retina — *see* Inflammation, chorioretinal
retrobulbar — *see* Abscess, orbit
retrocecal K65.1
retrolaryngeal J38.7
retromammary — *see* Abscess, breast
retroperitoneal NEC K68.19
postprocedural K68.11
retropharyngeal J39.0
retrouterine — *see* Peritonitis, pelvic, female
retrovesical — *see* Cystitis, specified type NEC
root, tooth K04.7
with sinus (alveolar) K04.6
round ligament — *see also* Disease, pelvis, inflammatory N73.2
rupture (spontaneous) NOS L02.91
sacrum (tuberculous) A18.01
nontuberculous M46.28
salivary (duct) (gland) K11.3
scalp (any part) L02.811
scapular — *see* Osteomyelitis, specified type NEC
sclera — *see* Scleritis
scrofulous (tuberculous) A18.2
scrotum N49.2
seminal vesicle N49.0
septal, dental K04.7
with sinus (alveolar) K04.6
serous — *see* Periostitis
shoulder (region) — *see* Abscess, upper limb
sigmoid K63.0
sinus (accessory) (chronic) (nasal) — *see also* Sinusitis
intracranial venous (any) G06.0
Skene's duct or gland N34.0
skin — *see* Abscess, by site
specified site NEC L02.818
spermatic cord N49.1
sphenoidal (sinus) (chronic) J32.3
spinal cord (any part) (staphylococcal) G06.1
tuberculous A17.81
spine (column) (tuberculous) A18.01
epidural G06.1
nontuberculous — *see* Osteomyelitis, vertebra
spleen D73.3
amebic A06.89
stitch T81.41
following an obstetrical procedure O86.01
subarachnoid G06.2
brain G06.0
spinal cord G06.1
subareolar — *see* Abscess, breast

Abscess (connective tissue) (embolic) (fistulous) (infective) (metastatic) (multiple) (pernicious) (pyogenic) (septic) - *continued*
subcecal K35.33
subcutaneous — *see also* Abscess, by site
following procedure T81.41
obstetrical O86.01
pheomycotic (chromomycotic) B43.2
subdiaphragmatic K65.1
subdural G06.2
brain G06.0
sequelae G09
spinal cord G06.1
sub-fascial, following an obstetrical procedure O86.02
subgaleal L02.811
subhepatic K65.1
sublingual K12.2
gland K11.3
submammary — *see* Abscess, breast
submandibular (region) (space) (triangle) K12.2
gland K11.3
submaxillary (region) L02.01
gland K11.3
submental L02.01
gland K11.3
subperiosteal — *see* Osteomyelitis, specified type NEC
subphrenic K65.1
following an obstetrical procedure O86.03
postoperative T81.43
suburethral N34.0
sudoriparous L75.8
supraclavicular (fossa) — *see* Abscess, upper limb
supralevator K61.5
suprapelvic, acute N73.0
suprarenal (capsule) (gland) E27.8
sweat gland L74.8
tear duct — *see* Inflammation, lacrimal, passages, acute
temple L02.01
temporal region L02.01
temporosphenoidal G06.0
tendon (sheath) M65.00
ankle M65.07-
foot M65.07-
forearm M65.03-
hand M65.04-
lower leg M65.06-
pelvic region M65.05-
shoulder region M65.01-
specified site NEC M65.08
thigh M65.05-
upper arm M65.02-
testis N45.4
thigh — *see* Abscess, lower limb
thorax J86.9
with fistula J86.0
throat J39.1
thumb — *see also* Abscess, hand
nail — *see* Cellulitis, finger
thymus (gland) E32.1
thyroid (gland) E06.0
toe (any) — *see also* Abscess, foot
nail — *see* Cellulitis, toe
tongue (staphylococcal) K14.0
tonsil (s) (lingual) J36
tonsillopharyngeal J36
tooth, teeth (root) K04.7
with sinus (alveolar) K04.6
supporting structures NEC — *see* Periodontitis, aggressive, localized
trachea J39.8
trunk L02.219
abdominal wall L02.211
back L02.212
chest wall L02.213
groin L02.214
perineum L02.215
umbilicus L02.216
tubal — *see* Salpingitis
tuberculous — *see* Tuberculosis, abscess
tubo-ovarian — *see* Salpingo-oophoritis

Abscess (connective tissue) (embolic) (fistulous) (infective) (metastatic) (multiple) (pernicious) (pyogenic) (septic) - *continued*
tunica vaginalis N49.1
umbilicus L02.216
upper
limb L02.41-
respiratory J39.8
urethral (gland) N34.0
urinary N34.0
uterus, uterine (wall) — *see also* Endometritis
ligament — *see also* Disease, pelvis, inflammatory N73.2
neck — *see* Cervicitis
uvula K12.2
vagina (wall) — *see* Vaginitis
vaginorectal — *see* Vaginitis
vas deferens N49.1
vermiform appendix K35.33
vertebra (column) (tuberculous) A18.01
nontuberculous — *see* Osteomyelitis, vertebra
vesical — *see* Cystitis, specified type NEC
vesico-uterine pouch — *see* Peritonitis, pelvic, female
vitreous (humor) — *see* Endophthalmitis, purulent
vocal cord J38.3
von Bezold's — *see* Mastoiditis, acute
vulva N76.4
vulvovaginal gland N75.1
web space — *see* Abscess, hand
wound T81.49
wrist — *see* Abscess, upper limb

Absence (of) (organ or part) (complete or partial)
adrenal (gland) (congenital) Q89.1
acquired E89.6
albumin in blood E88.09
alimentary tract (congenital) Q45.8
upper Q40.8
alveolar process (acquired) — *see* Anomaly, alveolar
ankle (acquired) Z89.44-
anus (congenital) Q42.3
with fistula Q42.2
aorta (congenital) Q25.41
appendix, congenital Q42.8
arm (acquired) Z89.20-
above elbow Z89.22-
congenital (with hand present) — *see* Agenesis, arm, with hand present
and hand — *see* Agenesis, forearm, and hand
below elbow Z89.21-
congenital (with hand present) — *see* Agenesis, arm, with hand present
and hand — *see* Agenesis, forearm, and hand
congenital — *see* Defect, reduction, upper limb
shoulder (following explantation of shoulder joint prosthesis) (joint) (with or without presence of antibiotic-impregnated cement spacer) Z89.23-
congenital (with hand present) — *see* Agenesis, arm, with hand present
artery (congenital) (peripheral) Q27.8
brain Q28.3
coronary Q24.5
pulmonary Q25.79
specified NEC Q27.8
umbilical Q27.0
atrial septum (congenital) Q21.1
auditory canal (congenital) (external) Q16.1
auricle (ear), congenital Q16.0
bile, biliary duct, congenital Q44.5
bladder (acquired) Z90.6
congenital Q64.5
bowel sounds R19.11
brain Q00.0
part of Q04.3
breast (s) (and nipple (s)) (acquired) Z90.1-
congenital Q83.8

Absence (of) (organ or part) (complete or partial) - *continued*
broad ligament Q50.6
bronchus (congenital) Q32.4
canaliculus lacrimalis, congenital Q10.4
cerebellum (vermis) Q04.3
cervix (acquired) (with uterus) Z90.710
with remaining uterus Z90.712
congenital Q51.5
chin, congenital Q18.8
cilia (congenital) Q10.3
acquired — *see* Madarosis
clitoris (congenital) Q52.6
coccyx, congenital Q76.49
cold sense R20.8
congenital
lumen — *see* Atresia
organ or site NEC — *see* Agenesis
septum — *see* Imperfect, closure
corpus callosum Q04.0
cricoid cartilage, congenital Q31.8
diaphragm (with hernia), congenital Q79.1
digestive organ (s) or tract, congenital Q45.8
acquired NEC Z90.49
upper Q40.8
ductus arteriosus Q28.8
duodenum (acquired) Z90.49
congenital Q41.0
ear, congenital Q16.9
acquired H93.8-
auricle Q16.0
external Q16.0
inner Q16.5
lobe, lobule Q17.8
middle, except ossicles Q16.4
ossicles Q16.3
ossicles Q16.3
ejaculatory duct (congenital) Q55.4
endocrine gland (congenital) NEC Q89.2
acquired E89.89
epididymis (congenital) Q55.4
acquired Z90.79
epiglottis, congenital Q31.8
esophagus (congenital) Q39.8
acquired (partial) Z90.49
eustachian tube (congenital) Q16.2
extremity (acquired) Z89.9
congenital Q73.0
knee (following explantation of knee joint prosthesis) (joint) (with or without presence of antibiotic-impregnated cement spacer) Z89.52-
lower (above knee) Z89.619
below knee Z89.51-
upper — *see* Absence, arm
eye (acquired) Z90.01
congenital Q11.1
muscle (congenital) Q10.3
eyeball (acquired) Z90.01
eyelid (fold) (congenital) Q10.3
acquired Z90.01
face, specified part NEC Q18.8
fallopian tube (s) (acquired) Z90.79
congenital Q50.6
family member (causing problem in home) NEC — *see also* Disruption, family Z63.32
femur, congenital — *see* Defect, reduction, lower limb, longitudinal, femur
fibrinogen (congenital) D68.2
acquired D65
finger (s) (acquired) Z89.02-
congenital — *see* Agenesis, hand
foot (acquired) Z89.43-
congenital — *see* Agenesis, foot
forearm (acquired) — *see* Absence, arm, below elbow
gallbladder (acquired) Z90.49
congenital Q44.0
gamma globulin in blood D80.1
hereditary D80.0
genital organs
acquired (female) (male) Z90.79
female, congenital Q52.8
external Q52.71

Absence (of) (organ or part) (complete or partial) - *continued*
genital organs - *continued*
female, congenital - *continued*
internal NEC Q52.8
male, congenital Q55.8
genitourinary organs, congenital NEC
female Q52.8
male Q55.8
globe (acquired) Z90.01
congenital Q11.1
glottis, congenital Q31.8
hand and wrist (acquired) Z89.11-
congenital — *see* Agenesis, hand
head, part (acquired) NEC Z90.09
heat sense R20.8
hip (following explantation of hip joint prosthesis) (joint) (with or without presence of antibiotic-impregnated cement spacer) Z89.62-
hymen (congenital) Q52.4
ileum (acquired) Z90.49
congenital Q41.2
immunoglobulin, isolated NEC D80.3
IgA D80.2
IgG D80.3
IgM D80.4
incus (acquired) — *see* Loss, ossicles, ear
congenital Q16.3
inner ear, congenital Q16.5
intestine (acquired) (small) Z90.49
congenital Q41.9
specified NEC Q41.8
large Z90.49
congenital Q42.9
specified NEC Q42.8
iris, congenital Q13.1
jejunum (acquired) Z90.49
congenital Q41.1
joint
acquired
hip (following explantation of hip joint prosthesis) (with or without presence of antibiotic-impregnated cement spacer) Z89.62-
knee (following explantation of knee joint prosthesis) (with or without presence of antibiotic-impregnated cement spacer) Z89.52-
shoulder (following explantation of shoulder joint prosthesis) (with or without presence of antibiotic-impregnated cement spacer) Z89.23-
congenital NEC Q74.8
kidney (s) (acquired) Z90.5
congenital Q60.2
bilateral Q60.1
unilateral Q60.0
knee (following explantation of knee joint prosthesis) (joint) (with or without presence of antibiotic-impregnated cement spacer) Z89.52-
labyrinth, membranous Q16.5
larynx (congenital) Q31.8
acquired Z90.02
leg (acquired) (above knee) Z89.61-
below knee (acquired) Z89.51-
congenital — *see* Defect, reduction, lower limb
lens (acquired) — *see also* Aphakia
congenital Q12.3
post cataract extraction Z98.4-
limb (acquired) — *see* Absence, extremity
lip Q38.6
liver (congenital) Q44.7
lung (fissure) (lobe) (bilateral) (unilateral) (congenital) Q33.3
acquired (any part) Z90.2
menstruation — *see* Amenorrhea
muscle (congenital) (pectoral) Q79.8
ocular Q10.3
neck, part Q18.8
neutrophil — *see* Agranulocytosis
nipple (s) (with breast (s)) (acquired) Z90.1-

Absence (of) (organ or part) (complete or partial) - *continued*
nipple (s) (with breast (s)) (acquired) - *continued*
congenital Q83.2
nose (congenital) Q30.1
acquired Z90.09
organ
of Corti, congenital Q16.5
or site, congenital NEC Q89.8
acquired NEC Z90.89
osseous meatus (ear) Q16.4
ovary (acquired)
bilateral Z90.722
congenital
bilateral Q50.02
unilateral Q50.01
unilateral Z90.721
oviduct (acquired)
bilateral Z90.722
congenital Q50.6
unilateral Z90.721
pancreas (congenital) Q45.0
acquired Z90.410
complete Z90.410
partial Z90.411
total Z90.410
parathyroid gland (acquired) E89.2
congenital Q89.2
patella, congenital Q74.1
penis (congenital) Q55.5
acquired Z90.79
pericardium (congenital) Q24.8
pituitary gland (congenital) Q89.2
acquired E89.3
prostate (acquired) Z90.79
congenital Q55.4
pulmonary valve Q22.0
punctum lacrimale (congenital) Q10.4
radius, congenital — *see* Defect, reduction, upper limb, longitudinal, radius
rectum (congenital) Q42.1
with fistula Q42.0
acquired Z90.49
respiratory organ NOS Q34.9
rib (acquired) Z90.89
congenital Q76.6
sacrum, congenital Q76.49
salivary gland (s) , congenital Q38.4
scrotum, congenital Q55.29
seminal vesicles (congenital) Q55.4
acquired Z90.79
septum
atrial (congenital) Q21.1
between aorta and pulmonary artery Q21.4
ventricular (congenital) Q20.4
sex chromosome
female phenotype Q97.8
male phenotype Q98.8
skull bone (congenital) Q75.8
with
anencephaly Q00.0
encephalocele — *see* Encephalocele
hydrocephalus Q03.9
with spina bifida — *see* Spina bifida, by site, with hydrocephalus
microcephaly Q02
spermatic cord, congenital Q55.4
spine, congenital Q76.49
spleen (congenital) Q89.01
acquired Z90.81
sternum, congenital Q76.7
stomach (acquired) (partial) Z90.3
congenital Q40.2
superior vena cava, congenital Q26.8
teeth, tooth (congenital) K00.0
acquired (complete) K08.109
class I K08.101
class II K08.102
class III K08.103
class IV K08.104
due to
caries K08.139
class I K08.131
class II K08.132

Absence (of) (organ or part) (complete or partial) - *continued*
teeth, tooth (congenital) - *continued*
acquired (complete) - *continued*
due to - *continued*
caries - *continued*
class III K08.133
class IV K08.134
periodontal disease K08.129
class I K08.121
class II K08.122
class III K08.123
class IV K08.124
specified NEC K08.199
class I K08.191
class II K08.192
class III K08.193
class IV K08.194
trauma K08.119
class I K08.111
class II K08.112
class III K08.113
class IV K08.114
partial K08.409
class I K08.401
class II K08.402
class III K08.403
class IV K08.404
due to
caries K08.439
class I K08.431
class II K08.432
class III K08.433
class IV K08.434
periodontal disease K08.429
class I K08.421
class II K08.422
class III K08.423
class IV K08.424
specified NEC K08.499
class I K08.491
class II K08.492
class III K08.493
class IV K08.494
trauma K08.419
class I K08.411
class II K08.412
class III K08.413
class IV K08.414
tendon (congenital) Q79.8
testis (congenital) Q55.0
acquired Z90.79
thumb (acquired) Z89.01-
congenital — *see* Agenesis, hand
thymus gland Q89.2
thyroid (gland) (acquired) E89.0
cartilage, congenital Q31.8
congenital E03.1
toe (s) (acquired) Z89.42-
with foot — *see* Absence, foot and ankle
congenital — *see* Agenesis, foot
great Z89.41-
tongue, congenital Q38.3
trachea (cartilage) , congenital Q32.1
transverse aortic arch, congenital Q25.49
tricuspid valve Q22.4
umbilical artery, congenital Q27.0
upper arm and forearm with hand present, congenital — *see* Agenesis, arm, with hand present
ureter (congenital) Q62.4
acquired Z90.6
urethra, congenital Q64.5
uterus (acquired) Z90.710
with cervix Z90.710
with remaining cervical stump Z90.711
congenital Q51.0
uvula, congenital Q38.5
vagina, congenital Q52.0
vas deferens (congenital) Q55.4
acquired Z90.79
vein (peripheral) congenital NEC Q27.8
cerebral Q28.3
digestive system Q27.8
great Q26.8

Absence (of) (organ or part) (complete or partial) - *continued*
vein (peripheral) congenital NEC - *continued*
lower limb Q27.8
portal Q26.5
precerebral Q28.1
specified site NEC Q27.8
upper limb Q27.8
vena cava (inferior) (superior) , congenital Q26.8
ventricular septum Q20.4
vertebra, congenital Q76.49
vulva, congenital Q52.71
wrist (acquired) Z89.12-
Absorbent system disease I87.8
Absorption
carbohydrate, disturbance K90.49
chemical — *see* Table of Drugs and Chemicals
through placenta (newborn) P04.9
environmental substance P04.6
nutritional substance P04.5
obstetric anesthetic or analgesic drug P04.0
drug NEC — *see* Table of Drugs and Chemicals
addictive
through placenta (newborn) — *see also* Newborn, affected by, maternal, use of P04.40
cocaine P04.41
hallucinogens P04.42
specified drug NEC P04.49
medicinal
through placenta (newborn) P04.19
through placenta (newborn) P04.19
obstetric anesthetic or analgesic drug P04.0
fat, disturbance K90.49
pancreatic K90.3
noxious substance — *see* Table of Drugs and Chemicals
protein, disturbance K90.49
starch, disturbance K90.49
toxic substance — *see* Table of Drugs and Chemicals
uremic — *see* Uremia
Abstinence symptoms, syndrome
alcohol F10.239
with delirium F10.231
cocaine F14.23
neonatal P96.1
nicotine — *see* Dependence, drug, nicotine, with, withdrawal
opioid F11.93
with dependence F11.23
psychoactive NEC F19.939
with
delirium F19.931
dependence F19.239
with
delirium F19.231
perceptual disturbance F19.232
uncomplicated F19.230
perceptual disturbance F19.932
uncomplicated F19.930
sedative F13.939
with
delirium F13.931
dependence F13.239
with
delirium F13.231
perceptual disturbance F13.232
uncomplicated F13.230
perceptual disturbance F13.932
uncomplicated F13.930
stimulant NEC F15.93
with dependence F15.23
Abulia R68.89
Abulomania F60.7
Abuse
adult — *see* Maltreatment, adult
as reason for
couple seeking advice (including offender) Z63.0

Abuse - *continued*
alcohol (non-dependent) F10.10
with
anxiety disorder F10.180
intoxication F10.129
with delirium F10.121
uncomplicated F10.120
mood disorder F10.14
other specified disorder F10.188
psychosis F10.159
delusions F10.150
hallucinations F10.151
sexual dysfunction F10.181
sleep disorder F10.182
unspecified disorder F10.19
withdrawal F10.139
with
perceptual disturbance F10.132
delirium F10.131
uncomplicated F10.130
counseling and surveillance Z71.41
in remission (early) (sustained) F10.11
amphetamine (or related substance) — *see also* Abuse, drug, stimulant NEC
stimulant NEC F15.10
with
anxiety disorder F15.180
intoxication F15.129
with
delirium F15.121
perceptual disturbance F15.122
withdrawal F15.13
analgesics (non-prescribed) (over the counter) F55.8
antacids F55.0
antidepressants — *see* Abuse, drug, psychoactive NEC
anxiolytic — *see* Abuse, drug, sedative
barbiturates — *see* Abuse, drug, sedative
caffeine — *see* Abuse, drug, stimulant NEC
cannabis, cannabinoids — *see* Abuse, drug, cannabis
child — *see* Maltreatment, child
cocaine — *see* Abuse, drug, cocaine
drug NEC (non-dependent) F19.10
with sleep disorder F19.182
amphetamine type — *see* Abuse, drug, stimulant NEC
analgesics (non-prescribed) (over the counter) F55.8
antacids F55.0
antidepressants — *see* Abuse, drug, psychoactive NEC
anxiolytics — *see* Abuse, drug, sedative
barbiturates — *see* Abuse, drug, sedative
caffeine — *see* Abuse, drug, stimulant NEC
cannabis F12.10
with
anxiety disorder F12.180
intoxication F12.129
with
delirium F12.121
perceptual disturbance F12.122
uncomplicated F12.120
other specified disorder F12.188
psychosis F12.159
delusions F12.150
hallucinations F12.151
unspecified disorder F12.19
withdrawal F12.13
in remission (early) (sustained) F12.11
cocaine F14.10
with
anxiety disorder F14.180
intoxication F14.129
with
delirium F14.121
perceptual disturbance F14.122
uncomplicated F14.120
mood disorder F14.14
other specified disorder F14.188
psychosis F14.159
delusions F14.150
hallucinations F14.151

Abuse - *continued*
drug NEC (non-dependent) - *continued*
cocaine - *continued*
with - *continued*
sexual dysfunction F14.181
sleep disorder F14.182
unspecified disorder F14.19
withdrawal F14.13
in remission (early) (sustained) F14.11
counseling and surveillance Z71.51
hallucinogen F16.10
with
anxiety disorder F16.180
flashbacks F16.183
intoxication F16.129
with
delirium F16.121
perceptual disturbance F16.122
uncomplicated F16.120
mood disorder F16.14
other specified disorder F16.188
perception disorder, persisting F16.183
psychosis F16.159
delusions F16.150
hallucinations F16.151
unspecified disorder F16.19
in remission (early) (sustained) F16.11
hashish — *see* Abuse, drug, cannabis
herbal or folk remedies F55.1
hormones F55.3
hypnotics — *see* Abuse, drug, sedative
inhalant F18.10
with
anxiety disorder F18.180
dementia, persisting F18.17
intoxication F18.129
with delirium F18.121
uncomplicated F18.120
mood disorder F18.14
other specified disorder F18.188
psychosis F18.159
delusions F18.150
hallucinations F18.151
unspecified disorder F18.19
in remission (early) (sustained) F18.11
in remission (early) (sustained) F19.11
laxatives F55.2
LSD — *see* Abuse, drug, hallucinogen
marihuana — *see* Abuse, drug, cannabis
morphine type (opioids) — *see* Abuse, drug, opioid
opioid F11.10
with
intoxication F11.129
with
delirium F11.121
perceptual disturbance F11.122
uncomplicated F11.120
mood disorder F11.14
other specified disorder F11.188
psychosis F11.159
delusions F11.150
hallucinations F11.151
sexual dysfunction F11.181
sleep disorder F11.182
unspecified disorder F11.19
withdrawal F11.13
in remission (early) (sustained) F11.11
PCP (phencyclidine) (or related substance) — *see* Abuse, drug, hallucinogen
psychoactive NEC F19.10
with
amnestic disorder F19.16
anxiety disorder F19.180
dementia F19.17
intoxication F19.129
with
delirium F19.121
perceptual disturbance F19.122
uncomplicated F19.120
mood disorder F19.14
other specified disorder F19.188
psychosis F19.159

ABSENCE - ABUSE

Addison-Biermer anemia (pernicious) D51.0

Addisonian crisis E27.2

Addison's
- anemia (pernicious) D51.0
- disease (bronze) or syndrome E27.1
  - tuberculous A18.7
- keloid L94.0

Addison-Schilder complex E71.528

Additional — *see also* Accessory
- chromosome (s) Q99.8
  - sex — *see* Abnormal, chromosome, sex
  - 21 — *see* Trisomy, 21

Adduction contracture, hip or other joint — *see* Contraction, joint

Adenitis — *see also* Lymphadenitis
- acute, unspecified site L04.9
- axillary I88.9
  - acute L04.2
  - chronic or subacute I88.1
- Bartholin's gland N75.8
- bulbourethral gland — *see* Urethritis
- cervical I88.9
  - acute L04.0
  - chronic or subacute I88.1
- chancroid (Hemophilus ducreyi) A57
- chronic, unspecified site I88.1
- Cowper's gland — *see* Urethritis
- due to Pasteurella multocida (P. septica) A28.0
- epidemic, acute B27.09
- gangrenous L04.9
- gonorrheal NEC A54.89
- groin I88.9
  - acute L04.1
  - chronic or subacute I88.1
- infectious (acute) (epidemic) B27.09
- inguinal I88.9
  - acute L04.1
  - chronic or subacute I88.1
- lymph gland or node, except mesenteric I88.9
  - acute — *see* Lymphadenitis, acute
  - chronic or subacute I88.1
- mesenteric (acute) (chronic) (nonspecific) (subacute) I88.0
- parotid gland (suppurative) — *see* Sialoadenitis
- salivary gland (any) (suppurative) — *see* Sialoadenitis
- scrofulous (tuberculous) A18.2
- Skene's duct or gland — *see* Urethritis
- strumous, tuberculous A18.2
- subacute, unspecified site I88.1
- sublingual gland (suppurative) — *see* Sialoadenitis
- submandibular gland (suppurative) — *see* Sialoadenitis
- submaxillary gland (suppurative) — *see* Sialoadenitis
- tuberculous — *see* Tuberculosis, lymph gland
- urethral gland — *see* Urethritis
- Wharton's duct (suppurative) — *see* Sialoadenitis

Adenoacanthoma — *see* Neoplasm, malignant, by site

Adenoameloblastoma — *see* Cyst, calcifying odontogenic

Adenocarcinoid (tumor) — *see* Neoplasm, malignant, by site

Adenocarcinoma — *see also* Neoplasm, malignant, by site
- acidophil
  - specified site — *see* Neoplasm, malignant, by site
  - unspecified site C75.1
- adrenal cortical C74.0-
- alveolar — *see* Neoplasm, lung, malignant
- apocrine
  - breast — *see* Neoplasm, breast, malignant
  - in situ
    - breast D05.8-
    - specified site NEC — *see* Neoplasm, skin, in situ
    - unspecified site D04.9

Adenocarcinoma - *continued*
- apocrine - *continued*
  - specified site NEC — *see* Neoplasm, skin, malignant
  - unspecified site C44.99
- basal cell
  - specified site — *see* Neoplasm, skin, malignant
  - unspecified site C08.9
- basophil
  - specified site — *see* Neoplasm, malignant, by site
  - unspecified site C75.1
- bile duct type C22.1
  - liver C22.1
  - specified site NEC — *see* Neoplasm, malignant, by site
  - unspecified site C22.1
- bronchiolar — *see* Neoplasm, lung, malignant
- bronchioloalveolar — *see* Neoplasm, lung, malignant
- ceruminous C44.29-
- cervix, in situ — *see also* Carcinoma, cervix uteri, in situ D06.9
- chromophobe
  - specified site — *see* Neoplasm, malignant, by site
  - unspecified site C75.1
- diffuse type
  - specified site — *see* Neoplasm, malignant, by site
  - unspecified site C16.9
- duct
  - infiltrating
    - with Paget's disease — *see* Neoplasm, breast, malignant
    - specified site — *see* Neoplasm, malignant, by site
    - unspecified site (female) C50.91-
      - male C50.92-
  - specified site — *see* Neoplasm, malignant, by site
  - unspecified site
    - female C56.9
    - male C61
- eosinophil
  - specified site — *see* Neoplasm, malignant, by site
  - unspecified site C75.1
- follicular
  - with papillary C73
  - moderately differentiated C73
  - specified site — *see* Neoplasm, malignant, by site
  - trabecular C73
  - unspecified site C73
  - well differentiated C73
- Hurthle cell C73
- in
  - adenomatous
    - polyposis coli C18.9
- infiltrating duct
  - with Paget's disease — *see* Neoplasm, breast, malignant
  - specified site — *see* Neoplasm, by site, malignant
  - unspecified site (female) C50.91-
    - male C50.92-
- inflammatory
  - specified site — *see* Neoplasm, by site, malignant
  - unspecified site (female) C50.91-
    - male C50.92-
- intestinal type
  - specified site — *see* Neoplasm, by site, malignant
  - unspecified site C16.9
- intracystic papillary
- intraductal
  - breast D05.1-
  - noninfiltrating
    - breast D05.1-
    - papillary
      - with invasion

Adenocarcinoma - *continued*
- intraductal - *continued*
  - noninfiltrating - *continued*
    - papillary - *continued*
      - with invasion - *continued*
        - specified site — *see* Neoplasm, by site, malignant
        - unspecified site (female) C50.91-
          - male C50.92-
      - breast D05.1-
      - specified site NEC — *see* Neoplasm, in situ, by site
      - unspecified site D05.1-
    - specified site NEC — *see* Neoplasm, in situ, by site
    - unspecified site D05.1-
  - papillary
    - with invasion
      - specified site — *see* Neoplasm, malignant, by site
      - unspecified site (female) C50.91-
        - male C50.92-
    - breast D05.1-
    - specified site — *see* Neoplasm, in situ, by site
    - unspecified site D05.1-
  - specified site NEC — *see* Neoplasm, in situ, by site
  - unspecified site D05.1-
- islet cell
  - with exocrine, mixed
    - specified site — *see* Neoplasm, malignant, by site
    - unspecified site C25.9
  - pancreas C25.4
  - specified site NEC — *see* Neoplasm, malignant, by site
  - unspecified site C25.4
- lobular
  - in situ
    - breast D05.0-
    - specified site NEC — *see* Neoplasm, in situ, by site
    - unspecified site D05.0-
  - specified site — *see* Neoplasm, malignant, by site
  - unspecified site (female) C50.91-
    - male C50.92-
- mucoid — *see also* Neoplasm, malignant, by site
  - cell
    - specified site — *see* Neoplasm, malignant, by site
    - unspecified site C75.1
- nonencapsulated sclerosing C73
- papillary
  - with follicular C73
  - follicular variant C73
  - intraductal (noninfiltrating)
    - with invasion
      - specified site — *see* Neoplasm, malignant, by site
      - unspecified site (female) C50.91-
        - male C50.92-
    - breast D05.1-
    - specified site NEC — *see* Neoplasm, in situ, by site
    - unspecified site D05.1-
  - serous
    - specified site — *see* Neoplasm, malignant, by site
    - unspecified site C56.9
- papillocystic
  - specified site — *see* Neoplasm, malignant, by site
  - unspecified site C56.9
- pseudomucinous
  - specified site — *see* Neoplasm, malignant, by site
  - unspecified site C56.9
- renal cell C64-
- sebaceous — *see* Neoplasm, skin, malignant
- serous — *see also* Neoplasm, malignant, by site
  - papillary

Adenocarcinoma - *continued*
  serous - *continued*
    papillary - *continued*
      specified site — *see* Neoplasm, malignant, by site
      unspecified site C56.9
  sweat gland — *see* Neoplasm, skin, malignant
  water-clear cell C75.0
Adenocarcinoma-in-situ — *see also* Neoplasm, in situ, by site
  breast D05.9-
Adenofibroma
  clear cell — *see* Neoplasm, benign, by site
  endometrioid D27.9
    borderline malignancy D39.10
    malignant C56-
  mucinous
    specified site — *see* Neoplasm, benign, by site
    unspecified site D27.9
  papillary
    specified site — *see* Neoplasm, benign, by site
    unspecified site D27.9
  prostate — *see* Enlargement, enlarged, prostate
  serous
    specified site — *see* Neoplasm, benign, by site
    unspecified site D27.9
  specified site — *see* Neoplasm, benign, by site
  unspecified site D27.9
Adenofibrosis
  breast — *see* Fibroadenosis, breast
  endometrioid N80.0
Adenoiditis (chronic) J35.02
  with tonsillitis J35.03
  acute J03.90
    recurrent J03.91
    specified organism NEC J03.80
      recurrent J03.81
    staphylococcal J03.80
      recurrent J03.81
    streptococcal J03.00
      recurrent J03.01
Adenoids — *see* condition
Adenolipoma — *see* Neoplasm, benign, by site
Adenolipomatosis, Launois-Bensaude E88.89
Adenolymphoma
  specified site — *see* Neoplasm, benign, by site
  unspecified site D11.9
Adenoma — *see also* Neoplasm, benign, by site
  acidophil
    specified site — *see* Neoplasm, benign, by site
    unspecified site D35.2
  acidophil-basophil, mixed
    specified site — *see* Neoplasm, benign, by site
    unspecified site D35.2
  adrenal (cortical) D35.00
    clear cell D35.00
    compact cell D35.00
    glomerulosa cell D35.00
    heavily pigmented variant D35.00
    mixed cell D35.00
  alpha-cell
    pancreas D13.7
    specified site NEC — *see* Neoplasm, benign, by site
    unspecified site D13.7
  alveolar D14.30
  apocrine
    breast D24-
    specified site NEC — *see* Neoplasm, skin, benign, by site
    unspecified site D23.9
  basal cell D11.9
  basophil
    specified site — *see* Neoplasm, benign, by site

Adenoma - *continued*
  basophil - *continued*
    unspecified site D35.2
  basophil-acidophil, mixed
    specified site — *see* Neoplasm, benign, by site
    unspecified site D35.2
  beta-cell
    pancreas D13.7
    specified site NEC — *see* Neoplasm, benign, by site
    unspecified site D13.7
  bile duct D13.4
    common D13.5
    extrahepatic D13.5
    intrahepatic D13.4
    specified site NEC — *see* Neoplasm, benign, by site
    unspecified site D13.4
  black D35.00
  bronchial D38.1
    cylindroid type — *see* Neoplasm, lung, malignant
  ceruminous D23.2-
  chief cell D35.1
  chromophobe
    specified site — *see* Neoplasm, benign, by site
    unspecified site D35.2
  colloid
    specified site — *see* Neoplasm, benign, by site
    unspecified site D34
  eccrine, papillary — *see* Neoplasm, skin, benign
  endocrine, multiple
    single specified site — *see* Neoplasm, uncertain behavior, by site
    two or more specified sites D44-
    unspecified site D44.9
  endometrioid — *see also* Neoplasm, benign
    borderline malignancy — *see* Neoplasm, uncertain behavior, by site
  eosinophil
    specified site — *see* Neoplasm, benign, by site
    unspecified site D35.2
  fetal
    specified site — *see* Neoplasm, benign, by site
    unspecified site D34
  follicular
    specified site — *see* Neoplasm, benign, by site
    unspecified site D34
  hepatocellular D13.4
  Hurthle cell D34
  islet cell
    pancreas D13.7
    specified site NEC — *see* Neoplasm, benign, by site
    unspecified site D13.7
  liver cell D13.4
  macrofollicular
    specified site — *see* Neoplasm, benign, by site
    unspecified site D34
  malignant, malignum — *see* Neoplasm, malignant, by site
  microcystic
    pancreas D13.6
    specified site NEC — *see* Neoplasm, benign, by site
    unspecified site D13.6
  microfollicular
    specified site — *see* Neoplasm, benign, by site
    unspecified site D34
  mucoid cell
    specified site — *see* Neoplasm, benign, by site
    unspecified site D35.2
  multiple endocrine
    single specified site — *see* Neoplasm, uncertain behavior, by site

Adenoma - *continued*
  multiple endocrine - *continued*
    two or more specified sites D44-
    unspecified site D44.9
  nipple D24-
  papillary — *see also* Neoplasm, benign, by site
    eccrine — *see* Neoplasm, skin, benign, by site
  Pick's tubular
    specified site — *see* Neoplasm, benign, by site
    unspecified site
      female D27.9
      male D29.20
  pleomorphic
    carcinoma in — *see* Neoplasm, salivary gland, malignant
      specified site — *see* Neoplasm, malignant, by site
      unspecified site C08.9
  polypoid — *see also* Neoplasm, benign
    adenocarcinoma in — *see* Neoplasm, malignant, by site
    adenocarcinoma in situ — *see* Neoplasm, in situ, by site
  prostate — *see* Neoplasm, benign, prostate
  rete cell D29.20
  sebaceous — *see* Neoplasm, skin, benign
  Sertoli cell
    specified site — *see* Neoplasm, benign, by site
    unspecified site
      female D27.9
      male D29.20
  skin appendage — *see* Neoplasm, skin, benign
  sudoriferous gland — *see* Neoplasm, skin, benign
  sweat gland — *see* Neoplasm, skin, benign
  testicular
    specified site — *see* Neoplasm, benign, by site
    unspecified site
      female D27.9
      male D29.20
  tubular — *see also* Neoplasm, benign, by site
    adenocarcinoma in — *see* Neoplasm, malignant, by site
    adenocarcinoma in situ — *see* Neoplasm, in situ, by site
    Pick's
      specified site — *see* Neoplasm, benign, by site
      unspecified site
        female D27.9
        male D29.20
  tubulovillous — *see also* Neoplasm, benign, by site
    adenocarcinoma in — *see* Neoplasm, malignant, by site
    adenocarcinoma in situ — *see* Neoplasm, in situ, by site
  villous — *see* Neoplasm, uncertain behavior, by site
    adenocarcinoma in — *see* Neoplasm, malignant, by site
    adenocarcinoma in situ — *see* Neoplasm, in situ, by site
  water-clear cell D35.1
Adenomatosis
  endocrine (multiple) E31.20
    single specified site — *see* Neoplasm, uncertain behavior, by site
  erosive of nipple D24-
  pluriendocrine — *see* Adenomatosis, endocrine
  pulmonary D38.1
    malignant — *see* Neoplasm, lung, malignant
  specified site — *see* Neoplasm, benign, by site
  unspecified site D12.6
Adenomatous
  goiter (nontoxic) E04.9

- **Adenomatous** - *continued*
  - goiter (nontoxic) - *continued*
    - with hyperthyroidism — *see* Hyperthyroidism, with, goiter, nodular
    - toxic — *see* Hyperthyroidism, with, goiter, nodular
- **Adenomyoma** — *see also* Neoplasm, benign, by site
  - prostate — *see* Enlarged, prostate
- **Adenomyometritis** N80.0
- **Adenomyosis** N80.0
- **Adenopathy (lymph gland)** R59.9
  - generalized R59.1
  - inguinal R59.0
  - localized R59.0
  - mediastinal R59.0
  - mesentery R59.0
  - syphilitic (secondary) A51.49
  - tracheobronchial R59.0
    - tuberculous A15.4
      - primary (progressive) A15.7
  - tuberculous — *see also* Tuberculosis, lymph gland
    - tracheobronchial A15.4
      - primary (progressive) A15.7
- **Adenosalpingitis** — *see* Salpingitis
- **Adenosarcoma** — *see* Neoplasm, malignant, by site
- **Adenosclerosis** I88.8
- **Adenosis (sclerosing) breast** — *see* Fibroadenosis, breast
- **Adenovirus, as cause of disease classified elsewhere** B97.0
- **Adentia (complete) (partial)** — *see* Absence, teeth
- **Adherent** — *see also* Adhesions
  - labia (minora) N90.89
  - pericardium (nonrheumatic) I31.0
    - rheumatic I09.2
  - placenta (with hemorrhage) O72.0
    - without hemorrhage O73.0
  - prepuce, newborn N47.0
  - scar (skin) L90.5
  - tendon in scar L90.5
- **Adhesions, adhesive (postinfective)** K66.0
  - with intestinal obstruction K56.50
    - complete K56.52
    - incomplete K56.51
    - partial K56.51
  - abdominal (wall) — *see* Adhesions, peritoneum
  - appendix K38.8
  - bile duct (common) (hepatic) K83.8
  - bladder (sphincter) N32.89
  - bowel — *see* Adhesions, peritoneum
  - cardiac I31.0
    - rheumatic I09.2
  - cecum — *see* Adhesions, peritoneum
  - cervicovaginal N88.1
    - congenital Q52.8
    - postpartal O90.89
      - old N88.1
  - cervix N88.1
  - ciliary body NEC — *see* Adhesions, iris
  - clitoris N90.89
  - colon — *see* Adhesions, peritoneum
  - common duct K83.8
  - congenital — *see also* Anomaly, by site
    - fingers — *see* Syndactylism, complex, fingers
    - omental, anomalous Q43.3
    - peritoneal Q43.3
    - tongue (to gum or roof of mouth) Q38.3
  - conjunctiva (acquired) H11.21-
    - congenital Q15.8
  - cystic duct K82.8
  - diaphragm — *see* Adhesions, peritoneum
  - due to foreign body — *see* Foreign body
  - duodenum — *see* Adhesions, peritoneum
  - ear
    - middle H74.1-
  - epididymis N50.89
  - epidural — *see* Adhesions, meninges
  - epiglottis J38.7

- **Adhesions, adhesive (postinfective)** - *continued*
  - eyelid H02.59
  - female pelvis N73.6
  - gallbladder K82.8
  - globe H44.89
  - heart I31.0
    - rheumatic I09.2
  - ileocecal (coil) — *see* Adhesions, peritoneum
  - ileum — *see* Adhesions, peritoneum
  - intestine — *see also* Adhesions, peritoneum
    - with obstruction K56.50
      - complete K56.52
      - incomplete K56.51
      - partial K56.51
  - intra-abdominal — *see* Adhesions, peritoneum
  - iris H21.50-
    - anterior H21.51-
    - goniosynechiae H21.52-
    - posterior H21.54-
    - to corneal graft T85.898
  - joint — *see* Ankylosis
    - knee M23.8X
    - temporomandibular M26.61-
  - labium (majus) (minus), congenital Q52.5
  - liver — *see* Adhesions, peritoneum
  - lung J98.4
  - mediastinum J98.59
  - meninges (cerebral) (spinal) G96.12
    - congenital Q07.8
    - tuberculous (cerebral) (spinal) A17.0
  - mesenteric — *see* Adhesions, peritoneum
  - nasal (septum) (to turbinates) J34.89
  - ocular muscle — *see* Strabismus, mechanical
  - omentum — *see* Adhesions, peritoneum
  - ovary N73.6
    - congenital (to cecum, kidney or omentum) Q50.39
  - paraovarian N73.6
  - pelvic (peritoneal)
    - female N73.6
      - postprocedural N99.4
    - male — *see* Adhesions, peritoneum
    - postpartal (old) N73.6
    - tuberculous A18.17
  - penis to scrotum (congenital) Q55.8
  - periappendiceal — *see also* Adhesions, peritoneum
  - pericardium (nonrheumatic) I31.0
    - focal I31.8
    - rheumatic I09.2
    - tuberculous A18.84
  - pericholecystic K82.8
  - perigastric — *see* Adhesions, peritoneum
  - periovarian N73.6
  - periprostatic N42.89
  - perirectal — *see* Adhesions, peritoneum
  - perirenal N28.89
  - peritoneum, peritoneal (postinfective) K66.0
    - with obstruction (intestinal) K56.50
      - complete K56.52
      - incomplete K56.51
      - partial K56.51
    - congenital Q43.3
    - pelvic, female N73.6
      - postprocedural N99.4
    - postpartal, pelvic N73.6
    - postprocedural K66.0
    - to uterus N73.6
  - peritubal N73.6
  - periureteral N28.89
  - periuterine N73.6
  - perivesical N32.89
  - perivesicular (seminal vesicle) N50.89
  - pleura, pleuritic J94.8
    - tuberculous NEC A15.6
  - pleuropericardial J94.8
  - postoperative (gastrointestinal tract) K66.0
    - with obstruction — *see also* Obstruction, intestine, postoperative K91.30
    - due to foreign body accidentally left in wound — *see* Foreign body, accidentally left during a procedure
    - pelvic peritoneal N99.4

- **Adhesions, adhesive (postinfective)** - *continued*
  - postoperative (gastrointestinal tract) - *continued*
    - urethra — *see* Stricture, urethra, postprocedural
    - vagina N99.2
  - postpartal, old (vulva or perineum) N90.89
  - preputial, prepuce N47.5
  - pulmonary J98.4
  - pylorus — *see* Adhesions, peritoneum
  - sciatic nerve — *see* Lesion, nerve, sciatic
  - seminal vesicle N50.89
  - shoulder (joint) — *see* Capsulitis, adhesive
  - sigmoid flexure — *see* Adhesions, peritoneum
  - spermatic cord (acquired) N50.89
    - congenital Q55.4
  - spinal canal G96.12
  - stomach — *see* Adhesions, peritoneum
  - subscapular — *see* Capsulitis, adhesive
  - temporomandibular M26.61-
  - tendinitis — *see also* Tenosynovitis, specified type NEC
    - shoulder — *see* Capsulitis, adhesive
  - testis N44.8
  - tongue, congenital (to gum or roof of mouth) Q38.3
    - acquired K14.8
  - trachea J39.8
  - tubo-ovarian N73.6
  - tunica vaginalis N44.8
  - uterus N73.6
    - internal N85.6
    - to abdominal wall N73.6
  - vagina (chronic) N89.5
    - postoperative N99.2
  - vitreomacular H43.82-
  - vitreous H43.89
  - vulva N90.89
- **Adiaspiromycosis** B48.8
- **Adie (-Holmes) pupil or syndrome** — *see* Anomaly, pupil, function, tonic pupil
- **Adiponecrosis neonatorum** P83.88
- **Adiposis** — *see also* Obesity
  - cerebralis E23.6
  - dolorosa E88.2
- **Adiposity** — *see also* Obesity
  - heart — *see* Degeneration, myocardial
  - localized E65
- **Adiposogenital dystrophy** E23.6
- **Adjustment**
  - disorder — *see* Disorder, adjustment
  - implanted device — *see* Encounter (for), adjustment (of)
  - prosthesis, external — *see* Fitting
  - reaction — *see* Disorder, adjustment
- **Administration of tPA (rtPA) in a different facility within the last 24 hours prior to admission to current facility** Z92.82
- **Admission (for)** — *see also* Encounter (for)
  - adjustment (of)
    - artificial
      - arm Z44.00-
        - complete Z44.01-
        - partial Z44.02-
      - eye Z44.2
      - leg Z44.10-
        - complete Z44.11-
        - partial Z44.12-
    - brain neuropacemaker Z46.2
      - implanted Z45.42
    - breast
      - implant Z45.81
      - prosthesis (external) Z44.3
    - colostomy belt Z46.89
    - contact lenses Z46.0
    - cystostomy device Z46.6
    - dental prosthesis Z46.3
    - device NEC
      - abdominal Z46.89
      - implanted Z45.89
        - cardiac Z45.09
          - defibrillator (with synchronous cardiac pacemaker) Z45.02

Admission (for) - *continued*
adjustment (of) - *continued*
device NEC - *continued*
implanted - *continued*
cardiac - *continued*
pacemaker (cardiac resynchronization therapy (CRT-P)) Z45.018
pulse generator Z45.010
resynchronization therapy defibrillator (CRT-D) Z45.02
hearing device Z45.328
bone conduction Z45.320
cochlear Z45.321
infusion pump Z45.1
nervous system Z45.49
CSF drainage Z45.41
hearing device — *see* Admission, adjustment, device, implanted, hearing device
neuropacemaker Z45.42
visual substitution Z45.31
specified NEC Z45.89
vascular access Z45.2
visual substitution Z45.31
nervous system Z46.2
implanted — *see* Admission, adjustment, device, implanted, nervous system
orthodontic Z46.4
prosthetic Z44.9
arm — *see* Admission, adjustment, artificial, arm
breast Z44.3
dental Z46.3
eye Z44.2
leg — *see* Admission, adjustment, artificial, leg
specified type NEC Z44.8
substitution
auditory Z46.2
implanted — *see* Admission, adjustment, device, implanted, hearing device
nervous system Z46.2
implanted — *see* Admission, adjustment, device, implanted, nervous system
visual Z46.2
implanted Z45.31
urinary Z46.6
hearing aid Z46.1
implanted — *see* Admission, adjustment, device, implanted, hearing device
ileostomy device Z46.89
intestinal appliance or device NEC Z46.89
neuropacemaker (brain) (peripheral nerve) (spinal cord) Z46.2
implanted Z45.42
orthodontic device Z46.4
orthopedic (brace) (cast) (device) (shoes) Z46.89
pacemaker (cardiac resynchronization therapy (CRT-P))
cardiac Z45.018
pulse generator Z45.010
nervous system Z46.2
implanted Z45.42
portacath (port-a-cath) Z45.2
prosthesis Z44.9
arm — *see* Admission, adjustment, artificial, arm
breast Z44.3
dental Z46.3
eye Z44.2
leg — *see* Admission, adjustment, artificial, leg
specified NEC Z44.8
spectacles Z46.0
aftercare — *see also* Aftercare Z51.89
postpartum
immediately after delivery Z39.0
routine follow-up Z39.2
radiation therapy (antineoplastic) Z51.0

Admission (for) - *continued*
attention to artificial opening (of) Z43.9
artificial vagina Z43.7
colostomy Z43.3
cystostomy Z43.5
enterostomy Z43.4
gastrostomy Z43.1
ileostomy Z43.2
jejunostomy Z43.4
nephrostomy Z43.6
specified site NEC Z43.8
intestinal tract Z43.4
urinary tract Z43.6
tracheostomy Z43.0
ureterostomy Z43.6
urethrostomy Z43.6
breast augmentation or reduction Z41.1
breast reconstruction following mastectomy Z42.1
change of
dressing (nonsurgical) Z48.00
neuropacemaker device (brain) (peripheral nerve) (spinal cord) Z46.2
implanted Z45.42
surgical dressing Z48.01
circumcision, ritual or routine (in absence of diagnosis) Z41.2
clinical research investigation (control) (normal comparison) (participant) Z00.6
contraceptive management Z30.9
cosmetic surgery NEC Z41.1
counseling — *see also* Counseling
dietary Z71.3
gestational carrier Z31.7
HIV Z71.7
human immunodeficiency virus Z71.7
nonattending third party Z71.0
procreative management NEC Z31.69
delivery, full-term, uncomplicated O80
cesarean, without indication O82
desensitization to allergens Z51.6
dietary surveillance and counseling Z71.3
ear piercing Z41.3
examination at health care facility (adult) — *see also* Examination Z00.00
with abnormal findings Z00.01
clinical research investigation (control) (normal comparison) (participant) Z00.6
dental Z01.20
with abnormal findings Z01.21
donor (potential) Z00.5
ear Z01.10
with abnormal findings NEC Z01.118
eye Z01.00
with abnormal findings Z01.01
following failed vision screening Z01.020
with abnormal findings Z01.021
general, specified reason NEC Z00.8
hearing Z01.10
with abnormal findings NEC Z01.118
infant or child (over 28 days old) Z00.129
with abnormal findings Z00.121
postpartum checkup Z39.2
psychiatric (general) Z00.8
requested by authority Z04.6
vision Z01.00
with abnormal findings Z01.01
following failed vision screening Z01.020
with abnormal findings Z01.021
infant or child (over 28 days old) Z00.129
with abnormal findings Z00.121
fitting (of)
artificial
arm — *see* Admission, adjustment, artificial, arm
eye Z44.2
leg — *see* Admission, adjustment, artificial, leg
brain neuropacemaker Z46.2
implanted Z45.42

Admission (for) - *continued*
fitting (of) - *continued*
breast prosthesis (external) Z44.3
colostomy belt Z46.89
contact lenses Z46.0
cystostomy device Z46.6
dental prosthesis Z46.3
dentures Z46.3
device NEC
abdominal Z46.89
nervous system Z46.2
implanted — *see* Admission, adjustment, device, implanted, nervous system
orthodontic Z46.4
prosthetic Z44.9
breast Z44.3
dental Z46.3
eye Z44.2
substitution
auditory Z46.2
implanted — *see* Admission, adjustment, device, implanted, hearing device
nervous system Z46.2
implanted — *see* Admission, adjustment, device, implanted, nervous system
visual Z46.2
implanted Z45.31
hearing aid Z46.1
ileostomy device Z46.89
intestinal appliance or device NEC Z46.89
neuropacemaker (brain) (peripheral nerve) (spinal cord) Z46.2
implanted Z45.42
orthodontic device Z46.4
orthopedic device (brace) (cast) (shoes) Z46.89
prosthesis Z44.9
arm — *see* Admission, adjustment, artificial, arm
breast Z44.3
dental Z46.3
eye Z44.2
leg — *see* Admission, adjustment, artificial, leg
specified type NEC Z44.8
spectacles Z46.0
follow-up examination Z09
intrauterine device management Z30.431
initial prescription Z30.014
mental health evaluation Z00.8
requested by authority Z04.6
observation — *see* Observation
Papanicolaou smear, cervix Z12.4
for suspected malignant neoplasm Z12.4
plastic and reconstructive surgery following medical procedure or healed injury NEC Z42.8
plastic surgery, cosmetic NEC Z41.1
postpartum observation
immediately after delivery Z39.0
routine follow-up Z39.2
poststerilization (for restoration) Z31.0
aftercare Z31.42
procreative management Z31.9
prophylactic (measure) — *see also* Encounter, prophylactic measures
organ removal Z40.00
breast Z40.01
fallopian tube (s) Z40.03
with ovary (s) Z40.02
ovary (s) Z40.02
specified organ NEC Z40.09
testes Z40.09
vaccination Z23
psychiatric examination (general) Z00.8
requested by authority Z04.6
radiation therapy (antineoplastic) Z51.0
reconstructive surgery following medical procedure or healed injury NEC Z42.8
removal of
cystostomy catheter Z43.5
drains Z48.03

Agenesis - *continued*
finger (complete) (partial) — *see* Agenesis, hand
foot (and toes) (complete) (partial) Q72.3-
forearm (with hand present) — *see* Agenesis, arm, with hand present
and hand Q71.2-
gallbladder Q44.0
gastric Q40.2
genitalia, genital (organ (s))
female Q52.8
external Q52.71
internal NEC Q52.8
male Q55.8
glottis Q31.8
hair Q84.0
hand (and fingers) (complete) (partial) Q71.3-
heart Q24.8
valve NEC Q24.8
pulmonary Q22.0
hepatic Q44.7
humerus — *see* Defect, reduction, upper limb
hymen Q52.4
ileum Q41.2
incus Q16.3
intestine (small) Q41.9
large Q42.9
specified NEC Q42.8
iris (dilator fibers) Q13.1
jaw M26.09
jejunum Q41.1
kidney (s) (partial) Q60.2
bilateral Q60.1
unilateral Q60.0
labium (majus) (minus) Q52.71
labyrinth, membranous Q16.5
lacrimal apparatus Q10.4
larynx Q31.8
leg (complete) Q72.0-
with foot present Q72.1-
lower leg (with foot present) — *see* Agenesis, leg, with foot present
and foot Q72.2-
lens Q12.3
limb (complete) Q73.0
lower — *see* Agenesis, leg
upper — *see* Agenesis, arm
lip Q38.0
liver Q44.7
lung (fissure) (lobe) (bilateral) (unilateral) Q33.3
mandible, maxilla M26.09
metacarpus — *see* Agenesis, hand
metatarsus — *see* Agenesis, foot
muscle Q79.8
eyelid Q10.3
ocular Q15.8
musculoskeletal system NEC Q79.8
nail (s) Q84.3
neck, part Q18.8
nerve Q07.8
nervous system, part NEC Q07.8
nipple Q83.2
nose Q30.1
nuclear Q07.8
organ
of Corti Q16.5
or site not listed — *see* Anomaly, by site
osseous meatus (ear) Q16.1
ovary
bilateral Q50.02
unilateral Q50.01
oviduct Q50.6
pancreas Q45.0
parathyroid (gland) Q89.2
parotid gland (s) Q38.4
patella Q74.1
pelvic girdle (complete) (partial) Q74.2
penis Q55.5
pericardium Q24.8
pituitary (gland) Q89.2
prostate Q55.4
punctum lacrimale Q10.4

Agenesis - *continued*
radioulnar — *see* Defect, reduction, upper limb
radius — *see* Defect, reduction, upper limb, longitudinal, radius
rectum Q42.1
with fistula Q42.0
renal Q60.2
bilateral Q60.1
unilateral Q60.0
respiratory organ NEC Q34.8
rib Q76.6
roof of orbit Q75.8
round ligament Q52.8
sacrum Q76.49
salivary gland Q38.4
scapula Q74.0
scrotum Q55.29
seminal vesicles Q55.4
septum
atrial Q21.1
between aorta and pulmonary artery Q21.4
ventricular Q20.4
shoulder girdle (complete) (partial) Q74.0
skull (bone) Q75.8
with
anencephaly Q00.0
encephalocele — *see* Encephalocele
hydrocephalus Q03.9
with spina bifida — *see* Spina bifida, by site, with hydrocephalus
microcephaly Q02
spermatic cord Q55.4
spinal cord Q06.0
spine Q76.49
spleen Q89.01
sternum Q76.7
stomach Q40.2
submaxillary gland (s) (congenital) Q38.4
tarsus — *see* Agenesis, foot
tendon Q79.8
testicle Q55.0
thymus (gland) Q89.2
thyroid (gland) E03.1
cartilage Q31.8
tibia — *see* Defect, reduction, lower limb, longitudinal, tibia
tibiofibular — *see* Defect, reduction, lower limb, specified type NEC
toe (and foot) (complete) (partial) — *see* Agenesis, foot
tongue Q38.3
trachea (cartilage) Q32.1
ulna — *see* Defect, reduction, upper limb, longitudinal, ulna
upper limb — *see* Agenesis, arm
ureter Q62.4
urethra Q64.5
urinary tract NEC Q64.8
uterus Q51.0
uvula Q38.5
vagina Q52.0
vas deferens Q55.4
vein (s) (peripheral) Q27.9
brain Q28.3
great NEC Q26.8
portal Q26.5
vena cava (inferior) (superior) Q26.8
vermis of cerebellum Q04.3
vertebra Q76.49
vulva Q52.71
Ageusia R43.2
Agitated — *see* condition
Agitation R45.1
Aglossia (congenital) Q38.3
Aglossia-adactylia syndrome Q87.0
Aglycogenosis E74.00
Agnosia (body image) (other senses) (tactile) R48.1
developmental F88
verbal R48.1
auditory R48.1
developmental F80.2
developmental F80.2
visual (object) R48.3

Agoraphobia F40.00
with panic disorder F40.01
without panic disorder F40.02
Agrammatism R48.8
Agranulocytopenia — *see* Agranulocytosis
Agranulocytosis (chronic) (cyclical) (genetic) (infantile) (periodic) (pernicious) — *see also* Neutropenia D70.9
congenital D70.0
cytoreductive cancer chemotherapy sequela D70.1
drug-induced D70.2
due to cytoreductive cancer chemotherapy D70.1
due to infection D70.3
secondary D70.4
drug-induced D70.2
due to cytoreductive cancer chemotherapy D70.1
Agraphia (absolute) R48.8
with alexia R48.0
developmental F81.81
Ague (dumb) — *see* Malaria
Agyria Q04.3
Ahumada-del Castillo syndrome E23.0
Aichomophobia F40.298
AIDS (related complex) B20
Ailment heart — *see* Disease, heart
Ailurophobia F40.218
AIN — *see* Neoplasia, intraepithelial, anal
Ainhum (disease) L94.6
AIPHI (acute idiopathic pulmonary hemorrhage in infants (over 28 days old)) R04.81
Air
anterior mediastinum J98.2
compressed, disease T70.3
conditioner lung or pneumonitis J67.7
embolism (artery) (cerebral) (any site) T79.0
with ectopic or molar pregnancy O08.2
due to implanted device NEC — *see* Complications, by site and type, specified NEC
following
abortion — *see* Abortion by type, complicated by, embolism
ectopic or molar pregnancy O08.2
infusion, therapeutic injection or transfusion T80.0
in pregnancy, childbirth or puerperium — *see* Embolism, obstetric
traumatic T79.0
hunger, psychogenic F45.8
rarefied, effects of — *see* Effect, adverse, high altitude
sickness T75.3
Airplane sickness T75.3
Akathisia (drug-induced) (treatment-induced) G25.71
neuroleptic induced (acute) G25.71
tardive G25.71
Akinesia R29.898
Akinetic mutism R41.89
Akureyri's disease G93.3
Alactasia, congenital E73.0
Alagille's syndrome Q44.7
Alastrim B03
Albers-Schönberg syndrome Q78.2
Albert's syndrome — *see* Tendinitis, Achilles
Albinism, albino E70.30
with hematologic abnormality E70.339
Chédiak-Higashi syndrome E70.330
Hermansky-Pudlak syndrome E70.331
other specified E70.338
I E70.320
II E70.321
ocular E70.319
autosomal recessive E70.311
other specified E70.318
X-linked E70.310
oculocutaneous E70.329
other specified E70.328
tyrosinase (ty) negative E70.320
tyrosinase (ty) positive E70.321
other specified E70.39

Albinismus E70.30
Albright (-McCune) (-Sternberg) syndrome Q78.1
Albuminous — *see* condition
Albuminuria, albuminuric (acute) (chronic) (subacute) — *see also* Proteinuria R80.9
  complicating pregnancy — *see* Proteinuria, gestational
    with
      gestational hypertension — *see* Pre-eclampsia
      pre-existing hypertension — *see* Hypertension, complicating pregnancy, pre-existing, with, pre-eclampsia
  gestational — *see* Proteinuria, gestational
    with
      gestational hypertension — *see* Pre-eclampsia
      pre-existing hypertension — *see* Hypertension, complicating pregnancy, pre-existing, with, pre-eclampsia
  orthostatic R80.2
  postural R80.2
  pre-eclamptic — *see* Pre-eclampsia
  scarlatinal A38.8
Albuminurophobia F40.298
Alcaptonuria E70.29
Alcohol, alcoholic, alcohol-induced
  addiction (without remission) F10.20
    with remission F10.21
  amnestic disorder, persisting F10.96
    with dependence F10.26
  anxiety disorder F10.980
  bipolar and related disorder F10.94
  depressive disorder F10.94
  major neurocognitive disorder, amnestic-confabulatory type F10.96
  major neurocognitive disorder, nonamnestic-confabulatory type F10.97
  mild neurocognitive disorder F10.988
  psychotic disorder F10.959
  sexual dysfunction F10.981
  sleep disorder F10.982
  brain syndrome, chronic F10.97
    with dependence F10.27
  cardiopathy I42.6
  counseling and surveillance Z71.41
    family member Z71.42
  delirium (acute) (tremens) (withdrawal) F10.231
    with intoxication F10.921
      in
        abuse F10.121
        dependence F10.221
  dementia F10.97
    with dependence F10.27
  deterioration F10.97
    with dependence F10.27
  hallucinosis (acute) F10.951
    in
      abuse F10.151
      dependence F10.251
  insanity F10.959
  intoxication (acute) (without dependence) F10.129
    with
      delirium F10.121
      dependence F10.229
        with delirium F10.221
        uncomplicated F10.220
    uncomplicated F10.120
  jealousy F10.988
  Korsakoff's, Korsakov's, Korsakow's F10.26
  liver K70.9
    acute — *see* Disease, liver, alcoholic, hepatitis
  mania (acute) (chronic) F10.959
  paranoia, paranoid (type) psychosis F10.950
  pellagra E52
  poisoning, accidental (acute) NEC — *see* Table of Drugs and Chemicals, alcohol, poisoning
  psychosis — *see* Psychosis, alcoholic

Alcohol, alcoholic, alcohol-induced - *continued*
  withdrawal (without convulsions) F10.239
    with delirium F10.231
Alcoholism (chronic) (without remission) F10.20
  with
    psychosis — *see* Psychosis, alcoholic
    remission F10.21
  Korsakov's F10.96
    with dependence F10.26
Alder (-Reilly) anomaly or syndrome (leukocyte granulation) D72.0
Aldosteronism E26.9
  familial (type I) E26.02
  glucocorticoid-remediable E26.02
  primary (due to (bilateral) adrenal hyperplasia) E26.09
  primary NEC E26.09
  secondary E26.1
  specified NEC E26.89
Aldosteronoma D44.10
Aldrich (-Wiskott) syndrome (eczema-thrombocytopenia) D82.0
Alektorophobia F40.218
Aleppo boil B55.1
Aleukemic — *see* condition
Aleukia
  congenital D70.0
  hemorrhagica D61.9
    congenital D61.09
  splenica D73.1
Alexia R48.0
  developmental F81.0
  secondary to organic lesion R48.0
Algoneurodystrophy M89.00
  ankle M89.07-
  foot M89.07-
  forearm M89.03-
  hand M89.04-
  lower leg M89.06-
  multiple sites M89.0-
  shoulder M89.01-
  specified site NEC M89.08
  thigh M89.05-
  upper arm M89.02-
Algophobia F40.298
Alienation, mental — *see* Psychosis
Alkalemia E87.3
Alkalosis E87.3
  metabolic E87.3
    with respiratory acidosis E87.4
    of newborn P74.41
  respiratory E87.3
Alkaptonuria E70.29
Allen-Masters syndrome N83.8
Allergy, allergic (reaction) (to) T78.40
  air-borne substance NEC (rhinitis) J30.89
  alveolitis (extrinsic) J67.9
    due to
      Aspergillus clavatus J67.4
      Cryptostroma corticale J67.6
      organisms (fungal, thermophilic actinomycete) growing in ventilation (air conditioning) systems J67.7
    specified type NEC J67.8
  anaphylactic reaction or shock T78.2
  angioneurotic edema T78.3
  animal (dander) (epidermal) (hair) (rhinitis) J30.81
  bee sting (anaphylactic shock) — *see* Toxicity, venom, arthropod, bee
  biological — *see* Allergy, drug
  colitis — *see also* Colitis, allergic K52.29
  dander (animal) (rhinitis) J30.81
  dandruff (rhinitis) J30.81
  dental restorative material (existing) K08.55
  dermatitis — *see* Dermatitis, contact, allergic
  diathesis — *see* History, allergy
  drug, medicament & biological (any) (external) (internal) T78.40

Allergy, allergic (reaction) (to) - *continued*
  drug, medicament & biological (any) (external) (internal) - *continued*
    correct substance properly administered — *see* Table of Drugs and Chemicals, by drug, adverse effect
    wrong substance given or taken NEC (by accident) — *see* Table of Drugs and Chemicals, by drug, poisoning
  due to pollen J30.1
  dust (house) (stock) (rhinitis) J30.89
    with asthma — *see* Asthma, allergic extrinsic
  eczema — *see* Dermatitis, contact, allergic
  epidermal (animal) (rhinitis) J30.81
  feathers (rhinitis) J30.89
  food (any) (ingested) NEC T78.1
    anaphylactic shock — *see* Shock, anaphylactic, due to food
    dermatitis — *see* Dermatitis, due to, food
    dietary counseling and surveillance Z71.3
    in contact with skin L23.6
    rhinitis J30.5
    status (without reaction) Z91.018
      beef Z91.014
      eggs Z91.012
      lamb Z91.014
      mammalian meats Z91.014
      milk products Z91.011
      peanuts Z91.010
      pork Z91.014
      red meats Z91.014
      seafood Z91.013
      specified NEC Z91.018
  gastrointestinal — *see also* specific type of allergic reaction
    meaning colitis — *see also* Colitis, allergic K52.29
    meaning gastroenteritis — *see also* Gastroenteritis, allergic K52.29
    meaning other adverse food reaction not elsewhere classified T78.1
  grain J30.1
  grass (hay fever) (pollen) J30.1
    asthma — *see* Asthma, allergic extrinsic
  hair (animal) (rhinitis) J30.81
  history (of) — *see* History, allergy
  horse serum — *see* Allergy, serum
  inhalant (rhinitis) J30.89
    pollen J30.1
  kapok (rhinitis) J30.89
  medicine — *see* Allergy, drug
  milk protein — *see also* Allergy, food Z91.011
    anaphylactic reaction T78.07
    dermatitis L27.2
    enterocolitis syndrome K52.21
    enteropathy K52.22
    gastroenteritis K52.29
    gastroesophageal reflux — *see also* Reaction, adverse, food K21.9
      with esophagitis (without bleeding) K21.00
        with bleeding K21.01
    proctocolitis K52.29
  nasal, seasonal due to pollen J30.1
  pneumonia J82.89
  pollen (any) (hay fever) J30.1
    asthma — *see* Asthma, allergic extrinsic
  primrose J30.1
  primula J30.1
  proctocolitis K52.29
  purpura D69.0
  ragweed (hay fever) (pollen) J30.1
    asthma — *see* Asthma, allergic extrinsic
  rose (pollen) J30.1
  seasonal NEC J30.2
  Senecio jacobae (pollen) J30.1
  serum — *see also* Reaction, serum T80.69
    anaphylactic shock T80.59
  shock (anaphylactic) T78.2
    due to
      administration of blood and blood products T80.51

Allergy, allergic (reaction) (to) - *continued*
shock (anaphylactic) - *continued*
due to - *continued*
adverse effect of correct medicinal substance properly administered T88.6
immunization T80.52
serum NEC T80.59
vaccination T80.52
specific NEC T78.49
tree (any) (hay fever) (pollen) J30.1
asthma — *see* Asthma, allergic extrinsic
upper respiratory J30.9
urticaria L50.0
vaccine — *see* Allergy, serum
wheat — *see* Allergy, food
Allescheriasis B48.2
Alligator skin disease Q80.9
Allocheiria, allochiria R20.8
Almeida's disease — *see* Paracoccidioidomycosis
Alopecia (hereditaria) (seborrheica) L65.9
androgenic L64.9
drug-induced L64.0
specified NEC L64.8
areata L63.9
ophiasis L63.2
specified NEC L63.8
totalis L63.0
universalis L63.1
cicatricial L66.9
specified NEC L66.8
circumscripta L63.9
congenital, congenitalis Q84.0
due to cytotoxic drugs NEC L65.8
mucinosa L65.2
postinfective NEC L65.8
postpartum L65.0
premature L64.8
specific (syphilitic) A51.32
specified NEC L65.8
syphilitic (secondary) A51.32
totalis (capitis) L63.0
universalis (entire body) L63.1
X-ray L58.1
Alpers' disease G31.81
Alpine sickness T70.29
Alport syndrome Q87.81
ALTE (apparent life threatening event) in newborn and infant R68.13
Alteration (of) , Altered
awareness
transient R40.4
unintended under general anesthesia, during procedureT88.53
mental status R41.82
pattern of family relationships affecting child Z62.898
sensation
following
cerebrovascular disease I69.998
cerebral infarction I69.398
intracerebral hemorrhage I69.198
nontraumatic intracranial hemorrhage NEC I69.298
specified disease NEC I69.898
subarachnoid hemorrhage I69.098
Alternating — *see* condition
Altitude, high (effects) — *see* Effect, adverse, high altitude
Aluminosis (of lung) J63.0
Alveolitis
allergic (extrinsic) — *see* Pneumonitis, hypersensitivity
due to
Aspergillus clavatus J67.4
Cryptostroma corticale J67.6
fibrosing (cryptogenic) (idiopathic) J84.112
jaw M27.3
sicca dolorosa M27.3
Alveolus, alveolar — *see* condition
Alymphocytosis D72.810
thymic (with immunodeficiency) D82.1
Alymphoplasia, thymic D82.1
Alzheimer's disease or sclerosis — *see* Disease, Alzheimer's
Amastia (with nipple present) Q83.8
with absent nipple Q83.0
Amathophobia F40.228
Amaurosis (acquired) (congenital) — *see also* Blindness
fugax G45.3
hysterical F44.6
Leber's congenital H35.50
uremic — *see* Uremia
Amaurotic idiocy (infantile) (juvenile) (late) E75.4
Amaxophobia F40.248
Ambiguous genitalia Q56.4
Amblyopia (congenital) (ex anopsia) (partial) (suppression) H53.00-
anisometropic — *see* Amblyopia, refractive
deprivation H53.01-
hysterical F44.6
nocturnal — *see also* Blindness, night
vitamin A deficiency E50.5
refractive H53.02-
strabismic H53.03-
suspect H53.04-
tobacco H53.8
toxic NEC H53.8
uremic — *see* Uremia
Ameba, amebic (histolytica) — *see also* Amebiasis
abscess (liver) A06.4
Amebiasis A06.9
with abscess — *see* Abscess, amebic
acute A06.0
chronic (intestine) A06.1
with abscess — *see* Abscess, amebic
cutaneous A06.7
cutis A06.7
cystitis A06.81
genitourinary tract NEC A06.82
hepatic — *see* Abscess, liver, amebic
intestine A06.0
nondysenteric colitis A06.2
skin A06.7
specified site NEC A06.89
Ameboma (of intestine) A06.3
Amelia Q73.0
lower limb — *see* Agenesis, leg
upper limb — *see* Agenesis, arm
Ameloblastoma — *see also* Cyst, calcifying odontogenic
long bones C40.9-
lower limb C40.2-
upper limb C40.0-
malignant C41.1
jaw (bone) (lower) C41.1
upper C41.0
tibial C40.2-
Amelogenesis imperfecta K00.5
nonhereditaria (segmentalis) K00.4
Amenorrhea N91.2
hyperhormonal E28.8
primary N91.0
secondary N91.1
Amentia — *see* Disability, intellectual
Meynert's (nonalcoholic) F04
American
leishmaniasis B55.2
mountain tick fever A93.2
Ametropia — *see* Disorder, refraction
AMH (asymptomatic microscopic hematuria) R31.21
Amianthosis J61
Amimia R48.8
Amino-acid disorder E72.9
anemia D53.0
Aminoacidopathy E72.9
Aminoaciduria E72.9
Amnes (t) ic syndrome (post-traumatic) F04
induced by
alcohol F10.96
with dependence F10.26
psychoactive NEC F19.96
with
abuse F19.16
Amnes (t) ic syndrome (post-traumatic) - *continued*
induced by - *continued*
psychoactive NEC - *continued*
with - *continued*
dependence F19.26
sedative F13.96
with dependence F13.26
Amnesia R41.3
anterograde R41.1
auditory R48.8
dissociative F44.0
with dissociative fugue F44.1
hysterical F44.0
postictal in epilepsy — *see* Epilepsy
psychogenic F44.0
retrograde R41.2
transient global G45.4
Amnion, amniotic — *see* condition
Amnionitis — *see* Pregnancy, complicated by
Amok F68.8
Amoral traits F60.89
Amphetamine (or other stimulant) -induced
anxiety disorder F15.980
bipolar and related disorder F15.94
delirium F15.921
depressive disorder F15.94
obsessive-compulsive and related disorder F15.988
psychotic disorder F15.959
sexual dysfunction F15.981
sleep disorder F15.982
stimulant withdrawal F15.23
Ampulla
lower esophagus K22.89
phrenic K22.89
Amputation — *see also* Absence, by site, acquired
neuroma (postoperative) (traumatic) — *see* Complications, amputation stump, neuroma
stump (surgical)
abnormal, painful, or with complication (late) — *see* Complications, amputation stump
healed or old NOS Z89.9
traumatic (complete) (partial)
arm (upper) (complete) S48.91-
at
elbow S58.01-
partial S58.02-
shoulder joint (complete) S48.01-
partial S48.02-
between
elbow and wrist (complete) S58.11-
partial S58.12-
shoulder and elbow (complete) S48.11-
partial S48.12-
partial S48.92-
breast (complete) S28.21-
partial S28.22-
clitoris (complete) S38.211
partial S38.212
ear (complete) S08.11-
partial S08.12-
finger (complete) (metacarpophalangeal) S68.11-
index S68.11-
little S68.11-
middle S68.11-
partial S68.12-
index S68.12-
little S68.12-
middle S68.12-
ring S68.12-
ring S68.11-
thumb — *see* Amputation, traumatic, thumb
transphalangeal (complete) S68.61-
index S68.61-
little S68.61-
middle S68.61-
partial S68.62-
index S68.62-

Amputation - *continued*
traumatic (complete) (partial) - *continued*
finger (complete) (metacarpophalangeal) - *continued*
transphalangeal (complete) - *continued*
partial - *continued*
little S68.62-
middle S68.62-
ring S68.62-
ring S68.61-
foot (complete) S98.91-
at ankle level S98.01-
partial S98.02-
midfoot S98.31-
partial S98.32-
partial S98.92-
forearm (complete) S58.91-
at elbow level (complete) S58.01-
partial S58.02-
between elbow and wrist (complete) S58.11-
partial S58.12-
partial S58.92-
genital organ (s) (external)
female (complete) S38.211
partial S38.212
male
penis (complete) S38.221
partial S38.222
scrotum (complete) S38.231
partial S38.232
testes (complete) S38.231
partial S38.232
hand (complete) (wrist level) S68.41-
finger (s) alone — *see* Amputation, traumatic, finger
partial S68.42-
thumb alone — *see* Amputation, traumatic, thumb
transmetacarpal (complete) S68.71-
partial S68.72-
head
ear — *see* Amputation, traumatic, ear
nose (partial) S08.812
complete S08.811
part S08.89
scalp S08.0
hip (and thigh) (complete) S78.91-
at hip joint (complete) S78.01-
partial S78.02-
between hip and knee (complete) S78.11-
partial S78.12-
partial S78.92-
labium (majus) (minus) (complete) S38.21-
partial S38.21-
leg (lower) S88.91-
at knee level S88.01-
partial S88.02-
between knee and ankle S88.11-
partial S88.12-
partial S88.92-
nose (partial) S08.812
complete S08.811
penis (complete) S38.221
partial S38.222
scrotum (complete) S38.231
partial S38.232
shoulder — *see* Amputation, traumatic, arm
at shoulder joint — *see* Amputation, traumatic, arm, at shoulder joint
testes (complete) S38.231
partial S38.232
thigh — *see* Amputation, traumatic, hip
thorax, part of S28.1
breast — *see* Amputation, traumatic, breast
thumb (complete) (metacarpophalangeal) S68.01-
partial S68.02-
transphalangeal (complete) S68.51-
partial S68.52-
toe (lesser) S98.13-

Amputation - *continued*
traumatic (complete) (partial) - *continued*
toe (lesser) - *continued*
great S98.11-
partial S98.12-
more than one S98.21-
partial S98.22-
partial S98.14-
vulva (complete) S38.211
partial S38.212
Amputee (bilateral) (old) Z89.9
Amsterdam dwarfism Q87.19
Amusia R48.8
developmental F80.89
Amyelencephalus, amyelencephaly Q00.0
Amyelia Q06.0
Amygdalitis — *see* Tonsillitis
Amygdalolith J35.8
Amyloid heart (disease) E85.4 *[I43]*
Amyloidosis (generalized) (primary) E85.9
with lung involvement E85.4 *[J99]*
familial E85.2
genetic E85.2
heart E85.4 *[I43]*
hemodialysis-associated E85.3
light chain (AL) E85.81
liver E85.4 *[K77]*
localized E85.4
neuropathic heredofamilial E85.1
non-neuropathic heredofamilial E85.0
organ limited E85.4
Portuguese E85.1
pulmonary E85.4 *[J99]*
secondary systemic E85.3
senile systemic (SSA) E85.82
skin (lichen) (macular) E85.4 *[L99]*
specified NEC E85.89
subglottic E85.4 *[J99]*
wild-type transthyretin-related (ATTR) E85.82
Amylopectinosis (brancher enzyme deficiency) E74.03
Amylophagia — *see* Pica
Amyoplasia congenita Q79.8
Amyotonia M62.89
congenita G70.2
Amyotrophia, amyotrophy, amyotrophic G71.8
congenita Q79.8
diabetic — *see* Diabetes, amyotrophy
lateral sclerosis G12.21
neuralgic G54.5
spinal progressive G12.25
Anacidity, gastric K31.83
psychogenic F45.8
Anaerosis of newborn P28.89
Analbuminemia E88.09
Analgesia — *see* Anesthesia
Analphalipoproteinemia E78.6
Anaphylactic
purpura D69.0
shock or reaction — *see* Shock, anaphylactic
Anaphylactoid shock or reaction — *see* Shock, anaphylactic
Anaphylactoid syndrome of pregnancy O88.01-
Anaphylaxis — *see* Shock, anaphylactic
Anaplasia cervix — *see also* Dysplasia, cervix N87.9
Anaplasmosis [A. phagocytophilum] (transfusion transmitted) A79.82
human A77.49
Anarthria R47.1
Anasarca R60.1
cardiac — *see* Failure, heart, congestive
lung J18.2
newborn P83.2
nutritional E43
pulmonary J18.2
renal N04.9
Anastomosis
aneurysmal — *see* Aneurysm
arteriovenous ruptured brain I60.8
intracerebral I61.8
intraparenchymal I61.8

Anastomosis - *continued*
arteriovenous ruptured brain - *continued*
intraventricular I61.5
subarachnoid I60.8
intestinal K63.89
complicated NEC K91.89
involving urinary tract N99.89
retinal and choroidal vessels (congenital) Q14.8
Anatomical narrow angle H40.03-
Ancylostoma, ancylostomiasis (braziliense) (caninum) (ceylanicum) (duodenale) B76.0
Necator americanus B76.1
Andersen's disease (glycogen storage) E74.09
Anderson-Fabry disease E75.21
Andes disease T70.29
Andrews' disease (bacterid) L08.89
Androblastoma
benign
specified site — *see* Neoplasm, benign, by site
unspecified site
female D27.9
male D29.20
malignant
specified site — *see* Neoplasm, malignant, by site
unspecified site
female C56.9
male C62.90
specified site — *see* Neoplasm, uncertain behavior, by site
tubular
with lipid storage
specified site — *see* Neoplasm, benign, by site
unspecified site
female D27.9
male D29.20
specified site — *see* Neoplasm, benign, by site
unspecified site
female D27.9
male D29.20
unspecified site
female D39.10
male D40.10
Androgen insensitivity syndrome — *see also* Syndrome, androgen insensitivity E34.50
Androgen resistance syndrome — *see also* Syndrome, androgen insensitivity E34.50
Android pelvis Q74.2
with disproportion (fetopelvic) O33.3
causing obstructed labor O65.3
Androphobia F40.290
Anectasis, pulmonary (newborn) — *see* Atelectasis
Anemia (essential) (general) (hemoglobin deficiency) (infantile) (primary) (profound) D64.9
with (due to) (in)
disorder of
anaerobic glycolysis D55.29
pentose phosphate pathway D55.1
koilonychia D50.9
achlorhydric D50.8
achrestic D53.1
Addison (-Biermer) (pernicious) D51.0
agranulocytic — *see* Agranulocytosis
amino-acid-deficiency D53.0
aplastic D61.9
congenital D61.09
drug-induced D61.1
due to
drugs D61.1
external agents NEC D61.2
infection D61.2
radiation D61.2
idiopathic D61.3
red cell (pure) D60.9
chronic D60.0
congenital D61.01

Anemia (essential) (general) (hemoglobin deficiency) (infantile) (primary) (profound) - *continued*

- aplastic - *continued*
  - red cell (pure) - *continued*
    - specified type NEC D60.8
    - transient D60.1
  - specified type NEC D61.89
  - toxic D61.2
- aregenerative
  - congenital D61.09
- asiderotic D50.9
- atypical (primary) D64.9
- Baghdad spring D55.0
- Balantidium coli A07.0
- Biermer's (pernicious) D51.0
- blood loss (chronic) D50.0
  - acute D62
- bothriocephalus B70.0 *[D63.8]*
- brickmaker's B76.9 *[D63.8]*
- cerebral I67.89
- childhood D58.9
- chlorotic D50.8
- chronic
  - blood loss D50.0
  - hemolytic D58.9
    - idiopathic D59.9
  - simple D53.9
- chronica congenita aregenerativa D61.09
- combined system disease NEC D51.0 *[G32.0]*
  - due to dietary vitamin B12 deficiency D51.3 *[G32.0]*
- complicating pregnancy, childbirth or puerperium — *see* Pregnancy, complicated by (management affected by), anemia
- congenital P61.4
  - aplastic D61.09
  - due to isoimmunization NOS P55.9
  - dyserythropoietic, dyshematopoietic D64.4
  - following fetal blood loss P61.3
  - Heinz body D58.2
  - hereditary hemolytic NOS D58.9
  - pernicious D51.0
  - spherocytic D58.0
- Cooley's (erythroblastic) D56.1
- cytogenic D51.0
- deficiency D53.9
  - 2, 3 diphosphoglycurate mutase D55.29
  - 2, 3 PG D55.29
  - 6 phosphogluconate dehydrogenase D55.1
  - 6-PGD D55.1
  - amino-acid D53.0
  - combined B12 and folate D53.1
  - enzyme D55.9
    - drug-induced (hemolytic) D59.2
    - glucose-6-phosphate dehydrogenase (G6PD) D55.0
    - glycolytic D55.29
    - nucleotide metabolism D55.3
    - related to hexose monophosphate (HMP) shunt pathway NEC D55.1
    - specified type NEC D55.8
  - erythrocytic glutathione D55.1
  - folate D52.9
    - dietary D52.0
    - drug-induced D52.1
  - folic acid D52.9
    - dietary D52.0
    - drug-induced D52.1
  - G SH D55.1
  - GGS-R D55.1
  - glucose-6-phosphate dehydrogenase D55.0
  - glutathione reductase D55.1
  - glyceraldehyde phosphate dehydrogenase D55.29
  - G6PD D55.0
  - hexokinase D55.29
  - iron D50.9
    - secondary to blood loss (chronic) D50.0
  - nutritional D53.9
    - with
      - poor iron absorption D50.8
      - specified deficiency NEC D53.8

Anemia (essential) (general) (hemoglobin deficiency) (infantile) (primary) (profound) - *continued*

- deficiency - *continued*
  - phosphofructo-aldolase D55.29
  - phosphoglycerate kinase D55.29
  - PK D55.21
  - protein D53.0
  - pyruvate kinase D55.21
  - transcobalamin II D51.2
  - triose-phosphate isomerase D55.29
  - vitamin B12 NOS D51.9
    - dietary D51.3
    - due to
      - intrinsic factor deficiency D51.0
      - selective vitamin B12 malabsorption with proteinuria D51.1
    - pernicious D51.0
    - specified type NEC D51.8
- Diamond-Blackfan (congenital hypoplastic) D61.01
- dibothriocephalus B70.0 *[D63.8]*
- dimorphic D53.1
- diphasic D53.1
- Diphyllobothrium (Dibothriocephalus) B70.0 *[D63.8]*
- due to (in) (with)
  - antineoplastic chemotherapy D64.81
  - blood loss (chronic) D50.0
    - acute D62
  - chemotherapy, antineoplastic D64.81
  - chronic disease classified elsewhere NEC D63.8
  - chronic kidney disease D63.1
  - deficiency
    - amino-acid D53.0
    - copper D53.8
    - folate (folic acid) D52.9
      - dietary D52.0
      - drug-induced D52.1
    - molybdenum D53.8
    - protein D53.0
    - zinc D53.8
  - dietary vitamin B12 deficiency D51.3
  - disorder of
    - glutathione metabolism D55.1
    - nucleotide metabolism D55.3
  - drug — *see* Anemia, by type — *see also* Table of Drugs and Chemicals
  - end stage renal disease D63.1
  - enzyme disorder D55.9
  - fetal blood loss P61.3
  - fish tapeworm (D.latum) infestation B70.0 *[D63.8]*
  - hemorrhage (chronic) D50.0
    - acute D62
  - impaired absorption D50.9
  - loss of blood (chronic) D50.0
    - acute D62
  - myxedema E03.9 *[D63.8]*
  - Necator americanus B76.1 *[D63.8]*
  - prematurity P61.2
  - selective vitamin B12 malabsorption with proteinuria D51.1
  - transcobalamin II deficiency D51.2
- Dyke-Young type (secondary) (symptomatic) D59.19
- dyserythropoietic (congenital) D64.4
- dyshematopoietic (congenital) D64.4
- Egyptian B76.9 *[D63.8]*
- elliptocytosis — *see* Elliptocytosis
- enzyme-deficiency, drug-induced D59.2
- epidemic — *see also* Ancylostomiasis B76.9 *[D63.8]*
- erythroblastic
  - familial D56.1
  - newborn — *see also* Disease, hemolytic P55.9
  - of childhood D56.1
- erythrocytic glutathione deficiency D55.1
- erythropoietin-resistant anemia (EPO resistant anemia) D63.1
- Faber's (achlorhydric anemia) D50.9
- factitious (self-induced blood letting) D50.0
- familial erythroblastic D56.1

Anemia (essential) (general) (hemoglobin deficiency) (infantile) (primary) (profound) - *continued*

- Fanconi's (congenital pancytopenia) D61.09
- favism D55.0
- fish tapeworm (D. latum) infestation B70.0 *[D63.8]*
- folate (folic acid) deficiency D52.9
- glucose-6-phosphate dehydrogenase (G6PD) deficiency D55.0
- glutathione-reductase deficiency D55.1
- goat's milk D52.0
- granulocytic — *see* Agranulocytosis
- Heinz body, congenital D58.2
- hemolytic D58.9
  - acquired D59.9
    - with hemoglobinuria NEC D59.6
    - autoimmune NEC D59.19
    - infectious D59.4
    - specified type NEC D59.8
    - toxic D59.4
  - acute D59.9
    - due to enzyme deficiency specified type NEC D55.8
    - Lederer's D59.19
  - autoimmune D59.10
    - cold D59.12
    - drug-induced D59.0
    - mixed D59.13
    - warm D59.11
  - chronic D58.9
    - idiopathic D59.9
  - cold type (primary) (secondary) (symptomatic) D59.12
  - congenital (spherocytic) — *see* Spherocytosis
  - due to
    - cardiac conditions D59.4
    - drugs (nonautoimmune) D59.2
      - autoimmune D59.0
    - enzyme disorder D55.9
      - drug-induced D59.2
    - presence of shunt or other internal prosthetic device D59.4
  - familial D58.9
  - hereditary D58.9
    - due to enzyme disorder D55.9
      - specified type NEC D55.8
    - specified type NEC D58.8
  - idiopathic (chronic) D59.9
  - mechanical D59.4
  - microangiopathic D59.4
  - mixed type (primary) (secondary) (symptomatic) D59.13
  - nonautoimmune D59.4
    - drug-induced D59.2
  - nonspherocytic
    - congenital or hereditary NEC D55.8
      - glucose-6-phosphate dehydrogenase deficiency D55.0
      - pyruvate kinase deficiency D55.21
      - type
        - I D55.1
        - II D55.29
    - type
      - I D55.1
      - II D55.29
  - primary
    - autoimmune
      - cold type D59.12
      - mixed type D59.13
      - warm type D59.11
  - secondary D59.4
    - autoimmune
      - cold type D59.12
      - mixed type D59.13
      - warm type D59.11
  - specified (hereditary) type NEC D58.8
  - Stransky-Regala type — *see also* Hemoglobinopathy D58.8
  - symptomatic D59.4
    - autoimmune
      - cold type D59.12
      - mixed type D59.13
      - warm type D59.11

Anemia (essential) (general) (hemoglobin deficiency) (infantile) (primary) (profound) - *continued*
hemolytic - *continued*
toxic D59.4
warm type (primary) (secondary) (symptomatic) D59.11
hemorrhagic (chronic) D50.0
acute D62
Herrick's D57.1
hexokinase deficiency D55.29
hookworm B76.9 *[D63.8]*
hypochromic (idiopathic) (microcytic) (normoblastic) D50.9
due to blood loss (chronic) D50.0
acute D62
familial sex-linked D64.0
pyridoxine-responsive D64.3
sideroblastic, sex-linked D64.0
hypoplasia, red blood cells D61.9
congenital or familial D61.01
hypoplastic (idiopathic) D61.9
congenital or familial (of childhood) D61.01
hypoproliferative (refractive) D61.9
idiopathic D64.9
aplastic D61.3
hemolytic, chronic D59.9
in (due to) (with)
chronic kidney disease D63.1
end stage renal disease D63.1
failure, kidney (renal) D63.1
neoplastic disease — *see also* Neoplasm D63.0
intertropical — *see also* Ancylostomiasis D63.8
iron deficiency D50.9
secondary to blood loss (chronic) D50.0
acute D62
specified type NEC D50.8
Joseph-Diamond-Blackfan (congenital hypoplastic) D61.01
Lederer's (hemolytic) D59.19
leukoerythroblastic D61.82
macrocytic D53.9
nutritional D52.0
tropical D52.8
malarial — *see also* Malaria B54 *[D63.8]*
malignant (progressive) D51.0
malnutrition D53.9
marsh — *see also* Malaria B54 *[D63.8]*
Mediterranean (with other hemoglobinopathy) D56.9
megaloblastic D53.1
combined B12 and folate deficiency D53.1
hereditary D51.1
nutritional D52.0
orotic aciduria D53.0
refractory D53.1
specified type NEC D53.1
megalocytic D53.1
microcytic (hypochromic) D50.9
due to blood loss (chronic) D50.0
acute D62
familial D56.8
microdrepanocytosis D57.40
microelliptopoikilocytic (Rietti-Greppi-Micheli) D56.9
miner's B76.9 *[D63.8]*
myelodysplastic D46.9
myelofibrosis D75.81
myelogenous D64.89
myelopathic D64.89
myelophthisic D61.82
myeloproliferative D47.Z9
newborn P61.4
due to
ABO (antibodies, isoimmunization, maternal/fetal incompatibility) P55.1
Rh (antibodies, isoimmunization, maternal/fetal incompatibility) P55.0
following fetal blood loss P61.3
posthemorrhagic (fetal) P61.3

Anemia (essential) (general) (hemoglobin deficiency) (infantile) (primary) (profound) - *continued*
nonspherocytic hemolytic — *see* Anemia, hemolytic, nonspherocytic
normocytic (infectional) D64.9
due to blood loss (chronic) D50.0
acute D62
myelophthisic D61.82
nutritional (deficiency) D53.9
with
poor iron absorption D50.8
specified deficiency NEC D53.8
megaloblastic D52.0
of prematurity P61.2
orotaciduric (congenital) (hereditary) D53.0
osteosclerotic D64.89
ovalocytosis (hereditary) — *see* Elliptocytosis
paludal — *see also* Malaria B54 *[D63.8]*
pernicious (congenital) (malignant) (progressive) D51.0
pleochromic D64.89
of sprue D52.8
posthemorrhagic (chronic) D50.0
acute D62
newborn P61.3
postoperative (postprocedural)
due to (acute) blood loss D62
chronic blood loss D50.0
specified NEC D64.89
postpartum O90.81
pressure D64.89
progressive D64.9
malignant D51.0
pernicious D51.0
protein-deficiency D53.0
pseudoleukemica infantum D64.89
pure red cell D60.9
congenital D61.01
pyridoxine-responsive D64.3
pyruvate kinase deficiency D55.21
refractory D46.4
with
excess of blasts D46.20
1 (RAEB 1) D46.21
2 (RAEB 2) D46.22
in transformation (RAEB T) — *see* Leukemia, acute myeloblastic
hemochromatosis D46.1
sideroblasts (ring) (RARS) D46.1
megaloblastic D53.1
sideroblastic D46.1
sideropenic D50.9
without ring sideroblasts, so stated D46.0
without sideroblasts without excess of blasts D46.0
Rietti-Greppi-Micheli D56.9
scorbutic D53.2
secondary to
blood loss (chronic) D50.0
acute D62
hemorrhage (chronic) D50.0
acute D62
semiplastic D61.89
sickle-cell — *see* Disease, sickle-cell
sideroblastic D64.3
hereditary D64.0
hypochromic, sex-linked D64.0
pyridoxine-responsive NEC D64.3
refractory D46.1
secondary (due to)
disease D64.1
drugs and toxins D64.2
specified type NEC D64.3
sideropenic (refractory) D50.9
due to blood loss (chronic) D50.0
acute D62
simple chronic D53.9
specified type NEC D64.89
spherocytic (hereditary) — *see* Spherocytosis
splenic D64.89
splenomegalic D64.89
stomatocytosis D58.8
syphilitic (acquired) (late) A52.79 *[D63.8]*

Anemia (essential) (general) (hemoglobin deficiency) (infantile) (primary) (profound) - *continued*
target cell D64.89
thalassemia D56.9
thrombocytopenic — *see* Thrombocytopenia
toxic D61.2
tropical B76.9 *[D63.8]*
macrocytic D52.8
tuberculous A18.89 *[D63.8]*
vegan D51.3
vitamin
B6-responsive D64.3
B12 deficiency (dietary) pernicious D51.0
von Jaksch's D64.89
Witts' (achlorhydric anemia) D50.8
Anemophobia F40.228
Anencephalus, anencephaly Q00.0
Anergasia — *see* Psychosis, organic
Anesthesia, anesthetic R20.0
complication or reaction NEC — *see also* Complications, anesthesia T88.59
due to
correct substance properly administered — *see* Table of Drugs and Chemicals, by drug, adverse effect
overdose or wrong substance given — *see* Table of Drugs and Chemicals, by drug, poisoning
unintended awareness under general anesthesia during procedure T88.53
personal history of Z92.84
cornea H18.81-
dissociative F44.6
functional (hysterical) F44.6
hyperesthetic, thalamic G89.0
hysterical F44.6
local skin lesion R20.0
sexual (psychogenic) F52.1
shock (due to) T88.2
skin R20.0
testicular N50.9
Anetoderma (maculosum) (of) L90.8
Jadassohn-Pellizzari L90.2
Schweniger-Buzzi L90.1
Aneurin deficiency E51.9
Aneurysm (anastomotic) (artery) (cirsoid) (diffuse) (false) (fusiform) (multiple) (saccular) I72.9
abdominal (aorta) I71.4
ruptured I71.3
syphilitic A52.01
aorta, aortic (nonsyphilitic) I71.9
abdominal I71.4
ruptured I71.3
arch I71.2
ruptured I71.1
arteriosclerotic I71.9
ruptured I71.8
ascending I71.2
ruptured I71.1
congenital Q25.43
descending I71.9
abdominal I71.4
ruptured I71.3
ruptured I71.8
thoracic I71.2
ruptured I71.1
root Q25.43
ruptured I71.8
sinus, congenital Q25.43
syphilitic A52.01
thoracic I71.2
ruptured I71.1
thoracoabdominal I71.6
ruptured I71.5
thorax, thoracic (arch) I71.2
ruptured I71.1
transverse I71.2
ruptured I71.1
valve (heart) — *see also* Endocarditis, aortic I35.8
arteriosclerotic I72.9
cerebral I67.1

Angina (attack) (cardiac) (chest) (heart) (pectoris) (syndrome) (vasomotor) - *continued*
spasm-induced — *see* Angina, with documented spasm
specified NEC I20.8
stable I20.8
stenocardia — *see* Angina, specified NEC
stridulous, diphtheritic A36.2
tonsil J36
trachealis J05.0
unstable I20.0
variant — *see* Angina, with documented spasm
Vincent's A69.1
worsening effort — *see* Angina, unstable
Angioblastoma — *see* Neoplasm, connective tissue, uncertain behavior
Angiocholecystitis — *see* Cholecystitis, acute
Angiocholitis — *see also* Cholecystitis, acute K83.09
Angiodysgenesis spinalis G95.19
Angiodysplasia (cecum) (colon) K55.20
with bleeding K55.21
duodenum (and stomach) K31.819
with bleeding K31.811
stomach (and duodenum) K31.819
with bleeding K31.811
Angioedema (allergic) (any site) (with urticaria) T78.3
episodic, with eosinophilia D72.118
hereditary D84.1
Angioendothelioma — *see* Neoplasm, uncertain behavior, by site
benign D18.00
intra-abdominal D18.03
intracranial D18.02
skin D18.01
specified site NEC D18.09
bone — *see* Neoplasm, bone, malignant
Ewing's — *see* Neoplasm, bone, malignant
Angioendotheliomatosis C85.8-
Angiofibroma — *see also* Neoplasm, benign, by site
juvenile
specified site — *see* Neoplasm, benign, by site
unspecified site D10.6
Angiohemophilia (A) (B) D68.0
Angioid streaks (choroid) (macula) (retina) H35.33
Angiokeratoma — *see* Neoplasm, skin, benign
corporis diffusum E75.21
Angioleiomyoma — *see* Neoplasm, connective tissue, benign
Angiolipoma — *see also* Lipoma
infiltrating — *see* Lipoma
Angioma — *see also* Hemangioma, by site
capillary I78.1
hemorrhagicum hereditaria I78.0
intra-abdominal D18.03
intracranial D18.02
malignant — *see* Neoplasm, connective tissue, malignant
plexiform D18.00
intra-abdominal D18.03
intracranial D18.02
skin D18.01
specified site NEC D18.09
senile I78.1
serpiginosum L81.7
skin D18.01
specified site NEC D18.09
spider I78.1
stellate I78.1
venous Q28.3
Angiomatosis Q82.8
bacillary A79.89
encephalotrigeminal Q85.8
hemorrhagic familial I78.0
hereditary familial I78.0
liver K76.4
Angiomyolipoma — *see* Lipoma
Angiomyoliposarcoma — *see* Neoplasm, connective tissue, malignant
Angiomyoma — *see* Neoplasm, connective tissue, benign
Angiomyosarcoma — *see* Neoplasm, connective tissue, malignant
Angiomyxoma — *see* Neoplasm, connective tissue, uncertain behavior
Angioneurosis F45.8
Angioneurotic edema (allergic) (any site) (with urticaria) T78.3
hereditary D84.1
Angiopathia, angiopathy I99.9
cerebral I67.9
amyloid E85.4 *[I68.0]*
diabetic (peripheral) — *see* Diabetes, angiopathy
peripheral I73.9
diabetic — *see* Diabetes, angiopathy
specified type NEC I73.89
retinae syphilitica A52.05
retinalis (juvenilis)
diabetic — *see* Diabetes, retinopathy
proliferative — *see* Retinopathy, proliferative
Angiosarcoma — *see also* Neoplasm, connective tissue, malignant
liver C22.3
Angiosclerosis — *see* Arteriosclerosis
Angiospasm (peripheral) (traumatic) (vessel) I73.9
brachial plexus G54.0
cerebral G45.9
cervical plexus G54.2
nerve
arm — *see* Mononeuropathy, upper limb
axillary G54.0
median — *see* Lesion, nerve, median
ulnar — *see* Lesion, nerve, ulnar
axillary G54.0
leg — *see* Mononeuropathy, lower limb
median — *see* Lesion, nerve, median
plantar — *see* Lesion, nerve, plantar
ulnar — *see* Lesion, nerve, ulnar
Angiospastic disease or edema I73.9
Angiostrongyliasis
due to
Parastrongylus
cantonensis B83.2
costaricensis B81.3
intestinal B81.3
Anguillulosis — *see* Strongyloidiasis
Angulation
cecum — *see* Obstruction, intestine
coccyx (acquired) (*see also* subcategory M43.8)
congenital NEC Q76.49
femur (acquired) — *see also* Deformity, limb, specified type NEC, thigh
congenital Q74.2
intestine (large) (small) — *see* Obstruction, intestine
sacrum (acquired) (*see also* subcategory M43.8)
congenital NEC Q76.49
sigmoid (flexure) — *see* Obstruction, intestine
spine — *see* Dorsopathy, deforming, specified NEC
tibia (acquired) — *see also* Deformity, limb, specified type NEC, lower leg
congenital Q74.2
ureter N13.5
with infection N13.6
wrist (acquired) — *see also* Deformity, limb, specified type NEC, forearm
congenital Q74.0
Angulus infectiosus (lips) K13.0
Anhedonia R45.84
sexual F52.0
Anhidrosis L74.4
Anhydration E86.0
Anhydremia E86.0
Anidrosis L74.4
Aniridia (congenital) Q13.1
Anisakiasis (infection) (infestation) B81.0
Anisakis larvae infestation B81.0
Aniseikonia H52.32
Anisocoria (pupil) H57.02
congenital Q13.2
Anisocytosis R71.8
Anisometropia (congenital) H52.31
Ankle — *see* condition
Ankyloblepharon (eyelid) (acquired) — *see also* Blepharophimosis
filiforme (adnatum) (congenital) Q10.3
total Q10.3
Ankyloglossia Q38.1
Ankylosis (fibrous) (osseous) (joint) M24.60
ankle M24.67-
arthrodesis status Z98.1
cricoarytenoid (cartilage) (joint) (larynx) J38.7
dental K03.5
ear ossicles H74.31-
elbow M24.62-
foot M24.67-
hand M24.64-
hip M24.65-
incostapedial joint (infectional) — *see* Ankylosis, ear ossicles
jaw (temporomandibular) M26.61-
knee M24.66-
lumbosacral (joint) M43.27
postoperative (status) Z98.1
produced by surgical fusion, status Z98.1
sacro-iliac (joint) M43.28
shoulder M24.61-
specified site NEC M24.69
spine (joint) — *see also* Fusion, spine
spondylitic — *see* Spondylitis, ankylosing
surgical Z98.1
temporomandibular M26.61-
tooth, teeth (hard tissues) K03.5
wrist M24.63-
Ankylostoma — *see* Ancylostoma
Ankylostomiasis — *see* Ancylostomiasis
Ankylurethria — *see* Stricture, urethra
Annular — *see also* condition
detachment, cervix N88.8
organ or site, congenital NEC — *see* Distortion
pancreas (congenital) Q45.1
Anodontia (complete) (partial) (vera) K00.0
acquired K08.10
Anomaly, anomalous (congenital) (unspecified type) Q89.9
abdominal wall NEC Q79.59
acoustic nerve Q07.8
adrenal (gland) Q89.1
Alder (-Reilly) (leukocyte granulation) D72.0
alimentary tract Q45.9
upper Q40.9
alveolar M26.70
hyperplasia M26.79
mandibular M26.72
maxillary M26.71
hypoplasia M26.79
mandibular M26.74
maxillary M26.73
ridge (process) M26.79
specified NEC M26.79
ankle (joint) Q74.2
anus Q43.9
aorta (arch) NEC Q25.40
coarctation (preductal) (postductal) Q25.1
aortic cusp or valve Q23.9
appendix Q43.8
apple peel syndrome Q41.1
aqueduct of Sylvius Q03.0
with spina bifida — *see* Spina bifida, with hydrocephalus
arm Q74.0
arteriovenous NEC
coronary Q24.5
gastrointestinal Q27.33
acquired — *see* Angiodysplasia
artery (peripheral) Q27.9
basilar NEC Q28.1
cerebral Q28.3
coronary Q24.5

Anomaly, anomalous (congenital) (unspecified type) - *continued*
renal Q63.9
artery Q27.2
pelvis Q63.9
specified NEC Q63.8
respiratory system Q34.9
specified NEC Q34.8
retina Q14.1
rib Q76.6
cervical Q76.5
Rieger's Q13.81
rotation — *see* Malrotation
hip or thigh Q65.89
round ligament Q52.8
sacroiliac (joint) NEC Q74.2
sacrum NEC Q76.49
kyphosis — *see* Kyphosis, congenital
lordosis — *see* Lordosis, congenital
saddle nose, syphilitic A50.57
salivary duct or gland Q38.4
scapula Q74.0
scrotum — *see* Malformation, testis and scrotum
sebaceous gland Q82.9
seminal vesicles Q55.4
sense organs NEC Q07.8
sex chromosomes NEC — *see also* Anomaly, chromosomes
female phenotype Q97.8
male phenotype Q98.9
shoulder (girdle) (joint) Q74.0
sigmoid (flexure) Q43.9
simian crease Q82.8
sinus of Valsalva Q25.49
skeleton generalized Q78.9
skin (appendage) Q82.9
skull Q75.9
with
anencephaly Q00.0
encephalocele — *see* Encephalocele
hydrocephalus Q03.9
with spina bifida — *see* Spina bifida, by site, with hydrocephalus
microcephaly Q02
specified organ or site NEC Q89.8
spermatic cord Q55.4
spine, spinal NEC Q76.49
column NEC Q76.49
kyphosis — *see* Kyphosis, congenital
lordosis — *see* Lordosis, congenital
cord Q06.9
nerve root Q07.8
spleen Q89.09
agenesis Q89.01
stenonian duct Q38.4
sternum NEC Q76.7
stomach Q40.3
submaxillary gland Q38.4
tarsus NEC Q74.2
tendon Q79.9
testis — *see* Malformation, testis and scrotum
thigh NEC Q74.2
thorax (wall) Q67.8
bony Q76.9
throat Q38.8
thumb Q74.0
thymus gland Q89.2
thyroid (gland) Q89.2
cartilage Q31.8
tibia NEC Q74.2
saber A50.56
toe Q74.2
tongue Q38.3
tooth, teeth K00.9
eruption K00.6
position, fully erupted M26.30
spacing, fully erupted M26.30
trachea (cartilage) Q32.1
tragus Q17.9
tricuspid (leaflet) (valve) Q22.9
atresia or stenosis Q22.4
Ebstein's Q22.5

Anomaly, anomalous (congenital) (unspecified type) - *continued*
Uhl's (hypoplasia of myocardium, right ventricle) Q24.8
ulna Q74.0
umbilical artery Q27.0
union
cricoid cartilage and thyroid cartilage Q31.8
thyroid cartilage and hyoid bone Q31.8
trachea with larynx Q31.8
upper limb Q74.0
urachus Q64.4
ureter Q62.8
obstructive NEC Q62.39
cecoureterocele Q62.32
orthotopic ureterocele Q62.31
urethra Q64.70
absence Q64.5
double Q64.74
fistula to rectum Q64.73
obstructive Q64.39
stricture Q64.32
prolapse Q64.71
specified type NEC Q64.79
urinary tract Q64.9
uterus Q51.9
with only one functioning horn Q51.4
uvula Q38.5
vagina Q52.4
valleculae Q31.8
valve (heart) NEC Q24.8
coronary sinus Q24.5
inferior vena cava Q24.8
pulmonary Q22.3
sinus coronario Q24.5
venae cavae inferioris Q24.8
vas deferens Q55.4
vascular Q27.9
brain Q28.3
ring Q25.45
vein (s) (peripheral) Q27.9
brain Q28.3
cerebral Q28.3
coronary Q24.5
developmental Q28.3
great Q26.9
specified NEC Q26.8
vena cava (inferior) (superior) Q26.9
venous — *see* Anomaly, vein(s)
venous return Q26.8
ventricular
bands or folds Q24.8
septa Q21.0
vertebra Q76.49
kyphosis — *see* Kyphosis, congenital
lordosis — *see* Lordosis, congenital
vesicourethral orifice Q64.79
vessel (s) Q27.9
optic papilla Q14.2
precerebral Q28.1
vitelline duct Q43.0
vitreous body or humor Q14.0
vulva Q52.70
wrist (joint) Q74.0
Anomia R48.8
Anonychia (congenital) Q84.3
acquired L60.8
Anophthalmos, anophthalmus (congenital) (globe) Q11.1
acquired Z90.01
Anopia, anopsia H53.46-
quadrant H53.46-
Anorchia, anorchism, anorchidism Q55.0
Anorexia R63.0
hysterical F44.89
nervosa F50.00
atypical F50.9
binge-eating type F50.2
with purging F50.02
restricting type F50.01
Anorgasmy, psychogenic (female) F52.31
male F52.32
Anosmia R43.0
hysterical F44.6

Anosmia - *continued*
postinfectional J39.8
Anosognosia R41.89
Anosteoplasia Q78.9
Anovulatory cycle N97.0
Anoxemia R09.02
newborn P84
Anoxia (pathological) R09.02
altitude T70.29
cerebral G93.1
complicating
anesthesia (general) (local) or other sedation T88.59
in labor and delivery O74.3
in pregnancy O29.21-
postpartum, puerperal O89.2
delivery (cesarean) (instrumental) O75.4
during a procedure G97.81
newborn P84
resulting from a procedure G97.82
due to
drowning T75.1
high altitude T70.29
heart — *see* Insufficiency, coronary
intrauterine P84
myocardial — *see* Insufficiency, coronary
newborn P84
spinal cord G95.11
systemic (by suffocation) (low content in atmosphere) — *see* Asphyxia, traumatic
Anteflexion — *see* Anteversion
Antenatal
care (normal pregnancy) Z34.90
screening (encounter for) of mother — *see also* Encounter, antenatal screening Z36.9
Antepartum — *see* condition
Anterior — *see* condition
Antero-occlusion M26.220
Anteversion
cervix — *see* Anteversion, uterus
femur (neck) , congenital Q65.89
uterus, uterine (cervix) (postinfectional) (postpartal, old) N85.4
congenital Q51.818
in pregnancy or childbirth — *see* Pregnancy, complicated by
Anthophobia F40.228
Anthracosilicosis J60
Anthracosis (lung) (occupational) J60
lingua K14.3
Anthrax A22.9
with pneumonia A22.1
cerebral A22.8
colitis A22.2
cutaneous A22.0
gastrointestinal A22.2
inhalation A22.1
intestinal A22.2
meningitis A22.8
pulmonary A22.1
respiratory A22.1
sepsis A22.7
specified manifestation NEC A22.8
Anthropoid pelvis Q74.2
with disproportion (fetopelvic) O33.0
Anthropophobia F40.10
generalized F40.11
Antibodies, maternal (blood group) — *see* Isoimmunization, affecting management of pregnancy
anti-D — *see* Isoimmunization, affecting management of pregnancy, Rh
newborn P55.0
Antibody
anticardiolipin R76.0
with
hemorrhagic disorder D68.312
hypercoagulable state D68.61
antiphosphatidylglycerol R76.0
with
hemorrhagic disorder D68.312
hypercoagulable state D68.61
antiphosphatidylinositol R76.0
with

Antibody - *continued*
antiphosphatidylinositol - *continued*
with - *continued*
hemorrhagic disorder D68.312
hypercoagulable state D68.61
antiphosphatidylserine R76.0
with
hemorrhagic disorder D68.312
hypercoagulable state D68.61
antiphospholipid R76.0
with
hemorrhagic disorder D68.312
hypercoagulable state D68.61
Anticardiolipin syndrome D68.61
Anticoagulant, circulating (intrinsic) — *see also* - Disorder, hemorrhagic D68.318
drug-induced (extrinsic) — *see also* - Disorder, hemorrhagic D68.32
iatrogenic D68.32
Antidiuretic hormone syndrome E22.2
Antimonial cholera — *see* Poisoning, antimony
Antiphospholipid
antibody
with hemorrhagic disorder D68.312
syndrome D68.61
Antisocial personality F60.2
Antithrombinemia — *see* Circulating anticoagulants
Antithromboplastinemia D68.318
Antithromboplastinogenemia D68.318
Antitoxin complication or reaction — *see* Complications, vaccination
Antlophobia F40.228
Antritis J32.0
maxilla J32.0
acute J01.00
recurrent J01.01
stomach K29.60
with bleeding K29.61
Antrum, antral — *see* condition
Anuria R34
calculous (impacted) (recurrent) — *see also* Calculus, urinary N20.9
following
abortion — *see* Abortion by type complicated by, renal failure
ectopic or molar pregnancy O08.4
newborn P96.0
postprocedural N99.0
postrenal N13.8
traumatic (following crushing) T79.5
Anus, anal — *see* condition
Anusitis K62.89
Anxiety F41.9
depression F41.8
episodic paroxysmal F41.0
generalized F41.1
hysteria F41.8
neurosis F41.1
panic type F41.0
reaction F41.1
separation, abnormal (of childhood) F93.0
specified NEC F41.8
state F41.1
Aorta, aortic — *see* condition
Aortectasia — *see* Ectasia, aorta
with aneurysm — *see* Aneurysm, aorta
Aortitis (nonsyphilitic) (calcific) I77.6
arteriosclerotic I70.0
Doehle-Heller A52.02
luetic A52.02
rheumatic — *see* Endocarditis, acute, rheumatic
specific (syphilitic) A52.02
syphilitic A52.02
congenital A50.54 *[I79.1]*
Apathetic thyroid storm — *see* Thyrotoxicosis
Apathy R45.3
Apeirophobia F40.228
Apepsia K30
psychogenic F45.8
Aperistalsis, esophagus K22.0
Apertognathia M26.29
Apert's syndrome Q87.0
Aphagia R13.0
psychogenic F50.9
Aphakia (acquired) (postoperative) H27.0-
congenital Q12.3
Aphasia (amnestic) (global) (nominal) (semantic) (syntactic) R47.01
acquired, with epilepsy (Landau-Kleffner syndrome) — *see* Epilepsy, specified NEC
auditory (developmental) F80.2
developmental (receptive type) F80.2
expressive type F80.1
Wernicke's F80.2
following
cerebrovascular disease I69.920
cerebral infarction I69.320
intracerebral hemorrhage I69.120
nontraumatic intracranial hemorrhage NEC I69.220
specified disease NEC I69.820
subarachnoid hemorrhage I69.020
primary progressive G31.01 *[F02.80]*
with behavioral disturbance G31.01 *[F02.81]*
progressive isolated G31.01 *[F02.80]*
with behavioral disturbance G31.01 *[F02.81]*
sensory F80.2
syphilis, tertiary A52.19
Wernicke's (developmental) F80.2
Aphonia (organic) R49.1
hysterical F44.4
psychogenic F44.4
Aphthae, aphthous — *see also* condition
Bednar's K12.0
cachectic K14.0
epizootic B08.8
fever B08.8
oral (recurrent) K12.0
stomatitis (major) (minor) K12.0
thrush B37.0
ulcer (oral) (recurrent) K12.0
genital organ (s) NEC
female N76.6
male N50.89
larynx J38.7
Apical — *see* condition
Apiphobia F40.218
Aplasia — *see also* Agenesis
abdominal muscle syndrome Q79.4
alveolar process (acquired) — *see* Anomaly, alveolar
congenital Q38.6
aorta (congenital) Q25.41
axialis extracorticalis (congenita) E75.29
bone marrow (myeloid) D61.9
congenital D61.01
brain Q00.0
part of Q04.3
bronchus Q32.4
cementum K00.4
cerebellum Q04.3
cervix (congenital) Q51.5
congenital pure red cell D61.01
corpus callosum Q04.0
cutis congenita Q84.8
erythrocyte congenital D61.01
extracortical axial E75.29
eye Q11.1
fovea centralis (congenital) Q14.1
gallbladder, congenital Q44.0
iris Q13.1
labyrinth, membranous Q16.5
limb (congenital) Q73.8
lower — *see* Defect, reduction, lower limb
upper — *see* Agenesis, arm
lung, congenital (bilateral) (unilateral) Q33.3
pancreas Q45.0
parathyroid-thymic D82.1
Pelizaeus-Merzbacher E75.29
penis Q55.5
prostate Q55.4
red cell (with thymoma) D60.9
acquired D60.9
Aplasia - *continued*
red cell (with thymoma) - *continued*
acquired - *continued*
due to drugs D60.9
adult D60.9
chronic D60.0
congenital D61.01
constitutional D61.01
due to drugs D60.9
hereditary D61.01
of infants D61.01
primary D61.01
pure D61.01
due to drugs D60.9
specified type NEC D60.8
transient D60.1
round ligament Q52.8
skin Q84.8
spermatic cord Q55.4
spleen Q89.01
testicle Q55.0
thymic, with immunodeficiency D82.1
thyroid (congenital) (with myxedema) E03.1
uterus Q51.0
ventral horn cell Q06.1
Apnea, apneic (of) (spells) R06.81
newborn NEC P28.4
obstructive P28.4
sleep (central) (obstructive) (primary) P28.3
prematurity P28.4
sleep G47.30
central (primary) G47.31
idiopathic G47.31
in conditions classified elsewhere G47.37
obstructive (adult) (pediatric) G47.33
hypopnea G47.33
primary central G47.31
specified NEC G47.39
Apneumatosis, newborn P28.0
Apocrine metaplasia (breast) — *see* Dysplasia, mammary, specified type NEC
Apophysitis (bone) — *see also* Osteochondropathy
calcaneus M92.8
juvenile M92.9
Apoplectiform convulsions (cerebral ischemia) I67.82
Apoplexia, apoplexy, apoplectic
adrenal A39.1
heart (auricle) (ventricle) — *see* Infarct, myocardium
heat T67.01
hemorrhagic (stroke) — *see* Hemorrhage, intracranial
meninges, hemorrhagic — *see* Hemorrhage, intracranial, subarachnoid
uremic N18.9 *[I68.8]*
Appearance
bizarre R46.1
specified NEC R46.89
very low level of personal hygiene R46.0
Appendage
epididymal (organ of Morgagni) Q55.4
intestine (epiploic) Q43.8
preauricular Q17.0
testicular (organ of Morgagni) Q55.29
Appendicitis (pneumococcal) (retrocecal) K37
with
gangrene K35.891
perforation NOS K35.32
peritoneal abscess K35.33
peritonitis NEC K35.33
generalized (with perforation or rupture) K35.20
with abscess K35.21
localized K35.30
with
gangrene K35.31
perforation K35.32
and abscess K35.33
rupture (with localized peritonitis) K35.32

APPENDICITIS - ARTERIOSCLEROSIS, ARTERIOSCLEROTIC

Arteriosclerosis, arteriosclerotic (diffuse) (obliterans) (of) (senile) (with calcification) - *continued*

- with - *continued*
  - critical limb ischemia - *continued*
    - bypass graft - *continued*
      - specified graft NEC - *continued*
        - leg - *continued*
          - left - *continued*
            - with - *continued*
              - ulceration (and intermittent claudication and rest pain) - *continued*
                - midfoot I70.744
                - thigh I70.741
          - right I70.721
            - with
              - gangrene (and intermittent claudication, rest pain, and ulcer) I70.761
              - rest pain (and intermittent claudication) I70.721
              - ulceration (and intermittent claudication and rest pain) I70.739
                - ankle I70.733
                - calf I70.732
                - foot site NEC I70.735
                - heel I70.734
                - lower leg NEC I70.738
                - midfoot I70.734
                - thigh I70.731
    - leg I70.229
      - with
        - gangrene (and intermittent claudication, rest pain, and ulcer) I70.269
        - rest pain (and intermittent claudication) I70.229
      - bilateral I70.223
        - with
          - gangrene (and intermittent claudication, rest pain, and ulcer) I70.263
          - rest pain (and intermittent claudication) I70.223
      - left I70.222
        - with
          - gangrene (and intermittent claudication, rest pain, and ulcer) I70.262
          - rest pain (and intermittent claudication) I70.222
          - ulceration (and intermittent claudication and rest pain) I70.249
            - ankle I70.243
            - calf I70.242
            - foot site NEC I70.245
            - heel I70.244
            - lower leg NEC I70.248
            - midfoot I70.244
            - thigh I70.241
      - right I70.221
        - with
          - gangrene (and intermittent claudication, rest pain, and ulcer) I70.261
          - rest pain (and intermittent claudication) I70.221
          - ulceration (and intermittent claudication and rest pain) I70.239
            - ankle I70.233
            - calf I70.232
            - foot site NEC I70.235
            - heel I70.234
            - lower leg NEC I70.238
            - midfoot I70.234
            - thigh I70.231
- aorta I70.0
- arteries of extremities — *see* Arteriosclerosis, extremities
  - with

Arteriosclerosis, arteriosclerotic (diffuse) (obliterans) (of) (senile) (with calcification) - *continued*

- arteries of extremities - *continued*
  - with - *continued*
    - chronic limb-threatening ischemia — *see* Arteriosclerosis, with critical limb ischemia
    - critical limb ischemia — *see* Arteriosclerosis, with critical limb ischemia
- brain I67.2
- bypass graft
  - with
    - chronic limb-threatening ischemia — *see* Arteriosclerosis, with critical limb ischemia
    - critical limb ischemia — *see* Arteriosclerosis, with critical limb ischemia
  - coronary — *see* Arteriosclerosis, coronary, bypass graft
  - extremities — *see* Arteriosclerosis, extremities, bypass graft
- cardiac — *see* Disease, heart, ischemic, atherosclerotic
- cardiopathy — *see* Disease, heart, ischemic, atherosclerotic
- cardiorenal — *see* Hypertension, cardiorenal
- cardiovascular — *see* Disease, heart, ischemic, atherosclerotic
- carotid — *see also* Occlusion, artery, carotid I65.2-
- central nervous system I67.2
- cerebral I67.2
- cerebrovascular I67.2
- coronary (artery) I25.10
  - due to
    - calcified coronary lesion (severely) I25.84
    - lipid rich plaque I25.83
  - bypass graft I25.810
    - with
      - angina pectoris I25.709
        - with documented spasm I25.701
        - specified type NEC I25.708
        - unstable I25.700
      - ischemic chest pain I25.709
    - autologous artery I25.810
      - with
        - angina pectoris I25.729
          - with documented spasm I25.721
          - specified type I25.728
          - unstable I25.720
        - ischemic chest pain I25.729
    - autologous vein I25.810
      - with
        - angina pectoris I25.719
          - with documented spasm I25.711
          - specified type I25.718
          - unstable I25.710
        - ischemic chest pain I25.719
    - nonautologous biological I25.810
      - with
        - angina pectoris I25.739
          - with documented spasm I25.731
          - specified type I25.738
          - unstable I25.730
        - ischemic chest pain I25.739
    - specified type NEC I25.810
      - with
        - angina pectoris I25.799
          - with documented spasm I25.791
          - specified type I25.798
          - unstable I25.790
        - ischemic chest pain I25.799
  - native vessel
    - with
      - angina pectoris I25.119
        - with documented spasm I25.111
        - specified type NEC I25.118
        - unstable I25.110
      - ischemic chest pain I25.119
  - transplanted heart I25.811
    - bypass graft I25.812

Arteriosclerosis, arteriosclerotic (diffuse) (obliterans) (of) (senile) (with calcification) - *continued*

- coronary (artery) - *continued*
  - transplanted heart - *continued*
    - bypass graft - *continued*
      - with
        - angina pectoris I25.769
          - with documented spasm I25.761
          - specified type I25.768
          - unstable I25.760
        - ischemic chest pain I25.769
    - native coronary artery I25.811
      - with
        - angina pectoris I25.759
          - with documented spasm I25.751
          - specified type I25.758
          - unstable I25.750
        - ischemic chest pain I25.759
- extremities (native arteries) I70.209
  - with
    - chronic limb-threatening ischemia — *see* Arteriosclerosis, with critical limb ischemia
    - critical limb ischemia — *see* Arteriosclerosis, with critical limb ischemia
  - bypass graft I70.309
    - with
      - chronic limb-threatening ischemia — *see* Arteriosclerosis, with critical limb ischemia
      - critical limb ischemia — *see* Arteriosclerosis, with critical limb ischemia
    - autologous vein graft I70.409
      - leg I70.409
        - with
          - gangrene (and intermittent claudication, rest pain and ulcer) I70.469
          - intermittent claudication I70.419
          - rest pain (and intermittent claudication) I70.429
        - bilateral I70.403
          - with
            - gangrene (and intermittent claudication, rest pain and ulcer) I70.463
            - intermittent claudication I70.413
            - rest pain (and intermittent claudication) I70.423
          - specified type NEC I70.493
        - left I70.402
          - with
            - gangrene (and intermittent claudication, rest pain and ulcer) I70.462
            - intermittent claudication I70.412
            - rest pain (and intermittent claudication) I70.422
            - ulceration (and intermittent claudication and rest pain) I70.449
              - ankle I70.443
              - calf I70.442
              - foot site NEC I70.445
              - heel I70.444
              - lower leg NEC I70.448
              - midfoot I70.444
              - thigh I70.441
          - specified type NEC I70.492
        - right I70.401
          - with
            - gangrene (and intermittent claudication, rest pain and ulcer) I70.461
            - intermittent claudication I70.411
            - rest pain (and intermittent claudication) I70.421

- **Arteriosclerosis, arteriosclerotic (diffuse) (obliterans) (of) (senile) (with calcification)** - *continued*
  - extremities (native arteries) - *continued*
    - bypass graft - *continued*
      - autologous vein graft - *continued*
        - leg - *continued*
          - right - *continued*
            - with - *continued*
              - ulceration (and intermittent claudication and rest pain) I70.439
                - ankle I70.433
                - calf I70.432
                - foot site NEC I70.435
                - heel I70.434
                - lower leg NEC I70.438
                - midfoot I70.434
                - thigh I70.431
            - specified type NEC I70.491
          - specified type NEC I70.499
        - specified NEC I70.408
          - with
            - gangrene (and intermittent claudication, rest pain and ulcer) I70.468
            - intermittent claudication I70.418
            - rest pain (and intermittent claudication) I70.428
            - ulceration (and intermittent claudication and rest pain) I70.45
          - specified type NEC I70.498
      - leg I70.309
        - with
          - gangrene (and intermittent claudication, rest pain and ulcer) I70.369
          - intermittent claudication I70.319
          - rest pain (and intermittent claudication) I70.329
        - bilateral I70.303
          - with
            - gangrene (and intermittent claudication, rest pain and ulcer) I70.363
            - intermittent claudication I70.313
            - rest pain (and intermittent claudication) I70.323
          - specified type NEC I70.393
        - left I70.302
          - with
            - gangrene (and intermittent claudication, rest pain and ulcer) I70.362
            - intermittent claudication I70.312
            - rest pain (and intermittent claudication) I70.322
            - ulceration (and intermittent claudication and rest pain) I70.349
              - ankle I70.343
              - calf I70.342
              - foot site NEC I70.345
              - heel I70.344
              - lower leg NEC I70.348
              - midfoot I70.344
              - thigh I70.341
          - specified type NEC I70.392
        - right I70.301
          - with
            - gangrene (and intermittent claudication, rest pain and ulcer) I70.361
            - intermittent claudication I70.311
            - rest pain (and intermittent claudication) I70.321
            - ulceration (and intermittent claudication and rest pain) I70.339
              - ankle I70.333
              - calf I70.332
              - foot site NEC I70.335
              - heel I70.334
              - lower leg NEC I70.338

- **Arteriosclerosis, arteriosclerotic (diffuse) (obliterans) (of) (senile) (with calcification)** - *continued*
  - extremities (native arteries) - *continued*
    - bypass graft - *continued*
      - leg - *continued*
        - right - *continued*
          - with - *continued*
            - ulceration (and intermittent claudication and rest pain) - *continued*
              - midfoot I70.334
              - thigh I70.331
          - specified type NEC I70.391
        - specified type NEC I70.399
      - nonautologous biological graft I70.509
        - leg I70.509
          - with
            - gangrene (and intermittent claudication, rest pain and ulcer) I70.569
            - intermittent claudication I70.519
            - rest pain (and intermittent claudication) I70.529
          - bilateral I70.503
            - with
              - gangrene (and intermittent claudication, rest pain and ulcer) I70.563
              - intermittent claudication I70.513
              - rest pain (and intermittent claudication) I70.523
            - specified type NEC I70.593
          - left I70.502
            - with
              - gangrene (and intermittent claudication, rest pain and ulcer) I70.562
              - intermittent claudication I70.512
              - rest pain (and intermittent claudication) I70.522
              - ulceration (and intermittent claudication and rest pain) I70.549
                - ankle I70.543
                - calf I70.542
                - foot site NEC I70.545
                - heel I70.544
                - lower leg NEC I70.548
                - midfoot I70.544
                - thigh I70.541
            - specified type NEC I70.592
          - right I70.501
            - with
              - gangrene (and intermittent claudication, rest pain and ulcer) I70.561
              - intermittent claudication I70.511
              - rest pain (and intermittent claudication) I70.521
              - ulceration (and intermittent claudication and rest pain) I70.539
                - ankle I70.533
                - calf I70.532
                - foot site NEC I70.535
                - heel I70.534
                - lower leg NEC I70.538
                - midfoot I70.534
                - thigh I70.531
            - specified type NEC I70.591
          - specified type NEC I70.599
        - specified NEC I70.508
          - with
            - gangrene (and intermittent claudication, rest pain and ulcer) I70.568
            - intermittent claudication I70.518
            - rest pain (and intermittent claudication) I70.528

- **Arteriosclerosis, arteriosclerotic (diffuse) (obliterans) (of) (senile) (with calcification)** - *continued*
  - extremities (native arteries) - *continued*
    - bypass graft - *continued*
      - nonautologous biological graft - *continued*
        - specified NEC - *continued*
          - with - *continued*
            - ulceration (and intermittent claudication and rest pain) I70.55
          - specified type NEC I70.598
      - nonbiological graft I70.609
        - leg I70.609
          - with
            - gangrene (and intermittent claudication, rest pain and ulcer) I70.669
            - intermittent claudication I70.619
            - rest pain (and intermittent claudication) I70.629
          - bilateral I70.603
            - with
              - gangrene (and intermittent claudication, rest pain and ulcer) I70.663
              - intermittent claudication I70.613
              - rest pain (and intermittent claudication) I70.623
            - specified type NEC I70.693
          - left I70.602
            - with
              - gangrene (and intermittent claudication, rest pain and ulcer) I70.662
              - intermittent claudication I70.612
              - rest pain (and intermittent claudication) I70.622
              - ulceration (and intermittent claudication and rest pain) I70.649
                - ankle I70.643
                - calf I70.642
                - foot site NEC I70.645
                - heel I70.644
                - lower leg NEC I70.648
                - midfoot I70.644
                - thigh I70.641
            - specified type NEC I70.692
          - right I70.601
            - with
              - gangrene (and intermittent claudication, rest pain and ulcer) I70.661
              - intermittent claudication I70.611
              - rest pain (and intermittent claudication) I70.621
              - ulceration (and intermittent claudication and rest pain) I70.639
                - ankle I70.633
                - calf I70.632
                - foot site NEC I70.635
                - heel I70.634
                - lower leg NEC I70.638
                - midfoot I70.634
                - thigh I70.631
            - specified type NEC I70.691
          - specified type NEC I70.699
        - specified NEC I70.608
          - with
            - gangrene (and intermittent claudication, rest pain and ulcer) I70.668
            - intermittent claudication I70.618
            - rest pain (and intermittent claudication) I70.628
            - ulceration (and intermittent claudication and rest pain) I70.65
          - specified type NEC I70.698

Arteriosclerosis, arteriosclerotic (diffuse) (obliterans) (of) (senile) (with calcification) - *continued*
extremities (native arteries) - *continued*
bypass graft - *continued*
specified graft NEC I70.709
leg I70.709
with
gangrene (and intermittent claudication, rest pain and ulcer) I70.769
intermittent claudication I70.719
rest pain (and intermittent claudication) I70.729
bilateral I70.703
with
gangrene (and intermittent claudication, rest pain and ulcer) I70.763
intermittent claudication I70.713
rest pain (and intermittent claudication) I70.723
specified type NEC I70.793
left I70.702
with
gangrene (and intermittent claudication, rest pain and ulcer) I70.762
intermittent claudication I70.712
rest pain (and intermittent claudication) I70.722
ulceration (and intermittent claudication and rest pain) I70.749
ankle I70.743
calf I70.742
foot site NEC I70.745
heel I70.744
lower leg NEC I70.748
midfoot I70.744
thigh I70.741
specified type NEC I70.792
right I70.701
with
gangrene (and intermittent claudication, rest pain and ulcer) I70.761
intermittent claudication I70.711
rest pain (and intermittent claudication) I70.721
ulceration (and intermittent claudication and rest pain) I70.739
ankle I70.733
calf I70.732
foot site NEC I70.735
heel I70.734
lower leg NEC I70.738
midfoot I70.734
thigh I70.731
specified type NEC I70.791
specified type NEC I70.799
specified NEC I70.708
with
gangrene (and intermittent claudication, rest pain and ulcer) I70.768
intermittent claudication I70.718
rest pain (and intermittent claudication) I70.728
ulceration (and intermittent claudication and rest pain) I70.75
specified type NEC I70.798
specified NEC I70.308
with
gangrene (and intermittent claudication, rest pain and ulcer) I70.368
intermittent claudication I70.318
rest pain (and intermittent claudication) I70.328

Arteriosclerosis, arteriosclerotic (diffuse) (obliterans) (of) (senile) (with calcification) - *continued*
extremities (native arteries) - *continued*
bypass graft - *continued*
specified NEC - *continued*
with - *continued*
ulceration (and intermittent claudication and rest pain) I70.35
specified type NEC I70.398
leg I70.209
with
gangrene (and intermittent claudication, rest pain and ulcer) I70.269
intermittent claudication I70.219
rest pain (and intermittent claudication) I70.229
bilateral I70.203
with
gangrene (and intermittent claudication, rest pain and ulcer) I70.263
intermittent claudication I70.213
rest pain (and intermittent claudication) I70.223
specified type NEC I70.293
left I70.202
with
gangrene (and intermittent claudication, rest pain and ulcer) I70.262
intermittent claudication I70.212
rest pain (and intermittent claudication) I70.222
ulceration (and intermittent claudication and rest pain) I70.249
ankle I70.243
calf I70.242
foot site NEC I70.245
heel I70.244
lower leg NEC I70.248
midfoot I70.244
thigh I70.241
specified type NEC I70.292
right I70.201
with
gangrene (and intermittent claudication, rest pain and ulcer) I70.261
intermittent claudication I70.211
rest pain (and intermittent claudication) I70.221
ulceration (and intermittent claudication and rest pain) I70.239
ankle I70.233
calf I70.232
foot site NEC I70.235
heel I70.234
lower leg NEC I70.238
midfoot I70.234
thigh I70.231
specified type NEC I70.291
specified type NEC I70.299
specified site NEC I70.208
with
gangrene (and intermittent claudication, rest pain and ulcer) I70.268
intermittent claudication I70.218
rest pain (and intermittent claudication) I70.228
ulceration (and intermittent claudication and rest pain) I70.25
specified type NEC I70.298
generalized I70.91
heart (disease) — *see* Arteriosclerosis, coronary (artery),
kidney — *see* Hypertension, kidney
medial — *see* Arteriosclerosis, extremities
mesenteric (artery) K55.1

Arteriosclerosis, arteriosclerotic (diffuse) (obliterans) (of) (senile) (with calcification) - *continued*
Mönckeberg's — *see* Arteriosclerosis, extremities
myocarditis I51.4
peripheral (of extremities) — *see* Arteriosclerosis, extremities
pulmonary (idiopathic) I27.0
renal (arterioles) — *see also* Hypertension, kidney
artery I70.1
retina (vascular) I70.8 *[H35.0-]*
specified artery NEC I70.8
spinal (cord) G95.19
vertebral (artery) I67.2
Arteriospasm I73.9
Arteriovenous — *see* condition
Arteritis I77.6
allergic M31.0
aorta (nonsyphilitic) I77.6
syphilitic A52.02
aortic arch M31.4
brachiocephalic M31.4
brain I67.7
syphilitic A52.04
cerebral I67.7
in
diseases classified elsewhere I68.2
systemic lupus erythematosus M32.19
listerial A32.89
syphilitic A52.04
tuberculous A18.89
coronary (artery) I25.89
rheumatic I01.8
chronic I09.89
syphilitic A52.06
cranial (left) (right) , giant cell M31.6
deformans — *see* Arteriosclerosis
giant cell NEC M31.6
with polymyalgia rheumatica M31.5
necrosing or necrotizing M31.9
specified NEC M31.8
nodosa M30.0
obliterans — *see* Arteriosclerosis
pulmonary I28.8
rheumatic — *see* Fever, rheumatic
senile — *see* Arteriosclerosis
suppurative I77.2
syphilitic (general) A52.09
brain A52.04
coronary A52.06
spinal A52.09
temporal, giant cell M31.6
young female aortic arch syndrome M31.4
Artery, arterial — *see also* condition
abscess I77.89
single umbilical Q27.0
Arthralgia (allergic) — *see also* Pain, joint
in caisson disease T70.3
temporomandibular M26.62-
Arthritis, arthritic (acute) (chronic) (nonpyogenic) (subacute) M19.90
allergic — *see* Arthritis, specified form NEC
ankylosing (crippling) (spine) — *see also* Spondylitis, ankylosing
sites other than spine — *see* Arthritis, specified form NEC
atrophic — *see* Osteoarthritis
spine — *see* Spondylitis, ankylosing
back — *see* Spondylopathy, inflammatory
blennorrhagic (gonococcal) A54.42
Charcot's — *see* Arthropathy, neuropathic
diabetic — *see* Diabetes, arthropathy, neuropathic
syringomyelic G95.0
chylous (filarial) (*see also* category M01) B74.9
climacteric (any site) NEC — *see* Arthritis, specified form NEC
crystal (-induced) — *see* Arthritis, in, crystals
deformans — *see* Osteoarthritis
degenerative — *see* Osteoarthritis
due to or associated with

Arthritis, arthritic (acute) (chronic) (nonpyogenic) (subacute) - *continued*
  due to or associated with - *continued*
    acromegaly E22.0
    brucellosis — *see* Brucellosis
    caisson disease T70.3
    diabetes — *see* Diabetes, arthropathy
    dracontiasis (*see also* category M01) B72
    enteritis NEC
      regional — *see* Enteritis, regional
    erysipelas (*see also* category M01) A46
    erythema
      epidemic A25.1
      nodosum L52
    filariasis NOS B74.9
    glanders A24.0
    helminthiasis (*see also* category M01) B83.9
    hemophilia D66 *[M36.2]*
    Henoch- (Schönlein) purpura D69.0 *[M36.4]*
    human parvovirus (*see also* category M01) B97.6
    infectious disease NEC — *see* category M01
    leprosy (see also category M01) — *see also* Leprosy A30.9
    Lyme disease A69.23
    mycobacteria (*see also* category M01) A31.8
    parasitic disease NEC (*see also* category M01) B89
    paratyphoid fever (see also category M01) — *see also* Fever, paratyphoid A01.4
    rat bite fever (*see also* category M01) A25.1
    regional enteritis — *see* Enteritis, regional
    respiratory disorder NOS J98.9
    serum sickness — *see also* Reaction, serum T80.69
    syringomyelia G95.0
    typhoid fever A01.04
  epidemic erythema A25.1
  facet joint — *see also* Spondylosis M47.819
  febrile — *see* Fever, rheumatic
  gonococcal A54.42
  gouty (acute) — *see* Gout
  in (due to)
    acromegaly (*see also* subcategory M14.8-) E22.0
    amyloidosis (*see also* subcategory M14.8-) E85.4
    bacterial disease (*see also* subcategory M01) A49.9
    Behçet's syndrome M35.2
    caisson disease (*see also* subcategory M14.8-) T70.3
    coliform bacilli (Escherichia coli) — *see* Arthritis, in, pyogenic organism NEC
    crystals M11.9
      dicalcium phosphate — *see* Arthritis, in, crystals, specified type NEC
      hydroxyapatite M11.0-
      pyrophosphate — *see* Arthritis, in, crystals, specified type NEC
      specified type NEC M11.80
        ankle M11.87-
        elbow M11.82-
        foot joint M11.87-
        hand joint M11.84-
        hip M11.85-
        knee M11.86-
        multiple sites M11.8-
        shoulder M11.81-
        vertebrae M11.88
        wrist M11.83-
    dermatoarthritis, lipoid E78.81
    dracontiasis (dracunculiasis) (*see also* category M01) B72
    endocrine disorder NEC (*see also* subcategory M14.8-) E34.9
    enteritis, infectious NEC (*see also* category M01) A09

Arthritis, arthritic (acute) (chronic) (nonpyogenic) (subacute) - *continued*
  in (due to) - *continued*
    enteritis, infectious NEC - *continued*
      specified organism NEC (*see also* category M01) A08.8
    erythema
      multiforme (*see also* subcategory M14.8-) L51.9
      nodosum (*see also* subcategory M14.8-) L52
    gout — *see* Gout
    helminthiasis NEC (*see also* category M01) B83.9
    hemochromatosis (*see also* subcategory M14.8-) E83.118
    hemoglobinopathy NEC D58.2 *[M36.3]*
    hemophilia NEC D66 *[M36.2]*
    Hemophilus influenzae M00.8- *[B96.3]*
    Henoch (-Schönlein) purpura D69.0 *[M36.4]*
    hyperparathyroidism NEC (*see also* subcategory M14.8-) E21.3
    hypersensitivity reaction NEC T78.49 *[M36.4]*
    hypogammaglobulinemia (*see also* subcategory M14.8-) D80.1
    hypothyroidism NEC (*see also* subcategory M14.8-) E03.9
    infection — *see* Arthritis, pyogenic or pyemic
      spine — *see* Spondylopathy, infective
    infectious disease NEC — *see* category M01
    leprosy (*see also* category M01) A30.9
    leukemia NEC C95.9- *[M36.1]*
    lipoid dermatoarthritis E78.81
    Lyme disease A69.23
    Mediterranean fever, familial (*see also* subcategory M14.8-) M04.1
    Meningococcus A39.83
    metabolic disorder NEC (*see also* subcategory M14.8-) E88.9
    multiple myelomatosis C90.0- *[M36.1]*
    mumps B26.85
    mycosis NEC (*see also* category M01) B49
    myelomatosis (multiple) C90.0- *[M36.1]*
    neurological disorder NEC G98.0
    ochronosis (*see also* subcategory M14.8-) E70.29
    O'nyong-nyong (*see also* category M01) A92.1
    parasitic disease NEC (*see also* category M01) B89
    paratyphoid fever (*see also* category M01) A01.4
    Pseudomonas — *see* Arthritis, pyogenic, bacterial NEC
    psoriasis L40.50
    pyogenic organism NEC — *see* Arthritis, pyogenic, bacterial NEC
    Reiter's disease — *see* Reiter's disease
    respiratory disorder NEC (*see also* subcategory M14.8-) J98.9
    reticulosis, malignant (*see also* subcategory M14.8-) C86.0
    rubella B06.82
    Salmonella (arizonae) (cholerae-suis) (enteritidis) (typhimurium) A02.23
    sarcoidosis D86.86
    specified bacteria NEC — *see* Arthritis, pyogenic, bacterial NEC
    sporotrichosis B42.82
    syringomyelia G95.0
    thalassemia NEC D56.9 *[M36.3]*
    tuberculosis — *see* Tuberculosis, arthritis
    typhoid fever A01.04
    urethritis, Reiter's — *see* Reiter's disease
    viral disease NEC (*see also* category M01) B34.9
  infectious or infective — *see also* Arthritis, pyogenic or pyemic
    spine — *see* Spondylopathy, infective
  juvenile M08.90
    with systemic onset — *see* Still's disease

Arthritis, arthritic (acute) (chronic) (nonpyogenic) (subacute) - *continued*
  juvenile - *continued*
    ankle M08.97-
    elbow M08.92-
    foot joint M08.97-
    hand joint M08.94-
    hip M08.95-
    knee M08.96-
    multiple site M08.99
    pauciarticular M08.40
      ankle M08.47-
      elbow M08.42-
      foot joint M08.47-
      hand joint M08.44-
      hip M08.45-
      knee M08.46-
      shoulder M08.41-
      specified site NEC M08.4A
      vertebrae M08.48
      wrist M08.43-
    psoriatic L40.54
    rheumatoid — *see* Arthritis, rheumatoid, juvenile
    shoulder M08.91-
    specified site NEC M08.9A
    vertebra M08.98
    specified type NEC M08.80
      ankle M08.87-
      elbow M08.82-
      foot joint M08.87-
      hand joint M08.84-
      hip M08.85-
      knee M08.86-
      multiple site M08.89
      shoulder M08.81-
      specified joint NEC M08.88
      vertebrae M08.88
      wrist M08.83-
    wrist M08.93-
  meaning osteoarthritis — *see* Osteoarthritis
  meningococcal A39.83
  menopausal (any site) NEC — *see* Arthritis, specified form NEC
  mutilans (psoriatic) L40.52
  mycotic NEC (*see also* category M01) B49
  neuropathic (Charcot) — *see* Arthropathy, neuropathic
    diabetic — *see* Diabetes, arthropathy, neuropathic
    nonsyphilitic NEC G98.0
    syringomyelic G95.0
  ochronotic (*see also* subcategory M14.8-) E70.29
  palindromic (any site) — *see* Rheumatism, palindromic
  pneumococcal M00.10
    ankle M00.17-
    elbow M00.12-
    foot joint — *see* Arthritis, pneumococcal, ankle
    hand joint M00.14-
    hip M00.15-
    knee M00.16-
    multiple site M00.19
    shoulder M00.11-
    vertebra M00.18
    wrist M00.13-
  postdysenteric — *see* Arthropathy, postdysenteric
  postmeningococcal A39.84
  postrheumatic, chronic — *see* Arthropathy, postrheumatic, chronic
  primary progressive — *see also* Arthritis, specified form NEC
    spine — *see* Spondylitis, ankylosing
  psoriatic L40.50
  purulent (any site except spine) — *see* Arthritis, pyogenic or pyemic
    spine — *see* Spondylopathy, infective
  pyogenic or pyemic (any site except spine) M00.9
    bacterial NEC M00.80
      ankle M00.87-
      elbow M00.82-

Arthritis, arthritic (acute) (chronic) (nonpyogenic) (subacute) - *continued*
pyogenic or pyemic (any site except spine) - *continued*
bacterial NEC - *continued*
foot joint — *see* Arthritis, pyogenic, bacterial NEC, ankle
hand joint M00.84-
hip M00.85-
knee M00.86-
multiple site M00.89
shoulder M00.81-
vertebra M00.88
wrist M00.83-
pneumococcal — *see* Arthritis, pneumococcal
spine — *see* Spondylopathy, infective
staphylococcal — *see* Arthritis, staphylococcal
streptococcal — *see* Arthritis, streptococcal NEC
pneumococcal — *see* Arthritis, pneumococcal
reactive — *see* Reiter's disease
rheumatic — *see also* Arthritis, rheumatoid
acute or subacute — *see* Fever, rheumatic
rheumatoid M06.9
with
carditis — *see* Rheumatoid, carditis
endocarditis — *see* Rheumatoid, carditis
heart involvement NEC — *see* Rheumatoid, carditis
lung involvement — *see* Rheumatoid, lung
myocarditis — *see* Rheumatoid, carditis
myopathy — *see* Rheumatoid, myopathy
pericarditis — *see* Rheumatoid, carditis
polyneuropathy — *see* Rheumatoid, polyneuropathy
rheumatoid factor — *see* Arthritis, rheumatoid, seropositive
splenoadenomegaly and leukopenia — *see* Felty's syndrome
vasculitis — *see* Rheumatoid, vasculitis
visceral involvement NEC — *see* Rheumatoid, arthritis, with involvement of organs NEC
juvenile (with or without rheumatoid factor) M08.00
with systemic onset — *see* Still's disease
ankle M08.07-
elbow M08.02-
foot joint M08.07-
hand joint M08.04-
hip M08.05-
knee M08.06-
multiple site M08.09
shoulder M08.01-
specified site NEC M08.0A
vertebra M08.08
wrist M08.03-
seronegative M06.00
ankle M06.07-
elbow M06.02-
foot joint M06.07-
hand joint M06.04-
hip M06.05-
knee M06.06-
multiple site M06.09
shoulder M06.01-
specified site NEC M06.0A
vertebra M06.08
wrist M06.03-
seropositive M05.9
specified NEC M05.80
ankle M05.87-
elbow M05.82-
foot joint M05.87-
hand joint M05.84-
hip M05.85-
knee M05.86-
multiple sites M05.89
shoulder M05.81-
specified site NEC M05.8A

Arthritis, arthritic (acute) (chronic) (nonpyogenic) (subacute) - *continued*
rheumatoid - *continued*
seropositive - *continued*
specified NEC - *continued*
vertebra — *see* Spondylitis, ankylosing
wrist M05.83-
without organ involvement M05.70
ankle M05.77-
elbow M05.72-
foot joint M05.77-
hand joint M05.74-
hip M05.75-
knee M05.76-
multiple sites M05.79
shoulder M05.71-
specified site NEC M05.7A
vertebra — *see* Spondylitis, ankylosing
wrist M05.73-
specified type NEC M06.80
ankle M06.87-
elbow M06.82-
foot joint M06.87-
hand joint M06.84-
hip M06.85-
knee M06.86-
multiple site M06.89
shoulder M06.81-
specified site NEC M06.8A
vertebra M06.88
wrist M06.83-
spine — *see* Spondylitis, ankylosing
rubella B06.82
scorbutic (*see also* subcategory M14.8-) E54
senile or senescent — *see* Osteoarthritis
septic (any site except spine) — *see* Arthritis, pyogenic or pyemic
spine — *see* Spondylopathy, infective
serum (nontherapeutic) (therapeutic) — *see* Arthropathy, postimmunization
specified form NEC M13.80
ankle M13.87-
elbow M13.82-
foot joint M13.87-
hand joint M13.84-
hip M13.85-
knee M13.86-
multiple site M13.89
shoulder M13.81-
specified joint NEC M13.88
wrist M13.83-
spine — *see also* Spondylosis
infectious or infective NEC — *see* Spondylopathy, infective
Marie-Strümpell — *see* Spondylitis, ankylosing
pyogenic — *see* Spondylopathy, infective
rheumatoid — *see* Spondylitis, ankylosing
traumatic (old) — *see* Spondylopathy, traumatic
tuberculous A18.01
staphylococcal M00.00
ankle M00.07-
elbow M00.02-
foot joint — *see* Arthritis, staphylococcal, ankle
hand joint M00.04-
hip M00.05-
knee M00.06-
multiple site M00.09
shoulder M00.01-
vertebra M00.08
wrist M00.03-
streptococcal NEC M00.20
ankle M00.27-
elbow M00.22-
foot joint — *see* Arthritis, streptococcal, ankle
hand joint M00.24-
hip M00.25-
knee M00.26-
multiple site M00.29
shoulder M00.21-

Arthritis, arthritic (acute) (chronic) (nonpyogenic) (subacute) - *continued*
streptococcal NEC - *continued*
vertebra M00.28
wrist M00.23-
suppurative — *see* Arthritis, pyogenic or pyemic
syphilitic (late) A52.16
congenital A50.55 *[M12.80]*
syphilitica deformans (Charcot) A52.16
temporomandibular joint M26.64-
toxic of menopause (any site) — *see* Arthritis, specified form NEC
transient — *see* Arthropathy, specified form NEC
traumatic (chronic) — *see* Arthropathy, traumatic
tuberculous A18.02
spine A18.01
uratic — *see* Gout
urethritica (Reiter's) — *see* Reiter's disease
vertebral — *see* Spondylopathy, inflammatory
villous (any site) — *see* Arthropathy, specified form NEC
Arthrocele — *see* Effusion, joint
Arthrodesis status Z98.1
Arthrodynia — *see also* Pain, joint
Arthrodysplasia Q74.9
Arthrofibrosis, joint — *see* Ankylosis
Arthrogryposis (congenital) Q68.8
multiplex congenita Q74.3
Arthrokatadysis M24.7
Arthropathy — *see also* Arthritis M12.9
Charcot's — *see* Arthropathy, neuropathic
diabetic — *see* Diabetes, arthropathy, neuropathic
syringomyelic G95.0
cricoarytenoid J38.7
crystal (-induced) — *see* Arthritis, in, crystals
diabetic NEC — *see* Diabetes, arthropathy
distal interphalangeal, psoriatic L40.51
enteropathic M07.60
ankle M07.67-
elbow M07.62-
foot joint M07.67-
hand joint M07.64-
hip M07.65-
knee M07.66-
multiple site M07.69
shoulder M07.61-
vertebra M07.68
wrist M07.63-
facet joint — *see also* Spondylosis M47.819
following intestinal bypass M02.00
ankle M02.07-
elbow M02.02-
foot joint M02.07-
hand joint M02.04-
hip M02.05-
knee M02.06-
multiple site M02.09
shoulder M02.01-
vertebra M02.08
wrist M02.03-
gouty — *see also* Gout
in (due to)
Lesch-Nyhan syndrome E79.1 *[M14.8-]*
sickle-cell disorders D57- *[M14.8-]*
hemophilic NEC D66 *[M36.2]*
in (due to)
hyperparathyroidism NEC E21.3 *[M14.8-]*
metabolic disease NOS E88.9 *[M14.8-]*
in (due to)
acromegaly E22.0 *[M14.8-]*
amyloidosis E85.4 *[M14.8-]*
blood disorder NOS D75.9 *[M36.3]*
diabetes — *see* Diabetes, arthropathy
endocrine disease NOS E34.9 *[M14.8-]*
erythema
multiforme L51.9 *[M14.8-]*
nodosum L52 *[M14.8-]*
hemochromatosis E83.118 *[M14.8-]*

Arthropathy - *continued*
in (due to) - *continued*
hemoglobinopathy NEC D58.2 *[M36.3]*
hemophilia NEC D66 *[M36.2]*
Henoch-Schönlein purpura D69.0 *[M36.4]*
hyperthyroidism E05.90 *[M14.8-]*
hypothyroidism E03.9 *[M14.8-]*
infective endocarditis I33.0 *[M12.80]*
leukemia NEC C95.9- *[M36.1]*
malignant histiocytosis C96.A *[M36.1]*
metabolic disease NOS E88.9 *[M14.8-]*
multiple myeloma C90.0- *[M36.1]*
neoplastic disease NOS (see also Neoplasm) D49.9 *[M36.1]*
nutritional deficiency (*see also* subcategory M14.8-) E63.9
psoriasis NOS L40.50
sarcoidosis D86.86
syphilis (late) A52.77
congenital A50.55 *[M12.80]*
thyrotoxicosis (*see also* subcategory M14.8-) E05.90
ulcerative colitis K51.90 *[M07.60]*
viral hepatitis (postinfectious) NEC B19.9 *[M12.80]*
Whipple's disease (*see also* subcategory M14.8-) K90.81
Jaccoud — *see* Arthropathy, postrheumatic, chronic
juvenile — *see* Arthritis, juvenile
psoriatic L40.54
mutilans (psoriatic) L40.52
neuropathic (Charcot) M14.60
ankle M14.67-
diabetic — *see* Diabetes, arthropathy, neuropathic
elbow M14.62-
foot joint M14.67-
hand joint M14.64-
hip M14.65-
knee M14.66-
multiple site M14.69
nonsyphilitic NEC G98.0
shoulder M14.61-
syringomyelic G95.0
vertebra M14.68
wrist M14.63-
osteopulmonary — *see* Osteoarthropathy, hypertrophic, specified NEC
postdysenteric M02.10
ankle M02.17-
elbow M02.12-
foot joint M02.17-
hand joint M02.14-
hip M02.15-
knee M02.16-
multiple site M02.19
shoulder M02.11-
vertebra M02.18
wrist M02.13-
postimmunization M02.20
ankle M02.27-
elbow M02.22-
foot joint M02.27-
hand joint M02.24-
hip M02.25-
knee M02.26-
multiple site M02.29
shoulder M02.21-
vertebra M02.28
wrist M02.23-
postinfectious NEC B99 *[M12.80]*
in (due to)
enteritis due to Yersinia enterocolitica A04.6 *[M12.80]*
syphilis A52.77
viral hepatitis NEC B19.9 *[M12.80]*
postrheumatic, chronic (Jaccoud) M12.00
ankle M12.07-
elbow M12.02-
foot joint M12.07-
hand joint M12.04-
hip M12.05-
knee M12.06-
multiple site M12.09

Arthropathy - *continued*
postrheumatic, chronic (Jaccoud) - *continued*
shoulder M12.01-
specified joint NEC M12.08
vertebrae M12.08
wrist M12.03-
psoriatic NEC L40.59
interphalangeal, distal L40.51
reactive M02.9
in (due to)
infective endocarditis I33.0 *[M02.9]*
specified type NEC M02.80
ankle M02.87-
elbow M02.82-
foot joint M02.87-
hand joint M02.84-
hip M02.85-
knee M02.86-
multiple site M02.89
shoulder M02.81-
vertebra M02.88
wrist M02.83-
specified form NEC M12.80
ankle M12.87-
elbow M12.82-
foot joint M12.87-
hand joint M12.84-
hip M12.85-
knee M12.86-
multiple site M12.89
shoulder M12.81-
specified joint NEC M12.88
vertebrae M12.88
wrist M12.83-
syringomyelic G95.0
tabes dorsalis A52.16
tabetic A52.16
temporomandibular joint M26.65-
transient — *see* Arthropathy, specified form NEC
traumatic M12.50
ankle M12.57-
elbow M12.52-
foot joint M12.57-
hand joint M12.54-
hip M12.55-
knee M12.56-
multiple site M12.59
shoulder M12.51-
specified joint NEC M12.58
vertebrae M12.58
wrist M12.53-
Arthropyosis — *see* Arthritis, pyogenic or pyemic
Arthrosis (deformans) (degenerative) (localized) — *see also* Osteoarthritis M19.90
spine — *see* Spondylosis
Arthus' phenomenon or reaction T78.41
due to
drug — *see* Table of Drugs and Chemicals, by drug
Articular — *see* condition
Articulation, reverse (teeth) M26.24
Artificial
insemination complication — *see* Complications, artificial, fertilization
opening status (functioning) (without complication) Z93.9
anus (colostomy) Z93.3
colostomy Z93.3
cystostomy Z93.50
appendico-vesicostomy Z93.52
cutaneous Z93.51
specified NEC Z93.59
enterostomy Z93.4
gastrostomy Z93.1
ileostomy Z93.2
intestinal tract NEC Z93.4
jejunostomy Z93.4
nephrostomy Z93.6
specified site NEC Z93.8
tracheostomy Z93.0
ureterostomy Z93.6
urethrostomy Z93.6

Artificial - *continued*
opening status (functioning) (without complication) - *continued*
urinary tract NEC Z93.6
vagina Z93.8
vagina status Z93.8
Arytenoid — *see* condition
Asbestosis (occupational) J61
Ascariasis B77.9
with
complications NEC B77.89
intestinal complications B77.0
pneumonia, pneumonitis B77.81
Ascaridosis, ascaridiasis — *see* Ascariasis
Ascaris (infection) (infestation) (lumbricoides) — *see* Ascariasis
Ascending — *see* condition
ASC-H (atypical squamous cells cannot exclude high grade squamous intraepithelial lesion on cytologic smear)
anus R85.611
cervix R87.611
vagina R87.621
Aschoff's bodies — *see* Myocarditis, rheumatic
Ascites (abdominal) R18.8
cardiac — *see also* Failure, heart, right I50.810
chylous (nonfilarial) I89.8
filarial — *see* Infestation, filarial
due to
cirrhosis, alcoholic K70.31
hepatitis
alcoholic K70.11
chronic active K71.51
S. japonicum B65.2
heart — *see also* Failure, heart, right I50.810
malignant R18.0
pseudochylous R18.8
syphilitic A52.74
tuberculous A18.31
ASC-US (atypical squamous cells of undetermined significance on cytologic smear)
anus R85.610
cervix R87.610
vagina R87.620
Aseptic — *see* condition
Asherman's syndrome N85.6
Asialia K11.7
Asiatic cholera — *see* Cholera
Asimultagnosia (simultanagnosia) R48.3
Askin's tumor — *see* Neoplasm, connective tissue, malignant
Asocial personality F60.2
Asomatognosia R41.4
Aspartylglucosaminuria E77.1
Asperger's disease or syndrome F84.5
Aspergilloma — *see* Aspergillosis
Aspergillosis (with pneumonia) B44.9
bronchopulmonary, allergic B44.81
disseminated B44.7
generalized B44.7
pulmonary NEC B44.1
allergic B44.81
invasive B44.0
specified NEC B44.89
tonsillar B44.2
Aspergillus (flavus) (fumigatus) (infection) (terreus) — *see* Aspergillosis
Aspermatogenesis — *see* Azoospermia
Aspermia (testis) — *see* Azoospermia
Asphyxia, asphyxiation (by) R09.01
antenatal P84
birth P84
bunny bag — *see* Asphyxia, due to, mechanical threat to breathing, trapped in bed clothes
crushing S28.0
drowning T75.1
gas, fumes, or vapor — *see* Table of Drugs and Chemicals
inhalation — *see* Inhalation
intrauterine P84

Asthma, asthmatic (bronchial) (catarrh) (spasmodic) - *continued*
mixed - *continued*
with - *continued*
status asthmaticus J45.902
moderate persistent J45.40
with
exacerbation (acute) J45.41
status asthmaticus J45.42
nervous — *see* Asthma, nonallergic
nonallergic (intrinsic) J45.909
with
exacerbation (acute) J45.901
status asthmaticus J45.902
persistent
mild J45.30
with
exacerbation (acute) J45.31
status asthmaticus J45.32
moderate J45.40
with
exacerbation (acute) J45.41
status asthmaticus J45.42
severe J45.50
with
exacerbation (acute) J45.51
status asthmaticus J45.52
platinum J45.998
pneumoconiotic NEC J64
potter's J62.8
predominantly allergic J45.909
psychogenic F54
pulmonary eosinophilic J82.83
red cedar J67.8
Rostan's I50.1
sandblaster's J62.8
sequoiosis J67.8
severe persistent J45.50
with
exacerbation (acute) J45.51
status asthmaticus J45.52
specified NEC J45.998
stonemason's J62.8
thymic E32.8
tuberculous — *see* Tuberculosis, pulmonary
Wichmann's (laryngismus stridulus) J38.5
wood J67.8
Astigmatism (compound) (congenital) H52.20-
irregular H52.21-
regular H52.22-
Astraphobia F40.220
Astroblastoma
specified site — *see* Neoplasm, malignant, by site
unspecified site C71.9
Astrocytoma (cystic)
anaplastic
specified site — *see* Neoplasm, malignant, by site
unspecified site C71.9
fibrillary
specified site — *see* Neoplasm, malignant, by site
unspecified site C71.9
fibrous
specified site — *see* Neoplasm, malignant, by site
unspecified site C71.9
gemistocytic
specified site — *see* Neoplasm, malignant, by site
unspecified site C71.9
juvenile
specified site — *see* Neoplasm, malignant, by site
unspecified site C71.9
pilocytic
specified site — *see* Neoplasm, malignant, by site
unspecified site C71.9
piloid
specified site — *see* Neoplasm, malignant, by site
unspecified site C71.9

Astrocytoma (cystic) - *continued*
protoplasmic
specified site — *see* Neoplasm, malignant, by site
unspecified site C71.9
specified site NEC — *see* Neoplasm, malignant, by site
subependymal D43.2
giant cell
specified site — *see* Neoplasm, uncertain behavior, by site
unspecified site D43.2
specified site — *see* Neoplasm, uncertain behavior, by site
unspecified site D43.2
unspecified site C71.9
Astroglioma
specified site — *see* Neoplasm, malignant, by site
unspecified site C71.9
Asymbolia R48.8
Asymmetry — *see also* Distortion
between native and reconstructed breast N65.1
face Q67.0
jaw (lower) — *see* Anomaly, dentofacial, jaw-cranial base relationship, asymmetry
Asynergia, asynergy R27.8
ventricular I51.89
Asystole (heart) — *see* Arrest, cardiac
At risk
for
dental caries Z91.849
high Z91.843
low Z91.841
moderate Z91.842
falling Z91.81
Ataxia, ataxy, ataxic R27.0
acute R27.8
autosomal recessive Friedreich G11.11
brain (hereditary) G11.9
cerebellar (hereditary) G11.9
with defective DNA repair G11.3
alcoholic G31.2
early-onset G11.10
with
essential tremor G11.19
myoclonus [Hunt's ataxia] G11.19
retained tendon reflexes G11.19
in
alcoholism G31.2
myxedema E03.9 *[G13.2]*
neoplastic disease — *see also* Neoplasm D49.9 *[G32.81]*
specified disease NEC G32.81
late-onset (Marie's) G11.2
cerebral (hereditary) G11.9
congenital nonprogressive G11.0
family, familial — *see* Ataxia, hereditary
following
cerebrovascular disease I69.993
cerebral infarction I69.393
intracerebral hemorrhage I69.193
nontraumatic intracranial hemorrhage NEC I69.293
specified disease NEC I69.893
subarachnoid hemorrhage I69.093
Friedreich's (heredofamilial) (cerebellar) (spinal) (with retained reflexes) G11.11
gait R26.0
hysterical F44.4
general R27.8
gluten M35.9 *[G32.81]*
with celiac disease K90.0 *[G32.81]*
hereditary G11.9
with neuropathy G60.2
cerebellar — *see* Ataxia, cerebellar
spastic G11.4
specified NEC G11.8
spinal (Friedreich's) G11.11
heredofamilial — *see* Ataxia, hereditary
Hunt's G11.19
hysterical F44.4

Ataxia, ataxy, ataxic - *continued*
locomotor (progressive) (syphilitic) (partial) (spastic) A52.11
diabetic — *see* Diabetes, ataxia
Marie's (cerebellar) (heredofamilial) (late-onset) G11.2
nonorganic origin F44.4
nonprogressive, congenital G11.0
psychogenic F44.4
Roussy-Lévy G60.0
Sanger-Brown's (hereditary) G11.2
spastic hereditary G11.4
spinal
hereditary (Friedreich's) G11.11
progressive (syphilitic) A52.11
spinocerebellar, X-linked recessive G11.19
telangiectasia (Louis-Bar) G11.3
Ataxia-telangiectasia (Louis-Bar) G11.3
Atelectasis (massive) (partial) (pressure) (pulmonary) J98.11
newborn P28.10
due to resorption P28.11
partial P28.19
primary P28.0
secondary P28.19
primary (newborn) P28.0
tuberculous — *see* Tuberculosis, pulmonary
Atelocardia Q24.9
Atelomyelia Q06.1
Atheroembolism
of
extremities
lower I75.02-
upper I75.01-
kidney I75.81
specified NEC I75.89
Atheroma, atheromatous — *see also* Arteriosclerosis I70.90
aorta, aortic I70.0
valve — *see also* Endocarditis, aortic I35.8
aorto-iliac I70.0
artery — *see* Arteriosclerosis
basilar (artery) I67.2
carotid (artery) (common) (internal) I67.2
cerebral (arteries) I67.2
coronary (artery) I25.10
with angina pectoris — *see* Arteriosclerosis, coronary (artery),
degeneration — *see* Arteriosclerosis
heart, cardiac — *see* Disease, heart, ischemic, atherosclerotic
mitral (valve) I34.8
myocardium, myocardial — *see* Disease, heart, ischemic, atherosclerotic
pulmonary valve (heart) — *see also* Endocarditis, pulmonary I37.8
tricuspid (heart) (valve) I36.8
valve, valvular — *see* Endocarditis
vertebral (artery) I67.2
Atheromatosis — *see* Arteriosclerosis
Atherosclerosis — *see also* Arteriosclerosis
coronary
artery I25.10
with angina pectoris — *see* Arteriosclerosis, coronary (artery),
due to
calcified coronary lesion (severely) I25.84
lipid rich plaque I25.83
transplanted heart I25.811
bypass graft I25.812
with angina pectoris — *see* Arteriosclerosis, coronary (artery),
native coronary artery I25.811
with angina pectoris — *see* Arteriosclerosis, coronary (artery),
Athetosis (acquired) R25.8
bilateral (congenital) G80.3
congenital (bilateral) (double) G80.3
double (congenital) G80.3
unilateral R25.8
Athlete's
foot B35.3
heart I51.7
Athrepsia E41

Athyrea (acquired) — *see also* Hypothyroidism
- congenital E03.1

Atonia, atony, atonic
- bladder (sphincter) (neurogenic) N31.2
- capillary I78.8
- cecum K59.89
  - psychogenic F45.8
- colon — *see* Atony, intestine
- congenital P94.2
- esophagus K22.89
- intestine K59.89
  - psychogenic F45.8
- stomach K31.89
  - neurotic or psychogenic F45.8
- uterus (during labor) O62.2
  - with hemorrhage (postpartum) O72.1
  - postpartum (with hemorrhage) O72.1
    - without hemorrhage O75.89

Atopy — *see* History, allergy

Atransferrinemia, congenital E88.09

Atresia, atretic
- alimentary organ or tract NEC Q45.8
  - upper Q40.8
- ani, anus, anal (canal) Q42.3
  - with fistula Q42.2
- aorta (ring) Q25.29
- aortic (orifice) (valve) Q23.0
  - arch Q25.21
  - congenital with hypoplasia of ascending aorta and defective development of left ventricle (with mitral stenosis) Q23.4
  - in hypoplastic left heart syndrome Q23.4
- aqueduct of Sylvius Q03.0
  - with spina bifida — *see* Spina bifida, with hydrocephalus
- artery NEC Q27.8
  - cerebral Q28.3
  - coronary Q24.5
  - digestive system Q27.8
  - eye Q15.8
  - lower limb Q27.8
  - pulmonary Q25.5
  - specified site NEC Q27.8
  - umbilical Q27.0
  - upper limb Q27.8
- auditory canal (external) Q16.1
- bile duct (common) (congenital) (hepatic) Q44.2
  - acquired — *see* Obstruction, bile duct
- bladder (neck) Q64.39
  - obstruction Q64.31
- bronchus Q32.4
- cecum Q42.8
- cervix (acquired) N88.2
  - congenital Q51.828
  - in pregnancy or childbirth — *see* Anomaly, cervix, in pregnancy or childbirth
    - causing obstructed labor O65.5
- choana Q30.0
- colon Q42.9
  - specified NEC Q42.8
- common duct Q44.2
- cricoid cartilage Q31.8
- cystic duct Q44.2
  - acquired K82.8
    - with obstruction K82.0
- digestive organs NEC Q45.8
- duodenum Q41.0
- ear canal Q16.1
- ejaculatory duct Q55.4
- epiglottis Q31.8
- esophagus Q39.0
  - with tracheoesophageal fistula Q39.1
- eustachian tube Q17.8
- fallopian tube (congenital) Q50.6
  - acquired N97.1
- follicular cyst N83.0-
- foramen of
  - Luschka Q03.1
    - with spina bifida — *see* Spina bifida, with hydrocephalus
  - Magendie Q03.1

Atresia, atretic - *continued*
- foramen of - *continued*
  - Magendie - *continued*
    - with spina bifida — *see* Spina bifida, with hydrocephalus
- gallbladder Q44.1
- genital organ
  - external
    - female Q52.79
    - male Q55.8
  - internal
    - female Q52.8
    - male Q55.8
- glottis Q31.8
- gullet Q39.0
  - with tracheoesophageal fistula Q39.1
- heart valve NEC Q24.8
  - pulmonary Q22.0
  - tricuspid Q22.4
- hymen Q52.3
  - acquired (postinfective) N89.6
- ileum Q41.2
- intestine (small) Q41.9
  - large Q42.9
    - specified NEC Q42.8
- iris, filtration angle Q15.0
- jejunum Q41.1
- lacrimal apparatus Q10.4
- larynx Q31.8
- meatus urinarius Q64.33
- mitral valve Q23.2
  - in hypoplastic left heart syndrome Q23.4
- nares (anterior) (posterior) Q30.0
- nasopharynx Q34.8
- nose, nostril Q30.0
  - acquired J34.89
- organ or site NEC Q89.8
- osseous meatus (ear) Q16.1
- oviduct (congenital) Q50.6
  - acquired N97.1
- parotid duct Q38.4
  - acquired K11.8
- pulmonary (artery) Q25.5
  - valve Q22.0
- pulmonic Q22.0
- pupil Q13.2
- rectum Q42.1
  - with fistula Q42.0
- salivary duct Q38.4
  - acquired K11.8
- sublingual duct Q38.4
  - acquired K11.8
- submandibular duct Q38.4
  - acquired K11.8
- submaxillary duct Q38.4
  - acquired K11.8
- thyroid cartilage Q31.8
- trachea Q32.1
- tricuspid valve Q22.4
- ureter Q62.10
  - pelvic junction Q62.11
  - vesical orifice Q62.12
- ureteropelvic junction Q62.11
- ureterovesical orifice Q62.12
- urethra (valvular) Q64.39
  - stricture Q64.32
- urinary tract NEC Q64.8
- uterus Q51.818
  - acquired N85.8
- vagina (congenital) Q52.4
  - acquired (postinfectional) (senile) N89.5
- vas deferens Q55.3
- vascular NEC Q27.8
  - cerebral Q28.3
  - digestive system Q27.8
  - lower limb Q27.8
  - specified site NEC Q27.8
  - upper limb Q27.8
- vein NEC Q27.8
  - digestive system Q27.8
  - great Q26.8
  - lower limb Q27.8
  - portal Q26.5
  - pulmonary Q26.4
    - partial Q26.3

Atresia, atretic - *continued*
- vein NEC - *continued*
  - pulmonary - *continued*
    - total Q26.2
  - specified site NEC Q27.8
  - upper limb Q27.8
- vena cava (inferior) (superior) Q26.8
- vesicourethral orifice Q64.31
- vulva Q52.79
  - acquired N90.5

Atrichia, atrichosis — *see* Alopecia

Atrophia — *see also* Atrophy
- cutis senilis L90.8
  - due to radiation L57.8
- gyrata of choroid and retina H31.23
- senilis R54
  - dermatological L90.8
    - due to radiation (nonionizing) (solar) L57.8
- unguium L60.3
  - congenita Q84.6

Atrophie blanche (en plaque) (de Milian) L95.0

Atrophoderma, atrophodermia (of) L90.9
- diffusum (idiopathic) L90.4
- maculatum L90.8
  - et striatum L90.8
    - due to syphilis A52.79
  - syphilitic A51.39
- neuriticum L90.8
- Pasini and Pierini L90.3
- pigmentosum Q82.1
- reticulatum symmetricum faciei L66.4
- senile L90.8
  - due to radiation (nonionizing) (solar) L57.8
- vermiculata (cheeks) L66.4

Atrophy, atrophic (of)
- adrenal (capsule) (gland) E27.49
  - primary (autoimmune) E27.1
- alveolar process or ridge (edentulous) K08.20
- anal sphincter (disuse) N81.84
- appendix K38.8
- arteriosclerotic — *see* Arteriosclerosis
- bile duct (common) (hepatic) K83.8
- bladder N32.89
  - neurogenic N31.8
- blanche (en plaque) (of Milian) L95.0
- bone (senile) NEC — *see also* Disorder, bone, specified type NEC
  - due to
    - tabes dorsalis (neurogenic) A52.11
- brain (cortex) (progressive) G31.9
  - frontotemporal circumscribed G31.01 *[F02.80]*
    - with behavioral disturbance G31.01 *[F02.81]*
  - senile NEC G31.1
- breast N64.2
  - obstetric — *see* Disorder, breast, specified type NEC
- buccal cavity K13.79
- cardiac — *see* Degeneration, myocardial
- cartilage (infectional) (joint) — *see* Disorder, cartilage, specified NEC
- cerebellar — *see* Atrophy, brain
- cerebral — *see* Atrophy, brain
- cervix (mucosa) (senile) (uteri) N88.8
  - menopausal N95.8
- Charcot-Marie-Tooth G60.0
- choroid (central) (macular) (myopic) (retina) H31.10-
  - diffuse secondary H31.12-
  - gyrate H31.23
  - senile H31.11-
- ciliary body — *see* Atrophy, iris
- conjunctiva (senile) H11.89
- corpus cavernosum N48.89
- cortical — *see* Atrophy, brain
- cystic duct K82.8
- Déjérine-Thomas G23.8
- disuse NEC — *see* Atrophy, muscle
- Duchenne-Aran G12.21
- ear H93.8-

ATHYREA - ATROPHY, ATROPHIC

Atrophy, atrophic (of) - *continued*
edentulous alveolar ridge K08.20
endometrium (senile) N85.8
cervix N88.8
enteric K63.89
epididymis N50.89
eyeball — *see* Disorder, globe, degenerated condition, atrophy
eyelid (senile) — *see* Disorder, eyelid, degenerative
facial (skin) L90.9
fallopian tube (senile) N83.32-
with ovary N83.33-
fascioscapulohumeral (Landouzy-Déjérine) G71.02
fatty, thymus (gland) E32.8
gallbladder K82.8
gastric K29.40
with bleeding K29.41
gastrointestinal K63.89
glandular I89.8
globe H44.52-
gum — *see* Recession, gingival
hair L67.8
heart (brown) — *see* Degeneration, myocardial
hemifacial Q67.4
Romberg G51.8
infantile E41
paralysis, acute — *see* Poliomyelitis, paralytic
intestine K63.89
iris (essential) (progressive) H21.26-
specified NEC H21.29
kidney (senile) (terminal) — *see also* Sclerosis, renal N26.1
congenital or infantile Q60.5
bilateral Q60.4
unilateral Q60.3
hydronephrotic — *see* Hydronephrosis
lacrimal gland (primary) H04.14-
secondary H04.15-
Landouzy-Déjérine G71.02
laryngitis, infective J37.0
larynx J38.7
Leber's optic (hereditary) H47.22
lip K13.0
liver (yellow) K72.90
with coma K72.91
acute, subacute K72.00
with coma K72.01
chronic K72.10
with coma K72.11
lung (senile) J98.4
macular (dermatological) L90.8
syphilitic, skin A51.39
striated A52.79
mandible (edentulous) K08.20
minimal K08.21
moderate K08.22
severe K08.23
maxilla K08.20
minimal K08.24
moderate K08.25
severe K08.26
muscle, muscular (diffuse) (general) (idiopathic) (primary) M62.50
ankle M62.57-
Duchenne-Aran G12.21
foot M62.57-
forearm M62.53-
hand M62.54-
infantile spinal G12.0
lower leg M62.56-
multiple sites M62.59
myelopathic — *see* Atrophy, muscle, spinal
myotonic G71.11
neuritic G58.9
neuropathic (peroneal) (progressive) G60.0
pelvic (disuse) N81.84
peroneal G60.0
progressive (bulbar) G12.21
adult G12.1
infantile (spinal) G12.0

Atrophy, atrophic (of) - *continued*
muscle, muscular (diffuse) (general) (idiopathic) (primary) - *continued*
progressive (bulbar) - *continued*
spinal G12.25
adult G12.1
infantile G12.0
pseudohypertrophic G71.02
shoulder region M62.51-
specified site NEC M62.58
spinal G12.9
adult form G12.1
Aran-Duchenne G12.21
childhood form, type II G12.1
distal G12.1
hereditary NEC G12.1
infantile, type I (Werdnig-Hoffmann) G12.0
juvenile form, type III (Kugelberg-Welander) G12.1
progressive G12.25
scapuloperoneal form G12.1
specified NEC G12.8
syphilitic A52.78
thigh M62.55-
upper arm M62.52-
myocardium — *see* Degeneration, myocardial
myometrium (senile) N85.8
cervix N88.8
myopathic NEC — *see* Atrophy, muscle
myotonia G71.11
nail L60.3
nasopharynx J31.1
nerve — *see also* Disorder, nerve
abducens — *see* Strabismus, paralytic, sixth nerve
accessory G52.8
acoustic or auditory — *see* subcategory H93.3
cranial G52.9
eighth (auditory) — *see* subcategory H93.3
eleventh (accessory) G52.8
fifth (trigeminal) G50.8
first (olfactory) G52.0
fourth (trochlear) — *see* Strabismus, paralytic, fourth nerve
second (optic) H47.20
sixth (abducens) — *see* Strabismus, paralytic, sixth nerve
tenth (pneumogastric) (vagus) G52.2
third (oculomotor) — *see* Strabismus, paralytic, third nerve
twelfth (hypoglossal) G52.3
hypoglossal G52.3
oculomotor — *see* Strabismus, paralytic, third nerve
olfactory G52.0
optic (papillomacular bundle)
syphilitic (late) A52.15
congenital A50.44
pneumogastric G52.2
trigeminal G50.8
trochlear — *see* Strabismus, paralytic, fourth nerve
vagus (pneumogastric) G52.2
neurogenic, bone, tabetic A52.11
nutritional E43
with marasmus E41
old age R54
olivopontocerebellar G23.8
optic (nerve) H47.20
glaucomatous H47.23-
hereditary H47.22
primary H47.21-
specified type NEC H47.29-
syphilitic (late) A52.15
congenital A50.44
orbit H05.31-
ovary (senile) N83.31-
with fallopian tube N83.33-
oviduct (senile) — *see* Atrophy, fallopian tube
palsy, diffuse (progressive) G12.22

Atrophy, atrophic (of) - *continued*
pancreas (duct) (senile) K86.89
parotid gland K11.0
pelvic muscle N81.84
penis N48.89
pharynx J39.2
pluriglandular E31.8
autoimmune E31.0
polyarthritis M15.9
prostate N42.89
pseudohypertrophic (muscle) G71.02
renal — *see also* Sclerosis, renal N26.1
retina, retinal (postinfectional) H35.89
rhinitis J31.0
salivary gland K11.0
scar L90.5
sclerosis, lobar (of brain) G31.09 *[F02.80]*
with behavioral disturbance G31.09 *[F02.81]*
scrotum N50.89
seminal vesicle N50.89
senile R54
due to radiation (nonionizing) (solar) L57.8
skin (patches) (spots) L90.9
degenerative (senile) L90.8
due to radiation (nonionizing) (solar) L57.8
senile L90.8
spermatic cord N50.89
spinal (acute) (cord) G95.89
muscular — *see* Atrophy, muscle, spinal
paralysis G12.20
acute — *see* Poliomyelitis, paralytic
meaning progressive muscular atrophy G12.25
spine (column) — *see* Spondylopathy, specified NEC
spleen (senile) D73.0
stomach K29.40
with bleeding K29.41
striate (skin) L90.6
syphilitic A52.79
subcutaneous L90.9
sublingual gland K11.0
submandibular gland K11.0
submaxillary gland K11.0
Sudeck's — *see* Algoneurodystrophy
suprarenal (capsule) (gland) E27.49
primary E27.1
systemic affecting central nervous system in
myxedema E03.9 *[G13.2]*
neoplastic disease — *see also* Neoplasm D49.9 *[G13.1]*
specified disease NEC G13.8
tarso-orbital fascia, congenital Q10.3
testis N50.0
thenar, partial — *see* Syndrome, carpal tunnel
thymus (fatty) E32.8
thyroid (gland) (acquired) E03.4
with cretinism E03.1
congenital (with myxedema) E03.1
tongue (senile) K14.8
papillae K14.4
trachea J39.8
tunica vaginalis N50.89
turbinate J34.89
tympanic membrane (nonflaccid) H73.82-
flaccid H73.81-
upper respiratory tract J39.8
uterus, uterine (senile) N85.8
cervix N88.8
due to radiation (intended effect) N85.8
adverse effect or misadventure N99.89
vagina (senile) N95.2
vas deferens N50.89
vascular I99.8
vertebra (senile) — *see* Spondylopathy, specified NEC
vulva (senile) N90.5
Werdnig-Hoffmann G12.0
yellow — *see* Failure, hepatic

Attack, attacks
- with alteration of consciousness (with automatisms) — *see* Epilepsy, localization-related, symptomatic, with complex partial seizures
- Adams-Stokes I45.9
- akinetic — *see* Epilepsy, generalized, specified NEC
- angina — *see* Angina
- atonic — *see* Epilepsy, generalized, specified NEC
- benign shuddering G25.83
- cataleptic — *see* Catalepsy
- coronary — *see* Infarct, myocardium
- cyanotic, newborn P28.2
- drop NEC R55
- epileptic — *see* Epilepsy
- heart — *see* infarct, myocardium
- hysterical F44.9
- jacksonian — *see* Epilepsy, localization-related, symptomatic, with simple partial seizures
- myocardium, myocardial — *see* Infarct, myocardium
- myoclonic — *see* Epilepsy, generalized, specified NEC
- panic F41.0
- psychomotor — *see* Epilepsy, localization-related, symptomatic, with complex partial seizures
- salaam — *see* Epilepsy, spasms
- schizophreniform, brief F23
- shuddering, benign G25.83
- Stokes-Adams I45.9
- syncope R55
- transient ischemic (TIA) G45.9
  - specified NEC G45.8
- unconsciousness R55
  - hysterical F44.89
- vasomotor R55
- vasovagal (paroxysmal) (idiopathic) R55
- without alteration of consciousness — *see* Epilepsy, localization-related, symptomatic, with simple partial seizures

Attention (to)
- artificial
  - opening (of) Z43.9
    - digestive tract NEC Z43.4
      - colon Z43.3
      - ilium Z43.2
      - stomach Z43.1
    - specified NEC Z43.8
    - trachea Z43.0
    - urinary tract NEC Z43.6
      - cystostomy Z43.5
      - nephrostomy Z43.6
      - ureterostomy Z43.6
      - urethrostomy Z43.6
  - vagina Z43.7
- colostomy Z43.3
- cystostomy Z43.5
- deficit disorder or syndrome F98.8
  - with hyperactivity — *see* Disorder, attention-deficit hyperactivity
- gastrostomy Z43.1
- ileostomy Z43.2
- jejunostomy Z43.4
- nephrostomy Z43.6
- surgical dressings Z48.01
- sutures Z48.02
- tracheostomy Z43.0
- ureterostomy Z43.6
- urethrostomy Z43.6

Attrition
- gum — *see* Recession, gingival
- tooth, teeth (excessive) (hard tissues) K03.0

Atypical, atypism — *see also* condition
- cells (on cytolgocial smear) (endocervical) (endometrial) (glandular)
  - cervix R87.619
  - vagina R87.629
- cervical N87.9
- endometrium N85.9
  - hyperplasia N85.00

Atypical, atypism - *continued*
- parenting situation Z62.9

Auditory — *see* condition
Aujeszky's disease B33.8
Aurantiasis, cutis E67.1
Auricle, auricular — *see also* condition
- cervical Q18.2

Auriculotemporal syndrome G50.8
Austin Flint murmur (aortic insufficiency) I35.1
Australian
- Q fever A78
- X disease A83.4

Autism, autistic (childhood) (infantile) F84.0
- atypical F84.9
- spectrum disorder F84.0

Autodigestion R68.89
Autoerythrocyte sensitization (syndrome) D69.2
Autographism L50.3
Autoimmune
- disease (systemic) M35.9
- inhibitors to clotting factors D68.311
- lymphoproliferative syndrome [ALPS] D89.82
- thyroiditis E06.3

Autointoxication R68.89
Automatism G93.89
- with temporal sclerosis G93.81
- epileptic — *see* Epilepsy, localization-related, symptomatic, with complex partial seizures
- paroxysmal, idiopathic — *see* Epilepsy, localization-related, symptomatic, with complex partial seizures

Autonomic, autonomous
- bladder (neurogenic) N31.2
- hysteria seizure F44.5

Autosensitivity, erythrocyte D69.2
Autosensitization, cutaneous L30.2
Autosome — *see* condition by chromosome involved
Autotopagnosia R48.1
Autotoxemia R68.89
Autumn — *see* condition
Avellis' syndrome G46.8
Aversion
- oral R63.39
  - newborn P92.-
  - nonorganic origin F98.2
- sexual F52.1

Aviator's
- disease or sickness — *see* Effect, adverse, high altitude
- ear T70.0

Avitaminosis (multiple) — *see also* Deficiency, vitamin E56.9
- B E53.9
  - with
    - beriberi E51.11
    - pellagra E52
- B2 E53.0
- B6 E53.1
- B12 E53.8
- D E55.9
  - with rickets E55.0
- G E53.0
- K E56.1
- nicotinic acid E52

AVNRT (atrioventricular nodal re-entrant tachycardia) I47.1
AVRT (atrioventricular nodal re-entrant tachycardia) I47.1
Avulsion (traumatic)
- blood vessel — *see* Injury, blood vessel
- bone — *see* Fracture, by site
- cartilage — *see also* Dislocation, by site
  - symphyseal (inner) , complicating delivery O71.6
- external site other than limb — *see* Wound, open, by site
- eye S05.7-
- head (intracranial)
  - external site NEC S08.89
  - scalp S08.0

Avulsion (traumatic) - *continued*
- internal organ or site — *see* Injury, by site
- joint — *see also* Dislocation, by site
  - capsule — *see* Sprain, by site
- kidney S37.06-
- ligament — *see* Sprain, by site
- limb — *see also* Amputation, traumatic, by site
  - skin and subcutaneous tissue — *see* Wound, open, by site
- muscle — *see* Injury, muscle
- nerve (root) — *see* Injury, nerve
- scalp S08.0
- skin and subcutaneous tissue — *see* Wound, open, by site
- spleen S36.032
- symphyseal cartilage (inner) , complicating delivery O71.6
- tendon — *see* Injury, muscle
- tooth S03.2

Awareness of heart beat R00.2
Axenfeld's
- anomaly or syndrome Q15.0
- degeneration (calcareous) Q13.4

Axilla, axillary — *see also* condition
- breast Q83.1

Axonotmesis — *see* Injury, nerve
Ayerza's disease or syndrome (pulmonary artery sclerosis with pulmonary hypertension) I27.0
Azoospermia (organic) N46.01
- due to
  - drug therapy N46.021
  - efferent duct obstruction N46.023
  - infection N46.022
  - radiation N46.024
  - specified cause NEC N46.029
  - systemic disease N46.025

Azotemia R79.89
- meaning uremia N19

Aztec ear Q17.3
Azygos
- continuation inferior vena cava Q26.8
- lobe (lung) Q33.1

B

Baastrup's disease — *see* Kissing spine
Babesiosis B60.00
- due to
  - Babesia
    - divergens B60.03
    - duncani B60.02
    - KO-1 B60.09
    - microti B60.01
    - MO-1 B60.03
    - species
      - unspecified B60.00
    - venatorum B60.09
  - specified NEC B60.09

Babington's disease (familial hemorrhagic telangiectasia) I78.0
Babinski's syndrome A52.79
Baby
- crying constantly R68.11
- floppy (syndrome) P94.2

Bacillary — *see* condition
Bacilluria R82.71
Bacillus — *see also* Infection, bacillus
- abortus infection A23.1
- anthracis infection A22.9
- coli infection — *see also* Escherichia coli B96.20
- Flexner's A03.1
- mallei infection A24.0
- Shiga's A03.0
- suipestifer infection — *see* Infection, salmonella

Back — *see* condition
Backache (postural) M54.9
- sacroiliac M53.3
- specified NEC M54.89

Backflow — *see* Reflux
Backward reading (dyslexia) F81.0
Bacteremia R78.81
- with sepsis — *see* Sepsis

Bactericholia — *see* Cholecystitis, acute

Bacterid, bacteride (pustular) L40.3
Bacterium, bacteria, bacterial
- agent NEC, as cause of disease classified elsewhere B96.89
- in blood — *see* Bacteremia
- in urine — *see* Bacteriuria

Bacteriuria, bacteruria R82.71
- asymptomatic R82.71

Bacteroides
- fragilis, as cause of disease classified elsewhere B96.6

Bad
- heart — *see* Disease, heart
- trip
  - due to drug abuse — *see* Abuse, drug, hallucinogen
  - due to drug dependence — *see* Dependence, drug, hallucinogen

Baelz's disease (cheilitis glandularis apostematosa) K13.0
Baerensprung's disease (eczema marginatum) B35.6
Bagasse disease or pneumonitis J67.1
Bagassosis J67.1
Baker's cyst — *see* Cyst, Baker's
Bakwin-Krida syndrome (metaphyseal dysplasia) Q78.5
Balancing side interference M26.56
Balanitis (circinata) (erosiva) (gangrenosa) (phagedenic) (vulgaris) N48.1
- amebic A06.82
- candidal B37.42
- due to Haemophilus ducreyi A57
- gonococcal (acute) (chronic) A54.23
- xerotica obliterans N48.0

Balanoposthitis N47.6
- gonococcal (acute) (chronic) A54.23
- ulcerative (specific) A63.8

Balanorrhagia — *see* Balanitis
Balantidiasis, balantidiosis A07.0
Bald tongue K14.4
Baldness — *see also* Alopecia
- male-pattern — *see* Alopecia, androgenic

Balkan grippe A78
Balloon disease — *see* Effect, adverse, high altitude
Balo's disease (concentric sclerosis) G37.5
Bamberger-Marie disease — *see* Osteoarthropathy, hypertrophic, specified type NEC
Bancroft's filariasis B74.0
Band (s)
- adhesive — *see* Adhesions, peritoneum
- anomalous or congenital — *see also* Anomaly, by site
  - heart (atrial) (ventricular) Q24.8
  - intestine Q43.3
  - omentum Q43.3
- cervix N88.1
- constricting, congenital Q79.8
- gallbladder (congenital) Q44.1
- intestinal (adhesive) — *see* Adhesions, peritoneum
- obstructive
  - intestine K56.50
    - complete K56.52
    - incomplete K56.51
    - partial K56.51
  - peritoneum K56.50
    - complete K56.52
    - incomplete K56.51
    - partial K56.51
- periappendiceal, congenital Q43.3
- peritoneal (adhesive) — *see* Adhesions, peritoneum
- uterus N73.6
  - internal N85.6
- vagina N89.5

Bandemia D72.825
Bandl's ring (contraction) , complicating delivery O62.4
Bangkok hemorrhagic fever A91
Bang's disease (brucella abortus) A23.1
Bankruptcy, anxiety concerning Z59.89
Bannister's disease T78.3
- hereditary D84.1

Banti's disease or syndrome (with cirrhosis) (with portal hypertension) K76.6
Bar, median, prostate — *see* Enlargement, enlarged, prostate
Barcoo disease or rot — *see* Ulcer, skin
Barlow's disease E54
Barodontalgia T70.29
Baron Münchausen syndrome — *see* Disorder, factitious
Barosinusitis T70.1
Barotitis T70.0
Barotrauma T70.29
- odontalgia T70.29
- otitic T70.0
- sinus T70.1

Barraquer (-Simons) disease or syndrome (progressive lipodystrophy) E88.1
Barré-Guillain disease or syndrome G61.0
Barrel chest M95.4
Barré-Liéou syndrome (posterior cervical sympathetic) M53.0
Barrett's
- disease — *see* Barrett's, esophagus
- esophagus K22.70
  - with dysplasia K22.719
    - high grade K22.711
    - low grade K22.710
  - without dysplasia K22.70
- syndrome — *see* Barrett's, esophagus
- ulcer K22.10
  - with bleeding K22.11
  - without bleeding K22.10

Bársony (-Polgár) (-Teschendorf) syndrome (corkscrew esophagus) K22.4
Barth syndrome E78.71
Bartholinitis (suppurating) N75.8
- gonococcal (acute) (chronic) (with abscess) A54.1

Bartonellosis A44.9
- cutaneous A44.1
- mucocutaneous A44.1
- specified NEC A44.8
- systemic A44.0

Barton's fracture S52.56-
Bartter's syndrome E26.81
Basal — *see* condition
Basan's (hidrotic) ectodermal dysplasia Q82.4
Baseball finger — *see* Dislocation, finger
Basedow's disease (exophthalmic goiter) — *see* Hyperthyroidism, with, goiter
Basic — *see* condition
Basilar — *see* condition
Bason's (hidrotic) ectodermal dysplasia Q82.4
Basopenia — *see* Agranulocytosis
Basophilia D72.824
Basophilism (cortico-adrenal) (Cushing's) (pituitary) E24.0
Bassen-Kornzweig disease or syndrome E78.6
Bat ear Q17.5
Bateman's
- disease B08.1
- purpura (senile) D69.2

Bathing cramp T75.1
Bathophobia F40.248
Batten (-Mayou) disease E75.4
- retina E75.4 *[H36]*

Batten-Steinert syndrome G71.11
Battered — *see* Maltreatment
Battey Mycobacterium infection A31.0
Battle exhaustion F43.0
Battledore placenta O43.19-
Baumgarten-Cruveilhier cirrhosis, disease or syndrome K74.69
Bauxite fibrosis (of lung) J63.1
Bayle's disease (general paresis) A52.17
Bazin's disease (primary) (tuberculous) A18.4
Beach ear — *see* Swimmer's, ear
Beaded hair (congenital) Q84.1
Béal conjunctivitis or syndrome B30.2
Beard's disease (neurasthenia) F48.8
Beat (s)
- atrial, premature I49.1
- ectopic I49.49
- elbow — *see* Bursitis, elbow
- escaped, heart I49.49
- hand — *see* Bursitis, hand
- knee — *see* Bursitis, knee
- premature I49.40
  - atrial I49.1
  - auricular I49.1
  - supraventricular I49.1

Beau's
- disease or syndrome — *see* Degeneration, myocardial
- lines (transverse furrows on fingernails) L60.4

Bechterev's syndrome — *see* Spondylitis, ankylosing
Becker's
- cardiomyopathy I42.8
- disease
  - idiopathic mural endomyocardial disease I42.3
  - myotonia congenita, recessive form G71.12
- dystrophy G71.01
- pigmented hairy nevus D22.5

Beck's syndrome (anterior spinal artery occlusion) I65.8
Beckwith-Wiedemann syndrome Q87.3
Bed confinement status Z74.01
Bed sore — *see* Ulcer, pressure, by site
Bedbug bite (s) — *see* Bite(s), by site, superficial, insect
Bedclothes, asphyxiation or suffocation by — *see* Asphyxia, traumatic, due to, mechanical, trapped
Bednar's
- aphthae K12.0
- tumor — *see* Neoplasm, malignant, by site

Bedridden Z74.01
Bedsore — *see* Ulcer, pressure, by site
Bedwetting — *see* Enuresis
Bee sting (with allergic or anaphylactic shock) — *see* Toxicity, venom, arthropod, bee
Beer drinker's heart (disease) I42.6
Begbie's disease (exophthalmic goiter) — *see* Hyperthyroidism, with, goiter
Behavior
- antisocial
  - adult Z72.811
  - child or adolescent Z72.810
- disorder, disturbance — *see* Disorder, conduct
- disruptive — *see* Disorder, conduct
- drug seeking Z76.5
- inexplicable R46.2
- marked evasiveness R46.5
- obsessive-compulsive R46.81
- overactivity R46.3
- poor responsiveness R46.4
- self-damaging (life-style) Z72.89
- sleep-incompatible Z72.821
- slowness R46.4
- specified NEC R46.89
- strange (and inexplicable) R46.2
- suspiciousness R46.5
- type A pattern Z73.1
- undue concern or preoccupation with stressful events R46.6
- verbosity and circumstantial detail obscuring reason for contact R46.7

Behçet's disease or syndrome M35.2
Behr's disease — *see* Degeneration, macula
Beigel's disease or morbus (white piedra) B36.2
Bejel A65
Bekhterev's syndrome — *see* Spondylitis, ankylosing
Belching — *see* Eructation
Bell's
- mania F30.8

- **Bell's** - *continued*
  - palsy, paralysis G51.0
    - infant or newborn P11.3
  - spasm G51.3-
- **Bence Jones albuminuria or proteinuria NEC** R80.3
- **Bends** T70.3
- **Benedikt's paralysis or syndrome** G46.3
- **Benign** — *see also* condition
  - prostatic hyperplasia — *see* Hyperplasia, prostate
- **Bennett's fracture (displaced)** S62.21-
- **Benson's disease** — *see* Deposit, crystalline
- **Bent**
  - back (hysterical) F44.4
  - nose M95.0
    - congenital Q67.4
- **Bereavement (uncomplicated)** Z63.4
- **Bergeron's disease (hysterical chorea)** F44.4
- **Berger's disease** — *see* Nephropathy, IgA
- **Beriberi (dry)** E51.11
  - heart (disease) E51.12
  - polyneuropathy E51.11
  - wet E51.12
    - involving circulatory system E51.11
- **Berlin's disease or edema (traumatic)** S05.8X-
- **Berlock (berloque) dermatitis** L56.2
- **Bernard-Horner syndrome** G90.2
- **Bernard-Soulier disease or thrombopathia** D69.1
- **Bernhardt (-Roth) disease** — *see* Mononeuropathy, lower limb, meralgia paresthetica
- **Bernheim's syndrome** — *see* Failure, heart, right
- **Bertielliasis** B71.8
- **Berylliosis (lung)** J63.2
- **Besnier-Boeck (-Schaumann) disease** — *see* Sarcoidosis
- **Besnier's**
  - lupus pernio D86.3
  - prurigo L20.0
- **Bestiality** F65.89
- **Best's disease** H35.50
- **Betalipoproteinemia, broad or floating** E78.2
- **Beta-mercaptolactate-cysteine disulfiduria** E72.09
- **Betting and gambling** Z72.6
  - pathological (compulsive) F63.0
- **Bezoar** T18.9
  - intestine T18.3
  - stomach T18.2
- **Bezold's abscess** — *see* Mastoiditis, acute
- **Bianchi's syndrome** R48.8
- **Bicornate or bicornis uterus** Q51.3
  - in pregnancy or childbirth O34.00
    - causing obstructed labor O65.5
- **Bicuspid aortic valve** Q23.1
- **Biedl-Bardet syndrome** Q87.89
- **Bielschowsky (-Jansky) disease** E75.4
- **Biermer's (pernicious) anemia or disease** D51.0
- **Biett's disease** L93.0
- **Bifid (congenital)**
  - apex, heart Q24.8
  - clitoris Q52.6
  - kidney Q63.8
  - nose Q30.2
  - patella Q74.1
  - scrotum Q55.29
  - toe NEC Q74.2
  - tongue Q38.3
  - ureter Q62.8
  - uterus Q51.3
  - uvula Q35.7
- **Biforis uterus (suprasimplex)** Q51.3
- **Bifurcation (congenital)**
  - gallbladder Q44.1
  - kidney pelvis Q63.8
  - renal pelvis Q63.8
  - rib Q76.6
  - tongue, congenital Q38.3
  - trachea Q32.1
  - ureter Q62.8
- **Bifurcation (congenital)** - *continued*
  - urethra Q64.74
  - vertebra Q76.49
- **Big spleen syndrome** D73.1
- **Bigeminal pulse** R00.8
- **Bilateral** — *see* condition
- **Bile**
  - duct — *see* condition
  - pigments in urine R82.2
- **Bilharziasis** — *see also* Schistosomiasis
  - chyluria B65.0
  - cutaneous B65.3
  - galacturia B65.0
  - hematochyluria B65.0
  - intestinal B65.1
  - lipemia B65.9
  - lipuria B65.0
  - oriental B65.2
  - piarhemia B65.9
  - pulmonary NOS B65.9 *[J99]*
    - pneumonia B65.9 *[J17]*
  - tropical hematuria B65.0
  - vesical B65.0
- **Biliary** — *see* condition
- **Bilirubin metabolism disorder** E80.7
  - specified NEC E80.6
- **Bilirubinemia, familial nonhemolytic** E80.4
- **Bilirubinuria** R82.2
- **Biliuria** R82.2
- **Bilocular stomach** K31.2
- **Binswanger's disease** I67.3
- **Biparta, bipartite**
  - carpal scaphoid Q74.0
  - patella Q74.1
  - vagina Q52.10
- **Bird**
  - face Q75.8
  - fancier's disease or lung J67.2
- **Birth**
  - complications in mother — *see* Delivery, complicated
  - compression during NOS P15.9
  - defect — *see* Anomaly
  - immature (less than 37 completed weeks) — *see* Preterm, newborn
    - extremely (less than 28 completed weeks) — *see* Immaturity, extreme
  - inattention, at or after — *see* Maltreatment, child, neglect
  - injury NOS P15.9
    - basal ganglia P11.1
    - brachial plexus NEC P14.3
    - brain (compression) (pressure) P11.2
    - central nervous system NOS P11.9
    - cerebellum P11.1
    - cerebral hemorrhage P10.1
    - external genitalia P15.5
    - eye P15.3
    - face P15.4
    - fracture
      - bone P13.9
        - specified NEC P13.8
      - clavicle P13.4
      - femur P13.2
      - humerus P13.3
      - long bone, except femur P13.3
      - radius and ulna P13.3
      - skull P13.0
      - spine P11.5
      - tibia and fibula P13.3
    - intracranial P11.2
      - laceration or hemorrhage P10.9
        - specified NEC P10.8
    - intraventricular hemorrhage P10.2
    - laceration
      - brain P10.1
      - by scalpel P15.8
      - peripheral nerve P14.9
    - liver P15.0
    - meninges
      - brain P11.1
      - spinal cord P11.5
    - nerve
      - brachial plexus P14.3
      - cranial NEC (except facial) P11.4
- **Birth** - *continued*
  - injury NOS - *continued*
    - nerve - *continued*
      - facial P11.3
      - peripheral P14.9
      - phrenic (paralysis) P14.2
    - paralysis
      - facial nerve P11.3
      - spinal P11.5
    - penis P15.5
    - rupture
      - spinal cord P11.5
    - scalp P12.9
    - scalpel wound P15.8
    - scrotum P15.5
    - skull NEC P13.1
      - fracture P13.0
    - specified type NEC P15.8
    - spinal cord P11.5
    - spine P11.5
    - spleen P15.1
    - sternomastoid (hematoma) P15.2
    - subarachnoid hemorrhage P10.3
    - subcutaneous fat necrosis P15.6
    - subdural hemorrhage P10.0
    - tentorial tear P10.4
    - testes P15.5
    - vulva P15.5
  - lack of care, at or after — *see* Maltreatment, child, neglect
  - neglect, at or after — *see* Maltreatment, child, neglect
  - palsy or paralysis, newborn, NOS (birth injury) P14.9
  - premature (infant) — *see* Preterm, newborn
  - shock, newborn P96.89
  - trauma — *see* Birth, injury
  - weight
    - low (2499 grams or less) — *see* Low, birthweight
      - extremely (999 grams or less) — *see* Low, birthweight, extreme
    - 4000 grams to 4499 grams P08.1
    - 4500 grams or more P08.0
- **Birthmark** Q82.5
- **Birt-Hogg-Dube syndrome** Q87.89
- **Bisalbuminemia** E88.09
- **Biskra's button** B55.1
- **Bite (s) (animal) (human)**
  - abdomen, abdominal
    - wall S31.159
      - with penetration into peritoneal cavity S31.659
      - epigastric region S31.152
        - with penetration into peritoneal cavity S31.652
      - left
        - lower quadrant S31.154
          - with penetration into peritoneal cavity S31.654
        - upper quadrant S31.151
          - with penetration into peritoneal cavity S31.651
      - periumbilic region S31.155
        - with penetration into peritoneal cavity S31.655
      - right
        - lower quadrant S31.153
          - with penetration into peritoneal cavity S31.653
        - upper quadrant S31.150
          - with penetration into peritoneal cavity S31.650
      - superficial NEC S30.871
        - insect S30.861
  - alveolar (process) — *see* Bite, oral cavity
  - amphibian (venomous) — *see* Venom, bite, amphibian
  - animal — *see also* Bite, by site
    - venomous — *see* Venom
  - ankle S91.05-
    - superficial NEC S90.57-
      - insect S90.56-
  - antecubital space — *see* Bite, elbow
  - anus S31.835

BITE - BLEPHARITIS

Blepharitis (angularis) (ciliaris) (eyelid) (marginal) (nonulcerative) - *continued*
- ulcerative - *continued*
  - left - *continued*
    - upper and lower H01.01B
  - right H01.013
    - lower H01.012
    - upper H01.011
    - upper and lower H01.01A

Blepharochalasis H02.30
- congenital Q10.0
- left H02.36
  - lower H02.35
  - upper H02.34
- right H02.33
  - lower H02.32
  - upper H02.31

Blepharoclonus H02.59

Blepharoconjunctivitis H10.50-
- angular H10.52-
- contact H10.53-
- ligneous H10.51-

Blepharophimosis (eyelid) H02.529
- congenital Q10.3
- left H02.526
  - lower H02.525
  - upper H02.524
- right H02.523
  - lower H02.522
  - upper H02.521

Blepharoptosis H02.40-
- congenital Q10.0
- mechanical H02.41-
- myogenic H02.42-
- neurogenic H02.43-
- paralytic H02.43-

Blepharopyorrhea, gonococcal A54.39

Blepharospasm G24.5
- drug induced G24.01

Blighted ovum O02.0

Blind — *see also* Blindness
- bronchus (congenital) Q32.4
- loop syndrome K90.2
  - congenital Q43.8
- sac, fallopian tube (congenital) Q50.6
- spot, enlarged — *see* Defect, visual field, localized, scotoma, blind spot area
- tract or tube, congenital NEC — *see* Atresia, by site

Blindness (acquired) (congenital) (both eyes) H54.0X-
- blast S05.8X-
- color — *see* Deficiency, color vision
- concussion S05.8X-
- cortical H47.619
  - left brain H47.612
  - right brain H47.611
- day H53.11
- due to injury (current episode) S05.9-
  - sequelae -- code to injury with seventh character S
- eclipse (total) — *see* Retinopathy, solar
- emotional (hysterical) F44.6
- face H53.16
- hysterical F44.6
- legal (both eyes) (USA definition) H54.8
- mind R48.8
- night H53.60
  - abnormal dark adaptation curve H53.61
  - acquired H53.62
  - congenital H53.63
  - specified type NEC H53.69
  - vitamin A deficiency E50.5
- one eye (other eye normal) H54.40
  - left (normal vision on right) H54.42-
    - low vision on right H54.12-
  - low vision, other eye H54.10
  - right (normal vision on left) H54.41-
    - low vision on left H54.11-
- psychic R48.8
- river B73.01
- snow — *see* Photokeratitis
- sun, solar — *see* Retinopathy, solar
- transient — *see* Disturbance, vision, subjective, loss, transient

Blindness (acquired) (congenital) (both eyes) - *continued*
- traumatic (current episode) S05.9-
- word (developmental) F81.0
  - acquired R48.0
  - secondary to organic lesion R48.0

Blister (nonthermal)
- abdominal wall S30.821
- alveolar process S00.522
- ankle S90.52-
- antecubital space — *see* Blister, elbow
- anus S30.827
- arm (upper) S40.82-
- auditory canal — *see* Blister, ear
- auricle — *see* Blister, ear
- axilla — *see* Blister, arm
- back, lower S30.820
- beetle dermatitis L24.89
- breast S20.12-
- brow S00.82
- calf — *see* Blister, leg
- canthus — *see* Blister, eyelid
- cheek S00.82
  - internal S00.522
- chest wall — *see* Blister, thorax
- chin S00.82
- costal region — *see* Blister, thorax
- digit (s)
  - foot — *see* Blister, toe
  - hand — *see* Blister, finger
- due to burn — *see* Burn, by site, second degree
- ear S00.42-
- elbow S50.32-
- epiglottis S10.12
- esophagus, cervical S10.12
- eyebrow — *see* Blister, eyelid
- eyelid S00.22-
- face S00.82
- fever B00.1
- finger (s) S60.429
  - index S60.42-
  - little S60.42-
  - middle S60.42-
  - ring S60.42-
- foot (except toe (s) alone) S90.82-
  - toe — *see* Blister, toe
- forearm S50.82-
  - elbow only — *see* Blister, elbow
- forehead S00.82
- fracture - omit code
- genital organ
  - female S30.826
  - male S30.825
- gum S00.522
- hand S60.52-
- head S00.92
  - ear — *see* Blister, ear
  - eyelid — *see* Blister, eyelid
  - lip S00.521
  - nose S00.32
  - oral cavity S00.522
  - scalp S00.02
  - specified site NEC S00.82
- heel — *see* Blister, foot
- hip S70.22-
- interscapular region S20.429
- jaw S00.82
- knee S80.22-
- larynx S10.12
- leg (lower) S80.82-
  - knee — *see* Blister, knee
  - upper — *see* Blister, thigh
- lip S00.521
- malar region S00.82
- mammary — *see* Blister, breast
- mastoid region S00.82
- mouth S00.522
- multiple, skin, nontraumatic R23.8
- nail
  - finger — *see* Blister, finger
  - toe — *see* Blister, toe
- nasal S00.32
- neck S10.92
  - specified site NEC S10.82

Blister (nonthermal) - *continued*
- neck - *continued*
  - throat S10.12
- nose S00.32
- occipital region S00.02
- oral cavity S00.522
- orbital region — *see* Blister, eyelid
- palate S00.522
- palm — *see* Blister, hand
- parietal region S00.02
- pelvis S30.820
- penis S30.822
- periocular area — *see* Blister, eyelid
- phalanges
  - finger — *see* Blister, finger
  - toe — *see* Blister, toe
- pharynx S10.12
- pinna — *see* Blister, ear
- popliteal space — *see* Blister, knee
- scalp S00.02
- scapular region — *see* Blister, shoulder
- scrotum S30.823
- shin — *see* Blister, leg
- shoulder S40.22-
- sternal region S20.329
- submaxillary region S00.82
- submental region S00.82
- subungual
  - finger (s) — *see* Blister, finger
  - toe (s) — *see* Blister, toe
- supraclavicular fossa S10.82
- supraorbital S00.82
- temple S00.82
- temporal region S00.82
- testis S30.823
- thermal — *see* Burn, second degree, by site
- thigh S70.32-
- thorax, thoracic (wall) S20.92
  - back S20.42-
  - front S20.32-
- throat S10.12
- thumb S60.32-
- toe (s) S90.42-
  - great S90.42-
- tongue S00.522
- trachea S10.12
- tympanum, tympanic membrane — *see* Blister, ear
- upper arm — *see* Blister, arm (upper)
- uvula S00.522
- vagina S30.824
- vocal cords S10.12
- vulva S30.824
- wrist S60.82-

Bloating R14.0

Bloch-Sulzberger disease or syndrome Q82.3

Block, blocked
- alveolocapillary J84.10
- arborization (heart) I45.5
- arrhythmic I45.9
- atrioventricular (incomplete) (partial) I44.30
  - with atrioventricular dissociation I44.2
  - complete I44.2
    - congenital Q24.6
  - congenital Q24.6
  - first degree I44.0
  - second degree (types I and II) I44.1
  - specified NEC I44.39
  - third degree I44.2
  - types I and II I44.1
- auriculoventricular — *see* Block, atrioventricular
- bifascicular (cardiac) I45.2
- bundle-branch (complete) (false) (incomplete) I45.4
  - bilateral I45.2
  - left I44.7
    - with right bundle branch block I45.2
    - hemiblock I44.60
      - anterior I44.4
      - posterior I44.5
    - incomplete I44.7
      - with right bundle branch block I45.2
  - right I45.10
    - with

BLEPHARITIS - BLOCK, BLOCKED

Block, blocked - *continued*
bundle-branch (complete) (false) (incomplete) - *continued*
right - *continued*
with - *continued*
left bundle branch block I45.2
left fascicular block I45.2
specified NEC I45.19
Wilson's type I45.19
cardiac I45.9
conduction I45.9
complete I44.2
fascicular (left) I44.60
anterior I44.4
posterior I44.5
right I45.0
specified NEC I44.69
foramen Magendie (acquired) G91.1
congenital Q03.1
with spina bifida — *see* Spina bifida, by site, with hydrocephalus
heart I45.9
bundle branch I45.4
bilateral I45.2
complete (atrioventricular) I44.2
congenital Q24.6
first degree (atrioventricular) I44.0
second degree (atrioventricular) I44.1
specified type NEC I45.5
third degree (atrioventricular) I44.2
hepatic vein I82.0
intraventricular (nonspecific) I45.4
bundle branch
bilateral I45.2
kidney N28.9
postcystoscopic or postprocedural N99.0
Mobitz (types I and II) I44.1
myocardial — *see* Block, heart
nodal I45.5
organ or site, congenital NEC — *see* Atresia, by site
portal (vein) I81
second degree (types I and II) I44.1
sinoatrial I45.5
sinoauricular I45.5
third degree I44.2
trifascicular I45.3
tubal N97.1
vein NOS I82.90
Wenckebach (types I and II) I44.1
Blockage — *see* Obstruction
Blocq's disease F44.4
Blood
constituents, abnormal R78.9
disease D75.9
donor — *see* Donor, blood
dyscrasia D75.9
with
abortion — *see* Abortion, by type, complicated by, hemorrhage
ectopic pregnancy O08.1
molar pregnancy O08.1
following ectopic or molar pregnancy O08.1
newborn P61.9
puerperal, postpartum O72.3
flukes NEC — *see* Schistosomiasis
in
feces K92.1
occult R19.5
urine — *see* Hematuria
mole O02.0
occult in feces R19.5
pressure
decreased, due to shock following injury T79.4
examination only Z01.30
fluctuating I99.8
high — *see* Hypertension
borderline R03.0
incidental reading, without diagnosis of hypertension R03.0
low — *see also* Hypotension
incidental reading, without diagnosis of hypotension R03.1

Blood - *continued*
spitting — *see* Hemoptysis
staining cornea — *see* Pigmentation, cornea, stromal
transfusion
reaction or complication — *see* Complications, transfusion
type
A (Rh positive) Z67.10
Rh negative Z67.11
AB (Rh positive) Z67.30
Rh negative Z67.31
B (Rh positive) Z67.20
Rh negative Z67.21
O (Rh positive) Z67.40
Rh negative Z67.41
Rh (positive) Z67.90
negative Z67.91
vessel rupture — *see* Hemorrhage
vomiting — *see* Hematemesis
Blood-forming organs, disease D75.9
Bloodgood's disease — *see* Mastopathy, cystic
Bloom (-Machacek) (-Torre) syndrome Q82.8
Blount disease or osteochondrosis M92.51-
Blue
baby Q24.9
diaper syndrome E72.09
dome cyst (breast) — *see* Cyst, breast
dot cataract Q12.0
nevus D22.9
sclera Q13.5
with fragility of bone and deafness Q78.0
toe syndrome I75.02-
Blueness — *see* Cyanosis
Blues, postpartal O90.6
baby O90.6
Blurring, visual H53.8
Blushing (abnormal) (excessive) R23.2
BMI — *see* Body, mass index
Boarder, hospital NEC Z76.4
accompanying sick person Z76.3
healthy infant or child Z76.2
foundling Z76.1
Bockhart's impetigo L01.02
Bodechtel-Guttman disease (subacute sclerosing panencephalitis) A81.1
Boder-Sedgwick syndrome (ataxia-telangiectasia) G11.3
Body, bodies
Aschoff's — *see* Myocarditis, rheumatic
asteroid, vitreous — *see* Deposit, crystalline
cytoid (retina) — *see* Occlusion, artery, retina
drusen (degenerative) (macula) (retinal) — *see also* Degeneration, macula, drusen
optic disc — *see* Drusen, optic disc
foreign — *see* Foreign body
loose
joint, except knee — *see* Loose, body, joint
knee M23.4-
sheath, tendon — *see* Disorder, tendon, specified type NEC
mass index (BMI)
adult
19.9 or less Z68.1
20.0-20.9 Z68.20
21.0-21.9 Z68.21
22.0-22.9 Z68.22
23.0-23.9 Z68.23
24.0-24.9 Z68.24
25.0-25.9 Z68.25
26.0-26.9 Z68.26
27.0-27.9 Z68.27
28.0-28.9 Z68.28
29.0-29.9 Z68.29
30.0-30.9 Z68.30
31.0-31.9 Z68.31
32.0-32.9 Z68.32
33.0-33.9 Z68.33
34.0-34.9 Z68.34
35.0-35.9 Z68.35
36.0-36.9 Z68.36
37.0-37.9 Z68.37
38.0-38.9 Z68.38

Body, bodies - *continued*
mass index (BMI) - *continued*
adult - *continued*
39.0-39.9 Z68.39
40.0-44.9 Z68.41
45.0-49.9 Z68.42
50.0-59.9 Z68.43
60.0-69.9 Z68.44
70 and over Z68.45
pediatric
5th percentile to less than 85th percentile for age Z68.52
85th percentile to less than 95th percentile for age Z68.53
greater than or equal to ninety-fifth percentile for age Z68.54
less than fifth percentile for age Z68.51
Mooser's A75.2
rice — *see also* Loose, body, joint
knee M23.4-
rocking F98.4
Boeck's
disease or sarcoid — *see* Sarcoidosis
lupoid (miliary) D86.3
Boerhaave's syndrome (spontaneous esophageal rupture) K22.3
Boggy
cervix N88.8
uterus N85.8
Boil — *see also* Furuncle, by site
Aleppo B55.1
Baghdad B55.1
Delhi B55.1
lacrimal
gland — *see* Dacryoadenitis
passages (duct) (sac) — *see* Inflammation, lacrimal, passages, acute
Natal B55.1
orbit, orbital — *see* Abscess, orbit
tropical B55.1
Bold hives — *see* Urticaria
Bombé, iris — *see* Membrane, pupillary
Bone — *see* condition
Bonnevie-Ullrich syndrome — *see also* Turner's syndrome Q87.19
Bonnier's syndrome — *see* subcategory H81.8
Bonvale dam fever T73.3
Bony block of joint — *see* Ankylosis
BOOP (bronchiolitis obliterans organized pneumonia) J84.89
Borderline
diabetes mellitus R73.03
hypertension R03.0
osteopenia M85.8-
pelvis, with obstruction during labor O65.1
personality F60.3
Borna disease A83.9
Bornholm disease B33.0
Boston exanthem A88.0
Botalli, ductus (patent) (persistent) Q25.0
Bothriocephalus latus infestation B70.0
Botulism (foodborne intoxication) A05.1
infant A48.51
non-foodborne A48.52
wound A48.52
Bouba — *see* Yaws
Bouchard's nodes (with arthropathy) M15.2
Bouffée délirante F23
Bouillaud's disease or syndrome (rheumatic heart disease) I01.9
Bourneville's disease Q85.1
Boutonniere deformity (finger) — *see* Deformity, finger, boutonniere
Bouveret (-Hoffmann) syndrome (paroxysmal tachycardia) I47.9
Bovine heart — *see* Hypertrophy, cardiac
Bowel — *see* condition
Bowen's
dermatosis (precancerous) — *see* Neoplasm, skin, in situ
disease — *see* Neoplasm, skin, in situ
epithelioma — *see* Neoplasm, skin, in situ
type
epidermoid carcinoma-in-situ — *see* Neoplasm, skin, in situ

Bowen's - *continued*
type - *continued*
intraepidermal squamous cell carcinoma — *see* Neoplasm, skin, in situ
Bowing
femur — *see also* Deformity, limb, specified type NEC, thigh
congenital Q68.3
fibula — *see also* Deformity, limb, specified type NEC, lower leg
congenital Q68.4
forearm — *see* Deformity, limb, specified type NEC, forearm
leg (s) , long bones, congenital Q68.5
radius — *see* Deformity, limb, specified type NEC, forearm
tibia — *see also* Deformity, limb, specified type NEC, lower leg
congenital Q68.4
Bowleg (s) (acquired) M21.16-
congenital Q68.5
rachitic E64.3
Boyd's dysentery A03.2
Brachial — *see* condition
Brachycardia R00.1
Brachycephaly Q75.0
Bradley's disease A08.19
Bradyarrhythmia, cardiac I49.8
Bradycardia (sinoatrial) (sinus) (vagal) R00.1
neonatal P29.12
reflex G90.09
tachycardia syndrome I49.5
Bradykinesia R25.8
Bradypnea R06.89
Bradytachycardia I49.5
Brailsford's disease or osteochondrosis — *see* Osteochondrosis, juvenile, radius
Brain — *see also* condition
death G93.82
syndrome — *see* Syndrome, brain
Branched-chain amino-acid disorder E71.2
Branchial — *see* condition
cartilage, congenital Q18.2
Branchiogenic remnant (in neck) Q18.0
Brandt's syndrome (acrodermatitis enteropathica) E83.2
Brash (water) R12
Bravais-jacksonian epilepsy — *see* Epilepsy, localization-related, symptomatic, with simple partial seizures
Braxton Hicks contractions — *see* False, labor
Brazilian leishmaniasis B55.2
BRBPR K62.5
Break, retina (without detachment) H33.30-
with retinal detachment — *see* Detachment, retina
horseshoe tear H33.31-
multiple H33.33-
round hole H33.32-
Breakdown
device, graft or implant — *see also* Complications, by site and type, mechanical T85.618
arterial graft NEC — *see* Complication, cardiovascular device, mechanical, vascular
breast (implant) T85.41
catheter NEC T85.618
cystostomy T83.010
Hopkins T83.018
ileostomy T83.018
dialysis (renal) T82.41
intraperitoneal T85.611
infusion NEC T82.514
cranial T85.610
epidural T85.610
intrathecal T85.610
spinal T85.610
subarachnoid T85.610
subdural T85.610
nephrostomy T83.012

Breakdown - *continued*
device, graft or implant - *continued*
catheter NEC - *continued*
urethral indwelling T83.011
urinary NEC T83.018
urostomy T83.018
electronic (electrode) (pulse generator) (stimulator)
bone T84.310
cardiac T82.119
electrode T82.110
pulse generator T82.111
specified type NEC T82.118
nervous system — *see* Complication, prosthetic device, mechanical, electronic nervous system stimulator
urinary — *see* Complication, genitourinary, device, urinary, mechanical
fixation, internal (orthopedic) NEC — *see* Complication, fixation device, mechanical
gastrointestinal — *see* Complications, prosthetic device, mechanical, gastrointestinal device
genital NEC T83.418
intrauterine contraceptive device T83.31
penile prosthesis (cylinder) (implanted) (pump) (resevoir) T83.410
testicular prosthesis T83.411
heart NEC — *see* Complication, cardiovascular device, mechanical
intrathecal infusion pump T85.615
joint prosthesis — *see* Complications..., joint prosthesis,internal, mechanical, by site
nervous system, specified device NEC T85.615
ocular NEC — *see* Complications, prosthetic device, mechanical, ocular device
orthopedic NEC — *see* Complication, orthopedic, device, mechanical
specified NEC T85.618
subcutaneous device pocket
nervous system prosthetic device, implant, or graft T85.890
other internal prosthetic device, implant, or graft T85.898
sutures, permanent T85.612
used in bone repair — *see* Complications, fixation device, internal (orthopedic), mechanical
urinary NEC T83.118
graft T83.21
sphincter, implanted T83.111
stent (ileal conduit) (nephroureteral) T83.113
ureteral indwelling T83.112
vascular NEC — *see* Complication, cardiovascular device, mechanical
ventricular intracranial shunt T85.01
nervous F48.8
perineum O90.1
respirator J95.850
specified NEC J95.859
ventilator J95.850
specified NEC J95.859
Breast — *see also* condition
buds E30.1
in newborn P96.89
dense R92.2
nodule — *see also* Lump, breast N63.0
Breath
foul R19.6
holder, child R06.89
holding spell R06.89
shortness R06.02
Breathing
labored — *see* Hyperventilation
mouth R06.5
causing malocclusion M26.5
periodic R06.3
high altitude G47.32

Breathlessness R06.81
Breda's disease — *see* Yaws
Breech presentation (mother) O32.1
causing obstructed labor O64.1
footling O32.8
causing obstructed labor O64.8
incomplete O32.8
causing obstructed labor O64.8
Breisky's disease N90.4
Brennemann's syndrome I88.0
Brenner
tumor (benign) D27.9
borderline malignancy D39.1-
malignant C56
proliferating D39.1-
Bretonneau's disease or angina A36.0
Breus' mole O02.0
Brevicollis Q76.49
Brickmakers' anemia B76.9 *[D63.8]*
Bridge, myocardial Q24.5
Bright red blood per rectum (BRBPR) K62.5
Bright's disease — *see also* Nephritis
arteriosclerotic — *see* Hypertension, kidney
Brill (-Zinsser) disease (recrudescent typhus) A75.1
Brill-Symmers' disease C82.90
Brion-Kayser disease — *see* Fever, parathyroid
Briquet's disorder or syndrome F45.0
Brissaud's
infantilism or dwarfism E23.0
motor-verbal tic F95.2
Brittle
bones disease Q78.0
nails L60.3
congenital Q84.6
Broad — *see also* condition
beta disease E78.2
ligament laceration syndrome N83.8
Broad- or floating -betalipoproteinemia E78.2
Brock's syndrome (atelectasis due to enlarged lymph nodes) J98.19
Brocq-Duhring disease (dermatitis herpetiformis) L13.0
Brodie's abscess or disease M86.8X-
Broken
arches — *see also* Deformity, limb, flat foot
arm (meaning upper limb) — *see* Fracture, arm
back — *see* Fracture, vertebra
bone — *see* Fracture
implant or internal device — *see* Complications, by site and type, mechanical
leg (meaning lower limb) — *see* Fracture, leg
nose S02.2
tooth, teeth — *see* Fracture, tooth
Bromhidrosis, bromidrosis L75.0
Bromidism, bromism G92.8
due to
correct substance properly administered — *see* Table of Drugs and Chemicals, by drug, adverse effect
overdose or wrong substance given or taken — *see* Table of Drugs and Chemicals, by drug, poisoning
chronic (dependence) F13.20
Bromidrosiphobia F40.298
Bronchi, bronchial — *see* condition
Bronchiectasis (cylindrical) (diffuse) (fusiform) (localized) (saccular) J47.9
with
acute
bronchitis J47.0
lower respiratory infection J47.0
exacerbation (acute) J47.1
congenital Q33.4
tuberculous NEC — *see* Tuberculosis, pulmonary
Bronchiolectasis — *see* Bronchiectasis
Bronchiolitis (acute) (infective) (subacute) J21.9
with

Bronchiolitis (acute) (infective) (subacute) - *continued*
- with - *continued*
  - bronchospasm or obstruction J21.9
  - influenza, flu or grippe — *see* Influenza, with, respiratory manifestations NEC
- chemical (chronic) J68.4
  - acute J68.0
- chronic (fibrosing) (obliterative) J44.9
- due to
  - external agent — *see* Bronchitis, acute, due to
  - human metapneumovirus J21.1
  - respiratory syncytial virus (RSV) J21.0
  - specified organism NEC J21.8
- fibrosa obliterans J44.9
- influenzal — *see* Influenza, with, respiratory manifestations NEC
- obliterans J42
  - with organizing pneumonia (BOOP) J84.89
- obliterative (chronic) (subacute) J44.9
  - due to fumes or vapors J68.4
  - due to chemicals, gases, fumes or vapors (inhalation) J68.4
- respiratory, interstitial lung disease J84.115

Bronchitis (diffuse) (fibrinous) (hypostatic) (infective) (membranous) J40
- with
  - influenza, flu or grippe — *see* Influenza, with, respiratory manifestations NEC
  - obstruction (airway) (lung) J44.9
  - tracheitis (15 years of age and above) J40
    - acute or subacute J20.9
    - chronic J42
    - under 15 years of age J20.9
- acute or subacute (with bronchospasm or obstruction) J20.9
  - with
    - bronchiectasis J47.0
    - chronic obstructive pulmonary disease J44.0
  - chemical (due to gases, fumes or vapors) J68.0
  - due to
    - fumes or vapors J68.0
    - Haemophilus influenzae J20.1
    - Mycoplasma pneumoniae J20.0
    - radiation J70.0
    - specified organism NEC J20.8
    - Streptococcus J20.2
    - virus
      - coxsackie J20.3
      - echovirus J20.7
      - parainfluenzae J20.4
      - respiratory syncytial (RSV) J20.5
      - rhinovirus J20.6
  - viral NEC J20.8
- allergic (acute) J45.909
  - with
    - exacerbation (acute) J45.901
    - status asthmaticus J45.902
- arachidic T17.528
- aspiration (due to food and vomit) J69.0
- asthmatic J45.9
  - chronic J44.9
    - with
      - acute lower respiratory infection J44.0
      - exacerbation (acute) J44.1
- capillary — *see* Pneumonia, broncho
- caseous (tuberculous) A15.5
- Castellani's A69.8
- catarrhal (15 years of age and above) J40
  - acute — *see* Bronchitis, acute
  - chronic J41.0
  - under 15 years of age J20.9
- chemical (acute) (subacute) J68.0
  - chronic J68.4
  - due to fumes or vapors J68.0
    - chronic J68.4
- chronic J42
  - with
    - airways obstruction J44.9
    - tracheitis (chronic) J42
  - asthmatic (obstructive) J44.9

Bronchitis (diffuse) (fibrinous) (hypostatic) (infective) (membranous) - *continued*
- chronic - *continued*
  - catarrhal J41.0
  - chemical (due to fumes or vapors) J68.4
  - due to
    - chemicals, gases, fumes or vapors (inhalation) J68.4
    - radiation J70.1
    - tobacco smoking J41.0
  - emphysematous J44.9
  - mucopurulent J41.1
  - non-obstructive J41.0
  - obliterans J44.9
  - obstructive J44.9
  - purulent J41.1
  - simple J41.0
- croupous — *see* Bronchitis, acute
- due to gases, fumes or vapors (chemical) J68.0
- emphysematous (obstructive) J44.9
- exudative — *see* Bronchitis, acute
- fetid J41.1
- grippal — *see* Influenza, with, respiratory manifestations NEC
- in those under 15 years age — *see* Bronchitis, acute
  - chronic — *see* Bronchitis, chronic
- influenzal — *see* Influenza, with, respiratory manifestations NEC
- mixed simple and mucopurulent J41.8
- moulder's J62.8
- mucopurulent (chronic) (recurrent) J41.1
  - acute or subacute J20.9
  - simple (mixed) J41.8
- obliterans (chronic) J44.9
- obstructive (chronic) (diffuse) J44.9
- pituitous J41.1
- pneumococcal, acute or subacute J20.2
- pseudomembranous, acute or subacute — *see* Bronchitis, acute
- purulent (chronic) (recurrent) J41.1
  - acute or subacute — *see* Bronchitis, acute
- putrid J41.1
- senile (chronic) J42
- simple and mucopurulent (mixed) J41.8
- smokers' J41.0
- spirochetal NEC A69.8
- subacute — *see* Bronchitis, acute
- suppurative (chronic) J41.1
  - acute or subacute — *see* Bronchitis, acute
- tuberculous A15.5
- under 15 years of age — *see* Bronchitis, acute
  - chronic — *see* Bronchitis, chronic
- viral NEC, acute or subacute — *see also* Bronchitis, acute J20.8

Bronchoalveolitis J18.0

Bronchoaspergillosis B44.1

Bronchocele meaning goiter E04.0

Broncholithiasis J98.09
- tuberculous NEC A15.5

Bronchomalacia J98.09
- congenital Q32.2

Bronchomycosis NOS B49 *[J99]*
- candidal B37.1

Bronchopleuropneumonia — *see* Pneumonia, broncho

Bronchopneumonia — *see* Pneumonia, broncho

Bronchopneumonitis — *see* Pneumonia, broncho

Bronchopulmonary — *see* condition

Bronchopulmonitis — *see* Pneumonia, broncho

Bronchorrhagia (see Hemoptysis)

Bronchorrhea J98.09
- acute J20.9
- chronic (infective) (purulent) J42

Bronchospasm (acute) J98.01
- with
  - bronchiolitis, acute J21.9
  - bronchitis, acute (conditions in J20) — *see* Bronchitis, acute
- due to external agent — *see* condition, respiratory, acute, due to

Bronchospasm (acute) - *continued*
- exercise induced J45.990

Bronchospirochetosis A69.8
- Castellani A69.8

Bronchostenosis J98.09

Bronchus — *see* condition

Brontophobia F40.220

Bronze baby syndrome P83.88

Brooke's tumor — *see* Neoplasm, skin, benign

Brown enamel of teeth (hereditary) K00.5

Brown's sheath syndrome H50.61-

Brown-Séquard disease, paralysis or syndrome G83.81

Bruce sepsis A23.0

Brucellosis (infection) A23.9
- abortus A23.1
- canis A23.3
- dermatitis A23.9
- melitensis A23.0
- mixed A23.8
- sepsis A23.9
  - melitensis A23.0
  - specified NEC A23.8
- suis A23.2

Bruck-de Lange disease Q87.19

Bruck's disease — *see* Deformity, limb

BRUE (brief resolved unexplained event) R68.13

Brugsch's syndrome Q82.8

Bruise (skin surface intact) — *see also* Contusion
- with
  - open wound — *see* Wound, open
- internal organ — *see* Injury, by site
- newborn P54.5
- scalp, due to birth injury, newborn P12.3
- umbilical cord O69.5

Bruit (arterial) R09.89
- cardiac R01.1

Brush burn — *see* Abrasion, by site

Bruton's X-linked agammaglobulinemia D80.0

Bruxism
- psychogenic F45.8
- sleep related G47.63

Bubbly lung syndrome P27.0

Bubo I88.8
- blennorrhagic (gonococcal) A54.89
- chancroidal A57
- climatic A55
- due to Haemophilus ducreyi A57
- gonococcal A54.89
- indolent (nonspecific) I88.8
- inguinal (nonspecific) I88.8
  - chancroidal A57
  - climatic A55
  - due to H. ducreyi A57
  - infective I88.8
- scrofulous (tuberculous) A18.2
- soft chancre A57
- suppurating — *see* Lymphadenitis, acute
- syphilitic (primary) A51.0
  - congenital A50.07
- tropical A55
- virulent (chancroidal) A57

Bubonic plague A20.0

Bubonocele — *see* Hernia, inguinal

Buccal — *see* condition

Buchanan's disease or osteochondrosis M91.0

Buchem's syndrome (hyperostosis corticalis) M85.2

Bucket-handle fracture or tear (semilunar cartilage) — *see* Tear, meniscus

Budd-Chiari syndrome (hepatic vein thrombosis) I82.0

Budgerigar fancier's disease or lung J67.2

Buds
- breast E30.1
  - in newborn P96.89

Buerger's disease (thromboangiitis obliterans) I73.1

Bulbar — *see* condition

Bulbus cordis (left ventricle) (persistent) Q21.8

Bulimia (nervosa) F50.2
atypical F50.9
normal weight F50.9
Bulky
stools R19.5
uterus N85.2
Bulla (e) R23.8
lung (emphysematous) (solitary) J43.9
newborn P25.8
Bullet wound — *see also* Wound, open
fracture - code as Fracture, by site
internal organ — *see* Injury, by site
Bundle
branch block (complete) (false) (incomplete) — *see* Block, bundle-branch
of His — *see* condition
Bunion M21.61-
tailor's M21.62-
Bunionette M21.62-
Buphthalmia, buphthalmos (congenital) Q15.0
Burdwan fever B55.0
Bürger-Grütz disease or syndrome E78.3
Buried
penis (congenital) Q55.64
acquired N48.83
roots K08.3
Burke's syndrome K86.89
Burkitt
cell leukemia C91.0-
lymphoma (malignant) C83.7-
small noncleaved, diffuse C83.7-
spleen C83.77
undifferentiated C83.7-
tumor C83.7-
type
acute lymphoblastic leukemia C91.0-
undifferentiated C83.7-
Burn (electricity) (flame) (hot gas, liquid or hot object) (radiation) (steam) (thermal) T30.0
abdomen, abdominal (muscle) (wall) T21.02
first degree T21.12
second degree T21.22
third degree T21.32
above elbow T22.039
first degree T22.139
left T22.032
first degree T22.132
second degree T22.232
third degree T22.332
right T22.031
first degree T22.131
second degree T22.231
third degree T22.331
second degree T22.239
third degree T22.339
acid (caustic) (external) (internal) — *see* Corrosion, by site
alimentary tract NEC T28.2
esophagus T28.1
mouth T28.0
pharynx T28.0
alkaline (caustic) (external) (internal) — *see* Corrosion, by site
ankle T25.019
first degree T25.119
left T25.012
first degree T25.112
second degree T25.212
third degree T25.312
multiple with foot — *see* Burn, lower, limb, multiple, ankle and foot
right T25.011
first degree T25.111
second degree T25.211
third degree T25.311
second degree T25.219
third degree T25.319
anus — *see* Burn, buttock
arm (lower) (upper) — *see* Burn, upper, limb
axilla T22.049
first degree T22.149
left T22.042

Burn (electricity) (flame) (hot gas, liquid or hot object) (radiation) (steam) (thermal) - *continued*
axilla - *continued*
left - *continued*
first degree T22.142
second degree T22.242
third degree T22.342
right T22.041
first degree T22.141
second degree T22.241
third degree T22.341
second degree T22.249
third degree T22.349
back (lower) T21.04
first degree T21.14
second degree T21.24
third degree T21.34
upper T21.03
first degree T21.13
second degree T21.23
third degree T21.33
blisters - code as Burn, second degree, by site
breast (s) — *see* Burn, chest wall
buttock (s) T21.05
first degree T21.15
second degree T21.25
third degree T21.35
calf T24.039
first degree T24.139
left T24.032
first degree T24.132
second degree T24.232
third degree T24.332
right T24.031
first degree T24.131
second degree T24.231
third degree T24.331
second degree T24.239
third degree T24.339
canthus (eye) — *see* Burn, eyelid
caustic acid or alkaline — *see* Corrosion, by site
cervix T28.3
cheek T20.06
first degree T20.16
second degree T20.26
third degree T20.36
chemical (acids) (alkalines) (caustics) (external) (internal) — *see* Corrosion, by site
chest wall T21.01
first degree T21.11
second degree T21.21
third degree T21.31
chin T20.03
first degree T20.13
second degree T20.23
third degree T20.33
colon T28.2
conjunctiva (and cornea) — *see* Burn, cornea
cornea (and conjunctiva) T26.1-
chemical — *see* Corrosion, cornea
corrosion (external) (internal) — *see* Corrosion, by site
deep necrosis of underlying tissue - code as Burn, third degree, by site
dorsum of hand T23.069
first degree T23.169
left T23.062
first degree T23.162
second degree T23.262
third degree T23.362
right T23.061
first degree T23.161
second degree T23.261
third degree T23.361
second degree T23.269
third degree T23.369
due to ingested chemical agent — *see* Corrosion, by site
ear (auricle) (external) (canal) T20.01
first degree T20.11
second degree T20.21
third degree T20.31

Burn (electricity) (flame) (hot gas, liquid or hot object) (radiation) (steam) (thermal) - *continued*
elbow T22.029
first degree T22.129
left T22.022
first degree T22.122
second degree T22.222
third degree T22.322
right T22.021
first degree T22.121
second degree T22.221
third degree T22.321
second degree T22.229
third degree T22.329
epidermal loss - code as Burn, second degree, by site
erythema, erythematous - code as Burn, first degree, by site
esophagus T28.1
extent (percentage of body surface)
less than 10 percent T31.0
10-19 percent T31.10
with 0-9 percent third degree burns T31.10
with 10-19 percent third degree burns T31.11
20-29 percent T31.20
with 0-9 percent third degree burns T31.20
with 10-19 percent third degree burns T31.21
with 20-29 percent third degree burns T31.22
30-39 percent T31.30
with 0-9 percent third degree burns T31.30
with 10-19 percent third degree burns T31.31
with 20-29 percent third degree burns T31.32
with 30-39 percent third degree burns T31.33
40-49 percent T31.40
with 0-9 percent third degree burns T31.40
with 10-19 percent third degree burns T31.41
with 20-29 percent third degree burns T31.42
with 30-39 percent third degree burns T31.43
with 40-49 percent third degree burns T31.44
50-59 percent T31.50
with 0-9 percent third degree burns T31.50
with 10-19 percent third degree burns T31.51
with 20-29 percent third degree burns T31.52
with 30-39 percent third degree burns T31.53
with 40-49 percent third degree burns T31.54
with 50-59 percent third degree burns T31.55
60-69 percent T31.60
with 0-9 percent third degree burns T31.60
with 10-19 percent third degree burns T31.61
with 20-29 percent third degree burns T31.62
with 30-39 percent third degree burns T31.63
with 40-49 percent third degree burns T31.64
with 50-59 percent third degree burns T31.65
with 60-69 percent third degree burns T31.66
70-79 percent T31.70
with 0-9 percent third degree burns T31.70

- **Burn (electricity) (flame) (hot gas, liquid or hot object) (radiation) (steam) (thermal)** - *continued*
  - extent (percentage of body surface) - *continued*
    - 70-79 percent - *continued*
      - with 10-19 percent third degree burns T31.71
      - with 20-29 percent third degree burns T31.72
      - with 30-39 percent third degree burns T31.73
      - with 40-49 percent third degree burns T31.74
      - with 50-59 percent third degree burns T31.75
      - with 60-69 percent third degree burns T31.76
      - with 70-79 percent third degree burns T31.77
    - 80-89 percent T31.80
      - with 0-9 percent third degree burns T31.80
      - with 10-19 percent third degree burns T31.81
      - with 20-29 percent third degree burns T31.82
      - with 30-39 percent third degree burns T31.83
      - with 40-49 percent third degree burns T31.84
      - with 50-59 percent third degree burns T31.85
      - with 60-69 percent third degree burns T31.86
      - with 70-79 percent third degree burns T31.87
      - with 80-89 percent third degree burns T31.88
    - 90 percent or more T31.90
      - with 0-9 percent third degree burns T31.90
      - with 10-19 percent third degree burns T31.91
      - with 20-29 percent third degree burns T31.92
      - with 30-39 percent third degree burns T31.93
      - with 40-49 percent third degree burns T31.94
      - with 50-59 percent third degree burns T31.95
      - with 60-69 percent third degree burns T31.96
      - with 70-79 percent third degree burns T31.97
      - with 80-89 percent third degree burns T31.98
      - with 90 percent or more third degree burns T31.99
  - extremity — *see* Burn, limb
  - eye (s) and adnexa T26.4-
    - with resulting rupture and destruction of eyeball T26.2-
    - conjunctival sac — *see* Burn, cornea
    - cornea — *see* Burn, cornea
    - lid — *see* Burn, eyelid
    - periocular area — *see* Burn, eyelid
    - specified site NEC T26.3-
  - eyeball — *see* Burn, eye
  - eyelid (s) T26.0-
    - chemical — *see* Corrosion, eyelid
  - face — *see* Burn, head
  - finger T23.029
    - first degree T23.129
    - left T23.022
      - first degree T23.122
      - second degree T23.222
      - third degree T23.322
    - multiple sites (without thumb) T23.039
      - with thumb T23.049
        - first degree T23.149
        - left T23.042
          - first degree T23.142
          - second degree T23.242

- **Burn (electricity) (flame) (hot gas, liquid or hot object) (radiation) (steam) (thermal)** - *continued*
  - finger - *continued*
    - multiple sites (without thumb) - *continued*
      - with thumb - *continued*
        - left - *continued*
          - third degree T23.342
        - right T23.041
          - first degree T23.141
          - second degree T23.241
          - third degree T23.341
        - second degree T23.249
        - third degree T23.349
      - first degree T23.139
      - left T23.032
        - first degree T23.132
        - second degree T23.232
        - third degree T23.332
      - right T23.031
        - first degree T23.131
        - second degree T23.231
        - third degree T23.331
      - second degree T23.239
      - third degree T23.339
    - right T23.021
      - first degree T23.121
      - second degree T23.221
      - third degree T23.321
    - second degree T23.229
    - third degree T23.329
  - flank — *see* Burn, abdominal wall
  - foot T25.029
    - first degree T25.129
    - left T25.022
      - first degree T25.122
      - second degree T25.222
      - third degree T25.322
    - multiple with ankle — *see* Burn, lower, limb, multiple, ankle and foot
    - right T25.021
      - first degree T25.121
      - second degree T25.221
      - third degree T25.321
    - second degree T25.229
    - third degree T25.329
  - forearm T22.019
    - first degree T22.119
    - left T22.012
      - first degree T22.112
      - second degree T22.212
      - third degree T22.312
    - right T22.011
      - first degree T22.111
      - second degree T22.211
      - third degree T22.311
    - second degree T22.219
    - third degree T22.319
  - forehead T20.06
    - first degree T20.16
    - second degree T20.26
    - third degree T20.36
  - fourth degree - code as Burn, third degree, by site
  - friction — *see* Burn, by site
  - from swallowing caustic or corrosive substance NEC — *see* Corrosion, by site
  - full thickness skin loss - code as Burn, third degree, by site
  - gastrointestinal tract NEC T28.2
    - from swallowing caustic or corrosive substance T28.7
  - genital organs
    - external
      - female T21.07
        - first degree T21.17
        - second degree T21.27
        - third degree T21.37
      - male T21.06
        - first degree T21.16
        - second degree T21.26
        - third degree T21.36
    - internal T28.3

- **Burn (electricity) (flame) (hot gas, liquid or hot object) (radiation) (steam) (thermal)** - *continued*
  - genital organs - *continued*
    - internal - *continued*
      - from caustic or corrosive substance T28.8
  - groin — *see* Burn, abdominal wall
  - hand (s) T23.009
    - back — *see* Burn, dorsum of hand
    - finger — *see* Burn, finger
    - first degree T23.109
    - left T23.002
      - first degree T23.102
      - second degree T23.202
      - third degree T23.302
    - multiple sites with wrist T23.099
      - first degree T23.199
      - left T23.092
        - first degree T23.192
        - second degree T23.292
        - third degree T23.392
      - right T23.091
        - first degree T23.191
        - second degree T23.291
        - third degree T23.391
      - second degree T23.299
      - third degree T23.399
    - palm — *see* Burn, palm
    - right T23.001
      - first degree T23.101
      - second degree T23.201
      - third degree T23.301
    - second degree T23.209
    - third degree T23.309
    - thumb — *see* Burn, thumb
  - head (and face) (and neck) T20.00
    - cheek — *see* Burn, cheek
    - chin — *see* Burn, chin
    - ear — *see* Burn, ear
    - eye (s) only — *see* Burn, eye
    - first degree T20.10
    - forehead — *see* Burn, forehead
    - lip — *see* Burn, lip
    - multiple sites T20.09
      - first degree T20.19
      - second degree T20.29
      - third degree T20.39
    - neck — *see* Burn, neck
    - nose — *see* Burn, nose
    - scalp — *see* Burn, scalp
    - second degree T20.20
    - third degree T20.30
  - hip (s) — *see* Burn, thigh
  - inhalation — *see* Burn, respiratory tract
    - caustic or corrosive substance (fumes) — *see* Corrosion, respiratory tract
  - internal organ (s) T28.40
    - alimentary tract T28.2
      - esophagus T28.1
    - eardrum T28.41
    - esophagus T28.1
    - from caustic or corrosive substance (swallowing) NEC — *see* Corrosion, by site
    - genitourinary T28.3
    - mouth T28.0
    - pharynx T28.0
    - respiratory tract — *see* Burn, respiratory tract
    - specified organ NEC T28.49
  - interscapular region — *see* Burn, back, upper
  - intestine (large) (small) T28.2
  - knee T24.029
    - first degree T24.129
    - left T24.022
      - first degree T24.122
      - second degree T24.222
      - third degree T24.322
    - right T24.021
      - first degree T24.121
      - second degree T24.221
      - third degree T24.321
    - second degree T24.229
    - third degree T24.329

Burn (electricity) (flame) (hot gas, liquid or hot object) (radiation) (steam) (thermal) - *continued*

- labium (majus) (minus) — *see* Burn, genital organs, external, female
- lacrimal apparatus, duct, gland or sac — *see* Burn, eye, specified site NEC
- larynx T27.0
  - with lung T27.1
- leg (s) (lower) (upper) — *see* Burn, lower, limb
- lightning — *see* Burn, by site
- limb (s)
  - lower (except ankle or foot alone) — *see* Burn, lower, limb
  - upper — *see* Burn, upper limb
- lip (s) T20.02
  - first degree T20.12
  - second degree T20.22
  - third degree T20.32
- lower
  - back — *see* Burn, back
  - limb T24.009
    - ankle — *see* Burn, ankle
    - calf — *see* Burn, calf
    - first degree T24.109
    - foot — *see* Burn, foot
    - hip — *see* Burn, thigh
    - knee — *see* Burn, knee
    - left T24.002
      - first degree T24.102
      - second degree T24.202
      - third degree T24.302
    - multiple sites, except ankle and foot T24.099
      - ankle and foot T25.099
        - first degree T25.199
        - left T25.092
          - first degree T25.192
          - second degree T25.292
          - third degree T25.392
        - right T25.091
          - first degree T25.191
          - second degree T25.291
          - third degree T25.391
        - second degree T25.299
        - third degree T25.399
      - first degree T24.199
      - left T24.092
        - first degree T24.192
        - second degree T24.292
        - third degree T24.392
      - right T24.091
        - first degree T24.191
        - second degree T24.291
        - third degree T24.391
      - second degree T24.299
      - third degree T24.399
    - right T24.001
      - first degree T24.101
      - second degree T24.201
      - third degree T24.301
    - second degree T24.209
    - thigh — *see* Burn, thigh
    - third degree T24.309
    - toe — *see* Burn, toe
- lung (with larynx and trachea) T27.1
- mouth T28.0
- neck T20.07
  - first degree T20.17
  - second degree T20.27
  - third degree T20.37
- nose (septum) T20.04
  - first degree T20.14
  - second degree T20.24
  - third degree T20.34
- ocular adnexa — *see* Burn, eye
- orbit region — *see* Burn, eyelid
- palm T23.059
  - first degree T23.159
  - left T23.052
    - first degree T23.152
    - second degree T23.252
    - third degree T23.352
  - right T23.051

Burn (electricity) (flame) (hot gas, liquid or hot object) (radiation) (steam) (thermal) - *continued*

- palm - *continued*
  - right - *continued*
    - first degree T23.151
    - second degree T23.251
    - third degree T23.351
  - second degree T23.259
  - third degree T23.359
- partial thickness - code as Burn, by site, second degree
- pelvis — *see* Burn, trunk
- penis — *see* Burn, genital organs, external, male
- perineum
  - female — *see* Burn, genital organs, external, female
  - male — *see* Burn, genital organs, external, male
- periocular area — *see* Burn, eyelid
- pharynx T28.0
- rectum T28.2
- respiratory tract T27.3
  - larynx — *see* Burn, larynx
  - specified part NEC T27.2
  - trachea — *see* Burn, trachea
- sac, lacrimal — *see* Burn, eye, specified site NEC
- scalp T20.05
  - first degree T20.15
  - second degree T20.25
  - third degree T20.35
- scapular region T22.069
  - first degree T22.169
  - left T22.062
    - first degree T22.162
    - second degree T22.262
    - third degree T22.362
  - right T22.061
    - first degree T22.161
    - second degree T22.261
    - third degree T22.361
  - second degree T22.269
  - third degree T22.369
- sclera — *see* Burn, eye, specified site NEC
- scrotum — *see* Burn, genital organs, external, male
- shoulder T22.059
  - first degree T22.159
  - left T22.052
    - first degree T22.152
    - second degree T22.252
    - third degree T22.352
  - right T22.051
    - first degree T22.151
    - second degree T22.251
    - third degree T22.351
  - second degree T22.259
  - third degree T22.359
- stomach T28.2
- temple — *see* Burn, head
- testis — *see* Burn, genital organs, external, male
- thigh T24.019
  - first degree T24.119
  - left T24.012
    - first degree T24.112
    - second degree T24.212
    - third degree T24.312
  - right T24.011
    - first degree T24.111
    - second degree T24.211
    - third degree T24.311
  - second degree T24.219
  - third degree T24.319
- thorax (external) — *see* Burn, trunk
- throat (meaning pharynx) T28.0
- thumb (s) T23.019
  - first degree T23.119
  - left T23.012
    - first degree T23.112
    - second degree T23.212
    - third degree T23.312
  - multiple sites with fingers T23.049

Burn (electricity) (flame) (hot gas, liquid or hot object) (radiation) (steam) (thermal) - *continued*

- thumb (s) - *continued*
  - multiple sites with fingers - *continued*
    - first degree T23.149
    - left T23.042
      - first degree T23.142
      - second degree T23.242
      - third degree T23.342
    - right T23.041
      - first degree T23.141
      - second degree T23.241
      - third degree T23.341
    - second degree T23.249
    - third degree T23.349
  - right T23.011
    - first degree T23.111
    - second degree T23.211
    - third degree T23.311
  - second degree T23.219
  - third degree T23.319
- toe T25.039
  - first degree T25.139
  - left T25.032
    - first degree T25.132
    - second degree T25.232
    - third degree T25.332
  - right T25.031
    - first degree T25.131
    - second degree T25.231
    - third degree T25.331
  - second degree T25.239
  - third degree T25.339
- tongue T28.0
- tonsil (s) T28.0
- trachea T27.0
  - with lung T27.1
- trunk T21.00
  - abdominal wall — *see* Burn, abdominal wall
  - anus — *see* Burn, buttock
  - axilla — *see* Burn, upper limb
  - back — *see* Burn, back
  - breast — *see* Burn, chest wall
  - buttock — *see* Burn, buttock
  - chest wall — *see* Burn, chest wall
  - first degree T21.10
  - flank — *see* Burn, abdominal wall
  - genital
    - female — *see* Burn, genital organs, external, female
    - male — *see* Burn, genital organs, external, male
  - groin — *see* Burn, abdominal wall
  - interscapular region — *see* Burn, back, upper
  - labia — *see* Burn, genital organs, external, female
  - lower back — *see* Burn, back
  - penis — *see* Burn, genital organs, external, male
  - perineum
    - female — *see* Burn, genital organs, external, female
    - male — *see* Burn, genital organs, external, male
  - scapula region — *see* Burn, scapular region
  - scrotum — *see* Burn, genital organs, external, male
  - second degree T21.20
  - specified site NEC T21.09
    - first degree T21.19
    - second degree T21.29
    - third degree T21.39
  - testes — *see* Burn, genital organs, external, male
  - third degree T21.30
  - upper back — *see* Burn, back, upper
  - vulva — *see* Burn, genital organs, external, female
- unspecified site with extent of body surface involved specified
  - less than 10 percent T31.0

Busse-Buschke disease — *see* Cryptococcosis by site

Buttock — *see* condition

Button
- Biskra B55.1
- Delhi B55.1
- oriental B55.1

Buttonhole deformity (finger) — *see* Deformity, finger, boutonniere

Bwamba fever A92.8

Byssinosis J66.0

Bywaters' syndrome T79.5

C

Cachexia R64
- cancerous R64
- cardiac — *see* Disease, heart
- dehydration E86.0
- due to malnutrition R64
- exophthalmic — *see* Hyperthyroidism
- heart — *see* Disease, heart
- hypophyseal E23.0
- hypopituitary E23.0
- lead — *see* Poisoning, lead
- malignant R64
- marsh — *see* Malaria
- nervous F48.8
- old age R54
- paludal — *see* Malaria
- pituitary E23.0
- pulmonary R64
- renal N28.9
- saturnine — *see* Poisoning, lead
- senile R54
- Simmonds' E23.0
- splenica D73.0
- strumipriva E03.4
- tuberculous NEC — *see* Tuberculosis

CADASIL (cerebral autosomal dominant arteriopathy with subcortical infarcts and leukoencephalopathy) I67.850

Café, au lait spots L81.3

Caffeine-induced
- anxiety disorder F15.980
- sleep disorder F15.982

Caffey's syndrome Q78.8

Caisson disease T70.3

Cake kidney Q63.1

Caked breast (puerperal, postpartum) O92.79

Calabar swelling B74.3

Calcaneal spur — *see* Spur, bone, calcaneal

Calcaneo-apophysitis M92.8

Calcareous — *see* condition

Calcicosis J62.8

Calciferol (vitamin D) deficiency E55.9
- with rickets E55.0

Calcification
- adrenal (capsule) (gland) E27.49
  - tuberculous E35 *[B90.8]*
- aorta I70.0
- artery (annular) — *see* Arteriosclerosis
- auricle (ear) — *see* Disorder, pinna, specified type NEC
- basal ganglia G23.8
- bladder N32.89
  - due to Schistosoma hematobium B65.0
- brain (cortex) — *see* Calcification, cerebral
- bronchus J98.09
- bursa M71.40
  - ankle M71.47-
  - elbow M71.42-
  - foot M71.47-
  - hand M71.44-
  - hip M71.45-
  - knee M71.46-
  - multiple sites M71.49
  - shoulder M75.3-
  - specified site NEC M71.48
  - wrist M71.43-
- cardiac — *see* Degeneration, myocardial
- cerebral (cortex) G93.89
  - artery I67.2
- cervix (uteri) N88.8
- choroid plexus G93.89
- conjunctiva — *see* Concretion, conjunctiva

Calcification - *continued*
- corpora cavernosa (penis) N48.89
- cortex (brain) — *see* Calcification, cerebral
- dental pulp (nodular) K04.2
- dentinal papilla K00.4
- fallopian tube N83.8
- falx cerebri G96.198
- gallbladder K82.8
- general E83.59
- heart — *see also* Degeneration, myocardial
  - valve — *see* Endocarditis
- idiopathic infantile arterial (IIAC) Q28.8
- intervertebral cartilage or disc (postinfective) — *see* Disorder, disc, specified NEC
- intracranial — *see* Calcification, cerebral
- joint — *see* Disorder, joint, specified type NEC
- kidney N28.89
  - tuberculous N29 *[B90.1]*
- larynx (senile) J38.7
- lens — *see* Cataract, specified NEC
- lung (active) (postinfectional) J98.4
  - tuberculous B90.9
- lymph gland or node (postinfectional) I89.8
  - tuberculous — *see also* Tuberculosis, lymph gland B90.8
- mammographic R92.1
- massive (paraplegic) — *see* Myositis, ossificans, in, quadriplegia
- medial — *see* Arteriosclerosis, extremities
- meninges (cerebral) (spinal) G96.198
- metastatic E83.59
- Mönckeberg's — *see* Arteriosclerosis, extremities
- muscle M61.9
  - due to burns — *see* Myositis, ossificans, in, burns
  - paralytic — *see* Myositis, ossificans, in, quadriplegia
  - specified type NEC M61.40
    - ankle M61.47-
    - foot M61.47-
    - forearm M61.43-
    - hand M61.44-
    - lower leg M61.46-
    - multiple sites M61.49
    - pelvic region M61.45-
    - shoulder region M61.41-
    - specified site NEC M61.48
    - thigh M61.45-
    - upper arm M61.42-
- myocardium, myocardial — *see* Degeneration, myocardial
- ovary N83.8
- pancreas K86.89
- penis N48.89
- periarticular — *see* Disorder, joint, specified type NEC
- pericardium — *see also* Pericarditis I31.1
- pineal gland E34.8
- pleura J94.8
  - postinfectional J94.8
  - tuberculous NEC B90.9
- pulpal (dental) (nodular) K04.2
- sclera H15.89
- spleen D73.89
- subcutaneous L94.2
- suprarenal (capsule) (gland) E27.49
- tendon (sheath) — *see also* Tenosynovitis, specified type NEC
  - with bursitis, synovitis or tenosynovitis — *see* Tendinitis, calcific
- trachea J39.8
- ureter N28.89
- uterus N85.8
- vitreous — *see* Deposit, crystalline

Calcified — *see* Calcification

Calcinosis (interstitial) (tumoral) (universalis) E83.59
- with Raynaud's phenomenon, esophageal dysfunction, sclerodactyly, telangiectasia (CREST syndrome) M34.1
- circumscripta (skin) L94.2

Calcinosis (interstitial) (tumoral) (universalis) - *continued*
- cutis L94.2

Calciphylaxis — *see also* Calcification, by site E83.59

Calcium
- deposits — *see* Calcification, by site
- metabolism disorder E83.50
- salts or soaps in vitreous — *see* Deposit, crystalline

Calciuria R82.994

Calculi — *see* Calculus

Calculosis, intrahepatic — *see* Calculus, bile duct

Calculus, calculi, calculous
- ampulla of Vater — *see* Calculus, bile duct
- anuria (impacted) (recurrent) — *see also* Calculus, urinary N20.9
- appendix K38.1
- bile duct (common) (hepatic) K80.50
  - with
    - calculus of gallbladder — *see* Calculus, gallbladder and bile duct
    - cholangitis K80.30
      - with
        - cholecystitis — *see* Calculus, bile duct, with cholecystitis
        - obstruction K80.31
      - acute K80.32
        - with
          - chronic cholangitis K80.36
            - with obstruction K80.37
          - obstruction K80.33
      - chronic K80.34
        - with
          - acute cholangitis K80.36
            - with obstruction K80.37
          - obstruction K80.35
    - cholecystitis (with cholangitis) K80.40
      - with obstruction K80.41
      - acute K80.42
        - with
          - chronic cholecystitis K80.46
            - with obstruction K80.47
          - obstruction K80.43
      - chronic K80.44
        - with
          - acute cholecystitis K80.46
            - with obstruction K80.47
          - obstruction K80.45
    - obstruction K80.51
- biliary — *see also* Calculus, gallbladder
  - specified NEC K80.80
    - with obstruction K80.81
- bilirubin, multiple — *see* Calculus, gallbladder
- bladder (encysted) (impacted) (urinary) (diverticulum) N21.0
- bronchus J98.09
- calyx (kidney) (renal) — *see* Calculus, kidney
- cholesterol (pure) (solitary) — *see* Calculus, gallbladder
- common duct (bile) — *see* Calculus, bile duct
- conjunctiva — *see* Concretion, conjunctiva
- cystic N21.0
  - duct — *see* Calculus, gallbladder
- dental (subgingival) (supragingival) K03.6
- diverticulum
  - bladder N21.0
  - kidney N20.0
- epididymis N50.89
- gallbladder K80.20
  - with
    - bile duct calculus — *see* Calculus, gallbladder and bile duct
    - cholecystitis K80.10
      - with obstruction K80.11
      - acute K80.00
        - with
          - chronic cholecystitis K80.12
            - with obstruction K80.13
          - obstruction K80.01
      - chronic K80.10

- **Calculus, calculi, calculous** - *continued*
  - gallbladder - *continued*
    - with - *continued*
      - cholecystitis - *continued*
        - chronic - *continued*
          - with
            - acute cholecystitis K80.12
              - with obstruction K80.13
            - obstruction K80.11
        - specified NEC K80.18
          - with obstruction K80.19
      - obstruction K80.21
  - gallbladder and bile duct K80.70
    - with
      - cholecystitis K80.60
        - with obstruction K80.61
        - acute K80.62
          - with
            - chronic cholecystitis K80.66
              - with obstruction K80.67
            - obstruction K80.63
        - chronic K80.64
          - with
            - acute cholecystitis K80.66
              - with obstruction K80.67
            - obstruction K80.65
      - obstruction K80.71
  - hepatic (duct) — *see* Calculus, bile duct
  - hepatobiliary K80.80
    - with obstruction K80.81
  - ileal conduit N21.8
  - intestinal (impaction) (obstruction) K56.49
  - kidney (impacted) (multiple) (pelvis) (recurrent) (staghorn) N20.0
    - with calculus, ureter N20.2
    - congenital Q63.8
  - lacrimal passages — *see* Dacryolith
  - liver (impacted) — *see* Calculus, bile duct
  - lung J98.4
  - mammographic R92.1
  - nephritic (impacted) (recurrent) — *see* Calculus, kidney
  - nose J34.89
  - pancreas (duct) K86.89
  - parotid duct or gland K11.5
  - pelvis, encysted — *see* Calculus, kidney
  - prostate N42.0
  - pulmonary J98.4
  - pyelitis (impacted) (recurrent) N20.0
    - with hydronephrosis N13.6
  - pyelonephritis (impacted) (recurrent) — *see* category N20
    - with hydronephrosis N13.6
  - renal (impacted) (recurrent) — *see* Calculus, kidney
  - salivary (duct) (gland) K11.5
  - seminal vesicle N50.89
  - staghorn — *see* Calculus, kidney
  - Stensen's duct K11.5
  - stomach K31.89
  - sublingual duct or gland K11.5
    - congenital Q38.4
  - submandibular duct, gland or region K11.5
  - submaxillary duct, gland or region K11.5
  - suburethral N21.8
  - tonsil J35.8
  - tooth, teeth (subgingival) (supragingival) K03.6
  - tunica vaginalis N50.89
  - ureter (impacted) (recurrent) N20.1
    - with calculus, kidney N20.2
      - with hydronephrosis N13.2
        - with infection N13.6
  - ureteropelvic junction N20.1
  - urethra (impacted) N21.1
  - urinary (duct) (impacted) (passage) (tract) N20.9
    - with hydronephrosis N13.2
      - with infection N13.6
    - in (due to)
    - lower N21.9
      - specified NEC N21.8
  - vagina N89.8
  - vesical (impacted) N21.0
  - Wharton's duct K11.5
- **Calculus, calculi, calculous** - *continued*
  - xanthine E79.8 *[N22]*
- **Calicectasis** N28.89
- **Caliectasis** N28.89
- **California**
  - disease B38.9
  - encephalitis A83.5
- **Caligo cornea** — *see* Opacity, cornea, central
- **Callositas, callosity (infected)** L84
- **Callus (infected)** L84
  - bone — *see* Osteophyte
    - excessive, following fracture - code as Sequelae of fracture
- **CALME (childhood asymmetric labium majus enlargement)** N90.61
- **Calorie deficiency or malnutrition** — *see also* Malnutrition E46
- **Calvé-Perthes disease** — *see* Legg-Calvé-Perthes disease
- **Calvé's disease** — *see* Osteochondrosis, juvenile, spine
- **Calvities** — *see* Alopecia, androgenic
- **Cameroon fever** — *see* Malaria
- **Camptocormia (hysterical)** F44.4
- **Camurati-Engelmann syndrome** Q78.3
- **Canal** — *see also* condition
  - atrioventricular common Q21.2
- **Canaliculitis (lacrimal) (acute) (subacute)** H04.33-
  - Actinomyces A42.89
  - chronic H04.42-
- **Canavan's disease** E75.29
- **Canceled procedure (surgical)** Z53.9
  - because of
    - contraindication Z53.09
      - smoking Z53.01
    - left against medical advice (AMA) Z53.29
    - patient's decision Z53.20
      - for reasons of belief or group pressure Z53.1
      - specified reason NEC Z53.29
    - specified reason NEC Z53.8
- **Cancer** — *see also* Neoplasm, by site, malignant
  - bile duct type liver C22.1
  - blood — *see* Leukemia
  - breast — *see also* Neoplasm, breast, malignant C50.91-
  - hepatocellular C22.0
  - lung — *see also* Neoplasm, lung, malignant C34.90-
  - ovarian — *see also* Neoplasm ovary, malignant C56.9-
  - unspecified site (primary) C80.1
- **Cancerous** — *see* Neoplasm, malignant, by site
- **Cancer (o) phobia** F45.29
- **Cancrum oris** A69.0
- **Candidiasis, candidal** B37.9
  - balanitis B37.42
  - bronchitis B37.1
  - cheilitis B37.83
  - congenital P37.5
  - cystitis B37.41
  - disseminated B37.7
  - endocarditis B37.6
  - enteritis B37.82
  - esophagitis B37.81
  - intertrigo B37.2
  - lung B37.1
  - meningitis B37.5
  - mouth B37.0
  - nails B37.2
  - neonatal P37.5
  - onychia B37.2
  - oral B37.0
  - osteomyelitis B37.89
  - otitis externa B37.84
  - paronychia B37.2
  - perionyxis B37.2
  - pneumonia B37.1
  - proctitis B37.82
  - pulmonary B37.1
  - pyelonephritis B37.49
  - sepsis B37.7
- **Candidiasis, candidal** - *continued*
  - skin B37.2
  - specified site NEC B37.89
  - stomatitis B37.0
  - systemic B37.7
  - urethritis B37.41
  - urogenital site NEC B37.49
  - vagina B37.3
  - vulva B37.3
  - vulvovaginitis B37.3
- **Candidid** L30.2
- **Candidosis** — *see* Candidiasis
- **Candiru infection or infestation** B88.8
- **Canities (premature)** L67.1
  - congenital Q84.2
- **Canker (mouth) (sore)** K12.0
  - rash A38.9
- **Cannabinosis** J66.2
- **Cannabis induced**
  - anxiety disorder F12.980
  - psychotic disorder F12.959
  - sleep disorder F12.988
- **Canton fever** A75.9
- **Cantrell's syndrome** Q87.89
- **Capillariasis (intestinal)** B81.1
  - hepatic B83.8
- **Capillary** — *see* condition
- **Caplan's syndrome** — *see* Rheumatoid, lung
- **Capsule** — *see* condition
- **Capsulitis (joint)** — *see also* Enthesopathy
  - adhesive (shoulder) M75.0-
  - hepatic K65.8
  - labyrinthine — *see* Otosclerosis, specified NEC
  - thyroid E06.9
- **Caput**
  - crepitus Q75.8
  - medusae I86.8
  - succedaneum P12.81
- **Car sickness** T75.3
- **Carapata (disease)** A68.0
- **Carate** — *see* Pinta
- **Carbon lung** J60
- **Carbuncle** L02.93
  - abdominal wall L02.231
  - anus K61.0
  - auditory canal, external — *see* Abscess, ear, external
  - auricle ear — *see* Abscess, ear, external
  - axilla L02.43-
  - back (any part) L02.232
  - breast N61.1
  - buttock L02.33
  - cheek (external) L02.03
  - chest wall L02.233
  - chin L02.03
  - corpus cavernosum N48.21
  - ear (any part) (external) (middle) — *see* Abscess, ear, external
  - external auditory canal — *see* Abscess, ear, external
  - eyelid — *see* Abscess, eyelid
  - face NEC L02.03
  - femoral (region) — *see* Carbuncle, lower limb
  - finger — *see* Carbuncle, hand
  - flank L02.231
  - foot L02.63-
  - forehead L02.03
  - genital — *see* Abscess, genital
  - gluteal (region) L02.33
  - groin L02.234
  - hand L02.53-
  - head NEC L02.831
  - heel — *see* Carbuncle, foot
  - hip — *see* Carbuncle, lower limb
  - kidney — *see* Abscess, kidney
  - knee — *see* Carbuncle, lower limb
  - labium (majus) (minus) N76.4
  - lacrimal
    - gland — *see* Dacryoadenitis
    - passages (duct) (sac) — *see* Inflammation, lacrimal, passages, acute
  - leg — *see* Carbuncle, lower limb
  - lower limb L02.43-

Carbuncle - *continued*
  malignant A22.0
  navel L02.236
  neck L02.13
  nose (external) (septum) J34.0
  orbit, orbital — *see* Abscess, orbit
  palmar (space) — *see* Carbuncle, hand
  partes posteriores L02.33
  pectoral region L02.233
  penis N48.21
  perineum L02.235
  pinna — *see* Abscess, ear, external
  popliteal — *see* Carbuncle, lower limb
  scalp L02.831
  seminal vesicle N49.0
  shoulder — *see* Carbuncle, upper limb
  specified site NEC L02.838
  temple (region) L02.03
  thumb — *see* Carbuncle, hand
  toe — *see* Carbuncle, foot
  trunk L02.239
    abdominal wall L02.231
    back L02.232
    chest wall L02.233
    groin L02.234
    perineum L02.235
    umbilicus L02.236
  umbilicus L02.236
  upper limb L02.43-
  urethra N34.0
  vulva N76.4
Carbunculus — *see* Carbuncle
Carcinoid (tumor) — *see* Tumor, carcinoid
Carcinoidosis E34.0
Carcinoma (malignant) — *see also* Neoplasm, by site, malignant
  acidophil
    specified site — *see* Neoplasm, malignant, by site
    unspecified site C75.1
  acidophil-basophil, mixed
    specified site — *see* Neoplasm, malignant, by site
    unspecified site C75.1
  adnexal (skin) — *see* Neoplasm, skin, malignant
  adrenal cortical C74.0-
  alveolar — *see* Neoplasm, lung, malignant
    cell — *see* Neoplasm, lung, malignant
  ameloblastic C41.1
    upper jaw (bone) C41.0
  apocrine
    breast — *see* Neoplasm, breast, malignant
    specified site NEC — *see* Neoplasm, skin, malignant
    unspecified site C44.99
  basal cell (pigmented) (see also Neoplasm, skin, malignant) C44.91
    fibro-epithelial — *see* Neoplasm, skin, malignant
    morphea — *see* Neoplasm, skin, malignant
    multicentric — *see* Neoplasm, skin, malignant
  basaloid
  basal-squamous cell, mixed — *see* Neoplasm, skin, malignant
  basophil
    specified site — *see* Neoplasm, malignant, by site
    unspecified site C75.1
  basophil-acidophil, mixed
    specified site — *see* Neoplasm, malignant, by site
    unspecified site C75.1
  basosquamous — *see* Neoplasm, skin, malignant
  bile duct
    with hepatocellular, mixed C22.0
    liver C22.1
    specified site NEC — *see* Neoplasm, malignant, by site
    unspecified site C22.1
  branchial or branchiogenic C10.4
  bronchial or bronchogenic — *see* Neoplasm, lung, malignant

Carcinoma (malignant) - *continued*
  bronchiolar — *see* Neoplasm, lung, malignant
  bronchioloalveolar — *see* Neoplasm, lung, malignant
  C cell
    specified site — *see* Neoplasm, malignant, by site
    unspecified site C73
  ceruminous C44.29-
  cervix uteri
    in situ D06.9
      endocervix D06.0
      exocervix D06.1
      specified site NEC D06.7
  chorionic
    specified site — *see* Neoplasm, malignant, by site
    unspecified site
      female C58
      male C62.90
  chromophobe
    specified site — *see* Neoplasm, malignant, by site
    unspecified site C75.1
  cloacogenic
    specified site — *see* Neoplasm, malignant, by site
    unspecified site C21.2
  diffuse type
    specified site — *see* Neoplasm, malignant, by site
    unspecified site C16.9
  duct (cell)
    with Paget's disease — *see* Neoplasm, breast, malignant
    infiltrating
      with lobular carcinoma (in situ)
        specified site — *see* Neoplasm, malignant, by site
        unspecified site (female) C50.91-
          male C50.92-
      specified site — *see* Neoplasm, malignant, by site
        unspecified site (female) C50.91-
          male C50.92-
  ductal
    with lobular
      specified site — *see* Neoplasm, malignant, by site
      unspecified site (female) C50.91-
        male C50.92-
  ductular, infiltrating
    specified site — *see* Neoplasm, malignant, by site
    unspecified site (female) C50.91-
      male C50.92-
  embryonal
    liver C22.7
  endometrioid
    specified site — *see* Neoplasm, malignant, by site
    unspecified site
      female C56.9
      male C61
  eosinophil
    specified site — *see* Neoplasm, malignant, by site
    unspecified site C75.1
  epidermoid — *see also* Neoplasm, skin malignant
    in situ, Bowen's type — *see* Neoplasm, skin, in situ
  fibroepithelial, basal cell — *see* Neoplasm, skin, malignant
  follicular
    with papillary (mixed) C73
    moderately differentiated C73
    pure follicle C73
    specified site — *see* Neoplasm, malignant, by site
    trabecular C73
    unspecified site C73
    well differentiated C73

Carcinoma (malignant) - *continued*
  generalized, with unspecified primary site C80.0
  glycogen-rich — *see* Neoplasm, breast, malignant
  granulosa cell C56-
  hepatic cell C22.0
  hepatocellular C22.0
    with bile duct, mixed C22.0
    fibrolamellar C22.0
  hepatocholangiolitic C22.0
  Hurthle cell C73
  in
    adenomatous
      polyposis coli C18.9
    pleomorphic adenoma — *see* Neoplasm, salivary glands, malignant
    situ — *see* Carcinoma-in-situ
  infiltrating
    duct
      with lobular
        specified site — *see* Neoplasm, malignant, by site
        unspecified site (female) C50.91-
          male C50.92-
      with Paget's disease — *see* Neoplasm, breast, malignant
      specified site — *see* Neoplasm, malignant
      unspecified site (female) C50.91-
        male C50.92-
    ductular
      specified site — *see* Neoplasm, malignant
      unspecified site (female) C50.91-
        male C50.92-
    lobular
      specified site — *see* Neoplasm, malignant
      unspecified site (female) C50.91-
        male C50.92-
  inflammatory
    specified site — *see* Neoplasm, malignant
    unspecified site (female) C50.91-
      male C50.92-
  intestinal type
    specified site — *see* Neoplasm, malignant, by site
    unspecified site C16.9
  intracystic
    noninfiltrating — *see* Neoplasm, in situ, by site
  intraductal (noninfiltrating)
    with Paget's disease — *see* Neoplasm, breast, malignant
    breast D05.1-
    papillary
      with invasion
        specified site — *see* Neoplasm, malignant, by site
        unspecified site (female) C50.91-
          male C50.92-
      breast D05.1-
      specified site NEC — *see* Neoplasm, in situ, by site
      unspecified site (female) D05.1-
    specified site NEC — *see* Neoplasm, in situ, by site
    unspecified site (female) D05.1-
  intraepidermal — *see* Neoplasm, in situ
    squamous cell, Bowen's type — *see* Neoplasm, skin, in situ
  intraepithelial — *see* Neoplasm, in situ, by site
    squamous cell — *see* Neoplasm, in situ, by site
  intraosseous C41.1
    upper jaw (bone) C41.0
  islet cell
    with exocrine, mixed
      specified site — *see* Neoplasm, malignant, by site
      unspecified site C25.9
    pancreas C25.4

Carcinoma (malignant) - *continued*
  islet cell - *continued*
    specified site NEC — *see* Neoplasm, malignant, by site
    unspecified site C25.4
  juvenile, breast — *see* Neoplasm, breast, malignant
  large cell
    small cell
      specified site — *see* Neoplasm, malignant, by site
      unspecified site C34.90
  Leydig cell (testis)
    specified site — *see* Neoplasm, malignant, by site
    unspecified site
      female C56.9
      male C62.90
  lipid-rich (female) C50.91-
    male C50.92-
  liver cell C22.0
  liver NEC C22.7
  lobular (infiltrating)
    with intraductal
      specified site — *see* Neoplasm, malignant, by site
      unspecified site (female) C50.91-
        male C50.92-
    noninfiltrating
      breast D05.0-
      specified site NEC — *see* Neoplasm, in situ, by site
      unspecified site D05.0-
    specified site — *see* Neoplasm, malignant, by site
    unspecified site (female) C50.91-
      male C50.92-
  medullary
    with
      amyloid stroma
        specified site — *see* Neoplasm, malignant, by site
        unspecified site C73
      lymphoid stroma
        specified site — *see* Neoplasm, malignant, by site
        unspecified site (female) C50.91-
          male C50.92-
  Merkel cell C4A.9
    anal margin C4A.51
    anal skin C4A.51
    canthus C4A.1-
    ear and external auricular canal C4A.2-
    external auricular canal C4A.2-
    eyelid, including canthus C4A.1-
    face C4A.30
      specified NEC C4A.39
    hip C4A.7-
    lip C4A.0
    lower limb, including hip C4A.7-
    neck C4A.4
    nodal presentation C7B.1
    nose C4A.31
    overlapping sites C4A.8
    perianal skin C4A.51
    scalp C4A.4
    secondary C7B.1
    shoulder C4A.6-
    skin of breast C4A.52
    trunk NEC C4A.59
    upper limb, including shoulder C4A.6-
    visceral metastatic C7B.1
  metastatic — *see* Neoplasm, secondary, by site
  metatypical — *see* Neoplasm, skin, malignant
  morphea, basal cell — *see* Neoplasm, skin, malignant
  mucoid
    cell
      specified site — *see* Neoplasm, malignant, by site
      unspecified site C75.1
  neuroendocrine — *see also* Tumor, neuroendocrine

Carcinoma (malignant) - *continued*
  neuroendocrine - *continued*
    high grade, any site C7A.1
    poorly differentiated, any site C7A.1
  nonencapsulated sclerosing C73
  noninfiltrating
    intracystic — *see* Neoplasm, in situ, by site
    intraductal
      breast D05.1-
      papillary
        breast D05.1-
        specified site NEC — *see* Neoplasm, in situ, by site
        unspecified site D05.1-
      specified site — *see* Neoplasm, in situ, by site
      unspecified site D05.1-
    lobular
      breast D05.0-
      specified site NEC — *see* Neoplasm, in situ, by site
      unspecified site (female) D05.0-
  oat cell
    specified site — *see* Neoplasm, malignant, by site
    unspecified site C34.90
  odontogenic C41.1
    upper jaw (bone) C41.0
  papillary
    with follicular (mixed) C73
    follicular variant C73
    intraductal (noninfiltrating)
      with invasion
        specified site — *see* Neoplasm, malignant, by site
        unspecified site (female) C50.91-
          male C50.92-
      breast D05.1-
      specified site NEC — *see* Neoplasm, in situ, by site
      unspecified site D05.1-
    serous
      specified site — *see* Neoplasm, malignant, by site
      surface
        specified site — *see* Neoplasm, malignant, by site
        unspecified site C56.9
      unspecified site C56.9
  papillocystic
    specified site — *see* Neoplasm, malignant, by site
    unspecified site C56.9
  parafollicular cell
    specified site — *see* Neoplasm, malignant, by site
    unspecified site C73
  pilomatrix — *see* Neoplasm, skin, malignant
  pseudomucinous
    specified site — *see* Neoplasm, malignant, by site
    unspecified site C56.9
  renal cell C64-
  Schmincke — *see* Neoplasm, nasopharynx, malignant
  Schneiderian
    specified site — *see* Neoplasm, malignant, by site
    unspecified site C30.0
  sebaceous — *see* Neoplasm, skin, malignant
  secondary — *see also* Neoplasm, secondary, by site
    Merkel cell C7B.1
  secretory, breast — *see* Neoplasm, breast, malignant
  serous
    papillary
      specified site — *see* Neoplasm, malignant, by site
      unspecified site C56.9
    surface, papillary
      specified site — *see* Neoplasm, malignant, by site
      unspecified site C56.9
  Sertoli cell

Carcinoma (malignant) - *continued*
  Sertoli cell - *continued*
    specified site — *see* Neoplasm, malignant, by site
    unspecified site C62.90
      female C56.9
      male C62.90
  skin appendage — *see* Neoplasm, skin, malignant
  small cell
    fusiform cell
      specified site — *see* Neoplasm, malignant, by site
      unspecified site C34.90
    intermediate cell
      specified site — *see* Neoplasm, malignant, by site
      unspecified site C34.90
    large cell
      specified site — *see* Neoplasm, malignant, by site
      unspecified site C34.90
  solid
    with amyloid stroma
      specified site — *see* Neoplasm, malignant, by site
      unspecified site C73
    microinvasive
      specified site — *see* Neoplasm, malignant, by site
      unspecified site C53.9
  sweat gland — *see* Neoplasm, skin, malignant
  theca cell C56.-
  thymic C37
  unspecified site (primary) C80.1
  water-clear cell C75.0
Carcinoma-in-situ — *see also* Neoplasm, in situ, by site
  breast NOS D05.9-
    specified type NEC D05.8-
  epidermoid — *see also* Neoplasm, in situ, by site
    with questionable stromal invasion
      cervix D06.9
      specified site NEC — *see* Neoplasm, in situ, by site
      unspecified site D06.9
    Bowen's type — *see* Neoplasm, skin, in situ
  intraductal
    breast D05.1-
    specified site NEC — *see* Neoplasm, in situ, by site
    unspecified site D05.1-
  lobular
    with
      infiltrating duct
        breast (female) C50.91-
          male C50.92-
        specified site NEC — *see* Neoplasm, malignant
        unspecified site (female) C50.91-
          male C50.92-
      intraductal
        breast D05.8-
        specified site NEC — *see* Neoplasm, in situ, by site
        unspecified site (female) D05.8-
    breast D05.0-
    specified site NEC — *see* Neoplasm, in situ, by site
    unspecified site D05.0-
  squamous cell — *see also* Neoplasm, in situ, by site
    with questionable stromal invasion
      cervix D06.9
      specified site NEC — *see* Neoplasm, in situ, by site
      unspecified site D06.9
Carcinomaphobia F45.29
Carcinomatosis C80.0
  peritonei C78.6
  unspecified site (primary) (secondary) C80.0

Carcinosarcoma — *see* Neoplasm, malignant, by site
embryonal — *see* Neoplasm, malignant, by site
Cardia, cardial — *see* condition
Cardiac — *see also* condition
death, sudden — *see* Arrest, cardiac
pacemaker
in situ Z95.0
management or adjustment Z45.018
tamponade I31.4
Cardialgia — *see* Pain, precordial
Cardiectasis — *see* Hypertrophy, cardiac
Cardiochalasia K21.9
Cardiomalacia I51.5
Cardiomegalia glycogenica diffusa E74.02 *[I43]*
Cardiomegaly — *see also* Hypertrophy, cardiac
congenital Q24.8
glycogen E74.02 *[I43]*
idiopathic I51.7
Cardiomyoliposis I51.5
Cardiomyopathy (familial) (idiopathic) I42.9
alcoholic I42.6
amyloid E85.4 *[I43]*
transthyretin-related (ATTR) familial E85.4 *[I43]*
arteriosclerotic — *see* Disease, heart, ischemic, atherosclerotic
beriberi E51.12
cobalt-beer I42.6
congenital I42.4
congestive I42.0
constrictive NOS I42.5
dilated I42.0
due to
alcohol I42.6
beriberi E51.12
cardiac glycogenosis E74.02 *[I43]*
drugs I42.7
external agents NEC I42.7
Friedreich's ataxia G11.11
myotonia atrophica G71.11 *[I43]*
progressive muscular dystrophy G71.09 *[I43]*
glycogen storage E74.02 *[I43]*
hypertensive — *see* Hypertension, heart
hypertrophic (nonobstructive) I42.2
obstructive I42.1
congenital Q24.8
in
Chagas' disease (chronic) B57.2
acute B57.0
sarcoidosis D86.85
ischemic I25.5
metabolic E88.9 *[I43]*
thyrotoxic E05.90 *[I43]*
with thyroid storm E05.91 *[I43]*
newborn I42.8
congenital I42.4
non-ischemic — *see also* by cause I42.8
nutritional E63.9 *[I43]*
beriberi E51.12
obscure of Africa I42.8
peripartum O90.3
postpartum O90.3
restrictive NEC I42.5
rheumatic I09.0
secondary I42.9
specified NEC I42.8
stress induced I51.81
takotsubo I51.81
thyrotoxic E05.90 *[I43]*
with thyroid storm E05.91 *[I43]*
toxic NEC I42.7
transthyretin-related (ATTR) familial amyloid E85.4
tuberculous A18.84
viral B33.24
Cardionephritis — *see* Hypertension, cardiorenal
Cardionephropathy — *see* Hypertension, cardiorenal
Cardionephrosis — *see* Hypertension, cardiorenal
Cardiopathia nigra I27.0
Cardiopathy — *see also* Disease, heart I51.9
idiopathic I42.9
mucopolysaccharidosis E76.3 *[I52]*
Cardiopericarditis — *see* Pericarditis
Cardiophobia F45.29
Cardiorenal — *see* condition
Cardiorrhexis — *see* Infarct, myocardium
Cardiosclerosis — *see* Disease, heart, ischemic, atherosclerotic
Cardiosis — *see* Disease, heart
Cardiospasm (esophagus) (reflex) (stomach) K22.0
congenital Q39.5
with megaesophagus Q39.5
Cardiostenosis — *see* Disease, heart
Cardiosymphysis I31.0
Cardiovascular — *see* condition
Carditis (acute) (bacterial) (chronic) (subacute) I51.89
meningococcal A39.50
rheumatic — *see* Disease, heart, rheumatic
rheumatoid — *see* Rheumatoid, carditis
viral B33.20
Care (of) (for) (following)
child (routine) Z76.2
family member (handicapped) (sick)
creating problem for family Z63.6
provided away from home for holiday relief Z75.5
unavailable, due to
absence (person rendering care) (sufferer) Z74.2
inability (any reason) of person rendering care Z74.2
foundling Z76.1
holiday relief Z75.5
improper — *see* Maltreatment
lack of (at or after birth) (infant) — *see* Maltreatment, child, neglect
lactating mother Z39.1
palliative Z51.5
postpartum
immediately after delivery Z39.0
routine follow-up Z39.2
respite Z75.5
unavailable, due to
absence of person rendering care Z74.2
inability (any reason) of person rendering care Z74.2
well-baby Z76.2
Caries
bone NEC A18.03
dental (dentino enamel junction) (early childhood) (of dentine) (pre-eruptive) (recurrent) (to the pulp) K02.9
arrested (coronal) (root) K02.3
chewing surface
limited to enamel K02.51
penetrating into dentin K02.52
penetrating into pulp K02.53
coronal surface
chewing surface
limited to enamel K02.51
penetrating into dentin K02.52
penetrating into pulp K02.53
pit and fissure surface
limited to enamel K02.51
penetrating into dentin K02.52
penetrating into pulp K02.53
smooth surface
limited to enamel K02.61
penetrating into dentin K02.62
penetrating into pulp K02.63
pit and fissure surface
limited to enamel K02.51
penetrating into dentin K02.52
penetrating into pulp K02.53
primary, cervical origin K02.52
root K02.7
smooth surface
limited to enamel K02.61
penetrating into dentin K02.62
Caries - *continued*
dental (dentino enamel junction) (early childhood) (of dentine) (pre-eruptive) (recurrent) (to the pulp) - *continued*
smooth surface - *continued*
penetrating into pulp K02.63
external meatus — *see* Disorder, ear, external, specified type NEC
hip (tuberculous) A18.02
initial (tooth)
chewing surface K02.51
pit and fissure surface K02.51
smooth surface K02.61
knee (tuberculous) A18.02
labyrinth — *see* subcategory H83.8
limb NEC (tuberculous) A18.03
mastoid process (chronic) — *see* Mastoiditis, chronic
tuberculous A18.03
middle ear — *see* subcategory H74.8
nose (tuberculous) A18.03
orbit (tuberculous) A18.03
ossicles, ear — *see* Abnormal, ear ossicles
petrous bone — *see* Petrositis
root (dental) (tooth) K02.7
sacrum (tuberculous) A18.01
spine, spinal (column) (tuberculous) A18.01
syphilitic A52.77
congenital (early) A50.02 *[M90.80]*
tooth, teeth — *see* Caries, dental
tuberculous A18.03
vertebra (column) (tuberculous) A18.01
Carious teeth — *see* Caries, dental
Carneous mole O02.0
Carnitine insufficiency E71.40
Carotenemia (dietary) E67.1
Carotenosis (cutis) (skin) E67.1
Carotid body or sinus syndrome G90.01
Carotidynia G90.01
Carpal tunnel syndrome — *see* Syndrome, carpal tunnel
Carpenter's syndrome Q87.0
Carpopedal spasm — *see* Tetany
Carr-Barr-Plunkett syndrome Q97.1
Carrier (suspected) of
amebiasis Z22.1
bacterial disease NEC Z22.39
diphtheria Z22.2
intestinal infectious NEC Z22.1
typhoid Z22.0
meningococcal Z22.31
sexually transmitted Z22.4
specified NEC Z22.39
staphylococcal (Methicillin susceptible) Z22.321
Methicillin resistant Z22.322
streptococcal Z22.338
group B Z22.330
complicating pregnancy or delivery O99.82-
typhoid Z22.0
cholera Z22.1
diphtheria Z22.2
gastrointestinal pathogens NEC Z22.1
genetic Z14.8
cystic fibrosis Z14.1
hemophilia A (asymptomatic) Z14.01
symptomatic Z14.02
gestational, pregnant Z33.1
gonorrhea Z22.4
HAA (hepatitis Australian-antigen) B18.8
HB (c) (s) -AG B18.1
hepatitis (viral) B18.9
Australia-antigen (HAA) B18.8
B surface antigen (HBsAg) B18.1
with acute delta- (super) infection B17.0
C B18.2
specified NEC B18.8
human T-cell lymphotropic virus type-1 (HTLV-1) infection Z22.6
infectious organism Z22.9
specified NEC Z22.8
meningococci Z22.31
Salmonella typhosa Z22.0
serum hepatitis — *see* Carrier, hepatitis

Carrier (suspected) of - *continued*
staphylococci (Methicillin susceptible) Z22.321
Methicillin resistant Z22.322
streptococci Z22.338
group B Z22.330
complicating pregnancy or delivery O99.82-
syphilis Z22.4
typhoid Z22.0
venereal disease NEC Z22.4
Carrion's disease A44.0
Carter's relapsing fever (Asiatic) A68.1
Cartilage — *see* condition
Caruncle (inflamed)
conjunctiva (acute) — *see* Conjunctivitis, acute
labium (majus) (minus) N90.89
lacrimal — *see* Inflammation, lacrimal, passages
myrtiform N89.8
urethral (benign) N36.2
Cascade stomach K31.2
Caseation lymphatic gland (tuberculous) A18.2
Cassidy (-Scholte) syndrome (malignant carcinoid) E34.0
Castellani's disease A69.8
Castration, traumatic, male S38.231
Casts in urine R82.998
Cat
cry syndrome Q93.4
ear Q17.3
eye syndrome Q92.8
Catabolism, senile R54
Catalepsy (hysterical) F44.2
schizophrenic F20.2
Cataplexy (idiopathic) — *see* - Narcolepsy
Cataract (cortical) (immature) (incipient) H26.9
with
neovascularization — *see* Cataract, complicated
age-related — *see* Cataract, senile
anterior
and posterior axial embryonal Q12.0
pyramidal Q12.0
associated with
galactosemia E74.21 *[H28]*
myotonic disorders G71.19 *[H28]*
blue Q12.0
central Q12.0
cerulean Q12.0
complicated H26.20
with
neovascularization H26.21-
ocular disorder H26.22-
glaucomatous flecks H26.23-
congenital Q12.0
coraliform Q12.0
coronary Q12.0
crystalline Q12.0
diabetic — *see* Diabetes, cataract
drug-induced H26.3-
due to
ocular disorder — *see* Cataract, complicated
radiation H26.8
electric H26.8
extraction status Z98.4-
glass-blower's H26.8
heat ray H26.8
heterochromic — *see* Cataract, complicated
hypermature — *see* Cataract, senile, morgagnian type
in (due to)
chronic iridocyclitis — *see* Cataract, complicated
diabetes — *see* Diabetes, cataract
endocrine disease E34.9 *[H28]*
eye disease — *see* Cataract, complicated
hypoparathyroidism E20.9 *[H28]*
malnutrition-dehydration E46 *[H28]*
metabolic disease E88.9 *[H28]*
myotonic disorders G71.19 *[H28]*

Cataract (cortical) (immature) (incipient) - *continued*
in (due to) - *continued*
nutritional disease E63.9 *[H28]*
infantile — *see* Cataract, presenile
irradiational — *see* Cataract, specified NEC
juvenile — *see* Cataract, presenile
malnutrition-dehydration E46 *[H28]*
morgagnian — *see* Cataract, senile, morgagnian type
myotonic G71.19 *[H28]*
myxedema E03.9 *[H28]*
nuclear
embryonal Q12.0
sclerosis — *see* Cataract, senile, nuclear
presenile H26.00-
combined forms H26.06-
cortical H26.01-
lamellar — *see* Cataract, presenile, cortical
nuclear H26.03-
specified NEC H26.09
subcapsular polar (anterior) H26.04-
posterior H26.05-
zonular — *see* Cataract, presenile, cortical
secondary H26.40
Soemmering's ring H26.41-
specified NEC H26.49-
to eye disease — *see* Cataract, complicated
senile H25.9
brunescens — *see* Cataract, senile, nuclear
combined forms H25.81-
coronary — *see* Cataract, senile, incipient
cortical H25.01-
hypermature — *see* Cataract, senile, morgagnian type
incipient (mature) (total) H25.09-
cortical — *see* Cataract, senile, cortical
subcapsular — *see* Cataract, senile, subcapsular
morgagnian type (hypermature) H25.2-
nuclear (sclerosis) H25.1-
polar subcapsular (anterior) (posterior) — *see* Cataract, senile, incipient
punctate — *see* Cataract, senile, incipient
specified NEC H25.89
subcapsular polar (anterior) H25.03-
posterior H25.04-
snowflake — *see* Diabetes, cataract
specified NEC H26.8
toxic — *see* Cataract, drug-induced
traumatic H26.10-
localized H26.11-
partially resolved H26.12-
total H26.13-
zonular (perinuclear) Q12.0
Cataracta — *see also* Cataract
brunescens — *see* Cataract, senile, nuclear
centralis pulverulenta Q12.0
cerulea Q12.0
complicata — *see* Cataract, complicated
congenita Q12.0
coralliformis Q12.0
coronaria Q12.0
diabetic — *see* Diabetes, cataract
membranacea
accreta — *see* Cataract, secondary
congenita Q12.0
nigra — *see* Cataract, senile, nuclear
sunflower — *see* Cataract, complicated
Catarrh, catarrhal (acute) (febrile) (infectious) (inflammation) — *see also* condition J00
bronchial — *see* Bronchitis
chest — *see* Bronchitis
chronic J31.0
due to congenital syphilis A50.03
enteric — *see* Enteritis
eustachian H68.009
fauces — *see* Pharyngitis
gastrointestinal — *see* Enteritis
gingivitis K05.00
nonplaque induced K05.01
plaque induced K05.00
hay — *see* Fever, hay
intestinal — *see* Enteritis

Catarrh, catarrhal (acute) (febrile) (infectious) (inflammation) - *continued*
larynx, chronic J37.0
liver B15.9
with hepatic coma B15.0
lung — *see* Bronchitis
middle ear, chronic — *see* Otitis, media, nonsuppurative, chronic, serous
mouth K12.1
nasal (chronic) — *see* Rhinitis
nasobronchial J31.1
nasopharyngeal (chronic) J31.1
acute J00
pulmonary — *see* Bronchitis
spring (eye) (vernal) — *see* Conjunctivitis, acute, atopic
summer (hay) — *see* Fever, hay
throat J31.2
tubotympanal — *see also* Otitis, media, nonsuppurative
chronic — *see* Otitis, media, nonsuppurative, chronic, serous
Catatonia (schizophrenic) F20.2
Catatonic
disorder due to known physiologic condition F06.1
schizophrenia F20.2
stupor R40.1
Cat-scratch — *see also* Abrasion
disease or fever A28.1
Cauda equina — *see* condition
Cauliflower ear M95.1-
Causalgia (upper limb) G56.4-
lower limb G57.7-
Cause
external, general effects T75.89
Caustic burn — *see* Corrosion, by site
Cavare's disease (familial periodic paralysis) G72.3
Cave-in, injury
crushing (severe) — *see* Crush
suffocation — *see* Asphyxia, traumatic, due to low oxygen, due to cave-in
Cavernitis (penis) N48.29
Cavernositis N48.29
Cavernous — *see* condition
Cavitation of lung — *see also* Tuberculosis, pulmonary
nontuberculous J98.4
Cavities, dental — *see* Caries, dental
Cavity
lung — *see* Cavitation of lung
optic papilla Q14.2
pulmonary — *see* Cavitation of lung
Cavovarus foot, congenital Q66.1-
Cavus foot (congenital) Q66.7-
acquired — *see* Deformity, limb, foot, specified NEC
Cazenave's disease L10.2
CDKL5 (Cyclin-Dependent Kinase-Like 5 Deficiency Disorder) G40.42
Cecitis K52.9
with perforation, peritonitis, or rupture K65.8
Cecoureterocele Q62.32
Cecum — *see* condition
Celiac
artery compression syndrome I77.4
disease (with steatorrhea) K90.0
infantilism K90.0
Cell (s) , cellular — *see also* condition
in urine R82.998
Cellulitis (diffuse) (phlegmonous) (septic) (suppurative) L03.90
abdominal wall L03.311
anaerobic A48.0
ankle — *see* Cellulitis, lower limb
anus K61.0
arm — *see* Cellulitis, upper limb
auricle (ear) — *see* Cellulitis, ear
axilla L03.11-
back (any part) L03.312
breast (acute) (nonpuerperal) (subacute) N61.0
nipple N61.0
broad ligament

Chancre (any genital site) (hard) (hunterian) (mixed) (primary) (seronegative) (seropositive) (syphilitic) A51.0
congenital A50.07
conjunctiva NEC A51.2
Ducrey's A57
extragenital A51.2
eyelid A51.2
lip A51.2
nipple A51.2
Nisbet's A57
of
carate A67.0
pinta A67.0
yaws A66.0
palate, soft A51.2
phagedenic A57
simple A57
soft A57
bubo A57
palate A51.2
urethra A51.0
yaws A66.0
Chancroid (anus) (genital) (penis) (perineum) (rectum) (urethra) (vulva) A57
Chandler's disease (osteochondritis dissecans, hip) — *see* Osteochondritis, dissecans, hip
Change (s) (in) (of) — *see also* Removal
arteriosclerotic — *see* Arteriosclerosis
bone — *see also* Disorder, bone
diabetic — *see* Diabetes, bone change
bowel habit R19.4
cardiorenal (vascular) — *see* Hypertension, cardiorenal
cardiovascular — *see* Disease, cardiovascular
circulatory I99.9
cognitive (mild) (organic) R41.89
color, tooth, teeth
during formation K00.8
posteruptive K03.7
contraceptive device Z30.433
corneal membrane H18.30
Bowman's membrane fold or rupture H18.31-
Descemet's membrane
fold H18.32-
rupture H18.33-
coronary — *see* Disease, heart, ischemic
degenerative, spine or vertebra — *see* Spondylosis
dental pulp, regressive K04.2
dressing (nonsurgical) Z48.00
surgical Z48.01
heart — *see* Disease, heart
hip joint — *see* Derangement, joint, hip
hyperplastic larynx J38.7
hypertrophic
nasal sinus J34.89
turbinate, nasal J34.3
upper respiratory tract J39.8
indwelling catheter Z46.6
inflammatory — *see also* Inflammation
sacroiliac M46.1
job, anxiety concerning Z56.1
joint — *see* Derangement, joint
life — *see* Menopause
mental status R41.82
minimal (glomerular) — *see also* N00-N07 with fourth character .0 N05.0
myocardium, myocardial — *see* Degeneration, myocardial
of life — *see* Menopause
pacemaker Z45.018
pulse generator Z45.010
personality (enduring) F68.8
due to (secondary to)
general medical condition F07.0
secondary (nonspecific) F60.89
regressive, dental pulp K04.2
renal — *see* Disease, renal
retina H35.9

Change (s) (in) (of) - *continued*
retina - *continued*
myopic — *see also* Myopia, degenerative H44.2-
sacroiliac joint M53.3
senile — *see also* condition R54
sensory R20.8
skin R23.9
acute, due to ultraviolet radiation L56.9
specified NEC L56.8
chronic, due to nonionizing radiation L57.9
specified NEC L57.8
cyanosis R23.0
flushing R23.2
pallor R23.1
petechiae R23.3
specified change NEC R23.8
swelling — *see* Mass, localized
texture R23.4
trophic
arm — *see* Mononeuropathy, upper limb
leg — *see* Mononeuropathy, lower limb
vascular I99.9
vasomotor I73.9
voice R49.9
psychogenic F44.4
specified NEC R49.8
Changing sleep-work schedule, affecting sleep G47.26
Changuinola fever A93.1
Chapping skin T69.8
Charcot-Marie-Tooth disease, paralysis or syndrome G60.0
Charcot's
arthropathy — *see* Arthropathy, neuropathic
cirrhosis K74.3
disease (tabetic arthropathy) A52.16
joint (disease) (tabetic) A52.16
diabetic — *see* Diabetes, with, arthropathy
syringomyelic G95.0
syndrome (intermittent claudication) I73.9
CHARGE association Q89.8
Charley-horse (quadriceps) M62.831
traumatic (quadriceps) S76.11-
Charlouis' disease — *see* Yaws
Cheadle's disease E54
Checking (of)
cardiac pacemaker (battery) (electrode (s)) Z45.018
pulse generator Z45.010
implantable subdermal contraceptive Z30.46
intrauterine contraceptive device Z30.431
wound Z48.0-
due to injury - code to Injury, by site, using appropriate seventh character for subsequent encounter
Check-up — *see* Examination
Chédiak-Higashi (-Steinbrinck) syndrome (congenital gigantism of peroxidase granules) E70.330
Cheek — *see* condition
Cheese itch B88.0
Cheese-washer's lung J67.8
Cheese-worker's lung J67.8
Cheilitis (acute) (angular) (catarrhal) (chronic) (exfoliative) (gangrenous) (glandular) (infectional) (suppurative) (ulcerative) (vesicular) K13.0
actinic (due to sun) L56.8
other than from sun L59.8
candidal B37.83
Cheilodynia K13.0
Cheiloschisis — *see* Cleft, lip
Cheilosis (angular) K13.0
with pellagra E52
due to
vitamin B2 (riboflavin) deficiency E53.0
Cheiromegaly M79.89
Cheiropompholyx L30.1
Cheloid — *see* Keloid
Chemical burn — *see* Corrosion, by site
Chemodectoma — *see* Paraganglioma, nonchromaffin

Chemosis, conjunctiva — *see* Edema, conjunctiva
Chemotherapy (session) (for)
cancer Z51.11
neoplasm Z51.11
Cherubism M27.8
Chest — *see* condition
Cheyne-Stokes breathing (respiration) R06.3
Chiari's
disease or syndrome (hepatic vein thrombosis) I82.0
malformation
type I G93.5
type II — *see* Spina bifida
net Q24.8
Chicago disease B40.9
Chickenpox — *see* Varicella
Chiclero ulcer or sore B55.1
Chigger (infestation) B88.0
Chignon (disease) B36.8
newborn (from vacuum extraction) (birth injury) P12.1
Chilaiditi's syndrome (subphrenic displacement, colon) Q43.3
Chilblain (s) (lupus) T69.1
Child
custody dispute Z65.3
Childbirth — *see* Delivery
Childhood
cerebral X-linked adrenoleukodystrophy E71.520
period of rapid growth Z00.2
Chill (s) R68.83
with fever R50.9
congestive in malarial regions B54
without fever R68.83
Chilomastigiasis A07.8
Chimera 46,XX/46,XY Q99.0
Chin — *see* condition
Chinese dysentery A03.9
Chionophobia F40.228
Chitral fever A93.1
Chlamydia, chlamydial A74.9
cervicitis A56.09
conjunctivitis A74.0
cystitis A56.01
endometritis A56.11
epididymitis A56.19
female
pelvic inflammatory disease A56.11
pelviperitonitis A56.11
orchitis A56.19
peritonitis A74.81
pharyngitis A56.4
proctitis A56.3
psittaci (infection) A70
salpingitis A56.11
sexually-transmitted infection NEC A56.8
specified NEC A74.89
urethritis A56.01
vulvovaginitis A56.02
Chlamydiosis — *see* Chlamydia
Chloasma (skin) (idiopathic) (symptomatic) L81.1
eyelid H02.719
hyperthyroid E05.90 *[H02.719]*
with thyroid storm E05.91 *[H02.719]*
left H02.716
lower H02.715
upper H02.714
right H02.713
lower H02.712
upper H02.711
Chloroma C92.3-
Chlorosis D50.9
Egyptian B76.9 *[D63.8]*
miner's B76.9 *[D63.8]*
Chlorotic anemia D50.8
Chocolate cyst (ovary) N80.1
Choked
disc or disk — *see* Papilledema
on food, phlegm, or vomitus NOS — *see* Foreign body, by site
while vomiting NOS — *see* Foreign body, by site

Cirrhosis, cirrhotic (hepatic) (liver) - *continued*
fatty K76.0
alcoholic K70.0
Hanot's (hypertrophic) K74.3
hepatic — *see* Cirrhosis, liver
hypertrophic K74.3
Indian childhood K74.69
kidney — *see* Sclerosis, renal
Laennec's K70.30
with ascites K70.31
alcoholic K70.30
with ascites K70.31
nonalcoholic K74.69
liver K74.60
alcoholic K70.30
with ascites K70.31
fatty K70.0
congenital P78.81
syphilitic A52.74
lung (chronic) J84.10
macronodular K74.69
alcoholic K70.30
with ascites K70.31
micronodular K74.69
alcoholic K70.30
with ascites K70.31
mixed type K74.69
monolobular K74.3
nephritis — *see* Sclerosis, renal
nutritional K74.69
alcoholic K70.30
with ascites K70.31
obstructive — *see* Cirrhosis, biliary
ovarian N83.8
pancreas (duct) K86.89
pigmentary E83.110
portal K74.69
alcoholic K70.30
with ascites K70.31
postnecrotic K74.69
alcoholic K70.30
with ascites K70.31
pulmonary J84.10
renal — *see* Sclerosis, renal
spleen D73.2
stasis K76.1
Todd's K74.3
unilobar K74.3
xanthomatous (biliary) K74.5
due to xanthomatosis (familial) (metabolic) (primary) E78.2
Cistern, subarachnoid R93.0
Citrullinemia E72.23
Citrullinuria E72.23
Civatte's disease or poikiloderma L57.3
Clam digger's itch B65.3
Clammy skin R23.1
Clap — *see* Gonorrhea
Clarke-Hadfield syndrome (pancreatic infantilism) K86.89
Clark's paralysis G80.9
Clastothrix L67.8
Claude Bernard-Horner syndrome G90.2
traumatic — *see* Injury, nerve, cervical sympathetic
Claude's disease or syndrome G46.3
Claudicatio venosa intermittens I87.8
Claudication (intermittent) I73.9
cerebral (artery) G45.9
spinal cord (arteriosclerotic) G95.19
syphilitic A52.09
venous (axillary) I87.8
Claustrophobia F40.240
Clavus (infected) L84
Clawfoot (congenital) Q66.89
acquired — *see* Deformity, limb, clawfoot
Clawhand (acquired) — *see also* Deformity, limb, clawhand
congenital Q68.1
Clawtoe (congenital) Q66.89
acquired — *see* Deformity, toe, specified NEC
Clay eating — *see* Pica
Cleansing of artificial opening — *see* Attention to, artificial, opening
Cleft (congenital) — *see also* Imperfect, closure
alveolar process M26.79
branchial (persistent) Q18.2
cyst Q18.0
fistula Q18.0
sinus Q18.0
cricoid cartilage, posterior Q31.8
foot Q72.7
hand Q71.6
lip (unilateral) Q36.9
with cleft palate Q37.9
hard Q37.1
with soft Q37.5
soft Q37.3
with hard Q37.5
bilateral Q36.0
with cleft palate Q37.8
hard Q37.0
with soft Q37.4
soft Q37.2
with hard Q37.4
median Q36.1
nose Q30.2
palate Q35.9
with cleft lip (unilateral) Q37.9
bilateral Q37.8
hard Q35.1
with
cleft lip (unilateral) Q37.1
bilateral Q37.0
soft Q35.5
with cleft lip (unilateral) Q37.5
bilateral Q37.4
medial Q35.5
soft Q35.3
with
cleft lip (unilateral) Q37.3
bilateral Q37.2
hard Q35.5
with cleft lip (unilateral) Q37.5
bilateral Q37.4
penis Q55.69
scrotum Q55.29
thyroid cartilage Q31.8
uvula Q35.7
Cleidocranial dysostosis Q74.0
Cleptomania F63.2
Clicking hip (newborn) R29.4
Climacteric (female) — *see also* Menopause
arthritis (any site) NEC — *see* Arthritis, specified form NEC
depression (single episode) F32.89
recurrent episode F33.8
melancholia (single episode) F32.89
recurrent episode F33.8
male (symptoms) (syndrome) NEC N50.89
paranoid state F22
polyarthritis NEC — *see* Arthritis, specified form NEC
symptoms (female) N95.1
Clinical research investigation (clinical trial) (control subject) (normal comparison) (participant) Z00.6
Clitoris — *see* condition
Cloaca (persistent) Q43.7
Clonorchiasis, clonorchis infection (liver) B66.1
Clonus R25.8
Closed bite M26.29
Clostridium (C.) perfringens, as cause of disease classified elsewhere B96.7
Closure
congenital, nose Q30.0
cranial sutures, premature Q75.0
defective or imperfect NEC — *see* Imperfect, closure
fistula, delayed — *see* Fistula
foramen ovale, imperfect Q21.1
hymen N89.6
interauricular septum, defective Q21.1
interventricular septum, defective Q21.0
Closure - *continued*
lacrimal duct — *see also* Stenosis, lacrimal, duct
congenital Q10.5
nose (congenital) Q30.0
acquired M95.0
of artificial opening — *see* Attention to, artificial, opening
primary angle, without glaucoma damage H40.06-
vagina N89.5
valve — *see* Endocarditis
vulva N90.5
Clot (blood) — *see also* Embolism
artery (obstruction) (occlusion) — *see* Embolism
bladder N32.89
brain (intradural or extradural) — *see* Occlusion, artery, cerebral
circulation I74.9
heart — *see also* Infarct, myocardium
not resulting in infarction I51.3
vein — *see* Thrombosis
Clouded state R40.1
epileptic — *see* Epilepsy, specified NEC
paroxysmal — *see* Epilepsy, specified NEC
Cloudy antrum, antra J32.0
Clouston's (hidrotic) ectodermal dysplasia Q82.4
Clubbed nail
pachydermoperiostosis M89.40 *[L62]*
Clubbing of finger (s) (nails) R68.3
Clubfinger R68.3
congenital Q68.1
Clubfoot (congenital) Q66.89
acquired — *see* Deformity, limb, clubfoot
equinovarus Q66.0-
paralytic — *see* Deformity, limb, clubfoot
Clubhand (congenital) (radial) Q71.4-
acquired — *see* Deformity, limb, clubhand
Clubnail R68.3
congenital Q84.6
Clump, kidney Q63.1
Clumsiness, clumsy child syndrome F82
Cluttering F80.81
Clutton's joints A50.51 *[M12.80]*
Coagulation, intravascular (diffuse) (disseminated) — *see also* Defibrination syndrome
complicating abortion — *see* Abortion, by type, complicated by, intravascular coagulation
following ectopic or molar pregnancy O08.1
Coagulopathy — *see also* Defect, coagulation
consumption D65
intravascular D65
newborn P60
Coalition
calcaneo-scaphoid Q66.89
tarsal Q66.89
Coalminer's
elbow — *see* Bursitis, elbow, olecranon
lung or pneumoconiosis J60
Coalworker's lung or pneumoconiosis J60
Coarctation
aorta (preductal) (postductal) Q25.1
pulmonary artery Q25.71
Coated tongue K14.3
Coats' disease (exudative retinopathy) — *see* Retinopathy, exudative
Cocaine-induced
anxiety disorder F14.980
bipolar and related disorder F14.94
depressive disorder F14.94
obsessive-compulsive and related disorder F14.988
psychotic disorder F14.959
sleep disorder F14.982
sexual dysfunction F14.981
Cocainism — *see* Disorder, cocaine use
Coccidioidomycosis B38.9
cutaneous B38.3
disseminated B38.7
generalized B38.7
meninges B38.4

Collapse - *continued*
vertebra M48.50-
cervical region M48.52-
cervicothoracic region M48.53-
in (due to)
metastasis — *see* Collapse, vertebra, in, specified disease NEC
osteoporosis — *see also* Osteoporosis M80.88
cervical region M80.88
cervicothoracic region M80.88
lumbar region M80.88
lumbosacral region M80.88
multiple sites M80.88
occipito-atlanto-axial region M80.88
sacrococcygeal region M80.88
thoracic region M80.88
thoracolumbar region M80.88
specified disease NEC M48.50-
cervical region M48.52-
cervicothoracic region M48.53-
lumbar region M48.56-
lumbosacral region M48.57-
occipito-atlanto-axial region M48.51-
sacrococcygeal region M48.58-
thoracic region M48.54-
thoracolumbar region M48.55-
lumbar region M48.56-
lumbosacral region M48.57-
occipito-atlanto-axial region M48.51-
sacrococcygeal region M48.58-
thoracic region M48.54-
thoracolumbar region M48.55-
Collateral — *see also* condition
circulation (venous) I87.8
dilation, veins I87.8
Colles' fracture S52.53-
Collet (-Sicard) syndrome G52.7
Collier's asthma or lung J60
Collodion baby Q80.2
Colloid nodule (of thyroid) (cystic) E04.1
Coloboma (iris) Q13.0
eyelid Q10.3
fundus Q14.8
lens Q12.2
optic disc (congenital) Q14.2
acquired H47.31-
Coloenteritis — *see* Enteritis
Colon — *see* condition
Colonization
MRSA (Methicillin resistant Staphylococcus aureus) Z22.322
MSSA (Methicillin susceptible Staphylococcus aureus) Z22.321
status — *see* Carrier (suspected) of
Coloptosis K63.4
Color blindness — *see* Deficiency, color vision
Colostomy
attention to Z43.3
fitting or adjustment Z46.89
malfunctioning K94.03
status Z93.3
Colpitis (acute) — *see* Vaginitis
Colpocele N81.5
Colpocystitis — *see* Vaginitis
Colpospasm N94.2
Column, spinal, vertebral — *see* condition
Coma R40.20
with
motor response (none) R40.231
abnormal R40.233
abnormal extensor posturing to pain or noxious stimuli (< 2 years of age) R40.232
abnormal flexure posturing to pain or noxious stimuli (0-5 years of age) R40.233
extension R40.232
extensor posturing to pain or noxious stimuli (2-5 years of age) R40.232
flexion/decorticate posturing (< 2 years of age) R40.233
flexion withdrawal R40.234
localizes pain (2-5 years of age) R40.235

Coma - *continued*
with - *continued*
motor response (none) - *continued*
normal or spontaneous movement (< 2 years of age) R40.236
obeys commands (2-5 years of age) R40.236
score of
1 R40.231
2 R40.232
3 R40.233
4 R40.234
5 R40.235
6 R40.236
withdraws from pain or noxious stimuli (0-5 years of age) R40.234
withdraws to touch (< 2 years of age) R40.235
opening of eyes (never) R40.211
in response to
pain R40.212
sound R40.213
score of
1 R40.211
2 R40.212
3 R40.213
4 R40.214
spontaneous R40.214
verbal response (none) R40.221
confused conversation R40.224
cooing or babbling or crying appropriately (< 2 years of age) R40.225
inappropriate crying or screaming (< 2 years of age) R40.223
inappropriate words R40.223
inappropriate words (2-5 years of age) R40.224
incomprehensible sounds (2-5 years of age) R40.222
incomprehensible words R40.222
irritable cries (< 2 years of age) R40.224
moans/grunts to pain; restless (< 2 years old) R40.222
oriented R40.225
score of
1 R40.221
2 R40.222
3 R40.223
4 R40.224
5 R40.225
screaming (2-5 years of age) R40.223
uses appropriate words (2- 5 years of age) R40.225
eclamptic — *see* Eclampsia
epileptic — *see* Epilepsy
Glasgow, scale score — *see* Glasgow coma scale
hepatic — *see* Failure, hepatic, by type, with coma
hyperglycemic (diabetic) — *see* Diabetes, by type, with hyperosmolarity, with coma
hyperosmolar (diabetic) — *see* Diabetes, by type, with hyperosmolarity, with coma
hypoglycemic (diabetic) — *see* Diabetes, by type, with hypoglycemia, with coma
nondiabetic E15
in diabetes — *see* Diabetes, coma
insulin-induced — *see* Coma, hypoglycemic
ketoacidotic (diabetic) — *see* Diabetes, by type, with ketoacidosis, with coma
myxedematous E03.5
newborn P91.5
persistent vegetative state R40.3
specified NEC, without documented Glasgow coma scale score, or with partial Glasgow coma scale score reported R40.244
Comatose — *see* Coma
Combat fatigue F43.0
Combined — *see* condition
Comedo, comedones (giant) L70.0
Comedocarcinoma — *see also* Neoplasm, breast, malignant
noninfiltrating

Comedocarcinoma - *continued*
noninfiltrating - *continued*
breast D05.8-
specified site — *see* Neoplasm, in situ, by site
unspecified site D05.8-
Comedomastitis — *see* Ectasia, mammary duct
Comminuted fracture - code as Fracture, closed
Common
arterial trunk Q20.0
atrioventricular canal Q21.2
atrium Q21.1
cold (head) J00
truncus (arteriosus) Q20.0
variable immunodeficiency — *see* Immunodeficiency, common variable
ventricle Q20.4
Commotio, commotion (current)
brain — *see* Injury, intracranial, concussion
cerebri — *see* Injury, intracranial, concussion
retinae S05.8X-
spinal cord — *see* Injury, spinal cord, by region
spinalis — *see* Injury, spinal cord, by region
Communication
between
base of aorta and pulmonary artery Q21.4
left ventricle and right atrium Q20.5
pericardial sac and pleural sac Q34.8
pulmonary artery and pulmonary vein, congenital Q25.72
congenital between uterus and digestive or urinary tract Q51.7
Compartment syndrome (deep) (posterior) (traumatic) T79.A0
abdomen T79.A3
lower extremity (hip, buttock, thigh, leg, foot, toes) T79.A2
nontraumatic
abdomen M79.A3
lower extremity (hip, buttock, thigh, leg, foot, toes) M79.A2-
specified site NEC M79.A9
upper extremity (shoulder, arm, forearm, wrist, hand, fingers) M79.A1-
specified site NEC T79.A9
upper extremity (shoulder, arm, forearm, wrist, hand, fingers) T79.A1
Compensation
failure — *see* Disease, heart
neurosis, psychoneurosis — *see* Disorder, factitious
Complaint — *see also* Disease
bowel, functional K59.9
psychogenic F45.8
intestine, functional K59.9
psychogenic F45.8
kidney — *see* Disease, renal
miners' J60
Complete — *see* condition
Complex
Addison-Schilder E71.528
cardiorenal — *see* Hypertension, cardiorenal
Costen's M26.69
disseminated mycobacterium avium-intracellulare (DMAC) A31.2
Eisenmenger's (ventricular septal defect) I27.83
hypersexual F52.8
jumped process, spine — *see* Dislocation, vertebra
primary, tuberculous A15.7
Schilder-Addison E71.528
subluxation (vertebral) M99.19
abdomen M99.19
acromioclavicular M99.17
cervical region M99.11
cervicothoracic M99.11
costochondral M99.18
costovertebral M99.18
head region M99.10
hip M99.15
lower extremity M99.16

- **Complication (s) (from) (of)** - *continued*
  - bone - *continued*
    - device NEC - *continued*
      - mechanical - *continued*
        - obstruction T84.398
        - perforation T84.398
        - protrusion T84.398
      - pain T84.84
      - specified type NEC T84.89
      - stenosis T84.85
      - thrombosis T84.86
    - graft — *see* Complications, graft, bone
    - growth stimulator (electrode) — *see* Complications, electronic stimulator device, bone
    - marrow transplant — *see* Complications, transplant, bone, marrow
  - brain neurostimulator (electrode) — *see* Complications, electronic stimulator device, brain
  - breast implant (prosthetic) T85.9
    - capsular contracture T85.44
    - embolism T85.818
    - fibrosis T85.828
    - hemorrhage T85.838
    - infection and inflammation T85.79
    - mechanical
      - breakdown T85.41
      - displacement T85.42
      - leakage T85.43
      - malposition T85.42
      - obstruction T85.49
      - perforation T85.49
      - protrusion T85.49
      - specified NEC T85.49
    - pain T85.848
    - specified type NEC T85.898
    - stenosis T85.858
    - thrombosis T85.868
  - bypass — *see also* Complications, prosthetic device or implant
    - aortocoronary — *see* Complications, coronary artery (bypass) graft
    - arterial — *see also* Complications, graft, vascular
      - extremity — *see* Complications, extremity artery (bypass) graft
  - cardiac — *see also* Disease, heart
    - device, implant or graft T82.9
      - embolism T82.817
      - fibrosis T82.827
      - hemorrhage T82.837
      - infection or inflammation T82.7
        - valve prosthesis T82.6
      - mechanical
        - breakdown T82.519
          - specified device NEC T82.518
        - displacement T82.529
          - specified device NEC T82.528
        - leakage T82.539
          - specified device NEC T82.538
        - malposition T82.529
          - specified device NEC T82.528
        - obstruction T82.599
          - specified device NEC T82.598
        - perforation T82.599
          - specified device NEC T82.598
        - protrusion T82.599
          - specified device NEC T82.598
      - pain T82.847
      - specified type NEC T82.897
      - stenosis T82.857
      - thrombosis T82.867
  - cardiovascular device, graft or implant T82.9
    - aortic graft — *see* Complications, graft, vascular
    - arteriovenous
      - fistula, artificial — *see* Complication, arteriovenous, fistula, surgically created
      - shunt — *see* Complication, arteriovenous, shunt, surgically created
    - artificial heart — *see* Complication, artificial, heart

- **Complication (s) (from) (of)** - *continued*
  - cardiovascular device, graft or implant - *continued*
    - balloon (counterpulsation) device — *see* Complication, balloon implant, vascular
    - carotid artery graft — *see* Complications, graft, vascular
    - coronary bypass graft — *see* Complication, coronary artery (bypass) graft
    - dialysis catheter (vascular) — *see* Complication, catheter, dialysis
    - electronic T82.9
      - electrode T82.9
        - embolism T82.817
        - fibrosis T82.827
        - hemorrhage T82.837
        - infection T82.7
        - mechanical
          - breakdown T82.110
          - displacement T82.120
          - leakage T82.190
          - obstruction T82.190
          - perforation T82.190
          - protrusion T82.190
          - specified type NEC T82.190
        - pain T82.847
        - specified NEC T82.897
        - stenosis T82.857
        - thrombosis T82.867
      - embolism T82.817
      - fibrosis T82.827
      - hemorrhage T82.837
      - infection T82.7
      - mechanical
        - breakdown T82.119
        - displacement T82.129
        - leakage T82.199
        - obstruction T82.199
        - perforation T82.199
        - protrusion T82.199
        - specified type NEC T82.199
      - pain T82.847
      - pulse generator T82.9
        - embolism T82.817
        - fibrosis T82.827
        - hemorrhage T82.837
        - infection T82.7
        - mechanical
          - breakdown T82.111
          - displacement T82.121
          - leakage T82.191
          - obstruction T82.191
          - perforation T82.191
          - protrusion T82.191
          - specified type NEC T82.191
        - pain T82.847
        - specified NEC T82.897
        - stenosis T82.857
        - thrombosis T82.867
      - specified condition NEC T82.897
      - specified device NEC T82.9
        - embolism T82.817
        - fibrosis T82.827
        - hemorrhage T82.837
        - infection T82.7
        - mechanical
          - breakdown T82.118
          - displacement T82.128
          - leakage T82.198
          - obstruction T82.198
          - perforation T82.198
          - protrusion T82.198
          - specified type NEC T82.198
        - pain T82.847
        - specified NEC T82.897
        - stenosis T82.857
        - thrombosis T82.867
      - stenosis T82.857
      - thrombosis T82.867
    - extremity artery graft — *see* Complication, extremity artery (bypass) graft
    - femoral artery graft — *see* Complication, extremity artery (bypass) graft

- **Complication (s) (from) (of)** - *continued*
  - cardiovascular device, graft or implant - *continued*
    - heart-lung transplant — *see* Complication, transplant, heart, with lung
    - heart
      - transplant — *see* Complication, transplant, heart
      - valve — *see* Complication, prosthetic device, heart valve
        - graft — *see* Complication, heart, valve, graft
    - infection or inflammation T82.7
    - umbrella device — *see* Complication, umbrella device, vascular
    - vascular graft (or anastomosis) — *see* Complication, graft, vascular
  - carotid artery (bypass) graft — *see* Complications, graft, vascular
  - catheter (device) NEC — *see also* Complications, prosthetic device or implant
    - cranial infusion
      - infection and inflammation T85.735
      - mechanical
        - breakdown T85.610
        - displacement T85.620
        - leakage T85.630
        - malfunction T85.690
        - malposition T85.620
        - obstruction T85.690
        - perforation T85.690
        - protrusion T85.690
        - specified NEC T85.690
    - cystostomy T83.9
      - embolism T83.81
      - fibrosis T83.82
      - hemorrhage T83.83
      - infection and inflammation T83.510
      - mechanical
        - breakdown T83.010
        - displacement T83.020
        - leakage T83.030
        - malposition T83.020
        - obstruction T83.090
        - perforation T83.090
        - protrusion T83.090
        - specified NEC T83.090
      - pain T83.84
      - specified type NEC T83.89
      - stenosis T83.85
      - thrombosis T83.86
    - dialysis (vascular) T82.9
      - embolism T82.818
      - fibrosis T82.828
      - hemorrhage T82.838
      - infection and inflammation T82.7
      - intraperitoneal — *see* Complications, catheter, intraperitoneal
      - mechanical
        - breakdown T82.41
        - displacement T82.42
        - leakage T82.43
        - malposition T82.42
        - obstruction T82.49
        - perforation T82.49
        - protrusion T82.49
      - pain T82.848
      - specified type NEC T82.898
      - stenosis T82.858
      - thrombosis T82.868
    - epidural infusion T85.9
      - embolism T85.810
      - fibrosis T85.820
      - hemorrhage T85.830
      - infection and inflammation T85.735
      - mechanical
        - breakdown T85.610
        - displacement T85.620
        - leakage T85.630
        - malfunction T85.610
        - malposition T85.620
        - obstruction T85.690
        - perforation T85.690
        - protrusion T85.690

Complication (s) (from) (of) - *continued*
catheter (device) NEC - *continued*
epidural infusion - *continued*
mechanical - *continued*
specified NEC T85.690
pain T85.840
specified type NEC T85.890
stenosis T85.850
thrombosis T85.860
intraperitoneal dialysis T85.9
embolism T85.818
fibrosis T85.828
hemorrhage T85.838
infection and inflammation T85.71
mechanical
breakdown T85.611
displacement T85.621
leakage T85.631
malfunction T85.611
malposition T85.621
obstruction T85.691
perforation T85.691
protrusion T85.691
specified NEC T85.691
pain T85.848
specified type NEC T85.898
stenosis T85.858
thrombosis T85.868
intrathecal infusion
infection and inflammation T85.735
mechanical
breakdown T85.610
displacement T85.620
leakage T85.630
malfunction T85.690
malposition T85.620
obstruction T85.690
perforation T85.690
protrusion T85.690
specified NEC T85.690
intravenous infusion T82.9
embolism T82.818
fibrosis T82.828
hemorrhage T82.838
infection or inflammation T82.7
mechanical
breakdown T82.514
displacement T82.524
leakage T82.534
malposition T82.524
obstruction T82.594
perforation T82.594
protrusion T82.594
pain T82.848
specified type NEC T82.898
stenosis T82.858
thrombosis T82.868
spinal infusion
infection and inflammation T85.735
mechanical
breakdown T85.610
displacement T85.620
leakage T85.630
malfunction T85.690
malposition T85.620
obstruction T85.690
perforation T85.690
protrusion T85.690
specified NEC T85.690
subarachnoid infusion
infection and inflammation T85.735
mechanical
breakdown T85.610
displacement T85.620
leakage T85.630
malfunction T85.690
malposition T85.620
obstruction T85.690
perforation T85.690
protrusion T85.690
specified NEC T85.690
subdural infusion T85.9
embolism T85.810
fibrosis T85.820
hemorrhage T85.830

Complication (s) (from) (of) - *continued*
catheter (device) NEC - *continued*
subdural infusion - *continued*
infection and inflammation T85.735
mechanical
breakdown T85.610
displacement T85.620
leakage T85.630
malfunction T85.610
malposition T85.620
obstruction T85.690
perforation T85.690
protrusion T85.690
specified NEC T85.690
pain T85.840
specified type NEC T85.890
stenosis T85.850
thrombosis T85.860
urethral T83.9
displacement T83.028
embolism T83.81
fibrosis T83.82
hemorrhage T83.83
indwelling
breakdown T83.011
displacement T83.021
infection and inflammation T83.511
leakage T83.031
specified complication NEC T83.091
infection and inflammation T83.511
leakage T83.038
malposition T83.028
mechanical
breakdown T83.011
obstruction (mechanical) T83.091
pain T83.84
perforation T83.091
protrusion T83.091
specified type NEC T83.091
stenosis T83.85
thrombosis T83.86
urinary NEC
breakdown T83.018
displacement T83.028
infection and inflammation T83.518
leakage T83.038
specified complication NEC T83.098
cecostomy (stoma) — *see* Complications, colostomy
cesarean delivery wound NEC O90.89
disruption O90.0
hematoma O90.2
infection (following delivery) O86.00
chemotherapy (antineoplastic) NEC T88.7
chimeric antigen receptor (CAR-T) cell therapy T80.82
chin implant (prosthetic) — *see* Complication, prosthetic device or implant, specified NEC
circulatory system I99.8
intraoperative I97.88
postprocedural I97.89
following cardiac surgery — *see also* Infarct, myocardium, associated with revascularization procedure I97.19-
postcardiotomy syndrome I97.0
hypertension I97.3
lymphedema after mastectomy I97.2
postcardiotomy syndrome I97.0
specified NEC I97.89
colostomy (stoma) K94.00
hemorrhage K94.01
infection K94.02
malfunction K94.03
mechanical K94.03
specified complication NEC K94.09
contraceptive device, intrauterine — *see* Complications, intrauterine, contraceptive device
cord (umbilical) — *see* Complications, umbilical cord
corneal graft — *see* Complications, graft, cornea
coronary artery (bypass) graft T82.9

Complication (s) (from) (of) - *continued*
coronary artery (bypass) graft - *continued*
atherosclerosis — *see* Arteriosclerosis, coronary (artery),
embolism T82.818
fibrosis T82.828
hemorrhage T82.838
infection and inflammation T82.7
mechanical
breakdown T82.211
displacement T82.212
leakage T82.213
malposition T82.212
obstruction T82.218
perforation T82.218
protrusion T82.218
specified NEC T82.218
pain T82.848
specified type NEC T82.898
stenosis T82.858
thrombosis T82.868
counterpulsation device (balloon), intra-aortic — *see* Complications, balloon implant, vascular
cystostomy (stoma) N99.518
catheter — *see* Complications, catheter, cystostomy
hemorrhage N99.510
infection N99.511
malfunction N99.512
specified type NEC N99.518
delivery — *see also* Complications, obstetric O75.9
procedure (instrumental) (manual) (surgical) O75.4
specified NEC O75.89
dialysis (peritoneal) (renal) — *see also* Complications, infusion
catheter (vascular) — *see* Complication, catheter, dialysis
peritoneal, intraperitoneal — *see* Complications, catheter, intraperitoneal
dorsal column (spinal) neurostimulator — *see* Complications, electronic stimulator device, spinal cord
drug NEC T88.7
ear procedure — *see also* Disorder, ear
intraoperative H95.88
hematoma — *see* Complications, intraoperative, hemorrhage (hematoma) (of), ear
hemorrhage — *see* Complications, intraoperative, hemorrhage (hematoma) (of), ear
laceration — *see* Complications, intraoperative, puncture or laceration..., ear
specified NEC H95.88
postoperative H95.89
external ear canal stenosis H95.81-
hematoma — *see* Complications, postprocedural, hematoma (of), ear
hemorrhage — *see* Complications, postprocedural, hemorrhage (of), ear
postmastoidectomy — *see* Complications, postmastoidectomy
seroma — *see* Complications, postprocedural, seroma (of), mastoid process
specified NEC H95.89
ectopic pregnancy O08.9
damage to pelvic organs O08.6
embolism O08.2
genital infection O08.0
hemorrhage (delayed) (excessive) O08.1
metabolic disorder O08.5
renal failure O08.4
shock O08.3
specified type NEC O08.0
venous complication NEC O08.7
electronic stimulator device
bladder (urinary) — *see* Complications, electronic stimulator device, urinary

Complication (s) (from) (of) - *continued*
- electronic stimulator device - *continued*
  - bone T84.9
    - breakdown T84.310
    - displacement T84.320
    - embolism T84.81
    - fibrosis T84.82
    - hemorrhage T84.83
    - infection or inflammation T84.7
    - malfunction T84.310
    - malposition T84.320
    - mechanical NEC T84.390
    - obstruction T84.390
    - pain T84.84
    - perforation T84.390
    - protrusion T84.390
    - specified type NEC T84.89
    - stenosis T84.85
    - thrombosis T84.86
  - brain T85.9
    - embolism T85.810
    - fibrosis T85.820
    - hemorrhage T85.830
    - infection and inflammation T85.731
    - mechanical
      - breakdown T85.110
      - displacement T85.120
      - leakage T85.190
      - malposition T85.120
      - obstruction T85.190
      - perforation T85.190
      - protrusion T85.190
      - specified NEC T85.190
    - pain T85.840
    - specified type NEC T85.890
    - stenosis T85.850
    - thrombosis T85.860
  - cardiac (defibrillator) (pacemaker) — *see* Complications, cardiovascular device or implant, electronic
  - generator (brain) (gastric) (peripheral) (sacral) (spinal)
    - breakdown T85.113
    - displacement T85.123
    - leakage T85.193
    - malposition T85.123
    - obstruction T85.193
    - perforation T85.193
    - protrusion T85.193
    - specified type NEC T85.193
  - muscle T84.9
    - breakdown T84.418
    - displacement T84.428
    - embolism T84.81
    - fibrosis T84.82
    - hemorrhage T84.83
    - infection or inflammation T84.7
    - mechanical NEC T84.498
    - pain T84.84
    - specified type NEC T84.89
    - stenosis T84.85
    - thrombosis T84.86
  - nervous system T85.9
    - brain — *see* Complications, electronic stimulator device, brain
    - cranial nerve — *see* Complications, electronic stimulator device, peripheral nerve
    - embolism T85.810
    - fibrosis T85.820
    - gastric nerve — *see* Complications, electronic stimulator device, peripheral nerve
    - hemorrhage T85.830
    - infection and inflammation T85.738
    - mechanical
      - breakdown T85.118
      - displacement T85.128
      - leakage T85.199
      - malposition T85.128
      - obstruction T85.199
      - perforation T85.199
      - protrusion T85.199
      - specified NEC T85.199
    - pain T85.840

Complication (s) (from) (of) - *continued*
- electronic stimulator device - *continued*
  - nervous system - *continued*
    - peripheral nerve — *see* Complications, electronic stimulator device, peripheral nerve
    - sacral nerve — *see* Complications, electronic stimulator device, peripheral nerve
    - specified type NEC T85.890
    - spinal cord — *see* Complications, electronic stimulator device, spinal cord
    - stenosis T85.850
    - thrombosis T85.860
    - vagal nerve — *see* Complications, electronic stimulator device, peripheral nerve
  - peripheral nerve T85.9
    - embolism T85.810
    - fibrosis T85.820
    - hemorrhage T85.830
    - infection and inflammation T85.732
    - mechanical
      - breakdown T85.111
      - displacement T85.121
      - leakage T85.191
      - malposition T85.121
      - obstruction T85.191
      - perforation T85.191
      - protrusion T85.191
      - specified NEC T85.191
    - pain T85.840
    - specified type NEC T85.890
    - stenosis T85.850
    - thrombosis T85.860
  - spinal cord T85.9
    - embolism T85.810
    - fibrosis T85.820
    - hemorrhage T85.830
    - infection and inflammation T85.733
    - mechanical
      - breakdown T85.112
      - displacement T85.122
      - leakage T85.192
      - malposition T85.122
      - obstruction T85.192
      - perforation T85.192
      - protrusion T85.192
      - specified NEC T85.192
    - pain T85.840
    - specified type NEC T85.890
    - stenosis T85.850
    - thrombosis T85.860
  - urinary T83.9
    - embolism T83.81
    - fibrosis T83.82
    - hemorrhage T83.83
    - infection and inflammation T83.598
    - mechanical
      - breakdown T83.110
      - displacement T83.120
      - malposition T83.120
      - perforation T83.190
      - protrusion T83.190
      - specified NEC T83.190
    - pain T83.84
    - specified type NEC T83.89
    - stenosis T83.85
    - thrombosis T83.86
- electroshock therapy T88.9
  - specified NEC T88.8
- endocrine E34.9
  - postprocedural
    - adrenal hypofunction E89.6
    - hypoinsulinemia E89.1
    - hypoparathyroidism E89.2
    - hypopituitarism E89.3
    - hypothyroidism E89.0
    - ovarian failure E89.40
      - asymptomatic E89.40
      - symptomatic E89.41
    - specified NEC E89.89
    - testicular hypofunction E89.5
- endodontic treatment NEC M27.59

Complication (s) (from) (of) - *continued*
- enterostomy (stoma) K94.10
  - hemorrhage K94.11
  - infection K94.12
  - malfunction K94.13
  - mechanical K94.13
  - specified complication NEC K94.19
- episiotomy, disruption O90.1
- esophageal anti-reflux device T85.9
  - embolism T85.818
  - fibrosis T85.828
  - hemorrhage T85.838
  - infection and inflammation T85.79
  - mechanical
    - breakdown T85.511
    - displacement T85.521
    - malfunction T85.511
    - malposition T85.521
    - obstruction T85.591
    - perforation T85.591
    - protrusion T85.591
    - specified NEC T85.591
  - pain T85.848
  - specified type NEC T85.898
  - stenosis T85.858
  - thrombosis T85.868
- esophagostomy K94.30
  - hemorrhage K94.31
  - infection K94.32
  - malfunction K94.33
  - mechanical K94.33
  - specified complication NEC K94.39
- extracorporeal circulation T80.90
- extremity artery (bypass) graft T82.9
  - arteriosclerosis — *see* Arteriosclerosis, extremities, bypass graft
  - embolism T82.818
  - fibrosis T82.828
  - hemorrhage T82.838
  - infection and inflammation T82.7
  - mechanical
    - breakdown T82.318
      - femoral artery T82.312
    - displacement T82.328
      - femoral artery T82.322
    - leakage T82.338
      - femoral artery T82.332
    - malposition T82.328
      - femoral artery T82.322
    - obstruction T82.398
      - femoral artery T82.392
    - perforation T82.398
      - femoral artery T82.392
    - protrusion T82.398
      - femoral artery T82.392
  - pain T82.848
  - specified type NEC T82.898
  - stenosis T82.858
  - thrombosis T82.868
- eye H57.9
  - corneal graft — *see* Complications, graft, cornea
  - implant (prosthetic) T85.9
    - embolism T85.818
    - fibrosis T85.828
    - hemorrhage T85.838
    - infection and inflammation T85.79
    - mechanical
      - breakdown T85.318
      - displacement T85.328
      - leakage T85.398
      - malposition T85.328
      - obstruction T85.398
      - perforation T85.398
      - protrusion T85.398
      - specified NEC T85.398
    - pain T85.848
    - specified type NEC T85.898
    - stenosis T85.858
    - thrombosis T85.868
  - intraocular lens — *see* Complications, intraocular lens
  - orbital prosthesis — *see* Complications, orbital prosthesis
- female genital N94.9

Complication (s) (from) (of) - *continued*
female genital - *continued*
device, implant or graft NEC — *see* Complications, genitourinary, device or implant, genital tract
femoral artery (bypass) graft — *see* Complication, extremity artery (bypass) graft
fixation device, internal (orthopedic) T84.9
infection and inflammation T84.60
arm T84.61-
humerus T84.61-
radius T84.61-
ulna T84.61-
leg T84.629
femur T84.62-
fibula T84.62-
tibia T84.62-
specified site NEC T84.69
spine T84.63
mechanical
breakdown
limb T84.119
carpal T84.210
femur T84.11-
fibula T84.11-
humerus T84.11-
metacarpal T84.210
metatarsal T84.213
phalanx
foot T84.213
hand T84.210
radius T84.11-
tarsal T84.213
tibia T84.11-
ulna T84.11-
specified bone NEC T84.218
spine T84.216
displacement
limb T84.129
carpal T84.220
femur T84.12-
fibula T84.12-
humerus T84.12-
metacarpal T84.220
metatarsal T84.223
phalanx
foot T84.223
hand T84.220
radius T84.12-
tarsal T84.223
tibia T84.12-
ulna T84.12-
specified bone NEC T84.228
spine T84.226
malposition — *see* Complications, fixation device, internal, mechanical, displacement
obstruction — *see* Complications, fixation device, internal, mechanical, specified type NEC
perforation — *see* Complications, fixation device, internal, mechanical, specified type NEC
protrusion — *see* Complications, fixation device, internal, mechanical, specified type NEC
specified type NEC
limb T84.199
carpal T84.290
femur T84.19-
fibula T84.19-
humerus T84.19-
metacarpal T84.290
metatarsal T84.293
phalanx
foot T84.293
hand T84.290
radius T84.19-
tarsal T84.293
tibia T84.19-
ulna T84.19-
specified bone NEC T84.298
vertebra T84.296
specified type NEC T84.89

Complication (s) (from) (of) - *continued*
fixation device, internal (orthopedic) - *continued*
specified type NEC - *continued*
embolism T84.81
fibrosis T84.82
hemorrhage T84.83
pain T84.84
specified complication NEC T84.89
stenosis T84.85
thrombosis T84.86
following
acute myocardial infarction NEC I23.8
aneurysm (false) (of cardiac wall) (of heart wall) (ruptured) I23.3
angina I23.7
atrial
septal defect I23.1
thrombosis I23.6
cardiac wall rupture I23.3
chordae tendinae rupture I23.4
defect
septal
atrial (heart) I23.1
ventricular (heart) I23.2
hemopericardium I23.0
papillary muscle rupture I23.5
rupture
cardiac wall I23.3
with hemopericardium I23.0
chordae tendineae I23.4
papillary muscle I23.5
specified NEC I23.8
thrombosis
atrium I23.6
auricular appendage I23.6
ventricle (heart) I23.6
ventricular
septal defect I23.2
thrombosis I23.6
ectopic or molar pregnancy O08.9
cardiac arrest O08.81
sepsis O08.82
specified type NEC O08.89
urinary tract infection O08.83
termination of pregnancy — *see* Abortion
gastrointestinal K92.9
bile duct prosthesis — *see* Complications, bile duct implant
esophageal anti-reflux device — *see* Complications, esophageal anti-reflux device
postoperative
colostomy — *see* Complications, colostomy
dumping syndrome K91.1
enterostomy — *see* Complications, enterostomy
gastrostomy — *see* Complications, gastrostomy
malabsorption NEC K91.2
obstruction — *see also* Obstruction, intestine, postoperative K91.30
postcholecystectomy syndrome K91.5
specified NEC K91.89
vomiting after GI surgery K91.0
prosthetic device or implant
bile duct prosthesis — *see* Complications, bile duct implant
esophageal anti-reflux device — *see* Complications, esophageal anti-reflux device
specified type NEC
embolism T85.818
fibrosis T85.828
hemorrhage T85.838
mechanical
breakdown T85.518
displacement T85.528
malfunction T85.518
malposition T85.528
obstruction T85.598
perforation T85.598
protrusion T85.598
specified NEC T85.598

Complication (s) (from) (of) - *continued*
gastrointestinal - *continued*
prosthetic device or implant - *continued*
specified type NEC - *continued*
pain T85.848
specified complication NEC T85.898
stenosis T85.858
thrombosis T85.868
gastrostomy (stoma) K94.20
hemorrhage K94.21
infection K94.22
malfunction K94.23
mechanical K94.23
specified complication NEC K94.29
genitourinary
device or implant T83.9
genital tract T83.9
infection or inflammation T83.69
intrauterine contraceptive device — *see* Complications, intrauterine, contraceptive device
mechanical — *see* Complications, by device, mechanical
mesh — *see* Complications, prosthetic device or implant, mesh
penile prosthesis — *see* Complications, prosthetic device, penile
specified type NEC T83.89
embolism T83.81
fibrosis T83.82
hemorrhage T83.83
pain T83.84
specified complication NEC T83.89
stenosis T83.85
thrombosis T83.86
vaginal mesh — *see* Complications, prosthetic device or implant, mesh
urinary system T83.9
cystostomy catheter — *see* Complication, catheter, cystostomy
electronic stimulator — *see* Complications, electronic stimulator device, urinary
indwelling urethral catheter — *see* Complications, catheter, urethral, indwelling
infection or inflammation T83.598
indwelling urethral catheter T83.511
kidney transplant — *see* Complication, transplant, kidney
organ graft — *see* Complication, graft, urinary organ
specified type NEC T83.89
embolism T83.81
fibrosis T83.82
hemorrhage T83.83
mechanical T83.198
breakdown T83.118
displacement T83.128
malfunction T83.118
malposition T83.128
obstruction T83.198
perforation T83.198
protrusion T83.198
specified NEC T83.198
sphincter, implanted T83.191
stent (ileal conduit) (nephroureteral) T83.193
ureteral indwelling T83.192
pain T83.84
specified complication NEC T83.89
stenosis T83.85
thrombosis T83.86
sphincter implant — *see* Complications, implant, urinary sphincter
postprocedural
pelvic peritoneal adhesions N99.4
renal failure N99.0
specified NEC N99.89
stoma — *see* Complications, stoma, urinary tract

- **Complication (s) (from) (of)** - *continued*
  - genitourinary - *continued*
    - postprocedural - *continued*
      - urethral stricture — *see* Stricture, urethra, postprocedural
      - vaginal
        - adhesions N99.2
        - vault prolapse N99.3
  - graft (bypass) (patch) — *see also* Complications, prosthetic device or implant
    - aorta — *see* Complications, graft, vascular
    - arterial — *see* Complication, graft, vascular
    - bone T86.839
      - failure T86.831
      - infection T86.832
      - mechanical T84.318
        - breakdown T84.318
        - displacement T84.328
        - protrusion T84.398
        - specified type NEC T84.398
      - rejection T86.830
      - specified type NEC T86.838
    - carotid artery — *see* Complications, graft, vascular
    - cornea T86.849-
      - failure T86.841-
      - infection T86.842-
      - mechanical T85.398
        - breakdown T85.318
        - displacement T85.328
        - protrusion T85.398
        - specified type NEC T85.398
      - rejection T86.840-
      - retroprosthetic membrane T85.398
      - specified type NEC T86.848-
    - femoral artery (bypass) — *see* Complication, extremity artery (bypass) graft
    - genital organ or tract — *see* Complications, genitourinary, device or implant, genital tract
    - muscle T84.9
      - breakdown T84.410
      - displacement T84.420
      - embolism T84.81
      - fibrosis T84.82
      - hemorrhage T84.83
      - infection and inflammation T84.7
      - mechanical NEC T84.490
      - pain T84.84
      - specified type NEC T84.89
      - stenosis T84.85
      - thrombosis T84.86
    - nerve — *see* Complication, prosthetic device or implant, specified NEC
    - skin — *see* Complications, prosthetic device or implant, skin graft
    - tendon T84.9
      - breakdown T84.410
      - displacement T84.420
      - embolism T84.81
      - fibrosis T84.82
      - hemorrhage T84.83
      - infection and inflammation T84.7
      - mechanical NEC T84.490
      - pain T84.84
      - specified type NEC T84.89
      - stenosis T84.85
      - thrombosis T84.86
    - urinary organ T83.9
      - embolism T83.81
      - fibrosis T83.82
      - hemorrhage T83.83
      - infection and inflammation T83.598
        - indwelling urethral catheter T83.511
      - mechanical
        - breakdown T83.21
        - displacement T83.22
        - erosion T83.24
        - exposure T83.25
        - leakage T83.23
        - malposition T83.22
        - obstruction T83.29

- **Complication (s) (from) (of)** - *continued*
  - graft (bypass) (patch) - *continued*
    - urinary organ - *continued*
      - mechanical - *continued*
        - perforation T83.29
        - protrusion T83.29
        - specified NEC T83.29
      - pain T83.84
      - specified type NEC T83.89
      - stenosis T83.85
      - thrombosis T83.86
    - vascular T82.9
      - embolism T82.818
      - femoral artery — *see* Complication, extremity artery (bypass) graft
      - fibrosis T82.828
      - hemorrhage T82.838
      - mechanical
        - breakdown T82.319
          - aorta (bifurcation) T82.310
          - carotid artery T82.311
          - specified vessel NEC T82.318
        - displacement T82.329
          - aorta (bifurcation) T82.320
          - carotid artery T82.321
          - specified vessel NEC T82.328
        - leakage T82.339
          - aorta (bifurcation) T82.330
          - carotid artery T82.331
          - specified vessel NEC T82.338
        - malposition T82.329
          - aorta (bifurcation) T82.320
          - carotid artery T82.321
          - specified vessel NEC T82.328
        - obstruction T82.399
          - aorta (bifurcation) T82.390
          - carotid artery T82.391
          - specified vessel NEC T82.398
        - perforation T82.399
          - aorta (bifurcation) T82.390
          - carotid artery T82.391
          - specified vessel NEC T82.398
        - protrusion T82.399
          - aorta (bifurcation) T82.390
          - carotid artery T82.391
          - specified vessel NEC T82.398
      - pain T82.848
      - specified complication NEC T82.898
      - stenosis T82.858
      - thrombosis T82.868
  - heart I51.9
    - assist device
      - infection and inflammation T82.7
    - following acute myocardial infarction — *see* Complications, following, acute myocardial infarction
    - postoperative — *see* Complications, circulatory system
    - transplant — *see* Complication, transplant, heart
      - and lung (s) — *see* Complications, transplant, heart, with lung
    - valve
      - graft (biological) T82.9
        - embolism T82.817
        - fibrosis T82.827
        - hemorrhage T82.837
        - infection and inflammation T82.7
        - mechanical T82.228
          - breakdown T82.221
          - displacement T82.222
          - leakage T82.223
          - malposition T82.222
          - obstruction T82.228
          - perforation T82.228
          - protrusion T82.228
        - pain T82.847
        - specified type NEC T82.897
        - stenosis T82.857
        - thrombosis T82.867
      - prosthesis T82.9
        - embolism T82.817
        - fibrosis T82.827
        - hemorrhage T82.837
        - infection or inflammation T82.6

- **Complication (s) (from) (of)** - *continued*
  - heart - *continued*
    - valve - *continued*
      - prosthesis - *continued*
        - mechanical T82.09
          - breakdown T82.01
          - displacement T82.02
          - leakage T82.03
          - malposition T82.02
          - obstruction T82.09
          - perforation T82.09
          - protrusion T82.09
        - pain T82.847
        - specified type NEC T82.897
          - mechanical T82.09
        - stenosis T82.857
        - thrombosis T82.867
  - hematoma
    - intraoperative — *see* Complication, intraoperative, hemorrhage
    - postprocedural — *see* Complication, postprocedural, hematoma
  - hemodialysis — *see* Complications, dialysis
  - hemorrhage
    - intraoperative — *see* Complication, intraoperative, hemorrhage
    - postprocedural — *see* Complication, postprocedural, hemorrhage
  - IEC (immune effector cellular) therapy T80.82
  - ileostomy (stoma) — *see* Complications, enterostomy
  - immune effector cellular (IEC) therapy T80.82
  - immunization (procedure) — *see* Complications, vaccination
  - implant — *see also* Complications, by site and type
    - urinary sphincter T83.9
      - embolism T83.81
      - fibrosis T83.82
      - hemorrhage T83.83
      - infection and inflammation T83.591
      - mechanical
        - breakdown T83.111
        - displacement T83.121
        - leakage T83.191
        - malposition T83.121
        - obstruction T83.191
        - perforation T83.191
        - protrusion T83.191
        - specified NEC T83.191
      - pain T83.84
      - specified type NEC T83.89
      - stenosis T83.85
      - thrombosis T83.86
  - infusion (procedure) T80.90
    - air embolism T80.0
    - blood — *see* Complications, transfusion
    - catheter — *see* Complications, catheter
    - infection T80.29
    - pump — *see* Complications, cardiovascular, device or implant
    - sepsis T80.29
    - serum reaction — *see also* Reaction, serum T80.69
      - anaphylactic shock — *see also* Shock, anaphylactic T80.59
    - specified type NEC T80.89
  - inhalation therapy NEC T81.81
  - injection (procedure) T80.90
    - drug reaction — *see* Reaction, drug
    - infection T80.29
    - sepsis T80.29
    - serum (prophylactic) (therapeutic) — *see* Complications, vaccination
    - specified type NEC T80.89
    - vaccine (any) — *see* Complications, vaccination
  - inoculation (any) — *see* Complications, vaccination
  - insulin pump
    - infection and inflammation T85.72
    - mechanical
      - breakdown T85.614

- **Complication (s) (from) (of)** - *continued*
  - insulin pump - *continued*
    - mechanical - *continued*
      - displacement T85.624
      - leakage T85.633
      - malposition T85.624
      - obstruction T85.694
      - perforation T85.694
      - protrusion T85.694
      - specified NEC T85.694
  - intestinal pouch NEC K91.858
  - intraocular lens (prosthetic) T85.9
    - embolism T85.818
    - fibrosis T85.828
    - hemorrhage T85.838
    - infection and inflammation T85.79
    - mechanical
      - breakdown T85.21
      - displacement T85.22
      - malposition T85.22
      - obstruction T85.29
      - perforation T85.29
      - protrusion T85.29
      - specified NEC T85.29
    - pain T85.848
    - specified type NEC T85.898
    - stenosis T85.858
    - thrombosis T85.868
  - intraoperative (intraprocedural)
    - cardiac arrest — *see also* Infarct, myocardium, associated with revascularization procedure
      - during cardiac surgery I97.710
      - during other surgery I97.711
    - cardiac functional disturbance NEC — *see also* Infarct, myocardium, associated with revascularization procedure
      - during cardiac surgery I97.790
      - during other surgery I97.791
    - hemorrhage (hematoma) (of)
      - circulatory system organ or structure
        - during cardiac bypass I97.411
        - during cardiac catheterization I97.410
        - during other circulatory system procedure I97.418
        - during other procedure I97.42
      - digestive system organ
        - during procedure on digestive system K91.61
        - during procedure on other organ K91.62
      - ear
        - during procedure on ear and mastoid process H95.21
        - during procedure on other organ H95.22
      - endocrine system organ or structure
        - during procedure on endocrine system organ or structure E36.01
        - during procedure on other organ E36.02
      - eye and adnexa
        - during ophthalmic procedure H59.11-
        - during other procedure H59.12-
      - genitourinary organ or structure
        - during procedure on genitourinary organ or structure N99.61
        - during procedure on other organ N99.62
      - mastoid process
        - during procedure on ear and mastoid process H95.21
        - during procedure on other organ H95.22
      - musculoskeletal structure
        - during musculoskeletal surgery M96.810
        - during non-orthopedic surgery M96.811
        - during orthopedic surgery M96.810
      - nervous system
        - during a nervous system procedure G97.31
        - during other procedure G97.32
      - respiratory system

- **Complication (s) (from) (of)** - *continued*
  - intraoperative (intraprocedural) - *continued*
    - hemorrhage (hematoma) (of) - *continued*
      - respiratory system - *continued*
        - during other procedure J95.62
        - during procedure on respiratory system organ or structure J95.61
      - skin and subcutaneous tissue
        - during a dermatologic procedure L76.01
        - during a procedure on other organ L76.02
      - spleen
        - during a procedure on other organ D78.02
        - during a procedure on the spleen D78.01
    - puncture or laceration (accidental) (unintentional) (of)
      - brain
        - during a nervous system procedure G97.48
        - during other procedure G97.49
      - circulatory system organ or structure
        - during circulatory system procedure I97.51
        - during other procedure I97.52
      - digestive system
        - during procedure on digestive system K91.71
        - during procedure on other organ K91.72
      - ear
        - during procedure on ear and mastoid process H95.31
        - during procedure on other organ H95.32
      - endocrine system organ or structure
        - during procedure on endocrine system organ or structure E36.11
        - during procedure on other organ E36.12
      - eye and adnexa
        - during ophthalmic procedure H59.21-
        - during other procedure H59.22-
      - genitourinary organ or structure
        - during procedure on genitourinary organ or structure N99.71
        - during procedure on other organ N99.72
      - mastoid process
        - during procedure on ear and mastoid process H95.31
        - during procedure on other organ H95.32
      - musculoskeletal structure
        - during musculoskeletal surgery M96.820
        - during non-orthopedic surgery M96.821
        - during orthopedic surgery M96.820
      - nervous system
        - during a nervous system procedure G97.48
        - during other procedure G97.49
      - respiratory system
        - during other procedure J95.72
        - during procedure on respiratory system organ or structure J95.71
      - skin and subcutaneous tissue
        - during a dermatologic procedure L76.11
        - during a procedure on other organ L76.12
      - spleen
        - during a procedure on other organ D78.12
        - during a procedure on the spleen D78.11
    - specified NEC
      - circulatory system I97.88
      - digestive system K91.81
      - ear H95.88
      - endocrine system E36.8
      - eye and adnexa H59.88

- **Complication (s) (from) (of)** - *continued*
  - intraoperative (intraprocedural) - *continued*
    - specified NEC - *continued*
      - genitourinary system N99.81
      - mastoid process H95.88
      - musculoskeletal structure M96.89
      - nervous system G97.81
      - respiratory system J95.88
      - skin and subcutaneous tissue L76.81
      - spleen D78.81
  - intraperitoneal catheter (dialysis) (infusion) — *see* Complication(s), catheter, intraperitoneal dialysis
  - intrathecal infusion pump
    - infection and inflammation T85.738
    - mechanical
      - breakdown T85.615
      - displacement T85.625
      - leakage T85.635
      - malfunction T85.695
      - malposition T85.625
      - obstruction T85.695
      - perforation T85.695
      - protrusion T85.695
      - specified NEC T85.695
  - intrauterine
    - contraceptive device
      - embolism T83.81
      - fibrosis T83.82
      - hemorrhage T83.83
      - infection and inflammation T83.69
      - mechanical
        - breakdown T83.31
        - displacement T83.32
        - malposition T83.32
        - obstruction T83.39
        - perforation T83.39
        - protrusion T83.39
        - specified NEC T83.39
      - pain T83.84
      - specified type NEC T83.89
      - stenosis T83.85
      - thrombosis T83.86
    - procedure (fetal) , to newborn P96.5
  - jejunostomy (stoma) — *see* Complications, enterostomy
  - joint prosthesis, internal T84.9
    - breakage (fracture) T84.01-
    - dislocation T84.02-
    - fracture T84.01-
    - infection or inflammation T84.50
      - hip T84.5-
      - knee T84.5-
      - specified joint NEC T84.59
    - instability T84.02-
    - malposition — *see* Complications, joint prosthesis, mechanical, displacement
    - mechanical
      - breakage, broken T84.01-
      - dislocation T84.02-
      - fracture T84.01-
      - instability T84.02-
      - leakage — *see* Complications, joint prosthesis, mechanical, specified NEC
      - loosening T84.039
        - hip T84.03-
        - knee T84.03-
        - specified joint NEC T84.038
      - obstruction — *see* Complications, joint prosthesis, mechanical, specified NEC
      - perforation — *see* Complications, joint prosthesis, mechanical, specified NEC
        - osteolysis T84.059
          - hip T84.05-
          - knee T84.05-
          - other specified joint T84.058
      - periprosthetic osteolysis T84.059
      - protrusion — *see* Complications, joint prosthesis, mechanical, specified NEC
      - specified complication NEC T84.099
        - hip T84.09-

COMPLICATION - COMPLICATION

COMPLICATION - COMPLICATION
subluxation T84.02-
 wear of articular bearing
 surface T84.069
 hip T84.06-
 knee T84.06-
transplant, kidney
labor O75.9
 specified NEC O75.89
liver transplant (immune or nonimmune) —
metabolic E88.9
 postoperative E89.89
 specified NEC E89.89
molar pregnancy NOS O08.9
postoperative (postprocedural) M96.89
 with osteoporosis — *see* Osteoporosis
 fracture following insertion of device —
 see Fracture, following insertion of
 orthopedic implant, joint prosthesis
 or bone plate
 joint instability after prosthesis
 removal M96.89
 lordosis M96.4
 postlaminectomy syndrome NEC M96.1
 kyphosis M96.3
 pseudarthrosis M96.0
 specified complication NEC M96.89
 post radiation M96.89
 kyphosis M96.2
 scoliosis M96.5
 specified complication NEC M96.89
nephrostomy (stoma) — *see* Complications,
 stoma, urinary tract, external NEC
nervous system G98.8
 central G96.9
 device, implant or graft — *see also*
device
 postprocedural G97.82
 intracranial hypotension G97.2
 specified NEC G97.82
 spinal fluid leak G97.0
newborn, due to intrauterine (fetal)
 procedure P96.5
nonabsorbable (permanent) sutures — *see*
 Complication, sutures, permanent
obstetric O75.9
joint prosthesis, internal
 malfunction T84.418
 malposition T84.428
 mechanical NEC T84.498
orthopedic implant, joint prosthesis or
 bone plate
 postprocedural M96.89
 fracture — *see* Fracture, following
 insertion of orthopedic implant,
 joint prosthesis or bone plate
 postlaminectomy syndrome NEC M96.1
 kyphosis M96.3
 lordosis M96.4
 postradiation
 kyphosis M96.2
 scoliosis M96.5
 pseudarthrosis post-fusion M96.0
 specified type NEC M96.89
postmastoidectomy NEC H95.19-
 cyst, mucosal H95.13-
 granulation H95.12-
 inflammation, chronic H95.11-
 recurrent cholesteatoma H95.0-

- **Complication (s) (from) (of)** - *continued*
  - postoperative — *see* Complications, postprocedural
    - circulatory — *see* Complications, circulatory system
    - ear — *see* Complications, ear
    - endocrine — *see* Complications, endocrine
    - eye — *see* Complications, eye
    - lumbar puncture G97.1
      - cerebrospinal fluid leak G97.0
    - nervous system (central) (peripheral) — *see* Complications, nervous system
    - respiratory system — *see* Complications, respiratory system
  - postprocedural — *see also* Complications, surgical procedure
    - cardiac arrest — *see also* Infarct, myocardium, associated with revascularization procedure
      - following cardiac surgery I97.120
      - following other surgery I97.121
    - cardiac functional disturbance NEC — *see also* Infarct, myocardium, associated with revascularization procedure
      - following cardiac surgery I97.190
      - following other surgery I97.191
    - cardiac insufficiency
      - following cardiac surgery I97.110
      - following other surgery I97.111
    - chorioretinal scars following retinal surgery H59.81-
    - following cataract surgery
      - cataract (lens) fragments H59.02-
      - cystoid macular edema H59.03-
      - specified NEC H59.09-
      - vitreous (touch) syndrome H59.01-
    - heart failure
      - following cardiac surgery I97.130
      - following other surgery I97.131
    - hematoma (of)
      - circulatory system organ or structure
        - following cardiac bypass I97.631
        - following cardiac catheterization I97.630
        - following other circulatory system procedure I97.638
        - following other procedure I97.621
      - digestive system
        - following procedure on digestive system K91.870
        - following procedure on other organ K91.871
      - ear
        - following other procedure H95.52
        - following procedure on ear and mastoid process H95.51
      - endocrine system
        - following endocrine system procedure E89.820
        - following other procedure E89.821
      - eye and adnexa
        - following ophthalmic procedure H59.33-
        - following other procedure H59.34-
      - genitourinary organ or structure
        - following procedure on genitourinary organ or structure N99.840
        - following procedure on other organ N99.841
      - mastoid process
        - following other procedure H95.52
        - following procedure on ear and mastoid process H95.51
      - musculoskeletal structure
        - following musculoskeletal surgery M96.840
        - following non-orthopedic surgery M96.841
        - following orthopedic surgery M96.840
      - nervous system
        - following nervous system procedure G97.61
        - following other procedure G97.62
      - respiratory system
        - following other procedure J95.861

- **Complication (s) (from) (of)** - *continued*
  - postprocedural - *continued*
    - hematoma (of) - *continued*
      - respiratory system - *continued*
        - following procedure on respiratory system organ or structure J95.860
      - skin and subcutaneous tissue
        - following dermatologic procedure L76.31
        - following procedure on other organ L76.32
      - spleen
        - following procedure on other organ D78.32
        - following procedure on the spleen D78.31
    - hemorrhage (of)
      - circulatory system organ or structure
        - following cardiac bypass I97.611
        - following cardiac catheterization I97.610
        - following other circulatory system procedure I97.618
        - following other procedure I97.620
      - digestive system
        - following procedure on digestive system K91.840
        - following procedure on other organ K91.841
      - ear
        - following other procedure H95.42
        - following procedure on ear and mastoid process H95.41
      - endocrine system
        - following endocrine system procedure E89.810
        - following other procedure E89.811
      - eye and adnexa
        - following ophthalmic procedure H59.31-
        - following other procedure H59.32-
      - genitourinary organ or structure
        - following procedure on genitourinary organ or structure N99.820
        - following procedure on other organ N99.821
      - mastoid process
        - following other procedure H95.42
        - following procedure on ear and mastoid process H95.41
      - musculoskeletal structure
        - following musculoskeletal surgery M96.830
        - following non-orthopedic surgery M96.831
        - following orthopedic surgery M96.830
      - nervous system
        - following nervous system procedure G97.51
        - following other procedure G97.52
      - respiratory system
        - following other procedure J95.831
        - following procedure on respiratory system organ or structure J95.830
      - skin and subcutaneous tissue
        - following dermatologic procedure L76.21
        - following a procedure on other organ L76.22
      - spleen
        - following procedure on other organ D78.22
        - following procedure on the spleen D78.21
    - seroma (of)
      - circulatory system organ or structure
        - following cardiac bypass I97.641
        - following cardiac catheterization I97.640
        - following other circulatory system procedure I97.648
        - following other procedure I97.622
      - digestive system
        - following procedure on digestive system K91.872

- **Complication (s) (from) (of)** - *continued*
  - postprocedural - *continued*
    - seroma (of) - *continued*
      - digestive system - *continued*
        - following procedure on other organ K91.873
      - ear
        - following other procedure H95.54
        - following procedure on ear and mastoid process H95.53
      - endocrine system
        - following endocrine system procedure E89.822
        - following other procedure E89.823
      - eye and adnexa
        - following ophthalmic procedure H59.35-
        - following other procedure H59.36-
      - genitourinary organ or structure
        - following procedure on genitourinary organ or structure N99.842
        - following procedure on other organ N99.843
      - mastoid process
        - following other procedure H95.54
        - following procedure on ear and mastoid process H95.53
      - musculoskeletal structure
        - following musculoskeletal surgery M96.842
        - following non-orthopedic surgery M96.843
        - following orthopedic surgery M96.842
      - nervous system
        - following nervous system procedure G97.63
        - following other procedure G97.64
      - respiratory system
        - following other procedure J95.863
        - following procedure on respiratory system organ or structure J95.862
      - skin and subcutaneous tissue
        - following dermatologic procedure L76.33
        - following procedure on other organ L76.34
      - spleen
        - following procedure on other organ D78.34
        - following procedure on the spleen D78.33
    - specified NEC
      - circulatory system I97.89
      - digestive K91.89
      - ear H95.89
      - endocrine E89.89
      - eye and adnexa H59.89
      - genitourinary N99.89
      - mastoid process H95.89
      - metabolic E89.89
      - musculoskeletal structure M96.89
      - nervous system G97.82
      - respiratory system J95.89
      - skin and subcutaneous tissue L76.82
      - spleen D78.89
  - pregnancy NEC — *see* Pregnancy, complicated by
  - prosthetic device or implant T85.9
    - bile duct — *see* Complications, bile duct implant
    - breast — *see* Complications, breast implant
    - bulking agent
      - ureteral
        - erosion T83.714
        - exposure T83.724
      - urethral
        - erosion T83.713
        - exposure T83.723
    - cardiac and vascular NEC — *see* Complications, cardiovascular device or implant
    - corneal transplant — *see* Complications, graft, cornea

COMPLICATION - COMPLICATION

Complication (s) (from) (of) - *continued*
prosthetic device or implant - *continued*
electronic nervous system stimulator — *see* Complications, electronic stimulator device
epidural infusion catheter — *see* Complications, catheter, epidural
esophageal anti-reflux device — *see* Complications, esophageal anti-reflux device
genital organ or tract — *see* Complications, genitourinary, device or implant, genital tract
specified NEC T83.79
heart valve — *see* Complications, heart, valve, prosthesis
infection or inflammation T85.79
intestine transplant T86.892
liver transplant T86.43
lung transplant T86.812
pancreas transplant T86.892
skin graft T86.822
intraocular lens — *see* Complications, intraocular lens
intraperitoneal (dialysis) catheter — *see* Complication(s), catheter, intraperitoneal dialysis
joint — *see* Complications, joint prosthesis, internal
mechanical NEC T85.698
dialysis catheter (vascular) — *see also* Complication, catheter, dialysis, mechanical
peritoneal — *see* Complication(s), catheter, intraperitoneal dialysis
gastrointestinal device T85.598
ocular device T85.398
subdural (infusion) catheter T85.690
suture, permanent T85.692
that for bone repair — *see* Complications, fixation device, internal (orthopedic), mechanical
ventricular shunt
breakdown T85.01
displacement T85.02
leakage T85.03
malposition T85.02
obstruction T85.09
perforation T85.09
protrusion T85.09
specified NEC T85.09
mesh
erosion (to surrounding organ or tissue) T83.718
urethral (into pelvic floor muscles) T83.712
vaginal (into pelvic floor muscles) T83.711
exposure (into surrounding organ or tissue) T83.728
urethral (through urethral wall) T83.722
vaginal (into vagina) (through vaginal wall) T83.721
orbital — *see* Complications, orbital prosthesis
penile T83.9
embolism T83.81
fibrosis T83.82
hemorrhage T83.83
infection and inflammation T83.61
mechanical
breakdown T83.410
displacement T83.420
leakage T83.490
malposition T83.420
obstruction T83.490
perforation T83.490
protrusion T83.490
specified NEC T83.490
pain T83.84
specified type NEC T83.89
stenosis T83.85
thrombosis T83.86
prosthetic materials NEC

Complication (s) (from) (of) - *continued*
prosthetic device or implant - *continued*
prosthetic materials NEC - *continued*
erosion (to surrounding organ or tissue) T83.718
exposure (into surrounding organ or tissue) T83.728
skin graft T86.829
artificial skin or decellularized allodermis
embolism T85.818
fibrosis T85.828
hemorrhage T85.838
infection and inflammation T85.79
mechanical
breakdown T85.613
displacement T85.623
malfunction T85.613
malposition T85.623
obstruction T85.693
perforation T85.693
protrusion T85.693
specified NEC T85.693
pain T85.848
specified type NEC T85.898
stenosis T85.858
thrombosis T85.868
failure T86.821
infection T86.822
rejection T86.820
specified NEC T86.828
sling
urethral (female) (male)
erosion T83.712
exposure T83.722
specified NEC T85.9
embolism T85.818
fibrosis T85.828
hemorrhage T85.838
infection and inflammation T85.79
mechanical
breakdown T85.618
displacement T85.628
leakage T85.638
malfunction T85.618
malposition T85.628
obstruction T85.698
perforation T85.698
protrusion T85.698
specified NEC T85.698
pain T85.848
specified type NEC T85.898
stenosis T85.858
thrombosis T85.868
subdural infusion catheter — *see* Complications, catheter, subdural
sutures — *see* Complications, sutures
urinary organ or tract NEC — *see* Complications, genitourinary, device or implant, urinary system
vascular — *see* Complications, cardiovascular device or implant
ventricular shunt — *see* Complications, ventricular shunt (device)
puerperium — *see* Puerperal
puncture, spinal G97.1
cerebrospinal fluid leak G97.0
headache or reaction G97.1
pyelogram N99.89
radiation
kyphosis M96.2
scoliosis M96.5
reattached
extremity (infection) (rejection)
lower T87.1X-
upper T87.0X-
specified body part NEC T87.2
reconstructed breast
asymmetry between native and reconstructed breast N65.1
deformity N65.0
disproportion between native and reconstructed breast N65.1
excess tissue N65.0
misshappen N65.0

Complication (s) (from) (of) - *continued*
reimplant NEC — *see also* Complications, prosthetic device or implant
limb (infection) (rejection) — *see* Complications, reattached, extremity
organ (partial) (total) — *see* Complications, transplant
prosthetic device NEC — *see* Complications, prosthetic device
renal N28.9
allograft — *see* Complications, transplant, kidney
dialysis — *see* Complications, dialysis
respirator
mechancial J95.850
specified NEC J95.859
respiratory system J98.9
device, implant or graft — *see* Complication, prosthetic device or implant, specified NEC
lung transplant — *see* Complications, prosthetic device or implant, lung transplant
postoperative J95.89
air leak J95.812
Mendelson's syndrome (chemical pneumonitis) J95.4
pneumothorax J95.811
pulmonary insufficiency (acute) (after nonthoracic surgery) J95.2
chronic J95.3
following thoracic surgery J95.1
respiratory failure (acute) J95.821
acute and chronic J95.822
specified NEC J95.89
subglottic stenosis J95.5
tracheostomy complication — *see* Complications, tracheostomy
therapy T81.89
sedation during labor and delivery O74.9
cardiac O74.2
central nervous system O74.3
pulmonary NEC O74.1
shunt — *see also* Complications, prosthetic device or implant
arteriovenous — *see* Complications, arteriovenous, shunt
ventricular (communicating) — *see* Complications, ventricular shunt
skin
graft T86.829
failure T86.821
infection T86.822
rejection T86.820
specified type NEC T86.828
spinal
anesthesia — *see* Complications, anesthesia, spinal
catheter (epidural) (subdural) — *see* Complications, catheter
puncture or tap G97.1
cerebrospinal fluid leak G97.0
headache or reaction G97.1
stent
bile duct — *see* Complications, bile duct prosthesis
ureteral indwelling
breakdown T83.112
displacement T83.122
leakage T83.192
malposition T83.122
obstruction T83.192
perforation T83.192
protrusion T83.192
specified NEC T83.192
urinary NEC (ileal conduit) (nephroureteral) T83.193
embolism T83.81
fibrosis T83.82
hemorrhage T83.83
infection and inflammation T83.593
mechanical
breakdown T83.113
displacement T83.123
leakage T83.193

Complication (s) (from) (of) - *continued*
transplant T86.90
bone T86.839
failure T86.831
infection T86.832
rejection T86.830
specified type NEC T86.838
bone marrow T86.00
failure T86.02
infection T86.03
rejection T86.01
specified type NEC T86.09
cornea T86.849-
failure T86.841-
infection T86.842-
rejection T86.840-
specified type NEC T86.848-
failure T86.92
heart T86.20
with lung T86.30
cardiac allograft vasculopathy T86.290
failure T86.32
infection T86.33
rejection T86.31
specified type NEC T86.39
failure T86.22
infection T86.23
rejection T86.21
specified type NEC T86.298
infection T86.93
intestine T86.859
failure T86.851
infection T86.852
rejection T86.850
specified type NEC T86.858
kidney T86.10
failure T86.12
infection T86.13
rejection T86.11
specified type NEC T86.19
liver T86.40
failure T86.42
infection T86.43
rejection T86.41
specified type NEC T86.49
lung T86.819
with heart T86.30
failure T86.32
infection T86.33
rejection T86.31
specified type NEC T86.39
failure T86.811
infection T86.812
rejection T86.810
specified type NEC T86.818
malignant neoplasm C80.2
pancreas T86.899
failure T86.891
infection T86.892
rejection T86.890
specified type NEC T86.898
peripheral blood stem cells T86.5
post-transplant lymphoproliferative disorder (PTLD) D47.Z1
rejection T86.91
skin T86.829
failure T86.821
infection T86.822
rejection T86.820
specified type NEC T86.828
specified
tissue T86.899
failure T86.891
infection T86.892
rejection T86.890
specified type NEC T86.898
type NEC T86.99
stem cell (from peripheral blood) (from umbilical cord) T86.5
umbilical cord stem cells T86.5
trauma (early) T79.9
specified NEC T79.8
ultrasound therapy NEC T88.9
umbilical cord NEC
complicating delivery O69.9

Complication (s) (from) (of) - *continued*
umbilical cord NEC - *continued*
complicating delivery - *continued*
specified NEC O69.89
umbrella device, vascular T82.9
embolism T82.818
fibrosis T82.828
hemorrhage T82.838
infection or inflammation T82.7
mechanical
breakdown T82.515
displacement T82.525
leakage T82.535
malposition T82.525
obstruction T82.595
perforation T82.595
protrusion T82.595
pain T82.848
specified type NEC T82.898
stenosis T82.858
thrombosis T82.868
urethral catheter — *see* Complications, catheter, urethral, indwelling
vaccination T88.1
anaphylaxis NEC T80.52
arthropathy — *see* Arthropathy, postimmunization
cellulitis T88.0
encephalitis or encephalomyelitis G04.02
infection (general) (local) NEC T88.0
meningitis G03.8
myelitis G04.02
protein sickness T80.62
rash T88.1
reaction (allergic) T88.1
serum T80.62
sepsis T88.0
serum intoxication, sickness, rash, or other serum reaction NEC T80.62
anaphylactic shock T80.52
shock (allergic) (anaphylactic) T80.52
vaccinia (generalized) (localized) T88.1
vas deferens device or implant — *see* Complications, genitourinary, device or implant, genital tract
vascular I99.9
device or implant T82.9
embolism T82.818
fibrosis T82.828
hemorrhage T82.838
infection or inflammation T82.7
mechanical
breakdown T82.519
specified device NEC T82.518
displacement T82.529
specified device NEC T82.528
leakage T82.539
specified device NEC T82.538
malposition T82.529
specified device NEC T82.528
obstruction T82.599
specified device NEC T82.598
perforation T82.599
specified device NEC T82.598
protrusion T82.599
specified device NEC T82.598
pain T82.848
specified type NEC T82.898
stenosis T82.858
thrombosis T82.868
dialysis catheter — *see* Complication, catheter, dialysis
following infusion, therapeutic injection or transfusion T80.1
graft T82.9
embolism T82.818
fibrosis T82.828
hemorrhage T82.838
mechanical
breakdown T82.319
aorta (bifurcation) T82.310
carotid artery T82.311
specified vessel NEC T82.318
displacement T82.329
aorta (bifurcation) T82.320

Complication (s) (from) (of) - *continued*
vascular - *continued*
graft - *continued*
mechanical - *continued*
displacement - *continued*
carotid artery T82.321
specified vessel NEC T82.328
leakage T82.339
aorta (bifurcation) T82.330
carotid artery T82.331
specified vessel NEC T82.338
malposition T82.329
aorta (bifurcation) T82.320
carotid artery T82.321
specified vessel NEC T82.328
obstruction T82.399
aorta (bifurcation) T82.390
carotid artery T82.391
specified vessel NEC T82.398
perforation T82.399
aorta (bifurcation) T82.390
carotid artery T82.391
specified vessel NEC T82.398
protrusion T82.399
aorta (bifurcation) T82.390
carotid artery T82.391
specified vessel NEC T82.398
pain T82.848
specified complication NEC T82.898
stenosis T82.858
thrombosis T82.868
postoperative — *see* Complications, postoperative, circulatory
vena cava device (filter) (sieve) (umbrella) — *see* Complications, umbrella device, vascular
ventilation therapy NEC T81.81
ventilator
mechanical J95.850
specified NEC J95.859
ventricular (communicating) shunt (device) T85.9
embolism T85.810
fibrosis T85.820
hemorrhage T85.830
infection and inflammation T85.730
mechanical
breakdown T85.01
displacement T85.02
leakage T85.03
malposition T85.02
obstruction T85.09
perforation T85.09
protrusion T85.09
specified NEC T85.09
pain T85.840
specified type NEC T85.890
stenosis T85.850
thrombosis T85.860
wire suture, permanent (implanted) — *see* Complications, suture, permanent
Compressed air disease T70.3
Compression
with injury - code by Nature of injury
artery I77.1
celiac, syndrome I77.4
brachial plexus G54.0
brain (stem) G93.5
due to
contusion (diffuse) — *see also* Injury, intracranial, diffuse S06.A0
with herniation S06.A1
focal — *see also* Injury, intracranial, focal S06.A0
with herniation S06.A1
injury NEC — *see also* Injury, intracranial, diffuse S06.A0
nontraumatic G93.5
traumatic — *see also* Injury, intracranial, diffuse S06.A0
with herniation S06.A1
bronchus J98.09
cauda equina G83.4
celiac (artery) (axis) I77.4
cerebral — *see* Compression, brain

- **Compression** - *continued*
  - cervical plexus G54.2
  - cord
    - spinal — *see* Compression, spinal
    - umbilical — *see* Compression, umbilical cord
  - cranial nerve G52.9
    - eighth — *see* subcategory H93.3
    - eleventh G52.8
    - fifth G50.8
    - first G52.0
    - fourth — *see* Strabismus, paralytic, fourth nerve
    - ninth G52.1
    - second — *see* Disorder, nerve, optic
    - seventh G51.8
    - sixth — *see* Strabismus, paralytic, sixth nerve
    - tenth G52.2
    - third — *see* Strabismus, paralytic, third nerve
    - twelfth G52.3
  - diver's squeeze T70.3
  - during birth (newborn) P15.9
  - esophagus K22.2
  - eustachian tube — *see* Obstruction, eustachian tube, cartilaginous
  - facies Q67.1
  - fracture
    - nontraumatic NOS — *see* Collapse, vertebra
    - pathological — *see* Fracture, pathological
    - traumatic — *see* Fracture, traumatic
  - heart — *see* Disease, heart
  - intestine — *see* Obstruction, intestine
  - laryngeal nerve, recurrent G52.2
    - with paralysis of vocal cords and larynx J38.00
      - bilateral J38.02
      - unilateral J38.01
  - lumbosacral plexus G54.1
  - lung J98.4
  - lymphatic vessel I89.0
  - medulla — *see* Compression, brain
  - nerve — *see also* Disorder, nerve G58.9
    - arm NEC — *see* Mononeuropathy, upper limb
    - axillary G54.0
    - cranial — *see* Compression, cranial nerve
    - leg NEC — *see* Mononeuropathy, lower limb
    - median (in carpal tunnel) — *see* Syndrome, carpal tunnel
    - optic — *see* Disorder, nerve, optic
    - plantar — *see* Lesion, nerve, plantar
    - posterior tibial (in tarsal tunnel) — *see* Syndrome, tarsal tunnel
    - root or plexus NOS (in) G54.9
      - intervertebral disc disorder NEC — *see* Disorder, disc, with, radiculopathy
        - with myelopathy — *see* Disorder, disc, with, myelopathy
      - neoplastic disease — *see also* Neoplasm D49.9 *[G55]*
      - spondylosis — *see* Spondylosis, with radiculopathy
    - sciatic (acute) — *see* Lesion, nerve, sciatic
    - sympathetic G90.8
    - traumatic — *see* Injury, nerve
    - ulnar — *see* Lesion, nerve, ulnar
    - upper extremity NEC — *see* Mononeuropathy, upper limb
  - spinal (cord) G95.20
    - by displacement of intervertebral disc NEC — *see also* Disorder, disc, with, myelopathy
    - nerve root NOS G54.9
      - due to displacement of intervertebral disc NEC — *see* Disorder, disc, with, radiculopathy
        - with myelopathy — *see* Disorder, disc, with, myelopathy
    - specified NEC G95.29

- **Compression** - *continued*
  - spinal (cord) - *continued*
    - spondylogenic (cervical) (lumbar, lumbosacral) (thoracic) — *see* Spondylosis, with myelopathy NEC
      - anterior — *see* Syndrome, anterior, spinal artery, compression
    - traumatic — *see* Injury, spinal cord, by region
  - subcostal nerve (syndrome) — *see* Mononeuropathy, upper limb, specified NEC
  - sympathetic nerve NEC G90.8
  - syndrome T79.5
  - trachea J39.8
  - ulnar nerve (by scar tissue) — *see* Lesion, nerve, ulnar
  - umbilical cord
    - complicating delivery O69.2
      - cord around neck O69.1
      - prolapse O69.0
      - specified NEC O69.2
  - ureter N13.5
  - vein I87.1
  - vena cava (inferior) (superior) I87.1
- **Compulsion, compulsive**
  - gambling F63.0
  - neurosis F42.8
  - personality F60.5
  - states F42.8
  - swearing F42.8
    - in Gilles de la Tourette's syndrome F95.2
  - tics and spasms F95.9
- **Concato's disease (pericardial polyserositis)** A19.9
  - nontubercular I31.1
  - pleural — *see* Pleurisy, with effusion
- **Concavity chest wall** M95.4
- **Concealed penis** Q55.64
- **Concern (normal) about sick person in family** Z63.6
- **Concrescence (teeth)** K00.2
- **Concretio cordis** I31.1
  - rheumatic I09.2
- **Concretion** — *see also* Calculus
  - appendicular K38.1
  - canaliculus — *see* Dacryolith
  - clitoris N90.89
  - conjunctiva H11.12-
  - eyelid — *see* Disorder, eyelid, specified type NEC
  - lacrimal passages — *see* Dacryolith
  - prepuce (male) N47.8
  - salivary gland (any) K11.5
  - seminal vesicle N50.89
  - tonsil J35.8
- **Concussion (brain) (cerebral) (current)** S06.0X9
  - with
    - loss of consciousness of 30 minutes or less S06.0X1
    - loss of consciousness of unspecified duration S06.0X9
  - blast (air) (hydraulic) (immersion) (underwater)
    - abdomen or thorax — *see* Injury, blast, by site
    - ear with acoustic nerve injury — *see* Injury, nerve, acoustic, specified type NEC
  - cauda equina S34.3
  - conus medullaris S34.02
  - ocular S05.8X-
  - spinal (cord)
    - cervical S14.0
    - lumbar S34.01
    - sacral S34.02
    - thoracic S24.0
  - syndrome F07.81
  - without loss of consciousness S06.0X0
- **Condition** — *see also* Disease
  - post COVID-19 U09.9
- **Conditions arising in the perinatal period** — *see* Newborn, affected by
- **Conduct disorder** — *see* Disorder, conduct

- **Condyloma** A63.0
  - acuminatum A63.0
  - gonorrheal A54.09
  - latum A51.31
  - syphilitic A51.31
    - congenital A50.07
  - venereal, syphilitic A51.31
- **Conflagration** — *see also* Burn
  - asphyxia (by inhalation of gases, fumes or vapors) — *see also* Table of Drugs and Chemicals T59.9-
- **Conflict (with)** — *see also* Discord
  - family Z73.9
  - marital Z63.0
    - involving divorce or estrangement Z63.5
  - parent-child Z62.820
    - parent-adopted child Z62.821
    - parent-biological child Z62.820
    - parent-foster child Z62.822
  - social role NEC Z73.5
- **Confluent** — *see* condition
- **Confusion, confused** R41.0
  - epileptic F05
  - mental state (psychogenic) F44.89
  - psychogenic F44.89
  - reactive (from emotional stress, psychological trauma) F44.89
- **Confusional arousals** G47.51
- **Congelation** T69.9
- **Congenital** — *see also* condition
  - aortic septum Q25.49
  - intrinsic factor deficiency D51.0
  - malformation — *see* Anomaly
- **Congestion, congestive**
  - bladder N32.89
  - bowel K63.89
  - brain G93.89
  - breast N64.59
  - bronchial J98.09
  - catarrhal J31.0
  - chest R09.89
  - chill, malarial — *see* Malaria
  - circulatory NEC I99.8
  - duodenum K31.89
  - eye — *see* Hyperemia, conjunctiva
  - facial, due to birth injury P15.4
  - general R68.89
  - glottis J37.0
  - heart — *see* Failure, heart, congestive
  - hepatic K76.1
  - hypostatic (lung) — *see* Edema, lung
  - intestine K63.89
  - kidney N28.89
  - labyrinth — *see* subcategory H83.8
  - larynx J37.0
  - liver K76.1
  - lung R09.89
    - active or acute — *see* Pneumonia
  - malaria, malarial — *see* Malaria
  - nasal R09.81
  - nose R09.81
  - orbit, orbital — *see also* Exophthalmos
    - inflammatory (chronic) — *see* Inflammation, orbit
  - ovary N83.8
  - pancreas K86.89
  - pelvic, female N94.89
  - pleural J94.8
  - prostate (active) N42.1
  - pulmonary — *see* Congestion, lung
  - renal N28.89
  - retina H35.81
  - seminal vesicle N50.1
  - spinal cord G95.19
  - spleen (chronic) D73.2
  - stomach K31.89
  - trachea — *see* Tracheitis
  - urethra N36.8
  - uterus N85.8
    - with subinvolution N85.3
  - venous (passive) I87.8
  - viscera R68.89
- **Congestive** — *see* Congestion
- **Conical**
  - cervix (hypertrophic elongation) N88.4

Conical - *continued*
- cornea — *see* Keratoconus
- teeth K00.2

Conjoined twins Q89.4
Conjugal maladjustment Z63.0
- involving divorce or estrangement Z63.5

Conjunctiva — *see* condition
Conjunctivitis (staphylococcal) (streptococcal) NOS H10.9
- Acanthamoeba B60.12
- acute H10.3-
  - atopic H10.1-
  - mucopurulent H10.02-
    - follicular H10.01-
  - chemical — *see also* Corrosion, cornea H10.21-
  - pseudomembranous H10.22-
  - serous except viral H10.23-
    - viral — *see* Conjunctivitis, viral
  - toxic H10.21-
- adenoviral (acute) (follicular) B30.1
- allergic (acute) — *see* Conjunctivitis, acute, atopic
  - chronic H10.45
    - vernal H10.44
- anaphylactic — *see* Conjunctivitis, acute, atopic
- Apollo B30.3
- atopic (acute) — *see* Conjunctivitis, acute, atopic
- Béal's B30.2
- blennorrhagic (gonococcal) (neonatorum) A54.31
- chemical (acute) — *see also* Corrosion, cornea H10.21-
- chlamydial A74.0
  - due to trachoma A71.1
  - neonatal P39.1
- chronic (nodosa) (petrificans) (phlyctenular) H10.40-
  - allergic H10.45
    - vernal H10.44
  - follicular H10.43-
  - giant papillary H10.41-
  - simple H10.42-
  - vernal H10.44
- coxsackievirus 24 B30.3
- diphtheritic A36.86
- due to
  - dust — *see* Conjunctivitis, acute, atopic
  - filariasis B74.9
  - mucocutaneous leishmaniasis B55.2
- enterovirus type 70 (hemorrhagic) B30.3
- epidemic (viral) B30.9
  - hemorrhagic B30.3
- gonococcal (neonatorum) A54.31
- granular (trachomatous) A71.1
  - sequelae (late effect) B94.0
- hemorrhagic (acute) (epidemic) B30.3
- herpes zoster B02.31
- in (due to)
  - Acanthamoeba B60.12
  - adenovirus (acute) (follicular) B30.1
  - Chlamydia A74.0
  - coxsackievirus 24 B30.3
  - diphtheria A36.86
  - enterovirus type 70 (hemorrhagic) B30.3
  - filariasis B74.9
  - gonococci A54.31
  - herpes (simplex) virus B00.53
    - zoster B02.31
  - infectious disease NEC B99
  - meningococci A39.89
  - mucocutaneous leishmaniasis B55.2
  - rosacea H10.82-
  - syphilis (late) A52.71
  - zoster B02.31
- inclusion A74.0
- infantile P39.1
  - gonococcal A54.31
- Koch-Weeks' — *see* Conjunctivitis, acute, mucopurulent
- light — *see* Conjunctivitis, acute, atopic
- ligneous — *see* Blepharoconjunctivitis, ligneous

Conjunctivitis (staphylococcal) (streptococcal) NOS - *continued*
- meningococcal A39.89
- mucopurulent — *see* Conjunctivitis, acute, mucopurulent
- neonatal P39.1
  - gonococcal A54.31
- Newcastle B30.8
- of Béal B30.2
- parasitic
  - filariasis B74.9
  - mucocutaneous leishmaniasis B55.2
- Parinaud's H10.89
- petrificans H10.89
- rosacea H10.82-
- specified NEC H10.89
- swimming-pool B30.1
- trachomatous A71.1
  - acute A71.0
  - sequelae (late effect) B94.0
- traumatic NEC H10.89
- tuberculous A18.59
- tularemic A21.1
- tularensis A21.1
- viral B30.9
  - due to
    - adenovirus B30.1
    - enterovirus B30.3
  - specified NEC B30.8

Conjunctivochalasis H11.82-
Connective tissue — *see* condition
Conn's syndrome E26.01
Conradi (-Hunermann) disease Q77.3
Consanguinity Z84.3
- counseling Z71.89

Conscious simulation (of illness) Z76.5
Consecutive — *see* condition
Consolidation lung (base) — *see* Pneumonia, lobar
Constipation (atonic) (neurogenic) (simple) (spastic) K59.00
- chronic K59.09
  - idiopathic K59.04
- drug-induced K59.03
- functional K59.04
- outlet dysfunction K59.02
- psychogenic F45.8
- slow transit K59.01
- specified NEC K59.09

Constitutional — *see also* condition
- substandard F60.7

Constitutionally substandard F60.7
Constriction — *see also* Stricture
- auditory canal — *see* Stenosis, external ear canal
- bronchial J98.09
- duodenum K31.5
- esophagus K22.2
- external
  - abdomen, abdominal (wall) S30.841
  - alveolar process S00.542
  - ankle S90.54-
  - antecubital space — *see* Constriction, external, forearm
  - arm (upper) S40.84-
  - auricle — *see* Constriction, external, ear
  - axilla — *see* Constriction, external, arm
  - back, lower S30.840
  - breast S20.14-
  - brow S00.84
  - buttock S30.840
  - calf — *see* Constriction, external, leg
  - canthus — *see* Constriction, external, eyelid
  - cheek S00.84
    - internal S00.542
  - chest wall — *see* Constriction, external, thorax
  - chin S00.84
  - clitoris S30.844
  - costal region — *see* Constriction, external, thorax
  - digit (s)
    - foot — *see* Constriction, external, toe

Constriction - *continued*
- external - *continued*
  - digit (s) - *continued*
    - hand — *see* Constriction, external, finger
  - ear S00.44-
  - elbow S50.34-
  - epididymis S30.843
  - epigastric region S30.841
  - esophagus, cervical S10.14
  - eyebrow — *see* Constriction, external, eyelid
  - eyelid S00.24-
  - face S00.84
  - finger (s) S60.44-
    - index S60.44-
    - little S60.44-
    - middle S60.44-
    - ring S60.44-
  - flank S30.841
  - foot (except toe (s) alone) S90.84-
    - toe — *see* Constriction, external, toe
  - forearm S50.84-
    - elbow only — *see* Constriction, external, elbow
  - forehead S00.84
  - genital organs, external
    - female S30.846
    - male S30.845
  - groin S30.841
  - gum S00.542
  - hand S60.54-
  - head S00.94
    - ear — *see* Constriction, external, ear
    - eyelid — *see* Constriction, external, eyelid
    - lip S00.541
    - nose S00.34
    - oral cavity S00.542
    - scalp S00.04
    - specified site NEC S00.84
  - heel — *see* Constriction, external, foot
  - hip S70.24-
  - inguinal region S30.841
  - interscapular region S20.449
  - jaw S00.84
  - knee S80.24-
  - labium (majus) (minus) S30.844
  - larynx S10.14
  - leg (lower) S80.84-
    - knee — *see* Constriction, external, knee
    - upper — *see* Constriction, external, thigh
  - lip S00.541
  - lower back S30.840
  - lumbar region S30.840
  - malar region S00.84
  - mammary — *see* Constriction, external, breast
  - mastoid region S00.84
  - mouth S00.542
  - nail
    - finger — *see* Constriction, external, finger
    - toe — *see* Constriction, external, toe
  - nasal S00.34
  - neck S10.94
    - specified site NEC S10.84
    - throat S10.14
  - nose S00.34
  - occipital region S00.04
  - oral cavity S00.542
  - orbital region — *see* Constriction, external, eyelid
  - palate S00.542
  - palm — *see* Constriction, external, hand
  - parietal region S00.04
  - pelvis S30.840
  - penis S30.842
  - perineum
    - female S30.844
    - male S30.840
  - periocular area — *see* Constriction, external, eyelid
  - phalanges

- **Constriction** - *continued*
  - external - *continued*
    - phalanges - *continued*
      - finger — *see* Constriction, external, finger
      - toe — *see* Constriction, external, toe
    - pharynx S10.14
    - pinna — *see* Constriction, external, ear
    - popliteal space — *see* Constriction, external, knee
    - prepuce S30.842
    - pubic region S30.840
    - pudendum
      - female S30.846
      - male S30.845
    - sacral region S30.840
    - scalp S00.04
    - scapular region — *see* Constriction, external, shoulder
    - scrotum S30.843
    - shin — *see* Constriction, external, leg
    - shoulder S40.24-
    - sternal region S20.349
    - submaxillary region S00.84
    - submental region S00.84
    - subungual
      - finger (s) — *see* Constriction, external, finger
      - toe (s) — *see* Constriction, external, toe
    - supraclavicular fossa S10.84
    - supraorbital S00.84
    - temple S00.84
    - temporal region S00.84
    - testis S30.843
    - thigh S70.34-
    - thorax, thoracic (wall) S20.94
      - back S20.44-
      - front S20.34-
    - throat S10.14
    - thumb S60.34-
    - toe (s) (lesser) S90.44-
      - great S90.44-
    - tongue S00.542
    - trachea S10.14
    - tunica vaginalis S30.843
    - uvula S00.542
    - vagina S30.844
    - vulva S30.844
    - wrist S60.84-
  - gallbladder — *see* Obstruction, gallbladder
  - intestine — *see* Obstruction, intestine
  - larynx J38.6
    - congenital Q31.8
      - specified NEC Q31.8
      - subglottic Q31.1
  - organ or site, congenital NEC — *see* Atresia, by site
  - prepuce (acquired) (congenital) N47.1
  - pylorus (adult hypertrophic) K31.1
    - congenital or infantile Q40.0
    - newborn Q40.0
  - ring dystocia (uterus) O62.4
  - spastic — *see also* Spasm
    - ureter N13.5
  - ureter N13.5
    - with infection N13.6
  - urethra — *see* Stricture, urethra
  - visual field (peripheral) (functional) — *see* Defect, visual field
- **Constrictive** — *see* condition
- **Consultation**
  - medical — *see* Counseling, medical
  - religious Z71.81
  - specified reason NEC Z71.89
  - spiritual Z71.81
  - without complaint or sickness Z71.9
    - feared complaint unfounded Z71.1
    - specified reason NEC Z71.89
- **Consumption** — *see* Tuberculosis
- **Contact (with)** — *see also* Exposure (to)
  - acariasis Z20.7
  - AIDS virus Z20.6
  - air pollution Z77.110
  - algae and algae toxins Z77.121
  - algae bloom Z77.121
  - anthrax Z20.810
  - aromatic amines Z77.020
  - aromatic (hazardous) compounds NEC Z77.028
  - aromatic dyes NOS Z77.028
  - arsenic Z77.010
  - asbestos Z77.090
  - bacterial disease NEC Z20.818
  - benzene Z77.021
  - blue-green algae bloom Z77.121
  - body fluids (potentially hazardous) Z77.21
  - brown tide Z77.121
  - chemicals (chiefly nonmedicinal) (hazardous) NEC Z77.098
  - cholera Z20.09
  - chromium compounds Z77.018
  - communicable disease Z20.9
    - bacterial NEC Z20.818
    - specified NEC Z20.89
    - viral NEC Z20.828
    - Zika virus Z20.821
  - coronavirus (disease) (novel) 2019 Z20.822
  - COVID-19 Z20.822
  - cyanobacteria bloom Z77.121
  - dyes Z77.098
  - Escherichia coli (E. coli) Z20.01
  - fiberglass — *see* Table of Drugs and Chemicals, fiberglass
  - German measles Z20.4
  - gonorrhea Z20.2
  - hazardous metals NEC Z77.018
  - hazardous substances NEC Z77.29
  - hazards in the physical environment NEC Z77.128
  - hazards to health NEC Z77.9
  - HIV Z20.6
  - HTLV-III/LAV Z20.6
  - human immunodeficiency virus (HIV) Z20.6
  - infection Z20.9
    - specified NEC Z20.89
  - infestation (parasitic) NEC Z20.7
  - intestinal infectious disease NEC Z20.09
    - Escherichia coli (E. coli) Z20.01
  - lead Z77.011
  - positive maternal group B streptococcus P00.82
  - meningococcus Z20.811
  - mold (toxic) Z77.120
  - nickel dust Z77.018
  - noise Z77.122
  - parasitic disease Z20.7
  - pediculosis Z20.7
  - pfiesteria piscicida Z77.121
  - poliomyelitis Z20.89
  - pollution
    - air Z77.110
    - environmental NEC Z77.118
    - soil Z77.112
    - water Z77.111
  - polycyclic aromatic hydrocarbons Z77.028
  - rabies Z20.3
  - radiation, naturally occurring NEC Z77.123
  - radon Z77.123
  - red tide (Florida) Z77.121
  - rubella Z20.4
  - SARS-CoV-2 Z20.822
  - sexually-transmitted disease Z20.2
  - smallpox (laboratory) Z20.89
  - syphilis Z20.2
  - tuberculosis Z20.1
  - uranium Z77.012
  - varicella Z20.820
  - venereal disease Z20.2
  - viral disease NEC Z20.828
  - viral hepatitis Z20.5
  - water pollution Z77.111
  - Zika virus Z20.821
- **Contamination, food** — *see* Intoxication, foodborne
- **Contraception, contraceptive**
  - advice Z30.09
  - counseling Z30.09
  - device (intrauterine) (in situ) Z97.5
    - causing menorrhagia T83.83
    - checking Z30.431
    - complications — *see* Complications, intrauterine, contraceptive device
    - in place Z97.5
    - initial prescription Z30.014
    - reinsertion Z30.433
    - removal Z30.432
    - replacement Z30.433
  - emergency (postcoital) Z30.012
  - initial prescription Z30.019
    - barrier Z30.018
    - diaphragm Z30.018
    - injectable Z30.013
    - intrauterine device Z30.014
    - pills Z30.011
    - postcoital (emergency) Z30.012
    - specified type NEC Z30.018
    - subdermal implantable Z30.017
    - transdermal patch hormonal Z30.016
    - vaginal ring hormonal Z30.015
  - maintenance Z30.40
    - barrier Z30.49
    - diaphragm Z30.49
    - examination Z30.8
    - injectable Z30.42
    - intrauterine device Z30.431
    - pills Z30.41
    - specified type NEC Z30.49
    - subdermal implantable Z30.46
    - transdermal patch hormonal Z30.45
    - vaginal ring hormonal Z30.44
  - management Z30.9
    - specified NEC Z30.8
  - postcoital (emergency) Z30.012
  - prescription Z30.019
    - repeat Z30.40
  - sterilization Z30.2
  - surveillance (drug) — *see* Contraception, maintenance
- **Contraction (s) , contracture, contracted**
  - Achilles tendon — *see also* Short, tendon, Achilles
    - congenital Q66.89
  - amputation stump (surgical) (flexion) (late) (next proximal joint) T87.89
  - anus K59.89
  - bile duct (common) (hepatic) K83.8
  - bladder N32.89
    - neck or sphincter N32.0
  - bowel, cecum, colon or intestine, any part — *see* Obstruction, intestine
  - Braxton Hicks — *see* False, labor
  - breast implant, capsular T85.44
  - bronchial J98.09
  - burn (old) — *see* Cicatrix
  - cervix — *see* Stricture, cervix
  - cicatricial — *see* Cicatrix
  - conjunctiva, trachomatous, active A71.1
    - sequelae (late effect) B94.0
  - Dupuytren's M72.0
  - eyelid — *see* Disorder, eyelid function
  - fascia (lata) (postural) M72.8
    - Dupuytren's M72.0
    - palmar M72.0
    - plantar M72.2
  - finger NEC — *see also* Deformity, finger
    - congenital Q68.1
    - joint — *see* Contraction, joint, hand
  - flaccid — *see* Contraction, paralytic
  - gallbladder K82.0
  - heart valve — *see* Endocarditis
  - hip — *see* Contraction, joint, hip
  - hourglass
    - bladder N32.89
      - congenital Q64.79
    - gallbladder K82.0
      - congenital Q44.1
    - stomach K31.89
      - congenital Q40.2
      - psychogenic F45.8
    - uterus (complicating delivery) O62.4
  - hysterical F44.4
  - internal os — *see* Stricture, cervix

- **Contraction (s) , contracture, contracted** - *continued*
  - joint (abduction) (acquired) (adduction) (flexion) (rotation) M24.50
    - ankle M24.57-
    - congenital NEC Q68.8
      - hip Q65.89
    - elbow M24.52-
    - foot joint M24.57-
    - hand joint M24.54-
    - hip M24.55-
      - congenital Q65.89
    - hysterical F44.4
    - knee M24.56-
    - shoulder M24.51-
    - specified site NEC M24.59
    - wrist M24.53-
  - kidney (granular) (secondary) N26.9
    - congenital Q63.8
    - hydronephritic — *see* Hydronephrosis Page N26.2
    - pyelonephritic — *see* Pyelitis, chronic
    - tuberculous A18.11
  - ligament — *see also* Disorder, ligament
    - congenital Q79.8
  - muscle (postinfective) (postural) NEC M62.40
    - with contracture of joint — *see* Contraction, joint
    - ankle M62.47-
    - congenital Q79.8
      - sternocleidomastoid Q68.0
    - extraocular — *see* Strabismus
    - eye (extrinsic) — *see* Strabismus
    - foot M62.47-
    - forearm M62.43-
    - hand M62.44-
    - hysterical F44.4
    - ischemic (Volkmann's) T79.6
    - lower leg M62.46-
    - multiple sites M62.49
    - pelvic region M62.45-
    - posttraumatic — *see* Strabismus, paralytic
    - psychogenic F45.8
      - conversion reaction F44.4
    - shoulder region M62.41-
    - specified site NEC M62.48
    - thigh M62.45-
    - upper arm M62.42-
  - neck — *see* Torticollis
  - ocular muscle — *see* Strabismus
  - organ or site, congenital NEC — *see* Atresia, by site
  - outlet (pelvis) — *see* Contraction, pelvis
  - palmar fascia M72.0
  - paralytic
    - joint — *see* Contraction, joint
    - muscle — *see also* Contraction, muscle NEC
      - ocular — *see* Strabismus, paralytic
  - pelvis (acquired) (general) M95.5
    - with disproportion (fetopelvic) O33.1
      - causing obstructed labor O65.1
      - inlet O33.2
      - mid-cavity O33.3
      - outlet O33.3
  - plantar fascia M72.2
  - premature
    - atrium I49.1
    - auriculoventricular I49.49
    - heart I49.49
    - junctional I49.2
    - supraventricular I49.1
    - ventricular I49.3
  - prostate N42.89
  - pylorus NEC — *see also* Pylorospasm
    - psychogenic F45.8
  - rectum, rectal (sphincter) K59.89
  - ring (Bandl's) (complicating delivery) O62.4
  - scar — *see* Cicatrix
  - spine — *see* Dorsopathy, deforming
  - sternocleidomastoid (muscle) , congenital Q68.0
  - stomach K31.89
    - hourglass K31.89

- **Contraction (s) , contracture, contracted** - *continued*
  - stomach - *continued*
    - hourglass - *continued*
      - congenital Q40.2
      - psychogenic F45.8
    - psychogenic F45.8
  - tendon (sheath) M62.40
    - with contracture of joint — *see* Contraction, joint
    - Achilles — *see* Short, tendon, Achilles
    - ankle M62.47-
      - Achilles — *see* Short, tendon, Achilles
    - foot M62.47-
    - forearm M62.43-
    - hand M62.44-
    - lower leg M62.46-
    - multiple sites M62.49
    - neck M62.48
    - pelvic region M62.45-
    - shoulder region M62.41-
    - specified site NEC M62.48
    - thigh M62.45-
    - thorax M62.48
    - trunk M62.48
    - upper arm M62.42-
  - toe — *see* Deformity, toe, specified NEC
  - ureterovesical orifice (postinfectional) N13.5
    - with infection N13.6
  - urethra — *see also* Stricture, urethra
    - orifice N32.0
  - uterus N85.8
    - abnormal NEC O62.9
    - clonic (complicating delivery) O62.4
    - dyscoordinate (complicating delivery) O62.4
    - hourglass (complicating delivery) O62.4
    - hypertonic O62.4
    - hypotonic NEC O62.2
    - inadequate
      - primary O62.0
      - secondary O62.1
    - incoordinate (complicating delivery) O62.4
    - poor O62.2
    - tetanic (complicating delivery) O62.4
  - vagina (outlet) N89.5
  - vesical N32.89
    - neck or urethral orifice N32.0
  - visual field — *see* Defect, visual field, generalized
  - Volkmann's (ischemic) T79.6
- **Contusion (skin surface intact)** T14.8
  - abdomen, abdominal (muscle) (wall) S30.1
  - adnexa, eye NEC S05.8X-
  - adrenal gland S37.812
  - alveolar process S00.532
  - ankle S90.0-
  - antecubital space — *see* Contusion, forearm
  - anus S30.3
  - arm (upper) S40.02-
    - lower (with elbow) — *see* Contusion, forearm
  - auditory canal — *see* Contusion, ear
  - auricle — *see* Contusion, ear
  - axilla — *see* Contusion, arm, upper
  - back — *see also* Contusion, thorax, back
    - lower S30.0
  - bile duct S36.13
  - bladder S37.22
  - bone NEC T14.8
  - brain (diffuse) — *see* Injury, intracranial, diffuse
    - focal — *see* Injury, intracranial, focal
  - brainstem S06.38-
  - breast S20.0-
  - broad ligament S37.892
  - brow S00.83
  - buttock S30.0
  - canthus, eye S00.1-
  - cauda equina S34.3
  - cerebellar, traumatic S06.37-
  - cerebral S06.33-
    - left side S06.32-
    - right side S06.31-
  - cheek S00.83

- **Contusion (skin surface intact)** - *continued*
  - cheek - *continued*
    - internal S00.532
  - chest (wall) — *see* Contusion, thorax
  - chin S00.83
  - clitoris S30.23
  - colon — *see* Injury, intestine, large, contusion
  - common bile duct S36.13
  - conjunctiva S05.1-
    - with foreign body (in conjunctival sac) — *see* Foreign body, conjunctival sac
  - conus medullaris (spine) S34.139
  - cornea — *see* Contusion, eyeball
    - with foreign body — *see* Foreign body, cornea
  - corpus cavernosum S30.21
  - cortex (brain) (cerebral) — *see* Injury, intracranial, diffuse
    - focal — *see* Injury, intracranial, focal
  - costal region — *see* Contusion, thorax
  - cystic duct S36.13
  - diaphragm S27.802
  - duodenum S36.420
  - ear S00.43-
  - elbow S50.0-
    - with forearm — *see* Contusion, forearm
  - epididymis S30.22
  - epigastric region S30.1
  - epiglottis S10.0
  - esophagus (thoracic) S27.812
    - cervical S10.0
  - eyeball S05.1-
  - eyebrow S00.1-
  - eyelid (and periocular area) S00.1-
  - face NEC S00.83
  - fallopian tube S37.529
    - bilateral S37.522
    - unilateral S37.521
  - femoral triangle S30.1
  - finger (s) S60.00
    - with damage to nail (matrix) S60.10
    - index S60.02-
      - with damage to nail S60.12-
    - little S60.05-
      - with damage to nail S60.15-
    - middle S60.03-
      - with damage to nail S60.13-
    - ring S60.04-
      - with damage to nail S60.14-
    - thumb — *see* Contusion, thumb
  - flank S30.1
  - foot (except toe (s) alone) S90.3-
    - toe — *see* Contusion, toe
  - forearm S50.1-
    - elbow only — *see* Contusion, elbow
  - forehead S00.83
  - gallbladder S36.122
  - genital organs, external
    - female S30.202
    - male S30.201
  - globe (eye) — *see* Contusion, eyeball
  - groin S30.1
  - gum S00.532
  - hand S60.22-
    - finger (s) — *see* Contusion, finger
    - wrist — *see* Contusion, wrist
  - head S00.93
    - ear — *see* Contusion, ear
    - eyelid — *see* Contusion, eyelid
    - lip S00.531
    - nose S00.33
    - oral cavity S00.532
    - scalp S00.03
    - specified part NEC S00.83
  - heart — *see also* Injury, heart S26.91
  - heel — *see* Contusion, foot
  - hepatic duct S36.13
  - hip S70.0-
  - ileum S36.428
  - iliac region S30.1
  - inguinal region S30.1
  - interscapular region S20.229
  - intra-abdominal organ S36.92

Contusion (skin surface intact) - *continued*
- intra-abdominal organ - *continued*
  - colon — *see* Injury, intestine, large, contusion
  - liver S36.112
  - pancreas — *see* Contusion, pancreas
  - rectum S36.62
  - small intestine — *see* Injury, intestine, small, contusion
  - specified organ NEC S36.892
  - spleen — *see* Contusion, spleen
  - stomach S36.32
- iris (eye) — *see* Contusion, eyeball
- jaw S00.83
- jejunum S36.428
- kidney S37.01-
  - major (greater than 2 cm) S37.02-
  - minor (less than 2 cm) S37.01-
- knee S80.0-
- labium (majus) (minus) S30.23
- lacrimal apparatus, gland or sac S05.8X-
- larynx S10.0
- leg (lower) S80.1-
  - knee — *see* Contusion, knee
- lens — *see* Contusion, eyeball
- lip S00.531
- liver S36.112
- lower back S30.0
- lumbar region S30.0
- lung S27.329
  - bilateral S27.322
  - unilateral S27.321
- malar region S00.83
- mastoid region S00.83
- membrane, brain — *see* Injury, intracranial, diffuse
  - focal — *see* Injury, intracranial, focal
- mesentery S36.892
- mesosalpinx S37.892
- mouth S00.532
- muscle — *see* Contusion, by site
- nail
  - finger — *see* Contusion, finger, with damage to nail
  - toe — *see* Contusion, toe, with damage to nail
- nasal S00.33
- neck S10.93
  - specified site NEC S10.83
  - throat S10.0
- nerve — *see* Injury, nerve
- newborn P54.5
- nose S00.33
- occipital
  - lobe (brain) — *see* Injury, intracranial, diffuse
    - focal — *see* Injury, intracranial, focal
  - region (scalp) S00.03
- orbit (region) (tissues) S05.1-
- ovary S37.429
  - bilateral S37.422
  - unilateral S37.421
- palate S00.532
- pancreas S36.229
  - body S36.221
  - head S36.220
  - tail S36.222
- parietal
  - lobe (brain) — *see* Injury, intracranial, diffuse
    - focal — *see* Injury, intracranial, focal
  - region (scalp) S00.03
- pelvic organ S37.92
  - adrenal gland S37.812
  - bladder S37.22
  - fallopian tube — *see* Contusion, fallopian tube
  - kidney — *see* Contusion, kidney
  - ovary — *see* Contusion, ovary
  - prostate S37.822
  - specified organ NEC S37.892
  - ureter S37.12
  - urethra S37.32
  - uterus S37.62
- pelvis S30.0

Contusion (skin surface intact) - *continued*
- penis S30.21
- perineum
  - female S30.23
  - male S30.0
- periocular area S00.1-
- peritoneum S36.81
- periurethral tissue — *see* Contusion, urethra
- pharynx S10.0
- pinna — *see* Contusion, ear
- popliteal space — *see* Contusion, knee
- prepuce S30.21
- prostate S37.822
- pubic region S30.1
- pudendum
  - female S30.202
  - male S30.201
- quadriceps femoris — *see* Contusion, thigh
- rectum S36.62
- retroperitoneum S36.892
- round ligament S37.892
- sacral region S30.0
- scalp S00.03
  - due to birth injury P12.3
- scapular region — *see* Contusion, shoulder
- sclera — *see* Contusion, eyeball
- scrotum S30.22
- seminal vesicle S37.892
- shoulder S40.01-
- skin NEC T14.8
- small intestine — *see* Injury, intestine, small, contusion
- spermatic cord S30.22
- spinal cord — *see* Injury, spinal cord, by region
  - cauda equina S34.3
  - conus medullaris S34.139
- spleen S36.029
  - major S36.021
  - minor S36.020
- sternal region S20.219
- stomach S36.32
- subconjunctival S05.1-
- subcutaneous NEC T14.8
- submaxillary region S00.83
- submental region S00.83
- subperiosteal NEC T14.8
- subungual
  - finger — *see* Contusion, finger, with damage to nail
  - toe — *see* Contusion, toe, with damage to nail
- supraclavicular fossa S10.83
- supraorbital S00.83
- suprarenal gland S37.812
- temple (region) S00.83
- temporal
  - lobe (brain) — *see* Injury, intracranial, diffuse
    - focal — *see* Injury, intracranial, focal
  - region S00.83
- testis S30.22
- thigh S70.1-
- thorax (wall) S20.20
  - back S20.22-
  - front S20.21-
- throat S10.0
- thumb S60.01-
  - with damage to nail S60.11-
- toe (s) (lesser) S90.12-
  - with damage to nail S90.22-
  - great S90.11-
    - with damage to nail S90.21-
- tongue S00.532
- trachea (cervical) S10.0
  - thoracic S27.52
- tunica vaginalis S30.22
- tympanum, tympanic membrane — *see* Contusion, ear
- ureter S37.12
- urethra S37.32
- urinary organ NEC S37.892
- uterus S37.62
- uvula S00.532
- vagina S30.23

Contusion (skin surface intact) - *continued*
- vas deferens S37.892
- vesical S37.22
- vocal cord (s) S10.0
- vulva S30.23
- wrist S60.21-

Conus (congenital) (any type) Q14.8
- cornea — *see* Keratoconus
- medullaris syndrome G95.81

Conversion hysteria, neurosis or reaction F44.9

Converter, tuberculosis (test reaction) R76.11

Conviction (legal) , anxiety concerning Z65.0
- with imprisonment Z65.1

Convulsions (idiopathic) — *see also* Seizure(s) R56.9
- apoplectiform (cerebral ischemia) I67.82
- dissociative F44.5
- epileptic — *see* Epilepsy
- epileptiform, epileptoid — *see* Seizure, epileptiform
- ether (anesthetic) — *see* Table of Drugs and Chemicals, by drug
- febrile R56.00
  - with status epilepticus G40.901
  - complex R56.01
    - with status epilepticus G40.901
  - simple R56.00
- hysterical F44.5
- infantile P90
  - epilepsy — *see* Epilepsy
- jacksonian — *see* Epilepsy, localization-related, symptomatic, with simple partial seizures
- myoclonic G25.3
- newborn P90
- obstetrical (nephritic) (uremic) — *see* Eclampsia
- paretic A52.17
- post traumatic R56.1
- psychomotor — *see* Epilepsy, localization-related, symptomatic, with complex partial seizures
- recurrent R56.9
- reflex R25.8
- scarlatinal A38.8
- tetanus, tetanic — *see* Tetanus
- thymic E32.8

Convulsive — *see also* Convulsions

Cooley's anemia D56.1

Coolie itch B76.9

Cooper's
- disease — *see* Mastopathy, cystic
- hernia — *see* Hernia, abdomen, specified site NEC

Copra itch B88.0

Coprophagy F50.89

Coprophobia F40.298

Coproporphyria, hereditary E80.29

Cor
- biloculare Q20.8
- bovis, bovinum — *see* Hypertrophy, cardiac
- pulmonale (chronic) I27.81
  - acute I26.09
- triatriatum, triatrium Q24.2
- triloculare Q20.8
  - biatrium Q20.4
  - biventriculare Q21.1

Corbus' disease (gangrenous balanitis) N48.1

Cord — *see also* condition
- around neck
  - complicating delivery O69.81
    - with compression O69.1
- bladder G95.89
  - tabetic A52.19

Cordis ectopia Q24.8

Corditis (spermatic) N49.1

Corectopia Q13.2

Cori's disease (glycogen storage) E74.03

Corkhandler's disease or lung J67.3

Corkscrew esophagus K22.4

Corkworker's disease or lung J67.3

Corn (infected) L84

- **Cornea** — *see also* condition
  - donor Z52.5
  - plana Q13.4
- **Cornelia de Lange syndrome** Q87.19
- **Cornu cutaneum** L85.8
- **Cornual gestation or pregnancy** O00.80
  - with intrauterine pregnancy O00.81
- **Coronary (artery)** — *see* condition
- **Coronavirus (infection)**
  - 2019 — *see also* COVID-19 U07.1
  - as cause of disease classified elsewhere B97.29
  - coronavirus-19 — *see also* COVID-19 U07.1
  - COVID-19 — *see also* COVID-19 U07.1
  - SARS-associated B97.21
- **Corpora** — *see also* condition
  - amylacea, prostate N42.89
  - cavernosa — *see* condition
- **Corpulence** — *see* Obesity
- **Corpus** — *see* condition
- **Corrected transposition** Q20.5
- **Corrosion (injury) (acid) (caustic) (chemical) (lime) (external) (internal)** T30.4
  - abdomen, abdominal (muscle) (wall) T21.42
    - first degree T21.52
    - second degree T21.62
    - third degree T21.72
  - above elbow T22.439
    - first degree T22.539
    - left T22.432
      - first degree T22.532
      - second degree T22.632
      - third degree T22.732
    - right T22.431
      - first degree T22.531
      - second degree T22.631
      - third degree T22.731
    - second degree T22.639
    - third degree T22.739
  - alimentary tract NEC T28.7
  - ankle T25.419
    - first degree T25.519
    - left T25.412
      - first degree T25.512
      - second degree T25.612
      - third degree T25.712
    - multiple with foot — *see* Corrosion, lower, limb, multiple, ankle and foot
    - right T25.411
      - first degree T25.511
      - second degree T25.611
      - third degree T25.711
    - second degree T25.619
    - third degree T25.719
  - anus — *see* Corrosion, buttock
  - arm (s) (meaning upper limb (s)) — *see* Corrosion, upper limb
  - axilla T22.449
    - first degree T22.549
    - left T22.442
      - first degree T22.542
      - second degree T22.642
      - third degree T22.742
    - right T22.441
      - first degree T22.541
      - second degree T22.641
      - third degree T22.741
    - second degree T22.649
    - third degree T22.749
  - back (lower) T21.44
    - first degree T21.54
    - second degree T21.64
    - third degree T21.74
    - upper T21.43
      - first degree T21.53
      - second degree T21.63
      - third degree T21.73
  - blisters - code as Corrosion, second degree, by site
  - breast (s) — *see* Corrosion, chest wall
  - buttock (s) T21.45
    - first degree T21.55
    - second degree T21.65
    - third degree T21.75
  - calf T24.439

Corrosion (injury) (acid) (caustic) (chemical) (lime) (external) (internal) - *continued*

  - calf - *continued*
    - first degree T24.539
    - left T24.432
      - first degree T24.532
      - second degree T24.632
      - third degree T24.732
    - right T24.431
      - first degree T24.531
      - second degree T24.631
      - third degree T24.731
    - second degree T24.639
    - third degree T24.739
  - canthus (eye) — *see* Corrosion, eyelid
  - cervix T28.8
  - cheek T20.46
    - first degree T20.56
    - second degree T20.66
    - third degree T20.76
  - chest wall T21.41
    - first degree T21.51
    - second degree T21.61
    - third degree T21.71
  - chin T20.43
    - first degree T20.53
    - second degree T20.63
    - third degree T20.73
  - colon T28.7
  - conjunctiva (and cornea) — *see* Corrosion, cornea
  - cornea (and conjunctiva) T26.6-
  - deep necrosis of underlying tissue - code as Corrosion, third degree, by site
  - dorsum of hand T23.469
    - first degree T23.569
    - left T23.462
      - first degree T23.562
      - second degree T23.662
      - third degree T23.762
    - right T23.461
      - first degree T23.561
      - second degree T23.661
      - third degree T23.761
    - second degree T23.669
    - third degree T23.769
  - ear (auricle) (external) (canal) T20.41
    - drum T28.91
    - first degree T20.51
    - second degree T20.61
    - third degree T20.71
  - elbow T22.429
    - first degree T22.529
    - left T22.422
      - first degree T22.522
      - second degree T22.622
      - third degree T22.722
    - right T22.421
      - first degree T22.521
      - second degree T22.621
      - third degree T22.721
    - second degree T22.629
    - third degree T22.729
  - entire body — *see* Corrosion, multiple body regions
  - epidermal loss - code as Corrosion, second degree, by site
  - epiglottis T27.4
  - erythema, erythematous - code as Corrosion, first degree, by site
  - esophagus T28.6
  - extent (percentage of body surface)
    - less than 10 percent T32.0
    - 10-19 percent (0-9 percent third degree) T32.10
      - with 10-19 percent third degree T32.11
    - 20-29 percent (0-9 percent third degree) T32.20
      - with
        - 10-19 percent third degree T32.21
        - 20-29 percent third degree T32.22
    - 30-39 percent (0-9 percent third degree) T32.30
      - with
        - 10-19 percent third degree T32.31

Corrosion (injury) (acid) (caustic) (chemical) (lime) (external) (internal) - *continued*

  - extent (percentage of body surface) - *continued*
    - 30-39 percent (0-9 percent third degree) - *continued*
      - with - *continued*
        - 20-29 percent third degree T32.32
        - 30-39 percent third degree T32.33
    - 40-49 percent (0-9 percent third degree) T32.40
      - with
        - 10-19 percent third degree T32.41
        - 20-29 percent third degree T32.42
        - 30-39 percent third degree T32.43
        - 40-49 percent third degree T32.44
    - 50-59 percent (0-9 percent third degree) T32.50
      - with
        - 10-19 percent third degree T32.51
        - 20-29 percent third degree T32.52
        - 30-39 percent third degree T32.53
        - 40-49 percent third degree T32.54
        - 50-59 percent third degree T32.55
    - 60-69 percent (0-9 percent third degree) T32.60
      - with
        - 10-19 percent third degree T32.61
        - 20-29 percent third degree T32.62
        - 30-39 percent third degree T32.63
        - 40-49 percent third degree T32.64
        - 50-59 percent third degree T32.65
        - 60-69 percent third degree T32.66
    - 70-79 percent (0-9 percent third degree) T32.70
      - with
        - 10-19 percent third degree T32.71
        - 20-29 percent third degree T32.72
        - 30-39 percent third degree T32.73
        - 40-49 percent third degree T32.74
        - 50-59 percent third degree T32.75
        - 60-69 percent third degree T32.76
        - 70-79 percent third degree T32.77
    - 80-89 percent (0-9 percent third degree) T32.80
      - with
        - 10-19 percent third degree T32.81
        - 20-29 percent third degree T32.82
        - 30-39 percent third degree T32.83
        - 40-49 percent third degree T32.84
        - 50-59 percent third degree T32.85
        - 60-69 percent third degree T32.86
        - 70-79 percent third degree T32.87
        - 80-89 percent third degree T32.88
    - 90 percent or more (0-9 percent third degree) T32.90
      - with
        - 10-19 percent third degree T32.91
        - 20-29 percent third degree T32.92
        - 30-39 percent third degree T32.93
        - 40-49 percent third degree T32.94
        - 50-59 percent third degree T32.95
        - 60-69 percent third degree T32.96
        - 70-79 percent third degree T32.97
        - 80-89 percent third degree T32.98
        - 90-99 percent third degree T32.99
  - extremity — *see* Corrosion, limb
  - eye (s) and adnexa T26.9-
    - with resulting rupture and destruction of eyeball T26.7-
    - conjunctival sac — *see* Corrosion, cornea
    - cornea — *see* Corrosion, cornea
    - lid — *see* Corrosion, eyelid
    - periocular area — *see* Corrosion eyelid
    - specified site NEC T26.8-
  - eyeball — *see* Corrosion, eye
  - eyelid (s) T26.5-
  - face — *see* Corrosion, head
  - finger T23.429
    - first degree T23.529
    - left T23.422
      - first degree T23.522
      - second degree T23.622
      - third degree T23.722
    - multiple sites (without thumb) T23.439

Corrosion (injury) (acid) (caustic) (chemical) (lime) (external) (internal) - *continued*
respiratory tract - *continued*
larynx — *see* Corrosion, larynx
specified part NEC T27.6
trachea — *see* Corrosion, larynx
sac, lacrimal — *see* Corrosion, eye, specified site NEC
scalp T20.45
first degree T20.55
second degree T20.65
third degree T20.75
scapular region T22.469
first degree T22.569
left T22.462
first degree T22.562
second degree T22.662
third degree T22.762
right T22.461
first degree T22.561
second degree T22.661
third degree T22.761
second degree T22.669
third degree T22.769
sclera — *see* Corrosion, eye, specified site NEC
scrotum — *see* Corrosion, genital organs, external, male
shoulder T22.459
first degree T22.559
left T22.452
first degree T22.552
second degree T22.652
third degree T22.752
right T22.451
first degree T22.551
second degree T22.651
third degree T22.751
second degree T22.659
third degree T22.759
stomach T28.7
temple — *see* Corrosion, head
testis — *see* Corrosion, genital organs, external, male
thigh T24.419
first degree T24.519
left T24.412
first degree T24.512
second degree T24.612
third degree T24.712
right T24.411
first degree T24.511
second degree T24.611
third degree T24.711
second degree T24.619
third degree T24.719
thorax (external) — *see* Corrosion, trunk
throat (meaning pharynx) T28.5
thumb (s) T23.419
first degree T23.519
left T23.412
first degree T23.512
second degree T23.612
third degree T23.712
multiple sites with fingers T23.449
first degree T23.549
left T23.442
first degree T23.542
second degree T23.642
third degree T23.742
right T23.441
first degree T23.541
second degree T23.641
third degree T23.741
second degree T23.649
third degree T23.749
right T23.411
first degree T23.511
second degree T23.611
third degree T23.711
second degree T23.619
third degree T23.719
toe T25.439
first degree T25.539
left T25.432

Corrosion (injury) (acid) (caustic) (chemical) (lime) (external) (internal) - *continued*
toe - *continued*
left - *continued*
first degree T25.532
second degree T25.632
third degree T25.732
right T25.431
first degree T25.531
second degree T25.631
third degree T25.731
second degree T25.639
third degree T25.739
tongue T28.5
tonsil (s) T28.5
total body — *see* Corrosion, multiple body regions
trachea T27.4
with lung T27.5
trunk T21.40
abdominal wall — *see* Corrosion, abdominal wall
anus — *see* Corrosion, buttock
axilla — *see* Corrosion, upper limb
back — *see* Corrosion, back
breast — *see* Corrosion, chest wall
buttock — *see* Corrosion, buttock
chest wall — *see* Corrosion, chest wall
first degree T21.50
flank — *see* Corrosion, abdominal wall
genital
female — *see* Corrosion, genital organs, external, female
male — *see* Corrosion, genital organs, external, male
groin — *see* Corrosion, abdominal wall
interscapular region — *see* Corrosion, back, upper
labia — *see* Corrosion, genital organs, external, female
lower back — *see* Corrosion, back
penis — *see* Corrosion, genital organs, external, male
perineum
female — *see* Corrosion, genital organs, external, female
male — *see* Corrosion, genital organs, external, male
scapular region — *see* Corrosion, upper limb
scrotum — *see* Corrosion, genital organs, external, male
second degree T21.60
shoulder — *see* Corrosion, upper limb
specified site NEC T21.49
first degree T21.59
second degree T21.69
third degree T21.79
testes — *see* Corrosion, genital organs, external, male
third degree T21.70
upper back — *see* Corrosion, back, upper
vagina T28.8
vulva — *see* Corrosion, genital organs, external, female
unspecified site with extent of body surface involved specified
less than 10 percent T32.0
10-19 percent (0-9 percent third degree) T32.10
with 10-19 percent third degree T32.11
20-29 percent (0-9 percent third degree) T32.20
with
10-19 percent third degree T32.21
20-29 percent third degree T32.22
30-39 percent (0-9 percent third degree) T32.30
with
10-19 percent third degree T32.31
20-29 percent third degree T32.32
30-39 percent third degree T32.33
40-49 percent (0-9 percent third degree) T32.40
with

Corrosion (injury) (acid) (caustic) (chemical) (lime) (external) (internal) - *continued*
unspecified site with extent of body surface involved specified - *continued*
40-49 percent (0-9 percent third degree) - *continued*
with - *continued*
10-19 percent third degree T32.41
20-29 percent third degree T32.42
30-39 percent third degree T32.43
40-49 percent third degree T32.44
50-59 percent (0-9 percent third degree) T32.50
with
10-19 percent third degree T32.51
20-29 percent third degree T32.52
30-39 percent third degree T32.53
40-49 percent third degree T32.54
50-59 percent third degree T32.55
60-69 percent (0-9 percent third degree) T32.60
with
10-19 percent third degree T32.61
20-29 percent third degree T32.62
30-39 percent third degree T32.63
40-49 percent third degree T32.64
50-59 percent third degree T32.65
60-69 percent third degree T32.66
70-79 percent (0-9 percent third degree) T32.70
with
10-19 percent third degree T32.71
20-29 percent third degree T32.72
30-39 percent third degree T32.73
40-49 percent third degree T32.74
50-59 percent third degree T32.75
60-69 percent third degree T32.76
70-79 percent third degree T32.77
80-89 percent (0-9 percent third degree) T32.80
with
10-19 percent third degree T32.81
20-29 percent third degree T32.82
30-39 percent third degree T32.83
40-49 percent third degree T32.84
50-59 percent third degree T32.85
60-69 percent third degree T32.86
70-79 percent third degree T32.87
80-89 percent third degree T32.88
90 percent or more (0-9 percent third degree) T32.90
with
10-19 percent third degree T32.91
20-29 percent third degree T32.92
30-39 percent third degree T32.93
40-49 percent third degree T32.94
50-59 percent third degree T32.95
60-69 percent third degree T32.96
70-79 percent third degree T32.97
80-89 percent third degree T32.98
90-99 percent third degree T32.99
upper limb (axilla) (scapular region) T22.40
above elbow — *see* Corrosion, above elbow
axilla — *see* Corrosion, axilla
elbow — *see* Corrosion, elbow
first degree T22.50
forearm — *see* Corrosion, forearm
hand — *see* Corrosion, hand
interscapular region — *see* Corrosion, back, upper
multiple sites T22.499
first degree T22.599
left T22.492
first degree T22.592
second degree T22.692
third degree T22.792
right T22.491
first degree T22.591
second degree T22.691
third degree T22.791
second degree T22.699
third degree T22.799
scapular region — *see* Corrosion, scapular region

Corrosion (injury) (acid) (caustic) (chemical) (lime) (external) (internal) - *continued*
upper limb (axilla) (scapular region) - *continued*
second degree T22.60
shoulder — *see* Corrosion, shoulder
third degree T22.70
wrist — *see* Corrosion, hand
uterus T28.8
vagina T28.8
vulva — *see* Corrosion, genital organs, external, female
wrist T23.479
first degree T23.579
left T23.472
first degree T23.572
second degree T23.672
third degree T23.772
multiple sites with hand T23.499
first degree T23.599
left T23.492
first degree T23.592
second degree T23.692
third degree T23.792
right T23.491
first degree T23.591
second degree T23.691
third degree T23.791
second degree T23.699
third degree T23.799
right T23.471
first degree T23.571
second degree T23.671
third degree T23.771
second degree T23.679
third degree T23.779
Corrosive burn — *see* Corrosion
Corsican fever — *see* Malaria
Cortical — *see* condition
Cortico-adrenal — *see* condition
Coryza (acute) J00
with grippe or influenza — *see* Influenza, with, respiratory manifestations NEC
syphilitic
congenital (chronic) A50.05
Costen's syndrome or complex M26.69
Costiveness — *see* Constipation
Costochondritis M94.0
Cot death R99
Cotard's syndrome F22
Cotia virus B08.8
Cotton wool spots (retinal) H35.81
Cotungo's disease — *see* Sciatica
Cough (affected) (epidemic) (nervous) R05.9
with hemorrhage — *see* Hemoptysis
acute R05.1
bronchial R05.8
with grippe or influenza — *see* Influenza, with, respiratory manifestations NEC
chronic R05.3
functional F45.8
hysterical F45.8
laryngeal, spasmodic R05.8
paroxysmal, due to Bordetella pertussis (without pneumonia) A37.00
with pneumonia A37.01
persistent R05.3
psychogenic F45.8
refractory R05.3
smokers' J41.0
specified NEC R05.8
subacute R05.2
syncope R05.4
tea taster's B49
unexplained R05.3
Counseling (for) Z71.9
abuse NEC
perpetrator Z69.82
victim Z69.81
alcohol abuser Z71.41
family Z71.42
child abuse
nonparental
perpetrator Z69.021
victim Z69.020

Counseling (for) - *continued*
child abuse - *continued*
parental
perpetrator Z69.011
victim Z69.010
consanguinity Z71.89
contraceptive Z30.09
dietary Z71.3
drug abuser Z71.51
family member Z71.52
exercise Z71.82
family Z71.89
fertility preservation (prior to cancer therapy) (prior to removal of gonads) Z31.62
for non-attending third party Z71.0
related to sexual behavior or orientation Z70.2
genetic
nonprocreative Z71.83
procreative NEC Z31.5
gestational carrier Z31.7
health (advice) (education) (instruction) — *see* Counseling, medical
risk for travel (international) Z71.84
human immunodeficiency virus (HIV) Z71.7
immunization safety Z71.85
impotence Z70.1
insulin pump use Z46.81
medical (for) Z71.9
boarding school resident Z59.3
consanguinity Z71.89
feared complaint and no disease found Z71.1
human immunodeficiency virus (HIV) Z71.7
institutional resident Z59.3
on behalf of another Z71.0
related to sexual behavior or orientation Z70.2
person living alone Z60.2
specified reason NEC Z71.89
natural family planning
procreative Z31.61
to avoid pregnancy Z30.02
perpetrator (of)
abuse NEC Z69.82
child abuse
non-parental Z69.021
parental Z69.011
rape NEC Z69.82
spousal abuse Z69.12
procreative NEC Z31.69
fertility preservation (prior to cancer therapy) (prior to removal of gonads) Z31.62
using natural family planning Z31.61
promiscuity Z70.1
rape victim Z69.81
religious Z71.81
safety for travel (international) Z71.84
sex, sexual (related to) Z70.9
attitude (s) Z70.0
behavior or orientation Z70.1
combined concerns Z70.3
non-responsiveness Z70.1
on behalf of third party Z70.2
specified reason NEC Z70.8
specified reason NEC Z71.89
spiritual Z71.81
spousal abuse (perpetrator) Z69.12
victim Z69.11
substance abuse Z71.89
alcohol Z71.41
drug Z71.51
tobacco Z71.6
tobacco use Z71.6
travel (international) Z71.84
use (of)
insulin pump Z46.81
vaccine product safety Z71.85
victim (of)
abuse Z69.81
child abuse
by parent Z69.010
non-parental Z69.020

Counseling (for) - *continued*
victim (of) - *continued*
rape NEC Z69.81
Coupled rhythm R00.8
Couvelaire syndrome or uterus (complicating delivery) O45.8X-
COVID-19 U07.1
condition post U09.9
contact (with) Z20.822
exposure (to) Z20.822
history of (personal) Z86.16
long (haul) U09.9
pneumonia J12.82
screening Z11.52
sequelae (post acute) U09.9
Cowperitis — *see* Urethritis
Cowper's gland — *see* condition
Cowpox B08.010
due to vaccination T88.1
Coxa
magna M91.4-
plana M91.2-
valga (acquired) — *see also* Deformity, limb, specified type NEC, thigh
congenital Q65.81
sequelae (late effect) of rickets E64.3
vara (acquired) — *see also* Deformity, limb, specified type NEC, thigh
congenital Q65.82
sequelae (late effect) of rickets E64.3
Coxalgia, coxalgic (nontuberculous) — *see also* Pain, joint, hip
tuberculous A18.02
Coxitis — *see* Monoarthritis, hip
Coxsackie (virus) (infection) B34.1
as cause of disease classified elsewhere B97.11
carditis B33.20
central nervous system NEC A88.8
endocarditis B33.21
enteritis A08.39
meningitis (aseptic) A87.0
myocarditis B33.22
pericarditis B33.23
pharyngitis B08.5
pleurodynia B33.0
specific disease NEC B33.8
Crabs, meaning pubic lice B85.3
Crack baby P04.41
Cracked nipple N64.0
associated with
lactation O92.13
pregnancy O92.11-
puerperium O92.12
Cracked tooth K03.81
Cradle cap L21.0
Craft neurosis F48.8
Cramp (s) R25.2
abdominal — *see* Pain, abdominal
bathing T75.1
colic R10.83
psychogenic F45.8
due to immersion T75.1
fireman T67.2
heat T67.2
immersion T75.1
intestinal — *see* Pain, abdominal
psychogenic F45.8
leg, sleep related G47.62
limb (lower) (upper) NEC R25.2
sleep related G47.62
linotypist's F48.8
organic G25.89
muscle (limb) (general) R25.2
due to immersion T75.1
psychogenic F45.8
occupational (hand) F48.8
organic G25.89
salt-depletion E87.1
sleep related, leg G47.62
stoker's T67.2
swimmer's T75.1
telegrapher's F48.8
organic G25.89
typist's F48.8

Cramp (s) - *continued*
typist's - *continued*
organic G25.89
uterus N94.89
menstrual — *see* Dysmenorrhea
writer's F48.8
organic G25.89
Cranial — *see* condition
Craniocleidodysostosis Q74.0
Craniofenestria (skull) Q75.8
Craniolacunia (skull) Q75.8
Craniopagus Q89.4
Craniopathy, metabolic M85.2
Craniopharyngeal — *see* condition
Craniopharyngioma D44.4
Craniorachischisis (totalis) Q00.1
Cranioschisis Q75.8
Craniostenosis Q75.0
Craniosynostosis Q75.0
Craniotabes (cause unknown) M83.8
neonatal P96.3
rachitic E64.3
syphilitic A50.56
Cranium — *see* condition
Craw-craw — *see* Onchocerciasis
Creaking joint — *see* Derangement, joint, specified type NEC
Creeping
eruption B76.9
palsy or paralysis G12.22
Crenated tongue K14.8
Creotoxism A05.9
Crepitus
caput Q75.8
joint — *see* Derangement, joint, specified type NEC
Crescent or conus choroid, congenital Q14.3
CREST syndrome M34.1
Cretin, cretinism (congenital) (endemic) (nongoitrous) (sporadic) E00.9
pelvis
with disproportion (fetopelvic) O33.0
causing obstructed labor O65.0
type
hypothyroid E00.1
mixed E00.2
myxedematous E00.1
neurological E00.0
Creutzfeldt-Jakob disease or syndrome (with dementia) A81.00
familial A81.09
iatrogenic A81.09
specified NEC A81.09
sporadic A81.09
variant (vCJD) A81.01
Crib death R99
Cribriform hymen Q52.3
Cri-du-chat syndrome Q93.4
Crigler-Najjar disease or syndrome E80.5
Crime, victim of Z65.4
Crimean hemorrhagic fever A98.0
Criminalism F60.2
Crisis
abdomen R10.0
acute reaction F43.0
addisonian E27.2
adrenal (cortical) E27.2
celiac K90.0
Dietl's N13.8
emotional — *see also* Disorder, adjustment
acute reaction to stress F43.0
specific to childhood and adolescence F93.8
glaucomatocyclitic — *see* Glaucoma, secondary, inflammation
heart — *see* Failure, heart
nitritoid I95.2
correct substance properly administered — *see* Table of Drugs and Chemicals, by drug, adverse effect
overdose or wrong substance given or taken — *see* Table of Drugs and Chemicals, by drug, poisoning
oculogyric H51.8

Crisis - *continued*
oculogyric - *continued*
psychogenic F45.8
Pel's (tabetic) A52.11
psychosexual identity F64.2
renal N28.0
sickle-cell D57.00
with
acute chest syndrome D57.01
cerebral vascular involvement D57.03
crisis (painful) D57.00
with complication specified NEC D57.09
splenic sequestration D57.02
vasoocclusive pain D57.00
state (acute reaction) F43.0
tabetic A52.11
thyroid — *see* Thyrotoxicosis with thyroid storm
thyrotoxic — *see* Thyrotoxicosis with thyroid storm
Crocq's disease (acrocyanosis) I73.89
Crohn's disease — *see* Enteritis, regional
Crooked septum, nasal J34.2
Cross syndrome E70.328
Crossbite (anterior) (posterior) M26.24
Cross-eye — *see* Strabismus, convergent concomitant
Croup, croupous (catarrhal) (infectious) (inflammatory) (nondiphtheritic) J05.0
bronchial J20.9
diphtheritic A36.2
false J38.5
spasmodic J38.5
diphtheritic A36.2
stridulous J38.5
diphtheritic A36.2
Crouzon's disease Q75.1
Crowding, tooth, teeth, fully erupted M26.31
CRST syndrome M34.1
Cruchet's disease A85.8
Cruelty in children — *see also* Disorder, conduct
Crural ulcer — *see* Ulcer, lower limb
Crush, crushed, crushing T14.8
abdomen S38.1
ankle S97.0-
arm (upper) (and shoulder) S47.-
axilla — *see* Crush, arm
back, lower S38.1
buttock S38.1
cheek S07.0
chest S28.0
cranium S07.1
ear S07.0
elbow S57.0-
extremity
lower
ankle — *see* Crush, ankle
below knee — *see* Crush, leg
foot — *see* Crush, foot
hip — *see* Crush, hip
knee — *see* Crush, knee
thigh — *see* Crush, thigh
toe — *see* Crush, toe
upper
below elbow S67.9-
elbow — *see* Crush, elbow
finger — *see* Crush, finger
forearm — *see* Crush, forearm
hand — *see* Crush, hand
thumb — *see* Crush, thumb
upper arm — *see* Crush, arm
wrist — *see* Crush, wrist
face S07.0
finger (s) S67.1-
with hand (and wrist) — *see* Crush, hand, specified site NEC
index S67.19-
little S67.19-
middle S67.19-
ring S67.19-
thumb — *see* Crush, thumb
foot S97.8-
toe — *see* Crush, toe

Crush, crushed, crushing - *continued*
forearm S57.8-
genitalia, external
female S38.002
vagina S38.03
vulva S38.03
male S38.001
penis S38.01
scrotum S38.02
testis S38.02
hand (except fingers alone) S67.2-
with wrist S67.4-
head S07.9
specified NEC S07.8
heel — *see* Crush, foot
hip S77.0-
with thigh S77.2-
internal organ (abdomen, chest, or pelvis) NEC T14.8
knee S87.0-
labium (majus) (minus) S38.03
larynx S17.0
leg (lower) S87.8-
knee — *see* Crush, knee
lip S07.0
lower
back S38.1
leg — *see* Crush, leg
neck S17.9
nerve — *see* Injury, nerve
nose S07.0
pelvis S38.1
penis S38.01
scalp S07.8
scapular region — *see* Crush, arm
scrotum S38.02
severe, unspecified site T14.8
shoulder (and upper arm) — *see* Crush, arm
skull S07.1
syndrome (complication of trauma) T79.5
testis S38.02
thigh S77.1-
with hip S77.2-
throat S17.8
thumb S67.0-
with hand (and wrist) — *see* Crush, hand, specified site NEC
toe (s) S97.10-
great S97.11-
lesser S97.12-
trachea S17.0
vagina S38.03
vulva S38.03
wrist S67.3-
with hand S67.4-
Crusta lactea L21.0
Crusts R23.4
Crutch paralysis — *see* Injury, brachial plexus
Cruveilhier-Baumgarten cirrhosis, disease or syndrome K74.69
Cruveilhier's atrophy or disease G12.8
Crying (constant) (continuous) (excessive)
child, adolescent, or adult R45.83
infant (baby) (newborn) R68.11
Cryofibrinogenemia D89.2
Cryoglobulinemia (essential) (idiopathic) (mixed) (primary) (purpura) (secondary) (vasculitis) D89.1
with lung involvement D89.1 *[J99]*
Cryptitis (anal) (rectal) K62.89
Cryptococcosis, cryptococcus (infection) (neoformans) B45.9
bone B45.3
cerebral B45.1
cutaneous B45.2
disseminated B45.7
generalized B45.7
meningitis B45.1
meningocerebralis B45.1
osseous B45.3
pulmonary B45.0
skin B45.2
specified NEC B45.8
Cryptopapillitis (anus) K62.89

Cryptophthalmos Q11.2
  syndrome Q87.0
Cryptorchid, cryptorchism, cryptorchidism Q53.9
  bilateral Q53.20
    abdominal Q53.211
    perineal Q53.22
  unilateral Q53.10
    abdominal Q53.111
    perineal Q53.12
Cryptosporidiosis A07.2
  hepatobiliary B88.8
  respiratory B88.8
Cryptostromosis J67.6
Crystalluria R82.998
Cubitus
  congenital Q68.8
  valgus (acquired) M21.0-
    congenital Q68.8
    sequelae (late effect) of rickets E64.3
  varus (acquired) M21.1-
    congenital Q68.8
    sequelae (late effect) of rickets E64.3
Cultural deprivation or shock Z60.3
Curling esophagus K22.4
Curling's ulcer — *see* Ulcer, peptic, acute
Curschmann (-Batten) (-Steinert) disease or syndrome G71.11
Curse, Ondine's — *see* Apnea, sleep
Curvature
  organ or site, congenital NEC — *see* Distortion
  penis (lateral) Q55.61
  Pott's (spinal) A18.01
  radius, idiopathic, progressive (congenital) Q74.0
  spine (acquired) (angular) (idiopathic) (incorrect) (postural) — *see* Dorsopathy, deforming
    congenital Q67.5
    due to or associated with
      Charcot-Marie-Tooth disease (see also subcategory M49.8) G60.0
      osteitis
        deformans M88.88
        fibrosa cystica (*see also* subcategory M49.8) E21.0
      tuberculosis (Pott's curvature) A18.01
    sequelae (late effect) of rickets E64.3
    tuberculous A18.01
Cushingoid due to steroid therapy E24.2
  correct substance properly administered — *see* Table of Drugs and Chemicals, by drug, adverse effect
  overdose or wrong substance given or taken — *see* Table of Drugs and Chemicals, by drug, poisoning
Cushing's
  syndrome or disease E24.9
    drug-induced E24.2
    iatrogenic E24.2
    pituitary-dependent E24.0
    specified NEC E24.8
  ulcer — *see* Ulcer, peptic, acute
Cusp, Carabelli - omit code
Cut (external) — *see also* Laceration
  muscle — *see* Injury, muscle
Cutaneous — *see also* condition
  hemorrhage R23.3
  larva migrans B76.9
Cutis — *see also* condition
  hyperelastica Q82.8
    acquired L57.4
  laxa (hyperelastica) — *see* Dermatolysis
  marmorata R23.8
  osteosis L94.2
  pendula — *see* Dermatolysis
  rhomboidalis nuchae L57.2
  verticis gyrata Q82.8
    acquired L91.8
Cyanosis R23.0
  due to
    patent foramen botalli Q21.1
    persistent foramen ovale Q21.1
  enterogenous D74.8

Cyanosis - *continued*
  paroxysmal digital — *see* Raynaud's disease
    with gangrene I73.01
  retina, retinal H35.89
Cyanotic heart disease I24.9
  congenital Q24.9
Cycle
  anovulatory N97.0
  menstrual, irregular N92.6
Cyclencephaly Q04.9
Cyclical vomiting, in migraine, — *see also* Vomiting, cyclical G43.A0
  psychogenic F50.89
Cyclitis — *see also* Iridocyclitis H20.9
  chronic — *see* Iridocyclitis, chronic
  Fuchs' heterochromic H20.81-
  granulomatous — *see* Iridocyclitis, chronic
  lens-induced — *see* Iridocyclitis, lens-induced
  posterior H30.2-
Cycloid personality F34.0
Cyclophoria H50.54
Cyclopia, cyclops Q87.0
Cyclopism Q87.0
Cyclosporiasis A07.4
Cyclothymia F34.0
Cyclothymic personality F34.0
Cyclotropia H50.41-
Cylindroma — *see also* Neoplasm, malignant, by site
  eccrine dermal — *see* Neoplasm, skin, benign
  skin — *see* Neoplasm, skin, benign
Cylindruria R82.998
Cynanche
  diphtheritic A36.2
  tonsillaris J36
Cynophobia F40.218
Cynorexia R63.2
Cyphosis — *see* Kyphosis
Cyprus fever — *see* Brucellosis
Cyst (colloid) (mucous) (simple) (retention)
  adenoid (infected) J35.8
  adrenal gland E27.8
    congenital Q89.1
  air, lung J98.4
  allantoic Q64.4
  alveolar process (jaw bone) M27.40
  amnion, amniotic O41.8X-
  aneurysmal M27.49
  anterior
    chamber (eye) — *see* Cyst, iris
    nasopalatine K09.1
  antrum J34.1
  anus K62.89
  apical (tooth) (periodontal) K04.8
  appendix K38.8
  arachnoid, brain (acquired) G93.0
    congenital Q04.6
  arytenoid J38.7
  Baker's M71.2-
    ruptured M66.0
    tuberculous A18.02
  Bartholin's gland N75.0
  bile duct (common) (hepatic) K83.5
  bladder (multiple) (trigone) N32.89
  blue dome (breast) — *see* Cyst, breast
  bone (local) NEC M85.60
    aneurysmal M85.50
      ankle M85.57-
      foot M85.57-
      forearm M85.53-
      hand M85.54-
      jaw M27.49
      lower leg M85.56-
      multiple site M85.59
      neck M85.58
      rib M85.58
      shoulder M85.51-
      skull M85.58
      specified site NEC M85.58
      thigh M85.55-
      toe M85.57-
      upper arm M85.52-
      vertebra M85.58

Cyst (colloid) (mucous) (simple) (retention) - *continued*
  bone (local) NEC - *continued*
    solitary M85.40
      ankle M85.47-
      fibula M85.46-
      foot M85.47-
      hand M85.44-
      humerus M85.42-
      jaw M27.49
      neck M85.48
      pelvis M85.45-
      radius M85.43-
      rib M85.48
      shoulder M85.41-
      skull M85.48
      specified site NEC M85.48
      tibia M85.46-
      toe M85.47-
      ulna M85.43-
      vertebra M85.48
    specified type NEC M85.60
      ankle M85.67-
      foot M85.67-
      forearm M85.63-
      hand M85.64-
      jaw M27.40
        developmental (nonodontogenic) K09.1
          odontogenic K09.0
        latent M27.0
      lower leg M85.66-
      multiple site M85.69
      neck M85.68
      rib M85.68
      shoulder M85.61-
      skull M85.68
      specified site NEC M85.68
      thigh M85.65-
      toe M85.67-
      upper arm M85.62-
      vertebra M85.68
  brain (acquired) G93.0
    congenital Q04.6
    hydatid B67.99 *[G94]*
    third ventricle (colloid) , congenital Q04.6
  branchial (cleft) Q18.0
  branchiogenic Q18.0
  breast (benign) (blue dome) (pedunculated) (solitary) N60.0-
    involution — *see* Dysplasia, mammary, specified type NEC
    sebaceous — *see* Dysplasia, mammary, specified type NEC
  broad ligament (benign) N83.8
  bronchogenic (mediastinal) (sequestration) J98.4
    congenital Q33.0
  buccal K09.8
  bulbourethral gland N36.8
  bursa, bursal NEC M71.30
    with rupture — *see* Rupture, synovium
    ankle M71.37-
    elbow M71.32-
    foot M71.37-
    hand M71.34-
    hip M71.35-
    multiple sites M71.39
    pharyngeal J39.2
    popliteal space — *see* Cyst, Baker's
    shoulder M71.31-
    specified site NEC M71.38
    wrist M71.33-
  calcifying odontogenic D16.5
    upper jaw (bone) (maxilla) D16.4
  canal of Nuck (female) N94.89
    congenital Q52.4
  canthus — *see* Cyst, conjunctiva
  carcinomatous — *see* Neoplasm, malignant, by site
  cauda equina G95.89
  cavum septi pellucidi — *see* Cyst, brain
  celomic (pericardium) Q24.8
  cerebellopontine (angle) — *see* Cyst, brain
  cerebellum — *see* Cyst, brain

Cyst (colloid) (mucous) (simple) (retention) - *continued*
  cerebral — *see* Cyst, brain
  cervical lateral Q18.0
  cervix NEC N88.8
    embryonic Q51.6
    nabothian N88.8
  chiasmal optic NEC — *see* Disorder, optic, chiasm
  chocolate (ovary) N80.1
  choledochus, congenital Q44.4
  chorion O41.8X-
  choroid plexus G93.0
    congenital Q04.6
  ciliary body — *see* Cyst, iris
  clitoris N90.7
  colon K63.89
  common (bile) duct K83.5
  congenital NEC Q89.8
    adrenal gland Q89.1
    epiglottis Q31.8
    esophagus Q39.8
    fallopian tube Q50.4
    kidney Q61.00
      more than one (multiple) Q61.02
        specified as polycystic Q61.3
          adult type Q61.2
          infantile type NEC Q61.19
            collecting duct dilation Q61.11
      solitary Q61.01
    larynx Q31.8
    liver Q44.6
    lung Q33.0
    mediastinum Q34.1
    ovary Q50.1
    oviduct Q50.4
    periurethral (tissue) Q64.79
    prepuce Q55.69
    salivary gland (any) Q38.4
    sublingual Q38.6
    submaxillary gland Q38.6
    thymus (gland) Q89.2
    tongue Q38.3
    ureterovesical orifice Q62.8
    vulva Q52.79
  conjunctiva H11.44-
  cornea H18.89-
  corpora quadrigemina G93.0
  corpus
    albicans N83.29-
    luteum (hemorrhagic) (ruptured) N83.1-
  Cowper's gland (benign) (infected) N36.8
  cranial meninges G93.0
  craniobuccal pouch E23.6
  craniopharyngeal pouch E23.6
  cystic duct K82.8
  Cysticercus — *see* Cysticercosis
  Dandy-Walker Q03.1
    with spina bifida — *see* Spina bifida
  dental (root) K04.8
    developmental K09.0
    eruption K09.0
    primordial K09.0
  dentigerous (mandible) (maxilla) K09.0
  dermoid — *see* Neoplasm, benign, by site
    with malignant transformation C56.-
    implantation
      external area or site (skin) NEC L72.0
      iris — *see* Cyst, iris, implantation
      vagina N89.8
      vulva N90.7
    mouth K09.8
    oral soft tissue K09.8
    sacrococcygeal — *see* Cyst, pilonidal
  developmental K09.1
    odontogenic K09.0
    oral region (nonodontogenic) K09.1
    ovary, ovarian Q50.1
  dura (cerebral) G93.0
    spinal G96.198
  ear (external) Q18.1
  echinococcal — *see* Echinococcus
  embryonic
    cervix uteri Q51.6
    fallopian tube Q50.4

Cyst (colloid) (mucous) (simple) (retention) - *continued*
  embryonic - *continued*
    vagina Q52.4
  endometrium, endometrial (uterus) N85.8
    ectopic — *see* Endometriosis
  enterogenous Q43.8
  epidermal, epidermoid (inclusion) (see also Cyst, skin) L72.0
    mouth K09.8
    oral soft tissue K09.8
  epididymis N50.3
  epiglottis J38.7
  epiphysis cerebri E34.8
  epithelial (inclusion) L72.0
  epoophoron Q50.5
  eruption K09.0
  esophagus K22.89
  ethmoid sinus J34.1
  external female genital organs NEC N90.7
  eye NEC H57.89
    congenital Q15.8
  eyelid (sebaceous) H02.829
    infected — *see* Hordeolum
    left H02.826
      lower H02.825
      upper H02.824
    right H02.823
      lower H02.822
      upper H02.821
  fallopian tube N83.8
    congenital Q50.4
  fimbrial (twisted) Q50.4
  fissural (oral region) K09.1
  follicle (graafian) (hemorrhagic) N83.0-
    nabothian N88.8
  follicular (atretic) (hemorrhagic) (ovarian) N83.0-
    dentigerous K09.0
    odontogenic K09.0
    skin L72.9
      specified NEC L72.8
  frontal sinus J34.1
  gallbladder K82.8
  ganglion — *see* Ganglion
  Gartner's duct Q52.4
  gingiva K09.0
  gland of Moll — *see* Cyst, eyelid
  globulomaxillary K09.1
  graafian follicle (hemorrhagic) N83.0-
  granulosal lutein (hemorrhagic) N83.1-
  hemangiomatous D18.00
    intra-abdominal D18.03
    intracranial D18.02
    skin D18.01
    specified site NEC D18.09
  hemorrhagic M27.49
  hydatid — *see also* Echinococcus B67.90
    brain B67.99 *[G94]*
    liver — *see also* Cyst, liver, hydatid B67.8
    lung NEC B67.99 *[J99]*
    Morgagni
      female Q50.5
      male (epididymal) Q55.4
        testicular Q55.29
    specified site NEC B67.99
  hymen N89.8
    embryonic Q52.4
  hypopharynx J39.2
  hypophysis, hypophyseal (duct) (recurrent) E23.6
    cerebri E23.6
  implantation (dermoid)
    external area or site (skin) NEC L72.0
    iris — *see* Cyst, iris, implantation
    vagina N89.8
    vulva N90.7
  incisive canal K09.1
  inclusion (epidermal) (epithelial) (epidermoid) (squamous) L72.0
    not of skin - code under Cyst, by site
  intestine (large) (small) K63.89
  intracranial — *see* Cyst, brain
  intraligamentous — *see also* Disorder, ligament

Cyst (colloid) (mucous) (simple) (retention) - *continued*
  intraligamentous - *continued*
    knee — *see* Derangement, knee
  intrasellar E23.6
  iris H21.309
    exudative H21.31-
    idiopathic H21.30-
    implantation H21.32-
    parasitic H21.33-
    pars plana (primary) H21.34-
      exudative H21.35-
  jaw (bone) M27.40
    aneurysmal M27.49
    hemorrhagic M27.49
    traumatic M27.49
    developmental (odontogenic) K09.0
    fissural K09.1
  joint NEC — *see* Disorder, joint, specified type NEC
  kidney (acquired) N28.1
    calyceal — *see* Hydronephrosis
    congenital Q61.00
    more than one (multiple) Q61.02
      specified as polycystic Q61.3
        adult type (autosomal dominant) Q61.2
        infantile type (autosomal recessive) NEC Q61.19
          collecting duct dilation Q61.11
    pyelogenic — *see* Hydronephrosis
    simple N28.1
    solitary (single) Q61.01
      acquired N28.1
  labium (majus) (minus) N90.7
    sebaceous N90.7
  lacrimal — *see also* Disorder, lacrimal system, specified NEC
    gland H04.13-
    passages or sac — *see* Disorder, lacrimal system, specified NEC
  larynx J38.7
  lateral periodontal K09.0
  lens H27.8
    congenital Q12.8
  lip (gland) K13.0
  liver (idiopathic) (simple) K76.89
    congenital Q44.6
    hydatid B67.8
      granulosus B67.0
      multilocularis B67.5
  lung J98.4
    congenital Q33.0
    giant bullous J43.9
  lutein N83.1-
  lymphangiomatous D18.1
  lymphoepithelial, oral soft tissue K09.8
  macula — *see* Degeneration, macula, hole
  malignant — *see* Neoplasm, malignant, by site
  mammary gland — *see* Cyst, breast
  mandible M27.40
    dentigerous K09.0
    radicular K04.8
  maxilla M27.40
    dentigerous K09.0
    radicular K04.8
  medial, face and neck Q18.8
  median
    anterior maxillary K09.1
    palatal K09.1
  mediastinum, congenital Q34.1
  meibomian (gland) — *see* Chalazion
    infected — *see* Hordeolum
  membrane, brain G93.0
  meninges (cerebral) G93.0
    spinal G96.198
  meniscus, knee — *see* Derangement, knee, meniscus, cystic
  mesentery, mesenteric K66.8
    chyle I89.8
  mesonephric duct
    female Q50.5
    male Q55.4
  milk N64.89

Cyst (colloid) (mucous) (simple) (retention) - *continued*
  wolffian - *continued*
    male Q55.4
Cystadenocarcinoma — *see* Neoplasm, malignant, by site
  bile duct C22.1
  endometrioid — *see* Neoplasm, malignant, by site
    specified site — *see* Neoplasm, malignant, by site
    unspecified site
      female C56.9
      male C61
  mucinous
    papillary
      specified site — *see* Neoplasm, malignant, by site
      unspecified site C56.9
    specified site — *see* Neoplasm, malignant, by site
    unspecified site C56.9
  papillary
    mucinous
      specified site — *see* Neoplasm, malignant, by site
      unspecified site C56.9
    pseudomucinous
      specified site — *see* Neoplasm, malignant, by site
      unspecified site C56.9
    serous
      specified site — *see* Neoplasm, malignant, by site
      unspecified site C56.9
    specified site — *see* Neoplasm, malignant, by site
    unspecified site C56.9
  pseudomucinous
    papillary
      specified site — *see* Neoplasm, malignant, by site
      unspecified site C56.9
    specified site — *see* Neoplasm, malignant, by site
    unspecified site C56.9
  serous
    papillary
      specified site — *see* Neoplasm, malignant, by site
      unspecified site C56.9
    specified site — *see* Neoplasm, malignant, by site
    unspecified site C56.9
Cystadenofibroma
  clear cell — *see* Neoplasm, benign, by site
  endometrioid D27.9
    borderline malignancy D39.1-
    malignant C56.-
  mucinous
    specified site — *see* Neoplasm, benign, by site
    unspecified site D27.9
  serous
    specified site — *see* Neoplasm, benign, by site
    unspecified site D27.9
  specified site — *see* Neoplasm, benign, by site
  unspecified site D27.9
Cystadenoma — *see also* Neoplasm, benign, by site
  bile duct D13.4
  endometrioid — *see* Neoplasm, benign, by site
    borderline malignancy — *see* Neoplasm, uncertain behavior, by site
  malignant — *see* Neoplasm, malignant, by site
  mucinous
    borderline malignancy
      ovary C56.-
      specified site NEC — *see* Neoplasm, uncertain behavior, by site
      unspecified site C56.9

Cystadenoma - *continued*
  mucinous - *continued*
    papillary
      borderline malignancy
        ovary C56.-
        specified site NEC — *see* Neoplasm, uncertain behavior, by site
        unspecified site C56.9
      specified site — *see* Neoplasm, benign, by site
      unspecified site D27.9
    specified site — *see* Neoplasm, benign, by site
    unspecified site D27.9
  papillary
    borderline malignancy
      ovary C56.-
      specified site NEC — *see* Neoplasm, uncertain behavior, by site
      unspecified site C56.9
    lymphomatosum
      specified site — *see* Neoplasm, benign, by site
      unspecified site D11.9
    mucinous
      borderline malignancy
        ovary C56.-
        specified site NEC — *see* Neoplasm, uncertain behavior, by site
        unspecified site C56.9
      specified site — *see* Neoplasm, benign, by site
      unspecified site D27.9
    pseudomucinous
      borderline malignancy
        ovary C56.-
        specified site NEC — *see* Neoplasm, uncertain behavior, by site
        unspecified site C56.9
      specified site — *see* Neoplasm, benign, by site
      unspecified site D27.9
    serous
      borderline malignancy
        ovary C56.-
        specified site NEC — *see* Neoplasm, uncertain behavior, by site
        unspecified site C56.9
      specified site — *see* Neoplasm, benign, by site
      unspecified site D27.9
    specified site — *see* Neoplasm, benign, by site
    unspecified site D27.9
  pseudomucinous
    borderline malignancy
      ovary C56.-
      specified site NEC — *see* Neoplasm, uncertain behavior, by site
      unspecified site C56.9
    papillary
      borderline malignancy
        ovary C56.-
        specified site NEC — *see* Neoplasm, uncertain behavior, by site
        unspecified site C56.9
      specified site — *see* Neoplasm, benign, by site
      unspecified site D27.9
    specified site — *see* Neoplasm, benign, by site
    unspecified site D27.9
  serous
    borderline malignancy
      ovary C56.-
      specified site NEC — *see* Neoplasm, uncertain behavior, by site
      unspecified site C56.9
    papillary
      borderline malignancy
        ovary C56.-
        specified site NEC — *see* Neoplasm, uncertain behavior, by site
        unspecified site C56.9

Cystadenoma - *continued*
  serous - *continued*
    papillary - *continued*
      specified site — *see* Neoplasm, benign, by site
      unspecified site D27.9
    specified site — *see* Neoplasm, benign, by site
    unspecified site D27.9
Cystathionine synthase deficiency E72.11
Cystathioninemia E72.19
Cystathioninuria E72.19
Cystic — *see also* condition
  breast (chronic) — *see* Mastopathy, cystic
  corpora lutea (hemorrhagic) N83.1-
  duct — *see* condition
  eyeball (congenital) Q11.0
  fibrosis — *see* Fibrosis, cystic
  kidney (congenital) Q61.9
    adult type Q61.2
    infantile type NEC Q61.19
      collecting duct dilatation Q61.11
    medullary Q61.5
  liver, congenital Q44.6
  lung disease J98.4
    congenital Q33.0
  mastitis, chronic — *see* Mastopathy, cystic
  medullary, kidney Q61.5
  meniscus — *see* Derangement, knee, meniscus, cystic
  ovary N83.20-
Cysticercosis, cysticerciasis B69.9
  with
    epileptiform fits B69.0
    myositis B69.81
  brain B69.0
  central nervous system B69.0
  cerebral B69.0
  ocular B69.1
  specified NEC B69.89
Cysticercus cellulose infestation — *see* Cysticercosis
Cystinosis (malignant) E72.04
Cystinuria E72.01
Cystitis (exudative) (hemorrhagic) (septic) (suppurative) N30.90
  with
    fibrosis — *see* Cystitis, chronic, interstitial
    hematuria N30.91
    leukoplakia — *see* Cystitis, chronic, interstitial
    malakoplakia — *see* Cystitis, chronic, interstitial
    metaplasia — *see* Cystitis, chronic, interstitial
    prostatitis N41.3
  acute N30.00
    with hematuria N30.01
    of trigone N30.30
      with hematuria N30.31
  allergic — *see* Cystitis, specified type NEC
  amebic A06.81
  bilharzial B65.9 *[N33]*
  blennorrhagic (gonococcal) A54.01
  bullous — *see* Cystitis, specified type NEC
  calculous N21.0
  chlamydial A56.01
  chronic N30.20
    with hematuria N30.21
    interstitial N30.10
      with hematuria N30.11
    of trigone N30.30
      with hematuria N30.31
    specified NEC N30.20
      with hematuria N30.21
  cystic (a) — *see* Cystitis, specified type NEC
  diphtheritic A36.85
  echinococcal
    granulosus B67.39
    multilocularis B67.69
  emphysematous — *see* Cystitis, specified type NEC
  encysted — *see* Cystitis, specified type NEC
  eosinophilic — *see* Cystitis, specified type NEC

CYST - CYSTITIS

Cystitis (exudative) (hemorrhagic) (septic) (suppurative) - *continued*
  follicular — *see* Cystitis, of trigone
  gangrenous — *see* Cystitis, specified type NEC
  glandularis — *see* Cystitis, specified type NEC
  gonococcal A54.01
  incrusted — *see* Cystitis, specified type NEC
  interstitial (chronic) — *see* Cystitis, chronic, interstitial
  irradiation N30.40
    with hematuria N30.41
  irritation — *see* Cystitis, specified type NEC
  malignant — *see* Cystitis, specified type NEC
  of trigone N30.30
    with hematuria N30.31
  panmural — *see* Cystitis, chronic, interstitial
  polyposa — *see* Cystitis, specified type NEC
  prostatic N41.3
  puerperal (postpartum) O86.22
  radiation — *see* Cystitis, irradiation
  specified type NEC N30.80
    with hematuria N30.81
  subacute — *see* Cystitis, chronic
  submucous — *see* Cystitis, chronic, interstitial
  syphilitic (late) A52.76
  trichomonal A59.03
  tuberculous A18.12
  ulcerative — *see* Cystitis, chronic, interstitial
Cystocele (-urethrocele)
  female N81.10
    with prolapse of uterus — *see* Prolapse, uterus
    lateral N81.12
    midline N81.11
    paravaginal N81.12
  in pregnancy or childbirth O34.8-
    causing obstructed labor O65.5
  male N32.89
Cystolithiasis N21.0
Cystoma — *see also* Neoplasm, benign, by site
  endometrial, ovary N80.1
  mucinous
    specified site — *see* Neoplasm, benign, by site
    unspecified site D27.9
  serous
    specified site — *see* Neoplasm, benign, by site
    unspecified site D27.9
  simple (ovary) N83.29-
Cystoplegia N31.2
Cystoptosis N32.89
Cystopyelitis — *see* Pyelonephritis
Cystorrhagia N32.89
Cystosarcoma phyllodes D48.6-
  benign D24-
  malignant — *see* Neoplasm, breast, malignant
Cystostomy
  attention to Z43.5
  complication — *see* Complications, cystostomy
  status Z93.50
    appendico-vesicostomy Z93.52
    cutaneous Z93.51
    specified NEC Z93.59
Cystourethritis — *see* Urethritis
Cystourethrocele — *see also* Cystocele
  female N81.10
    with uterine prolapse — *see* Prolapse, uterus
    lateral N81.12
    midline N81.11
    paravaginal N81.12
  male N32.89
Cytomegalic inclusion disease
  congenital P35.1
Cytomegalovirus infection B25.9
Cytomycosis (reticuloendothelial) B39.4
Cytopenia D75.9
  refractory

Cytopenia - *continued*
  refractory - *continued*
    with multilineage dysplasia D46.A
      and ring sideroblasts (RCMD RS) D46.B
Czerny's disease (periodic hydrarthrosis of the knee) — *see* Effusion, joint, knee

D

Da Costa's syndrome F45.8
Daae (-Finsen) disease (epidemic pleurodynia) B33.0
Dabney's grip B33.0
Dacryoadenitis, dacryadenitis H04.00-
  acute H04.01-
  chronic H04.02-
Dacryocystitis H04.30-
  acute H04.32-
  chronic H04.41-
  neonatal P39.1
  phlegmonous H04.31-
  syphilitic A52.71
    congenital (early) A50.01
  trachomatous, active A71.1
    sequelae (late effect) B94.0
Dacryocystoblenorrhea — *see* Inflammation, lacrimal, passages, chronic
Dacryocystocele — *see* Disorder, lacrimal system, changes
Dacryolith, dacryolithiasis H04.51-
Dacryoma — *see* Disorder, lacrimal system, changes
Dacryopericystitis — *see* Dacryocystitis
Dacryops H04.11-
Dacryostenosis — *see also* Stenosis, lacrimal
  congenital Q10.5
Dactylitis
  bone — *see* Osteomyelitis
  sickle-cell D57.00
    Hb C D57.219
    Hb SS D57.00
    specified NEC D57.819
  skin L08.9
  syphilitic A52.77
  tuberculous A18.03
Dactylolysis spontanea (ainhum) L94.6
Dactylosymphysis Q70.9
  fingers — *see* Syndactylism, complex, fingers
  toes — *see* Syndactylism, complex, toes
Damage
  arteriosclerotic — *see* Arteriosclerosis
  brain (nontraumatic) G93.9
    anoxic, hypoxic G93.1
      resulting from a procedure G97.82
    child NEC G80.9
    due to birth injury P11.2
  cardiorenal (vascular) — *see* Hypertension, cardiorenal
  cerebral NEC — *see* Damage, brain
  coccyx, complicating delivery O71.6
  coronary — *see* Disease, heart, ischemic
  deep tissue, pressure-induced — *see also* L89 with final character .6
  eye, birth injury P15.3
  liver (nontraumatic) K76.9
    alcoholic K70.9
    due to drugs — *see* Disease, liver, toxic
    toxic — *see* Disease, liver, toxic
  lung
    dabbing (related) U07.0
    electronic cigarette (related) U07.0
    vaping (associated) (device) (product) (use) U07.0
  medication T88.7
  organ
    dabbing (related) U07.0
    electronic cigarette (related) U07.0
    vaping (associated) (device) (product) (use) U07.0
  pelvic
    joint or ligament, during delivery O71.6
    organ NEC
      during delivery O71.5
      following ectopic or molar pregnancy O08.6

Damage - *continued*
  renal — *see* Disease, renal
  subendocardium, subendocardial — *see* Degeneration, myocardial
  vascular I99.9
Dana-Putnam syndrome (subacute combined sclerosis with pernicious anemia) — *see* Degeneration, combined
Danbolt (-Cross) syndrome (acrodermatitis enteropathica) E83.2
Dandruff L21.0
Dandy-Walker syndrome Q03.1
  with spina bifida — *see* Spina bifida
Danlos' syndrome — *see also* Syndrome, Ehlers-Danlos Q79.60
Darier (-White) disease (congenital) Q82.8
  meaning erythema annulare centrifugum L53.1
Darier-Roussy sarcoid D86.3
Darling's disease or histoplasmosis B39.4
Darwin's tubercle Q17.8
Dawson's (inclusion body) encephalitis A81.1
De Beurmann (-Gougerot) disease B42.1
De la Tourette's syndrome F95.2
De Lange's syndrome Q87.19
De Morgan's spots (senile angiomas) I78.1
De Quervain's
  disease (tendon sheath) M65.4
  syndrome E34.51
  thyroiditis (subacute granulomatous thyroiditis) E06.1
De Toni-Fanconi (-Debré) syndrome E72.09
  with cystinosis E72.04
Dead
  fetus, retained (mother) O36.4
    early pregnancy O02.1
  labyrinth — *see* subcategory H83.2
  ovum, retained O02.0
Deaf nonspeaking NEC H91.3
Deafmutism (acquired) (congenital) NEC H91.3
  hysterical F44.6
  syphilitic, congenital (*see also* subcategory H94.8) A50.09
Deafness (acquired) (complete) (hereditary) (partial) H91.9-
  with blue sclera and fragility of bone Q78.0
  auditory fatigue — *see* Deafness, specified type NEC
  aviation T70.0
    nerve injury — *see* Injury, nerve, acoustic, specified type NEC
  boilermaker's — *see* subcategory H83.3
  central — *see* Deafness, sensorineural
  conductive H90.2
    and sensorineural
      mixed H90.8
        bilateral H90.6
    bilateral H90.0
    unilateral H90.1-
      with restricted hearing on the contralateral side H90.A-
  congenital H90.5
    with blue sclera and fragility of bone Q78.0
  due to toxic agents — *see* Deafness, ototoxic
  emotional (hysterical) F44.6
  functional (hysterical) F44.6
  high frequency H91.9-
  hysterical F44.6
  low frequency H91.9-
  mental R48.8
  mixed conductive and sensorineural H90.8
    bilateral H90.6
    unilateral H90.7-
  nerve — *see* Deafness, sensorineural
  neural — *see* Deafness, sensorineural
  noise-induced (*see also* subcategory H83.3)
    nerve injury — *see* Injury, nerve, acoustic, specified type NEC
  nonspeaking H91.3
  ototoxic — *see* subcategory H91.0
  perceptive — *see* Deafness, sensorineural
  psychogenic (hysterical) F44.6
  sensorineural H90.5

- **Deafness (acquired) (complete) (hereditary) (partial)** - *continued*
  - sensorineural - *continued*
    - and conductive
      - mixed H90.8
        - bilateral H90.6
    - bilateral H90.3
    - unilateral H90.4-
      - with restricted hearing on the contralateral side H90.A-
  - sensory — *see* Deafness, sensorineural
  - specified type NEC — *see* subcategory H91.8
  - sudden (idiopathic) H91.2-
  - syphilitic A52.15
  - transient ischemic H93.01-
  - traumatic — *see* Injury, nerve, acoustic, specified type NEC
  - word (developmental) H93.25
- **Death (cause unknown) (of) (unexplained) (unspecified cause)** R99
  - brain G93.82
  - cardiac (sudden) (with successful resuscitation) - code to underlying disease
    - family history of Z82.41
    - personal history of Z86.74
  - family member (assumed) Z63.4
- **Debility (chronic) (general) (nervous)** R53.81
  - congenital or neonatal NOS P96.9
  - nervous R53.81
  - old age R54
  - senile R54
- **Débove's disease (splenomegaly)** R16.1
- **Decalcification**
  - bone — *see* Osteoporosis
  - teeth K03.89
- **Decapsulation, kidney** N28.89
- **Decay**
  - dental — *see* Caries, dental
  - senile R54
  - tooth, teeth — *see* Caries, dental
- **Deciduitis (acute)**
  - following ectopic or molar pregnancy O08.0
- **Decline (general)** — *see* Debility
  - cognitive, age-associated R41.81
- **Decompensation**
  - cardiac (acute) (chronic) — *see* Disease, heart
  - cardiovascular — *see* Disease, cardiovascular
  - heart — *see* Disease, heart
  - hepatic — *see* Failure, hepatic
  - myocardial (acute) (chronic) — *see* Disease, heart
  - respiratory J98.8
- **Decompression sickness** T70.3
- **Decrease (d)**
  - absolute neutrophile count — *see* Neutropenia
  - blood
    - platelets — *see* Thrombocytopenia
    - pressure R03.1
      - due to shock following
        - injury T79.4
        - operation T81.19
  - estrogen E28.39
    - postablative E89.40
      - asymptomatic E89.40
      - symptomatic E89.41
  - fragility of erythrocytes D58.8
  - function
    - lipase (pancreatic) K90.3
    - ovary in hypopituitarism E23.0
    - parenchyma of pancreas K86.89
    - pituitary (gland) (anterior) (lobe) E23.0
      - posterior (lobe) E23.0
  - functional activity R68.89
  - glucose R73.09
  - hematocrit R71.0
  - hemoglobin R71.0
  - leukocytes D72.819
    - specified NEC D72.818
  - libido R68.82
  - lymphocytes D72.810
- **Decrease (d)** - *continued*
  - platelets D69.6
  - respiration, due to shock following injury T79.4
  - sexual desire R68.82
  - tear secretion NEC — *see* Syndrome, dry eye
  - tolerance
    - fat K90.49
    - glucose R73.09
    - pancreatic K90.3
    - salt and water E87.8
  - vision NEC H54.7
  - white blood cell count D72.819
    - specified NEC D72.818
- **Decubitus (ulcer)** — *see* Ulcer, pressure, by site
  - cervix N86
- **Deepening acetabulum** — *see* Derangement, joint, specified type NEC, hip
- **Defect, defective** Q89.9
  - 3-beta-hydroxysteroid dehydrogenase E25.0
  - 11-hydroxylase E25.0
  - 21-hydroxylase E25.0
  - abdominal wall, congenital Q79.59
  - antibody immunodeficiency D80.9
  - aorticopulmonary septum Q21.4
  - atrial septal (ostium secundum type) Q21.1
    - following acute myocardial infarction (current complication) I23.1
    - ostium primum type Q21.2
  - atrioventricular
    - canal Q21.2
    - septum Q21.2
  - auricular septal Q21.1
  - bilirubin excretion NEC E80.6
  - biosynthesis, androgen (testicular) E29.1
  - bulbar septum Q21.0
  - catalase E80.3
  - cell membrane receptor complex (CR3) D71
  - circulation I99.9
    - congenital Q28.9
    - newborn Q28.9
  - coagulation (factor) — *see also* Deficiency, factor D68.9
    - with
      - ectopic pregnancy O08.1
      - molar pregnancy O08.1
    - acquired D68.4
    - antepartum with hemorrhage — *see* Hemorrhage, antepartum, with coagulation defect
    - due to
      - liver disease D68.4
      - vitamin K deficiency D68.4
    - hereditary NEC D68.2
    - intrapartum O67.0
    - newborn, transient P61.6
    - postpartum O99.13
      - with hemorrhage O72.3
    - specified type NEC D68.8
  - complement system D84.1
  - conduction (heart) I45.9
    - bone — *see* Deafness, conductive
  - congenital, organ or site not listed — *see* Anomaly, by site
  - coronary sinus Q21.1
  - cushion, endocardial Q21.2
  - degradation, glycoprotein E77.1
  - dental bridge, crown, fillings — *see* Defect, dental restoration
  - dental restoration K08.50
    - specified NEC K08.59
  - dentin (hereditary) K00.5
  - Descemet's membrane, congenital Q13.89
  - developmental — *see also* Anomaly
    - cauda equina Q06.3
  - diaphragm
    - with elevation, eventration or hernia — *see* Hernia, diaphragm
    - congenital Q79.1
      - with hernia Q79.0
      - gross (with hernia) Q79.0
  - ectodermal, congenital Q82.9
  - Eisenmenger's Q21.8
  - enzyme
- **Defect, defective** - *continued*
  - enzyme - *continued*
    - catalase E80.3
    - peroxidase E80.3
  - esophagus, congenital Q39.9
  - extensor retinaculum M62.89
  - fibrin polymerization D68.2
  - filling
    - bladder R93.41
    - kidney R93.42-
    - renal pelvis R93.41
    - stomach R93.3
    - ureter R93.41
    - urinary organs, specified NEC R93.49
  - GABA (gamma aminobutyric acid) metabolic E72.81
  - Gerbode Q21.0
  - glucose transport, blood-brain barrier E74.810
  - glycoprotein degradation E77.1
  - Hageman (factor) D68.2
  - hearing — *see* Deafness
  - high grade F70
  - interatrial septal Q21.1
  - interauricular septal Q21.1
  - interventricular septal Q21.0
    - with dextroposition of aorta, pulmonary stenosis and hypertrophy of right ventricle Q21.3
    - in tetralogy of Fallot Q21.3
  - learning (specific) — *see* Disorder, learning
  - lymphocyte function antigen-1 (LFA-1) D84.0
  - lysosomal enzyme, post-translational modification E77.0
  - major osseous M89.70
    - ankle M89.77-
    - carpus M89.74-
    - clavicle M89.71-
    - femur M89.75-
    - fibula M89.76-
    - fingers M89.74-
    - foot M89.77-
    - forearm M89.73-
    - hand M89.74-
    - humerus M89.72-
    - lower leg M89.76-
    - metacarpus M89.74-
    - metatarsus M89.77-
    - multiple sites M89.79
    - pelvic region M89.75-
    - pelvis M89.75-
    - radius M89.73-
    - scapula M89.71-
    - shoulder region M89.71-
    - specified NEC M89.78
    - tarsus M89.77-
    - thigh M89.75-
    - tibia M89.76-
    - toes M89.77-
    - ulna M89.73-
  - mental — *see* Disability, intellectual
  - modification, lysosomal enzymes, post-translational E77.0
  - obstructive, congenital
    - renal pelvis Q62.39
    - ureter Q62.39
      - atresia — *see* Atresia, ureter
      - cecoureterocele Q62.32
      - megaureter Q62.2
      - orthotopic ureterocele Q62.31
  - osseous, major M89.70
    - ankle M89.77-
    - carpus M89.74-
    - clavicle M89.71-
    - femur M89.75-
    - fibula M89.76-
    - fingers M89.74-
    - foot M89.77-
    - forearm M89.73-
    - hand M89.74-
    - humerus M89.72-
    - lower leg M89.76-
    - metacarpus M89.74-
    - metatarsus M89.77-

Defect, defective - *continued*
osseous, major - *continued*
multiple sites M89.9
pelvic region M89.75-
pelvis M89.75-
radius M89.73-
scapula M89.71-
shoulder region M89.71-
specified NEC M89.78
tarsus M89.77-
thigh M89.75-
tibia M89.76-
toes M89.77-
ulna M89.73-
osteochondral NEC — *see also* Deformity M95.8
ostium
primum Q21.2
secundum Q21.1
peroxidase E80.3
placental blood supply — *see* Insufficiency, placental
platelets, qualitative D69.1
constitutional D68.0
postural NEC, spine — *see* Dorsopathy, deforming
reduction
limb Q73.8
lower Q72.9-
absence — *see* Agenesis, leg
foot — *see* Agenesis, foot
longitudinal
femur Q72.4-
fibula Q72.6-
tibia Q72.5-
specified type NEC Q72.89-
split foot Q72.7-
specified type NEC Q73.8
upper Q71.9-
absence — *see* Agenesis, arm
forearm — *see* Agenesis, forearm
hand — *see* Agenesis, hand
lobster-claw hand Q71.6-
longitudinal
radius Q71.4-
ulna Q71.5-
specified type NEC Q71.89-
renal pelvis Q63.8
obstructive Q62.39
respiratory system, congenital Q34.9
restoration, dental K08.50
specified NEC K08.59
retinal nerve bundle fibers H35.89
septal (heart) NOS Q21.9
acquired (atrial) (auricular) (ventricular) (old) I51.0
atrial Q21.1
concurrent with acute myocardial infarction — *see* Infarct, myocardium
following acute myocardial infarction (current complication) I23.1
ventricular — *see also* Defect, ventricular septal Q21.0
sinus venosus Q21.1
speech — *see* Disorder, speech
developmental F80.9
specified NEC R47.89
Taussig-Bing (aortic transposition and overriding pulmonary artery) Q20.1
teeth, wedge K03.1
vascular (local) I99.9
congenital Q27.9
ventricular septal Q21.0
concurrent with acute myocardial infarction — *see* Infarct, myocardium
following acute myocardial infarction (current complication) I23.2
in tetralogy of Fallot Q21.3
vision NEC H54.7
visual field H53.40
bilateral
heteronymous H53.47
homonymous H53.46-
generalized contraction H53.48-

Defect, defective - *continued*
visual field - *continued*
localized
arcuate H53.43-
scotoma (central area) H53.41-
blind spot area H53.42-
sector H53.43-
specified type NEC H53.45-
voice R49.9
specified NEC R49.8
wedge, tooth, teeth (abrasion) K03.1
Deferentitis N49.1
gonorrheal (acute) (chronic) A54.23
Defibrination (syndrome) D65
antepartum — *see* Hemorrhage, antepartum, with coagulation defect, disseminated intravascular coagulation
following ectopic or molar pregnancy O08.1
intrapartum O67.0
newborn P60
postpartum O72.3
Deficiency, deficient
3-beta hydroxysteroid dehydrogenase E25.0
5-alpha reductase (with male pseudohermaphroditism) E29.1
11-hydroxylase E25.0
21-hydroxylase E25.0
AADC (aromatic L-amino acid decarboxylase) E70.81
abdominal muscle syndrome Q79.4
accelerator globulin (Ac G) (blood) D68.2
AC globulin (congenital) (hereditary) D68.2
acquired D68.4
acid phosphatase E83.39
acid sphingomyelinase (ASMD) E75.249
type
A E75.240
A/B E75.244
B E75.241
activating factor (blood) D68.2
ADA2 (adenosine deaminase 2) D81.32
adenosine deaminase (ADA) D81.30
with severe combined immunodeficiency (SCID) D81.31
partial (type 1) D81.39
specified NEC D81.39
type 1 (without SCID) (without severe combined immunodeficiency) D81.39
type 2 D81.32
aldolase (hereditary) E74.19
alpha-1-antitrypsin E88.01
amino-acids E72.9
anemia — *see* Anemia
aneurin E51.9
antibody with
hyperimmunoglobulinemia D80.6
near-normal immunoglobins D80.6
antidiuretic hormone E23.2
anti-hemophilic
factor (A) D66
B D67
C D68.1
globulin (AHG) NEC D66
antithrombin (antithrombin III) D68.59
aromatic L-amino acid decarboxylase (AADC) E70.81
ascorbic acid E54
attention (disorder) (syndrome) F98.8
with hyperactivity — *see* Disorder, attention-deficit hyperactivity
autoprothrombin
I D68.2
II D67
C D68.2
beta-glucuronidase E76.29
biotin E53.8
biotin-dependent carboxylase D81.819
biotinidase D81.810
brancher enzyme (amylopectinosis) E74.03
calciferol E55.9
with
adult osteomalacia M83.8
rickets — *see* Rickets
calcium (dietary) E58
calorie, severe E43

Deficiency, deficient - *continued*
calorie, severe - *continued*
with marasmus E41
and kwashiorkor E42
cardiac — *see* Insufficiency, myocardial
carnitine E71.40
due to
hemodialysis E71.43
inborn errors of metabolism E71.42
Valproic acid therapy E71.43
iatrogenic E71.43
muscle palmityltransferase E71.314
primary E71.41
secondary E71.448
carotene E50.9
central nervous system G96.89
ceruloplasmin (Wilson) E83.01
choline E53.8
Christmas factor D67
chromium E61.4
chronic neurovisceral acid sphingomyelinase E75.244
chronic visceral acid sphingomyelinase E75.241
clotting (blood) — *see also* Deficiency, coagulation factor D68.9
clotting factor NEC (hereditary) — *see also* Deficiency, factor D68.2
coagulation NOS D68.9
with
ectopic pregnancy O08.1
molar pregnancy O08.1
acquired (any) D68.4
antepartum hemorrhage — *see* Hemorrhage, antepartum, with coagulation defect
clotting factor NEC — *see also* Deficiency, factor D68.2
due to
hyperprothrombinemia D68.4
liver disease D68.4
vitamin K deficiency D68.4
newborn, transient P61.6
postpartum O72.3
specified NEC D68.8
cognitive F09
color vision H53.50
achromatopsia H53.51
acquired H53.52
deuteranomaly H53.53
protanomaly H53.54
specified type NEC H53.59
tritanomaly H53.55
combined glucocorticoid and mineralocorticoid E27.49
contact factor D68.2
copper (nutritional) E61.0
corticoadrenal E27.40
primary E27.1
craniofacial axis Q75.0
cyanocobalamin E53.8
C1 esterase inhibitor (C1-INH) D84.1
debrancher enzyme (limit dextrinosis) E74.03
dehydrogenase
long chain/very long chain acyl CoA E71.310
medium chain acyl CoA E71.311
short chain acyl CoA E71.312
diet E63.9
dihydropyrimidine dehydrogenase (DPD) E88.89
disaccharidase E73.9
edema — *see* Malnutrition, severe
endocrine E34.9
energy-supply — *see* Malnutrition
enzymes, circulating NEC E88.09
ergosterol E55.9
with
adult osteomalacia M83.8
rickets — *see* Rickets
essential fatty acid (EFA) E63.0
eye movements
saccadic H55.81
smooth pursuit H55.82

- **Deficiency, deficient** - *continued*
  - factor — *see also* Deficiency, coagulation
    - Hageman D68.2
    - I (congenital) (hereditary) D68.2
    - II (congenital) (hereditary) D68.2
    - IX (congenital) (functional) (hereditary) (with functional defect) D67
    - multiple (congenital) D68.8
      - acquired D68.4
    - V (congenital) (hereditary) D68.2
    - VII (congenital) (hereditary) D68.2
    - VIII (congenital) (functional) (hereditary) (with functional defect) D66
      - with vascular defect D68.0
    - X (congenital) (hereditary) D68.2
    - XI (congenital) (hereditary) D68.1
    - XII (congenital) (hereditary) D68.2
    - XIII (congenital) (hereditary) D68.2
  - femoral, proximal focal (congenital) — *see* Defect, reduction, lower limb, longitudinal, femur
  - fibrin-stabilizing factor (congenital) (hereditary) D68.2
    - acquired D68.4
  - fibrinase D68.2
  - fibrinogen (congenital) (hereditary) D68.2
    - acquired D65
  - folate E53.8
  - folic acid E53.8
  - foreskin N47.3
  - fructokinase E74.11
  - fructose 1,6-diphosphatase E74.19
  - fructose-1-phosphate aldolase E74.19
  - GABA (gamma aminobutyric acid) transaminase E72.81
  - GABA-T (gamma aminobutyric acid transaminase) E72.81
  - galactokinase E74.29
  - galactose-1-phosphate uridyl transferase E74.29
  - gammaglobulin in blood D80.1
    - hereditary D80.0
  - glass factor D68.2
  - glucocorticoid E27.49
    - mineralocorticoid E27.49
  - glucose-6-phosphatase E74.01
  - glucose-6-phosphate dehydrogenase
    - anemia D55.0
    - without anemia D75.A
  - glucose transporter protein type 1 E74.810
  - glucuronyl transferase E80.5
  - Glut1 E74.810
  - glycogen synthetase E74.09
  - gonadotropin (isolated) E23.0
  - growth hormone (idiopathic) (isolated) E23.0
  - Hageman factor D68.2
  - hemoglobin D64.9
  - hepatophosphorylase E74.09
  - homogentisate 1,2-dioxygenase E70.29
  - hormone
    - anterior pituitary (partial) NEC E23.0
      - growth E23.0
    - growth (isolated) E23.0
    - pituitary E23.0
    - testicular E29.1
  - hypoxanthine- (guanine) -phosphoribosyltransferase (HG- PRT) (total H-PRT) E79.1
  - immunity D84.9
    - cell-mediated D84.89
      - with thrombocytopenia and eczema D82.0
    - combined D81.9
    - humoral D80.9
    - IgA (secretory) D80.2
    - IgG D80.3
    - IgM D80.4
  - immuno — *see* Immunodeficiency
  - immunoglobulin, selective
    - A (IgA) D80.2
    - G (IgG) (subclasses) D80.3
    - M (IgM) D80.4
  - infantile neurovisceral acid sphingomyelinase E75.240
  - inositol (B complex) E53.8
- **Deficiency, deficient** - *continued*
  - intrinsic
    - factor (congenital) D51.0
    - sphincter N36.42
      - with urethral hypermobility N36.43
  - iodine E61.8
    - congenital syndrome — *see* Syndrome, iodine-deficiency, congenital
  - iron E61.1
    - anemia D50.9
  - kalium E87.6
  - kappa-light chain D80.8
  - labile factor (congenital) (hereditary) D68.2
    - acquired D68.4
  - lacrimal fluid (acquired) — *see also* Syndrome, dry eye
    - congenital Q10.6
  - lactase
    - congenital E73.0
    - secondary E73.1
  - Laki-Lorand factor D68.2
  - lecithin cholesterol acyltransferase E78.6
  - lipocaic K86.89
  - lipoprotein (familial) (high density) E78.6
  - liver phosphorylase E74.09
  - lysosomal alpha-1, 4 glucosidase E74.02
  - magnesium E61.2
  - major histocompatibility complex
    - class I D81.6
    - class II D81.7
  - manganese E61.3
  - menadione (vitamin K) E56.1
    - newborn P53
  - mental (familial) (hereditary) — *see* Disability, intellectual
  - methylenetetrahydrofolate reductase (MTHFR) E72.12
  - mevalonate kinase M04.1
  - mineral NEC E61.8
  - mineralocorticoid E27.49
    - with glucocorticoid E27.49
  - molybdenum (nutritional) E61.5
  - moral F60.2
  - multiple nutrient elements E61.7
  - multiple sulfatase (MSD) E75.26
  - muscle
    - carnitine (palmityltransferase) E71.314
    - phosphofructokinase E74.09
  - myoadenylate deaminase E79.2
  - myocardial — *see* Insufficiency, myocardial
  - myophosphorylase E74.04
  - NADH diaphorase or reductase (congenital) D74.0
  - NADH-methemoglobin reductase (congenital) D74.0
  - natrium E87.1
  - niacin (amide) (-tryptophan) E52
  - nicotinamide E52
  - nicotinic acid E52
  - number of teeth — *see* Anodontia
  - nutrient element E61.9
    - multiple E61.7
    - specified NEC E61.8
  - nutrition, nutritional E63.9
    - sequelae — *see* Sequelae, nutritional deficiency
    - specified NEC E63.8
  - of interleukin 1 receptor antagonist [DIRA] M04.8
  - ornithine transcarbamylase E72.4
  - ovarian E28.39
  - oxygen — *see* Anoxia
  - pantothenic acid E53.8
  - parathyroid (gland) E20.9
  - perineum (female) N81.89
  - phenylalanine hydroxylase E70.1
  - phosphoenolpyruvate carboxykinase E74.4
  - phosphofructokinase E74.19
  - phosphomannomutuse E74.818
  - phosphomannose isomerase E74.818
  - phosphomannosyl mutase E74.818
  - phosphorylase kinase, liver E74.09
  - pituitary hormone (isolated) E23.0
  - plasma thromboplastin
    - antecedent (PTA) D68.1
- **Deficiency, deficient** - *continued*
  - plasma thromboplastin - *continued*
    - component (PTC) D67
  - plasminogen (type 1) (type 2) E88.02
  - platelet NEC D69.1
    - constitutional D68.0
  - polyglandular E31.8
    - autoimmune E31.0
  - potassium (K) E87.6
  - prepuce N47.3
  - proaccelerin (congenital) (hereditary) D68.2
    - acquired D68.4
  - proconvertin factor (congenital) (hereditary) D68.2
    - acquired D68.4
  - protein — *see also* Malnutrition E46
    - anemia D53.0
    - C D68.59
    - S D68.59
  - prothrombin (congenital) (heredItary) D68.2
    - acquired D68.4
  - Prower factor D68.2
  - pseudocholinesterase E88.09
  - PTA (plasma thromboplastin antecedent) D68.1
  - PTC (plasma thromboplastin component) D67
  - purine nucleoside phosphorylase (PNP) D81.5
  - pyracin (alpha) (beta) E53.1
  - pyridoxal E53.1
  - pyridoxamine E53.1
  - pyridoxine (derivatives) E53.1
  - pyruvate
    - carboxylase E74.4
    - dehydrogenase E74.4
  - riboflavin (vitamin B2) E53.0
  - salt E87.1
  - secretion
    - ovary E28.39
    - salivary gland (any) K11.7
    - urine R34
  - selenium (dietary) E59
  - serum antitrypsin, familial E88.01
  - short stature homeobox gene (SHOX)
    - with
      - dyschondrosteosis Q78.8
      - short stature (idiopathic) E34.3
      - Turner's syndrome Q96.9
  - sodium (Na) E87.1
  - SPCA (factor VII) D68.2
  - sphincter, intrinsic N36.42
    - with urethral hypermobility N36.43
  - stable factor (congenital) (hereditary) D68.2
    - acquired D68.4
  - Stuart-Prower (factor X) D68.2
  - succinic semialdehyde dehydrogenase E72.81
  - sucrase E74.39
  - sulfatase E75.26
  - sulfite oxidase E72.19
  - thiamin, thiaminic (chloride) E51.9
    - beriberi (dry) E51.11
      - wet E51.12
  - thrombokinase D68.2
    - newborn P53
  - thyroid (gland) — *see* Hypothyroidism
  - tocopherol E56.0
  - tooth bud K00.0
  - transcobalamine II (anemia) D51.2
  - vanadium E61.6
  - vascular I99.9
  - vasopressin E23.2
  - vertical ridge K06.8
  - viosterol — *see* Deficiency, calciferol
  - vitamin (multiple) NOS E56.9
    - A E50.9
      - with
        - Bitot's spot (corneal) E50.1
        - follicular keratosis E50.8
        - keratomalacia E50.4
        - manifestations NEC E50.8
        - night blindness E50.5
        - scar of cornea, xerophthalmic E50.6
        - xeroderma E50.8

Deficiency, deficient - *continued*
vitamin (multiple) NOS - *continued*
A - *continued*
with - *continued*
xerophthalmia E50.7
xerosis
conjunctival E50.0
and Bitot's spot E50.1
cornea E50.2
and ulceration E50.3
sequelae E64.1
B (complex) NOS E53.9
with
beriberi (dry) E51.11
wet E51.12
pellagra E52
B1 NOS E51.9
beriberi (dry) E51.11
with circulatory system manifestations E51.11
wet E51.12
B12 E53.8
B2 (riboflavin) E53.0
B6 E53.1
C E54
sequelae E64.2
D E55.9
with
adult osteomalacia M83.8
rickets — *see* Rickets
25-hydroxylase E83.32
E E56.0
folic acid E53.8
G E53.0
group B E53.9
specified NEC E53.8
H (biotin) E53.8
K E56.1
of newborn P53
nicotinic E52
P E56.8
PP (pellagra-preventing) E52
specified NEC E56.8
thiamin E51.9
beriberi — *see* Beriberi
zinc, dietary E60
Deficit — *see also* Deficiency
attention and concentration R41.840
following
cerebral infarction I69.310
cerebrovascular disease I69.910
specified disease NEC I69.810
nontraumatic
intracerebral hemorrhage I69.110
specified intracranial hemorrhage NEC I69.210
subarachnoid hemorrhage I69.010
disorder — *see* Attention, deficit
cognitive
communication R41.841
emotional
following
cerebral infarction I69.315
cerebrovascular disease I69.915
specified disease NEC I69.815
nontraumatic
intracerebral hemorrhage I69.115
specified intracranial hemorrhage NEC I69.215
subarachnoid hemorrhage I69.015
following
cerebral infarction I69.319
cerebrovascular disease I69.919
specified disease NEC I69.819
nontraumatic
intracerebral hemorrhage I69.119
specified intracranial hemorrhage NEC I69.219
subarachnoid hemorrhage I69.019
social
following
cerebral infarction I69.315
cerebrovascular disease I69.915
specified disease NEC I69.815
nontraumatic

Deficit - *continued*
cognitive - *continued*
social - *continued*
following - *continued*
nontraumatic - *continued*
intracerebral hemorrhage I69.115
specified intracranial hemorrhage NEC I69.215
subarachnoid hemorrhage I69.015
cognitive NEC R41.89
following
cerebral infarction I69.318
cerebrovascular disease I69.918
specified disease NEC I69.818
nontraumatic
intracerebral hemorrhage I69.118
specified intracranial hemorrhage NEC I69.218
subarachnoid hemorrhage I69.018
concentration R41.840
executive function R41.844
following
cerebral infarction I69.314
cerebrovascular disease I69.914
specified disease NEC I69.814
nontraumatic
intracerebral hemorrhage I69.114
specified intracranial hemorrhage NEC I69.214
subarachnoid hemorrhage I69.014
frontal lobe R41.844
following
cerebral infarction I69.314
cerebrovascular disease I69.914
specified disease NEC I69.814
nontraumatic
intracerebral hemorrhage I69.114
specified intracranial hemorrhage NEC I69.214
subarachnoid hemorrhage I69.014
memory
following
cerebral infarction I69.311
cerebrovascular disease I69.911
specified disease NEC I69.811
nontraumatic
intracerebral hemorrhage I69.111
specified intracranial hemorrhage NEC I69.211
subarachnoid hemorrhage I69.011
neurologic NEC R29.818
ischemic
reversible (RIND) I63.9
prolonged (PRIND) I63.9
oxygen R09.02
prolonged reversible ischemic neurologic (PRIND) I63.9
psychomotor R41.843
following
cerebral infarction I69.313
cerebrovascular disease I69.913
specified disease NEC I69.813
nontraumatic
intracerebral hemorrhage I69.113
specified intracranial hemorrhage NEC I69.213
subarachnoid hemorrhage I69.013
visuospatial R41.842
following
cerebral infarction I69.312
cerebrovascular disease I69.912
specified disease NEC I69.812
nontraumatic
intracerebral hemorrhage I69.112
specified intracranial hemorrhage NEC I69.212
subarachnoid hemorrhage I69.012
Deflection
radius — *see* Deformity, limb, specified type NEC, forearm
septum (acquired) (nasal) (nose) J34.2
spine — *see* Curvature, spine
turbinate (nose) J34.2
Defluvium
capillorum — *see* Alopecia

Defluvium - *continued*
ciliorum — *see* Madarosis
unguium L60.8
Deformity Q89.9
abdomen, congenital Q89.9
abdominal wall
acquired M95.8
congenital Q79.59
acquired (unspecified site) M95.9
adrenal gland Q89.1
alimentary tract, congenital Q45.9
upper Q40.9
ankle (joint) (acquired) — *see also* Deformity, limb, lower leg
abduction — *see* Contraction, joint, ankle
congenital Q68.8
contraction — *see* Contraction, joint, ankle
specified type NEC — *see* Deformity, limb, foot, specified NEC
anus (acquired) K62.89
congenital Q43.9
aorta (arch) (congenital) Q25.40
acquired I77.89
aortic
arch, acquired I77.89
cusp or valve (congenital) Q23.8
acquired — *see also* Endocarditis, aortic I35.8
arm (acquired) (upper) — *see also* Deformity, limb, upper arm
congenital Q68.8
forearm — *see* Deformity, limb, forearm
artery (congenital) (peripheral) NOS Q27.9
acquired I77.89
coronary (acquired) I25.9
congenital Q24.5
umbilical Q27.0
atrial septal Q21.1
auditory canal (external) (congenital) — *see also* Malformation, ear, external
acquired — *see* Disorder, ear, external, specified type NEC
auricle
ear (congenital) — *see also* Malformation, ear, external
acquired — *see* Disorder, pinna, deformity
back — *see* Dorsopathy, deforming
bile duct (common) (congenital) (hepatic) Q44.5
acquired K83.8
biliary duct or passage (congenital) Q44.5
acquired K83.8
bladder (neck) (trigone) (sphincter) (acquired) N32.89
congenital Q64.79
bone (acquired) NOS M95.9
congenital Q79.9
turbinate M95.0
brain (congenital) Q04.9
acquired G93.89
reduction Q04.3
breast (acquired) N64.89
congenital Q83.9
reconstructed N65.0
bronchus (congenital) Q32.4
acquired NEC J98.09
bursa, congenital Q79.9
canaliculi (lacrimalis) (acquired) — *see also* Disorder, lacrimal system, changes
congenital Q10.6
canthus, acquired — *see* Disorder, eyelid, specified type NEC
capillary (acquired) I78.8
cardiovascular system, congenital Q28.9
caruncle, lacrimal (acquired) — *see also* Disorder, lacrimal system, changes
congenital Q10.6
cascade, stomach K31.2
cecum (congenital) Q43.9
acquired K63.89
cerebral, acquired G93.89
congenital Q04.9
cervix (uterus) (acquired) NEC N88.8
congenital Q51.9

Deformity - *continued*
- cheek (acquired) M95.2
  - congenital Q18.9
- chest (acquired) (wall) M95.4
  - congenital Q67.8
  - sequelae (late effect) of rickets E64.3
- chin (acquired) M95.2
  - congenital Q18.9
- choroid (congenital) Q14.3
  - acquired H31.8
  - plexus Q07.8
    - acquired G96.198
- cicatricial — *see* Cicatrix
- cilia, acquired — *see* Disorder, eyelid, specified type NEC
- clavicle (acquired) M95.8
  - congenital Q68.8
- clitoris (congenital) Q52.6
  - acquired N90.89
- clubfoot — *see* Clubfoot
- coccyx (acquired) — *see* subcategory M43.8
- colon (congenital) Q43.9
  - acquired K63.89
- concha (ear) , congenital — *see also* Malformation, ear, external
  - acquired — *see* Disorder, pinna, deformity
- cornea (acquired) H18.70
  - congenital Q13.4
  - descemetocele — *see* Descemetocele
  - ectasia — *see* Ectasia, cornea
  - specified NEC H18.79-
  - staphyloma — *see* Staphyloma, cornea
- coronary artery (acquired) I25.9
  - congenital Q24.5
- cranium (acquired) — *see* Deformity, skull
- cricoid cartilage (congenital) Q31.8
  - acquired J38.7
- cystic duct (congenital) Q44.5
  - acquired K82.8
- Dandy-Walker Q03.1
  - with spina bifida — *see* Spina bifida
- diaphragm (congenital) Q79.1
  - acquired J98.6
- digestive organ NOS Q45.9
- ductus arteriosus Q25.0
- duodenal bulb K31.89
- duodenum (congenital) Q43.9
  - acquired K31.89
- dura — *see* Deformity, meninges
- ear (acquired) — *see also* Disorder, pinna, deformity
  - congenital (external) Q17.9
    - internal Q16.5
    - middle Q16.4
      - ossicles Q16.3
    - ossicles Q16.3
- ectodermal (congenital) NEC Q84.9
- ejaculatory duct (congenital) Q55.4
  - acquired N50.89
- elbow (joint) (acquired) — *see also* Deformity, limb, upper arm
  - congenital Q68.8
  - contraction — *see* Contraction, joint, elbow
- endocrine gland NEC Q89.2
- epididymis (congenital) Q55.4
  - acquired N50.89
- epiglottis (congenital) Q31.8
  - acquired J38.7
- esophagus (congenital) Q39.9
  - acquired K22.89
- eustachian tube (congenital) NEC Q17.8
- eye, congenital Q15.9
- eyebrow (congenital) Q18.8
- eyelid (acquired) — *see also* Disorder, eyelid, specified type NEC
  - congenital Q10.3
- face (acquired) M95.2
  - congenital Q18.9
- fallopian tube, acquired N83.8
- femur (acquired) — *see* Deformity, limb, specified type NEC, thigh
- fetal
  - with fetopelvic disproportion O33.7
  - causing obstructed labor O66.3

Deformity - *continued*
- finger (acquired) M20.00-
  - boutonniere M20.02-
  - congenital Q68.1
  - flexion contracture — *see* Contraction, joint, hand
  - mallet finger M20.01-
  - specified NEC M20.09-
  - swan-neck M20.03-
- flexion (joint) (acquired) — *see also* Deformity, limb, flexion M21.20
  - congenital NOS Q74.9
    - hip Q65.89
- foot (acquired) — *see also* Deformity, limb, lower leg
  - cavovarus (congenital) Q66.1-
  - congenital NOS Q66.9-
    - specified type NEC Q66.89
  - specified type NEC — *see* Deformity, limb, foot, specified NEC
  - valgus (congenital) Q66.6
    - acquired — *see* Deformity, valgus, ankle
  - varus (congenital) NEC Q66.3-
    - acquired — *see* Deformity, varus, ankle
- forearm (acquired) — *see also* Deformity, limb, forearm
  - congenital Q68.8
- forehead (acquired) M95.2
  - congenital Q75.8
- frontal bone (acquired) M95.2
  - congenital Q75.8
- gallbladder (congenital) Q44.1
  - acquired K82.8
- gastrointestinal tract (congenital) NOS Q45.9
  - acquired K63.89
- genitalia, genital organ (s) or system NEC
  - female (congenital) Q52.9
    - acquired N94.89
    - external Q52.70
  - male (congenital) Q55.9
    - acquired N50.89
- globe (eye) (congenital) Q15.8
  - acquired H44.89
- gum, acquired NEC K06.8
- hand (acquired) — *see* Deformity, limb, hand
  - congenital Q68.1
- head (acquired) M95.2
  - congenital Q75.8
- heart (congenital) Q24.9
  - septum Q21.9
    - auricular Q21.1
    - ventricular Q21.0
  - valve (congenital) NEC Q24.8
    - acquired — *see* Endocarditis
- heel (acquired) — *see* Deformity, foot
- hepatic duct (congenital) Q44.5
  - acquired K83.8
- hip (joint) (acquired) — *see also* Deformity, limb, thigh
  - congenital Q65.9
  - due to (previous) juvenile osteochondrosis — *see* Coxa, plana
  - flexion — *see* Contraction, joint, hip
- hourglass — *see* Contraction, hourglass
- humerus (acquired) M21.82-
  - congenital Q74.0
- hypophyseal (congenital) Q89.2
- ileocecal (coil) (valve) (acquired) K63.89
  - congenital Q43.9
- ileum (congenital) Q43.9
  - acquired K63.89
- ilium (acquired) M95.5
  - congenital Q74.2
- integument (congenital) Q84.9
- intervertebral cartilage or disc (acquired) — *see* Disorder, disc, specified NEC
- intestine (large) (small) (congenital) NOS Q43.9
  - acquired K63.89
- intrinsic minus or plus (hand) — *see* Deformity, limb, specified type NEC, forearm
- iris (acquired) H21.89
  - congenital Q13.2
- ischium (acquired) M95.5

Deformity - *continued*
- ischium (acquired) - *continued*
  - congenital Q74.2
- jaw (acquired) (congenital) M26.9
- joint (acquired) NEC M21.90
  - congenital Q68.8
  - elbow M21.92-
  - hand M21.94-
  - hip M21.95-
  - knee M21.96-
  - shoulder M21.92-
  - wrist M21.93-
- kidney (s) (calyx) (pelvis) (congenital) Q63.9
  - acquired N28.89
  - artery (congenital) Q27.2
    - acquired I77.89
- Klippel-Feil (brevicollis) Q76.1
- knee (acquired) NEC — *see also* Deformity, limb, lower leg
  - congenital Q68.2
- labium (majus) (minus) (congenital) Q52.79
  - acquired N90.89
- lacrimal passages or duct (congenital) NEC Q10.6
  - acquired — *see* Disorder, lacrimal system, changes
- larynx (muscle) (congenital) Q31.8
  - acquired J38.7
  - web (glottic) Q31.0
- leg (upper) (acquired) NEC — *see also* Deformity, limb, thigh
  - congenital Q68.8
  - lower leg — *see* Deformity, limb, lower leg
- lens (acquired) H27.8
  - congenital Q12.9
- lid (fold) (acquired) — *see also* Disorder, eyelid, specified type NEC
  - congenital Q10.3
- ligament (acquired) — *see* Disorder, ligament
  - congenital Q79.9
- limb (acquired) M21.90
  - clawfoot M21.53-
  - clawhand M21.51-
  - clubfoot M21.54-
  - clubhand M21.52-
  - congenital, except reduction deformity Q74.9
  - flat foot M21.4-
  - flexion M21.20
    - ankle M21.27-
    - elbow M21.22-
    - finger M21.24-
    - hip M21.25-
    - knee M21.26-
    - shoulder M21.21-
    - toe M21.27-
    - wrist M21.23-
  - foot
    - claw — *see* Deformity, limb, clawfoot
    - club — *see* Deformity, limb, clubfoot
    - drop M21.37-
    - flat — *see* Deformity, limb, flat foot
    - specified NEC M21.6X-
  - forearm M21.93-
  - hand M21.94-
  - lower leg M21.96-
  - specified type NEC M21.80
    - forearm M21.83-
    - lower leg M21.86-
    - thigh M21.85-
    - upper arm M21.82-
  - thigh M21.95-
  - unequal length M21.70
    - short site is
      - femur M21.75-
      - fibula M21.76-
      - humerus M21.72-
      - radius M21.73-
      - tibia M21.76-
      - ulna M21.73-
  - upper arm M21.92-
  - valgus — *see* Deformity, valgus
  - varus — *see* Deformity, varus

Deformity - *continued*
- urinary tract (congenital) Q64.9
  - urachus Q64.4
- uterus (congenital) Q51.9
  - acquired N85.8
- uvula (congenital) Q38.5
- vagina (acquired) N89.8
  - congenital Q52.4
- valgus NEC M21.00
  - ankle M21.07-
  - elbow M21.02-
  - hip M21.05-
  - knee M21.06-
- valve, valvular (congenital) (heart) Q24.8
  - acquired — *see* Endocarditis
- varus NEC M21.10
  - ankle M21.17-
  - elbow M21.12-
  - hip M21.15
  - knee M21.16-
  - tibia — *see* Osteochondrosis, juvenile, tibia
- vas deferens (congenital) Q55.4
  - acquired N50.89
- vein (congenital) Q27.9
  - great Q26.9
- vertebra — *see* Dorsopathy, deforming
- vertical talus (congenital) Q66.80
  - left foot Q66.82
  - right foot Q66.81
- vesicourethral orifice (acquired) N32.89
  - congenital NEC Q64.79
- vessels of optic papilla (congenital) Q14.2
- visual field (contraction) — *see* Defect, visual field
- vitreous body, acquired H43.89
- vulva (congenital) Q52.79
  - acquired N90.89
- wrist (joint) (acquired) — *see also* Deformity, limb, forearm
  - congenital Q68.8
  - contraction — *see* Contraction, joint, wrist

Degeneration, degenerative
- adrenal (capsule) (fatty) (gland) (hyaline) (infectional) E27.8
- amyloid — *see also* Amyloidosis E85.9
- anterior cornua, spinal cord G12.29
- anterior labral S43.49-
- aorta, aortic I70.0
  - fatty I77.89
- aortic valve (heart) — *see* Endocarditis, aortic
- arteriovascular — *see* Arteriosclerosis
- artery, arterial (atheromatous) (calcareous) — *see also* Arteriosclerosis
  - cerebral, amyloid E85.4 *[I68.0]*
  - medial — *see* Arteriosclerosis, extremities
- articular cartilage NEC — *see* Derangement, joint, articular cartilage, by site
- atheromatous — *see* Arteriosclerosis
- basal nuclei or ganglia G23.9
  - specified NEC G23.8
- bone NEC — *see* Disorder, bone, specified type NEC
- brachial plexus G54.0
- brain (cortical) (progressive) G31.9
  - alcoholic G31.2
  - arteriosclerotic I67.2
  - childhood G31.9
    - specified NEC G31.89
  - cystic G31.89
    - congenital Q04.6
  - in
    - alcoholism G31.2
    - beriberi E51.2
    - cerebrovascular disease I67.9
    - congenital hydrocephalus Q03.9
      - with spina bifida — *see also* Spina bifida
    - Fabry-Anderson disease E75.21
    - Gaucher's disease E75.22
    - Hunter's syndrome E76.1
    - lipidosis
      - cerebral E75.4
      - generalized E75.6

Degeneration, degenerative - *continued*
- brain (cortical) (progressive) - *continued*
  - in - *continued*
    - mucopolysaccharidosis — *see* Mucopolysaccharidosis
    - myxedema E03.9 *[G32.89]*
    - neoplastic disease — *see also* Neoplasm D49.6 *[G32.89]*
    - Niemann-Pick disease E75.249 *[G32.89]*
    - sphingolipidosis E75.3 *[G32.89]*
    - vitamin B12 deficiency E53.8 *[G32.89]*
  - senile NEC G31.1
- breast N64.89
- Bruch's membrane — *see* Degeneration, choroid
- capillaries (fatty) I78.8
  - amyloid E85.89 *[I79.8]*
- cardiac — *see also* Degeneration, myocardial
  - valve, valvular — *see* Endocarditis
- cardiorenal — *see* Hypertension, cardiorenal
- cardiovascular — *see also* Disease, cardiovascular
  - renal — *see* Hypertension, cardiorenal
- cerebellar NOS G31.9
  - alcoholic G31.2
  - primary (hereditary) (sporadic) G11.9
- cerebral — *see* Degeneration, brain
- cerebrovascular I67.9
  - due to hypertension I67.4
- cervical plexus G54.2
- cervix N88.8
  - due to radiation (intended effect) N88.8
    - adverse effect or misadventure N99.89
- chamber angle H21.21-
- changes, spine or vertebra — *see* Spondylosis
- chorioretinal — *see also* Degeneration, choroid
  - hereditary H31.20
- choroid (colloid) (drusen) H31.10-
  - atrophy — *see* Atrophy, choroidal
  - hereditary — *see* Dystrophy, choroidal, hereditary
- ciliary body H21.22-
- cochlear — *see* subcategory H83.8
- combined (spinal cord) (subacute) E53.8 *[G32.0]*
  - with anemia (pernicious) D51.0 *[G32.0]*
    - due to dietary vitamin B12 deficiency D51.3 *[G32.0]*
  - in (due to)
    - vitamin B12 deficiency E53.8 *[G32.0]*
      - anemia D51.9 *[G32.0]*
- conjunctiva H11.10
  - concretions — *see* Concretion, conjunctiva
  - deposits — *see* Deposit, conjunctiva
  - pigmentations — *see* Pigmentation, conjunctiva
  - pinguecula — *see* Pinguecula
  - xerosis — *see* Xerosis, conjunctiva
- cornea H18.40
  - calcerous H18.43
    - band keratopathy H18.42-
  - familial, hereditary — *see* Dystrophy, cornea
  - hyaline (of old scars) H18.49
  - keratomalacia — *see* Keratomalacia
  - nodular H18.45-
  - peripheral H18.46-
  - senile H18.41-
  - specified type NEC H18.49
- cortical (cerebellar) (parenchymatous) G31.89
  - alcoholic G31.2
  - diffuse, due to arteriopathy I67.2
- corticobasal G31.85
- cutis L98.8
  - amyloid E85.4 *[L99]*
- dental pulp K04.2
- disc disease — *see* Degeneration, intervertebral disc NEC
- dorsolateral (spinal cord) — *see* Degeneration, combined
- extrapyramidal G25.9

Degeneration, degenerative - *continued*
- eye, macular — *see also* Degeneration, macula
  - congenital or hereditary — *see* Dystrophy, retina
- facet joints — *see* Spondylosis
- fatty
  - liver NEC K76.0
    - alcoholic K70.0
- grey matter (brain) (Alpers') G31.81
- heart — *see also* Degeneration, myocardial
  - amyloid E85.4 *[I43]*
  - atheromatous — *see* Disease, heart, ischemic, atherosclerotic
  - ischemic — *see* Disease, heart, ischemic
- hepatolenticular (Wilson's) E83.01
- hepatorenal K76.7
- hyaline (diffuse) (generalized)
  - localized — *see* Degeneration, by site
- infrapatellar fat pad M79.4
- intervertebral disc NOS
  - with
    - myelopathy — *see* Disorder, disc, with, myelopathy
    - radiculitis or radiculopathy — *see* Disorder, disc, with, radiculopathy
  - cervical, cervicothoracic — *see* Disorder, disc, cervical, degeneration
    - with
      - myelopathy — *see* Disorder, disc, cervical, with myelopathy
      - neuritis, radiculitis or radiculopathy — *see* Disorder, disc, cervical, with neuritis
  - lumbar region M51.36
    - with
      - myelopathy M51.06
      - neuritis, radiculitis, radiculopathy or sciatica M51.16
  - lumbosacral region M51.37
    - with
      - neuritis, radiculitis, radiculopathy or sciatica M51.17
  - sacrococcygeal region M53.3
  - thoracic region M51.34
    - with
      - myelopathy M51.04
      - neuritis, radiculitis, radiculopathy M51.14
  - thoracolumbar region M51.35
    - with
      - myelopathy M51.05
      - neuritis, radiculitis, radiculopathy M51.15
- intestine, amyloid E85.4
- iris (pigmentary) H21.23-
- ischemic — *see* Ischemia
- joint disease — *see* Osteoarthritis
- kidney N28.89
  - amyloid E85.4 *[N29]*
  - cystic, congenital Q61.9
  - fatty N28.89
  - polycystic Q61.3
    - adult type (autosomal dominant) Q61.2
    - infantile type (autosomal recessive) NEC Q61.19
      - collecting duct dilatation Q61.11
- Kuhnt-Junius — *see also* Degeneration, macula H35.32-
- lens — *see* Cataract
- lenticular (familial) (progressive) (Wilson's) (with cirrhosis of liver) E83.01
- liver (diffuse) NEC K76.89
  - amyloid E85.4 *[K77]*
  - cystic K76.89
    - congenital Q44.6
  - fatty NEC K76.0
    - alcoholic K70.0
  - hypertrophic K76.89
  - parenchymatous, acute or subacute K72.00
    - with coma K72.01
  - pigmentary K76.89
  - toxic (acute) K71.9
- iung J98.4
- lymph gland I89.8

Degeneration, degenerative - *continued*
lymph gland - *continued*
hyaline I89.8
macula, macular (acquired) (age-related) (senile) H35.30
angioid streaks H35.33
atrophic age-related H35.31-
congenital or hereditary — *see* Dystrophy, retina
cystoid H35.35-
drusen H35.36-
dry age-related H35.31-
exudative H35.32-
hole H35.34-
nonexudative H35.31-
puckering H35.37-
toxic H35.38-
wet age-related H35.32-
membranous labyrinth, congenital (causing impairment of hearing) Q16.5
meniscus — *see* Derangement, meniscus
mitral — *see* Insufficiency, mitral
Mönckeberg's — *see* Arteriosclerosis, extremities
motor centers, senile G31.1
multi-system G90.3
mural — *see* Degeneration, myocardial
muscle (fatty) (fibrous) (hyaline) (progressive) M62.89
heart — *see* Degeneration, myocardial
myelin, central nervous system G37.9
myocardial, myocardium (fatty) (hyaline) (senile) I51.5
with rheumatic fever (conditions in I00) I09.0
active, acute or subacute I01.2
with chorea I02.0
inactive or quiescent (with chorea) I09.0
hypertensive — *see* Hypertension, heart
rheumatic — *see* Degeneration, myocardial, with rheumatic fever
syphilitic A52.06
nasal sinus (mucosa) J32.9
frontal J32.1
maxillary J32.0
nerve — *see* Disorder, nerve
nervous system G31.9
alcoholic G31.2
amyloid E85.4 *[G99.8]*
autonomic G90.9
fatty G31.89
specified NEC G31.89
nipple N64.89
olivopontocerebellar (hereditary) (familial) G23.8
osseous labyrinth — *see* subcategory H83.8
ovary N83.8
cystic N83.20-
microcystic N83.20-
pallidal pigmentary (progressive) G23.0
pancreas K86.89
tuberculous A18.83
penis N48.89
pigmentary (diffuse) (general)
localized — *see* Degeneration, by site
pallidal (progressive) G23.0
pineal gland E34.8
pituitary (gland) E23.6
popliteal fat pad M79.4
posterolateral (spinal cord) — *see* Degeneration, combined
pulmonary valve (heart) I37.8
pulp (tooth) K04.2
pupillary margin H21.24-
renal — *see* Degeneration, kidney
retina H35.9
hereditary (cerebroretinal) (congenital) (juvenile) (macula) (peripheral) (pigmentary) — *see* Dystrophy, retina
Kuhnt-Junius — *see also* Degeneration, macula H35.32-
macula (cystic) (exudative) (hole) (nonexudative) (pseudohole) (senile) (toxic) — *see* Degeneration, macula
peripheral H35.40

Degeneration, degenerative - *continued*
retina - *continued*
peripheral - *continued*
lattice H35.41-
microcystoid H35.42-
paving stone H35.43-
secondary
pigmentary H35.45-
vitreoretinal H35.46-
senile reticular H35.44-
pigmentary (primary) — *see also* Dystrophy, retina
secondary — *see* Degeneration, retina, peripheral, secondary
posterior pole — *see* Degeneration, macula
saccule, congenital (causing impairment of hearing) Q16.5
senile R54
brain G31.1
cardiac, heart or myocardium — *see* Degeneration, myocardial
motor centers G31.1
vascular — *see* Arteriosclerosis
sinus (cystic) — *see also* Sinusitis
polypoid J33.1
skin L98.8
amyloid E85.4 *[L99]*
colloid L98.8
spinal (cord) G31.89
amyloid E85.4 *[G32.89]*
combined (subacute) — *see* Degeneration, combined
dorsolateral — *see* Degeneration, combined
familial NEC G31.89
fatty G31.89
funicular — *see* Degeneration, combined
posterolateral — *see* Degeneration, combined
subacute combined — *see* Degeneration, combined
tuberculous A17.81
spleen D73.0
amyloid E85.4 *[D77]*
stomach K31.89
striatonigral G23.2
suprarenal (capsule) (gland) E27.8
synovial membrane (pulpy) — *see* Disorder, synovium, specified type NEC
tapetoretinal — *see* Dystrophy, retina
thymus (gland) E32.8
fatty E32.8
thyroid (gland) E07.89
tricuspid (heart) (valve) I07.9
tuberculous NEC — *see* Tuberculosis
turbinate J34.89
uterus (cystic) N85.8
vascular (senile) — *see* Arteriosclerosis
hypertensive — *see* Hypertension
vitreoretinal, secondary — *see* Degeneration, retina, peripheral, secondary, vitreoretinal
vitreous (body) H43.81-
Wallerian — *see* Disorder, nerve
Wilson's hepatolenticular E83.01
Deglutition
paralysis R13.0
hysterical F44.4
pneumonia J69.0
Degos' disease I77.89
Dehiscence (of)
amputation stump T87.81
cesarean wound O90.0
closure of
cornea T81.31
craniotomy T81.32
fascia (muscular) (superficial) T81.32
internal organ or tissue T81.32
laceration (external) (internal) T81.33
ligament T81.32
mucosa T81.31
muscle or muscle flap T81.32
ribs or rib cage T81.32
skin and subcutaneous tissue (full-thickness) (superficial) T81.31

Dehiscence (of) - *continued*
closure of - *continued*
skull T81.32
sternum (sternotomy) T81.32
tendon T81.32
traumatic laceration (external) (internal) T81.33
episiotomy O90.1
operation wound NEC T81.31
external operation wound (superficial) T81.31
internal operation wound (deep) T81.32
perineal wound (postpartum) O90.1
traumatic injury wound repair T81.33
wound T81.30
traumatic repair T81.33
Dehydration E86.0
newborn P74.1
Déjérine-Roussy syndrome G89.0
Déjérine-Sottas disease or neuropathy (hypertrophic) G60.0
Déjérine-Thomas atrophy G23.8
Delay, delayed
any plane in pelvis
complicating delivery O66.9
birth or delivery NOS O63.9
closure, ductus arteriosus (Botalli) P29.38
coagulation — *see* Defect, coagulation
conduction (cardiac) (ventricular) I45.9
delivery, second twin, triplet, etc O63.2
development R62.50
global F88
intellectual (specific) F81.9
language F80.9
due to hearing loss F80.4
learning F81.9
pervasive F84.9
physiological R62.50
specified stage NEC R62.0
reading F81.0
sexual E30.0
speech F80.9
due to hearing loss F80.4
spelling F81.81
ejaculation F52.32
gastric emptying K30
menarche E30.0
menstruation (cause unknown) N91.0
milestone R62.0
passage of meconium (newborn) P76.0
primary respiration P28.9
puberty (constitutional) E30.0
separation of umbilical cord P96.82
sexual maturation, female E30.0
sleep phase syndrome G47.21
union, fracture — *see* Fracture, by site
vaccination Z28.9
Deletion (s)
autosome Q93.9
identified by fluorescence in situ hybridization (FISH) Q93.89
identified by in situ hybridization (ISH) Q93.89
chromosome
with complex rearrangements NEC Q93.7
part of NEC Q93.59
seen only at prometaphase Q93.89
short arm
4 Q93.3
5p Q93.4
22q11.2 Q93.81
specified NEC Q93.89
long arm chromosome 18 or 21 Q93.89
with complex rearrangements NEC Q93.7
microdeletions NEC Q93.88
Delhi boil or button B55.1
Delinquency (juvenile) (neurotic) F91.8
group Z72.810
Delinquent immunization status Z28.3
Delirium, delirious (acute or subacute) (not alcohol- or drug-induced) (with dementia) R41.0
alcoholic (acute) (tremens) (withdrawal) F10.921
with intoxication F10.921

- **Delirium, delirious (acute or subacute) (not alcohol- or drug-induced) (with dementia)** - *continued*
  - alcoholic (acute) (tremens) (withdrawal) - *continued*
    - with intoxication - *continued*
      - in
        - abuse F10.121
        - dependence F10.221
  - due to (secondary to)
    - alcohol
      - intoxication F10.921
        - in
          - abuse F10.121
          - dependence F10.221
      - withdrawal F10.231
    - amphetamine intoxication F15.921
      - in
        - abuse F15.121
        - dependence F15.221
    - anxiolytic
      - intoxication F13.921
        - in
          - abuse F13.121
          - dependence F13.221
      - withdrawal F13.231
    - cannabis intoxication (acute) F12.921
      - in
        - abuse F12.121
        - dependence F12.221
    - cocaine intoxication (acute) F14.921
      - in
        - abuse F14.121
        - dependence F14.221
    - general medical condition F05
    - hallucinogen intoxication F16.921
      - in
        - abuse F16.121
        - dependence F16.221
    - hypnotic
      - intoxication F13.921
        - in
          - abuse F13.121
          - dependence F13.221
      - withdrawal F13.231
    - inhalant intoxication (acute) F18.921
      - in
        - abuse F18.121
        - dependence F18.221
    - multiple etiologies F05
    - opioid intoxication (acute) F11.921
      - in
        - abuse F11.121
        - dependence F11.221
    - other (or unknown) substance F19.921
    - phencyclidine intoxication (acute) F16.921
      - in
        - abuse F16.121
        - dependence F16.221
    - psychoactive substance NEC intoxication (acute) F19.921
      - in
        - abuse F19.121
        - dependence F19.221
    - sedative
      - intoxication F13.921
        - in
          - abuse F13.121
          - dependence F13.221
      - withdrawal F13.231
    - unknown etiology R41.0
  - exhaustion F43.0
  - hysterical F44.89
  - postprocedural (postoperative) F05
  - puerperal F05
  - thyroid — *see* Thyrotoxicosis with thyroid storm
  - traumatic — *see* Injury, intracranial
  - tremens (alcohol-induced) F10.231
    - sedative-induced F13.231
- **Delivery (childbirth) (labor)**
  - arrested active phase O62.1
  - cesarean (for)
    - abnormal

- **Delivery (childbirth) (labor)** - *continued*
  - cesarean (for) - *continued*
    - abnormal - *continued*
      - pelvis (bony) (deformity) (major) NEC with disproportion (fetopelvic) O33.0
        - with obstructed labor O65.0
      - presentation or position O32.9
    - abruptio placentae — *see also* Abruptio placentae O45.9-
    - acromion presentation O32.2
    - atony, uterus O62.2
    - breech presentation O32.1
      - incomplete O32.8
    - brow presentation O32.3
    - cephalopelvic disproportion O33.9
    - cerclage O34.3-
    - chin presentation O32.3
    - cicatrix of cervix O34.4-
    - contracted pelvis (general)
      - inlet O33.2
      - outlet O33.3
    - cord presentation or prolapse O69.0
    - cystocele O34.8-
    - deformity (acquired) (congenital)
      - pelvic organs or tissues NEC O34.8-
      - pelvis (bony) NEC O33.0
    - disproportion NOS O33.9
    - eclampsia — *see* Eclampsia
    - face presentation O32.3
    - failed
      - forceps O66.5
      - induction of labor O61.9
        - instrumental O61.1
        - mechanical O61.1
        - medical O61.0
        - specified NEC O61.8
        - surgical O61.1
      - trial of labor NOS O66.40
        - following previous cesarean delivery O66.41
      - vacuum extraction O66.5
      - ventouse O66.5
    - fetal-maternal hemorrhage O43.01-
    - hemorrhage (intrapartum) O67.9
      - with coagulation defect O67.0
      - specified cause NEC O67.8
    - high head at term O32.4
    - hydrocephalic fetus O33.6
    - incarceration of uterus O34.51-
    - incoordinate uterine action O62.4
    - increased size, fetus O33.5
    - inertia, uterus O62.2
      - primary O62.0
      - secondary O62.1
    - isthmocele O34.22
    - lateroversion, uterus O34.59-
    - mal lie O32.9
    - malposition
      - fetus O32.9
      - pelvic organs or tissues NEC O34.8-
      - uterus NEC O34.59-
    - malpresentation NOS O32.9
    - oblique presentation O32.2
    - occurring after 37 completed weeks of gestation but before 39 completed weeks gestation due to (spontaneous) onset of labor O75.82
    - oversize fetus O33.5
    - pelvic tumor NEC O34.8-
    - placenta previa O44.0-
      - complete O44.0-
        - with hemorrhage O44.1-
    - placental insufficiency O36.51-
    - planned, occurring after 37 completed weeks of gestation but before 39 completed weeks gestation due to (spontaneous) onset of labor O75.82
    - polyp, cervix O34.4-
      - causing obstructed labor O65.5
    - poor dilatation, cervix O62.0
    - pre-eclampsia O14.94
      - mild O14.04
      - moderate O14.04
      - severe O14.14

- **Delivery (childbirth) (labor)** - *continued*
  - cesarean (for) - *continued*
    - pre-eclampsia - *continued*
      - severe - *continued*
        - with hemolysis, elevated liver enzymes and low platelet count (HELLP) O14.24
    - previous
      - cesarean delivery O34.219
        - classical (vertical) scar O34.212
        - isthmocele O34.22
        - low transverse scar O34.211
        - mid-transverse T incision O34.218
        - scar
          - defect (isthmocele) O34.22
          - specified type NEC O34.218
      - surgery (to)
        - cervix O34.4-
        - gynecological NEC O34.8-
        - rectum O34.7-
        - uterus O34.29
        - vagina O34.6-
    - prolapse
      - arm or hand O32.2
      - uterus O34.52-
    - prolonged labor NOS O63.9
    - rectocele O34.8-
    - retroversion
      - uterus O34.53-
    - rigid
      - cervix O34.4-
      - pelvic floor O34.8-
      - perineum O34.7-
      - vagina O34.6-
      - vulva O34.7-
    - sacculation, pregnant uterus O34.59-
    - scar (s)
      - cervix O34.4-
      - cesarean delivery O34.219
        - classical (vertical) O34.212
        - isthmocele O34.22
        - low transverse O34.211
        - mid-transverse T incision O34.218
        - scar
          - defect (isthmocele) O34.22
          - specified type NEC O34.218
      - defect (isthmocele) O34.22
      - transmural uterine O34.29
      - uterus O34.29
    - Shirodkar suture in situ O34.3-
    - shoulder presentation O32.2
    - stenosis or stricture, cervix O34.4-
    - streptococcus group B (GBS) carrier state O99.824
    - transmural uterine scar O34.29
    - transverse presentation or lie O32.2
    - tumor, pelvic organs or tissues NEC O34.8-
      - cervix O34.4-
    - umbilical cord presentation or prolapse O69.0
    - without indication O82
  - completely normal case O80
  - complicated O75.9
    - by
      - abnormal, abnormality (of)
        - forces of labor O62.9
          - specified type NEC O62.8
        - glucose O99.814
        - uterine contractions NOS O62.9
      - abruptio placentae — *see also* Abruptio placentae O45.9-
      - abuse
        - physical O9A.32
        - psychological O9A.52
        - sexual O9A.42
      - adherent placenta O72.0
        - without hemorrhage O73.0
      - alcohol use O99.314
      - anemia (pre-existing) O99.02
      - anesthetic death O74.8
      - annular detachment of cervix O71.3
      - atony, uterus O62.2
      - attempted vacuum extraction and forceps O66.5

DELIVERY - DELIVERY

- **Delivery (childbirth) (labor)** - *continued*
  - complicated - *continued*
    - by - *continued*
      - malposition, malpresentation - *continued*
        - without obstruction - *continued*
          - specified NEC O32.8
          - transverse O32.2
          - unstable lie O32.0
      - meconium in amniotic fluid O77.0
      - mental disorder NEC O99.344
      - metrorrhexis — *see* Delivery, complicated by, rupture, uterus
      - nervous system disorder O99.354
      - obesity (pre-existing) O99.214
      - obesity surgery status O99.844
      - obstetric trauma O71.9
        - specified NEC O71.89
      - obstructed labor
        - due to
          - breech (complete) (frank) presentation O64.1
            - incomplete O64.8
          - brow presentation O64.3
          - buttock presentation O64.1
          - chin presentation O64.2
          - compound presentation O64.5
          - contracted pelvis O65.1
          - deep transverse arrest O64.0
          - deformed pelvis O65.0
          - dystocia (fetal) O66.9
            - due to
              - conjoined twins O66.3
              - fetal
                - abnormality NEC O66.3
                - ascites O66.3
                - hydrops O66.3
                - meningomyelocele O66.3
                - sacral teratoma O66.3
                - tumor O66.3
              - hydrocephalic fetus O66.3
            - shoulder O66.0
          - face presentation O64.2
          - fetopelvic disproportion O65.4
          - footling presentation O64.8
          - impacted shoulders O66.0
          - incomplete rotation of fetal head O64.0
          - large fetus O66.2
          - locked twins O66.1
          - malposition O64.9
            - specified NEC O64.8
          - malpresentation O64.9
            - specified NEC O64.8
          - multiple fetuses NEC O66.6
          - pelvic
            - abnormality (maternal) O65.9
              - organ O65.5
                - specified NEC O65.8
            - contraction
              - inlet O65.2
              - mid-cavity O65.3
              - outlet O65.3
          - persistent (position)
            - occipitoiliac O64.0
            - occipitoposterior O64.0
            - occipitosacral O64.0
            - occipitotransverse O64.0
          - prolapsed arm O64.4
          - shoulder presentation O64.4
        - specified NEC O66.8
      - pathological retraction ring, uterus O62.4
      - penetration, pregnant uterus by instrument O71.1
      - perforation — *see* Delivery, complicated by, laceration
      - placenta, placental
        - ablatio — *see also* Abruptio placentae O45.9-
        - abnormality O43.9-
          - specified NEC O43.89-
        - abruptio — *see also* Abruptio placentae O45.9-
        - accreta O43.21-
        - adherent (with hemorrhage) O72.0

- **Delivery (childbirth) (labor)** - *continued*
  - complicated - *continued*
    - by - *continued*
      - placenta, placental - *continued*
        - adherent (with hemorrhage) - *continued*
          - without hemorrhage O73.0
        - detachment (premature) — *see also* Abruptio placentae O45.9-
        - disorder O43.9-
          - specified NEC O43.89-
        - hemorrhage NEC O67.8
        - increta O43.22-
        - low (implantation) (lying) O44.4-
          - with hemorrhage O44.5-
        - malformation O43.10-
        - malposition O44.0-
          - without hemorrhage O44.1-
        - percreta O43.23-
        - previa (central) (complete) (lateral) (total) O44.0-
          - with hemorrhage O44.1-
          - marginal O44.2-
            - with hemorrhage O44.3-
          - partial O44.2-
            - with hemorrhage O44.3-
        - retained (with hemorrhage) O72.0
          - without hemorrhage O73.0
        - separation (premature) O45.9-
          - specified NEC O45.8X-
        - vicious insertion O44.1-
      - precipitate labor O62.3
      - premature rupture, membranes — *see also* Pregnancy, complicated by, premature rupture of membranes O42.90
      - prolapse
        - arm or hand O32.2
        - cord (umbilical) O69.0
        - foot or leg O32.8
        - uterus O34.52-
      - prolonged labor O63.9
        - first stage O63.0
        - second stage O63.1
      - protozoal disease (maternal) O98.62
      - respiratory disease NEC O99.52
      - retained membranes or portions of placenta O72.2
        - without hemorrhage O73.1
      - retarded birth O63.9
      - retention of secundines (with hemorrhage) O72.0
        - without hemorrhage O73.0
        - partial O72.2
          - without hemorrhage O73.1
      - rupture
        - bladder (urinary) O71.5
        - cervix O71.3
        - pelvic organ NEC O71.5
        - urethra O71.5
        - uterus (during or after labor) O71.1
          - before labor O71.0-
      - separation, pubic bone (symphysis pubis) O71.6
      - shock O75.1
      - shoulder presentation O64.4
      - skin disorder NEC O99.72
      - spasm, cervix O62.4
      - stenosis or stricture, cervix O65.5
      - streptococcus group B (GBS) carrier state O99.824
      - subluxation of symphysis (pubis) O26.72
      - syphilis (maternal) O98.12
      - tear — *see* Delivery, complicated by, laceration
      - tetanic uterus O62.4
      - trauma (obstetrical) — *see also* Delivery, complicated, by, damage to O71.9
        - non-obstetric O9A.22
        - periurethral O71.82
        - specified NEC O71.89
      - tuberculosis (maternal) O98.02
      - tumor, pelvic organs or tissues NEC O65.5

- **Delivery (childbirth) (labor)** - *continued*
  - complicated - *continued*
    - by - *continued*
      - umbilical cord around neck
        - with compression O69.1
        - without compression O69.81
      - uterine inertia O62.2
        - during latent phase of labor O62.0
        - primary O62.0
        - secondary O62.1
      - vasa previa O69.4
      - velamentous insertion of cord O43.12-
    - specified complication NEC O75.89
  - delayed NOS O63.9
    - following rupture of membranes
      - artificial O75.5
    - second twin, triplet, etc. O63.2
  - forceps, low following failed vacuum extraction O66.5
  - missed (at or near term) O36.4
  - normal O80
  - obstructed — *see* Delivery, complicated by, obstructed labor
  - precipitate O62.3
  - preterm — *see also* Pregnancy, complicated by, preterm labor O60.10
  - spontaneous O80
  - term pregnancy NOS O80
  - uncomplicated O80
  - vaginal, following previous cesarean delivery O34.219
    - classical (vertical) scar O34.212
    - low transverse scar O34.211
    - mid-transverse T incision O34.218
    - scar
      - defect (isthmocele) O34.22
      - specified type NEC O34.218
- **Delusions (paranoid)** — *see* Disorder, delusional
- **Dementia (degenerative (primary)) (old age) (persisting)** F03.90
  - with
    - aggressive behavior F03.91
    - behavioral disturbance F03.91
    - combative behavior F03.91
    - Lewy bodies G31.83 *[F02.80]*
      - with behavioral disturbance G31.83 *[F02.81]*
    - Parkinsonism G31.83 *[F02.80]*
      - with behavioral disturbance G31.83 *[F02.81]*
    - Parkinson's disease G20 *[F02.80]*
      - with behavioral disturbance G20 *[F02.81]*
    - violent behavior F03.91
  - alcoholic F10.97
    - with dependence F10.27
  - Alzheimer's type — *see* Disease, Alzheimer's
  - arteriosclerotic — *see* Dementia, vascular
  - atypical, Alzheimer's type — *see* Disease, Alzheimer's, specified NEC
  - congenital — *see* Disability, intellectual
  - frontal (lobe) G31.09 *[F02.80]*
    - with behavioral disturbance G31.09 *[F02.81]*
  - frontotemporal G31.09 *[F02.80]*
    - with behavioral disturbance G31.09 *[F02.81]*
    - specified NEC G31.09 *[F02.80]*
      - with behavioral disturbance G31.09 *[F02.81]*
  - in (due to)
    - alcohol F10.97
      - with dependence F10.27
    - Alzheimer's disease — *see* Disease, Alzheimer's
    - arteriosclerotic brain disease — *see* Dementia, vascular
    - cerebral lipidoses E75.- *[F02.80]*
      - with behavioral disturbance E75.- *[F02.81]*
    - Creutzfeldt-Jakob disease — *see also* Creutzfeldt-Jakob disease or syndrome (with dementia) A81.00
    - epilepsy G40.- *[F02.80]*

Dementia (degenerative (primary)) (old age) (persisting) - *continued*
- in (due to) - *continued*
  - epilepsy - *continued*
    - with behavioral disturbance G40.- *[F02.81]*
  - hepatolenticular degeneration E83.01 *[F02.80]*
    - with behavioral disturbance E83.01 *[F02.81]*
  - human immunodeficiency virus (HIV) disease B20 *[F02.80]*
    - with behavioral disturbance B20 *[F02.81]*
  - Huntington's disease or chorea G10 *[F02.80]*
    - with behavioral disturbance G10 *[F02.81]*
  - hypercalcemia E83.52 *[F02.80]*
    - with behavioral disturbance E83.52 *[F02.81]*
  - hypothyroidism, acquired E03.9 *[F02.80]*
    - with behavioral disturbance E03.9 *[F02.81]*
    - due to iodine deficiency E01.8 *[F02.80]*
      - with behavioral disturbance E01.8 *[F02.81]*
  - inhalants F18.97
    - with dependence F18.27
  - multiple
    - etiologies F03
    - sclerosis G35 *[F02.80]*
      - with behavioral disturbance G35 *[F02.81]*
  - neurosyphilis A52.17 *[F02.80]*
    - with behavioral disturbance A52.17 *[F02.81]*
    - juvenile A50.49 *[F02.80]*
      - with behavioral disturbance A50.49 *[F02.81]*
  - niacin deficiency E52 *[F02.80]*
    - with behavioral disturbance E52 *[F02.81]*
  - paralysis agitans G20 *[F02.80]*
    - with behavioral disturbance G20 *[F02.81]*
  - Parkinson's disease G20 *[F02.80]*
  - pellagra E52 *[F02.80]*
    - with behavioral disturbance E52 *[F02.81]*
  - Pick's G31.01 *[F02.80]*
    - with behavioral disturbance G31.01 *[F02.81]*
  - polyarteritis nodosa M30.0 *[F02.80]*
    - with behavioral disturbance M30.0 *[F02.81]*
  - psychoactive drug F19.97
    - with dependence F19.27
    - inhalants F18.97
      - with dependence F18.27
    - sedatives, hypnotics or anxiolytics F13.97
      - with dependence F13.27
  - sedatives, hypnotics or anxiolytics F13.97
    - with dependence F13.27
  - systemic lupus erythematosus M32.- *[F02.80]*
    - with behavioral disturbance M32.- *[F02.81]*
  - trypanosomiasis
    - African B56.9 *[F02.80]*
      - with behavioral disturbance B56.9 *[F02.81]*
  - unknown etiology F03
  - vitamin B12 deficiency E53.8 *[F02.80]*
    - with behavioral disturbance E53.8 *[F02.81]*
  - volatile solvents F18.97
    - with dependence F18.27
  - with behavioral disturbance G31.83 *[F02.81]*
- infantile, infantilis F84.3
- Lewy body G31.83 *[F02.80]*
  - with behavioral disturbance G31.83 *[F02.81]*

Dementia (degenerative (primary)) (old age) (persisting) - *continued*
- multi-infarct — *see* Dementia, vascular
- paralytica, paralytic (syphilitic) A52.17 *[F02.80]*
  - with behavioral disturbance A52.17 *[F02.81]*
  - juvenilis A50.45
- paretic A52.17
- praecox — *see* Schizophrenia
- presenile F03
  - Alzheimer's type — *see* Disease, Alzheimer's, early onset
- primary degenerative F03
- progressive, syphilitic A52.17
- senile F03
  - with acute confusional state F05
  - Alzheimer's type — *see* Disease, Alzheimer's, late onset
  - depressed or paranoid type F03
- vascular (acute onset) (mixed) (multi-infarct) (subcortical) F01.50
  - with behavioral disturbance F01.51

Demineralization, bone — *see* Osteoporosis

Demodex folliculorum (infestation) B88.0

Demophobia F40.248

Demoralization R45.3

Demyelination, demyelinization
- central nervous system G37.9
  - specified NEC G37.8
- corpus callosum (central) G37.1
- disseminated, acute G36.9
  - specified NEC G36.8
- global G35
- in optic neuritis G36.0

Dengue (classical) (fever) A90
- hemorrhagic A91
- sandfly A93.1

Dennie-Marfan syphilitic syndrome A50.45

Dens evaginatus, in dente or invaginatus K00.2

Dense breasts R92.2

Density
- increased, bone (disseminated) (generalized) (spotted) — *see* Disorder, bone, density and structure, specified type NEC
- lung (nodular) J98.4

Dental — *see also* condition
- examination Z01.20
  - with abnormal findings Z01.21
- restoration
  - aesthetically inadequate or displeasing K08.56
  - defective K08.50
    - specified NEC K08.59
  - failure of marginal integrity K08.51
  - failure of periodontal anatomical integrity K08.54

Dentia praecox K00.6

Denticles (pulp) K04.2

Dentigerous cyst K09.0

Dentin
- irregular (in pulp) K04.3
- opalescent K00.5
- secondary (in pulp) K04.3
- sensitive K03.89

Dentinogenesis imperfecta K00.5

Dentinoma — *see* Cyst, calcifying odontogenic

Dentition (syndrome) K00.7
- delayed K00.6
- difficult K00.7
- precocious K00.6
- premature K00.6
- retarded K00.6

Dependence (on) (syndrome) F19.20
- with remission F19.21
- alcohol (ethyl) (methyl) (without remission) F10.20
  - with
    - amnestic disorder, persisting F10.26
    - anxiety disorder F10.280
    - dementia, persisting F10.27
    - intoxication F10.229
      - with delirium F10.221

Dependence (on) (syndrome) - *continued*
- alcohol (ethyl) (methyl) (without remission) - *continued*
  - with - *continued*
    - intoxication - *continued*
      - uncomplicated F10.220
    - mood disorder F10.24
    - psychotic disorder F10.259
      - with
        - delusions F10.250
        - hallucinations F10.251
    - remission F10.21
    - sexual dysfunction F10.281
    - sleep disorder F10.282
    - specified disorder NEC F10.288
    - withdrawal F10.239
      - with
        - delirium F10.231
        - perceptual disturbance F10.232
      - uncomplicated F10.230
  - counseling and surveillance Z71.41
  - in remission F10.21
- amobarbital — *see* Dependence, drug, sedative
- amphetamine (s) (type) — *see* Dependence, drug, stimulant NEC
- amytal (sodium) — *see* Dependence, drug, sedative
- analgesic NEC F55.8
- anesthetic (agent) (gas) (general) (local) NEC — *see* Dependence, drug, psychoactive NEC
- anxiolytic NEC — *see* Dependence, drug, sedative
- barbital (s) — *see* Dependence, drug, sedative
- barbiturate (s) (compounds) (drugs classifiable to T42) — *see* Dependence, drug, sedative
- benzedrine — *see* Dependence, drug, stimulant NEC
- bhang — *see* Dependence, drug, cannabis
- bromide (s) NEC — *see* Dependence, drug, sedative
- caffeine — *see* Dependence, drug, stimulant NEC
- cannabis (sativa) (indica) (resin) (derivatives) (type) — *see* Dependence, drug, cannabis
- chloral (betaine) (hydrate) — *see* Dependence, drug, sedative
- chlordiazepoxide — *see* Dependence, drug, sedative
- coca (leaf) (derivatives) — *see* Dependence, drug, cocaine
- cocaine — *see* Dependence, drug, cocaine
- codeine — *see* Dependence, drug, opioid
- combinations of drugs F19.20
- dagga — *see* Dependence, drug, cannabis
- demerol — *see* Dependence, drug, opioid
- dexamphetamine — *see* Dependence, drug, stimulant NEC
- dexedrine — *see* Dependence, drug, stimulant NEC
- dextromethorphan — *see* Dependence, drug, opioid
- dextromoramide — *see* Dependence, drug, opioid
- dextro-nor-pseudo-ephedrine — *see* Dependence, drug, stimulant NEC
- dextrorphan — *see* Dependence, drug, opioid
- diazepam — *see* Dependence, drug, sedative
- dilaudid — *see* Dependence, drug, opioid
- D-lysergic acid diethylamide — *see* Dependence, drug, hallucinogen
- drug NEC F19.20
  - with sleep disorder F19.282
  - cannabis F12.20
    - with
      - anxiety disorder F12.280
      - intoxication F12.229
        - with
          - delirium F12.221
          - perceptual disturbance F12.222
        - uncomplicated F12.220

DEMENTIA - DEPENDENCE

- **Dependence (on) (syndrome)** - *continued*
  - drug NEC - *continued*
    - cannabis - *continued*
      - with - *continued*
        - other specified disorder F12.288
        - psychosis F12.259
          - delusions F12.250
          - hallucinations F12.251
        - unspecified disorder F12.29
        - withdrawal F12.23
      - in remission F12.21
    - cocaine F14.20
      - with
        - anxiety disorder F14.280
        - intoxication F14.229
          - with
            - delirium F14.221
            - perceptual disturbance F14.222
          - uncomplicated F14.220
        - mood disorder F14.24
        - other specified disorder F14.288
        - psychosis F14.259
          - delusions F14.250
          - hallucinations F14.251
        - sexual dysfunction F14.281
        - sleep disorder F14.282
        - unspecified disorder F14.29
        - withdrawal F14.23
      - in remission F14.21
      - withdrawal symptoms in newborn P96.1
    - counseling and surveillance Z71.51
    - hallucinogen F16.20
      - with
        - anxiety disorder F16.280
        - flashbacks F16.283
        - intoxication F16.229
          - with delirium F16.221
          - uncomplicated F16.220
        - mood disorder F16.24
        - other specified disorder F16.288
        - perception disorder, persisting F16.283
        - psychosis F16.259
          - delusions F16.250
          - hallucinations F16.251
        - unspecified disorder F16.29
      - in remission F16.21
    - in remission F19.21
    - inhalant F18.20
      - with
        - anxiety disorder F18.280
        - dementia, persisting F18.27
        - intoxication F18.229
          - with delirium F18.221
          - uncomplicated F18.220
        - mood disorder F18.24
        - other specified disorder F18.288
        - psychosis F18.259
          - delusions F18.250
          - hallucinations F18.251
        - unspecified disorder F18.29
      - in remission F18.21
    - nicotine F17.200
      - with disorder F17.209
        - in remission F17.201
        - specified disorder NEC F17.208
        - withdrawal F17.203
      - chewing tobacco F17.220
        - with disorder F17.229
          - in remission F17.221
          - specified disorder NEC F17.228
          - withdrawal F17.223
      - cigarettes F17.210
        - with disorder F17.219
          - in remission F17.211
          - specified disorder NEC F17.218
          - withdrawal F17.213
      - specified product NEC F17.290
        - with disorder F17.299
          - remission F17.291
          - specified disorder NEC F17.298
          - withdrawal F17.293
    - opioid F11.20
      - with
        - intoxication F11.229

- **Dependence (on) (syndrome)** - *continued*
  - drug NEC - *continued*
    - opioid - *continued*
      - with - *continued*
        - intoxication - *continued*
          - with
            - delirium F11.221
            - perceptual disturbance F11.222
          - uncomplicated F11.220
        - mood disorder F11.24
        - other specified disorder F11.288
        - psychosis F11.259
          - delusions F11.250
          - hallucinations F11.251
        - sexual dysfunction F11.281
        - sleep disorder F11.282
        - unspecified disorder F11.29
        - withdrawal F11.23
      - in remission F11.21
    - psychoactive NEC F19.20
      - with
        - amnestic disorder F19.26
        - anxiety disorder F19.280
        - dementia F19.27
        - intoxication F19.229
          - with
            - delirium F19.221
            - perceptual disturbance F19.222
          - uncomplicated F19.220
        - mood disorder F19.24
        - other specified disorder F19.288
        - psychosis F19.259
          - delusions F19.250
          - hallucinations F19.251
        - sexual dysfunction F19.281
        - sleep disorder F19.282
        - unspecified disorder F19.29
        - withdrawal F19.239
          - with
            - delirium F19.231
            - perceptual disturbance F19.232
          - uncomplicated F19.230
    - sedative, hypnotic or anxiolytic F13.20
      - with
        - amnestic disorder F13.26
        - anxiety disorder F13.280
        - dementia, persisting F13.27
        - intoxication F13.229
          - with delirium F13.221
          - uncomplicated F13.220
        - mood disorder F13.24
        - other specified disorder F13.288
        - psychosis F13.259
          - delusions F13.250
          - hallucinations F13.251
        - sexual dysfunction F13.281
        - sleep disorder F13.282
        - unspecified disorder F13.29
        - withdrawal F13.239
          - with
            - delirium F13.231
            - perceptual disturbance F13.232
          - uncomplicated F13.230
      - in remission F13.21
    - stimulant NEC F15.20
      - with
        - anxiety disorder F15.280
        - intoxication F15.229
          - with
            - delirium F15.221
            - perceptual disturbance F15.222
          - uncomplicated F15.220
        - mood disorder F15.24
        - other specified disorder F15.288
        - psychosis F15.259
          - delusions F15.250
          - hallucinations F15.251
        - sexual dysfunction F15.281
        - sleep disorder F15.282
        - unspecified disorder F15.29
        - withdrawal F15.23
      - in remission F15.21
  - ethyl
    - alcohol (without remission) F10.20
      - with remission F10.21

- **Dependence (on) (syndrome)** - *continued*
  - ethyl - *continued*
    - bromide — *see* Dependence, drug, sedative
    - carbamate F19.20
    - chloride F19.20
    - morphine — *see* Dependence, drug, opioid
  - ganja — *see* Dependence, drug, cannabis
  - glue (airplane) (sniffing) — *see* Dependence, drug, inhalant
  - glutethimide — *see* Dependence, drug, sedative
  - hallucinogenics — *see* Dependence, drug, hallucinogen
  - hashish — *see* Dependence, drug, cannabis
  - hemp — *see* Dependence, drug, cannabis
  - heroin (salt) (any) — *see* Dependence, drug, opioid
  - hypnotic NEC — *see* Dependence, drug, sedative
  - Indian hemp — *see* Dependence, drug, cannabis
  - inhalants — *see* Dependence, drug, inhalant
  - khat — *see* Dependence, drug, stimulant NEC
  - laudanum — *see* Dependence, drug, opioid
  - LSD (-25) (derivatives) — *see* Dependence, drug, hallucinogen
  - luminal — *see* Dependence, drug, sedative
  - lysergic acid — *see* Dependence, drug, hallucinogen
  - maconha — *see* Dependence, drug, cannabis
  - marihuana — *see* Dependence, drug, cannabis
  - meprobamate — *see* Dependence, drug, sedative
  - mescaline — *see* Dependence, drug, hallucinogen
  - methadone — *see* Dependence, drug, opioid
  - methamphetamine (s) — *see* Dependence, drug, stimulant NEC
  - methaqualone — *see* Dependence, drug, sedative
  - methyl
    - alcohol (without remission) F10.20
      - with remission F10.21
    - bromide — *see* Dependence, drug, sedative
    - morphine — *see* Dependence, drug, opioid
    - phenidate — *see* Dependence, drug, stimulant NEC
    - sulfonal — *see* Dependence, drug, sedative
  - morphine (sulfate) (sulfite) (type) — *see* Dependence, drug, opioid
  - narcotic (drug) NEC — *see* Dependence, drug, opioid
  - nembutal — *see* Dependence, drug, sedative
  - neraval — *see* Dependence, drug, sedative
  - neravan — *see* Dependence, drug, sedative
  - neurobarb — *see* Dependence, drug, sedative
  - nicotine — *see* Dependence, drug, nicotine
  - nitrous oxide F19.20
  - nonbarbiturate sedatives and tranquilizers with similar effect — *see* Dependence, drug, sedative
  - on
    - artificial heart (fully implantable) (mechanical) Z95.812
    - aspirator Z99.0
    - care provider (because of) Z74.9
      - impaired mobility Z74.09
      - need for
        - assistance with personal care Z74.1
        - continuous supervision Z74.3
      - no other household member able to render care Z74.2
      - specified reason NEC Z74.8
    - machine Z99.89
      - enabling NEC Z99.89
      - specified type NEC Z99.89
    - renal dialysis (hemodialysis) (peritoneal) Z99.2
    - respirator Z99.11
    - ventilator Z99.11
    - wheelchair Z99.3

Derangement - *continued*
knee (recurrent) - *continued*
meniscus - *continued*
cystic - *continued*
medial - *continued*
anterior horn M23.01-
posterior horn M23.02-
specified NEC M23.03-
degenerate — *see* Derangement, knee, meniscus, specified NEC
detached — *see* Derangement, knee, meniscus, specified NEC
due to old tear or injury M23.20-
lateral M23.20-
anterior horn M23.24-
posterior horn M23.25-
specified NEC M23.26-
medial M23.20-
anterior horn M23.21-
posterior horn M23.22-
specified NEC M23.23-
retained — *see* Derangement, knee, meniscus, specified NEC
specified NEC M23.30-
lateral M23.30-
anterior horn M23.34-
posterior horn M23.35-
specified NEC M23.36-
medial M23.30-
anterior horn M23.31-
posterior horn M23.32-
specified NEC M23.33-
old M23.8X-
specified NEC — *see* subcategory M23.8
low back NEC — *see* Dorsopathy, specified NEC
meniscus — *see* Derangement, knee, meniscus
mental — *see* Psychosis
patella, specified NEC — *see* Disorder, patella, derangement NEC
semilunar cartilage (knee) — *see* Derangement, knee, meniscus, specified NEC
shoulder (internal) — *see* Derangement, joint, shoulder
Dercum's disease E88.2
Derealization (neurotic) F48.1
Dermal — *see* condition
Dermaphytid — *see* Dermatophytosis
Dermatitis (eczematous) L30.9
ab igne L59.0
acarine B88.0
actinic (due to sun) L57.8
other than from sun L59.8
allergic — *see* Dermatitis, contact, allergic
ambustionis, due to burn or scald — *see* Burn
amebic A06.7
ammonia L22
arsenical (ingested) L27.8
artefacta L98.1
psychogenic F54
atopic L20.9
psychogenic F54
specified NEC L20.89
autoimmune progesterone L30.8
berlock, berloque L56.2
blastomycotic B40.3
blister beetle L24.89
bullous, bullosa L13.9
mucosynechial, atrophic L12.1
seasonal L30.8
specified NEC L13.8
calorica L59.0
due to burn or scald — *see* Burn
caterpillar L24.89
cercarial B65.3
combustionis L59.0
due to burn or scald — *see* Burn
congelationis T69.1
contact (occupational) L25.9
allergic L23.9
due to
adhesives L23.1

Dermatitis (eczematous) - *continued*
contact (occupational) - *continued*
allergic - *continued*
due to - *continued*
cement L23.5
chemical products NEC L23.5
chromium L23.0
cosmetics L23.2
dander (cat) (dog) L23.81
drugs in contact with skin L23.3
dyes L23.4
food in contact with skin L23.6
hair (cat) (dog) L23.81
insecticide L23.5
metals L23.0
nickel L23.0
plants, non-food L23.7
plastic L23.5
rubber L23.5
specified agent NEC L23.89
due to
cement L25.3
chemical products NEC L25.3
cosmetics L25.0
dander (cat) (dog) L23.81
drugs in contact with skin L25.1
dyes L25.2
food in contact with skin L25.4
hair (cat) (dog) L23.81
plants, non-food L25.5
specified agent NEC L25.8
irritant L24.9
due to
body fluids L24.A0
incontinence (dual) (fecal) (urinary) L24.A2
saliva L24.A1
specified NEC L24.A9
cement L24.5
chemical products NEC L24.5
cosmetics L24.3
detergents L24.0
drugs in contact with skin L24.4
food in contact with skin L24.6
oils and greases L24.1
plants, non-food L24.7
solvents L24.2
specified agent NEC L24.89
related to
colostomy L24.B3
endotracheal tube L24.A9
enterocutaneous fistula L24.B3
gastrostomy L24.B1
ileostomy L24.B3
jejunostomy L24.B1
saliva or spit fistula L24.B1
stoma or fistula L24.B0
digestive L24.B1
fecal or urinary L24.B3
respiratory L24.B2
tracheostomy L24.B2
contusiformis L52
desquamative L30.8
diabetic — *see* E08-E13 with .620
diaper L22
diphtheritica A36.3
dry skin L85.3
due to
acetone (contact) (irritant) L24.2
acids (contact) (irritant) L24.5
adhesive (s) (allergic) (contact) (plaster) L23.1
irritant L24.5
alcohol (irritant) (skin contact) (substances in category T51) L24.2
taken internally L27.8
alkalis (contact) (irritant) L24.5
arsenic (ingested) L27.8
carbon disulfide (contact) (irritant) L24.2
caustics (contact) (irritant) L24.5
cement (contact) L25.3
cereal (ingested) L27.2
chemical (s) NEC L25.3
taken internally L27.8
chlorocompounds L24.2

Dermatitis (eczematous) - *continued*
due to - *continued*
chromium (contact) (irritant) L24.81
coffee (ingested) L27.2
cold weather L30.8
cosmetics (contact) L25.0
allergic L23.2
irritant L24.3
cyclohexanes L24.2
dander (cat) (dog) L23.81
Demodex species B88.0
Dermanyssus gallinae B88.0
detergents (contact) (irritant) L24.0
dichromate L24.81
drugs and medicaments (generalized) (internal use) L27.0
external — *see* Dermatitis, due to, drugs, in contact with skin
in contact with skin L25.1
allergic L23.3
irritant L24.4
localized skin eruption L27.1
specified substance — *see* Table of Drugs and Chemicals
dyes (contact) L25.2
allergic L23.4
irritant L24.89
epidermophytosis — *see* Dermatophytosis
esters L24.2
external irritant NEC L24.9
fish (ingested) L27.2
flour (ingested) L27.2
food (ingested) L27.2
in contact with skin L25.4
fruit (ingested) L27.2
furs (allergic) (contact) L23.81
glues — *see* Dermatitis, due to, adhesives
glycols L24.2
greases NEC (contact) (irritant) L24.1
hair (cat) (dog) L23.81
hot
objects and materials — *see* Burn
weather or places L59.0
hydrocarbons L24.2
infrared rays L59.8
ingestion, ingested substance L27.9
chemical NEC L27.8
drugs and medicaments — *see* Dermatitis, due to, drugs
food L27.2
specified NEC L27.8
insecticide in contact with skin L24.5
internal agent L27.9
drugs and medicaments (generalized) — *see* Dermatitis, due to, drugs
food L27.2
irradiation — *see* Dermatitis, due to, radioactive substance
ketones L24.2
lacquer tree (allergic) (contact) L23.7
light (sun) NEC L57.8
acute L56.8
other L59.8
Liponyssoides sanguineus B88.0
low temperature L30.8
meat (ingested) L27.2
metals, metal salts (contact) (irritant) L24.81
milk (ingested) L27.2
nickel (contact) (irritant) L24.81
nylon (contact) (irritant) L24.5
oils NEC (contact) (irritant) L24.1
paint solvent (contact) (irritant) L24.2
petroleum products (contact) (irritant) (substances in T52.0) L24.2
plants NEC (contact) L25.5
allergic L23.7
irritant L24.7
plasters (adhesive) (any) (allergic) (contact) L23.1
irritant L24.5
plastic (contact) L25.3
preservatives (contact) — *see* Dermatitis, due to, chemical, in contact with skin
primrose (allergic) (contact) L23.7

DERMATITIS - DERMATOSIS

Dermatosis - *continued*
herpetiformis L13.0
juvenile L12.2
linear IgA L13.8
menstrual NEC L98.8
neutrophilic, febrile L98.2
occupational — *see* Dermatitis, contact
papulosa nigra L82.1
pigmentary L81.9
progressive L81.7
Schamberg's L81.7
psychogenic F54
purpuric, pigmented L81.7
pustular, subcorneal L13.1
transient acantholytic L11.1
Dermographia, dermographism L50.3
Dermoid (cyst) — *see also* Neoplasm, benign, by site
with malignant transformation C56-
due to radiation (nonionizing) L57.8
Dermopathy
infiltrative with thyrotoxicosis — *see* Thyrotoxicosis
nephrogenic fibrosing L90.8
Dermophytosis — *see* Dermatophytosis
Descemetocele H18.73-
Descemet's membrane — *see* condition
Descending — *see* condition
Descensus uteri — *see* Prolapse, uterus
Desert
rheumatism B38.0
sore — *see* Ulcer, skin
Desertion (newborn) — *see* Maltreatment
Desmoid (extra-abdominal) (tumor) — *see* Neoplasm, connective tissue, uncertain behavior
abdominal D48.1
Despondency F32.A
Desquamation, skin R23.4
Destruction, destructive — *see also* Damage
articular facet — *see also* Derangement, joint, specified type NEC
knee M23.8X-
vertebra — *see* Spondylosis
bone — *see also* Disorder, bone, specified type NEC
syphilitic A52.77
joint — *see also* Derangement, joint, specified type NEC
sacroiliac M53.3
rectal sphincter K62.89
septum (nasal) J34.89
tuberculous NEC — *see* Tuberculosis
tympanum, tympanic membrane (nontraumatic) — *see* Disorder, tympanic membrane, specified NEC
vertebral disc — *see* Degeneration, intervertebral disc
Destructiveness — *see also* Disorder, conduct
adjustment reaction — *see* Disorder, adjustment
Desultory labor O62.2
Detachment
cartilage — *see* Sprain
cervix, annular N88.8
complicating delivery O71.3
choroid (old) (postinfectional) (simple) (spontaneous) H31.40-
hemorrhagic H31.41-
serous H31.42-
ligament — *see* Sprain
meniscus (knee) — *see also* Derangement, knee, meniscus, specified NEC
current injury — *see* Tear, meniscus
due to old tear or injury — *see* Derangement, knee, meniscus, due to old tear
retina (without retinal break) (serous) H33.2-
with retinal:
break H33.00-
giant H33.03-
multiple H33.02-
single H33.01-
dialysis H33.04-

Detachment - *continued*
retina (without retinal break) (serous) - *continued*
pigment epithelium — *see* Degeneration, retina, separation of layers, pigment epithelium detachment
rhegmatogenous — *see* Detachment, retina, with retinal, break
specified NEC H33.8
total H33.05-
traction H33.4-
vitreous (body) H43.81
Detergent asthma J69.8
Deterioration
epileptic F06.8
general physical R53.81
heart, cardiac — *see* Degeneration, myocardial
mental — *see* Psychosis
myocardial, myocardium — *see* Degeneration, myocardial
senile (simple) R54
Deuteranomaly (anomalous trichromat) H53.53
Deuteranopia (complete) (incomplete) H53.53
Development
abnormal, bone Q79.9
arrested R62.50
bone — *see* Arrest, development or growth, bone
child R62.50
due to malnutrition E45
defective, congenital — *see also* Anomaly, by site
cauda equina Q06.3
left ventricle Q24.8
in hypoplastic left heart syndrome Q23.4
valve Q24.8
pulmonary Q22.3
delayed — *see also* Delay, development R62.50
arithmetical skills F81.2
language (skills) (expressive) F80.1
learning skill F81.9
mixed skills F88
motor coordination F82
reading F81.0
specified learning skill NEC F81.89
speech F80.9
spelling F81.81
written expression F81.81
imperfect, congenital — *see also* Anomaly, by site
heart Q24.9
lungs Q33.6
incomplete
bronchial tree Q32.4
organ or site not listed — *see* Hypoplasia, by site
respiratory system Q34.9
sexual, precocious NEC E30.1
tardy, mental — *see also* Disability, intellectual F79
Developmental — *see* condition
testing, infant or child — *see* Examination, child
Devergie's disease (pityriasis rubra pilaris) L44.0
Deviation (in)
conjugate palsy (eye) (spastic) H51.0
esophagus (acquired) K22.89
eye, skew H51.8
midline (jaw) (teeth) (dental arch) M26.29
specified site NEC — *see* Malposition
nasal septum J34.2
congenital Q67.4
opening and closing of the mandible M26.53
organ or site, congenital NEC — *see* Malposition, congenital
septum (nasal) (acquired) J34.2
congenital Q67.4
sexual F65.9
bestiality F65.89
erotomania F52.8

Deviation (in) - *continued*
sexual - *continued*
exhibitionism F65.2
fetishism, fetishistic F65.0
transvestism F65.1
frotteurism F65.81
masochism F65.51
multiple F65.89
necrophilia F65.89
nymphomania F52.8
pederosis F65.4
pedophilia F65.4
sadism, sadomasochism F65.52
satyriasis F52.8
specified type NEC F65.89
transvestism F64.1
voyeurism F65.3
teeth, midline M26.29
trachea J39.8
ureter, congenital Q62.61
Device
cerebral ventricle (communicating) in situ Z98.2
contraceptive — *see* Contraceptive, device
drainage, cerebrospinal fluid, in situ Z98.2
Devic's disease G36.0
Devil's
grip B33.0
pinches (purpura simplex) D69.2
Devitalized tooth K04.99
Devonshire colic — *see* Poisoning, lead
Dextraposition, aorta Q20.3
in tetralogy of Fallot Q21.3
Dextrinosis, limit (debrancher enzyme deficiency) E74.03
Dextrocardia (true) Q24.0
with
complete transposition of viscera Q89.3
situs inversus Q89.3
Dextrotransposition, aorta Q20.3
d-glycericacidemia E72.59
Dhat syndrome F48.8
Dhobi itch B35.6
Di George's syndrome D82.1
Di Guglielmo's disease C94.0-
Diabetes, diabetic (mellitus) (sugar) E11.9
with
amyotrophy E11.44
arthropathy NEC E11.618
autonomic (poly) neuropathy E11.43
cataract E11.36
Charcot's joints E11.610
chronic kidney disease E11.22
circulatory complication NEC E11.59
coma due to
hyperosmolarity E11.01
hypoglycemia E11.641
ketoacidosis E11.11
complication E11.8
specified NEC E11.69
dermatitis E11.620
foot ulcer E11.621
gangrene E11.52
gastroparalysis E11.43
gastroparesis E11.43
glomerulonephrosis, intracapillary E11.21
glomerulosclerosis, intercapillary E11.21
hyperglycemia E11.65
hyperosmolarity E11.00
with coma E11.01
hypoglycemia E11.649
with coma E11.641
ketoacidosis E11.10
with coma E11.11
kidney complications NEC E11.29
Kimmelsteil-Wilson disease E11.21
loss of protective sensation (LOPS) — *see* Diabetes, by type, with neuropathy
mononeuropathy E11.41
myasthenia E11.44
necrobiosis lipoidica E11.620
nephropathy E11.21
neuralgia E11.42
neurologic complication NEC E11.49
neuropathic arthropathy E11.610

Diabetes, diabetic (mellitus) (sugar) - *continued*
- with - *continued*
  - neuropathy E11.40
  - ophthalmic complication NEC E11.39
  - oral complication NEC E11.638
  - osteomyelitis E11.69
  - periodontal disease E11.630
  - peripheral angiopathy E11.51
    - with gangrene E11.52
  - polyneuropathy E11.42
  - renal complication NEC E11.29
  - renal tubular degeneration E11.29
  - retinopathy E11.319
    - with macular edema E11.311
      - resolved following treatment E11.37
    - nonproliferative E11.329
      - with macular edema E11.321
      - mild E11.329
        - with macular edema E11.321
      - moderate E11.339
        - with macular edema E11.331
      - severe E11.349
        - with macular edema E11.341
    - proliferative E11.359
      - with
        - combined traction retinal detachment and rhegmatogenous retinal detachment E11.354
        - macular edema E11.351
        - stable proliferative diabetic retinopathy E11.355
        - traction retinal detachment involving the macula E11.352
        - traction retinal detachment not involving the macula E11.353
  - skin complication NEC E11.628
  - skin ulcer NEC E11.622
- brittle — *see* Diabetes, type 1
- bronzed E83.110
- complicating pregnancy — *see* Pregnancy, complicated by, diabetes
- dietary counseling and surveillance Z71.3
- due to
  - autoimmune process — *see* Diabetes, type 1
  - immune mediated pancreatic islet beta-cell destruction — *see* Diabetes, type 1
- due to drug or chemical E09.9
  - with
    - amyotrophy E09.44
    - arthropathy NEC E09.618
    - autonomic (poly) neuropathy E09.43
    - cataract E09.36
    - Charcot's joints E09.610
    - chronic kidney disease E09.22
    - circulatory complication NEC E09.59
    - complication E09.8
      - specified NEC E09.69
    - dermatitis E09.620
    - foot ulcer E09.621
    - gangrene E09.52
    - gastroparalysis E09.43
    - gastroparesis E09.43
    - glomerulonephrosis, intracapillary E09.21
    - glomerulosclerosis, intercapillary E09.21
    - hyperglycemia E09.65
    - hyperosmolarity E09.00
      - with coma E09.01
    - hypoglycemia E09.649
      - with coma E09.641
    - ketoacidosis E09.10
      - with coma E09.11
    - kidney complications NEC E09.29
    - Kimmelsteil-Wilson disease E09.21
    - mononeuropathy E09.41
    - myasthenia E09.44
    - necrobiosis lipoidica E09.620
    - nephropathy E09.21
    - neuralgia E09.42
    - neurologic complication NEC E09.49
    - neuropathic arthropathy E09.610

Diabetes, diabetic (mellitus) (sugar) - *continued*
- due to drug or chemical - *continued*
  - with - *continued*
    - neuropathy E09.40
    - ophthalmic complication NEC E09.39
    - oral complication NEC E09.638
    - periodontal disease E09.630
    - peripheral angiopathy E09.51
      - with gangrene E09.52
    - polyneuropathy E09.42
    - renal complication NEC E09.29
    - renal tubular degeneration E09.29
    - retinopathy E09.319
      - with macular edema E09.311
        - resolved following treatment E09.37
      - nonproliferative E09.329
        - with macular edema E09.321
        - mild E09.329
          - with macular edema E09.321
        - moderate E09.339
          - with macular edema E09.331
        - severe E09.349
          - with macular edema E09.341
      - proliferative E09.359
        - with
          - combined traction retinal detachment and rhegmatogenous retinal detachment E09.354
          - macular edema E09.351
          - stable proliferative diabetic retinopathy E09.355
          - traction retinal detachment involving the macula E09.352
          - traction retinal detachment not involving the macula E09.353
    - skin complication NEC E09.628
    - skin ulcer NEC E09.622
- due to underlying condition E08.9
  - with
    - amyotrophy E08.44
    - arthropathy NEC E08.618
    - autonomic (poly) neuropathy E08.43
    - cataract E08.36
    - Charcot's joints E08.610
    - chronic kidney disease E08.22
    - circulatory complication NEC E08.59
    - complication E08.8
      - specified NEC E08.69
    - dermatitis E08.620
    - foot ulcer E08.621
    - gangrene E08.52
    - gastroparalysis E08.43
    - gastroparesis E08.43
    - glomerulonephrosis, intracapillary E08.21
    - glomerulosclerosis, intercapillary E08.21
    - hyperglycemia E08.65
    - hyperosmolarity E08.00
      - with coma E08.01
    - hypoglycemia E08.649
      - with coma E08.641
    - ketoacidosis E08.10
      - with coma E08.11
    - kidney complications NEC E08.29
    - Kimmelsteil-WIlson disease E08.21
    - mononeuropathy E08.41
    - myasthenia E08.44
    - necrobiosis lipoidica E08.620
    - nephropathy E08.21
    - neuralgia E08.42
    - neurologic complication NEC E08.49
    - neuropathic arthropathy E08.610
    - neuropathy E08.40
    - ophthalmic complication NEC E08.39
    - oral complication NEC E08.638
    - periodontal disease E08.630
    - peripheral angiopathy E08.51
      - with gangrene E08.52
    - polyneuropathy E08.42
    - renal complication NEC E08.29

Diabetes, diabetic (mellitus) (sugar) - *continued*
- due to underlying condition - *continued*
  - with - *continued*
    - renal tubular degeneration E08.29
    - retinopathy E08.319
      - with macular edema E08.311
        - resolved following treatment E08.37
      - nonproliferative E08.329
        - with macular edema E08.321
        - mild E08.329
          - with macular edema E08.321
        - moderate E08.339
          - with macular edema E08.331
        - severe E08.349
          - with macular edema E08.341
      - proliferative E08.359
        - with
          - combined traction retinal detachment and rhegmatogenous retinal detachment E08.354
          - macular edema E08.351
          - stable proliferative diabetic retinopathy E08.355
          - traction retinal detachment involving the macula E08.352
          - traction retinal detachment not involving the macula E08.353
    - skin complication NEC E08.628
    - skin ulcer NEC E08.622
- gestational (in pregnancy) O24.419
  - affecting newborn P70.0
  - diet controlled O24.410
  - in childbirth O24.429
    - diet controlled O24.420
    - insulin (and diet) controlled O24.424
    - oral drug controlled (antidiabetic) (hypoglycemic) O24.425
  - insulin (and diet) controlled O24.414
  - oral drug controlled (antidiabetic) (hypoglycemic) O24.415
  - puerperal O24.439
    - diet controlled O24.430
    - insulin (and diet) controlled O24.434
    - oral drug controlled (antidiabetic) (hypoglycemic) O24.435
- hepatogenous E13.9
- idiopathic — *see* Diabetes, type 1
- inadequately controlled - code to Diabetes, by type, with hyperglycemia
- insipidus E23.2
  - nephrogenic N25.1
  - pituitary E23.2
  - vasopressin resistant N25.1
- insulin dependent - code to type of diabetes
- juvenile-onset — *see* Diabetes, type 1
- ketosis-prone — *see* Diabetes, type 1
- latent R73.03
- neonatal (transient) P70.2
- non-insulin dependent - code to type of diabetes
- out of control - code to Diabetes, by type, with hyperglycemia
- phosphate E83.39
- poorly controlled - code to Diabetes, by type, with hyperglycemia
- postpancreatectomy — *see* Diabetes, specified type NEC
- postprocedural — *see* Diabetes, specified type NEC
- secondary diabetes mellitus NEC — *see* Diabetes, specified type NEC
- specified type NEC E13.9
  - with
    - amyotrophy E13.44
    - arthropathy NEC E13.618
    - autonomic (poly) neuropathy E13.43
    - cataract E13.36
    - Charcot's joints E13.610
    - chronic kidney disease E13.22
    - circulatory complication NEC E13.59
    - complication E13.8

Diabetes, diabetic (mellitus) (sugar) - *continued*
- specified type NEC - *continued*
  - with - *continued*
    - complication - *continued*
      - specified NEC E13.69
    - dermatitis E13.620
    - foot ulcer E13.621
    - gangrene E13.52
    - gastroparalysis E13.43
    - gastroparesis E13.43
    - glomerulonephrosis, intracapillary E13.21
    - glomerulosclerosis, intercapillary E13.21
    - hyperglycemia E13.65
    - hyperosmolarity E13.00
      - with coma E13.01
    - hypoglycemia E13.649
      - with coma E13.641
    - ketoacidosis E13.10
      - with coma E13.11
    - kidney complications NEC E13.29
    - Kimmelsteil-Wilson disease E13.21
    - mononeuropathy E13.41
    - myasthenia E13.44
    - necrobiosis lipoidica E13.620
    - nephropathy E13.21
    - neuralgia E13.42
    - neurologic complication NEC E13.49
    - neuropathic arthropathy E13.610
    - neuropathy E13.40
    - ophthalmic complication NEC E13.39
    - oral complication NEC E13.638
    - periodontal disease E13.630
    - peripheral angiopathy E13.51
      - with gangrene E13.52
    - polyneuropathy E13.42
    - renal complication NEC E13.29
    - renal tubular degeneration E13.29
    - retinopathy E13.319
      - with macular edema E13.311
      - resolved following treatment E13.37
      - nonproliferative E13.329
        - with macular edema E13.321
        - mild E13.329
          - with macular edema E13.321
        - moderate E13.339
          - with macular edema E13.331
        - severe E13.349
          - with macular edema E13.341
      - proliferative E13.359
        - with
          - combined traction retinal detachment and rhegmatogenous retinal detachment E13.354
          - macular edema E13.351
          - stable proliferative diabetic retinopathy E13.355
          - traction retinal detachment involving the macula E13.352
          - traction retinal detachment not involving the macula E13.353
    - skin complication NEC E13.628
    - skin ulcer NEC E13.622
- steroid-induced — *see* Diabetes, due to, drug or chemical
- type 1 E10.9
  - with
    - amyotrophy E10.44
    - arthropathy NEC E10.618
    - autonomic (poly) neuropathy E10.43
    - cataract E10.36
    - Charcot's joints E10.610
    - chronic kidney disease E10.22
    - circulatory complication NEC E10.59
    - coma due to
      - hypoglycemia E10.641
      - ketoacidosis E10.11
    - complication E10.8
      - specified NEC E10.69
    - dermatitis E10.620

Diabetes, diabetic (mellitus) (sugar) - *continued*
- type 1 - *continued*
  - with - *continued*
    - foot ulcer E10.621
    - gangrene E10.52
    - gastroparalysis E10.43
    - gastroparesis E10.43
    - glomerulonephrosis, intracapillary E10.21
    - glomerulosclerosis, intercapillary E10.21
    - hyperglycemia E10.65
    - hypoglycemia E10.649
      - with coma E10.641
    - ketoacidosis E10.10
      - with coma E10.11
    - kidney complications NEC E10.29
    - Kimmelsteil-Wilson disease E10.21
    - mononeuropathy E10.41
    - myasthenia E10.44
    - necrobiosis lipoidica E10.620
    - nephropathy E10.21
    - neuralgia E10.42
    - neurologic complication NEC E10.49
    - neuropathic arthropathy E10.610
    - neuropathy E10.40
    - ophthalmic complication NEC E10.39
    - oral complication NEC E10.638
    - osteomyelitis E10.69
    - periodontal disease E10.630
    - peripheral angiopathy E10.51
      - with gangrene E10.52
    - polyneuropathy E10.42
    - renal complication NEC E10.29
    - renal tubular degeneration E10.29
    - retinopathy E10.319
      - with macular edema E10.311
      - resolved following treatment E10.37
      - nonproliferative E10.329
        - with macular edema E10.321
        - mild E10.329
          - with macular edema E10.321
        - moderate E10.339
          - with macular edema E10.331
        - severe E10.349
          - with macular edema E10.341
      - proliferative E10.359
        - with
          - combined traction retinal detachment and rhegmatogenous retinal detachment E10.354
          - macular edema E10.351
          - stable proliferative diabetic retinopathy E10.355
          - traction retinal detachment involving the macula E10.352
          - traction retinal detachment not involving the macula E10.353
    - skin complication NEC E10.628
    - skin ulcer NEC E10.622
- type 2 E11.9
  - with
    - amyotrophy E11.44
    - arthropathy NEC E11.618
    - autonomic (poly) neuropathy E11.43
    - cataract E11.36
    - Charcot's joints E11.610
    - chronic kidney disease E11.22
    - circulatory complication NEC E11.59
    - complication E11.8
      - specified NEC E11.69
    - coma due to
      - hyperosmolarity E11.01
      - hypoglycemia E11.641
      - ketoacidosis
    - dermatitis E11.620
    - foot ulcer E11.621
    - gangrene E11.52
    - gastroparalysis E11.43
    - gastroparesis E11.43

Diabetes, diabetic (mellitus) (sugar) - *continued*
- type 2 - *continued*
  - with - *continued*
    - glomerulonephrosis, intracapillary E11.21
    - glomerulosclerosis, intercapillary E11.21
    - hyperglycemia E11.65
    - hyperosmolarity E11.00
      - with coma E11.01
    - hypoglycemia E11.649
      - with coma E11.641
    - ketoacidosis E11.10
      - with coma E11.11
    - kidney complications NEC E11.29
    - Kimmelsteil-Wilson disease E11.21
    - mononeuropathy E11.41
    - myasthenia E11.44
    - necrobiosis lipoidica E11.620
    - nephropathy E11.21
    - neuralgia E11.42
    - neurologic complication NEC E11.49
    - neuropathic arthropathy E11.610
    - neuropathy E11.40
    - ophthalmic complication NEC E11.39
    - oral complication NEC E11.638
    - osteomyelitis E11.69
    - periodontal disease E11.630
    - peripheral angiopathy E11.51
      - with gangrene E11.52
    - polyneuropathy E11.42
    - renal complication NEC E11.29
    - renal tubular degeneration E11.29
    - retinopathy E11.319
      - with macular edema E11.311
      - resolved following treatment E11.37
      - nonproliferative E11.329
        - with macular edema E11.321
        - mild E11.329
          - with macular edema E11.321
        - moderate E11.339
          - with macular edema E11.331
        - severe E11.349
          - with macular edema E11.341
      - proliferative E11.359
        - with
          - combined traction retinal detachment and rhegmatogenous retinal detachment E11.354
          - macular edema E11.351
          - stable proliferative diabetic retinopathy E11.355
          - traction retinal detachment involving the macula E11.352
          - traction retinal detachment not involving the macula E11.353
    - skin complication NEC E11.628
    - skin ulcer NEC E11.622
- uncontrolled
  - meaning
    - hyperglycemia — *see* Diabetes, by type, with, hyperglycemia
    - hypoglycemia — *see* Diabetes, by type, with, hypoglycemia

Diacyclothrombopathia D69.1

Diagnosis deferred R69

Dialysis (intermittent) (treatment)
- noncompliance (with) Z91.15
- renal (hemodialysis) (peritoneal) , status Z99.2
- retina, retinal — *see* Detachment, retina, with retinal, dialysis

Diamond-Blackfan anemia (congenital hypoplastic) D61.01

Diamond-Gardener syndrome (autoerythrocyte sensitization) D69.2

Diaper rash L22

Diaphoresis (excessive) R61

Diaphragm — *see* condition

Diaphragmalgia R07.1

Diaphragmatitis, diaphragmitis J98.6

Diaphysial aclasis Q78.6

Dilatation - *continued*
- pulmonary
  - artery (idiopathic) I28.8
  - valve, congenital Q22.3
- pupil H57.04
- rectum K59.39
- saccule, congenital Q16.5
- salivary gland (duct) K11.8
- sphincter ani K62.89
- stomach K31.89
  - acute K31.0
  - psychogenic F45.8
- submaxillary duct K11.8
- trachea, congenital Q32.1
- ureter (idiopathic) N28.82
  - congenital Q62.2
  - due to obstruction N13.4
- urethra (acquired) N36.8
- vasomotor I73.9
- vein I86.8
- ventricular, ventricle (acute) (chronic) — *see also* Hypertrophy, cardiac
  - cerebral, congenital Q04.8
- venule NEC I86.8
- vesical orifice N32.89

Dilated, dilation — *see* Dilatation

Diminished, diminution
- hearing (acuity) — *see* Deafness
- sense or sensation (cold) (heat) (tactile) (vibratory) R20.8
- vision NEC H54.7
- vital capacity R94.2

Diminuta taenia B71.0

Dimitri-Sturge-Weber disease Q85.8

Dimple
- congenital sacral Q82.6
- parasacral Q82.6
- pilonidal or postanal — *see* Cyst, pilonidal

Dioctophyme renalis (infection) (infestation) B83.8

Dipetalonemiasis B74.4

Diphallus Q55.69

Diphtheria, diphtheritic (gangrenous) (hemorrhagic) A36.9
- carrier (suspected) Z22.2
- cutaneous A36.3
- faucial A36.0
- infection of wound A36.3
- laryngeal A36.2
- myocarditis A36.81
- nasal, anterior A36.89
- nasopharyngeal A36.1
- neurological complication A36.89
- pharyngeal A36.0
- specified site NEC A36.89
- tonsillar A36.0

Diphyllobothriasis (intestine) B70.0
- larval B70.1

Diplacusis H93.22-

Diplegia (upper limbs) G83.0
- congenital (cerebral) G80.8
- facial G51.0
- lower limbs G82.20
- spastic G80.1

Diplococcus, diplococcal — *see* condition

Diplopia H53.2

Dipsomania F10.20
- with
  - psychosis — *see* Psychosis, alcoholic
- remission F10.21

Dipylidiasis B71.1

DIRA (deficiency of interleukin 1 receptor antagonist) M04.8

Direction, teeth, abnormal, fully erupted M26.30

Dirofilariasis B74.8

Dirt-eating child F98.3

Disability, disabilities
- heart — *see* Disease, heart
- intellectual F79
  - with
    - autistic features F84.9
    - pathogenic CHAMP1 (genetic) (variant) F78.A9

Disability, disabilities - *continued*
- intellectual - *continued*
  - with - *continued*
    - pathogenic HNRNPH2 (genetic) (variant) F78.A9
    - pathogenic SATB2 (genetic) (variant) F78.A9
    - pathogenic SETBP1 (genetic) (variant) F78.A9
    - pathogenic STXBP1 (genetic) (variant) F78.A9
    - pathogenic SYNGAP1 (genetic) (variant) F78.A1
  - autosomal dominant F78.A9
  - autosomal recessive F78.A9
  - genetic related F78.A9
    - with
      - pathogenic CHAMP1 (variant) F78.A9
      - pathogenic HNRNPH2 (variant) F78.A9
      - pathogenic SATB2 (variant) F78.A9
      - pathogenic SETBP1 (variant) F78.A9
      - pathogenic STXBP1 (variant) F78.A9
      - pathogenic SYNGAP1 (variant) F78.A1
    - specified NEC F78.A9
    - SYNGAP1-related F78.A1
  - in
    - autosomal dominant mental retardation F78.A9
    - autosomal recessive mental retardation F78.A9
    - SATB2-associated syndrome F78.A9
    - SETBP1 disorder F78.A9
    - STXBP1 encephalopathy with epilepsy — *see also* Encephalopathy; and see also Epilepsy F78.A9
    - X-linked mental retardation (syndromic) (Bain type) F78.A9
  - mild (I.Q.50-69) F70
  - moderate (I.Q.35-49) F71
  - profound (I.Q. under 20) F73
  - severe (I.Q.20-34) F72
  - specified level NEC F78.A9
  - SYNGAP1-related F78.A1
  - X-linked (syndromic) (Bain type) F78.A9
- knowledge acquisition F81.9
- learning F81.9
- limiting activities Z73.6
- spelling, specific F81.81

Disappearance of family member Z63.4

Disarticulation — *see* Amputation
- meaning traumatic amputation — *see* Amputation, traumatic

Discharge (from)
- abnormal finding in — *see* Abnormal, specimen
- breast (female) (male) N64.52
- diencephalic autonomic idiopathic — *see* Epilepsy, specified NEC
- ear — *see also* Otorrhea
  - blood — *see* Otorrhagia
- excessive urine R35.89
- nipple N64.52
- penile R36.9
- postnasal R09.82
- prison, anxiety concerning Z65.2
- urethral R36.9
  - without blood R36.0
  - hematospermia R36.1
- vaginal N89.8

Discitis, diskitis M46.40
- cervical region M46.42
- cervicothoracic region M46.43
- lumbar region M46.46
- lumbosacral region M46.47
- multiple sites M46.49
- occipito-atlanto-axial region M46.41
- pyogenic — *see* Infection, intervertebral disc, pyogenic
- sacrococcygeal region M46.48
- thoracic region M46.44
- thoracolumbar region M46.45

Discoid
- meniscus (congenital) Q68.6
- semilunar cartilage (congenital) — *see* Derangement, knee, meniscus, specified NEC

Discoloration
- nails L60.8
- teeth (posteruptive) K03.7
  - during formation K00.8

Discomfort
- chest R07.89
- visual H53.14-

Discontinuity, ossicles, ear H74.2-

Discord (with)
- boss Z56.4
- classmates Z55.4
- counselor Z64.4
- employer Z56.4
- family Z63.8
- fellow employees Z56.4
- in-laws Z63.1
- landlord Z59.2
- lodgers Z59.2
- neighbors Z59.2
- probation officer Z64.4
- social worker Z64.4
- teachers Z55.4
- workmates Z56.4

Discordant connection
- atrioventricular (congenital) Q20.5
- ventriculoarterial Q20.3

Discrepancy
- centric occlusion maximum intercuspation M26.55
- leg length (acquired) — *see* Deformity, limb, unequal length
  - congenital — *see* Defect, reduction, lower limb
- uterine size date O26.84-

Discrimination
- ethnic Z60.5
- political Z60.5
- racial Z60.5
- religious Z60.5
- sex Z60.5

Disease, diseased — *see also* Syndrome
- absorbent system I87.8
- acid-peptic K30
- Acosta's T70.29
- Adams-Stokes (-Morgagni) (syncope with heart block) I45.9
- Addison's anemia (pernicious) D51.0
- adenoids (and tonsils) J35.9
- adrenal (capsule) (cortex) (gland) (medullary) E27.9
  - hyperfunction E27.0
  - specified NEC E27.8
- ainhum L94.6
- airway
  - obstructive, chronic J44.9
    - due to
      - cotton dust J66.0
      - specific organic dusts NEC J66.8
  - reactive — *see* Asthma
- akamushi (scrub typhus) A75.3
- Albers-Schönberg (marble bones) Q78.2
- Albert's — *see* Tendinitis, Achilles
- alimentary canal K63.9
- alligator-skin Q80.9
  - acquired L85.0
- alpha heavy chain C88.3
- alpine T70.29
- altitude T70.20
- alveolar ridge
  - edentulous K06.9
    - specified NEC K06.8
- alveoli, teeth K08.9
- Alzheimer's G30.9 *[F02.80]*
  - with behavioral disturbance G30.9 *[F02.81]*
  - early onset G30.0 *[F02.80]*
    - with behavioral disturbance G30.0 *[F02.81]*
  - late onset G30.1 *[F02.80]*

Disease, diseased - *continued*
Alzheimer's - *continued*
late onset - *continued*
with behavioral disturbance G30.1 *[F02.81]*
specified NEC G30.8 *[F02.80]*
with behavioral disturbance G30.8 *[F02.81]*
amyloid — *see* Amyloidosis
Andersen's (glycogenosis IV) E74.09
Andes T70.29
Andrews' (bacterid) L08.89
angiospastic I73.9
cerebral G45.9
vein I87.8
anterior
chamber H21.9
horn cell G12.29
antiglomerular basement membrane (anti-GBM) antibody M31.0
tubulo-interstitial nephritis N12
antral — *see* Sinusitis, maxillary
anus K62.9
specified NEC K62.89
aorta (nonsyphilitic) I77.9
syphilitic NEC A52.02
aortic (heart) (valve) I35.9
rheumatic I06.9
Apollo B30.3
aponeuroses — *see* Enthesopathy
appendix K38.9
specified NEC K38.8
aqueous (chamber) H21.9
Arnold-Chiari — *see* Arnold-Chiari disease
arterial I77.9
occlusive — *see* Occlusion, by site
due to stricture or stenosis I77.1
peripheral I73.9
arteriocardiorenal — *see* Hypertension, cardiorenal
arteriolar (generalized) (obliterative) I77.9
arteriorenal — *see* Hypertension, kidney
arteriosclerotic — *see also* Arteriosclerosis
cardiovascular — *see* Disease, heart, ischemic, atherosclerotic
coronary (artery) — *see* Disease, heart, ischemic, atherosclerotic
heart — *see* Disease, heart, ischemic, atherosclerotic
artery I77.9
cerebral I67.9
coronary I25.10
with angina pectoris — *see* Arteriosclerosis, coronary (artery)
peripheral I73.9
arthropod-borne NOS (viral) A94
specified type NEC A93.8
atticoantral, chronic H66.20
left H66.22
with right H66.23
right H66.21
with left H66.23
auditory canal — *see* Disorder, ear, external
auricle, ear NEC — *see* Disorder, pinna
Australian X A83.4
autoimmune (systemic) NOS M35.9
hemolytic D59.10
cold type (primary) (secondary) (symptomatic) D59.12
mixed type (primary) (secondary) (symptomatic) D59.13
warm type (primary) (secondary) (symptomatic) D59.11
drug-induced D59.0
thyroid E06.3
autoinflammatory M04.9
NOD2-associated M04.8
specified type NEC M04.8
aviator's — *see* Effect, adverse, high altitude
Ayerza's (pulmonary artery sclerosis with pulmonary hypertension) I27.0
Babington's (familial hemorrhagic telangiectasia) I78.0
bacterial A49.9
specified NEC A48.8

Disease, diseased - *continued*
bacterial - *continued*
zoonotic A28.9
specified type NEC A28.8
Baelz's (cheilitis glandularis apostematosa) K13.0
bagasse J67.1
balloon — *see* Effect, adverse, high altitude
Bang's (brucella abortus) A23.1
Bannister's T78.3
barometer makers' — *see* Poisoning, mercury
Barraquer (-Simons') (progressive lipodystrophy) E88.1
Barrett's — *see* Barrett's, esophagus
Bartholin's gland N75.9
basal ganglia G25.9
degenerative G23.9
specified NEC G23.8
specified NEC G25.89
Basedow's (exophthalmic goiter) — *see* Hyperthyroidism, with, goiter (diffuse)
Bateman's B08.1
Batten-Steinert G71.11
Battey A31.0
Beard's (neurasthenia) F48.8
Becker
idiopathic mural endomyocardial I42.3
myotonia congenita G71.12
Begbie's (exophthalmic goiter) — *see* Hyperthyroidism, with, goiter (diffuse)
behavioral, organic F07.9
Beigel's (white piedra) B36.2
Benson's — *see* Deposit, crystalline
Bernard-Soulier (thrombopathy) D69.1
Bernhardt (-Roth) — *see* Mononeuropathy, lower limb, meralgia paresthetica
Biermer's (pernicious anemia) D51.0
bile duct (common) (hepatic) K83.9
with calculus, stones — *see* Calculus, bile duct
specified NEC K83.8
biliary (tract) K83.9
specified NEC K83.8
Billroth's — *see* Spina bifida
bird fancier's J67.2
black lung J60
bladder N32.9
in (due to)
schistosomiasis (bilharziasis) B65.0 *[N33]*
specified NEC N32.89
bleeder's D66
blood D75.9
forming organs D75.9
vessel I99.9
Bloodgood's — *see* Mastopathy, cystic
Blount M92.51-
Bodechtel-Guttmann (subacute sclerosing panencephalitis) A81.1
bone — *see also* Disorder, bone
aluminum M83.4
fibrocystic NEC
jaw M27.49
bone-marrow D75.9
Borna A83.9
Bornholm (epidemic pleurodynia) B33.0
Bouchard's (myopathic dilatation of the stomach) K31.0
Bouillaud's (rheumatic heart disease) I01.9
Bourneville (-Brissaud) (tuberous sclerosis) Q85.1
Bouveret (-Hoffmann) (paroxysmal tachycardia) I47.9
bowel K63.9
functional K59.9
psychogenic F45.8
brain G93.9
arterial, artery I67.9
arteriosclerotic I67.2
congenital Q04.9
degenerative — *see* Degeneration, brain
inflammatory — *see* Encephalitis
organic G93.9
arteriosclerotic I67.2
parasitic NEC B71.9 *[G94]*

Disease, diseased - *continued*
brain - *continued*
senile NEC G31.1
specified NEC G93.89
breast — *see also* Disorder, breast N64.9
cystic (chronic) — *see* Mastopathy, cystic
fibrocystic — *see* Mastopathy, cystic
Paget's
female, unspecified side C50.91-
male, unspecified side C50.92-
specified NEC N64.89
Breda's — *see* Yaws
Bretonneau's (diphtheritic malignant angina) A36.0
Bright's — *see* Nephritis
arteriosclerotic — *see* Hypertension, kidney
Brill's (recrudescent typhus) A75.1
Brill-Zinsser (recrudescent typhus) A75.1
Brion-Kayser — *see* Fever, paratyphoid
broad
beta E78.2
ligament (noninflammatory) N83.9
inflammatory — *see* Disease, pelvis, inflammatory
specified NEC N83.8
Brocq-Duhring (dermatitis herpetiformis) L13.0
Brocq's
meaning
dermatitis herpetiformis L13.0
prurigo L28.2
bronchopulmonary J98.4
bronchus NEC J98.09
bronze Addison's E27.1
tuberculous A18.7
budgerigar fancier's J67.2
bullous L13.9
chronic of childhood L12.2
specified NEC L13.8
Buerger's (thromboangiitis obliterans) I73.1
Bürger-Grütz (essential familial hyperlipemia) E78.3
bursa — *see* Bursopathy
caisson T70.3
California — *see* Coccidioidomycosis
capillaries I78.9
specified NEC I78.8
Carapata A68.0
cardiac — *see* Disease, heart
cardiopulmonary, chronic I27.9
cardiorenal (hepatic) (hypertensive) (vascular) — *see* Hypertension, cardiorenal
cardiovascular (atherosclerotic) I25.10
with angina pectoris — *see* Arteriosclerosis, coronary (artery),
congenital Q28.9
newborn P29.9
specified NEC P29.89
hypertensive — *see* Hypertension, heart
renal (hypertensive) — *see* Hypertension, cardiorenal
syphilitic (asymptomatic) A52.00
cartilage — *see* Disorder, cartilage
Castellani's A69.8
Castleman (unicentric) (multicentric) D47.Z2
HHV-8-associated — *see also* Herpesvirus, human, 8 D47.Z2
cat-scratch A28.1
Cavare's (familial periodic paralysis) G72.3
cecum K63.9
celiac (adult) (infantile) (with steatorrhea) K90.0
cellular tissue L98.9
central core G71.29
cerebellar, cerebellum — *see* Disease, brain
cerebral — *see also* Disease, brain
degenerative — *see* Degeneration, brain
cerebrospinal G96.9
cerebrovascular I67.9
acute I67.89
embolic I63.4-
thrombotic I63.3-
arteriosclerotic I67.2

Disease, diseased - *continued*
  cerebrovascular - *continued*
    hereditary NEC I67.858
    specified NEC I67.89
  cervix (uteri) (noninflammatory) N88.9
    inflammatory — *see* Cervicitis
    specified NEC N88.8
  Chabert's A22.9
  Chandler's (osteochondritis dissecans, hip) — *see* Osteochondritis, dissecans, hip
  Charlouis — *see* Yaws
  Chédiak-Steinbrinck (-Higashi) (congenital gigantism of peroxidase granules) E70.330
  chest J98.9
  Chiari's (hepatic vein thrombosis) I82.0
  Chicago B40.9
  Chignon B36.8
  chigo, chigoe B88.1
  childhood granulomatous D71
  Chinese liver fluke B66.1
  chlamydial A74.9
    specified NEC A74.89
  cholecystic K82.9
  choroid H31.9
    specified NEC H31.8
  Christmas D67
  chronic bullous of childhood L12.2
  chylomicron retention E78.3
  ciliary body H21.9
    specified NEC H21.89
  circulatory (system) NEC I99.8
    newborn P29.9
    syphilitic A52.00
      congenital A50.54
  coagulation factor deficiency (congenital) — *see* Defect, coagulation
  coccidioidal — *see* Coccidioidomycosis
  cold
    agglutinin or hemoglobinuria D59.12
      paroxysmal D59.6
    hemagglutinin (chronic) D59.12
  collagen NOS (nonvascular) (vascular) M35.9
    specified NEC M35.89
  colon K63.9
    functional K59.9
      congenital Q43.2
    ischemic — *see also* Ischemia, intestine, acute K55.039
  colonic inflammatory bowel, unclassified (IBDU) K52.3
  combined system — *see* Degeneration, combined
  compressed air T70.3
  Concato's (pericardial polyserositis) A19.9
    nontubercular I31.1
    pleural — *see* Pleurisy, with effusion
  conjunctiva H11.9
    chlamydial A74.0
    specified NEC H11.89
    viral B30.9
      specified NEC B30.8
  connective tissue, systemic (diffuse) M35.9
    in (due to)
      hypogammaglobulinemia D80.1 *[M36.8]*
      ochronosis E70.29 *[M36.8]*
    specified NEC M35.89
  Conor and Bruch's (boutonneuse fever) A77.1
  Cooper's — *see* Mastopathy, cystic
  Cori's (glycogenosis III) E74.03
  corkhandler's or corkworker's J67.3
  cornea H18.9
    specified NEC H18.89-
  coronary (artery) — *see* Disease, heart, ischemic, atherosclerotic
    congenital Q24.5
    ostial, syphilitic (aortic) (mitral) (pulmonary) A52.03
  corpus cavernosum N48.9
    specified NEC N48.89
  Cotugno's — *see* Sciatica

Disease, diseased - *continued*
  COVID-19 U07.1
  coxsackie (virus) NEC B34.1
  cranial nerve NOS G52.9
  Creutzfeldt-Jakob — *see* Creutzfeldt-Jakob disease or syndrome
  Crocq's (acrocyanosis) I73.89
  Crohn's — *see* Enteritis, regional
  Curschmann G71.11
  cystic
    breast (chronic) — *see* Mastopathy, cystic
    kidney, congenital Q61.9
    liver, congenital Q44.6
    lung J98.4
      congenital Q33.0
  cytomegalic inclusion (generalized) B25.9
    with pneumonia B25.0
    congenital P35.1
  cytomegaloviral B25.9
    specified NEC B25.8
  Czerny's (periodic hydrarthrosis of the knee) — *see* Effusion, joint, knee
  Daae (-Finsen) (epidemic pleurodynia) B33.0
  Darling's — *see* Histoplasmosis capsulati
  Débove's (splenomegaly) R16.1
  deer fly — *see* Tularemia
  Degos' I77.89
  demyelinating, demyelinizating (nervous system) G37.9
    multiple sclerosis G35
    specified NEC G37.8
  dense deposit — *see also* N00-N07 with fourth character .6 N05.6
  deposition, hydroxyapatite — *see* Disease, hydroxyapatite deposition
  de Quervain's (tendon sheath) M65.4
    thyroid (subacute granulomatous thyroiditis) E06.1
  Devergie's (pityriasis rubra pilaris) L44.0
  Devic's G36.0
  diaphorase deficiency D74.0
  diaphragm J98.6
  diarrheal, infectious NEC A09
  digestive system K92.9
    specified NEC K92.89
  disc, degenerative — *see* Degeneration, intervertebral disc
  discogenic — *see also* Displacement, intervertebral disc NEC
    with myelopathy — *see* Disorder, disc, with, myelopathy
  diverticular — *see* Diverticula
  Dubois (thymus) A50.59 *[E35]*
  Duchenne-Griesinger G71.01
  Duchenne's
    muscular dystrophy G71.01
    pseudohypertrophy, muscles G71.01
  ductless glands E34.9
  Duhring's (dermatitis herpetiformis) L13.0
  duodenum K31.9
    specified NEC K31.89
  Dupré's (meningism) R29.1
  Dupuytren's (muscle contracture) M72.0
  Durand-Nicholas-Favre (climatic bubo) A55
  Duroziez's (congenital mitral stenosis) Q23.2
  ear — *see* Disorder, ear
  Eberth's — *see* Fever, typhoid
  Ebola (virus) A98.4
  Ebstein's heart Q22.5
  Echinococcus — *see* Echinococcus
  echovirus NEC B34.1
  Eddowes' (brittle bones and blue sclera) Q78.0
  edentulous (alveolar) ridge K06.9
    specified NEC K06.8
  Edsall's T67.2
  Eichstedt's (pityriasis versicolor) B36.0
  Eisenmenger's (irreversible) I27.83
  Ellis-van Creveld (chondroectodermal dysplasia) Q77.6
  end stage renal (ESRD) N18.6
    due to hypertension I12.0
  endocrine glands or system NEC E34.9
  endomyocardial (eosinophilic) I42.3
  English (rickets) E55.0

Disease, diseased - *continued*
  enteroviral, enterovirus NEC B34.1
    central nervous system NEC A88.8
  epidemic B99.9
    specified NEC B99.8
  epididymis N50.9
  Erb (-Landouzy) G71.02
  Erdheim-Chester (ECD) E88.89
  esophagus K22.9
    functional K22.4
    psychogenic F45.8
    specified NEC K22.89
  Eulenburg's (congenital paramyotonia) G71.19
  eustachian tube — *see* Disorder, eustachian tube
  external
    auditory canal — *see* Disorder, ear, external
    ear — *see* Disorder, ear, external
  extrapyramidal G25.9
    specified NEC G25.89
  eye H57.9
    anterior chamber H21.9
    inflammatory NEC H57.89
    muscle (external) — *see* Strabismus
    specified NEC H57.89
    syphilitic — *see* Oculopathy, syphilitic
  eyeball H44.9
    specified NEC H44.89
  eyelid — *see* Disorder, eyelid
    specified NEC — *see* Disorder, eyelid, specified type NEC
  eyeworm of Africa B74.3
  facial nerve (seventh) G51.9
    newborn (birth injury) P11.3
  Fahr (of brain) G23.8
  Fahr Volhard (of kidney) I12.-
  fallopian tube (noninflammatory) N83.9
    inflammatory — *see* Salpingo-oophoritis
    specified NEC N83.8
  familial periodic paralysis G72.3
  Fanconi's (congenital pancytopenia) D61.09
  fascia NEC — *see also* Disorder, muscle
    inflammatory — *see* Myositis
    specified NEC M62.89
  Fauchard's (periodontitis) — *see* Periodontitis
  Favre-Durand-Nicolas (climatic bubo) A55
  Fede's K14.0
  Feer's — *see* Poisoning, mercury
  female pelvic inflammatory — *see also* Disease, pelvis, inflammatory N73.9
    syphilitic (secondary) A51.42
    tuberculous A18.17
  Fernels' (aortic aneurysm) I71.9
  fibrocaseous of lung — *see* Tuberculosis, pulmonary
  fibrocystic — *see* Fibrocystic disease
  Fiedler's (leptospiral jaundice) A27.0
  fifth B08.3
  file-cutter's — *see* Poisoning, lead
  fish-skin Q80.9
    acquired L85.0
  Flajani (-Basedow) (exophthalmic goiter) — *see* Hyperthyroidism, with, goiter (diffuse)
  flax-dresser's J66.1
  fluke — *see* Infestation, fluke
  foot and mouth B08.8
  foot process N04.9
  Forbes' (glycogenosis III) E74.03
  Fordyce-Fox (apocrine miliaria) L75.2
  Fordyce's (ectopic sebaceous glands) (mouth) Q38.6
  Forestier's (rhizomelic pseudopolyarthritis) M35.3
    meaning ankylosing hyperostosis — *see* Hyperostosis, ankylosing
  Fothergill's
    neuralgia — *see* Neuralgia, trigeminal
    scarlatina anginosa A38.9
  Fournier (gangrene) N49.3
    female N76.89
  fourth B08.8

Disease, diseased - *continued*
- Fox (-Fordyce) (apocrine miliaria) L75.2
- Francis' — *see* Tularemia
- Franklin C88.2
- Frei's (climatic bubo) A55
- Friedreich's
  - combined systemic or ataxia G11.11
  - myoclonia G25.3
- frontal sinus — *see* Sinusitis, frontal
- fungus NEC B49
- Gaisböck's (polycythemia hypertonica) D75.1
- gallbladder K82.9
  - calculus — *see* Calculus, gallbladder
  - cholecystitis — *see* Cholecystitis
  - cholesterolosis K82.4
  - fistula — *see* Fistula, gallbladder
  - hydrops K82.1
  - obstruction — *see* Obstruction, gallbladder
  - perforation K82.2
  - specified NEC K82.8
- gamma heavy chain C88.2
- Gamna's (siderotic splenomegaly) D73.2
- Gamstorp's (adynamia episodica hereditaria) G72.3
- Gandy-Nanta (siderotic splenomegaly) D73.2
- ganister J62.8
- gastric — *see* Disease, stomach
- gastroesophageal reflux (GERD) K21.9
  - with esophagitis (without bleeding) K21.00
    - with bleeding K21.01
- gastrointestinal (tract) K92.9
  - amyloid E85.4
  - functional K59.9
    - psychogenic F45.8
  - specified NEC K92.89
- Gee (-Herter) (-Heubner) (-Thaysen) (nontropical sprue) K90.0
- genital organs
  - female N94.9
  - male N50.9
- Gerhardt's (erythromelalgia) I73.81
- Gibert's (pityriasis rosea) L42
- Gierke's (glycogenosis I) E74.01
- Gilles de la Tourette's (motor-verbal tic) F95.2
- gingiva K06.9
  - plaque induced K05.00
  - specified NEC K06.8
- gland (lymph) I89.9
- Glanzmann's (hereditary hemorrhagic thrombasthenia) D69.1
- glass-blower's (cataract) — *see* Cataract, specified NEC
  - salivary gland hypertrophy K11.1
- Glisson's — *see* Rickets
- globe H44.9
  - specified NEC H44.89
- glomerular — *see also* Glomerulonephritis
  - with edema — *see* Nephrosis
  - acute — *see* Nephritis, acute
  - chronic — *see* Nephritis, chronic
  - minimal change N05.0
  - rapidly progressive N01.9
- glycogen storage E74.00
  - Andersen's E74.09
  - Cori's E74.03
  - Forbes' E74.03
  - generalized E74.00
  - glucose-6-phosphatase deficiency E74.01
  - heart E74.02 *[I43]*
  - hepatorenal E74.09
  - Hers' E74.09
  - liver and kidney E74.09
  - McArdle's E74.04
  - muscle phosphofructokinase E74.09
  - myocardium E74.02 *[I43]*
  - Pompe's E74.02
  - Tauri's E74.09
  - type 0 E74.09
  - type I E74.01
  - type II E74.02
  - type III E74.03
  - type IV E74.09

Disease, diseased - *continued*
- glycogen storage - *continued*
  - type V E74.04
  - type VI-XI E74.09
  - Von Gierke's E74.01
- Goldstein's (familial hemorrhagic telangiectasia) I78.0
- gonococcal NOS A54.9
- graft-versus-host (GVH) D89.813
  - acute D89.810
  - acute on chronic D89.812
  - chronic D89.811
- grainhandler's J67.8
- granulomatous (childhood) (chronic) D71
- Graves' (exophthalmic goiter) — *see* Hyperthyroidism, with, goiter (diffuse)
- Griesinger's — *see* Ancylostomiasis
- Grisel's M43.6
- Gruby's (tinea tonsurans) B35.0
- Guillain-Barré G61.0
- Guinon's (motor-verbal tic) F95.2
- gum K06.9
- gynecological N94.9
- H (Hartnup's) E72.02
- Haff — *see* Poisoning, mercury
- Hageman (congenital factor XII deficiency) D68.2
- hair (color) (shaft) L67.9
  - follicles L73.9
    - specified NEC L73.8
- Hamman's (spontaneous mediastinal emphysema) J98.2
- hand, foot and mouth B08.4
- Hansen's — *see* Leprosy
- Hantavirus, with pulmonary manifestations B33.4
  - with renal manifestations A98.5
- Harada's H30.81-
- Hartnup (pellagra-cerebellar ataxia-renal aminoaciduria) E72.02
- Hart's (pellagra-cerebellar ataxia-renal aminoaciduria) E72.02
- Hashimoto's (struma lymphomatosa) E06.3
- Hb — *see* Disease, hemoglobin
- heart (organic) I51.9
  - with
    - pulmonary edema (acute) — *see also* Failure, ventricular, left I50.1
    - rheumatic fever (conditions in I00)
      - active I01.9
        - with chorea I02.0
        - specified NEC I01.8
      - inactive or quiescent (with chorea) I09.9
        - specified NEC I09.89
  - amyloid E85.4 *[I43]*
  - aortic (valve) I35.9
  - arteriosclerotic or sclerotic (senile) — *see* Disease, heart, ischemic, atherosclerotic
  - artery, arterial — *see* Disease, heart, ischemic, atherosclerotic
  - beer drinkers' I42.6
  - beriberi (wet) E51.12
  - black I27.0
  - congenital Q24.9
    - cyanotic Q24.9
    - specified NEC Q24.8
  - coronary — *see* Disease, heart, ischemic
  - cryptogenic I51.9
  - fibroid — *see* Myocarditis
  - functional I51.89
    - psychogenic F45.8
  - glycogen storage E74.02 *[I43]*
  - gonococcal A54.83
  - hypertensive — *see* Hypertension, heart
  - hyperthyroid — *see also* Hyperthyroidism E05.90 *[I43]*
    - with thyroid storm E05.91 *[I43]*
  - ischemic (chronic or with a stated duration of over 4 weeks) I25.9
    - atherosclerotic (of) I25.10
      - with angina pectoris — *see* Arteriosclerosis, coronary (artery)

Disease, diseased - *continued*
- heart (organic) - *continued*
  - ischemic (chronic or with a stated duration of over 4 weeks) - *continued*
    - atherosclerotic (of) - *continued*
      - coronary artery bypass graft — *see* Arteriosclerosis, coronary (artery),
    - cardiomyopathy I25.5
    - diagnosed on ECG or other special investigation, but currently presenting no symptoms I25.6
    - silent I25.6
    - specified form NEC I25.89
  - kyphoscoliotic I27.1
  - meningococcal A39.50
    - endocarditis A39.51
    - myocarditis A39.52
    - pericarditis A39.53
  - mitral I05.9
    - specified NEC I05.8
  - muscular — *see* Degeneration, myocardial
  - psychogenic (functional) F45.8
  - pulmonary (chronic) I27.9
    - in schistosomiasis B65.9 *[I52]*
    - specified NEC I27.89
  - rheumatic (chronic) (inactive) (old) (quiescent) (with chorea) I09.9
    - active or acute I01.9
      - with chorea (acute) (rheumatic) (Sydenham's) I02.0
    - specified NEC I09.89
  - senile — *see* Myocarditis
  - syphilitic A52.06
    - aortic A52.03
      - aneurysm A52.01
    - congenital A50.54 *[I52]*
  - thyrotoxic — *see also* Thyrotoxicosis E05.90 *[I43]*
    - with thyroid storm E05.91 *[I43]*
  - valve, valvular (obstructive) (regurgitant) — *see also* Endocarditis
    - congenital NEC Q24.8
      - pulmonary Q22.3
  - vascular — *see* Disease, cardiovascular
- heavy chain NEC C88.2
  - alpha C88.3
  - gamma C88.2
  - mu C88.2
- Hebra's
  - pityriasis
    - maculata et circinata L42
    - rubra pilaris L44.0
  - prurigo L28.2
- hematopoietic organs D75.9
- hemoglobin or Hb
  - abnormal (mixed) NEC D58.2
    - with thalassemia D56.9
  - AS genotype D57.3
  - Bart's D56.0
  - C (Hb-C) D58.2
    - with other abnormal hemoglobin NEC D58.2
    - elliptocytosis D58.1
    - Hb-S D57.2-
    - sickle-cell D57.2-
    - thalassemia D56.8
  - Constant Spring D58.2
  - D (Hb-D) D58.2
  - E (Hb-E) D58.2
  - E-beta thalassemia D56.5
  - elliptocytosis D58.1
  - H (Hb-H) (thalassemia) D56.0
    - with other abnormal hemoglobin NEC D56.9
    - Constant Spring D56.0
  - I thalassemia D56.9
  - M D74.0
  - S or SS D57.1
    - with
      - acute chest syndrome D57.01
      - cerebral vascular involvement D57.03
      - crisis (painful) D57.00
        - with complication specified NEC D57.09

Disease, diseased - *continued*
hemoglobin or Hb - *continued*
S or SS - *continued*
with - *continued*
splenic sequestration D57.02
vasoocclusive pain D57.00
beta plus D57.44
with
acute chest syndrome D57.451
cerebral vascular involvement D57.453
crisis D57.459
with specified complication NEC D57.458
splenic sequestration D57.452
vasoocclusive pain D57.459
without crisis D57.44
beta zero D57.42
with
acute chest syndrome D57.431
cerebral vascular involvement D57.433
crisis D57.439
with specified complication NEC D57.438
splenic sequestration D57.432
vasoocclusive pain D57.439
without crisis D57.42
SC D57.2-
SD D57.8-
SE D57.8-
spherocytosis D58.0
unstable, hemolytic D58.2
hemolytic (newborn) P55.9
autoimmune D59.10
cold type (primary) (secondary) (symptomatic) D59.12
mixed type (primary) (secondary) (symptomatic) D59.13
warm type (primary) (secondary) (symptomatic) D59.11
drug-induced D59.0
due to or with
incompatibility
ABO (blood group) P55.1
blood (group) (Duffy) (K) (Kell) (Kidd) (Lewis) (M) (S) NEC P55.8
Rh (blood group) (factor) P55.0
Rh negative mother P55.0
specified type NEC P55.8
unstable hemoglobin D58.2
hemorrhagic D69.9
newborn P53
Henoch (-Schönlein) (purpura nervosa) D69.0
hepatic — *see* Disease, liver
hepatobiliary K83.9
toxic K71.9
hepatolenticular E83.01
heredodegenerative NEC
spinal cord G95.89
herpesviral, disseminated B00.7
Hers' (glycogenosis VI) E74.09
Herter (-Gee) (-Heubner) (nontropical sprue) K90.0
Heubner-Herter (nontropical sprue) K90.0
high fetal gene or hemoglobin thalassemia D56.9
Hildenbrand's — *see* Typhus
hip (joint) M25.9
congenital Q65.89
suppurative M00.9
tuberculous A18.02
His (-Werner) (trench fever) A79.0
Hodgson's I71.2
ruptured I71.1
Holla — *see* Spherocytosis
hookworm B76.9
specified NEC B76.8
host-versus-graft D89.813
acute D89.810
acute on chronic D89.812
chronic D89.811
human immunodeficiency virus (HIV) B20

Disease, diseased - *continued*
Huntington's G10
with dementia G10 *[F02.80]*
Hutchinson's (cheiropompholyx) — *see* Hutchinson's disease
hyaline (diffuse) (generalized)
membrane (lung) (newborn) P22.0
adult J80
hydatid — *see* Echinococcus
hydroxyapatite deposition M11.00
ankle M11.07-
elbow M11.02-
foot joint M11.07-
hand joint M11.04-
hip M11.05-
knee M11.06-
multiple site M11.09
shoulder M11.01-
vertebra M11.08
wrist M11.03-
hyperkinetic — *see* Hyperkinesia
hypertensive — *see* Hypertension
hypophysis E23.7
Iceland G93.3
I-cell E77.0
immune D89.9
immunoproliferative (malignant) C88.9
small intestinal C88.3
specified NEC C88.8
inclusion B25.9
salivary gland B25.9
infectious, infective B99.9
congenital P37.9
specified NEC P37.8
viral P35.9
specified type NEC P35.8
specified NEC B99.8
inflammatory
penis N48.29
abscess N48.21
cellulitis N48.22
prepuce N47.7
balanoposthitis N47.6
tubo-ovarian — *see* Salpingo-oophoritis
intervertebral disc — *see also* Disorder, disc
with myelopathy — *see* Disorder, disc, with, myelopathy
cervical, cervicothoracic — *see* Disorder, disc, cervical
with
myelopathy — *see* Disorder, disc, cervical, with myelopathy
neuritis, radiculitis or radiculopathy — *see* Disorder, disc, cervical, with neuritis
specified NEC — *see* Disorder, disc, cervical, specified type NEC
lumbar (with)
myelopathy M51.06
neuritis, radiculitis, radiculopathy or sciatica M51.16
specified NEC M51.86
lumbosacral (with)
neuritis, radiculitis, radiculopathy or sciatica M51.17
specified NEC M51.87
specified NEC — *see* Disorder, disc, specified NEC
thoracic (with)
myelopathy M51.04
neuritis, radiculitis or radiculopathy M51.14
specified NEC M51.84
thoracolumbar (with)
myelopathy M51.05
neuritis, radiculitis or radiculopathy M51.15
specified NEC M51.85
intestine K63.9
functional K59.9
psychogenic F45.8
specified NEC K59.89
organic K63.9
protozoal A07.9
specified NEC K63.89

Disease, diseased - *continued*
iris H21.9
specified NEC H21.89
iron metabolism or storage E83.10
island (scrub typhus) A75.3
itai-itai — *see* Poisoning, cadmium
Jakob-Creutzfeldt — *see* Creutzfeldt-Jakob disease or syndrome
jaw M27.9
fibrocystic M27.49
specified NEC M27.8
jigger B88.1
joint — *see also* Disorder, joint
Charcot's — *see* Arthropathy, neuropathic (Charcot)
degenerative — *see* Osteoarthritis
multiple M15.9
spine — *see* Spondylosis
facet joint — *see also* Spondylosis M47.819
hypertrophic — *see* Osteoarthritis
sacroiliac M53.3
specified NEC — *see* Disorder, joint, specified type NEC
spine NEC — *see* Dorsopathy
suppurative — *see* Arthritis, pyogenic or pyemic
Jourdain's (acute gingivitis) K05.00
nonplaque induced K05.01
plaque induced K05.00
Kaschin-Beck (endemic polyarthritis) M12.10
ankle M12.17-
elbow M12.12-
foot joint M12.17-
hand joint M12.14-
hip M12.15-
knee M12.16-
multiple site M12.19
shoulder M12.11-
vertebra M12.18
wrist M12.13-
Katayama B65.2
Kedani (scrub typhus) A75.3
Keshan E59
kidney (functional) (pelvis) N28.9
chronic N18.9
hypertensive — *see* Hypertension, kidney
stage 1 N18.1
stage 2 (mild) N18.2
stage 3 (moderate) N18.30
stage 3a N18.31
stage 3b N18.32
stage 4 (severe) N18.4
stage 5 N18.5
complicating pregnancy — *see* Pregnancy, complicated by, renal disease
cystic (congenital) Q61.9
diabetic — *see* E08-E13 with .22
fibrocystic (congenital) Q61.8
hypertensive — *see* Hypertension, kidney
in (due to)
schistosomiasis (bilharziasis) B65.9 *[N29]*
multicystic Q61.4
polycystic Q61.3
adult type Q61.2
childhood type NEC Q61.19
collecting duct dilatation Q61.11
Kimmelstiel (-Wilson) (intercapillary polycystic (congenital) glomerulosclerosis) — *see* E08-E13 with .21
Kimura D21.9
specified site (see Neoplasm, connective tissue benign)
Kinnier Wilson's (hepatolenticular degeneration) E83.01
kissing — *see* Mononucleosis, infectious
Klebs' — *see also* Glomerulonephritis N05.-
Klippel-Feil (brevicollis) Q76.1
Köhler-Pellegrini-Stieda (calcification, knee joint) — *see* Bursitis, tibial collateral
Kok Q89.8

Disease, diseased - *continued*
König's (osteochondritis dissecans) — *see* Osteochondritis, dissecans
Korsakoff's (nonalcoholic) F04
alcoholic F10.96
with dependence F10.26
Kostmann's (infantile genetic agranulocytosis) D70.0
kuru A81.81
Kyasanur Forest A98.2
labyrinth, ear — *see* Disorder, ear, inner
lacrimal system — *see* Disorder, lacrimal system
Lafora's — *see* Epilepsy, generalized, idiopathic
Lancereaux-Mathieu (leptospiral jaundice) A27.0
Landry's G61.0
Larrey-Weil (leptospiral jaundice) A27.0
larynx J38.7
legionnaires' A48.1
nonpneumonic A48.2
Lenegre's I44.2
lens H27.9
specified NEC H27.8
Lev's (acquired complete heart block) I44.2
Lewy body (dementia) G31.83 *[F02.80]*
with behavioral disturbance G31.83 *[F02.81]*
Lichtheim's (subacute combined sclerosis with pernicious anemia) D51.0
Lightwood's (renal tubular acidosis) N25.89
Lignac's (cystinosis) E72.04
lip K13.0
lipid-storage E75.6
specified NEC E75.5
Lipschütz's N76.6
liver (chronic) (organic) K76.9
alcoholic (chronic) K70.9
acute — *see* Disease, liver, alcoholic, hepatitis
cirrhosis K70.30
with ascites K70.31
failure K70.40
with coma K70.41
fatty liver K70.0
fibrosis K70.2
hepatitis K70.10
with ascites K70.11
sclerosis K70.2
cystic, congenital Q44.6
drug-induced (idiosyncratic) (toxic) (predictable) (unpredictable) — *see* Disease, liver, toxic
end stage K72.10
with coma K72.11
due to hepatitis — *see* Hepatitis
fatty, nonalcoholic (NAFLD) K76.0
alcoholic K70.0
fibrocystic (congenital) Q44.6
fluke
Chinese B66.1
oriental B66.1
sheep B66.3
gestational alloimmune (GALD) P78.84
glycogen storage E74.09 *[K77]*
in (due to)
schistosomiasis (bilharziasis) B65.9 *[K77]*
inflammatory K75.9
alcoholic K70.1
specified NEC K75.89
polycystic (congenital) Q44.6
toxic K71.9
with
cholestasis K71.0
cirrhosis (liver) K71.7
fibrosis (liver) K71.7
focal nodular hyperplasia K71.8
hepatic granuloma K71.8
hepatic necrosis K71.10
with coma K71.11
hepatitis NEC K71.6
acute K71.2
chronic

Disease, diseased - *continued*
liver (chronic) (organic) - *continued*
toxic - *continued*
with - *continued*
hepatitis NEC - *continued*
chronic - *continued*
active K71.50
with ascites K71.51
lobular K71.4
persistent K71.3
lupoid K71.50
with ascites K71.51
peliosis hepatis K71.8
veno-occlusive disease (VOD) of liver K71.8
veno-occlusive K76.5
Lobo's (keloid blastomycosis) B48.0
Lobstein's (brittle bones and blue sclera) Q78.0
Ludwig's (submaxillary cellulitis) K12.2
lumbosacral region M53.87
lung J98.4
black J60
congenital Q33.9
cystic J98.4
congenital Q33.0
dabbing (related) U07.0
electronic cigarette (related) U07.0
fibroid (chronic) — *see* Fibrosis, lung
fluke B66.4
oriental B66.4
in
amyloidosis E85.4 *[J99]*
sarcoidosis D86.0
Sjögren's syndrome M35.02
systemic
lupus erythematosus M32.13
sclerosis M34.81
interstitial J84.9
with progressive fibrotic phenotype, in diseases classified elsewhere J84.170
of childhood, specified NEC J84.848
respiratory bronchiolitis J84.115
specified NEC J84.89
obstructive (chronic) J44.9
with
acute
bronchitis J44.0
exacerbation NEC J44.1
lower respiratory infection J44.0
alveolitis, allergic J67.9
asthma J44.9
bronchiectasis J47.9
with
exacerbation (acute) J47.1
lower respiratory infection J47.0
bronchitis J44.9
with
exacerbation (acute) J44.1
lower respiratory infection J44.0
emphysema J43.9
hypersensitivity pneumonitis J67.9
decompensated J44.1
with
exacerbation (acute) J44.1
polycystic J98.4
congenital Q33.0
rheumatoid (diffuse) (interstitial) — *see* Rheumatoid, lung
vaping (associated) (device) (product) (use) U07.0
Lutembacher's (atrial septal defect with mitral stenosis) Q21.1
Lyme A69.20
lymphatic (gland) (system) (channel) (vessel) I89.9
lymphoproliferative D47.9
specified NEC D47.Z9
T-gamma D47.Z9
X-linked D82.3
Magitot's M27.2
malarial — *see* Malaria
malignant — *see also* Neoplasm, malignant, by site

Disease, diseased - *continued*
Manson's B65.1
maple bark J67.6
maple-syrup-urine E71.0
Marburg (virus) A98.3
Marion's (bladder neck obstruction) N32.0
Marsh's (exophthalmic goiter) — *see* Hyperthyroidism, with, goiter (diffuse)
mastoid (process) — *see* Disorder, ear, middle
Mathieu's (leptospiral jaundice) A27.0
Maxcy's A75.2
McArdle (-Schmid-Pearson) (glycogenosis V) E74.04
mediastinum J98.59
medullary center (idiopathic) (respiratory) G93.89
Meige's (chronic hereditary edema) Q82.0
meningococcal — *see* Infection, meningococcal
mental F99
organic F09
mesenchymal M35.9
mesenteric embolic — *see also* Ischemia, intestine, acute K55.039
metabolic, metabolism E88.9
bilirubin E80.7
metal-polisher's J62.8
metastatic — *see also* Neoplasm, secondary, by site C79.9
microvascular - code to condition
microvillus
atrophy Q43.8
inclusion (MVD) Q43.8
middle ear — *see* Disorder, ear, middle
Mikulicz' (dryness of mouth, absent or decreased lacrimation) K11.8
Milroy's (chronic hereditary edema) Q82.0
Minamata — *see* Poisoning, mercury
minicore G71.29
Minor's G95.19
Minot's (hemorrhagic disease, newborn) P53
Minot-von Willebrand-Jürgens (angiohemophilia) D68.0
Mitchell's (erythromelalgia) I73.81
mitral (valve) I05.9
nonrheumatic I34.9
mixed connective tissue M35.1
moldy hay J67.0
Monge's T70.29
Morgagni-Adams-Stokes (syncope with heart block) I45.9
Morgagni's (syndrome) (hyperostosis frontalis interna) M85.2
Morton's (with metatarsalgia) — *see* Lesion, nerve, plantar
Morvan's G60.8
motor neuron (bulbar) (mixed type) (spinal) G12.20
amyotrophic lateral sclerosis G12.21
familial G12.24
progressive bulbar palsy G12.22
specified NEC G12.29
moyamoya I67.5
mu heavy chain disease C88.2
multicore G71.29
multiminicore G71.29
muscle — *see also* Disorder, muscle
inflammatory — *see* Myositis
ocular (external) — *see* Strabismus
musculoskeletal system, soft tissue — *see* also Disorder, soft tissue
specified NEC — *see* Disorder, soft tissue, specified type NEC
mushroom workers' J67.5
mycotic B49
myelodysplastic, not classified — *see also* Syndrome, myelodysplasia C94.6
myeloproliferative, not classified C94.6
chronic D47.1
myocardium, myocardial — *see also* Degeneration, myocardial I51.5
primary (idiopathic) I42.9
myoneural G70.9
Naegeli's D69.1

Disease, diseased - *continued*
renal (functional) (pelvis) - *continued*
polycystic (congenital) - *continued*
adult type Q61.2
childhood type NEC Q61.19
collecting duct dilatation Q61.11
rapidly progressive N01.9
subacute N01.9
Rendu-Osler-Weber (familial hemorrhagic telangiectasia) I78.0
renovascular (arteriosclerotic) — *see* Hypertension, kidney
respiratory (tract) J98.9
acute or subacute NOS J06.9
due to
chemicals, gases, fumes or vapors (inhalation) J68.3
external agent J70.9
specified NEC J70.8
radiation J70.0
smoke inhalation J70.5
noninfectious J39.8
chronic NOS J98.9
due to
chemicals, gases, fumes or vapors J68.4
external agent J70.9
specified NEC J70.8
radiation J70.1
newborn P27.9
specified NEC P27.8
due to
chemicals, gases, fumes or vapors J68.9
acute or subacute NEC J68.3
chronic J68.4
external agent J70.9
specified NEC J70.8
newborn P28.9
specified type NEC P28.89
upper J39.9
acute or subacute J06.9
noninfectious NEC J39.8
specified NEC J39.8
streptococcal J06.9
retina, retinal H35.9
Batten's or Batten-Mayou E75.4 *[H36]*
specified NEC H35.89
rheumatoid — *see* Arthritis, rheumatoid
rickettsial NOS A79.9
specified type NEC A79.89
Riga (-Fede) (cachectic aphthae) K14.0
Riggs' (compound periodontitis) — *see* Periodontitis
Ritter's L00
Rivalta's (cervicofacial actinomycosis) A42.2
Robles' (onchocerciasis) B73.01
rod body G71.21
Roger's (congenital interventricular septal defect) Q21.0
Rosenthal's (factor XI deficiency) D68.1
Rossbach's (hyperchlorhydria) K31.89
psychogenic F45.8
Ross River B33.1
Rotes Quérol — *see* Hyperostosis, ankylosing
Roth (-Bernhardt) — *see* Mononeuropathy, lower limb, meralgia paresthetica
Runeberg's (progressive pernicious anemia) D51.0
sacroiliac NEC M53.3
salivary gland or duct K11.9
inclusion B25.9
specified NEC K11.8
virus B25.9
sandworm B76.9
Schimmelbusch's — *see* Mastopathy, cystic
Schmorl's — *see* Schmorl's disease or nodes
Schönlein (-Henoch) (purpura rheumatica) D69.0
Schottmüller's — *see* Fever, paratyphoid
Schultz's (agranulocytosis) — *see* Agranulocytosis
Schwalbe-Ziehen-Oppenheim G24.1
Schwartz-Jampel G71.13
sclera H15.9

Disease, diseased - *continued*
sclera - *continued*
specified NEC H15.89
scrofulous (tuberculous) A18.2
scrotum N50.9
sebaceous glands L73.9
semilunar cartilage, cystic — *see also* Derangement, knee, meniscus, cystic
seminal vesicle N50.9
serum NEC — *see also* Reaction, serum T80.69
sexually transmitted A64
anogenital
herpesviral infection — *see* Herpes, anogenital
warts A63.0
chancroid A57
chlamydial infection — *see* Chlamydia
gonorrhea — *see* Gonorrhea
granuloma inguinale A58
specified organism NEC A63.8
syphilis — *see* Syphilis
trichomoniasis — *see* Trichomoniasis
Sézary C84.1-
shimamushi (scrub typhus) A75.3
shipyard B30.0
sickle-cell D57.1
with
acute chest syndrome D57.01
cerebral vascular involvement D57.03
crisis (painful) D57.00
with complication specified NEC D57.09
splenic sequestration D57.02
vasoocclusive pain D57.00
elliptocytosis D57.8-
Hb-C D57.20
with
acute chest syndrome D57.211
cerebral vascular involvement D57.213
crisis D57.219
with specified complication NEC D57.218
splenic sequestration D57.212
vasoocclusive pain D57.219
without crisis D57.20
Hb-SD D57.80
with
acute chest syndrome D57.811
cerebral vascular involvement D57.813
crisis D57.819
with complication specified NEC D57.818
splenic sequestration D57.812
vasoocclusive pain D57.819
without crisis D57.80
Hb-SE D57.80
with
acute chest syndrome D57.811
cerebral vascular involvement D57.813
crisis D57.819
with complication specified NEC D57.818
splenic sequestration D57.812
vasoocclusive pain D57.819
without crisis D57.80
specified NEC D57.80
with
acute chest syndrome D57.811
cerebral vascular involvement D57.813
crisis D57.819
with complication specified NEC D57.818
splenic sequestration D57.812
vasoocclusive pain D57.819
without crisis D57.80
spherocytosis D57.80
with
acute chest syndrome D57.811
cerebral vascular involvement D57.813

Disease, diseased - *continued*
sickle-cell - *continued*
spherocytosis - *continued*
with - *continued*
crisis D57.819
with complication specified NEC D57.818
splenic sequestration D57.812
vasoocclusive pain D57.819
without crisis D57.80
thalassemia D57.40
with
acute chest syndrome D57.411
cerebral vascular involvement D57.413
crisis (painful) D57.419
with specified complication NEC D57.418
splenic sequestration D57.412
vasoocclusive pain D57.419
beta plus D57.44
with
acute chest syndrome D57.451
cerebral vascular involvement D57.453
crisis D57.459
with specified complication NEC D57.458
splenic sequestration D57.452
vasoocclusive pain D57.459
without crisis D57.44
beta zero D57.42
with
acute chest syndrome D57.431
cerebral vascular involvement D57.433
crisis D57.439
with specified complication NEC D57.438
splenic sequestration D57.432
vasoocclusive pain D57.439
without crisis D57.42
without crisis D57.40
silo-filler's J68.8
bronchitis J68.0
pneumonitis J68.0
pulmonary edema J68.1
simian B B00.4
Simons' (progressive lipodystrophy) E88.1
sin nombre virus B33.4
sinus — *see* Sinusitis
Sirkari's B55.0
sixth B08.20
due to human herpesvirus 6 B08.21
due to human herpesvirus 7 B08.22
skin L98.9
due to metabolic disorder NEC E88.9 *[L99]*
specified NEC L98.8
slim (HIV) B20
small vessel I73.9
Sneddon-Wilkinson (subcorneal pustular dermatosis) L13.1
South African creeping B88.0
spinal (cord) G95.9
congenital Q06.9
specified NEC G95.89
spine — *see also* Spondylopathy
joint — *see* Dorsopathy
tuberculous A18.01
spinocerebellar (hereditary) G11.9
specified NEC G11.8
spleen D73.9
amyloid E85.4 *[D77]*
organic D73.9
polycystic Q89.09
postinfectional D73.89
sponge-diver's — *see* Toxicity, venom, marine animal, sea anemone
Startle Q89.8
Steinert's G71.11
Sticker's (erythema infectiosum) B08.3
Stieda's (calcification, knee joint) — *see* Bursitis, tibial collateral

DISLOCATION - DISLOCATION

Disorder (of) - *continued*
- amphetamine-type substance use - *continued*
  - severe F15.20
    - in remission (early) (sustained) F15.21
- amphetamine (or other stimulant) use
  - mild
    - with
      - amphetamine (or other stimulant) -induced
        - anxiety disorder F15.180
        - bipolar and related disorder F15.14
        - depressive disorder F15.14
        - obsessive-compulsive and related disorder F15.188
        - psychotic disorder F15.159
        - sexual dysfunction F15.181
      - amphetamine, cocaine, or other stimulant intoxication
        - with perceptual disturbances F15.122
        - without perceptual disturbances F15.129
      - intoxication delirium F15.121
  - moderate or severe
    - with
      - amphetamine (or other stimulant) -induced
        - anxiety disorder F15.280
        - obsessive-compulsive and related disorder F15.288
        - sexual dysfunction F15.281
        - bipolar and related disorder F15.24
        - depressive disorder F15.24
        - psychotic disorder F15.259
      - amphetamine, cocaine, or other stimulant intoxication
        - with perceptual disturbances F15.222
        - without perceptual disturbances F15.229
      - intoxication delirium F15.221
- anaerobic glycolysis with anemia D55.29
- anxiety F41.9
  - due to (secondary to)
    - alcohol F10.980
      - in
        - abuse F10.180
        - dependence F10.280
    - amphetamine F15.980
      - in
        - abuse F15.180
        - dependence F15.280
    - anxiolytic F13.980
      - in
        - abuse F13.180
        - dependence F13.280
    - caffeine F15.980
      - in
        - abuse F15.180
        - dependence F15.280
    - cannabis F12.980
      - in
        - abuse F12.180
        - dependence F12.280
    - cocaine F14.980
      - in
        - abuse F14.180
        - dependence F14.180
    - general medical condition F06.4
    - hallucinogen F16.980
      - in
        - abuse F16.180
        - dependence F16.280
    - hypnotic F13.980
      - in
        - abuse F13.180
        - dependence F13.280
    - inhalant F18.980
      - in
        - abuse F18.180
        - dependence F18.280
    - phencyclidine F16.980
      - in
        - abuse F16.180
        - dependence F16.280

Disorder (of) - *continued*
- anxiety - *continued*
  - due to (secondary to) - *continued*
    - psychoactive substance NEC F19.980
      - in
        - abuse F19.180
        - dependence F19.280
    - sedative F13.980
      - in
        - abuse F13.180
        - dependence F13.280
    - volatile solvents F18.980
      - in
        - abuse F18.180
        - dependence F18.280
  - generalized F41.1
  - illness F45.21
  - mixed
    - with depression (mild) F41.8
    - specified NEC F41.3
  - organic F06.4
  - phobic F40.9
    - of childhood F40.8
  - specified NEC F41.8
- aortic valve — *see* Endocarditis, aortic
- aromatic amino-acid metabolism E70.9
  - specified NEC E70.89
- arteriole NEC I77.89
- artery NEC I77.89
- articulation — *see* Disorder, joint
- attachment (childhood)
  - disinhibited F94.2
  - reactive F94.1
- attention-deficit hyperactivity (adolescent) (adult) (child) F90.9
  - combined
    - presentation F90.2
    - type F90.2
  - hyperactive
    - impulsive presentation F90.1
    - type F90.1
  - inattentive
    - presentation F90.0
    - type F90.0
  - specified type NEC F90.8
- attention-deficit without hyperactivity (adolescent) (adult) (child) F98.8
- auditory processing (central) H93.25
- autistic F84.0
- autism spectrum F84.0
- autoimmune D89.89
- autonomic nervous system G90.9
  - specified NEC G90.8
- avoidant
  - child or adolescent F40.10
  - restrictive food intake F50.82
- balance
  - acid-base E87.8
    - mixed E87.4
  - electrolyte E87.8
  - fluid NEC E87.8
- behavioral (disruptive) — *see* Disorder, conduct
- beta-amino-acid metabolism E72.89
- bile acid and cholesterol metabolism E78.70
  - Barth syndrome E78.71
  - other specified E78.79
  - Smith-Lemli-Opitz syndrome E78.72
- bilirubin excretion E80.6
- binge eating F50.81
- binocular
  - movement H51.9
    - convergence
      - excess H51.12
      - insufficiency H51.11
    - internuclear ophthalmoplegia — *see* Ophthalmoplegia, internuclear
    - palsy of conjugate gaze H51.0
    - specified type NEC H51.8
  - vision NEC — *see* Disorder, vision, binocular
- bipolar (I) (type 1) F31.9
  - and related due to a known physiological condition
    - with

Disorder (of) - *continued*
- bipolar (I) (type 1) - *continued*
  - and related due to a known physiological condition - *continued*
    - with - *continued*
      - manic features F06.33
      - manic- or hypomanic-like episodes F06.33
      - mixed features F06.34
  - current (or most recent) episode
    - depressed F31.9
      - with psychotic features F31.5
      - without psychotic features F31.30
        - mild F31.31
        - moderate F31.32
        - severe (without psychotic features) F31.4
          - with psychotic features F31.5
    - hypomanic F31.0
    - manic F31.9
      - with psychotic features F31.2
      - without psychotic features F31.10
        - mild F31.11
        - moderate F31.12
        - severe (without psychotic features) F31.13
          - with psychotic features F31.2
    - mixed F31.60
      - mild F31.61
      - moderate F31.62
      - severe (without psychotic features) F31.63
        - with psychotic features F31.64
    - severe depression (without psychotic features) F31.4
      - with psychotic features F31.5
  - in remission (currently) F31.70
    - in full remission
      - most recent episode
        - depressed F31.76
        - hypomanic F31.72
        - manic F31.74
        - mixed F31.78
    - in partial remission
      - most recent episode
        - depressed F31.75
        - hypomanic F31.71
        - manic F31.73
        - mixed F31.77
  - specified NEC F31.89
  - II (type 2) F31.81
  - organic F06.30
  - single manic episode F30.9
    - mild F30.11
    - moderate F30.12
    - severe (without psychotic symptoms) F30.13
      - with psychotic symptoms F30.2
- bladder N32.9
  - functional NEC N31.9
  - in schistosomiasis B65.0 *[N33]*
  - specified NEC N32.89
- bleeding D68.9
- blood D75.9
  - in congenital early syphilis A50.09 *[D77]*
- body dysmorphic F45.22
- bone M89.9
  - continuity M84.9
    - specified type NEC M84.80
      - ankle M84.87-
      - fibula M84.86-
      - foot M84.87-
      - hand M84.84-
      - humerus M84.82-
      - neck M84.88
      - pelvis M84.859
      - radius M84.83-
      - rib M84.88
      - shoulder M84.81-
      - skull M84.88
      - thigh M84.85-
      - tibia M84.86-
      - ulna M84.83-
      - vertebra M84.88
  - density and structure M85.9

- **Disorder (of)** - *continued*
  - ear - *continued*
    - middle - *continued*
      - specified NEC, in diseases classified elsewhere H75.8-
    - postprocedural — *see* Complications, ear, procedure
    - specified NEC, in diseases classified elsewhere H94.8-
  - eating (adult) (psychogenic) F50.9
    - anorexia — *see* Anorexia
    - binge F50.81
    - bulimia F50.2
    - child F98.29
      - pica F98.3
      - rumination disorder F98.21
    - pica F50.89
      - childhood F98.3
  - electrolyte (balance) NEC E87.8
    - with
      - abortion — *see* Abortion by type complicated by specified condition NEC
      - ectopic pregnancy O08.5
      - molar pregnancy O08.5
    - acidosis (metabolic) (respiratory) E87.2
    - alkalosis (metabolic) (respiratory) E87.3
  - elimination, transepidermal L87.9
    - specified NEC L87.8
  - emotional (persistent) F34.9
    - of childhood F93.9
      - specified NEC F93.8
  - endocrine E34.9
    - postprocedural E89.89
      - specified NEC E89.89
  - erectile (male) (organic) — *see also* Dysfunction, sexual, male, erectile N52.9
    - nonorganic F52.21
  - erythematous — *see* Erythema
  - esophagus K22.9
    - functional K22.4
    - psychogenic F45.8
  - eustachian tube H69.9-
    - infection — *see* Salpingitis, eustachian
    - obstruction — *see* Obstruction, eustachian tube
    - patulous — *see* Patulous, eustachian tube
    - specified NEC H69.8-
  - exhibitionistic F65.2
  - extrapyramidal G25.9
    - in diseases classified elsewhere — *see* category G26
    - specified type NEC G25.89
  - eye H57.9
    - postprocedural — *see* Complication, postprocedural, eye
  - eyelid H02.9
    - cyst — *see* Cyst, eyelid
    - degenerative H02.70
      - chloasma — *see* Chloasma, eyelid
      - madarosis — *see* Madarosis
      - specified type NEC H02.79
      - vitiligo — *see* Vitiligo, eyelid
      - xanthelasma — *see* Xanthelasma
    - dermatochalasis — *see* Dermatochalasis
    - edema — *see* Edema, eyelid
    - elephantiasis — *see* Elephantiasis, eyelid
    - foreign body, retained — *see* Foreign body, retained, eyelid
    - function H02.59
      - abnormal innervation syndrome — *see* Syndrome, abnormal innervation
      - blepharochalasis — *see* Blepharochalasis
      - blepharoclonus — *see* Blepharoclonus
      - blepharophimosis — *see* Blepharophimosis
      - blepharoptosis — *see* Blepharoptosis
      - lagophthalmos — *see* Lagophthalmos
      - lid retraction — *see* Retraction, lid
    - hypertrichosis — *see* Hypertrichosis, eyelid
    - specified type NEC H02.89
    - vascular H02.879

- **Disorder (of)** - *continued*
  - eyelid - *continued*
    - vascular - *continued*
      - left H02.876
        - lower H02.875
        - upper H02.874
      - right H02.873
        - lower H02.872
        - upper H02.871
  - factitious
    - by proxy F68.A
    - imposed on another F68.A
    - imposed on self F68.10
      - with predominantly
        - psychological symptoms F68.11
          - with physical symptoms F68.13
        - physical symptoms F68.12
          - with psychological symptoms F68.13
  - factor, coagulation — *see* Defect, coagulation
  - fatty acid
    - metabolism E71.30
      - specified NEC E71.39
    - oxidation
      - LCAD E71.310
      - MCAD E71.311
      - SCAD E71.312
      - specified deficiency NEC E71.318
  - feeding (infant or child) — *see also* Disorder, eating R63.30
    - pediatric
      - acute R63.31
      - chronic R63.32
    - or eating disorder F50.9
    - specified NEC F50.9
  - feigned (with obvious motivation) Z76.5
    - without obvious motivation — *see* Disorder, factitious
  - female
    - hypoactive sexual desire F52.0
    - orgasmic F52.31
    - sexual interest/arousal F52.22
  - fetishistic F65.0
  - fibroblastic M72.9
    - specified NEC M72.8
  - fluency
    - adult onset F98.5
    - childhood onset F80.81
    - following
      - cerebral infarction I69.323
      - cerebrovascular disease I69.923
        - specified disease NEC I69.823
      - intracerebral hemorrhage I69.123
      - nontraumatic intracranial hemorrhage NEC I69.223
      - subarachnoid hemorrhage I69.023
    - in conditions classified elsewhere R47.82
  - fluid balance E87.8
  - follicular (skin) L73.9
    - specified NEC L73.8
  - frotteuristic F65.81
  - fructose metabolism E74.10
    - essential fructosuria E74.11
    - fructokinase deficiency E74.11
    - fructose-1, 6-diphosphatase deficiency E74.19
    - hereditary fructose intolerance E74.12
    - other specified E74.19
  - functional polymorphonuclear neutrophils D71
  - gallbladder, biliary tract and pancreas in diseases classified elsewhere K87
  - gambling F63.0
  - gamma aminobutyric acid (GABA) metabolism E72.81
  - gamma-glutamyl cycle E72.89
  - gastric (functional) K31.9
    - motility K30
    - psychogenic F45.8
    - secretion K30
  - gastrointestinal (functional) NOS K92.9
    - newborn P78.9
    - psychogenic F45.8
  - gender-identity or -role F64.9

- **Disorder (of)** - *continued*
  - gender-identity or -role - *continued*
    - childhood F64.2
    - effect on relationship F66
    - of adolescence or adulthood F64.0
      - nontranssexual F64.8
    - specified NEC F64.8
    - uncertainty F66
  - genito-pelvic pain penetration F52.6
  - genitourinary system
    - female N94.9
    - male N50.9
    - psychogenic F45.8
  - globe H44.9
    - degenerated condition H44.50
      - absolute glaucoma H44.51-
      - atrophy H44.52-
      - leucocoria H44.53-
    - degenerative H44.30
      - chalcosis H44.31-
      - myopia — *see also* Myopia, degenerative H44.2-
      - siderosis H44.32-
      - specified type NEC H44.39-
    - endophthalmitis — *see* Endophthalmitis
    - foreign body, retained — *see* Foreign body, intraocular, old, retained
    - hemophthalmos — *see* Hemophthalmos
    - hypotony H44.40
      - due to
        - ocular fistula H44.42-
        - specified disorder NEC H44.43-
      - flat anterior chamber H44.41-
      - primary H44.44-
    - luxation — *see* Luxation, globe
    - specified type NEC H44.89
  - glomerular (in) N05.9
    - amyloidosis E85.4 *[N08]*
    - cryoglobulinemia D89.1 *[N08]*
    - disseminated intravascular coagulation D65 *[N08]*
    - Fabry's disease E75.21 *[N08]*
    - familial lecithin cholesterol acyltransferase deficiency E78.6 *[N08]*
    - Goodpasture's syndrome M31.0
    - hemolytic-uremic syndrome D59.3
    - Henoch (-Schönlein) purpura D69.0 *[N08]*
    - malariae malaria B52.0
    - microscopic polyangiitis M31.7 *[N08]*
    - multiple myeloma C90.0- *[N08]*
    - mumps B26.83
    - schistosomiasis B65.9 *[N08]*
    - sepsis NEC A41.- *[N08]*
      - streptococcal A40.- *[N08]*
    - sickle-cell disorders D57.- *[N08]*
    - strongyloidiasis B78.9 *[N08]*
    - subacute bacterial endocarditis I33.0 *[N08]*
    - syphilis A52.75
    - systemic lupus erythematosus M32.14
    - thrombotic thrombocytopenic purpura M31.19 *[N08]*
    - Waldenström macroglobulinemia C88.0 *[N08]*
    - Wegener's granulomatosis M31.31
  - gluconeogenesis E74.4
  - glucosaminoglycan metabolism — *see* Disorder, metabolism, glucosaminoglycan
  - glucose transport E74.819
    - specified NEC E74.818
  - glycine metabolism E72.50
    - d-glycericacidemia E72.59
    - hyperhydroxyprolinemia E72.59
    - hyperoxaluria R82.992
      - primary E72.53
    - hyperprolinemia E72.59
    - non-ketotic hyperglycinemia E72.51
    - oxalosis E72.53
    - oxaluria E72.53
    - sarcosinemia E72.59
    - trimethylaminuria E72.52
  - glycoprotein metabolism E77.9
    - specified NEC E77.8
  - habit (and impulse) F63.9
    - involving sexual behavior NEC F65.9

Disorder (of) - *continued*
habit (and impulse) - *continued*
specified NEC F63.89
hallucinogen use
mild F16.10
with
hallucinogen-induced
anxiety disorder F16.180
bipolar and related disorder F16.14
depressive disorder F16.14
psychotic disorder F16.159
hallucinogen intoxication delirium F16.121
other hallucinogen intoxication F16.129
in remission (early) (sustained) F16.11
moderate or severe F16.20
with
hallucinogen-induced
anxiety disorder F16.280
bipolar and related disorder F16.24
depressive disorder F16.24
psychotic disorder F16.259
hallucinogen intoxication delirium F16.221
other hallucinogen intoxication F16.229
in remission (early) (sustained) F16.21
heart action I49.9
hematological D75.9
newborn (transient) P61.9
specified NEC P61.8
hematopoietic organs D75.9
hemorrhagic NEC D69.9
drug-induced D68.32
due to
extrinsic circulating anticoagulants D68.32
increase in
anti-IIa D68.32
anti-Xa D68.32
intrinsic
circulating anticoagulants D68.318
increase in
antithrombin D68.318
anti-VIIIa D68.318
anti-IXa D68.318
anti-XIa D68.318
following childbirth O72.3
hemostasis — *see* Defect, coagulation
histidine metabolism E70.40
histidinemia E70.41
other specified E70.49
hoarding F42.3
hyperkinetic — *see* Disorder, attention-deficit hyperactivity
hyperleucine-isoleucinemia E71.19
hypervalinemia E71.19
hypoactive sexual desire F52.0
hypochondriacal F45.20
body dysmorphic F45.22
neurosis F45.21
other specified F45.29
identity
dissociative F44.81
of childhood F93.8
illness anxiety F45.21
immune mechanism (immunity) D89.9
specified type NEC D89.89
impaired renal tubular function N25.9
specified NEC N25.89
impulse (control) F63.9
inflammatory
pelvic, in diseases classified elsewhere — *see* category N74
penis N48.29
abscess N48.21
cellulitis N48.22
inhalant use
mild F18.10
with
inhalant-induced
anxiety disorder F18.180
depressive disorder F18.14

Disorder (of) - *continued*
inhalant use - *continued*
mild - *continued*
with - *continued*
inhalant-induced - *continued*
major neurocognitive disorder F18.17
mild neurocognitive disorder F18.188
psychotic disorder F18.159
inhalant intoxication F18.129
inhalant intoxication delirium F18.121
in remission (early) (sustained) F18.11
moderate or severe F18.20
with
inhalant-induced
anxiety disorder F18.280
depressive disorder F18.24
major neurocognitive disorder F18.27
mild neurocognitive disorder F18.288
psychotic disorder F18.259
inhalant intoxication F18.229
inhalant intoxication delirium F18.221
in remission (early) (sustained) F18.21
integument, newborn P83.9
specified NEC P83.88
intermittent explosive F63.81
internal secretion pancreas — *see* Increased, secretion, pancreas, endocrine
intestine, intestinal
carbohydrate absorption NEC E74.39
postoperative K91.2
functional NEC K59.9
postoperative K91.89
psychogenic F45.8
vascular K55.9
chronic K55.1
specified NEC K55.8
intraoperative (intraprocedural) — *see* Complications, intraoperative
involuntary emotional expression (IEED) F48.2
iris H21.9
adhesions — *see* Adhesions, iris
atrophy — *see* Atrophy, iris
chamber angle recession — *see* Recession, chamber angle
cyst — *see* Cyst, iris
degeneration — *see* Degeneration, iris
in diseases classified elsewhere H22
iridodialysis — *see* Iridodialysis
iridoschisis — *see* Iridoschisis
miotic pupillary cyst — *see* Cyst, pupillary
pupillary
abnormality — *see* Abnormality, pupillary
membrane — *see* Membrane, pupillary
specified type NEC H21.89
vascular NEC H21.1X-
iron metabolism E83.10
specified NEC E83.19
isovaleric acidemia E71.110
jaw, developmental M27.0
temporomandibular — *see also* Anomaly, dentofacial, temporomandibular joint M26.60-
joint M25.9
derangement — *see* Derangement, joint
effusion — *see* Effusion, joint
fistula — *see* Fistula, joint
hemarthrosis — *see* Hemarthrosis
instability — *see* Instability, joint
osteophyte — *see* Osteophyte
pain — *see* Pain, joint
psychogenic F45.8
specified type NEC M25.80
ankle M25.87-
elbow M25.82-
foot joint M25.87-
hand joint M25.84-
hip M25.85-
knee M25.86-
shoulder M25.81-

Disorder (of) - *continued*
joint - *continued*
specified type NEC - *continued*
wrist M25.83-
stiffness — *see* Stiffness, joint
ketone metabolism E71.32
kidney N28.9
functional (tubular) N25.9
in
schistosomiasis B65.9 *[N29]*
tubular function N25.9
specified NEC N25.89
lacrimal system H04.9
changes H04.69
fistula — *see* Fistula, lacrimal
gland H04.19
atrophy — *see* Atrophy, lacrimal gland
cyst — *see* Cyst, lacrimal, gland
dacryops — *see* Dacryops
dislocation — *see* Dislocation, lacrimal gland
dry eye syndrome — *see* Syndrome, dry eye
infection — *see* Dacryoadenitis
granuloma — *see* Granuloma, lacrimal
inflammation — *see* Inflammation, lacrimal
obstruction — *see* Obstruction, lacrimal
specified NEC H04.89
lactation NEC O92.79
language (developmental) F80.9
expressive F80.1
mixed receptive and expressive F80.2
receptive F80.2
late luteal phase dysphoric N94.89
learning (specific) F81.9
acalculia R48.8
alexia R48.0
mathematics F81.2
reading F81.0
specified
with impairment in
mathematics F81.2
reading F81.0
written expression F81.81
specified NEC F81.89
spelling F81.81
written expression F81.81
lens H27.9
aphakia — *see* Aphakia
cataract — *see* Cataract
dislocation — *see* Dislocation, lens
specified type NEC H27.8
ligament M24.20
ankle M24.27-
attachment, spine — *see* Enthesopathy, spinal
elbow M24.22-
foot joint M24.27-
hand joint M24.24-
hip M24.25-
knee — *see* Derangement, knee, specified NEC
shoulder M24.21-
specified site NEC M24.29
vertebra M24.28
wrist M24.23-
ligamentous attachments — *see also* Enthesopathy
spine — *see* Enthesopathy, spinal
lipid
metabolism, congenital E78.9
storage E75.6
specified NEC E75.5
lipoprotein
deficiency (familial) E78.6
metabolism E78.9
specified NEC E78.89
liver K76.9
malarial B54 *[K77]*
low back — *see also* Dorsopathy, specified NEC
lumbosacral
plexus G54.1
root (nerve) NEC G54.4

DISORDER - DISORDER

- **Disorder (of)** - *continued*
  - opioid use - *continued*
    - moderate or severe - *continued*
      - with - *continued*
        - opioid intoxication - *continued*
          - with perceptual disturbances F11.222
          - delirium F11.221
          - without perceptual disturbances F11.229
      - in remission (early) (sustained) F11.21
  - oppositional defiant F91.3
  - optic
    - chiasm H47.49
      - due to
        - inflammatory disorder H47.41
        - neoplasm H47.42
        - vascular disorder H47.43
    - disc H47.39-
      - coloboma — *see* Coloboma, optic disc
      - drusen — *see* Drusen, optic disc
      - pseudopapilledema — *see* Pseudopapilledema
    - radiations — *see* Disorder, visual, pathway
    - tracts — *see* Disorder, visual, pathway
  - orbit H05.9
    - cyst — *see* Cyst, orbit
    - deformity — *see* Deformity, orbit
    - edema — *see* Edema, orbit
    - enophthalmos — *see* Enophthalmos
    - exophthalmos — *see* Exophthalmos
    - hemorrhage — *see* Hemorrhage, orbit
    - inflammation — *see* Inflammation, orbit
    - myopathy — *see* Myopathy, extraocular muscles
    - retained foreign body — *see* Foreign body, orbit, old
    - specified type NEC H05.89
  - organic
    - anxiety F06.4
    - catatonic F06.1
    - delusional F06.2
    - dissociative F06.8
    - emotionally labile (asthenic) F06.8
    - mood (affective) F06.30
    - schizophrenia-like F06.2
  - orgasmic (female) F52.31
    - male F52.32
  - ornithine metabolism E72.4
  - overanxious F41.1
    - of childhood F93.8
  - pain
    - with related psychological factors F45.42
    - exclusively related to psychological factors F45.41
    - genito-pelvic penetration disorder F52.6
  - pancreatic internal secretion E16.9
    - specified NEC E16.8
  - panic F41.0
    - with agoraphobia F40.01
  - papulosquamous L44.9
    - in diseases classified elsewhere L45
    - specified NEC L44.8
  - paranoid F22
    - induced F24
    - shared F24
  - paraphilic F65.9
    - specified NEC F65.89
  - parathyroid (gland) E21.5
    - specified NEC E21.4
  - parietoalveolar NEC J84.09
  - paroxysmal, mixed R56.9
  - patella M22.9-
    - chondromalacia — *see* Chondromalacia, patella
    - derangement NEC M22.3X-
    - recurrent
      - dislocation — *see* Dislocation, patella, recurrent
      - subluxation — *see* Dislocation, patella, recurrent, incomplete
    - specified NEC M22.8X-
  - patellofemoral M22.2X-
  - pedophilic F65.4

- **Disorder (of)** - *continued*
  - pentose phosphate pathway with anemia D55.1
  - perception, due to hallucinogens F16.983
    - in
      - abuse F16.183
      - dependence F16.283
  - peripheral nervous system NEC G64
  - peroxisomal E71.50
    - biogenesis
      - neonatal adrenoleukodystrophy E71.511
      - specified disorder NEC E71.518
      - Zellweger syndrome E71.510
    - rhizomelic chondrodysplasia punctata E71.540
    - specified form NEC E71.548
      - group 1 E71.518
      - group 2 E71.53
      - group 3 E71.542
    - X-linked adrenoleukodystrophy E71.529
      - adolescent E71.521
      - adrenomyeloneuropathy E71.522
      - childhood E71.520
      - specified form NEC E71.528
    - Zellweger-like syndrome E71.541
  - persistent
    - (somatoform) pain F45.41
    - affective (mood) F34.9
  - personality — *see also* Personality F60.9
    - affective F34.0
    - aggressive F60.3
    - amoral F60.2
    - anankastic F60.5
    - antisocial F60.2
    - anxious F60.6
    - asocial F60.2
    - asthenic F60.7
    - avoidant F60.6
    - borderline F60.3
    - change (secondary) due to general medical condition F07.0
    - compulsive F60.5
    - cyclothymic F34.0
    - dependent (passive) F60.7
    - depressive F34.1
    - dissocial F60.2
    - emotional instability F60.3
    - expansive paranoid F60.0
    - explosive F60.3
    - following organic brain damage F07.9
    - histrionic F60.4
    - hyperthymic F34.0
    - hypothymic F34.1
    - hysterical F60.4
    - immature F60.89
    - inadequate F60.7
    - labile F60.3
    - mixed (nonspecific) F60.89
    - moral deficiency F60.2
    - narcissistic F60.81
    - negativistic F60.89
    - obsessional F60.5
    - obsessive (-compulsive) F60.5
    - organic F07.9
    - overconscientious F60.5
    - paranoid F60.0
    - passive (-dependent) F60.7
    - passive-aggressive F60.89
    - pathological NEC F60.9
    - pseudosocial F60.2
    - psychopathic F60.2
    - schizoid F60.1
    - schizotypal F21
    - self-defeating F60.7
    - specified NEC F60.89
    - type A F60.5
    - unstable (emotional) F60.3
  - pervasive, developmental F84.9
  - phencyclidine use
    - mild F16.10
      - with
        - phencyclidine-induced
          - anxiety disorder F16.180
          - bipolar and related disorder F16.14
          - depressive disorder F16.14

- **Disorder (of)** - *continued*
  - phencyclidine use - *continued*
    - mild - *continued*
      - with - *continued*
        - phencyclidine-induced - *continued*
          - psychotic disorder F16.159
        - phencyclidine intoxication F16.129
        - phencyclidine intoxication delirium F16.121
      - in remission (early) (sustained) F16.11
    - moderate or severe F16.20
      - with
        - phencyclidine-induced
          - anxiety disorder F16.280
          - bipolar and related disorder F16.24
          - depressive disorder F16.24
          - psychotic disorder F16.259
        - phencyclidine intoxication F16.229
        - phencyclidine intoxication delirium F16.221
      - in remission (early) (sustained) F16.21
  - phobic anxiety, childhood F40.8
  - phosphate-losing tubular N25.0
  - pigmentation L81.9
    - choroid, congenital Q14.3
    - diminished melanin formation L81.6
    - iron L81.8
    - specified NEC L81.8
  - pinna (noninfective) H61.10-
    - deformity, acquired H61.11-
    - hematoma H61.12-
    - perichondritis — *see* Perichondritis, ear
    - specified type NEC H61.19-
  - pituitary gland E23.7
    - iatrogenic (postprocedural) E89.3
    - specified NEC E23.6
  - platelets D69.1
  - plexus G54.9
    - specified NEC G54.8
  - polymorphonuclear neutrophils D71
  - porphyrin metabolism — *see* Porphyria
  - postconcussional F07.81
  - posthallucinogen perception F16.983
    - in
      - abuse F16.183
      - dependence F16.283
  - postmenopausal N95.9
    - specified NEC N95.8
  - postprocedural (postoperative) — *see* Complications, postprocedural
  - post-transplant lymphoproliferative D47.Z1
  - post-traumatic stress (PTSD) F43.10
    - acute F43.11
    - chronic F43.12
  - premenstrual dysphoric (PMDD) F32.81
  - prepuce N47.8
  - propionic acidemia E71.121
  - prostate N42.9
    - specified NEC N42.89
  - psychogenic NOS — *see also* condition F45.9
    - anxiety F41.8
    - appetite F50.9
    - asthenic F48.8
    - cardiovascular (system) F45.8
    - compulsive F42.8
    - cutaneous F54
    - depressive F32.9
    - digestive (system) F45.8
    - dysmenorrheic F45.8
    - dyspneic F45.8
    - endocrine (system) F54
    - eye NEC F45.8
    - feeding — *see* Disorder, eating
    - functional NEC F45.8
    - gastric F45.8
    - gastrointestinal (system) F45.8
    - genitourinary (system) F45.8
    - heart (function) (rhythm) F45.8
    - hyperventilatory F45.8
    - hypochondriacal — *see* Disorder, hypochondriacal
    - intestinal F45.8
    - joint F45.8
    - learning F81.9

Disorder (of) - *continued*
psychogenic NOS - *continued*
limb F45.8
lymphatic (system) F45.8
menstrual F45.8
micturition F45.8
monoplegic NEC F44.4
motor F44.4
muscle F45.8
musculoskeletal F45.8
neurocirculatory F45.8
obsessive F42.8
occupational F48.8
organ or part of body NEC F45.8
paralytic NEC F44.4
phobic F40.9
physical NEC F45.8
rectal F45.8
respiratory (system) F45.8
rheumatic F45.8
sexual (function) F52.9
skin (allergic) (eczematous) F54
sleep F51.9
specified part of body NEC F45.8
stomach F45.8
psychological F99
associated with
disease classified elsewhere F54
sexual
development F66
relationship F66
uncertainty about gender identity F64.9
psychomotor NEC F44.4
hysterical F44.4
psychoneurotic — *see also* Neurosis
mixed NEC F48.8
psychophysiologic — *see* Disorder, somatoform
psychosexual F65.9
development F66
identity of childhood F64.2
psychosomatic NOS — *see* Disorder, somatoform
multiple F45.0
undifferentiated F45.1
psychotic — *see* Psychosis
transient (acute) F23
puberty E30.9
specified NEC E30.8
pulmonary (valve) — *see* Endocarditis, pulmonary
purine metabolism E79.9
pyrimidine metabolism E79.9
pyruvate metabolism E74.4
reactive attachment (childhood) F94.1
reading R48.0
developmental (specific) F81.0
receptive language F80.2
receptor, hormonal, peripheral — *see also* Syndrome, androgen insensitivity E34.50
recurrent brief depressive F33.8
reflex R29.2
refraction H52.7
aniseikonia H52.32
anisometropia H52.31
astigmatism — *see* Astigmatism
hypermetropia — *see* Hypermetropia
myopia — *see* Myopia
presbyopia H52.4
specified NEC H52.6
relationship F68.8
due to sexual orientation F66
REM sleep behavior G47.52
renal function, impaired (tubular) N25.9
resonance R49.9
specified NEC R49.8
respiratory function, impaired — *see also* Failure, respiration
postprocedural — *see* Complication, postoperative, respiratory system
psychogenic F45.8
retina H35.9
angioid streaks H35.33
changes in vascular appearance H35.01-

Disorder (of) - *continued*
retina - *continued*
degeneration — *see* Degeneration, retina
dystrophy (hereditary) — *see* Dystrophy, retina
edema H35.81
hemorrhage — *see* Hemorrhage, retina
ischemia H35.82
macular degeneration — *see* Degeneration, macula
microaneurysms H35.04-
microvascular abnormality NEC H35.09
neovascularization — *see* Neovascularization, retina
retinopathy — *see* Retinopathy
separation of layers H35.70
central serous chorioretinopathy H35.71-
pigment epithelium detachment (serous) H35.72-
hemorrhagic H35.73-
specified type NEC H35.89
telangiectasis — *see* Telangiectasis, retina
vasculitis — *see* Vasculitis, retina
retroperitoneal K68.9
right hemisphere organic affective F07.89
rumination (infant or child) F98.21
sacrum, sacrococcygeal NEC M53.3
schizoaffective F25.9
bipolar type F25.0
depressive type F25.1
manic type F25.0
mixed type F25.0
specified NEC F25.8
schizoid of childhood F84.5
schizophrenia spectrum and other psychotic disorder F29
specified NEC F28
schizophreniform F20.81
brief F23
schizotypal (personality) F21
secretion, thyrocalcitonin E07.0
sedative, hypnotic, or anxiolytic use
mild F13.10
with
sedative, hypnotic, or anxiolytic-induced
anxiety disorder F13.180
bipolar and related disorder F13.14
depressive disorder F13.14
psychotic disorder F13.159
sexual dysfunction F13.181
sedative, hypnotic, or anxiolytic intoxication F13.129
sedative, hypnotic, or anxiolytic intoxication delirium F13.121
in remission (early) (sustained) F13.11
moderate or severe F13.20
with
sedative, hypnotic, or anxiolytic-induced
anxiety disorder F13.280
bipolar and related disorder F13.24
depressive disorder F13.24
major neurocognitive disorder F13.27
mild neurocognitive disorder F13.288
psychotic disorder F13.259
sexual dysfunction F13.281
sedative, hypnotic, or anxiolytic intoxication F13.229
sedative, hypnotic, or anxiolytic intoxication delirium F13.221
in remission (early) (sustained) F13.21
seizure — *see also* Epilepsy G40.909
intractable G40.919
with status epilepticus G40.911
semantic pragmatic F80.89
with autism F84.0
sense of smell R43.1
psychogenic F45.8
separation anxiety, of childhood F93.0
sexual
arousal, female F52.22
aversion F52.1

Disorder (of) - *continued*
sexual - *continued*
function, psychogenic F52.9
interest/arousal, female F52.22
masochism F65.51
maturation F66
nonorganic F52.9
preference — *see also* Deviation, sexual F65.9
fetishistic transvestism F65.1
relationship F66
sadism F65.52
shyness, of childhood and adolescence F40.10
sibling rivalry F93.8
sickle-cell (sickling) (homozygous) — *see* Disease, sickle-cell
heterozygous D57.3
specified type NEC D57.8-
trait D57.3
sinus (nasal) J34.9
specified NEC J34.89
skin L98.9
atrophic L90.9
specified NEC L90.8
granulomatous L92.9
specified NEC L92.8
hypertrophic L91.9
specified NEC L91.8
infiltrative NEC L98.6
newborn P83.9
specified NEC P83.88
picking F42.4
psychogenic (allergic) (eczematous) F54
sleep G47.9
breathing-related — *see* Apnea, sleep
circadian rhythm G47.20
advance sleep phase type G47.22
delayed sleep phase type G47.21
due to
alcohol
abuse F10.182
dependence F10.282
use F10.982
amphetamines
abuse F15.182
dependence F15.282
use F15.982
caffeine
abuse F15.182
dependence F15.282
use F15.982
cocaine
abuse F14.182
dependence F14.282
use F14.982
drug NEC
abuse F19.182
dependence F19.282
use F19.982
opioid
abuse F11.182
dependence F11.282
use F11.982
psychoactive substance NEC
abuse F19.182
dependence F19.282
use F19.982
sedative, hypnotic, or anxiolytic
abuse F13.182
dependence F13.282
use F13.982
stimulant NEC
abuse F15.182
dependence F15.282
use F15.982
free running type G47.24
in conditions classified elsewhere G47.27
irregular sleep wake type G47.23
jet lag type G47.25
non-24-hour sleep-wake type G47.24
shift work type G47.26
specified NEC G47.29
due to

- **Disorder (of)** - *continued*
  - sleep - *continued*
    - due to - *continued*
      - alcohol
        - abuse F10.182
        - dependence F10.282
        - use F10.982
      - amphetamine
        - abuse F15.182
        - dependence F15.282
        - use F15.982
      - anxiolytic
        - abuse F13.182
        - dependence F13.282
        - use F13.982
      - caffeine
        - abuse F15.182
        - dependence F15.282
        - use F15.982
      - cocaine
        - abuse F14.182
        - dependence F14.282
        - use F14.982
      - drug NEC
        - abuse F19.182
        - dependence F19.282
        - use F19.982
      - hypnotic
        - abuse F13.182
        - dependence F13.282
        - use F13.982
      - opioid
        - abuse F11.182
        - dependence F11.282
        - use F11.982
      - psychoactive substance NEC
        - abuse F19.182
        - dependence F19.282
        - use F19.982
      - sedative
        - abuse F13.182
        - dependence F13.282
        - use F13.982
      - stimulant NEC
        - abuse F15.182
        - dependence F15.282
        - use F15.982
    - emotional F51.9
    - excessive somnolence — *see* Hypersomnia
    - hypersomnia type — *see* Hypersomnia
    - initiating or maintaining — *see* Insomnia
    - nightmares F51.5
    - nonorganic F51.9
      - specified NEC F51.8
    - parasomnia type G47.50
    - specified NEC G47.8
    - terrors F51.4
    - walking F51.3
  - sleep-wake pattern or schedule — *see also* Disorder, sleep, circadian rhythm G47.9
    - specified NEC G47.8
  - social
    - anxiety (of childhood) F40.10
      - generalized F40.11
    - functioning in childhood F94.9
      - specified NEC F94.8
    - pragmatic F80.82
  - soft tissue M79.9
    - ankle M79.9
    - due to use, overuse and pressure M70.90
      - ankle M70.97-
      - bursitis — *see* Bursitis
      - foot M70.97-
      - forearm M70.93-
      - hand M70.94-
      - lower leg M70.96-
      - multiple sites M70.99
      - pelvic region M70.95-
      - shoulder region M70.91-
      - specified site NEC M70.98
      - specified type NEC M70.80
        - ankle M70.87-
        - foot M70.87-
        - forearm M70.83-

- **Disorder (of)** - *continued*
  - soft tissue - *continued*
    - due to use, overuse and pressure - *continued*
      - specified type NEC - *continued*
        - hand M70.84-
        - lower leg M70.86-
        - multiple sites M70.89
        - pelvic region M70.85-
        - shoulder region M70.81-
        - specified site NEC M70.88
        - thigh M70.85-
        - upper arm M70.82-
      - thigh M70.95-
      - upper arm M70.92-
    - foot M79.9
    - forearm M79.9
    - hand M79.9
    - lower leg M79.9
    - multiple sites M79.9
    - occupational — *see* Disorder, soft tissue, due to use, overuse and pressure
    - pelvic region M79.9
    - shoulder region M79.9
    - specified type NEC M79.89
    - thigh M79.9
    - upper arm M79.9
  - somatic symptom F45.1
  - somatization F45.0
  - somatoform F45.9
    - pain (persistent) F45.41
    - somatization (multiple) (long-lasting) F45.0
    - specified NEC F45.8
    - undifferentiated F45.1
  - somnolence, excessive — *see* Hypersomnia
  - specific
    - arithmetical F81.2
    - developmental, of motor F82
    - reading F81.0
    - speech and language F80.9
    - spelling F81.81
    - written expression F81.81
  - speech R47.9
    - articulation (functional) (specific) F80.0
    - developmental F80.9
    - specified NEC R47.89
  - speech-sound F80.0
  - spelling (specific) F81.81
  - spine — *see also* Dorsopathy
    - ligamentous or muscular attachments, peripheral — *see* Enthesopathy, spinal
    - specified NEC — *see* Dorsopathy, specified NEC
  - stereotyped, habit or movement F98.4
  - stimulant use (other) (unspecified)
    - mild F15.10
      - in remission (early) (sustained) F15.11
    - moderate or severe F15.20
      - in remission (early) (sustained) F15.21
  - stomach (functional) — *see* Disorder, gastric
  - stress F43.9
    - acute F43.0
    - post-traumatic F43.10
      - acute F43.11
      - chronic F43.12
  - substance use (other) (unknown)
    - mild F19.10
      - with substance-induced
        - anxiety disorder F19.180
        - bipolar and related disorder F19.14
        - depressive disorder F19.14
        - major neurocognitive disorder F19.17
        - mild neurocognitive disorder F19.188
        - obsessive-compulsive and related disorder F19.188
        - sexual dysfunction F19.181
      - substance intoxication F19.129
      - substance intoxication delirium F19.121
    - moderate or severe F19.20
      - with substance-induced
        - anxiety disorder F19.280
        - bipolar and related disorder F19.24
        - depressive disorder F19.24
        - major neurocognitive disorder F19.27

- **Disorder (of)** - *continued*
  - substance use (other) (unknown) - *continued*
    - moderate or severe - *continued*
      - with substance-induced - *continued*
        - mild neurocognitive disorder F19.288
        - obsessive-compulsive and related disorder F19.288
        - sexual dysfunction F19.281
      - in remission (early) (sustained) F19.21
      - substance intoxication F19.229
      - substance intoxication delirium F19.221
  - sulfur-bearing amino-acid metabolism E72.10
  - sweat gland (eccrine) L74.9
    - apocrine L75.9
      - specified NEC L75.8
    - specified NEC L74.8
  - synovium M67.90
    - acromioclavicular M67.91-
    - ankle M67.97-
    - elbow M67.92-
    - foot M67.97-
    - forearm M67.93-
    - hand M67.94-
    - hip M67.95-
    - knee M67.96-
    - multiple sites M67.99
    - rupture — *see* Rupture, synovium
    - shoulder M67.91-
    - specified type NEC M67.80
      - acromioclavicular M67.81-
      - ankle M67.87-
      - elbow M67.82-
      - foot M67.87-
      - hand M67.84-
      - hip M67.85-
      - knee M67.86-
      - multiple sites M67.89
      - wrist M67.83-
    - synovitis — *see* Synovitis
    - upper arm M67.92-
    - wrist M67.93-
  - temperature regulation, newborn P81.9
    - specified NEC P81.8
  - temporomandibular joint M26.60-
  - tendon M67.90
    - acromioclavicular M67.91-
    - ankle M67.97-
    - contracture — *see* Contracture, tendon
    - elbow M67.92-
    - foot M67.97-
    - forearm M67.93-
    - hand M67.94-
    - hip M67.95-
    - knee M67.96-
    - multiple sites M67.99
    - rupture — *see* Rupture, tendon
    - shoulder M67.91-
    - specified type NEC M67.80
      - acromioclavicular M67.81-
      - ankle M67.87-
      - elbow M67.82-
      - foot M67.87-
      - hand M67.84-
      - hip M67.85-
      - knee M67.86-
      - multiple sites M67.89
      - trunk M67.88
      - wrist M67.83-
    - synovitis — *see* Synovitis
    - tendinitis — *see* Tendinitis
    - tenosynovitis — *see* Tenosynovitis
    - trunk M67.98
    - upper arm M67.92-
    - wrist M67.93-
  - thoracic root (nerve) NEC G54.3
  - thyrocalcitonin hypersecretion E07.0
  - thyroid (gland) E07.9
    - function NEC, neonatal, transitory P72.2
    - iodine-deficiency related E01.8
    - specified NEC E07.89
  - tic — *see* Tic
  - tobacco use
    - chewing tobacco (mild) (moderate) (severe)

Disorder (of) - *continued*
tobacco use - *continued*
chewing tobacco (mild) (moderate) (severe) - *continued*
in remission (early) (sustained) F17.221
cigarettes (mild) (moderate) (severe)
in remission (early) (sustained) F17.211
mild F17.200
in remission (early) (sustained) F17.201
moderate F17.200
in remission (early) (sustained) F17.201
severe F17.200
in remission (early) (sustained) F17.201
specified product NEC (mild) (moderate) (severe)
in remission (early) (sustained) F17.291
tooth K08.9
development K00.9
specified NEC K00.8
eruption K00.6
Tourette's F95.2
trance and possession F44.89
transvestic F65.1
trauma and stressor-related F43.9
other specified F43.8
tricuspid (valve) — *see* Endocarditis, tricuspid
tryptophan metabolism E70.5
tubular, phosphate-losing N25.0
tubulo-interstitial (in)
brucellosis A23.9 *[N16]*
cystinosis E72.04
diphtheria A36.84
glycogen storage disease E74.00 *[N16]*
leukemia NEC C95.9- *[N16]*
lymphoma NEC C85.9- *[N16]*
mixed cryoglobulinemia D89.1 *[N16]*
multiple myeloma C90.0- *[N16]*
Salmonella infection A02.25
sarcoidosis D86.84
sepsis A41.9 *[N16]*
streptococcal A40.9 *[N16]*
systemic lupus erythematosus M32.15
toxoplasmosis B58.83
transplant rejection T86.91 *[N16]*
Wilson's disease E83.01 *[N16]*
tubulo-renal function, impaired N25.9
specified NEC N25.89
tympanic membrane H73.9-
atrophy — *see* Atrophy, tympanic membrane
infection — *see* Myringitis
perforation — *see* Perforation, tympanum
specified NEC H73.89-
unsocialized aggressive F91.1
urea cycle metabolism E72.20
argininemia E72.21
arginosuccinic aciduria E72.22
citrullinemia E72.23
ornithine transcarbamylase deficiency E72.4
other specified E72.29
ureter (in) N28.9
schistosomiasis B65.0 *[N29]*
tuberculosis A18.11
urethra N36.9
specified NEC N36.8
urinary system N39.9
specified NEC N39.8
valve, heart
aortic — *see* Endocarditis, aortic
mitral — *see* Endocarditis, mitral
pulmonary — *see* Endocarditis, pulmonary
rheumatic
aortic — *see* Endocarditis, aortic, rheumatic
mitral — *see* Endocarditis, mitral
pulmonary — *see* Endocarditis, pulmonary, rheumatic
tricuspid — *see* Endocarditis, tricuspid
tricuspid — *see* Endocarditis, tricuspid
vestibular function H81.9-
specified NEC — *see* subcategory H81.8
in diseases classified elsewhere H82.-
vertigo — *see* Vertigo

Disorder (of) - *continued*
vision, binocular H53.30
abnormal retinal correspondence H53.31
diplopia H53.2
fusion with defective stereopsis H53.32
simultaneous perception H53.33
suppression H53.34
visual
cortex
blindness H47.619
left brain H47.612
right brain H47.611
due to
inflammatory disorder H47.629
left brain H47.622
right brain H47.621
neoplasm H47.639
left brain H47.632
right brain H47.631
vascular disorder H47.649
left brain H47.642
right brain H47.641
pathway H47.9
due to
inflammatory disorder H47.51-
neoplasm H47.52-
vascular disorder H47.53-
optic chiasm — *see* Disorder, optic, chiasm
vitreous body H43.9
crystalline deposits — *see* Deposit, crystalline
degeneration — *see* Degeneration, vitreous
hemorrhage — *see* Hemorrhage, vitreous
opacities — *see* Opacity, vitreous
prolapse — *see* Prolapse, vitreous
specified type NEC H43.89
voice R49.9
specified type NEC R49.8
volatile solvent use
due to drug abuse — *see* Abuse, drug, inhalant
due to drug dependence — *see* Dependence, drug, inhalant
voyeuristic F65.3
white blood cells D72.9
specified NEC D72.89
withdrawing, child or adolescent F40.10

Disorientation R41.0

Displacement, displaced
acquired traumatic of bone, cartilage, joint, tendon NEC — *see* Dislocation
adrenal gland (congenital) Q89.1
appendix, retrocecal (congenital) Q43.8
auricle (congenital) Q17.4
bladder (acquired) N32.89
congenital Q64.19
brachial plexus (congenital) Q07.8
brain stem, caudal (congenital) Q04.8
canaliculus (lacrimalis) , congenital Q10.6
cardia through esophageal hiatus (congenital) Q40.1
cerebellum, caudal (congenital) Q04.8
cervix — *see* Malposition, uterus
colon (congenital) Q43.3
device, implant or graft — *see also* Complications, by site and type, mechanical T85.628
arterial graft NEC — *see* Complication, cardiovascular device, mechanical, vascular
breast (implant) T85.42
catheter NEC T85.628
dialysis (renal) T82.42
intraperitoneal T85.621
infusion NEC T82.524
spinal (epidural) (subdural) T85.620
urinary
cystostomy T83.020
Hopkins T83.028
ileostomy T83.028
indwelling T83.021
nephrostomy T83.022
specified NEC T83.028
urostomy T83.028

Displacement, displaced - *continued*
device, implant or graft - *continued*
electronic (electrode) (pulse generator) (stimulator) — *see* Complication, electronic stimulator
fixation, internal (orthopedic) NEC — *see* Complication, fixation device, mechanical
gastrointestinal — *see* Complications, prosthetic device, mechanical, gastrointestinal device
genital NEC T83.428
intrauterine contraceptive device (string) T83.32
penile prosthesis (cylinder) (implanted) (pump) (resevoir) T83.420
testicular prosthesis T83.421
heart NEC — *see* Complication, cardiovascular device, mechanical
joint prosthesis — *see* Complications, joint prosthesis, mechanical
ocular — *see* Complications, prosthetic device, mechanical, ocular device
orthopedic NEC — *see* Complication, orthopedic, device or graft, mechanical
specified NEC T85.628
urinary NEC T83.128
graft T83.22
sphincter, implanted T83.121
stent (ileal conduit) (nephroureteral) T83.123
ureteral indwelling T83.122
vascular NEC — *see* Complication, cardiovascular device, mechanical
ventricular intracranial shunt T85.02
electronic stimulator
bone T84.320
cardiac — *see* Complications, cardiac device, electronic
nervous system — *see* Complication, prosthetic device, mechanical, electronic nervous system stimulator
urinary — *see* Complications, electronic stimulator, urinary
esophageal mucosa into cardia of stomach, congenital Q39.8
esophagus (acquired) K22.89
congenital Q39.8
eyeball (acquired) (lateral) (old) — *see* Displacement, globe
congenital Q15.8
current — *see* Avulsion, eye
fallopian tube (acquired) N83.4-
congenital Q50.6
opening (congenital) Q50.6
gallbladder (congenital) Q44.1
gastric mucosa (congenital) Q40.2
globe (acquired) (old) (lateral) H05.21-
current — *see* Avulsion, eye
heart (congenital) Q24.8
acquired I51.89
hymen (upward) (congenital) Q52.4
intervertebral disc NEC
with myelopathy — *see* Disorder, disc, with, myelopathy
cervical, cervicothoracic (with) M50.20
myelopathy — *see* Disorder, disc, cervical, with myelopathy
neuritis, radiculitis or radiculopathy — *see* Disorder, disc, cervical, with neuritis
due to trauma — *see* Dislocation, vertebra
lumbar region M51.26
with
myelopathy M51.06
neuritis, radiculitis, radiculopathy or sciatica M51.16
lumbosacral region M51.27
with
neuritis, radiculitis, radiculopathy or sciatica M51.17
sacrococcygeal region M53.3
thoracic region M51.24
with

Distortion (s) (congenital) - *continued*
sacrum Q76.49
scapula Q74.0
shoulder girdle Q74.0
skull bone (s) NEC Q75.8
with
anencephalus Q00.0
encephalocele — *see* Encephalocele
hydrocephalus Q03.9
with spina bifida — *see* Spina bifida, with hydrocephalus
microcephaly Q02
spinal cord Q06.8
spine Q76.49
kyphosis — *see* Kyphosis, congenital
lordosis — *see* Lordosis, congenital
spleen Q89.09
sternum NEC Q76.7
thorax (wall) Q67.8
bony Q76.8
thymus (gland) Q89.2
thyroid (gland) Q89.2
tibia NEC Q68.8
toe (s) Q66.9-
tongue Q38.3
trachea (cartilage) Q32.1
ulna NEC Q68.8
ureter Q62.8
urethra Q64.79
causing obstruction Q64.39
uterus Q51.9
vagina Q52.4
vertebra Q76.49
kyphosis — *see* Kyphosis, congenital
lordosis — *see* Lordosis, congenital
visual — *see also* Disturbance, vision
shape and size H53.15
vulva Q52.79
wrist (bones) (joint) Q68.8
Distress
abdomen — *see* Pain, abdominal
acute respiratory R06.03
syndrome (adult) (child) J80
epigastric R10.13
fetal P84
complicating pregnancy — *see* Stress, fetal
gastrointestinal (functional) K30
psychogenic F45.8
intestinal (functional) NOS K59.9
psychogenic F45.8
maternal, during labor and delivery O75.0
relationship, with spouse or intimate partner Z63.0
respiratory (adult) (child) R06.03
newborn P22.9
specified NEC P22.8
orthopnea R06.01
psychogenic F45.8
shortness of breath R06.02
specified type NEC R06.09
Distribution vessel, atypical Q27.9
coronary artery Q24.5
precerebral Q28.1
Districhiasis L68.8
Disturbance (s) — *see also* Disease
absorption K90.9
calcium E58
carbohydrate K90.49
fat K90.49
pancreatic K90.3
protein K90.49
starch K90.49
vitamin — *see* Deficiency, vitamin
acid-base equilibrium E87.8
mixed E87.4
activity and attention (with hyperkinesis) — *see* Disorder, attention-deficit hyperactivity
amino acid transport E72.00
assimilation, food K90.9
auditory nerve, except deafness — *see* subcategory H93.3
behavior — *see* Disorder, conduct
blood clotting (mechanism) — *see also* Defect, coagulation D68.9

Disturbance (s) - *continued*
cerebral
nerve — *see* Disorder, nerve, cranial
status, newborn P91.9
specified NEC P91.88
circulatory I99.9
conduct — *see also* Disorder, conduct F91.9
adjustment reaction — *see* Disorder, adjustment
compulsive F63.9
disruptive F91.9
hyperkinetic — *see* Disorder, attention-deficit hyperactivity
socialized F91.2
specified NEC F91.8
unsocialized F91.1
coordination R27.8
cranial nerve — *see* Disorder, nerve, cranial
deep sensibility — *see* Disturbance, sensation
digestive K30
psychogenic F45.8
electrolyte — *see also* Imbalance, electrolyte
newborn, transitory P74.49
hyperammonemia P74.6
hyperchloremia P74.421
hyperchloremic metabolic acidosis P74.421
hypochloremia P74.422
potassium balance
hyperkalemia P74.31
hypokalemia P74.32
sodium balance
hypernatremia P74.21
hyponatremia P74.22
specified type NEC P74.49
emotions specific to childhood and adolescence F93.9
with
anxiety and fearfulness NEC F93.8
elective mutism F94.0
oppositional disorder F91.3
sensitivity (withdrawal) F40.10
shyness F40.10
social withdrawal F40.10
involving relationship problems F93.8
mixed F93.8
specified NEC F93.8
endocrine (gland) E34.9
neonatal, transitory P72.9
specified NEC P72.8
equilibrium R42
fructose metabolism E74.10
gait — *see* Gait
hysterical F44.4
psychogenic F44.4
gastrointestinal (functional) K30
psychogenic F45.8
habit, child F98.9
hearing, except deafness and tinnitus — *see* Abnormal, auditory perception
heart, functional (conditions in I44-I50)
due to presence of (cardiac) prosthesis I97.19-
postoperative I97.89
cardiac surgery — *see also* Infarct, myocardium, associated with revascularization procedure I97.19-
hormones E34.9
innervation uterus (parasympathetic) (sympathetic) N85.8
keratinization NEC
gingiva K05.10
nonplaque induced K05.11
plaque induced K05.10
lip K13.0
oral (mucosa) (soft tissue) K13.29
tongue K13.29
learning (specific) — *see* Disorder, learning
memory — *see* Amnesia
mild, following organic brain damage F06.8
mental F99
associated with diseases classified elsewhere F54

Disturbance (s) - *continued*
metabolism E88.9
with
abortion — *see* Abortion, by type with other specified complication
ectopic pregnancy O08.5
molar pregnancy O08.5
amino-acid E72.9
aromatic E70.9
branched-chain E71.2
straight-chain E72.89
sulfur-bearing E72.10
ammonia E72.20
arginine E72.21
arginosuccinic acid E72.22
carbohydrate E74.9
cholesterol E78.9
citrulline E72.23
cystathionine E72.19
general E88.9
glutamine E72.89
histidine E70.40
homocystine E72.19
hydroxylysine E72.3
in labor or delivery O75.89
iron E83.10
lipoid E78.9
lysine E72.3
methionine E72.19
neonatal, transitory P74.9
calcium and magnesium P71.9
specified type NEC P71.8
carbohydrate metabolism P70.9
specified type NEC P70.8
specified NEC P74.8
ornithine E72.4
phosphate E83.39
sodium NEC E87.8
threonine E72.89
tryptophan E70.5
tyrosine E70.20
urea cycle E72.20
motor R29.2
nervous, functional R45.0
neuromuscular mechanism (eye) , due to syphilis A52.15
nutritional E63.9
nail L60.3
ocular motion H51.9
psychogenic F45.8
oculogyric H51.8
psychogenic F45.8
oculomotor H51.9
psychogenic F45.8
olfactory nerve R43.1
optic nerve NEC — *see* Disorder, nerve, optic
oral epithelium, including tongue NEC K13.29
perceptual due to
alcohol withdrawal F10.232
amphetamine intoxication F15.922
in
abuse F15.122
dependence F15.222
anxiolytic withdrawal F13.232
cannabis intoxication (acute) F12.922
in
abuse F12.122
dependence F12.222
cocaine intoxication (acute) F14.922
in
abuse F14.122
dependence F14.222
hypnotic withdrawal F13.232
opioid intoxication (acute) F11.922
in
abuse F11.122
dependence F11.222
phencyclidine intoxication (acute) F16.122
sedative withdrawal F13.232
personality (pattern) (trait) — *see also* Disorder, personality F60.9
following organic brain damage F07.9
polyglandular E31.9

Disturbance (s) - *continued*
polyglandular - *continued*
specified NEC E31.8
potassium balance, newborn
hyperkalemia P74.31
hypokalemia P74.32
psychogenic F45.9
psychomotor F44.4
psychophysical visual H53.16
pupillary — *see* Anomaly, pupil, function
reflex R29.2
rhythm, heart I49.9
salivary secretion K11.7
sensation (cold) (heat) (localization) (tactile discrimination) (texture) (vibratory) NEC R20.9
hysterical F44.6
skin R20.9
anesthesia R20.0
hyperesthesia R20.3
hypoesthesia R20.1
paresthesia R20.2
specified type NEC R20.8
smell R43.9
and taste (mixed) R43.8
anosmia R43.0
parosmia R43.1
specified NEC R43.8
taste R43.9
and smell (mixed) R43.8
parageusia R43.2
specified NEC R43.8
sensory — *see* Disturbance, sensation
situational (transient) — *see also* Disorder, adjustment
acute F43.0
sleep G47.9
nonorganic origin F51.9
smell — *see* Disturbance, sensation, smell
sociopathic F60.2
sodium balance, newborn
hypernatremia P74.21
hyponatremia P74.22
speech R47.9
developmental F80.9
specified NEC R47.89
stomach (functional) K31.9
sympathetic (nerve) G90.9
taste — *see* Disturbance, sensation, taste
temperature
regulation, newborn P81.9
specified NEC P81.8
sense R20.8
hysterical F44.6
tooth
eruption K00.6
formation K00.4
structure, hereditary NEC K00.5
touch — *see* Disturbance, sensation
vascular I99.9
arteriosclerotic — *see* Arteriosclerosis
vasomotor I73.9
vasospastic I73.9
vision, visual H53.9
following
cerebral infarction I69.398
cerebrovascular disease I69.998
specified NEC I69.898
intracerebral hemorrhage I69.198
nontraumatic intracranial hemorrhage NEC I69.298
specified disease NEC I69.898
subarachnoid hemorrhage I69.098
psychophysical H53.16
specified NEC H53.8
subjective H53.10
day blindness H53.11
discomfort H53.14-
distortions of shape and size H53.15
loss
sudden H53.13-
transient H53.12-
specified type NEC H53.19
voice R49.9
psychogenic F44.4

Disturbance (s) - *continued*
voice - *continued*
specified NEC R49.8
Diuresis R35.89
Diver's palsy, paralysis or squeeze T70.3
Diverticulitis (acute) K57.92
bladder — *see* Cystitis
ileum — *see* Diverticulitis, intestine, small
intestine K57.92
with
abscess, perforation K57.80
with bleeding K57.81
bleeding K57.93
congenital Q43.8
large K57.32
with
abscess, perforation K57.20
with bleeding K57.21
bleeding K57.33
small intestine K57.52
with
abscess, perforation K57.40
with bleeding K57.41
bleeding K57.53
small K57.12
with
abscess, perforation K57.00
with bleeding K57.01
bleeding K57.13
large intestine K57.52
with
abscess, perforation K57.40
with bleeding K57.41
bleeding K57.53
Diverticulosis K57.90
with bleeding K57.91
large intestine K57.30
with
bleeding K57.31
small intestine K57.50
with bleeding K57.51
small intestine K57.10
with
bleeding K57.11
large intestine K57.50
with bleeding K57.51
Diverticulum, diverticula (multiple) K57.90
appendix (noninflammatory) K38.2
bladder (sphincter) N32.3
congenital Q64.6
bronchus (congenital) Q32.4
acquired J98.09
calyx, calyceal (kidney) N28.89
cardia (stomach) K31.4
cecum — *see* Diverticulosis, intestine, large
congenital Q43.8
colon — *see* Diverticulosis, intestine, large
congenital Q43.8
duodenum — *see* Diverticulosis, intestine, small
congenital Q43.8
epiphrenic (esophagus) K22.5
esophagus (congenital) Q39.6
acquired (epiphrenic) (pulsion) (traction) K22.5
eustachian tube — *see* Disorder, eustachian tube, specified NEC
fallopian tube N83.8
gastric K31.4
heart (congenital) Q24.8
ileum — *see* Diverticulosis, intestine, small
jejunum — *see* Diverticulosis, intestine, small
kidney (pelvis) (calyces) N28.89
with calculus — *see* Calculus, kidney
Meckel's (displaced) (hypertrophic) Q43.0
malignant — *see* Table of Neoplasms, small intestine, malignant
midthoracic K22.5
organ or site, congenital NEC — *see* Distortion
pericardium (congenital) (cyst) Q24.8
acquired I31.8
pharyngoesophageal (congenital) Q39.6
acquired K22.5

Diverticulum, diverticula (multiple) - *continued*
pharynx (congenital) Q38.7
rectosigmoid — *see* Diverticulosis, intestine, large
congenital Q43.8
rectum — *see* Diverticulosis, intestine, large
Rokitansky's K22.5
seminal vesicle N50.89
sigmoid — *see* Diverticulosis, intestine, large
congenital Q43.8
stomach (acquired) K31.4
congenital Q40.2
trachea (acquired) J39.8
ureter (acquired) N28.89
congenital Q62.8
ureterovesical orifice N28.89
urethra (acquired) N36.1
congenital Q64.79
ventricle, left (congenital) Q24.8
vesical N32.3
congenital Q64.6
Zenker's (esophagus) K22.5
Division
cervix uteri (acquired) N88.8
glans penis Q55.69
labia minora (congenital) Q52.79
ligament (partial or complete) (current) — *see also* Sprain
with open wound — *see* Wound, open
muscle (partial or complete) (current) — *see also* Injury, muscle
with open wound — *see* Wound, open
nerve (traumatic) — *see* Injury, nerve
spinal cord — *see* Injury, spinal cord, by region
vein I87.8
Divorce, causing family disruption Z63.5
Dix-Hallpike neurolabyrinthitis — *see* Neuronitis, vestibular
Dizziness R42
hysterical F44.89
psychogenic F45.8
DMAC (disseminated mycobacterium avium- intracellulare complex) A31.2
DNR (do not resuscitate) Z66
Doan-Wiseman syndrome (primary splenic neutropenia) — *see* Agranulocytosis
Doehle-Heller aortitis A52.02
Dog bite — *see* Bite
Dohle body panmyelopathic syndrome D72.0
Dolichocephaly Q67.2
Dolichocolon Q43.8
Dolichostenomelia — *see* Syndrome, Marfan's
Donohue's syndrome E34.8
Donor (organ or tissue) Z52.9
blood (whole) Z52.000
autologous Z52.010
specified component (lymphocytes) (platelets) NEC Z52.008
autologous Z52.018
specified donor NEC Z52.098
specified donor NEC Z52.090
stem cells Z52.001
autologous Z52.011
specified donor NEC Z52.091
bone Z52.20
autologous Z52.21
marrow Z52.3
specified type NEC Z52.29
cornea Z52.5
egg (Oocyte) Z52.819
age 35 and over Z52.812
anonymous recipient Z52.812
designated recipient Z52.813
under age 35 Z52.810
anonymous recipient Z52.810
designated recipient Z52.811
kidney Z52.4
liver Z52.6
lung Z52.89
lymphocyte — *see* Donor, blood, specified components NEC
Oocyte — *see* Donor, egg
platelets Z52.008

- **Dysadrenocortism** E27.9
  - hyperfunction E27.0
- **Dysarthria** R47.1
  - following
    - cerebral infarction I69.322
    - cerebrovascular disease I69.922
      - specified disease NEC I69.822
    - intracerebral hemorrhage I69.122
    - nontraumatic intracranial hemorrhage NEC I69.222
    - subarachnoid hemorrhage I69.022
- **Dysautonomia (familial)** G90.1
- **Dysbarism** T70.3
- **Dysbasia** R26.2
  - angiosclerotica intermittens I73.9
  - hysterical F44.4
  - lordotica (progressiva) G24.1
  - nonorganic origin F44.4
  - psychogenic F44.4
- **Dysbetalipoproteinemia (familial)** E78.2
- **Dyscalculia** R48.8
  - developmental F81.2
- **Dyschezia** K59.00
- **Dyschondroplasia (with hemangiomata)** Q78.4
- **Dyschromia (skin)** L81.9
- **Dyscollagenosis** M35.9
- **Dyscranio-pygo-phalangy** Q87.0
- **Dyscrasia**
  - blood (with) D75.9
    - antepartum hemorrhage — *see* Hemorrhage, antepartum, with coagulation defect
    - newborn P61.9
      - specified type NEC P61.8
    - intrapartum hemorrhage O67.0
    - puerperal, postpartum O72.3
  - polyglandular, pluriglandular E31.9
- **Dysendocrinism** E34.9
- **Dysentery, dysenteric (catarrhal) (diarrhea) (epidemic) (hemorrhagic) (infectious) (sporadic) (tropical)** A09
  - abscess, liver A06.4
  - amebic — *see also* Amebiasis A06.0
    - with abscess — *see* Abscess, amebic
    - acute A06.0
    - chronic A06.1
  - arthritis (*see also* category M01) A09
    - bacillary (*see also* category M01) A03.9
  - bacillary A03.9
    - arthritis (*see also* category M01) A03.9
    - Boyd A03.2
    - Flexner A03.1
    - Schmitz (-Stutzer) A03.0
    - Shiga (-Kruse) A03.0
    - Shigella A03.9
      - boydii A03.2
      - dysenteriae A03.0
      - flexneri A03.1
      - group A A03.0
      - group B A03.1
      - group C A03.2
      - group D A03.3
      - sonnei A03.3
      - specified type NEC A03.8
    - Sonne A03.3
    - specified type NEC A03.8
  - balantidial A07.0
  - Balantidium coli A07.0
  - Boyd's A03.2
  - candidal B37.82
  - Chilomastix A07.8
  - Chinese A03.9
  - coccidial A07.3
  - Dientamoeba (fragilis) A07.8
  - Embadomonas A07.8
  - Entamoeba, entamebic — *see* Dysentery, amebic
  - Flexner-Boyd A03.2
  - Flexner's A03.1
  - Giardia lamblia A07.1
  - Hiss-Russell A03.1
  - Lamblia A07.1
  - leishmanial B55.0
  - malarial — *see* Malaria

Dysentery, dysenteric (catarrhal) (diarrhea) (epidemic) (hemorrhagic) (infectious) (sporadic) (tropical) - *continued*

  - metazoal B82.0
  - monilial B37.82
  - protozoal A07.9
  - Salmonella A02.0
  - schistosomal B65.1
  - Schmitz (-Stutzer) A03.0
  - Shiga (-Kruse) A03.0
  - Shigella NOS — *see* Dysentery, bacillary
  - Sonne A03.3
  - strongyloidiasis B78.0
  - trichomonal A07.8
  - viral — *see also* Enteritis, viral A08.4
- **Dysequilibrium** R42
- **Dysesthesia** R20.8
  - hysterical F44.6
- **Dysfibrinogenemia (congenital)** D68.2
- **Dysfunction**
  - adrenal E27.9
    - hyperfunction E27.0
  - autonomic
    - due to alcohol G31.2
    - somatoform F45.8
  - bladder N31.9
    - neurogenic NOS — *see* Dysfunction, bladder, neuromuscular
    - neuromuscular NOS N31.9
      - atonic (motor) (sensory) N31.2
      - autonomous N31.2
      - flaccid N31.2
      - nonreflex N31.2
      - reflex N31.1
      - specified NEC N31.8
      - uninhibited N31.0
  - bleeding, uterus N93.8
  - cerebral G93.89
  - colon K59.9
    - psychogenic F45.8
  - colostomy K94.03
  - cystic duct K82.8
  - cystostomy (stoma) — *see* Complications, cystostomy
  - ejaculatory N53.19
    - anejaculatory orgasm N53.13
    - painful N53.12
    - premature F52.4
    - retarded N53.11
  - endocrine NOS E34.9
  - endometrium N85.8
  - enterostomy K94.13
  - erectile — *see* Dysfunction, sexual, male, erectile
  - feeding, pediatric
    - acute R63.31
    - chronic R63.32
  - gallbladder K82.8
  - gastrostomy (stoma) K94.23
  - gland, glandular NOS E34.9
    - meibomian, of eyelid — *see* Dysfunction, meibomian gland
  - heart I51.89
  - hemoglobin D75.89
  - hepatic K76.89
  - hypophysis E23.7
  - hypothalamic NEC E23.3
  - ileostomy (stoma) K94.13
  - jejunostomy (stoma) K94.13
  - kidney — *see* Disease, renal
  - labyrinthine — *see* subcategory H83.2
  - left ventricular, following sudden emotional stress I51.81
  - liver K76.89
  - male — *see* Dysfunction, sexual, male
  - meibomian gland, of eyelid H02.889
    - left H02.886
      - lower H02.885
      - upper H02.884
      - upper and lower eyelids H02.88B
    - right H02.883
      - lower H02.882
      - upper H02.881
      - upper and lower eyelids H02.88A
  - orgasmic (female) F52.31

Dysfunction - *continued*

  - orgasmic (female) - *continued*
    - male F52.32
  - ovary E28.9
    - specified NEC E28.8
  - papillary muscle I51.89
  - parathyroid E21.4
  - physiological NEC R68.89
    - psychogenic F59
  - pineal gland E34.8
  - pituitary (gland) E23.3
  - platelets D69.1
  - polyglandular E31.9
    - specified NEC E31.8
  - psychophysiologic F59
  - psychosexual F52.9
    - with
      - dyspareunia F52.6
      - premature ejaculation F52.4
      - vaginismus F52.5
  - pylorus K31.9
  - rectum K59.9
    - psychogenic F45.8
  - reflex (sympathetic) — *see* Syndrome, pain, complex regional I
  - segmental — *see* Dysfunction, somatic
  - senile R54
  - sexual (due to) R37
    - alcohol F10.981
    - amphetamine F15.981
      - in
        - abuse F15.181
        - dependence F15.281
    - anxiolytic F13.981
      - in
        - abuse F13.181
        - dependence F13.281
    - cocaine F14.981
      - in
        - abuse F14.181
        - dependence F14.281
    - excessive sexual drive F52.8
    - failure of genital response (male) F52.21
      - female F52.22
    - female N94.9
      - aversion F52.1
      - dyspareunia N94.10
        - psychogenic F52.6
      - frigidity F52.22
      - nymphomania F52.8
      - orgasmic F52.31
      - psychogenic F52.9
        - aversion F52.1
        - dyspareunia F52.6
        - frigidity F52.22
        - nymphomania F52.8
        - orgasmic F52.31
        - vaginismus F52.5
      - vaginismus N94.2
        - psychogenic F52.5
    - hypnotic F13.981
      - in
        - abuse F13.181
        - dependence F13.281
    - inhibited orgasm (female) F52.31
      - male F52.32
    - lack
      - of sexual enjoyment F52.1
      - or loss of sexual desire F52.0
    - male N53.9
      - anejaculatory orgasm N53.13
      - ejaculatory N53.19
        - painful N53.12
        - premature F52.4
        - retarded N53.11
      - erectile N52.9
        - drug induced N52.2
        - due to
          - disease classified elsewhere N52.1
          - drug N52.2
        - postoperative (postprocedural) N52.39
          - following
            - cryotherapy N52.37
            - interstitial seed therapy N52.36
            - prostate ablative therapy N52.37

Dysfunction - *continued*
sexual (due to) - *continued*
male - *continued*
erectile - *continued*
postoperative (postprocedural) - *continued*
following - *continued*
prostatectomy N52.34
radical N52.31
radiation therapy N52.35
radical cystectomy N52.32
ultrasound ablative therapy N52.37
urethral surgery N52.33
psychogenic F52.21
specified cause NEC N52.8
vasculogenic
arterial insufficiency N52.01
with corporo-venous occlusive N52.03
corporo-venous occlusive N52.02
with arterial insufficiency N52.03
impotence — *see* Dysfunction, sexual, male, erectile
psychogenic F52.9
aversion F52.1
erectile F52.21
orgasmic F52.32
premature ejaculation F52.4
satyriasis F52.8
specified type NEC F52.8
specified type NEC N53.8
nonorganic F52.9
specified NEC F52.8
opioid F11.981
in
abuse F11.181
dependence F11.281
orgasmic dysfunction (female) F52.31
male F52.32
premature ejaculation F52.4
psychoactive substances NEC F19.981
in
abuse F19.181
dependence F19.281
psychogenic F52.9
sedative F13.981
in
abuse F13.181
dependence F13.281
sexual aversion F52.1
vaginismus (nonorganic) (psychogenic) F52.5
sinoatrial node I49.5
somatic M99.09
abdomen M99.09
acromioclavicular M99.07
cervical region M99.01
cervicothoracic M99.01
costochondral M99.08
costovertebral M99.08
head region M99.00
hip M99.05
lower extremity M99.06
lumbar region M99.03
lumbosacral M99.03
occipitocervical M99.00
pelvic region M99.05
pubic M99.05
rib cage M99.08
sacral region M99.04
sacrococcygeal M99.04
sacroiliac M99.04
specified NEC M99.09
sternochondral M99.08
sternoclavicular M99.07
thoracic region M99.02
thoracolumbar M99.02
upper extremity M99.07
somatoform autonomic F45.8
stomach K31.89
psychogenic F45.8
suprarenal E27.9
hyperfunction E27.0
symbolic R48.9

Dysfunction - *continued*
symbolic - *continued*
specified type NEC R48.8
temporomandibular (joint) M26.69
joint-pain syndrome M26.62-
testicular (endocrine) E29.9
specified NEC E29.8
thymus E32.9
thyroid E07.9
ureterostomy (stoma) — *see* Complications, stoma, urinary tract
urethrostomy (stoma) — *see* Complications, stoma, urinary tract
uterus, complicating delivery O62.9
hypertonic O62.4
hypotonic O62.2
primary O62.0
secondary O62.1
ventricular I51.9
with congestive heart failure — *see also* Failure, heart I50.9
left, reversible, following sudden emotional stress I51.81
Dysgenesis
gonadal (due to chromosomal anomaly) Q96.9
pure Q99.1
renal Q60.5
bilateral Q60.4
unilateral Q60.3
reticular D72.0
tidal platelet D69.3
Dysgerminoma
specified site — *see* Neoplasm, malignant, by site
unspecified site
female C56.9
male C62.90
Dysgeusia R43.2
Dysgraphia R27.8
Dyshidrosis, dysidrosis L30.1
Dyskaryotic cervical smear R87.619
Dyskeratosis L85.8
cervix — *see* Dysplasia, cervix
congenital Q82.8
uterus NEC N85.8
Dyskinesia G24.9
biliary (cystic duct or gallbladder) K82.8
drug induced
orofacial G24.01
esophagus K22.4
hysterical F44.4
intestinal K59.89
nonorganic origin F44.4
orofacial (idiopathic) G24.4
drug induced G24.01
psychogenic F44.4
subacute, drug induced G24.01
tardive G24.01
neuroleptic induced G24.01
trachea J39.8
tracheobronchial J98.09
Dyslalia (developmental) F80.0
Dyslexia R48.0
developmental F81.0
Dyslipidemia E78.5
depressed HDL cholesterol E78.6
elevated fasting triglycerides E78.1
Dysmaturity — *see also* Light for dates
pulmonary (newborn) (Wilson-Mikity) P27.0
Dysmenorrhea (essential) (exfoliative) N94.6
congestive (syndrome) N94.6
primary N94.4
psychogenic F45.8
secondary N94.5
Dysmetabolic syndrome X E88.81
Dysmetria R27.8
Dysmorphism (due to)
alcohol Q86.0
exogenous cause NEC Q86.8
hydantoin Q86.1
warfarin Q86.2
Dysmorphophobia (nondelusional) F45.22
delusional F22
Dysnomia R47.01

Dysorexia R63.0
psychogenic F50.89
Dysostosis
cleidocranial, cleidocranialis Q74.0
craniofacial Q75.1
Fairbank's (idiopathic familial generalized osteophytosis) Q78.9
mandibulofacial (incomplete) Q75.4
multiplex E76.01
oculomandibular Q75.5
Dyspareunia (female) N94.10
deep N94.12
male N53.12
nonorganic F52.6
psychogenic F52.6
secondary N94.19
specified NEC N94.19
superficial (introital) N94.11
Dyspepsia R10.13
atonic K30
functional (allergic) (congenital) (gastrointestinal) (occupational) (reflex) K30
intestinal K59.89
nervous F45.8
neurotic F45.8
psychogenic F45.8
Dysphagia R13.10
cervical R13.19
following
cerebral infarction I69.391
cerebrovascular disease I69.991
specified NEC I69.891
intracerebral hemorrhage I69.191
nontraumatic intracranial hemorrhage NEC I69.291
specified disease NEC I69.891
subarachnoid hemorrhage I69.091
functional (hysterical) F45.8
hysterical F45.8
nervous (hysterical) F45.8
neurogenic R13.19
oral phase R13.11
oropharyngeal phase R13.12
pharyngeal phase R13.13
pharyngoesophageal phase R13.14
psychogenic F45.8
sideropenic D50.1
spastica K22.4
specified NEC R13.19
Dysphagocytosis, congenital D71
Dysphasia R47.02
developmental
expressive type F80.1
receptive type F80.2
following
cerebrovascular disease I69.921
cerebral infarction I69.321
intracerebral hemorrhage I69.121
nontraumatic intracranial hemorrhage NEC I69.221
specified disease NEC I69.821
subarachnoid hemorrhage I69.021
Dysphonia R49.0
functional F44.4
hysterical F44.4
psychogenic F44.4
spastica J38.3
Dysphoria
gender F64.9
in
adolescence and adulthood F64.0
children F64.2
specified NEC F64.8
postpartal O90.6
Dyspituitarism E23.3
Dysplasia — *see also* Anomaly
acetabular, congenital Q65.89
alveolar capillary, with vein misalignment J84.843
anus (histologically confirmed) (mild) (moderate) K62.82
severe D01.3
arrhythmogenic right ventricular I42.8
arterial, fibromuscular I77.3

Dysplasia - *continued*
- asphyxiating thoracic (congenital) Q77.2
- brain Q07.9
- bronchopulmonary, perinatal P27.1
- cervix (uteri) N87.9
  - mild N87.0
  - moderate N87.1
  - severe D06.9
- chondroectodermal Q77.6
- colon D12.6
- craniometaphyseal Q78.8
- dentinal K00.5
- diaphyseal, progressive Q78.3
- dystrophic Q77.5
- ectodermal (anhidrotic) (congenital) (hereditary) Q82.4
  - hydrotic Q82.8
- epithelial, uterine cervix — *see* Dysplasia, cervix
- eye (congenital) Q11.2
- fibrous
  - bone NEC (monostotic) M85.00
    - ankle M85.07-
    - foot M85.07-
    - forearm M85.03-
    - hand M85.04-
    - lower leg M85.06-
    - multiple site M85.09
    - neck M85.08
    - rib M85.08
    - shoulder M85.01-
    - skull M85.08
    - specified site NEC M85.08
    - thigh M85.05-
    - toe M85.07-
    - upper arm M85.02-
    - vertebra M85.08
  - diaphyseal, progressive Q78.3
  - jaw M27.8
  - polyostotic Q78.1
- florid osseous — *see also* Cyst, calcifying odontogenic
- high grade, focal D12.6
- hip, congenital Q65.89
- joint, congenital Q74.8
- kidney Q61.4
  - multicystic Q61.4
- leg Q74.2
- lung, congenital (not associated with short gestation) Q33.6
- mammary (gland) (benign) N60.9-
  - cyst (solitary) — *see* Cyst, breast
  - cystic — *see* Mastopathy, cystic
  - duct ectasia — *see* Ectasia, mammary duct
  - fibroadenosis — *see* Fibroadenosis, breast
  - fibrosclerosis — *see* Fibrosclerosis, breast
  - specified type NEC N60.8-
- metaphyseal Q78.5
- muscle Q79.8
- oculodentodigital Q87.0
- periapical (cemental) (cemento-osseous) — *see* Cyst, calcifying odontogenic
- periosteum — *see* Disorder, bone, specified type NEC
- polyostotic fibrous Q78.1
- prostate — *see also* Neoplasia, intraepithelial, prostate N42.30
  - severe D07.5
  - specified NEC N42.39
- renal Q61.4
  - multicystic Q61.4
- retinal, congenital Q14.1
- right ventricular, arrhythmogenic I42.8
- septo-optic Q04.4
- skin L98.8
- spinal cord Q06.1
- spondyloepiphyseal Q77.7
- thymic, with immunodeficiency D82.1
- vagina N89.3
  - mild N89.0
  - moderate N89.1
  - severe NEC D07.2
- vulva N90.3
  - mild N90.0
  - moderate N90.1

Dysplasia - *continued*
- vulva - *continued*
  - severe NEC D07.1

Dysplasminogenemia E88.02

Dyspnea (nocturnal) (paroxysmal) R06.00
- asthmatic (bronchial) J45.909
  - with
    - exacerbation (acute) J45.901
    - bronchitis J45.909
      - with
        - exacerbation (acute) J45.901
        - status asthmaticus J45.902
      - chronic J44.9
    - status asthmaticus J45.902
  - cardiac — *see* Failure, ventricular, left
- cardiac — *see* Failure, ventricular, left
- functional F45.8
- hyperventilation R06.4
- hysterical F45.8
- newborn P28.89
- orthopnea R06.01
- psychogenic F45.8
- shortness of breath R06.02
- specified type NEC R06.09

Dyspraxia R27.8
- developmental (syndrome) F82

Dysproteinemia E88.09

Dysreflexia, autonomic G90.4

Dysrhythmia
- cardiac I49.9
  - newborn
    - bradycardia P29.12
    - occurring before birth P03.819
      - before onset of labor P03.810
      - during labor P03.811
    - tachycardia P29.11
  - postoperative I97.89
- cerebral or cortical — *see* Epilepsy

Dyssomnia — *see* Disorder, sleep

Dyssynergia
- biliary K83.8
- bladder sphincter N36.44
- cerebellaris myoclonica (Hunt's ataxia) G11.19

Dysthymia F34.1

Dysthyroidism E07.9

Dystocia O66.9
- affecting newborn P03.1
- cervical (hypotonic) O62.2
  - affecting newborn P03.6
  - primary O62.0
  - secondary O62.1
- contraction ring O62.4
- fetal O66.9
  - abnormality NEC O66.3
  - conjoined twins O66.3
  - oversize O66.2
- maternal O66.9
- positional O64.9
- shoulder (girdle) O66.0
  - causing obstructed labor O66.0
- uterine NEC O62.4

Dystonia G24.9
- cervical G24.3
- deformans progressiva G24.1
- drug induced NEC G24.09
  - acute G24.02
  - specified NEC G24.09
- familial G24.1
- idiopathic G24.1
  - familial G24.1
  - nonfamilial G24.2
  - orofacial G24.4
- lenticularis G24.8
- musculorum deformans G24.1
- neuroleptic induced (acute) G24.02
- orofacial (idiopathic) G24.4
- oromandibular G24.4
  - due to drug G24.01
- specified NEC G24.8
- torsion (familial) (idiopathic) G24.1
  - acquired G24.8
  - genetic G24.1
  - symptomatic (nonfamilial) G24.2

Dystonic movements R25.8

Dystrophy, dystrophia
- adiposogenital E23.6
- autosomal recessive, childhood type, muscular dystrophy resembling Duchenne or Becker G71.01
- Becker's type G71.01
- cervical sympathetic G90.2
- choroid (hereditary) H31.20
  - central areolar H31.22
  - choroideremia H31.21
  - gyrate atrophy H31.23
  - specified type NEC H31.29
- cornea (hereditary) H18.50-
  - endothelial H18.51-
  - epithelial H18.52-
  - granular H18.53-
  - lattice H18.54-
  - macular H18.55-
  - specified type NEC H18.59-
- Duchenne's type G71.01
- due to malnutrition E45
- Erb's G71.02
- Fuchs' H18.51-
- Gower's muscular G71.01
- hair L67.8
- infantile neuraxonal G31.89
- Landouzy-Déjérine G71.02
- Leyden-Möbius G71.09
- muscular G71.00
  - autosomal recessive, childhood type, muscular dystrophy resembling Duchenne or Becker G71.01
  - benign (Becker type) G71.01
    - scapuloperoneal with early contractures [Emery-Dreifuss] G71.09
  - congenital (hereditary) (progressive) (with specific morphological abnormalities of the muscle fiber) G71.09
    - myotonic G71.11
  - distal G71.09
  - Duchenne type G71.01
  - Emery-Dreifuss G71.09
  - Erb type G71.02
  - facioscapulohumeral G71.02
  - Gower's G71.01
  - hereditary (progressive) G71.09
  - Landouzy-Déjérine type G71.02
  - limb-girdle G71.09
  - myotonic G71.11
  - progressive (hereditary) G71.09
    - Charcot-Marie (-Tooth) type G60.0
  - pseudohypertrophic (infantile) G71.01
  - scapulohumeral G71.02
  - scapuloperoneal G71.09
  - severe (Duchenne type) G71.01
  - specified type NEC G71.09
- myocardium, myocardial — *see* Degeneration, myocardial
- myotonic, myotonica G71.11
- nail L60.3
  - congenital Q84.6
- nutritional E45
- ocular G71.09
- oculocerebrorenal E72.03
- oculopharyngeal G71.09
- ovarian N83.8
- polyglandular E31.8
- reflex (neuromuscular) (sympathetic) — *see* Syndrome, pain, complex regional I
- retinal (hereditary) H35.50
  - in
    - lipid storage disorders E75.6 *[H36]*
    - systemic lipidoses E75.6 *[H36]*
  - involving
    - pigment epithelium H35.54
    - sensory area H35.53
  - pigmentary H35.52
  - vitreoretinal H35.51
- Salzmann's nodular — *see* Degeneration, cornea, nodular
- scapuloperoneal G71.09
- skin NEC L98.8
- sympathetic (reflex) — *see* Syndrome, pain, complex regional I
  - cervical G90.2

Dystrophy, dystrophia - *continued*
tapetoretinal H35.54
thoracic, asphyxiating Q77.2
unguium L60.3
congenital Q84.6
vitreoretinal H35.51
vulva N90.4
yellow (liver) — *see* Failure, hepatic
Dysuria R30.0
psychogenic F45.8

E

Eales' disease H35.06-
Ear — *see also* condition
piercing Z41.3
tropical NEC B36.9 *[H62.40]*
in
aspergillosis B44.89
candidiasis B37.84
moniliasis B37.84
wax (impacted) H61.20
left H61.22
with right H61.23
right H61.21
with left H61.23
Earache — *see* subcategory H92.0
Early satiety R68.81
Eaton-Lambert syndrome — *see* Syndrome, Lambert-Eaton
Eberth's disease (typhoid fever) A01.00
Ebola virus disease A98.4
Ebstein's anomaly or syndrome (heart) Q22.5
Eccentro-osteochondrodysplasia E76.29
Ecchondroma — *see* Neoplasm, bone, benign
Ecchondrosis D48.0
Ecchymosis R58
conjunctiva — *see* Hemorrhage, conjunctiva
eye (traumatic) — *see* Contusion, eyeball
eyelid (traumatic) — *see* Contusion, eyelid
newborn P54.5
spontaneous R23.3
traumatic — *see* Contusion
Echinococciasis — *see* Echinococcus
Echinococcosis — *see* Echinococcus
Echinococcus (infection) B67.90
granulosus B67.4
bone B67.2
liver B67.0
lung B67.1
multiple sites B67.32
specified site NEC B67.39
thyroid B67.31
liver NOS B67.8
granulosus B67.0
multilocularis B67.5
lung NEC B67.99
granulosus B67.1
multilocularis B67.69
multilocularis B67.7
liver B67.5
multiple sites B67.61
specified site NEC B67.69
specified site NEC B67.99
granulosus B67.39
multilocularis B67.69
thyroid NEC B67.99
granulosus B67.31
multilocularis B67.69 *[E35]*
Echinorhynchiasis B83.8
Echinostomiasis B66.8
Echolalia R48.8
Echovirus, as cause of disease classified elsewhere B97.12
Eclampsia, eclamptic (coma) (convulsions) (delirium) (with hypertension) NEC O15.9
complicating
labor and delivery O15.1
postpartum O15.2
pregnancy O15.0-
puerperium O15.2
Economic circumstances affecting care Z59.9
Economo's disease A85.8
Ectasia, ectasis
annuloaortic I35.8

Ectasia, ectasis - *continued*
aorta I77.819
with aneurysm — *see* Aneurysm, aorta
abdominal I77.811
thoracic I77.810
thoracoabdominal I77.812
breast — *see* Ectasia, mammary duct
capillary I78.8
cornea H18.71-
gastric antral vascular (GAVE) K31.819
with hemorrhage K31.811
without hemorrhage K31.819
mammary duct N60.4-
salivary gland (duct) K11.8
sclera — *see* Sclerectasia
Ecthyma L08.0
contagiosum B08.02
gangrenosum L08.0
infectiosum B08.02
Ectocardia Q24.8
Ectodermal dysplasia (anhidrotic) Q82.4
Ectodermosis erosiva pluriorificialis L51.1
Ectopic, ectopia (congenital)
abdominal viscera Q45.8
due to defect in anterior abdominal wall Q79.59
ACTH syndrome E24.3
adrenal gland Q89.1
anus Q43.5
atrial beats I49.1
beats I49.49
atrial I49.1
ventricular I49.3
bladder Q64.10
bone and cartilage in lung Q33.5
brain Q04.8
breast tissue Q83.8
cardiac Q24.8
cerebral Q04.8
cordis Q24.8
endometrium — *see* Endometriosis
gastric mucosa Q40.2
gestation — *see* Pregnancy, by site
heart Q24.8
hormone secretion NEC E34.2
kidney (crossed) (pelvis) Q63.2
lens, lentis Q12.1
mole — *see* Pregnancy, by site
organ or site NEC — *see* Malposition, congenital
pancreas Q45.3
pregnancy — *see* Pregnancy, ectopic
pupil — *see* Abnormality, pupillary
renal Q63.2
sebaceous glands of mouth Q38.6
spleen Q89.09
testis Q53.00
bilateral Q53.02
unilateral Q53.01
thyroid Q89.2
tissue in lung Q33.5
ureter Q62.63
ventricular beats I49.3
vesicae Q64.10
Ectromelia Q73.8
lower limb — *see* Defect, reduction, limb, lower, specified type NEC
upper limb — *see* Defect, reduction, limb, upper, specified type NEC
Ectropion H02.109
cervix N86
with cervicitis N72
congenital Q10.1
eyelid H02.109
cicatricial H02.119
left H02.116
lower H02.115
upper H02.114
right H02.113
lower H02.112
upper H02.111
congenital Q10.1
left H02.106
lower H02.105
upper H02.104

Ectropion - *continued*
eyelid - *continued*
mechanical H02.129
left H02.126
lower H02.125
upper H02.124
right H02.123
lower H02.122
upper H02.121
paralytic H02.159
left H02.156
lower H02.155
upper H02.154
right H02.153
lower H02.152
upper H02.151
right H02.103
lower H02.102
upper H02.101
senile H02.139
left H02.136
lower H02.135
upper H02.134
right H02.133
lower H02.132
upper H02.131
spastic H02.149
left H02.146
lower H02.145
upper H02.144
right H02.143
lower H02.142
upper H02.141
iris H21.89
lip (acquired) K13.0
congenital Q38.0
urethra N36.8
uvea H21.89
Eczema (acute) (chronic) (erythematous) (fissum) (rubrum) (squamous) — *see also* Dermatitis L30.9
contact — *see* Dermatitis, contact
dyshydrotic L30.1
external ear — *see* Otitis, externa, acute, eczematoid
flexural L20.82
herpeticum B00.0
hypertrophicum L28.0
hypostatic — *see* Varix, leg, with, inflammation
impetiginous L01.1
infantile (due to any substance) L20.83
intertriginous L21.1
seborrheic L21.1
intertriginous NEC L30.4
infantile L21.1
intrinsic (allergic) L20.84
lichenified NEC L28.0
marginatum (hebrae) B35.6
pustular L30.3
stasis I87.2
with varicose veins — *see* Varix, leg, with, inflammation
vaccination, vaccinatum T88.1
varicose — *see* Varix, leg, with, inflammation
Eczematid L30.2
Eddowes (-Spurway) syndrome Q78.0
Edema, edematous (infectious) (pitting) (toxic) R60.9
with nephritis — *see* Nephrosis
allergic T78.3
amputation stump (surgical) (sequelae (late effect)) T87.89
angioneurotic (allergic) (any site) (with urticaria) T78.3
hereditary D84.1
angiospastic I73.9
Berlin's (traumatic) S05.8X-
brain (cytotoxic) (vasogenic) G93.6
due to birth injury P11.0
newborn (anoxia or hypoxia) P52.4
birth injury P11.0
traumatic — *see* Injury, intracranial, cerebral edema

Edema, edematous (infectious) (pitting) (toxic) - *continued*
cardiac — *see* Failure, heart, congestive
cardiovascular — *see* Failure, heart, congestive
cerebral — *see* Edema, brain
cerebrospinal — *see* Edema, brain
cervix (uteri) (acute) N88.8
puerperal, postpartum O90.89
chronic hereditary Q82.0
circumscribed, acute T78.3
hereditary D84.1
conjunctiva H11.42-
cornea H18.2-
idiopathic H18.22-
secondary H18.23-
due to contact lens H18.21-
due to
lymphatic obstruction I89.0
salt retention E87.0
epiglottis — *see* Edema, glottis
essential, acute T78.3
hereditary D84.1
extremities, lower — *see* Edema, legs
eyelid NEC H02.849
left H02.846
lower H02.845
upper H02.844
right H02.843
lower H02.842
upper H02.841
familial, hereditary Q82.0
famine — *see* Malnutrition, severe
generalized R60.1
glottis, glottic, glottidis (obstructive) (passive) J38.4
allergic T78.3
hereditary D84.1
heart — *see* Failure, heart, congestive
heat T67.7
hereditary Q82.0
inanition — *see* Malnutrition, severe
intracranial G93.6
iris H21.89
joint — *see* Effusion, joint
larynx — *see* Edema, glottis
legs R60.0
due to venous obstruction I87.1
hereditary Q82.0
localized R60.0
due to venous obstruction I87.1
lower limbs — *see* Edema, legs
lung J81.1
with heart condition or failure — *see* Failure, ventricular, left
acute J81.0
chemical (acute) J68.1
chronic J68.1
chronic J81.1
due to
chemicals, gases, fumes or vapors (inhalation) J68.1
external agent J70.9
specified NEC J70.8
radiation J70.1
due to
chemicals, fumes or vapors (inhalation) J68.1
external agent J70.9
specified NEC J70.8
high altitude T70.29
near drowning T75.1
radiation J70.0
meaning failure, left ventricle I50.1
lymphatic I89.0
due to mastectomy I97.2
macula H35.81
cystoid, following cataract surgery — *see* Complications, postprocedural, following cataract surgery
diabetic — *see* Diabetes, by type, with, retinopathy, with macular edema
malignant — *see* Gangrene, gas
Milroy's Q82.0
nasopharynx J39.2

Edema, edematous (infectious) (pitting) (toxic) - *continued*
newborn P83.30
hydrops fetalis — *see* Hydrops, fetalis
specified NEC P83.39
nutritional — *see also* Malnutrition, severe with dyspigmentation, skin and hair E40
optic disc or nerve — *see* Papilledema
orbit H05.22-
pancreas K86.89
papilla, optic — *see* Papilledema
penis N48.89
periodic T78.3
hereditary D84.1
pharynx J39.2
pulmonary — *see* Edema, lung
Quincke's T78.3
hereditary D84.1
renal — *see* Nephrosis
retina H35.81
diabetic — *see* Diabetes, by type, with, retinopathy, with macular edema
salt E87.0
scrotum N50.89
seminal vesicle N50.89
spermatic cord N50.89
spinal (cord) (vascular) (nontraumatic) G95.19
starvation — *see* Malnutrition, severe
stasis — *see* Hypertension, venous, (chronic)
subglottic — *see* Edema, glottis
supraglottic — *see* Edema, glottis
testis N44.8
tunica vaginalis N50.89
vas deferens N50.89
vulva (acute) N90.89
Edentulism — *see* Absence, teeth, acquired
Edsall's disease T67.2
Educational handicap Z55.9
less than a high school diploma Z55.5
no general equivalence degree (GED) Z55.5
specified NEC Z55.8
Edward's syndrome — *see* Trisomy, 18
Effect (s) (of) (from) — *see* Effect, adverse NEC
Effect, adverse
abnormal gravitational (G) forces or states T75.81
abuse — *see* Maltreatment
air pressure T70.9
specified NEC T70.8
altitude (high) — *see* Effect, adverse, high altitude
anesthesia — *see also* Anesthesia T88.59
in labor and delivery O74.9
local, toxic
in labor and delivery O74.4
in pregnancy NEC O29.3-
postpartum, puerperal O89.3
postpartum, puerperal O89.9
specified NEC T88.59
in labor and delivery O74.8
postpartum, puerperal O89.8
spinal and epidural T88.59
headache T88.59
in labor and delivery O74.5
postpartum, puerperal O89.4
specified NEC
in labor and delivery O74.6
postpartum, puerperal O89.5
antitoxin — *see* Complications, vaccination
atmospheric pressure T70.9
due to explosion T70.8
high T70.3
low — *see* Effect, adverse, high altitude
specified effect NEC T70.8
biological, correct substance properly administered — *see* Effect, adverse, drug
blood (derivatives) (serum) (transfusion) — *see* Complications, transfusion
chemical substance — *see* Table of Drugs and Chemicals
cold (temperature) (weather) T69.9
chilblains T69.1

Effect, adverse - *continued*
cold (temperature) (weather) - *continued*
frostbite — *see* Frostbite
specified effect NEC T69.8
drugs and medicaments T88.7
specified drug — *see* Table of Drugs and Chemicals, by drug, adverse effect
specified effect - code to condition
electric current, electricity (shock) T75.4
burn — *see* Burn
exertion (excessive) T73.3
exposure — *see* Exposure
external cause NEC T75.89
foodstuffs T78.1
allergic reaction — *see* Allergy, food
causing anaphylaxis — *see* Shock, anaphylactic, due to food
noxious — *see* Poisoning, food, noxious
gases, fumes, or vapors T59.9-
specified agent — *see* Table of Drugs and Chemicals
glue (airplane) sniffing
due to drug abuse — *see* Abuse, drug, inhalant
due to drug dependence — *see* Dependence, drug, inhalant
heat — *see* Heat
high altitude NEC T70.29
anoxia T70.29
on
ears T70.0
sinuses T70.1
polycythemia D75.1
high pressure fluids T70.4
hot weather — *see* Heat
hunger T73.0
immersion, foot — *see* Immersion
immunization — *see* Complications, vaccination
immunological agents — *see* Complications, vaccination
infrared (radiation) (rays) NOS T66
dermatitis or eczema L59.8
infusion — *see* Complications, infusion
lack of care of infants — *see* Maltreatment, child
lightning — *see* Lightning
medical care T88.9
specified NEC T88.8
medicinal substance, correct, properly administered — *see* Effect, adverse, drug
motion T75.3
noise, on inner ear — *see* subcategory H83.3
overheated places — *see* Heat
psychosocial, of work environment Z56.5
radiation (diagnostic) (infrared) (natural source) (therapeutic) (ultraviolet) (X-ray) NOS T66
dermatitis or eczema — *see* Dermatitis, due to, radiation
fibrosis of lung J70.1
pneumonitis J70.0
pulmonary manifestations
acute J70.0
chronic J70.1
skin L59.9
radioactive substance NOS
dermatitis or eczema — *see* Radiodermatitis
reduced temperature T69.9
immersion foot or hand — *see* Immersion
specified effect NEC T69.8
serum NEC — *see also* Reaction, serum T80.69
specified NEC T78.8
external cause NEC T75.89
strangulation — *see* Asphyxia, traumatic
submersion T75.1
thirst T73.1
toxic — *see* Toxicity
transfusion — *see* Complications, transfusion
ultraviolet (radiation) (rays) NOS T66
burn — *see* Burn

Embolism (multiple) (paradoxical) - *continued*
- air (any site) (traumatic) - *continued*
  - following - *continued*
    - procedure NEC
      - artery T81.719
        - mesenteric T81.710
        - renal T81.711
        - specified NEC T81.718
      - vein T81.72
  - in pregnancy, childbirth or puerperium — *see* Embolism, obstetric
- amniotic fluid (pulmonary) — *see also* Embolism, obstetric
  - following
    - abortion — *see* Abortion by type complicated by embolism
    - ectopic pregnancy O08.2
    - molar pregnancy O08.2
- aorta, aortic I74.10
  - abdominal I74.09
    - saddle I74.01
  - bifurcation I74.09
  - saddle I74.01
  - thoracic I74.11
- artery I74.9
  - auditory, internal I65.8
  - basilar — *see* Occlusion, artery, basilar
  - carotid (common) (internal) — *see* Occlusion, artery, carotid
  - cerebellar (anterior inferior) (posterior inferior) (superior) I66.3
  - cerebral — *see* Occlusion, artery, cerebral
  - choroidal (anterior) I65.8
  - communicating posterior I65.8
  - coronary — *see also* Infarct, myocardium
    - not resulting in infarction I24.0
  - extremity I74.4
    - lower I74.3
    - upper I74.2
  - hypophyseal I65.8
  - iliac I74.5
  - limb I74.4
    - lower I74.3
    - upper I74.2
  - mesenteric (with gangrene) — *see also* Ischemia, intestine, acute K55.059
  - ophthalmic — *see* Occlusion, artery, retina
  - peripheral I74.4
  - pontine I65.8
  - precerebral — *see* Occlusion, artery, precerebral
  - pulmonary — *see* Embolism, pulmonary
  - renal N28.0
  - retinal — *see* Occlusion, artery, retina
  - septic I76
  - specified NEC I74.8
  - vertebral — *see* Occlusion, artery, vertebral
- basilar (artery) I65.1
- blood clot
  - following
    - abortion — *see* Abortion by type complicated by embolism
    - ectopic or molar pregnancy O08.2
  - in pregnancy, childbirth or puerperium — *see* Embolism, obstetric
- brain — *see also* Occlusion, artery, cerebral
  - following
    - abortion — *see* Abortion by type complicated by embolism
    - ectopic or molar pregnancy O08.2
  - puerperal, postpartum, childbirth — *see* Embolism, obstetric
- capillary I78.8
- cardiac — *see also* Infarct, myocardium
  - not resulting in infarction I51.3
- carotid (artery) (common) (internal) — *see* Occlusion, artery, carotid
- cavernous sinus (venous) — *see* Embolism, intracranial venous sinus
- cerebral — *see* Occlusion, artery, cerebral
- cholesterol — *see* Atheroembolism
- coronary (artery or vein) (systemic) — *see* Occlusion, coronary

Embolism (multiple) (paradoxical) - *continued*
- due to device, implant or graft — *see also* Complications, by site and type, specified NEC
  - arterial graft NEC T82.818
  - breast (implant) T85.818
  - catheter NEC T85.818
    - dialysis (renal) T82.818
      - intraperitoneal T85.818
    - infusion NEC T82.818
      - spinal (epidural) (subdural) T85.810
    - urinary (indwelling) T83.81
  - electronic (electrode) (pulse generator) (stimulator)
    - bone T84.81
    - cardiac T82.817
    - nervous system (brain) (peripheral nerve) (spinal) T85.810
    - urinary T83.81
  - fixation, internal (orthopedic) NEC T84.81
  - gastrointestinal (bile duct) (esophagus) T85.818
  - genital NEC T83.81
  - heart (graft) (valve) T82.817
  - joint prosthesis T84.81
  - ocular (corneal graft) (orbital implant) T85.818
  - orthopedic (bone graft) NEC T86.838
  - specified NEC T85.818
  - urinary (graft) NEC T83.81
  - vascular NEC T82.818
  - ventricular intracranial shunt T85.810
- extremities
  - lower — *see* Embolism, vein, lower extremity
    - arterial I74.3
  - upper I74.2
- eye H34.9
- fat (cerebral) (pulmonary) (systemic) T79.1
  - following
    - abortion — *see* Abortion by type complicated by embolism
    - ectopic or molar pregnancy O08.2
  - complicating delivery — *see* Embolism, obstetric
- following
  - abortion — *see* Abortion by type complicated by embolism
  - ectopic or molar pregnancy O08.2
  - infusion, therapeutic injection or transfusion
    - air T80.0
- heart (fatty) — *see also* Infarct, myocardium
  - not resulting in infarction I51.3
- hepatic (vein) I82.0
- in pregnancy, childbirth or puerperium — *see* Embolism, obstetric
- intestine (artery) (vein) (with gangrene) — *see also* Ischemia, intestine, acute K55.039
- intracranial — *see also* Occlusion, artery, cerebral
  - venous sinus (any) G08
    - nonpyogenic I67.6
- intraspinal venous sinuses or veins G08
  - nonpyogenic G95.19
- kidney (artery) N28.0
- lateral sinus (venous) — *see* Embolism, intracranial, venous sinus
- leg — *see* Embolism, vein, lower extremity
  - arterial I74.3
- longitudinal sinus (venous) — *see* Embolism, intracranial, venous sinus
- lung (massive) — *see* Embolism, pulmonary
- meninges I66.8
- mesenteric (artery) (vein) (with gangrene) — *see also* Ischemia, intestine, acute K55.059
- obstetric (in) (pulmonary)
  - childbirth O88.22
    - air O88.02
    - amniotic fluid O88.12
    - blood clot O88.22
    - fat O88.82

Embolism (multiple) (paradoxical) - *continued*
- obstetric (in) (pulmonary) - *continued*
  - childbirth - *continued*
    - pyemic O88.32
    - septic O88.32
    - specified type NEC O88.82
  - pregnancy O88.21-
    - air O88.01-
    - amniotic fluid O88.11-
    - blood clot O88.21-
    - fat O88.81-
    - pyemic O88.31-
    - septic O88.31-
    - specified type NEC O88.81-
  - puerperal O88.23
    - air O88.03
    - amniotic fluid O88.13
    - blood clot O88.23
    - fat O88.83
    - pyemic O88.33
    - septic O88.33
    - specified type NEC O88.83
- ophthalmic — *see* Occlusion, artery, retina
- penis N48.81
- peripheral artery NOS I74.4
- pituitary E23.6
- popliteal (artery) I74.3
- portal (vein) I81
- postoperative, postprocedural
  - artery T81.719
    - mesenteric T81.710
    - renal T81.711
    - specified NEC T81.718
  - vein T81.72
- precerebral artery — *see* Occlusion, artery, precerebral
- puerperal — *see* Embolism, obstetric
- pulmonary (acute) (artery) (vein) I26.99
  - with acute cor pulmonale I26.09
  - chronic I27.82
  - following
    - abortion — *see* Abortion by type complicated by embolism
    - ectopic or molar pregnancy O08.2
  - healed or old Z86.711
  - in pregnancy, childbirth or puerperium — *see* Embolism, obstetric
  - multiple subsegmental without acute cor pulmonale I26.94
  - personal history of Z86.711
  - saddle I26.92
    - with acute cor pulmonale I26.02
  - septic I26.90
    - with acute cor pulmonale I26.01
  - single subsegmental without acute cor pulmonale I26.93
  - subsegmental NOS I26.93
- pyemic (multiple) I76
  - following
    - abortion — *see* Abortion by type complicated by embolism
    - ectopic or molar pregnancy O08.2
  - Hemophilus influenzae A41.3
  - pneumococcal A40.3
    - with pneumonia J13
  - puerperal, postpartum, childbirth (any organism) — *see* Embolism, obstetric
  - specified organism NEC A41.89
  - staphylococcal A41.2
  - streptococcal A40.9
- renal (artery) N28.0
  - vein I82.3
- retina, retinal — *see* Occlusion, artery, retina
- saddle
  - abdominal aorta I74.01
  - pulmonary artery I26.92
    - with acute cor pulmonale I26.02
- septic (arterial) I76
  - complicating abortion — *see* Abortion, by type, complicated by, embolism
- sinus — *see* Embolism, intracranial, venous sinus
- soap complicating abortion — *see* Abortion, by type, complicated by, embolism

Embolism (multiple) (paradoxical) - *continued*
- spinal cord G95.19
  - pyogenic origin G06.1
- spleen, splenic (artery) I74.8
- upper extremity I74.2
- vein (acute) I82.90
  - antecubital I82.61-
    - chronic I82.71-
  - axillary I82.A1-
    - chronic I82.A2-
  - basilic I82.61-
    - chronic I82.71-
  - brachial I82.62-
    - chronic I82.72-
  - brachiocephalic (innominate) I82.290
    - chronic I82.291
  - cephalic I82.61-
    - chronic I82.71-
  - chronic I82.91
  - deep (DVT) I82.40-
    - calf I82.4Z-
      - chronic I82.5Z-
    - lower leg I82.4Z-
      - chronic I82.5Z-
    - thigh I82.4Y-
      - chronic I82.5Y-
    - upper leg I82.4Y
      - chronic I82.5y--
  - femoral I82.41-
    - chronic I82.51-
  - iliac (iliofemoral) I82.42-
    - chronic I82.52-
  - innominate I82.290
    - chronic I82.291
  - internal jugular I82.C1-
    - chronic I82.C2-
  - lower extremity
    - deep I82.40-
      - chronic I82.50-
      - specified NEC I82.49-
        - chronic NEC I82.59-
    - distal
      - deep I82.4Z-
    - proximal
      - deep I82.4Y-
        - chronic I82.5Y-
    - superficial I82.81-
  - popliteal I82.43-
    - chronic I82.53-
  - radial I82.62-
    - chronic I82.72-
  - renal I82.3
  - saphenous (greater) (lesser) I82.81-
  - specified NEC I82.890
    - chronic NEC I82.891
  - subclavian I82.B1-
    - chronic I82.B2-
  - thoracic NEC I82.290
    - chronic I82.291
  - tibial I82.44-
    - chronic I82.54-
  - ulnar I82.62-
    - chronic I82.72-
  - upper extremity I82.60-
    - chronic I82.70-
    - deep I82.62-
      - chronic I82.72-
    - superficial I82.61-
      - chronic I82.71-
  - vena cava
    - inferior (acute) I82.220
      - chronic I82.221
    - superior (acute) I82.210
      - chronic I82.211
- venous sinus G08
- vessels of brain — *see* Occlusion, artery, cerebral

Embolus — *see* Embolism

Embryoma — *see also* Neoplasm, uncertain behavior, by site
- benign — *see* Neoplasm, benign, by site
- kidney C64.-
- liver C22.0

Embryoma - *continued*
- malignant — *see also* Neoplasm, malignant, by site
  - kidney C64.-
  - liver C22.0
  - testis C62.9-
    - descended (scrotal) C62.1-
    - undescended C62.0-
- testis C62.9-
  - descended (scrotal) C62.1-
  - undescended C62.0-

Embryonic
- circulation Q28.9
- heart Q28.9
- vas deferens Q55.4

Embryopathia NOS Q89.9

Embryotoxon Q13.4

Emesis — *see* Vomiting

Emotional lability R45.86

Emotionality, pathological F60.3

Emotogenic disease — *see* Disorder, psychogenic

Emphysema (atrophic) (bullous) (chronic) (interlobular) (lung) (obstructive) (pulmonary) (senile) (vesicular) J43.9
- cellular tissue (traumatic) T79.7
  - surgical T81.82
- centrilobular J43.2
- compensatory J98.3
- congenital (interstitial) P25.0
- conjunctiva H11.89
- connective tissue (traumatic) T79.7
  - surgical T81.82
- due to chemicals, gases, fumes or vapors J68.4
- eyelid (s) — *see* Disorder, eyelid, specified type NEC
  - surgical T81.82
  - traumatic T79.7
- interstitial J98.2
  - congenital P25.0
  - perinatal period P25.0
- laminated tissue T79.7
  - surgical T81.82
- mediastinal J98.2
  - newborn P25.2
- orbit, orbital — *see* Disorder, orbit, specified type NEC
- panacinar J43.1
- panlobular J43.1
- specified NEC J43.8
- subcutaneous (traumatic) T79.7
  - nontraumatic J98.2
  - postprocedural T81.82
  - surgical T81.82
- surgical T81.82
- thymus (gland) (congenital) E32.8
- traumatic (subcutaneous) T79.7
- unilateral J43.0

Empty nest syndrome Z60.0

Empyema (acute) (chest) (double) (pleura) (supradiaphragmatic) (thorax) J86.9
- with fistula J86.0
- accessory sinus (chronic) — *see* Sinusitis
- antrum (chronic) — *see* Sinusitis, maxillary
- brain (any part) — *see* Abscess, brain
- ethmoidal (chronic) (sinus) — *see* Sinusitis, ethmoidal
- extradural — *see* Abscess, extradural
- frontal (chronic) (sinus) — *see* Sinusitis, frontal
- gallbladder K81.0
- mastoid (process) (acute) — *see* Mastoiditis, acute
- maxilla, maxillary M27.2
  - sinus (chronic) — *see* Sinusitis, maxillary
- nasal sinus (chronic) — *see* Sinusitis
- sinus (accessory) (chronic) (nasal) — *see* Sinusitis
- sphenoidal (sinus) (chronic) — *see* Sinusitis, sphenoidal
- subarachnoid — *see* Abscess, extradural
- subdural — *see* Abscess, subdural
- tuberculous A15.6
- ureter — *see* Ureteritis

Empyema (acute) (chest) (double) (pleura) (supradiaphragmatic) (thorax) - *continued*
- ventricular — *see* Abscess, brain

En coup de sabre lesion L94.1

Enamel pearls K00.2

Enameloma K00.2

Enanthema, viral B09

Encephalitis (chronic) (hemorrhagic) (idiopathic) (nonepidemic) (spurious) (subacute) G04.90
- acute — *see also* Encephalitis, viral A86
  - disseminated G04.00
    - infectious G04.01
    - noninfectious G04.81
    - postimmunization (postvaccination) G04.02
    - postinfectious G04.01
  - inclusion body A85.8
  - necrotizing hemorrhagic G04.30
    - postimmunization G04.32
    - postinfectious G04.31
    - specified NEC G04.39
- arboviral, arbovirus NEC A85.2
- arthropod-borne NEC (viral) A85.2
- Australian A83.4
- California (virus) A83.5
- Central European (tick-borne) A84.1
- Czechoslovakian A84.1
- Dawson's (inclusion body) A81.1
- diffuse sclerosing A81.1
- disseminated, acute G04.00
- due to
  - cat scratch disease A28.1
  - human immunodeficiency virus (HIV) disease B20 *[G05.3]*
  - malaria — *see* Malaria
  - rickettsiosis — *see* Rickettsiosis
  - smallpox inoculation G04.02
  - typhus — *see* Typhus
- Eastern equine A83.2
- endemic (viral) A86
- epidemic NEC (viral) A86
- equine (acute) (infectious) (viral) A83.9
  - Eastern A83.2
  - Venezuelan A92.2
  - Western A83.1
- Far Eastern (tick-borne) A84.0
- following vaccination or other immunization procedure G04.02
- herpes zoster B02.0
- herpesviral B00.4
  - due to herpesvirus 6 B10.01
  - due to herpesvirus 7 B10.09
  - specified NEC B10.09
- Ilheus (virus) A83.8
- inclusion body A81.1
- in (due to)
  - actinomycosis A42.82
  - adenovirus A85.1
  - African trypanosomiasis B56.9 *[G05.3]*
  - Chagas' disease (chronic) B57.42
  - cytomegalovirus B25.8
  - enterovirus A85.0
  - herpes (simplex) virus B00.4
    - due to herpesvirus 6 B10.01
    - due to herpesvirus 7 B10.09
    - specified NEC B10.09
  - infectious disease NEC B99 *[G05.3]*
  - influenza — *see* Influenza, with, encephalopathy
  - listeriosis A32.12
  - measles B05.0
  - mumps B26.2
  - naegleriasis B60.2
  - parasitic disease NEC B89 *[G05.3]*
  - poliovirus A80.9 *[G05.3]*
  - rubella B06.01
  - syphilis
    - congenital A50.42
    - late A52.14
  - systemic lupus erythematosus M32.19
  - toxoplasmosis (acquired) B58.2
    - congenital P37.1
  - tuberculosis A17.82
  - zoster B02.0

Encephalitis (chronic) (hemorrhagic) (idiopathic) (nonepidemic) (spurious) (subacute) - *continued*
- infectious (acute) (virus) NEC A86
- Japanese (B type) A83.0
- La Crosse A83.5
- lead — *see* Poisoning, lead
- lethargica (acute) (infectious) A85.8
- louping ill A84.89
- lupus erythematosus, systemic M32.19
- lymphatica A87.2
- Mengo A85.8
- meningococcal A39.81
- Murray Valley A83.4
- otitic NEC H66.40 *[G05.3]*
- parasitic NOS B71.9
- periaxial G37.0
- periaxialis (concentrica) (diffuse) G37.5
- postchickenpox B01.11
- postexanthematous NEC B09
- postimmunization G04.02
- postinfectious NEC G04.01
- postmeasles B05.0
- postvaccinal G04.02
- postvaricella B01.11
- postviral NEC A86
- Powassan A84.81
- Rasmussen G04.81
- Rio Bravo A85.8
- Russian
  - autumnal A83.0
  - spring-summer (taiga) A84.0
- saturnine — *see* Poisoning, lead
- specified NEC G04.81
- St. Louis A83.3
- subacute sclerosing A81.1
- summer A83.0
- suppurative G04.81
- tick-borne A84.9
- Torula, torular (cryptococcal) B45.1
- toxic NEC G92.8
- trichinosis B75 *[G05.3]*
- type
  - B A83.0
  - C A83.3
- van Bogaert's A81.1
- Venezuelan equine A92.2
- Vienna A85.8
- viral, virus A86
  - arthropod-borne NEC A85.2
    - mosquito-borne A83.9
      - Australian X disease A83.4
      - California virus A83.5
      - Eastern equine A83.2
      - Japanese (B type) A83.0
      - Murray Valley A83.4
      - specified NEC A83.8
      - St. Louis A83.3
      - type B A83.0
      - type C A83.3
      - Western equine A83.1
    - tick-borne A84.9
      - biundulant A84.1
      - central European A84.1
      - Czechoslovakian A84.1
      - diphasic meningoencephalitis A84.1
      - Far Eastern A84.0
      - Russian spring-summer (taiga) A84.0
      - specified NEC A84.89
  - specified type NEC A85.8
  - tick-borne, specified NEC A84.89
- Western equine A83.1

Encephalocele Q01.9
- frontal Q01.0
- nasofrontal Q01.1
- occipital Q01.2
- specified NEC Q01.8

Encephalocystocele — *see* Encephalocele

Encephaloduroarteriomyosynangiosis (EDAMS) I67.5

Encephalomalacia (brain) (cerebellar) (cerebral) — *see* Softening, brain

Encephalomeningitis — *see* Meningoencephalitis

Encephalomeningocele — *see* Encephalocele

Encephalomeningomyelitis — *see* Meningoencephalitis

Encephalomyelitis — *see also* Encephalitis G04.90
- acute disseminated G04.00
  - infectious G04.01
  - noninfectious G04.81
  - postimmunization G04.02
  - postinfectious G04.01
- acute necrotizing hemorrhagic G04.30
  - postimmunization G04.32
  - postinfectious G04.31
  - specified NEC G04.39
- benign myalgic G93.3
- equine A83.9
  - Eastern A83.2
  - Venezuelan A92.2
  - Western A83.1
- in diseases classified elsewhere G05.3
- myalgic, benign G93.3
- postchickenpox B01.11
- postinfectious NEC G04.01
- postmeasles B05.0
- postvaccinal G04.02
- postvaricella B01.11
- rubella B06.01
- specified NEC G04.81
- Venezuelan equine A92.2

Encephalomyelocele — *see* Encephalocele

Encephalomyclomeningitis — *see* Meningoencephalitis

Encephalomyelopathy G96.9

Encephalomyeloradiculitis (acute) G61.0

Encephalomyeloradiculoneuritis (acute) (Guillain-Barré) G61.0

Encephalomyeloradiculopathy G96.9

Encephalopathia hyperbilirubinemica, newborn P57.9
- due to isoimmunization (conditions in P55) P57.0

Encephalopathy (acute) G93.40
- acute necrotizing hemorrhagic G04.30
  - postimmunization G04.32
  - postinfectious G04.31
  - specified NEC G04.39
- alcoholic G31.2
- anoxic — *see* Damage, brain, anoxic
- arteriosclerotic I67.2
- centrolobar progressive (Schilder) G37.0
- congenital Q07.9
- degenerative, in specified disease NEC G32.89
- demyelinating callosal G37.1
- due to
  - drugs — *see also* Table of Drugs and Chemicals G92.8
- hepatic — *see* Failure, hepatic
- hyperbilirubinemic, newborn P57.9
  - due to isoimmunization (conditions in P55) P57.0
- hypertensive I67.4
- hypoglycemic E16.2
- hypoxic — *see* Damage, brain, anoxic
- hypoxic ischemic P91.60
  - mild P91.61
  - moderate P91.62
  - severe P91.63
- in (due to) (with)
  - birth injury P11.1
  - hyperinsulinism E16.1 *[G94]*
  - influenza — *see* Influenza, with, encephalopathy
  - lack of vitamin — *see also* Deficiency, vitamin E56.9 *[G32.89]*
  - neoplastic disease (see also Neoplasm) D49.9 *[G13.1]*
  - serum — *see also* Reaction, serum T80.69
  - syphilis A52.17
  - trauma (postconcussional) F07.81
    - current injury — *see* Injury, intracranial
  - vaccination G04.02
- lead — *see* Poisoning, lead
- metabolic G93.41
  - drug induced G92.8
  - toxic G92.8

Encephalopathy (acute) - *continued*
- myoclonic, early, symptomatic — *see* Epilepsy, generalized, specified NEC
- necrotizing, subacute (Leigh) G31.82
- neonatal P91.819
  - in diseases classified elsewhere P91.811
- pellagrous E52 *[G32.89]*
- portosystemic — *see* Failure, hepatic
- postcontusional F07.81
  - current injury — *see* Injury, intracranial, diffuse
- posthypoglycemic (coma) E16.1 *[G94]*
- postradiation G93.89
- saturnine — *see* Poisoning, lead
- septic G93.41
- specified NEC G93.49
- spongioform, subacute (viral) A81.09
- toxic G92.9
  - metabolic G92.8
- traumatic (postconcussional) F07.81
  - current injury — *see* Injury, intracranial
- vitamin B deficiency NEC E53.9 *[G32.89]*
  - vitamin B1 E51.2
- Wernicke's E51.2

Encephalorrhagia — *see* Hemorrhage, intracranial, intracerebral

Encephalosis, posttraumatic F07.81

Enchondroma — *see also* Neoplasm, bone, benign

Enchondromatosis (cartilaginous) (multiple) Q78.4

Encopresis R15.9
- functional F98.1
- nonorganic origin F98.1
- psychogenic F98.1

Encounter (with health service) (for) Z76.89
- adjustment and management (of)
  - breast implant Z45.81
  - implanted device NEC Z45.89
  - myringotomy device (stent) (tube) Z45.82
  - neurostimulator (brain) (gastric) (peripheral nerve) (sacral nerve) (spinal cord) (vagus nerve) Z45.42
- administrative purpose only Z02.9
  - examination for
    - adoption Z02.82
    - armed forces Z02.3
    - disability determination Z02.71
    - driving license Z02.4
    - employment Z02.1
    - insurance Z02.6
    - medical certificate NEC Z02.79
    - paternity testing Z02.81
    - residential institution admission Z02.2
    - school admission Z02.0
    - sports Z02.5
  - specified reason NEC Z02.89
- aftercare — *see* Aftercare
- antenatal screening Z36.9
  - cervical length Z36.86
  - chromosomal anomalies Z36.0
  - congenital cardiac abnormalities Z36.83
  - elevated maternal serum alphafetoprotein level Z36.1
  - fetal growth retardation Z36.4
  - fetal lung maturity Z36.84
  - fetal macrosomia Z36.88
  - hydrops fetalis Z36.81
  - intrauterine growth restriction (IUGR) /small-for-dates Z36.4
  - isoimmunization Z36.5
  - large-for-dates Z36.88
  - malformations Z36.3
  - non-visualized anatomy on a previous scan Z36.2
  - nuchal translucency Z36.82
  - raised alphafetoprotein level Z36.1
  - risk of pre-term labor Z36.86
  - specified type NEC Z36.89
  - specified follow-up NEC Z36.2
  - specified genetic defects NEC Z36.8A
  - Streptococcus B Z36.85
  - suspected anomaly Z36.3
  - uncertain dates Z36.87

Encounter (with health service) (for) - *continued*
- assisted reproductive fertility procedure cycle Z31.83
- blood typing Z01.83
  - Rh typing Z01.83
- breast augmentation or reduction Z41.1
- breast implant exchange (different material) (different size) Z45.81
- breast reconstruction following mastectomy Z42.1
- check-up — *see* Examination
- chemotherapy for neoplasm Z51.11
- colonoscopy, screening Z12.11
- counseling — *see* Counseling
- delivery, full-term, uncomplicated O80
  - cesarean, without indication O82
- desensitization to allergens Z51.6
- ear piercing Z41.3
- examination — *see* Examination
- expectant parent (s) (adoptive) pre-birth pediatrician visit Z76.81
- fertility preservation procedure (prior to cancer therapy) (prior to removal of gonads) Z31.84
- fitting (of) — *see* Fitting (and adjustment) (of)
- genetic
  - counseling
    - nonprocreative Z71.83
    - procreative Z31.5
  - testing — *see* Test, genetic
- hearing conservation and treatment Z01.12
- immunotherapy for neoplasm Z51.12
- in vitro fertilization cycle Z31.83
- instruction (in)
  - childbirth Z32.2
  - child care (postpartal) (prenatal) Z32.3
  - natural family planning
    - procreative Z31.61
    - to avoid pregnancy Z30.02
- insulin pump titration Z46.81
- joint prosthesis insertion following prior explantation of joint prosthesis (staged procedure)
  - hip Z47.32
  - knee Z47.33
  - shoulder Z47.31
- laboratory (as part of a general medical examination) Z00.00
  - with abnormal findings Z00.01
- mental health services (for)
  - abuse NEC
    - perpetrator Z69.82
    - victim Z69.81
  - child abuse
    - nonparental
      - perpetrator Z69.021
      - victim Z69.020
    - parental
      - perpetrator Z69.011
      - victim Z69.010
  - child neglect
    - nonparental
      - perpetrator Z69.021
      - victim Z69.020
    - parental
      - perpetrator Z69.011
      - victim Z69.010
  - child psychological abuse
    - nonparental
      - perpetrator Z69.021
      - victim Z69.020
    - parental
      - perpetrator Z69.011
      - victim Z69.010
  - child sexual abuse
    - nonparental
      - perpetrator Z69.021
      - victim Z69.020
    - parental
      - perpetrator Z69.011
      - victim Z69.010
  - non-spousal adult abuse
    - perpetrator Z69.82

Encounter (with health service) (for) - *continued*
- mental health services (for) - *continued*
  - non-spousal adult abuse - *continued*
    - victim Z69.81
  - spousal or partner
    - abuse
      - perpetrator Z69.12
      - victim Z69.11
    - neglect
      - perpetrator Z69.12
      - victim Z69.11
    - psychological abuse
      - perpetrator Z69.12
      - victim Z69.11
    - violence
      - perpetrator (physical) (sexual) Z69.12
      - victim (physical) Z69.11
        - sexual Z69.81
- observation (for) (ruled out)
  - exposure to (suspected)
    - anthrax Z03.810
    - biological agent NEC Z03.818
- pediatrician visit, by expectant parent (s) (adoptive) Z76.81
- placental sample (taken vaginally) — *see also* Encounter, antenatal screening Z36.9
- plastic and reconstructive surgery following medical procedure or healed injury NEC Z42.8
- pregnancy
  - supervision of — *see* Pregnancy, supervision of
  - test Z32.00
    - result negative Z32.02
    - result positive Z32.01
- procreative management and counseling for gestational carrier Z31.7
- prophylactic measures Z29.9
  - antivenin Z29.12
  - fluoride administration Z29.3
  - immunotherapy for respiratory syncytial virus (RSV) Z29.11
  - rabies immune globin Z29.14
  - Rho (D) immune globulin Z29.13
  - specified NEC Z29.8
- radiation therapy (antineoplastic) Z51.0
- radiological (as part of a general medical examination) Z00.00
  - with abnormal findings Z00.01
- reconstructive surgery following medical procedure or healed injury NEC Z42.8
- removal (of) — *see also* Removal
  - artificial
    - arm Z44.00-
      - complete Z44.01-
      - partial Z44.02-
    - eye Z44.2-
    - leg Z44.10-
      - complete Z44.11-
      - partial Z44.12-
  - breast implant Z45.81
    - tissue expander (with or without synchronous insertion of permanent implant) Z45.81
  - device Z46.9
    - specified NEC Z46.89
  - external
    - fixation device - code to fracture with seventh character D
    - prosthesis, prosthetic device Z44.9
      - breast Z44.3-
      - specified NEC Z44.8
  - implanted device NEC Z45.89
  - insulin pump Z46.81
  - internal fixation device Z47.2
  - myringotomy device (stent) (tube) Z45.82
  - nervous system device NEC Z46.2
    - brain neuropacemaker Z46.2
    - visual substitution device Z46.2
      - implanted Z45.31
  - non-vascular catheter Z46.82
  - orthodontic device Z46.4
  - stent

Encounter (with health service) (for) - *continued*
- removal (of) - *continued*
  - stent - *continued*
    - ureteral Z46.6
  - urinary device Z46.6
- repeat cervical smear to confirm findings of recent normal smear following initial abnormal smear Z01.42
- respirator [ventilator] use during power failure Z99.12
- Rh typing Z01.83
- screening — *see* Screening
- specified NEC Z76.89
- sterilization Z30.2
- suspected condition, ruled out
  - amniotic cavity and membrane Z03.71
  - cervical shortening Z03.75
  - fetal anomaly Z03.73
  - fetal growth Z03.74
  - maternal and fetal conditions NEC Z03.79
  - oligohydramnios Z03.71
  - placental problem Z03.72
  - polyhydramnios Z03.71
- suspected exposure (to) , ruled out
  - anthrax Z03.810
  - biological agents NEC Z03.818
- termination of pregnancy, elective Z33.2
- testing — *see* Test
- therapeutic drug level monitoring Z51.81
- titration, insulin pump Z46.81
- to determine fetal viability of pregnancy O36.80
- training
  - insulin pump Z46.81
- X-ray of chest (as part of a general medical examination) Z00.00
  - with abnormal findings Z00.01

Encystment — *see* Cyst

Endarteritis (bacterial, subacute) (infective) I77.6
- brain I67.7
- cerebral or cerebrospinal I67.7
- deformans — *see* Arteriosclerosis
- embolic — *see* Embolism
- obliterans — *see also* Arteriosclerosis
  - pulmonary I28.8
- pulmonary I28.8
- retina — *see* Vasculitis, retina
- senile — *see* Arteriosclerosis
- syphilitic A52.09
  - brain or cerebral A52.04
  - congenital A50.54 *[I79.8]*
- tuberculous A18.89

Endemic — *see* condition

Endocarditis (chronic) (marantic) (nonbacterial) (thrombotic) (valvular) I38
- with rheumatic fever (conditions in I00)
  - active — *see* Endocarditis, acute, rheumatic
  - inactive or quiescent (with chorea) I09.1
- acute or subacute I33.9
  - infective I33.0
  - rheumatic (aortic) (mitral) (pulmonary) (tricuspid) I01.1
    - with chorea (acute) (rheumatic) (Sydenham's) I02.0
- aortic (heart) (nonrheumatic) (valve) I35.8
  - with
    - mitral disease I08.0
      - with tricuspid (valve) disease I08.3
      - active or acute I01.1
        - with chorea (acute) (rheumatic) (Sydenham's) I02.0
    - rheumatic fever (conditions in I00)
      - active — *see* Endocarditis, acute, rheumatic
      - inactive or quiescent (with chorea) I06.9
    - tricuspid (valve) disease I08.2
      - with mitral (valve) disease I08.3
  - acute or subacute I33.9
  - arteriosclerotic I35.8
  - rheumatic I06.9

Endocarditis (chronic) (marantic) (nonbacterial) (thrombotic) (valvular) - *continued*
aortic (heart) (nonrheumatic) (valve) - *continued*
rheumatic - *continued*
with mitral disease I08.0
with tricuspid (valve) disease I08.3
active or acute I01.1
with chorea (acute) (rheumatic) (Sydenham's) I02.0
active or acute I01.1
with chorea (acute) (rheumatic) (Sydenham's) I02.0
specified NEC I06.8
specified cause NEC I35.8
syphilitic A52.03
arteriosclerotic I38
atypical verrucous (Libman-Sacks) M32.11
bacterial (acute) (any valve) (subacute) I33.0
candidal B37.6
congenital Q24.8
constrictive I33.0
Coxiella burnetii A78 *[I39]*
Coxsackie B33.21
due to
prosthetic cardiac valve T82.6
Q fever A78 *[I39]*
Serratia marcescens I33.0
typhoid (fever) A01.02
gonococcal A54.83
infectious or infective (acute) (any valve) (subacute) I33.0
lenta (acute) (any valve) (subacute) I33.0
Libman-Sacks M32.11
listerial A32.82
Löffler's I42.3
malignant (acute) (any valve) (subacute) I33.0
meningococcal A39.51
mitral (chronic) (double) (fibroid) (heart) (inactive) (valve) (with chorea) I05.9
with
aortic (valve) disease I08.0
with tricuspid (valve) disease I08.3
active or acute I01.1
with chorea (acute) (rheumatic) (Sydenham's) I02.0
rheumatic fever (conditions in I00)
active — *see* Endocarditis, acute, rheumatic
inactive or quiescent (with chorea) I05.9
tricuspid (valve) disease I08.1
with aortic (valve) disease I08.3
active or acute I01.1
with chorea (acute) (rheumatic) (Sydenham's) I02.0
bacterial I33.0
arteriosclerotic I34.8
nonrheumatic I34.8
acute or subacute I33.9
specified NEC I05.8
monilial B37.6
multiple valves I08.9
specified disorders I08.8
mycotic (acute) (any valve) (subacute) I33.0
pneumococcal (acute) (any valve) (subacute) I33.0
pulmonary (chronic) (heart) (valve) I37.8
with rheumatic fever (conditions in I00)
active — *see* Endocarditis, acute, rheumatic
inactive or quiescent (with chorea) I09.89
with aortic, mitral or tricuspid disease I08.8
acute or subacute I33.9
rheumatic I01.1
with chorea (acute) (rheumatic) (Sydenham's) I02.0
arteriosclerotic I37.8
congenital Q22.2
rheumatic (chronic) (inactive) (with chorea) I09.89

Endocarditis (chronic) (marantic) (nonbacterial) (thrombotic) (valvular) - *continued*
pulmonary (chronic) (heart) (valve) - *continued*
rheumatic (chronic) (inactive) (with chorea) - *continued*
active or acute I01.1
with chorea (acute) (rheumatic) (Sydenham's) I02.0
syphilitic A52.03
purulent (acute) (any valve) (subacute) I33.0
Q fever A78 *[I39]*
rheumatic (chronic) (inactive) (with chorea) I09.1
active or acute (aortic) (mitral) (pulmonary) (tricuspid) I01.1
with chorea (acute) (rheumatic) (Sydenham's) I02.0
rheumatoid — *see* Rheumatoid, carditis
septic (acute) (any valve) (subacute) I33.0
streptococcal (acute) (any valve) (subacute) I33.0
subacute — *see* Endocarditis, acute
suppurative (acute) (any valve) (subacute) I33.0
syphilitic A52.03
toxic I33.9
tricuspid (chronic) (heart) (inactive) (rheumatic) (valve) (with chorea) I07.9
with
aortic (valve) disease I08.2
mitral (valve) disease I08.3
mitral (valve) disease I08.1
aortic (valve) disease I08.3
rheumatic fever (conditions in I00)
active — *see* Endocarditis, acute, rheumatic
inactive or quiescent (with chorea) I07.8
active or acute I01.1
with chorea (acute) (rheumatic) (Sydenham's) I02.0
arteriosclerotic I36.8
nonrheumatic I36.8
acute or subacute I33.9
specified cause, except rheumatic I36.8
tuberculous — *see* Tuberculosis, endocarditis
typhoid A01.02
ulcerative (acute) (any valve) (subacute) I33.0
vegetative (acute) (any valve) (subacute) I33.0
verrucous (atypical) (nonbacterial) (nonrheumatic) M32.11
Endocardium, endocardial — *see also* condition
cushion defect Q21.2
Endocervicitis — *see also* Cervicitis
due to intrauterine (contraceptive) device T83.69
hyperplastic N72
Endocrine — *see* condition
Endocrinopathy, pluriglandular E31.9
Endodontic
overfill M27.52
underfill M27.53
Endodontitis K04.01
irreversible K04.02
reversible K04.01
Endomastoiditis — *see* Mastoiditis
Endometrioma N80.9
Endometriosis N80.9
appendix N80.5
bladder N80.8
bowel N80.5
broad ligament N80.3
cervix N80.0
colon N80.5
cul-de-sac (Douglas') N80.3
exocervix N80.0
fallopian tube N80.2
female genital organ NEC N80.8
gallbladder N80.8
in scar of skin N80.6

Endometriosis - *continued*
internal N80.0
intestine N80.5
lung N80.8
myometrium N80.0
ovary N80.1
parametrium N80.3
pelvic peritoneum N80.3
peritoneal (pelvic) N80.3
rectovaginal septum N80.4
rectum N80.5
round ligament N80.3
skin (scar) N80.6
specified site NEC N80.8
stromal D39.0
thorax N80.8
umbilicus N80.8
uterus (internal) N80.0
vagina N80.4
vulva N80.8
Endometritis (decidual) (nonspecific) (purulent) (senile) (atrophic) (suppurative) N71.9
with ectopic pregnancy O08.0
acute N71.0
blenorrhagic (gonococcal) (acute) (chronic) A54.24
cervix, cervical (with erosion or ectropion) — *see also* Cervicitis
hyperplastic N72
chlamydial A56.11
chronic N71.1
following
abortion — *see* Abortion by type complicated by genital infection
ectopic or molar pregnancy O08.0
gonococcal, gonorrheal (acute) (chronic) A54.24
hyperplastic — *see also* Hyperplasia, endometrial N85.00-
cervix N72
puerperal, postpartum, childbirth O86.12
subacute N71.0
tuberculous A18.17
Endometrium — *see* condition
Endomyocardiopathy, South African I42.3
Endomyocarditis — *see* Endocarditis
Endomyofibrosis I42.3
Endomyometritis — *see* Endometritis
Endopericarditis — *see* Endocarditis
Endoperineuritis — *see* Disorder, nerve
Endophlebitis — *see* Phlebitis
Endophthalmia — *see* Endophthalmitis, purulent
Endophthalmitis (acute) (infective) (metastatic) (subacute) H44.009
bleb associated H59.4 — *see* also Bleb, inflammed (infected), postprocedural
gonorrheal A54.39
in (due to)
cysticercosis B69.1
onchocerciasis B73.01
toxocariasis B83.0
panuveitis — *see* Panuveitis
parasitic H44.12-
purulent H44.00-
panophthalmitis — *see* Panophthalmitis
vitreous abscess H44.02-
specified NEC H44.19
sympathetic — *see* Uveitis, sympathetic
Endosalpingioma D28.2
Endosalpingiosis N94.89
Endosteitis — *see* Osteomyelitis
Endothelioma, bone — *see* Neoplasm, bone, malignant
Endotheliosis (hemorrhagic infectional) D69.8
Endotoxemia - code to condition
Endotrachelitis — *see* Cervicitis
Engelmann (-Camurati) syndrome Q78.3
English disease — *see* Rickets
Engman's disease L30.3
Engorgement
breast N64.59
newborn P83.4

Engorgement - *continued*
  breast - *continued*
    puerperal, postpartum O92.79
  lung (passive) — *see* Edema, lung
  pulmonary (passive) — *see* Edema, lung
  stomach K31.89
  venous, retina — *see* Occlusion, retina, vein, engorgement
Enlargement, enlarged — *see also* Hypertrophy
  adenoids J35.2
    with tonsils J35.3
  alveolar ridge K08.89
    congenital — *see* Anomaly, alveolar
  apertures of diaphragm (congenital) Q79.1
  gingival K06.1
  heart, cardiac — *see* Hypertrophy, cardiac
  labium majus, childhood asymmetric (CALME) N90.61
  lacrimal gland, chronic H04.03-
  liver — *see* Hypertrophy, liver
  lymph gland or node R59.9
    generalized R59.1
    localized R59.0
  orbit H05.34-
  organ or site, congenital NEC — *see* Anomaly, by site
  parathyroid (gland) E21.0
  pituitary fossa R93.0
  prostate N40.0
    with lower urinary tract symptoms (LUTS) N40.1
    without lower urinary tract symtpoms (LUTS) N40.0
  sella turcica R93.0
  spleen — *see* Splenomegaly
  thymus (gland) (congenital) E32.0
  thyroid (gland) — *see* Goiter
  tongue K14.8
  tonsils J35.1
    with adenoids J35.3
  uterus N85.2
  vestibular aqueduct Q16.5
Enophthalmos H05.40-
  due to
    orbital tissue atrophy H05.41-
    trauma or surgery H05.42-
Enostosis M27.8
Entamebic, entamebiasis — *see* Amebiasis
Entanglement
  umbilical cord (s) O69.82
    with compression O69.2
    around neck (with compression) O69.81
      with compression O69.1
      without compression O69.81
    of twins in monoamniotic sac O69.2
    without compression O69.82
Enteralgia — *see* Pain, abdominal
Enteric — *see* condition
Enteritis (acute) (diarrheal) (hemorrhagic) (noninfective) K52.9
  adenovirus A08.2
  aertrycke infection A02.0
  allergic K52.29
    with
      eosinophilic gastritis or gastroenteritis K52.81
      food protein-induced enterocolitis syndrome K52.21
      food protein-induced enteropathy K52.22
      FPIES K52.21
  amebic (acute) A06.0
    with abscess — *see* Abscess, amebic
    chronic A06.1
      with abscess — *see* Abscess, amebic
      nondysenteric A06.2
    nondysenteric A06.2
  astrovirus A08.32
  bacillary NOS A03.9
  bacterial A04.9
    specified NEC A04.8
  calicivirus A08.31
  candidal B37.82
  Chilomastix A07.8

Enteritis (acute) (diarrheal) (hemorrhagic) (noninfective) - *continued*
  choleriformis A00.1
  chronic (noninfectious) K52.9
    ulcerative — *see* Colitis, ulcerative
  cicatrizing (chronic) — *see* Enteritis, regional, small intestine
  Clostridium
    botulinum (food poisoning) A05.1
    difficile
      not specified as recurrent A04.72
      recurrent A04.71
  coccidial A07.3
  coxsackie virus A08.39
  dietetic — *see also* Enteritis, allergic K52.29
  drug-induced K52.1
  due to
    astrovirus A08.32
    calicivirus A08.31
    coxsackie virus A08.39
    drugs K52.1
    echovirus A08.39
    enterovirus NEC A08.39
    food hypersensitivity — *see also* Enteritis, allergic K52.29
    infectious organism (bacterial) (viral) — *see* Enteritis, infectious
    torovirus A08.39
    Yersinia enterocolitica A04.6
  echovirus A08.39
  eltor A00.1
  enterovirus NEC A08.39
  eosinophilic K52.81
  epidemic (infectious) A09
  fulminant — *see also* Ischemia, intestine, acute K55.019
  gangrenous — *see* Enteritis, infectious
  giardial A07.1
  infectious NOS A09
    due to
      adenovirus A08.2
      Aerobacter aerogenes A04.8
      Arizona (bacillus) A02.0
      bacteria NOS A04.9
        specified NEC A04.8
      Campylobacter A04.5
      Clostridium difficile
        not specified as recurrent A04.72
        recurrent A04.71
      Clostridium perfringens A04.8
      Enterobacter aerogenes A04.8
      enterovirus A08.39
      Escherichia coli A04.4
        enteroaggregative A04.4
        enterohemorrhagic A04.3
        enteroinvasive A04.2
        enteropathogenic A04.0
        enterotoxigenic A04.1
        specified NEC A04.4
      specified
        bacteria NEC A04.8
        virus NEC A08.39
      Staphylococcus A04.8
      virus NEC A08.4
        specified type NEC A08.39
      Yersinia enterocolitica A04.6
    specified organism NEC A08.8
  influenzal — *see* Influenza, with, digestive manifestations
  ischemic K55.9
    acute — *see also* Ischemia, intestine, acute K55.019
    chronic K55.1
  microsporidial A07.8
  mucomembranous, myxomembranous — *see* Syndrome, irritable bowel
  mucous — *see* Syndrome, irritable bowel
  necroticans A05.2
  necrotizing of newborn — *see* Enterocolitis, necrotizing, in newborn
  neurogenic — *see* Syndrome, irritable bowel
  newborn necrotizing — *see* Enterocolitis, necrotizing, in newborn
  noninfectious K52.9
  norovirus A08.11

Enteritis (acute) (diarrheal) (hemorrhagic) (noninfective) - *continued*
  parasitic NEC B82.9
  paratyphoid (fever) — *see* Fever, paratyphoid
  protozoal A07.9
    specified NEC A07.8
  radiation K52.0
  regional (of) K50.90
    with
      complication K50.919
        abscess K50.914
        fistula K50.913
        intestinal obstruction K50.912
        rectal bleeding K50.911
        specified complication NEC K50.918
    colon — *see* Enteritis, regional, large intestine
    duodenum — *see* Enteritis, regional, small intestine
    ileum — *see* Enteritis, regional, small intestine
    jejunum — *see* Enteritis, regional, small intestine
    large bowel — *see* Enteritis, regional, large intestine
    large intestine (colon) (rectum) K50.10
      with
        complication K50.119
          abscess K50.114
          fistula K50.113
          intestinal obstruction K50.112
          rectal bleeding K50.111
          small intestine (duodenum) (ileum) (jejunum) involvement K50.80
            with
              complication K50.819
                abscess K50.814
                fistula K50.813
                intestinal obstruction K50.812
                rectal bleeding K50.811
                specified complication NEC K50.818
          specified complication NEC K50.118
    rectum — *see* Enteritis, regional, large intestine
    small intestine (duodenum) (ileum) (jejunum) K50.00
      with
        complication K50.019
          abscess K50.014
          fistula K50.013
          intestinal obstruction K50.012
          large intestine (colon) (rectum) involvement K50.80
            with
              complication K50.819
                abscess K50.814
                fistula K50.813
                intestinal obstruction K50.812
                rectal bleeding K50.811
                specified complication NEC K50.818
          rectal bleeding K50.011
          specified complication NEC K50.018
  rotaviral A08.0
  Salmonella, salmonellosis (arizonae) (cholerae-suis) (enteritidis) (typhimurium) A02.0
  segmental — *see* Enteritis, regional
  septic A09
  Shigella — *see* Infection, Shigella
  small round structured NEC A08.19
  spasmodic, spastic — *see* Syndrome, irritable bowel
  staphylococcal A04.8
    due to food A05.0
  torovirus A08.39
  toxic NEC K52.1
    due to Clostridium difficile
      not specified as recurrent A04.72
      recurrent A04.71

Enteritis (acute) (diarrheal) (hemorrhagic) (noninfective) - *continued*
trichomonal A07.8
tuberculous A18.32
typhosa A01.00
ulcerative (chronic) — *see* Colitis, ulcerative
viral A08.4
adenovirus A08.2
enterovirus A08.39
Rotavirus A08.0
small round structured NEC A08.19
specified NEC A08.39
virus specified NEC A08.39
Enterobiasis B80
Enterobius vermicularis (infection) (infestation) B80
Enterocele — *see also* Hernia, abdomen
pelvic, pelvis (acquired) (congenital) N81.5
vagina, vaginal (acquired) (congenital) NEC N81.5
Enterocolitis — *see also* Enteritis K52.9
due to Clostridium difficile
not specified as recurrent A04.72
recurrent A04.71
fulminant ischemic — *see also* Ischemia, intestine, acute K55.059
granulomatous — *see* Enteritis, regional
hemorrhagic (acute) — *see also* Ischemia, intestine, acute K55.059
chronic K55.1
infectious NEC A09
ischemic K55.9
necrotizing K55.30
with
perforation K55.33
pneumatosis K55.32
and perforation K55.33
due to Clostridium difficile
not specified as recurrent A04.72
recurrent A04.71
in non-newborn K55.30
stage 1 (without pneumatosis, without perforation) K55.31
stage 2 (with pneumatosis, without perforation) K55.32
stage 3 (with pneumatosis, with perforation) K55.33
in newborn P77.9
stage 1 (without pneumatosis, without perforation) P77.1
stage 2 (with pneumatosis, without perforation) P77.2
stage 3 (with pneumatosis, with perforation) P77.3
without pneumatosis or perforation K55.31
noninfectious K52.9
newborn — *see* Enterocolitis, necrotizing, in newborn
pseudomembranous (newborn)
not specified as recurrent A04.72
recurrent A04.71
radiation K52.0
newborn — *see* Enterocolitis, necrotizing, in newborn
ulcerative (chronic) — *see* Pancolitis, ulcerative (chronic)
Enterogastritis — *see* Enteritis
Enteropathy K63.9
food protein-induced K52.22
celiac-gluten-sensitive K90.0
non-celiac K90.41
hemorrhagic, terminal — *see also* Ischemia, intestine, acute K55.059
protein-losing K90.49
Enteroperitonitis — *see* Peritonitis
Enteroptosis K63.4
Enterorrhagia K92.2
Enterospasm — *see also* Syndrome, irritable, bowel
psychogenic F45.8
Enterostenosis — *see also* Obstruction, intestine, specified NEC K56.699
Enterostomy
complication — *see* Complication, enterostomy
Enterostomy - *continued*
status Z93.4
Enterovirus, as cause of disease classified elsewhere B97.10
coxsackievirus B97.11
echovirus B97.12
other specified B97.19
Enthesopathy (peripheral) M77.9
Achilles tendinitis — *see* Tendinitis, Achilles
ankle and tarsus M77.5-
specified type NEC — *see* Enthesopathy, foot, specified type NEC
anterior tibial syndrome M76.81-
calcaneal spur — *see* Spur, bone, calcaneal
elbow region M77.8
lateral epicondylitis — *see* Epicondylitis, lateral
medial epicondylitis — *see* Epicondylitis, medial
foot NEC M77.8
metatarsalgia — *see* Metatarsalgia
specified type NEC M77.5-
forearm M77.8
gluteal tendinitis — *see* Tendinitis, gluteal
hand M77.8
hip — *see* Enthesopathy, lower limb, specified type NEC
iliac crest spur — *see* Spur, bone, iliac crest
iliotibial band syndrome — *see* Syndrome, iliotibial band
knee — *see* Enthesopathy, lower limb, lower leg, specified type NEC
lateral epicondylitis — *see* Epicondylitis, lateral
lower limb (excluding foot) M76.9
Achilles tendinitis — *see* Tendinitis, Achilles
ankle and tarsus M77.5-
specified type NEC — *see* Enthesopathy, foot, specified type NEC
anterior tibial syndrome M76.81-
gluteal tendinitis — *see* Tendinitis, gluteal
iliac crest spur — *see* Spur, bone, iliac crest
iliotibial band syndrome — *see* Syndrome, iliotibial band
patellar tendinitis — *see* Tendinitis, patellar
pelvic region — *see* Enthesopathy, lower limb, specified type NEC
peroneal tendinitis — *see* Tendinitis, peroneal
posterior tibial syndrome M76.82-
psoas tendinitis — *see* Tendinitis, psoas
specified type NEC M76.89-
tibial collateral bursitis — *see* Bursitis, tibial collateral
medial epicondylitis — *see* Epicondylitis, medial
metatarsalgia — *see* Metatarsalgia
multiple sites M77.8
patellar tendinitis — *see* Tendinitis, patellar
pelvis M77.8
periarthritis of wrist — *see* Periarthritis, wrist
peroneal tendinitis — *see* Tendinitis, peroneal
posterior tibial syndrome M76.82-
psoas tendinitis — *see* Tendinitis, psoas
shoulder M77.8
shoulder region — *see* Lesion, shoulder
specified type NEC M77.8
spinal M46.00
cervical region M46.02
cervicothoracic region M46.03
lumbar region M46.06
lumbosacral region M46.07
multiple sites M46.09
occipito-atlanto-axial region M46.01
sacrococcygeal region M46.08
thoracic region M46.04
thoracolumbar region M46.05
tibial collateral bursitis — *see* Bursitis, tibial collateral
upper arm M77.8
wrist and carpus NEC M77.8
Enthesopathy (peripheral) - *continued*
wrist and carpus NEC - *continued*
calcaneal spur — *see* Spur, bone, calcaneal
periarthritis of wrist — *see* Periarthritis, wrist
Entomophobia F40.218
Entomophthoromycosis B46.8
Entrance, air into vein — *see* Embolism, air
Entrapment, nerve — *see* Neuropathy, entrapment
Entropion (eyelid) (paralytic) H02.009
cicatricial H02.019
left H02.016
lower H02.015
upper H02.014
right H02.013
lower H02.012
upper H02.011
congenital Q10.2
left H02.006
lower H02.005
upper H02.004
mechanical H02.029
left H02.026
lower H02.025
upper H02.024
right H02.023
lower H02.022
upper H02.021
right H02.003
lower H02.002
upper H02.001
senile H02.039
left H02.036
lower H02.035
upper H02.034
right H02.033
lower H02.032
upper H02.031
spastic H02.049
left H02.046
lower H02.045
upper H02.044
right H02.043
lower H02.042
upper H02.041
Enucleated eye (traumatic, current) S05.7-
Enuresis R32
functional F98.0
habit disturbance F98.0
nocturnal N39.44
psychogenic F98.0
nonorganic origin F98.0
psychogenic F98.0
Eosinopenia — *see* Agranulocytosis
Eosinophilia (allergic) (idiopathic) (secondary) D72.10
with
angiolymphoid hyperplasia (ALHE) D18.01
familial D72.19
hereditary D72.19
in disease classified elsewhere D72.18
infiltrative — *see* Eosinophilia, pulmonary
Löffler's J82.89
peritoneal — *see* Peritonitis, eosinophilic
pulmonary NEC J82.89
acute J82.82
asthmatic J82.83
chronic J82.81
specified NEC D72.19
tropical (pulmonary) J82.89
Eosinophilia-myalgia syndrome M35.89
Ependymitis (acute) (cerebral) (chronic) (granular) — *see* Encephalomyelitis
Ependymoblastoma
specified site — *see* Neoplasm, malignant, by site
unspecified site C71.9
Ependymoma (epithelial) (malignant)
anaplastic
specified site — *see* Neoplasm, malignant, by site
unspecified site C71.9
benign

ENTERITIS - EPENDYMOMA

Ependymoma (epithelial) (malignant) - *continued*
benign - *continued*
specified site — *see* Neoplasm, benign, by site
unspecified site D33.2
myxopapillary D43.2
specified site — *see* Neoplasm, uncertain behavior, by site
unspecified site D43.2
papillary D43.2
specified site — *see* Neoplasm, uncertain behavior, by site
unspecified site D43.2
specified site — *see* Neoplasm, malignant, by site
unspecified site C71.9
Ependymopathy G93.89
Ephelis, ephelides L81.2
Epiblepharon (congenital) Q10.3
Epicanthus, epicanthic fold (eyelid) (congenital) Q10.3
Epicondylitis (elbow)
lateral M77.1-
medial M77.0-
Epicystitis — *see* Cystitis
Epidemic — *see* condition
Epidermidalization, cervix — *see* Dysplasia, cervix
Epidermis, epidermal — *see* condition
Epidermodysplasia verruciformis B07.8
Epidermolysis
bullosa (congenital) Q81.9
acquired L12.30
drug-induced L12.31
specified cause NEC L12.35
dystrophica Q81.2
letalis Q81.1
simplex Q81.0
specified NEC Q81.8
necroticans combustiformis L51.2
due to drug — *see* Table of Drugs and Chemicals, by drug
Epidermophytid — *see* Dermatophytosis
Epidermophytosis (infected) — *see* Dermatophytosis
Epididymis — *see* condition
Epididymitis (acute) (nonvenereal) (recurrent) (residual) N45.1
with orchitis N45.3
blennorrhagic (gonococcal) A54.23
caseous (tuberculous) A18.15
chlamydial A56.19
filarial — *see also* Infestation, filarial B74.9 *[N51]*
gonococcal A54.23
syphilitic A52.76
tuberculous A18.15
Epididymo-orchitis — *see also* Epididymitis N45.3
Epidural — *see* condition
Epigastrium, epigastric — *see* condition
Epigastrocele — *see* Hernia, ventral
Epiglottis — *see* condition
Epiglottitis, epiglottiditis (acute) J05.10
with obstruction J05.11
chronic J37.0
Epignathus Q89.4
Epilepsia partialis continua — *see also* Kozhevnikof's epilepsy G40.1-
Epilepsy, epileptic, epilepsia (attack) (cerebral) (convulsion) (fit) (seizure) G40.909
Note: the following terms are to be considered equivalent to intractable: pharmacoresistant (pharmacologically resistant) , treatment resistant, refractory (medically) and poorly controlled
with
complex partial seizures — *see* Epilepsy, localization-related, symptomatic, with complex partial seizures
grand mal seizures on awakening — *see* Epilepsy, generalized, specified NEC

Epilepsy, epileptic, epilepsia (attack) (cerebral) (convulsion) (fit) (seizure) - *continued*
with - *continued*
myoclonic absences — *see* Epilepsy, generalized, specified NEC
myoclonic-astatic seizures — *see* Epilepsy, generalized, specified NEC
simple partial seizures — *see* Epilepsy, localization-related, symptomatic, with simple partial seizures
akinetic — *see* Epilepsy, generalized, specified NEC
benign childhood with centrotemporal EEG spikes — *see* Epilepsy, localization-related, idiopathic
benign myoclonic in infancy G40.80-
Bravais-jacksonian — *see* Epilepsy, localization-related, symptomatic, with simple partial seizures
childhood
with occipital EEG paroxysms — *see* Epilepsy, localization-related, idiopathic
absence G40.A09
intractable G40.A19
with status epilepticus G40.A11
without status epilepticus G40.A19
not intractable G40.A09
with status epilepticus G40.A01
without status epilepticus G40.A09
climacteric — *see* Epilepsy, specified NEC
cysticercosis B69.0
deterioration (mental) F06.8
due to syphilis A52.19
focal — *see* Epilepsy, localization-related, symptomatic, with simple partial seizures
generalized
idiopathic G40.309
intractable G40.319
with status epilepticus G40.311
without status epilepticus G40.319
not intractable G40.309
with status epilepticus G40.301
without status epilepticus G40.309
specified NEC G40.409
intractable G40.419
with status epilepticus G40.411
without status epilepticus G40.419
not intractable G40.409
with status epilepticus G40.401
without status epilepticus G40.409
impulsive petit mal — *see* Epilepsy, juvenile myoclonic
intractable G40.919
with status epilepticus G40.911
without status epilepticus G40.919
juvenile absence G40.A09
intractable G40.A19
with status epilepticus G40.A11
without status epilepticus G40.A19
not intractable G40.A09
with status epilepticus G40.A01
without status epilepticus G40.A09
juvenile myoclonic G40.B09
intractable G40.B19
with status epilepticus G40.B11
without status epilepticus G40.B19
not intractable G40.B09
with status epilepticus G40.B01
without status epilepticus G40.B09
localization-related (focal) (partial)
idiopathic G40.009
with seizures of localized onset G40.009
intractable G40.019
with status epilepticus G40.011
without status epilepticus G40.019
not intractable G40.009
with status epilepticus G40.001
without status epilepticus G40.009
symptomatic
with complex partial seizures G40.209
intractable G40.219
with status epilepticus G40.211

Epilepsy, epileptic, epilepsia (attack) (cerebral) (convulsion) (fit) (seizure) - *continued*
localization-related (focal) (partial) - *continued*
symptomatic - *continued*
with complex partial seizures - *continued*
intractable - *continued*
without status epilepticus G40.219
not intractable G40.209
with status epilepticus G40.201
without status epilepticus G40.209
with simple partial seizures G40.109
intractable G40.119
with status epilepticus G40.111
without status epilepticus G40.119
not intractable G40.109
with status epilepticus G40.101
without status epilepticus G40.109
myoclonus, myoclonic — *see also* Epilepsy, generalized, specified NEC
progressive — *see* Epilepsy, generalized, idiopathic
severe, in infancy (SMEI) G40.83-
not intractable G40.909
with status epilepticus G40.901
without status epilepticus G40.909
on awakening — *see* Epilepsy, generalized, specified NEC
parasitic NOS B71.9 *[G94]*
partialis continua — *see also* Kozhevnikof's epilepsy G40.1-
peripheral — *see* Epilepsy, specified NEC
polymorphic, in infancy (PMEI) G40.83-
procursiva — *see* Epilepsy, localization-related, symptomatic, with simple partial seizures
progressive (familial) myoclonic — *see* Epilepsy, generalized, idiopathic
reflex — *see* Epilepsy, specified NEC
related to
alcohol G40.509
not intractable G40.509
with status epilepticus G40.501
without status eplepticus G40.509
drugs G40.509
not intractable G40.509
with status epilepticus G40.501
without status eplepticus G40.509
external causes G40.509
not intractable G40.509
with status epilepticus G40.501
without status eplepticus G40.509
hormonal changes G40.509
not intractable G40.509
with status epilepticus G40.501
without status eplepticus G40.509
sleep deprivation G40.509
not intractable G40.509
with status epilepticus G40.501
without status eplepticus G40.509
stress G40.509
not intractable G40.509
with status epilepticus G40.501
without status eplepticus G40.509
somatomotor — *see* Epilepsy, localization-related, symptomatic, with simple partial seizures
somatosensory — *see* Epilepsy, localization-related, symptomatic, with simple partial seizures
spasms G40.822
intractable G40.824
with status epilepticus G40.823
without status epilepticus G40.824
not intractable G40.822
with status epilepticus G40.821
without status epilepticus G40.822
specified NEC G40.802
intractable G40.804
with status epilepticus G40.803
without status epilepticus G40.804
not intractable G40.802
with status epilepticus G40.801

Epilepsy, epileptic, epilepsia (attack) (cerebral) (convulsion) (fit) (seizure) - *continued*
specified NEC - *continued*
not intractable - *continued*
without status epilepticus G40.802
syndromes
generalized
idiopathic G40.309
intractable G40.319
with status epilepticus G40.311
without status epilepticus G40.319
not intractable G40.309
with status epilepticus G40.301
without status epilepticus G40.309
specified NEC G40.409
intractable G40.419
with status epilepticus G40.411
without status epilepticus G40.419
not intractable G40.409
with status epilepticus G40.401
without status epilepticus G40.409
localization-related (focal) (partial)
idiopathic G40.009
with seizures of localized onset G40.009
intractable G40.019
with status epilepticus G40.011
without status epilepticus G40.019
not intractable G40.009
with status epilepticus G40.001
without status epilepticus G40.009
symptomatic
with complex partial seizures G40.209
intractable G40.219
with status epilepticus G40.211
without status epilepticus G40.219
not intractable G40.209
with status epilepticus G40.201
without status epilepticus G40.209
with simple partial seizures G40.109
intractable G40.119
with status epilepticus G40.111
without status epilepticus G40.119
not intractable G40.109
with status epilepticus G40.101
without status epilepticus G40.109
specified NEC G40.802
intractable G40.804
with status epilepticus G40.803
without status epilepticus G40.804
not intractable G40.802
with status epilepticus G40.801
without status epilepticus G40.802
tonic (-clonic) — *see* Epilepsy, generalized, specified NEC
twilight F05
uncinate (gyrus) — *see* Epilepsy, localization-related, symptomatic, with complex partial seizures
Unverricht (-Lundborg) (familial myoclonic) — *see* Epilepsy, generalized, idiopathic
visceral — *see* Epilepsy, specified NEC
visual — *see* Epilepsy, specified NEC
Epiloia Q85.1
Epimenorrhea N92.0
Epipharyngitis — *see* Nasopharyngitis
Epiphora H04.20-
due to
excess lacrimation H04.21-
insufficient drainage H04.22-
Epiphyseal arrest — *see* Arrest, epiphyseal
Epiphyseolysis, epiphysiolysis — *see* Osteochondropathy
Epiphysitis — *see also* Osteochondropathy
juvenile M92.9
syphilitic (congenital) A50.02
Epiplocele — *see* Hernia, abdomen
Epiploitis — *see* Peritonitis
Epiplosarcomphalocele — *see* Hernia, umbilicus
Episcleritis (suppurative) H15.10-
in (due to)
syphilis A52.71
tuberculosis A18.51
nodular H15.12-
periodica fugax H15.11-
angioneurotic — *see* Edema, angioneurotic
syphilitic (late) A52.71
tuberculous A18.51
Episode
affective, mixed F39
depersonalization (in neurotic state) F48.1
depressive F32.A
major F32.9
mild F32.0
moderate F32.1
severe (without psychotic symptoms) F32.2
with psychotic symptoms F32.3
recurrent F33.9
brief F33.8
specified NEC F32.89
hypomanic F30.8
manic F30.9
with
psychotic symptoms F30.2
remission (full) F30.4
partial F30.3
other specified F30.8
recurrent F31.89
without psychotic symptoms F30.10
mild F30.11
moderate F30.12
severe (without psychotic symptoms) F30.13
with psychotic symptoms F30.2
psychotic F23
organic F06.8
schizophrenic (acute) NEC, brief F23
Epispadias (female) (male) Q64.0
Episplenitis D73.89
Epistaxis (multiple) R04.0
hereditary I78.0
vicarious menstruation N94.89
Epithelioma (malignant) — *see* also Neoplasm, malignant, by site
adenoides cysticum — *see* Neoplasm, skin, benign
basal cell — *see* Neoplasm, skin, malignant
benign — *see* Neoplasm, benign, by site
Bowen's — *see* Neoplasm, skin, in situ
calcifying, of Malherbe — *see* Neoplasm, skin, benign
external site — *see* Neoplasm, skin, malignant
intraepidermal, Jadassohn — *see* Neoplasm, skin, benign
squamous cell — *see* Neoplasm, malignant, by site
Epitheliomatosis pigmented Q82.1
Epitheliopathy, multifocal placoid pigment H30.14-
Epithelium, epithelial — *see* condition
Epituberculosis (with atelectasis) (allergic) A15.7
Eponychia Q84.6
Epstein's
nephrosis or syndrome — *see* Nephrosis
pearl K09.8
Epulis (gingiva) (fibrous) (giant cell) K06.8
Equinia A24.0
Equinovarus (congenital) (talipes) Q66.0-
acquired — *see* Deformity, limb, clubfoot
Equivalent
convulsive (abdominal) — *see* Epilepsy, specified NEC
epileptic (psychic) — *see* Epilepsy, localization-related, symptomatic, with complex partial seizures
Erb (-Duchenne) paralysis (birth injury) (newborn) P14.0
Erb-Goldflam disease or syndrome G70.00
with exacerbation (acute) G70.01
in crisis G70.01
Erb's
disease G71.02
palsy, paralysis (brachial) (birth) (newborn) P14.0
spinal (spastic) syphilitic A52.17
pseudohypertrophic muscular dystrophy G71.02
Erdheim's syndrome (acromegalic macrospondylitis) E22.0
Erection, painful (persistent) — *see* Priapism
Ergosterol deficiency (vitamin D) E55.9
with
adult osteomalacia M83.8
rickets — *see* Rickets
Ergotism — *see also* Poisoning, food, noxious, plant
from ergot used as drug (migraine therapy) — *see* Table of Drugs and Chemicals
Erosio interdigitalis blastomycetica B37.2
Erosion
artery I77.2
without rupture I77.89
bone — *see* Disorder, bone, density and structure, specified NEC
bronchus J98.09
cartilage (joint) — *see* Disorder, cartilage, specified type NEC
cervix (uteri) (acquired) (chronic) (congenital) N86
with cervicitis N72
cornea (nontraumatic) — *see* Ulcer, cornea
recurrent H18.83-
traumatic — *see* Abrasion, cornea
dental (idiopathic) (occupational) (due to diet, drugs or vomiting) K03.2
duodenum, postpyloric — *see* Ulcer, duodenum
esophagus K22.10
with bleeding K22.11
gastric — *see* Ulcer, stomach
gastrojejunal — *see* Ulcer, gastrojejunal
implanted mesh — *see* Complications, prosthetic device or implant, mesh
intestine K63.3
lymphatic vessel I89.8
pylorus, pyloric (ulcer) — *see* Ulcer, stomach
spine, aneurysmal A52.09
stomach — *see* Ulcer, stomach
subcutaneous device pocket
nervous system prosthetic device, implant, or graft T85.890
other internal prosthetic device, implant, or graft T85.898
teeth (idiopathic) (occupational) (due to diet, drugs or vomiting) K03.2
urethra N36.8
uterus N85.8
Erotomania F52.8
Error
metabolism, inborn -- se Disorder, metabolism
refractive — *see* Disorder, refraction
Eructation R14.2
nervous or psychogenic F45.8
Eruption
creeping B76.9
drug (generalized) (taken internally) L27.0
fixed L27.1
in contact with skin — *see* Dermatitis, due to drugs
localized L27.1
Hutchinson, summer L56.4
Kaposi's varicelliform B00.0
napkin L22
polymorphous light (sun) L56.4
recalcitrant pustular L13.8
ringed R23.8
skin (nonspecific) R21
creeping (meaning hookworm) B76.9

Eruption - *continued*
  skin (nonspecific) - *continued*
    due to inoculation/vaccination (generalized) — *see also* Dermatitis, due to, vaccine L27.0
      localized L27.1
    erysipeloid A26.0
    feigned L98.1
    Kaposi's varicelliform B00.0
    lichenoid L28.0
    meaning dermatitis — *see* Dermatitis
    toxic NEC L53.0
  tooth, teeth, abnormal (incomplete) (late) (premature) (sequence) K00.6
  vesicular R23.8
Erysipelas (gangrenous) (infantile) (newborn) (phlegmonous) (suppurative) A46
  external ear A46 *[H62.40]*
  puerperal, postpartum O86.89
Erysipeloid A26.9
  cutaneous (Rosenbach's) A26.0
  disseminated A26.8
  sepsis A26.7
  specified NEC A26.8
Erythema, erythematous (infectional) (inflammation) L53.9
  ab igne L59.0
  annulare (centrifugum) (rheumaticum) L53.1
  arthriticum epidemicum A25.1
  brucellum — *see* Brucellosis
  chronic figurate NEC L53.3
  chronicum migrans (Borrelia burgdorferi) A69.20
  diaper L22
  due to
    chemical NEC L53.0
      in contact with skin L24.5
    drug (internal use) — *see* Dermatitis, due to, drugs
  elevatum diutinum L95.1
  endemic E52
  epidemic, arthritic A25.1
  figuratum perstans L53.3
  gluteal L22
  heat - code by site under Burn, first degree
  ichthyosiforme congenitum bullous Q80.3
  in diseases classified elsewhere L54
  induratum (nontuberculous) L52
    tuberculous A18.4
  infectiosum B08.3
  intertrigo L30.4
  iris L51.9
  marginatum L53.2
    in (due to) acute rheumatic fever I00
  medicamentosum — *see* Dermatitis, due to, drugs
  migrans A26.0
    chronicum A69.20
    tongue K14.1
  multiforme (major) (minor) L51.9
    bullous, bullosum L51.1
    conjunctiva L51.1
    nonbullous L51.0
    pemphigoides L12.0
    specified NEC L51.8
  napkin L22
  neonatorum P83.88
    toxic P83.1
  nodosum L52
    tuberculous A18.4
  palmar L53.8
  pernio T69.1
  rash, newborn P83.88
  scarlatiniform (recurrent) (exfoliative) L53.8
  solare L55.0
  specified NEC L53.8
  toxic, toxicum NEC L53.0
    newborn P83.1
  tuberculous (primary) A18.4
Erythematous, erythematosus — *see* condition
Erythermalgia (primary) I73.81
Erythralgia I73.81
Erythrasma L08.1
Erythredema (polyneuropathy) — *see* Poisoning, mercury
Erythremia (acute) C94.0-
  chronic D45
  secondary D75.1
Erythroblastopenia — *see also* Aplasia, red cell D60.9
  congenital D61.01
Erythroblastophthisis D61.09
Erythroblastosis (fetalis) (newborn) P55.9
  due to
    ABO (antibodies) (incompatibility) (isoimmunization) P55.1
    Rh (antibodies) (incompatibility) (isoimmunization) P55.0
Erythrocyanosis (crurum) I73.89
Erythrocythemia — *see* Erythremia
Erythrocytosis (megalosplenic) (secondary) D75.1
  familial D75.0
  oval, hereditary — *see* Elliptocytosis
  secondary D75.1
  stress D75.1
Erythroderma (secondary) — *see also* Erythema L53.9
  bullous ichthyosiform, congenital Q80.3
  desquamativum L21.1
  ichthyosiform, congenital (bullous) Q80.3
  neonatorum P83.88
  psoriaticum L40.8
Erythrodysesthesia, palmar plantar (PPE) L27.1
Erythrogenesis imperfecta D61.09
Erythroleukemia C94.0-
Erythromelalgia I73.81
Erythrophagocytosis D75.89
Erythrophobia F40.298
Erythroplakia, oral epithelium, and tongue K13.29
Erythroplasia (Queyrat) D07.4
  specified site — *see* Neoplasm, skin, in situ
  unspecified site D07.4
Escherichia coli (E. coli) , as cause of disease classified elsewhere B96.20
  non-O157 Shiga toxin-producing (with known O group) B96.22
  non-Shiga toxin-producing B96.29
  O157 B96.21
  O157 with confirmation of Shiga toxin when H antigen is unknown, or is not H7 B96.21
  O157:H- (nonmotile) with confirmation of Shiga toxin B96.21
  O157:H7 with or without confirmation of Shiga toxin-production B96.21
    specified NEC B96.22
  Shiga toxin-producing (with unspecified O group) (STEC) B96.23
  specified NEC B96.29
Esophagismus K22.4
Esophagitis (acute) (alkaline) (chemical) (chronic) (infectional) (necrotic) (peptic) (postoperative) (without bleeding) K20.90
  with bleeding K20.91
  candidal B37.81
  due to gastrointestinal reflux disease (without bleeding) K21.00
    with bleeding K21.01
  eosinophilic K20.0
  reflux K21.00
  specified NEC (without bleeding) K20.80
    with bleeding K20.81
  tuberculous A18.83
  ulcerative K22.10
    with bleeding K22.11
Esophagocele K22.5
Esophagomalacia K22.89
Esophagospasm K22.4
Esophagostenosis K22.2
Esophagostomiasis B81.8
Esophagotracheal — *see* condition
Esophagus — *see* condition
Esophoria H50.51
  convergence, excess H51.12
Esophoria - *continued*
  divergence, insufficiency H51.8
Esotropia — *see* Strabismus, convergent concomitant
Espundia B55.2
Essential — *see* condition
Esthesioneuroblastoma C30.0
Esthesioneurocytoma C30.0
Esthesioneuroepithelioma C30.0
Esthiomene A55
Estivo-autumnal malaria (fever) B50.9
Estrangement (marital) Z63.5
  parent-child NEC Z62.890
Estriasis — *see* Myiasis
Ethanolism — *see* Alcoholism
Etherism — *see* Dependence, drug, inhalant
Ethmoid, ethmoidal — *see* condition
Ethmoiditis (chronic) (nonpurulent) (purulent) — *see also* Sinusitis, ethmoidal
  influenzal — *see* Influenza, with, respiratory manifestations NEC
  Woakes' J33.1
Ethylism — *see* Alcoholism
Eulenburg's disease (congenital paramyotonia) G71.19
Eumycetoma B47.0
Eunuchoidism E29.1
  hypogonadotropic E23.0
European blastomycosis — *see* Cryptococcosis
Eustachian — *see* condition
Evaluation (for) (of)
  development state
    adolescent Z00.3
    period of
      delayed growth in childhood Z00.70
        with abnormal findings Z00.71
      rapid growth in childhood Z00.2
    puberty Z00.3
  growth and developmental state (period of rapid growth) Z00.2
    delayed growth Z00.70
      with abnormal findings Z00.71
  mental health (status) Z00.8
    requested by authority Z04.6
  period of
    delayed growth in childhood Z00.70
      with abnormal findings Z00.71
    rapid growth in childhood Z00.2
  suspected condition — *see* Observation
Evans syndrome D69.41
Event
  apparent life threatening in newborn and infant (ALTE) R68.13
  brief resolved unexplained event (BRUE) R68.13
Eventration — *see also* Hernia, ventral
  colon into chest — *see* Hernia, diaphragm
  diaphragm (congenital) Q79.1
Eversion
  bladder N32.89
  cervix (uteri) N86
    with cervicitis N72
  foot NEC — *see also* Deformity, valgus, ankle
    congenital Q66.6
  punctum lacrimale (postinfectional) (senile) H04.52-
  ureter (meatus) N28.89
  urethra (meatus) N36.8
  uterus N81.4
Evidence
  cytologic
    of malignancy on anal smear R85.614
    of malignancy on cervical smear R87.614
    of malignancy on vaginal smear R87.624
Evisceration
  birth injury P15.8
  traumatic NEC
    eye — *see* Enucleated eye
Evulsion — *see* Avulsion
Ewing's sarcoma or tumor — *see* Neoplasm, bone, malignant

Examination (for) (following) (general) (of) (routine) Z00.00
with abnormal findings Z00.01
abuse, physical (alleged) , ruled out
adult Z04.71
child Z04.72
adolescent (development state) Z00.3
alleged rape or sexual assault (victim) , ruled out
adult Z04.41
child Z04.42
allergy Z01.82
annual (adult) (periodic) (physical) Z00.00
with abnormal findings Z00.01
gynecological Z01.419
with abnormal findings Z01.411
antibody response Z01.84
blood — *see* Examination, laboratory
blood pressure Z01.30
with abnormal findings Z01.31
cancer staging — *see* Neoplasm, malignant, by site
cervical Papanicolaou smear Z12.4
as part of routine gynecological examination Z01.419
with abnormal findings Z01.411
child (over 28 days old) Z00.129
with abnormal findings Z00.121
under 28 days old — *see* Newborn, examination
clinical research control or normal comparison (control) (participant) Z00.6
contraceptive (drug) maintenance (routine) Z30.8
device (intrauterine) Z30.431
dental Z01.20
with abnormal findings Z01.21
developmental — *see* Examination, child
donor (potential) Z00.5
ear Z01.10
with abnormal findings NEC Z01.118
eye Z01.00
with abnormal findings Z01.01
following failed vision screening Z01.020
with abnormal findings Z01.021
following
accident NEC Z04.3
transport Z04.1
work Z04.2
assault, alleged, ruled out
adult Z04.71
child Z04.72
motor vehicle accident Z04.1
treatment (for) Z09
combined NEC Z09
fracture Z09
malignant neoplasm Z08
malignant neoplasm Z08
mental disorder Z09
specified condition NEC Z09
follow-up (routine) (following) Z09
chemotherapy NEC Z09
malignant neoplasm Z08
fracture Z09
malignant neoplasm Z08
postpartum Z39.2
psychotherapy Z09
radiotherapy NEC Z09
malignant neoplasm Z08
surgery NEC Z09
malignant neoplasm Z08
forced labor exploitation Z04.82
forced sexual exploitation Z04.81
gynecological Z01.419
with abnormal findings Z01.411
for contraceptive maintenance Z30.8
health — *see* Examination, medical
hearing Z01.10
with abnormal findings NEC Z01.118
infant or child (over 28 days old) Z00.129
with abnormal findings Z00.121
following failed hearing screening Z01.110
immunity status testing Z01.84
laboratory (as part of a general medical examination) Z00.00

Examination (for) (following) (general) (of) (routine) - *continued*
laboratory (as part of a general medical examination) - *continued*
with abnormal findings Z00.01
preprocedural Z01.812
lactating mother Z39.1
medical (adult) (for) (of) Z00.00
with abnormal findings Z00.01
administrative purpose only Z02.9
specified NEC Z02.89
admission to
armed forces Z02.3
old age home Z02.2
prison Z02.89
residential institution Z02.2
school Z02.0
following illness or medical treatment Z02.0
summer camp Z02.89
adoption Z02.82
blood alcohol or drug level Z02.83
camp (summer) Z02.89
clinical research, normal subject (control) (participant) Z00.6
control subject in clinical research (normal comparison) (participant) Z00.6
donor (potential) Z00.5
driving license Z02.4
general (adult) Z00.00
with abnormal findings Z00.01
immigration Z02.89
insurance purposes Z02.6
marriage Z02.89
medicolegal reasons NEC Z04.89
naturalization Z02.89
participation in sport Z02.5
paternity testing Z02.81
population survey Z00.8
pre-employment Z02.1
pre-operative — *see* Examination, pre-procedural
pre-procedural
cardiovascular Z01.810
respiratory Z01.811
specified NEC Z01.818
preschool children
for admission to school Z02.0
prisoners
for entrance into prison Z02.89
recruitment for armed forces Z02.3
specified NEC Z00.8
sport competition Z02.5
medicolegal reason NEC Z04.89
following
forced labor exploitation Z04.82
forced sexual exploitation Z04.81
newborn — *see* Newborn, examination
pelvic (annual) (periodic) Z01.419
with abnormal findings Z01.411
period of rapid growth in childhood Z00.2
periodic (adult) (annual) (routine) Z00.00
with abnormal findings Z00.01
physical (adult) — *see also* Examination, medical Z00.00
sports Z02.5
postpartum
immediately after delivery Z39.0
routine follow-up Z39.2
prenatal (normal pregnancy) — *see also* Pregnancy, normal Z34.9-
pre-chemotherapy (antineoplastic) Z01.818
pre-procedural (pre-operative)
cardiovascular Z01.810
laboratory Z01.812
respiratory Z01.811
specified NEC Z01.818
prior to chemotherapy (antineoplastic) Z01.818
psychiatric NEC Z00.8
follow-up not needing further care Z09
requested by authority Z04.6
radiological (as part of a general medical examination) Z00.00
with abnormal findings Z00.01

Examination (for) (following) (general) (of) (routine) - *continued*
repeat cervical smear to confirm findings of recent normal smear following initial abnormal smear Z01.42
skin (hypersensitivity) Z01.82
special — *see also* Examination, by type Z01.89
specified type NEC Z01.89
specified type or reason NEC Z04.89
teeth Z01.20
with abnormal findings Z01.21
urine — *see* Examination, laboratory
vision Z01.00
with abnormal findings Z01.01
following failed vision screening Z01.020
with abnormal findings Z01.021
infant or child (over 28 days old) Z00.129
with abnormal findings Z00.121

Exanthem, exanthema — *see also* Rash
with enteroviral vesicular stomatitis B08.4
Boston A88.0
epidemic with meningitis A88.0 *[G02]*
subitum B08.20
due to human herpesvirus 6 B08.21
due to human herpesvirus 7 B08.22
viral, virus B09
specified type NEC B08.8

Excess, excessive, excessively
alcohol level in blood R78.0
androgen (ovarian) E28.1
attrition, tooth, teeth K03.0
carotene, carotin (dietary) E67.1
cold, effects of T69.9
specified effect NEC T69.8
convergence H51.12
crying
in child, adolescent, or adult R45.83
in infant R68.11
development, breast N62
divergence H51.8
drinking (alcohol) NEC (without dependence) F10.10
habitual (continual) (without remission) F10.20
eating R63.2
estrogen E28.0
fat — *see also* Obesity
in heart — *see* Degeneration, myocardial
localized E65
foreskin N47.8
gas R14.0
glucagon E16.3
heat — *see* Heat
intermaxillary vertical dimension of fully erupted teeth M26.37
interocclusal distance of fully erupted teeth M26.37
kalium E87.5
large
colon K59.39
congenital Q43.8
infant P08.0
organ or site, congenital NEC — *see* Anomaly, by site
long
organ or site, congenital NEC — *see* Anomaly, by site
menstruation (with regular cycle) N92.0
with irregular cycle N92.1
napping Z72.821
natrium E87.0
number of teeth K00.1
nutrient (dietary) NEC R63.2
potassium (K) E87.5
salivation K11.7
secretion — *see also* Hypersecretion
milk O92.6
sputum R09.3
sweat R61
sexual drive F52.8
short
organ or site, congenital NEC — *see* Anomaly, by site
umbilical cord in labor or delivery O69.3

EXCESS, EXCESSIVE, EXCESSIVELY - EXPOSURE

Exposure (to) - *continued*
smallpox (laboratory) Z20.89
syphilis Z20.2
terrorism Z65.4
torture Z65.4
tuberculosis Z20.1
uranium Z77.012
varicella Z20.820
venereal disease Z20.2
viral disease NEC Z20.828
war Z65.5
water pollution Z77.111
Zika virus Z20.821
Exsanguination — *see* Hemorrhage
Exstrophy
abdominal contents Q45.8
bladder Q64.10
cloacal Q64.12
specified type NEC Q64.19
supravesical fissure Q64.11
Extensive — *see* condition
Extra — *see also* Accessory
marker chromosomes (normal individual) Q92.61
in abnormal individual Q92.62
rib Q76.6
cervical Q76.5
Extrasystoles (supraventricular) I49.49
atrial I49.1
auricular I49.1
junctional I49.2
ventricular I49.3
Extrauterine gestation or pregnancy — *see* Pregnancy, by site
Extravasation
blood R58
chyle into mesentery I89.8
pelvicalyceal N13.8
pyelosinus N13.8
urine (from ureter) R39.0
vesicant agent
antineoplastic chemotherapy T80.810
other agent NEC T80.818
Extremity — *see* condition, limb
Extrophy — *see* Exstrophy
Extroversion
bladder Q64.19
uterus N81.4
complicating delivery O71.2
postpartal (old) N81.4
Extruded tooth (teeth) M26.34
Extrusion
breast implant (prosthetic) T85.42
eye implant (globe) (ball) T85.328
intervertebral disc — *see* Displacement, intervertebral disc
ocular lens implant (prosthetic) — *see* Complications, intraocular lens
vitreous — *see* Prolapse, vitreous
Exudate
pleural — *see* Effusion, pleura
retina H35.89
wound fluids L24.A9
Exudative — *see* condition
Eye, eyeball, eyelid — *see* condition
Eyestrain — *see* Disturbance, vision, subjective
Eyeworm disease of Africa B74.3

F

Faber's syndrome (achlorhydric anemia) D50.9
Fabry (-Anderson) disease E75.21
Facet syndrome M47.89-
Faciocephalalgia, autonomic — *see also* Neuropathy, peripheral, autonomic G90.09
Factor (s)
psychic, associated with diseases classified elsewhere F54
psychological
affecting physical conditions F54
or behavioral
affecting general medical condition F54
associated with disorders or diseases classified elsewhere F54
Fahr disease (of brain) G23.8
Fahr Volhard disease (of kidney) I12.-
Failure, failed
abortion — *see* Abortion, attempted
aortic (valve) I35.8
rheumatic I06.8
attempted abortion — *see* Abortion, attempted
biventricular I50.82
due to left heart failure I50.814
bone marrow — *see* Anemia, aplastic
cardiac — *see* Failure, heart
cardiorenal (chronic) — *see also* Failure, renal, and Failure, heart I50.9
hypertensive I13.2
cardiorespiratory — *see also* Failure, heart R09.2
cardiovascular (chronic) — *see* Failure, heart
cerebrovascular I67.9
cervical dilatation in labor O62.0
circulation, circulatory (peripheral) R57.9
newborn P29.89
compensation — *see* Disease, heart
compliance with medical treatment or regimen — *see* Noncompliance
congestive — *see* Failure, heart, congestive
dental implant (endosseous) M27.69
due to
failure of dental prosthesis M27.63
lack of attached gingiva M27.62
occlusal trauma (poor prosthetic design) M27.62
parafunctional habits M27.62
periodontal infection (peri-implantitis) M27.62
poor oral hygiene M27.62
osseointegration M27.61
due to
complications of systemic disease M27.61
poor bone quality M27.61
iatrogenic M27.61
post-osseointegration
biological M27.62
due to complications of systemic disease M27.62
iatrogenic M27.62
mechanical M27.63
pre-integration M27.61
pre-osseointegration M27.61
specified NEC M27.69
descent of head (at term) of pregnancy (mother) O32.4
endosseous dental implant — *see* Failure, dental implant
engagement of head (term of pregnancy) (mother) O32.4
erection (penile) — *see also* Dysfunction, sexual, male, erectile N52.9
nonorganic F52.21
examination (s) , anxiety concerning Z55.2
expansion terminal respiratory units (newborn) (primary) P28.0
forceps NOS (with subsequent cesarean delivery) O66.5
gain weight (child over 28 days old) R62.51
adult R62.7
newborn P92.6
genital response (male) F52.21
female F52.22
heart (acute) (senile) (sudden) I50.9
with
acute pulmonary edema — *see* Failure, ventricular, left
decompensation I50.9
with
normal ejection fraction I50.33
preserved ejection fraction I50.33
reduced ejection fraction I50.23
with diastolic dysfunction I50.43
combined systolic and diastolic I50.43
diastolic I50.33
right I50.813
systolic I50.23
dilatation — *see* Disease, heart

Failure, failed - *continued*
heart (acute) (senile) (sudden) - *continued*
with - *continued*
hypertension — *see* Hypertension, heart
normal ejection fraction — *see* Failure, heart, diastolic
preserved ejection fraction — *see* Failure, heart, diastolic
reduced ejection fraction — *see* Failure, heart, systolic
arteriosclerotic I70.90
biventricular I50.82
due to left heart failure I50.814
combined left-right sided I50.82
due to left heart failure I50.814
compensated — *see also* Failure, heart, by type as diastolic or systolic, chronic I50.9
complicating
anesthesia (general) (local) or other sedation
in labor and delivery O74.2
in pregnancy O29.12-
postpartum, puerperal O89.1
delivery (cesarean) (instrumental) O75.4
congestive I50.9
with rheumatic fever (conditions in I00)
active I01.8
inactive or quiescent (with chorea) I09.81
newborn P29.0
rheumatic (chronic) (inactive) (with chorea) I09.81
active or acute I01.8
with chorea I02.0
decompensated — *see also* Failure, heart, by type as diastolic or systolic, acute and chronic I50.9
degenerative — *see* Degeneration, myocardial
diastolic (congestive) (left ventricular) I50.30
acute (congestive) I50.31
and (on) chronic (congestive) I50.33
chronic (congestive) I50.32
and (on) acute (congestive) I50.33
combined with systolic (congestive) I50.40
acute (congestive) I50.41
and (on) chronic (congestive) I50.43
chronic (congestive) I50.42
and (on) acute (congestive) I50.43
due to presence of cardiac prosthesis I97.13-
end stage — *see also* Failure, heart, by type as diastolic or systolic, chronic I50.84
following cardiac surgery I97.13-
high output NOS I50.83
hypertensive — *see* Hypertension, heart
left (ventricular) — *see also* Failure, ventricular, left
combined diastolic and systolic — *see* Failure, heart, diastolic, combined with systolic
diastolic — *see* Failure, heart, diastolic
systolic — *see* Failure, heart, systolic
low output (syndrome) NOS I50.9
newborn P29.0
organic — *see* Disease, heart
peripartum O90.3
postprocedural I97.13-
rheumatic (chronic) (inactive) I09.9
right (isolated) (ventricular) I50.810
acute I50.811
and (on) chronic I50.813
chronic I50.812
and acute I50.813
secondary to left heart failure I50.814
specified NEC I50.89

Failure, failed - *continued*
Note: heart failure stages A, B, C, and D are based on the American College of Cardiology and American Heart Association stages of heart failure, which complement and should not be confused with the New York Heart Association Classification of Heart Failure, into Class I, Class II, Class III, and Class IV
stage A Z91.89
stage B — *see also* Failure, heart, by type as diastolic or systolic I50.9
stage C — *see also* Failure, heart, by type as diastolic or systolic I50.9
stage D — *see also* Failure, heart, by type as diastolic or systolic, chronic I50.84
systolic (congestive) (left ventricular) I50.20
acute (congestive) I50.21
and (on) chronic (congestive) I50.23
chronic (congestive) I50.22
and (on) acute (congestive) I50.23
combined with diastolic (congestive) I50.40
acute (congestive) I50.41
and (on) chronic (congestive) I50.43
chronic (congestive) I50.42
and (on) acute (congestive) I50.43
thyrotoxic — *see also* Thyrotoxicosis E05.90 *[I43]*
with
high output — *see also* Thyrotoxicosis I50.83
thyroid storm E05.91 *[I43]*
high output — *see also* Thyrotoxicosis I50.83
valvular — *see* Endocarditis
hepatic K72.90
with coma K72.91
acute or subacute K72.00
with coma K72.01
due to drugs K71.10
with coma K71.11
alcoholic (acute) (chronic) (subacute) K70.40
with coma K70.41
chronic K72.10
with coma K72.11
due to drugs (acute) (subacute) (chronic) K71.10
with coma K71.11
due to drugs (acute) (subacute) (chronic) K71.10
with coma K71.11
postprocedural K91.82
hepatorenal K76.7
induction (of labor) O61.9
abortion — *see* Abortion, attempted
by
oxytocic drugs O61.0
prostaglandins O61.0
instrumental O61.1
mechanical O61.1
medical O61.0
specified NEC O61.8
surgical O61.1
intubation during anesthesia T88.4
in pregnancy O29.6-
labor and delivery O74.7
postpartum, puerperal O89.6
involution, thymus (gland) E32.0
kidney — *see also* Disease, kidney, chronic N19
acute — *see also* Failure, renal, acute N17.9-
diabetic — *see* E08-E13 with .22
lactation (complete) O92.3
partial O92.4
Leydig's cell, adult E29.1
liver — *see* Failure, hepatic
menstruation at puberty N91.0
mitral I05.8
myocardial, myocardium — *see also* Failure, heart I50.9

Failure, failed - *continued*
myocardial, myocardium - *continued*
chronic — *see also* Failure, heart, congestive I50.9
congestive — *see also* Failure, heart, congestive I50.9
newborn screening — *see* Abnormal, neonatal screening
neonatal congenital heart disease P09.5
orgasm (female) (psychogenic) F52.31
male F52.32
ovarian (primary) E28.39
iatrogenic E89.40
asymptomatic E89.40
symptomatic E89.41
postprocedural (postablative) (postirradiation) (postsurgical) E89.40
asymptomatic E89.40
symptomatic E89.41
ovulation causing infertility N97.0
polyglandular, autoimmune E31.0
prosthetic joint implant — *see* Complications, joint prosthesis, mechanical, breakdown, by site
renal N19
with
tubular necrosis (acute) N17.0
acute N17.9
with
cortical necrosis N17.1
medullary necrosis N17.2
tubular necrosis N17.0
specified NEC N17.8
chronic N18.9
hypertensive — *see* Hypertension, kidney
congenital P96.0
end stage (chronic) N18.6
due to hypertension I12.0
following
abortion — *see* Abortion by type complicated by specified condition NEC
crushing T79.5
ectopic or molar pregnancy O08.4
labor and delivery (acute) O90.4
hypertensive — *see* Hypertension, kidney
postprocedural N99.0
respiration, respiratory J96.90
with
hypercapnia J96.92
hypercarbia J96.92
hypoxia J96.91
acute J96.00
with
hypercapnia J96.02
hypercarbia J96.02
hypoxia J96.01
center G93.89
acute and (on) chronic J96.20
with
hypercapnia J96.22
hypercarbia J96.22
hypoxia J96.21
chronic J96.10
with
hypercapnia J96.12
hypercarbia J96.12
hypoxia J96.11
newborn P28.5
postprocedural (acute) J95.821
acute and chronic J95.822
rotation
cecum Q43.3
colon Q43.3
intestine Q43.3
kidney Q63.2
sedation (conscious) (moderate) during procedure T88.52
history of Z92.83
segmentation — *see also* Fusion
fingers — *see* Syndactylism, complex, fingers
vertebra Q76.49
with scoliosis Q76.3

Failure, failed - *continued*
seminiferous tubule, adult E29.1
senile (general) R54
sexual arousal (male) F52.21
female F52.22
testicular endocrine function E29.1
to thrive (child over 28 days old) R62.51
adult R62.7
newborn P92.6
transplant T86.92
bone T86.831
marrow T86.02
cornea T86.841-
heart T86.22
with lung (s) T86.32
intestine T86.851
kidney T86.12
liver T86.42
lung (s) T86.811
with heart T86.32
pancreas T86.891
skin (allograft) (autograft) T86.821
specified organ or tissue NEC T86.891
stem cell (peripheral blood) (umbilical cord) T86.5
trial of labor (with subsequent cesarean delivery) O66.40
following previous cesarean delivery O66.41
tubal ligation N99.89
urinary — *see* Disease, kidney, chronic
vacuum extraction NOS (with subsequent cesarean delivery) O66.5
vasectomy N99.89
ventouse NOS (with subsequent cesarean delivery) O66.5
ventricular — *see also* Failure, heart I50.9
left — *see also* Failure, heart, left I50.1
with rheumatic fever (conditions in I00)
active I01.8
with chorea I02.0
inactive or quiescent (with chorea) I09.81
rheumatic (chronic) (inactive) (with chorea) I09.81
active or acute I01.8
with chorea I02.0
right — *see* Failure, heart, right
vital centers, newborn P91.88
Fainting (fit) R55
Fallen arches — *see* Deformity, limb, flat foot
Falling, falls (repeated) R29.6
any organ or part — *see* Prolapse
Fallopian
insufflation Z31.41
tube — *see* condition
Fallot's
pentalogy Q21.8
tetrad or tetralogy Q21.3
triad or trilogy Q22.3
False — *see also* condition
croup J38.5
joint — *see* Nonunion, fracture
labor (pains) O47.9
at or after 37 completed weeks of gestation O47.1
before 37 completed weeks of gestation O47.0-
passage, urethra (prostatic) N36.5
pregnancy F45.8
Family, familial — *see also* condition
disruption Z63.8
involving divorce or separation Z63.5
Li-Fraumeni (syndrome) Z15.01
planning advice Z30.09
problem Z63.9
specified NEC Z63.8
retinoblastoma C69.2-
Famine (effects of) T73.0
edema — *see* Malnutrition, severe
Fanconi (-de Toni) (-Debré) syndrome E72.09
with cystinosis E72.04
Fanconi's anemia (congenital pancytopenia) D61.09

FAILURE, FAILED - FANCONI'S ANEMIA

Farber's disease or syndrome E75.29
Farcy A24.0
Farmer's
lung J67.0
skin L57.8
Farsightedness — *see* Hypermetropia
Fascia — *see* condition
Fasciculation R25.3
Fasciitis M72.9
diffuse (eosinophilic) M35.4
infective M72.8
necrotizing M72.6
necrotizing M72.6
nodular M72.4
perirenal (with ureteral obstruction) N13.5
with infection N13.6
plantar M72.2
specified NEC M72.8
traumatic (old) M72.8
current - code by site under Sprain
Fascioliasis B66.3
Fasciolopsis, fasciolopsiasis (intestinal) B66.5
Fascioscapulohumeral myopathy G71.02
Fast pulse R00.0
Fat
embolism — *see* Embolism, fat
excessive — *see also* Obesity
in heart — *see* Degeneration, myocardial
in stool R19.5
localized (pad) E65
heart — *see* Degeneration, myocardial
knee M79.4
retropatellar M79.4
necrosis
breast N64.1
mesentery K65.4
omentum K65.4
pad E65
knee M79.4
Fatigue R53.83
auditory deafness — *see* Deafness
chronic R53.82
combat F43.0
general R53.83
psychogenic F48.8
heat (transient) T67.6
muscle M62.89
myocardium — *see* Failure, heart
neoplasm-related R53.0
nervous, neurosis F48.8
operational F48.8
psychogenic (general) F48.8
senile R54
voice R49.8
Fatness — *see* Obesity
Fatty — *see also* condition
apron E65
degeneration — *see* Degeneration, fatty
heart (enlarged) — *see* Degeneration, myocardial
liver NEC K76.0
alcoholic K70.0
nonalcoholic K76.0
necrosis — *see* Degeneration, fatty
Fauces — *see* condition
Fauchard's disease (periodontitis) — *see* Periodontitis
Faucitis J02.9
Favism (anemia) D55.0
Favus — *see* Dermatophytosis
Fazio-Londe disease or syndrome G12.1
Fear complex or reaction F40.9
Fear of — *see* Phobia
Feared complaint unfounded Z71.1
Febris, febrile — *see also* Fever
flava — *see also* Fever, yellow A95.9
melitensis A23.0
pestis — *see* Plague
recurrens — *see* Fever, relapsing
rubra A38.9
Fecal
incontinence R15.9
smearing R15.1
soiling R15.1
urgency R15.2
Fecalith (impaction) K56.41
appendix K38.1
congenital P76.8
Fede's disease K14.0
Feeble rapid pulse due to shock following injury T79.4
Feeble-minded F70
Feeding
difficulties R63.30
problem (elderly) (infant) R63.39
newborn P92.9
specified NEC P92.8
nonorganic (adult) — *see* Disorder, eating
Feeling (of)
foreign body in throat R09.89
Feer's disease — *see* Poisoning, mercury
Feet — *see* condition
Feigned illness Z76.5
Feil-Klippel syndrome (brevicollis) Q76.1
Feinmesser's (hidrotic) ectodermal dysplasia Q82.4
Felinophobia F40.218
Felon — *see also* Cellulitis, digit
with lymphangitis — *see* Lymphangitis, acute, digit
Felty's syndrome M05.00
ankle M05.07-
elbow M05.02-
foot joint M05.07-
hand joint M05.04-
hip M05.05-
knee M05.06-
multiple site M05.09
shoulder M05.01-
vertebra — *see* Spondylitis, ankylosing
wrist M05.03-
Female genital cutting status — *see* Female genital mutilation status (FGM)
Female genital mutilation status (FGM) N90.810
specified NEC N90.818
type I (clitorectomy status) N90.811
type II (clitorectomy with excision of labia minora status) N90.812
type III (infibulation status) N90.813
type IV N90.818
Femur, femoral — *see* condition
Fenestration, fenestrated — *see also* Imperfect, closure
aortico-pulmonary Q21.4
cusps, heart valve NEC Q24.8
pulmonary Q22.3
pulmonic cusps Q22.3
Fernell's disease (aortic aneurysm) I71.9
Fertile eunuch syndrome E23.0
Fetid
breath R19.6
sweat L75.0
Fetishism F65.0
transvestic F65.1
Fetus, fetal — *see also* condition
alcohol syndrome (dysmorphic) Q86.0
compressus O31.0-
hydantoin syndrome Q86.1
lung tissue P28.0
papyraceous O31.0-
Fever (inanition) (of unknown origin) (persistent) (with chills) (with rigor) R50.9
abortus A23.1
Aden (dengue) A90
African tick bite A77.8
African tick-borne A68.1
American
mountain (tick) A93.2
spotted A77.0
aphthous B08.8
arbovirus, arboviral A94
hemorrhagic A94
specified NEC A93.8
Argentinian hemorrhagic A96.0
Assam B55.0
Australian Q A78
Bangkok hemorrhagic A91
Barmah forest A92.8
Fever (inanition) (of unknown origin) (persistent) (with chills) (with rigor) - *continued*
Bartonella A44.0
bilious, hemoglobinuric B50.8
blackwater B50.8
blister B00.1
Bolivian hemorrhagic A96.1
Bonvale dam T73.3
boutonneuse A77.1
brain — *see* Encephalitis
Brazilian purpuric A48.4
breakbone A90
Bullis A77.0
Bunyamwera A92.8
Burdwan B55.0
Bwamba A92.8
Cameroon — *see* Malaria
Canton A75.9
catarrhal (acute) J00
chronic J31.0
cat-scratch A28.1
Central Asian hemorrhagic A98.0
cerebral — *see* Encephalitis
cerebrospinal meningococcal A39.0
Chagres B50.9
Chandipura A92.8
Changuinola A93.1
Charcot's (biliary) (hepatic) (intermittent) — *see* Calculus, bile duct
Chikungunya (viral) (hemorrhagic) A92.0
Chitral A93.1
Colombo — *see* Fever, paratyphoid
Colorado tick (virus) A93.2
congestive (remittent) — *see* Malaria
Congo virus A98.0
continued malarial B50.9
Corsican — *see* Malaria
Crimean-Congo hemorrhagic A98.0
Cyprus — *see* Brucellosis
dandy A90
deer fly — *see* Tularemia
dengue (virus) A90
hemorrhagic A91
sandfly A93.1
desert B38.0
drug induced R50.2
due to
conditions classified elsewhere R50.81
heat T67.01
enteric A01.00
enteroviral exanthematous (Boston exanthem) A88.0
ephemeral (of unknown origin) R50.9
epidemic hemorrhagic A98.5
erysipelatous — *see* Erysipelas
estivo-autumnal (malarial) B50.9
famine A75.0
five day A79.0
following delivery O86.4
Fort Bragg A27.89
gastroenteric A01.00
gastromalarial — *see* Malaria
Gibraltar — *see* Brucellosis
glandular — *see* Mononucleosis, infectious
Guama (viral) A92.8
Haverhill A25.1
hay (allergic) J30.1
with asthma (bronchial) J45.909
with
exacerbation (acute) J45.901
status asthmaticus J45.902
due to
allergen other than pollen J30.89
pollen, any plant or tree J30.1
heat (effects) T67.01
hematuric, bilious B50.8
hemoglobinuric (malarial) (bilious) B50.8
hemorrhagic (arthropod-borne) NOS A94
with renal syndrome A98.5
arenaviral A96.9
specified NEC A96.8
Argentinian A96.0
Bangkok A91
Bolivian A96.1

Fever (inanition) (of unknown origin) (persistent) (with chills) (with rigor) - *continued*
hemorrhagic (arthropod-borne) NOS - *continued*
Central Asian A98.0
Chikungunya A92.0
Crimean-Congo A98.0
dengue (virus) A91
epidemic A98.5
Junin (virus) A96.0
Korean A98.5
Kyasanur forest A98.2
Machupo (virus) A96.1
mite-borne A93.8
mosquito-borne A92.8
Omsk A98.1
Philippine A91
Russian A98.5
Singapore A91
Southeast Asia A91
Thailand A91
tick-borne NEC A93.8
viral A99
specified NEC A98.8
hepatic — *see* Cholecystitis
herpetic — *see* Herpes
icterohemorrhagic A27.0
Indiana A93.8
infective B99.9
specified NEC B99.8
intermittent (bilious) — *see also* Malaria
of unknown origin R50.9
pernicious B50.9
iodide R50.2
Japanese river A75.3
jungle — *see also* Malaria
yellow A95.0
Junin (virus) hemorrhagic A96.0
Katayama B65.2
kedani A75.3
Kenya (tick) A77.1
Kew Garden A79.1
Korean hemorrhagic A98.5
Lassa A96.2
Lone Star A77.0
Machupo (virus) hemorrhagic A96.1
malaria, malarial — *see* Malaria
Malta A23.9
Marseilles A77.1
marsh — *see* Malaria
Mayaro (viral) A92.8
Mediterranean — *see also* Brucellosis A23.9
familial M04.1
tick A77.1
meningeal — *see* Meningitis
Meuse A79.0
Mexican A75.2
mianeh A68.1
miasmatic — *see* Malaria
mosquito-borne (viral) A92.9
hemorrhagic A92.8
mountain — *see also* Brucellosis
meaning Rocky Mountain spotted fever A77.0
tick (American) (Colorado) (viral) A93.2
Mucambo (viral) A92.8
mud A27.9
Neapolitan — *see* Brucellosis
neutropenic D70.9
newborn P81.9
environmental P81.0
Nine-Mile A78
non-exanthematous tick A93.2
North Asian tick-borne A77.2
Omsk hemorrhagic A98.1
O'nyong-nyong (viral) A92.1
Oropouche (viral) A93.0
Oroya A44.0
pacific coast tick A77.8
paludal — *see* Malaria
Panama (malarial) B50.9
Pappataci A93.1
paratyphoid A01.4
A A01.1

Fever (inanition) (of unknown origin) (persistent) (with chills) (with rigor) - *continued*
paratyphoid - *continued*
B A01.2
C A01.3
parrot A70
periodic (Mediterranean) M04.1
persistent (of unknown origin) R50.9
petechial A39.0
pharyngoconjunctival B30.2
Philippine hemorrhagic A91
phlebotomus A93.1
Piry (virus) A93.8
Pixuna (viral) A92.8
Plasmodium ovale B53.0
polioviral (nonparalytic) A80.4
Pontiac A48.2
postimmunization R50.83
postoperative R50.82
due to infection T81.40
posttransfusion R50.84
postvaccination R50.83
presenting with conditions classified elsewhere R50.81
pretibial A27.89
puerperal O86.4
Q A78
quadrilateral A78
quartan (malaria) B52.9
Queensland (coastal) (tick) A77.3
quintan A79.0
rabbit — *see* Tularemia
rat-bite A25.9
due to
Spirillum A25.0
Streptobacillus moniliformis A25.1
recurrent — *see* Fever, relapsing
relapsing (Borrelia) A68.9
Carter's (Asiatic) A68.1
Dutton's (West African) A68.1
Koch's A68.9
louse-borne A68.0
Novy's
louse-borne A68.0
tick-borne A68.1
Obermeyer's (European) A68.0
tick-borne A68.1
remittent (bilious) (congestive) (gastric) — *see* Malaria
rheumatic (active) (acute) (chronic) (subacute) I00
with central nervous system involvement I02.9
active with heart involvement — *see* category I01
inactive or quiescent with
cardiac hypertrophy I09.89
carditis I09.9
endocarditis I09.1
aortic (valve) I06.9
with mitral (valve) disease I08.0
mitral (valve) I05.9
with aortic (valve) disease I08.0
pulmonary (valve) I09.89
tricuspid (valve) I07.8
heart disease NEC I09.89
heart failure (congestive) (conditions in category I50.) I09.81
left ventricular failure (conditions in I50.1-I50.4-) I09.81
myocarditis, myocardial degeneration (conditions in I51.4) I09.0
pancarditis I09.9
pericarditis I09.2
Rift Valley (viral) A92.4
Rocky Mountain spotted A77.0
rose J30.1
Ross River B33.1
Russian hemorrhagic A98.5
San Joaquin (Valley) B38.0
sandfly A93.1
Sao Paulo A77.0
scarlet A38.9

Fever (inanition) (of unknown origin) (persistent) (with chills) (with rigor) - *continued*
seven day (leptospirosis) (autumnal) (Japanese) A27.89
dengue A90
shin-bone A79.0
Singapore hemorrhagic A91
solar A90
Songo A98.5
sore B00.1
South African tick-bite A68.1
Southeast Asia hemorrhagic A91
spinal — *see* Meningitis
spirillary A25.0
splenic — *see* Anthrax
spotted A77.9
American A77.0
Brazilian A77.0
cerebrospinal meningitis A39.0
Colombian A77.0
due to Rickettsia
africae (African tick bite fever) A77.8
australis A77.3
conorii A77.1
parkeri A77.8
rickettsii A77.0
sibirica A77.2
specified type NEC A77.8
Ehrlichiosis A77.40
due to
E. chafeensis A77.41
specified organism NEC A77.49
Rocky Mountain A77.0
steroid R50.2
streptobacillary A25.1
subtertian B50.9
Sumatran mite A75.3
sun A90
swamp A27.9
swine A02.8
sylvatic, yellow A95.0
Tahyna B33.8
tertian — *see* Malaria, tertian
Thailand hemorrhagic A91
thermic T67.01
three-day A93.1
tick
American mountain A93.2
Colorado A93.2
Kemerovo A93.8
Mediterranean A77.1
mountain A93.2
nonexanthematous A93.2
Quaranfil A93.8
tick-bite NEC A93.8
tick-borne (hemorrhagic) NEC A93.8
trench A79.0
tsutsugamushi A75.3
typhogastric A01.00
typhoid (abortive) (hemorrhagic) (intermittent) (malignant) A01.00
complicated by
arthritis A01.04
heart involvement A01.02
meningitis A01.01
osteomyelitis A01.05
pneumonia A01.03
specified NEC A01.09
typhomalarial — *see* Malaria
typhus — *see* Typhus (fever)
undulant — *see* Brucellosis
unknown origin R50.9
uveoparotid D86.89
valley B38.0
Venezuelan equine A92.2
vesicular stomatitis A93.8
viral hemorrhagic — *see* Fever, hemorrhagic, by type of virus
Volhynian A79.0
Wesselsbron (viral) A92.8
West
African B50.8
Nile (viral) A92.30
with

Fever (inanition) (of unknown origin) (persistent) (with chills) (with rigor) - *continued*
West - *continued*
Nile (viral) - *continued*
with - *continued*
complications NEC A92.39
cranial nerve disorders A92.32
encephalitis A92.31
encephalomyelitis A92.31
neurologic manifestation NEC A92.32
optic neuritis A92.32
polyradiculitis A92.32
Whitmore's — *see* Melioidosis
Wolhynian A79.0
worm B83.9
yellow A95.9
jungle A95.0
sylvatic A95.0
urban A95.1
Zika virus A92.5
Fibrillation
atrial or auricular (established) I48.91
chronic I48.20
persistent I48.19
paroxysmal I48.0
permanent I48.21
persistent (chronic) (NOS) (other) I48.19
longstanding I48.11
cardiac I49.8
heart I49.8
muscular M62.89
ventricular I49.01
Fibrin
ball or bodies, pleural (sac) J94.1
chamber, anterior (eye) (gelatinous exudate) — *see* Iridocyclitis, acute
Fibrinogenolysis — *see* Fibrinolysis
Fibrinogenopenia D68.8
acquired D65
congenital D68.2
Fibrinolysis (hemorrhagic) (acquired) D65
antepartum hemorrhage — *see* Hemorrhage, antepartum, with coagulation defect
following
abortion — *see* Abortion by type complicated by hemorrhage
ectopic or molar pregnancy O08.1
intrapartum O67.0
newborn, transient P60
postpartum O72.3
Fibrinopenia (hereditary) D68.2
acquired D68.4
Fibrinopurulent — *see* condition
Fibrinous — *see* condition
Fibroadenoma
cellular intracanalicular D24-
giant D24-
intracanalicular
cellular D24-
giant D24-
specified site — *see* Neoplasm, benign, by site
unspecified site D24-
juvenile D24-
pericanalicular
specified site — *see* Neoplasm, benign, by site
unspecified site D24-
phyllodes D24-
prostate D29.1
specified site NEC — *see* Neoplasm, benign, by site
unspecified site D24-
Fibroadenosis, breast (chronic) (cystic) (diffuse) (periodic) (segmental) N60.2-
Fibroangioma — *see also* Neoplasm, benign, by site
juvenile
specified site — *see* Neoplasm, benign, by site
unspecified site D10.6
Fibrochondrosarcoma — *see* Neoplasm, cartilage, malignant
Fibrocystic
disease — *see also* Fibrosis, cystic
breast — *see* Mastopathy, cystic
jaw M27.49
kidney (congenital) Q61.8
liver Q44.6
pancreas E84.9
kidney (congenital) Q61.8
Fibrodysplasia ossificans progressiva — *see* Myositis, ossificans, progressiva
Fibroelastosis (cordis) (endocardial) (endomyocardial) I42.4
Fibroid (tumor) — *see also* Neoplasm, connective tissue, benign
disease, lung (chronic) — *see* Fibrosis, lung
heart (disease) — *see* Myocarditis
in pregnancy or childbirth O34.1-
causing obstructed labor O65.5
induration, lung (chronic) — *see* Fibrosis, lung
lung — *see* Fibrosis, lung
pneumonia (chronic) — *see* Fibrosis, lung
uterus — *see also* Leiomyoma, uterus D25.9
Fibrolipoma — *see* Lipoma
Fibroliposarcoma — *see* Neoplasm, connective tissue, malignant
Fibroma — *see also* Neoplasm, connective tissue, benign
ameloblastic — *see* Cyst, calcifying odontogenic
bone (nonossifying) — *see* Disorder, bone, specified type NEC
ossifying — *see* Neoplasm, bone, benign
cementifying — *see* Neoplasm, bone, benign
chondromyxoid — *see* Neoplasm, bone, benign
desmoplastic — *see* Neoplasm, connective tissue, uncertain behavior
durum — *see* Neoplasm, connective tissue, benign
fascial — *see* Neoplasm, connective tissue, benign
invasive — *see* Neoplasm, connective tissue, uncertain behavior
molle — *see* Lipoma
myxoid — *see* Neoplasm, connective tissue, benign
nasopharynx, nasopharyngeal (juvenile) D10.6
nonosteogenic (nonossifying) — *see* Dysplasia, fibrous
odontogenic (central) — *see* Cyst, calcifying odontogenic
ossifying — *see* Neoplasm, bone, benign
periosteal — *see* Neoplasm, bone, benign
soft — *see* Lipoma
Fibromatosis M72.9
abdominal — *see* Neoplasm, connective tissue, uncertain behavior
aggressive — *see* Neoplasm, connective tissue, uncertain behavior
congenital generalized — *see* Neoplasm, connective tissue, uncertain behavior
Dupuytren's M72.0
gingival K06.1
palmar (fascial) M72.0
plantar (fascial) M72.2
pseudosarcomatous (proliferative) (subcutaneous) M72.4
retroperitoneal D48.3
specified NEC M72.8
Fibromyalgia M79.7
Fibromyoma — *see also* Neoplasm, connective tissue, benign
uterus (corpus) — *see also* Leiomyoma, uterus
in pregnancy or childbirth — *see* Fibroid, in pregnancy or childbirth
causing obstructed labor O65.5
Fibromyositis M79.7
Fibromyxolipoma D17.9
Fibromyxoma — *see* Neoplasm, connective tissue, benign
Fibromyxosarcoma — *see* Neoplasm, connective tissue, malignant
Fibro-odontoma, ameloblastic — *see* Cyst, calcifying odontogenic
Fibro-osteoma — *see* Neoplasm, bone, benign
Fibroplasia, retrolental H35.17-
Fibropurulent — *see* condition
Fibrosarcoma — *see also* Neoplasm, connective tissue, malignant
ameloblastic C41.1
upper jaw (bone) C41.0
congenital — *see* Neoplasm, connective tissue, malignant
fascial — *see* Neoplasm, connective tissue, malignant
infantile — *see* Neoplasm, connective tissue, malignant
odontogenic C41.1
upper jaw (bone) C41.0
periosteal — *see* Neoplasm, bone, malignant
Fibrosclerosis
breast N60.3-
multifocal M35.5
penis (corpora cavernosa) N48.6
Fibrosis, fibrotic
adrenal (gland) E27.8
amnion O41.8X-
anal papillae K62.89
arteriocapillary — *see* Arteriosclerosis
bladder N32.89
interstitial — *see* Cystitis, chronic, interstitial
localized submucosal — *see* Cystitis, chronic, interstitial
panmural — *see* Cystitis, chronic, interstitial
breast — *see* Fibrosclerosis, breast
capillary — *see also* Arteriosclerosis I70.90
lung (chronic) — *see* Fibrosis, lung
cardiac — *see* Myocarditis
cervix N88.8
chorion O41.8X-
corpus cavernosum (sclerosing) N48.6
cystic (of pancreas) E84.9
with
distal intestinal obstruction syndrome E84.19
fecal impaction E84.19
intestinal manifestations NEC E84.19
pulmonary manifestations E84.0
specified manifestations NEC E84.8
due to device, implant or graft — *see also* Complications, by site and type, specified NEC T85.828
arterial graft NEC T82.828
breast (implant) T85.828
catheter NEC T85.828
dialysis (renal) T82.828
intraperitoneal T85.828
infusion NEC T82.828
spinal (epidural) (subdural) T85.820
urinary (indwelling) T83.82
electronic (electrode) (pulse generator) (stimulator)
bone T84.82
cardiac T82.827
nervous system (brain) (peripheral nerve) (spinal) T85.820
urinary T83.82
fixation, internal (orthopedic) NEC T84.82
gastrointestinal (bile duct) (esophagus) T85.828
genital NEC T83.82
heart NEC T82.827
joint prosthesis T84.82
ocular (corneal graft) (orbital implant) NEC T85.828
orthopedic NEC T84.82
specified NEC T85.828
urinary NEC T83.82
vascular NEC T82.828
ventricular intracranial shunt T85.820
ejaculatory duct N50.89
endocardium — *see* Endocarditis
endomyocardial (tropical) I42.3
epididymis N50.89
eye muscle — *see* Strabismus, mechanical

FIBROSIS, FIBROTIC - FINDINGS, ABNORMAL, INCONCLUSIVE, WITHOUT DIAGNOSIS

Findings, abnormal, inconclusive, without diagnosis - *continued*
radiologic (X-ray) - *continued*
breast R92.8
gastrointestinal tract R93.3
genitourinary organs R93.89
head R93.0
inconclusive due to excess body fat of patient R93.9
intrathoracic organs NEC R93.1
musculoskeletal
limbs R93.6
other than limb R93.7
placenta R93.89
retroperitoneum R93.5
skin R93.89
skull R93.0
subcutaneous tissue R93.89
testis R93.81-
red blood cell (count) (morphology) (sickling) (volume) R71.8
scan NEC R94.8
bladder R94.8
bone R94.8
kidney R94.4
liver R93.2
lung R94.2
pancreas R94.8
placental R94.8
spleen R94.8
thyroid R94.6
sedimentation rate, elevated R70.0
SGOT R74.01
SGPT R74.01
sodium (deficiency) E87.1
excess E87.0
specified body fluid NEC R88.8
stress test R94.39
thyroid (function) (metabolic rate) (scan) (uptake) R94.6
transaminase (level) R74.01
triglycerides E78.9
high E78.1
with high cholesterol E78.2
tuberculin skin test (without active tuberculosis) R76.11
urine R82.90
acetone R82.4
bacteria R82.71
bile R82.2
casts or cells R82.998
chyle R82.0
culture positive R82.79
glucose R81
hemoglobin R82.3
ketone R82.4
sugar R81
vanillylmandelic acid (VMA), elevated R82.5
vectorcardiogram (VCG) R94.39
ventriculogram R93.0
white blood cell (count) (differential) (morphology) D72.9
xerography R92.8
Finger — *see* condition
Fire, Saint Anthony's — *see* Erysipelas
Fire-setting
pathological (compulsive) F63.1
Fish hook stomach K31.89
Fishmeal-worker's lung J67.8
Fissure, fissured
anus, anal K60.2
acute K60.0
chronic K60.1
congenital Q43.8
ear, lobule, congenital Q17.8
epiglottis (congenital) Q31.8
larynx J38.7
congenital Q31.8
lip K13.0
congenital — *see* Cleft, lip
nipple N64.0
associated with
lactation O92.13
pregnancy O92.11-

Fissure, fissured - *continued*
nipple - *continued*
associated with - *continued*
puerperium O92.12
nose Q30.2
palate (congenital) — *see* Cleft, palate
skin R23.4
spine (congenital) — *see also* Spina bifida
with hydrocephalus — *see* Spina bifida, by site, with hydrocephalus
tongue (acquired) K14.5
congenital Q38.3
Fistula (cutaneous) L98.8
abdomen (wall) K63.2
bladder N32.2
intestine NEC K63.2
ureter N28.89
uterus N82.5
abdominorectal K63.2
abdominosigmoidal K63.2
abdominothoracic J86.0
abdominouterine N82.5
congenital Q51.7
abdominovesical N32.2
accessory sinuses — *see* Sinusitis
actinomycotic — *see* Actinomycosis
alveolar antrum — *see* Sinusitis, maxillary
alveolar process K04.6
anorectal K60.5
antrobuccal — *see* Sinusitis, maxillary
antrum — *see* Sinusitis, maxillary
anus, anal (recurrent) (infectional) K60.3
congenital Q43.6
with absence, atresia and stenosis Q42.2
tuberculous A18.32
aorta-duodenal I77.2
appendix, appendicular K38.3
arteriovenous (acquired) (nonruptured) I77.0
brain I67.1
congenital Q28.2
ruptured — *see* Fistula, arteriovenous, brain, ruptured
ruptured I60.8
intracerebral I61.8
intraparenchymal I61.8
intraventricular I61.5
subarachnoid I60.8
cerebral — *see* Fistula, arteriovenous, brain
congenital (peripheral) — *see also* Malformation, arteriovenous
brain Q28.2
ruptured — *see* Fistula, arteriovenous, brain, ruptured
coronary Q24.5
pulmonary Q25.72
coronary I25.41
congenital Q24.5
pulmonary I28.0
congenital Q25.72
surgically created (for dialysis) Z99.2
complication — *see* Complication, arteriovenous, fistula, surgically created
traumatic — *see* Injury, blood vessel
artery I77.2
aural (mastoid) — *see* Mastoiditis, chronic
auricle — *see also* Disorder, pinna, specified type NEC
congenital Q18.1
Bartholin's gland N82.8
bile duct (common) (hepatic) K83.3
with calculus, stones — *see also* Calculus, bile duct K83.8
biliary (tract) — *see* Fistula, bile duct
bladder (sphincter) NEC — *see also* Fistula, vesico- N32.2
into seminal vesicle N32.2
bone — *see also* Disorder, bone, specified type NEC
with osteomyelitis, chronic — *see* Osteomyelitis, chronic, with draining sinus
brain G93.89

Fistula (cutaneous) - *continued*
brain - *continued*
arteriovenous (acquired) — *see also* Fistula, arteriovenous, brain I67.1
congenital Q28.2
branchial (cleft) Q18.0
branchiogenous Q18.0
breast N61.0
puerperal, postpartum or gestational, due to mastitis (purulent) — *see* Mastitis, obstetric, purulent
bronchial J86.0
bronchocutaneous, bronchomediastinal, bronchopleural, bronchopleuromediastinal (infective) J86.0
tuberculous NEC A15.5
bronchoesophageal J86.0
congenital Q39.2
with atresia of esophagus Q39.1
bronchovisceral J86.0
buccal cavity (infective) K12.2
cecosigmoidal K63.2
cecum K63.2
cerebrospinal (fluid) G96.08
cervical, lateral Q18.1
cervicoaural Q18.1
cervicosigmoidal N82.4
cervicovesical N82.1
cervix N82.8
chest (wall) J86.0
cholecystenteric — *see* Fistula, gallbladder
cholecystocolic — *see* Fistula, gallbladder
cholecystocolonic — *see* Fistula, gallbladder
cholecystoduodenal — *see* Fistula, gallbladder
cholecystogastric — *see* Fistula, gallbladder
cholecystointestinal — *see* Fistula, gallbladder
choledochoduodenal — *see* Fistula, bile duct
cholocolic K82.3
coccyx — *see* Sinus, pilonidal
colon K63.2
colostomy K94.09
colovesical N32.1
common duct — *see* Fistula, bile duct
congenital, site not listed — *see* Anomaly, by site
coronary, arteriovenous I25.41
congenital Q24.5
costal region J86.0
cul-de-sac, Douglas' N82.8
cystic duct — *see also* Fistula, gallbladder
congenital Q44.5
dental K04.6
diaphragm J86.0
duodenum K31.6
ear (external) (canal) — *see* Disorder, ear, external, specified type NEC
enterocolic K63.2
enterocutaneous K63.2
enterouterine N82.4
congenital Q51.7
enterovaginal N82.4
congenital Q52.2
large intestine N82.3
small intestine N82.2
enterovesical N32.1
epididymis N50.89
tuberculous A18.15
esophagobronchial J86.0
congenital Q39.2
with atresia of esophagus Q39.1
esophagocutaneous K22.89
esophagopleural-cutaneous J86.0
esophagotracheal J86.0
congenital Q39.2
with atresia of esophagus Q39.1
esophagus K22.89
congenital Q39.2
with atresia of esophagus Q39.1
ethmoid — *see* Sinusitis, ethmoidal
eyeball (cornea) (sclera) — *see* Disorder, globe, hypotony
eyelid H01.8

Fistula (cutaneous) - *continued*
fallopian tube, external N82.5
fecal K63.2
congenital Q43.6
from periapical abscess K04.6
frontal sinus — *see* Sinusitis, frontal
gallbladder K82.3
with calculus, cholelithiasis, stones — *see* Calculus, gallbladder
gastric K31.6
gastrocolic K31.6
congenital Q40.2
tuberculous A18.32
gastroenterocolic K31.6
gastroesophageal K31.6
gastrojejunal K31.6
gastrojejunocolic K31.6
genital tract (female) N82.9
specified NEC N82.8
to intestine NEC N82.4
to skin N82.5
hepatic artery-portal vein, congenital Q26.6
hepatopleural J86.0
hepatopulmonary J86.0
ileorectal or ileosigmoidal K63.2
ileovaginal N82.2
ileovesical N32.1
ileum K63.2
in ano K60.3
tuberculous A18.32
inner ear (labyrinth) — *see* subcategory H83.1
intestine NEC K63.2
intestinocolonic (abdominal) K63.2
intestinoureteral N28.89
intestinouterine N82.4
intestinovaginal N82.4
large intestine N82.3
small intestine N82.2
intestinovesical N32.1
ischiorectal (fossa) K61.39
jejunum K63.2
joint M25.10
ankle M25.17-
elbow M25.12-
foot joint M25.17-
hand joint M25.14-
hip M25.15-
knee M25.16-
shoulder M25.11-
specified joint NEC M25.18
tuberculous — *see* Tuberculosis, joint
vertebrae M25.18
wrist M25.13-
kidney N28.89
labium (majus) (minus) N82.8
labyrinth — *see* subcategory H83.1
lacrimal (gland) (sac) H04.61-
lacrimonasal duct — *see* Fistula, lacrimal
laryngotracheal, congenital Q34.8
larynx J38.7
lip K13.0
congenital Q38.0
lumbar, tuberculous A18.01
lung J86.0
lymphatic I89.8
mammary (gland) N61.0
mastoid (process) (region) — *see* Mastoiditis, chronic
maxillary J32.0
medial, face and neck Q18.8
mediastinal J86.0
mediastinobronchial J86.0
mediastinocutaneous J86.0
middle ear — *see* subcategory H74.8
mouth K12.2
nasal J34.89
sinus — *see* Sinusitis
nasopharynx J39.2
nipple N64.0
nose J34.89
oral (cutaneous) K12.2
maxillary J32.0
nasal (with cleft palate) — *see* Cleft, palate

Fistula (cutaneous) - *continued*
orbit, orbital — *see* Disorder, orbit, specified type NEC
oroantral J32.0
oviduct, external N82.5
palate (hard) M27.8
pancreatic K86.89
pancreaticoduodenal K86.89
parotid (gland) K11.4
region K12.2
penis N48.89
perianal K60.3
pericardium (pleura) (sac) — *see* Pericarditis
pericecal K63.2
perineorectal K60.4
perineosigmoidal K63.2
perineum, perineal (with urethral involvement) NEC N36.0
tuberculous A18.13
ureter N28.89
perirectal K60.4
tuberculous A18.32
peritoneum K65.9
pharyngoesophageal J39.2
pharynx J39.2
branchial cleft (congenital) Q18.0
pilonidal (infected) (rectum) — *see* Sinus, pilonidal
pleura, pleural, pleurocutaneous, pleuroperitoneal J86.0
tuberculous NEC A15.6
pleuropericardial I31.8
portal vein-hepatic artery, congenital Q26.6
postauricular H70.81-
postoperative, persistent T81.83
specified site — *see* Fistula, by site
preauricular (congenital) Q18.1
prostate N42.89
pulmonary J86.0
arteriovenous I28.0
congenital Q25.72
tuberculous — *see* Tuberculosis, pulmonary
pulmonoperitoneal J86.0
rectolabial N82.4
rectosigmoid (intercommunicating) K63.2
rectoureteral N28.89
rectourethral N36.0
congenital Q64.73
rectouterine N82.4
congenital Q51.7
rectovaginal N82.3
congenital Q52.2
tuberculous A18.18
rectovesical N32.1
congenital Q64.79
rectovesicovaginal N82.3
rectovulval N82.4
congenital Q52.79
rectum (to skin) K60.4
congenital Q43.6
with absence, atresia and stenosis Q42.0
tuberculous A18.32
renal N28.89
retroauricular — *see* Fistula, postauricular
salivary duct or gland (any) K11.4
congenital Q38.4
scrotum (urinary) N50.89
tuberculous A18.15
semicircular canals — *see* subcategory H83.1
sigmoid K63.2
to bladder N32.1
sinus — *see* Sinusitis
skin L98.8
to genital tract (female) N82.5
splenocolic D73.89
stercoral K63.2
stomach K31.6
sublingual gland K11.4
submandibular gland K11.4
submaxillary (gland) K11.4
region K12.2
thoracic J86.0
duct I89.8
thoracoabdominal J86.0

Fistula (cutaneous) - *continued*
thoracogastric J86.0
thoracointestinal J86.0
thorax J86.0
thyroglossal duct Q89.2
thyroid E07.89
trachea, congenital (external) (internal) Q32.1
tracheoesophageal J86.0
congenital Q39.2
with atresia of esophagus Q39.1
following tracheostomy J95.04
traumatic arteriovenous — *see* Injury, blood vessel, by site
tuberculous - code by site under Tuberculosis
typhoid A01.09
umbilicourinary Q64.8
urachus, congenital Q64.4
ureter (persistent) N28.89
ureteroabdominal N28.89
ureterorectal N28.89
ureterosigmoido-abdominal N28.89
ureterovaginal N82.1
ureterovesical N32.2
urethra N36.0
congenital Q64.79
tuberculous A18.13
urethroperineal N36.0
urethroperineovesical N32.2
urethrorectal N36.0
congenital Q64.73
urethroscrotal N50.89
urethrovaginal N82.1
urethrovesical N32.2
urinary (tract) (persistent) (recurrent) N36.0
uteroabdominal N82.5
congenital Q51.7
uteroenteric, uterointestinal N82.4
congenital Q51.7
uterorectal N82.4
congenital Q51.7
uteroureteric N82.1
uterourethral Q51.7
uterovaginal N82.8
uterovesical N82.1
congenital Q51.7
uterus N82.8
vagina (postpartal) (wall) N82.8
vaginocutaneous (postpartal) N82.5
vaginointestinal NEC N82.4
large intestine N82.3
small intestine N82.2
vaginoperineal N82.5
vasocutaneous, congenital Q55.7
vesical NEC N32.2
vesicoabdominal N32.2
vesicocervicovaginal N82.1
vesicocolic N32.1
vesicocutaneous N32.2
vesicoenteric N32.1
vesicointestinal N32.1
vesicometrorectal N82.4
vesicoperineal N32.2
vesicorectal N32.1
congenital Q64.79
vesicosigmoidal N32.1
vesicosigmoidovaginal N82.3
vesicoureteral N32.2
vesicoureterovaginal N82.1
vesicourethral N32.2
vesicourethrorectal N32.1
vesicouterine N82.1
congenital Q51.7
vesicovaginal N82.0
vulvorectal N82.4
congenital Q52.79
Fit R56.9
epileptic — *see* Epilepsy
fainting R55
hysterical F44.5
newborn P90
Fitting (and adjustment) (of)
artificial
arm — *see* Admission, adjustment, artificial, arm

- **Fitting (and adjustment) (of)** - *continued*
  - artificial - *continued*
    - breast Z44.3
    - eye Z44.2
    - leg — *see* Admission, adjustment, artificial, leg
  - automatic implantable cardiac defibrillator (with synchronous cardiac pacemaker) Z45.02
  - brain neuropacemaker Z46.2
    - implanted Z45.42
  - cardiac defibrillator — *see* Fitting (and adjustment) (of), automatic implantable cardiac defibrillator
  - catheter, non-vascular Z46.82
  - colostomy belt Z46.89
  - contact lenses Z46.0
  - CRT-D (resynchronization therapy defibrillator) Z45.02
  - CRT-P (cardiac resynchronization therapy pacemaker) Z45.018
    - pulse generator Z45.010
  - cystostomy device Z46.6
  - defibrillator, cardiac — *see* Fitting (and adjustment) (of), automatic implantable cardiac defibrillator
  - dentures Z46.3
  - device NOS Z46.9
    - abdominal Z46.89
    - gastrointestinal NEC Z46.59
    - implanted NEC Z45.89
    - nervous system Z46.2
      - implanted — *see* Admission, adjustment, device, implanted, nervous system
    - orthodontic Z46.4
    - orthoptic Z46.0
    - orthotic Z46.89
    - prosthetic (external) Z44.9
      - breast Z44.3
      - dental Z46.3
      - eye Z44.2
      - specified NEC Z44.8
    - specified NEC Z46.89
    - substitution
      - auditory Z46.2
        - implanted — *see* Admission, adjustment, device, implanted, hearing device
      - nervous system Z46.2
        - implanted — *see* Admission, adjustment, device, implanted, nervous system
      - visual Z46.2
        - implanted Z45.31
    - urinary Z46.6
  - gastric lap band Z46.51
  - gastrointestinal appliance NEC Z46.59
  - glasses (reading) Z46.0
  - hearing aid Z46.1
  - ileostomy device Z46.89
  - insulin pump Z46.81
  - intestinal appliance NEC Z46.89
  - myringotomy device (stent) (tube) Z45.82
  - neuropacemaker Z46.2
    - implanted Z45.42
  - non-vascular catheter Z46.82
  - orthodontic device Z46.4
  - orthopedic device (brace) (cast) (corset) (shoes) Z46.89
  - pacemaker (cardiac) (cardiac resynchronization therapy (CRT-P)) Z45.018
    - nervous system (brain) (peripheral nerve) (spinal cord) Z46.2
      - implanted Z45.42
    - pulse generator Z45.010
  - portacath (port-a-cath) Z45.2
  - prosthesis (external) Z44.9
    - arm — *see* Admission, adjustment, artificial, arm
    - breast Z44.3
    - dental Z46.3
    - eye Z44.2

- **Fitting (and adjustment) (of)** - *continued*
  - prosthesis (external) - *continued*
    - leg — *see* Admission, adjustment, artificial, leg
    - specified NEC Z44.8
  - spectacles Z46.0
  - wheelchair Z46.89
- **Fitzhugh-Curtis syndrome**
  - due to
    - Chlamydia trachomatis A74.81
    - Neisseria gonorrhorea (gonococcal peritonitis) A54.85
- **Fitz's syndrome (acute hemorrhagic pancreatitis)** — *see also* Pancreatitis, acute K85.80
- **Fixation**
  - joint — *see* Ankylosis
  - larynx J38.7
  - stapes — *see* Ankylosis, ear ossicles
    - deafness — *see* Deafness, conductive
  - uterus (acquired) — *see* Malposition, uterus
  - vocal cord J38.3
- **Flabby ridge** K06.8
- **Flaccid** — *see also* condition
  - palate, congenital Q38.5
- **Flail**
  - chest S22.5
    - newborn (birth injury) P13.8
  - joint (paralytic) M25.20
    - ankle M25.27-
    - elbow M25.22-
    - foot joint M25.27-
    - hand joint M25.24-
    - hip M25.25-
    - knee M25.26-
    - shoulder M25.21-
    - specified joint NEC M25.28
    - wrist M25.23-
- **Flajani's disease** — *see* Hyperthyroidism, with, goiter (diffuse)
- **Flap, liver** K71.3
- **Flashbacks (residual to hallucinogen use)** F16.283
- **Flat**
  - chamber (eye) — *see* Disorder, globe, hypotony, flat anterior chamber
  - chest, congenital Q67.8
  - foot (acquired) (fixed type) (painful) (postural) — *see also* Deformity, limb, flat foot
    - congenital (rigid) (spastic (everted)) Q66.5-
    - rachitic sequelae (late effect) E64.3
  - organ or site, congenital NEC — *see* Anomaly, by site
  - pelvis M95.5
    - with disproportion (fetopelvic) O33.0
      - causing obstructed labor O65.0
    - congenital Q74.2
- **Flatau-Schilder disease** G37.0
- **Flatback syndrome** M40.30
  - lumbar region M40.36
  - lumbosacral region M40.37
  - thoracolumbar region M40.35
- **Flattening**
  - head, femur M89.8X5
  - hip — *see* Coxa, plana
  - lip (congenital) Q18.8
  - nose (congenital) Q67.4
    - acquired M95.0
- **Flatulence** R14.3
  - psychogenic F45.8
- **Flatus** R14.3
  - vaginalis N89.8
- **Flax-dresser's disease** J66.1
- **Flea bite** — *see* Injury, bite, by site, superficial, insect
- **Flecks, glaucomatous (subcapsular)** — *see* Cataract, complicated
- **Fleischer (-Kayser) ring (cornea)** H18.04-
- **Fleshy mole** O02.0
- **Flexibilitas cerea** — *see* Catalepsy
- **Flexion**
  - amputation stump (surgical) T87.89
  - cervix — *see* Malposition, uterus

- **Flexion** - *continued*
  - contracture, joint — *see* Contraction, joint
  - deformity, joint — *see also* Deformity, limb, flexion M21.20
    - hip, congenital Q65.89
  - uterus — *see also* Malposition, uterus
    - lateral — *see* Lateroversion, uterus
- **Flexner-Boyd dysentery** A03.2
- **Flexner's dysentery** A03.1
- **Flexure** — *see* Flexion
- **Flint murmur (aortic insufficiency)** I35.1
- **Floater, vitreous** — *see* Opacity, vitreous
- **Floating**
  - cartilage (joint) — *see also* Loose, body, joint
    - knee — *see* Derangement, knee, loose body
  - gallbladder, congenital Q44.1
  - kidney N28.89
    - congenital Q63.8
  - spleen D73.89
- **Flooding** N92.0
- **Floor** — *see* condition
- **Floppy**
  - baby syndrome (nonspecific) P94.2
  - iris syndrome (intraoperative) (IFIS) H21.81
  - nonrheumatic mitral valve syndrome I34.1
- **Flu** — *see also* Influenza
  - avian — *see also* Influenza, due to, identified novel influenza A virus J09.X2
  - bird — *see also* Influenza, due to, identified novel influenza A virus J09.X2
  - intestinal NEC A08.4
  - swine (viruses that normally cause infections in pigs) — *see also* Influenza, due to, identified novel influenza A virus J09.X2
- **Fluctuating blood pressure** I99.8
- **Fluid**
  - abdomen R18.8
  - chest J94.8
  - heart — *see* Failure, heart, congestive
  - joint — *see* Effusion, joint
  - loss (acute) E86.9
  - lung — *see* Edema, lung
  - overload E87.70
    - specified NEC E87.79
  - peritoneal cavity R18.8
  - pleural cavity J94.8
  - retention R60.9
- **Flukes NEC** — *see also* Infestation, fluke
  - blood NEC — *see* Schistosomiasis
  - liver B66.3
- **Fluor (vaginalis)** N89.8
  - trichomonal or due to Trichomonas (vaginalis) A59.00
- **Fluorosis**
  - dental K00.3
  - skeletal M85.10
    - ankle M85.17-
    - foot M85.17-
    - forearm M85.13-
    - hand M85.14-
    - lower leg M85.16-
    - multiple site M85.19
    - neck M85.18
    - rib M85.18
    - shoulder M85.11-
    - skull M85.18
    - specified site NEC M85.18
    - thigh M85.15-
    - toe M85.17-
    - upper arm M85.12-
    - vertebra M85.18
- **Flush syndrome** E34.0
- **Flushing** R23.2
  - menopausal N95.1
- **Flutter**
  - atrial or auricular I48.92
    - atypical I48.4
    - type I I48.3
    - type II I48.4
    - typical I48.3
  - heart I49.8
    - atrial or auricular I48.92

FITTING - FLUTTER

Flutter - *continued*
  heart - *continued*
    atrial or auricular - *continued*
      atypical I48.4
      type I I48.3
      type II I48.4
      typical I48.3
    ventricular I49.02
  ventricular I49.02
FNHTR (febrile nonhemolytic transfusion reaction) R50.84
Fochier's abscess - code by site under Abscess
Focus, Assmann's — *see* Tuberculosis, pulmonary
Fogo selvagem L10.3
Foix-Alajouanine syndrome G95.19
Fold, folds (anomalous) — *see also* Anomaly, by site
  Descemet's membrane — *see* Change, corneal membrane, Descemet's, fold
  epicanthic Q10.3
  heart Q24.8
Folie à deux F24
Follicle
  cervix (nabothian) (ruptured) N88.8
  graafian, ruptured, with hemorrhage N83.0-
  nabothian N88.8
Follicular — *see* condition
Folliculitis (superficial) L73.9
  abscedens et suffodiens L66.3
  cyst N83.0-
  decalvans L66.2
  deep — *see* Furuncle, by site
  gonococcal (acute) (chronic) A54.01
  keloid, keloidalis L73.0
  pustular L01.02
  ulerythematosa reticulata L66.4
Folliculome lipidique
  specified site — *see* Neoplasm, benign, by site
  unspecified site
    female D27.9
    male D29.20
Følling's disease E70.0
Follow-up — *see* Examination, follow-up
Fong's syndrome (hereditary osteo-onychodysplasia) Q87.2
Food
  allergy L27.2
  asphyxia (from aspiration or inhalation) — *see* Foreign body, by site
  choked on — *see* Foreign body, by site
  deprivation T73.0
    specified kind of food NEC E63.8
  insecurity Z59.41
  intoxication — *see* Poisoning, food
  lack of T73.0
  poisoning — *see* Poisoning, food
  rejection NEC — *see* Disorder, eating
  strangulation or suffocation — *see* Foreign body, by site
  toxemia — *see* Poisoning, food
Foot — *see* condition
Foramen ovale (nonclosure) (patent) (persistent) Q21.1
Forbes' glycogen storage disease E74.03
Fordyce-Fox disease L75.2
Fordyce's disease (mouth) Q38.6
Forearm — *see* condition
Foreclosure on loan Z59.89
Foreign body
  with
    laceration — *see* Laceration, by site, with foreign body
    puncture wound — *see* Puncture, by site, with foreign body
  accidentally left following a procedure T81.509
    aspiration T81.506
      resulting in
        adhesions T81.516
        obstruction T81.526
        perforation T81.536
        specified complication NEC T81.596

Foreign body - *continued*
  accidentally left following a procedure - *continued*
    cardiac catheterization T81.505
      resulting in
        acute reaction T81.60
          aseptic peritonitis T81.61
          specified NEC T81.69
        adhesions T81.515
        obstruction T81.525
        perforation T81.535
        specified complication NEC T81.595
    causing
      acute reaction T81.60
        aseptic peritonitis T81.61
        specified complication NEC T81.69
      adhesions T81.519
      aseptic peritonitis T81.61
      obstruction T81.529
      perforation T81.539
      specified complication NEC T81.599
    endoscopy T81.504
      resulting in
        adhesions T81.514
        obstruction T81.524
        perforation T81.534
        specified complication NEC T81.594
    immunization T81.503
      resulting in
        adhesions T81.513
        obstruction T81.523
        perforation T81.533
        specified complication NEC T81.593
    infusion T81.501
      resulting in
        adhesions T81.511
        obstruction T81.521
        perforation T81.531
        specified complication NEC T81.591
    injection T81.503
      resulting in
        adhesions T81.513
        obstruction T81.523
        perforation T81.533
        specified complication NEC T81.593
    kidney dialysis T81.502
      resulting in
        adhesions T81.512
        obstruction T81.522
        perforation T81.532
        specified complication NEC T81.592
    packing removal T81.507
      resulting in
        acute reaction T81.60
          aseptic peritonitis T81.61
          specified NEC T81.69
        adhesions T81.517
        obstruction T81.527
        perforation T81.537
        specified complication NEC T81.597
    puncture T81.506
      resulting in
        adhesions T81.516
        obstruction T81.526
        perforation T81.536
        specified complication NEC T81.596
    specified procedure NEC T81.508
      resulting in
        acute reaction T81.60
          aseptic peritonitis T81.61
          specified NEC T81.69
        adhesions T81.518
        obstruction T81.528
        perforation T81.538
        specified complication NEC T81.598
    surgical operation T81.500
      resulting in
        acute reaction T81.60
          aseptic peritonitis T81.61
          specified NEC T81.69
        adhesions T81.510
        obstruction T81.520
        perforation T81.530
        specified complication NEC T81.590
    transfusion T81.501

Foreign body - *continued*
  accidentally left following a procedure - *continued*
    transfusion - *continued*
      resulting in
        adhesions T81.511
        obstruction T81.521
        perforation T81.531
        specified complication NEC T81.591
  alimentary tract T18.9
    anus T18.5
    colon T18.4
    esophagus — *see* Foreign body, esophagus
    mouth T18.0
    multiple sites T18.8
    rectosigmoid (junction) T18.5
    rectum T18.5
    small intestine T18.3
    specified site NEC T18.8
    stomach T18.2
  anterior chamber (eye) S05.5-
  auditory canal — *see* Foreign body, entering through orifice, ear
  bronchus T17.508
    causing
      asphyxiation T17.500
        food (bone) (seed) T17.520
        gastric contents (vomitus) T17.510
        specified type NEC T17.590
      injury NEC T17.508
        food (bone) (seed) T17.528
        gastric contents (vomitus) T17.518
        specified type NEC T17.598
  canthus — *see* Foreign body, conjunctival sac
  ciliary body (eye) S05.5-
  conjunctival sac T15.1-
  cornea T15.0-
  entering through orifice
    accessory sinus T17.0
    alimentary canal T18.9
      multiple parts T18.8
      specified part NEC T18.8
    alveolar process T18.0
    antrum (Highmore's) T17.0
    anus T18.5
    appendix T18.4
    auditory canal — *see* Foreign body, entering through orifice, ear
    auricle — *see* Foreign body, entering through orifice, ear
    bladder T19.1
    bronchioles — *see* Foreign body, respiratory tract, specified site NEC
    bronchus (main) — *see* Foreign body, bronchus
    buccal cavity T18.0
    canthus (inner) — *see* Foreign body, conjunctival sac
    cecum T18.4
    cervix (canal) (uteri) T19.3
    colon T18.4
    conjunctival sac — *see* Foreign body, conjunctival sac
    cornea — *see* Foreign body, cornea
    digestive organ or tract NOS T18.9
      multiple parts T18.8
      specified part NEC T18.8
    duodenum T18.3
    ear (external) T16.-
    esophagus — *see* Foreign body, esophagus
    eye (external) NOS T15.9-
      conjunctival sac — *see* Foreign body, conjunctival sac
      cornea — *see* Foreign body, cornea
      specified part NEC T15.8-
    eyeball — *see also* Foreign body, entering through orifice, eye, specified part NEC
      with penetrating wound — *see* Puncture, eyeball
    eyelid — *see also* Foreign body, conjunctival sac
      with

Foreign body - *continued*
entering through orifice - *continued*
eyelid - *continued*
with - *continued*
laceration — *see* Laceration, eyelid, with foreign body
puncture — *see* Puncture, eyelid, with foreign body
superficial injury — *see* Foreign body, superficial, eyelid
gastrointestinal tract T18.9
multiple parts T18.8
specified part NEC T18.8
genitourinary tract T19.9
multiple parts T19.8
specified part NEC T19.8
globe — *see* Foreign body, entering through orifice, eyeball
gum T18.0
Highmore's antrum T17.0
hypopharynx — *see* Foreign body, pharynx
ileum T18.3
intestine (small) T18.3
large T18.4
lacrimal apparatus (punctum) — *see* Foreign body, entering through orifice, eye, specified part NEC
large intestine T18.4
larynx — *see* Foreign body, larynx
lung — *see* Foreign body, respiratory tract, specified site NEC
maxillary sinus T17.0
mouth T18.0
nasal sinus T17.0
nasopharynx — *see* Foreign body, pharynx
nose (passage) T17.1
nostril T17.1
oral cavity T18.0
palate T18.0
penis T19.4
pharynx — *see* Foreign body, pharynx
piriform sinus — *see* Foreign body, pharynx
rectosigmoid (junction) T18.5
rectum T18.5
respiratory tract — *see* Foreign body, respiratory tract
sinus (accessory) (frontal) (maxillary) (nasal) T17.0
piriform — *see* Foreign body, pharynx
small intestine T18.3
stomach T18.2
suffocation by — *see* Foreign body, by site
tear ducts or glands — *see* Foreign body, entering through orifice, eye, specified part NEC
throat — *see* Foreign body, pharynx
tongue T18.0
tonsil, tonsillar (fossa) — *see* Foreign body, pharynx
trachea — *see* Foreign body, trachea
ureter T19.8
urethra T19.0
uterus (any part) T19.3
vagina T19.2
vulva T19.2
esophagus T18.108
causing
injury NEC T18.108
food (bone) (seed) T18.128
gastric contents (vomitus) T18.118
specified type NEC T18.198
tracheal compression T18.100
food (bone) (seed) T18.120
gastric contents (vomitus) T18.110
specified type NEC T18.190
feeling of, in throat R09.89
fragment — *see* Retained, foreign body fragments (type of)
genitourinary tract T19.9
bladder T19.1
multiple parts T19.8
penis T19.4
specified site NEC T19.8
urethra T19.0

Foreign body - *continued*
genitourinary tract - *continued*
uterus T19.3
IUD Z97.5
vagina T19.2
contraceptive device Z97.5
vulva T19.2
granuloma (old) (soft tissue) — *see also* Granuloma, foreign body
skin L92.3
in
laceration — *see* Laceration, by site, with foreign body
puncture wound — *see* Puncture, by site, with foreign body
soft tissue (residual) M79.5
inadvertently left in operation wound — *see* Foreign body, accidentally left during a procedure
ingestion, ingested NOS T18.9
inhalation or inspiration — *see* Foreign body, by site
internal organ, not entering through a natural orifice - code as specific injury with foreign body
intraocular S05.5-
old, retained (nonmagnetic) H44.70-
anterior chamber H44.71-
ciliary body H44.72-
iris H44.72-
lens H44.73-
magnetic H44.60-
anterior chamber H44.61-
ciliary body H44.62-
iris H44.62-
lens H44.63-
posterior wall H44.64-
specified site NEC H44.69-
vitreous body H44.65-
posterior wall H44.74-
specified site NEC H44.79-
vitreous body H44.75-
iris — *see* Foreign body, intraocular
lacrimal punctum — *see* Foreign body, entering through orifice, eye, specified part NEC
larynx T17.308
causing
asphyxiation T17.300
food (bone) (seed) T17.320
gastric contents (vomitus) T17.310
specified type NEC T17.390
injury NEC T17.308
food (bone) (seed) T17.328
gastric contents (vomitus) T17.318
specified type NEC T17.398
lens — *see* Foreign body, intraocular
ocular muscle S05.4-
old, retained — *see* Foreign body, orbit, old
old or residual
soft tissue (residual) M79.5
operation wound, left accidentally — *see* Foreign body, accidentally left during a procedure
orbit S05.4-
old, retained H05.5-
pharynx T17.208
causing
asphyxiation T17.200
food (bone) (seed) T17.220
gastric contents (vomitus) T17.210
specified type NEC T17.290
injury NEC T17.208
food (bone) (seed) T17.228
gastric contents (vomitus) T17.218
specified type NEC T17.298
respiratory tract T17.908
bronchioles — *see* Foreign body, respiratory tract, specified site NEC
bronchus — *see* Foreign body, bronchus
causing
asphyxiation T17.900
food (bone) (seed) T17.920
gastric contents (vomitus) T17.910

Foreign body - *continued*
respiratory tract - *continued*
causing - *continued*
asphyxiation - *continued*
specified type NEC T17.990
injury NEC T17.908
food (bone) (seed) T17.928
gastric contents (vomitus) T17.918
specified type NEC T17.998
larynx — *see* Foreign body, larynx
lung — *see* Foreign body, respiratory tract, specified site NEC
multiple parts — *see* Foreign body, respiratory tract, specified site NEC
nasal sinus T17.0
nasopharynx — *see* Foreign body, pharynx
nose T17.1
nostril T17.1
pharynx — *see* Foreign body, pharynx
specified site NEC T17.808
causing
asphyxiation T17.800
food (bone) (seed) T17.820
gastric contents (vomitus) T17.810
specified type NEC T17.890
injury NEC T17.808
food (bone) (seed) T17.828
gastric contents (vomitus) T17.818
specified type NEC T17.898
throat — *see* Foreign body, pharynx
trachea — *see* Foreign body, trachea
retained (old) (nonmagnetic) (in)
anterior chamber (eye) — *see* Foreign body, intraocular, old, retained, anterior chamber
magnetic — *see* Foreign body, intraocular, old, retained, magnetic, anterior chamber
ciliary body — *see* Foreign body, intraocular, old, retained, ciliary body
magnetic — *see* Foreign body, intraocular, old, retained, magnetic, ciliary body
eyelid H02.819
left H02.816
lower H02.815
upper H02.814
right H02.813
lower H02.812
upper H02.811
fragments — *see* Retained, foreign body fragments (type of)
globe — *see* Foreign body, intraocular, old, retained
magnetic — *see* Foreign body, intraocular, old, retained, magnetic
intraocular — *see* Foreign body, intraocular, old, retained
magnetic — *see* Foreign body, intraocular, old, retained, magnetic
iris — *see* Foreign body, intraocular, old, retained, iris
magnetic — *see* Foreign body, intraocular, old, retained, magnetic, iris
lens — *see* Foreign body, intraocular, old, retained, lens
magnetic — *see* Foreign body, intraocular, old, retained, magnetic, lens
muscle — *see* Foreign body, retained, soft tissue
orbit — *see* Foreign body, orbit, old
posterior wall of globe — *see* Foreign body, intraocular, old, retained, posterior wall
magnetic — *see* Foreign body, intraocular, old, retained, magnetic, posterior wall
retrobulbar — *see* Foreign body, orbit, old, retrobulbar
soft tissue M79.5
vitreous — *see* Foreign body, intraocular, old, retained, vitreous body

Foreign body - *continued*
  retained (old) (nonmagnetic) (in) - *continued*
    vitreous - *continued*
      magnetic — *see* Foreign body, intraocular, old, retained, magnetic, vitreous body
  retina S05.5-
  superficial, without open wound
    abdomen, abdominal (wall) S30.851
    alveolar process S00.552
    ankle S90.55-
    antecubital space — *see* Foreign body, superficial, forearm
    anus S30.857
    arm (upper) S40.85-
    auditory canal — *see* Foreign body, superficial, ear
    auricle — *see* Foreign body, superficial, ear
    axilla — *see* Foreign body, superficial, arm
    back, lower S30.850
    breast S20.15-
    brow S00.85
    buttock S30.850
    calf — *see* Foreign body, superficial, leg
    canthus — *see* Foreign body, superficial, eyelid
    cheek S00.85
      internal S00.552
    chest wall — *see* Foreign body, superficial, thorax
    chin S00.85
    clitoris S30.854
    costal region — *see* Foreign body, superficial, thorax
    digit (s)
      hand — *see* Foreign body, superficial, finger
      foot — *see* Foreign body, superficial, toe
    ear S00.45-
    elbow S50.35-
    epididymis S30.853
    epigastric region S30.851
    epiglottis S10.15
    esophagus, cervical S10.15
    eyebrow — *see* Foreign body, superficial, eyelid
    eyelid S00.25-
    face S00.85
    finger (s) S60.459
      index S60.45-
      little S60.45-
      middle S60.45-
      ring S60.45-
    flank S30.851
    foot (except toe (s) alone) S90.85-
      toe — *see* Foreign body, superficial, toe
    forearm S50.85-
      elbow only — *see* Foreign body, superficial, elbow
    forehead S00.85
    genital organs, external
      female S30.856
      male S30.855
    groin S30.851
    gum S00.552
    hand S60.55-
    head S00.95
      ear — *see* Foreign body, superficial, ear
      eyelid — *see* Foreign body, superficial, eyelid
      lip S00.551
      nose S00.35
      oral cavity S00.552
      scalp S00.05
      specified site NEC S00.85
    heel — *see* Foreign body, superficial, foot
    hip S70.25-
    inguinal region S30.851
    interscapular region S20.459
    jaw S00.85
    knee S80.25-
    labium (majus) (minus) S30.854
    larynx S10.15
    leg (lower) S80.85-

Foreign body - *continued*
  superficial, without open wound - *continued*
    leg (lower) - *continued*
      knee — *see* Foreign body, superficial, knee
      upper — *see* Foreign body, superficial, thigh
    lip S00.551
    lower back S30.850
    lumbar region S30.850
    malar region S00.85
    mammary — *see* Foreign body, superficial, breast
    mastoid region S00.85
    mouth S00.552
    nail
      finger — *see* Foreign body, superficial, finger
      toe — *see* Foreign body, superficial, toe
    nape S10.85
    nasal S00.35
    neck S10.95
      specified site NEC S10.85
      throat S10.15
    nose S00.35
    occipital region S00.05
    oral cavity S00.552
    orbital region — *see* Foreign body, superficial, eyelid
    palate S00.552
    palm — *see* Foreign body, superficial, hand
    parietal region S00.05
    pelvis S30.850
    penis S30.852
    perineum
      female S30.854
      male S30.850
    periocular area — *see* Foreign body, superficial, eyelid
    phalanges
      finger — *see* Foreign body, superficial, finger
      toe — *see* Foreign body, superficial, toe
    pharynx S10.15
    pinna — *see* Foreign body, superficial, ear
    popliteal space — *see* Foreign body, superficial, knee
    prepuce S30.852
    pubic region S30.850
    pudendum
      female S30.856
      male S30.855
    sacral region S30.850
    scalp S00.05
    scapular region — *see* Foreign body, superficial, shoulder
    scrotum S30.853
    shin — *see* Foreign body, superficial, leg
    shoulder S40.25-
    sternal region S20.359
    submaxillary region S00.85
    submental region S00.85
    subungual
      finger (s) — *see* Foreign body, superficial, finger
      toe (s) — *see* Foreign body, superficial, toe
    supraclavicular fossa S10.85
    supraorbital S00.85
    temple S00.85
    temporal region S00.85
    testis S30.853
    thigh S70.35-
    thorax, thoracic (wall) S20.95
      back S20.45-
      front S20.35-
    throat S10.15
    thumb S60.35-
    toe (s) (lesser) S90.456
      great S90.45-
    tongue S00.552
    trachea S10.15
    tunica vaginalis S30.853

Foreign body - *continued*
  superficial, without open wound - *continued*
    tympanum, tympanic membrane — *see* Foreign body, superficial, ear
    uvula S00.552
    vagina S30.854
    vocal cords S10.15
    vulva S30.854
    wrist S60.85-
  swallowed T18.9
  trachea T17.408
    causing
      asphyxiation T17.400
        food (bone) (seed) T17.420
        gastric contents (vomitus) T17.410
        specified type NEC T17.490
      injury NEC T17.408
        food (bone) (seed) T17.428
        gastric contents (vomitus) T17.418
        specified type NEC T17.498
  type of fragment — *see* Retained, foreign body fragments (type of)
  vitreous (humor) S05.5-
Forestier's disease (rhizomelic pseudopolyarthritis) M35.3
  meaning ankylosing hyperostosis — *see* Hyperostosis, ankylosing
Formation
  hyalin in cornea — *see* Degeneration, cornea
  sequestrum in bone (due to infection) — *see* Osteomyelitis, chronic
  valve
    colon, congenital Q43.8
    ureter (congenital) Q62.39
Formication R20.2
Fort Bragg fever A27.89
Fossa — *see also* condition
  pyriform — *see* condition
Foster-Kennedy syndrome H47.14-
Fothergill's
  disease (trigeminal neuralgia) — *see also* Neuralgia, trigeminal
  scarlatina anginosa A38.9
Foul breath R19.6
Foundling Z76.1
Fournier disease or gangrene N49.3
  female N76.89
Fourth
  cranial nerve — *see* condition
  molar K00.1
Foville's (peduncular) disease or syndrome G46.3
Fox (-Fordyce) disease (apocrine miliaria) L75.2
FPIES (food protein-induced enterocolitis syndrome) K52.21
Fracture, burst — *see* Fracture, traumatic, by site
Fracture, chronic — *see* Fracture, pathological, by site
Fracture, insufficiency — *see* Fracture, pathological, by site
Fracture, nontraumatic, NEC
  atypical
    femur M84.750-
      complete
        oblique M84.759
          left side M84.758
          right side M84.757
        transverse M84.756
          left side M84.755
          right side M84.754
      incomplete M84.753
        left side M84.752
        right side M84.751
Fracture, pathological (pathologic) — *see also* Fracture, traumatic M84.40
  ankle M84.47-
  carpus M84.44-
  clavicle M84.41-
  compression (not due to trauma) — *see also* Collapse, vertebra M48.50-
  dental implant M27.63
  dental restorative material K08.539
    with loss of material K08.531

Fracture, pathological (pathologic) - *continued*
- dental restorative material - *continued*
  - without loss of material K08.530
- due to
  - neoplastic disease NEC — *see also* Neoplasm M84.50
    - ankle M84.57-
    - carpus M84.54-
    - clavicle M84.51-
    - femur M84.55-
    - fibula M84.56-
    - finger M84.54-
    - hip M84.559
    - humerus M84.52-
    - ilium M84.550
    - ischium M84.550
    - metacarpus M84.54-
    - metatarsus M84.57-
    - neck M84.58
    - pelvis M84.550
    - radius M84.53-
    - rib M84.58
    - scapula M84.51-
    - skull M84.58
    - specified site NEC M84.58
    - tarsus M84.57-
    - tibia M84.56-
    - toe M84.57-
    - ulna M84.53-
    - vertebra M84.58
  - osteoporosis M80.00
    - disuse — *see* Osteoporosis, specified type NEC, with pathological fracture
    - drug-induced — *see* Osteoporosis, drug induced, with pathological fracture
    - idiopathic — *see* Osteoporosis, specified type NEC, with pathological fracture
    - postmenopausal — *see* Osteoporosis, postmenopausal, with pathological fracture
    - postoophorectomy — *see* Osteoporosis, postoophorectomy, with pathological fracture
    - postsurgical malabsorption — *see* Osteoporosis, specified type NEC, with pathological fracture
    - specified cause NEC — *see* Osteoporosis, specified type NEC, with pathological fracture
  - specified disease NEC M84.60
    - ankle M84.67-
    - carpus M84.64-
    - clavicle M84.61-
    - femur M84.65-
    - fibula M84.66-
    - finger M84.64-
    - hip M84.65-
    - humerus M84.62-
    - ilium M84.650
    - ischium M84.650
    - metacarpus M84.64-
    - metatarsus M84.67-
    - neck M84.68
    - radius M84.63-
    - rib M84.68
    - scapula M84.61-
    - skull M84.68
    - tarsus M84.67-
    - tibia M84.66-
    - toe M84.67-
    - ulna M84.63-
    - vertebra M84.68
- femur M84.45-
- fibula M84.46-
- finger M84.44-
- hip M84.459
- humerus M84.42-
- ilium M84.454
- ischium M84.454
- joint prosthesis — *see* Complications, joint prosthesis, mechanical, breakdown, by site

Fracture, pathological (pathologic) - *continued*
- joint prosthesis - *continued*
  - periprosthetic — *see* Fracture, pathological, periprosthetic
- metacarpus M84.44-
- metatarsus M84.47-
- neck M84.48
- pelvis M84.454
- periprosthetic M97.9
  - ankle M97.2-
  - elbow M97.4-
  - finger M97.8
  - hip M97.0-
  - knee M97.1-
  - other specified joint M97.8
  - shoulder M97.3-
  - spinal joint M97.8
  - toe joint M97.8
  - wrist joint M97.8
- radius M84.43-
- restorative material (dental) K08.539
  - with loss of material K08.531
  - without loss of material K08.530
- rib M84.48
- scapula M84.41-
- skull M84.48
- tarsus M84.47-
- tibia M84.46-
- toe M84.47-
- ulna M84.43-
- vertebra M84.48

Fracture, traumatic (abduction) (adduction) (separation) — *see also* Fracture, pathological T14.8
- acetabulum S32.40-
  - column
    - anterior (displaced) (iliopubic) S32.43-
      - nondisplaced S32.436
    - posterior (displaced) (ilioischial) S32.443
      - nondisplaced S32.44-
  - dome (displaced) S32.48-
    - nondisplaced S32.48
  - specified NEC S32.49-
  - transverse (displaced) S32.45-
    - with associated posterior wall fracture (displaced) S32.46-
      - nondisplaced S32.46-
    - nondisplaced S32.45-
  - wall
    - anterior (displaced) S32.41-
      - nondisplaced S32.41-
    - medial (displaced) S32.47-
      - nondisplaced S32.47-
    - posterior (displaced) S32.42-
      - with associated transverse fracture (displaced) S32.46-
        - nondisplaced S32.46-
      - nondisplaced S32.42-
- acromion — *see* Fracture, scapula, acromial process
- ankle S82.899
  - bimalleolar (displaced) S82.84-
    - nondisplaced S82.84-
  - lateral malleolus only (displaced) S82.6-
    - nondisplaced S82.6-
  - medial malleolus (displaced) S82.5-
    - associated with Maisonneuve's fracture — *see* Fracture, Maisonneuve's
    - nondisplaced S82.5-
  - talus — *see* Fracture, tarsal, talus
  - trimalleolar (displaced) S82.85-
    - nondisplaced S82.85-
- arm (upper) — *see also* Fracture, humerus, shaft
  - humerus — *see* Fracture, humerus
  - radius — *see* Fracture, radius
  - ulna — *see* Fracture, ulna
- astragalus — *see* Fracture, tarsal, talus
- atlas — *see* Fracture, neck, cervical vertebra, first
- axis — *see* Fracture, neck, cervical vertebra, second

Fracture, traumatic (abduction) (adduction) (separation) - *continued*
- back — *see* Fracture, vertebra
- Barton's — *see* Barton's fracture
- base of skull — *see* Fracture, skull, base
- basicervical (basal) (femoral) S72.0
- Bennett's — *see* Bennett's fracture
- bimalleolar — *see* Fracture, ankle, bimalleolar
- blow-out S02.3-
- bone NEC T14.8
  - birth injury P13.9
  - following insertion of orthopedic implant, joint prosthesis or bone plate — *see* Fracture, following insertion of orthopedic implant, joint prosthesis or bone plate
  - in (due to) neoplastic disease NEC — *see* Fracture, pathological, due to, neoplastic disease
  - pathological (cause unknown) — *see* Fracture, pathological
- breast bone — *see* Fracture, sternum
- bucket handle (semilunar cartilage) — *see* Tear, meniscus
- buckle — *see* Fracture, by site, torus
- burst — *see* Fracture, traumatic, by site
- calcaneus — *see* Fracture, tarsal, calcaneus
- carpal bone (s) S62.10-
  - capitate (displaced) S62.13-
    - nondisplaced S62.13-
  - cuneiform — *see* Fracture, carpal bone, triquetrum
  - hamate (body) (displaced) S62.143
    - hook process (displaced) S62.15-
      - nondisplaced S62.15-
    - nondisplaced S62.14-
  - larger multangular — *see* Fracture, carpal bones, trapezium
  - lunate (displaced) S62.12-
    - nondisplaced S62.12-
  - navicular S62.00-
    - distal pole (displaced) S62.01-
      - nondisplaced S62.01-
    - middle third (displaced) S62.02-
      - nondisplaced S62.02-
    - proximal third (displaced) S62.03-
      - nondisplaced S62.03-
    - volar tuberosity — *see* Fracture, carpal bones, navicular, distal pole
  - os magnum — *see* Fracture, carpal bones, capitate
  - pisiform (displaced) S62.16-
    - nondisplaced S62.16-
  - semilunar — *see* Fracture, carpal bones, lunate
  - smaller multangular — *see* Fracture, carpal bones, trapezoid
  - trapezium (displaced) S62.17-
    - nondisplaced S62.17-
  - trapezoid (displaced) S62.18-
    - nondisplaced S62.18-
  - triquetrum (displaced) S62.11-
    - nondisplaced S62.11-
  - unciform — *see* Fracture, carpal bones, hamate
- cervical — *see* Fracture, vertebra, cervical
- clavicle S42.00-
  - acromial end (displaced) S42.03-
    - nondisplaced S42.03-
  - birth injury P13.4
  - lateral end — *see* Fracture, clavicle, acromial end
  - shaft (displaced) S42.02-
    - nondisplaced S42.02-
  - sternal end (anterior) (displaced) S42.01-
    - nondisplaced S42.01-
    - posterior S42.01-
- coccyx S32.2
- collapsed — *see* Collapse, vertebra
- collar bone — *see* Fracture, clavicle
- Colles' — *see* Colles' fracture
- coronoid process — *see* Fracture, ulna, upper end, coronoid process
- corpus cavernosum penis S39.840

Fracture, traumatic (abduction) (adduction) (separation) - *continued*
- costochondral cartilage S23.41
- costochondral, costosternal junction — *see* Fracture, rib
- cranium — *see* Fracture, skull
- cricoid cartilage S12.8
- cuboid (ankle) — *see* Fracture, tarsal, cuboid
- cuneiform
  - foot — *see* Fracture, tarsal, cuneiform
  - wrist — *see* Fracture, carpal, triquetrum
- delayed union — *see* Delay, union, fracture
- dental restorative material K08.539
  - with loss of material K08.531
  - without loss of material K08.530
- due to
  - birth injury — *see* Birth, injury, fracture
  - osteoporosis — *see* Osteoporosis, with fracture
- Dupuytren's — *see* Fracture, ankle, lateral malleolus
- elbow S42.40-
- ethmoid (bone) (sinus) — *see* Fracture, skull, base
- face bone S02.92
- fatigue — *see also* Fracture, stress
  - vertebra M48.40
    - cervical region M48.42
    - cervicothoracic region M48.43
    - lumbar region M48.46
    - lumbosacral region M48.47
    - occipito-atlanto-axial region M48.41
    - sacrococcygeal region M48.48
    - thoracic region M48.44
    - thoracolumbar region M48.45
- femur, femoral S72.9-
  - basicervical (basal) S72.0
  - birth injury P13.2
  - capital epiphyseal S79.01-
  - condyles, epicondyles — *see* Fracture, femur, lower end
  - distal end — *see* Fracture, femur, lower end
  - epiphysis
    - head — *see* Fracture, femur, upper end, epiphysis
    - lower — *see* Fracture, femur, lower end, epiphysis
    - upper — *see* Fracture, femur, upper end, epiphysis
  - following insertion of implant, prosthesis or plate M96.66-
  - head — *see* Fracture, femur, upper end, head
  - intertrochanteric — *see* Fracture, femur, trochanteric
  - intratrochanteric — *see* Fracture, femur, trochanteric
  - lower end S72.40-
    - condyle (displaced) S72.41-
      - lateral (displaced) S72.42-
        - nondisplaced S72.42-
      - medial (displaced) S72.43-
        - nondisplaced S72.43-
      - nondisplaced S72.41-
    - epiphysis (displaced) S72.44-
      - nondisplaced S72.44-
    - physeal S79.10-
      - Salter-Harris
        - Type I S79.11-
        - Type II S79.12-
        - Type III S79.13-
        - Type IV S79.14-
      - specified NEC S79.19-
    - specified NEC S72.49-
    - supracondylar (displaced) S72.45-
      - with intracondylar extension (displaced) S72.46-
        - nondisplaced S72.46-
      - nondisplaced S72.45-
    - torus S72.47-
  - neck — *see* Fracture, femur, upper end, neck
  - pertrochanteric — *see* Fracture, femur, trochanteric

Fracture, traumatic (abduction) (adduction) (separation) - *continued*
- femur, femoral - *continued*
  - shaft (lower third) (middle third) (upper third) S72.30-
    - comminuted (displaced) S72.35-
      - nondisplaced S72.35-
    - oblique (displaced) S72.33-
      - nondisplaced S72.33-
    - segmental (displaced) S72.36-
      - nondisplaced S72.36-
    - specified NEC S72.39-
    - spiral (displaced) S72.34-
      - nondisplaced S72.34-
    - transverse (displaced) S72.32-
      - nondisplaced S72.32-
  - specified site NEC — *see* subcategory S72.8
  - subcapital (displaced) S72.01-
  - subtrochanteric (region) (section) (displaced) S72.2-
    - nondisplaced S72.2-
  - transcervical — *see* Fracture, femur, midcervical
  - transtrochanteric — *see* Fracture, femur, trochanteric
  - trochanteric S72.10-
    - apophyseal (displaced) S72.13-
      - nondisplaced S72.13-
    - greater trochanter (displaced) S72.11-
      - nondisplaced S72.11-
    - intertrochanteric (displaced) S72.14-
      - nondisplaced S72.14-
    - lesser trochanter (displaced) S72.12-
      - nondisplaced S72.12-
  - upper end S72.00-
    - apophyseal (displaced) S72.13-
      - nondisplaced S72.13-
    - cervicotrochanteric — *see* Fracture, femur, upper end, neck, base
    - epiphysis (displaced) S72.02-
      - nondisplaced S72.02-
    - head S72.05-
      - articular (displaced) S72.06-
        - nondisplaced S72.06-
      - specified NEC S72.09-
    - intertrochanteric (displaced) S72.14-
      - nondisplaced S72.14-
    - intracapsular S72.01-
    - midcervical (displaced) S72.03-
      - nondisplaced S72.03-
    - neck S72.00-
      - base (displaced) S72.04-
        - nondisplaced S72.04-
      - specified NEC S72.09-
    - pertrochanteric — *see* Fracture, femur, upper end, trochanteric
    - physeal S79.00-
      - Salter-Harris type I S79.01-
      - specified NEC S79.09-
    - subcapital (displaced) S72.01-
    - subtrochanteric (displaced) S72.2-
      - nondisplaced S72.2-
    - transcervical — *see* Fracture, femur, upper end, midcervical
    - trochanteric S72.10-
      - greater (displaced) S72.11-
        - nondisplaced S72.11-
      - lesser (displaced) S72.12-
        - nondisplaced S72.12-
- fibula (shaft) (styloid) S82.40-
  - comminuted (displaced) S82.45-
    - nondisplaced S82.45-
  - following insertion of implant, prosthesis or plate M96.67-
  - involving ankle or malleolus — *see* Fracture, fibula, lateral malleolus
  - lateral malleolus (displaced) S82.6-
    - nondisplaced S82.6-
  - lower end
    - physeal S89.30-
      - Salter-Harris
        - Type I S89.31-
        - Type II S89.32-
      - specified NEC S89.39-

Fracture, traumatic (abduction) (adduction) (separation) - *continued*
- fibula (shaft) (styloid) - *continued*
  - lower end - *continued*
    - specified NEC S82.83-
    - torus S82.82-
  - oblique (displaced) S82.43-
    - nondisplaced S82.43-
  - segmental (displaced) S82.46-
    - nondisplaced S82.46-
  - specified NEC S82.49-
  - spiral (displaced) S82.44-
    - nondisplaced S82.44-
  - transverse (displaced) S82.42-
    - nondisplaced S82.42-
  - upper end
    - physeal S89.20-
      - Salter-Harris
        - Type I S89.21-
        - Type II S89.22-
      - specified NEC S89.29-
    - specified NEC S82.83-
    - torus S82.81-
- finger (except thumb) S62.60-
  - distal phalanx (displaced) S62.63-
    - nondisplaced S62.66-
  - index S62.60-
    - distal phalanx (displaced) S62.63-
      - nondisplaced S62.66-
    - middle phalanx (displaced) S62.62-
      - nondisplaced S62.65-
    - proximal phalanx (displaced) S62.61-
      - nondisplaced S62.64-
  - little S62.60-
    - distal phalanx (displaced) S62.63-
      - nondisplaced S62.66-
    - middle phalanx (displaced) S62.62-
      - nondisplaced S62.65-
    - proximal phalanx (displaced) S62.61-
      - nondisplaced S62.64-
  - middle phalanx (displaced) S62.62-
    - nondisplaced S62.65-
  - middle S62.60-
    - distal phalanx (displaced) S62.63-
      - nondisplaced S62.66-
    - middle phalanx (displaced) S62.62-
      - nondisplaced S62.65-
    - proximal phalanx (displaced) S62.61-
      - nondisplaced S62.64-
  - proximal phalanx (displaced) S62.61-
    - nondisplaced S62.64-
  - ring S62.60-
    - distal phalanx (displaced) S62.63-
      - nondisplaced S62.66-
    - middle phalanx (displaced) S62.62-
      - nondisplaced S62.65-
    - proximal phalanx (displaced) S62.61-
      - nondisplaced S62.64-
  - thumb — *see* Fracture, thumb
- following insertion (intraoperative) (postoperative) of orthopedic implant, joint prosthesis or bone plate M96.69
  - femur M96.66-
  - fibula M96.67-
  - humerus M96.62-
  - pelvis M96.65
  - radius M96.63-
  - specified bone NEC M96.69
  - tibia M96.67-
  - ulna M96.63-
- foot S92.90-
  - astragalus — *see* Fracture, tarsal, talus
  - calcaneus — *see* Fracture, tarsal, calcaneus
  - cuboid — *see* Fracture, tarsal, cuboid
  - cuneiform — *see* Fracture, tarsal, cuneiform
  - metatarsal — *see* Fracture, metatarsal
  - navicular — *see* Fracture, tarsal, navicular
  - sesamoid S92.81-
  - specified NEC S92.81-
  - talus — *see* Fracture, tarsal, talus
  - tarsal — *see* Fracture, tarsal
  - toe — *see* Fracture, toe
- forearm S52.9-
  - radius — *see* Fracture, radius

Fracture, traumatic (abduction) (adduction) (separation) - *continued*
- forearm - *continued*
  - ulna — *see* Fracture, ulna
- fossa (anterior) (middle) (posterior) S02.19
- fragility — *see* Fracture, pathological, due to osteoporosis
- frontal (bone) (skull) S02.0
  - sinus S02.19
- glenoid (cavity) (scapula) — *see* Fracture, scapula, glenoid cavity
- greenstick — *see* Fracture, by site
- hallux — *see* Fracture, toe, great
- hand S62.9-
  - carpal — *see* Fracture, carpal bone
  - finger (except thumb) — *see* Fracture, finger
  - metacarpal — *see* Fracture, metacarpal
  - navicular (scaphoid) (hand) — *see* Fracture, carpal bone, navicular
  - thumb — *see* Fracture, thumb
- healed or old
  - with complications - code by Nature of the complication
- heel bone — *see* Fracture, tarsal, calcaneus
- Hill-Sachs S42.29-
- hip — *see* Fracture, femur, neck
- humerus S42.30-
  - anatomical neck — *see* Fracture, humerus, upper end
  - articular process — *see* Fracture, humerus, lower end
  - capitellum — *see* Fracture, humerus, lower end, condyle, lateral
  - distal end — *see* Fracture, humerus, lower end
  - epiphysis
    - lower — *see* Fracture, humerus, lower end, physeal
    - upper — *see* Fracture, humerus, upper end, physeal
  - external condyle — *see* Fracture, humerus, lower end, condyle, lateral
  - following insertion of implant, prosthesis or plate M96.62-
  - great tuberosity — *see* Fracture, humerus, upper end, greater tuberosity
  - intercondylar — *see* Fracture, humerus, lower end
  - internal epicondyle — *see* Fracture, humerus, lower end, epicondyle, medial
  - lesser tuberosity — *see* Fracture, humerus, upper end, lesser tuberosity
  - lower end S42.40-
    - condyle
      - lateral (displaced) S42.45-
        - nondisplaced S42.45-
      - medial (displaced) S42.46-
        - nondisplaced S42.46-
    - epicondyle
      - lateral (displaced) S42.43-
        - nondisplaced S42.43-
      - medial (displaced) S42.44-
        - incarcerated S42.44-
        - nondisplaced S42.44-
    - physeal S49.10-
      - Salter-Harris
        - Type I S49.11-
        - Type II S49.12-
        - Type III S49.13-
        - Type IV S49.14-
      - specified NEC S49.19-
    - specified NEC (displaced) S42.49-
      - nondisplaced S42.49-
    - supracondylar (simple) (displaced) S42.41-
      - with intercondylar fracture — *see* Fracture, humerus, lower end
      - comminuted (displaced) S42.42-
        - nondisplaced S42.42-
      - nondisplaced S42.41-
    - torus S42.48-
    - transcondylar (displaced) S42.47-
      - nondisplaced S42.47-

Fracture, traumatic (abduction) (adduction) (separation) - *continued*
- humerus - *continued*
  - proximal end — *see* Fracture, humerus, upper end
  - shaft S42.30-
    - comminuted (displaced) S42.35-
      - nondisplaced S42.35-
    - greenstick S42.31-
    - oblique (displaced) S42.33-
      - nondisplaced S42.33-
    - segmental (displaced) S42.36-
      - nondisplaced S42.36-
    - specified NEC S42.39-
    - spiral (displaced) S42.34-
      - nondisplaced S42.34-
    - transverse (displaced) S42.32-
      - nondisplaced S42.32-
  - supracondylar — *see* Fracture, humerus, lower end
  - surgical neck — *see* Fracture, humerus, upper end, surgical neck
  - trochlea — *see* Fracture, humerus, lower end, condyle, medial
  - tuberosity — *see* Fracture, humerus, upper end
  - upper end S42.20-
    - anatomical neck — *see* Fracture, humerus, upper end, specified NEC
    - articular head — *see* Fracture, humerus, upper end, specified NEC
    - epiphysis — *see* Fracture, humerus, upper end, physeal
    - greater tuberosity (displaced) S42.25-
      - nondisplaced S42.25-
    - lesser tuberosity (displaced) S42.26-
      - nondisplaced S42.26-
    - physeal S49.00-
      - Salter-Harris
        - Type I S49.01-
        - Type II S49.02-
        - Type III S49.03-
        - Type IV S49.04-
      - specified NEC S49.09-
    - specified NEC (displaced) S42.29-
      - nondisplaced S42.29-
    - surgical neck (displaced) S42.21-
      - four-part S42.24-
      - nondisplaced S42.21-
      - three-part S42.23-
      - two-part (displaced) S42.22-
        - nondisplaced S42.22-
    - torus S42.27-
    - transepiphyseal — *see* Fracture, humerus, upper end, physeal
- hyoid bone S12.8
- ilium S32.30-
  - with disruption of pelvic ring — *see* Disruption, pelvic ring
  - avulsion (displaced) S32.31-
    - nondisplaced S32.31-
  - specified NEC S32.39-
- impaction, impacted - code as Fracture, by site
- innominate bone — *see* Fracture, ilium
- instep — *see* Fracture, foot
- ischium S32.60-
  - with disruption of pelvic ring — *see* Disruption, pelvic ring
  - avulsion (displaced) S32.61-
    - nondisplaced S32.61-
  - specified NEC S32.69-
- jaw (bone) (lower) — *see* Fracture, mandible
  - upper — *see* Fracture, maxilla
- joint prosthesis — *see* Complications, joint prosthesis, mechanical, breakdown, by site
  - periprosthetic — *see* Fracture, traumatic, periprosthetic
- knee cap — *see* Fracture, patella
- larynx S12.8
- late effects — *see* Sequelae, fracture
- leg (lower) S82.9-
  - ankle — *see* Fracture, ankle
  - femur — *see* Fracture, femur

Fracture, traumatic (abduction) (adduction) (separation) - *continued*
- leg (lower) - *continued*
  - fibula — *see* Fracture, fibula
  - malleolus — *see* Fracture, ankle
  - patella — *see* Fracture, patella
  - specified site NEC S82.89-
  - tibia — *see* Fracture, tibia
- lumbar spine — *see* Fracture, vertebra, lumbar
- lumbosacral spine S32.9
- Maisonneuve's (displaced) S82.86-
  - nondisplaced S82.86-
- malar bone — *see also* Fracture, maxilla S02.400
  - left side S02.40B
  - right side S02.40A
- malleolus — *see* Fracture, ankle
- malunion — *see* Fracture, by site
- mandible (lower jaw (bone)) S02.609
  - alveolus S02.67-
  - angle (of jaw) S02.65-
  - body, unspecified S02.600
    - left side S02.602
    - right side S02.601
  - condylar process S02.61-
  - coronoid process S02.63-
  - ramus, unspecified S02.64-
  - specified site NEC S02.69
  - subcondylar process S02.62-
  - symphysis S02.66
- manubrium (sterni) S22.21
  - dissociation from sternum S22.23
- march — *see* Fracture, traumatic, stress, by site
- maxilla, maxillary (bone) (sinus) (superior) (upper jaw) S02.401
  - alveolus S02.42
  - inferior — *see* Fracture, mandible
  - LeFort I S02.411
  - LeFort II S02.412
  - LeFort III S02.413
  - left side S02.40D
  - right side S02.40C
- metacarpal S62.309
  - base (displaced) S62.319
    - nondisplaced S62.349
  - fifth S62.30-
    - base (displaced) S62.31-
      - nondisplaced S62.34-
    - neck (displaced) S62.33-
      - nondisplaced S62.36-
    - shaft (displaced) S62.32-
      - nondisplaced S62.35-
    - specified NEC S62.398
  - first S62.20-
    - base NEC (displaced) S62.23-
      - nondisplaced S62.23-
    - Bennett's — *see* Bennett's fracture
    - neck (displaced) S62.25-
      - nondisplaced S62.25-
    - shaft (displaced) S62.24-
      - nondisplaced S62.24-
    - specified NEC S62.29-
  - fourth S62.30-
    - base (displaced) S62.31-
      - nondisplaced S62.34-
    - neck (displaced) S62.33-
      - nondisplaced S62.36-
    - shaft (displaced) S62.32-
      - nondisplaced S62.35-
    - specified NEC S62.39-
  - neck (displaced) S62.33-
    - nondisplaced S62.36-
  - Rolando's — *see* Rolando's fracture
  - second S62.30-
    - base (displaced) S62.31-
      - nondisplaced S62.34-
    - neck (displaced) S62.33-
      - nondisplaced S62.36-
    - shaft (displaced) S62.32-
      - nondisplaced S62.35-
    - specified NEC S62.39-
  - shaft (displaced) S62.32-
    - nondisplaced S62.35-

Fracture, traumatic (abduction) (adduction) (separation) - *continued*
metacarpal - *continued*
third S62.30-
base (displaced) S62.31-
nondisplaced S62.34-
neck (displaced) S62.33-
nondisplaced S62.36-
shaft (displaced) S62.32-
nondisplaced S62.35-
specified NEC S62.39-
specified NEC S62.399
metaphyseal — *see* Fracture, traumatic, by site, shaft
metastatic — *see* Fracture, pathological, due to, neoplastic disease — *see also* Neoplasm
metatarsal bone S92.30-
fifth (displaced) S92.35-
nondisplaced S92.35-
first (displaced) S92.31-
nondisplaced S92.31-
fourth (displaced) S92.34-
nondisplaced S92.34-
physeal S99.10-
Salter-Harris
Type I S99.11-
Type II S99.12-
Type III S99.13-
Type IV S99.14-
specified NEC S99.19-
second (displaced) S92.32-
nondisplaced S92.32-
third (displaced) S92.33-
nondisplaced S92.33-
Monteggia's — *see* Monteggia's fracture
multiple
hand (and wrist) NEC — *see* Fracture, by site
ribs — *see* Fracture, rib, multiple
nasal (bone (s)) S02.2
navicular (scaphoid) (foot) — *see also* Fracture, tarsal, navicular
hand — *see* Fracture, carpal, navicular
neck S12.9
cervical vertebra S12.9
fifth (displaced) S12.400
nondisplaced S12.401
specified type NEC (displaced) S12.490
nondisplaced S12.491
first (displaced) S12.000
burst (stable) S12.01
unstable S12.02
lateral mass (displaced) S12.040
nondisplaced S12.041
nondisplaced S12.001
posterior arch (displaced) S12.030
nondisplaced S12.031
specified type NEC (displaced) S12.090
nondisplaced S12.091
fourth (displaced) S12.300
nondisplaced S12.301
specified type NEC (displaced) S12.390
nondisplaced S12.391
second (displaced) S12.100
nondisplaced S12.101
dens (anterior) (displaced) (type II) S12.110
nondisplaced S12.112
posterior S12.111
specified type NEC (displaced) S12.120
nondisplaced S12.121
specified type NEC (displaced) S12.190
nondisplaced S12.191
seventh (displaced) S12.600
nondisplaced S12.601
specified type NEC (displaced) S12.690
nondisplaced S12.691
sixth (displaced) S12.500

Fracture, traumatic (abduction) (adduction) (separation) - *continued*
neck - *continued*
cervical vertebra - *continued*
sixth (displaced) - *continued*
nondisplaced S12.501
specified type NEC (displaced) S12.590
nondisplaced S12.591
third (displaced) S12.200
nondisplaced S12.201
specified type NEC (displaced) S12.290
nondisplaced S12.291
hyoid bone S12.8
larynx S12.8
specified site NEC S12.8
thyroid cartilage S12.8
trachea S12.8
neoplastic NEC — *see* Fracture, pathological, due to, neoplastic disease
neural arch — *see* Fracture, vertebra
newborn — *see* Birth, injury, fracture
nontraumatic — *see* Fracture, pathological
nonunion — *see* Nonunion, fracture
nose, nasal (bone) (septum) S02.2
occiput — *see* Fracture, skull, base, occiput
odontoid process — *see* Fracture, neck, cervical vertebra, second
olecranon (process) (ulna) — *see* Fracture, ulna, upper end, olecranon process
orbit, orbital (bone) (region) S02.85
floor (blow-out) S02.3-
roof S02.12-
wall S02.85
lateral S02.84-
medial S02.83-
os
calcis — *see* Fracture, tarsal, calcaneus
magnum — *see* Fracture, carpal, capitate
pubis — *see* Fracture, pubis
palate S02.8-
parietal bone (skull) S02.0
patella S82.00-
comminuted (displaced) S82.04-
nondisplaced S82.04-
longitudinal (displaced) S82.02-
nondisplaced S82.02-
osteochondral (displaced) S82.01-
nondisplaced S82.01-
specified NEC S82.09-
transverse (displaced) S82.03-
nondisplaced S82.03-
pedicle (of vertebral arch) — *see* Fracture, vertebra
pelvis, pelvic (bone) S32.9
acetabulum — *see* Fracture, acetabulum
circle — *see* Disruption, pelvic ring
following insertion of implant, prosthesis or plate M96.65
ilium — *see* Fracture, ilium
ischium — *see* Fracture, ischium
multiple
with disruption of pelvic ring (circle) — *see* Disruption, pelvic ring
without disruption of pelvic ring (circle) S32.82
pubis — *see* Fracture, pubis
specified site NEC S32.89
sacrum — *see* Fracture, sacrum
periprosthetic, around internal prosthetic joint M97.9
ankle M97.2-
elbow M97.4-
finger M97.8
hip M97.0-
knee M97.1--
shoulder M97.3-
specified joint NEC M97.8
spine M97.8
toe M97.8
wrist M97.8
phalanx
foot — *see* Fracture, toe
hand — *see* Fracture, finger

Fracture, traumatic (abduction) (adduction) (separation) - *continued*
pisiform — *see* Fracture, carpal, pisiform
pond — *see* Fracture, skull
prosthetic device, internal — *see* Complications, prosthetic device, by site, mechanical
pubis S32.50-
with disruption of pelvic ring — *see* Disruption, pelvic ring
specified site NEC S32.59-
superior rim S32.51-
radius S52.9-
distal end — *see* Fracture, radius, lower end
following insertion of implant, prosthesis or plate M96.63-
head — *see* Fracture, radius, upper end, head
lower end S52.50-
Barton's — *see* Barton's fracture
Colles' — *see* Colles' fracture
extraarticular NEC S52.55-
intraarticular NEC S52.57-
physeal S59.20-
Salter-Harris
Type I S59.21-
Type II S59.22-
Type III S59.23-
Type IV S59.24-
specified NEC S59.29-
Smith's — *see* Smith's fracture
specified NEC S52.59-
styloid process (displaced) S52.51-
nondisplaced S52.51-
torus S52.52-
neck — *see* Fracture, radius, upper end
proximal end — *see* Fracture, radius, upper end
shaft S52.30-
bent bone S52.38-
comminuted (displaced) S52.35-
nondisplaced S52.35-
Galeazzi's — *see* Galeazzi's fracture
greenstick S52.31-
oblique (displaced) S52.33-
nondisplaced S52.33-
segmental (displaced) S52.36-
nondisplaced S52.36-
specified NEC S52.39-
spiral (displaced) S52.34-
nondisplaced S52.34-
transverse (displaced) S52.32-
nondisplaced S52.32-
upper end S52.10-
head (displaced) S52.12-
nondisplaced S52.12-
neck (displaced) S52.13-
nondisplaced S52.13-
specified NEC S52.18-
physeal S59.10-
Salter-Harris
Type I S59.11-
Type II S59.12-
Type III S59.13-
Type IV S59.14-
specified NEC S59.19-
torus S52.11-
ramus
inferior or superior, pubis — *see* Fracture, pubis
mandible — *see* Fracture, mandible
restorative material (dental) K08.539
with loss of material K08.531
without loss of material K08.530
rib S22.3-
with flail chest — *see* Flail, chest
multiple S22.4-
with flail chest — *see* Flail, chest
root, tooth — *see* Fracture, tooth
sacrum S32.10
specified NEC S32.19
Type
1 S32.14
2 S32.15

Fracture, traumatic (abduction) (adduction) (separation) - *continued*
- tibia (shaft) - *continued*
  - epiphysis - *continued*
    - lower — *see* Fracture, tibia, lower end
    - upper — *see* Fracture, tibia, upper end
  - following insertion of implant, prosthesis or plate M96.67-
  - head (involving knee joint) — *see* Fracture, tibia, upper end
  - intercondyloid eminence — *see* Fracture, tibia, upper end
  - involving ankle or malleolus — *see* Fracture, ankle, medial malleolus
  - lower end S82.30-
    - physeal S89.10-
      - Salter-Harris
        - Type I S89.11-
        - Type II S89.12-
        - Type III S89.13-
        - Type IV S89.14-
      - specified NEC S89.19-
    - pilon (displaced) S82.87-
      - nondisplaced S82.87-
    - specified NEC S82.39-
    - torus S82.31-
  - malleolus — *see* Fracture, ankle, medial malleolus
  - oblique (displaced) S82.23-
    - nondisplaced S82.23-
  - pilon — *see* Fracture, tibia, lower end, pilon
  - proximal end — *see* Fracture, tibia, upper end
  - segmental (displaced) S82.26-
    - nondisplaced S82.26-
  - specified NEC S82.29-
  - spine — *see* Fracture, tibia, upper end, spine
  - spiral (displaced) S82.24-
    - nondisplaced S82.24-
  - transverse (displaced) S82.22-
    - nondisplaced S82.22-
  - tuberosity — *see* Fracture, tibia, upper end, tuberosity
  - upper end S82.10-
    - bicondylar (displaced) S82.14-
      - nondisplaced S82.14-
    - lateral condyle (displaced) S82.12-
      - nondisplaced S82.12-
    - medial condyle (displaced) S82.13-
      - nondisplaced S82.13-
    - physeal S89.00-
      - Salter-Harris
        - Type I S89.01-
        - Type II S89.02-
        - Type III S89.03-
        - Type IV S89.04-
      - specified NEC S89.09-
    - plateau — *see* Fracture, tibia, upper end, bicondylar
    - spine (displaced) S82.11-
      - nondisplaced S82.11-
    - torus S82.16-
    - specified NEC S82.19-
    - tuberosity (displaced) S82.15-
      - nondisplaced S82.15-
- toe S92.91-
  - great (displaced) S92.40-
    - distal phalanx (displaced) S92.42-
      - nondisplaced S92.42-
    - nondisplaced S92.40-
    - proximal phalanx (displaced) S92.41-
      - nondisplaced S92.41-
    - specified NEC S92.49-
  - lesser (displaced) S92.50-
    - distal phalanx (displaced) S92.53-
      - nondisplaced S92.53-
    - middle phalanx (displaced) S92.52-
      - nondisplaced S92.52-
    - nondisplaced S92.50-
    - proximal phalanx (displaced) S92.51-
      - nondisplaced S92.51-
    - specified NEC S92.59-
  - physeal

Fracture, traumatic (abduction) (adduction) (separation) - *continued*
- toe - *continued*
  - physeal - *continued*
    - phalanx S99.20-
      - Salter-Harris
        - Type I S99.21-
        - Type II S99.22-
        - Type III S99.23-
        - Type IV S99.24-
      - specified NEC S99.29-
- tooth (root) S02.5
- trachea (cartilage) S12.8
- transverse process — *see* Fracture, vertebra
- trapezium or trapezoid bone — *see* Fracture, carpal
- trimalleolar — *see* Fracture, ankle, trimalleolar
- triquetrum (cuneiform of carpus) — *see* Fracture, carpal, triquetrum
- trochanter — *see* Fracture, femur, trochanteric
- tuberosity (external) — *see* Fracture, traumatic, by site
- ulna (shaft) S52.20-
  - bent bone S52.28-
  - coronoid process — *see* Fracture, ulna, upper end, coronoid process
  - distal end — *see* Fracture, ulna, lower end
  - following insertion of implant, prosthesis or plate M96.63-
  - head S52.60-
  - lower end S52.60-
    - physeal S59.00-
      - Salter-Harris
        - Type I S59.01-
        - Type II S59.02-
        - Type III S59.03-
        - Type IV S59.04-
      - specified NEC S59.09-
    - specified NEC S52.69-
    - styloid process (displaced) S52.61-
      - nondisplaced S52.61-
    - torus S52.62-
  - proximal end — *see* Fracture, ulna, upper end
  - shaft S52.20-
    - comminuted (displaced) S52.25-
      - nondisplaced S52.25-
    - greenstick S52.21-
    - Monteggia's — *see* Monteggia's fracture
    - oblique (displaced) S52.23-
      - nondisplaced S52.23-
    - segmental (displaced) S52.26-
      - nondisplaced S52.26-
    - specified NEC S52.29-
    - spiral (displaced) S52.24-
      - nondisplaced S52.24-
    - transverse (displaced) S52.22-
      - nondisplaced S52.22-
  - upper end S52.00-
    - coronoid process (displaced) S52.04-
      - nondisplaced S52.04-
    - olecranon process (displaced) S52.02-
      - with intraarticular extension S52.03-
      - nondisplaced S52.02-
        - with intraarticular extension S52.03-
    - specified NEC S52.09-
    - torus S52.01-
- unciform — *see* Fracture, carpal, hamate
- vault of skull S02.0
- vertebra, vertebral (arch) (body) (column) (neural arch) (pedicle) (spinous process) (transverse process)
  - atlas — *see* Fracture, neck, cervical vertebra, first
  - axis — *see* Fracture, neck, cervical vertebra, second
  - cervical (teardrop) S12.9
    - axis — *see* Fracture, neck, cervical vertebra, second
    - first (atlas) — *see* Fracture, neck, cervical vertebra, first
    - second (axis) — *see* Fracture, neck, cervical vertebra, second

Fracture, traumatic (abduction) (adduction) (separation) - *continued*
- vertebra, vertebral (arch) (body) (column) (neural arch) (pedicle) (spinous process) (transverse process) - *continued*
  - chronic M84.48
  - coccyx S32.2
  - dorsal — *see* Fracture, thorax, vertebra
  - lumbar S32.009
    - burst (stable) S32.001
      - unstable S32.002
    - fifth S32.059
      - burst (stable) S32.051
        - unstable S32.052
      - specified type NEC S32.058
      - wedge compression S32.050
    - first S32.019
      - burst (stable) S32.011
        - unstable S32.012
      - specified type NEC S32.018
      - wedge compression S32.010
    - fourth S32.049
      - burst (stable) S32.041
        - unstable S32.042
      - specified type NEC S32.048
      - wedge compression S32.040
    - second S32.029
      - burst (stable) S32.021
        - unstable S32.022
      - specified type NEC S32.028
      - wedge compression S32.020
    - specified type NEC S32.008
    - third S32.039
      - burst (stable) S32.031
        - unstable S32.032
      - specified type NEC S32.038
      - wedge compression S32.030
    - wedge compression S32.000
  - metastatic — *see* Collapse, vertebra, in, specified disease NEC — *see also* Neoplasm
  - newborn (birth injury) P11.5
  - sacrum S32.10
    - specified NEC S32.19
    - Type
      - 1 S32.14
      - 2 S32.15
      - 3 S32.16
      - 4 S32.17
    - Zone
      - I S32.119
        - displaced (minimally) S32.111
          - severely S32.112
        - nondisplaced S32.110
      - II S32.129
        - displaced (minimally) S32.121
          - severely S32.122
        - nondisplaced S32.120
      - III S32.139
        - displaced (minimally) S32.131
          - severely S32.132
        - nondisplaced S32.130
  - thoracic — *see* Fracture, thorax, vertebra
- vertex S02.0
- vomer (bone) S02.2
- wrist S62.10-
  - carpal — *see* Fracture, carpal bone
  - navicular (scaphoid) (hand) — *see* Fracture, carpal, navicular
- xiphisternum, xiphoid (process) S22.24
- zygoma S02.402
  - left side S02.40F
  - right side S02.40E

Fragile, fragility
- autosomal site Q95.5
- bone, congenital (with blue sclera) Q78.0
- capillary (hereditary) D69.8
- hair L67.8
- nails L60.3
- non-sex chromosome site Q95.5
- X chromosome Q99.2

Fragilitas
- crinium L67.8
- ossium (with blue sclerae) (hereditary) Q78.0
- unguium L60.3

Fragilitas - *continued*
unguium - *continued*
congenital Q84.6
Fragments, cataract (lens), following cataract surgery H59.02-
retained foreign body — *see* Retained, foreign body fragments (type of)
Frailty (frail) R54
mental R41.81
Frambesia, frambesial (tropica) — *see also* Yaws
initial lesion or ulcer A66.0
primary A66.0
Frambeside
gummatous A66.4
of early yaws A66.2
Frambesioma A66.1
Franceschetti-Klein (-Wildervanck) disease or syndrome Q75.4
Francis' disease — *see* Tularemia
Franklin disease C88.2
Frank's essential thrombocytopenia D69.3
Fraser's syndrome Q87.0
Freckle (s) L81.2
malignant melanoma in — *see* Melanoma
melanotic (Hutchinson's) — *see* Melanoma, in situ
retinal D49.81
Frederickson's hyperlipoproteinemia, type
I and V E78.3
IIA E78.00
IIB and III E78.2
IV E78.1
Freeman Sheldon syndrome Q87.0
Freezing — *see also* Effect, adverse, cold T69.9
Freiberg's disease (infraction of metatarsal head or osteochondrosis) — *see* Osteochondrosis, juvenile, metatarsus
Frei's disease A55
Fremitus, friction, cardiac R01.2
Frenum, frenulum
external os Q51.828
tongue (shortening) (congenital) Q38.1
Frequency micturition (nocturnal) R35.0
psychogenic F45.8
Frey's syndrome
auriculotemporal G50.8
hyperhidrosis L74.52
Friction
burn — *see* Burn, by site
fremitus, cardiac R01.2
precordial R01.2
sounds, chest R09.89
Friderichsen-Waterhouse syndrome or disease A39.1
Friedländer's B (bacillus) NEC — *see also* condition A49.8
Friedreich's
ataxia G11.11
combined systemic disease G11.11
facial hemihypertrophy Q67.4
sclerosis (cerebellum) (spinal cord) G11.11
Frigidity F52.22
Fröhlich's syndrome E23.6
Frontal — *see also* condition
lobe syndrome F07.0
Frostbite (superficial) T33.90
with
partial thickness skin loss — *see* Frostbite (superficial), by site
tissue necrosis T34.90
abdominal wall T33.3
with tissue necrosis T34.3
ankle T33.81-
with tissue necrosis T34.81-
arm T33.4-
with tissue necrosis T34.4-
finger (s) — *see* Frostbite, finger
hand — *see* Frostbite, hand
wrist — *see* Frostbite, wrist
ear T33.01-
with tissue necrosis T34.01-
face T33.09
with tissue necrosis T34.09

Frostbite (superficial) - *continued*
finger T33.53-
with tissue necrosis T34.53-
foot T33.82-
with tissue necrosis T34.82-
hand T33.52-
with tissue necrosis T34.52-
head T33.09
with tissue necrosis T34.09
ear — *see* Frostbite, ear
nose — *see* Frostbite, nose
hip (and thigh) T33.6-
with tissue necrosis T34.6-
knee T33.7-
with tissue necrosis T34.7-
leg T33.9-
with tissue necrosis T34.9-
ankle — *see* Frostbite, ankle
foot — *see* Frostbite, foot
knee — *see* Frostbite, knee
lower T33.7-
with tissue necrosis T34.7-
thigh — *see* Frostbite, hip
toe — *see* Frostbite, toe
limb
lower T33.99
with tissue necrosis T34.99
upper — *see* Frostbite, arm
neck T33.1
with tissue necrosis T34.1
nose T33.02
with tissue necrosis T34.02
pelvis T33.3
with tissue necrosis T34.3
specified site NEC T33.99
with tissue necrosis T34.99
thigh — *see* Frostbite, hip
thorax T33.2
with tissue necrosis T34.2
toes T33.83-
with tissue necrosis T34.83-
trunk T33.99
with tissue necrosis T34.99
wrist T33.51-
with tissue necrosis T34.51-
Frotteurism F65.81
Frozen — *see also* Effect, adverse, cold T69.9
pelvis (female) N94.89
male K66.8
shoulder — *see* Capsulitis, adhesive
Fructokinase deficiency E74.11
Fructose 1,6 diphosphatase deficiency E74.19
Fructosemia (benign) (essential) E74.12
Fructosuria (benign) (essential) E74.11
Fuchs'
black spot (myopic) — *see also* Myopia, degenerative H44.2-
dystrophy (corneal endothelium) H18.51-
heterochromic cyclitis — *see* Cyclitis, Fuchs' heterochromic
Fucosidosis E77.1
Fugue R68.89
dissociative F44.1
hysterical (dissociative) F44.1
postictal in epilepsy — *see* Epilepsy
reaction to exceptional stress (transient) F43.0
Fulminant, fulminating — *see* condition
Functional — *see also* condition
bleeding (uterus) N93.8
Functioning, intellectual, borderline R41.83
Fundus — *see* condition
Fungemia NOS B49
Fungus, fungous
cerebral G93.89
disease NOS B49
infection — *see* Infection, fungus
Funiculitis (acute) (chronic) (endemic) N49.1
gonococcal (acute) (chronic) A54.23
tuberculous A18.15
Funnel
breast (acquired) M95.4
congenital Q67.6
sequelae (late effect) of rickets E64.3

Funnel - *continued*
chest (acquired) M95.4
congenital Q67.6
sequelae (late effect) of rickets E64.3
pelvis (acquired) M95.5
with disproportion (fetopelvic) O33.3
causing obstructed labor O65.3
congenital Q74.2
FUO (fever of unknown origin) R50.9
Furfur L21.0
microsporon B36.0
Furrier's lung J67.8
Furrowed K14.5
nail (s) (transverse) L60.4
congenital Q84.6
tongue K14.5
congenital Q38.3
Furuncle L02.92
abdominal wall L02.221
ankle — *see* Furuncle, lower limb
anus K61.0
antecubital space — *see* Furuncle, upper limb
arm — *see* Furuncle, upper limb
auditory canal, external — *see* Abscess, ear, external
auricle (ear) — *see* Abscess, ear, external
axilla (region) L02.42-
back (any part) L02.222
breast N61.1
buttock L02.32
cheek (external) L02.02
chest wall L02.223
chin L02.02
corpus cavernosum N48.21
ear, external — *see* Abscess, ear, external
external auditory canal — *see* Abscess, ear, external
eyelid — *see* Abscess, eyelid
face L02.02
femoral (region) — *see* Furuncle, lower limb
finger — *see* Furuncle, hand
flank L02.221
foot L02.62-
forehead L02.02
gluteal (region) L02.32
groin L02.224
hand L02.52-
head L02.821
face L02.02
hip — *see* Furuncle, lower limb
kidney — *see* Abscess, kidney
knee — *see* Furuncle, lower limb
labium (majus) (minus) N76.4
lacrimal
gland — *see* Dacryoadenitis
passages (duct) (sac) — *see* Inflammation, lacrimal, passages, acute
leg (any part) — *see* Furuncle, lower limb
lower limb L02.42-
malignant A22.0
mouth K12.2
navel L02.226
neck L02.12
nose J34.0
orbit, orbital — *see* Abscess, orbit
palmar (space) — *see* Furuncle, hand
partes posteriores L02.32
pectoral region L02.223
penis N48.21
perineum L02.225
pinna — *see* Abscess, ear, external
popliteal — *see* Furuncle, lower limb
prepatellar — *see* Furuncle, lower limb
scalp L02.821
seminal vesicle N49.0
shoulder — *see* Furuncle, upper limb
specified site NEC L02.828
submandibular K12.2
temple (region) L02.02
thumb — *see* Furuncle, hand
toe — *see* Furuncle, foot
trunk L02.229
abdominal wall L02.221
back L02.222

G

Gangrene, gangrenous (connective tissue) (dropsical) (dry) (moist) (skin) (ulcer) - *continued*
- penis N48.29
  - noninfective N48.89
- perineum I96
- pharynx — *see also* Pharyngitis
  - Vincent's A69.1
- presenile I73.1
- progressive synergistic — *see* Ulcer, skin
- pulmonary J85.0
- pulpal (dental) K04.1
- quinsy J36
- Raynaud's (symmetric gangrene) I73.01
- retropharyngeal J39.2
- scrotum N49.3
  - noninfective N50.89
- senile (atherosclerotic) — *see* Arteriosclerosis, extremities, with, gangrene
- spermatic cord N49.1
  - noninfective N50.89
- spine I96
- spirochetal NEC A69.8
- spreading cutaneous I96
- stomatitis A69.0
- symmetrical I73.01
- testis (infectional) N45.2
  - noninfective N44.8
- throat — *see also* Pharyngitis
  - diphtheritic A36.0
  - Vincent's A69.1
- thyroid (gland) E07.89
- tooth (pulp) K04.1
- tuberculous NEC — *see* Tuberculosis
- tunica vaginalis N49.1
  - noninfective N50.89
- umbilicus I96
- uterus — *see* Endometritis
- uvulitis K12.2
- vas deferens N49.1
  - noninfective N50.89
- vulva N76.89

Ganister disease J62.8

Ganser's syndrome (hysterical) F44.89

Gardner-Diamond syndrome (autoerythrocyte sensitization) D69.2

Gargoylism E76.01

Garré's disease, osteitis (sclerosing), osteomyelitis — *see* Osteomyelitis, specified type NEC

Garrod's pad, knuckle M72.1

Gartner's duct
- cyst Q52.4
- persistent Q50.6

Gas R14.3
- asphyxiation, inhalation, poisoning, suffocation NEC — *see* Table of Drugs and Chemicals
- excessive R14.0
- gangrene A48.0
  - following
    - abortion — *see* Abortion by type complicated by infection
    - ectopic or molar pregnancy O08.0
- on stomach R14.0
- pains R14.1

Gastralgia — *see also* Pain, abdominal

Gastrectasis K31.0
- psychogenic F45.8

Gastric — *see* condition

Gastrinoma
- malignant
  - pancreas C25.4
  - specified site NEC — *see* Neoplasm, malignant, by site
  - unspecified site C25.4
- specified site — *see* Neoplasm, uncertain behavior
- unspecified site D37.9

Gastritis (simple) K29.70
- with bleeding K29.71
- acute (erosive) K29.00
  - with bleeding K29.01
- alcoholic K29.20

Gastritis (simple) - *continued*
- alcoholic - *continued*
  - with bleeding K29.21
- allergic K29.60
  - with bleeding K29.61
- atrophic (chronic) K29.40
  - with bleeding K29.41
- chronic (antral) (fundal) K29.50
  - with bleeding K29.51
  - atrophic K29.40
    - with bleeding K29.41
  - superficial K29.30
    - with bleeding K29.31
- dietary counseling and surveillance Z71.3
- due to diet deficiency E63.9
- eosinophilic K52.81
- giant hypertrophic K29.60
  - with bleeding K29.61
- granulomatous K29.60
  - with bleeding K29.61
- hypertrophic (mucosa) K29.60
  - with bleeding K29.61
- nervous F54
- spastic K29.60
  - with bleeding K29.61
- specified NEC K29.60
  - with bleeding K29.61
- superficial chronic K29.30
  - with bleeding K29.31
- tuberculous A18.83
- viral NEC A08.4

Gastrocarcinoma — *see* Neoplasm, malignant, stomach

Gastrocolic — *see* condition

Gastrodisciasis, gastrodiscoidiasis B66.8

Gastroduodenitis K29.90
- with bleeding K29.91
- virus, viral A08.4
  - specified type NEC A08.39

Gastrodynia — *see* Pain, abdominal

Gastroenteritis (acute) (chronic) (noninfectious) — *see also* Enteritis K52.9
- allergic K52.29
  - with
    - eosinophilic gastritis or gastroenteritis K52.81
    - food protein-induced enterocolitis syndrome K52.21
    - food protein-induced enteropathy K52.22
- dietetic — *see also* Gastroenteritis, allergic K52.29
- drug-induced K52.1
- due to
  - Cryptosporidium A07.2
  - drugs K52.1
  - food poisoning — *see* Intoxication, foodborne
  - radiation K52.0
- eosinophilic K52.81
- epidemic (infectious) A09
- food hypersensitivity — *see also* Gastroenteritis, allergic K52.29
- infectious — *see* Enteritis, infectious
- influenzal — *see* Influenza, with gastroenteritis
- noninfectious K52.9
  - specified NEC K52.89
- rotaviral A08.0
- Salmonella A02.0
- toxic K52.1
- viral NEC A08.4
  - acute infectious A08.39
    - type Norwalk A08.11
  - infantile (acute) A08.39
  - Norwalk agent A08.11
  - rotaviral A08.0
  - severe of infants A08.39
  - specified type NEC A08.39

Gastroenteropathy — *see also* Gastroenteritis K52.9
- acute, due to Norwalk agent A08.11
- acute, due to Norovirus A08.11
- infectious A09

Gastroenteroptosis K63.4

Gastroesophageal laceration- hemorrhage syndrome K22.6

Gastrointestinal — *see* condition

Gastrojejunal — *see* condition

Gastrojejunitis — *see also* Enteritis K52.9

Gastrojejunocolic — *see* condition

Gastroliths K31.89

Gastromalacia K31.89

Gastroparalysis K31.84
- diabetic — *see* Diabetes, gastroparalysis

Gastroparesis K31.84
- diabetic — *see* Diabetes, by type, with gastroparesis

Gastropathy K31.9
- congestive portal (see also, Hypertension, portal) K31.89
- erythematous K29.70
- exudative K90.89
- portal hypertensive (see also, Hypertension, portal) K31.89

Gastroptosis K31.89

Gastrorrhagia K92.2
- psychogenic F45.8

Gastroschisis (congenital) Q79.3

Gastrospasm (neurogenic) (reflex) K31.89
- neurotic F45.8
- psychogenic F45.8

Gastrostaxis — *see* Gastritis, with bleeding

Gastrostenosis K31.89

Gastrostomy
- attention to Z43.1
- status Z93.1

Gastrosuccorrhea (continuous) (intermittent) K31.89
- neurotic F45.8
- psychogenic F45.8

Gatophobia F40.218

Gaucher's disease or splenomegaly (adult) (infantile) E75.22

Gee (-Herter) (-Thaysen) disease (nontropical sprue) K90.0

Gélineau's syndrome G47.419
- with cataplexy G47.411

Gemination, tooth, teeth K00.2

Gemistocytoma
- specified site — *see* Neoplasm, malignant, by site
- unspecified site C71.9

General, generalized — *see* condition

Genetic
- carrier (status)
  - cystic fibrosis Z14.1
  - hemophilia A (asymptomatic) Z14.01
    - symptomatic Z14.02
  - specified NEC Z14.8
- susceptibility to disease NEC Z15.89
  - malignant neoplasm Z15.09
    - breast Z15.01
    - endometrium Z15.04
    - ovary Z15.02
    - prostate Z15.03
    - specified NEC Z15.09
  - multiple endocrine neoplasia Z15.81

Genital — *see* condition

Genito-anorectal syndrome A55

Genitourinary system — *see* condition

Genu
- congenital Q74.1
- extrorsum (acquired) — *see also* Deformity, varus, knee
  - congenital Q74.1
  - sequelae (late effect) of rickets E64.3
- introrsum (acquired) — *see also* Deformity, valgus, knee
  - congenital Q74.1
  - sequelae (late effect) of rickets E64.3
- rachitic (old) E64.3
- recurvatum (acquired) — *see also* Deformity, limb, specified type NEC, lower leg
  - congenital Q68.2
  - sequelae (late effect) of rickets E64.3
- valgum (acquired) (knock-knee) M21.06-
  - congenital Q74.1
  - sequelae (late effect) of rickets E64.3

Genu - *continued*
varum (acquired) (bowleg) M21.16-
congenital Q74.1
sequelae (late effect) of rickets E64.3
Geographic tongue K14.1
Geophagia — *see* Pica
Geotrichosis B48.3
stomatitis B48.3
Gephyrophobia F40.242
Gerbode defect Q21.0
GERD (gastroesophageal reflux disease) K21.9
Gerhardt's
disease (erythromelalgia) I73.81
syndrome (vocal cord paralysis) J38.00
bilateral J38.02
unilateral J38.01
German measles — *see also* Rubella
exposure to Z20.4
Germinoblastoma (diffuse) C85.9-
follicular C82.9-
Germinoma — *see* Neoplasm, malignant, by site
Gerontoxon — *see* Degeneration, cornea, senile
Gerstmann's syndrome R48.8
developmental F81.2
Gerstmann-Sträussler-Scheinker syndrome (GSS) A81.82
Gestation (period) — *see also* Pregnancy
ectopic — *see* Pregnancy, by site
multiple O30.9-
greater than quadruplets — *see* Pregnancy, multiple (gestation), specified NEC
specified NEC — *see* Pregnancy, multiple (gestation), specified NEC
Gestational
mammary abscess O91.11-
purulent mastitis O91.11-
subareolar abscess O91.11-
Ghon tubercle, primary infection A15.7
Ghost
teeth K00.4
vessels (cornea) H16.41-
Ghoul hand A66.3
Gianotti-Crosti disease L44.4
Giant
cell
epulis K06.8
peripheral granuloma K06.8
esophagus, congenital Q39.5
kidney, congenital Q63.3
urticaria T78.3
hereditary D84.1
Giardiasis A07.1
Gibert's disease or pityriasis L42
Giddiness R42
hysterical F44.89
psychogenic F45.8
Gierke's disease (glycogenosis I) E74.01
Gigantism (cerebral) (hypophyseal) (pituitary) E22.0
constitutional E34.4
Gilbert's disease or syndrome E80.4
Gilchrist's disease B40.9
Gilford-Hutchinson disease E34.8
Gilles de la Tourette's disease or syndrome (motor-verbal tic) F95.2
Gingivitis K05.10
acute (catarrhal) K05.00
necrotizing A69.1
nonplaque induced K05.01
plaque induced K05.00
chronic (desquamative) (hyperplastic) (simple marginal) (pregnancy associated) (ulcerative) K05.10
nonplaque induced K05.11
plaque induced K05.10
expulsiva — *see* Periodontitis
necrotizing ulcerative (acute) A69.1
pellagrous E52
acute necrotizing A69.1
Vincent's A69.1
Gingivoglossitis K14.0
Gingivopericementitis — *see* Periodontitis
Gingivosis — *see* Gingivitis, chronic
Gingivostomatitis K05.10
herpesviral B00.2
necrotizing ulcerative (acute) A69.1
Gland, glandular — *see* condition
Glanders A24.0
Glanzmann (-Naegeli) disease or thrombasthenia D69.1
Glasgow coma scale
total score
3-8 R40.243
9-12 R40.242
13-15 R40.241
Glass-blower's disease (cataract) — *see* Cataract, specified NEC
Glaucoma H40.9
with
increased episcleral venous pressure H40.81-
pseudoexfoliation of lens — *see* Glaucoma, open angle, primary, capsular
absolute H44.51-
angle-closure (primary) H40.20-
acute (attack) (crisis) H40.21-
chronic H40.22-
intermittent H40.23-
residual stage H40.24-
borderline H40.00-
capsular (with pseudoexfoliation of lens) — *see* Glaucoma, open angle, primary, capsular
childhood Q15.0
closed angle — *see* Glaucoma, angle-closure
congenital Q15.0
corticosteroid-induced — *see* Glaucoma, secondary, drugs
hypersecretion H40.82-
in (due to)
amyloidosis E85.4 *[H42]*
aniridia Q13.1 *[H42]*
concussion of globe — *see* Glaucoma, secondary, trauma
dislocation of lens — *see* Glaucoma, secondary
disorder of lens NEC — *see* Glaucoma, secondary
drugs — *see* Glaucoma, secondary, drugs
endocrine disease NOS E34.9 *[H42]*
eye
inflammation — *see* Glaucoma, secondary, inflammation
trauma — *see* Glaucoma, secondary, trauma
hypermature cataract — *see* Glaucoma, secondary
iridocyclitis — *see* Glaucoma, secondary, inflammation
lens disorder — *see* Glaucoma, secondary,
Lowe's syndrome E72.03 *[H42]*
metabolic disease NOS E88.9 *[H42]*
ocular disorders NEC — *see* Glaucoma, secondary
onchocerciasis B73.02
pupillary block — *see* Glaucoma, secondary
retinal vein occlusion — *see* Glaucoma, secondary
Rieger's anomaly Q13.81 *[H42]*
rubeosis of iris — *see* Glaucoma, secondary
tumor of globe — *see* Glaucoma, secondary
infantile Q15.0
low tension — *see* Glaucoma, open angle, primary, low-tension
malignant H40.83-
narrow angle — *see* Glaucoma, angle-closure
newborn Q15.0
noncongestive (chronic) — *see* Glaucoma, open angle
nonobstructive — *see* Glaucoma, open angle
obstructive — *see also* Glaucoma, angle-closure
Glaucoma - *continued*
obstructive - *continued*
due to lens changes — *see* Glaucoma, secondary
open angle H40.10-
primary H40.11-
capsular (with pseudoexfoliation of lens) H40.14-
low-tension H40.12-
pigmentary H40.13-
residual stage H40.15-
phacolytic — *see* Glaucoma, secondary
pigmentary — *see* Glaucoma, open angle, primary, pigmentary
postinfectious — *see* Glaucoma, secondary, inflammation
secondary (to) H40.5-
drugs H40.6-
inflammation H40.4-
trauma H40.3-
simple (chronic) H40.11-
simplex H40.11-
specified type NEC H40.89
suspect H40.00-
syphilitic A52.71
traumatic — *see also* Glaucoma, secondary, trauma
newborn (birth injury) P15.3
tuberculous A18.59
Glaucomatous flecks (subcapsular) — *see* Cataract, complicated
Glazed tongue K14.4
Gleet (gonococcal) A54.01
Glénard's disease K63.4
Glioblastoma (multiforme)
with sarcomatous component
specified site — *see* Neoplasm, malignant, by site
unspecified site C71.9
giant cell
specified site — *see* Neoplasm, malignant, by site
unspecified site C71.9
specified site — *see* Neoplasm, malignant, by site
unspecified site C71.9
Glioma (malignant)
astrocytic
specified site — *see* Neoplasm, malignant, by site
unspecified site C71.9
mixed
specified site — *see* Neoplasm, malignant, by site
unspecified site C71.9
nose Q30.8
specified site NEC — *see* Neoplasm, malignant, by site
subependymal D43.2
specified site — *see* Neoplasm, uncertain behavior, by site
unspecified site D43.2
unspecified site C71.9
Gliomatosis cerebri C71.0
Glioneuroma — *see* Neoplasm, uncertain behavior, by site
Gliosarcoma
specified site — *see* Neoplasm, malignant, by site
unspecified site C71.9
Gliosis (cerebral) G93.89
spinal G95.89
Glisson's disease — *see* Rickets
Globinuria R82.3
Globus (hystericus) F45.8
Glomangioma D18.00
intra-abdominal D18.03
intracranial D18.02
skin D18.01
specified site NEC D18.09
Glomangiomyoma D18.00
intra-abdominal D18.03
intracranial D18.02
skin D18.01
specified site NEC D18.09

- **Glomangiosarcoma** — *see* Neoplasm, connective tissue, malignant
- **Glomerular**
  - disease in syphilis A52.75
  - nephritis — *see* Glomerulonephritis
- **Glomerulitis** — *see* Glomerulonephritis
- **Glomerulonephritis** — *see also* Nephritis N05.9
  - with
    - C3
      - glomerulonephritis N05.A
      - glomerulopathy N05.A
        - with dense deposit disease N05.6
    - edema — *see* Nephrosis
    - minimal change N05.0
    - minor glomerular abnormality N05.0
  - acute N00.9
  - chronic N03.9
  - crescentic (diffuse) NEC — *see also* N00-N07 with fourth character .7 N05.7
  - dense deposit — *see also* N00-N07 with fourth character .6 N05.6
  - diffuse
    - crescentic — *see also* N00-N07 with fourth character .7 N05.7
    - endocapillary proliferative — *see also* N00-N07 with fourth character .4 N05.4
    - membranous — *see also* N00-N07 with fourth character .2 N05.2
    - mesangial proliferative — *see also* N00-N07 with fourth character .3 N05.3
    - mesangiocapillary — *see also* N00-N07 with fourth character .5 N05.5
    - sclerosing N18.9
  - endocapillary proliferative (diffuse) NEC — *see also* N00-N07 with fourth character .4 N05.4
  - extracapillary NEC — *see also* N00-N07 with fourth character .7 N05.7
  - focal (and segmental) — *see also* N00-N07 with fourth character .1 N05.1
  - hypocomplementemic — *see* Glomerulonephritis, membranoproliferative
  - IgA — *see* Nephropathy, IgA
  - immune complex (circulating) NEC N05.8
  - in (due to)
    - amyloidosis E85.4 *[N08]*
    - bilharziasis B65.9 *[N08]*
    - cryoglobulinemia D89.1 *[N08]*
    - defibrination syndrome D65 *[N08]*
    - diabetes mellitus — *see* Diabetes, glomerulosclerosis
    - disseminated intravascular coagulation D65 *[N08]*
    - Fabry (-Anderson) disease E75.21 *[N08]*
    - Goodpasture's syndrome M31.0
    - hemolytic-uremic syndrome D59.3
    - Henoch (-Schönlein) purpura D69.0 *[N08]*
    - lecithin cholesterol acyltransferase deficiency E78.6 *[N08]*
    - microscopic polyangiitis M31.7 *[N08]*
    - multiple myeloma C90.0- *[N08]*
    - Plasmodium malariae B52.0
    - schistosomiasis B65.9 *[N08]*
    - sepsis A41.9 *[N08]*
      - streptococcal A40- *[N08]*
    - sickle-cell disorders D57.- *[N08]*
    - strongyloidiasis B78.9 *[N08]*
    - subacute bacterial endocarditis I33.0 *[N08]*
    - syphilis (late) congenital A50.59 *[N08]*
    - systemic lupus erythematosus M32.14
    - thrombotic thrombocytopenic purpura M31.19 *[N08]*
    - typhoid fever A01.09
    - Waldenström macroglobulinemia C88.0 *[N08]*
    - Wegener's granulomatosis M31.31
  - latent or quiescent N03.9
  - lobular, lobulonodular — *see* Glomerulonephritis, membranoproliferative

Glomerulonephritis - *continued*

  - membranoproliferative (diffuse) (type 1 or 3) — *see also* N00-N07 with fourth character .5 N05.5
    - dense deposit (type 2) NEC — *see also* N00-N07 with fourth character .6 N05.6
  - membranous (diffuse) NEC — *see also* N00-N07 with fourth character .2 N05.2
  - mesangial
    - IgA/IgG — *see* Nephropathy, IgA
    - proliferative (diffuse) NEC — *see also* N00-N07 with fourth character .3 N05.3
  - mesangiocapillary (diffuse) NEC — *see also* N00-N07 with fourth character .5 N05.5
  - necrotic, necrotizing NEC — *see also* N00-N07 with fourth character .8 N05.8
  - nodular — *see* Glomerulonephritis, membranoproliferative
  - poststreptococcal NEC N05.9
    - acute N00.9
    - chronic N03.9
    - rapidly progressive N01.9
  - proliferative NEC — *see also* N00-N07 with fourth character .8 N05.8
    - diffuse (lupus) M32.14
  - rapidly progressive N01.9
  - sclerosing, diffuse N18.9
  - specified pathology NEC — *see also* N00-N07 with fourth character .8 N05.8
  - subacute N01.9
- **Glomerulopathy** — *see* Glomerulonephritis
- **Glomerulosclerosis** — *see also* Sclerosis, renal
  - intercapillary (nodular) (with diabetes) — *see* Diabetes, glomerulosclerosis
  - intracapillary — *see* Diabetes, glomerulosclerosis
- **Glossagra** K14.6
- **Glossalgia** K14.6
- **Glossitis (chronic superficial) (gangrenous) (Moeller's)** K14.0
  - areata exfoliativa K14.1
  - atrophic K14.4
  - benign migratory K14.1
  - cortical superficial, sclerotic K14.0
  - Hunter's D51.0
  - interstitial, sclerous K14.0
  - median rhomboid K14.2
  - pellagrous E52
  - superficial, chronic K14.0
- **Glossocele** K14.8
- **Glossodynia** K14.6
  - exfoliativa K14.4
- **Glossoncus** K14.8
- **Glossopathy** K14.9
- **Glossophytia** K14.3
- **Glossoplegia** K14.8
- **Glossoptosis** K14.8
- **Glossopyrosis** K14.6
- **Glossotrichia** K14.3
- **Glossy skin** L90.8
- **Glottis** — *see* condition
- **Glottitis** — *see also* Laryngitis J04.0
- **Glucagonoma**
  - pancreas
    - benign D13.7
    - malignant C25.4
    - uncertain behavior D37.8
  - specified site NEC
    - benign — *see* Neoplasm, benign, by site
    - malignant — *see* Neoplasm, malignant, by site
    - uncertain behavior — *see* Neoplasm, uncertain behavior, by site
  - unspecified site
    - benign D13.7
    - malignant C25.4
    - uncertain behavior D37.8
- **Glucoglycinuria** E72.51
- **Glucose-galactose malabsorption** E74.39
- **Glue**
  - ear — *see* Otitis, media, nonsuppurative, chronic, mucoid
  - sniffing (airplane) — *see* Abuse, drug, inhalant
    - dependence — *see* Dependence, drug, inhalant
- **GLUT1 deficiency syndrome 1, infantile onset** E74.810
- **GLUT1 deficiency syndrome 2, childhood onset** E74.810
- **Glutaric aciduria** E72.3
- **Glycinemia** E72.51
- **Glycinuria (renal) (with ketosis)** E72.09
- **Glycogen**
  - infiltration — *see* Disease, glycogen storage
  - storage disease — *see* Disease, glycogen storage
- **Glycogenosis (diffuse) (generalized)** — *see also* Disease, glycogen storage
  - cardiac E74.02 *[I43]*
  - diabetic, secondary — *see* Diabetes, glycogenosis, secondary
  - pulmonary interstitial J84.842
- **Glycopenia** E16.2
- **Glycosuria** R81
  - renal (familial) E74.818
- **Gnathostoma spinigerum (infection) (infestation) , gnathostomiasis (wandering swelling)** B83.1
- **Goiter (plunging) (substernal)** E04.9
  - with
    - hyperthyroidism (recurrent) — *see* Hyperthyroidism, with, goiter
    - thyrotoxicosis — *see* Hyperthyroidism, with, goiter
  - adenomatous — *see* Goiter, nodular
  - cancerous C73
  - congenital (nontoxic) E03.0
    - diffuse E03.0
    - parenchymatous E03.0
    - transitory, with normal functioning P72.0
  - cystic E04.2
    - due to iodine-deficiency E01.1
  - due to
    - enzyme defect in synthesis of thyroid hormone E07.1
    - iodine-deficiency (endemic) E01.2
  - dyshormonogenetic (familial) E07.1
  - endemic (iodine-deficiency) E01.2
    - diffuse E01.0
    - multinodular E01.1
  - exophthalmic — *see* Hyperthyroidism, with, goiter
  - iodine-deficiency (endemic) E01.2
    - diffuse E01.0
    - multinodular E01.1
    - nodular E01.1
  - lingual Q89.2
  - lymphadenoid E06.3
  - malignant C73
  - multinodular (cystic) (nontoxic) E04.2
    - toxic or with hyperthyroidism E05.20
      - with thyroid storm E05.21
  - neonatal NEC P72.0
  - nodular (nontoxic) (due to) E04.9
    - with
      - hyperthyroidism E05.20
        - with thyroid storm E05.21
      - thyrotoxicosis E05.20
        - with thyroid storm E05.21
    - endemic E01.1
    - iodine-deficiency E01.1
    - sporadic E04.9
    - toxic E05.20
      - with thyroid storm E05.21
  - nontoxic E04.9
    - diffuse (colloid) E04.0
    - multinodular E04.2
    - simple E04.0
    - specified NEC E04.8
    - uninodular E04.1
  - simple E04.0
  - toxic — *see* Hyperthyroidism, with, goiter
  - uninodular (nontoxic) E04.1

Headache - *continued*
  medication overuse - *continued*
    not intractable G44.40
  menstrual — *see* Migraine, menstrual
  migraine (type) — *see also*
      Migraine G43.909
  nasal septum R51.9
  neuralgiform, short lasting unilateral, with
      conjunctival injection and tearing
      (SUNCT) G44.059
    intractable G44.051
    not intractable G44.059
  new daily persistent (NDPH) G44.52
  orgasmic G44.82
  periodic syndromes in adults and
      children G43.C0
    with refractory migraine G43.C1
    intractable G43.C1
    not intractable G43.C0
    without refractory migraine G43.C0
  postspinal puncture G97.1
  post-traumatic G44.309
    acute G44.319
      intractable G44.311
      not intractable G44.319
    chronic G44.329
      intractable G44.321
      not intractable G44.329
    intractable G44.301
    not intractable G44.309
  pre-menstrual — *see* Migraine, menstrual
  preorgasmic G44.82
  primary
    cough G44.83
    exertional G44.84
    stabbing G44.85
    thunderclap G44.53
  rebound G44.40
    intractable G44.41
    not intractable G44.40
  short lasting unilateral neuralgiform, with
      conjunctival injection and tearing
      (SUNCT) G44.059
    intractable G44.051
    not intractable G44.059
  specified syndrome NEC G44.89
  spinal and epidural anesthesia -
      induced T88.59
    in labor and delivery O74.5
    in pregnancy O29.4-
    postpartum, puerperal O89.4
  spinal fluid loss (from puncture) G97.1
  stabbing (primary) G44.85
  tension (-type) G44.209
    chronic G44.229
      intractable G44.221
      not intractable G44.229
    episodic G44.219
      intractable G44.211
      not intractable G44.219
    intractable G44.201
    not intractable G44.209
  thunderclap (primary) G44.53
  vascular NEC G44.1
Healthy
  infant
    accompanying sick mother Z76.3
    receiving care Z76.2
  person accompanying sick person Z76.3
Hearing examination Z01.10
  with abnormal findings NEC Z01.118
  infant or child (over 28 days old) Z00.129
    with abnormal findings Z00.121
  following failed hearing screening Z01.110
  for hearing conservation and
      treatment Z01.12
Heart — *see* condition
Heart beat
  abnormality R00.9
    specified NEC R00.8
  awareness R00.2
  rapid R00.0
  slow R00.1
Heartburn R12
  psychogenic F45.8
Heartland virus disease A93.8
Heat (effects) T67.9
  apoplexy T67.01
  burn — *see also* Burn L55.9
  collapse T67.1
  cramps T67.2
  dermatitis or eczema L59.0
  edema T67.7
  erythema - code by site under Burn, first
      degree
  excessive T67.9
    specified effect NEC T67.8
  exhaustion T67.5
    anhydrotic T67.3
    due to
      salt (and water) depletion T67.4
      water depletion T67.3
        with salt depletion T67.4
  fatigue (transient) T67.6
  fever T67.01
  hyperpyrexia T67.01
  prickly L74.0
  prostration — *see* Heat, exhaustion
  pyrexia T67.01
  rash L74.0
  specified effect NEC T67.8
  stroke T67.01
    exertional T67.02
    specified NEC T67.09
  sunburn — *see* Sunburn
  syncope T67.1
**Heavy-for-dates NEC (infant) (4000g to
    4499g)** P08.1
  exceptionally (4500g or more) P08.0
**Hebephrenia, hebephrenic
    (schizophrenia)** F20.1
**Heberden's disease or nodes (with
    arthropathy)** M15.1
Hebra's
  pityriasis L26
  prurigo L28.2
Heel — *see* condition
Heerfordt's disease D86.89
Hegglin's anomaly or syndrome D72.0
Heilmeyer-Schoner disease D45
Heine-Medin disease A80.9
Heinz body anemia, congenital D58.2
Heliophobia F40.228
Heller's disease or syndrome F84.3
**HELLP syndrome (hemolysis, elevated liver
    enzymes and low platelet count)** O14.2-
  complicating
    childbirth O14.24
    puerperium O14.25
Helminthiasis — *see also* Infestation, helminth
  Ancylostoma B76.0
  intestinal B82.0
    mixed types (types classifiable to more
        than one of the titles B65.0-B81.3 and
        B81.8) B81.4
    specified type NEC B81.8
  mixed types (intestinal) (types classifiable to
      more than one of the titles B65.0-B81.3
      and B81.8) B81.4
  Necator (americanus) B76.1
  specified type NEC B83.8
Heloma L84
Hemangioblastoma — *see* Neoplasm,
    connective tissue, uncertain behavior
  malignant — *see* Neoplasm, connective
      tissue, malignant
Hemangioendothelioma — *see also*
    Neoplasm, uncertain behavior, by site
  benign D18.00
    intra-abdominal D18.03
    intracranial D18.02
    skin D18.01
    specified site NEC D18.09
  bone (diffuse) — *see* Neoplasm, bone,
      malignant
  epithelioid — *see also* Neoplasm, uncertain
      behavior, by site
    malignant — *see* Neoplasm, malignant, by
        site
Hemangioendothelioma - *continued*
  malignant — *see* Neoplasm, connective
      tissue, malignant
Hemangiofibroma — *see* Neoplasm, benign,
    by site
Hemangiolipoma — *see* Lipoma
Hemangioma D18.00
  arteriovenous D18.00
    intra-abdominal D18.03
    intracranial D18.02
    skin D18.01
    specified site NEC D18.09
  capillary I78.1
    intra-abdominal D18.03
    intracranial D18.02
    skin D18.01
    specified site NEC D18.09
  cavernous D18.00
    intra-abdominal D18.03
    intracranial D18.02
    skin D18.01
    specified site NEC D18.09
  epithelioid D18.00
    intra-abdominal D18.03
    intracranial D18.02
    skin D18.01
    specified site NEC D18.09
  histiocytoid D18.00
    intra-abdominal D18.03
    intracranial D18.02
    skin D18.01
    specified site NEC D18.09
  infantile D18.00
    intra-abdominal D18.03
    intracranial D18.02
    skin D18.01
    specified site NEC D18.09
  intra-abdominal D18.03
  intracranial D18.02
  intramuscular D18.00
    intra-abdominal D18.03
    intracranial D18.02
    skin D18.01
    specified site NEC D18.09
  intrathoracic structures D18.09
  juvenile D18.00
  malignant — *see* Neoplasm,connective
      tissue, malignant
  plexiform D18.00
    intra-abdominal D18.03
    intracranial D18.02
    skin D18.01
    specified site NEC D18.09
  racemose D18.00
    intra-abdominal D18.03
    intracranial D18.02
    skin D18.01
    specified site NEC D18.09
  sclerosing — *see* Neoplasm,skin, benign
  simplex D18.00
    intra-abdominal D18.03
    intracranial D18.02
    skin D18.01
    specified site NEC D18.09
  skin D18.01
  specified site NEC D18.09
  venous D18.00
    intra-abdominal D18.03
    intracranial D18.02
    skin D18.01
    specified site NEC D18.09
  verrucous keratotic D18.00
    intra-abdominal D18.03
    intracranial D18.02
    skin D18.01
    specified site NEC D18.09
Hemangiomatosis (systemic) I78.8
  involving single site — *see* Hemangioma
Hemangiopericytoma — *see also* Neoplasm,
    connective tissue, uncertain behavior
  benign — *see* Neoplasm, connective tissue,
      benign
  malignant — *see* Neoplasm, connective
      tissue, malignant

Hemianopia, hemianopsia (heteronymous) H53.47
- homonymous H53.46-
- syphilitic A52.71

Hemiathetosis R25.8

Hemiatrophy R68.89
- cerebellar G31.9
- face, facial, progressive (Romberg) G51.8
- tongue K14.8

Hemiballism (us) G25.5

Hemicardia Q24.8

Hemicephalus, hemicephaly Q00.0

Hemichorea G25.5

Hemicolitis, left — *see* Colitis, left sided

Hemicrania
- congenital malformation Q00.0
- continua G44.51
- meaning migraine — *see also* Migraine G43.909
- paroxysmal G44.039
  - chronic G44.049
    - intractable G44.041
    - not intractable G44.049
  - episodic G44.039
    - intractable G44.031
    - not intractable G44.039
  - intractable G44.031
  - not intractable G44.039

Hemidystrophy — *see* Hemiatrophy

Hemiectromelia Q73.8

Hemihypalgesia R20.8

Hemihypesthesia R20.1

Hemi-inattention R41.4

Hemimelia Q73.8
- lower limb — *see* Defect, reduction, lower limb, specified type NEC
- upper limb — *see* Defect, reduction, upper limb, specified type NEC

Hemiparalysis — *see* Hemiplegia

Hemiparesis — *see* Hemiplegia

Hemiparesthesia R20.2

Hemiparkinsonism G20

Hemiplegia G81.9-
- alternans facialis G83.89
- ascending NEC G81.90
  - spinal G95.89
- congenital (cerebral) G80.8
  - spastic G80.2
- embolic (current episode) I63.4-
- flaccid G81.0-
- following
  - cerebrovascular disease I69.959
    - cerebral infarction I69.35-
    - intracerebral hemorrhage I69.15-
    - nontraumatic intracranial hemorrhage NEC I69.25-
    - specified disease NEC I69.85-
    - stroke NOS I69.35-
    - subarachnoid hemorrhage I69.05-
- hysterical F44.4
- newborn NEC P91.88
  - birth injury P11.9
- spastic G81.1-
  - congenital G80.2
- thrombotic (current episode) I63.3-

Hemisection, spinal cord — *see* Injury, spinal cord, by region

Hemispasm (facial) R25.2

Hemisporosis B48.8

Hemitremor R25.1

Hemivertebra Q76.49
- failure of segmentation with scoliosis Q76.3
- fusion with scoliosis Q76.3

Hemochromatosis E83.119
- with refractory anemia D46.1
- due to repeated red blood cell transfusion E83.111
- hereditary (primary) E83.110
- neonatal P78.84
- primary E83.110
- specified NEC E83.118

Hemoglobin — *see also* condition
- abnormal (disease) — *see* Disease, hemoglobin
- AS genotype D57.3

Hemoglobin - *continued*
- Constant Spring D58.2
- E-beta thalassemia D56.5
- fetal, hereditary persistence (HPFH) D56.4
- H Constant Spring D56.0
- low NOS D64.9
- S (Hb S) , heterozygous D57.3

Hemoglobinemia D59.9
- due to blood transfusion T80.89
- paroxysmal D59.6
  - nocturnal D59.5

Hemoglobinopathy (mixed) D58.2
- with thalassemia D56.8
- sickle-cell D57.1
  - with thalassemia D57.40
    - with
      - acute chest syndrome D57.411
      - cerebral vascular involvement D57.413
      - crisis (painful) D57.419
        - with specified complication NEC D57.418
      - splenic sequestration D57.412
      - vasoocclusive pain D57.419
    - without crisis D57.40

Hemoglobinuria R82.3
- with anemia, hemolytic, acquired (chronic) NEC D59.6
- cold (paroxysmal) (with Raynaud's syndrome) D59.6
  - agglutinin D59.12
- due to exertion or hemolysis NEC D59.6
- intermittent D59.6
- malarial B50.8
- march D59.6
- nocturnal (paroxysmal) D59.5
- paroxysmal (cold) D59.6
  - nocturnal D59.5

Hemolymphangioma D18.1

Hemolysis
- intravascular
  - with
    - abortion — *see* Abortion, by type, complicated by, hemorrhage
    - ectopic or molar pregnancy O08.1
    - hemorrhage
      - antepartum — *see* Hemorrhage, antepartum, with coagulation defect
      - intrapartum — *see also* Hemorrhage, complicating, delivery O67.0
  - postpartum O72.3
- neonatal (excessive) P58.9
  - specified NEC P58.8

Hemolytic — *see* condition

Hemopericardium I31.2
- following acute myocardial infarction (current complication) I23.0
- newborn P54.8
- traumatic — *see* Injury, heart, with hemopericardium

Hemoperitoneum K66.1
- infectional K65.9
- traumatic S36.899
  - with open wound — *see* Wound, open, with penetration into peritoneal cavity

Hemophilia (classical) (familial) (hereditary) D66
- A D66
- B D67
- C D68.1
- acquired D68.311
- autoimmune D68.311
- calcipriva — *see also* Defect, coagulation D68.4
- nonfamilial — *see also* Defect, coagulation D68.4
- secondary D68.311
- vascular D68.0

Hemophthalmos H44.81-

Hemopneumothorax — *see also* Hemothorax
- traumatic S27.2

Hemoptysis R04.2
- newborn P26.9
- tuberculous — *see* Tuberculosis, pulmonary

Hemorrhage, hemorrhagic (concealed) R58
- abdomen R58
- accidental antepartum — *see* Hemorrhage, antepartum
- acute idiopathic pulmonary, in infants R04.81
- adenoid J35.8
- adrenal (capsule) (gland) E27.49
  - medulla E27.8
  - newborn P54.4
- after delivery — *see* Hemorrhage, postpartum
- alveolar
  - lung, newborn P26.8
  - process K08.89
- alveolus K08.89
- amputation stump (surgical) T87.89
- anemia (chronic) D50.0
  - acute D62
- antepartum (with) O46.90
  - with coagulation defect O46.00-
    - afibrinogenemia O46.01-
    - disseminated intravascular coagulation O46.02-
    - hypofibrinogenemia O46.01-
    - specified defect NEC O46.09-
  - before 20 weeks gestation O20.9
    - specified type NEC O20.8
    - threatened abortion O20.0
  - due to
    - abruptio placenta — *see also* Abruptio placentae O45.9-
    - leiomyoma, uterus — *see* Hemorrhage, antepartum, specified cause NEC
    - placenta previa O44.1-
  - specified cause NEC — *see* subcategory O46.8X-
- anus (sphincter) K62.5
- apoplexy (stroke) — *see* Hemorrhage, intracranial, intracerebral
- arachnoid — *see* Hemorrhage, intracranial, subarachnoid
- artery R58
  - brain — *see* Hemorrhage, intracranial, intracerebral
- basilar (ganglion) I61.0
- bladder N32.89
- bowel K92.2
  - newborn P54.3
- brain (miliary) (nontraumatic) — *see* Hemorrhage, intracranial, intracerebral
  - due to
    - birth injury P10.1
    - syphilis A52.05
  - epidural or extradural (traumatic) — *see* Injury, intracranial, epidural hemorrhage
  - newborn P52.4
    - birth injury P10.1
  - subarachnoid — *see* Hemorrhage, intracranial, subarachnoid
  - subdural — *see* Hemorrhage, intracranial, subdural
- brainstem (nontraumatic) I61.3
  - traumatic S06.38-
- breast N64.59
- bronchial tube — *see* Hemorrhage, lung
- bronchopulmonary — *see* Hemorrhage, lung
- bronchus — *see* Hemorrhage, lung
- bulbar I61.5
- capillary I78.8
  - primary D69.8
- cecum K92.2
- cerebellar, cerebellum (nontraumatic) I61.4
  - newborn P52.6
  - traumatic S06.37-
- cerebral, cerebrum — *see also* Hemorrhage, intracranial, intracerebral
  - newborn (anoxic) P52.4
    - birth injury P10.1
  - lobe I61.1
- cerebromeningeal I61.8
- cerebrospinal — *see* Hemorrhage, intracranial, intracerebral
- cervix (uteri) (stump) NEC N88.8

Hemorrhage, hemorrhagic (concealed) - *continued*
- chamber, anterior (eye) — *see* Hyphema
- childbirth — *see* Hemorrhage, complicating, delivery
- choroid H31.30-
  - expulsive H31.31-
- ciliary body — *see* Hyphema
- cochlea — *see* subcategory H83.8
- colon K92.2
- complicating
  - abortion — *see* Abortion, by type, complicated by, hemorrhage
  - delivery O67.9
    - associated with coagulation defect (afibrinogenemia) (DIC) (hyperfibrinolysis) O67.0
    - specified cause NEC O67.8
  - surgical procedure — *see* Hemorrhage, intraoperative
- conjunctiva H11.3-
  - newborn P54.8
- cord, newborn (stump) P51.9
- corpus luteum (ruptured) cyst N83.1-
- cortical (brain) I61.1
- cranial — *see* Hemorrhage, intracranial
- cutaneous R23.3
  - due to autosensitivity, erythrocyte D69.2
  - newborn P54.5
- delayed
  - following ectopic or molar pregnancy O08.1
  - postpartum O72.2
- diathesis (familial) D69.9
- disease D69.9
  - newborn P53
  - specified type NEC D69.8
- due to or associated with
  - afibrinogenemia or other coagulation defect (conditions in categories D65-D69)
    - antepartum — *see* Hemorrhage, antepartum, with coagulation defect
    - intrapartum O67.0
  - dental implant M27.61
  - device, implant or graft — *see also* Complications, by site and type, specified NEC T85.838
    - arterial graft NEC T82.838
    - breast T85.838
    - catheter NEC T85.838
      - dialysis (renal) T82.838
        - intraperitoneal T85.838
      - infusion NEC T82.838
        - spinal (epidural) (subdural) T85.830
      - urinary (indwelling) T83.83
    - electronic (electrode) (pulse generator) (stimulator)
      - bone T84.83
      - cardiac T82.837
      - nervous system (brain) (peripheral nerve) (spinal) T85.830
      - urinary T83.83
    - fixation, internal (orthopedic) NEC T84.83
    - gastrointestinal (bile duct) (esophagus) T85.838
    - genital NEC T83.83
    - heart NEC T82.837
    - joint prosthesis T84.83
    - ocular (corneal graft) (orbital implant) NEC T85.838
    - orthopedic NEC T84.83
      - bone graft T86.838
    - specified NEC T85.838
    - urinary NEC T83.83
    - vascular NEC T82.838
    - ventricular intracranial shunt T85.830
- duodenum, duodenal K92.2
  - ulcer — *see* Ulcer, duodenum, with hemorrhage
- dura mater — *see* Hemorrhage, intracranial, subdural
- endotracheal — *see* Hemorrhage, lung

Hemorrhage, hemorrhagic (concealed) - *continued*
- epicranial subaponeurotic (massive) , birth injury P12.2
- epidural (traumatic) — *see also* Injury, intracranial, epidural hemorrhage
  - nontraumatic I62.1
- esophagus K22.89
  - varix I85.01
    - secondary I85.11
- excessive, following ectopic gestation (subsequent episode) O08.1
- extradural (traumatic) — *see* Injury, intracranial, epidural hemorrhage
  - birth injury P10.8
  - newborn (anoxic) (nontraumatic) P52.8
  - nontraumatic I62.1
- eye NEC H57.89
  - fundus — *see* Hemorrhage, retina
  - lid — *see* Disorder, eyelid, specified type NEC
- fallopian tube N83.6
- fibrinogenolysis — *see* Fibrinolysis
- fibrinolytic (acquired) — *see* Fibrinolysis
- from
  - ear (nontraumatic) — *see* Otorrhagia
  - tracheostomy stoma J95.01
- fundus, eye — *see* Hemorrhage, retina
- funis — *see* Hemorrhage, umbilicus, cord
- gastric — *see* Hemorrhage, stomach
- gastroenteric K92.2
  - newborn P54.3
- gastrointestinal (tract) K92.2
  - newborn P54.3
- genital organ, male N50.1
- genitourinary (tract) NOS R31.9
- gingiva K06.8
- globe (eye) — *see* Hemophthalmos
- graafian follicle cyst (ruptured) N83.0-
- gum K06.8
- heart I51.89
- hypopharyngeal (throat) R04.1
- intermenstrual (regular) N92.3
  - irregular N92.1
- internal (organs) NEC R58
  - capsule I61.0
  - ear — *see* subcategory H83.8
  - newborn P54.8
- intestine K92.2
  - newborn P54.3
- intra-abdominal R58
- intra-alveolar (lung) , newborn P26.8
- intracerebral (nontraumatic) — *see* Hemorrhage, intracranial, intracerebral
- intracranial (nontraumatic) I62.9
  - birth injury P10.9
  - epidural, nontraumatic I62.1
  - extradural, nontraumatic I62.1
  - newborn P52.9
    - specified NEC P52.8
  - intracerebral (nontraumatic) (in) I61.9
    - brain stem I61.3
    - cerebellum I61.4
    - newborn P52.4
      - birth injury P10.1
    - hemisphere I61.2
      - cortical (superficial) I61.1
      - subcortical (deep) I61.0
    - intraoperative
      - during a nervous system procedure G97.31
      - during other procedure G97.32
    - intraventricular I61.5
    - multiple localized I61.6
    - postprocedural
      - following a nervous system procedure G97.51
      - following other procedure G97.52
    - specified NEC I61.8
    - superficial I61.1
    - traumatic (diffuse) — *see* Injury, intracranial, diffuse
      - focal — *see* Injury, intracranial, focal
  - subarachnoid (nontraumatic) (from) I60.9
    - newborn P52.5

Hemorrhage, hemorrhagic (concealed) - *continued*
- intracranial (nontraumatic) - *continued*
  - subarachnoid (nontraumatic) (from) - *continued*
    - newborn - *continued*
      - birth injury P10.3
    - intracranial (cerebral) artery I60.7
      - anterior communicating I60.2
      - basilar I60.4
      - carotid siphon and bifurcation I60.0-
      - communicating I60.7
        - anterior I60.2
        - posterior I60.3-
      - middle cerebral I60.1-
      - posterior communicating I60.3-
      - specified artery NEC I60.6
      - vertebral I60.5-
    - specified NEC I60.8
    - traumatic S06.6X-
  - subdural (nontraumatic) I62.00
    - acute I62.01
    - birth injury P10.0
    - chronic I62.03
    - newborn (anoxic) (hypoxic) P52.8
      - birth injury P10.0
    - spinal G95.19
    - subacute I62.02
    - traumatic — *see* Injury, intracranial, subdural hemorrhage
  - traumatic — *see* Injury, intracranial, focal brain injury
- intramedullary NEC G95.19
- intraocular — *see* Hemophthalmos
- intraoperative, intraprocedural — *see* Complication, hemorrhage (hematoma), intraoperative (intraprocedural), by site
- intrapartum — *see* Hemorrhage, complicating, delivery
- intrapelvic
  - female N94.89
  - male K66.1
- intraperitoneal K66.1
- intrapontine I61.3
- intraprocedural — *see* Complication, hemorrhage (hematoma), intraoperative (intraprocedural), by site
- intrauterine N85.7
  - complicating delivery — *see also* Hemorrhage, complicating, delivery O67.9
  - postpartum — *see* Hemorrhage, postpartum
- intraventricular I61.5
  - newborn (nontraumatic) — *see also* Newborn, affected by, hemorrhage P52.3
    - due to birth injury P10.2
    - grade
      - 1 P52.0
      - 2 P52.1
      - 3 P52.21
      - 4 P52.22
- intravesical N32.89
- iris (postinfectional) (postinflammatory) (toxic) — *see* Hyphema
- joint (nontraumatic) — *see* Hemarthrosis
- kidney N28.89
- knee (joint) (nontraumatic) — *see* Hemarthrosis, knee
- labyrinth — *see* subcategory H83.8
- lenticular striate artery I61.0
- ligature, vessel — *see* Hemorrhage, postoperative
- liver K76.89
- lung R04.89
  - newborn P26.9
    - massive P26.1
    - specified NEC P26.8
  - tuberculous — *see* Tuberculosis, pulmonary
- massive umbilical, newborn P51.0
- mediastinum — *see* Hemorrhage, lung
- medulla I61.3
- membrane (brain) I60.8

Hemorrhage, hemorrhagic (concealed) - *continued*
  membrane (brain) - *continued*
    spinal cord — *see* Hemorrhage, spinal cord
  meninges, meningeal (brain) (middle) I60.8
    spinal cord — *see* Hemorrhage, spinal cord
  mesentery K66.1
  metritis — *see* Endometritis
  mouth K13.79
  mucous membrane NEC R58
    newborn P54.8
  muscle M62.89
  nail (subungual) L60.8
  nasal turbinate R04.0
    newborn P54.8
  navel, newborn P51.9
  newborn P54.9
    specified NEC P54.8
  nipple N64.59
  nose R04.0
    newborn P54.8
  omentum K66.1
  optic nerve (sheath) H47.02-
  orbit, orbital H05.23-
  ovary NEC N83.8
  oviduct N83.6
  pancreas K86.89
  parathyroid (gland) (spontaneous) E21.4
  parturition — *see* Hemorrhage, complicating, delivery
  penis N48.89
  pericardium, pericarditis I31.2
  peritoneum, peritoneal K66.1
  peritonsillar tissue J35.8
    due to infection J36
  petechial R23.3
    due to autosensitivity, erythrocyte D69.2
  pituitary (gland) E23.6
  pleura — *see* Hemorrhage, lung
  polioencephalitis, superior E51.2
  polymyositis — *see* Polymyositis
  pons, pontine I61.3
  posterior fossa (nontraumatic) I61.8
    newborn P52.6
  postmenopausal N95.0
  postnasal R04.0
  postoperative — *see* Complications, postprocedural, hemorrhage, by site
  postpartum NEC (following delivery of placenta) O72.1
    delayed or secondary O72.2
    retained placenta O72.0
    third stage O72.0
  pregnancy — *see* Hemorrhage, antepartum
  preretinal — *see* Hemorrhage, retina
  prostate N42.1
  puerperal — *see* Hemorrhage, postpartum
    delayed or secondary O72.2
  pulmonary R04.89
    newborn P26.9
      massive P26.1
      specified NEC P26.8
    tuberculous — *see* Tuberculosis, pulmonary
  purpura (primary) D69.3
  rectum (sphincter) K62.5
    newborn P54.2
  recurring, following initial hemorrhage at time of injury T79.2
  renal N28.89
  respiratory passage or tract R04.9
    specified NEC R04.89
  retina, retinal (vessels) H35.6-
    diabetic — *see* Diabetes, retinal, hemorrhage
  retroperitoneal R58
  scalp R58
  scrotum N50.1
  secondary (nontraumatic) R58
    following initial hemorrhage at time of injury T79.2
  seminal vesicle N50.1
  skin R23.3
    newborn P54.5
  slipped umbilical ligature P51.8

Hemorrhage, hemorrhagic (concealed) - *continued*
  spermatic cord N50.1
  spinal (cord) G95.19
    newborn (birth injury) P11.5
  spleen D73.5
    intraoperative — *see* Complications, intraoperative, hemorrhage, spleen
    postprocedural — *see* Complications, postprocedural, hemorrhage, spleen
  stomach K92.2
    newborn P54.3
    ulcer — *see* Ulcer, stomach, with hemorrhage
  subarachnoid (nontraumatic) — *see* Hemorrhage, intracranial, subarachnoid
  subconjunctival — *see also* Hemorrhage, conjunctiva
    birth injury P15.3
  subcortical (brain) I61.0
  subcutaneous R23.3
  subdiaphragmatic R58
  subdural (acute) (nontraumatic) — *see* Hemorrhage, intracranial, subdural
  subependymal
    newborn P52.0
      with intraventricular extension P52.1
        and intracerebral extension P52.22
  subgaleal P12.2
  subhyaloid — *see* Hemorrhage, retina
  subperiosteal — *see* Disorder, bone, specified type NEC
  subretinal — *see* Hemorrhage, retina
  subtentorial — *see* Hemorrhage, intracranial, subdural
  subungual L60.8
  suprarenal (capsule) (gland) E27.49
    newborn P54.4
  tentorium (traumatic) NEC — *see* Hemorrhage, brain
    newborn (birth injury) P10.4
  testis N50.1
  third stage (postpartum) O72.0
  thorax — *see* Hemorrhage, lung
  throat R04.1
  thymus (gland) E32.8
  thyroid (cyst) (gland) E07.89
  tongue K14.8
  tonsil J35.8
  trachea — *see* Hemorrhage, lung
  tracheobronchial R04.89
    newborn P26.0
  traumatic - code to specific injury
    cerebellar — *see* Hemorrhage, brain
    intracranial — *see* Hemorrhage, brain
    recurring or secondary (following initial hemorrhage at time of injury) T79.2
  tuberculous NEC — *see also* Tuberculosis, pulmonary A15.0
  tunica vaginalis N50.1
  ulcer - code by site under Ulcer, with hemorrhage K27.4
  umbilicus, umbilical
    cord
      after birth, newborn P51.9
      complicating delivery O69.5
    newborn P51.9
      massive P51.0
      slipped ligature P51.8
    stump P51.9
  urethra (idiopathic) N36.8
  uterus, uterine (abnormal) N93.9
    climacteric N92.4
    complicating delivery — *see* Hemorrhage, complicating, delivery
    dysfunctional or functional N93.8
    intermenstrual (regular) N92.3
      irregular N92.1
    postmenopausal N95.0
    postpartum — *see* Hemorrhage, postpartum
    preclimacteric or premenopausal N92.4
    prepubertal N93.8
    pubertal N92.2
  vagina (abnormal) N93.9

Hemorrhage, hemorrhagic (concealed) - *continued*
  vagina (abnormal) - *continued*
    newborn P54.6
  vas deferens N50.1
  vasa previa O69.4
  ventricular I61.5
  vesical N32.89
  viscera NEC R58
    newborn P54.8
  vitreous (humor) (intraocular) H43.1-
  vulva N90.89

Hemorrhoids (bleeding) (without mention of degree) K64.9
  1st degree (grade/stage I) (without prolapse outside of anal canal) K64.0
  2nd degree (grade/stage II) (that prolapse with straining but retract spontaneously) K64.1
  3rd degree (grade/stage III) (that prolapse with straining and require manual replacement back inside anal canal) K64.2
  4th degree (grade/stage IV) (with prolapsed tissue that cannot be manually replaced) K64.3
  complicating
    pregnancy O22.4
    puerperium O87.2
  external K64.4
    with
      thrombosis K64.5
  internal (without mention of degree) K64.8
  prolapsed K64.8
  skin tags
    anus K64.4
    residual K64.4
  specified NEC K64.8
  strangulated — *see also* Hemorrhoids, by degree K64.8
  thrombosed — *see also* Hemorrhoids, by degree K64.5
  ulcerated — *see also* Hemorrhoids, by degree K64.8

Hemosalpinx N83.6
  with
    hematocolpos N89.7
    hematometra N85.7
      with hematocolpos N89.7

Hemosiderosis (dietary) E83.19
  pulmonary, idiopathic E83.1- *[J84.03]*
  transfusion T80.89

Hemothorax (bacterial) (nontuberculous) J94.2
  newborn P54.8
  traumatic S27.1
    with pneumothorax S27.2
  tuberculous NEC A15.6

Henoch (-Schönlein) disease or syndrome (purpura) D69.0

Henpue, henpuye A66.6

Hepar lobatum (syphilitic) A52.74

Hepatalgia K76.89

Hepatitis K75.9
  acute B17.9
    with coma K72.01
    with hepatic failure — *see* Failure, hepatic
    alcoholic — *see* Hepatitis, alcoholic
    infectious B17.9
    non-viral K72.0
    viral B17.9
  alcoholic (acute) (chronic) K70.10
    with ascites K70.11
  amebic — *see* Abscess, liver, amebic
  anicteric, (viral) — *see* Hepatitis, viral
  antigen-associated (HAA) — *see* Hepatitis, B
  Australia-antigen (positive) — *see* Hepatitis, B
  autoimmune K75.4
  B B19.10
    with hepatic coma B19.11
    acute B16.9
      with
        delta-agent (coinfection) (without hepatic coma) B16.1

Hepatitis - *continued*
B - *continued*
acute - *continued*
with - *continued*
delta-agent (coinfection) (without hepatic coma) - *continued*
with hepatic coma B16.0
hepatic coma (without delta-agent coinfection) B16.2
chronic B18.1
with delta-agent B18.0
bacterial NEC K75.89
C (viral) B19.20
with hepatic coma B19.21
acute B17.10
with hepatic coma B17.11
chronic B18.2
catarrhal (acute) B15.9
with hepatic coma B15.0
cholangiolitic K75.89
cholestatic K75.89
chronic K73.9
active NEC K73.2
lobular NEC K73.1
persistent NEC K73.0
specified NEC K73.8
cytomegaloviral B25.1
due to ethanol (acute) (chronic) — *see* Hepatitis, alcoholic
epidemic B15.9
with hepatic coma B15.0
fulminant NEC (viral) — *see* Hepatitis, viral
neonatal giant cell P59.29
granulomatous NEC K75.3
herpesviral B00.81
history of
B Z86.19
C Z86.19
homologous serum — *see* Hepatitis, viral, type B
in (due to)
mumps B26.81
toxoplasmosis (acquired) B58.1
congenital (active) P37.1 *[K77]*
infectious, infective B15.9
acute (subacute) B17.9
chronic B18.9
inoculation — *see* Hepatitis, viral, type B
interstitial (chronic) K74.69
ischemia, ischemic K72.00
lupoid NEC K75.4
malignant NEC (with hepatic failure) K72.90
with coma K72.91
neonatal (idiopathic) (toxic) P59.29
newborn P59.29
postimmunization — *see* Hepatitis, viral, type B
post-transfusion — *see* Hepatitis, viral, type B
reactive, nonspecific K75.2
serum — *see* Hepatitis, viral, type B
shock K72.00
specified type NEC
with hepatic failure — *see* Failure, hepatic
syphilitic (late) A52.74
congenital (early) A50.08 *[K77]*
late A50.59 *[K77]*
secondary A51.45
toxic — *see also* Disease, liver, toxic K71.6
tuberculous A18.83
viral, virus B19.9
with hepatic coma B19.0
acute B17.9
chronic B18.9
specified NEC B18.8
type
B B18.1
with delta-agent B18.0
C B18.2
congenital P35.3
coxsackie B33.8 *[K77]*
cytomegalic inclusion B25.1
in remission, any type - code to Hepatitis, chronic, by type
non-A, non-B B17.8

Hepatitis - *continued*
viral, virus - *continued*
specified type NEC (with or without coma) B17.8
type
A B15.9
with hepatic coma B15.0
B B19.10
with hepatic coma B19.11
acute B16.9
with
delta-agent (coinfection) (without hepatic coma) B16.1
with hepatic coma B16.0
hepatic coma (without delta-agent coinfection) B16.2
chronic B18.1
with delta-agent B18.0
C B19.20
with hepatic coma B19.21
acute B17.10
with hepatic coma B17.11
chronic B18.2
E B17.2
non-A, non-B B17.8
Hepatization lung (acute) — *see* Pneumonia, lobar
Hepatoblastoma C22.2
Hepatocarcinoma C22.0
Hepatocholangiocarcinoma C22.0
Hepatocholangioma, benign D13.4
Hepatocholangitis K75.89
Hepatolenticular degeneration E83.01
Hepatoma (malignant) C22.0
benign D13.4
embryonal C22.0
Hepatomegaly — *see also* Hypertrophy, liver
with splenomegaly R16.2
congenital Q44.7
in mononucleosis
gammaherpesviral B27.09
infectious specified NEC B27.89
Hepatoptosis K76.89
Hepatorenal syndrome following labor and delivery O90.4
Hepatosis K76.89
Hepatosplenomegaly R16.2
hyperlipemic (Bürger-Grütz type) E78.3 *[K77]*
Hereditary — *see* condition
Hereditary alpha tryptasemia (syndrome) D89.44
Heredodegeneration, macular — *see* Dystrophy, retina
Heredopathia atactica polyneuritiformis G60.1
Heredosyphilis — *see* Syphilis, congenital
Herlitz' syndrome Q81.1
Hermansky-Pudlak syndrome E70.331
Hermaphrodite, hermaphroditism (true) Q56.0
46,XX with streak gonads Q99.1
46,XX/46,XY Q99.0
46,XY with streak gonads Q99.1
chimera 46,XX/46,XY Q99.0
Hernia, hernial (acquired) (recurrent) K46.9
with
gangrene — *see* Hernia, by site, with, gangrene
incarceration — *see* Hernia, by site, with, obstruction
irreducible — *see* Hernia, by site, with, obstruction
obstruction — *see* Hernia, by site, with, obstruction
strangulation — *see* Hernia, by site, with, obstruction
abdomen, abdominal K46.9
with
gangrene (and obstruction) K46.1
obstruction K46.0
femoral — *see* Hernia, femoral
incisional — *see* Hernia, incisional
inguinal — *see* Hernia, inguinal
specified site NEC K45.8

Hernia, hernial (acquired) (recurrent) - *continued*
abdomen, abdominal - *continued*
specified site NEC - *continued*
with
gangrene (and obstruction) K45.1
obstruction K45.0
umbilical — *see* Hernia, umbilical
wall — *see* Hernia, ventral
appendix — *see* Hernia, abdomen
bladder (mucosa) (sphincter)
congenital (female) (male) Q79.51
female — *see* Cystocele
male N32.89
brain, congenital — *see* Encephalocele
cartilage, vertebra — *see* Displacement, intervertebral disc
cerebral, congenital — *see also* Encephalocele
endaural Q01.8
ciliary body (traumatic) S05.2-
colon — *see* Hernia, abdomen
Cooper's — *see* Hernia, abdomen, specified site NEC
crural — *see* Hernia, femoral
diaphragm, diaphragmatic K44.9
with
gangrene (and obstruction) K44.1
obstruction K44.0
congenital Q79.0
direct (inguinal) — *see* Hernia, inguinal
diverticulum, intestine — *see* Hernia, abdomen
double (inguinal) — *see* Hernia, inguinal, bilateral
due to adhesions (with obstruction) K56.50
epigastric — *see also* Hernia, ventral K43.9
esophageal hiatus — *see* Hernia, hiatal
external (inguinal) — *see* Hernia, inguinal
fallopian tube N83.4-
fascia M62.89
femoral K41.90
with
gangrene (and obstruction) K41.40
not specified as recurrent K41.40
recurrent K41.41
obstruction K41.30
not specified as recurrent K41.30
recurrent K41.31
bilateral K41.20
with
gangrene (and obstruction) K41.10
not specified as recurrent K41.10
recurrent K41.11
obstruction K41.00
not specified as recurrent K41.00
recurrent K41.01
not specified as recurrent K41.20
recurrent K41.21
unilateral K41.90
with
gangrene (and obstruction) K41.40
not specified as recurrent K41.40
recurrent K41.41
obstruction K41.30
not specified as recurrent K41.30
recurrent K41.31
not specified as recurrent K41.90
recurrent K41.91
not specified as recurrent K41.90
recurrent K41.91
foramen magnum G93.5
congenital Q01.8
funicular (umbilical) — *see also* Hernia, umbilicus
spermatic (cord) — *see* Hernia, inguinal
gastrointestinal tract — *see* Hernia, abdomen
Hesselbach's — *see* Hernia, femoral, specified site NEC
hiatal (esophageal) (sliding) K44.9
with
gangrene (and obstruction) K44.1
obstruction K44.0
congenital Q40.1
hypogastric — *see* Hernia, ventral

Hernia, hernial (acquired) (recurrent) - *continued*
incarcerated — *see also* Hernia, by site, with obstruction
with gangrene — *see* Hernia, by site, with gangrene
incisional K43.2
with
gangrene (and obstruction) K43.1
obstruction K43.0
indirect (inguinal) — *see* Hernia, inguinal
inguinal (direct) (external) (funicular) (indirect) (internal) (oblique) (scrotal) (sliding) K40.90
with
gangrene (and obstruction) K40.40
not specified as recurrent K40.40
recurrent K40.41
obstruction K40.30
not specified as recurrent K40.30
recurrent K40.31
not specified as recurrent K40.90
recurrent K40.91
bilateral K40.20
with
gangrene (and obstruction) K40.10
not specified as recurrent K40.10
recurrent K40.11
obstruction K40.00
not specified as recurrent K40.00
recurrent K40.01
not specified as recurrent K40.20
recurrent K40.21
unilateral K40.90
with
gangrene (and obstruction) K40.40
not specified as recurrent K40.40
recurrent K40.41
obstruction K40.30
not specified as recurrent K40.30
recurrent K40.31
not specified as recurrent K40.90
recurrent K40.91
internal — *see also* Hernia, abdomen
inguinal — *see* Hernia, inguinal
interstitial — *see* Hernia, abdomen
intervertebral cartilage or disc — *see* Displacement, intervertebral disc
intestine, intestinal — *see* Hernia, by site
intra-abdominal — *see* Hernia, abdomen
iris (traumatic) S05.2-
irreducible — *see also* Hernia, by site, with obstruction
with gangrene — *see* Hernia, by site, with gangrene
ischiatic — *see* Hernia, abdomen, specified site NEC
ischiorectal — *see* Hernia, abdomen, specified site NEC
lens (traumatic) S05.2-
linea (alba) (semilunaris) — *see* Hernia, ventral
Littre's — *see* Hernia, abdomen
lumbar — *see* Hernia, abdomen, specified site NEC
lung (subcutaneous) J98.4
mediastinum J98.59
mesenteric (internal) — *see* Hernia, abdomen
midline — *see* Hernia, ventral
muscle (sheath) M62.89
nucleus pulposus — *see* Displacement, intervertebral disc
oblique (inguinal) — *see* Hernia, inguinal
obstructive — *see also* Hernia, by site, with obstruction
with gangrene — *see* Hernia, by site, with gangrene
obturator — *see* Hernia, abdomen, specified site NEC
omental — *see* Hernia, abdomen
ovary N83.4-
oviduct N83.4-
paraesophageal — *see also* Hernia, diaphragm
congenital Q40.1

Hernia, hernial (acquired) (recurrent) - *continued*
parastomal K43.5
with
gangrene (and obstruction) K43.4
obstruction K43.3
paraumbilical — *see* Hernia, umbilicus
perineal — *see* Hernia, abdomen, specified site NEC
Petit's — *see* Hernia, abdomen, specified site NEC
postoperative — *see* Hernia, incisional
pregnant uterus — *see* Abnormal, uterus in pregnancy or childbirth
prevesical N32.89
properitoneal — *see* Hernia, abdomen, specified site NEC
pudendal — *see* Hernia, abdomen, specified site NEC
rectovaginal N81.6
retroperitoneal — *see* Hernia, abdomen, specified site NEC
Richter's — *see* Hernia, abdomen, with obstruction
Rieux's, Riex's — *see* Hernia, abdomen, specified site NEC
sac condition (adhesion) (dropsy) (inflammation) (laceration) (suppuration) - code by site under Hernia
sciatic — *see* Hernia, abdomen, specified site NEC
scrotum, scrotal — *see* Hernia, inguinal
sliding (inguinal) — *see also* Hernia, inguinal
hiatus — *see* Hernia, hiatal
spigelian — *see* Hernia, ventral
spinal — *see* Spina bifida
strangulated — *see also* Hernia, by site, with obstruction
with gangrene — *see* Hernia, by site, with gangrene
subxiphoid — *see* Hernia, ventral
supra-umbilicus — *see* Hernia, ventral
tendon — *see* Disorder, tendon, specified type NEC
Treitz's (fossa) — *see* Hernia, abdomen, specified site NEC
tunica vaginalis Q55.29
umbilicus, umbilical K42.9
with
gangrene (and obstruction) K42.1
obstruction K42.0
ureter N28.89
urethra, congenital Q64.79
urinary meatus, congenital Q64.79
uterus N81.4
pregnant — *see* Abnormal, uterus in pregnancy or childbirth
vaginal (anterior) (wall) — *see* Cystocele
Velpeau's — *see* Hernia, femoral
ventral K43.9
with
gangrene (and obstruction) K43.7
obstruction K43.6
recurrent — *see* Hernia, incisional
incisional K43.2
with
gangrene (and obstruction) K43.1
obstruction K43.0
specified NEC K43.9
with
gangrene (and obstruction) K43.7
obstruction K43.6
vesical
congenital (female) (male) Q79.51
female — *see* Cystocele
male N32.89
vitreous (into wound) S05.2-
into anterior chamber — *see* Prolapse, vitreous

Herniation — *see also* Hernia
brain (stem) G93.5
nontraumatic G93.5
traumatic S06.A1

Herniation - *continued*
brain (stem) - *continued*
traumatic - *continued*
cerebellar S06.A1
subfalcine (cingulate) S06.A1
tonsillar S06.A1
transtentorial (central) (upward cerebellar) S06.A1
uncal S06.A1
cerebral G93.5
nontraumatic G93.5
traumatic S06.A1
mediastinum J98.59
nucleus pulposus — *see* Displacement, intervertebral disc

Herpangina B08.5

Herpes, herpesvirus, herpetic B00.9
anogenital A60.9
perianal skin A60.1
rectum A60.1
urogenital tract A60.00
cervix A60.03
male genital organ NEC A60.02
penis A60.01
specified site NEC A60.09
vagina A60.04
vulva A60.04
blepharitis (zoster) B02.39
simplex B00.59
circinatus B35.4
bullosus L12.0
conjunctivitis (simplex) B00.53
zoster B02.31
cornea B02.33
encephalitis B00.4
due to herpesvirus 6 B10.01
due to herpesvirus 7 B10.09
specified NEC B10.09
eye (zoster) B02.30
simplex B00.50
eyelid (zoster) B02.39
simplex B00.59
facialis B00.1
febrilis B00.1
geniculate ganglionitis B02.21
genital, genitalis A60.00
female A60.09
male A60.02
gestational, gestationis O26.4-
gingivostomatitis B00.2
human B00.9
1 — *see* Herpes, simplex
2 — *see* Herpes, simplex
3 — *see* Varicella
4 — *see* Mononucleosis, Epstein-Barr (virus)
5 — *see* Disease, cytomegalic inclusion (generalized)
6
encephalitis B10.01
specified NEC B10.81
7
encephalitis B10.09
specified NEC B10.82
8 B10.89
infection NEC B10.89
Kaposi's sarcoma associated B10.89
iridocyclitis (simplex) B00.51
zoster B02.32
iris (vesicular erythema multiforme) L51.9
iritis (simplex) B00.51
Kaposi's sarcoma associated B10.89
keratitis (simplex) (dendritic) (disciform) (interstitial) B00.52
zoster (interstitial) B02.33
keratoconjunctivitis (simplex) B00.52
zoster B02.33
labialis B00.1
lip B00.1
meningitis (simplex) B00.3
zoster B02.1
ophthalmicus (zoster) NEC B02.30
simplex B00.50
penis A60.01
perianal skin A60.1

Herpes, herpesvirus, herpetic - *continued*
pharyngitis, pharyngotonsillitis B00.2
rectum A60.1
scrotum A60.02
sepsis B00.7
simplex B00.9
complicated NEC B00.89
congenital P35.2
conjunctivitis B00.53
external ear B00.1
eyelid B00.59
hepatitis B00.81
keratitis (interstitial) B00.52
myleitis B00.82
specified complication NEC B00.89
visceral B00.89
stomatitis B00.2
tonsurans B35.0
visceral B00.89
vulva A60.04
whitlow B00.89
zoster — *see also* condition B02.9
auricularis B02.21
complicated NEC B02.8
conjunctivitis B02.31
disseminated B02.7
encephalitis B02.0
eye (lid) B02.39
geniculate ganglionitis B02.21
keratitis (interstitial) B02.33
meningitis B02.1
myelitis B02.24
neuritis, neuralgia B02.29
ophthalmicus NEC B02.30
oticus B02.21
polyneuropathy B02.23
specified complication NEC B02.8
trigeminal neuralgia B02.22
Herpesvirus (human) — *see* Herpes
Herpetophobia F40.218
Herrick's anemia — *see* Disease, sickle-cell
Hers' disease E74.09
Herter-Gee syndrome K90.0
Herxheimer's reaction R68.89
Hesitancy
of micturition R39.11
urinary R39.11
Hesselbach's hernia — *see* Hernia, femoral, specified site NEC
Heterochromia (congenital) Q13.2
cataract — *see* Cataract, complicated
cyclitis (Fuchs) — *see* Cyclitis, Fuchs' heterochromic
hair L67.1
iritis — *see* Cyclitis, Fuchs' heterochromic
retained metallic foreign body (nonmagnetic) — *see* Foreign body, intraocular, old, retained
magnetic — *see* Foreign body, intraocular, old, retained, magnetic
uveitis — *see* Cyclitis, Fuchs' heterochromic
Heterophoria — *see* Strabismus, heterophoria
Heterophyes, heterophyiasis (small intestine) B66.8
Heterotopia, heterotopic — *see also* Malposition, congenital
cerebralis Q04.8
Heterotropia — *see* Strabismus
Heubner-Herter disease K90.0
Hexadactylism Q69.9
HGSIL (cytology finding) (high grade squamous intraepithelial lesion on cytologic smear) (Pap smear finding)
anus R85.613
cervix R87.613
biopsy (histology) finding — *see* Neoplasia, intraepithelial, cervix, grade II or grade III
vagina R87.623
biopsy (histology) finding — *see* Neoplasia, intraepithelial, vagina, grade II or grade III
Hibernoma — *see* Lipoma
Hiccup, hiccough R06.6
epidemic B33.0

Hiccup, hiccough - *continued*
psychogenic F45.8
Hidden penis (congenital) Q55.64
acquired N48.83
Hidradenitis (axillaris) (suppurative) L73.2
Hidradenoma (nodular) — *see also* Neoplasm, skin, benign
clear cell — *see* Neoplasm, skin, benign
papillary — *see* Neoplasm, skin, benign
Hidrocystoma — *see* Neoplasm, skin, benign
High
altitude effects T70.20
anoxia T70.29
on
ears T70.0
sinuses T70.1
polycythemia D75.1
arch
foot Q66.7-
palate, congenital Q38.5
arterial tension — *see* Hypertension
basal metabolic rate R94.8
blood pressure — *see also* Hypertension
borderline R03.0
reading (incidental) (isolated) (nonspecific) , without diagnosis of hypertension R03.0
cholesterol E78.00
with high triglycerides E78.2
diaphragm (congenital) Q79.1
expressed emotional level within family Z63.8
head at term O32.4
palate, congenital Q38.5
risk
infant NEC Z76.2
sexual behavior (heterosexual) Z72.51
bisexual Z72.53
homosexual Z72.52
scrotal testis, testes
bilateral Q53.23
unilateral Q53.13
temperature (of unknown origin) R50.9
thoracic rib Q76.6
triglycerides E78.1
with high cholesterol E78.2
Hildenbrand's disease A75.0
Hilum — *see* condition
Hip — *see* condition
Hippel's disease Q85.8
Hippophobia F40.218
Hippus H57.09
Hirschsprung's disease or megacolon Q43.1
Hirsutism, hirsuties L68.0
Hirudiniasis
external B88.3
internal B83.4
Hiss-Russell dysentery A03.1
Histidinemia, histidinuria E70.41
Histiocytoma — *see also* Neoplasm, skin, benign
fibrous — *see also* Neoplasm, skin, benign
atypical — *see* Neoplasm, connective tissue, uncertain behavior
malignant — *see* Neoplasm, connective tissue, malignant
Histiocytosis D76.3
acute differentiated progressive C96.0
Langerhans' cell NEC C96.6
multifocal X
multisystemic (disseminated) C96.0
unisystemic C96.5
pulmonary, adult (adult PLCH) J84.82
unifocal (X) C96.6
lipid, lipoid D76.3
essential E75.29
malignant C96.A
mononuclear phagocytes NEC D76.1
Langerhans' cells C96.6
non-Langerhans cell D76.3
polyostotic sclerosing D76.3
sinus, with massive lymphadenopathy D76.3
syndrome NEC D76.3
X NEC C96.6
acute (progressive) C96.0

Histiocytosis - *continued*
X NEC - *continued*
chronic C96.6
multifocal C96.5
multisystemic C96.0
unifocal C96.6
Histoplasmosis B39.9
with pneumonia NEC B39.2
African B39.5
American — *see* Histoplasmosis, capsulati
capsulati B39.4
disseminated B39.3
generalized B39.3
pulmonary B39.2
acute B39.0
chronic B39.1
Darling's B39.4
duboisii B39.5
lung NEC B39.2
History
family (of) — *see also* History, personal (of)
alcohol abuse Z81.1
allergy NEC Z84.89
anemia Z83.2
arthritis Z82.61
asthma Z82.5
blindness Z82.1
cardiac death (sudden) Z82.41
carrier of genetic disease Z84.81
chromosomal anomaly Z82.79
chronic
disabling disease NEC Z82.8
lower respiratory disease Z82.5
colonic polyps Z83.71
congenital malformations and deformations Z82.79
polycystic kidney Z82.71
consanguinity Z84.3
deafness Z82.2
diabetes mellitus Z83.3
disability NEC Z82.8
disease or disorder (of)
allergic NEC Z84.89
behavioral NEC Z81.8
blood and blood-forming organs Z83.2
cardiovascular NEC Z82.49
chronic disabling NEC Z82.8
digestive Z83.79
ear NEC Z83.52
endocrine NEC Z83.49
elevated lipoprotein (a) (Lp (a)) Z83.430
eye NEC Z83.518
glaucoma Z83.511
familial hypercholesterolemia Z83.42
genitourinary NEC Z84.2
glaucoma Z83.511
hematological Z83.2
immune mechanism Z83.2
infectious NEC Z83.1
ischemic heart Z82.49
kidney Z84.1
lipoprotein metabolism Z83.438
mental NEC Z81.8
metabolic Z83.49
musculoskeletal NEC Z82.69
neurological NEC Z82.0
nutritional Z83.49
parasitic NEC Z83.1
psychiatric NEC Z81.8
respiratory NEC Z83.6
skin and subcutaneous tissue NEC Z84.0
specified NEC Z84.89
drug abuse NEC Z81.3
elevated lipoprotein (a) (Lp (a)) Z83.430
epilepsy Z82.0
familial hypercholesterolemia Z83.42
genetic disease carrier Z84.81
glaucoma Z83.511
hearing loss Z82.2
human immunodeficiency virus (HIV) infection Z83.0
Huntington's chorea Z82.0
hyperlipidemia, familial combined Z83.438

History - *continued*
- personal (of) - *continued*
  - fracture (healed) - *continued*
    - stress Z87.312
    - traumatic Z87.81
  - gene therapy Z92.86
  - gestational diabetes Z86.32
  - hepatitis
    - B Z86.19
    - C Z86.19
  - Hodgkin disease Z85.71
  - hyperthermia, malignant Z88.4
  - hypospadias (corrected) Z87.710
  - hysterectomy Z90.710
  - immunosuppression therapy Z92.25
  - in situ neoplasm
    - breast Z86.000
    - cervix uteri Z86.001
    - digestive organs, specified NEC Z86.004
    - esophagus Z86.003
    - genital organs, specified NEC Z86.002
    - melanoma Z86.006
    - middle ear Z86.005
    - oral cavity Z86.003
    - respiratory system Z86.005
    - skin Z86.007
    - specified NEC Z86.008
    - stomach Z86.003
  - infection NEC Z86.19
    - central nervous system Z86.61
    - coronavirus (disease) (novel) 2019 Z86.16
    - COVID-19 Z86.16
    - latent tuberculosis Z86.15
    - Methicillin resistant Staphylococcus aureus (MRSA) Z86.14
    - SARS-CoV-2 Z86.16
    - urinary (recurrent) (tract) Z87.440
  - injury NEC Z87.828
  - in utero procedure during pregnancy Z98.870
  - in utero procedure while a fetus Z98.871
  - irradiation Z92.3
  - kidney stones Z87.442
  - latent tuberculosis infection Z86.15
  - leukemia Z85.6
  - lymphoma (non-Hodgkin) Z85.72
  - malignant melanoma (skin) Z85.820
  - malignant neoplasm (of) Z85.9
    - accessory sinuses Z85.22
    - anus NEC Z85.048
      - carcinoid Z85.040
    - bladder Z85.51
    - bone Z85.830
    - brain Z85.841
    - breast Z85.3
    - bronchus NEC Z85.118
      - carcinoid Z85.110
    - carcinoid — *see* History, personal (of), malignant neoplasm, by site, carcinioid
    - cervix Z85.41
    - colon NEC Z85.038
      - carcinoid Z85.030
    - digestive organ Z85.00
      - specified NEC Z85.09
    - endocrine gland NEC Z85.858
    - epididymis Z85.48
    - esophagus Z85.01
    - eye Z85.840
    - gastrointestinal tract — *see* History, malignant neoplasm, digestive organ
    - genital organ
      - female Z85.40
        - specified NEC Z85.44
      - male Z85.45
        - specified NEC Z85.49
    - hematopoietic NEC Z85.79
    - intrathoracic organ Z85.20
    - kidney NEC Z85.528
      - carcinoid Z85.520
    - large intestine NEC Z85.038
      - carcinoid Z85.030
    - larynx Z85.21

History - *continued*
- personal (of) - *continued*
  - malignant neoplasm (of) - *continued*
    - liver Z85.05
    - lung NEC Z85.118
      - carcinoid Z85.110
    - mediastinum Z85.29
    - Merkel cell Z85.821
    - middle ear Z85.22
    - nasal cavities Z85.22
    - nervous system NEC Z85.848
    - oral cavity Z85.819
      - specified site NEC Z85.818
    - ovary Z85.43
    - pancreas Z85.07
    - pharynx Z85.819
      - specified site NEC Z85.818
    - pelvis Z85.53
    - pleura Z85.29
    - prostate Z85.46
    - rectosigmoid junction NEC Z85.048
      - carcinoid Z85.040
    - rectum NEC Z85.048
      - carcinoid Z85.040
    - respiratory organ Z85.20
    - sinuses, accessory Z85.22
    - skin NEC Z85.828
      - melanoma Z85.820
      - Merkel cell Z85.821
    - small intestine NEC Z85.068
      - carcinoid Z85.060
    - soft tissue Z85.831
    - specified site NEC Z85.89
    - stomach NEC Z85.028
      - carcinoid Z85.020
    - testis Z85.47
    - thymus NEC Z85.238
      - carcinoid Z85.230
    - thyroid Z85.850
    - tongue Z85.810
    - trachea Z85.12
    - ureter Z85.54
    - urinary organ or tract Z85.50
      - specified NEC Z85.59
    - uterus Z85.42
  - maltreatment Z91.89
  - medical treatment NEC Z92.89
  - melanoma Z85.820
    - in situ Z86.006
    - malignant (skin) Z85.820
  - meningitis Z86.61
  - mental disorder Z86.59
  - Merkel cell carcinoma (skin) Z85.821
  - Methicillin resistant Staphylococcus aureus (MRSA) Z86.14
  - military deployment Z91.82
  - military war, peacekeeping and humanitarian deployment (current or past conflict) Z91.82
  - myocardial infarction (old) I25.2
  - neglect (in)
    - adult Z91.412
    - childhood Z62.812
  - neoplasia
    - anal intraepithelial, III [AIN III] Z86.004
    - high-grade prostatic intraepithelial, III [HGPIN III] Z86.002
    - vaginal intraepithelial, III [VAIN III] Z86.002
    - vulvar intraepithelial, III [VIN III] Z86.002
  - neoplasm
    - benign Z86.018
      - brain Z86.011
      - colon polyp Z86.010
    - in situ
      - breast Z86.000
      - cervix uteri Z86.001
      - digestive organs, specified NEC Z86.004
      - esophagus Z86.003
      - genital organs, specified NEC Z86.002
      - melanoma Z86.006
      - middle ear Z86.005

History - *continued*
- personal (of) - *continued*
  - neoplasm - *continued*
    - in situ - *continued*
      - oral cavity Z86.003
      - respiratory system Z86.005
      - skin Z86.007
      - specified NEC Z86.008
      - stomach Z86.003
    - malignant — *see* History of, malignant neoplasm
    - uncertain behavior Z86.03
  - nephrotic syndrome Z87.441
  - nicotine dependence Z87.891
  - noncompliance with medical treatment or regimen — *see* Noncompliance
  - nutritional deficiency Z86.39
  - obstetric complications Z87.59
    - childbirth Z87.59
    - pregnancy Z87.59
    - pre-term labor Z87.51
    - puerperium Z87.59
  - osteoporosis fractures Z87.31
  - parasuicide (attempt) Z91.51
  - physical trauma NEC Z87.828
    - self-harm or suicide attempt Z91.51
  - poisoning NEC Z91.89
    - self-harm or suicide attempt Z91.51
  - poor personal hygiene Z91.89
  - pneumonia (recurrent) Z87.01
  - preterm labor Z87.51
  - prolonged reversible ischemic neurologic deficit (PRIND) Z86.73
  - procedure during pregnancy Z98.870
  - procedure while a fetus Z98.871
  - prostatic dysplasia Z87.430
  - psychological
    - abuse
      - adult Z91.411
      - child Z62.811
    - trauma, specified NEC Z91.49
  - radiation therapy Z92.3
  - removal
    - implant
      - breast Z98.86
  - renal calculi Z87.442
  - respiratory condition NEC Z87.09
  - retained foreign body fully removed Z87.821
  - risk factors NEC Z91.89
  - SARS-CoV-2 infection Z86.16
  - self-harm
    - nonsuicidal Z91.52
    - suicidal Z91.51
  - self-inflicted injury without suicidal intent Z91.52
  - self-injury
    - nonsuicidal Z91.52
  - self-mutilation Z91.52
  - self-poisoning attempt Z91.51
  - sex reassignment Z87.890
  - sleep-wake cycle problem Z72.821
  - specified NEC Z87.898
  - steroid therapy (systemic) Z92.241
    - inhaled Z92.240
  - stroke without residual deficits Z86.73
  - substance abuse NEC F10-F19
  - sudden cardiac arrest Z86.74
  - sudden cardiac death successfully resuscitated Z86.74
  - suicidal behavior Z91.51
  - suicide attempt Z91.51
  - surgery NEC Z98.890
    - with uterine scar Z98.891
    - sex reassignment Z87.890
    - transplant — *see* Transplant
  - thrombophlebitis Z86.72
  - thrombosis (venous) Z86.718
    - pulmonary Z86.711
  - tobacco dependence Z87.891
  - transient ischemic attack (TIA) without residual deficits Z86.73
  - trauma (physical) NEC Z87.828
    - psychological NEC Z91.49
    - self-harm Z91.51

HISTORY - HISTORY

History - *continued*
personal (of) - *continued*
traumatic brain injury Z87.820
tuberculosis, latent infection Z86.15
unhealthy sleep-wake cycle Z72.821
unintended awareness under general anesthesia Z92.84
urinary calculi Z87.442
urinary (recurrent) (tract) infection (s) Z87.440
uterine scar from previous surgery Z98.891
vaginal dysplasia Z87.411
venous thrombosis or embolism Z86.718
pulmonary Z86.711
vulvar dysplasia Z87.412
His-Werner disease A79.0
HIV — *see also* Human, immunodeficiency virus B20
laboratory evidence (nonconclusive) R75
positive, seropositive Z21
nonconclusive test (in infants) R75
Hives (bold) — *see* Urticaria
Hoarseness R49.0
Hobo Z59.00
Hodgkin disease — *see* Lymphoma, Hodgkin
Hodgson's disease I71.2
ruptured I71.1
Hoffa-Kastert disease E88.89
Hoffa's disease E88.89
Hoffmann-Bouveret syndrome I47.9
Hoffmann's syndrome E03.9 *[G73.7]*
Hole (round)
macula H35.34-
retina (without detachment) — *see* Break, retina, round hole
with detachment — *see* Detachment, retina, with retinal, break
Holiday relief care Z75.5
Hollenhorst's plaque — *see* Occlusion, artery, retina
Hollow foot (congenital) Q66.7-
acquired — *see* Deformity, limb, foot, specified NEC
Holoprosencephaly Q04.2
Holt-Oram syndrome Q87.2
Homelessness Z59.00
sheltered Z59.01
unsheltered Z59.02
Homesickness — *see* Disorder, adjustment
Homocysteinemia R79.83
Homocystinemia, homocystinuria E72.11
Homogentisate 1,2-dioxygenase deficiency E70.29
Homologous serum hepatitis (prophylactic) (therapeutic) — *see* Hepatitis, viral, type B
Honeycomb lung J98.4
congenital Q33.0
Hooded
clitoris Q52.6
penis Q55.69
Hookworm (disease) (infection) (infestation) B76.9
with anemia B76.9 *[D63.8]*
specified NEC B76.8
Hordeolum (eyelid) (externum) (recurrent) H00.019
internum H00.029
left H00.026
lower H00.025
upper H00.024
right H00.023
lower H00.022
upper H00.021
left H00.016
lower H00.015
upper H00.014
right H00.013
lower H00.012
upper H00.011
Horn
cutaneous L85.8
nail L60.2
congenital Q84.6
Horner (-Claude Bernard) syndrome G90.2
traumatic — *see* Injury, nerve, cervical sympathetic
Horseshoe kidney (congenital) Q63.1
Horton's headache or neuralgia G44.099
intractable G44.091
not intractable G44.099
Hospital hopper syndrome — *see* Disorder, factitious
Hospitalism in children — *see* Disorder, adjustment
Hostility R45.5
towards child Z62.3
Hot flashes
menopausal N95.1
Hourglass (contracture) — *see also* Contraction, hourglass
stomach K31.89
congenital Q40.2
stricture K31.2
Household, housing circumstance affecting care Z59.9
specified NEC Z59.89
Housemaid's knee — *see* Bursitis, prepatellar
HSCT-TMA (hematopoietic stem cell transplantation-associated thrombotic microangiopathy) M31.11
Hudson (-Stähli) line (cornea) — *see* Pigmentation, cornea, anterior
Human
bite (open wound) — *see also* Bite
intact skin surface — *see* Bite, superficial
herpesvirus — *see* Herpes
immunodeficiency virus (HIV) disease (infection) B20
asymptomatic status Z21
contact Z20.6
counseling Z71.7
dementia B20 *[F02.80]*
with behavioral disturbance B20 *[F02.81]*
exposure to Z20.6
laboratory evidence R75
type-2 (HIV 2) as cause of disease classified elsewhere B97.35
papillomavirus (HPV)
DNA test positive
high risk
cervix R87.810
vagina R87.811
low risk
cervix R87.820
vagina R87.821
screening for Z11.51
T-cell lymphotropic virus
type-1 (HTLV-I) infection B33.3
as cause of disease classified elsewhere B97.33
carrier Z22.6
type-2 (HTLV-II) as cause of disease classified elsewhere B97.34
Humidifier lung or pneumonitis J67.7
Humiliation (experience) in childhood Z62.898
Humpback (acquired) — *see* Kyphosis
Hunchback (acquired) — *see* Kyphosis
Hunger T73.0
air, psychogenic F45.8
Hungry bone syndrome E83.81
Hunner's ulcer — *see* Cystitis, chronic, interstitial
Hunter's
glossitis D51.0
syndrome E76.1
Huntington's disease or chorea G10
with dementia G10 *[F02.80]*
with behavioral disturbance G10 *[F02.81]*
Hunt's
disease or syndrome (herpetic geniculate ganglionitis) B02.21
dyssynergia cerebellaris myoclonica G11.19
neuralgia B02.21
Hurler (-Scheie) disease or syndrome E76.02
Hurst's disease G36.1
Hurthle cell
adenocarcinoma C73
adenoma D34
carcinoma C73
tumor D34
Hutchinson-Boeck disease or syndrome — *see* Sarcoidosis
Hutchinson-Gilford disease or syndrome E34.8
Hutchinson's
disease, meaning
angioma serpiginosum L81.7
pompholyx (cheiropompholyx) L30.1
prurigo estivalis L56.4
summer eruption or summer prurigo L56.4
melanotic freckle — *see* Melanoma, in situ
malignant melanoma in — *see* Melanoma
teeth or incisors (congenital syphilis) A50.52
triad (congenital syphilis) A50.53
Hyalin plaque, sclera, senile H15.89
Hyaline membrane (disease) (lung) (pulmonary) (newborn) P22.0
Hyalinosis
cutis (et mucosae) E78.89
focal and segmental (glomerular) — *see also* N00-N07 with fourth character .1 N05.1
Hyalitis, hyalosis, asteroid — *see also* Deposit, crystalline
syphilitic (late) A52.71
Hydatid
cyst or tumor — *see* Echinococcus
mole — *see* Hydatidiform mole
Morgagni
female Q50.5
male (epididymal) Q55.4
testicular Q55.29
Hydatidiform mole (benign) (complicating pregnancy) (delivered) (undelivered) O01.9
classical O01.0
complete O01.0
incomplete O01.1
invasive D39.2
malignant D39.2
partial O01.1
Hydatidosis — *see* Echinococcus
Hydradenitis (axillaris) (suppurative) L73.2
Hydradenoma — *see* Hidradenoma
Hydramnios O40.-
Hydrancephaly, hydranencephaly Q04.3
with spina bifida — *see* Spina bifida, with hydrocephalus
Hydrargyrism NEC — *see* Poisoning, mercury
Hydrarthrosis — *see also* Effusion, joint
gonococcal A54.42
intermittent M12.40
ankle M12.47-
elbow M12.42-
foot joint M12.47-
hand joint M12.44-
hip M12.45-
knee M12.46-
multiple site M12.49
shoulder M12.41-
specified joint NEC M12.48
wrist M12.43-
of yaws (early) (late) (*see also* subcategory M14.8-) A66.6
syphilitic (late) A52.77
congenital A50.55 *[M12.80]*
Hydremia D64.89
Hydrencephalocele (congenital) — *see* Encephalocele
Hydrencephalomeningocele (congenital) — *see* Encephalocele
Hydroa R23.8
aestivale L56.4
vacciniforme L56.4
Hydroadenitis (axillaris) (suppurative) L73.2
Hydrocalycosis — *see* Hydronephrosis
Hydrocele (spermatic cord) (testis) (tunica vaginalis) N43.3
canal of Nuck N94.89

- **Hydrocele (spermatic cord) (testis) (tunica vaginalis)** - *continued*
  - communicating N43.2
    - congenital P83.5
  - congenital P83.5
  - encysted N43.0
  - female NEC N94.89
  - infected N43.1
  - newborn P83.5
  - round ligament N94.89
  - specified NEC N43.2
  - spinalis — *see* Spina bifida
  - vulva N90.89
- **Hydrocephalus (acquired) (external) (internal) (malignant) (recurrent)** G91.9
  - aqueduct Sylvius stricture Q03.0
  - causing disproportion O33.6
    - with obstructed labor O66.3
  - communicating G91.0
  - congenital (external) (internal) Q03.9
    - with spina bifida Q05.4
      - cervical Q05.0
      - dorsal Q05.1
      - lumbar Q05.2
      - lumbosacral Q05.2
      - sacral Q05.3
      - thoracic Q05.1
      - thoracolumbar Q05.1
    - specified NEC Q03.8
  - due to toxoplasmosis (congenital) P37.1
  - foramen Magendie block (acquired) G91.1
    - congenital — *see also* Hydrocephalus, congenital Q03.1
  - in (due to)
    - infectious disease NEC B89 *[G91.4]*
    - neoplastic disease NEC (see also Neoplasm) G91.4
    - parasitic disease B89 *[G91.4]*
  - newborn Q03.9
    - with spina bifida — *see* Spina bifida, with hydrocephalus
  - noncommunicating G91.1
  - normal pressure G91.2
    - secondary G91.0
  - obstructive G91.1
  - otitic G93.2
  - post-traumatic NEC G91.3
  - secondary G91.4
    - post-traumatic G91.3
  - specified NEC G91.8
  - syphilitic, congenital A50.49
- **Hydrocolpos (congenital)** N89.8
- **Hydrocystoma** — *see* Neoplasm, skin, benign
- **Hydroencephalocele (congenital)** — *see* Encephalocele
- **Hydroencephalomeningocele (congenital)** — *see* Encephalocele
- **Hydrohematopneumothorax** — *see* Hemothorax
- **Hydromeningitis** — *see* Meningitis
- **Hydromeningocele (spinal)** — *see also* Spina bifida
  - cranial — *see* Encephalocele
- **Hydrometra** N85.8
- **Hydrometrocolpos** N89.8
- **Hydromicrocephaly** Q02
- **Hydromphalos (since birth)** Q45.8
- **Hydromyelia** Q06.4
- **Hydromyelocele** — *see* Spina bifida
- **Hydronephrosis (atrophic) (early) (functionless) (intermittent) (primary) (secondary) NEC** N13.30
  - with
    - infection N13.6
    - obstruction (by) (of)
      - renal calculus N13.2
        - with infection N13.6
      - ureteral NEC N13.1
        - with infection N13.6
        - calculus N13.2
          - with infection N13.6
      - ureteropelvic junction (congenital) Q62.11
        - acquired N13.0
          - with infection N13.6
- **Hydronephrosis (atrophic) (early) (functionless) (intermittent) (primary) (secondary) NEC** - *continued*
  - with - *continued*
    - ureteral stricture NEC N13.1
      - with infection N13.6
  - congenital Q62.0
    - due to acquired occlusion of ureteropelvic junction N13.0
  - specified type NEC N13.39
  - tuberculous A18.11
- **Hydropericarditis** — *see* Pericarditis
- **Hydropericardium** — *see* Pericarditis
- **Hydroperitoneum** R18.8
- **Hydrophobia** — *see* Rabies
- **Hydrophthalmos** Q15.0
- **Hydropneumohemothorax** — *see* Hemothorax
- **Hydropneumopericarditis** — *see* Pericarditis
- **Hydropneumopericardium** — *see* Pericarditis
- **Hydropneumothorax** J94.8
  - traumatic — *see* Injury, intrathoracic, lung
  - tuberculous NEC A15.6
- **Hydrops** R60.9
  - abdominis R18.8
  - articulorum intermittens — *see* Hydrarthrosis, intermittent
  - cardiac — *see* Failure, heart, congestive
  - causing obstructed labor (mother) O66.3
  - endolymphatic H81.0-
  - fetal — *see* Pregnancy, complicated by, hydrops, fetalis
  - fetalis P83.2
    - due to
      - ABO isoimmunization P56.0
      - alpha thalassemia D56.0
      - hemolytic disease P56.90
        - specified NEC P56.99
      - isoimmunization (ABO) (Rh) P56.0
      - other specified nonhemolytic disease NEC P83.2
      - Rh incompatibility P56.0
    - during pregnancy — *see* Pregnancy, complicated by, hydrops, fetalis
  - gallbladder K82.1
  - joint — *see* Effusion, joint
  - labyrinth H81.0-
  - newborn (idiopathic) P83.2
    - due to
      - ABO isoimmunization P56.0
      - alpha thalassemia D56.0
      - hemolytic disease P56.90
        - specified NEC P56.99
      - isoimmunization (ABO) (Rh) P56.0
      - Rh incompatibility P56.0
  - nutritional — *see* Malnutrition, severe
  - pericardium — *see* Pericarditis
  - pleura — *see* Hydrothorax
  - spermatic cord — *see* Hydrocele
- **Hydropyonephrosis** N13.6
- **Hydrorachis** Q06.4
- **Hydrorrhea (nasal)** J34.89
  - pregnancy — *see* Rupture, membranes, premature
- **Hydrosadenitis (axillaris) (suppurative)** L73.2
- **Hydrosalpinx (fallopian tube) (follicularis)** N70.11
- **Hydrothorax (double) (pleura)** J94.8
  - chylous (nonfilarial) I89.8
    - filarial — *see also* Infestation, filarial B74.9 *[J91.8]*
  - traumatic — *see* Injury, intrathoracic
  - tuberculous NEC (non primary) A15.6
- **Hydroureter** — *see also* Hydronephrosis N13.4
  - with infection N13.6
  - congenital Q62.39
- **Hydroureteronephrosis** — *see* Hydronephrosis
- **Hydrourethra** N36.8
- **Hydroxykynureninuria** E70.89
- **Hydroxylysinemia** E72.3
- **Hydroxyprolinemia** E72.59
- **Hygiene, sleep**
  - abuse Z72.821
  - inadequate Z72.821
  - poor Z72.821
- **Hygroma (congenital) (cystic)** D18.1
  - praepatellare, prepatellar — *see* Bursitis, prepatellar
- **Hymen** — *see* condition
- **Hymenolepis, hymenolepiasis (diminuta) (infection) (infestation) (nana)** B71.0
- **Hypalgesia** R20.8
- **Hyperacidity (gastric)** K31.89
  - psychogenic F45.8
- **Hyperactive, hyperactivity** F90.9
  - basal cell, uterine cervix — *see* Dysplasia, cervix
  - bowel sounds R19.12
  - cervix epithelial (basal) — *see* Dysplasia, cervix
  - child F90.9
    - attention deficit — *see* Disorder, attention-deficit hyperactivity
  - detrusor muscle N32.81
  - gastrointestinal K31.89
    - psychogenic F45.8
  - nasal mucous membrane J34.3
  - stomach K31.89
  - thyroid (gland) — *see* Hyperthyroidism
- **Hyperacusis** H93.23-
- **Hyperadrenalism** E27.5
- **Hyperadrenocorticism** E24.9
  - congenital E25.0
  - iatrogenic E24.2
    - correct substance properly administered — *see* Table of Drugs and Chemicals, by drug, adverse effect
    - overdose or wrong substance given or taken — *see* Table of Drugs and Chemicals, by drug, poisoning
  - not associated with Cushing's syndrome E27.0
  - pituitary-dependent E24.0
- **Hyperaldosteronism** E26.9
  - familial (type I) E26.02
  - glucocorticoid-remediable E26.02
  - primary (due to (bilateral) adrenal hyperplasia) E26.09
  - primary NEC E26.09
  - secondary E26.1
  - specified NEC E26.89
- **Hyperalgesia** R20.8
- **Hyperalimentation** R63.2
  - carotene, carotin E67.1
  - specified NEC E67.8
  - vitamin
    - A E67.0
    - D E67.3
- **Hyperaminoaciduria**
  - arginine E72.21
  - cystine E72.01
  - lysine E72.3
  - ornithine E72.4
- **Hyperammonemia (congenital)** E72.20
- **Hyperazotemia** — *see* Uremia
- **Hyperbetalipoproteinemia (familial)** E78.00
  - with prebetalipoproteinemia E78.2
- **Hyperbicarbonatemia** P74.41
- **Hyperbilirubinemia**
  - constitutional E80.6
  - familial conjugated E80.6
  - neonatal (transient) — *see* Jaundice, newborn
- **Hypercalcemia, hypocalciuric, familial** E83.52
- **Hypercalciuria, idiopathic** R82.994
- **Hypercapnia** R06.89
  - newborn P84
- **Hypercarotenemia (dietary)** E67.1
- **Hypercementosis** K03.4
- **Hyperchloremia** E87.8
- **Hyperchlorhydria** K31.89
  - neurotic F45.8
  - psychogenic F45.8
- **Hypercholesterinemia** — *see* Hypercholesterolemia

Hypercholesterolemia (essential) (primary) (pure) E78.00
with hyperglyceridemia, endogenous E78.2
dietary counseling and surveillance Z71.3
familial E78.01
hereditary E78.01
Hyperchylia gastrica, psychogenic F45.8
Hyperchylomicronemia (familial) (primary) E78.3
with hyperbetalipoproteinemia E78.3
Hypercoagulable (state) D68.59
activated protein C resistance D68.51
antithrombin (III) deficiency D68.59
factor V Leiden mutation D68.51
primary NEC D68.59
protein C deficiency D68.59
protein S deficiency D68.59
prothrombin gene mutation D68.52
secondary D68.69
specified NEC D68.69
Hypercoagulation (state) D68.59
Hypercorticalism, pituitary-dependent E24.0
Hypercorticosolism — *see* Cushing's, syndrome
Hypercorticosteronism E24.2
correct substance properly administered — *see* Table of Drugs and Chemicals, by drug, adverse effect
overdose or wrong substance given or taken — *see* Table of Drugs and Chemicals, by drug, poisoning
Hypercortisonism E24.2
correct substance properly administered — *see* Table of Drugs and Chemicals, by drug, adverse effect
overdose or wrong substance given or taken — *see* Table of Drugs and Chemicals, by drug, poisoning
Hyperekplexia Q89.8
Hyperelectrolytemia E87.8
Hyperemesis R11.10
with nausea R11.2
gravidarum (mild) O21.0
with
carbohydrate depletion O21.1
dehydration O21.1
electrolyte imbalance O21.1
metabolic disturbance O21.1
severe (with metabolic disturbance) O21.1
projectile R11.12
psychogenic F45.8
Hyperemia (acute) (passive) R68.89
anal mucosa K62.89
bladder N32.89
cerebral I67.89
conjunctiva H11.43-
ear internal, acute — *see* subcategory H83.0
enteric K59.89
eye — *see* Hyperemia, conjunctiva
eyelid (active) (passive) — *see* Disorder, eyelid, specified type NEC
intestine K59.89
iris — *see* Disorder, iris, vascular
kidney N28.89
labyrinth — *see* subcategory H83.0
liver (active) K76.89
lung (passive) — *see* Edema, lung
pulmonary (passive) — *see* Edema, lung
renal N28.89
retina H35.89
stomach K31.89
Hyperesthesia (body surface) R20.3
larynx (reflex) J38.7
hysterical F44.89
pharynx (reflex) J39.2
hysterical F44.89
Hyperestrogenism (drug-induced) (iatrogenic) E28.0
Hyperexplexia Q89.8
Hyperfibrinolysis — *see* Fibrinolysis
Hyperfructosemia E74.19
Hyperfunction
adrenal cortex, not associated with Cushing's syndrome E27.0
medulla E27.5
Hyperfunction - *continued*
adrenal cortex, not associated with Cushing's syndrome - *continued*
medulla - *continued*
adrenomedullary E27.5
virilism E25.9
congenital E25.0
ovarian E28.8
pancreas K86.89
parathyroid (gland) E21.3
pituitary (gland) (anterior) E22.9
specified NEC E22.8
polyglandular E31.1
testicular E29.0
Hypergammaglobulinemia D89.2
polyclonal D89.0
Waldenström D89.0
Hypergastrinemia E16.4
Hyperglobulinemia R77.1
Hyperglycemia, hyperglycemic (transient) R73.9
coma — *see* Diabetes, by type, with coma
postpancreatectomy E89.1
Hyperglyceridemia (endogenous) (essential) (familial) (hereditary) (pure) E78.1
mixed E78.3
Hyperglycinemia (non-ketotic) E72.51
Hypergonadism
ovarian E28.8
testicular (primary) (infantile) E29.0
Hyperheparinemia D68.32
Hyperhidrosis, hyperidrosis R61
focal
primary L74.519
axilla L74.510
face L74.511
palms L74.512
soles L74.513
secondary L74.52
generalized R61
localized
primary L74.519
axilla L74.510
face L74.511
palms L74.512
soles L74.513
secondary L74.52
psychogenic F45.8
secondary R61
focal L74.52
Hyperhistidinemia E70.41
Hyperhomocysteinemia E72.11
Hyperhydroxyprolinemia E72.59
Hyperinsulinism (functional) E16.1
with
coma (hypoglycemic) E15
encephalopathy E16.1 *[G94]*
ectopic E16.1
therapeutic misadventure (from administration of insulin) — *see* subcategory T38.3
Hyperkalemia E87.5
Hyperkeratosis — *see also* Keratosis L85.9
cervix N88.0
due to yaws (early) (late) (palmar or plantar) A66.3
follicularis Q82.8
penetrans (in cutem) L87.0
palmoplantaris climacterica L85.1
pinta A67.1
senile (with pruritus) L57.0
universalis congenita Q80.8
vocal cord J38.3
vulva N90.4
Hyperkinesia, hyperkinetic (disease) (reaction) (syndrome) (childhood) (adolescence) — *see also* Disorder, attention-deficit hyperactivity
heart I51.89
Hyperleucine-isoleucinemia E71.19
Hyperlipemia, hyperlipidemia E78.5
combined E78.2
familial E78.49
group
A E78.00
Hyperlipemia, hyperlipidemia - *continued*
group - *continued*
B E78.1
C E78.2
D E78.3
mixed E78.2
specified NEC E78.49
Hyperlipidosis E75.6
hereditary NEC E75.5
Hyperlipoproteinemia E78.5
Fredrickson's type
I E78.3
IIa E78.00
IIb E78.2
III E78.2
IV E78.1
V E78.3
low-density-lipoprotein-type (LDL) E78.00
very-low-density-lipoprotein-type (VLDL) E78.1
Hyperlucent lung, unilateral J43.0
Hyperlysinemia E72.3
Hypermagnesemia E83.41
neonatal P71.8
Hypermenorrhea N92.0
Hypermethioninemia E72.19
Hypermetropia (congenital) H52.0-
Hypermobility, hypermotility
cecum — *see* Syndrome, irritable bowel
coccyx — *see* subcategory M53.2
colon — *see* Syndrome, irritable bowel
psychogenic F45.8
ileum K58.9
intestine — *see also* Syndrome, irritable bowel K58.9
psychogenic F45.8
meniscus (knee) — *see* Derangement, knee, meniscus
scapula — *see* Instability, joint, shoulder
stomach K31.89
psychogenic F45.8
syndrome M35.7
urethra N36.41
with intrinsic sphincter deficiency N36.43
Hypernasality R49.21
Hypernatremia E87.0
Hypernephroma C64.-
Hyperopia — *see* Hypermetropia
Hyperorexia nervosa F50.2
Hyperornithinemia E72.4
Hyperosmia R43.1
Hyperosmolality E87.0
Hyperostosis (monomelic) — *see also* Disorder, bone, density and structure, specified NEC
ankylosing (spine) M48.10
cervical region M48.12
cervicothoracic region M48.13
lumbar region M48.16
lumbosacral region M48.17
multiple sites M48.19
occipito-atlanto-axial region M48.11
sacrococcygeal region M48.18
thoracic region M48.14
thoracolumbar region M48.15
cortical (skull) M85.2
infantile M89.8X-
frontal, internal of skull M85.2
interna frontalis M85.2
skeletal, diffuse idiopathic — *see* Hyperostosis, ankylosing
skull M85.2
congenital Q75.8
vertebral, ankylosing — *see* Hyperostosis, ankylosing
Hyperovarism E28.8
Hyperoxaluria R82.992
primary E72.53
Hyperparathyroidism E21.3
primary E21.0
secondary (renal) N25.81
non-renal E21.1
specified NEC E21.2
tertiary E21.2
Hyperpathia R20.8

- **Hyperperistalsis** R19.2
  - psychogenic F45.8
- **Hyperpermeability, capillary** I78.8
- **Hyperphagia** R63.2
- **Hyperphenylalaninemia NEC** E70.1
- **Hyperphoria (alternating)** H50.53
- **Hyperphosphatemia** E83.39
- **Hyperpiesis, hyperpiesia** — *see* Hypertension
- **Hyperpigmentation** — *see also* Pigmentation
  - melanin NEC L81.4
  - postinflammatory L81.0
- **Hyperpinealism** E34.8
- **Hyperpituitarism** E22.9
- **Hyperplasia, hyperplastic**
  - adenoids J35.2
  - adrenal (capsule) (cortex) (gland) E27.8
    - with
      - sexual precocity (male) E25.9
        - congenital E25.0
      - virilism, adrenal E25.9
        - congenital E25.0
      - virilization (female) E25.9
        - congenital E25.0
    - congenital E25.0
      - salt-losing E25.0
  - adrenomedullary E27.5
  - angiolymphoid, eosinophilia (ALHE) D18.01
  - appendix (lymphoid) K38.0
  - artery, fibromuscular I77.3
  - bone — *see also* Hypertrophy, bone
    - marrow D75.89
  - breast — *see also* Hypertrophy, breast
    - atypical, atypia N60.9-
      - ductal N60.9-
      - lobular N60.9-
  - C-cell, thyroid E07.0
  - cementation (tooth) (teeth) K03.4
  - cervical gland R59.0
  - cervix (uteri) (basal cell) (endometrium) (polypoid) — *see also* Dysplasia, cervix
    - congenital Q51.828
  - clitoris, congenital Q52.6
  - denture K06.2
  - endocervicitis N72
  - endometrium, endometrial (adenomatous) (cystic) (glandular) (glandular-cystic) (polypoid) N85.00
    - with atypia N85.02
    - benign N85.01
    - cervix — *see* Dysplasia, cervix
    - complex (without atypia) N85.01
    - simple (without atypia) N85.01
  - epithelial L85.9
    - focal, oral, including tongue K13.29
    - nipple N62
    - skin L85.9
    - tongue K13.29
    - vaginal wall N89.3
  - erythroid D75.89
  - fibromuscular of artery (carotid) (renal) I77.3
  - genital
    - female NEC N94.89
    - male N50.89
  - gingiva K06.1
  - glandularis cystica uteri (interstitialis) — *see also* Hyperplasia, endometrial N85.00-
  - gum K06.1
  - hymen, congenital Q52.4
  - irritative, edentulous (alveolar) K06.2
  - jaw M26.09
    - alveolar M26.79
    - lower M26.03
      - alveolar M26.72
    - upper M26.01
      - alveolar M26.71
  - kidney (congenital) Q63.3
  - labia N90.69
    - epithelial N90.3
  - liver (congenital) Q44.7
    - nodular, focal K76.89
  - lymph gland or node R59.9
  - mandible, mandibular M26.03
    - alveolar M26.72
    - unilateral condylar M27.8
  - maxilla, maxillary M26.01

- **Hyperplasia, hyperplastic** - *continued*
  - maxilla, maxillary - *continued*
    - alveolar M26.71
  - myometrium, myometrial N85.2
  - neuroendocrine cell, of infancy J84.841
  - nose
    - lymphoid J34.89
    - polypoid J33.9
  - oral mucosa (irritative) K13.6
  - organ or site, congenital NEC — *see* Anomaly, by site
  - ovary N83.8
  - palate, papillary (irritative) K13.6
  - pancreatic islet cells E16.9
    - alpha E16.8
      - with excess
        - gastrin E16.4
        - glucagon E16.3
    - beta E16.1
  - parathyroid (gland) E21.0
  - pharynx (lymphoid) J39.2
  - prostate (adenofibromatous) (nodular) N40.0
    - with lower urinary tract symptoms (LUTS) N40.1
    - without lower urinary tract symtpoms (LUTS) N40.0
  - renal artery I77.89
  - reticulo-endothelial (cell) D75.89
  - salivary gland (any) K11.1
  - Schimmelbusch's — *see* Mastopathy, cystic
  - suprarenal capsule (gland) E27.8
  - thymus (gland) (persistent) E32.0
  - thyroid (gland) — *see* Goiter
  - tonsils (faucial) (infective) (lingual) (lymphoid) J35.1
    - with adenoids J35.3
  - unilateral condylar M27.8
  - uterus, uterine N85.2
    - endometrium (glandular) — *see also* Hyperplasia, endometrial N85.00-
  - vulva N90.69
    - epithelial N90.3
- **Hyperpnea** — *see* Hyperventilation
- **Hyperpotassemia** E87.5
- **Hyperprebetalipoproteinemia (familial)** E78.1
- **Hyperprolactinemia** E22.1
- **Hyperprolinemia (type I) (type II)** E72.59
- **Hyperproteinemia** E88.09
- **Hyperprothrombinemia, causing coagulation factor deficiency** D68.4
- **Hyperpyrexia** R50.9
  - heat (effects) T67.01
  - malignant, due to anesthetic T88.3
  - rheumatic — *see* Fever, rheumatic
  - unknown origin R50.9
- **Hyper-reflexia** R29.2
- **Hypersalivation** K11.7
- **Hypersecretion**
  - ACTH (not associated with Cushing's syndrome) E27.0
    - pituitary E24.0
  - adrenaline E27.5
  - adrenomedullary E27.5
  - androgen (testicular) E29.0
    - ovarian (drug-induced) (iatrogenic) E28.1
  - calcitonin E07.0
  - catecholamine E27.5
  - corticoadrenal E24.9
  - cortisol E24.9
  - epinephrine E27.5
  - estrogen E28.0
  - gastric K31.89
    - psychogenic F45.8
  - gastrin E16.4
  - glucagon E16.3
  - hormone (s)
    - ACTH (not associated with Cushing's syndrome) E27.0
      - pituitary E24.0
    - antidiuretic E22.2
    - growth E22.0
    - intestinal NEC E34.1
    - ovarian androgen E28.1
    - pituitary E22.9

- **Hypersecretion** - *continued*
  - hormone (s) - *continued*
    - testicular E29.0
    - thyroid stimulating E05.80
      - with thyroid storm E05.81
  - insulin — *see* Hyperinsulinism
  - lacrimal glands — *see* Epiphora
  - medulloadrenal E27.5
  - milk O92.6
  - ovarian androgens E28.1
  - salivary gland (any) K11.7
  - thyrocalcitonin E07.0
  - upper respiratory J39.8
- **Hypersegmentation, leukocytic, hereditary** D72.0
- **Hypersensitive, hypersensitiveness, hypersensitivity** — *see also* Allergy
  - carotid sinus G90.01
  - colon — *see* Irritable, colon
  - drug T88.7
  - gastrointestinal K52.29
    - immediate K52.29
    - psychogenic F45.8
  - labyrinth — *see* subcategory H83.2
  - pain R20.8
  - pneumonitis — *see* Pneumonitis, allergic
  - reaction T78.40
    - upper respiratory tract NEC J39.3
- **Hypersomnia (organic)** G47.10
  - due to
    - alcohol
      - abuse F10.182
      - dependence F10.282
      - use F10.982
    - amphetamines
      - abuse F15.182
      - dependence F15.282
      - use F15.982
    - caffeine
      - abuse F15.182
      - dependence F15.282
      - use F15.982
    - cocaine
      - abuse F14.182
      - dependence F14.282
      - use F14.982
    - drug NEC
      - abuse F19.182
      - dependence F19.282
      - use F19.982
    - medical condition G47.14
    - mental disorder F51.13
    - opioid
      - abuse F11.182
      - dependence F11.282
      - use F11.982
    - psychoactive substance NEC
      - abuse F19.182
      - dependence F19.282
      - use F19.982
    - sedative, hypnotic, or anxiolytic
      - abuse F13.182
      - dependence F13.282
      - use F13.982
    - stimulant NEC
      - abuse F15.182
      - dependence F15.282
      - use F15.982
  - idiopathic G47.11
    - with long sleep time G47.11
    - without long sleep time G47.12
  - menstrual related G47.13
  - nonorganic origin F51.11
    - specified NEC F51.19
  - not due to a substance or known physiological condition F51.11
    - specified NEC F51.19
  - primary F51.11
  - recurrent G47.13
  - specified NEC G47.19
- **Hyperspelnia, hypersplenism** D73.1
- **Hyperstimulation, ovaries (associated with induced ovulation)** N98.1
- **Hypersusceptibility** — *see* Allergy
- **Hypertelorism (ocular) (orbital)** Q75.2

Hypervitaminosis (dietary) NEC - *continued*
K - *continued*
overdose or wrong substance given or taken — *see* Table of Drugs and Chemicals, vitamins, poisoning
Hypervolemia E87.70
specified NEC E87.79
Hypesthesia R20.1
cornea — *see* Anesthesia, cornea
Hyphema H21.0-
traumatic S05.1-
Hypoacidity, gastric K31.89
psychogenic F45.8
Hypoadrenalism, hypoadrenia E27.40
primary E27.1
tuberculous A18.7
Hypoadrenocorticism E27.40
pituitary E23.0
primary E27.1
Hypoalbuminemia E88.09
Hypoaldosteronism E27.40
Hypoalphalipoproteinemia E78.6
Hypobarism T70.29
Hypobaropathy T70.29
Hypobetalipoproteinemia (familial) E78.6
Hypocalcemia E83.51
dietary E58
neonatal P71.1
due to cow's milk P71.0
phosphate-loading (newborn) P71.1
Hypochloremia E87.8
Hypochlorhydria K31.89
neurotic F45.8
psychogenic F45.8
Hypochondria, hypochondriac, hypochondriasis (reaction) F45.21
sleep F51.03
Hypochondrogenesis Q77.0
Hypochondroplasia Q77.4
Hypochromasia, blood cells D50.8
Hypocitraturia R82.991
Hypodontia — *see* Anodontia
Hypoeosinophilia D72.89
Hypoesthesia R20.1
Hypofibrinogenemia D68.8
acquired D65
congenital (hereditary) D68.2
Hypofunction
adrenocortical E27.40
drug-induced E27.3
postprocedural E89.6
primary E27.1
adrenomedullary, postprocedural E89.6
cerebral R29.818
corticoadrenal NEC E27.40
intestinal K59.89
labyrinth — *see* subcategory H83.2
ovary E28.39
pituitary (gland) (anterior) E23.0
testicular E29.1
postprocedural (postsurgical) (postirradiation) (iatrogenic) E89.5
Hypogalactia O92.4
Hypogammaglobulinemia — *see also* Agammaglobulinemia D80.1
hereditary D80.0
nonfamilial D80.1
transient, of infancy D80.7
Hypogenitalism (congenital) — *see* Hypogonadism
Hypoglossia Q38.3
Hypoglycemia (spontaneous) E16.2
coma E15
diabetic — *see* Diabetes, by type, with hypoglycemia, with coma
diabetic — *see* Diabetes, hypoglycemia
dietary counseling and surveillance Z71.3
drug-induced E16.0
with coma (nondiabetic) E15
due to insulin E16.0
with coma (nondiabetic) E15
therapeutic misadventure — *see* subcategory T38.3
functional, nonhyperinsulinemic E16.1
iatrogenic E16.0

Hypoglycemia (spontaneous) - *continued*
iatrogenic - *continued*
with coma (nondiabetic) E15
in infant of diabetic mother P70.1
gestational diabetes P70.0
infantile E16.1
leucine-induced E71.19
neonatal (transitory) P70.4
iatrogenic P70.3
reactive (not drug-induced) E16.1
transitory neonatal P70.4
Hypogonadism
female E28.39
hypogonadotropic E23.0
male E29.1
ovarian (primary) E28.39
pituitary E23.0
testicular (primary) E29.1
Hypohidrosis, hypoidrosis L74.4
Hypoinsulinemia, postprocedural E89.1
Hypokalemia E87.6
Hypoleukocytosis — *see* Agranulocytosis
Hypolipoproteinemia (alpha) (beta) E78.6
Hypomagnesemia E83.42
neonatal P71.2
Hypomania, hypomanic reaction F30.8
Hypomenorrhea — *see* Oligomenorrhea
Hypometabolism R63.8
Hypomotility
gastrointestinal (tract) K31.89
psychogenic F45.8
intestine K59.89
psychogenic F45.8
stomach K31.89
psychogenic F45.8
Hyponasality R49.22
Hyponatremia E87.1
Hypo-osmolality E87.1
Hypo-ovarianism, hypo-ovarism E28.39
Hypoparathyroidism E20.9
familial E20.8
idiopathic E20.0
neonatal, transitory P71.4
postprocedural E89.2
specified NEC E20.8
Hypoperfusion (in)
newborn P96.89
Hypopharyngitis — *see* Laryngopharyngitis
Hypophoria H50.53
Hypophosphatemia, hypophosphatasia (acquired) (congenital) (renal) E83.39
familial E83.31
Hypophyseal, hypophysis — *see also* condition
dwarfism E23.0
gigantism E22.0
Hypopiesis — *see* Hypotension
Hypopinealism E34.8
Hypopituitarism (juvenile) E23.0
drug-induced E23.1
due to
hypophysectomy E89.3
radiotherapy E89.3
iatrogenic NEC E23.1
postirradiation E89.3
postpartum O99.285
postprocedural E89.3
Hypoplasia, hypoplastic
adrenal (gland) , congenital Q89.1
alimentary tract, congenital Q45.8
upper Q40.8
anus, anal (canal) Q42.3
with fistula Q42.2
aorta, aortic Q25.42
ascending, in hypoplastic left heart syndrome Q23.4
valve Q23.1
in hypoplastic left heart syndrome Q23.4
areola, congenital Q83.8
arm (congenital) — *see* Defect, reduction, upper limb
artery (peripheral) Q27.8
brain (congenital) Q28.3
coronary Q24.5
digestive system Q27.8

Hypoplasia, hypoplastic - *continued*
artery (peripheral) - *continued*
lower limb Q27.8
pulmonary Q25.79
functional, unilateral J43.0
retinal (congenital) Q14.1
specified site NEC Q27.8
umbilical Q27.0
upper limb Q27.8
auditory canal Q17.8
causing impairment of hearing Q16.9
biliary duct or passage Q44.5
bone NOS Q79.9
face Q75.8
marrow D61.9
megakaryocytic D69.49
skull — *see* Hypoplasia, skull
brain Q02
gyri Q04.3
part of Q04.3
breast (areola) N64.82
bronchus Q32.4
cardiac Q24.8
carpus — *see* Defect, reduction, upper limb, specified type NEC
cartilage hair Q78.8
cecum Q42.8
cementum K00.4
cephalic Q02
cerebellum Q04.3
cervix (uteri) , congenital Q51.821
clavicle (congenital) Q74.0
coccyx Q76.49
colon Q42.9
specified NEC Q42.8
corpus callosum Q04.0
cricoid cartilage Q31.2
digestive organ (s) or tract NEC Q45.8
upper (congenital) Q40.8
ear (auricle) (lobe) Q17.2
middle Q16.4
enamel of teeth (neonatal) (postnatal) (prenatal) K00.4
endocrine (gland) NEC Q89.2
endometrium N85.8
epididymis (congenital) Q55.4
epiglottis Q31.2
erythroid, congenital D61.01
esophagus (congenital) Q39.8
eustachian tube Q17.8
eye Q11.2
eyelid (congenital) Q10.3
face Q18.8
bone (s) Q75.8
femur (congenital) — *see* Defect, reduction, lower limb, specified type NEC
fibula (congenital) — *see* Defect, reduction, lower limb, specified type NEC
finger (congenital) — *see* Defect, reduction, upper limb, specified type NEC
focal dermal Q82.8
foot — *see* Defect, reduction, lower limb, specified type NEC
gallbladder Q44.0
genitalia, genital organ (s)
female, congenital Q52.8
external Q52.79
internal NEC Q52.8
in adiposogenital dystrophy E23.6
glottis Q31.2
hair Q84.2
hand (congenital) — *see* Defect, reduction, upper limb, specified type NEC
heart Q24.8
humerus (congenital) — *see* Defect, reduction, upper limb, specified type NEC
intestine (small) Q41.9
large Q42.9
specified NEC Q42.8
jaw M26.09
alveolar M26.79
lower M26.04
alveolar M26.74
upper M26.02

Hypoplasia, hypoplastic - *continued*
jaw - *continued*
upper - *continued*
alveolar M26.73
kidney (s) Q60.5
bilateral Q60.4
unilateral Q60.3
labium (majus) (minus) , congenital Q52.79
larynx Q31.2
left heart syndrome Q23.4
leg (congenital) — *see* Defect, reduction, lower limb
limb Q73.8
lower (congenital) — *see* Defect, reduction, lower limb
upper (congenital) — *see* Defect, reduction, upper limb
liver Q44.7
lung (lobe) (not associated with short gestation) Q33.6
associated with immaturity, low birth weight, prematurity, or short gestation P28.0
mammary (areola) , congenital Q83.8
mandible, mandibular M26.04
alveolar M26.74
unilateral condylar M27.8
maxillary M26.02
alveolar M26.73
medullary D61.9
megakaryocytic D69.49
metacarpus — *see* Defect, reduction, upper limb, specified type NEC
metatarsus — *see* Defect, reduction, lower limb, specified type NEC
muscle Q79.8
nail (s) Q84.6
nose, nasal Q30.1
optic nerve H47.03-
osseous meatus (ear) Q17.8
ovary, congenital Q50.39
pancreas Q45.0
parathyroid (gland) Q89.2
parotid gland Q38.4
patella Q74.1
pelvis, pelvic girdle Q74.2
penis (congenital) Q55.62
peripheral vascular system Q27.8
digestive system Q27.8
lower limb Q27.8
specified site NEC Q27.8
upper limb Q27.8
pituitary (gland) (congenital) Q89.2
pulmonary (not associated with short gestation) Q33.6
artery, functional J43.0
associated with short gestation P28.0
radioulnar — *see* Defect, reduction, upper limb, specified type NEC
radius — *see* Defect, reduction, upper limb
rectum Q42.1
with fistula Q42.0
respiratory system NEC Q34.8
rib Q76.6
right heart syndrome Q22.6
sacrum Q76.49
scapula Q74.0
scrotum Q55.1
shoulder girdle Q74.0
skin Q82.8
skull (bone) Q75.8
with
anencephaly Q00.0
encephalocele — *see* Encephalocele
hydrocephalus Q03.9
with spina bifida — *see* Spina bifida, by site, with hydrocephalus
microcephaly Q02
spinal (cord) (ventral horn cell) Q06.1
spine Q76.49
sternum Q76.7
tarsus — *see* Defect, reduction, lower limb, specified type NEC
testis Q55.1
thymic, with immunodeficiency D82.1

Hypoplasia, hypoplastic - *continued*
thymus (gland) Q89.2
with immunodeficiency D82.1
thyroid (gland) E03.1
cartilage Q31.2
tibiofibular (congenital) — *see* Defect, reduction, lower limb, specified type NEC
toe — *see* Defect, reduction, lower limb, specified type NEC
tongue Q38.3
Turner's K00.4
ulna (congenital) — *see* Defect, reduction, upper limb
umbilical artery Q27.0
unilateral condylar M27.8
ureter Q62.8
uterus, congenital Q51.811
vagina Q52.4
vascular NEC peripheral Q27.8
brain Q28.3
digestive system Q27.8
lower limb Q27.8
specified site NEC Q27.8
upper limb Q27.8
vein (s) (peripheral) Q27.8
brain Q28.3
digestive system Q27.8
great Q26.8
lower limb Q27.8
specified site NEC Q27.8
upper limb Q27.8
vena cava (inferior) (superior) Q26.8
vertebra Q76.49
vulva, congenital Q52.79
zonule (ciliary) Q12.8
Hypoplasminogenemia E88.02
Hypopnea, obstructive sleep apnea G47.33
Hypopotassemia E87.6
Hypoproconvertinemia, congenital (hereditary) D68.2
Hypoproteinemia E77.8
Hypoprothrombinemia (congenital) (hereditary) (idiopathic) D68.2
acquired D68.4
newborn, transient P61.6
Hypoptyalism K11.7
Hypopyon (eye) (anterior chamber) — *see* Iridocyclitis, acute, hypopyon
Hypopyrexia R68.0
Hyporeflexia R29.2
Hyposecretion
ACTH E23.0
antidiuretic hormone E23.2
ovary E28.39
salivary gland (any) K11.7
vasopressin E23.2
Hyposegmentation, leukocytic, hereditary D72.0
Hyposiderinemia D50.9
Hypospadias Q54.9
balanic Q54.0
coronal Q54.0
glandular Q54.0
penile Q54.1
penoscrotal Q54.2
perineal Q54.3
specified NEC Q54.8
Hypospermatogenesis — *see* Oligospermia
Hyposplenism D73.0
Hypostasis pulmonary, passive — *see* Edema, lung
Hypostatic — *see* condition
Hyposthenuria N28.89
Hypotension (arterial) (constitutional) I95.9
chronic I95.89
due to (of) hemodialysis I95.3
drug-induced I95.2
iatrogenic I95.89
idiopathic (permanent) I95.0
intracranial G96.810
following
lumbar cerebrospinal fluid shunting G97.83
specified procedure NEC G97.84

Hypotension (arterial) (constitutional) - *continued*
intracranial - *continued*
following - *continued*
ventricular shunting (ventriculostomy) G97.2
specified NEC G96.819
spontaneous G96.811
intra-dialytic I95.3
maternal, syndrome (following labor and delivery) O26.5-
neurogenic, orthostatic G90.3
orthostatic (chronic) I95.1
due to drugs I95.2
neurogenic G90.3
postoperative I95.81
postural I95.1
specified NEC I95.89
Hypothermia (accidental) T68
due to anesthesia, anesthetic T88.51
low environmental temperature T68
neonatal P80.9
environmental (mild) NEC P80.8
mild P80.8
severe (chronic) (cold injury syndrome) P80.0
specified NEC P80.8
not associated with low environmental temperature R68.0
Hypothyroidism (acquired) E03.9
autoimmune — *see* Thyroiditis, autoimmune
congenital (without goiter) E03.1
with goiter (diffuse) E03.0
due to
exogenous substance NEC E03.2
iodine-deficiency, acquired E01.8
subclinical E02
irradiation therapy E89.0
medicament NEC E03.2
P-aminosalicylic acid (PAS) E03.2
phenylbutazone E03.2
resorcinol E03.2
sulfonamide E03.2
surgery E89.0
thiourea group drugs E03.2
iatrogenic NEC E03.2
iodine-deficiency (acquired) E01.8
congenital — *see* Syndrome, iodine-deficiency, congenital
subclinical E02
neonatal, transitory P72.2
postinfectious E03.3
postirradiation E89.0
postprocedural E89.0
postsurgical E89.0
specified NEC E03.8
subclinical, iodine-deficiency related E02
Hypotonia, hypotonicity, hypotony
bladder N31.2
congenital (benign) P94.2
eye — *see* Disorder, globe, hypotony
Hypotrichosis — *see* Alopecia
Hypotropia H50.2-
Hypoventilation R06.89
congenital central alveolar G47.35
sleep related
idiopathic nonobstructive alveolar G47.34
in conditions classified elsewhere G47.36
Hypovitaminosis — *see* Deficiency, vitamin
Hypovolemia E86.1
surgical shock T81.19
traumatic (shock) T79.4
Hypoxemia R09.02
newborn P84
sleep related, in conditions classified elsewhere G47.36
Hypoxia — *see also* Anoxia R09.02
cerebral, during a procedure NEC G97.81
postprocedural NEC G97.82
intrauterine P84
myocardial — *see* Insufficiency, coronary
newborn P84
sleep-related G47.34
Hypsarhythmia — *see* Epilepsy, generalized, specified NEC

HYSTERALGIA, PREGNANT UTERUS - IMMUNODEFICIENCY

- **Impetigo (any organism) (any site) (circinate) (contagiosa) (simplex) (vulgaris)** - *continued*
  - ulcerative L01.09
- **Impingement (on teeth)**
  - joint — *see* Disorder, joint, specified type NEC
  - soft tissue
    - anterior M26.81
    - posterior M26.82
- **Implant, endometrial** N80.9
- **Implantation**
  - anomalous — *see* Anomaly, by site
    - ureter Q62.63
  - cyst
    - external area or site (skin) NEC L72.0
    - iris — *see* Cyst, iris, implantation
    - vagina N89.8
    - vulva N90.7
  - dermoid (cyst) — *see* Implantation, cyst
- **Impotence (sexual)** N52.9
  - counseling Z70.1
  - organic origin — *see also* Dysfunction, sexual, male, erectile N52.9
  - psychogenic F52.21
- **Impression, basilar** Q75.8
- **Imprisonment, anxiety concerning** Z65.1
- **Improper care (child) (newborn)** — *see* Maltreatment
- **Improperly tied umbilical cord (causing hemorrhage)** P51.8
- **Impulsiveness (impulsive)** R45.87
- **Inability to swallow** — *see* Aphagia
- **Inaccessible, inaccessibility**
  - health care NEC Z75.3
    - due to
      - waiting period Z75.2
        - for admission to facility elsewhere Z75.1
  - other helping agencies Z75.4
- **Inactive** — *see* condition
- **Inadequate, inadequacy**
  - aesthetics of dental restoration K08.56
  - biologic, constitutional, functional, or social F60.7
  - development
    - child R62.50
    - genitalia
      - after puberty NEC E30.0
      - congenital
        - female Q52.8
          - external Q52.79
          - internal Q52.8
        - male Q55.8
    - lungs Q33.6
      - associated with short gestation P28.0
    - organ or site not listed — *see* Anomaly, by site
  - diet (causing nutritional deficiency) E63.9
  - drinking-water supply Z58.6
  - eating habits Z72.4
  - environment, household Z59.1
  - family support Z63.8
  - food (supply) NEC Z59.48
    - hunger effects T73.0
  - functional F60.7
  - household care, due to
    - family member
      - handicapped or ill Z74.2
      - on vacation Z75.5
      - temporarily away from home Z74.2
    - technical defects in home Z59.1
    - temporary absence from home of person rendering care Z74.2
  - housing (heating) (space) Z59.1
  - income (financial) Z59.6
  - intrafamilial communication Z63.8
  - material resources Z59.9
  - mental — *see* Disability, intellectual
  - parental supervision or control of child Z62.0
  - personality F60.7
  - pulmonary
    - function R06.89
      - newborn P28.5
    - ventilation, newborn P28.5
- **Inadequate, inadequacy** - *continued*
  - sample of cytologic smear
    - anus R85.615
    - cervix R87.615
    - vagina R87.625
  - social F60.7
    - insurance Z59.7
    - skills NEC Z73.4
  - supervision of child by parent Z62.0
  - teaching affecting education Z55.8
  - welfare support Z59.7
- **Inanition** R64
  - with edema — *see* Malnutrition, severe
  - due to
    - deprivation of food T73.0
    - malnutrition — *see* Malnutrition
  - fever R50.9
- **Inappropriate**
  - change in quantitative human chorionic gonadotropin (hCG) in early pregnancy O02.81
  - diet or eating habits Z72.4
  - level of quantitative human chorionic gonadotropin (hCG) for gestational age in early pregnancy O02.81
  - secretion
    - antidiuretic hormone (ADH) (excessive) E22.2
      - deficiency E23.2
    - pituitary (posterior) E22.2
- **Inattention at or after birth** — *see* Neglect
- **Incarceration, incarcerated**
  - enterocele K46.0
    - gangrenous K46.1
  - epiplocele K46.0
    - gangrenous K46.1
  - exomphalos K42.0
    - gangrenous K42.1
  - hernia — *see also* Hernia, by site, with obstruction
    - with gangrene — *see* Hernia, by site, with gangrene
  - iris, in wound — *see* Injury, eye, laceration, with prolapse
  - lens, in wound — *see* Injury, eye, laceration, with prolapse
  - omphalocele K42.0
  - prison, anxiety concerning Z65.1
  - rupture — *see* Hernia, by site
  - sarcoepiplocele K46.0
    - gangrenous K46.1
  - sarcoepiplomphalocele K42.0
    - with gangrene K42.1
  - uterus N85.8
    - gravid O34.51-
      - causing obstructed labor O65.5
- **Incised wound**
  - external — *see* Laceration
  - internal organs — *see* Injury, by site
- **Incision, incisional**
  - hernia K43.2
    - with
      - gangrene (and obstruction) K43.1
      - obstruction K43.0
  - surgical, complication — *see* Complications, surgical procedure
  - traumatic
    - external — *see* Laceration
    - internal organs — *see* Injury, by site
- **Inclusion**
  - azurophilic leukocytic D72.0
  - blennorrhea (neonatal) (newborn) P39.1
  - gallbladder in liver (congenital) Q44.1
- **Incompatibility**
  - ABO
    - affecting management of pregnancy O36.11-
      - anti-A sensitization O36.11-
      - anti-B sensitization O36.19-
      - specified NEC O36.19-
    - infusion or transfusion reaction — *see* Complication(s), transfusion, incompatibility reaction, ABO
    - newborn P55.1
- **Incompatibility** - *continued*
  - blood (group) (Duffy) (K) (Kell) (Kidd) (Lewis) (M) (S) NEC
    - affecting management of pregnancy O36.11-
      - anti-A sensitization O36.11-
      - anti-B sensitization O36.19-
    - infusion or transfusion reaction T80.89
    - newborn P55.8
  - divorce or estrangement Z63.5
  - Rh (blood group) (factor) Z31.82
    - affecting management of pregnancy NEC O36.09-
      - anti-D antibody O36.01-
    - infusion or transfusion reaction — *see* Complication(s), transfusion, incompatibility reaction, Rh (factor)
    - newborn P55.0
  - rhesus — *see* Incompatibility, Rh
- **Incompetency, incompetent, incompetence**
  - annular
    - aortic (valve) — *see* Insufficiency, aortic
    - mitral (valve) I34.0
    - pulmonary valve (heart) I37.1
  - aortic (valve) — *see* Insufficiency, aortic
  - cardiac valve — *see* Endocarditis
  - cervix, cervical (os) N88.3
    - in pregnancy O34.3-
  - chronotropic I45.89
    - with
      - autonomic dysfunction G90.8
      - ischemic heart disease I25.89
      - left ventricular dysfunction I51.89
      - sinus node dysfunction I49.8
  - esophagogastric (junction) (sphincter) K22.0
  - mitral (valve) — *see* Insufficiency, mitral
  - pelvic fundus N81.89
  - pubocervical tissue N81.82
  - pulmonary valve (heart) I37.1
    - congenital Q22.3
  - rectovaginal tissue N81.83
  - tricuspid (annular) (valve) — *see* Insufficiency, tricuspid
  - valvular — *see* Endocarditis
    - congenital Q24.8
  - vein, venous (saphenous) (varicose) — *see* Varix, leg
- **Incomplete** — *see also* condition
  - bladder, emptying R33.9
  - defecation R15.0
  - expansion lungs (newborn) NEC — *see* Atelectasis
  - rotation, intestine Q43.3
- **Inconclusive**
  - diagnostic imaging due to excess body fat of patient R93.9
  - findings on diagnostic imaging of breast NEC R92.8
  - mammogram (due to dense breasts) R92.2
- **Incontinence** R32
  - anal sphincter R15.9
  - coital N39.491
  - feces R15.9
    - nonorganic origin F98.1
  - insensible (urinary) N39.42
  - overflow N39.490
  - postural (urinary) N39.492
  - psychogenic F45.8
  - rectal R15.9
  - reflex N39.498
  - stress (female) (male) N39.3
    - and urge N39.46
  - urethral sphincter R32
  - urge N39.41
    - and stress (female) (male) N39.46
  - urine (urinary) R32
    - continuous N39.45
    - due to cognitive impairment, or severe physical disability or immobility R39.81
    - functional R39.81
    - insensible N39.42
    - mixed (stress and urge) N39.46
    - nocturnal N39.44
    - nonorganic origin F98.0

Incontinence - *continued*
urine (urinary) - *continued*
overflow N39.490
post dribbling N39.43
postural N39.492
reflex N39.498
specified NEC N39.498
stress (female) (male) N39.3
and urge N39.46
total N39.498
unaware N39.42
urge N39.41
and stress (female) (male) N39.46
Incontinentia pigmenti Q82.3
Incoordinate, incoordination
esophageal-pharyngeal (newborn) — *see* Dysphagia
muscular R27.8
uterus (action) (contractions) (complicating delivery) O62.4
Increase, increased
abnormal, in development R63.8
androgens (ovarian) E28.1
anticoagulants (antithrombin) (anti-VIIIa) (anti-IXa) (anti-Xa) (anti-XIa) — *see* Circulating anticoagulants
cold sense R20.8
estrogen E28.0
function
adrenal
cortex — *see* Cushing's, syndrome
medulla E27.5
pituitary (gland) (anterior) (lobe) E22.9
posterior E22.2
heat sense R20.8
intracranial pressure (benign) G93.2
permeability, capillaries I78.8
pressure, intracranial G93.2
secretion
gastrin E16.4
glucagon E16.3
pancreas, endocrine E16.9
growth hormone-releasing hormone E16.8
pancreatic polypeptide E16.8
somatostatin E16.8
vasoactive-intestinal polypeptide E16.8
sphericity, lens Q12.4
splenic activity D73.1
venous pressure I87.8
portal K76.6
Increta placenta O43.22-
Incrustation, cornea, foreign body (lead) (zinc) — *see* Foreign body, cornea
Incyclophoria H50.54
Incyclotropia — *see* Cyclotropia
Indeterminate sex Q56.4
India rubber skin Q82.8
Indigestion (acid) (bilious) (functional) K30
catarrhal K31.89
due to decomposed food NOS A05.9
nervous F45.8
psychogenic F45.8
Indirect — *see* condition
Induratio penis plastica N48.6
Induration, indurated
brain G93.89
breast (fibrous) N64.51
puerperal, postpartum O92.29
broad ligament N83.8
chancre
anus A51.1
congenital A50.07
extragenital NEC A51.2
corpora cavernosa (penis) (plastic) N48.6
liver (chronic) K76.89
lung (black) (chronic) (fibroid) — *see also* Fibrosis, lung J84.10
essential brown J84.03
penile (plastic) N48.6
phlebitic — *see* Phlebitis
skin R23.4
Inebriety (without dependence) — *see* Alcohol, intoxication
Inefficiency, kidney N28.9
Inelasticity, skin R23.4
Inequality, leg (length) (acquired) — *see also* Deformity, limb, unequal length
congenital — *see* Defect, reduction, lower limb
lower leg — *see* Deformity, limb, unequal length
Inertia
bladder (neurogenic) N31.2
stomach K31.89
psychogenic F45.8
uterus, uterine during labor O62.2
during latent phase of labor O62.0
primary O62.0
secondary O62.1
vesical (neurogenic) N31.2
Infancy, infantile, infantilism — *see also* condition
celiac K90.0
genitalia, genitals (after puberty) E30.0
Herter's (nontropical sprue) K90.0
intestinal K90.0
Lorain E23.0
pancreatic K86.89
pelvis M95.5
with disproportion (fetopelvic) O33.1
causing obstructed labor O65.1
pituitary E23.0
renal N25.0
uterus — *see* Infantile, genitalia
Infant (s) — *see also* Infancy
excessive crying R68.11
irritable child R68.12
lack of care — *see* Neglect
liveborn (singleton) Z38.2
born in hospital Z38.00
by cesarean Z38.01
born outside hospital Z38.1
multiple NEC Z38.8
born in hospital Z38.68
by cesarean Z38.69
born outside hospital Z38.7
quadruplet Z38.8
born in hospital Z38.63
by cesarean Z38.64
born outside hospital Z38.7
quintuplet Z38.8
born in hospital Z38.65
by cesarean Z38.66
born outside hospital Z38.7
triplet Z38.8
born in hospital Z38.61
by cesarean Z38.62
born outside hospital Z38.7
twin Z38.5
born in hospital Z38.30
by cesarean Z38.31
born outside hospital Z38.4
of diabetic mother (syndrome of) P70.1
gestational diabetes P70.0
Infantile — *see also* condition
genitalia, genitals E30.0
os, uterine E30.0
penis E30.0
testis E29.1
uterus E30.0
Infantilism — *see* Infancy
Infarct, infarction
adrenal (capsule) (gland) E27.49
appendices epiploicae — *see also* Infarct, intestine K55.069
bowel — *see also* Infarct, intestine K55.069
brain (stem) — *see* Infarct, cerebral
breast N64.89
brewer's (kidney) N28.0
cardiac — *see* Infarct, myocardium
cerebellar — *see* Infarct, cerebral
cerebral (acute) (chronic) — *see also* Occlusion, artery cerebral or precerebral, with infarction I63.9-
aborted I63.9
cortical I63.9
due to
cerebral venous thrombosis, nonpyogenic I63.6
Infarct, infarction - *continued*
cerebral (acute) (chronic) - *continued*
due to - *continued*
embolism
cerebral arteries I63.4-
precerebral arteries I63.1-
occlusion NEC
cerebral arteries I63.5-
precerebral arteries I63.2-
small artery I63.81
stenosis NEC
cerebral arteries I63.5-
precerebral arteries I63.2-
small artery I63.81
thrombosis
cerebral artery I63.3-
precerebral artery I63.0-
intraoperative
during cardiac surgery I97.810
during other surgery I97.811
neonatal P91.82-
perinatal (arterial ischemic) P91.82-
postprocedural
following cardiac surgery I97.820
following other surgery I97.821
specified NEC I63.89
colon (acute) (agnogenic) (embolic) (hemorrhagic) (nonocclusive) (nonthrombotic) (occlusive) (segmental) (thrombotic) (with gangrene) — *see also* Infarct, intestine K55.049
coronary artery — *see* Infarct, myocardium
embolic — *see* Embolism
fallopian tube N83.8
gallbladder K82.8
heart — *see* Infarct, myocardium
hepatic K76.3
hypophysis (anterior lobe) E23.6
impending (myocardium) I20.0
intestine (acute) (agnogenic) (embolic) (hemorrhagic) (nonocclusive) (nonthrombotic) (occlusive) (thrombotic) (with gangrene) K55.069
diffuse K55.062
focal K55.061
large K55.049
diffuse K55.042
focal K55.041
small K55.029
diffuse K55.022
focal K55.021
kidney N28.0
lacunar I63.81
liver K76.3
lung (embolic) (thrombotic) — *see* Embolism, pulmonary
lymph node I89.8
mesentery, mesenteric (embolic) (thrombotic) (with gangrene) — *see also* Infarct, intestine K55.069
muscle (ischemic) M62.20
ankle M62.27-
foot M62.27-
forearm M62.23-
hand M62.24-
lower leg M62.26-
pelvic region M62.25-
shoulder region M62.21-
specified site NEC M62.28
thigh M62.25-
upper arm M62.22-
myocardium, myocardial (acute) (with stated duration of 4 weeks or less) I21.9
associated with revascularization procedure I21.A9
diagnosed on ECG, but presenting no symptoms I25.2
due to
demand ischemia I21.A1
ischemic imbalance I21.A1
healed or old I25.2
intraoperative — *see also* Infarct, myocardium, associated with revascularization procedure
during cardiac surgery I97.790

Infarct, infarction - *continued*
myocardium, myocardial (acute) (with stated duration of 4 weeks or less) - *continued*
intraoperative - *continued*
during other surgery I97.791
non-Q wave I21.4
non-ST elevation (NSTEMI) I21.4
subsequent I22.2
nontransmural I21.4
past (diagnosed on ECG or other investigation, but currently presenting no symptoms) I25.2
postprocedural — *see also* Infarct, myocardium, associated with revascularization procedure
following cardiac surgery surgery — *see also* Infarct, myocardium, type 4 or type 5 I97.190
following other surgery I97.191
Q wave (see also, Infarct, myocardium, by site) I21.3
secondary to
demand ischemia I21.A1
ischemic imbalance I21.A1
ST elevation (STEMI) I21.3
anterior (anteroapical) (anterolateral) (anteroseptal) (Q wave) (wall) I21.09
subsequent I22.0
inferior (diaphragmatic) (inferolateral) (inferoposterior) (wall) NEC I21.19
subsequent I22.1
inferoposterior transmural (Q wave) I21.11
involving
coronary artery of anterior wall NEC I21.09
coronary artery of inferior wall NEC I21.19
diagonal coronary artery I21.02
left anterior descending coronary artery I21.02
left circumflex coronary artery I21.21
left main coronary artery I21.01
oblique marginal coronary artery I21.21
right coronary artery I21.11
lateral (apical-lateral) (basal-lateral) (high) I21.29
subsequent I22.8
posterior (posterobasal) (posterolateral) (posteroseptal) (true) I21.29
subsequent I22.8
septal I21.29
subsequent I22.8
specified NEC I21.29
subsequent I22.8
subsequent I22.9
subsequent (recurrent) (reinfarction) I22.9
anterior (anteroapical) (anterolateral) (anteroseptal) (wall) I22.0
diaphragmatic (wall) I22.1
inferior (diaphragmatic) (inferolateral) (inferoposterior) (wall) I22.1
lateral (apical-lateral) (basal-lateral) (high) I22.8
non-ST elevation (NSTEMI) I22.2
posterior (posterobasal) (posterolateral) (posteroseptal) (true) I22.8
septal I22.8
specified NEC I22.8
ST elevation I22.9
anterior (anteroapical) (anterolateral) (anteroseptal) (wall) I22.0
inferior (diaphragmatic) (inferolateral) (inferoposterior) (wall) I22.1
specified NEC I22.8
subendocardial I22.2
transmural I21.3
anterior (anteroapical) (anterolateral) (anteroseptal) (wall) I22.0
diaphragmatic (wall) I22.1
inferior (diaphragmatic) (inferolateral) (inferoposterior) (wall) I22.1

Infarct, infarction - *continued*
myocardium, myocardial (acute) (with stated duration of 4 weeks or less) - *continued*
subsequent (recurrent) (reinfarction) - *continued*
transmural - *continued*
lateral (apical-lateral) (basal-lateral) (high) I22.8
posterior (posterobasal) (posterolateral) (posteroseptal) (true) I22.8
specified NEC I22.8
type 1 — *see also* Infarction, myocardial, subsequent, by site, or by ST elevation or non-ST elevation I22.9
type 2 I21.A1
type 3 I21.A9
type 4 I21.A9
type 5 I21.A9
syphilitic A52.06
transmural I21.9
anterior (anteroapical) (anterolateral) (anteroseptal) (Q wave) (wall) NEC I21.09
inferior (diaphragmatic) (inferolateral) (inferoposterior) (Q wave) (wall) NEC I21.19
inferoposterior (Q wave) I21.11
lateral (apical-lateral) (basal-lateral) (high) NEC I21.29
posterior (posterobasal) (posterolateral) (posteroseptal) (true) NEC I21.29
septal NEC I21.29
specified NEC I21.29
type 1 — *see also* Infarction, myocardial, by site, or by ST elevation or non-ST elevation I21.9
type 2 I21.A1
type 3 I21.A9
type 4 (a) (b) (c) I21.A9
type 5 I21.A9
nontransmural I21.4
omentum — *see also* Infarct, intestine K55.069
ovary N83.8
pancreas K86.89
papillary muscle — *see* Infarct, myocardium
parathyroid gland E21.4
pituitary (gland) E23.6
placenta O43.81-
prostate N42.89
pulmonary (artery) (vein) (hemorrhagic) — *see* Embolism, pulmonary
renal (embolic) (thrombotic) N28.0
retina, retinal (artery) — *see* Occlusion, artery, retina
spinal (cord) (acute) (embolic) (nonembolic) G95.11
spleen D73.5
embolic or thrombotic I74.8
subendocardial (acute) (nontransmural) I21.4
suprarenal (capsule) (gland) E27.49
testis N50.1
thrombotic — *see also* Thrombosis
artery, arterial — *see* Embolism
thyroid (gland) E07.89
ventricle (heart) — *see* Infarct, myocardium
Infecting — *see* condition
Infection, infected, infective (opportunistic) B99.9
with
drug resistant organism — *see* Resistance (to), drug — *see also* specific organism
lymphangitis — *see* Lymphangitis
organ dysfunction (acute) R65.20
with septic shock R65.21
abscess (skin) - code by site under Abscess
Absidia — *see* Mucormycosis
Acanthamoeba — *see* Acanthamebiasis
Acanthocheilonema (perstans) (streptocerca) B74.4
accessory sinus (chronic) — *see* Sinusitis
achorion — *see* Dermatophytosis

Infection, infected, infective (opportunistic) - *continued*
Acremonium falciforme B47.0
acromioclavicular M00.9
Actinobacillus (actinomycetem-comitans) A28.8
mallei A24.0
muris A25.1
Actinomadura B47.1
Actinomyces (israelii) — *see also* Actinomycosis A42.9
Actinomycetales — *see* Actinomycosis
actinomycotic NOS — *see* Actinomycosis
adenoid (and tonsil) J03.90
chronic J35.02
adenovirus NEC
as cause of disease classified elsewhere B97.0
unspecified nature or site B34.0
aerogenes capsulatus A48.0
aertrycke — *see* Infection, salmonella
alimentary canal NOS — *see* Enteritis, infectious
Allescheria boydii B48.2
Alternaria B48.8
alveolus, alveolar (process) K04.7
Ameba, amebic (histolytica) — *see* Amebiasis
amniotic fluid, sac or cavity O41.10-
chorioamnionitis O41.12-
placentitis O41.14-
amputation stump (surgical) — *see* Complication, amputation stump, infection
Ancylostoma (duodenalis) B76.0
Anisakiasis, Anisakis larvae B81.0
anthrax — *see* Anthrax
antrum (chronic) — *see* Sinusitis, maxillary
anus, anal (papillae) (sphincter) K62.89
arbovirus (arbor virus) A94
specified type NEC A93.8
artificial insemination N98.0
Ascaris lumbricoides — *see* Ascariasis
Ascomycetes B47.0
Aspergillus (flavus) (fumigatus) (terreus) — *see* Aspergillosis
atypical
acid-fast (bacilli) — *see* Mycobacterium, atypical
mycobacteria — *see* Mycobacterium, atypical
virus A81.9
specified type NEC A81.89
auditory meatus (external) — *see* Otitis, externa, infective
auricle (ear) — *see* Otitis, externa, infective
axillary gland (lymph) L04.2
Bacillus A49.9
abortus A23.1
anthracis — *see* Anthrax
Ducrey's (any location) A57
Flexner's A03.1
Friedländer's NEC A49.8
gas (gangrene) A48.0
mallei A24.0
melitensis A23.0
paratyphoid, paratyphosus A01.4
A A01.1
B A01.2
C A01.3
Shiga (-Kruse) A03.0
suipestifer — *see* Infection, salmonella
swimming pool A31.1
typhosa A01.00
welchii — *see* Gangrene, gas
bacterial NOS A49.9
as cause of disease classified elsewhere B96.89
Clostridium perfringens [C. perfringens] B96.7
Bacteroides fragilis [B. fragilis] B96.6
Enterobacter sakazakii B96.89
Enterococcus B95.2
Escherichia coli [E. coli] — *see also* Escherichia coli B96.20

Infection, infected, infective (opportunistic) - *continued*
bacterial NOS - *continued*
as cause of disease classified elsewhere - *continued*
Helicobacter pylori [H.pylori] B96.81
Hemophilus influenzae [H. influenzae] B96.3
Klebsiella pneumoniae [K. pneumoniae] B96.1
Mycoplasma pneumoniae [M. pneumoniae] B96.0
Proteus (mirabilis) (morganii) B96.4
Pseudomonas (aeruginosa) (mallei) (pseudomallei) B96.5
Staphylococcus B95.8
aureus (methicillin susceptible) (MSSA) B95.61
methicillin resistant (MRSA) B95.62
specified NEC B95.7
Streptococcus B95.5
group A B95.0
group B B95.1
pneumoniae B95.3
specified NEC B95.4
Vibrio vulnificus B96.82
specified NEC A48.8
Bacterium
paratyphosum A01.4
A A01.1
B A01.2
C A01.3
typhosum A01.00
Bacteroides NEC A49.8
fragilis, as cause of disease classified elsewhere B96.6
Balantidium coli A07.0
Bartholin's gland N75.8
Basidiobolus B46.8
bile duct (common) (hepatic) — *see* Cholangitis
bladder — *see* Cystitis
Blastomyces, blastomycotic — *see also* Blastomycosis
brasiliensis — *see* Paracoccidioidomycosis
dermatitidis — *see* Blastomycosis
European — *see* Cryptococcosis
Loboi B48.0
North American B40.9
South American — *see* Paracoccidioidomycosis
bleb, postprocedure — *see* Blebitis
bone — *see* Osteomyelitis
Bordetella — *see* Whooping cough
Borrelia bergdorfi A69.20
brain — *see also* Encephalitis G04.90
membranes — *see* Meningitis
septic G06.0
meninges — *see* Meningitis, bacterial
branchial cyst Q18.0
breast — *see* Mastitis
bronchus — *see* Bronchitis
Brucella A23.9
abortus A23.1
canis A23.3
melitensis A23.0
mixed A23.8
specified NEC A23.8
suis A23.2
Brugia (malayi) B74.1
timori B74.2
bursa — *see* Bursitis, infective
buttocks (skin) L08.9
Campylobacter, intestinal A04.5
as cause of disease classified elsewhere B96.81
Candida (albicans) (tropicalis) — *see* Candidiasis
candiru B88.8
Capillaria (intestinal) B81.1
hepatica B83.8
philippinensis B81.1
cartilage — *see* Disorder, cartilage, specified type NEC

Infection, infected, infective (opportunistic) - *continued*
catheter-related bloodstream (CRBSI) T80.211
cat liver fluke B66.0
cellulitis - code by site under Cellulitis
central line-associated T80.219
bloodstream (CLABSI) T80.211
specified NEC T80.218
Cephalosporium falciforme B47.0
cerebrospinal — *see* Meningitis
cervical gland (lymph) L04.0
cervix — *see* Cervicitis
cesarean delivery wound (puerperal) O86.00
cestodes — *see* Infestation, cestodes
chest J22
Chilomastix (intestinal) A07.8
Chlamydia, chlamydial A74.9
anus A56.3
genitourinary tract A56.2
lower A56.00
specified NEC A56.19
lymphogranuloma A55
pharynx A56.4
psittaci A70
rectum A56.3
sexually transmitted NEC A56.8
cholera — *see* Cholera
Cladosporium
bantianum (brain abscess) B43.1
carrionii B43.0
castellanii B36.1
trichoides (brain abscess) B43.1
werneckii B36.1
Clonorchis (sinensis) (liver) B66.1
Clostridium NEC
bifermentans A48.0
botulinum (food poisoning) A05.1
infant A48.51
wound A48.52
difficile
as cause of disease classified elsewhere B96.89
foodborne (disease)
not specified as recurrent A04.72
recurrent A04.71
gas gangrene A48.0
necrotizing enterocolitis
not specified as recurrent A04.72
recurrent A04.71
sepsis A41.4
gas-forming NEC A48.0
histolyticum A48.0
novyi, causing gas gangrene A48.0
oedematiens A48.0
perfringens
as cause of disease classified elsewhere B96.7
due to food A05.2
foodborne (disease) A05.2
gas gangrene A48.0
sepsis A41.4
septicum, causing gas gangrene A48.0
sordellii, causing gas gangrene A48.0
welchii
as cause of disease classified elsewhere B96.7
foodborne (disease) A05.2
gas gangrene A48.0
necrotizing enteritis A05.2
sepsis A41.4
Coccidioides (immitis) — *see* Coccidioidomycosis
colon — *see* Enteritis, infectious
colostomy K94.02
common duct — *see* Cholangitis
congenital P39.9
Candida (albicans) P37.5
cytomegalovirus P35.1
hepatitis, viral P35.3
herpes simplex P35.2
infectious or parasitic disease P37.9
specified NEC P37.8
listeriosis (disseminated) P37.2
malaria NEC P37.4

Infection, infected, infective (opportunistic) - *continued*
congenital - *continued*
malaria NEC - *continued*
falciparum P37.3
Plasmodium falciparum P37.3
poliomyelitis P35.8
rubella P35.0
skin P39.4
toxoplasmosis (acute) (subacute) (chronic) P37.1
tuberculosis P37.0
urinary (tract) P39.3
vaccinia P35.8
virus P35.9
specified type NEC P35.8
Conidiobolus B46.8
coronavirus-2019 U07.1
coronavirus NEC B34.2
as cause of disease classified elsewhere B97.29
severe acute respiratory syndrome (SARS associated) B97.21
corpus luteum — *see* Salpingo-oophoritis
Corynebacterium diphtheriae — *see* Diphtheria
cotia virus B08.8
COVID-19 — *see also* COVID-19 U07.1
Coxiella burnetii A78
coxsackie — *see* Coxsackie
Cryptococcus neoformans — *see* Cryptococcosis
Cryptosporidium A07.2
Cunninghamella — *see* Mucormycosis
cyst — *see* Cyst
cystic duct — *see also* Cholecystitis K81.9
Cysticercus cellulosae — *see* Cysticercosis
cytomegalovirus, cytomegaloviral B25.9
congenital P35.1
maternal, maternal care for (suspected) damage to fetus O35.3
mononucleosis B27.10
with
complication NEC B27.19
meningitis B27.12
polyneuropathy B27.11
delta-agent (acute) , in hepatitis B carrier B17.0
dental (pulpal origin) K04.7
Deuteromycetes B47.0
Dicrocoelium dendriticum B66.2
Dipetalonema (perstans) (streptocerca) B74.4
diphtherial — *see* Diphtheria
Diphyllobothrium (adult) (latum) (pacificum) B70.0
larval B70.1
Diplogonoporus (grandis) B71.8
Dipylidium caninum B67.4
Dirofilaria B74.8
Dracunculus medinensis B72
Drechslera (hawaiiensis) B43.8
Ducrey Haemophilus (any location) A57
due to or resulting from
artificial insemination N98.0
Babesia
divergens (-like) strain B60.03
duncani (-type) species B60.02
microti B60.01
species
specified NEC B60.09
central venous catheter T80.219
bloodstream T80.211
exit or insertion site T80.212
localized T80.212
port or reservoir T80.212
specified NEC T80.218
tunnel T80.212
device, implant or graft — *see also* Complications, by site and type, infection or inflammation T85.79
arterial graft NEC T82.7
breast (implant) T85.79
catheter NEC T85.79
dialysis (renal) T82.7
central line T80.211

Infection, infected, infective (opportunistic) - *continued*
due to or resulting from - *continued*
device, implant or graft - *continued*
catheter NEC - *continued*
dialysis (renal) - *continued*
intraperitoneal T85.71
infusion NEC T82.7
cranial T85.735
intrathecal T85.735
spinal (epidural) (subdural) T85.735
subarachnoid T85.735
urinary T83.518
cystostomy T83.510
Hopkins T83.518
ileostomy T83.518
nephrostomy T83.512
specified NEC T83.518
urethral indwelling T83.511
urostomy T83.518
electronic (electrode) (pulse generator) (stimulator)
bone T84.7
cardiac T82.7
nervous system T85.738
brain T85.731
cranial nerve T85.732
gastric nerve T85.732
generator pocket T85.734
neurostimulator generator T85.734
peripheral nerve T85.732
sacral nerve T85.732
spinal cord T85.733
vagal nerve T85.732
urinary T83.590
fixation, internal (orthopedic) NEC — *see* Complication, fixation device, infection
gastrointestinal (bile duct) (esophagus) T85.79
neurostimulator electrode (lead) T85.732
genital NEC T83.69
heart NEC T82.7
valve (prosthesis) T82.6
graft T82.7
joint prosthesis — *see* Complication, joint prosthesis, infection
ocular (corneal graft) (orbital implant) NEC T85.79
orthopedic NEC T84.7
penile (cylinder) (pump) (resevoir) T83.61
specified NEC T85.79
testicular T83.62
urinary NEC T83.598
ileal conduit stent T83.593
implanted neurostimulation T83.590
implanted sphincter T83.591
indwelling ureteral stent T83.592
nephroureteral stent T83.593
specified stent NEC T83.593
vascular NEC T82.7
ventricular intracranial (communicating) shunt T85.730
Hickman catheter T80.219
bloodstream T80.211
localized T80.212
specified NEC T80.218
immunization or vaccination T88.0
infusion, injection or transfusion NEC T80.29
acute T80.22
injury NEC - code by site under Wound, open
peripherally inserted central catheter (PICC) T80.219
bloodstream T80.211
localized T80.212
specified NEC T80.218
portacath (port-a-cath) T80.219
bloodstream T80.211
localized T80.212
specified NEC T80.218

Infection, infected, infective (opportunistic) - *continued*
due to or resulting from - *continued*
protozoa of the order Piroplasmida NEC B60.09
pulmonary artery catheter — *see* Infection, due to or resulting from, central venous catheter
surgery T81.40
Swan Ganz catheter — *see* Infection, due to or resulting from, central venous catheter
triple lumen catheter T80.219
bloodstream T80.211
localized T80.212
specified NEC T80.218
umbilical venous catheter T80.219
bloodstream T80.211
localized T80.212
specified NEC T80.218
during labor NEC O75.3
ear (middle) — *see also* Otitis media
external — *see* Otitis, externa, infective
inner — *see* subcategory H83.0
Eberthella typhosa A01.00
Echinococcus — *see* Echinococcus
echovirus
as cause of disease classified elsewhere B97.12
unspecified nature or site B34.1
endocardium I33.0
endocervix — *see* Cervicitis
Entamoeba — *see* Amebiasis
enteric — *see* Enteritis, infectious
Enterobacter sakazakii B96.89
Enterobius vermicularis B80
enterostomy K94.12
enterovirus B34.1
as cause of disease classified elsewhere B97.10
coxsackievirus B97.11
echovirus B97.12
specified NEC B97.19
Entomophthora B46.8
Epidermophyton — *see* Dermatophytosis
epididymis — *see* Epididymitis
episiotomy (puerperal) O86.09
Erysipelothrix (insidiosa) (rhusiopathiae) — *see* Erysipeloid
erythema infectiosum B08.3
Escherichia (E.) coli NEC A49.8
as cause of disease classified elsewhere — *see also* Escherichia coli B96.20
congenital P39.8
sepsis P36.4
generalized A41.51
intestinal — *see* Enteritis, infectious, due to, Escherichia coli
ethmoidal (chronic) (sinus) — *see* Sinusitis, ethmoidal
eustachian tube (ear) — *see* Salpingitis, eustachian
external auditory canal (meatus) NEC — *see* Otitis, externa, infective
eye (purulent) — *see* Endophthalmitis, purulent
eyelid — *see* Inflammation, eyelid
fallopian tube — *see* Salpingo-oophoritis
Fasciola (gigantica) (hepatica) (indica) B66.3
Fasciolopsis (buski) B66.5
filarial — *see* Infestation, filarial
finger (skin) L08.9
nail L03.01-
fungus B35.1
fish tapeworm B70.0
larval B70.1
flagellate, intestinal A07.9
fluke — *see* Infestation, fluke
focal
teeth (pulpal origin) K04.7
tonsils J35.01
Fonsecaea (compactum) (pedrosoi) B43.0
food — *see* Intoxication, foodborne
foot (skin) L08.9
dermatophytic fungus B35.3

Infection, infected, infective (opportunistic) - *continued*
Francisella tularensis — *see* Tularemia
frontal (sinus) (chronic) — *see* Sinusitis, frontal
fungus NOS B49
beard B35.0
dermatophytic — *see* Dermatophytosis
foot B35.3
groin B35.6
hand B35.2
nail B35.1
pathogenic to compromised host only B48.8
perianal (area) B35.6
scalp B35.0
skin B36.9
foot B35.3
hand B35.2
toenails B35.1
Fusarium B48.8
gallbladder — *see* Cholecystitis
gas bacillus — *see* Gangrene, gas
gastrointestinal — *see* Enteritis, infectious
generalized NEC — *see* Sepsis
generator pocket, implanted electronic neurostimulator T85.734
genital organ or tract
female — *see* Disease, pelvis, inflammatory
male N49.9
multiple sites N49.8
specified NEC N49.8
Ghon tubercle, primary A15.7
Giardia lamblia A07.1
gingiva (chronic) K05.10
acute K05.00
nonplaque induced K05.01
plaque induced K05.00
nonplaque induced K05.11
plaque induced K05.10
glanders A24.0
glenosporopsis B48.0
Gnathostoma (spinigerum) B83.1
Gongylonema B83.8
gonococcal — *see* Gonococcus
gram-negative bacilli NOS A49.9
guinea worm B72
gum (chronic) K05.10
acute K05.00
nonplaque induced K05.01
plaque induced K05.00
nonplaque induced K05.11
plaque induced K05.10
Haemophilus — *see* Infection, Hemophilus
heart — *see* Carditis
Helicobacter pylori A04.8
as cause of disease classified elsewhere B96.81
helminths B83.9
intestinal B82.0
mixed (types classifiable to more than one of the titles B65.0-B81.3 and B81.8) B81.4
specified type NEC B81.8
specified type NEC B83.8
Hemophilus
aegyptius, systemic A48.4
ducrey (any location) A57
influenzae NEC A49.2
as cause of disease classified elsewhere B96.3
generalized A41.3
herpes (simplex) — *see also* Herpes
congenital P35.2
disseminated B00.7
zoster B02.9
herpesvirus, herpesviral — *see* Herpes
hip (joint) NEC M00.9
due to internal joint prosthesis
left T84.52
right T84.51
skin NEC L08.9
Heterophyes (heterophyes) B66.8
Histoplasma — *see* Histoplasmosis

Infection, infected, infective (opportunistic) - *continued*
Pasteurella NEC - *continued*
pseudotuberculosis A28.0
septica (cat bite) (dog bite) A28.0
tularensis — *see* Tularemia
pelvic, female — *see* Disease, pelvis, inflammatory
Penicillium (marneffei) B48.4
penis (glans) (retention) NEC N48.29
periapical K04.5
peridental, periodontal K05.20
generalized — *see* Periodontitis, aggressive, generalized
localized — *see* Periodontitis, aggressive, localized
perinatal period P39.9
specified type NEC P39.8
perineal repair (puerperal) O86.09
periorbital — *see* Inflammation, orbit
perirectal K62.89
perirenal — *see* Infection, kidney
peritoneal — *see* Peritonitis
periureteral N28.89
Petriellidium boydii B48.2
pharynx — *see also* Pharyngitis
coxsackievirus B08.5
posterior, lymphoid (chronic) J35.03
Phialophora
gougerotii (subcutaneous abscess or cyst) B43.2
jeanselmei (subcutaneous abscess or cyst) B43.2
verrucosa (skin) B43.0
Piedraia hortae B36.3
pinta A67.9
intermediate A67.1
late A67.2
mixed A67.3
primary A67.0
pinworm B80
pityrosporum furfur B36.0
pleuro-pneumonia-like organism (PPLO) NEC A49.3
as cause of disease classified elsewhere B96.0
pneumococcus, pneumococcal NEC A49.1
as cause of disease classified elsewhere B95.3
generalized (purulent) A40.3
with pneumonia J13
Pneumocystis carinii (pneumonia) B59
Pneumocystis jiroveci (pneumonia) B59
port or reservoir T80.212
postoperative T81.40
postoperative wound T81.49
surgical site
deep incisional T81.42
organ and space T81.43
specified NEC T81.49
superficial incisional T81.41
postprocedural T81.40
postvaccinal T88.0
prepuce NEC N47.7
with penile inflammation N47.6
prion — *see* Disease, prion, central nervous system
prostate (capsule) — *see* Prostatitis
Proteus (mirabilis) (morganii) (vulgaris) NEC A49.8
as cause of disease classified elsewhere B96.4
protozoal NEC B64
intestinal A07.9
specified NEC A07.8
specified NEC B60.8
Pseudoallescheria boydii B48.2
Pseudomonas NEC A49.8
as cause of disease classified elsewhere B96.5
mallei A24.0
pneumonia J15.1
pseudomallei — *see* Melioidosis
puerperal O86.4
genitourinary tract NEC O86.89

Infection, infected, infective (opportunistic) - *continued*
puerperal - *continued*
major or generalized O85
minor O86.4
specified NEC O86.89
pulmonary — *see* Infection, lung
purulent — *see* Abscess
Pyrenochaeta romeroi B47.0
Q fever A78
rectum (sphincter) K62.89
renal — *see also* Infection, kidney
pelvis and ureter (cystic) N28.85
reovirus, as cause of disease classified elsewhere B97.5
respiratory (tract) NEC J98.8
acute J22
chronic J98.8
influenzal (upper) (acute) — *see* Influenza, with, respiratory manifestations NEC
lower (acute) J22
chronic — *see* Bronchitis, chronic
rhinovirus J00
syncytial virus (RSV) — *see* Infection, virus, respiratory syncytial (RSV)
upper (acute) NOS J06.9
chronic J39.8
streptococcal J06.9
viral NOS J06.9
due to respiratory syncytial virus (RSV) J06.9 *[B97.4]*
resulting from
presence of internal prosthesis, implant, graft — *see* Complications, by site and type, infection
retortamoniasis A07.8
retroperitoneal NEC K68.9
retrovirus B33.3
as cause of disease classified elsewhere B97.30
human
immunodeficiency, type 2 (HIV 2) B97.35
T-cell lymphotropic
type I (HTLV-I) B97.33
type II (HTLV-II) B97.34
lentivirus B97.31
oncovirus B97.32
specified NEC B97.39
Rhinosporidium (seeberi) B48.1
rhinovirus
as cause of disease classified elsewhere B97.89
unspecified nature or site B34.8
Rhizopus — *see* Mucormycosis
rickettsial NOS A79.9
roundworm (large) NEC B82.0
Ascariasis — *see also* Ascariasis B77.9
rubella — *see* Rubella
Saccharomyces — *see* Candidiasis
salivary duct or gland (any) — *see* Sialoadenitis
Salmonella (aertrycke) (arizonae) (callinarum) (cholerae-suis) (enteritidis) (suipestifer) (typhimurium) A02.9
with
(gastro) enteritis A02.0
sepsis A02.1
specified manifestation NEC A02.8
due to food (poisoning) A02.9
hirschfeldii A01.3
localized A02.20
arthritis A02.23
meningitis A02.21
osteomyelitis A02.24
pneumonia A02.22
pyelonephritis A02.25
specified NEC A02.29
paratyphi A01.4
A A01.1
B A01.2
C A01.3
schottmuelleri A01.2
typhi, typhosa — *see* Typhoid
Sarcocystis A07.8

Infection, infected, infective (opportunistic) - *continued*
SARS-CoV-2 — *see* Infection, COVID-19
scabies B86
Schistosoma — *see* Infestation, Schistosoma
scrotum (acute) NEC N49.2
seminal vesicle — *see* Vesiculitis
septic
localized, skin — *see* Abscess
sheep liver fluke B66.3
Shigella A03.9
boydii A03.2
dysenteriae A03.0
flexneri A03.1
group
A A03.0
B A03.1
C A03.2
D A03.3
Schmitz (-Stutzer) A03.0
schmitzii A03.0
shigae A03.0
sonnei A03.3
specified NEC A03.8
shoulder (joint) NEC M00.9
due to internal joint prosthesis T84.59
skin NEC L08.9
sinus (accessory) (chronic) (nasal) — *see also* Sinusitis
pilonidal — *see* Sinus, pilonidal
skin NEC L08.89
Skene's duct or gland — *see* Urethritis
skin (local) (staphylococcal) (streptococcal) L08.9
abscess - code by site under Abscess
cellulitis - code by site under Cellulitis
due to fungus B36.9
specified type NEC B36.8
mycotic B36.9
specified type NEC B36.8
newborn P39.4
ulcer — *see* Ulcer, skin
slow virus A81.9
specified NEC A81.89
Sparganum (mansoni) (proliferum) (baxteri) B70.1
specific — *see also* Syphilis
to perinatal period — *see* Infection, congenital
specified NEC B99.8
spermatic cord NEC N49.1
sphenoidal (sinus) — *see* Sinusitis, sphenoidal
spinal cord NOS — *see also* Myelitis G04.91
abscess G06.1
meninges — *see* Meningitis
streptococcal G04.89
Spirillum A25.0
spirochetal NOS A69.9
lung A69.8
specified NEC A69.8
Spirometra larvae B70.1
spleen D73.89
Sporotrichum, Sporothrix (schenckii) — *see* Sporotrichosis
staphylococcal, unspecified site
aureus (methicillin susceptible) (MSSA) A49.01
methicillin resistant (MRSA) A49.02
as cause of disease classified elsewhere B95.8
aureus (methicillin susceptible) (MSSA) B95.61
methicillin resistant (MRSA) B95.62
specified NEC B95.7
food poisoning A05.0
generalized (purulent) A41.2
pneumonia — *see* Pneumonia, staphylococcal
Stellantchasmus falcatus B66.8
streptobacillus moniliformis A25.1
streptococcal NEC A49.1
as cause of disease classified elsewhere B95.5
B genitourinary complicating

Infection, infected, infective (opportunistic) - *continued*
streptococcal NEC - *continued*
B genitourinary complicating - *continued*
childbirth O98.82
pregnancy O98.81-
puerperium O98.83
congenital
sepsis P36.10
group B P36.0
specified NEC P36.19
generalized (purulent) A40.9
Streptomyces B47.1
Strongyloides (stercoralis) — *see* Strongyloidiasis
stump (amputation) (surgical) — *see* Complication, amputation stump, infection
subcutaneous tissue, local L08.9
suipestifer — *see* Infection, salmonella
swimming pool bacillus A31.1
Taenia — *see* Infestation, Taenia
Taeniarhynchus saginatus B68.1
tapeworm — *see* Infestation, tapeworm
tendon (sheath) — *see* Tenosynovitis, infective NEC
Ternidens diminutus B81.8
testis — *see* Orchitis
threadworm B80
throat — *see* Pharyngitis
thyroglossal duct K14.8
toe (skin) L08.9
cellulitis L03.03-
fungus B35.1
nail L03.03-
fungus B35.1
tongue NEC K14.0
parasitic B37.0
tonsil (and adenoid) (faucial) (lingual) (pharyngeal) — *see* Tonsillitis
tooth, teeth K04.7
periapical K04.7
peridental, periodontal K05.20
generalized — *see* Periodontitis, aggressive, generalized
localized — *see* Periodontitis, aggressive, localized
pulp K04.01
irreversible K04.02
reversible K04.01
socket M27.3
TORCH — *see* Infection, congenital
without active infection P00.2
Torula histolytica — *see* Cryptococcosis
Toxocara (canis) (cati) (felis) B83.0
Toxoplasma gondii — *see* Toxoplasma
trachea, chronic J42
trematode NEC — *see* Infestation, fluke
trench fever A79.0
Treponema pallidum — *see* Syphilis
Trichinella (spiralis) B75
Trichomonas A59.9
cervix A59.09
intestine A07.8
prostate A59.02
specified site NEC A59.8
urethra A59.03
urogenitalis A59.00
vagina A59.01
vulva A59.01
Trichophyton, trichophytic — *see* Dermatophytosis
Trichosporon (beigelii) cutaneum B36.2
Trichostrongylus B81.2
Trichuris (trichiura) B79
Trombicula (irritans) B88.0
Trypanosoma
brucei
gambiense B56.0
rhodesiense B56.1
cruzi — *see* Chagas' disease
tubal — *see* Salpingo-oophoritis
tuberculous
latent (LTBI) Z22.7
NEC — *see* Tuberculosis

Infection, infected, infective (opportunistic) - *continued*
tubo-ovarian — *see* Salpingo-oophoritis
tunnel T80.212
tunica vaginalis N49.1
tympanic membrane NEC — *see* Myringitis
typhoid (abortive) (ambulant) (bacillus) — *see* Typhoid
typhus A75.9
flea-borne A75.2
mite-borne A75.3
recrudescent A75.1
tick-borne A77.9
African A77.1
North Asian A77.2
umbilicus L08.82
ureter — *see* Ureteritis
urethra — *see* Urethritis
urinary (tract) N39.0
bladder — *see* Cystitis
complicating
pregnancy O23.4-
specified type NEC O23.3-
kidney — *see* Infection, kidney
newborn P39.3
puerperal (postpartum) O86.20
tuberculous A18.13
urethra — *see* Urethritis
uterus, uterine — *see* Endometritis
vaccination T88.0
vaccinia not from vaccination B08.011
vagina (acute) — *see* Vaginitis
varicella B01.9
varicose veins — *see* Varix
vas deferens NEC N49.1
vesical — *see* Cystitis
Vibrio
cholerae A00.0
El Tor A00.1
parahaemolyticus (food poisoning) A05.3
vulnificus
as cause of disease classified elsewhere B96.82
foodborne intoxication A05.5
Vincent's (gum) (mouth) (tonsil) A69.1
virus, viral NOS B34.9
adenovirus
as cause of disease classified elsewhere B97.0
unspecified nature or site B34.0
arborvirus, arbovirus arthropod-borne A94
as cause of disease classified elsewhere B97.89
adenovirus B97.0
coronavirus B97.29
SARS-associated B97.21
coxsackievirus B97.11
echovirus B97.12
enterovirus B97.10
coxsackievirus B97.11
echovirus B97.12
specified NEC B97.19
human
immunodeficiency, type 2 (HIV 2) B97.35
T-cell lymphotropic,
type I (HTLV-I) B97.33
type II (HTLV-II) B97.34
metapneumovirus B97.81
papillomavirus B97.7
parvovirus B97.6
reovirus B97.5
respiratory syncytial (RSV) — *see* Infection, virus, respiratory syncytial (RSV)
retrovirus B97.30
human
immunodeficiency, type 2 (HIV 2) B97.35
T-cell lymphotropic,
type I (HTLV-I) B97.33
type II (HTLV-II) B97.34
lentivirus B97.31
oncovirus B97.32
specified NEC B97.39

Infection, infected, infective (opportunistic) - *continued*
virus, viral NOS - *continued*
as cause of disease classified elsewhere - *continued*
specified NEC B97.89
central nervous system A89
atypical A81.9
specified NEC A81.89
enterovirus NEC A88.8
meningitis A87.0
slow virus A81.9
specified NEC A81.89
specified NEC A88.8
chest J98.8
cotia B08.8
COVID-19 U07.1
coxsackie — *see also* Infection, coxsackie B34.1
as cause of disease classified elsewhere B97.11
ECHO
as cause of disease classified elsewhere B97.12
unspecified nature or site B34.1
encephalitis, tick-borne A84.9
enterovirus, as cause of disease classified elsewhere B97.10
coxsackievirus B97.11
echovirus B97.12
specified NEC B97.19
exanthem NOS B09
human papilloma as cause of disease classified elsewhere B97.7
human metapneumovirus as cause of disease classified elsewhere B97.81
intestine — *see* Enteritis, viral
respiratory syncytial (RSV)
as cause of disease classified elsewhere B97.4
bronchiolitis J21.0
bronchitis J20.5
bronchopneumonia J12.1
otitis media H65.- *[B97.4]*
pneumonia J12.1
upper respiratory infection J06.9 *[B97.4]*
rhinovirus
as cause of disease classified elsewhere B97.89
unspecified nature or site B34.8
slow A81.9
specified NEC A81.89
specified type NEC B33.8
as cause of disease classified elsewhere B97.89
unspecified nature or site B34.8
unspecified nature or site B34.9
West Nile — *see* Virus, West Nile
vulva (acute) — *see* Vulvitis
West Nile — *see* Virus, West Nile
whipworm B79
worms B83.9
specified type NEC B83.8
Wuchereria (bancrofti) B74.0
malayi B74.1
yatapoxvirus B08.70
specified NEC B08.79
yeast — *see also* Candidiasis B37.9
yellow fever — *see* Fever, yellow
Yersinia
enterocolitica (intestinal) A04.6
pestis — *see* Plague
pseudotuberculosis A28.2
Zeis' gland — *see* Hordeolum
Zika virus A92.5
congenital P35.4
zoonotic bacterial NOS A28.9
Zopfia senegalensis B47.0
Infective, infectious — *see* condition
Infertility
female N97.9
age-related N97.8
associated with
anovulation N97.0

Infestation - *continued*
  parasite, parasitic - *continued*
    tongue B37.0
  Parastrongylus
    cantonensis B83.2
    costaricensis B81.3
  Pediculus B85.2
    body B85.1
    capitis (humanus) (any site) B85.0
    corporis (humanus) (any site) B85.1
    head B85.0
    mixed (classifiable to more than one of the titles B85.0-B85.3) B85.4
    pubis (any site) B85.3
  Pentastoma B88.8
  Phthirus (pubis) (any site) B85.3
    with any infestation classifiable to B85.0-B85.2 B85.4
  pinworm B80
  pork tapeworm (adult) B68.0
  protozoal NEC B64
    intestinal A07.9
      specified NEC A07.8
    specified NEC B60.8
  pubic, louse B85.3
  rat tapeworm B71.0
  red bug B88.0
  roundworm (large) NEC B82.0
    Ascariasis — *see also* Ascariasis B77.9
  sandflea B88.1
  Sarcoptes scabiei B86
  scabies B86
  Schistosoma B65.9
    bovis B65.8
    cercariae B65.3
    haematobium B65.0
    intercalatum B65.8
    japonicum B65.2
    mansoni B65.1
    mattheei B65.8
    mekongi B65.8
    specified type NEC B65.8
    spindale B65.8
  screw worms — *see* Myiasis
  skin NOS B88.9
  Sparganum (mansoni) (proliferum) (baxteri) B70.1
    larval B70.1
  specified type NEC B88.8
  Spirometra larvae B70.1
  Stellantchasmus falcatus B66.8
  Strongyloides stercoralis — *see* Strongyloidiasis
  Taenia B68.9
    diminuta B71.0
    echinococcus — *see* Echinococcus
    mediocanellata B68.1
    nana B71.0
    saginata B68.1
    solium (intestinal form) B68.0
      larval form — *see* Cysticercosis
  Taeniarhynchus saginatus B68.1
  tapeworm B71.9
    beef B68.1
    broad B70.0
      larval B70.1
    dog B67.4
    dwarf B71.0
    fish B70.0
      larval B70.1
    pork B68.0
    rat B71.0
  Ternidens diminutus B81.8
  Tetranychus molestissimus B88.0
  threadworm B80
  tongue B37.0
  Toxocara (canis) (cati) (felis) B83.0
  trematode (s) NEC — *see* Infestation, fluke
  Trichinella (spiralis) B75
  Trichocephalus B79
  Trichomonas — *see* Trichomoniasis
  Trichostrongylus B81.2
  Trichuris (trichiura) B79
  Trombicula (irritans) B88.0
  Tunga penetrans B88.1

Infestation - *continued*
  Uncinaria americana B76.1
  Vandellia cirrhosa B88.8
  whipworm B79
  worms B83.9
    intestinal B82.0
  Wuchereria (bancrofti) B74.0
Infiltrate, infiltration
  amyloid (generalized) (localized) — *see* Amyloidosis
  calcareous NEC R89.7
    localized — *see* Degeneration, by site
  calcium salt R89.7
  cardiac
    fatty — *see* Degeneration, myocardial
    glycogenic E74.02 *[I43]*
  corneal — *see* Edema, cornea
  eyelid — *see* Inflammation, eyelid
  glycogen, glycogenic — *see* Disease, glycogen storage
  heart, cardiac
    fatty — *see* Degeneration, myocardial
    glycogenic E74.02 *[I43]*
  inflammatory in vitreous H43.89
  kidney N28.89
  leukemic — *see* Leukemia
  liver K76.89
    fatty — *see* Fatty, liver NEC
    glycogen — *see also* Disease, glycogen storage E74.03 *[K77]*
  lung R91.8
    eosinophilic — *see* Eosinophilia, pulmonary
  lymphatic — *see also* Leukemia, lymphatic C91.9-
    gland I88.9
  muscle, fatty M62.89
  myocardium, myocardial
    fatty — *see* Degeneration, myocardial
    glycogenic E74.02 *[I43]*
  on chest x-ray R91.8
  pulmonary R91.8
    with eosinophilia — *see* Eosinophilia, pulmonary
  skin (lymphocytic) L98.6
  thymus (gland) (fatty) E32.8
  urine R39.0
  vesicant agent
    antineoplastic chemotherapy T80.810
    other agent NEC T80.818
  vitreous body H43.89
Infirmity R68.89
  senile R54
Inflammation, inflamed, inflammatory (with exudation)
  abducent (nerve) — *see* Strabismus, paralytic, sixth nerve
  accessory sinus (chronic) — *see* Sinusitis
  adrenal (gland) E27.8
  alveoli, teeth M27.3
    scorbutic E54
  anal canal, anus K62.89
  antrum (chronic) — *see* Sinusitis, maxillary
  appendix — *see* Appendicitis
  arachnoid — *see* Meningitis
  areola N61.0
    puerperal, postpartum or gestational — *see* Infection, nipple
  areolar tissue NOS L08.9
  artery — *see* Arteritis
  auditory meatus (external) — *see* Otitis, externa
  Bartholin's gland N75.8
  bile duct (common) (hepatic) or passage — *see* Cholangitis
  bladder — *see* Cystitis
  bone — *see* Osteomyelitis
  brain — *see also* Encephalitis
    membrane — *see* Meningitis
  breast N61.0
    puerperal, postpartum, gestational — *see* Mastitis, obstetric
  broad ligament — *see* Disease, pelvis, inflammatory
  bronchi — *see* Bronchitis

Inflammation, inflamed, inflammatory (with exudation) - *continued*
  catarrhal J00
  cecum — *see* Appendicitis
  cerebral — *see also* Encephalitis
    membrane — *see* Meningitis
  cerebrospinal
    meningococcal A39.0
  cervix (uteri) — *see* Cervicitis
  chest J98.8
  chorioretinal H30.9-
    cyclitis — *see* Cyclitis
    disseminated H30.10-
      generalized H30.13-
      peripheral H30.12-
      posterior pole H30.11-
    epitheliopathy — *see* Epitheliopathy
    focal H30.00-
      juxtapapillary H30.01-
      macular H30.04-
      paramacular — *see* Inflammation, chorioretinal, focal, macular
      peripheral H30.03-
      posterior pole H30.02-
    specified type NEC H30.89-
  choroid — *see* Inflammation, chorioretinal
  chronic, postmastoidectomy cavity — *see* Complications, postmastoidectomy, inflammation
  colon — *see* Enteritis
  connective tissue (diffuse) NEC — *see* Disorder, soft tissue, specified type NEC
  cornea — *see* Keratitis
  corpora cavernosa N48.29
  cranial nerve — *see* Disorder, nerve, cranial
  Douglas' cul-de-sac or pouch (chronic) N73.0
  due to device, implant or graft — *see also* Complications, by site and type, infection or inflammation
    arterial graft T82.7
    breast (implant) T85.79
    catheter T85.79
      dialysis (renal) T82.7
        intraperitoneal T85.71
      infusion T82.7
        cranial T85.735
        intrathecal T85.735
        spinal (epidural) (subdural) T85.735
        subarachnoid T85.735
      urinary T83.518
        cystostomy T83.510
        Hopkins T83.518
        ileostomy T83.518
        nephrostomy T83.512
        specified NEC T83.518
        urethral indwelling T83.511
        urostomy T83.518
    electronic (electrode) (pulse generator) (stimulator)
      bone T84.7
      cardiac T82.7
      nervous system T85.738
        brain T85.731
        cranial nerve T85.732
        gastric nerve T85.732
        neurostimulator generator T85.734
        peripheral nerve T85.732
        sacral nerve T85.732
        spinal cord T85.733
        vagal nerve T85.732
      urinary T83.590
    fixation, internal (orthopedic) NEC — *see* Complication, fixation device, infection
    gastrointestinal (bile duct) (esophagus) T85.79
      neurostimulator electrode (lead) T85.732
    genital NEC T83.69
    heart NEC T82.7
      valve (prosthesis) T82.6
        graft T82.7
    joint prosthesis — *see* Complication, joint prosthesis, infection

INFESTATION - INFLAMMATION, INFLAMED, INFLAMMATORY

Inflammation, inflamed, inflammatory (with exudation) - *continued*
due to device, implant or graft - *continued*
ocular (corneal graft) (orbital implant) NEC T85.79
orthopedic NEC T84.7
penile (cylinder) (pump) (resevoir) T83.61
specified NEC T85.79
testicular T83.62
urinary NEC T83.598
ileal conduit stent T83.593
implanted neurostimulation T83.590
implanted sphincter T83.591
indwelling ureteral stent T83.592
nephroureteral stent T83.593
specified stent NEC T83.593
vascular NEC T82.7
ventricular intracranial (communicating) shunt T85.730
duodenum K29.80
with bleeding K29.81
dura mater — *see* Meningitis
ear (middle) — *see also* Otitis, media
external — *see* Otitis, externa
inner — *see* subcategory H83.0
epididymis — *see* Epididymitis
esophagus — *see* Esophagitis
ethmoidal (sinus) (chronic) — *see* Sinusitis, ethmoidal
eustachian tube (catarrhal) — *see* Salpingitis, eustachian
eyelid H01.9
abscess — *see* Abscess, eyelid
blepharitis — *see* Blepharitis
chalazion — *see* Chalazion
dermatosis (noninfectious) — *see* Dermatosis, eyelid
hordeolum — *see* Hordeolum
specified NEC H01.8
fallopian tube — *see* Salpingo-oophoritis
fascia — *see* Myositis
follicular, pharynx J31.2
frontal (sinus) (chronic) — *see* Sinusitis, frontal
gallbladder — *see* Cholecystitis
gastric — *see* Gastritis
gastrointestinal — *see* Enteritis
genital organ (internal) (diffuse)
female — *see* Disease, pelvis, inflammatory
male N49.9
multiple sites N49.8
specified NEC N49.8
gland (lymph) — *see* Lymphadenitis
glottis — *see* Laryngitis
granular, pharynx J31.2
gum K05.10
nonplaque induced K05.11
plaque induced K05.10
heart — *see* Carditis
hepatic duct — *see* Cholangitis
ileoanal (internal) pouch K91.850
ileum — *see also* Enteritis
regional or terminal — *see* Enteritis, regional
intestine (any part) — *see* Enteritis
intestinal pouch K91.850
jaw (acute) (bone) (chronic) (lower) (suppurative) (upper) M27.2
joint NEC — *see* Arthritis
sacroiliac M46.1
kidney — *see* Nephritis
knee (joint) M13.169
tuberculous A18.02
labium (majus) (minus) — *see* Vulvitis
lacrimal
gland — *see* Dacryoadenitis
passages (duct) (sac) — *see also* Dacryocystitis
canaliculitis — *see* Canaliculitis, lacrimal
larynx — *see* Laryngitis
leg NOS L08.9
lip K13.0
liver (capsule) — *see also* Hepatitis

Inflammation, inflamed, inflammatory (with exudation) - *continued*
liver (capsule) - *continued*
chronic K73.9
suppurative K75.0
lung (acute) — *see also* Pneumonia
chronic J98.4
lymph gland or node — *see* Lymphadenitis
lymphatic vessel — *see* Lymphangitis
maxilla, maxillary M27.2
sinus (chronic) — *see* Sinusitis, maxillary
membranes of brain or spinal cord — *see* Meningitis
meninges — *see* Meningitis
mouth K12.1
muscle — *see* Myositis
myocardium — *see* Myocarditis
nasal sinus (chronic) — *see* Sinusitis
nasopharynx — *see* Nasopharyngitis
navel L08.82
nerve NEC — *see* Neuritis
nipple N61.0
puerperal, postpartum or gestational — *see* Infection, nipple
nose — *see* Rhinitis
oculomotor (nerve) — *see* Strabismus, paralytic, third nerve
optic nerve — *see* Neuritis, optic
orbit (chronic) H05.10
acute H05.00
abscess — *see* Abscess, orbit
cellulitis — *see* Cellulitis, orbit
osteomyelitis — *see* Osteomyelitis, orbit
periostitis — *see* Periostitis, orbital
tenonitis — *see* Tenonitis, eye
granuloma — *see* Granuloma, orbit
myositis — *see* Myositis, orbital
ovary — *see* Salpingo-oophoritis
oviduct — *see* Salpingo-oophoritis
pancreas (acute) — *see* Pancreatitis
parametrium N73.0
parotid region L08.9
pelvis, female — *see* Disease, pelvis, inflammatory
penis (corpora cavernosa) N48.29
perianal K62.89
pericardium — *see* Pericarditis
perineum (female) (male) L08.9
perirectal K62.89
peritoneum — *see* Peritonitis
periuterine — *see* Disease, pelvis, inflammatory
perivesical — *see* Cystitis
petrous bone (acute) (chronic) — *see* Petrositis
pharynx (acute) — *see* Pharyngitis
pia mater — *see* Meningitis
pleura — *see* Pleurisy
polyp, colon — *see also* Polyp, colon, inflammatory K51.40
prostate — *see also* Prostatitis
specified type NEC N41.8
rectosigmoid — *see* Rectosigmoiditis
rectum — *see also* Proctitis K62.89
respiratory, upper — *see also* Infection, respiratory, upper J06.9
acute, due to radiation J70.0
chronic, due to external agent — *see* condition, respiratory, chronic, due to
due to
chemicals, gases, fumes or vapors (inhalation) J68.2
radiation J70.1
retina — *see* Chorioretinitis
retrocecal — *see* Appendicitis
retroperitoneal — *see* Peritonitis
salivary duct or gland (any) (suppurative) — *see* Sialoadenitis
scorbutic, alveoli, teeth E54
scrotum N49.2
seminal vesicle — *see* Vesiculitis
sigmoid — *see* Enteritis
sinus — *see* Sinusitis
Skene's duct or gland — *see* Urethritis
skin L08.9

Inflammation, inflamed, inflammatory (with exudation) - *continued*
spermatic cord N49.1
sphenoidal (sinus) — *see* Sinusitis, sphenoidal
spinal
cord — *see* Encephalitis
membrane — *see* Meningitis
nerve — *see* Disorder, nerve
spine — *see* Spondylopathy, inflammatory
spleen (capsule) D73.89
stomach — *see* Gastritis
subcutaneous tissue L08.9
suprarenal (gland) E27.8
synovial — *see* Tenosynovitis
tendon (sheath) NEC — *see* Tenosynovitis
testis — *see* Orchitis
throat (acute) — *see* Pharyngitis
thymus (gland) E32.8
thyroid (gland) — *see* Thyroiditis
tongue K14.0
tonsil — *see* Tonsillitis
trachea — *see* Tracheitis
trochlear (nerve) — *see* Strabismus, paralytic, fourth nerve
tubal — *see* Salpingo-oophoritis
tuberculous NEC — *see* Tuberculosis
tubo-ovarian — *see* Salpingo-oophoritis
tunica vaginalis N49.1
tympanic membrane — *see* Tympanitis
umbilicus, umbilical L08.82
uterine ligament — *see* Disease, pelvis, inflammatory
uterus (catarrhal) — *see* Endometritis
uveal tract (anterior) NOS — *see also* Iridocyclitis
posterior — *see* Chorioretinitis
vagina — *see* Vaginitis
vas deferens N49.1
vein — *see also* Phlebitis
intracranial or intraspinal (septic) G08
thrombotic I80.9
leg — *see* Phlebitis, leg
lower extremity — *see* Phlebitis, leg
vocal cord J38.3
vulva — *see* Vulvitis
Wharton's duct (suppurative) — *see* Sialoadenitis

Inflation, lung, imperfect (newborn) — *see* Atelectasis

Influenza (bronchial) (epidemic) (respiratory (upper)) (unidentified influenza virus) J11.1
with
digestive manifestations J11.2
encephalopathy J11.81
enteritis J11.2
gastroenteritis J11.2
gastrointestinal manifestations J11.2
laryngitis J11.1
myocarditis J11.82
otitis media J11.83
pharyngitis J11.1
pneumonia J11.00
specified type J11.08
respiratory manifestations NEC J11.1
specified manifestation NEC J11.89
A (non-novel) J10-
A/H5N1 — *see also* Influenza, due to, identified novel influenza A virus J09.X2
avian — *see also* Influenza, due to, identified novel influenza A virus J09.X2
B J10-
bird — *see also* Influenza, due to, identified novel influenza A virus J09.X2
C J10-
due to
avian — *see also* Influenza, due to, identified novel influenza A virus J09.X2
identified influenza virus NEC J10.1
with
digestive manifestations J10.2
encephalopathy J10.81

Influenza (bronchial) (epidemic) (respiratory (upper)) (unidentified influenza virus) - *continued*
  due to - *continued*
    identified influenza virus NEC - *continued*
      with - *continued*
        enteritis J10.2
        gastroenteritis J10.2
        gastrointestinal manifestations J10.2
        laryngitis J10.1
        myocarditis J10.82
        otitis media J10.83
        pharyngitis J10.1
        pneumonia (unspecified type) J10.00
          with same identified influenza virus J10.01
          specified type NEC J10.08
        respiratory manifestations NEC J10.1
        specified manifestation NEC J10.89
    identified novel influenza A virus J09.X2
      with
        digestive manifestations J09.X3
        encephalopathy J09.X9
        enteritis J09.X3
        gastroenteritis J09.X3
        gastrointestinal manifestations J09.X3
        laryngitis J09.X2
        myocarditis J09.X9
        otitis media J09.X9
        pharyngitis J09.X2
        pneumonia J09.X1
        respiratory manifestations NEC J09.X2
        specified manifestation NEC J09.X9
        upper respiratory symptoms J09.X2
  novel (2009) H1N1 influenza — *see also* Influenza, due to, identified influenza virus NEC J10.1
  novel influenza A/H1N1 — *see also* Influenza, due to, identified influenza virus NEC J10.1
  of other animal origin, not bird or swine — *see also* Influenza, due to, identified novel influenza A virus J09.X2
  swine (viruses that normally cause infections in pigs) — *see also* Influenza, due to, identified novel influenza A virus J09.X2
Influenzal — *see* Influenza
Influenza-like disease — *see* Influenza
Infraction, Freiberg's (metatarsal head) — *see* Osteochondrosis, juvenile, metatarsus
Infraeruption of tooth (teeth) M26.34
Infusion complication, misadventure, or reaction — *see* Complications, infusion
Ingestion
  chemical — *see* Table of Drugs and Chemicals, by substance, poisoning
  drug or medicament
    correct substance properly administered — *see* Table of Drugs and Chemicals, by drug, adverse effect
    overdose or wrong substance given or taken — *see* Table of Drugs and Chemicals, by drug, poisoning
  foreign body — *see* Foreign body, alimentary tract
  multiple drug — *see* Table of Drugs and Chemicals, multiple
  tularemia A21.3
Ingrowing
  hair (beard) L73.1
  nail (finger) (toe) L60.0
Inguinal — *see also* condition
  testicle Q53.9
    bilateral Q53.212
    unilateral Q53.112
Inhalant-induced
  anxiety disorder F18.980
  depressive disorder F18.94
  major neurocognitive disorder F18.97
  mild neurocognitive disorder F18.988
  psychotic disorder F18.959
Inhalation
  anthrax A22.1
  flame T27.3
  food or foreign body — *see* Foreign body, by site
  gases, fumes, or vapors T59.9-
    specified agent NEC — *see* Table of Drugs and Chemicals, by substance T59.89-
  liquid or vomitus — *see* Asphyxia
  meconium (newborn) P24.00
    with
      pneumonia (pneumonitis) P24.01
      with respiratory symptoms P24.01
  mucus — *see* Asphyxia, mucus
  oil or gasoline (causing suffocation) — *see* Foreign body, by site
  smoke T59.81-
    with respiratory conditions J70.5
      due to chemicals, gases, fumes and vapors J68.9
  steam — *see also* Burn, respiratory tract T59.9-
  stomach contents or secretions — *see* Foreign body, by site
    due to anesthesia (general) (local) or other sedation T88.59
      in labor and delivery O74.0
      in pregnancy O29.01-
      postpartum, puerperal O89.01
Inhibition, orgasm
  female F52.31
  male F52.32
Inhibitor, systemic lupus erythematosus (presence of) D68.62
Iniencephalus, iniencephaly Q00.2
Injection, traumatic jet (air) (industrial) (water) (paint or dye) T70.4
Injury — *see also* specified injury type T14.90
  abdomen, abdominal S39.91
    blood vessel — *see* Injury, blood vessel, abdomen
    cavity — *see* Injury, intra-abdominal
    contusion S30.1
    internal — *see* Injury, intra-abdominal
    intra-abdominal organ — *see* Injury, intra-abdominal
    nerve — *see* Injury, nerve, abdomen
    open — *see* Wound, open, abdomen
    specified NEC S39.81
    superficial — *see* Injury, superficial, abdomen
  Achilles tendon S86.00-
    laceration S86.02-
    specified type NEC S86.09-
    strain S86.01-
  acoustic, resulting in deafness — *see* Injury, nerve, acoustic
  adrenal (gland) S37.819
    contusion S37.812
    laceration S37.813
    specified type NEC S37.818
  alveolar (process) S09.93
  ankle S99.91-
    contusion — *see* Contusion, ankle
    dislocation — *see* Dislocation, ankle
    fracture — *see* Fracture, ankle
    nerve — *see* Injury, nerve, ankle
    open — *see* Wound, open, ankle
    specified type NEC S99.81-
    sprain — *see* Sprain, ankle
    superficial — *see* Injury, superficial, ankle
  anterior chamber, eye — *see* Injury, eye, specified site NEC
  anus — *see* Injury, abdomen
  aorta (thoracic) S25.00
    abdominal S35.00
      laceration (minor) (superficial) S35.01
        major S35.02
      specified type NEC S35.09
    laceration (minor) (superficial) S25.01
      major S25.02
    specified type NEC S25.09
  arm (upper) S49.9-
    blood vessel — *see* Injury, blood vessel, arm
Injury - *continued*
  arm (upper) - *continued*
    contusion — *see* Contusion, arm, upper
    fracture — *see* Fracture, humerus
    lower — *see* Injury, forearm
    muscle — *see* Injury, muscle, shoulder
    nerve — *see* Injury, nerve, arm
    open — *see* Wound, open, arm
    specified type NEC S49.8-
    superficial — *see* Injury, superficial, arm
  artery (complicating trauma) — *see also* Injury, blood vessel, by site
    cerebral or meningeal — *see* Injury, intracranial
  auditory canal (external) (meatus) S09.91
  auricle, auris, ear S09.91
  axilla — *see* Injury, shoulder
  back — *see* Injury, back, lower
  bile duct S36.13
  birth — *see also* Birth, injury P15.9
  bladder (sphincter) S37.20
    at delivery O71.5
    contusion S37.22
    laceration S37.23
    obstetrical trauma O71.5
    specified type NEC S37.29
  blast (air) (hydraulic) (immersion) (underwater) NEC T14.8
    acoustic nerve trauma — *see* Injury, nerve, acoustic
    bladder — *see* Injury, bladder
    brain — *see* Concussion
    colon — *see* Injury, intestine, large, blast injury
    ear (primary) S09.31-
      secondary S09.39-
    generalized T70.8
    lung — *see* Injury, intrathoracic, lung, blast injury
    multiple body organs T70.8
    peritoneum S36.81
    rectum S36.61
    retroperitoneum S36.898
    small intestine S36.419
      duodenum S36.410
      specified site NEC S36.418
    specified
      intra-abdominal organ NEC S36.898
      pelvic organ NEC S37.899
  blood vessel NEC T14.8
    abdomen S35.9-
      aorta — *see* Injury, aorta, abdominal
      celiac artery — *see* Injury, blood vessel, celiac artery
      iliac vessel — *see* Injury, blood vessel, iliac
      laceration S35.91
      mesenteric vessel — *see* Injury, mesenteric
      portal vein — *see* Injury, blood vessel, portal vein
      renal vessel — *see* Injury, blood vessel, renal
      specified vessel NEC S35.8X-
      splenic vessel — *see* Injury, blood vessel, splenic
      vena cava — *see* Injury, vena cava, inferior
    ankle — *see* Injury, blood vessel, foot
    aorta (abdominal) (thoracic) — *see* Injury, aorta
    arm (upper) NEC S45.90-
      forearm — *see* Injury, blood vessel, forearm
      laceration S45.91-
      specified
        site NEC S45.80-
          laceration S45.81-
          specified type NEC S45.89-
        type NEC S45.99-
      superficial vein S45.30-
        laceration S45.31-
        specified type NEC S45.39-
    axillary
      artery S45.00-

INFLUENZA - INJURY

Injury - *continued*
blood vessel NEC - *continued*
axillary - *continued*
artery - *continued*
laceration S45.01-
specified type NEC S45.09-
vein S45.20-
laceration S45.21-
specified type NEC S45.29-
azygos vein — *see* Injury, blood vessel, thoracic, specified site NEC
brachial
artery S45.10-
laceration S45.11-
specified type NEC S45.19-
vein S45.20-
laceration S45.219
specified type NEC S45.29-
carotid artery (common) (external) (internal, extracranial) S15.00-
internal, intracranial S06.8-
laceration (minor) (superficial) S15.01-
major S15.02-
specified type NEC S15.09-
celiac artery S35.219
branch S35.299
laceration (minor) (superficial) S35.291
major S35.292
specified NEC S35.298
laceration (minor) (superficial) S35.211
major S35.212
specified type NEC S35.218
cerebral — *see* Injury, intracranial
deep plantar — *see* Injury, blood vessel, plantar artery
digital (hand) — *see* Injury, blood vessel, finger
dorsal
artery (foot) S95.00-
laceration S95.01-
specified type NEC S95.09-
vein (foot) S95.20-
laceration S95.21-
specified type NEC S95.29-
due to accidental laceration during procedure — *see* Laceration, accidental complicating surgery
extremity — *see* Injury, blood vessel, limb
femoral
artery (common) (superficial) S75.00-
laceration (minor) (superficial) S75.01-
major S75.02-
specified type NEC S75.09-
vein (hip level) (thigh level) S75.10-
laceration (minor) (superficial) S75.11-
major S75.12-
specified type NEC S75.19-
finger S65.50-
index S65.50-
laceration S65.51-
specified type NEC S65.59-
laceration S65.51-
little S65.50-
laceration S65.51-
specified type NEC S65.59-
middle S65.50-
laceration S65.51-
specified type NEC S65.59-
specified type NEC S65.59-
thumb — *see* Injury, blood vessel, thumb
foot S95.90-
dorsal
artery — *see* Injury, blood vessel, dorsal, artery
vein — *see* Injury, blood vessel, dorsal, vein
laceration S95.91-
plantar artery — *see* Injury, blood vessel, plantar artery
specified
site NEC S95.80-
laceration S95.81-

Injury - *continued*
blood vessel NEC - *continued*
foot - *continued*
specified - *continued*
site NEC - *continued*
specified type NEC S95.89-
specified type NEC S95.99-
forearm S55.90-
laceration S55.91-
radial artery — *see* Injury, blood vessel, radial artery
specified
site NEC S55.80-
laceration S55.81-
specified type NEC S55.89-
type NEC S55.99-
ulnar artery — *see* Injury, blood vessel, ulnar artery
vein S55.20-
laceration S55.21-
specified type NEC S55.29-
gastric
artery — *see* Injury, mesenteric, artery, branch
vein — *see* Injury, blood vessel, abdomen
gastroduodenal artery — *see* Injury, mesenteric, artery, branch
greater saphenous vein (lower leg level) S85.30-
hip (and thigh) level S75.20-
laceration (minor) (superficial) S75.21-
major S75.22-
specified type NEC S75.29-
laceration S85.31-
specified type NEC S85.39-
hand (level) S65.90-
finger — *see* Injury, blood vessel, finger
laceration S65.91-
palmar arch — *see* Injury, blood vessel, palmar arch
radial artery — *see* Injury, blood vessel, radial artery, hand
specified
site NEC S65.80-
laceration S65.81-
specified type NEC S65.89-
type NEC S65.99-
thumb — *see* Injury, blood vessel, thumb
ulnar artery — *see* Injury, blood vessel, ulnar artery, hand
head S09.0
intracranial — *see* Injury, intracranial
multiple S09.0
hepatic
artery — *see* Injury, mesenteric, artery
vein — *see* Injury, vena cava, inferior
hip S75.90-
femoral artery — *see* Injury, blood vessel, femoral, artery
femoral vein — *see* Injury, blood vessel, femoral, vein
greater saphenous vein — *see* Injury, blood vessel, greater saphenous, hip level
laceration S75.91-
specified
site NEC S75.80-
laceration S75.81-
specified type NEC S75.89-
type NEC S75.99-
hypogastric (artery) (vein) — *see* Injury, blood vessel, iliac
iliac S35.5-
artery S35.51-
specified vessel NEC S35.5-
uterine vessel — *see* Injury, blood vessel, uterine
vein S35.51-
innominate — *see* Injury, blood vessel, thoracic, innominate
intercostal (artery) (vein) — *see* Injury, blood vessel, thoracic, intercostal
jugular vein (external) S15.20-

Injury - *continued*
blood vessel NEC - *continued*
jugular vein (external) - *continued*
internal S15.30-
laceration (minor) (superficial) S15.31-
major S15.32-
specified type NEC S15.39-
laceration (minor) (superficial) S15.21-
major S15.22-
specified type NEC S15.29-
leg (level) (lower) S85.90-
greater saphenous — *see* Injury, blood vessel, greater saphenous
laceration S85.91-
lesser saphenous — *see* Injury, blood vessel, lesser saphenous
peroneal artery — *see* Injury, blood vessel, peroneal artery
popliteal
artery — *see* Injury, blood vessel, popliteal, artery
vein — *see* Injury, blood vessel, popliteal, vein
specified
site NEC S85.80-
laceration S85.81-
specified type NEC S85.89-
type NEC S85.99-
thigh — *see* Injury, blood vessel, hip
tibial artery — *see* Injury, blood vessel, tibial artery
lesser saphenous vein (lower leg level) S85.40-
laceration S85.41-
specified type NEC S85.49-
limb
lower — *see* Injury, blood vessel, leg
upper — *see* Injury, blood vessel, arm
lower back — *see* Injury, blood vessel, abdomen
specified NEC — *see* Injury, blood vessel, abdomen, specified, site NEC
mammary (artery) (vein) — *see* Injury, blood vessel, thoracic, specified site NEC
mesenteric (inferior) (superior)
artery — *see* Injury, mesenteric, artery
vein — *see* Injury, mesenteric, vein
neck S15.9
specified site NEC S15.8
ovarian (artery) (vein) — *see* subcategory S35.8
palmar arch (superficial) S65.20-
deep S65.30-
laceration S65.31-
specified type NEC S65.39-
laceration S65.21-
specified type NEC S65.29-
pelvis — *see* Injury, blood vessel, abdomen
specified NEC — *see* Injury, blood vessel, abdomen, specified, site NEC
peroneal artery S85.20-
laceration S85.21-
specified type NEC S85.29-
plantar artery (deep) (foot) S95.10-
laceration S95.11-
specified type NEC S95.19-
popliteal
artery S85.00-
laceration S85.01-
specified type NEC S85.09-
vein S85.50-
laceration S85.51-
specified type NEC S85.59-
portal vein S35.319
laceration S35.311
specified type NEC S35.318
precerebral — *see* Injury, blood vessel, neck
pulmonary (artery) (vein) — *see* Injury, blood vessel, thoracic, pulmonary

- **Injury** - *continued*
  - intestine - *continued*
    - large - *continued*
      - descending (left) - *continued*
        - blast injury (primary) S36.512
          - secondary S36.592
        - contusion S36.522
        - laceration S36.532
        - specified type NEC S36.592
      - laceration S36.539
        - ascending (right) S36.530
        - descending (left) S36.532
        - rectum S36.63
        - sigmoid S36.533
        - specified site NEC S36.538
        - transverse S36.531
      - rectum S36.60
        - blast injury (primary) S36.61
          - secondary S36.69
        - contusion S36.62
        - laceration S36.63
        - specified type NEC S36.69
      - sigmoid S36.503
        - blast injury (primary) S36.513
          - secondary S36.593
        - contusion S36.523
        - laceration S36.533
        - specified type NEC S36.593
      - specified
        - site NEC S36.508
          - blast injury (primary) S36.518
            - secondary S36.598
          - contusion S36.528
          - laceration S36.538
          - specified type NEC S36.598
        - type NEC S36.599
          - ascending (right) S36.590
          - descending (left) S36.592
          - rectum S36.69
          - sigmoid S36.593
          - specified site NEC S36.598
          - transverse S36.591
      - transverse S36.501
        - blast injury (primary) S36.511
          - secondary S36.591
        - contusion S36.521
        - laceration S36.531
        - specified type NEC S36.591
    - small S36.409
      - blast injury (primary) S36.419
        - duodenum S36.410
        - secondary S36.499
          - duodenum S36.490
          - specified site NEC S36.498
        - specified site NEC S36.418
      - contusion S36.429
        - duodenum S36.420
        - specified site NEC S36.428
      - duodenum S36.400
        - blast injury (primary) S36.410
          - secondary S36.490
        - contusion S36.420
        - laceration S36.430
        - specified NEC S36.490
      - laceration S36.439
        - duodenum S36.430
        - specified site NEC S36.438
      - specified
        - type NEC S36.499
          - duodenum S36.490
          - specified site NEC S36.498
        - site NEC S36.408
  - intra-abdominal S36.90
    - adrenal gland — *see* Injury, adrenal gland
    - bladder — *see* Injury, bladder
    - colon — *see* Injury, intestine, large
    - contusion S36.92
    - fallopian tube — *see* Injury, fallopian tube
    - gallbladder — *see* Injury, gallbladder
    - intestine — *see* Injury, intestine
    - laceration S36.93
    - liver — *see* Injury, liver
    - kidney — *see* Injury, kidney
    - ovary — *see* Injury, ovary
    - pancreas — *see* Injury, pancreas

- **Injury** - *continued*
  - intra-abdominal - *continued*
    - pelvic NOS S37.90
    - peritoneum — *see* Injury, intra-abdominal, specified, site NEC
    - prostate — *see* Injury, prostate
    - rectum — *see* Injury, intestine, large, rectum
    - retroperitoneum — *see* Injury, intra-abdominal, specified, site NEC
    - seminal vesicle — *see* Injury, pelvis, organ, specified site NEC
    - small intestine — *see* Injury, intestine, small
    - specified
      - site NEC S36.899
        - contusion S36.892
        - laceration S36.893
        - specified type NEC S36.898
      - type NEC S36.99
      - pelvic S37.90
        - specified
          - site NEC S37.899
            - specified type NEC S37.898
          - type NEC S37.99
    - spleen — *see* Injury, spleen
    - stomach — *see* Injury, stomach
    - ureter — *see* Injury, ureter
    - urethra — *see* Injury, urethra
    - uterus — *see* Injury, uterus
    - vas deferens — *see* Injury, pelvis, organ, specified site NEC
  - intracranial (traumatic) (see also, if applicable, Compression, brain, traumatic) S06.9-
    - cerebellar hemorrhage, traumatic — *see* Injury, intracranial, focal
    - cerebral edema, traumatic S06.1X-
      - diffuse S06.1X-
      - focal S06.1X-
    - diffuse (axonal) S06.2X-
    - epidural hemorrhage (traumatic) S06.4X-
    - focal brain injury S06.30-
      - contusion — *see* Contusion, cerebral
      - laceration — *see* Laceration, cerebral
    - intracerebral hemorrhage, traumatic S06.36-
      - left side S06.35-
      - right side S06.34-
    - subarachnoid hemorrhage, traumatic S06.6X-
    - subdural hemorrhage, traumatic S06.5X-
  - intraocular — *see* Injury, eyeball, penetrating
  - intrathoracic S27.9
    - bronchus S27.409
      - bilateral S27.402
      - blast injury (primary) S27.419
        - bilateral S27.412
        - secondary — *see* Injury, intrathoracic, bronchus, specified type NEC
        - unilateral S27.411
      - contusion S27.429
        - bilateral S27.422
        - unilateral S27.421
      - laceration S27.439
        - bilateral S27.432
        - unilateral S27.431
      - specified type NEC S27.499
        - bilateral S27.492
        - unilateral S27.491
      - unilateral S27.401
    - diaphragm S27.809
      - contusion S27.802
      - laceration S27.803
      - specified type NEC S27.808
    - esophagus (thoracic) S27.819
      - contusion S27.812
      - laceration S27.813
      - specified type NEC S27.818
    - heart — *see* Injury, heart
    - hemopneumothorax S27.2
    - hemothorax S27.1
    - lung S27.309
      - aspiration J69.0
      - bilateral S27.302

- **Injury** - *continued*
  - intrathoracic - *continued*
    - lung - *continued*
      - blast injury (primary) S27.319
        - bilateral S27.312
        - secondary — *see* Injury, intrathoracic, lung, specified type NEC
        - unilateral S27.311
      - contusion S27.329
        - bilateral S27.322
        - unilateral S27.321
      - laceration S27.339
        - bilateral S27.332
        - unilateral S27.331
      - specified type NEC S27.399
        - bilateral S27.392
        - unilateral S27.391
      - unilateral S27.301
    - pleura S27.60
      - laceration S27.63
      - specified type NEC S27.69
    - pneumothorax S27.0
    - specified organ NEC S27.899
      - contusion S27.892
      - laceration S27.893
      - specified type NEC S27.898
    - thoracic duct — *see* Injury, intrathoracic, specified organ NEC
    - thymus gland — *see* Injury, intrathoracic, specified organ NEC
    - trachea, thoracic S27.50
      - blast (primary) S27.51
      - contusion S27.52
      - laceration S27.53
      - specified type NEC S27.59
  - iris — *see* Injury, eye, specified site NEC
    - penetrating — *see* Injury, eyeball, penetrating
  - jaw S09.93
  - jejunum — *see* Injury, intestine, small
  - joint NOS T14.8
    - old or residual — *see* Disorder, joint, specified type NEC
  - kidney S37.00-
    - acute (nontraumatic) N17.9
    - contusion — *see* Contusion, kidney
    - laceration — *see* Laceration, kidney
    - specified NEC S37.09-
  - knee S89.9-
    - contusion — *see* Contusion, knee
    - dislocation — *see* Dislocation, knee
    - meniscus (lateral) (medial) — *see* Sprain, knee, specified site NEC
      - old injury or tear — *see* Derangement, knee, meniscus, due to old injury
    - open — *see* Wound, open, knee
    - specified NEC S89.8-
    - sprain — *see* Sprain, knee
    - superficial — *see* Injury, superficial, knee
  - labium (majus) (minus) S39.94
  - labyrinth, ear S09.30-
  - lacrimal apparatus, duct, gland, or sac — *see* Injury, eye, specified site NEC
  - larynx NEC S19.81
  - leg (lower) S89.9-
    - blood vessel — *see* Injury, blood vessel, leg
    - contusion — *see* Contusion, leg
    - fracture — *see* Fracture, leg
    - muscle — *see* Injury, muscle, leg
    - nerve — *see* Injury, nerve, leg
    - open — *see* Wound, open, leg
    - specified NEC S89.8-
    - superficial — *see* Injury, superficial, leg
  - lens, eye — *see* Injury, eye, specified site NEC
    - penetrating — *see* Injury, eyeball, penetrating
  - limb NEC T14.8
  - lip S09.93
  - liver S36.119
    - contusion S36.112
    - laceration S36.113
      - major (stellate) S36.116
      - minor S36.114

Injury - *continued*
muscle (and fascia) (and tendon) - *continued*
forearm (level) - *continued*
specified - *continued*
site NEC - *continued*
type NEC S56.89-
strain S56.91-
hand (level) S66.90-
laceration S66.92-
specified
site NEC S66.80-
laceration S66.82-
specified type NEC S66.89-
strain S66.81-
type NEC S66.99-
strain S66.91-
head S09.10
laceration S09.12
specified type NEC S09.19
strain S09.11
hip NEC S76.00-
laceration S76.02-
specified type NEC S76.09-
strain S76.01-
intrinsic
ankle and foot level — *see* Injury, muscle, foot, intrinsic
finger (other than thumb) — *see* Injury, muscle, finger by site, intrinsic
foot (level) — *see* Injury, muscle, foot, intrinsic
thumb — *see* Injury, muscle, thumb, intrinsic
leg (level) (lower) S86.90-
Achilles tendon — *see* Injury, Achilles tendon
anterior muscle group — *see* Injury, muscle, anterior muscle group
laceration S86.92-
peroneal muscle group — *see* Injury, muscle, peroneal muscle group
posterior muscle group — *see* Injury, muscle, posterior muscle group, leg level
specified
site NEC S86.80-
laceration S86.82-
specified type NEC S86.89-
strain S86.81-
type NEC S86.99-
strain S86.91-
long
extensor toe, at ankle and foot level — *see* Injury, muscle, toe, extensor
flexor, toe, at ankle and foot level — *see* Injury, muscle, toe, flexor
head, biceps — *see* Injury, muscle, biceps, long head
lower back S39.002
laceration S39.022
specified type NEC S39.092
strain S39.012
neck (level) S16.9
laceration S16.2
specified type NEC S16.8
strain S16.1
pelvis S39.003
laceration S39.023
specified type NEC S39.093
strain S39.013
peroneal muscle group, at leg level (lower) S86.30-
laceration S86.32-
specified type NEC S86.39-
strain S86.31-
posterior muscle (group)
leg level (lower) S86.10-
laceration S86.12-
specified type NEC S86.19-
strain S86.11-
thigh level S76.30-
laceration S76.32-
specified type NEC S76.39-
strain S76.31-
quadriceps (thigh) S76.10-

Injury - *continued*
muscle (and fascia) (and tendon) - *continued*
quadriceps (thigh) - *continued*
laceration S76.12-
specified type NEC S76.19-
strain S76.11-
shoulder S46.90-
laceration S46.92-
rotator cuff — *see* Injury, rotator cuff
specified site NEC S46.80-
laceration S46.82-
strain S46.81-
specified type NEC S46.89-
strain S46.91-
specified type NEC S46.99-
thigh NEC (level) S76.90-
adductor — *see* Injury, muscle, adductor, thigh
laceration S76.92-
posterior muscle (group) — *see* Injury, muscle, posterior muscle, thigh level
quadriceps — *see* Injury, muscle, quadriceps
specified
site NEC S76.80-
laceration S76.82-
specified type NEC S76.89-
strain S76.81-
type NEC S76.99-
strain S76.91-
thorax (level) S29.009
back wall S29.002
front wall S29.001
laceration S29.029
back wall S29.022
front wall S29.021
specified type NEC S29.099
back wall S29.092
front wall S29.091
strain S29.019
back wall S29.012
front wall S29.011
thumb
abductor (forearm level) S56.30-
laceration S56.32-
specified type NEC S56.39-
strain S56.31-
extensor (forearm level) S56.30-
hand level S66.20-
laceration S66.22-
specified type NEC S66.29-
strain S66.21-
laceration S56.32-
specified type NEC S56.39-
strain S56.31-
flexor (forearm level) S56.00-
hand level S66.00-
laceration S66.02-
specified type NEC S66.09-
strain S66.01-
laceration S56.02-
specified type NEC S56.09-
strain S56.01-
wrist level — *see* Injury, muscle, thumb, flexor, hand level
intrinsic S66.40-
laceration S66.42-
specified type NEC S66.49-
strain S66.41-
toe — *see also* Injury, muscle, foot
extensor, long S96.10-
laceration S96.12-
specified type NEC S96.19-
strain S96.11-
flexor, long S96.00-
laceration S96.02-
specified type NEC S96.09-
strain S96.01-
triceps S46.30-
laceration S46.32-
specified type NEC S46.39-
strain S46.31-
wrist (and hand) level — *see* Injury, muscle, hand

Injury - *continued*
musculocutaneous nerve — *see* Injury, nerve, musculocutaneous
myocardial (acute) (chronic) (non-ischemic) (non-traumatic) I5A
traumatic — *see* Injury, heart
myocardium — *see also* Injury, heart
non-traumatic — *see* Injury, myocardial
nape — *see* Injury, neck
nasal (septum) (sinus) S09.92
nasopharynx S09.92
neck S19.9
specified NEC S19.80
specified site NEC S19.89
nerve NEC T14.8
abdomen S34.9
peripheral S34.6
specified site NEC S34.8
abducens S04.4-
contusion S04.4-
laceration S04.4-
specified type NEC S04.4-
abducent — *see* Injury, nerve, abducens
accessory S04.7-
contusion S04.7-
laceration S04.7-
specified type NEC S04.7-
acoustic S04.6-
contusion S04.6-
laceration S04.6-
specified type NEC S04.6-
ankle S94.9-
cutaneous sensory S94.3-
specified site NEC — *see* subcategory S94.8
anterior crural, femoral — *see* Injury, nerve, femoral
arm (upper) S44.9-
axillary — *see* Injury, nerve, axillary
cutaneous — *see* Injury, nerve, cutaneous, arm
median — *see* Injury, nerve, median, upper arm
musculocutaneous — *see* Injury, nerve, musculocutaneous
radial — *see* Injury, nerve, radial, upper arm
specified site NEC — *see* subcategory S44.8
ulnar — *see* Injury, nerve, ulnar, arm
auditory — *see* Injury, nerve, acoustic
axillary S44.3-
brachial plexus — *see* Injury, brachial plexus
cervical sympathetic S14.5
cranial S04.9
contusion S04.9
eighth (acoustic or auditory) — *see* Injury, nerve, acoustic
eleventh (accessory) — *see* Injury, nerve, accessory
fifth (trigeminal) — *see* Injury, nerve, trigeminal
first (olfactory) — *see* Injury, nerve, olfactory
fourth (trochlear) — *see* Injury, nerve, trochlear
laceration S04.9
ninth (glossopharyngeal) — *see* Injury, nerve, glossopharyngeal
second (optic) — *see* Injury, nerve, optic
seventh (facial) — *see* Injury, nerve, facial
sixth (abducent) — *see* Injury, nerve, abducens
specified
nerve NEC S04.89-
contusion S04.89-
laceration S04.89-
specified type NEC S04.89-
type NEC S04.9
tenth (pneumogastric or vagus) — *see* Injury, nerve, vagus
third (oculomotor) — *see* Injury, nerve, oculomotor

INJURY - INJURY

- **Injury** - *continued*
  - spinal (cord) - *continued*
    - lumbar - *continued*
      - incomplete lesion - *continued*
        - L3 level S34.123
        - L4 level S34.124
        - L5 level S34.125
      - L1 level S34.101
      - L2 level S34.102
      - L3 level S34.103
      - L4 level S34.104
      - L5 level S34.105
    - nerve root NEC
      - cervical — *see* Injury, nerve, spinal, root, cervical
      - dorsal — *see* Injury, nerve, spinal, root, dorsal
      - lumbar S34.21
      - sacral S34.22
      - thoracic — *see* Injury, nerve, spinal, root, dorsal
    - plexus
      - brachial — *see* Injury, brachial plexus
      - lumbosacral — *see* Injury, lumbosacral plexus
    - sacral S34.139
      - complete lesion S34.131
      - incomplete lesion S34.132
    - thoracic S24.109
      - anterior cord syndrome S24.139
        - T1 level S24.131
        - T2-T6 level S24.132
        - T7-T10 level S24.133
        - T11-T12 level S24.134
      - Brown-Séquard syndrome S24.149
        - T1 level S24.141
        - T2-T6 level S24.142
        - T7-T10 level S24.143
        - T11-T12 level S24.144
      - complete lesion S24.119
        - T1 level S24.111
        - T2-T6 level S24.112
        - T7-T10 level S24.113
        - T11-T12 level S24.114
      - concussion S24.0
      - edema S24.0
      - incomplete lesion specified NEC S24.159
        - T1 level S24.151
        - T2-T6 level S24.152
        - T7-T10 level S24.153
        - T11-T12 level S24.154
      - posterior cord syndrome S24.159
        - T1 level S24.151
        - T2-T6 level S24.152
        - T7-T10 level S24.153
        - T11-T12 level S24.154
      - T1 level S24.101
      - T2-T6 level S24.102
      - T7-T10 level S24.103
      - T11-T12 level S24.104
  - splanchnic nerve — *see* Injury, nerve, lumbosacral, sympathetic
  - spleen S36.00
    - contusion S36.029
      - major S36.021
      - minor S36.020
    - laceration S36.039
      - major (massive) (stellate) S36.032
      - moderate S36.031
      - superficial (capsular) (minor) S36.030
    - specified type NEC S36.09
  - splenic artery — *see* Injury, blood vessel, celiac artery, branch
  - stellate ganglion — *see* Injury, nerve, thorax, sympathetic
  - sternal region S29.9
  - stomach S36.30
    - contusion S36.32
    - laceration S36.33
    - specified type NEC S36.39
  - subconjunctival — *see* Injury, eye, conjunctiva
  - subcutaneous NEC T14.8
  - submaxillary region S09.93

- **Injury** - *continued*
  - submental region S09.93
  - subungual
    - fingers — *see* Injury, hand
    - toes — *see* Injury, foot
  - superficial NEC T14.8
    - abdomen, abdominal (wall) S30.92
      - abrasion S30.811
      - bite S30.871
        - insect S30.861
      - contusion S30.1
      - external constriction S30.841
      - foreign body S30.851
    - abrasion — *see* Abrasion, by site
    - adnexa, eye NEC — *see* Injury, eye, specified site NEC
    - alveolar process — *see* Injury, superficial, oral cavity
    - ankle S90.91-
      - abrasion — *see* Abrasion, ankle
      - blister — *see* Blister, ankle
      - bite — *see* Bite, ankle
      - contusion — *see* Contusion, ankle
      - external constriction — *see* Constriction, external, ankle
      - foreign body — *see* Foreign body, superficial, ankle
    - anus S30.98
    - arm (upper) S40.92-
      - abrasion — *see* Abrasion, arm
      - bite — *see* Bite, superficial, arm
      - blister — *see* Blister, arm (upper)
      - contusion — *see* Contusion, arm
      - external constriction — *see* Constriction, external, arm
      - foreign body — *see* Foreign body, superficial, arm
    - auditory canal (external) (meatus) — *see* Injury, superficial, ear
    - auricle — *see* Injury, superficial, ear
    - axilla — *see* Injury, superficial, arm
    - back — *see also* Injury, superficial, thorax, back
      - lower S30.91
        - abrasion S30.810
        - contusion S30.0
        - external constriction S30.840
        - superficial
          - bite NEC S30.870
            - insect S30.860
          - foreign body S30.850
    - bite NEC — *see* Bite, superficial NEC, by site
    - blister — *see* Blister, by site
    - breast S20.10-
      - abrasion — *see* Abrasion, breast
      - bite — *see* Bite, superficial, breast
      - contusion — *see* Contusion, breast
      - external constriction — *see* Constriction, external, breast
      - foreign body — *see* Foreign body, superficial, breast
    - brow — *see* Injury, superficial, head, specified NEC
    - buttock S30.91
    - calf — *see* Injury, superficial, leg
    - canthus, eye — *see* Injury, superficial, periocular area
    - cheek (external) — *see* Injury, superficial, head, specified NEC
      - internal — *see* Injury, superficial, oral cavity
    - chest wall — *see* Injury, superficial, thorax
    - chin — *see* Injury, superficial, head NEC
    - clitoris S30.95
    - conjunctiva — *see* Injury, eye, conjunctiva
      - with foreign body (in conjunctival sac) — *see* Foreign body, conjunctival sac
    - contusion — *see* Contusion, by site
    - costal region — *see* Injury, superficial, thorax
    - digit (s)
      - hand — *see* Injury, superficial, finger
    - ear (auricle) (canal) (external) S00.40-

- **Injury** - *continued*
  - superficial NEC - *continued*
    - ear (auricle) (canal) (external) - *continued*
      - abrasion — *see* Abrasion, ear
      - bite — *see* Bite, superficial, ear
      - contusion — *see* Contusion, ear
      - external constriction — *see* Constriction, external, ear
      - foreign body — *see* Foreign body, superficial, ear
    - elbow S50.90-
      - abrasion — *see* Abrasion, elbow
      - bite — *see* Bite, superficial, elbow
      - blister — *see* Blister, elbow
      - contusion — *see* Contusion, elbow
      - external constriction — *see* Constriction, external, elbow
      - foreign body — *see* Foreign body, superficial, elbow
    - epididymis S30.94
    - epigastric region S30.92
    - epiglottis — *see* Injury, superficial, throat
    - esophagus
      - cervical — *see* Injury, superficial, throat
    - external constriction — *see* Constriction, external, by site
    - extremity NEC T14.8
    - eyeball NEC — *see* Injury, eye, specified site NEC
    - eyebrow — *see* Injury, superficial, periocular area
    - eyelid S00.20-
      - abrasion — *see* Abrasion, eyelid
      - bite — *see* Bite, superficial, eyelid
      - contusion — *see* Contusion, eyelid
      - external constriction — *see* Constriction, external, eyelid
      - foreign body — *see* Foreign body, superficial, eyelid
    - face NEC — *see* Injury, superficial, head, specified NEC
    - finger (s) S60.949
      - abrasion — *see* Abrasion, finger
      - bite — *see* Bite, superficial, finger
      - blister — *see* Blister, finger
      - contusion — *see* Contusion, finger
      - external constriction — *see* Constriction, external, finger
      - foreign body — *see* Foreign body, superficial, finger
      - insect bite — *see* Bite, by site, superficial, insect
      - index S60.94-
      - little S60.94-
      - middle S60.94-
      - ring S60.94-
    - flank S30.92
    - foot S90.92-
      - abrasion — *see* Abrasion, foot
      - bite — *see* Bite, foot
      - blister — *see* Blister, foot
      - contusion — *see* Contusion, foot
      - external constriction — *see* Constriction, external, foot
      - foreign body — *see* Foreign body, superficial, foot
    - forearm S50.91-
      - abrasion — *see* Abrasion, forearm
      - bite — *see* Bite, forearm, superficial
      - blister — *see* Blister, forearm
      - contusion — *see* Contusion, forearm
      - elbow only — *see* Injury, superficial, elbow
      - external constriction — *see* Constriction, external, forearm
      - foreign body — *see* Foreign body, superficial, forearm
    - forehead — *see* Injury, superficial, head NEC
    - foreign body — *see* Foreign body, superficial
    - genital organs, external
      - female S30.97
      - male S30.96

INJURY - INJURY

Injury - *continued*
- superficial NEC - *continued*
  - globe (eye) — *see* Injury, eye, specified site NEC
  - groin S30.92
  - gum — *see* Injury, superficial, oral cavity
  - hand S60.92-
    - abrasion — *see* Abrasion, hand
    - bite — *see* Bite, superficial, hand
    - contusion — *see* Contusion, hand
    - external constriction — *see* Constriction, external, hand
    - foreign body — *see* Foreign body, superficial, hand
  - head S00.90
    - ear — *see* Injury, superficial, ear
    - eyelid — *see* Injury, superficial, eyelid
    - nose S00.30
    - oral cavity S00.502
    - scalp S00.00
    - specified site NEC S00.80
  - heel — *see* Injury, superficial, foot
  - hip S70.91-
    - abrasion — *see* Abrasion, hip
    - bite — *see* Bite, superficial, hip
    - blister — *see* Blister, hip
    - contusion — *see* Contusion, hip
    - external constriction — *see* Constriction, external, hip
    - foreign body — *see* Foreign body, superficial, hip
  - iliac region — *see* Injury, superficial, abdomen
  - inguinal region — *see* Injury, superficial, abdomen
  - insect bite — *see* Bite, by site, superficial, insect
  - interscapular region — *see* Injury, superficial, thorax, back
  - jaw — *see* Injury, superficial, head, specified NEC
  - knee S80.91-
    - abrasion — *see* Abrasion, knee
    - bite — *see* Bite, superficial, knee
    - blister — *see* Blister, knee
    - contusion — *see* Contusion, knee
    - external constriction — *see* Constriction, external, knee
    - foreign body — *see* Foreign body, superficial, knee
  - labium (majus) (minus) S30.95
  - lacrimal (apparatus) (gland) (sac) — *see* Injury, eye, specified site NEC
  - larynx — *see* Injury, superficial, throat
  - leg (lower) S80.92-
    - abrasion — *see* Abrasion, leg
    - bite — *see* Bite, superficial, leg
    - contusion — *see* Contusion, leg
    - external constriction — *see* Constriction, external, leg
    - foreign body — *see* Foreign body, superficial, leg
    - knee — *see* Injury, superficial, knee
  - limb NEC T14.8
  - lip S00.501
  - lower back S30.91
  - lumbar region S30.91
  - malar region — *see* Injury, superficial, head, specified NEC
  - mammary — *see* Injury, superficial, breast
  - mastoid region — *see* Injury, superficial, head, specified NEC
  - mouth — *see* Injury, superficial, oral cavity
  - muscle NEC T14.8
  - nail NEC T14.8
    - finger — *see* Injury, superficial, finger
    - toe — *see* Injury, superficial, toe
  - nasal (septum) — *see* Injury, superficial, nose
  - neck S10.90
    - specified site NEC S10.80
  - nose (septum) S00.30
  - occipital region — *see* Injury, superficial, scalp

Injury - *continued*
- superficial NEC - *continued*
  - oral cavity S00.502
  - orbital region — *see* Injury, superficial, periocular area
  - palate — *see* Injury, superficial, oral cavity
  - palm — *see* Injury, superficial, hand
  - parietal region — *see* Injury, superficial, scalp
  - pelvis S30.91
    - girdle — *see* Injury, superficial, hip
  - penis S30.93
  - perineum
    - female S30.95
    - male S30.91
  - periocular area S00.20-
    - abrasion — *see* Abrasion, eyelid
    - bite — *see* Bite, superficial, eyelid
    - contusion — *see* Contusion, eyelid
    - external constriction — *see* Constriction, external, eyelid
    - foreign body — *see* Foreign body, superficial, eyelid
  - phalanges
    - finger — *see* Injury, superficial, finger
    - toe — *see* Injury, superficial, toe
  - pharynx — *see* Injury, superficial, throat
  - pinna — *see* Injury, superficial, ear
  - popliteal space — *see* Injury, superficial, knee
  - prepuce S30.93
  - pubic region S30.91
  - pudendum
    - female S30.97
    - male S30.96
  - sacral region S30.91
  - scalp S00.00
  - scapular region — *see* Injury, superficial, shoulder
  - sclera — *see* Injury, eye, specified site NEC
  - scrotum S30.94
  - shin — *see* Injury, superficial, leg
  - shoulder S40.91-
    - abrasion — *see* Abrasion, shoulder
    - bite — *see* Bite, superficial, shoulder
    - blister — *see* Blister, shoulder
    - contusion — *see* Contusion, shoulder
    - external constriction — *see* Constriction, external, shoulder
    - foreign body — *see* Foreign body, superficial, shoulder
  - skin NEC T14.8
  - sternal region — *see* Injury, superficial, thorax, front
  - subconjunctival — *see* Injury, eye, specified site NEC
  - subcutaneous NEC T14.8
  - submaxillary region — *see* Injury, superficial, head, specified NEC
  - submental region — *see* Injury, superficial, head, specified NEC
  - subungual
    - finger (s) — *see* Injury, superficial, finger
    - toe (s) — *see* Injury, superficial, toe
  - supraclavicular fossa — *see* Injury, superficial, neck
  - supraorbital — *see* Injury, superficial, head, specified NEC
  - temple — *see* Injury, superficial, head, specified NEC
  - temporal region — *see* Injury, superficial, head, specified NEC
  - testis S30.94
  - thigh S70.92-
    - abrasion — *see* Abrasion, thigh
    - bite — *see* Bite, superficial, thigh
    - blister — *see* Blister, thigh
    - contusion — *see* Contusion, thigh
    - external constriction — *see* Constriction, external, thigh
    - foreign body — *see* Foreign body, superficial, thigh
  - thorax, thoracic (wall) S20.90

Injury - *continued*
- superficial NEC - *continued*
  - thorax, thoracic (wall) - *continued*
    - abrasion — *see* Abrasion, thorax
    - back S20.40-
    - bite — *see* Bite, thorax, superficial
    - blister — *see* Blister, thorax
    - contusion — *see* Contusion, thorax
    - external constriction — *see* Constriction, external, thorax
    - foreign body — *see* Foreign body, superficial, thorax
    - front S20.30-
  - throat S10.10
    - abrasion S10.11
    - bite S10.17
      - insect S10.16
    - blister S10.12
    - contusion S10.0
    - external constriction S10.14
    - foreign body S10.15
  - thumb S60.93-
    - abrasion — *see* Abrasion, thumb
    - bite — *see* Bite, superficial, thumb
    - blister — *see* Blister, thumb
    - contusion — *see* Contusion, thumb
    - external constriction — *see* Constriction, external, thumb
    - foreign body — *see* Foreign body, superficial, thumb
    - insect bite — *see* Bite, by site, superficial, insect
    - specified type NEC S60.39-
  - toe (s) S90.93-
    - abrasion — *see* Abrasion, toe
    - bite — *see* Bite, toe
    - blister — *see* Blister, toe
    - contusion — *see* Contusion, toe
    - external constriction — *see* Constriction, external, toe
    - foreign body — *see* Foreign body, superficial, toe
    - great S90.93-
  - tongue — *see* Injury, superficial, oral cavity
  - tooth, teeth — *see* Injury, superficial, oral cavity
  - trachea S10.10
  - tunica vaginalis S30.94
  - tympanum, tympanic membrane — *see* Injury, superficial, ear
  - uvula — *see* Injury, superficial, oral cavity
  - vagina S30.95
  - vocal cords — *see* Injury, superficial, throat
  - vulva S30.95
  - wrist S60.91-
- supraclavicular region — *see* Injury, neck
- supraorbital S09.93
- suprarenal gland (multiple) — *see* Injury, adrenal
- surgical complication (external or internal site) — *see* Laceration, accidental complicating surgery
- temple S09.90
- temporal region S09.90
- tendon — *see also* Injury, muscle, by site
  - abdomen — *see* Injury, muscle, abdomen
  - Achilles — *see* Injury, Achilles tendon
  - lower back — *see* Injury, muscle, lower back
  - pelvic organs — *see* Injury, muscle, pelvis
- tenth cranial nerve (pneumogastric or vagus) — *see* Injury, nerve, vagus
- testis S39.94
- thigh S79.92-
  - blood vessel — *see* Injury, blood vessel, hip
  - contusion — *see* Contusion, thigh
  - fracture — *see* Fracture, femur
  - muscle — *see* Injury, muscle, thigh
  - nerve — *see* Injury, nerve, thigh
  - open — *see* Wound, open, thigh
  - specified NEC S79.82-
  - superficial — *see* Injury, superficial, thigh

Injury - *continued*
third cranial nerve (oculomotor) — *see* Injury, nerve, oculomotor
thorax, thoracic S29.9
blood vessel — *see* Injury, blood vessel, thorax
cavity — *see* Injury, intrathoracic
dislocation — *see* Dislocation, thorax
external (wall) S29.9
contusion — *see* Contusion, thorax
nerve — *see* Injury, nerve, thorax
open — *see* Wound, open, thorax
specified NEC S29.8
sprain — *see* Sprain, thorax
superficial — *see* Injury, superficial, thorax
fracture — *see* Fracture, thorax
internal — *see* Injury, intrathoracic
intrathoracic organ — *see* Injury, intrathoracic
sympathetic ganglion — *see* Injury, nerve, thorax, sympathetic
throat — *see also* Injury, neck S19.9
thumb S69.9-
blood vessel — *see* Injury, blood vessel, thumb
contusion — *see* Contusion, thumb
dislocation — *see* Dislocation, thumb
fracture — *see* Fracture, thumb
muscle — *see* Injury, muscle, thumb
nerve — *see* Injury, nerve, digital, thumb
open — *see* Wound, open, thumb
specified NEC S69.8-
sprain — *see* Sprain, thumb
superficial — *see* Injury, superficial, thumb
thymus (gland) — *see* Injury, intrathoracic, specified organ NEC
thyroid (gland) NEC S19.84
toe S99.92-
contusion — *see* Contusion, toe
dislocation — *see* Dislocation, toe
fracture — *see* Fracture, toe
muscle — *see* Injury, muscle, toe
open — *see* Wound, open, toe
specified type NEC S99.82-
sprain — *see* Sprain, toe
superficial — *see* Injury, superficial, toe
tongue S09.93
tonsil S09.93
tooth S09.93
trachea (cervical) NEC S19.82
thoracic — *see* Injury, intrathoracic, trachea, thoracic
transfusion-related acute lung (TRALI) J95.84
tunica vaginalis S39.94
twelfth cranial nerve (hypoglossal) — *see* Injury, nerve, hypoglossal
ureter S37.10
contusion S37.12
laceration S37.13
specified type NEC S37.19
urethra (sphincter) S37.30
at delivery O71.5
contusion S37.32
laceration S37.33
specified type NEC S37.39
urinary organ S37.90
contusion S37.92
laceration S37.93
specified
site NEC S37.899
contusion S37.892
laceration S37.893
specified type NEC S37.898
type NEC S37.99
uterus, uterine S37.60
with ectopic or molar pregnancy O08.6
blood vessel — *see* Injury, blood vessel, iliac
contusion S37.62
laceration S37.63
cervix at delivery O71.3

Injury - *continued*
uterus, uterine - *continued*
rupture associated with obstetrics — *see* Rupture, uterus
specified type NEC S37.69
uvula S09.93
vagina S39.93
abrasion S30.814
bite S31.45
insect S30.864
superficial NEC S30.874
contusion S30.23
crush S38.03
during delivery — *see* Laceration, vagina, during delivery
external constriction S30.844
insect bite S30.864
laceration S31.41
with foreign body S31.42
open wound S31.40
puncture S31.43
with foreign body S31.44
superficial S30.95
foreign body S30.854
vas deferens — *see* Injury, pelvic organ, specified site NEC
vascular NEC T14.8
vein — *see* Injury, blood vessel
vena cava (superior) S25.20
inferior S35.10
laceration (minor) (superficial) S35.11
major S35.12
specified type NEC S35.19
laceration (minor) (superficial) S25.21
major S25.22
specified type NEC S25.29
vesical (sphincter) — *see* Injury, bladder
visual cortex S04.04-
vitreous (humor) S05.90
specified NEC S05.8X-
vocal cord NEC S19.83
vulva S39.94
abrasion S30.814
bite S31.45
insect S30.864
superficial NEC S30.874
contusion S30.23
crush S38.03
during delivery — *see* Laceration, perineum, female, during delivery
external constriction S30.844
insect bite S30.864
laceration S31.41
with foreign body S31.42
open wound S31.40
puncture S31.43
with foreign body S31.44
superficial S30.95
foreign body S30.854
whiplash (cervical spine) S13.4
wrist S69.9-
blood vessel — *see* Injury, blood vessel, hand
contusion — *see* Contusion, wrist
dislocation — *see* Dislocation, wrist
fracture — *see* Fracture, wrist
muscle — *see* Injury, muscle, hand
nerve — *see* Injury, nerve, hand
open — *see* Wound, open, wrist
specified NEC S69.8-
sprain — *see* Sprain, wrist
superficial — *see* Injury, superficial, wrist
Inoculation — *see also* Vaccination
complication or reaction — *see* Complications, vaccination
Insanity, insane — *see also* Psychosis
adolescent — *see* Schizophrenia
confusional F28
acute or subacute F05
delusional F22
senile F03
Insect
bite — *see* Bite, by site, superficial, insect
venomous, poisoning NEC (by) — *see* Venom, arthropod

Insecurity, food Z59.41
Insensitivity
adrenocorticotropin hormone (ACTH) E27.49
androgen E34.50
complete E34.51
partial E34.52
Insertion
cord (umbilical) lateral or velamentous O43.12-
intrauterine contraceptive device (encounter for) — *see* Intrauterine contraceptive device
Insolation (sunstroke) T67.01
Insomnia (organic) G47.00
adjustment F51.02
adjustment disorder F51.02
behavioral, of childhood Z73.819
combined type Z73.812
limit setting type Z73.811
sleep-onset association type Z73.810
childhood Z73.819
chronic F51.04
somatized tension F51.04
conditioned F51.04
due to
alcohol
abuse F10.182
dependence F10.282
use F10.982
amphetamines
abuse F15.182
dependence F15.282
use F15.982
anxiety disorder F51.05
caffeine
abuse F15.182
dependence F15.282
use F15.982
cocaine
abuse F14.182
dependence F14.282
use F14.982
depression F51.05
drug NEC
abuse F19.182
dependence F19.282
use F19.982
medical condition G47.01
mental disorder NEC F51.05
opioid
abuse F11.182
dependence F11.282
use F11.982
psychoactive substance NEC
abuse F19.182
dependence F19.282
use F19.982
sedative, hypnotic, or anxiolytic
abuse F13.182
dependence F13.282
use F13.982
stimulant NEC
abuse F15.182
dependence F15.282
use F15.982
fatal familial (FFI) A81.83
idiopathic F51.01
learned F51.3
nonorganic origin F51.01
not due to a substance or known physiological condition F51.01
specified NEC F51.09
paradoxical F51.03
primary F51.01
psychiatric F51.05
psychophysiologic F51.04
related to psychopathology F51.05
short-term F51.02
specified NEC G47.09
stress-related F51.02
transient F51.02
without objective findings F51.02

Inspiration
- food or foreign body — *see* Foreign body, by site
- mucus — *see* Asphyxia, mucus

Inspissated bile syndrome (newborn) P59.1

Instability
- emotional (excessive) F60.3
- housing
  - housed Z59.819
    - with risk of homelessness Z59.811
    - homelessness in past 12 months Z59.812
- joint (post-traumatic) M25.30
  - ankle M25.37-
  - due to old ligament injury — *see* Disorder, ligament
  - elbow M25.32-
  - flail — *see* Flail, joint
  - foot M25.37-
  - hand M25.34-
  - hip M25.35-
  - knee M25.36-
  - lumbosacral — *see* subcategory M53.2
  - prosthesis — *see* Complications, joint prosthesis, mechanical, displacement, by site
  - sacroiliac — *see* subcategory M53.2
  - secondary to
    - old ligament injury — *see* Disorder, ligament
    - removal of joint prosthesis M96.89
  - shoulder (region) M25.31-
  - specified site NEC M25.39
  - spine — *see* subcategory M53.2
  - wrist M25.33-
- knee (chronic) M23.5-
- lumbosacral — *see* subcategory M53.2
- nervous F48.8
- personality (emotional) F60.3
- spine — *see* Instability, joint, spine
- vasomotor R55

Institutional syndrome (childhood) F94.2

Institutionalization, affecting child Z62.22
- disinhibited attachment F94.2

Insufficiency, insufficient
- accommodation, old age H52.4
- adrenal (gland) E27.40
  - primary E27.1
- adrenocortical E27.40
  - drug-induced E27.3
  - iatrogenic E27.3
  - primary E27.1
- anatomic crown height K08.89
- anterior (occlusal) guidance M26.54
- anus K62.89
- aortic (valve) I35.1
  - with
    - mitral (valve) disease I08.0
      - with tricuspid (valve) disease I08.3
    - stenosis I35.2
    - tricuspid (valve) disease I08.2
      - with mitral (valve) disease I08.3
  - congenital Q23.1
  - rheumatic I06.1
    - with
      - mitral (valve) disease I08.0
        - with tricuspid (valve) disease I08.3
      - stenosis I06.2
        - with mitral (valve) disease I08.0
          - with tricuspid (valve) disease I08.3
      - tricuspid (valve) disease I08.2
        - with mitral (valve) disease I08.3
  - specified cause NEC I35.1
  - syphilitic A52.03
- arterial I77.1
  - basilar G45.0
  - carotid (hemispheric) G45.1
  - cerebral I67.81
  - coronary (acute or subacute) I24.8
  - mesenteric K55.1
  - peripheral I73.9
  - precerebral (multiple) (bilateral) G45.2
  - vertebral G45.0
- arteriovenous I99.8
- biliary K83.8

Insufficiency, insufficient - *continued*
- cardiac — *see also* Insufficiency, myocardial
  - due to presence of (cardiac) prosthesis I97.11-
  - postprocedural I97.11-
- cardiorenal, hypertensive I13.2
- cardiovascular — *see* Disease, cardiovascular
- cerebrovascular (acute) I67.81
  - with transient focal neurological signs and symptoms G45.8
- circulatory NEC I99.8
  - newborn P29.89
- clinical crown length K08.89
- convergence H51.11
- coronary (acute or subacute) I24.8
  - chronic or with a stated duration of over 4 weeks I25.89
- corticoadrenal E27.40
  - primary E27.1
- dietary E63.9
- divergence H51.8
- food T73.0
- gastroesophageal K22.89
- gonadal
  - ovary E28.39
  - testis E29.1
- heart — *see also* Insufficiency, myocardial
  - newborn P29.0
  - valve — *see* Endocarditis
- hepatic — *see* Failure, hepatic
- idiopathic autonomic G90.09
- interocclusal distance of fully erupted teeth (ridge) M26.36
- kidney N28.9
  - acute N28.9
  - chronic N18.9
- lacrimal (secretion) H04.12-
  - passages — *see* Stenosis, lacrimal
- liver — *see* Failure, hepatic
- lung — *see* Insufficiency, pulmonary
- mental (congenital) — *see* Disability, intellectual
- mesenteric K55.1
- mitral (valve) I34.0
  - with
    - aortic valve disease I08.0
      - with tricuspid (valve) disease I08.3
    - obstruction or stenosis I05.2
      - with aortic valve disease I08.0
    - tricuspid (valve) disease I08.1
      - with aortic (valve) disease I08.3
  - congenital Q23.3
  - rheumatic I05.1
    - with
      - aortic valve disease I08.0
        - with tricuspid (valve) disease I08.3
      - obstruction or stenosis I05.2
        - with aortic valve disease I08.0
          - with tricuspid (valve) disease I08.3
      - tricuspid (valve) disease I08.1
        - with aortic (valve) disease I08.3
    - active or acute I01.1
      - with chorea, rheumatic (Sydenham's) I02.0
  - specified cause, except rheumatic I34.0
- muscle — *see also* Disease, muscle
  - heart — *see* Insufficiency, myocardial
  - ocular NEC H50.9
- myocardial, myocardium (with arteriosclerosis) — *see also* Failure, heart I50.9
  - with
    - rheumatic fever (conditions in I00) I09.0
      - active, acute or subacute I01.2
        - with chorea I02.0
      - inactive or quiescent (with chorea) I09.0
  - congenital Q24.8
  - hypertensive — *see* Hypertension, heart
  - newborn P29.0
  - rheumatic I09.0
    - active, acute, or subacute I01.2
  - syphilitic A52.06

Insufficiency, insufficient - *continued*
- nourishment T73.0
- pancreatic K86.89
  - exocrine K86.81
- parathyroid (gland) E20.9
- peripheral vascular (arterial) I73.9
- pituitary E23.0
- placental (mother) O36.51-
- platelets D69.6
- prenatal care affecting management of pregnancy O09.3-
- progressive pluriglandular E31.0
- pulmonary J98.4
  - acute, following surgery (nonthoracic) J95.2
    - thoracic J95.1
  - chronic, following surgery J95.3
  - following
    - shock J98.4
    - trauma J98.4
  - newborn P28.89
  - valve I37.1
    - with stenosis I37.2
    - congenital Q22.2
    - rheumatic I09.89
      - with aortic, mitral or tricuspid (valve) disease I08.8
- pyloric K31.89
- renal (acute) N28.9
  - chronic N18.9
- respiratory R06.89
  - newborn P28.5
- rotation — *see* Malrotation
- sleep syndrome F51.12
- social insurance Z59.7
- suprarenal E27.40
  - primary E27.1
- tarso-orbital fascia, congenital Q10.3
- testis E29.1
- thyroid (gland) (acquired) E03.9
  - congenital E03.1
- tricuspid (valve) (rheumatic) I07.1
  - with
    - aortic (valve) disease I08.2
      - with mitral (valve) disease I08.3
    - mitral (valve) disease I08.1
      - with aortic (valve) disease I08.3
    - obstruction or stenosis I07.2
      - with aortic (valve) disease I08.2
        - with mitral (valve) disease I08.3
  - congenital Q22.8
  - nonrheumatic I36.1
    - with stenosis I36.2
- urethral sphincter R32
- valve, valvular (heart) I38
  - aortic — *see* Insufficiency, aortic (valve)
  - mitral — *see* Insufficiency, mitral (valve)
  - pulmonary — *see* Insufficiency, pulmonary, valve
  - tricuspid — *see* Insufficiency, tricuspid (valve)
  - congenital Q24.8
- vascular I99.8
  - intestine K55.9
    - acute — *see also* Ischemia, intestine, acute K55.059
  - mesenteric K55.1
  - peripheral I73.9
  - renal — *see* Hypertension, kidney
- velopharyngeal
  - acquired K13.79
  - congenital Q38.8
- venous (chronic) (peripheral) I87.2
- ventricular — *see* Insufficiency, myocardial
- welfare support Z59.7

Insufflation, fallopian Z31.41

Insular — *see* condition

Insulinoma
- pancreas
  - benign D13.7
  - malignant C25.4
  - uncertain behavior D37.8
- specified site
  - benign — *see* Neoplasm, by site, benign

- **Ischialgia** — *see* Sciatica
- **Ischiopagus** Q89.4
- **Ischium, ischial** — *see* condition
- **Ischuria** R34
- **Iselin's disease or osteochondrosis** — *see* Osteochondrosis, juvenile, metatarsus
- **Islands of**
  - parotid tissue in
    - lymph nodes Q38.6
    - neck structures Q38.6
  - submaxillary glands in
    - fascia Q38.6
    - lymph nodes Q38.6
    - neck muscles Q38.6
- **Islet cell tumor, pancreas** D13.7
- **Isoimmunization NEC** — *see also* Incompatibility
  - affecting management of pregnancy (ABO) (with hydrops fetalis) O36.11-
    - anti-A sensitization O36.11-
    - anti-B sensitization O36.19-
    - anti-c sensitization O36.09-
    - anti-C sensitization O36.09-
    - anti-e sensitization O36.09-
    - anti-E sensitization O36.09-
    - Rh NEC O36.09-
      - anti-D antibody O36.01-
    - specified NEC O36.19-
  - newborn P55.9
    - with
      - hydrops fetalis P56.0
      - kernicterus P57.0
    - ABO (blood groups) P55.1
    - Rhesus (Rh) factor P55.0
    - specified type NEC P55.8
- **Isolation, isolated**
  - dwelling Z59.89
  - family Z63.79
  - social Z60.4
- **Isoleucinosis** E71.19
- **Isomerism atrial appendages (with asplenia or polysplenia)** Q20.6
- **Isosporiasis, isosporosis** A07.3
- **Isovaleric acidemia** E71.110
- **Issue of**
  - medical certificate Z02.79
    - for disability determination Z02.71
  - repeat prescription (appliance) (glasses) (medicinal substance, medicament, medicine) Z76.0
    - contraception — *see* Contraception
- **Itch, itching** — *see also* Pruritus
  - baker's L23.6
  - barber's B35.0
  - bricklayer's L24.5
  - cheese B88.0
  - clam digger's B65.3
  - coolie B76.9
  - copra B88.0
  - dew B76.9
  - dhobi B35.6
  - filarial — *see* Infestation, filarial
  - grain B88.0
  - grocer's B88.0
  - ground B76.9
  - harvest B88.0
  - jock B35.6
  - Malabar B35.5
    - beard B35.0
    - foot B35.3
    - scalp B35.0
  - meaning scabies B86
  - Norwegian B86
  - perianal L29.0
  - poultrymen's B88.0
  - sarcoptic B86
  - scabies B86
  - scrub B88.0
  - straw B88.0
  - swimmer's B65.3
  - water B76.9
  - winter L29.8
- **Ivemark's syndrome (asplenia with congenital heart disease)** Q89.01
- **Ivory bones** Q78.2
- **Ixodiasis NEC** B88.8

J

- **Jaccoud's syndrome** — *see* Arthropathy, postrheumatic, chronic
- **Jackson's**
  - membrane Q43.3
  - paralysis or syndrome G83.89
  - veil Q43.3
- **Jacquet's dermatitis (diaper dermatitis)** L22
- **Jadassohn-Pellizari's disease or anetoderma** L90.2
- **Jadassohn's**
  - blue nevus — *see* Nevus
  - intraepidermal epithelioma — *see* Neoplasm, skin, benign
- **Jaffe-Lichtenstein (-Uehlinger) syndrome** — *see* Dysplasia, fibrous, bone NEC
- **Jakob-Creutzfeldt disease or syndrome** — *see* Creutzfeldt-Jakob disease or syndrome
- **Jaksch-Luzet disease** D64.89
- **Jamaican**
  - neuropathy G92.8
  - paraplegic tropical ataxic-spastic syndrome G92.8
- **Janet's disease** F48.8
- **Janiceps** Q89.4
- **Jansky-Bielschowsky amaurotic idiocy** E75.4
- **Japanese**
  - B-type encephalitis A83.0
  - river fever A75.3
- **Jaundice (yellow)** R17
  - acholuric (familial) (splenomegalic) — *see also* Spherocytosis
    - acquired D59.8
  - breast-milk (inhibitor) P59.3
  - catarrhal (acute) B15.9
    - with hepatic coma B15.0
  - cholestatic (benign) R17
  - due to or associated with
    - delayed conjugation P59.8
      - associated with (due to) preterm delivery P59.0
    - preterm delivery P59.0
  - epidemic (catarrhal) B15.9
    - with hepatic coma B15.0
    - leptospiral A27.0
    - spirochetal A27.0
  - familial nonhemolytic (congenital) (Gilbert) E80.4
    - Crigler-Najjar E80.5
  - febrile (acute) B15.9
    - with hepatic coma B15.0
    - leptospiral A27.0
    - spirochetal A27.0
  - hematogenous D59.9
  - hemolytic (acquired) D59.9
    - congenital — *see* Spherocytosis
  - hemorrhagic (acute) (leptospiral) (spirochetal) A27.0
  - infectious (acute) (subacute) B15.9
    - with hepatic coma B15.0
    - leptospiral A27.0
    - spirochetal A27.0
  - leptospiral (hemorrhagic) A27.0
  - malignant (without coma) K72.90
    - with coma K72.91
  - newborn P59.9
    - due to or associated with
      - ABO
        - antibodies P55.1
        - incompatibility, maternal/fetal P55.1
        - isoimmunization P55.1
      - absence or deficiency of enzyme system for bilirubin conjugation (congenital) P59.8
      - bleeding P58.1
      - breast milk inhibitors to conjugation P59.3
        - associated with preterm delivery P59.0
      - bruising P58.0
      - Crigler-Najjar syndrome E80.5
      - delayed conjugation P59.8
        - associated with preterm delivery P59.0

Jaundice (yellow) - *continued*

- newborn - *continued*
  - due to or associated with - *continued*
    - drugs or toxins
      - given to newborn P58.42
      - transmitted from mother P58.41
    - excessive hemolysis P58.9
      - due to
        - bleeding P58.1
        - bruising P58.0
        - drugs or toxins
          - given to newborn P58.42
          - transmitted from mother P58.41
        - infection P58.2
        - polycythemia P58.3
        - swallowed maternal blood P58.5
      - specified type NEC P58.8
    - galactosemia E74.21
    - Gilbert syndrome E80.4
    - hemolytic disease P55.9
      - ABO isoimmunization P55.1
      - Rh isoimmunization P55.0
      - specified NEC P55.8
    - hepatocellular damage P59.20
      - specified NEC P59.29
    - hereditary hemolytic anemia P58.8
    - hypothyroidism, congenital E03.1
    - incompatibility, maternal/fetal NOS P55.9
    - infection P58.2
    - inspissated bile syndrome P59.1
    - isoimmunization NOS P55.9
    - mucoviscidosis E84.9
    - polycythemia P58.3
    - preterm delivery P59.0
    - Rh
      - antibodies P55.0
      - incompatibility, maternal/fetal P55.0
      - isoimmunization P55.0
    - specified cause NEC P59.8
    - swallowed maternal blood P58.5
  - spherocytosis (congenital) D58.0
- neonatal — *see* Jaundice, newborn
- nonhemolytic congenital familial (Gilbert) E80.4
- nuclear, newborn — *see also* Kernicterus of newborn P57.9
- obstructive — *see also* Obstruction, bile duct K83.1
- post-immunization — *see* Hepatitis, viral, type, B
- post-transfusion — *see* Hepatitis, viral, type, B
- regurgitation — *see also* Obstruction, bile duct K83.1
- serum (homologous) (prophylactic) (therapeutic) — *see* Hepatitis, viral, type, B
- spirochetal (hemorrhagic) A27.0
- symptomatic R17
  - newborn P59.9

- **Jaw** — *see* condition
- **Jaw-winking phenomenon or syndrome** Q07.8
- **Jealousy**
  - alcoholic F10.988
  - childhood F93.8
  - sibling F93.8
- **Jejunitis** — *see* Enteritis
- **Jejunostomy status** Z93.4
- **Jejunum, jejunal** — *see* condition
- **Jensen's disease** — *see* Inflammation, chorioretinal, focal, juxtapapillary
- **Jerks, myoclonic** G25.3
- **Jervell-Lange-Nielsen syndrome** I45.81
- **Jeune's disease** Q77.2
- **Jigger disease** B88.1
- **Job's syndrome (chronic granulomatous disease)** D71
- **Joint** — *see also* condition
  - mice — *see* Loose, body, joint
    - knee M23.4-
- **Jordan's anomaly or syndrome** D72.0
- **Joseph-Diamond-Blackfan anemia (congenital hypoplastic)** D61.01

Jungle yellow fever A95.0
Jüngling's disease — *see* Sarcoidosis
Juvenile — *see* condition

K

Kahler's disease C90.0-
Kakke E51.11
Kala-azar B55.0
Kallmann's syndrome E23.0
Kanner's syndrome (autism) — *see* Psychosis, childhood
Kaposi's
  dermatosis (xeroderma pigmentosum) Q82.1
  lichen ruber L44.0
    acuminatus L44.0
  sarcoma
    colon C46.4
    connective tissue C46.1
    gastrointestinal organ C46.4
    lung C46.5-
    lymph node (multiple) C46.3
    palate (hard) (soft) C46.2
    rectum C46.4
    skin (multiple sites) C46.0
    specified site NEC C46.7
    stomach C46.4
    unspecified site C46.9
  varicelliform eruption B00.0
    vaccinia T88.1
Kartagener's syndrome or triad (sinusitis, bronchiectasis, situs inversus) Q89.3
Karyotype
  with abnormality except iso (Xq) Q96.2
  45,X Q96.0
  46,X
    iso (Xq) Q96.1
  46,XX Q98.3
    with streak gonads Q50.32
    hermaphrodite (true) Q99.1
    male Q98.3
  46,XY
    with streak gonads Q56.1
    female Q97.3
    hermaphrodite (true) Q99.1
  47,XXX Q97.0
  47,XXY Q98.0
  47,XYY Q98.5
Kaschin-Beck disease — *see* Disease, Kaschin-Beck
Katayama's disease or fever B65.2
Kawasaki's syndrome M30.3
Kayser-Fleischer ring (cornea) (pseudosclerosis) H18.04-
Kaznelson's syndrome (congenital hypoplastic anemia) D61.01
Kearns-Sayre syndrome H49.81-
Kedani fever A75.3
Kelis L91.0
Kelly (-Patterson) syndrome (sideropenic dysphagia) D50.1
Keloid, cheloid L91.0
  acne L73.0
  Addison's L94.0
  cornea — *see* Opacity, cornea
  Hawkin's L91.0
  scar L91.0
Keloma L91.0
Kenya fever A77.1
Keratectasia — *see also* Ectasia, cornea
  congenital Q13.4
Keratinization of alveolar ridge mucosa
  excessive K13.23
  minimal K13.22
Keratinized residual ridge mucosa
  excessive K13.23
  minimal K13.22
Keratitis (nodular) (nonulcerative) (simple) (zonular) H16.9
  with ulceration (central) (marginal) (perforated) (ring) — *see* Ulcer, cornea
  actinic — *see* Photokeratitis
  arborescens (herpes simplex) B00.52
  areolar H16.11-
  bullosa H16.8
  deep H16.309
    specified type NEC H16.399

Keratitis (nodular) (nonulcerative) (simple) (zonular) - *continued*
  dendritic (a) (herpes simplex) B00.52
  disciform (is) (herpes simplex) B00.52
    varicella B01.81
  filamentary H16.12-
  gonococcal (congenital or prenatal) A54.33
  herpes, herpetic (simplex) B00.52
    zoster B02.33
  in (due to)
    acanthamebiasis B60.13
    adenovirus B30.0
    exanthema — *see also* Exanthem B09
    herpes (simplex) virus B00.52
    measles B05.81
    syphilis A50.31
    tuberculosis A18.52
    zoster B02.33
  interstitial (nonsyphilitic) H16.30-
    diffuse H16.32-
    herpes, herpetic (simplex) B00.52
      zoster B02.33
    sclerosing H16.33-
    specified type NEC H16.39-
    syphilitic (congenital) (late) A50.31
    tuberculous A18.52
  macular H16.11-
  nummular H16.11-
  oyster shuckers' H16.8
  parenchymatous — *see* Keratitis, interstitial
  petrificans H16.8
  postmeasles B05.81
  punctata
    leprosa A30.9 *[H16.14-]*
    syphilitic (profunda) A50.31
  punctate H16.14-
  purulent H16.8
  rosacea L71.8
  sclerosing H16.33-
  specified type NEC H16.8
  stellate H16.11-
  striate H16.11-
  superficial H16.10-
    with conjunctivitis — *see* Keratoconjunctivitis
    due to light — *see* Photokeratitis
  suppurative H16.8
  syphilitic (congenital) (prenatal) A50.31
  trachomatous A71.1
    sequelae B94.0
  tuberculous A18.52
  vesicular H16.8
  xerotic — *see also* Keratomalacia H16.8
    vitamin A deficiency E50.4
Keratoacanthoma L85.8
Keratocele — *see* Descemetocele
Keratoconjunctivitis H16.20-
  Acanthamoeba B60.13
  adenoviral B30.0
  epidemic B30.0
  exposure H16.21-
  herpes, herpetic (simplex) B00.52
    zoster B02.33
  in exanthema — *see also* Exanthem B09
  infectious B30.0
  lagophthalmic — *see* Keratoconjunctivitis, specified type NEC
  neurotrophic H16.23-
  phlyctenular H16.25-
  postmeasles B05.81
  shipyard B30.0
  sicca (Sjogren's) M35.0-
    not Sjogren's H16.22-
  specified type NEC H16.29-
  tuberculous (phlyctenular) A18.52
  vernal H16.26-
Keratoconus H18.60-
  congenital Q13.4
  stable H18.61-
  unstable H18.62-
Keratocyst (dental) (odontogenic) — *see* Cyst, calcifying odontogenic

Keratoderma, keratodermia (congenital) (palmaris et plantaris) (symmetrical) Q82.8
  acquired L85.1
    in diseases classified elsewhere L86
  climactericum L85.1
  gonococcal A54.89
  gonorrheal A54.89
  punctata L85.2
  Reiter's — *see* Reiter's disease
Keratodermatocele — *see* Descemetocele
Keratoglobus H18.79
  congenital Q15.8
    with glaucoma Q15.0
Keratohemia — *see* Pigmentation, cornea, stromal
Keratoiritis — *see also* Iridocyclitis
  syphilitic A50.39
  tuberculous A18.54
Keratoma L57.0
  palmaris and plantaris hereditarium Q82.8
  senile L57.0
Keratomalacia H18.44-
  vitamin A deficiency E50.4
Keratomegaly Q13.4
Keratomycosis B49
  nigrans, nigricans (palmaris) B36.1
Keratopathy H18.9
  band H18.42-
  bullous H18.1-
  bullous (aphakic) , following cataract surgery H59.01-
Keratoscleritis, tuberculous A18.52
Keratosis L57.0
  actinic L57.0
  arsenical L85.8
  congenital, specified NEC Q80.8
  female genital NEC N94.89
  follicularis Q82.8
    acquired L11.0
    congenita Q82.8
    et parafollicularis in cutem penetrans L87.0
    spinulosa (decalvans) Q82.8
    vitamin A deficiency E50.8
  gonococcal A54.89
  male genital (external) N50.89
  nigricans L83
  obturans, external ear (canal) — *see* Cholesteatoma, external ear
  palmaris et plantaris (inherited) (symmetrical) Q82.8
    acquired L85.1
  penile N48.89
  pharynx J39.2
  pilaris, acquired L85.8
  punctata (palmaris et plantaris) L85.2
  scrotal N50.89
  seborrheic L82.1
    inflamed L82.0
  senile L57.0
  solar L57.0
  tonsillaris J35.8
  vagina N89.4
  vegetans Q82.8
  vitamin A deficiency E50.8
  vocal cord J38.3
Kerato-uveitis — *see* Iridocyclitis
Kerion (celsi) B35.0
Kernicterus of newborn (not due to isoimmunization) P57.9
  due to isoimmunization (conditions in P55.0-P55.9) P57.0
  specified type NEC P57.8
Kerunoparalysis T75.09
Keshan disease E59
Ketoacidosis E87.2
  diabetic — *see* Diabetes, by type, with ketoacidosis
Ketonuria R82.4
Ketosis NEC E88.89
  diabetic — *see* Diabetes, by type, with ketoacidosis
Kew Garden fever A79.1
Kidney — *see* condition

Kienböck's disease — *see also* Osteochondrosis, juvenile, hand, carpal lunate
adult M93.1
Kimmelstiel (-Wilson) disease — *see* Diabetes, Kimmelstiel (-Wilson) disease
Kimura disease D21.9
specified site (see Neoplasm, connective tissue benign)
Kink, kinking
artery I77.1
hair (acquired) L67.8
ileum or intestine — *see* Obstruction, intestine
Lane's — *see* Obstruction, intestine
organ or site, congenital NEC — *see* Anomaly, by site
ureter (pelvic junction) N13.5
with
hydronephrosis N13.1
with infection N13.6
pyelonephritis (chronic) N11.1
congenital Q62.39
vein (s) I87.8
caval I87.1
peripheral I87.1
Kinnier Wilson's disease (hepatolenticular degeneration) E83.01
Kissing spine M48.20
cervical region M48.22
cervicothoracic region M48.23
lumbar region M48.26
lumbosacral region M48.27
occipito-atlanto-axial region M48.21
thoracic region M48.24
thoracolumbar region M48.25
Klatskin's tumor C24.0
Klauder's disease A26.8
Klebs' disease — *see also* Glomerulonephritis N05.-
Klebsiella (K.) pneumoniae, as cause of disease classified elsewhere B96.1
Klein (e) -Levin syndrome G47.13
Kleptomania F63.2
Klinefelter's syndrome Q98.4
karyotype 47,XXY Q98.0
male with more than two X chromosomes Q98.1
Klippel-Feil deficiency, disease, or syndrome (brevicollis) Q76.1
Klippel's disease I67.2
Klippel-Trenaunay (-Weber) syndrome Q87.2
Klumpke (-Déjerine) palsy, paralysis (birth) (newborn) P14.1
Knee — *see* condition
Knock knee (acquired) M21.06-
congenital Q74.1
Knot (s)
intestinal, syndrome (volvulus) K56.2
surfer S89.8-
umbilical cord (true) O69.2
Knotting (of)
hair L67.8
intestine K56.2
Knuckle pad (Garrod's) M72.1
Koch's
infection — *see* Tuberculosis
relapsing fever A68.9
Koch-Weeks' conjunctivitis — *see* Conjunctivitis, acute, mucopurulent
Köebner's syndrome Q81.8
Köenig's disease (osteochondritis dissecans) — *see* Osteochondritis, dissecans
Köhler-Pellegrini-Steida disease or syndrome (calcification, knee joint) — *see* Bursitis, tibial collateral
Köhler's disease
patellar — *see* Osteochondrosis, juvenile, patella
tarsal navicular — *see* Osteochondrosis, juvenile, tarsus
Koilonychia L60.3
congenital Q84.6
Kojevnikov's, epilepsy — *see* Kozhevnikof's epilepsy
Koplik's spots B05.9
Kopp's asthma E32.8
Korsakoff's (Wernicke) disease, psychosis or syndrome (alcoholic) F10.96
with dependence F10.26
drug-induced
due to drug abuse — *see* Abuse, drug, by type, with amnestic disorder
due to drug dependence — *see* Dependence, drug, by type, with amnestic disorder
nonalcoholic F04
Korsakov's disease, psychosis or syndrome — *see* Korsakoff's disease
Korsakow's disease, psychosis or syndrome — *see* Korsakoff's disease
Kostmann's disease or syndrome (infantile genetic agranulocytosis) — *see* Agranulocytosis
Kozhevnikof's epilepsy G40.109
intractable G40.119
with status epilepticus G40.111
without status epilepticus G40.119
not intractable G40.109
with status epilepticus G40.101
without status epilepticus G40.109
Krabbe's
disease E75.23
syndrome, congenital muscle hypoplasia Q79.8
Kraepelin-Morel disease — *see* Schizophrenia
Kraft-Weber-Dimitri disease Q85.8
Kraurosis
ani K62.89
penis N48.0
vagina N89.8
vulva N90.4
Kreotoxism A05.9
Krukenberg's
spindle — *see* Pigmentation, cornea, posterior
tumor C79.6-
Kufs' disease E75.4
Kugelberg-Welander disease G12.1
Kuhnt-Junius degeneration — *see also* Degeneration, macula H35.32-
Kümmell's disease or spondylitis — *see* Spondylopathy, traumatic
Kupffer cell sarcoma C22.3
Kuru A81.81
Kussmaul's
disease M30.0
respiration E87.2
in diabetic acidosis — *see* Diabetes, by type, with ketoacidosis
Kwashiorkor E40
marasmic, marasmus type E42
Kyasanur Forest disease A98.2
Kyphoscoliosis, kyphoscoliotic (acquired) — *see also* Scoliosis M41.9
congenital Q67.5
heart (disease) I27.1
sequelae of rickets E64.3
tuberculous A18.01
Kyphosis, kyphotic (acquired) M40.209
cervical region M40.202
cervicothoracic region M40.203
congenital Q76.419
cervical region Q76.412
cervicothoracic region Q76.413
occipito-atlanto-axial region Q76.411
thoracic region Q76.414
thoracolumbar region Q76.415
Morquio-Brailsford type (spinal) (*see also* subcategory M49.8) E76.219
postlaminectomy M96.3
postradiation therapy M96.2
postural (adolescent) M40.00
cervicothoracic region M40.03
thoracic region M40.04
thoracolumbar region M40.05
secondary NEC M40.10
Kyphosis, kyphotic (acquired) - *continued*
secondary NEC - *continued*
cervical region M40.12
cervicothoracic region M40.13
thoracic region M40.14
thoracolumbar region M40.15
sequelae of rickets E64.3
specified type NEC M40.299
cervical region M40.292
cervicothoracic region M40.293
thoracic region M40.294
thoracolumbar region M40.295
syphilitic, congenital A50.56
thoracic region M40.204
thoracolumbar region M40.205
tuberculous A18.01
Kyrle disease L87.0

L

Labia, labium — *see* condition
Labile
blood pressure R09.89
vasomotor system I73.9
Labioglossal paralysis G12.29
Labium leporinum — *see* Cleft, lip
Labor — *see* Delivery
Labored breathing — *see* Hyperventilation
Labyrinthitis (circumscribed) (destructive) (diffuse) (inner ear) (latent) (purulent) (suppurative) (*see also* subcategory H83.0)
syphilitic A52.79
Laceration
with abortion — *see* Abortion, by type, complicated by laceration of pelvic organs
abdomen, abdominal
wall S31.119
with
foreign body S31.129
penetration into peritoneal cavity S31.619
with foreign body S31.629
epigastric region S31.112
with
foreign body S31.122
penetration into peritoneal cavity S31.612
with foreign body S31.622
left
lower quadrant S31.114
with
foreign body S31.124
penetration into peritoneal cavity S31.614
with foreign body S31.624
upper quadrant S31.111
with
foreign body S31.121
penetration into peritoneal cavity S31.611
with foreign body S31.621
periumbilic region S31.115
with
foreign body S31.125
penetration into peritoneal cavity S31.615
with foreign body S31.625
right
lower quadrant S31.113
with
foreign body S31.123
penetration into peritoneal cavity S31.613
with foreign body S31.623
upper quadrant S31.110
with
foreign body S31.120
penetration into peritoneal cavity S31.610
with foreign body S31.620
accidental, complicating surgery — *see* Complications, surgical, accidental puncture or laceration
Achilles tendon S86.02-
adrenal gland S37.813

Laceration - *continued*
alveolar (process) — *see* Laceration, oral cavity
ankle S91.01-
with
foreign body S91.02-
antecubital space — *see* Laceration, elbow
anus (sphincter) S31.831
with
ectopic or molar pregnancy O08.6
foreign body S31.832
complicating delivery — *see* Delivery, complicated, by, laceration, anus (sphincter)
following ectopic or molar pregnancy O08.6
nontraumatic, nonpuerperal — *see* Fissure, anus
arm (upper) S41.11-
with foreign body S41.12-
lower — *see* Laceration, forearm
auditory canal (external) (meatus) — *see* Laceration, ear
auricle, ear — *see* Laceration, ear
axilla — *see* Laceration, arm
back — *see also* Laceration, thorax, back
lower S31.010
with
foreign body S31.020
with penetration into retroperitoneal space S31.021
penetration into retroperitoneal space S31.011
bile duct S36.13
bladder S37.23
with ectopic or molar pregnancy O08.6
following ectopic or molar pregnancy O08.6
obstetrical trauma O71.5
blood vessel — *see* Injury, blood vessel
bowel — *see also* Laceration, intestine
with ectopic or molar pregnancy O08.6
complicating abortion — *see* Abortion, by type, complicated by, specified condition NEC
following ectopic or molar pregnancy O08.6
obstetrical trauma O71.5
brain (any part) (cortex) (diffuse) (membrane) — *see also* Injury, intracranial, diffuse
during birth P10.8
with hemorrhage P10.1
focal — *see* Injury, intracranial, focal brain injury
brainstem S06.38-
breast S21.01-
with foreign body S21.02-
broad ligament S37.893
with ectopic or molar pregnancy O08.6
following ectopic or molar pregnancy O08.6
laceration syndrome N83.8
obstetrical trauma O71.6
syndrome (laceration) N83.8
buttock S31.801
with foreign body S31.802
left S31.821
with foreign body S31.822
right S31.811
with foreign body S31.812
calf — *see* Laceration, leg
canaliculus lacrimalis — *see* Laceration, eyelid
canthus, eye — *see* Laceration, eyelid
capsule, joint — *see* Sprain
causing eversion of cervix uteri (old) N86
central (perineal) , complicating delivery O70.9
cerebellum, traumatic S06.37-
cerebral S06.33-
left side S06.32-
during birth P10.8
with hemorrhage P10.1
right side S06.31-

Laceration - *continued*
cervix (uteri)
with ectopic or molar pregnancy O08.6
following ectopic or molar pregnancy O08.6
nonpuerperal, nontraumatic N88.1
obstetrical trauma (current) O71.3
old (postpartal) N88.1
traumatic S37.63
cheek (external) S01.41-
with foreign body S01.42-
internal — *see* Laceration, oral cavity
chest wall — *see* Laceration, thorax
chin — *see* Laceration, head, specified site NEC
chordae tendinae NEC I51.1
concurrent with acute myocardial infarction — *see* Infarct, myocardium
following acute myocardial infarction (current complication) I23.4
clitoris — *see* Laceration, vulva
colon — *see* Laceration, intestine, large, colon
common bile duct S36.13
cortex (cerebral) — *see* Injury, intracranial, diffuse
costal region — *see* Laceration, thorax
cystic duct S36.13
diaphragm S27.803
digit (s)
hand — *see* Laceration, finger
foot — *see* Laceration, toe
duodenum S36.430
ear (canal) (external) S01.31-
with foreign body S01.32-
drum S09.2-
elbow S51.01-
with
foreign body S51.02-
epididymis — *see* Laceration, testis
epigastric region — *see* Laceration, abdomen, wall, epigastric region
esophagus K22.89
traumatic
cervical S11.21
with foreign body S11.22
thoracic S27.813
eye (ball) S05.3-
with prolapse or loss of intraocular tissue S05.2-
penetrating S05.6-
eyebrow — *see* Laceration, eyelid
eyelid S01.11-
with foreign body S01.12-
face NEC — *see* Laceration, head, specified site NEC
fallopian tube S37.539
bilateral S37.532
unilateral S37.531
finger (s) S61.219
with
damage to nail S61.319
with
foreign body S61.329
foreign body S61.229
index S61.218
with
damage to nail S61.318
with
foreign body S61.328
foreign body S61.228
left S61.211
with
damage to nail S61.311
with
foreign body S61.321
foreign body S61.221
right S61.210
with
damage to nail S61.310
with
foreign body S61.320
foreign body S61.220
little S61.218
with

Laceration - *continued*
finger (s) - *continued*
little - *continued*
with - *continued*
damage to nail S61.318
with
foreign body S61.328
foreign body S61.228
left S61.217
with
damage to nail S61.317
with
foreign body S61.327
foreign body S61.227
right S61.216
with
damage to nail S61.316
with
foreign body S61.326
foreign body S61.226
middle S61.218
with
damage to nail S61.318
with
foreign body S61.328
foreign body S61.228
left S61.213
with
damage to nail S61.313
with
foreign body S61.323
foreign body S61.223
right S61.212
with
damage to nail S61.312
with
foreign body S61.322
foreign body S61.222
ring S61.218
with
damage to nail S61.318
with
foreign body S61.328
foreign body S61.228
left S61.215
with
damage to nail S61.315
with
foreign body S61.325
foreign body S61.225
right S61.214
with
damage to nail S61.314
with
foreign body S61.324
foreign body S61.224
flank S31.119
with foreign body S31.129
foot (except toe (s) alone) S91.319
with foreign body S91.329
left S91.312
with foreign body S91.322
right S91.311
with foreign body S91.321
toe — *see* Laceration, toe
forearm S51.819
with
foreign body S51.829
elbow only — *see* Laceration, elbow
left S51.812
with
foreign body S51.822
right S51.811
with
foreign body S51.821
forehead S01.81
with foreign body S01.82
fourchette O70.0
with ectopic or molar pregnancy O08.6
complicating delivery O70.0
following ectopic or molar pregnancy O08.6
gallbladder S36.123
genital organs, external
female S31.512

LACERATION - LACERATION

- **Laceration** - *continued*
  - genital organs, external - *continued*
    - female - *continued*
      - with foreign body S31.522
      - vagina — *see* Laceration, vagina
      - vulva — *see* Laceration, vulva
    - male S31.511
      - with foreign body S31.521
      - penis — *see* Laceration, penis
      - scrotum — *see* Laceration, scrotum
      - testis — *see* Laceration, testis
  - groin — *see* Laceration, abdomen, wall
  - gum — *see* Laceration, oral cavity
  - hand S61.419
    - with
      - foreign body S61.429
    - finger — *see* Laceration, finger
    - left S61.412
      - with
        - foreign body S61.422
    - right S61.411
      - with
        - foreign body S61.421
    - thumb — *see* Laceration, thumb
  - head S01.91
    - with foreign body S01.92
    - cheek — *see* Laceration, cheek
    - ear — *see* Laceration, ear
    - eyelid — *see* Laceration, eyelid
    - lip — *see* Laceration, lip
    - nose — *see* Laceration, nose
    - oral cavity — *see* Laceration, oral cavity
    - scalp S01.01
      - with foreign body S01.02
    - specified site NEC S01.81
      - with foreign body S01.82
    - temporomandibular area — *see* Laceration, cheek
  - heart — *see* Injury, heart, laceration
  - heel — *see* Laceration, foot
  - hepatic duct S36.13
  - hip S71.019
    - with foreign body S71.029
    - left S71.012
      - with foreign body S71.022
    - right S71.011
      - with foreign body S71.021
  - hymen — *see* Laceration, vagina
  - hypochondrium — *see* Laceration, abdomen, wall
  - hypogastric region — *see* Laceration, abdomen, wall
  - ileum S36.438
  - inguinal region — *see* Laceration, abdomen, wall
  - instep — *see* Laceration, foot
  - internal organ — *see* Injury, by site
  - interscapular region — *see* Laceration, thorax, back
  - intestine
    - large
      - colon S36.539
        - ascending S36.530
        - descending S36.532
        - sigmoid S36.533
        - specified site NEC S36.538
      - rectum S36.63
        - transverse S36.531
    - small S36.439
      - duodenum S36.430
      - specified site NEC S36.438
  - intra-abdominal organ S36.93
    - intestine — *see* Laceration, intestine
    - liver — *see* Laceration, liver
    - pancreas — *see* Laceration, pancreas
    - peritoneum S36.81
    - specified site NEC S36.893
    - spleen — *see* Laceration, spleen
    - stomach — *see* Laceration, stomach
  - intracranial NEC — *see also* Injury, intracranial, diffuse
    - birth injury P10.9
  - jaw — *see* Laceration, head, specified site NEC
  - jejunum S36.438

- **Laceration** - *continued*
  - joint capsule — *see* Sprain, by site
  - kidney S37.03-
    - major (greater than 3 cm) (massive) (stellate) S37.06-
    - minor (less than 1 cm) S37.04-
    - moderate (1 to 3 cm) S37.05-
      - multiple S37.06-
  - knee S81.01-
    - with foreign body S81.02-
  - labium (majus) (minus) — *see* Laceration, vulva
  - lacrimal duct — *see* Laceration, eyelid
  - large intestine — *see* Laceration, intestine, large
  - larynx S11.011
    - with foreign body S11.012
  - leg (lower) S81.819
    - with foreign body S81.829
    - foot — *see* Laceration, foot
    - knee — *see* Laceration, knee
    - left S81.812
      - with foreign body S81.822
    - right S81.811
      - with foreign body S81.821
    - upper — *see* Laceration, thigh
  - ligament — *see* Sprain
  - lip S01.511
    - with foreign body S01.521
  - liver S36.113
    - major (stellate) S36.116
    - minor S36.114
    - moderate S36.115
  - loin — *see* Laceration, abdomen, wall
  - lower back — *see* Laceration, back, lower
  - lumbar region — *see* Laceration, back, lower
  - lung S27.339
    - bilateral S27.332
    - unilateral S27.331
  - malar region — *see* Laceration, head, specified site NEC
  - mammary — *see* Laceration, breast
  - mastoid region — *see* Laceration, head, specified site NEC
  - meninges — *see* Injury, intracranial, diffuse
  - meniscus — *see* Tear, meniscus
  - mesentery S36.893
  - mesosalpinx S37.893
  - mouth — *see* Laceration, oral cavity
  - muscle — *see* Injury, muscle, by site, laceration
  - nail
    - finger — *see* Laceration, finger, with damage to nail
    - toe — *see* Laceration, toe, with damage to nail
  - nasal (septum) (sinus) — *see* Laceration, nose
  - nasopharynx — *see* Laceration, head, specified site NEC
  - neck S11.91
    - with foreign body S11.92
    - involving
      - cervical esophagus S11.21
        - with foreign body S11.22
      - larynx — *see* Laceration, larynx
      - pharynx — *see* Laceration, pharynx
      - thyroid gland — *see* Laceration, thyroid gland
      - trachea — *see* Laceration, trachea
    - specified site NEC S11.81
      - with foreign body S11.82
  - nerve — *see* Injury, nerve
  - nose (septum) (sinus) S01.21
    - with foreign body S01.22
  - ocular NOS S05.3-
    - adnexa NOS S01.11-
  - oral cavity S01.512
    - with foreign body S01.522
  - orbit (eye) — *see* Wound, open, ocular, orbit
  - ovary S37.439
    - bilateral S37.432
    - unilateral S37.431
  - palate — *see* Laceration, oral cavity
  - palm — *see* Laceration, hand

- **Laceration** - *continued*
  - pancreas S36.239
    - body S36.231
      - major S36.261
      - minor S36.241
      - moderate S36.251
    - head S36.230
      - major S36.260
      - minor S36.240
      - moderate S36.250
    - major S36.269
    - minor S36.249
    - moderate S36.259
    - tail S36.232
      - major S36.262
      - minor S36.242
      - moderate S36.252
  - pelvic S31.010
    - with
      - foreign body S31.020
        - penetration into retroperitoneal cavity S31.021
      - penetration into retroperitoneal cavity S31.011
    - floor — *see also* Laceration, back, lower
      - with ectopic or molar pregnancy O08.6
      - complicating delivery O70.1
      - following ectopic or molar pregnancy O08.6
      - old (postpartal) N81.89
    - organ S37.93
      - with ectopic or molar pregnancy O08.6
      - adrenal gland S37.813
      - bladder S37.23
      - fallopian tube — *see* Laceration, fallopian tube
      - following ectopic or molar pregnancy O08.6
      - kidney — *see* Laceration, kidney
      - obstetrical trauma O71.5
      - ovary — *see* Laceration, ovary
      - prostate S37.823
      - specified site NEC S37.893
      - ureter S37.13
      - urethra S37.33
      - uterus S37.63
  - penis S31.21
    - with foreign body S31.22
  - perineum
    - female S31.41
      - with
        - ectopic or molar pregnancy O08.6
        - foreign body S31.42
      - during delivery O70.9
        - first degree O70.0
        - fourth degree O70.3
        - second degree O70.1
        - third degree — *see also* Delivery, complicated, by, laceration, perineum, third degree O70.20
      - old (postpartal) N81.89
      - postpartal N81.89
      - secondary (postpartal) O90.1
    - male S31.119
      - with foreign body S31.129
  - periocular area (with or without lacrimal passages) — *see* Laceration, eyelid
  - peritoneum S36.893
  - periumbilic region — *see* Laceration, abdomen, wall, periumbilic
  - periurethral tissue — *see* Laceration, urethra
  - phalanges
    - finger — *see* Laceration, finger
    - toe — *see* Laceration, toe
  - pharynx S11.21
    - with foreign body S11.22
  - pinna — *see* Laceration, ear
  - popliteal space — *see* Laceration, knee
  - prepuce — *see* Laceration, penis
  - prostate S37.823
  - pubic region S31.119
    - with foreign body S31.129
  - pudendum — *see* Laceration, genital organs, external

Laceration - *continued*
rectovaginal septum — *see* Laceration, vagina
rectum S36.63
retroperitoneum S36.893
round ligament S37.893
sacral region — *see* Laceration, back, lower
sacroiliac region — *see* Laceration, back, lower
salivary gland — *see* Laceration, oral cavity
scalp S01.01
  with foreign body S01.02
scapular region — *see* Laceration, shoulder
scrotum S31.31
  with foreign body S31.32
seminal vesicle S37.893
shin — *see* Laceration, leg
shoulder S41.019
  with foreign body S41.029
  left S41.012
    with foreign body S41.022
  right S41.011
    with foreign body S41.021
small intestine — *see* Laceration, intestine, small
spermatic cord — *see* Laceration, testis
spinal cord (meninges) — *see also* Injury, spinal cord, by region
  due to injury at birth P11.5
  newborn (birth injury) P11.5
spleen S36.039
  major (massive) (stellate) S36.032
  moderate S36.031
  superficial (minor) S36.030
sternal region — *see* Laceration, thorax, front
stomach S36.33
submaxillary region — *see* Laceration, head, specified site NEC
submental region — *see* Laceration, head, specified site NEC
subungual
  finger (s) — *see* Laceration, finger, with damage to nail
  toe (s) — *see* Laceration, toe, with damage to nail
suprarenal gland — *see* Laceration, adrenal gland
temple, temporal region — *see* Laceration, head, specified site NEC
temporomandibular area — *see* Laceration, cheek
tendon — *see* Injury, muscle, by site, laceration
  Achilles S86.02-
tentorium cerebelli — *see* Injury, intracranial, diffuse
testis S31.31
  with foreign body S31.32
thigh S71.11-
  with foreign body S71.12-
thorax, thoracic (wall) S21.91
  with foreign body S21.92
    back S21.22-
      with penetration into thoracic cavity S21.42-
    front S21.12-
      with penetration into thoracic cavity S21.32-
  back S21.21-
    with
      foreign body S21.22-
        with penetration into thoracic cavity S21.42-
      penetration into thoracic cavity S21.41-
  breast — *see* Laceration, breast
  front S21.11-
    with
      foreign body S21.12-
        with penetration into thoracic cavity S21.32-
      penetration into thoracic cavity S21.31-
thumb S61.019
  with

Laceration - *continued*
thumb - *continued*
  with - *continued*
    damage to nail S61.119
      with
        foreign body S61.129
    foreign body S61.029
  left S61.012
    with
      damage to nail S61.112
        with
          foreign body S61.122
      foreign body S61.022
  right S61.011
    with
      damage to nail S61.111
        with
          foreign body S61.121
      foreign body S61.021
thyroid gland S11.11
  with foreign body S11.12
toe (s) S91.119
  with
    damage to nail S91.219
      with
        foreign body S91.229
    foreign body S91.129
  great S91.113
    with
      damage to nail S91.213
        with
          foreign body S91.223
      foreign body S91.123
    left S91.112
      with
        damage to nail S91.212
          with
            foreign body S91.222
        foreign body S91.122
    right S91.111
      with
        damage to nail S91.211
          with
            foreign body S91.221
        foreign body S91.121
  lesser S91.116
    with
      damage to nail S91.216
        with
          foreign body S91.226
      foreign body S91.126
    left S91.115
      with
        damage to nail S91.215
          with
            foreign body S91.225
        foreign body S91.125
    right S91.114
      with
        damage to nail S91.214
          with
            foreign body S91.224
        foreign body S91.124
tongue — *see* Laceration, oral cavity
trachea S11.021
  with foreign body S11.022
tunica vaginalis — *see* Laceration, testis
tympanum, tympanic membrane — *see* Laceration, ear, drum
umbilical region S31.115
  with foreign body S31.125
ureter S37.13
urethra S37.33
  with or following ectopic or molar pregnancy O08.6
  obstetrical trauma O71.5
urinary organ NEC S37.893
uterus S37.63
  with ectopic or molar pregnancy O08.6
  following ectopic or molar pregnancy O08.6
  nonpuerperal, nontraumatic N85.8
  obstetrical trauma NEC O71.81
  old (postpartal) N85.8
uvula — *see* Laceration, oral cavity

Laceration - *continued*
vagina S31.41
  with
    ectopic or molar pregnancy O08.6
    foreign body S31.42
  during delivery O71.4
    with perineal laceration — *see* Laceration, perineum, female, during delivery
  following ectopic or molar pregnancy O08.6
  nonpuerperal, nontraumatic N89.8
  old (postpartal) N89.8
vas deferens S37.893
vesical — *see* Laceration, bladder
vocal cords S11.031
  with foreign body S11.032
vulva S31.41
  with
    ectopic or molar pregnancy O08.6
    foreign body S31.42
  complicating delivery O70.0
  following ectopic or molar pregnancy O08.6
  nonpuerperal, nontraumatic N90.89
  old (postpartal) N90.89
wrist S61.519
  with
    foreign body S61.529
  left S61.512
    with
      foreign body S61.522
  right S61.511
    with
      foreign body S61.521

Lack of
achievement in school Z55.3
adequate
  food Z59.48
  intermaxillary vertical dimension of fully erupted teeth M26.36
  sleep Z72.820
appetite (see Anorexia) R63.0
awareness R41.9
care
  in home Z74.2
  of infant (at or after birth) T76.02
    confirmed T74.02
cognitive functions R41.9
coordination R27.9
  ataxia R27.0
  specified type NEC R27.8
development (physiological) R62.50
  failure to thrive (child over 28 days old) R62.51
    adult R62.7
    newborn P92.6
  short stature R62.52
  specified type NEC R62.59
energy R53.83
financial resources Z59.6
food Z59.48
growth R62.52
heating Z59.1
housing (permanent) (temporary) Z59.00
  adequate Z59.1
learning experiences in childhood Z62.898
leisure time (affecting life-style) Z73.2
material resources Z59.9
memory — *see also* Amnesia
  mild, following organic brain damage F06.8
ovulation N97.0
parental supervision or control of child Z62.0
person able to render necessary care Z74.2
physical exercise Z72.3
play experience in childhood Z62.898
posterior occlusal support M26.57
relaxation (affecting life-style) Z73.2
safe drinking water Z58.6
sexual
  desire F52.0
  enjoyment F52.1
shelter Z59.02
sleep (adequate) Z72.820

Lack of - *continued*
supervision of child by parent Z62.0
support, posterior occlusal M26.57
water T73.1
safe drinking Z58.6
Lacrimal — *see* condition
Lacrimation, abnormal — *see* Epiphora
Lacrimonasal duct — *see* condition
Lactation, lactating (breast) (puerperal, postpartum)
associated
cracked nipple O92.13
retracted nipple O92.03
defective O92.4
disorder NEC O92.79
excessive O92.6
failed (complete) O92.3
partial O92.4
mastitis NEC — *see* Mastitis, obstetric
mother (care and/or examination) Z39.1
nonpuerperal N64.3
Lacticemia, excessive E87.2
Lacunar skull Q75.8
Laennec's cirrhosis K70.30
with ascites K70.31
nonalcoholic K74.69
Lafora's disease — *see* Epilepsy, generalized, idiopathic
Lag, lid (nervous) — *see* Retraction, lid
Lagophthalmos (eyelid) (nervous) H02.209
bilateral, upper and lower eyelids H02.20C
cicatricial H02.219
bilateral, upper and lower eyelids H02.21C
left H02.216
lower H02.215
upper H02.214
upper and lower eyelids H02.21B
right H02.213
lower H02.212
upper H02.211
upper and lower eyelids H02.21A
keratoconjunctivitis — *see* Keratoconjunctivitis
left H02.206
lower H02.205
upper H02.204
upper and lower eyelids H02.20B
mechanical H02.229
bilateral, upper and lower eyelids H02.22C
left H02.226
lower H02.225
upper H02.224
upper and lower eyelids H02.22B
right H02.223
lower H02.222
upper H02.221
upper and lower eyelids H02.22A
paralytic H02.239
bilateral, upper and lower eyelids H02.23C
left H02.236
lower H02.235
upper H02.234
upper and lower eyelids H02.23B
right H02.233
lower H02.232
upper H02.231
upper and lower eyelids H02.23A
right H02.203
lower H02.202
upper H02.201
upper and lower eyelids H02.20A
Laki-Lorand factor deficiency — *see* Defect, coagulation, specified type NEC
Lalling F80.0
Lambert-Eaton syndrome — *see* Syndrome, Lambert-Eaton
Lambliasis, lambliosis A07.1
Landau-Kleffner syndrome — *see* Epilepsy, specified NEC
Landouzy-Déjérine dystrophy or facioscapulohumeral atrophy G71.02
Landouzy's disease (icterohemorrhagic leptospirosis) A27.0
Landry-Guillain-Barré, syndrome or paralysis G61.0
Landry's disease or paralysis G61.0
Lane's
band Q43.3
kink — *see* Obstruction, intestine
syndrome K90.2
Langdon Down syndrome — *see* Trisomy, 21
Lapsed immunization schedule status Z28.3
Large
baby (regardless of gestational age) (4000g to 4499g) P08.1
ear, congenital Q17.1
physiological cup Q14.2
stature R68.89
Large-for-dates NEC (infant) (4000g to 4499g) P08.1
affecting management of pregnancy O36.6-
exceptionally (4500g or more) P08.0
Larsen-Johansson disease orosteochondrosis — *see* Osteochondrosis, juvenile, patella
Larsen's syndrome (flattened facies and multiple congenital dislocations) Q74.8
Larva migrans
cutaneous B76.9
Ancylostoma B76.0
visceral B83.0
Laryngeal — *see* condition
Laryngismus (stridulus) J38.5
congenital P28.89
diphtheritic A36.2
Laryngitis (acute) (edematous) (fibrinous) (infective) (infiltrative) (malignant) (membranous) (phlegmonous) (pneumococcal) (pseudomembranous) (septic) (subglottic) (suppurative) (ulcerative) J04.0
with
influenza, flu, or grippe — *see* Influenza, with, laryngitis
tracheitis (acute) — *see* Laryngotracheitis
atrophic J37.0
catarrhal J37.0
chronic J37.0
with tracheitis (chronic) J37.1
diphtheritic A36.2
due to external agent — *see* Inflammation, respiratory, upper, due to
Hemophilus influenzae J04.0
H. influenzae J04.0
hypertrophic J37.0
influenzal — *see* Influenza, with, respiratory manifestations NEC
obstructive J05.0
sicca J37.0
spasmodic J05.0
acute J04.0
streptococcal J04.0
stridulous J05.0
syphilitic (late) A52.73
congenital A50.59 *[J99]*
early A50.03 *[J99]*
tuberculous A15.5
Vincent's A69.1
Laryngocele (congenital) (ventricular) Q31.3
Laryngofissure J38.7
congenital Q31.8
Laryngomalacia (congenital) Q31.5
Laryngopharyngitis (acute) J06.0
chronic J37.0
due to external agent — *see* Inflammation, respiratory, upper, due to
Laryngoplegia J38.00
bilateral J38.02
unilateral J38.01
Laryngoptosis J38.7
Laryngospasm J38.5
Laryngostenosis J38.6
Laryngotracheitis (acute) (Infectional) (infective) (viral) J04.2
atrophic J37.1
catarrhal J37.1
chronic J37.1
diphtheritic A36.2
due to external agent — *see* Inflammation, respiratory, upper, due to
Laryngotracheitis (acute) (Infectional) (infective) (viral) - *continued*
Hemophilus influenzae J04.2
hypertrophic J37.1
influenzal — *see* Influenza, with, respiratory manifestations NEC
pachydermic J38.7
sicca J37.1
spasmodic J38.5
acute J05.0
streptococcal J04.2
stridulous J38.5
syphilitic (late) A52.73
congenital A50.59 *[J99]*
early A50.03 *[J99]*
tuberculous A15.5
Vincent's A69.1
Laryngotracheobronchitis — *see* Bronchitis
Larynx, laryngeal — *see* condition
Lassa fever A96.2
Lassitude — *see* Weakness
Late
talker R62.0
walker R62.0
Late effect (s) — *see* Sequelae
Latent — *see* condition
Laterocession — *see* Lateroversion
Lateroflexion — *see* Lateroversion
Lateroversion
cervix — *see* Lateroversion, uterus
uterus, uterine (cervix) (postinfectional) (postpartal, old) N85.4
congenital Q51.818
in pregnancy or childbirth O34.59-
Lathyrism — *see* Poisoning, food, noxious, plant
Launois' syndrome (pituitary gigantism) E22.0
Launois-Bensaude adenolipomatosis E88.89
Laurence-Moon (-Bardet) -Biedl syndrome Q87.89
Lax, laxity — *see also* Relaxation
ligament (ous) — *see also* Disorder, ligament
familial M35.7
knee — *see* Derangement, knee
skin (acquired) L57.4
congenital Q82.8
Laxative habit F55.2
Lazy leukocyte syndrome D70.8
Lead miner's lung J63.6
Leak, leakage
air NEC J93.82
postprocedural J95.812
amniotic fluid — *see* Rupture, membranes, premature
blood (microscopic) , fetal, into maternal circulation affecting management of pregnancy — *see* Pregnancy, complicated by
cerebrospinal fluid G96.00
cranial
postoperative G96.08
specified NEC G96.08
spontaneous G96.01
traumatic G96.08
from spinal (lumbar) puncture G97.0
spinal
postoperative G96.09
post-traumatic G96.09
specified NEC G96.09
spontaneous G96.02
spontaneous
from
skull base G96.01
spine G96.02
CSF — *see* Leak, cerebrospinal fluid
device, implant or graft — *see also* Complications, by site and type, mechanical
arterial graft NEC — *see* Complication, cardiovascular device, mechanical, vascular
breast (implant) T85.43
catheter NEC T85.638
urinary T83.038

Leak, leakage - *continued*
device, implant or graft - *continued*
catheter NEC - *continued*
urinary - *continued*
cystostomy T83.030
Hopkins T83.038
ileostomy T83.038
indwelling T83.031
nephrostomy T83.032
specified NEC T83.038
urostomy T83.038
dialysis (renal) T82.43
intraperitoneal T85.631
infusion NEC T82.534
spinal (epidural) (subdural) T85.630
gastrointestinal — *see* Complications, prosthetic device, mechanical, gastrointestinal device
genital NEC T83.498
penile prosthesis (cylinder) (implanted) (pump) (resevoir) T83.490
testicular prosthesis T83.491
heart NEC — *see* Complication, cardiovascular device, mechanical
joint prosthesis — *see* Complications, joint prosthesis, mechanical, specified NEC, by site
ocular NEC — *see* Complications, prosthetic device, mechanical, ocular device
orthopedic NEC — *see* Complication, orthopedic, device, mechanical
persistent air J93.82
specified NEC T85.638
urinary NEC — *see also* Complication, genitourinary, device, urinary, mechanical
graft T83.23
vascular NEC — *see* Complication, cardiovascular device, mechanical
ventricular intracranial shunt T85.03
urine — *see* Incontinence
Leaky heart — *see* Endocarditis
Learning defect (specific) F81.9
Leather bottle stomach C16.9
Leber's
congenital amaurosis H35.50
optic atrophy (hereditary) H47.22
Lederer's anemia D59.19
Leeches (external) — *see* Hirudiniasis
Leg — *see* condition
Legg (-Calvé) -Perthes disease, syndrome or osteochondrosis M91.1-
Legionellosis A48.1
nonpneumonic A48.2
Legionnaires'
disease A48.1
nonpneumonic A48.2
pneumonia A48.1
Leigh's disease G31.82
Leiner's disease L21.1
Leiofibromyoma — *see* Leiomyoma
Leiomyoblastoma — *see* Neoplasm, connective tissue, benign
Leiomyofibroma — *see also* Neoplasm, connective tissue, benign
uterus (cervix) (corpus) D25.9
Leiomyoma — *see also* Neoplasm, connective tissue, benign
bizarre — *see* Neoplasm, connective tissue, benign
cellular — *see* Neoplasm, connective tissue, benign
epithelioid — *see* Neoplasm, connective tissue, benign
uterus (cervix) (corpus) D25.9
intramural D25.1
submucous D25.0
subserosal D25.2
vascular — *see* Neoplasm, connective tissue, benign
Leiomyoma, leiomyomatosis (intravascular) — *see* Neoplasm, connective tissue, uncertain behavior
Leiomyosarcoma — *see also* Neoplasm, connective tissue, malignant
epithelioid — *see* Neoplasm, connective tissue, malignant
myxoid — *see* Neoplasm, connective tissue, malignant
Leishmaniasis B55.9
American (mucocutaneous) B55.2
cutaneous B55.1
Asian Desert B55.1
Brazilian B55.2
cutaneous (any type) B55.1
dermal — *see also* Leishmaniasis, cutaneous
post-kala-azar B55.0
eyelid B55.1
infantile B55.0
Mediterranean B55.0
mucocutaneous (American) (New World) B55.2
naso-oral B55.2
nasopharyngeal B55.2
old world B55.1
tegumentaria diffusa B55.1
visceral B55.0
Leishmanoid, dermal — *see also* Leishmaniasis, cutaneous
post-kala-azar B55.0
Lenegre's disease I44.2
Lengthening, leg — *see* Deformity, limb, unequal length
Lennert's lymphoma — *see* Lymphoma, Lennert's
Lennox-Gastaut syndrome G40.812
intractable G40.814
with status epilepticus G40.813
without status epilepticus G40.814
not intractable G40.812
with status epilepticus G40.811
without status epilepticus G40.812
Lens — *see* condition
Lenticonus (anterior) (posterior) (congenital) Q12.8
Lenticular degeneration, progressive E83.01
Lentiglobus (posterior) (congenital) Q12.8
Lentigo (congenital) L81.4
maligna — *see also* Melanoma, in situ
melanoma — *see* Melanoma
Lentivirus, as cause of disease classified elsewhere B97.31
Leontiasis
ossium M85.2
syphilitic (late) A52.78
congenital A50.59
Lepothrix A48.8
Lepra — *see* Leprosy
Leprechaunism E34.8
Leprosy A30.-
with muscle disorder A30.9 *[M63.80]*
ankle A30.9 *[M63.87-]*
foot A30.9 *[M63.87-]*
forearm A30.9 *[M63.83-]*
hand A30.9 *[M63.84-]*
lower leg A30.9 *[M63.86-]*
multiple sites A30.9 *[M63.89]*
pelvic region A30.9 *[M63.85-]*
shoulder region A30.9 *[M63.81-]*
specified site NEC A30.9 *[M63.88]*
thigh A30.9 *[M63.85-]*
upper arm A30.9 *[M63.82-]*
anesthetic A30.9
BB A30.3
BL A30.4
borderline (infiltrated) (neuritic) A30.3
lepromatous A30.4
tuberculoid A30.2
BT A30.2
dimorphous (infiltrated) (neuritic) A30.3
I A30.0
indeterminate (macular) (neuritic) A30.0
lepromatous (diffuse) (infiltrated) (macular) (neuritic) (nodular) A30.5
LL A30.5
macular (early) (neuritic) (simple) A30.9
maculoanesthetic A30.9
mixed A30.3
Leprosy - *continued*
neural A30.9
nodular A30.5
primary neuritic A30.3
specified type NEC A30.8
TT A30.1
tuberculoid (major) (minor) A30.1
Leptocytosis, hereditary D56.9
Leptomeningitis (chronic) (circumscribed) (hemorrhagic) (nonsuppurative) — *see* Meningitis
Leptomeningopathy G96.198
Leptospiral — *see* condition
Leptospirochetal — *see* condition
Leptospirosis A27.9
canicola A27.89
due to Leptospira interrogans serovar icterohaemorrhagiae A27.0
icterohemorrhagica A27.0
pomona A27.89
Weil's disease A27.0
Leptus dermatitis B88.0
Leriche's syndrome (aortic bifurcation occlusion) I74.09
Leri's pleonosteosis Q78.8
Leri-Weill syndrome Q77.8
Lermoyez' syndrome — *see* Vertigo, peripheral NEC
Lesch-Nyhan syndrome E79.1
Leser-Trélat disease L82.1
inflamed L82.0
Lesion (s) (nontraumatic)
abducens nerve — *see* Strabismus, paralytic, sixth nerve
alveolar process K08.9
angiocentric immunoproliferative D47.Z9
anorectal K62.9
aortic (valve) I35.9
auditory nerve — *see* subcategory H93.3
basal ganglion G25.9
bile duct — *see* Disease, bile duct
biomechanical M99.9
specified type NEC M99.89
abdomen M99.89
acromioclavicular M99.87
cervical region M99.81
cervicothoracic M99.81
costochondral M99.88
costovertebral M99.88
head region M99.80
hip M99.85
lower extremity M99.86
lumbar region M99.83
lumbosacral M99.83
occipitocervical M99.80
pelvic region M99.85
pubic M99.85
rib cage M99.88
sacral region M99.84
sacrococcygeal M99.84
sacroiliac M99.84
specified NEC M99.89
sternochondral M99.88
sternoclavicular M99.87
thoracic region M99.82
thoracolumbar M99.82
upper extremity M99.87
bladder N32.9
bone — *see* Disorder, bone
brachial plexus G54.0
brain G93.9
congenital Q04.9
vascular I67.9
degenerative I67.9
hypertensive I67.4
buccal cavity K13.79
calcified — *see* Calcification
canthus — *see* Disorder, eyelid
carate — *see* Pinta, lesions
cardia K31.9
cardiac — *see also* Disease, heart I51.9
congenital Q24.9
valvular — *see* Endocarditis
cauda equina G83.4
cecum K63.9

Lesion (s) (nontraumatic) - *continued*
- cerebral — *see* Lesion, brain
- cerebrovascular I67.9
  - degenerative I67.9
  - hypertensive I67.4
- cervical (nerve) root NEC G54.2
- chiasmal — *see* Disorder, optic, chiasm
- chorda tympani G51.8
- coin, lung R91.1
- colon K63.9
- combined periodontic - endodontic K05.5
- congenital — *see* Anomaly, by site
- conjunctiva H11.9
- conus medullaris — *see* Injury, conus medullaris
- coronary artery — *see* Ischemia, heart
- cranial nerve G52.9
  - eighth — *see* Disorder, ear
  - eleventh G52.9
  - fifth G50.9
  - first G52.0
  - fourth — *see* Strabismus, paralytic, fourth nerve
  - seventh G51.9
  - sixth — *see* Strabismus, paralytic, sixth nerve
  - tenth G52.2
  - twelfth G52.3
- cystic — *see* Cyst
- degenerative — *see* Degeneration
- duodenum K31.9
- edentulous (alveolar) ridge, associated with trauma, due to traumatic occlusion K06.2
- en coup de sabre L94.1
- eyelid — *see* Disorder, eyelid
- gasserian ganglion G50.8
- gastric K31.9
- gastroduodenal K31.9
- gastrointestinal K63.9
- gingiva, associated with trauma K06.2
- glomerular
  - focal and segmental — *see also* N00-N07 with fourth character .1 N05.1
  - minimal change — *see also* N00-N07 with fourth character .0 N05.0
- heart (organic) — *see* Disease, heart
- hyperchromic, due to pinta (carate) A67.1
- hyperkeratotic — *see* Hyperkeratosis
- hypothalamic E23.7
- ileocecal K63.9
- ileum K63.9
- iliohypogastric nerve G57.8-
- inflammatory — *see* Inflammation
- intestine K63.9
- intracerebral — *see* Lesion, brain
- intrachiasmal (optic) — *see* Disorder, optic, chiasm
- intracranial, space-occupying R90.0
- joint — *see* Disorder, joint
  - sacroiliac (old) M53.3
- keratotic — *see* Keratosis
- kidney — *see* Disease, renal
- laryngeal nerve (recurrent) G52.2
- lip K13.0
- liver K76.9
- lumbosacral
  - plexus G54.1
  - root (nerve) NEC G54.4
- lung (coin) R91.1
- maxillary sinus J32.0
- mitral I05.9
- Morel-Lavallée — *see* Hematoma, by site
- motor cortex NEC G93.89
- mouth K13.79
- nerve G58.9
  - femoral G57.2-
  - median G56.1-
    - carpal tunnel syndrome — *see* Syndrome, carpal tunnel
  - plantar G57.6-
  - popliteal (lateral) G57.3-
    - medial G57.4-
  - radial G56.3-
  - sciatic G57.0-

Lesion (s) (nontraumatic) - *continued*
- nerve - *continued*
  - spinal — *see* Injury, nerve, spinal
  - ulnar G56.2-
- nervous system, congenital Q07.9
- nonallopathic — *see* Lesion, biomechanical
- nose (internal) J34.89
- obstructive — *see* Obstruction
- obturator nerve G57.8-
- oral mucosa K13.70
- organ or site NEC — *see* Disease, by site
- osteolytic — *see* Osteolysis
- peptic K27.9
- periodontal, due to traumatic occlusion K05.5
- pharynx J39.2
- pigment, pigmented (skin) L81.9
- pinta — *see* Pinta, lesions
- polypoid — *see* Polyp
- prechiasmal (optic) — *see* Disorder, optic, chiasm
- primary — *see also* Syphilis, primary A51.0
  - carate A67.0
  - pinta A67.0
  - yaws A66.0
- pulmonary J98.4
  - valve I37.9
- pylorus K31.9
- rectosigmoid K63.9
- retina, retinal H35.9
- sacroiliac (joint) (old) M53.3
- salivary gland K11.9
  - benign lymphoepithelial K11.8
- saphenous nerve G57.8-
- sciatic nerve G57.0-
- secondary — *see* Syphilis, secondary
- shoulder (region) M75.9-
  - specified NEC M75.8-
- sigmoid K63.9
- sinus (accessory) (nasal) J34.89
- skin L98.9
  - suppurative L08.0
- SLAP S43.43-
- spinal cord G95.9
  - congenital Q06.9
- spleen D73.89
- stomach K31.9
- superior glenoid labrum S43.43-
- syphilitic — *see* Syphilis
- tertiary — *see* Syphilis, tertiary
- thoracic root (nerve) NEC G54.3
- tonsillar fossa J35.9
- tooth, teeth K08.9
  - white spot
    - chewing surface K02.51
    - pit and fissure surface K02.51
    - smooth surface K02.61
- traumatic — *see* specific type of injury by site
- tricuspid (valve) I07.9
  - nonrheumatic I36.9
- trigeminal nerve G50.9
- ulcerated or ulcerative — *see* Ulcer, skin
- uterus N85.9
- vagina N89.8
- vulva N90.89
- vagus nerve G52.2
- valvular — *see* Endocarditis
- vascular I99.9
  - affecting central nervous system I67.9
  - following trauma NEC T14.8
  - umbilical cord, complicating delivery O69.5
- warty — *see* Verruca
- white spot (tooth)
  - chewing surface K02.51
  - pit and fissure surface K02.51
  - smooth surface K02.61

Less than a high school diploma Z55.5

Lethargic — *see* condition

Lethargy R53.83

Letterer-Siwe's disease C96.0

Leukemia, leukemic C95.9-
- acute basophilic C94.8-
- acute bilineal C95.0-

Leukemia, leukemic - *continued*
- acute erythroid C94.0-
- acute lymphoblastic C91.0-
- acute megakaryoblastic C94.2-
- acute megakaryocytic C94.2-
- acute mixed lineage C95.0-
- acute monoblastic (monoblastic/monocytic) C93.0-
- acute monocytic (monoblastic/monocytic) C93.0-
- acute myeloblastic (minimal differentiation) (with maturation) C92.0-
- acute myeloid, NOS C92.0-
  - with
    - 11q23-abnormality C92.6-
    - dysplasia of remaining hematopoesis and/or myelodysplastic disease in its history C92.A-
    - multilineage dysplasia C92.A-
    - variation of MLL-gene C92.6-
  - M6 (a) (b) C94.0-
  - M7 C94.2-
- acute myelomonocytic C92.5-
- acute promyelocytic C92.4-
- adult T-cell (HTLV-1-associated) (acute variant) (chronic variant) (lymphomatoid variant) (smouldering variant) C91.5-
- aggressive NK-cell C94.8-
- AML (1/ETO) (M0) (M1) (M2) (without a FAB classification) C92.0-
- AML M3 C92.4-
- AML M4 (Eo with inv (16) or t (16;16)) C92.5-
- AML M5 C93.0-
- AML M5a C93.0-
- AML M5b C93.0-
- AML Me with t (15;17) and variants C92.4-
- atypical chronic myeloid, BCR/ABL-negative C92.2-
- biphenotypic acute C95.0-
- blast cell C95.0-
- Burkitt-type, mature B-cell C91.A-
- chronic eosinophilic — *see also* Syndrome, hypereosinophilic, myeloid C94.8-
- chronic lymphocytic, of B-cell type C91.1-
- chronic monocytic C93.1-
- chronic myelogenous (Philadelphia chromosome (Ph1) positive) (t (9;22)) (q34;q11) (with crisis of blast cells) C92.1-
- chronic myeloid, BCR/ABL-positive C92.1-
  - atypical, BCR/ABL-negative C92.2-
- chronic myelomonocytic C93.1-
- chronic neutrophilic D47.1
- CMML (-1) (-2) (with eosinophilia) C93.1-
- granulocytic (*see also* Category C92) C92.9-
- hairy cell C91.4-
- juvenile myelomonocytic C93.3-
- lymphoid C91.9-
  - specified NEC C91.Z-
- mast cell C94.3-
- mature B-cell, Burkitt-type C91.A-
- monocytic (subacute) C93.9-
  - specified NEC C93.Z-
- myelogenous (*see also* Category C92) C92.9-
- myeloid C92.9-
  - acute C92.0-
  - specified NEC C92.Z-
- plasma cell C90.1-
- plasmacytic C90.1-
- prolymphocytic
  - of B-cell type C91.3-
  - of T-cell type C91.6-
- specified NEC C94.8-
- stem cell, of unclear lineage C95.0-
- subacute lymphocytic C91.9-
- T-cell large granular lymphocytic C91.Z-
- unspecified cell type C95.9-
  - acute C95.0-
  - chronic C95.1-

Leukemoid reaction — *see also* Reaction, leukemoid D72.823-

Leukoaraiosis (hypertensive) I67.81

Leukoariosis — *see* Leukoaraiosis

Leukocoria — *see* Disorder, globe, degenerated condition, leucocoria
Leukocytopenia D72.819
Leukocytosis D72.829
eosinophilic D72.19
Leukoderma, leukodermia NEC L81.5
syphilitic A51.39
late A52.79
Leukodystrophy E75.29
Leukoedema, oral epithelium K13.29
Leukoencephalitis G04.81
acute (subacute) hemorrhagic G36.1
postimmunization or postvaccinal G04.02
postinfectious G04.01
subacute sclerosing A81.1
van Bogaert's (sclerosing) A81.1
Leukoencephalopathy — *see also* Encephalopathy G93.49
Binswanger's I67.3
heroin vapor G92.8
metachromatic E75.25
multifocal (progressive) A81.2
postimmunization and postvaccinal G04.02
progressive multifocal A81.2
reversible, posterior G93.6
van Bogaert's (sclerosing) A81.1
vascular, progressive I67.3
Leukoerythroblastosis D75.9
Leukokeratosis — *see also* Leukoplakia
mouth K13.21
nicotina palati K13.24
oral mucosa K13.21
tongue K13.21
vocal cord J38.3
Leukokraurosis vulva (e) N90.4
Leukoma (cornea) — *see also* Opacity, cornea
adherent H17.0-
interfering with central vision — *see* Opacity, cornea, central
Leukomalacia, cerebral, newborn P91.2
periventricular P91.2
Leukomelanopathy, hereditary D72.0
Leukonychia (punctata) (striata) L60.8
congenital Q84.4
Leukopathia unguium L60.8
congenital Q84.4
Leukopenia D72.819
basophilic D72.818
chemotherapy (cancer) induced D70.1
congenital D70.0
cyclic D70.0
drug induced NEC D70.2
due to cytoreductive cancer chemotherapy D70.1
eosinophilic D72.818
familial D70.0
infantile genetic D70.0
malignant D70.9
periodic D70.0
transitory neonatal P61.5
Leukopenic — *see* condition
Leukoplakia
anus K62.89
bladder (postinfectional) N32.89
buccal K13.21
cervix (uteri) N88.0
esophagus K22.89
gingiva K13.21
hairy (oral mucosa) (tongue) K13.3
kidney (pelvis) N28.89
larynx J38.7
lip K13.21
mouth K13.21
oral epithelium, including tongue (mucosa) K13.21
palate K13.21
pelvis (kidney) N28.89
penis (infectional) N48.0
rectum K62.89
syphilitic (late) A52.79
tongue K13.21
ureter (postinfectional) N28.89
urethra (postinfectional) N36.8
uterus N85.8
vagina N89.4
Leukoplakia - *continued*
vocal cord J38.3
vulva N90.4
Leukorrhea N89.8
due to Trichomonas (vaginalis) A59.00
trichomonal A59.00
Leukosarcoma C85.9-
Levocardia (isolated) Q24.1
with situs inversus Q89.3
Levotransposition Q20.5
Lev's disease or syndrome (acquired complete heart block) I44.2
Levulosuria — *see* Fructosuria
Levurid L30.2
Lewy body (ies) (dementia) (disease) G31.83
Leyden-Moebius dystrophy G71.09
Leydig cell
carcinoma
specified site — *see* Neoplasm, malignant, by site
unspecified site
female C56.9
male C62.9-
tumor
benign
specified site — *see* Neoplasm, benign, by site
unspecified site
female D27.-
male D29.2-
malignant
specified site — *see* Neoplasm, malignant, by site
unspecified site
female C56.-
male C62.9-
specified site — *see* Neoplasm, uncertain behavior, by site
unspecified site
female D39.1-
male D40.1-
Leydig-Sertoli cell tumor
specified site — *see* Neoplasm, benign, by site
unspecified site
female D27.-
male D29.2-
LGSIL (Low grade squamous intraepithelial lesion on cytologic smear of)
anus R85.612
cervix R87.612
vagina R87.622
Liar, pathologic F60.2
Libido
decreased R68.82
Libman-Sacks disease M32.11
Lice (infestation) B85.2
body (Pediculus corporis) B85.1
crab B85.3
head (Pediculus capitis) B85.0
mixed (classifiable to more than one of the titles B85.0-B85.3) B85.4
pubic (Phthirus pubis) B85.3
Lichen L28.0
albus L90.0
penis N48.0
vulva N90.4
amyloidosis E85.4 *[L99]*
atrophicus L90.0
penis N48.0
vulva N90.4
congenital Q82.8
myxedematosus L98.5
nitidus L44.1
pilaris Q82.8
acquired L85.8
planopilaris L66.1
planus (chronicus) L43.9
annularis L43.8
bullous L43.1
follicular L66.1
hypertrophic L43.0
moniliformis L44.3
of Wilson L43.9
specified NEC L43.8
Lichen - *continued*
planus (chronicus) - *continued*
subacute (active) L43.3
tropicus L43.3
ruber
acuminatus L44.0
moniliformis L44.3
planus L43.9
sclerosus (et atrophicus) L90.0
penis N48.0
vulva N90.4
scrofulosus (primary) (tuberculous) A18.4
simplex (chronicus) (circumscriptus) L28.0
striatus L44.2
urticatus L28.2
Lichenification L28.0
Lichenoides tuberculosis (primary) A18.4
Lichtheim's disease or syndrome D51.0
Lien migrans D73.89
Ligament — *see* condition
Light
for gestational age — *see* Light for dates
headedness R42
Light-for-dates (infant) P05.00
with weight of
499 grams or less P05.01
500-749 grams P05.02
750-999 grams P05.03
1000-1249 grams P05.04
1250-1499 grams P05.05
1500-1749 grams P05.06
1750-1999 grams P05.07
2000-2499 grams P05.08
2500 grams and over P05.09
specified NEC P05.09
and small-for-dates — *see* Small for dates
affecting management of pregnancy O36.59-
Lightning (effects) (stroke) (struck by) T75.00
burn — *see* Burn
foot E53.8
shock T75.01
specified effect NEC T75.09
Lightwood-Albright syndrome N25.89
Lightwood's disease or syndrome (renal tubular acidosis) N25.89
Lignac (-de Toni) (-Fanconi) (-Debré) disease or syndrome E72.09
with cystinosis E72.04
Ligneous thyroiditis E06.5
Likoff's syndrome I20.8
Limb — *see* condition
Limbic epilepsy personality syndrome F07.0
Limitation, limited
activities due to disability Z73.6
cardiac reserve — *see* Disease, heart
eye muscle duction, traumatic — *see* Strabismus, mechanical
mandibular range of motion M26.52
Lindau (-von Hippel) disease Q85.8
Line (s)
Beau's L60.4
Harris' — *see* Arrest, epiphyseal
Hudson's (cornea) — *see* Pigmentation, cornea, anterior
Stähli's (cornea) — *see* Pigmentation, cornea, anterior
Linea corneae senilis — *see* Change, cornea, senile
Lingua
geographica K14.1
nigra (villosa) K14.3
plicata K14.5
tylosis K13.29
Lingual — *see* condition
Linguatulosis B88.8
Linitis (gastric) plastica C16.9
Lip — *see* condition
Lipedema — *see* Edema
Lipemia — *see also* Hyperlipidemia
retina, retinalis E78.3
Lipidosis E75.6
cerebral (infantile) (juvenile) (late) E75.4
cerebroretinal E75.4
cerebroside E75.22

LIPIDOSIS - LOOSENING

- **Lupus** - *continued*
  - erythematosus (discoid) (local) - *continued*
    - systemic - *continued*
      - with organ or system involvement - *continued*
        - specified organ or system NEC M32.19
      - drug-induced M32.0
      - inhibitor (presence of) D68.62
        - with
          - hemorrhagic disorder D68.312
          - hypercoagulable state D68.62
        - finding without diagnosis R76.0
      - specified NEC M32.8
  - exedens A18.4
  - hydralazine M32.0
    - correct substance properly administered — *see* Table of Drugs and Chemicals, by drug, adverse effect
    - overdose or wrong substance given or taken — *see* Table of Drugs and Chemicals, by drug, poisoning
  - nephritis (chronic) M32.14
  - nontuberculous, not disseminated L93.0
  - panniculitis L93.2
  - pernio (Besnier) D86.3
  - systemic — *see* Lupus, erythematosus, systemic
  - tuberculous A18.4
    - eyelid A18.4
  - vulgaris A18.4
    - eyelid A18.4
- **Luteinoma** D27.-
- **Lutembacher's disease or syndrome (atrial septal defect with mitral stenosis)** Q21.1
- **Luteoma** D27.-
- **Lutz (-Splendore-de Almeida) disease** — *see* Paracoccidioidomycosis
- **Luxation** — *see also* Dislocation
  - eyeball (nontraumatic) — *see* Luxation, globe
    - birth injury P15.3
  - globe, nontraumatic H44.82-
  - lacrimal gland — *see* Dislocation, lacrimal gland
  - lens (old) (partial) (spontaneous)
    - congenital Q12.1
      - syphilitic A50.39
- **Lycanthropy** F22
- **Lyell's syndrome** L51.2
  - due to drug L51.2
    - correct substance properly administered — *see* Table of Drugs and Chemicals, by drug, adverse effect
    - overdose or wrong substance given or taken — *see* Table of Drugs and Chemicals, by drug, poisoning
- **Lyme disease** A69.20
- **Lymph**
  - gland or node — *see* condition
  - scrotum — *see* Infestation, filarial
- **Lymphadenitis** I88.9
  - with ectopic or molar pregnancy O08.0
  - acute L04.9
    - axilla L04.2
    - face L04.0
    - head L04.0
    - hip L04.3
    - limb
      - lower L04.3
      - upper L04.2
    - neck L04.0
    - shoulder L04.2
    - specified site NEC L04.8
    - trunk L04.1
  - anthracosis (occupational) J60
  - any site, except mesenteric I88.9
    - chronic I88.1
    - subacute I88.1
  - breast
    - gestational — *see* Mastitis, obstetric
    - puerperal, postpartum (nonpurulent) O91.22
- **Lymphadenitis** - *continued*
  - chancroidal (congenital) A57
  - chronic I88.1
    - mesenteric I88.0
  - due to
    - Brugia (malayi) B74.1
      - timori B74.2
    - chlamydial lymphogranuloma A55
    - diphtheria (toxin) A36.89
    - lymphogranuloma venereum A55
    - Wuchereria bancrofti B74.0
  - following ectopic or molar pregnancy O08.0
  - gonorrheal A54.89
  - infective — *see* Lymphadenitis, acute
  - mesenteric (acute) (chronic) (nonspecific) (subacute) I88.0
    - due to Salmonella typhi A01.09
    - tuberculous A18.39
  - mycobacterial A31.8
  - purulent — *see* Lymphadenitis, acute
  - pyogenic — *see* Lymphadenitis, acute
  - regional, nonbacterial I88.8
  - septic — *see* Lymphadenitis, acute
  - subacute, unspecified site I88.1
  - suppurative — *see* Lymphadenitis, acute
  - syphilitic (early) (secondary) A51.49
    - late A52.79
  - tuberculous — *see* Tuberculosis, lymph gland
  - venereal (chlamydial) A55
- **Lymphadenoid goiter** E06.3
- **Lymphadenopathy (generalized)** R59.1
  - angioimmunoblastic, with dysproteinemia (AILD) C86.5
  - due to toxoplasmosis (acquired) B58.89
    - congenital (acute) (subacute) (chronic) P37.1
  - localized R59.0
  - syphilitic (early) (secondary) A51.49
- **Lymphadenosis** R59.1
- **Lymphangiectasis** I89.0
  - conjunctiva H11.89
  - postinfectional I89.0
  - scrotum I89.0
- **Lymphangiectatic elephantiasis, nonfilarial** I89.0
- **Lymphangioendothelioma** D18.1
  - malignant — *see* Neoplasm, connective tissue, malignant
- **Lymphangioleiomyomatosis** J84.81
- **Lymphangioma** D18.1
  - capillary D18.1
  - cavernous D18.1
  - cystic D18.1
  - malignant — *see* Neoplasm, connective tissue, malignant
- **Lymphangiomyoma** D18.1
- **Lymphangiomyomatosis** J84.81
- **Lymphangiosarcoma** — *see* Neoplasm, connective tissue, malignant
- **Lymphangitis** I89.1
  - with
    - abscess - code by site under Abscess
    - cellulitis - code by site under Cellulitis
    - ectopic or molar pregnancy O08.0
  - acute L03.91
    - abdominal wall L03.321
    - ankle — *see* Lymphangitis, acute, lower limb
    - arm — *see* Lymphangitis, acute, upper limb
    - auricle (ear) — *see* Lymphangitis, acute, ear
    - axilla L03.12-
    - back (any part) L03.322
    - buttock L03.327
    - cervical (meaning neck) L03.222
    - cheek (external) L03.212
    - chest wall L03.323
    - digit
      - finger — *see* Lymphangitis, acute, finger
      - toe — *see* Lymphangitis, acute, toe
    - ear (external) H60.1-
      - external auditory canal — *see* Lymphangitis, acute, ear
- **Lymphangitis** - *continued*
  - acute - *continued*
    - eyelid — *see* Abscess, eyelid
    - face NEC L03.212
    - finger (intrathecal) (periosteal) (subcutaneous) (subcuticular) L03.02-
    - foot — *see* Lymphangitis, acute, lower limb
    - gluteal (region) L03.327
    - groin L03.324
    - hand — *see* Lymphangitis, acute, upper limb
    - head NEC L03.891
      - face (any part, except ear, eye and nose) L03.212
    - heel — *see* Lymphangitis, acute, lower limb
    - hip — *see* Lymphangitis, acute, lower limb
    - jaw (region) L03.212
    - knee — *see* Lymphangitis, acute, lower limb
    - leg — *see* Lymphangitis, acute, lower limb
    - lower limb L03.12-
      - toe — *see* Lymphangitis, acute, toe
    - navel L03.326
    - neck (region) L03.222
    - orbit, orbital — *see* Cellulitis, orbit
    - pectoral (region) L03.323
    - perineal, perineum L03.325
    - scalp (any part) L03.891
    - shoulder — *see* Lymphangitis, acute, upper limb
    - specified site NEC L03.898
    - thigh — *see* Lymphangitis, acute, lower limb
    - thumb (intrathecal) (periosteal) (subcutaneous) (subcuticular) — *see* Lymphangitis, acute, finger
    - toe (intrathecal) (periosteal) (subcutaneous) (subcuticular) L03.04-
    - trunk L03.329
      - abdominal wall L03.321
      - back (any part) L03.322
      - buttock L03.327
      - chest wall L03.323
      - groin L03.324
      - perineal, perineum L03.325
      - umbilicus L03.326
    - umbilicus L03.326
    - upper limb L03.12-
      - axilla — *see* Lymphangitis, acute, axilla
      - finger — *see* Lymphangitis, acute, finger
      - thumb — *see* Lymphangitis, acute, finger
    - wrist — *see* Lymphangitis, acute, upper limb
  - breast
    - gestational — *see* Mastitis, obstetric
  - chancroidal A57
  - chronic (any site) I89.1
  - due to
    - Brugia (malayi) B74.1
      - timori B74.2
    - Wuchereria bancrofti B74.0
  - following ectopic or molar pregnancy O08.89
  - penis
    - acute N48.29
    - gonococcal (acute) (chronic) A54.09
  - puerperal, postpartum, childbirth O86.89
  - strumous, tuberculous A18.2
  - subacute (any site) I89.1
  - tuberculous — *see* Tuberculosis, lymph gland
- **Lymphatic (vessel)** — *see* condition
- **Lymphatism** E32.8
- **Lymphectasia** I89.0
- **Lymphedema (acquired)** — *see also* Elephantiasis
  - congenital Q82.0
  - hereditary (chronic) (idiopathic) Q82.0
  - postmastectomy I97.2
  - praecox I89.0
  - secondary I89.0
  - surgical NEC I97.89

Malabsorption - *continued*
  postsurgical K91.2
  protein K90.49
  starch K90.49
  sucrose E74.39
  syndrome K90.9
    postsurgical K91.2
Malacia, bone (adult) M83.9
  juvenile — *see* Rickets
Malacoplakia
  bladder N32.89
  pelvis (kidney) N28.89
  ureter N28.89
  urethra N36.8
Malacosteon, juvenile — *see* Rickets
Maladaptation — *see* Maladjustment
Maladie de Roger Q21.0
Maladjustment
  conjugal Z63.0
    involving divorce or estrangement Z63.5
  educational Z55.4
  family Z63.9
  marital Z63.0
    involving divorce or estrangement Z63.5
  occupational NEC Z56.89
  simple, adult — *see* Disorder, adjustment
  situational — *see* Disorder, adjustment
  social Z60.9
    due to
      acculturation difficulty Z60.3
      discrimination and persecution (perceived) Z60.5
      exclusion and isolation Z60.4
      life-cycle (phase of life) transition Z60.0
      rejection Z60.4
      specified reason NEC Z60.8
Malaise R53.81
Malakoplakia — *see* Malacoplakia
Malaria, malarial (fever) B54
  with
    blackwater fever B50.8
      hemoglobinuric (bilious) B50.8
    hemoglobinuria B50.8
  accidentally induced (therapeutically) - code by type under Malaria
  algid B50.9
  cerebral B50.0 *[G94]*
  clinically diagnosed (without parasitological confirmation) B54
  congenital NEC P37.4
    falciparum P37.3
  congestion, congestive B54
  continued (fever) B50.9
  estivo-autumnal B50.9
  falciparum B50.9
    with complications NEC B50.8
      cerebral B50.0 *[G94]*
    severe B50.8
  hemorrhagic B54
  malariae B52.9
    with
      complications NEC B52.8
      glomerular disorder B52.0
  malignant (tertian) — *see* Malaria, falciparum
  mixed infections - code to first listed type in B50-B53
  ovale B53.0
  parasitologically confirmed NEC B53.8
  pernicious, acute — *see* Malaria, falciparum
  Plasmodium (P.)
    falciparum NEC — *see* Malaria, falciparum
    malariae NEC B52.9
      with Plasmodium
        falciparum (and or vivax) — *see* Malaria, falciparum
        vivax — *see also* Malaria, vivax
          and falciparum — *see* Malaria, falciparum
    ovale B53.0
      with Plasmodium malariae — *see also* Malaria, malariae
        and vivax — *see also* Malaria, vivax

Malaria, malarial (fever) - *continued*
  Plasmodium (P.) - *continued*
    ovale - *continued*
      with Plasmodium malariae - *continued*
        and vivax - *continued*
          and falciparum — *see* Malaria, falciparum
    simian B53.1
      with Plasmodium malariae — *see also* Malaria, malariae
        and vivax — *see also* Malaria, vivax
          and falciparum — *see* Malaria, falciparum
    vivax NEC B51.9
      with Plasmodium falciparum — *see* Malaria, falciparum
  quartan — *see* Malaria, malariae
  quotidian — *see* Malaria, falciparum
  recurrent B54
  remittent B54
  specified type NEC (parasitologically confirmed) B53.8
  spleen B54
  subtertian (fever) — *see* Malaria, falciparum
  tertian (benign) — *see also* Malaria, vivax
    malignant B50.9
  tropical B50.9
  typhoid B54
  vivax B51.9
    with
      complications NEC B51.8
      ruptured spleen B51.0
Malassez's disease (cystic) N50.89
Malassimilation K90.9
Maldescent, testis Q53.9
  bilateral Q53.20
    abdominal Q53.211
    perineal Q53.22
  unilateral Q53.10
    abdominal Q53.111
    perineal Q53.12
Maldevelopment — *see also* Anomaly
  brain Q07.9
  colon Q43.9
  hip Q74.2
    congenital dislocation Q65.2
      bilateral Q65.1
      unilateral Q65.0-
  mastoid process Q75.8
  middle ear Q16.4
    except ossicles Q16.4
    ossicles Q16.3
  ossicles Q16.3
  spine Q76.49
  toe Q74.2
Male type pelvis Q74.2
  with disproportion (fetopelvic) O33.3
    causing obstructed labor O65.3
Malformation (congenital) — *see also* Anomaly
  adrenal gland Q89.1
  affecting multiple systems with skeletal changes NEC Q87.5
  alimentary tract Q45.9
    specified type NEC Q45.8
    upper Q40.9
      specified type NEC Q40.8
  aorta Q25.40
    absence Q25.41
    aneurysm, congenital Q25.43
    aplasia Q25.41
    atresia Q25.29
      aortic arch Q25.21
    coarctation (preductal) (postductal) Q25.1
    dilatation, congenital Q25.44
    hypoplasia Q25.42
    patent ductus arteriosus Q25.0
    specified type NEC Q25.49
    stenosis Q25.1
      supravalvular Q25.3
  aortic valve Q23.9
    specified NEC Q23.8
  arteriovenous, aneurysmatic (congenital) Q27.30
    brain Q28.2

Malformation (congenital) - *continued*
  arteriovenous, aneurysmatic (congenital) - *continued*
    brain - *continued*
      ruptured I60.8
        intracerebral I61.8
        intraparenchymal I61.8
        intraventricular I61.5
        subarachnoid I60.8
    cerebral — *see also* Malformation, arteriovenous, brain Q28.2
    peripheral Q27.30
      digestive system — *see* Angiodysplasia
        congenital Q27.33
      lower limb Q27.32
      other specified site Q27.39
      renal vessel Q27.34
      upper limb Q27.31
    precerebral vessels (nonruptured) Q28.0
  auricle
    ear (congenital) Q17.3
      acquired H61.119
        left H61.112
          with right H61.113
        right H61.111
          with left H61.113
  bile duct Q44.5
  bladder Q64.79
    aplasia Q64.5
    diverticulum Q64.6
    exstrophy — *see* Exstrophy, bladder
    neck obstruction Q64.31
  bone Q79.9
    face Q75.9
      specified type NEC Q75.8
    skull Q75.9
      specified type NEC Q75.8
  brain (multiple) Q04.9
    arteriovenous Q28.2
    specified type NEC Q04.8
  branchial cleft Q18.2
  breast Q83.9
    specified type NEC Q83.8
  broad ligament Q50.6
  bronchus Q32.4
  bursa Q79.9
  cardiac
    chambers Q20.9
      specified type NEC Q20.8
    septum Q21.9
      specified type NEC Q21.8
  cerebral Q04.9
    vessels Q28.3
  cervix uteri Q51.9
    specified type NEC Q51.828
  Chiari
    Type I G93.5
    Type II Q07.01
  choroid (congenital) Q14.3
    plexus Q07.8
  circulatory system Q28.9
  cochlea Q16.5
  cornea Q13.4
  coronary vessels Q24.5
  corpus callosum (congenital) Q04.0
  diaphragm Q79.1
  digestive system NEC, specified type NEC Q45.8
  dura Q07.9
    brain Q04.9
    spinal Q06.9
  ear Q17.9
    causing impairment of hearing Q16.9
    external Q17.9
      accessory auricle Q17.0
      causing impairment of hearing Q16.9
        absence of
          auditory canal Q16.1
          auricle Q16.0
      macrotia Q17.1
      microtia Q17.2
      misplacement Q17.4
      misshapen NEC Q17.3
      prominence Q17.5
      specified type NEC Q17.8

MALFORMATION - MALNUTRITION

Malnutrition - *continued*
protein - *continued*
calorie - *continued*
severe E43
intermediate form E42
with
kwashiorkor (and marasmus) E42
marasmus E41
energy E46
mild E44.1
moderate E44.0
severe E43
intermediate form E42
with
kwashiorkor (and marasmus) E42
marasmus E41
severe (protein-energy) E43
with
kwashiorkor (and marasmus) E42
marasmus E41
Malocclusion (teeth) M26.4
Angle's M26.219
class I M26.211
class II M26.212
class III M26.213
due to
abnormal swallowing M26.59
mouth breathing M26.59
tongue, lip or finger habits M26.59
temporomandibular (joint) M26.69
Malposition
cervix — *see* Malposition, uterus
congenital
adrenal (gland) Q89.1
alimentary tract Q45.8
lower Q43.8
upper Q40.8
aorta Q25.49
appendix Q43.8
arterial trunk Q20.0
artery (peripheral) Q27.8
coronary Q24.5
digestive system Q27.8
lower limb Q27.8
pulmonary Q25.79
specified site NEC Q27.8
upper limb Q27.8
auditory canal Q17.8
causing impairment of hearing Q16.9
auricle (ear) Q17.4
causing impairment of hearing Q16.9
cervical Q18.2
biliary duct or passage Q44.5
bladder (mucosa) — *see* Exstrophy, bladder
brachial plexus Q07.8
brain tissue Q04.8
breast Q83.8
bronchus Q32.4
cecum Q43.8
clavicle Q74.0
colon Q43.8
digestive organ or tract NEC Q45.8
lower Q43.8
upper Q40.8
ear (auricle) (external) Q17.4
ossicles Q16.3
endocrine (gland) NEC Q89.2
epiglottis Q31.8
eustachian tube Q17.8
eye Q15.8
facial features Q18.8
fallopian tube Q50.6
finger (s) Q68.1
supernumerary Q69.0
foot Q66.9-
gallbladder Q44.1
gastrointestinal tract Q45.8
genitalia, genital organ (s) or tract
female Q52.8
external Q52.79
internal NEC Q52.8
male Q55.8
glottis Q31.8
hand Q68.1

Malposition - *continued*
congenital - *continued*
heart Q24.8
dextrocardia Q24.0
with complete transposition of viscera Q89.3
hepatic duct Q44.5
hip (joint) Q65.89
intestine (large) (small) Q43.8
with anomalous adhesions, fixation or malrotation Q43.3
joint NEC Q68.8
kidney Q63.2
larynx Q31.8
limb Q68.8
lower Q68.8
upper Q68.8
liver Q44.7
lung (lobe) Q33.8
nail (s) Q84.6
nerve Q07.8
nervous system NEC Q07.8
nose, nasal (septum) Q30.8
organ or site not listed — *see* Anomaly, by site
ovary Q50.39
pancreas Q45.3
parathyroid (gland) Q89.2
patella Q74.1
peripheral vascular system Q27.8
pituitary (gland) Q89.2
respiratory organ or system NEC Q34.8
rib (cage) Q76.6
supernumerary in cervical region Q76.5
scapula Q74.0
shoulder Q74.0
spinal cord Q06.8
spleen Q89.09
sternum NEC Q76.7
stomach Q40.2
symphysis pubis Q74.2
thymus (gland) Q89.2
thyroid (gland) (tissue) Q89.2
cartilage Q31.8
toe (s) Q66.9-
supernumerary Q69.2
tongue Q38.3
trachea Q32.1
ureter Q62.60
deviation Q62.61
displacement Q62.62
ectopia Q62.63
specified type NEC Q62.69
uterus Q51.818
vein (s) (peripheral) Q27.8
great Q26.8
vena cava (inferior) (superior) Q26.8
device, implant or graft — *see also* Complications, by site and type, mechanical T85.628
arterial graft NEC — *see* Complication, cardiovascular device, mechanical, vascular
breast (implant) T85.42
catheter NEC T85.628
cystostomy T83.020
dialysis (renal) T82.42
intraperitoneal T85.621
infusion NEC T82.524
spinal (epidural) (subdural) T85.620
urinary — *see also* Displacement, device, catheter, urinary T83.028
electronic (electrode) (pulse generator) (stimulator)
bone T84.320
cardiac T82.129
electrode T82.120
pulse generator T82.121
specified type NEC T82.128
nervous system — *see* Complication, prosthetic device, mechanical, electronic nervous system stimulator

Malposition - *continued*
device, implant or graft - *continued*
electronic (electrode) (pulse generator) (stimulator) - *continued*
urinary — *see* Complication, genitourinary, device, urinary, mechanical
fixation, internal (orthopedic) NEC — *see* Complication, fixation device, mechanical
gastrointestinal — *see* Complications, prosthetic device, mechanical, gastrointestinal device
genital NEC T83.428
intrauterine contraceptive device (string) T83.32
penile prosthesis (cylinder) (implanted) (pump) (resevoir) T83.420
testicular prosthesis T83.421
heart NEC — *see* Complication, cardiovascular device, mechanical
joint prosthesis — *see* Complication, joint prosthesis, mechanical
ocular NEC — *see* Complications, prosthetic device, mechanical, ocular device
orthopedic NEC — *see* Complication, orthopedic, device, mechanical
specified NEC T85.628
urinary NEC — *see also* Complication, genitourinary, device, urinary, mechanical
graft T83.22
vascular NEC — *see* Complication, cardiovascular device, mechanical
ventricular intracranial shunt T85.02
fetus — *see* Pregnancy, complicated by (management affected by), presentation, fetal
gallbladder K82.8
gastrointestinal tract, congenital Q45.8
heart, congenital NEC Q24.8
joint prosthesis — *see* Complications, joint prosthesis, mechanical, displacement, by site
stomach K31.89
congenital Q40.2
tooth, teeth, fully erupted M26.30
uterus (acute) (acquired) (adherent) (asymptomatic) (postinfectional) (postpartal, old) N85.4
anteflexion or anteversion N85.4
congenital Q51.818
flexion N85.4
lateral — *see* Lateroversion, uterus
inversion N85.5
lateral (flexion) (version) — *see* Lateroversion, uterus
in pregnancy or childbirth — *see* subcategory O34.5
retroflexion or retroversion — *see* Retroversion, uterus
Malposture R29.3
Malrotation
cecum Q43.3
colon Q43.3
intestine Q43.3
kidney Q63.2
Malta fever — *see* Brucellosis
Maltreatment
adult
abandonment
confirmed T74.01
suspected T76.01
bullying
confirmed T74.31
suspected T76.31
confirmed T74.91
history of Z91.419
intimidation (through social media)
confirmed T74.31
suspected T76.31
neglect
confirmed T74.01
suspected T76.01

Maltreatment - *continued*
  adult - *continued*
    physical abuse
      confirmed T74.11
      suspected T76.11
    psychological abuse
      confirmed T74.31
      suspected T76.31
      history of Z91.411
    sexual abuse
      confirmed T74.21
      suspected T76.21
    suspected T76.91
  child
    abandonment
      confirmed T74.02
      suspected T76.02
    bullying
      confirmed T74.32
      suspected T76.32
    confirmed T74.92
    history of — *see* History, personal (of), abuse
    intimidation (through social media)
      confirmed T74.32
      suspected T76.32
    neglect
      confirmed T74.02
      history of — *see* History, personal (of), abuse
      suspected T76.02
    physical abuse
      confirmed T74.12
      history of — *see* History, personal (of), abuse
      suspected T76.12
    psychological abuse
      confirmed T74.32
      history of — *see* History, personal (of), abuse
      suspected T76.32
    sexual abuse
      confirmed T74.22
      history of — *see* History, personal (of), abuse
      suspected T76.22
    suspected T76.92
  personal history of Z91.89
Maltworker's lung J67.4
Malunion, fracture — *see* Fracture, by site
Mammillitis N61.0
  puerperal, postpartum O91.02
Mammitis — *see* Mastitis
Mammogram (examination) Z12.39
  routine Z12.31
Mammoplasia N62
Management (of)
  bone conduction hearing device (implanted) Z45.320
  cardiac pacemaker NEC Z45.018
  cerebrospinal fluid drainage device Z45.41
  cochlear device (implanted) Z45.321
  contraceptive Z30.9
    specified NEC Z30.8
  implanted device Z45.9
    specified NEC Z45.89
  infusion pump Z45.1
  procreative Z31.9
    male factor infertility in female Z31.81
    specified NEC Z31.89
  prosthesis (external) — *see also* Fitting Z44.9
    implanted Z45.9
      specified NEC Z45.89
  renal dialysis catheter Z49.01
  vascular access device Z45.2
Mangled — *see* specified injury by site
Mania (monopolar) — *see also* Disorder, mood, manic episode
  with psychotic symptoms F30.2
  without psychotic symptoms F30.10
    mild F30.11
    moderate F30.12
    severe F30.13
  Bell's F30.8
Mania (monopolar) - *continued*
  chronic (recurrent) F31.89
  hysterical F44.89
  puerperal F30.8
  recurrent F31.89
Manic depression F31.9
Manic-depressive insanity, psychosis, or syndrome — *see* Disorder, bipolar
Mannosidosis E77.1
Mansonelliasis, mansonellosis B74.4
Manson's
  disease B65.1
  schistosomiasis B65.1
Manual — *see* condition
Maple-bark-stripper's lung (disease) J67.6
Maple-syrup-urine disease E71.0
Marable's syndrome (celiac artery compression) I77.4
Marasmus E41
  due to malnutrition E41
  intestinal E41
  nutritional E41
  senile R54
  tuberculous NEC — *see* Tuberculosis
Marble
  bones Q78.2
  skin R23.8
Marburg virus disease A98.3
March
  fracture — *see* Fracture, traumatic, stress, by site
  hemoglobinuria D59.6
Marchesani (-Weill) syndrome Q87.0
Marchiafava (-Bignami) syndrome or disease G37.1
Marchiafava-Micheli syndrome D59.5
Marcus Gunn's syndrome Q07.8
Marfan's syndrome — *see* Syndrome, Marfan's
Marie-Bamberger disease — *see* Osteoarthropathy, hypertrophic, specified NEC
Marie-Charcot-Tooth neuropathic muscular atrophy G60.0
Marie's
  cerebellar ataxia (late-onset) G11.2
  disease or syndrome (acromegaly) E22.0
Marie-Strümpell arthritis, disease or spondylitis — *see* Spondylitis, ankylosing
Marion's disease (bladder neck obstruction) N32.0
Marital conflict Z63.0
Mark
  port wine Q82.5
  raspberry Q82.5
  strawberry Q82.5
  stretch L90.6
  tattoo L81.8
Marker heterochromatin — *see* Extra, marker chromosomes
Maroteaux-Lamy syndrome (mild) (severe) E76.29
Marrow (bone)
  arrest D61.9
  poor function D75.89
Marseilles fever A77.1
Marsh fever — *see* Malaria
Marshall's (hidrotic) ectodermal dysplasia Q82.4
Marsh's disease (exophthalmic goiter) E05.00
  with storm E05.01
Masculinization (female) with adrenal hyperplasia E25.9
  congenital E25.0
Masculinovoblastoma D27.-
Masochism (sexual) F65.51
Mason's lung J62.8
Mass
  abdominal R19.00
    epigastric R19.06
    generalized R19.07
    left lower quadrant R19.04
    left upper quadrant R19.02
    periumbilic R19.05
Mass - *continued*
  abdominal - *continued*
    right lower quadrant R19.03
    right upper quadrant R19.01
    specified site NEC R19.09
  breast — *see also* Lump, breast N63.0
  chest R22.2
  cystic — *see* Cyst
  ear H93.8-
  head R22.0
  intra-abdominal (diffuse) (generalized) — *see* Mass, abdominal
  kidney N28.89
  liver R16.0
  localized (skin) R22.9
    chest R22.2
    head R22.0
    limb
      lower R22.4-
      upper R22.3-
    neck R22.1
    trunk R22.2
  lung R91.8
  malignant — *see* Neoplasm, malignant, by site
  neck R22.1
  pelvic (diffuse) (generalized) — *see* Mass, abdominal
  specified organ NEC — *see* Disease, by site
  splenic R16.1
  substernal thyroid — *see* Goiter
  superficial (localized) R22.9
  umbilical (diffuse) (generalized) R19.09
Massive — *see* condition
Mast cell
  disease, systemic tissue D47.02
  leukemia C94.3-
  neoplasm
    malignant C96.20
      specified type NEC C96.29
    of uncertain behavior NEC D47.09
  sarcoma C96.22
  tumor D47.09
Mastalgia N64.4
Masters-Allen syndrome N83.8
Mastitis (acute) (diffuse) (nonpuerperal) (subacute) N61.0
  with abscess N61.1
  chronic (cystic) — *see* Mastopathy, cystic
  cystic (Schimmelbusch's type) — *see* Mastopathy, cystic
  fibrocystic — *see* Mastopathy, cystic
  granulomatous N61.2-
  infective N61.0
    newborn P39.0
  interstitial, gestational or puerperal — *see* Mastitis, obstetric
  neonatal (noninfective) P83.4
    infective P39.0
  obstetric (interstitial) (nonpurulent)
    associated with
      lactation O91.23
      pregnancy O91.21-
      puerperium O91.22
    purulent
      associated with
        lactation O91.13
        pregnancy O91.11-
        puerperium O91.12
  periductal — *see* Ectasia, mammary duct
  phlegmonous — *see* Mastopathy, cystic
  plasma cell — *see* Ectasia, mammary duct
  without abscess N61.0
Mastocytoma (extracutaneous) D47.09
  malignant C96.29
  solitary D47.01
Mastocytosis D47.09
  aggressive systemic C96.21
  cutaneous (diffuse) (maculopapular) D47.01
    congenital Q82.2
    of neonatal onset Q82.2
    of newborn onset Q82.2
  indolent systemic D47.02
  isolated bone marrow D47.02
  malignant C96.29

Mastocytosis - *continued*
- systemic (indolent) (smoldering)
  - with an associated hematological non-mast cell lineage disease (SM-AHNMD) D47.02

Mastodynia N64.4
Mastoid — *see* condition
Mastoidalgia — *see* subcategory H92.0
Mastoiditis (coalescent) (hemorrhagic) (suppurative) H70.9-
- acute, subacute H70.00-
  - complicated NEC H70.09-
  - subperiosteal H70.01-
- chronic (necrotic) (recurrent) H70.1-
- in (due to)
  - infectious disease NEC B99 *[H75.0-]*
  - parasitic disease NEC B89 *[H75.0-]*
  - tuberculosis A18.03
- petrositis — *see* Petrositis
- postauricular fistula — *see* Fistula, postauricular
- specified NEC H70.89-
- tuberculous A18.03

Mastopathy, mastopathia N64.9
- chronica cystica — *see* Mastopathy, cystic
- cystic (chronic) (diffuse) N60.1-
  - with epithelial proliferation N60.3-
- diffuse cystic — *see* Mastopathy, cystic
- estrogenic, oestrogenica N64.89
- ovarian origin N64.89

Mastoplasia, mastoplastia N62
Masturbation (excessive) F98.8
Maternal care (for) — *see* Pregnancy (complicated by) (management affected by)
Matheiu's disease (leptospiral jaundice) A27.0
Mauclaire's disease or osteochondrosis — *see* Osteochondrosis, juvenile, hand, metacarpal
Maxcy's disease A75.2
Maxilla, maxillary — *see* condition
May (-Hegglin) anomaly or syndrome D72.0
McArdle (-Schmid) (-Pearson) disease (glycogen storage) E74.04
McCune-Albright syndrome Q78.1
McQuarrie's syndrome (idiopathic familial hypoglycemia) E16.2
Meadow's syndrome Q86.1
Measles (black) (hemorrhagic) (suppressed) B05.9
- with
  - complications NEC B05.89
  - encephalitis B05.0
  - intestinal complications B05.4
  - keratitis (keratoconjunctivitis) B05.81
  - meningitis B05.1
  - otitis media B05.3
  - pneumonia B05.2
- French — *see* Rubella
- German — *see* Rubella
- Liberty — *see* Rubella

Meatitis, urethral — *see* Urethritis
Meatus, meatal — *see* condition
Meat-wrappers' asthma J68.9
Meckel-Gruber syndrome Q61.9
Meckel's diverticulitis, diverticulum (displaced) (hypertrophic) Q43.0
- malignant — *see* Table of Neoplasms, small intestine, malignant

Meconium
- ileus, newborn P76.0
  - in cystic fibrosis E84.11
  - meaning meconium plug (without cystic fibrosis) P76.0
- obstruction, newborn P76.0
  - due to fecaliths P76.0
  - in mucoviscidosis E84.11
- peritonitis P78.0
- plug syndrome (newborn) NEC P76.0

Median — *see also* condition
- arcuate ligament syndrome I77.4
- bar (prostate) (vesical orifice) — *see* Hyperplasia, prostate
- rhomboid glossitis K14.2

Mediastinal shift R93.89
Mediastinitis (acute) (chronic) J98.51
- syphilitic A52.73
- tuberculous A15.8

Mediastinopericarditis — *see also* Pericarditis
- acute I30.9
- adhesive I31.0
- chronic I31.8
  - rheumatic I09.2

Mediastinum, mediastinal — *see* condition
Medicine poisoning — *see* Table of Drugs and Chemicals, by drug, poisoning
Mediterranean
- fever — *see* Brucellosis
  - familial M04.1
  - tick A77.1
- kala-azar B55.0
- leishmaniasis B55.0
- tick fever A77.1

Medulla — *see* condition
Medullary cystic kidney Q61.5
Medullated fibers
- optic (nerve) Q14.8
- retina Q14.1

Medulloblastoma
- desmoplastic C71.6
- specified site — *see* Neoplasm, malignant, by site
- unspecified site C71.6

Medulloepithelioma — *see also* Neoplasm, malignant, by site
- teratoid — *see* Neoplasm, malignant, by site

Medullomyoblastoma
- specified site — *see* Neoplasm, malignant, by site
- unspecified site C71.6

Meekeren-Ehlers-Danlos syndrome — *see also* Syndrome, Ehlers-Danlos Q79.69
Megacolon (acquired) (functional) (not Hirschsprung's disease) (in) K59.39
- Chagas' disease B57.32
- congenital, congenitum (aganglionic) Q43.1
- Hirschsprung's (disease) Q43.1
- toxic NEC K59.31
  - due to Clostridium difficile
    - not specified as recurrent A04.72
    - recurrent A04.71

Megaesophagus (functional) K22.0
- congenital Q39.5
- in (due to) Chagas' disease B57.31

Megalencephaly Q04.5
Megalerythema (epidemic) B08.3
Megaloappendix Q43.8
Megalocephalus, megalocephaly NEC Q75.3
Megalocornea Q15.8
- with glaucoma Q15.0

Megalocytic anemia D53.1
Megalodactylia (fingers) (thumbs) (congenital) Q74.0
- toes Q74.2

Megaloduodenum Q43.8
Megaloesophagus (functional) K22.0
- congenital Q39.5

Megalogastria (acquired) K31.89
- congenital Q40.2

Megalophthalmos Q11.3
Megalopsia H53.15
Megalosplenia — *see* Splenomegaly
Megaloureter N28.82
- congenital Q62.2

Megarectum K62.89
Megasigmoid K59.39
- congenital Q43.2

Megaureter N28.82
- congenital Q62.2

Megavitamin-B6 syndrome E67.2
Megrim — *see* Migraine
Meibomian
- cyst, infected — *see* Hordeolum
- gland — *see* condition
- sty, stye — *see* Hordeolum

Meibomitis — *see* Hordeolum
Meige-Milroy disease (chronic hereditary edema) Q82.0
Meige's syndrome Q82.0
Melalgia, nutritional E53.8
Melancholia F32.A
- climacteric (single episode) F32.89
  - recurrent episode F33.8
- hypochondriac F45.29
- intermittent (single episode) F32.89
  - recurrent episode F33.8
- involutional (single episode) F32.89
  - recurrent episode F33.8
- menopausal (single episode) F32.89
  - recurrent episode F33.8
- puerperal F32.89
- reactive (emotional stress or trauma) F32.3
- recurrent F33.9
- senile F03
- stuporous (single episode) F32.89
  - recurrent episode F33.8

Melanemia R79.89
Melanoameloblastoma — *see* Neoplasm, bone, benign
Melanoblastoma — *see* Melanoma
Melanocarcinoma — *see* Melanoma
Melanocytoma, eyeball D31.9-
Melanocytosis, neurocutaneous Q82.8
Melanoderma, melanodermia L81.4
Melanodontia, infantile K03.89
Melanodontoclasia K03.89
Melanoepithelioma — *see* Melanoma
Melanoma (malignant) C43.9
- acral lentiginous, malignant — *see* Melanoma, skin, by site
- amelanotic — *see* Melanoma, skin, by site
- balloon cell — *see* Melanoma, skin, by site
- benign — *see* Nevus
- desmoplastic, malignant — *see* Melanoma, skin, by site
- epithelioid cell — *see* Melanoma, skin, by site
  - with spindle cell, mixed — *see* Melanoma, skin, by site
- in
  - giant pigmented nevus — *see* Melanoma, skin, by site
  - Hutchinson's melanotic freckle — *see* Melanoma, skin, by site
  - junctional nevus — *see* Melanoma, skin, by site
  - precancerous melanosis — *see* Melanoma, skin, by site
- in situ D03.9
  - abdominal wall D03.59
  - ala nasi D03.39
  - ankle D03.7-
  - anus, anal (margin) (skin) D03.51
  - arm D03.6-
  - auditory canal D03.2-
  - auricle (ear) D03.2-
  - auricular canal (external) D03.2-
  - axilla, axillary fold D03.59
  - back D03.59
  - breast D03.52
  - brow D03.39
  - buttock D03.59
  - canthus (eye) D03.1-
  - cheek (external) D03.39
  - chest wall D03.59
  - chin D03.39
  - choroid D03.8
  - conjunctiva D03.8
  - ear (external) D03.2-
  - external meatus (ear) D03.2-
  - eye D03.8
  - eyebrow D03.39
  - eyelid (lower) (upper) D03.1-
  - face D03.30
    - specified NEC D03.39
  - female genital organ (external) NEC D03.8
  - finger D03.6-
  - flank D03.59
  - foot D03.7-
  - forearm D03.6-
  - forehead D03.39
  - foreskin D03.8
  - gluteal region D03.59

Melanoma (malignant) - *continued*
- in situ - *continued*
  - groin D03.59
  - hand D03.6-
  - heel D03.7-
  - helix D03.2-
  - hip D03.7-
  - interscapular region D03.59
  - iris D03.8
  - jaw D03.39
  - knee D03.7-
  - labium (majus) (minus) D03.8
  - lacrimal gland D03.8
  - leg D03.7-
  - lip (lower) (upper) D03.0
  - lower limb NEC D03.7-
  - male genital organ (external) NEC D03.8
  - nail D03.9
    - finger D03.6-
    - toe D03.7-
  - neck D03.4
  - nose (external) D03.39
  - orbit D03.8
  - penis D03.8
  - perianal skin D03.51
  - perineum D03.51
  - pinna D03.2-
  - popliteal fossa or space D03.7-
  - prepuce D03.8
  - pudendum D03.8
  - retina D03.8
  - retrobulbar D03.8
  - scalp D03.4
  - scrotum D03.8
  - shoulder D03.6-
  - specified site NEC D03.8
  - submammary fold D03.52
  - temple D03.39
  - thigh D03.7-
  - toe D03.7-
  - trunk NEC D03.59
  - umbilicus D03.59
  - upper limb NEC D03.6-
  - vulva D03.8
- juvenile — *see* Nevus
- malignant, of soft parts except skin — *see* Neoplasm, connective tissue, malignant
- metastatic
  - breast C79.81
  - genital organ C79.82
  - specified site NEC C79.89
- neurotropic, malignant — *see* Melanoma, skin, by site
- nodular — *see* Melanoma, skin, by site
- regressing, malignant — *see* Melanoma, skin, by site
- skin C43.9
  - abdominal wall C43.59
  - ala nasi C43.31
  - ankle C43.7-
  - anus, anal (skin) C43.51
  - arm C43.6-
  - auditory canal (external) C43.2-
  - auricle (ear) C43.2-
  - auricular canal (external) C43.2-
  - axilla, axillary fold C43.59
  - back C43.59
  - breast (female) (male) C43.52
  - brow C43.39
  - buttock C43.59
  - canthus (eye) C43.1-
  - cheek (external) C43.39
  - chest wall C43.59
  - chin C43.39
  - ear (external) C43.2-
  - elbow C43.6-
  - external meatus (ear) C43.2-
  - eyebrow C43.39
  - eyelid (lower) (upper) C43.1-
  - face C43.30
    - specified NEC C43.39
  - female genital organ (external) NEC C51.9
  - finger C43.6-
  - flank C43.59
  - foot C43.7-

Melanoma (malignant) - *continued*
- skin - *continued*
  - forearm C43.6-
  - forehead C43.39
  - foreskin C60.0
  - glabella C43.39
  - gluteal region C43.59
  - groin C43.59
  - hand C43.6-
  - heel C43.7-
  - helix C43.2-
  - hip C43.7-
  - interscapular region C43.59
  - jaw (external) C43.39
  - knee C43.7-
  - labium C51.9
    - majus C51.0
    - minus C51.1
  - leg C43.7-
  - lip (lower) (upper) C43.0
  - lower limb NEC C43.7-
  - male genital organ (external) NEC C63.9
  - nail
    - finger C43.6-
    - toe C43.7-
  - nasolabial groove C43.39
  - nates C43.59
  - neck C43.4
  - nose (external) C43.31
  - overlapping site C43.8
  - palpebra C43.1-
  - penis C60.9
  - perianal skin C43.51
  - perineum C43.51
  - pinna C43.2-
  - popliteal fossa or space C43.7-
  - prepuce C60.0
  - pudendum C51.9
  - scalp C43.4
  - scrotum C63.2
  - shoulder C43.6-
  - skin NEC C43.9
  - submammary fold C43.52
  - temple C43.39
  - thigh C43.7-
  - toe C43.7-
  - trunk NEC C43.59
  - umbilicus C43.59
  - upper limb NEC C43.6-
  - vulva C51.9
    - overlapping sites C51.8
- spindle cell
  - with epithelioid, mixed — *see* Melanoma, skin, by site
  - type A C69.4-
  - type B C69.4-
- superficial spreading — *see* Melanoma, skin, by site

Melanosarcoma — *see also* Melanoma
- epithelioid cell — *see* Melanoma

Melanosis L81.4
- addisonian E27.1
  - tuberculous A18.7
- adrenal E27.1
- colon K63.89
- conjunctiva — *see* Pigmentation, conjunctiva
  - congenital Q13.89
- cornea (presenile) (senile) — *see also* Pigmentation, cornea
  - congenital Q13.4
- eye NEC H57.89
  - congenital Q15.8
- lenticularis progressiva Q82.1
- liver K76.89
- precancerous — *see also* Melanoma, in situ
  - malignant melanoma in — *see* Melanoma
- Riehl's L81.4
- sclera H15.89
  - congenital Q13.89
- suprarenal E27.1
- tar L81.4
- toxic L81.4

Melanuria R82.998

MELAS syndrome E88.41

Melasma L81.1
- adrenal (gland) E27.1
- suprarenal (gland) E27.1

Melena K92.1
- with ulcer - code by site under Ulcer, with hemorrhage K27.4
- due to swallowed maternal blood P78.2
- newborn, neonatal P54.1
  - due to swallowed maternal blood P78.2

Meleney's
- gangrene (cutaneous) — *see* Ulcer, skin
- ulcer (chronic undermining) — *see* Ulcer, skin

Melioidosis A24.9
- acute A24.1
- chronic A24.2
- fulminating A24.1
- pneumonia A24.1
- pulmonary (chronic) A24.2
  - acute A24.1
  - subacute A24.2
- sepsis A24.1
- specified NEC A24.3
- subacute A24.2

Melitensis, febris A23.0

Melkersson (-Rosenthal) syndrome G51.2

Mellitus, diabetes — *see* Diabetes

Melorheostosis (bone) — *see* Disorder, bone, density and structure, specified NEC

Meloschisis Q18.4

Melotia Q17.4

Membrana
- capsularis lentis posterior Q13.89
- epipapillaris Q14.2

Membranacea placenta O43.19-

Membranaceous uterus N85.8

Membrane (s) , membranous — *see also* condition
- cyclitic — *see* Membrane, pupillary
- folds, congenital — *see* Web
- Jackson's Q43.3
- over face of newborn P28.9
- premature rupture — *see* Rupture, membranes, premature
- pupillary H21.4-
  - persistent Q13.89
- retained (with hemorrhage) (complicating delivery) O72.2
  - without hemorrhage O73.1
- secondary cataract — *see* Cataract, secondary
- unruptured (causing asphyxia) — *see* Asphyxia, newborn
- vitreous — *see* Opacity, vitreous, membranes and strands

Membranitis — *see* Chorioamnionitis

Memory disturbance, lack or loss — *see also* Amnesia
- mild, following organic brain damage F06.8

Menadione deficiency E56.1

Menarche
- delayed E30.0
- precocious E30.1

Mendacity, pathologic F60.2

Mendelson's syndrome (due to anesthesia) J95.4
- in labor and delivery O74.0
- in pregnancy O29.01-
- obstetric O74.0
- postpartum, puerperal O89.01

Ménétrier's disease or syndrome K29.60
- with bleeding K29.61

Ménière's disease, syndrome or vertigo H81.0-

Meninges, meningeal — *see* condition

Meningioma — *see also* Neoplasm, meninges, benign
- angioblastic — *see* Neoplasm, meninges, benign
- angiomatous — *see* Neoplasm, meninges, benign
- atypical — *see* Neoplasm, meninges, uncertain behavior
- endotheliomatous — *see* Neoplasm, meninges, benign

Meningomyeloneuritis — *see* Meningoencephalitis
Meningoradiculitis — *see* Meningitis
Meningovascular — *see* condition
Menkes' disease or syndrome E83.09
meaning maple-syrup-urine disease E71.0
Menometrorrhagia N92.1
Menopause, menopausal (asymptomatic) (state) Z78.0
arthritis (any site) NEC — *see* Arthritis, specified form NEC
bleeding N92.4
depression (single episode) F32.89
agitated (single episode) F32.2
recurrent episode F33.9
psychotic (single episode) F32.89
recurrent episode F33.9
recurrent episode F33.8
melancholia (single episode) F32.89
recurrent episode F33.8
paranoid state F22
premature E28.319
asymptomatic E28.319
postirradiation E89.40
postsurgical E89.40
symptomatic E28.310
postirradiation E89.41
postsurgical E89.41
psychosis NEC F28
symptomatic N95.1
toxic polyarthritis NEC — *see* Arthritis, specified form NEC
Menorrhagia (primary) N92.0
climacteric N92.4
menopausal N92.4
menopausal N92.4
perimenopausal N92.4
postclimacteric N95.0
postmenopausal N95.0
preclimacteric or premenopausal N92.4
pubertal (menses retained) N92.2
Menostaxis N92.0
Menses, retention N94.89
Menstrual — *see* Menstruation
Menstruation
absent — *see* Amenorrhea
anovulatory N97.0
cycle, irregular N92.6
delayed N91.0
disorder N93.9
psychogenic F45.8
during pregnancy O20.8
excessive (with regular cycle) N92.0
with irregular cycle N92.1
at puberty N92.2
frequent N92.0
infrequent — *see* Oligomenorrhea
irregular N92.6
specified NEC N92.5
latent N92.5
membranous N92.5
painful — *see also* Dysmenorrhea N94.6
primary N94.4
psychogenic F45.8
secondary N94.5
passage of clots N92.0
precocious E30.1
protracted N92.5
rare — *see* Oligomenorrhea
retained N94.89
retrograde N92.5
scanty — *see* Oligomenorrhea
suppression N94.89
vicarious (nasal) N94.89
Mental — *see also* condition
deficiency — *see* Disability, intellectual
deterioration — *see* Psychosis
disorder — *see* Disorder, mental
exhaustion F48.8
insufficiency (congenital) — *see* Disability, intellectual
observation without need for further medical care Z03.89
retardation — *see* Disability, intellectual
subnormality — *see* Disability, intellectuall
Mental - *continued*
upset — *see* Disorder, mental
Meralgia paresthetica G57.1-
Mercurial — *see* condition
Mercurialism — *see* subcategory T56.1
Merkel cell tumor — *see* Carcinoma, Merkel cell
Merocele — *see* Hernia, femoral
Meromelia
lower limb — *see* Defect, reduction, lower limb
intercalary
femur — *see* Defect, reduction, lower limb, specified type NEC
tibiofibular (complete) (incomplete) — *see* Defect, reduction, lower limb
upper limb — *see* Defect, reduction, upper limb
intercalary, humeral, radioulnar — *see* Agenesis, arm, with hand present
MERRF syndrome (myoclonic epilepsy associated with ragged-red fiber) E88.42
Merzbacher-Pelizaeus disease E75.29
Mesaortitis — *see* Aortitis
Mesarteritis — *see* Arteritis
Mesencephalitis — *see* Encephalitis
Mesenchymoma — *see also* Neoplasm, connective tissue, uncertain behavior
benign — *see* Neoplasm, connective tissue, benign
malignant — *see* Neoplasm, connective tissue, malignant
Mesenteritis
retractile K65.4
sclerosing K65.4
Mesentery, mesenteric — *see* condition
Mesiodens, mesiodentes K00.1
Mesio-occlusion M26.213
Mesocolon — *see* condition
Mesonephroma (malignant) — *see* Neoplasm, malignant, by site
benign — *see* Neoplasm, benign, by site
Mesophlebitis — *see* Phlebitis
Mesostromal dysgenesia Q13.89
Mesothelioma (malignant) C45.9
benign
mesentery D19.1
mesocolon D19.1
omentum D19.1
peritoneum D19.1
pleura D19.0
specified site NEC D19.7
unspecified site D19.9
biphasic C45.9
benign
mesentery D19.1
mesocolon D19.1
omentum D19.1
peritoneum D19.1
pleura D19.0
specified site NEC D19.7
unspecified site D19.9
cystic D48.4
epithelioid C45.9
benign
mesentery D19.1
mesocolon D19.1
omentum D19.1
peritoneum D19.1
pleura D19.0
specified site NEC D19.7
unspecified site D19.9
fibrous C45.9
benign
mesentery D19.1
mesocolon D19.1
omentum D19.1
peritoneum D19.1
pleura D19.0
specified site NEC D19.7
unspecified site D19.9
site classification
liver C45.7
Mesothelioma (malignant) - *continued*
site classification - *continued*
lung C45.7
mediastinum C45.7
mesentery C45.1
mesocolon C45.1
omentum C45.1
pericardium C45.2
peritoneum C45.1
pleura C45.0
parietal C45.0
retroperitoneum C45.7
specified site NEC C45.7
unspecified C45.9
Metabolic syndrome E88.81
Metagonimiasis B66.8
Metagonimus infestation (intestine) B66.8
Metal
pigmentation L81.8
polisher's disease J62.8
Metamorphopsia H53.15
Metaplasia
apocrine (breast) — *see* Dysplasia, mammary, specified type NEC
cervix (squamous) — *see* Dysplasia, cervix
endometrium (squamous) (uterus) N85.8
esophagus K22.7-
gastric intestinal K31.A0
with dysplasia K31.A29
high grade K31.A22
low grade K31.A21
indefinite for dysplasia K31.A0
without dysplasia K31.A19
involving
antrum K31.A11
body (corpus) K31.A12
cardia K31.A14
fundus K31.A13
multiple sites K31.A15
kidney (pelvis) (squamous) N28.89
myelogenous D73.1
myeloid (agnogenic) (megakaryocytic) D73.1
spleen D73.1
squamous cell, bladder N32.89
Metastasis, metastatic
abscess — *see* Abscess
calcification E83.59
cancer
from specified site — *see* Neoplasm, malignant, by site
to specified site — *see* Neoplasm, secondary, by site
deposits (in) — *see* Neoplasm, secondary, by site
disease — *see also* Neoplasm, secondary, by site C79.9
spread (to) — *see* Neoplasm, secondary, by site
Metastrongyliasis B83.8
Metatarsalgia M77.4-
anterior G57.6-
Morton's G57.6-
Metatarsus, metatarsal — *see also* condition
adductus, congenital Q66.22-
valgus (abductus) , congenital Q66.6
varus (congenital) Q66.22-
primus Q66.21-
Methadone use — *see* Use, opioid
Methemoglobinemia D74.9
acquired (with sulfhemoglobinemia) D74.8
congenital D74.0
enzymatic (congenital) D74.0
Hb M disease D74.0
hereditary D74.0
toxic D74.8
Methemoglobinuria — *see* Hemoglobinuria
Methioninemia E72.19
Methylmalonic acidemia E71.120
Metritis (catarrhal) (hemorrhagic) (septic) (suppurative) — *see also* Endometritis
cervical — *see* Cervicitis
Metropathia hemorrhagica N93.8
Metroperitonitis — *see* Peritonitis, pelvic, female

Metrorrhagia N92.1
climacteric N92.4
menopausal N92.4
perimenopausal N92.4
postpartum NEC (atonic) (following delivery of placenta) O72.1
delayed or secondary O72.2
preclimacteric or premenopausal N92.4
psychogenic F45.8
Metrorrhexis — *see* Rupture, uterus
Metrosalpingitis N70.91
Metrostaxis N93.8
Metrovaginitis — *see* Endometritis
Meyer-Schwickerath and Weyers syndrome Q87.0
Meynert's amentia (nonalcoholic) F04
alcoholic F10.96
with dependence F10.26
Mibelli's disease (porokeratosis) Q82.8
Mice, joint — *see* Loose, body, joint
knee M23.4-
Micrencephalon, micrencephaly Q02
Microalbuminuria R80.9
Microaneurysm, retinal — *see also* Disorder, retina, microaneurysms
diabetic — *see* E08-E13 with .31
Microangiopathy (peripheral) I73.9
thrombotic M31.10
hematopoietic stem cell transplantation-associated [HSCT-TMA] M31.10
Microcalcifications, breast R92.0
Microcephalus, microcephalic, microcephaly Q02
due to toxoplasmosis (congenital) P37.1
Microcheilia Q18.7
Microcolon (congenital) Q43.8
Microcornea (congenital) Q13.4
Microcytic — *see* condition
Microdeletions NEC Q93.88
Microdontia K00.2
Microdrepanocytosis D57.40
with
acute chest syndrome D57.411
cerebral vascular involvement D57.413
crisis (painful) D57.419
with specified complication NEC D57.418
splenic sequestration D57.412
vasoocclusive pain D57.419
Microembolism
atherothrombotic — *see* Atheroembolism
retinal — *see* Occlusion, artery, retina
Microencephalon Q02
Microfilaria streptocerca infestation — *see* Onchocerciasis
Microgastria (congenital) Q40.2
Microgenia M26.06
Microgenitalia, congenital
female Q52.8
male Q55.8
Microglioma — *see* Lymphoma, non-Hodgkin, specified NEC
Microglossia (congenital) Q38.3
Micrognathia, micrognathism (congenital) (mandibular) (maxillary) M26.09
Microgyria (congenital) Q04.3
Microinfarct of heart — *see* Insufficiency, coronary
Microlentia (congenital) Q12.8
Microlithiasis, alveolar, pulmonary J84.02
Micromastia N64.82
Micromyelia (congenital) Q06.8
Micropenis Q55.62
Microphakia (congenital) Q12.8
Microphthalmos, microphthalmia (congenital) Q11.2
due to toxoplasmosis P37.1
Micropsia H53.15
Microscopic polyangiitis (polyarteritis) M31.7
Microsporidiosis B60.8
intestinal A07.8
Microsporon furfur infestation B36.0
Microsporosis — *see also* Dermatophytosis
nigra B36.1
Microstomia (congenital) Q18.5
Microtia (congenital) (external ear) Q17.2
Microtropia H50.40
Microvillus inclusion disease (MVD) (MVID) Q43.8
Micturition
disorder NEC — *see also* Difficulty, micturition R39.198
psychogenic F45.8
frequency R35.0
psychogenic F45.8
hesitancy R39.11
incomplete emptying R39.14
nocturnal R35.1
painful R30.9
dysuria R30.0
psychogenic F45.8
tenesmus R30.1
poor stream R39.12
position dependent R39.192
split stream R39.13
straining R39.16
urgency R39.15
Mid plane — *see* condition
Middle
ear — *see* condition
lobe (right) syndrome J98.19
Miescher's elastoma L87.2
Mietens' syndrome Q87.2
Migraine (idiopathic) G43.909
with refractory migraine G43.919
with status migrainosus G43.911
without status migrainosus G43.919
with aura (acute-onset) (prolonged) (typical) (without headache) G43.109
with refractory migraine G43.119
with status migrainosus G43.111
without status migrainosus G43.119
intractable G43.119
with status migrainosus G43.111
without status migrainosus G43.119
not intractable G43.109
with status migrainosus G43.101
without status migrainosus G43.109
persistent G43.509
with cerebral infarction G43.609
with refractory migraine G43.619
with status migrainosus G43.611
without status migrainosus G43.619
intractable G43.619
with status migrainosus G43.611
without status migrainosus G43.619
not intractable G43.609
with status migrainosus G43.601
without status migrainosus G43.609
without refractory migraine G43.609
with status migrainosus G43.601
without status migrainosus G43.609
without cerebral infarction G43.509
with refractory migraine G43.519
with status migrainosus G43.511
without status migrainosus G43.519
intractable G43.519
with status migrainosus G43.511
without status migrainosus G43.519
not intractable G43.509
with status migrainosus G43.501
without status migrainosus G43.509
without refractory migraine G43.509
with status migrainosus G43.501
without status migrainosus G43.509
without mention of refractory migraine G43.109
with status migrainosus G43.101
without status migrainosus G43.109
abdominal G43.D0
with refractory migraine G43.D1
intractable G43.D1
not intractable G43.D0
without refractory migraine G43.D0
basilar — *see* Migraine, with aura
classical — *see* Migraine, with aura
common — *see* Migraine, without aura
complicated G43.109
equivalents — *see* Migraine, with aura

Migraine (idiopathic) - *continued*
familiar — *see* Migraine, hemiplegic
hemiplegic G43.409
with refractory migraine G43.419
with status migrainosus G43.411
without status migrainosus G43.419
intractable G43.419
with status migrainosus G43.411
without status migrainosus G43.419
not intractable G43.409
with status migrainosus G43.401
without status migrainosus G43.409
without refractory migraine G43.409
with status migrainosus G43.401
without status migrainosus G43.409
intractable G43.919
with status migrainosus G43.911
without status migrainosus G43.919
menstrual G43.829
with refractory migraine G43.839
with status migrainosus G43.831
without status migrainosus G43.839
intractable G43.839
with status migrainosus G43.831
without status migrainosus G43.839
not intractable G43.829
with status migrainosus G43.821
without status migrainosus G43.829
without refractory migraine G43.829
with status migrainosus G43.821
without status migrainosus G43.829
menstrually related — *see* Migraine, menstrual
not intractable G43.909
with status migrainosus G43.901
without status migrainosus G43.919
ophthalmoplegic G43.B0
with refractory migraine G43.B1
intractable G43.B1
not intractable G43.B0
without refractory migraine G43.B0
persistent aura (with, without) cerebral infarction — *see* Migraine, with aura, persistent
preceded or accompanied by transient focal neurological phenomena — *see* Migraine, with aura
pre-menstrual — *see* Migraine, menstrual
pure menstrual — *see* Migraine, menstrual
retinal — *see* Migraine, with aura
specified NEC G43.809
intractable G43.819
with status migrainosus G43.811
without status migrainosus G43.819
not intractable G43.809
with status migrainosus G43.801
without status migrainosus G43.809
sporadic — *see* Migraine, hemiplegic
transformed — *see* Migraine, without aura, chronic
triggered seizures — *see* Migraine, with aura
without aura G43.009
with refractory migraine G43.019
with status migrainosus G43.011
without status migrainosus G43.019
chronic G43.709
with refractory migraine G43.719
with status migrainosus G43.711
without status migrainosus G43.719
intractable
with status migrainosus G43.711
without status migrainosus G43.719
not intractable
with status migrainosus G43.701
without status migrainosus G43.709
without refractory migraine G43.709
with status migrainosus G43.701
without status migrainosus G43.709
intractable
with status migrainosus G43.011
without status migrainosus G43.019
not intractable
with status migrainosus G43.001
without status migrainosus G43.009

Migraine (idiopathic) - *continued*
without aura - *continued*
without mention of refractory migraine G43.009
with status migrainosus G43.001
without status migrainosus G43.009
without refractory migraineG43.909
with status migrainosus G43.901
without status migrainosus G43.919
Migrant, social Z59.00
Migration, anxiety concerning Z60.3
Migratory, migrating — *see also* condition
person Z59.00
testis Q55.29
Mikity-Wilson disease or syndrome P27.0
Mikulicz' disease or syndrome K11.8
Miliaria L74.3
alba L74.1
apocrine L75.2
crystallina L74.1
profunda L74.2
rubra L74.0
tropicalis L74.2
Miliary — *see* condition
Milium L72.0
colloid L57.8
Milk
crust L21.0
excessive secretion O92.6
poisoning — *see* Poisoning, food, noxious
retention O92.79
sickness — *see* Poisoning, food, noxious
spots I31.0
Milk-alkali disease or syndrome E83.52
Milk-leg (deep vessels) (nonpuerperal) — *see* Embolism, vein, lower extremity
complicating pregnancy O22.3-
puerperal, postpartum, childbirth O87.1
Milkman's disease or syndrome M83.8
Milky urine — *see* Chyluria
Millard-Gubler (-Foville) paralysis or syndrome G46.3
Millar's asthma J38.5
Miller Fisher syndrome G61.0
Mills' disease — *see* Hemiplegia
Millstone maker's pneumoconiosis J62.8
Milroy's disease (chronic hereditary edema) Q82.0
Minamata disease T56.1
Miners' asthma or lung J60
Minkowski-Chauffard syndrome — *see* Spherocytosis
Minor — *see* condition
Minor's disease (hematomyelia) G95.19
Minot's disease (hemorrhagic disease), newborn P53
Minot-von Willebrand-Jurgens disease or syndrome (angiohemophilia) D68.0
Minus (and plus) hand (intrinsic) — *see* Deformity, limb, specified type NEC, forearm
Miosis (pupil) H57.03
Mirizzi's syndrome (hepatic duct stenosis) K83.1
Mirror writing F81.0
MIS-A M35.81
Misadventure (of) (prophylactic) (therapeutic) — *see also* Complications T88.9
administration of insulin (by accident) — *see* subcategory T38.3
infusion — *see* Complications, infusion
local applications (of fomentations, plasters, etc.) T88.9
burn or scald — *see* Burn
specified NEC T88.8
medical care (early) (late) T88.9
adverse effect of drugs or chemicals — *see* Table of Drugs and Chemicals
medical care (early) (late)
burn or scald — *see* Burn
specified NEC T88.8
specified NEC T88.8
surgical procedure (early) (late) — *see* Complications, surgical procedure

Misadventure (of) (prophylactic) (therapeutic) - *continued*
transfusion — *see* Complications, transfusion
vaccination or other immunological procedure — *see* Complications, vaccination
MIS-C M35.81
Miscarriage O03.9
Misdirection, aqueous H40.83-
Misperception, sleep state F51.02
Misplaced, misplacement
ear Q17.4
kidney (acquired) N28.89
congenital Q63.2
organ or site, congenital NEC — *see* Malposition, congenital
Missed
abortion O02.1
delivery O36.4
Missing — *see also* Absence
string of intrauterine contraceptive device T83.32
Misuse of drugs F19.99
Mitchell's disease (erythromelalgia) I73.81
Mite (s) (infestation) B88.9
diarrhea B88.0
grain (itch) B88.0
hair follicle (itch) B88.0
in sputum B88.0
Mitral — *see* condition
Mittelschmerz N94.0
Mixed — *see* condition
MMN (multifocal motor neuropathy) G61.82
MNGIE (Mitochondrial Neurogastrointestinal Encephalopathy) syndrome E88.49
Mobile, mobility
cecum Q43.3
excessive — *see* Hypermobility
gallbladder, congenital Q44.1
kidney N28.89
organ or site, congenital NEC — *see* Malposition, congenital
Mobitz heart block (atrioventricular) I44.1
Moebius, Möbius
disease (ophthalmoplegic migraine) — *see* Migraine, ophthalmoplegic
syndrome Q87.0
congenital oculofacial paralysis (with other anomalies) Q87.0
ophthalmoplegic migraine — *see* Migraine, ophthalmoplegic
Moeller's glossitis K14.0
Mohr's syndrome (Types I and II) Q87.0
Mola destruens D39.2
Molar pregnancy O02.0
Molarization of premolars K00.2
Molding, head (during birth) - omit code
Mole (pigmented) — *see also* Nevus
blood O02.0
Breus' O02.0
cancerous — *see* Melanoma
carneous O02.0
destructive D39.2
fleshy O02.0
hydatid, hydatidiform (benign) (complicating pregnancy) (delivered) (undelivered) O01.9
classical O01.0
complete O01.0
incomplete O01.1
invasive D39.2
malignant D39.2
partial O01.1
intrauterine O02.0
invasive (hydatidiform) D39.2
malignant
meaning
malignant hydatidiform mole D39.2
melanoma — *see* Melanoma
nonhydatidiform O02.0
nonpigmented — *see* Nevus
pregnancy NEC O02.0
skin — *see* Nevus
tubal O00.10-

Mole (pigmented) - *continued*
tubal - *continued*
with intrauterine pregnancy O00.11-
vesicular — *see* Mole, hydatidiform
Molimen, molimina (menstrual) N94.3
Molluscum contagiosum (epitheliale) B08.1
Mönckeberg's arteriosclerosis, disease, or sclerosis — *see* Arteriosclerosis, extremities
Mondini's malformation (cochlea) Q16.5
Mondor's disease I80.8
Monge's disease T70.29
Monilethrix (congenital) Q84.1
Moniliasis — *see also* Candidiasis B37.9
neonatal P37.5
Monitoring (encounter for)
therapeutic drug level Z51.81
Monkey malaria B53.1
Monkeypox B04
Monoarthritis M13.10
ankle M13.17-
elbow M13.12-
foot joint M13.17-
hand joint M13.14-
hip M13.15-
knee M13.16-
shoulder M13.11-
wrist M13.13-
Monoblastic — *see* condition
Monochromat (ism), monochromatopsia (acquired) (congenital) H53.51
Monocytic — *see* condition
Monocytopenia D72.818
Monocytosis (symptomatic) D72.821
Monomania — *see* Psychosis
Mononeuritis G58.9
cranial nerve — *see* Disorder, nerve, cranial
femoral nerve G57.2-
lateral
cutaneous nerve of thigh G57.1-
popliteal nerve G57.3-
lower limb G57.9-
specified nerve NEC G57.8-
medial popliteal nerve G57.4-
median nerve G56.1-
multiplex G58.7
plantar nerve G57.6-
posterior tibial nerve G57.5-
radial nerve G56.3-
sciatic nerve G57.0-
specified NEC G58.8
tibial nerve G57.4-
ulnar nerve G56.2-
upper limb G56.9-
specified nerve NEC G56.8-
vestibular — *see* subcategory H93.3
Mononeuropathy G58.9
carpal tunnel syndrome — *see* Syndrome, carpal tunnel
diabetic NEC — *see* E08-E13 with .41
femoral nerve — *see* Lesion, nerve, femoral
ilioinguinal nerve G57.8-
in diseases classified elsewhere — *see* category G59
intercostal G58.0
lower limb G57.9-
causalgia — *see* Causalgia, lower limb
femoral nerve — *see* Lesion, nerve, femoral
meralgia paresthetica G57.1-
plantar nerve — *see* Lesion, nerve, plantar
popliteal nerve — *see* Lesion, nerve, popliteal
sciatic nerve — *see* Lesion, nerve, sciatic
specified NEC G57.8-
tarsal tunnel syndrome — *see* Syndrome, tarsal tunnel
median nerve — *see* Lesion, nerve, median
multiplex G58.7
obturator nerve G57.8-
popliteal nerve — *see* Lesion, nerve, popliteal
radial nerve — *see* Lesion, nerve, radial
saphenous nerve G57.8-
specified NEC G58.8

- **Mononeuropathy** - *continued*
  - tarsal tunnel syndrome — *see* Syndrome, tarsal tunnel
  - tuberculous A17.83
  - ulnar nerve — *see* Lesion, nerve, ulnar
  - upper limb G56.9-
    - carpal tunnel syndrome — *see* Syndrome, carpal tunnel
    - causalgia — *see* Causalgia
    - median nerve — *see* Lesion, nerve, median
    - radial nerve — *see* Lesion, nerve, radial
    - specified site NEC G56.8-
    - ulnar nerve — *see* Lesion, nerve, ulnar
- **Mononucleosis, infectious** B27.90
  - with
    - complication NEC B27.99
    - meningitis B27.92
    - polyneuropathy B27.91
  - cytomegaloviral B27.10
    - with
      - complication NEC B27.19
      - meningitis B27.12
      - polyneuropathy B27.11
  - Epstein-Barr (virus) B27.00
    - with
      - complication NEC B27.09
      - meningitis B27.02
      - polyneuropathy B27.01
  - gammaherpesviral B27.00
    - with
      - complication NEC B27.09
      - meningitis B27.02
      - polyneuropathy B27.01
  - specified NEC B27.80
    - with
      - complication NEC B27.89
      - meningitis B27.82
      - polyneuropathy B27.81
- **Monoplegia** G83.3-
  - congenital (cerebral) G80.8
    - spastic G80.1
  - embolic (current episode) I63.4-
  - following
    - cerebrovascular disease
      - cerebral infarction
        - lower limb I69.34-
        - upper limb I69.33-
      - intracerebral hemorrhage
        - lower limb I69.14-
        - upper limb I69.13-
      - lower limb I69.94-
      - nontraumatic intracranial hemorrhage NEC
        - lower limb I69.24-
        - upper limb I69.23-
      - specified disease NEC
        - lower limb I69.84-
        - upper limb I69.83-
      - stroke NOS
        - lower limb I69.34-
        - upper limb I69.33-
      - subarachnoid hemorrhage
        - lower limb I69.04-
        - upper limb I69.03-
      - upper limb I69.93-
  - hysterical (transient) F44.4
  - lower limb G83.1-
  - psychogenic (conversion reaction) F44.4
  - thrombotic (current episode) I63.3-
  - transient R29.818
  - upper limb G83.2-
- **Monorchism, monorchidism** Q55.0
- **Monosomy** — *see also* Deletion, chromosome Q93.9
  - specified NEC Q93.89
  - whole chromosome
    - meiotic nondisjunction Q93.0
    - mitotic nondisjunction Q93.1
    - mosaicism Q93.1
  - X Q96.9
- **Monster, monstrosity (single)** Q89.7
  - acephalic Q00.0
  - twin Q89.4
- **Monteggia's fracture (-dislocation)** S52.27-
- **Mooren's ulcer (cornea)** — *see* Ulcer, cornea, Mooren's
- **Moore's syndrome** — *see* Epilepsy, specified NEC
- **Mooser-Neill reaction** A75.2
- **Mooser's bodies** A75.2
- **Morbidity not stated or unknown** R69
- **Morbilli** — *see* Measles
- **Morbus** — *see also* Disease
  - angelicus, anglorum E55.0
  - Beigel B36.2
  - caducus — *see* Epilepsy
  - celiacus K90.0
  - comitialis — *see* Epilepsy
  - cordis — *see also* Disease, heart I51.9
    - valvulorum — *see* Endocarditis
  - coxae senilis M16.9
    - tuberculous A18.02
  - hemorrhagicus neonatorum P53
  - maculosus neonatorum P54.5
- **Morel (-Stewart) (-Morgagni) syndrome** M85.2
- **Morel-Kraepelin disease** — *see* Schizophrenia
- **Morel-Moore syndrome** M85.2
- **Morgagni's**
  - cyst, organ, hydatid, or appendage
    - female Q50.5
    - male (epididymal) Q55.4
      - testicular Q55.29
  - syndrome M85.2
- **Morgagni-Stewart-Morel syndrome** M85.2
- **Morgagni-Stokes-Adams syndrome** I45.9
- **Morgagni-Turner (-Albright) syndrome** Q96.9
- **Moria** F07.0
- **Moron (I.Q.50-69)** F70
- **Morphea** L94.0
- **Morphinism (without remission)** F11.20
  - with remission F11.21
- **Morphinomania (without remission)** F11.20
  - with remission F11.21
- **Morquio (-Ullrich) (-Brailsford) disease or syndrome** — *see* Mucopolysaccharidosis
- **Mortification (dry) (moist)** — *see* Gangrene
- **Morton's metatarsalgia (neuralgia) (neuroma) (syndrome)** G57.6-
- **Morvan's disease or syndrome** G60.8
- **Mosaicism, mosaic (autosomal) (chromosomal)**
  - 45,X/other cell lines NEC with abnormal sex chromosome Q96.4
  - 45,X/46,XX Q96.3
  - sex chromosome
    - female Q97.8
    - lines with various numbers of X chromosomes Q97.2
    - male Q98.7
  - XY Q96.3
- **Moschowitz' disease** M31.19
- **Mother yaw** A66.0
- **Motion sickness (from travel, any vehicle) (from roundabouts or swings)** T75.3
- **Mottled, mottling, teeth (enamel) (endemic) (nonendemic)** K00.3
- **Mounier-Kuhn syndrome** Q32.4
  - with bronchiectasis J47.9
    - exacerbation (acute) J47.1
    - lower respiratory infection J47.0
  - acquired J98.09
    - with bronchiectasis J47.9
      - with
        - exacerbation (acute) J47.1
        - lower respiratory infection J47.0
- **Mountain**
  - sickness T70.29
    - with polycythemia , acquired (acute) D75.1
  - tick fever A93.2
- **Mouse, joint** — *see* Loose, body, joint
  - knee M23.4-
- **Mouth** — *see* condition
- **Movable**
  - coccyx — *see* subcategory M53.2
  - kidney N28.89
- **Movable** - *continued*
  - kidney - *continued*
    - congenital Q63.8
  - spleen D73.89
- **Movements, dystonic** R25.8
- **Moyamoya disease** I67.5
- **MRSA (Methicillin resistant Staphylococcus aureus)**
  - infection A49.02
    - as the cause of diseases classified elsewhere B95.62
  - sepsis A41.02
- **MSD (multiple sulfatase deficiency)** E75.26
- **MSSA (Methicillin susceptible Staphylococcus aureus)**
  - infection A49.01
    - as the cause of diseases classified elsewhere B95.61
  - sepsis A41.01
- **Mucha-Habermann disease** L41.0
- **Mucinosis (cutaneous) (focal) (papular) (reticular erythematous) (skin)** L98.5
  - oral K13.79
- **Mucocele**
  - appendix K38.8
  - buccal cavity K13.79
  - gallbladder K82.1
  - lacrimal sac, chronic H04.43-
  - nasal sinus J34.1
  - nose J34.1
  - salivary gland (any) K11.6
  - sinus (accessory) (nasal) J34.1
  - turbinate (bone) (middle) (nasal) J34.1
  - uterus N85.8
- **Mucolipidosis**
  - I E77.1
  - II, III E77.0
  - IV E75.11
- **Mucopolysaccharidosis** E76.3
  - beta-gluduronidase deficiency E76.29
  - cardiopathy E76.3 *[I52]*
  - Hunter's syndrome E76.1
  - Hurler's syndrome E76.01
  - Hurler-Scheie syndrome E76.02
  - Maroteaux-Lamy syndrome E76.29
  - Morquio syndrome E76.219
    - A E76.210
    - B E76.211
    - classic E76.210
  - Sanfilippo syndrome E76.22
  - Scheie's syndrome E76.03
  - specified NEC E76.29
  - type
    - I
      - Hurler's syndrome E76.01
      - Hurler-Scheie syndrome E76.02
      - Scheie's syndrome E76.03
    - II E76.1
    - III E76.22
    - IV E76.219
    - IVA E76.210
    - IVB E76.211
    - VI E76.29
    - VII E76.29
- **Mucormycosis** B46.5
  - cutaneous B46.3
  - disseminated B46.4
  - gastrointestinal B46.2
  - generalized B46.4
  - pulmonary B46.0
  - rhinocerebral B46.1
  - skin B46.3
  - subcutaneous B46.3
- **Mucositis (ulcerative)** K12.30
  - due to drugs NEC K12.32
  - gastrointestinal K92.81
  - mouth (oral) (oropharyngeal) K12.30
    - due to antineoplastic therapy K12.31
    - due to drugs NEC K12.32
    - due to radiation K12.33
    - specified NEC K12.39
    - viral K12.39
  - nasal J34.81
  - oral cavity — *see* Mucositis, mouth
  - oral soft tissues — *see* Mucositis, mouth

Mucositis (ulcerative) - *continued*
  vagina and vulva N76.81
Mucositis necroticans agranulocytica — *see* Agranulocytosis
Mucous — *see also* condition
  patches (syphilitic) A51.39
    congenital A50.07
Mucoviscidosis E84.9
  with meconium obstruction E84.11
Mucus
  asphyxia or suffocation — *see* Asphyxia, mucus
  in stool R19.5
  plug — *see* Asphyxia, mucus
Muguet B37.0
Mulberry molars (congenital syphilis) A50.52
Müllerian mixed tumor
  specified site — *see* Neoplasm, malignant, by site
  unspecified site C54.9
Multicystic kidney (development) Q61.4
Multiparity (grand) Z64.1
  affecting management of pregnancy, labor and delivery (supervision only) O09.4-
  requiring contraceptive management — *see* Contraception
Multipartita placenta O43.19-
Multiple, multiplex — *see also* condition
  digits (congenital) Q69.9
  endocrine neoplasia — *see* Neoplasia, endocrine, multiple (MEN)
  personality F44.81
Multisystem inflammatory syndrome (in adult) (in children) M35.81
Mumps B26.9
  arthritis B26.85
  complication NEC B26.89
  encephalitis B26.2
  hepatitis B26.81
  meningitis (aseptic) B26.1
  meningoencephalitis B26.2
  myocarditis B26.82
  oophoritis B26.89
  orchitis B26.0
  pancreatitis B26.3
  polyneuropathy B26.84
Mumu — *see also* Infestation, filarial B74.9 *[N51]*
Münchhausen's syndrome — *see* Disorder, factitious
Münchmeyer's syndrome — *see* Myositis, ossificans, progressiva
Mural — *see* condition
Murmur (cardiac) (heart) (organic) R01.1
  abdominal R19.15
  aortic (valve) — *see* Endocarditis, aortic
  benign R01.0
  diastolic — *see* Endocarditis
  Flint I35.1
  functional R01.0
  Graham Steell I37.1
  innocent R01.0
  mitral (valve) — *see* Insufficiency, mitral
  nonorganic R01.0
  presystolic, mitral — *see* Insufficiency, mitral
  pulmonic (valve) I37.8
  systolic R01.1
  tricuspid (valve) I07.9
  valvular — *see* Endocarditis
Murri's disease (intermittent hemoglobinuria) D59.6
Muscle, muscular — *see also* condition
  carnitine (palmityltransferase) deficiency E71.314
Musculoneuralgia — *see* Neuralgia
Mushrooming hip — *see* Derangement, joint, specified NEC, hip
Mushroom-workers' (pickers') disease or lung J67.5
Mutation (s)
  factor V Leiden D68.51
  surfactant, of lung J84.83
  prothrombin gene D68.52
Mutism — *see also* Aphasia
  deaf (acquired) (congenital) NEC H91.3
  elective (adjustment reaction) (childhood) F94.0
  hysterical F44.4
  selective (childhood) F94.0
MVD (microvillus inclusion disease) Q43.8
MVID (microvillus inclusion disease) Q43.8
Myalgia M79.10
  auxiliary muscles, head and neck M79.12
  epidemic (cervical) B33.0
  mastication muscle M79.11
  site specified NEC M79.18
  traumatic NEC T14.8
Myasthenia G70.9
  congenital G70.2
  cordis — *see* Failure, heart
  developmental G70.2
  gravis G70.00
    with exacerbation (acute) G70.01
    in crisis G70.01
    neonatal, transient P94.0
    pseudoparalytica G70.00
      with exacerbation (acute) G70.01
      in crisis G70.01
  stomach, psychogenic F45.8
  syndrome
    in
      diabetes mellitus — *see* E08-E13 with .44
      neoplastic disease — *see also* Neoplasm D49.9 *[G73.3]*
      pernicious anemia D51.0 *[G73.3]*
      thyrotoxicosis E05.90 *[G73.3]*
        with thyroid storm E05.91 *[G73.3]*
Myasthenic M62.81
Mycelium infection B49
Mycetismus — *see* Poisoning, food, noxious, mushroom
Mycetoma B47.9
  actinomycotic B47.1
  bone (mycotic) B47.9 *[M90.80]*
  eumycotic B47.0
  foot B47.9
    actinomycotic B47.1
    mycotic B47.0
  madurae NEC B47.9
    mycotic B47.0
  maduromycotic B47.0
  mycotic B47.0
  nocardial B47.1
Mycobacteriosis — *see* Mycobacterium
Mycobacterium, mycobacterial (infection) A31.9
  anonymous A31.9
  atypical A31.9
    cutaneous A31.1
    pulmonary A31.0
      tuberculous — *see* Tuberculosis, pulmonary
    specified site NEC A31.8
  avium (intracellulare complex) A31.0
  balnei A31.1
  Battey A31.0
  chelonei A31.8
  cutaneous A31.1
  extrapulmonary systemic A31.8
  fortuitum A31.8
  intracellulare (Battey bacillus) A31.0
  kansasii (yellow bacillus) A31.0
  kakaferifu A31.8
  kasongo A31.8
  leprae — *see also* Leprosy A30.9
  luciflavum A31.1
  marinum (M. balnei) A31.1
  nonspecific — *see* Mycobacterium, atypical
  pulmonary (atypical) A31.0
    tuberculous — *see* Tuberculosis, pulmonary
  scrofulaceum A31.8
  simiae A31.8
  systemic, extrapulmonary A31.8
  szulgai A31.8
  terrae A31.8
  triviale A31.8
Mycobacterium, mycobacterial (infection) - *continued*
  tuberculosis (human, bovine) — *see* Tuberculosis
  ulcerans A31.1
  xenopi A31.8
Mycoplasma (M.) pneumoniae, as cause of disease classified elsewhere B96.0
Mycosis, mycotic B49
  cutaneous NEC B36.9
  ear B36.9
    in
      aspergillosis B44.89
      candidiasis B37.84
      moniliasis B37.84
  fungoides (extranodal) (solid organ) C84.0-
  mouth B37.0
  nails B35.1
  opportunistic B48.8
  skin NEC B36.9
  specified NEC B48.8
  stomatitis B37.0
  vagina, vaginitis (candidal) B37.3
Mydriasis (pupil) H57.04
Myelatelia Q06.1
Myelinolysis, pontine, central G37.2
Myelitis (acute) (ascending) (childhood) (chronic) (descending) (diffuse) (disseminated) (idiopathic) (pressure) (progressive) (spinal cord) (subacute) — *see also* Encephalitis G04.91
  flaccid G04.82
  herpes simplex B00.82
  herpes zoster B02.24
  in diseases classified elsewhere G05.4
  necrotizing, subacute G37.4
  optic neuritis in G36.0
  postchickenpox B01.12
  postherpetic B02.24
  postimmunization G04.02
  postinfectious NEC G04.89
  postvaccinal G04.02
  specified NEC G04.89
  syphilitic (transverse) A52.14
  toxic G92.9
  transverse (in demyelinating diseases of central nervous system) G37.3
  tuberculous A17.82
  varicella B01.12
Myeloblastic — *see* condition
Myeloblastoma
  granular cell — *see also* Neoplasm, connective tissue
    malignant — *see* Neoplasm, connective tissue, malignant
    tongue D10.1
Myelocele — *see* Spina bifida
Myelocystocele — *see* Spina bifida
Myelocytic — *see* condition
Myelodysplasia D46.9
  specified NEC D46.Z
  spinal cord (congenital) Q06.1
Myelodysplastic syndrome — *see also* Syndrome, myelodysplastic D46.9
  with
    5q deletion D46.C
    isolated del (5q) chromosomal abnormality D46.C
  specified NEC D46.Z
Myeloencephalitis — *see* Encephalitis
Myelofibrosis D75.81
  with myeloid metaplasia D47.4
  acute C94.4-
  idiopathic (chronic) D47.4
  primary D47.1
  secondary D75.81
    in myeloproliferative disease D47.4
Myelogenous — *see* condition
Myeloid — *see* condition
Myelokathexis D70.9
Myeloleukodystrophy E75.29
Myelolipoma — *see* Lipoma
Myeloma (multiple) C90.0-
  monostotic C90.3
    plasma cell C90.0-

Myeloma (multiple) - *continued*
plasma cell C90.0-
solitary — *see also* Plasmacytoma, solitary C90.3-
Myelomalacia G95.89
Myelomatosis C90.0-
Myelomeningitis — *see* Meningoencephalitis
Myelomeningocele (spinal cord) — *see* Spina bifida
Myelo-osteo-musculodysplasia hereditaria Q79.8
Myelopathic
anemia D64.89
muscle atrophy — *see* Atrophy, muscle, spinal
pain syndrome G89.0
Myelopathy (spinal cord) G95.9
drug-induced G95.89
in (due to)
degeneration or displacement, intervertebral disc NEC — *see* Disorder, disc, with, myelopathy
infection — *see* Encephalitis
intervertebral disc disorder — *see also* Disorder, disc, with, myelopathy
mercury — *see* subcategory T56.1
neoplastic disease — *see also* Neoplasm D49.9 *[G99.2]*
pernicious anemia D51.0 *[G99.2]*
spondylosis — *see* Spondylosis, with myelopathy NEC
necrotic (subacute) (vascular) G95.19
radiation-induced G95.89
spondylogenic NEC — *see* Spondylosis, with myelopathy NEC
toxic G95.89
transverse, acute G37.3
vascular G95.19
vitamin B12 E53.8 *[G32.0]*
Myelophthisis D61.82
Myeloradiculitis G04.91
Myeloradiculodysplasia (spinal) Q06.1
Myelosarcoma C92.3-
Myelosclerosis D75.89
with myeloid metaplasia D47.4
disseminated, of nervous system G35
megakaryocytic D47.4
with myeloid metaplasia D47.4
Myelosis
acute C92.0-
aleukemic C92.9-
chronic D47.1
erythremic (acute) C94.0-
megakaryocytic C94.2-
nonleukemic D72.828
subacute C92.9-
Myiasis (cavernous) B87.9
aural B87.4
creeping B87.0
cutaneous B87.0
dermal B87.0
ear (external) (middle) B87.4
eye B87.2
genitourinary B87.81
intestinal B87.82
laryngeal B87.3
nasopharyngeal B87.3
ocular B87.2
orbit B87.2
skin B87.0
specified site NEC B87.89
traumatic B87.1
wound B87.1
Myoadenoma, prostate — *see* Hyperplasia, prostate
Myoblastoma
granular cell — *see also* Neoplasm, connective tissue, benign
malignant — *see* Neoplasm, connective tissue, malignant
tongue D10.1
Myocardial — *see* condition
Myocardiopathy (congestive) (constrictive) (familial) (hypertrophic nonobstructive) (idiopathic) (infiltrative) (obstructive) (primary) (restrictive) (sporadic) — *see also* Cardiomyopathy I42.9
alcoholic I42.6
cobalt-beer I42.6
glycogen storage E74.02 *[I43]*
hypertrophic obstructive I42.1
in (due to)
beriberi E51.12
cardiac glycogenosis E74.02 *[I43]*
Friedreich's ataxia G11.11 *[I43]*
myotonia atrophica G71.11 *[I43]*
progressive muscular dystrophy G71.09 *[I43]*
obscure (African) I42.8
secondary I42.9
thyrotoxic E05.90 *[I43]*
with storm E05.91 *[I43]*
toxic NEC I42.7
Myocarditis (with arteriosclerosis) (chronic) (fibroid) (interstitial) (old) (progressive) (senile) I51.4
with
rheumatic fever (conditions in I00) I09.0
active — *see* Myocarditis, acute, rheumatic
inactive or quiescent (with chorea) I09.0
active I40.9
rheumatic I01.2
with chorea (acute) (rheumatic) (Sydenham's) I02.0
acute or subacute (interstitial) I40.9
due to
streptococcus (beta-hemolytic) I01.2
idiopathic I40.1
rheumatic I01.2
with chorea (acute) (rheumatic) (Sydenham's) I02.0
specified NEC I40.8
aseptic of newborn B33.22
bacterial (acute) I40.0
Coxsackie (virus) B33.22
diphtheritic A36.81
eosinophilic I40.1
epidemic of newborn (Coxsackie) B33.22
Fiedler's (acute) (isolated) I40.1
giant cell (acute) (subacute) I40.1
gonococcal A54.83
granulomatous (idiopathic) (isolated) (nonspecific) I40.1
hypertensive — *see* Hypertension, heart
idiopathic (granulomatous) I40.1
in (due to)
diphtheria A36.81
epidemic louse-borne typhus A75.0 *[I41]*
Lyme disease A69.29
sarcoidosis D86.85
scarlet fever A38.1
toxoplasmosis (acquired) B58.81
typhoid A01.02
typhus NEC A75.9 *[I41]*
infective I40.0
influenzal — *see* Influenza, with, myocarditis
isolated (acute) I40.1
meningococcal A39.52
mumps B26.82
nonrheumatic, active I40.9
parenchymatous I40.9
pneumococcal I40.0
rheumatic (chronic) (inactive) (with chorea) I09.0
active or acute I01.2
with chorea (acute) (rheumatic) (Sydenham's) I02.0
rheumatoid — *see* Rheumatoid, carditis
septic I40.0
staphylococcal I40.0
suppurative I40.0
syphilitic (chronic) A52.06
toxic I40.8
rheumatic — *see* Myocarditis, acute, rheumatic
Myocarditis (with arteriosclerosis) (chronic) (fibroid) (interstitial) (old) (progressive) (senile) - *continued*
tuberculous A18.84
typhoid A01.02
valvular — *see* Endocarditis
virus, viral I40.0
of newborn (Coxsackie) B33.22
Myocardium, myocardial — *see* condition
Myocardosis — *see* Cardiomyopathy
Myoclonus, myoclonic, myoclonia (familial) (essential) (multifocal) (simplex) G25.3
drug-induced G25.3
epilepsy — *see also* Epilepsy, generalized, specified NEC G40.4-
familial (progressive) G25.3
epileptica G40.409
with status epilepticus G40.401
facial G51.3-
familial progressive G25.3
Friedreich's G25.3
jerks G25.3
massive G25.3
palatal G25.3
pharyngeal G25.3
Myocytolysis I51.5
Myodiastasis — *see* Diastasis, muscle
Myoendocarditis — *see* Endocarditis
Myoepithelioma — *see* Neoplasm, benign, by site
Myofasciitis (acute) — *see* Myositis
Myofibroma — *see also* Neoplasm, connective tissue, benign
uterus (cervix) (corpus) — *see* Leiomyoma
Myofibromatosis D48.1
infantile Q89.8
Myofibrosis M62.89
heart — *see* Myocarditis
scapulohumeral — *see* Lesion, shoulder, specified NEC
Myofibrositis M79.7
scapulohumeral — *see* Lesion, shoulder, specified NEC
Myoglobulinuria, myoglobinuria (primary) R82.1
Myokymia, facial G51.4
Myolipoma — *see* Lipoma
Myoma — *see also* Neoplasm, connective tissue, benign
malignant — *see* Neoplasm, connective tissue, malignant
prostate D29.1
uterus (cervix) (corpus) — *see* Leiomyoma
Myomalacia M62.89
Myometritis — *see* Endometritis
Myometrium — *see* condition
Myonecrosis, clostridial A48.0
Myopathy G72.9
acute
necrotizing G72.81
quadriplegic G72.81
alcoholic G72.1
benign congenital G71.20
central core G71.29
centronuclear G71.228
autosomal (dominant) (recessive) G71.228
other specified NEC G71.228
congenital (benign) G71.20
critical illness G72.81
distal G71.09
drug-induced G72.0
endocrine NEC E34.9 *[G73.7]*
extraocular muscles H05.82-
facioscapulohumeral G71.02
hereditary G71.9
specified NEC G71.8
hyaline body G71.29
immune NEC G72.49
in (due to)
Addison's disease E27.1 *[G73.7]*
alcohol G72.1
amyloidosis E85.0 *[G73.7]*
cretinism E00.9 *[G73.7]*
Cushing's syndrome E24.9 *[G73.7]*
drugs G72.0

Myopathy - *continued*
- in (due to) - *continued*
  - endocrine disease NEC E34.9 *[G73.7]*
  - giant cell arteritis M31.6 *[G73.7]*
  - glycogen storage disease E74.00 *[G73.7]*
  - hyperadrenocorticism E24.9 *[G73.7]*
  - hyperparathyroidism NEC E21.3 *[G73.7]*
  - hypoparathyroidism E20.9 *[G73.7]*
  - hypopituitarism E23.0 *[G73.7]*
  - hypothyroidism E03.9 *[G73.7]*
  - infectious disease NEC B99 *[G73.7]*
  - lipid storage disease E75.6 *[G73.7]*
  - metabolic disease NEC E88.9 *[G73.7]*
  - myxedema E03.9 *[G73.7]*
  - parasitic disease NEC B89 *[G73.7]*
  - polyarteritis nodosa M30.0 *[G73.7]*
  - rheumatoid arthritis — *see* Rheumatoid, myopathy
  - sarcoidosis D86.87
  - scleroderma M34.82
  - sicca syndrome M35.03
  - Sjögren's syndrome M35.03
  - systemic lupus erythematosus M32.19
  - thyrotoxicosis (hyperthyroidism) E05.90 *[G73.7]*
    - with thyroid storm E05.91 *[G73.7]*
  - toxic agent NEC G72.2
- inflammatory NEC G72.49
- intensive care (ICU) G72.81
- limb-girdle G71.09
- mitochondrial NEC G71.3
- myosin storage G71.29
- mytonic, proximal (PROMM) G71.11
- myotubular (centronuclear) G71.220
  - X-linked G71.220
- nemaline G71.21
- ocular G71.09
- oculopharyngeal G71.09
- of critical illness G72.81
- primary G71.9
  - specified NEC G71.8
- progressive NEC G72.89
- proximal myotonic (PROMM) G71.11
- rod (body) G71.21
- scapulohumeral G71.02
- specified NEC G72.89
- toxic G72.2

Myopericarditis — *see also* Pericarditis
- chronic rheumatic I09.2

Myopia (axial) (congenital) H52.1-
- degenerative (malignant) H44.20
  - with
    - choroidal neovascularization H44.2A-
    - foveoschisis H44.2D-
    - macular hole H44.2B-
    - retinal detachment H44.2C-
    - specified maculopathy NEC H44.2E-
  - bilateral H44.23
  - left eye H44.22
  - right eye H44.21
- malignant — *see also* Myopia, degenerative H44.2-
- pernicious — *see also* Myopia, degenerative H44.2-
- progressive high (degenerative) — *see also* Myopia, degenerative H44.2-

Myosarcoma — *see* Neoplasm, connective tissue, malignant

Myosis (pupil) H57.03
- stromal (endolymphatic) D39.0

Myositis M60.9
- clostridial A48.0
- due to posture — *see* Myositis, specified type NEC
- epidemic B33.0
- fibrosa or fibrous (chronic) , Volkmann's T79.6
- foreign body granuloma — *see* Granuloma, foreign body
- in (due to)
  - bilharziasis B65.9 *[M63.8-]*
  - cysticercosis B69.81
  - leprosy A30.9 *[M63.8-]*
  - mycosis B49 *[M63.8-]*
  - sarcoidosis D86.87

Myositis - *continued*
- in (due to) - *continued*
  - schistosomiasis B65.9 *[M63.8-]*
  - syphilis
    - late A52.78
    - secondary A51.49
  - toxoplasmosis (acquired) B58.82
  - trichinellosis B75 *[M63.8-]*
  - tuberculosis A18.09
- inclusion body [IBM] G72.41
- infective M60.009
  - arm M60.002
    - left M60.001
    - right M60.000
  - leg M60.005
    - left M60.004
    - right M60.003
  - lower limb M60.005
    - ankle M60.07-
    - foot M60.07-
    - lower leg M60.06-
    - thigh M60.05-
    - toe M60.07-
  - multiple sites M60.09
  - specified site NEC M60.08
  - upper limb M60.002
    - finger M60.04-
    - forearm M60.03-
    - hand M60.04-
    - shoulder region M60.01-
    - upper arm M60.02-
- interstitial M60.10
  - ankle M60.17-
  - foot M60.17-
  - forearm M60.13-
  - hand M60.14-
  - lower leg M60.16-
  - multiple sites M60.19
  - shoulder region M60.11-
  - specified site NEC M60.18
  - thigh M60.15-
  - upper arm M60.12-
- mycotic B49 *[M63.8-]*
- orbital, chronic H05.12-
- ossificans or ossifying (circumscripta) — *see also* Ossification, muscle, specified NEC
  - in (due to)
    - burns M61.30
      - ankle M61.37-
      - foot M61.37-
      - forearm M61.33-
      - hand M61.34-
      - lower leg M61.36-
      - multiple sites M61.39
      - pelvic region M61.35-
      - shoulder region M61.31-
      - specified site NEC M61.38
      - thigh M61.35-
      - upper arm M61.32-
    - quadriplegia or paraplegia M61.20
      - ankle M61.27-
      - foot M61.27-
      - forearm M61.23-
      - hand M61.24-
      - lower leg M61.26-
      - multiple sites M61.29
      - pelvic region M61.25-
      - shoulder region M61.21-
      - specified site NEC M61.28
      - thigh M61.25-
      - upper arm M61.22-
  - progressiva M61.10
    - ankle M61.17-
    - finger M61.14-
    - foot M61.17-
    - forearm M61.13-
    - hand M61.14-
    - lower leg M61.16-
    - multiple sites M61.19
    - pelvic region M61.15-
    - shoulder region M61.11-
    - specified site NEC M61.18
    - thigh M61.15-
    - toe M61.17-

Myositis - *continued*
- ossificans or ossifying (circumscripta) - *continued*
  - progressiva - *continued*
    - upper arm M61.12-
  - traumatica M61.00
    - ankle M61.07-
    - foot M61.07-
    - forearm M61.03-
    - hand M61.04-
    - lower leg M61.06-
    - multiple sites M61.09
    - pelvic region M61.05-
    - shoulder region M61.01-
    - specified site NEC M61.08
    - thigh M61.05-
    - upper arm M61.02-
- purulent — *see* Myositis, infective
- specified type NEC M60.80
  - ankle M60.87-
  - foot M60.87-
  - forearm M60.83-
  - hand M60.84-
  - lower leg M60.86-
  - multiple sites M60.89
  - pelvic region M60.85-
  - shoulder region M60.81-
  - specified site NEC M60.88
  - thigh M60.85-
  - upper arm M60.82-
- suppurative — *see* Myositis, infective
- traumatic (old) — *see* Myositis, specified type NEC

Myospasia impulsiva F95.2

Myotonia (acquisita) (intermittens) M62.89
- atrophica G71.11
- chondrodystrophic G71.13
- congenita (acetazolamide responsive) (dominant) (recessive) G71.12
- drug-induced G71.14
- dystrophica G71.11
- fluctuans G71.19
- levior G71.12
- permanens G71.19
- symptomatic G71.19

Myotonic pupil — *see* Anomaly, pupil, function, tonic pupil

Myriapodiasis B88.2

Myringitis H73.2-
- with otitis media — *see* Otitis, media
- acute H73.00-
  - bullous H73.01-
  - specified NEC H73.09-
- bullous — *see* Myringitis, acute, bullous
- chronic H73.1-

Mysophobia F40.228

Mytilotoxism — *see* Poisoning, fish

Myxadenitis labialis K13.0

Myxedema (adult) (idiocy) (infantile) (juvenile) — *see also* Hypothyroidism E03.9
- circumscribed E05.90
  - with storm E05.91
- coma E03.5
- congenital E00.1
- cutis L98.5
- localized (pretibial) E05.90
  - with storm E05.91
- papular L98.5

Myxochondrosarcoma — *see* Neoplasm, cartilage, malignant

Myxofibroma — *see* Neoplasm, connective tissue, benign
- odontogenic — *see* Cyst, calcifying odontogenic

Myxofibrosarcoma — *see* Neoplasm, connective tissue, malignant

Myxolipoma D17.9

Myxoliposarcoma — *see* Neoplasm, connective tissue, malignant

Myxoma — *see also* Neoplasm, connective tissue, benign
- nerve sheath — *see* Neoplasm, nerve, benign
- odontogenic — *see* Cyst, calcifying odontogenic

Myxosarcoma — *see* Neoplasm, connective tissue, malignant

N

Naegeli's
- disease Q82.8
- leukemia, monocytic C93.1-

Naegleriasis (with meningoencephalitis) B60.2
Naffziger's syndrome G54.0
Naga sore — *see* Ulcer, skin
Nägele's pelvis M95.5
- with disproportion (fetopelvic) O33.0
  - causing obstructed labor O65.0

Nail — *see also* condition
- biting F98.8
- patella syndrome Q87.2

Nanism, nanosomia — *see* Dwarfism
Nanophyetiasis B66.8
Nanukayami A27.89
Napkin rash L22
Narcolepsy G47.419
- with cataplexy G47.411
- in conditions classified elsewhere G47.429
  - with cataplexy G47.421

Narcosis R06.89
Narcotism — *see* Dependence
NARP (Neuropathy, Ataxia and Retinitis pigmentosa) syndrome E88.49
Narrow
- anterior chamber angle H40.03-
- gingival width (of periodontal soft tissue) K05.5
- pelvis — *see* Contraction, pelvis

Narrowing — *see also* Stenosis
- artery I77.1
  - auditory, internal I65.8
  - basilar — *see* Occlusion, artery, basilar
  - carotid — *see* Occlusion, artery, carotid
  - cerebellar — *see* Occlusion, artery, cerebellar
  - cerebral — *see* Occlusion artery, cerebral
  - choroidal — *see* Occlusion, artery, precerebral, specified NEC
  - communicating posterior — *see* Occlusion, artery, precerebral, specified NEC
  - coronary — *see also* Disease, heart, ischemic, atherosclerotic
    - congenital Q24.5
      - syphilitic A50.54 *[I52]*
    - due to syphilis NEC A52.06
  - hypophyseal — *see* Occlusion, artery, precerebral, specified NEC
  - pontine — *see* Occlusion, artery, precerebral, specified NEC
  - precerebral — *see* Occlusion, artery, precerebral
  - vertebral — *see* Occlusion, artery, vertebral
- auditory canal (external) — *see* Stenosis, external ear canal
- eustachian tube — *see* Obstruction, eustachian tube
- eyelid — *see* Disorder, eyelid function
- larynx J38.6
- mesenteric artery — *see also* Ischemia, intestine, acute K55.059
- palate M26.89
- palpebral fissure — *see* Disorder, eyelid function
- ureter N13.5
  - with infection N13.6
- urethra — *see* Stricture, urethra

Narrowness, abnormal, eyelid Q10.3
Nasal — *see* condition
Nasolachrymal, nasolacrimal — *see* condition
Nasopharyngeal — *see also* condition
- pituitary gland Q89.2
- torticollis M43.6

Nasopharyngitis (acute) (infective) (streptococcal) (subacute) J00
- chronic (suppurative) (ulcerative) J31.1

Nasopharynx, nasopharyngeal — *see* condition
Natal tooth, teeth K00.6
Nausea (without vomiting) R11.0
- with vomiting R11.2
- gravidarum — *see* Hyperemesis, gravidarum
- marina T75.3
- navalis T75.3

Navel — *see* condition
Neapolitan fever — *see* Brucellosis
Near drowning T75.1
Nearsightedness — *see* Myopia
Near-syncope R55
Nebula, cornea — *see* Opacity, cornea
Necator americanus infestation B76.1
Necatoriasis B76.1
Neck — *see* condition
Necrobiosis R68.89
- lipoidica NEC L92.1
  - with diabetes — *see* E08-E13 with .620

Necrolysis, toxic epidermal L51.2
- due to drug
  - correct substance properly administered — *see* Table of Drugs and Chemicals, by drug, adverse effect
  - overdose or wrong substance given or taken — *see* Table of Drugs and Chemicals, by drug, poisoning

Necrophilia F65.89
Necrosis, necrotic (ischemic) — *see also* Gangrene
- adrenal (capsule) (gland) E27.49
- amputation stump (surgical) (late) T87.50
  - arm T87.5-
  - leg T87.5-
- antrum J32.0
- aorta (hyaline) — *see also* Aneurysm, aorta
  - cystic medial — *see* Dissection, aorta
- artery I77.5
- bladder (aseptic) (sphincter) N32.89
- bone — *see also* Osteonecrosis M87.9
  - aseptic or avascular — *see* Osteonecrosis
    - idiopathic M87.00
  - ethmoid J32.2
  - jaw M27.2
  - tuberculous — *see* Tuberculosis, bone
- brain I67.89
- breast (aseptic) (fat) (segmental) N64.1
- bronchus J98.09
- central nervous system NEC I67.89
- cerebellar I67.89
- cerebral I67.89
- colon — *see also* Infarct, intestine K55.049
- cornea H18.89-
- cortical (acute) (renal) N17.1
- cystic medial (aorta) — *see* Dissection, aorta
- dental pulp K04.1
- esophagus K22.89
- ethmoid (bone) J32.2
- eyelid — *see* Disorder, eyelid, degenerative
- fat, fatty (generalized) — *see also* Disorder, soft tissue, specified type NEC
  - abdominal wall K65.4
  - breast (aseptic) (segmental) N64.1
  - localized — *see* Degeneration, by site, fatty
  - mesentery K65.4
  - omentum K65.4
  - pancreas K86.89
  - peritoneum K65.4
  - skin (subcutaneous) , newborn P83.0
  - subcutaneous, due to birth injury P15.6
- gallbladder — *see* Cholecystitis, acute
- heart — *see* Infarct, myocardium
- hip, aseptic or avascular — *see* Osteonecrosis, by type, femur
- intestine (acute) (hemorrhagic) (massive) — *see also* Infarct, intestine K55.069
- jaw M27.2
- kidney (bilateral) N28.0
  - acute N17.9
  - cortical (acute) (bilateral) N17.1
    - with ectopic or molar pregnancy O08.4
  - medullary (bilateral) (in acute renal failure) (papillary) N17.2
  - papillary (bilateral) (in acute renal failure) N17.2

Necrosis, necrotic (ischemic) - *continued*
- kidney (bilateral) - *continued*
  - tubular N17.0
    - with ectopic or molar pregnancy O08.4
    - complicating
      - abortion — *see* Abortion, by type, complicated by, tubular necrosis
      - ectopic or molar pregnancy O08.4
      - pregnancy — *see* Pregnancy, complicated by, diseases of, specified type or system NEC
    - following ectopic or molar pregnancy O08.4
    - traumatic T79.5
- larynx J38.7
- liver (with hepatic failure) (cell) — *see* Failure, hepatic
  - hemorrhagic, central K76.2
- lung J85.0
- lymphatic gland — *see* Lymphadenitis, acute
- mammary gland (fat) (segmental) N64.1
- mastoid (chronic) — *see* Mastoiditis, chronic
- medullary (acute) (renal) N17.2
- mesentery — *see also* Infarct, intestine K55.069
  - fat K65.4
- mitral valve — *see* Insufficiency, mitral
- myocardium, myocardial — *see* Infarct, myocardium
- nose J34.0
- omentum (with mesenteric infarction) — *see also* Infarct, intestine K55.069
  - fat K65.4
- orbit, orbital — *see* Osteomyelitis, orbit
- ossicles, ear — *see* Abnormal, ear ossicles
- ovary N70.92
- pancreas (aseptic) (duct) (fat) K86.89
  - acute (infective) — *see* Pancreatitis, acute
  - infective — *see* Pancreatitis, acute
- papillary (acute) (renal) N17.2
- perineum N90.89
- peritoneum (with mesenteric infarction) — *see also* Infarct, intestine K55.069
  - fat K65.4
- pharynx J02.9
  - in granulocytopenia — *see* Neutropenia
  - Vincent's A69.1
- phosphorus — *see* subcategory T54.2
- pituitary (gland) E23.0
  - postpartum O99.285
  - Sheehan O99.285
- pressure — *see* Ulcer, pressure, by site
- pulmonary J85.0
- pulp (dental) K04.1
- radiation — *see* Necrosis, by site
- radium — *see* Necrosis, by site
- renal — *see* Necrosis, kidney
- sclera H15.89
- scrotum N50.89
- skin or subcutaneous tissue NEC I96
- spine, spinal (column) — *see also* Osteonecrosis, by type, vertebra
  - cord G95.19
- spleen D73.5
- stomach K31.89
- stomatitis (ulcerative) A69.0
- subcutaneous fat, newborn P83.88
- subendocardial (acute) I21.4
  - chronic I25.89
- suprarenal (capsule) (gland) E27.49
- testis N50.89
- thymus (gland) E32.8
- tonsil J35.8
- trachea J39.8
- tuberculous NEC — *see* Tuberculosis
- tubular (acute) (anoxic) (renal) (toxic) N17.0
  - postprocedural N99.0
- vagina N89.8
- vertebra — *see also* Osteonecrosis, by type, vertebra
  - tuberculous A18.01
- vulva N90.89
- X-ray — *see* Necrosis, by site

Necrospermia — *see* Infertility, male

- **Need (for)**
  - care provider because (of)
    - assistance with personal care Z74.1
    - continuous supervision required Z74.3
    - impaired mobility Z74.09
    - no other household member able to render care Z74.2
    - specified reason NEC Z74.8
  - immunization — *see* Vaccination
  - vaccination — *see* Vaccination
- **Neglect**
  - adult
    - confirmed T74.01
    - history of Z91.412
    - suspected T76.01
  - child (childhood)
    - confirmed T74.02
    - history of Z62.812
    - suspected T76.02
  - emotional, in childhood Z62.898
  - hemispatial R41.4
  - left-sided R41.4
  - sensory R41.4
  - visuospatial R41.4
- **Neisserian infection NEC** — *see* Gonococcus
- **Nelaton's syndrome** G60.8
- **Nelson's syndrome** E24.1
- **Nematodiasis (intestinal)** B82.0
  - Ancylostoma B76.0
- **Neonatal** — *see also* Newborn
  - acne L70.4
  - bradycardia P29.12
  - tachycardia P29.11
  - screening, abnormal findings on — *see* Abnormal, neonatal screening
  - tooth, teeth K00.6
- **Neonatorum** — *see* condition
- **Neoplasia**
  - endocrine, multiple (MEN) E31.20
    - type I E31.21
    - type IIA E31.22
    - type IIB E31.23
  - intraepithelial (histologically confirmed)
    - anal (AIN) (histologically confirmed) K62.82
      - grade I K62.82
      - grade II K62.82
      - severe D01.3
    - cervical glandular (histologically confirmed) D06.9
    - cervix (uteri) (CIN) (histologically confirmed) N87.9
      - glandular D06.9
      - grade I N87.0
      - grade II N87.1
      - grade III (severe dysplasia) — *see also* Carcinoma, cervix uteri, in situ D06.9
    - prostate (histologically confirmed) (PIN) N42.31
      - grade I N42.31
      - grade II N42.31
      - grade III (severe dysplasia) D07.5
    - vagina (histologically confirmed) (VAIN) N89.3
      - grade I N89.0
      - grade II N89.1
      - grade III (severe dysplasia) D07.2
    - vulva (histologically confirmed) (VIN) N90.3
      - grade I N90.0
      - grade II N90.1
      - grade III (severe dysplasia) D07.1
- **Neoplasm, neoplastic** — *see also* Table of Neoplasms
  - lipomatous, benign — *see* Lipoma
  - malignant mast cell C96.20
    - specified type NEC C96.29
  - mast cell, of uncertain behavior NEC D47.09
- **Neovascularization**
  - ciliary body — *see* Disorder, iris, vascular
  - cornea H16.40-
    - deep H16.44-
    - ghost vessels — *see* Ghost, vessels
    - localized H16.43-
- **Neovascularization** - *continued*
  - cornea - *continued*
    - pannus — *see* Pannus
  - iris — *see* Disorder, iris, vascular
  - retina H35.05-
- **Nephralgia** N23
- **Nephritis, nephritic (albuminuric) (azotemic) (congenital) (disseminated) (epithelial) (familial) (focal) (granulomatous) (hemorrhagic) (infantile) (nonsuppurative, excretory) (uremic)** N05.9
  - with
    - C3
      - glomerulonephritis N05.A
      - glomerulopathy N05.A
        - with dense deposit disease N05.6
    - dense deposit disease N05.6
    - diffuse
      - crescentic glomerulonephritis N05.7
      - endocapillary proliferative glomerulonephritis N05.4
      - membranous glomerulonephritis N05.2
      - mesangial proliferative glomerulonephritis N05.3
      - mesangiocapillary glomerulonephritis N05.5
    - edema — *see* Nephrosis
    - focal and segmental glomerular lesions N05.1
    - foot process disease N04.9
    - glomerular lesion
      - diffuse sclerosing N05.8
      - hypocomplementemic — *see* Nephritis, membranoproliferative
      - IgA — *see* Nephropathy, IgA
      - lobular, lobulonodular — *see* Nephritis, membranoproliferative
      - nodular — *see* Nephritis, membranoproliferative
    - lesion of
      - glomerulonephritis, proliferative N05.8
      - renal necrosis N05.9
    - minor glomerular abnormality N05.0
    - specified morphological changes NEC N05.8
  - acute N00.9
    - with
      - C3
        - glomerulonephritis N00.A
        - glomerulopathy N00.A
          - with dense deposit disease N00.6
      - dense deposit disease N00.6
      - diffuse
        - crescentic glomerulonephritis N00.7
        - endocapillary proliferative glomerulonephritis N00.4
        - membranous glomerulonephritis N00.2
        - mesangial proliferative glomerulonephritis N00.3
        - mesangiocapillary glomerulonephritis N00.5
      - focal and segmental glomerular lesions N00.1
      - minor glomerular abnormality N00.0
      - specified morphological changes NEC N00.8
  - amyloid E85.4 *[N08]*
  - antiglomerular basement membrane (anti-GBM) antibody NEC
    - in Goodpasture's syndrome M31.0
  - antitubular basement membrane (tubulo-interstitial) NEC N12
    - toxic — *see* Nephropathy, toxic
  - arteriolar — *see* Hypertension, kidney
  - arteriosclerotic — *see* Hypertension, kidney
  - ascending — *see* Nephritis, tubulo-interstitial
  - atrophic N03.9
  - Balkan (endemic) N15.0
  - calculous, calculus — *see* Calculus, kidney
  - cardiac — *see* Hypertension, kidney
  - cardiovascular — *see* Hypertension, kidney
  - chronic N03.9
    - with
- **Nephritis, nephritic (albuminuric) (azotemic) (congenital) (disseminated) (epithelial) (familial) (focal) (granulomatous) (hemorrhagic) (infantile) (nonsuppurative, excretory) (uremic)** - *continued*
  - chronic - *continued*
    - with - *continued*
      - C3
        - glomerulonephritis N03.A
        - glomerulopathy N03.A
          - with dense deposit disease N03.6
      - dense deposit disease N03.6
      - diffuse
        - crescentic glomerulonephritis N03.7
        - endocapillary proliferative glomerulonephritis N03.4
        - membranous glomerulonephritis N03.2
        - mesangial proliferative glomerulonephritis N03.3
        - mesangiocapillary glomerulonephritis N03.5
      - focal and segmental glomerular lesions N03.1
      - minor glomerular abnormality N03.0
      - specified morphological changes NEC N03.8
    - arteriosclerotic — *see* Hypertension, kidney
  - cirrhotic N26.9
  - complicating pregnancy O26.83-
  - croupous N00.9
  - degenerative — *see* Nephrosis
  - diffuse sclerosing N05.8
  - due to
    - diabetes mellitus — *see* E08-E13 with .21
    - subacute bacterial endocarditis I33.0
    - systemic lupus erythematosus (chronic) M32.14
    - typhoid fever A01.09
  - gonococcal (acute) (chronic) A54.21
  - hypocomplementemic — *see* Nephritis, membranoproliferative
  - IgA — *see* Nephropathy, IgA
  - immune complex (circulating) NEC N05.8
  - infective — *see* Nephritis, tubulo-interstitial
  - interstitial — *see* Nephritis, tubulo-interstitial
  - lead N14.3
  - membranoproliferative (diffuse) (type 1 or 3) — *see also* N00-N07 with fourth character .5 N05.5
    - type 2 — *see also* N00-N07 with fourth character .6 N05.6
  - minimal change N05.0
  - necrotic, necrotizing NEC — *see also* N00-N07 with fourth character .8 N05.8
  - nephrotic — *see* Nephrosis
  - nodular — *see* Nephritis, membranoproliferative
  - polycystic Q61.3
    - adult type Q61.2
    - autosomal
      - dominant Q61.2
      - recessive NEC Q61.19
    - childhood type NEC Q61.19
    - infantile type NEC Q61.19
  - poststreptococcal N05.9
    - acute N00.9
    - chronic N03.9
    - rapidly progressive N01.9
  - proliferative NEC — *see also* N00-N07 with fourth character .8 N05.8
  - purulent — *see* Nephritis, tubulo-interstitial
  - rapidly progressive N01.9
    - with
      - C3
        - glomerulonephritis N01.A
        - glomerulopathy N01.A
          - with dense deposit disease N01.6
      - dense deposit disease N01.6
      - diffuse
        - crescentic glomerulonephritis N01.7
        - endocapillary proliferative glomerulonephritis N01.4

Neurasthenia - *continued*
gastric F45.8
heart F45.8
Neurilemmoma — *see also* Neoplasm, nerve, benign
acoustic (nerve) D33.3
malignant — *see also* Neoplasm, nerve, malignant
acoustic (nerve) C72.4-
Neurilemmosarcoma — *see* Neoplasm, nerve, malignant
Neurinoma — *see* Neoplasm, nerve, benign
Neurinomatosis — *see* Neoplasm, nerve, uncertain behavior
Neuritis (rheumatoid) M79.2
abducens (nerve) — *see* Strabismus, paralytic, sixth nerve
accessory (nerve) G52.8
acoustic (nerve) (*see also* subcategory H93.3)
in (due to)
infectious disease NEC B99 *[H94.0-]*
parasitic disease NEC B89 *[H94.0-]*
syphilitic A52.15
alcoholic G62.1
with psychosis — *see* Psychosis, alcoholic
amyloid, any site E85.4 *[G63]*
auditory (nerve) — *see* subcategory H93.3
brachial — *see* Radiculopathy
due to displacement, intervertebral disc — *see* Disorder, disc, cervical, with neuritis
cranial nerve
due to Lyme disease A69.22
eighth or acoustic or auditory — *see* subcategory H93.3
eleventh or accessory G52.8
fifth or trigeminal G51.0
first or olfactory G52.0
fourth or trochlear — *see* Strabismus, paralytic, fourth nerve
second or optic — *see* Neuritis, optic
seventh or facial G51.8
newborn (birth injury) P11.3
sixth or abducent — *see* Strabismus, paralytic, sixth nerve
tenth or vagus G52.2
third or oculomotor — *see* Strabismus, paralytic, third nerve
twelfth or hypoglossal G52.3
Déjérine-Sottas G60.0
diabetic (mononeuropathy) — *see* E08-E13 with .41
polyneuropathy — *see* E08-E13 with .42
due to
beriberi E51.11
displacement, prolapse or rupture, intervertebral disc — *see* Disorder, disc, with, radiculopathy
herniation, nucleus pulposus M51.9 *[G55]*
endemic E51.11
facial G51.8
newborn (birth injury) P11.3
general — *see* Polyneuropathy
geniculate ganglion G51.1
due to herpes (zoster) B02.21
gouty — *see also* Gout, by type M10.9 *[G63]*
hypoglossal (nerve) G52.3
ilioinguinal (nerve) G57.9-
infectious (multiple) NEC G61.0
interstitial hypertrophic progressive G60.0
lumbar M54.16
lumbosacral M54.17
multiple — *see also* Polyneuropathy
endemic E51.11
infective, acute G61.0
multiplex endemica E51.11
nerve root — *see* Radiculopathy
oculomotor (nerve) — *see* Strabismus, paralytic, third nerve
olfactory nerve G52.0
optic (nerve) (hereditary) (sympathetic) H46.9
with demyelination G36.0
in myelitis G36.0

Neuritis (rheumatoid) - *continued*
optic (nerve) (hereditary) (sympathetic) - *continued*
nutritional H46.2
papillitis — *see* Papillitis, optic
retrobulbar H46.1-
specified type NEC H46.8
toxic H46.3
peripheral (nerve) G62.9
multiple — *see* Polyneuropathy
single — *see* Mononeuritis
pneumogastric (nerve) G52.2
postherpetic, postzoster B02.29
progressive hypertrophic interstitial G60.0
retrobulbar — *see also* Neuritis, optic, retrobulbar
in (due to)
late syphilis A52.15
meningococcal infection A39.82
meningococcal A39.82
syphilitic A52.15
sciatic (nerve) — *see also* Sciatica
due to displacement of intervertebral disc — *see* Disorder, disc, with, radiculopathy
serum — *see also* Reaction, serum T80.69
shoulder-girdle G54.5
specified nerve NEC G58.8
spinal (nerve) root — *see* Radiculopathy
syphilitic A52.15
thenar (median) G56.1-
thoracic M54.14
toxic NEC G62.2
trochlear (nerve) — *see* Strabismus, paralytic, fourth nerve
vagus (nerve) G52.2
Neuroastrocytoma — *see* Neoplasm, uncertain behavior, by site
Neuroavitaminosis E56.9 *[G99.8]*
Neuroblastoma
olfactory C30.0
specified site — *see* Neoplasm, malignant, by site
unspecified site C74.90
Neurochorioretinitis — *see* Chorioretinitis
Neurocirculatory asthenia F45.8
Neurocysticercosis B69.0
Neurocytoma — *see* Neoplasm, benign, by site
Neurodermatitis (circumscribed) (circumscripta) (local) L28.0
atopic L20.81
diffuse (Brocq) L20.81
disseminated L20.81
Neuroencephalomyelopathy, optic G36.0
Neuroepithelioma — *see also* Neoplasm, malignant, by site
olfactory C30.0
Neurofibroma — *see also* Neoplasm, nerve, benign
melanotic — *see* Neoplasm, nerve, benign
multiple — *see* Neurofibromatosis
plexiform — *see* Neoplasm, nerve, benign
Neurofibromatosis (multiple) (nonmalignant) Q85.00
acoustic Q85.02
malignant — *see* Neoplasm, nerve, malignant
specified NEC Q85.09
type 1 (von Recklinghausen) Q85.01
type 2 Q85.02
Neurofibrosarcoma — *see* Neoplasm, nerve, malignant
Neurogenic — *see also* condition
bladder — *see also* Dysfunction, bladder, neuromuscular N31.9
cauda equina syndrome G83.4
bowel NEC K59.2
heart F45.8
Neuroglioma — *see* Neoplasm, uncertain behavior, by site
Neurolabyrinthitis (of Dix and Hallpike) — *see* Neuronitis, vestibular
Neurolathyrism — *see* Poisoning, food, noxious, plant

Neuroleprosy A30.9
Neuroma — *see also* Neoplasm, nerve, benign
acoustic (nerve) D33.3
amputation (stump) (traumatic) (surgical complication) (late) T87.3-
arm T87.3-
leg T87.3-
digital (toe) G57.6-
interdigital G58.8
lower limb (toe) G57.8-
upper limb G56.8-
intermetatarsal G57.8-
Morton's G57.6-
nonneoplastic
arm G56.9-
leg G57.9-
lower extremity G57.9-
upper extremity G56.9-
optic (nerve) D33.3
plantar G57.6-
plexiform — *see* Neoplasm, nerve, benign
surgical (nonneoplastic)
arm G56.9-
leg G57.9-
lower extremity G57.9-
upper extremity G56.9-
Neuromyalgia — *see* Neuralgia
Neuromyasthenia (epidemic) (postinfectious) G93.3
Neuromyelitis G36.9
ascending G61.0
optica G36.0
Neuromyopathy G70.9
paraneoplastic D49.9 *[G13.0]*
Neuromyotonia (Isaacs) G71.19
Neuronevus — *see* Nevus
Neuronitis G58.9
ascending (acute) G57.2-
vestibular H81.2-
Neuroparalytic — *see* condition
Neuropathy, neuropathic G62.9
acute motor G62.81
alcoholic G62.1
with psychosis — *see* Psychosis, alcoholic
arm G56.9-
autonomic, peripheral — *see* Neuropathy, peripheral, autonomic
axillary G56.9-
bladder N31.9
atonic (motor) (sensory) N31.2
autonomous N31.2
flaccid N31.2
nonreflex N31.2
reflex N31.1
uninhibited N31.0
brachial plexus G54.0
cervical plexus G54.2
chronic
progressive segmentally demyelinating G62.89
relapsing demyelinating G62.89
Déjérine-Sottas G60.0
diabetic — *see* E08-E13 with .40
mononeuropathy — *see* E08-E13 with .41
polyneuropathy — *see* E08-E13 with .42
entrapment G58.9
iliohypogastric nerve G57.8-
ilioinguinal nerve G57.8-
lateral cutaneous nerve of thigh G57.1-
median nerve G56.0-
obturator nerve G57.8-
peroneal nerve G57.3-
posterior tibial nerve G57.5-
saphenous nerve G57.8-
ulnar nerve G56.2-
facial nerve G51.9
hereditary G60.9
motor and sensory (types I-IV) G60.0
sensory G60.8
specified NEC G60.8
hypertrophic G60.0
Charcot-Marie-Tooth G60.0
Déjérine-Sottas G60.0
interstitial progressive G60.0
of infancy G60.0

Neuropathy, neuropathic - *continued*
hypertrophic - *continued*
Refsum G60.1
idiopathic G60.9
progressive G60.3
specified NEC G60.8
in association with hereditary ataxia G60.2
intercostal G58.0
ischemic — *see* Disorder, nerve
Jamaica (ginger) G62.2
leg NEC G57.9-
lower extremity G57.9-
lumbar plexus G54.1
median nerve G56.1-
motor and sensory — *see also* Polyneuropathy
hereditary (types I-IV) G60.0
multifocal motor (MMN) G61.82
multiple (acute) (chronic) — *see* Polyneuropathy
optic (nerve) — *see also* Neuritis, optic
ischemic H47.01-
paraneoplastic (sensorial) (Denny Brown) D49.9 *[G13.0]*
peripheral (nerve) — *see also* Polyneuropathy G62.9
autonomic G90.9
idiopathic G90.09
in (due to)
amyloidosis E85.4 *[G99.0]*
diabetes mellitus — *see* E08-E13 with .43
endocrine disease NEC E34.9 *[G99.0]*
gout M10.00 *[G99.0]*
hyperthyroidism E05.90 *[G99.0]*
with thyroid storm E05.91 *[G99.0]*
metabolic disease NEC E88.9 *[G99.0]*
idiopathic G60.9
progressive G60.3
in (due to)
antitetanus serum G62.0
arsenic G62.2
drugs NEC G62.0
lead G62.2
organophosphate compounds G62.2
toxic agent NEC G62.2
plantar nerves G57.6-
progressive
hypertrophic interstitial G60.0
inflammatory G62.81
radicular NEC — *see* Radiculopathy
sacral plexus G54.1
sciatic G57.0-
serum G61.1
toxic NEC G62.2
trigeminal sensory G50.8
ulnar nerve G56.2-
uremic N18.9 *[G63]*
vitamin B12 E53.8 *[G63]*
with anemia (pernicious) D51.0 *[G63]*
due to dietary deficiency D51.3 *[G63]*
Neurophthisis — *see also* Disorder, nerve
peripheral, diabetic — *see* E08-E13 with .42
Neuroretinitis — *see* Chorioretinitis
Neuroretinopathy, hereditary optic H47.22
Neurosarcoma — *see* Neoplasm, nerve, malignant
Neurosclerosis — *see* Disorder, nerve
Neurosis, neurotic F48.9
anankastic F42.8
anxiety (state) F41.1
panic type F41.0
asthenic F48.8
bladder F45.8
cardiac (reflex) F45.8
cardiovascular F45.8
character F60.9
colon F45.8
compensation F68.10
compulsive, compulsion F42.8
conversion F44.9
craft F48.8
cutaneous F45.8
depersonalization F48.1
depressive (reaction) (type) F34.1

Neurosis, neurotic - *continued*
environmental F48.8
excoriation L98.1
fatigue F48.8
functional — *see* Disorder, somatoform
gastric F45.8
gastrointestinal F45.8
heart F45.8
hypochondriacal F45.21
hysterical F44.9
incoordination F45.8
larynx F45.8
vocal cord F45.8
intestine F45.8
larynx (sensory) F45.8
hysterical F44.4
mixed NEC F48.8
musculoskeletal F45.8
obsessional F42.8
obsessive-compulsive F42.8
occupational F48.8
ocular NEC F45.8
organ — *see* Disorder, somatoform
pharynx F45.8
phobic F40.9
posttraumatic (situational) F43.10
acute F43.11
chronic F43.12
psychasthenic (type) F48.8
railroad F48.8
rectum F45.8
respiratory F45.8
rumination F45.8
sexual F65.9
situational F48.8
social F40.10
generalized F40.11
specified type NEC F48.8
state F48.9
with depersonalization episode F48.1
stomach F45.8
traumatic F43.10
acute F43.11
chronic F43.12
vasomotor F45.8
visceral F45.8
war F48.8
Neurospongioblastosis diffusa Q85.1
Neurosyphilis (arrested) (early) (gumma) (late) (latent) (recurrent) (relapse) A52.3
with ataxia (cerebellar) (locomotor) (spastic) (spinal) A52.19
aneurysm (cerebral) A52.05
arachnoid (adhesive) A52.13
arteritis (any artery) (cerebral) A52.04
asymptomatic A52.2
congenital A50.40
dura (mater) A52.13
general paresis A52.17
hemorrhagic A52.05
juvenile (asymptomatic) (meningeal) A50.40
leptomeninges (aseptic) A52.13
meningeal, meninges (adhesive) A52.13
meningitis A52.13
meningovascular (diffuse) A52.13
optic atrophy A52.15
parenchymatous (degenerative) A52.19
paresis, paretic A52.17
juvenile A50.45
remission in (sustained) A52.3
serological (without symptoms) A52.2
specified nature or site NEC A52.19
tabes, tabetic (dorsalis) A52.11
juvenile A50.45
taboparesis A52.17
juvenile A50.45
thrombosis (cerebral) A52.05
vascular (cerebral) NEC A52.05
Neurothekeoma — *see* Neoplasm, nerve, benign
Neurotic — *see* Neurosis
Neurotoxemia — *see* Toxemia
Neutroclusion M26.211

Neutropenia, neutropenic (chronic) (genetic) (idiopathic) (immune) (infantile) (malignant) (pernicious) (splenic) D70.9
congenital (primary) D70.0
cyclic D70.4
cytoreductive cancer chemotherapy sequela D70.1
drug-induced D70.2
due to cytoreductive cancer chemotherapy D70.1
due to infection D70.3
fever D70.9
neonatal, transitory (isoimmune) (maternal transfer) P61.5
periodic D70.4
secondary (cyclic) (periodic) (splenic) D70.4
drug-induced D70.2
due to cytoreductive cancer chemotherapy D70.1
toxic D70.8
Neutrophilia, hereditary giant D72.0
Nevocarcinoma — *see* Melanoma
Nevus D22.9
achromic — *see* Neoplasm, skin, benign
amelanotic — *see* Neoplasm, skin, benign
angiomatousD18.00
intra-abdominal D18.03
intracranial D18.02
skin D18.01
specified site NEC D18.09
araneus I78.1
balloon cell — *see* Neoplasm, skin, benign
bathing trunk D48.5
blue — *see* Neoplasm, skin, benign
cellular — *see* Neoplasm, skin, benign
giant — *see* Neoplasm, skin, benign
Jadassohn's — *see* Neoplasm, skin, benign
malignant — *see* Melanoma
capillary D18.00
intra-abdominal D18.03
intracranial D18.02
skin D18.01
specified site NEC D18.09
cavernous D18.00
intra-abdominal D18.03
intracranial D18.02
skin D18.01
specified site NEC D18.09
cellular — *see* Neoplasm, skin, benign
blue — *see* Neoplasm, skin, benign
choroid D31.3-
comedonicus Q82.5
conjunctiva D31.0-
dermal — *see* Neoplasm, skin, benign
with epidermal nevus — *see* Neoplasm, skin, benign
dysplastic — *see* Neoplasm, skin, benign
eye D31.9-
flammeus Q82.5
hemangiomatous D18.00
intra-abdominal D18.03
intracranial D18.02
skin D18.01
specified site NEC D18.09
iris D31.4-
lacrimal gland D31.5-
lymphatic D18.1
magnocellular
specified site — *see* Neoplasm, benign, by site
unspecified site D31.40
malignant — *see* Melanoma
meaning hemangioma D18.00
intra-abdominal D18.03
intracranial D18.02
skin D18.01
specified site NEC D18.09
mouth (mucosa) D10.30
specified site NEC D10.39
white sponge Q38.6
multiplex Q85.1
non-neoplastic I78.1
oral mucosa D10.30
specified site NEC D10.39
white sponge Q38.6

Newborn (infant) (liveborn) (singleton) - *continued*
affected by - *continued*
maternal (complication of) (use of) - *continued*
sedative-hypnotics P04.17
surgical procedure P00.6
tranquilizers administered for procedures during pregnancy or labor and delivery P04.0
urinary tract disease P00.1
uterine contraction (abnormal) P03.6
meconium peritonitis P78.0
medication (legal) (maternal use) (prescribed) P04.19
membrane abnormalities P02.9
specified NEC P02.8
membranitis P02.78
methamphetamine (s) P04.49
mixed metabolic and respiratory acidosis P84
neonatal abstinence syndrome P96.1
noxious substances transmitted via placenta or breast milk P04.9
cannabis P04.81
specified NEC P04.89
nutritional supplements P04.5
placenta previa P02.0
placental
abnormality (functional) (morphological) P02.20
specified NEC P02.29
dysfunction P02.29
infarction P02.29
insufficiency P02.29
separation NEC P02.1
transfusion syndromes P02.3
placentitis P02.78
precipitate delivery P03.5
prolapsed cord P02.4
respiratory arrest P28.81
slow intrauterine growth P05.9
tobacco P04.2
twin to twin transplacental transfusion P02.3
umbilical cord (tightly) around neck P02.5
umbilical cord condition P02.60
short cord P02.69
specified NEC P02.69
uterine contractions (abnormal) P03.6
vasa previa P02.69
from intrauterine blood loss P50.0
apnea P28.4
primary P28.3
obstructive P28.4
sleep (central) (obstructive) (primary) P28.3
born in hospital Z38.00
by cesarean Z38.01
born outside hospital Z38.1
breast buds P96.89
breast engorgement P83.4
check-up — *see* Newborn, examination
convulsion P90
dehydration P74.1
examination
8 to 28 days old Z00.111
under 8 days old Z00.110
fever P81.9
environmentally-induced P81.0
hyperbilirubinemia P59.9
of prematurity P59.0
hypernatremia P74.21
hyponatremia P74.22
infection P39.9
candidal P37.5
specified NEC P39.8
urinary tract P39.3
jaundice P59.9
due to
breast milk inhibitor P59.3
hepatocellular damage P59.20
specified NEC P59.29
preterm delivery P59.0
of prematurity P59.0

Newborn (infant) (liveborn) (singleton) - *continued*
jaundice - *continued*
specified NEC P59.8
late metabolic acidosis P74.0
mastitis P39.0
infective P39.0
noninfective P83.4
multiple born NEC Z38.8
born in hospital Z38.68
by cesarean Z38.69
born outside hospital Z38.7
omphalitis P38.9
with mild hemorrhage P38.1
without hemorrhage P38.9
post-term P08.21
prolonged gestation (over 42 completed weeks) P08.22
quadruplet Z38.8
born in hospital Z38.63
by cesarean Z38.64
born outside hospital Z38.7
quintuplet Z38.8
born in hospital Z38.65
by cesarean Z38.66
born outside hospital Z38.7
seizure P90
sepsis (congenital) P36.9
due to
anaerobes NEC P36.5
Escherichia coli P36.4
Staphylococcus P36.30
aureus P36.2
specified NEC P36.39
Streptococcus P36.10
group B P36.0
specified NEC P36.19
specified NEC P36.8
triplet Z38.8
born in hospital Z38.61
by cesarean Z38.62
born outside hospital Z38.7
twin Z38.5
born in hospital Z38.30
by cesarean Z38.31
born outside hospital Z38.4
vomiting P92.09
bilious P92.01
weight check Z00.111

Newcastle conjunctivitis or disease B30.8
Nezelof's syndrome (pure alymphocytosis) D81.4
Niacin (amide) deficiency E52
Nicolas (-Durand) -Favre disease A55
Nicotine — *see* Tobacco
Nicotinic acid deficiency E52
Niemann-Pick disease or syndrome E75.249
specified NEC E75.248
type
A E75.240
A/B E75.244
B E75.241
C E75.242
D E75.243
Night
blindness — *see* Blindness, night
sweats R61
terrors (child) F51.4
Nightmares (REM sleep type) F51.5
NIHSS (National Institutes of Health Stroke Scale) score R29.7-
Nipple — *see* condition
Nisbet's chancre A57
Nishimoto (-Takeuchi) disease I67.5
Nitritoid crisis or reaction — *see* Crisis, nitritoid
Nitrosohemoglobinemia D74.8
Njovera A65
No general equivalence degree (GED) Z55.5
Nocardiosis, nocardiasis A43.9
cutaneous A43.1
lung A43.0
pneumonia A43.0
pulmonary A43.0
specified site NEC A43.8

Nocturia R35.1
psychogenic F45.8
Nocturnal — *see* condition
Nodal rhythm I49.8
Node (s) — *see also* Nodule
Bouchard's (with arthropathy) M15.2
Haygarth's M15.8
Heberden's (with arthropathy) M15.1
larynx J38.7
lymph — *see* condition
milker's B08.03
Osler's I33.0
Schmorl's — *see* Schmorl's disease
singer's J38.2
teacher's J38.2
tuberculous — *see* Tuberculosis, lymph gland
vocal cord J38.2
Nodule (s) , nodular
actinomycotic — *see* Actinomycosis
breast NEC — *see also* Lump, breast N63.0
colloid (cystic) , thyroid E04.1
cutaneous — *see* Swelling, localized
endometrial (stromal) D26.1
Haygarth's M15.8
inflammatory — *see* Inflammation
juxta-articular
syphilitic A52.77
yaws A66.7
larynx J38.7
lung, solitary (subsegmental branch of the bronchial tree) R91.1
multiple R91.8
milker's B08.03
prostate N40.2
with lower urinary tract symptoms (LUTS) N40.3
without lower urinary tract symtpoms (LUTS) N40.2
pulmonary, solitary (subsegmental branch of the bronchial tree) R91.1
retrocardiac R09.89
rheumatoid M06.30
ankle M06.37-
elbow M06.32-
foot joint M06.37-
hand joint M06.34-
hip M06.35-
knee M06.36-
multiple site M06.39
shoulder M06.31-
vertebra M06.38
wrist M06.33-
scrotum (inflammatory) N49.2
singer's J38.2
solitary, lung (subsegmental branch of the bronchial tree) R91.1
multiple R91.8
subcutaneous — *see* Swelling, localized
teacher's J38.2
thyroid (cold) (gland) (nontoxic) E04.1
with thyrotoxicosis E05.20
with thyroid storm E05.21
toxic or with hyperthyroidism E05.20
with thyroid storm E05.21
vocal cord J38.2
Noma (gangrenous) (hospital) (infective) A69.0
auricle I96
mouth A69.0
pudendi N76.89
vulvae N76.89
Nomad, nomadism Z59.00
NOMID (neonatal onset multisystemic inflammatory disorder) M04.2
Nonadherence to medical treatment Z91.19
Nonautoimmune hemolytic anemia D59.4
drug-induced D59.2
Nonclosure — *see also* Imperfect, closure
ductus arteriosus (Botallo's) Q25.0
foramen
botalli Q21.1
ovale Q21.1
Noncompliance Z91.19
with

O

NONCOMPLIANCE - OBSERVATION

Observation (following) (for) (without need for further medical care) - *continued*
suspected, ruled out - *continued*
foreign body
aspirated (inhaled) Z03.822
ingested Z03.821
inserted (injected) , in (eye) (orifice) (skin) Z03.823
suicide attempt, alleged Z03.89
self-poisoning Z03.6
toxic effects from ingested substance (drug) (poison) Z03.6
toxic effects from ingested substance (drug) (poison) Z03.6
Obsession, obsessional state F42.8
mixed thoughts and acts F42.2
Obsessive-compulsive neurosis or reaction F42.8
Obstetric embolism, septic — *see* Embolism, obstetric, septic
Obstetrical trauma (complicating delivery) O71.9
with or following ectopic or molar pregnancy O08.6
specified type NEC O71.89
Obstipation — *see* Constipation
Obstruction, obstructed, obstructive
airway J98.8
with
allergic alveolitis J67.9
asthma J45.909
with
exacerbation (acute) J45.901
status asthmaticus J45.902
bronchiectasis J47.9
with
exacerbation (acute) J47.1
lower respiratory infection J47.0
bronchitis (chronic) J44.9
emphysema J43.9
chronic J44.9
with
allergic alveolitis — *see* Pneumonitis, hypersensitivity
bronchiectasis J47.9
with
exacerbation (acute) J47.1
lower respiratory infection J47.0
due to
foreign body — *see* Foreign body, by site, causing asphyxia
inhalation of fumes or vapors J68.9
laryngospasm J38.5
ampulla of Vater K83.1
aortic (heart) (valve) — *see* Stenosis, aortic
aortoiliac I74.09
aqueduct of Sylvius G91.1
congenital Q03.0
with spina bifida — *see* Spina bifida, by site, with hydrocephalus
Arnold-Chiari — *see* Arnold-Chiari disease
artery — *see also* Atherosclerosis, artery I70.9
stent — *see* Restenosis, stent
basilar (complete) (partial) — *see* Occlusion, artery, basilar
carotid (complete) (partial) — *see* Occlusion, artery, carotid
cerebellar — *see* Occlusion, artery, cerebellar
cerebral (anterior) (middle) (posterior) — *see* Occlusion, artery, cerebral
precerebral — *see* Occlusion, artery, precerebral
renal N28.0
retinal NEC — *see* Occlusion, artery, retina
vertebral (complete) (partial) — *see* Occlusion, artery, vertebral
band (intestinal) — *see also* Obstruction, intestine, specified NEC K56.699
bile duct or passage (common) (hepatic) (noncalculous) K83.1
with calculus K80.51
congenital (causing jaundice) Q44.3

Obstruction, obstructed, obstructive - *continued*
biliary (duct) (tract) K83.1
gallbladder K82.0
bladder-neck (acquired) N32.0
congenital Q64.31
due to hyperplasia (hypertrophy) of prostate — *see* Hyperplasia, prostate
bowel — *see* Obstruction, intestine
bronchus J98.09
canal, ear — *see* Stenosis, external ear canal
cardia K22.2
caval veins (inferior) (superior) I87.1
cecum — *see* Obstruction, intestine
circulatory I99.8
colon — *see* Obstruction, intestine
common duct (noncalculous) K83.1
coronary (artery) — *see* Occlusion, coronary
cystic duct — *see also* Obstruction, gallbladder
with calculus K80.21
device, implant or graft — *see also* Complications, by site and type, mechanical T85.698
arterial graft NEC — *see* Complication, cardiovascular device, mechanical, vascular
catheter NEC T85.628
cystostomy T83.090
dialysis (renal) T82.49
intraperitoneal T85.691
Hopkins T83.098
ileostomy T83.098
infusion NEC T82.594
spinal (epidural) (subdural) T85.690
nephrostomy T83.092
urethral indwelling T83.091
urinary T83.098
urostomy T83.098
due to infection T85.79
gastrointestinal — *see* Complications, prosthetic device, mechanical, gastrointestinal device
genital NEC T83.498
intrauterine contraceptive device T83.39
penile prosthesis (cylinder) (implanted) (pump) (resevoir) T83.490
testicular prosthesis T83.491
heart NEC — *see* Complication, cardiovascular device, mechanical
joint prosthesis — *see* Complications, joint prosthesis, mechanical, specified NEC, by site
orthopedic NEC — *see* Complication, orthopedic, device, mechanical
specified NEC T85.628
urinary NEC — *see also* Complication, genitourinary, device, urinary, mechanical
graft T83.29
vascular NEC — *see* Complication, cardiovascular device, mechanical
ventricular intracranial shunt T85.09
due to foreign body accidentally left in operative wound T81.529
duodenum K31.5
ejaculatory duct N50.89
esophagus K22.2
eustachian tube (complete) (partial) H68.10-
cartilagenous (extrinsic) H68.13-
intrinsic H68.12-
osseous H68.11-
fallopian tube (bilateral) N97.1
fecal K56.41
with hernia — *see* Hernia, by site, with obstruction
foramen of Monro (congenital) Q03.8
with spina bifida — *see* Spina bifida, by site, with hydrocephalus
foreign body — *see* Foreign body
gallbladder K82.0
with calculus, stones K80.21
congenital Q44.1
gastric outlet K31.1
gastrointestinal — *see* Obstruction, intestine

Obstruction, obstructed, obstructive - *continued*
hepatic K76.89
duct (noncalculous) K83.1
hepatobiliary K83.1
ileum — *see* Obstruction, intestine
iliofemoral (artery) I74.5
intestine K56.609
complete K56.601
incomplete K56.600
partial K56.600
with
adhesions (intestinal) (peritoneal) K56.50
complete K56.52
incomplete K56.51
partial K56.51
adynamic K56.0
by gallstone K56.3
congenital (small) Q41.9
large Q42.9
specified part NEC Q42.8
neurogenic K56.0
Hirschsprung's disease or megacolon Q43.1
newborn P76.9
due to
fecaliths P76.8
inspissated milk P76.2
meconium (plug) P76.0
in mucoviscidosis E84.11
specified NEC P76.8
postoperative K91.30
complete K91.32
incomplete K91.31
partial K91.31
reflex K56.0
specified NEC K56.699
complete K56.691
incomplete K56.690
partial K56.690
volvulus K56.2
intracardiac ball valve prosthesis T82.09
jejunum — *see* Obstruction, intestine
joint prosthesis — *see* Complications, joint prosthesis, mechanical, specified NEC, by site
kidney (calices) — *see also* Hydronephrosis N28.89
labor — *see* Delivery
lacrimal (passages) (duct)
by
dacryolith — *see* Dacryolith
stenosis — *see* Stenosis, lacrimal
congenital Q10.5
neonatal H04.53-
lacrimonasal duct — *see* Obstruction, lacrimal
lacteal, with steatorrhea K90.2
laryngitis — *see* Laryngitis
larynx NEC J38.6
congenital Q31.8
lung J98.4
disease, chronic J44.9
lymphatic I89.0
meconium (plug)
newborn P76.0
due to fecaliths P76.0
in mucoviscidosis E84.11
mitral — *see* Stenosis, mitral
nasal J34.89
nasolacrimal duct — *see also* Obstruction, lacrimal
congenital Q10.5
nasopharynx J39.2
nose J34.89
organ or site, congenital NEC — *see* Atresia, by site
pancreatic duct K86.89
parotid duct or gland K11.8
pelviureteral junction N13.5
with hydronephrosis N13.0
congenital Q62.39
pharynx J39.2
portal (circulation) (vein) I81

Obstruction, obstructed, obstructive - *continued*
  prostate — *see also* Hyperplasia, prostate
    valve (urinary) N32.0
  pulmonary valve (heart) I37.0
  pyelonephritis (chronic) N11.1
  pylorus
    adult K31.1
    congenital or infantile Q40.0
  rectosigmoid — *see* Obstruction, intestine
  rectum K62.4
  renal — *see also* Hydronephrosis N28.89
    outflow N13.8
    pelvis, congenital Q62.39
  respiratory J98.8
    chronic J44.9
  retinal (vessels) H34.9
  salivary duct (any) K11.8
    with calculus K11.5
  sigmoid — *see* Obstruction, intestine
  sinus (accessory) (nasal) J34.89
  Stensen's duct K11.8
  stomach NEC K31.89
    acute K31.0
    congenital Q40.2
    due to pylorospasm K31.3
  submandibular duct K11.8
  submaxillary gland K11.8
    with calculus K11.5
  thoracic duct I89.0
  thrombotic — *see* Thrombosis
  trachea J39.8
  tracheostomy airway J95.03
  tricuspid (valve) — *see* Stenosis, tricuspid
  upper respiratory, congenital Q34.8
  ureter (functional) (pelvic junction)
      NEC N13.5
    with
      hydronephrosis N13.1
        with infection N13.6
        congenital Q62.39
      pyelonephritis (chronic) N11.1
    congenital Q62.39
    due to calculus — *see* Calculus, ureter
  urethra NEC N36.8
    congenital Q64.39
  urinary (moderate) N13.9
    due to hyperplasia (hypertrophy) of
        prostate — *see* Hyperplasia, prostate
    organ or tract (lower) N13.9
    prostatic valve N32.0
    specified NEC N13.8
  uropathy N13.9
  uterus N85.8
  vagina N89.5
  valvular — *see* Endocarditis
  vein, venous I87.1
    caval (inferior) (superior) I87.1
    thrombotic — *see* Thrombosis
  vena cava (inferior) (superior) I87.1
  vesical NEC N32.0
  vesicourethral orifice N32.0
    congenital Q64.31
  vessel NEC I99.8
    stent — *see* Restenosis, stent
Obturator — *see* condition
Occlusal wear, teeth K03.0
Occlusio pupillae — *see* Membrane, pupillary
Occlusion, occluded
  anus K62.4
    congenital Q42.3
      with fistula Q42.2
  aortoiliac (chronic) I74.09
  aqueduct of Sylvius G91.1
    congenital Q03.0
      with spina bifida — *see* Spina bifida, by
          site, with hydrocephalus
  artery — *see also* Atherosclerosis,
      artery I70.9
    auditory, internal I65.8
    basilar I65.1
      with
        infarction I63.22
          due to
            embolism I63.12

Occlusion, occluded - *continued*
  artery - *continued*
    basilar - *continued*
      with - *continued*
        infarction - *continued*
          due to - *continued*
            thrombosis I63.02
    brain or cerebral I66.9
      with infarction (due to) I63.5-
        embolism I63.4-
        thrombosis I63.3-
    carotid I65.2-
      with
        infarction I63.23-
          due to
            embolism I63.13-
            thrombosis I63.03-
    cerebellar (anterior inferior) (posterior
        inferior) (superior) I66.3
      with infarction I63.54-
        due to
          embolism I63.44-
          thrombosis I63.34-
    cerebral I66.9
      with infarction I63.50
        due to
          embolism I63.40
            specified NEC I63.49
          thrombosis I63.30
            specified NEC I63.39
      anterior I66.1-
        with infarction I63.52-
          due to
            embolism I63.42-
            thrombosis I63.32-
      middle I66.0-
        with infarction I63.51-
          due to
            embolism I63.41-
            thrombosis I63.31-
      posterior I66.2-
        with infarction I63.53-
          due to
            embolism I63.43-
            thrombosis I63.33-
      specified NEC I66.8
        with infarction I63.59
          due to
            embolism I63.4-
            thrombosis I63.3-
    choroidal (anterior) — *see* Occlusion,
        artery, precerebral, specified NEC
    communicating posterior — *see* Occlusion,
        artery, precerebral, specified NEC
    complete
      coronary I25.82
      extremities I70.92
    coronary (acute) (thrombotic) (without
        myocardial infarction) I24.0
      with myocardial infarction — *see*
          Infarction, myocardium
      chronic total I25.82
      complete I25.82
      healed or old I25.2
      total (chronic) I25.82
    hypophyseal — *see* Occlusion, artery,
        precerebral, specified NEC
    iliac I74.5
    lower extremities due to stenosis or
        stricture I77.1
    mesenteric (embolic) (thrombotic) — *see
        also* Infarct, intestine K55.069
    perforating — *see* Occlusion, artery,
        cerebral, specified NEC
    peripheral I77.9
      thrombotic or embolic I74.4
    pontine — *see* Occlusion, artery,
        precerebral, specified NEC
    precerebral I65.9
      with infarction I63.20
        specified NEC I63.29
        due to
          embolism I63.10
            specified NEC I63.19
          thrombosis I63.00

Occlusion, occluded - *continued*
  artery - *continued*
    precerebral - *continued*
      with infarction - *continued*
        due to - *continued*
          thrombosis - *continued*
            specified NEC I63.09
      basilar — *see* Occlusion, artery, basilar
      carotid — *see* Occlusion, artery, carotid
      puerperal O88.23
      specified NEC I65.8
        with infarction I63.29
          due to
            embolism I63.19
            thrombosis I63.09
      vertebral — *see* Occlusion, artery,
          vertebral
    renal N28.0
    retinal
      central H34.1-
      partial H34.21-
      branch H34.23-
      transient H34.0-
    spinal — *see* Occlusion, artery,
        precerebral, vertebral
    total (chronic)
      coronary I25.82
      extremities I70.92
    vertebral I65.0-
      with
        infarction I63.21-
          due to
            embolism I63.11-
            thrombosis I63.01-
  basilar artery — *see* Occlusion, artery, basilar
  bile duct (common) (hepatic)
      (noncalculous) K83.1
  bowel — *see* Obstruction, intestine
  carotid (artery) (common) (internal) — *see*
      Occlusion, artery, carotid
  centric (of teeth) M26.59
    maximum intercuspation
        discrepancy M26.55
  cerebellar (artery) — *see* Occlusion, artery,
      cerebellar
  cerebral (artery) — *see* Occlusion, artery,
      cerebral
  cerebrovascular — *see also* Occlusion,
      artery, cerebral
    with infarction I63.5-
  cervical canal — *see* Stricture, cervix
  cervix (uteri) — *see* Stricture, cervix
  choanal Q30.0
  choroidal (artery) — *see* Occlusion, artery,
      precerebral, specified NEC
  colon — *see* Obstruction, intestine
  communicating posterior artery — *see*
      Occlusion, artery, precerebral, specified
      NEC
  coronary (artery) (vein) (thrombotic) — *see
      also* Infarct, myocardium
    chronic total I25.82
    healed or old I25.2
    not resulting in infarction I24.0
    total (chronic) I25.82
  cystic duct — *see* Obstruction, gallbladder
  embolic — *see* Embolism
  fallopian tube N97.1
    congenital Q50.6
  gallbladder — *see also* Obstruction,
      gallbladder
    congenital (causing jaundice) Q44.1
  gingiva, traumatic K06.2
  hymen N89.6
    congenital Q52.3
  hypophyseal (artery) — *see* Occlusion,
      artery, precerebral, specified NEC
  iliac artery I74.5
  intestine — *see* Obstruction, intestine
  lacrimal passages — *see* Obstruction,
      lacrimal
  lung J98.4
  lymph or lymphatic channel I89.0
  mammary duct N64.89

Occlusion, occluded - *continued*
- mesenteric artery (embolic) (thrombotic) — *see also* Infarct, intestine K55.069
- nose J34.89
  - congenital Q30.0
- organ or site, congenital NEC — *see* Atresia, by site
- oviduct N97.1
  - congenital Q50.6
- peripheral arteries
  - due to stricture or stenosis I77.1
  - upper extremity I74.2
- pontine (artery) — *see* Occlusion, artery, precerebral, specified NEC
- posterior lingual, of mandibular teeth M26.29
- precerebral artery — *see* Occlusion, artery, precerebral
- punctum lacrimale — *see* Obstruction, lacrimal
- pupil — *see* Membrane, pupillary
- pylorus, adult — *see also* Stricture, pylorus K31.1
- renal artery N28.0
- retina, retinal
  - artery — *see* Occlusion, artery, retinal
  - vein (central) H34.81-
    - engorgement H34.82-
    - tributary H34.83-
  - vessels H34.9
- spinal artery — *see* Occlusion, artery, precerebral, vertebral
- teeth (mandibular) (posterior lingual) M26.29
- thoracic duct I89.0
- thrombotic — *see* Thrombosis, artery
- traumatic
  - edentulous (alveolar) ridge K06.2
  - gingiva K06.2
  - periodontal K05.5
- tubal N97.1
- ureter (complete) (partial) N13.5
  - congenital Q62.10
- ureteropelvic junction N13.5
  - congenital Q62.11
- ureterovesical orifice N13.5
  - congenital Q62.12
- urethra — *see* Stricture, urethra
- uterus N85.8
- vagina N89.5
- vascular NEC I99.8
- vein — *see* Thrombosis
  - retinal — *see* Occlusion, retinal, vein
- vena cava (inferior) (superior) — *see* Embolism, vena cava
- ventricle (brain) NEC G91.1
- vertebral (artery) — *see* Occlusion, artery, vertebral
- vessel (blood) I99.8
- vulva N90.5

Occult
- blood in feces (stools) R19.5

Occupational
- problems NEC Z56.89

Ochlophobia — *see* Agoraphobia
Ochronosis (endogenous) E70.29
Ocular muscle — *see* condition
Oculogyric crisis or disturbance H51.8
- psychogenic F45.8

Oculomotor syndrome H51.9
Oculopathy
- syphilitic NEC A52.71
  - congenital
    - early A50.01
    - late A50.30
  - early (secondary) A51.43
  - late A52.71

Oddi's sphincter spasm K83.4
Odontalgia K08.89
Odontoameloblastoma — *see* Cyst, calcifying odontogenic
Odontoclasia K03.89
Odontodysplasia, regional K00.4
Odontogenesis imperfecta K00.5
Odontoma (ameloblastic) (complex) (compound) (fibroameloblastic) — *see* Cyst, calcifying odontogenic
Odontomyelitis (closed) (open) K04.01
- irreversible K04.02
- reversible K04.01

Odontorrhagia K08.89
Odontosarcoma, ameloblastic C41.1
- upper jaw (bone) C41.0

Oestriasis — *see* Myiasis
Oguchi's disease H53.63
Ohara's disease — *see* Tularemia
OHS (obesity hypoventilation syndrome) E66.2
Oidiomycosis — *see* Candidiasis
Oidium albicans infection — *see* Candidiasis
Old age (without mention of debility) R54
- dementia F03

Old (previous) myocardial infarction I25.2
Olfactory — *see* condition
Oligemia — *see* Anemia
Oligoastrocytoma
- specified site — *see* Neoplasm, malignant, by site
- unspecified site C71.9

Oligocythemia D64.9
Oligodendroblastoma
- specified site — *see* Neoplasm, malignant
- unspecified site C71.9

Oligodendroglioma
- anaplastic type
  - specified site — *see* Neoplasm, malignant, by site
  - unspecified site C71.9
- specified site — *see* Neoplasm, malignant, by site
- unspecified site C71.9

Oligodontia — *see* Anodontia
Oligoencephalon Q02
Oligohidrosis L74.4
Oligohydramnios O41.0-
Oligohydrosis L74.4
Oligomenorrhea N91.5
- primary N91.3
- secondary N91.4

Oligophrenia — *see also* Disability, intellectual
- phenylpyruvic E70.0

Oligospermia N46.11
- due to
  - drug therapy N46.121
  - efferent duct obstruction N46.123
  - infection N46.122
  - radiation N46.124
  - specified cause NEC N46.129
  - systemic disease N46.125

Oligotrichia — *see* Alopecia
Oliguria R34
- with, complicating or following ectopic or molar pregnancy O08.4
- postprocedural N99.0

Ollier's disease Q78.4
Omenotocele — *see* Hernia, abdomen, specified site NEC
Omentitis — *see* Peritonitis
Omentum, omental — *see* condition
Omphalitis (congenital) (newborn) P38.9
- with mild hemorrhage P38.1
- without hemorrhage P38.9
- not of newborn L08.82
- tetanus A33

Omphalocele Q79.2
Omphalomesenteric duct, persistent Q43.0
Omphalorrhagia, newborn P51.9
Omsk hemorrhagic fever A98.1
Onanism (excessive) F98.8
Onchocerciasis, onchocercosis B73.1
- with
  - eye disease B73.00
    - endophthalmitis B73.01
    - eyelid B73.09
    - glaucoma B73.02
    - specified NEC B73.09
- eye NEC B73.00
- eyelid B73.09

Oncocytoma — *see* Neoplasm, benign, by site
Oncovirus, as cause of disease classified elsewhere B97.32
Ondine's curse — *see* Apnea, sleep
Oneirophrenia F23
Onychauxis L60.2
- congenital Q84.5

Onychia — *see also* Cellulitis, digit
- with lymphangitis — *see* Lymphangitis, acute, digit
- candidal B37.2
- dermatophytic B35.1

Onychitis — *see also* Cellulitis, digit
- with lymphangitis — *see* Lymphangitis, acute, digit

Onychocryptosis L60.0
Onychodystrophy L60.3
- congenital Q84.6

Onychogryphosis, onychogryposis L60.2
Onycholysis L60.1
Onychomadesis L60.8
Onychomalacia L60.3
Onychomycosis (finger) (toe) B35.1
Onycho-osteodysplasia Q87.2
Onychophagia F98.8
Onychophosis L60.8
Onychoptosis L60.8
Onychorrhexis L60.3
- congenital Q84.6

Onychoschizia L60.3
Onyxis (finger) (toe) L60.0
Onyxitis — *see also* Cellulitis, digit
- with lymphangitis — *see* Lymphangitis, acute, digit

Oophoritis (cystic) (infectional) (interstitial) N70.92
- with salpingitis N70.93
- acute N70.02
  - with salpingitis N70.03
- chronic N70.12
  - with salpingitis N70.13
- complicating abortion — *see* Abortion, by type, complicated by, oophoritis

Oophorocele N83.4-
Opacity, opacities
- cornea H17.-
  - central H17.1-
  - congenital Q13.3
  - degenerative — *see* Degeneration, cornea
  - hereditary — *see* Dystrophy, cornea
  - inflammatory — *see* Keratitis
  - minor H17.81-
  - peripheral H17.82-
  - sequelae of trachoma (healed) B94.0
  - specified NEC H17.89
- enamel (teeth) (fluoride) (nonfluoride) K00.3
- lens — *see* Cataract
- snowball — *see* Deposit, crystalline
- vitreous (humor) NEC H43.39-
  - congenital Q14.0
  - membranes and strands H43.31-

Opalescent dentin (hereditary) K00.5
Open, opening
- abnormal, organ or site, congenital — *see* Imperfect, closure
- angle with
  - borderline
    - findings
      - high risk H40.02-
      - low risk H40.01-
    - intraocular pressure H40.00-
  - cupping of discs H40.01-
  - glaucoma (primary) — *see* Glaucoma, open angle
- bite
  - anterior M26.220
  - posterior M26.221
- false — *see* Imperfect, closure
- margin on tooth restoration K08.51
- restoration margins of tooth K08.51
- wound — *see* Wound, open

Operational fatigue F48.8
Operative — *see* condition
Operculitis — *see* Periodontitis
Operculum — *see* Break, retina

Ophiasis L63.2
Ophthalmia — *see also* Conjunctivitis H10.9
actinic rays — *see* Photokeratitis
allergic (acute) — *see* Conjunctivitis, acute, atopic
blennorrhagic (gonococcal) (neonatorum) A54.31
diphtheritic A36.86
Egyptian A71.1
electrica — *see* Photokeratitis
gonococcal (neonatorum) A54.31
metastatic — *see* Endophthalmitis, purulent
migraine — *see* Migraine, ophthalmoplegic
neonatorum, newborn P39.1
gonococcal A54.31
nodosa H16.24-
purulent — *see* Conjunctivitis, acute, mucopurulent
spring — *see* Conjunctivitis, acute, atopic
sympathetic — *see* Uveitis, sympathetic
Ophthalmitis — *see* Ophthalmia
Ophthalmocele (congenital) Q15.8
Ophthalmoneuromyelitis G36.0
Ophthalmoplegia — *see also* Strabismus, paralytic
anterior internuclear — *see* Ophthalmoplegia, internuclear
ataxia-areflexia G61.0
diabetic — *see* E08-E13 with .39
exophthalmic E05.00
with thyroid storm E05.01
external H49.88-
progressive H49.4-
with pigmentary retinopathy — *see* Kearns-Sayre syndrome
total H49.3-
internal (complete) (total) H52.51-
internuclear H51.2-
migraine — *see* Migraine, ophthalmoplegic
Parinaud's H49.88-
progressive external — *see* Ophthalmoplegia, external, progressive
supranuclear, progressive G23.1
total (external) — *see* Ophthalmoplegia, external, total
Opioid (s)
abuse — *see* Abuse, drug, opioids
dependence — *see* Dependence, drug, opioids
induced, without use disorder
anxiety disorder F11.988
delirium F11.921
depressive disorder F11.94
sexual dysfunction F11.981
sleep disorder F11.982
Opisthognathism M26.09
Opisthorchiasis (felineus) (viverrini) B66.0
Opitz' disease D73.2
Opiumism — *see* Dependence, drug, opioid
Oppenheim's disease G70.2
Oppenheim-Urbach disease (necrobiosis lipoidica diabeticorum) — *see* E08-E13 with .620
Optic nerve — *see* condition
Orbit — *see* condition
Orchioblastoma C62.9-
Orchitis (gangrenous) (nonspecific) (septic) (suppurative) N45.2
blennorrhagic (gonococcal) (acute) (chronic) A54.23
chlamydial A56.19
filarial — *see also* Infestation, filarial B74.9 *[N51]*
gonococcal (acute) (chronic) A54.23
mumps B26.0
syphilitic A52.76
tuberculous A18.15
Orf (virus disease) B08.02
Organic — *see also* condition
brain syndrome F09
heart — *see* Disease, heart
mental disorder F09
psychosis F09
Orgasm
anejaculatory N53.13
Oriental
bilharziasis B65.2
schistosomiasis B65.2
Orifice — *see* condition
Origin of both great vessels from right ventricle Q20.1
Ormond's disease (with ureteral obstruction) N13.5
with infection N13.6
Ornithine metabolism disorder E72.4
Ornithinemia (Type I) (Type II) E72.4
Ornithosis A70
Orotaciduria, oroticaciduria (congenital) (hereditary) (pyrimidine deficiency) E79.8
anemia D53.0
Orthodontics
adjustment Z46.4
fitting Z46.4
Orthopnea R06.01
Orthopoxvirus B08.09
Os, uterus — *see* condition
Osgood-Schlatter disease or osteochondrosis M92.52-
Osler (-Weber) -Rendu disease I78.0
Osler's nodes I33.0
Osmidrosis L75.0
Osseous — *see* condition
Ossification
artery — *see* Arteriosclerosis
auricle (ear) — *see* Disorder, pinna, specified type NEC
bronchial J98.09
cardiac — *see* Degeneration, myocardial
cartilage (senile) — *see* Disorder, cartilage, specified type NEC
coronary (artery) — *see* Disease, heart, ischemic, atherosclerotic
diaphragm J98.6
ear, middle — *see* Otosclerosis
falx cerebri G96.198
fontanel, premature Q75.0
heart — *see also* Degeneration, myocardial
valve — *see* Endocarditis
larynx J38.7
ligament — *see* Disorder, tendon, specified type NEC
posterior longitudinal — *see* Spondylopathy, specified NEC
meninges (cerebral) (spinal) G96.198
multiple, eccentric centers — *see* Disorder, bone, development or growth
muscle — *see also* Calcification, muscle
due to burns — *see* Myositis, ossificans, in, burns
paralytic — *see* Myositis, ossificans, in, quadriplegia
progressive — *see* Myositis, ossificans, progressiva
specified NEC M61.50
ankle M61.57-
foot M61.57-
forearm M61.53-
hand M61.54-
lower leg M61.56-
multiple sites M61.59
pelvic region M61.55-
shoulder region M61.51-
specified site NEC M61.58
thigh M61.55-
upper arm M61.52-
traumatic — *see* Myositis, ossificans, traumatica
myocardium, myocardial — *see* Degeneration, myocardial
penis N48.89
periarticular — *see* Disorder, joint, specified type NEC
pinna — *see* Disorder, pinna, specified type NEC
rider's bone — *see* Ossification, muscle, specified NEC
sclera H15.89
subperiosteal, post-traumatic M89.8X-
Ossification - *continued*
tendon — *see* Disorder, tendon, specified type NEC
trachea J39.8
tympanic membrane — *see* Disorder, tympanic membrane, specified NEC
vitreous (humor) — *see* Deposit, crystalline
Osteitis — *see also* Osteomyelitis
alveolar M27.3
condensans M85.30
ankle M85.37-
foot M85.37-
forearm M85.33-
hand M85.34-
lower leg M85.36-
multiple site M85.39
neck M85.38
rib M85.38
shoulder M85.31-
skull M85.38
specified site NEC M85.38
thigh M85.35-
toe M85.37-
upper arm M85.32-
vertebra M85.38
deformans M88.9
in (due to)
malignant neoplasm of bone C41.9 *[M90.60]*
neoplastic disease — *see also* Neoplasm D49.9 *[M90.60]*
carpus D49.9 *[M90.64-]*
clavicle D49.9 *[M90.61-]*
femur D49.9 *[M90.65-]*
fibula D49.9 *[M90.66-]*
finger D49.9 *[M90.64-]*
humerus D49.9 *[M90.62-]*
ilium D49.9 *[M90.65-]*
ischium D49.9 *[M90.65-]*
metacarpus D49.9 *[M90.64-]*
metatarsus D49.9 *[M90.67-]*
multiple sites D49.9 *[M90.69]*
neck D49.9 *[M90.68]*
radius D49.9 *[M90.63-]*
rib D49.9 *[M90.68]*
scapula D49.9 *[M90.61-]*
skull D49.9 *[M90.68]*
tarsus D49.9 *[M90.67-]*
tibia D49.9 *[M90.66-]*
toe D49.9 *[M90.67-]*
ulna D49.9 *[M90.63-]*
vertebra D49.9 *[M90.68]*
skull M88.0
specified NEC — *see* Paget's disease, bone, by site
vertebra M88.1
due to yaws A66.6
fibrosa NEC — *see* Cyst, bone, by site
circumscripta — *see* Dysplasia, fibrous, bone NEC
cystica (generalisata) E21.0
disseminata Q78.1
osteoplastica E21.0
fragilitans Q78.0
Garr's (sclerosing) — *see* Osteomyelitis, specified type NEC
jaw (acute) (chronic) (lower) (suppurative) (upper) M27.2
parathyroid E21.0
petrous bone (acute) (chronic) — *see* Petrositis
sclerotic, nonsuppurative — *see* Osteomyelitis, specified type NEC
tuberculosa A18.09
cystica D86.89
multiplex cystoides D86.89
Osteoarthritis M19.90
ankle M19.07-
elbow M19.02-
foot joint M19.07-
generalized (multiple joints) M15.9
erosive M15.4
primary M15.0
specified NEC M15.8
hand joint M19.04-

Osteoarthritis - *continued*
- hand joint - *continued*
  - first carpometacarpal joint M18.9
- hip M16.1-
  - bilateral M16.0
  - due to hip dysplasia (unilateral) M16.3-
    - bilateral M16.2
- interphalangeal
  - distal (Heberden) M15.1
  - proximal (Bouchard) M15.2
- knee M17.1-
  - bilateral M17.0
- shoulder M19.01-
- specified site NEC M19.09
- spine — *see* Spondylosis
- wrist M19.03-
- post-traumatic NEC M19.92
  - ankle M19.17-
  - elbow M19.12-
  - foot joint M19.17-
  - hand joint M19.14-
    - first carpometacarpal joint M18.3-
      - bilateral M18.2
  - hip M16.5-
    - bilateral M16.4
  - knee M17.3-
    - bilateral M17.2
  - shoulder M19.11-
  - specified site NEC M19.19
  - wrist M19.13-
- primary M19.91
  - ankle M19.07-
  - elbow M19.02-
  - foot joint M19.07-
  - hand joint M19.04-
    - first carpometacarpal joint M18.1-
      - bilateral M18.0
  - hip M16.1-
    - bilateral M16.0
  - knee M17.1-
    - bilateral M17.0
  - multiple sites M15.9
  - shoulder M19.01-
  - spine — *see* Spondylosis
  - wrist M19.03-
- secondary M19.93
  - ankle M19.27-
  - elbow M19.22-
  - foot joint M19.27-
  - hand joint M19.24-
    - first carpometacarpal joint M18.5-
      - bilateral M18.4
  - hip M16.7
    - bilateral M16.6
  - knee M17.5
    - bilateral M17.4
  - multiple M15.3
  - shoulder M19.21-
  - specified site NEC M19.29
  - spine — *see* Spondylosis
  - wrist M19.23-

Osteoarthropathy (hypertrophic) M19.90
- ankle — *see* Osteoarthritis, primary, ankle
- elbow — *see* Osteoarthritis, primary, elbow
- foot joint — *see* Osteoarthritis, primary, foot
- hand joint — *see* Osteoarthritis, primary, hand joint
- knee joint — *see* Osteoarthritis, primary, knee
- multiple site — *see* Osteoarthritis, primary, multiple joint
- pulmonary — *see also* Osteoarthropathy, specified type NEC
  - hypertrophic — *see* Osteoarthropathy, hypertrophic, specified type NEC
- secondary hypertrophic — *see* Osteoarthropathy, specified type NEC
- shoulder — *see* Osteoarthritis, primary, shoulder
- specified joint NEC — *see* Osteoarthritis, primary, specified joint NEC
- specified type NEC M89.40
  - carpus M89.44-
  - clavicle M89.41-
  - femur M89.45-

Osteoarthropathy (hypertrophic) - *continued*
- specified type NEC - *continued*
  - fibula M89.46-
  - finger M89.44-
  - humerus M89.42-
  - ilium M89.459
  - ischium M89.459
  - metacarpus M89.44-
  - metatarsus M89.47-
  - multiple sites M89.49
  - neck M89.48
  - radius M89.43-
  - rib M89.48
  - scapula M89.41-
  - skull M89.48
  - tarsus M89.47-
  - tibia M89.46-
  - toe M89.47-
  - ulna M89.43-
  - vertebra M89.48
- secondary — *see* Osteoarthropathy, specified type NEC
- spine — *see* Spondylosis
- wrist — *see* Osteoarthritis, primary, wrist

Osteoarthrosis (degenerative) (hypertrophic) (joint) — *see also* Osteoarthritis
- deformans alkaptonurica E70.29 *[M36.8]*
- erosive M15.4
- generalized M15.9
  - primary M15.0
- polyarticular M15.9
- spine — *see* Spondylosis

Osteoblastoma — *see* Neoplasm, bone, benign
- aggressive — *see* Neoplasm, bone, uncertain behavior

Osteochondritis — *see also* Osteochondropathy, by site
- Brailsford's — *see* Osteochondrosis, juvenile, radius
- dissecans M93.20
  - ankle M93.27-
  - elbow M93.22-
  - foot M93.27-
  - hand M93.24-
  - hip M93.25-
  - knee M93.26-
  - multiple sites M93.29
  - shoulder joint M93.21-
  - specified site NEC M93.28
  - wrist M93.23-
- juvenile M92.9
  - patellar — *see* Osteochondrosis, juvenile, patella
- syphilitic (congenital) (early) A50.02 *[M90.80]*
  - ankle A50.02 *[M90.87-]*
  - elbow A50.02 *[M90.82-]*
  - foot A50.02 *[M90.87-]*
  - forearm A50.02 *[M90.83-]*
  - hand A50.02 *[M90.84-]*
  - hip A50.02 *[M90.85-]*
  - knee A50.02 *[M90.86-]*
  - multiple sites A50.02 *[M90.89]*
  - shoulder joint A50.02 *[M90.81-]*
  - specified site NEC A50.02 *[M90.88]*

Osteochondroarthrosis deformans endemica — *see* Disease, Kaschin-Beck

Osteochondrodysplasia Q78.9
- with defects of growth of tubular bones and spine Q77.9
  - specified NEC Q77.8
- specified NEC Q78.8

Osteochondrodystrophy E78.9

Osteochondrolysis — *see* Osteochondritis, dissecans

Osteochondroma — *see* Neoplasm, bone, benign

Osteochondromatosis D48.0
- syndrome Q78.4

Osteochondromyxosarcoma — *see* Neoplasm, bone, malignant

Osteochondropathy M93.90
- ankle M93.97-
- elbow M93.92-
- foot M93.97-

Osteochondropathy - *continued*
- hand M93.94-
- hip M93.95-
- Kienböck's disease of adults M93.1
- knee M93.96-
- multiple joints M93.99
- osteochondritis dissecans — *see* Osteochondritis, dissecans
- osteochondrosis — *see* Osteochondrosis
- shoulder region M93.91-
- slipped upper femoral epiphysis — *see* Slipped, epiphysis, upper femoral
- specified joint NEC M93.98
- specified type NEC M93.80
  - ankle M93.87-
  - elbow M93.82-
  - foot M93.87-
  - hand M93.84-
  - hip M93.85-
  - knee M93.86-
  - multiple joints M93.89
  - shoulder region M93.81-
  - specified joint NEC M93.88
  - wrist M93.83-
- syphilitic, congenital
  - early A50.02 *[M90.80]*
  - late A50.56 *[M90.80]*
- wrist M93.93-

Osteochondrosarcoma — *see* Neoplasm, bone, malignant

Osteochondrosis — *see also* Osteochondropathy, by site
- acetabulum (juvenile) M91.0
- adult — *see* Osteochondropathy, specified type NEC, by site
- astragalus (juvenile) — *see* Osteochondrosis, juvenile, tarsus
- Blount M92.51-
- Buchanan's M91.0
- Burns' — *see* Osteochondrosis, juvenile, ulna
- calcaneus (juvenile) — *see* Osteochondrosis, juvenile, tarsus
- capitular epiphysis (femur) (juvenile) — *see* Legg-Calvé-Perthes disease
- carpal (juvenile) (lunate) (scaphoid) — *see* Osteochondrosis, juvenile, hand, carpal lunate
  - adult M93.1
- coxae juvenilis — *see* Legg-Calvé-Perthes disease
- deformans juvenilis, coxae — *see* Legg-Calvé-Perthes disease
- Diaz's — *see* Osteochondrosis, juvenile, tarsus
- dissecans (knee) (shoulder) — *see* Osteochondritis, dissecans
- femoral capital epiphysis (juvenile) — *see* Legg-Calvé-Perthes disease
- femur (head) , juvenile — *see* Legg-Calvé-Perthes disease
- fibula (juvenile) — *see* Osteochondrosis, juvenile, fibula
- foot NEC (juvenile) M92.8
- Freiberg's — *see* Osteochondrosis, juvenile, metatarsus
- Haas' (juvenile) — *see* Osteochondrosis, juvenile, humerus
- Haglund's — *see* Osteochondrosis, juvenile, tarsus
- hip (juvenile) — *see* Legg-Calvé-Perthes disease
- humerus (capitulum) (head) (juvenile) — *see* Osteochondrosis, juvenile, humerus
- ilium, iliac crest (juvenile) M91.0
- ischiopubic synchondrosis M91.0
- Iselin's — *see* Osteochondrosis, juvenile, metatarsus
- juvenile, juvenilis M92.9
  - after congenital dislocation of hip reduction — *see* Osteochondrosis, juvenile, hip, specified NEC
  - arm — *see* Osteochondrosis, juvenile, upper limb NEC
  - capitular epiphysis (femur) — *see* Legg-Calvé-Perthes disease

Osteochondrosis - *continued*
- juvenile, juvenilis - *continued*
  - clavicle, sternal epiphysis — *see* Osteochondrosis, juvenile, upper limb NEC
  - coxae — *see* Legg-Calvé-Perthes disease
  - deformans M92.9
  - fibula M92.50-
  - foot NEC M92.8
  - hand M92.20-
    - carpal lunate M92.21-
    - metacarpal head M92.22-
    - specified site NEC M92.29-
  - head of femur — *see* Legg-Calvé-Perthes disease
  - hip and pelvis M91.9-
    - coxa plana — *see* Coxa, plana
    - femoral head — *see* Legg-Calvé-Perthes disease
    - pelvis M91.0
    - pseudocoxalgia — *see* Pseudocoxalgia
    - specified NEC M91.8-
  - humerus M92.0-
  - limb
    - lower NEC M92.8
    - upper NEC — *see* Osteochondrosis, juvenile, upper limb NEC
  - medial cuneiform bone — *see* Osteochondrosis, juvenile, tarsus
  - metatarsus M92.7-
  - patella M92.4-
  - radius M92.1-
  - specified
    - site NEC M92.8
    - type NEC M92.8
      - tibia and fibula M92.59-
  - spine M42.00
    - cervical region M42.02
    - cervicothoracic region M42.03
    - lumbar region M42.06
    - lumbosacral region M42.07
    - multiple sites M42.09
    - occipito-atlanto-axial region M42.01
    - sacrococcygeal region M42.08
    - thoracic region M42.04
    - thoracolumbar region M42.05
  - tarsus M92.6-
  - tibia M92.50-
    - proximal M92.51-
    - tubercle M92.52-
  - ulna M92.1-
  - upper limb NEC M92.3-
  - vertebra (body) (epiphyseal plates) (Calvé's) (Scheuermann's) — *see* Osteochondrosis, juvenile, spine
- Kienböck's — *see* Osteochondrosis, juvenile, hand, carpal lunate
  - adult M93.1
- Köhler's
  - patellar — *see* Osteochondrosis, juvenile, patella
  - tarsal navicular — *see* Osteochondrosis, juvenile, tarsus
- Legg-Perthes (-Calvé) (-Waldenström) — *see* Legg-Calvé-Perthes disease
- limb
  - lower NEC (juvenile) M92.8
    - tibia and fibula M92.59-
  - upper NEC (juvenile) — *see* Osteochondrosis, juvenile, upper limb NEC
- lunate bone (carpal) (juvenile) — *see also* Osteochondrosis, juvenile, hand, carpal lunate
  - adult M93.1
- Mauclaire's — *see* Osteochondrosis, juvenile, hand, metacarpal
- metacarpal (head) (juvenile) — *see* Osteochondrosis, juvenile, hand, metacarpal
- metatarsus (fifth) (head) (juvenile) (second) — *see* Osteochondrosis, juvenile, metatarsus
- navicular (juvenile) — *see* Osteochondrosis, juvenile, tarsus

Osteochondrosis - *continued*
- os
  - calcis (juvenile) — *see* Osteochondrosis, juvenile, tarsus
  - tibiale externum (juvenile) — *see* Osteochondrosis, juvenile, tarsus
- Osgood-Schlatter M92.52-
- Panner's — *see* Osteochondrosis, juvenile, humerus
- patellar center (juvenile) (primary) (secondary) — *see* Osteochondrosis, juvenile, patella
- pelvis (juvenile) M91.0
- Pierson's M91.0
- radius (head) (juvenile) — *see* Osteochondrosis, juvenile, radius
- Scheuermann's — *see* Osteochondrosis, juvenile, spine
- Sever's — *see* Osteochondrosis, juvenile, tarsus
- Sinding-Larsen — *see* Osteochondrosis, juvenile, patella
- spine M42.9
  - adult M42.10
    - cervical region M42.12
    - cervicothoracic region M42.13
    - lumbar region M42.16
    - lumbosacral region M42.17
    - multiple sites M42.19
    - occipito-atlanto-axial region M42.11
    - sacrococcygeal region M42.18
    - thoracic region M42.14
    - thoracolumbar region M42.15
  - juvenile — *see* Osteochondrosis, juvenile, spine
- symphysis pubis (juvenile) M91.0
- syphilitic (congenital) A50.02
- talus (juvenile) — *see* Osteochondrosis, juvenile, tarsus
- tarsus (navicular) (juvenile) — *see* Osteochondrosis, juvenile, tarsus
- tibia (proximal) (tubercle) (juvenile) — *see* Osteochondrosis, juvenile, tibia
- tuberculous — *see* Tuberculosis, bone
- ulna (lower) (juvenile) — *see* Osteochondrosis, juvenile, ulna
- van Neck's M91.0
- vertebral — *see* Osteochondrosis, spine

Osteoclastoma D48.0
- malignant — *see* Neoplasm, bone, malignant

Osteodynia — *see* Disorder, bone, specified type NEC

Osteodystrophy Q78.9
- azotemic N25.0
- congenital Q78.9
- parathyroid, secondary E21.1
- renal N25.0

Osteofibroma — *see* Neoplasm, bone, benign

Osteofibrosarcoma — *see* Neoplasm, bone, malignant

Osteogenesis imperfecta Q78.0

Osteogenic — *see* condition

Osteolysis M89.50
- carpus M89.54-
- clavicle M89.51-
- femur M89.55-
- fibula M89.56-
- finger M89.54-
- humerus M89.52-
- ilium M89.559
- ischium M89.559
- joint prosthesis (periprosthetic) — *see* Complications, joint prosthesis, mechanical, periprosthetic, osteolysis, by site
- metacarpus M89.54-
- metatarsus M89.57-
- multiple sites M89.59
- neck M89.58
- periprosthetic — *see* Complications, joint prosthesis, mechanical, periprosthetic, osteolysis, by site
- radius M89.53-
- rib M89.58
- scapula M89.51-

Osteolysis - *continued*
- skull M89.58
- tarsus M89.57-
- tibia M89.56-
- toe M89.57-
- ulna M89.53-
- vertebra M89.58

Osteoma — *see also* Neoplasm, bone, benign
- osteoid — *see also* Neoplasm, bone, benign
  - giant — *see* Neoplasm, bone, benign

Osteomalacia M83.9
- adult M83.9
  - drug-induced NEC M83.5
  - due to
    - malabsorption (postsurgical) M83.2
    - malnutrition M83.3
  - specified NEC M83.8
- aluminium-induced M83.4
- infantile — *see* Rickets
- juvenile — *see* Rickets
- oncogenic E83.89
- pelvis M83.8
- puerperal M83.0
- senile M83.1
- vitamin-D-resistant in adults E83.31 *[M90.8-]*
  - carpus E83.31 *[M90.84-]*
  - clavicle E83.31 *[M90.81-]*
  - femur E83.31 *[M90.85-]*
  - fibula E83.31 *[M90.86-]*
  - finger E83.31 *[M90.84-]*
  - humerus E83.31 *[M90.82-]*
  - ilium E83.31 *[M90.859]*
  - ischium E83.31 *[M90.859]*
  - metacarpus E83.31 *[M90.84-]*
  - metatarsus E83.31 *[M90.87-]*
  - multiple sites E83.31 *[M90.89]*
  - neck E83.31 *[M90.88]*
  - radius E83.31 *[M90.83-]*
  - rib E83.31 *[M90.88]*
  - scapula E83.31 *[M90.819]*
  - skull E83.31 *[M90.88]*
  - tarsus E83.31 *[M90.879]*
  - tibia E83.31 *[M90.869]*
  - toe E83.31 *[M90.879]*
  - ulna E83.31 *[M90.839]*
  - vertebra E83.31 *[M90.88]*

Osteomyelitis (general) (infective) (localized) (neonatal) (purulent) (septic) (staphylococcal) (streptococcal) (suppurative) (with periostitis) M86.9
- acute M86.10
  - carpus M86.14-
  - clavicle M86.11-
  - femur M86.15-
  - fibula M86.16-
  - finger M86.14-
  - hematogenous M86.00
    - carpus M86.04-
    - clavicle M86.01-
    - femur M86.05-
    - fibula M86.06-
    - finger M86.04-
    - humerus M86.02-
    - ilium M86.08
    - ischium M86.08
    - mandible M27.2
    - metacarpus M86.04-
    - metatarsus M86.07-
    - multiple sites M86.09
    - neck M86.08
    - orbit H05.02-
    - petrous bone — *see* Petrositis
    - radius M86.03-
    - rib M86.08
    - scapula M86.01-
    - skull M86.08
    - tarsus M86.07-
    - tibia M86.06-
    - toe M86.07-
    - ulna M86.03-
    - vertebra — *see* Osteomyelitis, vertebra
  - humerus M86.12-
  - ilium M86.18
  - ischium M86.18

- **Osteomyelitis (general) (infective) (localized) (neonatal) (purulent) (septic) (staphylococcal) (streptococcal) (suppurative) (with periostitis)** - *continued*
  - acute - *continued*
    - mandible M27.2
    - metacarpus M86.14-
    - metatarsus M86.17-
    - multiple sites M86.19
    - neck M86.18
    - orbit H05.02-
    - petrous bone — *see* Petrositis
    - radius M86.13-
    - rib M86.18
    - scapula M86.11-
    - skull M86.18
    - tarsus M86.17-
    - tibia M86.16-
    - toe M86.17-
    - ulna M86.13-
    - vertebra — *see* Osteomyelitis, vertebra
  - chronic (or old) M86.60
    - with draining sinus M86.40
      - carpus M86.44-
      - clavicle M86.41-
      - femur M86.45-
      - fibula M86.46-
      - finger M86.44-
      - humerus M86.42-
      - ilium M86.459
      - ischium M86.459
      - mandible M27.2
      - metacarpus M86.44-
      - metatarsus M86.47-
      - multiple sites M86.49
      - neck M86.48
      - orbit H05.02-
      - petrous bone — *see* Petrositis
      - radius M86.43-
      - rib M86.48
      - scapula M86.41-
      - skull M86.48
      - tarsus M86.47-
      - tibia M86.46-
      - toe M86.47-
      - ulna M86.43-
      - vertebra — *see* Osteomyelitis, vertebra
    - carpus M86.64-
    - clavicle M86.61-
    - femur M86.65-
    - fibula M86.66-
    - finger M86.64-
    - hematogenous NEC M86.50
      - carpus M86.54-
      - clavicle M86.51-
      - femur M86.55-
      - fibula M86.56-
      - finger M86.54-
      - humerus M86.52-
      - ilium M86.559
      - ischium M86.559
      - mandible M27.2
      - metacarpus M86.54-
      - metatarsus M86.57-
      - multifocal M86.30
        - carpus M86.34-
        - clavicle M86.31-
        - femur M86.35-
        - fibula M86.36-
        - finger M86.34-
        - humerus M86.32-
        - ilium M86.359
        - ischium M86.359
        - metacarpus M86.34-
        - metatarsus M86.37-
        - multiple sites M86.39
        - neck M86.38
        - radius M86.33-
        - rib M86.38
        - scapula M86.31-
        - skull M86.38
        - tarsus M86.37-
        - tibia M86.36-
        - toe M86.37-
        - ulna M86.33-

- **Osteomyelitis (general) (infective) (localized) (neonatal) (purulent) (septic) (staphylococcal) (streptococcal) (suppurative) (with periostitis)** - *continued*
  - chronic (or old) - *continued*
    - hematogenous NEC - *continued*
      - multifocal - *continued*
        - vertebra — *see* Osteomyelitis, vertebra
      - multiple sites M86.59
      - neck M86.58
      - orbit H05.02-
      - petrous bone — *see* Petrositis
      - radius M86.53-
      - rib M86.58
      - scapula M86.51-
      - skull M86.58
      - tarsus M86.57-
      - tibia M86.56-
      - toe M86.57-
      - ulna M86.53-
      - vertebra — *see* Osteomyelitis, vertebra
    - humerus M86.62-
    - ilium M86.659
    - ischium M86.659
    - mandible M27.2
    - metacarpus M86.64-
    - metatarsus M86.67-
    - multifocal — *see* Osteomyelitis, chronic, hematogenous, multifocal
    - multiple sites M86.69
    - neck M86.68
    - orbit H05.02-
    - petrous bone — *see* Petrositis
    - radius M86.63-
    - rib M86.68
    - scapula M86.61-
    - skull M86.68
    - tarsus M86.67-
    - tibia M86.66-
    - toe M86.67-
    - ulna M86.63-
    - vertebra — *see* Osteomyelitis, vertebra
  - echinococcal B67.2
  - Garr's — *see* Osteomyelitis, specified type NEC
  - in diabetes mellitus — *see* E08-E13 with .69
  - jaw (acute) (chronic) (lower) (neonatal) (suppurative) (upper) M27.2
  - nonsuppurating — *see* Osteomyelitis, specified type NEC
  - orbit H05.02-
  - petrous bone — *see* Petrositis
  - Salmonella (arizonae) (cholerae-suis) (enteritidis) (typhimurium) A02.24
  - sclerosing, nonsuppurative — *see* Osteomyelitis, specified type NEC
  - specified type NEC (*see also* subcategory M86.8X-)
    - mandible M27.2
    - orbit H05.02-
    - petrous bone — *see* Petrositis
    - vertebra — *see* Osteomyelitis, vertebra
  - subacute M86.20
    - carpus M86.24-
    - clavicle M86.21-
    - femur M86.25-
    - fibula M86.26-
    - finger M86.24-
    - humerus M86.22-
    - mandible M27.2
    - metacarpus M86.24-
    - metatarsus M86.27-
    - multiple sites M86.29
    - neck M86.28
    - orbit H05.02-
    - petrous bone — *see* Petrositis
    - radius M86.23-
    - rib M86.28
    - scapula M86.21-
    - skull M86.28
    - tarsus M86.27-
    - tibia M86.26-
    - toe M86.27-
    - ulna M86.23-

- **Osteomyelitis (general) (infective) (localized) (neonatal) (purulent) (septic) (staphylococcal) (streptococcal) (suppurative) (with periostitis)** - *continued*
  - subacute - *continued*
    - vertebra — *see* Osteomyelitis, vertebra
  - syphilitic A52.77
    - congenital (early) A50.02 *[M90.80]*
  - tuberculous — *see* Tuberculosis, bone
  - typhoid A01.05
  - vertebra M46.20
    - cervical region M46.22
    - cervicothoracic region M46.23
    - lumbar region M46.26
    - lumbosacral region M46.27
    - occipito-atlanto-axial region M46.21
    - sacrococcygeal region M46.28
    - thoracic region M46.24
    - thoracolumbar region M46.25
- **Osteomyelofibrosis** D47.4
- **Osteomyelosclerosis** D75.89
- **Osteonecrosis** M87.9
  - due to
    - drugs — *see* Osteonecrosis, secondary, due to, drugs
    - trauma — *see* Osteonecrosis, secondary, due to, trauma
  - idiopathic aseptic M87.00
    - ankle M87.07-
    - carpus M87.03-
    - clavicle M87.01-
    - femur M87.05-
    - fibula M87.06-
    - finger M87.04-
    - humerus M87.02-
    - ilium M87.050
    - ischium M87.050
    - metacarpus M87.04-
    - metatarsus M87.07-
    - multiple sites M87.09
    - neck M87.08
    - pelvis M87.050
    - radius M87.03-
    - rib M87.08
    - scapula M87.01-
    - skull M87.08
    - tarsus M87.07-
    - tibia M87.06-
    - toe M87.07-
    - ulna M87.03-
    - vertebra M87.08
  - secondary NEC M87.30
    - carpus M87.33-
    - clavicle M87.31-
    - due to
      - drugs M87.10
        - carpus M87.13-
        - clavicle M87.11-
        - femur M87.15-
        - fibula M87.16-
        - finger M87.14-
        - humerus M87.12-
        - ilium M87.159
        - ischium M87.159
        - jaw M87.180
        - metacarpus M87.14-
        - metatarsus M87.17-
        - multiple sites M87.19
        - neck M87.18
        - radius M87.13-
        - rib M87.18
        - scapula M87.11-
        - skull M87.18
        - tarsus M87.17-
        - tibia M87.16-
        - toe M87.17-
        - ulna M87.13-
        - vertebra M87.18
      - hemoglobinopathy NEC D58.2 *[M90.50]*
        - carpus D58.2 *[M90.54-]*
        - clavicle D58.2 *[M90.51-]*
        - femur D58.2 *[M90.55-]*
        - fibula D58.2 *[M90.56-]*
        - finger D58.2 *[M90.54-]*

Osteoporosis (female) (male) - *continued*
specified type NEC - *continued*
with pathological fracture - *continued*
vertebra M80.88
Osteopsathyrosis (idiopathica) Q78.0
Osteoradionecrosis, jaw (acute) (chronic) (lower) (suppurative) (upper) M27.2
Osteosarcoma (any form) — *see* Neoplasm, bone, malignant
Osteosclerosis Q78.2
acquired M85.8-
congenita Q77.4
fragilitas (generalisata) Q78.2
myelofibrosis D75.81
Osteosclerotic anemia D64.89
Osteosis
cutis L94.2
renal fibrocystic N25.0
Österreicher-Turner syndrome Q87.2
Ostium
atrioventriculare commune Q21.2
primum (arteriosum) (defect) (persistent) Q21.2
secundum (arteriosum) (defect) (patent) (persistent) Q21.1
Ostrum-Furst syndrome Q75.8
Otalgia — *see* subcategory H92.0
Otitis (acute) H66.90
with effusion — *see also* Otitis, media, nonsuppurative
purulent — *see* Otitis, media, suppurative
adhesive — *see* subcategory H74.1
chronic — *see also* Otitis, media, chronic
with effusion — *see also* Otitis, media, nonsuppurative, chronic
externa H60.9-
abscess — *see* Abscess, ear, external
acute (noninfective) H60.50-
actinic H60.51-
chemical H60.52-
contact H60.53-
eczematoid H60.54-
infective — *see* Otitis, externa, infective
reactive H60.55-
specified NEC H60.59-
cellulitis — *see* Cellulitis, ear
chronic H60.6-
diffuse — *see* Otitis, externa, infective, diffuse
hemorrhagic — *see* Otitis, externa, infective, hemorrhagic
in (due to)
aspergillosis B44.89
candidiasis B37.84
erysipelas A46 *[H62.40]*
herpes (simplex) virus infection B00.1
zoster B02.8
impetigo L01.00 *[H62.40]*
infectious disease NEC B99 *[H62.4-]*
mycosis NEC B36.9 *[H62.40]*
parasitic disease NEC B89 *[H62.40]*
viral disease NEC B34.9 *[H62.40]*
zoster B02.8
infective NEC H60.39-
abscess — *see* Abscess, ear, external
cellulitis — *see* Cellulitis, ear
diffuse H60.31-
hemorrhagic H60.32-
swimmer's ear — *see* Swimmer's, ear
malignant H60.2-
mycotic NEC B36.9 *[H62.40]*
in
aspergillosis B44.89
candidiasis B37.84
moniliasis B37.84
necrotizing — *see* Otitis, externa, malignant
Pseudomonas aeruginosa — *see* Otitis, externa, malignant
reactive — *see* Otitis, externa, acute, reactive
specified NEC — *see* subcategory H60.8
tropical NEC B36.9 *[H62.40]*
in
aspergillosis B44.89

Otitis (acute) - *continued*
externa - *continued*
tropical NEC - *continued*
in - *continued*
candidiasis B37.84
moniliasis B37.84
insidiosa — *see* Otosclerosis
interna — *see* subcategory H83.0
media (hemorrhagic) (staphylococcal) (streptococcal) H66.9-
with effusion (nonpurulent) — *see* Otitis, media, nonsuppurative
acute, subacute H66.90
allergic — *see* Otitis, media, nonsuppurative, acute, allergic
exudative — *see* Otitis, media, suppurative, acute
mucoid — *see* Otitis, media, nonsuppurative, acute
necrotizing — *see also* Otitis, media, suppurative, acute
in
measles B05.3
scarlet fever A38.0
nonsuppurative NEC — *see* Otitis, media, nonsuppurative, acute
purulent — *see* Otitis, media, suppurative, acute
sanguinous — *see* Otitis, media, nonsuppurative, acute
secretory — *see* Otitis, media, nonsuppurative, acute, serous
seromucinous — *see* Otitis, media, nonsuppurative, acute
serous — *see* Otitis, media, nonsuppurative, acute, serous
suppurative — *see* Otitis, media, suppurative, acute
allergic — *see* Otitis, media, nonsuppurative
catarrhal — *see* Otitis, media, nonsuppurative
chronic H66.90
with effusion (nonpurulent) — *see* Otitis, media, nonsuppurative, chronic
allergic — *see* Otitis, media, nonsuppurative, chronic, allergic
benign suppurative — *see* Otitis, media, suppurative, chronic, tubotympanic
catarrhal — *see* Otitis, media, nonsuppurative, chronic, serous
exudative — *see* Otitis, media, nonsuppurative, chronic
mucinous — *see* Otitis, media, nonsuppurative, chronic, mucoid
mucoid — *see* Otitis, media, nonsuppurative, chronic, mucoid
nonsuppurative NEC — *see* Otitis, media, nonsuppurative, chronic
purulent — *see* Otitis, media, suppurative, chronic
secretory — *see* Otitis, media, nonsuppurative, chronic, mucoid
seromucinous — *see* Otitis, media, nonsuppurative, chronic
serous — *see* Otitis, media, nonsuppurative, chronic, serous
suppurative — *see* Otitis, media, suppurative, chronic
transudative — *see* Otitis, media, nonsuppurative, chronic, mucoid
exudative — *see* Otitis, media, suppurative
in (due to) (with)
influenza — *see* Influenza, with, otitis media
measles B05.3
scarlet fever A38.0
tuberculosis A18.6
viral disease NEC B34.- *[H67.-]*
mucoid — *see* Otitis, media, nonsuppurative
nonsuppurative H65.9-
acute or subacute NEC H65.19-
allergic H65.11-

Otitis (acute) - *continued*
media (hemorrhagic) (staphylococcal) (streptococcal) - *continued*
nonsuppurative - *continued*
acute or subacute NEC - *continued*
allergic - *continued*
recurrent H65.11-
recurrent H65.19-
secretory — *see* Otitis, media, nonsuppurative, serous
serous H65.0-
recurrent H65.0-
chronic H65.49-
allergic H65.41-
mucoid H65.3-
serous H65.2-
postmeasles B05.3
purulent — *see* Otitis, media, suppurative
secretory — *see* Otitis, media, nonsuppurative
seromucinous — *see* Otitis, media, nonsuppurative
serous — *see* Otitis, media, nonsuppurative
suppurative H66.4-
acute H66.00-
with rupture of ear drum H66.01-
recurrent H66.00-
with rupture of ear drum H66.01-
chronic (*see also* subcategory H66.3)
atticoantral H66.2-
benign — *see* Otitis, media, suppurative, chronic, tubotympanic
tubotympanic H66.1-
transudative — *see* Otitis, media, nonsuppurative
tuberculous A18.6
Otocephaly Q18.2
Otolith syndrome — *see* subcategory H81.8
Otomycosis (diffuse) NEC B36.9 *[H62.40]*
in
aspergillosis B44.89
candidiasis B37.84
moniliasis B37.84
Otoporosis — *see* Otosclerosis
Otorrhagia (nontraumatic) H92.2-
traumatic - code by Type of injury
Otorrhea H92.1-
cerebrospinal (fluid) G96.01
postoperative G96.08
specified NEC G96.08
spontaneous G96.01
traumatic G96.08
Otosclerosis (general) H80.9-
cochlear (endosteal) H80.2-
involving
otic capsule — *see* Otosclerosis, cochlear
oval window
nonobliterative H80.0-
obliterative H80.1-
round window — *see* Otosclerosis, cochlear
nonobliterative — *see* Otosclerosis, involving, oval window, nonobliterative
obliterative — *see* Otosclerosis, involving, oval window, obliterative
specified NEC H80.8-
Otospongiosis — *see* Otosclerosis
Otto's disease or pelvis M24.7
Outcome of delivery Z37.9
multiple births Z37.9
all liveborn Z37.50
quadruplets Z37.52
quintuplets Z37.53
sextuplets Z37.54
specified number NEC Z37.59
triplets Z37.51
all stillborn Z37.7
some liveborn Z37.60
quadruplets Z37.62
quintuplets Z37.63
sextuplets Z37.64
specified number NEC Z37.69
triplets Z37.61

Pain (s) - *continued*
  due to device, implant or graft - *continued*
    infusion NEC T85.848
    joint prosthesis T84.84
    ocular (corneal graft) (orbital implant) NEC T85.848
    orthopedic NEC T84.84
    specified NEC T85.848
    urinary NEC T83.84
    vascular NEC T82.848
    ventricular intracranial shunt T85.840
  due to malignancy (primary) (secondary) G89.3
  ear — *see* subcategory H92.0
  epigastric, epigastrium R10.13
  eye — *see* Pain, ocular
  face, facial R51.9
    atypical G50.1
  female genital organs NEC N94.89
  finger — *see* Pain, limb, upper
  flank — *see* Pain, abdominal
  foot — *see* Pain, limb, lower
  gallbladder K82.9
  gas (intestinal) R14.1
  gastric — *see* Pain, abdominal
  generalized NOS R52
  genital organ
    female N94.89
    male N50.89
  groin — *see* Pain, abdominal, lower
  hand — *see* Pain, limb, upper
  head — *see* Headache
  heart — *see* Pain, precordial
  infra-orbital — *see* Neuralgia, trigeminal
  intercostal R07.82
  intermenstrual N94.0
  jaw R68.84
  joint M25.50
    ankle M25.57-
    elbow M25.52-
    finger M25.54-
    foot M25.57-
    hand M25.54-
    hip M25.55-
    knee M25.56-
    shoulder M25.51-
    specified site NEC M25.59
    toe M25.57-
    wrist M25.53-
  kidney N23
  laryngeal R07.0
  leg — *see* Pain, limb, lower
  limb M79.609
    lower M79.60-
      foot M79.67-
      lower leg M79.66-
      thigh M79.65-
      toe M79.67-
    upper M79.60-
      axilla M79.62-
      finger M79.64-
      forearm M79.63-
      hand M79.64-
      upper arm M79.62-
  loin M54.50
  low back M54.50
    specified NEC M54.59
    vertebral end plate M54.51
    vertebrogenic M54.51
  lumbar region M54.50
    vertebral end plate M54.51
    vertebrogenic M54.51
  mandibular R68.84
  mastoid — *see* subcategory H92.0
  maxilla R68.84
  menstrual — *see also* Dysmenorrhea N94.6
  metacarpophalangeal (joint) — *see* Pain, joint, hand
  metatarsophalangeal (joint) — *see* Pain, joint, foot
  mouth K13.79
  muscle — *see* Myalgia
  musculoskeletal — *see also* Pain, by site M79.18
  myofascial M79.18

Pain (s) - *continued*
  nasal J34.89
  nasopharynx J39.2
  neck NEC M54.2
  nerve NEC — *see* Neuralgia
  neuromuscular — *see* Neuralgia
  nose J34.89
  ocular H57.1-
  ophthalmic — *see* Pain, ocular
  orbital region — *see* Pain, ocular
  ovary N94.89
  over heart — *see* Pain, precordial
  ovulation N94.0
  pelvic (female) R10.2
  penis N48.89
  pericardial — *see* Pain, precordial
  perineal, perineum R10.2
  pharynx J39.2
  pleura, pleural, pleuritic R07.81
  postoperative NOS G89.18
  postprocedural NOS G89.18
  post-thoracotomy G89.12
  precordial (region) R07.2
  premenstrual N94.3
  psychogenic (persistent) (any site) F45.41
  radicular (spinal) — *see* Radiculopathy
  rectum K62.89
  respiration R07.1
  retrosternal R07.2
  rheumatoid, muscular — *see* Myalgia
  rib R07.81
  root (spinal) — *see* Radiculopathy
  round ligament (stretch) R10.2
  sacroiliac M53.3
  sciatic — *see* Sciatica
  scrotum N50.82
  seminal vesicle N50.89
  shoulder M25.51-
  spermatic cord N50.89
  spinal root — *see* Radiculopathy
  spine M54.9
    cervical M54.2
    low back M54.50
      with sciatica M54.4-
    thoracic M54.6
  stomach — *see* Pain, abdominal
  substernal R07.2
  temporomandibular (joint) M26.62-
  testis N50.81-
  thoracic spine M54.6
    with radicular and visceral pain M54.14
  throat R07.0
  tibia — *see* Pain, limb, lower
  toe — *see* Pain, limb, lower
  tongue K14.6
  tooth K08.89
  trigeminal — *see* Neuralgia, trigeminal
  tumor associated G89.3
  ureter N23
  urinary (organ) (system) N23
  uterus NEC N94.89
  vagina R10.2
  vertebral end plate — *see* Pain, vertebrogenic
  vertebrogenic M54.89
    low back M54.51
    lumbar M54.51
    syndrome M54.89
  vesical R39.89
    associated with micturition — *see* Micturition, painful
  vulva R10.2
Painful — *see also* Pain
  coitus
    female N94.10
    male N53.12
    psychogenic F52.6
  ejaculation (semen) N53.12
    psychogenic F52.6
  erection — *see* Priapism
  feet syndrome E53.8
  joint replacement (hip) (knee) T84.84
  menstruation — *see* Dysmenorrhea
    psychogenic F45.8
  micturition — *see* Micturition, painful
  respiration R07.1

Painful - *continued*
  scar NEC L90.5
  wire sutures T81.89
Painter's colic — *see* subcategory T56.0
Palate — *see* condition
Palatoplegia K13.79
Palatoschisis — *see* Cleft, palate
Palilalia R48.8
Palliative care Z51.5
Pallor R23.1
  optic disc, temporal — *see* Atrophy, optic
Palmar — *see also* condition
  fascia — *see* condition
Palpable
  cecum K63.89
  kidney N28.89
  ovary N83.8
  prostate N42.9
  spleen — *see* Splenomegaly
Palpitations (heart) R00.2
  psychogenic F45.8
Palsy — *see also* Paralysis G83.9
  atrophic diffuse (progressive) G12.22
  Bell's — *see also* Palsy, facial
    newborn P11.3
  brachial plexus NEC G54.0
    newborn (birth injury) P14.3
  brain — *see* Palsy, cerebral
  bulbar (progressive) (chronic) G12.22
    of childhood (Fazio-Londe) G12.1
    pseudo NEC G12.29
    supranuclear (progressive) G23.1
  cerebral (congenital) G80.9
    ataxic G80.4
    athetoid G80.3
    choreathetoid G80.3
    diplegic G80.8
      spastic G80.1
    dyskinetic G80.3
      athetoid G80.3
      choreathetoid G80.3
      distonic G80.3
    dystonic G80.3
    hemiplegic G80.8
      spastic G80.2
    mixed G80.8
    monoplegic G80.8
      spastic G80.1
    paraplegic G80.8
      spastic G80.1
    quadriplegic G80.8
      spastic G80.0
    spastic G80.1
      diplegic G80.1
      hemiplegic G80.2
      monoplegic G80.1
      quadriplegic G80.0
      specified NEC G80.1
      tetrapelgic G80.0
    specified NEC G80.8
    syphilitic A52.12
      congenital A50.49
    tetraplegic G80.8
      spastic G80.0
  cranial nerve — *see also* Disorder, nerve, cranial
    multiple G52.7
      in
        infectious disease B99 *[G53]*
        neoplastic disease — *see also* Neoplasm D49.9 *[G53]*
        parasitic disease B89 *[G53]*
        sarcoidosis D86.82
  creeping G12.22
  diver's T70.3
  Erb's P14.0
  facial G51.0
    newborn (birth injury) P11.3
  glossopharyngeal G52.1
  Klumpke (-Déjérine) P14.1
  lead — *see* subcategory T56.0
  median nerve (tardy) G56.1-
  nerve G58.9
    specified NEC G58.8
  peroneal nerve (acute) (tardy) G57.3-

Palsy - *continued*
  progressive supranuclear G23.1
  pseudobulbar NEC G12.29
  radial nerve (acute) G56.3-
  seventh nerve — *see also* Palsy, facial
    newborn P11.3
  shaking — *see* Parkinsonism
  spastic (cerebral) (spinal) G80.1
  ulnar nerve (tardy) G56.2-
  wasting G12.29
Paludism — *see* Malaria
Panangiitis M30.0
Panaris, panaritium — *see also* Cellulitis, digit
  with lymphangitis — *see* Lymphangitis, acute, digit
Panarteritis nodosa M30.0
  brain or cerebral I67.7
Pancake heart R93.1
  with cor pulmonale (chronic) I27.81
Pancarditis (acute) (chronic) I51.89
  rheumatic I09.89
    active or acute I01.8
Pancoast's syndrome or tumor C34.1-
Pancolitis, ulcerative (chronic) K51.00
  with
    complication K51.019
    abscess K51.014
    fistula K51.013
    obstruction K51.012
    rectal bleeding K51.011
    specified complication NEC K51.018
Pancreas, pancreatic — *see* condition
Pancreatitis (annular) (apoplectic) (calcareous) (edematous) (hemorrhagic) (malignant) (subacute) (suppurative) K85.90
  with necrosis (uninfected) K85.91
    infected K85.92
  acute (without necrosis or infection) K85.90
    with necrosis (uninfected) K85.91
      infected K85.92
    alcohol induced (without necrosis or infection) K85.20
      with necrosis (uninfected) K85.21
        infected K85.22
    biliary (without necrosis or infection) K85.10
      with necrosis (uninfected) K85.11
        infected K85.12
    drug induced (without necrosis or infection) K85.30
      with necrosis (uninfected) K85.31
        infected K85.32
    gallstone (without necrosis or infection) K85.10
      with necrosis (uninfected) K85.11
        infected K85.12
    idiopathic (without necrosis or infection) K85.00
      with necrosis (uninfected) K85.01
        infected K85.02
    specified NEC (without necrosis or infection) K85.80
      with necrosis (uninfected) K85.81
        infected K85.82
  chronic (infectious) K86.1
    alcohol-induced K86.0
    recurrent K86.1
    relapsing K86.1
  cystic (chronic) K86.1
  cytomegaloviral B25.2
  fibrous (chronic) K86.1
  gangrenous — *see* Pancreatitis, acute
  gallstone (without necrosis or infection) K85.10
    with necrosis (uninfected) K85.11
      infected K85.12
  interstitial (chronic) K86.1
    acute — *see also* Pancreatitis, acute K85.80
  mumps B26.3
  recurrent
    acute — *see* Pancreatitis, acute by type
    chronic K86.1

Pancreatitis (annular) (apoplectic) (calcareous) (edematous) (hemorrhagic) (malignant) (subacute) (suppurative) - *continued*
  relapsing, chronic K86.1
  syphilitic A52.74
Pancreatoblastoma — *see* Neoplasm, pancreas, malignant
Pancreolithiasis K86.89
Pancytolysis D75.89
Pancytopenia (acquired) D61.818
  with
    malformations D61.09
    myelodysplastic syndrome — *see* Syndrome, myelodysplastic
  antineoplastic chemotherapy induced D61.810
  congenital D61.09
  drug-induced NEC D61.811
PANDAS (pediatric autoimmune neuropsychiatric disorders associated with streptococcal infections syndrome) D89.89
Panencephalitis, subacute, sclerosing A81.1
Panhematopenia D61.9
  congenital D61.09
  constitutional D61.09
  splenic, primary D73.1
Panhemocytopenia D61.9
  congenital D61.09
  constitutional D61.09
Panhypogonadism E29.1
Panhypopituitarism E23.0
  prepubertal E23.0
Panic (attack) (state) F41.0
  reaction to exceptional stress (transient) F43.0
Panmyelopathy, familial, constitutional D61.09
Panmyelophthisis D61.82
  congenital D61.09
Panmyelosis (acute) (with myelofibrosis) C94.4-
Panner's disease — *see* Osteochondrosis, juvenile, humerus
Panneuritis endemica E51.11
Panniculitis (nodular) (nonsuppurative) M79.3
  back M54.00
    cervical region M54.02
    cervicothoracic region M54.03
    lumbar region M54.06
    lumbosacral region M54.07
    multiple sites M54.09
    occipito-atlanto-axial region M54.01
    sacrococcygeal region M54.08
    thoracic region M54.04
    thoracolumbar region M54.05
  lupus L93.2
  mesenteric K65.4
  neck M54.02
    cervicothoracic region M54.03
    occipito-atlanto-axial region M54.01
  relapsing M35.6
Panniculus adiposus (abdominal) E65
Pannus (allergic) (cornea) (degenerativus) (keratic) H16.42-
  abdominal (symptomatic) E65
  trachomatosus, trachomatous (active) A71.1
Panophthalmitis H44.01-
Pansinusitis (chronic) (hyperplastic) (nonpurulent) (purulent) J32.4
  acute J01.40
    recurrent J01.41
  tuberculous A15.8
Panuveitis (sympathetic) H44.11-
Panvalvular disease I08.9
  specified NEC I08.8
PAPA (pyogenic arthritis, pyoderma gangrenosum, and acne syndrome) M04.8
Papanicolaou smear, cervix Z12.4
  as part of routine gynecological examination Z01.419
    with abnormal findings Z01.411

Papanicolaou smear, cervix - *continued*
  for suspected neoplasm Z12.4
  nonspecific abnormal finding R87.619
  routine Z01.419
    with abnormal findings Z01.411
Papilledema (choked disc) H47.10
  associated with
    decreased ocular pressure H47.12
    increased intracranial pressure H47.11
    retinal disorder H47.13
  Foster-Kennedy syndrome H47.14-
Papillitis H46.00
  anus K62.89
  chronic lingual K14.4
  necrotizing, kidney N17.2
  optic H46.0-
  rectum K62.89
  renal, necrotizing N17.2
  tongue K14.0
Papilloma — *see also* Neoplasm, benign, by site
  acuminatum (female) (male) (anogenital) A63.0
  basal cell L82.1
    inflamed L82.0
  benign pinta (primary) A67.0
  bladder (urinary) (transitional cell) D41.4
  choroid plexus (lateral ventricle) (third ventricle) D33.0
    anaplastic C71.5
    fourth ventricle D33.1
    malignant C71.5
  renal pelvis (transitional cell) D41.1-
    benign D30.1-
  Schneiderian
    specified site — *see* Neoplasm, benign, by site
    unspecified site D14.0
  serous surface
    borderline malignancy
      specified site — *see* Neoplasm, uncertain behavior, by site
      unspecified site D39.10
    specified site — *see* Neoplasm, benign, by site
    unspecified site D27.9
  transitional (cell)
    bladder (urinary) D41.4
    inverted type — *see* Neoplasm, uncertain behavior, by site
    renal pelvis D41.1-
    ureter D41.2-
  ureter (transitional cell) D41.2-
    benign D30.2-
  urothelial — *see* Neoplasm, uncertain behavior, by site
  villous — *see* Neoplasm, uncertain behavior, by site
    adenocarcinoma in — *see* Neoplasm, malignant, by site
    in situ — *see* Neoplasm, in situ
  yaws, plantar or palmar A66.1
Papillomata, multiple, of yaws A66.1
Papillomatosis — *see also* Neoplasm, benign, by site
  confluent and reticulated L83
  cystic, breast — *see* Mastopathy, cystic
  ductal, breast — *see* Mastopathy, cystic
  intraductal (diffuse) — *see* Neoplasm, benign, by site
  subareolar duct D24-
Papillomavirus, as cause of disease classified elsewhere B97.7
Papillon-Léage and Psaume syndrome Q87.0
Papule (s) R23.8
  carate (primary) A67.0
  fibrous, of nose D22.39
  Gottron's L94.4
  pinta (primary) A67.0
Papulosis
  lymphomatoid C86.6
  malignant I77.89
Papyraceous fetus O31.0-
Para-albuminemia E88.09
Paracephalus Q89.7

PALSY - PARACEPHALUS

Parachute mitral valve Q23.2
Paracoccidioidomycosis B41.9
  disseminated B41.7
  generalized B41.7
  mucocutaneous-lymphangitic B41.8
  pulmonary B41.0
  specified NEC B41.8
  visceral B41.8
Paradentosis K05.4
Paraffinoma T88.8
Paraganglioma D44.7
  adrenal D35.0-
    malignant C74.1-
  aortic body D44.7
    malignant C75.5
  carotid body D44.6
    malignant C75.4
  chromaffin — *see also* Neoplasm, benign, by site
    malignant — *see* Neoplasm, malignant, by site
  extra-adrenal D44.7
    malignant C75.5
      specified site — *see* Neoplasm, malignant, by site
      unspecified site C75.5
    specified site — *see* Neoplasm, uncertain behavior, by site
    unspecified site D44.7
  gangliocytic D13.2
    specified site — *see* Neoplasm, benign, by site
    unspecified site D13.2
  glomus jugulare D44.7
    malignant C75.5
  jugular D44.7
  malignant C75.5
    specified site — *see* Neoplasm, malignant, by site
    unspecified site C75.5
  nonchromaffin D44.7
    malignant C75.5
      specified site — *see* Neoplasm, malignant, by site
      unspecified site C75.5
    specified site — *see* Neoplasm, uncertain behavior, by site
    unspecified site D44.7
  parasympathetic D44.7
    specified site — *see* Neoplasm, uncertain behavior, by site
    unspecified site D44.7
  specified site — *see* Neoplasm, uncertain behavior, by site
  sympathetic D44.7
    specified site — *see* Neoplasm, uncertain behavior, by site
    unspecified site D44.7
  unspecified site D44.7
Parageusia R43.2
  psychogenic F45.8
Paragonimiasis B66.4
Paragranuloma, Hodgkin — *see* Lymphoma, Hodgkin, specified NEC
Parahemophilia — *see also* Defect, coagulation D68.2
Parakeratosis R23.4
  variegata L41.0
Paralysis, paralytic (complete) (incomplete) G83.9
  with
    syphilis A52.17
  abducens, abducent (nerve) — *see* Strabismus, paralytic, sixth nerve
  abductor, lower extremity G57.9-
  accessory nerve G52.8
  accommodation — *see also* Paresis, of accommodation
    hysterical F44.89
  acoustic nerve (except Deafness) — *see* subcategory H93.3
  agitans — *see also* Parkinsonism G20
    arteriosclerotic G21.4
  alternating (oculomotor) G83.89
  amyotrophic G12.21

Paralysis, paralytic (complete) (incomplete) - *continued*
  ankle G57.9-
  anus (sphincter) K62.89
  arm — *see* Monoplegia, upper limb
  ascending (spinal) , acute G61.0
  association G12.29
  asthenic bulbar G70.00
    with exacerbation (acute) G70.01
    in crisis G70.01
  ataxic (hereditary) G11.9
    general (syphilitic) A52.17
  atrophic G58.9
    infantile, acute — *see* Poliomyelitis, paralytic
    progressive G12.22
    spinal (acute) — *see* Poliomyelitis, paralytic
  axillary G54.0
  Babinski-Nageotte's G83.89
  Bell's G51.0
    newborn P11.3
  Benedikt's G46.3
  birth injury P14.9
    spinal cord P11.5
  bladder (neurogenic) (sphincter) N31.2
  bowel, colon or intestine K56.0
  brachial plexus G54.0
    birth injury P14.3
    newborn (birth injury) P14.3
  brain G83.9
    diplegia G83.0
    triplegia G83.89
  bronchial J98.09
  Brown-Séquard G83.81
  bulbar (chronic) (progressive) G12.22
    infantile — *see* Poliomyelitis, paralytic
    poliomyelitic — *see* Poliomyelitis, paralytic
    pseudo G12.29
  bulbospinal G70.00
    with exacerbation (acute) G70.01
    in crisis G70.01
  cardiac — *see also* Failure, heart I50.9
  cerebrocerebellar, diplegic G80.1
  cervical
    plexus G54.2
    sympathetic G90.09
  Céstan-Chenais G46.3
  Charcot-Marie-Tooth type G60.0
  Clark's G80.9
  colon K56.0
  compressed air T70.3
  compression
    arm G56.9-
    leg G57.9-
    lower extremity G57.9-
    upper extremity G56.9-
  congenital (cerebral) — *see* Palsy, cerebral
  conjugate movement (gaze) (of eye) H51.0
    cortical (nuclear) (supranuclear) H51.0
  cordis — *see* Failure, heart
  cranial or cerebral nerve G52.9
  creeping G12.22
  crossed leg G83.89
  crutch — *see* Injury, brachial plexus
  deglutition R13.0
    hysterical F44.4
  dementia A52.17
  descending (spinal) NEC G12.29
  diaphragm (flaccid) J98.6
    due to accidental dissection of phrenic nerve during procedure — *see* Puncture, accidental complicating surgery
  digestive organs NEC K59.89
  diplegic — *see* Diplegia
  divergence (nuclear) H51.8
  diver's T70.3
  Duchenne's
    birth injury P14.0
    due to or associated with
      motor neuron disease G12.22
      muscular dystrophy G71.01

Paralysis, paralytic (complete) (incomplete) - *continued*
  due to intracranial or spinal birth injury — *see* Palsy, cerebral
  embolic (current episode) I63.4-
  Erb (-Duchenne) (birth) (newborn) P14.0
  Erb's syphilitic spastic spinal A52.17
  esophagus K22.89
  eye muscle (extrinsic) H49.9
    intrinsic — *see also* Paresis, of accommodation
  facial (nerve) G51.0
    birth injury P11.3
    congenital P11.3
    following operation NEC — *see* Puncture, accidental complicating surgery
    newborn (birth injury) P11.3
  familial (recurrent) (periodic) G72.3
    spastic G11.4
  fauces J39.2
  finger G56.9-
  gait R26.1
  gastric nerve (nondiabetic) G52.2
  gaze, conjugate H51.0
  general (progressive) (syphilitic) A52.17
    juvenile A50.45
  glottis J38.00
    bilateral J38.02
    unilateral J38.01
  gluteal G54.1
  Gubler (-Millard) G46.3
  hand — *see* Monoplegia, upper limb
  heart — *see* Arrest, cardiac
  hemiplegic — *see* Hemiplegia
  hyperkalemic periodic (familial) G72.3
  hypoglossal (nerve) G52.3
  hypokalemic periodic G72.3
  hysterical F44.4
  ileus K56.0
  infantile — *see also* Poliomyelitis, paralytic A80.30
    bulbar — *see* Poliomyelitis, paralytic
    cerebral — *see* Palsy, cerebral
    spastic — *see* Palsy, cerebral, spastic
  infective — *see* Poliomyelitis, paralytic
  inferior nuclear G83.9
  internuclear — *see* Ophthalmoplegia, internuclear
  intestine K56.0
  iris H57.09
    due to diphtheria (toxin) A36.89
  ischemic, Volkmann's (complicating trauma) T79.6
  Jackson's G83.89
  jake — *see* Poisoning, food, noxious, plant
  Jamaica ginger (jake) G62.2
  juvenile general A50.45
  Klumpke (-Déjérine) (birth) (newborn) P14.1
  labioglossal (laryngeal) (pharyngeal) G12.29
  Landry's G61.0
  laryngeal nerve (recurrent) (superior) (unilateral) J38.00
    bilateral J38.02
    unilateral J38.01
  larynx J38.00
    bilateral J38.02
    due to diphtheria (toxin) A36.2
    unilateral J38.01
  lateral G12.23
  lead — *see* subcategory T56.0
  left side — *see* Hemiplegia
  leg G83.1-
    both — *see* Paraplegia
    crossed G83.89
    hysterical F44.4
    psychogenic F44.4
    transient or transitory R29.818
      traumatic NEC — *see* Injury, nerve, leg
  levator palpebrae superioris — *see* Blepharoptosis, paralytic
  limb — *see* Monoplegia
  lip K13.0
  Lissauer's A52.17
  lower limb — *see* Monoplegia, lower limb
    both — *see* Paraplegia

Paralysis, paralytic (complete) (incomplete) - *continued*
- lung J98.4
- median nerve G56.1-
- medullary (tegmental) G83.89
- mesencephalic NEC G83.89
  - tegmental G83.89
- middle alternating G83.89
- Millard-Gubler-Foville G46.3
- monoplegic — *see* Monoplegia
- motor G83.9
- muscle, muscular NEC G72.89
  - due to nerve lesion G58.9
  - eye (extrinsic) H49.9
    - intrinsic — *see* Paresis, of accommodation
    - oblique — *see* Strabismus, paralytic, fourth nerve
  - iris sphincter H21.9
  - ischemic (Volkmann's) (complicating trauma) T79.6
  - progressive G12.21
  - progressive, spinal G12.25
  - spinal progressive G12.25
  - pseudohypertrophic G71.02
- musculocutaneous nerve G56.9-
- musculospiral G56.9-
- nerve — *see also* Disorder, nerve
  - abducent — *see* Strabismus, paralytic, sixth nerve
  - accessory G52.8
  - auditory (except Deafness) — *see* subcategory H93.3
  - birth injury P14.9
  - cranial or cerebral G52.9
  - facial G51.0
    - birth injury P11.3
    - congenital P11.3
    - newborn (birth injury) P11.3
  - fourth or trochlear — *see* Strabismus, paralytic, fourth nerve
  - newborn (birth injury) P14.9
  - oculomotor — *see* Strabismus, paralytic, third nerve
  - phrenic (birth injury) P14.2
  - radial G56.3-
  - seventh or facial G51.0
    - newborn (birth injury) P11.3
  - sixth or abducent — *see* Strabismus, paralytic, sixth nerve
  - syphilitic A52.15
  - third or oculomotor — *see* Strabismus, paralytic, third nerve
  - trigeminal G50.9
  - trochlear — *see* Strabismus, paralytic, fourth nerve
  - ulnar G56.2-
- normokalemic periodic G72.3
- ocular H49.9
  - alternating G83.89
- oculofacial, congenital (Moebius) Q87.0
- oculomotor (external bilateral) (nerve) — *see* Strabismus, paralytic, third nerve
- palate (soft) K13.79
- paratrigeminal G50.9
- periodic (familial) (hyperkalemic) (hypokalemic) (myotonic) (normokalemic) (potassium sensitive) (secondary) G72.3
- peripheral autonomic nervous system — *see* Neuropathy, peripheral, autonomic
- peroneal (nerve) G57.3-
- pharynx J39.2
- phrenic nerve G56.8-
- plantar nerve (s) G57.6-
- pneumogastric nerve G52.2
- poliomyelitis (current) — *see* Poliomyelitis, paralytic
- popliteal nerve G57.3-
- postepileptic transitory G83.84
- progressive (atrophic) (bulbar) (spinal) G12.22
  - general A52.17
  - infantile acute — *see* Poliomyelitis, paralytic

Paralysis, paralytic (complete) (incomplete) - *continued*
- progressive (atrophic) (bulbar) (spinal) - *continued*
  - supranuclear G23.1
- pseudobulbar G12.29
- pseudohypertrophic (muscle) G71.09
- psychogenic F44.4
- quadriceps G57.9-
- quadriplegic — *see* Tetraplegia
- radial nerve G56.3-
- rectus muscle (eye) H49.9
- recurrent isolated sleep G47.53
- respiratory (muscle) (system) (tract) R06.81
  - center NEC G93.89
  - congenital P28.89
  - newborn P28.89
- right side — *see* Hemiplegia
- saturnine — *see* subcategory T56.0
- sciatic nerve G57.0-
- senile G83.9
- shaking — *see* Parkinsonism
- shoulder G56.9-
- sleep, recurrent isolated G47.53
- spastic G83.9
  - cerebral — *see* Palsy, cerebral, spastic
  - congenital (cerebral) — *see* Palsy, cerebral, spastic
  - familial G11.4
  - hereditary G11.4
  - quadriplegic G80.0
  - syphilitic (spinal) A52.17
- sphincter, bladder — *see* Paralysis, bladder
- spinal (cord) G83.9
  - accessory nerve G52.8
  - acute — *see* Poliomyelitis, paralytic
  - ascending acute G61.0
  - atrophic (acute) — *see also* Poliomyelitis, paralytic
    - spastic, syphilitic A52.17
  - congenital NEC — *see* Palsy, cerebral
  - infantile — *see* Poliomyelitis, paralytic
  - hereditary G95.89
  - progressive G12.21
    - muscle G12.25
  - sequelae NEC G83.89
- sternomastoid G52.8
- stomach K31.84
  - diabetic — *see* Diabetes, by type, with gastroparesis
  - nerve G52.2
    - diabetic — *see* Diabetes, by type, with gastroparesis
- stroke — *see* Infarct, brain
- subcapsularis G56.8-
- supranuclear (progressive) G23.1
- sympathetic G90.8
  - cervical G90.09
  - nervous system — *see* Neuropathy, peripheral, autonomic
- syndrome G83.9
  - specified NEC G83.89
- syphilitic spastic spinal (Erb's) A52.17
- thigh G57.9-
- throat J39.2
  - diphtheritic A36.0
  - muscle J39.2
- thrombotic (current episode) I63.3-
- thumb G56.9-
- tick — *see* Toxicity, venom, arthropod, specified NEC
- Todd's (postepileptic transitory paralysis) G83.84
- toe G57.6-
- tongue K14.8
- transient R29.5
  - arm or leg NEC R29.818
  - traumatic NEC — *see* Injury, nerve
- trapezius G52.8
- traumatic, transient NEC — *see* Injury, nerve
- trembling — *see* Parkinsonism
- triceps brachii G56.9-
- trigeminal nerve G50.9
- trochlear (nerve) — *see* Strabismus, paralytic, fourth nerve

Paralysis, paralytic (complete) (incomplete) - *continued*
- ulnar nerve G56.2-
- upper limb — *see* Monoplegia, upper limb
- uremic N18.9 *[G99.8]*
- uveoparotitic D86.89
- uvula K13.79
  - postdiphtheritic A36.0
- vagus nerve G52.2
- vasomotor NEC G90.8
- velum palati K13.79
- vesical — *see* Paralysis, bladder
- vestibular nerve (except Vertigo) — *see* subcategory H93.3
- vocal cords J38.00
  - bilateral J38.02
  - unilateral J38.01
- Volkmann's (complicating trauma) T79.6
- wasting G12.29
- Weber's G46.3
- wrist G56.9-

Paramedial urethrovesical orifice Q64.79

Paramenia N92.6

Parametritis — *see also* Disease, pelvis, inflammatory N73.2
- acute N73.0
- complicating abortion — *see* Abortion, by type, complicated by, parametritis

Parametrium, parametric — *see* condition

Paramnesia — *see* Amnesia

Paramolar K00.1

Paramyloidosis E85.89

Paramyoclonus multiplex G25.3

Paramyotonia (congenita) G71.19

Parangi — *see* Yaws

Paranoia (querulans) F22
- senile F03

Paranoid
- dementia (senile) F03
  - praecox — *see* Schizophrenia
- personality F60.0
- psychosis (climacteric) (involutional) (menopausal) F22
  - psychogenic (acute) F23
  - senile F03
- reaction (acute) F23
  - chronic F22
- schizophrenia F20.0
- state (climacteric) (involutional) (menopausal) (simple) F22
  - senile F03
- tendencies F60.0
- traits F60.0
- trends F60.0
- type, psychopathic personality F60.0

Paraparesis — *see* Paraplegia

Paraphasia R47.02

Paraphilia F65.9

Paraphimosis (congenital) N47.2
- chancroidal A57

Paraphrenia, paraphrenic (late) F22
- schizophrenia F20.0

Paraplegia (lower) G82.20
- ataxic — *see* Degeneration, combined, spinal cord
- complete G82.21
- congenital (cerebral) G80.8
  - spastic G80.1
- familial spastic G11.4
- functional (hysterical) F44.4
- hereditary, spastic G11.4
- hysterical F44.4
- incomplete G82.22
- Pott's A18.01
- psychogenic F44.4
- spastic
  - Erb's spinal, syphilitic A52.17
  - hereditary G11.4
  - tropical G04.1
- syphilitic (spastic) A52.17
- traumatic
  - current injury - code to injury with seventh character A
    - sequela of previous injury - code to injury with seventh character S

PARAPLEGIA - PEDIATRIC INFLAMMATORY MULTISYSTEM SYNDROME

Pediculosis (infestation) B85.2
- capitis (head-louse) (any site) B85.0
- corporis (body-louse) (any site) B85.1
- eyelid B85.0
- mixed (classifiable to more than one of the titles B85.0-B85.3) B85.4
- pubis (pubic louse) (any site) B85.3
- vestimenti B85.1
- vulvae B85.3

Pediculus (infestation) — *see* Pediculosis
Pedophilia F65.4
Peg-shaped teeth K00.2
Pelade — *see* Alopecia, areata
Pelger-Huët anomaly or syndrome D72.0
Peliosis (rheumatica) D69.0
- hepatis K76.4
  - with toxic liver disease K71.8

Pelizaeus-Merzbacher disease E75.29
Pellagra (alcoholic) (with polyneuropathy) E52
Pellagra-cerebellar-ataxia-renal aminoaciduria syndrome E72.02
Pellegrini (-Stieda) disease or syndrome — *see* Bursitis, tibial collateral
Pellizzi's syndrome E34.8
Pel's crisis A52.11
Pelvic — *see also* condition
- examination (periodic) (routine) Z01.419
  - with abnormal findings Z01.411
- kidney, congenital Q63.2

Pelviolithiasis — *see* Calculus, kidney
Pelviperitonitis — *see also* Peritonitis, pelvic
- gonococcal A54.24
- puerperal O85

Pelvis — *see* condition or type
Pemphigoid L12.9
- benign, mucous membrane L12.1
- bullous L12.0
- cicatricial L12.1
- juvenile L12.2
- ocular L12.1
- specified NEC L12.8

Pemphigus L10.9
- benign familial (chronic) Q82.8
- Brazilian L10.3
- circinatus L13.0
- conjunctiva L12.1
- drug-induced L10.5
- erythematosus L10.4
- foliaceous L10.2
- gangrenous — *see* Gangrene
- neonatorum L01.03
- ocular L12.1
- paraneoplastic L10.81
- specified NEC L10.89
- syphilitic (congenital) A50.06
- vegetans L10.1
- vulgaris L10.0
- wildfire L10.3

Pendred's syndrome E07.1
Pendulous
- abdomen, in pregnancy — *see* Pregnancy, complicated by, abnormal, pelvic organs or tissues NEC
- breast N64.89

Penetrating wound — *see also* Puncture
- with internal injury — *see* Injury, by site
- eyeball — *see* Puncture, eyeball
- orbit (with or without foreign body) — *see* Puncture, orbit
- uterus by instrument with or following ectopic or molar pregnancy O08.6

Penicillosis B48.4
Penis — *see* condition
Penitis N48.29
Pentalogy of Fallot Q21.8
Pentasomy X syndrome Q97.1
Pentosuria (essential) E74.89
Percreta placenta O43.23-
Peregrinating patient — *see* Disorder, factitious
Perforation, perforated (nontraumatic) (of)
- accidental during procedure (blood vessel) (nerve) (organ) — *see* Complication, accidental puncture or laceration

Perforation, perforated (nontraumatic) (of) - *continued*
- antrum — *see* Sinusitis, maxillary
- appendix K35.32
  - with localized peritonitis K35.32
- atrial septum, multiple Q21.1
- attic, ear — *see* Perforation, tympanum, attic
- bile duct (common) (hepatic) K83.2
  - cystic K82.2
- bladder (urinary)
  - with or following ectopic or molar pregnancy O08.6
  - obstetrical trauma O71.5
  - traumatic S37.29
    - at delivery O71.5
- bowel K63.1
  - with or following ectopic or molar pregnancy O08.6
  - newborn P78.0
  - obstetrical trauma O71.5
  - traumatic — *see* Laceration, intestine
- broad ligament N83.8
  - with or following ectopic or molar pregnancy O08.6
  - obstetrical trauma O71.6
- by
  - device, implant or graft — *see also* Complications, by site and type, mechanical T85.628
    - arterial graft NEC — *see* Complication, cardiovascular device, mechanical, vascular
    - breast (implant) T85.49
    - catheter NEC T85.698
      - cystostomy T83.090
      - dialysis (renal) T82.49
        - intraperitoneal T85.691
      - infusion NEC T82.594
        - spinal (epidural) (subdural) T85.690
      - urinary — *see also* Complications, catheter, urinary T83.098
    - electronic (electrode) (pulse generator) (stimulator)
      - bone T84.390
      - cardiac T82.199
        - electrode T82.190
        - pulse generator T82.191
        - specified type NEC T82.198
      - nervous system — *see* Complication, prosthetic device, mechanical, electronic nervous system stimulator
      - urinary — *see* Complication, genitourinary, device, urinary, mechanical
    - fixation, internal (orthopedic) NEC — *see* Complication, fixation device, mechanical
    - gastrointestinal — *see* Complications, prosthetic device, mechanical, gastrointestinal device
    - genital NEC T83.498
      - intrauterine contraceptive device T83.39
      - penile prosthesis T83.490
    - heart NEC — *see* Complication, cardiovascular device, mechanical
    - joint prosthesis — *see* Complications, joint prosthesis, mechanical, specified NEC, by site
    - ocular NEC — *see* Complications, prosthetic device, mechanical, ocular device
    - orthopedic NEC — *see* Complication, orthopedic, device, mechanical
    - specified NEC T85.628
    - urinary NEC — *see also* Complication, genitourinary, device, urinary, mechanical
      - graft T83.29
    - vascular NEC — *see* Complication, cardiovascular device, mechanical
    - ventricular intracranial shunt T85.09
  - foreign body left accidentally in operative wound T81.539

Perforation, perforated (nontraumatic) (of) - *continued*
- by - *continued*
  - instrument (any) during a procedure, accidental — *see* Puncture, accidental complicating surgery
- cecum K35.32
  - with localized peritonitis K35.32
- cervix (uteri) N88.8
  - with or following ectopic or molar pregnancy O08.6
  - obstetrical trauma O71.3
- colon K63.1
  - newborn P78.0
  - obstetrical trauma O71.5
  - traumatic — *see* Laceration, intestine, large
- common duct (bile) K83.2
- cornea (due to ulceration) — *see* Ulcer, cornea, perforated
- cystic duct K82.2
- diverticulum (intestine) K57.80
  - with bleeding K57.81
  - large intestine K57.20
    - with
      - bleeding K57.21
      - small intestine K57.40
        - with bleeding K57.41
  - small intestine K57.00
    - with
      - bleeding K57.01
      - large intestine K57.40
        - with bleeding K57.41
- ear drum — *see* Perforation, tympanum
- esophagus K22.3
- ethmoidal sinus — *see* Sinusitis, ethmoidal
- frontal sinus — *see* Sinusitis, frontal
- gallbladder K82.2
- heart valve — *see* Endocarditis
- ileum K63.1
  - newborn P78.0
  - obstetrical trauma O71.5
  - traumatic — *see* Laceration, intestine, small
- instrumental, surgical (accidental) (blood vessel) (nerve) (organ) — *see* Puncture, accidental complicating surgery
- intestine NEC K63.1
  - with ectopic or molar pregnancy O08.6
  - newborn P78.0
  - obstetrical trauma O71.5
  - traumatic — *see* Laceration, intestine
  - ulcerative NEC K63.1
    - newborn P78.0
- jejunum, jejunal K63.1
  - obstetrical trauma O71.5
  - traumatic — *see* Laceration, intestine, small
  - ulcer — *see* Ulcer, gastrojejunal, with perforation
- joint prosthesis — *see* Complications, joint prosthesis, mechanical, specified NEC, by site
- mastoid (antrum) (cell) — *see* Disorder, mastoid, specified NEC
- maxillary sinus — *see* Sinusitis, maxillary
- membrana tympani — *see* Perforation, tympanum
- nasal
  - septum J34.89
    - congenital Q30.3
    - syphilitic A52.73
  - sinus J34.89
    - congenital Q30.8
    - due to sinusitis — *see* Sinusitis
- palate — *see also* Cleft, palate Q35.9
  - syphilitic A52.79
- palatine vault — *see also* Cleft, palate, hard Q35.1
  - syphilitic A52.79
    - congenital A50.59
- pars flaccida (ear drum) — *see* Perforation, tympanum, attic
- pelvic
  - floor S31.030

Perforation, perforated (nontraumatic) (of) - *continued*
pelvic - *continued*
floor - *continued*
with
ectopic or molar pregnancy O08.6
penetration into retroperitoneal space S31.031
retained foreign body S31.040
with penetration into retroperitoneal space S31.041
following ectopic or molar pregnancy O08.6
obstetrical trauma O70.1
organ S37.99
adrenal gland S37.818
bladder — *see* Perforation, bladder
fallopian tube S37.599
bilateral S37.592
unilateral S37.591
kidney S37.09-
obstetrical trauma O71.5
ovary S37.499
bilateral S37.492
unilateral S37.491
prostate S37.828
specified organ NEC S37.898
ureter — *see* Perforation, ureter
urethra — *see* Perforation, urethra
uterus — *see* Perforation, uterus
perineum — *see* Laceration, perineum
pharynx J39.2
rectum K63.1
newborn P78.0
obstetrical trauma O71.5
traumatic S36.63
root canal space due to endodontic treatment M27.51
sigmoid K63.1
newborn P78.0
obstetrical trauma O71.5
traumatic S36.533
sinus (accessory) (chronic) (nasal) J34.89
sphenoidal sinus — *see* Sinusitis, sphenoidal
surgical (accidental) (by instrument) (blood vessel) (nerve) (organ) — *see* Puncture, accidental complicating surgery
traumatic
external — *see* Puncture
eye — *see* Puncture, eyeball
internal organ — *see* Injury, by site
tympanum, tympanic (membrane) (persistent post-traumatic) (postinflammatory) H72.9-
attic H72.1-
multiple — *see* Perforation, tympanum, multiple
total — *see* Perforation, tympanum, total
central H72.0-
multiple — *see* Perforation, tympanum, multiple
total — *see* Perforation, tympanum, total
marginal NEC — *see* subcategory H72.2
multiple H72.81-
pars flaccida — *see* Perforation, tympanum, attic
total H72.82-
traumatic, current episode S09.2-
typhoid, gastrointestinal — *see* Typhoid
ulcer — *see* Ulcer, by site, with perforation
ureter N28.89
traumatic S37.19
urethra N36.8
with ectopic or molar pregnancy O08.6
following ectopic or molar pregnancy O08.6
obstetrical trauma O71.5
traumatic S37.39
at delivery O71.5
uterus
with ectopic or molar pregnancy O08.6
by intrauterine contraceptive device T83.39
following ectopic or molar pregnancy O08.6

Perforation, perforated (nontraumatic) (of) - *continued*
uterus - *continued*
obstetrical trauma O71.1
traumatic S37.69
obstetric O71.1
uvula K13.79
syphilitic A52.79
vagina
obstetrical trauma O71.4
other trauma — *see* Puncture, vagina
Periadenitis mucosa necrotica recurrens K12.0
Periappendicitis (acute) — *see* Appendicitis
Periarteritis nodosa (disseminated) (infectious) (necrotizing) M30.0
Periarthritis (joint) — *see also* Enthesopathy
Duplay's M75.0-
gonococcal A54.42
humeroscapularis — *see* Capsulitis, adhesive
scapulohumeral — *see* Capsulitis, adhesive
shoulder — *see* Capsulitis, adhesive
wrist M77.2-
Periarthrosis (angioneural) — *see* Enthesopathy
Pericapsulitis, adhesive (shoulder) — *see* Capsulitis, adhesive
Pericarditis (with decompensation) (with effusion) I31.9
with rheumatic fever (conditions in I00)
active — *see* Pericarditis, rheumatic
inactive or quiescent I09.2
acute (hemorrhagic) (nonrheumatic) (Sicca) I30.9
with chorea (acute) (rheumatic) (Sydenham's) I02.0
benign I30.8
nonspecific I30.0
rheumatic I01.0
with chorea (acute) (Sydenham's) I02.0
adhesive or adherent (chronic) (external) (internal) I31.0
acute — *see* Pericarditis, acute
rheumatic I09.2
bacterial (acute) (subacute) (with serous or seropurulent effusion) I30.1
calcareous I31.1
cholesterol (chronic) I31.8
acute I30.9
chronic (nonrheumatic) I31.9
rheumatic I09.2
constrictive (chronic) I31.1
coxsackie B33.23
fibrinocaseous (tuberculous) A18.84
fibrinopurulent I30.1
fibrinous I30.8
fibrous I31.0
gonococcal A54.83
idiopathic I30.0
in systemic lupus erythematosus M32.12
infective I30.1
meningococcal A39.53
neoplastic (chronic) I31.8
acute I30.9
obliterans, obliterating I31.0
plastic I31.0
pneumococcal I30.1
postinfarction I24.1
purulent I30.1
rheumatic (active) (acute) (with effusion) (with pneumonia) I01.0
with chorea (acute) (rheumatic) (Sydenham's) I02.0
chronic or inactive (with chorea) I09.2
rheumatoid — *see* Rheumatoid, carditis
septic I30.1
serofibrinous I30.8
staphylococcal I30.1
streptococcal I30.1
suppurative I30.1
syphilitic A52.06
tuberculous A18.84
uremic N18.9 *[I32]*
viral I30.1
Pericardium, pericardial — *see* condition

Pericellulitis — *see* Cellulitis
Pericementitis (chronic) (suppurative) — *see also* Periodontitis
acute K05.20
generalized — *see* Periodontitis, aggressive, generalized
localized — *see* Periodontitis, aggressive, localized
Perichondritis
auricle — *see* Perichondritis, ear
bronchus J98.09
ear (external) H61.00-
acute H61.01-
chronic H61.02-
external auditory canal — *see* Perichondritis, ear
larynx J38.7
syphilitic A52.73
typhoid A01.09
nose J34.89
pinna — *see* Perichondritis, ear
trachea J39.8
Periclasia K05.4
Pericoronitis — *see* Periodontitis
Pericystitis N30.90
with hematuria N30.91
Peridiverticulitis (intestine) K57.92
cecum — *see* Diverticulitis, intestine, large
colon — *see* Diverticulitis, intestine, large
duodenum — *see* Diverticulitis, intestine, small
intestine — *see* Diverticulitis, intestine
jejunum — *see* Diverticulitis, intestine, small
rectosigmoid — *see* Diverticulitis, intestine, large
rectum — *see* Diverticulitis, intestine, large
sigmoid — *see* Diverticulitis, intestine, large
Periendocarditis — *see* Endocarditis
Periepididymitis N45.1
Perifolliculitis L01.02
abscedens, caput, scalp L66.3
capitis, abscedens (et suffodiens) L66.3
superficial pustular L01.02
Perihepatitis K65.8
Perilabyrinthitis (acute) — *see* subcategory H83.0
Perimeningitis — *see* Meningitis
Perimetritis — *see* Endometritis
Perimetrosalpingitis — *see* Salpingo-oophoritis
Perineocele N81.81
Perinephric, perinephritic — *see* condition
Perinephritis — *see also* Infection, kidney
purulent — *see* Abscess, kidney
Perineum, perineal — *see* condition
Perineuritis NEC — *see* Neuralgia
Periodic — *see* condition
Periodontitis (chronic) (complex) (compound) (local) (simplex) K05.30
acute K05.20
generalized K05.229
moderate K05.222
severe K05.223
slight K05.221
localized K05.219
moderate K05.212
severe K05.213
slight K05.211
apical K04.5
acute (pulpal origin) K04.4
generalized K05.329
moderate K05.322
severe K05.323
slight K05.321
localized K05.319
moderate K05.312
severe K05.313
slight K05.311
Periodontoclasia K05.4
Periodontosis (juvenile) K05.4
Periods — *see also* Menstruation
heavy N92.0
irregular N92.6
shortened intervals (irregular) N92.1

PERFORATION, PERFORATED - PERIODS

Perionychia — *see also* Cellulitis, digit
with lymphangitis — *see* Lymphangitis, acute, digit
Perioophoritis — *see* Salpingo-oophoritis
Periorchitis N45.2
Periosteum, periosteal — *see* condition
Periostitis (albuminosa) (circumscribed) (diffuse) (infective) (monomelic) — *see also* Osteomyelitis
alveolar M27.3
alveolodental M27.3
dental M27.3
gonorrheal A54.43
jaw (lower) (upper) M27.2
orbit H05.03-
syphilitic A52.77
congenital (early) A50.02 *[M90.80]*
secondary A51.46
tuberculous — *see* Tuberculosis, bone
yaws (hypertrophic) (early) (late) A66.6 *[M90.80]*
Periostosis (hyperplastic) — *see also* Disorder, bone, specified type NEC
with osteomyelitis — *see* Osteomyelitis, specified type NEC
Peripartum
cardiomyopathy O90.3
Periphlebitis — *see* Phlebitis
Periproctitis K62.89
Periprostatitis — *see* Prostatitis
Perirectal — *see* condition
Perirenal — *see* condition
Perisalpingitis — *see* Salpingo-oophoritis
Perisplenitis (infectional) D73.89
Peristalsis, visible or reversed R19.2
Peritendinitis — *see* Enthesopathy
Peritoneum, peritoneal — *see* condition
Peritonitis (adhesive) (bacterial) (fibrinous) (hemorrhagic) (idiopathic) (localized) (perforative) (primary) (with adhesions) (with effusion) K65.9
with or following
abscess K65.1
appendicitis
with perforation or rupture K35.32
generalized — *see also* Appendicitis K35.20
localized — *see also* Appendicitis K35.30
diverticular disease (intestine) K57.80
with bleeding K57.81
large intestine K57.20
with
bleeding K57.21
small intestine K57.40
with bleeding K57.41
small intestine K57.00
with
bleeding K57.01
large intestine K57.40
with bleeding K57.41
ectopic or molar pregnancy O08.0
acute (generalized) K65.0
aseptic T81.61
bile, biliary K65.3
chemical T81.61
chlamydial A74.81
complicating abortion — *see* Abortion, by type, complicated by, pelvic peritonitis
congenital P78.1
chronic proliferative K65.8
diaphragmatic K65.0
diffuse K65.0
diphtheritic A36.89
disseminated K65.0
due to
bile K65.3
foreign
body or object accidentally left during a procedure (instrument) (sponge) (swab) T81.599
substance accidentally left during a procedure (chemical) (powder) (talc) T81.61
talc T81.61

Peritonitis (adhesive) (bacterial) (fibrinous) (hemorrhagic) (idiopathic) (localized) (perforative) (primary) (with adhesions) (with effusion) - *continued*
due to - *continued*
urine K65.8
eosinophilic K65.8
acute K65.0
fibrocaseous (tuberculous) A18.31
fibropurulent K65.0
following ectopic or molar pregnancy O08.0
general (ized) K65.0
gonococcal A54.85
meconium (newborn) P78.0
neonatal P78.1
meconium P78.0
pancreatic K65.0
paroxysmal, familial E85.0
benign E85.0
pelvic
female N73.5
acute N73.3
chronic N73.4
with adhesions N73.6
male K65.0
periodic, familial E85.0
proliferative, chronic K65.8
puerperal, postpartum, childbirth O85
purulent K65.0
septic K65.0
specified NEC K65.8
spontaneous bacterial K65.2
subdiaphragmatic K65.0
subphrenic K65.0
suppurative K65.0
syphilitic A52.74
congenital (early) A50.08 *[K67]*
talc T81.61
tuberculous A18.31
urine K65.8
Peritonsillar — *see* condition
Peritonsillitis J36
Perityphlitis K37
Periureteritis N28.89
Periurethral — *see* condition
Periurethritis (gangrenous) — *see* Urethritis
Periuterine — *see* condition
Perivaginitis — *see* Vaginitis
Perivasculitis, retinal H35.06-
Perivasitis (chronic) N49.1
Perivesiculitis (seminal) — *see* Vesiculitis
Perlèche NEC K13.0
due to
candidiasis B37.83
moniliasis B37.83
riboflavin deficiency E53.0
vitamin B2 (riboflavin) deficiency E53.0
Pernicious — *see* condition
Pernio, perniosis T69.1
Perpetrator (of abuse) — *see* Index to External Causes of Injury, Perpetrator
Persecution
delusion F22
social Z60.5
Perseveration (tonic) R48.8
Persistence, persistent (congenital)
anal membrane Q42.3
with fistula Q42.2
arteria stapedia Q16.3
atrioventricular canal Q21.2
branchial cleft NOS Q18.2
cyst Q18.0
fistula Q18.0
sinus Q18.0
bulbus cordis in left ventricle Q21.8
canal of Cloquet Q14.0
capsule (opaque) Q12.8
cilioretinal artery or vein Q14.8
cloaca Q43.7
communication — *see* Fistula, congenital
convolutions
aortic arch Q25.46
fallopian tube Q50.6
oviduct Q50.6
uterine tube Q50.6

Persistence, persistent (congenital) - *continued*
double aortic arch Q25.45
ductus arteriosus (Botalli) Q25.0
fetal
circulation P29.38
form of cervix (uteri) Q51.828
hemoglobin, hereditary (HPFH) D56.4
foramen
Botalli Q21.1
ovale Q21.1
Gartner's duct Q52.4
hemoglobin, fetal (hereditary) (HPFH) D56.4
hyaloid
artery (generally incomplete) Q14.0
system Q14.8
hymen, in pregnancy or childbirth — *see* Pregnancy, complicated by, abnormal, vulva
lanugo Q84.2
left
posterior cardinal vein Q26.8
root with right arch of aorta Q25.49
superior vena cava Q26.1
Meckel's diverticulum Q43.0
malignant — *see* Table of Neoplasms, small intestine, malignant
mucosal disease (middle ear) — *see* Otitis, media, suppurative, chronic, tubotympanic
nail (s) , anomalous Q84.6
omphalomesenteric duct Q43.0
organ or site not listed — *see* Anomaly, by site
ostium
atrioventriculare commune Q21.2
primum Q21.2
secundum Q21.1
ovarian rests in fallopian tube Q50.6
pancreatic tissue in intestinal tract Q43.8
primary (deciduous)
teeth K00.6
vitreous hyperplasia Q14.0
pupillary membrane Q13.89
right aortic arch Q25.47
rhesus (Rh) titer — *see* Complication(s), transfusion, incompatibility reaction, Rh (factor)
sinus
urogenitalis
female Q52.8
male Q55.8
venosus with imperfect incorporation in right auricle Q26.8
thymus (gland) (hyperplasia) E32.0
thyroglossal duct Q89.2
thyrolingual duct Q89.2
truncus arteriosus or communis Q20.0
tunica vasculosa lentis Q12.2
umbilical sinus Q64.4
urachus Q64.4
vitelline duct Q43.0
Person (with)
admitted for clinical research, as a control subject (normal comparison) (participant) Z00.6
awaiting admission to adequate facility elsewhere Z75.1
concern (normal) about sick person in family Z63.6
consulting on behalf of another Z71.0
feigning illness Z76.5
living (in)
alone Z60.2
boarding school Z59.3
residential institution Z59.3
without
adequate housing (heating) (space) Z59.1
housing (permanent) (temporary) Z59.00
person able to render necessary care Z74.2
shelter Z59.02
on waiting list Z75.1
sick or handicapped in family Z63.6

Personality (disorder) F60.9
  accentuation of traits (type A pattern) Z73.1
  affective F34.0
  aggressive F60.3
  amoral F60.2
  anacastic, anankastic F60.5
  antisocial F60.2
  anxious F60.6
  asocial F60.2
  asthenic F60.7
  avoidant F60.6
  borderline F60.3
  change due to organic condition (enduring) F07.0
  compulsive F60.5
  cycloid F34.0
  cyclothymic F34.0
  dependent F60.7
  depressive F34.1
  dissocial F60.2
  dual F44.81
  eccentric F60.89
  emotionally unstable F60.3
  expansive paranoid F60.0
  explosive F60.3
  fanatic F60.0
  haltlose type F60.89
  histrionic F60.4
  hyperthymic F34.0
  hypothymic F34.1
  hysterical F60.4
  immature F60.89
  inadequate F60.7
  labile (emotional) F60.3
  mixed (nonspecific) F60.89
  morally defective F60.2
  multiple F44.81
  narcissistic F60.81
  obsessional F60.5
  obsessive (-compulsive) F60.5
  organic F07.0
  overconscientious F60.5
  paranoid F60.0
  passive (-dependent) F60.7
  passive-aggressive F60.89
  pathologic F60.9
  pattern defect or disturbance F60.9
  pseudopsychopathic (organic) F07.0
  pseudoretarded (organic) F07.0
  psychoinfantile F60.4
  psychoneurotic NEC F60.89
  psychopathic F60.2
  querulant F60.0
  sadistic F60.89
  schizoid F60.1
  self-defeating F60.89
  sensitive paranoid F60.0
  sociopathic (amoral) (antisocial) (asocial) (dissocial) F60.2
  specified NEC F60.89
  type A Z73.1
  unstable (emotional) F60.3
Perthes' disease — *see* Legg-Calvé-Perthes disease
Pertussis — *see also* Whooping cough A37.90
Perversion, perverted
  appetite F50.89
    psychogenic F50.89
  function
    pituitary gland E23.2
      posterior lobe E22.2
  sense of smell and taste R43.8
    psychogenic F45.8
  sexual — *see* Deviation, sexual
Pervious, congenital — *see also* Imperfect, closure
  ductus arteriosus Q25.0
Pes (congenital) — *see also* Talipes
  acquired — *see also* Deformity, limb, foot, specified NEC
    planus — *see* Deformity, limb, flat foot
  adductus Q66.89
  cavus Q66.7-
  deformity NEC, acquired — *see* Deformity, limb, foot, specified NEC
Pes (congenital) - *continued*
  planus (acquired) (any degree) — *see also* Deformity, limb, flat foot
    rachitic sequelae (late effect) E64.3
  valgus Q66.6
Pest, pestis — *see* Plague
Petechia, petechiae R23.3
  newborn P54.5
Petechial typhus A75.9
Peter's anomaly Q13.4
Petit mal seizure — *see* Epilepsy, childhood, absence
Petit's hernia — *see* Hernia, abdomen, specified site NEC
Petrellidosis B48.2
Petrositis H70.20-
  acute H70.21-
  chronic H70.22-
Peutz-Jeghers disease or syndrome Q85.8
Peyronie's disease N48.6
PFAPA (periodic fever, aphthous stomatitis, pharyngitis, and adenopathy syndrome) M04.8
Pfeiffer's disease — *see* Mononucleosis, infectious
Phagedena (dry) (moist) (sloughing) — *see also* Gangrene
  geometric L88
  penis N48.29
  tropical — *see* Ulcer, skin
  vulva N76.6
Phagedenic — *see* condition
Phakoma H35.89
Phakomatosis — *see also* specific eponymous syndromes Q85.9
  Bourneville's Q85.1
  specified NEC Q85.8
Phantom limb syndrome (without pain) G54.7
  with pain G54.6
Pharyngeal pouch syndrome D82.1
Pharyngitis (acute) (catarrhal) (gangrenous) (infective) (malignant) (membranous) (phlegmonous) (pseudomembranous) (simple) (subacute) (suppurative) (ulcerative) (viral) J02.9
  with influenza, flu, or grippe — *see* Influenza, with, pharyngitis
  aphthous B08.5
  atrophic J31.2
  chlamydial A56.4
  chronic (atrophic) (granular) (hypertrophic) J31.2
  coxsackievirus B08.5
  diphtheritic A36.0
  enteroviral vesicular B08.5
  follicular (chronic) J31.2
  fusospirochetal A69.1
  gonococcal A54.5
  granular (chronic) J31.2
  herpesviral B00.2
  hypertrophic J31.2
  infectional, chronic J31.2
  influenzal — *see* Influenza, with, respiratory manifestations NEC
  lymphonodular, acute (enteroviral) B08.8
  pneumococcal J02.8
  purulent J02.9
  putrid J02.9
  septic J02.0
  sicca J31.2
  specified organism NEC J02.8
  staphylococcal J02.8
  streptococcal J02.0
  syphilitic, congenital (early) A50.03
  tuberculous A15.8
  vesicular, enteroviral B08.5
  viral NEC J02.8
Pharyngoconjunctivitis, viral B30.2
Pharyngolaryngitis (acute) J06.0
  chronic J37.0
Pharyngoplegia J39.2
Pharyngotonsillitis, herpesviral B00.2
Pharyngotracheitis, chronic J42
Pharynx, pharyngeal — *see* condition
Phencyclidine-induced
  anxiety disorder F16.980
  bipolar and related disorder F16.94
  depressive disorder F16.94
  psychotic disorder F16.959
Phenomenon
  Arthus' — *see* Arthus' phenomenon
  jaw-winking Q07.8
  lupus erythematosus (LE) cell M32.9
  Raynaud's (secondary) I73.00
    with gangrene I73.01
  vasomotor R55
  vasospastic I73.9
  vasovagal R55
  Wenckebach's I44.1
Phenylketonuria E70.1
  classical E70.0
  maternal E70.1
Pheochromoblastoma
  specified site — *see* Neoplasm, malignant, by site
  unspecified site C74.10
Pheochromocytoma
  malignant
    specified site — *see* Neoplasm, malignant, by site
    unspecified site C74.10
  specified site — *see* Neoplasm, benign, by site
  unspecified site D35.00
Pheohyphomycosis — *see* Chromomycosis
Pheomycosis — *see* Chromomycosis
Phimosis (congenital) (due to infection) N47.1
  chancroidal A57
Phlebectasia — *see also* Varix
  congenital Q27.4
Phlebitis (infective) (pyemic) (septic) (suppurative) I80.9
  antepartum — *see* Thrombophlebitis, antepartum
  blue — *see* Phlebitis, leg, deep
  breast, superficial I80.8
  cavernous (venous) sinus — *see* Phlebitis, intracranial (venous) sinus
  calf muscular vein (NOS) I80.25-
  cerebral (venous) sinus — *see* Phlebitis, intracranial (venous) sinus
  chest wall, superficial I80.8
  cranial (venous) sinus — *see* Phlebitis, intracranial (venous) sinus
  deep (vessels) — *see* Phlebitis, leg, deep
  due to implanted device — *see* Complications, by site and type, specified NEC
  during or resulting from a procedure T81.72
  femoral vein (superficial) I80.1-
  femoropopliteal vein I80.0-
  gastrocnemial vein I80.25-
  gestational — *see* Phlebopathy, gestational
  hepatic veins I80.8
  iliac vein (common) (external) (internal) I80.21-
  iliofemoral — *see* Phlebitis, femoral vein
  intracranial (venous) sinus (any) G08
    nonpyogenic I67.6
  intraspinal venous sinuses and veins G08
    nonpyogenic G95.19
  lateral (venous) sinus — *see* Phlebitis, intracranial (venous) sinus
  leg I80.3
    antepartum — *see* Thrombophlebitis, antepartum
    deep (vessels) NEC I80.20-
      iliac I80.21-
      popliteal vein I80.22-
      specified vessel NEC I80.29-
      tibial vein (anterior) (posterior) I80.23-
    femoral vein (superficial) I80.1-
    superficial (vessels) I80.0-
  longitudinal sinus — *see* Phlebitis, intracranial (venous) sinus
  lower limb — *see* Phlebitis, leg
  migrans, migrating (superficial) I82.1
  pelvic

Phlebitis (infective) (pyemic) (septic) (suppurative) - *continued*
pelvic - *continued*
with ectopic or molar pregnancy O08.0
following ectopic or molar pregnancy O08.0
puerperal, postpartum O87.1
peroneal vein I80.24-
popliteal vein — *see* Phlebitis, leg, deep, popliteal
portal (vein) K75.1
postoperative T81.72
pregnancy — *see* Thrombophlebitis, antepartum
puerperal, postpartum, childbirth O87.0
deep O87.1
pelvic O87.1
superficial O87.0
retina — *see* Vasculitis, retina
saphenous (accessory) (great) (long) (small) — *see* Phlebitis, leg, superficial
sinus (meninges) — *see* Phlebitis, intracranial (venous) sinus
soleal vein I80.25-
specified site NEC I80.8
syphilitic A52.09
tibial vein — *see* Phlebitis, leg, deep, tibial
ulcerative I80.9
leg — *see* Phlebitis, leg
umbilicus I80.8
uterus (septic) — *see* Endometritis
varicose (leg) (lower limb) — *see* Varix, leg, with, inflammation
Phlebofibrosis I87.8
Phleboliths I87.8
Phlebopathy,
gestational O22.9-
puerperal O87.9
Phlebosclerosis I87.8
Phlebothrombosis — *see also* Thrombosis
antepartum — *see* Thrombophlebitis, antepartum
pregnancy — *see* Thrombophlebitis, antepartum
puerperal — *see* Thrombophlebitis, puerperal
Phlebotomus fever A93.1
Phlegmasia
alba dolens O87.1
nonpuerperal — *see* Phlebitis, femoral vein
cerulea dolens — *see* Phlebitis, leg, deep
Phlegmon — *see* Abscess
Phlegmonous — *see* condition
Phlyctenulosis (allergic) (keratoconjunctivitis) (nontuberculous) — *see also* Keratoconjunctivitis
cornea — *see* Keratoconjunctivitis
tuberculous A18.52
Phobia, phobic F40.9
animal F40.218
spiders F40.210
examination F40.298
reaction F40.9
simple F40.298
social F40.10
generalized F40.11
specific (isolated) F40.298
animal F40.218
spiders F40.210
blood F40.230
injection F40.231
injury F40.233
men F40.290
natural environment F40.228
thunderstorms F40.220
situational F40.248
bridges F40.242
closed in spaces F40.240
flying F40.243
heights F40.241
specified focus NEC F40.298
transfusion F40.231
women F40.291
specified NEC F40.8
medical care NEC F40.232
state F40.9
Phocas' disease — *see* Mastopathy, cystic
Phocomelia Q73.1
lower limb — *see* Agenesis, leg, with foot present
upper limb — *see* Agenesis, arm, with hand present
Phoria H50.50
Phosphate-losing tubular disorder N25.0
Phosphatemia E83.39
Phosphaturia E83.39
Photodermatitis (sun) L56.8
chronic L57.8
due to drug L56.8
light other than sun L59.8
Photokeratitis H16.13-
Photophobia H53.14-
Photophthalmia — *see* Photokeratitis
Photopsia H53.19
Photoretinitis — *see* Retinopathy, solar
Photosensitivity, photosensitization (sun) skin L56.8
light other than sun L59.8
Phrenitis — *see* Encephalitis
Phrynoderma (vitamin A deficiency) E50.8
Phthiriasis (pubis) B85.3
with any infestation classifiable to B85.0-B85.2 B85.4
Phthirus infestation — *see* Phthiriasis
Phthisis — *see also* Tuberculosis
bulbi (infectional) — *see* Disorder, globe, degenerated condition, atrophy
eyeball (due to infection) — *see* Disorder, globe, degenerated condition, atrophy
Phycomycosis — *see* Zygomycosis
Physalopteriasis B81.8
Physical restraint status Z78.1
Phytobezoar T18.9
intestine T18.3
stomach T18.2
Pian — *see* Yaws
Pianoma A66.1
Pica F50.89
in adults F50.89
infant or child F98.3
Picking, nose F98.8
Pick-Niemann disease — *see* Niemann-Pick disease or syndrome
Pick's
cerebral atrophy G31.01 *[F02.80]*
with behavioral disturbance G31.01 *[F02.81]*
disease or syndrome (brain) G31.01 *[F02.80]*
with behavioral disturbance G31.01 *[F02.81]*
brain G31.01 *[F02.80]*
with behavioral disturbance G31.01 *[F02.81]*
pericardium (pericardial pseudocirrhosis of liver) I31.1
syndrome
brain G31.01 *[F02.80]*
with behavioral disturbance G31.01 *[F02.81]*
of heart (pericardial pseudocirrhosis of liver) I31.1
Pickwickian syndrome E66.2
Piebaldism E70.39
Piedra (beard) (scalp) B36.8
black B36.3
white B36.2
Pierre Robin deformity or syndrome Q87.0
Pierson's disease or osteochondrosis M91.0
Pig-bel A05.2
Pigeon
breast or chest (acquired) M95.4
congenital Q67.7
rachitic sequelae (late effect) E64.3
breeder's disease or lung J67.2
fancier's disease or lung J67.2
toe — *see* Deformity, toe, specified NEC
Pigmentation (abnormal) (anomaly) L81.9
conjunctiva H11.13-
cornea (anterior) H18.01-
posterior H18.05-
stromal H18.06-
Pigmentation (abnormal) (anomaly) - *continued*
diminished melanin formation NEC L81.6
iron L81.8
lids, congenital Q82.8
limbus corneae — *see* Pigmentation, cornea
metals L81.8
optic papilla, congenital Q14.2
retina, congenital (grouped) (nevoid) Q14.1
scrotum, congenital Q82.8
tattoo L81.8
Piles — *see also* Hemorrhoids K64.9
Pili
annulati or torti (congenital) Q84.1
incarnati L73.1
Pill roller hand (intrinsic) — *see* Parkinsonism
Pilomatrixoma — *see* Neoplasm, skin, benign
malignant — *see* Neoplasm, skin, malignant
Pilonidal — *see* condition
Pimple R23.8
PIMS M35.81
PIN — *see* Neoplasia, intraepithelial, prostate
Pinched nerve — *see* Neuropathy, entrapment
Pindborg tumor — *see* Cyst, calcifying odontogenic
Pineal body or gland — *see* condition
Pinealoblastoma C75.3
Pinealoma D44.5
malignant C75.3
Pineoblastoma C75.3
Pineocytoma D44.5
Pinguecula H11.15-
Pingueculitis H10.81-
Pinhole meatus — *see also* Stricture, urethra N35.919
Pink
disease — *see* subcategory T56.1
eye — *see* Conjunctivitis, acute, mucopurulent
Pinkus' disease (lichen nitidus) L44.1
Pinpoint
meatus — *see* Stricture, urethra
os (uteri) — *see* Stricture, cervix
Pins and needles R20.2
Pinta A67.9
cardiovascular lesions A67.2
chancre (primary) A67.0
erythematous plaques A67.1
hyperchromic lesions A67.1
hyperkeratosis A67.1
lesions A67.9
cardiovascular A67.2
hyperchromic A67.1
intermediate A67.1
late A67.2
mixed A67.3
primary A67.0
skin (achromic) (cicatricial) (dyschromic) A67.2
hyperchromic A67.1
mixed (achromic and hyperchromic) A67.3
papule (primary) A67.0
skin lesions (achromic) (cicatricial) (dyschromic) A67.2
hyperchromic A67.1
mixed (achromic and hyperchromic) A67.3
vitiligo A67.2
Pintids A67.1
Pinworm (disease) (infection) (infestation) B80
Piroplasmosis — *see also* Babesiosis B60.00
specified NEC B60.09
Pistol wound — *see* Gunshot wound
Pitchers' elbow — *see* Derangement, joint, specified type NEC, elbow
Pithecoid pelvis Q74.2
with disproportion (fetopelvic) O33.0
causing obstructed labor O65.0
Pithiatism F48.8
Pitted — *see* Pitting
Pitting — *see also* Edema R60.9
lip R60.0
nail L60.8

PHLEBITIS - PITTING

Pitting - *continued*
- teeth K00.4

Pituitary gland — *see* condition
Pituitary-snuff-taker's disease J67.8
Pityriasis (capitis) L21.0
- alba L30.5
- circinata (et maculata) L42
- furfuracea L21.0
- Hebra's L26
- lichenoides L41.0
  - chronica L41.1
  - et varioliformis (acuta) L41.0
- maculata (et circinata) L30.5
- nigra B36.1
- pilaris, Hebra's L44.0
- rosea L42
- rotunda L44.8
- rubra (Hebra) pilaris L44.0
- simplex L30.5
- specified type NEC L30.5
- streptogenes L30.5
- versicolor (scrotal) B36.0

Placenta, placental — *see* Pregnancy, complicated by (care of) (management affected by), specified condition
Placentitis O41.14-
Plagiocephaly Q67.3
Plague A20.9
- abortive A20.8
- ambulatory A20.8
- asymptomatic A20.8
- bubonic A20.0
- cellulocutaneous A20.1
- cutaneobubonic A20.1
- lymphatic gland A20.0
- meningitis A20.3
- pharyngeal A20.8
- pneumonic (primary) (secondary) A20.2
- pulmonary, pulmonic A20.2
- septicemic A20.7
- tonsillar A20.8
  - septicemic A20.7

Planning, family
- contraception Z30.9
- procreation Z31.69

Plaque (s)
- artery, arterial — *see* Arteriosclerosis
- calcareous — *see* Calcification
- coronary, lipid rich I25.83
- epicardial I31.8
- erythematous, of pinta A67.1
- Hollenhorst's — *see* Occlusion, artery, retina
- lipid rich, coronary I25.83
- pleural (without asbestos) J92.9
  - with asbestos J92.0
- tongue K13.29

Plasmacytoma C90.3-
- extramedullary C90.2-
- medullary C90.0-
- solitary C90.3-

Plasmacytopenia D72.818
Plasmacytosis D72.822
Plaster ulcer — *see* Ulcer, pressure, by site
Plateau iris syndrome (post-iridectomy) (postprocedural) (without glaucoma) H21.82
- with glaucoma H40.22-

Platybasia Q75.8
Platyonychia (congenital) Q84.6
- acquired L60.8

Platypelloid pelvis M95.5
- with disproportion (fetopelvic) O33.0
  - causing obstructed labor O65.0
- congenital Q74.2

Platyspondylisis Q76.49
Plaut (-Vincent) disease — *see also* Vincent's A69.1
Plethora R23.2
- newborn P61.1

Pleura, pleural — *see* condition
Pleuralgia R07.81
Pleurisy (acute) (adhesive) (chronic) (costal) (diaphragmatic) (double) (dry) (fibrinous) (fibrous) (interlobar) (latent) (plastic) (primary) (residual) (sicca) (sterile) (subacute) (unresolved) R09.1
- with
  - adherent pleura J86.0
  - effusion J90
    - chylous, chyliform J94.0
    - tuberculous (non primary) A15.6
      - primary (progressive) A15.7
  - tuberculosis — *see* Pleurisy, tuberculous (non primary)
- encysted — *see* Pleurisy, with effusion
- exudative — *see* Pleurisy, with effusion
- fibrinopurulent, fibropurulent — *see* Pyothorax
- hemorrhagic — *see* Hemothorax
- pneumococcal J90
- purulent — *see* Pyothorax
- septic — *see* Pyothorax
- serofibrinous — *see* Pleurisy, with effusion
- seropurulent — *see* Pyothorax
- serous — *see* Pleurisy, with effusion
- staphylococcal J86.9
- streptococcal J90
- suppurative — *see* Pyothorax
- traumatic (post) (current) — *see* Injury, intrathoracic, pleura
- tuberculous (with effusion) (non primary) A15.6
  - primary (progressive) A15.7

Pleuritis sicca — *see* Pleurisy
Pleurobronchopneumonia — *see* Pneumonia, broncho-
Pleurodynia R07.81
- epidemic B33.0
- viral B33.0

Pleuropericarditis — *see also* Pericarditis
- acute I30.9

Pleuropneumonia (acute) (bilateral) (double) (septic) — *see also* Pneumonia J18.8
- chronic — *see* Fibrosis, lung

Pleuro-pneumonia-like-organism (PPLO) , as cause of disease classified elsewhere B96.0
Pleurorrhea — *see* Pleurisy, with effusion
Plexitis, brachial G54.0
Plica
- polonica B85.0
- syndrome, knee M67.5-
- tonsil J35.8

Plicated tongue K14.5
Plug
- bronchus NEC J98.09
- meconium (newborn) NEC syndrome P76.0
- mucus — *see* Asphyxia, mucus

Plumbism — *see* subcategory T56.0
Plummer's disease E05.20
- with thyroid storm E05.21

Plummer-Vinson syndrome D50.1
Pluricarential syndrome of infancy E40
Plus (and minus) hand (intrinsic) — *see* Deformity, limb, specified type NEC, forearm
PMEI (polymorphic epilepsy in infancy) G40.83-
Pneumathemia — *see* Air, embolism
Pneumatic hammer (drill) syndrome T75.21
Pneumatocele (lung) J98.4
- intracranial G93.89
- tension J44.9

Pneumatosis
- cystoides intestinalis K63.89
- intestinalis K63.89
- peritonei K66.8

Pneumaturia R39.89
Pneumoblastoma — *see* Neoplasm, lung, malignant
Pneumocephalus G93.89
Pneumococcemia A40.3
Pneumococcus, pneumococcal — *see* condition
Pneumoconiosis (due to) (inhalation of) J64
- with tuberculosis (any type in A15) J65

Pneumoconiosis (due to) (inhalation of) - *continued*
- aluminum J63.0
- asbestos J61
- bagasse, bagassosis J67.1
- bauxite J63.1
- beryllium J63.2
- coal miners' (simple) J60
- coalworkers' (simple) J60
- collier's J60
- cotton dust J66.0
- diatomite (diatomaceous earth) J62.8
- dust
  - inorganic NEC J63.6
  - lime J62.8
  - marble J62.8
  - organic NEC J66.8
- fumes or vapors (from silo) J68.9
- graphite J63.3
- grinder's J62.8
- kaolin J62.8
- mica J62.8
- millstone maker's J62.8
- mineral fibers NEC J61
- miner's J60
- moldy hay J67.0
- potter's J62.8
- rheumatoid — *see* Rheumatoid, lung
- sandblaster's J62.8
- silica, silicate NEC J62.8
  - with carbon J60
- stonemason's J62.8
- talc (dust) J62.0

Pneumocystis carinii pneumonia B59
Pneumocystis jiroveci (pneumonia) B59
Pneumocystosis (with pneumonia) B59
Pneumohemopericardium I31.2
Pneumohemothorax J94.2
- traumatic S27.2

Pneumohydropericardium — *see* Pericarditis
Pneumohydrothorax — *see* Hydrothorax
Pneumomediastinum J98.2
- congenital or perinatal P25.2

Pneumomycosis B49 *[J99]*
Pneumonia (acute) (double) (migratory) (purulent) (septic) (unresolved) J18.9
- with
  - lung abscess J85.1
    - due to specified organism — *see* Pneumonia, in (due to)
  - influenza — *see* Influenza, with, pneumonia
- 2019 (novel) coronavirus J12.82
- adenoviral J12.0
- adynamic J18.2
- alba A50.04
- allergic — *see also* Pneumonitis, hypersensitivity J82.89
- alveolar — *see* Pneumonia, lobar
- anaerobes J15.8
- anthrax A22.1
- apex, apical — *see* Pneumonia, lobar
- Ascaris B77.81
- aspiration J69.0
  - due to
    - aspiration of microorganisms
      - bacterial J15.9
      - viral J12.9
    - food (regurgitated) J69.0
    - gastric secretions J69.0
    - milk (regurgitated) J69.0
    - oils, essences J69.1
    - solids, liquids NEC J69.8
    - vomitus J69.0
  - newborn P24.81
    - amniotic fluid (clear) P24.11
    - blood P24.21
    - liquor (amnii) P24.11
    - meconium P24.01
    - milk P24.31
    - mucus P24.11
    - food (regurgitated) P24.31
    - specified NEC P24.81
    - stomach contents P24.31
  - postprocedural J95.4

Pneumonia (acute) (double) (migratory) (purulent) (septic) (unresolved) - *continued*
  neonatal - *continued*
    aspiration — *see* Aspiration, by substance, with pneumonia
  nitrogen dioxide J68.0
  organizing J84.89
    due to
      collagen vascular disease J84.178
      known underlying cause J84.178
    in diseases classified elsewhere J84.178
  orthostatic J18.2
  parainfluenza virus J12.2
  parenchymatous — *see* Fibrosis, lung
  passive J18.2
  patchy — *see* Pneumonia, broncho
  Peptococcus J15.8
  Peptostreptococcus J15.8
  plasma cell (of infants) B59
  pleurolobar — *see* Pneumonia, lobar
  pleuro-pneumonia-like organism (PPLO) J15.7
  pneumococcal (broncho) (lobar) J13
  Pneumocystis (carinii) (jiroveci) B59
  postinfectional NEC B99 *[J17]*
  postmeasles B05.2
  Proteus J15.6
  Pseudomonas J15.1
  psittacosis A70
  radiation J70.0
  respiratory syncytial virus (RSV) J12.1
  resulting from a procedure J95.89
  rheumatic I00 *[J17]*
  Salmonella (arizonae) (cholerae-suis) (enteritidis) (typhimurium) A02.22
    typhi A01.03
    typhoid fever A01.03
  SARS-associated coronavirus J12.81
  SARS-CoV-2 J12.82
  segmented, segmental — *see* Pneumonia, broncho-
  Serratia marcescens J15.6
  specified NEC J18.8
    bacterium NEC J15.8
    organism NEC J16.8
    virus NEC J12.89
  spirochetal NEC A69.8
  staphylococcal (broncho) (lobar) J15.20
    aureus (methicillin susceptible) (MSSA) J15.211
      methicillin resistant (MRSA) J15.212
    specified NEC J15.29
  static, stasis J18.2
  streptococcal NEC (broncho) (lobar) J15.4
    group
      A J15.4
      B J15.3
      specified NEC J15.4
  Streptococcus pneumoniae J13
  syphilitic, congenital (early) A50.04
  traumatic (complication) (early) (secondary) T79.8
  tuberculous (any) — *see* Tuberculosis, pulmonary
  tularemic A21.2
  varicella B01.2
  Veillonella J15.8
  ventilator associated J95.851
  viral, virus (broncho) (interstitial) (lobar) J12.9
    adenoviral J12.0
    congenital P23.0
    human metapneumovirus J12.3
    parainfluenza J12.2
    respiratory syncytial (RSV) J12.1
    SARS-associated coronavirus J12.81
    specified NEC J12.89
  white (congenital) A50.04
Pneumonic — *see* condition
Pneumonitis (acute) (primary) — *see also* Pneumonia
  air-conditioner J67.7
  allergic (due to) J67.9
    organic dust NEC J67.8
    red cedar dust J67.8
Pneumonitis (acute) (primary) - *continued*
  allergic (due to) - *continued*
    sequoiosis J67.8
    wood dust J67.8
  aspiration J69.0
    due to
      anesthesia J95.4
        during
          labor and delivery O74.0
          pregnancy O29.01-
          puerperium O89.01
      fumes or gases J68.0
    obstetric O74.0
  chemical (due to gases, fumes or vapors) (inhalation) J68.0
    due to anesthesia J95.4
  cholesterol J84.89
  crack (cocaine) J68.0
  chronic — *see* Fibrosis, lung
  congenital rubella P35.0
  due to
    beryllium J68.0
    cadmium J68.0
    crack (cocaine) J68.0
    detergent J69.8
    fluorocarbon-polymer J68.0
    food, vomit (aspiration) J69.0
    fumes or vapors J68.0
    gases, fumes or vapors (inhalation) J68.0
    inhalation
      blood J69.8
      essences J69.1
      food (regurgitated) , milk, vomit J69.0
      oils, essences J69.1
      saliva J69.0
      solids, liquids NEC J69.8
    manganese J68.0
    nitrogen dioxide J68.0
    oils, essences J69.1
    solids, liquids NEC J69.8
    toxoplasmosis (acquired) B58.3
      congenital P37.1
    vanadium J68.0
    ventilator J95.851
  eosinophilic J82.81
    acute J82.82
    chronic J82.81
  hypersensitivity J67.9
    air conditioner lung J67.7
    bagassosis J67.1
    bird fancier's lung J67.2
    farmer's lung J67.0
    maltworker's lung J67.4
    maple bark-stripper's lung J67.6
    mushroom worker's lung J67.5
    specified organic dust NEC J67.8
    suberosis J67.3
  interstitial (chronic) J84.89
    acute J84.114
    lymphoid J84.2
    non-specific J84.89
      idiopathic J84.113
  lymphoid, interstitial J84.2
  meconium P24.01
  postanesthetic J95.4
    correct substance properly administered — *see* Table of Drugs and Chemicals, by drug, adverse effect
    in labor and delivery O74.0
    in pregnancy O29.01-
    obstetric O74.0
    overdose or wrong substance given or taken (by accident) — *see* Table of Drugs and Chemicals, by drug, poisoning
    postpartum, puerperal O89.01
  postoperative J95.4
    obstetric O74.0
  radiation J70.0
  rubella, congenital P35.0
  ventilation (air-conditioning) J67.7
  ventilator associated J95.851
  wood-dust J67.8
Pneumonoconiosis — *see* Pneumoconiosis
Pneumoparotid K11.8
Pneumopathy NEC J98.4
  alveolar J84.09
  due to organic dust NEC J66.8
  parietoalveolar J84.09
Pneumopericarditis — *see also* Pericarditis
  acute I30.9
Pneumopericardium — *see also* Pericarditis
  congenital P25.3
  newborn P25.3
  traumatic (post) — *see* Injury, heart
Pneumophagia (psychogenic) F45.8
Pneumopleurisy, pneumopleuritis — *see also* Pneumonia J18.8
Pneumopyopericardium I30.1
Pneumopyothorax — *see* Pyopneumothorax
  with fistula J86.0
Pneumorrhagia — *see also* Hemorrhage, lung
  tuberculous — *see* Tuberculosis, pulmonary
Pneumothorax NOS J93.9
  acute J93.83
  chronic J93.81
  congenital P25.1
  perinatal period P25.1
  postprocedural J95.811
  specified NEC J93.83
  spontaneous NOS J93.83
    newborn P25.1
    primary J93.11
    secondary J93.12
    tension J93.0
  tense valvular, infectional J93.0
  tension (spontaneous) J93.0
  traumatic S27.0
    with hemothorax S27.2
  tuberculous — *see* Tuberculosis, pulmonary
Podagra — *see also* Gout M10.9
Podencephalus Q01.9
Poikilocytosis R71.8
Poikiloderma L81.6
  Civatte's L57.3
  congenital Q82.8
  vasculare atrophicans L94.5
Poikilodermatomyositis M33.10
  with
    myopathy M33.12
    respiratory involvement M33.11
    specified organ involvement NEC M33.19
Pointed ear (congenital) Q17.3
Poison ivy, oak, sumac or other plant dermatitis (allergic) (contact) L23.7
Poisoning (acute) — *see also* Table of Drugs and Chemicals
  algae and toxins T65.82-
  Bacillus B (aertrycke) (cholerae (suis)) (paratyphosus) (suipestifer) A02.9
    botulinus A05.1
  bacterial toxins A05.9
  berries, noxious — *see* Poisoning, food, noxious, berries
  botulism A05.1
  ciguatera fish T61.0-
  Clostridium botulinum A05.1
  death-cap (Amanita phalloides) (Amanita verna) — *see* Poisoning, food, noxious, mushrooms
  drug — *see* Table of Drugs and Chemicals, by drug, poisoning
  epidemic, fish (noxious) — *see* Poisoning, seafood
    bacterial A05.9
  fava bean D55.0
  fish (noxious) T61.9-
    bacterial — *see* Intoxication, foodborne, by agent
    ciguatera fish — *see* Poisoning, ciguatera fish
    scombroid fish — *see* Poisoning, scombroid fish
    specified type NEC T61.77-
  food NEC A05.9
    bacterial — *see* Intoxication, foodborne, by agent
    due to

Polyneuropathy (peripheral) - *continued*
- in (due to) - *continued*
  - amyloidosis, familial (Portuguese) E85.1 *[G63]*
  - antitetanus serum G61.1
  - arsenic G62.2
    - sequelae G65.2
  - avitaminosis NEC E56.9 *[G63]*
  - beriberi E51.11
  - collagen vascular disease NEC M35.9 *[G63]*
  - deficiency (of)
    - B (-complex) vitamins E53.9 *[G63]*
    - vitamin B6 E53.1 *[G63]*
  - diabetes — *see* Diabetes, polyneuropathy
  - diphtheria A36.83
  - drug or medicament G62.0
    - correct substance properly administered — *see* Table of Drugs and Chemicals, by drug, adverse effect
    - overdose or wrong substance given or taken — *see* Table of Drugs and Chemicals, by drug, poisoning
  - endocrine disease NEC E34.9 *[G63]*
  - herpes zoster B02.23
  - hypoglycemia E16.2 *[G63]*
  - infectious
    - disease NEC B99 *[G63]*
    - mononucleosis B27.91
  - lack of vitamin NEC E56.9 *[G63]*
  - lead G62.2
    - sequelae G65.2
  - leprosy A30.9 *[G63]*
  - Lyme disease A69.22
  - metabolic disease NEC E88.9 *[G63]*
  - microscopic polyangiitis M31.7 *[G63]*
  - mumps B26.84
  - neoplastic disease — *see also* Neoplasm D49.9 *[G63]*
  - nutritional deficiency NEC E63.9 *[G63]*
  - organophosphate compounds G62.2
    - sequelae G65.2
  - parasitic disease NEC B89 *[G63]*
  - pellagra E52 *[G63]*
  - polyarteritis nodosa M30.0
  - porphyria E80.20 *[G63]*
  - radiation G62.82
  - rheumatoid arthritis — *see* Rheumatoid, polyneuropathy
  - sarcoidosis D86.89
  - serum G61.1
  - syphilis (late) A52.15
    - congenital A50.43
  - systemic
    - connective tissue disorder M35.9 *[G63]*
    - lupus erythematosus M32.19
  - toxic agent NEC G62.2
    - sequelae G65.2
  - transthyretin-related (ATTR) familial amyloid E85.1
  - triorthocresyl phosphate G62.2
    - sequelae G65.2
  - tuberculosis A17.89
  - uremia N18.9 *[G63]*
  - vitamin B12 deficiency E53.8 *[G63]*
    - with anemia (pernicious) D51.0 *[G63]*
      - due to dietary deficiency D51.3 *[G63]*
  - zoster B02.23
- inflammatory G61.9
  - chronic demyelinating (CIDP) G61.81
  - sequelae G65.1
  - specified NEC G61.89
- lead G62.2
  - sequelae G65.2
- nutritional NEC E63.9 *[G63]*
- postherpetic (zoster) B02.23
- progressive G60.3
- radiation-induced G62.82
- sensory (hereditary) (idiopathic) G60.8
- specified NEC G62.89
- syphilitic (late) A52.15
  - congenital A50.43

Polyopia H53.8

Polyorchism, polyorchidism Q55.21

Polyosteoarthritis — *see also* Osteoarthritis, generalized M15.9-
- post-traumatic M15.3
- specified NEC M15.8

Polyostotic fibrous dysplasia Q78.1

Polyotia Q17.0

Polyp, polypus
- accessory sinus J33.8
- adenocarcinoma in — *see* Neoplasm, malignant, by site
- adenocarcinoma in situ in — *see* Neoplasm, in situ, by site
- adenoid tissue J33.0
- adenomatous — *see also* Neoplasm, benign, by site
  - adenocarcinoma in — *see* Neoplasm, malignant, by site
  - adenocarcinoma in situ in — *see* Neoplasm, in situ, by site
  - carcinoma in — *see* Neoplasm, malignant, by site
  - carcinoma in situ in — *see* Neoplasm, in situ, by site
  - multiple — *see* Neoplasm, benign
    - adenocarcinoma in — *see* Neoplasm, malignant, by site
    - adenocarcinoma in situ in — *see* Neoplasm, in situ, by site
- antrum J33.8
- anus, anal (canal) K62.0
- Bartholin's gland N84.3
- bladder D41.4
- carcinoma in — *see* Neoplasm, malignant, by site
- carcinoma in situ in — *see* Neoplasm, in situ, by site
- cecum D12.0
- cervix (uteri) N84.1
  - in pregnancy or childbirth — *see* Pregnancy, complicated by, abnormal, cervix
  - mucous N84.1
  - nonneoplastic N84.1
- choanal J33.0
- cholesterol K82.4
- clitoris N84.3
- colon K63.5
  - adenomatous D12.6
    - ascending D12.2
    - cecum D12.0
    - descending D12.4
    - sigmoid D12.5
    - transverse D12.3
  - ascending K63.5
  - cecum K63.5
  - descending K63.5
  - hyperplastic, (any site) K63.5
  - inflammatory K51.40
    - with
      - abscess K51.414
      - complication K51.419
        - specified NEC K51.418
      - fistula K51.413
      - intestinal obstruction K51.412
      - rectal bleeding K51.411
  - sigmoid K63.5
  - transverse K63.5
- corpus uteri N84.0
- dental K04.01
  - irreversible K04.02
  - reversible K04.01
- duodenum K31.7
- ear (middle) H74.4-
- endometrium N84.0
- esophageal K22.81
- esophagogastric junction K22.82
- ethmoidal (sinus) J33.8
- fallopian tube N84.8
- female genital tract N84.9
  - specified NEC N84.8
- frontal (sinus) J33.8
- gallbladder K82.4
- gingiva, gum K06.8
- labia, labium (majus) (minus) N84.3
- larynx (mucous) J38.1

Polyp, polypus - *continued*
- larynx (mucous) - *continued*
  - adenomatous D14.1
- malignant — *see* Neoplasm, malignant, by site
- maxillary (sinus) J33.8
- middle ear — *see* Polyp, ear (middle)
- myometrium N84.0
- nares
  - anterior J33.9
  - posterior J33.0
- nasal (mucous) J33.9
  - cavity J33.0
  - septum J33.0
- nasopharyngeal J33.0
- nose (mucous) J33.9
- oviduct N84.8
- pharynx J39.2
- placenta O90.89
- prostate — *see* Enlargement, enlarged, prostate
- pudenda, pudendum N84.3
- pulpal (dental) K04.01
  - irreversible K04.02
  - reversible K04.01
- rectum (nonadenomatous) K62.1
  - adenomatous — *see* Polyp, adenomatous
- septum (nasal) J33.0
- sinus (accessory) (ethmoidal) (frontal) (maxillary) (sphenoidal) J33.8
- sphenoidal (sinus) J33.8
- stomach K31.7
  - adenomatous D13.1
- tube, fallopian N84.8
- turbinate, mucous membrane J33.8
- umbilical, newborn P83.6
- ureter N28.89
- urethra N36.2
- uterus (body) (corpus) (mucous) N84.0
  - cervix N84.1
  - in pregnancy or childbirth — *see* Pregnancy, complicated by, tumor, uterus
- vagina N84.2
- vocal cord (mucous) J38.1
- vulva N84.3

Polyphagia R63.2

Polyploidy Q92.7

Polypoid — *see* condition

Polyposis — *see also* Polyp
- coli (adenomatous) D12.6
  - adenocarcinoma in C18.9
  - adenocarcinoma in situ in — *see* Neoplasm, in situ, by site
  - carcinoma in C18.9
- colon (adenomatous) D12.6
- familial D12.6
  - adenocarcinoma in situ in — *see* Neoplasm, in situ, by site
- intestinal (adenomatous) D12.6
- malignant lymphomatous C83.1-
- multiple, adenomatous — *see also* Neoplasm, benign D36.9

Polyradiculitis — *see* Polyneuropathy

Polyradiculoneuropathy (acute) (postinfective) (segmentally demyelinating) G61.0

Polyserositis
- due to pericarditis I31.1
- pericardial I31.1
- periodic, familial E85.0
- tuberculous A19.9
  - acute A19.1
  - chronic A19.8

Polysplenia syndrome Q89.09

Polysyndactyly — *see also* Syndactylism, syndactyly Q70.4

Polytrichia L68.3

Polyunguia Q84.6

Polyuria R35.89
- nocturnal R35.81
- psychogenic F45.8
- specified NEC R35.89

Pompe's disease (glycogen storage) E74.02

Pompholyx L30.1

- **Pre-eclampsia** - *continued*
  - severe - *continued*
    - with hemolysis, elevated liver enzymes and low platelet count (HELLP) - *continued*
      - complicating
        - childbirth O14.24
        - puerperium O14.25
    - complicating
      - childbirth O14.14
      - puerperium O14.15
- **Pre-eruptive color change, teeth, tooth** K00.8
- **Pre-excitation atrioventricular conduction** I45.6
- **Preglaucoma** H40.00-
- **Pregnancy (single) (uterine)** — *see also* Delivery and Puerperal Z33.1
  - Note: The Tabular must be reviewed for assignment of the appropriate character indicating the trimester of the pregnancy
  - Note: The Tabular must be reviewed for assignment of appropriate seventh character for multiple gestation codes in Chapter 15
  - abdominal (ectopic) O00.00
    - with intrauterine pregnancy O00.01
    - with viable fetus O36.7-
  - ampullar O00.10-
    - with intrauterine pregnancy O00.11-
  - biochemical O02.81
  - broad ligament O00.80
    - with intrauterine pregnancy O00.81
  - cervical O00.80
    - with intrauterine pregnancy O00.81
  - chemical O02.81
  - complicated NOS O26.9-
  - complicated by (care of) (management affected by)
    - abnormal, abnormality
      - cervix O34.4-
        - causing obstructed labor O65.5
      - cord (umbilical) O69.9
      - fetal heart rate or rhythm O36.83-
      - findings on antenatal screening of mother O28.9
        - biochemical O28.1
        - cytological O28.2
        - chromosomal O28.5
        - genetic O28.5
        - hematological O28.0
        - radiological O28.4
        - specified NEC O28.8
        - ultrasonic O28.3
      - glucose (tolerance) NEC O99.810
      - pelvic organs O34.9-
        - specified NEC O34.8-
          - causing obstructed labor O65.5
      - pelvis (bony) (major) NEC O33.0
      - perineum O34.7-
      - position
        - placenta O44.0-
          - with hemorrhage O44.1-
        - uterus O34.59-
      - uterus O34.59-
        - causing obstructed labor O65.5
        - congenital O34.0-
      - vagina O34.6-
        - causing obstructed labor O65.5
      - vulva O34.7-
        - causing obstructed labor O65.5
    - abruptio placentae — *see* Abruptio placentae
    - abscess or cellulitis
      - bladder O23.1-
      - breast O91.11-
      - genital organ or tract O23.9-
    - abuse
      - physical O9A.31-
      - psychological O9A.51-
      - sexual O9A.41-
    - adverse effect anesthesia O29.9-
      - aspiration pneumonitis O29.01-
      - cardiac arrest O29.11-
      - cardiac complication NEC O29.19-
      - cardiac failure O29.12-

- **Pregnancy (single) (uterine)** - *continued*
  - complicated by (care of) (management affected by) - *continued*
    - adverse effect anesthesia - *continued*
      - central nervous system complication NEC O29.29-
      - cerebral anoxia O29.21-
      - failed or difficult intubation O29.6-
      - inhalation of stomach contents or secretions NOS O29.01-
      - local, toxic reaction O29.3X
      - Mendelson's syndrome O29.01-
      - pressure collapse of lung O29.02-
      - pulmonary complications NEC O29.09-
      - specified NEC O29.8X-
      - spinal and epidural type NEC O29.5X
        - induced headache O29.4-
    - albuminuria — *see also* Proteinuria, gestational O12.1-
    - alcohol use O99.31-
    - amnionitis O41.12-
    - anaphylactoid syndrome of pregnancy O88.01-
    - anemia (conditions in D50-D64) (pre-existing) O99.01-
      - complicating the puerperium O99.03
    - antepartum hemorrhage O46.9-
      - with coagulation defect — *see* Hemorrhage, antepartum, with coagulation defect
      - specified NEC O46.8X-
    - appendicitis O99.61-
    - atrophy (yellow) (acute) liver (subacute) O26.61-
    - bariatric surgery status O99.84-
    - bicornis or bicornuate uterus O34.0-
    - biliary tract problems O26.61-
    - breech presentation O32.1
    - cardiovascular diseases (conditions in I00-I09, I20-I52, I70-I99) O99.41-
    - cerebrovascular disorders (conditions in I60-I69) O99.41-
    - cervical shortening O26.87-
    - cervicitis O23.51-
    - cesarean scar defect (isthmocele) O34.22
    - chloasma (gravidarum) O26.89-
    - cholestasis (intrahepatic) O26.61-
    - cholecystitis O99.61-
    - chorioamnionitis O41.12-
    - circulatory system disorder (conditions in I00-I09, I20-I99, O99.41-)
    - compound presentation O32.6
    - conjoined twins O30.02-
    - connective system disorders (conditions in M00-M99) O99.891
    - contracted pelvis (general) O33.1
      - inlet O33.2
      - outlet O33.3
    - convulsions (eclamptic) (uremic) — *see also* Eclampsia O15.9-
    - cracked nipple O92.11-
    - cystitis O23.1-
    - cystocele O34.8-
    - death of fetus (near term) O36.4
      - early pregnancy O02.1
      - of one fetus or more in multiple gestation O31.2-
    - deciduitis O41.14-
    - decreased fetal movement O36.81-
    - dental problems O99.61-
    - diabetes (mellitus) O24.91-
      - gestational (pregnancy induced) — *see* Diabetes, gestational
      - pre-existing O24.31-
        - specified NEC O24.81-
        - type 1 O24.01-
        - type 2 O24.11-
    - digestive system disorders (conditions in K00-K93) O99.61-
    - diseases of — *see* Pregnancy, complicated by, specified body system disease
      - biliary tract O26.61-
      - blood NEC (conditions in D65-D77) O99.11-
      - liver O26.61-

- **Pregnancy (single) (uterine)** - *continued*
  - complicated by (care of) (management affected by) - *continued*
    - diseases of - *continued*
      - specified NEC O99.891
    - disorders of — *see* Pregnancy, complicated by, specified body system disorder
      - amniotic fluid and membranes O41.9-
        - specified NEC O41.8X-
      - biliary tract O26.61-
      - ear and mastoid process (conditions in H60-H95) O99.891
      - eye and adnexa (conditions in H00-H59) O99.891
      - liver O26.61-
      - skin (conditions in L00-L99) O99.71-
      - specified NEC O99.891
    - displacement, uterus NEC O34.59-
      - causing obstructed labor O65.5
    - disproportion (due to) O33.9
      - fetal (ascites) (hydrops) (meningomyelocele) (sacral teratoma) (tumor) deformities NEC O33.7
      - generally contracted pelvis O33.1
      - hydrocephalic fetus O33.6
      - inlet contraction of pelvis O33.2
      - mixed maternal and fetal origin O33.4
      - specified NEC O33.8
    - double uterus O34.0-
      - causing obstructed labor O65.5
    - drug use (conditions in F11-F19) O99.32-
    - eclampsia, eclamptic (coma) (convulsions) (delirium) (nephritis) (uremia) — *see also* Eclampsia O15.-
    - ectopic pregnancy — *see* Pregnancy, ectopic
    - edema O12.0-
      - with
        - gestational hypertension, mild — *see also* Pre-eclampsia O14.0-
      - proteinuria O12.2-
    - effusion, amniotic fluid — *see* Pregnancy, complicated by, premature rupture of membranes
    - elderly
      - multigravida O09.52-
      - primigravida O09.51-
    - embolism — *see also* Embolism, obstetric, pregnancy O88.-
    - endocrine diseases NEC O99.28-
    - endometritis O86.12
    - excessive weight gain O26.0-
    - exhaustion O26.81-
      - during labor and delivery O75.81
    - face presentation O32.3
    - failed induction of labor O61.9
      - instrumental O61.1
      - mechanical O61.1
      - medical O61.0
      - specified NEC O61.8
      - surgical O61.1
    - failed or difficult intubation for anesthesia O29.6-
    - false labor (pains) O47.9
      - at or after 37 completed weeks of pregnancy O47.1
      - before 37 completed weeks of pregnancy O47.0-
    - fatigue O26.81-
      - during labor and delivery O75.81
    - fatty metamorphosis of liver O26.61-
    - female genital mutilation O34.8- *[N90.81-]*
    - fetal (maternal care for)
      - abnormality or damage O35.9
        - acid-base balance O68
        - specified type NEC O35.8
      - acidemia O68
      - acidosis O68
      - alkalosis O68
      - anemia and thrombocytopenia O36.82-
      - anencephaly O35.0
      - bradycardia O36.83-
      - chromosomal abnormality (conditions in Q90-Q99) O35.1

Pregnancy (single) (uterine) - *continued*
- complicated by (care of) (management affected by) - *continued*
  - fetal (maternal care for) - *continued*
    - conjoined twins O30.02-
    - damage from
      - amniocentesis O35.7
      - biopsy procedures O35.7
      - drug addiction O35.5
      - hematological investigation O35.7
      - intrauterine contraceptive device O35.7
      - maternal
        - alcohol addiction O35.4
        - cytomegalovirus infection O35.3
        - disease NEC O35.8
        - drug addiction O35.5
        - listeriosis O35.8
        - rubella O35.3
        - toxoplasmosis O35.8
        - viral infection O35.3
      - medical procedure NEC O35.7
      - radiation O35.6
    - death (near term) O36.4
      - early pregnancy O02.1
    - decreased movement O36.81-
    - depressed heart rate tones O36.83-
    - disproportion due to deformity (fetal) O33.7
    - excessive growth (large for dates) O36.6-
    - growth retardation O36.59-
      - light for dates O36.59-
      - small for dates O36.59-
    - heart rate irregularity (abnormal variability) (bradycardia) (decelerations) (tachycardia) O36.83-
    - hereditary disease O35.2
    - hydrocephalus O35.0
    - intrauterine death O36.4
    - non-reassuring heart rate or rhythm O36.83-
    - poor growth O36.59-
      - light for dates O36.59-
      - small for dates O36.59-
    - problem O36.9-
      - specified NEC O36.89-
    - reduction (elective) O31.3-
    - selective termination O31.3-
    - spina bifida O35.0
    - thrombocytopenia O36.82-
  - fibroid (tumor) (uterus) O34.1-
  - fissure of nipple O92.11-
  - gallstones O99.61-
  - gastric banding status O99.84-
  - gastric bypass status O99.84-
  - genital herpes (asymptomatic) (history of) (inactive) O98.3-
  - genital tract infection O23.9-
  - glomerular diseases (conditions in N00-N07) O26.83-
    - with hypertension, pre-existing — *see* Hypertension, complicating, pregnancy, pre-existing, with, renal disease
  - gonorrhea O98.21-
  - grand multiparity O09.4
  - habitual aborter — *see* Pregnancy, complicated by, recurrent pregnancy loss
  - HELLP syndrome (hemolysis, elevated liver enzymes and low platelet count) O14.2-
  - hemorrhage
    - antepartum — *see* Hemorrhage, antepartum
    - before 20 completed weeks gestation O20.9
      - specified NEC O20.8
    - due to premature separation, placenta — *see also* Abruptio placentae O45.9-
    - early O20.9
      - specified NEC O20.8
    - threatened abortion O20.0

Pregnancy (single) (uterine) - *continued*
- complicated by (care of) (management affected by) - *continued*
  - hemorrhoids O22.4-
  - hepatitis (viral) O98.41-
  - herniation of uterus O34.59-
  - high
    - head at term O32.4
    - risk — *see* Supervision (of) (for), high-risk
  - history of in utero procedure during previous pregnancy O09.82-
  - HIV O98.71-
  - human immunodeficiency virus (HIV) disease O98.71-
  - hydatidiform mole — *see also* Mole, hydatidiform O01.9-
  - hydramnios O40.-
  - hydrocephalic fetus (disproportion) O33.6
  - hydrops
    - amnii O40.-
    - fetalis O36.2-
      - associated with isoimmunization — *see also* Pregnancy, complicated by, isoimmunization O36.11-
  - hydrorrhea O42.90
  - hyperemesis (gravidarum) (mild) — *see also* Hyperemesis, gravidarum O21.0-
  - hypertension — *see* Hypertension, complicating pregnancy
  - hypertensive
    - heart and renal disease, pre-existing — *see* Hypertension, complicating, pregnancy, pre-existing, with, heart disease, with renal disease
    - heart disease, pre-existing — *see* Hypertension, complicating, pregnancy, pre-existing, with, heart disease
    - renal disease, pre-existing — *see* Hypertension, complicating, pregnancy, pre-existing, with, renal disease
  - hypotension O26.5-
  - immune disorders NEC (conditions in D80-D89) O99.11-
  - incarceration, uterus O34.51-
  - incompetent cervix O34.3-
  - inconclusive fetal viability O36.80
  - infection (s) O98.91-
    - amniotic fluid or sac O41.10-
    - bladder O23.1-
    - carrier state NEC O99.830
      - streptococcus B O99.820
    - genital organ or tract O23.9-
      - specified NEC O23.59-
    - genitourinary tract O23.9-
    - gonorrhea O98.21-
    - hepatitis (viral) O98.41-
    - HIV O98.71-
    - human immunodeficiency virus (HIV) O98.71-
    - intrauterine O41.12
    - kidney O23.0-
    - nipple O91.01-
    - parasitic disease O98.91-
      - specified NEC O98.81-
    - protozoal disease O98.61-
    - sexually transmitted NEC O98.31-
    - specified type NEC O98.81-
    - syphilis O98.11-
    - tuberculosis O98.01-
    - urethra O23.2-
    - urinary (tract) O23.4-
      - specified NEC O23.3-
    - viral disease O98.51-
  - inflammation
    - intrauterine O41.12
  - injury or poisoning (conditions in S00-T88) O9A.21-
    - due to abuse
      - physical O9A.31-
      - psychological O9A.51-
      - sexual O9A.41-
  - insufficient

Pregnancy (single) (uterine) - *continued*
- complicated by (care of) (management affected by) - *continued*
  - insufficient - *continued*
    - prenatal care O09.3-
    - weight gain O26.1-
  - insulin resistance O26.89
  - intrauterine fetal death (near term) O36.4
    - early pregnancy O02.1
    - multiple gestation (one fetus or more) O31.2-
  - isoimmunization O36.11-
    - anti-A sensitization O36.11-
    - anti-B sensitization O36.19-
    - Rh O36.09-
      - anti-D antibody O36.01-
    - specified NEC O36.19-
  - laceration of uterus NEC O71.81
  - malformation
    - placenta, placental (vessel) O43.10-
      - specified NEC O43.19-
    - uterus (congenital) O34.0-
  - malnutrition (conditions in E40-E46) O25.1-
  - maternal hypotension syndrome O26.5-
  - mental disorders (conditions in F01-F09, F20-F52 and F54-F99) O99.34-
    - alcohol use O99.31-
    - drug use O99.32-
    - smoking O99.33-
  - mentum presentation O32.3
  - metabolic disorders O99.28-
  - missed
    - abortion O02.1
    - delivery O36.4
  - multiple gestations O30.9-
    - conjoined twins O30.02-
    - specified number of multiples NEC — *see* Pregnancy, multiple (gestation), specified NEC
    - quadruplet — *see* Pregnancy, quadruplet
    - specified complication NEC O31.8X-
    - triplet — *see* Pregnancy, triplet
    - twin — *see* Pregnancy, twin
  - musculoskeletal condition (conditions is M00-M99) O99.891
  - necrosis, liver (conditions in K72) O26.61-
  - neoplasm
    - benign
      - cervix O34.4-
      - corpus uteri O34.1-
      - uterus O34.1-
    - malignant O9A.11-
  - nephropathy NEC O26.83-
  - nervous system condition (conditions in G00-G99) O99.35-
  - nutritional diseases NEC O99.28-
  - obesity (pre-existing) O99.21-
  - obesity surgery status O99.84-
  - oblique lie or presentation O32.2
  - older mother — *see* Pregnancy, complicated by, elderly
  - oligohydramnios O41.0-
    - with premature rupture of membranes — *see also* Pregnancy, complicated by, premature rupture of membranes O42.-
  - onset (spontaneous) of labor after 37 completed weeks of gestation but before 39 completed weeks gestation, with delivery by (planned) cesarean section O75.82
  - oophoritis O23.52-
  - overdose, drug — *see also* Table of Drugs and Chemicals, by drug, poisoning O9A.21-
  - oversize fetus O33.5
  - papyraceous fetus O31.0-
  - pelvic inflammatory disease O99.891
  - periodontal disease O99.61-
  - peripheral neuritis O26.82-
  - peritoneal (pelvic) adhesions O99.891
  - phlebitis O22.9-
  - phlebopathy O22.9-
  - phlebothrombosis (superficial) O22.2-

PREGNANCY - PREGNANCY

Pregnancy (single) (uterine) - *continued*
complicated by (care of) (management affected by) - *continued*
phlebothrombosis (superficial) - *continued*
deep O22.3-
placenta accreta O43.21-
placenta increta O43.22-
placenta percreta O43.23-
placenta previa O44.0-
complete O44.0-
with hemorrhage O44.1-
marginal O44.2-
with hemorrhage O44.3-
partial O44.2-
with hemorrhage O44.3-
placental disorder O43.9-
specified NEC O43.89-
placental dysfunction O43.89-
placental infarction O43.81-
placental insufficiency O36.51-
placental transfusion syndromes
fetomaternal O43.01-
fetus to fetus O43.02-
maternofetal O43.01-
placentitis O41.14-
pneumonia O99.51-
poisoning — *see also* Table of Drugs and Chemicals O9A.21-
polyhydramnios O40-
polymorphic eruption of pregnancy O26.86
poor obstetric history NEC O09.29-
postmaturity (post-term) (40 to 42 weeks) O48.0
more than 42 completed weeks gestation (prolonged) O48.1
pre-eclampsia O14.9-
mild O14.0-
moderate O14.0-
severe O14.1-
with hemolysis, elevated liver enzymes and low platelet count (HELLP) O14.2-
premature labor — *see* Pregnancy, complicated by, preterm labor
premature rupture of membranes O42.90
full-term, unspecified as to length of time between rupture and onset of labor O42.92
with onset of labor
within 24 hours O42.00
at or after 37 weeks gestation, onset of labor within 24 hours of rupture O42.02
pre-term (before 37 completed weeks of gestation) O42.01-
after 24 hours O42.10
at or after 37 weeks gestation, onset of labor more than 24 hours following rupture O42.12
pre-term (before 37 completed weeks of gestation) O42.11-
at or after 37 weeks gestation, unspecified as to length of time between rupture and onset of labor O42.92
pre-term (before 37 completed weeks of gestation) O42.91-
premature separation of placenta — *see also* Abruptio placentae O45.9-
presentation, fetal — *see* Delivery, complicated by, malposition
preterm delivery O60.10
preterm labor
with delivery O60.10
preterm O60.10
term O60.20
second trimester
with term delivery O60.22
without delivery O60.02
with preterm delivery
second trimester O60.12
third trimester O60.13
third trimester
with term delivery O60.23

Pregnancy (single) (uterine) - *continued*
complicated by (care of) (management affected by) - *continued*
preterm labor - *continued*
third trimester - *continued*
without delivery O60.03
with third trimester preterm delivery O60.14
without delivery O60.00
second trimester O60.02
third trimester O60.03
previous history of — *see* Pregnancy, supervision of, high-risk
prolapse, uterus O34.52-
proteinuria (gestational) — *see also* Proteinuria, gestational O12.1-
with edema O12.2-
pruritic urticarial papules and plaques of pregnancy (PUPPP) O26.86
pruritus (neurogenic) O26.89-
psychosis or psychoneurosis (puerperal) F53.1
ptyalism O26.89-
PUPPP (pruritic urticarial papules and plaques of pregnancy) O26.86
pyelitis O23.0-
recurrent pregnancy loss O26.2-
renal disease or failure NEC O26.83-
with secondary hypertension, pre-existing — *see* Hypertension, complicating, pregnancy, pre-existing, secondary
hypertensive, pre-existing — *see* Hypertension, complicating, pregnancy, pre-existing, with, renal disease
respiratory condition (conditions in J00-J99) O99.51-
retained, retention
dead ovum O02.0
intrauterine contraceptive device O26.3-
retroversion, uterus O34.53-
Rh immunization, incompatibility or sensitization NEC O36.09-
anti-D antibody O36.01-
rupture
amnion (premature) — *see also* Pregnancy, complicated by, premature rupture of membranes O42-
membranes (premature) — *see also* Pregnancy, complicated by, premature rupture of membranes O42-
uterus (during labor) O71.1
before onset of labor O71.0-
salivation (excessive) O26.89-
salpingitis O23.52-
salpingo-oophoritis O23.52-
sepsis (conditions in A40, A41) O98.81-
size date discrepancy (uterine) O26.84-
skin condition (conditions in L00-L99) O99.71-
smoking (tobacco) O99.33-
social problem O09.7-
specified condition NEC O26.89-
spotting O26.85-
streptococcus group B (GBS) carrier state O99.820
subluxation of symphysis (pubis) O26.71-
syphilis (conditions in A50-A53) O98.11-
threatened
abortion O20.0
labor O47.9
at or after 37 completed weeks of gestation O47.1
before 37 completed weeks of gestation O47.0-
thrombophlebitis (superficial) O22.2-
thrombosis O22.9-
cerebral venous O22.5-
cerebrovenous sinus O22.5-
deep O22.3-
tobacco use disorder (smoking) O99.33-
torsion of uterus O34.59-

Pregnancy (single) (uterine) - *continued*
complicated by (care of) (management affected by) - *continued*
toxemia O14.9-
transverse lie or presentation O32.2
tuberculosis (conditions in A15-A19) O98.01-
tumor (benign)
cervix O34.4-
malignant O9A.11-
uterus O34.1-
unstable lie O32.0
upper respiratory infection O99.51-
urethritis O23.2-
uterine size date discrepancy O26.84-
vaginitis or vulvitis O23.59-
varicose veins (lower extremities) O22.0-
genitals O22.1-
legs O22.0-
perineal O22.1-
vaginal or vulval O22.1-
venereal disease NEC (conditions in A63.8) O98.31-
venous disorders O22.9-
specified NEC O22.8X-
viral diseases (conditions in A80-B09, B25-B34) O98.51-
very young mother — *see* Pregnancy, complicated by, young mother
vomiting O21.9
due to diseases classified elsewhere O21.8
hyperemesis gravidarum (mild) — *see also* Hyperemesis, gravidarum O21.0-
late (occurring after 20 weeks of gestation) O21.2
young mother
multigravida O09.62-
primigravida O09.61-
concealed O09.3-
continuing following
elective fetal reduction of one or more fetus O31.3-
intrauterine death of one or more fetus O31.2-
spontaneous abortion of one or more fetus O31.1-
cornual O00.80
with intrauterine pregnancy O00.81
ectopic (ruptured) O00.90
with intrauterine pregnancy O00.91
abdominal O00.00
with
intrauterine pregnancy O00.01
viable fetus O36.7-
cervical O00.80
with intrauterine pregnancy O00.81
complicated (by) O08.9
afibrinogenemia O08.1
cardiac arrest O08.81
chemical damage of pelvic organ (s) O08.6
circulatory collapse O08.3
defibrination syndrome O08.1
electrolyte imbalance O08.5
embolism (amniotic fluid) (blood clot) (pulmonary) (septic) O08.2
endometritis O08.0
genital tract and pelvic infection O08.0
hemorrhage (delayed) (excessive) O08.1
infection
genital tract or pelvic O08.0
kidney 008.83
urinary tract O08.83
intravascular coagulation O08.1
laceration of pelvic organ (s) O08.6
metabolic disorder O08.5
oliguria O08.4
oophoritis O08.0
parametritis O08.0
pelvic peritonitis O08.0
perforation of pelvic organ (s) O08.6
renal failure or shutdown O08.4
salpingitis or salpingo-oophoritis O08.0

PREGNANCY - PREGNANCY

- **Pregnancy (single) (uterine)** - *continued*
  - ectopic (ruptured) - *continued*
    - complicated (by) - *continued*
      - sepsis O08.82
      - shock O08.83
        - septic O08.82
      - specified condition NEC O08.89
      - tubular necrosis (renal) O08.4
      - uremia O08.4
      - urinary infection O08.83
      - venous complication NEC O08.7
        - embolism O08.2
    - cornual O00.80
      - with intrauterine pregnancy O00.81
    - intraligamentous O00.80
      - with intrauterine pregnancy O00.81
    - mural O00.80
      - with intrauterine pregnancy O00.81
    - ovarian O00.20-
      - with intrauterine pregnancy O00.21-
    - specified site NEC O00.80
      - with intrauterine pregnancy O00.81
    - tubal (ruptured) O00.10-
      - with intrauterine pregnancy O00.11-
  - examination (normal) Z34.9-
    - high-risk — *see* Pregnancy, supervision of, high-risk
    - first Z34.0-
    - specified Z34.8-
  - extrauterine — *see* Pregnancy, ectopic
  - fallopian O00.10-
    - with intrauterine pregnancy O00.11-
  - false F45.8
  - gestational carrier Z33.3
  - heptachorionic, hepta-amniotic (septuplets) O30.83-
  - hexachorionic, hexa-amniotic (sextuplets) O30.83-
  - hidden O09.3-
  - high-risk — *see* Pregnancy, supervision of, high-risk
  - incidental finding Z33.1
  - interstitial O00.80
    - with intrauterine pregnancy O00.81
  - intraligamentous O00.80
    - with intrauterine pregnancy O00.81
  - intramural O00.80
    - with intrauterine pregnancy O00.81
  - intraperitoneal O00.00
    - with intrauterine pregnancy O00.01
  - isthmian O00.10-
    - with intrauterine pregnancy O00.11-
  - mesometric (mural) O00.80
    - with intrauterine pregnancy O00.81
  - molar NEC O02.0
    - complicated (by) O08.9
      - afibrinogenemia O08.1
      - cardiac arrest O08.81
      - chemical damage of pelvic organ (s) O08.6
      - circulatory collapse O08.3
      - defibrination syndrome O08.1
      - electrolyte imbalance O08.5
      - embolism (amniotic fluid) (blood clot) (pulmonary) (septic) O08.2
      - endometritis O08.0
      - genital tract and pelvic infection O08.0
      - hemorrhage (delayed) (excessive) O08.1
      - infection
        - genital tract or pelvic O08.0
        - kidney O08.83
        - urinary tract O08.83
      - intravascular coagulation O08.1
      - laceration of pelvic organ (s) O08.6
      - metabolic disorder O08.5
      - oliguria O08.4
      - oophoritis O08.0
      - parametritis O08.0
      - pelvic peritonitis O08.0
      - perforation of pelvic organ (s) O08.6
      - renal failure or shutdown O08.4
      - salpingitis or salpingo-oophoritis O08.0
      - sepsis O08.82
      - shock O08.3
        - septic O08.82

- **Pregnancy (single) (uterine)** - *continued*
  - molar NEC - *continued*
    - complicated (by) - *continued*
      - specified condition NEC O08.89
      - tubular necrosis (renal) O08.4
      - uremia O08.4
      - urinary infection O08.83
      - venous complication NEC O08.7
        - embolism O08.2
    - hydatidiform — *see also* Mole, hydatidiform O01.9-
  - multiple (gestation) O30.9-
    - greater than quadruplets — *see* Pregnancy, multiple (gestation), specified NEC
    - specified NEC O30.80-
      - with
        - two or more monoamniotic fetuses O30.82-
        - two or more monochorionic fetuses O30.81-
      - number of chorions and amnions are both equal to the number of fetuses O30.83-
      - two or more monoamniotic fetuses O30.82-
      - two or more monochorionic fetuses O30.81-
      - unable to determine number of placenta and number of amniotic sacs O30.89-
      - unspecified number of placenta and unspecified number of amniotic sacs O30.80-
  - mural O00.80
    - with intrauterine pregnancy O00.81
  - normal (supervision of) Z34.9-
    - high-risk — *see* Pregnancy, supervision of, high-risk
    - first Z34.0-
    - specified Z34.8-
  - ovarian O00.20-
    - with intrauterine pregnancy O00.21-
  - pentachorionic, penta-amniotic (quintuplets) O30.83-
  - postmature (40 to 42 weeks) O48.0
    - more than 42 weeks gestation O48.1
  - post-term (40 to 42 weeks) O48.0
  - prenatal care only Z34.9-
    - high-risk — *see* Pregnancy, supervision of, high-risk
    - first Z34.0-
    - specified Z34.8-
  - prolonged (more than 42 weeks gestation) O48.1
  - quadruplet O30.20-
    - with
      - two or more monoamniotic fetuses O30.22-
      - two or more monochorionic fetuses O30.21-
    - quadrachorionic/quadra-amniotic O30.23-
    - two or more monoamniotic fetuses O30.22-
    - two or more monochorionic fetuses O30.21-
    - unable to determine number of placenta and number of amniotic sacs O30.29-
    - unspecified number of placenta and unspecified number of amniotic sacs O30.20-
  - quintuplet — *see* Pregnancy, multiple (gestation), specified NEC
  - sextuplet — *see* Pregnancy, multiple (gestation), specified NEC
  - supervision of
    - concealed pregnancy O09.3-
    - elderly mother
      - multigravida O09.52-
      - primigravida O09.51-
    - hidden pregnancy O09.3-
    - high-risk O09.9-
      - due to (history of)
        - ectopic pregnancy O09.1-
        - elderly — *see* Pregnancy, supervision, elderly mother

- **Pregnancy (single) (uterine)** - *continued*
  - supervision of - *continued*
    - high-risk - *continued*
      - due to (history of) - *continued*
        - grand multiparity O09.4
        - infertility O09.0-
        - insufficient prenatal care O09.3-
        - in utero procedure during previous pregnancy O09.82-
        - in vitro fertilization O09.81-
        - molar pregnancy O09.A-
        - multiple previous pregnancies O09.4-
        - older mother — *see* Pregnancy, supervision of, elderly mother
        - poor reproductive or obstetric history NEC O09.29-
        - pre-term labor O09.21-
        - previous
          - neonatal death O09.29-
        - social problems O09.7-
        - specified NEC O09.89-
        - very young mother — *see* Pregnancy, supervision, young mother
      - resulting from in vitro fertilization O09.81-
    - normal Z34.9-
      - first Z34.0-
      - specified NEC Z34.8-
    - young mother
      - multigravida O09.62-
      - primigravida O09.61-
  - triplet O30.10-
    - with
      - two or more monoamniotic fetuses O30.12-
      - two or more monochorionic fetuses O30.11-
    - trichorionic/triamniotic O30.13-
    - two or more monoamniotic fetuses O30.12-
    - two or more monochorionic fetuses O30.11-
    - unable to determine number of placenta and number of amniotic sacs O30.19-
    - unspecified number of placenta and unspecified number of amniotic sacs O30.10-
  - tubal (with abortion) (with rupture) O00.10-
    - with intrauterine pregnancy O00.11-
  - twin O30.00-
    - conjoined O30.02-
    - dichorionic/diamniotic (two placenta, two amniotic sacs) O30.04-
    - monochorionic/diamniotic (one placenta, two amniotic sacs) O30.03-
    - monochorionic/monoamniotic (one placenta, one amniotic sac) O30.01-
    - unable to determine number of placenta and number of amniotic sacs O30.09-
    - unspecified number of placenta and unspecified number of amniotic sacs O30.00-
  - unwanted Z64.0
  - weeks of gestation
    - 8 weeks Z3A.08
    - 9 weeks Z3A.09
    - 10 weeks Z3A.10
    - 11 weeks Z3A.11
    - 12 weeks Z3A.12
    - 13 weeks Z3A.13
    - 14 weeks Z3A.14
    - 15 weeks Z3A.15
    - 16 weeks Z3A.16
    - 17 weeks Z3A.17
    - 18 weeks Z3A.18
    - 19 weeks Z3A.19
    - 20 weeks Z3A.20
    - 21 weeks Z3A.21
    - 22 weeks Z3A.22
    - 23 weeks Z3A.23
    - 24 weeks Z3A.24
    - 25 weeks Z3A.25
    - 26 weeks Z3A.26
    - 27 weeks Z3A.27
    - 28 weeks Z3A.28

Pregnancy (single) (uterine) - *continued*
weeks of gestation - *continued*
29 weeks Z3A.29
30 weeks Z3A.30
31 weeks Z3A.31
32 weeks Z3A.32
33 weeks Z3A.33
34 weeks Z3A.34
35 weeks Z3A.35
36 weeks Z3A.36
37 weeks Z3A.37
38 weeks Z3A.38
39 weeks Z3A.39
40 weeks Z3A.40
41 weeks Z3A.41
42 weeks Z3A.42
greater than 42 weeks Z3A.49
less than 8 weeks Z3A.01
not specified Z3A.00
Preiser's disease — *see* Osteonecrosis, secondary, due to, trauma, metacarpus
Pre-kwashiorkor — *see* Malnutrition, severe
Preleukemia (syndrome) D46.9
Preluxation, hip, congenital Q65.6
Premature — *see also* condition
adrenarche E27.0
aging E34.8
beats I49.40
atrial I49.1
auricular I49.1
supraventricular I49.1
birth NEC — *see* Preterm, newborn
closure, foramen ovale Q21.8
contraction
atrial I49.1
atrioventricular I49.2
auricular I49.1
auriculoventricular I49.49
heart (extrasystole) I49.49
junctional I49.2
ventricular I49.3
delivery — *see also* Pregnancy, complicated by, preterm labor O60.10
ejaculation F52.4
infant NEC — *see* Preterm, newborn
light-for-dates — *see* Light for dates
labor — *see* Pregnancy, complicated by, preterm labor
lungs P28.0
menopause E28.319
asymptomatic E28.319
symptomatic E28.310
newborn
extreme (less than 28 completed weeks) — *see* Immaturity, extreme
less than 37 completed weeks — *see* Preterm, newborn
puberty E30.1
rupture membranes or amnion — *see* Pregnancy, complicated by, premature rupture of membranes
senility E34.8
thelarche E30.8
ventricular systole I49.3
Prematurity NEC (less than 37 completed weeks) — *see* Preterm, newborn
extreme (less than 28 completed weeks) — *see* Immaturity, extreme
Premenstrual
dysphoric disorder (PMDD) F32.81
tension (syndrome) N94.3
Premolarization, cuspids K00.2
Prenatal
care, normal pregnancy — *see* Pregnancy, normal
screening of mother — *see also* Encounter, antenatal screening Z36.9
teeth K00.6
Preparatory care for subsequent treatment NEC
for dialysis Z49.01
peritoneal Z49.02
Prepartum — *see* condition
Preponderance, left or right ventricular I51.7
Prepuce — *see* condition
PRES (posterior reversible encephalopathy syndrome) I67.83
Presbycardia R54
Presbycusis, presbyacusia H91.1-
Presbyesophagus K22.89
Presbyophrenia F03
Presbyopia H52.4
Prescription of contraceptives (initial) Z30.019
barrier Z30.018
diaphragm Z30.018
emergency (postcoital) Z30.012
implantable subdermal Z30.017
injectable Z30.013
intrauterine contraceptive device Z30.014
pills Z30.011
postcoital (emergency) Z30.012
repeat Z30.40
barrier Z30.49
diaphragm Z30.49
implantable subdermal Z30.46
injectable Z30.42
pills Z30.41
specified type NEC Z30.49
transdermal patch hormonal Z30.45
vaginal ring hormonal Z30.44
specified type NEC Z30.018
transdermal patch hormonal Z30.016
vaginal ring hormonal Z30.015
Presence (of)
ankle-joint implant (functional) (prosthesis) Z96.66-
aortocoronary (bypass) graft Z95.1
arterial-venous shunt (dialysis) Z99.2
artificial
eye (globe) Z97.0
heart (fully implantable) (mechanical) Z95.812
valve Z95.2
larynx Z96.3
lens (intraocular) Z96.1
limb (complete) (partial) Z97.1-
arm Z97.1-
bilateral Z97.15
leg Z97.1-
bilateral Z97.16
audiological implant (functional) Z96.29
bladder implant (functional) Z96.0
bone
conduction hearing device Z96.29
implant (functional) NEC Z96.7
joint (prosthesis) — *see* Presence, joint implant
cardiac
defibrillator (functional) (with synchronous cardiac pacemaker) Z95.810
implant or graft Z95.9
specified type NEC Z95.818
pacemaker Z95.0
resynchronization therapy
defibrillator Z95.810
pacemaker Z95.0
cerebrospinal fluid drainage device Z98.2
cochlear implant (functional) Z96.21
contact lens (es) Z97.3
coronary artery graft or prosthesis Z95.5
CRT-D (cardiac resynchronization therapy defibrillator) Z95.810
CRT-P (cardiac resynchronization therapy pacemaker) Z95.0
cardioverter-defribrillator (ICD) Z95.810
CSF shunt Z98.2
dental prosthesis device Z97.2
dentures Z97.2
device (external) NEC Z97.8
cardiac NEC Z95.818
heart assist Z95.811
implanted (functional) Z96.9
specified NEC Z96.89
prosthetic Z97.8
ear implant Z96.20
cochlear implant Z96.21
myringotomy tube Z96.22

Presence (of) - *continued*
ear implant - *continued*
specified type NEC Z96.29
elbow-joint implant (functional) (prosthesis) Z96.62-
endocrine implant (functional) NEC Z96.49
eustachian tube stent or device (functional) Z96.29
external hearing-aid or device Z97.4
finger-joint implant (functional) (prosthetic) Z96.69-
functional implant Z96.9
specified NEC Z96.89
graft
cardiac NEC Z95.818
vascular NEC Z95.828
hearing-aid or device (external) Z97.4
implant (bone) (cochlear) (functional) Z96.21
heart assist device Z95.811
heart valve implant (functional) Z95.2
prosthetic Z95.2
specified type NEC Z95.4
xenogenic Z95.3
hip-joint implant (functional) (prosthesis) Z96.64-
ICD (cardioverter-defibrillator) Z95.810
implanted device (artificial) (functional) (prosthetic) Z96.9
automatic cardiac defibrillator (with synchronous cardiac pacemaker) Z95.810
cardiac pacemaker Z95.0
cochlear Z96.21
dental Z96.5
heart Z95.812
heart valve Z95.2
prosthetic Z95.2
specified NEC Z95.4
xenogenic Z95.3
insulin pump Z96.41
intraocular lens Z96.1
joint Z96.60
ankle Z96.66-
elbow Z96.62-
finger Z96.69-
hip Z96.64-
knee Z96.65-
shoulder Z96.61-
specified NEC Z96.698
wrist Z96.63-
larynx Z96.3
myringotomy tube Z96.22
otological Z96.20
cochlear Z96.21
eustachian stent Z96.29
myringotomy Z96.22
specified NEC Z96.29
stapes Z96.29
skin Z96.81
skull plate Z96.7
specified NEC Z96.89
urogenital Z96.0
insulin pump (functional) Z96.41
intestinal bypass or anastomosis Z98.0
intraocular lens (functional) Z96.1
intrauterine contraceptive device (IUD) Z97.5
intravascular implant (functional) (prosthetic) NEC Z95.9
coronary artery Z95.5
defibrillator (with synchronous cardiac pacemaker) Z95.810
peripheral vessel (with angioplasty) Z95.820
joint implant (prosthetic) (any) Z96.60
ankle — *see* Presence, ankle joint implant
elbow — *see* Presence, elbow joint implant
finger — *see* Presence, finger joint implant
hip — *see* Presence, hip joint implant
knee — *see* Presence, knee joint implant
shoulder — *see* Presence, shoulder joint implant
specified joint NEC Z96.698
wrist — *see* Presence, wrist joint implant

Presence (of) - *continued*
knee-joint implant (functional) (prosthesis) Z96.65-
laryngeal implant (functional) Z96.3
mandibular implant (dental) Z96.5
myringotomy tube (s) Z96.22
neurostimulator (brain) (gastric) (peripheral nerve) (sacral nerve) (spinal cord) (vagus nerve) Z96.82
orthopedic-joint implant (prosthetic) (any) — *see* Presence, joint implant
otological implant (functional) Z96.29
shoulder-joint implant (functional) (prosthesis) Z96.61-
skull-plate implant Z96.7
spectacles Z97.3
stapes implant (functional) Z96.29
systemic lupus erythematosus [SLE] inhibitor D68.62
tendon implant (functional) (graft) Z96.7
tooth root (s) implant Z96.5
ureteral stent Z96.0
urethral stent Z96.0
urogenital implant (functional) Z96.0
vascular implant or device Z95.9
access port device Z95.828
specified type NEC Z95.828
wrist-joint implant (functional) (prosthesis) Z96.63-
Presenile — *see also* condition
dementia F03
premature aging E34.8
Presentation, fetal — *see* Delivery , complicated by, malposition
Prespondylolisthesis (congenital) Q76.2
Pressure
area, skin — *see* Ulcer, pressure, by site
brachial plexus G54.0
brain G93.5
injury at birth NEC P11.1
cerebral — *see* Pressure, brain
chest R07.89
cone, tentorial G93.5
hyposystolic — *see also* Hypotension
incidental reading, without diagnosis of hypotension R03.1
increased
intracranial benign, G93.2
injury at birth P11.0
intraocular H40.05-
injury — *see* Ulcer, pressure, by site
lumbosacral plexus G54.1
mediastinum J98.59
necrosis (chronic) — *see* Ulcer, pressure, by site
parental, inappropriate (excessive) Z62.6
sore (chronic) — *see* Ulcer, pressure, by site
spinal cord G95.20
ulcer (chronic) — *see* Ulcer, pressure, by site
venous, increased I87.8
Pre-syncope R55
Preterm
delivery — *see also* Pregnancy, complicated by, preterm labor O60.10
labor — *see* Pregnancy, complicated by, preterm labor
newborn (infant) P07.30
gestational age
28 completed weeks (28 weeks, 0 days through 28 weeks, 6 days) P07.31
29 completed weeks (29 weeks, 0 days through 29 weeks, 6 days) P07.32
30 completed weeks (30 weeks, 0 days through 30 weeks, 6 days) P07.33
31 completed weeks (31 weeks, 0 days through 31 weeks, 6 days) P07.34
32 completed weeks (32 weeks, 0 days through 32 weeks, 6 days) P07.35
33 completed weeks (33 weeks, 0 days through 33 weeks, 6 days) P07.36
34 completed weeks (34 weeks, 0 days through 34 weeks, 6 days) P07.37
35 completed weeks (35 weeks, 0 days through 35 weeks, 6 days) P07.38

Preterm - *continued*
newborn (infant) - *continued*
gestational age - *continued*
36 completed weeks (36 weeks, 0 days through 36 weeks, 6 days) P07.39
Previa
placenta (total) (without hemorrhage) O44.0-
with hemorrhage O44.1-
complete O44.0-
with hemorrhage O44.1-
low — *see also* Delivery, complicated, by, placenta, low O44.4-
with hemorrhage O44.5-
marginal O44.2-
with hemorrhage O44.3-
partial O44.2-
with hemorrhage O44.3-
vasa O69.4
Priapism N48.30
due to
disease classified elsewhere N48.32
drug N48.33
specified cause NEC N48.39
trauma N48.31
Prickling sensation (skin) R20.2
Prickly heat L74.0
Primary — *see* condition
Primigravida
elderly, affecting management of pregnancy, labor and delivery (supervision only) — *see* Pregnancy, complicated by, elderly, primigravida
older, affecting management of pregnancy, labor and delivery (supervision only) — *see* Pregnancy, complicated by, elderly, primigravida
very young, affecting management of pregnancy, labor and delivery (supervision only) — *see* Pregnancy, complicated by, young mother, primigravida
Primipara
elderly, affecting management of pregnancy, labor and delivery (supervision only) — *see* Pregnancy, complicated by, elderly, primigravida
older, affecting management of pregnancy, labor and delivery (supervision only) — *see* Pregnancy, complicated by, elderly, primigravida
very young, affecting management of pregnancy, labor and delivery (supervision only) — *see* Pregnancy, complicated by, young mother, primigravida
Primus varus Q66.21-
PRIND (Prolonged reversible ischemic neurologic deficit) I63.9
Pringle's disease (tuberous sclerosis) Q85.1
Prinzmetal angina I20.1
Prizefighter ear — *see* Cauliflower ear
Problem (with) (related to)
academic Z55.8
acculturation Z60.3
adjustment (to)
change of job Z56.1
life-cycle transition Z60.0
pension Z60.0
retirement Z60.0
adopted child Z62.821
alcoholism in family Z63.72
atypical parenting situation Z62.9
bankruptcy Z59.89
behavioral (adult) F69
drug seeking Z76.5
birth of sibling affecting child Z62.898
care (of)
provider dependency Z74.9
specified NEC Z74.8
sick or handicapped person in family or household Z63.6
child
abuse (affecting the child) — *see* Maltreatment, child
custody or support proceedings Z65.3

Problem (with) (related to) - *continued*
child - *continued*
in welfare custody Z62.21
in care of non-parental family member Z62.21
in foster care Z62.21
living in orphanage or group home Z62.22
child-rearing Z62.9
specified NEC Z62.898
communication (developmental) F80.9
conflict or discord (with)
boss Z56.4
classmates Z55.4
counselor Z64.4
employer Z56.4
family Z63.9
specified NEC Z63.8
probation officer Z64.4
social worker Z64.4
teachers Z55.4
workmates Z56.4
conviction in legal proceedings Z65.0
with imprisonment Z65.1
counselor Z64.4
creditors Z59.89
digestive K92.9
drug addict in family Z63.72
ear — *see* Disorder, ear
economic Z59.9
affecting care Z59.9
specified NEC Z59.89
education Z55.9
specified NEC Z55.8
employment Z56.9
change of job Z56.1
discord Z56.4
environment Z56.5
sexual harassment Z56.81
specified NEC Z56.89
stress NEC Z56.6
stressful schedule Z56.3
threat of job loss Z56.2
unemployment Z56.0
enuresis, child F98.0
eye H57.9
failed examinations (school) Z55.2
falling Z91.81
family — *see also* Disruption, family Z63.9-
specified NEC Z63.8
feeding (elderly) (infant) R63.39
newborn P92.9
breast P92.5
overfeeding P92.4
slow P92.2
specified NEC P92.8
underfeeding P92.3
nonorganic F50.89
finance Z59.9
specified NEC Z59.89
foreclosure on loan Z59.89
foster child Z62.822
frightening experience (s) in childhood Z62.898
genital NEC
female N94.9
male N50.9
health care Z75.9
specified NEC Z75.8
hearing — *see* Deafness
homelessness Z59.00
housing Z59.9
inadequate Z59.1
isolated Z59.89
specified NEC Z59.89
identity (of childhood) F93.8
illegitimate pregnancy (unwanted) Z64.0
illiteracy Z55.0
impaired mobility Z74.09
imprisonment or incarceration Z65.1
inadequate teaching affecting education Z55.8
inappropriate (excessive) parental pressure Z62.6
influencing health status NEC Z78.9
in-law Z63.1

Problem (with) (related to) - *continued*
  institutionalization, affecting child Z62.22
  intrafamilial communication Z63.8
  jealousy, child F93.8
  landlord Z59.2
  language (developmental) F80.9
  learning (developmental) F81.9
  legal Z65.3
    conviction without imprisonment Z65.0
    imprisonment Z65.1
    release from prison Z65.2
  life-management Z73.9
    specified NEC Z73.89
  life-style Z72.9
    gambling Z72.6
    high-risk sexual behavior (heterosexual) Z72.51
      bisexual Z72.53
      homosexual Z72.52
    inappropriate eating habits Z72.4
    self-damaging behavior NEC Z72.89
    specified NEC Z72.89
    tobacco use Z72.0
  literacy Z55.9
    low level Z55.0
    specified NEC Z55.8
  living alone Z60.2
  lodgers Z59.2
  loss of love relationship in childhood Z62.898
  marital Z63.0
    involving
      divorce Z63.5
      estrangement Z63.5
      gender identity F66
  mastication K08.89
  medical
    care, within family Z63.6
    facilities Z75.9
      specified NEC Z75.8
  mental F48.9
  multiparity Z64.1
  negative life events in childhood Z62.9
    altered pattern of family relationships Z62.898
    frightening experience Z62.898
    loss of
      love relationship Z62.898
      self-esteem Z62.898
    physical abuse (alleged) — *see* Maltreatment, child
    removal from home Z62.29
    specified event NEC Z62.898
  neighbor Z59.2
  neurological NEC R29.818
  new step-parent affecting child Z62.898
  none (feared complaint unfounded) Z71.1
  occupational NEC Z56.89
  parent-child — *see* Conflict, parent-child
  personal hygiene Z91.89
  personality F69
  phase-of-life transition, adjustment Z60.0
  presence of sick or disabled person in family or household Z63.79
    needing care Z63.6
  primary support group (family) Z63.9
    specified NEC Z63.8
  probation officer Z64.4
  psychiatric F99
  psychosexual (development) F66
  psychosocial Z65.9
    religious or spiritual Z65.8
    specified NEC Z65.8
  relationship Z63.9
    childhood F93.8
  release from prison Z65.2
    religious or spiritual Z65.8
  removal from home affecting child Z62.29
  seeking and accepting known hazardous and harmful
    behavioral or psychological interventions Z65.8
    chemical, nutritional or physical interventions Z65.8
  sexual function (nonorganic) F52.9

Problem (with) (related to) - *continued*
  sight H54.7
  sleep disorder, child F51.9
  smell — *see* Disturbance, sensation, smell
  social
    environment Z60.9
      specified NEC Z60.8
    exclusion and rejection Z60.4
    worker Z64.4
  speech R47.9
    developmental F80.9
    specified NEC R47.89
  swallowing — *see* Dysphagia
  taste — *see* Disturbance, sensation, taste
  tic, child F95.0
  underachievement in school Z55.3
  unemployment Z56.0
    threatened Z56.2
  unwanted pregnancy Z64.0
  upbringing Z62.9
    specified NEC Z62.898
  urinary N39.9
  voice production R47.89
  work schedule (stressful) Z56.3
Procedure (surgical)
  converted
    arthroscopic to open Z53.33
    laparoscopic to open Z53.31
    specified procedure NEC to open Z53.39
    thoracoscopic to open Z53.32
  for purpose other than remedying health state Z41.9
    specified NEC Z41.8
  not done Z53.9
    because of
      administrative reasons Z53.8
      contraindication Z53.09
        smoking Z53.01
      patient's decision Z53.20
        for reasons of belief or group pressure Z53.1
        left against medical advice (AMA) Z53.29
        left without being seen Z53.21
        specified reason NEC Z53.29
      specified reason NEC Z53.8
Procidentia (uteri) N81.3
Proctalgia K62.89
  fugax K59.4
  spasmodic K59.4
Proctitis K62.89
  amebic (acute) A06.0
  chlamydial A56.3
  gonococcal A54.6
  granulomatous — *see* Enteritis, regional, large intestine
  herpetic A60.1
  radiation K62.7
  tuberculous A18.32
  ulcerative (chronic) K51.20
    with
      complication K51.219
        abscess K51.214
        fistula K51.213
        obstruction K51.212
        rectal bleeding K51.211
        specified NEC K51.218
Proctocele
  female (without uterine prolapse) N81.6
    with uterine prolapse N81.2
      complete N81.3
  male K62.3
Proctocolitis
  allergic K52.29
  food-induced eosinophilic K52.29
  food protein-induced K52.29
  milk protein-induced K52.29
  mucosal — *see* Rectosigmoiditis, ulcerative
Proctoptosis K62.3
Proctorrhagia K62.5
Proctosigmoiditis K63.89
  ulcerative (chronic) — *see* Rectosigmoiditis, ulcerative
Proctospasm K59.4
  psychogenic F45.8

Profichet's disease — *see* Disorder, soft tissue, specified type NEC
Progeria E34.8
Prognathism (mandibular) (maxillary) M26.19
Progonoma (melanotic) — *see* Neoplasm, benign, by site
Progressive — *see* condition
Prolactinoma
  specified site — *see* Neoplasm, benign, by site
  unspecified site D35.2
Prolapse, prolapsed
  anus, anal (canal) (sphincter) K62.2
  arm or hand O32.2
    causing obstructed labor O64.4
  bladder (mucosa) (sphincter) (acquired)
    congenital Q79.4
    female — *see* Cystocele
    male N32.89
  breast implant (prosthetic) T85.49
  cecostomy K94.09
  cecum K63.4
  cervix, cervical (hypertrophied) N81.2
    anterior lip, obstructing labor O65.5
    congenital Q51.828
    postpartal, old N81.2
    stump N81.85
  ciliary body (traumatic) — *see* Laceration, eye(ball), with prolapse or loss of interocular tissue
  colon (pedunculated) K63.4
  colostomy K94.09
  disc (intervertebral) — *see* Displacement, intervertebral disc
  eye implant (orbital) T85.398
    lens (ocular) — *see* Complications, intraocular lens
  fallopian tube N83.4-
  gastric (mucosa) K31.89
  genital, female N81.9
    specified NEC N81.89
  globe, nontraumatic — *see* Luxation, globe
  ileostomy bud K94.19
  intervertebral disc — *see* Displacement, intervertebral disc
  intestine (small) K63.4
  iris (traumatic) — *see* Laceration, eye(ball), with prolapse or loss of interocular tissue
    nontraumatic H21.89
  kidney N28.83
    congenital Q63.2
  laryngeal muscles or ventricle J38.7
  liver K76.89
  meatus urinarius N36.8
  mitral (valve) I34.1
  ocular lens implant — *see* Complications, intraocular lens
  organ or site, congenital NEC — *see* Malposition, congenital
  ovary N83.4-
  pelvic floor, female N81.89
  perineum, female N81.89
  rectum (mucosa) (sphincter) K62.3
    due to trichuris trichuria B79
  spleen D73.89
  stomach K31.89
  umbilical cord
    complicating delivery O69.0
  urachus, congenital Q64.4
  ureter N28.89
    with obstruction N13.5
      with infection N13.6
  ureterovesical orifice N28.89
  urethra (acquired) (infected) (mucosa) N36.8
    congenital Q64.71
  urinary meatus N36.8
    congenital Q64.72
  uterovaginal N81.4
    complete N81.3
    incomplete N81.2
  uterus (with prolapse of vagina) N81.4
    complete N81.3
    congenital Q51.818

Prolapse, prolapsed - *continued*
uterus (with prolapse of vagina) - *continued*
first degree N81.2
in pregnancy or childbirth — *see* Pregnancy, complicated by, abnormal, uterus
incomplete N81.2
postpartal (old) N81.4
second degree N81.2
third degree N81.3
uveal (traumatic) — *see* Laceration, eye(ball), with prolapse or loss of interocular tissue
vagina (anterior) (wall) — *see* Cystocele
with prolapse of uterus N81.4
complete N81.3
incomplete N81.2
posterior wall N81.6
posthysterectomy N99.3
vitreous (humor) H43.0-
in wound — *see* Laceration, eye(ball), with prolapse or loss of interocular tissue
womb — *see* Prolapse, uterus
Prolapsus, female N81.9
specified NEC N81.89
Proliferation (s)
prostate, atypical small acinar N42.32
primary cutaneous CD30-positive large T-cell C86.6
Proliferative — *see* condition
Prolonged, prolongation (of)
bleeding (time) (idiopathic) R79.1
coagulation (time) R79.1
gestation (over 42 completed weeks)
mother O48.1
newborn P08.22
interval I44.0
labor O63.9
first stage O63.0
second stage O63.1
partial thromboplastin time (PTT) R79.1
pregnancy (more than 42 weeks gestation) O48.1
prothrombin time R79.1
QT interval R94.31
uterine contractions in labor O62.4
Prominence, prominent
auricle (congenital) (ear) Q17.5
ischial spine or sacral promontory with disproportion (fetopelvic) O33.0
causing obstructed labor O65.0
nose (congenital) acquired M95.0
Promiscuity — *see* High, risk, sexual behavior
Pronation
ankle — *see* Deformity, limb, foot, specified NEC
foot — *see also* Deformity, limb, foot, specified NEC
congenital Q74.2
Prophylactic
administration of
antibiotics, long-term Z79.2
short-term use - omit code
drug — *see also* Long-term (current) drug therapy (use of) Z79.899-
medication Z79.899
organ removal (for neoplasia management) Z40.00
breast Z40.01
fallopian tube (s) Z40.03
with ovary (s) Z40.02
ovary (s) Z40.02
specified site NEC Z40.09
surgery Z40.9
for risk factors related to malignant neoplasm — *see* Prophylactic, organ removal
specified NEC Z40.8
vaccination Z23
Propionic acidemia E71.121
Proptosis (ocular) — *see also* Exophthalmos
thyroid — *see* Hyperthyroidism, with goiter
Prosecution, anxiety concerning Z65.3
Prosopagnosia R48.3
Prostadynia N42.81
Prostate, prostatic — *see* condition
Prostatism — *see* Hyperplasia, prostate
Prostatitis (congestive) (suppurative) (with cystitis) N41.9
acute N41.0
cavitary N41.8
chronic N41.1
diverticular N41.8
due to Trichomonas (vaginalis) A59.02
fibrous N41.1
gonococcal (acute) (chronic) A54.22
granulomatous N41.4
hypertrophic N41.1
subacute N41.1
trichomonal A59.02
tuberculous A18.14
Prostatocystitis N41.3
Prostatorrhea N42.89
Prostatosis N42.82
Prostration R53.83
heat — *see also* Heat, exhaustion
anhydrotic T67.3
due to
salt (and water) depletion T67.4
water depletion T67.3
nervous F48.8
senile R54
Protanomaly (anomalous trichromat) H53.54
Protanopia (complete) (incomplete) H53.54
Protection (against) (from) — *see* Prophylactic
Protein
deficiency NEC — *see* Malnutrition
malnutrition — *see* Malnutrition
sickness — *see also* Reaction, serum T80.69
Proteinemia R77.9
Proteinosis
alveolar (pulmonary) J84.01
lipid or lipoid (of Urbach) E78.89
Proteinuria R80.9
Bence Jones R80.3
complicating pregnancy — *see* Proteinuria, gestational
gestational
complicating
childbirth O12.14
pregnancy O12.1-
with edema O12.2-
puerperium O12.15
idiopathic R80.0
isolated R80.0
with glomerular lesion N06.9
C3
glomerulonephritis N06.A
glomerulopathy N06.A
with dense deposit disease N06.6
dense deposit disease N06.6
diffuse
crescentic glomerulonephritis N06.7
endocapillary proliferative glomerulonephritis N06.4
mesangiocapillary glomerulonephritis N06.5
focal and segmental hyalinosis or sclerosis N06.1
membranous (diffuse) N06.2
mesangial proliferative (diffuse) N06.3
minimal change N06.0
specified pathology NEC N06.8
orthostatic R80.2
with glomerular lesion — *see* Proteinuria, isolated, with glomerular lesion
persistent R80.1
with glomerular lesion — *see* Proteinuria, isolated, with glomerular lesion
postural R80.2
with glomerular lesion — *see* Proteinuria, isolated, with glomerular lesion
pre-eclamptic — *see* Pre-eclampsia
puerperal O12.15
specified type NEC R80.8
Proteolysis, pathologic D65
Proteus (mirabilis) (morganii) , as cause of disease classified elsewhere B96.4
Prothrombin gene mutation D68.52
Protoporphyria, erythropoietic E80.0
Protozoal — *see also* condition
disease B64
specified NEC B60.8
Protrusion, protrusio
acetabuli M24.7
acetabulum (into pelvis) M24.7
device, implant or graft — *see also* Complications, by site and type, mechanical T85.698
arterial graft NEC — *see* Complication, cardiovascular device, mechanical, vascular
breast (implant) T85.49
catheter NEC T85.698
cystostomy T83.090
dialysis (renal) T82.49
intraperitoneal T85.691
infusion NEC T82.594
spinal (epidural) (subdural) T85.690
urinary — *see also* Complications, catheter, urinary T83.098
electronic (electrode) (pulse generator) (stimulator)
bone T84.390
nervous system — *see* Complication, prosthetic device, mechanical, electronic nervous system stimulator
fixation, internal (orthopedic) NEC — *see* Complication, fixation device, mechanical
gastrointestinal — *see* Complications, prosthetic device, mechanical, gastrointestinal device
genital NEC T83.498
intrauterine contraceptive device T83.39
penile prosthesis (cylinder) (implanted) (pump) (resevoir) T83.490
testicular prosthesis T83.491
heart NEC — *see* Complication, cardiovascular device, mechanical
joint prosthesis — *see* Complications, joint prosthesis, mechanical, specified NEC, by site
ocular NEC — *see* Complications, prosthetic device, mechanical, ocular device
orthopedic NEC — *see* Complication, orthopedic, device, mechanical
specified NEC T85.628
urinary NEC — *see also* Complication, genitourinary, device, urinary, mechanical
graft T83.29
vascular NEC — *see* Complication, cardiovascular device, mechanical
ventricular intracranial shunt T85.09
intervertebral disc — *see* Displacement, intervertebral disc
joint prosthesis — *see* Complications, joint prosthesis, mechanical, specified NEC, by site
nucleus pulposus — *see* Displacement, intervertebral disc
Prune belly (syndrome) Q79.4
Prurigo (ferox) (gravis) (Hebrae) (Hebra's) (mitis) (simplex) L28.2
Besnier's L20.0
estivalis L56.4
nodularis L28.1
psychogenic F45.8
Pruritus, pruritic (essential) L29.9
ani, anus L29.0
psychogenic F45.8
anogenital L29.3
psychogenic F45.8
due to onchocerca volvulus B73.1
gravidarum — *see* Pregnancy, complicated by, specified pregnancy-related condition NEC
hiemalis L29.8
neurogenic (any site) F45.8
perianal L29.0
psychogenic (any site) F45.8

Pruritus, pruritic (essential) - *continued*
  scroti, scrotum L29.1
    psychogenic F45.8
  senile, senilis L29.8
  specified NEC L29.8
    psychogenic F45.8
  Trichomonas A59.9
  vulva, vulvae L29.2
    psychogenic F45.8
Pseudarthrosis, pseudoarthrosis (bone) — *see* Nonunion, fracture
  clavicle, congenital Q74.0
  joint, following fusion or arthrodesis M96.0
Pseudoaneurysm — *see* Aneurysm
Pseudoangina (pectoris) — *see* Angina
Pseudoangioma I81
Pseudoarteriosus Q28.8
Pseudoarthrosis — *see* Pseudarthrosis
Pseudobulbar affect (PBA) F48.2
Pseudochromhidrosis L67.8
Pseudocirrhosis, liver, pericardial I31.1
Pseudocowpox B08.03
Pseudocoxalgia M91.3-
Pseudocroup J38.5
Pseudo-Cushing's syndrome, alcohol-induced E24.4
Pseudocyesis F45.8
Pseudocyst
  lung J98.4
  pancreas K86.3
  retina — *see* Cyst, retina
Pseudoelephantiasis neuroarthritica Q82.0
Pseudoexfoliation, capsule (lens) — *see* Cataract, specified NEC
Pseudofolliculitis barbae L73.1
Pseudoglioma H44.89
Pseudohemophilia (Bernuth's) (hereditary) (type B) D68.0
  Type A D69.8
  vascular D69.8
Pseudohermaphroditism Q56.3
  adrenal E25.8
  female Q56.2
    with adrenocortical disorder E25.8
    without adrenocortical disorder Q56.2
    adrenal (congenital) E25.0
    unspecified E25.9
  male Q56.1
    with
      adrenocortical disorder E25.8
      androgen resistance E34.51
      cleft scrotum Q56.1
      feminizing testis E34.51
      5-alpha-reductase deficiency E29.1
    without gonadal disorder Q56.1
    adrenal E25.8
    unspecified E25.9
Pseudo-Hurler's polydystrophy E77.0
Pseudohydrocephalus G93.2
Pseudohypertrophic muscular dystrophy (Erb's) G71.02
Pseudohypertrophy, muscle G71.09
Pseudohypoparathyroidism E20.1
Pseudoinsomnia F51.03
Pseudoleukemia, infantile D64.89
Pseudomembranous — *see* condition
Pseudomeningocele (cerebral) (infective) (post-traumatic) G96.198
  postprocedural (spinal) G97.82
Pseudomenses (newborn) P54.6
Pseudomenstruation (newborn) P54.6
Pseudomonas
  aeruginosa, as cause of disease classified elsewhere B96.5
  mallei infection A24.0
    as cause of disease classified elsewhere B96.5
  pseudomallei, as cause of disease classified elsewhere B96.5
Pseudomyotonia G71.19
Pseudomyxoma peritonei C78.6
Pseudoneuritis, optic (nerve) (disc) (papilla), congenital Q14.2
Pseudo-obstruction intestine (acute) (chronic) (idiopathic) (intermittent secondary) (primary) K59.89
  colonic K59.81
Pseudopapilledema H47.33-
  congenital Q14.2
Pseudoparalysis
  arm or leg R29.818
  atonic, congenital P94.2
Pseudopelade L66.0
Pseudophakia Z96.1
Pseudopolyarthritis, rhizomelic M35.3
Pseudopolycythemia D75.1
Pseudopseudohypoparathyroidism E20.1
Pseudopterygium H11.81-
Pseudoptosis (eyelid) — *see* Blepharochalasis
Pseudopuberty, precocious
  female heterosexual E25.8
  male isosexual E25.8
Pseudorickets (renal) N25.0
Pseudorubella B08.20
Pseudosclerema, newborn P83.88
Pseudosclerosis (brain)
  of Westphal (Strümpell) E83.01
  Jakob's — *see* Creutzfeldt-Jakob disease or syndrome
  spastic — *see* Creutzfeldt-Jakob disease or syndrome
Pseudotetanus — *see* Convulsions
Pseudotetany R29.0
  hysterical F44.5
Pseudotruncus arteriosus Q25.49
Pseudotuberculosis A28.2
  enterocolitis A04.8
  pasteurella (infection) A28.0
Pseudotumor G93.2
  cerebri G93.2
  orbital H05.11-
Pseudoxanthoma elasticum Q82.8
Psilosis (sprue) (tropical) K90.1
  nontropical K90.0
Psittacosis A70
Psoitis M60.88
Psoriasis L40.9
  arthropathic L40.50
    arthritis mutilans L40.52
    distal interphalangeal L40.51
    juvenile L40.54
    other specified L40.59
    spondylitis L40.53
  buccal K13.29
  flexural L40.8
  guttate L40.4
  mouth K13.29
  nummular L40.0
  plaque L40.0
  psychogenic F54
  pustular (generalized) L40.1
    palmaris et plantaris L40.3
  specified NEC L40.8
  vulgaris L40.0
Psychasthenia F48.8
Psychiatric disorder or problem F99
Psychogenic — *see also* condition
  factors associated with physical conditions F54
Psychological and behavioral factors affecting medical condition F59
Psychoneurosis, psychoneurotic — *see also* Neurosis
  anxiety (state) F41.1
  depersonalization F48.1
  hypochondriacal F45.21
  hysteria F44.9
  neurasthenic F48.8
  personality NEC F60.89
Psychopathy, psychopathic
  affectionless F94.2
  autistic F84.5
  constitution, post-traumatic F07.81
  personality — *see* Disorder, personality
  sexual — *see* Deviation, sexual
  state F60.2
Psychosexual identity disorder of childhood F64.2
Psychosis, psychotic F29
  acute (transient) F23
    hysterical F44.9
  affective — *see* Disorder, mood
  alcoholic F10.959
    with
      abuse F10.159
      anxiety disorder F10.980
        with
          abuse F10.180
          dependence F10.280
      delirium tremens F10.231
      delusions F10.950
        with
          abuse F10.150
          dependence F10.250
      dementia F10.97
        with dependence F10.27
      dependence F10.259
      hallucinosis F10.951
        with
          abuse F10.151
          dependence F10.251
      mood disorder F10.94
        with
          abuse F10.14
          dependence F10.24
      paranoia F10.950
        with
          abuse F10.150
          dependence F10.250
      persisting amnesia F10.96
        with dependence F10.26
    amnestic confabulatory F10.96
      with dependence F10.26
    delirium tremens F10.231
    Korsakoff's, Korsakov's, Korsakow's F10.26
    paranoid type F10.950
      with
        abuse F10.150
        dependence F10.250
  anergastic — *see* Psychosis, organic
  arteriosclerotic (simple type) (uncomplicated) F01.50
    with behavioral disturbance F01.51
  childhood F84.0
    atypical F84.8
  climacteric — *see* Psychosis, involutional
  confusional F29
    acute or subacute F05
    reactive F23
  cycloid F23
  depressive — *see* Disorder, depressive
  disintegrative (childhood) F84.3
  drug-induced — *see* F11-F19 with .x59
    paranoid and hallucinatory states — *see* F11-F19 with .x50 or .x51
  due to or associated with
    addiction, drug — *see* F11-F19 with .x59
    dependence
      alcohol F10.259
      drug — *see* F11-F19 with .x59
    epilepsy F06.8
    Huntington's chorea F06.8
    ischemia, cerebrovascular (generalized) F06.8
    multiple sclerosis F06.8
    physical disease F06.8
    presenile dementia F03
    senile dementia F03
    vascular disease (arteriosclerotic) (cerebral) F01.50
      with behavioral disturbance F01.51
  epileptic F06.8
  episode F23
    due to or associated with physical condition F06.8
  exhaustive F43.0
  hallucinatory, chronic F28
  hypomanic F30.8
  hysterical (acute) F44.9
  induced F24
  infantile F84.0
    atypical F84.8

Psychosis, psychotic - *continued*
infective (acute) (subacute) F05
involutional F28
depressive — *see* Disorder, depressive
melancholic — *see* Disorder, depressive
paranoid (state) F22
Korsakoff's, Korsakov's, Korsakow's (nonalcoholic) F04
alcoholic F10.96
in dependence F10.26
induced by other psychoactive substance — *see* categories F11-F19 with .x5x
mania, manic (single episode) F30.2
recurrent type F31.89
manic-depressive — *see* Disorder, bipolar
menopausal — *see* Psychosis, involutional
mixed schizophrenic and affective F25.8
multi-infarct (cerebrovascular) F01.50
with behavioral disturbance F01.51
nonorganic F29
specified NEC F28
organic F09
due to or associated with
arteriosclerosis (cerebral) — *see* Psychosis, arteriosclerotic
cerebrovascular disease, arteriosclerotic — *see* Psychosis, arteriosclerotic
childbirth — *see* Psychosis, puerperal
Creutzfeldt-Jakob disease or syndrome — *see* Creutzfeldt-Jakob disease or syndrome
dependence, alcohol F10.259
disease
alcoholic liver F10.259
brain, arteriosclerotic — *see* Psychosis, arteriosclerotic
cerebrovascular F01.50
with behavioral disturbance F01.51
Creutzfeldt-Jakob — *see* Creutzfeldt-Jakob disease or syndrome
endocrine or metabolic F06.8
acute or subacute F05
liver, alcoholic F10.259
epilepsy transient (acute) F05
infection
brain (intracranial) F06.8
acute or subacute F05
intoxication
alcoholic (acute) F10.259
drug F11-F19 with .x59
ischemia, cerebrovascular (generalized) — *see* Psychosis, arteriosclerotic
puerperium — *see* Psychosis, puerperal
trauma, brain (birth) (from electric current) (surgical) F06.8
acute or subacute F05
infective F06.8
acute or subacute F05
post-traumatic F06.8
acute or subacute F05
paranoiac F22
paranoid (climacteric) (involutional) (menopausal) F22
psychogenic (acute) F23
schizophrenic F20.0
senile F03
postpartum (NOS) F53.1
presbyophrenic (type) F03
presenile F03
psychogenic (paranoid) F23
depressive F32.3
puerperal (NOS) F53.1
specified type — *see* Psychosis, by type
reactive (brief) (transient) (emotional stress) (psychological trauma) F23
depressive F32.3
recurrent F33.3
excitative type F30.8
schizoaffective F25.9
depressive type F25.1
manic type F25.0

Psychosis, psychotic - *continued*
schizophrenia, schizophrenic — *see* Schizophrenia
schizophrenia-like, in epilepsy F06.2
schizophreniform F20.81
affective type F25.9
brief F23
confusional type F23
mixed type F25.0
senile NEC F03
depressed or paranoid type F03
simple deterioration F03
specified type - code to condition
shared F24
situational (reactive) F23
symbiotic (childhood) F84.3
symptomatic F09
Psychosomatic — *see* Disorder, psychosomatic
Psychosyndrome, organic F07.9
Psychotic episode due to or associated with physical condition F06.8
Pterygium (eye) H11.00-
amyloid H11.01-
central H11.02-
colli Q18.3
double H11.03-
peripheral
progressive H11.05-
stationary H11.04-
recurrent H11.06-
Ptilosis (eyelid) — *see* Madarosis
Ptomaine (poisoning) — *see* Poisoning, food
Ptosis — *see also* Blepharoptosis
adiposa (false) — *see* Blepharoptosis
breast N64.81
brow H57.81-
cecum K63.4
colon K63.4
congenital (eyelid) Q10.0
specified site NEC — *see* Anomaly, by site
eyebrow H57.81-
eyelid — *see* Blepharoptosis
congenital Q10.0
gastric K31.89
intestine K63.4
kidney N28.83
liver K76.89
renal N28.83
splanchnic K63.4
spleen D73.89
stomach K31.89
viscera K63.4
PTP D69.51
Ptyalism (periodic) K11.7
hysterical F45.8
pregnancy — *see* Pregnancy, complicated by, specified pregnancy-related condition NEC
psychogenic F45.8
Ptyalolithiasis K11.5
Pubarche, precocious E30.1
Pubertas praecox E30.1
Puberty (development state) Z00.3
bleeding (excessive) N92.2
delayed E30.0
precocious (constitutional) (cryptogenic) (idiopathic) E30.1
central E22.8
due to
ovarian hyperfunction E28.1
estrogen E28.0
testicular hyperfunction E29.0
premature E30.1
due to
adrenal cortical hyperfunction E25.8
pineal tumor E34.8
pituitary (anterior) hyperfunction E22.8
Puckering, macula — *see* Degeneration, macula, puckering
Pudenda, pudendum — *see* condition
Puente's disease (simple glandular cheilitis) K13.0

Puerperal, puerperium (complicated by, complications)
abnormal glucose (tolerance test) O99.815
abscess
areola O91.02
associated with lactation O91.03
Bartholin's gland O86.19
breast O91.12
associated with lactation O91.13
cervix (uteri) O86.11
genital organ NEC O86.19
kidney O86.21
mammary O91.12
associated with lactation O91.13
nipple O91.02
associated with lactation O91.03
peritoneum O85
subareolar O91.12
associated with lactation O91.13
urinary tract — *see* Puerperal, infection, urinary
uterus O86.12
vagina (wall) O86.13
vaginorectal O86.13
vulvovaginal gland O86.13
adnexitis O86.19
afibrinogenemia, or other coagulation defect O72.3
albuminuria (acute) (subacute) — *see* Proteinuria, gestational
alcohol use O99.315
anemia O90.81
pre-existing (pre-pregnancy) O99.03
anesthetic death O89.8
apoplexy O99.43
bariatric surgery status O99.845
blood disorder NEC O99.13
blood dyscrasia O72.3
cardiomyopathy O90.3
cerebrovascular disorder (conditions in I60-I69) O99.43
cervicitis O86.11
circulatory system disorder O99.43
coagulopathy (any) O99.13
with hemorrhage O72.3
complications O90.9
specified NEC O90.89
convulsions — *see* Eclampsia
cystitis O86.22
cystopyelitis O86.29
delirium NEC F05
diabetes O24.93
gestational — *see* Puerperal, gestational diabetes
pre-existing O24.33
specified NEC O24.83
type 1 O24.03
type 2 O24.13
digestive system disorder O99.63
disease O90.9
breast NEC O92.29
cerebrovascular (acute) O99.43
nonobstetric NEC O99.893
tubo-ovarian O86.19
Valsuani's O99.03
disorder O90.9
biliary tract O26.63
lactation O92.70
liver O26.63
nonobstetric NEC O99.893
disruption
cesarean wound O90.0
episiotomy wound O90.1
perineal laceration wound O90.1
drug use O99.325
eclampsia (with pre-existing hypertension) O15.2
embolism (pulmonary) (blood clot) — *see* Embolism, obstetric, puerperal
endocrine, nutritional or metabolic disease NEC O99.285
endophlebitis — *see* Puerperal, phlebitis
endotrachelitis O86.11
failure
lactation (complete) O92.3

Puerperal, puerperium (complicated by, complications) - *continued*
- failure - *continued*
  - lactation (complete) - *continued*
    - partial O92.4
  - renal, acute O90.4
- fever (of unknown origin) O86.4
  - septic O85
- fissure, nipple O92.12
  - associated with lactation O92.13
- fistula
  - breast (due to mastitis) O91.12
    - associated with lactation O91.13
  - nipple O91.02
    - associated with lactation O91.03
- galactophoritis O91.22
  - associated with lactation O91.23
- galactorrhea O92.6
- gastric banding status O99.845
- gastric bypass status O99.845
- gastrointestinal disease NEC O99.63
- gestational
  - diabetes O24.439
    - diet controlled O24.430
    - insulin (and diet) controlled O24.434
    - oral drug controlled (antidiabetic) (hypoglycemic) O24.435
  - edema O12.05
    - with proteinuria O12.25
  - proteinuria O12.15
- gonorrhea O98.23
- hematoma, subdural O99.43
- hemiplegia, cerebral O99.355
  - due to cerbrovascular disorder O99.43
- hemorrhage O72.1
  - brain O99.43
  - bulbar O99.43
  - cerebellar O99.43
  - cerebral O99.43
  - cortical O99.43
  - delayed or secondary O72.2
  - extradural O99.43
  - internal capsule O99.43
  - intracranial O99.43
  - intrapontine O99.43
  - meningeal O99.43
  - pontine O99.43
  - retained placenta O72.0
  - subarachnoid O99.43
  - subcortical O99.43
  - subdural O99.43
  - third stage O72.0
  - uterine, delayed O72.2
  - ventricular O99.43
- hemorrhoids O87.2
- hepatorenal syndrome O90.4
- hypertension — *see* Hypertension, complicating, puerperium
- hypertrophy, breast O92.29
- induration breast (fibrous) O92.29
- infection O86.4
  - cervix O86.11
  - generalized O85
  - genital tract NEC O86.19
    - obstetric surgical wound O86.09
  - kidney (bacillus coli) O86.21
  - maternal O98.93
    - carrier state NEC O99.835
    - gonorrhea O98.23
    - human immunodeficiency virus (HIV) O98.73
    - protozoal O98.63
    - sexually transmitted NEC O98.33
    - specified NEC O98.83
    - streptococcus group B (GBS) carrier state O99.825
    - syphilis O98.13
    - tuberculosis O98.03
    - viral hepatitis O98.43
    - viral NEC O98.53
  - nipple O91.02
    - associated with lactation O91.03
  - peritoneum O85
  - renal O86.21
  - specified NEC O86.89

Puerperal, puerperium (complicated by, complications) - *continued*
- infection - *continued*
  - urinary (asymptomatic) (tract) NEC O86.20
    - bladder O86.22
    - kidney O86.21
    - specified site NEC O86.29
    - urethra O86.22
  - vagina O86.13
  - vein — *see* Puerperal, phlebitis
- ischemia, cerebral O99.43
- lymphangitis O86.89
  - breast O91.22
    - associated with lactation O91.23
- malignancy O9A.13
- malnutrition O25.3
- mammillitis O91.02
  - associated with lactation O91.03
- mammitis O91.22
  - associated with lactation O91.23
- mania F30.8
- mastitis O91.22
  - associated with lactation O91.23
  - purulent O91.12
    - associated with lactation O91.13
- melancholia — *see* Disorder, depressive
- mental disorder NEC O99.345
- metroperitonitis O85
- metrorrhagia — *see* Hemorrhage, postpartum
- metrosalpingitis O86.19
- metrovaginitis O86.13
- milk leg O87.1
- monoplegia, cerebral O99.43
- mood disturbance O90.6
- necrosis, liver (acute) (subacute) (conditions in subcategory K72.0) O26.63
  - with renal failure O90.4
- nervous system disorder O99.355
- neuritis O90.89
- obesity (pre-existing prior to pregnancy) O99.215
- obesity surgery status O99.845
- occlusion, precerebral artery O99.43
- paralysis
  - bladder (sphincter) O90.89
  - cerebral O99.43
- paralytic stroke O99.43
- parametritis O85
- paravaginitis O86.13
- pelviperitonitis O85
- perimetritis O86.12
- perimetrosalpingitis O86.19
- perinephritis O86.21
- periphlebitis — *see* Puerperal phlebitis
- peritoneal infection O85
- peritonitis (pelvic) O85
- perivaginitis O86.13
- phlebitis O87.0
  - deep O87.1
  - pelvic O87.1
  - superficial O87.0
- phlebothrombosis, deep O87.1
- phlegmasia alba dolens O87.1
- placental polyp O90.89
- pneumonia, embolic — *see* Embolism, obstetric, puerperal
- pre-eclampsia — *see* Pre-eclampsia
- psychosis (NOS) F53.1
- pyelitis O86.21
- pyelocystitis O86.29
- pyelonephritis O86.21
- pyelonephrosis O86.21
- pyemia O85
- pyocystitis O86.29
- pyohemia O85
- pyometra O86.12
- pyonephritis O86.21
- pyosalpingitis O86.19
- pyrexia (of unknown origin) O86.4
- renal
  - disease NEC O90.89
  - failure O90.4
- respiratory disease NEC O99.53
- retention

Puerperal, puerperium (complicated by, complications) - *continued*
- retention - *continued*
  - decidua — *see* Retention, decidua
  - placenta O72.0
  - secundines — *see* Retention, secundines
- retrated nipple O92.02
- salpingo-ovaritis O86.19
- salpingoperitonitis O85
- secondary perineal tear O90.1
- sepsis (pelvic) O85
- sepsis O85
- septic thrombophlebitis O86.81
- skin disorder NEC O99.73
- specified condition NEC O99.893
- stroke O99.43
- subinvolution (uterus) O90.89
- subluxation of symphysis (pubis) O26.73
- suppuration — *see* Puerperal, abscess
- tetanus A34
- thelitis O91.02
  - associated with lactation O91.03
- thrombocytopenia O72.3
- thrombophlebitis (superficial) O87.0
  - deep O87.1
  - pelvic O87.1
  - septic O86.81
- thrombosis (venous) — *see* Thrombosis, puerperal
- thyroiditis O90.5
- toxemia (eclamptic) (pre-eclamptic) (with convulsions) O15.2
- trauma, non-obstetric O9A.23
  - caused by abuse (physical) (suspected) O9A.33
    - confirmed O9A.33
    - psychological (suspected) O9A.53
      - confirmed O9A.53
    - sexual (suspected) O9A.43
      - confirmed O9A.43
- uremia (due to renal failure) O90.4
- urethritis O86.22
- vaginitis O86.13
- varicose veins (legs) O87.4
  - vulva or perineum O87.8
- venous O87.9
- vulvitis O86.19
- vulvovaginitis O86.13
- white leg O87.1

Puerperium — *see* Puerperal

Pulmolithiasis J98.4

Pulmonary — *see* condition

Pulpitis (acute) (anachoretic) (chronic) (hyperplastic) (putrescent) (suppurative) (ulcerative) K04.01
- irreversible K04.02
- reversible K04.01

Pulpless tooth K04.99

Pulse
- alternating R00.8
- bigeminal R00.8
- fast R00.0
- feeble, rapid due to shock following injury T79.4
- rapid R00.0
- weak R09.89

Pulsus alternans or trigeminus R00.8

Punch drunk F07.81

Punctum lacrimale occlusion — *see* Obstruction, lacrimal

Puncture
- abdomen, abdominal
  - wall S31.139
    - with
      - foreign body S31.149
      - penetration into peritoneal cavity S31.639
        - with foreign body S31.649
    - epigastric region S31.132
      - with
        - foreign body S31.142
        - penetration into peritoneal cavity S31.632
          - with foreign body S31.642
    - left

PUNCTURE - PUNCTURE

Puncture - *continued*
genital organs, external - *continued*
female S31.532
with foreign body S31.542
vagina — *see* Puncture, vagina
vulva — *see* Puncture, vulva
male S31.531
with foreign body S31.541
penis — *see* Puncture, penis
scrotum — *see* Puncture, scrotum
testis — *see* Puncture, testis
groin — *see* Puncture, abdomen, wall
gum — *see* Puncture, oral cavity
hand S61.439
with
foreign body S61.449
finger — *see* Puncture, finger
left S61.432
with
foreign body S61.442
right S61.431
with
foreign body S61.441
thumb — *see* Puncture, thumb
head S01.93
with foreign body S01.94
cheek — *see* Puncture, cheek
ear — *see* Puncture, ear
eyelid — *see* Puncture, eyelid
lip — *see* Puncture, oral cavity
nose — *see* Puncture, nose
oral cavity — *see* Puncture, oral cavity
scalp S01.03
with foreign body S01.04
specified site NEC S01.83
with foreign body S01.84
temporomandibular area — *see* Puncture, cheek
heart S26.99
with hemopericardium S26.09
without hemopericardium S26.19
heel — *see* Puncture, foot
hip S71.039
with foreign body S71.049
left S71.032
with foreign body S71.042
right S71.031
with foreign body S71.041
hymen — *see* Puncture, vagina
hypochondrium — *see* Puncture, abdomen, wall
hypogastric region — *see* Puncture, abdomen, wall
inguinal region — *see* Puncture, abdomen, wall
instep — *see* Puncture, foot
internal organs — *see* Injury, by site
interscapular region — *see* Puncture, thorax, back
intestine
large
colon S36.599
ascending S36.590
descending S36.592
sigmoid S36.593
specified site NEC S36.598
transverse S36.591
rectum S36.69
small S36.499
duodenum S36.490
specified site NEC S36.498
intra-abdominal organ S36.99
gallbladder S36.128
intestine — *see* Puncture, intestine
liver S36.118
pancreas — *see* Puncture, pancreas
peritoneum S36.81
specified site NEC S36.898
spleen S36.09
stomach S36.39
jaw — *see* Puncture, head, specified site NEC
knee S81.039
with foreign body S81.049
left S81.032

Puncture - *continued*
knee - *continued*
left - *continued*
with foreign body S81.042
right S81.031
with foreign body S81.041
labium (majus) (minus) — *see* Puncture, vulva
lacrimal duct — *see* Puncture, eyelid
larynx S11.013
with foreign body S11.014
leg (lower) S81.839
with foreign body S81.849
foot — *see* Puncture, foot
knee — *see* Puncture, knee
left S81.832
with foreign body S81.842
right S81.831
with foreign body S81.841
upper — *see* Puncture, thigh
lip S01.531
with foreign body S01.541
loin — *see* Puncture, abdomen, wall
lower back — *see* Puncture, back, lower
lumbar region — *see* Puncture, back, lower
malar region — *see* Puncture, head, specified site NEC
mammary — *see* Puncture, breast
mastoid region — *see* Puncture, head, specified site NEC
mouth — *see* Puncture, oral cavity
nail
finger — *see* Puncture, finger, with damage to nail
toe — *see* Puncture, toe, with damage to nail
nasal (septum) (sinus) — *see* Puncture, nose
nasopharynx — *see* Puncture, head, specified site NEC
neck S11.93
with foreign body S11.94
involving
cervical esophagus — *see* Puncture, cervical esophagus
larynx — *see* Puncture, larynx
pharynx — *see* Puncture, pharynx
thyroid gland — *see* Puncture, thyroid gland
trachea — *see* Puncture, trachea
specified site NEC S11.83
with foreign body S11.84
nose (septum) (sinus) S01.23
with foreign body S01.24
ocular — *see* Puncture, eyeball
oral cavity S01.532
with foreign body S01.542
orbit S05.4-
palate — *see* Puncture, oral cavity
palm — *see* Puncture, hand
pancreas S36.299
body S36.291
head S36.290
tail S36.292
pelvis — *see* Puncture, back, lower
penis S31.23
with foreign body S31.24
perineum
female S31.43
with foreign body S31.44
male S31.139
with foreign body S31.149
periocular area (with or without lacrimal passages) — *see* Puncture, eyelid
phalanges
finger — *see* Puncture, finger
toe — *see* Puncture, toe
pharynx S11.23
with foreign body S11.24
pinna — *see* Puncture, ear
popliteal space — *see* Puncture, knee
prepuce — *see* Puncture, penis
pubic region S31.139
with foreign body S31.149
pudendum — *see* Puncture, genital organs, external

Puncture - *continued*
rectovaginal septum — *see* Puncture, vagina
sacral region — *see* Puncture, back, lower
sacroiliac region — *see* Puncture, back, lower
salivary gland — *see* Puncture, oral cavity
scalp S01.03
with foreign body S01.04
scapular region — *see* Puncture, shoulder
scrotum S31.33
with foreign body S31.34
shin — *see* Puncture, leg
shoulder S41.039
with foreign body S41.049
left S41.032
with foreign body S41.042
right S41.031
with foreign body S41.041
spermatic cord — *see* Puncture, testis
sternal region — *see* Puncture, thorax, front
submaxillary region — *see* Puncture, head, specified site NEC
submental region — *see* Puncture, head, specified site NEC
subungual
finger (s) — *see* Puncture, finger, with damage to nail
toe — *see* Puncture, toe, with damage to nail
supraclavicular fossa — *see* Puncture, neck, specified site NEC
temple, temporal region — *see* Puncture, head, specified site NEC
temporomandibular area — *see* Puncture, cheek
testis S31.33
with foreign body S31.34
thigh S71.139
with foreign body S71.149
left S71.132
with foreign body S71.142
right S71.131
with foreign body S71.141
thorax, thoracic (wall) S21.93
with foreign body S21.94
back S21.23-
with
foreign body S21.24-
with penetration S21.44
penetration S21.43
breast — *see* Puncture, breast
front S21.13-
with
foreign body S21.14-
with penetration S21.34
penetration S21.33
throat — *see* Puncture, neck
thumb S61.039
with
damage to nail S61.139
with
foreign body S61.149
foreign body S61.049
left S61.032
with
damage to nail S61.132
with
foreign body S61.142
foreign body S61.042
right S61.031
with
damage to nail S61.131
with
foreign body S61.141
foreign body S61.041
thyroid gland S11.13
with foreign body S11.14
toe (s) S91.139
with
damage to nail S91.239
with
foreign body S91.249
foreign body S91.149
great S91.133
with

Puncture - *continued*
toe (s) - *continued*
great - *continued*
with - *continued*
damage to nail S91.233
with
foreign body S91.243
foreign body S91.143
left S91.132
with
damage to nail S91.232
with
foreign body S91.242
foreign body S91.142
right S91.131
with
damage to nail S91.231
with
foreign body S91.241
foreign body S91.141
lesser S91.136
with
damage to nail S91.236
with
foreign body S91.246
foreign body S91.146
left S91.135
with
damage to nail S91.235
with
foreign body S91.245
foreign body S91.145
right S91.134
with
damage to nail S91.234
with
foreign body S91.244
foreign body S91.144
tongue — *see* Puncture, oral cavity
trachea S11.023
with foreign body S11.024
tunica vaginalis — *see* Puncture, testis
tympanum, tympanic membrane S09.2-
umbilical region S31.135
with foreign body S31.145
uvula — *see* Puncture, oral cavity
vagina S31.43
with foreign body S31.44
vocal cords S11.033
with foreign body S11.034
vulva S31.43
with foreign body S31.44
wrist S61.539
with
foreign body S61.549
left S61.532
with
foreign body S61.542
right S61.531
with
foreign body S61.541
PUO (pyrexia of unknown origin) R50.9
Pupillary membrane (persistent) Q13.89
Pupillotonia — *see* Anomaly, pupil, function, tonic pupil
Purpura D69.2
abdominal D69.0
allergic D69.0
anaphylactoid D69.0
annularis telangiectodes L81.7
arthritic D69.0
autoerythrocyte sensitization D69.2
autoimmune D69.0
bacterial D69.0
Bateman's (senile) D69.2
capillary fragility (hereditary) (idiopathic) D69.8
cryoglobulinemic D89.1
Devil's pinches D69.2
fibrinolytic — *see* Fibrinolysis
fulminans, fulminous D65
gangrenous D65
hemorrhagic, hemorrhagica D69.3
not due to thrombocytopenia D69.0
Henoch (-Schönlein) (allergic) D69.0

Purpura - *continued*
hypergammaglobulinemic (benign) (Waldenström) D89.0
idiopathic (thrombocytopenic) D69.3
nonthrombocytopenic D69.0
immune thrombocytopenic D69.3
infectious D69.0
malignant D69.0
neonatorum P54.5
nervosa D69.0
newborn P54.5
nonthrombocytopenic D69.2
hemorrhagic D69.0
idiopathic D69.0
nonthrombopenic D69.2
peliosis rheumatica D69.0
posttransfusion (post-transfusion) (from (fresh) whole blood or blood products) D69.51
primary D69.49
red cell membrane sensitivity D69.2
rheumatica D69.0
Schönlein (-Henoch) (allergic) D69.0
scorbutic E54 *[D77]*
senile D69.2
simplex D69.2
symptomatica D69.0
telangiectasia annularis L81.7
thrombocytopenic D69.49
congenital D69.42
hemorrhagic D69.3
hereditary D69.42
idiopathic D69.3
immune D69.3
neonatal, transitory P61.0
thrombotic M31.19
thrombohemolytic — *see* Fibrinolysis
thrombolytic — *see* Fibrinolysis
thrombopenic D69.49
thrombotic, thrombocytopenic M31.19
toxic D69.0
vascular D69.0
visceral symptoms D69.0
Purpuric spots R23.3
Purulent — *see* condition
Pus
in
stool R19.5
urine N39.0
tube (rupture) — *see* Salpingo-oophoritis
Pustular rash L08.0
Pustule (nonmalignant) L08.9
malignant A22.0
Pustulosis palmaris et plantaris L40.3
Putnam (-Dana) disease or syndrome — *see* Degeneration, combined
Putrescent pulp (dental) K04.1
Pyarthritis, pyarthrosis — *see* Arthritis, pyogenic or pyemic
tuberculous — *see* Tuberculosis, joint
Pyelectasis — *see* Hydronephrosis
Pyelitis (congenital) (uremic) — *see also* Pyelonephritis
with
calculus — *see* category N20
with hydronephrosis N13.6
contracted kidney N11.9
acute N10
chronic N11.9
with calculus — *see* category N20
with hydronephrosis N13.6
cystica N28.84
puerperal (postpartum) O86.21
tuberculous A18.11
Pyelocystitis — *see* Pyelonephritis
Pyelonephritis — *see also* Nephritis, tubulo-interstitial
with
calculus — *see* category N20
with hydronephrosis N13.6
contracted kidney N11.9
acute N10
calculous — *see* category N20
with hydronephrosis N13.6
chronic N11.9

Pyelonephritis - *continued*
chronic - *continued*
with calculus — *see* category N20
with hydronephrosis N13.6
associated with ureteral obstruction or stricture N11.1
nonobstructive N11.8
with reflux (vesicoureteral) N11.0
obstructive N11.1
specified NEC N11.8
in (due to)
brucellosis A23.9 *[N16]*
cryoglobulinemia (mixed) D89.1 *[N16]*
cystinosis E72.04
diphtheria A36.84
glycogen storage disease E74.09 *[N16]*
leukemia NEC C95.9- *[N16]*
lymphoma NEC C85.90 *[N16]*
multiple myeloma C90.0- *[N16]*
obstruction N11.1
Salmonella infection A02.25
sarcoidosis D86.84
sepsis A41.9 *[N16]*
Sjögren's disease M35.04
toxoplasmosis B58.83
transplant rejection T86.91 *[N16]*
Wilson's disease E83.01 *[N16]*
nonobstructive N12
with reflux (vesicoureteral) N11.0
chronic N11.8
syphilitic A52.75
Pyelonephrosis (obstructive) N11.1
chronic N11.9
Pyelophlebitis I80.8
Pyeloureteritis cystica N28.85
Pyemia, pyemic (fever) (infection) (purulent) — *see also* Sepsis
joint — *see* Arthritis, pyogenic or pyemic
liver K75.1
pneumococcal A40.3
portal K75.1
postvaccinal T88.0
puerperal, postpartum, childbirth O85
specified organism NEC A41.89
tuberculous — *see* Tuberculosis, miliary
Pygopagus Q89.4
Pyknoepilepsy (idiopathic) — *see* Pyknolepsy
Pyknolepsy G40.A09
intractable G40.A19
with status epilepticus G40.A11
without status epilepticus G40.A19
not intractable G40.A09
with status epilepticus G40.A01
without status epilepticus G40.A09
Pylephlebitis K75.1
Pyle's syndrome Q78.5
Pylethrombophlebitis K75.1
Pylethrombosis K75.1
Pyloritis K29.90
with bleeding K29.91
Pylorospasm (reflex) NEC K31.3
congenital or infantile Q40.0
newborn Q40.0
neurotic F45.8
psychogenic F45.8
Pylorus, pyloric — *see* condition
Pyoarthrosis — *see* Arthritis, pyogenic or pyemic
Pyocele
mastoid — *see* Mastoiditis, acute
sinus (accessory) — *see* Sinusitis
turbinate (bone) J32.9
urethra — *see also* Urethritis N34.0
Pyocolpos — *see* Vaginitis
Pyocystitis N30.80
with hematuria N30.81
Pyoderma, pyodermia L08.0
gangrenosum L88
newborn P39.4
phagedenic L88
vegetans L08.81
Pyodermatitis L08.0
vegetans L08.81
Pyogenic — *see* condition
Pyohydronephrosis N13.6

Pyometra, pyometrium, pyometritis — *see* Endometritis
Pyomyositis (tropical) — *see* Myositis, infective
Pyonephritis N12
Pyonephrosis N13.6
tuberculous A18.11
Pyo-oophoritis — *see* Salpingo-oophoritis
Pyo-ovarium — *see* Salpingo-oophoritis
Pyopericarditis, pyopericardium I30.1
Pyophlebitis — *see* Phlebitis
Pyopneumopericardium I30.1
Pyopneumothorax (infective) J86.9
with fistula J86.0
tuberculous NEC A15.6
Pyosalpinx, pyosalpingitis — *see also* Salpingo-oophoritis
Pyothorax J86.9
with fistula J86.0
tuberculous NEC A15.6
Pyoureter N28.89
tuberculous A18.11
Pyramidopallidonigral syndrome G20
Pyrexia (of unknown origin) R50.9
atmospheric T67.01
during labor NEC O75.2
heat T67.01
newborn P81.9
environmentally-induced P81.0
persistent R50.9
puerperal O86.4
Pyroglobulinemia NEC E88.09
Pyromania F63.1
Pyrosis R12
Pyuria (bacterial) (sterile) R82.81

Q

Q fever A78
with pneumonia A78
Quadricuspid aortic valve Q23.8
Quadrilateral fever A78
Quadriparesis — *see* Quadriplegia
meaning muscle weakness M62.81
Quadriplegia G82.50
complete
C1-C4 level G82.51
C5-C7 level G82.53
congenital (cerebral) (spinal) G80.8
spastic G80.0
embolic (current episode) I63.4-
functional R53.2
incomplete
C1-C4 level G82.52
C5-C7 level G82.54
thrombotic (current episode) I63.3-
traumatic -- code to injury with seventh character S
current episode — *see* Injury, spinal (cord), cervical
Quadruplet, pregnancy — *see* Pregnancy, quadruplet
Quarrelsomeness F60.3
Queensland fever A77.3
Quervain's disease M65.4
thyroid E06.1
Queyrat's erythroplasia D07.4
penis D07.4
specified site — *see* Neoplasm, skin, in situ
unspecified site D07.4
Quincke's disease or edema T78.3
hereditary D84.1
Quinsy (gangrenous) J36
Quintan fever A79.0
Quintuplet, pregnancy — *see* Pregnancy, quintuplet

R

Rabbit fever — *see* Tularemia
Rabies A82.9
contact Z20.3
exposure to Z20.3
inoculation reaction — *see* Complications, vaccination
sylvatic A82.0
urban A82.1
Rachischisis — *see* Spina bifida
Rachitic — *see also* condition
deformities of spine (late effect) (sequelae) E64.3
pelvis (late effect) (sequelae) E64.3
with disproportion (fetopelvic) O33.0
causing obstructed labor O65.0
Rachitis, rachitism (acute) (tarda) — *see also* Rickets
renalis N25.0
sequelae E64.3
Radial nerve — *see* condition
Radiation
burn — *see* Burn
effects NOS T66
sickness NOS T66
therapy, encounter for Z51.0
Radiculitis (pressure) (vertebrogenic) — *see* Radiculopathy
Radiculomyelitis — *see also* Encephalitis
toxic, due to
Clostridium tetani A35
Corynebacterium diphtheriae A36.82
Radiculopathy M54.10
cervical region M54.12
cervicothoracic region M54.13
due to
disc disorder
C3 M50.11
C4 M50.11
C5 M50.121
C6 M50.122
C7 M50.123
C8 M50.13
displacement of intervertebral disc — *see* Disorder, disc, with, radiculopathy
leg M54.1-
lumbar region M54.16
lumbosacral region M54.17
occipito-atlanto-axial region M54.11
postherpetic B02.29
sacrococcygeal region M54.18
syphilitic A52.11
thoracic region (with visceral pain) M54.14
thoracolumbar region M54.15
Radiodermal burns (acute, chronic, or occupational) — *see* Burn
Radiodermatitis L58.9
acute L58.0
chronic L58.1
Radiotherapy session Z51.0
RAEB (refractory anemia with excess blasts) D46.2-
Rage, meaning rabies — *see* Rabies
Ragpicker's disease A22.1
Ragsorter's disease A22.1
Raillietiniasis B71.8
Railroad neurosis F48.8
Railway spine F48.8
Raised — *see also* Elevated
antibody titer R76.0
Rake teeth, tooth M26.39
Rales R09.89
Ramifying renal pelvis Q63.8
Ramsay-Hunt disease or syndrome — *see also* Hunt's disease B02.21
meaning dyssynergia cerebellaris myoclonica G11.19
Ranula K11.6
congenital Q38.4
Rape
adult
confirmed T74.21
suspected T76.21
alleged, observation or examination, ruled out
adult Z04.41
child Z04.42
child
confirmed T74.22
suspected T76.22
Rapid
feeble pulse, due to shock, following injury T79.4
heart (beat) R00.0
psychogenic F45.8
Rapid - *continued*
second stage (delivery) O62.3
time-zone change syndrome G47.25
Rarefaction, bone — *see* Disorder, bone, density and structure, specified NEC
Rash (toxic) R21
canker A38.9
diaper L22
drug (internal use) L27.0
contact — *see also* Dermatitis, due to, drugs, external L25.1
following immunization T88.1
food — *see* Dermatitis, due to, food
heat L74.0
napkin (psoriasiform) L22
nettle — *see* Urticaria
pustular L08.0
rose R21
epidemic B06.9
scarlet A38.9
serum — *see also* Reaction, serum T80.69
wandering tongue K14.1
Rasmussen aneurysm — *see* Tuberculosis, pulmonary
Rasmussen encephalitis G04.81
Rat-bite fever A25.9
due to Streptobacillus moniliformis A25.1
spirochetal (morsus muris) A25.0
Rathke's pouch tumor D44.3
Raymond (-Céstan) syndrome I65.8
Raynaud's disease, phenomenon or syndrome (secondary) I73.00
with gangrene (symmetric) I73.01
RDS (newborn) (type I) P22.0
type II P22.1
Reaction — *see also* Disorder
adaptation — *see* Disorder, adjustment
adjustment (anxiety) (conduct disorder) (depressiveness) (distress) — *see* Disorder, adjustment
with
mutism, elective (child) (adolescent) F94.0
adverse
food (any) (ingested) NEC T78.1
anaphylactic — *see* Shock, anaphylactic, due to food
affective — *see* Disorder, mood
allergic — *see* Allergy
anaphylactic — *see* Shock, anaphylactic
anaphylactoid — *see* Shock, anaphylactic
anesthesia — *see* Anesthesia, complication
antitoxin (prophylactic) (therapeutic) — *see* Complications, vaccination
anxiety F41.1
Arthus — *see* Arthus' phenomenon
asthenic F48.8
combat and operational stress F43.0
compulsive F42.8
conversion F44.9
crisis, acute F43.0
deoxyribonuclease (DNA) (DNase) hypersensitivity D69.2
depressive (single episode) F32.9
affective (single episode) F31.4
recurrent episode F33.9
neurotic F34.1
psychoneurotic F34.1
psychotic F32.3
recurrent — *see* Disorder, depressive, recurrent
dissociative F44.9
drug NEC T88.7
addictive — *see* Dependence, drug
transmitted via placenta or breast milk — *see* Absorption, drug, addictive, through placenta
allergic — *see* Allergy, drug
lichenoid L43.2
newborn P93.8
gray baby syndrome P93.0
overdose or poisoning (by accident) — *see* Table of Drugs and Chemicals, by drug, poisoning
photoallergic L56.1

- **Reflux** - *continued*
  - esophageal - *continued*
    - newborn P78.83
  - gastroesophageal K21.9
    - with esophagitis (without bleeding) K21.00
      - with bleeding K21.01
  - mitral — *see* Insufficiency, mitral
  - ureteral — *see* Reflux, vesicoureteral
  - vesicoureteral (with scarring) N13.70
    - with
      - nephropathy N13.729
        - with hydroureter N13.739
          - bilateral N13.732
          - unilateral N13.731
        - bilateral N13.722
        - unilateral N13.721
        - without hydroureter N13.729
          - bilateral N13.722
          - unilateral N13.721
      - pyelonephritis (chronic) N11.0
    - congenital Q62.7
    - without nephropathy N13.71
- **Reforming, artificial openings** — *see* Attention to, artificial, opening
- **Refractive error** — *see* Disorder, refraction
- **Refsum's disease or syndrome** G60.1
- **Refusal of**
  - food, psychogenic F50.89
  - treatment (because of) Z53.20
    - left against medical advice (AMA) Z53.29
    - left without being seen Z53.21
    - patient's decision NEC Z53.29
    - reasons of belief or group pressure Z53.1
- **Regional** — *see* condition
- **Regurgitation** R11.10
  - aortic (valve) — *see* Insufficiency, aortic
  - food — *see also* Vomiting
    - with reswallowing — *see* Rumination
    - newborn P92.1
  - gastric contents — *see* Vomiting
  - heart — *see* Endocarditis
  - mitral (valve) — *see* Insufficiency, mitral
    - congenital Q23.3
  - myocardial — *see* Endocarditis
  - pulmonary (valve) (heart) I37.1
    - congenital Q22.2
    - syphilitic A52.03
  - tricuspid — *see* Insufficiency, tricuspid
  - valve, valvular — *see* Endocarditis
    - congenital Q24.8
  - vesicoureteral — *see* Reflux, vesicoureteral
- **Reichmann's disease or syndrome** K31.89
- **Reifenstein syndrome** E34.52
- **Reinsertion**
  - implantable subdermal contraceptive Z30.46
  - intrauterine contraceptive device Z30.433
- **Reiter's disease, syndrome, or urethritis** M02.30
  - ankle M02.37-
  - elbow M02.32-
  - foot joint M02.37-
  - hand joint M02.34-
  - hip M02.35-
  - knee M02.36-
  - multiple site M02.39
  - shoulder M02.31-
  - vertebra M02.38
  - wrist M02.33-
- **Rejection**
  - food, psychogenic F50.89
  - transplant T86.91
    - bone T86.830
      - marrow T86.01
    - cornea T86.840-
    - heart T86.21
      - with lung (s) T86.31
    - intestine T86.850
    - kidney T86.11
    - liver T86.41
    - lung (s) T86.810
      - with heart T86.31
    - organ (immune or nonimmune cause) T86.91
    - pancreas T86.890
- **Rejection** - *continued*
  - transplant - *continued*
    - skin (allograft) (autograft) T86.820
    - specified NEC T86.890
    - stem cell (peripheral blood) (umbilical cord) T86.5
- **Relapsing fever** A68.9
  - Carter's (Asiatic) A68.1
  - Dutton's (West African) A68.1
  - Koch's A68.9
  - louse-borne (epidemic) A68.0
  - Novy's (American) A68.1
  - Obermeyers's (European) A68.0
  - Spirillum A68.9
  - tick-borne (endemic) A68.1
- **Relationship**
  - occlusal
    - open anterior M26.220
    - open posterior M26.221
- **Relaxation**
  - anus (sphincter) K62.89
    - psychogenic F45.8
  - arch (foot) — *see also* Deformity, limb, flat foot
  - back ligaments — *see* Instability, joint, spine
  - bladder (sphincter) N31.2
  - cardioesophageal K21.9
  - cervix — *see* Incompetency, cervix
  - diaphragm J98.6
  - joint (capsule) (ligament) (paralytic) — *see* Flail, joint
    - congenital NEC Q74.8
  - lumbosacral (joint) — *see* subcategory M53.2
  - pelvic floor N81.89
  - perineum N81.89
  - posture R29.3
  - rectum (sphincter) K62.89
  - sacroiliac (joint) — *see* subcategory M53.2
  - scrotum N50.89
  - urethra (sphincter) N36.44
  - vesical N31.2
- **Release from prison, anxiety concerning** Z65.2
- **Remains**
  - canal of Cloquet Q14.0
  - capsule (opaque) Q14.8
- **Remittent fever (malarial)** B54
- **Remnant**
  - canal of Cloquet Q14.0
  - capsule (opaque) Q14.8
  - cervix, cervical stump (acquired) (postoperative) N88.8
  - cystic duct, postcholecystectomy K91.5
  - fingernail L60.8
    - congenital Q84.6
  - meniscus, knee — *see* Derangement, knee, meniscus, specified NEC
  - thyroglossal duct Q89.2
  - tonsil J35.8
    - infected (chronic) J35.01
  - urachus Q64.4
- **Removal (from) (of)**
  - artificial
    - arm Z44.00-
      - complete Z44.01-
      - partial Z44.02-
    - eye Z44.2-
    - leg Z44.10-
      - complete Z44.11-
      - partial Z44.12-
  - breast implant Z45.81
  - cardiac pulse generator (battery) (end-of-life) Z45.010
  - catheter (urinary) (indwelling) Z46.6
    - from artificial opening — *see* Attention to, artificial, opening
    - non-vascular Z46.82
    - vascular NEC Z45.2
  - drains Z48.03
  - device Z46.9
    - contraceptive Z30.432
      - implantable subdermal Z30.46
    - implanted NEC Z45.89
    - specified NEC Z46.89
- **Removal (from) (of)** - *continued*
  - dressing (nonsurgical) Z48.00
    - surgical Z48.01
  - external
    - fixation device - code to fracture with seventh character D
    - prosthesis, prosthetic device Z44.9
      - breast Z44.3-
      - specified NEC Z44.8
  - home in childhood (to foster home or institution) Z62.29
  - ileostomy Z43.2
  - insulin pump Z46.81
  - myringotomy device (stent) (tube) Z45.82
  - nervous system device NEC Z46.2
    - brain neuropacemaker Z46.2
    - visual substitution device Z46.2
      - implanted Z45.31
  - non-vascular catheter Z46.82
  - orthodontic device Z46.4
  - organ, prophylactic (for neoplasia management) — *see* Prophylactic, organ removal
  - staples Z48.02
  - stent
    - ureteral Z46.6
  - suture Z48.02
  - urinary device Z46.6
  - vascular access device or catheter Z45.2
- **Ren**
  - arcuatus Q63.1
  - mobile, mobilis N28.89
    - congenital Q63.8
  - unguliformis Q63.1
- **Renal** — *see* condition
- **Rendu-Osler-Weber disease or syndrome** I78.0
- **Reninoma** D41.0-
- **Renon-Delille syndrome** E23.3
- **Reovirus, as cause of disease classified elsewhere** B97.5
- **Repeated falls NEC** R29.6
- **Replaced chromosome by dicentric ring** Q93.2
- **Replacement by artificial or mechanical device or prosthesis of**
  - bladder Z96.0
  - blood vessel NEC Z95.828
  - bone NEC Z96.7
  - cochlea Z96.21
  - coronary artery Z95.5
  - eustachian tube Z96.29
  - eye globe Z97.0
  - heart Z95.812
    - valve Z95.2
      - prosthetic Z95.2
      - specified NEC Z95.4
      - xenogenic Z95.3
  - intestine Z96.89
  - joint Z96.60
    - hip — *see* Presence, hip joint implant
    - knee — *see* Presence, knee joint implant
    - specified site NEC Z96.698
  - larynx Z96.3
  - lens Z96.1
  - limb (s) — *see* Presence, artificial, limb
  - mandible NEC (for tooth root implant (s)) Z96.5
  - organ NEC Z96.89
  - peripheral vessel NEC Z95.828
  - stapes Z96.29
  - teeth Z97.2
  - tendon Z96.7
  - tissue NEC Z96.89
  - tooth root (s) Z96.5
  - vessel NEC Z95.828
    - coronary (artery) Z95.5
- **Request for expert evidence** Z04.89
- **Reserve, decreased or low**
  - cardiac — *see* Disease, heart
  - kidney N28.89
- **Residing**
  - in place not meant for human habitation (abandoned building) (car) (park) (sidewalk) Z59.02

RETENTION - RHEUMATOID

Rheumatoid - *continued*
arthritis - *continued*
seronegative — *see* Arthritis, rheumatoid, seronegative
seropositive — *see* Arthritis, rheumatoid, seropositive
carditis M05.30
ankle M05.37-
elbow M05.32-
foot joint M05.37-
hand joint M05.34-
hip M05.35-
knee M05.36-
multiple site M05.39
shoulder M05.31-
vertebra — *see* Spondylitis, ankylosing
wrist M05.33-
endocarditis — *see* Rheumatoid, carditis
lung (disease) M05.10
ankle M05.17-
elbow M05.12-
foot joint M05.17-
hand joint M05.14-
hip M05.15-
knee M05.16-
multiple site M05.19
shoulder M05.11-
vertebra — *see* Spondylitis, ankylosing
wrist M05.13-
myocarditis — *see* Rheumatoid, carditis
myopathy M05.40
ankle M05.47-
elbow M05.42-
foot joint M05.47-
hand joint M05.44-
hip M05.45-
knee M05.46-
multiple site M05.49
shoulder M05.41-
vertebra — *see* Spondylitis, ankylosing
wrist M05.43-
pericarditis — *see* Rheumatoid, carditis
polyarthritis — *see* Arthritis, rheumatoid
polyneuropathy M05.50
ankle M05.57-
elbow M05.52-
foot joint M05.57-
hand joint M05.54-
hip M05.55-
knee M05.56-
multiple site M05.59
shoulder M05.51-
vertebra — *see* Spondylitis, ankylosing
wrist M05.53-
vasculitis M05.20
ankle M05.27-
elbow M05.22-
foot joint M05.27-
hand joint M05.24-
hip M05.25-
knee M05.26-
multiple site M05.29
shoulder M05.21-
vertebra — *see* Spondylitis, ankylosing
wrist M05.23-
Rhinitis (atrophic) (catarrhal) (chronic) (croupous) (fibrinous) (granulomatous) (hyperplastic) (hypertrophic) (membranous) (obstructive) (purulent) (suppurative) (ulcerative) J31.0
with
sore throat — *see* Nasopharyngitis
acute J00
allergic J30.9
with asthma J45.909
with
exacerbation (acute) J45.901
status asthmaticus J45.902
due to
food J30.5
pollen J30.1
nonseasonal J30.89
perennial J30.89
seasonal NEC J30.2
specified NEC J30.89
Rhinitis (atrophic) (catarrhal) (chronic) (croupous) (fibrinous) (granulomatous) (hyperplastic) (hypertrophic) (membranous) (obstructive) (purulent) (suppurative) (ulcerative) - *continued*
infective J00
pneumococcal J00
syphilitic A52.73
congenital A50.05 *[J99]*
tuberculous A15.8
vasomotor J30.0
Rhinoantritis (chronic) — *see* Sinusitis, maxillary
Rhinodacryolith — *see* Dacryolith
Rhinolith (nasal sinus) J34.89
Rhinomegaly J34.89
Rhinopharyngitis (acute) (subacute) — *see also* Nasopharyngitis
chronic J31.1
destructive ulcerating A66.5
mutilans A66.5
Rhinophyma L71.1
Rhinorrhea J34.89
cerebrospinal (fluid) G96.01
postoperative G96.08
specified NEC G96.08
spontaneous G96.01
traumatic G96.08
paroxysmal — *see* Rhinitis, allergic
spasmodic — *see* Rhinitis, allergic
Rhinosalpingitis — *see* Salpingitis, eustachian
Rhinoscleroma A48.8
Rhinosporidiosis B48.1
Rhinovirus infection NEC B34.8
Rhizomelic chondrodysplasia punctata E71.540
Rhythm
atrioventricular nodal I49.8
disorder I49.9
coronary sinus I49.8
ectopic I49.8
nodal I49.8
escape I49.9
heart, abnormal I49.9
idioventricular I44.2
nodal I49.8
sleep, inversion G47.2-
nonorganic origin — *see* Disorder, sleep, circadian rhythm, psychogenic
Rhytidosis facialis L98.8
Rib — *see also* condition
cervical Q76.5
Riboflavin deficiency E53.0
Rice bodies — *see also* Loose, body, joint
knee M23.4-
Richter syndrome — *see* Leukemia, chronic lymphocytic, B-cell type
Richter's hernia — *see* Hernia, abdomen, with obstruction
Ricinism — *see* Poisoning, food, noxious, plant
Rickets (active) (acute) (adolescent) (chest wall) (congenital) (current) (infantile) (intestinal) E55.0
adult — *see* Osteomalacia
celiac K90.0
hypophosphatemic with nephrotic-glycosuric dwarfism E72.09
inactive E64.3
kidney N25.0
renal N25.0
sequelae, any E64.3
vitamin-D-resistant E83.31 *[M90.80]*
Rickettsia 364D/R. philipii (Pacific Coast tick fever) A77.8
Rickettsial disease A79.9
specified type NEC A79.89
Rickettsialpox (Rickettsia akari) A79.1
Rickettsiosis A79.9
due to
Ehrlichia sennetsu A79.81
Neorickettsia sennetsu A79.81
Rickettsia akari (rickettsialpox) A79.1
specified type NEC A79.89
tick-borne A77.9
Rickettsiosis - *continued*
vesicular A79.1
Rider's bone — *see* Ossification, muscle, specified NEC
Ridge, alveolus — *see also* condition
flabby K06.8
Ridged ear, congenital Q17.3
Riedel's
lobe, liver Q44.7
struma, thyroiditis or disease E06.5
Rieger's anomaly or syndrome Q13.81
Riehl's melanosis L81.4
Rietti-Greppi-Micheli anemia D56.9
Rieux's hernia — *see* Hernia, abdomen, specified site NEC
Riga (-Fede) disease K14.0
Riggs' disease — *see* Periodontitis
Right aortic arch Q25.47
Right middle lobe syndrome J98.11
Rigid, rigidity — *see also* condition
abdominal R19.30
with severe abdominal pain R10.0
epigastric R19.36
generalized R19.37
left lower quadrant R19.34
left upper quadrant R19.32
periumbilic R19.35
right lower quadrant R19.33
right upper quadrant R19.31
articular, multiple, congenital Q68.8
cervix (uteri) in pregnancy — *see* Pregnancy, complicated by, abnormal, cervix
hymen (acquired) (congenital) N89.6
nuchal R29.1
pelvic floor in pregnancy — *see* Pregnancy, complicated by, abnormal, pelvic organs or tissues NEC
perineum or vulva in pregnancy — *see* Pregnancy, complicated by, abnormal, vulva
spine — *see* Dorsopathy, specified NEC
vagina in pregnancy — *see* Pregnancy, complicated by, abnormal, vagina
Rigors R68.89
with fever R50.9
Riley-Day syndrome G90.1
RIND (reversible ischemic neurologic deficit) I63.9
Ring (s)
aorta (vascular) Q25.45
Bandl's O62.4
contraction, complicating delivery O62.4
esophageal, lower (muscular) K22.2
Fleischer's (cornea) H18.04-
hymenal, tight (acquired) (congenital) N89.6
Kayser-Fleischer (cornea) H18.04-
retraction, uterus, pathological O62.4
Schatzki's (esophagus) (lower) K22.2
congenital Q39.3
Soemmerring's — *see* Cataract, secondary
vascular (congenital) Q25.8
aorta Q25.45
Ringed hair (congenital) Q84.1
Ringworm B35.9
beard B35.0
black dot B35.0
body B35.4
Burmese B35.5
corporeal B35.4
foot B35.3
groin B35.6
hand B35.2
honeycomb B35.0
nails B35.1
perianal (area) B35.6
scalp B35.0
specified NEC B35.8
Tokelau B35.5
Rise, venous pressure I87.8
Rising, PSA following treatment for malignant neoplasm of prostate R97.21
Risk
for
dental caries Z91.849
high Z91.843

Risk - *continued*
- for - *continued*
  - dental caries - *continued*
    - low Z91.841
    - moderate Z91.842
  - homelessness, imminent Z59.811
- suicidal
  - meaning personal history of attempted suicide Z91.51
  - meaning suicidal ideation — *see* Ideation, suicidal

Ritter's disease L00
Rivalry, sibling Z62.891
Rivalta's disease A42.2
River blindness B73.01
Robert's pelvis Q74.2
- with disproportion (fetopelvic) O33.0
  - causing obstructed labor O65.0

Robin (-Pierre) syndrome Q87.0
Robinow-Silvermann-Smith syndrome Q87.19
Robinson's (hidrotic) ectodermal dysplasia or syndrome Q82.4
Robles' disease B73.01
Rocky Mountain (spotted) fever A77.0
Roetheln — *see* Rubella
Roger's disease Q21.0
Rokitansky-Aschoff sinuses (gallbladder) K82.8
Rolando's fracture (displaced) S62.22-
- nondisplaced S62.22-

Romano-Ward (prolonged QT interval) syndrome I45.81
Romberg's disease or syndrome G51.8
Roof, mouth — *see* condition
Rosacea L71.9
- acne L71.9
- keratitis L71.8
- specified NEC L71.8

Rosary, rachitic E55.0
Rose
- cold J30.1
- fever J30.1
- rash R21
  - epidemic B06.9

Rosenbach's erysipeloid A26.0
Rosenthal's disease or syndrome D68.1
Roseola B09
- infantum B08.20
  - due to human herpesvirus 6 B08.21
  - due to human herpesvirus 7 B08.22

Ross River disease or fever B33.1
Rossbach's disease K31.89
- psychogenic F45.8

Rostan's asthma (cardiac) — *see* Failure, ventricular, left
Rotation
- anomalous, incomplete or insufficient, intestine Q43.3
- cecum (congenital) Q43.3
- colon (congenital) Q43.3
- spine, incomplete or insufficient — *see* Dorsopathy, deforming, specified NEC
- tooth, teeth, fully erupted M26.35
- vertebra, incomplete or insufficient — *see* Dorsopathy, deforming, specified NEC

Rotes Quérol disease or syndrome — *see* Hyperostosis, ankylosing
Roth (-Bernhardt) disease or syndrome — *see* Meralgia paraesthetica
Rothmund (-Thomson) syndrome Q82.8
Rotor's disease or syndrome E80.6
Round
- back (with wedging of vertebrae) — *see* Kyphosis
  - sequelae (late effect) of rickets E64.3
- worms (large) (infestation) NEC B82.0
  - Ascariasis — *see also* Ascariasis B77.9

Roussy-Lévy syndrome G60.0
Rubella (German measles) B06.9
- complication NEC B06.09
  - neurological B06.00
- congenital P35.0
- contact Z20.4
- exposure to Z20.4

Rubella (German measles) - *continued*
- maternal
  - manifest rubella in infant P35.0
  - care for (suspected) damage to fetus O35.3
  - suspected damage to fetus affecting management of pregnancy O35.3
- specified complications NEC B06.89

Rubeola (meaning measles) — *see* Measles
- meaning rubella — *see* Rubella

Rubeosis, iris — *see* Disorder, iris, vascular
Rubinstein-Taybi syndrome Q87.2
Rudimentary (congenital) — *see also* Agenesis
- arm — *see* Defect, reduction, upper limb
- bone Q79.9
- cervix uteri Q51.828
- eye Q11.2
- lobule of ear Q17.3
- patella Q74.1
- respiratory organs in thoracopagus Q89.4
- tracheal bronchus Q32.4
- uterus Q51.818
  - in male Q56.1
- vagina Q52.0

Ruled out condition — *see* Observation, suspected
Rumination R11.10
- with nausea R11.2
- disorder of infancy F98.21
- neurotic F42.8
- newborn P92.1
- obsessional F42.8
- psychogenic F42.8

Runeberg's disease D51.0
Runny nose R09.89
Rupia (syphilitic) A51.39
- congenital A50.06
- tertiary A52.79

Rupture, ruptured
- abscess (spontaneous) - code by site under Abscess
- aneurysm — *see* Aneurysm
- anus (sphincter) — *see* Laceration, anus
- aorta, aortic I71.8
  - abdominal I71.3
  - arch I71.1
  - ascending I71.1
  - descending I71.8
    - abdominal I71.3
    - thoracic I71.1
  - syphilitic A52.01
  - thoracoabdominal I71.5
  - thorax, thoracic I71.1
  - transverse I71.1
  - traumatic — *see* Injury, aorta, laceration, major
  - valve or cusp — *see also* Endocarditis, aortic I35.8
- appendix (with peritonitis) — *see also* Appendicitis K35.32
  - with localized peritonitis — *see also* Appendicitis K35.32
- arteriovenous fistula, brain — *see* Fistula, arteriovenous, brain, ruptured
- artery I77.2
  - brain — *see* Hemorrhage, intracranial, intracerebral
  - coronary — *see* Infarct, myocardium
  - heart — *see* Infarct, myocardium
  - pulmonary I28.8
  - traumatic (complication) — *see* Injury, blood vessel
- bile duct (common) (hepatic) K83.2
  - cystic K82.2
- bladder (sphincter) (nontraumatic) (spontaneous) N32.89
  - following ectopic or molar pregnancy O08.6
  - obstetrical trauma O71.5
  - traumatic S37.29
- blood vessel — *see also* Hemorrhage
  - brain — *see* Hemorrhage, intracranial, intracerebral
  - heart — *see* Infarct, myocardium

Rupture, ruptured - *continued*
- blood vessel - *continued*
  - traumatic (complication) — *see* Injury, blood vessel, laceration, major, by site
- bone — *see* Fracture
- bowel (nontraumatic) K63.1
- brain
  - aneurysm (congenital) — *see also* Hemorrhage, intracranial, subarachnoid
    - syphilitic A52.05
  - hemorrhagic — *see* Hemorrhage, intracranial, intracerebral
- capillaries I78.8
- cardiac (auricle) (ventricle) (wall) I23.3
  - with hemopericardium I23.0
  - infectional I40.9
  - traumatic — *see* Injury, heart
- cartilage (articular) (current) — *see also* Sprain
  - knee S83.3-
  - semilunar — *see* Tear, meniscus
- cecum (with peritonitis) K65.0
  - with peritoneal abscess K35.33
  - traumatic S36.598
- celiac artery, traumatic — *see* Injury, blood vessel, celiac artery, laceration, major
- cerebral aneurysm (congenital) (see Hemorrhage, intracranial, subarachnoid)
- cervix (uteri)
  - with ectopic or molar pregnancy O08.6
  - following ectopic or molar pregnancy O08.6
  - obstetrical trauma O71.3
  - traumatic S37.69
- chordae tendineae NEC I51.1
  - concurrent with acute myocardial infarction — *see* Infarct, myocardium
  - following acute myocardial infarction (current complication) I23.4
- choroid (direct) (indirect) (traumatic) H31.32-
- circle of Willis I60.6
- colon (nontraumatic) K63.1
  - traumatic — *see* Injury, intestine, large
- cornea (traumatic) — *see* Injury, eye, laceration
- coronary (artery) (thrombotic) — *see* Infarct, myocardium
- corpus luteum (infected) (ovary) N83.1-
- cyst — *see* Cyst
- cystic duct K82.2
- Descemet's membrane — *see* Change, corneal membrane, Descemet's, rupture
  - traumatic — *see* Injury, eye, laceration
- diaphragm, traumatic — *see* Injury, intrathoracic, diaphragm
- disc — *see* Rupture, intervertebral disc
- diverticulum (intestine) K57.80
  - with bleeding K57.81
  - bladder N32.3
  - large intestine K57.20
    - with
      - bleeding K57.21
      - small intestine K57.40
        - with bleeding K57.41
  - small intestine K57.00
    - with
      - bleeding K57.01
      - large intestine K57.40
        - with bleeding K57.41
- duodenal stump K31.89
- ear drum (nontraumatic) — *see also* Perforation, tympanum
  - traumatic S09.2-
    - due to blast injury — *see* Injury, blast, ear
- esophagus K22.3
- eye (without prolapse or loss of intraocular tissue) — *see* Injury, eye, laceration
- fallopian tube NEC (nonobstetric) (nontraumatic) N83.8
  - due to pregnancy O00.10-
    - with intrauterine pregnancy O00.11-
- fontanel P13.1

Rupture, ruptured - *continued*
- gallbladder K82.2
  - traumatic S36.128
- gastric — *see also* Rupture, stomach
  - vessel K92.2
- globe (eye) (traumatic) — *see* Injury, eye, laceration
- graafian follicle (hematoma) N83.0-
- heart — *see* Rupture, cardiac
- hymen (nontraumatic) (nonintentional) N89.8
- internal organ, traumatic — *see* Injury, by site
- intervertebral disc — *see* Displacement, intervertebral disc
  - traumatic — *see* Rupture, traumatic, intervertebral disc
- intestine NEC (nontraumatic) K63.1
  - traumatic — *see* Injury, intestine
- iris — *see also* Abnormality, pupillary
  - traumatic — *see* Injury, eye, laceration
- joint capsule, traumatic — *see* Sprain
- kidney (traumatic) S37.06-
  - birth injury P15.8
  - nontraumatic N28.89
- lacrimal duct (traumatic) — *see* Injury, eye, specified site NEC
- lens (cataract) (traumatic) — *see* Cataract, traumatic
- ligament, traumatic — *see* Rupture, traumatic, ligament, by site
- liver S36.116
  - birth injury P15.0
- lymphatic vessel I89.8
- marginal sinus (placental) (with hemorrhage) — *see* Hemorrhage, antepartum, specified cause NEC
- membrana tympani (nontraumatic) — *see* Perforation, tympanum
- membranes (spontaneous)
  - artificial
    - delayed delivery following O75.5
  - delayed delivery following — *see* Pregnancy, complicated by, premature rupture of membranes
- meningeal artery I60.8
- meniscus (knee) — *see also* Tear, meniscus
  - old — *see* Derangement, meniscus
  - site other than knee - code as Sprain
- mesenteric artery, traumatic — *see* Injury, mesenteric, artery, laceration, major
- mesentery (nontraumatic) K66.8
  - traumatic — *see* Injury, intra-abdominal, specified, site NEC
- mitral (valve) I34.8
- muscle (traumatic) — *see also* Strain
  - diastasis — *see* Diastasis, muscle
  - nontraumatic M62.10
    - ankle M62.17-
    - foot M62.17-
    - forearm M62.13-
    - hand M62.14-
    - lower leg M62.16-
    - pelvic region M62.15-
    - shoulder region M62.11-
    - specified site NEC M62.18
    - thigh M62.15-
    - upper arm M62.12-
  - traumatic — *see* Strain, by site
- musculotendinous junction NEC, nontraumatic — *see* Rupture, tendon, spontaneous
- mycotic aneurysm causing cerebral hemorrhage — *see* Hemorrhage, intracranial, subarachnoid
- myocardium, myocardial — *see* Rupture, cardiac
  - traumatic — *see* Injury, heart
- nontraumatic, meaning hernia — *see* Hernia
- obstructed — *see* Hernia, by site, obstructed
- operation wound — *see* Disruption, wound, operation
- ovary, ovarian N83.8
  - corpus luteum cyst N83.1-
  - follicle (graafian) N83.0-

Rupture, ruptured - *continued*
- oviduct (nonobstetric) (nontraumatic) N83.8
  - due to pregnancy O00.10-
    - with intrauterine pregnancy O00.11-
- pancreas (nontraumatic) K86.89
  - traumatic S36.299
- papillary muscle NEC I51.2
  - following acute myocardial infarction (current complication) I23.5
- pelvic
  - floor, complicating delivery O70.1
  - organ NEC, obstetrical trauma O71.5
- perineum (nonobstetric) (nontraumatic) N90.89
  - complicating delivery — *see* Delivery, complicated, by, laceration, anus (sphincter)
- postoperative wound — *see* Disruption, wound, operation
- prostate (traumatic) S37.828
- pulmonary
  - artery I28.8
  - valve (heart) I37.8
  - vein I28.8
  - vessel I28.8
- pus tube — *see* Salpingitis
- pyosalpinx — *see* Salpingitis
- rectum (nontraumatic) K63.1
  - traumatic S36.69
- retina, retinal (traumatic) (without detachment) — *see also* Break, retina
  - with detachment — *see* Detachment, retina, with retinal, break
- rotator cuff (nontraumatic) M75.10-
  - complete M75.12-
  - incomplete M75.11-
- sclera — *see* Injury, eye, laceration
- sigmoid (nontraumatic) K63.1
  - traumatic S36.593
- spinal cord — *see also* Injury, spinal cord, by region
  - due to injury at birth P11.5
  - newborn (birth injury) P11.5
- spleen (traumatic) S36.09
  - birth injury P15.1
  - congenital (birth injury) P15.1
  - due to P. vivax malaria B51.0
  - nontraumatic D73.5
  - spontaneous D73.5
- splenic vein R58
  - traumatic — *see* Injury, blood vessel, splenic vein
- stomach (nontraumatic) (spontaneous) K31.89
  - traumatic S36.39
- supraspinatus (complete) (incomplete) (nontraumatic) — *see* Tear, rotator cuff
- symphysis pubis
  - obstetric O71.6
  - traumatic S33.4
- synovium (cyst) M66.10
  - ankle M66.17-
  - elbow M66.12-
  - finger M66.14-
  - foot M66.17-
  - forearm M66.13-
  - hand M66.14-
  - pelvic region M66.15-
  - shoulder region M66.11-
  - specified site NEC M66.18
  - thigh M66.15-
  - toe M66.17-
  - upper arm M66.12-
  - wrist M66.13-
- tendon (traumatic) — *see* Strain
  - nontraumatic (spontaneous) M66.9
    - ankle M66.87-
    - extensor M66.20
      - ankle M66.27-
      - foot M66.27-
      - forearm M66.23-
      - hand M66.24-
      - lower leg M66.26-
      - multiple sites M66.29
      - pelvic region M66.25-

Rupture, ruptured - *continued*
- tendon (traumatic) - *continued*
  - nontraumatic (spontaneous) - *continued*
    - extensor - *continued*
      - shoulder region M66.21-
      - specified site NEC M66.28
      - thigh M66.25-
      - upper arm M66.22-
    - flexor M66.30
      - ankle M66.37-
      - foot M66.37-
      - forearm M66.33-
      - hand M66.34-
      - lower leg M66.36-
      - multiple sites M66.39
      - pelvic region M66.35-
      - shoulder region M66.31-
      - specified site NEC M66.38
      - thigh M66.35-
      - upper arm M66.32-
    - foot M66.87-
    - forearm M66.83-
    - hand M66.84-
    - lower leg M66.86-
    - multiple sites M66.89
    - pelvic region M66.85-
    - shoulder region M66.81-
    - specified
      - site NEC M66.88
      - tendon M66.80
    - thigh M66.85-
    - upper arm M66.82-
- thoracic duct I89.8
- tonsil J35.8
- traumatic
  - aorta — *see* Injury, aorta, laceration, major
  - diaphragm — *see* Injury, intrathoracic, diaphragm
  - external site — *see* Wound, open, by site
  - eye — *see* Injury, eye, laceration
  - internal organ — *see* Injury, by site
  - intervertebral disc
    - cervical S13.0
    - lumbar S33.0
    - thoracic S23.0
  - kidney S37.06-
  - ligament — *see also* Sprain
    - ankle — *see* Sprain, ankle
    - carpus — *see* Rupture, traumatic, ligament, wrist
    - collateral (hand) — *see* Rupture, traumatic, ligament, finger, collateral
    - finger (metacarpophalangeal) (interphalangeal) S63.40-
      - collateral S63.41-
        - index S63.41-
        - little S63.41-
        - middle S63.41-
        - ring S63.41-
      - index S63.40-
      - little S63.40-
      - middle S63.40-
      - palmar S63.42-
        - index S63.42-
        - little S63.42-
        - middle S63.42-
        - ring S63.42-
      - ring S63.40-
      - specified site NEC S63.499
        - index S63.49-
        - little S63.49-
        - middle S63.49-
        - ring S63.49-
      - volar plate S63.43-
        - index S63.43-
        - little S63.43-
        - middle S63.43-
        - ring S63.43-
    - foot — *see* Sprain, foot
    - radial collateral S53.2-
    - radiocarpal — *see* Rupture, traumatic, ligament, wrist, radiocarpal
    - ulnar collateral S53.3-

Rupture, ruptured - *continued*
- traumatic - *continued*
  - ligament - *continued*
    - ulnocarpal — *see* Rupture, traumatic, ligament, wrist, ulnocarpal
    - wrist S63.30-
      - collateral S63.31-
      - radiocarpal S63.32-
      - specified site NEC S63.39-
      - ulnocarpal (palmar) S63.33-
  - liver S36.116
  - membrana tympani — *see* Rupture, ear drum, traumatic
  - muscle or tendon — *see* Strain
  - myocardium — *see* Injury, heart
  - pancreas S36.299
  - rectum S36.69
  - sigmoid S36.593
  - spleen S36.09
  - stomach S36.39
  - symphysis pubis S33.4
  - tympanum, tympanic (membrane) — *see* Rupture, ear drum, traumatic
  - ureter S37.19
  - uterus S37.69
  - vagina — *see* Injury, vagina
  - vena cava — *see* Injury, vena cava, laceration, major
- tricuspid (heart) (valve) I07.8
- tube, tubal (nonobstetric) (nontraumatic) N83.8
  - abscess — *see* Salpingitis
  - due to pregnancy O00.10-
    - with intrauterine pregnancy O00.11-
- tympanum, tympanic (membrane) (nontraumatic) — *see also* Perforation, tympanic membrane H72.9-
  - traumatic — *see* Rupture, ear drum, traumatic
- umbilical cord, complicating delivery O69.89
- ureter (traumatic) S37.19
  - nontraumatic N28.89
- urethra (nontraumatic) N36.8
  - with ectopic or molar pregnancy O08.6
  - following ectopic or molar pregnancy O08.6
  - obstetrical trauma O71.5
  - traumatic S37.39
- uterosacral ligament (nonobstetric) (nontraumatic) N83.8
- uterus (traumatic) S37.69
  - before labor O71.0-
  - during or after labor O71.1
  - nonpuerperal, nontraumatic N85.8
  - pregnant (during labor) O71.1
    - before labor O71.0-
- vagina — *see* Injury, vagina
- valve, valvular (heart) — *see* Endocarditis
- varicose vein — *see* Varix
- varix — *see* Varix
- vena cava R58
  - traumatic — *see* Injury, vena cava, laceration, major
- vesical (urinary) N32.89
- vessel (blood) R58
  - pulmonary I28.8
  - traumatic — *see* Injury, blood vessel
- viscus R19.8
- vulva complicating delivery O70.0

Russell-Silver syndrome Q87.19
Russian spring-summer type encephalitis A84.0
Rust's disease (tuberculous cervical spondylitis) A18.01
Ruvalcaba-Myhre-Smith syndrome E71.440
Rytand-Lipsitch syndrome I44.2

S

Saber, sabre shin or tibia (syphilitic) A50.56 *[M90.8-]*
Sac lacrimal — *see* condition
Saccharomyces infection B37.9
Saccharopinuria E72.3
Saccular — *see* condition
Sacculation
- aorta (nonsyphilitic) — *see* Aneurysm, aorta

Sacculation - *continued*
- bladder N32.3
- intralaryngeal (congenital) (ventricular) Q31.3
- larynx (congenital) (ventricular) Q31.3
- organ or site, congenital — *see* Distortion
- pregnant uterus — *see* Pregnancy, complicated by, abnormal, uterus
- ureter N28.89
- urethra N36.1
- vesical N32.3

Sachs' amaurotic familial idiocy or disease E75.02
Sachs-Tay disease E75.02
Sacks-Libman disease M32.11
Sacralgia M53.3
Sacralization Q76.49
Sacrodynia M53.3
Sacroiliac joint — *see* condition
Sacroiliitis NEC M46.1
Sacrum — *see* condition
Saddle
- back — *see* Lordosis
- embolus
  - abdominal aorta I74.01
  - pulmonary artery I26.92
    - with acute cor pulmonale I26.02
- injury - code to condition
- nose M95.0
  - due to syphilis A50.57

Sadism (sexual) F65.52
Sadness, postpartal O90.6
Sadomasochism F65.50
Saemisch's ulcer (cornea) — *see* Ulcer, cornea, central
Sagging
- skin and subcutaneous tissue (following bariatric surgery weight loss) (following dietary weight loss) L98.7

Sahib disease B55.0
Sailors' skin L57.8
Saint
- Anthony's fire — *see* Erysipelas
- triad — *see* Hernia, diaphragm
- Vitus' dance — *see* Chorea, Sydenham's

Salaam
- attack (s) — *see* Epilepsy, spasms
- tic R25.8

Salicylism
- abuse F55.8
- overdose or wrong substance given — *see* Table of Drugs and Chemicals, by drug, poisoning

Salivary duct or gland — *see* condition
Salivation, excessive K11.7
Salmonella — *see* Infection, Salmonella
Salmonellosis A02.0
Salpingitis (catarrhal) (fallopian tube) (nodular) (pseudofollicular) (purulent) (septic) N70.91
- with oophoritis N70.93
- acute N70.01
  - with oophoritis N70.03
- chlamydial A56.11
- chronic N70.11
  - with oophoritis N70.13
- complicating abortion — *see* Abortion, by type, complicated by, salpingitis
- ear — *see* Salpingitis, eustachian
- eustachian (tube) H68.00-
  - acute H68.01-
  - chronic H68.02-
- follicularis N70.11
  - with oophoritis N70.13
- gonococcal (acute) (chronic) A54.24
- interstitial, chronic N70.11
  - with oophoritis N70.13
- isthmica nodosa N70.11
  - with oophoritis N70.13
- specific (gonococcal) (acute) (chronic) A54.24
- tuberculous (acute) (chronic) A18.17
- venereal (gonococcal) (acute) (chronic) A54.24

Salpingocele N83.4-
Salpingo-oophoritis (catarrhal) (purulent) (ruptured) (septic) (suppurative) N70.93
- acute N70.03
  - with ectopic or molar pregnancy O08.0
  - following ectopic or molar pregnancy O08.0
  - gonococcal A54.24
- chronic N70.13
- following ectopic or molar pregnancy O08.0
- gonococcal (acute) (chronic) A54.24
- puerperal O86.19
- specific (gonococcal) (acute) (chronic) A54.24
- subacute N70.03
- tuberculous (acute) (chronic) A18.17
- venereal (gonococcal) (acute) (chronic) A54.24

Salpingo-ovaritis — *see* Salpingo-oophoritis
Salpingoperitonitis — *see* Salpingo-oophoritis
Salzmann's nodular dystrophy — *see* Degeneration, cornea, nodular
Sampson's cyst or tumor N80.1
San Joaquin (Valley) fever B38.0
Sandblaster's asthma, lung or pneumoconiosis J62.8
Sander's disease (paranoia) F22
Sandfly fever A93.1
Sandhoff's disease E75.01
Sanfilippo (Type B) (Type C) (Type D) syndrome E76.22
Sanger-Brown ataxia G11.2
Sao Paulo fever or typhus A77.0
Saponification, mesenteric K65.8
Sarcocele (benign)
- syphilitic A52.76
  - congenital A50.59

Sarcocystosis A07.8
Sarcoepiplocele — *see* Hernia
Sarcoepiplomphalocele Q79.2
Sarcoid — *see also* Sarcoidosis
- arthropathy D86.86
- Boeck's D86.9
- Darier-Roussy D86.3
- iridocyclitis D86.83
- meningitis D86.81
- myocarditis D86.85
- myositis D86.87
- pyelonephritis D86.84
- Spiegler-Fendt L08.89

Sarcoidosis D86.9
- with
  - cranial nerve palsies D86.82
  - hepatic granuloma D86.89
  - polyarthritis D86.86
  - tubulo-interstitial nephropathy D86.84
- combined sites NEC D86.89
- lung D86.0
  - and lymph nodes D86.2
- lymph nodes D86.1
  - and lung D86.2
- meninges D86.81
- skin D86.3
- specified type NEC D86.89

Sarcoma (of) — *see also* Neoplasm, connective tissue, malignant
- alveolar soft part — *see* Neoplasm, connective tissue, malignant
- ameloblastic C41.1
  - upper jaw (bone) C41.0
- botryoid — *see* Neoplasm, connective tissue, malignant
- botryoides — *see* Neoplasm, connective tissue, malignant
- cerebellar C71.6
  - circumscribed (arachnoidal) C71.6
- circumscribed (arachnoidal) cerebellar C71.6
- clear cell — *see also* Neoplasm, connective tissue, malignant
  - kidney C64.-
- dendritic cells (accessory cells) C96.4
- embryonal — *see* Neoplasm, connective tissue, malignant
- endometrial (stromal) C54.1
  - isthmus C54.0

Sarcoma (of) - *continued*
epithelioid (cell) — *see* Neoplasm, connective tissue, malignant
Ewing's — *see* Neoplasm, bone, malignant
follicular dendritic cell C96.4
germinoblastic (diffuse) — *see* Lymphoma, diffuse large cell
follicular — *see* Lymphoma, follicular, specified NEC
giant cell (except of bone) — *see also* Neoplasm, connective tissue, malignant
bone — *see* Neoplasm, bone, malignant
glomoid — *see* Neoplasm, connective tissue, malignant
granulocytic C92.3-
hemangioendothelial — *see* Neoplasm, connective tissue, malignant
hemorrhagic, multiple — *see* Sarcoma, Kaposi's
histiocytic C96.A
Hodgkin — *see* Lymphoma, Hodgkin
immunoblastic (diffuse) — *see* Lymphoma, diffuse large cell
interdigitating dendritic cell C96.4
Kaposi's
colon C46.4
connective tissue C46.1
gastrointestinal organ C46.4
lung C46.5-
lymph node (s) C46.3
palate (hard) (soft) C46.2
rectum C46.4
skin C46.0
specified site NEC C46.7
stomach C46.4
unspecified site C46.9
Kupffer cell C22.3
Langerhans cell C96.4
leptomeningeal — *see* Neoplasm, meninges, malignant
liver NEC C22.4
lymphangioendothelial — *see* Neoplasm, connective tissue, malignant
lymphoblastic — *see* Lymphoma, lymphoblastic (diffuse)
lymphocytic — *see* Lymphoma, small cell B-cell
mast cell C96.22
melanotic — *see* Melanoma
meningeal — *see* Neoplasm, meninges, malignant
meningothelial — *see* Neoplasm, meninges, malignant
mesenchymal — *see also* Neoplasm, connective tissue, malignant
mixed — *see* Neoplasm, connective tissue, malignant
mesothelial — *see* Mesothelioma
monstrocellular
specified site — *see* Neoplasm, malignant, by site
unspecified site C71.9
myeloid C92.3-
neurogenic — *see* Neoplasm, nerve, malignant
odontogenic C41.1
upper jaw (bone) C41.0
osteoblastic — *see* Neoplasm, bone, malignant
osteogenic — *see also* Neoplasm, bone, malignant
juxtacortical — *see* Neoplasm, bone, malignant
periosteal — *see* Neoplasm, bone, malignant
periosteal — *see also* Neoplasm, bone, malignant
osteogenic — *see* Neoplasm, bone, malignant
pleomorphic cell — *see* Neoplasm, connective tissue, malignant
reticulum cell (diffuse) — *see* Lymphoma, diffuse large cell
nodular — *see* Lymphoma, follicular

Sarcoma (of) - *continued*
reticulum cell (diffuse) - *continued*
pleomorphic cell type — *see* Lymphoma, diffuse large cell
rhabdoid — *see* Neoplasm, malignant, by site
round cell — *see* Neoplasm, connective tissue, malignant
small cell — *see* Neoplasm, connective tissue, malignant
soft tissue — *see* Neoplasm, connective tissue, malignant
spindle cell — *see* Neoplasm, connective tissue, malignant
stromal (endometrial) C54.1
isthmus C54.0
synovial — *see also* Neoplasm, connective tissue, malignant
biphasic — *see* Neoplasm, connective tissue, malignant
epithelioid cell — *see* Neoplasm, connective tissue, malignant
spindle cell — *see* Neoplasm, connective tissue, malignant
Sarcomatosis
meningeal — *see* Neoplasm, meninges, malignant
specified site NEC — *see* Neoplasm, connective tissue, malignant
unspecified site C80.1
Sarcopenia (age-related) M62.84
Sarcosinemia E72.59
Sarcosporidiosis (intestinal) A07.8
SARS-CoV-2 — *see also* COVID-19
sequelae (post acute) U09.9
Satiety, early R68.81
Saturnine — *see* condition
Saturnism
overdose or wrong substance given or taken — *see* Table of Drugs and Chemicals, by drug, poisoning
Satyriasis F52.8
Sauriasis — *see* Ichthyosis
SBE (subacute bacterial endocarditis) I33.0
Scabies (any site) B86
Scabs R23.4
Scaglietti-Dagnini syndrome E22.0
Scald — *see* Burn
Scalenus anticus (anterior) syndrome G54.0
Scales R23.4
Scaling, skin R23.4
Scalp — *see* condition
Scapegoating affecting child Z62.3
Scaphocephaly Q75.0
Scapulalgia M89.8X1
Scapulohumeral myopathy G71.02
Scar, scarring — *see also* Cicatrix L90.5
adherent L90.5
atrophic L90.5
cervix
in pregnancy or childbirth — *see* Pregnancy, complicated by, abnormal cervix
cheloid L91.0
chorioretinal H31.00-
posterior pole macula H31.01-
postsurgical H59.81-
solar retinopathy H31.02-
specified type NEC H31.09-
choroid — *see* Scar, chorioretinal
conjunctiva H11.24-
cornea H17.9
xerophthalmic — *see also* Opacity, cornea
vitamin A deficiency E50.6
defect (isthmocele) O34.22
duodenum, obstructive K31.5
hypertrophic L91.0
keloid L91.0
labia N90.89
lung (base) J98.4
macula — *see* Scar, chorioretinal, posterior pole
muscle M62.89
myocardium, myocardial I25.2
painful L90.5

Scar, scarring - *continued*
posterior pole (eye) — *see* Scar, chorioretinal, posterior pole
retina — *see* Scar, chorioretinal
trachea J39.8
transmural uterine, in pregnancy O34.29
uterus N85.8
in pregnancy O34.29
vagina N89.8
postoperative N99.2
vulva N90.89
Scarabiasis B88.2
Scarlatina (anginosa) (maligna) A38.9
myocarditis (acute) A38.1
old — *see* Myocarditis
otitis media A38.0
ulcerosa A38.8
Scarlet fever (albuminuria) (angina) A38.9
Schamberg's disease (progressive pigmentary dermatosis) L81.7
Schatzki's ring (acquired) (esophagus) (lower) K22.2
congenital Q39.3
Schaufenster krankheit I20.8
Schaumann's
benign lymphogranulomatosis D86.1
disease or syndrome — *see* Sarcoidosis
Scheie's syndrome E76.03
Schenck's disease B42.1
Scheuermann's disease or osteochondrosis — *see* Osteochondrosis, juvenile, spine
Schilder (-Flatau) disease G37.0
Schilling-type monocytic leukemia C93.0-
Schimmelbusch's disease, cystic mastitis, or hyperplasia — *see* Mastopathy, cystic
Schistosoma infestation — *see* Infestation, Schistosoma
Schistosomiasis B65.9
with muscle disorder B65.9 *[M63.80]*
ankle B65.9 *[M63.87-]*
foot B65.9 *[M63.87-]*
forearm B65.9 *[M63.83-]*
hand B65.9 *[M63.84-]*
lower leg B65.9 *[M63.86-]*
multiple sites B65.9 *[M63.89]*
pelvic region B65.9 *[M63.85-]*
shoulder region B65.9 *[M63.81-]*
specified site NEC B65.9 *[M63.88]*
thigh B65.9 *[M63.85-]*
upper arm B65.9 *[M63.82-]*
Asiatic B65.2
bladder B65.0
chestermani B65.8
colon B65.1
cutaneous B65.3
due to
S. haematobium B65.0
S. japonicum B65.2
S. mansoni B65.1
S. mattheii B65.8
Eastern B65.2
genitourinary tract B65.0
intestinal B65.1
lung NEC B65.9 *[J99]*
pneumonia B65.9 *[J17]*
Manson's (intestinal) B65.1
oriental B65.2
pulmonary NEC B65.9 *[J99]*
pneumonia B65.9
Schistosoma
haematobium B65.0
japonicum B65.2
mansoni B65.1
specified type NEC B65.8
urinary B65.0
vesical B65.0
Schizencephaly Q04.6
Schizoaffective psychosis F25.9
Schizodontia K00.2
Schizoid personality F60.1
Schizophrenia, schizophrenic F20.9
acute (brief) (undifferentiated) F23
atypical (form) F20.3
borderline F21

Schizophrenia, schizophrenic - *continued*
- catalepsy F20.2
- catatonic (type) (excited) (withdrawn) F20.2
- cenesthopathic, cenesthesiopathic F20.89
- childhood type F84.5
- chronic undifferentiated F20.9
- cyclic F25.0
- disorganized (type) F20.1
- flexibilitas cerea F20.2
- hebephrenic (type) F20.1
- incipient F21
- latent F21
- negative type F20.5
- paranoid (type) F20.0
- paraphrenic F20.0
- post-psychotic depression F32.89
- prepsychotic F21
- prodromal F21
- pseudoneurotic F21
- pseudopsychopathic F21
- reaction F23
- residual (state) (type) F20.5
- restzustand F20.5
- schizoaffective (type) — *see* Psychosis, schizoaffective
- simple (type) F20.89
- simplex F20.89
- specified type NEC F20.89
- spectrum and other psychotic disorder F29
  - specified NEC F28
- stupor F20.2
- syndrome of childhood F84.5
- undifferentiated (type) F20.3
  - chronic F20.5

Schizothymia (persistent) F60.1

Schlatter-Osgood disease or osteochondrosis M92.52-

Schlatter's tibia — *see* Osteochondrosis, juvenile, tibia

Schmidt's syndrome (polyglandular, autoimmune) E31.0

Schmincke's carcinoma or tumor — *see* Neoplasm, nasopharynx, malignant

Schmitz (-Stutzer) dysentery A03.0

Schmorl's disease or nodes
- lumbar region M51.46
- lumbosacral region M51.47
- sacrococcygeal region M53.3
- thoracic region M51.44
- thoracolumbar region M51.45

Schneiderian
- papilloma — *see* Neoplasm, nasopharynx, benign
  - specified site — *see* Neoplasm, benign, by site
  - unspecified site D14.0
- specified site — *see* Neoplasm, malignant, by site
  - unspecified site C30.0

Scholte's syndrome (malignant carcinoid) E34.0

Scholz (-Bielchowsky-Henneberg) disease or syndrome E75.25

Schönlein (-Henoch) disease or purpura (primary) (rheumatic) D69.0

Schottmuller's disease A01.4

Schroeder's syndrome (endocrine hypertensive) E27.0

Schüller-Christian disease or syndrome C96.5

Schultze's type acroparesthesia, simple I73.89

Schultz's disease or syndrome — *see* Agranulocytosis

Schwalbe-Ziehen-Oppenheim disease G24.1

Schwannoma — *see also* Neoplasm, nerve, benign
- malignant — *see also* Neoplasm, nerve, malignant
  - with rhabdomyoblastic differentiation — *see* Neoplasm, nerve, malignant
- melanocytic — *see* Neoplasm, nerve, benign
- pigmented — *see* Neoplasm, nerve, benign

Schwannomatosis Q85.03

Schwartz (-Jampel) syndrome G71.13

Schwartz-Bartter syndrome E22.2

Schweniger-Buzzi anetoderma L90.1

Sciatic — *see* condition

Sciatica (infective) M54.3
- with lumbago M54.4-
  - due to intervertebral disc disorder — *see* Disorder, disc, with, radiculopathy
- due to displacement of intervertebral disc (with lumbago) — *see* Disorder, disc, with, radiculopathy
- wallet M54.3-

Scimitar syndrome Q26.8

Sclera — *see* condition

Sclerectasia H15.84-

Scleredema
- adultorum — *see* Sclerosis, systemic
- Buschke's — *see* Sclerosis, systemic
- newborn P83.0

Sclerema (adiposum) (edematosum) (neonatorum) (newborn) P83.0
- adultorum — *see* Sclerosis, systemic

Scleriasis — *see* Scleroderma

Scleritis H15.00-
- with corneal involvement H15.04-
- anterior H15.01-
- brawny H15.02-
- in (due to) zoster B02.34
- posterior H15.03-
- specified type NEC H15.09-
- syphilitic A52.71
- tuberculous (nodular) A18.51

Sclerochoroiditis H31.8

Scleroconjunctivitis — *see* Scleritis

Sclerocystic ovary syndrome E28.2

Sclerodactyly, sclerodactylia L94.3

Scleroderma, sclerodermia (acrosclerotic) (diffuse) (generalized) (progressive) (pulmonary) — *see also* Sclerosis, systemic M34.9-
- circumscribed L94.0
- linear L94.1
- localized L94.0
- newborn P83.88
- systemic M34.9

Sclerokeratitis H16.8
- tuberculous A18.52

Scleroma nasi A48.8

Scleromalacia (perforans) H15.05-

Scleromyxedema L98.5

Sclérose en plaques G35

Sclerosis, sclerotic
- adrenal (gland) E27.8
- Alzheimer's — *see* Disease, Alzheimer's
- amyotrophic (lateral) G12.21
- aorta, aortic I70.0
  - valve — *see* Endocarditis, aortic
- artery, arterial, arteriolar, arteriovascular — *see* Arteriosclerosis
- ascending multiple G35
- brain (generalized) (lobular) G37.9
  - artery, arterial I67.2
  - diffuse G37.0
  - disseminated G35
  - insular G35
  - Krabbe's E75.23
  - miliary G35
  - multiple G35
  - presenile (Alzheimer's) — *see* Disease, Alzheimer's, early onset
  - senile (arteriosclerotic) I67.2
  - stem, multiple G35
  - tuberous Q85.1
- bulbar, multiple G35
- bundle of His I44.39
- cardiac — *see* Disease, heart, ischemic, atherosclerotic
- cardiorenal — *see* Hypertension, cardiorenal
- cardiovascular — *see also* Disease, cardiovascular
  - renal — *see* Hypertension, cardiorenal
- cerebellar — *see* Sclerosis, brain
- cerebral — *see* Sclerosis, brain
- cerebrospinal (disseminated) (multiple) G35
- cerebrovascular I67.2
- choroid — *see* Degeneration, choroid

Sclerosis, sclerotic - *continued*
- combined (spinal cord) — *see also* Degeneration, combined
  - multiple G35
- concentric (Balo) G37.5
- cornea — *see* Opacity, cornea
- coronary (artery) I25.10
  - with angina pectoris — *see* Arteriosclerosis, coronary (artery),
- corpus cavernosum
  - female N90.89
  - male N48.6
- diffuse (brain) (spinal cord) G37.0
- disseminated G35
- dorsal G35
- dorsolateral (spinal cord) — *see* Degeneration, combined
- endometrium N85.5
- extrapyramidal G25.9
- eye, nuclear (senile) — *see* Cataract, senile, nuclear
- focal and segmental (glomerular) — *see also* N00-N07 with fourth character .1 N05.1
- Friedreich's (spinal cord) G11.11
- funicular (spermatic cord) N50.89
- general (vascular) — *see* Arteriosclerosis
- gland (lymphatic) I89.8
- hepatic K74.1
  - alcoholic K70.2
- hereditary
  - cerebellar G11.9
  - spinal (Friedreich's ataxia) G11.11
- hippocampal G93.81
- insular G35
- kidney — *see* Sclerosis, renal
- larynx J38.7
- lateral (amyotrophic) (descending) (spinal) G12.21
  - primary G12.23
- lens, senile nuclear — *see* Cataract, senile, nuclear
- liver K74.1
  - with fibrosis K74.2
    - alcoholic K70.2
  - alcoholic K70.2
  - cardiac K76.1
- lung — *see* Fibrosis, lung
- mastoid — *see* Mastoiditis, chronic
- mesial temporal G93.81
- mitral I05.8
- Mönckeberg's (medial) — *see* Arteriosclerosis, extremities
- multiple (brain stem) (cerebral) (generalized) (spinal cord) G35
- myocardium, myocardial — *see* Disease, heart, ischemic, atherosclerotic
- nuclear (senile) , eye — *see* Cataract, senile, nuclear
- ovary N83.8
- pancreas K86.89
- penis N48.6
- peripheral arteries — *see* Arteriosclerosis, extremities
- plaques G35
- pluriglandular E31.8
- polyglandular E31.8
- posterolateral (spinal cord) — *see* Degeneration, combined
- presenile (Alzheimer's) — *see* Disease, Alzheimer's, early onset
- primary, lateral G12.23
- progressive, systemic M34.0
- pulmonary — *see* Fibrosis, lung
  - artery I27.0
  - valve (heart) — *see* Endocarditis, pulmonary
- renal N26.9
  - with
    - cystine storage disease E72.09
    - hypertensive heart disease (conditions in I11) — *see* Hypertension, cardiorenal
  - arteriolar (hyaline) (hyperplastic) — *see* Hypertension, kidney

Sclerosis, sclerotic - *continued*
- retina (senile) (vascular) H35.00
- senile (vascular) — *see* Arteriosclerosis
- spinal (cord) (progressive) G95.89
  - ascending G61.0
  - combined — *see also* Degeneration, combined
    - multiple G35
    - syphilitic A52.11
  - disseminated G35
  - dorsolateral — *see* Degeneration, combined
  - hereditary (Friedreich's) (mixed form) G11.11
  - lateral (amyotrophic) G12.21
    - progressive G12.23
  - multiple G35
  - posterior (syphilitic) A52.11
- stomach K31.89
- subendocardial, congenital I42.4
- systemic M34.9
  - with
    - lung involvement M34.81
    - myopathy M34.82
    - polyneuropathy M34.83
  - drug-induced M34.2
  - due to chemicals NEC M34.2
  - progressive M34.0
  - specified NEC M34.89
- temporal (mesial) G93.81
- tricuspid (heart) (valve) I07.8
- tuberous (brain) Q85.1
- tympanic membrane — *see* Disorder, tympanic membrane, specified NEC
- valve, valvular (heart) — *see* Endocarditis
- vascular — *see* Arteriosclerosis
- vein I87.8

Scoliosis (acquired) (postural) M41.9
- adolescent (idiopathic) — *see* Scoliosis, idiopathic, adolescent
- congenital Q67.5
  - due to bony malformation Q76.3
  - failure of segmentation (hemivertebra) Q76.3
  - hemivertebra fusion Q76.3
  - postural Q67.5
- degenerative M41.8-
- idiopathic M41.20
  - adolescent M41.129
    - cervical region M41.122
    - cervicothoracic region M41.123
    - lumbar region M41.126
    - lumbosacral region M41.127
    - thoracic region M41.124
    - thoracolumbar region M41.125
  - cervical region M41.22
  - cervicothoracic region M41.23
  - infantile M41.00
    - cervical region M41.02
    - cervicothoracic region M41.03
    - lumbar region M41.06
    - lumbosacral region M41.07
    - sacrococcygeal region M41.08
    - thoracic region M41.04
    - thoracolumbar region M41.05
  - juvenile M41.119
    - cervical region M41.112
    - cervicothoracic region M41.113
    - lumbar region M41.116
    - lumbosacral region M41.117
    - thoracic region M41.114
    - thoracolumbar region M41.115
  - lumbar region M41.26
  - lumbosacral region M41.27
  - thoracic region M41.24
  - thoracolumbar region M41.25
- infantile — *see* Scoliosis, idiopathic, infantile
- neuromuscular M41.40
  - cervical region M41.42
  - cervicothoracic region M41.43
  - lumbar region M41.46
  - lumbosacral region M41.47
  - occipito-atlanto-axial region M41.41
  - thoracic region M41.44

Scoliosis (acquired) (postural) - *continued*
- neuromuscular - *continued*
  - thoracolumbar region M41.45
- paralytic — *see* Scoliosis, neuromuscular
- postradiation therapy M96.5
- rachitic (late effect or sequelae) E64.3 *[M49.80]*
  - cervical region E64.3 *[M49.82]*
  - cervicothoracic region E64.3 *[M49.83]*
  - lumbar region E64.3 *[M49.86]*
  - lumbosacral region E64.3 *[M49.87]*
  - multiple sites E64.3 *[M49.89]*
  - occipito-atlanto-axial region E64.3 *[M49.81]*
  - sacrococcygeal region E64.3 *[M49.88]*
  - thoracic region E64.3 *[M49.84]*
  - thoracolumbar region E64.3 *[M49.85]*
- sciatic M54.4-
- secondary (to) NEC M41.50
  - cerebral palsy, Friedreich's ataxia, poliomyelitis, neuromuscular disorders — *see* Scoliosis, neuromuscular
  - cervical region M41.52
  - cervicothoracic region M41.53
  - lumbar region M41.56
  - lumbosacral region M41.57
  - thoracic region M41.54
  - thoracolumbar region M41.55
- specified form NEC M41.80
  - cervical region M41.82
  - cervicothoracic region M41.83
  - lumbar region M41.86
  - lumbosacral region M41.87
  - thoracic region M41.84
  - thoracolumbar region M41.85
- thoracogenic M41.30
  - thoracic region M41.34
  - thoracolumbar region M41.35
- tuberculous A18.01

Scoliotic pelvis
- with disproportion (fetopelvic) O33.0
  - causing obstructed labor O65.0

Scorbutus, scorbutic — *see also* Scurvy
- anemia D53.2

Score, NIHSS (National Institutes of Health Stroke Scale) R29.7-

Scotoma (arcuate) (Bjerrum) (central) (ring) — *see also* Defect, visual field, localized, scotoma
- scintillating H53.19

Scratch — *see* Abrasion

Scratchy throat R09.89

Screening (for) Z13.9
- alcoholism Z13.39
- anemia Z13.0
- anomaly, congenital Z13.89
- antenatal, of mother — *see also* Encounter, antenatal screening Z36.9
- arterial hypertension Z13.6
- arthropod-borne viral disease NEC Z11.59
- autism Z13.41
- bacteriuria, asymptomatic Z13.89
- behavioral disorder Z13.30
  - specified NEC Z13.39
- brain injury, traumatic Z13.850
- bronchitis, chronic Z13.83
- brucellosis Z11.2
- cardiovascular disorder Z13.6
- cataract Z13.5
- chlamydial diseases Z11.8
- cholera Z11.0
- chromosomal abnormalities (nonprocreative) NEC Z13.79
- colonoscopy Z12.11
- congenital
  - dislocation of hip Z13.89
  - eye disorder Z13.5
  - malformation or deformation Z13.89
- contamination NEC Z13.88
- coronavirus (disease) (novel) 2019 Z11.52
- COVID-19 Z11.52
- cystic fibrosis Z13.228
- dengue fever Z11.59
- dental disorder Z13.84

Screening (for) - *continued*
- depression (adult) (adolescent) (child) Z13.31
  - maternal Z13.32
  - perinatal Z13.32
- developmental
  - delays Z13.40
    - global (milestones) Z13.42
    - specified NEC Z13.49
  - handicap Z13.42
    - in early childhood Z13.42
- diabetes mellitus Z13.1
- diphtheria Z11.2
- disability, intellectual Z13.39
- disease or disorder Z13.9
  - bacterial NEC Z11.2
    - intestinal infectious Z11.0
    - respiratory tuberculosis Z11.1
  - behavioral Z13.30
    - specified NEC Z13.39
  - blood or blood-forming organ Z13.0
  - cardiovascular Z13.6
  - Chagas' Z11.6
  - chlamydial Z11.8
  - coronavirus (novel) 2019 Z11.52
  - COVID-19 Z11.52
  - dental Z13.89
  - developmental delays Z13.40
    - global (milestones) Z13.42
    - specified NEC Z13.49
  - digestive tract NEC Z13.818
    - lower GI Z13.811
    - upper GI Z13.810
  - ear Z13.5
  - endocrine Z13.29
  - eye Z13.5
  - genitourinary Z13.89
  - heart Z13.6
  - human immunodeficiency virus (HIV) infection Z11.4
  - immunity Z13.0
  - infection
    - intestinal Z11.0
      - specified NEC Z11.6
  - infectious Z11.9
  - mental health and behavioral Z13.30
    - specified NEC Z13.39
  - metabolic Z13.228
  - neurological Z13.89
  - nutritional Z13.21
    - metabolic Z13.228
      - lipoid disorders Z13.220
  - protozoal Z11.6
    - intestinal Z11.0
  - respiratory Z13.83
  - rheumatic Z13.828
  - rickettsial Z11.8
  - sexually-transmitted NEC Z11.3
    - human immunodeficiency virus (HIV) Z11.4
  - sickle-cell (trait) Z13.0
  - skin Z13.89
  - specified NEC Z13.89
  - spirochetal Z11.8
  - thyroid Z13.29
  - vascular Z13.6
  - venereal Z11.3
  - viral NEC Z11.59
    - coronavirus (novel) 2019 Z11.52
    - COVID-19 Z11.52
    - human immunodeficiency virus (HIV) Z11.4
    - intestinal Z11.0
    - SARS-CoV-2 Z11.52
- elevated titer Z13.89
- emphysema Z13.83
- encephalitis, viral (mosquito- or tick-borne) Z11.59
- exposure to contaminants (toxic) Z13.88
- fever
  - dengue Z11.59
  - hemorrhagic Z11.59
  - yellow Z11.59
- filariasis Z11.6
- galactosemia Z13.228

SCLEROSIS, SCLEROTIC - SCREENING

Screening (for) - *continued*
gastrointestinal condition Z13.818
genetic (nonprocreative) - for procreative management — *see* Testing, genetic, for procreative management
disease carrier status (nonprocreative) Z13.71
specified NEC (nonprocreative) Z13.79
genitourinary condition Z13.89
glaucoma Z13.5
gonorrhea Z11.3
gout Z13.89
helminthiasis (intestinal) Z11.6
hematopoietic malignancy Z12.89
hemoglobinopathies NEC Z13.0
hemorrhagic fever Z11.59
Hodgkin disease Z12.89
human immunodeficiency virus (HIV) Z11.4
human papillomavirus Z11.51
hypertension Z13.6
immunity disorders Z13.0
infant or child (over 28 days old) Z00.129
with abnormal findings Z00.121
infection
mycotic Z11.8
parasitic Z11.8
ingestion of radioactive substance Z13.88
intellectual disability Z13.39
intestinal
helminthiasis Z11.6
infectious disease Z11.0
leishmaniasis Z11.6
leprosy Z11.2
leptospirosis Z11.8
leukemia Z12.89
lymphoma Z12.89
malaria Z11.6
malnutrition Z13.29
metabolic Z13.228
nutritional Z13.21
measles Z11.59
mental health disorder Z13.30
specified NEC Z13.39
metabolic errors, inborn Z13.228
multiphasic Z13.89
musculoskeletal disorder Z13.828
osteoporosis Z13.820
mycoses Z11.8
myocardial infarction (acute) Z13.6
neoplasm (malignant) (of) Z12.9
bladder Z12.6
blood Z12.89
breast Z12.39
routine mammogram Z12.31
cervix Z12.4
colon Z12.11
genitourinary organs NEC Z12.79
bladder Z12.6
cervix Z12.4
ovary Z12.73
prostate Z12.5
testis Z12.71
vagina Z12.72
hematopoietic system Z12.89
intestinal tract Z12.10
colon Z12.11
rectum Z12.12
small intestine Z12.13
lung Z12.2
lymph (glands) Z12.89
nervous system Z12.82
oral cavity Z12.81
prostate Z12.5
rectum Z12.12
respiratory organs Z12.2
skin Z12.83
small intestine Z12.13
specified site NEC Z12.89
stomach Z12.0
nephropathy Z13.89
nervous system disorders NEC Z13.858
neurological condition Z13.89
osteoporosis Z13.820
parasitic infestation Z11.9
specified NEC Z11.8

Screening (for) - *continued*
phenylketonuria Z13.228
plague Z11.2
poisoning (chemical) (heavy metal) Z13.88
poliomyelitis Z11.59
postnatal, chromosomal abnormalities Z13.89
prenatal, of mother — *see also* Encounter, antenatal screening Z36.9
protozoal disease Z11.6
intestinal Z11.0
pulmonary tuberculosis Z11.1
radiation exposure Z13.88
respiratory condition Z13.83
respiratory tuberculosis Z11.1
rheumatoid arthritis Z13.828
rubella Z11.59
SARS-CoV-2 Z11.52
schistosomiasis Z11.6
sexually-transmitted disease NEC Z11.3
human immunodeficiency virus (HIV) Z11.4
sickle-cell disease or trait Z13.0
skin condition Z13.89
sleeping sickness Z11.6
special Z13.9
specified NEC Z13.89
syphilis Z11.3
tetanus Z11.2
trachoma Z11.8
traumatic brain injury Z13.850
trypanosomiasis Z11.6
tuberculosis, respiratory Z11.1
active Z11.1
latent Z11.7
venereal disease Z11.3
viral encephalitis (mosquito- or tick-borne) Z11.59
whooping cough Z11.2
worms, intestinal Z11.6
yaws Z11.8
yellow fever Z11.59
Scrofula, scrofulosis (tuberculosis of cervical lymph glands) A18.2
Scrofulide (primary) (tuberculous) A18.4
Scrofuloderma, scrofulodermia (any site) (primary) A18.4
Scrofulosus lichen (primary) (tuberculous) A18.4
Scrofulous — *see* condition
Scrotal tongue K14.5
Scrotum — *see* condition
Scurvy, scorbutic E54
anemia D53.2
gum E54
infantile E54
rickets E55.0 *[M90.80]*
Sealpox B08.62
Seasickness T75.3
Seatworm (infection) (infestation) B80
Sebaceous — *see also* condition
cyst — *see* Cyst, sebaceous
Seborrhea, seborrheic L21.9
capillitii R23.8
capitis L21.0
dermatitis L21.9
infantile L21.1
eczema L21.9
infantile L21.1
sicca L21.0
Seckel's syndrome Q87.19
Seclusion, pupil — *see* Membrane, pupillary
Second hand tobacco smoke exposure (acute) (chronic) Z77.22
in the perinatal period P96.81
Secondary
dentin (in pulp) K04.3
neoplasm, secondaries — *see* Table of Neoplasms, secondary
Secretion
antidiuretic hormone, inappropriate E22.2
catecholamine, by pheochromocytoma E27.5
hormone
antidiuretic, inappropriate (syndrome) E22.2

Secretion - *continued*
hormone - *continued*
by
carcinoid tumor E34.0
pheochromocytoma E27.5
ectopic NEC E34.2
urinary
excessive R35.89
suppression R34
Section
nerve, traumatic — *see* Injury, nerve
Sedative, hypnotic, or anxiolytic-induced
anxiety disorder F13.980
bipolar and related disorder F13.94
delirium F13.921
depressive disorder F13.94
major neurocognitive disorder F13.97
mild neurocognitive disorder F13.988
psychotic disorder F13.959
sexual dysfunction F13.981
sleep disorder F13.982
Segmentation, incomplete (congenital) — *see also* Fusion
bone NEC Q78.8
lumbosacral (joint) (vertebra) Q76.49
Seitelberger's syndrome (infantile neuraxonal dystrophy) G31.89
Seizure (s) — *see also* Convulsions R56.9
absence G40.A-
akinetic — *see* Epilepsy, generalized, specified NEC
atonic — *see* Epilepsy, generalized, specified NEC
autonomic (hysterical) F44.5
convulsive — *see* Convulsions
cortical (focal) (motor) — *see* Epilepsy, localization-related, symptomatic, with simple partial seizures
disorder — *see also* Epilepsy G40.909
due to stroke — *see* Sequelae (of), disease, cerebrovascular, by type, specified NEC
epileptic — *see* Epilepsy
febrile (simple) R56.00
with status epilepticus G40.901
complex (atypical) (complicated) R56.01
with status epilepticus G40.901
grand mal G40.409
intractable G40.419
with status epilepticus G40.411
without status epilepticus G40.419
not intractable G40.409
with status epilepticus G40.401
without status epilepticus G40.409
heart — *see* Disease, heart
hysterical F44.5
intractable G40.919
with status epilepticus G40.911
Jacksonian (focal) (motor type) (sensory type) — *see* Epilepsy, localization-related, symptomatic, with simple partial seizures
newborn P90
nonspecific epileptic
atonic — *see* Epilepsy, generalized, specified NEC
clonic — *see* Epilepsy, generalized, specified NEC
myoclonic — *see* Epilepsy, generalized, specified NEC
tonic — *see* Epilepsy, generalized, specified NEC
tonic-clonic — *see* Epilepsy, generalized, specified NEC
partial, developing into secondarily generalized seizures
complex — *see* Epilepsy, localization-related, symptomatic, with complex partial seizures
simple — *see* Epilepsy, localization-related, symptomatic, with simple partial seizures
petit mal G40.A-
intractable G40.A1-
with status epilepticus G40.A11
without status epilepticus G40.A19

Septic — *see* condition
  arm — *see* Cellulitis, upper limb
    with lymphangitis — *see* Lymphangitis, acute, upper limb
  embolus — *see* Embolism
  finger — *see* Cellulitis, digit
    with lymphangitis — *see* Lymphangitis, acute, digit
  foot — *see* Cellulitis, lower limb
    with lymphangitis — *see* Lymphangitis, acute, lower limb
  gallbladder (acute) K81.0
  hand — *see* Cellulitis, upper limb
    with lymphangitis — *see* Lymphangitis, acute, upper limb
  joint — *see* Arthritis, pyogenic or pyemic
  leg — *see* Cellulitis, lower limb
    with lymphangitis — *see* Lymphangitis, acute, lower limb
  nail — *see also* Cellulitis, digit
    with lymphangitis — *see* Lymphangitis, acute, digit
  sore — *see also* Abscess
    throat J02.0
      streptococcal J02.0
  spleen (acute) D73.89
  teeth, tooth (pulpal origin) K04.4
  throat — *see* Pharyngitis
  thrombus — *see* Thrombosis
  toe — *see* Cellulitis, digit
    with lymphangitis — *see* Lymphangitis, acute, digit
  tonsils, chronic J35.01
    with adenoiditis J35.03
  uterus — *see* Endometritis
Septicemia A41.9
  meaning sepsis — *see* Sepsis
Septum, septate (congenital) — *see also* Anomaly, by site
  anal Q42.3
    with fistula Q42.2
  aqueduct of Sylvius Q03.0
    with spina bifida — *see* Spina bifida, by site, with hydrocephalus
  uterus Q51.28
    complete Q51.21
    partial Q51.22
    specified NEC Q51.28
  vagina Q52.10
    in pregnancy — *see* Pregnancy, complicated by, abnormal vagina
      causing obstructed labor O65.5
    longitudinal Q52.129
      microperforate
        left side Q52.124
        right side Q52.123
      nonobstruction Q52.120
      obstructing Q52.129
        left side Q52.122
        right side Q52.121
    transverse Q52.11
Sequelae (of) — *see also* condition
  abscess, intracranial or intraspinal (conditions in G06) G09
  amputation -- code to injury with seventh character S
  burn and corrosion -- code to injury with seventh character S
  calcium deficiency E64.8
  cerebrovascular disease — *see* Sequelae, disease, cerebrovascular
  childbirth O94
  contusion -- code to injury with seventh character S
  corrosion — *see* Sequelae, burn and corrosion
  COVID-19 (post acute) U09.9
  crushing injury -- code to injury with seventh character S
  disease
    cerebrovascular I69.90
      alteration of sensation I69.998
      aphasia I69.920
      apraxia I69.990
      ataxia I69.993

Sequelae (of) - *continued*
  disease - *continued*
    cerebrovascular - *continued*
      cognitive deficits I69.91
      disturbance of vision I69.998
      dysarthria I69.922
      dysphagia I69.991
      dysphasia I69.921
      facial droop I69.992
      facial weakness I69.992
      fluency disorder I69.923
      hemiplegia I69.95-
      hemorrhage
        intracerebral — *see* Sequelae, hemorrhage, intracerebral
        intracranial, nontraumatic NEC — *see* Sequelae, hemorrhage, intracranial, nontraumatic
        subarachnoid — *see* Sequelae, hemorrhage, subarachnoid
      language deficit I69.928
      monoplegia
        lower limb I69.94-
        upper limb I69.93-
      paralytic syndrome I69.96-
      specified effect NEC I69.998
      specified type NEC I69.80
        alteration of sensation I69.898
        aphasia I69.820
        apraxia I69.890
        ataxia I69.893
        cognitive deficits I69.81
        disturbance of vision I69.898
        dysarthria I69.822
        dysphagia I69.891
        dysphasia I69.821
        facial droop I69.892
        facial weakness I69.892
        fluency disorder I69.823
        hemiplegia I69.85-
        language deficit I69.828
        monoplegia
          lower limb I69.84-
          upper limb I69.83-
        paralytic syndrome I69.86-
        specified effect NEC I69.898
      speech deficit I69.928
        speech deficit I69.828
      stroke NOS — *see* Sequelae, stroke NOS
  dislocation -- code to injury with seventh character S
  encephalitis or encephalomyelitis (conditions in G04) G09
    in infectious disease NEC B94.8
    viral B94.1
  external cause -- code to injury with seventh character S
  foreign body entering natural orifice -- code to injury with seventh character S
  fracture -- code to injury with seventh character S
  frostbite -- code to injury with seventh character S
  Hansen's disease B92
  hemorrhage
    intracerebral I69.10
      alteration of sensation I69.198
      aphasia I69.120
      apraxia I69.190
      ataxia I69.193
      cognitive deficits I69.11
      disturbance of vision I69.198
      dysarthria I69.122
      dysphagia I69.191
      dysphasia I69.121
      facial droop I69.192
      facial weakness I69.192
      fluency disorder I69.123
      hemiplegia I69.15-
      language deficit NEC I69.128
      monoplegia
        lower limb I69.14-
        upper limb I69.13-
      paralytic syndrome I69.16-

Sequelae (of) - *continued*
  hemorrhage - *continued*
    intracerebral - *continued*
      specified effect NEC I69.198
      speech deficit NEC I69.128
    intracranial, nontraumatic NEC I69.20
      alteration of sensation I69.298
      aphasia I69.220
      apraxia I69.290
      ataxia I69.293
      cognitive deficits I69.21
      disturbance of vision I69.298
      dysarthria I69.222
      dysphagia I69.291
      dysphasia I69.221
      facial droop I69.292
      facial weakness I69.292
      fluency disorder I69.223
      hemiplegia I69.25-
      language deficit NEC I69.228
      monoplegia
        lower limb I69.24-
        upper limb I69.23-
      paralytic syndrome I69.26-
      specified effect NEC I69.298
      speech deficit NEC I69.228
    subarachnoid I69.00
      alteration of sensation I69.098
      aphasia I69.020
      apraxia I69.090
      ataxia I69.093
      cognitive deficits — *see* subcategory I69.01-
      disturbance of vision I69.098
      dysarthria I69.022
      dysphagia I69.091
      dysphasia I69.021
      facial droop I69.092
      facial weakness I69.092
      fluency disorder I69.023
      hemiplegia I69.05-
      language deficit NEC I69.028
      monoplegia
        lower limb I69.04-
        upper limb I69.03-
      paralytic syndrome I69.06-
      specified effect NEC I69.098
      speech deficit NEC I69.028
  hepatitis, viral B94.2
  hyperalimentation E68
  infarction
    cerebral I69.30
      alteration of sensation I69.398
      aphasia I69.320
      apraxia I69.390
      ataxia I69.393
      cognitive deficits I69.31
      disturbance of vision I69.398
      dysarthria I69.322
      dysphagia I69.391
      dysphasia I69.321
      facial droop I69.392
      facial weakness I69.392
      fluency disorder I69.323
      hemiplegia I69.35-
      language deficit NEC I69.328
      monoplegia
        lower limb I69.34-
        upper limb I69.33-
      paralytic syndrome I69.36-
      specified effect NEC I69.398
      speech deficit NEC I69.328
  infection, pyogenic, intracranial or intraspinal G09
  infectious disease B94.9
    specified NEC B94.8
  injury -- code to injury with seventh character S
  leprosy B92
  meningitis
    bacterial (conditions in G00) G09
    other or unspecified cause (conditions in G03) G09
  muscle (and tendon) injury -- code to injury with seventh character S

Shock - *continued*
- anesthetic - *continued*
  - overdose or wrong substance given or taken — *see* Table of Drugs and Chemicals, by drug, poisoning
    - specified anesthetic — *see* Table of Drugs and Chemicals, by drug, poisoning
- cardiogenic R57.0
- chemical substance — *see* Table of Drugs and Chemicals
- complicating ectopic or molar pregnancy O08.3
- culture — *see* Disorder, adjustment
- drug
  - due to correct substance properly administered T88.6
  - overdose or wrong substance given or taken (by accident) — *see* Table of Drugs and Chemicals, by drug, poisoning
- during or after labor and delivery O75.1
- electric T75.4
- (taser) T75.4
- endotoxic R65.21
  - postprocedural (resulting from a procedure, not elsewhere classified) T81.12
- following
  - ectopic or molar pregnancy O08.3
  - injury (immediate) (delayed) T79.4
  - labor and delivery O75.1
- food (anaphylactic) — *see* Shock, anaphylactic, due to food
- from electroshock gun (taser) T75.4
- gram-negative R65.21
  - postprocedural (resulting from a procedure, not elsewhere classified) T81.12
- hematologic R57.8
- hemorrhagic R57.8
  - surgery (intraoperative) (postoperative) T81.19
  - trauma T79.4
- hypovolemic R57.1
  - surgical T81.19
  - traumatic T79.4
- insulin E15
  - therapeutic misadventure — *see* subcategory T38.3
- kidney N17.0
  - traumatic (following crushing) T79.5
- liver K72.00
- lightning T75.01
- lung J80
- obstetric O75.1
  - with ectopic or molar pregnancy O08.3
  - following ectopic or molar pregnancy O08.3
- pleural (surgical) T81.19
  - due to trauma T79.4
- postprocedural (postoperative) T81.10
  - with ectopic or molar pregnancy O08.3
  - cardiogenic T81.11
  - endotoxic T81.12
  - following ectopic or molar pregnancy O08.3
  - gram-negative T81.12
  - hypovolemic T81.19
  - septic T81.12
  - specified type NEC T81.19
- psychic F43.0
- septic (due to severe sepsis) R65.21
- specified NEC R57.8
- surgical T81.10
- taser gun (taser) T75.4
- therapeutic misadventure NEC T81.10
- thyroxin
  - overdose or wrong substance given or taken — *see* Table of Drugs and Chemicals, by drug, poisoning
- toxic, syndrome A48.3
- transfusion — *see* Complications, transfusion
- traumatic (immediate) (delayed) T79.4

Shoemaker's chest M95.4

Short, shortening, shortness
- arm (acquired) — *see also* Deformity, limb, unequal length
  - congenital Q71.81-
  - forearm — *see* Deformity, limb, unequal length
- bowel syndrome K91.2
- breath R06.02
- cervical (complicating pregnancy) O26.87-
  - non-gravid uterus N88.3
- common bile duct, congenital Q44.5
- cord (umbilical) , complicating delivery O69.3
- cystic duct, congenital Q44.5
- esophagus (congenital) Q39.8
- femur (acquired) — *see* Deformity, limb, unequal length, femur
  - congenital — *see* Defect, reduction, lower limb, longitudinal, femur
- frenum, frenulum, linguae (congenital) Q38.1
- hip (acquired) — *see also* Deformity, limb, unequal length
  - congenital Q65.89
- leg (acquired) — *see also* Deformity, limb, unequal length
  - congenital Q72.81-
  - lower leg — *see also* Deformity, limb, unequal length
- limbed stature, with immunodeficiency D82.2
- lower limb (acquired) — *see also* Deformity, limb, unequal length
  - congenital Q72.81-
- organ or site, congenital NEC — *see* Distortion
- palate, congenital Q38.5
- radius (acquired) — *see also* Deformity, limb, unequal length
  - congenital — *see* Defect, reduction, upper limb, longitudinal, radius
- rib syndrome Q77.2
- stature (child) (hereditary) (idiopathic) NEC R62.52
  - constitutional E34.3
  - due to endocrine disorder E34.3
  - Laron-type E34.3
- tendon — *see also* Contraction, tendon
  - with contracture of joint — *see* Contraction, joint
  - Achilles (acquired) M67.0-
    - congenital Q66.89
  - congenital Q79.8
- thigh (acquired) — *see also* Deformity, limb, unequal length, femur
  - congenital — *see* Defect, reduction, lower limb, longitudinal, femur
- tibialis anterior (tendon) — *see* Contraction, tendon
- umbilical cord
  - complicating delivery O69.3
- upper limb, congenital — *see* Defect, reduction, upper limb, specified type NEC
- urethra N36.8
- uvula, congenital Q38.5
- vagina (congenital) Q52.4

Shortsightedness — *see* Myopia

Shoshin (acute fulminating beriberi) E51.11

Shoulder — *see* condition

Shovel-shaped incisors K00.2

Shower, thromboembolic — *see* Embolism

Shunt
- arterial-venous (dialysis) Z99.2
- arteriovenous, pulmonary (acquired) I28.0
  - congenital Q25.72
- cerebral ventricle (communicating) in situ Z98.2
- surgical, prosthetic, with complications — *see* Complications, cardiovascular, device or implant

Shutdown, renal N28.9

Shy-Drager syndrome G90.3

Sialadenitis, sialadenosis (any gland) (chronic) (periodic) (suppurative) — *see* Sialoadenitis

Sialectasia K11.8

Sialidosis E77.1

Sialitis, silitis (any gland) (chronic) (suppurative) — *see* Sialoadenitis

Sialoadenitis (any gland) (periodic) (suppurative) K11.20
- acute K11.21
  - recurrent K11.22
- chronic K11.23

Sialoadenopathy K11.9

Sialoangitis — *see* Sialoadenitis

Sialodochitis (fibrinosa) — *see* Sialoadenitis

Sialodocholithiasis K11.5

Sialolithiasis K11.5

Sialometaplasia, necrotizing K11.8

Sialorrhea — *see also* Ptyalism
- periodic — *see* Sialoadenitis

Sialosis K11.7

Siamese twin Q89.4

Sibling rivalry Z62.891

Sicard's syndrome G52.7

Sicca syndrome — *see* Syndrome, Sjögren

Sick R69
- or handicapped person in family Z63.79
  - needing care at home Z63.6
- sinus (syndrome) I49.5

Sick-euthyroid syndrome E07.81

Sickle-cell
- anemia — *see* Disease, sickle-cell
- beta plus — *see* Disease, sickle-cell, thalassemia, beta plus
- beta zero — *see* Disease, sickle-cell, thalassemia, beta zero
- trait D57.3

Sicklemia — *see also* Disease, sickle-cell
- trait D57.3

Sickness
- air (travel) T75.3
- airplane T75.3
- alpine T70.29
- altitude T70.20
- Andes T70.29
- aviator's T70.29
- balloon T70.29
- car T75.3
- compressed air T70.3
- decompression T70.3
- green D50.8
- milk — *see* Poisoning, food, noxious
- motion T75.3
- mountain T70.29
  - acute D75.1
- protein — *see also* Reaction, serum T80.69
- radiation T66
- roundabout (motion) T75.3
- sea T75.3
- serum NEC — *see also* Reaction, serum T80.69
- sleeping (African) B56.9
  - by Trypanosoma B56.9
    - brucei
      - gambiense B56.0
      - rhodesiense B56.1
  - East African B56.1
  - Gambian B56.0
  - Rhodesian B56.1
  - West African B56.0
- swing (motion) T75.3
- train (railway) (travel) T75.3
- travel (any vehicle) T75.3

Sideropenia — *see* Anemia, iron deficiency

Siderosilicosis J62.8

Siderosis (lung) J63.4
- brain G93.89
- eye (globe) — *see* Disorder, globe, degenerative, siderosis

Siemens' syndrome (ectodermal dysplasia) Q82.8

Sighing R06.89
- psychogenic F45.8

Sigmoid — *see also* condition
- flexure — *see* condition

Sigmoid - *continued*
  kidney Q63.1
Sigmoiditis — *see also* Enteritis K52.9
  infectious A09
  noninfectious K52.9
Silfversköld's syndrome Q78.9
Silicosiderosis J62.8
Silicosis, silicotic (simple) (complicated) J62.8
  with tuberculosis J65
Silicotuberculosis J65
Silo-fillers' disease J68.8
  bronchitis J68.0
  pneumonitis J68.0
  pulmonary edema J68.1
Silver's syndrome Q87.19
Simian malaria B53.1
Simmonds' cachexia or disease E23.0
Simons' disease or syndrome (progressive lipodystrophy) E88.1
Simple, simplex — *see* condition
Simulation, conscious (of illness) Z76.5
Simultanagnosia (asimultagnosia) R48.3
Sin Nombre virus disease (Hantavirus) (cardio) -pulmonary syndrome) B33.4
Sinding-Larsen disease or osteochondrosis — *see* Osteochondrosis, juvenile, patella
Singapore hemorrhagic fever A91
Singer's node or nodule J38.2
Single
  atrium Q21.2
  coronary artery Q24.5
  umbilical artery Q27.0
  ventricle Q20.4
Singultus R06.6
  epidemicus B33.0
Sinus — *see also* Fistula
  abdominal K63.89
  arrest I45.5
  arrhythmia I49.8
  bradycardia R00.1
  branchial cleft (internal) (external) Q18.0
  coccygeal — *see* Sinus, pilonidal
  dental K04.6
  dermal (congenital) Q06.8
    with abscess Q06.8
    coccygeal, pilonidal — *see* Sinus, coccygeal
  infected, skin NEC L08.89
  marginal, ruptured or bleeding — *see* Hemorrhage, antepartum, specified cause NEC
  medial, face and neck Q18.8
  pause I45.5
  pericranii Q01.9
  pilonidal (infected) (rectum) L05.92
    with abscess L05.02
  preauricular Q18.1
  rectovaginal N82.3
  Rokitansky-Aschoff (gallbladder) K82.8
  sacrococcygeal (dermoid) (infected) — *see* Sinus, pilonidal
  tachycardia R00.0
    paroxysmal I47.1
  tarsi syndrome M25.57-
  testis N50.89
  tract (postinfective) — *see* Fistula
  urachus Q64.4
Sinusitis (accessory) (chronic) (hyperplastic) (nasal) (nonpurulent) (purulent) J32.9
  acute J01.90
    ethmoidal J01.20
      recurrent J01.21
    frontal J01.10
      recurrent J01.11
    involving more than one sinus, other than pansinusitis J01.80
      recurrent J01.81
    maxillary J01.00
      recurrent J01.01
    pansinusitis J01.40
      recurrent J01.41
    recurrent J01.91
    specified NEC J01.80

Sinusitis (accessory) (chronic) (hyperplastic) (nasal) (nonpurulent) (purulent) - *continued*
  acute - *continued*
    specified NEC - *continued*
      recurrent J01.81
    sphenoidal J01.30
      recurrent J01.31
  allergic — *see* Rhinitis, allergic
  due to high altitude T70.1
  ethmoidal J32.2
    acute J01.20
      recurrent J01.21
  frontal J32.1
    acute J01.10
      recurrent J01.11
  influenzal — *see* Influenza, with, respiratory manifestations NEC
  involving more than one sinus but not pansinusitis J32.8
    acute J01.80
      recurrent J01.81
  maxillary J32.0
    acute J01.00
      recurrent J01.01
  sphenoidal J32.3
    acute J01.30
      recurrent J01.31
  tuberculous, any sinus A15.8
Sinusitis-bronchiectasis-situs inversus (syndrome) (triad) Q89.3
Sipple's syndrome E31.22
Sirenomelia (syndrome) Q87.2
Siriasis T67.01
Sirkari's disease B55.0
Siti A65
Situation, psychiatric F99
Situational
  disturbance (transient) — *see* Disorder, adjustment
    acute F43.0
  maladjustment — *see* Disorder, adjustment
  reaction — *see* Disorder, adjustment
    acute F43.0
Situs inversus or transversus (abdominalis) (thoracis) Q89.3
Sixth disease B08.20
  due to human herpesvirus 6 B08.21
  due to human herpesvirus 7 B08.22
Sjögren-Larsson syndrome Q87.19
Sjögren's syndrome or disease — *see* Syndrome, Sjögren
Skeletal — *see* condition
Skene's gland — *see* condition
Skenitis — *see* Urethritis
Skerljevo A65
Skevas-Zerfus disease — *see* Toxicity, venom, marine animal, sea anemone
Skin — *see also* condition
  clammy R23.1
  donor — *see* Donor, skin
  dry L85.3
  hidebound M35.9
Slate-dressers' or slate-miners' lung J62.8
Sleep
  apnea — *see* Apnea, sleep
  deprivation Z72.820
  disorder or disturbance G47.9
    child F51.9
    nonorganic origin F51.9
    specified NEC G47.8
  disturbance G47.9
    nonorganic origin F51.9
  drunkenness F51.9
  rhythm inversion G47.2-
  terrors F51.4
  walking F51.3
    hysterical F44.89
Sleep hygiene
  abuse Z72.821
  inadequate Z72.821
  poor Z72.821
Sleeping sickness — *see* Sickness, sleeping
Sleeplessness — *see* Insomnia
  menopausal N95.1
Sleep-wake schedule disorder G47.20

Slim disease (in HIV infection) B20
Slipped, slipping
  epiphysis (traumatic) — *see also* Osteochondropathy, specified type NEC
    capital femoral (traumatic)
      acute (on chronic) S79.01-
    current traumatic - code as Fracture, by site
    upper femoral (nontraumatic) M93.00-
      acute M93.01-
        on chronic M93.03-
      chronic M93.02-
  intervertebral disc — *see* Displacement, intervertebral disc
  ligature, umbilical P51.8
  patella — *see* Disorder, patella, derangement NEC
  rib M89.8X8
  sacroiliac joint — *see* subcategory M53.2
  tendon — *see* Disorder, tendon
  ulnar nerve, nontraumatic — *see* Lesion, nerve, ulnar
  vertebra NEC — *see* Spondylolisthesis
Slocumb's syndrome E27.0
Sloughing (multiple) (phagedena) (skin) — *see also* Gangrene
  abscess — *see* Abscess
  appendix K38.8
  fascia — *see* Disorder, soft tissue, specified type NEC
  scrotum N50.89
  tendon — *see* Disorder, tendon
  transplanted organ — *see* Rejection, transplant
  ulcer — *see* Ulcer, skin
Slow
  feeding, newborn P92.2
  flow syndrome, coronary I20.8
  heart (beat) R00.1
Slowing, urinary stream R39.198
Sluder's neuralgia (syndrome) G44.89
Slurred, slurring speech R47.81
Small (ness)
  for gestational age — *see* Small for dates
  introitus, vagina N89.6
  kidney (unknown cause) N27.9
    bilateral N27.1
    unilateral N27.0
  ovary (congenital) Q50.39
  pelvis
    with disproportion (fetopelvic) O33.1
      causing obstructed labor O65.1
  uterus N85.8
  white kidney N03.9
Small-and-light-for-dates — *see* Small for dates
Small-for-dates (infant) P05.10
  with weight of
    499 grams or less P05.11
    500-749 grams P05.12
    750-999 grams P05.13
    1000-1249 grams P05.14
    1250-1499 grams P05.15
    1500-1749 grams P05.16
    1750-1999 grams P05.17
    2000-2499 grams P05.18
    2500 grams and over P05.19
  specified NEC P05.19
Smallpox B03
Smearing, fecal R15.1
SMEI (severe myoclonic epilepsy in infancy) G40.83-
Smith-Lemli-Opitz syndrome E78.72
Smith's fracture S52.54-
Smoker — *see* Dependence, drug, nicotine
Smoker's
  bronchitis J41.0
  cough J41.0
  palate K13.24
  throat J31.2
  tongue K13.24
Smoking
  passive Z77.22
Smothering spells R06.81
Snaggle teeth, tooth M26.39

Snapping
- finger — *see* Trigger finger
- hip — *see* Derangement, joint, specified type NEC, hip
  - involving the iliotiblial band M76.3-
- knee — *see* Derangement, knee
  - involving the iliotiblial band M76.3-

Sneddon-Wilkinson disease or syndrome (sub-corneal pustular dermatosis) L13.1

Sneezing (intractable) R06.7

Sniffing
- cocaine
  - abuse — *see* Abuse, drug, cocaine
  - dependence — *see* Dependence, drug, cocaine
- gasoline
  - abuse — *see* Abuse, drug, inhalant
  - dependence — *see* Dependence, drug, inhalant
- glue (airplane)
  - abuse — *see* Abuse, drug, inhalant
  - drug dependence — *see* Dependence, drug, inhalant

Sniffles
- newborn P28.89

Snoring R06.83

Snow blindness — *see* Photokeratitis

Snuffles (non-syphilitic) R06.5
- newborn P28.89
- syphilitic (infant) A50.05 *[J99]*

Social
- exclusion Z60.4
  - due to discrimination or persecution (perceived) Z60.5
- migrant Z59.00
  - acculturation difficulty Z60.3
- rejection Z60.4
  - due to discrimination or persecution Z60.5
- role conflict NEC Z73.5
- skills inadequacy NEC Z73.4
- transplantation Z60.3

Sodoku A25.0

Soemmerring's ring — *see* Cataract, secondary

Soft — *see also* condition
- nails L60.3

Softening
- bone — *see* Osteomalacia
- brain (necrotic) (progressive) G93.89
  - congenital Q04.8
  - embolic I63.4-
  - hemorrhagic — *see* Hemorrhage, intracranial, intracerebral
  - occlusive I63.5-
  - thrombotic I63.3-
- cartilage M94.2-
  - patella M22.4-
- cerebellar — *see* Softening, brain
- cerebral — *see* Softening, brain
- cerebrospinal — *see* Softening, brain
- myocardial, heart — *see* Degeneration, myocardial
- spinal cord G95.89
- stomach K31.89

Soldier's
- heart F45.8
- patches I31.0

Solitary
- cyst, kidney N28.1
- kidney, congenital Q60.0

Solvent abuse — *see* Abuse, drug, inhalant
- dependence — *see* Dependence, drug, inhalant

Somatization reaction, somatic reaction — *see* Disorder, somatoform

Somnambulism F51.3
- hysterical F44.89

Somnolence R40.0
- nonorganic origin F51.11

Sonne dysentery A03.3

Soor B37.0

Sore
- bed — *see* Ulcer, pressure, by site
- chiclero B55.1
- Delhi B55.1
- desert — *see* Ulcer, skin
- eye H57.1-
- Lahore B55.1
- mouth K13.79
  - canker K12.0
- muscle M79.10
- Naga — *see* Ulcer, skin
- of skin — *see* Ulcer, skin
- oriental B55.1
- pressure — *see* Ulcer, pressure, by site
- skin L98.9
- soft A57
- throat (acute) — *see also* Pharyngitis
  - with influenza, flu, or grippe — *see* Influenza, with, respiratory manifestations NEC
  - chronic J31.2
  - coxsackie (virus) B08.5
  - diphtheritic A36.0
  - herpesviral B00.2
  - influenzal — *see* Influenza, with, respiratory manifestations NEC
  - septic J02.0
  - streptococcal (ulcerative) J02.0
  - viral NEC J02.8
    - coxsackie B08.5
- tropical — *see* Ulcer, skin
- veldt — *see* Ulcer, skin

Soto's syndrome (cerebral gigantism) Q87.3

South African cardiomyopathy syndrome I42.8

Southeast Asian hemorrhagic fever A91

Spacing
- abnormal, tooth, teeth, fully erupted M26.30
- excessive, tooth, fully erupted M26.32

Spade-like hand (congenital) Q68.1

Spading nail L60.8
- congenital Q84.6

Spanish collar N47.1

Sparganosis B70.1

Spasm (s) , spastic, spasticity — *see also* condition R25.2
- accommodation — *see* Spasm, of accommodation
- ampulla of Vater K83.4
- anus, ani (sphincter) (reflex) K59.4
  - psychogenic F45.8
- artery I73.9
  - cerebral G45.9
- Bell's G51.3-
- bladder (sphincter, external or internal) N32.89
  - psychogenic F45.8
- bronchus, bronchiole J98.01
- cardia K22.0
- cardiac I20.1
- carpopedal — *see* Tetany
- cerebral (arteries) (vascular) G45.9
- cervix, complicating delivery O62.4
- ciliary body (of accommodation) — *see* Spasm, of accommodation
- colon — *see also* Irritable, bowel K58.9
  - with diarrhea K58.0
  - psychogenic F45.8
- common duct K83.8
- compulsive — *see* Tic
- conjugate H51.8
- coronary (artery) I20.1
- diaphragm (reflex) R06.6
  - epidemic B33.0
  - psychogenic F45.8
- duodenum K59.89
- epidemic diaphragmatic (transient) B33.0
- esophagus (diffuse) K22.4
  - psychogenic F45.8
- facial G51.3-
- fallopian tube N83.8
- gastrointestinal (tract) K31.89
  - psychogenic F45.8
- glottis J38.5
  - hysterical F44.4
  - psychogenic F45.8
    - conversion reaction F44.4

Spasm (s) , spastic, spasticity - *continued*
- glottis - *continued*
  - reflex through recurrent laryngeal nerve J38.5
- habit — *see* Tic
- heart I20.1
- hemifacial (clonic) G51.3-
- hourglass — *see* Contraction, hourglass
- hysterical F44.4
- infantile — *see* Epilepsy, spasms
- inferior oblique, eye H51.8
- intestinal — *see also* Syndrome, irritable bowel K58.9
  - psychogenic F45.8
- larynx, laryngeal J38.5
  - hysterical F44.4
  - psychogenic F45.8
    - conversion reaction F44.4
- levator palpebrae superioris — *see* Disorder, eyelid function
- muscle NEC M62.838
  - back M62.830
- nerve, trigeminal G51.0
- nervous F45.8
- nodding F98.4
- occupational F48.8
- oculogyric H51.8
  - psychogenic F45.8
- of accommodation H52.53-
- ophthalmic artery — *see* Occlusion, artery, retina
- perineal, female N94.89
- peroneo-extensor — *see also* Deformity, limb, flat foot
- pharynx (reflex) J39.2
  - hysterical F45.8
  - psychogenic F45.8
- psychogenic F45.8
- pylorus NEC K31.3
  - adult hypertrophic K31.89
  - congenital or infantile Q40.0
  - psychogenic F45.8
- rectum (sphincter) K59.4
  - psychogenic F45.8
- retinal (artery) — *see* Occlusion, artery, retina
- sigmoid — *see also* Syndrome, irritable bowel K58.9
  - psychogenic F45.8
- sphincter of Oddi K83.4
- stomach K31.89
  - neurotic F45.8
- throat J39.2
  - hysterical F45.8
  - psychogenic F45.8
- tic F95.9
  - chronic F95.1
  - transient of childhood F95.0
- tongue K14.8
- torsion (progressive) G24.1
- trigeminal nerve — *see* Neuralgia, trigeminal
- ureter N13.5
- urethra (sphincter) N35.919
- uterus N85.8
  - complicating labor O62.4
- vagina N94.2
  - psychogenic F52.5
- vascular I73.9
- vasomotor I73.9
- vein NEC I87.8
- viscera — *see* Pain, abdominal

Spasmodic — *see* condition

Spasmophilia — *see* Tetany

Spasmus nutans F98.4

Spastic, spasticity — *see also* Spasm
- child (cerebral) (congenital) (paralysis) G80.1

Speaker's throat R49.8

Specific, specified — *see* condition

Speech
- defect, disorder, disturbance, impediment — *see* Disorder, speech R47.9
  - psychogenic, in childhood and adolescence F98.8
  - slurring R47.81

Speech - *continued*
- defect, disorder, disturbance, impediment - *continued*
  - specified NEC R47.89

Spencer's disease A08.19

Spens' syndrome (syncope with heart block) I45.9

Sperm counts (fertility testing) Z31.41
- postvasectomy Z30.8
  - reversal Z31.42

Spermatic cord — *see* condition

Spermatocele N43.40
- congenital Q55.4
- multiple N43.42
- single N43.41

Spermatocystitis N49.0

Spermatocytoma C62.9-
- specified site — *see* Neoplasm, malignant, by site

Spermatorrhea N50.89

Sphacelus — *see* Gangrene

Sphenoidal — *see* condition

Sphenoiditis (chronic) — *see* Sinusitis, sphenoidal

Sphenopalatine ganglion neuralgia G90.09

Sphericity, increased, lens (congenital) Q12.4

Spherocytosis (congenital) (familial) (hereditary) D58.0
- hemoglobin disease D58.0
- sickle-cell (disease) D57.8-

Spherophakia Q12.4

Sphincter — *see* condition

Sphincteritis, sphincter of Oddi — *see* Cholangitis

Sphingolipidosis E75.3
- specified NEC E75.29

Sphingomyelinosis E75.3

Spicule tooth K00.2

Spider
- bite — *see* Toxicity, venom, spider
  - nonvenomous — *see* Bite, by site, superficial, insect
- fingers — *see* Syndrome, Marfan's
- nevus I78.1
- toes — *see* Syndrome, Marfan's
- vascular I78.1

Spiegler-Fendt
- benign lymphocytoma L98.8
- sarcoid L08.89

Spielmeyer-Vogt disease E75.4

Spina bifida (aperta) Q05.9
- with hydrocephalus NEC Q05.4
- cervical Q05.5
  - with hydrocephalus Q05.0
- dorsal Q05.6
  - with hydrocephalus Q05.1
- lumbar Q05.7
  - with hydrocephalus Q05.2
- lumbosacral Q05.7
  - with hydrocephalus Q05.2
- occulta Q76.0
- sacral Q05.8
  - with hydrocephalus Q05.3
- thoracic Q05.6
  - with hydrocephalus Q05.1
- thoracolumbar Q05.6
  - with hydrocephalus Q05.1

Spindle, Krukenberg's — *see* Pigmentation, cornea, posterior

Spine, spinal — *see* condition

Spiradenoma (eccrine) — *see* Neoplasm, skin, benign

Spirillosis A25.0

Spirillum
- minus A25.0
- obermeieri infection A68.0

Spirochetal — *see* condition

Spirochetosis A69.9
- arthritic, arthritica A69.9
- bronchopulmonary A69.8
- icterohemorrhagic A27.0
- lung A69.8

Spirometrosis B70.1

Spitting blood — *see* Hemoptysis

Splanchnoptosis K63.4

Spleen, splenic — *see* condition

Splenectasis — *see* Splenomegaly

Splenitis (interstitial) (malignant) (nonspecific) D73.89
- malarial — *see also* Malaria B54 *[D77]*
- tuberculous A18.85

Splenocele D73.89

Splenomegaly, splenomegalia (Bengal) (cryptogenic) (idiopathic) (tropical) R16.1
- with hepatomegaly R16.2
- cirrhotic D73.2
- congenital Q89.09
- congestive, chronic D73.2
- Egyptian B65.1
- Gaucher's E75.22
- malarial — *see also* Malaria B54 *[D77]*
- neutropenic D73.81
- Niemann-Pick — *see* Niemann-Pick disease or syndrome
- siderotic D73.2
- syphilitic A52.79
  - congenital (early) A50.08 *[D77]*

Splenopathy D73.9

Splenoptosis D73.89

Splenosis D73.89

Splinter — *see* Foreign body, superficial, by site

Split, splitting
- foot Q72.7-
- hand Q71.6
- heart sounds R01.2
- lip, congenital — *see* Cleft, lip
- nails L60.3
- urinary stream R39.13

Spondylarthrosis — *see* Spondylosis

Spondylitis (chronic) — *see also* Spondylopathy, inflammatory
- ankylopoietica — *see* Spondylitis, ankylosing
- ankylosing (chronic) M45.9
  - with lung involvement M45.9 *[J99]*
  - cervical region M45.2
  - cervicothoracic region M45.3
  - juvenile M08.1
  - lumbar region M45.6
  - lumbosacral region M45.7
  - multiple sites M45.0
  - occipito-atlanto-axial region M45.1
  - sacrococcygeal region M45.8
  - thoracic region M45.4
  - thoracolumbar region M45.5
- atrophic (ligamentous) — *see* Spondylitis, ankylosing
- deformans (chronic) — *see* Spondylosis
- gonococcal A54.41
- gouty — *see also* Gout, by type, vertebrae M10.08
- in (due to)
  - brucellosis A23.9 *[M49.80]*
    - cervical region A23.9 *[M49.82]*
    - cervicothoracic region A23.9 *[M49.83]*
    - lumbar region A23.9 *[M49.86]*
    - lumbosacral region A23.9 *[M49.87]*
    - multiple sites A23.9 *[M49.89]*
    - occipito-atlanto-axial region A23.9 *[M49.81]*
    - sacrococcygeal region A23.9 *[M49.88]*
    - thoracic region A23.9 *[M49.84]*
    - thoracolumbar region A23.9 *[M49.85]*
  - enterobacteria (*see also* subcategory M49.8) A04.9
  - tuberculosis A18.01
- infectious NEC — *see* Spondylopathy, infective
- juvenile ankylosing (chronic) M08.1
- Kümmell's — *see* Spondylopathy, traumatic
- Marie-Strümpell — *see* Spondylitis, ankylosing
- muscularis — *see* Spondylopathy, specified NEC
- psoriatic L40.53
- rheumatoid — *see* Spondylitis, ankylosing
- rhizomelica — *see* Spondylitis, ankylosing
- sacroiliac NEC M46.1

Spondylitis (chronic) - *continued*
- senescent, senile — *see* Spondylosis
- traumatic (chronic) or post-traumatic — *see* Spondylopathy, traumatic
- tuberculous A18.01
- typhosa A01.05

Spondyloarthritis
- axial — *see also* Spondlyitis, ankylosing
  - non-radiographic M45.A0
    - cervical M45.A2
    - cervicothoracic M45.A3
    - lumbar M45.A6
    - lumbosacral M45.A7
    - multiple sites M45.AB
    - occipito-atlanto-axial region M45.A1
    - sacral and sacrococcygeal M45.A8
    - thoracic M45.A4
    - thoracolumbar M45.A5

Spondylolisthesis (acquired) (degenerative) M43.10
- with disproportion (fetopelvic) O33.0
  - causing obstructed labor O65.0
- cervical region M43.12
- cervicothoracic region M43.13
- congenital Q76.2
- lumbar region M43.16
- lumbosacral region M43.17
- multiple sites M43.19
- occipito-atlanto-axial region M43.11
- sacrococcygeal region M43.18
- thoracic region M43.14
- thoracolumbar region M43.15
- traumatic (old) M43.10
  - acute
    - fifth cervical (displaced) S12.430
      - nondisplaced S12.431
      - specified type NEC (displaced) S12.450
        - nondisplaced S12.451
      - type III S12.44
    - fourth cervical (displaced) S12.330
      - nondisplaced S12.331
      - specified type NEC (displaced) S12.350
        - nondisplaced S12.351
      - type III S12.34
    - second cervical (displaced) S12.130
      - nondisplaced S12.131
      - specified type NEC (displaced) S12.150
        - nondisplaced S12.151
      - type III S12.14
    - seventh cervical (displaced) S12.630
      - nondisplaced S12.631
      - specified type NEC (displaced) S12.650
        - nondisplaced S12.651
      - type III S12.64
    - sixth cervical (displaced) S12.530
      - nondisplaced S12.531
      - specified type NEC (displaced) S12.550
        - nondisplaced S12.551
      - type III S12.54
    - third cervical (displaced) S12.230
      - nondisplaced S12.231
      - specified type NEC (displaced) S12.250
        - nondisplaced S12.251
      - type III S12.24

Spondylolysis (acquired) M43.00
- cervical region M43.02
- cervicothoracic region M43.03
- congenital Q76.2
- lumbar region M43.06
- lumbosacral region M43.07
  - with disproportion (fetopelvic) O33.0
    - causing obstructed labor O65.8
- multiple sites M43.09
- occipito-atlanto-axial region M43.01
- sacrococcygeal region M43.08
- thoracic region M43.04
- thoracolumbar region M43.05

Spondylopathy M48.9
- infective NEC M46.50

Spondylopathy - *continued*
infective NEC - *continued*
cervical region M46.52
cervicothoracic region M46.53
lumbar region M46.56
lumbosacral region M46.57
multiple sites M46.59
occipito-atlanto-axial region M46.51
sacrococcygeal region M46.58
thoracic region M46.54
thoracolumbar region M46.55
inflammatory M46.90
cervical region M46.92
cervicothoracic region M46.93
lumbar region M46.96
lumbosacral region M46.97
multiple sites M46.99
occipito-atlanto-axial region M46.91
sacrococcygeal region M46.98
specified type NEC M46.80
cervical region M46.82
cervicothoracic region M46.83
lumbar region M46.86
lumbosacral region M46.87
multiple sites M46.89
occipito-atlanto-axial region M46.81
sacrococcygeal region M46.88
thoracic region M46.84
thoracolumbar region M46.85
thoracic region M46.94
thoracolumbar region M46.95
neuropathic, in
syringomyelia and syringobulbia G95.0
tabes dorsalis A52.11
specified NEC — *see* subcategory M48.8
traumatic M48.30
cervical region M48.32
cervicothoracic region M48.33
lumbar region M48.36
lumbosacral region M48.37
occipito-atlanto-axial region M48.31
sacrococcygeal region M48.38
thoracic region M48.34
thoracolumbar region M48.35

Spondylosis M47.9
with
disproportion (fetopelvic) O33.0
causing obstructed labor O65.0
myelopathy NEC M47.10
cervical region M47.12
cervicothoracic region M47.13
lumbar region M47.16
occipito-atlanto-axial region M47.11
thoracic region M47.14
thoracolumbar region M47.15
radiculopathy M47.20
cervical region M47.22
cervicothoracic region M47.23
lumbar region M47.26
lumbosacral region M47.27
occipito-atlanto-axial region M47.21
sacrococcygeal region M47.28
thoracic region M47.24
thoracolumbar region M47.25
specified NEC M47.899
cervical region M47.892
cervicothoracic region M47.893
facet joint — *see also* Spondylosis M47.819
lumbar region M47.896
lumbosacral region M47.897
occipito-atlanto-axial region M47.891
sacrococcygeal region M47.898
thoracic region M47.894
thoracolumbar region M47.895
traumatic — *see* Spondylopathy, traumatic
without myelopathy or radiculopathy M47.819
cervical region M47.812
cervicothoracic region M47.813
lumbar region M47.816
lumbosacral region M47.817
occipito-atlanto-axial region M47.811
sacrococcygeal region M47.818
thoracic region M47.814

Spondylosis - *continued*
without myelopathy or radiculopathy - *continued*
thoracolumbar region M47.815

Sponge
inadvertently left in operation wound — *see* Foreign body, accidentally left during a procedure
kidney (medullary) Q61.5

Sponge-diver's disease — *see* Toxicity, venom, marine animal, sea anemone

Spongioblastoma (any type) — *see* Neoplasm, malignant, by site
specified site — *see* Neoplasm, malignant, by site
unspecified site C71.9

Spongioneuroblastoma — *see* Neoplasm, malignant, by site

Spontaneous — *see also* condition
fracture (cause unknown) — *see* Fracture, pathological

Spoon nail L60.3
congenital Q84.6

Sporadic — *see* condition

Sporothrix schenckii infection — *see* Sporotrichosis

Sporotrichosis B42.9
arthritis B42.82
disseminated B42.7
generalized B42.7
lymphocutaneous (fixed) (progressive) B42.1
pulmonary B42.0
specified NEC B42.89

Spots, spotting (in) (of)
Bitot's — *see also* Pigmentation, conjunctiva
in the young child E50.1
vitamin A deficiency E50.1
café, au lait L81.3
Cayenne pepper I78.1
cotton wool, retina — *see* Occlusion, artery, retina
de Morgan's (senile angiomas) I78.1
Fuchs' black (myopic) — *see also* Myopia, degenerative H44.2-
intermenstrual (regular) N92.0
irregular N92.1
Koplik's B05.9
liver L81.4
pregnancy O26.85-
purpuric R23.3
ruby I78.1

Spotted fever — *see* Fever, spotted A77.9

Sprain (joint) (ligament)
acromioclavicular joint or ligament S43.5-
ankle S93.40-
calcaneofibular ligament S93.41-
deltoid ligament S93.42-
internal collateral ligament — *see* Sprain, ankle, specified ligament NEC
specified ligament NEC S93.49-
talofibular ligament — *see* Sprain, ankle, specified ligament NEC
tibiofibular ligament S93.43-
anterior longitudinal, cervical S13.4
atlas, atlanto-axial, atlanto-occipital S13.4
breast bone — *see* Sprain, sternum
calcaneofibular — *see* Sprain, ankle
carpal — *see* Sprain, wrist
carpometacarpal — *see* Sprain, hand, specified site NEC
cartilage
costal S23.41
semilunar (knee) — *see* Sprain, knee, specified site NEC
with current tear — *see* Tear, meniscus
thyroid region S13.5
xiphoid — *see* Sprain, sternum
cervical, cervicodorsal, cervicothoracic S13.4
chondrosternal S23.421
coracoclavicular S43.8-
coracohumeral S43.41-
coronary, knee — *see* Sprain, knee, specified site NEC
costal cartilage S23.41
cricoarytenoid articulation or ligament S13.5

Sprain (joint) (ligament) - *continued*
cricothyroid articulation S13.5
cruciate, knee — *see* Sprain, knee, cruciate
deltoid, ankle — *see* Sprain, ankle
dorsal (spine) S23.3
elbow S53.40-
radial collateral ligament S53.43-
radiohumeral S53.41-
rupture
radial collateral ligament — *see* Rupture, traumatic, ligament, radial collateral
ulnar collateral ligament — *see* Rupture, traumatic, ligament, ulnar collateral
specified type NEC S53.49-
ulnar collateral ligament S53.44-
ulnohumeral S53.42-
femur, head — *see* Sprain, hip
fibular collateral, knee — *see* Sprain, knee, collateral
fibulocalcaneal — *see* Sprain, ankle
finger (s) S63.61-
index S63.61-
interphalangeal (joint) S63.63-
index S63.63-
little S63.63-
middle S63.63-
ring S63.63-
little S63.61-
middle S63.61-
ring S63.61-
metacarpophalangeal (joint) S63.65-
specified site NEC S63.69-
index S63.69-
little S63.69-
middle S63.69-
ring S63.69-
foot S93.60-
specified ligament NEC S93.69-
tarsal ligament S93.61-
tarsometatarsal ligament S93.62-
toe — *see* Sprain, toe
hand S63.9-
finger — *see* Sprain, finger
specified site NEC — *see* subcategory S63.8
thumb — *see* Sprain, thumb
head S03.9
hip S73.10-
iliofemoral ligament S73.11-
ischiocapsular (ligament) S73.12-
specified NEC S73.19-
iliofemoral — *see* Sprain, hip
innominate
acetabulum — *see* Sprain, hip
sacral junction S33.6
internal
collateral, ankle — *see* Sprain, ankle
semilunar cartilage — *see* Sprain, knee, specified site NEC
interphalangeal
finger — *see* Sprain, finger, interphalangeal (joint)
toe — *see* Sprain, toe, interphalangeal joint
ischiocapsular — *see* Sprain, hip
ischiofemoral — *see* Sprain, hip
jaw (articular disc) (cartilage) (meniscus) S03.4-
old M26.69
knee S83.9-
collateral ligament S83.40-
lateral (fibular) S83.42-
medial (tibial) S83.41-
cruciate ligament S83.50-
anterior S83.51-
posterior S83.52-
lateral (fibular) collateral ligament S83.42-
medial (tibial) collateral ligament S83.41-
patellar ligament S76.11-
specified site NEC S83.8X-
superior tibiofibular joint (ligament) S83.6-
lateral collateral, knee — *see* Sprain, knee, collateral
lumbar (spine) S33.5

Sprain (joint) (ligament) - *continued*
lumbosacral S33.9
mandible (articular disc) S03.4-
old M26.69
medial collateral, knee — *see* Sprain, knee, collateral
meniscus
jaw S03.4-
old M26.69
knee — *see* Sprain, knee, specified site NEC
with current tear — *see* Tear, meniscus
old — *see* Derangement, knee, meniscus, due to old tear
mandible S03.4-
old M26.69
metacarpal (distal) (proximal) — *see* Sprain, hand, specified site NEC
metacarpophalangeal — *see* Sprain, finger, metacarpophalangeal (joint)
metatarsophalangeal — *see* Sprain, toe, metatarsophalangeal joint
midcarpal — *see* Sprain, hand, specified site NEC
midtarsal — *see* Sprain, foot, specified site NEC
neck S13.9
anterior longitudinal cervical ligament S13.4
atlanto-axial joint S13.4
atlanto-occipital joint S13.4
cervical spine S13.4
cricoarytenoid ligament S13.5
cricothyroid ligament S13.5
specified site NEC S13.8
thyroid region (cartilage) S13.5
nose S03.8
orbicular, hip — *see* Sprain, hip
patella — *see* Sprain, knee, specified site NEC
patellar ligament S76.11-
pelvis NEC S33.8
phalanx
finger — *see* Sprain, finger
toe — *see* Sprain, toe
pubofemoral — *see* Sprain, hip
radiocarpal — *see* Sprain, wrist
radiohumeral — *see* Sprain, elbow
radius, collateral — *see* Rupture, traumatic, ligament, radial collateral
rib (cage) S23.41
rotator cuff (capsule) S43.42-
sacroiliac (region)
chronic or old — *see* subcategory M53.2
joint S33.6
scaphoid (hand) — *see* Sprain, hand, specified site NEC
scapula (r) — *see* Sprain, shoulder girdle, specified site NEC
semilunar cartilage (knee) — *see* Sprain, knee, specified site NEC
with current tear — *see* Tear, meniscus
old — *see* Derangement, knee, meniscus, due to old tear
shoulder joint S43.40-
acromioclavicular joint (ligament) — *see* Sprain, acromioclavicular joint
blade — *see* Sprain, shoulder, girdle, specified site NEC
coracoclavicular joint (ligament) — *see* Sprain, coracoclavicular joint
coracohumeral ligament — *see* Sprain, coracohumeral joint
girdle S43.9-
specified site NEC S43.8-
rotator cuff — *see* Sprain, rotator cuff
specified site NEC S43.49-
sternoclavicular joint (ligament) — *see* Sprain, sternoclavicular joint
spine
cervical S13.4
lumbar S33.5
thoracic S23.3
sternoclavicular joint S43.6-
sternum S23.429

Sprain (joint) (ligament) - *continued*
sternum - *continued*
chondrosternal joint S23.421
specified site NEC S23.428
sternoclavicular (joint) (ligament) S23.420
symphysis
jaw S03.4-
old M26.69
mandibular S03.4-
old M26.69
talofibular — *see* Sprain, ankle
tarsal — *see* Sprain, foot, specified site NEC
tarsometatarsal — *see* Sprain, foot, specified site NEC
temporomandibular S03.4-
old M26.69
thorax S23.9
ribs S23.41
specified site NEC S23.8
spine S23.3
sternum — *see* Sprain, sternum
thumb S63.60-
interphalangeal (joint) S63.62-
metacarpophalangeal (joint) S63.64-
specified site NEC S63.68-
thyroid cartilage or region S13.5
tibia (proximal end) — *see* Sprain, knee, specified site NEC
tibial collateral, knee — *see* Sprain, knee, collateral
tibiofibular
distal — *see* Sprain, ankle
superior — *see* Sprain, knee, specified site NEC
toe (s) S93.50-
great S93.50-
interphalangeal joint S93.51-
great S93.51-
lesser S93.51-
lesser S93.50-
metatarsophalangeal joint S93.52-
great S93.52-
lesser S93.52-
ulna, collateral — *see* Rupture, traumatic, ligament, ulnar collateral
ulnohumeral — *see* Sprain, elbow
wrist S63.50-
carpal S63.51-
radiocarpal S63.52-
specified site NEC S63.59-
xiphoid cartilage — *see* Sprain, sternum
Sprengel's deformity (congenital) Q74.0
Sprue (tropical) K90.1
celiac K90.0
idiopathic K90.49
meaning thrush B37.0
nontropical K90.0
Spur, bone — *see also* Enthesopathy
calcaneal M77.3-
iliac crest M76.2-
nose (septum) J34.89
Spurway's syndrome Q78.0
Sputum
abnormal (amount) (color) (odor) (purulent) R09.3
blood-stained R04.2
excessive (cause unknown) R09.3
Squamous — *see also* condition
epithelium in
cervical canal (congenital) Q51.828
uterine mucosa (congenital) Q51.818
Squashed nose M95.0
congenital Q67.4
Squeeze, diver's T70.3
Squint — *see also* Strabismus
accommodative — *see* Strabismus, convergent concomitant
SSADHD (succinic semialdehyde dehydrogenase deficiency) E72.81
St. Hubert's disease A82.9
Stab — *see also* Laceration
internal organs — *see* Injury, by site
Stafne's cyst or cavity M27.0
Staggering gait R26.0
hysterical F44.4

Staghorn calculus — *see* Calculus, kidney
Stähli's line (cornea) (pigment) — *see* Pigmentation, cornea, anterior
Stain, staining
meconium (newborn) P96.83
port wine Q82.5
tooth, teeth (hard tissues) (extrinsic) K03.6
due to
accretions K03.6
deposits (betel) (black) (green) (materia alba) (orange) (soft) (tobacco) K03.6
metals (copper) (silver) K03.7
nicotine K03.6
pulpal bleeding K03.7
tobacco K03.6
intrinsic K00.8
Stammering — *see also* Disorder, fluency F80.81
Standstill
auricular I45.5
cardiac — *see* Arrest, cardiac
sinoatrial I45.5
ventricular — *see* Arrest, cardiac
Stannosis J63.5
Stanton's disease — *see* Melioidosis
Staphylitis (acute) (catarrhal) (chronic) (gangrenous) (membranous) (suppurative) (ulcerative) K12.2
Staphylococcal scalded skin syndrome L00
Staphylococcemia A41.2
Staphylococcus, staphylococcal — *see also* condition
as cause of disease classified elsewhere B95.8
aureus (methicillin susceptible) (MSSA) B95.61
methicillin resistant (MRSA) B95.62
specified NEC, as cause of disease classified elsewhere B95.7
Staphyloma (sclera)
cornea H18.72-
equatorial H15.81-
localized (anterior) H15.82-
posticum H15.83-
ring H15.85-
Stargardt's disease — *see* Dystrophy, retina
Starvation (inanition) (due to lack of food) T73.0
edema — *see* Malnutrition, severe
Stasis
bile (noncalculous) K83.1
bronchus J98.09
with infection — *see* Bronchitis
cardiac — *see* Failure, heart, congestive
cecum K59.89
colon K59.89
dermatitis I87.2
with
varicose ulcer — *see* Varix, leg, with ulcer, with inflammation
varicose veins — *see* Varix, leg, with, inflammation
due to postthrombotic syndrome — *see* Syndrome, postthrombotic
duodenal K31.5
eczema — *see* Varix, leg, with, inflammation
edema — *see* Hypertension, venous (chronic), idiopathic
foot T69.0-
ileocecal coil K59.89
ileum K59.89
intestinal K59.89
jejunum K59.89
kidney N19
liver (cirrhotic) K76.1
lymphatic I89.8
pneumonia J18.2
pulmonary — *see* Edema, lung
rectal K59.89
renal N19
tubular N17.0
ulcer — *see* Varix, leg, with, ulcer
without varicose veins I87.2
urine — *see* Retention, urine

STATUS - STENOSIS, STENOTIC

Stenosis, stenotic (cicatricial) - *continued*
  lacrimal (passage) - *continued*
    duct H04.55-
    punctum H04.56-
    sac H04.57-
  lacrimonasal duct — *see* Stenosis, lacrimal, duct
    congenital Q10.5
  larynx J38.6
    congenital NEC Q31.8
      subglottic Q31.1
    syphilitic A52.73
      congenital A50.59 *[J99]*
  mitral (chronic) (inactive) (valve) I05.0
    with
      aortic valve disease I08.0
      incompetency, insufficiency or regurgitation I05.2
    active or acute I01.1
      with rheumatic or Sydenham's chorea I02.0
    congenital Q23.2
    specified cause, except rheumatic I34.2
    syphilitic A52.03
  myocardium, myocardial — *see also* Degeneration, myocardial
    hypertrophic subaortic (idiopathic) I42.1
  nares (anterior) (posterior) J34.89
    congenital Q30.0
  nasal duct — *see also* Stenosis, lacrimal, duct
    congenital Q10.5
  nasolacrimal duct — *see also* Stenosis, lacrimal, duct
    congenital Q10.5
  neural canal — *see also* Lesion, biomechanical, specified NEC
    connective tissue M99.49
      abdomen M99.49
      cervical region M99.41
      cervicothoracic M99.41
      head region M99.40
      lower extremity M99.46
      lumbar region M99.43
      lumbosacral M99.43
      occipitocervical M99.40
      pelvic M99.45
      rib cage M99.48
      sacral region M99.44
      sacrococcygeal M99.44
      sacroiliac M99.44
      specified NEC M99.49
      thoracic region M99.42
      thoracolumbar M99.42
      upper extremity M99.47
    intervertebral disc M99.59
      abdomen M99.59
      cervical region M99.51
      cervicothoracic M99.51
      head region M99.50
      lower extremity M99.56
      lumbar region M99.53
      lumbosacral M99.53
      occipitocervical M99.50
      pelvic M99.55
      rib cage M99.58
      sacral region M99.54
      sacrococcygeal M99.54
      sacroiliac M99.54
      specified NEC M99.59
      thoracic region M99.52
      thoracolumbar M99.52
      upper extremity M99.57
    osseous M99.39
      abdomen M99.39
      cervical region M99.31
      cervicothoracic M99.31
      head region M99.30
      lower extremity M99.36
      lumbar region M99.33
      lumbosacral M99.33
      pelvic M99.35
      rib cage M99.38
      occipitocervical M99.30
      sacral region M99.34

Stenosis, stenotic (cicatricial) - *continued*
  neural canal - *continued*
    osseous - *continued*
      sacrococcygeal M99.34
      sacroiliac M99.34
      specified NEC M99.39
      thoracic region M99.32
      thoracolumbar M99.32
      upper extremity M99.37
    subluxation M99.29
      cervical region M99.21
      cervicothoracic M99.21
      head region M99.20
      lower extremity M99.26
      lumbar region M99.23
      lumbosacral M99.23
      occipitocervical M99.20
      pelvic M99.25
      rib cage M99.28
      sacral region M99.24
      sacrococcygeal M99.24
      sacroiliac M99.24
      specified NEC M99.29
      thoracic region M99.22
      thoracolumbar M99.22
      upper extremity M99.27
  organ or site, congenital NEC — *see* Atresia, by site
  papilla of Vater K83.1
  pulmonary (artery) (congenital) Q25.6
    with ventricular septal defect, transposition of aorta, and hypertrophy of right ventricle Q21.3
    acquired I28.8
    in tetralogy of Fallot Q21.3
    infundibular Q24.3
    subvalvular Q24.3
    supravalvular Q25.6
    valve I37.0
      with insufficiency I37.2
      congenital Q22.1
      rheumatic I09.89
        with aortic, mitral or tricuspid (valve) disease I08.8
    vein, acquired I28.8
    vessel NEC I28.8
  pulmonic (congenital) Q22.1
    infundibular Q24.3
    subvalvular Q24.3
  pylorus (hypertrophic) (acquired) K31.1
    adult K31.1
    congenital Q40.0
    infantile Q40.0
  rectum (sphincter) — *see* Stricture, rectum
  renal artery I70.1
    congenital Q27.1
  salivary duct (any) K11.8
  sphincter of Oddi K83.1
  spinal M48.00
    cervical region M48.02
    cervicothoracic region M48.03
    lumbar region (NOS) (without neurogenic claudication) M48.061
      with neurogenic claudication M48.062
    lumbosacral region M48.07
    occipito-atlanto-axial region M48.01
    sacrococcygeal region M48.08
    thoracic region M48.04
    thoracolumbar region M48.05
  stent
    vascular
      end stent
        adjacent to stent — *see* Arteriosclerosis
        within the stent
          coronary T82.855
          peripheral T82.856
      in stent
        coronary vessel T82.855
        peripheral vessel T82.856
  stomach, hourglass K31.2
  subaortic (congenital) Q24.4
    hypertrophic (idiopathic) I42.1
  subglottic J38.6
    congenital Q31.1

Stenosis, stenotic (cicatricial) - *continued*
  subglottic - *continued*
    postprocedural J95.5
  trachea J39.8
    congenital Q32.1
    syphilitic A52.73
    tuberculous NEC A15.5
  tracheostomy J95.03
  tricuspid (valve) I07.0
    with
      aortic (valve) disease I08.2
      incompetency, insufficiency or regurgitation I07.2
        with aortic (valve) disease I08.2
          with mitral (valve) disease I08.3
      mitral (valve) disease I08.1
        with aortic (valve) disease I08.3
    congenital Q22.4
    nonrheumatic I36.0
      with insufficiency I36.2
  tubal N97.1
  ureter — *see* Atresia, ureter
  ureteropelvic junction, congenital Q62.11
  ureterovesical orifice, congenital Q62.12
  urethra (valve) — *see also* Stricture, urethra
    congenital Q64.32
  urinary meatus, congenital Q64.33
  vagina N89.5
    congenital Q52.4
    in pregnancy — *see* Pregnancy, complicated by, abnormal vagina
      causing obstructed labor O65.5
  valve (cardiac) (heart) — *see also* Endocarditis I38
    congenital Q24.8
      aortic Q23.0
      mitral Q23.2
      pulmonary Q22.1
      tricuspid Q22.4
  vena cava (inferior) (superior) I87.1
    congenital Q26.0
  vesicourethral orifice Q64.31
  vulva N90.5
Stent jail T82.897
Stercolith (impaction) K56.41
  appendix K38.1
Stercoraceous, stercoral ulcer K63.3
  anus or rectum K62.6
Stereotypies NEC F98.4
Sterility — *see* Infertility
Sterilization — *see* Encounter (for), sterilization
Sternalgia — *see* Angina
Sternopagus Q89.4
Sternum bifidum Q76.7
Steroid
  effects (adverse) (adrenocortical) (iatrogenic)
    cushingoid E24.2
      correct substance properly administered — *see* Table of Drugs and Chemicals, by drug, adverse effect
      overdose or wrong substance given or taken — *see* Table of Drugs and Chemicals, by drug, poisoning
    diabetes — *see* category E09
      correct substance properly administered — *see* Table of Drugs and Chemicals, by drug, adverse effect
      overdose or wrong substance given or taken — *see* Table of Drugs and Chemicals, by drug, poisoning
    fever R50.2
    insufficiency E27.3
      correct substance properly administered — *see* Table of Drugs and Chemicals, by drug, adverse effect
      overdose or wrong substance given or taken — *see* Table of Drugs and Chemicals, by drug, poisoning
  responder H40.04-
Stevens-Johnson disease or syndrome L51.1
  toxic epidermal necrolysis overlap L51.3

- **Streptobacillary fever** A25.1
- **Streptobacillosis** A25.1
- **Streptobacillus moniliformis** A25.1
- **Streptococcus, streptococcal** — *see also* condition
  - as cause of disease classified elsewhere B95.5
  - group
    - A, as cause of disease classified elsewhere B95.0
    - B, as cause of disease classified elsewhere B95.1
    - D, as cause of disease classified elsewhere B95.2
  - pneumoniae, as cause of disease classified elsewhere B95.3
  - specified NEC, as cause of disease classified elsewhere B95.4
- **Streptomycosis** B47.1
- **Streptotrichosis** A48.8
- **Stress** F43.9
  - family — *see* Disruption, family
  - fetal P84
    - complicating pregnancy O77.9
      - due to drug administration O77.1
  - mental NEC Z73.3
    - work-related Z56.6
  - physical NEC Z73.3
    - work-related Z56.6
  - polycythemia D75.1
  - reaction — *see also* Reaction, stress F43.9
  - work schedule Z56.3
- **Stretching, nerve** — *see* Injury, nerve
- **Striae albicantes, atrophicae or distensae (cutis)** L90.6
- **Stricture** — *see also* Stenosis
  - ampulla of Vater K83.1
  - anus (sphincter) K62.4
    - congenital Q42.3
      - with fistula Q42.2
    - infantile Q42.3
      - with fistula Q42.2
  - aorta (ascending) (congenital) Q25.1
    - arteriosclerotic I70.0
    - calcified I70.0
    - supravalvular, congenital Q25.3
  - aortic (valve) — *see* Stenosis, aortic
  - aqueduct of Sylvius (congenital) Q03.0
    - with spina bifida — *see* Spina bifida, by site, with hydrocephalus
    - acquired G91.1
  - artery I77.1
    - basilar — *see* Occlusion, artery, basilar
    - carotid — *see* Occlusion, artery, carotid
    - celiac I77.4
    - congenital (peripheral) Q27.8
      - cerebral Q28.3
      - coronary Q24.5
      - digestive system Q27.8
      - lower limb Q27.8
      - retinal Q14.1
      - specified site NEC Q27.8
      - umbilical Q27.0
      - upper limb Q27.8
    - coronary — *see* Disease, heart, ischemic, atherosclerotic
      - congenital Q24.5
    - precerebral — *see* Occlusion, artery, precerebral
    - pulmonary (congenital) Q25.6
      - acquired I28.8
    - renal I70.1
    - vertebral — *see* Occlusion, artery, vertebral
  - auditory canal (external) (congenital)
    - acquired — *see* Stenosis, external ear canal
  - bile duct (common) (hepatic) K83.1
    - congenital Q44.3
    - postoperative K91.89
  - bladder N32.89
    - neck N32.0
  - bowel — *see* Obstruction, intestine
  - brain G93.89
  - bronchus J98.09
    - congenital Q32.3

- **Stricture** - *continued*
  - bronchus - *continued*
    - syphilitic A52.72
  - cardia (stomach) K22.2
    - congenital Q39.3
  - cardiac — *see also* Disease, heart
    - orifice (stomach) K22.2
  - cecum — *see* Obstruction, intestine
  - cervix, cervical (canal) N88.2
    - congenital Q51.828
    - in pregnancy — *see* Pregnancy, complicated by, abnormal cervix
      - causing obstructed labor O65.5
  - colon — *see also* Obstruction, intestine
    - congenital Q42.9
      - specified NEC Q42.8
  - colostomy K94.03
  - common (bile) duct K83.1
  - coronary (artery) — *see* Disease, heart, ischemic, atherosclerotic
  - cystic duct — *see* Obstruction, gallbladder
  - digestive organs NEC, congenital Q45.8
  - duodenum K31.5
    - congenital Q41.0
  - ear canal (external) (congenital) Q16.1
    - acquired — *see* Stricture, auditory canal, acquired
  - ejaculatory duct N50.89
  - enterostomy K94.13
  - esophagus K22.2
    - congenital Q39.3
    - syphilitic A52.79
      - congenital A50.59 *[K23]*
  - eustachian tube — *see also* Obstruction, eustachian tube
    - congenital Q17.8
  - fallopian tube N97.1
    - gonococcal A54.24
    - tuberculous A18.17
  - gallbladder — *see* Obstruction, gallbladder
  - glottis J38.6
  - heart — *see also* Disease, heart
    - valve — *see also* Endocarditis I38
      - aortic Q23.0
      - mitral Q23.2
      - pulmonary Q22.1
      - tricuspid Q22.4
  - hepatic duct K83.1
  - hourglass, of stomach K31.2
  - hymen N89.6
  - hypopharynx J39.2
  - ileum — *see also* Obstruction, intestine, specified NEC K56.699
    - congenital Q41.2
  - intestine — *see also* Obstruction, intestine
    - congenital (small) Q41.9
      - large Q42.9
        - specified NEC Q42.8
      - specified NEC Q41.8
    - ischemic K55.1
  - jejunum — *see also* Obstruction, intestine, specified NEC K56.699
    - congenital Q41.1
  - lacrimal passages — *see also* Stenosis, lacrimal
    - congenital Q10.5
  - larynx J38.6
    - congenital NEC Q31.8
      - subglottic Q31.1
    - syphilitic A52.73
      - congenital A50.59 *[J99]*
  - meatus
    - ear (congenital) Q16.1
      - acquired — *see* Stricture, auditory canal, acquired
    - osseous (ear) (congenital) Q16.1
      - acquired — *see* Stricture, auditory canal, acquired
    - urinarius — *see also* Stricture, urethra
      - congenital Q64.33
  - mitral (valve) — *see* Stenosis, mitral
  - myocardium, myocardial I51.5
    - hypertrophic subaortic (idiopathic) I42.1
  - nares (anterior) (posterior) J34.89
    - congenital Q30.0

- **Stricture** - *continued*
  - nasal duct — *see also* Stenosis, lacrimal, duct
    - congenital Q10.5
  - nasolacrimal duct — *see also* Stenosis, lacrimal, duct
    - congenital Q10.5
  - nasopharynx J39.2
    - syphilitic A52.73
  - nose J34.89
    - congenital Q30.0
  - nostril (anterior) (posterior) J34.89
    - congenital Q30.0
    - syphilitic A52.73
      - congenital A50.59 *[J99]*
  - organ or site, congenital NEC — *see* Atresia, by site
  - os uteri — *see* Stricture, cervix
  - osseous meatus (ear) (congenital) Q16.1
    - acquired — *see* Stricture, auditory canal, acquired
  - oviduct — *see* Stricture, fallopian tube
  - pelviureteric junction (congenital) Q62.11
    - acquired, with hydronephrosis N13.0
  - penis, by foreign body T19.4
  - pharynx J39.2
  - prostate N42.89
  - pulmonary, pulmonic
    - artery (congenital) Q25.6
      - acquired I28.8
      - noncongenital I28.8
    - infundibulum (congenital) Q24.3
    - valve I37.0
      - congenital Q22.1
    - vein, acquired I28.8
    - vessel NEC I28.8
  - punctum lacrimale — *see also* Stenosis, lacrimal, punctum
    - congenital Q10.5
  - pylorus (hypertrophic) K31.1
    - adult K31.1
    - congenital Q40.0
    - infantile Q40.0
  - rectosigmoid — *see also* Obstruction, intestine, specified NEC K56.699
  - rectum (sphincter) K62.4
    - congenital Q42.1
      - with fistula Q42.0
    - due to
      - chlamydial lymphogranuloma A55
      - irradiation K91.89
      - lymphogranuloma venereum A55
    - gonococcal A54.6
    - inflammatory (chlamydial) A55
    - syphilitic A52.74
    - tuberculous A18.32
  - renal artery I70.1
    - congenital Q27.1
  - salivary duct or gland (any) K11.8
  - sigmoid (flexure) — *see* Obstruction, intestine
  - spermatic cord N50.89
  - stoma (following) (of)
    - colostomy K94.03
    - enterostomy K94.13
    - gastrostomy K94.23
    - ileostomy K94.13
    - tracheostomy J95.03
  - stomach K31.89
    - congenital Q40.2
    - hourglass K31.2
  - subaortic Q24.4
    - hypertrophic (acquired) (idiopathic) I42.1
  - subglottic J38.6
  - syphilitic NEC A52.79
  - trachea J39.8
    - congenital Q32.1
    - syphilitic A52.73
    - tuberculous NEC A15.5
  - tracheostomy J95.03
  - tricuspid (valve) — *see* Stenosis, tricuspid
  - tunica vaginalis N50.89
  - ureter (postoperative) N13.5
    - with
      - hydronephrosis N13.1

Stricture - *continued*
  ureter (postoperative) - *continued*
    with - *continued*
      hydronephrosis - *continued*
        with infection N13.6
      pyelonephritis (chronic) N11.1
    congenital — *see* Atresia, ureter
    tuberculous A18.11
  ureteropelvic junction (congenital) Q62.11
    acquired, with hydronephrosis N13.0
  ureterovesical orifice N13.5
    with infection N13.6
  urethra (organic) (spasmodic) — *see also* Stricture, urethra, male N35.919
    associated with schistosomiasis B65.0 *[N37]*
    congenital Q64.39
      valvular (posterior) Q64.2
    due to
      infection — *see* Stricture, urethra, postinfective
      trauma — *see* Stricture, urethra, post-traumatic
    female N35.92
    gonococcal, gonorrheal A54.01
    infective NEC — *see* Stricture, urethra, postinfective
    late effect (sequelae) of injury — *see* Stricture, urethra, post-traumatic
    male N35.919
      anterior urethra N35.914
      bulbous urethra N35.912
      meatal N35.911
      membranous urethra N35.913
      overlapping sites N35.916
    postcatheterization — *see* Stricture, urethra, postprocedural
    postinfective NEC
      female N35.12
      male N35.119
        anterior urethra N35.114
        bulbous urethra N35.112
        meatal N35.111
        membranous urethra N35.113
        overlapping sites N35.116
    postobstetric N35.021
    postoperative — *see* Stricture, urethra, postprocedural
    postprocedural
      female N99.12
      male N99.114
        anterior bulbous urethra N99.113
        bulbous urethra N99.111
        fossa navicularis N99.115
        meatal N99.110
        membranous urethra N99.112
        overlapping sites N99.116
    post-traumatic
      female N35.028
        due to childbirth N35.021
      male N35.014
        anterior urethra N35.013
        bulbous urethra N35.011
        meatal N35.010
        membranous urethra N35.012
        overlapping sites N35.016
    sequela (late effect) of
      childbirth N35.021
      injury — *see* Stricture, urethra, post-traumatic
    specified cause NEC
      female N35.82
      male N35.819
        anterior urethra N35.814
        bulbous urethra N35.812
        meatal N35.811
        membranous urethra N35.813
        overlapping sites N35.816
    syphilitic A52.76
    traumatic — *see* Stricture, urethra, post-traumatic
    valvular (posterior) , congenital Q64.2
  urinary meatus — *see* Stricture, urethra
  uterus, uterine (synechiae) N85.6

Stricture - *continued*
  uterus, uterine (synechiae) - *continued*
    os (external) (internal) — *see* Stricture, cervix
  vagina (outlet) — *see* Stenosis, vagina
  valve (cardiac) (heart) — *see also* Endocarditis
    congenital
      aortic Q23.0
      mitral Q23.2
      pulmonary Q22.1
      tricuspid Q22.4
  vas deferens N50.89
    congenital Q55.4
  vein I87.1
  vena cava (inferior) (superior) NEC I87.1
    congenital Q26.0
  vesicourethral orifice N32.0
    congenital Q64.31
  vulva (acquired) N90.5
Stridor R06.1
  congenital (larynx) P28.89
Stridulous — *see* condition
Stroke (apoplectic) (brain) (embolic) (ischemic) (paralytic) (thrombotic) I63.9
  cerebral, perinatal P91.82-
  cryptogenic — *see also* infarction, cerebral I63.9
  epileptic — *see* Epilepsy
  heat T67.01
    exertional T67.02
    specified NEC T67.09
  in evolution I63.9
  intraoperative
    during cardiac surgery I97.810
    during other surgery I97.811
  ischemic, perinatal arterial P91.82-
  lightning — *see* Lightning
  meaning
    cerebral hemorrhage - code to Hemorrhage, intracranial
    cerebral infarction - code to Infarction, cerebral
  neonatal P91.82-
  postprocedural
    following cardiac surgery I97.820
    following other surgery I97.821
  sun T67.01
    specified NEC T67.09
  unspecified (NOS) I63.9
Stromatosis, endometrial D39.0
Strongyloidiasis, strongyloidosis B78.9
  cutaneous B78.1
  disseminated B78.7
  intestinal B78.0
Strophulus pruriginosus L28.2
Struck by lightning — *see* Lightning
Struma — *see also* Goiter
  Hashimoto E06.3
  lymphomatosa E06.3
  nodosa (simplex) E04.9
    endemic E01.2
      multinodular E01.1
    multinodular E04.2
      iodine-deficiency related E01.1
    toxic or with hyperthyroidism E05.20
      with thyroid storm E05.21
      multinodular E05.20
        with thyroid storm E05.21
      uninodular E05.10
        with thyroid storm E05.11
    toxicosa E05.20
      with thyroid storm E05.21
      multinodular E05.20
        with thyroid storm E05.21
      uninodular E05.10
        with thyroid storm E05.11
    uninodular E04.1
  ovarii D27.-
  Riedel's E06.5
Strumipriva cachexia E03.4
Strümpell-Marie spine — *see* Spondylitis, ankylosing
Strümpell-Westphal pseudosclerosis E83.01
Stuart deficiency disease (factor X) D68.2

Stuart-Prower factor deficiency (factor X) D68.2
Student's elbow — *see* Bursitis, elbow, olecranon
Stump — *see* Amputation
Stunting, nutritional E45
Stupor (catatonic) R40.1
  depressive (single episode) F32.89
    recurrent episode F33.8
  dissociative F44.2
  manic F30.2
  manic-depressive F31.89
  psychogenic (anergic) F44.2
  reaction to exceptional stress (transient) F43.0
Sturge (-Weber) (-Dimitri) (-Kalischer) disease or syndrome Q85.8
Stuttering F80.81
  adult onset F98.5
  childhood onset F80.81
  following cerebrovascular disease — *see* Disorder, fluency. following cerebrovascular disease
  in conditions classified elsewhere R47.82
Sty, stye (external) (internal) (meibomian) (zeisian) — *see* Hordeolum
Subacidity, gastric K31.89
  psychogenic F45.8
Subacute — *see* condition
Subarachnoid — *see* condition
Subcortical — *see* condition
Subcostal syndrome, nerve compression — *see* Mononeuropathy, upper limb, specified site NEC
Subcutaneous, subcuticular — *see* condition
Subdural — *see* condition
Subendocardium — *see* condition
Subependymoma
  specified site — *see* Neoplasm, uncertain behavior, by site
  unspecified site D43.2
Suberosis J67.3
Subglossitis — *see* Glossitis
Subhemophilia D66
Subinvolution
  breast (postlactational) (postpuerperal) N64.89
  puerperal O90.89
  uterus (chronic) (nonpuerperal) N85.3
    puerperal O90.89
Sublingual — *see* condition
Sublinguitis — *see* Sialoadenitis
Subluxatable hip Q65.6
Subluxation — *see also* Dislocation
  acromioclavicular S43.11-
  ankle S93.0-
  atlantoaxial, recurrent M43.4
    with myelopathy M43.3
  carpometacarpal (joint) NEC S63.05-
    thumb S63.04-
  complex, vertebral — *see* Complex, subluxation
  congenital — *see also* Malposition, congenital
    hip — *see* Dislocation, hip, congenital, partial
    joint (excluding hip)
      lower limb Q68.8
      shoulder Q68.8
      upper limb Q68.8
  elbow (traumatic) S53.10-
    anterior S53.11-
    lateral S53.14-
    medial S53.13-
    posterior S53.12-
    specified type NEC S53.19-
  finger S63.20-
    index S63.20-
    interphalangeal S63.22-
      distal S63.24-
        index S63.24-
        little S63.24-
        middle S63.24-
        ring S63.24-
      index S63.22-

- **Subluxation** - *continued*
  - finger - *continued*
    - interphalangeal - *continued*
      - little S63.22-
      - middle S63.22-
      - proximal S63.23-
        - index S63.23-
        - little S63.23-
        - middle S63.23-
        - ring S63.23-
      - ring S63.22-
    - little S63.20-
    - metacarpophalangeal S63.21-
      - index S63.21-
      - little S63.21-
      - middle S63.21-
      - ring S63.21-
    - middle S63.20-
    - ring S63.20-
  - foot S93.30-
    - specified site NEC S93.33-
    - tarsal joint S93.31-
    - tarsometatarsal joint S93.32-
    - toe — *see* Subluxation, toe
  - hip S73.00-
    - anterior S73.03-
      - obturator S73.02-
    - central S73.04-
    - posterior S73.01-
  - interphalangeal (joint)
    - finger S63.22-
      - distal joint S63.24-
        - index S63.24-
        - little S63.24-
        - middle S63.24-
        - ring S63.24-
      - index S63.22-
      - little S63.22-
      - middle S63.22-
      - proximal joint S63.23-
        - index S63.23-
        - little S63.23-
        - middle S63.23-
        - ring S63.23-
      - ring S63.22-
    - thumb S63.12-
    - toe S93.13-
      - great S93.13-
      - lesser S93.13-
  - joint prosthesis — *see* Complications, joint prosthesis, mechanical, displacement, by site
  - knee S83.10-
    - cap — *see* Subluxation, patella
    - patella — *see* Subluxation, patella
    - proximal tibia
      - anteriorly S83.11-
      - laterally S83.14-
      - medially S83.13-
      - posteriorly S83.12-
    - specified type NEC S83.19-
  - lens — *see* Dislocation, lens, partial
  - ligament, traumatic — *see* Sprain, by site
  - metacarpal (bone)
    - proximal end S63.06-
  - metacarpophalangeal (joint)
    - finger S63.21-
      - index S63.21-
      - little S63.21-
      - middle S63.21-
      - ring S63.21-
    - thumb S63.11-
  - metatarsophalangeal joint S93.14-
    - great toe S93.14-
    - lesser toe S93.14-
  - midcarpal (joint) S63.03-
  - patella S83.00-
    - lateral S83.01-
    - recurrent (nontraumatic) — *see* Dislocation, patella, recurrent, incomplete
    - specified type NEC S83.09-
  - pathological — *see* Dislocation, pathological
  - radial head S53.00-
    - anterior S53.01-
- **Subluxation** - *continued*
  - radial head - *continued*
    - nursemaid's elbow S53.03-
    - posterior S53.02-
    - specified type NEC S53.09-
  - radiocarpal (joint) S63.02-
  - radioulnar (joint)
    - distal S63.01-
    - proximal — *see* Subluxation, elbow
  - shoulder
    - congenital Q68.8
    - girdle S43.30-
      - scapula S43.31-
      - specified site NEC S43.39-
    - traumatic S43.00-
      - anterior S43.01-
      - inferior S43.03-
      - posterior S43.02-
      - specified type NEC S43.08-
  - sternoclavicular (joint) S43.20-
    - anterior S43.21-
    - posterior S43.22-
  - symphysis (pubis)
  - thumb S63.103
    - interphalangeal joint — *see* Subluxation, interphalangeal (joint), thumb
    - metacarpophalangeal joint — *see* Subluxation, metacarpophalangeal (joint), thumb
  - toe (s) S93.10-
    - great S93.10-
      - interphalangeal joint S93.13-
      - metatarsophalangeal joint S93.14-
    - interphalangeal joint S93.13-
    - lesser S93.10-
      - interphalangeal joint S93.13-
      - metatarsophalangeal joint S93.14-
    - metatarsophalangeal joint S93.149
  - ulnohumeral joint — *see* Subluxation, elbow
  - vertebral
    - recurrent NEC — *see* subcategory M43.5
    - traumatic
      - cervical S13.100
        - atlantoaxial joint S13.120
        - atlantooccipital joint S13.110
        - atloidooccipital joint S13.110
        - joint between
          - C0 and C1 S13.110
          - C1 and C2 S13.120
          - C2 and C3 S13.130
          - C3 and C4 S13.140
          - C4 and C5 S13.150
          - C5and C6 S13.160
          - C6and C7 S13.170
          - C7and T1 S13.180
        - occipitoatloid joint S13.110
      - lumbar S33.100
        - joint between
          - L1and L2 S33.110
          - L2and L3 S33.120
          - L3 and L4 S33.130
          - L4and L5 S33.140
      - thoracic S23.100
        - joint between
          - T1and T2 S23.110
          - T2and T3 S23.120
          - T3 and T4 S23.122
          - T4 and T5 S23.130
          - T5 and T6 S23.132
          - T6 and T7 S23.140
          - T7 and T8 S23.142
          - T8 and T9 S23.150
          - T9 and T10 S23.152
          - T10 and T11 S23.160
          - T11 and T12 S23.162
          - T12 and L1 S23.170
  - ulna
    - distal end S63.07-
    - proximal end — *see* Subluxation, elbow
  - wrist (carpal bone) S63.00-
    - carpometacarpal joint — *see* Subluxation, carpometacarpal (joint)
    - distal radioulnar joint — *see* Subluxation, radioulnar (joint), distal
- **Subluxation** - *continued*
  - wrist (carpal bone) - *continued*
    - metacarpal bone, proximal — *see* Subluxation, metacarpal (bone), proximal end
    - midcarpal — *see* Subluxation, midcarpal (joint)
    - radiocarpal joint — *see* Subluxation, radiocarpal (joint)
    - recurrent — *see* Dislocation, recurrent, wrist
    - specified site NEC S63.09-
    - ulna — *see* Subluxation, ulna, distal end
- **Submaxillary** — *see* condition
- **Submersion (fatal) (nonfatal)** T75.1
- **Submucous** — *see* condition
- **Subnormal, subnormality**
  - accommodation (old age) H52.4
  - mental — *see* Disability, intellectual
  - temperature (accidental) T68
- **Subphrenic** — *see* condition
- **Subscapular nerve** — *see* condition
- **Subseptus uterus** Q51.28
- **Subsiding appendicitis** K36
- **Substance (other psychoactive) -induced**
  - anxiety disorder F19.980
  - bipolar and related disorder F19.94
  - delirium F19.921
  - depressive disorder F19.94
  - major neurocognitive disorder F19.97
  - mild neurocognitive disorder F19.988
  - obsessive-compulsive and related disorder F19.988
  - psychotic disorder F19.959
  - sexual dysfunction F19.981
  - sleep disorder F19.982
- **Substernal thyroid** E04.9
  - congenital Q89.2
- **Substitution disorder** F44.9
- **Subtentorial** — *see* condition
- **Subthyroidism (acquired)** — *see also* Hypothyroidism
  - congenital E03.1
- **Succenturiate placenta** O43.19-
- **Sucking thumb, child (excessive)** F98.8
- **Sudamen, sudamina** L74.1
- **Sudanese kala-azar** B55.0
- **Sudden**
  - heart failure — *see* Failure, heart
  - hearing loss — *see* Deafness, sudden
- **Sudeck's atrophy, disease, or syndrome** — *see* Algoneurodystrophy
- **Suffocation** — *see* Asphyxia, traumatic
- **Sugar**
  - blood
    - high (transient) R73.9
    - low (transient) E16.2
  - in urine R81
- **Suicide, suicidal (attempted)** T14.91
  - by poisoning — *see* Table of Drugs and Chemicals
  - history of (personal) Z91.51
    - in family Z81.8
  - ideation — *see* Ideation, suicidal
  - risk
    - meaning personal history of attempted suicide Z91.51
    - meaning suicidal ideation — *see* Ideation, suicidal
  - tendencies
    - meaning personal history of attempted suicide Z91.51
    - meaning suicidal ideation — *see* Ideation, suicidal
  - trauma — *see* nature of injury by site
- **Suipestifer infection** — *see* Infection, salmonella
- **Sulfhemoglobinemia, sulphemoglobinemia (acquired) (with methemoglobinemia)** D74.8
- **Sumatran mite fever** A75.3
- **Summer** — *see* condition
- **Sunburn** L55.9
  - due to
    - tanning bed (acute) L56.8

Sunburn - *continued*
due to - *continued*
tanning bed (acute) - *continued*
chronic L57.8
ultraviolet radiation (acute) L56.8
chronic L57.8
first degree L55.0
second degree L55.1
third degree L55.2
SUNCT (short lasting unilateral neuralgiform headache with conjunctival injection and tearing) G44.059
intractable G44.051
not intractable G44.059
Sundowning F05
Sunken acetabulum — *see* Derangement, joint, specified type NEC, hip
Sunstroke T67.01
specified NEC T67.09
Superfecundation — *see* Pregnancy, multiple
Superfetation — *see* Pregnancy, multiple
Superinvolution (uterus) N85.8
Supernumerary (congenital)
aortic cusps Q23.8
auditory ossicles Q16.3
bone Q79.8
breast Q83.1
carpal bones Q74.0
cusps, heart valve NEC Q24.8
aortic Q23.8
mitral Q23.2
pulmonary Q22.3
digit (s) Q69.9
ear (lobule) Q17.0
fallopian tube Q50.6
finger Q69.0
hymen Q52.4
kidney Q63.0
lacrimonasal duct Q10.6
lobule (ear) Q17.0
mitral cusps Q23.2
muscle Q79.8
nipple (s) Q83.3
organ or site not listed — *see* Accessory
ossicles, auditory Q16.3
ovary Q50.31
oviduct Q50.6
pulmonary, pulmonic cusps Q22.3
rib Q76.6
cervical or first (syndrome) Q76.5
roots (of teeth) K00.2
spleen Q89.09
tarsal bones Q74.2
teeth K00.1
testis Q55.29
thumb Q69.1
toe Q69.2
uterus Q51.28
vagina Q52.1
vertebra Q76.49
Supervision (of)
contraceptive — *see* Prescription, contraceptives
dietary (for) Z71.3
allergy (food) Z71.3
colitis Z71.3
diabetes mellitus Z71.3
food allergy or intolerance Z71.3
gastritis Z71.3
hypercholesterolemia Z71.3
hypoglycemia Z71.3
intolerance (food) Z71.3
obesity Z71.3
specified NEC Z71.3
healthy infant or child Z76.2
foundling Z76.1
high-risk pregnancy — *see* Pregnancy, complicated by, high, risk
lactation Z39.1
pregnancy — *see* Pregnancy, supervision of
Supplemental teeth K00.1
Suppression
binocular vision H53.34
lactation O92.5

Suppression - *continued*
menstruation N94.89
ovarian secretion E28.39
renal N28.9
urine, urinary secretion R34
Suppuration, suppurative — *see also* condition
accessory sinus (chronic) — *see* Sinusitis
adrenal gland
antrum (chronic) — *see* Sinusitis, maxillary
bladder — *see* Cystitis
brain G06.0
sequelae G09
breast N61.1
puerperal, postpartum or gestational — *see* Mastitis, obstetric, purulent
dental periosteum M27.3
ear (middle) — *see also* Otitis, media
external NEC — *see* Otitis, externa, infective
internal — *see* subcategory H83.0
ethmoidal (chronic) (sinus) — *see* Sinusitis, ethmoidal
fallopian tube — *see* Salpingo-oophoritis
frontal (chronic) (sinus) — *see* Sinusitis, frontal
gallbladder (acute) K81.0
gum K05.20
generalized — *see* Periodontitis, aggressive, generalized
localized — *see* Periodontitis, aggressive, localized
intracranial G06.0
joint — *see* Arthritis, pyogenic or pyemic
labyrinthine — *see* subcategory H83.0
lung — *see* Abscess, lung
mammary gland N61.1
puerperal, postpartum O91.12
associated with lactation O91.13
maxilla, maxillary M27.2
sinus (chronic) — *see* Sinusitis, maxillary
muscle — *see* Myositis, infective
nasal sinus (chronic) — *see* Sinusitis
pancreas, acute — *see also* Pancreatitis, acute K85.80
parotid gland — *see* Sialoadenitis
pelvis, pelvic
female — *see* Disease, pelvis, inflammatory
male K65.0
pericranial — *see* Osteomyelitis
salivary duct or gland (any) — *see* Sialoadenitis
sinus (accessory) (chronic) (nasal) — *see* Sinusitis
sphenoidal sinus (chronic) — *see* Sinusitis, sphenoidal
thymus (gland) E32.1
thyroid (gland) E06.0
tonsil — *see* Tonsillitis
uterus — *see* Endometritis
Supraeruption of tooth (teeth) M26.34
Supraglottitis J04.30
with obstruction J04.31
Suprarenal (gland) — *see* condition
Suprascapular nerve — *see* condition
Suprasellar — *see* condition
Surfer's knots or nodules S89.8-
Surgical
emphysema T81.82
procedures, complication or misadventure — *see* Complications, surgical procedures
shock T81.10
Surveillance (of) (for) — *see also* Observation
alcohol abuse Z71.41
contraceptive — *see* Prescription, contraceptives
dietary Z71.3
drug abuse Z71.51
Susceptibility to disease, genetic Z15.89
malignant neoplasm Z15.09
breast Z15.01
endometrium Z15.04
ovary Z15.02

Susceptibility to disease, genetic - *continued*
malignant neoplasm - *continued*
prostate Z15.03
specified NEC Z15.09
multiple endocrine neoplasia Z15.81
Suspected condition, ruled out — *see also* Observation, suspected
amniotic cavity and membrane Z03.71
cervical shortening Z03.75
fetal anomaly Z03.73
fetal growth Z03.74
maternal and fetal conditions NEC Z03.79
newborn — *see also* Observation, newborn, suspected condition ruled out Z05.9
oligohydramnios Z03.71
placental problem Z03.72
polyhydramnios Z03.71
Suspended uterus
in pregnancy or childbirth — *see* Pregnancy, complicated by, abnormal uterus
Sutton's nevus D22.9
Suture
burst (in operation wound) T81.31
external operation wound T81.31
internal operation wound T81.32
inadvertently left in operation wound — *see* Foreign body, accidentally left during a procedure
removal Z48.02
Swab inadvertently left in operation wound — *see* Foreign body, accidentally left during a procedure
Swallowed, swallowing
difficulty — *see* Dysphagia
foreign body — *see* Foreign body, alimentary tract
Swan-neck deformity (finger) — *see* Deformity, finger, swan-neck
Swearing, compulsive F42.8
in Gilles de la Tourette's syndrome F95.2
Sweat, sweats
fetid L75.0
night R61
Sweating, excessive R61
Sweeley-Klionsky disease E75.21
Sweet's disease or dermatosis L98.2
Swelling (of) R60.9
abdomen, abdominal (not referable to any particular organ) — *see* Mass, abdominal
ankle — *see* Effusion, joint, ankle
arm M79.89
forearm M79.89
breast — *see also* Lump, breast N63.0
Calabar B74.3
cervical gland R59.0
chest, localized R22.2
ear H93.8-
extremity (lower) (upper) — *see* Disorder, soft tissue, specified type NEC
finger M79.89
foot M79.89
glands R59.9
generalized R59.1
localized R59.0
hand M79.89
head (localized) R22.0
inflammatory — *see* Inflammation
intra-abdominal — *see* Mass, abdominal
joint — *see* Effusion, joint
leg M79.89
lower M79.89
limb — *see* Disorder, soft tissue, specified type NEC
localized (skin) R22.9
chest R22.2
head R22.0
limb
lower — *see* Mass, localized, limb, lower
upper — *see* Mass, localized, limb, upper
neck R22.1
trunk R22.2
neck (localized) R22.1

Swelling (of) - *continued*
  pelvic — *see* Mass, abdominal
  scrotum N50.89
  splenic — *see* Splenomegaly
  testis N50.89
  toe M79.89
  umbilical R19.09
  wandering, due to Gnathostoma (spinigerum) B83.1
  white — *see* Tuberculosis, arthritis
Swift (-Feer) disease
  overdose or wrong substance given or taken — *see* Table of Drugs and Chemicals, by drug, poisoning
Swimmer's
  cramp T75.1
  ear H60.33-
  itch B65.3
Swimming in the head R42
Swollen — *see* Swelling
Swyer syndrome Q99.1
Sycosis L73.8
  barbae (not parasitic) L73.8
  contagiosa (mycotic) B35.0
  lupoides L73.8
  mycotic B35.0
  parasitic B35.0
  vulgaris L73.8
Sydenham's chorea — *see* Chorea, Sydenham's
Sylvatic yellow fever A95.0
Sylvest's disease B33.0
Symblepharon H11.23-
  congenital Q10.3
Symond's syndrome G93.2
Sympathetic — *see* condition
Sympatheticotonia G90.8
Sympathicoblastoma
  specified site — *see* Neoplasm, malignant, by site
  unspecified site C74.90
Sympathogonioma — *see* Sympathicoblastoma
Symphalangy (fingers) (toes) Q70.9
Symptoms NEC R68.89
  breast NEC N64.59
  cold J00
  development NEC R63.8
  factitious, self-induced — *see* Disorder, factitious
  genital organs, female R10.2
  involving
    abdomen NEC R19.8
    appearance NEC R46.89
    awareness R41.9
      altered mental status R41.82
      amnesia — *see* Amnesia
      borderline intellectual functioning R41.83
      coma — *see* Coma
      disorientation R41.0
      neurologic neglect syndrome R41.4
      senile cognitive decline R41.81
      specified symptom NEC R41.89
    behavior NEC R46.89
    cardiovascular system NEC R09.89
    chest NEC R09.89
    circulatory system NEC R09.89
    cognitive functions R41.9
      altered mental status R41.82
      amnesia — *see* Amnesia
      borderline intellectual functioning R41.83
      coma — *see* Coma
      disorientation R41.0
      neurologic neglect syndrome R41.4
      senile cognitive decline R41.81
      specified symptom NEC R41.89
    development NEC R62.50
    digestive system NEC R19.8
    emotional state NEC R45.89
      emotional lability R45.86
    food and fluid intake R63.8
    general perceptions and sensations R44.9
      specified NEC R44.8

Symptoms NEC - *continued*
  involving - *continued*
    musculoskeletal system R29.91
      specified NEC R29.898
    nervous system R29.90
      specified NEC R29.818
    pelvis NEC R19.8
    respiratory system NEC R09.89
    skin and integument R23.9
    urinary system R39.9
  menopausal N95.1
  metabolism NEC R63.8
  neurotic F48.8
  of infancy R68.19
  pelvis NEC, female R10.2
  skin and integument NEC R23.9
  subcutaneous tissue NEC R23.9
  viral cold J00
Sympus Q74.2
Syncephalus Q89.4
Synchondrosis
  abnormal (congenital) Q78.8
  ischiopubic M91.0
Synchysis (scintillans) (senile) (vitreous body) H43.89
Syncope (near) (pre-) R55
  anginosa I20.8
  bradycardia R00.1
  cardiac R55
  carotid sinus G90.01
  due to spinal (lumbar) puncture G97.1
  heart R55
  heat T67.1
  laryngeal R05.4
  psychogenic F48.8
  tussive R05.8
  vasoconstriction R55
  vasodepressor R55
  vasomotor R55
  vasovagal R55
Syndactylism, syndactyly Q70.9
  complex (with synostosis)
    fingers Q70.0-
    toes Q70.2-
  simple (without synostosis)
    fingers Q70.1-
    toes Q70.3-
Syndrome — *see also* Disease
  5q minus NOS D46.C
  48,XXXX Q97.1
  49,XXXXX Q97.1
  abdominal
    acute R10.0
    muscle deficiency Q79.4
  abnormal innervation H02.519
    left H02.516
      lower H02.515
      upper H02.514
    right H02.513
      lower H02.512
      upper H02.511
  abstinence, neonatal P96.1
  acid pulmonary aspiration, obstetric O74.0
  acquired immunodeficiency — *see* Human, immunodeficiency virus (HIV) disease
  acute abdominal R10.0
  acute respiratory distress (adult) (child) J80
    idiopathic J84.114
  Adair-Dighton Q78.0
  Adams-Stokes (-Morgagni) I45.9
  adiposogenital E23.6
  adrenal
    hemorrhage (meningococcal) A39.1
    meningococcic A39.1
  adrenocortical — *see* Cushing's, syndrome
  adrenogenital E25.9
    congenital, associated with enzyme deficiency E25.0
  afferent loop NEC K91.89
  Alagille's Q44.7
  alcohol withdrawal (without convulsions) — *see* Dependence, alcohol, with, withdrawal
  Alder's D72.0
  Aldrich (-Wiskott) D82.0

Syndrome - *continued*
  alien hand R41.4
  Alport Q87.81
  alveolar hypoventilation E66.2
  alveolocapillary block J84.10
  amnesic, amnestic (confabulatory) (due to) — *see* Disorder, amnesic
  amyostatic (Wilson's disease) E83.01
  androgen insensitivity E34.50
    complete E34.51
    partial E34.52
  androgen resistance — *see also* Syndrome, androgen insensitivity E34.50
  Angelman Q93.51
  anginal — *see* Angina
  ankyloglossia superior Q38.1
  anterior
    chest wall R07.89
    cord G83.82
    spinal artery G95.19
      compression M47.019
        cervical region M47.012
        cervicothoracic region M47.013
        lumbar region M47.016
        occipito-atlanto-axial region M47.011
        thoracic region M47.014
        thoracolumbar region M47.015
    tibial M76.81-
  antibody deficiency D80.9
    agammaglobulinemic D80.1
      hereditary D80.0
    congenital D80.0
    hypogammaglobulinemic D80.1
      hereditary D80.0
  anticardiolipin (-antibody) D68.61
  antidepressant discontinuation T43.205
  antiphospholipid (-antibody) D68.61
  aortic
    arch M31.4
    bifurcation I74.09
  aortomesenteric duodenum occlusion K31.5
  apical ballooning (transient left ventricular) I51.81
  arcuate ligament I77.4
  argentaffin, argintaffinoma E34.0
  Arnold-Chiari — *see* Arnold-Chiari disease
  Arrillaga-Ayerza I27.0
  arterial tortuosity Q87.82
  arteriovenous steal T82.898-
  Asherman's N85.6
  aspiration, of newborn — *see* Aspiration, by substance, with pneumonia
    meconium P24.01
  ataxia-telangiectasia G11.3
  auriculotemporal G50.8
  autoerythrocyte sensitization (Gardner-Diamond) D69.2
  autoimmune polyglandular E31.0
  autoimmune lymphoproliferative [ALPS] D89.82
  autoinflammatory M04.9
    specified type NEC M04.8
  autosomal — *see* Abnormal, autosomes
  Avellis' G46.8
  Ayerza (-Arrillaga) I27.0
  Babinski-Nageotte G83.89
  Bakwin-Krida Q78.5
  bare lymphocyte D81.6
  Barré-Guillain G61.0
  Barré-Liéou M53.0
  Barrett's — *see* Barrett's, esophagus
  Barsony-Polgar K22.4
  Barsony-Teschendorf K22.4
  Barth E78.71
  Bartter's E26.81
  basal cell nevus Q87.89
  Basedow's E05.00
    with thyroid storm E05.01
  basilar artery G45.0
  Batten-Steinert G71.11
  battered
    baby or child — *see* Maltreatment, child, physical abuse
    spouse — *see* Maltreatment, adult, physical abuse

Syndrome - *continued*
myasthenic - *continued*
in - *continued*
diabetes mellitus — *see* Diabetes, amyotrophy
endocrine disease NEC E34.9 *[G73.3]*
neoplastic disease — *see also* Neoplasm D49.9 *[G73.3]*
thyrotoxicosis (hyperthyroidism) E05.90 *[G73.3]*
with thyroid storm E05.91 *[G73.3]*
myelodysplastic D46.9
with
5q deletion D46.C
isolated del (5q) chromosomal abnormality D46.C
multilineage dysplasia D46.A
with ringed sideroblasts D46.B
lesions, low grade D46.20
specified NEC D46.Z
myeloid hypereosinophilic D72.118
myelopathic pain G89.0
myeloproliferative (chronic) D47.1
myofascial pain M79.18
Naffziger's G54.0
nail patella Q87.2
NARP (Neuropathy, Ataxia and Retinitis pigmentosa) E88.49
neonatal abstinence P96.1
nephritic — *see also* Nephritis
with edema — *see* Nephrosis
acute N00.9
chronic N03.9
rapidly progressive N01.9
nephrotic (congenital) — *see also* Nephrosis N04.9
with
C3
glomerulonephritis N04.A
glomerulopathy N04.A
with dense deposit disease N04.6
dense deposit disease N04.6
diffuse
crescentic glomerulonephritis N04.7
endocapillary proliferative glomerulonephritis N04.4
membranous glomerulonephritis N04.2
mesangial proliferative glomerulonephritis N04.3
mesangiocapillary glomerulonephritis N04.5
focal and segmental glomerular lesions N04.1
minor glomerular abnormality N04.0
specified morphological changes NEC N04.8
diabetic — *see* Diabetes, nephrosis
neurologic neglect R41.4
Nezelof's D81.4
Nonne-Milroy-Meige Q82.0
Nothnagel's vasomotor acroparesthesia I73.89
obesity hypoventilation (OHS) E66.2
oculomotor H51.9
Ogilvie K59.81
ophthalmoplegia-cerebellar ataxia — *see* Strabismus, paralytic, third nerve
oral allergy T78.1
oral-facial-digital Q87.0
organic
affective F06.30
amnesic (not alcohol- or drug-induced) F04
brain F09
depressive F06.31
hallucinosis F06.0
personality F07.0
Ormond's N13.5
oro-facial-digital Q87.0
os trigonum Q68.8
Osler-Weber-Rendu I78.0
osteoporosis-osteomalacia M83.8
Osterreicher-Turner Q87.2
otolith — *see* subcategory H81.8

Syndrome - *continued*
oto-palatal-digital Q87.0
outlet (thoracic) G54.0
ovary
polycystic E28.2
resistant E28.39
sclerocystic E28.2
Owren's D68.2
Paget-Schroetter I82.890
pain — *see also* Pain
complex regional I G90.50
lower limb G90.52-
specified site NEC G90.59
upper limb G90.51-
complex regional II — *see* Causalgia
painful
bruising D69.2
feet E53.8
prostate N42.81
paralysis agitans — *see* Parkinsonism
paralytic G83.9
specified NEC G83.89
Parinaud's H51.0
parkinsonian — *see* Parkinsonism
Parkinson's — *see* Parkinsonism
paroxysmal facial pain G50.0
Parry's E05.00
with thyroid storm E05.01
Parsonage (-Aldren) -Turner G54.5
patella clunk M25.86-
Paterson (-Brown) (-Kelly) D50.1
pectoral girdle I77.89
pectoralis minor I77.89
pediatric autoimmune neuropsychiatric disorders associated with streptococcal infections (PANDAS) D89.89
pediatric inflammatory multisystem M35.81
Pelger-Huet D72.0
pellagra-cerebellar ataxia-renal aminoaciduria E72.02
pellagroid E52
Pellegrini-Stieda — *see* Bursitis, tibial collateral
pelvic congestion-fibrosis, female N94.89
penta X Q97.1
peptic ulcer — *see* Ulcer, peptic
perabduction I77.89
periodic fever M04.1
periodic fever, aphthous stomatitis, pharyngitis, and adenopathy [PFAPA] M04.8
periodic headache, in adults and children — *see* Headache, periodic syndromes in adults and children
periurethral fibrosis N13.5
phantom limb (without pain) G54.7
with pain G54.6
pharyngeal pouch D82.1
Pick's — *see* Disease, Pick's
Pickwickian E66.2
PIE (pulmonary infiltration with eosinophilia) — *see also* Eosinophilia, pulmonary J82.89
pigmentary pallidal degeneration (progressive) G23.0
pineal E34.8
pituitary E22.0
plantar fascia M72.2
placental transfusion — *see* Pregnancy, complicated by, placental transfusion syndromes
plateau iris (post-iridectomy) (postprocedural) H21.82
Plummer-Vinson D50.1
pluricarential of infancy E40
plurideficiency E40
pluriglandular (compensatory) E31.8
autoimmune E31.0
pneumatic hammer T75.21
polyangiitis overlap M30.8
polycarential of infancy E40
polyglandular E31.8
autoimmune E31.0
polysplenia Q89.09
pontine NEC G93.89

Syndrome - *continued*
popliteal
artery entrapment I77.89
web Q87.89
postcardiac injury
postcardiotomy I97.0
postmyocardial infarction I24.1
postcardiotomy I97.0
post chemoembolization - code to associated conditions
postcholecystectomy K91.5
postcommissurotomy I97.0
postconcussional F07.81
postcontusional F07.81
post-COVID (-19) U09.9
postencephalitic F07.89
post endometrial ablation N99.85
posterior
cervical sympathetic M53.0
cord G83.83
fossa compression G93.5
reversible encephalopathy (PRES) I67.83
postgastrectomy (dumping) K91.1
postgastric surgery K91.1
postinfarction I24.1
postlaminectomy NEC M96.1
postleukotomy F07.0
postmastectomy lymphedema I97.2
postmyocardial infarction I24.1
postoperative NEC T81.9
blind loop K90.2
postpartum panhypopituitary (Sheehan) E23.0
postpolio (myelitic) G14
postthrombotic I87.009
with
inflammation I87.02-
with ulcer I87.03-
specified complication NEC I87.09-
ulcer I87.01-
with inflammation I87.03-
asymptomatic I87.00-
postvagotomy K91.1
postvalvulotomy I97.0
postviral NEC G93.3
fatigue G93.3
Potain's K31.0
potassium intoxication E87.5
Prader-Willi Q87.11
Prader-Willi-like Q87.19
precerebral artery (multiple) (bilateral) G45.2
preinfarction I20.0
preleukemic D46.9
premature senility E34.8
premenstrual dysphoric F32.81
premenstrual tension N94.3
Prinzmetal-Massumi R07.1
prune belly Q79.4
pseudocarpal tunnel (sublimis) — *see* Syndrome, carpal tunnel
pseudoparalytica G70.00
with exacerbation (acute) G70.01
in crisis G70.01
pseudo -Turner's Q87.19
psycho-organic (nonpsychotic severity) F07.9
acute or subacute F05
depressive type F06.31
hallucinatory type F06.0
nonpsychotic severity F07.0
specified NEC F07.89
pulmonary
arteriosclerosis I27.0
dysmaturity (Wilson-Mikity) P27.0
hypoperfusion (idiopathic) P22.0
renal (hemorrhagic) (Goodpasture's) M31.0
pure
motor lacunar G46.5
sensory lacunar G46.6
Putnam-Dana D51.0
pyogenic arthritis, pyoderma gangrenosum, and acne [PAPA] M04.8
pyramidopallidonigral G20
pyriformis — *see* Lesion, nerve, sciatic

- **Syndrome** - *continued*
  - QT interval prolongation I45.81
  - radicular NEC — *see* Radiculopathy
    - upper limbs, newborn (birth injury) P14.3
  - rapid time-zone change G47.25
  - Rasmussen G04.81
  - Raymond (-Céstan) I65.8
  - Raynaud's I73.00
    - with gangrene I73.01
  - RDS (respiratory distress syndrome, newborn) P22.0
  - reactive airways dysfunction J68.3
  - Refsum's G60.1
  - Reifenstein E34.52
  - renal glomerulohyalinosis-diabetic — *see* Diabetes, nephrosis
  - Rendu-Osler-Weber I78.0
  - residual ovary N99.83
  - resistant ovary E28.39
  - respiratory
    - distress
      - acute J80
        - adult J80
        - child J80
        - idiopathic J84.114
      - newborn (idiopathic) (type I) P22.0
        - type II P22.1
  - restless legs G25.81
  - retinoblastoma (familial) C69.2
  - retroperitoneal fibrosis N13.5
  - retroviral seroconversion (acute) Z21
  - Reye's G93.7
  - Richter — *see* Leukemia, chronic lymphocytic, B-cell type
  - Ridley's I50.1
  - right
    - heart, hypoplastic Q22.6
    - ventricular obstruction — *see* Failure, heart, right
  - Romano-Ward (prolonged QT interval) I45.81
  - rotator cuff, shoulder — *see also* Tear, rotator cuff M75.10-
  - Rotes Quérol — *see* Hyperostosis, ankylosing
  - Roth — *see* Meralgia paresthetica
  - rubella (congenital) P35.0
  - Ruvalcaba-Myhre-Smith E71.440
  - Rytand-Lipsitch I44.2
  - salt
    - depletion E87.1
      - due to heat NEC T67.8
        - causing heat exhaustion or prostration T67.4
    - low E87.1
  - salt-losing N28.89
  - SATB2-associated Q87.89
  - Scaglietti-Dagnini E22.0
  - scalenus anticus (anterior) G54.0
  - scapulocostal — *see* Mononeuropathy, upper limb, specified site NEC
  - scapuloperoneal G71.09
  - schizophrenic, of childhood NEC F84.5
  - Schnitzler D47.2
  - Scholte's E34.0
  - Schroeder's E27.0
  - Schüller-Christian C96.5
  - Schwachman's — *see* Syndrome, Shwachman's
  - Schwartz (-Jampel) G71.13
  - Schwartz-Bartter E22.2
  - scimitar Q26.8
  - sclerocystic ovary E28.2
  - Seitelberger's G31.89
  - septicemic adrenal hemorrhage A39.1
  - seroconversion, retroviral (acute) Z21
  - serous meningitis G93.2
  - severe acute respiratory (SARS) J12.81
    - coronavirus 2 — *see also* COVID-19 U07.1
      - pneumonia J12.82
  - shaken infant T74.4
  - shock (traumatic) T79.4
    - kidney N17.0
      - following crush injury T79.5

- **Syndrome** - *continued*
  - shock (traumatic) - *continued*
    - toxic A48.3
  - shock-lung J80
  - Shone's - code to specific anomalies
  - short
    - bowel K91.2
    - rib Q77.2
  - shoulder-hand — *see* Algoneurodystrophy
  - Shwachman's D70.4
  - sicca — *see* Syndrome, Sjögren
  - sick
    - cell E87.1
    - sinus I49.5
  - sick-euthyroid E07.81
  - sideropenic D50.1
  - Siemens' ectodermal dysplasia Q82.4
  - Silfverskjöld's Q78.9
  - Simons' E88.1
  - sinus tarsi M25.57-
  - sinusitis-bronchiectasis-situs inversus Q89.3
  - Sipple's E31.22
  - sirenomelia Q87.2
  - Sjögren M35.00
    - with
      - central nervous system involvement M35.07
      - dental involvement M35.0C
      - gastrointestinal involvement M35.08
      - glomerular disease M35.0A
      - inflammatory arthritis M35.05
      - keratoconjunctivitis M35.01
      - lung involvement M35.02
      - myopathy M35.03
      - peripheral nervous system involvement M35.06
      - renal tubular acidosis M35.04
      - specified organ involvement, NEC M35.09
      - tubulo-interstitial nephropathy M35.04
      - vasculitis M35.0B
  - Slocumb's E27.0
  - slow flow, coronary I20.8
  - Sluder's G44.89
  - Smith-Magenis Q93.88
  - Sneddon-Wilkinson L13.1
  - Soto's Q87.3
  - South African cardiomyopathy I42.8
  - spasmodic
    - upward movement, eyes H51.8
    - winking F95.8
  - Spen's I45.9
  - splenic
    - agenesis Q89.01
    - flexure K59.89
    - neutropenia D73.81
  - Spurway's Q78.0
  - staphylococcal scalded skin L00
  - steal
    - arteriovenous T82.898-
    - ischemic T82.898-
    - subclavian G45.8
  - Stein-Leventhal E28.2
  - Stein's E28.2
  - Stevens-Johnson syndrome L51.1
    - toxic epidermal necrolysis overlap L51.3
  - Stewart-Morel M85.2
  - Stickler Q89.8
  - stiff baby Q89.8
  - stiff man G25.82
  - Still-Felty — *see* Felty's syndrome
  - Stokes (-Adams) I45.9
  - stone heart I50.1
  - straight back, congenital Q76.49
  - subclavian steal G45.8
  - subcoracoid-pectoralis minor G54.0
  - subcostal nerve compression I77.89
  - subphrenic interposition Q43.3
  - superior
    - cerebellar artery I63.89
    - mesenteric artery K55.1
    - semi-circular canal dehiscence H83.8X-
    - vena cava I87.1
  - supine hypotensive (maternal) — *see* Syndrome, hypotension, maternal

- **Syndrome** - *continued*
  - suprarenal cortical E27.0
  - supraspinatus — *see also* Tear, rotator cuff M75.10-
  - Susac G93.49
  - swallowed blood P78.2
  - sweat retention L74.0
  - Swyer Q99.1
  - Symond's G93.2
  - sympathetic
    - cervical paralysis G90.2
    - pelvic, female N94.89
  - systemic inflammatory response (SIRS) , of non-infectious origin (without organ dysfunction) R65.10
    - with acute organ dysfunction R65.11
  - tachycardia-bradycardia I49.5
  - takotsubo I51.81
  - TAR (thrombocytopenia with absent radius) Q87.2
  - tarsal tunnel G57.5-
  - teething K00.7
  - tegmental G93.89
  - telangiectasic-pigmentation-cataract Q82.8
  - temporal pyramidal apex — *see* Otitis, media, suppurative, acute
  - temporomandibular joint-pain-dysfunction M26.62-
  - Terry's — *see also* Myopia, degenerative H44.2-
  - testicular feminization — *see also* Syndrome, androgen insensitivity E34.51
  - thalamic pain (hyperesthetic) G89.0
  - thoracic outlet (compression) G54.0
  - Thorson-Björck E34.0
  - thrombocytopenia with absent radius (TAR) Q87.2
  - thyroid-adrenocortical insufficiency E31.0
  - tibial
    - anterior M76.81-
    - posterior M76.82-
  - Tietze's M94.0
  - time-zone (rapid) G47.25
  - Toni-Fanconi E72.09
    - with cystinosis E72.04
  - Touraine's Q79.8
  - tourniquet — *see* Constriction, external, by site
  - toxic shock A48.3
  - transient left ventricular apical ballooning I51.81
  - traumatic vasospastic T75.22
  - Treacher Collins Q75.4
  - triple X, female Q97.0
  - trisomy Q92.9
    - 13 Q91.7
      - meiotic nondisjunction Q91.4
      - mitotic nondisjunction Q91.5
      - mosaicism Q91.5
      - translocation Q91.6
    - 18 Q91.3
      - meiotic nondisjunction Q91.0
      - mitotic nondisjunction Q91.1
      - mosaicism Q91.1
      - translocation Q91.2
    - 20 (q) (p) Q92.8
    - 21 Q90.9
      - meiotic nondisjunction Q90.0
      - mitotic nondisjunction Q90.1
      - mosaicism Q90.1
      - translocation Q90.2
    - 22 Q92.8
  - tropical wet feet T69.0-
  - Trousseau's I82.1
  - tumor lysis (following antineoplastic chemotherapy) (spontaneous) NEC E88.3
  - tumor necrosis factor receptor associated periodic (TRAPS) M04.1
  - Twiddler's (due to)
    - automatic implantable defibrillator T82.198
    - cardiac pacemaker T82.198
  - Unverricht (-Lundborg) — *see* Epilepsy, generalized, idiopathic

- **Syndrome** - *continued*
  - upward gaze H51.8
  - uremia, chronic — *see also* Disease, kidney, chronic N18.9
  - urethral N34.3
  - urethro-oculo-articular — *see* Reiter's disease
  - urohepatic K76.7
  - vago-hypoglossal G52.7
  - vascular NEC in cerebrovascular disease G46.8
  - vasoconstriction, reversible cerebrovascular I67.841
  - vasomotor I73.9
  - vasospastic (traumatic) T75.22
  - vasovagal R55
  - van Buchem's M85.2
  - van der Hoeve's Q78.0
  - VATER Q87.2
  - velo-cardio-facial Q93.81
  - vena cava (inferior) (superior) (obstruction) I87.1
  - vertebral
    - artery G45.0
      - compression — *see* Syndrome, anterior, spinal artery, compression
    - steal G45.0
  - vertebro-basilar artery G45.0
  - vertebrogenic (pain) — *see also* Pain, vertebrogenic M54.89
  - vertiginous — *see* Disorder, vestibular function
  - Vinson-Plummer D50.1
  - virus B34.9
  - visceral larva migrans B83.0
  - visual disorientation H53.8
  - vitamin B6 deficiency E53.1
  - vitreal corneal H59.01-
  - vitreous (touch) H59.01-
  - Vogt-Koyanagi H20.82-
  - Volkmann's T79.6
  - von Schroetter's I82.890
  - von Willebrand (-Jürgen) D68.0
  - Waldenström-Kjellberg D50.1
  - Wallenberg's G46.3
  - water retention E87.79
  - Waterhouse (-Friderichsen) A39.1
  - Weber-Gubler G46.3
  - Weber-Leyden G46.3
  - Weber's G46.3
  - Wegener's M31.30
    - with
      - kidney involvement M31.31
      - lung involvement M31.30
        - with kidney involvement M31.31
  - Weingarten's (tropical eosinophilia) J82.89
  - Weiss-Baker G90.09
  - Werdnig-Hoffman G12.0
  - Wermer's E31.21
  - Werner's E34.8
  - Wernicke-Korsakoff (nonalcoholic) F04
    - alcoholic F10.26
  - West's — *see* Epilepsy, spasms
  - Westphal-Strümpell E83.01
  - wet
    - feet (maceration) (tropical) T69.0-
    - lung, newborn P22.1
  - whiplash S13.4
  - whistling face Q87.0
  - Wilkie's K55.1
  - Wilkinson-Sneddon L13.1
  - Williams Q93.82
  - Willebrand (-Jürgens) D68.0
  - Wilson's (hepatolenticular degeneration) E83.01
  - Wiskott-Aldrich D82.0
  - withdrawal — *see* Withdrawal, state
    - drug
      - infant of dependent mother P96.1
      - therapeutic use, newborn P96.2
  - Woakes' (ethmoiditis) J33.1
  - Wright's (hyperabduction) G54.0
  - X I20.9
  - XXXX Q97.1
  - XXXXX Q97.1
  - XXXXY Q98.1
- **Syndrome** - *continued*
  - XXY Q98.0
  - Yao M04.8
  - yellow nail L60.5
  - Zahorsky's B08.5
  - Zellweger syndrome E71.510
  - Zellweger-like syndrome E71.541
- **Synechia (anterior) (iris) (posterior) (pupil)** — *see also* Adhesions, iris
  - intra-uterine (traumatic) N85.6
- **Synesthesia** R20.8
- **Syngamiasis, syngamosis** B83.3
- **Synodontia** K00.2
- **Synorchidism, synorchism** Q55.1
- **Synostosis (congenital)** Q78.8
  - astragalo-scaphoid Q74.2
  - radioulnar Q74.0
- **Synovial sarcoma** — *see* Neoplasm, connective tissue, malignant
- **Synovioma (malignant)** — *see also* Neoplasm, connective tissue, malignant
  - benign — *see* Neoplasm, connective tissue, benign
- **Synoviosarcoma** — *see* Neoplasm, connective tissue, malignant
- **Synovitis** — *see also* Tenosynovitis M65.9
  - crepitant
    - hand M70.0-
    - wrist M70.03-
  - gonococcal A54.49
  - gouty — *see* Gout
  - in (due to)
    - crystals M65.8-
    - gonorrhea A54.49
    - syphilis (late) A52.78
    - use, overuse, pressure — *see* Disorder, soft tissue, due to use
  - infective NEC — *see* Tenosynovitis, infective NEC
  - specified NEC — *see* Tenosynovitis, specified type NEC
  - syphilitic A52.78
    - congenital (early) A50.02
  - toxic — *see* Synovitis, transient
  - transient M67.3-
    - ankle M67.37-
    - elbow M67.32-
    - foot joint M67.37-
    - hand joint M67.34-
    - hip M67.35-
    - knee M67.36-
    - multiple site M67.39
    - pelvic region M67.35-
    - shoulder M67.31-
    - specified joint NEC M67.38
    - wrist M67.33-
  - traumatic, current — *see* Sprain
  - tuberculous — *see* Tuberculosis, synovitis
  - villonodular (pigmented) M12.2-
    - ankle M12.27-
    - elbow M12.22-
    - foot joint M12.27-
    - hand joint M12.24-
    - hip M12.25-
    - knee M12.26-
    - multiple site M12.29
    - pelvic region M12.25-
    - shoulder M12.21-
    - specified joint NEC M12.28
    - vertebrae M12.28
    - wrist M12.23-
- **Syphilid** A51.39
  - congenital A50.06
  - newborn A50.06
  - tubercular (late) A52.79
- **Syphilis, syphilitic (acquired)** A53.9
  - abdomen (late) A52.79
  - acoustic nerve A52.15
  - adenopathy (secondary) A51.49
  - adrenal (gland) (with cortical hypofunction) A52.79
  - age under 2 years NOS — *see also* Syphilis, congenital, early
    - acquired A51.9
  - alopecia (secondary) A51.32
- **Syphilis, syphilitic (acquired)** - *continued*
  - anemia (late) A52.79 *[D63.8]*
  - aneurysm (aorta) (ruptured) A52.01
    - central nervous system A52.05
    - congenital A50.54 *[I79.0]*
  - anus (late) A52.74
    - primary A51.1
    - secondary A51.39
  - aorta (arch) (abdominal) (thoracic) A52.02
    - aneurysm A52.01
  - aortic (insufficiency) (regurgitation) (stenosis) A52.03
    - aneurysm A52.01
  - arachnoid (adhesive) (cerebral) (spinal) A52.13
  - asymptomatic — *see* Syphilis, latent
  - ataxia (locomotor) A52.11
  - atrophoderma maculatum A51.39
  - auricular fibrillation A52.06
  - bladder (late) A52.76
  - bone A52.77
    - secondary A51.46
  - brain A52.17
  - breast (late) A52.79
  - bronchus (late) A52.72
  - bubo (primary) A51.0
  - bulbar palsy A52.19
  - bursa (late) A52.78
  - cardiac decompensation A52.06
  - cardiovascular A52.00
  - central nervous system (late) (recurrent) (relapse) (tertiary) A52.3
    - with
      - ataxia A52.11
      - general paralysis A52.17
        - juvenile A50.45
      - paresis (general) A52.17
        - juvenile A50.45
      - tabes (dorsalis) A52.11
        - juvenile A50.45
      - taboparesis A52.17
        - juvenile A50.45
    - aneurysm A52.05
    - congenital A50.40
    - juvenile A50.40
    - remission in (sustained) A52.3
    - serology doubtful, negative, or positive A52.3
    - specified nature or site NEC A52.19
    - vascular A52.05
  - cerebral A52.17
    - meningovascular A52.13
    - nerves (multiple palsies) A52.15
    - sclerosis A52.17
    - thrombosis A52.05
  - cerebrospinal (tabetic type) A52.12
  - cerebrovascular A52.05
  - cervix (late) A52.76
  - chancre (multiple) A51.0
    - extragenital A51.2
    - Rollet's A51.0
  - Charcot's joint A52.16
  - chorioretinitis A51.43
    - congenital A50.01
    - late A52.71
    - prenatal A50.01
  - choroiditis — *see* Syphilitic chorioretinitis
  - choroidoretinitis — *see* Syphilitic chorioretinitis
  - ciliary body (secondary) A51.43
    - late A52.71
  - colon (late) A52.74
  - combined spinal sclerosis A52.11
  - condyloma (latum) A51.31
  - congenital A50.9
    - with
      - paresis (general) A50.45
      - tabes (dorsalis) A50.45
      - taboparesis A50.45
    - chorioretinitis, choroiditis A50.01 *[H32]*
    - early, or less than 2 years after birth NEC A50.2
      - with manifestations — *see* Syphilis, congenital, early, symptomatic
      - latent (without manifestations) A50.1

Syphilis, syphilitic (acquired) - *continued*
- peripheral nerve A52.79
- petrous bone (late) A52.77
- pharynx (late) A52.73
  - secondary A51.39
- pituitary (gland) A52.79
- pleura (late) A52.73
- pneumonia, white A50.04
- pontine lesion A52.17
- portal vein A52.09
- primary A51.0
  - anal A51.1
  - and secondary — *see* Syphilis, secondary
  - central nervous system A52.3
  - extragenital chancre NEC A51.2
  - fingers A51.2
  - genital A51.0
  - lip A51.2
  - specified site NEC A51.2
  - tonsils A51.2
- prostate (late) A52.76
- ptosis (eyelid) A52.71
- pulmonary (late) A52.72
  - artery A52.09
- pyelonephritis (late) A52.75
- recently acquired, symptomatic A51.9
- rectum (late) A52.74
- respiratory tract (late) A52.73
- retina, late A52.71
- retrobulbar neuritis A52.15
- salpingitis A52.76
- sclera (late) A52.71
- sclerosis
  - cerebral A52.17
  - coronary A52.06
  - multiple A52.11
- scotoma (central) A52.71
- scrotum (late) A52.76
- secondary (and primary) A51.49
  - adenopathy A51.49
  - anus A51.39
  - bone A51.46
  - chorioretinitis, choroiditis A51.43
  - hepatitis A51.45
  - liver A51.45
  - lymphadenitis A51.49
  - meningitis (acute) A51.41
  - mouth A51.39
  - mucous membranes A51.39
  - periosteum, periostitis A51.46
  - pharynx A51.39
  - relapse (treated, untreated) A51.49
  - skin A51.39
  - specified form NEC A51.49
  - tonsil A51.39
  - ulcer A51.39
  - viscera NEC A51.49
  - vulva A51.39
- seminal vesicle (late) A52.76
- seronegative with signs or symptoms - code by site and stage under Syphilis
- seropositive
  - with signs or symptoms - code by site and stage under Syphilis
  - follow-up of latent syphilis — *see* Syphilis, latent
  - only finding — *see* Syphilis, latent
- seventh nerve (paralysis) A52.15
- sinus, sinusitis (late) A52.73
- skeletal system A52.77
- skin (with ulceration) (early) (secondary) A51.39
  - late or tertiary A52.79
- small intestine A52.74
- spastic spinal paralysis A52.17
- spermatic cord (late) A52.76
- spinal (cord) A52.12
- spleen A52.79
- splenomegaly A52.79
- spondylitis A52.77
- staphyloma A52.71
- stigmata (congenital) A50.59
- stomach A52.74
- synovium A52.78
- tabes dorsalis (late) A52.11

Syphilis, syphilitic (acquired) - *continued*
- tabes dorsalis (late) - *continued*
  - juvenile A50.45
- tabetic type A52.11
  - juvenile A50.45
- taboparesis A52.17
  - juvenile A50.45
- tachycardia A52.06
- tendon (late) A52.78
- tertiary A52.9
  - with symptoms NEC A52.79
  - cardiovascular A52.00
  - central nervous system A52.3
  - multiple NEC A52.79
  - specified site NEC A52.79
- testis A52.76
- thorax A52.73
- throat A52.73
- thymus (gland) (late) A52.79
- thyroid (late) A52.79
- tongue (late) A52.79
- tonsil (lingual) (late) A52.73
  - primary A51.2
  - secondary A51.39
- trachea (late) A52.73
- tunica vaginalis (late) A52.76
- ulcer (any site) (early) (secondary) A51.39
  - late A52.79
  - perforating A52.79
    - foot A52.11
- urethra (late) A52.76
- urogenital (late) A52.76
- uterus (late) A52.76
- uveal tract (secondary) A51.43
  - late A52.71
- uveitis (secondary) A51.43
  - late A52.71
- uvula (late) (perforated) A52.79
- vagina A51.0
  - late A52.76
- valvulitis NEC A52.03
- vascular A52.00
  - brain (cerebral) A52.05
- ventriculi A52.74
- vesicae urinariae (late) A52.76
- viscera (abdominal) (late) A52.74
  - secondary A51.49
- vitreous (opacities) (late) A52.71
  - hemorrhage A52.71
- vulva A51.0
  - late A52.76
  - secondary A51.39

Syphiloma A52.79
- cardiovascular system A52.00
- central nervous system A52.3
- circulatory system A52.00
- congenital A50.59

Syphilophobia F45.29

Syringadenoma — *see also* Neoplasm, skin, benign
- papillary — *see* Neoplasm, skin, benign

Syringobulbia G95.0

Syringocystadenoma — *see* Neoplasm, skin, benign
- papillary — *see* Neoplasm, skin, benign

Syringoma — *see also* Neoplasm, skin, benign
- chondroid — *see* Neoplasm, skin, benign

Syringomyelia G95.0

Syringomyelitis — *see* Encephalitis

Syringomyelocele — *see* Spina bifida

Syringopontia G95.0

System, systemic — *see also* condition
- disease, combined — *see* Degeneration, combined
- inflammatory response syndrome (SIRS) of non-infectious origin (without organ dysfunction) R65.10
  - with acute organ dysfunction R65.11
- lupus erythematosus M32.9
  - inhibitor present D68.62

T

Tabacism, tabacosis, tabagism — *see also* Poisoning, tobacco
- meaning dependence (without remission) F17.200

Tabacism, tabacosis, tabagism - *continued*
- meaning dependence (without remission) - *continued*
  - with
    - disorder F17.299
      - in remission F17.211
      - specified disorder NEC F17.298
    - withdrawal F17.203

Tabardillo A75.9
- flea-borne A75.2
- louse-borne A75.0

Tabes, tabetic A52.10
- with
  - central nervous system syphilis A52.10
  - Charcot's joint A52.16
  - cord bladder A52.19
  - crisis, viscera (any) A52.19
  - paralysis, general A52.17
  - paresis (general) A52.17
  - perforating ulcer (foot) A52.19
- arthropathy (Charcot) A52.16
- bladder A52.19
- bone A52.11
- cerebrospinal A52.12
- congenital A50.45
- conjugal A52.10
- dorsalis A52.11
  - juvenile A50.49
- juvenile A50.49
- latent A52.19
- mesenterica A18.39
- paralysis, insane, general A52.17
- spasmodic A52.17
- syphilis (cerebrospinal) A52.12

Taboparalysis A52.17

Taboparesis (remission) A52.17
- juvenile A50.45

TAC (trigeminal autonomic cephalgia) NEC G44.099
- intractable G44.091
- not intractable G44.099

Tache noir S60.22-

Tachyalimentation K91.2

Tachyarrhythmia, tachyrhythmia — *see* Tachycardia

Tachycardia R00.0
- atrial (paroxysmal) I47.1
- auricular I47.1
- AV nodal re-entry (re-entrant) I47.1
- junctional (paroxysmal) I47.1
- newborn P29.11
- nodal (paroxysmal) I47.1
- non-paroxysmal AV nodal I45.89
- paroxysmal (sustained) (nonsustained) I47.9
  - with sinus bradycardia I49.5
  - atrial (PAT) I47.1
  - atrioventricular (AV) (re-entrant) I47.1
    - psychogenic F54
  - junctional I47.1
    - ectopic I47.1
  - nodal I47.1
  - psychogenic (atrial) (supraventricular) (ventricular) F54
  - supraventricular (sustained) I47.1
    - psychogenic F54
  - ventricular I47.2
    - psychogenic F54
- psychogenic F45.8
- sick sinus I49.5
- sinoauricular NOS R00.0
  - paroxysmal I47.1
- sinus [sinusal] NOS R00.0
  - paroxysmal I47.1
- supraventricular I47.1
- ventricular (paroxysmal) (sustained) I47.2
  - psychogenic F54

Tachygastria K31.89

Tachypnea R06.82
- hysterical F45.8
- newborn (idiopathic) (transitory) P22.1
- psychogenic F45.8
- transitory, of newborn P22.1

TACO (transfusion associated circulatory overload) E87.71

Tendinitis, tendonitis — *see also* Enthesopathy
- Achilles M76.6-
- adhesive — *see* Tenosynovitis, specified type NEC
  - shoulder — *see* Capsulitis, adhesive
- bicipital M75.2-
- calcific M65.2-
  - ankle M65.27-
  - foot M65.27-
  - forearm M65.23-
  - hand M65.24-
  - lower leg M65.26-
  - multiple sites M65.29
  - pelvic region M65.25-
  - shoulder M75.3-
  - specified site NEC M65.28
  - thigh M65.25-
  - upper arm M65.22-
- due to use, overuse, pressure — *see also* Disorder, soft tissue, due to use
  - specified NEC — *see* Disorder, soft tissue, due to use, specified NEC
- gluteal M76.0-
- patellar M76.5-
- peroneal M76.7-
- psoas M76.1-
- tibial (posterior) M76.82-
  - anterior M76.81-
- trochanteric — *see* Bursitis, hip, trochanteric

Tendon — *see* condition

Tendosynovitis — *see* Tenosynovitis

Tenesmus (rectal) R19.8
- vesical R30.1

Tennis elbow — *see* Epicondylitis, lateral

Tenonitis — *see also* Tenosynovitis
- eye (capsule) H05.04-

Tenontosynovitis — *see* Tenosynovitis

Tenontothecitis — *see* Tenosynovitis

Tenophyte — *see* Disorder, synovium, specified type NEC

Tenosynovitis — *see also* Synovitis M65.9
- adhesive — *see* Tenosynovitis, specified type NEC
  - shoulder — *see* Capsulitis, adhesive
- bicipital (calcifying) — *see* Tendinitis, bicipital
- gonococcal A54.49
- in (due to)
  - crystals M65.8-
  - gonorrhea A54.49
  - syphilis (late) A52.78
  - use, overuse, pressure — *see also* Disorder, soft tissue, due to use
    - specified NEC — *see* Disorder, soft tissue, due to use, specified NEC
- infective NEC M65.1-
  - ankle M65.17-
  - foot M65.17-
  - forearm M65.13-
  - hand M65.14-
  - lower leg M65.16-
  - multiple sites M65.19
  - pelvic region M65.15-
  - shoulder region M65.11-
  - specified site NEC M65.18
  - thigh M65.15-
  - upper arm M65.12-
- radial styloid M65.4
- shoulder region M65.81-
  - adhesive — *see* Capsulitis, adhesive
- specified type NEC M65.88
  - ankle M65.87-
  - foot M65.87-
  - forearm M65.83-
  - hand M65.84-
  - lower leg M65.86-
  - multiple sites M65.89
  - pelvic region M65.85-
  - shoulder region M65.81-
  - specified site NEC M65.88
  - thigh M65.85-
  - upper arm M65.82-
- tuberculous — *see* Tuberculosis, tenosynovitis

Tenovaginitis — *see* Tenosynovitis

Tension
- arterial, high — *see also* Hypertension
  - without diagnosis of hypertension R03.0
- headache G44.209
  - intractable G44.201
  - not intractable G44.209
- nervous R45.0
- pneumothorax J93.0
- premenstrual N94.3
- state (mental) F48.9

Tentorium — *see* condition

Teratencephalus Q89.8

Teratism Q89.7

Teratoblastoma (malignant) — *see* Neoplasm, malignant, by site

Teratocarcinoma — *see also* Neoplasm, malignant, by site
- liver C22.7

Teratoma (solid) — *see also* Neoplasm, uncertain behavior, by site
- with embryonal carcinoma, mixed — *see* Neoplasm, malignant, by site
- with malignant transformation — *see* Neoplasm, malignant, by site
- adult (cystic) — *see* Neoplasm, benign, by site
- benign — *see* Neoplasm, benign, by site
- combined with choriocarcinoma — *see* Neoplasm, malignant, by site
- cystic (adult) — *see* Neoplasm, benign, by site
- differentiated — *see* Neoplasm, benign, by site
- embryonal — *see also* Neoplasm, malignant, by site
  - liver C22.7
- immature — *see* Neoplasm, malignant, by site
- liver C22.7
  - adult, benign, cystic, differentiated type or mature D13.4
- malignant — *see also* Neoplasm, malignant, by site
  - anaplastic — *see* Neoplasm, malignant, by site
  - intermediate — *see* Neoplasm, malignant, by site
    - specified site — *see* Neoplasm, malignant, by site
    - unspecified site C62.90
  - undifferentiated — *see* Neoplasm, malignant, by site
- mature — *see* Neoplasm, uncertain behavior, by site
  - malignant — *see* Neoplasm, by site, malignant, by site
- ovary D27.-
  - embryonal, immature or malignant C56-
- solid — *see* Neoplasm, uncertain behavior, by site
- testis C62.9-
  - adult, benign, cystic, differentiated type or mature D29.2-
  - scrotal C62.1-
  - undescended C62.0-

Termination
- anomalous — *see also* Malposition, congenital
  - right pulmonary vein Q26.3
- pregnancy, elective Z33.2

Ternidens diminutus infestation B81.8

Ternidensiasis B81.8

Terror (s) night (child) F51.4

Terrorism, victim of Z65.4

Terry's syndrome — *see also* Myopia, degenerative H44.2-

Tertiary — *see* condition

Test, tests, testing (for)
- adequacy (for dialysis)
  - hemodialysis Z49.31
  - peritoneal Z49.32
- blood-alcohol Z02.83
  - positive — *see* Findings, abnormal, in blood

Test, tests, testing (for) - *continued*
- blood-drug Z02.83
  - positive — *see* Findings, abnormal, in blood
- blood pressure Z01.30
  - abnormal reading — *see* Blood, pressure
- blood typing Z01.83
  - Rh typing Z01.83
- cardiac pulse generator (battery) Z45.010
- fertility Z31.41
- genetic
  - disease carrier status for procreative management
    - female Z31.430
    - male Z31.440
  - male partner of patient with recurrent pregnancy loss Z31.441
  - procreative management NEC
    - female Z31.438
    - male Z31.448
- hearing Z01.10
  - with abnormal findings NEC Z01.118
  - infant or child (over 28 days old) Z00.129
    - with abnormal findings Z00.121
- HIV (human immunodeficiency virus)
  - nonconclusive (in infants) R75
  - positive Z21
  - seropositive Z21
- immunity status Z01.84
- intelligence NEC Z01.89
- laboratory (as part of a general medical examination) Z00.00
  - with abnormal finding Z00.01
  - for medicolegal reason NEC Z04.89
- male partner of patient with recurrent pregnancy loss Z31.441
- Mantoux (for tuberculosis) Z11.1
  - abnormal result R76.11
- pregnancy, positive first pregnancy — *see* Pregnancy, normal, first
- procreative Z31.49
  - fertility Z31.41
- skin, diagnostic
  - allergy Z01.82
    - special screening examination — *see* Screening, by name of disease
  - Mantoux Z11.1
  - tuberculin Z11.1
- specified NEC Z01.89
- tuberculin Z11.1
  - abnormal result R76.11
- vision Z01.00
  - with abnormal findings Z01.01
  - following failed vision screening Z01.020
    - with abnormal findings Z01.021
  - infant or child (over 28 days old) Z00.129
    - with abnormal findings Z00.121
- Wassermann Z11.3
  - positive — *see* Serology for syphilis, positive

Testicle, testicular, testis — *see also* condition
- feminization syndrome — *see also* Syndrome, androgen insensitivity E34.51
- migrans Q55.29

Tetanus, tetanic (cephalic) (convulsions) A35
- with
  - abortion A34
  - ectopic or molar pregnancy O08.0
- following ectopic or molar pregnancy O08.0
- inoculation reaction (due to serum) — *see* Complications, vaccination
- neonatorum A33
- obstetrical A34
- puerperal, postpartum, childbirth A34

Tetany (due to) R29.0
- alkalosis E87.3
- associated with rickets E55.0
- convulsions R29.0
  - hysterical F44.5
- functional (hysterical) F44.5
- hyperkinetic R29.0
  - hysterical F44.5
- hyperpnea R06.4
  - hysterical F44.5

Tetany (due to) - *continued*
- hyperpnea - *continued*
  - psychogenic F45.8
- hyperventilation — *see also* Hyperventilation R06.4
  - hysterical F44.5
- neonatal (without calcium or magnesium deficiency) P71.3
- parathyroid (gland) E20.9
- parathyroprival E89.2
- post- (para) thyroidectomy E89.2
- postoperative E89.2
- pseudotetany R29.0
- psychogenic (conversion reaction) F44.5

Tetralogy of Fallot Q21.3

Tetraplegia (chronic) — *see also* Quadriplegia G82.50

Thailand hemorrhagic fever A91

Thalassanemia — *see* Thalassemia

Thalassemia (anemia) (disease) D56.9
- with other hemoglobinopathy D56.8
- alpha (major) (severe) (triple gene defect) D56.0
  - minor D56.3
  - silent carrier D56.3
  - trait D56.3
- beta (severe) D56.1
  - homozygous D56.1
  - major D56.1
  - minor D56.3
  - trait D56.3
- delta-beta (homozygous) D56.2
  - minor D56.3
  - trait D56.3
- dominant D56.8
- hemoglobin
  - C D56.8
  - E-beta D56.5
- intermedia D56.1
- major D56.1
- minor D56.3
- mixed D56.8
- sickle-cell — *see* Disease, sickle-cell, thalassemia
- specified type NEC D56.8
- trait D56.3
- variants D56.8

Thanatophoric dwarfism or short stature Q77.1

Thaysen-Gee disease (nontropical sprue) K90.0

Thaysen's disease K90.0

Thecoma D27-
- luteinized D27-
- malignant C56-

Thelarche, premature E30.8

Thelaziasis B83.8

Thelitis N61.0
- puerperal, postpartum or gestational — *see* Infection, nipple

Therapeutic — *see* condition

Therapy
- drug, long-term (current) (prophylactic)
  - agents affecting estrogen receptors and estrogen levels NEC Z79.818
  - anastrozole (Arimidex) Z79.811
  - antibiotics Z79.2
    - short-term use - omit code
  - anticoagulants Z79.01
  - anti-inflammatory Z79.1
  - antiplatelet Z79.02
  - antithrombotics Z79.02
  - aromatase inhibitors Z79.811
  - aspirin Z79.82
  - birth control pill or patch Z79.3
  - bisphosphonates Z79.83
  - contraceptive, oral Z79.3
  - drug, specified NEC Z79.899
  - estrogen receptor downregulators Z79.818
  - Evista Z79.810
  - exemestane (Aromasin) Z79.811
  - Fareston Z79.810
  - fulvestrant (Faslodex) Z79.818
  - gonadotropin-releasing hormone (GnRH) agonist Z79.818

Therapy - *continued*
- drug, long-term (current) (prophylactic) - *continued*
  - goserelin acetate (Zoladex) Z79.818
  - hormone replacement Z79.890
  - insulin Z79.4
  - letrozole (Femara) Z79.811
  - leuprolide acetate (leuprorelin) (Lupron) Z79.818
  - megestrol acetate (Megace) Z79.818
  - methadone
    - for pain management Z79.891
    - maintenance therapy F11.20
  - Nolvadex Z79.810
  - opiate analgesic Z79.891
  - oral contraceptive Z79.3
  - raloxifene (Evista) Z79.810
  - selective estrogen receptor modulators (SERMs) Z79.810
  - short term - omit code
  - steroids
    - inhaled Z79.51
    - systemic Z79.52
  - tamoxifen (Nolvadex) Z79.810
  - toremifene (Fareston) Z79.810

Thermic — *see* condition

Thermography (abnormal) — *see also* Abnormal, diagnostic imaging R93.89
- breast R92.8

Thermoplegia T67.01

Thesaurismosis, glycogen — *see* Disease, glycogen storage

Thiamin deficiency E51.9
- specified NEC E51.8

Thiaminic deficiency with beriberi E51.11

Thibierge-Weissenbach syndrome — *see* Sclerosis, systemic

Thickening
- bone — *see* Hypertrophy, bone
- breast N64.59
- endometrium R93.89
- epidermal L85.9
  - specified NEC L85.8
- hymen N89.6
- larynx J38.7
- nail L60.2
  - congenital Q84.5
- periosteal — *see* Hypertrophy, bone
- pleura J92.9
  - with asbestos J92.0
- skin R23.4
- subepiglottic J38.7
- tongue K14.8
- valve, heart — *see* Endocarditis

Thigh — *see* condition

Thinning vertebra — *see* Spondylopathy, specified NEC

Thirst, excessive R63.1
- due to deprivation of water T73.1

Thomsen disease G71.12

Thoracic — *see also* condition
- kidney Q63.2
- outlet syndrome G54.0

Thoracogastroschisis (congenital) Q79.8

Thoracopagus Q89.4

Thorax — *see* condition

Thorn's syndrome N28.89

Thorson-Björck syndrome E34.0

Threadworm (infection) (infestation) B80

Threatened
- abortion O20.0
  - with subsequent abortion O03.9
- job loss, anxiety concerning Z56.2
- labor (without delivery) O47.9
  - at or after 37 completed weeks of gestation O47.1
  - before 37 completed weeks of gestation O47.0-
- loss of job, anxiety concerning Z56.2
- miscarriage O20.0
- unemployment, anxiety concerning Z56.2

Three-day fever A93.1

Threshers' lung J67.0

Thrix annulata (congenital) Q84.1

Throat — *see* condition

Thrombasthenia (Glanzmann) (hemorrhagic) (hereditary) D69.1

Thromboangiitis I73.1
- obliterans (general) I73.1
  - cerebral I67.89
  - vessels
    - brain I67.89
    - spinal cord I67.89

Thromboarteritis — *see* Arteritis

Thromboasthenia (Glanzmann) (hemorrhagic) (hereditary) D69.1

Thrombocytasthenia (Glanzmann) D69.1

Thrombocythemia (hemorrhagic) — *see also* Thrombocytosis D75.839
- essential D47.3
- idiopathic D47.3
- primary D47.3

Thrombocytopathy (dystrophic) (granulopenic) D69.1

Thrombocytopenia, thrombocytopenic D69.6
- with absent radius (TAR) Q87.2
- congenital D69.42
- dilutional D69.59
- due to
  - drugs D69.59
  - extracorporeal circulation of blood D69.59
  - (massive) blood transfusion D69.59
  - platelet alloimmunization D69.59
- essential D69.3
- heparin induced (HIT) D75.82
- hereditary D69.42
- idiopathic D69.3
- neonatal, transitory P61.0
  - due to
    - exchange transfusion P61.0
    - idiopathic maternal thrombocytopenia P61.0
    - isoimmunization P61.0
- primary NEC D69.49
  - idiopathic D69.3
- puerperal, postpartum O72.3
- secondary D69.59
- transient neonatal P61.0

Thrombocytosis D75.839
- essential D47.3
- idiopathic D47.3
- primary D47.3
- reactive D75.838
- secondary D75.838
- specified NEC D75.838

Thromboembolism — *see* Embolism

Thrombopathy (Bernard-Soulier) D69.1
- constitutional D68.0
- Willebrand-Jurgens D68.0

Thrombopenia — *see* Thrombocytopenia

Thrombophilia D68.59
- primary NEC D68.59
- secondary NEC D68.69
- specified NEC D68.69

Thrombophlebitis I80.9
- antepartum O22.2-
  - deep O22.3-
  - superficial O22.2-
- calf muscular vein (NOS) I80.25-
- cavernous (venous) sinus G08
  - complicating pregnancy O22.5-
  - nonpyogenic I67.6
- cerebral (sinus) (vein) G08
  - nonpyogenic I67.6
  - sequelae G09
- due to implanted device — *see* Complications, by site and type, specified NEC
- during or resulting from a procedure NEC T81.72
- femoral vein (superficial) I80.1-
- femoropopliteal vein I80.0-
- gastrocnemial vein I80.25-
- hepatic (vein) I80.8
- idiopathic, recurrent I82.1
- iliac vein (common) (external) (internal) I80.21-
- iliofemoral I80.1-
- intracranial venous sinus (any) G08
  - nonpyogenic I67.6

Thrombophlebitis - *continued*
- intracranial venous sinus (any) - *continued*
  - sequelae G09
- intraspinal venous sinuses and veins G08
  - nonpyogenic G95.19
- lateral (venous) sinus G08
  - nonpyogenic I67.6
- leg I80.3
  - superficial I80.0-
- longitudinal (venous) sinus G08
  - nonpyogenic I67.6
- lower extremity I80.299
- migrans, migrating I82.1
- pelvic
  - with ectopic or molar pregnancy O08.0
  - following ectopic or molar pregnancy O08.0
  - puerperal O87.1
- peroneal vein I80.24-
- popliteal vein — *see* Phlebitis, leg, deep, popliteal
- portal (vein) K75.1
- postoperative T81.72
- pregnancy — *see* Thrombophlebitis, antepartum
- puerperal, postpartum, childbirth O87.0
  - deep O87.1
  - pelvic O87.1
  - septic O86.81
  - superficial O87.0
- saphenous (greater) (lesser) I80.0-
- sinus (intracranial) G08
  - nonpyogenic I67.6
- soleal vein I80.25-
- specified site NEC I80.8
- tibial vein (anterior) (posterior) I80.23-

Thrombosis, thrombotic (bland) (multiple) (progressive) (silent) (vessel) I82.90
- anal K64.5
- antepartum — *see* Thrombophlebitis, antepartum
- aorta, aortic I74.10
  - abdominal I74.09
    - saddle I74.01
  - bifurcation I74.09
  - saddle I74.01
  - specified site NEC I74.19
  - terminal I74.09
  - thoracic I74.11
  - valve — *see* Endocarditis, aortic
- apoplexy I63.3-
- artery, arteries (postinfectional) I74.9
  - auditory, internal — *see* Occlusion, artery, precerebral, specified NEC
  - basilar — *see* Occlusion, artery, basilar
  - carotid (common) (internal) — *see* Occlusion, artery, carotid
  - cerebellar (anterior inferior) (posterior inferior) (superior) — *see* Occlusion, artery, cerebellar
  - cerebral — *see* Occlusion, artery, cerebral
  - choroidal (anterior) — *see* Occlusion, artery, precerebral, specified NEC
  - communicating, posterior — *see* Occlusion, artery, precerebral, specified NEC
  - coronary — *see also* Infarct, myocardium
    - not resulting in infarction I24.0
  - hepatic I74.8
  - hypophyseal — *see* Occlusion, artery, precerebral, specified NEC
  - iliac I74.5
  - limb I74.4
    - lower I74.3
    - upper I74.2
  - meningeal, anterior or posterior — *see* Occlusion, artery, cerebral, specified NEC
  - mesenteric (with gangrene) — *see also* Infarct, intestine K55.069
  - ophthalmic — *see* Occlusion, artery, retina
  - pontine — *see* Occlusion, artery, precerebral, specified NEC
  - precerebral — *see* Occlusion, artery, precerebral

Thrombosis, thrombotic (bland) (multiple) (progressive) (silent) (vessel) - *continued*
- artery, arteries (postinfectional) - *continued*
  - pulmonary (iatrogenic) — *see* Embolism, pulmonary
  - renal N28.0
  - retinal — *see* Occlusion, artery, retina
  - spinal, anterior or posterior G95.11
  - traumatic NEC T14.8
  - vertebral — *see* Occlusion, artery, vertebral
- atrium, auricular — *see also* Infarct, myocardium
  - following acute myocardial infarction (current complication) I23.6
  - not resulting in infarction I51.3
  - old I51.3
- basilar (artery) — *see* Occlusion, artery, basilar
- brain (artery) (stem) — *see also* Occlusion, artery, cerebral
  - due to syphilis A52.05
  - puerperal O99.43
  - sinus — *see* Thrombosis, intracranial venous sinus
- capillary I78.8
- cardiac — *see also* Infarct, myocardium
  - not resulting in infarction I51.3
  - old I51.3
  - valve — *see* Endocarditis
- carotid (artery) (common) (internal) — *see* Occlusion, artery, carotid
- cavernous (venous) sinus — *see* Thrombosis, intracranial venous sinus
- cerebellar artery (anterior inferior) (posterior inferior) (superior) I66.3
- cerebral (artery) — *see* Occlusion, artery, cerebral
- cerebrovenous sinus — *see also* Thrombosis, intracranial venous sinus
  - puerperium O87.3
- chronic I82.91
- coronary (artery) (vein) — *see also* Infarct, myocardium
  - not resulting in infarction I24.0
- corpus cavernosum N48.89
- cortical I66.9
- deep — *see* Embolism, vein, lower extremity
- due to device, implant or graft — *see also* Complications, by site and type, specified NEC T85.868
  - arterial graft NEC T82.868
  - breast (implant) T85.868
  - catheter NEC T85.868
    - dialysis (renal) T82.868
      - intraperitoneal T85.868
    - infusion NEC T82.868
      - spinal (epidural) (subdural) T85.860
    - urinary (indwelling) T83.86
  - electronic (electrode) (pulse generator) (stimulator)
    - bone T84.86
    - cardiac T82.867
    - nervous system (brain) (peripheral nerve) (spinal) T85.860
    - urinary T83.86
  - fixation, internal (orthopedic) NEC T84.86
  - gastrointestinal (bile duct) (esophagus) T85.868
  - genital NEC T83.86
  - heart T82.867
  - joint prosthesis T84.86
  - ocular (corneal graft) (orbital implant) NEC T85.868
  - orthopedic NEC T84.86
  - specified NEC T85.868
  - urinary NEC T83.86
  - vascular NEC T82.868
  - ventricular intracranial shunt T85.860
- during the puerperium — *see* Thrombosis, puerperal
- endocardial — *see also* Infarct, myocardium
  - not resulting in infarction I51.3
- eye — *see* Occlusion, retina
- genital organ

Thrombosis, thrombotic (bland) (multiple) (progressive) (silent) (vessel) - *continued*
- genital organ - *continued*
  - female NEC N94.89
    - pregnancy — *see* Thrombophlebitis, antepartum
  - male N50.1
- gestational — *see* Phlebopathy, gestational
- heart (chamber) — *see also* Infarct, myocardium
  - not resulting in infarction I51.3
  - old I51.3
- hepatic (vein) I82.0
  - artery I74.8
- history (of) Z86.718
- intestine (with gangrene) — *see also* Infarct, intestine K55.069
- intracardiac NEC (apical) (atrial) (auricular) (ventricular) (old) I51.3
- intracranial (arterial) I66.9
  - venous sinus (any) G08
    - nonpyogenic origin I67.6
    - puerperium O87.3
- intramural — *see also* Infarct, myocardium
  - not resulting in infarction I51.3
  - old I51.3
- intraspinal venous sinuses and veins G08
  - nonpyogenic G95.19
- kidney (artery) N28.0
- lateral (venous) sinus — *see* Thrombosis, intracranial venous sinus
- leg — *see* Thrombosis, vein, lower extremity
  - arterial I74.3
- liver (venous) I82.0
  - artery I74.8
  - portal vein I81
- longitudinal (venous) sinus — *see* Thrombosis, intracranial venous sinus
- lower limb — *see* Thrombosis, vein, lower extremity
- lung (iatrogenic) (postoperative) — *see* Embolism, pulmonary
- meninges (brain) (arterial) I66.8
- mesenteric (artery) (with gangrene) — *see also* Infarct, intestine K55.069
  - vein (inferior) (superior) K55.0-
- mitral I34.8
- mural — *see also* Infarct, myocardium
  - due to syphilis A52.06
  - not resulting in infarction I51.3
  - old I51.3
- omentum (with gangrene) — *see also* Infarct, intestine K55.069
- ophthalmic — *see* Occlusion, retina
- pampiniform plexus (male) N50.1
- parietal — *see also* Infarct, myocardium
  - not resulting in infarction I24.0
- penis, superficial vein N48.81
- perianal venous K64.5
- peripheral arteries I74.4
  - upper I74.2
- personal history (of) Z86.718
- portal I81
  - due to syphilis A52.09
- precerebral artery — *see* Occlusion, artery, precerebral
- puerperal, postpartum O87.0
  - brain (artery) O99.43
    - venous (sinus) O87.3
  - cardiac O99.43
  - cerebral (artery) O99.43
    - venous (sinus) O87.3
  - superficial O87.0
- pulmonary (artery) (iatrogenic) (postoperative) (vein) — *see* Embolism, pulmonary
- renal (artery) N28.0
  - vein I82.3
- resulting from presence of device, implant or graft — *see* Complications, by site and type, specified NEC
- retina, retinal — *see* Occlusion, retina
- scrotum N50.1
- seminal vesicle N50.1

Thrombosis, thrombotic (bland) (multiple) (progressive) (silent) (vessel) - *continued*
- sigmoid (venous) sinus — *see* Thrombosis, intracranial venous sinus
- sinus, intracranial (any) — *see* Thrombosis, intracranial venous sinus
- specified site NEC I82.890
  - chronic I82.891
- spermatic cord N50.1
- spinal cord (arterial) G95.11
  - due to syphilis A52.09
  - pyogenic origin G06.1
- spleen, splenic D73.5
  - artery I74.8
- testis N50.1
- tumor — *see* Neoplasm, unspecified behavior, by site
- traumatic NEC T14.8
- tricuspid I07.8
- tunica vaginalis N50.1
- umbilical cord (vessels), complicating delivery O69.5
- vas deferens N50.1
- vein (acute) I82.90
  - antecubital I82.61-
    - chronic I82.71-
  - axillary I82.A1-
    - chronic I82.A2-
  - basilic I82.61-
    - chronic I82.71-
  - brachial I82.62-
    - chronic I82.72-
  - brachiocephalic (innominate) I82.290
    - chronic I82.291
  - cerebral, nonpyogenic I67.6
  - cephalic I82.61-
    - chronic I82.71-
  - chronic I82.91
  - deep (DVT) I82.40-
    - calf I82.4Z-
      - chronic I82.5Z-
    - lower leg I82.4Z-
      - chronic I82.5Z-
    - thigh I82.4Y-
      - chronic I82.5Y-
    - upper leg I82.4Y-
      - chronic I82.5Y-
  - femoral I82.41-
    - chronic I82.51-
  - iliac (iliofemoral) I82.42-
    - chronic I82.52-
  - innominate I82.290
    - chronic I82.291
  - internal jugular I82.C1-
    - chronic I82.C2-
  - lower extremity
    - deep I82.40-
      - chronic I82.50-
      - specified NEC I82.49-
        - chronic NEC I82.59-
    - distal
      - deep I82.4Z-
    - proximal
      - deep I82.4Y-
        - chronic I82.5Y-
    - superficial I82.81-
  - perianal K64.5
  - popliteal I82.43-
    - chronic I82.53-
  - radial I82.62-
    - chronic I82.72-
  - renal I82.3
  - saphenous (greater) (lesser) I82.81-
  - specified NEC I82.890
    - chronic NEC I82.891
  - subclavian I82.B1-
    - chronic I82.B2-
  - thoracic NEC I82.290
    - chronic I82.291
  - tibial I82.44-
    - chronic I82.54-
  - ulnar I82.62-
    - chronic I82.72-
  - upper extremity I82.60-
    - chronic I82.70-

Thrombosis, thrombotic (bland) (multiple) (progressive) (silent) (vessel) - *continued*
- vein (acute) - *continued*
  - upper extremity - *continued*
    - deep I82.62-
      - chronic I82.72-
    - superficial I82.61-
      - chronic I82.71-
- vena cava
  - inferior I82.220
    - chronic I82.221
  - superior I82.210
    - chronic I82.211
- venous, perianal K64.5
- ventricle — *see also* Infarct, myocardium
  - following acute myocardial infarction (current complication) I23.6
  - not resulting in infarction I24.0
  - old I51.3

Thrombus — *see* Thrombosis

Thrush — *see also* Candidiasis
- oral B37.0
  - newborn P37.5
- vaginal B37.3

Thumb — *see also* condition
- sucking (child problem) F98.8

Thymitis E32.8

Thymoma — *see also* Neoplasm, thymus, by type
- malignant C37
- metaplastic C37
- microscopic D15.0
- sclerosing C37
- type A C37
- type AB C37
- type B1 C37
- type B2 C37
- type B3 C37

Thymus, thymic (gland) — *see* condition

Thyrocele — *see* Goiter

Thyroglossal — *see also* condition
- cyst Q89.2
- duct, persistent Q89.2

Thyroid (gland) (body) — *see also* condition
- hormone resistance E07.89
- lingual Q89.2
- nodule (cystic) (nontoxic) (single) E04.1

Thyroiditis E06.9
- acute (nonsuppurative) (pyogenic) (suppurative) E06.0
- autoimmune E06.3
- chronic (nonspecific) (sclerosing) E06.5
  - with thyrotoxicosis, transient E06.2
  - fibrous E06.5
  - lymphadenoid E06.3
  - lymphocytic E06.3
  - lymphoid E06.3
- de Quervain's E06.1
- drug-induced E06.4
- fibrous (chronic) E06.5
- giant-cell (follicular) E06.1
- granulomatous (de Quervain) (subacute) E06.1
- Hashimoto's (struma lymphomatosa) E06.3
- iatrogenic E06.4
- ligneous E06.5
- lymphocytic (chronic) E06.3
- lymphoid E06.3
- lymphomatous E06.3
- nonsuppurative E06.1
- postpartum, puerperal O90.5
- pseudotuberculous E06.1
- pyogenic E06.0
- radiation E06.4
- Riedel's E06.5
- subacute (granulomatous) E06.1
- suppurative E06.0
- tuberculous A18.81
- viral E06.1
- woody E06.5

Thyrolingual duct, persistent Q89.2

Thyromegaly E01.0

Thyrotoxic
- crisis — *see* Thyrotoxicosis

Thyrotoxic - *continued*
- heart disease or failure — *see also* Thyrotoxicosis E05.90 *[I43]*
  - with thyroid storm E05.91 *[I43]*
- storm — *see* Thyrotoxicosis

Thyrotoxicosis (recurrent) E05.90
- with
  - goiter (diffuse) E05.00
    - with thyroid storm E05.01
    - adenomatous uninodular E05.10
      - with thyroid storm E05.11
    - multinodular E05.20
      - with thyroid storm E05.21
    - nodular E05.20
      - with thyroid storm E05.21
    - uninodular E05.10
      - with thyroid storm E05.11
  - infiltrative
    - dermopathy E05.00
      - with thyroid storm E05.01
    - ophthalmopathy E05.00
      - with thyroid storm E05.01
  - single thyroid nodule E05.10
    - with thyroid storm E05.11
  - thyroid storm E05.91
- due to
  - ectopic thyroid nodule or tissue E05.30
    - with thyroid storm E05.31
  - ingestion of (excessive) thyroid material E05.40
    - with thyroid storm E05.41
  - overproduction of thyroid-stimulating hormone E05.80
    - with thyroid storm E05.81
  - specified cause NEC E05.80
    - with thyroid storm E05.81
- factitia E05.40
  - with thyroid storm E05.41
- heart — *see also* Failure, heart, high-output E05.90 *[I43]*
  - with thyroid storm — *see also* Failure, heart, high-output E05.91 *[I43]*
  - failure — *see also* Failure, heart, high-output E05.90 *[I43]*
- neonatal (transient) P72.1
- transient with chronic thyroiditis E06.2

Tibia vara M92.51-

Tic (disorder) F95.9
- breathing F95.8
- child problem F95.0
- compulsive F95.1
- de la Tourette F95.2
- degenerative (generalized) (localized) G25.69
  - facial G25.69
- disorder
  - chronic
    - motor F95.1
    - vocal F95.1
  - combined vocal and multiple motor F95.2
  - transient F95.0
- douloureux G50.0
  - atypical G50.1
  - postherpetic, postzoster B02.22
- drug-induced G25.61
- eyelid F95.8
- habit F95.9
  - chronic F95.1
  - transient of childhood F95.0
- lid, transient of childhood F95.0
- motor-verbal F95.2
- occupational F48.8
- orbicularis F95.8
  - transient of childhood F95.0
- organic origin G25.69
- provisional F95.0
- postchoreic G25.69
- psychogenic, compulsive F95.1
- salaam R25.8
- spasm (motor or vocal) F95.9
  - chronic F95.1
  - transient of childhood F95.0
- specified NEC F95.8

Tick-borne — *see* condition

Tietze's disease or syndrome M94.0

Tight, tightness
- anus K62.89
- chest R07.89
- fascia (lata) M62.89
- foreskin (congenital) N47.1
- hymen, hymenal ring N89.6
- introitus (acquired) (congenital) N89.6
- rectal sphincter K62.89
- tendon — *see* Short, tendon
- urethral sphincter N35.919

Tilting vertebra — *see* Dorsopathy, deforming, specified NEC

Timidity, child F93.8

Tinea (intersecta) (tarsi) B35.9
- amiantacea L44.8
- asbestina B35.0
- barbae B35.0
- beard B35.0
- black dot B35.0
- blanca B36.2
- capitis B35.0
- corporis B35.4
- cruris B35.6
- flava B36.0
- foot B35.3
- furfuracea B36.0
- imbricata (Tokelau) B35.5
- kerion B35.0
- manuum B35.2
- microsporic — *see* Dermatophytosis
- nigra B36.1
- nodosa — *see* Piedra
- pedis B35.3
- scalp B35.0
- specified NEC B35.8
- sycosis B35.0
- tonsurans B35.0
- trichophytic — *see* Dermatophytosis
- unguium B35.1
- versicolor B36.0

Tingling sensation (skin) R20.2

Tin-miner's lung J63.5

Tinnitus NOS H93.1-
- audible H93.1-
- aurium H93.1-
- pulsatile H93.A-
- subjective H93.1-

Tipped tooth (teeth) M26.33

Tipping
- pelvis M95.5
  - with disproportion (fetopelvic) O33.0
    - causing obstructed labor O65.0
- tooth (teeth) , fully erupted M26.33

Tiredness R53.83

Tissue — *see* condition

Tobacco (nicotine)
- abuse — *see* Tobacco, use
- dependence — *see* Dependence, drug, nicotine
- harmful use Z72.0
- heart — *see* Tobacco, toxic effect
- maternal use, affecting newborn P04.2
- toxic effect — *see* Table of Drugs and Chemicals, by substance, poisoning
  - chewing tobacco — *see* Table of Drugs and Chemicals, by substance, poisoning
  - cigarettes — *see* Table of Drugs and Chemicals, by substance, poisoning
- use Z72.0
  - complicating
    - childbirth O99.334
    - pregnancy O99.33-
    - puerperium O99.335
  - counseling and surveillance Z71.6
  - history Z87.891
- withdrawal state — *see also* Dependence, drug, nicotine F17.203

Tocopherol deficiency E56.0

Todd's
- cirrhosis K74.3
- paralysis (postepileptic) (transitory) G83.84

Toe — *see* condition

Toilet, artificial opening — *see* Attention to, artificial, opening

Tokelau (ringworm) B35.5

Tollwut — *see* Rabies

Tommaselli's disease R31.9
- correct substance properly administered — *see* Table of Drugs and Chemicals, by drug, adverse effect
- overdose or wrong substance given or taken — *see* Table of Drugs and Chemicals, by drug, poisoning

Tongue — *see also* condition
- tie Q38.1

Tonic pupil — *see* Anomaly, pupil, function, tonic pupil

Toni-Fanconi syndrome (cystinosis) E72.09
- with cystinosis E72.04

Tonsil — *see* condition

Tonsillitis (acute) (catarrhal) (croupous) (follicular) (gangrenous) (infective) (lacunar) (lingual) (malignant) (membranous) (parenchymatous) (phlegmonous) (pseudomembranous) (purulent) (septic) (subacute) (suppurative) (toxic) (ulcerative) (vesicular) (viral) J03.90
- chronic J35.01
  - with adenoiditis J35.03
- diphtheritic A36.0
- hypertrophic J35.01
  - with adenoiditis J35.03
- recurrent J03.91
- specified organism NEC J03.80
  - recurrent J03.81
- staphylococcal J03.80
  - recurrent J03.81
- streptococcal J03.00
  - recurrent J03.01
- tuberculous A15.8
- Vincent's A69.1

Tooth, teeth — *see* condition

Toothache K08.89

Topagnosis R20.8

Tophi — *see* Gout, chronic

TORCH infection — *see* Infection, congenital
- without active infection P00.2

Torn — *see* Tear

Tornwaldt's cyst or disease J39.2

Torsion
- accessory tube — *see* Torsion, fallopian tube
- adnexa (female) — *see* Torsion, fallopian tube
- aorta, acquired I77.1
- appendix epididymis N44.04
- appendix testis N44.03
- bile duct (common) (hepatic) K83.8
  - congenital Q44.5
- bowel, colon or intestine K56.2
- cervix — *see* Malposition, uterus
- cystic duct K82.8
- dystonia — *see* Dystonia, torsion
- epididymis (appendix) N44.04
- fallopian tube N83.52-
  - with ovary N83.53
- gallbladder K82.8
  - congenital Q44.1
- hydatid of Morgagni
  - female N83.52-
  - male N44.03
- kidney (pedicle) (leading to infarction) N28.0
- Meckel's diverticulum (congenital) Q43.0
  - malignant — *see* Table of Neoplasms, small intestine, malignant
- mesentery K56.2
- omentum K56.2
- organ or site, congenital NEC — *see* Anomaly, by site
- ovary (pedicle) N83.51-
  - with fallopian tube N83.53
  - congenital Q50.2
- oviduct — *see* Torsion, fallopian tube
- penis (acquired) N48.82
  - congenital Q55.63
- spasm — *see* Dystonia, torsion
- spermatic cord N44.02
  - extravaginal N44.01
  - intravaginal N44.02

Torsion - *continued*
- spleen D73.5
- testis, testicle N44.00
  - appendix N44.03
- tibia — *see* Deformity, limb, specified type NEC, lower leg
- uterus — *see* Malposition, uterus

Torticollis (intermittent) (spastic) M43.6
- congenital (sternomastoid) Q68.0
- due to birth injury P15.8
- hysterical F44.4
- ocular R29.891
- psychogenic F45.8
  - conversion reaction F44.4
- rheumatic M43.6
- rheumatoid M06.88
- spasmodic G24.3
- traumatic, current S13.4

Tortipelvis G24.1

Tortuous
- aortic arch Q25.46
- artery I77.1
- organ or site, congenital NEC — *see* Distortion
- retinal vessel, congenital Q14.1
- ureter N13.8
- urethra N36.8
- vein — *see* Varix

Torture, victim of Z65.4

Torula, torular (histolytica) (infection) — *see* Cryptococcosis

Torulosis — *see* Cryptococcosis

Torus (mandibularis) (palatinus) M27.0
- fracture — *see* Fracture, by site, torus

Touraine's syndrome Q79.8

Tourette's syndrome F95.2

Tourniquet syndrome — *see* Constriction, external, by site

Tower skull Q75.0
- with exophthalmos Q87.0

Toxemia R68.89
- bacterial — *see* Sepsis
- burn — *see* Burn
- eclamptic (with pre-existing hypertension) — *see* Eclampsia
- erysipelatous — *see* Erysipelas
- fatigue R68.89
- food — *see* Poisoning, food
- gastrointestinal K52.1
- intestinal K52.1
- kidney — *see* Uremia
- malarial — *see* Malaria
- myocardial — *see* Myocarditis, toxic
- of pregnancy — *see* Pre-eclampsia
- pre-eclamptic — *see* Pre-eclampsia
- small intestine K52.1
- staphylococcal, due to food A05.0
- stasis R68.89
- uremic — *see* Uremia
- urinary — *see* Uremia

Toxemica cerebropathia psychica (nonalcoholic) F04
- alcoholic — *see* Alcohol, amnestic disorder

Toxic (poisoning) — *see also* condition T65.91
- effect — *see* Table of Drugs and Chemicals, by substance, poisoning
- shock syndrome A48.3
- thyroid (gland) — *see* Thyrotoxicosis

Toxicemia — *see* Toxemia

Toxicity — *see* Table of Drugs and Chemicals, by substance, poisoning
- fava bean D55.0
- food, noxious — *see* Poisoning, food
- from drug or nonmedicinal substance — *see* Table of Drugs and Chemicals, by drug

Toxicosis — *see also* Toxemia
- capillary, hemorrhagic D69.0

Toxinfection, gastrointestinal K52.1

Toxocariasis B83.0

Toxoplasma, toxoplasmosis (acquired) B58.9
- with
  - hepatitis B58.1
  - meningoencephalitis B58.2
  - ocular involvement B58.00
  - other organ involvement B58.89

Toxoplasma, toxoplasmosis (acquired) - *continued*
with - *continued*
pneumonia, pneumonitis B58.3
congenital (acute) (subacute) (chronic) P37.1
maternal, manifest toxoplasmosis in infant (acute) (subacute) (chronic) P37.1
tPA (rtPA) administation in a different facility within the last 24 hours prior to admission to current facility Z92.82
Trabeculation, bladder N32.89
Trachea — *see* condition
Tracheitis (catarrhal) (infantile) (membranous) (plastic) (septal) (suppurative) (viral) J04.10
with
bronchitis (15 years of age and above) J40
acute or subacute — *see* Bronchitis, acute
chronic J42
tuberculous NEC A15.5
under 15 years of age J20.9
laryngitis (acute) J04.2
chronic J37.1
tuberculous NEC A15.5
acute J04.10
with obstruction J04.11
chronic J42
with
bronchitis (chronic) J42
laryngitis (chronic) J37.1
diphtheritic (membranous) A36.89
due to external agent — *see* Inflammation, respiratory, upper, due to
syphilitic A52.73
tuberculous A15.5
Trachelitis (nonvenereal) — *see* Cervicitis
Tracheobronchial — *see* condition
Tracheobronchitis (15 years of age and above) — *see also* Bronchitis
due to
Bordetella bronchiseptica A37.80
with pneumonia A37.81
Francisella tularensis A21.8
Tracheobronchomegaly Q32.4
with bronchiectasis J47.9
with
exacerbation (acute) J47.1
lower respiratory infection J47.0
acquired J98.09
with bronchiectasis J47.9
with
exacerbation (acute) J47.1
lower respiratory infection J47.0
Tracheobronchopneumonitis — *see* Pneumonia, broncho-
Tracheocele (external) (internal) J39.8
congenital Q32.1
Tracheomalacia J39.8
congenital Q32.0
Tracheopharyngitis (acute) J06.9
chronic J42
due to external agent — *see* Inflammation, respiratory, upper, due to
Tracheostenosis J39.8
Tracheostomy
complication — *see* Complication, tracheostomy
status Z93.0
attention to Z43.0
malfunctioning J95.03
Trachoma, trachomatous A71.9
active (stage) A71.1
contraction of conjunctiva A71.1
dubium A71.0
initial (stage) A71.0
healed or sequelae B94.0
pannus A71.1
Türck's J37.0
Traction, vitreomacular H43.82-
Train sickness T75.3
Trait (s)
Hb-S D57.3
hemoglobin
abnormal NEC D58.2

Trait (s) - *continued*
hemoglobin - *continued*
abnormal NEC - *continued*
with thalassemia D56.3
C — *see* Disease, hemoglobin C
S (Hb-S) D57.3
Lepore D56.3
personality, accentuated Z73.1
sickle-cell D57.3
with elliptocytosis or spherocytosis D57.3
type A personality Z73.1
Tramp Z59.00
Trance R41.89
hysterical F44.89
Transaminasemia R74.01
Transection
abdomen (partial) S38.3
aorta (incomplete) — *see also* Injury, aorta
complete — *see* Injury, aorta, laceration, major
carotid artery (incomplete) — *see also* Injury, blood vessel, carotid, laceration
complete — *see* Injury, blood vessel, carotid, laceration, major
celiac artery (incomplete) S35.211
branch (incomplete) S35.291
complete S35.292
complete S35.212
innominate
artery (incomplete) — *see also* Injury, blood vessel, thoracic, innominate, artery, laceration
complete — *see* Injury, blood vessel, thoracic, innominate, artery, laceration, major
vein (incomplete) — *see also* Injury, blood vessel, thoracic, innominate, vein, laceration
complete — *see* Injury, blood vessel, thoracic, innominate, vein, laceration, major
jugular vein (external) (incomplete) — *see also* Injury, blood vessel, jugular vein, laceration
complete — *see* Injury, blood vessel, jugular vein, laceration, major
internal (incomplete) — *see also* Injury, blood vessel, jugular vein, internal, laceration
complete — *see* Injury, blood vessel, jugular vein, internal, laceration, major
mesenteric artery (incomplete) — *see also* Injury, mesenteric, artery, laceration
complete — *see* Injury, mesenteric artery, laceration, major
pulmonary vessel (incomplete) — *see also* Injury, blood vessel, thoracic, pulmonary, laceration
complete — *see* Injury, blood vessel, thoracic, pulmonary, laceration, major
subclavian — *see* Transection, innominate
vena cava (incomplete) — *see also* Injury, vena cava
complete — *see* Injury, vena cava, laceration, major
vertebral artery (incomplete) — *see also* Injury, blood vessel, vertebral, laceration
complete — *see* Injury, blood vessel, vertebral, laceration, major
Transfusion
associated (red blood cell) hemochromatosis E83.111
blood
ABO incompatible — *see* Complication(s), transfusion, incompatibility reaction, ABO
minor blood group (Duffy) (E) (K) (Kell) (Kidd) (Lewis) (M) (N) (P) (S) T80.89
reaction or complication — *see* Complications, transfusion

Transfusion - *continued*
fetomaternal (mother) — *see* Pregnancy, complicated by, placenta, transfusion syndrome
maternofetal (mother) — *see* Pregnancy, complicated by, placenta, transfusion syndrome
placental (syndrome) (mother) — *see* Pregnancy, complicated by, placenta, transfusion syndrome
reaction (adverse) — *see* Complications, transfusion
related acute lung injury (TRALI) J95.84
twin-to-twin — *see* Pregnancy, complicated by, placenta, transfusion syndrome, fetus to fetus
Transient (meaning homeless) — *see also* condition Z59.00
Translocation
balanced autosomal Q95.9
in normal individual Q95.0
chromosomes NEC Q99.8
balanced and insertion in normal individual Q95.0
Down syndrome Q90.2
trisomy
13 Q91.6
18 Q91.2
21 Q90.2
Translucency, iris — *see* Degeneration, iris
Transmission of chemical substances through the placenta — *see* Absorption, chemical, through placenta
Transparency, lung, unilateral J43.0
Transplant (ed) (status) Z94.9
awaiting organ Z76.82
bone Z94.6
marrow Z94.81
candidate Z76.82
complication — *see* Complication, transplant
cornea Z94.7
heart Z94.1
and lung (s) Z94.3
valve Z95.2
prosthetic Z95.2
specified NEC Z95.4
xenogenic Z95.3
intestine Z94.82
kidney Z94.0
liver Z94.4
lung (s) Z94.2
and heart Z94.3
organ (failure) (infection) (rejection) Z94.9
removal status Z98.85
pancreas Z94.83
skin Z94.5
social Z60.3
specified organ or tissue NEC Z94.89
stem cells Z94.84
tissue Z94.9
Transplants, ovarian, endometrial N80.1
Transposed — *see* Transposition
Transposition (congenital) — *see also* Malposition, congenital
abdominal viscera Q89.3
aorta (dextra) Q20.3
appendix Q43.8
colon Q43.8
corrected Q20.5
great vessels (complete) (partial) Q20.3
heart Q24.0
with complete transposition of viscera Q89.3
intestine (large) (small) Q43.8
reversed jejunal (for bypass) (status) Z98.0
scrotum Q55.23
stomach Q40.2
with general transposition of viscera Q89.3
tooth, teeth, fully erupted M26.30
vessels, great (complete) (partial) Q20.3
viscera (abdominal) (thoracic) Q89.3
Transsexualism F64.0
Transverse — *see also* condition
arrest (deep) , in labor O64.0
lie (mother) O32.2

- **Transverse** - *continued*
  - lie (mother) - *continued*
    - causing obstructed labor O64.8
- **Transvestism, transvestitism (dual-role)** F64.1
  - fetishistic F65.1
- **Trapped placenta (with hemorrhage)** O72.0
  - without hemorrhage O73.0
- **TRAPS (tumor necrosis factor receptor associated periodic syndrome)** M04.1
- **Trauma, traumatism** — *see also* Injury
  - acoustic — *see* subcategory H83.3
  - birth — *see* Birth, injury
  - complicating ectopic or molar pregnancy O08.6
  - during delivery O71.9
  - following ectopic or molar pregnancy O08.6
  - obstetric O71.9
    - specified NEC O71.89
  - occlusal
    - primary K08.81
    - secondary K08.82
- **Traumatic** — *see also* condition
  - brain injury S06.9
- **Treacher Collins syndrome** Q75.4
- **Treitz's hernia** — *see* Hernia, abdomen, specified site NEC
- **Trematode infestation** — *see* Infestation, fluke
- **Trematodiasis** — *see* Infestation, fluke
- **Trembling paralysis** — *see* Parkinsonism
- **Tremor (s)** R25.1
  - drug induced G25.1
  - essential (benign) G25.0
  - familial G25.0
  - hereditary G25.0
  - hysterical F44.4
  - intention G25.2
  - medication induced postural G25.1
  - mercurial — *see* subcategory T56.1
  - Parkinson's — *see* Parkinsonism
  - psychogenic (conversion reaction) F44.4
  - senilis R54
  - specified type NEC G25.2
- **Trench**
  - fever A79.0
  - foot — *see* Immersion, foot
  - mouth A69.1
- **Treponema pallidum infection** — *see* Syphilis
- **Treponematosis**
  - due to
    - T. pallidum — *see* Syphilis
    - T. pertenue — *see* Yaws
- **Triad**
  - Hutchinson's (congenital syphilis) A50.53
  - Kartagener's Q89.3
  - Saint's — *see* Hernia, diaphragm
- **Trichiasis (eyelid)** H02.059
  - with entropion — *see* Entropion
  - left H02.056
    - lower H02.055
    - upper H02.054
  - right H02.053
    - lower H02.052
    - upper H02.051
- **Trichinella spiralis (infection) (infestation)** B75
- **Trichinellosis, trichiniasis, trichinelliasis, trichinosis** B75
  - with muscle disorder B75 *[M63.80]*
    - ankle B75 *[M63.87-]*
    - foot B75 *[M63.87-]*
    - forearm B75 *[M63.83-]*
    - hand B75 *[M63.84-]*
    - lower leg B75 *[M63.86-]*
    - multiple sites B75 *[M63.89]*
    - pelvic region B75 *[M63.85-]*
    - shoulder region B75 *[M63.81-]*
    - specified site NEC B75 *[M63.88]*
    - thigh B75 *[M63.85-]*
    - upper arm B75 *[M63.82-]*
- **Trichobezoar** T18.9
  - intestine T18.3
  - stomach T18.2
- **Trichocephaliasis, trichocephalosis** B79
- **Trichocephalus infestation** B79
- **Trichoclasis** L67.8
- **Trichoepithelioma** — *see also* Neoplasm, skin, benign
  - malignant — *see* Neoplasm, skin, malignant
- **Trichofolliculoma** — *see* Neoplasm, skin, benign
- **Tricholemmoma** — *see* Neoplasm, skin, benign
- **Trichomoniasis** A59.9
  - bladder A59.03
  - cervix A59.09
  - intestinal A07.8
  - prostate A59.02
  - seminal vesicles A59.09
  - specified site NEC A59.8
  - urethra A59.03
  - urogenitalis A59.00
  - vagina A59.01
  - vulva A59.01
- **Trichomycosis**
  - axillaris A48.8
  - nodosa, nodularis B36.8
- **Trichonodosis** L67.8
- **Trichophytid, trichophyton infection** — *see* Dermatophytosis
- **Trichophytobezoar** T18.9
  - intestine T18.3
  - stomach T18.2
- **Trichophytosis** — *see* Dermatophytosis
- **Trichoptilosis** L67.8
- **Trichorrhexis (nodosa) (invaginata)** L67.0
- **Trichosis axillaris** A48.8
- **Trichosporosis nodosa** B36.2
- **Trichostasis spinulosa (congenital)** Q84.1
- **Trichostrongyliasis, trichostrongylosis (small intestine)** B81.2
- **Trichostrongylus infection** B81.2
- **Trichotillomania** F63.3
- **Trichromat, trichromatopsia, anomalous (congenital)** H53.55
- **Trichuriasis** B79
- **Trichuris trichiura (infection) (infestation) (any site)** B79
- **Tricuspid (valve)** — *see* condition
- **Trifid** — *see also* Accessory
  - kidney (pelvis) Q63.8
  - tongue Q38.3
- **Trigeminal neuralgia** — *see* Neuralgia, trigeminal
- **Trigeminy** R00.8
- **Trigger finger (acquired)** M65.30
  - congenital Q74.0
  - index finger M65.32-
  - little finger M65.35-
  - middle finger M65.33-
  - ring finger M65.34-
  - thumb M65.31-
- **Trigonitis (bladder) (chronic) (pseudomembranous)** N30.30
  - with hematuria N30.31
- **Trigonocephaly** Q75.0
- **Trilocular heart** — *see* Cor triloculare
- **Trimethylaminuria** E72.52
- **Tripartite placenta** O43.19-
- **Triphalangeal thumb** Q74.0
- **Triple** — *see also* Accessory
  - kidneys Q63.0
  - uteri Q51.818
  - X, female Q97.0
- **Triple I** O41.12-
- **Triplegia** G83.89
  - congenital G80.8
- **Triplet (newborn)** — *see also* Newborn, triplet
  - complicating pregnancy — *see* Pregnancy, triplet
- **Triplication** — *see* Accessory
- **Triploidy** Q92.7
- **Trismus** R25.2
  - neonatorum A33
  - newborn A33
- **Trisomy (syndrome)** Q92.9
  - autosomes Q92.9
  - chromosome specified NEC Q92.8
- **Trisomy (syndrome)** - *continued*
  - chromosome specified NEC - *continued*
    - partial Q92.2
      - due to unbalanced translocation Q92.5
    - whole (nonsex chromosome)
      - meiotic nondisjunction Q92.0
      - mitotic nondisjunction Q92.1
      - mosaicism Q92.1
    - specified NEC Q92.8
  - due to
    - dicentrics — *see* Extra, marker chromosomes
    - extra rings — *see* Extra, marker chromosomes
    - isochromosomes — *see* Extra, marker chromosomes
  - specified NEC Q92.8
  - whole chromosome Q92.9
    - meiotic nondisjunction Q92.0
    - mitotic nondisjunction Q92.1
    - mosaicism Q92.1
    - partial Q92.9
    - specified NEC Q92.8
  - 13 (partial) Q91.7
    - meiotic nondisjunction Q91.4
    - mitotic nondisjunction Q91.5
    - mosaicism Q91.5
    - translocation Q91.6
  - 18 (partial) Q91.3
    - meiotic nondisjunction Q91.0
    - mitotic nondisjunction Q91.1
    - mosaicism Q91.1
    - translocation Q91.2
  - 20 Q92.8
  - 21 (partial) Q90.9
    - meiotic nondisjunction Q90.0
    - mitotic nondisjunction Q90.1
    - mosaicism Q90.1
    - translocation Q90.2
  - 22 Q92.8
- **Tritanomaly, tritanopia** H53.55
- **Trombiculosis, trombiculiasis, trombidiosis** B88.0
- **Trophedema (congenital) (hereditary)** Q82.0
- **Trophoblastic disease** — *see also* Mole, hydatidiform O01.9
- **Tropholymphedema** Q82.0
- **Trophoneurosis NEC** G96.89
  - disseminated M34.9
- **Tropical** — *see* condition
- **Trouble** — *see also* Disease
  - heart — *see* Disease, heart
  - kidney — *see* Disease, renal
  - nervous R45.0
  - sinus — *see* Sinusitis
- **Trousseau's syndrome (thrombophlebitis migrans)** I82.1
- **Truancy, childhood**
  - from school Z72.810
- **Truncus**
  - arteriosus (persistent) Q20.0
  - communis Q20.0
- **Trunk** — *see* condition
- **Trypanosomiasis**
  - African B56.9
    - by Trypanosoma brucei
      - gambiense B56.0
      - rhodesiense B56.1
  - American — *see* Chagas' disease
  - Brazilian — *see* Chagas' disease
  - by Trypanosoma
    - brucei gambiense B56.0
    - brucei rhodesiense B56.1
    - cruzi — *see* Chagas' disease
  - gambiensis, Gambian B56.0
  - rhodesiensis, Rhodesian B56.1
  - South American — *see* Chagas' disease
  - where
    - African trypanosomiasis is prevalent B56.9
    - Chagas' disease is prevalent B57.2
- **Tryptasemia, hereditary alpha** D89.44
- **T-shaped incisors** K00.2
- **Tsutsugamushi (disease) (fever)** A75.3
- **Tube, tubal, tubular** — *see* condition

Tubercle — *see also* Tuberculosis
  brain, solitary A17.81
  Darwin's Q17.8
  Ghon, primary infection A15.7
Tuberculid, tuberculide (indurating, subcutaneous) (lichenoid) (miliary) (papulonecrotic) (primary) (skin) A18.4
Tuberculoma — *see also* Tuberculosis
  brain A17.81
  meninges (cerebral) (spinal) A17.1
  spinal cord A17.81
Tuberculosis, tubercular, tuberculous (calcification) (calcified) (caseous) (chromogenic acid-fast bacilli) (degeneration) (fibrocaseous) (fistula) (interstitial) (isolated circumscribed lesions) (necrosis) (parenchymatous) (ulcerative) A15.9
  with pneumoconiosis (any condition in J60-J64) J65
  abdomen (lymph gland) A18.39
  abscess (respiratory) A15.9
    bone A18.03
      hip A18.02
      knee A18.02
      sacrum A18.01
      specified site NEC A18.03
      spinal A18.01
      vertebra A18.01
    brain A17.81
    breast A18.89
    Cowper's gland A18.15
    dura (mater) (cerebral) (spinal) A17.81
    epidural (cerebral) (spinal) A17.81
    female pelvis A18.17
    frontal sinus A15.8
    genital organs NEC A18.10
    genitourinary A18.10
    gland (lymphatic) — *see* Tuberculosis, lymph gland
    hip A18.02
    intestine A18.32
    ischiorectal A18.32
    joint NEC A18.02
      hip A18.02
      knee A18.02
      specified NEC A18.02
      vertebral A18.01
    kidney A18.11
    knee A18.02
    latent Z22.7
    lumbar (spine) A18.01
    lung — *see* Tuberculosis, pulmonary
    meninges (cerebral) (spinal) A17.0
    muscle A18.09
    perianal (fistula) A18.32
    perinephritic A18.11
    perirectal A18.32
    rectum A18.32
    retropharyngeal A15.8
    sacrum A18.01
    scrofulous A18.2
    scrotum A18.15
    skin (primary) A18.4
    spinal cord A17.81
    spine or vertebra (column) A18.01
    subdiaphragmatic A18.31
    testis A18.15
    urinary A18.13
    uterus A18.17
  accessory sinus — *see* Tuberculosis, sinus
  Addison's disease A18.7
  adenitis — *see* Tuberculosis, lymph gland
  adenoids A15.8
  adenopathy — *see* Tuberculosis, lymph gland
  adherent pericardium A18.84
  adnexa (uteri) A18.17
  adrenal (capsule) (gland) A18.7
  alimentary canal A18.32
  anemia A18.89
  ankle (joint) (bone) A18.02
  anus A18.32
  apex, apical — *see* Tuberculosis, pulmonary
  appendicitis, appendix A18.32

Tuberculosis, tubercular, tuberculous (calcification) (calcified) (caseous) (chromogenic acid-fast bacilli) (degeneration) (fibrocaseous) (fistula) (interstitial) (isolated circumscribed lesions) (necrosis) (parenchymatous) (ulcerative) - *continued*
  arachnoid A17.0
  artery, arteritis A18.89
    cerebral A18.89
  arthritis (chronic) (synovial) A18.02
    spine or vertebra (column) A18.01
  articular — *see* Tuberculosis, joint
  ascites A18.31
  asthma — *see* Tuberculosis, pulmonary
  axilla, axillary (gland) A18.2
  bladder A18.12
  bone A18.03
    hip A18.02
    knee A18.02
    limb NEC A18.03
    sacrum A18.01
    spine or vertebral column A18.01
  bowel (miliary) A18.32
  brain A17.81
  breast A18.89
  broad ligament A18.17
  bronchi, bronchial, bronchus A15.5
    ectasia, ectasis (bronchiectasis) — *see* Tuberculosis, pulmonary
    fistula A15.5
      primary (progressive) A15.7
    gland or node A15.4
      primary (progressive) A15.7
    lymph gland or node A15.4
      primary (progressive) A15.7
  bronchiectasis — *see* Tuberculosis, pulmonary
  bronchitis A15.5
  bronchopleural A15.6
  bronchopneumonia, bronchopneumonic — *see* Tuberculosis, pulmonary
  bronchorrhagia A15.5
  bronchotracheal A15.5
  bronze disease A18.7
  buccal cavity A18.83
  bulbourethral gland A18.15
  bursa A18.09
  cachexia A15.9
  cardiomyopathy A18.84
  caries — *see* Tuberculosis, bone
  cartilage A18.02
    intervertebral A18.01
  catarrhal — *see* Tuberculosis, respiratory
  cecum A18.32
  cellulitis (primary) A18.4
  cerebellum A17.81
  cerebral, cerebrum A17.81
  cerebrospinal A17.81
    meninges A17.0
  cervical (lymph gland or node) A18.2
  cervicitis, cervix (uteri) A18.16
  chest — *see* Tuberculosis, respiratory
  chorioretinitis A18.53
  choroid, choroiditis A18.53
  ciliary body A18.54
  colitis A18.32
  collier's J65
  colliquativa (primary) A18.4
  colon A18.32
  complex, primary A15.7
  congenital P37.0
  conjunctiva A18.59
  connective tissue (systemic) A18.89
  contact Z20.1
  cornea (ulcer) A18.52
  Cowper's gland A18.15
  coxae A18.02
  coxalgia A18.02
  cul-de-sac of Douglas A18.17
  curvature, spine A18.01
  cutis (colliquativa) (primary) A18.4
  cyst, ovary A18.18
  cystitis A18.12
  dactylitis A18.03

Tuberculosis, tubercular, tuberculous (calcification) (calcified) (caseous) (chromogenic acid-fast bacilli) (degeneration) (fibrocaseous) (fistula) (interstitial) (isolated circumscribed lesions) (necrosis) (parenchymatous) (ulcerative) - *continued*
  diarrhea A18.32
  diffuse — *see* Tuberculosis, miliary
  digestive tract A18.32
  disseminated — *see* Tuberculosis, miliary
  duodenum A18.32
  dura (mater) (cerebral) (spinal) A17.0
    abscess (cerebral) (spinal) A17.81
  dysentery A18.32
  ear (inner) (middle) A18.6
    bone A18.03
    external (primary) A18.4
    skin (primary) A18.4
  elbow A18.02
  emphysema — *see* Tuberculosis, pulmonary
  empyema A15.6
  encephalitis A17.82
  endarteritis A18.89
  endocarditis A18.84
    aortic A18.84
    mitral A18.84
    pulmonary A18.84
    tricuspid A18.84
  endocrine glands NEC A18.82
  endometrium A18.17
  enteric, enterica, enteritis A18.32
  enterocolitis A18.32
  epididymis, epididymitis A18.15
  epidural abscess (cerebral) (spinal) A17.81
  epiglottis A15.5
  episcleritis A18.51
  erythema (induratum) (nodosum) (primary) A18.4
  esophagus A18.83
  eustachian tube A18.6
  exposure (to) Z20.1
  exudative — *see* Tuberculosis, pulmonary
  eye A18.50
  eyelid (primary) (lupus) A18.4
  fallopian tube (acute) (chronic) A18.17
  fascia A18.09
  fauces A15.8
  female pelvic inflammatory disease A18.17
  finger A18.03
  first infection A15.7
  gallbladder A18.83
  ganglion A18.09
  gastritis A18.83
  gastrocolic fistula A18.32
  gastroenteritis A18.32
  gastrointestinal tract A18.32
  general, generalized — *see* Tuberculosis, miliary
  genital organs A18.10
  genitourinary A18.10
  genu A18.02
  glandula suprarenalis A18.7
  glandular, general A18.2
  glottis A15.5
  grinder's J65
  gum A18.83
  hand A18.03
  heart A18.84
  hematogenous — *see* Tuberculosis, miliary
  hemoptysis — *see* Tuberculosis, pulmonary
  hemorrhage NEC — *see* Tuberculosis, pulmonary
  hemothorax A15.6
  hepatitis A18.83
  hilar lymph nodes A15.4
    primary (progressive) A15.7
  hip (joint) (disease) (bone) A18.02
  hydropneumothorax A15.6
  hydrothorax A15.6
  hypoadrenalism A18.7
  hypopharynx A15.8
  ileocecal (hyperplastic) A18.32
  ileocolitis A18.32
  ileum A18.32

Tuberculosis, tubercular, tuberculous (calcification) (calcified) (caseous) (chromogenic acid-fast bacilli) (degeneration) (fibrocaseous) (fistula) (interstitial) (isolated circumscribed lesions) (necrosis) (parenchymatous) (ulcerative) - *continued*

- iliac spine (superior) A18.03
- immunological findings only A15.7
- indurativa (primary) A18.4
- infantile A15.7
- infection A15.9
  - without clinical manifestations A15.7
- infraclavicular gland A18.2
- inguinal gland A18.2
- inguinalis A18.2
- intestine (any part) A18.32
- iridocyclitis A18.54
- iris, iritis A18.54
- ischiorectal A18.32
- jaw A18.03
- jejunum A18.32
- joint A18.02
  - vertebral A18.01
- keratitis (interstitial) A18.52
- keratoconjunctivitis A18.52
- kidney A18.11
- knee (joint) A18.02
- kyphosis, kyphoscoliosis A18.01
- laryngitis A15.5
- larynx A15.5
- latent Z22.7
- leptomeninges, leptomeningitis (cerebral) (spinal) A17.0
- lichenoides (primary) A18.4
- linguae A18.83
- lip A18.83
- liver A18.83
- lordosis A18.01
- lung — *see* Tuberculosis, pulmonary
- lupus vulgaris A18.4
- lymph gland or node (peripheral) A18.2
  - abdomen A18.39
  - bronchial A15.4
    - primary (progressive) A15.7
  - cervical A18.2
  - hilar A15.4
    - primary (progressive) A15.7
  - intrathoracic A15.4
    - primary (progressive) A15.7
  - mediastinal A15.4
    - primary (progressive) A15.7
  - mesenteric A18.39
  - retroperitoneal A18.39
  - tracheobronchial A15.4
    - primary (progressive) A15.7
- lymphadenitis — *see* Tuberculosis, lymph gland
- lymphangitis — *see* Tuberculosis, lymph gland
- lymphatic (gland) (vessel) — *see* Tuberculosis, lymph gland
- mammary gland A18.89
- marasmus A15.9
- mastoiditis A18.03
- mediastinal lymph gland or node A15.4
  - primary (progressive) A15.7
- mediastinitis A15.8
  - primary (progressive) A15.7
- mediastinum A15.8
  - primary (progressive) A15.7
- medulla A17.81
- melanosis, Addisonian A18.7
- meninges, meningitis (basilar) (cerebral) (cerebrospinal) (spinal) A17.0
- meningoencephalitis A17.82
- mesentery, mesenteric (gland or node) A18.39
- miliary A19.9
  - acute A19.2
    - multiple sites A19.1
    - single specified site A19.0
  - chronic A19.8
  - specified NEC A19.8
- millstone makers' J65
- miner's J65
- molder's J65
- mouth A18.83
- multiple A19.9
  - acute A19.1
  - chronic A19.8
- muscle A18.09
- myelitis A17.82
- myocardium, myocarditis A18.84
- nasal (passage) (sinus) A15.8
- nasopharynx A15.8
- neck gland A18.2
- nephritis A18.11
- nerve (mononeuropathy) A17.83
- nervous system A17.9
- nose (septum) A15.8
- ocular A18.50
- omentum A18.31
- oophoritis (acute) (chronic) A18.17
- optic (nerve trunk) (papilla) A18.59
- orbit A18.59
- orchitis A18.15
- organ, specified NEC A18.89
- osseous — *see* Tuberculosis, bone
- osteitis — *see* Tuberculosis, bone
- osteomyelitis — *see* Tuberculosis, bone
- otitis media A18.6
- ovary, ovaritis (acute) (chronic) A18.17
- oviduct (acute) (chronic) A18.17
- pachymeningitis A17.0
- palate (soft) A18.83
- pancreas A18.83
- papulonecrotic (a) (primary) A18.4
- parathyroid glands A18.82
- paronychia (primary) A18.4
- parotid gland or region A18.83
- pelvis (bony) A18.03
- penis A18.15
- peribronchitis A15.5
- pericardium, pericarditis A18.84
- perichondritis, larynx A15.5
- periostitis — *see* Tuberculosis, bone
- perirectal fistula A18.32
- peritoneum NEC A18.31
- peritonitis A18.31
- pharynx, pharyngitis A15.8
- phlyctenulosis (keratoconjunctivitis) A18.52
- phthisis NEC — *see* Tuberculosis, pulmonary
- pituitary gland A18.82
- pleura, pleural, pleurisy, pleuritis (fibrinous) (obliterative) (purulent) (simple plastic) (with effusion) A15.6
  - primary (progressive) A15.7
- pneumonia, pneumonic — *see* Tuberculosis, pulmonary
- pneumothorax (spontaneous) (tense valvular) — *see* Tuberculosis, pulmonary
- polyneuropathy A17.89
- polyserositis A19.9
  - acute A19.1
  - chronic A19.8
- potter's J65
- prepuce A18.15
- primary (complex) A15.7
- proctitis A18.32
- prostate, prostatitis A18.14
- pulmonalis — *see* Tuberculosis, pulmonary
- pulmonary (cavitated) (fibrotic) (infiltrative) (nodular) A15.0
  - childhood type or first infection A15.7
  - primary (complex) A15.7
- pyelitis A18.11
- pyelonephritis A18.11
- pyemia — *see* Tuberculosis, miliary
- pyonephrosis A18.11
- pyopneumothorax A15.6
- pyothorax A15.6
- rectum (fistula) (with abscess) A18.32
- reinfection stage — *see* Tuberculosis, pulmonary
- renal A18.11
- renis A18.11
- respiratory A15.9
  - primary A15.7
  - specified site NEC A15.8
- retina, retinitis A18.53
- retroperitoneal (lymph gland or node) A18.39
- rheumatism NEC A18.09
- rhinitis A15.8
- sacroiliac (joint) A18.01
- sacrum A18.01
- salivary gland A18.83
- salpingitis (acute) (chronic) A18.17
- sandblaster's J65
- sclera A18.51
- scoliosis A18.01
- scrofulous A18.2
- scrotum A18.15
- seminal tract or vesicle A18.15
- senile A15.9
- septic — *see* Tuberculosis, miliary
- shoulder (joint) A18.02
  - blade A18.03
- sigmoid A18.32
- sinus (any nasal) A15.8
  - bone A18.03
  - epididymis A18.15
- skeletal NEC A18.03
- skin (any site) (primary) A18.4
- small intestine A18.32
- soft palate A18.83
- spermatic cord A18.15
- spine, spinal (column) A18.01
  - cord A17.81
  - medulla A17.81
  - membrane A17.0
  - meninges A17.0
- spleen, splenitis A18.85
- spondylitis A18.01
- sternoclavicular joint A18.02
- stomach A18.83
- stonemason's J65
- subcutaneous tissue (cellular) (primary) A18.4
- subcutis (primary) A18.4
- subdeltoid bursa A18.83
- submaxillary (region) A18.83
- supraclavicular gland A18.2
- suprarenal (capsule) (gland) A18.7
- swelling, joint (see also category M01) — *see also* Tuberculosis, joint A18.02
- symphysis pubis A18.02
- synovitis A18.09
  - articular A18.02
  - spine or vertebra A18.01
- systemic — *see* Tuberculosis, miliary
- tarsitis A18.4
- tendon (sheath) — *see* Tuberculosis, tenosynovitis
- tenosynovitis A18.09
  - spine or vertebra A18.01
- testis A18.15
- throat A15.8
- thymus gland A18.82
- thyroid gland A18.81
- tongue A18.83
- tonsil, tonsillitis A15.8
- trachea, tracheal A15.5
  - lymph gland or node A15.4
    - primary (progressive) A15.7
- tracheobronchial A15.5
  - lymph gland or node A15.4
    - primary (progressive) A15.7
- tubal (acute) (chronic) A18.17

Tumor - *continued*
glomus - *continued*
intra-abdominal D18.03
intracranial D18.02
jugulare D44.7
malignant C75.5
skin D18.01
specified site NEC D18.09
gonadal stromal — *see* Neoplasm, uncertain behavior, by site
granular cell — *see also* Neoplasm, connective tissue, benign
malignant — *see* Neoplasm, connective tissue, malignant
granulosa cell D39.1-
juvenile D39.1-
malignant C56-
granulosa cell-theca cell D39.1-
malignant C56-
Grawitz's C64-
hemorrhoidal — *see* Hemorrhoids
hilar cell D27-
hilus cell D27-
Hurthle cell (benign) D34
malignant C73
hydatid — *see* Echinococcus
hypernephroid — *see also* Neoplasm, uncertain behavior, by site
interstitial cell — *see also* Neoplasm, uncertain behavior, by site
benign — *see* Neoplasm, benign, by site
malignant — *see* Neoplasm, malignant, by site
intravascular bronchial alveolar D38.1
islet cell — *see* Neoplasm, benign, by site
malignant — *see* Neoplasm, malignant, by site
pancreas C25.4
specified site NEC — *see* Neoplasm, malignant, by site
unspecified site C25.4
pancreas D13.7
specified site NEC — *see* Neoplasm, benign, by site
unspecified site D13.7
juxtaglomerular D41.0-
Klatskin's C24.0
Krukenberg's C79.6-
Leydig cell — *see* Neoplasm, uncertain behavior, by site
benign — *see* Neoplasm, benign, by site
specified site — *see* Neoplasm, benign, by site
unspecified site
female D27.9
male D29.20
malignant — *see* Neoplasm, malignant, by site
specified site — *see* Neoplasm, malignant, by site
unspecified site
female C56.9
male C62.90
specified site — *see* Neoplasm, uncertain behavior, by site
unspecified site
female D39.10
male D40.10
lipid cell, ovary D27-
lipoid cell, ovary D27-
malignant — *see also* Neoplasm, malignant, by site C80.1
fusiform cell (type) C80.1
giant cell (type) C80.1
localized, plasma cell — *see* Plasmacytoma, solitary
mixed NEC C80.1
small cell (type) C80.1
spindle cell (type) C80.1
unclassified C80.1
mast cell D47.09
melanotic, neuroectodermal — *see* Neoplasm, benign, by site
Merkel cell — *see* Carcinoma, Merkel cell
mesenchymal

Tumor - *continued*
mesenchymal - *continued*
malignant — *see* Neoplasm, connective tissue, malignant
mixed — *see* Neoplasm, connective tissue, uncertain behavior
mesodermal, mixed — *see also* Neoplasm, malignant, by site
liver C22.4
mesonephric — *see also* Neoplasm, uncertain behavior, by site
malignant — *see* Neoplasm, malignant, by site
metastatic
from specified site — *see* Neoplasm, malignant, by site
of specified site — *see* Neoplasm, malignant, by site
to specified site — *see* Neoplasm, secondary, by site
mixed NEC — *see also* Neoplasm, benign, by site
malignant — *see* Neoplasm, malignant, by site
mucinous of low malignant potential
specified site — *see* Neoplasm, malignant, by site
unspecified site C56.9
mucocarcinoid
specified site — *see* Neoplasm, malignant, by site
unspecified site C18.1
mucoepidermoid — *see* Neoplasm, uncertain behavior, by site
Müllerian, mixed
specified site — *see* Neoplasm, malignant, by site
unspecified site C54.9
myoepithelial — *see* Neoplasm, benign, by site
neuroectodermal (peripheral) — *see* Neoplasm, malignant, by site
primitive
specified site — *see* Neoplasm, malignant, by site
unspecified site C71.9
neuroendocrine D3A.8
malignant poorly differentiated C7A.1
secondary NEC C7B.8
specified NEC C7A.8
neurogenic olfactory C30.0
nonencapsulated sclerosing C73
odontogenic (adenomatoid) (benign) (calcifying epithelial) (keratocystic) (squamous) — *see* Cyst, calcifying odontogenic
malignant C41.1
upper jaw (bone) C41.0
ovarian stromal D39.1-
ovary, in pregnancy — *see* Pregnancy, complicated by
pacinian — *see* Neoplasm, skin, benign
Pancoast's — *see* Pancoast's syndrome
papillary — *see also* Papilloma
cystic D37.9
mucinous of low malignant potential C56-
specified site — *see* Neoplasm, malignant, by site
unspecified site C56.9
serous of low malignant potential
specified site — *see* Neoplasm, malignant, by site
unspecified site C56.9
pelvic, in pregnancy or childbirth — *see* Pregnancy, complicated by
phantom F45.8
phyllodes D48.6-
benign D24-
malignant — *see* Neoplasm, breast, malignant
Pindborg — *see* Cyst, calcifying odontogenic
placental site trophoblastic D39.2
plasma cell (malignant) (localized) — *see* Plasmacytoma, solitary
polyvesicular vitelline

Tumor - *continued*
polyvesicular vitelline - *continued*
specified site — *see* Neoplasm, malignant, by site
unspecified site
female C56.9
male C62.90
Pott's puffy — *see* Osteomyelitis, specified NEC
Rathke's pouch D44.3
retinal anlage — *see* Neoplasm, benign, by site
salivary gland type, mixed — *see* Neoplasm, salivary gland, benign
malignant — *see* Neoplasm, salivary gland, malignant
Sampson's N80.1
Schmincke's — *see* Neoplasm, nasopharynx, malignant
sclerosing stromal D27-
sebaceous — *see* Cyst, sebaceous
secondary — *see* Neoplasm, secondary, by site
carcinoid C7B.00
bone C7B.03
distant lymph nodes C7B.01
liver C7B.02
peritoneum C7B.04
specified NEC C7B.09
neuroendocrine NEC C7B.8
serous of low malignant potential
specified site — *see* Neoplasm, malignant, by site
unspecified site C56.9
Sertoli cell — *see* Neoplasm, benign, by site
with lipid storage
specified site — *see* Neoplasm, benign, by site
unspecified site
female D27.9
male D29.20
specified site — *see* Neoplasm, benign, by site
unspecified site
female D27.9
male D29.20
Sertoli-Leydig cell — *see* Neoplasm, benign, by site
specified site — *see* Neoplasm, benign, by site
unspecified site
female D27.9
male D29.20
sex cord (-stromal) — *see* Neoplasm, uncertain behavior, by site
with annular tubules D39.1-
skin appendage — *see* Neoplasm, skin, benign
smooth muscle — *see* Neoplasm, connective tissue, uncertain behavior
soft tissue
benign — *see* Neoplasm, connective tissue, benign
malignant — *see* Neoplasm, connective tissue, malignant
sternomastoid (congenital) Q68.0
stromal
endometrial D39.0
gastric D48.1
benign D21.4
malignant C16.9
uncertain behavior D48.1
gastrointestinal C49.A-
benign D21.4
esophagus C49.A1
large intestine C49.A4
malignant C49.A0
colon C49.A4
duodenum C49.A3
esophagus C49.A1
ileum C49.A3
jejunum C49.A3
large intestine C49.A4
Meckel diverticulum C49.A3
omentum C49.A9

U

ULCER, ULCERATED, ULCERATING, ULCERATION, ULCERATIVE - ULCER, ULCERATED, ULCERATING, ULCERATION, ULCERATIVE

Ulcer, ulcerated, ulcerating, ulceration, ulcerative - *continued*
- colon — *see* Ulcer, intestine
- conjunctiva H10.89
- cornea H16.00-
  - with hypopyon H16.03-
  - central H16.01-
  - dendritic (herpes simplex) B00.52
  - marginal H16.04-
  - Mooren's H16.05-
  - mycotic H16.06-
  - perforated H16.07-
  - ring H16.02-
  - tuberculous (phlyctenular) A18.52
- corpus cavernosum (chronic) N48.5
- crural — *see* Ulcer, lower limb
- Curling's — *see* Ulcer, peptic, acute
- Cushing's — *see* Ulcer, peptic, acute
- cystic duct K82.8
- cystitis (interstitial) — *see* Cystitis, interstitial
- decubitus — *see* Ulcer, pressure, by site
- dendritic, cornea (herpes simplex) B00.52
- diabetes, diabetic — *see* Diabetes, ulcer
- Dieulafoy's K25.0
- due to
  - infection NEC — *see* Ulcer, skin
  - radiation NEC L59.8
  - trophic disturbance (any region) — *see* Ulcer, skin
  - X-ray L58.1
- duodenum, duodenal (eroded) (peptic) K26.9
  - with
    - hemorrhage K26.4
      - and perforation K26.6
    - perforation K26.5
  - acute K26.3
    - with
      - hemorrhage K26.0
        - and perforation K26.2
      - perforation K26.1
  - chronic K26.7
    - with
      - hemorrhage K26.4
        - and perforation K26.6
      - perforation K26.5
- dysenteric A09
- elusive — *see* Cystitis, interstitial
- endocarditis (acute) (chronic) (subacute) I28.8
- epiglottis J38.7
- esophagus (peptic) K22.10
  - with bleeding K22.11
  - due to
    - aspirin K22.10
      - with bleeding K22.11
    - gastrointestinal reflux disease (without bleeding) K21.00
      - with bleeding K21.01
    - ingestion of chemical or medicament K22.10
      - with bleeding K22.11
  - fungal K22.10
    - with bleeding K22.11
  - infective K22.10
    - with bleeding K22.11
  - varicose — *see* Varix, esophagus
- eyelid (region) H01.8
- fauces J39.2
- Fenwick (-Hunner) (solitary) — *see* Cystitis, interstitial
- fistulous — *see* Ulcer, skin
- foot (indolent) (trophic) — *see* Ulcer, lower limb
- frambesial, initial A66.0
- frenum (tongue) K14.0
- gallbladder or duct K82.8
- gangrenous — *see* Gangrene
- gastric — *see* Ulcer, stomach
- gastrocolic — *see* Ulcer, gastrojejunal
- gastroduodenal — *see* Ulcer, peptic
- gastroesophageal — *see* Ulcer, stomach
- gastrointestinal — *see* Ulcer, gastrojejunal
- gastrojejunal (peptic) K28.9
  - with

Ulcer, ulcerated, ulcerating, ulceration, ulcerative - *continued*
- gastrojejunal (peptic) - *continued*
  - with - *continued*
    - hemorrhage K28.4
      - and perforation K28.6
    - perforation K28.5
  - acute K28.3
    - with
      - hemorrhage K28.0
        - and perforation K28.2
      - perforation K28.1
  - chronic K28.7
    - with
      - hemorrhage K28.4
        - and perforation K28.6
      - perforation K28.5
- gastrojejunocolic — *see* Ulcer, gastrojejunal
- gingiva K06.8
- gingivitis K05.10
  - nonplaque induced K05.11
  - plaque induced K05.10
- glottis J38.7
- granuloma of pudenda A58
- gum K06.8
- gumma, due to yaws A66.4
- heel — *see* Ulcer, lower limb
- hemorrhoid — *see also* Hemorrhoids, by degree K64.8
- Hunner's — *see* Cystitis, interstitial
- hypopharynx J39.2
- hypopyon (chronic) (subacute) — *see* Ulcer, cornea, with hypopyon
- hypostaticum — *see* Ulcer, varicose
- ileum — *see* Ulcer, intestine
- intestine, intestinal K63.3
  - with perforation K63.1
  - amebic A06.1
  - duodenal — *see* Ulcer, duodenum
  - granulocytopenic (with hemorrhage) — *see* Neutropenia
  - marginal — *see* Ulcer, gastrojejunal
  - perforating K63.1
    - newborn P78.0
  - primary, small intestine K63.3
  - rectum K62.6
  - stercoraceous, stercoral K63.3
  - tuberculous A18.32
  - typhoid (fever) — *see* Typhoid
  - varicose I86.8
- jejunum, jejunal — *see* Ulcer, gastrojejunal
- keratitis — *see* Ulcer, cornea
- knee — *see* Ulcer, lower limb
- labium (majus) (minus) N76.6
- laryngitis — *see* Laryngitis
- larynx (aphthous) (contact) J38.7
  - diphtheritic A36.2
- leg — *see* Ulcer, lower limb
- lip K13.0
- Lipschütz's N76.6
- lower limb (atrophic) (chronic) (neurogenic) (perforating) (pyogenic) (trophic) (tropical) L97.909
  - with
    - bone involvement without evidence of necrosis L97.906
    - bone necrosis L97.904
    - exposed fat layer L97.902
    - muscle involvement without evidence of necrosis L97.905
    - muscle necrosis L97.903
    - skin breakdown only L97.901
    - specified severity NEC L97.908
  - ankle L97.309
    - with
      - bone involvement without evidence of necrosis L97.306
      - bone necrosis L97.304
      - exposed fat layer L97.302
      - muscle involvement without evidence of necrosis L97.305
      - muscle necrosis L97.303
      - skin breakdown only L97.301
      - specified severity NEC L97.308
    - left L97.329

Ulcer, ulcerated, ulcerating, ulceration, ulcerative - *continued*
- lower limb (atrophic) (chronic) (neurogenic) (perforating) (pyogenic) (trophic) (tropical) - *continued*
  - ankle - *continued*
    - left - *continued*
      - with
        - bone involvement without evidence of necrosis L97.326
        - bone necrosis L97.324
        - exposed fat layer L97.322
        - muscle involvement without evidence of necrosis L97.325
        - muscle necrosis L97.323
        - skin breakdown only L97.321
        - specified severity NEC L97.328
    - right L97.319
      - with
        - bone involvement without evidence of necrosis L97.316
        - bone necrosis L97.314
        - exposed fat layer L97.312
        - muscle involvement without evidence of necrosis L97.315
        - muscle necrosis L97.313
        - skin breakdown only L97.311
        - specified severity NEC L97.318
  - calf L97.209
    - with
      - bone involvement without evidence of necrosis L97.206
      - bone necrosis L97.204
      - exposed fat layer L97.202
      - muscle involvement without evidence of necrosis L97.205
      - muscle necrosis L97.203
      - skin breakdown only L97.201
      - specified severity NEC L97.208
    - left L97.229
      - with
        - bone involvement without evidence of necrosis L97.226
        - bone necrosis L97.224
        - exposed fat layer L97.222
        - muscle involvement without evidence of necrosis L97.225
        - muscle necrosis L97.223
        - skin breakdown only L97.221
        - specified severity NEC L97.228
    - right L97.219
      - with
        - bone involvement without evidence of necrosis L97.216
        - bone necrosis L97.214
        - exposed fat layer L97.212
        - muscle involvement without evidence of necrosis L97.215
        - muscle necrosis L97.213
        - skin breakdown only L97.211
        - specified severity NEC L97.218
  - decubitus — *see* Ulcer, pressure, by site
  - foot specified NEC L97.509
    - with
      - bone involvement without evidence of necrosis L97.506
      - bone necrosis L97.504
      - exposed fat layer L97.502
      - muscle involvement without evidence of necrosis L97.505
      - muscle necrosis L97.503
      - skin breakdown only L97.501
      - specified severity NEC L97.508
    - left L97.529
      - with
        - bone involvement without evidence of necrosis L97.526
        - bone necrosis L97.524
        - exposed fat layer L97.522
        - muscle involvement without evidence of necrosis L97.525
        - muscle necrosis L97.523
        - skin breakdown only L97.521
        - specified severity NEC L97.528
    - right L97.519

Ulcer, ulcerated, ulcerating, ulceration, ulcerative - *continued*
lower limb (atrophic) (chronic) (neurogenic) (perforating) (pyogenic) (trophic) (tropical) - *continued*
foot specified NEC - *continued*
right - *continued*
with
bone involvement without evidence of necrosis L97.516
bone necrosis L97.514
exposed fat layer L97.512
muscle involvement without evidence of necrosis L97.515
muscle necrosis L97.513
skin breakdown only L97.511
specified severity NEC L97.518
heel L97.409
with
bone involvement without evidence of necrosis L97.406
bone necrosis L97.404
exposed fat layer L97.402
muscle involvement without evidence of necrosis L97.405
muscle necrosis L97.403
skin breakdown only L97.401
specified severity NEC L97.408
left L97.429
with
bone involvement without evidence of necrosis L97.426
bone necrosis L97.424
exposed fat layer L97.422
muscle involvement without evidence of necrosis L97.425
muscle necrosis L97.423
skin breakdown only L97.421
specified severity NEC L97.428
right L97.419
with
bone involvement without evidence of necrosis L97.416
bone necrosis L97.414
exposed fat layer L97.412
muscle involvement without evidence of necrosis L97.415
muscle necrosis L97.413
skin breakdown only L97.411
specified severity NEC L97.418
left L97.929
with
bone involvement without evidence of necrosis L97.926
bone necrosis L97.924
exposed fat layer L97.922
muscle involvement without evidence of necrosis L97.925
muscle necrosis L97.923
skin breakdown only L97.921
specified severity NEC L97.928
lower leg NOS L97.909
with
bone involvement without evidence of necrosis L97.906
bone necrosis L97.904
exposed fat layer L97.902
muscle involvement without evidence of necrosis L97.905
muscle necrosis L97.903
skin breakdown only L97.901
specified severity NEC L97.908
left L97.929
with
bone involvement without evidence of necrosis L97.926
bone necrosis L97.924
exposed fat layer L97.922
muscle involvement without evidence of necrosis L97.925
muscle necrosis L97.923
skin breakdown only L97.921
specified severity NEC L97.928
right L97.919
with

Ulcer, ulcerated, ulcerating, ulceration, ulcerative - *continued*
lower limb (atrophic) (chronic) (neurogenic) (perforating) (pyogenic) (trophic) (tropical) - *continued*
lower leg NOS - *continued*
right - *continued*
with - *continued*
bone involvement without evidence of necrosis L97.916
bone necrosis L97.914
exposed fat layer L97.912
muscle involvement without evidence of necrosis L97.915
muscle necrosis L97.913
skin breakdown only L97.911
specified severity NEC L97.918
specified site NEC L97.809
with
bone involvement without evidence of necrosis L97.806
bone necrosis L97.804
exposed fat layer L97.802
muscle involvement without evidence of necrosis L97.805
muscle necrosis L97.803
skin breakdown only L97.801
specified severity NEC L97.808
left L97.829
with
bone involvement without evidence of necrosis L97.826
bone necrosis L97.824
exposed fat layer L97.822
muscle involvement without evidence of necrosis L97.825
muscle necrosis L97.823
skin breakdown only L97.821
specified severity NEC L97.828
right L97.819
with
bone involvement without evidence of necrosis L97.816
bone necrosis L97.814
exposed fat layer L97.812
muscle involvement without evidence of necrosis L97.815
muscle necrosis L97.813
skin breakdown only L97.811
specified severity NEC L97.818
midfoot L97.409
with
bone involvement without evidence of necrosis L97.406
bone necrosis L97.404
exposed fat layer L97.402
muscle involvement without evidence of necrosis L97.405
muscle necrosis L97.403
skin breakdown only L97.401
specified severity NEC L97.408
left L97.429
with
bone involvement without evidence of necrosis L97.426
bone necrosis L97.424
exposed fat layer L97.422
muscle involvement without evidence of necrosis L97.425
muscle necrosis L97.423
skin breakdown only L97.421
specified severity NEC L97.428
right L97.419
with
bone involvement without evidence of necrosis L97.416
bone necrosis L97.414
exposed fat layer L97.412
muscle involvement without evidence of necrosis L97.415
muscle necrosis L97.413

Ulcer, ulcerated, ulcerating, ulceration, ulcerative - *continued*
lower limb (atrophic) (chronic) (neurogenic) (perforating) (pyogenic) (trophic) (tropical) - *continued*
midfoot - *continued*
right - *continued*
with - *continued*
skin breakdown only L97.411
specified severity NEC L97.418
right L97.919
with
bone involvement without evidence of necrosis L97.916
bone necrosis L97.914
exposed fat layer L97.912
muscle involvement without evidence of necrosis L97.915
muscle necrosis L97.913
skin breakdown only L97.911
specified severity NEC L97.918
thigh L97.109
with
bone involvement without evidence of necrosis L97.106
bone necrosis L97.104
muscle involvement without evidence of necrosis L97.105
exposed fat layer L97.102
muscle necrosis L97.103
skin breakdown only L97.101
specified severity NEC L97.108
left L97.129
with
bone involvement without evidence of necrosis L97.126
bone necrosis L97.124
exposed fat layer L97.122
muscle involvement without evidence of necrosis L97.125
muscle necrosis L97.123
skin breakdown only L97.121
specified severity NEC L97.128
right L97.119
with
bone involvement without evidence of necrosis L97.116
bone necrosis L97.114
exposed fat layer L97.112
muscle involvement without evidence of necrosis L97.115
muscle necrosis L97.113
skin breakdown only L97.111
specified severity NEC L97.118
toe L97.509
with
bone involvement without evidence of necrosis L97.506
bone necrosis L97.504
exposed fat layer L97.502
muscle involvement without evidence of necrosis L97.505
muscle necrosis L97.503
skin breakdown only L97.501
specified severity NEC L97.508
left L97.529
with
bone involvement without evidence of necrosis L97.526
bone necrosis L97.524
exposed fat layer L97.522
muscle involvement without evidence of necrosis L97.525
muscle necrosis L97.523
skin breakdown only L97.521
specified severity NEC L97.528
right L97.519
with
bone involvement without evidence of necrosis L97.516
bone necrosis L97.514
exposed fat layer L97.512
muscle involvement without evidence of necrosis L97.515
muscle necrosis L97.513

Ulcer, ulcerated, ulcerating, ulceration, ulcerative - *continued*
lower limb (atrophic) (chronic) (neurogenic) (perforating) (pyogenic) (trophic) (tropical) - *continued*
toe - *continued*
right - *continued*
with - *continued*
skin breakdown only L97.511
specified severity NEC L97.518
leprous A30.1
syphilitic A52.19
varicose — *see* Varix, leg, with, ulcer
luetic — *see* Ulcer, syphilitic
lung J98.4
tuberculous — *see* Tuberculosis, pulmonary
malignant — *see* Neoplasm, malignant, by site
marginal NEC — *see* Ulcer, gastrojejunal
meatus (urinarius) N34.2
Meckel's diverticulum Q43.0
malignant — *see* Table of Neoplasms, small intestine, malignant
Meleney's (chronic undermining) — *see* Ulcer, skin
Mooren's (cornea) — *see* Ulcer, cornea, Mooren's
mycobacterial (skin) A31.1
nasopharynx J39.2
neck, uterus N86
neurogenic NEC — *see* Ulcer, skin
nose, nasal (passage) (infective) (septum) J34.0
skin — *see* Ulcer, skin
spirochetal A69.8
varicose (bleeding) I86.8
oral mucosa (traumatic) K12.1
palate (soft) K12.1
penis (chronic) N48.5
peptic (site unspecified) K27.9
with
hemorrhage K27.4
and perforation K27.6
perforation K27.5
acute K27.3
with
hemorrhage K27.0
and perforation K27.2
perforation K27.1
chronic K27.7
with
hemorrhage K27.4
and perforation K27.6
perforation K27.5
esophagus K22.10
with bleeding K22.11
newborn P78.82
perforating K27.5
skin — *see* Ulcer, skin
peritonsillar J35.8
phagedenic (tropical) — *see* Ulcer, skin
pharynx J39.2
phlebitis — *see* Phlebitis
plaster — *see* Ulcer, pressure, by site
popliteal space — *see* Ulcer, lower limb
postpyloric — *see* Ulcer, duodenum
prepuce N47.7
prepyloric — *see* Ulcer, stomach
pressure (pressure area) L89.9-
ankle L89.5-
back L89.1-
buttock L89.3-
coccyx L89.15-
contiguous site of back, buttock, hip L89.4-
elbow L89.0-
face L89.81-
head L89.81-
heel L89.6-
hip L89.2-
sacral region (tailbone) L89.15-
specified site NEC L89.89-
stage 1 (healing) (pre-ulcer skin changes limited to persistent focal edema)

Ulcer, ulcerated, ulcerating, ulceration, ulcerative - *continued*
pressure (pressure area) - *continued*
stage 1 (healing) (pre-ulcer skin changes limited to persistent focal edema) - *continued*
ankle L89.5-
back L89.1-
buttock L89.3-
coccyx L89.15-
contiguous site of back, buttock, hip L89.4-
elbow L89.0-
face L89.81-
head L89.81-
heel L89.6-
hip L89.2-
sacral region (tailbone) L89.15-
specified site NEC L89.89-
stage 2 (healing) (abrasion, blister, partial thickness skin loss involving epidermis and/or dermis)
ankle L89.5-
back L89.1-
buttock L89.3-
coccyx L89.15-
contiguous site of back, buttock, hip L89.4-
elbow L89.0-
face L89.81-
head L89.81-
heel L89.6-
hip L89.2-
sacral region (tailbone) L89.15-
specified site NEC L89.89-
stage 3 (healing) (full thickness skin loss involving damage or necrosis of subcutaneous tissue)
ankle L89.5-
back L89.1-
buttock L89.3-
coccyx L89.15-
contiguous site of back, buttock, hip L89.4-
elbow L89.0-
face L89.81-
head L89.81-
heel L89.6-
hip L89.2-
sacral region (tailbone) L89.15-
specified site NEC L89.89-
stage 4 (healing) (necrosis of soft tissues through to underlying muscle, tendon, or bone)
ankle L89.5-
back L89.1-
buttock L89.3-
coccyx L89.15-
contiguous site of back, buttock, hip L89.4-
elbow L89.0-
face L89.81-
head L89.81-
heel L89.6-
hip L89.2-
sacral region (tailbone) L89.15-
specified site NEC L89.89-
unspecified stage
ankle L89.5-
back L89.1-
buttock L89.3-
coccyx L89.15-
contiguous site of back, buttock, hip L89.4-
elbow L89.0-
face L89.81-
head L89.81-
heel L89.6-
hip L89.2-
sacral region (tailbone) L89.15-
specified site NEC L89.89-
unstageable
ankle L89.5-
back L89.1-
buttock L89.3-

Ulcer, ulcerated, ulcerating, ulceration, ulcerative - *continued*
pressure (pressure area) - *continued*
unstageable - *continued*
coccyx L89.15-
contiguous site of back, buttock, hip L89.4-
elbow L89.0-
face L89.81-
head L89.81-
heel L89.6-
hip L89.2-
sacral region (tailbone) L89.15-
specified site NEC L89.89-
primary of intestine K63.3
with perforation K63.1
prostate N41.9
pyloric — *see* Ulcer, stomach
rectosigmoid K63.3
with perforation K63.1
rectum (sphincter) (solitary) K62.6
stercoraceous, stercoral K62.6
retina — *see* Inflammation, chorioretinal
rodent — *see also* Neoplasm, skin, malignant
sclera — *see* Scleritis
scrofulous (tuberculous) A18.2
scrotum N50.89
tuberculous A18.15
varicose I86.1
seminal vesicle N50.89
sigmoid — *see* Ulcer, intestine
skin (atrophic) (chronic) (neurogenic) (non-healing) (perforating) (pyogenic) (trophic) (tropical) L98.499
with gangrene — *see* Gangrene
amebic A06.7
back — *see* Ulcer, back
buttock — *see* Ulcer, buttock
decubitus — *see* Ulcer, pressure
lower limb — *see* Ulcer, lower limb
mycobacterial A31.1
specified site NEC L98.499
with
bone involvement without evidence of necrosis L98.496
bone necrosis L98.494
exposed fat layer L98.492
muscle involvement without evidence of necrosis L98.495
muscle necrosis L98.493
skin breakdown only L98.491
specified severity NEC L98.498
tuberculous (primary) A18.4
varicose — *see* Ulcer, varicose
sloughing — *see* Ulcer, skin
solitary, anus or rectum (sphincter) K62.6
sore throat J02.9
streptococcal J02.0
spermatic cord N50.89
spine (tuberculous) A18.01
stasis (venous) — *see* Varix, leg, with, ulcer
without varicose veins I87.2
stercoraceous, stercoral K63.3
with perforation K63.1
anus or rectum K62.6
stoma, stomal — *see* Ulcer, gastrojejunal
stomach (eroded) (peptic) (round) K25.9
with
hemorrhage K25.4
and perforation K25.6
perforation K25.5
acute K25.3
with
hemorrhage K25.0
and perforation K25.2
perforation K25.1
chronic K25.7
with
hemorrhage K25.4
and perforation K25.6
perforation K25.5
stomal — *see* Ulcer, gastrojejunal
stomatitis K12.1
stress — *see* Ulcer, peptic
strumous (tuberculous) A18.2

Ulcer, ulcerated, ulcerating, ulceration, ulcerative - *continued*
submucosal, bladder — *see* Cystitis, interstitial
syphilitic (any site) (early) (secondary) A51.39
late A52.79
perforating A52.79
foot A52.11
testis N50.89
thigh — *see* Ulcer, lower limb
throat J39.2
diphtheritic A36.0
toe — *see* Ulcer, lower limb
tongue (traumatic) K14.0
tonsil J35.8
diphtheritic A36.0
trachea J39.8
trophic — *see* Ulcer, skin
tropical — *see* Ulcer, skin
tuberculous — *see* Tuberculosis, ulcer
tunica vaginalis N50.89
turbinate J34.89
typhoid (perforating) — *see* Typhoid
unspecified site — *see* Ulcer, skin
urethra (meatus) — *see* Urethritis
uterus N85.8
cervix N86
with cervicitis N72
neck N86
with cervicitis N72
vagina N76.5
in Behçet's disease M35.2 *[N77.0]*
pessary N89.8
valve, heart I33.0
varicose (lower limb, any part) — *see also* Varix, leg, with, ulcer
broad ligament I86.2
esophagus — *see* Varix, esophagus
inflamed or infected — *see* Varix, leg, with ulcer, with inflammation
nasal septum I86.8
perineum I86.3
scrotum I86.1
specified site NEC I86.8
sublingual I86.0
vulva I86.3
vas deferens N50.89
vulva (acute) (infectional) N76.6
in (due to)
Behçet's disease M35.2 *[N77.0]*
herpesviral (herpes simplex) infection A60.04
tuberculosis A18.18
vulvobuccal, recurring N76.6
X-ray L58.1
yaws A66.4
Ulcerosa scarlatina A38.8
Ulcus — *see also* Ulcer
cutis tuberculosum A18.4
duodeni — *see* Ulcer, duodenum
durum (syphilitic) A51.0
extragenital A51.2
gastrojejunale — *see* Ulcer, gastrojejunal
hypostaticum — *see* Ulcer, varicose
molle (cutis) (skin) A57
serpens corneae — *see* Ulcer, cornea, central
ventriculi — *see* Ulcer, stomach
Ulegyria Q04.8
Ulerythema
ophryogenes, congenital Q84.2
sycosiforme L73.8
Ullrich (-Bonnevie) (-Turner) syndrome — *see also* Turner's syndrome Q87.19
Ullrich-Feichtiger syndrome Q87.0
Ulnar — *see* condition
Ulorrhagia, ulorrhea K06.8
Umbilicus, umbilical — *see* condition
Unacceptable
contours of tooth K08.54
morphology of tooth K08.54
Unavailability (of)
bed at medical facility Z75.1
health service-related agencies Z75.4
Unavailability (of) - *continued*
medical facilities (at) Z75.3
due to
investigation by social service agency Z75.2
lack of services at home Z75.0
remoteness from facility Z75.3
waiting list Z75.1
home Z75.0
outpatient clinic Z75.3
schooling Z55.1
social service agencies Z75.4
Uncinaria americana infestation B76.1
Uncinariasis B76.9
Uncongenial work Z56.5
Unconscious (ness) — *see* Coma
Under observation — *see* Observation
Underachievement in school Z55.3
Underdevelopment — *see also* Undeveloped
nose Q30.1
sexual E30.0
Underdosing — *see also* Table of Drugs and Chemicals, categories T36-T50, with final character 6 Z91.14
intentional NEC Z91.128
due to financial hardship of patient Z91.120
unintentional NEC Z91.138
due to patient's age related debility Z91.130
Underfeeding, newborn P92.3
Underfill, endodontic M27.53
Underimmunization status Z28.3
Undernourishment — *see* Malnutrition
Undernutrition — *see* Malnutrition
Underweight R63.6
for gestational age — *see* Light for dates
Underwood's disease P83.0
Undescended — *see also* Malposition, congenital
cecum Q43.3
colon Q43.3
testicle — *see* Cryptorchid
Undeveloped, undevelopment — *see also* Hypoplasia
brain (congenital) Q02
cerebral (congenital) Q02
heart Q24.8
lung Q33.6
testis E29.1
uterus E30.0
Undiagnosed (disease) R69
Undulant fever — *see* Brucellosis
Unemployment, anxiety concerning Z56.0
threatened Z56.2
Unequal length (acquired) (limb) — *see also* Deformity, limb, unequal length
leg — *see also* Deformity, limb, unequal length
congenital Q72.9-
Unextracted dental root K08.3
Unguis incarnatus L60.0
Unhappiness R45.2
Unicornate uterus Q51.4
in pregnancy or childbirth O34.00
Unilateral — *see also* condition
development, breast N64.89
organ or site, congenital NEC — *see* Agenesis, by site
Unilocular heart Q20.8
Union, abnormal — *see also* Fusion
larynx and trachea Q34.8
Universal mesentery Q43.3
Unrepairable overhanging of dental restorative materials K08.52
Unsatisfactory
restoration of tooth K08.50
specified NEC K08.59
sample of cytologic smear
anus R85.615
cervix R87.615
vagina R87.625
surroundings Z59.1
work Z56.5
Unsoundness of mind — *see* Psychosis
Unstable
back NEC — *see* Instability, joint, spine
hip (congenital) Q65.6
acquired — *see* Derangement, joint, specified type NEC, hip
joint — *see* Instability, joint
secondary to removal of joint prosthesis M96.89
lie (mother) O32.0
lumbosacral joint (congenital) — *see* subcategory M53.2
sacroiliac — *see* subcategory M53.2
spine NEC — *see* Instability, joint, spine
Unsteadiness on feet R26.81
Untruthfulness, child problem F91.8
Unverricht (-Lundborg) disease or epilepsy — *see* Epilepsy, generalized, idiopathic
Unwanted
multiple moves in the last 12 months Z59.81-
pregnancy Z64.0
Upbringing, institutional Z62.22
away from parents NEC Z62.29
in care of non-parental family member Z62.21
in foster care Z62.21
in orphanage or group home Z62.22
in welfare custody Z62.21
Upper respiratory — *see* condition
Upset
gastric K30
gastrointestinal K30
psychogenic F45.8
intestinal (large) (small) K59.9
psychogenic F45.8
menstruation N93.9
mental F48.9
stomach K30
psychogenic F45.8
Urachus — *see also* condition
patent or persistent Q64.4
Urbach-Oppenheim disease (necrobiosis lipoidica diabeticorum) — *see* E08-E13 with .620
Urbach's lipoid proteinosis E78.89
Urbach-Wiethe disease E78.89
Urban yellow fever A95.1
Urea
blood, high — *see* Uremia
cycle metabolism disorder — *see* Disorder, urea cycle metabolism
Uremia, uremic N19
with
ectopic or molar pregnancy O08.4
polyneuropathy N18.9 *[G63]*
chronic NOS — *see also* Disease, kidney, chronic N18.9
due to hypertension — *see* Hypertensive, kidney
complicating
ectopic or molar pregnancy O08.4
congenital P96.0
extrarenal R39.2
following ectopic or molar pregnancy O08.4
newborn P96.0
prerenal R39.2
Ureter, ureteral — *see* condition
Ureteralgia N23
Ureterectasis — *see* Hydroureter
Ureteritis N28.89
cystica N28.86
due to calculus N20.1
with calculus, kidney N20.2
with hydronephrosis N13.2
gonococcal (acute) (chronic) A54.21
nonspecific N28.89
Ureterocele N28.89
congenital (orthotopic) Q62.31
ectopic Q62.32
Ureterolith, ureterolithiasis — *see* Calculus, ureter
Ureterostomy
attention to Z43.6
status Z93.6
Urethra, urethral — *see* condition

Use (of) - *continued*
sedative, hypnotic, or anxiolytic - *continued*
with - *continued*
intoxication - *continued*
uncomplicated F13.920
other specified disorder F13.988
persisting
amnestic disorder F13.96
dementia F13.97
psychosis F13.959
delusions F13.950
hallucinations F13.951
sexual dysfunction F13.981
sleep disorder F13.982
unspecified disorder F13.99
harmful — *see* Abuse, drug, sedative, hypnotic, or anxiolytic
stimulant NEC F15.90
with
anxiety disorder F15.980
intoxication F15.929
with
delirium F15.921
perceptual disturbance F15.922
uncomplicated F15.920
mood disorder F15.94
other specified disorder F15.988
psychosis F15.959
delusions F15.950
hallucinations F15.951
sexual dysfunction F15.981
sleep disorder F15.982
unspecified disorder F15.99
withdrawal F15.93
harmful — *see* Abuse, drug, stimulant NEC
tobacco Z72.0
with dependence — *see* Dependence, drug, nicotine
volatile solvents — *see also* Use, inhalant F18.90
harmful — *see* Abuse, drug, inhalant
Usher-Senear disease or syndrome L10.4
Uta B55.1
Uteromegaly N85.2
Uterovaginal — *see* condition
Uterovesical — *see* condition
Uveal — *see* condition
Uveitis (anterior) — *see also* Iridocyclitis
acute — *see* Iridocyclitis, acute
chronic — *see* Iridocyclitis, chronic
due to toxoplasmosis (acquired) B58.09
congenital P37.1
granulomatous — *see* Iridocyclitis, chronic
heterochromic — *see* Cyclitis, Fuchs' heterochromic
lens-induced — *see* Iridocyclitis, lens-induced
posterior — *see* Chorioretinitis
sympathetic H44.13-
syphilitic (secondary) A51.43
congenital (early) A50.01
late A52.71
tuberculous A18.54
Uveoencephalitis — *see* Inflammation, chorioretinal
Uveokeratitis — *see* Iridocyclitis
Uveoparotitis D86.89
Uvula — *see* condition
Uvulitis (acute) (catarrhal) (chronic) (membranous) (suppurative) (ulcerative) K12.2

V

Vaccination (prophylactic)
complication or reaction — *see* Complications, vaccination
delayed Z28.9
encounter for Z23
not done — *see* Immunization, not done, because (of)
Vaccinia (generalized) (localized) T88.1
congenital P35.8
without vaccination B08.011
Vacuum, in sinus (accessory) (nasal) J34.89
Vagabond, vagabondage Z59.00
Vagabond's disease B85.1
Vagina, vaginal — *see* condition
Vaginalitis (tunica) (testis) N49.1
Vaginismus (reflex) N94.2
functional F52.5
nonorganic F52.5
psychogenic F52.5
secondary N94.2
Vaginitis (acute) (circumscribed) (diffuse) (emphysematous) (nonvenereal) (ulcerative) N76.0
with ectopic or molar pregnancy O08.0
amebic A06.82
atrophic, postmenopausal N95.2
bacterial N76.0
blennorrhagic (gonococcal) A54.02
candidal B37.3
chlamydial A56.02
chronic N76.1
due to Trichomonas (vaginalis) A59.01
following ectopic or molar pregnancy O08.0
gonococcal A54.02
with abscess (accessory gland) (periurethral) A54.1
granuloma A58
in (due to)
candidiasis B37.3
herpesviral (herpes simplex) infection A60.04
pinworm infection B80 *[N77.1]*
monilial B37.3
mycotic (candidal) B37.3
postmenopausal atrophic N95.2
puerperal (postpartum) O86.13
senile (atrophic) N95.2
subacute or chronic N76.1
syphilitic (early) A51.0
late A52.76
trichomonal A59.01
tuberculous A18.18
Vaginosis — *see* Vaginitis
Vagotonia G52.2
Vagrancy Z59.00
VAIN — *see* Neoplasia, intraepithelial, vagina
Vallecula — *see* condition
Valley fever B38.0
Valsuani's disease — *see* Anemia, obstetric
Valve, valvular (formation) — *see also* condition
cerebral ventricle (communicating) in situ Z98.2
cervix, internal os Q51.828
congenital NEC — *see* Atresia, by site
ureter (pelvic junction) (vesical orifice) Q62.39
urethra (congenital) (posterior) Q64.2
Valvulitis (chronic) — *see* Endocarditis
Valvulopathy — *see* Endocarditis
Van Bogaert's leukoencephalopathy (sclerosing) (subacute) A81.1
Van Bogaert-Scherer-Epstein disease or syndrome E75.5
Van Buchem's syndrome M85.2
Van Creveld-von Gierke disease E74.01
Van der Hoeve (-de Kleyn) syndrome Q78.0
Van der Woude's syndrome Q38.0
Van Neck's disease or osteochondrosis M91.0
Vanishing lung J44.9
Vapor asphyxia or suffocation T59.9
specified agent — *see* Table of Drugs and Chemicals
Variance, lethal ball, prosthetic heart valve T82.09
Variants, thalassemic D56.8
Variations in hair color L67.1
Varicella B01.9
with
complications NEC B01.89
encephalitis B01.11
encephalomyelitis B01.11
meningitis B01.0
myelitis B01.12
pneumonia B01.2
congenital P35.8
Varices — *see* Varix
Varicocele (scrotum) (thrombosed) I86.1
ovary I86.2
perineum I86.3
spermatic cord (ulcerated) I86.1
Varicose
aneurysm (ruptured) I77.0
dermatitis — *see* Varix, leg, with, inflammation
eczema — *see* Varix, leg, with, inflammation
phlebitis — *see* Varix, with, inflammation
tumor — *see* Varix
ulcer (lower limb, any part) — *see also* Varix, leg, with, ulcer
anus — *see also* Hemorrhoids K64.8
esophagus — *see* Varix, esophagus
inflamed or infected — *see* Varix, leg, with ulcer, with inflammation
nasal septum I86.8
perineum I86.3
scrotum I86.1
specified site NEC I86.8
vein — *see* Varix
vessel — *see* Varix, leg
Varicosis, varicosities, varicosity — *see* Varix
Variola (major) (minor) B03
Varioloid B03
Varix (lower limb) I83.90
with
bleeding I83.899
edema I83.899
inflammation I83.10
with ulcer (venous) I83.209
pain I83.819
rupture I83.899
specified complication NEC I83.899
stasis dermatitis I83.10
with ulcer (venous) I83.209
swelling I83.899
ulcer I83.009
with inflammation I83.209
aneurysmal I77.0
asymptomatic I83.9-
bladder I86.2
broad ligament I86.2
complicating
childbirth (lower extremity) O87.4
anus or rectum O87.2
genital (vagina, vulva or perineum) O87.8
pregnancy (lower extremity) O22.0-
anus or rectum O22.4-
genital (vagina, vulva or perineum) O22.1-
puerperium (lower extremity) O87.4
anus or rectum O87.2
genital (vagina, vulva, perineum) O87.8
congenital (any site) Q27.8
esophagus (idiopathic) (primary) (ulcerated) I85.00
bleeding I85.01
congenital Q27.8
in (due to)
alcoholic liver disease I85.10
bleeding I85.11
cirrhosis of liver I85.10
bleeding I85.11
portal hypertension I85.10
bleeding I85.11
schistosomiasis I85.10
bleeding I85.11
toxic liver disease I85.10
bleeding I85.11
secondary I85.10
bleeding I85.11
gastric I86.4
inflamed or infected I83.10
ulcerated I83.209
labia (majora) I86.3
leg (asymptomatic) I83.9-
with
edema I83.899
inflammation I83.10
with ulcer — *see* Varix, leg, with, ulcer, with inflammation by site
pain I83.819

Varix (lower limb) - *continued*
leg (asymptomatic) - *continued*
with - *continued*
specified complication NEC I83.899
swelling I83.899
ulcer I83.0-
with inflammation I83.2-
ankle I83.003
with inflammation I83.203
calf I83.002
with inflammation I83.202
foot NEC I83.005
with inflammation I83.205
heel I83.004
with inflammation I83.204
lower leg NEC I83.008
with inflammation I83.208
midfoot I83.004
with inflammation I83.204
thigh I83.001
with inflammation I83.201
bilateral (asymptomatic) I83.93
with
edema I83.893
pain I83.813
specified complication NEC I83.893
swelling I83.893
ulcer I83.0-
with inflammation I83.209
left (asymptomatic) I83.92
with
edema I83.892
pain I83.812
specified complication NEC I83.892
swelling I83.892
inflammation I83.12
with ulcer — *see* Varix, leg, with, ulcer, with inflammation by site
ulcer I83.029
with inflammation I83.229
ankle I83.023
with inflammation I83.223
calf I83.022
with inflammation I83.222
foot NEC I83.025
with inflammation I83.225
heel I83.024
with inflammation I83.224
lower leg NEC I83.028
with inflammation I83.228
midfoot I83.024
with inflammation I83.224
thigh I83.021
with inflammation I83.221
right (asymptomatic) I83.91
with
edema I83.891
pain I83.811
specified complication NEC I83.891
swelling I83.891
inflammation I83.11
with ulcer — *see* Varix, leg, with, ulcer, with inflammation by site
ulcer I83.019
with inflammation I83.219
ankle I83.013
with inflammation I83.213
calf I83.012
with inflammation I83.212
foot NEC I83.015
with inflammation I83.215
heel I83.014
with inflammation I83.214
lower leg NEC I83.018
with inflammation I83.218
midfoot I83.014
with inflammation I83.214
thigh I83.011
with inflammation I83.211
nasal septum I86.8
orbit I86.8
congenital Q27.8
ovary I86.2

Varix (lower limb) - *continued*
papillary I78.1
pelvis I86.2
perineum I86.3
pharynx I86.8
placenta O43.89-
renal papilla I86.8
retina H35.09
scrotum (ulcerated) I86.1
sigmoid colon I86.8
specified site NEC I86.8
spinal (cord) (vessels) I86.8
spleen, splenic (vein) (with phlebolith) I86.8
stomach I86.4
sublingual I86.0
ulcerated I83.009
inflamed or infected I83.209
uterine ligament I86.2
vagina I86.8
vocal cord I86.8
vulva I86.3
Vas deferens — *see* condition
Vas deferentitis N49.1
Vasa previa O69.4
hemorrhage from, affecting newborn P50.0
Vascular — *see also* condition
loop on optic papilla Q14.2
spasm I73.9
spider I78.1
Vascularization, cornea — *see* Neovascularization, cornea
Vasculitis I77.6
allergic D69.0
cryoglobulinemic D89.1
disseminated I77.6
hypocomplementemic M31.8
kidney I77.89
leukocytoclastic M31.0
livedoid L95.0
nodular L95.8
retina H35.06-
rheumatic — *see* Fever, rheumatic
rheumatoid — *see* Rheumatoid, vasculitis
skin (limited to) L95.9
specified NEC L95.8
systemic M31.8
Vasculopathy, necrotizing M31.9
cardiac allograft T86.290
specified NEC M31.8
Vasitis (nodosa) N49.1
tuberculous A18.15
Vasodilation I73.9
Vasomotor — *see* condition
Vasoplasty, after previous sterilization Z31.0
aftercare Z31.42
Vasospasm (vasoconstriction) I73.9
cerebral (cerebrovascular) (artery) I67.848
reversible I67.841
coronary I20.1
nerve
arm — *see* Mononeuropathy, upper limb
brachial plexus G54.0
cervical plexus G54.2
leg — *see* Mononeuropathy, lower limb
peripheral NOS I73.9
retina (artery) — *see* Occlusion, artery, retina
Vasospastic — *see* condition
Vasovagal attack (paroxysmal) R55
psychogenic F45.8
VATER syndrome Q87.2
Vater's ampulla — *see* condition
Vegetation, vegetative
adenoid (nasal fossa) J35.8
endocarditis (acute) (any valve) (subacute) I33.0
heart (mycotic) (valve) I33.0
Veil
Jackson's Q43.3
Vein, venous — *see* condition
Veldt sore — *see* Ulcer, skin
Velpeau's hernia — *see* Hernia, femoral
Venereal
bubo A55
disease A64
granuloma inguinale A58

Venereal - *continued*
lymphogranuloma (Durand-Nicolas-Favre) A55
Venofibrosis I87.8
Venom, venomous — *see* Table of Drugs and Chemicals, by animal or substance, poisoning
Venous — *see* condition
Ventilator lung, newborn P27.8
Ventral — *see* condition
Ventricle, ventricular — *see also* condition
escape I49.3
inversion Q20.5
Ventriculitis (cerebral) — *see also* Encephalitis G04.90
Ventriculostomy status Z98.2
Vernet's syndrome G52.7
Verneuil's disease (syphilitic bursitis) A52.78
Verruca (due to HPV) (filiformis) (simplex) (viral) (vulgaris) B07.9
acuminata A63.0
necrogenica (primary) (tuberculosa) A18.4
plana B07.8
plantaris B07.0
seborrheica L82.1
inflamed L82.0
senile (seborrheic) L82.1
inflamed L82.0
tuberculosa (primary) A18.4
venereal A63.0
Verrucosities — *see* Verruca
Verruga peruana, peruviana A44.1
Version
cervix — *see* Malposition, uterus
uterus (postinfectional) (postpartal, old) — *see* Malposition, uterus
Vertebra, vertebral — *see* condition
Vertical talus (congenital) Q66.80
left foot Q66.82
right foot Q66.81
Vertigo R42
auditory — *see* Vertigo, aural
aural H81.31-
benign paroxysmal (positional) H81.1-
central (origin) H81.4
cerebral H81.4
Dix and Hallpike (epidemic) — *see* Neuronitis, vestibular
due to infrasound T75.23
epidemic A88.1
Dix and Hallpike — *see* Neuronitis, vestibular
Pedersen's — *see* Neuronitis, vestibular
vestibular neuronitis — *see* Neuronitis, vestibular
hysterical F44.89
infrasound T75.23
labyrinthine — *see* subcategory H81.0
laryngeal R05.4
malignant positional H81.4
Ménière's — *see* subcategory H81.0
menopausal N95.1
otogenic — *see* Vertigo, aural
paroxysmal positional, benign — *see* Vertigo, benign paroxysmal
Pedersen's (epidemic) — *see* Neuronitis, vestibular
peripheral NEC H81.39-
positional
benign paroxysmal — *see* Vertigo, benign paroxysmal
malignant H81.4
Very-low-density-lipoprotein-type (VLDL) hyperlipoproteinemia E78.1
Vesania — *see* Psychosis
Vesical — *see* condition
Vesicle
cutaneous R23.8
seminal — *see* condition
skin R23.8
Vesicocolic — *see* condition
Vesicoperineal — *see* condition
Vesicorectal — *see* condition
Vesicourethrorectal — *see* condition
Vesicovaginal — *see* condition

Vesicular — *see* condition
Vesiculitis (seminal) N49.0
amebic A06.82
gonorrheal (acute) (chronic) A54.23
trichomonal A59.09
tuberculous A18.15
Vestibulitis (ear) (*see also* subcategory H83.0)
nose (external) J34.89
vulvar N94.810
Vestibulopathy , acute peripheral (recurrent) — *see* Neuronitis, vestibular
Vestige, vestigial — *see also* Persistence
branchial Q18.0
structures in vitreous Q14.0
Vibration
adverse effects T75.20
pneumatic hammer syndrome T75.21
specified effect NEC T75.29
vasospastic syndrome T75.22
vertigo from infrasound T75.23
exposure (occupational) Z57.7
vertigo T75.23
Vibriosis A28.9
Victim (of)
crime Z65.4
disaster Z65.5
terrorism Z65.4
torture Z65.4
war Z65.5
Vidal's disease L28.0
Villaret's syndrome G52.7
Villous — *see* condition
VIN — *see* Neoplasia, intraepithelial, vulva
Vincent's infection (angina) (gingivitis) A69.1
stomatitis NEC A69.1
Vinson-Plummer syndrome D50.1
Violence, physical R45.6
Viosterol deficiency — *see* Deficiency, calciferol
Vipoma — *see* Neoplasm, malignant, by site
Viremia B34.9
Virilism (adrenal) E25.9
congenital E25.0
Virilization (female) (suprarenal) E25.9
congenital E25.0
isosexual E28.2
Virulent bubo A57
Virus, viral — *see also* condition
as cause of disease classified elsewhere B97.89
respiratory syncytial virus (RSV) — *see* Virus, respiratory syncytial (RSV)
cytomegalovirus B25.9
human immunodeficiency (HIV) — *see* Human, immunodeficiency virus (HIV) disease
infection — *see* Infection, virus
respiratory syncytial (RSV)
as cause of disease classified elsewhere B97.4
bronchiolitis J21.0
bronchitis J20.5
bronchopneumonia J12.1
otitis media H65.- *[B97.4]*
pneumonia J12.1
upper respiratory infection J06.9 *[B97.4]*
specified NEC B34.8
swine influenza (viruses that normally cause infections in pigs) — *see also* Influenza, due to, identified novel influenza A virus J09.X2
West Nile (fever) A92.30
with
complications NEC A92.39
cranial nerve disorders A92.32
encephalitis A92.31
encephalomyelitis A92.31
neurologic manifestation NEC A92.32
optic neuritis A92.32
polyradiculitis A92.32
Viscera, visceral — *see* condition
Visceroptosis K63.4
Visible peristalsis R19.2
Vision, visual
binocular, suppression H53.34
blurred, blurring H53.8
hysterical F44.6
defect, defective NEC H54.7
disorientation (syndrome) H53.8
disturbance H53.9
hysterical F44.6
double H53.2
examination Z01.00
with abnormal findings Z01.01
following failed vision screening Z01.020
with abnormal findings Z01.021
field, limitation (defect) — *see* Defect, visual field
hallucinations R44.1
halos H53.19
loss — *see* Loss, vision
sudden — *see* Disturbance, vision, subjective, loss, sudden
low (both eyes) — *see* Low, vision
perception, simultaneous without fusion H53.33
Vitality, lack or want of R53.83
newborn P96.89
Vitamin deficiency — *see* Deficiency, vitamin
Vitelline duct, persistent Q43.0
Vitiligo L80
eyelid H02.739
left H02.736
lower H02.735
upper H02.734
right H02.733
lower H02.732
upper H02.731
pinta A67.2
vulva N90.89
Vitreal corneal syndrome H59.01-
Vitreoretinopathy, proliferative — *see also* Retinopathy, proliferative
with retinal detachment — *see* Detachment, retina, traction
Vitreous — *see also* condition
touch syndrome — *see* Complication, postprocedural, following cataract surgery
Vocal cord — *see* condition
Vogt-Koyanagi syndrome H20.82-
Vogt's disease or syndrome G80.3
Vogt-Spielmeyer amaurotic idiocy or disease E75.4
Voice
change R49.9
specified NEC R49.8
loss — *see* Aphonia
Volhynian fever A79.0
Volkmann's ischemic contracture or paralysis (complicating trauma) T79.6
Volvulus (bowel) (colon) (intestine) K56.2
with perforation K56.2
congenital Q43.8
duodenum K31.5
fallopian tube — *see* Torsion, fallopian tube
oviduct — *see* Torsion, fallopian tube
stomach (due to absence of gastrocolic ligament) K31.89
Vomiting R11.10
with nausea R11.2
asphyxia — *see* Foreign body, by site, causing asphyxia, gastric contents
bilious (cause unknown) R11.14
in newborn P92.01
following gastro-intestinal surgery K91.0
blood — *see* Hematemesis
causing asphyxia, choking, or suffocation — *see* Foreign body, by site
cyclical, in migraine, G43.A0
with refractory migraine G43.A1
intractable G43.A1
not intractable G43.A0
psychogenic F50.89
without refractory migraine G43.A0
cyclical syndrome NOS (unrelated to migraine) R11.15
fecal mater R11.13
Vomiting - *continued*
following gastrointestinal surgery K91.0
psychogenic F50.89
functional K31.89
hysterical F50.89
nervous F50.89
neurotic F50.89
newborn NEC P92.09
bilious P92.01
periodic R11.10
psychogenic F50.89
persistent R11.15
projectile R11.12
psychogenic F50.89
uremic — *see* Uremia
without nausea R11.11
Vomito negro — *see* Fever, yellow
Von Bezold's abscess — *see* Mastoiditis, acute
Von Economo-Cruchet disease A85.8
Von Eulenburg's disease G71.19
Von Gierke's disease E74.01
Von Hippel (-Lindau) disease or syndrome Q85.8
Von Jaksch's anemia or disease D64.89
Von Recklinghausen
disease (neurofibromatosis) Q85.01
bones E21.0
Von Schroetter's syndrome I82.890
Von Willebrand (-Jurgens) (-Minot) disease or syndrome D68.0
Von Zumbusch's disease L40.1
Voyeurism F65.3
Vrolik's disease Q78.0
Vulva — *see* condition
Vulvismus N94.2
Vulvitis (acute) (allergic) (atrophic) (hypertrophic) (intertriginous) (senile) N76.2
with ectopic or molar pregnancy O08.0
adhesive, congenital Q52.79
blennorrhagic (gonococcal) A54.02
candidal B37.3
chlamydial A56.02
due to Haemophilus ducreyi A57
following ectopic or molar pregnancy O08.0
gonococcal A54.02
with abscess (accessory gland) (periurethral) A54.1
herpesviral A60.04
leukoplakic N90.4
monilial B37.3
puerperal (postpartum) O86.19
subacute or chronic N76.3
syphilitic (early) A51.0
late A52.76
trichomonal A59.01
tuberculous A18.18
Vulvodynia N94.819
specified NEC N94.818
Vulvorectal — *see* condition
Vulvovaginitis (acute) — *see* Vaginitis

W

Waiting list, person on Z75.1
for organ transplant Z76.82
undergoing social agency investigation Z75.2
Waldenström
hypergammaglobulinemia D89.0
syndrome or macroglobulinemia C88.0
Waldenström-Kjellberg syndrome D50.1
Walking
difficulty R26.2
psychogenic F44.4
sleep F51.3
hysterical F44.89
Wall, abdominal — *see* condition
Wallenberg's disease or syndrome G46.3
Wallgren's disease I87.8
Wandering
gallbladder, congenital Q44.1
in diseases classified elsewhere Z91.83
kidney, congenital Q63.8
organ or site, congenital NEC — *see* Malposition, congenital, by site
pacemaker (heart) I49.8
spleen D73.89

War neurosis F48.8
Wart (due to HPV) (filiform) (infectious) (viral) B07.9
anogenital region (venereal) A63.0
common B07.8
external genital organs (venereal) A63.0
flat B07.8
Hassal-Henle's (of cornea) H18.49
Peruvian A44.1
plantar B07.0
prosector (tuberculous) A18.4
seborrheic L82.1
inflamed L82.0
senile (seborrheic) L82.1
inflamed L82.0
tuberculous A18.4
venereal A63.0
Warthin's tumor — *see* Neoplasm, salivary gland, benign
Wassilieff's disease A27.0
Wasting
disease R64
due to malnutrition E43
with marasmus E41
extreme (due to malnutrition) E43
with marasmus E41
muscle NEC — *see* Atrophy, muscle
Water
clefts (senile cataract) — *see* Cataract, senile, incipient
deprivation of T73.1
intoxication E87.79
itch B76.9
lack of T73.1
safe drinking Z58.6
loading E87.70
on
brain — *see* Hydrocephalus
chest J94.8
poisoning E87.79
Waterbrash R12
Waterhouse (-Friderichsen) syndrome or disease (meningococcal) A39.1
Water-losing nephritis N25.89
Watermelon stomach K31.819
with hemorrhage K31.811
without hemorrhage K31.819
Watsoniasis B66.8
Wax in ear — *see* Impaction, cerumen
Weak, weakening, weakness (generalized) R53.1
arches (acquired) — *see also* Deformity, limb, flat foot
bladder (sphincter) R32
facial R29.810
following
cerebrovascular disease I69.992
cerebral infarction I69.392
intracerebral hemorrhage I69.192
nontraumatic intracranial hemorrhage NEC I69.292
specified disease NEC I69.892
stroke I69.392
subarachnoid hemorrhage I69.092
foot (double) — *see also* Weak, arches
heart, cardiac — *see* Failure, heart
mind F70
muscle M62.81
myocardium — *see* Failure, heart
newborn P96.89
pelvic fundus N81.89
pubocervical tissue N81.82
senile R54
rectovaginal tissue N81.83
urinary stream R39.12
valvular — *see* Endocarditis
Wear, worn (with normal or routine use)
articular bearing surface of internal joint prosthesis — *see* Complications, joint prosthesis, mechanical, wear of articular bearing surfaces, by site
device, implant or graft — *see* Complications, by site, mechanical complication

Wear, worn (with normal or routine use) - *continued*
tooth, teeth (approximal) (hard tissues) (interproximal) (occlusal) K03.0
Weather, weathered
effects of
cold T69.9
specified effect NEC T69.8
hot — *see* Heat
skin L57.8
Weaver's syndrome Q87.3
Web, webbed (congenital)
duodenal Q43.8
esophagus Q39.4
fingers Q70.1-
larynx (glottic) (subglottic) Q31.0
neck (pterygium colli) Q18.3
Paterson-Kelly D50.1
popliteal syndrome Q87.89
toes Q70.3-
Weber-Christian disease M35.6
Weber-Cockayne syndrome (epidermolysis bullosa) Q81.8
Weber-Gubler syndrome G46.3
Weber-Leyden syndrome G46.3
Weber-Osler syndrome I78.0
Weber's paralysis or syndrome G46.3
Wedge-shaped or wedging vertebra — *see* Collapse, vertebra NEC
Wegener's granulomatosis or syndrome M31.30
with
kidney involvement M31.31
lung involvement M31.30
with kidney involvement M31.31
Wegner's disease A50.02
Weight
1000-2499 grams at birth (low) — *see* Low, birthweight
999 grams or less at birth (extremely low) — *see* Low, birthweight, extreme
and length below 10th percentile for gestational age P05.1-
below but length above 10th percentile for gestational age P05.0-
gain (abnormal) (excessive) R63.5
in pregnancy — *see* Pregnancy, complicated by, excessive weight gain
low — *see* Pregnancy, complicated by, insufficient, weight gain
loss (abnormal) (cause unknown) R63.4
Weightlessness (effect of) T75.82
Weil (l) -Marchesani syndrome Q87.19
Weil's disease A27.0
Weingarten's syndrome J82.89
Weir Mitchell's disease I73.81
Weiss-Baker syndrome G90.09
Wells' disease L98.3
Wen — *see* Cyst, sebaceous
Wenckebach's block or phenomenon I44.1
Werdnig-Hoffmann syndrome (muscular atrophy) G12.0
Werlhof's disease D69.3
Wermer's disease or syndrome E31.21
Werner-His disease A79.0
Werner's disease or syndrome E34.8
Wernicke-Korsakoff's syndrome or psychosis (alcoholic) F10.96
with dependence F10.26
drug-induced
due to drug abuse — *see* Abuse, drug, by type, with amnestic disorder
due to drug dependence — *see* Dependence, drug, by type, with amnestic disorder
nonalcoholic F04
Wernicke-Posadas disease B38.9
Wernicke's
developmental aphasia F80.2
disease or syndrome E51.2
encephalopathy E51.2
polioencephalitis, superior E51.2
West African fever B50.8
Westphal-Strümpell syndrome E83.01
West's syndrome — *see* Epilepsy, spasms

Wet
feet, tropical (maceration) (syndrome) — *see* Immersion, foot
lung (syndrome) , newborn P22.1
Wharton's duct — *see* condition
Wheal — *see* Urticaria
Wheezing R06.2
Whiplash injury S13.4
Whipple's disease (*see also* subcategory M14.8-) K90.81
Whipworm (disease) (infection) (infestation) B79
Whistling face Q87.0
White — *see also* condition
kidney, small N03.9
leg, puerperal, postpartum, childbirth O87.1
mouth B37.0
patches of mouth K13.29
spot lesions, teeth
chewing surface K02.51
pit and fissure surface K02.51
smooth surface K02.61
Whitehead L70.0
Whitlow — *see also* Cellulitis, digit
with lymphangitis — *see* Lymphangitis, acute, digit
herpesviral B00.89
Whitmore's disease or fever — *see* Melioidosis
Whooping cough A37.90
with pneumonia A37.91
due to Bordetella
bronchiseptica A37.81
parapertussis A37.11
pertussis A37.01
specified organism NEC A37.81
due to
Bordetella
bronchiseptica A37.80
with pneumonia A37.81
parapertussis A37.10
with pneumonia A37.11
pertussis A37.00
with pneumonia A37.01
specified NEC A37.80
with pneumonia A37.81
Wichman's asthma J38.5
Wide cranial sutures, newborn P96.3
Widening aorta — *see* Ectasia, aorta
with aneurysm — *see* Aneurysm, aorta
Wilkie's disease or syndrome K55.1
Wilkinson-Sneddon disease or syndrome L13.1
Willebrand (-Jürgens) thrombopathy D68.0
Williams syndrome Q93.82
Willige-Hunt disease or syndrome G23.1
Wilms' tumor C64-
Wilson-Mikity syndrome P27.0
Wilson's
disease or syndrome E83.01
hepatolenticular degeneration E83.01
lichen ruber L43.9
Window — *see also* Imperfect, closure
aorticopulmonary Q21.4
Winter — *see* condition
Wiskott-Aldrich syndrome D82.0
Withdrawal state — *see also* Dependence, drug by type, with withdrawal
alcohol
with perceptual disturbances F10.232
without perceptual disturbances F10.239
caffeine F15.93
cannabis F12.23
newborn
correct therapeutic substance properly administered P96.2
infant of dependent mother P96.1
therapeutic substance, neonatal P96.2
Witts' anemia D50.8
Witzelsucht F07.0
Woakes' ethmoiditis or syndrome J33.1
Wolff-Hirschorn syndrome Q93.3
Wolff-Parkinson-White syndrome I45.6
Wolhynian fever A79.0
Wolman's disease E75.5

Wood lung or pneumonitis J67.8
Woolly, wooly hair (congenital) (nevus) Q84.1
Woolsorter's disease A22.1
Word
- blindness (congenital) (developmental) F81.0
- deafness (congenital) (developmental) H93.25

Worm (s) (infection) (infestation) — *see also* Infestation, helminth
- guinea B72
- in intestine NEC B82.0

Worm-eaten soles A66.3
Worn out — *see* Exhaustion
- cardiac
  - defibrillator (with synchronous cardiac pacemaker) Z45.02
  - pacemaker
    - battery Z45.010
    - lead Z45.018
- device, implant or graft — *see* Complications, by site, mechanical

Worried well Z71.1
Worries R45.82
Wound check Z48.0-
- due to injury - code to Injury, by site, using appropriate seventh character for subsequent encounter

Wound, open T14.8-
- abdomen, abdominal
  - wall S31.109
    - with penetration into peritoneal cavity S31.609
    - bite — *see* Bite, abdomen, wall
    - epigastric region S31.102
      - with penetration into peritoneal cavity S31.602
      - bite — *see* Bite, abdomen, wall, epigastric region
      - laceration — *see* Laceration, abdomen, wall, epigastric region
      - puncture — *see* Puncture, abdomen, wall, epigastric region
    - laceration — *see* Laceration, abdomen, wall
    - left
      - lower quadrant S31.104
        - with penetration into peritoneal cavity S31.604
        - bite — *see* Bite, abdomen, wall, left, lower quadrant
        - laceration — *see* Laceration, abdomen, wall, left, lower quadrant
        - puncture — *see* Puncture, abdomen, wall, left, lower quadrant
      - upper quadrant S31.101
        - with penetration into peritoneal cavity S31.601
        - bite — *see* Bite, abdomen, wall, left, upper quadrant
        - laceration — *see* Laceration, abdomen, wall, left, upper quadrant
        - puncture — *see* Puncture, abdomen, wall, left, upper quadrant
    - periumbilic region S31.105
      - with penetration into peritoneal cavity S31.605
      - bite — *see* Bite, abdomen, wall, periumbilic region
      - laceration — *see* Laceration, abdomen, wall, periumbilic region
      - puncture — *see* Puncture, abdomen, wall, periumbilic region
    - puncture — *see* Puncture, abdomen, wall
    - right
      - lower quadrant S31.103
        - with penetration into peritoneal cavity S31.603
        - bite — *see* Bite, abdomen, wall, right, lower quadrant

Wound, open - *continued*
- abdomen, abdominal - *continued*
  - wall - *continued*
    - right - *continued*
      - lower quadrant - *continued*
        - laceration — *see* Laceration, abdomen, wall, right, lower quadrant
        - puncture — *see* Puncture, abdomen, wall, right, lower quadrant
      - upper quadrant S31.100
        - with penetration into peritoneal cavity S31.600
        - bite — *see* Bite, abdomen, wall, right, upper quadrant
        - laceration — *see* Laceration, abdomen, wall, right, upper quadrant
        - puncture — *see* Puncture, abdomen, wall, right, upper quadrant
- alveolar (process) — *see* Wound, open, oral cavity
- ankle S91.00-
  - bite — *see* Bite, ankle
  - laceration — *see* Laceration, ankle
  - puncture — *see* Puncture, ankle
- antecubital space — *see* Wound, open, elbow
- anterior chamber, eye — *see* Wound, open, ocular
- anus S31.839
  - bite S31.835
  - laceration — *see* Laceration, anus
  - puncture — *see* Puncture, anus
- arm (upper) S41.10-
  - with amputation — *see* Amputation, traumatic, arm
  - bite — *see* Bite, arm
  - forearm — *see* Wound, open, forearm
  - laceration — *see* Laceration, arm
  - puncture — *see* Puncture, arm
- auditory canal (external) (meatus) — *see* Wound, open, ear
- auricle, ear — *see* Wound, open, ear
- axilla — *see* Wound, open, arm
- back — *see also* Wound, open, thorax, back
  - lower S31.000
    - with penetration into retroperitoneal space S31.001
    - bite — *see* Bite, back, lower
    - laceration — *see* Laceration, back, lower
    - puncture — *see* Puncture, back, lower
- bite — *see* Bite
- blood vessel — *see* Injury, blood vessel
- breast S21.00-
  - with amputation — *see* Amputation, traumatic, breast
  - bite — *see* Bite, breast
  - laceration — *see* Laceration, breast
  - puncture — *see* Puncture, breast
- buttock S31.809
  - bite — *see* Bite, buttock
  - laceration — *see* Laceration, buttock
  - left S31.829
  - puncture — *see* Puncture, buttock
  - right S31.819
- calf — *see* Wound, open, leg
- canaliculus lacrimalis — *see* Wound, open, eyelid
- canthus, eye — *see* Wound, open, eyelid
- cervical esophagus S11.20
  - bite S11.25
  - laceration — *see* Laceration, esophagus, traumatic, cervical
  - puncture — *see* Puncture, cervical esophagus
- cheek (external) S01.40-
  - bite — *see* Bite, cheek
  - laceration — *see* Laceration, cheek
  - puncture — *see* Puncture, cheek
  - internal — *see* Wound, open, oral cavity
- chest wall — *see* Wound, open, thorax
- chin — *see* Wound, open, head, specified site NEC
- choroid — *see* Wound, open, ocular

Wound, open - *continued*
- ciliary body (eye) — *see* Wound, open, ocular
- clitoris S31.40
  - with amputation — *see* Amputation, traumatic, clitoris
  - bite S31.45
  - laceration — *see* Laceration, vulva
  - puncture — *see* Puncture, vulva
- conjunctiva — *see* Wound, open, ocular
- cornea — *see* Wound, open, ocular
- costal region — *see* Wound, open, thorax
- Descemet's membrane — *see* Wound, open, ocular
- digit (s)
  - foot — *see* Wound, open, toe
  - hand — *see* Wound, open, finger
- ear (canal) (external) S01.30-
  - with amputation — *see* Amputation, traumatic, ear
  - bite — *see* Bite, ear
  - laceration — *see* Laceration, ear
  - puncture — *see* Puncture, ear
  - drum S09.2-
- elbow S51.00-
  - bite — *see* Bite, elbow
  - laceration — *see* Laceration, elbow
  - puncture — *see* Puncture, elbow
- epididymis — *see* Wound, open, testis
- epigastric region S31.102
  - with penetration into peritoneal cavity S31.602
  - bite — *see* Bite, abdomen, wall, epigastric region
  - laceration — *see* Laceration, abdomen, wall, epigastric region
  - puncture — *see* Puncture, abdomen, wall, epigastric region
- epiglottis — *see* Wound, open, neck, specified site NEC
- esophagus (thoracic) S27.819
  - cervical — *see* Wound, open, cervical esophagus
  - laceration S27.813
  - specified type NEC S27.818
- eye — *see* Wound, open, ocular
- eyeball — *see* Wound, open, ocular
- eyebrow — *see* Wound, open, eyelid
- eyelid S01.10-
  - bite — *see* Bite, eyelid
  - laceration — *see* Laceration, eyelid
  - puncture — *see* Puncture, eyelid
- face NEC — *see* Wound, open, head, specified site NEC
- finger (s) S61.209
  - with
    - amputation — *see* Amputation, traumatic, finger
    - damage to nail S61.309
  - bite — *see* Bite, finger
  - index S61.208
    - with
      - damage to nail S61.308
    - left S61.201
      - with
        - damage to nail S61.301
    - right S61.200
      - with
        - damage to nail S61.300
  - laceration — *see* Laceration, finger
  - little S61.208
    - with
      - damage to nail S61.308
    - left S61.207
      - with damage to nail S61.307
    - right S61.206
      - with damage to nail S61.306
  - middle S61.208
    - with
      - damage to nail S61.308
    - left S61.203
      - with damage to nail S61.303
    - right S61.202
      - with damage to nail S61.302
  - puncture — *see* Puncture, finger

Wound, open - *continued*
pudendum — *see* Wound, open, genital organs, external
puncture wound — *see* Puncture
rectovaginal septum — *see* Wound, open, vagina
right
lower quadrant S31.103
with penetration into peritoneal cavity S31.603
bite — *see* Bite, abdomen, wall, right, lower quadrant
laceration — *see* Laceration, abdomen, wall, right, lower quadrant
puncture — *see* Puncture, abdomen, wall, right, lower quadrant
upper quadrant S31.100
with penetration into peritoneal cavity S31.600
bite — *see* Bite, abdomen, wall, right, upper quadrant
laceration — *see* Laceration, abdomen, wall, right, upper quadrant
puncture — *see* Puncture, abdomen, wall, right, upper quadrant
sacral region — *see* Wound, open, back, lower
sacroiliac region — *see* Wound, open, back, lower
salivary gland — *see* Wound, open, oral cavity
scalp S01.00
bite S01.05
laceration — *see* Laceration, scalp
puncture — *see* Puncture, scalp
scalpel, newborn (birth injury) P15.8
scapular region — *see* Wound, open, shoulder
sclera — *see* Wound, open, ocular
scrotum S31.30
with amputation — *see* Amputation, traumatic, scrotum
bite S31.35
laceration — *see* Laceration, scrotum
puncture — *see* Puncture, scrotum
shin — *see* Wound, open, leg
shoulder S41.00-
with amputation — *see* Amputation, traumatic, arm
bite — *see* Bite, shoulder
laceration — *see* Laceration, shoulder
puncture — *see* Puncture, shoulder
skin NOS T14.8
spermatic cord — *see* Wound, open, testis
sternal region — *see* Wound, open, thorax, front wall
submaxillary region — *see* Wound, open, head, specified site NEC
submental region — *see* Wound, open, head, specified site NEC
subungual
finger (s) — *see* Wound, open, finger
toe (s) — *see* Wound, open, toe
supraclavicular region — *see* Wound, open, neck, specified site NEC
temple, temporal region — *see* Wound, open, head, specified site NEC
temporomandibular area — *see* Wound, open, cheek
testis S31.30
with amputation — *see* Amputation, traumatic, testes
bite S31.35
laceration — *see* Laceration, testis
puncture — *see* Puncture, testis
thigh S71.10-
with amputation — *see* Amputation, traumatic, hip
bite — *see* Bite, thigh
laceration — *see* Laceration, thigh
puncture — *see* Puncture, thigh
thorax, thoracic (wall) S21.90
back S21.20-
with penetration S21.40
bite — *see* Bite, thorax

Wound, open - *continued*
thorax, thoracic (wall) - *continued*
breast — *see* Wound, open, breast
front S21.10-
with penetration S21.30
laceration — *see* Laceration, thorax
puncture — *see* Puncture, thorax
throat — *see* Wound, open, neck
thumb S61.009
with
amputation — *see* Amputation, traumatic, thumb
damage to nail S61.109
bite — *see* Bite, thumb
laceration — *see* Laceration, thumb
left S61.002
with
damage to nail S61.102
puncture — *see* Puncture, thumb
right S61.001
with
damage to nail S61.101
thyroid (gland) — *see* Wound, open, neck, thyroid
toe (s) S91.109
with
amputation — *see* Amputation, traumatic, toe
damage to nail S91.209
bite — *see* Bite, toe
great S91.103
with
damage to nail S91.203
left S91.102
with
damage to nail S91.202
right S91.101
with
damage to nail S91.201
laceration — *see* Laceration, toe
lesser S91.106
with
damage to nail S91.206
left S91.105
with
damage to nail S91.205
right S91.104
with
damage to nail S91.204
puncture — *see* Puncture, toe
tongue — *see* Wound, open, oral cavity
trachea (cervical region) — *see* Wound, open, neck, trachea
tunica vaginalis — *see* Wound, open, testis
tympanum, tympanic membrane S09.2-
laceration — *see* Laceration, ear, drum
puncture — *see* Puncture, tympanum
umbilical region — *see* Wound, open, abdomen, wall, periumbilic region
uvula — *see* Wound, open, oral cavity
vagina S31.40
bite S31.45
laceration — *see* Laceration, vagina
puncture — *see* Puncture, vagina
vocal cord S11.039
bite — *see* Bite, vocal cord
laceration S11.031
with foreign body S11.032
puncture S11.033
with foreign body S11.034
vitreous (humor) — *see* Wound, open, ocular
vulva S31.40
with amputation — *see* Amputation, traumatic, vulva
bite S31.45
laceration — *see* Laceration, vulva
puncture — *see* Puncture, vulva
wrist S61.50-
bite — *see* Bite, wrist
laceration — *see* Laceration, wrist
puncture — *see* Puncture, wrist
Wound, superficial — *see* Injury — *see also* specified injury type
Wright's syndrome G54.0
Wrist — *see* condition

Wrong drug (by accident) (given in error) — *see* Table of Drugs and Chemicals, by drug, poisoning
Wry neck — *see* Torticollis
Wuchereria (bancrofti) infestation B74.0
Wuchereriasis B74.0
Wucherende Struma Langhans C73

X

Xanthelasma (eyelid) (palpebrarum) H02.60
left H02.66
lower H02.65
upper H02.64
right H02.63
lower H02.62
upper H02.61
Xanthelasmatosis (essential) E78.2
Xanthinuria, hereditary E79.8
Xanthoastrocytoma
specified site — *see* Neoplasm, malignant, by site
unspecified site C71.9
Xanthofibroma — *see* Neoplasm, connective tissue, benign
Xanthogranuloma D76.3
Xanthoma (s) , xanthomatosis (primary) (familial) (hereditary) E75.5
with
hyperlipoproteinemia
Type I E78.3
Type III E78.2
Type IV E78.1
Type V E78.3
bone (generalisata) C96.5
cerebrotendinous E75.5
cutaneotendinous E75.5
disseminatum (skin) E78.2
eruptive E78.2
hypercholesterinemic E78.00
hypercholesterolemic E78.00
hyperlipidemic E78.5
joint E75.5
multiple (skin) E78.2
tendon (sheath) E75.5
tubo-eruptive E78.2
tuberosum E78.2
tuberous E78.2
verrucous, oral mucosa K13.4
Xanthosis R23.8
Xenophobia F40.10
Xeroderma — *see also* Ichthyosis
acquired L85.0
eyelid H01.149
left H01.146
lower H01.145
upper H01.144
right H01.143
lower H01.142
upper H01.141
pigmentosum Q82.1
vitamin A deficiency E50.8
Xerophthalmia (vitamin A deficiency) E50.7
unrelated to vitamin A deficiency — *see* Keratoconjunctivitis
Xerosis
conjunctiva H11.14-
with Bitot's spots — *see also* Pigmentation, conjunctiva
vitamin A deficiency E50.1
vitamin A deficiency E50.0
cornea H18.89-
with ulceration — *see* Ulcer, cornea
vitamin A deficiency E50.3
vitamin A deficiency E50.2
cutis (dry skin) L85.3
skin L85.3
Xerostomia K11.7
Xiphopagus Q89.4
XO syndrome Q96.9
X-ray (of)
abnormal findings — *see* Abnormal, diagnostic imaging
breast (mammogram) (routine) Z12.31
chest
routine (as part of a general medical examination) Z00.00

Neoplasm Table

1. The list below gives the code numbers for neoplasms by anatomical site. For each site there are six possible code numbers according to whether the neoplasm in question is malignant, benign, in situ, of uncertain behavior, or of unspecified nature. The description of the neoplasm will often indicate which of the six columns is appropriate; e.g., malignant melanoma of skin, benign fibroadenoma of breast, carcinoma in situ of cervix uteri. Where such descriptors are not present, the remainder of the Index should be consulted where guidance is given to the appropriate column for each morphological (histological) variety listed; e.g., Mesonephroma -- see Neoplasm, malignant; Embryoma -- see also Neoplasm, uncertain behavior; Disease, Bowen's -- see Neoplasm, skin, in situ. However, the guidance in the Index can be overridden if one of the descriptors mentioned above is present; e.g., malignant adenoma of colon to C18.9 and not to D12.6 as the adjective "malignant" overrides the Index entry "Adenoma - see also Neoplasm, benign."

2. Codes listed with a dash -, following the code have a required additional character for laterality. The tabular must be reviewed for the complete code.

	Malignant Primary	Malignant Secondary	Ca in situ	Benign	Uncertain Behavior	Unspecified Behavior
Neoplasm, neoplastic	**C80.1**	**C79.9**	**D09.9**	**D36.9**	**D48.9**	**D49.9**
abdomen, abdominal	C76.2	C79.8-	D09.8	D36.7	D48.7	D49.89
cavity	C76.2	C79.8-	D09.8	D36.7	D48.7	D49.89
organ	C76.2	C79.8-	D09.8	D36.7	D48.7	D49.89
viscera	C76.2	C79.8-	D09.8	D36.7	D48.7	D49.89
wall — *see also Neoplasm, abdomen, wall, skin*	C44.509	C79.2-	D04.5	D23.5	D48.5	D49.2
connective tissue	C49.4	C79.8-	-	D21.4	D48.1	D49.2
skin	C44.509					
basal cell carcinoma	C44.519	-	-	-	-	-
specified type NEC	C44.599	-	-	-	-	-
squamous cell carcinoma	C44.529	-	-	-	-	-
abdominopelvic	C76.8	C79.8-	-	D36.7	D48.7	D49.89
accessory sinus — *see Neoplasm, sinus*						
acoustic nerve	C72.4-	C79.49	-	D33.3	D43.3	D49.7
adenoid (pharynx) (tissue)	C11.1	C79.89	D00.08	D10.6	D37.05	D49.0
adipose tissue — *see also Neoplasm, connective tissue*	C49.4	C79.89	-	D21.9	D48.1	D49.2
adnexa (uterine)	C57.4	C79.89	D07.39	D28.7	D39.8	D49.59
adrenal	C74.9-	C79.7-	D09.3	D35.0-	D44.1-	D49.7
capsule	C74.9-	C79.7-	D09.3	D35.0-	D44.1-	D49.7
cortex	C74.0-	C79.7-	D09.3	D35.0-	D44.1-	D49.7
gland	C74.9-	C79.7-	D09.3	D35.0-	D44.1-	D49.7
medulla	C74.1-	C79.7-	D09.3	D35.0-	D44.1-	D49.7
ala nasi (external) — *see also Neoplasm, skin, nose*	C44.301	C79.2	D04.39	D23.39	D48.5	D49.2
alimentary canal or tract NEC	C26.9	C78.80	D01.9	D13.9	D37.9	D49.0
alveolar	C03.9	C79.89	D00.03	D10.39	D37.09	D49.0
mucosa	C03.9	C79.89	D00.03	D10.39	D37.09	D49.0
lower	C03.1	C79.89	D00.03	D10.39	D37.09	D49.0
upper	C03.0	C79.89	D00.03	D10.39	D37.09	D49.0
ridge or process	C41.1	C79.51	-	D16.5-	D48.0	D49.2
carcinoma	C03.9	C79.8-	-	-	-	-
lower	C03.1	C79.8-	-	-	-	-
upper	C03.0	C79.8-	-	-	-	-
lower	C41.1	C79.51	-	D16.5-	D48.0	D49.2
mucosa	C03.9	C79.89	D00.03	D10.39	D37.09	D49.0
lower	C03.1	C79.89	D00.03	D10.39	D37.09	D49.0
upper	C03.0	C79.89	D00.03	D10.39	D37.09	D49.0
upper	C41.0	C79.51	-	D16.4-	D48.0	D49.2
sulcus	C06.1	C79.89	D00.02	D10.39	D37.09	D49.0
alveolus	C03.9	C79.89	D00.03	D10.39	D37.09	D49.0
lower	C03.1	C79.89	D00.03	D10.39	D37.09	D49.0
upper	C03.0	C79.89	D00.03	D10.39	D37.09	D49.0
ampulla of Vater	C24.1	C78.89	D01.5	D13.5	D37.6	D49.0
ankle NEC	C76.5-	C79.89	D04.7-	D36.7	D48.7	D49.89
anorectum, anorectal (junction)	C21.8	C78.5	D01.3	D12.9	D37.8	D49.0
antecubital fossa or space	C76.4-	C79.89	D04.6-	D36.7	D48.7	D49.89
antrum (Highmore) (maxillary)	C31.0	C78.39	D02.3	D14.0	D38.5	D49.1

Neoplasm, neoplastic	Malignant Primary	Malignant Secondary	Ca in situ	Benign	Uncertain Behavior	Unspecified Behavior
pyloric	C16.3	C78.89	D00.2	D13.1	D37.1	D49.0
tympanicum	C30.1	C78.39	D02.3	D14.0	D38.5	D49.1
anus, anal	C21.0	C78.5	D01.3	D12.9	D37.8	D49.0
canal	C21.1	C78.5	D01.3	D12.9	D37.8	D49.0
cloacogenic zone	C21.2	C78.5	D01.3	D12.9	D37.8	D49.0
margin — *see also Neoplasm, anus, skin*	C44.500	C79.2	D04.5	D23.5	D48.5	D49.2
overlapping lesion with rectosigmoid junction or rectum	C21.8	-	-	-	-	-
skin	C44.500	C79.2	D04.5	D23.5	D48.5	D49.2
basal cell carcinoma	C44.510	-	-	-	-	-
specified type NEC	C44.590	-	-	-	-	-
squamous cell carcinoma	C44.520	-	-	-	-	-
sphincter	C21.1	C78.5	D01.3	D12.9	D37.8	D49.0
aorta (thoracic)	C49.3	C79.89	-	D21.3	D48.1	D49.2
abdominal	C49.4	C79.89	-	D21.4	D48.1	D49.2
aortic body	C75.5	C79.89	-	D35.6	D44.7	D49.7
aponeurosis	C49.9	C79.89	-	D21.9	D48.1	D49.2
palmar	C49.1-	C79.89	-	D21.1-	D48.1	D49.2
plantar	C49.2-	C79.89	-	D21.2-	D48.1	D49.2
appendix	C18.1	C78.5	D01.0	D12.1	D37.3	D49.0
arachnoid	C70.9	C79.49	-	D32.9	D42.9	D49.7
cerebral	C70.0	C79.32	-	D32.0	D42.0	D49.7
spinal	C70.1	C79.49	-	D32.1	D42.1	D49.7
areola	C50.0-	C79.81	D05.-	D24.-	D48.6-	D49.3
arm NEC	C76.4-	C79.89	D04.6-	D36.7	D48.7	D49.89
artery — *see Neoplasm, connective tissue*						
aryepiglottic fold	C13.1	C79.89	D00.08	D10.7	D37.05	D49.0
hypopharyngeal aspect	C13.1	C79.89	D00.08	D10.7	D37.05	D49.0
laryngeal aspect	C32.1	C78.39	D02.0	D14.1	D38.0	D49.1
marginal zone	C13.1	C79.89	D00.08	D10.7	D37.05	D49.0
arytenoid (cartilage)	C32.3	C78.39	D02.0	D14.1	D38.0	D49.1
fold — *see Neoplasm, aryepiglottic*						
associated with transplanted organ	C80.2	-	-	-	-	-
atlas	C41.2	C79.51	-	D16.6	D48.0	D49.2
atrium, cardiac	C38.0	C79.89	-	D15.1	D48.7	D49.89
auditory						
canal (external) (skin)	C44.20-	C79.2	D04.2-	D23.2-	D48.5	D49.2
internal	C30.1	C78.39	D02.3	D14.0	D38.5	D49.1
nerve	C72.4-	C79.49	-	D33.3	D43.3	D49.7
tube	C30.1	C78.39	D02.3	D14.0	D38.5	D49.1
opening	C11.2	C79.89	D00.08	D10.6	D37.05	D49.0
auricle, ear — *see also Neoplasm, skin, ear*	C44.20-	C79.2	D04.2-	D23.2-	D48.5	D49.2
auricular canal (external) — *see also Neoplasm, skin, ear*	C44.20-	C79.2	D04.2-	D23.2-	D48.5	D49.2
internal	C30.1	C78.39	D02.3	D14.0	D38.5	D49.2
autonomic nerve or nervous system NEC (see Neoplasm, nerve, peripheral)						
axilla, axillary	C76.1	C79.89	D09.8	D36.7	D48.7	D49.89
fold — *see also Neoplasm, skin, trunk*	C44.509	C79.2	D04.5	D23.5	D48.5	D49.2
back NEC	C76.8	C79.89	D04.5	D36.7	D48.7	D49.89
Bartholin's gland	C51.0	C79.82	D07.1	D28.0	D39.8	D49.59
basal ganglia	C71.0	C79.31	-	D33.0	D43.0	D49.6
basis pedunculi	C71.7	C79.31	-	D33.1	D43.1	D49.6
bile or biliary (tract)	C24.9	C78.89	D01.5	D13.5	D37.6	D49.0
canaliculi (biliferi) (intrahepatic)	C22.1	C78.7	D01.5	D13.4	D37.6	D49.0
canals, interlobular	C22.1	C78.89	D01.5	D13.4	D37.6	D49.0

Neoplasm, neoplastic	Malignant Primary	Malignant Secondary	Ca in situ	Benign	Uncertain Behavior	Unspecified Behavior
duct or passage (common) (cystic) (extrahepatic)	C24.0	C78.89	D01.5	D13.5	D37.6	D49.0
interlobular	C22.1	C78.89	D01.5	D13.4	D37.6	D49.0
intrahepatic	C22.1	C78.7	D01.5	D13.4	D37.6	D49.0
and extrahepatic	C24.8	C78.89	D01.5	D13.5	D37.6	D49.0
bladder (urinary)	C67.9	C79.11	D09.0	D30.3	D41.4	D49.4
dome	C67.1	C79.11	D09.0	D30.3	D41.4	D49.4
neck	C67.5	C79.11	D09.0	D30.3	D41.4	D49.4
orifice	C67.9	C79.11	D09.0	D30.3	D41.4	D49.4
ureteric	C67.6	C79.11	D09.0	D30.3	D41.4	D49.4
urethral	C67.5	C79.11	D09.0	D30.3	D41.4	D49.4
overlapping lesion	C67.8	-	-	-	-	-
sphincter	C67.8	C79.11	D09.0	D30.3	D41.4	D49.4
trigone	C67.0	C79.11	D09.0	D30.3	D41.4	D49.4
urachus	C67.7	C79.11	D09.0	D30.3	D41.4	D49.4
wall	C67.9	C79.11	D09.0	D30.3	D41.4	D49.4
anterior	C67.3	C79.11	D09.0	D30.3	D41.4	D49.4
lateral	C67.2	C79.11	D09.0	D30.3	D41.4	D49.4
posterior	C67.4	C79.11	D09.0	D30.3	D41.4	D49.4
blood vessel — *see Neoplasm, connective tissue*						
bone (periosteum)	C41.9	C79.51	-	D16.9-	D48.0	D49.2
acetabulum	C41.4	C79.51	-	D16.8-	D48.0	D49.2
ankle	C40.3-	C79.51	-	D16.3-	-	-
arm NEC	C40.0-	C79.51	-	D16.0-	-	-
astragalus	C40.3-	C79.51	-	D16.3-	-	-
atlas	C41.2	C79.51	-	D16.6-	D48.0	D49.2
axis	C41.2	C79.51	-	D16.6-	D48.0	D49.2
back NEC	C41.2	C79.51	-	D16.6-	D48.0	D49.2
calcaneus	C40.3-	C79.51	-	D16.3-	-	-
calvarium	C41.0	C79.51	-	D16.4-	D48.0	D49.2
carpus (any)	C40.1-	C79.51	-	D16.1-	-	-
cartilage NEC	C41.9	C79.51	-	D16.9-	D48.0	D49.2
clavicle	C41.3	C79.51	-	D16.7-	D48.0	D49.2
clivus	C41.0	C79.51	-	D16.4-	D48.0	D49.2
coccygeal vertebra	C41.4	C79.51	-	D16.8-	D48.0	D49.2
coccyx	C41.4	C79.51	-	D16.8-	D48.0	D49.2
costal cartilage	C41.3	C79.51	-	D16.7-	D48.0	D49.2
costovertebral joint	C41.3	C79.51	-	D16.7-	D48.0	D49.2
cranial	C41.0	C79.51	-	D16.4-	D48.0	D49.2
cuboid	C40.3-	C79.51	-	D16.3-	-	-
cuneiform	C41.9	C79.51	-	D16.9-	D48.0	D49.2
elbow	C40.0-	C79.51	-	D16.0-	-	-
ethmoid (labyrinth)	C41.0	C79.51	-	D16.4-	D48.0	D49.2
face	C41.0	C79.51	-	D16.4-	D48.0	D49.2
femur (any part)	C40.2-	C79.51	-	D16.2-	-	-
fibula (any part)	C40.2-	C79.51	-	D16.2-	-	-
finger (any)	C40.1-	C79.51	-	D16.1-	-	-
foot	C40.3-	C79.51	-	D16.3-	-	-
forearm	C40.0-	C79.51	-	D16.0-	-	-
frontal	C41.0	C79.51	-	D16.4-	D48.0	D49.2
hand	C40.1-	C79.51	-	D16.1-	-	-
heel	C40.3-	C79.51	-	D16.3-	-	-
hip	C41.4	C79.51	-	D16.8-	D48.0	D49.2
humerus (any part)	C40.0-	C79.51	-	D16.0-	-	-
hyoid	C41.0	C79.51	-	D16.4-	D48.0	D49.2
ilium	C41.4	C79.51	-	D16.8-	D48.0	D49.2
innominate	C41.4	C79.51	-	D16.8-	D48.0	D49.2
intervertebral cartilage or disc	C41.2	C79.51	-	D16.6-	D48.0	D49.2
ischium	C41.4	C79.51	-	D16.8-	D48.0	D49.2

	Malignant Primary	Malignant Secondary	Ca in situ	Benign	Uncertain Behavior	Unspecified Behavior
Neoplasm, neoplastic						
jaw (lower)	C41.1	C79.51	-	D16.5-	D48.0	D49.2
knee	C40.2-	C79.51	-	D16.2-	-	-
leg NEC	C40.2-	C79.51	-	D16.2-	-	-
limb NEC	C40.9-	C79.51	-	D16.9-	-	-
lower (long bones)	C40.2-	C79.51	-	D16.2-	-	-
short bones	C40.3-	C79.51	-	D16.3-	-	-
upper (long bones)	C40.0-	C79.51	-	D16.0-	-	-
short bones	C40.1-	C79.51	-	D16.1-	-	-
malar	C41.0	C79.51	-	D16.4-	D48.0	D49.2
mandible	C41.1	C79.51	-	D16.5-	D48.0	D49.2
marrow NEC (any bone)	C96.9	C79.52	-	-	D47.9	D49.89
mastoid	C41.0	C79.51	-	D16.4-	D48.0	D49.2
maxilla, maxillary (superior)	C41.0	C79.51	-	D16.4-	D48.0	D49.2
inferior	C41.1	C79.51	-	D16.5-	D48.0	D49.2
metacarpus (any)	C40.1-	C79.51	-	D16.1-	-	-
metatarsus (any)	C40.3-	C79.51	-	D16.3-	-	-
overlapping sites	C40.8-	-	-	-	-	-
navicular						
ankle	C40.3-	C79.51	-	-	-	-
hand	C40.1-	C79.51	-	-	-	-
nose, nasal	C41.0	C79.51	-	D16.4-	D48.0	D49.2
occipital	C41.0	C79.51	-	D16.4-	D48.0	D49.2
orbit	C41.0	C79.51	-	D16.4-	D48.0	D49.2
parietal	C41.0	C79.51	-	D16.4-	D48.0	D49.2
patella	C40.2-	C79.51	-	-	-	-
pelvic	C41.4	C79.51	-	D16.8	D48.0	D49.2
phalanges						
foot	C40.3-	C79.51	-	-	-	-
hand	C40.1-	C79.51	-	-	-	-
pubic	C41.4	C79.51	-	D16.8	D48.0	D49.2
radius (any part)	C40.0-	C79.51	-	D16.0-	-	-
rib	C41.3	C79.51	-	D16.7	D48.0	D49.2
sacral vertebra	C41.4	C79.51	-	D16.8	D48.0	D49.2
sacrum	C41.4	C79.51	-	D16.8	D48.0	D49.2
scaphoid						
of ankle	C40.3-	C79.51	-	-	-	-
of hand	C40.1-	C79.51	-	-	-	-
scapula (any part)	C40.0-	C79.51	-	D16.0-	-	-
sella turcica	C41.0	C79.51	-	D16.4-	D48.0	D49.2
shoulder	C40.0-	C79.51	-	D16.0-	-	-
skull	C41.0	C79.51	-	D16.4-	D48.0	D49.2
sphenoid	C41.0	C79.51	-	D16.4-	D48.0	D49.2
spine, spinal (column)	C41.2	C79.51	-	D16.6	D48.0	D49.2
coccyx	C41.4	C79.51	-	D16.8	D48.0	D49.2
sacrum	C41.4	C79.51	-	D16.8	D48.0	D49.2
sternum	C41.3	C79.51	-	D16.7	D48.0	D49.2
tarsus (any)	C40.3-	C79.51	-	-	-	-
temporal	C41.0	C79.51	-	D16.4-	D48.0	D49.2
thumb	C40.1-	C79.51	-	-	-	-
tibia (any part)	C40.2-	C79.51	-	-	-	-
toe (any)	C40.3-	C79.51	-	-	-	-
trapezium	C40.1-	C79.51	-	-	-	-
trapezoid	C40.1-	C79.51	-	-	-	-
turbinate	C41.0	C79.51	-	D16.4-	D48.0	D49.2
ulna (any part)	C40.0-	C79.51	-	D16.0-	-	-
unciform	C40.1-	C79.51	-	-	-	-
vertebra (column)	C41.2	C79.51	-	D16.6	D48.0	D49.2
coccyx	C41.4	C79.51	-	D16.8	D48.0	D49.2
sacrum	C41.4	C79.51	-	D16.8	D48.0	D49.2

Neoplasm, neoplastic	Malignant Primary	Malignant Secondary	Ca in situ	Benign	Uncertain Behavior	Unspecified Behavior
vomer	C41.0	C79.51	-	D16.4-	D48.0	D49.2
wrist	C40.1-	C79.51	-	-	-	-
xiphoid process	C41.3	C79.51	-	D16.7	D48.0	D49.2
zygomatic	C41.0	C79.51	-	D16.4-	D48.0	D49.2
book-leaf (mouth)	C06.89	C79.89	D00.00	D10.39	D37.09	D49.0
bowel — *see Neoplasm, intestine*						
brachial plexus	C47.1-	C79.89	-	D36.12	D48.2	D49.2
brain NEC	C71.9	C79.31	-	D33.2	D43.2	D49.6
basal ganglia	C71.0	C79.31	-	D33.0	D43.0	D49.6
cerebellopontine angle	C71.6	C79.31	-	D33.1	D43.1	D49.6
cerebellum NOS	C71.6	C79.31	-	D33.1	D43.1	D49.6
cerebrum	C71.0	C79.31	-	D33.0	D43.0	D49.6
choroid plexus	C71.7	C79.31	-	D33.1	D43.1	D49.6
corpus callosum	C71.8	C79.31	-	D33.2	D43.2	D49.6
corpus striatum	C71.0	C79.31	-	D33.0	D43.0	D49.6
cortex (cerebral)	C71.0	C79.31	-	D33.0	D43.0	D49.6
frontal lobe	C71.1	C79.31	-	D33.0	D43.0	D49.6
globus pallidus	C71.0	C79.31	-	D33.0	D43.0	D49.6
hippocampus	C71.2	C79.31	-	D33.0	D43.0	D49.6
hypothalamus	C71.0	C79.31	-	D33.0	D43.0	D49.6
internal capsule	C71.0	C79.31	-	D33.0	D43.0	D49.6
medulla oblongata	C71.7	C79.31	-	D33.1	D43.1	D49.6
meninges	C70.0	C79.32	-	D32.0	D42.0	D49.7
midbrain	C71.7	C79.31	-	D33.1	D43.1	D49.6
occipital lobe	C71.4	C79.31	-	D33.0	D43.0	D49.6
overlapping lesion	C71.8	C79.31	-	-	-	-
parietal lobe	C71.3	C79.31	-	D33.0	D43.0	D49.6
peduncle	C71.7	C79.31	-	D33.1	D43.1	D49.6
pons	C71.7	C79.31	-	D33.1	D43.1	D49.6
stem	C71.7	C79.31	-	D33.1	D43.1	D49.6
tapetum	C71.8	C79.31	-	D33.2	D43.2	D49.6
temporal lobe	C71.2	C79.31	-	D33.0	D43.0	D49.6
thalamus	C71.0	C79.31	-	D33.0	D43.0	D49.6
uncus	C71.2	C79.31	-	D33.0	D43.0	D49.6
ventricle (floor)	C71.5	C79.31	-	D33.0	D43.0	D49.6
fourth	C71.7	C79.31	-	D33.1	D43.1	D49.6
branchial (cleft) (cyst) (vestiges)	C10.4	C79.89	D00.08	D10.5	D37.05	D49.0
breast (connective tissue) (glandular tissue) (soft parts)	C50.9-	C79.81	D05.-	D24.-	D48.6-	D49.3
areola	C50.0-	C79.81	D05.-	D24.-	D48.6-	D49.3
axillary tail	C50.6-	C79.81	D05.-	D24.-	D48.6-	D49.3
central portion	C50.1-	C79.81	D05.-	D24.-	D48.6-	D49.3
inner	C50.8-	C79.81	D05.-	D24.-	D48.6-	D49.3
lower	C50.8-	C79.81	D05.-	D24.-	D48.6-	D49.3
lower-inner quadrant	C50.3-	C79.81	D05.-	D24.-	D48.6-	D49.3
lower-outer quadrant	C50.5-	C79.81	D05.-	D24.-	D48.6-	D49.3
mastectomy site (skin) — *see also Neoplasm, breast, skin*	C44.501	C79.2	-	-	-	-
specified as breast tissue	C50.8-	C79.81	-	-	-	-
midline	C50.8-	C79.81	D05.-	D24.-	D48.6-	D49.3
nipple	C50.0-	C79.81	D05.-	D24.-	D48.6-	D49.3
outer	C50.8-	C79.81	D05.-	D24.-	D48.6-	D49.3
overlapping lesion	C50.8-	-	-	-	-	-
skin	C44.501	C79.2	D04.5	D23.5	D48.5	D49.2
basal cell carcinoma	C44.511	-	-	-	-	-
specified type NEC	C44.591	-	-	-	-	-
squamous cell carcinoma	C44.521	-	-	-	-	-
tail (axillary)	C50.6-	C79.81	D05.-	D24.-	D48.6-	D49.3
upper	C50.8-	C79.81	D05.-	D24.-	D48.6-	D49.3
upper-inner quadrant	C50.2-	C79.81	D05.-	D24.-	D48.6-	D49.3

Neoplasm, neoplastic	Malignant Primary	Malignant Secondary	Ca in situ	Benign	Uncertain Behavior	Unspecified Behavior
upper-outer quadrant	C50.4-	C79.81	D05.-	D24.-	D48.6-	D49.3
broad ligament	C57.1	C79.82	D07.39	D28.2	D39.8	D49.59
bronchiogenic, bronchogenic (lung)	C34.9-	C78.0-	D02.2-	D14.3-	D38.1	D49.1
bronchiole	C34.9-	C78.0-	D02.2-	D14.3-	D38.1	D49.1
bronchus	C34.9-	C78.0-	D02.2-	D14.3-	D38.1	D49.1
carina	C34.0-	C78.0-	D02.2-	D14.3-	D38.1	D49.1
lower lobe of lung	C34.3-	C78.0-	D02.2-	D14.3-	D38.1	D49.1
main	C34.0-	C78.0-	D02.2-	D14.3-	D38.1	D49.1
middle lobe of lung	C34.2	C78.0-	D02.21	D14.31	D38.1	D49.1
overlapping lesion	C34.8-	-	-	-	-	-
upper lobe of lung	C34.1-	C78.0-	D02.2-	D14.3-	D38.1	D49.1
brow	C44.309	C79.2	D04.39	D23.39	D48.5	D49.2
basal cell carcinoma	C44.319	-	-	-	-	-
specified type NEC	C44.399	-	-	-	-	-
squamous cell carcinoma	C44.329	-	-	-	-	-
buccal (cavity)	C06.9	C79.89	D00.00	D10.39	D37.09	D49.0
commissure	C06.0	C79.89	D00.02	D10.39	D37.09	D49.0
groove (lower) (upper)	C06.1	C79.89	D00.02	D10.39	D37.09	D49.0
mucosa	C06.0	C79.89	D00.02	D10.39	D37.09	D49.0
sulcus (lower) (upper)	C06.1	C79.89	D00.02	D10.39	D37.09	D49.0
bulbourethral gland	C68.0	C79.19	D09.19	D30.4	D41.3	D49.59
bursa — *see Neoplasm, connective tissue*						
buttock NEC	C76.3	C79.89	D04.5	D36.7	D48.7	D49.89
calf	C76.5-	C79.89	D04.7-	D36.7	D48.7	D49.89
calvarium	C41.0	C79.51	-	D16.4-	D48.0	D49.2
calyx, renal	C65.-	C79.0-	D09.19	D30.1-	D41.1-	D49.51-
canal						
anal	C21.1	C78.5	D01.3	D12.9	D37.8	D49.0
auditory (external) — *see also Neoplasm, skin, ear*	C44.20-	C79.2	D04.2-	D23.2-	D48.5	D49.2
auricular (external) — *see also Neoplasm, skin, ear*	C44.20-	C79.2	D04.2-	D23.2-	D48.5	D49.2
canaliculi, biliary (biliferi) (intrahepatic)	C22.1	C78.7	D01.5	D13.4	D37.6	D49.0
canthus (eye) (inner) (outer)	C44.10-	C79.2	D04.1-	D23.1-	D48.5	D49.2
basal cell carcinoma	C44.11-	-	-	-	-	-
sebaceous cell	C44.13-	-	-	-	-	-
specified type NEC	C44.19-	-	-	-	-	-
squamous cell carcinoma	C44.12-	-	-	-	-	-
capillary — *see Neoplasm, connective tissue*						
caput coli	C18.0	C78.5	D01.0	D12.0	D37.4	D49.0
carcinoid — *see Tumor, carcinoid*						
cardia (gastric)	C16.0	C78.89	D00.2	D13.1	D37.1	D49.0
cardiac orifice (stomach)	C16.0	C78.89	D00.2	D13.1	D37.1	D49.0
cardio-esophageal junction	C16.0	C78.89	D00.2	D13.1	D37.1	D49.0
cardio-esophagus	C16.0	C78.89	D00.2	D13.1	D37.1	D49.0
carina (bronchus)	C34.0-	C78.0-	D02.2-	D14.3-	D38.1	D49.1
carotid (artery)	C49.0	C79.89	-	D21.0	D48.1	D49.2
body	C75.4	C79.89	-	D35.5	D44.6	D49.7
carpus (any bone)	C40.1-	C79.51	-	D16.1-	-	-
cartilage (articular) (joint) NEC — *see also Neoplasm, bone*	C41.9	C79.51	-	D16.9-	D48.0	D49.2
arytenoid	C32.3	C78.39	D02.0	D14.1	D38.0	D49.1
auricular	C49.0	C79.89	-	D21.0	D48.1	D49.2
bronchi	C34.0-	C78.39	-	D14.3-	D38.1	D49.1
costal	C41.3	C79.51	-	D16.7	D48.0	D49.2
cricoid	C32.3	C78.39	D02.0	D14.1	D38.0	D49.1
cuneiform	C32.3	C78.39	D02.0	D14.1	D38.0	D49.1
ear (external)	C49.0	C79.89	-	D21.0	D48.1	D49.2

Neoplasm, neoplastic	Malignant Primary	Malignant Secondary	Ca in situ	Benign	Uncertain Behavior	Unspecified Behavior
ensiform	C41.3	C79.51	-	D16.7	D48.0	D49.2
epiglottis	C32.1	C78.39	D02.0	D14.1	D38.0	D49.1
anterior surface	C10.1	C79.89	D00.08	D10.5	D37.05	D49.0
eyelid	C49.0	C79.89	-	D21.0	D48.1	D49.2
intervertebral	C41.2	C79.51	-	D16.6	D48.0	D49.2
larynx, laryngeal	C32.3	C78.39	D02.0	D14.1	D38.0	D49.1
nose, nasal	C30.0	C78.39	D02.3	D14.0	D38.5	D49.1
pinna	C49.0	C79.89	-	D21.0	D48.1	D49.2
rib	C41.3	C79.51	-	D16.7	D48.0	D49.2
semilunar (knee)	C40.2-	C79.51	-	D16.2-	D48.0	D49.2
thyroid	C32.3	C78.39	D02.0	D14.1	D38.0	D49.1
trachea	C33	C78.39	D02.1	D14.2	D38.1	D49.1
cauda equina	C72.1	C79.49	-	D33.4	D43.4	D49.7
cavity						
buccal	C06.9	C79.89	D00.00	D10.30	D37.09	D49.0
nasal	C30.0	C78.39	D02.3	D14.0	D38.5	D49.1
oral	C06.9	C79.89	D00.00	D10.30	D37.09	D49.0
peritoneal	C48.2	C78.6	-	D20.1	D48.4	D49.0
tympanic	C30.1	C78.39	D02.3	D14.0	D38.5	D49.1
cecum	C18.0	C78.5	D01.0	D12.0	D37.4	D49.0
central nervous system	C72.9	C79.40	-	-	-	-
cerebellopontine (angle)	C71.6	C79.31	-	D33.1	D43.1	D49.6
cerebellum, cerebellar	C71.6	C79.31	-	D33.1	D43.1	D49.6
cerebrum, cerebra (cortex) (hemisphere) (white matter)	C71.0	C79.31	-	D33.0	D43.0	D49.6
meninges	C70.0	C79.32	-	D32.0	D42.0	D49.7
peduncle	C71.7	C79.31	-	D33.1	D43.1	D49.6
ventricle	C71.5	C79.31	-	D33.0	D43.0	D49.6
fourth	C71.7	C79.31	-	D33.1	D43.1	D49.6
cervical region	C76.0	C79.89	D09.8	D36.7	D48.7	D49.89
cervix (cervical) (uteri) (uterus)	C53.9	C79.82	D06.9	D26.0	D39.0	D49.59
canal	C53.0	C79.82	D06.0	D26.0	D39.0	D49.59
endocervix (canal) (gland)	C53.0	C79.82	D06.0	D26.0	D39.0	D49.59
exocervix	C53.1	C79.82	D06.1	D26.0	D39.0	D49.59
external os	C53.1	C79.82	D06.1	D26.0	D39.0	D49.59
internal os	C53.0	C79.82	D06.0	D26.0	D39.0	D49.59
nabothian gland	C53.0	C79.82	D06.0	D26.0	D39.0	D49.59
overlapping lesion	C53.8	-	-	-	-	-
squamocolumnar junction	C53.8	C79.82	D06.7	D26.0	D39.0	D49.59
stump	C53.8	C79.82	D06.7	D26.0	D39.0	D49.59
cheek	C76.0	C79.89	D09.8	D36.7	D48.7	D49.89
external	C44.309	C79.2	D04.39	D23.39	D48.5	D49.2
basal cell carcinoma	C44.319	-	-	-	-	-
specified type NEC	C44.399	-	-	-	-	-
squamous cell carcinoma	C44.329	-	-	-	-	-
inner aspect	C06.0	C79.89	D00.02	D10.39	D37.09	D49.0
internal	C06.0	C79.89	D00.02	D10.39	D37.09	D49.0
mucosa	C06.0	C79.89	D00.02	D10.39	D37.09	D49.0
chest (wall) NEC	C76.1	C79.89	D09.8	D36.7	D48.7	D49.89
chiasma opticum	C72.3-	C79.49	-	D33.3	D43.3	D49.7
chin	C44.309	C79.2	D04.39	D23.39	D48.5	D49.2
basal cell carcinoma	C44.319	-	-	-	-	-
specified type NEC	C44.399	-	-	-	-	-
squamous cell carcinoma	C44.329	-	-	-	-	-
choana	C11.3	C79.89	D00.08	D10.6	D37.05	D49.0
cholangiole	C22.1	C78.89	D01.5	D13.4	D37.6	D49.0
choledochal duct	C24.0	C78.89	D01.5	D13.5	D37.6	D49.0
choroid	C69.3-	C79.49	D09.2-	D31.3-	D48.7	D49.81
plexus	C71.5	C79.31	-	D33.0	D43.0	D49.6
ciliary body	C69.4-	C79.49	D09.2-	D31.4-	D48.7	D49.89

Neoplasm, neoplastic	Malignant Primary	Malignant Secondary	Ca in situ	Benign	Uncertain Behavior	Unspecified Behavior
clavicle	C41.3	C79.51	-	D16.7	D48.0	D49.2
clitoris	C51.2	C79.82	D07.1	D28.0	D39.8	D49.59
clivus	C41.0	C79.51	-	D16.4-	D48.0	D49.2
cloacogenic zone	C21.2	C78.5	D01.3	D12.9	D37.8	D49.0
coccygeal						
body or glomus	C49.5	C79.89	-	D21.5	D48.1	D49.2
vertebra	C41.4	C79.51	-	D16.8	D48.0	D49.2
coccyx	C41.4	C79.51	-	D16.8	D48.0	D49.2
colon — *see also Neoplasm, intestine, large*	C18.9	C78.5	-	-	-	-
with rectum	C19	C78.5	D01.1	D12.7	D37.5	D49.0
column, spinal — *see Neoplasm, spine*						
columnella — *see also Neoplasm, skin, face*	C44.390	C79.2	D04.39	D23.39	D48.5	D49.2
commissure						
labial, lip	C00.6	C79.89	D00.01	D10.39	D37.01	D49.0
laryngeal	C32.0	C78.39	D02.0	D14.1	D38.0	D49.1
common (bile) duct	C24.0	C78.89	D01.5	D13.5	D37.6	D49.0
concha — *see also Neoplasm, skin, ear*	C44.20-	C79.2	D04.2-	D23.2-	D48.5	D49.2
nose	C30.0	C78.39	D02.3	D14.0	D38.5	D49.1
conjunctiva	C69.0-	C79.49	D09.2-	D31.0-	D48.7	D49.89
connective tissue NEC	C49.9	C79.89	-	D21.9	D48.1	D49.2
Note: For neoplasms of connective tissue (blood vessel, bursa, fascia, ligament, muscle, peripheral nerves, sympathetic and parasympathetic nerves and ganglia, synovia, tendon, etc.) or of morphological types that indicate connective tissue, code according to the list under "Neoplasm, connective tissue". For sites that do not appear in this list, code to neoplasm of that site; e.g., fibrosarcoma, pancreas (C25.9)						
Note: Morphological types that indicate connective tissue appear in their proper place in the alphabetic index with the instruction "see Neoplasm, connective tissue ...."						
abdomen	C49.4	C79.89	-	D21.4	D48.1	D49.2
abdominal wall	C49.4	C79.89	-	D21.4	D48.1	D49.2
ankle	C49.2-	C79.89	-	D21.2-	D48.1	D49.2
antecubital fossa or space	C49.1-	C79.89	-	D21.1-	D48.1	D49.2
arm	C49.1-	C79.89	-	D21.1-	D48.1	D49.2
auricle (ear)	C49.0	C79.89	-	D21.0	D48.1	D49.2
axilla	C49.3	C79.89	-	D21.3	D48.1	D49.2
back	C49.6	C79.89	-	D21.6	D48.1	D49.2
breast — *see Neoplasm, breast*						
buttock	C49.5	C79.89	-	D21.5	D48.1	D49.2
calf	C49.2-	C79.89	-	D21.2-	D48.1	D49.2
cervical region	C49.0	C79.89	-	D21.0	D48.1	D49.2
cheek	C49.0	C79.89	-	D21.0	D48.1	D49.2
chest (wall)	C49.3	C79.89	-	D21.3	D48.1	D49.2
chin	C49.0	C79.89	-	D21.0	D48.1	D49.2
diaphragm	C49.3	C79.89	-	D21.3	D48.1	D49.2
ear (external)	C49.0	C79.89	-	D21.0	D48.1	D49.2
elbow	C49.1-	C79.89	-	D21.1-	D48.1	D49.2
extrarectal	C49.5	C79.89	-	D21.5	D48.1	D49.2
extremity	C49.9	C79.89	-	D21.9	D48.1	D49.2
lower	C49.2-	C79.89	-	D21.2-	D48.1	D49.2
upper	C49.1-	C79.89	-	D21.1-	D48.1	D49.2
eyelid	C49.0	C79.89	-	D21.0	D48.1	D49.2

Neoplasm, neoplastic	Malignant Primary	Malignant Secondary	Ca in situ	Benign	Uncertain Behavior	Unspecified Behavior
face	C49.0	C79.89	-	D21.0	D48.1	D49.2
finger	C49.1-	C79.89	-	D21.1-	D48.1	D49.2
flank	C49.6	C79.89	-	D21.6	D48.1	D49.2
foot	C49.2-	C79.89	-	D21.2-	D48.1	D49.2
forearm	C49.1-	C79.89	-	D21.1-	D48.1	D49.2
forehead	C49.0	C79.89	-	D21.0	D48.1	D49.2
gastric	C49.4	C79.89	-	D21.4	D48.1	D49.2
gastrointestinal	C49.4	C79.89	-	D21.4	D48.1	D49.2
gluteal region	C49.5	C79.89	-	D21.5	D48.1	D49.2
great vessels NEC	C49.3	C79.89	-	D21.3	D48.1	D49.2
groin	C49.5	C79.89	-	D21.5	D48.1	D49.2
hand	C49.1-	C79.89	-	D21.1-	D48.1	D49.2
head	C49.0	C79.89	-	D21.0	D48.1	D49.2
heel	C49.2-	C79.89	-	D21.2-	D48.1	D49.2
hip	C49.2-	C79.89	-	D21.2-	D48.1	D49.2
hypochondrium	C49.4	C79.89	-	D21.4	D48.1	D49.2
iliopsoas muscle	C49.5	C79.89	-	D21.5	D48.1	D49.2
infraclavicular region	C49.3	C79.89	-	D21.3	D48.1	D49.2
inguinal (canal) (region)	C49.5	C79.89	-	D21.5	D48.1	D49.2
intestinal	C49.4	C79.89	-	D21.4	D48.1	D49.2
intrathoracic	C49.3	C79.89	-	D21.3	D48.1	D49.2
ischiorectal fossa	C49.5	C79.89	-	D21.5	D48.1	D49.2
jaw	C03.9	C79.89	D00.03	D10.39	D48.1	D49.0
knee	C49.2-	C79.89	-	D21.2-	D48.1	D49.2
leg	C49.2-	C79.89	-	D21.2-	D48.1	D49.2
limb NEC	C49.9	C79.89	-	D21.9	D48.1	D49.2
lower	C49.2-	C79.89	-	D21.2-	D48.1	D49.2
upper	C49.1-	C79.89	-	D21.1-	D48.1	D49.2
nates	C49.5	C79.89	-	D21.5	D48.1	D49.2
neck	C49.0	C79.89	-	D21.0	D48.1	D49.2
orbit	C69.6-	C79.49	D09.2-	D31.6-	D48.1	D49.89
overlapping lesion	C49.8	-	-	-	-	-
pararectal	C49.5	C79.89	-	D21.5	D48.1	D49.2
para-urethral	C49.5	C79.89	-	D21.5	D48.1	D49.2
paravaginal	C49.5	C79.89	-	D21.5	D48.1	D49.2
pelvis (floor)	C49.5	C79.89	-	D21.5	D48.1	D49.2
pelvo-abdominal	C49.8	C79.89	-	D21.6	D48.1	D49.2
perineum	C49.5	C79.89	-	D21.5	D48.1	D49.2
perirectal (tissue)	C49.5	C79.89	-	D21.5	D48.1	D49.2
periurethral (tissue)	C49.5	C79.89	-	D21.5	D48.1	D49.2
popliteal fossa or space	C49.2-	C79.89	-	D21.2-	D48.1	D49.2
presacral	C49.5	C79.89	-	D21.5	D48.1	D49.2
psoas muscle	C49.4	C79.89	-	D21.4	D48.1	D49.2
pterygoid fossa	C49.0	C79.89	-	D21.0	D48.1	D49.2
rectovaginal septum or wall	C49.5	C79.89	-	D21.5	D48.1	D49.2
rectovesical	C49.5	C79.89	-	D21.5	D48.1	D49.2
retroperitoneum	C48.0	C78.6	-	D20.0	D48.3	D49.0
sacrococcygeal region	C49.5	C79.89	-	D21.5	D48.1	D49.2
scalp	C49.0	C79.89	-	D21.0	D48.1	D49.2
scapular region	C49.3	C79.89	-	D21.3	D48.1	D49.2
shoulder	C49.1-	C79.89	-	D21.1-	D48.1	D49.2
skin (dermis) NEC — *see also Neoplasm, skin, by site*	C44.90	C79.2	D04.9	D23.9	D48.5	D49.2
stomach	C49.4	C79.89	-	D21.4	D48.1	D49.2
submental	C49.0	C79.89	-	D21.0	D48.1	D49.2
supraclavicular region	C49.0	C79.89	-	D21.0	D48.1	D49.2
temple	C49.0	C79.89	-	D21.0	D48.1	D49.2
temporal region	C49.0	C79.89	-	D21.0	D48.1	D49.2
thigh	C49.2-	C79.89	-	D21.2-	D48.1	D49.2
thoracic (duct) (wall)	C49.3	C79.89	-	D21.3	D48.1	D49.2

	Malignant Primary	Malignant Secondary	Ca in situ	Benign	Uncertain Behavior	Unspecified Behavior
Neoplasm, neoplastic						
thorax	C49.3	C79.89	-	D21.3	D48.1	D49.2
thumb	C49.1-	C79.89	-	D21.1-	D48.1	D49.2
toe	C49.2-	C79.89	-	D21.2-	D48.1	D49.2
trunk	C49.6	C79.89	-	D21.6	D48.1	D49.2
umbilicus	C49.4	C79.89	-	D21.4	D48.1	D49.2
vesicorectal	C49.5	C79.89	-	D21.5	D48.1	D49.2
wrist	C49.1-	C79.89	-	D21.1-	D48.1	D49.2
conus medullaris	C72.0	C79.49	-	D33.4	D43.4	D49.7
cord (true) (vocal)	C32.0	C78.39	D02.0	D14.1	D38.0	D49.1
false	C32.1	C78.39	D02.0	D14.1	D38.0	D49.1
spermatic	C63.1-	C79.82	D07.69	D29.8	D40.8	D49.59
spinal (cervical) (lumbar) (thoracic)	C72.0	C79.49	-	D33.4	D43.4	D49.7
cornea (limbus)	C69.1-	C79.49	D09.2-	D31.1-	D48.7	D49.89
corpus						
albicans	C56.-	C79.6-	D07.39	D27.-	D39.1-	D49.59
callosum, brain	C71.0	C79.31	-	D33.2	D43.2	D49.6
cavernosum	C60.2	C79.82	D07.4	D29.0	D40.8	D49.59
gastric	C16.2	C78.89	D00.2	D13.1	D37.1	D49.0
overlapping sites	C54.8	-	-	-	-	-
penis	C60.2	C79.82	D07.4	D29.0	D40.8	D49.59
striatum, cerebrum	C71.0	C79.31	-	D33.0	D43.0	D49.6
uteri	C54.9	C79.82	D07.0	D26.1	D39.0	D49.59
isthmus	C54.0	C79.82	D07.0	D26.1	D39.0	D49.59
cortex						
adrenal	C74.0-	C79.7-	D09.3	D35.0-	D44.1-	D49.7
cerebral	C71.0	C79.31	-	D33.0	D43.0	D49.6
costal cartilage	C41.3	C79.51	-	D16.7	D48.0	D49.2
costovertebral joint	C41.3	C79.51	-	D16.7	D48.0	D49.2
Cowper's gland	C68.0	C79.19	D09.19	D30.4	D41.3	D49.59
cranial (fossa, any)	C71.9	C79.31	-	D33.2	D43.2	D49.6
meninges	C70.0	C79.32	-	D32.0	D42.0	D49.7
nerve	C72.50	C79.49	-	D33.3	D43.3	D49.7
specified NEC	C72.59	C79.49	-	D33.3	D43.3	D49.7
craniobuccal pouch	C75.2	C79.89	D09.3	D35.2	D44.3	D49.7
craniopharyngeal (duct) (pouch)	C75.2	C79.89	D09.3	D35.3	D44.4	D49.7
cricoid	C13.0	C79.89	D00.08	D10.7	D37.05	D49.0
cartilage	C32.3	C78.39	D02.0	D14.1	D38.0	D49.1
cricopharynx	C13.0	C79.89	D00.08	D10.7	D37.05	D49.0
crypt of Morgagni	C21.8	C78.5	D01.3	D12.9	D37.8	D49.0
crystalline lens	C69.4-	C79.49	D09.2-	D31.4-	D48.7	D49.89
cul-de-sac (Douglas')	C48.1	C78.6	-	D20.1	D48.4	D49.0
cuneiform cartilage	C32.3	C78.39	D02.0	D14.1	D38.0	D49.1
cutaneous — *see Neoplasm, skin*						
cutis — *see Neoplasm, skin*						
cystic (bile) duct (common)	C24.0	C78.89	D01.5	D13.5	D37.6	D49.0
dermis — *see Neoplasm, skin*						
diaphragm	C49.3	C79.89	-	D21.3	D48.1	D49.2
digestive organs, system, tube, or tract NEC	C26.9	C78.89	D01.9	D13.9	D37.9	D49.0
disc, intervertebral	C41.2	C79.51	-	D16.6	D48.0	D49.2
disease, generalized	C80.0	-	-	-	-	-
disseminated	C80.0	-	-	-	-	-
Douglas' cul-de-sac or pouch	C48.1	C78.6	-	D20.1	D48.4	D49.0
duodenojejunal junction	C17.8	C78.4	D01.49	D13.39	D37.2	D49.0
duodenum	C17.0	C78.4	D01.49	D13.2	D37.2	D49.0
dura (cranial) (mater)	C70.9	C79.49	-	D32.9	D42.9	D49.7
cerebral	C70.0	C79.32	-	D32.0	D42.0	D49.7
spinal	C70.1	C79.49	-	D32.1	D42.1	D49.7
ear (external) — *see also Neoplasm, skin, ear*	C44.20-	C79.2	D04.2-	D23.2-	D48.5	D49.2

NEOPLASM CONNECTIVE TISSUE NEC - EAR

Neoplasm, neoplastic	Malignant Primary	Malignant Secondary	Ca in situ	Benign	Uncertain Behavior	Unspecified Behavior
auricle or auris — *see also Neoplasm, skin, ear*	C44.20-	C79.2	D04.2-	D23.2-	D48.5	D49.2
canal, external — *see also Neoplasm, skin, ear*	C44.20-	C79.2	D04.2-	D23.2-	D48.5	D49.2
cartilage	C49.0	C79.89	-	D21.0	D48.1	D49.2
external meatus — *see also Neoplasm, skin, ear*	C44.20-	C79.2	D04.2-	D23.2-	D48.5	D49.2
inner	C30.1	C78.39	D02.3	D14.0	D38.5	D49.1
lobule — *see also Neoplasm, skin, ear*	C44.20-	C79.2	D04.2-	D23.2-	D48.5	D49.2
middle	C30.1	C78.39	D02.3	D14.0	D38.5	D49.1
overlapping lesion with accessory sinuses	C31.8	-	-	-	-	-
skin	C44.20-	C79.2	D04.2-	D23.2-	D48.5	D49.2
basal cell carcinoma	C44.21-	-	-	-	-	-
specified type NEC	C44.29-	-	-	-	-	-
squamous cell carcinoma	C44.22-	-	-	-	-	-
earlobe	C44.20-	C79.2	D04.2-	D23.2-	D48.5	D49.2
basal cell carcinoma	C44.21-	-	-	-	-	-
specified type NEC	C44.29-	-	-	-	-	-
squamous cell carcinoma	C44.22-	-	-	-	-	-
ejaculatory duct	C63.7	C79.82	D07.69	D29.8	D40.8	D49.59
elbow NEC	C76.4-	C79.89	D04.6-	D36.7	D48.7	D49.89
endocardium	C38.0	C79.89	-	D15.1	D48.7	D49.89
endocervix (canal) (gland)	C53.0	C79.82	D06.0	D26.0	D39.0	D49.59
endocrine gland NEC	C75.9	C79.89	D09.3	D35.9	D44.9	D49.7
pluriglandular	C75.8	C79.89	D09.3	D35.7	D44.9	D49.7
endometrium (gland) (stroma)	C54.1	C79.82	D07.0	D26.1	D39.0	D49.59
ensiform cartilage	C41.3	C79.51	-	D16.7	D48.0	D49.2
enteric — *see Neoplasm, intestine*						
ependyma (brain)	C71.5	C79.31	-	D33.0	D43.0	D49.6
fourth ventricle	C71.7	C79.31	-	D33.1	D43.1	D49.6
epicardium	C38.0	C79.89	-	D15.1	D48.7	D49.89
epididymis	C63.0-	C79.82	D07.69	D29.3-	D40.8	D49.59
epidural	C72.9	C79.49	-	D33.9	D43.9	D49.7
epiglottis	C32.1	C78.39	D02.0	D14.1	D38.0	D49.1
anterior aspect or surface	C10.1	C79.89	D00.08	D10.5	D37.05	D49.0
cartilage	C32.3	C78.39	D02.0	D14.1	D38.0	D49.1
free border (margin)	C10.1	C79.89	D00.08	D10.5	D37.05	D49.0
junctional region	C10.8	C79.89	D00.08	D10.5	D37.05	D49.0
posterior (laryngeal) surface	C32.1	C78.39	D02.0	D14.1	D38.0	D49.1
suprahyoid portion	C32.1	C78.39	D02.0	D14.1	D38.0	D49.1
esophagogastric junction	C16.0	C78.89	D00.2	D13.1	D37.1	D49.0
esophagus	C15.9	C78.89	D00.1	D13.0	D37.8	D49.0
abdominal	C15.5	C78.89	D00.1	D13.0	D37.8	D49.0
cervical	C15.3	C78.89	D00.1	D13.0	D37.8	D49.0
distal (third)	C15.5	C78.89	D00.1	D13.0	D37.8	D49.0
lower (third)	C15.5	C78.89	D00.1	D13.0	D37.8	D49.0
middle (third)	C15.4	C78.89	D00.1	D13.0	D37.8	D49.0
overlapping lesion	C15.8	-	-	-	-	-
proximal (third)	C15.3	C78.89	D00.1	D13.0	D37.8	D49.0
thoracic	C15.4	C78.89	D00.1	D13.0	D37.8	D49.0
upper (third)	C15.3	C78.89	D00.1	D13.0	D37.8	D49.0
ethmoid (sinus)	C31.1	C78.39	D02.3	D14.0	D38.5	D49.1
bone or labyrinth	C41.0	C79.51	-	D16.4-	D48.0	D49.2
eustachian tube	C30.1	C78.39	D02.3	D14.0	D38.5	D49.1
exocervix	C53.1	C79.82	D06.1	D26.0	D39.0	D49.59
external						
meatus (ear) — *see also Neoplasm, skin, ear*	C44.20-	C79.2	D04.2-	D23.2-	D48.5	D49.2
os, cervix uteri	C53.1	C79.82	D06.1	D26.0	D39.0	D49.59

Neoplasm, neoplastic	Malignant Primary	Malignant Secondary	Ca in situ	Benign	Uncertain Behavior	Unspecified Behavior
extradural	C72.9	C79.49	-	D33.9	D43.9	D49.7
extrahepatic (bile) duct	C24.0	C78.89	D01.5	D13.5	D37.6	D49.0
overlapping lesion with gallbladder	C24.8	-	-	-	-	-
extraocular muscle	C69.6-	C79.49	D09.2-	D31.6-	D48.7	D49.89
extrarectal	C76.3	C79.89	D09.8	D36.7	D48.7	D49.89
extremity	C76.8	C79.89	D04.8	D36.7	D48.7	D49.89
lower	C76.5-	C79.89	D04.7-	D36.7	D48.7	D49.89
upper	C76.4-	C79.89	D04.6-	D36.7	D48.7	D49.89
eye NEC	C69.9-	C79.49	D09.2	D31.9	D48.7	D49.89
overlapping sites	C69.8	-	-	-	-	-
eyeball	C69.9-	C79.49	D09.2-	D31.9-	D48.7	D49.89
eyebrow	C44.309	C79.2	D04.39	D23.39	D48.5	D49.2
basal cell carcinoma	C44.319	-	-	-	-	-
specified type NEC	C44.399	-	-	-	-	-
squamous cell carcinoma	C44.329	-	-	-	-	-
eyelid (lower) (skin) (upper)	C44.10-	-	-	-	-	-
basal cell carcinoma	C44.11-	-	-	-	-	-
sebaceous cell	C44.13-	-	-	-	-	-
specified type NEC	C44.19-	-	-	-	-	-
squamous cell carcinoma	C44.12-	-	-	-	-	-
cartilage	C49.0	C79.89	-	D21.0	D48.1	D49.2
face NEC	C76.0	C79.89	D04.39	D36.7	D48.7	D49.89
fallopian tube (accessory)	C57.0-	C79.82	D07.39	D28.2	D39.8	D49.59
falx (cerebella) (cerebri)	C70.0	C79.32	-	D32.0	D42.0	D49.7
fascia — *see also Neoplasm, connective tissue*						
palmar	C49.1-	C79.89	-	D21.1-	D48.1	D49.2
plantar	C49.2-	C79.89	-	D21.2-	D48.1	D49.2
fatty tissue — *see Neoplasm, connective tissue*						
fauces, faucial NEC	C10.9	C79.89	D00.08	D10.5	D37.05	D49.0
pillars	C09.1	C79.89	D00.08	D10.5	D37.05	D49.0
tonsil	C09.9	C79.89	D00.08	D10.4	D37.05	D49.0
femur (any part)	C40.2-	-	-	D16.2-	-	-
fetal membrane	C58	C79.82	D07.0	D26.7	D39.2	D49.59
fibrous tissue — *see Neoplasm, connective tissue*						
fibula (any part)	C40.2-	C79.51	-	D16.2-	-	-
filum terminale	C72.0	C79.49	-	D33.4	D43.4	D49.7
finger NEC	C76.4-	C79.89	D04.6-	D36.7	D48.7	D49.89
flank NEC	C76.8	C79.89	D04.5	D36.7	D48.7	D49.89
follicle, nabothian	C53.0	C79.82	D06.0	D26.0	D39.0	D49.59
foot NEC	C76.5-	C79.89	D04.7-	D36.7	D48.7	D49.89
forearm NEC	C76.4-	C79.89	D04.6-	D36.7	D48.7	D49.89
forehead (skin)	C44.309	C79.2	D04.39	D23.39	D48.5	D49.2
basal cell carcinoma	C44.319	-	-	-	-	-
specified type NEC	C44.399	-	-	-	-	-
squamous cell carcinoma	C44.329	-	-	-	-	-
foreskin	C60.0	C79.82	D07.4	D29.0	D40.8	D49.59
fornix						
pharyngeal	C11.3	C79.89	D00.08	D10.6	D37.05	D49.0
vagina	C52	C79.82	D07.2	D28.1	D39.8	D49.59
fossa (of)						
anterior (cranial)	C71.9	C79.31	-	D33.2	D43.2	D49.6
cranial	C71.9	C79.31	-	D33.2	D43.2	D49.6
ischiorectal	C76.3	C79.89	D09.8	D36.7	D48.7	D49.89
middle (cranial)	C71.9	C79.31	-	D33.2	D43.2	D49.6
piriform	C12	C79.89	D00.08	D10.7	D37.05	D49.0
pituitary	C75.1	C79.89	D09.3	D35.2	D44.3	D49.7
posterior (cranial)	C71.9	C79.31	-	D33.2	D43.2	D49.6

Neoplasm, neoplastic	Malignant Primary	Malignant Secondary	Ca in situ	Benign	Uncertain Behavior	Unspecified Behavior
pterygoid	C49.0	C79.89	-	D21.0	D48.1	D49.2
pyriform	C12	C79.89	D00.08	D10.7	D37.05	D49.0
Rosenmuller	C11.2	C79.89	D00.08	D10.6	D37.05	D49.0
tonsillar	C09.0	C79.89	D00.08	D10.5	D37.05	D49.0
fourchette	C51.9	C79.82	D07.1	D28.0	D39.8	D49.59
frenulum						
labii — *see Neoplasm, lip, internal*						
linguae	C02.2	C79.89	D00.07	D10.1	D37.02	D49.0
frontal						
bone	C41.0	C79.51	-	D16.4-	D48.0	D49.2
lobe, brain	C71.1	C79.31	-	D33.0	D43.0	D49.6
pole	C71.1	C79.31	-	D33.0	D43.0	D49.6
sinus	C31.2	C78.39	D02.3	D14.0	D38.5	D49.1
fundus						
stomach	C16.1	C78.89	D00.2	D13.1	D37.1	D49.0
uterus	C54.3	C79.82	D07.0	D26.1	D39.0	D49.59
gall duct (extrahepatic)	C24.0	C78.89	D01.5	D13.5	D37.6	D49.0
intrahepatic	C22.1	C78.7	D01.5	D13.4	D37.6	D49.0
gallbladder	C23	C78.89	D01.5	D13.5	D37.6	D49.0
overlapping lesion with extrahepatic bile ducts	C24.8	-	-	-	-	-
ganglia — *see also Neoplasm, nerve, peripheral*	C47.9	C79.89	-	D36.10	D48.2	D49.2
basal	C71.0	C79.31	-	D33.0	D43.0	D49.6
cranial nerve	C72.50	C79.49	-	D33.3	D43.3	D49.7
Gartner's duct	C52	C79.82	D07.2	D28.1	D39.8	D49.59
gastric — *see Neoplasm, stomach*						
gastrocolic	C26.9	C78.89	D01.9	D13.9	D37.9	D49.0
gastroesophageal junction	C16.0	C78.89	D00.2	D13.1	D37.1	D49.0
gastrointestinal (tract) NEC	C26.9	C78.89	D01.9	D13.9	D37.9	D49.0
generalized	C80.0	-	-	-	-	-
genital organ or tract						
female NEC	C57.9	C79.82	D07.30	D28.9	D39.9	D49.59
overlapping lesion	C57.8	-	-	-	-	-
specified site NEC	C57.7	C79.82	D07.39	D28.7	D39.8	D49.59
male NEC	C63.9	C79.82	D07.60	D29.9	D40.9	D49.59
overlapping lesion	C63.8	-	-	-	-	-
specified site NEC	C63.7	C79.82	D07.69	D29.8	D40.8	D49.59
genitourinary tract						
female	C57.9	C79.82	D07.30	D28.9	D39.9	D49.59
male	C63.9	C79.82	D07.60	D29.9	D40.9	D49.59
gingiva (alveolar) (marginal)	C03.9	C79.89	D00.03	D10.39	D37.09	D49.0
lower	C03.1	C79.89	D00.03	D10.39	D37.09	D49.0
mandibular	C03.1	C79.89	D00.03	D10.39	D37.09	D49.0
maxillary	C03.0	C79.89	D00.03	D10.39	D37.09	D49.0
upper	C03.0	C79.89	D00.03	D10.39	D37.09	D49.0
gland, glandular (lymphatic) (system) — *see also Neoplasm, lymph gland*						
endocrine NEC	C75.9	C79.89	D09.3	D35.9	D44.9	D49.7
salivary — *see Neoplasm, salivary gland*						
glans penis	C60.1	C79.82	D07.4	D29.0	D40.8	D49.59
globus pallidus	C71.0	C79.31	-	D33.0	D43.0	D49.6
glomus						
coccygeal	C49.5	C79.89	-	D21.5	D48.1	D49.2
jugularis	C75.5	C79.89	-	D35.6	D44.7	D49.7
glosso-epiglottic fold (s)	C10.1	C79.89	D00.08	D10.5	D37.05	D49.0
glossopalatine fold	C09.1	C79.89	D00.08	D10.5	D37.05	D49.0
glossopharyngeal sulcus	C09.0	C79.89	D00.08	D10.5	D37.05	D49.0
glottis	C32.0	C78.39	D02.0	D14.1	D38.0	D49.1

Neoplasm, neoplastic	Malignant Primary	Malignant Secondary	Ca in situ	Benign	Uncertain Behavior	Unspecified Behavior
gluteal region	C76.3	C79.89	D04.5	D36.7	D48.7	D49.89
great vessels NEC	C49.3	C79.89	-	D21.3	D48.1	D49.2
groin NEC	C76.3	C79.89	D04.5	D36.7	D48.7	D49.89
gum	C03.9	C79.89	D00.03	D10.39	D37.09	D49.0
lower	C03.1	C79.89	D00.03	D10.39	D37.09	D49.0
upper	C03.0	C79.89	D00.03	D10.39	D37.09	D49.0
hand NEC	C76.4-	C79.89	D04.6-	D36.7	D48.7	D49.89
head NEC	C76.0	C79.89	D04.4	D36.7	D48.7	D49.89
heart	C38.0	C79.89	-	D15.1	D48.7	D49.89
heel NEC	C76.5-	C79.89	D04.7-	D36.7	D48.7	D49.89
helix — *see also Neoplasm, skin, ear*	C44.20-	C79.2	D04.2-	D23.2-	D48.5	D49.2
hematopoietic, hemopoietic tissue NEC	C96.9	-	-	-	-	-
specified NEC	C96.Z	-	-	-	-	-
hemisphere, cerebral	C71.0	C79.31	-	D33.0	D43.0	D49.6
hemorrhoidal zone	C21.1	C78.5	D01.3	D12.9	D37.8	D49.0
hepatic — *see also Index to disease, by histology*	C22.9	C78.7	D01.5	D13.4	D37.6	D49.0
duct (bile)	C24.0	C78.89	D01.5	D13.5	D37.6	D49.0
flexure (colon)	C18.3	C78.5	D01.0	D12.3	D37.4	D49.0
primary	C22.8	C78.7	D01.5	D13.4	D37.6	D49.0
hepatobiliary	C24.9	C78.89	D01.5	D13.5	D37.6	D49.0
hepatoblastoma	C22.2	C78.7	D01.5	D13.4	D37.6	D49.0
hepatoma	C22.0	C78.7	D01.5	D13.4	D37.6	D49.0
hilus of lung	C34.0-	C78.0-	D02.2-	D14.3-	D38.1	D49.1
hip NEC	C76.5-	C79.89	D04.7-	D36.7	D48.7	D49.89
hippocampus, brain	C71.2	C79.31	-	D33.0	D43.0	D49.6
humerus (any part)	C40.0-	C79.51	-	D16.0-	-	-
hymen	C52	C79.82	D07.2	D28.1	D39.8	D49.59
hypopharynx, hypopharyngeal NEC	C13.9	C79.89	D00.08	D10.7	D37.05	D49.0
overlapping lesion	C13.8	-	-	-	-	-
postcricoid region	C13.0	C79.89	D00.08	D10.7	D37.05	D49.0
posterior wall	C13.2	C79.89	D00.08	D10.7	D37.05	D49.0
pyriform fossa (sinus)	C12	C79.89	D00.08	D10.7	D37.05	D49.0
hypophysis	C75.1	C79.89	D09.3	D35.2	D44.3	D49.7
hypothalamus	C71.0	C79.31	-	D33.0	D43.0	D49.6
ileocecum, ileocecal (coil) (junction) (valve)	C18.0	C78.5	D01.0	D12.0	D37.4	D49.0
ileum	C17.2	C78.4	D01.49	D13.39	D37.2	D49.0
ilium	C41.4	C79.51	-	D16.8	D48.0	D49.2
immunoproliferative NEC	C88.9	-	-	-	-	-
infraclavicular (region)	C76.1	C79.89	D04.5	D36.7	D48.7	D49.89
inguinal (region)	C76.3	C79.89	D04.5	D36.7	D48.7	D49.89
insula	C71.0	C79.31	-	D33.0	D43.0	D49.6
insular tissue (pancreas)	C25.4	C78.89	D01.7	D13.7	D37.8	D49.0
brain	C71.0	C79.31	-	D33.0	D43.0	D49.6
interarytenoid fold	C13.1	C79.89	D00.08	D10.7	D37.05	D49.0
hypopharyngeal aspect	C13.1	C79.89	D00.08	D10.7	D37.05	D49.0
laryngeal aspect	C32.1	C78.39	D02.0	D14.1	D38.0	D49.1
marginal zone	C13.1	C79.89	D00.08	D10.7	D37.05	D49.0
interdental papillae	C03.9	C79.89	D00.03	D10.39	D37.09	D49.0
lower	C03.1	C79.89	D00.03	D10.39	D37.09	D49.0
upper	C03.0	C79.89	D00.03	D10.39	D37.09	D49.0
internal						
capsule	C71.0	C79.31	-	D33.0	D43.0	D49.6
os (cervix)	C53.0	C79.82	D06.0	D26.0	D39.0	D49.59
intervertebral cartilage or disc	C41.2	C79.51	-	D16.6	D48.0	D49.2
intestine, intestinal	C26.0	C78.80	D01.40	D13.9	D37.8	D49.0
large	C18.9	C78.5	D01.0	D12.6	D37.4	D49.0
appendix	C18.1	C78.5	D01.0	D12.1	D37.3	D49.0

Neoplasm, neoplastic	Malignant Primary	Malignant Secondary	Ca in situ	Benign	Uncertain Behavior	Unspecified Behavior
caput coli	C18.0	C78.5	D01.0	D12.0	D37.4	D49.0
cecum	C18.0	C78.5	D01.0	D12.0	D37.4	D49.0
colon	C18.9	C78.5	D01.0	D12.6	D37.4	D49.0
and rectum	C19	C78.5	D01.1	D12.7	D37.5	D49.0
ascending	C18.2	C78.5	D01.0	D12.2	D37.4	D49.0
caput	C18.0	C78.5	D01.0	D12.0	D37.4	D49.0
descending	C18.6	C78.5	D01.0	D12.4	D37.4	D49.0
distal	C18.6	C78.5	D01.0	D12.4	D37.4	D49.0
left	C18.6	C78.5	D01.0	D12.4	D37.4	D49.0
overlapping lesion	C18.8	-	-	-	-	-
pelvic	C18.7	C78.5	D01.0	D12.5	D37.4	D49.0
right	C18.2	C78.5	D01.0	D12.2	D37.4	D49.0
sigmoid (flexure)	C18.7	C78.5	D01.0	D12.5	D37.4	D49.0
transverse	C18.4	C78.5	D01.0	D12.3	D37.4	D49.0
hepatic flexure	C18.3	C78.5	D01.0	D12.3	D37.4	D49.0
ileocecum, ileocecal (coil) (valve)	C18.0	C78.5	D01.0	D12.0	D37.4	D49.0
overlapping lesion	C18.8	-	-	-	-	-
sigmoid flexure (lower) (upper)	C18.7	C78.5	D01.0	D12.5	D37.4	D49.0
splenic flexure	C18.5	C78.5	D01.0	D12.3	D37.4	D49.0
small	C17.9	C78.4	D01.40	D13.30	D37.2	D49.0
duodenum	C17.0	C78.4	D01.49	D13.2	D37.2	D49.0
ileum	C17.2	C78.4	D01.49	D13.39	D37.2	D49.0
jejunum	C17.1	C78.4	D01.49	D13.39	D37.2	D49.0
overlapping lesion	C17.8	-	-	-	-	-
tract NEC	C26.0	C78.89	D01.40	D13.9	D37.8	D49.0
intra-abdominal	C76.2	C79.89	D09.8	D36.7	D48.7	D49.89
intracranial NEC	C71.9	C79.31	-	D33.2	D43.2	D49.6
intrahepatic (bile) duct	C22.1	C78.7	D01.5	D13.4	D37.6	D49.0
intraocular	C69.9-	C79.49	D09.2-	D31.9-	D48.7	D49.89
intraorbital	C69.6-	C79.49	D09.2-	D31.6-	D48.7	D49.89
intrasellar	C75.1	C79.89	D09.3	D35.2	D44.3	D49.7
intrathoracic (cavity) (organs)	C76.1	C79.89	D09.8	D15.9	D48.7	D49.89
specified NEC	C76.1	C79.89	D09.8	D15.7	-	-
iris	C69.4-	C79.49	D09.2-	D31.4-	D48.7	D49.89
ischiorectal (fossa)	C76.3	C79.89	D09.8	D36.7	D48.7	D49.89
ischium	C41.4	C79.51	-	D16.8	D48.0	D49.2
island of Reil	C71.0	C79.31	-	D33.0	D43.0	D49.6
islands or islets of Langerhans	C25.4	C78.89	D01.7	D13.7	D37.8	D49.0
isthmus uteri	C54.0	C79.82	D07.0	D26.1	D39.0	D49.59
jaw	C76.0	C79.89	D09.8	D36.7	D48.7	D49.89
bone	C41.1	C79.51	-	D16.5-	D48.0	D49.2
lower	C41.1	C79.51	-	D16.5-	-	-
upper	C41.0	C79.51	-	D16.4-	-	-
carcinoma (any type) (lower) (upper)	C76.0	C79.89	-	-	-	-
skin — *see also Neoplasm, skin, face*	C44.309	C79.2	D04.39	D23.39	D48.5	D49.2
soft tissues	C03.9	C79.89	D00.03	D10.39	D37.09	D49.0
lower	C03.1	C79.89	D00.03	D10.39	D37.09	D49.0
upper	C03.0	C79.89	D00.03	D10.39	D37.09	D49.0
jejunum	C17.1	C78.4	D01.49	D13.39	D37.2	D49.0
joint NEC — *see also Neoplasm, bone*	C41.9	C79.51	-	D16.9-	D48.0	D49.2
acromioclavicular	C40.0-	C79.51	-	D16.0-	-	-
bursa or synovial membrane — *see Neoplasm, connective tissue*						
costovertebral	C41.3	C79.51	-	D16.7	D48.0	D49.2
sternocostal	C41.3	C79.51	-	D16.7	D48.0	D49.2
temporomandibular	C41.1	C79.51	-	D16.5-	D48.0	D49.2
junction						
anorectal	C21.8	C78.5	D01.3	D12.9	D37.8	D49.0
cardioesophageal	C16.0	C78.89	D00.2	D13.1	D37.1	D49.0

Neoplasm, neoplastic	Malignant Primary	Malignant Secondary	Ca in situ	Benign	Uncertain Behavior	Unspecified Behavior
esophagogastric	C16.0	C78.89	D00.2	D13.1	D37.1	D49.0
gastroesophageal	C16.0	C78.89	D00.2	D13.1	D37.1	D49.0
hard and soft palate	C05.9	C79.89	D00.00	D10.39	D37.09	D49.0
ileocecal	C18.0	C78.5	D01.0	D12.0	D37.4	D49.0
pelvirectal	C19	C78.5	D01.1	D12.7	D37.5	D49.0
pelviureteric	C65.-	C79.0-	D09.19	D30.1-	D41.1-	D49.59
rectosigmoid	C19	C78.5	D01.1	D12.7	D37.5	D49.0
squamocolumnar, of cervix	C53.8	C79.82	D06.7	D26.0	D39.0	D49.59
Kaposi's sarcoma — *see Kaposi's, sarcoma*						
kidney (parenchymal)	C64.-	C79.0-	D09.19	D30.0-	D41.0-	D49.51-
calyx	C65.-	C79.0-	D09.19	D30.1-	D41.1-	D49.51-
hilus	C65.-	C79.0-	D09.19	D30.1-	D41.1-	D49.51-
pelvis	C65.-	C79.0-	D09.19	D30.1-	D41.1-	D49.51-
knee NEC	C76.5-	C79.89	D04.7-	D36.7	D48.7	D49.89
labia (skin)	C51.9	C79.82	D07.1	D28.0	D39.8	D49.59
majora	C51.0	C79.82	D07.1	D28.0	D39.8	D49.59
minora	C51.1	C79.82	D07.1	D28.0	D39.8	D49.59
labial — *see also Neoplasm, lip*	C00.9	C79.89	D00.01	D10.0	D37.01	D49.0
sulcus (lower) (upper)	C06.1	C79.89	D00.02	D10.39	D37.09	D49.0
labium (skin)	C51.9	C79.82	D07.1	D28.0	D39.8	D49.59
majus	C51.0	C79.82	D07.1	D28.0	D39.8	D49.59
minus	C51.1	C79.82	D07.1	D28.0	D39.8	D49.59
lacrimal						
canaliculi	C69.5-	C79.49	D09.2-	D31.5-	D48.7	D49.89
duct (nasal)	C69.5-	C79.49	D09.2-	D31.5-	D48.7	D49.89
gland	C69.5-	C79.49	D09.2-	D31.5-	D48.7	D49.89
punctum	C69.5-	C79.49	D09.2-	D31.5-	D48.7	D49.89
sac	C69.5-	C79.49	D09.2-	D31.5-	D48.7	D49.89
Langerhans, islands or islets	C25.4	C78.89	D01.7	D13.7	D37.8	D49.0
laryngopharynx	C13.9	C79.89	D00.08	D10.7	D37.05	D49.0
larynx, laryngeal NEC	C32.9	C78.39	D02.0	D14.1	D38.0	D49.1
aryepiglottic fold	C32.1	C78.39	D02.0	D14.1	D38.0	D49.1
cartilage (arytenoid) (cricoid) (cuneiform) (thyroid)	C32.3	C78.39	D02.0	D14.1	D38.0	D49.1
commissure (anterior) (posterior)	C32.0	C78.39	D02.0	D14.1	D38.0	D49.1
extrinsic NEC	C32.1	C78.39	D02.0	D14.1	D38.0	D49.1
meaning hypopharynx	C13.9	C79.89	D00.08	D10.7	D37.05	D49.0
interarytenoid fold	C32.1	C78.39	D02.0	D14.1	D38.0	D49.1
intrinsic	C32.0	C78.39	D02.0	D14.1	D38.0	D49.1
overlapping lesion	C32.8	-	-	-	-	-
ventricular band	C32.1	C78.39	D02.0	D14.1	D38.0	D49.1
leg NEC	C76.5-	C79.89	D04.7-	D36.7	D48.7	D49.89
lens, crystalline	C69.4-	C79.49	D09.2-	D31.4-	D48.7	D49.89
lid (lower) (upper)	C44.10-	C79.2	D04.1-	D23.1-	D48.5	D49.2
basal cell carcinoma	C44.11-	-	-	-	-	-
sebaceous cell	C44.13-	-	-	-	-	-
specified type NEC	C44.19-	-	-	-	-	-
squamous cell carcinoma	C44.12-	-	-	-	-	-
ligament — *see also Neoplasm, connective tissue*						
broad	C57.1	C79.82	D07.39	D28.2	D39.8	D49.59
Mackenrodt's	C57.7	C79.82	D07.39	D28.7	D39.8	D49.59
non-uterine — *see Neoplasm, connective tissue*						
round	C57.2	C79.82	-	D28.2	D39.8	D49.59
sacro-uterine	C57.3	C79.82	-	D28.2	D39.8	D49.59
uterine	C57.3	C79.82	-	D28.2	D39.8	D49.59
utero-ovarian	C57.7	C79.82	D07.39	D28.2	D39.8	D49.59
uterosacral	C57.3	C79.82	-	D28.2	D39.8	D49.59

Neoplasm, neoplastic	Malignant Primary	Malignant Secondary	Ca in situ	Benign	Uncertain Behavior	Unspecified Behavior
limb	C76.8	C79.89	D04.8	D36.7	D48.7	D49.89
lower	C76.5-	C79.89	D04.7-	D36.7	D48.7	D49.89
upper	C76.4-	C79.89	D04.6-	D36.7	D48.7	D49.89
limbus of cornea	C69.1-	C79.49	D09.2-	D31.1-	D48.7	D49.89
lingual NEC — *see also Neoplasm, tongue*	C02.9	C79.89	D00.07	D10.1	D37.02	D49.0
lingula, lung	C34.1-	C78.0-	D02.2-	D14.3-	D38.1	D49.1
lip	C00.9	C79.89	D00.01	D10.0	D37.01	D49.0
buccal aspect — *see Neoplasm, lip, internal*						
commissure	C00.6	C79.89	D00.01	D10.0	D37.01	D49.0
external	C00.2	C79.89	D00.01	D10.0	D37.01	D49.0
lower	C00.1	C79.89	D00.01	D10.0	D37.01	D49.0
upper	C00.0	C79.89	D00.01	D10.0	D37.01	D49.0
frenulum — *see Neoplasm, lip, internal*						
inner aspect — *see Neoplasm, lip, internal*						
internal	C00.5	C79.89	D00.01	D10.0	D37.01	D49.0
lower	C00.4	C79.89	D00.01	D10.0	D37.01	D49.0
upper	C00.3	C79.89	D00.01	D10.0	D37.01	D49.0
lipstick area	C00.2	C79.89	D00.01	D10.0	D37.01	D49.0
lower	C00.1	C79.89	D00.01	D10.0	D37.01	D49.0
upper	C00.0	C79.89	D00.01	D10.0	D37.01	D49.0
lower	C00.1	C79.89	D00.01	D10.0	D37.01	D49.0
internal	C00.4	C79.89	D00.01	D10.0	D37.01	D49.0
mucosa — *see Neoplasm, lip, internal*						
oral aspect — *see Neoplasm, lip, internal*						
overlapping lesion	C00.8	-	-	-	-	-
with oral cavity or pharynx	C14.8	-	-	-	-	-
skin (commissure) (lower) (upper)	C44.00	C79.2	D04.0	D23.0	D48.5	D49.2
basal cell carcinoma	C44.01	-	-	-	-	-
specified type NEC	C44.09	-	-	-	-	-
squamous cell carcinoma	C44.02	-	-	-	-	-
upper	C00.0	C79.89	D00.01	D10.0	D37.01	D49.0
internal	C00.3	C79.89	D00.01	D10.0	D37.01	D49.0
vermilion border	C00.2	C79.89	D00.01	D10.0	D37.01	D49.0
lower	C00.1	C79.89	D00.01	D10.0	D37.01	D49.0
upper	C00.0	C79.89	D00.01	D10.0	D37.01	D49.0
lipomatous — *see Lipoma, by site*						
liver — *see also Index to disease, by histology*	C22.9	C78.7	D01.5	D13.4	D37.6	D49.0
primary	C22.8	C78.7	D01.5	D13.4	D37.6	D49.0
lumbosacral plexus	C47.5	C79.89	-	D36.16	D48.2	D49.2
lung	C34.9-	C78.0-	D02.2-	D14.3-	D38.1	D49.1
azygos lobe	C34.1-	C78.0-	D02.2-	D14.3-	D38.1	D49.1
carina	C34.0-	C78.0-	D02.2-	D14.3-	D38.1	D49.1
hilus	C34.0-	C78.0-	D02.2-	D14.3-	D38.1	D49.1
linqula	C34.1-	C78.0-	D02.2-	D14.3-	D38.1	D49.1
lobe NEC	C34.9-	C78.0-	D02.2-	D14.3-	D38.1	D49.1
lower lobe	C34.3-	C78.0-	D02.2-	D14.3-	D38.1	D49.1
main bronchus	C34.0-	C78.0-	D02.2-	D14.3-	D38.1	D49.1
mesothelioma — *see Mesothelioma*						
middle lobe	C34.2	C78.0-	D02.21	D14.31	D38.1	D49.1
overlapping lesion	C34.8-	-	-	-	-	-
upper lobe	C34.1-	C78.0-	D02.2-	D14.3-	D38.1	D49.1
lymph, lymphatic channel NEC	C49.9	C79.89	-	D21.9	D48.1	D49.2
gland (secondary)	-	C77.9	-	D36.0	D48.7	D49.89
abdominal	-	C77.2	-	D36.0	D48.7	D49.89

	Malignant Primary	Malignant Secondary	Ca in situ	Benign	Uncertain Behavior	Unspecified Behavior
Neoplasm, neoplastic						
aortic	-	C77.2	-	D36.0	D48.7	D49.89
arm	-	C77.3	-	D36.0	D48.7	D49.89
auricular (anterior) (posterior)	-	C77.0	-	D36.0	D48.7	D49.89
axilla, axillary	-	C77.3	-	D36.0	D48.7	D49.89
brachial	-	C77.3	-	D36.0	D48.7	D49.89
bronchial	-	C77.1	-	D36.0	D48.7	D49.89
bronchopulmonary	-	C77.1	-	D36.0	D48.7	D49.89
celiac	-	C77.2	-	D36.0	D48.7	D49.89
cervical	-	C77.0	-	D36.0	D48.7	D49.89
cervicofacial	-	C77.0	-	D36.0	D48.7	D49.89
Cloquet	-	C77.4	-	D36.0	D48.7	D49.89
colic	-	C77.2	-	D36.0	D48.7	D49.89
common duct	-	C77.2	-	D36.0	D48.7	D49.89
cubital	-	C77.3	-	D36.0	D48.7	D49.89
diaphragmatic	-	C77.1	-	D36.0	D48.7	D49.89
epigastric, inferior	-	C77.1	-	D36.0	D48.7	D49.89
epitrochlear	-	C77.3	-	D36.0	D48.7	D49.89
esophageal	-	C77.1	-	D36.0	D48.7	D49.89
face	-	C77.0	-	D36.0	D48.7	D49.89
femoral	-	C77.4	-	D36.0	D48.7	D49.89
gastric	-	C77.2	-	D36.0	D48.7	D49.89
groin	-	C77.4	-	D36.0	D48.7	D49.89
head	-	C77.0	-	D36.0	D48.7	D49.89
hepatic	-	C77.2	-	D36.0	D48.7	D49.89
hilar (pulmonary)	-	C77.1	-	D36.0	D48.7	D49.89
splenic	-	C77.2	-	D36.0	D48.7	D49.89
hypogastric	-	C77.5	-	D36.0	D48.7	D49.89
ileocolic	-	C77.2	-	D36.0	D48.7	D49.89
iliac	-	C77.5	-	D36.0	D48.7	D49.89
infraclavicular	-	C77.3	-	D36.0	D48.7	D49.89
inguina, inguinal	-	C77.4	-	D36.0	D48.7	D49.89
innominate	-	C77.1	-	D36.0	D48.7	D49.89
intercostal	-	C77.1	-	D36.0	D48.7	D49.89
intestinal	-	C77.2	-	D36.0	D48.7	D49.89
intrabdominal	-	C77.2	-	D36.0	D48.7	D49.89
intrapelvic	-	C77.5	-	D36.0	D48.7	D49.89
intrathoracic	-	C77.1	-	D36.0	D48.7	D49.89
jugular	-	C77.0	-	D36.0	D48.7	D49.89
leg	-	C77.4	-	D36.0	D48.7	D49.89
limb						
lower	-	C77.4	-	D36.0	D48.7	D49.89
upper	-	C77.3	-	D36.0	D48.7	D49.89
lower limb	-	C77.4	-	D36.0	D48.7	D49.89
lumbar	-	C77.2	-	D36.0	D48.7	D49.89
mandibular	-	C77.0	-	D36.0	D48.7	D49.89
mediastinal	-	C77.1	-	D36.0	D48.7	D49.89
mesenteric (inferior) (superior)	-	C77.2	-	D36.0	D48.7	D49.89
midcolic	-	C77.2	-	D36.0	D48.7	D49.89
multiple sites in categories C77.0 - C77.5	-	C77.8	-	D36.0	D48.7	D49.89
neck	-	C77.0	-	D36.0	D48.7	D49.89
obturator	-	C77.5	-	D36.0	D48.7	D49.89
occipital	-	C77.0	-	D36.0	D48.7	D49.89
pancreatic	-	C77.2	-	D36.0	D48.7	D49.89
para-aortic	-	C77.2	-	D36.0	D48.7	D49.89
paracervical	-	C77.5	-	D36.0	D48.7	D49.89
parametrial	-	C77.5	-	D36.0	D48.7	D49.89
parasternal	-	C77.1	-	D36.0	D48.7	D49.89
parotid	-	C77.0	-	D36.0	D48.7	D49.89
pectoral	-	C77.3	-	D36.0	D48.7	D49.89

Neoplasm, neoplastic	Malignant Primary	Malignant Secondary	Ca in situ	Benign	Uncertain Behavior	Unspecified Behavior
pelvic	-	C77.5	-	D36.0	D48.7	D49.89
peri-aortic	-	C77.2	-	D36.0	D48.7	D49.89
peripancreatic	-	C77.2	-	D36.0	D48.7	D49.89
popliteal	-	C77.4	-	D36.0	D48.7	D49.89
porta hepatis	-	C77.2	-	D36.0	D48.7	D49.89
portal	-	C77.2	-	D36.0	D48.7	D49.89
preauricular	-	C77.0	-	D36.0	D48.7	D49.89
prelaryngeal	-	C77.0	-	D36.0	D48.7	D49.89
presymphysial	-	C77.5	-	D36.0	D48.7	D49.89
pretracheal	-	C77.0	-	D36.0	D48.7	D49.89
primary (any site) NEC	C96.9	-	-	-	-	-
pulmonary (hiler)	-	C77.1	-	D36.0	D48.7	D49.89
pyloric	-	C77.2	-	D36.0	D48.7	D49.89
retroperitoneal	-	C77.2	-	D36.0	D48.7	D49.89
retropharyngeal	-	C77.0	-	D36.0	D48.7	D49.89
Rosenmuller's	-	C77.4	-	D36.0	D48.7	D49.89
sacral	-	C77.5	-	D36.0	D48.7	D49.89
scalene	-	C77.0	-	D36.0	D48.7	D49.89
site NEC	-	C77.9	-	D36.0	D48.7	D49.89
splenic (hilar)	-	C77.2	-	D36.0	D48.7	D49.89
subclavicular	-	C77.3	-	D36.0	D48.7	D49.89
subinguinal	-	C77.4	-	D36.0	D48.7	D49.89
sublingual	-	C77.0	-	D36.0	D48.7	D49.89
submandibular	-	C77.0	-	D36.0	D48.7	D49.89
submaxillary	-	C77.0	-	D36.0	D48.7	D49.89
submental	-	C77.0	-	D36.0	D48.7	D49.89
subscapular	-	C77.3	-	D36.0	D48.7	D49.89
supraclavicular	-	C77.0	-	D36.0	D48.7	D49.89
thoracic	-	C77.1	-	D36.0	D48.7	D49.89
tibial	-	C77.4	-	D36.0	D48.7	D49.89
tracheal	-	C77.1	-	D36.0	D48.7	D49.89
tracheobronchial	-	C77.1	-	D36.0	D48.7	D49.89
upper limb	-	C77.3	-	D36.0	D48.7	D49.89
Virchow's	-	C77.0	-	D36.0	D48.7	D49.89
node — *see also Neoplasm, lymph gland*						
primary NEC	C96.9	-	-	-	-	-
vessel — *see also Neoplasm, connective tissue*	C49.9	C79.89	-	D21.9	D48.1	D49.2
Mackenrodt's ligament	C57.7	C79.82	D07.39	D28.7	D39.8	D49.59
malar	C41.0	C79.51	-	D16.4-	D48.0	D49.2
region — *see Neoplasm, cheek*						
mammary gland — *see Neoplasm, breast*						
mandible	C41.1	C79.51	-	D16.5-	D48.0	D49.2
alveolar						
mucosa (carcinoma)	C03.1	C79.89	D00.03	D10.39	D37.09	D49.0
ridge or process	C41.1	C79.51	-	D16.5-	D48.0	D49.2
marrow (bone) NEC	C96.9	C79.52	-	-	D47.9	D49.89
mastectomy site (skin) — *see also Neoplasm, breast, skin*	C44.501	C79.2	-	-	-	-
specified as breast tissue	C50.8-	C79.81	-	-	-	-
mastoid (air cells) (antrum) (cavity)	C30.1	C78.39	D02.3	D14.0	D38.5	D49.1
bone or process	C41.0	C79.51	-	D16.4-	D48.0	D49.2
maxilla, maxillary (superior)	C41.0	C79.51	-	D16.4-	D48.0	D49.2
alveolar						
mucosa	C03.0	C79.89	D00.03	D10.39	D37.09	D49.0
ridge or process (carcinoma)	C41.0	C79.51	-	D16.4-	D48.0	D49.2
antrum	C31.0	C78.39	D02.3	D14.0	D38.5	D49.1
carcinoma	C03.0	C79.51	-	-	-	-

Neoplasm, neoplastic	Malignant Primary	Malignant Secondary	Ca in situ	Benign	Uncertain Behavior	Unspecified Behavior
inferior — *see Neoplasm, mandible*						
sinus	C31.0	C78.39	D02.3	D14.0	D38.5	D49.1
meatus external (ear) — *see also Neoplasm, skin, ear*	C44.20-	C79.2	D04.2-	D23.2-	D48.5	D49.2
Meckel diverticulum, malignant	C17.3	C78.4	D01.49	D13.39	D37.2	D49.0
mediastinum, mediastinal	C38.3	C78.1	-	D15.2	D38.3	D49.89
anterior	C38.1	C78.1	-	D15.2	D38.3	D49.89
posterior	C38.2	C78.1	-	D15.2	D38.3	D49.89
medulla						
adrenal	C74.1-	C79.7-	D09.3	D35.0-	D44.1-	D49.7
oblongata	C71.7	C79.31	-	D33.1	D43.1	D49.6
meibomian gland	C44.10-	C79.2	D04.1-	D23.1-	D48.5	D49.2
basal cell carcinoma	C44.11-	-	-	-	-	-
sebaceous cell	C44.13-	-	-	-	-	-
specified type NEC	C44.19-	-	-	-	-	-
squamous cell carcinoma	C44.12-	-	-	-	-	-
melanoma — *see Melanoma*						
meninges	C70.9	C79.49	-	D32.9	D42.9	D49.7
brain	C70.0	C79.32	-	D32.0	D42.0	D49.7
cerebral	C70.0	C79.32	-	D32.0	D42.0	D49.7
crainial	C70.0	C79.32	-	D32.0	D42.0	D49.7
intracranial	C70.0	C79.32	-	D32.0	D42.0	D49.7
spinal (cord)	C70.1	C79.49	-	D32.1	D42.1	D49.7
meniscus, knee joint (lateral) (medial)	C40.2-	C79.51	-	D16.2-	D48.0	D49.2
Merkel cell — *see Carcinoma, Merkel cell*						
mesentery, mesenteric	C48.1	C78.6	-	D20.1	D48.4	D49.0
mesoappendix	C48.1	C78.6	-	D20.1	D48.4	D49.0
mesocolon	C48.1	C78.6	-	D20.1	D48.4	D49.0
mesopharynx — *see Neoplasm, oropharynx*						
mesosalpinx	C57.1	C79.82	D07.39	D28.2	D39.8	D49.59
mesothelial tissue — *see Mesothelioma*						
mesothelioma — *see Mesothelioma*						
mesovarium	C57.1	C79.82	D07.39	D28.2	D39.8	D49.59
metacarpus (any bone)	C40.1-	C79.51	-	D16.1-	-	-
metastatic NEC — *see also Neoplasm, by site, secondary*	-	C79.9	-	-	-	-
metatarsus (any bone)	C40.3-	C79.51	-	D16.3-	-	-
midbrain	C71.7	C79.31	-	D33.1	D43.1	D49.6
milk duct — *see Neoplasm, breast*						
mons						
pubis	C51.9	C79.82	D07.1	D28.0	D39.8	D49.59
veneris	C51.9	C79.82	D07.1	D28.0	D39.8	D49.59
motor tract	C72.9	C79.49	-	D33.9	D43.9	D49.7
brain	C71.9	C79.31	-	D33.2	D43.2	D49.6
cauda equina	C72.1	C79.49	-	D33.4	D43.4	D49.7
spinal	C72.0	C79.49	-	D33.4	D43.4	D49.7
mouth	C06.9	C79.89	D00.00	D10.30	D37.09	D49.0
book-leaf	C06.89	C79.89	-	-	-	-
floor	C04.9	C79.89	D00.06	D10.2	D37.09	D49.0
anterior portion	C04.0	C79.89	D00.06	D10.2	D37.09	D49.0
lateral portion	C04.1	C79.89	D00.06	D10.2	D37.09	D49.0
overlapping lesion	C04.8	-	-	-	-	-
overlapping NEC	C06.80	-	-	-	-	-
roof	C05.9	C79.89	D00.00	D10.39	D37.09	D49.0
specified part NEC	C06.89	C79.89	D00.00	D10.39	D37.09	D49.0
vestibule	C06.1	C79.89	D00.00	D10.39	D37.09	D49.0
mucosa						
alveolar (ridge or process)	C03.9	C79.89	D00.03	D10.39	D37.09	D49.0

Neoplasm, neoplastic	Malignant Primary	Malignant Secondary	Ca in situ	Benign	Uncertain Behavior	Unspecified Behavior
lower	C03.1	C79.89	D00.03	D10.39	D37.09	D49.0
upper	C03.0	C79.89	D00.03	D10.39	D37.09	D49.0
buccal	C06.0	C79.89	D00.02	D10.39	D37.09	D49.0
cheek	C06.0	C79.89	D00.02	D10.39	D37.09	D49.0
lip — *see Neoplasm, lip, internal*						
nasal	C30.0	C78.39	D02.3	D14.0	D38.5	D49.1
oral	C06.0	C79.89	D00.02	D10.39	D37.09	D49.0
Mullerian duct						
female	C57.7	C79.82	D07.39	D28.7	D39.8	D49.59
male	C63.7	C79.82	D07.69	D29.8	D40.8	D49.59
muscle — *see also Neoplasm, connective tissue*						
extraocular	C69.6-	C79.49	D09.2-	D31.6-	D48.7	D49.89
myocardium	C38.0	C79.89	-	D15.1	D48.7	D49.89
myometrium	C54.2	C79.82	D07.0	D26.1	D39.0	D49.59
myopericardium	C38.0	C79.89	-	D15.1	D48.7	D49.89
nabothian gland (follicle)	C53.0	C79.82	D06.0	D26.0	D39.0	D49.59
nail — *see also Neoplasm, skin, limb*	C44.90	C79.2	D04.9	D23.9	D48.5	D49.2
finger — *see also Neoplasm, skin, limb, upper*	C44.60-	C79.2	D04.6-	D23.6-	D48.5	D49.2
toe — *see also Neoplasm, skin, limb, lower*	C44.70-	C79.2	D04.7-	D23.7-	D48.5	D49.2
nares, naris (anterior) (posterior)	C30.0	C78.39	D02.3	D14.0	D38.5	D49.1
nasal — *see Neoplasm, nose*						
nasolabial groove — *see also Neoplasm, skin, face*	C44.309	C79.2	D04.39	D23.39	D48.5	D49.2
nasolacrimal duct	C69.5-	C79.49	D09.2-	D31.5-	D48.7	D49.89
nasopharynx, nasopharyngeal	C11.9	C79.89	D00.08	D10.6	D37.05	D49.0
floor	C11.3	C79.89	D00.08	D10.6	D37.05	D49.0
overlapping lesion	C11.8	-	-	-	-	-
roof	C11.0	C79.89	D00.08	D10.6	D37.05	D49.0
wall	C11.9	C79.89	D00.08	D10.6	D37.05	D49.0
anterior	C11.3	C79.89	D00.08	D10.6	D37.05	D49.0
lateral	C11.2	C79.89	D00.08	D10.6	D37.05	D49.0
posterior	C11.1	C79.89	D00.08	D10.6	D37.05	D49.0
superior	C11.0	C79.89	D00.08	D10.6	D37.05	D49.0
nates — *see also Neoplasm, skin, trunk*	C44.509	C79.2	D04.5	D23.5	D48.5	D49.2
neck NEC	C76.0	C79.89	D09.8	D36.7	D48.7	D49.89
skin	C44.40	-	-	-	-	-
basal cell carcinoma	C44.41	-	-	-	-	-
specified type NEC	C44.49	-	-	-	-	-
squamous cell carcinoma	C44.42	-	-	-	-	-
nerve (ganglion)	C47.9	C79.89	-	D36.10	D48.2	D49.2
abducens	C72.59	C79.49	-	D33.3	D43.3	D49.7
accessory (spinal)	C72.59	C79.49	-	D33.3	D43.3	D49.7
acoustic	C72.4-	C79.49	-	D33.3	D43.3	D49.7
auditory	C72.4-	C79.49	-	D33.3	D43.3	D49.7
autonomic NEC — *see also Neoplasm, nerve, peripheral*	C47.9	C79.89	-	D36.10	D48.2	D49.2
brachial	C47.1-	C79.89	-	D36.12	D48.2	D49.2
cranial	C72.50	C79.49	-	D33.3	D43.3	D49.7
specified NEC	C72.59	C79.49	-	D33.3	D43.3	D49.7
facial	C72.59	C79.49	-	D33.3	D43.3	D49.7
femoral	C47.2-	C79.89	-	D36.13	D48.2	D49.2
ganglion NEC — *see also Neoplasm, nerve, peripheral*	C47.9	C79.89	-	D36.10	D48.2	D49.2
glossopharyngeal	C72.59	C79.49	-	D33.3	D43.3	D49.7
hypoglossal	C72.59	C79.49	-	D33.3	D43.3	D49.7
intercostal	C47.3	C79.89	-	D36.14	D48.2	D49.2
lumbar	C47.6	C79.89	-	D36.17	D48.2	D49.2

Neoplasm, neoplastic	Malignant Primary	Malignant Secondary	Ca in situ	Benign	Uncertain Behavior	Unspecified Behavior
median	C47.1-	C79.89	-	D36.12	D48.2	D49.2
obturator	C47.2-	C79.89	-	D36.13	D48.2	D49.2
oculomotor	C72.59	C79.49	-	D33.3	D43.3	D49.7
olfactory	C47.2-	C79.49	-	D33.3	D43.3	D49.7
optic	C72.3-	C79.49	-	D33.3	D43.3	D49.7
parasympathetic NEC	C47.9	C79.89	-	D36.10	D48.2	D49.2
peripheral NEC	C47.9	C79.89	-	D36.10	D48.2	D49.2
abdomen	C47.4	C79.89	-	D36.15	D48.2	D49.2
abdominal wall	C47.4	C79.89	-	D36.15	D48.2	D49.2
ankle	C47.2-	C79.89	-	D36.13	D48.2	D49.2
antecubital fossa or space	C47.1-	C79.89	-	D36.12	D48.2	D49.2
arm	C47.1-	C79.89	-	D36.12	D48.2	D49.2
auricle (ear)	C47.0	C79.89	-	D36.11	D48.2	D49.2
axilla	C47.3	C79.89	-	D36.12	D48.2	D49.2
back	C47.6	C79.89	-	D36.17	D48.2	D49.2
buttock	C47.5	C79.89	-	D36.16	D48.2	D49.2
calf	C47.2-	C79.89	-	D36.13	D48.2	D49.2
cervical region	C47.0	C79.89	-	D36.11	D48.2	D49.2
cheek	C47.0	C79.89	-	D36.11	D48.2	D49.2
chest (wall)	C47.3	C79.89	-	D36.14	D48.2	D49.2
chin	C47.0	C79.89	-	D36.11	D48.2	D49.2
ear (external)	C47.0	C79.89	-	D36.11	D48.2	D49.2
elbow	C47.1-	C79.89	-	D36.12	D48.2	D49.2
extrarectal	C47.5	C79.89	-	D36.16	D48.2	D49.2
extremity	C47.9	C79.89	-	D36.10	D48.2	D49.2
lower	C47.2-	C79.89	-	D36.13	D48.2	D49.2
upper	C47.1-	C79.89	-	D36.12	D48.2	D49.2
eyelid	C47.0	C79.89	-	D36.11	D48.2	D49.2
face	C47.0	C79.89	-	D36.11	D48.2	D49.2
finger	C47.1-	C79.89	-	D36.12	D48.2	D49.2
flank	C47.6	C79.89	-	D36.17	D48.2	D49.2
foot	C47.2-	C79.89	-	D36.13	D48.2	D49.2
forearm	C47.1-	C79.89	-	D36.12	D48.2	D49.2
forehead	C47.0	C79.89	-	D36.11	D48.2	D49.2
gluteal region	C47.5	C79.89	-	D36.16	D48.2	D49.2
groin	C47.5	C79.89	-	D36.16	D48.2	D49.2
hand	C47.1-	C79.89	-	D36.12	D48.2	D49.2
head	C47.0	C79.89	-	D36.11	D48.2	D49.2
heel	C47.2-	C79.89	-	D36.13	D48.2	D49.2
hip	C47.2-	C79.89	-	D36.13	D48.2	D49.2
infraclavicular region	C47.3	C79.89	-	D36.14	D48.2	D49.2
inguinal (canal) (region)	C47.5	C79.89	-	D36.16	D48.2	D49.2
intrathoracic	C47.3	C79.89	-	D36.14	D48.2	D49.2
ischiorectal fossa	C47.5	C79.89	-	D36.16	D48.2	D49.2
knee	C47.2-	C79.89	-	D36.13	D48.2	D49.2
leg	C47.2-	C79.89	-	D36.13	D48.2	D49.2
limb NEC	C47.9	C79.89	-	D36.10	D48.2	D49.2
lower	C47.2-	C79.89	-	D36.13	D48.2	D49.2
upper	C47.1-	C79.89	-	D36.12	D48.2	D49.2
nates	C47.5	C79.89	-	D36.16	D48.2	D49.2
neck	C47.0	C79.89	-	D36.11	D48.2	D49.2
orbit	C69.6-	C79.49	-	D31.6-	D48.7	D49.2
pararectal	C47.5	C79.89	-	D36.16	D48.2	D49.2
paraurethral	C47.5	C79.89	-	D36.16	D48.2	D49.2
paravaginal	C47.5	C79.89	-	D36.16	D48.2	D49.2
pelvis (floor)	C47.5	C79.89	-	D36.16	D48.2	D49.2
pelvoabdominal	C47.8	C79.89	-	D36.17	D48.2	D49.2
perineum	C47.5	C79.89	-	D36.16	D48.2	D49.2
perirectal (tissue)	C47.5	C79.89	-	D36.16	D48.2	D49.2

Neoplasm, neoplastic	Malignant Primary	Malignant Secondary	Ca in situ	Benign	Uncertain Behavior	Unspecified Behavior
periurethral (tissue)	C47.5	C79.89	-	D36.16	D48.2	D49.2
popliteal fossa or space	C47.2-	C79.89	-	D36.13	D48.2	D49.2
presacral	C47.5	C79.89	-	D36.16	D48.2	D49.2
pterygoid fossa	C47.0	C79.89	-	D36.11	D48.2	D49.2
rectovaginal septum or wall	C47.5	C79.89	-	D36.16	D48.2	D49.2
rectovesical	C47.5	C79.89	-	D36.16	D48.2	D49.2
sacrococcygeal region	C47.5	C79.89	-	D36.16	D48.2	D49.2
scalp	C47.0	C79.89	-	D36.11	D48.2	D49.2
scapular region	C47.3	C79.89	-	D36.14	D48.2	D49.2
shoulder	C47.1-	C79.89	-	D36.12	D48.2	D49.2
submental	C47.0	C79.89	-	D36.11	D48.2	D49.2
supraclavicular region	C47.0	C79.89	-	D36.11	D48.2	D49.2
temple	C47.0	C79.89	-	D36.11	D48.2	D49.2
temporal region	C47.0	C79.89	-	D36.11	D48.2	D49.2
thigh	C47.2-	C79.89	-	D36.13	D48.2	D49.2
thoracic (duct) (wall)	C47.3	C79.89	-	D36.14	D48.2	D49.2
thorax	C47.3	C79.89	-	D36.14	D48.2	D49.2
thumb	C47.1-	C79.89	-	D36.12	D48.2	D49.2
toe	C47.2-	C79.89	-	D36.13	D48.2	D49.2
trunk	C47.6	C79.89	-	D36.17	D48.2	D49.2
umbilicus	C47.4	C79.89	-	D36.15	D48.2	D49.2
vesicorectal	C47.5	C79.89	-	D36.16	D48.2	D49.2
wrist	C47.1-	C79.89	-	D36.12	D48.2	D49.2
radial	C47.1-	C79.89	-	D36.12	D48.2	D49.2
sacral	C47.5	C79.89	-	D36.16	D48.2	D49.2
sciatic	C47.2-	C79.89	-	D36.13	D48.2	D49.2
spinal NEC	C47.9	C79.89	-	D36.10	D48.2	D49.2
accessory	C72.59	C79.49	-	D33.3	D43.3	D49.7
sympathetic NEC — *see also Neoplasm, nerve, peripheral*	C47.9	C79.89	-	D36.10	D48.2	D49.2
trigeminal	C72.59	C79.49	-	D33.3	D43.3	D49.7
trochlear	C72.59	C79.49	-	D33.3	D43.3	D49.7
ulnar	C47.1-	C79.89	-	D36.12	D48.2	D49.2
vagus	C72.59	C79.49	-	D33.3	D43.3	D49.7
nervous system (central)	C72.9	C79.40	-	D33.9	D43.9	D49.7
autonomic — *see Neoplasm, nerve, peripheral*						
parasympathetic — *see Neoplasm, nerve, peripheral*						
specified site NEC	-	C79.49	-	D33.7	D43.8	-
sympathetic — *see Neoplasm, nerve, peripheral*						
nevus — *see Nevus*						
nipple	C50.0-	C79.81	D05.-	D24.-	-	-
nose, nasal	C76.0	C79.89	D09.8	D36.7	D48.7	D49.89
ala (external) (nasi) — *see also Neoplasm, nose, skin*	C44.301	C79.2	D04.39	D23.39	D48.5	D49.2
bone	C41.0	C79.51	-	D16.4-	D48.0	D49.2
cartilage	C30.0	C78.39	D02.3	D14.0	D38.5	D49.1
cavity	C30.0	C78.39	D02.3	D14.0	D38.5	D49.1
choana	C11.3	C79.89	D00.08	D10.6	D37.05	D49.0
external (skin) — *see also Neoplasm, nose, skin*	C44.301	C79.2	D04.39	D23.39	D48.5	D49.2
fossa	C30.0	C78.39	D02.3	D14.0	D38.5	D49.1
internal	C30.0	C78.39	D02.3	D14.0	D38.5	D49.1
mucosa	C30.0	C78.39	D02.3	D14.0	D38.5	D49.1
septum	C30.0	C78.39	D02.3	D14.0	D38.5	D49.1
posterior margin	C11.3	C79.89	D00.08	D10.6	D37.05	D49.0
sinus — *see Neoplasm, sinus*						
skin	C44.301	C79.2	D04.39	D23.39	D48.5	D49.2

	Malignant Primary	Malignant Secondary	Ca in situ	Benign	Uncertain Behavior	Unspecified Behavior
Neoplasm, neoplastic						
basal cell carcinoma	C44.311	-	-	-	-	-
specified type NEC	C44.391	-	-	-	-	-
squamous cell carcinoma	C44.321	-	-	-	-	-
turbinate (mucosa)	C30.0	C78.39	D02.3	D14.0	D38.5	D49.1
bone	C41.0	C79.51	-	D16.4-	D48.0	D49.2
vestibule	C30.0	C78.39	D02.3	D14.0	D38.5	D49.1
nostril	C30.0	C78.39	D02.3	D14.0	D38.5	D49.1
nucleus pulposus	C41.2	C79.51	-	D16.6	D48.0	D49.2
occipital						
bone	C41.0	C79.51	-	D16.4-	D48.0	D49.2
lobe or pole, brain	C71.4	C79.31	-	D33.0	D43.0	D49.6
odontogenic — *see Neoplasm, jaw bone*						
olfactory nerve or bulb	C72.2-	C79.49	-	D33.3	D43.3	D49.7
olive (brain)	C71.7	C79.31	-	D33.1	D43.1	D49.6
omentum	C48.1	C78.6	-	D20.1	D48.4	D49.0
operculum (brain)	C71.0	C79.31	-	D33.0	D43.0	D49.6
optic nerve, chiasm, or tract	C72.3-	C79.49	-	D33.3	D43.3	D49.7
oral (cavity)	C06.9	C79.89	D00.00	D10.30	D37.09	D49.0
ill-defined	C14.8	C79.89	D00.00	D10.30	D37.09	D49.0
mucosa	C06.0	C79.89	D00.02	D10.39	D37.09	D49.0
orbit	C69.6-	C79.49	D09.2-	D31.6-	D48.7	D49.89
autonomic nerve	C69.6-	C79.49	-	D31.6-	D48.7	D49.2
bone	C41.0	C79.51	-	D16.4-	D48.0	D49.2
eye	C69.6-	C79.49	D09.2-	D31.6-	D48.7	D49.89
peripheral nerves	C69.6-	C79.49	-	D31.6-	D48.7	D49.2
soft parts	C69.6-	C79.49	D09.2-	D31.6-	D48.7	D49.89
organ of Zuckerkandl	C75.5	C79.89	-	D35.6	D44.7	D49.7
oropharynx	C10.9	C79.89	D00.08	D10.5	D37.05	D49.0
branchial cleft (vestige)	C10.4	C79.89	D00.08	D10.5	D37.05	D49.0
junctional region	C10.8	C79.89	D00.08	D10.5	D37.05	D49.0
lateral wall	C10.2	C79.89	D00.08	D10.5	D37.05	D49.0
overlapping lesion	C10.8	-	-	-	-	-
pillars or fauces	C09.1	C79.89	D00.08	D10.5	D37.05	D49.0
posterior wall	C10.3	C79.89	D00.08	D10.5	D37.05	D49.0
vallecula	C10.0	C79.89	D00.08	D10.5	D37.05	D49.0
os						
external	C53.1	C79.82	D06.1	D26.0	D39.0	D49.59
internal	C53.0	C79.82	D06.0	D26.0	D39.0	D49.59
ovary	C56.-	C79.6-	D07.39	D27.-	D39.1-	D49.59
oviduct	C57.0-	C79.82	D07.39	D28.2	D39.8	D49.59
palate	C05.9	C79.89	D00.00	D10.39	D37.09	D49.0
hard	C05.0	C79.89	D00.05	D10.39	D37.09	D49.0
junction of hard and soft palate	C05.9	C79.89	D00.00	D10.39	D37.09	D49.0
overlapping lesions	C05.8	-	-	-	-	-
soft	C05.1	C79.89	D00.04	D10.39	D37.09	D49.0
nasopharyngeal surface	C11.3	C79.89	D00.08	D10.6	D37.05	D49.0
posterior surface	C11.3	C79.89	D00.08	D10.6	D37.05	D49.0
superior surface	C11.3	C79.89	D00.08	D10.6	D37.05	D49.0
palatoglossal arch	C09.1	C79.89	D00.00	D10.5	D37.09	D49.0
palatopharyngeal arch	C09.1	C79.89	D00.00	D10.5	D37.09	D49.0
pallium	C71.0	C79.31	-	D33.0	D43.0	D49.6
palpebra	C44.10-	C79.2	D04.1-	D23.1-	D48.5	D49.2
basal cell carcinoma	C44.11-	-	-	-	-	-
sebaceous cell	C44.13-	-	-	-	-	-
specified type NEC	C44.19-	-	-	-	-	-
squamous cell carcinoma	C44.12-	-	-	-	-	-
pancreas	C25.9	C78.89	D01.7	D13.6	D37.8	D49.0
body	C25.1	C78.89	D01.7	D13.6	D37.8	D49.0
duct (of Santorini) (of Wirsung)	C25.3	C78.89	D01.7	D13.6	D37.8	D49.0

Neoplasm, neoplastic	Malignant Primary	Malignant Secondary	Ca in situ	Benign	Uncertain Behavior	Unspecified Behavior
ectopic tissue	C25.7	C78.89	-	D13.6	D37.8	D49.0
head	C25.0	C78.89	D01.7	D13.6	D37.8	D49.0
islet cells	C25.4	C78.89	D01.7	D13.7	D37.8	D49.0
neck	C25.7	C78.89	D01.7	D13.6	D37.8	D49.0
overlapping lesion	C25.8	-	-	-	-	-
tail	C25.2	C78.89	D01.7	D13.6	D37.8	D49.0
para-aortic body	C75.5	C79.89	-	D35.6	D44.7	D49.7
paraganglion NEC	C75.5	C79.89	-	D35.6	D44.7	D49.7
parametrium	C57.3	C79.82	-	D28.2	D39.8	D49.59
paranephric	C48.0	C78.6	-	D20.0	D48.3	D49.0
pararectal	C76.3	C79.89	-	D36.7	D48.7	D49.89
parasagittal (region)	C76.0	C79.89	D09.8	D36.7	D48.7	D49.89
parasellar	C72.9	C79.49	-	D33.9	D43.8	D49.7
parathyroid (gland)	C75.0	C79.89	D09.3	D35.1	D44.2	D49.7
paraurethral	C76.3	C79.89	-	D36.7	D48.7	D49.89
gland	C68.1	C79.19	D09.19	D30.8	D41.8	D49.59
paravaginal	C76.3	C79.89	-	D36.7	D48.7	D49.89
parenchyma, kidney	C64.-	C79.0-	D09.19	D30.0-	D41.0-	D49.51-
parietal						
bone	C41.0	C79.51	-	D16.4-	D48.0	D49.2
lobe, brain	C71.3	C79.31	-	D33.0	D43.0	D49.6
paroophoron	C57.1	C79.82	D07.39	D28.2	D39.8	D49.59
parotid (duct) (gland)	C07	C79.89	D00.00	D11.0	D37.030	D49.0
parovarium	C57.1	C79.82	D07.39	D28.2	D39.8	D49.59
patella	C40.20	C79.51	-	-	-	-
peduncle, cerebral	C71.7	C79.31	-	D33.1	D43.1	D49.6
pelvirectal junction	C19	C78.5	D01.1	D12.7	D37.5	D49.0
pelvis, pelvic	C76.3	C79.89	D09.8	D36.7	D48.7	D49.89
bone	C41.4	C79.51	-	D16.8	D48.0	D49.2
floor	C76.3	C79.89	D09.8	D36.7	D48.7	D49.89
renal	C65.-	C79.0-	D09.19	D30.1-	D41.1-	D49.51-
viscera	C76.3	C79.89	D09.8	D36.7	D48.7	D49.89
wall	C76.3	C79.89	D09.8	D36.7	D48.7	D49.89
pelvo-abdominal	C76.8	C79.89	D09.8	D36.7	D48.7	D49.89
penis	C60.9	C79.82	D07.4	D29.0	D40.8	D49.59
body	C60.2	C79.82	D07.4	D29.0	D40.8	D49.59
corpus (cavernosum)	C60.2	C79.82	D07.4	D29.0	D40.8	D49.59
glans	C60.1	C79.82	D07.4	D29.0	D40.8	D49.59
overlapping sites	C60.8	-	-	-	-	-
skin NEC	C60.9	C79.82	D07.4	D29.0	D40.8	D49.59
periadrenal (tissue)	C48.0	C78.6	-	D20.0	D48.3	D49.0
perianal (skin) — *see also Neoplasm, anus, skin*	C44.500	C79.2	D04.5	D23.5	D48.5	D49.2
pericardium	C38.0	C79.89	-	D15.1	D48.7	D49.89
perinephric	C48.0	C78.6	-	D20.0	D48.3	D49.0
perineum	C76.3	C79.89	D09.8	D36.7	D48.7	D49.89
periodontal tissue NEC	C03.9	C79.89	D00.03	D10.39	D37.09	D49.0
periosteum — *see Neoplasm, bone*						
peripancreatic	C48.0	C78.6	-	D20.0	D48.3	D49.0
peripheral nerve NEC	C47.9	C79.89	-	D36.10	D48.2	D49.2
perirectal (tissue)	C76.3	C79.89	-	D36.7	D48.7	D49.89
perirenal (tissue)	C48.0	C78.6	-	D20.0	D48.3	D49.0
peritoneum, peritoneal (cavity)	C48.2	C78.6	-	D20.1	D48.4	D49.0
benign mesothelial tissue — *see Mesothelioma, benign*						
overlapping lesion	C48.8	-	-	-	-	-
with digestive organs	C26.9	-	-	-	-	-
parietal	C48.1	C78.6	-	D20.1	D48.4	D49.0
pelvic	C48.1	C78.6	-	D20.1	D48.4	D49.0

Neoplasm, neoplastic	Malignant Primary	Malignant Secondary	Ca in situ	Benign	Uncertain Behavior	Unspecified Behavior
specified part NEC	C48.1	C78.6	-	D20.1	D48.4	D49.0
peritonsillar (tissue)	C76.0	C79.89	D09.8	D36.7	D48.7	D49.89
periurethral tissue	C76.3	C79.89	-	D36.7	D48.7	D49.89
phalanges						
foot	C40.3-	C79.51	-	D16.3-	-	-
hand	C40.1-	C79.51	-	D16.1-	-	-
pharynx, pharyngeal	C14.0	C79.89	D00.08	D10.9	D37.05	D49.0
bursa	C11.1	C79.89	D00.08	D10.6	D37.05	D49.0
fornix	C11.3	C79.89	D00.08	D10.6	D37.05	D49.0
recess	C11.2	C79.89	D00.08	D10.6	D37.05	D49.0
region	C14.0	C79.89	D00.08	D10.9	D37.05	D49.0
tonsil	C11.1	C79.89	D00.08	D10.6	D37.05	D49.0
wall (lateral) (posterior)	C14.0	C79.89	D00.08	D10.9	D37.05	D49.0
pia mater	C70.9	C79.40	-	D32.9	D42.9	D49.7
cerebral	C70.0	C79.32	-	D32.0	D42.0	D49.7
cranial	C70.0	C79.32	-	D32.0	D42.0	D49.7
spinal	C70.1	C79.49	-	D32.1	D42.1	D49.7
pillars of fauces	C09.1	C79.89	D00.08	D10.5	D37.05	D49.0
pineal (body) (gland)	C75.3	C79.89	D09.3	D35.4	D44.5	D49.7
pinna (ear) NEC — *see also Neoplasm, skin, ear*	C44.20-	C79.2	D04.2-	D23.2-	D48.5	D49.2
piriform fossa or sinus	C12	C79.89	D00.08	D10.7	D37.05	D49.0
pituitary (body) (fossa) (gland) (lobe)	C75.1	C79.89	D09.3	D35.2	D44.3	D49.7
placenta	C58	C79.82	D07.0	D26.7	D39.2	D49.59
pleura, pleural (cavity)	C38.4	C78.2	-	D19.0	D38.2	D49.1
overlapping lesion with heart or mediastinum	C38.8	-	-	-	-	-
parietal	C38.4	C78.2	-	D19.0	D38.2	D49.1
visceral	C38.4	C78.2	-	D19.0	D38.2	D49.1
plexus						
brachial	C47.1-	C79.89	-	D36.12	D48.2	D49.2
cervical	C47.0	C79.89	-	D36.11	D48.2	D49.2
choroid	C71.5	C79.31	-	D33.0	D43.0	D49.6
lumbosacral	C47.5	C79.89	-	D36.16	D48.2	D49.2
sacral	C47.5	C79.89	-	D36.16	D48.2	D49.2
pluriendocrine	C75.8	C79.89	D09.3	D35.7	D44.9	D49.7
pole						
frontal	C71.1	C79.31	-	D33.0	D43.0	D49.6
occipital	C71.4	C79.31	-	D33.0	D43.0	D49.6
pons (varolii)	C71.7	C79.31	-	D33.1	D43.1	D49.6
popliteal fossa or space	C76.5-	C79.89	D04.7-	D36.7	D48.7	D49.89
postcricoid (region)	C13.0	C79.89	D00.08	D10.7	D37.05	D49.0
posterior fossa (cranial)	C71.9	C79.31	-	D33.2	D43.2	D49.6
postnasal space	C11.9	C79.89	D00.08	D10.6	D37.05	D49.0
prepuce	C60.0	C79.82	D07.4	D29.0	D40.8	D49.59
prepylorus	C16.4	C78.89	D00.2	D13.1	D37.1	D49.0
presacral (region)	C76.3	C79.89	-	D36.7	D48.7	D49.89
prostate (gland)	C61	C79.82	D07.5	D29.1	D40.0	D49.59
utricle	C68.0	C79.19	D09.19	D30.4	D41.3	D49.59
pterygoid fossa	C49.0	C79.89	-	D21.0	D48.1	D49.2
pubic bone	C41.4	C79.51	-	D16.8	D48.0	D49.2
pudenda, pudendum (femaie)	C51.9	C79.82	D07.1	D28.0	D39.8	D49.59
pulmonary — *see also Neoplasm, lung*	C34.9-	C78.0-	D02.2-	D14.3-	D38.1	D49.1
putamen	C71.0	C79.31	-	D33.0	D43.0	D49.6
pyloric						
antrum	C16.3	C78.89	D00.2	D13.1	D37.1	D49.0
canal	C16.4	C78.89	D00.2	D13.1	D37.1	D49.0
pylorus	C16.4	C78.89	D00.2	D13.1	D37.1	D49.0
pyramid (brain)	C71.7	C79.31	-	D33.1	D43.1	D49.6
pyriform fossa or sinus	C12	C79.89	D00.08	D10.7	D37.05	D49.0

Neoplasm, neoplastic	Malignant Primary	Malignant Secondary	Ca in situ	Benign	Uncertain Behavior	Unspecified Behavior
radius (any part)	C40.0-	C79.51	-	D16.0-	-	-
Rathke's pouch	C75.1	C79.89	D09.3	D35.2	D44.3	D49.7
rectosigmoid (junction)	C19	C78.5	D01.1	D12.7	D37.5	D49.0
overlapping lesion with anus or rectum	C21.8	-	-	-	-	-
rectouterine pouch	C48.1	C78.6	-	D20.1	D48.4	D49.0
rectovaginal septum or wall	C76.3	C79.89	D09.8	D36.7	D48.7	D49.89
rectovesical septum	C76.3	C79.89	D09.8	D36.7	D48.7	D49.89
rectum (ampulla)	C20	C78.5	D01.2	D12.8	D37.5	D49.0
and colon	C19	C78.5	D01.1	D12.7	D37.5	D49.0
overlapping lesion with anus or rectosigmoid junction	C21.8	-	-	-	-	-
renal	C64.-	C79.0-	D09.19	D30.0-	D41.0-	D49.51-
calyx	C65.-	C79.0-	D09.19	D30.1-	D41.1-	D49.51-
hilus	C65.-	C79.0-	D09.19	D30.1-	D41.1-	D49.51-
parenchyma	C64.-	C79.0-	D09.19	D30.0-	D41.0-	D49.51-
pelvis	C65.-	C79.0-	D09.19	D30.1-	D41.1-	D49.51-
respiratory						
organs or system NEC	C39.9	C78.30	D02.4	D14.4	D38.6	D49.1
tract NEC	C39.9	C78.30	D02.4	D14.4	D38.5	D49.1
upper	C39.0	C78.30	D02.4	D14.4	D38.5	D49.1
retina	C69.2-	C79.49	D09.2-	D31.2-	D48.7	D49.81
retrobulbar	C69.6-	C79.49	-	D31.6-	D48.7	D49.89
retrocecal	C48.0	C78.6	-	D20.0	D48.3	D49.0
retromolar (area) (triangle) (trigone)	C06.2	C79.89	D00.00	D10.39	D37.09	D49.0
retro-orbital	C76.0	C79.89	D09.8	D36.7	D48.7	D49.89
retroperitoneal (space) (tissue)	C48.0	C78.6	-	D20.0	D48.3	D49.0
retroperitoneum	C48.0	C78.6	-	D20.0	D48.3	D49.0
retropharyngeal	C14.0	C79.89	D00.08	D10.9	D37.05	D49.0
retrovesical (septum)	C76.3	C79.89	D09.8	D36.7	D48.7	D49.89
rhinencephalon	C71.0	C79.31	-	D33.0	D43.0	D49.6
rib	C41.3	C79.51	-	D16.7	D48.0	D49.2
Rosenmuller's fossa	C11.2	C79.89	D00.08	D10.6	D37.05	D49.0
round ligament	C57.2	C79.82	-	D28.2	D39.8	D49.59
sacrococcyx, sacrococcygeal	C41.4	C79.51		D16.8	D48.0	D49.2
region	C76.3	C79.89	D09.8	D36.7	D48.7	D49.89
sacrouterine ligament	C57.3	C79.82	-	D28.2	D39.8	D49.59
sacrum, sacral (vertebra)	C41.4	C79.51	-	D16.8	D48.0	D49.2
salivary gland or duct (major)	C08.9	C79.89	D00.00	D11.9	D37.039	D49.0
minor NEC	C06.9	C79.89	D00.00	D10.39	D37.04	D49.0
overlapping lesion	C08.9	-	-	-	-	-
parotid	C07	C79.89	D00.00	D11.0	D37.030	D49.0
pluriglandular	C08.9	C79.89	D00.00	D11.9	D37.039	D49.0
sublingual	C08.1	C79.89	D00.00	D11.7	D37.031	D49.0
submandibular	C08.0	C79.89	D00.00	D11.7	D37.032	D49.0
submaxillary	C08.0	C79.89	D00.00	D11.7	D37.032	D49.0
salpinx (uterine)	C57.0-	C79.82	D07.39	D28.2	D39.8	D49.59
Santorini's duct	C25.3	C78.89	D01.7	D13.6	D37.8	D49.0
scalp	C44.40	C79.2	D04.4	D23.4	D48.5	D49.2
basal cell carcinoma	C44.41	-	-	-	-	-
specified type NEC	C44.49	-	-	-	-	-
squamous cell carcinoma	C44.42	-	-	-	-	-
scapula (any part)	C40.0-	C79.51	-	D16.0-	-	-
scapular region	C76.1	C79.89	D09.8	D36.7	D48.7	D49.89
scar NEC — *see also Neoplasm, skin, by site*	C44.90	C79.2	D04.9	D23.9	D48.5	D49.2
sciatic nerve	C47.2-	C79.89	-	D36.13	D48.2	D49.2
sclera	C69.4-	C79.49	D09.2-	D31.4-	D48.7	D49.89
scrotum (skin)	C63.2	C79.82	D07.61	D29.4	D40.8	D49.59
sebaceous gland — *see Neoplasm, skin*						

Neoplasm, neoplastic	Malignant Primary	Malignant Secondary	Ca in situ	Benign	Uncertain Behavior	Unspecified Behavior
sella turcica	C75.1	C79.89	D09.3	D35.2	D44.3	D49.7
bone	C41.0	C79.51	-	D16.4-	D48.0	D49.2
semilunar cartilage (knee)	C40.2-	C79.51	-	D16.2-	D48.0	D49.2
seminal vesicle	C63.7	C79.82	D07.69	D29.8	D40.8	D49.59
septum						
nasal	C30.0	C78.39	D02.3	D14.0	D38.5	D49.1
posterior margin	C11.3	C79.89	D00.08	D10.6	D37.05	D49.0
rectovaginal	C76.3	C79.89	D09.8	D36.7	D48.7	D49.89
rectovesical	C76.3	C79.89	D09.8	D36.7	D48.7	D49.89
urethrovaginal	C57.9	C79.82	D07.30	D28.9	D39.9	D49.59
vesicovaginal	C57.9	C79.82	D07.30	D28.9	D39.9	D49.59
shoulder NEC	C76.4-	C79.89	D04.6-	D36.7	D48.7	D49.89
sigmoid flexure (lower) (upper)	C18.7	C78.5	D01.0	D12.5	D37.4	D49.0
sinus (accessory)	C31.9	C78.39	D02.3	D14.0	D38.5	D49.1
bone (any)	C41.0	C79.51	-	D16.4-	D48.0	D49.2
ethmoidal	C31.1	C78.39	D02.3	D14.0	D38.5	D49.1
frontal	C31.2	C78.39	D02.3	D14.0	D38.5	D49.1
maxillary	C31.0	C78.39	D02.3	D14.0	D38.5	D49.1
nasal, paranasal NEC	C31.9	C78.39	D02.3	D14.0	D38.5	D49.1
overlapping lesion	C31.8	-	-	-	-	-
pyriform	C12	C79.89	D00.08	D10.7	D37.05	D49.0
sphenoid	C31.3	C78.39	D02.3	D14.0	D38.5	D49.1
skeleton, skeletal NEC	C41.9	C79.51	-	D16.9-	D48.0	D49.2
Skene's gland	C68.1	C79.19	D09.19	D30.8	D41.8	D49.59
skin NOS	C44.90	C79.2	D04.9	D23.9	D48.5	D49.2
abdominal wall	C44.509	C79.2	D04.5	D23.5	D48.5	D49.2
basal cell carcinoma	C44.519	-	-	-	-	-
specified type NEC	C44.599	-	-	-	-	-
squamous cell carcinoma	C44.529	-	-	-	-	-
ala nasi — *see also Neoplasm, nose, skin*	C44.301	C79.2	D04.39	D23.39	D48.5	D49.2
ankle — *see also Neoplasm, skin, limb, lower*	C44.70-	C79.2	D04.7-	D23.7-	D48.5	D49.2
antecubital space — *see also Neoplasm, skin, limb, upper*	C44.60-	C79.2	D04.6-	D23.6-	D48.5	D49.2
anus	C44.500	C79.2	D04.5	D23.5	D48.5	D49.2
basal cell carcinoma	C44.510	-	-	-	-	-
specified type NEC	C44.590	-	-	-	-	-
squamous cell carcinoma	C44.520	-	-	-	-	-
arm — *see also Neoplasm, skin, limb, upper*	C44.60-	C79.2	D04.6-	D23.6-	D48.5	D49.2
auditory canal (external) — *see also Neoplasm, skin, ear*	C44.20-	C79.2	D04.2-	D23.2-	D48.5	D49.2
auricle (ear) — *see also Neoplasm, skin, ear*	C44.20-	C79.2	D04.2-	D23.2-	D48.5	D49.2
auricular canal (external) — *see also Neoplasm, skin, ear*	C44.20-	C79.2	D04.2-	D23.2-	D48.5	D49.2
axilla, axillary fold — *see also Neoplasm, skin, trunk*	C44.509	C79.2	D04.5	D23.5	D48.5	D49.2
back — *see also Neoplasm, skin, trunk*	C44.509	C79.2	D04.5	D23.5	D48.5	D49.2
basal cell carcinoma	C44.91					
breast	C44.501	C79.2	D04.5	D23.5	D48.5	D49.2
basal cell carcinoma	C44.511	-	-	-	-	-
specified type NEC	C44.591	-	-	-	-	-
squamous cell carcinoma	C44.521	-	-	-	-	-
brow — *see also Neoplasm, skin, face*	C44.309	C79.2	D04.39	D23.39	D48.5	D49.2
buttock — *see also Neoplasm, skin, trunk*	C44.509	C79.2	D04.5	D23.5	D48.5	D49.2
calf — *see also Neoplasm, skin, limb, lower*	C44.70-	C79.2	D04.7-	D23.7-	D48.5	D49.2

Neoplasm, neoplastic	Malignant Primary	Malignant Secondary	Ca in situ	Benign	Uncertain Behavior	Unspecified Behavior
canthus (eye) (inner) (outer)	C44.10-	C79.2	D04.1-	D23.1-	D48.5	D49.2
basal cell carcinoma	C44.11-	-	-	-	-	-
sebaceous cell	C44.13-	-	-	-	-	-
specified type NEC	C44.19-	-	-	-	-	-
squamous cell carcinoma	C44.12-	-	-	-	-	-
cervical region — *see also Neoplasm, skin, neck*	C44.40	C79.2	D04.4	D23.4	D48.5	D49.2
cheek (external) — *see also Neoplasm, skin, face*	C44.309	C79.2	D04.39	D23.39	D48.5	D49.2
chest (wall) — *see also Neoplasm, skin, trunk*	C44.509	C79.2	D04.5	D23.5	D48.5	D49.2
chin — *see also Neoplasm, skin, face*	C44.309	C79.2	D04.39	D23.39	D48.5	D49.2
clavicular area — *see also Neoplasm, skin, trunk*	C44.509	C79.2	D04.5	D23.5	D48.5	D49.2
clitoris	C51.2	C79.82	D07.1	D28.0	D39.8	D49.59
columnella — *see also Neoplasm, skin, face*	C44.309	C79.2	D04.39	D23.39	D48.5	D49.2
concha — *see also Neoplasm, skin, ear*	C44.20-	C79.2	D04.2-	D23.2-	D48.5	D49.2
ear (external)	C44.20-	C79.2	D04.2-	D23.2-	D48.5	D49.2
basal cell carcinoma	C44.21-	-	-	-	-	-
specified type NEC	C44.29-	-	-	-	-	-
squamous cell carcinoma	C44.22-	-	-	-	-	-
elbow — *see also Neoplasm, skin, limb, upper*	C44.60-	C79.2	D04.6-	D23.6-	D48.5	D49.2
eyebrow — *see also Neoplasm, skin, face*	C44.309	C79.2	D04.39	D23.39	D48.5	D49.2
eyelid	C44.10-	C79.2	D04.1-	D23.1-	D48.5	D49.2
basal cell carcinoma	C44.11-	-	-	-	-	-
sebaceous cell	C44.13-	-	-	-	-	-
specified type NEC	C44.19-	-	-	-	-	-
squamous cell carcinoma	C44.12-	-	-	-	-	-
face NOS	C44.300	C79.2	D04.30	D23.30	D48.5	D49.2
basal cell carcinoma	C44.310	-	-	-	-	-
specified type NEC	C44.390	-	-	-	-	-
squamous cell carcinoma	C44.320	-	-	-	-	-
female genital organs (external)	C51.9	C79.82	D07.1	D28.0	D39.8	D49.59
clitoris	C51.2	C79.82	D07.1	D28.0	D39.8	D49.59
labium NEC	C51.9	C79.82	D07.1	D28.0	D39.8	D49.59
majus	C51.0	C79.82	D07.1	D28.0	D39.8	D49.59
minus	C51.1	C79.82	D07.1	D28.0	D39.8	D49.59
pudendum	C51.9	C79.82	D07.1	D28.0	D39.8	D49.59
vulva	C51.9	C79.82	D07.1	D28.0	D39.8	D49.59
finger — *see also Neoplasm, skin, limb, upper*	C44.60-	C79.2	D04.6-	D23.6-	D48.5	D49.2
flank — *see also Neoplasm, skin, trunk*	C44.509	C79.2	D04.5	D23.5	D48.5	D49.2
foot — *see also Neoplasm, skin, limb, lower*	C44.70-	C79.2	D04.7-	D23.7-	D48.5	D49.2
forearm — *see also Neoplasm, skin, limb, upper*	C44.60-	C79.2	D04.6-	D23.6-	D48.5	D49.2
forehead — *see also Neoplasm, skin, face*	C44.309	C79.2	D04.39	D23.39	D48.5	D49.2
glabella — *see also Neoplasm, skin, face*	C44.309	C79.2	D04.39	D23.39	D48.5	D49.2
gluteal region — *see also Neoplasm, skin, trunk*	C44.509	C79.2	D04.5	D23.5	D48.5	D49.2
groin — *see also Neoplasm, skin, trunk*	C44.509	C79.2	D04.5	D23.5	D48.5	D49.2
hand — *see also Neoplasm, skin, limb, upper*	C44.60-	C79.2	D04.6-	D23.6-	D48.5	D49.2
head NEC — *see also Neoplasm, skin, scalp*	C44.40	C79.2	D04.4	D23.4	D48.5	D49.2

Neoplasm, neoplastic	Malignant Primary	Malignant Secondary	Ca in situ	Benign	Uncertain Behavior	Unspecified Behavior
heel — *see also Neoplasm, skin, limb, lower*	C44.70-	C79.2	D04.7-	D23.7-	D48.5	D49.2
helix — *see also Neoplasm, skin, ear*	C44.20-	C79.2	D04.2-	D23.2-	D48.5	D49.2
hip — *see also Neoplasm, skin, limb, lower*	C44.70-	C79.2	D04.7-	D23.7-	D48.5	D49.2
infraclavicular region — *see also Neoplasm, skin, trunk*	C44.509	C79.2	D04.5	D23.5	D48.5	D49.2
inguinal region — *see also Neoplasm, skin, trunk*	C44.509	C79.2	D04.5	D23.5	D48.5	D49.2
jaw — *see also Neoplasm, skin, face*	C44.309	C79.2	D04.39	D23.39	D48.5	D49.2
Kaposi's sarcoma — *see Kaposi's, sarcoma, skin*						
knee — *see also Neoplasm, skin, limb, lower*	C44.70-	C79.2	D04.7-	D23.7-	D48.5	D49.2
labia						
majora	C51.0	C79.82	D07.1	D28.0	D39.8	D49.59
minora	C51.1	C79.82	D07.1	D28.0	D39.8	D49.59
leg — *see also Neoplasm, skin, limb, lower*	C44.70-	C79.2	D04.7-	D23.7-	D48.5	D49.2
lid (lower) (upper)	C44.10-	C79.2	D04.1-	D23.1-	D48.5	D49.2
basal cell carcinoma	C44.11-	-	-	-	-	-
sebaceous cell	C44.13-	-	-	-	-	-
specified type NEC	C44.19-	-	-	-	-	-
squamous cell carcinoma	C44.12-	-	-	-	-	-
limb NEC	C44.90	C79.2	D04.9	D23.9	D48.5	D49.2
basal cell carcinoma	C44.91					
lower	C44.70-	C79.2	D04.7-	D23.7-	D48.5	D49.2
basal cell carcinoma	C44.71-	-	-	-	-	-
specified type NEC	C44.79-	-	-	-	-	-
squamous cell carcinoma	C44.72-	-	-	-	-	-
upper	C44.60-	C79.2	D04.6-	D23.6-	D48.5	D49.2
basal cell carcinoma	C44.61-	-	-	-	-	-
specified type NEC	C44.69-	-	-	-	-	-
squamous cell carcinoma	C44.62-	-	-	-	-	-
lip (lower) (upper)	C44.00	C79.2	D04.0	D23.0	D48.5	D49.2
basal cell carcinoma	C44.01	-	-	-	-	-
specified type NEC	C44.09	-	-	-	-	-
squamous cell carcinoma	C44.02	-	-	-	-	-
male genital organs	C63.9	C79.82	D07.60	D29.9	D40.8	D49.59
penis	C60.9	C79.82	D07.4	D29.0	D40.8	D49.59
prepuce	C60.0	C79.82	D07.4	D29.0	D40.8	D49.59
scrotum	C63.2	C79.82	D07.61	D29.4	D40.8	D49.59
mastectomy site (skin) — *see also Neoplasm, skin, breast*	C44.501	C79.2	-	-	-	-
specified as breast tissue	C50.8-	C79.81	-	-	-	-
meatus, acoustic (external) — *see also Neoplasm, skin, ear*	C44.20-	C79.2	D04.2-	D23.2-	D48.5	D49.2
melanotic — *see Melanoma*						
Merkel cell — *see Carcinoma, Merkel cell*						
nates — *see also Neoplasm, skin, trunk*	C44.509	C79.2	D04.5	D23.5	D48.5	D49.2
neck	C44.40	C79.2	D04.4	D23.4	D48.5	D49.2
basal cell carcinoma	C44.41	-	-	-	-	-
specified type NEC	C44.49	-	-	-	-	-
squamous cell carcinoma	C44.42	-	-	-	-	-
nevus — *see Nevus, skin*						
nose (external) — *see also Neoplasm, nose, skin*	C44.301	C79.2	D04.39	D23.39	D48.5	D49.2
overlapping lesion	C44.80	-	-	-	-	-
basal cell carcinoma	C44.81	-	-	-	-	-
specified type NEC	C44.89	-	-	-	-	-
squamous cell carcinoma	C44.82	-	-	-	-	-

Neoplasm, neoplastic	Malignant Primary	Malignant Secondary	Ca in situ	Benign	Uncertain Behavior	Unspecified Behavior
palm — *see also Neoplasm, skin, limb, upper*	C44.60-	C79.2	D04.6-	D23.6-	D48.5	D49.2
palpebra	C44.10-	C79.2	D04.1-	D23.1-	D48.5	D49.2
basal cell carcinoma	C44.11-	-	-	-	-	-
sebaceous cell	C44.13-	-	-	-	-	-
specified type NEC	C44.19-	-	-	-	-	-
squamous cell carcinoma	C44.12-	-	-	-	-	-
penis NEC	C60.9	C79.82	D07.4	D29.0	D40.8	D49.59
perianal — *see also Neoplasm, skin, anus*	C44.500	C79.2	D04.5	D23.5	D48.5	D49.2
perineum — *see also Neoplasm, skin, anus*	C44.500	C79.2	D04.5	D23.5	D48.5	D49.2
pinna — *see also Neoplasm, skin, ear*	C44.20-	C79.2	D04.2-	D23.2-	D48.5	D49.2
plantar — *see also Neoplasm, skin, limb, lower*	C44.70-	C79.2	D04.7-	D23.7-	D48.5	D49.2
popliteal fossa or space — *see also Neoplasm, skin, limb, lower*	C44.70-	C79.2	D04.7-	D23.7-	D48.5	D49.2
prepuce	C60.0	C79.82	D07.4	D29.0	D40.8	D49.59
pubes — *see also Neoplasm, skin, trunk*	C44.509	C79.2	D04.5	D23.5	D48.5	D49.2
sacrococcygeal region — *see also Neoplasm, skin, trunk*	C44.509	C79.2	D04.5	D23.5	D48.5	D49.2
scalp	C44.40	C79.2	D04.4	D23.4	D48.5	D49.2
basal cell carcinoma	C44.41	-	-	-	-	-
specified type NEC	C44.49	-	-	-	-	-
squamous cell carcinoma	C44.42	-	-	-	-	-
scapular region — *see also Neoplasm, skin, trunk*	C44.509	C79.2	D04.5	D23.5	D48.5	D49.2
scrotum	C63.2	C79.82	D07.61	D29.4	D40.8	D49.59
shoulder — *see also Neoplasm, skin, limb, upper*	C44.60-	C79.2	D04.6-	D23.6-	D48.5	D49.2
sole (foot) — *see also Neoplasm, skin, limb, lower*	C44.70-	C79.2	D04.7-	D23.7-	D48.5	D49.2
specified sites NEC	C44.80	C79.2	D04.8	D23.9	D48.5	D49.2
basal cell carcinoma	C44.81	-	-	-	-	-
specified type NEC	C44.89	-	-	-	-	-
squamous cell carcinoma	C44.82	-	-	-	-	-
specified type NEC	C44.99	-	-	-	-	-
squamous cell carcinoma	C44.92	-	-	-	-	-
submammary fold — *see also Neoplasm, skin, trunk*	C44.509	C79.2	D04.5	D23.5	D48.5	D49.2
supraclavicular region — *see also Neoplasm, skin, neck*	C44.40	C79.2	D04.4	D23.4	D48.5	D49.2
temple — *see also Neoplasm, skin, face*	C44.309	C79.2	D04.39	D23.39	D48.5	D49.2
thigh — *see also Neoplasm, skin, limb, lower*	C44.70-	C79.2	D04.7-	D23.7-	D48.5	D49.2
thoracic wall — *see also Neoplasm, skin, trunk*	C44.509	C79.2	D04.5	D23.5	D48.5	D49.2
thumb — *see also Neoplasm, skin, limb, upper*	C44.60-	C79.2	D04.6-	D23.6-	D48.5	D49.2
toe — *see also Neoplasm, skin, limb, lower*	C44.70-	C79.2	D04.7-	D23.7-	D48.5	D49.2
tragus — *see also Neoplasm, skin, ear*	C44.20-	C79.2	D04.2-	D23.2-	D48.5	D49.2
trunk	C44.509	C79.2	D04.5	D23.5	D48.5	D49.2
basal cell carcinoma	C44.519	-	-	-	-	-
specified type NEC	C44.599	-	-	-	-	-
squamous cell carcinoma	C44.529	-	-	-	-	-
umbilicus — *see also Neoplasm, skin, trunk*	C44.509	C79.2	D04.5	D23.5	D48.5	D49.2
vulva	C51.9	C79.82	D07.1	D28.0	D39.8	D49.59
overlapping lesion	C51.8	-	-	-	-	-

Neoplasm, neoplastic

	Malignant Primary	Malignant Secondary	Ca in situ	Benign	Uncertain Behavior	Unspecified Behavior
wrist — *see also Neoplasm, skin, limb, upper*	C44.60-	C79.2	D04.6-	D23.6-	D48.5	D49.2
skull	C41.0	C79.51	-	D16.4-	D48.0	D49.2
soft parts or tissues — *see Neoplasm, connective tissue*						
specified site NEC	C76.8	C79.89	D09.8	D36.7	D48.7	D49.89
spermatic cord	C63.1-	C79.82	D07.69	D29.8	D40.8	D49.59
sphenoid	C31.3	C78.39	D02.3	D14.0	D38.5	D49.1
bone	C41.0	C79.51	-	D16.4-	D48.0	D49.2
sinus	C31.3	C78.39	D02.3	D14.0	D38.5	D49.1
sphincter						
anal	C21.1	C78.5	D01.3	D12.9	D37.8	D49.0
of Oddi	C24.0	C78.89	D01.5	D13.5	D37.6	D49.0
spine, spinal (column)	C41.2	C79.51	-	D16.6	D48.0	D49.2
bulb	C71.7	C79.31	-	D33.1	D43.1	D49.6
coccyx	C41.4	C79.51	-	D16.8	D48.0	D49.2
cord (cervical) (lumbar) (sacral) (thoracic)	C72.0	C79.49	-	D33.4	D43.4	D49.7
dura mater	C70.1	C79.49	-	D32.1	D42.1	D49.7
lumbosacral	C41.2	C79.51	-	D16.6	D48.0	D49.2
marrow NEC	C96.9	C79.52	-	-	D47.9	D49.89
membrane	C70.1	C79.49	-	D32.1	D42.1	D49.7
meninges	C70.1	C79.49	-	D32.1	D42.1	D49.7
nerve (root)	C47.9	C79.89	-	D36.10	D48.2	D49.2
pia mater	C70.1	C79.49	-	D32.1	D42.1	D49.7
root	C47.9	C79.89	-	D36.10	D48.2	D49.2
sacrum	C41.4	C79.51	-	D16.8	D48.0	D49.2
spleen, splenic NEC	C26.1	C78.89	D01.7	D13.9	D37.8	D49.0
flexure (colon)	C18.5	C78.5	D01.0	D12.3	D37.4	D49.0
stem, brain	C71.7	C79.31	-	D33.1	D43.1	D49.6
Stensen's duct	C07	C79.89	D00.00	D11.0	D37.030	D49.0
sternum	C41.3	C79.51	-	D16.7	D48.0	D49.2
stomach	C16.9	C78.89	D00.2	D13.1	D37.1	D49.0
antrum (pyloric)	C16.3	C78.89	D00.2	D13.1	D37.1	D49.0
body	C16.2	C78.89	D00.2	D13.1	D37.1	D49.0
cardia	C16.0	C78.89	D00.2	D13.1	D37.1	D49.0
cardiac orifice	C16.0	C78.89	D00.2	D13.1	D37.1	D49.0
corpus	C16.2	C78.89	D00.2	D13.1	D37.1	D49.0
fundus	C16.1	C78.89	D00.2	D13.1	D37.1	D49.0
greater curvature NEC	C16.6	C78.89	D00.2	D13.1	D37.1	D49.0
lesser curvature NEC	C16.5	C78.89	D00.2	D13.1	D37.1	D49.0
overlapping lesion	C16.8	-	-	-	-	-
prepylorus	C16.4	C78.89	D00.2	D13.1	D37.1	D49.0
pylorus	C16.4	C78.89	D00.2	D13.1	D37.1	D49.0
wall NEC	C16.9	C78.89	D00.2	D13.1	D37.1	D49.0
anterior NEC	C16.8	C78.89	D00.2	D13.1	D37.1	D49.0
posterior NEC	C16.8	C78.89	D00.2	D13.1	D37.1	D49.0
stroma, endometrial	C54.1	C79.82	D07.0	D26.1	D39.0	D49.59
stump, cervical	C53.8	C79.82	D06.7	D26.0	D39.0	D49.59
subcutaneous (nodule) (tissue) NEC — *see Neoplasm, connective tissue*						
subdural	C70.9	C79.32	-	D32.9	D42.9	D49.7
subglottis, subglottic	C32.2	C78.39	D02.0	D14.1	D38.0	D49.1
sublingual	C04.9	C79.89	D00.06	D10.2	D37.09	D49.0
gland or duct	C08.1	C79.89	D00.00	D11.7	D37.031	D49.0
submandibular gland	C08.0	C79.89	D00.00	D11.7	D37.032	D49.0
submaxillary gland or duct	C08.0	C79.89	D00.00	D11.7	D37.032	D49.0
submental	C76.0	C79.89	D09.8	D36.7	D48.7	D49.89
subpleural	C34.9-	C78.0-	D02.2-	D14.3-	D38.1	D49.1
substernal	C38.1	C78.1	-	D15.2	D38.3	D49.89

Neoplasm, neoplastic	Malignant Primary	Malignant Secondary	Ca in situ	Benign	Uncertain Behavior	Unspecified Behavior
sudoriferous, sudoriparous gland, site unspecified	C44.90	C79.2	D04.9	D23.9	D48.5	D49.2
specified site — *see Neoplasm, skin*						
supraclavicular region	C76.0	C79.89	D09.8	D36.7	D48.7	D49.89
supraglottis	C32.1	C78.39	D02.0	D14.1	D38.0	D49.1
suprarenal	C74.9-	C79.7-	D09.3	D35.0-	D44.1-	D49.7
capsule	C74.9-	C79.7-	D09.3	D35.0-	D44.1-	D49.7
cortex	C74.0-	C79.7-	D09.3	D35.0-	D44.1-	D49.7
gland	C74.9-	C79.7-	D09.3	D35.0-	D44.1-	D49.7
medulla	C74.1-	C79.7-	D09.3	D35.0-	D44.1-	D49.7
suprasellar (region)	C71.9	C79.31	-	D33.2	D43.2	D49.6
supratentorial (brain) NEC	C71.0	C79.31	-	D33.0	D43.0	D49.6
sweat gland (apocrine) (eccrine) , site unspecified	C44.90	C79.2	D04.9	D23.9	D48.5	D49.2
specified site — *see Neoplasm, skin*						
sympathetic nerve or nervous system NEC	C47.9	C79.89	-	D36.10	D48.2	D49.2
symphysis pubis	C41.4	C79.51	-	D16.8	D48.0	D49.2
synovial membrane — *see Neoplasm, connective tissue*						
tapetum, brain	C71.8	C79.31	-	D33.2	D43.2	D49.6
tarsus (any bone)	C40.3-	C79.51	-	D16.3-	-	-
temple (skin) — *see also Neoplasm, skin, face*	C44.309	C79.2	D04.39	D23.39	D48.5	D49.2
temporal						
bone	C41.0	C79.51	-	D16.4-	D48.0	D49.2
lobe or pole	C71.2	C79.31	-	D33.0	D43.0	D49.6
region	C76.0	C79.89	D09.8	D36.7	D48.7	D49.89
skin — *see also Neoplasm, skin, face*	C44.309	C79.2	D04.39	D23.39	D48.5	D49.2
tendon (sheath) — *see Neoplasm, connective tissue*						
tentorium (cerebelli)	C70.0	C79.32	-	D32.0	D42.0	D49.7
testis, testes	C62.9-	C79.82	D07.69	D29.2-	D40.1-	D49.59
descended	C62.1-	C79.82	D07.69	D29.2-	D40.1-	D49.59
ectopic	C62.0-	C79.82	D07.69	D29.2-	D40.1-	D49.59
retained	C62.0-	C79.82	D07.69	D29.2-	D40.1-	D49.59
scrotal	C62.1-	C79.82	D07.69	D29.2-	D40.1-	D49.59
undescended	C62.0-	C79.82	D07.69	D29.2-	D40.1-	D49.59
unspecified whether descended or undescended	C62.9-	C79.82	D07.69	D29.2-	D40.1-	D49.59
thalamus	C71.0	C79.31	-	D33.0	D43.0	D49.6
thigh NEC	C76.5-	C79.89	D04.7-	D36.7	D48.7	D49.89
thorax, thoracic (cavity) (organs NEC)	C76.1	C79.89	D09.8	D36.7	D48.7	D49.89
duct	C49.3	C79.89	-	D21.3	D48.1	D49.2
wall NEC	C76.1	C79.89	D09.8	D36.7	D48.7	D49.89
throat	C14.0	C79.89	D00.08	D10.9	D37.05	D49.0
thumb NEC	C76.4-	C79.89	D04.6-	D36.7	D48.7	D49.89
thymus (gland)	C37	C79.89	D09.3	D15.0	D38.4	D49.89
thyroglossal duct	C73	C79.89	D09.3	D34	D44.0	D49.7
thyroid (gland)	C73	C79.89	D09.3	D34	D44.0	D49.7
cartilage	C32.3	C78.39	D02.0	D14.1	D38.0	D49.1
tibia (any part)	C40.2-	C79.51	-	D16.2-	-	-
toe NEC	C76.5-	C79.89	D04.7-	D36.7	D48.7	D49.89
tongue	C02.9	C79.89	D00.07	D10.1	D37.02	D49.0
anterior (two-thirds) NEC	C02.3	C79.89	D00.07	D10.1	D37.02	D49.0
dorsal surface	C02.0	C79.89	D00.07	D10.1	D37.02	D49.0
ventral surface	C02.2	C79.89	D00.07	D10.1	D37.02	D49.0
base (dorsal surface)	C01	C79.89	D00.07	D10.1	D37.02	D49.0
border (lateral)	C02.1	C79.89	D00.07	D10.1	D37.02	D49.0
dorsal surface NEC	C02.0	C79.89	D00.07	D10.1	D37.02	D49.0
fixed part NEC	C01	C79.89	D00.07	D10.1	D37.02	D49.0

	Malignant Primary	Malignant Secondary	Ca in situ	Benign	Uncertain Behavior	Unspecified Behavior
Neoplasm, neoplastic						
foreamen cecum	C02.0	C79.89	D00.07	D10.1	D37.02	D49.0
frenulum linguae	C02.2	C79.89	D00.07	D10.1	D37.02	D49.0
junctional zone	C02.8	C79.89	D00.07	D10.1	D37.02	D49.0
margin (lateral)	C02.1	C79.89	D00.07	D10.1	D37.02	D49.0
midline NEC	C02.0	C79.89	D00.07	D10.1	D37.02	D49.0
mobile part NEC	C02.3	C79.89	D00.07	D10.1	D37.02	D49.0
overlapping lesion	C02.8	-	-	-	-	-
posterior (third)	C01	C79.89	D00.07	D10.1	D37.02	D49.0
root	C01	C79.89	D00.07	D10.1	D37.02	D49.0
surface (dorsal)	C02.0	C79.89	D00.07	D10.1	D37.02	D49.0
base	C01	C79.89	D00.07	D10.1	D37.02	D49.0
ventral	C02.2	C79.89	D00.07	D10.1	D37.02	D49.0
tip	C02.1	C79.89	D00.07	D10.1	D37.02	D49.0
tonsil	C02.4	C79.89	D00.07	D10.1	D37.02	D49.0
tonsil	C09.9	C79.89	D00.08	D10.4	D37.05	D49.0
fauces, faucial	C09.9	C79.89	D00.08	D10.4	D37.05	D49.0
lingual	C02.4	C79.89	D00.07	D10.1	D37.02	D49.0
overlapping sites	C09.8	-	-	-	-	-
palatine	C09.9	C79.89	D00.08	D10.4	D37.05	D49.0
pharyngeal	C11.1	C79.89	D00.08	D10.6	D37.05	D49.0
pillar (anterior) (posterior)	C09.1	C79.89	D00.08	D10.5	D37.05	D49.0
tonsillar fossa	C09.0	C79.89	D00.08	D10.5	D37.05	D49.0
tooth socket NEC	C03.9	C79.89	D00.03	D10.39	D37.09	D49.0
trachea (cartilage) (mucosa)	C33	C78.39	D02.1	D14.2	D38.1	D49.1
overlapping lesion with bronchus or lung	C34.8-	-	-	-	-	-
tracheobronchial	C34.8-	C78.39	D02.1	D14.2	D38.1	D49.1
overlapping lesion with lung	C34.8-	-	-	-	-	-
tragus — *see also Neoplasm, skin, ear*	C44.20-	C79.2	D04.2-	D23.2-	D48.5	D49.2
trunk NEC	C76.8	C79.89	D04.5	D36.7	D48.7	D49.89
tubo-ovarian	C57.8	C79.82	D07.39	D28.7	D39.8	D49.59
tunica vaginalis	C63.7	C79.82	D07.69	D29.8	D40.8	D49.59
turbinate (bone)	C41.0	C79.51	-	D16.4-	D48.0	D49.2
nasal	C30.0	C78.39	D02.3	D14.0	D38.5	D49.1
tympanic cavity	C30.1	C78.39	D02.3	D14.0	D38.5	D49.1
ulna (any part)	C40.0-	C79.51	-	D16.0-	-	-
umbilicus, umbilical — *see also Neoplasm, skin, trunk*	C44.509	C79.2	D04.5	D23.5	D48.5	D49.2
uncus, brain	C71.2	C79.31	-	D33.0	D43.0	D49.6
unknown site or unspecified	C80.1	C79.9	D09.9	D36.9	D48.9	D49.9
urachus	C67.7	C79.11	D09.0	D30.3	D41.4	D49.4
ureter, ureteral	C66.-	C79.19	D09.19	D30.2-	D41.2-	D49.59
orifice (bladder)	C67.6	C79.11	D09.0	D30.3	D41.4	D49.4
ureter-bladder (junction)	C67.6	C79.11	D09.0	D30.3	D41.4	D49.4
urethra, urethral (gland)	C68.0	C79.19	D09.19	D30.4	D41.3	D49.59
orifice, internal	C67.5	C79.11	D09.0	D30.3	D41.4	D49.4
urethrovaginal (septum)	C57.9	C79.82	D07.30	D28.9	D39.8	D49.59
urinary organ or system	C68.9	C79.10	D09.10	D30.9	D41.9	D49.59
bladder — *see Neoplasm, bladder*						
overlapping lesion	C68.8	-	-	-	-	-
specified sites NEC	C68.8	C79.19	D09.19	D30.8	D41.8	D49.59
utero-ovarian	C57.8	C79.82	D07.39	D28.7	D39.8	D49.59
ligament	C57.1	C79.82	D07.39	D28.2	D39.8	D49.59
uterosacral ligament	C57.3	C79.82	-	D28.2	D39.8	D49.59
uterus, uteri, uterine	C55	C79.82	D07.0	D26.9	D39.0	D49.59
adnexa NEC	C57.4	C79.82	D07.39	D28.7	D39.8	D49.59
body	C54.9	C79.82	D07.0	D26.1	D39.0	D49.59
cervix	C53.9	C79.82	D06.9	D26.0	D39.0	D49.59
cornu	C54.9	C79.82	D07.0	D26.1	D39.0	D49.59
corpus	C54.9	C79.82	D07.0	D26.1	D39.0	D49.59

Neoplasm, neoplastic	Malignant Primary	Malignant Secondary	Ca in situ	Benign	Uncertain Behavior	Unspecified Behavior
endocervix (canal) (gland)	C53.0	C79.82	D06.0	D26.0	D39.0	D49.59
endometrium	C54.1	C79.82	D07.0	D26.1	D39.0	D49.59
exocervix	C53.1	C79.82	D06.1	D26.0	D39.0	D49.59
external os	C53.1	C79.82	D06.1	D26.0	D39.0	D49.59
fundus	C54.3	C79.82	D07.0	D26.1	D39.0	D49.59
internal os	C53.0	C79.82	D06.0	D26.0	D39.0	D49.59
isthmus	C54.0	C79.82	D07.0	D26.1	D39.0	D49.59
ligament	C57.3	C79.82	-	D28.2	D39.8	D49.59
broad	C57.1	C79.82	D07.39	D28.2	D39.8	D49.59
round	C57.2	C79.82	-	D28.2	D39.8	D49.59
lower segment	C54.0	C79.82	D07.0	D26.1	D39.0	D49.59
myometrium	C54.2	C79.82	D07.0	D26.1	D39.0	D49.59
overlapping sites	C54.8	-	-	-	-	-
squamocolumnar junction	C53.8	C79.82	D06.7	D26.0	D39.0	D49.59
tube	C57.0-	C79.82	D07.39	D28.2	D39.8	D49.59
utricle, prostatic	C68.0	C79.19	D09.19	D30.4	D41.3	D49.59
uveal tract	C69.4-	C79.49	D09.2-	D31.4-	D48.7	D49.89
uvula	C05.2	C79.89	D00.04	D10.39	D37.09	D49.0
vagina, vaginal (fornix) (vault) (wall)	C52	C79.82	D07.2	D28.1	D39.8	D49.59
vaginovesical	C57.9	C79.82	D07.30	D28.9	D39.9	D49.59
septum	C57.9	C79.82	D07.30	D28.9	D39.9	D49.59
vallecula (epigiottis)	C10.0	C79.89	D00.08	D10.5	D37.05	D49.0
vas deferens	C63.1-	C79.82	D07.69	D29.8	D40.8	D49.59
vascular — *see Neoplasm, connective tissue*						
Vater's ampulla	C24.1	C78.89	D01.5	D13.5	D37.6	D49.0
vein, venous — *see Neoplasm, connective tissue*						
vena cava (abdominal) (inferior)	C49.4	C79.89	-	D21.4	D48.1	D49.2
superior	C49.3	C79.89	-	D21.3	D48.1	D49.2
ventricle (cerebral) (floor) (lateral) (third)	C71.5	C79.31	-	D33.0	D43.0	D49.6
cardiac (left) (right)	C38.0	C79.89	-	D15.1	D48.7	D49.89
fourth	C71.7	C79.31	-	D33.1	D43.1	D49.6
ventricular band of larynx	C32.1	C78.39	D02.0	D14.1	D38.0	D49.1
ventriculus — *see Neoplasm, stomach*						
vermillion border — *see Neoplasm, lip*						
vermis, cerebellum	C71.6	C79.31	-	D33.1	D43.1	D49.6
vertebra (column)	C41.2	C79.51	-	D16.6	D48.0	D49.2
coccyx	C41.4	C79.51	-	D16.8-	D48.0	D49.2
marrow NEC	C96.9	C79.52	-	-	D47.9	D49.89
sacrum	C41.4	C79.51	-	D16.8-	D48.0	D49.2
vesical — *see Neoplasm, bladder*						
vesicle, seminal	C63.7	C79.82	D07.69	D29.8	D40.8	D49.59
vesicocervical tissue	C57.9	C79.82	D07.30	D28.9	D39.9	D49.59
vesicorectal	C76.3	C79.82	D09.8	D36.7	D48.7	D49.89
vesicovaginal	C57.9	C79.82	D07.30	D28.9	D39.9	D49.59
septum	C57.9	C79.82	D07.30	D28.9	D39.8	D49.59
vessel (blood) — *see Neoplasm, connective tissue*						
vestibular gland, greater	C51.0	C79.82	D07.1	D28.0	D39.8	D49.59
vestibule						
mouth	C06.1	C79.89	D00.00	D10.39	D37.09	D49.0
nose	C30.0	C78.39	D02.3	D14.0	D38.5	D49.1
Virchow's gland	C77.0	C77.0	-	D36.0	D48.7	D49.89
viscera NEC	C76.8	C79.89	D09.8	D36.7	D48.7	D49.89
vocal cords (true)	C32.0	C78.39	D02.0	D14.1	D38.0	D49.1
false	C32.1	C78.39	D02.0	D14.1	D38.0	D49.1
vomer	C41.0	C79.51	-	D16.4-	D48.0	D49.2
vulva	C51.9	C79.82	D07.1	D28.0	D39.8	D49.59

	Malignant Primary	Malignant Secondary	Ca in situ	Benign	Uncertain Behavior	Unspecified Behavior
Neoplasm, neoplastic						
vulvovaginal gland	C51.0	C79.82	D07.1	D28.0	D39.8	D49.59
Waldeyer's ring	C14.2	C79.89	D00.08	D10.9	D37.05	D49.0
Wharton's duct	C08.0	C79.89	D00.00	D11.7	D37.032	D49.0
white matter (central) (cerebral)	C71.0	C79.31	-	D33.0	D43.0	D49.6
windpipe	C33	C78.39	D02.1	D14.2	D38.1	D49.1
Wirsung's duct	C25.3	C78.89	D01.7	D13.6	D37.8	D49.0
wolffian (body) (duct)						
female	C57.7	C79.82	D07.39	D28.7	D39.8	D49.59
male	C63.7	C79.82	D07.69	D29.8	D40.8	D49.59
womb — *see Neoplasm, uterus*						
wrist NEC	C76.4-	C79.89	D04.6-	D36.7	D48.7	D49.89
xiphoid process	C41.3	C79.51	-	D16.7	D48.0	D49.2
Zuckerkandl organ	C75.5	C79.89	-	D35.6	D44.7	D49.7

Table of Drugs and Chemicals

Substance	Poisoning Accidental (unintentional)	Poisoning Intentional self-harm	Poisoning Assault	Poisoning Undetermined	Adverse effect	Underdosing
1-propanol	T51.3X1-	T51.3X2-	T51.3X3-	T51.3X4-	-	-
2-propanol	T51.2X1-	T51.2X2-	T51.2X3-	T51.2X4-	-	-
2,4-D (dichlorophen-oxyacetic acid)	T60.3X1-	T60.3X2-	T60.3X3-	T60.3X4-	-	-
2,4-toluene diisocyanate	T65.0X1-	T65.0X2-	T65.0X3-	T65.0X4-	-	-
2,4,5-T (trichloro-phenoxyacetic acid)	T60.1X1-	T60.1X2-	T60.1X3-	T60.1X4-	-	-
3,4-methylenedioxymethamphetamine	T43.641-	T43.642-	T43.643-	T43.644-	-	-
14-hydroxydihydro-morphinone	T40.2X1-	T40.2X2-	T40.2X3-	T40.2X4-	T40.2X5-	T40.2X6-
ABOB	T37.5X1-	T37.5X2-	T37.5X3-	T37.5X4-	T37.5X5-	T37.5X6-
Abrine	T62.2X1-	T62.2X2-	T62.2X3-	T62.2X4-	-	-
Abrus (seed)	T62.2X1-	T62.2X2-	T62.2X3-	T62.2X4-	-	-
Absinthe	T51.0X1-	T51.0X2-	T51.0X3-	T51.0X4-	-	
beverage	T51.0X1-	T51.0X2-	T51.0X3-	T51.0X4-	-	-
Acaricide	T60.8X1-	T60.8X2-	T60.8X3-	T60.8X4-	-	-
Acebutolol	T44.7X1-	T44.7X2-	T44.7X3-	T44.7X4-	T44.7X5-	T44.7X6-
Acecarbromal	T42.6X1-	T42.6X2-	T42.6X3-	T42.6X4-	T42.6X5-	T42.6X6-
Aceclidine	T44.1X1-	T44.1X2-	T44.1X3-	T44.1X4-	T44.1X5-	T44.1X6-
Acedapsone	T37.0X1-	T37.0X2-	T37.0X3-	T37.0X4-	T37.0X5-	T37.0X6-
Acefylline piperazine	T48.6X1-	T48.6X2-	T48.6X3-	T48.6X4-	T48.6X5-	T48.6X6-
Acemorphan	T40.2X1-	T40.2X2-	T40.2X3-	T40.2X4-	T40.2X5-	T40.2X6-
Acenocoumarin	T45.511-	T45.512-	T45.513-	T45.514-	T45.515-	T45.516-
Acenocoumarol	T45.511-	T45.512-	T45.513-	T45.514-	T45.515-	T45.516-
Acepifylline	T48.6X1-	T48.6X2-	T48.6X3-	T48.6X4-	T48.6X5-	T48.6X6-
Acepromazine	T43.3X1-	T43.3X2-	T43.3X3-	T43.3X4-	T43.3X5-	T43.3X6-
Acesulfamethoxypyridazine	T37.0X1-	T37.0X2-	T37.0X3-	T37.0X4-	T37.0X5-	T37.0X6-
Acetal	T52.8X1-	T52.8X2-	T52.8X3-	T52.8X4-	-	-
Acetaldehyde (vapor)	T52.8X1-	T52.8X2-	T52.8X3-	T52.8X4-	-	-
liquid	T65.891-	T65.892-	T65.893-	T65.894-	-	-
P-Acetamidophenol	T39.1X1-	T39.1X2-	T39.1X3-	T39.1X4-	T39.1X5-	T39.1X6-
Acetaminophen	T39.1X1-	T39.1X2-	T39.1X3-	T39.1X4-	T39.1X5-	T39.1X6-
Acetaminosalol	T39.1X1-	T39.1X2-	T39.1X3-	T39.1X4-	T39.1X5-	T39.1X6-
Acetanilide	T39.1X1-	T39.1X2-	T39.1X3-	T39.1X4-	T39.1X5-	T39.1X6-
Acetarsol	T37.3X1-	T37.3X2-	T37.3X3-	T37.3X4-	T37.3X5-	T37.3X6-
Acetazolamide	T50.2X1-	T50.2X2-	T50.2X3-	T50.2X4-	T50.2X5-	T50.2X6-
Acetiamine	T45.2X1-	T45.2X2-	T45.2X3-	T45.2X4-	T45.2X5-	T45.2X6-
Acetic						
acid	T54.2X1-	T54.2X2-	T54.2X3-	T54.2X4-	-	-
with sodium acetate (ointment)	T49.3X1-	T49.3X2-	T49.3X3-	T49.3X4-	T49.3X5-	T49.3X6-
ester (solvent) (vapor)	T52.8X1-	T52.8X2-	T52.8X3-	T52.8X4-	-	-
irrigating solution	T50.3X1-	T50.3X2-	T50.3X3-	T50.3X4-	T50.3X5-	T50.3X6-
medicinal (lotion)	T49.2X1-	T49.2X2-	T49.2X3-	T49.2X4-	T49.2X5-	T49.2X6-
anhydride	T65.891-	T65.892-	T65.893-	T65.894-	-	-
ether (vapor)	T52.8X1-	T52.8X2-	T52.8X3-	T52.8X4-	-	-
Acetohexamide	T38.3X1-	T38.3X2-	T38.3X3-	T38.3X4-	T38.3X5-	T38.3X6-
Acetohydroxamic acid	T50.991-	T50.992-	T50.993-	T50.994-	T50.995-	T50.996-
Acetomenaphthone	T45.7X1-	T45.7X2-	T45.7X3-	T45.7X4-	T45.7X5-	T45.7X6-
Acetomorphine	T40.1X1-	T40.1X2-	T40.1X3-	T40.1X4-	-	-
Acetone (oils)	T52.4X1-	T52.4X2-	T52.4X3-	T52.4X4-	-	-
chlorinated	T52.4X1-	T52.4X2-	T52.4X3-	T52.4X4-	-	-
vapor	T52.4X1-	T52.4X2-	T52.4X3-	T52.4X4-	-	-
Acetonitrile	T52.8X1-	T52.8X2-	T52.8X3-	T52.8X4-	-	-
Acetophenazine	T43.3X1-	T43.3X2-	T43.3X3-	T43.3X4-	T43.3X5-	T43.3X6-
Acetophenetedin	T39.1X1-	T39.1X2-	T39.1X3-	T39.1X4-	T39.1X5-	T39.1X6-
Acetophenone	T52.4X1-	T52.4X2-	T52.4X3-	T52.4X4-	-	-
Acetorphine	T40.2X1-	T40.2X2-	T40.2X3-	T40.2X4-	-	-
Acetosulfone (sodium)	T37.1X1-	T37.1X2-	T37.1X3-	T37.1X4-	T37.1X5-	T37.1X6-
Acetrizoate (sodium)	T50.8X1-	T50.8X2-	T50.8X3-	T50.8X4-	T50.8X5-	T50.8X6-

Substance	Poisoning Accidental (unintentional)	Poisoning Intentional self-harm	Poisoning Assault	Poisoning Undetermined	Adverse effect	Underdosing
Acetrizoic acid	T50.8X1-	T50.8X2-	T50.8X3-	T50.8X4-	T50.8X5-	T50.8X6-
Acetyl						
bromide	T53.6X1-	T53.6X2-	T53.6X3-	T53.6X4-	-	-
chloride	T53.6X1-	T53.6X2-	T53.6X3-	T53.6X4-	-	-
Acetylcarbromal	T42.6X1-	T42.6X2-	T42.6X3-	T42.6X4-	T42.6X5-	T42.6X6-
Acetylcholine						
chloride	T44.1X1-	T44.1X2-	T44.1X3-	T44.1X4-	T44.1X5-	T44.1X6-
derivative	T44.1X1-	T44.1X2-	T44.1X3-	T44.1X4-	T44.1X5-	T44.1X6-
Acetylcysteine	T48.4X1-	T48.4X2-	T48.4X3-	T48.4X4-	T48.4X5-	T48.4X6-
Acetyldigitoxin	T46.0X1-	T46.0X2-	T46.0X3-	T46.0X4-	T46.0X5-	T46.0X6-
Acetyldigoxin	T46.0X1-	T46.0X2-	T46.0X3-	T46.0X4-	T46.0X5-	T46.0X6-
Acetyldihydrocodeine	T40.2X1-	T40.2X2-	T40.2X3-	T40.2X4-	-	-
Acetyldihydrocodeinone	T40.2X1-	T40.2X2-	T40.2X3-	T40.2X4-	-	-
Acetylene (gas)	T59.891-	T59.892-	T59.893-	T59.894-	-	-
dichloride	T53.6X1-	T53.6X2-	T53.6X3-	T53.6X4-	-	-
incomplete combustion of	T58.11X-	T58.12X-	T58.13X-	T58.14X-	-	-
industrial	T59.891-	T59.892-	T59.893-	T59.894-	-	-
tetrachloride	T53.6X1-	T53.6X2-	T53.6X3-	T53.6X4-	-	-
vapor	T53.6X1-	T53.6X2-	T53.6X3-	T53.6X4-	-	-
Acetylpheneturide	T42.6X1-	T42.6X2-	T42.6X3-	T42.6X4-	T42.6X5-	T42.6X6-
Acetylphenylhydrazine	T39.8X1-	T39.8X2-	T39.8X3-	T39.8X4-	T39.8X5-	T39.8X6-
Acetylsalicylic acid (salts)	T39.011-	T39.012-	T39.013-	T39.014-	T39.015-	T39.016-
enteric coated	T39.011-	T39.012-	T39.013-	T39.014-	T39.015-	T39.016-
Acetylsulfamethoxypyridazine	T37.0X1-	T37.0X2-	T37.0X3-	T37.0X4-	T37.0X5-	T37.0X6-
Achromycin	T36.4X1-	T36.4X2-	T36.4X3-	T36.4X4-	T36.4X5-	T36.4X6-
ophthalmic preparation	T49.5X1-	T49.5X2-	T49.5X3-	T49.5X4-	T49.5X5-	T49.5X6-
topical NEC	T49.0X1-	T49.0X2-	T49.0X3-	T49.0X4-	T49.0X5-	T49.0X6-
Aciclovir	T37.5X1-	T37.5X2-	T37.5X3-	T37.5X4-	T37.5X5-	T37.5X6-
Acid (corrosive) NEC	T54.2X1-	T54.2X2-	T54.2X3-	T54.2X4-	-	-
Acidifying agent NEC	T50.901-	T50.902-	T50.903-	T50.904-	T50.905-	T50.906-
Acipimox	T46.6X1-	T46.6X2-	T46.6X3-	T46.6X4-	T46.6X5-	T46.6X6-
Acitretin	T50.991-	T50.992-	T50.993-	T50.994-	T50.995-	T50.996-
Aclarubicin	T45.1X1-	T45.1X2-	T45.1X3-	T45.1X4-	T45.1X5-	T45.1X6-
Aclatonium napadisilate	T48.1X1-	T48.1X2-	T48.1X3-	T48.1X4-	T48.1X5-	T48.1X6-
Aconite (wild)	T46.991-	T46.992-	T46.993-	T46.994-	T46.995-	T46.996-
Aconitine	T46.991-	T46.992-	T46.993-	T46.994-	T46.995-	T46.996-
Aconitum ferox	T46.991-	T46.992-	T46.993-	T46.994-	T46.995-	T46.996-
Acridine	T65.6X1-	T65.6X2-	T65.6X3-	T65.6X4-	-	-
vapor	T59.891-	T59.892-	T59.893-	T59.894-	-	-
Acriflavine	T37.91X-	T37.92X-	T37.93X-	T37.94X-	T37.95X-	T37.96X-
Acriflavinium chloride	T49.0X1-	T49.0X2-	T49.0X3-	T49.0X4-	T49.0X5-	T49.0X6-
Acrinol	T49.0X1-	T49.0X2-	T49.0X3-	T49.0X4-	T49.0X5-	T49.0X6-
Acrisorcin	T49.0X1-	T49.0X2-	T49.0X3-	T49.0X4-	T49.0X5-	T49.0X6-
Acrivastine	T45.0X1-	T45.0X2-	T45.0X3-	T45.0X4-	T45.0X5-	T45.0X6-
Acrolein (gas)	T59.891-	T59.892-	T59.893-	T59.894-	-	-
liquid	T54.1X1-	T54.1X2-	T54.1X3-	T54.1X4-	-	-
Acrylamide	T65.891-	T65.892-	T65.893-	T65.894-	-	-
Acrylic resin	T49.3X1-	T49.3X2-	T49.3X3-	T49.3X4-	T49.3X5-	T49.3X6-
Acrylonitrile	T65.891-	T65.892-	T65.893-	T65.894-	-	-
Actaea spicata	T62.2X1-	T62.2X2-	T62.2X3-	T62.2X4-	-	-
berry	T62.1X1-	T62.1X2-	T62.1X3-	T62.1X4-	-	-
Acterol	T37.3X1-	T37.3X2-	T37.3X3-	T37.3X4-	T37.3X5-	T37.3X6-
ACTH	T38.811-	T38.812-	T38.813-	T38.814-	T38.815-	T38.816-
Actinomycin C	T45.1X1-	T45.1X2-	T45.1X3-	T45.1X4-	T45.1X5-	T45.1X6-
Actinomycin D	T45.1X1-	T45.1X2-	T45.1X3-	T45.1X4-	T45.1X5-	T45.1X6-
Activated charcoal — *see also Charcoal, medicinal*	T47.6X1-	T47.6X2-	T47.6X3-	T47.6X4-	T47.6X5-	T47.6X6-
Acyclovir	T37.5X1-	T37.5X2-	T37.5X3-	T37.5X4-	T37.5X5-	T37.5X6-

Substance	Poisoning Accidental (unintentional)	Poisoning Intentional self-harm	Poisoning Assault	Poisoning Undetermined	Adverse effect	Underdosing
Adenine	T45.2X1-	T45.2X2-	T45.2X3-	T45.2X4-	T45.2X5-	T45.2X6-
arabinoside	T37.5X1-	T37.5X2-	T37.5X3-	T37.5X4-	T37.5X5-	T37.5X6-
Adenosine (phosphate)	T46.2X1-	T46.2X2-	T46.2X3-	T46.2X4-	T46.2X5-	T46.2X6-
ADH	T38.891-	T38.892-	T38.893-	T38.894-	T38.895-	T38.896-
Adhesive NEC	T65.891-	T65.892-	T65.893-	T65.894-	-	-
Adicillin	T36.0X1-	T36.0X2-	T36.0X3-	T36.0X4-	T36.0X5-	T36.0X6-
Adiphenine	T44.3X1-	T44.3X2-	T44.3X3-	T44.3X4-	T44.3X5-	T44.3X6-
Adipiodone	T50.8X1-	T50.8X2-	T50.8X3-	T50.8X4-	T50.8X5-	T50.8X6-
Adjunct, pharmaceutical	T50.901-	T50.902-	T50.903-	T50.904-	T50.905-	T50.906-
Adrenal (extract, cortex or medulla) (glucocorticoids) (hormones) (mineralocorticoids)	T38.0X1-	T38.0X2-	T38.0X3-	T38.0X4-	T38.0X5-	T38.0X6-
ENT agent	T49.6X1-	T49.6X2-	T49.6X3-	T49.6X4-	T49.6X5-	T49.6X6-
ophthalmic preparation	T49.5X1-	T49.5X2-	T49.5X3-	T49.5X4-	T49.5X5-	T49.5X6-
topical NEC	T49.0X1-	T49.0X2-	T49.0X3-	T49.0X4-	T49.0X5-	T49.0X6-
Adrenaline	T44.5X1-	T44.5X2-	T44.5X3-	T44.5X4-	T44.5X5-	T44.5X6-
Adrenalin — *see Adrenaline*						
Adrenergic NEC	T44.901-	T44.902-	T44.903-	T44.904-	T44.905-	T44.906-
blocking agent NEC	T44.8X1-	T44.8X2-	T44.8X3-	T44.8X4-	T44.8X5-	T44.8X6-
beta, heart	T44.7X1-	T44.7X2-	T44.7X3-	T44.7X4-	T44.7X5-	T44.7X6-
specified NEC	T44.991-	T44.992-	T44.993-	T44.994-	T44.995-	T44.996-
Adrenochrome						
(mono) semicarbazone	T46.991-	T46.992-	T46.993-	T46.994-	T46.995-	T46.996-
derivative	T46.991-	T46.992-	T46.993-	T46.994-	T46.995-	T46.996-
Adrenocorticotrophic hormone	T38.811-	T38.812-	T38.813-	T38.814-	T38.815-	T38.816-
Adrenocorticotrophin	T38.811-	T38.812-	T38.813-	T38.814-	T38.815-	T38.816-
Adriamycin	T45.1X1-	T45.1X2-	T45.1X3-	T45.1X4-	T45.1X5-	T45.1X6-
Aerosol spray NEC	T65.91X-	T65.92X-	T65.93X-	T65.94X-	-	-
Aerosporin	T36.8X1-	T36.8X2-	T36.8X3-	T36.8X4-	T36.8X5-	T36.8X6-
ENT agent	T49.6X1-	T49.6X2-	T49.6X3-	T49.6X4-	T49.6X5-	T49.6X6-
ophthalmic preparation	T49.5X1-	T49.5X2-	T49.5X3-	T49.5X4-	T49.5X5-	T49.5X6-
topical NEC	T49.0X1-	T49.0X2-	T49.0X3-	T49.0X4-	T49.0X5-	T49.0X6-
Aethusa cynapium	T62.2X1-	T62.2X2-	T62.2X3-	T62.2X4-	-	-
Afghanistan black	T40.711-	T40.712-	T40.713-	T40.714-	T40.715-	T40.716-
Aflatoxin	T64.01X-	T64.02X-	T64.03X-	T64.04X-	-	-
Afloqualone	T42.8X1-	T42.8X2-	T42.8X3-	T42.8X4-	T42.8X5-	T42.8X6-
African boxwood	T62.2X1-	T62.2X2-	T62.2X3-	T62.2X4-	-	-
Agar	T47.4X1-	T47.4X2-	T47.4X3-	T47.4X4-	T47.4X5-	T47.4X6-
Agonist						
predominantly						
alpha-adrenoreceptor	T44.4X1-	T44.4X2-	T44.4X3-	T44.4X4-	T44.4X5-	T44.4X6-
beta-adrenoreceptor	T44.5X1-	T44.5X2-	T44.5X3-	T44.5X4-	T44.5X5-	T44.5X6-
Agricultural agent NEC	T65.91X-	T65.92X-	T65.93X-	T65.94X-	-	-
Agrypnal	T42.3X1-	T42.3X2-	T42.3X3-	T42.3X4-	T42.3X5-	T42.3X6-
AHLG	T50.Z11-	T50.Z12-	T50.Z13-	T50.Z14-	T50.Z15-	T50.Z16-
Air contaminant (s) , source/type NOS	T65.91X-	T65.92X-	T65.93X-	T65.94X-	-	-
Ajmaline	T46.2X1-	T46.2X2-	T46.2X3-	T46.2X4-	T46.2X5-	T46.2X6-
Akee	T62.1X1-	T62.1X2-	T62.1X3-	T62.1X4-	-	-
Akrinol	T49.0X1-	T49.0X2-	T49.0X3-	T49.0X4-	T49.0X5-	T49.0X6-
Akritoin	T37.8X1-	T37.8X2-	T37.8X3-	T37.8X4-	T37.8X5-	T37.8X6-
Alacepril	T46.4X1-	T46.4X2-	T46.4X3-	T46.4X4-	T46.4X5-	T46.4X6-
Alantolactone	T37.4X1-	T37.4X2-	T37.4X3-	T37.4X4-	T37.4X5-	T37.4X6-
Albamycin	T36.8X1-	T36.8X2-	T36.8X3-	T36.8X4-	T36.8X5-	T36.8X6-
Albendazole	T37.4X1-	T37.4X2-	T37.4X3-	T37.4X4-	T37.4X5-	T37.4X6-
Albumin						
bovine	T45.8X1-	T45.8X2-	T45.8X3-	T45.8X4-	T45.8X5-	T45.8X6-
human serum	T45.8X1-	T45.8X2-	T45.8X3-	T45.8X4-	T45.8X5-	T45.8X6-
salt-poor	T45.8X1-	T45.8X2-	T45.8X3-	T45.8X4-	T45.8X5-	T45.8X6-

Substance	Poisoning Accidental (unintentional)	Poisoning Intentional self-harm	Poisoning Assault	Poisoning Undetermined	Adverse effect	Underdosing
Albumin (continued)						
normal human serum	T45.8X1-	T45.8X2-	T45.8X3-	T45.8X4-	T45.8X5-	T45.8X6-
Albuterol	T48.6X1-	T48.6X2-	T48.6X3-	T48.6X4-	T48.6X5-	T48.6X6-
Albutoin	T42.0X1-	T42.0X2-	T42.0X3-	T42.0X4-	T42.0X5-	T42.0X6-
Alclometasone	T49.0X1-	T49.0X2-	T49.0X3-	T49.0X4-	T49.0X5-	T49.0X6-
Alcohol	T51.91X-	T51.92X-	T51.93X-	T51.94X-	-	-
absolute	T51.0X1-	T51.0X2-	T51.0X3-	T51.0X4-	-	-
beverage	T51.0X1-	T51.0X2-	T51.0X3-	T51.0X4-	-	-
allyl	T51.8X1-	T51.8X2-	T51.8X3-	T51.8X4-	-	-
amyl	T51.3X1-	T51.3X2-	T51.3X3-	T51.3X4-	-	-
antifreeze	T51.1X1-	T51.1X2-	T51.1X3-	T51.1X4-	-	-
beverage	T51.0X1-	T51.0X2-	T51.0X3-	T51.0X4-	-	-
butyl	T51.3X1-	T51.3X2-	T51.3X3-	T51.3X4-	-	-
dehydrated	T51.0X1-	T51.0X2-	T51.0X3-	T51.0X4-	-	-
beverage	T51.0X1-	T51.0X2-	T51.0X3-	T51.0X4-	-	-
denatured	T51.0X1-	T51.0X2-	T51.0X3-	T51.0X4-	-	-
deterrent NEC	T50.6X1-	T50.6X2-	T50.6X3-	T50.6X4-	T50.6X5-	T50.6X6-
diagnostic (gastric function)	T50.8X1-	T50.8X2-	T50.8X3-	T50.8X4-	T50.8X5-	T50.8X6-
ethyl	T51.0X1-	T51.0X2-	T51.0X3-	T51.0X4-	-	-
beverage	T51.0X1-	T51.0X2-	T51.0X3-	T51.0X4-	-	-
grain	T51.0X1-	T51.0X2-	T51.0X3-	T51.0X4-	-	-
beverage	T51.0X1-	T51.0X2-	T51.0X3-	T51.0X4-	-	-
industrial	T51.0X1-	T51.0X2-	T51.0X3-	T51.0X4-	-	-
isopropyl	T51.2X1-	T51.2X2-	T51.2X3-	T51.2X4-	-	-
methyl	T51.1X1-	T51.1X2-	T51.1X3-	T51.1X4-	-	-
preparation for consumption	T51.0X1-	T51.0X2-	T51.0X3-	T51.0X4-	-	-
propyl	T51.3X1-	T51.3X2-	T51.3X3-	T51.3X4-	-	-
secondary	T51.2X1-	T51.2X2-	T51.2X3-	T51.2X4-	-	-
radiator	T51.1X1-	T51.1X2-	T51.1X3-	T51.1X4-	-	-
rubbing	T51.2X1-	T51.2X2-	T51.2X3-	T51.2X4-	-	-
specified type NEC	T51.8X1-	T51.8X2-	T51.8X3-	T51.8X4-	-	-
surgical	T51.0X1-	T51.0X2-	T51.0X3-	T51.0X4-	-	-
vapor (from any type of Alcohol)	T59.891-	T59.892-	T59.893-	T59.894-	-	-
wood	T51.1X1-	T51.1X2-	T51.1X3-	T51.1X4-	-	-
Alcuronium (chloride)	T48.1X1-	T48.1X2-	T48.1X3-	T48.1X4-	T48.1X5-	T48.1X6-
Aldactone	T50.0X1-	T50.0X2-	T50.0X3-	T50.0X4-	T50.0X5-	T50.0X6-
Aldesulfone sodium	T37.1X1-	T37.1X2-	T37.1X3-	T37.1X4-	T37.1X5-	T37.1X6-
Aldicarb	T60.0X1-	T60.0X2-	T60.0X3-	T60.0X4-	-	-
Aldomet	T46.5X1-	T46.5X2-	T46.5X3-	T46.5X4-	T46.5X5-	T46.5X6-
Aldosterone	T50.0X1-	T50.0X2-	T50.0X3-	T50.0X4-	T50.0X5-	T50.0X6-
Aldrin (dust)	T60.1X1-	T60.1X2-	T60.1X3-	T60.1X4-	-	-
Aleve — *see Naproxen*						
Alexitol sodium	T47.1X1-	T47.1X2-	T47.1X3-	T47.1X4-	T47.1X5-	T47.1X6-
Alfacalcidol	T45.2X1-	T45.2X2-	T45.2X3-	T45.2X4-	T45.2X5-	T45.2X6-
Alfadolone	T41.1X1-	T41.1X2-	T41.1X3-	T41.1X4-	T41.1X5-	T41.1X6-
Alfaxalone	T41.1X1-	T41.1X2-	T41.1X3-	T41.1X4-	T41.1X5-	T41.1X6-
Alfentanil	T40.411-	T40.412-	T40.413-	T40.414-	T40.415-	T40.416-
Alfuzosin (hydrochloride)	T44.8X1-	T44.8X2-	T44.8X3-	T44.8X4-	T44.8X5-	T44.8X6-
Algae (harmful) (toxin)	T65.821-	T65.822-	T65.823-	T65.824-	-	-
Algeldrate	T47.1X1-	T47.1X2-	T47.1X3-	T47.1X4-	T47.1X5-	T47.1X6-
Algin	T47.8X1-	T47.8X2-	T47.8X3-	T47.8X4-	T47.8X5-	T47.8X6-
Alglucerase	T45.3X1-	T45.3X2-	T45.3X3-	T45.3X4-	T45.3X5-	T45.3X6-
Alidase	T45.3X1-	T45.3X2-	T45.3X3-	T45.3X4-	T45.3X5-	T45.3X6-
Alimemazine	T43.3X1-	T43.3X2-	T43.3X3-	T43.3X4-	T43.3X5-	T43.3X6-
Aliphatic thiocyanates	T65.0X1-	T65.0X2-	T65.0X3-	T65.0X4-	-	-
Alizapride	T45.0X1-	T45.0X2-	T45.0X3-	T45.0X4-	T45.0X5-	T45.0X6-
Alkali (caustic)	T54.3X1-	T54.3X2-	T54.3X3-	T54.3X4-	-	-
Alkaline antiseptic solution (aromatic)	T49.6X1-	T49.6X2-	T49.6X3-	T49.6X4-	T49.6X5-	T49.6X6-
Alkalinizing agents (medicinal)	T50.901-	T50.902-	T50.903-	T50.904-	T50.905-	T50.906-

Substance	Poisoning Accidental (unintentional)	Poisoning Intentional self-harm	Poisoning Assault	Poisoning Undetermined	Adverse effect	Underdosing
Alkalizing agent NEC	T50.901-	T50.902-	T50.903-	T50.904-	T50.905-	T50.906-
Alka-seltzer	T39.011-	T39.012-	T39.013-	T39.014-	T39.015-	T39.016-
Alkavervir	T46.5X1-	T46.5X2-	T46.5X3-	T46.5X4-	T46.5X5-	T46.5X6-
Alkonium (bromide)	T49.0X1-	T49.0X2-	T49.0X3-	T49.0X4-	T49.0X5-	T49.0X6-
Alkylating drug NEC	T45.1X1-	T45.1X2-	T45.1X3-	T45.1X4-	T45.1X5-	T45.1X6-
antimyeloproliferative	T45.1X1-	T45.1X2-	T45.1X3-	T45.1X4-	T45.1X5-	T45.1X6-
lymphatic	T45.1X1-	T45.1X2-	T45.1X3-	T45.1X4-	T45.1X5-	T45.1X6-
Alkylisocyanate	T65.0X1-	T65.0X2-	T65.0X3-	T65.0X4-	-	-
Allantoin	T49.4X1-	T49.4X2-	T49.4X3-	T49.4X4-	T49.4X5-	T49.4X6-
Allegron	T43.011-	T43.012-	T43.013-	T43.014-	T43.015-	T43.016-
Allethrin	T49.0X1-	T49.0X2-	T49.0X3-	T49.0X4-	T49.0X5-	T49.0X6-
Allobarbital	T42.3X1-	T42.3X2-	T42.3X3-	T42.3X4-	T42.3X5-	T42.3X6-
Allopurinol	T50.4X1-	T50.4X2-	T50.4X3-	T50.4X4-	T50.4X5-	T50.4X6-
Allyl						
Alcohol	T51.8X1-	T51.8X2-	T51.8X3-	T51.8X4-	-	-
disulfide	T46.6X1-	T46.6X2-	T46.6X3-	T46.6X4-	T46.6X5-	T46.6X6-
Allylestrenol	T38.5X1-	T38.5X2-	T38.5X3-	T38.5X4-	T38.5X5-	T38.5X6-
Allylisopropylacetylurea	T42.6X1-	T42.6X2-	T42.6X3-	T42.6X4-	T42.6X5-	T42.6X6-
Allylisopropylmalonylurea	T42.3X1-	T42.3X2-	T42.3X3-	T42.3X4-	T42.3X5-	T42.3X6-
Allylthiourea	T49.3X1-	T49.3X2-	T49.3X3-	T49.3X4-	T49.3X5-	T49.3X6-
Allyltribromide	T42.6X1-	T42.6X2-	T42.6X3-	T42.6X4-	T42.6X5-	T42.6X6-
Allypropymal	T42.3X1-	T42.3X2-	T42.3X3-	T42.3X4-	T42.3X5-	T42.3X6-
Almagate	T47.1X1-	T47.1X2-	T47.1X3-	T47.1X4-	T47.1X5-	T47.1X6-
Almasilate	T47.1X1-	T47.1X2-	T47.1X3-	T47.1X4-	T47.1X5-	T47.1X6-
Almitrine	T50.7X1-	T50.7X2-	T50.7X3-	T50.7X4-	T50.7X5-	T50.7X6-
Aloes	T47.2X1-	T47.2X2-	T47.2X3-	T47.2X4-	T47.2X5-	T47.2X6-
Aloglutamol	T47.1X1-	T47.1X2-	T47.1X3-	T47.1X4-	T47.1X5-	T47.1X6-
Aloin	T47.2X1-	T47.2X2-	T47.2X3-	T47.2X4-	T47.2X5-	T47.2X6-
Aloxidone	T42.2X1-	T42.2X2-	T42.2X3-	T42.2X4-	T42.2X5-	T42.2X6-
Alpha						
acetyldigoxin	T46.0X1-	T46.0X2-	T46.0X3-	T46.0X4-	T46.0X5-	T46.0X6-
adrenergic blocking drug	T44.6X1-	T44.6X2-	T44.6X3-	T44.6X4-	T44.6X5-	T44.6X6-
amylase	T45.3X1-	T45.3X2-	T45.3X3-	T45.3X4-	T45.3X5-	T45.3X6-
tocoferol (acetate)	T45.2X1-	T45.2X2-	T45.2X3-	T45.2X4-	T45.2X5-	T45.2X6-
tocopherol	T45.2X1-	T45.2X2-	T45.2X3-	T45.2X4-	T45.2X5-	T45.2X6-
Alphadolone	T41.1X1-	T41.1X2-	T41.1X3-	T41.1X4-	T41.1X5-	T41.1X6-
Alphaprodine	T40.491-	T40.492-	T40.493-	T40.494-	T40.495-	T40.496-
Alphaxalone	T41.1X1-	T41.1X2-	T41.1X3-	T41.1X4-	T41.1X5-	T41.1X6-
Alprazolam	T42.4X1-	T42.4X2-	T42.4X3-	T42.4X4-	T42.4X5-	T42.4X6-
Alprenolol	T44.7X1-	T44.7X2-	T44.7X3-	T44.7X4-	T44.7X5-	T44.7X6-
Alprostadil	T46.7X1-	T46.7X2-	T46.7X3-	T46.7X4-	T46.7X5-	T46.7X6-
Alsactide	T38.811-	T38.812-	T38.813-	T38.814-	T38.815-	T38.816-
Alseroxylon	T46.5X1-	T46.5X2-	T46.5X3-	T46.5X4-	T46.5X5-	T46.5X6-
Alteplase	T45.611-	T45.612-	T45.613-	T45.614-	T45.615-	T45.616-
Altizide	T50.2X1-	T50.2X2-	T50.2X3-	T50.2X4-	T50.2X5-	T50.2X6-
Altretamine	T45.1X1-	T45.1X2-	T45.1X3-	T45.1X4-	T45.1X5-	T45.1X6-
Alum (medicinal)	T49.4X1-	T49.4X2-	T49.4X3-	T49.4X4-	T49.4X5-	T49.4X6-
nonmedicinal (ammonium) (potassium)	T56.891-	T56.892-	T56.893-	T56.894-	-	-
Aluminium, aluminum						
acetate	T49.2X1-	T49.2X2-	T49.2X3-	T49.2X4-	T49.2X5-	T49.2X6-
solution	T49.0X1-	T49.0X2-	T49.0X3-	T49.0X4-	T49.0X5-	T49.0X6-
aspirin	T39.011-	T39.012-	T39.013-	T39.014-	T39.015-	T39.016-
bis (acetylsalicylate)	T39.011-	T39.012-	T39.013-	T39.014-	T39.015-	T39.016-
carbonate (gel, basic)	T47.1X1-	T47.1X2-	T47.1X3-	T47.1X4-	T47.1X5-	T47.1X6-
chlorhydroxide-complex	T47.1X1-	T47.1X2-	T47.1X3-	T47.1X4-	T47.1X5-	T47.1X6-
chloride	T49.2X1-	T49.2X2-	T49.2X3-	T49.2X4-	T49.2X5-	T49.2X6-
clofibrate	T46.6X1-	T46.6X2-	T46.6X3-	T46.6X4-	T46.6X5-	T46.6X6-
diacetate	T49.2X1-	T49.2X2-	T49.2X3-	T49.2X4-	T49.2X5-	T49.2X6-

Substance	Poisoning Accidental (unintentional)	Poisoning Intentional self-harm	Poisoning Assault	Poisoning Undetermined	Adverse effect	Underdosing
Aluminium, aluminum (continued)						
glycinate	T47.1X1-	T47.1X2-	T47.1X3-	T47.1X4-	T47.1X5-	T47.1X6-
hydroxide (gel)	T47.1X1-	T47.1X2-	T47.1X3-	T47.1X4-	T47.1X5-	T47.1X6-
hydroxide-magnesium carb. gel	T47.1X1-	T47.1X2-	T47.1X3-	T47.1X4-	T47.1X5-	T47.1X6-
magnesium silicate	T47.1X1-	T47.1X2-	T47.1X3-	T47.1X4-	T47.1X5-	T47.1X6-
nicotinate	T46.7X1-	T46.7X2-	T46.7X3-	T46.7X4-	T46.7X5-	T46.7X6-
ointment (surgical) (topical)	T49.3X1-	T49.3X2-	T49.3X3-	T49.3X4-	T49.3X5-	T49.3X6-
phosphate	T47.1X1-	T47.1X2-	T47.1X3-	T47.1X4-	T47.1X5-	T47.1X6-
salicylate	T39.091-	T39.092-	T39.093-	T39.094-	T39.095-	T39.096-
silicate	T47.1X1-	T47.1X2-	T47.1X3-	T47.1X4-	T47.1X5-	T47.1X6-
sodium silicate	T47.1X1-	T47.1X2-	T47.1X3-	T47.1X4-	T47.1X5-	T47.1X6-
subacetate	T49.2X1-	T49.2X2-	T49.2X3-	T49.2X4-	T49.2X5-	T49.2X6-
sulfate	T49.0X1-	T49.0X2-	T49.0X3-	T49.0X4-	T49.0X5-	T49.0X6-
tannate	T47.6X1-	T47.6X2-	T47.6X3-	T47.6X4-	T47.6X5-	T47.6X6-
topical NEC	T49.3X1-	T49.3X2-	T49.3X3-	T49.3X4-	T49.3X5-	T49.3X6-
Alurate	T42.3X1-	T42.3X2-	T42.3X3-	T42.3X4-	T42.3X5-	T42.3X6-
Alverine	T44.3X1-	T44.3X2-	T44.3X3-	T44.3X4-	T44.3X5-	T44.3X6-
Alvodine	T40.2X1-	T40.2X2-	T40.2X3-	T40.2X4-	T40.2X5-	T40.2X6-
Amanita phalloides	T62.0X1-	T62.0X2-	T62.0X3-	T62.0X4-	-	-
Amanitine	T62.0X1-	T62.0X2-	T62.0X3-	T62.0X4-	-	-
Amantadine	T42.8X1-	T42.8X2-	T42.8X3-	T42.8X4-	T42.8X5-	T42.8X6-
Ambazone	T49.6X1-	T49.6X2-	T49.6X3-	T49.6X4-	T49.6X5-	T49.6X6-
Ambenonium (chloride)	T44.0X1-	T44.0X2-	T44.0X3-	T44.0X4-	T44.0X5-	T44.0X6-
Ambroxol	T48.4X1-	T48.4X2-	T48.4X3-	T48.4X4-	T48.4X5-	T48.4X6-
Ambuphylline	T48.6X1-	T48.6X2-	T48.6X3-	T48.6X4-	T48.6X5-	T48.6X6-
Ambutonium bromide	T44.3X1-	T44.3X2-	T44.3X3-	T44.3X4-	T44.3X5-	T44.3X6-
Amcinonide	T49.0X1-	T49.0X2-	T49.0X3-	T49.0X4-	T49.0X5-	T49.0X6-
Amdinocilline	T36.0X1-	T36.0X2-	T36.0X3-	T36.0X4-	T36.0X5-	T36.0X6-
Ametazole	T50.8X1-	T50.8X2-	T50.8X3-	T50.8X4-	T50.8X5-	T50.8X6-
Amethocaine	T41.3X1-	T41.3X2-	T41.3X3-	T41.3X4-	T41.3X5-	T41.3X6-
regional	T41.3X1-	T41.3X2-	T41.3X3-	T41.3X4-	T41.3X5-	T41.3X6-
spinal	T41.3X1-	T41.3X2-	T41.3X3-	T41.3X4-	T41.3X5-	T41.3X6-
Amethopterin	T45.1X1-	T45.1X2-	T45.1X3-	T45.1X4-	T45.1X5-	T45.1X6-
Amezinium metilsulfate	T44.991-	T44.992-	T44.993-	T44.994-	T44.995-	T44.996-
Amfebutamone	T43.291-	T43.292-	T43.293-	T43.294-	T43.295-	T43.296-
Amfepramone	T50.5X1-	T50.5X2-	T50.5X3-	T50.5X4-	T50.5X5-	T50.5X6-
Amfetamine	T43.621-	T43.622-	T43.623-	T43.624-	T43.625-	T43.626-
Amfetaminil	T43.621-	T43.622-	T43.623-	T43.624-	T43.625-	T43.626-
Amfomycin	T36.8X1-	T36.8X2-	T36.8X3-	T36.8X4-	T36.8X5-	T36.8X6-
Amidefrine mesilate	T48.5X1-	T48.5X2-	T48.5X3-	T48.5X4-	T48.5X5-	T48.5X6-
Amidone	T40.3X1-	T40.3X2-	T40.3X3-	T40.3X4-	T40.3X5-	T40.3X6-
Amidopyrine	T39.2X1-	T39.2X2-	T39.2X3-	T39.2X4-	T39.2X5-	T39.2X6-
Amidotrizoate	T50.8X1-	T50.8X2-	T50.8X3-	T50.8X4-	T50.8X5-	T50.8X6-
Amiflamine	T43.1X1-	T43.1X2-	T43.1X3-	T43.1X4-	T43.1X5-	T43.1X6-
Amikacin	T36.5X1-	T36.5X2-	T36.5X3-	T36.5X4-	T36.5X5-	T36.5X6-
Amikhelline	T46.3X1-	T46.3X2-	T46.3X3-	T46.3X4-	T46.3X5-	T46.3X6-
Amiloride	T50.2X1-	T50.2X2-	T50.2X3-	T50.2X4-	T50.2X5-	T50.2X6-
Aminacrine	T49.0X1-	T49.0X2-	T49.0X3-	T49.0X4-	T49.0X5-	T49.0X6-
Amineptine	T43.011-	T43.012-	T43.013-	T43.014-	T43.015-	T43.016-
Aminitrozole	T37.3X1-	T37.3X2-	T37.3X3-	T37.3X4-	T37.3X5-	T37.3X6-
Amino acids	T50.3X1-	T50.3X2-	T50.3X3-	T50.3X4-	T50.3X5-	T50.3X6-
Aminoacetic acid (derivatives)	T50.3X1-	T50.3X2-	T50.3X3-	T50.3X4-	T50.3X5-	T50.3X6-
Aminoacridine	T49.0X1-	T49.0X2-	T49.0X3-	T49.0X4-	T49.0X5-	T49.0X6-
Aminobenzoic acid (-p)	T49.3X1-	T49.3X2-	T49.3X3-	T49.3X4-	T49.3X5-	T49.3X6-
4-Aminobutyric acid	T43.8X1-	T43.8X2-	T43.8X3-	T43.8X4-	T43.8X5-	T43.8X6-
Aminocaproic acid	T45.621-	T45.622-	T45.623-	T45.624-	T45.625-	T45.626-
Aminoethylisothiourium	T45.8X1-	T45.8X2-	T45.8X3-	T45.8X4-	T45.8X5-	T45.8X6-
Aminofenazone	T39.2X1-	T39.2X2-	T39.2X3-	T39.2X4-	T39.2X5-	T39.2X6-
Aminoglutethimide	T45.1X1-	T45.1X2-	T45.1X3-	T45.1X4-	T45.1X5-	T45.1X6-

Substance	Poisoning Accidental (unintentional)	Poisoning Intentional self-harm	Poisoning Assault	Poisoning Undetermined	Adverse effect	Underdosing
Aminohippuric acid	T50.8X1-	T50.8X2-	T50.8X3-	T50.8X4-	T50.8X5-	T50.8X6-
Aminomethylbenzoic acid	T45.691-	T45.692-	T45.693-	T45.694-	T45.695-	T45.696-
Aminometradine	T50.2X1-	T50.2X2-	T50.2X3-	T50.2X4-	T50.2X5-	T50.2X6-
Aminopentamide	T44.3X1-	T44.3X2-	T44.3X3-	T44.3X4-	T44.3X5-	T44.3X6-
Aminophenazone	T39.2X1-	T39.2X2-	T39.2X3-	T39.2X4-	T39.2X5-	T39.2X6-
Aminophenol	T54.0X1-	T54.0X2-	T54.0X3-	T54.0X4-	-	-
4-Aminophenol derivatives	T39.1X1-	T39.1X2-	T39.1X3-	T39.1X4-	T39.1X5-	T39.1X6-
Aminophenylpyridone	T43.591-	T43.592-	T43.593-	T43.594-	T43.595-	T43.596-
Aminophylline	T48.6X1-	T48.6X2-	T48.6X3-	T48.6X4-	T48.6X5-	T48.6X6-
Aminopterin sodium	T45.1X1-	T45.1X2-	T45.1X3-	T45.1X4-	T45.1X5-	T45.1X6-
Aminopyrine	T39.2X1-	T39.2X2-	T39.2X3-	T39.2X4-	T39.2X5-	T39.2X6-
8-Aminoquinoline drugs	T37.2X1-	T37.2X2-	T37.2X3-	T37.2X4-	T37.2X5-	T37.2X6-
Aminorex	T50.5X1-	T50.5X2-	T50.5X3-	T50.5X4-	T50.5X5-	T50.5X6-
Aminosalicylic acid	T37.1X1-	T37.1X2-	T37.1X3-	T37.1X4-	T37.1X5-	T37.1X6-
Aminosalylum	T37.1X1-	T37.1X2-	T37.1X3-	T37.1X4-	T37.1X5-	T37.1X6-
Amiodarone	T46.2X1-	T46.2X2-	T46.2X3-	T46.2X4-	T46.2X5-	T46.2X6-
Amiphenazole	T50.7X1-	T50.7X2-	T50.7X3-	T50.7X4-	T50.7X5-	T50.7X6-
Amiquinsin	T46.5X1-	T46.5X2-	T46.5X3-	T46.5X4-	T46.5X5-	T46.5X6-
Amisometradine	T50.2X1-	T50.2X2-	T50.2X3-	T50.2X4-	T50.2X5-	T50.2X6-
Amisulpride	T43.591-	T43.592-	T43.593-	T43.594-	T43.595-	T43.596-
Amitriptyline	T43.011-	T43.012-	T43.013-	T43.014-	T43.015-	T43.016-
Amitriptylinoxide	T43.011-	T43.012-	T43.013-	T43.014-	T43.015-	T43.016-
Amlexanox	T48.6X1-	T48.6X2-	T48.6X3-	T48.6X4-	T48.6X5-	T48.6X6-
Ammonia (fumes) (gas) (vapor)	T59.891-	T59.892-	T59.893-	T59.894-	-	-
aromatic spirit	T48.991-	T48.992-	T48.993-	T48.994-	T48.995-	T48.996-
liquid (household)	T54.3X1-	T54.3X2-	T54.3X3-	T54.3X4-	-	-
Ammoniated mercury	T49.0X1-	T49.0X2-	T49.0X3-	T49.0X4-	T49.0X5-	T49.0X6-
Ammonium						
acid tartrate	T49.5X1-	T49.5X2-	T49.5X3-	T49.5X4-	T49.5X5-	T49.5X6-
bromide	T42.6X1-	T42.6X2-	T42.6X3-	T42.6X4-	T42.6X5-	T42.6X6-
carbonate	T54.3X1-	T54.3X2-	T54.3X3-	T54.3X4-	-	-
chloride	T50.991-	T50.992-	T50.993-	T50.994-	T50.995-	T50.996-
expectorant	T48.4X1-	T48.4X2-	T48.4X3-	T48.4X4-	T48.4X5-	T48.4X6-
compounds (household) NEC	T54.3X1-	T54.3X2-	T54.3X3-	T54.3X4-	-	-
fumes (any usage)	T59.891-	T59.892-	T59.893-	T59.894-	-	-
industrial	T54.3X1-	T54.3X2-	T54.3X3-	T54.3X4-	-	-
ichthyosulronate	T49.4X1-	T49.4X2-	T49.4X3-	T49.4X4-	T49.4X5-	T49.4X6-
mandelate	T37.91X-	T37.92X-	T37.93X-	T37.94X-	T37.95X-	T37.96X-
sulfamate	T60.3X1-	T60.3X2-	T60.3X3-	T60.3X4-	-	-
sulfonate resin	T47.8X1-	T47.8X2-	T47.8X3-	T47.8X4-	T47.8X5-	T47.8X6-
Amobarbital (sodium)	T42.3X1-	T42.3X2-	T42.3X3-	T42.3X4-	T42.3X5-	T42.3X6-
Amodiaquine	T37.2X1-	T37.2X2-	T37.2X3-	T37.2X4-	T37.2X5-	T37.2X6-
Amopyroquin (e)	T37.2X1-	T37.2X2-	T37.2X3-	T37.2X4-	T37.2X5-	T37.2X6-
Amoxapine	T43.011-	T43.012-	T43.013-	T43.014-	T43.015-	T43.016-
Amoxicillin	T36.0X1-	T36.0X2-	T36.0X3-	T36.0X4-	T36.0X5-	T36.0X6-
Amperozide	T43.591-	T43.592-	T43.593-	T43.594-	T43.595-	T43.596-
Amphenidone	T43.591-	T43.592-	T43.593-	T43.594-	T43.595-	T43.596-
Amphetamine NEC	T43.621-	T43.622-	T43.623-	T43.624-	T43.625-	T43.626-
Amphomycin	T36.8X1-	T36.8X2-	T36.8X3-	T36.8X4-	T36.8X5-	T36.8X6-
Amphotalide	T37.4X1-	T37.4X2-	T37.4X3-	T37.4X4-	T37.4X5-	T37.4X6-
Amphotericin B	T36.7X1-	T36.7X2-	T36.7X3-	T36.7X4-	T36.7X5-	T36.7X6-
topical	T49.0X1-	T49.0X2-	T49.0X3-	T49.0X4-	T49.0X5-	T49.0X6-
Ampicillin	T36.0X1-	T36.0X2-	T36.0X3-	T36.0X4-	T36.0X5-	T36.0X6-
Amprotropine	T44.3X1-	T44.3X2-	T44.3X3-	T44.3X4-	T44.3X5-	T44.3X6-
Amsacrine	T45.1X1-	T45.1X2-	T45.1X3-	T45.1X4-	T45.1X5-	T45.1X6-
Amygdaline	T62.2X1-	T62.2X2-	T62.2X3-	T62.2X4-	-	-
Amyl						
acetate	T52.8X1-	T52.8X2-	T52.8X3-	T52.8X4-	-	-
vapor	T59.891-	T59.892-	T59.893-	T59.894-	-	-

AMINOHIPPURIC ACID - AMYL

Substance	Poisoning Accidental (unintentional)	Poisoning Intentional self-harm	Poisoning Assault	Poisoning Undetermined	Adverse effect	Underdosing
Amyl (continued)						
alcohol	T51.3X1-	T51.3X2-	T51.3X3-	T51.3X4-	-	-
chloride	T53.6X1-	T53.6X2-	T53.6X3-	T53.6X4-	-	-
formate	T52.8X1-	T52.8X2-	T52.8X3-	T52.8X4-	-	-
nitrite	T46.3X1-	T46.3X2-	T46.3X3-	T46.3X4-	T46.3X5-	T46.3X6-
propionate	T65.891-	T65.892-	T65.893-	T65.894-	-	-
Amylase	T47.5X1-	T47.5X2-	T47.5X3-	T47.5X4-	T47.5X5-	T47.5X6-
Amyleine, regional	T41.3X1-	T41.3X2-	T41.3X3-	T41.3X4-	T41.3X5-	T41.3X6-
Amylene						
dichloride	T53.6X1-	T53.6X2-	T53.6X3-	T53.6X4-	-	-
hydrate	T51.3X1-	T51.3X2-	T51.3X3-	T51.3X4-	-	-
Amylmetacresol	T49.6X1-	T49.6X2-	T49.6X3-	T49.6X4-	T49.6X5-	T49.6X6-
Amylobarbitone	T42.3X1-	T42.3X2-	T42.3X3-	T42.3X4-	T42.3X5-	T42.3X6-
Amylocaine, regional	T41.3X1-	T41.3X2-	T41.3X3-	T41.3X4-	T41.3X5-	T41.3X6-
infiltration (subcutaneous)	T41.3X1-	T41.3X2-	T41.3X3-	T41.3X4-	T41.3X5-	T41.3X6-
nerve block (peripheral) (plexus)	T41.3X1-	T41.3X2-	T41.3X3-	T41.3X4-	T41.3X5-	T41.3X6-
spinal	T41.3X1-	T41.3X2-	T41.3X3-	T41.3X4-	T41.3X5-	T41.3X6-
topical (surface)	T41.3X1-	T41.3X2-	T41.3X3-	T41.3X4-	T41.3X5-	T41.3X6-
Amylopectin	T47.6X1-	T47.6X2-	T47.6X3-	T47.6X4-	T47.6X5-	T47.6X6-
Amytal (sodium)	T42.3X1-	T42.3X2-	T42.3X3-	T42.3X4-	T42.3X5-	T42.3X6-
Anabolic steroid	T38.7X1-	T38.7X2-	T38.7X3-	T38.7X4-	T38.7X5-	T38.7X6-
Analeptic NEC	T50.7X1-	T50.7X2-	T50.7X3-	T50.7X4-	T50.7X5-	T50.7X6-
Analgesic	T39.91X-	T39.92X-	T39.93X-	T39.94X-	T39.95X-	T39.96X-
anti-inflammatory NEC	T39.91X-	T39.92X-	T39.93X-	T39.94X-	T39.95X-	T39.96X-
propionic acid derivative	T39.311-	T39.312-	T39.313-	T39.314-	T39.315-	T39.316-
antirheumatic NEC	T39.4X1-	T39.4X2-	T39.4X3-	T39.4X4-	T39.4X5-	T39.4X6-
aromatic NEC	T39.1X1-	T39.1X2-	T39.1X3-	T39.1X4-	T39.1X5-	T39.1X6-
narcotic NEC	T40.601-	T40.602-	T40.603-	T40.604-	T40.605-	T40.606-
combination	T40.601-	T40.602-	T40.603-	T40.604-	T40.605-	T40.606-
obstetric	T40.601-	T40.602-	T40.603-	T40.604-	T40.605-	T40.606-
non-narcotic NEC	T39.91X-	T39.92X-	T39.93X-	T39.94X-	T39.95X-	T39.96X-
combination	T39.91X-	T39.92X-	T39.93X-	T39.94X-	T39.95X-	T39.96X-
pyrazole	T39.2X1-	T39.2X2-	T39.2X3-	T39.2X4-	T39.2X5-	T39.2X6-
specified NEC	T39.8X1-	T39.8X2-	T39.8X3-	T39.8X4-	T39.8X5-	T39.8X6-
Analgin	T39.2X1-	T39.2X2-	T39.2X3-	T39.2X4-	T39.2X5-	T39.2X6-
Anamirta cocculus	T62.1X1-	T62.1X2-	T62.1X3-	T62.1X4-	-	-
Ancillin	T36.0X1-	T36.0X2-	T36.0X3-	T36.0X4-	T36.0X5-	T36.0X6-
Ancrod	T45.691-	T45.692-	T45.693-	T45.694-	T45.695-	T45.696-
Androgen	T38.7X1-	T38.7X2-	T38.7X3-	T38.7X4-	T38.7X5-	T38.7X6-
Androgen-estrogen mixture	T38.7X1-	T38.7X2-	T38.7X3-	T38.7X4-	T38.7X5-	T38.7X6-
Androstalone	T38.7X1-	T38.7X2-	T38.7X3-	T38.7X4-	T38.7X5-	T38.7X6-
Androstanolone	T38.7X1-	T38.7X2-	T38.7X3-	T38.7X4-	T38.7X5-	T38.7X6-
Androsterone	T38.7X1-	T38.7X2-	T38.7X3-	T38.7X4-	T38.7X5-	T38.7X6-
Anemone pulsatilla	T62.2X1-	T62.2X2-	T62.2X3-	T62.2X4-	-	-
Anesthesia						
caudal	T41.3X1-	T41.3X2-	T41.3X3-	T41.3X4-	T41.3X5-	T41.3X6-
endotracheal	T41.0X1-	T41.0X2-	T41.0X3-	T41.0X4-	T41.0X5-	T41.0X6-
epidural	T41.3X1-	T41.3X2-	T41.3X3-	T41.3X4-	T41.3X5-	T41.3X6-
inhalation	T41.0X1-	T41.0X2-	T41.0X3-	T41.0X4-	T41.0X5-	T41.0X6-
local	T41.3X1-	T41.3X2-	T41.3X3-	T41.3X4-	T41.3X5-	T41.3X6-
mucosal	T41.3X1-	T41.3X2-	T41.3X3-	T41.3X4-	T41.3X5-	T41.3X6-
muscle relaxation	T48.1X1-	T48.1X2-	T48.1X3-	T48.1X4-	T48.1X5-	T48.1X6-
nerve blocking	T41.3X1-	T41.3X2-	T41.3X3-	T41.3X4-	T41.3X5-	T41.3X6-
plexus blocking	T41.3X1-	T41.3X2-	T41.3X3-	T41.3X4-	T41.3X5-	T41.3X6-
potentiated	T41.201-	T41.202-	T41.203-	T41.204-	T41.205-	T41.206-
rectal	T41.201-	T41.202-	T41.203-	T41.204-	T41.205-	T41.206-
general	T41.201-	T41.202-	T41.203-	T41.204-	T41.205-	T41.206-
local	T41.3X1-	T41.3X2-	T41.3X3-	T41.3X4-	T41.3X5-	T41.3X6-
regional	T41.3X1-	T41.3X2-	T41.3X3-	T41.3X4-	T41.3X5-	T41.3X6-

Substance	Poisoning Accidental (unintentional)	Poisoning Intentional self-harm	Poisoning Assault	Poisoning Undetermined	Adverse effect	Underdosing
Anesthesia (continued)						
surface	T41.3X1-	T41.3X2-	T41.3X3-	T41.3X4-	T41.3X5-	T41.3X6-
Anesthetic NEC — *see also Anesthesia*	T41.41X-	T41.42X-	T41.43X-	T41.44X-	T41.45X-	T41.46X-
with muscle relaxant	T41.201-	T41.202-	T41.203-	T41.204-	T41.205-	T41.206-
general	T41.201-	T41.202-	T41.203-	T41.204-	T41.205-	T41.206-
local	T41.3X1-	T41.3X2-	T41.3X3-	T41.3X4-	T41.3X5-	T41.3X6-
gaseous NEC	T41.0X1-	T41.0X2-	T41.0X3-	T41.0X4-	T41.0X5-	T41.0X6-
general NEC	T41.201-	T41.202-	T41.203-	T41.204-	T41.205-	T41.206-
halogenated hydrocarbon derivatives NEC	T41.0X1-	T41.0X2-	T41.0X3-	T41.0X4-	T41.0X5-	T41.0X6-
infiltration NEC	T41.3X1-	T41.3X2-	T41.3X3-	T41.3X4-	T41.3X5-	T41.3X6-
intravenous NEC	T41.1X1-	T41.1X2-	T41.1X3-	T41.1X4-	T41.1X5-	T41.1X6-
local NEC	T41.3X1-	T41.3X2-	T41.3X3-	T41.3X4-	T41.3X5-	T41.3X6-
rectal	T41.201-	T41.202-	T41.203-	T41.204-	T41.205-	T41.206-
general	T41.201-	T41.202-	T41.203-	T41.204-	T41.205-	T41.206-
local	T41.3X1-	T41.3X2-	T41.3X3-	T41.3X4-	T41.3X5-	T41.3X6-
regional NEC	T41.3X1-	T41.3X2-	T41.3X3-	T41.3X4-	T41.3X5-	T41.3X6-
spinal NEC	T41.3X1-	T41.3X2-	T41.3X3-	T41.3X4-	T41.3X5-	T41.3X6-
thiobarbiturate	T41.1X1-	T41.1X2-	T41.1X3-	T41.1X4-	T41.1X5-	T41.1X6-
topical	T41.3X1-	T41.3X2-	T41.3X3-	T41.3X4-	T41.3X5-	T41.3X6-
Aneurine	T45.2X1-	T45.2X2-	T45.2X3-	T45.2X4-	T45.2X5-	T45.2X6-
Angio-Conray	T50.8X1-	T50.8X2-	T50.8X3-	T50.8X4-	T50.8X5-	T50.8X6-
Angiotensin	T44.5X1-	T44.5X2-	T44.5X3-	T44.5X4-	T44.5X5-	T44.5X6-
Angiotensinamide	T44.991-	T44.992-	T44.993-	T44.994-	T44.995-	T44.996-
Anhydrohydroxy-progesterone	T38.5X1-	T38.5X2-	T38.5X3-	T38.5X4-	T38.5X5-	T38.5X6-
Anhydron	T50.2X1-	T50.2X2-	T50.2X3-	T50.2X4-	T50.2X5-	T50.2X6-
Anileridine	T40.491-	T40.492-	T40.493-	T40.494-	T40.495-	T40.496-
Aniline (dye) (liquid)	T65.3X1-	T65.3X2-	T65.3X3-	T65.3X4-	-	-
analgesic	T39.1X1-	T39.1X2-	T39.1X3-	T39.1X4-	T39.1X5-	T39.1X6-
derivatives, therapeutic NEC	T39.1X1-	T39.1X2-	T39.1X3-	T39.1X4-	T39.1X5-	T39.1X6-
vapor	T65.3X1-	T65.3X2-	T65.3X3-	T65.3X4-	-	-
Aniscoropine	T44.3X1-	T44.3X2-	T44.3X3-	T44.3X4-	T44.3X5-	T44.3X6-
Anise oil	T47.5X1-	T47.5X2-	T47.5X3-	T47.5X4-	T47.5X5-	T47.5X6-
Anisidine	T65.3X1-	T65.3X2-	T65.3X3-	T65.3X4-	-	-
Anisindione	T45.511-	T45.512-	T45.513-	T45.514-	T45.515-	T45.516-
Anisotropine methyl-bromide	T44.3X1-	T44.3X2-	T44.3X3-	T44.3X4-	T44.3X5-	T44.3X6-
Anistreplase	T45.611-	T45.612-	T45.613-	T45.614-	T45.615-	T45.616-
Anorexiant (central)	T50.5X1-	T50.5X2-	T50.5X3-	T50.5X4-	T50.5X5-	T50.5X6-
Anorexic agents	T50.5X1-	T50.5X2-	T50.5X3-	T50.5X4-	T50.5X5-	T50.5X6-
Ansamycin	T36.6X1-	T36.6X2-	T36.6X3-	T36.6X4-	T36.6X5-	T36.6X6-
Ant (bite) (sting)	T63.421-	T63.422-	T63.423-	T63.424-	-	-
Ant poison — *see Insecticide*						
Antabuse	T50.6X1-	T50.6X2-	T50.6X3-	T50.6X4-	T50.6X5-	T50.6X6-
Antacid NEC	T47.1X1-	T47.1X2-	T47.1X3-	T47.1X4-	T47.1X5-	T47.1X6-
Antagonist						
Aldosterone	T50.0X1-	T50.0X2-	T50.0X3-	T50.0X4-	T50.0X5-	T50.0X6-
alpha-adrenoreceptor	T44.6X1-	T44.6X2-	T44.6X3-	T44.6X4-	T44.6X5-	T44.6X6-
anticoagulant	T45.7X1-	T45.7X2-	T45.7X3-	T45.7X4-	T45.7X5-	T45.7X6-
beta-adrenoreceptor	T44.7X1-	T44.7X2-	T44.7X3-	T44.7X4-	T44.7X5-	T44.7X6-
extrapyramidal NEC	T44.3X1-	T44.3X2-	T44.3X3-	T44.3X4-	T44.3X5-	T44.3X6-
folic acid	T45.1X1-	T45.1X2-	T45.1X3-	T45.1X4-	T45.1X5-	T45.1X6-
H2 receptor	T47.0X1-	T47.0X2-	T47.0X3-	T47.0X4-	T47.0X5-	T47.0X6-
heavy metal	T45.8X1-	T45.8X2-	T45.8X3-	T45.8X4-	T45.8X5-	T45.8X6-
narcotic analgesic	T50.7X1-	T50.7X2-	T50.7X3-	T50.7X4-	T50.7X5-	T50.7X6-
opiate	T50.7X1-	T50.7X2-	T50.7X3-	T50.7X4-	T50.7X5-	T50.7X6-
pyrimidine	T45.1X1-	T45.1X2-	T45.1X3-	T45.1X4-	T45.1X5-	T45.1X6-
serotonin	T46.5X1-	T46.5X2-	T46.5X3-	T46.5X4-	T46.5X5-	T46.5X6-
Antazolin (e)	T45.0X1-	T45.0X2-	T45.0X3-	T45.0X4-	T45.0X5-	T45.0X6-
Anterior pituitary hormone NEC	T38.811-	T38.812-	T38.813-	T38.814-	T38.815-	T38.816-

Substance	Poisoning Accidental (unintentional)	Poisoning Intentional self-harm	Poisoning Assault	Poisoning Undetermined	Adverse effect	Underdosing
Anthelmintic NEC	T37.4X1-	T37.4X2-	T37.4X3-	T37.4X4-	T37.4X5-	T37.4X6-
Anthiolimine	T37.4X1-	T37.4X2-	T37.4X3-	T37.4X4-	T37.4X5-	T37.4X6-
Anthralin	T49.4X1-	T49.4X2-	T49.4X3-	T49.4X4-	T49.4X5-	T49.4X6-
Anthramycin	T45.1X1-	T45.1X2-	T45.1X3-	T45.1X4-	T45.1X5-	T45.1X6-
Antiadrenergic NEC	T44.8X1-	T44.8X2-	T44.8X3-	T44.8X4-	T44.8X5-	T44.8X6-
Antiallergic NEC	T45.0X1-	T45.0X2-	T45.0X3-	T45.0X4-	T45.0X5-	T45.0X6-
Anti-anemic (drug) (preparation)	T45.8X1-	T45.8X2-	T45.8X3-	T45.8X4-	T45.8X5-	T45.8X6-
Antiandrogen NEC	T38.6X1-	T38.6X2-	T38.6X3-	T38.6X4-	T38.6X5-	T38.6X6-
Antianxiety drug NEC	T43.501-	T43.502-	T43.503-	T43.504-	T43.505-	T43.506-
Antiaris toxicaria	T65.891-	T65.892-	T65.893-	T65.894-	-	-
Antiarteriosclerotic drug	T46.6X1-	T46.6X2-	T46.6X3-	T46.6X4-	T46.6X5-	T46.6X6-
Antiasthmatic drug NEC	T48.6X1-	T48.6X2-	T48.6X3-	T48.6X4-	T48.6X5-	T48.6X6-
Antibiotic NEC	T36.91X-	T36.92X-	T36.93X-	T36.94X-	T36.95X-	T36.96X-
aminoglycoside	T36.5X1-	T36.5X2-	T36.5X3-	T36.5X4-	T36.5X5-	T36.5X6-
anticancer	T45.1X1-	T45.1X2-	T45.1X3-	T45.1X4-	T45.1X5-	T45.1X6-
antifungal	T36.7X1-	T36.7X2-	T36.7X3-	T36.7X4-	T36.7X5-	T36.7X6-
antimycobacterial	T36.5X1-	T36.5X2-	T36.5X3-	T36.5X4-	T36.5X5-	T36.5X6-
antineoplastic	T45.1X1-	T45.1X2-	T45.1X3-	T45.1X4-	T45.1X5-	T45.1X6-
cephalosporin (group)	T36.1X1-	T36.1X2-	T36.1X3-	T36.1X4-	T36.1X5-	T36.1X6-
chloramphenicol (group)	T36.2X1-	T36.2X2-	T36.2X3-	T36.2X4-	T36.2X5-	T36.2X6-
ENT	T49.6X1-	T49.6X2-	T49.6X3-	T49.6X4-	T49.6X5-	T49.6X6-
eye	T49.5X1-	T49.5X2-	T49.5X3-	T49.5X4-	T49.5X5-	T49.5X6-
fungicidal (local)	T49.0X1-	T49.0X2-	T49.0X3-	T49.0X4-	T49.0X5-	T49.0X6-
intestinal	T36.8X1-	T36.8X2-	T36.8X3-	T36.8X4-	T36.8X5-	T36.8X6-
b-lactam NEC	T36.1X1-	T36.1X2-	T36.1X3-	T36.1X4-	T36.1X5-	T36.1X6-
local	T49.0X1-	T49.0X2-	T49.0X3-	T49.0X4-	T49.0X5-	T49.0X6-
macrolides	T36.3X1-	T36.3X2-	T36.3X3-	T36.3X4-	T36.3X5-	T36.3X6-
polypeptide	T36.8X1-	T36.8X2-	T36.8X3-	T36.8X4-	T36.8X5-	T36.8X6-
specified NEC	T36.8X1-	T36.8X2-	T36.8X3-	T36.8X4-	T36.8X5-	T36.8X6-
tetracycline (group)	T36.4X1-	T36.4X2-	T36.4X3-	T36.4X4-	T36.4X5-	T36.4X6-
throat	T49.6X1-	T49.6X2-	T49.6X3-	T49.6X4-	T49.6X5-	T49.6X6-
Anticancer agents NEC	T45.1X1-	T45.1X2-	T45.1X3-	T45.1X4-	T45.1X5-	T45.1X6-
Anticholesterolemic drug NEC	T46.6X1-	T46.6X2-	T46.6X3-	T46.6X4-	T46.6X5-	T46.6X6-
Anticholinergic NEC	T44.3X1-	T44.3X2-	T44.3X3-	T44.3X4-	T44.3X5-	T44.3X6-
Anticholinesterase	T44.0X1-	T44.0X2-	T44.0X3-	T44.0X4-	T44.0X5-	T44.0X6-
organophosphorus	T44.0X1-	T44.0X2-	T44.0X3-	T44.0X4-	T44.0X5-	T44.0X6-
insecticide	T60.0X1-	T60.0X2-	T60.0X3-	T60.0X4-	-	-
nerve gas	T59.891-	T59.892-	T59.893-	T59.894-	-	-
reversible	T44.0X1-	T44.0X2-	T44.0X3-	T44.0X4-	T44.0X5-	T44.0X6-
ophthalmological	T49.5X1-	T49.5X2-	T49.5X3-	T49.5X4-	T49.5X5-	T49.5X6-
Anticoagulant NEC	T45.511-	T45.512-	T45.513-	T45.514-	T45.515-	T45.516-
Antagonist	T45.7X1-	T45.7X2-	T45.7X3-	T45.7X4-	T45.7X5-	T45.7X6-
Anti-common-cold drug NEC	T48.5X1-	T48.5X2-	T48.5X3-	T48.5X4-	T48.5X5-	T48.5X6-
Anticonvulsant	T42.71X-	T42.72X-	T42.73X-	T42.74X-	T42.75X-	T42.76X-
barbiturate	T42.3X1-	T42.3X2-	T42.3X3-	T42.3X4-	T42.3X5-	T42.3X6-
combination (with barbiturate)	T42.3X1-	T42.3X2-	T42.3X3-	T42.3X4-	T42.3X5-	T42.3X6-
hydantoin	T42.0X1-	T42.0X2-	T42.0X3-	T42.0X4-	T42.0X5-	T42.0X6-
hypnotic NEC	T42.6X1-	T42.6X2-	T42.6X3-	T42.6X4-	T42.6X5-	T42.6X6-
oxazolidinedione	T42.2X1-	T42.2X2-	T42.2X3-	T42.2X4-	T42.2X5-	T42.2X6-
pyrimidinedione	T42.6X1-	T42.6X2-	T42.6X3-	T42.6X4-	T42.6X5-	T42.6X6-
specified NEC	T42.6X1-	T42.6X2-	T42.6X3-	T42.6X4-	T42.6X5-	T42.6X6-
succinimide	T42.2X1-	T42.2X2-	T42.2X3-	T42.2X4-	T42.2X5-	T42.2X6-
Anti-D immunoglobulin (human)	T50.Z11-	T50.Z12-	T50.Z13-	T50.Z14-	T50.Z15-	T50.Z16-
Antidepressant	T43.201-	T43.202-	T43.203-	T43.204-	T43.205-	T43.206-
monoamine oxidase inhibitor	T43.1X1-	T43.1X2-	T43.1X3-	T43.1X4-	T43.1X5-	T43.1X6-
selective serotonin norepinephrine reuptake inhibitor	T43.211-	T43.212-	T43.213-	T43.214-	T43.215-	T43.216-
selective serotonin reuptake inhibitor	T43.221-	T43.222-	T43.223-	T43.224-	T43.225-	T43.226-
specified NEC	T43.291-	T43.292-	T43.293-	T43.294-	T43.295-	T43.296-

Substance	Poisoning Accidental (unintentional)	Poisoning Intentional self-harm	Poisoning Assault	Poisoning Undetermined	Adverse effect	Underdosing
Antidepressant (continued)						
tetracyclic	T43.021-	T43.022-	T43.023-	T43.024-	T43.025-	T43.026-
triazolopyridine	T43.211-	T43.212-	T43.213-	T43.214-	T43.215-	T43.216-
tricyclic	T43.011-	T43.012-	T43.013-	T43.014-	T43.015-	T43.016-
Antidiabetic NEC	T38.3X1-	T38.3X2-	T38.3X3-	T38.3X4-	T38.3X5-	T38.3X6-
biguanide	T38.3X1-	T38.3X2-	T38.3X3-	T38.3X4-	T38.3X5-	T38.3X6-
and sulfonyl combined	T38.3X1-	T38.3X2-	T38.3X3-	T38.3X4-	T38.3X5-	T38.3X6-
combined	T38.3X1-	T38.3X2-	T38.3X3-	T38.3X4-	T38.3X5-	T38.3X6-
sulfonylurea	T38.3X1-	T38.3X2-	T38.3X3-	T38.3X4-	T38.3X5-	T38.3X6-
Antidiarrheal drug NEC	T47.6X1-	T47.6X2-	T47.6X3-	T47.6X4-	T47.6X5-	T47.6X6-
absorbent	T47.6X1-	T47.6X2-	T47.6X3-	T47.6X4-	T47.6X5-	T47.6X6-
Antidiphtheria serum	T50.Z11-	T50.Z12-	T50.Z13-	T50.Z14-	T50.Z15-	T50.Z16-
Antidiuretic hormone	T38.891-	T38.892-	T38.893-	T38.894-	T38.895-	T38.896-
Antidote NEC	T50.6X1-	T50.6X2-	T50.6X3-	T50.6X4-	T50.6X5-	T50.6X6-
heavy metal	T45.8X1-	T45.8X2-	T45.8X3-	T45.8X4-	T45.8X5-	T45.8X6-
Antidysrhythmic NEC	T46.2X1-	T46.2X2-	T46.2X3-	T46.2X4-	T46.2X5-	T46.2X6-
Antiemetic drug	T45.0X1-	T45.0X2-	T45.0X3-	T45.0X4-	T45.0X5-	T45.0X6-
Antiepilepsy agent	T42.71X-	T42.72X-	T42.73X-	T42.74X-	T42.75X-	T42.76X-
combination	T42.5X1-	T42.5X2-	T42.5X3-	T42.5X4-	T42.5X5-	T42.5X6-
mixed	T42.5X1-	T42.5X2-	T42.5X3-	T42.5X4-	T42.5X5-	T42.5X6-
specified, NEC	T42.6X1-	T42.6X2-	T42.6X3-	T42.6X4-	T42.6X5-	T42.6X6-
Antiestrogen NEC	T38.6X1-	T38.6X2-	T38.6X3-	T38.6X4-	T38.6X5-	T38.6X6-
Antifertility pill	T38.4X1-	T38.4X2-	T38.4X3-	T38.4X4-	T38.4X5-	T38.4X6-
Antifibrinolytic drug	T45.621-	T45.622-	T45.623-	T45.624-	T45.625-	T45.626-
Antifilarial drug	T37.4X1-	T37.4X2-	T37.4X3-	T37.4X4-	T37.4X5-	T37.4X6-
Antiflatulent	T47.5X1-	T47.5X2-	T47.5X3-	T47.5X4-	T47.5X5-	T47.5X6-
Antifreeze	T65.91X-	T65.92X-	T65.93X-	T65.94X-	-	-
alcohol	T51.1X1-	T51.1X2-	T51.1X3-	T51.1X4-	-	-
ethylene glycol	T51.8X1-	T51.8X2-	T51.8X3-	T51.8X4-	-	-
Antifungal						
antibiotic (systemic)	T36.7X1-	T36.7X2-	T36.7X3-	T36.7X4-	T36.7X5-	T36.7X6-
anti-infective NEC	T37.91X-	T37.92X-	T37.93X-	T37.94X-	T37.95X-	T37.96X-
disinfectant, local	T49.0X1-	T49.0X2-	T49.0X3-	T49.0X4-	T49.0X5-	T49.0X6-
nonmedicinal (spray)	T60.3X1-	T60.3X2-	T60.3X3-	T60.3X4-	-	-
topical	T49.0X1-	T49.0X2-	T49.0X3-	T49.0X4-	T49.0X5-	T49.0X6-
Anti-gastric-secretion drug NEC	T47.1X1-	T47.1X2-	T47.1X3-	T47.1X4-	T47.1X5-	T47.1X6-
Antigonadotrophin NEC	T38.6X1-	T38.6X2-	T38.6X3-	T38.6X4-	T38.6X5-	T38.6X6-
Antihallucinogen	T43.501-	T43.502-	T43.503-	T43.504-	T43.505-	T43.506-
Antihelmintics	T37.4X1-	T37.4X2-	T37.4X3-	T37.4X4-	T37.4X5-	T37.4X6-
Antihemophilic						
factor	T45.8X1-	T45.8X2-	T45.8X3-	T45.8X4-	T45.8X5-	T45.8X6-
fraction	T45.8X1-	T45.8X2-	T45.8X3-	T45.8X4-	T45.8X5-	T45.8X6-
globulin concentrate	T45.7X1-	T45.7X2-	T45.7X3-	T45.7X4-	T45.7X5-	T45.7X6-
human plasma	T45.8X1-	T45.8X2-	T45.8X3-	T45.8X4-	T45.8X5-	T45.8X6-
plasma, dried	T45.7X1-	T45.7X2-	T45.7X3-	T45.7X4-	T45.7X5-	T45.7X6-
Antihemorrhoidal preparation	T49.2X1-	T49.2X2-	T49.2X3-	T49.2X4-	T49.2X5-	T49.2X6-
Antiheparin drug	T45.7X1-	T45.7X2-	T45.7X3-	T45.7X4-	T45.7X5-	T45.7X6-
Antihistamine	T45.0X1-	T45.0X2-	T45.0X3-	T45.0X4-	T45.0X5-	T45.0X6-
Antihookworm drug	T37.4X1-	T37.4X2-	T37.4X3-	T37.4X4-	T37.4X5-	T37.4X6-
Anti-human lymphocytic globulin	T50.Z11-	T50.Z12-	T50.Z13-	T50.Z14-	T50.Z15-	T50.Z16-
Antihyperlipidemic drug	T46.6X1-	T46.6X2-	T46.6X3-	T46.6X4-	T46.6X5-	T46.6X6-
Antihypertensive drug NEC	T46.5X1-	T46.5X2-	T46.5X3-	T46.5X4-	T46.5X5-	T46.5X6-
Anti-infective NEC	T37.91X-	T37.92X-	T37.93X-	T37.94X-	T37.95X-	T37.96X-
anthelmintic	T37.4X1-	T37.4X2-	T37.4X3-	T37.4X4-	T37.4X5-	T37.4X6-
antibiotics	T36.91X-	T36.92X-	T36.93X-	T36.94X-	T36.95X-	T36.96X-
specified NEC	T36.8X1-	T36.8X2-	T36.8X3-	T36.8X4-	T36.8X5-	T36.8X6-
antimalarial	T37.2X1-	T37.2X2-	T37.2X3-	T37.2X4-	T37.2X5-	T37.2X6-
antimycobacterial NEC	T37.1X1-	T37.1X2-	T37.1X3-	T37.1X4-	T37.1X5-	T37.1X6-

ANTIDEPRESSANT - ANTI-INFECTIVE NEC

Substance	Poisoning Accidental (unintentional)	Poisoning Intentional self-harm	Poisoning Assault	Poisoning Undetermined	Adverse effect	Underdosing
Anti-infective NEC (continued)						
antibiotics	T36.5X1-	T36.5X2-	T36.5X3-	T36.5X4-	T36.5X5-	T36.5X6-
antiprotozoal NEC	T37.3X1-	T37.3X2-	T37.3X3-	T37.3X4-	T37.3X5-	T37.3X6-
blood	T37.2X1-	T37.2X2-	T37.2X3-	T37.2X4-	T37.2X5-	T37.2X6-
antiviral	T37.5X1-	T37.5X2-	T37.5X3-	T37.5X4-	T37.5X5-	T37.5X6-
arsenical	T37.8X1-	T37.8X2-	T37.8X3-	T37.8X4-	T37.8X5-	T37.8X6-
bismuth, local	T49.0X1-	T49.0X2-	T49.0X3-	T49.0X4-	T49.0X5-	T49.0X6-
ENT	T49.6X1-	T49.6X2-	T49.6X3-	T49.6X4-	T49.6X5-	T49.6X6-
eye NEC	T49.5X1-	T49.5X2-	T49.5X3-	T49.5X4-	T49.5X5-	T49.5X6-
heavy metals NEC	T37.8X1-	T37.8X2-	T37.8X3-	T37.8X4-	T37.8X5-	T37.8X6-
local NEC	T49.0X1-	T49.0X2-	T49.0X3-	T49.0X4-	T49.0X5-	T49.0X6-
specified NEC	T49.0X1-	T49.0X2-	T49.0X3-	T49.0X4-	T49.0X5-	T49.0X6-
mixed	T37.91X-	T37.92X-	T37.93X-	T37.94X-	T37.95X-	T37.96X-
ophthalmic preparation	T49.5X1-	T49.5X2-	T49.5X3-	T49.5X4-	T49.5X5-	T49.5X6-
topical NEC	T49.0X1-	T49.0X2-	T49.0X3-	T49.0X4-	T49.0X5-	T49.0X6-
Anti-inflammatory drug NEC	T39.391-	T39.392-	T39.393-	T39.394-	T39.395-	T39.396-
local	T49.0X1-	T49.0X2-	T49.0X3-	T49.0X4-	T49.0X5-	T49.0X6-
nonsteroidal NEC	T39.391-	T39.392-	T39.393-	T39.394-	T39.395-	T39.396-
propionic acid derivative	T39.311-	T39.312-	T39.313-	T39.314-	T39.315-	T39.316-
specified NEC	T39.391-	T39.392-	T39.393-	T39.394-	T39.395-	T39.396-
Antikaluretic	T50.3X1-	T50.3X2-	T50.3X3-	T50.3X4-	T50.3X5-	T50.3X6-
Antiknock (tetraethyl lead)	T56.0X1-	T56.0X2-	T56.0X3-	T56.0X4-	-	-
Antilipemic drug NEC	T46.6X1-	T46.6X2-	T46.6X3-	T46.6X4-	T46.6X5-	T46.6X6-
Antimalarial	T37.2X1-	T37.2X2-	T37.2X3-	T37.2X4-	T37.2X5-	T37.2X6-
prophylactic NEC	T37.2X1-	T37.2X2-	T37.2X3-	T37.2X4-	T37.2X5-	T37.2X6-
pyrimidine derivative	T37.2X1-	T37.2X2-	T37.2X3-	T37.2X4-	T37.2X5-	T37.2X6-
Antimetabolite	T45.1X1-	T45.1X2-	T45.1X3-	T45.1X4-	T45.1X5-	T45.1X6-
Antimitotic agent	T45.1X1-	T45.1X2-	T45.1X3-	T45.1X4-	T45.1X5-	T45.1X6-
Antimony (compounds) (vapor) NEC	T56.891-	T56.892-	T56.893-	T56.894-	-	-
anti-infectives	T37.8X1-	T37.8X2-	T37.8X3-	T37.8X4-	T37.8X5-	T37.8X6-
dimercaptosuccinate	T37.3X1-	T37.3X2-	T37.3X3-	T37.3X4-	T37.3X5-	T37.3X6-
hydride	T56.891-	T56.892-	T56.893-	T56.894-	-	-
pesticide (vapor)	T60.8X1-	T60.8X2-	T60.8X3-	T60.8X4-	-	-
potassium (sodium) tartrate	T37.8X1-	T37.8X2-	T37.8X3-	T37.8X4-	T37.8X5-	T37.8X6-
sodium dimercaptosuccinate	T37.3X1-	T37.3X2-	T37.3X3-	T37.3X4-	T37.3X5-	T37.3X6-
tartrated	T37.8X1-	T37.8X2-	T37.8X3-	T37.8X4-	T37.8X5-	T37.8X6-
Antimuscarinic NEC	T44.3X1-	T44.3X2-	T44.3X3-	T44.3X4-	T44.3X5-	T44.3X6-
Antimycobacterial drug NEC	T37.1X1-	T37.1X2-	T37.1X3-	T37.1X4-	T37.1X5-	T37.1X6-
antibiotics	T36.5X1-	T36.5X2-	T36.5X3-	T36.5X4-	T36.5X5-	T36.5X6-
combination	T37.1X1-	T37.1X2-	T37.1X3-	T37.1X4-	T37.1X5-	T37.1X6-
Antinausea drug	T45.0X1-	T45.0X2-	T45.0X3-	T45.0X4-	T45.0X5-	T45.0X6-
Antinematode drug	T37.4X1-	T37.4X2-	T37.4X3-	T37.4X4-	T37.4X5-	T37.4X6-
Antineoplastic NEC	T45.1X1-	T45.1X2-	T45.1X3-	T45.1X4-	T45.1X5-	T45.1X6-
alkaloidal	T45.1X1-	T45.1X2-	T45.1X3-	T45.1X4-	T45.1X5-	T45.1X6-
antibiotics	T45.1X1-	T45.1X2-	T45.1X3-	T45.1X4-	T45.1X5-	T45.1X6-
combination	T45.1X1-	T45.1X2-	T45.1X3-	T45.1X4-	T45.1X5-	T45.1X6-
estrogen	T38.5X1-	T38.5X2-	T38.5X3-	T38.5X4-	T38.5X5-	T38.5X6-
steroid	T38.7X1-	T38.7X2-	T38.7X3-	T38.7X4-	T38.7X5-	T38.7X6-
Antiparasitic drug (systemic)	T37.91X-	T37.92X-	T37.93X-	T37.94X-	T37.95X-	T37.96X-
local	T49.0X1-	T49.0X2-	T49.0X3-	T49.0X4-	T49.0X5-	T49.0X6-
specified NEC	T37.8X1-	T37.8X2-	T37.8X3-	T37.8X4-	T37.8X5-	T37.8X6-
Antiparkinsonism drug NEC	T42.8X1-	T42.8X2-	T42.8X3-	T42.8X4-	T42.8X5-	T42.8X6-
Antiperspirant NEC	T49.2X1-	T49.2X2-	T49.2X3-	T49.2X4-	T49.2X5-	T49.2X6-
Antiphlogistic NEC	T39.4X1-	T39.4X2-	T39.4X3-	T39.4X4-	T39.4X5-	T39.4X6-
Antiplatyhelmintic drug	T37.4X1-	T37.4X2-	T37.4X3-	T37.4X4-	T37.4X5-	T37.4X6-
Antiprotozoal drug NEC	T37.3X1-	T37.3X2-	T37.3X3-	T37.3X4-	T37.3X5-	T37.3X6-
blood	T37.2X1-	T37.2X2-	T37.2X3-	T37.2X4-	T37.2X5-	T37.2X6-
local	T49.0X1-	T49.0X2-	T49.0X3-	T49.0X4-	T49.0X5-	T49.0X6-

Substance	Poisoning Accidental (unintentional)	Poisoning Intentional self-harm	Poisoning Assault	Poisoning Undetermined	Adverse effect	Underdosing
Antipruritic drug NEC	T49.1X1-	T49.1X2-	T49.1X3-	T49.1X4-	T49.1X5-	T49.1X6-
Antipsychotic drug	T43.501-	T43.502-	T43.503-	T43.504-	T43.505-	T43.506-
specified NEC	T43.591-	T43.592-	T43.593-	T43.594-	T43.595-	T43.596-
Antipyretic	T39.91X-	T39.92X-	T39.93X-	T39.94X-	T39.95X-	T39.96X-
specified NEC	T39.8X1-	T39.8X2-	T39.8X3-	T39.8X4-	T39.8X5-	T39.8X6-
Antipyrine	T39.2X1-	T39.2X2-	T39.2X3-	T39.2X4-	T39.2X5-	T39.2X6-
Antirabies hyperimmune serum	T50.Z11-	T50.Z12-	T50.Z13-	T50.Z14-	T50.Z15-	T50.Z16-
Antirheumatic NEC	T39.4X1-	T39.4X2-	T39.4X3-	T39.4X4-	T39.4X5-	T39.4X6-
Antirigidity drug NEC	T42.8X1-	T42.8X2-	T42.8X3-	T42.8X4-	T42.8X5-	T42.8X6-
Antischistosomal drug	T37.4X1-	T37.4X2-	T37.4X3-	T37.4X4-	T37.4X5-	T37.4X6-
Antiscorpion sera	T50.Z11-	T50.Z12-	T50.Z13-	T50.Z14-	T50.Z15-	T50.Z16-
Antiseborrheics	T49.4X1-	T49.4X2-	T49.4X3-	T49.4X4-	T49.4X5-	T49.4X6-
Antiseptics (external) (medicinal)	T49.0X1-	T49.0X2-	T49.0X3-	T49.0X4-	T49.0X5-	T49.0X6-
Antistine	T45.0X1-	T45.0X2-	T45.0X3-	T45.0X4-	T45.0X5-	T45.0X6-
Antitapeworm drug	T37.4X1-	T37.4X2-	T37.4X3-	T37.4X4-	T37.4X5-	T37.4X6-
Antitetanus immunoglobulin	T50.Z11-	T50.Z12-	T50.Z13-	T50.Z14-	T50.Z15-	T50.Z16-
Antithrombotic	T45.521-	T45.522-	T45.523-	T45.524-	T45.525-	T45.526-
Antithyroid drug NEC	T38.2X1-	T38.2X2-	T38.2X3-	T38.2X4-	T38.2X5-	T38.2X6-
Antitoxin	T50.Z11-	T50.Z12-	T50.Z13-	T50.Z14-	T50.Z15-	T50.Z16-
diphtheria	T50.Z11-	T50.Z12-	T50.Z13-	T50.Z14-	T50.Z15-	T50.Z16-
gas gangrene	T50.Z11-	T50.Z12-	T50.Z13-	T50.Z14-	T50.Z15-	T50.Z16-
tetanus	T50.Z11-	T50.Z12-	T50.Z13-	T50.Z14-	T50.Z15-	T50.Z16-
Antitrichomonal drug	T37.3X1-	T37.3X2-	T37.3X3-	T37.3X4-	T37.3X5-	T37.3X6-
Antituberculars	T37.1X1-	T37.1X2-	T37.1X3-	T37.1X4-	T37.1X5-	T37.1X6-
antibiotics	T36.5X1-	T36.5X2-	T36.5X3-	T36.5X4-	T36.5X5-	T36.5X6-
Antitussive NEC	T48.3X1-	T48.3X2-	T48.3X3-	T48.3X4-	T48.3X5-	T48.3X6-
codeine mixture	T40.2X1-	T40.2X2-	T40.2X3-	T40.2X4-	T40.2X5-	T40.2X6-
opiate	T40.2X1-	T40.2X2-	T40.2X3-	T40.2X4-	T40.2X5-	T40.2X6-
Antivaricose drug	T46.8X1-	T46.8X2-	T46.8X3-	T46.8X4-	T46.8X5-	T46.8X6-
Antivenin, antivenom (sera)	T50.Z11-	T50.Z12-	T50.Z13-	T50.Z14-	T50.Z15-	T50.Z16-
crotaline	T50.Z11-	T50.Z12-	T50.Z13-	T50.Z14-	T50.Z15-	T50.Z16-
spider bite	T50.Z11-	T50.Z12-	T50.Z13-	T50.Z14-	T50.Z15-	T50.Z16-
Antivertigo drug	T45.0X1-	T45.0X2-	T45.0X3-	T45.0X4-	T45.0X5-	T45.0X6-
Antiviral drug NEC	T37.5X1-	T37.5X2-	T37.5X3-	T37.5X4-	T37.5X5-	T37.5X6-
eye	T49.5X1-	T49.5X2-	T49.5X3-	T49.5X4-	T49.5X5-	T49.5X6-
Antiwhipworm drug	T37.4X1-	T37.4X2-	T37.4X3-	T37.4X4-	T37.4X5-	T37.4X6-
Antrol — *see also by specific chemical substance*	T60.91X-	T60.92X-	T60.93X-	T60.94X-	-	-
fungicide	T60.91X-	T60.92X-	T60.93X-	T60.94X-	-	-
ANTU (alpha naphthylthiourea)	T60.4X1-	T60.4X2-	T60.4X3-	T60.4X4-	-	-
Apalcillin	T36.0X1-	T36.0X2-	T36.0X3-	T36.0X4-	T36.0X5-	T36.0X6-
APC	T48.5X1-	T48.5X2-	T48.5X3-	T48.5X4-	T48.5X5-	T48.5X6-
Aplonidine	T44.4X1-	T44.4X2-	T44.4X3-	T44.4X4-	T44.4X5-	T44.4X6-
Apomorphine	T47.7X1-	T47.7X2-	T47.7X3-	T47.7X4-	T47.7X5-	T47.7X6-
Appetite depressants, central	T50.5X1-	T50.5X2-	T50.5X3-	T50.5X4-	T50.5X5-	T50.5X6-
Apraclonidine (hydrochloride)	T44.4X1-	T44.4X2-	T44.4X3-	T44.4X4-	T44.4X5-	T44.4X6-
Apresoline	T46.5X1-	T46.5X2-	T46.5X3-	T46.5X4-	T46.5X5-	T46.5X6-
Aprindine	T46.2X1-	T46.2X2-	T46.2X3-	T46.2X4-	T46.2X5-	T46.2X6-
Aprobarbital	T42.3X1-	T42.3X2-	T42.3X3-	T42.3X4-	T42.3X5-	T42.3X6-
Apronalide	T42.6X1-	T42.6X2-	T42.6X3-	T42.6X4-	T42.6X5-	T42.6X6-
Aprotinin	T45.621-	T45.622-	T45.623-	T45.624-	T45.625-	T45.626-
Aptocaine	T41.3X1-	T41.3X2-	T41.3X3-	T41.3X4-	T41.3X5-	T41.3X6-
Aqua fortis	T54.2X1-	T54.2X2-	T54.2X3-	T54.2X4-	-	-
Ara-A	T37.5X1-	T37.5X2-	T37.5X3-	T37.5X4-	T37.5X5-	T37.5X6-
Ara-C	T45.1X1-	T45.1X2-	T45.1X3-	T45.1X4-	T45.1X5-	T45.1X6-
Arachis oil	T49.3X1-	T49.3X2-	T49.3X3-	T49.3X4-	T49.3X5-	T49.3X6-
cathartic	T47.4X1-	T47.4X2-	T47.4X3-	T47.4X4-	T47.4X5-	T47.4X6-
Aralen	T37.2X1-	T37.2X2-	T37.2X3-	T37.2X4-	T37.2X5-	T37.2X6-

Substance	Poisoning Accidental (unintentional)	Poisoning Intentional self-harm	Poisoning Assault	Poisoning Undetermined	Adverse effect	Underdosing
Arecoline	T44.1X1-	T44.1X2-	T44.1X3-	T44.1X4-	T44.1X5-	T44.1X6-
Arginine	T50.991-	T50.992-	T50.993-	T50.994-	T50.995-	T50.996-
glutamate	T50.991-	T50.992-	T50.993-	T50.994-	T50.995-	T50.996-
Argyrol	T49.0X1-	T49.0X2-	T49.0X3-	T49.0X4-	T49.0X5-	T49.0X6-
ENT agent	T49.6X1-	T49.6X2-	T49.6X3-	T49.6X4-	T49.6X5-	T49.6X6-
ophthalmic preparation	T49.5X1-	T49.5X2-	T49.5X3-	T49.5X4-	T49.5X5-	T49.5X6-
Aristocort	T38.0X1-	T38.0X2-	T38.0X3-	T38.0X4-	T38.0X5-	T38.0X6-
ENT agent	T49.6X1-	T49.6X2-	T49.6X3-	T49.6X4-	T49.6X5-	T49.6X6-
ophthalmic preparation	T49.5X1-	T49.5X2-	T49.5X3-	T49.5X4-	T49.5X5-	T49.5X6-
topical NEC	T49.0X1-	T49.0X2-	T49.0X3-	T49.0X4-	T49.0X5-	T49.0X6-
Aromatics, corrosive	T54.1X1-	T54.1X2-	T54.1X3-	T54.1X4-	-	-
disinfectants	T54.1X1-	T54.1X2-	T54.1X3-	T54.1X4-	-	-
Arsenate of lead	T57.0X1-	T57.0X2-	T57.0X3-	T57.0X4-	-	-
herbicide	T57.0X1-	T57.0X2-	T57.0X3-	T57.0X4-	-	-
Arsenic, arsenicals (compounds) (dust) (vapor) NEC	T57.0X1-	T57.0X2-	T57.0X3-	T57.0X4-	-	-
anti-infectives	T37.8X1-	T37.8X2-	T37.8X3-	T37.8X4-	T37.8X5-	T37.8X6-
pesticide (dust) (fumes)	T57.0X1-	T57.0X2-	T57.0X3-	T57.0X4-	-	-
Arsine (gas)	T57.0X1-	T57.0X2-	T57.0X3-	T57.0X4-	-	-
Arsphenamine (silver)	T37.8X1-	T37.8X2-	T37.8X3-	T37.8X4-	T37.8X5-	T37.8X6-
Arsthinol	T37.3X1-	T37.3X2-	T37.3X3-	T37.3X4-	T37.3X5-	T37.3X6-
Artane	T44.3X1-	T44.3X2-	T44.3X3-	T44.3X4-	T44.3X5-	T44.3X6-
Arthropod (venomous) NEC	T63.481-	T63.482-	T63.483-	T63.484-	-	-
Articaine	T41.3X1-	T41.3X2-	T41.3X3-	T41.3X4-	T41.3X5-	T41.3X6-
Asbestos	T57.8X1-	T57.8X2-	T57.8X3-	T57.8X4-	-	-
Ascaridole	T37.4X1-	T37.4X2-	T37.4X3-	T37.4X4-	T37.4X5-	T37.4X6-
Ascorbic acid	T45.2X1-	T45.2X2-	T45.2X3-	T45.2X4-	T45.2X5-	T45.2X6-
Asiaticoside	T49.0X1-	T49.0X2-	T49.0X3-	T49.0X4-	T49.0X5-	T49.0X6-
Asparaginase	T45.1X1-	T45.1X2-	T45.1X3-	T45.1X4-	T45.1X5-	T45.1X6-
Aspidium (oleoresin)	T37.4X1-	T37.4X2-	T37.4X3-	T37.4X4-	T37.4X5-	T37.4X6-
Aspirin (aluminum) (soluble)	T39.011-	T39.012-	T39.013-	T39.014-	T39.015-	T39.016-
Aspoxicillin	T36.0X1-	T36.0X2-	T36.0X3-	T36.0X4-	T36.0X5-	T36.0X6-
Astemizole	T45.0X1-	T45.0X2-	T45.0X3-	T45.0X4-	T45.0X5-	T45.0X6-
Astringent (local)	T49.2X1-	T49.2X2-	T49.2X3-	T49.2X4-	T49.2X5-	T49.2X6-
specified NEC	T49.2X1-	T49.2X2-	T49.2X3-	T49.2X4-	T49.2X5-	T49.2X6-
Astromicin	T36.5X1-	T36.5X2-	T36.5X3-	T36.5X4-	T36.5X5-	T36.5X6-
Ataractic drug NEC	T43.501-	T43.502-	T43.503-	T43.504-	T43.505-	T43.506-
Atenolol	T44.7X1-	T44.7X2-	T44.7X3-	T44.7X4-	T44.7X5-	T44.7X6-
Atonia drug, intestinal	T47.4X1-	T47.4X2-	T47.4X3-	T47.4X4-	T47.4X5-	T47.4X6-
Atophan	T50.4X1-	T50.4X2-	T50.4X3-	T50.4X4-	T50.4X5-	T50.4X6-
Atracurium besilate	T48.1X1-	T48.1X2-	T48.1X3-	T48.1X4-	T48.1X5-	T48.1X6-
Atropine	T44.3X1-	T44.3X2-	T44.3X3-	T44.3X4-	T44.3X5-	T44.3X6-
derivative	T44.3X1-	T44.3X2-	T44.3X3-	T44.3X4-	T44.3X5-	T44.3X6-
methonitrate	T44.3X1-	T44.3X2-	T44.3X3-	T44.3X4-	T44.3X5-	T44.3X6-
Attapulgite	T47.6X1-	T47.6X2-	T47.6X3-	T47.6X4-	T47.6X5-	T47.6X6-
Auramine	T65.891-	T65.892-	T65.893-	T65.894-	-	-
dye	T65.6X1-	T65.6X2-	T65.6X3-	T65.6X4-	-	-
fungicide	T60.3X1-	T60.3X2-	T60.3X3-	T60.3X4-	-	-
Auranofin	T39.4X1-	T39.4X2-	T39.4X3-	T39.4X4-	T39.4X5-	T39.4X6-
Aurantiin	T46.991-	T46.992-	T46.993-	T46.994-	T46.995-	T46.996-
Aureomycin	T36.4X1-	T36.4X2-	T36.4X3-	T36.4X4-	T36.4X5-	T36.4X6-
ophthalmic preparation	T49.5X1-	T49.5X2-	T49.5X3-	T49.5X4-	T49.5X5-	T49.5X6-
topical NEC	T49.0X1-	T49.0X2-	T49.0X3-	T49.0X4-	T49.0X5-	T49.0X6-
Aurothioglucose	T39.4X1-	T39.4X2-	T39.4X3-	T39.4X4-	T39.4X5-	T39.4X6-
Aurothioglycanide	T39.4X1-	T39.4X2-	T39.4X3-	T39.4X4-	T39.4X5-	T39.4X6-
Aurothiomalate sodium	T39.4X1-	T39.4X2-	T39.4X3-	T39.4X4-	T39.4X5-	T39.4X6-
Aurotioprol	T39.4X1-	T39.4X2-	T39.4X3-	T39.4X4-	T39.4X5-	T39.4X6-

Substance	Poisoning Accidental (unintentional)	Poisoning Intentional self-harm	Poisoning Assault	Poisoning Undetermined	Adverse effect	Underdosing
Automobile fuel	T52.0X1-	T52.0X2-	T52.0X3-	T52.0X4-	-	-
Autonomic nervous system agent NEC	T44.901-	T44.902-	T44.903-	T44.904-	T44.905-	T44.906-
Avlosulfon	T37.1X1-	T37.1X2-	T37.1X3-	T37.1X4-	T37.1X5-	T37.1X6-
Avomine	T42.6X1-	T42.6X2-	T42.6X3-	T42.6X4-	T42.6X5-	T42.6X6-
Axerophthol	T45.2X1-	T45.2X2-	T45.2X3-	T45.2X4-	T45.2X5-	T45.2X6-
Azacitidine	T45.1X1-	T45.1X2-	T45.1X3-	T45.1X4-	T45.1X5-	T45.1X6-
Azacyclonol	T43.591-	T43.592-	T43.593-	T43.594-	T43.595-	T43.596-
Azadirachta	T60.2X1-	T60.2X2-	T60.2X3-	T60.2X4-	-	-
Azanidazole	T37.3X1-	T37.3X2-	T37.3X3-	T37.3X4-	T37.3X5-	T37.3X6-
Azapetine	T46.7X1-	T46.7X2-	T46.7X3-	T46.7X4-	T46.7X5-	T46.7X6-
Azapropazone	T39.2X1-	T39.2X2-	T39.2X3-	T39.2X4-	T39.2X5-	T39.2X6-
Azaribine	T45.1X1-	T45.1X2-	T45.1X3-	T45.1X4-	T45.1X5-	T45.1X6-
Azaserine	T45.1X1-	T45.1X2-	T45.1X3-	T45.1X4-	T45.1X5-	T45.1X6-
Azatadine	T45.0X1-	T45.0X2-	T45.0X3-	T45.0X4-	T45.0X5-	T45.0X6-
Azatepa	T45.1X1-	T45.1X2-	T45.1X3-	T45.1X4-	T45.1X5-	T45.1X6-
Azathioprine	T45.1X1-	T45.1X2-	T45.1X3-	T45.1X4-	T45.1X5-	T45.1X6-
Azelaic acid	T49.0X1-	T49.0X2-	T49.0X3-	T49.0X4-	T49.0X5-	T49.0X6-
Azelastine	T45.0X1-	T45.0X2-	T45.0X3-	T45.0X4-	T45.0X5-	T45.0X6-
Azidocillin	T36.0X1-	T36.0X2-	T36.0X3-	T36.0X4-	T36.0X5-	T36.0X6-
Azidothymidine	T37.5X1-	T37.5X2-	T37.5X3-	T37.5X4-	T37.5X5-	T37.5X6-
Azinphos (ethyl) (methyl)	T60.0X1-	T60.0X2-	T60.0X3-	T60.0X4-	-	-
Aziridine (chelating)	T54.1X1-	T54.1X2-	T54.1X3-	T54.1X4-	-	-
Azithromycin	T36.3X1-	T36.3X2-	T36.3X3-	T36.3X4-	T36.3X5-	T36.3X6-
Azlocillin	T36.0X1-	T36.0X2-	T36.0X3-	T36.0X4-	T36.0X5-	T36.0X6-
Azobenzene smoke	T65.3X1-	T65.3X2-	T65.3X3-	T65.3X4-	-	-
acaricide	T60.8X1-	T60.8X2-	T60.8X3-	T60.8X4-	-	-
Azosulfamide	T37.0X1-	T37.0X2-	T37.0X3-	T37.0X4-	T37.0X5-	T37.0X6-
AZT	T37.5X1-	T37.5X2-	T37.5X3-	T37.5X4-	T37.5X5-	T37.5X6-
Aztreonam	T36.1X1-	T36.1X2-	T36.1X3-	T36.1X4-	T36.1X5-	T36.1X6-
Azulfidine	T37.0X1-	T37.0X2-	T37.0X3-	T37.0X4-	T37.0X5-	T37.0X6-
Azuresin	T50.8X1-	T50.8X2-	T50.8X3-	T50.8X4-	T50.8X5-	T50.8X6-
Bacampicillin	T36.0X1-	T36.0X2-	T36.0X3-	T36.0X4-	T36.0X5-	T36.0X6-
Bacillus						
lactobacillus	T47.8X1-	T47.8X2-	T47.8X3-	T47.8X4-	T47.8X5-	T47.8X6-
subtilis	T47.6X1-	T47.6X2-	T47.6X3-	T47.6X4-	T47.6X5-	T47.6X6-
Bacimycin	T49.0X1-	T49.0X2-	T49.0X3-	T49.0X4-	T49.0X5-	T49.0X6-
ophthalmic preparation	T49.5X1-	T49.5X2-	T49.5X3-	T49.5X4-	T49.5X5-	T49.5X6-
Bacitracin zinc	T49.0X1-	T49.0X2-	T49.0X3-	T49.0X4-	T49.0X5-	T49.0X6-
with neomycin	T49.0X1-	T49.0X2-	T49.0X3-	T49.0X4-	T49.0X5-	T49.0X6-
ENT agent	T49.6X1-	T49.6X2-	T49.6X3-	T49.6X4-	T49.6X5-	T49.6X6-
ophthalmic preparation	T49.5X1-	T49.5X2-	T49.5X3-	T49.5X4-	T49.5X5-	T49.5X6-
topical NEC	T49.0X1-	T49.0X2-	T49.0X3-	T49.0X4-	T49.0X5-	T49.0X6-
Baclofen	T42.8X1-	T42.8X2-	T42.8X3-	T42.8X4-	T42.8X5-	T42.8X6-
Baking soda	T50.991-	T50.992-	T50.993-	T50.994-	T50.995-	T50.996-
BAL	T45.8X1-	T45.8X2-	T45.8X3-	T45.8X4-	T45.8X5-	T45.8X6-
Bambuterol	T48.6X1-	T48.6X2-	T48.6X3-	T48.6X4-	T48.6X5-	T48.6X6-
Bamethan (sulfate)	T46.7X1-	T46.7X2-	T46.7X3-	T46.7X4-	T46.7X5-	T46.7X6-
Bamifylline	T48.6X1-	T48.6X2-	T48.6X3-	T48.6X4-	T48.6X5-	T48.6X6-
Bamipine	T45.0X1-	T45.0X2-	T45.0X3-	T45.0X4-	T45.0X5-	T45.0X6-
Baneberry — *see Actaea spicata*						
Banewort — *see Belladonna*						
Barbenyl	T42.3X1-	T42.3X2-	T42.3X3-	T42.3X4-	T42.3X5-	T42.3X6-
Barbexaclone	T42.6X1-	T42.6X2-	T42.6X3-	T42.6X4-	T42.6X5-	T42.6X6-
Barbital	T42.3X1-	T42.3X2-	T42.3X3-	T42.3X4-	T42.3X5-	T42.3X6-
sodium	T42.3X1-	T42.3X2-	T42.3X3-	T42.3X4-	T42.3X5-	T42.3X6-
Barbitone	T42.3X1-	T42.3X2-	T42.3X3-	T42.3X4-	T42.3X5-	T42.3X6-
Barbiturate NEC	T42.3X1-	T42.3X2-	T42.3X3-	T42.3X4-	T42.3X5-	T42.3X6-
with tranquilizer	T42.3X1-	T42.3X2-	T42.3X3-	T42.3X4-	T42.3X5-	T42.3X6-

Substance	Poisoning Accidental (unintentional)	Poisoning Intentional self-harm	Poisoning Assault	Poisoning Undetermined	Adverse effect	Underdosing
Barbiturate NEC (continued)						
anesthetic (intravenous)	T41.1X1-	T41.1X2-	T41.1X3-	T41.1X4-	T41.1X5-	T41.1X6-
Barium (carbonate) (chloride) (sulfite)	T57.8X1-	T57.8X2-	T57.8X3-	T57.8X4-	-	-
diagnostic agent	T50.8X1-	T50.8X2-	T50.8X3-	T50.8X4-	T50.8X5-	T50.8X6-
pesticide	T60.4X1-	T60.4X2-	T60.4X3-	T60.4X4-	-	-
rodenticide	T60.4X1-	T60.4X2-	T60.4X3-	T60.4X4-	-	-
sulfate (medicinal)	T50.8X1-	T50.8X2-	T50.8X3-	T50.8X4-	T50.8X5-	T50.8X6-
Barrier cream	T49.3X1-	T49.3X2-	T49.3X3-	T49.3X4-	T49.3X5-	T49.3X6-
Basic fuchsin	T49.0X1-	T49.0X2-	T49.0X3-	T49.0X4-	T49.0X5-	T49.0X6-
Battery acid or fluid	T54.2X1-	T54.2X2-	T54.2X3-	T54.2X4-	-	-
Bay rum	T51.8X1-	T51.8X2-	T51.8X3-	T51.8X4-	-	-
BCG (vaccine)	T50.A91-	T50.A92-	T50.A93-	T50.A94-	T50.A95-	T50.A96-
BCNU	T45.1X1-	T45.1X2-	T45.1X3-	T45.1X4-	T45.1X5-	T45.1X6-
Bearsfoot	T62.2X1-	T62.2X2-	T62.2X3-	T62.2X4-	-	-
Beclamide	T42.6X1-	T42.6X2-	T42.6X3-	T42.6X4-	T42.6X5-	T42.6X6-
Beclomethasone	T44.5X1-	T44.5X2-	T44.5X3-	T44.5X4-	T44.5X5-	T44.5X6-
Bee (sting) (venom)	T63.441-	T63.442-	T63.443-	T63.444-	-	-
Befunolol	T49.5X1-	T49.5X2-	T49.5X3-	T49.5X4-	T49.5X5-	T49.5X6-
Bekanamycin	T36.5X1-	T36.5X2-	T36.5X3-	T36.5X4-	T36.5X5-	T36.5X6-
Belladonna — *see also Nightshade*						
alkaloids	T44.3X1-	T44.3X2-	T44.3X3-	T44.3X4-	T44.3X5-	T44.3X6-
extract	T44.3X1-	T44.3X2-	T44.3X3-	T44.3X4-	T44.3X5-	T44.3X6-
herb	T44.3X1-	T44.3X2-	T44.3X3-	T44.3X4-	T44.3X5-	T44.3X6-
Bemegride	T50.7X1-	T50.7X2-	T50.7X3-	T50.7X4-	T50.7X5-	T50.7X6-
Benactyzine	T44.3X1-	T44.3X2-	T44.3X3-	T44.3X4-	T44.3X5-	T44.3X6-
Benadryl	T45.0X1-	T45.0X2-	T45.0X3-	T45.0X4-	T45.0X5-	T45.0X6-
Benaprizine	T44.3X1-	T44.3X2-	T44.3X3-	T44.3X4-	T44.3X5-	T44.3X6-
Benazepril	T46.4X1-	T46.4X2-	T46.4X3-	T46.4X4-	T46.4X5-	T46.4X6-
Bencyclane	T46.7X1-	T46.7X2-	T46.7X3-	T46.7X4-	T46.7X5-	T46.7X6-
Bendazol	T46.3X1-	T46.3X2-	T46.3X3-	T46.3X4-	T46.3X5-	T46.3X6-
Bendrofluazide	T50.2X1-	T50.2X2-	T50.2X3-	T50.2X4-	T50.2X5-	T50.2X6-
Bendroflumethiazide	T50.2X1-	T50.2X2-	T50.2X3-	T50.2X4-	T50.2X5-	T50.2X6-
Benemid	T50.4X1-	T50.4X2-	T50.4X3-	T50.4X4-	T50.4X5-	T50.4X6-
Benethamine penicillin	T36.0X1-	T36.0X2-	T36.0X3-	T36.0X4-	T36.0X5-	T36.0X6-
Benexate	T47.1X1-	T47.1X2-	T47.1X3-	T47.1X4-	T47.1X5-	T47.1X6-
Benfluorex	T46.6X1-	T46.6X2-	T46.6X3-	T46.6X4-	T46.6X5-	T46.6X6-
Benfotiamine	T45.2X1-	T45.2X2-	T45.2X3-	T45.2X4-	T45.2X5-	T45.2X6-
Benisone	T49.0X1-	T49.0X2-	T49.0X3-	T49.0X4-	T49.0X5-	T49.0X6-
Benomyl	T60.0X1-	T60.0X2-	T60.0X3-	T60.0X4-	-	-
Benoquin	T49.8X1-	T49.8X2-	T49.8X3-	T49.8X4-	T49.8X5-	T49.8X6-
Benoxinate	T41.3X1-	T41.3X2-	T41.3X3-	T41.3X4-	T41.3X5-	T41.3X6-
Benperidol	T43.4X1-	T43.4X2-	T43.4X3-	T43.4X4-	T43.4X5-	T43.4X6-
Benproperine	T48.3X1-	T48.3X2-	T48.3X3-	T48.3X4-	T48.3X5-	T48.3X6-
Benserazide	T42.8X1-	T42.8X2-	T42.8X3-	T42.8X4-	T42.8X5-	T42.8X6-
Bentazepam	T42.4X1-	T42.4X2-	T42.4X3-	T42.4X4-	T42.4X5-	T42.4X6-
Bentiromide	T50.8X1-	T50.8X2-	T50.8X3-	T50.8X4-	T50.8X5-	T50.8X6-
Bentonite	T49.3X1-	T49.3X2-	T49.3X3-	T49.3X4-	T49.3X5-	T49.3X6-
Benzalbutyramide	T46.6X1-	T46.6X2-	T46.6X3-	T46.6X4-	T46.6X5-	T46.6X6-
Benzalkonium (chloride)	T49.0X1-	T49.0X2-	T49.0X3-	T49.0X4-	T49.0X5-	T49.0X6-
ophthalmic preparation	T49.5X1-	T49.5X2-	T49.5X3-	T49.5X4-	T49.5X5-	T49.5X6-
Benzamidosalicylate (calcium)	T37.1X1-	T37.1X2-	T37.1X3-	T37.1X4-	T37.1X5-	T37.1X6-
Benzamine	T41.3X1-	T41.3X2-	T41.3X3-	T41.3X4-	T41.3X5-	T41.3X6-
lactate	T49.1X1-	T49.1X2-	T49.1X3-	T49.1X4-	T49.1X5-	T49.1X6-
Benzamphetamine	T50.5X1-	T50.5X2-	T50.5X3-	T50.5X4-	T50.5X5-	T50.5X6-
Benzapril hydrochloride	T46.5X1-	T46.5X2-	T46.5X3-	T46.5X4-	T46.5X5-	T46.5X6-
Benzathine benzylpenicillin	T36.0X1-	T36.0X2-	T36.0X3-	T36.0X4-	T36.0X5-	T36.0X6-
Benzathine penicillin	T36.0X1-	T36.0X2-	T36.0X3-	T36.0X4-	T36.0X5-	T36.0X6-
Benzatropine	T42.8X1-	T42.8X2-	T42.8X3-	T42.8X4-	T42.8X5-	T42.8X6-
Benzbromarone	T50.4X1-	T50.4X2-	T50.4X3-	T50.4X4-	T50.4X5-	T50.4X6-

Substance	Poisoning Accidental (unintentional)	Poisoning Intentional self-harm	Poisoning Assault	Poisoning Undetermined	Adverse effect	Underdosing
Benzcarbimine	T45.1X1-	T45.1X2-	T45.1X3-	T45.1X4-	T45.1X5-	T45.1X6-
Benzedrex	T44.991-	T44.992-	T44.993-	T44.994-	T44.995-	T44.996-
Benzedrine (amphetamine)	T43.621-	T43.622-	T43.623-	T43.624-	T43.625-	T43.626-
Benzenamine	T65.3X1-	T65.3X2-	T65.3X3-	T65.3X4-	-	-
Benzene	T52.1X1-	T52.1X2-	T52.1X3-	T52.1X4-	-	-
homologues (acetyl) (dimethyl) (methyl) (solvent)	T52.2X1-	T52.2X2-	T52.2X3-	T52.2X4-	-	-
Benzethonium (chloride)	T49.0X1-	T49.0X2-	T49.0X3-	T49.0X4-	T49.0X5-	T49.0X6-
Benzfetamine	T50.5X1-	T50.5X2-	T50.5X3-	T50.5X4-	T50.5X5-	T50.5X6-
Benzhexol	T44.3X1-	T44.3X2-	T44.3X3-	T44.3X4-	T44.3X5-	T44.3X6-
Benzhydramine (chloride)	T45.0X1-	T45.0X2-	T45.0X3-	T45.0X4-	T45.0X5-	T45.0X6-
Benzidine	T65.891-	T65.892-	T65.893-	T65.894-	-	-
Benzilonium bromide	T44.3X1-	T44.3X2-	T44.3X3-	T44.3X4-	T44.3X5-	T44.3X6-
Benzimidazole	T60.3X1-	T60.3X2-	T60.3X3-	T60.3X4-	-	-
Benzin (e) — *see Ligroin*						
Benziodarone	T46.3X1-	T46.3X2-	T46.3X3-	T46.3X4-	T46.3X5-	T46.3X6-
Benznidazole	T37.3X1-	T37.3X2-	T37.3X3-	T37.3X4-	T37.3X5-	T37.3X6-
Benzocaine	T41.3X1-	T41.3X2-	T41.3X3-	T41.3X4-	T41.3X5-	T41.3X6-
Benzodiapin	T42.4X1-	T42.4X2-	T42.4X3-	T42.4X4-	T42.4X5-	T42.4X6-
Benzodiazepine NEC	T42.4X1-	T42.4X2-	T42.4X3-	T42.4X4-	T42.4X5-	T42.4X6-
Benzoic acid	T49.0X1	T49.0X2-	T49.0X3-	T49.0X4-	T49.0X5-	T49.0X6-
with salicylic acid	T49.0X1-	T49.0X2-	T49.0X3-	T49.0X4-	T49.0X5-	T49.0X6-
Benzoin (tincture)	T48.5X1-	T48.5X2-	T48.5X3-	T48.5X4-	T48.5X5-	T48.5X6-
Benzol (benzene)	T52.1X1-	T52.1X2-	T52.1X3-	T52.1X4-	-	-
vapor	T52.0X1-	T52.0X2-	T52.0X3-	T52.0X4-	-	-
Benzomorphan	T40.2X1-	T40.2X2-	T40.2X3-	T40.2X4-	T40.2X5-	T40.2X6-
Benzonatate	T48.3X1-	T48.3X2-	T48.3X3-	T48.3X4-	T48.3X5-	T48.3X6-
Benzophenones	T49.3X1-	T49.3X2-	T49.3X3-	T49.3X4-	T49.3X5-	T49.3X6-
Benzopyrone	T46.991-	T46.992-	T46.993-	T46.994-	T46.995-	T46.996-
Benzothiadiazides	T50.2X1-	T50.2X2-	T50.2X3-	T50.2X4-	T50.2X5-	T50.2X6-
Benzoxonium chloride	T49.0X1-	T49.0X2-	T49.0X3-	T49.0X4-	T49.0X5-	T49.0X6-
Benzoyl peroxide	T49.0X1-	T49.0X2-	T49.0X3-	T49.0X4-	T49.0X5-	T49.0X6-
Benzoylpas calcium	T37.1X1-	T37.1X2-	T37.1X3-	T37.1X4-	T37.1X5-	T37.1X6-
Benzperidin	T43.591-	T43.592-	T43.593-	T43.594-	T43.595-	T43.596-
Benzperidol	T43.591-	T43.592-	T43.593-	T43.594-	T43.595-	T43.596-
Benzphetamine	T50.5X1-	T50.5X2-	T50.5X3-	T50.5X4-	T50.5X5-	T50.5X6-
Benzpyrinium bromide	T44.1X1-	T44.1X2-	T44.1X3-	T44.1X4-	T44.1X5-	T44.1X6-
Benzquinamide	T45.0X1-	T45.0X2-	T45.0X3-	T45.0X4-	T45.0X5-	T45.0X6-
Benzthiazide	T50.2X1-	T50.2X2-	T50.2X3-	T50.2X4-	T50.2X5-	T50.2X6-
Benztropine						
anticholinergic	T44.3X1-	T44.3X2-	T44.3X3-	T44.3X4-	T44.3X5-	T44.3X6-
antiparkinson	T42.8X1-	T42.8X2-	T42.8X3-	T42.8X4-	T42.8X5-	T42.8X6-
Benzydamine	T49.0X1-	T49.0X2-	T49.0X3-	T49.0X4-	T49.0X5-	T49.0X6-
Benzyl						
acetate	T52.8X1-	T52.8X2-	T52.8X3-	T52.8X4-	-	-
alcohol	T49.0X1-	T49.0X2-	T49.0X3-	T49.0X4-	T49.0X5-	T49.0X6-
benzoate	T49.0X1-	T49.0X2-	T49.0X3-	T49.0X4-	T49.0X5-	T49.0X6-
Benzoic acid	T49.0X1-	T49.0X2-	T49.0X3-	T49.0X4-	T49.0X5-	T49.0X6-
morphine	T40.2X1-	T40.2X2-	T40.2X3-	T40.2X4-	-	-
nicotinate	T46.6X1-	T46.6X2-	T46.6X3-	T46.6X4-	T46.6X5-	T46.6X6-
penicillin	T36.0X1-	T36.0X2-	T36.0X3-	T36.0X4-	T36.0X5-	T36.0X6-
Benzylhydrochlorthia-zide	T50.2X1-	T50.2X2-	T50.2X3-	T50.2X4-	T50.2X5-	T50.2X6-
Benzylpenicillin	T36.0X1-	T36.0X2-	T36.0X3-	T36.0X4-	T36.0X5-	T36.0X6-
Benzylthiouracil	T38.2X1-	T38.2X2-	T38.2X3-	T38.2X4-	T38.2X5-	T38.2X6-
Bephenium hydroxy-naphthoate	T37.4X1-	T37.4X2-	T37.4X3-	T37.4X4-	T37.4X5-	T37.4X6-
Bepridil	T46.1X1-	T46.1X2-	T46.1X3-	T46.1X4-	T46.1X5-	T46.1X6-
Bergamot oil	T65.891-	T65.892-	T65.893-	T65.894-	-	-
Bergapten	T50.991-	T50.992-	T50.993-	T50.994-	T50.995-	T50.996-
Berries, poisonous	T62.1X1-	T62.1X2-	T62.1X3-	T62.1X4-	-	-

Substance	Poisoning Accidental (unintentional)	Poisoning Intentional self-harm	Poisoning Assault	Poisoning Undetermined	Adverse effect	Underdosing
Beryllium (compounds)	T56.7X1-	T56.7X2-	T56.7X3-	T56.7X4-	-	-
b-acetyldigoxin	T46.0X1-	T46.0X2-	T46.0X3-	T46.0X4-	T46.0X5-	T46.0X6-
beta adrenergic blocking agent, heart	T44.7X1-	T44.7X2-	T44.7X3-	T44.7X4-	T44.7X5-	T44.7X6-
b-benzalbutyramide	T46.6X1-	T46.6X2-	T46.6X3-	T46.6X4-	T46.6X5-	T46.6X6-
Betacarotene	T45.2X1-	T45.2X2-	T45.2X3-	T45.2X4-	T45.2X5-	T45.2X6-
b-eucaine	T49.1X1-	T49.1X2-	T49.1X3-	T49.1X4-	T49.1X5-	T49.1X6-
Beta-Chlor	T42.6X1-	T42.6X2-	T42.6X3-	T42.6X4-	T42.6X5-	T42.6X6-
b-galactosidase	T47.5X1-	T47.5X2-	T47.5X3-	T47.5X4-	T47.5X5-	T47.5X6-
Betahistine	T46.7X1-	T46.7X2-	T46.7X3-	T46.7X4-	T46.7X5-	T46.7X6-
Betaine	T47.5X1-	T47.5X2-	T47.5X3-	T47.5X4-	T47.5X5-	T47.5X6-
Betamethasone	T49.0X1-	T49.0X2-	T49.0X3-	T49.0X4-	T49.0X5-	T49.0X6-
topical	T49.0X1-	T49.0X2-	T49.0X3-	T49.0X4-	T49.0X5-	T49.0X6-
Betamicin	T36.8X1-	T36.8X2-	T36.8X3-	T36.8X4-	T36.8X5-	T36.8X6-
Betanidine	T46.5X1-	T46.5X2-	T46.5X3-	T46.5X4-	T46.5X5-	T46.5X6-
b-sitosterol (s)	T46.6X1-	T46.6X2-	T46.6X3-	T46.6X4-	T46.6X5-	T46.6X6-
Betaxolol	T44.7X1-	T44.7X2-	T44.7X3-	T44.7X4-	T44.7X5-	T44.7X6-
Betazole	T50.8X1-	T50.8X2-	T50.8X3-	T50.8X4-	T50.8X5-	T50.8X6-
Bethanechol	T44.1X1-	T44.1X2-	T44.1X3-	T44.1X4-	T44.1X5-	T44.1X6-
chloride	T44.1X1-	T44.1X2-	T44.1X3-	T44.1X4-	T44.1X5-	T44.1X6-
Bethanidine	T46.5X1-	T46.5X2-	T46.5X3-	T46.5X4-	T46.5X5-	T46.5X6-
Betoxycaine	T41.3X1-	T41.3X2-	T41.3X3-	T41.3X4-	T41.3X5-	T41.3X6-
Betula oil	T49.3X1-	T49.3X2-	T49.3X3-	T49.3X4-	T49.3X5-	T49.3X6-
Bevantolol	T44.7X1-	T44.7X2-	T44.7X3-	T44.7X4-	T44.7X5-	T44.7X6-
Bevonium metilsulfate	T44.3X1-	T44.3X2-	T44.3X3-	T44.3X4-	T44.3X5-	T44.3X6-
Bezafibrate	T46.6X1-	T46.6X2-	T46.6X3-	T46.6X4-	T46.6X5-	T46.6X6-
Bezitramide	T40.491-	T40.492-	T40.493-	T40.494-	T40.495-	T40.496-
BHA	T50.991-	T50.992-	T50.993-	T50.994-	T50.995-	T50.996-
Bhang	T40.711-	T40.712-	T40.713-	T40.714-	T40.715-	T40.716-
BHC (medicinal)	T49.0X1-	T49.0X2-	T49.0X3-	T49.0X4-	T49.0X5-	T49.0X6-
nonmedicinal (vapor)	T53.6X1-	T53.6X2-	T53.6X3-	T53.6X4-	-	-
Bialamicol	T37.3X1-	T37.3X2-	T37.3X3-	T37.3X4-	T37.3X5-	T37.3X6-
Bibenzonium bromide	T48.3X1-	T48.3X2-	T48.3X3-	T48.3X4-	T48.3X5-	T48.3X6-
Bibrocathol	T49.5X1-	T49.5X2-	T49.5X3-	T49.5X4-	T49.5X5-	T49.5X6-
Bichloride of mercury — *see Mercury, chloride*						
Bichromates (calcium) (potassium) (sodium) (crystals)	T57.8X1-	T57.8X2-	T57.8X3-	T57.8X4-	-	-
fumes	T56.2X1-	T56.2X2-	T56.2X3-	T56.2X4-	-	-
Biclotymol	T49.6X1-	T49.6X2-	T49.6X3-	T49.6X4-	T49.6X5-	T49.6X6-
Bicucculine	T50.7X1-	T50.7X2-	T50.7X3-	T50.7X4-	T50.7X5-	T50.7X6-
Bifemelane	T43.291-	T43.292-	T43.293-	T43.294-	T43.295-	T43.296-
Biguanide derivatives, oral	T38.3X1-	T38.3X2-	T38.3X3-	T38.3X4-	T38.3X5-	T38.3X6-
Bile salts	T47.5X1-	T47.5X2-	T47.5X3-	T47.5X4-	T47.5X5-	T47.5X6-
Biligrafin	T50.8X1-	T50.8X2-	T50.8X3-	T50.8X4-	T50.8X5-	T50.8X6-
Bilopaque	T50.8X1-	T50.8X2-	T50.8X3-	T50.8X4-	T50.8X5-	T50.8X6-
Binifibrate	T46.6X1-	T46.6X2-	T46.6X3-	T46.6X4-	T46.6X5-	T46.6X6-
Binitrobenzol	T65.3X1-	T65.3X2-	T65.3X3-	T65.3X4-	-	-
Bioflavonoid (s)	T46.991-	T46.992-	T46.993-	T46.994-	T46.995-	T46.996-
Biological substance NEC	T50.901-	T50.902-	T50.903-	T50.904-	T50.905-	T50.906-
Biotin	T45.2X1-	T45.2X2-	T45.2X3-	T45.2X4-	T45.2X5-	T45.2X6-
Biperiden	T44.3X1-	T44.3X2-	T44.3X3-	T44.3X4-	T44.3X5-	T44.3X6-
Bisacodyl	T47.2X1-	T47.2X2-	T47.2X3-	T47.2X4-	T47.2X5-	T47.2X6-
Bisbentiamine	T45.2X1-	T45.2X2-	T45.2X3-	T45.2X4-	T45.2X5-	T45.2X6-
Bisbutiamine	T45.2X1-	T45.2X2-	T45.2X3-	T45.2X4-	T45.2X5-	T45.2X6-
Bisdequalinium (salts) (diacetate)	T49.6X1-	T49.6X2-	T49.6X3-	T49.6X4-	T49.6X5-	T49.6X6-
Bishydroxycoumarin	T45.511-	T45.512-	T45.513-	T45.514-	T45.515-	T45.516-
Bismarsen	T37.8X1-	T37.8X2-	T37.8X3-	T37.8X4-	T37.8X5-	T37.8X6-
Bismuth salts	T47.6X1-	T47.6X2-	T47.6X3-	T47.6X4-	T47.6X5-	T47.6X6-
aluminate	T47.1X1-	T47.1X2-	T47.1X3-	T47.1X4-	T47.1X5-	T47.1X6-

Substance	Poisoning Accidental (unintentional)	Poisoning Intentional self-harm	Poisoning Assault	Poisoning Undetermined	Adverse effect	Underdosing
Bismuth salts (continued)						
anti-infectives	T37.8X1-	T37.8X2-	T37.8X3-	T37.8X4-	T37.8X5-	T37.8X6-
formic iodide	T49.0X1-	T49.0X2-	T49.0X3-	T49.0X4-	T49.0X5-	T49.0X6-
glycolylarsenate	T49.0X1-	T49.0X2-	T49.0X3-	T49.0X4-	T49.0X5-	T49.0X6-
nonmedicinal (compounds) NEC	T65.91X-	T65.92X-	T65.93X-	T65.94X-	-	-
subcarbonate	T47.6X1-	T47.6X2-	T47.6X3-	T47.6X4-	T47.6X5-	T47.6X6-
subsalicylate	T37.8X1-	T37.8X2-	T37.8X3-	T37.8X4-	T37.8X5-	T37.8X6-
sulfarsphenamine	T37.8X1-	T37.8X2-	T37.8X3-	T37.8X4-	T37.8X5-	T37.8X6-
Bisoprolol	T44.7X1-	T44.7X2-	T44.7X3-	T44.7X4-	T44.7X5-	T44.7X6-
Bisoxatin	T47.2X1-	T47.2X2-	T47.2X3-	T47.2X4-	T47.2X5-	T47.2X6-
Bisulepin (hydrochloride)	T45.0X1-	T45.0X2-	T45.0X3-	T45.0X4-	T45.0X5-	T45.0X6-
Bithionol	T37.8X1-	T37.8X2-	T37.8X3-	T37.8X4-	T37.8X5-	T37.8X6-
anthelminthic	T37.4X1-	T37.4X2-	T37.4X3-	T37.4X4-	T37.4X5-	T37.4X6-
Bitolterol	T48.6X1-	T48.6X2-	T48.6X3-	T48.6X4-	T48.6X5-	T48.6X6-
Bitoscanate	T37.4X1-	T37.4X2-	T37.4X3-	T37.4X4-	T37.4X5-	T37.4X6-
Bitter almond oil	T62.8X1-	T62.8X2-	T62.8X3-	T62.8X4-	-	-
Bittersweet	T62.2X1-	T62.2X2-	T62.2X3-	T62.2X4-	-	-
Black						
flag	T60.91X-	T60.92X-	T60.93X-	T60.94X-	-	-
henbane	T62.2X1-	T62.2X2-	T62.2X3-	T62.2X4-	-	-
leaf (40)	T60.91X-	T60.92X-	T60.93X-	T60.94X-	-	-
widow spider (bite)	T63.311-	T63.312-	T63.313-	T63.314-	-	-
antivenin	T50.Z11-	T50.Z12-	T50.Z13-	T50.Z14-	T50.Z15-	T50.Z16-
Blast furnace gas (carbon monoxide from)	T58.8X1-	T58.8X2-	T58.8X3-	T58.8X4-	-	-
Bleach	T54.91X-	T54.92X-	T54.93X-	T54.94X-	-	-
Bleaching agent (medicinal)	T49.4X1-	T49.4X2-	T49.4X3-	T49.4X4-	T49.4X5-	T49.4X6-
Bleomycin	T45.1X1-	T45.1X2-	T45.1X3-	T45.1X4-	T45.1X5-	T45.1X6-
Blockain	T41.3X1-	T41.3X2-	T41.3X3-	T41.3X4-	T41.3X5-	T41.3X6-
infiltration (subcutaneous)	T41.3X1-	T41.3X2-	T41.3X3-	T41.3X4-	T41.3X5-	T41.3X6-
nerve block (peripheral) (plexus)	T41.3X1-	T41.3X2-	T41.3X3-	T41.3X4-	T41.3X5-	T41.3X6-
topical (surface)	T41.3X1-	T41.3X2-	T41.3X3-	T41.3X4-	T41.3X5-	T41.3X6-
Blockers, calcium channel	T46.1X1-	T46.1X2-	T46.1X3-	T46.1X4-	T46.1X5-	T46.1X6-
Blood (derivatives) (natural) (plasma) (whole)	T45.8X1-	T45.8X2-	T45.8X3-	T45.8X4-	T45.8X5-	T45.8X6-
dried	T45.8X1-	T45.8X2-	T45.8X3-	T45.8X4-	T45.8X5-	T45.8X6-
drug affecting NEC	T45.91X-	T45.92X-	T45.93X-	T45.94X-	T45.95X-	T45.96X-
expander NEC	T45.8X1-	T45.8X2-	T45.8X3-	T45.8X4-	T45.8X5-	T45.8X6-
fraction NEC	T45.8X1-	T45.8X2-	T45.8X3-	T45.8X4-	T45.8X5-	T45.8X6-
substitute (macromolecular)	T45.8X1-	T45.8X2-	T45.8X3-	T45.8X4-	T45.8X5-	T45.8X6-
Blue velvet	T40.2X1-	T40.2X2-	T40.2X3-	T40.2X4-	-	-
Bone meal	T62.8X1-	T62.8X2-	T62.8X3-	T62.8X4-	-	-
Bonine	T45.0X1-	T45.0X2-	T45.0X3-	T45.0X4-	T45.0X5-	T45.0X6-
Bopindolol	T44.7X1-	T44.7X2-	T44.7X3-	T44.7X4-	T44.7X5-	T44.7X6-
Boracic acid	T49.0X1-	T49.0X2-	T49.0X3-	T49.0X4-	T49.0X5-	T49.0X6-
ENT agent	T49.6X1-	T49.6X2-	T49.6X3-	T49.6X4-	T49.6X5-	T49.6X6-
ophthalmic preparation	T49.5X1-	T49.5X2-	T49.5X3-	T49.5X4-	T49.5X5-	T49.5X6-
Borane complex	T57.8X1-	T57.8X2-	T57.8X3-	T57.8X4-	-	-
Borate (s)	T57.8X1-	T57.8X2-	T57.8X3-	T57.8X4-	-	-
buffer	T50.991-	T50.992-	T50.993-	T50.994-	T50.995-	T50.996-
cleanser	T54.91X-	T54.92X-	T54.93X-	T54.94X-	-	-
sodium	T57.8X1-	T57.8X2-	T57.8X3-	T57.8X4-	-	-
Borax (cleanser)	T54.91X-	T54.92X-	T54.93X-	T54.94X-	-	-
Bordeaux mixture	T60.3X1-	T60.3X2-	T60.3X3-	T60.3X4-	-	-
Boric acid	T49.0X1-	T49.0X2-	T49.0X3-	T49.0X4-	T49.0X5-	T49.0X6-
ENT agent	T49.6X1-	T49.6X2-	T49.6X3-	T49.6X4-	T49.6X5-	T49.6X6-
ophthalmic preparation	T49.5X1-	T49.5X2-	T49.5X3-	T49.5X4-	T49.5X5-	T49.5X6-
Bornaprine	T44.3X1-	T44.3X2-	T44.3X3-	T44.3X4-	T44.3X5-	T44.3X6-

Substance	Poisoning Accidental (unintentional)	Poisoning Intentional self-harm	Poisoning Assault	Poisoning Undetermined	Adverse effect	Underdosing
Boron	T57.8X1-	T57.8X2-	T57.8X3-	T57.8X4-	-	-
hydride NEC	T57.8X1-	T57.8X2-	T57.8X3-	T57.8X4-	-	-
fumes or gas	T57.8X1-	T57.8X2-	T57.8X3-	T57.8X4-	-	-
trifluoride	T59.891-	T59.892-	T59.893-	T59.894-	-	-
Botox	T48.291-	T48.292-	T48.293-	T48.294-	T48.295-	T48.296-
Botulinus anti-toxin (type A, B)	T50.Z11-	T50.Z12-	T50.Z13-	T50.Z14-	T50.Z15-	T50.Z16-
Brake fluid vapor	T59.891-	T59.892-	T59.893-	T59.894-	-	-
Brallobarbital	T42.3X1-	T42.3X2-	T42.3X3-	T42.3X4-	T42.3X5-	T42.3X6-
Bran (wheat)	T47.4X1-	T47.4X2-	T47.4X3-	T47.4X4-	T47.4X5-	T47.4X6-
Brass (fumes)	T56.891-	T56.892-	T56.893-	T56.894-	-	-
Brasso	T52.0X1-	T52.0X2-	T52.0X3-	T52.0X4-	-	-
Bretylium tosilate	T46.2X1-	T46.2X2-	T46.2X3-	T46.2X4-	T46.2X5-	T46.2X6-
Brevital (sodium)	T41.1X1-	T41.1X2-	T41.1X3-	T41.1X4-	T41.1X5-	T41.1X6-
Brinase	T45.3X1-	T45.3X2-	T45.3X3-	T45.3X4-	T45.3X5-	T45.3X6-
British antilewisite	T45.8X1-	T45.8X2-	T45.8X3-	T45.8X4-	T45.8X5-	T45.8X6-
Brodifacoum	T60.4X1-	T60.4X2-	T60.4X3-	T60.4X4-	-	-
Bromal (hydrate)	T42.6X1-	T42.6X2-	T42.6X3-	T42.6X4-	T42.6X5-	T42.6X6-
Bromazepam	T42.4X1-	T42.4X2-	T42.4X3-	T42.4X4-	T42.4X5-	T42.4X6-
Bromazine	T45.0X1-	T45.0X2-	T45.0X3-	T45.0X4-	T45.0X5-	T45.0X6-
Brombenzylcyanide	T59.3X1-	T59.3X2-	T59.3X3-	T59.3X4-	-	-
Bromelains	T45.3X1-	T45.3X2-	T45.3X3-	T45.3X4-	T45.3X5-	T45.3X6-
Bromethalin	T60.4X1-	T60.4X2-	T60.4X3-	T60.4X4-	-	-
Bromhexine	T48.4X1-	T48.4X2-	T48.4X3-	T48.4X4-	T48.4X5-	T48.4X6-
Bromide salts	T42.6X1-	T42.6X2-	T42.6X3-	T42.6X4-	T42.6X5-	T42.6X6-
Bromindione	T45.511-	T45.512-	T45.513-	T45.514-	T45.515-	T45.516-
Bromine						
compounds (medicinal)	T42.6X1-	T42.6X2-	T42.6X3-	T42.6X4-	T42.6X5-	T42.6X6-
sedative	T42.6X1-	T42.6X2-	T42.6X3-	T42.6X4-	T42.6X5-	T42.6X6-
vapor	T59.891-	T59.892-	T59.893-	T59.894-	-	-
Bromisoval	T42.6X1-	T42.6X2-	T42.6X3-	T42.6X4-	T42.6X5-	T42.6X6-
Bromisovalum	T42.6X1-	T42.6X2-	T42.6X3-	T42.6X4-	T42.6X5-	T42.6X6-
Bromobenzylcyanide	T59.3X1-	T59.3X2-	T59.3X3-	T59.3X4-	-	-
Bromochlorosalicylani-lide	T49.0X1-	T49.0X2-	T49.0X3-	T49.0X4-	T49.0X5-	T49.0X6-
Bromocriptine	T42.8X1-	T42.8X2-	T42.8X3-	T42.8X4-	T42.8X5-	T42.8X6-
Bromodiphenhydramine	T45.0X1-	T45.0X2-	T45.0X3-	T45.0X4-	T45.0X5-	T45.0X6-
Bromoform	T42.6X1-	T42.6X2-	T42.6X3-	T42.6X4-	T42.6X5-	T42.6X6-
Bromophenol blue reagent	T50.991-	T50.992-	T50.993-	T50.994-	T50.995-	T50.996-
Bromopride	T47.8X1-	T47.8X2-	T47.8X3-	T47.8X4-	T47.8X5-	T47.8X6-
Bromosalicylchloranitide	T49.0X1-	T49.0X2-	T49.0X3-	T49.0X4-	T49.0X5-	T49.0X6-
Bromosalicylhydroxamic acid	T37.1X1-	T37.1X2-	T37.1X3-	T37.1X4-	T37.1X5-	T37.1X6-
Bromo-seltzer	T39.1X1-	T39.1X2-	T39.1X3-	T39.1X4-	T39.1X5-	T39.1X6-
Bromoxynil	T60.3X1-	T60.3X2-	T60.3X3-	T60.3X4-	-	-
Bromperidol	T43.4X1-	T43.4X2-	T43.4X3-	T43.4X4-	T43.4X5-	T43.4X6-
Brompheniramine	T45.0X1-	T45.0X2-	T45.0X3-	T45.0X4-	T45.0X5-	T45.0X6-
Bromsulfophthalein	T50.8X1-	T50.8X2-	T50.8X3-	T50.8X4-	T50.8X5-	T50.8X6-
Bromural	T42.6X1-	T42.6X2-	T42.6X3-	T42.6X4-	T42.6X5-	T42.6X6-
Bromvaletone	T42.6X1-	T42.6X2-	T42.6X3-	T42.6X4-	T42.6X5-	T42.6X6-
Bronchodilator NEC	T48.6X1-	T48.6X2-	T48.6X3-	T48.6X4-	T48.6X5-	T48.6X6-
Brotizolam	T42.4X1-	T42.4X2-	T42.4X3-	T42.4X4-	T42.4X5-	T42.4X6-
Brovincamine	T46.7X1-	T46.7X2-	T46.7X3-	T46.7X4-	T46.7X5-	T46.7X6-
Brown recluse spider (bite) (venom)	T63.331-	T63.332-	T63.333-	T63.334-	-	-
Brown spider (bite) (venom)	T63.391-	T63.392-	T63.393-	T63.394-	-	-
Broxaterol	T48.6X1-	T48.6X2-	T48.6X3-	T48.6X4-	T48.6X5-	T48.6X6-
Broxuridine	T45.1X1-	T45.1X2-	T45.1X3-	T45.1X4-	T45.1X5-	T45.1X6-
Broxyquinoline	T37.8X1-	T37.8X2-	T37.8X3-	T37.8X4-	T37.8X5-	T37.8X6-
Bruceine	T48.291-	T48.292-	T48.293-	T48.294-	T48.295-	T48.296-
Brucia	T62.2X1-	T62.2X2-	T62.2X3-	T62.2X4-	-	-
Brucine	T65.1X1-	T65.1X2-	T65.1X3-	T65.1X4-	-	-
Brunswick green — *see Copper*						

Substance	Poisoning Accidental (unintentional)	Poisoning Intentional self-harm	Poisoning Assault	Poisoning Undetermined	Adverse effect	Underdosing
Bruten — *see Ibuprofen*						
Bryonia	T47.2X1-	T47.2X2-	T47.2X3-	T47.2X4-	T47.2X5-	T47.2X6-
Buclizine	T45.0X1-	T45.0X2-	T45.0X3-	T45.0X4-	T45.0X5-	T45.0X6-
Buclosamide	T49.0X1-	T49.0X2-	T49.0X3-	T49.0X4-	T49.0X5-	T49.0X6-
Budesonide	T44.5X1-	T44.5X2-	T44.5X3-	T44.5X4-	T44.5X5-	T44.5X6-
Budralazine	T46.5X1-	T46.5X2-	T46.5X3-	T46.5X4-	T46.5X5-	T46.5X6-
Bufferin	T39.011-	T39.012-	T39.013-	T39.014-	T39.015-	T39.016-
Buflomedil	T46.7X1-	T46.7X2-	T46.7X3-	T46.7X4-	T46.7X5-	T46.7X6-
Buformin	T38.3X1-	T38.3X2-	T38.3X3-	T38.3X4-	T38.3X5-	T38.3X6-
Bufotenine	T40.991-	T40.992-	T40.993-	T40.994-	-	-
Bufrolin	T48.6X1-	T48.6X2-	T48.6X3-	T48.6X4-	T48.6X5-	T48.6X6-
Bufylline	T48.6X1-	T48.6X2-	T48.6X3-	T48.6X4-	T48.6X5-	T48.6X6-
Bulk filler	T50.5X1-	T50.5X2-	T50.5X3-	T50.5X4-	T50.5X5-	T50.5X6-
cathartic	T47.4X1-	T47.4X2-	T47.4X3-	T47.4X4-	T47.4X5-	T47.4X6-
Bumetanide	T50.1X1-	T50.1X2-	T50.1X3-	T50.1X4-	T50.1X5-	T50.1X6-
Bunaftine	T46.2X1-	T46.2X2-	T46.2X3-	T46.2X4-	T46.2X5-	T46.2X6-
Bunamiodyl	T50.8X1-	T50.8X2-	T50.8X3-	T50.8X4-	T50.8X5-	T50.8X6-
Bunazosin	T44.6X1-	T44.6X2-	T44.6X3-	T44.6X4-	T44.6X5-	T44.6X6-
Bunitrolol	T44.7X1-	T44.7X2-	T44.7X3-	T44.7X4-	T44.7X5-	T44.7X6-
Buphenine	T46.7X1-	T46.7X2-	T46.7X3-	T46.7X4-	T46.7X5-	T46.7X6-
Bupivacaine	T41.3X1-	T41.3X2-	T41.3X3-	T41.3X4-	T41.3X5-	T41.3X6-
infiltration (subcutaneous)	T41.3X1-	T41.3X2-	T41.3X3-	T41.3X4-	T41.3X5-	T41.3X6-
nerve block (peripheral) (plexus)	T41.3X1-	T41.3X2-	T41.3X3-	T41.3X4-	T41.3X5-	T41.3X6-
spinal	T41.3X1-	T41.3X2-	T41.3X3-	T41.3X4-	T41.3X5-	T41.3X6-
Bupranolol	T44.7X1-	T44.7X2-	T44.7X3-	T44.7X4-	T44.7X5-	T44.7X6-
Buprenorphine	T40.491-	T40.492-	T40.493-	T40.494-	T40.495-	T40.496-
Bupropion	T43.291-	T43.292-	T43.293-	T43.294-	T43.295-	T43.296-
Burimamide	T47.1X1-	T47.1X2-	T47.1X3-	T47.1X4-	T47.1X5-	T47.1X6-
Buserelin	T38.891-	T38.892-	T38.893-	T38.894-	T38.895-	T38.896-
Buspirone	T43.591-	T43.592-	T43.593-	T43.594-	T43.595-	T43.596-
Busulfan, busulphan	T45.1X1-	T45.1X2-	T45.1X3-	T45.1X4-	T45.1X5-	T45.1X6-
Butabarbital (sodium)	T42.3X1-	T42.3X2-	T42.3X3-	T42.3X4-	T42.3X5-	T42.3X6-
Butabarbitone	T42.3X1-	T42.3X2-	T42.3X3-	T42.3X4-	T42.3X5-	T42.3X6-
Butabarpal	T42.3X1-	T42.3X2-	T42.3X3-	T42.3X4-	T42.3X5-	T42.3X6-
Butacaine	T41.3X1-	T41.3X2-	T41.3X3-	T41.3X4-	T41.3X5-	T41.3X6-
Butalamine	T46.7X1-	T46.7X2-	T46.7X3-	T46.7X4-	T46.7X5-	T46.7X6-
Butalbital	T42.3X1-	T42.3X2-	T42.3X3-	T42.3X4-	T42.3X5-	T42.3X6-
Butallylonal	T42.3X1-	T42.3X2-	T42.3X3-	T42.3X4-	T42.3X5-	T42.3X6-
Butamben	T41.3X1-	T41.3X2-	T41.3X3-	T41.3X4-	T41.3X5-	T41.3X6-
Butamirate	T48.3X1-	T48.3X2-	T48.3X3-	T48.3X4-	T48.3X5-	T48.3X6-
Butane (distributed in mobile container)	T59.891-	T59.892-	T59.893-	T59.894-	-	-
distributed through pipes	T59.891-	T59.892-	T59.893-	T59.894-	-	-
incomplete combustion	T58.11X-	T58.12X-	T58.13X-	T58.14X-	-	-
Butanilicaine	T41.3X1-	T41.3X2-	T41.3X3-	T41.3X4-	T41.3X5-	T41.3X6-
Butanol	T51.3X1-	T51.3X2-	T51.3X3-	T51.3X4-	-	-
Butanone, 2-butanone	T52.4X1-	T52.4X2-	T52.4X3-	T52.4X4-	-	-
Butantrone	T49.4X1-	T49.4X2-	T49.4X3-	T49.4X4-	T49.4X5-	T49.4X6-
Butaperazine	T43.3X1-	T43.3X2-	T43.3X3-	T43.3X4-	T43.3X5-	T43.3X6-
Butazolidin	T39.2X1-	T39.2X2-	T39.2X3-	T39.2X4-	T39.2X5-	T39.2X6-
Butetamate	T48.6X1-	T48.6X2-	T48.6X3-	T48.6X4-	T48.6X5-	T48.6X6-
Butethal	T42.3X1-	T42.3X2-	T42.3X3-	T42.3X4-	T42.3X5-	T42.3X6-
Butethamate	T44.3X1-	T44.3X2-	T44.3X3-	T44.3X4-	T44.3X5-	T44.3X6-
Buthalitone (sodium)	T41.1X1-	T41.1X2-	T41.1X3-	T41.1X4-	T41.1X5-	T41.1X6-
Butisol (sodium)	T42.3X1-	T42.3X2-	T42.3X3-	T42.3X4-	T42.3X5-	T42.3X6-
Butizide	T50.2X1-	T50.2X2-	T50.2X3-	T50.2X4-	T50.2X5-	T50.2X6-
Butobarbital	T42.3X1-	T42.3X2-	T42.3X3-	T42.3X4-	T42.3X5-	T42.3X6-
sodium	T42.3X1-	T42.3X2-	T42.3X3-	T42.3X4-	T42.3X5-	T42.3X6-
Butobarbitone	T42.3X1-	T42.3X2-	T42.3X3-	T42.3X4-	T42.3X5-	T42.3X6-

Substance	Poisoning Accidental (unintentional)	Poisoning Intentional self-harm	Poisoning Assault	Poisoning Undetermined	Adverse effect	Underdosing
Butoconazole (nitrate)	T49.0X1-	T49.0X2-	T49.0X3-	T49.0X4-	T49.0X5-	T49.0X6-
Butorphanol	T40.491-	T40.492-	T40.493-	T40.494-	T40.495-	T40.496-
Butriptyline	T43.011-	T43.012-	T43.013-	T43.014-	T43.015-	T43.016-
Butropium bromide	T44.3X1-	T44.3X2-	T44.3X3-	T44.3X4-	T44.3X5-	T44.3X6-
Butter of antimony — *see Antimony*						
Buttercups	T62.2X1-	T62.2X2-	T62.2X3-	T62.2X4-	-	-
Butyl						
acetate (secondary)	T52.8X1-	T52.8X2-	T52.8X3-	T52.8X4-	-	-
alcohol	T51.3X1-	T51.3X2-	T51.3X3-	T51.3X4-	-	-
aminobenzoate	T41.3X1-	T41.3X2-	T41.3X3-	T41.3X4-	T41.3X5-	T41.3X6-
butyrate	T52.8X1-	T52.8X2-	T52.8X3-	T52.8X4-	-	-
carbinol	T51.3X1-	T51.3X2-	T51.3X3-	T51.3X4-	-	-
carbitol	T52.3X1-	T52.3X2-	T52.3X3-	T52.3X4-	-	-
cellosolve	T52.3X1-	T52.3X2-	T52.3X3-	T52.3X4-	-	-
chloral (hydrate)	T42.6X1-	T42.6X2-	T42.6X3-	T42.6X4-	T42.6X5-	T42.6X6-
formate	T52.8X1-	T52.8X2-	T52.8X3-	T52.8X4-	-	-
lactate	T52.8X1-	T52.8X2-	T52.8X3-	T52.8X4-	-	-
propionate	T52.8X1-	T52.8X2-	T52.8X3-	T52.8X4-	-	-
scopolamine bromide	T44.3X1-	T44.3X2-	T44.3X3-	T44.3X4-	T44.3X5-	T44.3X6-
thiobarbital sodium	T41.1X1-	T41.1X2-	T41.1X3-	T41.1X4-	T41.1X5-	T41.1X6-
Butylated hydroxy-anisole	T50.991-	T50.992-	T50.993-	T50.994-	T50.995-	T50.996-
Butylchloral hydrate	T42.6X1-	T42.6X2-	T42.6X3-	T42.6X4-	T42.6X5-	T42.6X6-
Butyltoluene	T52.2X1-	T52.2X2-	T52.2X3-	T52.2X4-	-	-
Butyn	T41.3X1-	T41.3X2-	T41.3X3-	T41.3X4-	T41.3X5-	T41.3X6-
Butyrophenone (-based tranquilizers)	T43.4X1-	T43.4X2-	T43.4X3-	T43.4X4-	T43.4X5-	T43.4X6-
Cabergoline	T42.8X1-	T42.8X2-	T42.8X3-	T42.8X4-	T42.8X5-	T42.8X6-
Cacodyl, cacodylic acid	T57.0X1-	T57.0X2-	T57.0X3-	T57.0X4-	-	-
Cactinomycin	T45.1X1-	T45.1X2-	T45.1X3-	T45.1X4-	T45.1X5-	T45.1X6-
Cade oil	T49.4X1-	T49.4X2-	T49.4X3-	T49.4X4-	T49.4X5-	T49.4X6-
Cadexomer iodine	T49.0X1-	T49.0X2-	T49.0X3-	T49.0X4-	T49.0X5-	T49.0X6-
Cadmium (chloride) (fumes) (oxide)	T56.3X1-	T56.3X2-	T56.3X3-	T56.3X4-	-	-
sulfide (medicinal) NEC	T49.4X1-	T49.4X2-	T49.4X3-	T49.4X4-	T49.4X5-	T49.4X6-
Cadralazine	T46.5X1-	T46.5X2-	T46.5X3-	T46.5X4-	T46.5X5-	T46.5X6-
Caffeine	T43.611-	T43.612-	T43.613-	T43.614-	T43.615-	T43.616-
Calabar bean	T62.2X1-	T62.2X2-	T62.2X3-	T62.2X4-	-	-
Caladium seguinum	T62.2X1-	T62.2X2-	T62.2X3-	T62.2X4-	-	-
Calamine (lotion)	T49.3X1-	T49.3X2-	T49.3X3-	T49.3X4-	T49.3X5-	T49.3X6-
Calcifediol	T45.2X1-	T45.2X2-	T45.2X3-	T45.2X4-	T45.2X5-	T45.2X6-
Calciferol	T45.2X1-	T45.2X2-	T45.2X3-	T45.2X4-	T45.2X5-	T45.2X6-
Calcitonin	T50.991-	T50.992-	T50.993-	T50.994-	T50.995-	T50.996-
Calcitriol	T45.2X1-	T45.2X2-	T45.2X3-	T45.2X4-	T45.2X5-	T45.2X6-
Calcium	T50.3X1-	T50.3X2-	T50.3X3-	T50.3X4-	T50.3X5-	T50.3X6-
actylsalicylate	T39.011-	T39.012-	T39.013-	T39.014-	T39.015-	T39.016-
benzamidosalicylate	T37.1X1-	T37.1X2-	T37.1X3-	T37.1X4-	T37.1X5-	T37.1X6-
bromide	T42.6X1-	T42.6X2-	T42.6X3-	T42.6X4-	T42.6X5-	T42.6X6-
bromolactobionate	T42.6X1-	T42.6X2-	T42.6X3-	T42.6X4-	T42.6X5-	T42.6X6-
carbaspirin	T39.011-	T39.012-	T39.013-	T39.014-	T39.015-	T39.016-
carbimide	T50.6X1-	T50.6X2-	T50.6X3-	T50.6X4-	T50.6X5-	T50.6X6-
carbonate	T47.1X1-	T47.1X2-	T47.1X3-	T47.1X4-	T47.1X5-	T47.1X6-
chloride	T50.991-	T50.992-	T50.993-	T50.994-	T50.995-	T50.996-
anhydrous	T50.991-	T50.992-	T50.993-	T50.994-	T50.995-	T50.996-
cyanide	T57.8X1-	T57.8X2-	T57.8X3-	T57.8X4-	-	-
dioctyl sulfosuccinate	T47.4X1-	T47.4X2-	T47.4X3-	T47.4X4-	T47.4X5-	T47.4X6-
disodium edathamil	T45.8X1-	T45.8X2-	T45.8X3-	T45.8X4-	T45.8X5-	T45.8X6-
disodium edetate	T45.8X1-	T45.8X2-	T45.8X3-	T45.8X4-	T45.8X5-	T45.8X6-
dobesilate	T46.991-	T46.992-	T46.993-	T46.994-	T46.995-	T46.996-
EDTA	T45.8X1-	T45.8X2-	T45.8X3-	T45.8X4-	T45.8X5-	T45.8X6-
ferrous citrate	T45.4X1-	T45.4X2-	T45.4X3-	T45.4X4-	T45.4X5-	T45.4X6-
folinate	T45.8X1-	T45.8X2-	T45.8X3-	T45.8X4-	T45.8X5-	T45.8X6-

Substance	Poisoning Accidental (unintentional)	Poisoning Intentional self-harm	Poisoning Assault	Poisoning Undetermined	Adverse effect	Underdosing
Calcium (continued)						
glubionate	T50.3X1-	T50.3X2-	T50.3X3-	T50.3X4-	T50.3X5-	T50.3X6-
gluconate	T50.3X1-	T50.3X2-	T50.3X3-	T50.3X4-	T50.3X5-	T50.3X6-
gluconogalactogluc-onate	T50.3X1-	T50.3X2-	T50.3X3-	T50.3X4-	T50.3X5-	T50.3X6-
hydrate, hydroxide	T54.3X1-	T54.3X2-	T54.3X3-	T54.3X4-	-	-
hypochlorite	T54.3X1-	T54.3X2-	T54.3X3-	T54.3X4-	-	-
iodide	T48.4X1-	T48.4X2-	T48.4X3-	T48.4X4-	T48.4X5-	T48.4X6-
ipodate	T50.8X1-	T50.8X2-	T50.8X3-	T50.8X4-	T50.8X5-	T50.8X6-
lactate	T50.3X1-	T50.3X2-	T50.3X3-	T50.3X4-	T50.3X5-	T50.3X6-
leucovorin	T45.8X1-	T45.8X2-	T45.8X3-	T45.8X4-	T45.8X5-	T45.8X6-
mandelate	T37.91X-	T37.92X-	T37.93X-	T37.94X-	T37.95X-	T37.96X-
oxide	T54.3X1-	T54.3X2-	T54.3X3-	T54.3X4-	-	-
pantothenate	T45.2X1-	T45.2X2-	T45.2X3-	T45.2X4-	T45.2X5-	T45.2X6-
phosphate	T50.3X1-	T50.3X2-	T50.3X3-	T50.3X4-	T50.3X5-	T50.3X6-
salicylate	T39.091-	T39.092-	T39.093-	T39.094-	T39.095-	T39.096-
salts	T50.3X1-	T50.3X2-	T50.3X3-	T50.3X4-	T50.3X5-	T50.3X6-
Calculus-dissolving drug	T50.991-	T50.992-	T50.993-	T50.994-	T50.995-	T50.996-
Calomel	T49.0X1-	T49.0X2-	T49.0X3-	T49.0X4-	T49.0X5-	T49.0X6-
Caloric agent	T50.3X1-	T50.3X2-	T50.3X3-	T50.3X4-	T50.3X5-	T50.3X6-
Calusterone	T38.7X1-	T38.7X2-	T38.7X3-	T38.7X4-	T38.7X5-	T38.7X6-
Camazepam	T42.4X1-	T42.4X2-	T42.4X3-	T42.4X4-	T42.4X5-	T42.4X6-
Camomile	T49.0X1-	T49.0X2-	T49.0X3-	T49.0X4-	T49.0X5-	T49.0X6-
Camoquin	T37.2X1-	T37.2X2-	T37.2X3-	T37.2X4-	T37.2X5-	T37.2X6-
Camphor						
insecticide	T60.2X1-	T60.2X2-	T60.2X3-	T60.2X4-	-	-
medicinal	T49.8X1-	T49.8X2-	T49.8X3-	T49.8X4-	T49.8X5-	T49.8X6-
Camylofin	T44.3X1-	T44.3X2-	T44.3X3-	T44.3X4-	T44.3X5-	T44.3X6-
Cancer chemotherapy drug regimen	T45.1X1-	T45.1X2-	T45.1X3-	T45.1X4-	T45.1X5-	T45.1X6-
Candeptin	T49.0X1-	T49.0X2-	T49.0X3-	T49.0X4-	T49.0X5-	T49.0X6-
Candicidin	T49.0X1-	T49.0X2-	T49.0X3-	T49.0X4-	T49.0X5-	T49.0X6-
Cannabinoids, synthetic	T40.721-	T40.722-	T40.723-	T40.724-	T40.725-	T40.726-
Cannabinol	T40.711-	T40.712-	T40.713-	T40.714-	T40.715-	T40.716-
Cannabis (derivatives)	T40.711-	T40.712-	T40.713-	T40.714-	T40.715-	T40.716-
Canned heat	T51.1X1-	T51.1X2-	T51.1X3-	T51.1X4-	-	-
Canrenoic acid	T50.0X1-	T50.0X2-	T50.0X3-	T50.0X4-	T50.0X5-	T50.0X6-
Canrenone	T50.0X1-	T50.0X2-	T50.0X3-	T50.0X4-	T50.0X5-	T50.0X6-
Cantharides, cantharidin, cantharis	T49.8X1-	T49.8X2-	T49.8X3-	T49.8X4-	T49.8X5-	T49.8X6-
Canthaxanthin	T50.991-	T50.992-	T50.993-	T50.994-	T50.995-	T50.996-
Capillary-active drug NEC	T46.901-	T46.902-	T46.903-	T46.904-	T46.905-	T46.906-
Capreomycin	T36.8X1-	T36.8X2-	T36.8X3-	T36.8X4-	T36.8X5-	T36.8X6-
Capsicum	T49.4X1-	T49.4X2-	T49.4X3-	T49.4X4-	T49.4X5-	T49.4X6-
Captafol	T60.3X1-	T60.3X2-	T60.3X3-	T60.3X4-	-	-
Captan	T60.3X1-	T60.3X2-	T60.3X3-	T60.3X4-	-	-
Captodiame, captodiamine	T43.591-	T43.592-	T43.593-	T43.594-	T43.595-	T43.596-
Captopril	T46.4X1-	T46.4X2-	T46.4X3-	T46.4X4-	T46.4X5-	T46.4X6-
Caramiphen	T44.3X1-	T44.3X2-	T44.3X3-	T44.3X4-	T44.3X5-	T44.3X6-
Carazolol	T44.7X1-	T44.7X2-	T44.7X3-	T44.7X4-	T44.7X5-	T44.7X6-
Carbachol	T44.1X1-	T44.1X2-	T44.1X3-	T44.1X4-	T44.1X5-	T44.1X6-
Carbacrylamine (resin)	T50.3X1-	T50.3X2-	T50.3X3-	T50.3X4-	T50.3X5-	T50.3X6-
Carbamate (insecticide)	T60.0X1-	T60.0X2-	T60.0X3-	T60.0X4-	-	-
Carbamate (sedative)	T42.6X1-	T42.6X2-	T42.6X3-	T42.6X4-	T42.6X5-	T42.6X6-
herbicide	T60.0X1-	T60.0X2-	T60.0X3-	T60.0X4-	-	-
insecticide	T60.0X1-	T60.0X2-	T60.0X3-	T60.0X4-	-	-
Carbamazepine	T42.1X1-	T42.1X2-	T42.1X3-	T42.1X4-	T42.1X5-	T42.1X6-
Carbamide	T47.3X1-	T47.3X2-	T47.3X3-	T47.3X4-	T47.3X5-	T47.3X6-
peroxide	T49.0X1-	T49.0X2-	T49.0X3-	T49.0X4-	T49.0X5-	T49.0X6-
topical	T49.8X1-	T49.8X2-	T49.8X3-	T49.8X4-	T49.8X5-	T49.8X6-
Carbamylcholine chloride	T44.1X1-	T44.1X2-	T44.1X3-	T44.1X4-	T44.1X5-	T44.1X6-
Carbaril	T60.0X1-	T60.0X2-	T60.0X3-	T60.0X4-	-	-

Substance	Poisoning Accidental (unintentional)	Poisoning Intentional self-harm	Poisoning Assault	Poisoning Undetermined	Adverse effect	Underdosing
Carbarsone	T37.3X1-	T37.3X2-	T37.3X3-	T37.3X4-	T37.3X5-	T37.3X6-
Carbaryl	T60.0X1-	T60.0X2-	T60.0X3-	T60.0X4-	-	-
Carbaspirin	T39.011-	T39.012-	T39.013-	T39.014-	T39.015-	T39.016-
Carbazochrome (salicylate) (sodium sulfonate)	T49.4X1-	T49.4X2-	T49.4X3-	T49.4X4-	T49.4X5-	T49.4X6-
Carbenicillin	T36.0X1-	T36.0X2-	T36.0X3-	T36.0X4-	T36.0X5-	T36.0X6-
Carbenoxolone	T47.1X1-	T47.1X2-	T47.1X3-	T47.1X4-	T47.1X5-	T47.1X6-
Carbetapentane	T48.3X1-	T48.3X2-	T48.3X3-	T48.3X4-	T48.3X5-	T48.3X6-
Carbethyl salicylate	T39.091-	T39.092-	T39.093-	T39.094-	T39.095-	T39.096-
Carbidopa (with levodopa)	T42.8X1-	T42.8X2-	T42.8X3-	T42.8X4-	T42.8X5-	T42.8X6-
Carbimazole	T38.2X1-	T38.2X2-	T38.2X3-	T38.2X4-	T38.2X5-	T38.2X6-
Carbinol	T51.1X1-	T51.1X2-	T51.1X3-	T51.1X4-	-	-
Carbinoxamine	T45.0X1-	T45.0X2-	T45.0X3-	T45.0X4-	T45.0X5-	T45.0X6-
Carbiphene	T39.8X1-	T39.8X2-	T39.8X3-	T39.8X4-	T39.8X5-	T39.8X6-
Carbitol	T52.3X1-	T52.3X2-	T52.3X3-	T52.3X4-	-	-
Carbo medicinalis	T47.6X1-	T47.6X2-	T47.6X3-	T47.6X4-	T47.6X5-	T47.6X6-
Carbocaine	T41.3X1-	T41.3X2-	T41.3X3-	T41.3X4-	T41.3X5-	T41.3X6-
infiltration (subcutaneous)	T41.3X1-	T41.3X2-	T41.3X3-	T41.3X4-	T41.3X5-	T41.3X6-
nerve block (peripheral) (plexus)	T41.3X1-	T41.3X2-	T41.3X3-	T41.3X4-	T41.3X5-	T41.3X6-
topical (surface)	T41.3X1-	T41.3X2-	T41.3X3-	T41.3X4-	T41.3X5-	T41.3X6-
Carbocisteine	T48.4X1-	T48.4X2-	T48.4X3-	T48.4X4-	T48.4X5-	T48.4X6-
Carbocromen	T46.3X1-	T46.3X2-	T46.3X3-	T46.3X4-	T46.3X5-	T46.3X6-
Carbol fuchsin	T49.0X1-	T49.0X2-	T49.0X3-	T49.0X4-	T49.0X5-	T49.0X6-
Carbolic acid — *see also Phenol*	T54.0X1-	T54.0X2-	T54.0X3-	T54.0X4-	-	-
Carbolonium (bromide)	T48.1X1-	T48.1X2-	T48.1X3-	T48.1X4-	T48.1X5-	T48.1X6-
Carbomycin	T36.8X1-	T36.8X2-	T36.8X3-	T36.8X4-	T36.8X5-	T36.8X6-
Carbon						
bisulfide (liquid)	T65.4X1-	T65.4X2-	T65.4X3-	T65.4X4-	-	-
vapor	T65.4X1-	T65.4X2-	T65.4X3-	T65.4X4-	-	-
dioxide (gas)	T59.7X1-	T59.7X2-	T59.7X3-	T59.7X4-	-	-
medicinal	T41.5X1-	T41.5X2-	T41.5X3-	T41.5X4-	T41.5X5-	T41.5X6-
nonmedicinal	T59.7X1-	T59.7X2-	T59.7X3-	T59.7X4-	-	-
snow	T49.4X1-	T49.4X2-	T49.4X3-	T49.4X4-	T49.4X5-	T49.4X6-
disulfide (liquid)	T65.4X1-	T65.4X2-	T65.4X3-	T65.4X4-	-	-
vapor	T65.4X1-	T65.4X2-	T65.4X3-	T65.4X4-	-	-
monoxide (from incomplete combustion)	T58.91X-	T58.92X-	T58.93X-	T58.94X-	-	-
blast furnace gas	T58.8X1-	T58.8X2-	T58.8X3-	T58.8X4-	-	-
butane (distributed in mobile container)	T58.11X-	T58.12X-	T58.13X-	T58.14X-	-	-
distributed through pipes	T58.11X-	T58.12X-	T58.13X-	T58.14X-	-	-
charcoal fumes	T58.2X1-	T58.2X2-	T58.2X3-	T58.2X4-	-	-
coal	T58.2X1-	T58.2X2-	T58.2X3-	T58.2X4-	-	-
coke (in domestic stoves, fireplaces)	T58.2X1-	T58.2X2-	T58.2X3-	T58.2X4-	-	-
gas (piped)	T58.11X-	T58.12X-	T58.13X-	T58.14X-	-	-
solid (in domestic stoves, fireplaces)	T58.2X1-	T58.2X2-	T58.2X3-	T58.2X4-	-	-
exhaust gas (motor) not in transit	T58.01X-	T58.02X-	T58.03X-	T58.04X-	-	-
combustion engine, any not in watercraft	T58.01X-	T58.02X-	T58.03X-	T58.04X-	-	-
farm tractor, not in transit	T58.01X-	T58.02X-	T58.03X-	T58.04X-	-	-
gas engine	T58.01X-	T58.02X-	T58.03X-	T58.04X-	-	-
motor pump	T58.01X-	T58.02X-	T58.03X-	T58.04X-	-	-
motor vehicle, not in transit	T58.01X-	T58.02X-	T58.03X-	T58.04X-	-	-
fuel (in domestic use)	T58.2X1-	T58.2X2-	T58.2X3-	T58.2X4-	-	-
gas (piped)	T58.11X-	T58.12X-	T58.13X-	T58.14X-	-	-
in mobile container	T58.11X-	T58.12X-	T58.13X-	T58.14X-	-	-
piped (natural)	T58.11X-	T58.12X-	T58.13X-	T58.14X-	-	-
utility	T58.11X-	T58.12X-	T58.13X-	T58.14X-	-	-
in mobile container	T58.11X-	T58.12X-	T58.13X-	T58.14X-	-	-
illuminating gas	T58.11X-	T58.12X-	T58.13X-	T58.14X-	-	-

CARBARSONE - CARBON

Substance	Poisoning Accidental (unintentional)	Poisoning Intentional self-harm	Poisoning Assault	Poisoning Undetermined	Adverse effect	Underdosing
Carbon (continued)						
industrial fuels or gases, any	T58.8X1-	T58.8X2-	T58.8X3-	T58.8X4-	-	-
kerosene (in domestic stoves, fireplaces)	T58.2X1-	T58.2X2-	T58.2X3-	T58.2X4-	-	-
kiln gas or vapor	T58.8X1-	T58.8X2-	T58.8X3-	T58.8X4-	-	-
motor exhaust gas, not in transit	T58.01X-	T58.02X-	T58.03X-	T58.04X-	-	-
piped gas (manufactured) (natural)	T58.11X-	T58.12X-	T58.13X-	T58.14X-	-	-
producer gas	T58.8X1-	T58.8X2-	T58.8X3-	T58.8X4-	-	-
propane (distributed in mobile container)	T58.11X-	T58.12X-	T58.13X-	T58.14X-	-	-
distributed through pipes	T58.11X-	T58.12X-	T58.13X-	T58.14X-	-	-
specified source NEC	T58.8X1-	T58.8X2-	T58.8X3-	T58.8X4-	-	-
stove gas	T58.11X-	T58.12X-	T58.13X-	T58.14X-	-	-
piped	T58.11X-	T58.12X-	T58.13X-	T58.14X-	-	-
utility gas	T58.11X-	T58.12X-	T58.13X-	T58.14X-	-	-
piped	T58.11X-	T58.12X-	T58.13X-	T58.14X-	-	-
water gas	T58.11X-	T58.12X-	T58.13X-	T58.14X-	-	-
wood (in domestic stoves, fireplaces)	T58.2X1-	T58.2X2-	T58.2X3-	T58.2X4-	-	-
tetrachloride (vapor) NEC	T53.0X1-	T53.0X2-	T53.0X3-	T53.0X4-	-	-
liquid (cleansing agent) NEC	T53.0X1-	T53.0X2-	T53.0X3-	T53.0X4-	-	-
solvent	T53.0X1-	T53.0X2-	T53.0X3-	T53.0X4-	-	-
Carbonic acid gas	T59.7X1-	T59.7X2-	T59.7X3-	T59.7X4-	-	-
anhydrase inhibitor NEC	T50.2X1-	T50.2X2-	T50.2X3-	T50.2X4-	T50.2X5-	T50.2X6-
Carbophenothion	T60.0X1-	T60.0X2-	T60.0X3-	T60.0X4-	-	-
Carboplatin	T45.1X1-	T45.1X2-	T45.1X3-	T45.1X4-	T45.1X5-	T45.1X6-
Carboprost	T48.0X1-	T48.0X2-	T48.0X3-	T48.0X4-	T48.0X5-	T48.0X6-
Carboquone	T45.1X1-	T45.1X2-	T45.1X3-	T45.1X4-	T45.1X5-	T45.1X6-
Carbowax	T49.3X1-	T49.3X2-	T49.3X3-	T49.3X4-	T49.3X5-	T49.3X6-
Carboxymethyl-cellulose	T47.4X1-	T47.4X2-	T47.4X3-	T47.4X4-	T47.4X5-	T47.4X6-
S-Carboxymethyl-cysteine	T48.4X1-	T48.4X2-	T48.4X3-	T48.4X4-	T48.4X5-	T48.4X6-
Carbrital	T42.3X1-	T42.3X2-	T42.3X3-	T42.3X4-	T42.3X5-	T42.3X6-
Carbromal	T42.6X1-	T42.6X2-	T42.6X3-	T42.6X4-	T42.6X5-	T42.6X6-
Carbutamide	T38.3X1-	T38.3X2-	T38.3X3-	T38.3X4-	T38.3X5-	T38.3X6-
Carbuterol	T48.6X1-	T48.6X2-	T48.6X3-	T48.6X4-	T48.6X5-	T48.6X6-
Cardiac						
depressants	T46.2X1-	T46.2X2-	T46.2X3-	T46.2X4-	T46.2X5-	T46.2X6-
rhythm regulator	T46.2X1-	T46.2X2-	T46.2X3-	T46.2X4-	T46.2X5-	T46.2X6-
specified NEC	T46.2X1-	T46.2X2-	T46.2X3-	T46.2X4-	T46.2X5-	T46.2X6-
Cardiografin	T50.8X1-	T50.8X2-	T50.8X3-	T50.8X4-	T50.8X5-	T50.8X6-
Cardio-green	T50.8X1-	T50.8X2-	T50.8X3-	T50.8X4-	T50.8X5-	T50.8X6-
Cardiotonic (glycoside) NEC	T46.0X1-	T46.0X2-	T46.0X3-	T46.0X4-	T46.0X5-	T46.0X6-
Cardiovascular drug NEC	T46.901-	T46.902-	T46.903-	T46.904-	T46.905-	T46.906-
Cardrase	T50.2X1-	T50.2X2-	T50.2X3-	T50.2X4-	T50.2X5-	T50.2X6-
Carfecillin	T36.0X1-	T36.0X2-	T36.0X3-	T36.0X4-	T36.0X5-	T36.0X6-
Carfenazine	T43.3X1-	T43.3X2-	T43.3X3-	T43.3X4-	T43.3X5-	T43.3X6-
Carfusin	T49.0X1-	T49.0X2-	T49.0X3-	T49.0X4-	T49.0X5-	T49.0X6-
Carindacillin	T36.0X1-	T36.0X2-	T36.0X3-	T36.0X4-	T36.0X5-	T36.0X6-
Carisoprodol	T42.8X1-	T42.8X2-	T42.8X3-	T42.8X4-	T42.8X5-	T42.8X6-
Carmellose	T47.4X1-	T47.4X2-	T47.4X3-	T47.4X4-	T47.4X5-	T47.4X6-
Carminative	T47.5X1-	T47.5X2-	T47.5X3-	T47.5X4-	T47.5X5-	T47.5X6-
Carmofur	T45.1X1-	T45.1X2-	T45.1X3-	T45.1X4-	T45.1X5-	T45.1X6-
Carmustine	T45.1X1-	T45.1X2-	T45.1X3-	T45.1X4-	T45.1X5-	T45.1X6-
Carotene	T45.2X1-	T45.2X2-	T45.2X3-	T45.2X4-	T45.2X5-	T45.2X6-
Carphenazine	T43.3X1-	T43.3X2-	T43.3X3-	T43.3X4-	T43.3X5-	T43.3X6-
Carpipramine	T42.4X1-	T42.4X2-	T42.4X3-	T42.4X4-	T42.4X5-	T42.4X6-
Carprofen	T39.311-	T39.312-	T39.313-	T39.314-	T39.315-	T39.316-
Carpronium chloride	T44.3X1-	T44.3X2-	T44.3X3-	T44.3X4-	T44.3X5-	T44.3X6-
Carrageenan	T47.8X1-	T47.8X2-	T47.8X3-	T47.8X4-	T47.8X5-	T47.8X6-
Carteolol	T44.7X1-	T44.7X2-	T44.7X3-	T44.7X4-	T44.7X5-	T44.7X6-
Carter's Little Pills	T47.2X1-	T47.2X2-	T47.2X3-	T47.2X4-	T47.2X5-	T47.2X6-

Substance	Poisoning Accidental (unintentional)	Poisoning Intentional self-harm	Poisoning Assault	Poisoning Undetermined	Adverse effect	Underdosing
Cascara (sagrada)	T47.2X1-	T47.2X2-	T47.2X3-	T47.2X4-	T47.2X5-	T47.2X6-
Cassava	T62.2X1-	T62.2X2-	T62.2X3-	T62.2X4-	-	-
Castellani's paint	T49.0X1-	T49.0X2-	T49.0X3-	T49.0X4-	T49.0X5-	T49.0X6-
Castor						
bean	T62.2X1-	T62.2X2-	T62.2X3-	T62.2X4-	-	-
oil	T47.2X1-	T47.2X2-	T47.2X3-	T47.2X4-	T47.2X5-	T47.2X6-
Catalase	T45.3X1-	T45.3X2-	T45.3X3-	T45.3X4-	T45.3X5-	T45.3X6-
Caterpillar (sting)	T63.431-	T63.432-	T63.433-	T63.434-	-	-
Catha (edulis) (tea)	T43.691-	T43.692-	T43.693-	T43.694-	-	-
Cathartic NEC	T47.4X1-	T47.4X2-	T47.4X3-	T47.4X4-	T47.4X5-	T47.4X6-
anthacene derivative	T47.2X1-	T47.2X2-	T47.2X3-	T47.2X4-	T47.2X5-	T47.2X6-
bulk	T47.4X1-	T47.4X2-	T47.4X3-	T47.4X4-	T47.4X5-	T47.4X6-
contact	T47.2X1-	T47.2X2-	T47.2X3-	T47.2X4-	T47.2X5-	T47.2X6-
emollient NEC	T47.4X1-	T47.4X2-	T47.4X3-	T47.4X4-	T47.4X5-	T47.4X6-
irritant NEC	T47.2X1-	T47.2X2-	T47.2X3-	T47.2X4-	T47.2X5-	T47.2X6-
mucilage	T47.4X1-	T47.4X2-	T47.4X3-	T47.4X4-	T47.4X5-	T47.4X6-
saline	T47.3X1-	T47.3X2-	T47.3X3-	T47.3X4-	T47.3X5-	T47.3X6-
vegetable	T47.2X1-	T47.2X2-	T47.2X3-	T47.2X4-	T47.2X5-	T47.2X6-
Cathine	T50.5X1-	T50.5X2-	T50.5X3-	T50.5X4-	T50.5X5-	T50.5X6-
Cathomycin	T36.8X1-	T36.8X2-	T36.8X3-	T36.8X4-	T36.8X5-	T36.8X6-
Cation exchange resin	T50.3X1-	T50.3X2-	T50.3X3-	T50.3X4-	T50.3X5-	T50.3X6-
Caustic (s) NEC	T54.91X-	T54.92X-	T54.93X-	T54.94X-	-	-
alkali	T54.3X1-	T54.3X2-	T54.3X3-	T54.3X4-	-	-
hydroxide	T54.3X1-	T54.3X2-	T54.3X3-	T54.3X4-	-	-
potash	T54.3X1-	T54.3X2-	T54.3X3-	T54.3X4-	-	-
soda	T54.3X1-	T54.3X2-	T54.3X3-	T54.3X4-	-	-
specified NEC	T54.91X-	T54.92X-	T54.93X-	T54.94X-	-	-
Ceepryn	T49.0X1-	T49.0X2-	T49.0X3-	T49.0X4-	T49.0X5-	T49.0X6-
ENT agent	T49.6X1-	T49.6X2-	T49.6X3-	T49.6X4-	T49.6X5-	T49.6X6-
lozenges	T49.6X1-	T49.6X2-	T49.6X3-	T49.6X4-	T49.6X5-	T49.6X6-
Cefacetrile	T36.1X1-	T36.1X2-	T36.1X3-	T36.1X4-	T36.1X5-	T36.1X6-
Cefaclor	T36.1X1-	T36.1X2-	T36.1X3-	T36.1X4-	T36.1X5-	T36.1X6-
Cefadroxil	T36.1X1-	T36.1X2-	T36.1X3-	T36.1X4-	T36.1X5-	T36.1X6-
Cefalexin	T36.1X1-	T36.1X2-	T36.1X3-	T36.1X4-	T36.1X5-	T36.1X6-
Cefaloglycin	T36.1X1-	T36.1X2-	T36.1X3-	T36.1X4-	T36.1X5-	T36.1X6-
Cefaloridine	T36.1X1-	T36.1X2-	T36.1X3-	T36.1X4-	T36.1X5-	T36.1X6-
Cefalosporins	T36.1X1-	T36.1X2-	T36.1X3-	T36.1X4-	T36.1X5-	T36.1X6-
Cefalotin	T36.1X1-	T36.1X2-	T36.1X3-	T36.1X4-	T36.1X5-	T36.1X6-
Cefamandole	T36.1X1-	T36.1X2-	T36.1X3-	T36.1X4-	T36.1X5-	T36.1X6-
Cefamycin antibiotic	T36.1X1-	T36.1X2-	T36.1X3-	T36.1X4-	T36.1X5-	T36.1X6-
Cefapirin	T36.1X1-	T36.1X2-	T36.1X3-	T36.1X4-	T36.1X5-	T36.1X6-
Cefatrizine	T36.1X1-	T36.1X2-	T36.1X3-	T36.1X4-	T36.1X5-	T36.1X6-
Cefazedone	T36.1X1-	T36.1X2-	T36.1X3-	T36.1X4-	T36.1X5-	T36.1X6-
Cefazolin	T36.1X1-	T36.1X2-	T36.1X3-	T36.1X4-	T36.1X5-	T36.1X6-
Cefbuperazone	T36.1X1-	T36.1X2-	T36.1X3-	T36.1X4-	T36.1X5-	T36.1X6-
Cefetamet	T36.1X1-	T36.1X2-	T36.1X3-	T36.1X4-	T36.1X5-	T36.1X6-
Cefixime	T36.1X1-	T36.1X2-	T36.1X3-	T36.1X4-	T36.1X5-	T36.1X6-
Cefmenoxime	T36.1X1-	T36.1X2-	T36.1X3-	T36.1X4-	T36.1X5-	T36.1X6-
Cefmetazole	T36.1X1-	T36.1X2-	T36.1X3-	T36.1X4-	T36.1X5-	T36.1X6-
Cefminox	T36.1X1-	T36.1X2-	T36.1X3-	T36.1X4-	T36.1X5-	T36.1X6-
Cefonicid	T36.1X1-	T36.1X2-	T36.1X3-	T36.1X4-	T36.1X5-	T36.1X6-
Cefoperazone	T36.1X1-	T36.1X2-	T36.1X3-	T36.1X4-	T36.1X5-	T36.1X6-
Ceforanide	T36.1X1-	T36.1X2-	T36.1X3-	T36.1X4-	T36.1X5-	T36.1X6-
Cefotaxime	T36.1X1-	T36.1X2-	T36.1X3-	T36.1X4-	T36.1X5-	T36.1X6-
Cefotetan	T36.1X1-	T36.1X2-	T36.1X3-	T36.1X4-	T36.1X5-	T36.1X6-
Cefotiam	T36.1X1-	T36.1X2-	T36.1X3-	T36.1X4-	T36.1X5-	T36.1X6-
Cefoxitin	T36.1X1-	T36.1X2-	T36.1X3-	T36.1X4-	T36.1X5-	T36.1X6-
Cefpimizole	T36.1X1-	T36.1X2-	T36.1X3-	T36.1X4-	T36.1X5-	T36.1X6-
Cefpiramide	T36.1X1-	T36.1X2-	T36.1X3-	T36.1X4-	T36.1X5-	T36.1X6-

Substance	Poisoning Accidental (unintentional)	Poisoning Intentional self-harm	Poisoning Assault	Poisoning Undetermined	Adverse effect	Underdosing
Cefradine	T36.1X1-	T36.1X2-	T36.1X3-	T36.1X4-	T36.1X5-	T36.1X6-
Cefroxadine	T36.1X1-	T36.1X2-	T36.1X3-	T36.1X4-	T36.1X5-	T36.1X6-
Cefsulodin	T36.1X1-	T36.1X2-	T36.1X3-	T36.1X4-	T36.1X5-	T36.1X6-
Ceftazidime	T36.1X1-	T36.1X2-	T36.1X3-	T36.1X4-	T36.1X5-	T36.1X6-
Cefteram	T36.1X1-	T36.1X2-	T36.1X3-	T36.1X4-	T36.1X5-	T36.1X6-
Ceftezole	T36.1X1-	T36.1X2-	T36.1X3-	T36.1X4-	T36.1X5-	T36.1X6-
Ceftizoxime	T36.1X1-	T36.1X2-	T36.1X3-	T36.1X4-	T36.1X5-	T36.1X6-
Ceftriaxone	T36.1X1-	T36.1X2-	T36.1X3-	T36.1X4-	T36.1X5-	T36.1X6-
Cefuroxime	T36.1X1-	T36.1X2-	T36.1X3-	T36.1X4-	T36.1X5-	T36.1X6-
Cefuzonam	T36.1X1-	T36.1X2-	T36.1X3-	T36.1X4-	T36.1X5-	T36.1X6-
Celestone	T38.0X1-	T38.0X2-	T38.0X3-	T38.0X4-	T38.0X5-	T38.0X6-
topical	T49.0X1-	T49.0X2-	T49.0X3-	T49.0X4-	T49.0X5-	T49.0X6-
Celiprolol	T44.7X1-	T44.7X2-	T44.7X3-	T44.7X4-	T44.7X5-	T44.7X6-
Cell stimulants and proliferants	T49.8X1-	T49.8X2-	T49.8X3-	T49.8X4-	T49.8X5-	T49.8X6-
Cellosolve	T52.91X-	T52.92X-	T52.93X-	T52.94X-	-	-
Cellulose						
cathartic	T47.4X1-	T47.4X2-	T47.4X3-	T47.4X4-	T47.4X5-	T47.4X6-
hydroxyethyl	T47.4X1-	T47.4X2-	T47.4X3-	T47.4X4-	T47.4X5-	T47.4X6-
nitrates (topical)	T49.3X1-	T49.3X2-	T49.3X3-	T49.3X4-	T49.3X5-	T49.3X6-
oxidized	T49.4X1-	T49.4X2-	T49.4X3-	T49.4X4-	T49.4X5-	T49.4X6-
Centipede (bite)	T63.411-	T63.412-	T63.413-	T63.414-	-	-
Central nervous system						
depressants	T42.71X-	T42.72X-	T42.73X-	T42.74X-	T42.75X-	T42.76X-
anesthetic (general) NEC	T41.201-	T41.202-	T41.203-	T41.204-	T41.205-	T41.206-
gases NEC	T41.0X1-	T41.0X2-	T41.0X3-	T41.0X4-	T41.0X5-	T41.0X6-
intravenous	T41.1X1-	T41.1X2-	T41.1X3-	T41.1X4-	T41.1X5-	T41.1X6-
barbiturates	T42.3X1-	T42.3X2-	T42.3X3-	T42.3X4-	T42.3X5-	T42.3X6-
benzodiazepines	T42.4X1-	T42.4X2-	T42.4X3-	T42.4X4-	T42.4X5-	T42.4X6-
bromides	T42.6X1-	T42.6X2-	T42.6X3-	T42.6X4-	T42.6X5-	T42.6X6-
cannabis sativa	T40.711-	T40.712-	T40.713-	T40.714-	T40.715-	T40.716-
chloral hydrate	T42.6X1-	T42.6X2-	T42.6X3-	T42.6X4-	T42.6X5-	T42.6X6-
ethanol	T51.0X1-	T51.0X2-	T51.0X3-	T51.0X4-	-	-
hallucinogenics	T40.901-	T40.902-	T40.903-	T40.904-	T40.905-	T40.906-
hypnotics	T42.71X-	T42.72X-	T42.73X-	T42.74X-	T42.75X-	T42.76X-
specified NEC	T42.6X1-	T42.6X2-	T42.6X3-	T42.6X4-	T42.6X5-	T42.6X6-
muscle relaxants	T42.8X1-	T42.8X2-	T42.8X3-	T42.8X4-	T42.8X5-	T42.8X6-
paraldehyde	T42.6X1-	T42.6X2-	T42.6X3-	T42.6X4-	T42.6X5-	T42.6X6-
sedatives; sedative-hypnotics	T42.71X-	T42.72X-	T42.73X-	T42.74X-	T42.75X-	T42.76X-
mixed NEC	T42.6X1-	T42.6X2-	T42.6X3-	T42.6X4-	T42.6X5-	T42.6X6-
specified NEC	T42.6X1-	T42.6X2-	T42.6X3-	T42.6X4-	T42.6X5-	T42.6X6-
muscle-tone depressants	T42.8X1-	T42.8X2-	T42.8X3-	T42.8X4-	T42.8X5-	T42.8X6-
stimulants	T43.601-	T43.602-	T43.603-	T43.604-	T43.605-	T43.606-
amphetamines	T43.621-	T43.622-	T43.623-	T43.624-	T43.625-	T43.626-
analeptics	T50.7X1-	T50.7X2-	T50.7X3-	T50.7X4-	T50.7X5-	T50.7X6-
antidepressants	T43.201-	T43.202-	T43.203-	T43.204-	T43.205-	T43.206-
opiate antagonists	T50.7X1-	T50.7X2-	T50.7X3-	T50.7X4-	T50.7X5-	T50.7X6-
specified NEC	T43.691-	T43.692-	T43.693-	T43.694-	T43.695-	T43.696-
Cephalexin	T36.1X1-	T36.1X2-	T36.1X3-	T36.1X4-	T36.1X5-	T36.1X6-
Cephaloglycin	T36.1X1-	T36.1X2-	T36.1X3-	T36.1X4-	T36.1X5-	T36.1X6-
Cephaloridine	T36.1X1-	T36.1X2-	T36.1X3-	T36.1X4-	T36.1X5-	T36.1X6-
Cephalosporins	T36.1X1-	T36.1X2-	T36.1X3-	T36.1X4-	T36.1X5-	T36.1X6-
N (adicillin)	T36.0X1-	T36.0X2-	T36.0X3-	T36.0X4-	T36.0X5-	T36.0X6-
Cephalothin	T36.1X1-	T36.1X2-	T36.1X3-	T36.1X4-	T36.1X5-	T36.1X6-
Cephalotin	T36.1X1-	T36.1X2-	T36.1X3-	T36.1X4-	T36.1X5-	T36.1X6-
Cephradine	T36.1X1-	T36.1X2-	T36.1X3-	T36.1X4-	T36.1X5-	T36.1X6-
Cerbera (odallam)	T62.2X1-	T62.2X2-	T62.2X3-	T62.2X4-	-	-
Cerberin	T46.0X1-	T46.0X2-	T46.0X3-	T46.0X4-	T46.0X5-	T46.0X6-

CEFRADINE - CERBERIN

Substance	Poisoning Accidental (unintentional)	Poisoning Intentional self-harm	Poisoning Assault	Poisoning Undetermined	Adverse effect	Underdosing
Cerebral stimulants	T43.601-	T43.602-	T43.603-	T43.604-	T43.605-	T43.606-
psychotherapeutic	T43.601-	T43.602-	T43.603-	T43.604-	T43.605-	T43.606-
specified NEC	T43.691-	T43.692-	T43.693-	T43.694-	T43.695-	T43.696-
Cerium oxalate	T45.0X1-	T45.0X2-	T45.0X3-	T45.0X4-	T45.0X5-	T45.0X6-
Cerous oxalate	T45.0X1-	T45.0X2-	T45.0X3-	T45.0X4-	T45.0X5-	T45.0X6-
Ceruletide	T50.8X1-	T50.8X2-	T50.8X3-	T50.8X4-	T50.8X5-	T50.8X6-
Cetalkonium (chloride)	T49.0X1-	T49.0X2-	T49.0X3-	T49.0X4-	T49.0X5-	T49.0X6-
Cethexonium chloride	T49.0X1-	T49.0X2-	T49.0X3-	T49.0X4-	T49.0X5-	T49.0X6-
Cetiedil	T46.7X1-	T46.7X2-	T46.7X3-	T46.7X4-	T46.7X5-	T46.7X6-
Cetirizine	T45.0X1-	T45.0X2-	T45.0X3-	T45.0X4-	T45.0X5-	T45.0X6-
Cetomacrogol	T50.991-	T50.992-	T50.993-	T50.994-	T50.995-	T50.996-
Cetotiamine	T45.2X1-	T45.2X2-	T45.2X3-	T45.2X4-	T45.2X5-	T45.2X6-
Cetoxime	T45.0X1-	T45.0X2-	T45.0X3-	T45.0X4-	T45.0X5-	T45.0X6-
Cetraxate	T47.1X1-	T47.1X2-	T47.1X3-	T47.1X4-	T47.1X5-	T47.1X6-
Cetrimide	T49.0X1-	T49.0X2-	T49.0X3-	T49.0X4-	T49.0X5-	T49.0X6-
Cetrimonium (bromide)	T49.0X1-	T49.0X2-	T49.0X3-	T49.0X4-	T49.0X5-	T49.0X6-
Cetylpyridinium chloride	T49.0X1-	T49.0X2-	T49.0X3-	T49.0X4-	T49.0X5-	T49.0X6-
ENT agent	T49.6X1-	T49.6X2-	T49.6X3-	T49.6X4-	T49.6X5-	T49.6X6-
lozenges	T49.6X1-	T49.6X2-	T49.6X3-	T49.6X4-	T49.6X5-	T49.6X6-
Cevadilla — *see Sabadilla*						
Cevitamic acid	T45.2X1-	T45.2X2-	T45.2X3-	T45.2X4-	T45.2X5-	T45.2X6-
Chalk, precipitated	T47.1X1-	T47.1X2-	T47.1X3-	T47.1X4-	T47.1X5-	T47.1X6-
Chamomile	T49.0X1-	T49.0X2-	T49.0X3-	T49.0X4-	T49.0X5-	T49.0X6-
Ch'an su	T46.0X1-	T46.0X2-	T46.0X3-	T46.0X4-	T46.0X5-	T46.0X6-
Charcoal	T47.6X1-	T47.6X2-	T47.6X3-	T47.6X4-	T47.6X5-	T47.6X6-
activated — *see also Charcoal, medicinal*	T47.6X1-	T47.6X2-	T47.6X3-	T47.6X4-	T47.6X5-	T47.6X6-
fumes (Carbon monoxide)	T58.2X1-	T58.2X2-	T58.2X3-	T58.2X4-	-	-
industrial	T58.8X1-	T58.8X2-	T58.8X3-	T58.8X4-	-	-
medicinal (activated)	T47.6X1-	T47.6X2-	T47.6X3-	T47.6X4-	T47.6X5-	T47.6X6-
antidiarrheal	T47.6X1-	T47.6X2-	T47.6X3-	T47.6X4-	T47.6X5-	T47.6X6-
poison control	T47.8X1-	T47.8X2-	T47.8X3-	T47.8X4-	T47.8X5-	T47.8X6-
specified use other than for diarrhea	T47.8X1-	T47.8X2-	T47.8X3-	T47.8X4-	T47.8X5-	T47.8X6-
topical	T49.8X1-	T49.8X2-	T49.8X3-	T49.8X4-	T49.8X5-	T49.8X6-
Chaulmosulfone	T37.1X1-	T37.1X2-	T37.1X3-	T37.1X4-	T37.1X5-	T37.1X6-
Chelating agent NEC	T50.6X1-	T50.6X2-	T50.6X3-	T50.6X4-	T50.6X5-	T50.6X6-
Chelidonium majus	T62.2X1-	T62.2X2-	T62.2X3-	T62.2X4-	-	-
Chemical substance NEC	T65.91X-	T65.92X-	T65.93X-	T65.94X-	-	-
Chenodeoxycholic acid	T47.5X1-	T47.5X2-	T47.5X3-	T47.5X4-	T47.5X5-	T47.5X6-
Chenodiol	T47.5X1-	T47.5X2-	T47.5X3-	T47.5X4-	T47.5X5-	T47.5X6-
Chenopodium	T37.4X1-	T37.4X2-	T37.4X3-	T37.4X4-	T37.4X5-	T37.4X6-
Cherry laurel	T62.2X1-	T62.2X2-	T62.2X3-	T62.2X4-	-	-
Chinidin (e)	T46.2X1-	T46.2X2-	T46.2X3-	T46.2X4-	T46.2X5-	T46.2X6-
Chiniofon	T37.8X1-	T37.8X2-	T37.8X3-	T37.8X4-	T37.8X5-	T37.8X6-
Chlophedianol	T48.3X1-	T48.3X2-	T48.3X3-	T48.3X4-	T48.3X5-	T48.3X6-
Chloral	T42.6X1-	T42.6X2-	T42.6X3-	T42.6X4-	T42.6X5-	T42.6X6-
derivative	T42.6X1-	T42.6X2-	T42.6X3-	T42.6X4-	T42.6X5-	T42.6X6-
hydrate	T42.6X1-	T42.6X2-	T42.6X3-	T42.6X4-	T42.6X5-	T42.6X6-
Chloralamide	T42.6X1-	T42.6X2-	T42.6X3-	T42.6X4-	T42.6X5-	T42.6X6-
Chloralodol	T42.6X1-	T42.6X2-	T42.6X3-	T42.6X4-	T42.6X5-	T42.6X6-
Chloralose	T60.4X1-	T60.4X2-	T60.4X3-	T60.4X4-	-	-
Chlorambucil	T45.1X1-	T45.1X2-	T45.1X3-	T45.1X4-	T45.1X5-	T45.1X6-
Chloramine	T57.8X1-	T57.8X2-	T57.8X3-	T57.8X4-	-	-
T	T49.0X1-	T49.0X2-	T49.0X3-	T49.0X4-	T49.0X5-	T49.0X6-
topical	T49.0X1-	T49.0X2-	T49.0X3-	T49.0X4-	T49.0X5-	T49.0X6-
Chloramphenicol	T36.2X1-	T36.2X2-	T36.2X3-	T36.2X4-	T36.2X5-	T36.2X6-
ENT agent	T49.6X1-	T49.6X2-	T49.6X3-	T49.6X4-	T49.6X5-	T49.6X6-
ophthalmic preparation	T49.5X1-	T49.5X2-	T49.5X3-	T49.5X4-	T49.5X5-	T49.5X6-

Substance	Poisoning Accidental (unintentional)	Poisoning Intentional self-harm	Poisoning Assault	Poisoning Undetermined	Adverse effect	Underdosing
Chloramphenicol (continued)						
topical NEC	T49.0X1-	T49.0X2-	T49.0X3-	T49.0X4-	T49.0X5-	T49.0X6-
Chlorate (potassium) (sodium) NEC	T60.3X1-	T60.3X2-	T60.3X3-	T60.3X4-	-	-
herbicide	T60.3X1-	T60.3X2-	T60.3X3-	T60.3X4-	-	-
Chlorazanil	T50.2X1-	T50.2X2-	T50.2X3-	T50.2X4-	T50.2X5-	T50.2X6-
Chlorbenzene, chlorbenzol	T53.7X1-	T53.7X2-	T53.7X3-	T53.7X4-	-	-
Chlorbenzoxamine	T44.3X1-	T44.3X2-	T44.3X3-	T44.3X4-	T44.3X5-	T44.3X6-
Chlorbutol	T42.6X1-	T42.6X2-	T42.6X3-	T42.6X4-	T42.6X5-	T42.6X6-
Chlorcyclizine	T45.0X1-	T45.0X2-	T45.0X3-	T45.0X4-	T45.0X5-	T45.0X6-
Chlordan (e) (dust)	T60.1X1-	T60.1X2-	T60.1X3-	T60.1X4-	-	-
Chlordantoin	T49.0X1-	T49.0X2-	T49.0X3-	T49.0X4-	T49.0X5-	T49.0X6-
Chlordiazepoxide	T42.4X1-	T42.4X2-	T42.4X3-	T42.4X4-	T42.4X5-	T42.4X6-
Chlordiethyl benzamide	T49.3X1-	T49.3X2-	T49.3X3-	T49.3X4-	T49.3X5-	T49.3X6-
Chloresium	T49.8X1-	T49.8X2-	T49.8X3-	T49.8X4-	T49.8X5-	T49.8X6-
Chlorethiazol	T42.6X1-	T42.6X2-	T42.6X3-	T42.6X4-	T42.6X5-	T42.6X6-
Chlorethyl — *see Ethyl chloride*						
Chloretone	T42.6X1-	T42.6X2-	T42.6X3-	T42.6X4-	T42.6X5-	T42.6X6-
Chlorex	T53.6X1-	T53.6X2-	T53.6X3-	T53.6X4-	-	-
insecticide	T60.1X1-	T60.1X2-	T60.1X3-	T60.1X4-	-	-
Chlorfenvinphos	T60.0X1-	T60.0X2-	T60.0X3-	T60.0X4-	-	-
Chlorhexadol	T42.6X1-	T42.6X2-	T42.6X3-	T42.6X4-	T42.6X5-	T42.6X6-
Chlorhexamide	T45.1X1-	T45.1X2-	T45.1X3-	T45.1X4-	T45.1X5-	T45.1X6-
Chlorhexidine	T49.0X1-	T49.0X2-	T49.0X3-	T49.0X4-	T49.0X5-	T49.0X6-
Chlorhydroxyquinolin	T49.0X1-	T49.0X2-	T49.0X3-	T49.0X4-	T49.0X5-	T49.0X6-
Chloride of lime (bleach)	T54.3X1-	T54.3X2-	T54.3X3-	T54.3X4-	-	-
Chlorimipramine	T43.011-	T43.012-	T43.013-	T43.014-	T43.015-	T43.016-
Chlorinated						
camphene	T53.6X1-	T53.6X2-	T53.6X3-	T53.6X4-	-	-
diphenyl	T53.7X1-	T53.7X2-	T53.7X3-	T53.7X4-	-	-
hydrocarbons NEC	T53.91X-	T53.92X-	T53.93X-	T53.94X-	-	-
solvents	T53.91X-	T53.92X-	T53.93X-	T53.94X-	-	-
lime (bleach)	T54.3X1-	T54.3X2-	T54.3X3-	T54.3X4-	-	-
and boric acid solution	T49.0X1-	T49.0X2-	T49.0X3-	T49.0X4-	T49.0X5-	T49.0X6-
naphthalene (insecticide)	T60.1X1-	T60.1X2-	T60.1X3-	T60.1X4-	-	-
industrial (non-pesticide)	T53.7X1-	T53.7X2-	T53.7X3-	T53.7X4-	-	-
pesticide NEC	T60.8X1-	T60.8X2-	T60.8X3-	T60.8X4-	-	-
soda — *see also sodium hypochlorite*						
solution	T49.0X1-	T49.0X2-	T49.0X3-	T49.0X4-	T49.0X5-	T49.0X6-
Chlorine (fumes) (gas)	T59.4X1-	T59.4X2-	T59.4X3-	T59.4X4-	-	-
bleach	T54.3X1-	T54.3X2-	T54.3X3-	T54.3X4-	-	-
compound gas NEC	T59.4X1-	T59.4X2-	T59.4X3-	T59.4X4-	-	-
disinfectant	T59.4X1-	T59.4X2-	T59.4X3-	T59.4X4-	-	-
releasing agents NEC	T59.4X1-	T59.4X2-	T59.4X3-	T59.4X4-	-	-
Chlorisondamine chloride	T46.991-	T46.992-	T46.993-	T46.994-	T46.995-	T46.996-
Chlormadinone	T38.5X1-	T38.5X2-	T38.5X3-	T38.5X4-	T38.5X5-	T38.5X6-
Chlormephos	T60.0X1-	T60.0X2-	T60.0X3-	T60.0X4-	-	-
Chlormerodrin	T50.2X1-	T50.2X2-	T50.2X3-	T50.2X4-	T50.2X5-	T50.2X6-
Chlormethiazole	T42.6X1-	T42.6X2-	T42.6X3-	T42.6X4-	T42.6X5-	T42.6X6-
Chlormethine	T45.1X1-	T45.1X2-	T45.1X3-	T45.1X4-	T45.1X5-	T45.1X6-
Chlormethylenecycline	T36.4X1-	T36.4X2-	T36.4X3-	T36.4X4-	T36.4X5-	T36.4X6-
Chlormezanone	T42.6X1-	T42.6X2-	T42.6X3-	T42.6X4-	T42.6X5-	T42.6X6-
Chloroacetic acid	T60.3X1-	T60.3X2-	T60.3X3-	T60.3X4-	-	-
Chloroacetone	T59.3X1-	T59.3X2-	T59.3X3-	T59.3X4-	-	-
Chloroacetophenone	T59.3X1-	T59.3X2-	T59.3X3-	T59.3X4-	-	-
Chloroaniline	T53.7X1-	T53.7X2-	T53.7X3-	T53.7X4-	-	-
Chlorobenzene, chlorobenzol	T53.7X1-	T53.7X2-	T53.7X3-	T53.7X4-	-	-
Chlorobromomethane (fire extinguisher)	T53.6X1-	T53.6X2-	T53.6X3-	T53.6X4-	-	-
Chlorobutanol	T49.0X1-	T49.0X2-	T49.0X3-	T49.0X4-	T49.0X5-	T49.0X6-

Substance	Poisoning Accidental (unintentional)	Poisoning Intentional self-harm	Poisoning Assault	Poisoning Undetermined	Adverse effect	Underdosing
Chlorocresol	T49.0X1-	T49.0X2-	T49.0X3-	T49.0X4-	T49.0X5-	T49.0X6-
Chlorodehydro-methyltestosterone	T38.7X1-	T38.7X2-	T38.7X3-	T38.7X4-	T38.7X5-	T38.7X6-
Chlorodinitrobenzene	T53.7X1-	T53.7X2-	T53.7X3-	T53.7X4-	-	-
dust or vapor	T53.7X1-	T53.7X2-	T53.7X3-	T53.7X4-	-	-
Chlorodiphenyl	T53.7X1-	T53.7X2-	T53.7X3-	T53.7X4-	-	-
Chloroethane — *see Ethyl chloride*						
Chloroethylene	T53.6X1-	T53.6X2-	T53.6X3-	T53.6X4-	-	-
Chlorofluorocarbons	T53.5X1-	T53.5X2-	T53.5X3-	T53.5X4-	-	-
Chloroform (fumes) (vapor)	T53.1X1-	T53.1X2-	T53.1X3-	T53.1X4-	-	-
anesthetic	T41.0X1-	T41.0X2-	T41.0X3-	T41.0X4-	T41.0X5-	T41.0X6-
solvent	T53.1X1-	T53.1X2-	T53.1X3-	T53.1X4-	-	-
water, concentrated	T41.0X1-	T41.0X2-	T41.0X3-	T41.0X4-	T41.0X5-	T41.0X6-
Chloroguanide	T37.2X1-	T37.2X2-	T37.2X3-	T37.2X4-	T37.2X5-	T37.2X6-
Chloromycetin	T36.2X1-	T36.2X2-	T36.2X3-	T36.2X4-	T36.2X5-	T36.2X6-
ENT agent	T49.6X1-	T49.6X2-	T49.6X3-	T49.6X4-	T49.6X5-	T49.6X6-
ophthalmic preparation	T49.5X1-	T49.5X2-	T49.5X3-	T49.5X4-	T49.5X5-	T49.5X6-
otic solution	T49.6X1-	T49.6X2-	T49.6X3-	T49.6X4-	T49.6X5-	T49.6X6-
topical NEC	T49.0X1-	T49.0X2-	T49.0X3-	T49.0X4-	T49.0X5-	T49.0X6-
Chloronitrobenzene	T53.7X1-	T53.7X2-	T53.7X3-	T53.7X4-	-	-
dust or vapor	T53.7X1-	T53.7X2-	T53.7X3-	T53.7X4-	-	-
Chlorophacinone	T60.4X1-	T60.4X2-	T60.4X3-	T60.4X4-	-	-
Chlorophenol	T53.7X1-	T53.7X2-	T53.7X3-	T53.7X4-	-	-
Chlorophenothane	T60.1X1-	T60.1X2-	T60.1X3-	T60.1X4-	-	-
Chlorophyll	T50.991-	T50.992-	T50.993-	T50.994-	T50.995-	T50.996-
Chloropicrin (fumes)	T53.6X1-	T53.6X2-	T53.6X3-	T53.6X4-	-	-
fumigant	T60.8X1-	T60.8X2-	T60.8X3-	T60.8X4-	-	-
fungicide	T60.3X1-	T60.3X2-	T60.3X3-	T60.3X4-	-	-
pesticide	T60.8X1-	T60.8X2-	T60.8X3-	T60.8X4-	-	-
Chloroprocaine	T41.3X1-	T41.3X2-	T41.3X3-	T41.3X4-	T41.3X5-	T41.3X6-
infiltration (subcutaneous)	T41.3X1-	T41.3X2-	T41.3X3-	T41.3X4-	T41.3X5-	T41.3X6-
nerve block (peripheral) (plexus)	T41.3X1-	T41.3X2-	T41.3X3-	T41.3X4-	T41.3X5-	T41.3X6-
spinal	T41.3X1-	T41.3X2-	T41.3X3-	T41.3X4-	T41.3X5-	T41.3X6-
Chloroptic	T49.5X1-	T49.5X2-	T49.5X3-	T49.5X4-	T49.5X5-	T49.5X6-
Chloropurine	T45.1X1-	T45.1X2-	T45.1X3-	T45.1X4-	T45.1X5-	T45.1X6-
Chloropyramine	T45.0X1-	T45.0X2-	T45.0X3-	T45.0X4-	T45.0X5-	T45.0X6-
Chloropyrifos	T60.0X1-	T60.0X2-	T60.0X3-	T60.0X4-	-	-
Chloropyrilene	T45.0X1-	T45.0X2-	T45.0X3-	T45.0X4-	T45.0X5-	T45.0X6-
Chloroquine	T37.2X1-	T37.2X2-	T37.2X3-	T37.2X4-	T37.2X5-	T37.2X6-
Chlorothalonil	T60.3X1-	T60.3X2-	T60.3X3-	T60.3X4-	-	-
Chlorothen	T45.0X1-	T45.0X2-	T45.0X3-	T45.0X4-	T45.0X5-	T45.0X6-
Chlorothiazide	T50.2X1-	T50.2X2-	T50.2X3-	T50.2X4-	T50.2X5-	T50.2X6-
Chlorothymol	T49.4X1-	T49.4X2-	T49.4X3-	T49.4X4-	T49.4X5-	T49.4X6-
Chlorotrianisene	T38.5X1-	T38.5X2-	T38.5X3-	T38.5X4-	T38.5X5-	T38.5X6-
Chlorovinyldichloro-arsine, not in war	T57.0X1-	T57.0X2-	T57.0X3-	T57.0X4-	-	-
Chloroxine	T49.4X1-	T49.4X2-	T49.4X3-	T49.4X4-	T49.4X5-	T49.4X6-
Chloroxylenol	T49.0X1-	T49.0X2-	T49.0X3-	T49.0X4-	T49.0X5-	T49.0X6-
Chlorphenamine	T45.0X1-	T45.0X2-	T45.0X3-	T45.0X4-	T45.0X5-	T45.0X6-
Chlorphenesin	T42.8X1-	T42.8X2-	T42.8X3-	T42.8X4-	T42.8X5-	T42.8X6-
topical (antifungal)	T49.0X1-	T49.0X2-	T49.0X3-	T49.0X4-	T49.0X5-	T49.0X6-
Chlorpheniramine	T45.0X1-	T45.0X2-	T45.0X3-	T45.0X4-	T45.0X5-	T45.0X6-
Chlorphenoxamine	T45.0X1-	T45.0X2-	T45.0X3-	T45.0X4-	T45.0X5-	T45.0X6-
Chlorphentermine	T50.5X1-	T50.5X2-	T50.5X3-	T50.5X4-	T50.5X5-	T50.5X6-
Chlorprocaine — *see Chloroprocaine*						
Chlorproguanil	T37.2X1-	T37.2X2-	T37.2X3-	T37.2X4-	T37.2X5-	T37.2X6-
Chlorpromazine	T43.3X1-	T43.3X2-	T43.3X3-	T43.3X4-	T43.3X5-	T43.3X6-
Chlorpropamide	T38.3X1-	T38.3X2-	T38.3X3-	T38.3X4-	T38.3X5-	T38.3X6-
Chlorprothixene	T43.4X1-	T43.4X2-	T43.4X3-	T43.4X4-	T43.4X5-	T43.4X6-
Chlorquinaldol	T49.0X1-	T49.0X2-	T49.0X3-	T49.0X4-	T49.0X5-	T49.0X6-

Substance	Poisoning Accidental (unintentional)	Poisoning Intentional self-harm	Poisoning Assault	Poisoning Undetermined	Adverse effect	Underdosing
Chlorquinol	T49.0X1-	T49.0X2-	T49.0X3-	T49.0X4-	T49.0X5-	T49.0X6-
Chlortalidone	T50.2X1-	T50.2X2-	T50.2X3-	T50.2X4-	T50.2X5-	T50.2X6-
Chlortetracycline	T36.4X1-	T36.4X2-	T36.4X3-	T36.4X4-	T36.4X5-	T36.4X6-
Chlorthalidone	T50.2X1-	T50.2X2-	T50.2X3-	T50.2X4-	T50.2X5-	T50.2X6-
Chlorthiophos	T60.0X1-	T60.0X2-	T60.0X3-	T60.0X4-	-	-
Chlortrianisene	T38.5X1-	T38.5X2-	T38.5X3-	T38.5X4-	T38.5X5-	T38.5X6-
Chlor-Trimeton	T45.0X1-	T45.0X2-	T45.0X3-	T45.0X4-	T45.0X5-	T45.0X6-
Chlorthion	T60.0X1-	T60.0X2-	T60.0X3-	T60.0X4-	-	-
Chlorzoxazone	T42.8X1-	T42.8X2-	T42.8X3-	T42.8X4-	T42.8X5-	T42.8X6-
Choke damp	T59.7X1-	T59.7X2-	T59.7X3-	T59.7X4-	-	-
Cholagogues	T47.5X1-	T47.5X2-	T47.5X3-	T47.5X4-	T47.5X5-	T47.5X6-
Cholebrine	T50.8X1-	T50.8X2-	T50.8X3-	T50.8X4-	T50.8X5-	T50.8X6-
Cholecalciferol	T45.2X1-	T45.2X2-	T45.2X3-	T45.2X4-	T45.2X5-	T45.2X6-
Cholecystokinin	T50.8X1-	T50.8X2-	T50.8X3-	T50.8X4-	T50.8X5-	T50.8X6-
Cholera vaccine	T50.A91-	T50.A92-	T50.A93-	T50.A94-	T50.A95-	T50.A96-
Choleretic	T47.5X1-	T47.5X2-	T47.5X3-	T47.5X4-	T47.5X5-	T47.5X6-
Cholesterol-lowering agents	T46.6X1-	T46.6X2-	T46.6X3-	T46.6X4-	T46.6X5-	T46.6X6-
Cholestyramine (resin)	T46.6X1-	T46.6X2-	T46.6X3-	T46.6X4-	T46.6X5-	T46.6X6-
Cholic acid	T47.5X1-	T47.5X2-	T47.5X3-	T47.5X4-	T47.5X5-	T47.5X6-
Choline	T48.6X1-	T48.6X2-	T48.6X3-	T48.6X4-	T48.6X5-	T48.6X6-
chloride	T50.991-	T50.992-	T50.993-	T50.994-	T50.995-	T50.996-
dihydrogen citrate	T50.991-	T50.992-	T50.993-	T50.994-	T50.995-	T50.996-
salicylate	T39.091-	T39.092-	T39.093-	T39.094-	T39.095-	T39.096-
theophyllinate	T48.6X1-	T48.6X2-	T48.6X3-	T48.6X4-	T48.6X5-	T48.6X6-
Cholinergic (drug) NEC	T44.1X1-	T44.1X2-	T44.1X3-	T44.1X4-	T44.1X5-	T44.1X6-
muscle tone enhancer	T44.1X1-	T44.1X2-	T44.1X3-	T44.1X4-	T44.1X5-	T44.1X6-
organophosphorus	T44.0X1-	T44.0X2-	T44.0X3-	T44.0X4-	T44.0X5-	T44.0X6-
insecticide	T60.0X1-	T60.0X2-	T60.0X3-	T60.0X4-	-	-
nerve gas	T59.891-	T59.892-	T59.893-	T59.894-	-	-
trimethyl ammonium propanediol	T44.1X1-	T44.1X2-	T44.1X3-	T44.1X4-	T44.1X5-	T44.1X6-
Cholinesterase reactivator	T50.6X1-	T50.6X2-	T50.6X3-	T50.6X4-	T50.6X5-	T50.6X6-
Cholografin	T50.8X1-	T50.8X2-	T50.8X3-	T50.8X4-	T50.8X5-	T50.8X6-
Chorionic gonadotropin	T38.891-	T38.892-	T38.893-	T38.894-	T38.895-	T38.896-
Chromate	T56.2X1-	T56.2X2-	T56.2X3-	T56.2X4-	-	-
dust or mist	T56.2X1-	T56.2X2-	T56.2X3-	T56.2X4-	-	-
lead — *see also lead*	T56.0X1-	T56.0X2-	T56.0X3-	T56.0X4-	-	-
paint	T56.0X1-	T56.0X2-	T56.0X3-	T56.0X4-	-	-
Chromic						
acid	T56.2X1-	T56.2X2-	T56.2X3-	T56.2X4-	-	-
dust or mist	T56.2X1-	T56.2X2-	T56.2X3-	T56.2X4-	-	-
phosphate 32P	T45.1X1-	T45.1X2-	T45.1X3-	T45.1X4-	T45.1X5-	T45.1X6-
Chromium	T56.2X1-	T56.2X2-	T56.2X3-	T56.2X4-	-	-
compounds — *see Chromate*						
sesquioxide	T50.8X1-	T50.8X2-	T50.8X3-	T50.8X4-	T50.8X5-	T50.8X6-
Chromomycin A3	T45.1X1-	T45.1X2-	T45.1X3-	T45.1X4-	T45.1X5-	T45.1X6-
Chromonar	T46.3X1-	T46.3X2-	T46.3X3-	T46.3X4-	T46.3X5-	T46.3X6-
Chromyl chloride	T56.2X1-	T56.2X2-	T56.2X3-	T56.2X4-	-	-
Chrysarobin	T49.4X1-	T49.4X2-	T49.4X3-	T49.4X4-	T49.4X5-	T49.4X6-
Chrysazin	T47.2X1-	T47.2X2-	T47.2X3-	T47.2X4-	T47.2X5-	T47.2X6-
Chymar	T45.3X1-	T45.3X2-	T45.3X3-	T45.3X4-	T45.3X5-	T45.3X6-
ophthalmic preparation	T49.5X1-	T49.5X2-	T49.5X3-	T49.5X4-	T49.5X5-	T49.5X6-
Chymopapain	T45.3X1-	T45.3X2-	T45.3X3-	T45.3X4-	T45.3X5-	T45.3X6-
Chymotrypsin	T45.3X1-	T45.3X2-	T45.3X3-	T45.3X4-	T45.3X5-	T45.3X6-
ophthalmic preparation	T49.5X1-	T49.5X2-	T49.5X3-	T49.5X4-	T49.5X5-	T49.5X6-
Cianidanol	T50.991-	T50.992-	T50.993-	T50.994-	T50.995-	T50.996-
Cianopramine	T43.011-	T43.012-	T43.013-	T43.014-	T43.015-	T43.016-
Cibenzoline	T46.2X1-	T46.2X2-	T46.2X3-	T46.2X4-	T46.2X5-	T46.2X6-
Ciclacillin	T36.0X1-	T36.0X2-	T36.0X3-	T36.0X4-	T36.0X5-	T36.0X6-

Substance	Poisoning Accidental (unintentional)	Poisoning Intentional self-harm	Poisoning Assault	Poisoning Undetermined	Adverse effect	Underdosing
Ciclobarbital — *see Hexobarbital*						
Ciclonicate	T46.7X1-	T46.7X2-	T46.7X3-	T46.7X4-	T46.7X5-	T46.7X6-
Ciclopirox (olamine)	T49.0X1-	T49.0X2-	T49.0X3-	T49.0X4-	T49.0X5-	T49.0X6-
Ciclosporin	T45.1X1-	T45.1X2-	T45.1X3-	T45.1X4-	T45.1X5-	T45.1X6-
Cicuta maculata or virosa	T62.2X1-	T62.2X2-	T62.2X3-	T62.2X4-	-	-
Cicutoxin	T62.2X1-	T62.2X2-	T62.2X3-	T62.2X4-	-	-
Cigarette lighter fluid	T52.0X1-	T52.0X2-	T52.0X3-	T52.0X4-	-	-
Cigarettes (tobacco)	T65.221-	T65.222-	T65.223-	T65.224-	-	-
Ciguatoxin	T61.01X-	T61.02X-	T61.03X-	T61.04X-	-	-
Cilazapril	T46.4X1-	T46.4X2-	T46.4X3-	T46.4X4-	T46.4X5-	T46.4X6-
Cimetidine	T47.0X1-	T47.0X2-	T47.0X3-	T47.0X4-	T47.0X5-	T47.0X6-
Cimetropium bromide	T44.3X1-	T44.3X2-	T44.3X3-	T44.3X4-	T44.3X5-	T44.3X6-
Cinchocaine	T41.3X1-	T41.3X2-	T41.3X3-	T41.3X4-	T41.3X5-	T41.3X6-
topical (surface)	T41.3X1-	T41.3X2-	T41.3X3-	T41.3X4-	T41.3X5-	T41.3X6-
Cinchona	T37.2X1-	T37.2X2-	T37.2X3-	T37.2X4-	T37.2X5-	T37.2X6-
Cinchonine alkaloids	T37.2X1-	T37.2X2-	T37.2X3-	T37.2X4-	T37.2X5-	T37.2X6-
Cinchophen	T50.4X1-	T50.4X2-	T50.4X3-	T50.4X4-	T50.4X5-	T50.4X6-
Cinepazide	T46.7X1-	T46.7X2-	T46.7X3-	T46.7X4-	T46.7X5-	T46.7X6-
Cinnamedrine	T48.5X1-	T48.5X2-	T48.5X3-	T48.5X4-	T48.5X5-	T48.5X6-
Cinnarizine	T45.0X1-	T45.0X2-	T45.0X3-	T45.0X4-	T45.0X5-	T45.0X6-
Cinoxacin	T37.8X1-	T37.8X2-	T37.8X3-	T37.8X4-	T37.8X5-	T37.8X6-
Ciprofibrate	T46.6X1-	T46.6X2-	T46.6X3-	T46.6X4-	T46.6X5-	T46.6X6-
Ciprofloxacin	T36.8X1-	T36.8X2-	T36.8X3-	T36.8X4-	T36.8X5-	T36.8X6-
Cisapride	T47.8X1-	T47.8X2-	T47.8X3-	T47.8X4-	T47.8X5-	T47.8X6-
Cisplatin	T45.1X1-	T45.1X2-	T45.1X3-	T45.1X4-	T45.1X5-	T45.1X6-
Citalopram	T43.221-	T43.222-	T43.223-	T43.224-	T43.225-	T43.226-
Citanest	T41.3X1-	T41.3X2-	T41.3X3-	T41.3X4-	T41.3X5-	T41.3X6-
infiltration (subcutaneous)	T41.3X1-	T41.3X2-	T41.3X3-	T41.3X4-	T41.3X5-	T41.3X6-
nerve block (peripheral) (plexus)	T41.3X1-	T41.3X2-	T41.3X3-	T41.3X4-	T41.3X5-	T41.3X6-
Citric acid	T47.5X1-	T47.5X2-	T47.5X3-	T47.5X4-	T47.5X5-	T47.5X6-
Citrovorum (factor)	T45.8X1-	T45.8X2-	T45.8X3-	T45.8X4-	T45.8X5-	T45.8X6-
Claviceps purpurea	T62.2X1-	T62.2X2-	T62.2X3-	T62.2X4-	-	-
Clavulanic acid	T36.1X1-	T36.1X2-	T36.1X3-	T36.1X4-	T36.1X5-	T36.1X6-
Cleaner, cleansing agent, type not specified	T65.891-	T65.892-	T65.893-	T65.894-	-	-
of paint or varnish	T52.91X-	T52.92X-	T52.93X-	T52.94X-	-	-
specified type NEC	T65.891-	T65.892-	T65.893-	T65.894-	-	-
Clebopride	T47.8X1-	T47.8X2-	T47.8X3-	T47.8X4-	T47.8X5-	T47.8X6-
Clefamide	T37.3X1-	T37.3X2-	T37.3X3-	T37.3X4-	T37.3X5-	T37.3X6-
Clemastine	T45.0X1-	T45.0X2-	T45.0X3-	T45.0X4-	T45.0X5-	T45.0X6-
Clematis vitalba	T62.2X1-	T62.2X2-	T62.2X3-	T62.2X4-	-	-
Clemizole	T45.0X1-	T45.0X2-	T45.0X3-	T45.0X4-	T45.0X5-	T45.0X6-
penicillin	T36.0X1-	T36.0X2-	T36.0X3-	T36.0X4-	T36.0X5-	T36.0X6-
Clenbuterol	T48.6X1-	T48.6X2-	T48.6X3-	T48.6X4-	T48.6X5-	T48.6X6-
Clidinium bromide	T44.3X1-	T44.3X2-	T44.3X3-	T44.3X4-	T44.3X5-	T44.3X6-
Clindamycin	T36.8X1-	T36.8X2-	T36.8X3-	T36.8X4-	T36.8X5-	T36.8X6-
Clinofibrate	T46.6X1-	T46.6X2-	T46.6X3-	T46.6X4-	T46.6X5-	T46.6X6-
Clioquinol	T37.8X1-	T37.8X2-	T37.8X3-	T37.8X4-	T37.8X5-	T37.8X6-
Cliradon	T40.2X1-	T40.2X2-	T40.2X3-	T40.2X4-	-	-
Clobazam	T42.4X1-	T42.4X2-	T42.4X3-	T42.4X4-	T42.4X5-	T42.4X6-
Clobenzorex	T50.5X1-	T50.5X2-	T50.5X3-	T50.5X4-	T50.5X5-	T50.5X6-
Clobetasol	T49.0X1-	T49.0X2-	T49.0X3-	T49.0X4-	T49.0X5-	T49.0X6-
Clobetasone	T49.0X1-	T49.0X2-	T49.0X3-	T49.0X4-	T49.0X5-	T49.0X6-
Clobutinol	T48.3X1-	T48.3X2-	T48.3X3-	T48.3X4-	T48.3X5-	T48.3X6-
Clocortolone	T38.0X1-	T38.0X2-	T38.0X3-	T38.0X4-	T38.0X5-	T38.0X6-
Clodantoin	T49.0X1-	T49.0X2-	T49.0X3-	T49.0X4-	T49.0X5-	T49.0X6-
Clodronic acid	T50.991-	T50.992-	T50.993-	T50.994-	T50.995-	T50.996-
Clofazimine	T37.1X1-	T37.1X2-	T37.1X3-	T37.1X4-	T37.1X5-	T37.1X6-
Clofedanol	T48.3X1-	T48.3X2-	T48.3X3-	T48.3X4-	T48.3X5-	T48.3X6-

Substance	Poisoning Accidental (unintentional)	Poisoning Intentional self-harm	Poisoning Assault	Poisoning Undetermined	Adverse effect	Underdosing
Clofenamide	T50.2X1-	T50.2X2-	T50.2X3-	T50.2X4-	T50.2X5-	T50.2X6-
Clofenotane	T49.0X1-	T49.0X2-	T49.0X3-	T49.0X4-	T49.0X5-	T49.0X6-
Clofezone	T39.2X1-	T39.2X2-	T39.2X3-	T39.2X4-	T39.2X5-	T39.2X6-
Clofibrate	T46.6X1-	T46.6X2-	T46.6X3-	T46.6X4-	T46.6X5-	T46.6X6-
Clofibride	T46.6X1-	T46.6X2-	T46.6X3-	T46.6X4-	T46.6X5-	T46.6X6-
Cloforex	T50.5X1-	T50.5X2-	T50.5X3-	T50.5X4-	T50.5X5-	T50.5X6-
Clomethiazole	T42.6X1-	T42.6X2-	T42.6X3-	T42.6X4-	T42.6X5-	T42.6X6-
Clometocillin	T36.0X1-	T36.0X2-	T36.0X3-	T36.0X4-	T36.0X5-	T36.0X6-
Clomifene	T38.5X1-	T38.5X2-	T38.5X3-	T38.5X4-	T38.5X5-	T38.5X6-
Clomiphene	T38.5X1-	T38.5X2-	T38.5X3-	T38.5X4-	T38.5X5-	T38.5X6-
Clomipramine	T43.011-	T43.012-	T43.013-	T43.014-	T43.015-	T43.016-
Clomocycline	T36.4X1-	T36.4X2-	T36.4X3-	T36.4X4-	T36.4X5-	T36.4X6-
Clonazepam	T42.4X1-	T42.4X2-	T42.4X3-	T42.4X4-	T42.4X5-	T42.4X6-
Clonidine	T46.5X1-	T46.5X2-	T46.5X3-	T46.5X4-	T46.5X5-	T46.5X6-
Clonixin	T39.8X1-	T39.8X2-	T39.8X3-	T39.8X4-	T39.8X5-	T39.8X6-
Clopamide	T50.2X1-	T50.2X2-	T50.2X3-	T50.2X4-	T50.2X5-	T50.2X6-
Clopenthixol	T43.4X1-	T43.4X2-	T43.4X3-	T43.4X4-	T43.4X5-	T43.4X6-
Cloperastine	T48.3X1-	T48.3X2-	T48.3X3-	T48.3X4-	T48.3X5-	T48.3X6-
Clophedianol	T48.3X1-	T48.3X2-	T48.3X3-	T48.3X4-	T48.3X5-	T48.3X6-
Cloponone	T36.2X1-	T36.2X2-	T36.2X3-	T36.2X4-	T36.2X5-	T36.2X6-
Cloprednol	T38.0X1-	T38.0X2-	T38.0X3-	T38.0X4-	T38.0X5-	T38.0X6-
Cloral betaine	T42.6X1-	T42.6X2-	T42.6X3-	T42.6X4-	T42.6X5-	T42.6X6-
Cloramfenicol	T36.2X1-	T36.2X2-	T36.2X3-	T36.2X4-	T36.2X5-	T36.2X6-
Clorazepate (dipotassium)	T42.4X1-	T42.4X2-	T42.4X3-	T42.4X4-	T42.4X5-	T42.4X6-
Clorexolone	T50.2X1-	T50.2X2-	T50.2X3-	T50.2X4-	T50.2X5-	T50.2X6-
Clorfenamine	T45.0X1-	T45.0X2-	T45.0X3-	T45.0X4-	T45.0X5-	T45.0X6-
Clorgiline	T43.1X1-	T43.1X2-	T43.1X3-	T43.1X4-	T43.1X5-	T43.1X6-
Clorotepine	T44.3X1-	T44.3X2-	T44.3X3-	T44.3X4-	T44.3X5-	T44.3X6-
Clorox (bleach)	T54.91X-	T54.92X-	T54.93X-	T54.94X-	-	-
Clorprenaline	T48.6X1-	T48.6X2-	T48.6X3-	T48.6X4-	T48.6X5-	T48.6X6-
Clortermine	T50.5X1-	T50.5X2-	T50.5X3-	T50.5X4-	T50.5X5-	T50.5X6-
Clotiapine	T43.591-	T43.592-	T43.593-	T43.594-	T43.595-	T43.596-
Clotiazepam	T42.4X1-	T42.4X2-	T42.4X3-	T42.4X4-	T42.4X5-	T42.4X6-
Clotibric acid	T46.6X1-	T46.6X2-	T46.6X3-	T46.6X4-	T46.6X5-	T46.6X6-
Clotrimazole	T49.0X1-	T49.0X2-	T49.0X3-	T49.0X4-	T49.0X5-	T49.0X6-
Cloxacillin	T36.0X1-	T36.0X2-	T36.0X3-	T36.0X4-	T36.0X5-	T36.0X6-
Cloxazolam	T42.4X1-	T42.4X2-	T42.4X3-	T42.4X4-	T42.4X5-	T42.4X6-
Cloxiquine	T49.0X1-	T49.0X2-	T49.0X3-	T49.0X4-	T49.0X5-	T49.0X6-
Clozapine	T42.4X1-	T42.4X2-	T42.4X3-	T42.4X4-	T42.4X5-	T42.4X6-
Coagulant NEC	T45.7X1-	T45.7X2-	T45.7X3-	T45.7X4-	T45.7X5-	T45.7X6-
Coal (carbon monoxide from) — *see also Carbon, monoxide, coal*	T58.2X1-	T58.2X2-	T58.2X3-	T58.2X4-	-	-
oil — *see Kerosene*						
tar	T49.1X1-	T49.1X2-	T49.1X3-	T49.1X4-	T49.1X5-	T49.1X6-
fumes	T59.891-	T59.892-	T59.893-	T59.894-	-	-
medicinal (ointment)	T49.4X1-	T49.4X2-	T49.4X3-	T49.4X4-	T49.4X5-	T49.4X6-
analgesics NEC	T39.2X1-	T39.2X2-	T39.2X3-	T39.2X4-	T39.2X5-	T39.2X6-
naphtha (solvent)	T52.0X1-	T52.0X2-	T52.0X3-	T52.0X4-	-	-
Cobalamine	T45.2X1-	T45.2X2-	T45.2X3-	T45.2X4-	T45.2X5-	T45.2X6-
Cobalt (nonmedicinal) (fumes) (industrial)	T56.891-	T56.892-	T56.893-	T56.894-	-	-
medicinal (trace) (chloride)	T45.8X1-	T45.8X2-	T45.8X3-	T45.8X4-	T45.8X5-	T45.8X6-
Cobra (venom)	T63.041-	T63.042-	T63.043-	T63.044-	-	-
Coca (leaf)	T40.5X1-	T40.5X2-	T40.5X3-	T40.5X4-	T40.5X5-	T40.5X6-
Cocaine	T40.5X1-	T40.5X2-	T40.5X3-	T40.5X4-	T40.5X5-	T40.5X6-
topical anesthetic	T41.3X1-	T41.3X2-	T41.3X3-	T41.3X4-	T41.3X5-	T41.3X6-
Cocarboxylase	T45.3X1-	T45.3X2-	T45.3X3-	T45.3X4-	T45.3X5-	T45.3X6-
Coccidioidin	T50.8X1-	T50.8X2-	T50.8X3-	T50.8X4-	T50.8X5-	T50.8X6-
Cocculus indicus	T62.1X1-	T62.1X2-	T62.1X3-	T62.1X4-	-	-

Substance	Poisoning Accidental (unintentional)	Poisoning Intentional self-harm	Poisoning Assault	Poisoning Undetermined	Adverse effect	Underdosing
Cochineal	T65.6X1-	T65.6X2-	T65.6X3-	T65.6X4-	-	-
medicinal products	T50.991-	T50.992-	T50.993-	T50.994-	T50.995-	T50.996-
Codeine	T40.2X1-	T40.2X2-	T40.2X3-	T40.2X4-	T40.2X5-	T40.2X6-
Cod-liver oil	T45.2X1-	T45.2X2-	T45.2X3-	T45.2X4-	T45.2X5-	T45.2X6-
Coenzyme A	T50.991-	T50.992-	T50.993-	T50.994-	T50.995-	T50.996-
Coffee	T62.8X1-	T62.8X2-	T62.8X3-	T62.8X4-	-	-
Cogalactoiso-merase	T50.991-	T50.992-	T50.993-	T50.994-	T50.995-	T50.996-
Cogentin	T44.3X1-	T44.3X2-	T44.3X3-	T44.3X4-	T44.3X5-	T44.3X6-
Coke fumes or gas (carbon monoxide)	T58.2X1-	T58.2X2-	T58.2X3-	T58.2X4-	-	-
industrial use	T58.8X1-	T58.8X2-	T58.8X3-	T58.8X4-	-	-
Colace	T47.4X1-	T47.4X2-	T47.4X3-	T47.4X4-	T47.4X5-	T47.4X6-
Colaspase	T45.1X1-	T45.1X2-	T45.1X3-	T45.1X4-	T45.1X5-	T45.1X6-
Colchicine	T50.4X1-	T50.4X2-	T50.4X3-	T50.4X4-	T50.4X5-	T50.4X6-
Colchicum	T62.2X1-	T62.2X2-	T62.2X3-	T62.2X4-	-	-
Cold cream	T49.3X1-	T49.3X2-	T49.3X3-	T49.3X4-	T49.3X5-	T49.3X6-
Colecalciferol	T45.2X1-	T45.2X2-	T45.2X3-	T45.2X4-	T45.2X5-	T45.2X6-
Colestipol	T46.6X1-	T46.6X2-	T46.6X3-	T46.6X4-	T46.6X5-	T46.6X6-
Colestyramine	T46.6X1-	T46.6X2-	T46.6X3-	T46.6X4-	T46.6X5-	T46.6X6-
Colimycin	T36.8X1-	T36.8X2-	T36.8X3-	T36.8X4-	T36.8X5-	T36.8X6-
Colistimethate	T36.8X1-	T36.8X2-	T36.8X3-	T36.8X4-	T36.8X5-	T36.8X6-
Colistin	T36.8X1-	T36.8X2-	T36.8X3-	T36.8X4-	T36.8X5-	T36.8X6-
sulfate (eye preparation)	T49.5X1-	T49.5X2-	T49.5X3-	T49.5X4-	T49.5X5-	T49.5X6-
Collagen	T50.991-	T50.992-	T50.993-	T50.994-	T50.995-	T50.996-
Collagenase	T49.4X1-	T49.4X2-	T49.4X3-	T49.4X4-	T49.4X5-	T49.4X6-
Collodion	T49.3X1-	T49.3X2-	T49.3X3-	T49.3X4-	T49.3X5-	T49.3X6-
Colocynth	T47.2X1-	T47.2X2-	T47.2X3-	T47.2X4-	T47.2X5-	T47.2X6-
Colophony adhesive	T49.3X1-	T49.3X2-	T49.3X3-	T49.3X4-	T49.3X5-	T49.3X6-
Colorant — *see also Dye*	T50.991-	T50.992-	T50.993-	T50.994-	T50.995-	T50.996-
Coloring matter — *see Dye(s)*						
Combustion gas (after combustion) — *see Carbon, monoxide*						
prior to combustion	T59.891-	T59.892-	T59.893-	T59.894-	-	-
Compazine	T43.3X1-	T43.3X2-	T43.3X3-	T43.3X4-	T43.3X5-	T43.3X6-
Compound						
42 (warfarin)	T60.4X1-	T60.4X2-	T60.4X3-	T60.4X4-	-	-
269 (endrin)	T60.1X1-	T60.1X2-	T60.1X3-	T60.1X4-	-	-
497 (dieldrin)	T60.1X1-	T60.1X2-	T60.1X3-	T60.1X4-	-	-
1080 (sodium fluoroacetate)	T60.4X1-	T60.4X2-	T60.4X3-	T60.4X4-	-	-
3422 (parathion)	T60.0X1-	T60.0X2-	T60.0X3-	T60.0X4-	-	-
3911 (phorate)	T60.0X1-	T60.0X2-	T60.0X3-	T60.0X4-	-	-
3956 (toxaphene)	T60.1X1-	T60.1X2-	T60.1X3-	T60.1X4-	-	-
4049 (malathion)	T60.0X1-	T60.0X2-	T60.0X3-	T60.0X4-	-	-
4069 (malathion)	T60.0X1-	T60.0X2-	T60.0X3-	T60.0X4-	-	-
4124 (dicapthon)	T60.0X1-	T60.0X2-	T60.0X3-	T60.0X4-	-	-
E (cortisone)	T38.0X1-	T38.0X2-	T38.0X3-	T38.0X4-	T38.0X5-	T38.0X6-
F (hydrocortisone)	T38.0X1-	T38.0X2-	T38.0X3-	T38.0X4-	T38.0X5-	T38.0X6-
Congener, anabolic	T38.7X1-	T38.7X2-	T38.7X3-	T38.7X4-	T38.7X5-	T38.7X6-
Congo red	T50.8X1-	T50.8X2-	T50.8X3-	T50.8X4-	T50.8X5-	T50.8X6-
Coniine, conine	T62.2X1-	T62.2X2-	T62.2X3-	T62.2X4-	-	-
Conium (maculatum)	T62.2X1-	T62.2X2-	T62.2X3-	T62.2X4-	-	-
Conjugated estrogenic substances	T38.5X1-	T38.5X2-	T38.5X3-	T38.5X4-	T38.5X5-	T38.5X6-
Contac	T48.5X1-	T48.5X2-	T48.5X3-	T48.5X4-	T48.5X5-	T48.5X6-
Contact lens solution	T49.5X1-	T49.5X2-	T49.5X3-	T49.5X4-	T49.5X5-	T49.5X6-
Contraceptive (oral)	T38.4X1-	T38.4X2-	T38.4X3-	T38.4X4-	T38.4X5-	T38.4X6-
vaginal	T49.8X1-	T49.8X2-	T49.8X3-	T49.8X4-	T49.8X5-	T49.8X6-
Contrast medium, radiography	T50.8X1-	T50.8X2-	T50.8X3-	T50.8X4-	T50.8X5-	T50.8X6-
Convallaria glycosides	T46.0X1-	T46.0X2-	T46.0X3-	T46.0X4-	T46.0X5-	T46.0X6-

Substance	Poisoning Accidental (unintentional)	Poisoning Intentional self-harm	Poisoning Assault	Poisoning Undetermined	Adverse effect	Underdosing
Convallaria majalis	T62.2X1-	T62.2X2-	T62.2X3-	T62.2X4-	-	-
berry	T62.1X1-	T62.1X2-	T62.1X3-	T62.1X4-	-	-
Copper (dust) (fumes) (nonmedicinal) NEC	T56.4X1-	T56.4X2-	T56.4X3-	T56.4X4-	-	-
arsenate, arsenite	T57.0X1-	T57.0X2-	T57.0X3-	T57.0X4-	-	-
insecticide	T60.2X1-	T60.2X2-	T60.2X3-	T60.2X4-	-	-
emetic	T47.7X1-	T47.7X2-	T47.7X3-	T47.7X4-	T47.7X5-	T47.7X6-
fungicide	T60.3X1-	T60.3X2-	T60.3X3-	T60.3X4-	-	-
gluconate	T49.0X1-	T49.0X2-	T49.0X3-	T49.0X4-	T49.0X5-	T49.0X6-
insecticide	T60.2X1-	T60.2X2-	T60.2X3-	T60.2X4-	-	-
medicinal (trace)	T45.8X1-	T45.8X2-	T45.8X3-	T45.8X4-	T45.8X5-	T45.8X6-
oleate	T49.0X1-	T49.0X2-	T49.0X3-	T49.0X4-	T49.0X5-	T49.0X6-
sulfate	T56.4X1-	T56.4X2-	T56.4X3-	T56.4X4-	-	-
cupric	T56.4X1-	T56.4X2-	T56.4X3-	T56.4X4-	-	-
fungicide	T60.3X1-	T60.3X2-	T60.3X3-	T60.3X4-	-	-
medicinal						
ear	T49.6X1-	T49.6X2-	T49.6X3-	T49.6X4-	T49.6X5-	T49.6X6-
emetic	T47.7X1-	T47.7X2-	T47.7X3-	T47.7X4-	T47.7X5-	T47.7X6-
eye	T49.5X1-	T49.5X2-	T49.5X3-	T49.5X4-	T49.5X5-	T49.5X6-
cuprous	T56.4X1-	T56.4X2-	T56.4X3-	T56.4X4-	-	-
fungicide	T60.3X1-	T60.3X2-	T60.3X3-	T60.3X4-	-	-
medicinal						
ear	T49.6X1-	T49.6X2-	T49.6X3-	T49.6X4-	T49.6X5-	T49.6X6-
emetic	T47.7X1-	T47.7X2-	T47.7X3-	T47.7X4-	T47.7X5-	T47.7X6-
eye	T49.5X1-	T49.5X2-	T49.5X3-	T49.5X4-	T49.5X5-	T49.5X6-
Copperhead snake (bite) (venom)	T63.061-	T63.062-	T63.063-	T63.064-	-	-
Coral (sting)	T63.691-	T63.692-	T63.693-	T63.694-	-	-
snake (bite) (venom)	T63.021-	T63.022-	T63.023-	T63.024-	-	-
Corbadrine	T49.6X1-	T49.6X2-	T49.6X3-	T49.6X4-	T49.6X5-	T49.6X6-
Cordite	T65.891-	T65.892-	T65.893-	T65.894-	-	-
vapor	T59.891-	T59.892-	T59.893-	T59.894-	-	-
Cordran	T49.0X1-	T49.0X2-	T49.0X3-	T49.0X4-	T49.0X5-	T49.0X6-
Corn cures	T49.4X1-	T49.4X2-	T49.4X3-	T49.4X4-	T49.4X5-	T49.4X6-
Corn starch	T49.3X1-	T49.3X2-	T49.3X3-	T49.3X4-	T49.3X5-	T49.3X6-
Cornhusker's lotion	T49.3X1-	T49.3X2-	T49.3X3-	T49.3X4-	T49.3X5-	T49.3X6-
Coronary vasodilator NEC	T46.3X1-	T46.3X2-	T46.3X3-	T46.3X4-	T46.3X5-	T46.3X6-
Corrosive NEC	T54.91X-	T54.92X-	T54.93X-	T54.94X-	-	-
acid NEC	T54.2X1-	T54.2X2-	T54.2X3-	T54.2X4-	-	-
aromatics	T54.1X1-	T54.1X2-	T54.1X3-	T54.1X4-	-	-
disinfectant	T54.1X1-	T54.1X2-	T54.1X3-	T54.1X4-	-	-
fumes NEC	T54.91X-	T54.92X-	T54.93X-	T54.94X-	-	-
specified NEC	T54.91X-	T54.92X-	T54.93X-	T54.94X-	-	-
sublimate	T56.1X1-	T56.1X2-	T56.1X3-	T56.1X4-	-	-
Cortate	T38.0X1-	T38.0X2-	T38.0X3-	T38.0X4-	T38.0X5-	T38.0X6-
Cort-Dome	T38.0X1-	T38.0X2-	T38.0X3-	T38.0X4-	T38.0X5-	T38.0X6-
ENT agent	T49.6X1-	T49.6X2-	T49.6X3-	T49.6X4-	T49.6X5-	T49.6X6-
ophthalmic preparation	T49.5X1-	T49.5X2-	T49.5X3-	T49.5X4-	T49.5X5-	T49.5X6-
topical NEC	T49.0X1-	T49.0X2-	T49.0X3-	T49.0X4-	T49.0X5-	T49.0X6-
Cortef	T38.0X1-	T38.0X2-	T38.0X3-	T38.0X4-	T38.0X5-	T38.0X6-
ENT agent	T49.6X1-	T49.6X2-	T49.6X3-	T49.6X4-	T49.6X5-	T49.6X6-
ophthalmic preparation	T49.5X1-	T49.5X2-	T49.5X3-	T49.5X4-	T49.5X5-	T49.5X6-
topical NEC	T49.0X1-	T49.0X2-	T49.0X3-	T49.0X4-	T49.0X5-	T49.0X6-
Corticosteroid	T38.0X1-	T38.0X2-	T38.0X3-	T38.0X4-	T38.0X5-	T38.0X6-
ENT agent	T49.6X1-	T49.6X2-	T49.6X3-	T49.6X4-	T49.6X5-	T49.6X6-
mineral	T50.0X1-	T50.0X2-	T50.0X3-	T50.0X4-	T50.0X5-	T50.0X6-
ophthalmic	T49.5X1-	T49.5X2-	T49.5X3-	T49.5X4-	T49.5X5-	T49.5X6-
topical NEC	T49.0X1-	T49.0X2-	T49.0X3-	T49.0X4-	T49.0X5-	T49.0X6-
Corticotropin	T38.811-	T38.812-	T38.813-	T38.814-	T38.815-	T38.816-

Substance	Poisoning Accidental (unintentional)	Poisoning Intentional self-harm	Poisoning Assault	Poisoning Undetermined	Adverse effect	Underdosing
Cortisol	T49.0X1-	T49.0X2-	T49.0X3-	T49.0X4-	T49.0X5-	T49.0X6-
ENT agent	T49.6X1-	T49.6X2-	T49.6X3-	T49.6X4-	T49.6X5-	T49.6X6-
ophthalmic preparation	T49.5X1-	T49.5X2-	T49.5X3-	T49.5X4-	T49.5X5-	T49.5X6-
topical NEC	T49.0X1-	T49.0X2-	T49.0X3-	T49.0X4-	T49.0X5-	T49.0X6-
Cortisone (acetate)	T38.0X1-	T38.0X2-	T38.0X3-	T38.0X4-	T38.0X5-	T38.0X6-
ENT agent	T49.6X1-	T49.6X2-	T49.6X3-	T49.6X4-	T49.6X5-	T49.6X6-
ophthalmic preparation	T49.5X1-	T49.5X2-	T49.5X3-	T49.5X4-	T49.5X5-	T49.5X6-
topical NEC	T49.0X1-	T49.0X2-	T49.0X3-	T49.0X4-	T49.0X5-	T49.0X6-
Cortivazol	T38.0X1-	T38.0X2-	T38.0X3-	T38.0X4-	T38.0X5-	T38.0X6-
Cortogen	T38.0X1-	T38.0X2-	T38.0X3-	T38.0X4-	T38.0X5-	T38.0X6-
ENT agent	T49.6X1-	T49.6X2-	T49.6X3-	T49.6X4-	T49.6X5-	T49.6X6-
ophthalmic preparation	T49.5X1-	T49.5X2-	T49.5X3-	T49.5X4-	T49.5X5-	T49.5X6-
Cortone	T38.0X1-	T38.0X2-	T38.0X3-	T38.0X4-	T38.0X5-	T38.0X6-
ENT agent	T49.6X1-	T49.6X2-	T49.6X3-	T49.6X4-	T49.6X5-	T49.6X6-
ophthalmic preparation	T49.5X1-	T49.5X2-	T49.5X3-	T49.5X4-	T49.5X5-	T49.5X6-
Cortril	T38.0X1-	T38.0X2-	T38.0X3-	T38.0X4-	T38.0X5-	T38.0X6-
ENT agent	T49.6X1-	T49.6X2-	T49.6X3-	T49.6X4-	T49.6X5-	T49.6X6-
ophthalmic preparation	T49.5X1-	T49.5X2-	T49.5X3-	T49.5X4-	T49.5X5-	T49.5X6-
topical NEC	T49.0X1-	T49.0X2-	T49.0X3-	T49.0X4-	T49.0X5-	T49.0X6-
Corynebacterium parvum	T45.1X1-	T45.1X2-	T45.1X3-	T45.1X4-	T45.1X5-	T45.1X6-
Cosmetic preparation	T49.8X1-	T49.8X2-	T49.8X3-	T49.8X4-	T49.8X5-	T49.8X6-
Cosmetics	T49.8X1-	T49.8X2-	T49.8X3-	T49.8X4-	T49.8X5-	T49.8X6-
Cosyntropin	T38.811-	T38.812-	T38.813-	T38.814-	T38.815-	T38.816-
Cotarnine	T45.7X1-	T45.7X2-	T45.7X3-	T45.7X4-	T45.7X5-	T45.7X6-
Co-trimoxazole	T36.8X1-	T36.8X2-	T36.8X3-	T36.8X4-	T36.8X5-	T36.8X6-
Cottonseed oil	T49.3X1-	T49.3X2-	T49.3X3-	T49.3X4-	T49.3X5-	T49.3X6-
Cough mixture (syrup)	T48.4X1-	T48.4X2-	T48.4X3-	T48.4X4-	T48.4X5-	T48.4X6-
containing opiates	T40.2X1-	T40.2X2-	T40.2X3-	T40.2X4-	T40.2X5-	T40.2X6-
expectorants	T48.4X1-	T48.4X2-	T48.4X3-	T48.4X4-	T48.4X5-	T48.4X6-
Coumadin	T45.511-	T45.512-	T45.513-	T45.514-	T45.515-	T45.516-
rodenticide	T60.4X1-	T60.4X2-	T60.4X3-	T60.4X4-	-	-
Coumaphos	T60.0X1-	T60.0X2-	T60.0X3-	T60.0X4-	-	-
Coumarin	T45.511-	T45.512-	T45.513-	T45.514-	T45.515-	T45.516-
Coumetarol	T45.511-	T45.512-	T45.513-	T45.514-	T45.515-	T45.516-
Cowbane	T62.2X1-	T62.2X2-	T62.2X3-	T62.2X4-	-	-
Cozyme	T45.2X1-	T45.2X2-	T45.2X3-	T45.2X4-	T45.2X5-	T45.2X6-
Crack	T40.5X1-	T40.5X2-	T40.5X3-	T40.5X4-	-	-
Crataegus extract	T46.0X1-	T46.0X2-	T46.0X3-	T46.0X4-	T46.0X5-	T46.0X6-
Creolin	T54.1X1-	T54.1X2-	T54.1X3-	T54.1X4-	-	-
disinfectant	T54.1X1-	T54.1X2-	T54.1X3-	T54.1X4-	-	-
Creosol (compound)	T49.0X1-	T49.0X2-	T49.0X3-	T49.0X4-	T49.0X5-	T49.0X6-
Creosote (coal tar) (beechwood)	T49.0X1-	T49.0X2-	T49.0X3-	T49.0X4-	T49.0X5-	T49.0X6-
medicinal (expectorant)	T48.4X1-	T48.4X2-	T48.4X3-	T48.4X4-	T48.4X5-	T48.4X6-
syrup	T48.4X1-	T48.4X2-	T48.4X3-	T48.4X4-	T48.4X5-	T48.4X6-
Cresol (s)	T49.0X1-	T49.0X2-	T49.0X3-	T49.0X4-	T49.0X5-	T49.0X6-
and soap solution	T49.0X1-	T49.0X2-	T49.0X3-	T49.0X4-	T49.0X5-	T49.0X6-
Cresyl acetate	T49.0X1-	T49.0X2-	T49.0X3-	T49.0X4-	T49.0X5-	T49.0X6-
Cresylic acid	T49.0X1-	T49.0X2-	T49.0X3-	T49.0X4-	T49.0X5-	T49.0X6-
Crimidine	T60.4X1-	T60.4X2-	T60.4X3-	T60.4X4-	-	-
Croconazole	T37.8X1-	T37.8X2-	T37.8X3-	T37.8X4-	T37.8X5-	T37.8X6-
Cromoglicic acid	T48.6X1-	T48.6X2-	T48.6X3-	T48.6X4-	T48.6X5-	T48.6X6-
Cromolyn	T48.6X1-	T48.6X2-	T48.6X3-	T48.6X4-	T48.6X5-	T48.6X6-
Cromonar	T46.3X1-	T46.3X2-	T46.3X3-	T46.3X4-	T46.3X5-	T46.3X6-
Cropropamide	T39.8X1-	T39.8X2-	T39.8X3-	T39.8X4-	T39.8X5-	T39.8X6-
with crotethamide	T50.7X1-	T50.7X2-	T50.7X3-	T50.7X4-	T50.7X5-	T50.7X6-
Crotamiton	T49.0X1-	T49.0X2-	T49.0X3-	T49.0X4-	T49.0X5-	T49.0X6-

Substance	Poisoning Accidental (unintentional)	Poisoning Intentional self-harm	Poisoning Assault	Poisoning Undetermined	Adverse effect	Underdosing
Crotethamide	T39.8X1-	T39.8X2-	T39.8X3-	T39.8X4-	T39.8X5-	T39.8X6-
with cropropamide	T50.7X1-	T50.7X2-	T50.7X3-	T50.7X4-	T50.7X5-	T50.7X6-
Croton (oil)	T47.2X1-	T47.2X2-	T47.2X3-	T47.2X4-	T47.2X5-	T47.2X6-
chloral	T42.6X1-	T42.6X2-	T42.6X3-	T42.6X4-	T42.6X5-	T42.6X6-
Crude oil	T52.0X1-	T52.0X2-	T52.0X3-	T52.0X4-	-	-
Cryogenine	T39.8X1-	T39.8X2-	T39.8X3-	T39.8X4-	T39.8X5-	T39.8X6-
Cryolite (vapor)	T60.1X1-	T60.1X2-	T60.1X3-	T60.1X4-	-	-
insecticide	T60.1X1-	T60.1X2-	T60.1X3-	T60.1X4-	-	-
Cryptenamine (tannates)	T46.5X1-	T46.5X2-	T46.5X3-	T46.5X4-	T46.5X5-	T46.5X6-
Crystal violet	T49.0X1-	T49.0X2-	T49.0X3-	T49.0X4-	T49.0X5-	T49.0X6-
Cuckoopint	T62.2X1-	T62.2X2-	T62.2X3-	T62.2X4-	-	-
Cumetharol	T45.511-	T45.512-	T45.513-	T45.514-	T45.515-	T45.516-
Cupric						
acetate	T60.3X1-	T60.3X2-	T60.3X3-	T60.3X4-	-	-
acetoarsenite	T57.0X1-	T57.0X2-	T57.0X3-	T57.0X4-	-	-
arsenate	T57.0X1-	T57.0X2-	T57.0X3-	T57.0X4-	-	-
gluconate	T49.0X1-	T49.0X2-	T49.0X3-	T49.0X4-	T49.0X5-	T49.0X6-
oleate	T49.0X1-	T49.0X2-	T49.0X3-	T49.0X4-	T49.0X5-	T49.0X6-
sulfate	T56.4X1-	T56.4X2-	T56.4X3-	T56.4X4-	-	-
Cuprous sulfate — *see also Copper sulfate*	T56.4X1-	T56.4X2-	T56.4X3-	T56.4X4-	-	-
Curare, curarine	T48.1X1-	T48.1X2-	T48.1X3-	T48.1X4-	T48.1X5-	T48.1X6-
Cyamemazine	T43.3X1-	T43.3X2-	T43.3X3-	T43.3X4-	T43.3X5-	T43.3X6-
Cyamopsis tetragono-loba	T46.6X1-	T46.6X2-	T46.6X3-	T46.6X4-	T46.6X5-	T46.6X6-
Cyanacetyl hydrazide	T37.1X1-	T37.1X2-	T37.1X3-	T37.1X4-	T37.1X5-	T37.1X6-
Cyanic acid (gas)	T59.891-	T59.892-	T59.893-	T59.894-	-	-
Cyanide (s) (compounds) (potassium) (sodium) NEC	T65.0X1-	T65.0X2-	T65.0X3-	T65.0X4-	-	-
dust or gas (inhalation) NEC	T57.3X1-	T57.3X2-	T57.3X3-	T57.3X4-	-	-
fumigant	T65.0X1-	T65.0X2-	T65.0X3-	T65.0X4-	-	-
hydrogen	T57.3X1-	T57.3X2-	T57.3X3-	T57.3X4-	-	-
mercuric — *see Mercury*						
pesticide (dust) (fumes)	T65.0X1-	T65.0X2-	T65.0X3-	T65.0X4-	-	-
Cyanoacrylate adhesive	T49.3X1-	T49.3X2-	T49.3X3-	T49.3X4-	T49.3X5-	T49.3X6-
Cyanocobalamin	T45.8X1-	T45.8X2-	T45.8X3-	T45.8X4-	T45.8X5-	T45.8X6-
Cyanogen (chloride) (gas) NEC	T59.891-	T59.892-	T59.893-	T59.894-	-	-
Cyclacillin	T36.0X1-	T36.0X2-	T36.0X3-	T36.0X4-	T36.0X5-	T36.0X6-
Cyclaine	T41.3X1-	T41.3X2-	T41.3X3-	T41.3X4-	T41.3X5-	T41.3X6-
Cyclamate	T50.991-	T50.992-	T50.993-	T50.994-	T50.995-	T50.996-
Cyclamen europaeum	T62.2X1-	T62.2X2-	T62.2X3-	T62.2X4-	-	-
Cyclandelate	T46.7X1-	T46.7X2-	T46.7X3-	T46.7X4-	T46.7X5-	T46.7X6-
Cyclazocine	T50.7X1-	T50.7X2-	T50.7X3-	T50.7X4-	T50.7X5-	T50.7X6-
Cyclizine	T45.0X1-	T45.0X2-	T45.0X3-	T45.0X4-	T45.0X5-	T45.0X6-
Cyclobarbital	T42.3X1-	T42.3X2-	T42.3X3-	T42.3X4-	T42.3X5-	T42.3X6-
Cyclobarbitone	T42.3X1-	T42.3X2-	T42.3X3-	T42.3X4-	T42.3X5-	T42.3X6-
Cyclobenzaprine	T48.1X1-	T48.1X2-	T48.1X3-	T48.1X4-	T48.1X5-	T48.1X6-
Cyclodrine	T44.3X1-	T44.3X2-	T44.3X3-	T44.3X4-	T44.3X5-	T44.3X6-
Cycloguanil embonate	T37.2X1-	T37.2X2-	T37.2X3-	T37.2X4-	T37.2X5-	T37.2X6-
Cyclohexane	T52.8X1-	T52.8X2-	T52.8X3-	T52.8X4-	-	-
Cyclohexanol	T51.8X1-	T51.8X2-	T51.8X3-	T51.8X4-	-	-
Cyclohexanone	T52.4X1-	T52.4X2-	T52.4X3-	T52.4X4-	-	-
Cycloheximide	T60.3X1-	T60.3X2-	T60.3X3-	T60.3X4-	-	-
Cyclohexyl acetate	T52.8X1-	T52.8X2-	T52.8X3-	T52.8X4-	-	-
Cycloleucin	T45.1X1-	T45.1X2-	T45.1X3-	T45.1X4-	T45.1X5-	T45.1X6-
Cyclomethycaine	T41.3X1-	T41.3X2-	T41.3X3-	T41.3X4-	T41.3X5-	T41.3X6-
Cyclopentamine	T44.4X1-	T44.4X2-	T44.4X3-	T44.4X4-	T44.4X5-	T44.4X6-
Cyclopenthiazide	T50.2X1-	T50.2X2-	T50.2X3-	T50.2X4-	T50.2X5-	T50.2X6-
Cyclopentolate	T44.3X1-	T44.3X2-	T44.3X3-	T44.3X4-	T44.3X5-	T44.3X6-
Cyclophosphamide	T45.1X1-	T45.1X2-	T45.1X3-	T45.1X4-	T45.1X5-	T45.1X6-

Substance	Poisoning Accidental (unintentional)	Poisoning Intentional self-harm	Poisoning Assault	Poisoning Undetermined	Adverse effect	Underdosing
Cycloplegic drug	T49.5X1-	T49.5X2-	T49.5X3-	T49.5X4-	T49.5X5-	T49.5X6-
Cyclopropane	T41.291-	T41.292-	T41.293-	T41.294-	T41.295-	T41.296-
Cyclopyrabital	T39.8X1-	T39.8X2-	T39.8X3-	T39.8X4-	T39.8X5-	T39.8X6-
Cycloserine	T37.1X1-	T37.1X2-	T37.1X3-	T37.1X4-	T37.1X5-	T37.1X6-
Cyclosporin	T45.1X1-	T45.1X2-	T45.1X3-	T45.1X4-	T45.1X5-	T45.1X6-
Cyclothiazide	T50.2X1-	T50.2X2-	T50.2X3-	T50.2X4-	T50.2X5-	T50.2X6-
Cycrimine	T44.3X1-	T44.3X2-	T44.3X3-	T44.3X4-	T44.3X5-	T44.3X6-
Cyhalothrin	T60.1X1-	T60.1X2-	T60.1X3-	T60.1X4-	-	-
Cymarin	T46.0X1-	T46.0X2-	T46.0X3-	T46.0X4-	T46.0X5-	T46.0X6-
Cypermethrin	T60.1X1-	T60.1X2-	T60.1X3-	T60.1X4-	-	-
Cyphenothrin	T60.2X1-	T60.2X2-	T60.2X3-	T60.2X4-	-	-
Cyproheptadine	T45.0X1-	T45.0X2-	T45.0X3-	T45.0X4-	T45.0X5-	T45.0X6-
Cyproterone	T38.6X1-	T38.6X2-	T38.6X3-	T38.6X4-	T38.6X5-	T38.6X6-
Cysteamine	T50.6X1-	T50.6X2-	T50.6X3-	T50.6X4-	T50.6X5-	T50.6X6-
Cytarabine	T45.1X1-	T45.1X2-	T45.1X3-	T45.1X4-	T45.1X5-	T45.1X6-
Cytisus						
laburnum	T62.2X1-	T62.2X2-	T62.2X3-	T62.2X4-	-	-
scoparius	T62.2X1-	T62.2X2-	T62.2X3-	T62.2X4-	-	-
Cytochrome C	T47.5X1-	T47.5X2-	T47.5X3-	T47.5X4-	T47.5X5-	T47.5X6-
Cytomel	T38.1X1-	T38.1X2-	T38.1X3-	T38.1X4-	T38.1X5-	T38.1X6-
Cytosine arabinoside	T45.1X1-	T45.1X2-	T45.1X3-	T45.1X4-	T45.1X5-	T45.1X6-
Cytoxan	T45.1X1-	T45.1X2-	T45.1X3-	T45.1X4-	T45.1X5-	T45.1X6-
Cytozyme	T45.7X1-	T45.7X2-	T45.7X3-	T45.7X4-	T45.7X5-	T45.7X6-
2,4-D	T60.3X1-	T60.3X2-	T60.3X3-	T60.3X4-	-	-
Dacarbazine	T45.1X1-	T45.1X2-	T45.1X3-	T45.1X4-	T45.1X5-	T45.1X6-
Dactinomycin	T45.1X1-	T45.1X2-	T45.1X3-	T45.1X4-	T45.1X5-	T45.1X6-
DADPS	T37.1X1-	T37.1X2-	T37.1X3-	T37.1X4-	T37.1X5-	T37.1X6-
Dakin's solution	T49.0X1-	T49.0X2-	T49.0X3-	T49.0X4-	T49.0X5-	T49.0X6-
Dalapon (sodium)	T60.3X1-	T60.3X2-	T60.3X3-	T60.3X4-	-	-
Dalmane	T42.4X1-	T42.4X2-	T42.4X3-	T42.4X4-	T42.4X5-	T42.4X6-
Danazol	T38.6X1-	T38.6X2-	T38.6X3-	T38.6X4-	T38.6X5-	T38.6X6-
Danilone	T45.511-	T45.512-	T45.513-	T45.514-	T45.515-	T45.516-
Danthron	T47.2X1-	T47.2X2-	T47.2X3-	T47.2X4-	T47.2X5-	T47.2X6-
Dantrolene	T42.8X1-	T42.8X2-	T42.8X3-	T42.8X4-	T42.8X5-	T42.8X6-
Dantron	T47.2X1-	T47.2X2-	T47.2X3-	T47.2X4-	T47.2X5-	T47.2X6-
Daphne (gnidium) (mezereum)	T62.2X1-	T62.2X2-	T62.2X3-	T62.2X4-	-	-
berry	T62.1X1-	T62.1X2-	T62.1X3-	T62.1X4-	-	-
Dapsone	T37.1X1-	T37.1X2-	T37.1X3-	T37.1X4-	T37.1X5-	T37.1X6-
Daraprim	T37.2X1-	T37.2X2-	T37.2X3-	T37.2X4-	T37.2X5-	T37.2X6-
Darnel	T62.2X1-	T62.2X2-	T62.2X3-	T62.2X4-	-	-
Darvon	T39.8X1-	T39.8X2-	T39.8X3-	T39.8X4-	T39.8X5-	T39.8X6-
Daunomycin	T45.1X1-	T45.1X2-	T45.1X3-	T45.1X4-	T45.1X5-	T45.1X6-
Daunorubicin	T45.1X1-	T45.1X2-	T45.1X3-	T45.1X4-	T45.1X5-	T45.1X6-
DBI	T38.3X1-	T38.3X2-	T38.3X3-	T38.3X4-	T38.3X5-	T38.3X6-
D-Con	T60.91X-	T60.92X-	T60.93X-	T60.94X-	-	-
insecticide	T60.2X1-	T60.2X2-	T60.2X3-	T60.2X4-	-	-
rodenticide	T60.4X1-	T60.4X2-	T60.4X3-	T60.4X4-	-	-
DDAVP	T38.891-	T38.892-	T38.893-	T38.894-	T38.895-	T38.896-
DDE (bis (chlorophenyl) -dichloroethylene)	T60.2X1-	T60.2X2-	T60.2X3-	T60.2X4-	-	-
DDS	T37.1X1-	T37.1X2-	T37.1X3-	T37.1X4-	T37.1X5-	T37.1X6-
DDT (dust)	T60.1X1-	T60.1X2-	T60.1X3-	T60.1X4-	-	-
Deadly nightshade — *see also Belladonna*	T62.2X1-	T62.2X2-	T62.2X3-	T62.2X4-	-	-
berry	T62.1X1-	T62.1X2-	T62.1X3-	T62.1X4-	-	-
Deamino-D-arginine vasopressin	T38.891-	T38.892-	T38.893-	T38.894-	T38.895-	T38.896-
Deanol (aceglumate)	T50.991-	T50.992-	T50.993-	T50.994-	T50.995-	T50.996-
Debrisoquine	T46.5X1-	T46.5X2-	T46.5X3-	T46.5X4-	T46.5X5-	T46.5X6-

Substance	Poisoning Accidental (unintentional)	Poisoning Intentional self-harm	Poisoning Assault	Poisoning Undetermined	Adverse effect	Underdosing
Decaborane	T57.8X1-	T57.8X2-	T57.8X3-	T57.8X4-	-	-
fumes	T59.891-	T59.892-	T59.893-	T59.894-	-	-
Decadron	T38.0X1-	T38.0X2-	T38.0X3-	T38.0X4-	T38.0X5-	T38.0X6-
ENT agent	T49.6X1-	T49.6X2-	T49.6X3-	T49.6X4-	T49.6X5-	T49.6X6-
ophthalmic preparation	T49.5X1-	T49.5X2-	T49.5X3-	T49.5X4-	T49.5X5-	T49.5X6-
topical NEC	T49.0X1-	T49.0X2-	T49.0X3-	T49.0X4-	T49.0X5-	T49.0X6-
Decahydronaphthalene	T52.8X1-	T52.8X2-	T52.8X3-	T52.8X4-	-	-
Decalin	T52.8X1-	T52.8X2-	T52.8X3-	T52.8X4-	-	-
Decamethonium (bromide)	T48.1X1-	T48.1X2-	T48.1X3-	T48.1X4-	T48.1X5-	T48.1X6-
Decholin	T47.5X1-	T47.5X2-	T47.5X3-	T47.5X4-	T47.5X5-	T47.5X6-
Declomycin	T36.4X1-	T36.4X2-	T36.4X3-	T36.4X4-	T36.4X5-	T36.4X6-
Decongestant, nasal (mucosa)	T48.5X1-	T48.5X2-	T48.5X3-	T48.5X4-	T48.5X5-	T48.5X6-
combination	T48.5X1-	T48.5X2-	T48.5X3-	T48.5X4-	T48.5X5-	T48.5X6-
Deet	T60.8X1-	T60.8X2-	T60.8X3-	T60.8X4-	-	-
Deferoxamine	T45.8X1-	T45.8X2-	T45.8X3-	T45.8X4-	T45.8X5-	T45.8X6-
Deflazacort	T38.0X1-	T38.0X2-	T38.0X3-	T38.0X4-	T38.0X5-	T38.0X6-
Deglycyrrhizinized extract of licorice	T48.4X1-	T48.4X2-	T48.4X3-	T48.4X4-	T48.4X5-	T48.4X6-
Dehydrocholic acid	T47.5X1-	T47.5X2-	T47.5X3-	T47.5X4-	T47.5X5-	T47.5X6-
Dehydroemetine	T37.3X1-	T37.3X2-	T37.3X3-	T37.3X4-	T37.3X5-	T37.3X6-
Dekalin	T52.8X1-	T52.8X2-	T52.8X3-	T52.8X4-	-	-
Delalutin	T38.5X1-	T38.5X2-	T38.5X3-	T38.5X4-	T38.5X5-	T38.5X6-
Delorazepam	T42.4X1-	T42.4X2-	T42.4X3-	T42.4X4-	T42.4X5-	T42.4X6-
Delphinium	T62.2X1-	T62.2X2-	T62.2X3-	T62.2X4-	-	-
Deltamethrin	T60.1X1-	T60.1X2-	T60.1X3-	T60.1X4-	-	-
Deltasone	T38.0X1-	T38.0X2-	T38.0X3-	T38.0X4-	T38.0X5-	T38.0X6-
Deltra	T38.0X1-	T38.0X2-	T38.0X3-	T38.0X4-	T38.0X5-	T38.0X6-
Delvinal	T42.3X1-	T42.3X2-	T42.3X3-	T42.3X4-	T42.3X5-	T42.3X6-
Demecarium (bromide)	T49.5X1-	T49.5X2-	T49.5X3-	T49.5X4-	T49.5X5-	T49.5X6-
Demeclocycline	T36.4X1-	T36.4X2-	T36.4X3-	T36.4X4-	T36.4X5-	T36.4X6-
Demecolcine	T45.1X1-	T45.1X2-	T45.1X3-	T45.1X4-	T45.1X5-	T45.1X6-
Demegestone	T38.5X1-	T38.5X2-	T38.5X3-	T38.5X4-	T38.5X5-	T38.5X6-
Demelanizing agents	T49.8X1-	T49.8X2-	T49.8X3-	T49.8X4-	T49.8X5-	T49.8X6-
Demephion -O and -S	T60.0X1-	T60.0X2-	T60.0X3-	T60.0X4-	-	-
Demerol	T40.2X1-	T40.2X2-	T40.2X3-	T40.2X4-	T40.2X5-	T40.2X6-
Demethylchlortetracycline	T36.4X1-	T36.4X2-	T36.4X3-	T36.4X4-	T36.4X5-	T36.4X6-
Demethyltetracycline	T36.4X1-	T36.4X2-	T36.4X3-	T36.4X4-	T36.4X5-	T36.4X6-
Demeton -O and -S	T60.0X1-	T60.0X2-	T60.0X3-	T60.0X4-	-	-
Demulcent (external)	T49.3X1-	T49.3X2-	T49.3X3-	T49.3X4-	T49.3X5-	T49.3X6-
specified NEC	T49.3X1-	T49.3X2-	T49.3X3-	T49.3X4-	T49.3X5-	T49.3X6-
Demulen	T38.4X1-	T38.4X2-	T38.4X3-	T38.4X4-	T38.4X5-	T38.4X6-
Denatured alcohol	T51.0X1-	T51.0X2-	T51.0X3-	T51.0X4-	-	-
Dendrid	T49.5X1-	T49.5X2-	T49.5X3-	T49.5X4-	T49.5X5-	T49.5X6-
Dental drug, topical application NEC	T49.7X1-	T49.7X2-	T49.7X3-	T49.7X4-	T49.7X5-	T49.7X6-
Dentifrice	T49.7X1-	T49.7X2-	T49.7X3-	T49.7X4-	T49.7X5-	T49.7X6-
Deodorant spray (feminine hygiene)	T49.8X1-	T49.8X2-	T49.8X3-	T49.8X4-	T49.8X5-	T49.8X6-
Deoxycortone	T50.0X1-	T50.0X2-	T50.0X3-	T50.0X4-	T50.0X5-	T50.0X6-
2-Deoxy-5-fluorouridine	T45.1X1-	T45.1X2-	T45.1X3-	T45.1X4-	T45.1X5-	T45.1X6-
5-Deoxy-5-fluorouridine	T45.1X1-	T45.1X2-	T45.1X3-	T45.1X4-	T45.1X5-	T45.1X6-
Deoxyribonuclease (pancreatic)	T45.3X1-	T45.3X2-	T45.3X3-	T45.3X4-	T45.3X5-	T45.3X6-
Depilatory	T49.4X1-	T49.4X2-	T49.4X3-	T49.4X4-	T49.4X5-	T49.4X6-
Deprenalin	T42.8X1-	T42.8X2-	T42.8X3-	T42.8X4-	T42.8X5-	T42.8X6-
Deprenyl	T42.8X1-	T42.8X2-	T42.8X3-	T42.8X4-	T42.8X5-	T42.8X6-
Depressant, appetite	T50.5X1-	T50.5X2-	T50.5X3-	T50.5X4-	T50.5X5-	T50.5X6-
Depressant						
appetite (central)	T50.5X1-	T50.5X2-	T50.5X3-	T50.5X4-	T50.5X5-	T50.5X6-
cardiac	T46.2X1-	T46.2X2-	T46.2X3-	T46.2X4-	T46.2X5-	T46.2X6-
central nervous system (anesthetic) — *see also Central nervous system, depressants*	T42.71X-	T42.72X-	T42.73X-	T42.74X-	T42.75X-	T42.76X-

DECABORANE - DEPRESSANT

Substance	Poisoning Accidental (unintentional)	Poisoning Intentional self-harm	Poisoning Assault	Poisoning Undetermined	Adverse effect	Underdosing
Depressant (continued)						
general anesthetic	T41.201-	T41.202-	T41.203-	T41.204-	T41.205-	T41.206-
muscle tone	T42.8X1-	T42.8X2-	T42.8X3-	T42.8X4-	T42.8X5-	T42.8X6-
muscle tone, central	T42.8X1-	T42.8X2-	T42.8X3-	T42.8X4-	T42.8X5-	T42.8X6-
psychotherapeutic	T43.501-	T43.502-	T43.503-	T43.504-	T43.505-	T43.506-
Deptropine	T45.0X1-	T45.0X2-	T45.0X3-	T45.0X4-	T45.0X5-	T45.0X6-
Dequalinium (chloride)	T49.0X1-	T49.0X2-	T49.0X3-	T49.0X4-	T49.0X5-	T49.0X6-
Derris root	T60.2X1-	T60.2X2-	T60.2X3-	T60.2X4-	-	-
Deserpidine	T46.5X1-	T46.5X2-	T46.5X3-	T46.5X4-	T46.5X5-	T46.5X6-
Desferrioxamine	T45.8X1-	T45.8X2-	T45.8X3-	T45.8X4-	T45.8X5-	T45.8X6-
Desipramine	T43.011-	T43.012-	T43.013-	T43.014-	T43.015-	T43.016-
Deslanoside	T46.0X1-	T46.0X2-	T46.0X3-	T46.0X4-	T46.0X5-	T46.0X6-
Desloughing agent	T49.4X1-	T49.4X2-	T49.4X3-	T49.4X4-	T49.4X5-	T49.4X6-
Desmethylimipramine	T43.011-	T43.012-	T43.013-	T43.014-	T43.015-	T43.016-
Desmopressin	T38.891-	T38.892-	T38.893-	T38.894-	T38.895-	T38.896-
Desocodeine	T40.2X1-	T40.2X2-	T40.2X3-	T40.2X4-	T40.2X5-	T40.2X6-
Desogestrel	T38.5X1-	T38.5X2-	T38.5X3-	T38.5X4-	T38.5X5-	T38.5X6-
Desomorphine	T40.2X1-	T40.2X2-	T40.2X3-	T40.2X4-	-	-
Desonide	T49.0X1-	T49.0X2-	T49.0X3-	T49.0X4-	T49.0X5-	T49.0X6-
Desoximetasone	T49.0X1-	T49.0X2-	T49.0X3-	T49.0X4-	T49.0X5-	T49.0X6-
Desoxycorticosteroid	T50.0X1-	T50.0X2-	T50.0X3-	T50.0X4-	T50.0X5-	T50.0X6-
Desoxycortone	T50.0X1-	T50.0X2-	T50.0X3-	T50.0X4-	T50.0X5-	T50.0X6-
Desoxyephedrine	T43.621-	T43.622-	T43.623-	T43.624-	T43.625-	T43.626-
Detaxtran	T46.6X1-	T46.6X2-	T46.6X3-	T46.6X4-	T46.6X5-	T46.6X6-
Detergent	T49.2X1-	T49.2X2-	T49.2X3-	T49.2X4-	T49.2X5-	T49.2X6-
external medication	T49.2X1-	T49.2X2-	T49.2X3-	T49.2X4-	T49.2X5-	T49.2X6-
local	T49.2X1-	T49.2X2-	T49.2X3-	T49.2X4-	T49.2X5-	T49.2X6-
medicinal	T49.2X1-	T49.2X2-	T49.2X3-	T49.2X4-	T49.2X5-	T49.2X6-
nonmedicinal	T55.1X1-	T55.1X2-	T55.1X3-	T55.1X4-	-	-
specified NEC	T55.1X1-	T55.1X2-	T55.1X3-	T55.1X4-	-	-
Deterrent, alcohol	T50.6X1-	T50.6X2-	T50.6X3-	T50.6X4-	T50.6X5-	T50.6X6-
Detoxifying agent	T50.6X1-	T50.6X2-	T50.6X3-	T50.6X4-	T50.6X5-	T50.6X6-
Detrothyronine	T38.1X1-	T38.1X2-	T38.1X3-	T38.1X4-	T38.1X5-	T38.1X6-
Dettol (external medication)	T49.0X1-	T49.0X2-	T49.0X3-	T49.0X4-	T49.0X5-	T49.0X6-
Dexamethasone	T38.0X1-	T38.0X2-	T38.0X3-	T38.0X4-	T38.0X5-	T38.0X6-
ENT agent	T49.6X1-	T49.6X2-	T49.6X3-	T49.6X4-	T49.6X5-	T49.6X6-
ophthalmic preparation	T49.5X1-	T49.5X2-	T49.5X3-	T49.5X4-	T49.5X5-	T49.5X6-
topical NEC	T49.0X1-	T49.0X2-	T49.0X3-	T49.0X4-	T49.0X5-	T49.0X6-
Dexamfetamine	T43.621-	T43.622-	T43.623-	T43.624-	T43.625-	T43.626-
Dexamphetamine	T43.621-	T43.622-	T43.623-	T43.624-	T43.625-	T43.626-
Dexbrompheniramine	T45.0X1-	T45.0X2-	T45.0X3-	T45.0X4-	T45.0X5-	T45.0X6-
Dexchlorpheniramine	T45.0X1-	T45.0X2-	T45.0X3-	T45.0X4-	T45.0X5-	T45.0X6-
Dexedrine	T43.621-	T43.622-	T43.623-	T43.624-	T43.625-	T43.626-
Dexetimide	T44.3X1-	T44.3X2-	T44.3X3-	T44.3X4-	T44.3X5-	T44.3X6-
Dexfenfluramine	T50.5X1-	T50.5X2-	T50.5X3-	T50.5X4-	T50.5X5-	T50.5X6-
Dexpanthenol	T45.2X1-	T45.2X2-	T45.2X3-	T45.2X4-	T45.2X5-	T45.2X6-
Dextran (40) (70) (150)	T45.8X1-	T45.8X2-	T45.8X3-	T45.8X4-	T45.8X5-	T45.8X6-
Dextriferron	T45.4X1-	T45.4X2-	T45.4X3-	T45.4X4-	T45.4X5-	T45.4X6-
Dextro calcium pantothenate	T45.2X1-	T45.2X2-	T45.2X3-	T45.2X4-	T45.2X5-	T45.2X6-
Dextro pantothenyl alcohol	T45.2X1-	T45.2X2-	T45.2X3-	T45.2X4-	T45.2X5-	T45.2X6-
Dextroamphetamine	T43.621-	T43.622-	T43.623-	T43.624-	T43.625-	T43.626-
Dextromethorphan	T48.3X1-	T48.3X2-	T48.3X3-	T48.3X4-	T48.3X5-	T48.3X6-
Dextromoramide	T40.491-	T40.492-	T40.493-	T40.494-	-	-
topical	T49.8X1-	T49.8X2-	T49.8X3-	T49.8X4-	T49.8X5-	T49.8X6-
Dextropropoxyphene	T40.491-	T40.492-	T40.493-	T40.494-	T40.495-	T40.496-
Dextrorphan	T40.2X1-	T40.2X2-	T40.2X3-	T40.2X4-	T40.2X5-	T40.2X6-
Dextrose	T50.3X1-	T50.3X2-	T50.3X3-	T50.3X4-	T50.3X5-	T50.3X6-
concentrated solution, intravenous	T46.8X1-	T46.8X2-	T46.8X3-	T46.8X4-	T46.8X5-	T46.8X6-
Dextrothyroxin	T38.1X1-	T38.1X2-	T38.1X3-	T38.1X4-	T38.1X5-	T38.1X6-

Substance	Poisoning Accidental (unintentional)	Poisoning Intentional self-harm	Poisoning Assault	Poisoning Undetermined	Adverse effect	Underdosing
Dextrothyroxine sodium	T38.1X1-	T38.1X2-	T38.1X3-	T38.1X4-	T38.1X5-	T38.1X6-
DFP	T44.0X1-	T44.0X2-	T44.0X3-	T44.0X4-	T44.0X5-	T44.0X6-
DHE	T37.3X1-	T37.3X2-	T37.3X3-	T37.3X4-	T37.3X5-	T37.3X6-
45	T46.5X1-	T46.5X2-	T46.5X3-	T46.5X4-	T46.5X5-	T46.5X6-
Diabinese	T38.3X1-	T38.3X2-	T38.3X3-	T38.3X4-	T38.3X5-	T38.3X6-
Diacetone alcohol	T52.4X1-	T52.4X2-	T52.4X3-	T52.4X4-	-	-
Diacetyl monoxime	T50.991-	T50.992-	T50.993-	T50.994-	-	-
Diacetylmorphine	T40.1X1-	T40.1X2-	T40.1X3-	T40.1X4-	-	-
Diachylon plaster	T49.4X1-	T49.4X2-	T49.4X3-	T49.4X4-	T49.4X5-	T49.4X6-
Diaethylstilboestrolum	T38.5X1-	T38.5X2-	T38.5X3-	T38.5X4-	T38.5X5-	T38.5X6-
Diagnostic agent NEC	T50.8X1-	T50.8X2-	T50.8X3-	T50.8X4-	T50.8X5-	T50.8X6-
Dial (soap)	T49.2X1-	T49.2X2-	T49.2X3-	T49.2X4-	T49.2X5-	T49.2X6-
sedative	T42.3X1-	T42.3X2-	T42.3X3-	T42.3X4-	T42.3X5-	T42.3X6-
Dialkyl carbonate	T52.91X-	T52.92X-	T52.93X-	T52.94X-	-	-
Diallylbarbituric acid	T42.3X1-	T42.3X2-	T42.3X3-	T42.3X4-	T42.3X5-	T42.3X6-
Diallymal	T42.3X1-	T42.3X2-	T42.3X3-	T42.3X4-	T42.3X5-	T42.3X6-
Dialysis solution (intraperitoneal)	T50.3X1-	T50.3X2-	T50.3X3-	T50.3X4-	T50.3X5-	T50.3X6-
Diaminodiphenylsulfone	T37.1X1-	T37.1X2-	T37.1X3-	T37.1X4-	T37.1X5-	T37.1X6-
Diamorphine	T40.1X1-	T40.1X2-	T40.1X3-	T40.1X4-	-	-
Diamox	T50.2X1-	T50.2X2-	T50.2X3-	T50.2X4-	T50.2X5-	T50.2X6-
Diamthazole	T49.0X1-	T49.0X2-	T49.0X3-	T49.0X4-	T49.0X5-	T49.0X6-
Dianthone	T47.2X1-	T47.2X2-	T47.2X3-	T47.2X4-	T47.2X5-	T47.2X6-
Diaphenylsulfone	T37.0X1-	T37.0X2-	T37.0X3-	T37.0X4-	T37.0X5-	T37.0X6-
Diasone (sodium)	T37.1X1-	T37.1X2-	T37.1X3-	T37.1X4-	T37.1X5-	T37.1X6-
Diastase	T47.5X1-	T47.5X2-	T47.5X3-	T47.5X4-	T47.5X5-	T47.5X6-
Diatrizoate	T50.8X1-	T50.8X2-	T50.8X3-	T50.8X4-	T50.8X5-	T50.8X6-
Diazepam	T42.4X1-	T42.4X2-	T42.4X3-	T42.4X4-	T42.4X5-	T42.4X6-
Diazinon	T60.0X1-	T60.0X2-	T60.0X3-	T60.0X4-	-	-
Diazomethane (gas)	T59.891-	T59.892-	T59.893-	T59.894-	-	-
Diazoxide	T46.5X1-	T46.5X2-	T46.5X3-	T46.5X4-	T46.5X5-	T46.5X6-
Dibekacin	T36.5X1-	T36.5X2-	T36.5X3-	T36.5X4-	T36.5X5-	T36.5X6-
Dibenamine	T44.6X1-	T44.6X2-	T44.6X3-	T44.6X4-	T44.6X5-	T44.6X6-
Dibenzepin	T43.011-	T43.012-	T43.013-	T43.014-	T43.015-	T43.016-
Dibenzheptropine	T45.0X1-	T45.0X2-	T45.0X3-	T45.0X4-	T45.0X5-	T45.0X6-
Dibenzyline	T44.6X1-	T44.6X2-	T44.6X3-	T44.6X4-	T44.6X5-	T44.6X6-
Diborane (gas)	T59.891-	T59.892-	T59.893-	T59.894-	-	-
Dibromochloropropane	T60.8X1-	T60.8X2-	T60.8X3-	T60.8X4-	-	-
Dibromodulcitol	T45.1X1-	T45.1X2-	T45.1X3-	T45.1X4-	T45.1X5-	T45.1X6-
Dibromoethane	T53.6X1-	T53.6X2-	T53.6X3-	T53.6X4-	-	-
Dibromomannitol	T45.1X1-	T45.1X2-	T45.1X3-	T45.1X4-	T45.1X5-	T45.1X6-
Dibromopropamidine isethionate	T49.0X1-	T49.0X2-	T49.0X3-	T49.0X4-	T49.0X5-	T49.0X6-
Dibrompropamidine	T49.0X1-	T49.0X2-	T49.0X3-	T49.0X4-	T49.0X5-	T49.0X6-
Dibucaine	T41.3X1-	T41.3X2-	T41.3X3-	T41.3X4-	T41.3X5-	T41.3X6-
topical (surface)	T41.3X1-	T41.3X2-	T41.3X3-	T41.3X4-	T41.3X5-	T41.3X6-
Dibunate sodium	T48.3X1-	T48.3X2-	T48.3X3-	T48.3X4-	T48.3X5-	T48.3X6-
Dibutoline sulfate	T44.3X1-	T44.3X2-	T44.3X3-	T44.3X4-	T44.3X5-	T44.3X6-
Dicamba	T60.3X1-	T60.3X2-	T60.3X3-	T60.3X4-	-	-
Dicapthon	T60.0X1-	T60.0X2-	T60.0X3-	T60.0X4-	-	-
Dichlobenil	T60.3X1-	T60.3X2-	T60.3X3-	T60.3X4-	-	-
Dichlone	T60.3X1-	T60.3X2-	T60.3X3-	T60.3X4-	-	-
Dichloralphenozone	T42.6X1-	T42.6X2-	T42.6X3-	T42.6X4-	T42.6X5-	T42.6X6-
Dichlorbenzidine	T65.3X1-	T65.3X2-	T65.3X3-	T65.3X4-	-	-
Dichlorhydrin	T52.8X1-	T52.8X2-	T52.8X3-	T52.8X4-	-	-
Dichlorhydroxyquinoline	T37.8X1-	T37.8X2-	T37.8X3-	T37.8X4-	T37.8X5-	T37.8X6-
Dichlorobenzene	T53.7X1-	T53.7X2-	T53.7X3-	T53.7X4-	-	-
Dichlorobenzyl alcohol	T49.6X1-	T49.6X2-	T49.6X3-	T49.6X4-	T49.6X5-	T49.6X6-
Dichlorodifluoromethane	T53.5X1-	T53.5X2-	T53.5X3-	T53.5X4-	-	-
Dichloroethane	T52.8X1-	T52.8X2-	T52.8X3-	T52.8X4-	-	-
Sym-Dichloroethyl ether	T53.6X1-	T53.6X2-	T53.6X3-	T53.6X4-	-	-

Substance	Poisoning Accidental (unintentional)	Poisoning Intentional self-harm	Poisoning Assault	Poisoning Undetermined	Adverse effect	Underdosing
Dichloroethyl sulfide, not in war	T59.891-	T59.892-	T59.893-	T59.894-	-	-
Dichloroethylene	T53.6X1-	T53.6X2-	T53.6X3-	T53.6X4-	-	-
Dichloroformoxine, not in war	T59.891-	T59.892-	T59.893-	T59.894-	-	-
Dichlorohydrin, alpha-dichlorohydrin	T52.8X1-	T52.8X2-	T52.8X3-	T52.8X4-	-	-
Dichloromethane (solvent)	T53.4X1-	T53.4X2-	T53.4X3-	T53.4X4-	-	-
vapor	T53.4X1-	T53.4X2-	T53.4X3-	T53.4X4-	-	-
Dichloronaphthoquinone	T60.3X1-	T60.3X2-	T60.3X3-	T60.3X4-	-	-
Dichlorophen	T37.4X1-	T37.4X2-	T37.4X3-	T37.4X4-	T37.4X5-	T37.4X6-
2,4-Dichlorophenoxyacetic acid	T60.3X1-	T60.3X2-	T60.3X3-	T60.3X4-	-	-
Dichloropropene	T60.3X1-	T60.3X2-	T60.3X3-	T60.3X4-	-	-
Dichloropropionic acid	T60.3X1-	T60.3X2-	T60.3X3-	T60.3X4-	-	-
Dichlorphenamide	T50.2X1-	T50.2X2-	T50.2X3-	T50.2X4-	T50.2X5-	T50.2X6-
Dichlorvos	T60.0X1-	T60.0X2-	T60.0X3-	T60.0X4-	-	-
Diclofenac	T39.391-	T39.392-	T39.393-	T39.394-	T39.395-	T39.396-
Diclofenamide	T50.2X1-	T50.2X2-	T50.2X3-	T50.2X4-	T50.2X5-	T50.2X6-
Diclofensine	T43.291-	T43.292-	T43.293-	T43.294-	T43.295-	T43.296-
Diclonixine	T39.8X1-	T39.8X2-	T39.8X3-	T39.8X4-	T39.8X5-	T39.8X6-
Dicloxacillin	T36.0X1-	T36.0X2-	T36.0X3-	T36.0X4-	T36.0X5-	T36.0X6-
Dicophane	T49.0X1-	T49.0X2-	T49.0X3-	T49.0X4-	T49.0X5-	T49.0X6-
Dicoumarol, dicoumarin, dicumarol	T45.511-	T45.512-	T45.513-	T45.514-	T45.515-	T45.516-
Dicrotophos	T60.0X1-	T60.0X2-	T60.0X3-	T60.0X4-	-	-
Dicyanogen (gas)	T65.0X1-	T65.0X2-	T65.0X3-	T65.0X4-	-	-
Dicyclomine	T44.3X1-	T44.3X2-	T44.3X3-	T44.3X4-	T44.3X5-	T44.3X6-
Dicycloverine	T44.3X1-	T44.3X2-	T44.3X3-	T44.3X4-	T44.3X5-	T44.3X6-
Dideoxycytidine	T37.5X1-	T37.5X2-	T37.5X3-	T37.5X4-	T37.5X5-	T37.5X6-
Dideoxyinosine	T37.5X1-	T37.5X2-	T37.5X3-	T37.5X4-	T37.5X5-	T37.5X6-
Dieldrin (vapor)	T60.1X1-	T60.1X2-	T60.1X3-	T60.1X4-	-	-
Diemal	T42.3X1-	T42.3X2-	T42.3X3-	T42.3X4-	T42.3X5-	T42.3X6-
Dienestrol	T38.5X1-	T38.5X2-	T38.5X3-	T38.5X4-	T38.5X5-	T38.5X6-
Dienoestrol	T38.5X1-	T38.5X2-	T38.5X3-	T38.5X4-	T38.5X5-	T38.5X6-
Dietetic drug NEC	T50.901-	T50.902-	T50.903-	T50.904-	T50.905-	T50.906-
Diethazine	T42.8X1-	T42.8X2-	T42.8X3-	T42.8X4-	T42.8X5-	T42.8X6-
Diethyl						
barbituric acid	T42.3X1-	T42.3X2-	T42.3X3-	T42.3X4-	T42.3X5-	T42.3X6-
carbamazine	T37.4X1-	T37.4X2-	T37.4X3-	T37.4X4-	T37.4X5-	T37.4X6-
carbinol	T51.3X1-	T51.3X2-	T51.3X3-	T51.3X4-	-	-
carbonate	T52.8X1-	T52.8X2-	T52.8X3-	T52.8X4-	-	-
ether (vapor) — *see also ether*	T41.0X1-	T41.0X2-	T41.0X3-	T41.0X4-	T41.0X5-	T41.0X6-
oxide	T52.8X1-	T52.8X2-	T52.8X3-	T52.8X4-	-	-
propion	T50.5X1-	T50.5X2-	T50.5X3-	T50.5X4-	T50.5X5-	T50.5X6-
stilbestrol	T38.5X1-	T38.5X2-	T38.5X3-	T38.5X4-	T38.5X5-	T38.5X6-
toluamide (nonmedicinal)	T60.8X1-	T60.8X2-	T60.8X3-	T60.8X4-	-	-
medicinal	T49.3X1-	T49.3X2-	T49.3X3-	T49.3X4-	T49.3X5-	T49.3X6-
Diethylcarbamazine	T37.4X1-	T37.4X2-	T37.4X3-	T37.4X4-	T37.4X5-	T37.4X6-
Diethylene						
dioxide	T52.8X1-	T52.8X2-	T52.8X3-	T52.8X4-	-	-
glycol (monoacetate) (monobutyl ether) (monoethyl ether)	T52.3X1-	T52.3X2-	T52.3X3-	T52.3X4-	-	-
Diethylhexylphthalate	T65.891-	T65.892-	T65.893-	T65.894-	-	-
Diethylpropion	T50.5X1-	T50.5X2-	T50.5X3-	T50.5X4-	T50.5X5-	T50.5X6-
Diethylstilbestrol	T38.5X1-	T38.5X2-	T38.5X3-	T38.5X4-	T38.5X5-	T38.5X6-
Diethylstilboestrol	T38.5X1-	T38.5X2-	T38.5X3-	T38.5X4-	T38.5X5-	T38.5X6-
Diethylsulfone-diethylmethane	T42.6X1-	T42.6X2-	T42.6X3-	T42.6X4-	T42.6X5-	T42.6X6-
Diethyltoluamide	T49.0X1-	T49.0X2-	T49.0X3-	T49.0X4-	T49.0X5-	T49.0X6-
Diethyltryptamine (DET)	T40.991-	T40.992-	T40.993-	T40.994-	-	-
Difebarbamate	T42.3X1-	T42.3X2-	T42.3X3-	T42.3X4-	T42.3X5-	T42.3X6-
Difencloxazine	T40.2X1-	T40.2X2-	T40.2X3-	T40.2X4-	T40.2X5-	T40.2X6-
Difenidol	T45.0X1-	T45.0X2-	T45.0X3-	T45.0X4-	T45.0X5-	T45.0X6-
Difenoxin	T47.6X1-	T47.6X2-	T47.6X3-	T47.6X4-	T47.6X5-	T47.6X6-

Substance	Poisoning Accidental (unintentional)	Poisoning Intentional self-harm	Poisoning Assault	Poisoning Undetermined	Adverse effect	Underdosing
Difetarsone	T37.3X1-	T37.3X2-	T37.3X3-	T37.3X4-	T37.3X5-	T37.3X6-
Diffusin	T45.3X1-	T45.3X2-	T45.3X3-	T45.3X4-	T45.3X5-	T45.3X6-
Diflorasone	T49.0X1-	T49.0X2-	T49.0X3-	T49.0X4-	T49.0X5-	T49.0X6-
Diflos	T44.0X1-	T44.0X2-	T44.0X3-	T44.0X4-	T44.0X5-	T44.0X6-
Diflubenzuron	T60.1X1-	T60.1X2-	T60.1X3-	T60.1X4-	-	-
Diflucortolone	T49.0X1-	T49.0X2-	T49.0X3-	T49.0X4-	T49.0X5-	T49.0X6-
Diflunisal	T39.091-	T39.092-	T39.093-	T39.094-	T39.095-	T39.096-
Difluoromethyldopa	T42.8X1-	T42.8X2-	T42.8X3-	T42.8X4-	T42.8X5-	T42.8X6-
Difluorophate	T44.0X1-	T44.0X2-	T44.0X3-	T44.0X4-	T44.0X5-	T44.0X6-
Digestant NEC	T47.5X1-	T47.5X2-	T47.5X3-	T47.5X4-	T47.5X5-	T47.5X6-
Digitalin (e)	T46.0X1-	T46.0X2-	T46.0X3-	T46.0X4-	T46.0X5-	T46.0X6-
Digitalis (leaf) (glycoside)	T46.0X1-	T46.0X2-	T46.0X3-	T46.0X4-	T46.0X5-	T46.0X6-
lanata	T46.0X1-	T46.0X2-	T46.0X3-	T46.0X4-	T46.0X5-	T46.0X6-
purpurea	T46.0X1-	T46.0X2-	T46.0X3-	T46.0X4-	T46.0X5-	T46.0X6-
Digitoxin	T46.0X1-	T46.0X2-	T46.0X3-	T46.0X4-	T46.0X5-	T46.0X6-
Digitoxose	T46.0X1-	T46.0X2-	T46.0X3-	T46.0X4-	T46.0X5-	T46.0X6-
Digoxin	T46.0X1-	T46.0X2-	T46.0X3-	T46.0X4-	T46.0X5-	T46.0X6-
Digoxine	T46.0X1-	T46.0X2-	T46.0X3-	T46.0X4-	T46.0X5-	T46.0X6-
Dihydralazine	T46.5X1-	T46.5X2-	T46.5X3-	T46.5X4-	T46.5X5-	T46.5X6-
Dihydrazine	T46.5X1-	T46.5X2-	T46.5X3-	T46.5X4-	T46.5X5-	T46.5X6-
Dihydrocodeine	T40.2X1-	T40.2X2-	T40.2X3-	T40.2X4-	T40.2X5-	T40.2X6-
Dihydrocodeinone	T40.2X1-	T40.2X2-	T40.2X3-	T40.2X4-	T40.2X5-	T40.2X6-
Dihydroergocornine	T46.7X1-	T46.7X2-	T46.7X3-	T46.7X4-	T46.7X5-	T46.7X6-
Dihydroergocristine (mesilate)	T46.7X1-	T46.7X2-	T46.7X3-	T46.7X4-	T46.7X5-	T46.7X6-
Dihydroergokryptine	T46.7X1-	T46.7X2-	T46.7X3-	T46.7X4-	T46.7X5-	T46.7X6-
Dihydroergotamine	T46.5X1-	T46.5X2-	T46.5X3-	T46.5X4-	T46.5X5-	T46.5X6-
Dihydroergotoxine	T46.7X1-	T46.7X2-	T46.7X3-	T46.7X4-	T46.7X5-	T46.7X6-
mesilate	T46.7X1-	T46.7X2-	T46.7X3-	T46.7X4-	T46.7X5-	T46.7X6-
Dihydrohydroxycodeinone	T40.2X1-	T40.2X2-	T40.2X3-	T40.2X4-	T40.2X5-	T40.2X6-
Dihydrohydroxymorphinone	T40.2X1-	T40.2X2-	T40.2X3-	T40.2X4-	T40.2X5-	T40.2X6-
Dihydroisocodeine	T40.2X1-	T40.2X2-	T40.2X3-	T40.2X4-	T40.2X5-	T40.2X6-
Dihydromorphine	T40.2X1-	T40.2X2-	T40.2X3-	T40.2X4-	-	-
Dihydromorphinone	T40.2X1-	T40.2X2-	T40.2X3-	T40.2X4-	T40.2X5-	T40.2X6-
Dihydrostreptomycin	T36.5X1-	T36.5X2-	T36.5X3-	T36.5X4-	T36.5X5-	T36.5X6-
Dihydrotachysterol	T45.2X1-	T45.2X2-	T45.2X3-	T45.2X4-	T45.2X5-	T45.2X6-
Dihydroxyaluminum aminoacetate	T47.1X1-	T47.1X2-	T47.1X3-	T47.1X4-	T47.1X5-	T47.1X6-
Dihydroxyaluminum sodium carbonate	T47.1X1-	T47.1X2-	T47.1X3-	T47.1X4-	T47.1X5-	T47.1X6-
Dihydroxyanthraquinone	T47.2X1-	T47.2X2-	T47.2X3-	T47.2X4-	T47.2X5-	T47.2X6-
Dihydroxycodeinone	T40.2X1-	T40.2X2-	T40.2X3-	T40.2X4-	T40.2X5-	T40.2X6-
Dihydroxypropyl theophylline	T50.2X1-	T50.2X2-	T50.2X3-	T50.2X4-	T50.2X5-	T50.2X6-
Diiodohydroxyquin	T37.8X1-	T37.8X2-	T37.8X3-	T37.8X4-	T37.8X5-	T37.8X6-
topical	T49.0X1-	T49.0X2-	T49.0X3-	T49.0X4-	T49.0X5-	T49.0X6-
Diiodohydroxyquinoline	T37.8X1-	T37.8X2-	T37.8X3-	T37.8X4-	T37.8X5-	T37.8X6-
Diiodotyrosine	T38.2X1-	T38.2X2-	T38.2X3-	T38.2X4-	T38.2X5-	T38.2X6-
Diisopromine	T44.3X1-	T44.3X2-	T44.3X3-	T44.3X4-	T44.3X5-	T44.3X6-
Diisopropylamine	T46.3X1-	T46.3X2-	T46.3X3-	T46.3X4-	T46.3X5-	T46.3X6-
Diisopropylfluorophos-phonate	T44.0X1-	T44.0X2-	T44.0X3-	T44.0X4-	T44.0X5-	T44.0X6-
Dilantin	T42.0X1-	T42.0X2-	T42.0X3-	T42.0X4-	T42.0X5-	T42.0X6-
Dilaudid	T40.2X1-	T40.2X2-	T40.2X3-	T40.2X4-	T40.2X5-	T40.2X6-
Dilazep	T46.3X1-	T46.3X2-	T46.3X3-	T46.3X4-	T46.3X5-	T46.3X6-
Dill	T47.5X1-	T47.5X2-	T47.5X3-	T47.5X4-	T47.5X5-	T47.5X6-
Diloxanide	T37.3X1-	T37.3X2-	T37.3X3-	T37.3X4-	T37.3X5-	T37.3X6-
Diltiazem	T46.1X1-	T46.1X2-	T46.1X3-	T46.1X4-	T46.1X5-	T46.1X6-
Dimazole	T49.0X1-	T49.0X2-	T49.0X3-	T49.0X4-	T49.0X5-	T49.0X6-
Dimefline	T50.7X1-	T50.7X2-	T50.7X3-	T50.7X4-	T50.7X5-	T50.7X6-
Dimefox	T60.0X1-	T60.0X2-	T60.0X3-	T60.0X4-	-	-
Dimemorfan	T48.3X1-	T48.3X2-	T48.3X3-	T48.3X4-	T48.3X5-	T48.3X6-
Dimenhydrinate	T45.0X1-	T45.0X2-	T45.0X3-	T45.0X4-	T45.0X5-	T45.0X6-

Substance	Poisoning Accidental (unintentional)	Poisoning Intentional self-harm	Poisoning Assault	Poisoning Undetermined	Adverse effect	Underdosing
Dimercaprol (British anti-lewisite)	T45.8X1-	T45.8X2-	T45.8X3-	T45.8X4-	T45.8X5-	T45.8X6-
Dimercaptopropanol	T45.8X1-	T45.8X2-	T45.8X3-	T45.8X4-	T45.8X5-	T45.8X6-
Dimestrol	T38.5X1-	T38.5X2-	T38.5X3-	T38.5X4-	T38.5X5-	T38.5X6-
Dimetane	T45.0X1-	T45.0X2-	T45.0X3-	T45.0X4-	T45.0X5-	T45.0X6-
Dimethicone	T47.1X1-	T47.1X2-	T47.1X3-	T47.1X4-	T47.1X5-	T47.1X6-
Dimethindene	T45.0X1-	T45.0X2-	T45.0X3-	T45.0X4-	T45.0X5-	T45.0X6-
Dimethisoquin	T49.1X1-	T49.1X2-	T49.1X3-	T49.1X4-	T49.1X5-	T49.1X6-
Dimethisterone	T38.5X1-	T38.5X2-	T38.5X3-	T38.5X4-	T38.5X5-	T38.5X6-
Dimethoate	T60.0X1-	T60.0X2-	T60.0X3-	T60.0X4-	-	-
Dimethocaine	T41.3X1-	T41.3X2-	T41.3X3-	T41.3X4-	T41.3X5-	T41.3X6-
Dimethoxanate	T48.3X1-	T48.3X2-	T48.3X3-	T48.3X4-	T48.3X5-	T48.3X6-
Dimethyl						
arsine, arsinic acid	T57.0X1-	T57.0X2-	T57.0X3-	T57.0X4-	-	-
carbinol	T51.2X1-	T51.2X2-	T51.2X3-	T51.2X4-	-	-
carbonate	T52.8X1-	T52.8X2-	T52.8X3-	T52.8X4-	-	-
diguanide	T38.3X1-	T38.3X2-	T38.3X3-	T38.3X4-	T38.3X5-	T38.3X6-
ketone	T52.4X1-	T52.4X2-	T52.4X3-	T52.4X4-	-	-
vapor	T52.4X1-	T52.4X2-	T52.4X3-	T52.4X4-	-	-
meperidine	T40.2X1-	T40.2X2-	T40.2X3-	T40.2X4-	T40.2X5-	T40.2X6-
parathion	T60.0X1-	T60.0X2-	T60.0X3-	T60.0X4-	-	-
phthlate	T49.3X1-	T49.3X2-	T49.3X3-	T49.3X4-	T49.3X5-	T49.3X6-
polysiloxane	T47.8X1-	T47.8X2-	T47.8X3-	T47.8X4-	T47.8X5-	T47.8X6-
sulfate (fumes)	T59.891-	T59.892-	T59.893-	T59.894-	-	-
liquid	T65.891-	T65.892-	T65.893-	T65.894-	-	-
sulfoxide (nonmedicinal)	T52.8X1-	T52.8X2-	T52.8X3-	T52.8X4-	-	-
medicinal	T49.4X1-	T49.4X2-	T49.4X3-	T49.4X4-	T49.4X5-	T49.4X6-
tryptamine	T40.991-	T40.992-	T40.993-	T40.994-	-	-
tubocurarine	T48.1X1-	T48.1X2-	T48.1X3-	T48.1X4-	T48.1X5-	T48.1X6-
Dimethylamine sulfate	T49.4X1-	T49.4X2-	T49.4X3-	T49.4X4-	T49.4X5-	T49.4X6-
Dimethylformamide	T52.8X1-	T52.8X2-	T52.8X3-	T52.8X4-	-	-
Dimethyltubocurarinium chloride	T48.1X1-	T48.1X2-	T48.1X3-	T48.1X4-	T48.1X5-	T48.1X6-
Dimeticone	T47.1X1-	T47.1X2-	T47.1X3-	T47.1X4-	T47.1X5-	T47.1X6-
Dimetilan	T60.0X1-	T60.0X2-	T60.0X3-	T60.0X4-	-	-
Dimetindene	T45.0X1-	T45.0X2-	T45.0X3-	T45.0X4-	T45.0X5-	T45.0X6-
Dimetotiazine	T43.3X1-	T43.3X2-	T43.3X3-	T43.3X4-	T43.3X5-	T43.3X6-
Dimorpholamine	T50.7X1-	T50.7X2-	T50.7X3-	T50.7X4-	T50.7X5-	T50.7X6-
Dimoxyline	T46.3X1-	T46.3X2-	T46.3X3-	T46.3X4-	T46.3X5-	T46.3X6-
Dinitrobenzene	T65.3X1-	T65.3X2-	T65.3X3-	T65.3X4-	-	-
vapor	T59.891-	T59.892-	T59.893-	T59.894-	-	-
Dinitrobenzol	T65.3X1-	T65.3X2-	T65.3X3-	T65.3X4-	-	-
vapor	T59.891-	T59.892-	T59.893-	T59.894-	-	-
Dinitrobutylphenol	T65.3X1-	T65.3X2-	T65.3X3-	T65.3X4-	-	-
Dinitro (-ortho-) cresol (pesticide) (spray)	T65.3X1-	T65.3X2-	T65.3X3-	T65.3X4-	-	-
Dinitrocyclohexylphenol	T65.3X1-	T65.3X2-	T65.3X3-	T65.3X4-	-	-
Dinitrophenol	T65.3X1-	T65.3X2-	T65.3X3-	T65.3X4-	-	-
Dinoprost	T48.0X1-	T48.0X2-	T48.0X3-	T48.0X4-	T48.0X5-	T48.0X6-
Dinoprostone	T48.0X1-	T48.0X2-	T48.0X3-	T48.0X4-	T48.0X5-	T48.0X6-
Dinoseb	T60.3X1-	T60.3X2-	T60.3X3-	T60.3X4-	-	-
Dioctyl sulfosuccinate (calcium) (sodium)	T47.4X1-	T47.4X2-	T47.4X3-	T47.4X4-	T47.4X5-	T47.4X6-
Diodone	T50.8X1-	T50.8X2-	T50.8X3-	T50.8X4-	T50.8X5-	T50.8X6-
Diodoquin	T37.8X1-	T37.8X2-	T37.8X3-	T37.8X4-	T37.8X5-	T37.8X6-
Dionin	T40.2X1-	T40.2X2-	T40.2X3-	T40.2X4-	T40.2X5-	T40.2X6-
Diosmin	T46.991-	T46.992-	T46.993-	T46.994-	T46.995-	T46.996-
Dioxane	T52.8X1-	T52.8X2-	T52.8X3-	T52.8X4-	-	-
Dioxathion	T60.0X1-	T60.0X2-	T60.0X3-	T60.0X4-	-	-
Dioxin	T53.7X1-	T53.7X2-	T53.7X3-	T53.7X4-	-	-
Dioxopromethazine	T43.3X1-	T43.3X2-	T43.3X3-	T43.3X4-	T43.3X5-	T43.3X6-

Substance	Poisoning Accidental (unintentional)	Poisoning Intentional self-harm	Poisoning Assault	Poisoning Undetermined	Adverse effect	Underdosing
Dioxyline	T46.3X1-	T46.3X2-	T46.3X3-	T46.3X4-	T46.3X5-	T46.3X6-
Dipentene	T52.8X1-	T52.8X2-	T52.8X3-	T52.8X4-	-	-
Diperodon	T41.3X1-	T41.3X2-	T41.3X3-	T41.3X4-	T41.3X5-	T41.3X6-
Diphacinone	T60.4X1-	T60.4X2-	T60.4X3-	T60.4X4-	-	-
Diphemanil	T44.3X1-	T44.3X2-	T44.3X3-	T44.3X4-	T44.3X5-	T44.3X6-
metilsulfate	T44.3X1-	T44.3X2-	T44.3X3-	T44.3X4-	T44.3X5-	T44.3X6-
Diphenadione	T45.511-	T45.512-	T45.513-	T45.514-	T45.515-	T45.516-
rodenticide	T60.4X1-	T60.4X2-	T60.4X3-	T60.4X4-	-	-
Diphenhydramine	T45.0X1-	T45.0X2-	T45.0X3-	T45.0X4-	T45.0X5-	T45.0X6-
Diphenidol	T45.0X1-	T45.0X2-	T45.0X3-	T45.0X4-	T45.0X5-	T45.0X6-
Diphenoxylate	T47.6X1-	T47.6X2-	T47.6X3-	T47.6X4-	T47.6X5-	T47.6X6-
Diphenylamine	T65.3X1-	T65.3X2-	T65.3X3-	T65.3X4-	-	-
Diphenylbutazone	T39.2X1-	T39.2X2-	T39.2X3-	T39.2X4-	T39.2X5-	T39.2X6-
Diphenylchloroarsine, not in war	T57.0X1-	T57.0X2-	T57.0X3-	T57.0X4-	-	-
Diphenylhydantoin	T42.0X1-	T42.0X2-	T42.0X3-	T42.0X4-	T42.0X5-	T42.0X6-
Diphenylmethane dye	T52.1X1-	T52.1X2-	T52.1X3-	T52.1X4-	-	-
Diphenylpyraline	T45.0X1-	T45.0X2-	T45.0X3-	T45.0X4-	T45.0X5-	T45.0X6-
Diphtheria						
antitoxin	T50.Z11-	T50.Z12-	T50.Z13-	T50.Z14-	T50.Z15-	T50.Z16-
toxoid	T50.A91-	T50.A92-	T50.A93-	T50.A94-	T50.A95-	T50.A96-
with tetanus toxoid	T50.A21-	T50.A22-	T50.A23-	T50.A24-	T50.A25-	T50.A26-
with pertussis component	T50.A11-	T50.A12-	T50.A13-	T50.A14-	T50.A15-	T50.A16-
vaccine	T50.A91-	T50.A92-	T50.A93-	T50.A94-	T50.A95-	T50.A96-
combination						
including pertussis	T50.A11-	T50.A12-	T50.A13-	T50.A14-	T50.A15-	T50.A16-
without pertussis	T50.A21-	T50.A22-	T50.A23-	T50.A24-	T50.A25-	T50.A26-
Diphylline	T50.2X1-	T50.2X2-	T50.2X3-	T50.2X4-	T50.2X5-	T50.2X6-
Dipipanone	T40.491-	T40.492-	T40.493-	T40.494-	-	-
Dipivefrine	T49.5X1-	T49.5X2-	T49.5X3-	T49.5X4-	T49.5X5-	T49.5X6-
Diplovax	T50.B91-	T50.B92-	T50.B93-	T50.B94-	T50.B95-	T50.B96-
Diprophylline	T50.2X1-	T50.2X2-	T50.2X3-	T50.2X4-	T50.2X5-	T50.2X6-
Dipropyline	T48.291-	T48.292-	T48.293-	T48.294-	T48.295-	T48.296-
Dipyridamole	T46.3X1-	T46.3X2-	T46.3X3-	T46.3X4-	T46.3X5-	T46.3X6-
Dipyrone	T39.2X1-	T39.2X2-	T39.2X3-	T39.2X4-	T39.2X5-	T39.2X6-
Diquat (dibromide)	T60.3X1-	T60.3X2-	T60.3X3-	T60.3X4-	-	-
Disinfectant	T65.891-	T65.892-	T65.893-	T65.894-	-	-
alkaline	T54.3X1-	T54.3X2-	T54.3X3-	T54.3X4-	-	-
aromatic	T54.1X1-	T54.1X2-	T54.1X3-	T54.1X4-	-	-
intestinal	T37.8X1-	T37.8X2-	T37.8X3-	T37.8X4-	T37.8X5-	T37.8X6-
Disipal	T42.8X1-	T42.8X2-	T42.8X3-	T42.8X4-	T42.8X5-	T42.8X6-
Disodium edetate	T50.6X1-	T50.6X2-	T50.6X3-	T50.6X4-	T50.6X5-	T50.6X6-
Disoprofol	T41.291-	T41.292-	T41.293-	T41.294-	T41.295-	T41.296-
Disopyramide	T46.2X1-	T46.2X2-	T46.2X3-	T46.2X4-	T46.2X5-	T46.2X6-
Distigmine (bromide)	T44.0X1-	T44.0X2-	T44.0X3-	T44.0X4-	T44.0X5-	T44.0X6-
Disulfamide	T50.2X1-	T50.2X2-	T50.2X3-	T50.2X4-	T50.2X5-	T50.2X6-
Disulfanilamide	T37.0X1-	T37.0X2-	T37.0X3-	T37.0X4-	T37.0X5-	T37.0X6-
Disulfiram	T50.6X1-	T50.6X2-	T50.6X3-	T50.6X4-	T50.6X5-	T50.6X6-
Disulfoton	T60.0X1-	T60.0X2-	T60.0X3-	T60.0X4-	-	-
Dithiazanine iodide	T37.4X1-	T37.4X2-	T37.4X3-	T37.4X4-	T37.4X5-	T37.4X6-
Dithiocarbamate	T60.0X1-	T60.0X2-	T60.0X3-	T60.0X4-	-	-
Dithranol	T49.4X1-	T49.4X2-	T49.4X3-	T49.4X4-	T49.4X5-	T49.4X6-
Diucardin	T50.2X1-	T50.2X2-	T50.2X3-	T50.2X4-	T50.2X5-	T50.2X6-
Diupres	T50.2X1-	T50.2X2-	T50.2X3-	T50.2X4-	T50.2X5-	T50.2X6-
Diuretic NEC	T50.2X1-	T50.2X2-	T50.2X3-	T50.2X4-	T50.2X5-	T50.2X6-
benzothiadiazine	T50.2X1-	T50.2X2-	T50.2X3-	T50.2X4-	T50.2X5-	T50.2X6-
carbonic acid anhydrase inhibitors	T50.2X1-	T50.2X2-	T50.2X3-	T50.2X4-	T50.2X5-	T50.2X6-
furfuryl NEC	T50.2X1-	T50.2X2-	T50.2X3-	T50.2X4-	T50.2X5-	T50.2X6-
loop (high-ceiling)	T50.1X1-	T50.1X2-	T50.1X3-	T50.1X4-	T50.1X5-	T50.1X6-

Substance	Poisoning Accidental (unintentional)	Poisoning Intentional self-harm	Poisoning Assault	Poisoning Undetermined	Adverse effect	Underdosing
Diuretic NEC (continued)						
mercurial NEC	T50.2X1-	T50.2X2-	T50.2X3-	T50.2X4-	T50.2X5-	T50.2X6-
osmotic	T50.2X1-	T50.2X2-	T50.2X3-	T50.2X4-	T50.2X5-	T50.2X6-
purine NEC	T50.2X1-	T50.2X2-	T50.2X3-	T50.2X4-	T50.2X5-	T50.2X6-
saluretic NEC	T50.2X1-	T50.2X2-	T50.2X3-	T50.2X4-	T50.2X5-	T50.2X6-
sulfonamide	T50.2X1-	T50.2X2-	T50.2X3-	T50.2X4-	T50.2X5-	T50.2X6-
thiazide NEC	T50.2X1-	T50.2X2-	T50.2X3-	T50.2X4-	T50.2X5-	T50.2X6-
xanthine	T50.2X1-	T50.2X2-	T50.2X3-	T50.2X4-	T50.2X5-	T50.2X6-
Diurgin	T50.2X1-	T50.2X2-	T50.2X3-	T50.2X4-	T50.2X5-	T50.2X6-
Diuril	T50.2X1-	T50.2X2-	T50.2X3-	T50.2X4-	T50.2X5-	T50.2X6-
Diuron	T60.3X1-	T60.3X2-	T60.3X3-	T60.3X4-	-	-
Divalproex	T42.6X1-	T42.6X2-	T42.6X3-	T42.6X4-	T42.6X5-	T42.6X6-
Divinyl ether	T41.0X1-	T41.0X2-	T41.0X3-	T41.0X4-	T41.0X5-	T41.0X6-
Dixanthogen	T49.0X1-	T49.0X2-	T49.0X3-	T49.0X4-	T49.0X5-	T49.0X6-
Dixyrazine	T43.3X1-	T43.3X2-	T43.3X3-	T43.3X4-	T43.3X5-	T43.3X6-
D-lysergic acid diethylamide	T40.8X1-	T40.8X2-	T40.8X3-	T40.8X4-	-	-
DMCT	T36.4X1-	T36.4X2-	T36.4X3-	T36.4X4-	T36.4X5-	T36.4X6-
DMSO — *see Dimethyl sulfoxide*						
DNBP	T60.3X1-	T60.3X2-	T60.3X3-	T60.3X4-	-	-
DNOC	T65.3X1-	T65.3X2-	T65.3X3-	T65.3X4-	-	-
Dobutamine	T44.5X1-	T44.5X2-	T44.5X3-	T44.5X4-	T44.5X5-	T44.5X6-
DOCA	T38.0X1-	T38.0X2-	T38.0X3-	T38.0X4-	T38.0X5-	T38.0X6-
Docusate sodium	T47.4X1-	T47.4X2-	T47.4X3-	T47.4X4-	T47.4X5-	T47.4X6-
Dodicin	T49.0X1-	T49.0X2-	T49.0X3-	T49.0X4-	T49.0X5-	T49.0X6-
Dofamium chloride	T49.0X1-	T49.0X2-	T49.0X3-	T49.0X4-	T49.0X5-	T49.0X6-
Dolophine	T40.3X1-	T40.3X2-	T40.3X3-	T40.3X4-	T40.3X5-	T40.3X6-
Doloxene	T39.8X1-	T39.8X2-	T39.8X3-	T39.8X4-	T39.8X5-	T39.8X6-
Domestic gas (after combustion) — *see Gas, utility*						
prior to combustion	T59.891-	T59.892-	T59.893-	T59.894-	-	-
Domiodol	T48.4X1-	T48.4X2-	T48.4X3-	T48.4X4-	T48.4X5-	T48.4X6-
Domiphen (bromide)	T49.0X1-	T49.0X2-	T49.0X3-	T49.0X4-	T49.0X5-	T49.0X6-
Domperidone	T45.0X1-	T45.0X2-	T45.0X3-	T45.0X4-	T45.0X5-	T45.0X6-
Dopa	T42.8X1-	T42.8X2-	T42.8X3-	T42.8X4-	T42.8X5-	T42.8X6-
Dopamine	T44.991-	T44.992-	T44.993-	T44.994-	T44.995-	T44.996-
Doriden	T42.6X1-	T42.6X2-	T42.6X3-	T42.6X4-	T42.6X5-	T42.6X6-
Dormiral	T42.3X1-	T42.3X2-	T42.3X3-	T42.3X4-	T42.3X5-	T42.3X6-
Dormison	T42.6X1-	T42.6X2-	T42.6X3-	T42.6X4-	T42.6X5-	T42.6X6-
Dornase	T48.4X1-	T48.4X2-	T48.4X3-	T48.4X4-	T48.4X5-	T48.4X6-
Dorsacaine	T41.3X1-	T41.3X2-	T41.3X3-	T41.3X4-	T41.3X5-	T41.3X6-
Dosulepin	T43.011-	T43.012-	T43.013-	T43.014-	T43.015-	T43.016-
Dothiepin	T43.011-	T43.012-	T43.013-	T43.014-	T43.015-	T43.016-
Doxantrazole	T48.6X1-	T48.6X2-	T48.6X3-	T48.6X4-	T48.6X5-	T48.6X6-
Doxapram	T50.7X1-	T50.7X2-	T50.7X3-	T50.7X4-	T50.7X5-	T50.7X6-
Doxazosin	T44.6X1-	T44.6X2-	T44.6X3-	T44.6X4-	T44.6X5-	T44.6X6-
Doxepin	T43.011-	T43.012-	T43.013-	T43.014-	T43.015-	T43.016-
Doxifluridine	T45.1X1-	T45.1X2-	T45.1X3-	T45.1X4-	T45.1X5	T45.1X6-
Doxorubicin	T45.1X1-	T45.1X2-	T45.1X3-	T45.1X4-	T45.1X5-	T45.1X6-
Doxycycline	T36.4X1-	T36.4X2-	T36.4X3-	T36.4X4-	T36.4X5-	T36.4X6-
Doxylamine	T45.0X1-	T45.0X2-	T45.0X3-	T45.0X4-	T45.0X5-	T45.0X6-
Dramamine	T45.0X1-	T45.0X2-	T45.0X3-	T45.0X4-	T45.0X5-	T45.0X6-
Drano (drain cleaner)	T54.3X1-	T54.3X2-	T54.3X3-	T54.3X4-	-	-
Dressing, live pulp	T49.7X1-	T49.7X2-	T49.7X3-	T49.7X4-	T49.7X5-	T49.7X6-
Drocode	T40.2X1-	T40.2X2-	T40.2X3-	T40.2X4-	T40.2X5-	T40.2X6-
Dromoran	T40.2X1-	T40.2X2-	T40.2X3-	T40.2X4-	T40.2X5-	T40.2X6-
Dromostanolone	T38.7X1-	T38.7X2-	T38.7X3-	T38.7X4-	T38.7X5-	T38.7X6-
Dronabinol	T40.711-	T40.712-	T40.713-	T40.714-	T40.715-	T40.716-
Droperidol	T43.591-	T43.592-	T43.593-	T43.594-	T43.595-	T43.596-
Dropropizine	T48.3X1-	T48.3X2-	T48.3X3-	T48.3X4-	T48.3X5-	T48.3X6-
Drostanolone	T38.7X1-	T38.7X2-	T38.7X3-	T38.7X4-	T38.7X5-	T38.7X6-

Substance	Poisoning Accidental (unintentional)	Poisoning Intentional self-harm	Poisoning Assault	Poisoning Undetermined	Adverse effect	Underdosing
Drotaverine	T44.3X1-	T44.3X2-	T44.3X3-	T44.3X4-	T44.3X5-	T44.3X6-
Drotrecogin alfa	T45.511-	T45.512-	T45.513-	T45.514-	T45.515-	T45.516-
Drug NEC	T50.901-	T50.902-	T50.903-	T50.904-	T50.905-	T50.906-
specified NEC	T50.991-	T50.992-	T50.993-	T50.994-	T50.995-	T50.996-
DTIC	T45.1X1-	T45.1X2-	T45.1X3-	T45.1X4-	T45.1X5-	T45.1X6-
Duboisine	T44.3X1-	T44.3X2-	T44.3X3-	T44.3X4-	T44.3X5-	T44.3X6-
Dulcolax	T47.2X1-	T47.2X2-	T47.2X3-	T47.2X4-	T47.2X5-	T47.2X6-
Duponol (C) (EP)	T49.2X1-	T49.2X2-	T49.2X3-	T49.2X4-	T49.2X5-	T49.2X6-
Durabolin	T38.7X1-	T38.7X2-	T38.7X3-	T38.7X4-	T38.7X5-	T38.7X6-
Dyclone	T41.3X1-	T41.3X2-	T41.3X3-	T41.3X4-	T41.3X5-	T41.3X6-
Dyclonine	T41.3X1-	T41.3X2-	T41.3X3-	T41.3X4-	T41.3X5-	T41.3X6-
Dydrogesterone	T38.5X1-	T38.5X2-	T38.5X3-	T38.5X4-	T38.5X5-	T38.5X6-
Dye NEC	T65.6X1-	T65.6X2-	T65.6X3-	T65.6X4-	-	-
antiseptic	T49.0X1-	T49.0X2-	T49.0X3-	T49.0X4-	T49.0X5-	T49.0X6-
diagnostic agents	T50.8X1-	T50.8X2-	T50.8X3-	T50.8X4-	T50.8X5-	T50.8X6-
pharmaceutical NEC	T50.901-	T50.902-	T50.903-	T50.904-	T50.905-	T50.906-
Dyflos	T44.0X1-	T44.0X2-	T44.0X3-	T44.0X4-	T44.0X5-	T44.0X6-
Dymelor	T38.3X1-	T38.3X2-	T38.3X3-	T38.3X4-	T38.3X5-	T38.3X6-
Dynamite	T65.3X1-	T65.3X2-	T65.3X3-	T65.3X4-	-	-
fumes	T59.891-	T59.892-	T59.893-	T59.894-	-	-
Dyphylline	T44.3X1-	T44.3X2-	T44.3X3-	T44.3X4-	T44.3X5-	T44.3X6-
Ear drug NEC	T49.6X1-	T49.6X2-	T49.6X3-	T49.6X4-	T49.6X5-	T49.6X6-
Ear preparations	T49.6X1-	T49.6X2-	T49.6X3-	T49.6X4-	T49.6X5-	T49.6X6-
Echothiophate, echothiopate, ecothiopate	T49.5X1-	T49.5X2-	T49.5X3-	T49.5X4-	T49.5X5-	T49.5X6-
Econazole	T49.0X1-	T49.0X2-	T49.0X3-	T49.0X4-	T49.0X5-	T49.0X6-
Ecothiopate iodide	T49.5X1-	T49.5X2-	T49.5X3-	T49.5X4-	T49.5X5-	T49.5X6-
Ecstasy	T43.641-	T43.642-	T43.643-	T43.644-	-	-
Ectylurea	T42.6X1-	T42.6X2-	T42.6X3-	T42.6X4-	T42.6X5-	T42.6X6-
Edathamil disodium	T45.8X1-	T45.8X2-	T45.8X3-	T45.8X4-	T45.8X5-	T45.8X6-
Edecrin	T50.1X1-	T50.1X2-	T50.1X3-	T50.1X4-	T50.1X5-	T50.1X6-
Edetate, disodium (calcium)	T45.8X1-	T45.8X2-	T45.8X3-	T45.8X4-	T45.8X5-	T45.8X6-
Edoxudine	T49.5X1-	T49.5X2-	T49.5X3-	T49.5X4-	T49.5X5-	T49.5X6-
Edrophonium	T44.0X1-	T44.0X2-	T44.0X3-	T44.0X4-	T44.0X5-	T44.0X6-
chloride	T44.0X1-	T44.0X2-	T44.0X3-	T44.0X4-	T44.0X5-	T44.0X6-
EDTA	T50.6X1-	T50.6X2-	T50.6X3-	T50.6X4-	T50.6X5-	T50.6X6-
Eflornithine	T37.2X1-	T37.2X2-	T37.2X3-	T37.2X4-	T37.2X5-	T37.2X6-
Efloxate	T46.3X1-	T46.3X2-	T46.3X3-	T46.3X4-	T46.3X5-	T46.3X6-
Elase	T49.8X1-	T49.8X2-	T49.8X3-	T49.8X4-	T49.8X5-	T49.8X6-
Elastase	T47.5X1-	T47.5X2-	T47.5X3-	T47.5X4-	T47.5X5-	T47.5X6-
Elaterium	T47.2X1-	T47.2X2-	T47.2X3-	T47.2X4-	T47.2X5-	T47.2X6-
Elcatonin	T50.991-	T50.992-	T50.993-	T50.994-	T50.995-	T50.996-
Elder	T62.2X1-	T62.2X2-	T62.2X3-	T62.2X4-	-	-
berry, (unripe)	T62.1X1-	T62.1X2-	T62.1X3-	T62.1X4-	-	-
Electrolyte balance drug	T50.3X1-	T50.3X2-	T50.3X3-	T50.3X4-	T50.3X5-	T50.3X6-
Electrolytes NEC	T50.3X1-	T50.3X2-	T50.3X3-	T50.3X4-	T50.3X5-	T50.3X6-
Electrolytic agent NEC	T50.3X1-	T50.3X2-	T50.3X3-	T50.3X4-	T50.3X5-	T50.3X6-
Elemental diet	T50.901-	T50.902-	T50.903-	T50.904-	T50.905-	T50.906-
Elliptinium acetate	T45.1X1-	T45.1X2-	T45.1X3-	T45.1X4-	T45.1X5-	T45.1X6-
Embramine	T45.0X1-	T45.0X2-	T45.0X3-	T45.0X4-	T45.0X5-	T45.0X6-
Emepronium (salts)	T44.3X1-	T44.3X2-	T44.3X3-	T44.3X4-	T44.3X5-	T44.3X6-
bromide	T44.3X1-	T44.3X2-	T44.3X3-	T44.3X4-	T44.3X5-	T44.3X6-
Emetic NEC	T47.7X1-	T47.7X2-	T47.7X3-	T47.7X4-	T47.7X5-	T47.7X6-
Emetine	T37.3X1-	T37.3X2-	T37.3X3-	T37.3X4-	T37.3X5-	T37.3X6-
Emollient NEC	T49.3X1-	T49.3X2-	T49.3X3-	T49.3X4-	T49.3X5-	T49.3X6-
Emorfazone	T39.8X1-	T39.8X2-	T39.8X3-	T39.8X4-	T39.8X5-	T39.8X6-
Emylcamate	T43.591-	T43.592-	T43.593-	T43.594-	T43.595-	T43.596-
Enalapril	T46.4X1-	T46.4X2-	T46.4X3-	T46.4X4-	T46.4X5-	T46.4X6-

Substance	Poisoning Accidental (unintentional)	Poisoning Intentional self-harm	Poisoning Assault	Poisoning Undetermined	Adverse effect	Underdosing
Enalaprilat	T46.4X1-	T46.4X2-	T46.4X3-	T46.4X4-	T46.4X5-	T46.4X6-
Encainide	T46.2X1-	T46.2X2-	T46.2X3-	T46.2X4-	T46.2X5-	T46.2X6-
Endocaine	T41.3X1-	T41.3X2-	T41.3X3-	T41.3X4-	T41.3X5-	T41.3X6-
Endosulfan	T60.2X1-	T60.2X2-	T60.2X3-	T60.2X4-	-	-
Endothall	T60.3X1-	T60.3X2-	T60.3X3-	T60.3X4-	-	-
Endralazine	T46.5X1-	T46.5X2-	T46.5X3-	T46.5X4-	T46.5X5-	T46.5X6-
Endrin	T60.1X1-	T60.1X2-	T60.1X3-	T60.1X4-	-	-
Enflurane	T41.0X1-	T41.0X2-	T41.0X3-	T41.0X4-	T41.0X5-	T41.0X6-
Enhexymal	T42.3X1-	T42.3X2-	T42.3X3-	T42.3X4-	T42.3X5-	T42.3X6-
Enocitabine	T45.1X1-	T45.1X2-	T45.1X3-	T45.1X4-	T45.1X5-	T45.1X6-
Enovid	T38.4X1-	T38.4X2-	T38.4X3-	T38.4X4-	T38.4X5-	T38.4X6-
Enoxacin	T36.8X1-	T36.8X2-	T36.8X3-	T36.8X4-	T36.8X5-	T36.8X6-
Enoxaparin (sodium)	T45.511-	T45.512-	T45.513-	T45.514-	T45.515-	T45.516-
Enpiprazole	T43.591-	T43.592-	T43.593-	T43.594-	T43.595-	T43.596-
Enprofylline	T48.6X1-	T48.6X2-	T48.6X3-	T48.6X4-	T48.6X5-	T48.6X6-
Enprostil	T47.1X1-	T47.1X2-	T47.1X3-	T47.1X4-	T47.1X5-	T47.1X6-
ENT preparations (anti-infectives)	T49.6X1-	T49.6X2-	T49.6X3-	T49.6X4-	T49.6X5-	T49.6X6-
Enterogastrone	T38.891-	T38.892-	T38.893-	T38.894-	T38.895-	T38.896-
Enviomycin	T36.8X1-	T36.8X2-	T36.8X3-	T36.8X4-	T36.8X5-	T36.8X6-
Enzodase	T45.3X1-	T45.3X2-	T45.3X3-	T45.3X4-	T45.3X5-	T45.3X6-
Enzyme NEC	T45.3X1-	T45.3X2-	T45.3X3-	T45.3X4-	T45.3X5-	T45.3X6-
depolymerizing	T49.8X1-	T49.8X2-	T49.8X3-	T49.8X4-	T49.8X5-	T49.8X6-
fibrolytic	T45.3X1-	T45.3X2-	T45.3X3-	T45.3X4-	T45.3X5-	T45.3X6-
gastric	T47.5X1-	T47.5X2-	T47.5X3-	T47.5X4-	T47.5X5-	T47.5X6-
intestinal	T47.5X1-	T47.5X2-	T47.5X3-	T47.5X4-	T47.5X5-	T47.5X6-
local action	T49.4X1-	T49.4X2-	T49.4X3-	T49.4X4-	T49.4X5-	T49.4X6-
proteolytic	T49.4X1-	T49.4X2-	T49.4X3-	T49.4X4-	T49.4X5-	T49.4X6-
thrombolytic	T45.3X1-	T45.3X2-	T45.3X3-	T45.3X4-	T45.3X5-	T45.3X6-
EPAB	T41.3X1-	T41.3X2-	T41.3X3-	T41.3X4-	T41.3X5-	T41.3X6-
Epanutin	T42.0X1-	T42.0X2-	T42.0X3-	T42.0X4-	T42.0X5-	T42.0X6-
Ephedra	T44.991-	T44.992-	T44.993-	T44.994-	T44.995-	T44.996-
Ephedrine	T44.991-	T44.992-	T44.993-	T44.994-	T44.995-	T44.996-
Epichlorhydrin, epichlorohydrin	T52.8X1-	T52.8X2-	T52.8X3-	T52.8X4-	-	-
Epicillin	T36.0X1-	T36.0X2-	T36.0X3-	T36.0X4-	T36.0X5-	T36.0X6-
Epiestriol	T38.5X1-	T38.5X2-	T38.5X3-	T38.5X4-	T38.5X5-	T38.5X6-
Epilim — *see Sodium valproate*						
Epimestrol	T38.5X1-	T38.5X2-	T38.5X3-	T38.5X4-	T38.5X5-	T38.5X6-
Epinephrine	T44.5X1-	T44.5X2-	T44.5X3-	T44.5X4-	T44.5X5-	T44.5X6-
Epirubicin	T45.1X1-	T45.1X2-	T45.1X3-	T45.1X4-	T45.1X5-	T45.1X6-
Epitiostanol	T38.7X1-	T38.7X2-	T38.7X3-	T38.7X4-	T38.7X5-	T38.7X6-
Epitizide	T50.2X1-	T50.2X2-	T50.2X3-	T50.2X4-	T50.2X5-	T50.2X6-
EPN	T60.0X1-	T60.0X2-	T60.0X3-	T60.0X4-	-	-
EPO	T45.8X1-	T45.8X2-	T45.8X3-	T45.8X4-	T45.8X5-	T45.8X6-
Epoetin alpha	T45.8X1-	T45.8X2-	T45.8X3-	T45.8X4-	T45.8X5-	T45.8X6-
Epomediol	T50.991-	T50.992-	T50.993-	T50.994-	T50.995-	T50.996-
Epoprostenol	T45.521-	T45.522-	T45.523-	T45.524-	T45.525-	T45.526-
Epoxy resin	T65.891-	T65.892-	T65.893-	T65.894-	-	-
Eprazinone	T48.4X1-	T48.4X2-	T48.4X3-	T48.4X4-	T48.4X5-	T48.4X6-
Epsilon amino-caproic acid	T45.621-	T45.622-	T45.623-	T45.624-	T45.625-	T45.626-
Epsom salt	T47.3X1-	T47.3X2-	T47.3X3-	T47.3X4-	T47.3X5-	T47.3X6-
Eptazocine	T40.491-	T40.492-	T40.493-	T40.494-	T40.495-	T40.496-
Equanil	T43.591-	T43.592-	T43.593-	T43.594-	T43.595-	T43.596-
Equisetum	T62.2X1-	T62.2X2-	T62.2X3-	T62.2X4-	-	-
diuretic	T50.2X1-	T50.2X2-	T50.2X3-	T50.2X4-	T50.2X5-	T50.2X6-
Ergobasine	T48.0X1-	T48.0X2-	T48.0X3-	T48.0X4-	T48.0X5-	T48.0X6-
Ergocalciferol	T45.2X1-	T45.2X2-	T45.2X3-	T45.2X4-	T45.2X5-	T45.2X6-
Ergoloid mesylates	T46.7X1-	T46.7X2-	T46.7X3-	T46.7X4-	T46.7X5-	T46.7X6-
Ergometrine	T48.0X1-	T48.0X2-	T48.0X3-	T48.0X4-	T48.0X5-	T48.0X6-
Ergonovine	T48.0X1-	T48.0X2-	T48.0X3-	T48.0X4-	T48.0X5-	T48.0X6-

Substance	Poisoning Accidental (unintentional)	Poisoning Intentional self-harm	Poisoning Assault	Poisoning Undetermined	Adverse effect	Underdosing
Ergot NEC	T64.81X-	T64.82X-	T64.83X-	T64.84X-	-	-
derivative	T48.0X1-	T48.0X2-	T48.0X3-	T48.0X4-	T48.0X5-	T48.0X6-
medicinal (alkaloids)	T48.0X1-	T48.0X2-	T48.0X3-	T48.0X4-	T48.0X5-	T48.0X6-
prepared	T48.0X1-	T48.0X2-	T48.0X3-	T48.0X4-	T48.0X5-	T48.0X6-
Ergotamine	T46.5X1-	T46.5X2-	T46.5X3-	T46.5X4-	T46.5X5-	T46.5X6-
Ergotocine	T48.0X1-	T48.0X2-	T48.0X3-	T48.0X4-	T48.0X5-	T48.0X6-
Ergotrate	T48.0X1-	T48.0X2-	T48.0X3-	T48.0X4-	T48.0X5-	T48.0X6-
Eritrityl tetranitrate	T46.3X1-	T46.3X2-	T46.3X3-	T46.3X4-	T46.3X5-	T46.3X6-
Erythrityl tetranitrate	T46.3X1-	T46.3X2-	T46.3X3-	T46.3X4-	T46.3X5-	T46.3X6-
Erythrol tetranitrate	T46.3X1-	T46.3X2-	T46.3X3-	T46.3X4-	T46.3X5-	T46.3X6-
Erythromycin (salts)	T36.3X1-	T36.3X2-	T36.3X3-	T36.3X4-	T36.3X5-	T36.3X6-
ophthalmic preparation	T49.5X1-	T49.5X2-	T49.5X3-	T49.5X4-	T49.5X5-	T49.5X6-
topical NEC	T49.0X1-	T49.0X2-	T49.0X3-	T49.0X4-	T49.0X5-	T49.0X6-
Erythropoietin	T45.8X1-	T45.8X2-	T45.8X3-	T45.8X4-	T45.8X5-	T45.8X6-
human	T45.8X1-	T45.8X2-	T45.8X3-	T45.8X4-	T45.8X5-	T45.8X6-
Escin	T46.991-	T46.992-	T46.993-	T46.994-	T46.995-	T46.996-
Esculin	T45.2X1-	T45.2X2-	T45.2X3-	T45.2X4-	T45.2X5-	T45.2X6-
Esculoside	T45.2X1-	T45.2X2-	T45.2X3-	T45.2X4-	T45.2X5-	T45.2X6-
ESDT (ether-soluble tar distillate)	T49.1X1-	T49.1X2-	T49.1X3-	T49.1X4-	T49.1X5-	T49.1X6-
Eserine	T49.5X1-	T49.5X2-	T49.5X3-	T49.5X4-	T49.5X5-	T49.5X6-
Esflurbiprofen	T39.311-	T39.312-	T39.313-	T39.314-	T39.315-	T39.316-
Eskabarb	T42.3X1-	T42.3X2-	T42.3X3-	T42.3X4-	T42.3X5-	T42.3X6-
Eskalith	T43.8X1-	T43.8X2-	T43.8X3-	T43.8X4-	T43.8X5-	T43.8X6-
Esmolol	T44.7X1-	T44.7X2-	T44.7X3-	T44.7X4-	T44.7X5-	T44.7X6-
Estanozolol	T38.7X1-	T38.7X2-	T38.7X3-	T38.7X4-	T38.7X5-	T38.7X6-
Estazolam	T42.4X1-	T42.4X2-	T42.4X3-	T42.4X4-	T42.4X5-	T42.4X6-
Estradiol	T38.5X1-	T38.5X2-	T38.5X3-	T38.5X4-	T38.5X5-	T38.5X6-
with testosterone	T38.7X1-	T38.7X2-	T38.7X3-	T38.7X4-	T38.7X5-	T38.7X6-
benzoate	T38.5X1-	T38.5X2-	T38.5X3-	T38.5X4-	T38.5X5-	T38.5X6-
Estramustine	T45.1X1-	T45.1X2-	T45.1X3-	T45.1X4-	T45.1X5-	T45.1X6-
Estriol	T38.5X1-	T38.5X2-	T38.5X3-	T38.5X4-	T38.5X5-	T38.5X6-
Estrogen	T38.5X1-	T38.5X2-	T38.5X3-	T38.5X4-	T38.5X5-	T38.5X6-
with progesterone	T38.5X1-	T38.5X2-	T38.5X3-	T38.5X4-	T38.5X5-	T38.5X6-
conjugated	T38.5X1-	T38.5X2-	T38.5X3-	T38.5X4-	T38.5X5-	T38.5X6-
Estrone	T38.5X1-	T38.5X2-	T38.5X3-	T38.5X4-	T38.5X5-	T38.5X6-
Estropipate	T38.5X1-	T38.5X2-	T38.5X3-	T38.5X4-	T38.5X5-	T38.5X6-
Etacrynate sodium	T50.1X1-	T50.1X2-	T50.1X3-	T50.1X4-	T50.1X5-	T50.1X6-
Etacrynic acid	T50.1X1-	T50.1X2-	T50.1X3-	T50.1X4-	T50.1X5-	T50.1X6-
Etafedrine	T48.6X1-	T48.6X2-	T48.6X3-	T48.6X4-	T48.6X5-	T48.6X6-
Etafenone	T46.3X1-	T46.3X2-	T46.3X3-	T46.3X4-	T46.3X5-	T46.3X6-
Etambutol	T37.1X1-	T37.1X2-	T37.1X3-	T37.1X4-	T37.1X5-	T37.1X6-
Etamiphyllin	T48.6X1-	T48.6X2-	T48.6X3-	T48.6X4-	T48.6X5-	T48.6X6-
Etamivan	T50.7X1-	T50.7X2-	T50.7X3-	T50.7X4-	T50.7X5-	T50.7X6-
Etamsylate	T45.7X1-	T45.7X2-	T45.7X3-	T45.7X4-	T45.7X5-	T45.7X6-
Etebenecid	T50.4X1-	T50.4X2-	T50.4X3-	T50.4X4-	T50.4X5-	T50.4X6-
Ethacridine	T49.0X1-	T49.0X2-	T49.0X3-	T49.0X4-	T49.0X5-	T49.0X6-
Ethacrynic acid	T50.1X1-	T50.1X2-	T50.1X3-	T50.1X4-	T50.1X5-	T50.1X6-
Ethadione	T42.2X1-	T42.2X2-	T42.2X3-	T42.2X4-	T42.2X5-	T42.2X6-
Ethambutol	T37.1X1-	T37.1X2-	T37.1X3-	T37.1X4-	T37.1X5-	T37.1X6-
Ethamide	T50.2X1-	T50.2X2-	T50.2X3-	T50.2X4-	T50.2X5-	T50.2X6-
Ethamivan	T50.7X1-	T50.7X2-	T50.7X3-	T50.7X4-	T50.7X5-	T50.7X6-
Ethamsylate	T45.7X1-	T45.7X2-	T45.7X3-	T45.7X4-	T45.7X5-	T45.7X6-
Ethanol	T51.0X1-	T51.0X2-	T51.0X3-	T51.0X4-	-	-
beverage	T51.0X1-	T51.0X2-	T51.0X3-	T51.0X4-	-	-
Ethanolamine oleate	T46.8X1-	T46.8X2-	T46.8X3-	T46.8X4-	T46.8X5-	T46.8X6-
Ethaverine	T44.3X1-	T44.3X2-	T44.3X3-	T44.3X4-	T44.3X5-	T44.3X6-
Ethchlorvynol	T42.6X1-	T42.6X2-	T42.6X3-	T42.6X4-	T42.6X5-	T42.6X6-
Ethebenecid	T50.4X1-	T50.4X2-	T50.4X3-	T50.4X4-	T50.4X5-	T50.4X6-

Substance	Poisoning Accidental (unintentional)	Poisoning Intentional self-harm	Poisoning Assault	Poisoning Undetermined	Adverse effect	Underdosing
Ether (vapor)	T41.0X1-	T41.0X2-	T41.0X3-	T41.0X4-	T41.0X5-	T41.0X6-
anesthetic	T41.0X1-	T41.0X2-	T41.0X3-	T41.0X4-	T41.0X5-	T41.0X6-
divinyl	T41.0X1-	T41.0X2-	T41.0X3-	T41.0X4-	T41.0X5-	T41.0X6-
ethyl (medicinal)	T41.0X1-	T41.0X2-	T41.0X3-	T41.0X4-	T41.0X5-	T41.0X6-
nonmedicinal	T52.8X1-	T52.8X2-	T52.8X3-	T52.8X4-	-	-
petroleum — *see Ligroin*						
solvent	T52.8X1-	T52.8X2-	T52.8X3-	T52.8X4-	-	-
Ethiazide	T50.2X1-	T50.2X2-	T50.2X3-	T50.2X4-	T50.2X5-	T50.2X6-
Ethidium chloride (vapor)	T59.891-	T59.892-	T59.893-	T59.894-	-	-
Ethinamate	T42.6X1-	T42.6X2-	T42.6X3-	T42.6X4-	T42.6X5-	T42.6X6-
Ethinylestradiol, ethinyloestradiol	T38.5X1-	T38.5X2-	T38.5X3-	T38.5X4-	T38.5X5-	T38.5X6-
with						
levonorgestrel	T38.4X1-	T38.4X2-	T38.4X3-	T38.4X4-	T38.4X5-	T38.4X6-
norethisterone	T38.4X1-	T38.4X2-	T38.4X3-	T38.4X4-	T38.4X5-	T38.4X6-
Ethiodized oil (131 I)	T50.8X1-	T50.8X2-	T50.8X3-	T50.8X4-	T50.8X5-	T50.8X6-
Ethion	T60.0X1-	T60.0X2-	T60.0X3-	T60.0X4-	-	-
Ethionamide	T37.1X1-	T37.1X2-	T37.1X3-	T37.1X4-	T37.1X5-	T37.1X6-
Ethioniamide	T37.1X1-	T37.1X2-	T37.1X3-	T37.1X4-	T37.1X5-	T37.1X6-
Ethisterone	T38.5X1-	T38.5X2-	T38.5X3-	T38.5X4-	T38.5X5-	T38.5X6-
Ethobral	T42.3X1-	T42.3X2-	T42.3X3-	T42.3X4-	T42.3X5-	T42.3X6-
Ethocaine (infiltration) (topical)	T41.3X1-	T41.3X2-	T41.3X3-	T41.3X4-	T41.3X5-	T41.3X6-
nerve block (peripheral) (plexus)	T41.3X1-	T41.3X2-	T41.3X3-	T41.3X4-	T41.3X5-	T41.3X6-
spinal	T41.3X1-	T41.3X2-	T41.3X3-	T41.3X4-	T41.3X5-	T41.3X6-
Ethoheptazine	T40.491-	T40.492-	T40.493-	T40.494-	T40.495-	T40.496-
Ethopropazine	T44.3X1-	T44.3X2-	T44.3X3-	T44.3X4-	T44.3X5-	T44.3X6-
Ethosuximide	T42.2X1-	T42.2X2-	T42.2X3-	T42.2X4-	T42.2X5-	T42.2X6-
Ethotoin	T42.0X1-	T42.0X2-	T42.0X3-	T42.0X4-	T42.0X5-	T42.0X6-
Ethoxazene	T37.91X-	T37.92X-	T37.93X-	T37.94X-	T37.95X-	T37.96X-
Ethoxazorutoside	T46.991-	T46.992-	T46.993-	T46.994-	T46.995-	T46.996-
2-Ethoxyethanol	T52.3X1-	T52.3X2-	T52.3X3-	T52.3X4-	-	-
Ethoxzolamide	T50.2X1-	T50.2X2-	T50.2X3-	T50.2X4-	T50.2X5-	T50.2X6-
Ethyl						
acetate	T52.8X1-	T52.8X2-	T52.8X3-	T52.8X4-	-	-
alcohol	T51.0X1-	T51.0X2-	T51.0X3-	T51.0X4-	-	-
beverage	T51.0X1-	T51.0X2-	T51.0X3-	T51.0X4-	-	-
aldehyde (vapor)	T59.891-	T59.892-	T59.893-	T59.894-	-	-
liquid	T52.8X1-	T52.8X2-	T52.8X3-	T52.8X4-	-	-
aminobenzoate	T41.3X1-	T41.3X2-	T41.3X3-	T41.3X4-	T41.3X5-	T41.3X6-
aminophenothiazine	T43.3X1-	T43.3X2-	T43.3X3-	T43.3X4-	T43.3X5-	T43.3X6-
benzoate	T52.8X1-	T52.8X2-	T52.8X3-	T52.8X4-	-	-
biscoumacetate	T45.511-	T45.512-	T45.513-	T45.514-	T45.515-	T45.516-
bromide (anesthetic)	T41.0X1-	T41.0X2-	T41.0X3-	T41.0X4-	T41.0X5-	T41.0X6-
carbamate	T45.1X1-	T45.1X2-	T45.1X3-	T45.1X4-	T45.1X5-	T45.1X6-
carbinol	T51.3X1-	T51.3X2-	T51.3X3-	T51.3X4-	-	-
carbonate	T52.8X1-	T52.8X2-	T52.8X3-	T52.8X4-	-	-
chaulmoograte	T37.1X1-	T37.1X2-	T37.1X3-	T37.1X4-	T37.1X5-	T37.1X6-
chloride (anesthetic)	T41.0X1-	T41.0X2-	T41.0X3-	T41.0X4-	T41.0X5-	T41.0X6-
anesthetic (local)	T41.3X1-	T41.3X2-	T41.3X3-	T41.3X4-	T41.3X5-	T41.3X6-
inhaled	T41.0X1-	T41.0X2-	T41.0X3-	T41.0X4-	T41.0X5-	T41.0X6-
local	T49.4X1-	T49.4X2-	T49.4X3-	T49.4X4-	T49.4X5-	T49.4X6-
solvent	T53.6X1-	T53.6X2-	T53.6X3-	T53.6X4-	-	-
dibunate	T48.3X1-	T48.3X2-	T48.3X3-	T48.3X4-	T48.3X5-	T48.3X6-
dichloroarsine (vapor)	T57.0X1-	T57.0X2-	T57.0X3-	T57.0X4-	-	-
estranol	T38.7X1-	T38.7X2-	T38.7X3-	T38.7X4-	T38.7X5-	T38.7X6-
ether — *see also ether*	T52.8X1-	T52.8X2-	T52.8X3-	T52.8X4-	-	-
formate NEC (solvent)	T52.0X1-	T52.0X2-	T52.0X3-	T52.0X4-	-	-
fumarate	T49.4X1-	T49.4X2-	T49.4X3-	T49.4X4-	T49.4X5-	T49.4X6-
hydroxyisobutyrate NEC (solvent)	T52.8X1-	T52.8X2-	T52.8X3-	T52.8X4-	-	-
iodoacetate	T59.3X1-	T59.3X2-	T59.3X3-	T59.3X4-	-	-

Substance	Poisoning Accidental (unintentional)	Poisoning Intentional self-harm	Poisoning Assault	Poisoning Undetermined	Adverse effect	Underdosing
Ethyl (continued)						
lactate NEC (solvent)	T52.8X1-	T52.8X2-	T52.8X3-	T52.8X4-	-	-
loflazepate	T42.4X1-	T42.4X2-	T42.4X3-	T42.4X4-	T42.4X5-	T42.4X6-
mercuric chloride	T56.1X1-	T56.1X2-	T56.1X3-	T56.1X4-	-	-
methylcarbinol	T51.8X1-	T51.8X2-	T51.8X3-	T51.8X4-	-	-
morphine	T40.2X1-	T40.2X2-	T40.2X3-	T40.2X4-	T40.2X5-	T40.2X6-
noradrenaline	T48.6X1-	T48.6X2-	T48.6X3-	T48.6X4-	T48.6X5-	T48.6X6-
oxybutyrate NEC (solvent)	T52.8X1-	T52.8X2-	T52.8X3-	T52.8X4-	-	-
Ethylene (gas)	T59.891-	T59.892-	T59.893-	T59.894-	-	-
anesthetic (general)	T41.0X1-	T41.0X2-	T41.0X3-	T41.0X4-	T41.0X5-	T41.0X6-
chlorohydrin	T52.8X1-	T52.8X2-	T52.8X3-	T52.8X4-	-	-
vapor	T53.6X1-	T53.6X2-	T53.6X3-	T53.6X4-	-	-
dichloride	T52.8X1-	T52.8X2-	T52.8X3-	T52.8X4-	-	-
vapor	T53.6X1-	T53.6X2-	T53.6X3-	T53.6X4-	-	-
dinitrate	T52.3X1-	T52.3X2-	T52.3X3-	T52.3X4-	-	-
glycol (s)	T52.8X1-	T52.8X2-	T52.8X3-	T52.8X4-	-	-
dinitrate	T52.3X1-	T52.3X2-	T52.3X3-	T52.3X4-	-	-
monobutyl ether	T52.3X1-	T52.3X2-	T52.3X3-	T52.3X4-	-	-
imine	T54.1X1-	T54.1X2-	T54.1X3-	T54.1X4-	-	-
oxide (fumigant) (nonmedicinal)	T59.891-	T59.892-	T59.893-	T59.894-	-	-
medicinal	T49.0X1-	T49.0X2-	T49.0X3-	T49.0X4-	T49.0X5-	T49.0X6-
Ethylenediamine theophylline	T48.6X1-	T48.6X2-	T48.6X3-	T48.6X4-	T48.6X5-	T48.6X6-
Ethylenediaminetetra-acetic acid	T50.6X1-	T50.6X2-	T50.6X3-	T50.6X4-	T50.6X5-	T50.6X6-
Ethylenedinitrilotetra-acetate	T50.6X1-	T50.6X2-	T50.6X3-	T50.6X4-	T50.6X5-	T50.6X6-
Ethylestrenol	T38.7X1-	T38.7X2-	T38.7X3-	T38.7X4-	T38.7X5-	T38.7X6-
Ethylhydroxycellulose	T47.4X1-	T47.4X2-	T47.4X3-	T47.4X4-	T47.4X5-	T47.4X6-
Ethylidene						
chloride NEC	T53.6X1-	T53.6X2-	T53.6X3-	T53.6X4-	-	-
diacetate	T60.3X1-	T60.3X2-	T60.3X3-	T60.3X4-	-	-
dicoumarin	T45.511-	T45.512-	T45.513-	T45.514-	T45.515-	T45.516-
dicoumarol	T45.511-	T45.512-	T45.513-	T45.514-	T45.515-	T45.516-
diethyl ether	T52.0X1-	T52.0X2-	T52.0X3-	T52.0X4-	-	-
Ethylmorphine	T40.2X1-	T40.2X2-	T40.2X3-	T40.2X4-	T40.2X5-	T40.2X6-
Ethylnorepinephrine	T48.6X1-	T48.6X2-	T48.6X3-	T48.6X4-	T48.6X5-	T48.6X6-
Ethylparachlorophen-oxyisobutyrate	T46.6X1-	T46.6X2-	T46.6X3-	T46.6X4-	T46.6X5-	T46.6X6-
Ethynodiol	T38.4X1-	T38.4X2-	T38.4X3-	T38.4X4-	T38.4X5-	T38.4X6-
with mestranol diacetate	T38.4X1-	T38.4X2-	T38.4X3-	T38.4X4-	T38.4X5-	T38.4X6-
Etidocaine	T41.3X1-	T41.3X2-	T41.3X3-	T41.3X4-	T41.3X5-	T41.3X6-
infiltration (subcutaneous)	T41.3X1-	T41.3X2-	T41.3X3-	T41.3X4-	T41.3X5-	T41.3X6-
nerve (peripheral) (plexus)	T41.3X1-	T41.3X2-	T41.3X3-	T41.3X4-	T41.3X5-	T41.3X6-
Etidronate	T50.991-	T50.992-	T50.993-	T50.994-	T50.995-	T50.996-
Etidronic acid (disodium salt)	T50.991-	T50.992-	T50.993-	T50.994-	T50.995-	T50.996-
Etifoxine	T42.6X1-	T42.6X2-	T42.6X3-	T42.6X4-	T42.6X5-	T42.6X6-
Etilefrine	T44.4X1-	T44.4X2-	T44.4X3-	T44.4X4-	T44.4X5-	T44.4X6-
Etilfen	T42.3X1-	T42.3X2-	T42.3X3-	T42.3X4-	T42.3X5-	T42.3X6-
Etinodiol	T38.4X1-	T38.4X2-	T38.4X3-	T38.4X4-	T38.4X5-	T38.4X6-
Etiroxate	T46.6X1-	T46.6X2-	T46.6X3-	T46.6X4-	T46.6X5-	T46.6X6-
Etizolam	T42.4X1-	T42.4X2-	T42.4X3-	T42.4X4-	T42.4X5-	T42.4X6-
Etodolac	T39.391-	T39.392-	T39.393-	T39.394-	T39.395-	T39.396-
Etofamide	T37.3X1-	T37.3X2-	T37.3X3-	T37.3X4-	T37.3X5-	T37.3X6-
Etofibrate	T46.6X1-	T46.6X2-	T46.6X3-	T46.6X4-	T46.6X5-	T46.6X6-
Etofylline	T46.7X1-	T46.7X2-	T46.7X3-	T46.7X4-	T46.7X5-	T46.7X6-
clofibrate	T46.6X1-	T46.6X2-	T46.6X3-	T46.6X4-	T46.6X5-	T46.6X6-
Etoglucid	T45.1X1-	T45.1X2-	T45.1X3-	T45.1X4-	T45.1X5-	T45.1X6-
Etomidate	T41.1X1-	T41.1X2-	T41.1X3-	T41.1X4-	T41.1X5-	T41.1X6-
Etomide	T39.8X1-	T39.8X2-	T39.8X3-	T39.8X4-	T39.8X5-	T39.8X6-
Etomidoline	T44.3X1-	T44.3X2-	T44.3X3-	T44.3X4-	T44.3X5-	T44.3X6-
Etoposide	T45.1X1-	T45.1X2-	T45.1X3-	T45.1X4-	T45.1X5-	T45.1X6-

Substance	Poisoning Accidental (unintentional)	Poisoning Intentional self-harm	Poisoning Assault	Poisoning Undetermined	Adverse effect	Underdosing
Etorphine	T40.2X1-	T40.2X2-	T40.2X3-	T40.2X4-	T40.2X5-	T40.2X6-
Etoval	T42.3X1-	T42.3X2-	T42.3X3-	T42.3X4-	T42.3X5-	T42.3X6-
Etozolin	T50.1X1-	T50.1X2-	T50.1X3-	T50.1X4-	T50.1X5-	T50.1X6-
Etretinate	T50.991-	T50.992-	T50.993-	T50.994-	T50.995-	T50.996-
Etryptamine	T43.691-	T43.692-	T43.693-	T43.694-	T43.695-	T43.696-
Etybenzatropine	T44.3X1-	T44.3X2-	T44.3X3-	T44.3X4-	T44.3X5-	T44.3X6-
Etynodiol	T38.4X1-	T38.4X2-	T38.4X3-	T38.4X4-	T38.4X5-	T38.4X6-
Eucaine	T41.3X1-	T41.3X2-	T41.3X3-	T41.3X4-	T41.3X5-	T41.3X6-
Eucalyptus oil	T49.7X1-	T49.7X2-	T49.7X3-	T49.7X4-	T49.7X5-	T49.7X6-
Eucatropine	T49.5X1-	T49.5X2-	T49.5X3-	T49.5X4-	T49.5X5-	T49.5X6-
Eucodal	T40.2X1-	T40.2X2-	T40.2X3-	T40.2X4-	T40.2X5-	T40.2X6-
Euneryl	T42.3X1-	T42.3X2-	T42.3X3-	T42.3X4-	T42.3X5-	T42.3X6-
Euphthalmine	T44.3X1-	T44.3X2-	T44.3X3-	T44.3X4-	T44.3X5-	T44.3X6-
Eurax	T49.0X1-	T49.0X2-	T49.0X3-	T49.0X4-	T49.0X5-	T49.0X6-
Euresol	T49.4X1-	T49.4X2-	T49.4X3-	T49.4X4-	T49.4X5-	T49.4X6-
Euthroid	T38.1X1-	T38.1X2-	T38.1X3-	T38.1X4-	T38.1X5-	T38.1X6-
Evans blue	T50.8X1-	T50.8X2-	T50.8X3-	T50.8X4-	T50.8X5-	T50.8X6-
Evipal	T42.3X1-	T42.3X2-	T42.3X3-	T42.3X4-	T42.3X5-	T42.3X6-
sodium	T41.1X1-	T41.1X2-	T41.1X3-	T41.1X4-	T41.1X5-	T41.1X6-
Evipan	T42.3X1-	T42.3X2-	T42.3X3-	T42.3X4-	T42.3X5-	T42.3X6-
sodium	T41.1X1-	T41.1X2-	T41.1X3-	T41.1X4-	T41.1X5-	T41.1X6-
Exalamide	T49.0X1-	T49.0X2-	T49.0X3-	T49.0X4-	T49.0X5-	T49.0X6-
Exalgin	T39.1X1-	T39.1X2-	T39.1X3-	T39.1X4-	T39.1X5-	T39.1X6-
Excipients, pharmaceutical	T50.901-	T50.902-	T50.903-	T50.904-	T50.905-	T50.906-
Exhaust gas (engine) (motor vehicle)	T58.01X-	T58.02X-	T58.03X-	T58.04X-	-	-
Ex-Lax (phenolphthalein)	T47.2X1-	T47.2X2-	T47.2X3-	T47.2X4-	T47.2X5-	T47.2X6-
Expectorant NEC	T48.4X1-	T48.4X2-	T48.4X3-	T48.4X4-	T48.4X5-	T48.4X6-
Extended insulin zinc suspension	T38.3X1-	T38.3X2-	T38.3X3-	T38.3X4-	T38.3X5-	T38.3X6-
External medications (skin) (mucous membrane)	T49.91X-	T49.92X-	T49.93X-	T49.94X-	T49.95X-	T49.96X-
dental agent	T49.7X1-	T49.7X2-	T49.7X3-	T49.7X4-	T49.7X5-	T49.7X6-
ENT agent	T49.6X1-	T49.6X2-	T49.6X3-	T49.6X4-	T49.6X5-	T49.6X6-
ophthalmic preparation	T49.5X1-	T49.5X2-	T49.5X3-	T49.5X4-	T49.5X5-	T49.5X6-
specified NEC	T49.8X1-	T49.8X2-	T49.8X3-	T49.8X4-	T49.8X5-	T49.8X6-
Extrapyramidal antagonist NEC	T44.3X1-	T44.3X2-	T44.3X3-	T44.3X4-	T44.3X5-	T44.3X6-
Eye agents (anti-infective)	T49.5X1-	T49.5X2-	T49.5X3-	T49.5X4-	T49.5X5-	T49.5X6-
Eye drug NEC	T49.5X1-	T49.5X2-	T49.5X3-	T49.5X4-	T49.5X5-	T49.5X6-
FAC (fluorouracil + doxorubicin + cyclophosphamide)	T45.1X1-	T45.1X2-	T45.1X3-	T45.1X4-	T45.1X5-	T45.1X6-
Factor						
I (fibrinogen)	T45.8X1-	T45.8X2-	T45.8X3-	T45.8X4-	T45.8X5-	T45.8X6-
III (thromboplastin)	T45.8X1-	T45.8X2-	T45.8X3-	T45.8X4-	T45.8X5-	T45.8X6-
VIII (antihemophilic Factor) (concentrate)	T45.8X1-	T45.8X2-	T45.8X3-	T45.8X4-	T45.8X5-	T45.8X6-
IX complex	T45.7X1-	T45.7X2-	T45.7X3-	T45.7X4-	T45.7X5-	T45.7X6-
human	T45.8X1-	T45.8X2-	T45.8X3-	T45.8X4-	T45.8X5-	T45.8X6-
Famotidine	T47.0X1-	T47.0X2-	T47.0X3-	T47.0X4-	T47.0X5-	T47.0X6-
Fat suspension, intravenous	T50.991-	T50.992-	T50.993-	T50.994-	T50.995-	T50.996-
Fazadinium bromide	T48.1X1-	T48.1X2-	T48.1X3-	T48.1X4-	T48.1X5-	T48.1X6-
Febarbamate	T42.3X1-	T42.3X2-	T42.3X3-	T42.3X4-	T42.3X5-	T42.3X6-
Fecal softener	T47.4X1-	T47.4X2-	T47.4X3-	T47.4X4-	T47.4X5-	T47.4X6-
Fedrilate	T48.3X1-	T48.3X2-	T48.3X3-	T48.3X4-	T48.3X5-	T48.3X6-
Felodipine	T46.1X1-	T46.1X2-	T46.1X3-	T46.1X4-	T46.1X5-	T46.1X6-
Felypressin	T38.891-	T38.892-	T38.893-	T38.894-	T38.895-	T38.896-
Femoxetine	T43.221-	T43.222-	T43.223-	T43.224-	T43.225-	T43.226-
Fenalcomine	T46.3X1-	T46.3X2-	T46.3X3-	T46.3X4-	T46.3X5-	T46.3X6-
Fenamisal	T37.1X1-	T37.1X2-	T37.1X3-	T37.1X4-	T37.1X5-	T37.1X6-
Fenazone	T39.2X1-	T39.2X2-	T39.2X3-	T39.2X4-	T39.2X5-	T39.2X6-
Fenbendazole	T37.4X1-	T37.4X2-	T37.4X3-	T37.4X4-	T37.4X5-	T37.4X6-

Substance	Poisoning Accidental (unintentional)	Poisoning Intentional self-harm	Poisoning Assault	Poisoning Undetermined	Adverse effect	Underdosing
Fenbutrazate	T50.5X1-	T50.5X2-	T50.5X3-	T50.5X4-	T50.5X5-	T50.5X6-
Fencamfamine	T43.691-	T43.692-	T43.693-	T43.694-	T43.695-	T43.696-
Fendiline	T46.1X1-	T46.1X2-	T46.1X3-	T46.1X4-	T46.1X5-	T46.1X6-
Fenetylline	T43.691-	T43.692-	T43.693-	T43.694-	T43.695-	T43.696-
Fenflumizole	T39.391-	T39.392-	T39.393-	T39.394-	T39.395-	T39.396-
Fenfluramine	T50.5X1-	T50.5X2-	T50.5X3-	T50.5X4-	T50.5X5-	T50.5X6-
Fenobarbital	T42.3X1-	T42.3X2-	T42.3X3-	T42.3X4-	T42.3X5-	T42.3X6-
Fenofibrate	T46.6X1-	T46.6X2-	T46.6X3-	T46.6X4-	T46.6X5-	T46.6X6-
Fenoprofen	T39.311-	T39.312-	T39.313-	T39.314-	T39.315-	T39.316-
Fenoterol	T48.6X1-	T48.6X2-	T48.6X3-	T48.6X4-	T48.6X5-	T48.6X6-
Fenoverine	T44.3X1-	T44.3X2-	T44.3X3-	T44.3X4-	T44.3X5-	T44.3X6-
Fenoxazoline	T48.5X1-	T48.5X2-	T48.5X3-	T48.5X4-	T48.5X5-	T48.5X6-
Fenproporex	T50.5X1-	T50.5X2-	T50.5X3-	T50.5X4-	T50.5X5-	T50.5X6-
Fenquizone	T50.2X1-	T50.2X2-	T50.2X3-	T50.2X4-	T50.2X5-	T50.2X6-
Fentanyl (analogs)	T40.411-	T40.412-	T40.413-	T40.414-	T40.415-	T40.416-
Fentazin	T43.3X1-	T43.3X2-	T43.3X3-	T43.3X4-	T43.3X5-	T43.3X6-
Fenthion	T60.0X1-	T60.0X2-	T60.0X3-	T60.0X4-	-	-
Fenticlor	T49.0X1-	T49.0X2-	T49.0X3-	T49.0X4-	T49.0X5-	T49.0X6-
Fenylbutazone	T39.2X1-	T39.2X2-	T39.2X3-	T39.2X4-	T39.2X5-	T39.2X6-
Feprazone	T39.2X1-	T39.2X2-	T39.2X3-	T39.2X4-	T39.2X5-	T39.2X6-
Fer de lance (bite) (venom)	T63.061-	T63.062-	T63.063-	T63.064-	-	-
Ferric — *see also Iron*						
chloride	T45.4X1-	T45.4X2-	T45.4X3-	T45.4X4-	T45.4X5-	T45.4X6-
citrate	T45.4X1-	T45.4X2-	T45.4X3-	T45.4X4-	T45.4X5-	T45.4X6-
hydroxide						
colloidal	T45.4X1-	T45.4X2-	T45.4X3-	T45.4X4-	T45.4X5-	T45.4X6-
polymaltose	T45.4X1-	T45.4X2-	T45.4X3-	T45.4X4-	T45.4X5-	T45.4X6-
pyrophosphate	T45.4X1-	T45.4X2-	T45.4X3-	T45.4X4-	T45.4X5-	T45.4X6-
Ferritin	T45.4X1-	T45.4X2-	T45.4X3-	T45.4X4-	T45.4X5-	T45.4X6-
Ferrocholinate	T45.4X1-	T45.4X2-	T45.4X3-	T45.4X4-	T45.4X5-	T45.4X6-
Ferrodextrane	T45.4X1-	T45.4X2-	T45.4X3-	T45.4X4-	T45.4X5-	T45.4X6-
Ferropolimaler	T45.4X1-	T45.4X2-	T45.4X3-	T45.4X4-	T45.4X5-	T45.4X6-
Ferrous — *see also Iron*						
phosphate	T45.4X1-	T45.4X2-	T45.4X3-	T45.4X4-	T45.4X5-	T45.4X6-
salt	T45.4X1-	T45.4X2-	T45.4X3-	T45.4X4-	T45.4X5-	T45.4X6-
with folic acid	T45.4X1-	T45.4X2-	T45.4X3-	T45.4X4-	T45.4X5-	T45.4X6-
Ferrous fumerate, gluconate, lactate, salt NEC, sulfate (medicinal)	T45.4X1-	T45.4X2-	T45.4X3-	T45.4X4-	T45.4X5-	T45.4X6-
Ferrovanadium (fumes)	T59.891-	T59.892-	T59.893-	T59.894-	-	-
Ferrum — *see Iron*						
Fertilizers NEC	T65.891-	T65.892-	T65.893-	T65.894-	-	-
with herbicide mixture	T60.3X1-	T60.3X2-	T60.3X3-	T60.3X4-	-	-
Fetoxilate	T47.6X1-	T47.6X2-	T47.6X3-	T47.6X4-	T47.6X5-	T47.6X6-
Fiber, dietary	T47.4X1-	T47.4X2-	T47.4X3-	T47.4X4-	T47.4X5-	T47.4X6-
Fiberglass	T65.831-	T65.832-	T65.833-	T65.834-	-	-
Fibrinogen (human)	T45.8X1-	T45.8X2-	T45.8X3-	T45.8X4-	T45.8X5-	T45.8X6-
Fibrinolysin (human)	T45.691-	T45.692-	T45.693-	T45.694-	T45.695-	T45.696-
Fibrinolysis						
affecting drug	T45.601-	T45.602-	T45.603-	T45.604-	T45.605-	T45.606-
inhibitor NEC	T45.621-	T45.622-	T45.623-	T45.624-	T45.625-	T45.626-
Fibrinolytic drug	T45.611-	T45.612-	T45.613-	T45.614-	T45.615-	T45.616-
Filix mas	T37.4X1-	T37.4X2-	T37.4X3-	T37.4X4-	T37.4X5-	T37.4X6-
Filtering cream	T49.3X1-	T49.3X2-	T49.3X3-	T49.3X4-	T49.3X5-	T49.3X6-
Fiorinal	T39.011-	T39.012-	T39.013-	T39.014-	T39.015-	T39.016-
Firedamp	T59.891-	T59.892-	T59.893-	T59.894-	-	-
Fish, noxious, nonbacterial	T61.91X-	T61.92X-	T61.93X-	T61.94X-	-	-
ciguatera	T61.01X-	T61.02X-	T61.03X-	T61.04X-	-	-
scombroid	T61.11X-	T61.12X-	T61.13X-	T61.14X-	-	-
shell	T61.781-	T61.782-	T61.783-	T61.784-	-	-

Substance	Poisoning Accidental (unintentional)	Poisoning Intentional self-harm	Poisoning Assault	Poisoning Undetermined	Adverse effect	Underdosing
Fish, noxious, nonbacterial (continued)						
specified NEC	T61.771-	T61.772-	T61.773-	T61.774-	-	-
Flagyl	T37.3X1-	T37.3X2-	T37.3X3-	T37.3X4-	T37.3X5-	T37.3X6-
Flavine adenine dinucleotide	T45.2X1-	T45.2X2-	T45.2X3-	T45.2X4-	T45.2X5-	T45.2X6-
Flavodic acid	T46.991-	T46.992-	T46.993-	T46.994-	T46.995-	T46.996-
Flavoxate	T44.3X1-	T44.3X2-	T44.3X3-	T44.3X4-	T44.3X5-	T44.3X6-
Flaxedil	T48.1X1-	T48.1X2-	T48.1X3-	T48.1X4-	T48.1X5-	T48.1X6-
Flaxseed (medicinal)	T49.3X1-	T49.3X2-	T49.3X3-	T49.3X4-	T49.3X5-	T49.3X6-
Flecainide	T46.2X1-	T46.2X2-	T46.2X3-	T46.2X4-	T46.2X5-	T46.2X6-
Fleroxacin	T36.8X1-	T36.8X2-	T36.8X3-	T36.8X4-	T36.8X5-	T36.8X6-
Floctafenine	T39.8X1-	T39.8X2-	T39.8X3-	T39.8X4-	T39.8X5-	T39.8X6-
Flomax	T44.6X1-	T44.6X2-	T44.6X3-	T44.6X4-	T44.6X5-	T44.6X6-
Flomoxef	T36.1X1-	T36.1X2-	T36.1X3-	T36.1X4-	T36.1X5-	T36.1X6-
Flopropione	T44.3X1-	T44.3X2-	T44.3X3-	T44.3X4-	T44.3X5-	T44.3X6-
Florantyrone	T47.5X1-	T47.5X2-	T47.5X3-	T47.5X4-	T47.5X5-	T47.5X6-
Floraquin	T37.8X1-	T37.8X2-	T37.8X3-	T37.8X4-	T37.8X5-	T37.8X6-
Florinef	T38.0X1-	T38.0X2-	T38.0X3-	T38.0X4-	T38.0X5-	T38.0X6-
ENT agent	T49.6X1-	T49.6X2-	T49.6X3-	T49.6X4-	T49.6X5-	T49.6X6-
ophthalmic preparation	T49.5X1-	T49.5X2-	T49.5X3-	T49.5X4-	T49.5X5-	T49.5X6-
topical NEC	T49.0X1-	T49.0X2-	T49.0X3-	T49.0X4-	T49.0X5-	T49.0X6-
Flowers of sulfur	T49.4X1-	T49.4X2-	T49.4X3-	T49.4X4-	T49.4X5-	T49.4X6-
Floxuridine	T45.1X1-	T45.1X2-	T45.1X3-	T45.1X4-	T45.1X5-	T45.1X6-
Fluanisone	T43.4X1-	T43.4X2-	T43.4X3-	T43.4X4-	T43.4X5-	T43.4X6-
Flubendazole	T37.4X1-	T37.4X2-	T37.4X3-	T37.4X4-	T37.4X5-	T37.4X6-
Fluclorolone acetonide	T49.0X1-	T49.0X2-	T49.0X3-	T49.0X4-	T49.0X5-	T49.0X6-
Flucloxacillin	T36.0X1-	T36.0X2-	T36.0X3-	T36.0X4-	T36.0X5-	T36.0X6-
Fluconazole	T37.8X1-	T37.8X2-	T37.8X3-	T37.8X4-	T37.8X5-	T37.8X6-
Flucytosine	T37.8X1-	T37.8X2-	T37.8X3-	T37.8X4-	T37.8X5-	T37.8X6-
Fludeoxyglucose (18F)	T50.8X1-	T50.8X2-	T50.8X3-	T50.8X4-	T50.8X5-	T50.8X6-
Fludiazepam	T42.4X1-	T42.4X2-	T42.4X3-	T42.4X4-	T42.4X5-	T42.4X6-
Fludrocortisone	T50.0X1-	T50.0X2-	T50.0X3-	T50.0X4-	T50.0X5-	T50.0X6-
ENT agent	T49.6X1-	T49.6X2-	T49.6X3-	T49.6X4-	T49.6X5-	T49.6X6-
ophthalmic preparation	T49.5X1-	T49.5X2-	T49.5X3-	T49.5X4-	T49.5X5-	T49.5X6-
topical NEC	T49.0X1-	T49.0X2-	T49.0X3-	T49.0X4-	T49.0X5-	T49.0X6-
Fludroxycortide	T49.0X1-	T49.0X2-	T49.0X3-	T49.0X4-	T49.0X5-	T49.0X6-
Flufenamic acid	T39.391-	T39.392-	T39.393-	T39.394-	T39.395-	T39.396-
Fluindione	T45.511-	T45.512-	T45.513-	T45.514-	T45.515-	T45.516-
Flumequine	T37.8X1-	T37.8X2-	T37.8X3-	T37.8X4-	T37.8X5-	T37.8X6-
Flumethasone	T49.0X1-	T49.0X2-	T49.0X3-	T49.0X4-	T49.0X5-	T49.0X6-
Flumethiazide	T50.2X1-	T50.2X2-	T50.2X3-	T50.2X4-	T50.2X5-	T50.2X6-
Flumidin	T37.5X1-	T37.5X2-	T37.5X3-	T37.5X4-	T37.5X5-	T37.5X6-
Flunarizine	T46.7X1-	T46.7X2-	T46.7X3-	T46.7X4-	T46.7X5-	T46.7X6-
Flunidazole	T37.8X1-	T37.8X2-	T37.8X3-	T37.8X4-	T37.8X5-	T37.8X6-
Flunisolide	T48.6X1-	T48.6X2-	T48.6X3-	T48.6X4-	T48.6X5-	T48.6X6-
Flunitrazepam	T42.4X1-	T42.4X2-	T42.4X3-	T42.4X4-	T42.4X5-	T42.4X6-
Fluocinolone (acetonide)	T49.0X1-	T49.0X2-	T49.0X3-	T49.0X4-	T49.0X5-	T49.0X6-
Fluocinonide	T49.0X1-	T49.0X2-	T49.0X3-	T49.0X4-	T49.0X5-	T49.0X6-
Fluocortin (butyl)	T49.0X1-	T49.0X2-	T49.0X3-	T49.0X4-	T49.0X5-	T49.0X6-
Fluocortolone	T49.0X1-	T49.0X2-	T49.0X3-	T49.0X4-	T49.0X5-	T49.0X6-
Fluohydrocortisone	T38.0X1-	T38.0X2-	T38.0X3-	T38.0X4-	T38.0X5-	T38.0X6-
ENT agent	T49.6X1-	T49.6X2-	T49.6X3-	T49.6X4-	T49.6X5-	T49.6X6-
ophthalmic preparation	T49.5X1-	T49.5X2-	T49.5X3-	T49.5X4-	T49.5X5-	T49.5X6-
topical NEC	T49.0X1-	T49.0X2-	T49.0X3-	T49.0X4-	T49.0X5-	T49.0X6-
Fluonid	T49.0X1-	T49.0X2-	T49.0X3-	T49.0X4-	T49.0X5-	T49.0X6-
Fluopromazine	T43.3X1-	T43.3X2-	T43.3X3-	T43.3X4-	T43.3X5-	T43.3X6-
Fluoracetate	T60.8X1-	T60.8X2-	T60.8X3-	T60.8X4-	-	-
Fluorescein	T50.8X1-	T50.8X2-	T50.8X3-	T50.8X4-	T50.8X5-	T50.8X6-
Fluorhydrocortisone	T50.0X1-	T50.0X2-	T50.0X3-	T50.0X4-	T50.0X5-	T50.0X6-

Substance	Poisoning Accidental (unintentional)	Poisoning Intentional self-harm	Poisoning Assault	Poisoning Undetermined	Adverse effect	Underdosing
Fluoride (nonmedicinal) (pesticide) (sodium) NEC	T60.8X1-	T60.8X2-	T60.8X3-	T60.8X4-	-	-
hydrogen — *see Hydrofluoric acid*						
medicinal NEC	T50.991-	T50.992-	T50.993-	T50.994-	T50.995-	T50.996-
dental use	T49.7X1-	T49.7X2-	T49.7X3-	T49.7X4-	T49.7X5-	T49.7X6-
not pesticide NEC	T54.91X-	T54.92X-	T54.93X-	T54.94X-	-	-
stannous	T49.7X1-	T49.7X2-	T49.7X3-	T49.7X4-	T49.7X5-	T49.7X6-
Fluorinated corticosteroids	T38.0X1-	T38.0X2-	T38.0X3-	T38.0X4-	T38.0X5-	T38.0X6-
Fluorine (gas)	T59.5X1-	T59.5X2-	T59.5X3-	T59.5X4-	-	-
salt — *see Fluoride(s)*						
Fluoristan	T49.7X1-	T49.7X2-	T49.7X3-	T49.7X4-	T49.7X5-	T49.7X6-
Fluormetholone	T49.0X1-	T49.0X2-	T49.0X3-	T49.0X4-	T49.0X5-	T49.0X6-
Fluoroacetate	T60.8X1-	T60.8X2-	T60.8X3-	T60.8X4-	-	-
Fluorocarbon monomer	T53.6X1-	T53.6X2-	T53.6X3-	T53.6X4-	-	-
Fluorocytosine	T37.8X1-	T37.8X2-	T37.8X3-	T37.8X4-	T37.8X5-	T37.8X6-
Fluorodeoxyuridine	T45.1X1-	T45.1X2-	T45.1X3-	T45.1X4-	T45.1X5-	T45.1X6-
Fluorometholone	T49.0X1-	T49.0X2-	T49.0X3-	T49.0X4-	T49.0X5-	T49.0X6-
ophthalmic preparation	T49.5X1-	T49.5X2-	T49.5X3-	T49.5X4-	T49.5X5-	T49.5X6-
Fluorophosphate insecticide	T60.0X1-	T60.0X2-	T60.0X3-	T60.0X4-	-	-
Fluorosol	T46.3X1-	T46.3X2-	T46.3X3-	T46.3X4-	T46.3X5-	T46.3X6-
Fluorouracil	T45.1X1-	T45.1X2-	T45.1X3-	T45.1X4-	T45.1X5-	T45.1X6-
Fluorphenylalanine	T49.5X1-	T49.5X2-	T49.5X3-	T49.5X4-	T49.5X5-	T49.5X6-
Fluothane	T41.0X1-	T41.0X2-	T41.0X3-	T41.0X4-	T41.0X5-	T41.0X6-
Fluoxetine	T43.221-	T43.222-	T43.223-	T43.224-	T43.225-	T43.226-
Fluoxymesterone	T38.7X1-	T38.7X2-	T38.7X3-	T38.7X4-	T38.7X5-	T38.7X6-
Flupenthixol	T43.4X1-	T43.4X2-	T43.4X3-	T43.4X4-	T43.4X5-	T43.4X6-
Flupentixol	T43.4X1-	T43.4X2-	T43.4X3-	T43.4X4-	T43.4X5-	T43.4X6-
Fluphenazine	T43.3X1-	T43.3X2-	T43.3X3-	T43.3X4-	T43.3X5-	T43.3X6-
Fluprednidene	T49.0X1-	T49.0X2-	T49.0X3-	T49.0X4-	T49.0X5-	T49.0X6-
Fluprednisolone	T38.0X1-	T38.0X2-	T38.0X3-	T38.0X4-	T38.0X5-	T38.0X6-
Fluradoline	T39.8X1-	T39.8X2-	T39.8X3-	T39.8X4-	T39.8X5-	T39.8X6-
Flurandrenolide	T49.0X1-	T49.0X2-	T49.0X3-	T49.0X4-	T49.0X5-	T49.0X6-
Flurandrenolone	T49.0X1-	T49.0X2-	T49.0X3-	T49.0X4-	T49.0X5-	T49.0X6-
Flurazepam	T42.4X1-	T42.4X2-	T42.4X3-	T42.4X4-	T42.4X5-	T42.4X6-
Flurbiprofen	T39.311-	T39.312-	T39.313-	T39.314-	T39.315-	T39.316-
Flurobate	T49.0X1-	T49.0X2-	T49.0X3-	T49.0X4-	T49.0X5-	T49.0X6-
Fluroxene	T41.0X1-	T41.0X2-	T41.0X3-	T41.0X4-	T41.0X5-	T41.0X6-
Fluspirilene	T43.591-	T43.592-	T43.593-	T43.594-	T43.595-	T43.596-
Flutamide	T38.6X1-	T38.6X2-	T38.6X3-	T38.6X4-	T38.6X5-	T38.6X6-
Flutazolam	T42.4X1-	T42.4X2-	T42.4X3-	T42.4X4-	T42.4X5-	T42.4X6-
Fluticasone propionate	T38.0X1-	T38.0X2-	T38.0X3-	T38.0X4-	T38.0X5-	T38.0X6-
Flutoprazepam	T42.4X1-	T42.4X2-	T42.4X3-	T42.4X4-	T42.4X5-	T42.4X6-
Flutropium bromide	T48.6X1-	T48.6X2-	T48.6X3-	T48.6X4-	T48.6X5-	T48.6X6-
Fluvoxamine	T43.221-	T43.222-	T43.223-	T43.224-	T43.225-	T43.226-
Folacin	T45.8X1-	T45.8X2-	T45.8X3-	T45.8X4-	T45.8X5-	T45.8X6-
Folic acid	T45.8X1-	T45.8X2-	T45.8X3-	T45.8X4-	T45.8X5-	T45.8X6-
with ferrous salt	T45.2X1-	T45.2X2-	T45.2X3-	T45.2X4-	T45.2X5-	T45.2X6-
antagonist	T45.1X1-	T45.1X2-	T45.1X3-	T45.1X4-	T45.1X5-	T45.1X6-
Folinic acid	T45.8X1-	T45.8X2-	T45.8X3-	T45.8X4-	T45.8X5-	T45.8X6-
Folium stramoniae	T48.6X1-	T48.6X2-	T48.6X3-	T48.6X4-	T48.6X5-	T48.6X6-
Follicle-stimulating hormone, human	T38.811-	T38.812-	T38.813-	T38.814-	T38.815-	T38.816-
Folpet	T60.3X1-	T60.3X2-	T60.3X3-	T60.3X4-	-	-
Fominoben	T48.3X1-	T48.3X2-	T48.3X3-	T48.3X4-	T48.3X5-	T48.3X6-
Food, foodstuffs, noxious, nonbacterial, NEC	T62.91X-	T62.92X-	T62.93X-	T62.94X-	-	-
berries	T62.1X1-	T62.1X2-	T62.1X3-	T62.1X4-	-	-
fish — *see also Fish*	T61.91X-	T61.92X-	T61.93X-	T61.94X-	-	-
mushrooms	T62.0X1-	T62.0X2-	T62.0X3-	T62.0X4-	-	-
plants	T62.2X1-	T62.2X2-	T62.2X3-	T62.2X4-	-	-

Substance	Poisoning Accidental (unintentional)	Poisoning Intentional self-harm	Poisoning Assault	Poisoning Undetermined	Adverse effect	Underdosing
Food, foodstuffs, noxious, nonbacterial, NEC (continued)						
seafood	T61.91X-	T61.92X-	T61.93X-	T61.94X-	-	-
specified NEC	T61.8X1-	T61.8X2-	T61.8X3-	T61.8X4-	-	-
seeds	T62.2X1-	T62.2X2-	T62.2X3-	T62.2X4-	-	-
shellfish	T61.781-	T61.782-	T61.783-	T61.784-	-	-
specified NEC	T62.8X1-	T62.8X2-	T62.8X3-	T62.8X4-	-	-
Fool's parsley	T62.2X1-	T62.2X2-	T62.2X3-	T62.2X4-	-	-
Formaldehyde (solution) , gas or vapor	T59.2X1-	T59.2X2-	T59.2X3-	T59.2X4-	-	-
fungicide	T60.3X1-	T60.3X2-	T60.3X3-	T60.3X4-	-	-
Formalin	T59.2X1-	T59.2X2-	T59.2X3-	T59.2X4-	-	-
fungicide	T60.3X1-	T60.3X2-	T60.3X3-	T60.3X4-	-	-
vapor	T59.2X1-	T59.2X2-	T59.2X3-	T59.2X4-	-	-
Formic acid	T54.2X1-	T54.2X2-	T54.2X3-	T54.2X4-	-	-
vapor	T59.891-	T59.892-	T59.893-	T59.894-	-	-
Foscarnet sodium	T37.5X1-	T37.5X2-	T37.5X3-	T37.5X4-	T37.5X5-	T37.5X6-
Fosfestrol	T38.5X1-	T38.5X2-	T38.5X3-	T38.5X4-	T38.5X5-	T38.5X6-
Fosfomycin	T36.8X1-	T36.8X2-	T36.8X3-	T36.8X4-	T36.8X5-	T36.8X6-
Fosfonet sodium	T37.5X1-	T37.5X2-	T37.5X3-	T37.5X4-	T37.5X5-	T37.5X6-
Fosinopril	T46.4X1-	T46.4X2-	T46.4X3-	T46.4X4-	T46.4X5-	T46.4X6-
sodium	T46.4X1-	T46.4X2-	T46.4X3-	T46.4X4-	T46.4X5-	T46.4X6-
Fowler's solution	T57.0X1-	T57.0X2-	T57.0X3-	T57.0X4-	-	-
Foxglove	T62.2X1-	T62.2X2-	T62.2X3-	T62.2X4-	-	-
Framycetin	T36.5X1-	T36.5X2-	T36.5X3-	T36.5X4-	T36.5X5-	T36.5X6-
Frangula	T47.2X1-	T47.2X2-	T47.2X3-	T47.2X4-	T47.2X5-	T47.2X6-
extract	T47.2X1-	T47.2X2-	T47.2X3-	T47.2X4-	T47.2X5-	T47.2X6-
Frei antigen	T50.8X1-	T50.8X2-	T50.8X3-	T50.8X4-	T50.8X5-	T50.8X6-
Freon	T53.5X1-	T53.5X2-	T53.5X3-	T53.5X4-	-	-
Fructose	T50.3X1-	T50.3X2-	T50.3X3-	T50.3X4-	T50.3X5-	T50.3X6-
Frusemide	T50.1X1-	T50.1X2-	T50.1X3-	T50.1X4-	T50.1X5-	T50.1X6-
FSH	T38.811-	T38.812-	T38.813-	T38.814-	T38.815-	T38.816-
Ftorafur	T45.1X1-	T45.1X2-	T45.1X3-	T45.1X4-	T45.1X5-	T45.1X6-
Fuel						
automobile	T52.0X1-	T52.0X2-	T52.0X3-	T52.0X4-	-	-
exhaust gas, not in transit	T58.01X-	T58.02X-	T58.03X-	T58.04X-	-	-
vapor NEC	T52.0X1-	T52.0X2-	T52.0X3-	T52.0X4-	-	-
gas (domestic use) — *see also Carbon, monoxide, fuel, utility*	T59.891-	T59.892-	T59.893-	T59.894-	-	-
utility	T59.891-	T59.892-	T59.893-	T59.894-	-	-
in mobile container	T59.891-	T59.892-	T59.893-	T59.894-	-	-
incomplete combustion of — *see Carbon, monoxide, fuel, utility*						
piped (natural)	T59.891-	T59.892-	T59.893-	T59.894-	-	-
industrial, incomplete combustion	T58.8X1-	T58.8X2-	T58.8X3-	T58.8X4-	-	-
Fugillin	T36.8X1-	T36.8X2-	T36.8X3-	T36.8X4-	T36.8X5-	T36.8X6-
Fulminate of mercury	T56.1X1-	T56.1X2-	T56.1X3-	T56.1X4-	-	-
Fulvicin	T36.7X1-	T36.7X2-	T36.7X3-	T36.7X4-	T36.7X5-	T36.7X6-
Fumadil	T36.8X1-	T36.8X2-	T36.8X3-	T36.8X4-	T36.8X5-	T36.8X6-
Fumagillin	T36.8X1-	T36.8X2-	T36.8X3-	T36.8X4-	T36.8X5-	T36.8X6-
Fumaric acid	T49.4X1-	T49.4X2-	T49.4X3-	T49.4X4-	T49.4X5-	T49.4X6-
Fumes (from)	T59.91X-	T59.92X-	T59.93X-	T59.94X-	-	-
carbon monoxide — *see Carbon, monoxide*						
charcoal (domestic use) — *see Charcoal, fumes*						
chloroform — *see Chloroform*						
coke (in domestic stoves, fireplaces) — *see Coke fumes*						
corrosive NEC	T54.91X-	T54.92X-	T54.93X-	T54.94X-	-	-

Substance	Poisoning Accidental (unintentional)	Poisoning Intentional self-harm	Poisoning Assault	Poisoning Undetermined	Adverse effect	Underdosing
Fumes (from) (continued)						
ether — *see ether*						
freons	T53.5X1-	T53.5X2-	T53.5X3-	T53.5X4-	-	-
hydrocarbons	T59.891-	T59.892-	T59.893-	T59.894-	-	-
petroleum (liquefied)	T59.891-	T59.892-	T59.893-	T59.894-	-	-
distributed through pipes (pure or mixed with air)	T59.891-	T59.892-	T59.893-	T59.894-	-	-
lead — *see lead*						
metal — *see Metals, or the specified metal*						
nitrogen dioxide	T59.0X1-	T59.0X2-	T59.0X3-	T59.0X4-	-	-
pesticides — *see Pesticides*						
petroleum (liquefied)	T59.891-	T59.892-	T59.893-	T59.894-	-	-
distributed through pipes (pure or mixed with air)	T59.891-	T59.892-	T59.893-	T59.894-	-	-
polyester	T59.891-	T59.892-	T59.893-	T59.894-	-	-
specified source NEC — *see also substance specified*	T59.891-	T59.892-	T59.893-	T59.894-	-	-
sulfur dioxide	T59.1X1-	T59.1X2-	T59.1X3-	T59.1X4-	-	-
Fumigant NEC	T60.91X-	T60.92X-	T60.93X-	T60.94X-	-	-
Fungi, noxious, used as food	T62.0X1-	T62.0X2-	T62.0X3-	T62.0X4-	-	-
Fungicide NEC (nonmedicinal)	T60.3X1-	T60.3X2-	T60.3X3-	T60.3X4-	-	-
Fungizone	T36.7X1-	T36.7X2-	T36.7X3-	T36.7X4-	T36.7X5-	T36.7X6-
topical	T49.0X1-	T49.0X2-	T49.0X3-	T49.0X4-	T49.0X5-	T49.0X6-
Furacin	T49.0X1-	T49.0X2-	T49.0X3-	T49.0X4-	T49.0X5-	T49.0X6-
Furadantin	T37.91X-	T37.92X-	T37.93X-	T37.94X-	T37.95X-	T37.96X-
Furazolidone	T37.8X1-	T37.8X2-	T37.8X3-	T37.8X4-	T37.8X5-	T37.8X6-
Furazolium chloride	T49.0X1-	T49.0X2-	T49.0X3-	T49.0X4-	T49.0X5-	T49.0X6-
Furfural	T52.8X1-	T52.8X2-	T52.8X3-	T52.8X4-	-	-
Furnace (coal burning) (domestic) , gas from	T58.2X1-	T58.2X2-	T58.2X3-	T58.2X4-	-	-
industrial	T58.8X1-	T58.8X2-	T58.8X3-	T58.8X4-	-	-
Furniture polish	T65.891-	T65.892-	T65.893-	T65.894-	-	-
Furosemide	T50.1X1-	T50.1X2-	T50.1X3-	T50.1X4-	T50.1X5-	T50.1X6-
Furoxone	T37.91X-	T37.92X-	T37.93X-	T37.94X-	T37.95X-	T37.96X-
Fursultiamine	T45.2X1-	T45.2X2-	T45.2X3-	T45.2X4-	T45.2X5-	T45.2X6-
Fusafungine	T36.8X1-	T36.8X2-	T36.8X3-	T36.8X4-	T36.8X5-	T36.8X6-
Fusel oil (any) (amyl) (butyl) (propyl) , vapor	T51.3X1-	T51.3X2-	T51.3X3-	T51.3X4-	-	-
Fusidate (ethanolamine) (sodium)	T36.8X1-	T36.8X2-	T36.8X3-	T36.8X4-	T36.8X5-	T36.8X6-
Fusidic acid	T36.8X1-	T36.8X2-	T36.8X3-	T36.8X4-	T36.8X5-	T36.8X6-
Fytic acid, nonasodium	T50.6X1-	T50.6X2-	T50.6X3-	T50.6X4-	T50.6X5-	T50.6X6-
GABA	T43.8X1-	T43.8X2-	T43.8X3-	T43.8X4-	T43.8X5-	T43.8X6-
Gadopentetic acid	T50.8X1-	T50.8X2-	T50.8X3-	T50.8X4-	T50.8X5-	T50.8X6-
Galactose	T50.3X1-	T50.3X2-	T50.3X3-	T50.3X4-	T50.3X5-	T50.3X6-
b-Galactosidase	T47.5X1-	T47.5X2-	T47.5X3-	T47.5X4-	T47.5X5-	T47.5X6-
Galantamine	T44.0X1-	T44.0X2-	T44.0X3-	T44.0X4-	T44.0X5-	T44.0X6-
Gallamine (triethiodide)	T48.1X1-	T48.1X2-	T48.1X3-	T48.1X4-	T48.1X5-	T48.1X6-
Gallium citrate	T50.991-	T50.992-	T50.993-	T50.994-	T50.995-	T50.996-
Gallopamil	T46.1X1-	T46.1X2-	T46.1X3-	T46.1X4-	T46.1X5-	T46.1X6-
Gamboge	T47.2X1-	T47.2X2-	T47.2X3-	T47.2X4-	T47.2X5-	T47.2X6-
Gamimune	T50.Z11-	T50.Z12-	T50.Z13-	T50.Z14-	T50.Z15-	T50.Z16-
Gamma globulin	T50.Z11-	T50.Z12-	T50.Z13-	T50.Z14-	T50.Z15-	T50.Z16-
Gamma-aminobutyric acid	T43.8X1-	T43.8X2-	T43.8X3-	T43.8X4-	T43.8X5-	T43.8X6-
Gamma-benzene hexachloride (medicinal)	T49.0X1-	T49.0X2-	T49.0X3-	T49.0X4-	T49.0X5-	T49.0X6-
nonmedicinal, vapor	T53.6X1-	T53.6X2-	T53.6X3-	T53.6X4-	-	-
Gamma-BHC (medicinal) — *see also Gamma-benzene hexachloride*	T49.0X1-	T49.0X2-	T49.0X3-	T49.0X4-	T49.0X5-	T49.0X6-
Gamulin	T50.Z11-	T50.Z12-	T50.Z13-	T50.Z14-	T50.Z15-	T50.Z16-
Ganciclovir (sodium)	T37.5X1-	T37.5X2-	T37.5X3-	T37.5X4-	T37.5X5-	T37.5X6-

Substance	Poisoning Accidental (unintentional)	Poisoning Intentional self-harm	Poisoning Assault	Poisoning Undetermined	Adverse effect	Underdosing
Ganglionic blocking drug NEC	T44.2X1-	T44.2X2-	T44.2X3-	T44.2X4-	T44.2X5-	T44.2X6-
specified NEC	T44.2X1-	T44.2X2-	T44.2X3-	T44.2X4-	T44.2X5-	T44.2X6-
Ganja	T40.711-	T40.712-	T40.713-	T40.714-	T40.715-	T40.716-
Garamycin	T36.5X1-	T36.5X2-	T36.5X3-	T36.5X4-	T36.5X5-	T36.5X6-
ophthalmic preparation	T49.5X1-	T49.5X2-	T49.5X3-	T49.5X4-	T49.5X5-	T49.5X6-
topical NEC	T49.0X1-	T49.0X2-	T49.0X3-	T49.0X4-	T49.0X5-	T49.0X6-
Gardenal	T42.3X1-	T42.3X2-	T42.3X3-	T42.3X4-	T42.3X5-	T42.3X6-
Gardepanyl	T42.3X1-	T42.3X2-	T42.3X3-	T42.3X4-	T42.3X5-	T42.3X6-
Gas NEC	T59.91X-	T59.92X-	T59.93X-	T59.94X-	-	-
acetylene	T59.891-	T59.892-	T59.893-	T59.894-	-	-
incomplete combustion of	T58.11X-	T58.12X-	T58.13X-	T58.14X-	-	-
air contaminants, source or type not specified	T59.91X-	T59.92X-	T59.93X-	T59.94X-	-	-
anesthetic	T41.0X1-	T41.0X2-	T41.0X3-	T41.0X4-	T41.0X5-	T41.0X6-
blast furnace	T58.8X1-	T58.8X2-	T58.8X3-	T58.8X4-	-	-
butane — *see butane*						
carbon monoxide — *see Carbon, monoxide*						
chlorine	T59.4X1-	T59.4X2-	T59.4X3-	T59.4X4-	-	-
coal	T58.2X1-	T58.2X2-	T58.2X3-	T58.2X4-	-	-
cyanide	T57.3X1-	T57.3X2-	T57.3X3-	T57.3X4-	-	-
dicyanogen	T65.0X1-	T65.0X2-	T65.0X3-	T65.0X4-	-	-
domestic — *see Domestic gas*						
exhaust	T58.01X-	T58.02X-	T58.03X-	T58.04X-	-	-
from utility (for cooking, heating, or lighting) (after combustion) — *see Carbon, monoxide, fuel, utility*						
prior to combustion	T59.891-	T59.892-	T59.893-	T59.894-	-	-
from wood- or coal-burning stove or fireplace	T58.2X1-	T58.2X2-	T58.2X3-	T58.2X4-	-	-
fuel (domestic use) (after combustion) — *see also Carbon, monoxide, fuel*						
industrial use	T58.8X1-	T58.8X2-	T58.8X3-	T58.8X4-	-	-
prior to combustion	T59.891-	T59.892-	T59.893-	T59.894-	-	-
utility	T59.891-	T59.892-	T59.893-	T59.894-	-	-
in mobile container	T59.891-	T59.892-	T59.893-	T59.894-	-	-
incomplete combustion of — *see Carbon, monoxide, fuel, utility*						
piped (natural)	T59.891-	T59.892-	T59.893-	T59.894-	-	-
garage	T58.01X-	T58.02X-	T58.03X-	T58.04X-	-	-
hydrocarbon NEC	T59.891-	T59.892-	T59.893-	T59.894-	-	-
incomplete combustion of — *see Carbon, monoxide, fuel, utility*						
liquefied — *see butane*						
piped	T59.891-	T59.892-	T59.893-	T59.894-	-	-
hydrocyanic acid	T65.0X1-	T65.0X2-	T65.0X3-	T65.0X4-	-	-
illuminating (after combustion)	T58.11X-	T58.12X-	T58.13X-	T58.14X-	-	-
prior to combustion	T59.891-	T59.892-	T59.893-	T59.894-	-	-
incomplete combustion, any — *see Carbon, monoxide*						
kiln	T58.8X1-	T58.8X2-	T58.8X3-	T58.8X4-	-	-
lacrimogenic	T59.3X1-	T59.3X2-	T59.3X3-	T59.3X4-	-	-
liquefied petroleum — *see butane*						
marsh	T59.891-	T59.892-	T59.893-	T59.894-	-	-
motor exhaust, not in transit	T58.01X-	T58.02X-	T58.03X-	T58.04X-	-	-
mustard, not in war	T59.891-	T59.892-	T59.893-	T59.894-	-	-
natural	T59.891-	T59.892-	T59.893-	T59.894-	-	-
nerve, not in war	T59.91X-	T59.92X-	T59.93X-	T59.94X-	-	-

GANGLIONIC BLOCKING DRUG NEC - GAS NEC

Substance	Poisoning Accidental (unintentional)	Poisoning Intentional self-harm	Poisoning Assault	Poisoning Undetermined	Adverse effect	Underdosing
Gas NEC (continued)						
oil	T52.0X1-	T52.0X2-	T52.0X3-	T52.0X4-	-	-
petroleum (liquefied) (distributed in mobile containers)	T59.891-	T59.892-	T59.893-	T59.894-	-	-
piped (pure or mixed with air)	T59.891-	T59.892-	T59.893-	T59.894-	-	-
piped (manufactured) (natural) NEC	T59.891-	T59.892-	T59.893-	T59.894-	-	-
producer	T58.8X1-	T58.8X2-	T58.8X3-	T58.8X4-	-	-
propane — *see propane*						
refrigerant (chlorofluoro-carbon)	T53.5X1-	T53.5X2-	T53.5X3-	T53.5X4-	-	-
not chlorofluoro-carbon	T59.891-	T59.892-	T59.893-	T59.894-	-	-
sewer	T59.91X-	T59.92X-	T59.93X-	T59.94X-	-	-
specified source NEC	T59.91X-	T59.92X-	T59.93X-	T59.94X-	-	-
stove (after combustion)	T58.11X-	T58.12X-	T58.13X-	T58.14X-	-	-
prior to combustion	T59.891-	T59.892-	T59.893-	T59.894-	-	-
tear	T59.3X1-	T59.3X2-	T59.3X3-	T59.3X4-	-	-
therapeutic	T41.5X1-	T41.5X2-	T41.5X3-	T41.5X4-	T41.5X5-	T41.5X6-
utility (for cooking, heating, or lighting) (piped) NEC	T59.891-	T59.892-	T59.893-	T59.894-	-	-
in mobile container	T59.891-	T59.892-	T59.893-	T59.894-	-	-
incomplete combustion of — *see Carbon, monoxide, fuel, utility*						
piped (natural)	T59.891-	T59.892-	T59.893-	T59.894-	-	-
water	T58.11X-	T58.12X-	T58.13X-	T58.14X-	-	-
incomplete combustion of — *see Carbon, monoxide, fuel, utility*						
Gaseous substance — *see Gas*						
Gasoline	T52.0X1-	T52.0X2-	T52.0X3-	T52.0X4-	-	-
vapor	T52.0X1-	T52.0X2-	T52.0X3-	T52.0X4-	-	-
Gastric enzymes	T47.5X1-	T47.5X2-	T47.5X3-	T47.5X4-	T47.5X5-	T47.5X6-
Gastrografin	T50.8X1-	T50.8X2-	T50.8X3-	T50.8X4-	T50.8X5-	T50.8X6-
Gastrointestinal drug	T47.91X-	T47.92X-	T47.93X-	T47.94X-	T47.95X-	T47.96X-
biological	T47.8X1-	T47.8X2-	T47.8X3-	T47.8X4-	T47.8X5-	T47.8X6-
specified NEC	T47.8X1-	T47.8X2-	T47.8X3-	T47.8X4-	T47.8X5-	T47.8X6-
Gaultheria procumbens	T62.2X1-	T62.2X2-	T62.2X3-	T62.2X4-	-	-
Gefarnate	T44.3X1-	T44.3X2-	T44.3X3-	T44.3X4-	T44.3X5-	T44.3X6-
Gelatin (intravenous)	T45.8X1-	T45.8X2-	T45.8X3-	T45.8X4-	T45.8X5-	T45.8X6-
absorbable (sponge)	T45.7X1-	T45.7X2-	T45.7X3-	T45.7X4-	T45.7X5-	T45.7X6-
Gelfilm	T49.8X1-	T49.8X2-	T49.8X3-	T49.8X4-	T49.8X5-	T49.8X6-
Gelfoam	T45.7X1-	T45.7X2-	T45.7X3-	T45.7X4-	T45.7X5-	T45.7X6-
Gelsemine	T50.991-	T50.992-	T50.993-	T50.994-	T50.995-	T50.996-
Gelsemium (sempervirens)	T62.2X1-	T62.2X2-	T62.2X3-	T62.2X4-	-	-
Gemeprost	T48.0X1-	T48.0X2-	T48.0X3-	T48.0X4-	T48.0X5-	T48.0X6-
Gemfibrozil	T46.6X1-	T46.6X2-	T46.6X3-	T46.6X4-	T46.6X5-	T46.6X6-
Gemonil	T42.3X1-	T42.3X2-	T42.3X3-	T42.3X4-	T42.3X5-	T42.3X6-
Gentamicin	T36.5X1-	T36.5X2-	T36.5X3-	T36.5X4-	T36.5X5-	T36.5X6-
ophthalmic preparation	T49.5X1-	T49.5X2-	T49.5X3-	T49.5X4-	T49.5X5-	T49.5X6-
topical NEC	T49.0X1-	T49.0X2-	T49.0X3-	T49.0X4-	T49.0X5-	T49.0X6-
Gentian	T47.5X1-	T47.5X2-	T47.5X3-	T47.5X4-	T47.5X5-	T47.5X6-
violet	T49.0X1-	T49.0X2-	T49.0X3-	T49.0X4-	T49.0X5-	T49.0X6-
Gepefrine	T44.4X1-	T44.4X2-	T44.4X3-	T44.4X4-	T44.4X5-	T44.4X6-
Gestonorone caproate	T38.5X1-	T38.5X2-	T38.5X3-	T38.5X4-	T38.5X5-	T38.5X6-
Gexane	T49.0X1-	T49.0X2-	T49.0X3-	T49.0X4-	T49.0X5-	T49.0X6-
Gila monster (venom)	T63.111-	T63.112-	T63.113-	T63.114-	-	-
Ginger	T47.5X1-	T47.5X2-	T47.5X3-	T47.5X4-	T47.5X5-	T47.5X6-
Jamaica — *see Jamaica, ginger*						
Gitalin	T46.0X1-	T46.0X2-	T46.0X3-	T46.0X4-	T46.0X5-	T46.0X6-
amorphous	T46.0X1-	T46.0X2-	T46.0X3-	T46.0X4-	T46.0X5-	T46.0X6-

Substance	Poisoning Accidental (unintentional)	Poisoning Intentional self-harm	Poisoning Assault	Poisoning Undetermined	Adverse effect	Underdosing
Gitaloxin	T46.0X1-	T46.0X2-	T46.0X3-	T46.0X4-	T46.0X5-	T46.0X6-
Gitoxin	T46.0X1-	T46.0X2-	T46.0X3-	T46.0X4-	T46.0X5-	T46.0X6-
Glafenine	T39.8X1-	T39.8X2-	T39.8X3-	T39.8X4-	T39.8X5-	T39.8X6-
Glandular extract (medicinal) NEC	T50.Z91-	T50.Z92-	T50.Z93-	T50.Z94-	T50.Z95-	T50.Z96-
Glaucarubin	T37.3X1-	T37.3X2-	T37.3X3-	T37.3X4-	T37.3X5-	T37.3X6-
Glibenclamide	T38.3X1-	T38.3X2-	T38.3X3-	T38.3X4-	T38.3X5-	T38.3X6-
Glibornuride	T38.3X1-	T38.3X2-	T38.3X3-	T38.3X4-	T38.3X5-	T38.3X6-
Gliclazide	T38.3X1-	T38.3X2-	T38.3X3-	T38.3X4-	T38.3X5-	T38.3X6-
Glimidine	T38.3X1-	T38.3X2-	T38.3X3-	T38.3X4-	T38.3X5-	T38.3X6-
Glipizide	T38.3X1-	T38.3X2-	T38.3X3-	T38.3X4-	T38.3X5-	T38.3X6-
Gliquidone	T38.3X1-	T38.3X2-	T38.3X3-	T38.3X4-	T38.3X5-	T38.3X6-
Glisolamide	T38.3X1-	T38.3X2-	T38.3X3-	T38.3X4-	T38.3X5-	T38.3X6-
Glisoxepide	T38.3X1-	T38.3X2-	T38.3X3-	T38.3X4-	T38.3X5-	T38.3X6-
Globin zinc insulin	T38.3X1-	T38.3X2-	T38.3X3-	T38.3X4-	T38.3X5-	T38.3X6-
Globulin						
antilymphocytic	T50.Z11-	T50.Z12-	T50.Z13-	T50.Z14-	T50.Z15-	T50.Z16-
antirhesus	T50.Z11-	T50.Z12-	T50.Z13-	T50.Z14-	T50.Z15-	T50.Z16-
antivenin	T50.Z11-	T50.Z12-	T50.Z13-	T50.Z14-	T50.Z15-	T50.Z16-
antiviral	T50.Z11-	T50.Z12-	T50.Z13-	T50.Z14-	T50.Z15-	T50.Z16-
Glucagon	T38.3X1-	T38.3X2-	T38.3X3-	T38.3X4-	T38.3X5-	T38.3X6-
Glucocorticoids	T38.0X1-	T38.0X2-	T38.0X3-	T38.0X4-	T38.0X5-	T38.0X6-
Glucocorticosteroid	T38.0X1-	T38.0X2-	T38.0X3-	T38.0X4-	T38.0X5-	T38.0X6-
Gluconic acid	T50.991-	T50.992-	T50.993-	T50.994-	T50.995-	T50.996-
Glucosamine sulfate	T39.4X1-	T39.4X2-	T39.4X3-	T39.4X4-	T39.4X5-	T39.4X6-
Glucose	T50.3X1-	T50.3X2-	T50.3X3-	T50.3X4-	T50.3X5-	T50.3X6-
with sodium chloride	T50.3X1-	T50.3X2-	T50.3X3-	T50.3X4-	T50.3X5-	T50.3X6-
Glucosulfone sodium	T37.1X1-	T37.1X2-	T37.1X3-	T37.1X4-	T37.1X5-	T37.1X6-
Glucurolactone	T47.8X1-	T47.8X2-	T47.8X3-	T47.8X4-	T47.8X5-	T47.8X6-
Glue NEC	T52.8X1-	T52.8X2-	T52.8X3-	T52.8X4-	-	-
Glutamic acid	T47.5X1-	T47.5X2-	T47.5X3-	T47.5X4-	T47.5X5-	T47.5X6-
Glutaral (medicinal)	T49.0X1-	T49.0X2-	T49.0X3-	T49.0X4-	T49.0X5-	T49.0X6-
nonmedicinal	T65.891-	T65.892-	T65.893-	T65.894-	-	-
Glutaraldehyde (nonmedicinal)	T65.891-	T65.892-	T65.893-	T65.894-	-	-
medicinal	T49.0X1-	T49.0X2-	T49.0X3-	T49.0X4-	T49.0X5-	T49.0X6-
Glutathione	T50.6X1-	T50.6X2-	T50.6X3-	T50.6X4-	T50.6X5-	T50.6X6-
Glutethimide	T42.6X1-	T42.6X2-	T42.6X3-	T42.6X4-	T42.6X5-	T42.6X6-
Glyburide	T38.3X1-	T38.3X2-	T38.3X3-	T38.3X4-	T38.3X5-	T38.3X6-
Glycerin	T47.4X1-	T47.4X2-	T47.4X3-	T47.4X4-	T47.4X5-	T47.4X6-
Glycerol	T47.4X1-	T47.4X2-	T47.4X3-	T47.4X4-	T47.4X5-	T47.4X6-
borax	T49.6X1-	T49.6X2-	T49.6X3-	T49.6X4-	T49.6X5-	T49.6X6-
intravenous	T50.3X1-	T50.3X2-	T50.3X3-	T50.3X4-	T50.3X5-	T50.3X6-
iodinated	T48.4X1-	T48.4X2-	T48.4X3-	T48.4X4-	T48.4X5-	T48.4X6-
Glycerophosphate	T50.991-	T50.992-	T50.993-	T50.994-	T50.995-	T50.996-
Glyceryl						
gualacolate	T48.4X1-	T48.4X2-	T48.4X3-	T48.4X4-	T48.4X5-	T48.4X6-
nitrate	T46.3X1-	T46.3X2-	T46.3X3-	T46.3X4-	T46.3X5-	T46.3X6-
triacetate (topical)	T49.0X1-	T49.0X2-	T49.0X3-	T49.0X4-	T49.0X5-	T49.0X6-
trinitrate	T46.3X1-	T46.3X2-	T46.3X3-	T46.3X4-	T46.3X5-	T46.3X6-
Glycine	T50.3X1-	T50.3X2-	T50.3X3-	T50.3X4-	T50.3X5-	T50.3X6-
Glyclopyramide	T38.3X1-	T38.3X2-	T38.3X3-	T38.3X4-	T38.3X5-	T38.3X6-
Glycobiarsol	T37.3X1-	T37.3X2-	T37.3X3-	T37.3X4-	T37.3X5-	T37.3X6-
Glycols (ether)	T52.3X1-	T52.3X2-	T52.3X3-	T52.3X4-	-	-
Glyconiazide	T37.1X1-	T37.1X2-	T37.1X3-	T37.1X4-	T37.1X5-	T37.1X6-
Glycopyrrolate	T44.3X1-	T44.3X2-	T44.3X3-	T44.3X4-	T44.3X5-	T44.3X6-
Glycopyrronium	T44.3X1-	T44.3X2-	T44.3X3-	T44.3X4-	T44.3X5-	T44.3X6-
bromide	T44.3X1-	T44.3X2-	T44.3X3-	T44.3X4-	T44.3X5-	T44.3X6-
Glycoside, cardiac (stimulant)	T46.0X1-	T46.0X2-	T46.0X3-	T46.0X4-	T46.0X5-	T46.0X6-
Glycyclamide	T38.3X1-	T38.3X2-	T38.3X3-	T38.3X4-	T38.3X5-	T38.3X6-

Substance	Poisoning Accidental (unintentional)	Poisoning Intentional self-harm	Poisoning Assault	Poisoning Undetermined	Adverse effect	Underdosing
Glycyrrhiza extract	T48.4X1-	T48.4X2-	T48.4X3-	T48.4X4-	T48.4X5-	T48.4X6-
Glycyrrhizic acid	T48.4X1-	T48.4X2-	T48.4X3-	T48.4X4-	T48.4X5-	T48.4X6-
Glycyrrhizinate potassium	T48.4X1-	T48.4X2-	T48.4X3-	T48.4X4-	T48.4X5-	T48.4X6-
Glymidine sodium	T38.3X1-	T38.3X2-	T38.3X3-	T38.3X4-	T38.3X5-	T38.3X6-
Glyphosate	T60.3X1-	T60.3X2-	T60.3X3-	T60.3X4-	-	-
Glyphylline	T48.6X1-	T48.6X2-	T48.6X3-	T48.6X4-	T48.6X5-	T48.6X6-
Gold						
colloidal (l98Au)	T45.1X1-	T45.1X2-	T45.1X3-	T45.1X4-	T45.1X5-	T45.1X6-
salts	T39.4X1-	T39.4X2-	T39.4X3-	T39.4X4-	T39.4X5-	T39.4X6-
Golden sulfide of antimony	T56.891-	T56.892-	T56.893-	T56.894-	-	-
Goldylocks	T62.2X1-	T62.2X2-	T62.2X3-	T62.2X4-	-	-
Gonadal tissue extract	T38.901-	T38.902-	T38.903-	T38.904-	T38.905-	T38.906-
female	T38.5X1-	T38.5X2-	T38.5X3-	T38.5X4-	T38.5X5-	T38.5X6-
male	T38.7X1-	T38.7X2-	T38.7X3-	T38.7X4-	T38.7X5-	T38.7X6-
Gonadorelin	T38.891-	T38.892-	T38.893-	T38.894-	T38.895-	T38.896-
Gonadotropin	T38.891-	T38.892-	T38.893-	T38.894-	T38.895-	T38.896-
chorionic	T38.891-	T38.892-	T38.893-	T38.894-	T38.895-	T38.896-
pituitary	T38.811-	T38.812-	T38.813-	T38.814-	T38.815-	T38.816-
Goserelin	T45.1X1-	T45.1X2-	T45.1X3-	T45.1X4-	T45.1X5-	T45.1X6-
Grain alcohol	T51.0X1-	T51.0X2-	T51.0X3-	T51.0X4-	-	-
Gramicidin	T49.0X1-	T49.0X2-	T49.0X3-	T49.0X4-	T49.0X5-	T49.0X6-
Granisetron	T45.0X1-	T45.0X2-	T45.0X3-	T45.0X4-	T45.0X5-	T45.0X6-
Gratiola officinalis	T62.2X1-	T62.2X2-	T62.2X3-	T62.2X4-	-	-
Grease	T65.891-	T65.892-	T65.893-	T65.894-	-	-
Green hellebore	T62.2X1-	T62.2X2-	T62.2X3-	T62.2X4-	-	-
Green soap	T49.2X1-	T49.2X2-	T49.2X3-	T49.2X4-	T49.2X5-	T49.2X6-
Grifulvin	T36.7X1-	T36.7X2-	T36.7X3-	T36.7X4-	T36.7X5-	T36.7X6-
Griseofulvin	T36.7X1-	T36.7X2-	T36.7X3-	T36.7X4-	T36.7X5-	T36.7X6-
Growth hormone	T38.811-	T38.812-	T38.813-	T38.814-	T38.815-	T38.816-
Guaiac reagent	T50.991-	T50.992-	T50.993-	T50.994-	T50.995-	T50.996-
Guaiacol derivatives	T48.4X1-	T48.4X2-	T48.4X3-	T48.4X4-	T48.4X5-	T48.4X6-
Guaifenesin	T48.4X1-	T48.4X2-	T48.4X3-	T48.4X4-	T48.4X5-	T48.4X6-
Guaimesal	T48.4X1-	T48.4X2-	T48.4X3-	T48.4X4-	T48.4X5-	T48.4X6-
Guaiphenesin	T48.4X1-	T48.4X2-	T48.4X3-	T48.4X4-	T48.4X5-	T48.4X6-
Guamecycline	T36.4X1-	T36.4X2-	T36.4X3-	T36.4X4-	T36.4X5-	T36.4X6-
Guanabenz	T46.5X1-	T46.5X2-	T46.5X3-	T46.5X4-	T46.5X5-	T46.5X6-
Guanacline	T46.5X1-	T46.5X2-	T46.5X3-	T46.5X4-	T46.5X5-	T46.5X6-
Guanadrel	T46.5X1-	T46.5X2-	T46.5X3-	T46.5X4-	T46.5X5-	T46.5X6-
Guanatol	T37.2X1-	T37.2X2-	T37.2X3-	T37.2X4-	T37.2X5-	T37.2X6-
Guanethidine	T46.5X1-	T46.5X2-	T46.5X3-	T46.5X4-	T46.5X5-	T46.5X6-
Guanfacine	T46.5X1-	T46.5X2-	T46.5X3-	T46.5X4-	T46.5X5-	T46.5X6-
Guano	T65.891-	T65.892-	T65.893-	T65.894-	-	-
Guanochlor	T46.5X1-	T46.5X2-	T46.5X3-	T46.5X4-	T46.5X5-	T46.5X6-
Guanoclor	T46.5X1-	T46.5X2-	T46.5X3-	T46.5X4-	T46.5X5-	T46.5X6-
Guanoctine	T46.5X1-	T46.5X2-	T46.5X3-	T46.5X4-	T46.5X5-	T46.5X6-
Guanoxabenz	T46.5X1-	T46.5X2-	T46.5X3-	T46.5X4-	T46.5X5-	T46.5X6-
Guanoxan	T46.5X1-	T46.5X2-	T46.5X3-	T46.5X4-	T46.5X5-	T46.5X6-
Guar gum (medicinal)	T46.6X1-	T46.6X2-	T46.6X3-	T46.6X4-	T46.6X5-	T46.6X6-
Hachimycin	T36.7X1-	T36.7X2-	T36.7X3-	T36.7X4-	T36.7X5-	T36.7X6-
Hair						
dye	T49.4X1-	T49.4X2-	T49.4X3-	T49.4X4-	T49.4X5-	T49.4X6-
preparation NEC	T49.4X1-	T49.4X2-	T49.4X3-	T49.4X4-	T49.4X5-	T49.4X6-
Halazepam	T42.4X1-	T42.4X2-	T42.4X3-	T42.4X4-	T42.4X5-	T42.4X6-
Halcinolone	T49.0X1-	T49.0X2-	T49.0X3-	T49.0X4-	T49.0X5-	T49.0X6-
Halcinonide	T49.0X1-	T49.0X2-	T49.0X3-	T49.0X4-	T49.0X5-	T49.0X6-
Halethazole	T49.0X1-	T49.0X2-	T49.0X3-	T49.0X4-	T49.0X5-	T49.0X6-
Hallucinogen NOS	T40.901-	T40.902-	T40.903-	T40.904-	T40.905-	T40.906-
specified NEC	T40.991-	T40.992-	T40.993-	T40.994-	T40.995-	T40.996-

Substance	Poisoning Accidental (unintentional)	Poisoning Intentional self-harm	Poisoning Assault	Poisoning Undetermined	Adverse effect	Underdosing
Halofantrine	T37.2X1-	T37.2X2-	T37.2X3-	T37.2X4-	T37.2X5-	T37.2X6-
Halofenate	T46.6X1-	T46.6X2-	T46.6X3-	T46.6X4-	T46.6X5-	T46.6X6-
Halometasone	T49.0X1-	T49.0X2-	T49.0X3-	T49.0X4-	T49.0X5-	T49.0X6-
Haloperidol	T43.4X1-	T43.4X2-	T43.4X3-	T43.4X4-	T43.4X5-	T43.4X6-
Haloprogin	T49.0X1-	T49.0X2-	T49.0X3-	T49.0X4-	T49.0X5-	T49.0X6-
Halotex	T49.0X1-	T49.0X2-	T49.0X3-	T49.0X4-	T49.0X5-	T49.0X6-
Halothane	T41.0X1-	T41.0X2-	T41.0X3-	T41.0X4-	T41.0X5-	T41.0X6-
Haloxazolam	T42.4X1-	T42.4X2-	T42.4X3-	T42.4X4-	T42.4X5-	T42.4X6-
Halquinols	T49.0X1-	T49.0X2-	T49.0X3-	T49.0X4-	T49.0X5-	T49.0X6-
Hamamelis	T49.2X1-	T49.2X2-	T49.2X3-	T49.2X4-	T49.2X5-	T49.2X6-
Haptendextran	T45.8X1-	T45.8X2-	T45.8X3-	T45.8X4-	T45.8X5-	T45.8X6-
Harmonyl	T46.5X1-	T46.5X2-	T46.5X3-	T46.5X4-	T46.5X5-	T46.5X6-
Hartmann's solution	T50.3X1-	T50.3X2-	T50.3X3-	T50.3X4-	T50.3X5-	T50.3X6-
Hashish	T40.711-	T40.712-	T40.713-	T40.714-	T40.715-	T40.716-
Hawaiian Woodrose seeds	T40.991-	T40.992-	T40.993-	T40.994-	-	-
HCB	T60.3X1-	T60.3X2-	T60.3X3-	T60.3X4-	-	-
HCH	T53.6X1-	T53.6X2-	T53.6X3-	T53.6X4-	-	-
medicinal	T49.0X1-	T49.0X2-	T49.0X3-	T49.0X4-	T49.0X5-	T49.0X6-
HCN	T57.3X1-	T57.3X2-	T57.3X3-	T57.3X4-	-	-
Headache cures, drugs, powders NEC	T50.901-	T50.902-	T50.903-	T50.904-	T50.905-	T50.906-
Heavenly Blue (morning glory)	T40.991-	T40.992-	T40.993-	T40.994-	-	-
Heavy metal antidote	T45.8X1-	T45.8X2-	T45.8X3-	T45.8X4-	T45.8X5-	T45.8X6-
Hedaquinium	T49.0X1-	T49.0X2-	T49.0X3-	T49.0X4-	T49.0X5-	T49.0X6-
Hedge hyssop	T62.2X1-	T62.2X2-	T62.2X3-	T62.2X4-	-	-
Heet	T49.8X1-	T49.8X2-	T49.8X3-	T49.8X4-	T49.8X5-	T49.8X6-
Helenin	T37.4X1-	T37.4X2-	T37.4X3-	T37.4X4-	T37.4X5-	T37.4X6-
Helium (nonmedicinal) NEC	T59.891-	T59.892-	T59.893-	T59.894-	-	-
medicinal	T48.991-	T48.992-	T48.993-	T48.994-	T48.995-	T48.996-
Hellebore (black) (green) (white)	T62.2X1-	T62.2X2-	T62.2X3-	T62.2X4-	-	-
Hematin	T45.8X1-	T45.8X2-	T45.8X3-	T45.8X4-	T45.8X5-	T45.8X6-
Hematinic preparation	T45.8X1-	T45.8X2-	T45.8X3-	T45.8X4-	T45.8X5-	T45.8X6-
Hematological agent	T45.91X-	T45.92X-	T45.93X-	T45.94X-	T45.95X-	T45.96X-
specified NEC	T45.8X1-	T45.8X2-	T45.8X3-	T45.8X4-	T45.8X5-	T45.8X6-
Hemlock	T62.2X1-	T62.2X2-	T62.2X3-	T62.2X4-	-	-
Hemostatic	T45.621-	T45.622-	T45.623-	T45.624-	T45.625-	T45.626-
drug, systemic	T45.621-	T45.622-	T45.623-	T45.624-	T45.625-	T45.626-
Hemostyptic	T49.4X1-	T49.4X2-	T49.4X3-	T49.4X4-	T49.4X5-	T49.4X6-
Henbane	T62.2X1-	T62.2X2-	T62.2X3-	T62.2X4-	-	-
Heparin (sodium)	T45.511-	T45.512-	T45.513-	T45.514-	T45.515-	T45.516-
action reverser	T45.7X1-	T45.7X2-	T45.7X3-	T45.7X4-	T45.7X5-	T45.7X6-
Heparin-fraction	T45.511-	T45.512-	T45.513-	T45.514-	T45.515-	T45.516-
Heparinoid (systemic)	T45.511-	T45.512-	T45.513-	T45.514-	T45.515-	T45.516-
Hepatic secretion stimulant	T47.8X1-	T47.8X2-	T47.8X3-	T47.8X4-	T47.8X5-	T47.8X6-
Hepatitis B						
immune globulin	T50.Z11-	T50.Z12-	T50.Z13-	T50.Z14-	T50.Z15-	T50.Z16-
vaccine	T50.B91-	T50.B92-	T50.B93-	T50.B94-	T50.B95-	T50.B96-
Hepronicate	T46.7X1-	T46.7X2-	T46.7X3-	T46.7X4-	T46.7X5-	T46.7X6-
Heptabarb	T42.3X1-	T42.3X2-	T42.3X3-	T42.3X4-	T42.3X5-	T42.3X6-
Heptabarbital	T42.3X1-	T42.3X2-	T42.3X3-	T42.3X4-	T42.3X5-	T42.3X6-
Heptabarbitone	T42.3X1-	T42.3X2-	T42.3X3-	T42.3X4-	T42.3X5-	T42.3X6-
Heptachlor	T60.1X1-	T60.1X2-	T60.1X3-	T60.1X4-	-	-
Heptalgin	T40.2X1-	T40.2X2-	T40.2X3-	T40.2X4-	T40.2X5-	T40.2X6-
Heptaminol	T46.3X1-	T46.3X2-	T46.3X3-	T46.3X4-	T46.3X5-	T46.3X6-
Herbicide NEC	T60.3X1-	T60.3X2-	T60.3X3-	T60.3X4-	-	-
Heroin	T40.1X1-	T40.1X2-	T40.1X3-	T40.1X4-	-	-
Herplex	T49.5X1-	T49.5X2-	T49.5X3-	T49.5X4-	T49.5X5-	T49.5X6-
HES	T45.8X1-	T45.8X2-	T45.8X3-	T45.8X4-	T45.8X5-	T45.8X6-
Hesperidin	T46.991-	T46.992-	T46.993-	T46.994-	T46.995-	T46.996-

Substance	Poisoning Accidental (unintentional)	Poisoning Intentional self-harm	Poisoning Assault	Poisoning Undetermined	Adverse effect	Underdosing
Hetacillin	T36.0X1-	T36.0X2-	T36.0X3-	T36.0X4-	T36.0X5-	T36.0X6-
Hetastarch	T45.8X1-	T45.8X2-	T45.8X3-	T45.8X4-	T45.8X5-	T45.8X6-
HETP	T60.0X1-	T60.0X2-	T60.0X3-	T60.0X4-	-	-
Hexachlorobenzene (vapor)	T60.3X1-	T60.3X2-	T60.3X3-	T60.3X4-	-	-
Hexachlorocyclohexane	T53.6X1-	T53.6X2-	T53.6X3-	T53.6X4-	-	-
Hexachlorophene	T49.0X1-	T49.0X2-	T49.0X3-	T49.0X4-	T49.0X5-	T49.0X6-
Hexadiline	T46.3X1-	T46.3X2-	T46.3X3-	T46.3X4-	T46.3X5-	T46.3X6-
Hexadimethrine (bromide)	T45.7X1-	T45.7X2-	T45.7X3-	T45.7X4-	T45.7X5-	T45.7X6-
Hexadylamine	T46.3X1-	T46.3X2-	T46.3X3-	T46.3X4-	T46.3X5-	T46.3X6-
Hexaethyl tetraphos-phate	T60.0X1-	T60.0X2-	T60.0X3-	T60.0X4-	-	-
Hexafluorenium bromide	T48.1X1-	T48.1X2-	T48.1X3-	T48.1X4-	T48.1X5-	T48.1X6-
Hexafluronium (bromide)	T48.1X1-	T48.1X2-	T48.1X3-	T48.1X4-	T48.1X5-	T48.1X6-
Hexa-germ	T49.2X1-	T49.2X2-	T49.2X3-	T49.2X4-	T49.2X5-	T49.2X6-
Hexahydrobenzol	T52.8X1-	T52.8X2-	T52.8X3-	T52.8X4-	-	-
Hexahydrocresol (s)	T51.8X1-	T51.8X2-	T51.8X3-	T51.8X4-	-	-
arsenide	T57.0X1-	T57.0X2-	T57.0X3-	T57.0X4-	-	-
arseniurated	T57.0X1-	T57.0X2-	T57.0X3-	T57.0X4-	-	-
cyanide	T57.3X1-	T57.3X2-	T57.3X3-	T57.3X4-	-	-
gas	T59.891-	T59.892-	T59.893-	T59.894-	-	-
Fluoride (liquid)	T57.8X1-	T57.8X2-	T57.8X3-	T57.8X4-	-	-
vapor	T59.891-	T59.892-	T59.893-	T59.894-	-	-
phophorated	T60.0X1-	T60.0X2-	T60.0X3-	T60.0X4-	-	-
sulfate	T57.8X1-	T57.8X2-	T57.8X3-	T57.8X4-	-	-
sulfide (gas)	T59.6X1-	T59.6X2-	T59.6X3-	T59.6X4-	-	-
arseniurated	T57.0X1-	T57.0X2-	T57.0X3-	T57.0X4-	-	-
sulfurated	T57.8X1-	T57.8X2-	T57.8X3-	T57.8X4-	-	-
Hexahydrophenol	T51.8X1-	T51.8X2-	T51.8X3-	T51.8X4-	-	-
Hexalen	T51.8X1-	T51.8X2-	T51.8X3-	T51.8X4-	-	-
Hexamethonium bromide	T44.2X1-	T44.2X2-	T44.2X3-	T44.2X4-	T44.2X5-	T44.2X6-
Hexamethylene	T52.8X1-	T52.8X2-	T52.8X3-	T52.8X4-	-	-
Hexamethylmelamine	T45.1X1-	T45.1X2-	T45.1X3-	T45.1X4-	T45.1X5-	T45.1X6-
Hexamidine	T49.0X1-	T49.0X2-	T49.0X3-	T49.0X4-	T49.0X5-	T49.0X6-
Hexamine (mandelate)	T37.8X1-	T37.8X2-	T37.8X3-	T37.8X4-	T37.8X5-	T37.8X6-
Hexanone, 2-hexanone	T52.4X1-	T52.4X2-	T52.4X3-	T52.4X4-	-	-
Hexanuorenium	T48.1X1-	T48.1X2-	T48.1X3-	T48.1X4-	T48.1X5-	T48.1X6-
Hexapropymate	T42.6X1-	T42.6X2-	T42.6X3-	T42.6X4-	T42.6X5-	T42.6X6-
Hexasonium iodide	T44.3X1-	T44.3X2-	T44.3X3-	T44.3X4-	T44.3X5-	T44.3X6-
Hexcarbacholine bromide	T48.1X1-	T48.1X2-	T48.1X3-	T48.1X4-	T48.1X5-	T48.1X6-
Hexemal	T42.3X1-	T42.3X2-	T42.3X3-	T42.3X4-	T42.3X5-	T42.3X6-
Hexestrol	T38.5X1-	T38.5X2-	T38.5X3-	T38.5X4-	T38.5X5-	T38.5X6-
Hexethal (sodium)	T42.3X1-	T42.3X2-	T42.3X3-	T42.3X4-	T42.3X5-	T42.3X6-
Hexetidine	T37.8X1-	T37.8X2-	T37.8X3-	T37.8X4-	T37.8X5-	T37.8X6-
Hexobarbital	T42.3X1-	T42.3X2-	T42.3X3-	T42.3X4-	T42.3X5-	T42.3X6-
rectal	T41.291-	T41.292-	T41.293-	T41.294-	T41.295-	T41.296-
sodium	T41.1X1-	T41.1X2-	T41.1X3-	T41.1X4-	T41.1X5-	T41.1X6-
Hexobendine	T46.3X1-	T46.3X2-	T46.3X3-	T46.3X4-	T46.3X5-	T46.3X6-
Hexocyclium	T44.3X1-	T44.3X2-	T44.3X3-	T44.3X4-	T44.3X5-	T44.3X6-
metilsulfate	T44.3X1-	T44.3X2-	T44.3X3-	T44.3X4-	T44.3X5-	T44.3X6-
Hexoestrol	T38.5X1-	T38.5X2-	T38.5X3-	T38.5X4-	T38.5X5-	T38.5X6-
Hexone	T52.4X1-	T52.4X2-	T52.4X3-	T52.4X4-	-	-
Hexoprenaline	T48.6X1-	T48.6X2-	T48.6X3-	T48.6X4-	T48.6X5-	T48.6X6-
Hexylcaine	T41.3X1-	T41.3X2-	T41.3X3-	T41.3X4-	T41.3X5-	T41.3X6-
Hexylresorcinol	T52.2X1-	T52.2X2-	T52.2X3-	T52.2X4-	-	-
HGH (human growth hormone)	T38.811-	T38.812-	T38.813-	T38.814-	T38.815-	T38.816-
Hinkle's pills	T47.2X1-	T47.2X2-	T47.2X3-	T47.2X4-	T47.2X5-	T47.2X6-
Histalog	T50.8X1-	T50.8X2-	T50.8X3-	T50.8X4-	T50.8X5-	T50.8X6-
Histamine (phosphate)	T50.8X1-	T50.8X2-	T50.8X3-	T50.8X4-	T50.8X5-	T50.8X6-
Histoplasmin	T50.8X1-	T50.8X2-	T50.8X3-	T50.8X4-	T50.8X5-	T50.8X6-
Holly berries	T62.2X1-	T62.2X2-	T62.2X3-	T62.2X4-	-	-

Substance	Poisoning Accidental (unintentional)	Poisoning Intentional self-harm	Poisoning Assault	Poisoning Undetermined	Adverse effect	Underdosing
Homatropine	T44.3X1-	T44.3X2-	T44.3X3-	T44.3X4-	T44.3X5-	T44.3X6-
methylbromide	T44.3X1-	T44.3X2-	T44.3X3-	T44.3X4-	T44.3X5-	T44.3X6-
Homochlorcyclizine	T45.0X1-	T45.0X2-	T45.0X3-	T45.0X4-	T45.0X5-	T45.0X6-
Homosalate	T49.3X1-	T49.3X2-	T49.3X3-	T49.3X4-	T49.3X5-	T49.3X6-
Homo-tet	T50.Z11-	T50.Z12-	T50.Z13-	T50.Z14-	T50.Z15-	T50.Z16-
Hormone	T38.801-	T38.802-	T38.803-	T38.804-	T38.805-	T38.806-
adrenal cortical steroids	T38.0X1-	T38.0X2-	T38.0X3-	T38.0X4-	T38.0X5-	T38.0X6-
androgenic	T38.7X1-	T38.7X2-	T38.7X3-	T38.7X4-	T38.7X5-	T38.7X6-
anterior pituitary NEC	T38.811-	T38.812-	T38.813-	T38.814-	T38.815-	T38.816-
antidiabetic agents	T38.3X1-	T38.3X2-	T38.3X3-	T38.3X4-	T38.3X5-	T38.3X6-
antidiuretic	T38.891-	T38.892-	T38.893-	T38.894-	T38.895-	T38.896-
cancer therapy	T45.1X1-	T45.1X2-	T45.1X3-	T45.1X4-	T45.1X5-	T45.1X6-
follicle stimulating	T38.811-	T38.812-	T38.813-	T38.814-	T38.815-	T38.816-
gonadotropic	T38.891-	T38.892-	T38.893-	T38.894-	T38.895-	T38.896-
pituitary	T38.811-	T38.812-	T38.813-	T38.814-	T38.815-	T38.816-
growth	T38.811-	T38.812-	T38.813-	T38.814-	T38.815-	T38.816-
luteinizing	T38.811-	T38.812-	T38.813-	T38.814-	T38.815-	T38.816-
ovarian	T38.5X1-	T38.5X2-	T38.5X3-	T38.5X4-	T38.5X5-	T38.5X6-
oxytocic	T48.0X1-	T48.0X2-	T48.0X3-	T48.0X4-	T48.0X5-	T48.0X6-
parathyroid (derivatives)	T50.991-	T50.992-	T50.993-	T50.994-	T50.995-	T50.996-
pituitary (posterior) NEC	T38.891-	T38.892-	T38.893-	T38.894-	T38.895-	T38.896-
anterior	T38.811-	T38.812-	T38.813-	T38.814-	T38.815-	T38.816-
specified, NEC	T38.891-	T38.892-	T38.893-	T38.894-	T38.895-	T38.896-
thyroid	T38.1X1-	T38.1X2-	T38.1X3-	T38.1X4-	T38.1X5-	T38.1X6-
Hornet (sting)	T63.451-	T63.452-	T63.453-	T63.454-	-	-
Horse anti-human lymphocytic serum	T50.Z11-	T50.Z12-	T50.Z13-	T50.Z14-	T50.Z15-	T50.Z16-
Horticulture agent NEC	T65.91X-	T65.92X-	T65.93X-	T65.94X-	-	-
with pesticide	T60.91X-	T60.92X-	T60.93X-	T60.94X-	-	-
Human						
albumin	T45.8X1-	T45.8X2-	T45.8X3-	T45.8X4-	T45.8X5-	T45.8X6-
growth hormone (HGH)	T38.811-	T38.812-	T38.813-	T38.814-	T38.815-	T38.816-
immune serum	T50.Z11-	T50.Z12-	T50.Z13-	T50.Z14-	T50.Z15-	T50.Z16-
Hyaluronidase	T45.3X1-	T45.3X2-	T45.3X3-	T45.3X4-	T45.3X5-	T45.3X6-
Hyazyme	T45.3X1-	T45.3X2-	T45.3X3-	T45.3X4-	T45.3X5-	T45.3X6-
Hycodan	T40.2X1-	T40.2X2-	T40.2X3-	T40.2X4-	T40.2X5-	T40.2X6-
Hydantoin derivative NEC	T42.0X1-	T42.0X2-	T42.0X3-	T42.0X4-	T42.0X5-	T42.0X6-
Hydeltra	T38.0X1-	T38.0X2-	T38.0X3-	T38.0X4-	T38.0X5-	T38.0X6-
Hydergine	T44.6X1-	T44.6X2-	T44.6X3-	T44.6X4-	T44.6X5-	T44.6X6-
Hydrabamine penicillin	T36.0X1-	T36.0X2-	T36.0X3-	T36.0X4-	T36.0X5-	T36.0X6-
Hydralazine	T46.5X1-	T46.5X2-	T46.5X3-	T46.5X4-	T46.5X5-	T46.5X6-
Hydrargaphen	T49.0X1-	T49.0X2-	T49.0X3-	T49.0X4-	T49.0X5-	T49.0X6-
Hydrargyri amino-chloridum	T49.0X1-	T49.0X2-	T49.0X3-	T49.0X4-	T49.0X5-	T49.0X6-
Hydrastine	T48.291-	T48.292-	T48.293-	T48.294-	T48.295-	T48.296-
Hydrazine	T54.1X1-	T54.1X2-	T54.1X3-	T54.1X4-	-	-
monoamine oxidase inhibitors	T43.1X1-	T43.1X2-	T43.1X3-	T43.1X4-	T43.1X5-	T43.1X6-
Hydrazoic acid, azides	T54.2X1-	T54.2X2-	T54.2X3-	T54.2X4-	-	-
Hydriodic acid	T48.4X1-	T48.4X2-	T48.4X3-	T48.4X4-	T48.4X5-	T48.4X6-
Hydrocarbon gas	T59.891-	T59.892-	T59.893-	T59.894-	-	-
incomplete combustion of — *see Carbon, monoxide, fuel, utility*						
liquefied (mobile container)	T59.891-	T59.892-	T59.893-	T59.894-	-	-
piped (natural)	T59.891-	T59.892-	T59.893-	T59.894-	-	-
Hydrochloric acid (liquid)	T54.2X1-	T54.2X2-	T54.2X3-	T54.2X4-	-	-
medicinal (digestant)	T47.5X1-	T47.5X2-	T47.5X3-	T47.5X4-	T47.5X5-	T47.5X6-
vapor	T59.891-	T59.892-	T59.893-	T59.894-	-	-
Hydrochlorothiazide	T50.2X1-	T50.2X2-	T50.2X3-	T50.2X4-	T50.2X5-	T50.2X6-
Hydrocodone	T40.2X1-	T40.2X2-	T40.2X3-	T40.2X4-	T40.2X5-	T40.2X6-

Substance	Poisoning Accidental (unintentional)	Poisoning Intentional self-harm	Poisoning Assault	Poisoning Undetermined	Adverse effect	Underdosing
Hydrocortisone (derivatives)	T38.0X1-	T38.0X2-	T38.0X3-	T38.0X4-	T38.0X5-	T38.0X6-
aceponate	T49.0X1-	T49.0X2-	T49.0X3-	T49.0X4-	T49.0X5-	T49.0X6-
ENT agent	T49.6X1-	T49.6X2-	T49.6X3-	T49.6X4-	T49.6X5-	T49.6X6-
ophthalmic preparation	T49.5X1-	T49.5X2-	T49.5X3-	T49.5X4-	T49.5X5-	T49.5X6-
topical NEC	T49.0X1-	T49.0X2-	T49.0X3-	T49.0X4-	T49.0X5-	T49.0X6-
Hydrocortone	T38.0X1-	T38.0X2-	T38.0X3-	T38.0X4-	T38.0X5-	T38.0X6-
ENT agent	T49.6X1-	T49.6X2-	T49.6X3-	T49.6X4-	T49.6X5-	T49.6X6-
ophthalmic preparation	T49.5X1-	T49.5X2-	T49.5X3-	T49.5X4-	T49.5X5-	T49.5X6-
topical NEC	T49.0X1-	T49.0X2-	T49.0X3-	T49.0X4-	T49.0X5-	T49.0X6-
Hydrocyanic acid (liquid)	T57.3X1-	T57.3X2-	T57.3X3-	T57.3X4-	-	-
gas	T65.0X1-	T65.0X2-	T65.0X3-	T65.0X4-	-	-
Hydroflumethiazide	T50.2X1-	T50.2X2-	T50.2X3-	T50.2X4-	T50.2X5-	T50.2X6-
Hydrofluoric acid (liquid)	T54.2X1-	T54.2X2-	T54.2X3-	T54.2X4-	-	-
vapor	T59.891-	T59.892-	T59.893-	T59.894-	-	-
Hydrogen	T59.891-	T59.892-	T59.893-	T59.894-	-	-
arsenide	T57.0X1-	T57.0X2-	T57.0X3-	T57.0X4-	-	-
arseniureted	T57.0X1-	T57.0X2-	T57.0X3-	T57.0X4-	-	-
chloride	T57.8X1-	T57.8X2-	T57.8X3-	T57.8X4-	-	-
cyanide (salts)	T57.3X1-	T57.3X2-	T57.3X3-	T57.3X4-	-	-
gas	T57.3X1-	T57.3X2-	T57.3X3-	T57.3X4-	-	-
Fluoride	T59.5X1-	T59.5X2-	T59.5X3-	T59.5X4-	-	-
vapor	T59.5X1-	T59.5X2-	T59.5X3-	T59.5X4-	-	-
peroxide	T49.0X1-	T49.0X2-	T49.0X3-	T49.0X4-	T49.0X5-	T49.0X6-
phosphureted	T57.1X1-	T57.1X2-	T57.1X3-	T57.1X4-	-	-
sulfide	T59.6X1-	T59.6X2-	T59.6X3-	T59.6X4-	-	-
arseniureted	T57.0X1-	T57.0X2-	T57.0X3-	T57.0X4-	-	-
sulfureted	T59.6X1-	T59.6X2-	T59.6X3-	T59.6X4-	-	-
Hydromethylpyridine	T46.7X1-	T46.7X2-	T46.7X3-	T46.7X4-	T46.7X5-	T46.7X6-
Hydromorphinol	T40.2X1-	T40.2X2-	T40.2X3-	T40.2X4-	-	-
Hydromorphinone	T40.2X1-	T40.2X2-	T40.2X3-	T40.2X4-	T40.2X5-	T40.2X6-
Hydromorphone	T40.2X1-	T40.2X2-	T40.2X3-	T40.2X4-	T40.2X5-	T40.2X6-
Hydromox	T50.2X1-	T50.2X2-	T50.2X3-	T50.2X4-	T50.2X5-	T50.2X6-
Hydrophilic lotion	T49.3X1-	T49.3X2-	T49.3X3-	T49.3X4-	T49.3X5-	T49.3X6-
Hydroquinidine	T46.2X1-	T46.2X2-	T46.2X3-	T46.2X4-	T46.2X5-	T46.2X6-
Hydroquinone	T52.2X1-	T52.2X2-	T52.2X3-	T52.2X4-	-	-
vapor	T59.891-	T59.892-	T59.893-	T59.894-	-	-
Hydrosulfuric acid (gas)	T59.6X1-	T59.6X2-	T59.6X3-	T59.6X4-	-	-
Hydrotalcite	T47.1X1-	T47.1X2-	T47.1X3-	T47.1X4-	T47.1X5-	T47.1X6-
Hydrous wool fat	T49.3X1-	T49.3X2-	T49.3X3-	T49.3X4-	T49.3X5-	T49.3X6-
Hydroxide, caustic	T54.3X1-	T54.3X2-	T54.3X3-	T54.3X4-	-	-
Hydroxocobalamin	T45.8X1-	T45.8X2-	T45.8X3-	T45.8X4-	T45.8X5-	T45.8X6-
Hydroxyamphetamine	T49.5X1-	T49.5X2-	T49.5X3-	T49.5X4-	T49.5X5-	T49.5X6-
Hydroxycarbamide	T45.1X1-	T45.1X2-	T45.1X3-	T45.1X4-	T45.1X5-	T45.1X6-
Hydroxychloroquine	T37.8X1-	T37.8X2-	T37.8X3-	T37.8X4-	T37.8X5-	T37.8X6-
Hydroxydihydrocodeinone	T40.2X1-	T40.2X2-	T40.2X3-	T40.2X4-	T40.2X5-	T40.2X6-
Hydroxyestrone	T38.5X1-	T38.5X2-	T38.5X3-	T38.5X4-	T38.5X5-	T38.5X6-
Hydroxyethyl starch	T45.8X1-	T45.8X2-	T45.8X3-	T45.8X4-	T45.8X5-	T45.8X6-
Hydroxymethylpenta-none	T52.4X1-	T52.4X2-	T52.4X3-	T52.4X4-	-	-
Hydroxyphenamate	T43.591-	T43.592-	T43.593-	T43.594-	T43.595-	T43.596-
Hydroxyphenylbutazone	T39.2X1-	T39.2X2-	T39.2X3-	T39.2X4-	T39.2X5-	T39.2X6-
Hydroxyprogesterone	T38.5X1-	T38.5X2-	T38.5X3-	T38.5X4-	T38.5X5-	T38.5X6-
caproate	T38.5X1-	T38.5X2-	T38.5X3-	T38.5X4-	T38.5X5-	T38.5X6-
Hydroxyquinoline (derivatives) NEC	T37.8X1-	T37.8X2-	T37.8X3-	T37.8X4-	T37.8X5-	T37.8X6-
Hydroxystilbamidine	T37.3X1-	T37.3X2-	T37.3X3-	T37.3X4-	T37.3X5-	T37.3X6-
Hydroxytoluene (nonmedicinal)	T54.0X1-	T54.0X2-	T54.0X3-	T54.0X4-	-	-
medicinal	T49.0X1-	T49.0X2-	T49.0X3-	T49.0X4-	T49.0X5-	T49.0X6-
Hydroxyurea	T45.1X1-	T45.1X2-	T45.1X3-	T45.1X4-	T45.1X5-	T45.1X6-
Hydroxyzine	T43.591-	T43.592-	T43.593-	T43.594-	T43.595-	T43.596-

Substance	Poisoning Accidental (unintentional)	Poisoning Intentional self-harm	Poisoning Assault	Poisoning Undetermined	Adverse effect	Underdosing
Hyoscine	T44.3X1-	T44.3X2-	T44.3X3-	T44.3X4-	T44.3X5-	T44.3X6-
Hyoscyamine	T44.3X1-	T44.3X2-	T44.3X3-	T44.3X4-	T44.3X5-	T44.3X6-
Hyoscyamus	T44.3X1-	T44.3X2-	T44.3X3-	T44.3X4-	T44.3X5-	T44.3X6-
dry extract	T44.3X1-	T44.3X2-	T44.3X3-	T44.3X4-	T44.3X5-	T44.3X6-
Hypaque	T50.8X1-	T50.8X2-	T50.8X3-	T50.8X4-	T50.8X5-	T50.8X6-
Hypertussis	T50.Z11-	T50.Z12-	T50.Z13-	T50.Z14-	T50.Z15-	T50.Z16-
Hypnotic	T42.71X-	T42.72X-	T42.73X-	T42.74X-	T42.75X-	T42.76X-
anticonvulsant	T42.71X-	T42.72X-	T42.73X-	T42.74X-	T42.75X-	T42.76X-
specified NEC	T42.6X1-	T42.6X2-	T42.6X3-	T42.6X4-	T42.6X5-	T42.6X6-
Hypochlorite	T49.0X1-	T49.0X2-	T49.0X3-	T49.0X4-	T49.0X5-	T49.0X6-
Hypophysis, posterior	T38.891-	T38.892-	T38.893-	T38.894-	T38.895-	T38.896-
Hypotensive NEC	T46.5X1-	T46.5X2-	T46.5X3-	T46.5X4-	T46.5X5-	T46.5X6-
Hypromellose	T49.5X1-	T49.5X2-	T49.5X3-	T49.5X4-	T49.5X5-	T49.5X6-
Ibacitabine	T37.5X1-	T37.5X2-	T37.5X3-	T37.5X4-	T37.5X5-	T37.5X6-
Ibopamine	T44.991-	T44.992-	T44.993-	T44.994-	T44.995-	T44.996-
Ibufenac	T39.311-	T39.312-	T39.313-	T39.314-	T39.315-	T39.316-
Ibuprofen	T39.311-	T39.312-	T39.313-	T39.314-	T39.315-	T39.316-
Ibuproxam	T39.311-	T39.312-	T39.313-	T39.314-	T39.315-	T39.316-
Ibuterol	T48.6X1-	T48.6X2-	T48.6X3-	T48.6X4-	T48.6X5-	T48.6X6-
Ichthammol	T49.0X1-	T49.0X2-	T49.0X3-	T49.0X4-	T49.0X5-	T49.0X6-
Ichthyol	T49.4X1-	T49.4X2-	T49.4X3-	T49.4X4-	T49.4X5-	T49.4X6-
Idarubicin	T45.1X1-	T45.1X2-	T45.1X3-	T45.1X4-	T45.1X5-	T45.1X6-
Idrocilamide	T42.8X1-	T42.8X2-	T42.8X3-	T42.8X4-	T42.8X5-	T42.8X6-
Ifenprodil	T46.7X1-	T46.7X2-	T46.7X3-	T46.7X4-	T46.7X5-	T46.7X6-
Ifosfamide	T45.1X1-	T45.1X2-	T45.1X3-	T45.1X4-	T45.1X5-	T45.1X6-
Iletin	T38.3X1-	T38.3X2-	T38.3X3-	T38.3X4-	T38.3X5-	T38.3X6-
Ilex	T62.2X1-	T62.2X2-	T62.2X3-	T62.2X4-	-	-
Illuminating gas (after combustion)	T58.11X-	T58.12X-	T58.13X-	T58.14X-	-	-
prior to combustion	T59.891-	T59.892-	T59.893-	T59.894-	-	-
Ilopan	T45.2X1-	T45.2X2-	T45.2X3-	T45.2X4-	T45.2X5-	T45.2X6-
Iloprost	T46.7X1-	T46.7X2-	T46.7X3-	T46.7X4-	T46.7X5-	T46.7X6-
Ilotycin	T36.3X1-	T36.3X2-	T36.3X3-	T36.3X4-	T36.3X5-	T36.3X6-
ophthalmic preparation	T49.5X1-	T49.5X2-	T49.5X3-	T49.5X4-	T49.5X5-	T49.5X6-
topical NEC	T49.0X1-	T49.0X2-	T49.0X3-	T49.0X4-	T49.0X5-	T49.0X6-
Imidazole-4-carboxamide	T45.1X1-	T45.1X2-	T45.1X3-	T45.1X4-	T45.1X5-	T45.1X6-
Imipenem	T36.0X1-	T36.0X2-	T36.0X3-	T36.0X4-	T36.0X5-	T36.0X6-
Imipramine	T43.011-	T43.012-	T43.013-	T43.014-	T43.015-	T43.016-
Iminostilbene	T42.1X1-	T42.1X2-	T42.1X3-	T42.1X4-	T42.1X5-	T42.1X6-
Immu-G	T50.Z11-	T50.Z12-	T50.Z13-	T50.Z14-	T50.Z15-	T50.Z16-
Immuglobin	T50.Z11-	T50.Z12-	T50.Z13-	T50.Z14-	T50.Z15-	T50.Z16-
Immune						
globulin	T50.Z11-	T50.Z12-	T50.Z13-	T50.Z14-	T50.Z15-	T50.Z16-
serum globulin	T50.Z11-	T50.Z12-	T50.Z13-	T50.Z14-	T50.Z15-	T50.Z16-
Immunoglobin human (intravenous) (normal)	T50.Z11-	T50.Z12-	T50.Z13-	T50.Z14-	T50.Z15-	T50.Z16-
unmodified	T50.Z11-	T50.Z12-	T50.Z13-	T50.Z14-	T50.Z15-	T50.Z16-
Immunosuppressive drug	T45.1X1-	T45.1X2-	T45.1X3-	T45.1X4-	T45.1X5-	T45.1X6-
Immu-tetanus	T50.Z11-	T50.Z12-	T50.Z13-	T50.Z14-	T50.Z15-	T50.Z16-
Indalpine	T43.221-	T43.222-	T43.223-	T43.224-	T43.225-	T43.226-
Indanazoline	T48.5X1-	T48.5X2-	T48.5X3-	T48.5X4-	T48.5X5-	T48.5X6-
Indandione (derivatives)	T45.511-	T45.512-	T45.513-	T45.514-	T45.515-	T45.516-
Indapamide	T46.5X1-	T46.5X2-	T46.5X3-	T46.5X4-	T46.5X5-	T46.5X6-
Indendione (derivatives)	T45.511-	T45.512-	T45.513-	T45.514-	T45.515-	T45.516-
Indenolol	T44.7X1-	T44.7X2-	T44.7X3-	T44.7X4-	T44.7X5-	T44.7X6-
Inderal	T44.7X1-	T44.7X2-	T44.7X3-	T44.7X4-	T44.7X5-	T44.7X6-
Indian						
hemp	T40.711-	T40.712-	T40.713-	T40.714-	T40.715-	T40.716-
tobacco	T62.2X1-	T62.2X2-	T62.2X3-	T62.2X4-	-	-

Substance	Poisoning Accidental (unintentional)	Poisoning Intentional self-harm	Poisoning Assault	Poisoning Undetermined	Adverse effect	Underdosing
Indigo carmine	T50.8X1-	T50.8X2-	T50.8X3-	T50.8X4-	T50.8X5-	T50.8X6-
Indobufen	T45.521-	T45.522-	T45.523-	T45.524-	T45.525-	T45.526-
Indocin	T39.2X1-	T39.2X2-	T39.2X3-	T39.2X4-	T39.2X5-	T39.2X6-
Indocyanine green	T50.8X1-	T50.8X2-	T50.8X3-	T50.8X4-	T50.8X5-	T50.8X6-
Indometacin	T39.391-	T39.392-	T39.393-	T39.394-	T39.395-	T39.396-
Indomethacin	T39.391-	T39.392-	T39.393-	T39.394-	T39.395-	T39.396-
farnesil	T39.4X1-	T39.4X2-	T39.4X3-	T39.4X4-	T39.4X5-	T39.4X6-
Indoramin	T44.6X1-	T44.6X2-	T44.6X3-	T44.6X4-	T44.6X5-	T44.6X6-
Industrial						
alcohol	T51.0X1-	T51.0X2-	T51.0X3-	T51.0X4-	-	-
fumes	T59.891-	T59.892-	T59.893-	T59.894-	-	-
solvents (fumes) (vapors)	T52.91X-	T52.92X-	T52.93X-	T52.94X-	-	-
Influenza vaccine	T50.B91-	T50.B92-	T50.B93-	T50.B94-	T50.B95-	T50.B96-
Ingested substance NEC	T65.91X-	T65.92X-	T65.93X-	T65.94X-	-	-
INH	T37.1X1-	T37.1X2-	T37.1X3-	T37.1X4-	T37.1X5-	T37.1X6-
Inhalation, gas (noxious) — *see Gas*						
Inhibitor						
angiotensin-converting enzyme	T46.4X1-	T46.4X2-	T46.4X3-	T46.4X4-	T46.4X5-	T46.4X6-
carbonic anhydrase	T50.2X1-	T50.2X2-	T50.2X3-	T50.2X4-	T50.2X5-	T50.2X6-
fibrinolysis	T45.621-	T45.622-	T45.623-	T45.624-	T45.625-	T45.626-
monoamine oxidase NEC	T43.1X1-	T43.1X2-	T43.1X3-	T43.1X4-	T43.1X5-	T43.1X6-
hydrazine	T43.1X1-	T43.1X2-	T43.1X3-	T43.1X4-	T43.1X5-	T43.1X6-
postsynaptic	T43.8X1-	T43.8X2-	T43.8X3-	T43.8X4-	T43.8X5-	T43.8X6-
prothrombin synthesis	T45.511-	T45.512-	T45.513-	T45.514-	T45.515-	T45.516-
Ink	T65.891-	T65.892-	T65.893-	T65.894-	-	-
Inorganic substance NEC	T57.91X-	T57.92X-	T57.93X-	T57.94X-	-	-
Inosine pranobex	T37.5X1-	T37.5X2-	T37.5X3-	T37.5X4-	T37.5X5-	T37.5X6-
Inositol	T50.991-	T50.992-	T50.993-	T50.994-	T50.995-	T50.996-
nicotinate	T46.7X1-	T46.7X2-	T46.7X3-	T46.7X4-	T46.7X5-	T46.7X6-
Inproquone	T45.1X1-	T45.1X2-	T45.1X3-	T45.1X4-	T45.1X5-	T45.1X6-
Insect (sting) , venomous	T63.481-	T63.482-	T63.483-	T63.484-	-	-
ant	T63.421-	T63.422-	T63.423-	T63.424-	-	-
bee	T63.441-	T63.442-	T63.443-	T63.444-	-	-
caterpillar	T63.431-	T63.432-	T63.433-	T63.434-	-	-
hornet	T63.451-	T63.452-	T63.453-	T63.454-	-	-
wasp	T63.461-	T63.462-	T63.463-	T63.464-	-	-
Insecticide NEC	T60.91X-	T60.92X-	T60.93X-	T60.94X-	-	-
carbamate	T60.0X1-	T60.0X2-	T60.0X3-	T60.0X4-	-	-
chlorinated	T60.1X1-	T60.1X2-	T60.1X3-	T60.1X4-	-	-
mixed	T60.91X-	T60.92X-	T60.93X-	T60.94X-	-	-
organochlorine	T60.1X1-	T60.1X2-	T60.1X3-	T60.1X4-	-	-
organophosphorus	T60.0X1-	T60.0X2-	T60.0X3-	T60.0X4-	-	-
Insular tissue extract	T38.3X1-	T38.3X2-	T38.3X3-	T38.3X4-	T38.3X5-	T38.3X6-
Insulin (amorphous) (globin) (isophane) (Lente) (NPH) (Semilente) (Ultralente)	T38.3X1-	T38.3X2-	T38.3X3-	T38.3X4-	T38.3X5-	T38.3X6-
defalan	T38.3X1-	T38.3X2-	T38.3X3-	T38.3X4-	T38.3X5-	T38.3X6-
human	T38.3X1-	T38.3X2-	T38.3X3-	T38.3X4-	T38.3X5-	T38.3X6-
injection, soluble	T38.3X1-	T38.3X2-	T38.3X3-	T38.3X4-	T38.3X5-	T38.3X6-
biphasic	T38.3X1-	T38.3X2-	T38.3X3-	T38.3X4-	T38.3X5-	T38.3X6-
intermediate acting	T38.3X1-	T38.3X2-	T38.3X3-	T38.3X4-	T38.3X5-	T38.3X6-
protamine zinc	T38.3X1-	T38.3X2-	T38.3X3-	T38.3X4-	T38.3X5-	T38.3X6-
slow acting	T38.3X1-	T38.3X2-	T38.3X3-	T38.3X4-	T38.3X5-	T38.3X6-
zinc						
protamine injection	T38.3X1-	T38.3X2-	T38.3X3-	T38.3X4-	T38.3X5-	T38.3X6-
suspension (amorphous) (crystalline)	T38.3X1-	T38.3X2-	T38.3X3-	T38.3X4-	T38.3X5-	T38.3X6-
Interferon (alpha) (beta) (gamma)	T37.5X1-	T37.5X2-	T37.5X3-	T37.5X4-	T37.5X5-	T37.5X6-

Substance	Poisoning Accidental (unintentional)	Poisoning Intentional self-harm	Poisoning Assault	Poisoning Undetermined	Adverse effect	Underdosing
Intestinal motility control drug	T47.6X1-	T47.6X2-	T47.6X3-	T47.6X4-	T47.6X5-	T47.6X6-
biological	T47.8X1-	T47.8X2-	T47.8X3-	T47.8X4-	T47.8X5-	T47.8X6-
Intranarcon	T41.1X1-	T41.1X2-	T41.1X3-	T41.1X4-	T41.1X5-	T41.1X6-
Intravenous						
amino acids	T50.991-	T50.992-	T50.993-	T50.994-	T50.995-	T50.996-
fat suspension	T50.991-	T50.992-	T50.993-	T50.994-	T50.995-	T50.996-
Inulin	T50.8X1-	T50.8X2-	T50.8X3-	T50.8X4-	T50.8X5-	T50.8X6-
Invert sugar	T50.3X1-	T50.3X2-	T50.3X3-	T50.3X4-	T50.3X5-	T50.3X6-
Inza — *see Naproxen*						
Iobenzamic acid	T50.8X1-	T50.8X2-	T50.8X3-	T50.8X4-	T50.8X5-	T50.8X6-
Iocarmic acid	T50.8X1-	T50.8X2-	T50.8X3-	T50.8X4-	T50.8X5-	T50.8X6-
Iocetamic acid	T50.8X1-	T50.8X2-	T50.8X3-	T50.8X4-	T50.8X5-	T50.8X6-
Iodamide	T50.8X1-	T50.8X2-	T50.8X3-	T50.8X4-	T50.8X5-	T50.8X6-
Iodide NEC — *see also Iodine*	T49.0X1-	T49.0X2-	T49.0X3-	T49.0X4-	T49.0X5-	T49.0X6-
mercury (ointment)	T49.0X1-	T49.0X2-	T49.0X3-	T49.0X4-	T49.0X5-	T49.0X6-
methylate	T49.0X1-	T49.0X2-	T49.0X3-	T49.0X4-	T49.0X5-	T49.0X6-
potassium (expectorant) NEC	T48.4X1-	T48.4X2-	T48.4X3-	T48.4X4-	T48.4X5-	T48.4X6-
Iodinated						
contrast medium	T50.8X1-	T50.8X2-	T50.8X3-	T50.8X4-	T50.8X5-	T50.8X6-
glycerol	T48.4X1-	T48.4X2-	T48.4X3-	T48.4X4-	T48.4X5-	T48.4X6-
human serum albumin (131I)	T50.8X1-	T50.8X2-	T50.8X3-	T50.8X4-	T50.8X5-	T50.8X6-
Iodine (antiseptic, external) (tincture) NEC	T49.0X1-	T49.0X2-	T49.0X3-	T49.0X4-	T49.0X5-	T49.0X6-
125 — *see also Radiation sickness, and Exposure to radioactivce isotopes*	T50.8X1-	T50.8X2-	T50.8X3-	T50.8X4-	T50.8X5-	T50.8X6-
therapeutic	T50.991-	T50.992-	T50.993-	T50.994-	T50.995-	T50.996-
131 — *see also Radiation sickness, and Exposure to radioactivce isotopes*	T50.8X1-	T50.8X2-	T50.8X3-	T50.8X4-	T50.8X5-	T50.8X6-
therapeutic	T38.2X1-	T38.2X2-	T38.2X3-	T38.2X4-	T38.2X5-	T38.2X6-
diagnostic	T50.8X1-	T50.8X2-	T50.8X3-	T50.8X4-	T50.8X5-	T50.8X6-
for thyroid conditions (antithyroid)	T38.2X1-	T38.2X2-	T38.2X3-	T38.2X4-	T38.2X5-	T38.2X6-
solution	T49.0X1-	T49.0X2-	T49.0X3-	T49.0X4-	T49.0X5-	T49.0X6-
vapor	T59.891-	T59.892-	T59.893-	T59.894-	-	-
Iodipamide	T50.8X1-	T50.8X2-	T50.8X3-	T50.8X4-	T50.8X5-	T50.8X6-
Iodized (poppy seed) oil	T50.8X1-	T50.8X2-	T50.8X3-	T50.8X4-	T50.8X5-	T50.8X6-
Iodobismitol	T37.8X1-	T37.8X2-	T37.8X3-	T37.8X4-	T37.8X5-	T37.8X6-
Iodochlorhydroxyquin	T37.8X1-	T37.8X2-	T37.8X3-	T37.8X4-	T37.8X5-	T37.8X6-
topical	T49.0X1-	T49.0X2-	T49.0X3-	T49.0X4-	T49.0X5-	T49.0X6-
Iodochlorhydroxyquinoline	T37.8X1-	T37.8X2-	T37.8X3-	T37.8X4-	T37.8X5-	T37.8X6-
Iodocholesterol (131I)	T50.8X1-	T50.8X2-	T50.8X3-	T50.8X4-	T50.8X5-	T50.8X6-
Iodoform	T49.0X1-	T49.0X2-	T49.0X3-	T49.0X4-	T49.0X5-	T49.0X6-
Iodohippuric acid	T50.8X1-	T50.8X2-	T50.8X3-	T50.8X4-	T50.8X5-	T50.8X6-
Iodopanoic acid	T50.8X1-	T50.8X2-	T50.8X3-	T50.8X4-	T50.8X5-	T50.8X6-
Iodophthalein (sodium)	T50.8X1-	T50.8X2-	T50.8X3-	T50.8X4-	T50.8X5-	T50.8X6-
Iodopyracet	T50.8X1-	T50.8X2-	T50.8X3-	T50.8X4-	T50.8X5-	T50.8X6-
Iodoquinol	T37.8X1-	T37.8X2-	T37.8X3-	T37.8X4-	T37.8X5-	T37.8X6-
Iodoxamic acid	T50.8X1-	T50.8X2-	T50.8X3-	T50.8X4-	T50.8X5-	T50.8X6-
Iofendylate	T50.8X1-	T50.8X2-	T50.8X3-	T50.8X4-	T50.8X5-	T50.8X6-
Ioglycamic acid	T50.8X1-	T50.8X2-	T50.8X3-	T50.8X4-	T50.8X5-	T50.8X6-
Iohexol	T50.8X1-	T50.8X2-	T50.8X3-	T50.8X4-	T50.8X5-	T50.8X6-
Ion exchange resin						
anion	T47.8X1-	T47.8X2-	T47.8X3-	T47.8X4-	T47.8X5-	T47.8X6-
cation	T50.3X1-	T50.3X2-	T50.3X3-	T50.3X4-	T50.3X5-	T50.3X6-
cholestyramine	T46.6X1-	T46.6X2-	T46.6X3-	T46.6X4-	T46.6X5-	T46.6X6-
intestinal	T47.8X1-	T47.8X2-	T47.8X3-	T47.8X4-	T47.8X5-	T47.8X6-
Iopamidol	T50.8X1-	T50.8X2-	T50.8X3-	T50.8X4-	T50.8X5-	T50.8X6-
Iopanoic acid	T50.8X1-	T50.8X2-	T50.8X3-	T50.8X4-	T50.8X5-	T50.8X6-
Iophenoic acid	T50.8X1-	T50.8X2-	T50.8X3-	T50.8X4-	T50.8X5-	T50.8X6-
Iopodate, sodium	T50.8X1-	T50.8X2-	T50.8X3-	T50.8X4-	T50.8X5-	T50.8X6-

Substance	Poisoning Accidental (unintentional)	Poisoning Intentional self-harm	Poisoning Assault	Poisoning Undetermined	Adverse effect	Underdosing
Iopodic acid	T50.8X1-	T50.8X2-	T50.8X3-	T50.8X4-	T50.8X5-	T50.8X6-
Iopromide	T50.8X1-	T50.8X2-	T50.8X3-	T50.8X4-	T50.8X5-	T50.8X6-
Iopydol	T50.8X1-	T50.8X2-	T50.8X3-	T50.8X4-	T50.8X5-	T50.8X6-
Iotalamic acid	T50.8X1-	T50.8X2-	T50.8X3-	T50.8X4-	T50.8X5-	T50.8X6-
Iothalamate	T50.8X1-	T50.8X2-	T50.8X3-	T50.8X4-	T50.8X5-	T50.8X6-
Iothiouracil	T38.2X1-	T38.2X2-	T38.2X3-	T38.2X4-	T38.2X5-	T38.2X6-
Iotrol	T50.8X1-	T50.8X2-	T50.8X3-	T50.8X4-	T50.8X5-	T50.8X6-
Iotrolan	T50.8X1-	T50.8X2-	T50.8X3-	T50.8X4-	T50.8X5-	T50.8X6-
Iotroxate	T50.8X1-	T50.8X2-	T50.8X3-	T50.8X4-	T50.8X5-	T50.8X6-
Iotroxic acid	T50.8X1-	T50.8X2-	T50.8X3-	T50.8X4-	T50.8X5-	T50.8X6-
Ioversol	T50.8X1-	T50.8X2-	T50.8X3-	T50.8X4-	T50.8X5-	T50.8X6-
Ioxaglate	T50.8X1-	T50.8X2-	T50.8X3-	T50.8X4-	T50.8X5-	T50.8X6-
Ioxaglic acid	T50.8X1-	T50.8X2-	T50.8X3-	T50.8X4-	T50.8X5-	T50.8X6-
Ioxitalamic acid	T50.8X1-	T50.8X2-	T50.8X3-	T50.8X4-	T50.8X5-	T50.8X6-
Ipecac	T47.7X1-	T47.7X2-	T47.7X3-	T47.7X4-	T47.7X5-	T47.7X6-
Ipecacuanha	T48.4X1-	T48.4X2-	T48.4X3-	T48.4X4-	T48.4X5-	T48.4X6-
Ipodate, calcium	T50.8X1-	T50.8X2-	T50.8X3-	T50.8X4-	T50.8X5-	T50.8X6-
Ipral	T42.3X1-	T42.3X2-	T42.3X3-	T42.3X4-	T42.3X5-	T42.3X6-
Ipratropium (bromide)	T48.6X1-	T48.6X2-	T48.6X3-	T48.6X4-	T48.6X5-	T48.6X6-
Ipriflavone	T46.3X1-	T46.3X2-	T46.3X3-	T46.3X4-	T46.3X5-	T46.3X6-
Iprindole	T43.011-	T43.012-	T43.013-	T43.014-	T43.015-	T43.016-
Iproclozide	T43.1X1-	T43.1X2-	T43.1X3-	T43.1X4-	T43.1X5-	T43.1X6-
Iprofenin	T50.8X1-	T50.8X2-	T50.8X3-	T50.8X4-	T50.8X5-	T50.8X6-
Iproheptine	T49.2X1-	T49.2X2-	T49.2X3-	T49.2X4-	T49.2X5-	T49.2X6-
Iproniazid	T43.1X1-	T43.1X2-	T43.1X3-	T43.1X4-	T43.1X5-	T43.1X6-
Iproplatin	T45.1X1-	T45.1X2-	T45.1X3-	T45.1X4-	T45.1X5-	T45.1X6-
Iproveratril	T46.1X1-	T46.1X2-	T46.1X3-	T46.1X4-	T46.1X5-	T46.1X6-
Iron (compounds) (medicinal) NEC	T45.4X1-	T45.4X2-	T45.4X3-	T45.4X4-	T45.4X5-	T45.4X6-
ammonium	T45.4X1-	T45.4X2-	T45.4X3-	T45.4X4-	T45.4X5-	T45.4X6-
dextran injection	T45.4X1-	T45.4X2-	T45.4X3-	T45.4X4-	T45.4X5-	T45.4X6-
nonmedicinal	T56.891-	T56.892-	T56.893-	T56.894-	-	-
salts	T45.4X1-	T45.4X2-	T45.4X3-	T45.4X4-	T45.4X5-	T45.4X6-
sorbitex	T45.4X1-	T45.4X2-	T45.4X3-	T45.4X4-	T45.4X5-	T45.4X6-
sorbitol citric acid complex	T45.4X1-	T45.4X2-	T45.4X3-	T45.4X4-	T45.4X5-	T45.4X6-
Irrigating fluid (vaginal)	T49.8X1-	T49.8X2-	T49.8X3-	T49.8X4-	T49.8X5-	T49.8X6-
eye	T49.5X1-	T49.5X2-	T49.5X3-	T49.5X4-	T49.5X5-	T49.5X6-
Isepamicin	T36.5X1-	T36.5X2-	T36.5X3-	T36.5X4-	T36.5X5-	T36.5X6-
Isoaminile (citrate)	T48.3X1-	T48.3X2-	T48.3X3-	T48.3X4-	T48.3X5-	T48.3X6-
Isoamyl nitrite	T46.3X1-	T46.3X2-	T46.3X3-	T46.3X4-	T46.3X5-	T46.3X6-
Isobenzan	T60.1X1-	T60.1X2-	T60.1X3-	T60.1X4-	-	-
Isobutyl acetate	T52.8X1-	T52.8X2-	T52.8X3-	T52.8X4-	-	-
Isocarboxazid	T43.1X1-	T43.1X2-	T43.1X3-	T43.1X4-	T43.1X5-	T43.1X6-
Isoconazole	T49.0X1-	T49.0X2-	T49.0X3-	T49.0X4-	T49.0X5-	T49.0X6-
Isocyanate	T65.0X1-	T65.0X2-	T65.0X3-	T65.0X4-	-	-
Isoephedrine	T44.991-	T44.992-	T44.993-	T44.994-	T44.995-	T44.996-
Isoetarine	T48.6X1-	T48.6X2-	T48.6X3-	T48.6X4-	T48.6X5-	T48.6X6-
Isoethadione	T42.2X1-	T42.2X2-	T42.2X3-	T42.2X4-	T42.2X5-	T42.2X6-
Isoetharine	T44.5X1-	T44.5X2-	T44.5X3-	T44.5X4-	T44.5X5-	T44.5X6-
Isoflurane	T41.0X1-	T41.0X2-	T41.0X3-	T41.0X4-	T41.0X5-	T41.0X6-
Isoflurophate	T44.0X1-	T44.0X2-	T44.0X3-	T44.0X4-	T44.0X5-	T44.0X6-
Isomaltose, ferric complex	T45.4X1-	T45.4X2-	T45.4X3-	T45.4X4-	T45.4X5-	T45.4X6-
Isometheptene	T44.3X1-	T44.3X2-	T44.3X3-	T44.3X4-	T44.3X5-	T44.3X6-
Isoniazid	T37.1X1-	T37.1X2-	T37.1X3-	T37.1X4-	T37.1X5-	T37.1X6-
with						
rifampicin	T36.6X1-	T36.6X2-	T36.6X3-	T36.6X4-	T36.6X5-	T36.6X6-
thioacetazone	T37.1X1-	T37.1X2-	T37.1X3-	T37.1X4-	T37.1X5-	T37.1X6-
Isonicotinic acid hydrazide	T37.1X1-	T37.1X2-	T37.1X3-	T37.1X4-	T37.1X5-	T37.1X6-
Isonipecaine	T40.491-	T40.492-	T40.493-	T40.494-	T40.495-	T40.496-
Isopentaquine	T37.2X1-	T37.2X2-	T37.2X3-	T37.2X4-	T37.2X5-	T37.2X6-

Substance	Poisoning Accidental (unintentional)	Poisoning Intentional self-harm	Poisoning Assault	Poisoning Undetermined	Adverse effect	Underdosing
Isophane insulin	T38.3X1-	T38.3X2-	T38.3X3-	T38.3X4-	T38.3X5-	T38.3X6-
Isophorone	T65.891-	T65.892-	T65.893-	T65.894-	-	-
Isophosphamide	T45.1X1-	T45.1X2-	T45.1X3-	T45.1X4-	T45.1X5-	T45.1X6-
Isopregnenone	T38.5X1-	T38.5X2-	T38.5X3-	T38.5X4-	T38.5X5-	T38.5X6-
Isoprenaline	T48.6X1-	T48.6X2-	T48.6X3-	T48.6X4-	T48.6X5-	T48.6X6-
Isopromethazine	T43.3X1-	T43.3X2-	T43.3X3-	T43.3X4-	T43.3X5-	T43.3X6-
Isopropamide	T44.3X1-	T44.3X2-	T44.3X3-	T44.3X4-	T44.3X5-	T44.3X6-
iodide	T44.3X1-	T44.3X2-	T44.3X3-	T44.3X4-	T44.3X5-	T44.3X6-
Isopropanol	T51.2X1-	T51.2X2-	T51.2X3-	T51.2X4-	-	-
Isopropyl						
acetate	T52.8X1-	T52.8X2-	T52.8X3-	T52.8X4-	-	-
alcohol	T51.2X1-	T51.2X2-	T51.2X3-	T51.2X4-	-	-
medicinal	T49.4X1-	T49.4X2-	T49.4X3-	T49.4X4-	T49.4X5-	T49.4X6-
ether	T52.8X1-	T52.8X2-	T52.8X3-	T52.8X4-	-	-
Isopropylaminophenazone	T39.2X1-	T39.2X2-	T39.2X3-	T39.2X4-	T39.2X5-	T39.2X6-
Isoproterenol	T48.6X1-	T48.6X2-	T48.6X3-	T48.6X4-	T48.6X5-	T48.6X6-
Isosorbide dinitrate	T46.3X1-	T46.3X2-	T46.3X3-	T46.3X4-	T46.3X5-	T46.3X6-
Isothipendyl	T45.0X1-	T45.0X2-	T45.0X3-	T45.0X4-	T45.0X5-	T45.0X6-
Isotretinoin	T50.991-	T50.992-	T50.993-	T50.994-	T50.995-	T50.996-
Isoxazolyl penicillin	T36.0X1-	T36.0X2-	T36.0X3-	T36.0X4-	T36.0X5-	T36.0X6-
Isoxicam	T39.391-	T39.392-	T39.393-	T39.394-	T39.395-	T39.396-
Isoxsuprine	T46.7X1-	T46.7X2-	T46.7X3-	T46.7X4-	T46.7X5-	T46.7X6-
Ispagula	T47.4X1-	T47.4X2-	T47.4X3-	T47.4X4-	T47.4X5-	T47.4X6-
husk	T47.4X1-	T47.4X2-	T47.4X3-	T47.4X4-	T47.4X5-	T47.4X6-
Isradipine	T46.1X1-	T46.1X2-	T46.1X3-	T46.1X4-	T46.1X5-	T46.1X6-
I-thyroxine sodium	T38.1X1-	T38.1X2-	T38.1X3-	T38.1X4-	T38.1X5-	T38.1X6-
Itraconazole	T37.8X1-	T37.8X2-	T37.8X3-	T37.8X4-	T37.8X5-	T37.8X6-
Itramin tosilate	T46.3X1-	T46.3X2-	T46.3X3-	T46.3X4-	T46.3X5-	T46.3X6-
Ivermectin	T37.4X1-	T37.4X2-	T37.4X3-	T37.4X4-	T37.4X5-	T37.4X6-
Izoniazid	T37.1X1-	T37.1X2-	T37.1X3-	T37.1X4-	T37.1X5-	T37.1X6-
with thioacetazone	T37.1X1-	T37.1X2-	T37.1X3-	T37.1X4-	T37.1X5-	T37.1X6-
Jalap	T47.2X1-	T47.2X2-	T47.2X3-	T47.2X4-	T47.2X5-	T47.2X6-
Jamaica						
dogwood (bark)	T39.8X1-	T39.8X2-	T39.8X3-	T39.8X4-	T39.8X5-	T39.8X6-
ginger	T65.891-	T65:892-	T65.893-	T65.894-	-	-
root	T62.2X1-	T62.2X2-	T62.2X3-	T62.2X4-	-	-
Jatropha	T62.2X1-	T62.2X2-	T62.2X3-	T62.2X4-	-	-
curcas	T62.2X1-	T62.2X2-	T62.2X3-	T62.2X4-	-	-
Jectofer	T45.4X1-	T45.4X2-	T45.4X3-	T45.4X4-	T45.4X5-	T45.4X6-
Jellyfish (sting)	T63.621-	T63.622-	T63.623-	T63.624-	-	-
Jequirity (bean)	T62.2X1-	T62.2X2-	T62.2X3-	T62.2X4-	-	-
Jimson weed (stramonium)	T62.2X1-	T62.2X2-	T62.2X3-	T62.2X4-	-	-
seeds	T62.2X1-	T62.2X2-	T62.2X3-	T62.2X4-	-	-
Josamycin	T36.3X1-	T36.3X2-	T36.3X3-	T36.3X4-	T36.3X5-	T36.3X6-
Juniper tar	T49.1X1-	T49.1X2-	T49.1X3-	T49.1X4-	T49.1X5-	T49.1X6-
Kallidinogenase	T46.7X1-	T46.7X2-	T46.7X3-	T46.7X4-	T46.7X5-	T46.7X6-
Kallikrein	T46.7X1-	T46.7X2-	T46.7X3-	T46.7X4-	T46.7X5-	T46.7X6-
Kanamycin	T36.5X1-	T36.5X2-	T36.5X3-	T36.5X4-	T36.5X5-	T36.5X6-
Kantrex	T36.5X1-	T36.5X2-	T36.5X3-	T36.5X4-	T36.5X5-	T36.5X6-
Kaolin	T47.6X1-	T47.6X2-	T47.6X3-	T47.6X4-	T47.6X5-	T47.6X6-
light	T47.6X1-	T47.6X2-	T47.6X3-	T47.6X4-	T47.6X5-	T47.6X6-
Karaya (gum)	T47.4X1-	T47.4X2-	T47.4X3-	T47.4X4-	T47.4X5-	T47.4X6-
Kebuzone	T39.2X1-	T39.2X2-	T39.2X3-	T39.2X4-	T39.2X5-	T39.2X6-
Kelevan	T60.1X1-	T60.1X2-	T60.1X3-	T60.1X4-	-	-
Kemithal	T41.1X1-	T41.1X2-	T41.1X3-	T41.1X4-	T41.1X5-	T41.1X6-
Kenacort	T38.0X1-	T38.0X2-	T38.0X3-	T38.0X4-	T38.0X5-	T38.0X6-

Substance	Poisoning Accidental (unintentional)	Poisoning Intentional self-harm	Poisoning Assault	Poisoning Undetermined	Adverse effect	Underdosing
Keratolytic drug NEC	T49.4X1-	T49.4X2-	T49.4X3-	T49.4X4-	T49.4X5-	T49.4X6-
anthracene	T49.4X1-	T49.4X2-	T49.4X3-	T49.4X4-	T49.4X5-	T49.4X6-
Keratoplastic NEC	T49.4X1-	T49.4X2-	T49.4X3-	T49.4X4-	T49.4X5-	T49.4X6-
Kerosene, kerosine (fuel) (solvent) NEC	T52.0X1-	T52.0X2-	T52.0X3-	T52.0X4-	-	-
insecticide	T52.0X1-	T52.0X2-	T52.0X3-	T52.0X4-	-	-
vapor	T52.0X1-	T52.0X2-	T52.0X3-	T52.0X4-	-	-
Ketamine	T41.291-	T41.292-	T41.293-	T41.294-	T41.295-	T41.296-
Ketazolam	T42.4X1-	T42.4X2-	T42.4X3-	T42.4X4-	T42.4X5-	T42.4X6-
Ketazon	T39.2X1-	T39.2X2-	T39.2X3-	T39.2X4-	T39.2X5-	T39.2X6-
Ketobemidone	T40.491-	T40.492-	T40.493-	T40.494-	-	-
Ketoconazole	T49.0X1-	T49.0X2-	T49.0X3-	T49.0X4-	T49.0X5-	T49.0X6-
Ketols	T52.4X1-	T52.4X2-	T52.4X3-	T52.4X4-	-	-
Ketone oils	T52.4X1-	T52.4X2-	T52.4X3-	T52.4X4-	-	-
Ketoprofen	T39.311-	T39.312-	T39.313-	T39.314-	T39.315-	T39.316-
Ketorolac	T39.8X1-	T39.8X2-	T39.8X3-	T39.8X4-	T39.8X5-	T39.8X6-
Ketotifen	T45.0X1-	T45.0X2-	T45.0X3-	T45.0X4-	T45.0X5-	T45.0X6-
Khat	T43.691-	T43.692-	T43.693-	T43.694-	-	-
Khellin	T46.3X1-	T46.3X2-	T46.3X3-	T46.3X4-	T46.3X5-	T46.3X6-
Khelloside	T46.3X1-	T46.3X2-	T46.3X3-	T46.3X4-	T46.3X5-	T46.3X6-
Kiln gas or vapor (carbon monoxide)	T58.8X1-	T58.8X2-	T58.8X3-	T58.8X4-	-	-
Kitasamycin	T36.3X1-	T36.3X2-	T36.3X3-	T36.3X4-	T36.3X5-	T36.3X6-
Konsyl	T47.4X1-	T47.4X2-	T47.4X3-	T47.4X4-	T47.4X5-	T47.4X6-
Kosam seed	T62.2X1-	T62.2X2-	T62.2X3-	T62.2X4-	-	-
Krait (venom)	T63.091-	T63.092-	T63.093-	T63.094-	-	-
Kwell (insecticide)	T60.1X1-	T60.1X2-	T60.1X3-	T60.1X4-	-	-
anti-infective (topical)	T49.0X1-	T49.0X2-	T49.0X3-	T49.0X4-	T49.0X5-	T49.0X6-
Labetalol	T44.8X1-	T44.8X2-	T44.8X3-	T44.8X4-	T44.8X5-	T44.8X6-
Laburnum (seeds)	T62.2X1-	T62.2X2-	T62.2X3-	T62.2X4-	-	-
leaves	T62.2X1-	T62.2X2-	T62.2X3-	T62.2X4-	-	-
Lachesine	T49.5X1-	T49.5X2-	T49.5X3-	T49.5X4-	T49.5X5-	T49.5X6-
Lacidipine	T46.5X1-	T46.5X2-	T46.5X3-	T46.5X4-	T46.5X5-	T46.5X6-
Lacquer	T65.6X1-	T65.6X2-	T65.6X3-	T65.6X4-	-	-
Lacrimogenic gas	T59.3X1-	T59.3X2-	T59.3X3-	T59.3X4-	-	-
Lactated potassic saline	T50.3X1-	T50.3X2-	T50.3X3-	T50.3X4-	T50.3X5-	T50.3X6-
Lactic acid	T49.8X1-	T49.8X2-	T49.8X3-	T49.8X4-	T49.8X5-	T49.8X6-
Lactobacillus						
acidophilus	T47.6X1-	T47.6X2-	T47.6X3-	T47.6X4-	T47.6X5-	T47.6X6-
compound	T47.6X1-	T47.6X2-	T47.6X3-	T47.6X4-	T47.6X5-	T47.6X6-
bifidus, lyophilized	T47.6X1-	T47.6X2-	T47.6X3-	T47.6X4-	T47.6X5-	T47.6X6-
bulgaricus	T47.6X1-	T47.6X2-	T47.6X3-	T47.6X4-	T47.6X5-	T47.6X6-
sporogenes	T47.6X1-	T47.6X2-	T47.6X3-	T47.6X4-	T47.6X5-	T47.6X6-
Lactoflavin	T45.2X1-	T45.2X2-	T45.2X3-	T45.2X4-	T45.2X5-	T45.2X6-
Lactose (as excipient)	T50.901-	T50.902-	T50.903-	T50.904-	T50.905-	T50.906-
Lactuca (virosa) (extract)	T42.6X1-	T42.6X2-	T42.6X3-	T42.6X4-	T42.6X5-	T42.6X6-
Lactucarium	T42.6X1-	T42.6X2-	T42.6X3-	T42.6X4-	T42.6X5-	T42.6X6-
Lactulose	T47.3X1-	T47.3X2-	T47.3X3-	T47.3X4-	T47.3X5-	T47.3X6-
Laevo — *see Levo-*						
Lanatosides	T46.0X1-	T46.0X2-	T46.0X3-	T46.0X4-	T46.0X5-	T46.0X6-
Lanolin	T49.3X1-	T49.3X2-	T49.3X3-	T49.3X4-	T49.3X5-	T49.3X6-
Largactil	T43.3X1-	T43.3X2-	T43.3X3-	T43.3X4-	T43.3X5-	T43.3X6-
Larkspur	T62.2X1-	T62.2X2-	T62.2X3-	T62.2X4-	-	-
Laroxyl	T43.011-	T43.012-	T43.013-	T43.014-	T43.015-	T43.016-
Lasix	T50.1X1-	T50.1X2-	T50.1X3-	T50.1X4-	T50.1X5-	T50.1X6-
Lassar's paste	T49.4X1-	T49.4X2-	T49.4X3-	T49.4X4-	T49.4X5-	T49.4X6-
Latamoxef	T36.1X1-	T36.1X2-	T36.1X3-	T36.1X4-	T36.1X5-	T36.1X6-
Latex	T65.811-	T65.812-	T65.813-	T65.814-	-	-
Lathyrus (seed)	T62.2X1-	T62.2X2-	T62.2X3-	T62.2X4-	-	-
Laudanum	T40.0X1-	T40.0X2-	T40.0X3-	T40.0X4-	T40.0X5-	T40.0X6-

KERATOLYTIC DRUG NEC - LAUDANUM

Substance	Poisoning Accidental (unintentional)	Poisoning Intentional self-harm	Poisoning Assault	Poisoning Undetermined	Adverse effect	Underdosing
Laudexium	T48.1X1-	T48.1X2-	T48.1X3-	T48.1X4-	T48.1X5-	T48.1X6-
Laughing gas	T41.0X1-	T41.0X2-	T41.0X3-	T41.0X4-	T41.0X5-	T41.0X6-
Laurel, black or cherry	T62.2X1-	T62.2X2-	T62.2X3-	T62.2X4-	-	-
Laurolinium	T49.0X1-	T49.0X2-	T49.0X3-	T49.0X4-	T49.0X5-	T49.0X6-
Lauryl sulfoacetate	T49.2X1-	T49.2X2-	T49.2X3-	T49.2X4-	T49.2X5-	T49.2X6-
Laxative NEC	T47.4X1-	T47.4X2-	T47.4X3-	T47.4X4-	T47.4X5-	T47.4X6-
osmotic	T47.3X1-	T47.3X2-	T47.3X3-	T47.3X4-	T47.3X5-	T47.3X6-
saline	T47.3X1-	T47.3X2-	T47.3X3-	T47.3X4-	T47.3X5-	T47.3X6-
stimulant	T47.2X1-	T47.2X2-	T47.2X3-	T47.2X4-	T47.2X5-	T47.2X6-
L-dopa	T42.8X1-	T42.8X2-	T42.8X3-	T42.8X4-	T42.8X5-	T42.8X6-
Lead (dust) (fumes) (vapor) NEC	T56.0X1-	T56.0X2-	T56.0X3-	T56.0X4-	-	-
acetate	T49.2X1-	T49.2X2-	T49.2X3-	T49.2X4-	T49.2X5-	T49.2X6-
alkyl (fuel additive)	T56.0X1-	T56.0X2-	T56.0X3-	T56.0X4-	-	-
anti-infectives	T37.8X1-	T37.8X2-	T37.8X3-	T37.8X4-	T37.8X5-	T37.8X6-
antiknock compound (tetraethyl)	T56.0X1-	T56.0X2-	T56.0X3-	T56.0X4-	-	-
arsenate, arsenite (dust) (herbicide) (insecticide) (vapor)	T57.0X1-	T57.0X2-	T57.0X3-	T57.0X4-	-	-
carbonate	T56.0X1-	T56.0X2-	T56.0X3-	T56.0X4-	-	-
paint	T56.0X1-	T56.0X2-	T56.0X3-	T56.0X4-	-	-
chromate	T56.0X1-	T56.0X2-	T56.0X3-	T56.0X4-	-	-
paint	T56.0X1-	T56.0X2-	T56.0X3-	T56.0X4-	-	-
dioxide	T56.0X1-	T56.0X2-	T56.0X3-	T56.0X4-	-	-
inorganic	T56.0X1-	T56.0X2-	T56.0X3-	T56.0X4-	-	-
iodide	T56.0X1-	T56.0X2-	T56.0X3-	T56.0X4-	-	-
pigment (paint)	T56.0X1-	T56.0X2-	T56.0X3-	T56.0X4-	-	-
monoxide (dust)	T56.0X1-	T56.0X2-	T56.0X3-	T56.0X4-	-	-
paint	T56.0X1-	T56.0X2-	T56.0X3-	T56.0X4-	-	-
organic	T56.0X1-	T56.0X2-	T56.0X3-	T56.0X4-	-	-
oxide	T56.0X1-	T56.0X2-	T56.0X3-	T56.0X4-	-	-
paint	T56.0X1-	T56.0X2-	T56.0X3-	T56.0X4-	-	-
paint	T56.0X1-	T56.0X2-	T56.0X3-	T56.0X4-	-	-
salts	T56.0X1-	T56.0X2-	T56.0X3-	T56.0X4-	-	-
specified compound NEC	T56.0X1-	T56.0X2-	T56.0X3-	T56.0X4-	-	-
tetra-ethyl	T56.0X1-	T56.0X2-	T56.0X3-	T56.0X4-	-	-
Lebanese red	T40.711-	T40.712-	T40.713-	T40.714-	T40.715-	T40.716-
Lefetamine	T39.8X1-	T39.8X2-	T39.8X3-	T39.8X4-	T39.8X5-	T39.8X6-
Lenperone	T43.4X1-	T43.4X2-	T43.4X3-	T43.4X4-	T43.4X5-	T43.4X6-
Lente lietin (insulin)	T38.3X1-	T38.3X2-	T38.3X3-	T38.3X4-	T38.3X5-	T38.3X6-
Leptazol	T50.7X1-	T50.7X2-	T50.7X3-	T50.7X4-	T50.7X5-	T50.7X6-
Leptophos	T60.0X1-	T60.0X2-	T60.0X3-	T60.0X4-	-	-
Leritine	T40.2X1-	T40.2X2-	T40.2X3-	T40.2X4-	T40.2X5-	T40.2X6-
Letosteine	T48.4X1-	T48.4X2-	T48.4X3-	T48.4X4-	T48.4X5-	T48.4X6-
Letter	T38.1X1-	T38.1X2-	T38.1X3-	T38.1X4-	T38.1X5-	T38.1X6-
Lettuce opium	T42.6X1-	T42.6X2-	T42.6X3-	T42.6X4-	T42.6X5-	T42.6X6-
Leucinocaine	T41.3X1-	T41.3X2-	T41.3X3-	T41.3X4-	T41.3X5-	T41.3X6-
Leucocianidol	T46.991-	T46.992-	T46.993-	T46.994-	T46.995-	T46.996-
Leucovorin (factor)	T45.8X1-	T45.8X2-	T45.8X3-	T45.8X4-	T45.8X5-	T45.8X6-
Leukeran	T45.1X1-	T45.1X2-	T45.1X3-	T45.1X4-	T45.1X5-	T45.1X6-
Leuprolide	T38.891-	T38.892-	T38.893-	T38.894-	T38.895-	T38.896-
Levalbuterol	T48.6X1-	T48.6X2-	T48.6X3-	T48.6X4-	T48.6X5-	T48.6X6-
Levallorphan	T50.7X1-	T50.7X2-	T50.7X3-	T50.7X4-	T50.7X5-	T50.7X6-
Levamisole	T37.4X1-	T37.4X2-	T37.4X3-	T37.4X4-	T37.4X5-	T37.4X6-
Levanil	T42.6X1-	T42.6X2-	T42.6X3-	T42.6X4-	T42.6X5-	T42.6X6-
Levarterenol	T44.4X1-	T44.4X2-	T44.4X3-	T44.4X4-	T44.4X5-	T44.4X6-
Levdropropizine	T48.3X1-	T48.3X2-	T48.3X3-	T48.3X4-	T48.3X5-	T48.3X6-
Levobunolol	T49.5X1-	T49.5X2-	T49.5X3-	T49.5X4-	T49.5X5-	T49.5X6-
Levocabastine (hydrochloride)	T45.0X1-	T45.0X2-	T45.0X3-	T45.0X4-	T45.0X5-	T45.0X6-
Levocarnitine	T50.991-	T50.992-	T50.993-	T50.994-	T50.995-	T50.996-

Substance	Poisoning Accidental (unintentional)	Poisoning Intentional self-harm	Poisoning Assault	Poisoning Undetermined	Adverse effect	Underdosing
Levodopa	T42.8X1-	T42.8X2-	T42.8X3-	T42.8X4-	T42.8X5-	T42.8X6-
with carbidopa	T42.8X1-	T42.8X2-	T42.8X3-	T42.8X4-	T42.8X5-	T42.8X6-
Levo-dromoran	T40.2X1-	T40.2X2-	T40.2X3-	T40.2X4-	T40.2X5-	T40.2X6-
Levoglutamide	T50.991-	T50.992-	T50.993-	T50.994-	T50.995-	T50.996-
Levoid	T38.1X1-	T38.1X2-	T38.1X3-	T38.1X4-	T38.1X5-	T38.1X6-
Levo-iso-methadone	T40.3X1-	T40.3X2-	T40.3X3-	T40.3X4-	T40.3X5-	T40.3X6-
Levomepromazine	T43.3X1-	T43.3X2-	T43.3X3-	T43.3X4-	T43.3X5-	T43.3X6-
Levonordefrin	T49.6X1-	T49.6X2-	T49.6X3-	T49.6X4-	T49.6X5-	T49.6X6-
Levonorgestrel	T38.4X1-	T38.4X2-	T38.4X3-	T38.4X4-	T38.4X5-	T38.4X6-
with ethinylestradiol	T38.5X1-	T38.5X2-	T38.5X3-	T38.5X4-	T38.5X5-	T38.5X6-
Levopromazine	T43.3X1-	T43.3X2-	T43.3X3-	T43.3X4-	T43.3X5-	T43.3X6-
Levoprome	T42.6X1-	T42.6X2-	T42.6X3-	T42.6X4-	T42.6X5-	T42.6X6-
Levopropoxyphene	T40.491-	T40.492-	T40.493-	T40.494-	T40.495-	T40.496-
Levopropylhexedrine	T50.5X1-	T50.5X2-	T50.5X3-	T50.5X4-	T50.5X5-	T50.5X6-
Levoproxyphylline	T48.6X1-	T48.6X2-	T48.6X3-	T48.6X4-	T48.6X5-	T48.6X6-
Levorphanol	T40.491-	T40.492-	T40.493-	T40.494-	T40.495-	T40.496-
Levothyroxine	T38.1X1-	T38.1X2-	T38.1X3-	T38.1X4-	T38.1X5-	T38.1X6-
sodium	T38.1X1-	T38.1X2-	T38.1X3-	T38.1X4-	T38.1X5-	T38.1X6-
Levsin	T44.3X1-	T44.3X2-	T44.3X3-	T44.3X4-	T44.3X5-	T44.3X6-
Levulose	T50.3X1-	T50.3X2-	T50.3X3-	T50.3X4-	T50.3X5-	T50.3X6-
Lewisite (gas) , not in war	T57.0X1-	T57.0X2-	T57.0X3-	T57.0X4-	-	-
Librium	T42.4X1-	T42.4X2-	T42.4X3-	T42.4X4-	T42.4X5-	T42.4X6-
Lidex	T49.0X1-	T49.0X2-	T49.0X3-	T49.0X4-	T49.0X5-	T49.0X6-
Lidocaine	T41.3X1-	T41.3X2-	T41.3X3-	T41.3X4-	T41.3X5-	T41.3X6-
regional	T41.3X1-	T41.3X2-	T41.3X3-	T41.3X4-	T41.3X5-	T41.3X6-
spinal	T41.3X1-	T41.3X2-	T41.3X3-	T41.3X4-	T41.3X5-	T41.3X6-
Lidofenin	T50.8X1-	T50.8X2-	T50.8X3-	T50.8X4-	T50.8X5-	T50.8X6-
Lidoflazine	T46.1X1-	T46.1X2-	T46.1X3-	T46.1X4-	T46.1X5-	T46.1X6-
Lighter fluid	T52.0X1-	T52.0X2-	T52.0X3-	T52.0X4-	-	-
Lignin hemicellulose	T47.6X1-	T47.6X2-	T47.6X3-	T47.6X4-	T47.6X5-	T47.6X6-
Lignocaine	T41.3X1-	T41.3X2-	T41.3X3-	T41.3X4-	T41.3X5-	T41.3X6-
regional	T41.3X1-	T41.3X2-	T41.3X3-	T41.3X4-	T41.3X5-	T41.3X6-
spinal	T41.3X1-	T41.3X2-	T41.3X3-	T41.3X4-	T41.3X5-	T41.3X6-
Ligroin (e) (solvent)	T52.0X1-	T52.0X2-	T52.0X3-	T52.0X4-	-	-
vapor	T59.891-	T59.892-	T59.893-	T59.894-	-	-
Ligustrum vulgare	T62.2X1-	T62.2X2-	T62.2X3-	T62.2X4-	-	-
Lily of the valley	T62.2X1-	T62.2X2-	T62.2X3-	T62.2X4-	-	-
Lime (chloride)	T54.3X1-	T54.3X2-	T54.3X3-	T54.3X4-	-	-
Limonene	T52.8X1-	T52.8X2-	T52.8X3-	T52.8X4-	-	-
Lincomycin	T36.8X1-	T36.8X2-	T36.8X3-	T36.8X4-	T36.8X5-	T36.8X6-
Lindane (insecticide) (nonmedicinal) (vapor)	T53.6X1-	T53.6X2-	T53.6X3-	T53.6X4-	-	-
medicinal	T49.0X1-	T49.0X2-	T49.0X3-	T49.0X4-	T49.0X5-	T49.0X6-
Liniments NEC	T49.91X-	T49.92X-	T49.93X-	T49.94X-	T49.95X-	T49.96X-
Linoleic acid	T46.6X1-	T46.6X2-	T46.6X3-	T46.6X4-	T46.6X5-	T46.6X6-
Linolenic acid	T46.6X1-	T46.6X2-	T46.6X3-	T46.6X4-	T46.6X5-	T46.6X6-
Linseed	T47.4X1-	T47.4X2-	T47.4X3-	T47.4X4-	T47.4X5-	T47.4X6-
Liothyronine	T38.1X1-	T38.1X2-	T38.1X3-	T38.1X4-	T38.1X5-	T38.1X6-
Liotrix	T38.1X1-	T38.1X2-	T38.1X3-	T38.1X4-	T38.1X5-	T38.1X6-
Lipancreatin	T47.5X1-	T47.5X2-	T47.5X3-	T47.5X4-	T47.5X5-	T47.5X6-
Lipo-alprostadil	T46.7X1-	T46.7X2-	T46.7X3-	T46.7X4-	T46.7X5-	T46.7X6-
Lipo-Lutin	T38.5X1-	T38.5X2-	T38.5X3-	T38.5X4-	T38.5X5-	T38.5X6-
Lipotropic drug NEC	T50.901-	T50.902-	T50.903-	T50.904-	T50.905-	T50.906-
Liquefied petroleum gases	T59.891-	T59.892-	T59.893-	T59.894-	-	-
piped (pure or mixed with air)	T59.891-	T59.892-	T59.893-	T59.894-	-	-
Liquid						
paraffin	T47.4X1-	T47.4X2-	T47.4X3-	T47.4X4-	T47.4X5-	T47.4X6-
petrolatum	T47.4X1-	T47.4X2-	T47.4X3-	T47.4X4-	T47.4X5-	T47.4X6-

Substance	Poisoning Accidental (unintentional)	Poisoning Intentional self-harm	Poisoning Assault	Poisoning Undetermined	Adverse effect	Underdosing
Liquid (continued)						
topical	T49.3X1-	T49.3X2-	T49.3X3-	T49.3X4-	T49.3X5-	T49.3X6-
specified NEC	T65.891-	T65.892-	T65.893-	T65.894-	-	-
substance	T65.91X-	T65.92X-	T65.93X-	T65.94X-	-	-
Liquor creosolis compositus	T65.891-	T65.892-	T65.893-	T65.894-	-	-
Liquorice	T48.4X1-	T48.4X2-	T48.4X3-	T48.4X4-	T48.4X5-	T48.4X6-
extract	T47.8X1-	T47.8X2-	T47.8X3-	T47.8X4-	T47.8X5-	T47.8X6-
Lisinopril	T46.4X1-	T46.4X2-	T46.4X3-	T46.4X4-	T46.4X5-	T46.4X6-
Lisuride	T42.8X1-	T42.8X2-	T42.8X3-	T42.8X4-	T42.8X5-	T42.8X6-
Lithane	T43.8X1-	T43.8X2-	T43.8X3-	T43.8X4-	T43.8X5-	T43.8X6-
Lithium	T56.891-	T56.892-	T56.893-	T56.894-	-	-
gluconate	T43.591-	T43.592-	T43.593-	T43.594-	T43.595-	T43.596-
salts (carbonate)	T43.591-	T43.592-	T43.593-	T43.594-	T43.595-	T43.596-
Lithonate	T43.8X1-	T43.8X2-	T43.8X3-	T43.8X4-	T43.8X5-	T43.8X6-
Liver						
extract	T45.8X1-	T45.8X2-	T45.8X3-	T45.8X4-	T45.8X5-	T45.8X6-
for parenteral use	T45.8X1-	T45.8X2-	T45.8X3-	T45.8X4-	T45.8X5-	T45.8X6-
fraction 1	T45.8X1-	T45.8X2-	T45.8X3-	T45.8X4-	T45.8X5-	T45.8X6-
hydrolysate	T45.8X1-	T45.8X2-	T45.8X3-	T45.8X4-	T45.8X5-	T45.8X6-
Lizard (bite) (venom)	T63.121-	T63.122-	T63.123-	T63.124-	-	-
LMD	T45.8X1-	T45.8X2-	T45.8X3-	T45.8X4-	T45.8X5-	T45.8X6-
Lobelia	T62.2X1-	T62.2X2-	T62.2X3-	T62.2X4-	-	-
Lobeline	T50.7X1-	T50.7X2-	T50.7X3-	T50.7X4-	T50.7X5-	T50.7X6-
Local action drug NEC	T49.8X1-	T49.8X2-	T49.8X3-	T49.8X4-	T49.8X5-	T49.8X6-
Locorten	T49.0X1-	T49.0X2-	T49.0X3-	T49.0X4-	T49.0X5-	T49.0X6-
Lofepramine	T43.011-	T43.012-	T43.013-	T43.014-	T43.015-	T43.016-
Lolium temulentum	T62.2X1-	T62.2X2-	T62.2X3-	T62.2X4-	-	-
Lomotil	T47.6X1-	T47.6X2-	T47.6X3-	T47.6X4-	T47.6X5-	T47.6X6-
Lomustine	T45.1X1-	T45.1X2-	T45.1X3-	T45.1X4-	T45.1X5-	T45.1X6-
Lonidamine	T45.1X1-	T45.1X2-	T45.1X3-	T45.1X4-	T45.1X5-	T45.1X6-
Loperamide	T47.6X1-	T47.6X2-	T47.6X3-	T47.6X4-	T47.6X5-	T47.6X6-
Loprazolam	T42.4X1-	T42.4X2-	T42.4X3-	T42.4X4-	T42.4X5-	T42.4X6-
Lorajmine	T46.2X1-	T46.2X2-	T46.2X3-	T46.2X4-	T46.2X5-	T46.2X6-
Loratidine	T45.0X1-	T45.0X2-	T45.0X3-	T45.0X4-	T45.0X5-	T45.0X6-
Lorazepam	T42.4X1-	T42.4X2-	T42.4X3-	T42.4X4-	T42.4X5-	T42.4X6-
Lorcainide	T46.2X1-	T46.2X2-	T46.2X3-	T46.2X4-	T46.2X5-	T46.2X6-
Lormetazepam	T42.4X1-	T42.4X2-	T42.4X3-	T42.4X4-	T42.4X5-	T42.4X6-
Lotions NEC	T49.91X-	T49.92X-	T49.93X-	T49.94X-	T49.95X-	T49.96X-
Lotusate	T42.3X1-	T42.3X2-	T42.3X3-	T42.3X4-	T42.3X5-	T42.3X6-
Lovastatin	T46.6X1-	T46.6X2-	T46.6X3-	T46.6X4-	T46.6X5-	T46.6X6-
Lowila	T49.2X1-	T49.2X2-	T49.2X3-	T49.2X4-	T49.2X5-	T49.2X6-
Loxapine	T43.591-	T43.592-	T43.593-	T43.594-	T43.595-	T43.596-
Lozenges (throat)	T49.6X1-	T49.6X2-	T49.6X3-	T49.6X4-	T49.6X5-	T49.6X6-
LSD	T40.8X1-	T40.8X2-	T40.8X3-	T40.8X4-	-	-
L-Tryptophan — *see amino acid*						
Lubricant, eye	T49.5X1-	T49.5X2-	T49.5X3-	T49.5X4-	T49.5X5-	T49.5X6-
Lubricating oil NEC	T52.0X1-	T52.0X2-	T52.0X3-	T52.0X4-	-	-
Lucanthone	T37.4X1-	T37.4X2-	T37.4X3-	T37.4X4-	T37.4X5-	T37.4X6-
Luminal	T42.3X1-	T42.3X2-	T42.3X3-	T42.3X4-	T42.3X5-	T42.3X6-
Lung irritant (gas) NEC	T59.91X-	T59.92X-	T59.93X-	T59.94X-	-	-
Luteinizing hormone	T38.811-	T38.812-	T38.813-	T38.814-	T38.815-	T38.816-
Lutocylol	T38.5X1-	T38.5X2-	T38.5X3-	T38.5X4-	T38.5X5-	T38.5X6-
Lutromone	T38.5X1-	T38.5X2-	T38.5X3-	T38.5X4-	T38.5X5-	T38.5X6-
Lututrin	T48.291-	T48.292-	T48.293-	T48.294-	T48.295-	T48.296-
Lye (concentrated)	T54.3X1-	T54.3X2-	T54.3X3-	T54.3X4-	-	-
Lygranum (skin test)	T50.8X1-	T50.8X2-	T50.8X3-	T50.8X4-	T50.8X5-	T50.8X6-
Lymecycline	T36.4X1-	T36.4X2-	T36.4X3-	T36.4X4-	T36.4X5-	T36.4X6-
Lymphogranuloma venereum antigen	T50.8X1-	T50.8X2-	T50.8X3-	T50.8X4-	T50.8X5-	T50.8X6-
Lynestrenol	T38.4X1-	T38.4X2-	T38.4X3-	T38.4X4-	T38.4X5-	T38.4X6-

Substance	Poisoning Accidental (unintentional)	Poisoning Intentional self-harm	Poisoning Assault	Poisoning Undetermined	Adverse effect	Underdosing
Lyovac Sodium Edecrin	T50.1X1-	T50.1X2-	T50.1X3-	T50.1X4-	T50.1X5-	T50.1X6-
Lypressin	T38.891-	T38.892-	T38.893-	T38.894-	T38.895-	T38.896-
Lysergic acid diethylamide	T40.8X1-	T40.8X2-	T40.8X3-	T40.8X4-	-	-
Lysergide	T40.8X1-	T40.8X2-	T40.8X3-	T40.8X4-	-	-
Lysine vasopressin	T38.891-	T38.892-	T38.893-	T38.894-	T38.895-	T38.896-
Lysol	T54.1X1-	T54.1X2-	T54.1X3-	T54.1X4-	-	-
Lysozyme	T49.0X1-	T49.0X2-	T49.0X3-	T49.0X4-	T49.0X5-	T49.0X6-
Lytta (vitatta)	T49.8X1-	T49.8X2-	T49.8X3-	T49.8X4-	T49.8X5-	T49.8X6-
Mace	T59.3X1-	T59.3X2-	T59.3X3-	T59.3X4-	-	-
Macrogol	T50.991-	T50.992-	T50.993-	T50.994-	T50.995-	T50.996-
Macrolide						
anabolic drug	T38.7X1-	T38.7X2-	T38.7X3-	T38.7X4-	T38.7X5-	T38.7X6-
antibiotic	T36.3X1-	T36.3X2-	T36.3X3-	T36.3X4-	T36.3X5-	T36.3X6-
Mafenide	T49.0X1-	T49.0X2-	T49.0X3-	T49.0X4-	T49.0X5-	T49.0X6-
Magaldrate	T47.1X1-	T47.1X2-	T47.1X3-	T47.1X4-	T47.1X5-	T47.1X6-
Magic mushroom	T40.991-	T40.992-	T40.993-	T40.994-	-	-
Magnamycin	T36.8X1-	T36.8X2-	T36.8X3-	T36.8X4-	T36.8X5-	T36.8X6-
Magnesia magma	T47.1X1-	T47.1X2-	T47.1X3-	T47.1X4-	T47.1X5-	T47.1X6-
Magnesium NEC	T56.891-	T56.892-	T56.893-	T56.894-	-	-
carbonate	T47.1X1-	T47.1X2-	T47.1X3-	T47.1X4-	T47.1X5-	T47.1X6-
citrate	T47.4X1-	T47.4X2-	T47.4X3-	T47.4X4-	T47.4X5-	T47.4X6-
hydroxide	T47.1X1-	T47.1X2-	T47.1X3-	T47.1X4-	T47.1X5-	T47.1X6-
oxide	T47.1X1-	T47.1X2-	T47.1X3-	T47.1X4-	T47.1X5-	T47.1X6-
peroxide	T49.0X1-	T49.0X2-	T49.0X3-	T49.0X4-	T49.0X5-	T49.0X6-
salicylate	T39.091-	T39.092-	T39.093-	T39.094-	T39.095-	T39.096-
silicofluoride	T50.3X1-	T50.3X2-	T50.3X3-	T50.3X4-	T50.3X5-	T50.3X6-
sulfate	T47.4X1-	T47.4X2-	T47.4X3-	T47.4X4-	T47.4X5-	T47.4X6-
thiosulfate	T45.0X1-	T45.0X2-	T45.0X3-	T45.0X4-	T45.0X5-	T45.0X6-
trisilicate	T47.1X1-	T47.1X2-	T47.1X3-	T47.1X4-	T47.1X5-	T47.1X6-
Malathion (medicinal)	T49.0X1-	T49.0X2-	T49.0X3-	T49.0X4-	T49.0X5-	T49.0X6-
insecticide	T60.0X1-	T60.0X2-	T60.0X3-	T60.0X4-	-	-
Male fern extract	T37.4X1-	T37.4X2-	T37.4X3-	T37.4X4-	T37.4X5-	T37.4X6-
M-AMSA	T45.1X1-	T45.1X2-	T45.1X3-	T45.1X4-	T45.1X5-	T45.1X6-
Mandelic acid	T37.8X1-	T37.8X2-	T37.8X3-	T37.8X4-	T37.8X5-	T37.8X6-
Manganese (dioxide) (salts)	T57.2X1-	T57.2X2-	T57.2X3-	T57.2X4-	-	-
medicinal	T50.991-	T50.992-	T50.993-	T50.994-	T50.995-	T50.996-
Mannitol	T47.3X1-	T47.3X2-	T47.3X3-	T47.3X4-	T47.3X5-	T47.3X6-
hexanitrate	T46.3X1-	T46.3X2-	T46.3X3-	T46.3X4-	T46.3X5-	T46.3X6-
Mannomustine	T45.1X1-	T45.1X2-	T45.1X3-	T45.1X4-	T45.1X5-	T45.1X6-
MAO inhibitors	T43.1X1-	T43.1X2-	T43.1X3-	T43.1X4-	T43.1X5-	T43.1X6-
Mapharsen	T37.8X1-	T37.8X2-	T37.8X3-	T37.8X4-	T37.8X5-	T37.8X6-
Maphenide	T49.0X1-	T49.0X2-	T49.0X3-	T49.0X4-	T49.0X5-	T49.0X6-
Maprotiline	T43.021-	T43.022-	T43.023-	T43.024-	T43.025-	T43.026-
Marcaine	T41.3X1-	T41.3X2-	T41.3X3-	T41.3X4-	T41.3X5-	T41.3X6-
infiltration (subcutaneous)	T41.3X1-	T41.3X2-	T41.3X3-	T41.3X4-	T41.3X5-	T41.3X6-
nerve block (peripheral) (plexus)	T41.3X1-	T41.3X2-	T41.3X3-	T41.3X4-	T41.3X5-	T41.3X6-
Marezine	T45.0X1-	T45.0X2-	T45.0X3-	T45.0X4-	T45.0X5-	T45.0X6-
Marihuana	T40.711-	T40.712-	T40.713-	T40.714-	T40.715-	T40.716-
Marijuana	T40.711-	T40.712-	T40.713-	T40.714-	T40.715-	T40.716-
Marine (sting)	T63.691-	T63.692-	T63.693-	T63.694-	-	-
animals (sting)	T63.691-	T63.692-	T63.693-	T63.694-	-	-
plants (sting)	T63.711-	T63.712-	T63.713-	T63.714-	-	-
Marplan	T43.1X1-	T43.1X2-	T43.1X3-	T43.1X4-	T43.1X5-	T43.1X6-
Marsh gas	T59.891-	T59.892-	T59.893-	T59.894-	-	-
Marsilid	T43.1X1-	T43.1X2-	T43.1X3-	T43.1X4-	T43.1X5-	T43.1X6-
Matulane	T45.1X1-	T45.1X2-	T45.1X3-	T45.1X4-	T45.1X5-	T45.1X6-
Mazindol	T50.5X1-	T50.5X2-	T50.5X3-	T50.5X4-	T50.5X5-	T50.5X6-
MCPA	T60.3X1-	T60.3X2-	T60.3X3-	T60.3X4-	-	-

Substance	Poisoning Accidental (unintentional)	Poisoning Intentional self-harm	Poisoning Assault	Poisoning Undetermined	Adverse effect	Underdosing
MDMA	T43.641-	T43.642-	T43.643-	T43.644-	-	-
Meadow saffron	T62.2X1-	T62.2X2-	T62.2X3-	T62.2X4-	-	-
Measles virus vaccine (attenuated)	T50.B91-	T50.B92-	T50.B93-	T50.B94-	T50.B95-	T50.B96-
Meat, noxious	T62.8X1-	T62.8X2-	T62.8X3-	T62.8X4-	-	-
Meballymal	T42.3X1-	T42.3X2-	T42.3X3-	T42.3X4-	T42.3X5-	T42.3X6-
Mebanazine	T43.1X1-	T43.1X2-	T43.1X3-	T43.1X4-	T43.1X5-	T43.1X6-
Mebaral	T42.3X1-	T42.3X2-	T42.3X3-	T42.3X4-	T42.3X5-	T42.3X6-
Mebendazole	T37.4X1-	T37.4X2-	T37.4X3-	T37.4X4-	T37.4X5-	T37.4X6-
Mebeverine	T44.3X1-	T44.3X2-	T44.3X3-	T44.3X4-	T44.3X5-	T44.3X6-
Mebhydrolin	T45.0X1-	T45.0X2-	T45.0X3-	T45.0X4-	T45.0X5-	T45.0X6-
Mebumal	T42.3X1-	T42.3X2-	T42.3X3-	T42.3X4-	T42.3X5-	T42.3X6-
Mebutamate	T43.591-	T43.592-	T43.593-	T43.594-	T43.595-	T43.596-
Mecamylamine	T44.2X1-	T44.2X2-	T44.2X3-	T44.2X4-	T44.2X5-	T44.2X6-
Mechlorethamine	T45.1X1-	T45.1X2-	T45.1X3-	T45.1X4-	T45.1X5-	T45.1X6-
Mecillinam	T36.0X1-	T36.0X2-	T36.0X3-	T36.0X4-	T36.0X5-	T36.0X6-
Meclizine (hydrochloride)	T45.0X1-	T45.0X2-	T45.0X3-	T45.0X4-	T45.0X5-	T45.0X6-
Meclocycline	T36.4X1-	T36.4X2-	T36.4X3-	T36.4X4-	T36.4X5-	T36.4X6-
Meclofenamate	T39.391-	T39.392-	T39.393-	T39.394-	T39.395-	T39.396-
Meclofenamic acid	T39.391-	T39.392-	T39.393-	T39.394-	T39.395-	T39.396-
Meclofenoxate	T43.691-	T43.692-	T43.693-	T43.694-	T43.695-	T43.696-
Meclozine	T45.0X1-	T45.0X2-	T45.0X3-	T45.0X4-	T45.0X5-	T45.0X6-
Mecobalamin	T45.8X1-	T45.8X2-	T45.8X3-	T45.8X4-	T45.8X5-	T45.8X6-
Mecoprop	T60.3X1-	T60.3X2-	T60.3X3-	T60.3X4-	-	-
Mecrilate	T49.3X1-	T49.3X2-	T49.3X3-	T49.3X4-	T49.3X5-	T49.3X6-
Mecysteine	T48.4X1-	T48.4X2-	T48.4X3-	T48.4X4-	T48.4X5-	T48.4X6-
Medazepam	T42.4X1-	T42.4X2-	T42.4X3-	T42.4X4-	T42.4X5-	T42.4X6-
Medicament NEC	T50.901-	T50.902-	T50.903-	T50.904-	T50.905-	T50.906-
Medinal	T42.3X1-	T42.3X2-	T42.3X3-	T42.3X4-	T42.3X5-	T42.3X6-
Medomin	T42.3X1-	T42.3X2-	T42.3X3-	T42.3X4-	T42.3X5-	T42.3X6-
Medrogestone	T38.5X1-	T38.5X2-	T38.5X3-	T38.5X4-	T38.5X5-	T38.5X6-
Medroxalol	T44.8X1-	T44.8X2-	T44.8X3-	T44.8X4-	T44.8X5-	T44.8X6-
Medroxyprogesterone acetate (depot)	T38.5X1-	T38.5X2-	T38.5X3-	T38.5X4-	T38.5X5-	T38.5X6-
Medrysone	T49.0X1-	T49.0X2-	T49.0X3-	T49.0X4-	T49.0X5-	T49.0X6-
Mefenamic acid	T39.391-	T39.392-	T39.393-	T39.394-	T39.395-	T39.396-
Mefenorex	T50.5X1-	T50.5X2-	T50.5X3-	T50.5X4-	T50.5X5-	T50.5X6-
Mefloquine	T37.2X1-	T37.2X2-	T37.2X3-	T37.2X4-	T37.2X5-	T37.2X6-
Mefruside	T50.2X1-	T50.2X2-	T50.2X3-	T50.2X4-	T50.2X5-	T50.2X6-
Megahallucinogen	T40.901-	T40.902-	T40.903-	T40.904-	T40.905-	T40.906-
Megestrol	T38.5X1-	T38.5X2-	T38.5X3-	T38.5X4-	T38.5X5-	T38.5X6-
Meglumine						
antimoniate	T37.8X1-	T37.8X2-	T37.8X3-	T37.8X4-	T37.8X5-	T37.8X6-
diatrizoate	T50.8X1-	T50.8X2-	T50.8X3-	T50.8X4-	T50.8X5-	T50.8X6-
iodipamide	T50.8X1-	T50.8X2-	T50.8X3-	T50.8X4-	T50.8X5-	T50.8X6-
iotroxate	T50.8X1-	T50.8X2-	T50.8X3-	T50.8X4-	T50.8X5-	T50.8X6-
MEK (methyl ethyl ketone)	T52.4X1-	T52.4X2-	T52.4X3-	T52.4X4-	-	-
Meladinin	T49.3X1-	T49.3X2-	T49.3X3-	T49.3X4-	T49.3X5-	T49.3X6-
Meladrazine	T44.3X1-	T44.3X2-	T44.3X3-	T44.3X4-	T44.3X5-	T44.3X6-
Melaleuca alternifolia oil	T49.0X1-	T49.0X2-	T49.0X3-	T49.0X4-	T49.0X5-	T49.0X6-
Melanizing agents	T49.3X1-	T49.3X2-	T49.3X3-	T49.3X4-	T49.3X5-	T49.3X6-
Melanocyte-stimulating hormone	T38.891-	T38.892-	T38.893-	T38.894-	T38.895-	T38.896-
Melarsonyl potassium	T37.3X1-	T37.3X2-	T37.3X3-	T37.3X4-	T37.3X5-	T37.3X6-
Melarsoprol	T37.3X1-	T37.3X2-	T37.3X3-	T37.3X4-	T37.3X5-	T37.3X6-
Melia azedarach	T62.2X1-	T62.2X2-	T62.2X3-	T62.2X4-	-	-
Melitracen	T43.011-	T43.012-	T43.013-	T43.014-	T43.015-	T43.016-
Mellaril	T43.3X1-	T43.3X2-	T43.3X3-	T43.3X4-	T43.3X5-	T43.3X6-
Meloxine	T49.3X1-	T49.3X2-	T49.3X3-	T49.3X4-	T49.3X5-	T49.3X6-
Melperone	T43.4X1-	T43.4X2-	T43.4X3-	T43.4X4-	T43.4X5-	T43.4X6-
Melphalan	T45.1X1-	T45.1X2-	T45.1X3-	T45.1X4-	T45.1X5-	T45.1X6-
Memantine	T43.8X1-	T43.8X2-	T43.8X3-	T43.8X4-	T43.8X5-	T43.8X6-

Substance	Poisoning Accidental (unintentional)	Poisoning Intentional self-harm	Poisoning Assault	Poisoning Undetermined	Adverse effect	Underdosing
Menadiol	T45.7X1-	T45.7X2-	T45.7X3-	T45.7X4-	T45.7X5-	T45.7X6-
sodium sulfate	T45.7X1-	T45.7X2-	T45.7X3-	T45.7X4-	T45.7X5-	T45.7X6-
Menadione	T45.7X1-	T45.7X2-	T45.7X3-	T45.7X4-	T45.7X5-	T45.7X6-
sodium bisulfite	T45.7X1-	T45.7X2-	T45.7X3-	T45.7X4-	T45.7X5-	T45.7X6-
Menaphthone	T45.7X1-	T45.7X2-	T45.7X3-	T45.7X4-	T45.7X5-	T45.7X6-
Menaquinone	T45.7X1-	T45.7X2-	T45.7X3-	T45.7X4-	T45.7X5-	T45.7X6-
Menatetrenone	T45.7X1-	T45.7X2-	T45.7X3-	T45.7X4-	T45.7X5-	T45.7X6-
Meningococcal vaccine	T50.A91-	T50.A92-	T50.A93-	T50.A94-	T50.A95-	T50.A96-
Menningovax (-AC) (-C)	T50.A91-	T50.A92-	T50.A93-	T50.A94-	T50.A95-	T50.A96-
Menotropins	T38.811-	T38.812-	T38.813-	T38.814-	T38.815-	T38.816-
Menthol	T48.5X1-	T48.5X2-	T48.5X3-	T48.5X4-	T48.5X5-	T48.5X6-
Mepacrine	T37.2X1-	T37.2X2-	T37.2X3-	T37.2X4-	T37.2X5-	T37.2X6-
Meparfynol	T42.6X1-	T42.6X2-	T42.6X3-	T42.6X4-	T42.6X5-	T42.6X6-
Mepartricin	T36.7X1-	T36.7X2-	T36.7X3-	T36.7X4-	T36.7X5-	T36.7X6-
Mepazine	T43.3X1-	T43.3X2-	T43.3X3-	T43.3X4-	T43.3X5-	T43.3X6-
Mepenzolate	T44.3X1-	T44.3X2-	T44.3X3-	T44.3X4-	T44.3X5-	T44.3X6-
bromide	T44.3X1-	T44.3X2-	T44.3X3-	T44.3X4-	T44.3X5-	T44.3X6-
Meperidine	T40.491-	T40.492-	T40.493-	T40.494-	T40.495-	T40.496-
Mephebarbital	T42.3X1-	T42.3X2-	T42.3X3-	T42.3X4-	T42.3X5-	T42.3X6-
Mephenamin (e)	T42.8X1-	T42.8X2-	T42.8X3-	T42.8X4-	T42.8X5-	T42.8X6-
Mephenesin	T42.8X1-	T42.8X2-	T42.8X3-	T42.8X4-	T42.8X5-	T42.8X6-
Mephenhydramine	T45.0X1-	T45.0X2-	T45.0X3-	T45.0X4-	T45.0X5-	T45.0X6-
Mephenoxalone	T42.8X1-	T42.8X2-	T42.8X3-	T42.8X4-	T42.8X5-	T42.8X6-
Mephentermine	T44.991-	T44.992-	T44.993-	T44.994-	T44.995-	T44.996-
Mephenytoin	T42.0X1-	T42.0X2-	T42.0X3-	T42.0X4-	T42.0X5-	T42.0X6-
with phenobarbital	T42.3X1-	T42.3X2-	T42.3X3-	T42.3X4-	T42.3X5-	T42.3X6-
Mephobarbital	T42.3X1-	T42.3X2-	T42.3X3-	T42.3X4-	T42.3X5-	T42.3X6-
Mephosfolan	T60.0X1-	T60.0X2-	T60.0X3-	T60.0X4-	-	-
Mepindolol	T44.7X1-	T44.7X2-	T44.7X3-	T44.7X4-	T44.7X5-	T44.7X6-
Mepiperphenidol	T44.3X1-	T44.3X2-	T44.3X3-	T44.3X4-	T44.3X5-	T44.3X6-
Mepitiostane	T38.7X1-	T38.7X2-	T38.7X3-	T38.7X4-	T38.7X5-	T38.7X6-
Mepivacaine	T41.3X1-	T41.3X2-	T41.3X3-	T41.3X4-	T41.3X5-	T41.3X6-
epidural	T41.3X1-	T41.3X2-	T41.3X3-	T41.3X4-	T41.3X5-	T41.3X6-
Meprednisone	T38.0X1-	T38.0X2-	T38.0X3-	T38.0X4-	T38.0X5-	T38.0X6-
Meprobam	T43.591-	T43.592-	T43.593-	T43.594-	T43.595-	T43.596-
Meprobamate	T43.591-	T43.592-	T43.593-	T43.594-	T43.595-	T43.596-
Meproscillarin	T46.0X1-	T46.0X2-	T46.0X3-	T46.0X4-	T46.0X5-	T46.0X6-
Meprylcaine	T41.3X1-	T41.3X2-	T41.3X3-	T41.3X4-	T41.3X5-	T41.3X6-
Meptazinol	T39.8X1-	T39.8X2-	T39.8X3-	T39.8X4-	T39.8X5-	T39.8X6-
Mepyramine	T45.0X1-	T45.0X2-	T45.0X3-	T45.0X4-	T45.0X5-	T45.0X6-
Mequitazine	T43.3X1-	T43.3X2-	T43.3X3-	T43.3X4-	T43.3X5-	T43.3X6-
Meralluride	T50.2X1-	T50.2X2-	T50.2X3-	T50.2X4-	T50.2X5-	T50.2X6-
Merbaphen	T50.2X1-	T50.2X2-	T50.2X3-	T50.2X4-	T50.2X5-	T50.2X6-
Merbromin	T49.0X1-	T49.0X2-	T49.0X3-	T49.0X4-	T49.0X5-	T49.0X6-
Mercaptobenzothiazole salts	T49.0X1-	T49.0X2-	T49.0X3-	T49.0X4-	T49.0X5-	T49.0X6-
Mercaptomerin	T50.2X1-	T50.2X2-	T50.2X3-	T50.2X4-	T50.2X5-	T50.2X6-
Mercaptopurine	T45.1X1-	T45.1X2-	T45.1X3-	T45.1X4-	T45.1X5-	T45.1X6-
Mercumatilin	T50.2X1-	T50.2X2-	T50.2X3-	T50.2X4-	T50.2X5-	T50.2X6-
Mercuramide	T50.2X1-	T50.2X2-	T50.2X3-	T50.2X4-	T50.2X5-	T50.2X6-
Mercurochrome	T49.0X1-	T49.0X2-	T49.0X3-	T49.0X4-	T49.0X5-	T49.0X6-
Mercurophylline	T50.2X1-	T50.2X2-	T50.2X3-	T50.2X4-	T50.2X5-	T50.2X6-
Mercury, mercurial, mercuric, mercurous (compounds) (cyanide) (fumes) (nonmedicinal) (vapor) NEC	T56.1X1-	T56.1X2-	T56.1X3-	T56.1X4-	-	-
ammoniated	T49.0X1-	T49.0X2-	T49.0X3-	T49.0X4-	T49.0X5-	T49.0X6-
anti-infective						
local	T49.0X1-	T49.0X2-	T49.0X3-	T49.0X4-	T49.0X5-	T49.0X6-
systemic	T37.8X1-	T37.8X2-	T37.8X3-	T37.8X4-	T37.8X5-	T37.8X6-

Substance	Poisoning Accidental (unintentional)	Poisoning Intentional self-harm	Poisoning Assault	Poisoning Undetermined	Adverse effect	Underdosing
Mercury, mercurial, mercuric, mercurous (compounds) (cyanide) (fumes) (nonmedicinal) (vapor) NEC (continued)						
topical	T49.0X1-	T49.0X2-	T49.0X3-	T49.0X4-	T49.0X5-	T49.0X6-
chloride (ammoniated)	T49.0X1-	T49.0X2-	T49.0X3-	T49.0X4-	T49.0X5-	T49.0X6-
fungicide	T56.1X1-	T56.1X2-	T56.1X3-	T56.1X4-	-	-
diuretic NEC	T50.2X1-	T50.2X2-	T50.2X3-	T50.2X4-	T50.2X5-	T50.2X6-
fungicide	T56.1X1-	T56.1X2-	T56.1X3-	T56.1X4-	-	-
organic (fungicide)	T56.1X1-	T56.1X2-	T56.1X3-	T56.1X4-	-	-
oxide, yellow	T49.0X1-	T49.0X2-	T49.0X3-	T49.0X4-	T49.0X5-	T49.0X6-
Mersalyl	T50.2X1-	T50.2X2-	T50.2X3-	T50.2X4-	T50.2X5-	T50.2X6-
Merthiolate	T49.0X1-	T49.0X2-	T49.0X3-	T49.0X4-	T49.0X5-	T49.0X6-
ophthalmic preparation	T49.5X1-	T49.5X2-	T49.5X3-	T49.5X4-	T49.5X5-	T49.5X6-
Meruvax	T50.B91-	T50.B92-	T50.B93-	T50.B94-	T50.B95-	T50.B96-
Mesalazine	T47.8X1-	T47.8X2-	T47.8X3-	T47.8X4-	T47.8X5-	T47.8X6-
Mescal buttons	T40.991-	T40.992-	T40.993-	T40.994-	-	-
Mescaline	T40.991-	T40.992-	T40.993-	T40.994-	-	-
Mesna	T48.4X1-	T48.4X2-	T48.4X3-	T48.4X4-	T48.4X5-	T48.4X6-
Mesoglycan	T46.6X1-	T46.6X2-	T46.6X3-	T46.6X4-	T46.6X5-	T46.6X6-
Mesoridazine	T43.3X1-	T43.3X2-	T43.3X3-	T43.3X4-	T43.3X5-	T43.3X6-
Mestanolone	T38.7X1-	T38.7X2-	T38.7X3-	T38.7X4-	T38.7X5-	T38.7X6-
Mesterolone	T38.7X1-	T38.7X2-	T38.7X3-	T38.7X4-	T38.7X5-	T38.7X6-
Mestranol	T38.5X1-	T38.5X2-	T38.5X3-	T38.5X4-	T38.5X5-	T38.5X6-
Mesulergine	T42.8X1-	T42.8X2-	T42.8X3-	T42.8X4-	T42.8X5-	T42.8X6-
Mesulfen	T49.0X1-	T49.0X2-	T49.0X3-	T49.0X4-	T49.0X5-	T49.0X6-
Mesuximide	T42.2X1-	T42.2X2-	T42.2X3-	T42.2X4-	T42.2X5-	T42.2X6-
Metabutethamine	T41.3X1-	T41.3X2-	T41.3X3-	T41.3X4-	T41.3X5-	T41.3X6-
Metactesylacetate	T49.0X1-	T49.0X2-	T49.0X3-	T49.0X4-	T49.0X5-	T49.0X6-
Metacycline	T36.4X1-	T36.4X2-	T36.4X3-	T36.4X4-	T36.4X5-	T36.4X6-
Metaldehyde (snail killer) NEC	T60.8X1-	T60.8X2-	T60.8X3-	T60.8X4-	-	-
Metals (heavy) (nonmedicinal)	T56.91X-	T56.92X-	T56.93X-	T56.94X-	-	-
dust, fumes, or vapor NEC	T56.91X-	T56.92X-	T56.93X-	T56.94X-	-	-
light NEC	T56.91X-	T56.92X-	T56.93X-	T56.94X-	-	-
dust, fumes, or vapor NEC	T56.91X-	T56.92X-	T56.93X-	T56.94X-	-	-
specified NEC	T56.891-	T56.892-	T56.893-	T56.894-	-	-
thallium	T56.811-	T56.812-	T56.813-	T56.814-	-	-
Metamfetamine	T43.621-	T43.622-	T43.623-	T43.624-	T43.625-	T43.626-
Metamizole sodium	T39.2X1-	T39.2X2-	T39.2X3-	T39.2X4-	T39.2X5-	T39.2X6-
Metampicillin	T36.0X1-	T36.0X2-	T36.0X3-	T36.0X4-	T36.0X5-	T36.0X6-
Metamucil	T47.4X1-	T47.4X2-	T47.4X3-	T47.4X4-	T47.4X5-	T47.4X6-
Metandienone	T38.7X1-	T38.7X2-	T38.7X3-	T38.7X4-	T38.7X5-	T38.7X6-
Metandrostenolone	T38.7X1-	T38.7X2-	T38.7X3-	T38.7X4-	T38.7X5-	T38.7X6-
Metaphen	T49.0X1-	T49.0X2-	T49.0X3-	T49.0X4-	T49.0X5-	T49.0X6-
Metaphos	T60.0X1-	T60.0X2-	T60.0X3-	T60.0X4-	-	-
Metapramine	T43.011-	T43.012-	T43.013-	T43.014-	T43.015-	T43.016-
Metaproterenol	T48.291-	T48.292-	T48.293-	T48.294-	T48.295-	T48.296-
Metaraminol	T44.4X1-	T44.4X2-	T44.4X3-	T44.4X4-	T44.4X5-	T44.4X6-
Metaxalone	T42.8X1-	T42.8X2-	T42.8X3-	T42.8X4-	T42.8X5-	T42.8X6-
Metenolone	T38.7X1-	T38.7X2-	T38.7X3-	T38.7X4-	T38.7X5-	T38.7X6-
Metergoline	T42.8X1-	T42.8X2-	T42.8X3-	T42.8X4-	T42.8X5-	T42.8X6-
Metescufylline	T46.991-	T46.992-	T46.993-	T46.994-	T46.995-	T46.996-
Metetoin	T42.0X1-	T42.0X2-	T42.0X3-	T42.0X4-	T42.0X5-	T42.0X6-
Metformin	T38.3X1-	T38.3X2-	T38.3X3-	T38.3X4-	T38.3X5-	T38.3X6-
Methacholine	T44.1X1-	T44.1X2-	T44.1X3-	T44.1X4-	T44.1X5-	T44.1X6-
Methacycline	T36.4X1-	T36.4X2-	T36.4X3-	T36.4X4-	T36.4X5-	T36.4X6-
Methadone	T40.3X1-	T40.3X2-	T40.3X3-	T40.3X4-	T40.3X5-	T40.3X6-
Methallenestril	T38.5X1-	T38.5X2-	T38.5X3-	T38.5X4-	T38.5X5-	T38.5X6-
Methallenoestril	T38.5X1-	T38.5X2-	T38.5X3-	T38.5X4-	T38.5X5-	T38.5X6-
Methamphetamine	T43.621-	T43.622-	T43.623-	T43.624-	T43.625-	T43.626-

Substance	Poisoning Accidental (unintentional)	Poisoning Intentional self-harm	Poisoning Assault	Poisoning Undetermined	Adverse effect	Underdosing
Methampyrone	T39.2X1-	T39.2X2-	T39.2X3-	T39.2X4-	T39.2X5-	T39.2X6-
Methandienone	T38.7X1-	T38.7X2-	T38.7X3-	T38.7X4-	T38.7X5-	T38.7X6-
Methandriol	T38.7X1-	T38.7X2-	T38.7X3-	T38.7X4-	T38.7X5-	T38.7X6-
Methandrostenolone	T38.7X1-	T38.7X2-	T38.7X3-	T38.7X4-	T38.7X5-	T38.7X6-
Methane	T59.891-	T59.892-	T59.893-	T59.894-	-	-
Methanethiol	T59.891-	T59.892-	T59.893-	T59.894-	-	-
Methaniazide	T37.1X1-	T37.1X2-	T37.1X3-	T37.1X4-	T37.1X5-	T37.1X6-
Methanol (vapor)	T51.1X1-	T51.1X2-	T51.1X3-	T51.1X4-	-	-
Methantheline	T44.3X1-	T44.3X2-	T44.3X3-	T44.3X4-	T44.3X5-	T44.3X6-
Methanthelinium bromide	T44.3X1-	T44.3X2-	T44.3X3-	T44.3X4-	T44.3X5-	T44.3X6-
Methaphenilene	T45.0X1-	T45.0X2-	T45.0X3-	T45.0X4-	T45.0X5-	T45.0X6-
Methapyrilene	T45.0X1-	T45.0X2-	T45.0X3-	T45.0X4-	T45.0X5-	T45.0X6-
Methaqualone (compound)	T42.6X1-	T42.6X2-	T42.6X3-	T42.6X4-	T42.6X5-	T42.6X6-
Metharbital	T42.3X1-	T42.3X2-	T42.3X3-	T42.3X4-	T42.3X5-	T42.3X6-
Methazolamide	T50.2X1-	T50.2X2-	T50.2X3-	T50.2X4-	T50.2X5-	T50.2X6-
Methdilazine	T43.3X1-	T43.3X2-	T43.3X3-	T43.3X4-	T43.3X5-	T43.3X6-
Methedrine	T43.621-	T43.622-	T43.623-	T43.624-	T43.625-	T43.626-
Methenamine (mandelate)	T37.8X1-	T37.8X2-	T37.8X3-	T37.8X4-	T37.8X5-	T37.8X6-
Methenolone	T38.7X1-	T38.7X2-	T38.7X3-	T38.7X4-	T38.7X5-	T38.7X6-
Methergine	T48.0X1-	T48.0X2-	T48.0X3-	T48.0X4-	T48.0X5-	T48.0X6-
Methetoin	T42.0X1-	T42.0X2-	T42.0X3-	T42.0X4-	T42.0X5-	T42.0X6-
Methiacil	T38.2X1-	T38.2X2-	T38.2X3-	T38.2X4-	T38.2X5-	T38.2X6-
Methicillin	T36.0X1-	T36.0X2-	T36.0X3-	T36.0X4-	T36.0X5-	T36.0X6-
Methimazole	T38.2X1-	T38.2X2-	T38.2X3-	T38.2X4-	T38.2X5-	T38.2X6-
Methiodal sodium	T50.8X1-	T50.8X2-	T50.8X3-	T50.8X4-	T50.8X5-	T50.8X6-
Methionine	T50.991-	T50.992-	T50.993-	T50.994-	T50.995-	T50.996-
Methisazone	T37.5X1-	T37.5X2-	T37.5X3-	T37.5X4-	T37.5X5-	T37.5X6-
Methisoprinol	T37.5X1-	T37.5X2-	T37.5X3-	T37.5X4-	T37.5X5-	T37.5X6-
Methitural	T42.3X1-	T42.3X2-	T42.3X3-	T42.3X4-	T42.3X5-	T42.3X6-
Methixene	T44.3X1-	T44.3X2-	T44.3X3-	T44.3X4-	T44.3X5-	T44.3X6-
Methobarbital, methobarbitone	T42.3X1-	T42.3X2-	T42.3X3-	T42.3X4-	T42.3X5-	T42.3X6-
Methocarbamol	T42.8X1-	T42.8X2-	T42.8X3-	T42.8X4-	T42.8X5-	T42.8X6-
skeletal muscle relaxant	T48.1X1-	T48.1X2-	T48.1X3-	T48.1X4-	T48.1X5-	T48.1X6-
Methohexital	T41.1X1-	T41.1X2-	T41.1X3-	T41.1X4-	T41.1X5-	T41.1X6-
Methohexitone	T41.1X1-	T41.1X2-	T41.1X3-	T41.1X4-	T41.1X5-	T41.1X6-
Methoin	T42.0X1-	T42.0X2-	T42.0X3-	T42.0X4-	T42.0X5-	T42.0X6-
Methopholine	T39.8X1-	T39.8X2-	T39.8X3-	T39.8X4-	T39.8X5-	T39.8X6-
Methopromazine	T43.3X1-	T43.3X2-	T43.3X3-	T43.3X4-	T43.3X5-	T43.3X6-
Methorate	T48.3X1-	T48.3X2-	T48.3X3-	T48.3X4-	T48.3X5-	T48.3X6-
Methoserpidine	T46.5X1-	T46.5X2-	T46.5X3-	T46.5X4-	T46.5X5-	T46.5X6-
Methotrexate	T45.1X1-	T45.1X2-	T45.1X3-	T45.1X4-	T45.1X5-	T45.1X6-
Methotrimeprazine	T43.3X1-	T43.3X2-	T43.3X3-	T43.3X4-	T43.3X5-	T43.3X6-
Methoxa-Dome	T49.3X1-	T49.3X2-	T49.3X3-	T49.3X4-	T49.3X5-	T49.3X6-
Methoxamine	T44.4X1-	T44.4X2-	T44.4X3-	T44.4X4-	T44.4X5-	T44.4X6-
Methoxsalen	T50.991-	T50.992-	T50.993-	T50.994-	T50.995-	T50.996-
Methoxyaniline	T65.3X1-	T65.3X2-	T65.3X3-	T65.3X4-	-	-
Methoxybenzyl penicillin	T36.0X1-	T36.0X2-	T36.0X3-	T36.0X4-	T36.0X5-	T36.0X6-
Methoxychlor	T53.7X1-	T53.7X2-	T53.7X3-	T53.7X4-	-	-
Methoxy-DDT	T53.7X1-	T53.7X2-	T53.7X3-	T53.7X4-	-	-
2-Methoxyethanol	T52.3X1-	T52.3X2-	T52.3X3-	T52.3X4-	-	-
Methoxyflurane	T41.0X1-	T41.0X2-	T41.0X3-	T41.0X4-	T41.0X5-	T41.0X6-
Methoxyphenamine	T48.6X1-	T48.6X2-	T48.6X3-	T48.6X4-	T48.6X5-	T48.6X6-
Methoxypromazine	T43.3X1-	T43.3X2-	T43.3X3-	T43.3X4-	T43.3X5-	T43.3X6-
5-Methoxypsoralen (5-MOP)	T50.991-	T50.992-	T50.993-	T50.994-	T50.995-	T50.996-
8-Methoxypsoralen (8-MOP)	T50.991-	T50.992-	T50.993-	T50.994-	T50.995-	T50.996-
Methscopolamine bromide	T44.3X1-	T44.3X2-	T44.3X3-	T44.3X4-	T44.3X5-	T44.3X6-
Methsuximide	T42.2X1-	T42.2X2-	T42.2X3-	T42.2X4-	T42.2X5-	T42.2X6-
Methyclothiazide	T50.2X1-	T50.2X2-	T50.2X3-	T50.2X4-	T50.2X5-	T50.2X6-

Substance	Poisoning Accidental (unintentional)	Poisoning Intentional self-harm	Poisoning Assault	Poisoning Undetermined	Adverse effect	Underdosing
Methyl						
acetate	T52.4X1-	T52.4X2-	T52.4X3-	T52.4X4-	-	-
acetone	T52.4X1-	T52.4X2-	T52.4X3-	T52.4X4-	-	-
acrylate	T65.891-	T65.892-	T65.893-	T65.894-	-	-
alcohol	T51.1X1-	T51.1X2-	T51.1X3-	T51.1X4-	-	-
aminophenol	T65.3X1-	T65.3X2-	T65.3X3-	T65.3X4-	-	-
amphetamine	T43.621-	T43.622-	T43.623-	T43.624-	T43.625-	T43.626-
androstanolone	T38.7X1-	T38.7X2-	T38.7X3-	T38.7X4-	T38.7X5-	T38.7X6-
atropine	T44.3X1-	T44.3X2-	T44.3X3-	T44.3X4-	T44.3X5-	T44.3X6-
benzene	T52.2X1-	T52.2X2-	T52.2X3-	T52.2X4-	-	-
benzoate	T52.8X1-	T52.8X2-	T52.8X3-	T52.8X4-	-	-
benzol	T52.2X1-	T52.2X2-	T52.2X3-	T52.2X4-	-	-
bromide (gas)	T59.891-	T59.892-	T59.893-	T59.894-	-	-
fumigant	T60.8X1-	T60.8X2-	T60.8X3-	T60.8X4-	-	-
butanol	T51.3X1-	T51.3X2-	T51.3X3-	T51.3X4-	-	-
carbinol	T51.1X1-	T51.1X2-	T51.1X3-	T51.1X4-	-	-
carbonate	T52.8X1-	T52.8X2-	T52.8X3-	T52.8X4-	-	-
CCNU	T45.1X1-	T45.1X2-	T45.1X3-	T45.1X4-	T45.1X5-	T45.1X6-
cellosolve	T52.91X-	T52.92X-	T52.93X-	T52.94X-	-	-
cellulose	T47.4X1-	T47.4X2-	T47.4X3-	T47.4X4-	T47.4X5-	T47.4X6-
chloride (gas)	T59.891-	T59.892-	T59.893-	T59.894-	-	-
chloroformate	T59.3X1-	T59.3X2-	T59.3X3-	T59.3X4-	-	-
cyclohexane	T52.8X1-	T52.8X2-	T52.8X3-	T52.8X4-	-	-
cyclohexanol	T51.8X1-	T51.8X2-	T51.8X3-	T51.8X4-	-	-
cyclohexanone	T52.8X1-	T52.8X2-	T52.8X3-	T52.8X4-	-	-
cyclohexyl acetate	T52.8X1-	T52.8X2-	T52.8X3-	T52.8X4-	-	-
demeton	T60.0X1-	T60.0X2-	T60.0X3-	T60.0X4-	-	-
dihydromorphinone	T40.2X1-	T40.2X2-	T40.2X3-	T40.2X4-	T40.2X5-	T40.2X6-
ergometrine	T48.0X1-	T48.0X2-	T48.0X3-	T48.0X4-	T48.0X5-	T48.0X6-
ergonovine	T48.0X1-	T48.0X2-	T48.0X3-	T48.0X4-	T48.0X5-	T48.0X6-
ethyl ketone	T52.4X1-	T52.4X2-	T52.4X3-	T52.4X4-	-	-
glucamine antimonate	T37.8X1-	T37.8X2-	T37.8X3-	T37.8X4-	T37.8X5-	T37.8X6-
hydrazine	T65.891-	T65.892-	T65.893-	T65.894-	-	-
iodide	T65.891-	T65.892-	T65.893-	T65.894-	-	-
isobutyl ketone	T52.4X1-	T52.4X2-	T52.4X3-	T52.4X4-	-	-
isothiocyanate	T60.3X1-	T60.3X2-	T60.3X3-	T60.3X4-	-	-
mercaptan	T59.891-	T59.892-	T59.893-	T59.894-	-	-
morphine NEC	T40.2X1-	T40.2X2-	T40.2X3-	T40.2X4-	T40.2X5-	T40.2X6-
nicotinate	T49.4X1-	T49.4X2-	T49.4X3-	T49.4X4-	T49.4X5-	T49.4X6-
paraben	T49.0X1-	T49.0X2-	T49.0X3-	T49.0X4-	T49.0X5-	T49.0X6-
parafynol	T42.6X1-	T42.6X2-	T42.6X3-	T42.6X4-	T42.6X5-	T42.6X6-
parathion	T60.0X1-	T60.0X2-	T60.0X3-	T60.0X4-	-	-
peridol	T43.4X1-	T43.4X2-	T43.4X3-	T43.4X4-	T43.4X5-	T43.4X6-
phenidate	T43.631-	T43.632-	T43.633-	T43.634-	T43.635-	T43.636-
prednisolone	T38.0X1-	T38.0X2-	T38.0X3-	T38.0X4-	T38.0X5-	T38.0X6-
ENT agent	T49.6X1-	T49.6X2-	T49.6X3-	T49.6X4-	T49.6X5-	T49.6X6-
ophthalmic preparation	T49.5X1-	T49.5X2-	T49.5X3-	T49.5X4-	T49.5X5-	T49.5X6-
topical NEC	T49.0X1-	T49.0X2-	T49.0X3-	T49.0X4-	T49.0X5-	T49.0X6-
propylcarbinol	T51.3X1-	T51.3X2-	T51.3X3-	T51.3X4-	-	-
rosaniline NEC	T49.0X1-	T49.0X2-	T49.0X3-	T49.0X4-	T49.0X5-	T49.0X6-
salicylate	T49.2X1-	T49.2X2-	T49.2X3-	T49.2X4-	T49.2X5-	T49.2X6-
sulfate (fumes)	T59.891-	T59.892-	T59.893-	T59.894-	-	-
liquid	T52.8X1-	T52.8X2-	T52.8X3-	T52.8X4-	-	-
sulfonal	T42.6X1-	T42.6X2-	T42.6X3-	T42.6X4-	T42.6X5-	T42.6X6-
testosterone	T38.7X1-	T38.7X2-	T38.7X3-	T38.7X4-	T38.7X5-	T38.7X6-
thiouracil	T38.2X1-	T38.2X2-	T38.2X3-	T38.2X4-	T38.2X5-	T38.2X6-
Methylamphetamine	T43.621-	T43.622-	T43.623-	T43.624-	T43.625-	T43.626-
Methylated spirit	T51.1X1-	T51.1X2-	T51.1X3-	T51.1X4-	-	-
Methylatropine nitrate	T44.3X1-	T44.3X2-	T44.3X3-	T44.3X4-	T44.3X5-	T44.3X6-

Substance	Poisoning Accidental (unintentional)	Poisoning Intentional self-harm	Poisoning Assault	Poisoning Undetermined	Adverse effect	Underdosing
Methylbenactyzium bromide	T44.3X1-	T44.3X2-	T44.3X3-	T44.3X4-	T44.3X5-	T44.3X6-
Methylbenzethonium chloride	T49.0X1-	T49.0X2-	T49.0X3-	T49.0X4-	T49.0X5-	T49.0X6-
Methylcellulose	T47.4X1-	T47.4X2-	T47.4X3-	T47.4X4-	T47.4X5-	T47.4X6-
laxative	T47.4X1-	T47.4X2-	T47.4X3-	T47.4X4-	T47.4X5-	T47.4X6-
Methylchlorophenoxy-acetic acid	T60.3X1-	T60.3X2-	T60.3X3-	T60.3X4-	-	-
Methyldopa	T46.5X1-	T46.5X2-	T46.5X3-	T46.5X4-	T46.5X5-	T46.5X6-
Methyldopate	T46.5X1-	T46.5X2-	T46.5X3-	T46.5X4-	T46.5X5-	T46.5X6-
Methylene						
blue	T50.6X1-	T50.6X2-	T50.6X3-	T50.6X4-	T50.6X5-	T50.6X6-
chloride or dichloride (solvent) NEC	T53.4X1-	T53.4X2-	T53.4X3-	T53.4X4-	-	-
Methylenedioxyamphetamine	T43.621-	T43.622-	T43.623-	T43.624-	T43.625-	T43.626-
Methylenedioxymethamphetamine	T43.641-	T43.642-	T43.643-	T43.644-	-	-
Methylergometrine	T48.0X1-	T48.0X2-	T48.0X3-	T48.0X4-	T48.0X5-	T48.0X6-
Methylergonovine	T48.0X1-	T48.0X2-	T48.0X3-	T48.0X4-	T48.0X5-	T48.0X6-
Methylestrenolone	T38.5X1-	T38.5X2-	T38.5X3-	T38.5X4-	T38.5X5-	T38.5X6-
Methylethyl cellulose	T50.991-	T50.992-	T50.993-	T50.994-	T50.995-	T50.996-
Methylhexabital	T42.3X1-	T42.3X2-	T42.3X3-	T42.3X4-	T42.3X5-	T42.3X6-
Methylmorphine	T40.2X1-	T40.2X2-	T40.2X3-	T40.2X4-	T40.2X5-	T40.2X6-
Methylparaben (ophthalmic)	T49.5X1-	T49.5X2-	T49.5X3-	T49.5X4-	T49.5X5-	T49.5X6-
Methylparafynol	T42.6X1-	T42.6X2-	T42.6X3-	T42.6X4-	T42.6X5-	T42.6X6-
Methylpentynol, methylpenthynol	T42.6X1-	T42.6X2-	T42.6X3-	T42.6X4-	T42.6X5-	T42.6X6-
Methylphenidate	T43.631-	T43.632-	T43.633-	T43.634-	T43.635-	T43.636-
Methylphenobarbital	T42.3X1-	T42.3X2-	T42.3X3-	T42.3X4-	T42.3X5-	T42.3X6-
Methylpolysiloxane	T47.1X1-	T47.1X2-	T47.1X3-	T47.1X4-	T47.1X5-	T47.1X6-
Methylprednisolone — *see Methyl, prednisolone*						
Methylrosaniline	T49.0X1-	T49.0X2-	T49.0X3-	T49.0X4-	T49.0X5-	T49.0X6-
Methylrosanilinium chloride	T49.0X1-	T49.0X2-	T49.0X3-	T49.0X4-	T49.0X5-	T49.0X6-
Methyltestosterone	T38.7X1-	T38.7X2-	T38.7X3-	T38.7X4-	T38.7X5-	T38.7X6-
Methylthionine chloride	T50.6X1-	T50.6X2-	T50.6X3-	T50.6X4-	T50.6X5-	T50.6X6-
Methylthioninium chloride	T50.6X1-	T50.6X2-	T50.6X3-	T50.6X4-	T50.6X5-	T50.6X6-
Methylthiouracil	T38.2X1-	T38.2X2-	T38.2X3-	T38.2X4-	T38.2X5-	T38.2X6-
Methyprylon	T42.6X1-	T42.6X2-	T42.6X3-	T42.6X4-	T42.6X5-	T42.6X6-
Methysergide	T46.5X1-	T46.5X2-	T46.5X3-	T46.5X4-	T46.5X5-	T46.5X6-
Metiamide	T47.1X1-	T47.1X2-	T47.1X3-	T47.1X4-	T47.1X5-	T47.1X6-
Meticillin	T36.0X1-	T36.0X2-	T36.0X3-	T36.0X4-	T36.0X5-	T36.0X6-
Meticrane	T50.2X1-	T50.2X2-	T50.2X3-	T50.2X4-	T50.2X5-	T50.2X6-
Metildigoxin	T46.0X1-	T46.0X2-	T46.0X3-	T46.0X4-	T46.0X5-	T46.0X6-
Metipranolol	T49.5X1-	T49.5X2-	T49.5X3-	T49.5X4-	T49.5X5-	T49.5X6-
Metirosine	T46.5X1-	T46.5X2-	T46.5X3-	T46.5X4-	T46.5X5-	T46.5X6-
Metisazone	T37.5X1-	T37.5X2-	T37.5X3-	T37.5X4-	T37.5X5-	T37.5X6-
Metixene	T44.3X1-	T44.3X2-	T44.3X3-	T44.3X4-	T44.3X5-	T44.3X6-
Metizoline	T48.5X1-	T48.5X2-	T48.5X3-	T48.5X4-	T48.5X5-	T48.5X6-
Metoclopramide	T45.0X1-	T45.0X2-	T45.0X3-	T45.0X4-	T45.0X5-	T45.0X6-
Metofenazate	T43.3X1-	T43.3X2-	T43.3X3-	T43.3X4-	T43.3X5-	T43.3X6-
Metofoline	T39.8X1-	T39.8X2-	T39.8X3-	T39.8X4-	T39.8X5-	T39.8X6-
Metolazone	T50.2X1-	T50.2X2-	T50.2X3-	T50.2X4-	T50.2X5-	T50.2X6-
Metopon	T40.2X1-	T40.2X2-	T40.2X3-	T40.2X4-	T40.2X5-	T40.2X6-
Metoprine	T45.1X1-	T45.1X2-	T45.1X3-	T45.1X4-	T45.1X5-	T45.1X6-
Metoprolol	T44.7X1-	T44.7X2-	T44.7X3-	T44.7X4-	T44.7X5-	T44.7X6-
Metrifonate	T60.0X1-	T60.0X2-	T60.0X3-	T60.0X4-	-	-
Metrizamide	T50.8X1-	T50.8X2-	T50.8X3-	T50.8X4-	T50.8X5-	T50.8X6-
Metrizoic acid	T50.8X1-	T50.8X2-	T50.8X3-	T50.8X4-	T50.8X5-	T50.8X6-
Metronidazole	T37.8X1-	T37.8X2-	T37.8X3-	T37.8X4-	T37.8X5-	T37.8X6-
Metycaine	T41.3X1-	T41.3X2-	T41.3X3-	T41.3X4-	T41.3X5-	T41.3X6-
infiltration (subcutaneous)	T41.3X1-	T41.3X2-	T41.3X3-	T41.3X4-	T41.3X5-	T41.3X6-
nerve block (peripheral) (plexus)	T41.3X1-	T41.3X2-	T41.3X3-	T41.3X4-	T41.3X5-	T41.3X6-
topical (surface)	T41.3X1-	T41.3X2-	T41.3X3-	T41.3X4-	T41.3X5-	T41.3X6-
Metyrapone	T50.8X1-	T50.8X2-	T50.8X3-	T50.8X4-	T50.8X5-	T50.8X6-

Substance	Poisoning Accidental (unintentional)	Poisoning Intentional self-harm	Poisoning Assault	Poisoning Undetermined	Adverse effect	Underdosing
Mevinphos	T60.0X1-	T60.0X2-	T60.0X3-	T60.0X4-	-	-
Mexazolam	T42.4X1-	T42.4X2-	T42.4X3-	T42.4X4-	T42.4X5-	T42.4X6-
Mexenone	T49.3X1-	T49.3X2-	T49.3X3-	T49.3X4-	T49.3X5-	T49.3X6-
Mexiletine	T46.2X1-	T46.2X2-	T46.2X3-	T46.2X4-	T46.2X5-	T46.2X6-
Mezereon	T62.2X1-	T62.2X2-	T62.2X3-	T62.2X4-	-	-
berries	T62.1X1-	T62.1X2-	T62.1X3-	T62.1X4-	-	-
Mezlocillin	T36.0X1-	T36.0X2-	T36.0X3-	T36.0X4-	T36.0X5-	T36.0X6-
Mianserin	T43.021-	T43.022-	T43.023-	T43.024-	T43.025-	T43.026-
Micatin	T49.0X1-	T49.0X2-	T49.0X3-	T49.0X4-	T49.0X5-	T49.0X6-
Miconazole	T49.0X1-	T49.0X2-	T49.0X3-	T49.0X4-	T49.0X5-	T49.0X6-
Micronomicin	T36.5X1-	T36.5X2-	T36.5X3-	T36.5X4-	T36.5X5-	T36.5X6-
Midazolam	T42.4X1-	T42.4X2-	T42.4X3-	T42.4X4-	T42.4X5-	T42.4X6-
Midecamycin	T36.3X1-	T36.3X2-	T36.3X3-	T36.3X4-	T36.3X5-	T36.3X6-
Mifepristone	T38.6X1-	T38.6X2-	T38.6X3-	T38.6X4-	T38.6X5-	T38.6X6-
Milk of magnesia	T47.1X1-	T47.1X2-	T47.1X3-	T47.1X4-	T47.1X5-	T47.1X6-
Millipede (tropical) (venomous)	T63.411-	T63.412-	T63.413-	T63.414-	-	-
Miltown	T43.591-	T43.592-	T43.593-	T43.594-	T43.595-	T43.596-
Milverine	T44.3X1-	T44.3X2-	T44.3X3-	T44.3X4-	T44.3X5-	T44.3X6-
Minaprine	T43.291-	T43.292-	T43.293-	T43.294-	T43.295-	T43.296-
Minaxolone	T41.291-	T41.292-	T41.293-	T41.294-	T41.295-	T41.296-
Mineral						
acids	T54.2X1-	T54.2X2-	T54.2X3-	T54.2X4-	-	-
oil (laxative) (medicinal)	T47.4X1-	T47.4X2-	T47.4X3-	T47.4X4-	T47.4X5-	T47.4X6-
emulsion	T47.2X1-	T47.2X2-	T47.2X3-	T47.2X4-	T47.2X5-	T47.2X6-
nonmedicinal	T52.0X1-	T52.0X2-	T52.0X3-	T52.0X4-	-	-
topical	T49.3X1-	T49.3X2-	T49.3X3-	T49.3X4-	T49.3X5-	T49.3X6-
salt NEC	T50.3X1-	T50.3X2-	T50.3X3-	T50.3X4-	T50.3X5-	T50.3X6-
spirits	T52.0X1-	T52.0X2-	T52.0X3-	T52.0X4-	-	-
Mineralocorticosteroid	T50.0X1-	T50.0X2-	T50.0X3-	T50.0X4-	T50.0X5-	T50.0X6-
Minocycline	T36.4X1-	T36.4X2-	T36.4X3-	T36.4X4-	T36.4X5-	T36.4X6-
Minoxidil	T46.7X1-	T46.7X2-	T46.7X3-	T46.7X4-	T46.7X5-	T46.7X6-
Miokamycin	T36.3X1-	T36.3X2-	T36.3X3-	T36.3X4-	T36.3X5-	T36.3X6-
Miotic drug	T49.5X1-	T49.5X2-	T49.5X3-	T49.5X4-	T49.5X5-	T49.5X6-
Mipafox	T60.0X1-	T60.0X2-	T60.0X3-	T60.0X4-	-	-
Mirex	T60.1X1-	T60.1X2-	T60.1X3-	T60.1X4-	-	-
Mirtazapine	T43.021-	T43.022-	T43.023-	T43.024-	T43.025-	T43.026-
Misonidazole	T37.3X1-	T37.3X2-	T37.3X3-	T37.3X4-	T37.3X5-	T37.3X6-
Misoprostol	T47.1X1-	T47.1X2-	T47.1X3-	T47.1X4-	T47.1X5-	T47.1X6-
Mithramycin	T45.1X1-	T45.1X2-	T45.1X3-	T45.1X4-	T45.1X5-	T45.1X6-
Mitobronitol	T45.1X1-	T45.1X2-	T45.1X3-	T45.1X4-	T45.1X5-	T45.1X6-
Mitoguazone	T45.1X1-	T45.1X2-	T45.1X3-	T45.1X4-	T45.1X5-	T45.1X6-
Mitolactol	T45.1X1-	T45.1X2-	T45.1X3-	T45.1X4-	T45.1X5-	T45.1X6-
Mitomycin	T45.1X1-	T45.1X2-	T45.1X3-	T45.1X4-	T45.1X5-	T45.1X6-
Mitopodozide	T45.1X1-	T45.1X2-	T45.1X3-	T45.1X4-	T45.1X5-	T45.1X6-
Mitotane	T45.1X1-	T45.1X2-	T45.1X3-	T45.1X4-	T45.1X5-	T45.1X6-
Mitoxantrone	T45.1X1-	T45.1X2-	T45.1X3-	T45.1X4-	T45.1X5-	T45.1X6-
Mivacurium chloride	T48.1X1-	T48.1X2-	T48.1X3-	T48.1X4-	T48.1X5-	T48.1X6-
Miyari bacteria	T47.6X1-	T47.6X2-	T47.6X3-	T47.6X4-	T47.6X5-	T47.6X6-
Moclobemide	T43.1X1-	T43.1X2-	T43.1X3-	T43.1X4-	T43.1X5-	T43.1X6-
Moderil	T46.5X1-	T46.5X2-	T46.5X3-	T46.5X4-	T46.5X5-	T46.5X6-
Mofebutazone	T39.2X1-	T39.2X2-	T39.2X3-	T39.2X4-	T39.2X5-	T39.2X6-
Mogadon — *see Nitrazepam*						
Molindone	T43.591-	T43.592-	T43.593-	T43.594-	T43.595-	T43.596-
Molsidomine	T46.3X1-	T46.3X2-	T46.3X3-	T46.3X4-	T46.3X5-	T46.3X6-
Mometasone	T49.0X1-	T49.0X2-	T49.0X3-	T49.0X4-	T49.0X5-	T49.0X6-
Monistat	T49.0X1-	T49.0X2-	T49.0X3-	T49.0X4-	T49.0X5-	T49.0X6-
Monkshood	T62.2X1-	T62.2X2-	T62.2X3-	T62.2X4-	-	-
Monoamine oxidase inhibitor NEC	T43.1X1-	T43.1X2-	T43.1X3-	T43.1X4-	T43.1X5-	T43.1X6-
hydrazine	T43.1X1-	T43.1X2-	T43.1X3-	T43.1X4-	T43.1X5-	T43.1X6-

Substance	Poisoning Accidental (unintentional)	Poisoning Intentional self-harm	Poisoning Assault	Poisoning Undetermined	Adverse effect	Underdosing
Monobenzone	T49.4X1-	T49.4X2-	T49.4X3-	T49.4X4-	T49.4X5-	T49.4X6-
Monochloroacetic acid	T60.3X1-	T60.3X2-	T60.3X3-	T60.3X4-	-	-
Monochlorobenzene	T53.7X1-	T53.7X2-	T53.7X3-	T53.7X4-	-	-
Monoethanolamine	T46.8X1-	T46.8X2-	T46.8X3-	T46.8X4-	T46.8X5-	T46.8X6-
oleate	T46.8X1-	T46.8X2-	T46.8X3-	T46.8X4-	T46.8X5-	T46.8X6-
Monooctanoin	T50.991-	T50.992-	T50.993-	T50.994-	T50.995-	T50.996-
Monophenylbutazone	T39.2X1-	T39.2X2-	T39.2X3-	T39.2X4-	T39.2X5-	T39.2X6-
Monosodium glutamate	T65.891-	T65.892-	T65.893-	T65.894-	-	-
Monosulfiram	T49.0X1-	T49.0X2-	T49.0X3-	T49.0X4-	T49.0X5-	T49.0X6-
Monoxide, carbon — *see Carbon, monoxide*						
Monoxidine hydrochloride	T46.1X1-	T46.1X2-	T46.1X3-	T46.1X4-	T46.1X5-	T46.1X6-
Monuron	T60.3X1-	T60.3X2-	T60.3X3-	T60.3X4-	-	-
Moperone	T43.4X1-	T43.4X2-	T43.4X3-	T43.4X4-	T43.4X5-	T43.4X6-
Mopidamol	T45.1X1-	T45.1X2-	T45.1X3-	T45.1X4-	T45.1X5-	T45.1X6-
MOPP (mechloreth-amine + vincristine + prednisone + procarba-zine)	T45.1X1-	T45.1X2-	T45.1X3-	T45.1X4-	T45.1X5-	T45.1X6-
Morfin	T40.2X1-	T40.2X2-	T40.2X3-	T40.2X4-	T40.2X5-	T40.2X6-
Morinamide	T37.1X1-	T37.1X2-	T37.1X3-	T37.1X4-	T37.1X5-	T37.1X6-
Morning glory seeds	T40.991-	T40.992-	T40.993-	T40.994-	-	-
Moroxydine	T37.5X1-	T37.5X2-	T37.5X3-	T37.5X4-	T37.5X5-	T37.5X6-
Morphazinamide	T37.1X1-	T37.1X2-	T37.1X3-	T37.1X4-	T37.1X5-	T37.1X6-
Morphine	T40.2X1-	T40.2X2-	T40.2X3-	T40.2X4-	T40.2X5-	T40.2X6-
antagonist	T50.7X1-	T50.7X2-	T50.7X3-	T50.7X4-	T50.7X5-	T50.7X6-
Morpholinylethylmorphine	T40.2X1-	T40.2X2-	T40.2X3-	T40.2X4-	-	-
Morsuximide	T42.2X1-	T42.2X2-	T42.2X3-	T42.2X4-	T42.2X5-	T42.2X6-
Mosapramine	T43.591-	T43.592-	T43.593-	T43.594-	T43.595-	T43.596-
Moth balls — *see also Pesticides*	T60.2X1-	T60.2X2-	T60.2X3-	T60.2X4-	-	-
naphthalene	T60.2X1-	T60.2X2-	T60.2X3-	T60.2X4-	-	-
paradichlorobenzene	T60.1X1-	T60.1X2-	T60.1X3-	T60.1X4-	-	-
Motor exhaust gas	T58.01X-	T58.02X-	T58.03X-	T58.04X-	-	-
Mouthwash (antiseptic) (zinc chloride)	T49.6X1-	T49.6X2-	T49.6X3-	T49.6X4-	T49.6X5-	T49.6X6-
Moxastine	T45.0X1-	T45.0X2-	T45.0X3-	T45.0X4-	T45.0X5-	T45.0X6-
Moxaverine	T44.3X1-	T44.3X2-	T44.3X3-	T44.3X4-	T44.3X5-	T44.3X6-
Moxisylyte	T46.7X1-	T46.7X2-	T46.7X3-	T46.7X4-	T46.7X5-	T46.7X6-
Mucilage, plant	T47.4X1-	T47.4X2-	T47.4X3-	T47.4X4-	T47.4X5-	T47.4X6-
Mucolytic drug	T48.4X1-	T48.4X2-	T48.4X3-	T48.4X4-	T48.4X5-	T48.4X6-
Mucomyst	T48.4X1-	T48.4X2-	T48.4X3-	T48.4X4-	T48.4X5-	T48.4X6-
Mucous membrane agents (external)	T49.91X-	T49.92X-	T49.93X-	T49.94X-	T49.95X-	T49.96X-
specified NEC	T49.8X1-	T49.8X2-	T49.8X3-	T49.8X4-	T49.8X5-	T49.8X6-
Multiple unspecified drugs, medicaments and biological substances	T50.911-	T50.912-	T50.913-	T50.914-	T50.915-	T50.916-
Mumps						
immune globulin (human)	T50.Z11-	T50.Z12-	T50.Z13-	T50.Z14-	T50.Z15-	T50.Z16-
skin test antigen	T50.8X1-	T50.8X2-	T50.8X3-	T50.8X4-	T50.8X5-	T50.8X6-
vaccine	T50.B91-	T50.B92-	T50.B93-	T50.B94-	T50.B95-	T50.B96-
Mumpsvax	T50.B91-	T50.B92-	T50.B93-	T50.B94-	T50.B95-	T50.B96-
Mupirocin	T49.0X1-	T49.0X2-	T49.0X3-	T49.0X4-	T49.0X5-	T49.0X6-
Muriatic acid — *see Hydrochloric acid*						
Muromonab-CD3	T45.1X1-	T45.1X2-	T45.1X3-	T45.1X4-	T45.1X5-	T45.1X6-
Muscle-action drug NEC	T48.201-	T48.202-	T48.203-	T48.204-	T48.205-	T48.206-
Muscle affecting agents NEC	T48.201-	T48.202-	T48.203-	T48.204-	T48.205-	T48.206-
oxytocic	T48.0X1-	T48.0X2-	T48.0X3-	T48.0X4-	T48.0X5-	T48.0X6-
relaxants	T48.201-	T48.202-	T48.203-	T48.204-	T48.205-	T48.206-
central nervous system	T42.8X1-	T42.8X2-	T42.8X3-	T42.8X4-	T42.8X5-	T42.8X6-
skeletal	T48.1X1-	T48.1X2-	T48.1X3-	T48.1X4-	T48.1X5-	T48.1X6-
smooth	T44.3X1-	T44.3X2-	T44.3X3-	T44.3X4-	T44.3X5-	T44.3X6-

Substance	Poisoning Accidental (unintentional)	Poisoning Intentional self-harm	Poisoning Assault	Poisoning Undetermined	Adverse effect	Underdosing
Muscle relaxant — *see Relaxant, muscle*						
Muscle-tone depressant, central NEC	T42.8X1-	T42.8X2-	T42.8X3-	T42.8X4-	T42.8X5-	T42.8X6-
specified NEC	T42.8X1-	T42.8X2-	T42.8X3-	T42.8X4-	T42.8X5-	T42.8X6-
Mushroom, noxious	T62.0X1-	T62.0X2-	T62.0X3-	T62.0X4-	-	-
Mussel, noxious	T61.781-	T61.782-	T61.783-	T61.784-	-	-
Mustard (emetic)	T47.7X1-	T47.7X2-	T47.7X3-	T47.7X4-	T47.7X5-	T47.7X6-
black	T47.7X1-	T47.7X2-	T47.7X3-	T47.7X4-	T47.7X5-	T47.7X6-
gas, not in war	T59.91X-	T59.92X-	T59.93X-	T59.94X-	-	-
nitrogen	T45.1X1-	T45.1X2-	T45.1X3-	T45.1X4-	T45.1X5-	T45.1X6-
Mustine	T45.1X1-	T45.1X2-	T45.1X3-	T45.1X4-	T45.1X5-	T45.1X6-
M-vac	T45.1X1-	T45.1X2-	T45.1X3-	T45.1X4-	T45.1X5-	T45.1X6-
Mycifradin	T36.5X1-	T36.5X2-	T36.5X3-	T36.5X4-	T36.5X5-	T36.5X6-
topical	T49.0X1-	T49.0X2-	T49.0X3-	T49.0X4-	T49.0X5-	T49.0X6-
Mycitracin	T36.8X1-	T36.8X2-	T36.8X3-	T36.8X4-	T36.8X5-	T36.8X6-
ophthalmic preparation	T49.5X1-	T49.5X2-	T49.5X3-	T49.5X4-	T49.5X5-	T49.5X6-
Mycostatin	T36.7X1-	T36.7X2-	T36.7X3-	T36.7X4-	T36.7X5-	T36.7X6-
topical	T49.0X1-	T49.0X2-	T49.0X3-	T49.0X4-	T49.0X5-	T49.0X6-
Mycotoxins	T64.81X-	T64.82X-	T64.83X-	T64.84X-	-	-
aflatoxin	T64.01X-	T64.02X-	T64.03X-	T64.04X-	-	-
specified NEC	T64.81X-	T64.82X-	T64.83X-	T64.84X-	-	-
Mydriacyl	T44.3X1-	T44.3X2-	T44.3X3-	T44.3X4-	T44.3X5-	T44.3X6-
Mydriatic drug	T49.5X1-	T49.5X2-	T49.5X3-	T49.5X4-	T49.5X5-	T49.5X6-
Myelobromal	T45.1X1-	T45.1X2-	T45.1X3-	T45.1X4-	T45.1X5-	T45.1X6-
Myleran	T45.1X1-	T45.1X2-	T45.1X3-	T45.1X4-	T45.1X5-	T45.1X6-
Myochrysin (e)	T39.2X1-	T39.2X2-	T39.2X3-	T39.2X4-	T39.2X5-	T39.2X6-
Myoneural blocking agents	T48.1X1-	T48.1X2-	T48.1X3-	T48.1X4-	T48.1X5-	T48.1X6-
Myralact	T49.0X1-	T49.0X2-	T49.0X3-	T49.0X4-	T49.0X5-	T49.0X6-
Myristica fragrans	T62.2X1-	T62.2X2-	T62.2X3-	T62.2X4-	-	-
Myristicin	T65.891-	T65.892-	T65.893-	T65.894-	-	-
Mysoline	T42.3X1-	T42.3X2-	T42.3X3-	T42.3X4-	T42.3X5-	T42.3X6-
Nabilone	T40.711-	T40.712-	T40.713-	T40.714-	T40.715-	T40.716-
Nabumetone	T39.391-	T39.392-	T39.393-	T39.394-	T39.395-	T39.396-
Nadolol	T44.7X1-	T44.7X2-	T44.7X3-	T44.7X4-	T44.7X5-	T44.7X6-
Nafcillin	T36.0X1-	T36.0X2-	T36.0X3-	T36.0X4-	T36.0X5-	T36.0X6-
Nafoxidine	T38.6X1-	T38.6X2-	T38.6X3-	T38.6X4-	T38.6X5-	T38.6X6-
Naftazone	T46.991-	T46.992-	T46.993-	T46.994-	T46.995-	T46.996-
Naftidrofuryl (oxalate)	T46.7X1-	T46.7X2-	T46.7X3-	T46.7X4-	T46.7X5-	T46.7X6-
Naftifine	T49.0X1-	T49.0X2-	T49.0X3-	T49.0X4-	T49.0X5-	T49.0X6-
Nail polish remover	T52.91X-	T52.92X-	T52.93X-	T52.94X-	-	-
Nalbuphine	T40.491-	T40.492-	T40.493-	T40.494-	T40.495-	T40.496-
Naled	T60.0X1-	T60.0X2-	T60.0X3-	T60.0X4-	-	-
Nalidixic acid	T37.8X1-	T37.8X2-	T37.8X3-	T37.8X4-	T37.8X5-	T37.8X6-
Nalorphine	T50.7X1-	T50.7X2-	T50.7X3-	T50.7X4-	T50.7X5-	T50.7X6-
Naloxone	T50.7X1-	T50.7X2-	T50.7X3-	T50.7X4-	T50.7X5-	T50.7X6-
Naltrexone	T50.7X1-	T50.7X2-	T50.7X3-	T50.7X4-	T50.7X5-	T50.7X6-
Namenda	T43.8X1-	T43.8X2-	T43.8X3-	T43.8X4-	T43.8X5-	T43.8X6-
Nandrolone	T38.7X1-	T38.7X2-	T38.7X3-	T38.7X4-	T38.7X5-	T38.7X6-
Naphazoline	T48.5X1-	T48.5X2-	T48.5X3-	T48.5X4-	T48.5X5-	T48.5X6-
Naphtha (painters') (petroleum)	T52.0X1-	T52.0X2-	T52.0X3-	T52.0X4-	-	-
solvent	T52.0X1-	T52.0X2-	T52.0X3-	T52.0X4-	-	-
vapor	T52.0X1-	T52.0X2-	T52.0X3-	T52.0X4-	-	-
Naphthalene (non-chlorinated)	T60.2X1-	T60.2X2-	T60.2X3-	T60.2X4-	-	-
chlorinated	T60.1X1-	T60.1X2-	T60.1X3-	T60.1X4-	-	-
vapor	T60.1X1-	T60.1X2-	T60.1X3-	T60.1X4-	-	-
insecticide or moth repellent	T60.2X1-	T60.2X2-	T60.2X3-	T60.2X4-	-	-
chlorinated	T60.1X1-	T60.1X2-	T60.1X3-	T60.1X4-	-	-
vapor	T60.2X1-	T60.2X2-	T60.2X3-	T60.2X4-	-	-
chlorinated	T60.1X1-	T60.1X2-	T60.1X3-	T60.1X4-	-	-

Substance	Poisoning Accidental (unintentional)	Poisoning Intentional self-harm	Poisoning Assault	Poisoning Undetermined	Adverse effect	Underdosing
Naphthol	T65.891-	T65.892-	T65.893-	T65.894-	-	-
Naphthylamine	T65.891-	T65.892-	T65.893-	T65.894-	-	-
Naphthylthiourea (ANTU)	T60.4X1-	T60.4X2-	T60.4X3-	T60.4X4-	-	-
Naprosyn — *see Naproxen*						
Naproxen	T39.311-	T39.312-	T39.313-	T39.314-	T39.315-	T39.316-
Narcotic (drug)	T40.601-	T40.602-	T40.603-	T40.604-	T40.605-	T40.606-
analgesic NEC	T40.601-	T40.602-	T40.603-	T40.604-	T40.605-	T40.606-
antagonist	T50.7X1-	T50.7X2-	T50.7X3-	T50.7X4-	T50.7X5-	T50.7X6-
specified NEC	T40.691-	T40.692-	T40.693-	T40.694-	T40.695-	T40.696-
synthetic	T40.491-	T40.492-	T40.493-	T40.494-	T40.495-	T40.496-
Narcotine	T48.3X1-	T48.3X2-	T48.3X3-	T48.3X4-	T48.3X5-	T48.3X6-
Nardil	T43.1X1-	T43.1X2-	T43.1X3-	T43.1X4-	T43.1X5-	T43.1X6-
Nasal drug NEC	T49.6X1-	T49.6X2-	T49.6X3-	T49.6X4-	T49.6X5-	T49.6X6-
Natamycin	T49.0X1-	T49.0X2-	T49.0X3-	T49.0X4-	T49.0X5-	T49.0X6-
Natrium cyanide — *see Cyanide(s)*						
Natural						
blood (product)	T45.8X1-	T45.8X2-	T45.8X3-	T45.8X4-	T45.8X5-	T45.8X6-
gas (piped)	T59.891-	T59.892-	T59.893-	T59.894-	-	-
incomplete combustion	T58.11X-	T58.12X-	T58.13X-	T58.14X-	-	-
Nealbarbital	T42.3X1-	T42.3X2-	T42.3X3-	T42.3X4-	T42.3X5-	T42.3X6-
Nectadon	T48.3X1-	T48.3X2-	T48.3X3-	T48.3X4-	T48.3X5-	T48.3X6-
Nedocromil	T48.6X1-	T48.6X2-	T48.6X3-	T48.6X4-	T48.6X5-	T48.6X6-
Nefopam	T39.8X1-	T39.8X2-	T39.8X3-	T39.8X4-	T39.8X5-	T39.8X6-
Nematocyst (sting)	T63.691-	T63.692-	T63.693-	T63.694-	-	-
Nembutal	T42.3X1-	T42.3X2-	T42.3X3-	T42.3X4-	T42.3X5-	T42.3X6-
Nemonapride	T43.591-	T43.592-	T43.593-	T43.594-	T43.595-	T43.596-
Neoarsphenamine	T37.8X1-	T37.8X2-	T37.8X3-	T37.8X4-	T37.8X5-	T37.8X6-
Neocinchophen	T50.4X1-	T50.4X2-	T50.4X3-	T50.4X4-	T50.4X5-	T50.4X6-
Neomycin (derivatives)	T36.5X1-	T36.5X2-	T36.5X3-	T36.5X4-	T36.5X5-	T36.5X6-
with						
bacitracin	T49.0X1-	T49.0X2-	T49.0X3-	T49.0X4-	T49.0X5-	T49.0X6-
neostigmine	T44.0X1-	T44.0X2-	T44.0X3-	T44.0X4-	T44.0X5-	T44.0X6-
ENT agent	T49.6X1-	T49.6X2-	T49.6X3-	T49.6X4-	T49.6X5-	T49.6X6-
ophthalmic preparation	T49.5X1-	T49.5X2-	T49.5X3-	T49.5X4-	T49.5X5-	T49.5X6-
topical NEC	T49.0X1-	T49.0X2-	T49.0X3-	T49.0X4-	T49.0X5-	T49.0X6-
Neonal	T42.3X1-	T42.3X2-	T42.3X3-	T42.3X4-	T42.3X5-	T42.3X6-
Neoprontosil	T37.0X1-	T37.0X2-	T37.0X3-	T37.0X4-	T37.0X5-	T37.0X6-
Neosalvarsan	T37.8X1-	T37.8X2-	T37.8X3-	T37.8X4-	T37.8X5-	T37.8X6-
Neosilversalvarsan	T37.8X1-	T37.8X2-	T37.8X3-	T37.8X4-	T37.8X5-	T37.8X6-
Neosporin	T36.8X1-	T36.8X2-	T36.8X3-	T36.8X4-	T36.8X5-	T36.8X6-
ENT agent	T49.6X1-	T49.6X2-	T49.6X3-	T49.6X4-	T49.6X5-	T49.6X6-
opthalmic preparation	T49.5X1-	T49.5X2-	T49.5X3-	T49.5X4-	T49.5X5-	T49.5X6-
topical NEC	T49.0X1-	T49.0X2-	T49.0X3-	T49.0X4-	T49.0X5-	T49.0X6-
Neostigmine bromide	T44.0X1-	T44.0X2-	T44.0X3-	T44.0X4-	T44.0X5-	T44.0X6-
Neraval	T42.3X1-	T42.3X2-	T42.3X3-	T42.3X4-	T42.3X5-	T42.3X6-
Neravan	T42.3X1-	T42.3X2-	T42.3X3-	T42.3X4-	T42.3X5-	T42.3X6-
Nerium oleander	T62.2X1-	T62.2X2-	T62.2X3-	T62.2X4-	-	-
Nerve gas, not in war	T59.91X-	T59.92X-	T59.93X-	T59.94X-	-	-
Nesacaine	T41.3X1-	T41.3X2-	T41.3X3-	T41.3X4-	T41.3X5-	T41.3X6-
infiltration (subcutaneous)	T41.3X1-	T41.3X2-	T41.3X3-	T41.3X4-	T41.3X5-	T41.3X6-
nerve block (peripheral) (plexus)	T41.3X1-	T41.3X2-	T41.3X3-	T41.3X4-	T41.3X5-	T41.3X6-
Netilmicin	T36.5X1-	T36.5X2-	T36.5X3-	T36.5X4-	T36.5X5-	T36.5X6-
Neurobarb	T42.3X1-	T42.3X2-	T42.3X3-	T42.3X4-	T42.3X5-	T42.3X6-
Neuroleptic drug NEC	T43.501-	T43.502-	T43.503-	T43.504-	T43.505-	T43.506-
Neuromuscular blocking drug	T48.1X1-	T48.1X2-	T48.1X3-	T48.1X4-	T48.1X5-	T48.1X6-
Neutral insulin injection	T38.3X1-	T38.3X2-	T38.3X3-	T38.3X4-	T38.3X5-	T38.3X6-
Neutral spirits	T51.0X1-	T51.0X2-	T51.0X3-	T51.0X4-	-	-
beverage	T51.0X1-	T51.0X2-	T51.0X3-	T51.0X4-	-	-

Substance	Poisoning Accidental (unintentional)	Poisoning Intentional self-harm	Poisoning Assault	Poisoning Undetermined	Adverse effect	Underdosing
Niacin	T46.7X1-	T46.7X2-	T46.7X3-	T46.7X4-	T46.7X5-	T46.7X6-
Niacinamide	T45.2X1-	T45.2X2-	T45.2X3-	T45.2X4-	T45.2X5-	T45.2X6-
Nialamide	T43.1X1-	T43.1X2-	T43.1X3-	T43.1X4-	T43.1X5-	T43.1X6-
Niaprazine	T42.6X1-	T42.6X2-	T42.6X3-	T42.6X4-	T42.6X5-	T42.6X6-
Nicametate	T46.7X1-	T46.7X2-	T46.7X3-	T46.7X4-	T46.7X5-	T46.7X6-
Nicardipine	T46.1X1-	T46.1X2-	T46.1X3-	T46.1X4-	T46.1X5-	T46.1X6-
Nicergoline	T46.7X1-	T46.7X2-	T46.7X3-	T46.7X4-	T46.7X5-	T46.7X6-
Nickel (carbonyl) (tetra-carbonyl) (fumes) (vapor)	T56.891-	T56.892-	T56.893-	T56.894-	-	-
Nickelocene	T56.891-	T56.892-	T56.893-	T56.894-	-	-
Niclosamide	T37.4X1-	T37.4X2-	T37.4X3-	T37.4X4-	T37.4X5-	T37.4X6-
Nicofuranose	T46.7X1-	T46.7X2-	T46.7X3-	T46.7X4-	T46.7X5-	T46.7X6-
Nicomorphine	T40.2X1-	T40.2X2-	T40.2X3-	T40.2X4-	-	-
Nicorandil	T46.3X1-	T46.3X2-	T46.3X3-	T46.3X4-	T46.3X5-	T46.3X6-
Nicotiana (plant)	T62.2X1-	T62.2X2-	T62.2X3-	T62.2X4-	-	-
Nicotinamide	T45.2X1-	T45.2X2-	T45.2X3-	T45.2X4-	T45.2X5-	T45.2X6-
Nicotine (insecticide) (spray) (sulfate) NEC	T60.2X1-	T60.2X2-	T60.2X3-	T60.2X4-	-	-
from tobacco	T65.291-	T65.292-	T65.293-	T65.294-	-	-
cigarettes	T65.221-	T65.222-	T65.223-	T65.224-	-	-
not insecticide	T65.291-	T65.292-	T65.293-	T65.294-	-	-
Nicotinic acid	T46.7X1-	T46.7X2-	T46.7X3-	T46.7X4-	T46.7X5-	T46.7X6-
Nicotinyl alcohol	T46.7X1-	T46.7X2-	T46.7X3-	T46.7X4-	T46.7X5-	T46.7X6-
Nicoumalone	T45.511-	T45.512-	T45.513-	T45.514-	T45.515-	T45.516-
Nifedipine	T46.1X1-	T46.1X2-	T46.1X3-	T46.1X4-	T46.1X5-	T46.1X6-
Nifenazone	T39.2X1-	T39.2X2-	T39.2X3-	T39.2X4-	T39.2X5-	T39.2X6-
Nifuraldezone	T37.91X-	T37.92X-	T37.93X-	T37.94X-	T37.95X-	T37.96X-
Nifuratel	T37.8X1-	T37.8X2-	T37.8X3-	T37.8X4-	T37.8X5-	T37.8X6-
Nifurtimox	T37.3X1-	T37.3X2-	T37.3X3-	T37.3X4-	T37.3X5-	T37.3X6-
Nifurtoinol	T37.8X1-	T37.8X2-	T37.8X3-	T37.8X4-	T37.8X5-	T37.8X6-
Nightshade, deadly (solanum) — *see also Belladonna*	T62.2X1-	T62.2X2-	T62.2X3-	T62.2X4-	-	-
berry	T62.1X1-	T62.1X2-	T62.1X3-	T62.1X4-	-	-
Nikethamide	T50.7X1-	T50.7X2-	T50.7X3-	T50.7X4-	T50.7X5-	T50.7X6-
Nilstat	T36.7X1-	T36.7X2-	T36.7X3-	T36.7X4-	T36.7X5-	T36.7X6-
topical	T49.0X1-	T49.0X2-	T49.0X3-	T49.0X4-	T49.0X5-	T49.0X6-
Nilutamide	T38.6X1-	T38.6X2-	T38.6X3-	T38.6X4-	T38.6X5-	T38.6X6-
Nimesulide	T39.391-	T39.392-	T39.393-	T39.394-	T39.395-	T39.396-
Nimetazepam	T42.4X1-	T42.4X2-	T42.4X3-	T42.4X4-	T42.4X5-	T42.4X6-
Nimodipine	T46.1X1-	T46.1X2-	T46.1X3-	T46.1X4-	T46.1X5-	T46.1X6-
Nimorazole	T37.3X1-	T37.3X2-	T37.3X3-	T37.3X4-	T37.3X5-	T37.3X6-
Nimustine	T45.1X1-	T45.1X2-	T45.1X3-	T45.1X4-	T45.1X5-	T45.1X6-
Niridazole	T37.4X1-	T37.4X2-	T37.4X3-	T37.4X4-	T37.4X5-	T37.4X6-
Nisentil	T40.2X1-	T40.2X2-	T40.2X3-	T40.2X4-	T40.2X5-	T40.2X6-
Nisoldipine	T46.1X1-	T46.1X2-	T46.1X3-	T46.1X4-	T46.1X5-	T46.1X6-
Nitramine	T65.3X1-	T65.3X2-	T65.3X3-	T65.3X4-	-	-
Nitrate, organic	T46.3X1-	T46.3X2-	T46.3X3-	T46.3X4-	T46.3X5-	T46.3X6-
Nitrazepam	T42.4X1-	T42.4X2-	T42.4X3-	T42.4X4-	T42.4X5-	T42.4X6-
Nitrefazole	T50.6X1-	T50.6X2-	T50.6X3-	T50.6X4-	T50.6X5-	T50.6X6-
Nitrendipine	T46.1X1-	T46.1X2-	T46.1X3-	T46.1X4-	T46.1X5-	T46.1X6-
Nitric						
acid (liquid)	T54.2X1-	T54.2X2-	T54.2X3-	T54.2X4-	-	-
vapor	T59.891-	T59.892-	T59.893-	T59.894-	-	-
oxide (gas)	T59.0X1-	T59.0X2-	T59.0X3-	T59.0X4-	-	-
Nitrimidazine	T37.3X1-	T37.3X2-	T37.3X3-	T37.3X4-	T37.3X5-	T37.3X6-
Nitrite, amyl (medicinal) (vapor)	T46.3X1-	T46.3X2-	T46.3X3-	T46.3X4-	T46.3X5-	T46.3X6-
Nitroaniline	T65.3X1-	T65.3X2-	T65.3X3-	T65.3X4-	-	-
vapor	T59.891-	T59.892-	T59.893-	T59.894-	-	-

Substance	Poisoning Accidental (unintentional)	Poisoning Intentional self-harm	Poisoning Assault	Poisoning Undetermined	Adverse effect	Underdosing
Nitrobenzene, nitrobenzol	T65.3X1-	T65.3X2-	T65.3X3-	T65.3X4-	-	-
vapor	T65.3X1-	T65.3X2-	T65.3X3-	T65.3X4-	-	-
Nitrocellulose	T65.891-	T65.892-	T65.893-	T65.894-	-	-
lacquer	T65.891-	T65.892-	T65.893-	T65.894-	-	-
Nitrodiphenyl	T65.3X1-	T65.3X2-	T65.3X3-	T65.3X4-	-	-
Nitrofural	T49.0X1-	T49.0X2-	T49.0X3-	T49.0X4-	T49.0X5-	T49.0X6-
Nitrofurantoin	T37.8X1-	T37.8X2-	T37.8X3-	T37.8X4-	T37.8X5-	T37.8X6-
Nitrofurazone	T49.0X1-	T49.0X2-	T49.0X3-	T49.0X4-	T49.0X5-	T49.0X6-
Nitrogen	T59.0X1-	T59.0X2-	T59.0X3-	T59.0X4-	-	-
mustard	T45.1X1-	T45.1X2-	T45.1X3-	T45.1X4-	T45.1X5-	T45.1X6-
Nitroglycerin, nitro-glycerol (medicinal)	T46.3X1-	T46.3X2-	T46.3X3-	T46.3X4-	T46.3X5-	T46.3X6-
nonmedicinal	T65.5X1-	T65.5X2-	T65.5X3-	T65.5X4-	-	-
fumes	T65.5X1-	T65.5X2-	T65.5X3-	T65.5X4-	-	-
Nitroglycol	T52.3X1-	T52.3X2-	T52.3X3-	T52.3X4-	-	-
Nitrohydrochloric acid	T54.2X1-	T54.2X2-	T54.2X3-	T54.2X4-	-	-
Nitromersol	T49.0X1-	T49.0X2-	T49.0X3-	T49.0X4-	T49.0X5-	T49.0X6-
Nitronaphthalene	T65.891-	T65.892-	T65.893-	T65.894-	-	-
Nitrophenol	T54.0X1-	T54.0X2-	T54.0X3-	T54.0X4-	-	-
Nitropropane	T52.8X1-	T52.8X2-	T52.8X3-	T52.8X4-	-	-
Nitroprusside	T46.5X1-	T46.5X2-	T46.5X3-	T46.5X4-	T46.5X5-	T46.5X6-
Nitrosodimethylamine	T65.3X1-	T65.3X2-	T65.3X3-	T65.3X4-	-	-
Nitrothiazol	T37.4X1-	T37.4X2-	T37.4X3-	T37.4X4-	T37.4X5-	T37.4X6-
Nitrotoluene, nitrotoluol	T65.3X1-	T65.3X2-	T65.3X3-	T65.3X4-	-	-
vapor	T65.3X1-	T65.3X2-	T65.3X3-	T65.3X4-	-	-
Nitrous						
acid (liquid)	T54.2X1-	T54.2X2-	T54.2X3-	T54.2X4-	-	-
fumes	T59.891-	T59.892-	T59.893-	T59.894-	-	-
ether spirit	T46.3X1-	T46.3X2-	T46.3X3-	T46.3X4-	T46.3X5-	T46.3X6-
oxide	T41.0X1-	T41.0X2-	T41.0X3-	T41.0X4-	T41.0X5-	T41.0X6-
Nitroxoline	T37.8X1-	T37.8X2-	T37.8X3-	T37.8X4-	T37.8X5-	T37.8X6-
Nitrozone	T49.0X1-	T49.0X2-	T49.0X3-	T49.0X4-	T49.0X5-	T49.0X6-
Nizatidine	T47.0X1-	T47.0X2-	T47.0X3-	T47.0X4-	T47.0X5-	T47.0X6-
Nizofenone	T43.8X1-	T43.8X2-	T43.8X3-	T43.8X4-	T43.8X5-	T43.8X6-
Noctec	T42.6X1-	T42.6X2-	T42.6X3-	T42.6X4-	T42.6X5-	T42.6X6-
Noludar	T42.6X1-	T42.6X2-	T42.6X3-	T42.6X4-	T42.6X5-	T42.6X6-
Nomegestrol	T38.5X1-	T38.5X2-	T38.5X3-	T38.5X4-	T38.5X5-	T38.5X6-
Nomifensine	T43.291-	T43.292-	T43.293-	T43.294-	T43.295-	T43.296-
Nonoxinol	T49.8X1-	T49.8X2-	T49.8X3-	T49.8X4-	T49.8X5-	T49.8X6-
Nonylphenoxy (polyethoxy-ethanol)	T49.8X1-	T49.8X2-	T49.8X3-	T49.8X4-	T49.8X5-	T49.8X6-
Noptil	T42.3X1-	T42.3X2-	T42.3X3-	T42.3X4-	T42.3X5-	T42.3X6-
Noradrenaline	T44.4X1-	T44.4X2-	T44.4X3-	T44.4X4-	T44.4X5-	T44.4X6-
Noramidopyrine	T39.2X1-	T39.2X2-	T39.2X3-	T39.2X4-	T39.2X5-	T39.2X6-
methanesulfonate sodium	T39.2X1-	T39.2X2-	T39.2X3-	T39.2X4-	T39.2X5-	T39.2X6-
Norbormide	T60.4X1-	T60.4X2-	T60.4X3-	T60.4X4-	-	-
Nordazepam	T42.4X1-	T42.4X2-	T42.4X3-	T42.4X4-	T42.4X5-	T42.4X6-
Norepinephrine	T44.4X1-	T44.4X2-	T44.4X3-	T44.4X4-	T44.4X5-	T44.4X6-
Norethandrolone	T38.7X1-	T38.7X2-	T38.7X3-	T38.7X4-	T38.7X5-	T38.7X6-
Norethindrone	T38.4X1-	T38.4X2-	T38.4X3-	T38.4X4-	T38.4X5-	T38.4X6-
Norethisterone (acetate) (enantate)	T38.4X1-	T38.4X2-	T38.4X3-	T38.4X4-	T38.4X5-	T38.4X6-
with ethinylestradiol	T38.5X1-	T38.5X2-	T38.5X3-	T38.5X4-	T38.5X5-	T38.5X6-
Noretynodrel	T38.5X1-	T38.5X2-	T38.5X3-	T38.5X4-	T38.5X5-	T38.5X6-
Norfenefrine	T44.4X1-	T44.4X2-	T44.4X3-	T44.4X4-	T44.4X5-	T44.4X6-
Norfloxacin	T36.8X1-	T36.8X2-	T36.8X3-	T36.8X4-	T36.8X5-	T36.8X6-
Norgestrel	T38.4X1-	T38.4X2-	T38.4X3-	T38.4X4-	T38.4X5-	T38.4X6-
Norgestrienone	T38.4X1-	T38.4X2-	T38.4X3-	T38.4X4-	T38.4X5-	T38.4X6-
Norlestrin	T38.4X1-	T38.4X2-	T38.4X3-	T38.4X4-	T38.4X5-	T38.4X6-
Norlutin	T38.4X1-	T38.4X2-	T38.4X3-	T38.4X4-	T38.4X5-	T38.4X6-

Substance	Poisoning Accidental (unintentional)	Poisoning Intentional self-harm	Poisoning Assault	Poisoning Undetermined	Adverse effect	Underdosing
Normal serum albumin (human), salt-poor	T45.8X1-	T45.8X2-	T45.8X3-	T45.8X4-	T45.8X5-	T45.8X6-
Normethandrone	T38.5X1-	T38.5X2-	T38.5X3-	T38.5X4-	T38.5X5-	T38.5X6-
Normison — *see Benzodiazepines*						
Normorphine	T40.2X1-	T40.2X2-	T40.2X3-	T40.2X4-	-	-
Norpseudoephedrine	T50.5X1-	T50.5X2-	T50.5X3-	T50.5X4-	T50.5X5-	T50.5X6-
Nortestosterone (furanpropionate)	T38.7X1-	T38.7X2-	T38.7X3-	T38.7X4-	T38.7X5-	T38.7X6-
Nortriptyline	T43.011-	T43.012-	T43.013-	T43.014-	T43.015-	T43.016-
Noscapine	T48.3X1-	T48.3X2-	T48.3X3-	T48.3X4-	T48.3X5-	T48.3X6-
Nose preparations	T49.6X1-	T49.6X2-	T49.6X3-	T49.6X4-	T49.6X5-	T49.6X6-
Novobiocin	T36.5X1-	T36.5X2-	T36.5X3-	T36.5X4-	T36.5X5-	T36.5X6-
Novocain (infiltration) (topical)	T41.3X1-	T41.3X2-	T41.3X3-	T41.3X4-	T41.3X5-	T41.3X6-
nerve block (peripheral) (plexus)	T41.3X1-	T41.3X2-	T41.3X3-	T41.3X4-	T41.3X5-	T41.3X6-
spinal	T41.3X1-	T41.3X2-	T41.3X3-	T41.3X4-	T41.3X5-	T41.3X6-
Noxious foodstuff	T62.91X-	T62.92X-	T62.93X-	T62.94X-	-	-
specified NEC	T62.8X1-	T62.8X2-	T62.8X3-	T62.8X4-	-	-
Noxiptiline	T43.011-	T43.012-	T43.013-	T43.014-	T43.015-	T43.016-
Noxytiolin	T49.0X1-	T49.0X2-	T49.0X3-	T49.0X4-	T49.0X5-	T49.0X6-
NPH Iletin (insulin)	T38.3X1-	T38.3X2-	T38.3X3-	T38.3X4-	T38.3X5-	T38.3X6-
Numorphan	T40.2X1-	T40.2X2-	T40.2X3-	T40.2X4-	T40.2X5-	T40.2X6-
Nunol	T42.3X1-	T42.3X2-	T42.3X3-	T42.3X4-	T42.3X5-	T42.3X6-
Nupercaine (spinal anesthetic)	T41.3X1-	T41.3X2-	T41.3X3-	T41.3X4-	T41.3X5-	T41.3X6-
topical (surface)	T41.3X1-	T41.3X2-	T41.3X3-	T41.3X4-	T41.3X5-	T41.3X6-
Nutmeg oil (liniment)	T49.3X1-	T49.3X2-	T49.3X3-	T49.3X4-	T49.3X5-	T49.3X6-
Nutritional supplement	T50.901-	T50.902-	T50.903-	T50.904-	T50.905-	T50.906-
Nux vomica	T65.1X1-	T65.1X2-	T65.1X3-	T65.1X4-	-	-
Nydrazid	T37.1X1-	T37.1X2-	T37.1X3-	T37.1X4-	T37.1X5-	T37.1X6-
Nylidrin	T46.7X1-	T46.7X2-	T46.7X3-	T46.7X4-	T46.7X5-	T46.7X6-
Nystatin	T36.7X1-	T36.7X2-	T36.7X3-	T36.7X4-	T36.7X5-	T36.7X6-
topical	T49.0X1-	T49.0X2-	T49.0X3-	T49.0X4-	T49.0X5-	T49.0X6-
Nytol	T45.0X1-	T45.0X2-	T45.0X3-	T45.0X4-	T45.0X5-	T45.0X6-
Obidoxime chloride	T50.6X1-	T50.6X2-	T50.6X3-	T50.6X4-	T50.6X5-	T50.6X6-
Octafonium (chloride)	T49.3X1-	T49.3X2-	T49.3X3-	T49.3X4-	T49.3X5-	T49.3X6-
Octamethyl pyrophos-phoramide	T60.0X1-	T60.0X2-	T60.0X3-	T60.0X4-	-	-
Octanoin	T50.991-	T50.992-	T50.993-	T50.994-	T50.995-	T50.996-
Octatropine methyl-bromide	T44.3X1-	T44.3X2-	T44.3X3-	T44.3X4-	T44.3X5-	T44.3X6-
Octotiamine	T45.2X1-	T45.2X2-	T45.2X3-	T45.2X4-	T45.2X5-	T45.2X6-
Octoxinol (9)	T49.8X1-	T49.8X2-	T49.8X3-	T49.8X4-	T49.8X5-	T49.8X6-
Octreotide	T38.991-	T38.992-	T38.993-	T38.994-	T38.995-	T38.996-
Octyl nitrite	T46.3X1-	T46.3X2-	T46.3X3-	T46.3X4-	T46.3X5-	T46.3X6-
Oestradiol	T38.5X1-	T38.5X2-	T38.5X3-	T38.5X4-	T38.5X5-	T38.5X6-
Oestriol	T38.5X1-	T38.5X2-	T38.5X3-	T38.5X4-	T38.5X5-	T38.5X6-
Oestrogen	T38.5X1-	T38.5X2-	T38.5X3-	T38.5X4-	T38.5X5-	T38.5X6-
Oestrone	T38.5X1-	T38.5X2-	T38.5X3-	T38.5X4-	T38.5X5-	T38.5X6-
Ofloxacin	T36.8X1-	T36.8X2-	T36.8X3-	T36.8X4-	T36.8X5-	T36.8X6-
Oil (of)	T65.891-	T65.892-	T65.893-	T65.894-	-	-
bitter almond	T62.8X1-	T62.8X2-	T62.8X3-	T62.8X4-	-	-
cloves	T49.7X1-	T49.7X2-	T49.7X3-	T49.7X4-	T49.7X5-	T49.7X6-
colors	T65.6X1-	T65.6X2-	T65.6X3-	T65.6X4-	-	-
fumes	T59.891-	T59.892-	T59.893-	T59.894-	-	-
lubricating	T52.0X1-	T52.0X2-	T52.0X3-	T52.0X4-	-	-
Niobe	T52.8X1-	T52.8X2-	T52.8X3-	T52.8X4-	-	-
vitriol (liquid)	T54.2X1-	T54.2X2-	T54.2X3-	T54.2X4-	-	-
fumes	T54.2X1-	T54.2X2-	T54.2X3-	T54.2X4-	-	-
wintergreen (bitter) NEC	T49.3X1-	T49.3X2-	T49.3X3-	T49.3X4-	T49.3X5-	T49.3X6-
Oily preparation (for skin)	T49.3X1-	T49.3X2-	T49.3X3-	T49.3X4-	T49.3X5-	T49.3X6-
Ointment NEC	T49.3X1-	T49.3X2-	T49.3X3-	T49.3X4-	T49.3X5-	T49.3X6-
Olanzapine	T43.591-	T43.592-	T43.593-	T43.594-	T43.595-	T43.596-
Oleander	T62.2X1-	T62.2X2-	T62.2X3-	T62.2X4-	-	-

Substance	Poisoning Accidental (unintentional)	Poisoning Intentional self-harm	Poisoning Assault	Poisoning Undetermined	Adverse effect	Underdosing
Oleandomycin	T36.3X1-	T36.3X2-	T36.3X3-	T36.3X4-	T36.3X5-	T36.3X6-
Oleandrin	T46.0X1-	T46.0X2-	T46.0X3-	T46.0X4-	T46.0X5-	T46.0X6-
Oleic acid	T46.6X1-	T46.6X2-	T46.6X3-	T46.6X4-	T46.6X5-	T46.6X6-
Oleovitamin A	T45.2X1-	T45.2X2-	T45.2X3-	T45.2X4-	T45.2X5-	T45.2X6-
Oleum ricini	T47.2X1-	T47.2X2-	T47.2X3-	T47.2X4-	T47.2X5-	T47.2X6-
Olive oil (medicinal) NEC	T47.4X1-	T47.4X2-	T47.4X3-	T47.4X4-	T47.4X5-	T47.4X6-
Olivomycin	T45.1X1-	T45.1X2-	T45.1X3-	T45.1X4-	T45.1X5-	T45.1X6-
Olsalazine	T47.8X1-	T47.8X2-	T47.8X3-	T47.8X4-	T47.8X5-	T47.8X6-
Omeprazole	T47.1X1-	T47.1X2-	T47.1X3-	T47.1X4-	T47.1X5-	T47.1X6-
OMPA	T60.0X1-	T60.0X2-	T60.0X3-	T60.0X4-	-	-
Oncovin	T45.1X1-	T45.1X2-	T45.1X3-	T45.1X4-	T45.1X5-	T45.1X6-
Ondansetron	T45.0X1-	T45.0X2-	T45.0X3-	T45.0X4-	T45.0X5-	T45.0X6-
Ophthaine	T41.3X1-	T41.3X2-	T41.3X3-	T41.3X4-	T41.3X5-	T41.3X6-
Ophthetic	T41.3X1-	T41.3X2-	T41.3X3-	T41.3X4-	T41.3X5-	T41.3X6-
Opiate NEC	T40.601-	T40.602-	T40.603-	T40.604-	T40.605-	T40.606-
antagonists	T50.7X1-	T50.7X2-	T50.7X3-	T50.7X4-	T50.7X5-	T50.7X6-
Opioid NEC	T40.2X1-	T40.2X2-	T40.2X3-	T40.2X4-	T40.2X5-	T40.2X6-
Opipramol	T43.011-	T43.012-	T43.013-	T43.014-	T43.015-	T43.016-
Opium alkaloids (total)	T40.0X1-	T40.0X2-	T40.0X3-	T40.0X4-	T40.0X5-	T40.0X6-
standardized powdered	T40.0X1-	T40.0X2-	T40.0X3-	T40.0X4-	T40.0X5-	T40.0X6-
tincture (camphorated)	T40.0X1-	T40.0X2-	T40.0X3-	T40.0X4-	T40.0X5-	T40.0X6-
Oracon	T38.4X1-	T38.4X2-	T38.4X3-	T38.4X4-	T38.4X5-	T38.4X6-
Oragrafin	T50.8X1-	T50.8X2-	T50.8X3-	T50.8X4-	T50.8X5-	T50.8X6-
Oral contraceptives	T38.4X1-	T38.4X2-	T38.4X3-	T38.4X4-	T38.4X5-	T38.4X6-
Oral rehydration salts	T50.3X1-	T50.3X2-	T50.3X3-	T50.3X4-	T50.3X5-	T50.3X6-
Orazamide	T50.991-	T50.992-	T50.993-	T50.994-	T50.995-	T50.996-
Orciprenaline	T48.291-	T48.292-	T48.293-	T48.294-	T48.295-	T48.296-
Organidin	T48.4X1-	T48.4X2-	T48.4X3-	T48.4X4-	T48.4X5-	T48.4X6-
Organonitrate NEC	T46.3X1-	T46.3X2-	T46.3X3-	T46.3X4-	T46.3X5-	T46.3X6-
Organophosphates	T60.0X1-	T60.0X2-	T60.0X3-	T60.0X4-	-	-
Orimune	T50.B91-	T50.B92-	T50.B93-	T50.B94-	T50.B95-	T50.B96-
Orinase	T38.3X1-	T38.3X2-	T38.3X3-	T38.3X4-	T38.3X5-	T38.3X6-
Ormeloxifene	T38.6X1-	T38.6X2-	T38.6X3-	T38.6X4-	T38.6X5-	T38.6X6-
Ornidazole	T37.3X1-	T37.3X2-	T37.3X3-	T37.3X4-	T37.3X5-	T37.3X6-
Ornithine aspartate	T50.991-	T50.992-	T50.993-	T50.994-	T50.995-	T50.996-
Ornoprostil	T47.1X1-	T47.1X2-	T47.1X3-	T47.1X4-	T47.1X5-	T47.1X6-
Orphenadrine (hydrochloride)	T42.8X1-	T42.8X2-	T42.8X3-	T42.8X4-	T42.8X5-	T42.8X6-
Ortal (sodium)	T42.3X1-	T42.3X2-	T42.3X3-	T42.3X4-	T42.3X5-	T42.3X6-
Orthoboric acid	T49.0X1-	T49.0X2-	T49.0X3-	T49.0X4-	T49.0X5-	T49.0X6-
ENT agent	T49.6X1-	T49.6X2-	T49.6X3-	T49.6X4-	T49.6X5-	T49.6X6-
ophthalmic preparation	T49.5X1-	T49.5X2-	T49.5X3-	T49.5X4-	T49.5X5-	T49.5X6-
Orthocaine	T41.3X1-	T41.3X2-	T41.3X3-	T41.3X4-	T41.3X5-	T41.3X6-
Orthodichlorobenzene	T53.7X1-	T53.7X2-	T53.7X3-	T53.7X4-	-	-
Ortho-Novum	T38.4X1-	T38.4X2-	T38.4X3-	T38.4X4-	T38.4X5-	T38.4X6-
Orthotolidine (reagent)	T54.2X1-	T54.2X2-	T54.2X3-	T54.2X4-	-	-
Osmic acid (liquid)	T54.2X1-	T54.2X2-	T54.2X3-	T54.2X4-	-	-
fumes	T54.2X1-	T54.2X2-	T54.2X3-	T54.2X4-	-	-
Osmotic diuretics	T50.2X1-	T50.2X2-	T50.2X3-	T50.2X4-	T50.2X5-	T50.2X6-
Otilonium bromide	T44.3X1-	T44.3X2-	T44.3X3-	T44.3X4-	T44.3X5-	T44.3X6-
Otorhinolaryngological drug NEC	T49.6X1-	T49.6X2-	T49.6X3-	T49.6X4-	T49.6X5-	T49.6X6-
Ouabain (e)	T46.0X1-	T46.0X2-	T46.0X3-	T46.0X4-	T46.0X5-	T46.0X6-
Ovarian						
hormone	T38.5X1-	T38.5X2-	T38.5X3-	T38.5X4-	T38.5X5-	T38.5X6-
stimulant	T38.5X1-	T38.5X2-	T38.5X3-	T38.5X4-	T38.5X5-	T38.5X6-
Ovral	T38.4X1-	T38.4X2-	T38.4X3-	T38.4X4-	T38.4X5-	T38.4X6-
Ovulen	T38.4X1-	T38.4X2-	T38.4X3-	T38.4X4-	T38.4X5-	T38.4X6-
Oxacillin	T36.0X1-	T36.0X2-	T36.0X3-	T36.0X4-	T36.0X5-	T36.0X6-

Substance	Poisoning Accidental (unintentional)	Poisoning Intentional self-harm	Poisoning Assault	Poisoning Undetermined	Adverse effect	Underdosing
Oxalic acid	T54.2X1-	T54.2X2-	T54.2X3-	T54.2X4-	-	-
ammonium salt	T50.991-	T50.992-	T50.993-	T50.994-	T50.995-	T50.996-
Oxamniquine	T37.4X1-	T37.4X2-	T37.4X3-	T37.4X4-	T37.4X5-	T37.4X6-
Oxanamide	T43.591-	T43.592-	T43.593-	T43.594-	T43.595-	T43.596-
Oxandrolone	T38.7X1-	T38.7X2-	T38.7X3-	T38.7X4-	T38.7X5-	T38.7X6-
Oxantel	T37.4X1-	T37.4X2-	T37.4X3-	T37.4X4-	T37.4X5-	T37.4X6-
Oxapium iodide	T44.3X1-	T44.3X2-	T44.3X3-	T44.3X4-	T44.3X5-	T44.3X6-
Oxaprotiline	T43.021-	T43.022-	T43.023-	T43.024-	T43.025-	T43.026-
Oxaprozin	T39.311-	T39.312-	T39.313-	T39.314-	T39.315-	T39.316-
Oxatomide	T45.0X1-	T45.0X2-	T45.0X3-	T45.0X4-	T45.0X5-	T45.0X6-
Oxazepam	T42.4X1-	T42.4X2-	T42.4X3-	T42.4X4-	T42.4X5-	T42.4X6-
Oxazimedrine	T50.5X1-	T50.5X2-	T50.5X3-	T50.5X4-	T50.5X5-	T50.5X6-
Oxazolam	T42.4X1-	T42.4X2-	T42.4X3-	T42.4X4-	T42.4X5-	T42.4X6-
Oxazolidine derivatives	T42.2X1-	T42.2X2-	T42.2X3-	T42.2X4-	T42.2X5-	T42.2X6-
Oxazolidinedione (derivative)	T42.2X1-	T42.2X2-	T42.2X3-	T42.2X4-	T42.2X5-	T42.2X6-
Ox bile extract	T47.5X1-	T47.5X2-	T47.5X3-	T47.5X4-	T47.5X5-	T47.5X6-
Oxcarbazepine	T42.1X1-	T42.1X2-	T42.1X3-	T42.1X4-	T42.1X5-	T42.1X6-
Oxedrine	T44.4X1-	T44.4X2-	T44.4X3-	T44.4X4-	T44.4X5-	T44.4X6-
Oxeladin (citrate)	T48.3X1-	T48.3X2-	T48.3X3-	T48.3X4-	T48.3X5-	T48.3X6-
Oxendolone	T38.5X1-	T38.5X2-	T38.5X3-	T38.5X4-	T38.5X5-	T38.5X6-
Oxetacaine	T41.3X1-	T41.3X2-	T41.3X3-	T41.3X4-	T41.3X5-	T41.3X6-
Oxethazine	T41.3X1-	T41.3X2-	T41.3X3-	T41.3X4-	T41.3X5-	T41.3X6-
Oxetorone	T39.8X1-	T39.8X2-	T39.8X3-	T39.8X4-	T39.8X5-	T39.8X6-
Oxiconazole	T49.0X1-	T49.0X2-	T49.0X3-	T49.0X4-	T49.0X5-	T49.0X6-
Oxidizing agent NEC	T54.91X-	T54.92X-	T54.93X-	T54.94X-	-	-
Oxipurinol	T50.4X1-	T50.4X2-	T50.4X3-	T50.4X4-	T50.4X5-	T50.4X6-
Oxitriptan	T43.291-	T43.292-	T43.293-	T43.294-	T43.295-	T43.296-
Oxitropium bromide	T48.6X1-	T48.6X2-	T48.6X3-	T48.6X4-	T48.6X5-	T48.6X6-
Oxodipine	T46.1X1-	T46.1X2-	T46.1X3-	T46.1X4-	T46.1X5-	T46.1X6-
Oxolamine	T48.3X1-	T48.3X2-	T48.3X3-	T48.3X4-	T48.3X5-	T48.3X6-
Oxolinic acid	T37.8X1-	T37.8X2-	T37.8X3-	T37.8X4-	T37.8X5-	T37.8X6-
Oxomemazine	T43.3X1-	T43.3X2-	T43.3X3-	T43.3X4-	T43.3X5-	T43.3X6-
Oxophenarsine	T37.3X1-	T37.3X2-	T37.3X3-	T37.3X4-	T37.3X5-	T37.3X6-
Oxprenolol	T44.7X1-	T44.7X2-	T44.7X3-	T44.7X4-	T44.7X5-	T44.7X6-
Oxsoralen	T49.3X1-	T49.3X2-	T49.3X3-	T49.3X4-	T49.3X5-	T49.3X6-
Oxtriphylline	T48.6X1-	T48.6X2-	T48.6X3-	T48.6X4-	T48.6X5-	T48.6X6-
Oxybate sodium	T41.291-	T41.292-	T41.293-	T41.294-	T41.295-	T41.296-
Oxybuprocaine	T41.3X1-	T41.3X2-	T41.3X3-	T41.3X4-	T41.3X5-	T41.3X6-
Oxybutynin	T44.3X1-	T44.3X2-	T44.3X3-	T44.3X4-	T44.3X5-	T44.3X6-
Oxychlorosene	T49.0X1-	T49.0X2-	T49.0X3-	T49.0X4-	T49.0X5-	T49.0X6-
Oxycodone	T40.2X1-	T40.2X2-	T40.2X3-	T40.2X4-	T40.2X5-	T40.2X6-
Oxyfedrine	T46.3X1-	T46.3X2-	T46.3X3-	T46.3X4-	T46.3X5-	T46.3X6-
Oxygen	T41.5X1-	T41.5X2-	T41.5X3-	T41.5X4-	T41.5X5-	T41.5X6-
Oxylone	T49.0X1-	T49.0X2-	T49.0X3-	T49.0X4-	T49.0X5-	T49.0X6-
ophthalmic preparation	T49.5X1-	T49.5X2-	T49.5X3-	T49.5X4-	T49.5X5-	T49.5X6-
Oxymesterone	T38.7X1-	T38.7X2-	T38.7X3-	T38.7X4-	T38.7X5-	T38.7X6-
Oxymetazoline	T48.5X1-	T48.5X2-	T48.5X3-	T48.5X4-	T48.5X5-	T48.5X6-
Oxymetholone	T38.7X1-	T38.7X2-	T38.7X3-	T38.7X4-	T38.7X5-	T38.7X6-
Oxymorphone	T40.2X1-	T40.2X2-	T40.2X3-	T40.2X4-	T40.2X5-	T40.2X6-
Oxypertine	T43.591-	T43.592-	T43.593-	T43.594-	T43.595-	T43.596-
Oxyphenbutazone	T39.2X1-	T39.2X2-	T39.2X3-	T39.2X4-	T39.2X5-	T39.2X6-
Oxyphencyclimine	T44.3X1-	T44.3X2-	T44.3X3-	T44.3X4-	T44.3X5-	T44.3X6-
Oxyphenisatine	T47.2X1-	T47.2X2-	T47.2X3-	T47.2X4-	T47.2X5-	T47.2X6-
Oxyphenonium bromide	T44.3X1-	T44.3X2-	T44.3X3-	T44.3X4-	T44.3X5-	T44.3X6-
Oxypolygelatin	T45.8X1-	T45.8X2-	T45.8X3-	T45.8X4-	T45.8X5-	T45.8X6-
Oxyquinoline (derivatives)	T37.8X1-	T37.8X2-	T37.8X3-	T37.8X4-	T37.8X5-	T37.8X6-
Oxytetracycline	T36.4X1-	T36.4X2-	T36.4X3-	T36.4X4-	T36.4X5-	T36.4X6-
Oxytocic drug NEC	T48.0X1-	T48.0X2-	T48.0X3-	T48.0X4-	T48.0X5-	T48.0X6-
Oxytocin (synthetic)	T48.0X1-	T48.0X2-	T48.0X3-	T48.0X4-	T48.0X5-	T48.0X6-

Substance	Poisoning Accidental (unintentional)	Poisoning Intentional self-harm	Poisoning Assault	Poisoning Undetermined	Adverse effect	Underdosing
Ozone	T59.891-	T59.892-	T59.893-	T59.894-	-	-
PABA	T49.3X1-	T49.3X2-	T49.3X3-	T49.3X4-	T49.3X5-	T49.3X6-
Packed red cells	T45.8X1-	T45.8X2-	T45.8X3-	T45.8X4-	T45.8X5-	T45.8X6-
Padimate	T49.3X1-	T49.3X2-	T49.3X3-	T49.3X4-	T49.3X5-	T49.3X6-
Paint NEC	T65.6X1-	T65.6X2-	T65.6X3-	T65.6X4-	-	-
cleaner	T52.91X-	T52.92X-	T52.93X-	T52.94X-	-	-
fumes NEC	T59.891-	T59.892-	T59.893-	T59.894-	-	-
lead (fumes)	T56.0X1-	T56.0X2-	T56.0X3-	T56.0X4-	-	-
solvent NEC	T52.8X1-	T52.8X2-	T52.8X3-	T52.8X4-	-	-
stripper	T52.8X1-	T52.8X2-	T52.8X3-	T52.8X4-	-	-
Palfium	T40.2X1-	T40.2X2-	T40.2X3-	T40.2X4-	-	-
Palm kernel oil	T50.991-	T50.992-	T50.993-	T50.994-	T50.995-	T50.996-
Paludrine	T37.2X1-	T37.2X2-	T37.2X3-	T37.2X4-	T37.2X5-	T37.2X6-
PAM (pralidoxime)	T50.6X1-	T50.6X2-	T50.6X3-	T50.6X4-	T50.6X5-	T50.6X6-
Pamaquine (naphthoute)	T37.2X1-	T37.2X2-	T37.2X3-	T37.2X4-	T37.2X5-	T37.2X6-
Panadol	T39.1X1-	T39.1X2-	T39.1X3-	T39.1X4-	T39.1X5-	T39.1X6-
Pancreatic						
digestive secretion stimulant	T47.8X1-	T47.8X2-	T47.8X3-	T47.8X4-	T47.8X5-	T47.8X6-
dornase	T45.3X1-	T45.3X2-	T45.3X3-	T45.3X4-	T45.3X5-	T45.3X6-
Pancreatin	T47.5X1-	T47.5X2-	T47.5X3-	T47.5X4-	T47.5X5-	T47.5X6-
Pancrelipase	T47.5X1-	T47.5X2-	T47.5X3-	T47.5X4-	T47.5X5-	T47.5X6-
Pancuronium (bromide)	T48.1X1-	T48.1X2-	T48.1X3-	T48.1X4-	T48.1X5-	T48.1X6-
Pangamic acid	T45.2X1-	T45.2X2-	T45.2X3-	T45.2X4-	T45.2X5-	T45.2X6-
Panthenol	T45.2X1-	T45.2X2-	T45.2X3-	T45.2X4-	T45.2X5-	T45.2X6-
topical	T49.8X1-	T49.8X2-	T49.8X3-	T49.8X4-	T49.8X5-	T49.8X6-
Pantopon	T40.0X1-	T40.0X2-	T40.0X3-	T40.0X4-	T40.0X5-	T40.0X6-
Pantothenic acid	T45.2X1-	T45.2X2-	T45.2X3-	T45.2X4-	T45.2X5-	T45.2X6-
Panwarfin	T45.511-	T45.512-	T45.513-	T45.514-	T45.515-	T45.516-
Papain	T47.5X1-	T47.5X2-	T47.5X3-	T47.5X4-	T47.5X5-	T47.5X6-
digestant	T47.5X1-	T47.5X2-	T47.5X3-	T47.5X4-	T47.5X5-	T47.5X6-
Papaveretum	T40.0X1-	T40.0X2-	T40.0X3-	T40.0X4-	T40.0X5-	T40.0X6-
Papaverine	T44.3X1-	T44.3X2-	T44.3X3-	T44.3X4-	T44.3X5-	T44.3X6-
Para-acetamidophenol	T39.1X1-	T39.1X2-	T39.1X3-	T39.1X4-	T39.1X5-	T39.1X6-
Para-aminobenzoic acid	T49.3X1-	T49.3X2-	T49.3X3-	T49.3X4-	T49.3X5-	T49.3X6-
Para-aminophenol derivatives	T39.1X1-	T39.1X2-	T39.1X3-	T39.1X4-	T39.1X5-	T39.1X6-
Para-aminosalicylic acid	T37.1X1-	T37.1X2-	T37.1X3-	T37.1X4-	T37.1X5-	T37.1X6-
Paracetaldehyde	T42.6X1-	T42.6X2-	T42.6X3-	T42.6X4-	T42.6X5-	T42.6X6-
Paracetamol	T39.1X1-	T39.1X2-	T39.1X3-	T39.1X4-	T39.1X5-	T39.1X6-
Parachlorophenol (camphorated)	T49.0X1-	T49.0X2-	T49.0X3-	T49.0X4-	T49.0X5-	T49.0X6-
Paracodin	T40.2X1-	T40.2X2-	T40.2X3-	T40.2X4-	T40.2X5-	T40.2X6-
Paradione	T42.2X1-	T42.2X2-	T42.2X3-	T42.2X4-	T42.2X5-	T42.2X6-
Paraffin (s) (wax)	T52.0X1-	T52.0X2-	T52.0X3-	T52.0X4-	-	-
liquid (medicinal)	T47.4X1-	T47.4X2-	T47.4X3-	T47.4X4-	T47.4X5-	T47.4X6-
nonmedicinal	T52.0X1-	T52.0X2-	T52.0X3-	T52.0X4-	-	-
Paraformaldehyde	T60.3X1-	T60.3X2-	T60.3X3-	T60.3X4-	-	-
Paraldehyde	T42.6X1-	T42.6X2-	T42.6X3-	T42.6X4-	T42.6X5-	T42.6X6-
Paramethadione	T42.2X1-	T42.2X2-	T42.2X3-	T42.2X4-	T42.2X5-	T42.2X6-
Paramethasone	T38.0X1-	T38.0X2-	T38.0X3-	T38.0X4-	T38.0X5-	T38.0X6-
acetate	T49.0X1-	T49.0X2-	T49.0X3-	T49.0X4-	T49.0X5-	T49.0X6-
Paraoxon	T60.0X1-	T60.0X2-	T60.0X3-	T60.0X4-	-	-
Paraquat	T60.3X1-	T60.3X2-	T60.3X3-	T60.3X4-	-	-
Parasympatholytic NEC	T44.3X1-	T44.3X2-	T44.3X3-	T44.3X4-	T44.3X5-	T44.3X6-
Parasympathomimetic drug NEC	T44.1X1-	T44.1X2-	T44.1X3-	T44.1X4-	T44.1X5-	T44.1X6-
Parathion	T60.0X1-	T60.0X2-	T60.0X3-	T60.0X4-	-	-
Parathormone	T50.991-	T50.992-	T50.993-	T50.994-	T50.995-	T50.996-
Parathyroid extract	T50.991-	T50.992-	T50.993-	T50.994-	T50.995-	T50.996-
Paratyphoid vaccine	T50.A91-	T50.A92-	T50.A93-	T50.A94-	T50.A95-	T50.A96-
Paredrine	T44.4X1-	T44.4X2-	T44.4X3-	T44.4X4-	T44.4X5-	T44.4X6-

Substance	Poisoning Accidental (unintentional)	Poisoning Intentional self-harm	Poisoning Assault	Poisoning Undetermined	Adverse effect	Underdosing
Paregoric	T40.0X1-	T40.0X2-	T40.0X3-	T40.0X4-	T40.0X5-	T40.0X6-
Pargyline	T46.5X1-	T46.5X2-	T46.5X3-	T46.5X4-	T46.5X5-	T46.5X6-
Paris green	T57.0X1-	T57.0X2-	T57.0X3-	T57.0X4-	-	-
insecticide	T57.0X1-	T57.0X2-	T57.0X3-	T57.0X4-	-	-
Parnate	T43.1X1-	T43.1X2-	T43.1X3-	T43.1X4-	T43.1X5-	T43.1X6-
Paromomycin	T36.5X1-	T36.5X2-	T36.5X3-	T36.5X4-	T36.5X5-	T36.5X6-
Paroxypropione	T45.1X1-	T45.1X2-	T45.1X3-	T45.1X4-	T45.1X5-	T45.1X6-
Parzone	T40.2X1-	T40.2X2-	T40.2X3-	T40.2X4-	T40.2X5-	T40.2X6-
PAS	T37.1X1-	T37.1X2-	T37.1X3-	T37.1X4-	T37.1X5-	T37.1X6-
Pasiniazid	T37.1X1-	T37.1X2-	T37.1X3-	T37.1X4-	T37.1X5-	T37.1X6-
PBB (polybrominated biphenyls)	T65.891-	T65.892-	T65.893-	T65.894-	-	-
PCB	T65.891-	T65.892-	T65.893-	T65.894-	-	-
PCP						
meaning pentachlorophenol	T60.1X1-	T60.1X2-	T60.1X3-	T60.1X4-	-	-
fungicide	T60.3X1-	T60.3X2-	T60.3X3-	T60.3X4-	-	-
herbicide	T60.3X1-	T60.3X2-	T60.3X3-	T60.3X4-	-	-
insecticide	T60.1X1-	T60.1X2-	T60.1X3-	T60.1X4-	-	-
meaning phencyclidine	T40.991-	T40.992-	T40.993-	T40.994-	-	-
Peach kernel oil (emulsion)	T47.4X1-	T47.4X2-	T47.4X3-	T47.4X4-	T47.4X5-	T47.4X6-
Peanut oil (emulsion) NEC	T47.4X1-	T47.4X2-	T47.4X3-	T47.4X4-	T47.4X5-	T47.4X6-
topical	T49.3X1-	T49.3X2-	T49.3X3-	T49.3X4-	T49.3X5-	T49.3X6-
Pearly Gates (morning glory seeds)	T40.991-	T40.992-	T40.993-	T40.994-	-	-
Pecazine	T43.3X1-	T43.3X2-	T43.3X3-	T43.3X4-	T43.3X5-	T43.3X6-
Pectin	T47.6X1-	T47.6X2-	T47.6X3-	T47.6X4-	T47.6X5-	T47.6X6-
Pefloxacin	T37.8X1-	T37.8X2-	T37.8X3-	T37.8X4-	T37.8X5-	T37.8X6-
Pegademase, bovine	T50.Z91-	T50.Z92-	T50.Z93-	T50.Z94-	T50.Z95-	T50.Z96-
Pelletierine tannate	T37.4X1-	T37.4X2-	T37.4X3-	T37.4X4-	T37.4X5-	T37.4X6-
Pemirolast (potassium)	T48.6X1-	T48.6X2-	T48.6X3-	T48.6X4-	T48.6X5-	T48.6X6-
Pemoline	T50.7X1-	T50.7X2-	T50.7X3-	T50.7X4-	T50.7X5-	T50.7X6-
Pempidine	T44.2X1-	T44.2X2-	T44.2X3-	T44.2X4-	T44.2X5-	T44.2X6-
Penamecillin	T36.0X1-	T36.0X2-	T36.0X3-	T36.0X4-	T36.0X5-	T36.0X6-
Penbutolol	T44.7X1-	T44.7X2-	T44.7X3-	T44.7X4-	T44.7X5-	T44.7X6-
Penethamate	T36.0X1-	T36.0X2-	T36.0X3-	T36.0X4-	T36.0X5-	T36.0X6-
Penfluridol	T43.591-	T43.592-	T43.593-	T43.594-	T43.595-	T43.596-
Penflutizide	T50.2X1-	T50.2X2-	T50.2X3-	T50.2X4-	T50.2X5-	T50.2X6-
Pengitoxin	T46.0X1-	T46.0X2-	T46.0X3-	T46.0X4-	T46.0X5-	T46.0X6-
Penicillamine	T50.6X1-	T50.6X2-	T50.6X3-	T50.6X4-	T50.6X5-	T50.6X6-
Penicillin (any)	T36.0X1-	T36.0X2-	T36.0X3-	T36.0X4-	T36.0X5-	T36.0X6-
Penicillinase	T45.3X1-	T45.3X2-	T45.3X3-	T45.3X4-	T45.3X5-	T45.3X6-
Penicilloyl polylysine	T50.8X1-	T50.8X2-	T50.8X3-	T50.8X4-	T50.8X5-	T50.8X6-
Penimepicycline	T36.4X1-	T36.4X2-	T36.4X3-	T36.4X4-	T36.4X5-	T36.4X6-
Pentachloroethane	T53.6X1-	T53.6X2-	T53.6X3-	T53.6X4-	-	-
Pentachloronaphthalene	T53.7X1-	T53.7X2-	T53.7X3-	T53.7X4-	-	-
Pentachlorophenol (pesticide)	T60.1X1-	T60.1X2-	T60.1X3-	T60.1X4-	-	-
fungicide	T60.3X1-	T60.3X2-	T60.3X3-	T60.3X4-	-	-
herbicide	T60.3X1-	T60.3X2-	T60.3X3-	T60.3X4-	-	-
insecticide	T60.1X1-	T60.1X2-	T60.1X3-	T60.1X4-	-	-
Pentaerythritol	T46.3X1-	T46.3X2-	T46.3X3-	T46.3X4-	T46.3X5-	T46.3X6-
chloral	T42.6X1-	T42.6X2-	T42.6X3-	T42.6X4-	T42.6X5-	T42.6X6-
tetranitrate NEC	T46.3X1-	T46.3X2-	T46.3X3-	T46.3X4-	T46.3X5-	T46.3X6-
Pentaerythrityl tetranitrate	T46.3X1-	T46.3X2-	T46.3X3-	T46.3X4-	T46.3X5-	T46.3X6-
Pentagastrin	T50.8X1-	T50.8X2-	T50.8X3-	T50.8X4-	T50.8X5-	T50.8X6-
Pentalin	T53.6X1-	T53.6X2-	T53.6X3-	T53.6X4-	-	-
Pentamethonium bromide	T44.2X1-	T44.2X2-	T44.2X3-	T44.2X4-	T44.2X5-	T44.2X6-
Pentamidine	T37.3X1-	T37.3X2-	T37.3X3-	T37.3X4-	T37.3X5-	T37.3X6-
Pentanol	T51.3X1-	T51.3X2-	T51.3X3-	T51.3X4-	-	-
Pentapyrrolinium (bitartrate)	T44.2X1-	T44.2X2-	T44.2X3-	T44.2X4-	T44.2X5-	T44.2X6-
Pentaquine	T37.2X1-	T37.2X2-	T37.2X3-	T37.2X4-	T37.2X5-	T37.2X6-

Substance	Poisoning Accidental (unintentional)	Poisoning Intentional self-harm	Poisoning Assault	Poisoning Undetermined	Adverse effect	Underdosing
Pentazocine	T40.491-	T40.492-	T40.493-	T40.494-	T40.495-	T40.496-
Pentetrazole	T50.7X1-	T50.7X2-	T50.7X3-	T50.7X4-	T50.7X5-	T50.7X6-
Penthienate bromide	T44.3X1-	T44.3X2-	T44.3X3-	T44.3X4-	T44.3X5-	T44.3X6-
Pentifylline	T46.7X1-	T46.7X2-	T46.7X3-	T46.7X4-	T46.7X5-	T46.7X6-
Pentobarbital	T42.3X1-	T42.3X2-	T42.3X3-	T42.3X4-	T42.3X5-	T42.3X6-
sodium	T42.3X1-	T42.3X2-	T42.3X3-	T42.3X4-	T42.3X5-	T42.3X6-
Pentobarbitone	T42.3X1-	T42.3X2-	T42.3X3-	T42.3X4-	T42.3X5-	T42.3X6-
Pentolonium tartrate	T44.2X1-	T44.2X2-	T44.2X3-	T44.2X4-	T44.2X5-	T44.2X6-
Pentosan polysulfate (sodium)	T39.8X1-	T39.8X2-	T39.8X3-	T39.8X4-	T39.8X5-	T39.8X6-
Pentostatin	T45.1X1-	T45.1X2-	T45.1X3-	T45.1X4-	T45.1X5-	T45.1X6-
Pentothal	T41.1X1-	T41.1X2-	T41.1X3-	T41.1X4-	T41.1X5-	T41.1X6-
Pentoxifylline	T46.7X1-	T46.7X2-	T46.7X3-	T46.7X4-	T46.7X5-	T46.7X6-
Pentoxyverine	T48.3X1-	T48.3X2-	T48.3X3-	T48.3X4-	T48.3X5-	T48.3X6-
Pentrinat	T46.3X1-	T46.3X2-	T46.3X3-	T46.3X4-	T46.3X5-	T46.3X6-
Pentylenetetrazole	T50.7X1-	T50.7X2-	T50.7X3-	T50.7X4-	T50.7X5-	T50.7X6-
Pentylsalicylamide	T37.1X1-	T37.1X2-	T37.1X3-	T37.1X4-	T37.1X5-	T37.1X6-
Pentymal	T42.3X1-	T42.3X2-	T42.3X3-	T42.3X4-	T42.3X5-	T42.3X6-
Peplomycin	T45.1X1-	T45.1X2-	T45.1X3-	T45.1X4-	T45.1X5-	T45.1X6-
Peppermint (oil)	T47.5X1-	T47.5X2-	T47.5X3-	T47.5X4-	T47.5X5-	T47.5X6-
Pepsin	T47.5X1-	T47.5X2-	T47.5X3-	T47.5X4-	T47.5X5-	T47.5X6-
digestant	T47.5X1-	T47.5X2-	T47.5X3-	T47.5X4-	T47.5X5-	T47.5X6-
Pepstatin	T47.1X1-	T47.1X2-	T47.1X3-	T47.1X4-	T47.1X5-	T47.1X6-
Peptavlon	T50.8X1-	T50.8X2-	T50.8X3-	T50.8X4-	T50.8X5-	T50.8X6-
Perazine	T43.3X1-	T43.3X2-	T43.3X3-	T43.3X4-	T43.3X5-	T43.3X6-
Percaine (spinal)	T41.3X1-	T41.3X2-	T41.3X3-	T41.3X4-	T41.3X5-	T41.3X6-
topical (surface)	T41.3X1-	T41.3X2-	T41.3X3-	T41.3X4-	T41.3X5-	T41.3X6-
Perchloroethylene	T53.3X1-	T53.3X2-	T53.3X3-	T53.3X4-	-	-
medicinal	T37.4X1-	T37.4X2-	T37.4X3-	T37.4X4-	T37.4X5-	T37.4X6-
vapor	T53.3X1-	T53.3X2-	T53.3X3-	T53.3X4-	-	-
Percodan	T40.2X1-	T40.2X2-	T40.2X3-	T40.2X4-	T40.2X5-	T40.2X6-
Percogesic — *see also acetaminophen*	T45.0X1-	T45.0X2-	T45.0X3-	T45.0X4-	T45.0X5-	T45.0X6-
Percorten	T38.0X1-	T38.0X2-	T38.0X3-	T38.0X4-	T38.0X5-	T38.0X6-
Pergolide	T42.8X1-	T42.8X2-	T42.8X3-	T42.8X4-	T42.8X5-	T42.8X6-
Pergonal	T38.811-	T38.812-	T38.813-	T38.814-	T38.815-	T38.816-
Perhexilene	T46.3X1-	T46.3X2-	T46.3X3-	T46.3X4-	T46.3X5-	T46.3X6-
Perhexiline (maleate)	T46.3X1-	T46.3X2-	T46.3X3-	T46.3X4-	T46.3X5-	T46.3X6-
Periactin	T45.0X1-	T45.0X2-	T45.0X3-	T45.0X4-	T45.0X5-	T45.0X6-
Periciazine	T43.3X1-	T43.3X2-	T43.3X3-	T43.3X4-	T43.3X5-	T43.3X6-
Periclor	T42.6X1-	T42.6X2-	T42.6X3-	T42.6X4-	T42.6X5-	T42.6X6-
Perindopril	T46.4X1-	T46.4X2-	T46.4X3-	T46.4X4-	T46.4X5-	T46.4X6-
Perisoxal	T39.8X1-	T39.8X2-	T39.8X3-	T39.8X4-	T39.8X5-	T39.8X6-
Peritoneal dialysis solution	T50.3X1-	T50.3X2-	T50.3X3-	T50.3X4-	T50.3X5-	T50.3X6-
Peritrate	T46.3X1-	T46.3X2-	T46.3X3-	T46.3X4-	T46.3X5-	T46.3X6-
Perlapine	T42.4X1-	T42.4X2-	T42.4X3-	T42.4X4-	T42.4X5-	T42.4X6-
Permanganate	T65.891-	T65.892-	T65.893-	T65.894-	-	-
Permethrin	T60.1X1-	T60.1X2-	T60.1X3-	T60.1X4-	-	-
Pernocton	T42.3X1-	T42.3X2-	T42.3X3-	T42.3X4-	T42.3X5-	T42.3X6-
Pernoston	T42.3X1-	T42.3X2-	T42.3X3-	T42.3X4-	T42.3X5-	T42.3X6-
Peronine	T40.2X1-	T40.2X2-	T40.2X3-	T40.2X4-	-	-
Perphenazine	T43.3X1-	T43.3X2-	T43.3X3-	T43.3X4-	T43.3X5-	T43.3X6-
Pertofrane	T43.011-	T43.012-	T43.013-	T43.014-	T43.015-	T43.016-
Pertussis						
immune serum (human)	T50.Z11-	T50.Z12-	T50.Z13-	T50.Z14-	T50.Z15-	T50.Z16-
vaccine (with diphtheria toxoid) (with tetanus toxoid)	T50.A11-	T50.A12-	T50.A13-	T50.A14-	T50.A15-	T50.A16-
Peruvian balsam	T49.0X1-	T49.0X2-	T49.0X3-	T49.0X4-	T49.0X5-	T49.0X6-
Peruvoside	T46.0X1-	T46.0X2-	T46.0X3-	T46.0X4-	T46.0X5-	T46.0X6-

Substance	Poisoning Accidental (unintentional)	Poisoning Intentional self-harm	Poisoning Assault	Poisoning Undetermined	Adverse effect	Underdosing
Pesticide (dust) (fumes) (vapor) NEC	T60.91X-	T60.92X-	T60.93X-	T60.94X-	-	-
arsenic	T57.0X1-	T57.0X2-	T57.0X3-	T57.0X4-	-	-
chlorinated	T60.1X1-	T60.1X2-	T60.1X3-	T60.1X4-	-	-
cyanide	T65.0X1-	T65.0X2-	T65.0X3-	T65.0X4-	-	-
kerosene	T52.0X1-	T52.0X2-	T52.0X3-	T52.0X4-	-	-
mixture (of compounds)	T60.91X-	T60.92X-	T60.93X-	T60.94X-	-	-
naphthalene	T60.2X1-	T60.2X2-	T60.2X3-	T60.2X4-	-	-
organochlorine (compounds)	T60.1X1-	T60.1X2-	T60.1X3-	T60.1X4-	-	-
petroleum (distillate) (products) NEC	T60.8X1-	T60.8X2-	T60.8X3-	T60.8X4-	-	-
specified ingredient NEC	T60.8X1-	T60.8X2-	T60.8X3-	T60.8X4-	-	-
strychnine	T65.1X1-	T65.1X2-	T65.1X3-	T65.1X4-	-	-
thallium	T60.4X1-	T60.4X2-	T60.4X3-	T60.4X4-	-	-
Pethidine	T40.491-	T40.492-	T40.493-	T40.494-	T40.495-	T40.496-
Petrichloral	T42.6X1-	T42.6X2-	T42.6X3-	T42.6X4-	T42.6X5-	T42.6X6-
Petrol	T52.0X1-	T52.0X2-	T52.0X3-	T52.0X4-	-	-
vapor	T52.0X1-	T52.0X2-	T52.0X3-	T52.0X4-	-	-
Petrolatum	T49.3X1-	T49.3X2-	T49.3X3-	T49.3X4-	T49.3X5-	T49.3X6-
hydrophilic	T49.3X1-	T49.3X2-	T49.3X3-	T49.3X4-	T49.3X5-	T49.3X6-
liquid	T47.4X1-	T47.4X2-	T47.4X3-	T47.4X4-	T47.4X5-	T47.4X6-
topical	T49.3X1-	T49.3X2-	T49.3X3-	T49.3X4-	T49.3X5-	T49.3X6-
nonmedicinal	T52.0X1-	T52.0X2-	T52.0X3-	T52.0X4-	-	-
red veterinary	T49.3X1-	T49.3X2-	T49.3X3-	T49.3X4-	T49.3X5-	T49.3X6-
white	T49.3X1-	T49.3X2-	T49.3X3-	T49.3X4-	T49.3X5-	T49.3X6-
Petroleum (products) NEC	T52.0X1-	T52.0X2-	T52.0X3-	T52.0X4-	-	-
benzine (s) — *see Ligroin*						
ether — *see Ligroin*						
jelly — *see Petrolatum*						
naphtha — *see Ligroin*						
pesticide	T60.8X1-	T60.8X2-	T60.8X3-	T60.8X4-	-	-
solids	T52.0X1-	T52.0X2-	T52.0X3-	T52.0X4-	-	-
solvents	T52.0X1-	T52.0X2-	T52.0X3-	T52.0X4-	-	-
vapor	T52.0X1-	T52.0X2-	T52.0X3-	T52.0X4-	-	-
Peyote	T40.991-	T40.992-	T40.993-	T40.994-	-	-
Phanodorm, phanodorn	T42.3X1-	T42.3X2-	T42.3X3-	T42.3X4-	T42.3X5-	T42.3X6-
Phanquinone	T37.3X1-	T37.3X2-	T37.3X3-	T37.3X4-	T37.3X5-	T37.3X6-
Phanquone	T37.3X1-	T37.3X2-	T37.3X3-	T37.3X4-	T37.3X5-	T37.3X6-
Pharmaceutical						
adjunct NEC	T50.901-	T50.902-	T50.903-	T50.904-	T50.905-	T50.906-
excipient NEC	T50.901-	T50.902-	T50.903-	T50.904-	T50.905-	T50.906-
sweetener	T50.901-	T50.902-	T50.903-	T50.904-	T50.905-	T50.906-
viscous agent	T50.901-	T50.902-	T50.903-	T50.904-	T50.905-	T50.906-
Phemitone	T42.3X1-	T42.3X2-	T42.3X3-	T42.3X4-	T42.3X5-	T42.3X6-
Phenacaine	T41.3X1-	T41.3X2-	T41.3X3-	T41.3X4-	T41.3X5-	T41.3X6-
Phenacemide	T42.6X1-	T42.6X2-	T42.6X3-	T42.6X4-	T42.6X5-	T42.6X6-
Phenacetin	T39.1X1-	T39.1X2-	T39.1X3-	T39.1X4-	T39.1X5-	T39.1X6-
Phenadoxone	T40.2X1-	T40.2X2-	T40.2X3-	T40.2X4-	-	-
Phenaglycodol	T43.591-	T43.592-	T43.593-	T43.594-	T43.595-	T43.596-
Phenantoin	T42.0X1-	T42.0X2-	T42.0X3-	T42.0X4-	T42.0X5-	T42.0X6-
Phenaphthazine reagent	T50.991-	T50.992-	T50.993-	T50.994-	T50.995-	T50.996-
Phenazocine	T40.491-	T40.492-	T40.493-	T40.494-	T40.495-	T40.496-
Phenazone	T39.2X1-	T39.2X2-	T39.2X3-	T39.2X4-	T39.2X5-	T39.2X6-
Phenazopyridine	T39.8X1-	T39.8X2-	T39.8X3-	T39.8X4-	T39.8X5-	T39.8X6-
Phenbenicillin	T36.0X1-	T36.0X2-	T36.0X3-	T36.0X4-	T36.0X5-	T36.0X6-
Phenbutrazate	T50.5X1-	T50.5X2-	T50.5X3-	T50.5X4-	T50.5X5-	T50.5X6-
Phencyclidine	T40.991-	T40.992-	T40.993-	T40.994-	T40.995-	T40.996-
Phendimetrazine	T50.5X1-	T50.5X2-	T50.5X3-	T50.5X4-	T50.5X5-	T50.5X6-
Phenelzine	T43.1X1-	T43.1X2-	T43.1X3-	T43.1X4-	T43.1X5-	T43.1X6-
Phenemal	T42.3X1-	T42.3X2-	T42.3X3-	T42.3X4-	T42.3X5-	T42.3X6-

Substance	Poisoning Accidental (unintentional)	Poisoning Intentional self-harm	Poisoning Assault	Poisoning Undetermined	Adverse effect	Underdosing
Phenergan	T42.6X1-	T42.6X2-	T42.6X3-	T42.6X4-	T42.6X5-	T42.6X6-
Pheneticillin	T36.0X1-	T36.0X2-	T36.0X3-	T36.0X4-	T36.0X5-	T36.0X6-
Pheneturide	T42.6X1-	T42.6X2-	T42.6X3-	T42.6X4-	T42.6X5-	T42.6X6-
Phenformin	T38.3X1-	T38.3X2-	T38.3X3-	T38.3X4-	T38.3X5-	T38.3X6-
Phenglutarimide	T44.3X1-	T44.3X2-	T44.3X3-	T44.3X4-	T44.3X5-	T44.3X6-
Phenicarbazide	T39.8X1-	T39.8X2-	T39.8X3-	T39.8X4-	T39.8X5-	T39.8X6-
Phenindamine	T45.0X1-	T45.0X2-	T45.0X3-	T45.0X4-	T45.0X5-	T45.0X6-
Phenindione	T45.511-	T45.512-	T45.513-	T45.514-	T45.515-	T45.516-
Pheniprazine	T43.1X1-	T43.1X2-	T43.1X3-	T43.1X4-	T43.1X5-	T43.1X6-
Pheniramine	T45.0X1-	T45.0X2-	T45.0X3-	T45.0X4-	T45.0X5-	T45.0X6-
Phenisatin	T47.2X1-	T47.2X2-	T47.2X3-	T47.2X4-	T47.2X5-	T47.2X6-
Phenmetrazine	T50.5X1-	T50.5X2-	T50.5X3-	T50.5X4-	T50.5X5-	T50.5X6-
Phenobal	T42.3X1-	T42.3X2-	T42.3X3-	T42.3X4-	T42.3X5-	T42.3X6-
Phenobarbital	T42.3X1-	T42.3X2-	T42.3X3-	T42.3X4-	T42.3X5-	T42.3X6-
with						
mephenytoin	T42.3X1-	T42.3X2-	T42.3X3-	T42.3X4-	T42.3X5-	T42.3X6-
phenytoin	T42.3X1-	T42.3X2-	T42.3X3-	T42.3X4-	T42.3X5-	T42.3X6-
sodium	T42.3X1-	T42.3X2-	T42.3X3-	T42.3X4-	T42.3X5-	T42.3X6-
Phenobarbitone	T42.3X1-	T42.3X2-	T42.3X3-	T42.3X4-	T42.3X5-	T42.3X6-
Phenobutiodil	T50.8X1-	T50.8X2-	T50.8X3-	T50.8X4-	T50.8X5-	T50.8X6-
Phenoctide	T49.0X1-	T49.0X2-	T49.0X3-	T49.0X4-	T49.0X5-	T49.0X6-
Phenol	T49.0X1-	T49.0X2-	T49.0X3-	T49.0X4-	T49.0X5-	T49.0X6-
disinfectant	T54.0X1-	T54.0X2-	T54.0X3-	T54.0X4-	-	-
in oil injection	T46.8X1-	T46.8X2-	T46.8X3-	T46.8X4-	T46.8X5-	T46.8X6-
medicinal	T49.1X1-	T49.1X2-	T49.1X3-	T49.1X4-	T49.1X5-	T49.1X6-
nonmedicinal NEC	T54.0X1-	T54.0X2-	T54.0X3-	T54.0X4-	-	-
pesticide	T60.8X1-	T60.8X2-	T60.8X3-	T60.8X4-	-	-
red	T50.8X1-	T50.8X2-	T50.8X3-	T50.8X4-	T50.8X5-	T50.8X6-
Phenolic preparation	T49.1X1-	T49.1X2-	T49.1X3-	T49.1X4-	T49.1X5-	T49.1X6-
Phenolphthalein	T47.2X1-	T47.2X2-	T47.2X3-	T47.2X4-	T47.2X5-	T47.2X6-
Phenolsulfonphthalein	T50.8X1-	T50.8X2-	T50.8X3-	T50.8X4-	T50.8X5-	T50.8X6-
Phenomorphan	T40.2X1-	T40.2X2-	T40.2X3-	T40.2X4-	-	-
Phenonyl	T42.3X1-	T42.3X2-	T42.3X3-	T42.3X4-	T42.3X5-	T42.3X6-
Phenoperidine	T40.491-	T40.492-	T40.493-	T40.494-	-	-
Phenopyrazone	T46.991-	T46.992-	T46.993-	T46.994-	T46.995-	T46.996-
Phenoquin	T50.4X1-	T50.4X2-	T50.4X3-	T50.4X4-	T50.4X5-	T50.4X6-
Phenothiazine (psychotropic) NEC	T43.3X1-	T43.3X2-	T43.3X3-	T43.3X4-	T43.3X5-	T43.3X6-
insecticide	T60.2X1-	T60.2X2-	T60.2X3-	T60.2X4-	-	-
Phenothrin	T49.0X1-	T49.0X2-	T49.0X3-	T49.0X4-	T49.0X5-	T49.0X6-
Phenoxybenzamine	T46.7X1-	T46.7X2-	T46.7X3-	T46.7X4-	T46.7X5-	T46.7X6-
Phenoxyethanol	T49.0X1-	T49.0X2-	T49.0X3-	T49.0X4-	T49.0X5-	T49.0X6-
Phenoxymethyl penicillin	T36.0X1-	T36.0X2-	T36.0X3-	T36.0X4-	T36.0X5-	T36.0X6-
Phenprobamate	T42.8X1-	T42.8X2-	T42.8X3-	T42.8X4-	T42.8X5-	T42.8X6-
Phenprocoumon	T45.511-	T45.512-	T45.513-	T45.514-	T45.515-	T45.516-
Phensuximide	T42.2X1-	T42.2X2-	T42.2X3-	T42.2X4-	T42.2X5-	T42.2X6-
Phentermine	T50.5X1-	T50.5X2-	T50.5X3-	T50.5X4-	T50.5X5-	T50.5X6-
Phenthicillin	T36.0X1-	T36.0X2-	T36.0X3-	T36.0X4-	T36.0X5-	T36.0X6-
Phentolamine	T46.7X1-	T46.7X2-	T46.7X3-	T46.7X4-	T46.7X5-	T46.7X6-
Phenyl						
butazone	T39.2X1-	T39.2X2-	T39.2X3-	T39.2X4-	T39.2X5-	T39.2X6-
enediamine	T65.3X1-	T65.3X2-	T65.3X3-	T65.3X4-	-	-
hydrazine	T65.3X1-	T65.3X2-	T65.3X3-	T65.3X4-	-	-
antineoplastic	T45.1X1-	T45.1X2-	T45.1X3-	T45.1X4-	T45.1X5-	T45.1X6-
mercuric compounds — see *Mercury*						
salicylate	T49.3X1-	T49.3X2-	T49.3X3-	T49.3X4-	T49.3X5-	T49.3X6-
Phenylalanine mustard	T45.1X1-	T45.1X2-	T45.1X3-	T45.1X4-	T45.1X5-	T45.1X6-
Phenylbutazone	T39.2X1-	T39.2X2-	T39.2X3-	T39.2X4-	T39.2X5-	T39.2X6-
Phenylenediamine	T65.3X1-	T65.3X2-	T65.3X3-	T65.3X4-	-	-
Phenylephrine	T44.4X1-	T44.4X2-	T44.4X3-	T44.4X4-	T44.4X5-	T44.4X6-

Substance	Poisoning Accidental (unintentional)	Poisoning Intentional self-harm	Poisoning Assault	Poisoning Undetermined	Adverse effect	Underdosing
Phenylethylbiguanide	T38.3X1-	T38.3X2-	T38.3X3-	T38.3X4-	T38.3X5-	T38.3X6-
Phenylmercuric						
acetate	T49.0X1-	T49.0X2-	T49.0X3-	T49.0X4-	T49.0X5-	T49.0X6-
borate	T49.0X1-	T49.0X2-	T49.0X3-	T49.0X4-	T49.0X5-	T49.0X6-
nitrate	T49.0X1-	T49.0X2-	T49.0X3-	T49.0X4-	T49.0X5-	T49.0X6-
Phenylmethylbarbitone	T42.3X1-	T42.3X2-	T42.3X3-	T42.3X4-	T42.3X5-	T42.3X6-
Phenylpropanol	T47.5X1-	T47.5X2-	T47.5X3-	T47.5X4-	T47.5X5-	T47.5X6-
Phenylpropanolamine	T44.991-	T44.992-	T44.993-	T44.994-	T44.995-	T44.996-
Phenylsulfthion	T60.0X1-	T60.0X2-	T60.0X3-	T60.0X4-	-	-
Phenyltoloxamine	T45.0X1-	T45.0X2-	T45.0X3-	T45.0X4-	T45.0X5-	T45.0X6-
Phenyramidol, phenyramidon	T39.8X1-	T39.8X2-	T39.8X3-	T39.8X4-	T39.8X5-	T39.8X6-
Phenytoin	T42.0X1-	T42.0X2-	T42.0X3-	T42.0X4-	T42.0X5-	T42.0X6-
with Phenobarbital	T42.3X1-	T42.3X2-	T42.3X3-	T42.3X4-	T42.3X5-	T42.3X6-
pHisoHex	T49.2X1-	T49.2X2-	T49.2X3-	T49.2X4-	T49.2X5-	T49.2X6-
Pholcodine	T48.3X1-	T48.3X2-	T48.3X3-	T48.3X4-	T48.3X5-	T48.3X6-
Pholedrine	T46.991-	T46.992-	T46.993-	T46.994-	T46.995-	T46.996-
Phorate	T60.0X1-	T60.0X2-	T60.0X3-	T60.0X4-	-	-
Phosdrin	T60.0X1-	T60.0X2-	T60.0X3-	T60.0X4-	-	-
Phosfolan	T60.0X1-	T60.0X2-	T60.0X3-	T60.0X4-	-	-
Phosgene (gas)	T59.891-	T59.892-	T59.893-	T59.894-	-	-
Phosphamidon	T60.0X1-	T60.0X2-	T60.0X3-	T60.0X4-	-	-
Phosphate	T65.891-	T65.892-	T65.893-	T65.894-	-	-
laxative	T47.4X1-	T47.4X2-	T47.4X3-	T47.4X4-	T47.4X5-	T47.4X6-
organic	T60.0X1-	T60.0X2-	T60.0X3-	T60.0X4-	-	-
solvent	T52.91X-	T52.92X-	T52.93X-	T52.94X-	-	-
tricresyl	T65.891-	T65.892-	T65.893-	T65.894-	-	-
Phosphine	T57.1X1-	T57.1X2-	T57.1X3-	T57.1X4-	-	-
fumigant	T57.1X1-	T57.1X2-	T57.1X3-	T57.1X4-	-	-
Phospholine	T49.5X1-	T49.5X2-	T49.5X3-	T49.5X4-	T49.5X5-	T49.5X6-
Phosphoric acid	T54.2X1-	T54.2X2-	T54.2X3-	T54.2X4-	-	-
Phosphorus (compound) NEC	T57.1X1-	T57.1X2-	T57.1X3-	T57.1X4-	-	-
pesticide	T60.0X1-	T60.0X2-	T60.0X3-	T60.0X4-	-	-
Phthalates	T65.891-	T65.892-	T65.893-	T65.894-	-	-
Phthalic anhydride	T65.891-	T65.892-	T65.893-	T65.894-	-	-
Phthalimidoglutarimide	T42.6X1-	T42.6X2-	T42.6X3-	T42.6X4-	T42.6X5-	T42.6X6-
Phthalylsulfathiazole	T37.0X1-	T37.0X2-	T37.0X3-	T37.0X4-	T37.0X5-	T37.0X6-
Phylloquinone	T45.7X1-	T45.7X2-	T45.7X3-	T45.7X4-	T45.7X5-	T45.7X6-
Physeptone	T40.3X1-	T40.3X2-	T40.3X3-	T40.3X4-	T40.3X5-	T40.3X6-
Physostigma venenosum	T62.2X1-	T62.2X2-	T62.2X3-	T62.2X4-	-	-
Physostigmine	T49.5X1-	T49.5X2-	T49.5X3-	T49.5X4-	T49.5X5-	T49.5X6-
Phytolacca decandra	T62.2X1-	T62.2X2-	T62.2X3-	T62.2X4-	-	-
berries	T62.1X1-	T62.1X2-	T62.1X3-	T62.1X4-	-	-
Phytomenadione	T45.7X1-	T45.7X2-	T45.7X3-	T45.7X4-	T45.7X5-	T45.7X6-
Phytonadione	T45.7X1-	T45.7X2-	T45.7X3-	T45.7X4-	T45.7X5-	T45.7X6-
Picoperine	T48.3X1-	T48.3X2-	T48.3X3-	T48.3X4-	T48.3X5-	T48.3X6-
Picosulfate (sodium)	T47.2X1-	T47.2X2-	T47.2X3-	T47.2X4-	T47.2X5-	T47.2X6-
Picric (acid)	T54.2X1-	T54.2X2-	T54.2X3-	T54.2X4-	-	-
Picrotoxin	T50.7X1-	T50.7X2-	T50.7X3-	T50.7X4-	T50.7X5-	T50.7X6-
Piketoprofen	T49.0X1-	T49.0X2-	T49.0X3-	T49.0X4-	T49.0X5-	T49.0X6-
Pilocarpine	T44.1X1-	T44.1X2-	T44.1X3-	T44.1X4-	T44.1X5-	T44.1X6-
Pilocarpus (jaborandi) extract	T44.1X1-	T44.1X2-	T44.1X3-	T44.1X4-	T44.1X5-	T44.1X6-
Pilsicainide (hydrochloride)	T46.2X1-	T46.2X2-	T46.2X3-	T46.2X4-	T46.2X5-	T46.2X6-
Pimaricin	T36.7X1-	T36.7X2-	T36.7X3-	T36.7X4-	T36.7X5-	T36.7X6-
Pimeclone	T50.7X1-	T50.7X2-	T50.7X3-	T50.7X4-	T50.7X5-	T50.7X6-
Pimelic ketone	T52.8X1-	T52.8X2-	T52.8X3-	T52.8X4-	-	-
Pimethixene	T45.0X1-	T45.0X2-	T45.0X3-	T45.0X4-	T45.0X5-	T45.0X6-
Piminodine	T40.2X1-	T40.2X2-	T40.2X3-	T40.2X4-	T40.2X5-	T40.2X6-
Pimozide	T43.591-	T43.592-	T43.593-	T43.594-	T43.595-	T43.596-

Substance	Poisoning Accidental (unintentional)	Poisoning Intentional self-harm	Poisoning Assault	Poisoning Undetermined	Adverse effect	Underdosing
Pinacidil	T46.5X1-	T46.5X2-	T46.5X3-	T46.5X4-	T46.5X5-	T46.5X6-
Pinaverium bromide	T44.3X1-	T44.3X2-	T44.3X3-	T44.3X4-	T44.3X5-	T44.3X6-
Pinazepam	T42.4X1-	T42.4X2-	T42.4X3-	T42.4X4-	T42.4X5-	T42.4X6-
Pindolol	T44.7X1-	T44.7X2-	T44.7X3-	T44.7X4-	T44.7X5-	T44.7X6-
Pindone	T60.4X1-	T60.4X2-	T60.4X3-	T60.4X4-	-	-
Pine oil (disinfectant)	T65.891-	T65.892-	T65.893-	T65.894-	-	-
Pinkroot	T37.4X1-	T37.4X2-	T37.4X3-	T37.4X4-	T37.4X5-	T37.4X6-
Pipadone	T40.2X1-	T40.2X2-	T40.2X3-	T40.2X4-	-	-
Pipamazine	T45.0X1-	T45.0X2-	T45.0X3-	T45.0X4-	T45.0X5-	T45.0X6-
Pipamperone	T43.4X1-	T43.4X2-	T43.4X3-	T43.4X4-	T43.4X5-	T43.4X6-
Pipazetate	T48.3X1-	T48.3X2-	T48.3X3-	T48.3X4-	T48.3X5-	T48.3X6-
Pipemidic acid	T37.8X1-	T37.8X2-	T37.8X3-	T37.8X4-	T37.8X5-	T37.8X6-
Pipenzolate bromide	T44.3X1-	T44.3X2-	T44.3X3-	T44.3X4-	T44.3X5-	T44.3X6-
Piperacetazine	T43.3X1-	T43.3X2-	T43.3X3-	T43.3X4-	T43.3X5-	T43.3X6-
Piperacillin	T36.0X1-	T36.0X2-	T36.0X3-	T36.0X4-	T36.0X5-	T36.0X6-
Piperazine	T37.4X1-	T37.4X2-	T37.4X3-	T37.4X4-	T37.4X5-	T37.4X6-
estrone sulfate	T38.5X1-	T38.5X2-	T38.5X3-	T38.5X4-	T38.5X5-	T38.5X6-
Piper cubeba	T62.2X1-	T62.2X2-	T62.2X3-	T62.2X4-	-	-
Piperidione	T48.3X1-	T48.3X2-	T48.3X3-	T48.3X4-	T48.3X5-	T48.3X6-
Piperidolate	T44.3X1-	T44.3X2-	T44.3X3-	T44.3X4-	T44.3X5-	T44.3X6-
Piperocaine	T41.3X1-	T41.3X2-	T41.3X3-	T41.3X4-	T41.3X5-	T41.3X6-
infiltration (subcutaneous)	T41.3X1-	T41.3X2-	T41.3X3-	T41.3X4-	T41.3X5-	T41.3X6-
nerve block (peripheral) (plexus)	T41.3X1-	T41.3X2-	T41.3X3-	T41.3X4-	T41.3X5-	T41.3X6-
topical (surface)	T41.3X1-	T41.3X2-	T41.3X3-	T41.3X4-	T41.3X5-	T41.3X6-
Piperonyl butoxide	T60.8X1-	T60.8X2-	T60.8X3-	T60.8X4-	-	-
Pipethanate	T44.3X1-	T44.3X2-	T44.3X3-	T44.3X4-	T44.3X5-	T44.3X6-
Pipobroman	T45.1X1-	T45.1X2-	T45.1X3-	T45.1X4-	T45.1X5-	T45.1X6-
Pipotiazine	T43.3X1-	T43.3X2-	T43.3X3-	T43.3X4-	T43.3X5-	T43.3X6-
Pipoxizine	T45.0X1-	T45.0X2-	T45.0X3-	T45.0X4-	T45.0X5-	T45.0X6-
Pipradrol	T43.691-	T43.692-	T43.693-	T43.694-	T43.695-	T43.696-
Piprinhydrinate	T45.0X1-	T45.0X2-	T45.0X3-	T45.0X4-	T45.0X5-	T45.0X6-
Pirarubicin	T45.1X1-	T45.1X2-	T45.1X3-	T45.1X4-	T45.1X5-	T45.1X6-
Pirazinamide	T37.1X1-	T37.1X2-	T37.1X3-	T37.1X4-	T37.1X5-	T37.1X6-
Pirbuterol	T48.6X1-	T48.6X2-	T48.6X3-	T48.6X4-	T48.6X5-	T48.6X6-
Pirenzepine	T47.1X1-	T47.1X2-	T47.1X3-	T47.1X4-	T47.1X5-	T47.1X6-
Piretanide	T50.1X1-	T50.1X2-	T50.1X3-	T50.1X4-	T50.1X5-	T50.1X6-
Piribedil	T42.8X1-	T42.8X2-	T42.8X3-	T42.8X4-	T42.8X5-	T42.8X6-
Piridoxilate	T46.3X1-	T46.3X2-	T46.3X3-	T46.3X4-	T46.3X5-	T46.3X6-
Piritramide	T40.491-	T40.492-	T40.493-	T40.494-	-	-
Piromidic acid	T37.8X1-	T37.8X2-	T37.8X3-	T37.8X4-	T37.8X5-	T37.8X6-
Piroxicam	T39.391-	T39.392-	T39.393-	T39.394-	T39.395-	T39.396-
beta-cyclodextrin complex	T39.8X1-	T39.8X2-	T39.8X3-	T39.8X4-	T39.8X5-	T39.8X6-
Pirozadil	T46.6X1-	T46.6X2-	T46.6X3-	T46.6X4-	T46.6X5-	T46.6X6-
Piscidia (bark) (erythrina)	T39.8X1-	T39.8X2-	T39.8X3-	T39.8X4-	T39.8X5-	T39.8X6-
Pitch	T65.891-	T65.892-	T65.893-	T65.894-	-	-
Pitkin's solution	T41.3X1-	T41.3X2-	T41.3X3-	T41.3X4-	T41.3X5-	T41.3X6-
Pitocin	T48.0X1-	T48.0X2-	T48.0X3-	T48.0X4-	T48.0X5-	T48.0X6-
Pitressin (tannate)	T38.891-	T38.892-	T38.893-	T38.894-	T38.895-	T38.896-
Pituitary extracts (posterior)	T38.891-	T38.892-	T38.893-	T38.894-	T38.895-	T38.896-
anterior	T38.811-	T38.812-	T38.813-	T38.814-	T38.815-	T38.816-
Pituitrin	T38.891-	T38.892-	T38.893-	T38.894-	T38.895-	T38.896-
Pivampicillin	T36.0X1-	T36.0X2-	T36.0X3-	T36.0X4-	T36.0X5-	T36.0X6-
Pivmecillinam	T36.0X1-	T36.0X2-	T36.0X3-	T36.0X4-	T36.0X5-	T36.0X6-
Placental hormone	T38.891-	T38.892-	T38.893-	T38.894-	T38.895-	T38.896-
Placidyl	T42.6X1-	T42.6X2-	T42.6X3-	T42.6X4-	T42.6X5-	T42.6X6-
Plague vaccine	T50.A91-	T50.A92-	T50.A93-	T50.A94-	T50.A95-	T50.A96-
Plant						
food or fertilizer NEC	T65.891-	T65.892-	T65.893-	T65.894-	-	-

Substance	Poisoning Accidental (unintentional)	Poisoning Intentional self-harm	Poisoning Assault	Poisoning Undetermined	Adverse effect	Underdosing
Plant (continued)						
containing herbicide	T60.3X1-	T60.3X2-	T60.3X3-	T60.3X4-	-	-
noxious, used as food	T62.2X1-	T62.2X2-	T62.2X3-	T62.2X4-	-	-
berries	T62.1X1-	T62.1X2-	T62.1X3-	T62.1X4-	-	-
seeds	T62.2X1-	T62.2X2-	T62.2X3-	T62.2X4-	-	-
specified type NEC	T62.2X1-	T62.2X2-	T62.2X3-	T62.2X4-	-	-
Plasma	T45.8X1-	T45.8X2-	T45.8X3-	T45.8X4-	T45.8X5-	T45.8X6-
expander NEC	T45.8X1-	T45.8X2-	T45.8X3-	T45.8X4-	T45.8X5-	T45.8X6-
protein fraction (human)	T45.8X1-	T45.8X2-	T45.8X3-	T45.8X4-	T45.8X5-	T45.8X6-
Plasmanate	T45.8X1-	T45.8X2-	T45.8X3-	T45.8X4-	T45.8X5-	T45.8X6-
Plasminogen (tissue) activator	T45.611-	T45.612-	T45.613-	T45.614-	T45.615-	T45.616-
Plaster dressing	T49.3X1-	T49.3X2-	T49.3X3-	T49.3X4-	T49.3X5-	T49.3X6-
Plastic dressing	T49.3X1-	T49.3X2-	T49.3X3-	T49.3X4-	T49.3X5-	T49.3X6-
Plegicil	T43.3X1-	T43.3X2-	T43.3X3-	T43.3X4-	T43.3X5-	T43.3X6-
Plicamycin	T45.1X1-	T45.1X2-	T45.1X3-	T45.1X4-	T45.1X5-	T45.1X6-
Podophyllotoxin	T49.8X1-	T49.8X2-	T49.8X3-	T49.8X4-	T49.8X5-	T49.8X6-
Podophyllum (resin)	T49.4X1-	T49.4X2-	T49.4X3-	T49.4X4-	T49.4X5-	T49.4X6-
Poison NEC	T65.91X-	T65.92X-	T65.93X-	T65.94X-	-	-
Poisonous berries	T62.1X1-	T62.1X2-	T62.1X3-	T62.1X4-	-	-
Pokeweed (any part)	T62.2X1-	T62.2X2-	T62.2X3-	T62.2X4-	-	-
Poldine metilsulfate	T44.3X1-	T44.3X2-	T44.3X3-	T44.3X4-	T44.3X5-	T44.3X6-
Polidexide (sulfate)	T46.6X1-	T46.6X2-	T46.6X3-	T46.6X4-	T46.6X5-	T46.6X6-
Polidocanol	T46.8X1-	T46.8X2-	T46.8X3-	T46.8X4-	T46.8X5-	T46.8X6-
Poliomyelitis vaccine	T50.B91-	T50.B92-	T50.B93-	T50.B94-	T50.B95-	T50.B96-
Polish (car) (floor) (furni-ture) (metal) (porcelain) (silver)	T65.891-	T65.892-	T65.893-	T65.894-	-	-
abrasive	T65.891-	T65.892-	T65.893-	T65.894-	-	-
porcelain	T65.891-	T65.892-	T65.893-	T65.894-	-	-
Poloxalkol	T47.4X1-	T47.4X2-	T47.4X3-	T47.4X4-	T47.4X5-	T47.4X6-
Poloxamer	T47.4X1-	T47.4X2-	T47.4X3-	T47.4X4-	T47.4X5-	T47.4X6-
Polyaminostyrene resins	T50.3X1-	T50.3X2-	T50.3X3-	T50.3X4-	T50.3X5-	T50.3X6-
Polycarbophil	T47.4X1-	T47.4X2-	T47.4X3-	T47.4X4-	T47.4X5-	T47.4X6-
Polychlorinated biphenyl	T65.891-	T65.892-	T65.893-	T65.894-	-	-
Polycycline	T36.4X1-	T36.4X2-	T36.4X3-	T36.4X4-	T36.4X5-	T36.4X6-
Polyester fumes	T59.891-	T59.892-	T59.893-	T59.894-	-	-
Polyester resin hardener	T52.91X-	T52.92X-	T52.93X-	T52.94X-	-	-
fumes	T59.891-	T59.892-	T59.893-	T59.894-	-	-
Polyestradiol phosphate	T38.5X1-	T38.5X2-	T38.5X3-	T38.5X4-	T38.5X5-	T38.5X6-
Polyethanolamine alkyl sulfate	T49.2X1-	T49.2X2-	T49.2X3-	T49.2X4-	T49.2X5-	T49.2X6-
Polyethylene adhesive	T49.3X1-	T49.3X2-	T49.3X3-	T49.3X4-	T49.3X5-	T49.3X6-
Polyferose	T45.4X1-	T45.4X2-	T45.4X3-	T45.4X4-	T45.4X5-	T45.4X6-
Polygeline	T45.8X1-	T45.8X2-	T45.8X3-	T45.8X4-	T45.8X5-	T45.8X6-
Polymyxin	T36.8X1-	T36.8X2-	T36.8X3-	T36.8X4-	T36.8X5-	T36.8X6-
B	T36.8X1-	T36.8X2-	T36.8X3-	T36.8X4-	T36.8X5-	T36.8X6-
ENT agent	T49.6X1-	T49.6X2-	T49.6X3-	T49.6X4-	T49.6X5-	T49.6X6-
ophthalmic preparation	T49.5X1-	T49.5X2-	T49.5X3-	T49.5X4-	T49.5X5-	T49.5X6-
topical NEC	T49.0X1-	T49.0X2-	T49.0X3-	T49.0X4-	T49.0X5-	T49.0X6-
E sulfate (eye preparation)	T49.5X1-	T49.5X2-	T49.5X3-	T49.5X4-	T49.5X5-	T49.5X6-
Polynoxylin	T49.0X1-	T49.0X2-	T49.0X3-	T49.0X4-	T49.0X5-	T49.0X6-
Polyoestradiol phosphate	T38.5X1-	T38.5X2-	T38.5X3-	T38.5X4-	T38.5X5-	T38.5X6-
Polyoxymethyleneurea	T49.0X1-	T49.0X2-	T49.0X3-	T49.0X4-	T49.0X5-	T49.0X6-
Polysilane	T47.8X1-	T47.8X2-	T47.8X3-	T47.8X4-	T47.8X5-	T47.8X6-
Polytetrafluoroethylene (inhaled)	T59.891-	T59.892-	T59.893-	T59.894-	-	-
Polythiazide	T50.2X1-	T50.2X2-	T50.2X3-	T50.2X4-	T50.2X5-	T50.2X6-
Polyvidone	T45.8X1-	T45.8X2-	T45.8X3-	T45.8X4-	T45.8X5-	T45.8X6-
Polyvinylpyrrolidone	T45.8X1-	T45.8X2-	T45.8X3-	T45.8X4-	T45.8X5-	T45.8X6-
Pontocaine (hydrochloride) (infiltration) (topical)	T41.3X1-	T41.3X2-	T41.3X3-	T41.3X4-	T41.3X5-	T41.3X6-
nerve block (peripheral) (plexus)	T41.3X1-	T41.3X2-	T41.3X3-	T41.3X4-	T41.3X5-	T41.3X6-

Substance	Poisoning Accidental (unintentional)	Poisoning Intentional self-harm	Poisoning Assault	Poisoning Undetermined	Adverse effect	Underdosing
Pontocaine (hydrochloride) (infiltration) (topical) (continued)						
spinal	T41.3X1-	T41.3X2-	T41.3X3-	T41.3X4-	T41.3X5-	T41.3X6-
Porfiromycin	T45.1X1-	T45.1X2-	T45.1X3-	T45.1X4-	T45.1X5-	T45.1X6-
Posterior pituitary hormone NEC	T38.891-	T38.892-	T38.893-	T38.894-	T38.895-	T38.896-
Pot	T40.711-	T40.712-	T40.713-	T40.714-	T40.715-	T40.716-
Potash (caustic)	T54.3X1-	T54.3X2-	T54.3X3-	T54.3X4-	-	-
Potassic saline injection (lactated)	T50.3X1-	T50.3X2-	T50.3X3-	T50.3X4-	T50.3X5-	T50.3X6-
Potassium (salts) NEC	T50.3X1-	T50.3X2-	T50.3X3-	T50.3X4-	T50.3X5-	T50.3X6-
aminobenzoate	T45.8X1-	T45.8X2-	T45.8X3-	T45.8X4-	T45.8X5-	T45.8X6-
aminosalicylate	T37.1X1-	T37.1X2-	T37.1X3-	T37.1X4-	T37.1X5-	T37.1X6-
antimony ' tartrate'	T37.8X1-	T37.8X2-	T37.8X3-	T37.8X4-	T37.8X5-	T37.8X6-
arsenite (solution)	T57.0X1-	T57.0X2-	T57.0X3-	T57.0X4-	-	-
bichromate	T56.2X1-	T56.2X2-	T56.2X3-	T56.2X4-	-	-
bisulfate	T47.3X1-	T47.3X2-	T47.3X3-	T47.3X4-	T47.3X5-	T47.3X6-
bromide	T42.6X1-	T42.6X2-	T42.6X3-	T42.6X4-	T42.6X5-	T42.6X6-
canrenoate	T50.0X1-	T50.0X2-	T50.0X3-	T50.0X4-	T50.0X5-	T50.0X6-
carbonate	T54.3X1-	T54.3X2-	T54.3X3-	T54.3X4-	-	-
chlorate NEC	T65.891-	T65.892-	T65.893-	T65.894-	-	-
chloride	T50.3X1-	T50.3X2-	T50.3X3-	T50.3X4-	T50.3X5-	T50.3X6-
citrate	T50.991-	T50.992-	T50.993-	T50.994-	T50.995-	T50.996-
cyanide	T65.0X1-	T65.0X2-	T65.0X3-	T65.0X4-	-	-
ferric hexacyanoferrate (medicinal)	T50.6X1-	T50.6X2-	T50.6X3-	T50.6X4-	T50.6X5-	T50.6X6-
nonmedicinal	T65.891-	T65.892-	T65.893-	T65.894-	-	-
Fluoride	T57.8X1-	T57.8X2-	T57.8X3-	T57.8X4-	-	-
glucaldrate	T47.1X1-	T47.1X2-	T47.1X3-	T47.1X4-	T47.1X5-	T47.1X6-
hydroxide	T54.3X1-	T54.3X2-	T54.3X3-	T54.3X4-	-	-
iodate	T49.0X1-	T49.0X2-	T49.0X3-	T49.0X4-	T49.0X5-	T49.0X6-
iodide	T48.4X1-	T48.4X2-	T48.4X3-	T48.4X4-	T48.4X5-	T48.4X6-
nitrate	T57.8X1-	T57.8X2-	T57.8X3-	T57.8X4-	-	-
oxalate	T65.891-	T65.892-	T65.893-	T65.894-	-	-
perchlorate (nonmedicinal) NEC	T65.891-	T65.892-	T65.893-	T65.894-	-	-
antithyroid	T38.2X1-	T38.2X2-	T38.2X3-	T38.2X4-	T38.2X5-	T38.2X6-
medicinal	T38.2X1-	T38.2X2-	T38.2X3-	T38.2X4-	T38.2X5-	T38.2X6-
Permanganate (nonmedicinal)	T65.891-	T65.892-	T65.893-	T65.894-	-	-
medicinal	T49.0X1-	T49.0X2-	T49.0X3-	T49.0X4-	T49.0X5-	T49.0X6-
sulfate	T47.2X1-	T47.2X2-	T47.2X3-	T47.2X4-	T47.2X5-	T47.2X6-
Potassium-removing resin	T50.3X1-	T50.3X2-	T50.3X3-	T50.3X4-	T50.3X5-	T50.3X6-
Potassium-retaining drug	T50.3X1-	T50.3X2-	T50.3X3-	T50.3X4-	T50.3X5-	T50.3X6-
Povidone	T45.8X1-	T45.8X2-	T45.8X3-	T45.8X4-	T45.8X5-	T45.8X6-
iodine	T49.0X1-	T49.0X2-	T49.0X3-	T49.0X4-	T49.0X5-	T49.0X6-
Practolol	T44.7X1-	T44.7X2-	T44.7X3-	T44.7X4-	T44.7X5-	T44.7X6-
Prajmalium bitartrate	T46.2X1-	T46.2X2-	T46.2X3-	T46.2X4-	T46.2X5-	T46.2X6-
Pralidoxime (iodide)	T50.6X1-	T50.6X2-	T50.6X3-	T50.6X4-	T50.6X5-	T50.6X6-
chloride	T50.6X1-	T50.6X2-	T50.6X3-	T50.6X4-	T50.6X5-	T50.6X6-
Pramiverine	T44.3X1-	T44.3X2-	T44.3X3-	T44.3X4-	T44.3X5-	T44.3X6-
Pramocaine	T49.1X1-	T49.1X2-	T49.1X3-	T49.1X4-	T49.1X5-	T49.1X6-
Pramoxine	T49.1X1-	T49.1X2-	T49.1X3-	T49.1X4-	T49.1X5-	T49.1X6-
Prasterone	T38.7X1-	T38.7X2-	T38.7X3-	T38.7X4-	T38.7X5-	T38.7X6-
Pravastatin	T46.6X1-	T46.6X2-	T46.6X3-	T46.6X4-	T46.6X5-	T46.6X6-
Prazepam	T42.4X1-	T42.4X2-	T42.4X3-	T42.4X4-	T42.4X5-	T42.4X6-
Praziquantel	T37.4X1-	T37.4X2-	T37.4X3-	T37.4X4-	T37.4X5-	T37.4X6-
Prazitone	T43.291-	T43.292-	T43.293-	T43.294-	T43.295-	T43.296-
Prazosin	T44.6X1-	T44.6X2-	T44.6X3-	T44.6X4-	T44.6X5-	T44.6X6-
Prednicarbate	T49.0X1-	T49.0X2-	T49.0X3-	T49.0X4-	T49.0X5-	T49.0X6-
Prednimustine	T45.1X1-	T45.1X2-	T45.1X3-	T45.1X4-	T45.1X5-	T45.1X6-
Prednisolone	T38.0X1-	T38.0X2-	T38.0X3-	T38.0X4-	T38.0X5-	T38.0X6-
ENT agent	T49.6X1-	T49.6X2-	T49.6X3-	T49.6X4-	T49.6X5-	T49.6X6-
ophthalmic preparation	T49.5X1-	T49.5X2-	T49.5X3-	T49.5X4-	T49.5X5-	T49.5X6-

Substance	Poisoning Accidental (unintentional)	Poisoning Intentional self-harm	Poisoning Assault	Poisoning Undetermined	Adverse effect	Underdosing
Prednisolone (continued)						
steaglate	T49.0X1-	T49.0X2-	T49.0X3-	T49.0X4-	T49.0X5-	T49.0X6-
topical NEC	T49.0X1-	T49.0X2-	T49.0X3-	T49.0X4-	T49.0X5-	T49.0X6-
Prednisone	T38.0X1-	T38.0X2-	T38.0X3-	T38.0X4-	T38.0X5-	T38.0X6-
Prednylidene	T38.0X1-	T38.0X2-	T38.0X3-	T38.0X4-	T38.0X5-	T38.0X6-
Pregnandiol	T38.5X1-	T38.5X2-	T38.5X3-	T38.5X4-	T38.5X5-	T38.5X6-
Pregneninolone	T38.5X1-	T38.5X2-	T38.5X3-	T38.5X4-	T38.5X5-	T38.5X6-
Preludin	T43.691-	T43.692-	T43.693-	T43.694-	T43.695-	T43.696-
Premarin	T38.5X1-	T38.5X2-	T38.5X3-	T38.5X4-	T38.5X5-	T38.5X6-
Premedication anesthetic	T41.201-	T41.202-	T41.203-	T41.204-	T41.205-	T41.206-
Prenalterol	T44.5X1-	T44.5X2-	T44.5X3-	T44.5X4-	T44.5X5-	T44.5X6-
Prenoxdiazine	T48.3X1-	T48.3X2-	T48.3X3-	T48.3X4-	T48.3X5-	T48.3X6-
Prenylamine	T46.3X1-	T46.3X2-	T46.3X3-	T46.3X4-	T46.3X5-	T46.3X6-
Preparation H	T49.8X1-	T49.8X2-	T49.8X3-	T49.8X4-	T49.8X5-	T49.8X6-
Preparation, local	T49.4X1-	T49.4X2-	T49.4X3-	T49.4X4-	T49.4X5-	T49.4X6-
Preservative (nonmedicinal)	T65.891-	T65.892-	T65.893-	T65.894-	-	-
medicinal	T50.901-	T50.902-	T50.903-	T50.904-	T50.905-	T50.906-
wood	T60.91X-	T60.92X-	T60.93X-	T60.94X-	-	-
Prethcamide	T50.7X1-	T50.7X2-	T50.7X3-	T50.7X4-	T50.7X5-	T50.7X6-
Pride of China	T62.2X1-	T62.2X2-	T62.2X3-	T62.2X4-	-	-
Pridinol	T44.3X1-	T44.3X2-	T44.3X3-	T44.3X4-	T44.3X5-	T44.3X6-
Prifinium bromide	T44.3X1-	T44.3X2-	T44.3X3-	T44.3X4-	T44.3X5-	T44.3X6-
Prilocaine	T41.3X1-	T41.3X2-	T41.3X3-	T41.3X4-	T41.3X5-	T41.3X6-
infiltration (subcutaneous)	T41.3X1-	T41.3X2-	T41.3X3-	T41.3X4-	T41.3X5-	T41.3X6-
nerve block (peripheral) (plexus)	T41.3X1-	T41.3X2-	T41.3X3-	T41.3X4-	T41.3X5-	T41.3X6-
regional	T41.3X1-	T41.3X2-	T41.3X3-	T41.3X4-	T41.3X5-	T41.3X6-
Primaquine	T37.2X1-	T37.2X2-	T37.2X3-	T37.2X4-	T37.2X5-	T37.2X6-
Primidone	T42.6X1-	T42.6X2-	T42.6X3-	T42.6X4-	T42.6X5-	T42.6X6-
Primula (veris)	T62.2X1-	T62.2X2-	T62.2X3-	T62.2X4-	-	-
Prinadol	T40.2X1-	T40.2X2-	T40.2X3-	T40.2X4-	T40.2X5-	T40.2X6-
Priscol, Priscoline	T44.6X1-	T44.6X2-	T44.6X3-	T44.6X4-	T44.6X5-	T44.6X6-
Pristinamycin	T36.3X1-	T36.3X2-	T36.3X3-	T36.3X4-	T36.3X5-	T36.3X6-
Privet	T62.2X1-	T62.2X2-	T62.2X3-	T62.2X4-	-	-
berries	T62.1X1-	T62.1X2-	T62.1X3-	T62.1X4-	-	-
Privine	T44.4X1-	T44.4X2-	T44.4X3-	T44.4X4-	T44.4X5-	T44.4X6-
Pro-Banthine	T44.3X1-	T44.3X2-	T44.3X3-	T44.3X4-	T44.3X5-	T44.3X6-
Probarbital	T42.3X1-	T42.3X2-	T42.3X3-	T42.3X4-	T42.3X5-	T42.3X6-
Probenecid	T50.4X1-	T50.4X2-	T50.4X3-	T50.4X4-	T50.4X5-	T50.4X6-
Probucol	T46.6X1-	T46.6X2-	T46.6X3-	T46.6X4-	T46.6X5-	T46.6X6-
Procainamide	T46.2X1-	T46.2X2-	T46.2X3-	T46.2X4-	T46.2X5-	T46.2X6-
Procaine	T41.3X1-	T41.3X2-	T41.3X3-	T41.3X4-	T41.3X5-	T41.3X6-
benzylpenicillin	T36.0X1-	T36.0X2-	T36.0X3-	T36.0X4-	T36.0X5-	T36.0X6-
nerve block (periphreal) (plexus)	T41.3X1-	T41.3X2-	T41.3X3-	T41.3X4-	T41.3X5-	T41.3X6-
penicillin G	T36.0X1-	T36.0X2-	T36.0X3-	T36.0X4-	T36.0X5-	T36.0X6-
regional	T41.3X1-	T41.3X2-	T41.3X3-	T41.3X4-	T41.3X5-	T41.3X6-
spinal	T41.3X1-	T41.3X2-	T41.3X3-	T41.3X4-	T41.3X5-	T41.3X6-
Procalmidol	T43.591-	T43.592-	T43.593-	T43.594-	T43.595-	T43.596-
Procarbazine	T45.1X1-	T45.1X2-	T45.1X3-	T45.1X4-	T45.1X5-	T45.1X6-
Procaterol	T44.5X1-	T44.5X2-	T44.5X3-	T44.5X4-	T44.5X5-	T44.5X6-
Prochlorperazine	T43.3X1-	T43.3X2-	T43.3X3-	T43.3X4-	T43.3X5-	T43.3X6-
Procyclidine	T44.3X1-	T44.3X2-	T44.3X3-	T44.3X4-	T44.3X5-	T44.3X6-
Producer gas	T58.8X1-	T58.8X2-	T58.8X3-	T58.8X4-	-	-
Profadol	T40.491-	T40.492-	T40.493-	T40.494-	T40.495-	T40.496-
Profenamine	T44.3X1-	T44.3X2-	T44.3X3-	T44.3X4-	T44.3X5-	T44.3X6-
Profenil	T44.3X1-	T44.3X2-	T44.3X3-	T44.3X4-	T44.3X5-	T44.3X6-
Proflavine	T49.0X1-	T49.0X2-	T49.0X3-	T49.0X4-	T49.0X5-	T49.0X6-
Progabide	T42.6X1-	T42.6X2-	T42.6X3-	T42.6X4-	T42.6X5-	T42.6X6-
Progesterone	T38.5X1-	T38.5X2-	T38.5X3-	T38.5X4-	T38.5X5-	T38.5X6-

Substance	Poisoning Accidental (unintentional)	Poisoning Intentional self-harm	Poisoning Assault	Poisoning Undetermined	Adverse effect	Underdosing
Progestin	T38.5X1-	T38.5X2-	T38.5X3-	T38.5X4-	T38.5X5-	T38.5X6-
oral contraceptive	T38.4X1-	T38.4X2-	T38.4X3-	T38.4X4-	T38.4X5-	T38.4X6-
Progestogen NEC	T38.5X1-	T38.5X2-	T38.5X3-	T38.5X4-	T38.5X5-	T38.5X6-
Progestone	T38.5X1-	T38.5X2-	T38.5X3-	T38.5X4-	T38.5X5-	T38.5X6-
Proglumide	T47.1X1-	T47.1X2-	T47.1X3-	T47.1X4-	T47.1X5-	T47.1X6-
Proguanil	T37.2X1-	T37.2X2-	T37.2X3-	T37.2X4-	T37.2X5-	T37.2X6-
Prolactin	T38.811-	T38.812-	T38.813-	T38.814-	T38.815-	T38.816-
Prolintane	T43.691-	T43.692-	T43.693-	T43.694-	T43.695-	T43.696-
Proloid	T38.1X1-	T38.1X2-	T38.1X3-	T38.1X4-	T38.1X5-	T38.1X6-
Proluton	T38.5X1-	T38.5X2-	T38.5X3-	T38.5X4-	T38.5X5-	T38.5X6-
Promacetin	T37.1X1-	T37.1X2-	T37.1X3-	T37.1X4-	T37.1X5-	T37.1X6-
Promazine	T43.3X1-	T43.3X2-	T43.3X3-	T43.3X4-	T43.3X5-	T43.3X6-
Promedol	T40.2X1-	T40.2X2-	T40.2X3-	T40.2X4-	-	-
Promegestone	T38.5X1-	T38.5X2-	T38.5X3-	T38.5X4-	T38.5X5-	T38.5X6-
Promethazine (teoclate)	T43.3X1-	T43.3X2-	T43.3X3-	T43.3X4-	T43.3X5-	T43.3X6-
Promin	T37.1X1-	T37.1X2-	T37.1X3-	T37.1X4-	T37.1X5-	T37.1X6-
Pronase	T45.3X1-	T45.3X2-	T45.3X3-	T45.3X4-	T45.3X5-	T45.3X6-
Pronestyl (hydrochloride)	T46.2X1-	T46.2X2-	T46.2X3-	T46.2X4-	T46.2X5-	T46.2X6-
Pronetalol	T44.7X1-	T44.7X2-	T44.7X3-	T44.7X4-	T44.7X5-	T44.7X6-
Prontosil	T37.0X1-	T37.0X2-	T37.0X3-	T37.0X4-	T37.0X5-	T37.0X6-
Propachlor	T60.3X1-	T60.3X2-	T60.3X3-	T60.3X4-	-	-
Propafenone	T46.2X1-	T46.2X2-	T46.2X3-	T46.2X4-	T46.2X5-	T46.2X6-
Propallylonal	T42.3X1-	T42.3X2-	T42.3X3-	T42.3X4-	T42.3X5-	T42.3X6-
Propamidine	T49.0X1-	T49.0X2-	T49.0X3-	T49.0X4-	T49.0X5-	T49.0X6-
Propane (distributed in mobile container)	T59.891-	T59.892-	T59.893-	T59.894-	-	-
distributed through pipes	T59.891-	T59.892-	T59.893-	T59.894-	-	-
incomplete combustion	T58.11X-	T58.12X-	T58.13X-	T58.14X-	-	-
Propanidid	T41.291-	T41.292-	T41.293-	T41.294-	T41.295-	T41.296-
Propanil	T60.3X1-	T60.3X2-	T60.3X3-	T60.3X4-	-	-
1-Propanol	T51.3X1-	T51.3X2-	T51.3X3-	T51.3X4-	-	-
2-Propanol	T51.2X1-	T51.2X2-	T51.2X3-	T51.2X4-	-	-
Propantheline	T44.3X1-	T44.3X2-	T44.3X3-	T44.3X4-	T44.3X5-	T44.3X6-
bromide	T44.3X1-	T44.3X2-	T44.3X3-	T44.3X4-	T44.3X5-	T44.3X6-
Proparacaine	T41.3X1-	T41.3X2-	T41.3X3-	T41.3X4-	T41.3X5-	T41.3X6-
Propatylnitrate	T46.3X1-	T46.3X2-	T46.3X3-	T46.3X4-	T46.3X5-	T46.3X6-
Propicillin	T36.0X1-	T36.0X2-	T36.0X3-	T36.0X4-	T36.0X5-	T36.0X6-
Propiolactone	T49.0X1-	T49.0X2-	T49.0X3-	T49.0X4-	T49.0X5-	T49.0X6-
Propiomazine	T45.0X1-	T45.0X2-	T45.0X3-	T45.0X4-	T45.0X5-	T45.0X6-
Propionaldehyde (medicinal)	T42.6X1-	T42.6X2-	T42.6X3-	T42.6X4-	T42.6X5-	T42.6X6-
Propionate (calcium) (sodium)	T49.0X1-	T49.0X2-	T49.0X3-	T49.0X4-	T49.0X5-	T49.0X6-
Propion gel	T49.0X1-	T49.0X2-	T49.0X3-	T49.0X4-	T49.0X5-	T49.0X6-
Propitocaine	T41.3X1-	T41.3X2-	T41.3X3-	T41.3X4-	T41.3X5-	T41.3X6-
infiltration (subcutaneous)	T41.3X1-	T41.3X2-	T41.3X3-	T41.3X4-	T41.3X5-	T41.3X6-
nerve block (peripheral) (plexus)	T41.3X1-	T41.3X2-	T41.3X3-	T41.3X4-	T41.3X5-	T41.3X6-
Propofol	T41.291-	T41.292-	T41.293-	T41.294-	T41.295-	T41.296-
Propoxur	T60.0X1-	T60.0X2-	T60.0X3-	T60.0X4-	-	-
Propoxycaine	T41.3X1-	T41.3X2-	T41.3X3-	T41.3X4-	T41.3X5-	T41.3X6-
infiltration (subcutaneous)	T41.3X1-	T41.3X2-	T41.3X3-	T41.3X4-	T41.3X5-	T41.3X6-
nerve block (peripheral) (plexus)	T41.3X1-	T41.3X2-	T41.3X3-	T41.3X4-	T41.3X5-	T41.3X6-
topical (surface)	T41.3X1-	T41.3X2-	T41.3X3-	T41.3X4-	T41.3X5-	T41.3X6-
Propoxyphene	T40.491-	T40.492-	T40.493-	T40.494-	T40.495-	T40.496-
Propranolol	T44.7X1-	T44.7X2-	T44.7X3-	T44.7X4-	T44.7X5-	T44.7X6-
Propyl						
alcohol	T51.3X1-	T51.3X2-	T51.3X3-	T51.3X4-	-	-
carbinol	T51.3X1-	T51.3X2-	T51.3X3-	T51.3X4-	-	-
hexadrine	T44.4X1-	T44.4X2-	T44.4X3-	T44.4X4-	T44.4X5-	T44.4X6-
iodone	T50.8X1-	T50.8X2-	T50.8X3-	T50.8X4-	T50.8X5-	T50.8X6-

Substance	Poisoning Accidental (unintentional)	Poisoning Intentional self-harm	Poisoning Assault	Poisoning Undetermined	Adverse effect	Underdosing
Propyl (continued)						
thiouracil	T38.2X1-	T38.2X2-	T38.2X3-	T38.2X4-	T38.2X5-	T38.2X6-
Propylaminopheno-thiazine	T43.3X1-	T43.3X2-	T43.3X3-	T43.3X4-	T43.3X5-	T43.3X6-
Propylene	T59.891-	T59.892-	T59.893-	T59.894-	-	-
Propylhexedrine	T48.5X1-	T48.5X2-	T48.5X3-	T48.5X4-	T48.5X5-	T48.5X6-
Propyliodone	T50.8X1-	T50.8X2-	T50.8X3-	T50.8X4-	T50.8X5-	T50.8X6-
Propylparaben (ophthalmic)	T49.5X1-	T49.5X2-	T49.5X3-	T49.5X4-	T49.5X5-	T49.5X6-
Propylthiouracil	T38.2X1-	T38.2X2-	T38.2X3-	T38.2X4-	T38.2X5-	T38.2X6-
Propyphenazone	T39.2X1-	T39.2X2-	T39.2X3-	T39.2X4-	T39.2X5-	T39.2X6-
Proquazone	T39.391-	T39.392-	T39.393-	T39.394-	T39.395-	T39.396-
Proscillaridin	T46.0X1-	T46.0X2-	T46.0X3-	T46.0X4-	T46.0X5-	T46.0X6-
Prostacyclin	T45.521-	T45.522-	T45.523-	T45.524-	T45.525-	T45.526-
Prostaglandin (I2)	T45.521-	T45.522-	T45.523-	T45.524-	T45.525-	T45.526-
E1	T46.7X1-	T46.7X2-	T46.7X3-	T46.7X4-	T46.7X5-	T46.7X6-
E2	T48.0X1-	T48.0X2-	T48.0X3-	T48.0X4-	T48.0X5-	T48.0X6-
F2 alpha	T48.0X1-	T48.0X2-	T48.0X3-	T48.0X4-	T48.0X5-	T48.0X6-
Prostigmin	T44.0X1-	T44.0X2-	T44.0X3-	T44.0X4-	T44.0X5-	T44.0X6-
Prosultiamine	T45.2X1-	T45.2X2-	T45.2X3-	T45.2X4-	T45.2X5-	T45.2X6-
Protamine sulfate	T45.7X1-	T45.7X2-	T45.7X3-	T45.7X4-	T45.7X5-	T45.7X6-
zinc insulin	T38.3X1-	T38.3X2-	T38.3X3-	T38.3X4-	T38.3X5-	T38.3X6-
Protease	T47.5X1-	T47.5X2-	T47.5X3-	T47.5X4-	T47.5X5-	T47.5X6-
Protectant, skin NEC	T49.3X1-	T49.3X2-	T49.3X3-	T49.3X4-	T49.3X5-	T49.3X6-
Protein hydrolysate	T50.991-	T50.992-	T50.993-	T50.994-	T50.995-	T50.996-
Prothiaden — *see Dothiepin hydrochloride*						
Prothionamide	T37.1X1-	T37.1X2-	T37.1X3-	T37.1X4-	T37.1X5-	T37.1X6-
Prothipendyl	T43.591-	T43.592-	T43.593-	T43.594-	T43.595-	T43.596-
Prothoate	T60.0X1-	T60.0X2-	T60.0X3-	T60.0X4-	-	-
Prothrombin						
activator	T45.7X1-	T45.7X2-	T45.7X3-	T45.7X4-	T45.7X5-	T45.7X6-
synthesis inhibitor	T45.511-	T45.512-	T45.513-	T45.514-	T45.515-	T45.516-
Protionamide	T37.1X1-	T37.1X2-	T37.1X3-	T37.1X4-	T37.1X5-	T37.1X6-
Protirelin	T38.891-	T38.892-	T38.893-	T38.894-	T38.895-	T38.896-
Protokylol	T48.6X1-	T48.6X2-	T48.6X3-	T48.6X4-	T48.6X5-	T48.6X6-
Protopam	T50.6X1-	T50.6X2-	T50.6X3-	T50.6X4-	T50.6X5-	T50.6X6-
Protoveratrine (s) (A) (B)	T46.5X1-	T46.5X2-	T46.5X3-	T46.5X4-	T46.5X5-	T46.5X6-
Protriptyline	T43.011-	T43.012-	T43.013-	T43.014-	T43.015-	T43.016-
Provera	T38.5X1-	T38.5X2-	T38.5X3-	T38.5X4-	T38.5X5-	T38.5X6-
Provitamin A	T45.2X1-	T45.2X2-	T45.2X3-	T45.2X4-	T45.2X5-	T45.2X6-
Proxibarbal	T42.3X1-	T42.3X2-	T42.3X3-	T42.3X4-	T42.3X5-	T42.3X6-
Proxymetacaine	T41.3X1-	T41.3X2-	T41.3X3-	T41.3X4-	T41.3X5-	T41.3X6-
Proxyphylline	T48.6X1-	T48.6X2-	T48.6X3-	T48.6X4-	T48.6X5-	T48.6X6-
Prozac — *see Fluoxetine hydrochloride*						
Prunus						
laurocerasus	T62.2X1-	T62.2X2-	T62.2X3-	T62.2X4-	-	-
virginiana	T62.2X1-	T62.2X2-	T62.2X3-	T62.2X4-	-	-
Prussian blue						
commercial	T65.891-	T65.892-	T65.893-	T65.894-	-	-
therapeutic	T50.6X1-	T50.6X2-	T50.6X3-	T50.6X4-	T50.6X5-	T50.6X6-
Prussic acid	T65.0X1-	T65.0X2-	T65.0X3-	T65.0X4-	-	-
vapor	T57.3X1-	T57.3X2-	T57.3X3-	T57.3X4-	-	-
Pseudoephedrine	T44.991-	T44.992-	T44.993-	T44.994-	T44.995-	T44.996-
Psilocin	T40.991-	T40.992-	T40.993-	T40.994-	-	-
Psilocybin	T40.991-	T40.992-	T40.993-	T40.994-	-	-
Psilocybine	T40.991-	T40.992-	T40.993-	T40.994-	-	-
Psoralene (nonmedicinal)	T65.891-	T65.892-	T65.893-	T65.894-	-	-
Psoralens (medicinal)	T50.991-	T50.992-	T50.993-	T50.994-	T50.995-	T50.996-
PSP (phenolsulfonphthalein)	T50.8X1-	T50.8X2-	T50.8X3-	T50.8X4-	T50.8X5-	T50.8X6-

Substance	Poisoning Accidental (unintentional)	Poisoning Intentional self-harm	Poisoning Assault	Poisoning Undetermined	Adverse effect	Underdosing
Psychodysleptic drug NOS	T40.901-	T40.902-	T40.903-	T40.904-	T40.905-	T40.906-
specified NEC	T40.991-	T40.992-	T40.993-	T40.994-	T40.995-	T40.996-
Psychostimulant	T43.601-	T43.602-	T43.603-	T43.604-	T43.605-	T43.606-
amphetamine	T43.621-	T43.622-	T43.623-	T43.624-	T43.625-	T43.626-
caffeine	T43.611-	T43.612-	T43.613-	T43.614-	T43.615-	T43.616-
methylphenidate	T43.631-	T43.632-	T43.633-	T43.634-	T43.635-	T43.636-
specified NEC	T43.691-	T43.692-	T43.693-	T43.694-	T43.695-	T43.696-
Psychotherapeutic drug NEC	T43.91X-	T43.92X-	T43.93X-	T43.94X-	T43.95X-	T43.96X-
antidepressants — *see also Antidepressant*	T43.201-	T43.202-	T43.203-	T43.204-	T43.205-	T43.206-
specified NEC	T43.8X1-	T43.8X2-	T43.8X3-	T43.8X4-	T43.8X5-	T43.8X6-
tranquilizers NEC	T43.501-	T43.502-	T43.503-	T43.504-	T43.505-	T43.506-
Psychotomimetic agents	T40.901-	T40.902-	T40.903-	T40.904-	T40.905-	T40.906-
Psychotropic drug NEC	T43.91X-	T43.92X-	T43.93X-	T43.94X-	T43.95X-	T43.96X-
specified NEC	T43.8X1-	T43.8X2-	T43.8X3-	T43.8X4-	T43.8X5-	T43.8X6-
Psyllium hydrophilic mucilloid	T47.4X1-	T47.4X2-	T47.4X3-	T47.4X4-	T47.4X5-	T47.4X6-
Pteroylglutamic acid	T45.8X1-	T45.8X2-	T45.8X3-	T45.8X4-	T45.8X5-	T45.8X6-
Pteroyltriglutamate	T45.1X1-	T45.1X2-	T45.1X3-	T45.1X4-	T45.1X5-	T45.1X6-
PTFE — *see Polytetrafluoroethylene*						
Pulp						
devitalizing paste	T49.7X1-	T49.7X2-	T49.7X3-	T49.7X4-	T49.7X5-	T49.7X6-
dressing	T49.7X1-	T49.7X2-	T49.7X3-	T49.7X4-	T49.7X5-	T49.7X6-
Pulsatilla	T62.2X1-	T62.2X2-	T62.2X3-	T62.2X4-	-	-
Pumpkin seed extract	T37.4X1-	T37.4X2-	T37.4X3-	T37.4X4-	T37.4X5-	T37.4X6-
Purex (bleach)	T54.91X-	T54.92X-	T54.93X-	T54.94X-	-	-
Purgative NEC — *see also Cathartic*	T47.4X1-	T47.4X2-	T47.4X3-	T47.4X4-	T47.4X5-	T47.4X6-
Purine analogue (antineoplastic)	T45.1X1-	T45.1X2-	T45.1X3-	T45.1X4-	T45.1X5-	T45.1X6-
Purine diuretics	T50.2X1-	T50.2X2-	T50.2X3-	T50.2X4-	T50.2X5-	T50.2X6-
Purinethol	T45.1X1-	T45.1X2-	T45.1X3-	T45.1X4-	T45.1X5-	T45.1X6-
PVP	T45.8X1-	T45.8X2-	T45.8X3-	T45.8X4-	T45.8X5-	T45.8X6-
Pyrabital	T39.8X1-	T39.8X2-	T39.8X3-	T39.8X4-	T39.8X5-	T39.8X6-
Pyramidon	T39.2X1-	T39.2X2-	T39.2X3-	T39.2X4-	T39.2X5-	T39.2X6-
Pyrantel	T37.4X1-	T37.4X2-	T37.4X3-	T37.4X4-	T37.4X5-	T37.4X6-
Pyrathiazine	T45.0X1-	T45.0X2-	T45.0X3-	T45.0X4-	T45.0X5-	T45.0X6-
Pyrazinamide	T37.1X1-	T37.1X2-	T37.1X3-	T37.1X4-	T37.1X5-	T37.1X6-
Pyrazinoic acid (amide)	T37.1X1-	T37.1X2-	T37.1X3-	T37.1X4-	T37.1X5-	T37.1X6-
Pyrazole (derivatives)	T39.2X1-	T39.2X2-	T39.2X3-	T39.2X4-	T39.2X5-	T39.2X6-
Pyrazolone analgesic NEC	T39.2X1-	T39.2X2-	T39.2X3-	T39.2X4-	T39.2X5-	T39.2X6-
Pyrethrin, pyrethrum (nonmedicinal)	T60.2X1-	T60.2X2-	T60.2X3-	T60.2X4-	-	-
Pyrethrum extract	T49.0X1-	T49.0X2-	T49.0X3-	T49.0X4-	T49.0X5-	T49.0X6-
Pyribenzamine	T45.0X1-	T45.0X2-	T45.0X3-	T45.0X4-	T45.0X5-	T45.0X6-
Pyridine	T52.8X1-	T52.8X2-	T52.8X3-	T52.8X4-	-	-
aldoxime methiodide	T50.6X1-	T50.6X2-	T50.6X3-	T50.6X4-	T50.6X5-	T50.6X6-
aldoxime methyl chloride	T50.6X1-	T50.6X2-	T50.6X3-	T50.6X4-	T50.6X5-	T50.6X6-
vapor	T59.891-	T59.892-	T59.893-	T59.894-	-	-
Pyridium	T39.8X1-	T39.8X2-	T39.8X3-	T39.8X4-	T39.8X5-	T39.8X6-
Pyridostigmine bromide	T44.0X1-	T44.0X2-	T44.0X3-	T44.0X4-	T44.0X5-	T44.0X6-
Pyridoxal phosphate	T45.2X1-	T45.2X2-	T45.2X3-	T45.2X4-	T45.2X5-	T45.2X6-
Pyridoxine	T45.2X1-	T45.2X2-	T45.2X3-	T45.2X4-	T45.2X5-	T45.2X6-
Pyrilamine	T45.0X1-	T45.0X2-	T45.0X3-	T45.0X4-	T45.0X5-	T45.0X6-
Pyrimethamine	T37.2X1-	T37.2X2-	T37.2X3-	T37.2X4-	T37.2X5-	T37.2X6-
with sulfadoxine	T37.2X1-	T37.2X2-	T37.2X3-	T37.2X4-	T37.2X5-	T37.2X6-
Pyrimidine antagonist	T45.1X1-	T45.1X2-	T45.1X3-	T45.1X4-	T45.1X5-	T45.1X6-
Pyriminil	T60.4X1-	T60.4X2-	T60.4X3-	T60.4X4-	-	-
Pyrithione zinc	T49.4X1-	T49.4X2-	T49.4X3-	T49.4X4-	T49.4X5-	T49.4X6-
Pyrithyldione	T42.6X1-	T42.6X2-	T42.6X3-	T42.6X4-	T42.6X5-	T42.6X6-
Pyrogallic acid	T49.0X1-	T49.0X2-	T49.0X3-	T49.0X4-	T49.0X5-	T49.0X6-
Pyrogallol	T49.0X1-	T49.0X2-	T49.0X3-	T49.0X4-	T49.0X5-	T49.0X6-

Substance	Poisoning Accidental (unintentional)	Poisoning Intentional self-harm	Poisoning Assault	Poisoning Undetermined	Adverse effect	Underdosing
Pyroxylin	T49.3X1-	T49.3X2-	T49.3X3-	T49.3X4-	T49.3X5-	T49.3X6-
Pyrrobutamine	T45.0X1-	T45.0X2-	T45.0X3-	T45.0X4-	T45.0X5-	T45.0X6-
Pyrrolizidine alkaloids	T62.8X1-	T62.8X2-	T62.8X3-	T62.8X4-	-	-
Pyrvinium chloride	T37.4X1-	T37.4X2-	T37.4X3-	T37.4X4-	T37.4X5-	T37.4X6-
PZI	T38.3X1-	T38.3X2-	T38.3X3-	T38.3X4-	T38.3X5-	T38.3X6-
Quaalude	T42.6X1-	T42.6X2-	T42.6X3-	T42.6X4-	T42.6X5-	T42.6X6-
Quarternary ammonium						
anti-infective	T49.0X1-	T49.0X2-	T49.0X3-	T49.0X4-	T49.0X5-	T49.0X6-
ganglion blocking	T44.2X1-	T44.2X2-	T44.2X3-	T44.2X4-	T44.2X5-	T44.2X6-
parasympatholytic	T44.3X1-	T44.3X2-	T44.3X3-	T44.3X4-	T44.3X5-	T44.3X6-
Quazepam	T42.4X1-	T42.4X2-	T42.4X3-	T42.4X4-	T42.4X5-	T42.4X6-
Quicklime	T54.3X1-	T54.3X2-	T54.3X3-	T54.3X4-	-	-
Quillaja extract	T48.4X1-	T48.4X2-	T48.4X3-	T48.4X4-	T48.4X5-	T48.4X6-
Quinacrine	T37.2X1-	T37.2X2-	T37.2X3-	T37.2X4-	T37.2X5-	T37.2X6-
Quinaglute	T46.2X1-	T46.2X2-	T46.2X3-	T46.2X4-	T46.2X5-	T46.2X6-
Quinalbarbital	T42.3X1-	T42.3X2-	T42.3X3-	T42.3X4-	T42.3X5-	T42.3X6-
Quinalbarbitone sodium	T42.3X1-	T42.3X2-	T42.3X3-	T42.3X4-	T42.3X5-	T42.3X6-
Quinalphos	T60.0X1-	T60.0X2-	T60.0X3-	T60.0X4-	-	-
Quinapril	T46.4X1-	T46.4X2-	T46.4X3-	T46.4X4-	T46.4X5-	T46.4X6-
Quinestradiol	T38.5X1-	T38.5X2-	T38.5X3-	T38.5X4-	T38.5X5-	T38.5X6-
Quinestradol	T38.5X1-	T38.5X2-	T38.5X3-	T38.5X4-	T38.5X5-	T38.5X6-
Quinestrol	T38.5X1-	T38.5X2-	T38.5X3-	T38.5X4-	T38.5X5-	T38.5X6-
Quinethazone	T50.2X1-	T50.2X2-	T50.2X3-	T50.2X4-	T50.2X5-	T50.2X6-
Quingestanol	T38.4X1-	T38.4X2-	T38.4X3-	T38.4X4-	T38.4X5-	T38.4X6-
Quinidine	T46.2X1-	T46.2X2-	T46.2X3-	T46.2X4-	T46.2X5-	T46.2X6-
Quinine	T37.2X1-	T37.2X2-	T37.2X3-	T37.2X4-	T37.2X5-	T37.2X6-
Quiniobine	T37.8X1-	T37.8X2-	T37.8X3-	T37.8X4-	T37.8X5-	T37.8X6-
Quinisocaine	T49.1X1-	T49.1X2-	T49.1X3-	T49.1X4-	T49.1X5-	T49.1X6-
Quinocide	T37.2X1-	T37.2X2-	T37.2X3-	T37.2X4-	T37.2X5-	T37.2X6-
Quinoline (derivatives) NEC	T37.8X1-	T37.8X2-	T37.8X3-	T37.8X4-	T37.8X5-	T37.8X6-
Quinupramine	T43.011-	T43.012-	T43.013-	T43.014-	T43.015-	T43.016-
Quotane	T41.3X1-	T41.3X2-	T41.3X3-	T41.3X4-	T41.3X5-	T41.3X6-
Rabies						
immune globulin (human)	T50.Z11-	T50.Z12-	T50.Z13-	T50.Z14-	T50.Z15-	T50.Z16-
vaccine	T50.B91-	T50.B92-	T50.B93-	T50.B94-	T50.B95-	T50.B96-
Racemoramide	T40.2X1-	T40.2X2-	T40.2X3-	T40.2X4-	-	-
Racemorphan	T40.2X1-	T40.2X2-	T40.2X3-	T40.2X4-	T40.2X5-	T40.2X6-
Racepinefrin	T44.5X1-	T44.5X2-	T44.5X3-	T44.5X4-	T44.5X5-	T44.5X6-
Raclopride	T43.591-	T43.592-	T43.593-	T43.594-	T43.595-	T43.596-
Radiator alcohol	T51.1X1-	T51.1X2-	T51.1X3-	T51.1X4-	-	-
Radioactive drug NEC	T50.8X1-	T50.8X2-	T50.8X3-	T50.8X4-	T50.8X5-	T50.8X6-
Radio-opaque (drugs) (materials)	T50.8X1-	T50.8X2-	T50.8X3-	T50.8X4-	T50.8X5-	T50.8X6-
Ramifenazone	T39.2X1-	T39.2X2-	T39.2X3-	T39.2X4-	T39.2X5-	T39.2X6-
Ramipril	T46.4X1-	T46.4X2-	T46.4X3-	T46.4X4-	T46.4X5-	T46.4X6-
Ranitidine	T47.0X1-	T47.0X2-	T47.0X3-	T47.0X4-	T47.0X5-	T47.0X6-
Ranunculus	T62.2X1-	T62.2X2-	T62.2X3-	T62.2X4-	-	-
Rat poison NEC	T60.4X1-	T60.4X2-	T60.4X3-	T60.4X4-	-	-
Rattlesnake (venom)	T63.011-	T63.012-	T63.013-	T63.014-	-	-
Raubasine	T46.7X1-	T46.7X2-	T46.7X3-	T46.7X4-	T46.7X5-	T46.7X6-
Raudixin	T46.5X1-	T46.5X2-	T46.5X3-	T46.5X4-	T46.5X5-	T46.5X6-
Rautensin	T46.5X1-	T46.5X2-	T46.5X3-	T46.5X4-	T46.5X5-	T46.5X6-
Rautina	T46.5X1-	T46.5X2-	T46.5X3-	T46.5X4-	T46.5X5-	T46.5X6-
Rautotal	T46.5X1-	T46.5X2-	T46.5X3-	T46.5X4-	T46.5X5-	T46.5X6-
Rauwiloid	T46.5X1-	T46.5X2-	T46.5X3-	T46.5X4-	T46.5X5-	T46.5X6-
Rauwoldin	T46.5X1-	T46.5X2-	T46.5X3-	T46.5X4-	T46.5X5-	T46.5X6-
Rauwolfia (alkaloids)	T46.5X1-	T46.5X2-	T46.5X3-	T46.5X4-	T46.5X5-	T46.5X6-
Razoxane	T45.1X1-	T45.1X2-	T45.1X3-	T45.1X4-	T45.1X5-	T45.1X6-
Realgar	T57.0X1-	T57.0X2-	T57.0X3-	T57.0X4-	-	-
Recombinant (R) — *see specific protein*						

Substance	Poisoning Accidental (unintentional)	Poisoning Intentional self-harm	Poisoning Assault	Poisoning Undetermined	Adverse effect	Underdosing
Red blood cells, packed	T45.8X1-	T45.8X2-	T45.8X3-	T45.8X4-	T45.8X5-	T45.8X6-
Red squill (scilliroside)	T60.4X1-	T60.4X2-	T60.4X3-	T60.4X4-	-	-
Reducing agent, industrial NEC	T65.891-	T65.892-	T65.893-	T65.894-	-	-
Refrigerant gas (chlorofluoro-carbon)	T53.5X1-	T53.5X2-	T53.5X3-	T53.5X4-	-	-
not chlorofluoro-carbon	T59.891-	T59.892-	T59.893-	T59.894-	-	-
Regroton	T50.2X1-	T50.2X2-	T50.2X3-	T50.2X4-	T50.2X5-	T50.2X6-
Rehydration salts (oral)	T50.3X1-	T50.3X2-	T50.3X3-	T50.3X4-	T50.3X5-	T50.3X6-
Rela	T42.8X1-	T42.8X2-	T42.8X3-	T42.8X4-	T42.8X5-	T42.8X6-
Relaxant, muscle						
anesthetic	T48.1X1-	T48.1X2-	T48.1X3-	T48.1X4-	T48.1X5-	T48.1X6-
central nervous system	T42.8X1-	T42.8X2-	T42.8X3-	T42.8X4-	T42.8X5-	T42.8X6-
skeletal NEC	T48.1X1-	T48.1X2-	T48.1X3-	T48.1X4-	T48.1X5-	T48.1X6-
smooth NEC	T44.3X1-	T44.3X2-	T44.3X3-	T44.3X4-	T44.3X5-	T44.3X6-
Remoxipride	T43.591-	T43.592-	T43.593-	T43.594-	T43.595-	T43.596-
Renese	T50.2X1-	T50.2X2-	T50.2X3-	T50.2X4-	T50.2X5-	T50.2X6-
Renografin	T50.8X1-	T50.8X2-	T50.8X3-	T50.8X4-	T50.8X5-	T50.8X6-
Replacement solution	T50.3X1-	T50.3X2-	T50.3X3-	T50.3X4-	T50.3X5-	T50.3X6-
Reproterol	T48.6X1-	T48.6X2-	T48.6X3-	T48.6X4-	T48.6X5-	T48.6X6-
Rescinnamine	T46.5X1-	T46.5X2-	T46.5X3-	T46.5X4-	T46.5X5-	T46.5X6-
Reserpin (e)	T46.5X1-	T46.5X2-	T46.5X3-	T46.5X4-	T46.5X5-	T46.5X6-
Resorcin, resorcinol (nonmedicinal)	T65.891-	T65.892-	T65.893-	T65.894-	-	-
medicinal	T49.4X1-	T49.4X2-	T49.4X3-	T49.4X4-	T49.4X5-	T49.4X6-
Respaire	T48.4X1-	T48.4X2-	T48.4X3-	T48.4X4-	T48.4X5-	T48.4X6-
Respiratory drug NEC	T48.901-	T48.902-	T48.903-	T48.904-	T48.905-	T48.906-
antiasthmatic NEC	T48.6X1-	T48.6X2-	T48.6X3-	T48.6X4-	T48.6X5-	T48.6X6-
anti-common-cold NEC	T48.5X1-	T48.5X2-	T48.5X3-	T48.5X4-	T48.5X5-	T48.5X6-
expectorant NEC	T48.4X1-	T48.4X2-	T48.4X3-	T48.4X4-	T48.4X5-	T48.4X6-
stimulant	T48.901-	T48.902-	T48.903-	T48.904-	T48.905-	T48.906-
Retinoic acid	T49.0X1-	T49.0X2-	T49.0X3-	T49.0X4-	T49.0X5-	T49.0X6-
Retinol	T45.2X1-	T45.2X2-	T45.2X3-	T45.2X4-	T45.2X5-	T45.2X6-
Rh (D) immune globulin (human)	T50.Z11-	T50.Z12-	T50.Z13-	T50.Z14-	T50.Z15-	T50.Z16-
Rhodine	T39.011-	T39.012-	T39.013-	T39.014-	T39.015-	T39.016-
RhoGAM	T50.Z11-	T50.Z12-	T50.Z13-	T50.Z14-	T50.Z15-	T50.Z16-
Rhubarb						
dry extract	T47.2X1-	T47.2X2-	T47.2X3-	T47.2X4-	T47.2X5-	T47.2X6-
tincture, compound	T47.2X1-	T47.2X2-	T47.2X3-	T47.2X4-	T47.2X5-	T47.2X6-
Ribavirin	T37.5X1-	T37.5X2-	T37.5X3-	T37.5X4-	T37.5X5-	T37.5X6-
Riboflavin	T45.2X1-	T45.2X2-	T45.2X3-	T45.2X4-	T45.2X5-	T45.2X6-
Ribostamycin	T36.5X1-	T36.5X2-	T36.5X3-	T36.5X4-	T36.5X5-	T36.5X6-
Ricin	T62.2X1-	T62.2X2-	T62.2X3-	T62.2X4-	-	-
Ricinus communis	T62.2X1-	T62.2X2-	T62.2X3-	T62.2X4-	-	-
Rickettsial vaccine NEC	T50.A91-	T50.A92-	T50.A93-	T50.A94-	T50.A95-	T50.A96-
Rifabutin	T36.6X1-	T36.6X2-	T36.6X3-	T36.6X4-	T36.6X5-	T36.6X6-
Rifamide	T36.6X1-	T36.6X2-	T36.6X3-	T36.6X4-	T36.6X5-	T36.6X6-
Rifampicin	T36.6X1-	T36.6X2-	T36.6X3-	T36.6X4-	T36.6X5-	T36.6X6-
with isoniazid	T37.1X1-	T37.1X2-	T37.1X3-	T37.1X4-	T37.1X5-	T37.1X6-
Rifampin	T36.6X1-	T36.6X2-	T36.6X3-	T36.6X4-	T36.6X5-	T36.6X6-
Rifamycin	T36.6X1-	T36.6X2-	T36.6X3-	T36.6X4-	T36.6X5-	T36.6X6-
Rifaximin	T36.6X1-	T36.6X2-	T36.6X3-	T36.6X4-	T36.6X5-	T36.6X6-
Rimantadine	T37.5X1-	T37.5X2-	T37.5X3-	T37.5X4-	T37.5X5-	T37.5X6-
Rimazolium metilsulfate	T39.8X1-	T39.8X2-	T39.8X3-	T39.8X4-	T39.8X5-	T39.8X6-
Rimifon	T37.1X1-	T37.1X2-	T37.1X3-	T37.1X4-	T37.1X5-	T37.1X6-
Rimiterol	T48.6X1-	T48.6X2-	T48.6X3-	T48.6X4-	T48.6X5-	T48.6X6-
Ringer (lactate) solution	T50.3X1-	T50.3X2-	T50.3X3-	T50.3X4-	T50.3X5-	T50.3X6-
Ristocetin	T36.8X1-	T36.8X2-	T36.8X3-	T36.8X4-	T36.8X5-	T36.8X6-
Ritalin	T43.631-	T43.632-	T43.633-	T43.634-	T43.635-	T43.636-
Ritodrine	T44.5X1-	T44.5X2-	T44.5X3-	T44.5X4-	T44.5X5-	T44.5X6-
Roach killer — *see Insecticide*						

Substance	Poisoning Accidental (unintentional)	Poisoning Intentional self-harm	Poisoning Assault	Poisoning Undetermined	Adverse effect	Underdosing
Rociverine	T44.3X1-	T44.3X2-	T44.3X3-	T44.3X4-	T44.3X5-	T44.3X6-
Rocky Mountain spotted fever vaccine	T50.A91-	T50.A92-	T50.A93-	T50.A94-	T50.A95-	T50.A96-
Rodenticide NEC	T60.4X1-	T60.4X2-	T60.4X3-	T60.4X4-	-	-
Rohypnol	T42.4X1-	T42.4X2-	T42.4X3-	T42.4X4-	T42.4X5-	T42.4X6-
Rokitamycin	T36.3X1-	T36.3X2-	T36.3X3-	T36.3X4-	T36.3X5-	T36.3X6-
Rolaids	T47.1X1-	T47.1X2-	T47.1X3-	T47.1X4-	T47.1X5-	T47.1X6-
Rolitetracycline	T36.4X1-	T36.4X2-	T36.4X3-	T36.4X4-	T36.4X5-	T36.4X6-
Romilar	T48.3X1-	T48.3X2-	T48.3X3-	T48.3X4-	T48.3X5-	T48.3X6-
Ronifibrate	T46.6X1-	T46.6X2-	T46.6X3-	T46.6X4-	T46.6X5-	T46.6X6-
Rosaprostol	T47.1X1-	T47.1X2-	T47.1X3-	T47.1X4-	T47.1X5-	T47.1X6-
Rose bengal sodium (131I)	T50.8X1-	T50.8X2-	T50.8X3-	T50.8X4-	T50.8X5-	T50.8X6-
Rose water ointment	T49.3X1-	T49.3X2-	T49.3X3-	T49.3X4-	T49.3X5-	T49.3X6-
Rosoxacin	T37.8X1-	T37.8X2-	T37.8X3-	T37.8X4-	T37.8X5-	T37.8X6-
Rotenone	T60.2X1-	T60.2X2-	T60.2X3-	T60.2X4-	-	-
Rotoxamine	T45.0X1-	T45.0X2-	T45.0X3-	T45.0X4-	T45.0X5-	T45.0X6-
Rough-on-rats	T60.4X1-	T60.4X2-	T60.4X3-	T60.4X4-	-	-
Roxatidine	T47.0X1-	T47.0X2-	T47.0X3-	T47.0X4-	T47.0X5-	T47.0X6-
Roxithromycin	T36.3X1-	T36.3X2-	T36.3X3-	T36.3X4-	T36.3X5-	T36.3X6-
Rt-PA	T45.611-	T45.612-	T45.613-	T45.614-	T45.615-	T45.616-
Rubbing alcohol	T51.2X1-	T51.2X2-	T51.2X3-	T51.2X4-	-	-
Rubefacient	T49.4X1-	T49.4X2-	T49.4X3-	T49.4X4-	T49.4X5-	T49.4X6-
Rubella vaccine	T50.B91-	T50.B92-	T50.B93-	T50.B94-	T50.B95-	T50.B96-
Rubeola vaccine	T50.B91-	T50.B92-	T50.B93-	T50.B94-	T50.B95-	T50.B96-
Rubidium chloride Rb82	T50.8X1-	T50.8X2-	T50.8X3-	T50.8X4-	T50.8X5-	T50.8X6-
Rubidomycin	T45.1X1-	T45.1X2-	T45.1X3-	T45.1X4-	T45.1X5-	T45.1X6-
Rue	T62.2X1-	T62.2X2-	T62.2X3-	T62.2X4-	-	-
Rufocromomycin	T45.1X1-	T45.1X2-	T45.1X3-	T45.1X4-	T45.1X5-	T45.1X6-
Russel's viper venin	T45.7X1-	T45.7X2-	T45.7X3-	T45.7X4-	T45.7X5-	T45.7X6-
Ruta (graveolens)	T62.2X1-	T62.2X2-	T62.2X3-	T62.2X4-	-	-
Rutinum	T46.991-	T46.992-	T46.993-	T46.994-	T46.995-	T46.996-
Rutoside	T46.991-	T46.992-	T46.993-	T46.994-	T46.995-	T46.996-
Sabadilla (plant)	T62.2X1-	T62.2X2-	T62.2X3-	T62.2X4-	-	-
pesticide	T60.2X1-	T60.2X2-	T60.2X3-	T60.2X4-	-	-
Saccharated iron oxide	T45.8X1-	T45.8X2-	T45.8X3-	T45.8X4-	T45.8X5-	T45.8X6-
Saccharin	T50.901-	T50.902-	T50.903-	T50.904-	T50.905-	T50.906-
Saccharomyces boulardii	T47.6X1-	T47.6X2-	T47.6X3-	T47.6X4-	T47.6X5-	T47.6X6-
Safflower oil	T46.6X1-	T46.6X2-	T46.6X3-	T46.6X4-	T46.6X5-	T46.6X6-
Safrazine	T43.1X1-	T43.1X2-	T43.1X3-	T43.1X4-	T43.1X5-	T43.1X6-
Salazosulfapyridine	T37.0X1-	T37.0X2-	T37.0X3-	T37.0X4-	T37.0X5-	T37.0X6-
Salbutamol	T48.6X1-	T48.6X2-	T48.6X3-	T48.6X4-	T48.6X5-	T48.6X6-
Salicylamide	T39.091-	T39.092-	T39.093-	T39.094-	T39.095-	T39.096-
Salicylate NEC	T39.091-	T39.092-	T39.093-	T39.094-	T39.095-	T39.096-
methyl	T49.3X1-	T49.3X2-	T49.3X3-	T49.3X4-	T49.3X5-	T49.3X6-
theobromine calcium	T50.2X1-	T50.2X2-	T50.2X3-	T50.2X4-	T50.2X5-	T50.2X6-
Salicylazosulfapyridine	T37.0X1-	T37.0X2-	T37.0X3-	T37.0X4-	T37.0X5-	T37.0X6-
Salicylhydroxamic acid	T49.0X1-	T49.0X2-	T49.0X3-	T49.0X4-	T49.0X5-	T49.0X6-
Salicylic acid	T49.4X1-	T49.4X2-	T49.4X3-	T49.4X4-	T49.4X5-	T49.4X6-
with benzoic acid	T49.4X1-	T49.4X2-	T49.4X3-	T49.4X4-	T49.4X5-	T49.4X6-
congeners	T39.091-	T39.092-	T39.093-	T39.094-	T39.095-	T39.096-
derivative	T39.091-	T39.092-	T39.093-	T39.094-	T39.095-	T39.096-
salts	T39.091-	T39.092-	T39.093-	T39.094-	T39.095-	T39.096-
Salinazid	T37.1X1-	T37.1X2-	T37.1X3-	T37.1X4-	T37.1X5-	T37.1X6-
Salmeterol	T48.6X1-	T48.6X2-	T48.6X3-	T48.6X4-	T48.6X5-	T48.6X6-
Salol	T49.3X1-	T49.3X2-	T49.3X3-	T49.3X4-	T49.3X5-	T49.3X6-
Salsalate	T39.091-	T39.092-	T39.093-	T39.094-	T39.095-	T39.096-
Salt substitute	T50.901-	T50.902-	T50.903-	T50.904-	T50.905-	T50.906-
Salt-replacing drug	T50.901-	T50.902-	T50.903-	T50.904-	T50.905-	T50.906-
Salt-retaining mineralocorticoid	T50.0X1-	T50.0X2-	T50.0X3-	T50.0X4-	T50.0X5-	T50.0X6-
Saluretic NEC	T50.2X1-	T50.2X2-	T50.2X3-	T50.2X4-	T50.2X5-	T50.2X6-

Substance	Poisoning Accidental (unintentional)	Poisoning Intentional self-harm	Poisoning Assault	Poisoning Undetermined	Adverse effect	Underdosing
Saluron	T50.2X1-	T50.2X2-	T50.2X3-	T50.2X4-	T50.2X5-	T50.2X6-
Salvarsan 606 (neosilver) (silver)	T37.8X1-	T37.8X2-	T37.8X3-	T37.8X4-	T37.8X5-	T37.8X6-
Sambucus canadensis	T62.2X1-	T62.2X2-	T62.2X3-	T62.2X4-	-	-
berry	T62.1X1-	T62.1X2-	T62.1X3-	T62.1X4-	-	-
Sandril	T46.5X1-	T46.5X2-	T46.5X3-	T46.5X4-	T46.5X5-	T46.5X6-
Sanguinaria canadensis	T62.2X1-	T62.2X2-	T62.2X3-	T62.2X4-	-	-
Saniflush (cleaner)	T54.2X1-	T54.2X2-	T54.2X3-	T54.2X4-	-	-
Santonin	T37.4X1-	T37.4X2-	T37.4X3-	T37.4X4-	T37.4X5-	T37.4X6-
Santyl	T49.8X1-	T49.8X2-	T49.8X3-	T49.8X4-	T49.8X5-	T49.8X6-
Saralasin	T46.5X1-	T46.5X2-	T46.5X3-	T46.5X4-	T46.5X5-	T46.5X6-
Sarcolysin	T45.1X1-	T45.1X2-	T45.1X3-	T45.1X4-	T45.1X5-	T45.1X6-
Sarkomycin	T45.1X1-	T45.1X2-	T45.1X3-	T45.1X4-	T45.1X5-	T45.1X6-
Saroten	T43.011-	T43.012-	T43.013-	T43.014-	T43.015-	T43.016-
Saturnine — *see Lead*						
Savin (oil)	T49.4X1-	T49.4X2-	T49.4X3-	T49.4X4-	T49.4X5-	T49.4X6-
Scammony	T47.2X1-	T47.2X2-	T47.2X3-	T47.2X4-	T47.2X5-	T47.2X6-
Scarlet red	T49.8X1-	T49.8X2-	T49.8X3-	T49.8X4-	T49.8X5-	T49.8X6-
Scheele's green	T57.0X1-	T57.0X2-	T57.0X3-	T57.0X4-	-	-
insecticide	T57.0X1-	T57.0X2-	T57.0X3-	T57.0X4-	-	-
Schizontozide (blood) (tissue)	T37.2X1-	T37.2X2-	T37.2X3-	T37.2X4-	T37.2X5-	T37.2X6-
Schradan	T60.0X1-	T60.0X2-	T60.0X3-	T60.0X4-	-	-
Schweinfurth green	T57.0X1-	T57.0X2-	T57.0X3-	T57.0X4-	-	-
insecticide	T57.0X1-	T57.0X2-	T57.0X3-	T57.0X4-	-	-
Scilla, rat poison	T60.4X1-	T60.4X2-	T60.4X3-	T60.4X4-	-	-
Scillaren	T60.4X1-	T60.4X2-	T60.4X3-	T60.4X4-	-	-
Sclerosing agent	T46.8X1-	T46.8X2-	T46.8X3-	T46.8X4-	T46.8X5-	T46.8X6-
Scombrotoxin	T61.11X-	T61.12X-	T61.13X-	T61.14X-	-	-
Scopolamine	T44.3X1-	T44.3X2-	T44.3X3-	T44.3X4-	T44.3X5-	T44.3X6-
Scopolia extract	T44.3X1-	T44.3X2-	T44.3X3-	T44.3X4-	T44.3X5-	T44.3X6-
Scouring powder	T65.891-	T65.892-	T65.893-	T65.894-	-	-
Sea						
anemone (sting)	T63.631-	T63.632-	T63.633-	T63.634-	-	-
cucumber (sting)	T63.691-	T63.692-	T63.693-	T63.694-	-	-
snake (bite) (venom)	T63.091-	T63.092-	T63.093-	T63.094-	-	-
urchin spine (puncture)	T63.691-	T63.692-	T63.693-	T63.694-	-	-
Seafood	T61.91X-	T61.92X-	T61.93X-	T61.94X-	-	-
specified NEC	T61.8X1-	T61.8X2-	T61.8X3-	T61.8X4-	-	-
Secbutabarbital	T42.3X1-	T42.3X2-	T42.3X3-	T42.3X4-	T42.3X5-	T42.3X6-
Secbutabarbitone	T42.3X1-	T42.3X2-	T42.3X3-	T42.3X4-	T42.3X5-	T42.3X6-
Secnidazole	T37.3X1-	T37.3X2-	T37.3X3-	T37.3X4-	T37.3X5-	T37.3X6-
Secobarbital	T42.3X1-	T42.3X2-	T42.3X3-	T42.3X4-	T42.3X5-	T42.3X6-
Seconal	T42.3X1-	T42.3X2-	T42.3X3-	T42.3X4-	T42.3X5-	T42.3X6-
Secretin	T50.8X1-	T50.8X2-	T50.8X3-	T50.8X4-	T50.8X5-	T50.8X6-
Sedative NEC	T42.71X-	T42.72X-	T42.73X-	T42.74X-	T42.75X-	T42.76X-
mixed NEC	T42.6X1-	T42.6X2-	T42.6X3-	T42.6X4-	T42.6X5-	T42.6X6-
Sedormid	T42.6X1-	T42.6X2-	T42.6X3-	T42.6X4-	T42.6X5-	T42.6X6-
Seed disinfectant or dressing	T60.8X1-	T60.8X2-	T60.8X3-	T60.8X4-	-	-
Seeds (poisonous)	T62.2X1-	T62.2X2-	T62.2X3-	T62.2X4-	-	-
Selegiline	T42.8X1-	T42.8X2-	T42.8X3-	T42.8X4-	T42.8X5-	T42.8X6-
Selenium NEC	T56.891-	T56.892-	T56.893-	T56.894-	-	-
disulfide or sulfide	T49.4X1-	T49.4X2-	T49.4X3-	T49.4X4-	T49.4X5-	T49.4X6-
fumes	T59.891-	T59.892-	T59.893-	T59.894-	-	-
sulfide	T49.4X1-	T49.4X2-	T49.4X3-	T49.4X4-	T49.4X5-	T49.4X6-
Selenomethionine (75Se)	T50.8X1-	T50.8X2-	T50.8X3-	T50.8X4-	T50.8X5-	T50.8X6-
Selsun	T49.4X1-	T49.4X2-	T49.4X3-	T49.4X4-	T49.4X5-	T49.4X6-
Semustine	T45.1X1-	T45.1X2-	T45.1X3-	T45.1X4-	T45.1X5-	T45.1X6-
Senega syrup	T48.4X1-	T48.4X2-	T48.4X3-	T48.4X4-	T48.4X5-	T48.4X6-
Senna	T47.2X1-	T47.2X2-	T47.2X3-	T47.2X4-	T47.2X5-	T47.2X6-

Substance	Poisoning Accidental (unintentional)	Poisoning Intentional self-harm	Poisoning Assault	Poisoning Undetermined	Adverse effect	Underdosing
Sennoside A+B	T47.2X1-	T47.2X2-	T47.2X3-	T47.2X4-	T47.2X5-	T47.2X6-
Septisol	T49.2X1-	T49.2X2-	T49.2X3-	T49.2X4-	T49.2X5-	T49.2X6-
Seractide	T38.811-	T38.812-	T38.813-	T38.814-	T38.815-	T38.816-
Serax	T42.4X1-	T42.4X2-	T42.4X3-	T42.4X4-	T42.4X5-	T42.4X6-
Serenesil	T42.6X1-	T42.6X2-	T42.6X3-	T42.6X4-	T42.6X5-	T42.6X6-
Serenium (hydrochloride)	T37.91X-	T37.92X-	T37.93X-	T37.94X-	T37.95X-	T37.96X-
Serepax — *see Oxazepam*						
Sermorelin	T38.891-	T38.892-	T38.893-	T38.894-	T38.895-	T38.896-
Sernyl	T41.1X1-	T41.1X2-	T41.1X3-	T41.1X4-	T41.1X5-	T41.1X6-
Serotonin	T50.991-	T50.992-	T50.993-	T50.994-	T50.995-	T50.996-
Serpasil	T46.5X1-	T46.5X2-	T46.5X3-	T46.5X4-	T46.5X5-	T46.5X6-
Serrapeptase	T45.3X1-	T45.3X2-	T45.3X3-	T45.3X4-	T45.3X5-	T45.3X6-
Serum						
antibotulinus	T50.Z11-	T50.Z12-	T50.Z13-	T50.Z14-	T50.Z15-	T50.Z16-
anticytotoxic	T50.Z11-	T50.Z12-	T50.Z13-	T50.Z14-	T50.Z15-	T50.Z16-
antidiphtheria	T50.Z11-	T50.Z12-	T50.Z13-	T50.Z14-	T50.Z15-	T50.Z16-
antimeningococcus	T50.Z11-	T50.Z12-	T50.Z13-	T50.Z14-	T50.Z15-	T50.Z16-
anti-Rh	T50.Z11-	T50.Z12-	T50.Z13-	T50.Z14-	T50.Z15-	T50.Z16-
anti-snake-bite	T50.Z11-	T50.Z12-	T50.Z13-	T50.Z14-	T50.Z15-	T50.Z16-
antitetanic	T50.Z11-	T50.Z12-	T50.Z13-	T50.Z14-	T50.Z15-	T50.Z16-
antitoxic	T50.Z11-	T50.Z12-	T50.Z13-	T50.Z14-	T50.Z15-	T50.Z16-
complement (inhibitor)	T45.8X1-	T45.8X2-	T45.8X3-	T45.8X4-	T45.8X5-	T45.8X6-
convalescent	T50.Z11-	T50.Z12-	T50.Z13-	T50.Z14-	T50.Z15-	T50.Z16-
hemolytic complement	T45.8X1-	T45.8X2-	T45.8X3-	T45.8X4-	T45.8X5-	T45.8X6-
immune (human)	T50.Z11-	T50.Z12-	T50.Z13-	T50.Z14-	T50.Z15-	T50.Z16-
protective NEC	T50.Z11-	T50.Z12-	T50.Z13-	T50.Z14-	T50.Z15-	T50.Z16-
Setastine	T45.0X1-	T45.0X2-	T45.0X3-	T45.0X4-	T45.0X5-	T45.0X6-
Setoperone	T43.591-	T43.592-	T43.593-	T43.594-	T43.595-	T43.596-
Sewer gas	T59.91X-	T59.92X-	T59.93X-	T59.94X-	-	-
Shampoo	T55.0X1-	T55.0X2-	T55.0X3-	T55.0X4-	-	-
Shellfish, noxious, nonbacterial	T61.781-	T61.782-	T61.783-	T61.784-	-	-
Sildenafil	T46.7X1-	T46.7X2-	T46.7X3-	T46.7X4-	T46.7X5-	T46.7X6-
Silibinin	T50.991-	T50.992-	T50.993-	T50.994-	T50.995-	T50.996-
Silicone NEC	T65.891-	T65.892-	T65.893-	T65.894-	-	-
medicinal	T49.3X1-	T49.3X2-	T49.3X3-	T49.3X4-	T49.3X5-	T49.3X6-
Silvadene	T49.0X1-	T49.0X2-	T49.0X3-	T49.0X4-	T49.0X5-	T49.0X6-
Silver	T49.0X1-	T49.0X2-	T49.0X3-	T49.0X4-	T49.0X5-	T49.0X6-
anti-infectives	T49.0X1-	T49.0X2-	T49.0X3-	T49.0X4-	T49.0X5-	T49.0X6-
arsphenamine	T37.8X1-	T37.8X2-	T37.8X3-	T37.8X4-	T37.8X5-	T37.8X6-
colloidal	T49.0X1-	T49.0X2-	T49.0X3-	T49.0X4-	T49.0X5-	T49.0X6-
nitrate	T49.0X1-	T49.0X2-	T49.0X3-	T49.0X4-	T49.0X5-	T49.0X6-
ophthalmic preparation	T49.5X1-	T49.5X2-	T49.5X3-	T49.5X4-	T49.5X5-	T49.5X6-
toughened (keratolytic)	T49.4X1-	T49.4X2-	T49.4X3-	T49.4X4-	T49.4X5-	T49.4X6-
nonmedicinal (dust)	T56.891-	T56.892-	T56.893-	T56.894-	-	-
protein	T49.5X1-	T49.5X2-	T49.5X3-	T49.5X4-	T49.5X5-	T49.5X6-
salvarsan	T37.8X1-	T37.8X2-	T37.8X3-	T37.8X4-	T37.8X5-	T37.8X6-
sulfadiazine	T49.4X1-	T49.4X2-	T49.4X3-	T49.4X4-	T49.4X5-	T49.4X6-
Silymarin	T50.991-	T50.992-	T50.993-	T50.994-	T50.995-	T50.996-
Simaldrate	T47.1X1-	T47.1X2-	T47.1X3-	T47.1X4-	T47.1X5-	T47.1X6-
Simazine	T60.3X1-	T60.3X2-	T60.3X3-	T60.3X4-	-	-
Simethicone	T47.1X1-	T47.1X2-	T47.1X3-	T47.1X4-	T47.1X5-	T47.1X6-
Simfibrate	T46.6X1-	T46.6X2-	T46.6X3-	T46.6X4-	T46.6X5-	T46.6X6-
Simvastatin	T46.6X1-	T46.6X2-	T46.6X3-	T46.6X4-	T46.6X5-	T46.6X6-
Sincalide	T50.8X1-	T50.8X2-	T50.8X3-	T50.8X4-	T50.8X5-	T50.8X6-
Sinequan	T43.011-	T43.012-	T43.013-	T43.014-	T43.015-	T43.016-
Singoserp	T46.5X1-	T46.5X2-	T46.5X3-	T46.5X4-	T46.5X5-	T46.5X6-
Sintrom	T45.511-	T45.512-	T45.513-	T45.514-	T45.515-	T45.516-
Sisomicin	T36.5X1-	T36.5X2-	T36.5X3-	T36.5X4-	T36.5X5-	T36.5X6-
Sitosterols	T46.6X1-	T46.6X2-	T46.6X3-	T46.6X4-	T46.6X5-	T46.6X6-

Substance	Poisoning Accidental (unintentional)	Poisoning Intentional self-harm	Poisoning Assault	Poisoning Undetermined	Adverse effect	Underdosing
Skeletal muscle relaxants	T48.1X1-	T48.1X2-	T48.1X3-	T48.1X4-	T48.1X5-	T48.1X6-
Skin						
agents (external)	T49.91X-	T49.92X-	T49.93X-	T49.94X-	T49.95X-	T49.96X-
specified NEC	T49.8X1-	T49.8X2-	T49.8X3-	T49.8X4-	T49.8X5-	T49.8X6-
test antigen	T50.8X1-	T50.8X2-	T50.8X3-	T50.8X4-	T50.8X5-	T50.8X6-
Sleep-eze	T45.0X1-	T45.0X2-	T45.0X3-	T45.0X4-	T45.0X5-	T45.0X6-
Sleeping draught, pill	T42.71X-	T42.72X-	T42.73X-	T42.74X-	T42.75X-	T42.76X-
Smallpox vaccine	T50.B11-	T50.B12-	T50.B13-	T50.B14-	T50.B15-	T50.B16-
Smelter fumes NEC	T56.91X-	T56.92X-	T56.93X-	T56.94X-	-	-
Smog	T59.1X1-	T59.1X2-	T59.1X3-	T59.1X4-	-	-
Smoke NEC	T59.811-	T59.812-	T59.813-	T59.814-	-	-
Smooth muscle relaxant	T44.3X1-	T44.3X2-	T44.3X3-	T44.3X4-	T44.3X5-	T44.3X6-
Snail killer NEC	T60.8X1-	T60.8X2-	T60.8X3-	T60.8X4-	-	-
Snake venom or bite	T63.001-	T63.002-	T63.003-	T63.004-	-	-
hemocoagulase	T45.7X1-	T45.7X2-	T45.7X3-	T45.7X4-	T45.7X5-	T45.7X6-
Snuff	T65.211-	T65.212-	T65.213-	T65.214-	-	-
Soap (powder) (product)	T55.0X1-	T55.0X2-	T55.0X3-	T55.0X4-	-	-
enema	T47.4X1-	T47.4X2-	T47.4X3-	T47.4X4-	T47.4X5-	T47.4X6-
medicinal, soft	T49.2X1-	T49.2X2-	T49.2X3-	T49.2X4-	T49.2X5-	T49.2X6-
superfatted	T49.2X1-	T49.2X2-	T49.2X3-	T49.2X4-	T49.2X5-	T49.2X6-
Sobrerol	T48.4X1-	T48.4X2-	T48.4X3-	T48.4X4-	T48.4X5-	T48.4X6-
Soda (caustic)	T54.3X1-	T54.3X2-	T54.3X3-	T54.3X4-	-	-
bicarb	T47.1X1-	T47.1X2-	T47.1X3-	T47.1X4-	T47.1X5-	T47.1X6-
chlorinated — *see Sodium, hypochlorite*						
Sodium						
acetosulfone	T37.1X1-	T37.1X2-	T37.1X3-	T37.1X4-	T37.1X5-	T37.1X6-
acetrizoate	T50.8X1-	T50.8X2-	T50.8X3-	T50.8X4-	T50.8X5-	T50.8X6-
acid phosphate	T50.3X1-	T50.3X2-	T50.3X3-	T50.3X4-	T50.3X5-	T50.3X6-
alginate	T47.8X1-	T47.8X2-	T47.8X3-	T47.8X4-	T47.8X5-	T47.8X6-
amidotrizoate	T50.8X1-	T50.8X2-	T50.8X3-	T50.8X4-	T50.8X5-	T50.8X6-
aminopterin	T45.1X1-	T45.1X2-	T45.1X3-	T45.1X4-	T45.1X5-	T45.1X6-
amylosulfate	T47.8X1-	T47.8X2-	T47.8X3-	T47.8X4-	T47.8X5-	T47.8X6-
amytal	T42.3X1-	T42.3X2-	T42.3X3-	T42.3X4-	T42.3X5-	T42.3X6-
antimony gluconate	T37.3X1-	T37.3X2-	T37.3X3-	T37.3X4-	T37.3X5-	T37.3X6-
arsenate	T57.0X1-	T57.0X2-	T57.0X3-	T57.0X4-	-	-
aurothiomalate	T39.4X1-	T39.4X2-	T39.4X3-	T39.4X4-	T39.4X5-	T39.4X6-
aurothiosulfate	T39.4X1-	T39.4X2-	T39.4X3-	T39.4X4-	T39.4X5-	T39.4X6-
barbiturate	T42.3X1-	T42.3X2-	T42.3X3-	T42.3X4-	T42.3X5-	T42.3X6-
basic phosphate	T47.4X1-	T47.4X2-	T47.4X3-	T47.4X4-	T47.4X5-	T47.4X6-
bicarbonate	T47.1X1-	T47.1X2-	T47.1X3-	T47.1X4-	T47.1X5-	T47.1X6-
bichromate	T57.8X1-	T57.8X2-	T57.8X3-	T57.8X4-	-	-
biphosphate	T50.3X1-	T50.3X2-	T50.3X3-	T50.3X4-	T50.3X5-	T50.3X6-
bisulfate	T65.891-	T65.892-	T65.893-	T65.894-	-	-
borate						
cleanser	T57.8X1-	T57.8X2-	T57.8X3-	T57.8X4-	-	-
eye	T49.5X1-	T49.5X2-	T49.5X3-	T49.5X4-	T49.5X5-	T49.5X6-
therapeutic	T49.8X1-	T49.8X2-	T49.8X3-	T49.8X4-	T49.8X5-	T49.8X6-
bromide	T42.6X1-	T42.6X2-	T42.6X3-	T42.6X4-	T42.6X5-	T42.6X6-
cacodylate (nonmedicinal) NEC	T50.8X1-	T50.8X2-	T50.8X3-	T50.8X4-	T50.8X5-	T50.8X6-
anti-infective	T37.8X1-	T37.8X2-	T37.8X3-	T37.8X4-	T37.8X5-	T37.8X6-
herbicide	T60.3X1-	T60.3X2-	T60.3X3-	T60.3X4-	-	-
calcium edetate	T45.8X1-	T45.8X2-	T45.8X3-	T45.8X4-	T45.8X5-	T45.8X6-
carbonate NEC	T54.3X1-	T54.3X2-	T54.3X3-	T54.3X4-	-	-
chlorate NEC	T65.891-	T65.892-	T65.893-	T65.894-	-	-
herbicide	T54.91X-	T54.92X-	T54.93X-	T54.94X-	-	-
chloride	T50.3X1-	T50.3X2-	T50.3X3-	T50.3X4-	T50.3X5-	T50.3X6-
with glucose	T50.3X1-	T50.3X2-	T50.3X3-	T50.3X4-	T50.3X5-	T50.3X6-
chromate	T65.891-	T65.892-	T65.893-	T65.894-	-	-

Substance	Poisoning Accidental (unintentional)	Poisoning Intentional self-harm	Poisoning Assault	Poisoning Undetermined	Adverse effect	Underdosing
Sodium (continued)						
citrate	T50.991-	T50.992-	T50.993-	T50.994-	T50.995-	T50.996-
cromoglicate	T48.6X1-	T48.6X2-	T48.6X3-	T48.6X4-	T48.6X5-	T48.6X6-
cyanide	T65.0X1-	T65.0X2-	T65.0X3-	T65.0X4-	-	-
cyclamate	T50.3X1-	T50.3X2-	T50.3X3-	T50.3X4-	T50.3X5-	T50.3X6-
dehydrocholate	T45.8X1-	T45.8X2-	T45.8X3-	T45.8X4-	T45.8X5-	T45.8X6-
diatrizoate	T50.8X1-	T50.8X2-	T50.8X3-	T50.8X4-	T50.8X5-	T50.8X6-
dibunate	T48.4X1-	T48.4X2-	T48.4X3-	T48.4X4-	T48.4X5-	T48.4X6-
dioctyl sulfosuccinate	T47.4X1-	T47.4X2-	T47.4X3-	T47.4X4-	T47.4X5-	T47.4X6-
dipantoyl ferrate	T45.8X1-	T45.8X2-	T45.8X3-	T45.8X4-	T45.8X5-	T45.8X6-
edetate	T45.8X1-	T45.8X2-	T45.8X3-	T45.8X4-	T45.8X5-	T45.8X6-
ethacrynate	T50.1X1-	T50.1X2-	T50.1X3-	T50.1X4-	T50.1X5-	T50.1X6-
feredetate	T45.8X1-	T45.8X2-	T45.8X3-	T45.8X4-	T45.8X5-	T45.8X6-
Fluoride — *see Fluoride*						
fluoroacetate (dust) (pesticide)	T60.4X1-	T60.4X2-	T60.4X3-	T60.4X4-	-	-
free salt	T50.3X1-	T50.3X2-	T50.3X3-	T50.3X4-	T50.3X5-	T50.3X6-
fusidate	T36.8X1-	T36.8X2-	T36.8X3-	T36.8X4-	T36.8X5-	T36.8X6-
glucaldrate	T47.1X1-	T47.1X2-	T47.1X3-	T47.1X4-	T47.1X5-	T47.1X6-
glucosulfone	T37.1X1-	T37.1X2-	T37.1X3-	T37.1X4-	T37.1X5-	T37.1X6-
glutamate	T45.8X1-	T45.8X2-	T45.8X3-	T45.8X4-	T45.8X5-	T45.8X6-
hydrogen carbonate	T50.3X1-	T50.3X2-	T50.3X3-	T50.3X4-	T50.3X5-	T50.3X6-
hydroxide	T54.3X1-	T54.3X2-	T54.3X3-	T54.3X4-	-	-
hypochlorite (bleach) NEC	T54.3X1-	T54.3X2-	T54.3X3-	T54.3X4-	-	-
disinfectant	T54.3X1-	T54.3X2-	T54.3X3-	T54.3X4-	-	-
medicinal (anti-infective) (external)	T49.0X1-	T49.0X2-	T49.0X3-	T49.0X4-	T49.0X5-	T49.0X6-
vapor	T54.3X1-	T54.3X2-	T54.3X3-	T54.3X4-	-	-
hyposulfite	T49.0X1-	T49.0X2-	T49.0X3-	T49.0X4-	T49.0X5-	T49.0X6-
indigotin disulfonate	T50.8X1-	T50.8X2-	T50.8X3-	T50.8X4-	T50.8X5-	T50.8X6-
iodide	T50.991-	T50.992-	T50.993-	T50.994-	T50.995-	T50.996-
I-131	T50.8X1-	T50.8X2-	T50.8X3-	T50.8X4-	T50.8X5-	T50.8X6-
therapeutic	T38.2X1-	T38.2X2-	T38.2X3-	T38.2X4-	T38.2X5-	T38.2X6-
iodohippurate (131I)	T50.8X1-	T50.8X2-	T50.8X3-	T50.8X4-	T50.8X5-	T50.8X6-
iopodate	T50.8X1-	T50.8X2-	T50.8X3-	T50.8X4-	T50.8X5-	T50.8X6-
iothalamate	T50.8X1-	T50.8X2-	T50.8X3-	T50.8X4-	T50.8X5-	T50.8X6-
iron edetate	T45.4X1-	T45.4X2-	T45.4X3-	T45.4X4-	T45.4X5-	T45.4X6-
lactate (compound solution)	T45.8X1-	T45.8X2-	T45.8X3-	T45.8X4-	T45.8X5-	T45.8X6-
lauryl (sulfate)	T49.2X1-	T49.2X2-	T49.2X3-	T49.2X4-	T49.2X5-	T49.2X6-
L-triiodothyronine	T38.1X1-	T38.1X2-	T38.1X3-	T38.1X4-	T38.1X5-	T38.1X6-
magnesium citrate	T50.991-	T50.992-	T50.993-	T50.994-	T50.995-	T50.996-
mersalate	T50.2X1-	T50.2X2-	T50.2X3-	T50.2X4-	T50.2X5-	T50.2X6-
metasilicate	T65.891-	T65.892-	T65.893-	T65.894-	-	-
metrizoate	T50.8X1-	T50.8X2-	T50.8X3-	T50.8X4-	T50.8X5-	T50.8X6-
monofluoroacetate (pesticide)	T60.1X1-	T60.1X2-	T60.1X3-	T60.1X4-	-	-
morrhuate	T46.8X1-	T46.8X2-	T46.8X3-	T46.8X4-	T46.8X5-	T46.8X6-
nafcillin	T36.0X1-	T36.0X2-	T36.0X3-	T36.0X4-	T36.0X5-	T36.0X6-
nitrate (oxidizing agent)	T65.891-	T65.892-	T65.893-	T65.894-	-	-
nitrite	T50.6X1-	T50.6X2-	T50.6X3-	T50.6X4-	T50.6X5-	T50.6X6-
nitroferricyanide	T46.5X1-	T46.5X2-	T46.5X3-	T46.5X4-	T46.5X5-	T46.5X6-
nitroprusside	T46.5X1-	T46.5X2-	T46.5X3-	T46.5X4-	T46.5X5-	T46.5X6-
oxalate	T65.891-	T65.892-	T65.893-	T65.894-	-	-
oxide/peroxide	T65.891-	T65.892-	T65.893-	T65.894-	-	-
oxybate	T41.291-	T41.292-	T41.293-	T41.294-	T41.295-	T41.296-
para-aminohippurate	T50.8X1-	T50.8X2-	T50.8X3-	T50.8X4-	T50.8X5-	T50.8X6-
perborate (nonmedicinal) NEC	T65.891-	T65.892-	T65.893-	T65.894-	-	-
medicinal	T49.0X1-	T49.0X2-	T49.0X3-	T49.0X4-	T49.0X5-	T49.0X6-
soap	T55.0X1-	T55.0X2-	T55.0X3-	T55.0X4-	-	-
percarbonate — *see Sodium, perborate*						
pertechnetate Tc99m	T50.8X1-	T50.8X2-	T50.8X3-	T50.8X4-	T50.8X5-	T50.8X6-
phosphate						
cellulose	T45.8X1-	T45.8X2-	T45.8X3-	T45.8X4-	T45.8X5-	T45.8X6-

Substance	Poisoning Accidental (unintentional)	Poisoning Intentional self-harm	Poisoning Assault	Poisoning Undetermined	Adverse effect	Underdosing
Sodium (continued)						
dibasic	T47.2X1-	T47.2X2-	T47.2X3-	T47.2X4-	T47.2X5-	T47.2X6-
monobasic	T47.2X1-	T47.2X2-	T47.2X3-	T47.2X4-	T47.2X5-	T47.2X6-
phytate	T50.6X1-	T50.6X2-	T50.6X3-	T50.6X4-	T50.6X5-	T50.6X6-
picosulfate	T47.2X1-	T47.2X2-	T47.2X3-	T47.2X4-	T47.2X5-	T47.2X6-
polyhydroxyaluminium monocarbonate	T47.1X1-	T47.1X2-	T47.1X3-	T47.1X4-	T47.1X5-	T47.1X6-
polystyrene sulfonate	T50.3X1-	T50.3X2-	T50.3X3-	T50.3X4-	T50.3X5-	T50.3X6-
propionate	T49.0X1-	T49.0X2-	T49.0X3-	T49.0X4-	T49.0X5-	T49.0X6-
propyl hydroxybenzoate	T50.991-	T50.992-	T50.993-	T50.994-	T50.995-	T50.996-
psylliate	T46.8X1-	T46.8X2-	T46.8X3-	T46.8X4-	T46.8X5-	T46.8X6-
removing resins	T50.3X1-	T50.3X2-	T50.3X3-	T50.3X4-	T50.3X5-	T50.3X6-
salicylate	T39.091-	T39.092-	T39.093-	T39.094-	T39.095-	T39.096-
salt NEC	T50.3X1-	T50.3X2-	T50.3X3-	T50.3X4-	T50.3X5-	T50.3X6-
selenate	T60.2X1-	T60.2X2-	T60.2X3-	T60.2X4-	-	-
stibogluconate	T37.3X1-	T37.3X2-	T37.3X3-	T37.3X4-	T37.3X5-	T37.3X6-
sulfate	T47.4X1-	T47.4X2-	T47.4X3-	T47.4X4-	T47.4X5-	T47.4X6-
sulfoxone	T37.1X1-	T37.1X2-	T37.1X3-	T37.1X4-	T37.1X5-	T37.1X6-
tetradecyl sulfate	T46.8X1-	T46.8X2-	T46.8X3-	T46.8X4-	T46.8X5-	T46.8X6-
thiopental	T41.1X1-	T41.1X2-	T41.1X3-	T41.1X4-	T41.1X5-	T41.1X6-
thiosalicylate	T39.091-	T39.092-	T39.093-	T39.094-	T39.095-	T39.096-
thiosulfate	T50.6X1-	T50.6X2-	T50.6X3-	T50.6X4-	T50.6X5-	T50.6X6-
tolbutamide	T38.3X1-	T38.3X2-	T38.3X3-	T38.3X4-	T38.3X5-	T38.3X6-
(L) -triiodothyronine	T38.1X1-	T38.1X2-	T38.1X3-	T38.1X4-	T38.1X5-	T38.1X6-
tyropanoate	T50.8X1-	T50.8X2-	T50.8X3-	T50.8X4-	T50.8X5-	T50.8X6-
valproate	T42.6X1-	T42.6X2-	T42.6X3-	T42.6X4-	T42.6X5-	T42.6X6-
versenate	T50.6X1-	T50.6X2-	T50.6X3-	T50.6X4-	T50.6X5-	T50.6X6-
Sodium-free salt	T50.901-	T50.902-	T50.903-	T50.904-	T50.905-	T50.906-
Sodium-removing resin	T50.3X1-	T50.3X2-	T50.3X3-	T50.3X4-	T50.3X5-	T50.3X6-
Soft soap	T55.0X1-	T55.0X2-	T55.0X3-	T55.0X4-	-	-
Solanine	T62.2X1-	T62.2X2-	T62.2X3-	T62.2X4-	-	-
berries	T62.1X1-	T62.1X2-	T62.1X3-	T62.1X4-	-	-
Solanum dulcamara	T62.2X1-	T62.2X2-	T62.2X3-	T62.2X4-	-	-
berries	T62.1X1-	T62.1X2-	T62.1X3-	T62.1X4-	-	-
Solapsone	T37.1X1-	T37.1X2-	T37.1X3-	T37.1X4-	T37.1X5-	T37.1X6-
Solar lotion	T49.3X1-	T49.3X2-	T49.3X3-	T49.3X4-	T49.3X5-	T49.3X6-
Solasulfone	T37.1X1-	T37.1X2-	T37.1X3-	T37.1X4-	T37.1X5-	T37.1X6-
Soldering fluid	T65.891-	T65.892-	T65.893-	T65.894-	-	-
Solid substance	T65.91X-	T65.92X-	T65.93X-	T65.94X-	-	-
specified NEC	T65.891-	T65.892-	T65.893-	T65.894-	-	-
Solvent, industrial NEC	T52.91X-	T52.92X-	T52.93X-	T52.94X-	-	-
naphtha	T52.0X1-	T52.0X2-	T52.0X3-	T52.0X4-	-	-
petroleum	T52.0X1-	T52.0X2-	T52.0X3-	T52.0X4-	-	-
specified NEC	T52.8X1-	T52.8X2-	T52.8X3-	T52.8X4-	-	-
Soma	T42.8X1-	T42.8X2-	T42.8X3-	T42.8X4-	T42.8X5-	T42.8X6-
Somatorelin	T38.891-	T38.892-	T38.893-	T38.894-	T38.895-	T38.896-
Somatostatin	T38.991-	T38.992-	T38.993-	T38.994-	T38.995-	T38.996-
Somatotropin	T38.811-	T38.812-	T38.813-	T38.814-	T38.815-	T38.816-
Somatrem	T38.811-	T38.812-	T38.813-	T38.814-	T38.815-	T38.816-
Somatropin	T38.811-	T38.812-	T38.813-	T38.814-	T38.815-	T38.816-
Sominex	T45.0X1-	T45.0X2-	T45.0X3-	T45.0X4-	T45.0X5-	T45.0X6-
Somnos	T42.6X1-	T42.6X2-	T42.6X3-	T42.6X4-	T42.6X5-	T42.6X6-
Somonal	T42.3X1-	T42.3X2-	T42.3X3-	T42.3X4-	T42.3X5-	T42.3X6-
Soneryl	T42.3X1-	T42.3X2-	T42.3X3-	T42.3X4-	T42.3X5-	T42.3X6-
Soothing syrup	T50.901-	T50.902-	T50.903-	T50.904-	T50.905-	T50.906-
Sopor	T42.6X1-	T42.6X2-	T42.6X3-	T42.6X4-	T42.6X5-	T42.6X6-
Soporific	T42.71X-	T42.72X-	T42.73X-	T42.74X-	T42.75X-	T42.76X-
Soporific drug	T42.71X-	T42.72X-	T42.73X-	T42.74X-	T42.75X-	T42.76X-
specified type NEC	T42.6X1-	T42.6X2-	T42.6X3-	T42.6X4-	T42.6X5-	T42.6X6-

Substance	Poisoning Accidental (unintentional)	Poisoning Intentional self-harm	Poisoning Assault	Poisoning Undetermined	Adverse effect	Underdosing
Sorbide nitrate	T46.3X1-	T46.3X2-	T46.3X3-	T46.3X4-	T46.3X5-	T46.3X6-
Sorbitol	T47.4X1-	T47.4X2-	T47.4X3-	T47.4X4-	T47.4X5-	T47.4X6-
Sotalol	T44.7X1-	T44.7X2-	T44.7X3-	T44.7X4-	T44.7X5-	T44.7X6-
Sotradecol	T46.8X1-	T46.8X2-	T46.8X3-	T46.8X4-	T46.8X5-	T46.8X6-
Soysterol	T46.6X1-	T46.6X2-	T46.6X3-	T46.6X4-	T46.6X5-	T46.6X6-
Spacoline	T44.3X1-	T44.3X2-	T44.3X3-	T44.3X4-	T44.3X5-	T44.3X6-
Spanish fly	T49.8X1-	T49.8X2-	T49.8X3-	T49.8X4-	T49.8X5-	T49.8X6-
Sparine	T43.3X1-	T43.3X2-	T43.3X3-	T43.3X4-	T43.3X5-	T43.3X6-
Sparteine	T48.0X1-	T48.0X2-	T48.0X3-	T48.0X4-	T48.0X5-	T48.0X6-
Spasmolytic						
anticholinergics	T44.3X1-	T44.3X2-	T44.3X3-	T44.3X4-	T44.3X5-	T44.3X6-
autonomic	T44.3X1-	T44.3X2-	T44.3X3-	T44.3X4-	T44.3X5-	T44.3X6-
bronchial NEC	T48.6X1-	T48.6X2-	T48.6X3-	T48.6X4-	T48.6X5-	T48.6X6-
quaternary ammonium	T44.3X1-	T44.3X2-	T44.3X3-	T44.3X4-	T44.3X5-	T44.3X6-
skeletal muscle NEC	T48.1X1-	T48.1X2-	T48.1X3-	T48.1X4-	T48.1X5-	T48.1X6-
Spectinomycin	T36.5X1-	T36.5X2-	T36.5X3-	T36.5X4-	T36.5X5-	T36.5X6-
Speed	T43.621-	T43.622-	T43.623-	T43.624-	T43.625-	T43.626-
Spermicide	T49.8X1-	T49.8X2-	T49.8X3-	T49.8X4-	T49.8X5-	T49.8X6-
Spider (bite) (venom)	T63.391-	T63.392-	T63.393-	T63.394-	-	-
antivenin	T50.Z11-	T50.Z12-	T50.Z13-	T50.Z14-	T50.Z15-	T50.Z16-
Spigelia (root)	T37.4X1-	T37.4X2-	T37.4X3-	T37.4X4-	T37.4X5-	T37.4X6-
Spindle inactivator	T50.4X1-	T50.4X2-	T50.4X3-	T50.4X4-	T50.4X5-	T50.4X6-
Spiperone	T43.4X1-	T43.4X2-	T43.4X3-	T43.4X4-	T43.4X5-	T43.4X6-
Spiramycin	T36.3X1-	T36.3X2-	T36.3X3-	T36.3X4-	T36.3X5-	T36.3X6-
Spirapril	T46.4X1-	T46.4X2-	T46.4X3-	T46.4X4-	T46.4X5-	T46.4X6-
Spirilene	T43.591-	T43.592-	T43.593-	T43.594-	T43.595-	T43.596-
Spirit (s) (neutral) NEC	T51.0X1-	T51.0X2-	T51.0X3-	T51.0X4-	-	-
beverage	T51.0X1-	T51.0X2-	T51.0X3-	T51.0X4-	-	-
industrial	T51.0X1-	T51.0X2-	T51.0X3-	T51.0X4-	-	-
mineral	T52.0X1-	T52.0X2-	T52.0X3-	T52.0X4-	-	-
of salt — *see Hydrochloric acid*						
surgical	T51.0X1-	T51.0X2-	T51.0X3-	T51.0X4-	-	-
Spironolactone	T50.0X1-	T50.0X2-	T50.0X3-	T50.0X4-	T50.0X5-	T50.0X6-
Spiroperidol	T43.4X1-	T43.4X2-	T43.4X3-	T43.4X4-	T43.4X5-	T43.4X6-
Sponge, absorbable (gelatin)	T45.7X1-	T45.7X2-	T45.7X3-	T45.7X4-	T45.7X5-	T45.7X6-
Sporostacin	T49.0X1-	T49.0X2-	T49.0X3-	T49.0X4-	T49.0X5-	T49.0X6-
Spray (aerosol)	T65.91X-	T65.92X-	T65.93X-	T65.94X-	-	-
cosmetic	T65.891-	T65.892-	T65.893-	T65.894-	-	-
medicinal NEC	T50.901-	T50.902-	T50.903-	T50.904-	T50.905-	T50.906-
pesticides — *see Pesticides*						
specified content — *see specific substance*						
Spurge flax	T62.2X1-	T62.2X2-	T62.2X3-	T62.2X4-	-	-
Spurges	T62.2X1-	T62.2X2-	T62.2X3-	T62.2X4-	-	-
Sputum viscosity-lowering drug	T48.4X1-	T48.4X2-	T48.4X3-	T48.4X4-	T48.4X5-	T48.4X6-
Squill	T46.0X1-	T46.0X2-	T46.0X3-	T46.0X4-	T46.0X5-	T46.0X6-
rat poison	T60.4X1-	T60.4X2-	T60.4X3-	T60.4X4-	-	-
Squirting cucumber (cathartic)	T47.2X1-	T47.2X2-	T47.2X3-	T47.2X4-	T47.2X5-	T47.2X6-
Stains	T65.6X1-	T65.6X2-	T65.6X3-	T65.6X4-	-	-
Stannous fluoride	T49.7X1-	T49.7X2-	T49.7X3-	T49.7X4-	T49.7X5-	T49.7X6-
Stanolone	T38.7X1-	T38.7X2-	T38.7X3-	T38.7X4-	T38.7X5-	T38.7X6-
Stanozolol	T38.7X1-	T38.7X2-	T38.7X3-	T38.7X4-	T38.7X5-	T38.7X6-
Staphisagria or stavesacre (pediculicide)	T49.0X1-	T49.0X2-	T49.0X3-	T49.0X4-	T49.0X5-	T49.0X6-
Starch	T50.901-	T50.902-	T50.903-	T50.904-	T50.905-	T50.906-
Stelazine	T43.3X1-	T43.3X2-	T43.3X3-	T43.3X4-	T43.3X5-	T43.3X6-
Stemetil	T43.3X1-	T43.3X2-	T43.3X3-	T43.3X4-	T43.3X5-	T43.3X6-
Stepronin	T48.4X1-	T48.4X2-	T48.4X3-	T48.4X4-	T48.4X5-	T48.4X6-
Sterculia	T47.4X1-	T47.4X2-	T47.4X3-	T47.4X4-	T47.4X5-	T47.4X6-

Substance	Poisoning Accidental (unintentional)	Poisoning Intentional self-harm	Poisoning Assault	Poisoning Undetermined	Adverse effect	Underdosing
Sternutator gas	T59.891-	T59.892-	T59.893-	T59.894-	-	-
Steroid	T38.0X1-	T38.0X2-	T38.0X3-	T38.0X4-	T38.0X5-	T38.0X6-
anabolic	T38.7X1-	T38.7X2-	T38.7X3-	T38.7X4-	T38.7X5-	T38.7X6-
androgenic	T38.7X1-	T38.7X2-	T38.7X3-	T38.7X4-	T38.7X5-	T38.7X6-
antineoplastic, hormone	T38.7X1-	T38.7X2-	T38.7X3-	T38.7X4-	T38.7X5-	T38.7X6-
estrogen	T38.5X1-	T38.5X2-	T38.5X3-	T38.5X4-	T38.5X5-	T38.5X6-
ENT agent	T49.6X1-	T49.6X2-	T49.6X3-	T49.6X4-	T49.6X5-	T49.6X6-
ophthalmic preparation	T49.5X1-	T49.5X2-	T49.5X3-	T49.5X4-	T49.5X5-	T49.5X6-
topical NEC	T49.0X1-	T49.0X2-	T49.0X3-	T49.0X4-	T49.0X5-	T49.0X6-
Stibine	T56.891-	T56.892-	T56.893-	T56.894-	-	-
Stibogluconate	T37.3X1-	T37.3X2-	T37.3X3-	T37.3X4-	T37.3X5-	T37.3X6-
Stibophen	T37.4X1-	T37.4X2-	T37.4X3-	T37.4X4-	T37.4X5-	T37.4X6-
Stilbamidine (isetionate)	T37.3X1-	T37.3X2-	T37.3X3-	T37.3X4-	T37.3X5-	T37.3X6-
Stilbestrol	T38.5X1-	T38.5X2-	T38.5X3-	T38.5X4-	T38.5X5-	T38.5X6-
Stilboestrol	T38.5X1-	T38.5X2-	T38.5X3-	T38.5X4-	T38.5X5-	T38.5X6-
Stimulant						
central nervous system — *see also Psychostimulant*	T43.601-	T43.602-	T43.603-	T43.604-	T43.605-	T43.606-
analeptics	T50.7X1-	T50.7X2-	T50.7X3-	T50.7X4-	T50.7X5-	T50.7X6-
opiate antagonist	T50.7X1-	T50.7X2-	T50.7X3-	T50.7X4-	T50.7X5-	T50.7X6-
psychotherapeutic NEC — *see also Psychotherapeutic drug*	T43.601-	T43.602-	T43.603-	T43.604-	T43.605-	T43.606-
specified NEC	T43.691-	T43.692-	T43.693-	T43.694-	T43.695-	T43.696-
respiratory	T48.901-	T48.902-	T48.903-	T48.904-	T48.905-	T48.906-
Stone-dissolving drug	T50.901-	T50.902-	T50.903-	T50.904-	T50.905-	T50.906-
Storage battery (cells) (acid)	T54.2X1-	T54.2X2-	T54.2X3-	T54.2X4-	-	-
Stovaine	T41.3X1-	T41.3X2-	T41.3X3-	T41.3X4-	T41.3X5-	T41.3X6-
infiltration (subcutaneous)	T41.3X1-	T41.3X2-	T41.3X3-	T41.3X4-	T41.3X5-	T41.3X6-
nerve block (peripheral) (plexus)	T41.3X1-	T41.3X2-	T41.3X3-	T41.3X4-	T41.3X5-	T41.3X6-
spinal	T41.3X1-	T41.3X2-	T41.3X3-	T41.3X4-	T41.3X5-	T41.3X6-
topical (surface)	T41.3X1-	T41.3X2-	T41.3X3-	T41.3X4-	T41.3X5-	T41.3X6-
Stovarsal	T37.8X1-	T37.8X2-	T37.8X3-	T37.8X4-	T37.8X5-	T37.8X6-
Stove gas — *see Gas, stove*						
Stoxil	T49.5X1-	T49.5X2-	T49.5X3-	T49.5X4-	T49.5X5-	T49.5X6-
Stramonium	T48.6X1-	T48.6X2-	T48.6X3-	T48.6X4-	T48.6X5-	T48.6X6-
natural state	T62.2X1-	T62.2X2-	T62.2X3-	T62.2X4-	-	-
Streptodornase	T45.3X1-	T45.3X2-	T45.3X3-	T45.3X4-	T45.3X5-	T45.3X6-
Streptoduocin	T36.5X1-	T36.5X2-	T36.5X3-	T36.5X4-	T36.5X5-	T36.5X6-
Streptokinase	T45.611-	T45.612-	T45.613-	T45.614-	T45.615-	T45.616-
Streptomycin (derivative)	T36.5X1-	T36.5X2-	T36.5X3-	T36.5X4-	T36.5X5-	T36.5X6-
Streptonivicin	T36.5X1-	T36.5X2-	T36.5X3-	T36.5X4-	T36.5X5-	T36.5X6-
Streptovarycin	T36.5X1-	T36.5X2-	T36.5X3-	T36.5X4-	T36.5X5-	T36.5X6-
Streptozocin	T45.1X1-	T45.1X2-	T45.1X3-	T45.1X4-	T45.1X5-	T45.1X6-
Streptozotocin	T45.1X1-	T45.1X2-	T45.1X3-	T45.1X4-	T45.1X5-	T45.1X6-
Stripper (paint) (solvent)	T52.8X1-	T52.8X2-	T52.8X3-	T52.8X4-	-	-
Strobane	T60.1X1-	T60.1X2-	T60.1X3-	T60.1X4-	-	-
Strofantina	T46.0X1-	T46.0X2-	T46.0X3-	T46.0X4-	T46.0X5-	T46.0X6-
Strophanthin (g) (k)	T46.0X1-	T46.0X2-	T46.0X3-	T46.0X4-	T46.0X5-	T46.0X6-
Strophanthus	T46.0X1-	T46.0X2-	T46.0X3-	T46.0X4-	T46.0X5-	T46.0X6-
Strophantin	T46.0X1-	T46.0X2-	T46.0X3-	T46.0X4-	T46.0X5-	T46.0X6-
Strophantin-g	T46.0X1-	T46.0X2-	T46.0X3-	T46.0X4-	T46.0X5-	T46.0X6-
Strychnine (nonmedicinal) (pesticide) (salts)	T65.1X1-	T65.1X2-	T65.1X3-	T65.1X4-	-	-
medicinal	T48.291-	T48.292-	T48.293-	T48.294-	T48.295-	T48.296-
Strychnos (ignatii) — *see Strychnine*						
Styramate	T42.8X1-	T42.8X2-	T42.8X3-	T42.8X4-	T42.8X5-	T42.8X6-
Styrene	T65.891-	T65.892-	T65.893-	T65.894-	-	-

Substance	Poisoning Accidental (unintentional)	Poisoning Intentional self-harm	Poisoning Assault	Poisoning Undetermined	Adverse effect	Underdosing
Succinimide, antiepileptic or anticonvulsant	T42.2X1-	T42.2X2-	T42.2X3-	T42.2X4-	T42.2X5-	T42.2X6-
mercuric — *see Mercury*						
Succinylcholine	T48.1X1-	T48.1X2-	T48.1X3-	T48.1X4-	T48.1X5-	T48.1X6-
Succinylsulfathiazole	T37.0X1-	T37.0X2-	T37.0X3-	T37.0X4-	T37.0X5-	T37.0X6-
Sucralfate	T47.1X1-	T47.1X2-	T47.1X3-	T47.1X4-	T47.1X5-	T47.1X6-
Sucrose	T50.3X1-	T50.3X2-	T50.3X3-	T50.3X4-	T50.3X5-	T50.3X6-
Sufentanil	T40.411-	T40.412-	T40.413-	T40.414-	T40.415-	T40.416-
Sulbactam	T36.0X1-	T36.0X2-	T36.0X3-	T36.0X4-	T36.0X5-	T36.0X6-
Sulbenicillin	T36.0X1-	T36.0X2-	T36.0X3-	T36.0X4-	T36.0X5-	T36.0X6-
Sulbentine	T49.0X1-	T49.0X2-	T49.0X3-	T49.0X4-	T49.0X5-	T49.0X6-
Sulfacetamide	T49.0X1-	T49.0X2-	T49.0X3-	T49.0X4-	T49.0X5-	T49.0X6-
ophthalmic preparation	T49.5X1-	T49.5X2-	T49.5X3-	T49.5X4-	T49.5X5-	T49.5X6-
Sulfachlorpyridazine	T37.0X1-	T37.0X2-	T37.0X3-	T37.0X4-	T37.0X5-	T37.0X6-
Sulfacitine	T37.0X1-	T37.0X2-	T37.0X3-	T37.0X4-	T37.0X5-	T37.0X6-
Sulfadiasulfone sodium	T37.0X1-	T37.0X2-	T37.0X3-	T37.0X4-	T37.0X5-	T37.0X6-
Sulfadiazine	T37.0X1-	T37.0X2-	T37.0X3-	T37.0X4-	T37.0X5-	T37.0X6-
silver (topical)	T49.0X1-	T49.0X2-	T49.0X3-	T49.0X4-	T49.0X5-	T49.0X6-
Sulfadimethoxine	T37.0X1-	T37.0X2-	T37.0X3-	T37.0X4-	T37.0X5-	T37.0X6-
Sulfadimidine	T37.0X1-	T37.0X2-	T37.0X3-	T37.0X4-	T37.0X5-	T37.0X6-
Sulfadoxine	T37.0X1-	T37.0X2-	T37.0X3-	T37.0X4-	T37.0X5-	T37.0X6-
with pyrimethamine	T37.2X1-	T37.2X2-	T37.2X3-	T37.2X4-	T37.2X5-	T37.2X6-
Sulfaethidole	T37.0X1-	T37.0X2-	T37.0X3-	T37.0X4-	T37.0X5-	T37.0X6-
Sulfafurazole	T37.0X1-	T37.0X2-	T37.0X3-	T37.0X4-	T37.0X5-	T37.0X6-
Sulfaguanidine	T37.0X1-	T37.0X2-	T37.0X3-	T37.0X4-	T37.0X5-	T37.0X6-
Sulfalene	T37.0X1-	T37.0X2-	T37.0X3-	T37.0X4-	T37.0X5-	T37.0X6-
Sulfaloxate	T37.0X1-	T37.0X2-	T37.0X3-	T37.0X4-	T37.0X5-	T37.0X6-
Sulfaloxic acid	T37.0X1-	T37.0X2-	T37.0X3-	T37.0X4-	T37.0X5-	T37.0X6-
Sulfamazone	T39.2X1-	T39.2X2-	T39.2X3-	T39.2X4-	T39.2X5-	T39.2X6-
Sulfamerazine	T37.0X1-	T37.0X2-	T37.0X3-	T37.0X4-	T37.0X5-	T37.0X6-
Sulfameter	T37.0X1-	T37.0X2-	T37.0X3-	T37.0X4-	T37.0X5-	T37.0X6-
Sulfamethazine	T37.0X1-	T37.0X2-	T37.0X3-	T37.0X4-	T37.0X5-	T37.0X6-
Sulfamethizole	T37.0X1-	T37.0X2-	T37.0X3-	T37.0X4-	T37.0X5-	T37.0X6-
Sulfamethoxazole	T37.0X1-	T37.0X2-	T37.0X3-	T37.0X4-	T37.0X5-	T37.0X6-
with trimethoprim	T36.8X1-	T36.8X2-	T36.8X3-	T36.8X4-	T36.8X5-	T36.8X6-
Sulfamethoxydiazine	T37.0X1-	T37.0X2-	T37.0X3-	T37.0X4-	T37.0X5-	T37.0X6-
Sulfamethoxypyridazine	T37.0X1-	T37.0X2-	T37.0X3-	T37.0X4-	T37.0X5-	T37.0X6-
Sulfamethylthiazole	T37.0X1-	T37.0X2-	T37.0X3-	T37.0X4-	T37.0X5-	T37.0X6-
Sulfametoxydiazine	T37.0X1-	T37.0X2-	T37.0X3-	T37.0X4-	T37.0X5-	T37.0X6-
Sulfamidopyrine	T39.2X1-	T39.2X2-	T39.2X3-	T39.2X4-	T39.2X5-	T39.2X6-
Sulfamonomethoxine	T37.0X1-	T37.0X2-	T37.0X3-	T37.0X4-	T37.0X5-	T37.0X6-
Sulfamoxole	T37.0X1-	T37.0X2-	T37.0X3-	T37.0X4-	T37.0X5-	T37.0X6-
Sulfamylon	T49.0X1-	T49.0X2-	T49.0X3-	T49.0X4-	T49.0X5-	T49.0X6-
Sulfan blue (diagnostic dye)	T50.8X1-	T50.8X2-	T50.8X3-	T50.8X4-	T50.8X5-	T50.8X6-
Sulfanilamide	T37.0X1-	T37.0X2-	T37.0X3-	T37.0X4-	T37.0X5-	T37.0X6-
Sulfanilylguanidine	T37.0X1-	T37.0X2-	T37.0X3-	T37.0X4-	T37.0X5-	T37.0X6-
Sulfaperin	T37.0X1-	T37.0X2-	T37.0X3-	T37.0X4-	T37.0X5-	T37.0X6-
Sulfaphenazole	T37.0X1-	T37.0X2-	T37.0X3-	T37.0X4-	T37.0X5-	T37.0X6-
Sulfaphenylthiazole	T37.0X1-	T37.0X2-	T37.0X3-	T37.0X4-	T37.0X5-	T37.0X6-
Sulfaproxyline	T37.0X1-	T37.0X2-	T37.0X3-	T37.0X4-	T37.0X5-	T37.0X6-
Sulfapyridine	T37.0X1-	T37.0X2-	T37.0X3-	T37.0X4-	T37.0X5-	T37.0X6-
Sulfapyrimidine	T37.0X1-	T37.0X2-	T37.0X3-	T37.0X4-	T37.0X5-	T37.0X6-
Sulfarsphenamine	T37.8X1-	T37.8X2-	T37.8X3-	T37.8X4-	T37.8X5-	T37.8X6-
Sulfasalazine	T37.0X1-	T37.0X2-	T37.0X3-	T37.0X4-	T37.0X5-	T37.0X6-
Sulfasuxidine	T37.0X1-	T37.0X2-	T37.0X3-	T37.0X4-	T37.0X5-	T37.0X6-
Sulfasymazine	T37.0X1-	T37.0X2-	T37.0X3-	T37.0X4-	T37.0X5-	T37.0X6-
Sulfated amylopectin	T47.8X1-	T47.8X2-	T47.8X3-	T47.8X4-	T47.8X5-	T47.8X6-
Sulfathiazole	T37.0X1-	T37.0X2-	T37.0X3-	T37.0X4-	T37.0X5-	T37.0X6-
Sulfatostearate	T49.2X1-	T49.2X2-	T49.2X3-	T49.2X4-	T49.2X5-	T49.2X6-

Substance	Poisoning Accidental (unintentional)	Poisoning Intentional self-harm	Poisoning Assault	Poisoning Undetermined	Adverse effect	Underdosing
Sulfinpyrazone	T50.4X1-	T50.4X2-	T50.4X3-	T50.4X4-	T50.4X5-	T50.4X6-
Sulfiram	T49.0X1-	T49.0X2-	T49.0X3-	T49.0X4-	T49.0X5-	T49.0X6-
Sulfisomidine	T37.0X1-	T37.0X2-	T37.0X3-	T37.0X4-	T37.0X5-	T37.0X6-
Sulfisoxazole	T37.0X1-	T37.0X2-	T37.0X3-	T37.0X4-	T37.0X5-	T37.0X6-
ophthalmic preparation	T49.5X1-	T49.5X2-	T49.5X3-	T49.5X4-	T49.5X5-	T49.5X6-
Sulfobromophthalein (sodium)	T50.8X1-	T50.8X2-	T50.8X3-	T50.8X4-	T50.8X5-	T50.8X6-
Sulfobromphthalein	T50.8X1-	T50.8X2-	T50.8X3-	T50.8X4-	T50.8X5-	T50.8X6-
Sulfogaiacol	T48.4X1-	T48.4X2-	T48.4X3-	T48.4X4-	T48.4X5-	T48.4X6-
Sulfomyxin	T36.8X1-	T36.8X2-	T36.8X3-	T36.8X4-	T36.8X5-	T36.8X6-
Sulfonal	T42.6X1-	T42.6X2-	T42.6X3-	T42.6X4-	T42.6X5-	T42.6X6-
Sulfonamide NEC	T37.0X1-	T37.0X2-	T37.0X3-	T37.0X4-	T37.0X5-	T37.0X6-
eye	T49.5X1-	T49.5X2-	T49.5X3-	T49.5X4-	T49.5X5-	T49.5X6-
Sulfonazide	T37.1X1-	T37.1X2-	T37.1X3-	T37.1X4-	T37.1X5-	T37.1X6-
Sulfones	T37.1X1-	T37.1X2-	T37.1X3-	T37.1X4-	T37.1X5-	T37.1X6-
Sulfonethylmethane	T42.6X1-	T42.6X2-	T42.6X3-	T42.6X4-	T42.6X5-	T42.6X6-
Sulfonmethane	T42.6X1-	T42.6X2-	T42.6X3-	T42.6X4-	T42.6X5-	T42.6X6-
Sulfonphthal, sulfonphthol	T50.8X1-	T50.8X2-	T50.8X3-	T50.8X4-	T50.8X5-	T50.8X6-
Sulfonylurea derivatives, oral	T38.3X1-	T38.3X2-	T38.3X3-	T38.3X4-	T38.3X5-	T38.3X6-
Sulforidazine	T43.3X1-	T43.3X2-	T43.3X3-	T43.3X4-	T43.3X5-	T43.3X6-
Sulfoxone	T37.1X1-	T37.1X2-	T37.1X3-	T37.1X4-	T37.1X5-	T37.1X6-
Sulfur, sulfurated, sulfuric, sulfurous, sulfuryl (compounds NEC) (medicinal)	T49.4X1-	T49.4X2-	T49.4X3-	T49.4X4-	T49.4X5-	T49.4X6-
acid	T54.2X1-	T54.2X2-	T54.2X3-	T54.2X4-	-	-
dioxide (gas)	T59.1X1-	T59.1X2-	T59.1X3-	T59.1X4-	-	-
ether — *see Ether(s)*						
hydrogen	T59.6X1-	T59.6X2-	T59.6X3-	T59.6X4-	-	-
medicinal (keratolytic) (ointment) NEC	T49.4X1-	T49.4X2-	T49.4X3-	T49.4X4-	T49.4X5-	T49.4X6-
ointment	T49.0X1-	T49.0X2-	T49.0X3-	T49.0X4-	T49.0X5-	T49.0X6-
pesticide (vapor)	T60.91X-	T60.92X-	T60.93X-	T60.94X-	-	-
vapor NEC	T59.891-	T59.892-	T59.893-	T59.894-	-	-
Sulfuric acid	T54.2X1-	T54.2X2-	T54.2X3-	T54.2X4-	-	-
Sulglicotide	T47.1X1-	T47.1X2-	T47.1X3-	T47.1X4-	T47.1X5-	T47.1X6-
Sulindac	T39.391-	T39.392-	T39.393-	T39.394-	T39.395-	T39.396-
Sulisatin	T47.2X1-	T47.2X2-	T47.2X3-	T47.2X4-	T47.2X5-	T47.2X6-
Sulisobenzone	T49.3X1-	T49.3X2-	T49.3X3-	T49.3X4-	T49.3X5-	T49.3X6-
Sulkowitch's reagent	T50.8X1-	T50.8X2-	T50.8X3-	T50.8X4-	T50.8X5-	T50.8X6-
Sulmetozine	T44.3X1-	T44.3X2-	T44.3X3-	T44.3X4-	T44.3X5-	T44.3X6-
Suloctidil	T46.7X1-	T46.7X2-	T46.7X3-	T46.7X4-	T46.7X5-	T46.7X6-
Sulph- — *see also Sulf-*						
Sulphadiazine	T37.0X1-	T37.0X2-	T37.0X3-	T37.0X4-	T37.0X5-	T37.0X6-
Sulphadimethoxine	T37.0X1-	T37.0X2-	T37.0X3-	T37.0X4-	T37.0X5-	T37.0X6-
Sulphadimidine	T37.0X1-	T37.0X2-	T37.0X3-	T37.0X4-	T37.0X5-	T37.0X6-
Sulphadione	T37.1X1-	T37.1X2-	T37.1X3-	T37.1X4-	T37.1X5-	T37.1X6-
Sulphafurazole	T37.0X1-	T37.0X2-	T37.0X3-	T37.0X4-	T37.0X5-	T37.0X6-
Sulphamethizole	T37.0X1-	T37.0X2-	T37.0X3-	T37.0X4-	T37.0X5-	T37.0X6-
Sulphamethoxazole	T37.0X1-	T37.0X2-	T37.0X3-	T37.0X4-	T37.0X5-	T37.0X6-
Sulphan blue	T50.8X1-	T50.8X2-	T50.8X3-	T50.8X4-	T50.8X5-	T50.8X6-
Sulphaphenazole	T37.0X1-	T37.0X2-	T37.0X3-	T37.0X4-	T37.0X5-	T37.0X6-
Sulphapyridine	T37.0X1-	T37.0X2-	T37.0X3-	T37.0X4-	T37.0X5-	T37.0X6-
Sulphasalazine	T37.0X1-	T37.0X2-	T37.0X3-	T37.0X4-	T37.0X5-	T37.0X6-
Sulphinpyrazone	T50.4X1-	T50.4X2-	T50.4X3-	T50.4X4-	T50.4X5-	T50.4X6-
Sulpiride	T43.591-	T43.592-	T43.593-	T43.594-	T43.595-	T43.596-
Sulprostone	T48.0X1-	T48.0X2-	T48.0X3-	T48.0X4-	T48.0X5-	T48.0X6-
Sulpyrine	T39.2X1-	T39.2X2-	T39.2X3-	T39.2X4-	T39.2X5-	T39.2X6-
Sultamicillin	T36.0X1-	T36.0X2-	T36.0X3-	T36.0X4-	T36.0X5-	T36.0X6-
Sulthiame	T42.6X1-	T42.6X2-	T42.6X3-	T42.6X4-	T42.6X5-	T42.6X6-
Sultiame	T42.6X1-	T42.6X2-	T42.6X3-	T42.6X4-	T42.6X5-	T42.6X6-
Sultopride	T43.591-	T43.592-	T43.593-	T43.594-	T43.595-	T43.596-

Substance	Poisoning Accidental (unintentional)	Poisoning Intentional self-harm	Poisoning Assault	Poisoning Undetermined	Adverse effect	Underdosing
Sumatriptan	T39.8X1-	T39.8X2-	T39.8X3-	T39.8X4-	T39.8X5-	T39.8X6-
Sunflower seed oil	T46.6X1-	T46.6X2-	T46.6X3-	T46.6X4-	T46.6X5-	T46.6X6-
Superinone	T48.4X1-	T48.4X2-	T48.4X3-	T48.4X4-	T48.4X5-	T48.4X6-
Suprofen	T39.311-	T39.312-	T39.313-	T39.314-	T39.315-	T39.316-
Suramin (sodium)	T37.4X1-	T37.4X2-	T37.4X3-	T37.4X4-	T37.4X5-	T37.4X6-
Surfacaine	T41.3X1-	T41.3X2-	T41.3X3-	T41.3X4-	T41.3X5-	T41.3X6-
Surital	T41.1X1-	T41.1X2-	T41.1X3-	T41.1X4-	T41.1X5-	T41.1X6-
Sutilains	T45.3X1-	T45.3X2-	T45.3X3-	T45.3X4-	T45.3X5-	T45.3X6-
Suxamethonium (chloride)	T48.1X1-	T48.1X2-	T48.1X3-	T48.1X4-	T48.1X5-	T48.1X6-
Suxethonium (chloride)	T48.1X1-	T48.1X2-	T48.1X3-	T48.1X4-	T48.1X5-	T48.1X6-
Suxibuzone	T39.2X1-	T39.2X2-	T39.2X3-	T39.2X4-	T39.2X5-	T39.2X6-
Sweet niter spirit	T46.3X1-	T46.3X2-	T46.3X3-	T46.3X4-	T46.3X5-	T46.3X6-
Sweet oil (birch)	T49.3X1-	T49.3X2-	T49.3X3-	T49.3X4-	T49.3X5-	T49.3X6-
Sweetener	T50.901-	T50.902-	T50.903-	T50.904-	T50.905-	T50.906-
Sym-dichloroethyl ether	T53.6X1-	T53.6X2-	T53.6X3-	T53.6X4-	-	-
Sympatholytic NEC	T44.8X1-	T44.8X2-	T44.8X3-	T44.8X4-	T44.8X5-	T44.8X6-
haloalkylamine	T44.8X1-	T44.8X2-	T44.8X3-	T44.8X4-	T44.8X5-	T44.8X6-
Sympathomimetic NEC	T44.901-	T44.902-	T44.903-	T44.904-	T44.905-	T44.906-
anti-common-cold	T48.5X1-	T48.5X2-	T48.5X3-	T48.5X4-	T48.5X5-	T48.5X6-
bronchodilator	T48.6X1-	T48.6X2-	T48.6X3-	T48.6X4-	T48.6X5-	T48.6X6-
specified NEC	T44.991-	T44.992-	T44.993-	T44.994-	T44.995-	T44.996-
Synagis	T50.B91-	T50.B92-	T50.B93-	T50.B94-	T50.B95-	T50.B96-
Synalar	T49.0X1-	T49.0X2-	T49.0X3-	T49.0X4-	T49.0X5-	T49.0X6-
Synthetic cannabinoids	T40.721-	T40.722-	T40.723-	T40.724-	T40.725-	T40.726-
Synthroid	T38.1X1-	T38.1X2-	T38.1X3-	T38.1X4-	T38.1X5-	T38.1X6-
Syntocinon	T48.0X1-	T48.0X2-	T48.0X3-	T48.0X4-	T48.0X5-	T48.0X6-
Syrosingopine	T46.5X1-	T46.5X2-	T46.5X3-	T46.5X4-	T46.5X5-	T46.5X6-
Systemic drug	T45.91X-	T45.92X-	T45.93X-	T45.94X-	T45.95X-	T45.96X-
specified NEC	T45.8X1-	T45.8X2-	T45.8X3-	T45.8X4-	T45.8X5-	T45.8X6-
2,4,5-T	T60.3X1-	T60.3X2-	T60.3X3-	T60.3X4-	-	-
Tablets — *see also specified substance*	T50.901-	T50.902-	T50.903-	T50.904-	T50.905-	T50.906-
Tace	T38.5X1-	T38.5X2-	T38.5X3-	T38.5X4-	T38.5X5-	T38.5X6-
Tacrine	T44.0X1-	T44.0X2-	T44.0X3-	T44.0X4-	T44.0X5-	T44.0X6-
Tadalafil	T46.7X1-	T46.7X2-	T46.7X3-	T46.7X4-	T46.7X5-	T46.7X6-
Talampicillin	T36.0X1-	T36.0X2-	T36.0X3-	T36.0X4-	T36.0X5-	T36.0X6-
Talbutal	T42.3X1-	T42.3X2-	T42.3X3-	T42.3X4-	T42.3X5-	T42.3X6-
Talc powder	T49.3X1-	T49.3X2-	T49.3X3-	T49.3X4-	T49.3X5-	T49.3X6-
Talcum	T49.3X1-	T49.3X2-	T49.3X3-	T49.3X4-	T49.3X5-	T49.3X6-
Taleranol	T38.6X1-	T38.6X2-	T38.6X3-	T38.6X4-	T38.6X5-	T38.6X6-
Tamoxifen	T38.6X1-	T38.6X2-	T38.6X3-	T38.6X4-	T38.6X5-	T38.6X6-
Tamsulosin	T44.6X1-	T44.6X2-	T44.6X3-	T44.6X4-	T44.6X5-	T44.6X6-
Tandearil, tanderil	T39.2X1-	T39.2X2-	T39.2X3-	T39.2X4-	T39.2X5-	T39.2X6-
Tannic acid	T49.2X1-	T49.2X2-	T49.2X3-	T49.2X4-	T49.2X5-	T49.2X6-
medicinal (astringent)	T49.2X1-	T49.2X2-	T49.2X3-	T49.2X4-	T49.2X5-	T49.2X6-
Tannin — *see Tannic acid*						
Tansy	T62.2X1-	T62.2X2-	T62.2X3-	T62.2X4-	-	-
TAO	T36.3X1-	T36.3X2-	T36.3X3-	T36.3X4-	T36.3X5-	T36.3X6-
Tapazole	T38.2X1-	T38.2X2-	T38.2X3-	T38.2X4-	T38.2X5-	T38.2X6-
Tar NEC	T52.0X1-	T52.0X2-	T52.0X3-	T52.0X4-	-	-
camphor	T60.1X1-	T60.1X2-	T60.1X3-	T60.1X4-	-	-
distillate	T49.1X1-	T49.1X2-	T49.1X3-	T49.1X4-	T49.1X5-	T49.1X6-
fumes	T59.891-	T59.892-	T59.893-	T59.894-	-	-
medicinal	T49.1X1-	T49.1X2-	T49.1X3-	T49.1X4-	T49.1X5-	T49.1X6-
ointment	T49.1X1-	T49.1X2-	T49.1X3-	T49.1X4-	T49.1X5-	T49.1X6-
Taractan	T43.591-	T43.592-	T43.593-	T43.594-	T43.595-	T43.596-
Tarantula (venomous)	T63.321-	T63.322-	T63.323-	T63.324-	-	-
Tartar emetic	T37.8X1-	T37.8X2-	T37.8X3-	T37.8X4-	T37.8X5-	T37.8X6-
Tartaric acid	T65.891-	T65.892-	T65.893-	T65.894-	-	-

Substance	Poisoning Accidental (unintentional)	Poisoning Intentional self-harm	Poisoning Assault	Poisoning Undetermined	Adverse effect	Underdosing
Tartrate, laxative	T47.4X1-	T47.4X2-	T47.4X3-	T47.4X4-	T47.4X5-	T47.4X6-
Tartrated antimony (anti-infective)	T37.8X1-	T37.8X2-	T37.8X3-	T37.8X4-	T37.8X5-	T37.8X6-
Tauromustine	T45.1X1-	T45.1X2-	T45.1X3-	T45.1X4-	T45.1X5-	T45.1X6-
TCA — *see Trichloroacetic acid*						
TCDD	T53.7X1-	T53.7X2-	T53.7X3-	T53.7X4-	-	-
TDI (vapor)	T65.0X1-	T65.0X2-	T65.0X3-	T65.0X4-	-	-
Tear						
gas	T59.3X1-	T59.3X2-	T59.3X3-	T59.3X4-	-	-
solution	T49.5X1-	T49.5X2-	T49.5X3-	T49.5X4-	T49.5X5-	T49.5X6-
Teclothiazide	T50.2X1-	T50.2X2-	T50.2X3-	T50.2X4-	T50.2X5-	T50.2X6-
Teclozan	T37.3X1-	T37.3X2-	T37.3X3-	T37.3X4-	T37.3X5-	T37.3X6-
Tegafur	T45.1X1-	T45.1X2-	T45.1X3-	T45.1X4-	T45.1X5-	T45.1X6-
Tegretol	T42.1X1-	T42.1X2-	T42.1X3-	T42.1X4-	T42.1X5-	T42.1X6-
Teicoplanin	T36.8X1-	T36.8X2-	T36.8X3-	T36.8X4-	T36.8X5-	T36.8X6-
Telepaque	T50.8X1-	T50.8X2-	T50.8X3-	T50.8X4-	T50.8X5-	T50.8X6-
Tellurium	T56.891-	T56.892-	T56.893-	T56.894-	-	-
fumes	T56.891-	T56.892-	T56.893-	T56.894-	-	-
TEM	T45.1X1-	T45.1X2-	T45.1X3-	T45.1X4-	T45.1X5-	T45.1X6-
Temazepam	T42.4X1-	T42.4X2-	T42.4X3-	T42.4X4-	T42.4X5-	T42.4X6-
Temocillin	T36.0X1-	T36.0X2-	T36.0X3-	T36.0X4-	T36.0X5-	T36.0X6-
Tenamfetamine	T43.621-	T43.622-	T43.623-	T43.624-	T43.625-	T43.626-
Teniposide	T45.1X1-	T45.1X2-	T45.1X3-	T45.1X4-	T45.1X5-	T45.1X6-
Tenitramine	T46.3X1-	T46.3X2-	T46.3X3-	T46.3X4-	T46.3X5-	T46.3X6-
Tenoglicin	T48.4X1-	T48.4X2-	T48.4X3-	T48.4X4-	T48.4X5-	T48.4X6-
Tenonitrozole	T37.3X1-	T37.3X2-	T37.3X3-	T37.3X4-	T37.3X5-	T37.3X6-
Tenoxicam	T39.391-	T39.392-	T39.393-	T39.394-	T39.395-	T39.396-
TEPA	T45.1X1-	T45.1X2-	T45.1X3-	T45.1X4-	T45.1X5-	T45.1X6-
TEPP	T60.0X1-	T60.0X2-	T60.0X3-	T60.0X4-	-	-
Teprotide	T46.5X1-	T46.5X2-	T46.5X3-	T46.5X4-	T46.5X5-	T46.5X6-
Terazosin	T44.6X1-	T44.6X2-	T44.6X3-	T44.6X4-	T44.6X5-	T44.6X6-
Terbufos	T60.0X1-	T60.0X2-	T60.0X3-	T60.0X4-	-	-
Terbutaline	T48.6X1-	T48.6X2-	T48.6X3-	T48.6X4-	T48.6X5-	T48.6X6-
Terconazole	T49.0X1-	T49.0X2-	T49.0X3-	T49.0X4-	T49.0X5-	T49.0X6-
Terfenadine	T45.0X1-	T45.0X2-	T45.0X3-	T45.0X4-	T45.0X5-	T45.0X6-
Teriparatide (acetate)	T50.991-	T50.992-	T50.993-	T50.994-	T50.995-	T50.996-
Terizidone	T37.1X1-	T37.1X2-	T37.1X3-	T37.1X4-	T37.1X5-	T37.1X6-
Terlipressin	T38.891-	T38.892-	T38.893-	T38.894-	T38.895-	T38.896-
Terodiline	T46.3X1-	T46.3X2-	T46.3X3-	T46.3X4-	T46.3X5-	T46.3X6-
Teroxalene	T37.4X1-	T37.4X2-	T37.4X3-	T37.4X4-	T37.4X5-	T37.4X6-
Terpin (cis) hydrate	T48.4X1-	T48.4X2-	T48.4X3-	T48.4X4-	T48.4X5-	T48.4X6-
Terramycin	T36.4X1-	T36.4X2-	T36.4X3-	T36.4X4-	T36.4X5-	T36.4X6-
Tertatolol	T44.7X1-	T44.7X2-	T44.7X3-	T44.7X4-	T44.7X5-	T44.7X6-
Tessalon	T48.3X1-	T48.3X2-	T48.3X3-	T48.3X4-	T48.3X5-	T48.3X6-
Testolactone	T38.7X1-	T38.7X2-	T38.7X3-	T38.7X4-	T38.7X5-	T38.7X6-
Testosterone	T38.7X1-	T38.7X2-	T38.7X3-	T38.7X4-	T38.7X5-	T38.7X6-
Tetanus toxoid or vaccine	T50.A91-	T50.A92-	T50.A93-	T50.A94-	T50.A95-	T50.A96-
antitoxin	T50.Z11-	T50.Z12-	T50.Z13-	T50.Z14-	T50.Z15-	T50.Z16-
immune globulin (human)	T50.Z11-	T50.Z12-	T50.Z13-	T50.Z14-	T50.Z15-	T50.Z16-
toxoid	T50.A91-	T50.A92-	T50.A93-	T50.A94-	T50.A95-	T50.A96-
with diphtheria toxoid	T50.A21-	T50.A22-	T50.A23-	T50.A24-	T50.A25-	T50.A26-
with pertussis	T50.A11-	T50.A12-	T50.A13-	T50.A14-	T50.A15-	T50.A16-
Tetrabenazine	T43.591-	T43.592-	T43.593-	T43.594-	T43.595-	T43.596-
Tetracaine	T41.3X1-	T41.3X2-	T41.3X3-	T41.3X4-	T41.3X5-	T41.3X6-
nerve block (peripheral) (plexus)	T41.3X1-	T41.3X2-	T41.3X3-	T41.3X4-	T41.3X5-	T41.3X6-
regional	T41.3X1-	T41.3X2-	T41.3X3-	T41.3X4-	T41.3X5-	T41.3X6-
spinal	T41.3X1-	T41.3X2-	T41.3X3-	T41.3X4-	T41.3X5-	T41.3X6-
Tetrachlorethylene — *see Tetrachloroethylene*						
Tetrachlormethiazide	T50.2X1-	T50.2X2-	T50.2X3-	T50.2X4-	T50.2X5-	T50.2X6-

Substance	Poisoning Accidental (unintentional)	Poisoning Intentional self-harm	Poisoning Assault	Poisoning Undetermined	Adverse effect	Underdosing
2,3,7,8-Tetrachlorodibenzo-p-dioxin	T53.7X1-	T53.7X2-	T53.7X3-	T53.7X4-	-	-
Tetrachloroethane	T53.6X1-	T53.6X2-	T53.6X3-	T53.6X4-	-	-
vapor	T53.6X1-	T53.6X2-	T53.6X3-	T53.6X4-	-	-
paint or varnish	T53.6X1-	T53.6X2-	T53.6X3-	T53.6X4-	-	-
Tetrachloroethylene (liquid)	T53.3X1-	T53.3X2-	T53.3X3-	T53.3X4-	-	-
medicinal	T37.4X1-	T37.4X2-	T37.4X3-	T37.4X4-	T37.4X5-	T37.4X6-
vapor	T53.3X1-	T53.3X2-	T53.3X3-	T53.3X4-	-	-
Tetrachloromethane — *see Carbon tetrachloride*						
Tetracosactide	T38.811-	T38.812-	T38.813-	T38.814-	T38.815-	T38.816-
Tetracosactrin	T38.811-	T38.812-	T38.813-	T38.814-	T38.815-	T38.816-
Tetracycline	T36.4X1-	T36.4X2-	T36.4X3-	T36.4X4-	T36.4X5-	T36.4X6-
ophthalmic preparation	T49.5X1-	T49.5X2-	T49.5X3-	T49.5X4-	T49.5X5-	T49.5X6-
topical NEC	T49.0X1-	T49.0X2-	T49.0X3-	T49.0X4-	T49.0X5-	T49.0X6-
Tetradifon	T60.8X1-	T60.8X2-	T60.8X3-	T60.8X4-	-	-
Tetradotoxin	T61.771-	T61.772-	T61.773-	T61.774-	-	-
Tetraethyl						
lead	T56.0X1-	T56.0X2-	T56.0X3-	T56.0X4-	-	-
pyrophosphate	T60.0X1-	T60.0X2-	T60.0X3-	T60.0X4-	-	-
Tetraethylammonium chloride	T44.2X1-	T44.2X2-	T44.2X3-	T44.2X4-	T44.2X5-	T44.2X6-
Tetraethylthiuram disulfide	T50.6X1-	T50.6X2-	T50.6X3-	T50.6X4-	T50.6X5-	T50.6X6-
Tetrahydroaminoacridine	T44.0X1-	T44.0X2-	T44.0X3-	T44.0X4-	T44.0X5-	T44.0X6-
Tetrahydrocannabinol	T40.711-	T40.712-	T40.713-	T40.714-	T40.715-	T40.716-
Tetrahydrofuran	T52.8X1-	T52.8X2-	T52.8X3-	T52.8X4-	-	-
Tetrahydronaphthalene	T52.8X1-	T52.8X2-	T52.8X3-	T52.8X4-	-	-
Tetrahydrozoline	T49.5X1-	T49.5X2-	T49.5X3-	T49.5X4-	T49.5X5-	T49.5X6-
Tetralin	T52.8X1-	T52.8X2-	T52.8X3-	T52.8X4-	-	-
Tetramethrin	T60.2X1-	T60.2X2-	T60.2X3-	T60.2X4-	-	-
Tetramethylthiuram (disulfide) NEC	T60.3X1-	T60.3X2-	T60.3X3-	T60.3X4-	-	-
medicinal	T49.0X1-	T49.0X2-	T49.0X3-	T49.0X4-	T49.0X5-	T49.0X6-
Tetramisole	T37.4X1-	T37.4X2-	T37.4X3-	T37.4X4-	T37.4X5-	T37.4X6-
Tetranicotinoyl fructose	T46.7X1-	T46.7X2-	T46.7X3-	T46.7X4-	T46.7X5-	T46.7X6-
Tetrazepam	T42.4X1-	T42.4X2-	T42.4X3-	T42.4X4-	T42.4X5-	T42.4X6-
Tetronal	T42.6X1-	T42.6X2-	T42.6X3-	T42.6X4-	T42.6X5-	T42.6X6-
Tetryl	T65.3X1-	T65.3X2-	T65.3X3-	T65.3X4-	-	-
Tetrylammonium chloride	T44.2X1-	T44.2X2-	T44.2X3-	T44.2X4-	T44.2X5-	T44.2X6-
Tetryzoline	T49.5X1-	T49.5X2-	T49.5X3-	T49.5X4-	T49.5X5-	T49.5X6-
Thalidomide	T45.1X1-	T45.1X2-	T45.1X3-	T45.1X4-	T45.1X5-	T45.1X6-
Thallium (compounds) (dust) NEC	T56.811-	T56.812-	T56.813-	T56.814-	-	-
pesticide	T60.4X1-	T60.4X2-	T60.4X3-	T60.4X4-	-	-
THC	T40.711-	T40.712-	T40.713-	T40.714-	T40.715-	T40.716-
Thebacon	T48.3X1-	T48.3X2-	T48.3X3-	T48.3X4-	T48.3X5-	T48.3X6-
Thebaine	T40.2X1-	T40.2X2-	T40.2X3-	T40.2X4-	T40.2X5-	T40.2X6-
Thenoic acid	T49.6X1-	T49.6X2-	T49.6X3-	T49.6X4-	T49.6X5-	T49.6X6-
Thenyldiamine	T45.0X1-	T45.0X2-	T45.0X3-	T45.0X4-	T45.0X5-	T45.0X6-
Theobromine (calcium salicylate)	T48.6X1-	T48.6X2-	T48.6X3-	T48.6X4-	T48.6X5-	T48.6X6-
sodium salicylate	T48.6X1-	T48.6X2-	T48.6X3-	T48.6X4-	T48.6X5-	T48.6X6-
Theophyllamine	T48.6X1-	T48.6X2-	T48.6X3-	T48.6X4-	T48.6X5-	T48.6X6-
Theophylline	T48.6X1-	T48.6X2-	T48.6X3-	T48.6X4-	T48.6X5-	T48.6X6-
aminobenzoic acid	T48.6X1-	T48.6X2-	T48.6X3-	T48.6X4-	T48.6X5-	T48.6X6-
ethylenediamine	T48.6X1-	T48.6X2-	T48.6X3-	T48.6X4-	T48.6X5-	T48.6X6-
piperazine p-amino-benzoate	T48.6X1-	T48.6X2-	T48.6X3-	T48.6X4-	T48.6X5-	T48.6X6-
Thiabendazole	T37.4X1-	T37.4X2-	T37.4X3-	T37.4X4-	T37.4X5-	T37.4X6-
Thialbarbital	T41.1X1-	T41.1X2-	T41.1X3-	T41.1X4-	T41.1X5-	T41.1X6-
Thiamazole	T38.2X1-	T38.2X2-	T38.2X3-	T38.2X4-	T38.2X5-	T38.2X6-
Thiambutosine	T37.1X1-	T37.1X2-	T37.1X3-	T37.1X4-	T37.1X5-	T37.1X6-
Thiamine	T45.2X1-	T45.2X2-	T45.2X3-	T45.2X4-	T45.2X5-	T45.2X6-
Thiamphenicol	T36.2X1-	T36.2X2-	T36.2X3-	T36.2X4-	T36.2X5-	T36.2X6-

Substance	Poisoning Accidental (unintentional)	Poisoning Intentional self-harm	Poisoning Assault	Poisoning Undetermined	Adverse effect	Underdosing
Thiamylal	T41.1X1-	T41.1X2-	T41.1X3-	T41.1X4-	T41.1X5-	T41.1X6-
sodium	T41.1X1-	T41.1X2-	T41.1X3-	T41.1X4-	T41.1X5-	T41.1X6-
Thiazesim	T43.291-	T43.292-	T43.293-	T43.294-	T43.295-	T43.296-
Thiazides (diuretics)	T50.2X1-	T50.2X2-	T50.2X3-	T50.2X4-	T50.2X5-	T50.2X6-
Thiazinamium metilsulfate	T43.3X1-	T43.3X2-	T43.3X3-	T43.3X4-	T43.3X5-	T43.3X6-
Thiethylperazine	T43.3X1-	T43.3X2-	T43.3X3-	T43.3X4-	T43.3X5-	T43.3X6-
Thimerosal	T49.0X1-	T49.0X2-	T49.0X3-	T49.0X4-	T49.0X5-	T49.0X6-
ophthalmic preparation	T49.5X1-	T49.5X2-	T49.5X3-	T49.5X4-	T49.5X5-	T49.5X6-
Thioacetazone	T37.1X1-	T37.1X2-	T37.1X3-	T37.1X4-	T37.1X5-	T37.1X6-
with isoniazid	T37.1X1-	T37.1X2-	T37.1X3-	T37.1X4-	T37.1X5-	T37.1X6-
Thiobarbital sodium	T41.1X1-	T41.1X2-	T41.1X3-	T41.1X4-	T41.1X5-	T41.1X6-
Thiobarbiturate anesthetic	T41.1X1-	T41.1X2-	T41.1X3-	T41.1X4-	T41.1X5-	T41.1X6-
Thiobismol	T37.8X1-	T37.8X2-	T37.8X3-	T37.8X4-	T37.8X5-	T37.8X6-
Thiobutabarbital sodium	T41.1X1-	T41.1X2-	T41.1X3-	T41.1X4-	T41.1X5-	T41.1X6-
Thiocarbamate (insecticide)	T60.0X1-	T60.0X2-	T60.0X3-	T60.0X4-	-	-
Thiocarbamide	T38.2X1-	T38.2X2-	T38.2X3-	T38.2X4-	T38.2X5-	T38.2X6-
Thiocarbarsone	T37.8X1-	T37.8X2-	T37.8X3-	T37.8X4-	T37.8X5-	T37.8X6-
Thiocarlide	T37.1X1-	T37.1X2-	T37.1X3-	T37.1X4-	T37.1X5-	T37.1X6-
Thioctamide	T50.991-	T50.992-	T50.993-	T50.994-	T50.995-	T50.996-
Thioctic acid	T50.991-	T50.992-	T50.993-	T50.994-	T50.995-	T50.996-
Thiofos	T60.0X1-	T60.0X2-	T60.0X3-	T60.0X4-	-	-
Thioglycolate	T49.4X1-	T49.4X2-	T49.4X3-	T49.4X4-	T49.4X5-	T49.4X6-
Thioglycolic acid	T65.891-	T65.892-	T65.893-	T65.894-	-	-
Thioguanine	T45.1X1-	T45.1X2-	T45.1X3-	T45.1X4-	T45.1X5-	T45.1X6-
Thiomercaptomerin	T50.2X1-	T50.2X2-	T50.2X3-	T50.2X4-	T50.2X5-	T50.2X6-
Thiomerin	T50.2X1-	T50.2X2-	T50.2X3-	T50.2X4-	T50.2X5-	T50.2X6-
Thiomersal	T49.0X1-	T49.0X2-	T49.0X3-	T49.0X4-	T49.0X5-	T49.0X6-
Thionazin	T60.0X1-	T60.0X2-	T60.0X3-	T60.0X4-	-	-
Thiopental (sodium)	T41.1X1-	T41.1X2-	T41.1X3-	T41.1X4-	T41.1X5-	T41.1X6-
Thiopentone (sodium)	T41.1X1-	T41.1X2-	T41.1X3-	T41.1X4-	T41.1X5-	T41.1X6-
Thiopropazate	T43.3X1-	T43.3X2-	T43.3X3-	T43.3X4-	T43.3X5-	T43.3X6-
Thioproperazine	T43.3X1-	T43.3X2-	T43.3X3-	T43.3X4-	T43.3X5-	T43.3X6-
Thioridazine	T43.3X1-	T43.3X2-	T43.3X3-	T43.3X4-	T43.3X5-	T43.3X6-
Thiosinamine	T49.3X1-	T49.3X2-	T49.3X3-	T49.3X4-	T49.3X5-	T49.3X6-
Thiotepa	T45.1X1-	T45.1X2-	T45.1X3-	T45.1X4-	T45.1X5-	T45.1X6-
Thiothixene	T43.4X1-	T43.4X2-	T43.4X3-	T43.4X4-	T43.4X5-	T43.4X6-
Thiouracil (benzyl) (methyl) (propyl)	T38.2X1-	T38.2X2-	T38.2X3-	T38.2X4-	T38.2X5-	T38.2X6-
Thiourea	T38.2X1-	T38.2X2-	T38.2X3-	T38.2X4-	T38.2X5-	T38.2X6-
Thiphenamil	T44.3X1-	T44.3X2-	T44.3X3-	T44.3X4-	T44.3X5-	T44.3X6-
Thiram	T60.3X1-	T60.3X2-	T60.3X3-	T60.3X4-	-	-
medicinal	T49.2X1-	T49.2X2-	T49.2X3-	T49.2X4-	T49.2X5-	T49.2X6-
Thonzylamine (systemic)	T45.0X1-	T45.0X2-	T45.0X3-	T45.0X4-	T45.0X5-	T45.0X6-
mucosal decongestant	T48.5X1-	T48.5X2-	T48.5X3-	T48.5X4-	T48.5X5-	T48.5X6-
Thorazine	T43.3X1-	T43.3X2-	T43.3X3-	T43.3X4-	T43.3X5-	T43.3X6-
Thorium dioxide suspension	T50.8X1-	T50.8X2-	T50.8X3-	T50.8X4-	T50.8X5-	T50.8X6-
Thornapple	T62.2X1-	T62.2X2-	T62.2X3-	T62.2X4-	-	-
Throat drug NEC	T49.6X1-	T49.6X2-	T49.6X3-	T49.6X4-	T49.6X5-	T49.6X6-
Thrombin	T45.7X1-	T45.7X2-	T45.7X3-	T45.7X4-	T45.7X5-	T45.7X6-
Thrombolysin	T45.611-	T45.612-	T45.613-	T45.614-	T45.615-	T45.616-
Thromboplastin	T45.7X1-	T45.7X2-	T45.7X3-	T45.7X4-	T45.7X5-	T45.7X6-
Thurfyl nicotinate	T46.7X1-	T46.7X2-	T46.7X3-	T46.7X4-	T46.7X5-	T46.7X6-
Thymol	T49.0X1-	T49.0X2-	T49.0X3-	T49.0X4-	T49.0X5-	T49.0X6-
Thymopentin	T37.5X1-	T37.5X2-	T37.5X3-	T37.5X4-	T37.5X5-	T37.5X6-
Thymoxamine	T46.7X1-	T46.7X2-	T46.7X3-	T46.7X4-	T46.7X5-	T46.7X6-
Thymus extract	T38.891-	T38.892-	T38.893-	T38.894-	T38.895-	T38.896-
Thyreotrophic hormone	T38.811-	T38.812-	T38.813-	T38.814-	T38.815-	T38.816-
Thyroglobulin	T38.1X1-	T38.1X2-	T38.1X3-	T38.1X4-	T38.1X5-	T38.1X6-
Thyroid (hormone)	T38.1X1-	T38.1X2-	T38.1X3-	T38.1X4-	T38.1X5-	T38.1X6-

Substance	Poisoning Accidental (unintentional)	Poisoning Intentional self-harm	Poisoning Assault	Poisoning Undetermined	Adverse effect	Underdosing
Thyrolar	T38.1X1-	T38.1X2-	T38.1X3-	T38.1X4-	T38.1X5-	T38.1X6-
Thyrotrophin	T38.811-	T38.812-	T38.813-	T38.814-	T38.815-	T38.816-
Thyrotropic hormone	T38.811-	T38.812-	T38.813-	T38.814-	T38.815-	T38.816-
Thyroxine	T38.1X1-	T38.1X2-	T38.1X3-	T38.1X4-	T38.1X5-	T38.1X6-
Tiabendazole	T37.4X1-	T37.4X2-	T37.4X3-	T37.4X4-	T37.4X5-	T37.4X6-
Tiamizide	T50.2X1-	T50.2X2-	T50.2X3-	T50.2X4-	T50.2X5-	T50.2X6-
Tianeptine	T43.291-	T43.292-	T43.293-	T43.294-	T43.295-	T43.296-
Tiapamil	T46.1X1-	T46.1X2-	T46.1X3-	T46.1X4-	T46.1X5-	T46.1X6-
Tiapride	T43.591-	T43.592-	T43.593-	T43.594-	T43.595-	T43.596-
Tiaprofenic acid	T39.311-	T39.312-	T39.313-	T39.314-	T39.315-	T39.316-
Tiaramide	T39.8X1-	T39.8X2-	T39.8X3-	T39.8X4-	T39.8X5-	T39.8X6-
Ticarcillin	T36.0X1-	T36.0X2-	T36.0X3-	T36.0X4-	T36.0X5-	T36.0X6-
Ticlatone	T49.0X1-	T49.0X2-	T49.0X3-	T49.0X4-	T49.0X5-	T49.0X6-
Ticlopidine	T45.521-	T45.522-	T45.523-	T45.524-	T45.525-	T45.526-
Ticrynafen	T50.1X1-	T50.1X2-	T50.1X3-	T50.1X4-	T50.1X5-	T50.1X6-
Tidiacic	T50.991-	T50.992-	T50.993-	T50.994-	T50.995-	T50.996-
Tiemonium	T44.3X1-	T44.3X2-	T44.3X3-	T44.3X4-	T44.3X5-	T44.3X6-
iodide	T44.3X1-	T44.3X2-	T44.3X3-	T44.3X4-	T44.3X5-	T44.3X6-
Tienilic acid	T50.1X1-	T50.1X2-	T50.1X3-	T50.1X4-	T50.1X5-	T50.1X6-
Tifenamil	T44.3X1-	T44.3X2-	T44.3X3-	T44.3X4-	T44.3X5-	T44.3X6-
Tigan	T45.0X1-	T45.0X2-	T45.0X3-	T45.0X4-	T45.0X5-	T45.0X6-
Tigloidine	T44.3X1-	T44.3X2-	T44.3X3-	T44.3X4-	T44.3X5-	T44.3X6-
Tilactase	T47.5X1-	T47.5X2-	T47.5X3-	T47.5X4-	T47.5X5-	T47.5X6-
Tiletamine	T41.291-	T41.292-	T41.293-	T41.294-	T41.295-	T41.296-
Tilidine	T40.491-	T40.492-	T40.493-	T40.494-	-	-
Timepidium bromide	T44.3X1-	T44.3X2-	T44.3X3-	T44.3X4-	T44.3X5-	T44.3X6-
Timiperone	T43.4X1-	T43.4X2-	T43.4X3-	T43.4X4-	T43.4X5-	T43.4X6-
Timolol	T44.7X1-	T44.7X2-	T44.7X3-	T44.7X4-	T44.7X5-	T44.7X6-
Tin (chloride) (dust) (oxide) NEC	T56.6X1-	T56.6X2-	T56.6X3-	T56.6X4-	-	-
anti-infectives	T37.8X1-	T37.8X2-	T37.8X3-	T37.8X4-	T37.8X5-	T37.8X6-
Tincture, iodine — *see Iodine*						
Tindal	T43.3X1-	T43.3X2-	T43.3X3-	T43.3X4-	T43.3X5-	T43.3X6-
Tinidazole	T37.3X1-	T37.3X2-	T37.3X3-	T37.3X4-	T37.3X5-	T37.3X6-
Tinoridine	T39.8X1-	T39.8X2-	T39.8X3-	T39.8X4-	T39.8X5-	T39.8X6-
Tiocarlide	T37.1X1-	T37.1X2-	T37.1X3-	T37.1X4-	T37.1X5-	T37.1X6-
Tioclomarol	T45.511-	T45.512-	T45.513-	T45.514-	T45.515-	T45.516-
Tioconazole	T49.0X1-	T49.0X2-	T49.0X3-	T49.0X4-	T49.0X5-	T49.0X6-
Tioguanine	T45.1X1-	T45.1X2-	T45.1X3-	T45.1X4-	T45.1X5-	T45.1X6-
Tiopronin	T50.991-	T50.992-	T50.993-	T50.994-	T50.995-	T50.996-
Tiotixene	T43.4X1-	T43.4X2-	T43.4X3-	T43.4X4-	T43.4X5-	T43.4X6-
Tioxolone	T49.4X1-	T49.4X2-	T49.4X3-	T49.4X4-	T49.4X5-	T49.4X6-
Tipepidine	T48.3X1-	T48.3X2-	T48.3X3-	T48.3X4-	T48.3X5-	T48.3X6-
Tiquizium bromide	T44.3X1-	T44.3X2-	T44.3X3-	T44.3X4-	T44.3X5-	T44.3X6-
Tiratricol	T38.1X1-	T38.1X2-	T38.1X3-	T38.1X4-	T38.1X5-	T38.1X6-
Tisopurine	T50.4X1-	T50.4X2-	T50.4X3-	T50.4X4-	T50.4X5-	T50.4X6-
Titanium (compounds) (vapor)	T56.891-	T56.892-	T56.893-	T56.894-	-	-
dioxide	T49.3X1-	T49.3X2-	T49.3X3-	T49.3X4-	T49.3X5-	T49.3X6-
ointment	T49.3X1-	T49.3X2-	T49.3X3-	T49.3X4-	T49.3X5-	T49.3X6-
oxide	T49.3X1-	T49.3X2-	T49.3X3-	T49.3X4-	T49.3X5-	T49.3X6-
tetrachloride	T56.891-	T56.892-	T56.893-	T56.894-	-	-
Titanocene	T56.891-	T56.892-	T56.893-	T56.894-	-	-
Titroid	T38.1X1-	T38.1X2-	T38.1X3-	T38.1X4-	T38.1X5-	T38.1X6-
Tizanidine	T42.8X1-	T42.8X2-	T42.8X3-	T42.8X4-	T42.8X5-	T42.8X6-
TMTD	T60.3X1-	T60.3X2-	T60.3X3-	T60.3X4-	-	-
TNT (fumes)	T65.3X1-	T65.3X2-	T65.3X3-	T65.3X4-	-	-
Toadstool	T62.0X1-	T62.0X2-	T62.0X3-	T62.0X4-	-	-
Tobacco NEC	T65.291-	T65.292-	T65.293-	T65.294-	-	-
cigarettes	T65.221-	T65.222-	T65.223-	T65.224-	-	-
Indian	T62.2X1-	T62.2X2-	T62.2X3-	T62.2X4-	-	-

Substance	Poisoning Accidental (unintentional)	Poisoning Intentional self-harm	Poisoning Assault	Poisoning Undetermined	Adverse effect	Underdosing
Tobacco NEC (continued)						
smoke, second-hand	T65.221-	T65.222-	T65.223-	T65.224-	-	-
Tobramycin	T36.5X1-	T36.5X2-	T36.5X3-	T36.5X4-	T36.5X5-	T36.5X6-
Tocainide	T46.2X1-	T46.2X2-	T46.2X3-	T46.2X4-	T46.2X5-	T46.2X6-
Tocoferol	T45.2X1-	T45.2X2-	T45.2X3-	T45.2X4-	T45.2X5-	T45.2X6-
Tocopherol	T45.2X1-	T45.2X2-	T45.2X3-	T45.2X4-	T45.2X5-	T45.2X6-
acetate	T45.2X1-	T45.2X2-	T45.2X3-	T45.2X4-	T45.2X5-	T45.2X6-
Tocosamine	T48.0X1-	T48.0X2-	T48.0X3-	T48.0X4-	T48.0X5-	T48.0X6-
Todralazine	T46.5X1-	T46.5X2-	T46.5X3-	T46.5X4-	T46.5X5-	T46.5X6-
Tofisopam	T42.4X1-	T42.4X2-	T42.4X3-	T42.4X4-	T42.4X5-	T42.4X6-
Tofranil	T43.011-	T43.012-	T43.013-	T43.014-	T43.015-	T43.016-
Toilet deodorizer	T65.891-	T65.892-	T65.893-	T65.894-	-	-
Tolamolol	T44.7X1-	T44.7X2-	T44.7X3-	T44.7X4-	T44.7X5-	T44.7X6-
Tolazamide	T38.3X1-	T38.3X2-	T38.3X3-	T38.3X4-	T38.3X5-	T38.3X6-
Tolazoline	T46.7X1-	T46.7X2-	T46.7X3-	T46.7X4-	T46.7X5-	T46.7X6-
Tolbutamide (sodium)	T38.3X1-	T38.3X2-	T38.3X3-	T38.3X4-	T38.3X5-	T38.3X6-
Tolciclate	T49.0X1-	T49.0X2-	T49.0X3-	T49.0X4-	T49.0X5-	T49.0X6-
Tolmetin	T39.391-	T39.392-	T39.393-	T39.394-	T39.395-	T39.396-
Tolnaftate	T49.0X1-	T49.0X2-	T49.0X3-	T49.0X4-	T49.0X5-	T49.0X6-
Tolonidine	T46.5X1-	T46.5X2-	T46.5X3-	T46.5X4-	T46.5X5-	T46.5X6-
Toloxatone	T42.6X1-	T42.6X2-	T42.6X3-	T42.6X4-	T42.6X5-	T42.6X6-
Tolperisone	T44.3X1-	T44.3X2-	T44.3X3-	T44.3X4-	T44.3X5-	T44.3X6-
Tolserol	T42.8X1-	T42.8X2-	T42.8X3-	T42.8X4-	T42.8X5-	T42.8X6-
Toluene (liquid)	T52.2X1-	T52.2X2-	T52.2X3-	T52.2X4-	-	-
diisocyanate	T65.0X1-	T65.0X2-	T65.0X3-	T65.0X4-	-	-
Toluidine	T65.891-	T65.892-	T65.893-	T65.894-	-	-
vapor	T59.891-	T59.892-	T59.893-	T59.894-	-	-
Toluol (liquid)	T52.2X1-	T52.2X2-	T52.2X3-	T52.2X4-	-	-
vapor	T52.2X1-	T52.2X2-	T52.2X3-	T52.2X4-	-	-
Toluylenediamine	T65.3X1-	T65.3X2-	T65.3X3-	T65.3X4-	-	-
Tolylene-2,4-diisocyanate	T65.0X1-	T65.0X2-	T65.0X3-	T65.0X4-	-	-
Tonic NEC	T50.901-	T50.902-	T50.903-	T50.904-	T50.905-	T50.906-
Topical action drug NEC	T49.91X-	T49.92X-	T49.93X-	T49.94X-	T49.95X-	T49.96X-
ear, nose or throat	T49.6X1-	T49.6X2-	T49.6X3-	T49.6X4-	T49.6X5-	T49.6X6-
eye	T49.5X1-	T49.5X2-	T49.5X3-	T49.5X4-	T49.5X5-	T49.5X6-
skin	T49.91X-	T49.92X-	T49.93X-	T49.94X-	T49.95X-	T49.96X-
specified NEC	T49.8X1-	T49.8X2-	T49.8X3-	T49.8X4-	T49.8X5-	T49.8X6-
Toquizine	T44.3X1-	T44.3X2-	T44.3X3-	T44.3X4-	T44.3X5-	T44.3X6-
Toremifene	T38.6X1-	T38.6X2-	T38.6X3-	T38.6X4-	T38.6X5-	T38.6X6-
Tosylchloramide sodium	T49.8X1-	T49.8X2-	T49.8X3-	T49.8X4-	T49.8X5-	T49.8X6-
Toxaphene (dust) (spray)	T60.1X1-	T60.1X2-	T60.1X3-	T60.1X4-	-	-
Toxin, diphtheria (Schick Test)	T50.8X1-	T50.8X2-	T50.8X3-	T50.8X4-	T50.8X5-	T50.8X6-
Toxoid						
combined	T50.A21-	T50.A22-	T50.A23-	T50.A24-	T50.A25-	T50.A26-
diphtheria	T50.A91-	T50.A92-	T50.A93-	T50.A94-	T50.A95-	T50.A96-
tetanus	T50.A91-	T50.A92-	T50.A93-	T50.A94-	T50.A95-	T50.A96-
Trace element NEC	T45.8X1-	T45.8X2-	T45.8X3-	T45.8X4-	T45.8X5-	T45.8X6-
Tractor fuel NEC	T52.0X1-	T52.0X2-	T52.0X3-	T52.0X4-	-	-
Tragacanth	T50.991-	T50.992-	T50.993-	T50.994-	T50.995-	T50.996-
Tramadol	T40.421-	T40.422-	T40.423-	T40.424-	T40.425-	T40.426-
Tramazoline	T48.5X1-	T48.5X2-	T48.5X3-	T48.5X4-	T48.5X5-	T48.5X6-
Tranexamic acid	T45.621-	T45.622-	T45.623-	T45.624-	T45.625-	T45.626-
Tranilast	T45.0X1-	T45.0X2-	T45.0X3-	T45.0X4-	T45.0X5-	T45.0X6-
Tranquilizer NEC	T43.501-	T43.502-	T43.503-	T43.504-	T43.505-	T43.506-
with hypnotic or sedative	T42.6X1-	T42.6X2-	T42.6X3-	T42.6X4-	T42.6X5-	T42.6X6-
benzodiazepine NEC	T42.4X1-	T42.4X2-	T42.4X3-	T42.4X4-	T42.4X5-	T42.4X6-
butyrophenone NEC	T43.4X1-	T43.4X2-	T43.4X3-	T43.4X4-	T43.4X5-	T43.4X6-
carbamate	T43.591-	T43.592-	T43.593-	T43.594-	T43.595-	T43.596-

Substance	Poisoning Accidental (unintentional)	Poisoning Intentional self-harm	Poisoning Assault	Poisoning Undetermined	Adverse effect	Underdosing
Tranquilizer NEC (continued)						
dimethylamine	T43.3X1-	T43.3X2-	T43.3X3-	T43.3X4-	T43.3X5-	T43.3X6-
ethylamine	T43.3X1-	T43.3X2-	T43.3X3-	T43.3X4-	T43.3X5-	T43.3X6-
hydroxyzine	T43.591-	T43.592-	T43.593-	T43.594-	T43.595-	T43.596-
major NEC	T43.501-	T43.502-	T43.503-	T43.504-	T43.505-	T43.506-
penothiazine NEC	T43.3X1-	T43.3X2-	T43.3X3-	T43.3X4-	T43.3X5-	T43.3X6-
phenothiazine-based	T43.3X1-	T43.3X2-	T43.3X3-	T43.3X4-	T43.3X5-	T43.3X6-
piperazine NEC	T43.3X1-	T43.3X2-	T43.3X3-	T43.3X4-	T43.3X5-	T43.3X6-
piperidine	T43.3X1-	T43.3X2-	T43.3X3-	T43.3X4-	T43.3X5-	T43.3X6-
propylamine	T43.3X1-	T43.3X2-	T43.3X3-	T43.3X4-	T43.3X5-	T43.3X6-
specified NEC	T43.591-	T43.592-	T43.593-	T43.594-	T43.595-	T43.596-
thioxanthene NEC	T43.591-	T43.592-	T43.593-	T43.594-	T43.595-	T43.596-
Tranxene	T42.4X1-	T42.4X2-	T42.4X3-	T42.4X4-	T42.4X5-	T42.4X6-
Tranylcypromine	T43.1X1-	T43.1X2-	T43.1X3-	T43.1X4-	T43.1X5-	T43.1X6-
Trapidil	T46.3X1-	T46.3X2-	T46.3X3-	T46.3X4-	T46.3X5-	T46.3X6-
Trasentine	T44.3X1-	T44.3X2-	T44.3X3-	T44.3X4-	T44.3X5-	T44.3X6-
Travert	T50.3X1-	T50.3X2-	T50.3X3-	T50.3X4-	T50.3X5-	T50.3X6-
Trazodone	T43.211-	T43.212-	T43.213-	T43.214-	T43.215-	T43.216-
Trecator	T37.1X1-	T37.1X2-	T37.1X3-	T37.1X4-	T37.1X5-	T37.1X6-
Treosulfan	T45.1X1-	T45.1X2-	T45.1X3-	T45.1X4-	T45.1X5-	T45.1X6-
Tretamine	T45.1X1-	T45.1X2-	T45.1X3-	T45.1X4-	T45.1X5-	T45.1X6-
Tretinoin	T49.0X1-	T49.0X2-	T49.0X3-	T49.0X4-	T49.0X5-	T49.0X6-
Tretoquinol	T48.6X1-	T48.6X2-	T48.6X3-	T48.6X4-	T48.6X5-	T48.6X6-
Triacetin	T49.0X1-	T49.0X2-	T49.0X3-	T49.0X4-	T49.0X5-	T49.0X6-
Triacetoxyanthracene	T49.4X1-	T49.4X2-	T49.4X3-	T49.4X4-	T49.4X5-	T49.4X6-
Triacetyloleandomycin	T36.3X1-	T36.3X2-	T36.3X3-	T36.3X4-	T36.3X5-	T36.3X6-
Triamcinolone	T38.0X1-	T38.0X2-	T38.0X3-	T38.0X4-	T38.0X5-	T38.0X6-
ENT agent	T49.6X1-	T49.6X2-	T49.6X3-	T49.6X4-	T49.6X5-	T49.6X6-
hexacetonide	T49.0X1-	T49.0X2-	T49.0X3-	T49.0X4-	T49.0X5-	T49.0X6-
ophthalmic preparation	T49.5X1-	T49.5X2-	T49.5X3-	T49.5X4-	T49.5X5-	T49.5X6-
topical NEC	T49.0X1-	T49.0X2-	T49.0X3-	T49.0X4-	T49.0X5-	T49.0X6-
Triampyzine	T44.3X1-	T44.3X2-	T44.3X3-	T44.3X4-	T44.3X5-	T44.3X6-
Triamterene	T50.2X1-	T50.2X2-	T50.2X3-	T50.2X4-	T50.2X5-	T50.2X6-
Triazine (herbicide)	T60.3X1-	T60.3X2-	T60.3X3-	T60.3X4-	-	-
Triaziquone	T45.1X1-	T45.1X2-	T45.1X3-	T45.1X4-	T45.1X5-	T45.1X6-
Triazolam	T42.4X1-	T42.4X2-	T42.4X3-	T42.4X4-	T42.4X5-	T42.4X6-
Triazole (herbicide)	T60.3X1-	T60.3X2-	T60.3X3-	T60.3X4-	-	-
Tribenoside	T46.991-	T46.992-	T46.993-	T46.994-	T46.995-	T46.996-
Tribromacetaldehyde	T42.6X1-	T42.6X2-	T42.6X3-	T42.6X4-	T42.6X5-	T42.6X6-
Tribromoethanol, rectal	T41.291-	T41.292-	T41.293-	T41.294-	T41.295-	T41.296-
Tribromomethane	T42.6X1-	T42.6X2-	T42.6X3-	T42.6X4-	T42.6X5-	T42.6X6-
Trichlorethane	T53.2X1-	T53.2X2-	T53.2X3-	T53.2X4-	-	-
Trichlorethylene	T53.2X1-	T53.2X2-	T53.2X3-	T53.2X4-	-	-
Trichlorfon	T60.0X1-	T60.0X2-	T60.0X3-	T60.0X4-	-	-
Trichlormethiazide	T50.2X1-	T50.2X2-	T50.2X3-	T50.2X4-	T50.2X5-	T50.2X6-
Trichlormethine	T45.1X1-	T45.1X2-	T45.1X3-	T45.1X4-	T45.1X5-	T45.1X6-
Trichloroacetic acid, Trichloracetic acid	T54.2X1-	T54.2X2-	T54.2X3-	T54.2X4-	-	-
medicinal	T49.4X1-	T49.4X2-	T49.4X3-	T49.4X4-	T49.4X5-	T49.4X6-
Trichloroethane	T53.2X1-	T53.2X2-	T53.2X3-	T53.2X4-	-	-
Trichloroethanol	T42.6X1-	T42.6X2-	T42.6X3-	T42.6X4-	T42.6X5-	T42.6X6-
Trichloroethyl phosphate	T42.6X1-	T42.6X2-	T42.6X3-	T42.6X4-	T42.6X5-	T42.6X6-
Trichloroethylene (liquid) (vapor)	T53.2X1-	T53.2X2-	T53.2X3-	T53.2X4-	-	-
anesthetic (gas)	T41.0X1-	T41.0X2-	T41.0X3-	T41.0X4-	T41.0X5-	T41.0X6-
vapor NEC	T53.2X1-	T53.2X2-	T53.2X3-	T53.2X4-	-	-
Trichlorofluoromethane NEC	T53.5X1-	T53.5X2-	T53.5X3-	T53.5X4-	-	-
Trichloronate	T60.0X1-	T60.0X2-	T60.0X3-	T60.0X4-	-	-
2,4,5-Trichlorophen-oxyacetic acid	T60.3X1-	T60.3X2-	T60.3X3-	T60.3X4-	-	-
Trichloropropane	T53.6X1-	T53.6X2-	T53.6X3-	T53.6X4-	-	-

Substance	Poisoning Accidental (unintentional)	Poisoning Intentional self-harm	Poisoning Assault	Poisoning Undetermined	Adverse effect	Underdosing
Trichlorotriethylamine	T45.1X1-	T45.1X2-	T45.1X3-	T45.1X4-	T45.1X5-	T45.1X6-
Trichomonacides NEC	T37.3X1-	T37.3X2-	T37.3X3-	T37.3X4-	T37.3X5-	T37.3X6-
Trichomycin	T36.7X1-	T36.7X2-	T36.7X3-	T36.7X4-	T36.7X5-	T36.7X6-
Triclobisonium chloride	T49.0X1-	T49.0X2-	T49.0X3-	T49.0X4-	T49.0X5-	T49.0X6-
Triclocarban	T49.0X1-	T49.0X2-	T49.0X3-	T49.0X4-	T49.0X5-	T49.0X6-
Triclofos	T42.6X1-	T42.6X2-	T42.6X3-	T42.6X4-	T42.6X5-	T42.6X6-
Triclosan	T49.0X1-	T49.0X2-	T49.0X3-	T49.0X4-	T49.0X5-	T49.0X6-
Tricresyl phosphate	T65.891-	T65.892-	T65.893-	T65.894-	-	-
solvent	T52.91X-	T52.92X-	T52.93X-	T52.94X-	-	-
Tricyclamol chloride	T44.3X1-	T44.3X2-	T44.3X3-	T44.3X4-	T44.3X5-	T44.3X6-
Tridesilon	T49.0X1-	T49.0X2-	T49.0X3-	T49.0X4-	T49.0X5-	T49.0X6-
Tridihexethyl iodide	T44.3X1-	T44.3X2-	T44.3X3-	T44.3X4-	T44.3X5-	T44.3X6-
Tridione	T42.2X1-	T42.2X2-	T42.2X3-	T42.2X4-	T42.2X5-	T42.2X6-
Trientine	T45.8X1-	T45.8X2-	T45.8X3-	T45.8X4-	T45.8X5-	T45.8X6-
Triethanolamine NEC	T54.3X1-	T54.3X2-	T54.3X3-	T54.3X4-	-	-
detergent	T54.3X1-	T54.3X2-	T54.3X3-	T54.3X4-	-	-
trinitrate (biphosphate)	T46.3X1-	T46.3X2-	T46.3X3-	T46.3X4-	T46.3X5-	T46.3X6-
Triethanomelamine	T45.1X1-	T45.1X2-	T45.1X3-	T45.1X4-	T45.1X5-	T45.1X6-
Triethylenemelamine	T45.1X1-	T45.1X2-	T45.1X3-	T45.1X4-	T45.1X5-	T45.1X6-
Triethylenephosphoramide	T45.1X1-	T45.1X2-	T45.1X3-	T45.1X4-	T45.1X5-	T45.1X6-
Triethylenethiophosphoramide	T45.1X1-	T45.1X2-	T45.1X3-	T45.1X4-	T45.1X5-	T45.1X6-
Trifluoperazine	T43.3X1-	T43.3X2-	T43.3X3-	T43.3X4-	T43.3X5-	T43.3X6-
Trifluoroethyl vinyl ether	T41.0X1-	T41.0X2-	T41.0X3-	T41.0X4-	T41.0X5-	T41.0X6-
Trifluperidol	T43.4X1-	T43.4X2-	T43.4X3-	T43.4X4-	T43.4X5-	T43.4X6-
Triflupromazine	T43.3X1-	T43.3X2-	T43.3X3-	T43.3X4-	T43.3X5-	T43.3X6-
Trifluridine	T37.5X1-	T37.5X2-	T37.5X3-	T37.5X4-	T37.5X5-	T37.5X6-
Triflusal	T45.521-	T45.522-	T45.523-	T45.524-	T45.525-	T45.526-
Trihexyphenidyl	T44.3X1-	T44.3X2-	T44.3X3-	T44.3X4-	T44.3X5-	T44.3X6-
Triiodothyronine	T38.1X1-	T38.1X2-	T38.1X3-	T38.1X4-	T38.1X5-	T38.1X6-
Trilene	T41.0X1-	T41.0X2-	T41.0X3-	T41.0X4-	T41.0X5-	T41.0X6-
Trilostane	T38.991-	T38.992-	T38.993-	T38.994-	T38.995-	T38.996-
Trimebutine	T44.3X1-	T44.3X2-	T44.3X3-	T44.3X4-	T44.3X5-	T44.3X6-
Trimecaine	T41.3X1-	T41.3X2-	T41.3X3-	T41.3X4-	T41.3X5-	T41.3X6-
Trimeprazine (tartrate)	T44.3X1-	T44.3X2-	T44.3X3-	T44.3X4-	T44.3X5-	T44.3X6-
Trimetaphan camsilate	T44.2X1-	T44.2X2-	T44.2X3-	T44.2X4-	T44.2X5-	T44.2X6-
Trimetazidine	T46.7X1-	T46.7X2-	T46.7X3-	T46.7X4-	T46.7X5-	T46.7X6-
Trimethadione	T42.2X1-	T42.2X2-	T42.2X3-	T42.2X4-	T42.2X5-	T42.2X6-
Trimethaphan	T44.2X1-	T44.2X2-	T44.2X3-	T44.2X4-	T44.2X5-	T44.2X6-
Trimethidinium	T44.2X1-	T44.2X2-	T44.2X3-	T44.2X4-	T44.2X5-	T44.2X6-
Trimethobenzamide	T45.0X1-	T45.0X2-	T45.0X3-	T45.0X4-	T45.0X5-	T45.0X6-
Trimethoprim	T37.8X1-	T37.8X2-	T37.8X3-	T37.8X4-	T37.8X5-	T37.8X6-
with sulfamethoxazole	T36.8X1-	T36.8X2-	T36.8X3-	T36.8X4-	T36.8X5-	T36.8X6-
Trimethylcarbinol	T51.3X1-	T51.3X2-	T51.3X3-	T51.3X4-	-	-
Trimethylpsoralen	T49.3X1-	T49.3X2-	T49.3X3-	T49.3X4-	T49.3X5-	T49.3X6-
Trimeton	T45.0X1-	T45.0X2-	T45.0X3-	T45.0X4-	T45.0X5-	T45.0X6-
Trimetrexate	T45.1X1-	T45.1X2-	T45.1X3-	T45.1X4-	T45.1X5-	T45.1X6-
Trimipramine	T43.011-	T43.012-	T43.013-	T43.014-	T43.015-	T43.016-
Trimustine	T45.1X1-	T45.1X2-	T45.1X3-	T45.1X4-	T45.1X5-	T45.1X6-
Trinitrine	T46.3X1-	T46.3X2-	T46.3X3-	T46.3X4-	T46.3X5-	T46.3X6-
Trinitrobenzol	T65.3X1-	T65.3X2-	T65.3X3-	T65.3X4-	-	-
Trinitrophenol	T65.3X1-	T65.3X2-	T65.3X3-	T65.3X4-	-	-
Trinitrotoluene (fumes)	T65.3X1-	T65.3X2-	T65.3X3-	T65.3X4-	-	-
Trional	T42.6X1-	T42.6X2-	T42.6X3-	T42.6X4-	T42.6X5-	T42.6X6-
Triorthocresyl phosphate	T65.891-	T65.892-	T65.893-	T65.894-	-	-
Trioxide of arsenic	T57.0X1-	T57.0X2-	T57.0X3-	T57.0X4-	-	-
Trioxysalen	T49.4X1-	T49.4X2-	T49.4X3-	T49.4X4-	T49.4X5-	T49.4X6-
Tripamide	T50.2X1-	T50.2X2-	T50.2X3-	T50.2X4-	T50.2X5-	T50.2X6-
Triparanol	T46.6X1-	T46.6X2-	T46.6X3-	T46.6X4-	T46.6X5-	T46.6X6-
Tripelennamine	T45.0X1-	T45.0X2-	T45.0X3-	T45.0X4-	T45.0X5-	T45.0X6-

Substance	Poisoning Accidental (unintentional)	Poisoning Intentional self-harm	Poisoning Assault	Poisoning Undetermined	Adverse effect	Underdosing
Triperiden	T44.3X1-	T44.3X2-	T44.3X3-	T44.3X4-	T44.3X5-	T44.3X6-
Triperidol	T43.4X1-	T43.4X2-	T43.4X3-	T43.4X4-	T43.4X5-	T43.4X6-
Triphenylphosphate	T65.891-	T65.892-	T65.893-	T65.894-	-	-
Triple						
bromides	T42.6X1-	T42.6X2-	T42.6X3-	T42.6X4-	T42.6X5-	T42.6X6-
carbonate	T47.1X1-	T47.1X2-	T47.1X3-	T47.1X4-	T47.1X5-	T47.1X6-
vaccine						
DPT	T50.A11-	T50.A12-	T50.A13-	T50.A14-	T50.A15-	T50.A16-
including pertussis	T50.A11-	T50.A12-	T50.A13-	T50.A14-	T50.A15-	T50.A16-
MMR	T50.B91-	T50.B92-	T50.B93-	T50.B94-	T50.B95-	T50.B96-
Triprolidine	T45.0X1-	T45.0X2-	T45.0X3-	T45.0X4-	T45.0X5-	T45.0X6-
Trisodium hydrogen edetate	T50.6X1-	T50.6X2-	T50.6X3-	T50.6X4-	T50.6X5-	T50.6X6-
Trisoralen	T49.3X1-	T49.3X2-	T49.3X3-	T49.3X4-	T49.3X5-	T49.3X6-
Trisulfapyrimidines	T37.0X1-	T37.0X2-	T37.0X3-	T37.0X4-	T37.0X5-	T37.0X6-
Trithiozine	T44.3X1-	T44.3X2-	T44.3X3-	T44.3X4-	T44.3X5-	T44.3X6-
Tritiozine	T44.3X1-	T44.3X2-	T44.3X3-	T44.3X4-	T44.3X5-	T44.3X6-
Tritoqualine	T45.0X1-	T45.0X2-	T45.0X3-	T45.0X4-	T45.0X5-	T45.0X6-
Trofosfamide	T45.1X1-	T45.1X2-	T45.1X3-	T45.1X4-	T45.1X5-	T45.1X6-
Troleandomycin	T36.3X1-	T36.3X2-	T36.3X3-	T36.3X4-	T36.3X5-	T36.3X6-
Trolnitrate (phosphate)	T46.3X1-	T46.3X2-	T46.3X3-	T46.3X4-	T46.3X5-	T46.3X6-
Tromantadine	T37.5X1-	T37.5X2-	T37.5X3-	T37.5X4-	T37.5X5-	T37.5X6-
Trometamol	T50.2X1-	T50.2X2-	T50.2X3-	T50.2X4-	T50.2X5-	T50.2X6-
Tromethamine	T50.2X1-	T50.2X2-	T50.2X3-	T50.2X4-	T50.2X5-	T50.2X6-
Tronothane	T41.3X1-	T41.3X2-	T41.3X3-	T41.3X4-	T41.3X5-	T41.3X6-
Tropacine	T44.3X1-	T44.3X2-	T44.3X3-	T44.3X4-	T44.3X5-	T44.3X6-
Tropatepine	T44.3X1-	T44.3X2-	T44.3X3-	T44.3X4-	T44.3X5-	T44.3X6-
Tropicamide	T44.3X1-	T44.3X2-	T44.3X3-	T44.3X4-	T44.3X5-	T44.3X6-
Trospium chloride	T44.3X1-	T44.3X2-	T44.3X3-	T44.3X4-	T44.3X5-	T44.3X6-
Troxerutin	T46.991-	T46.992-	T46.993-	T46.994-	T46.995-	T46.996-
Troxidone	T42.2X1-	T42.2X2-	T42.2X3-	T42.2X4-	T42.2X5-	T42.2X6-
Tryparsamide	T37.3X1-	T37.3X2-	T37.3X3-	T37.3X4-	T37.3X5-	T37.3X6-
Trypsin	T45.3X1-	T45.3X2-	T45.3X3-	T45.3X4-	T45.3X5-	T45.3X6-
Tryptizol	T43.011-	T43.012-	T43.013-	T43.014-	T43.015-	T43.016-
TSH	T38.811-	T38.812-	T38.813-	T38.814-	T38.815-	T38.816-
Tuaminoheptane	T48.5X1-	T48.5X2-	T48.5X3-	T48.5X4-	T48.5X5-	T48.5X6-
Tuberculin, purified protein derivative (PPD)	T50.8X1-	T50.8X2-	T50.8X3-	T50.8X4-	T50.8X5-	T50.8X6-
Tubocurare	T48.1X1-	T48.1X2-	T48.1X3-	T48.1X4-	T48.1X5-	T48.1X6-
Tubocurarine (chloride)	T48.1X1-	T48.1X2-	T48.1X3-	T48.1X4-	T48.1X5-	T48.1X6-
Tulobuterol	T48.6X1-	T48.6X2-	T48.6X3-	T48.6X4-	T48.6X5-	T48.6X6-
Turpentine (spirits of)	T52.8X1-	T52.8X2-	T52.8X3-	T52.8X4-	-	-
vapor	T52.8X1-	T52.8X2-	T52.8X3-	T52.8X4-	-	-
Tybamate	T43.591-	T43.592-	T43.593-	T43.594-	T43.595-	T43.596-
Tyloxapol	T48.4X1-	T48.4X2-	T48.4X3-	T48.4X4-	T48.4X5-	T48.4X6-
Tymazoline	T48.5X1-	T48.5X2-	T48.5X3-	T48.5X4-	T48.5X5-	T48.5X6-
Typhoid-paratyphoid vaccine	T50.A91-	T50.A92-	T50.A93-	T50.A94-	T50.A95-	T50.A96-
Typhus vaccine	T50.A91-	T50.A92-	T50.A93-	T50.A94-	T50.A95-	T50.A96-
Tyropanoate	T50.8X1-	T50.8X2-	T50.8X3-	T50.8X4-	T50.8X5-	T50.8X6-
Tyrothricin	T49.6X1-	T49.6X2-	T49.6X3-	T49.6X4-	T49.6X5-	T49.6X6-
ENT agent	T49.6X1-	T49.6X2-	T49.6X3-	T49.6X4-	T49.6X5-	T49.6X6-
ophthalmic preparation	T49.5X1-	T49.5X2-	T49.5X3-	T49.5X4-	T49.5X5-	T49.5X6-
Ufenamate	T39.391-	T39.392-	T39.393-	T39.394-	T39.395-	T39.396-
Ultraviolet light protectant	T49.3X1-	T49.3X2-	T49.3X3-	T49.3X4-	T49.3X5-	T49.3X6-
Undecenoic acid	T49.0X1-	T49.0X2-	T49.0X3-	T49.0X4-	T49.0X5-	T49.0X6-
Undecoylium	T49.0X1-	T49.0X2-	T49.0X3-	T49.0X4-	T49.0X5-	T49.0X6-
Undecylenic acid (derivatives)	T49.0X1-	T49.0X2-	T49.0X3-	T49.0X4-	T49.0X5-	T49.0X6-
Unna's boot	T49.3X1-	T49.3X2-	T49.3X3-	T49.3X4-	T49.3X5-	T49.3X6-
Unsaturated fatty acid	T46.6X1-	T46.6X2-	T46.6X3-	T46.6X4-	T46.6X5-	T46.6X6-
Uracil mustard	T45.1X1-	T45.1X2-	T45.1X3-	T45.1X4-	T45.1X5-	T45.1X6-

Substance	Poisoning Accidental (unintentional)	Poisoning Intentional self-harm	Poisoning Assault	Poisoning Undetermined	Adverse effect	Underdosing
Uramustine	T45.1X1-	T45.1X2-	T45.1X3-	T45.1X4-	T45.1X5-	T45.1X6-
Urapidil	T46.5X1-	T46.5X2-	T46.5X3-	T46.5X4-	T46.5X5-	T46.5X6-
Urari	T48.1X1-	T48.1X2-	T48.1X3-	T48.1X4-	T48.1X5-	T48.1X6-
Urate oxidase	T50.4X1-	T50.4X2-	T50.4X3-	T50.4X4-	T50.4X5-	T50.4X6-
Urea	T47.3X1-	T47.3X2-	T47.3X3-	T47.3X4-	T47.3X5-	T47.3X6-
peroxide	T49.0X1-	T49.0X2-	T49.0X3-	T49.0X4-	T49.0X5-	T49.0X6-
stibamine	T37.4X1-	T37.4X2-	T37.4X3-	T37.4X4-	T37.4X5-	T37.4X6-
topical	T49.8X1-	T49.8X2-	T49.8X3-	T49.8X4-	T49.8X5-	T49.8X6-
Urethane	T45.1X1-	T45.1X2-	T45.1X3-	T45.1X4-	T45.1X5-	T45.1X6-
Urginea (maritima) (scilla) — *see Squill*						
Uric acid metabolism drug NEC	T50.4X1-	T50.4X2-	T50.4X3-	T50.4X4-	T50.4X5-	T50.4X6-
Uricosuric agent	T50.4X1-	T50.4X2-	T50.4X3-	T50.4X4-	T50.4X5-	T50.4X6-
Urinary anti-infective	T37.8X1-	T37.8X2-	T37.8X3-	T37.8X4-	T37.8X5-	T37.8X6-
Urofollitropin	T38.811-	T38.812-	T38.813-	T38.814-	T38.815-	T38.816-
Urokinase	T45.611-	T45.612-	T45.613-	T45.614-	T45.615-	T45.616-
Urokon	T50.8X1-	T50.8X2-	T50.8X3-	T50.8X4-	T50.8X5-	T50.8X6-
Ursodeoxycholic acid	T50.991-	T50.992-	T50.993-	T50.994-	T50.995-	T50.996-
Ursodiol	T50.991-	T50.992-	T50.993-	T50.994-	T50.995-	T50.996-
Urtica	T62.2X1-	T62.2X2-	T62.2X3-	T62.2X4-	-	-
Utility gas — *see Gas, utility*						
Vaccine NEC	T50.Z91-	T50.Z92-	T50.Z93-	T50.Z94-	T50.Z95-	T50.Z96-
antineoplastic	T50.Z91-	T50.Z92-	T50.Z93-	T50.Z94-	T50.Z95-	T50.Z96-
bacterial NEC	T50.A91-	T50.A92-	T50.A93-	T50.A94-	T50.A95-	T50.A96-
with						
other bacterial component	T50.A21-	T50.A22-	T50.A23-	T50.A24-	T50.A25-	T50.A26-
pertussis component	T50.A11-	T50.A12-	T50.A13-	T50.A14-	T50.A15-	T50.A16-
viral-rickettsial component	T50.A21-	T50.A22-	T50.A23-	T50.A24-	T50.A25-	T50.A26-
mixed NEC	T50.A21-	T50.A22-	T50.A23-	T50.A24-	T50.A25-	T50.A26-
BCG	T50.A91-	T50.A92-	T50.A93-	T50.A94-	T50.A95-	T50.A96-
cholera	T50.A91-	T50.A92-	T50.A93-	T50.A94-	T50.A95-	T50.A96-
diphtheria	T50.A91-	T50.A92-	T50.A93-	T50.A94-	T50.A95-	T50.A96-
with tetanus	T50.A21-	T50.A22-	T50.A23-	T50.A24-	T50.A25-	T50.A26-
and pertussis	T50.A11-	T50.A12-	T50.A13-	T50.A14-	T50.A15-	T50.A16-
influenza	T50.B91-	T50.B92-	T50.B93-	T50.B94-	T50.B95-	T50.B96-
measles	T50.B91-	T50.B92-	T50.B93-	T50.B94-	T50.B95-	T50.B96-
with mumps and rubella	T50.B91-	T50.B92-	T50.B93-	T50.B94-	T50.B95-	T50.B96-
meningococcal	T50.A91-	T50.A92-	T50.A93-	T50.A94-	T50.A95-	T50.A96-
mumps	T50.B91-	T50.B92-	T50.B93-	T50.B94-	T50.B95-	T50.B96-
paratyphoid	T50.A91-	T50.A92-	T50.A93-	T50.A94-	T50.A95-	T50.A96-
pertussis	T50.A11-	T50.A12-	T50.A13-	T50.A14-	T50.A15-	T50.A16-
with diphtheria	T50.A11-	T50.A12-	T50.A13-	T50.A14-	T50.A15-	T50.A16-
and tetanus	T50.A11-	T50.A12-	T50.A13-	T50.A14-	T50.A15-	T50.A16-
with other component	T50.A11-	T50.A12-	T50.A13-	T50.A14-	T50.A15-	T50.A16-
plague	T50.A91-	T50.A92-	T50.A93-	T50.A94-	T50.A95-	T50.A96-
poliomyelitis	T50.B91-	T50.B92-	T50.B93-	T50.B94-	T50.B95-	T50.B96-
poliovirus	T50.B91-	T50.B92-	T50.B93-	T50.B94-	T50.B95-	T50.B96-
rabies	T50.B91-	T50.B92-	T50.B93-	T50.B94-	T50.B95-	T50.B96-
respiratory syncytial virus	T50.B91-	T50.B92-	T50.B93-	T50.B94-	T50.B95-	T50.B96-
rickettsial NEC	T50.A91-	T50.A92-	T50.A93-	T50.A94-	T50.A95-	T50.A96-
with						
bacterial component	T50.A21-	T50.A22-	T50.A23-	T50.A24-	T50.A25-	T50.A26-
Rocky Mountain spotted fever	T50.A91-	T50.A92-	T50.A93-	T50.A94-	T50.A95-	T50.A96-
rubella	T50.B91-	T50.B92-	T50.B93-	T50.B94-	T50.B95-	T50.B96-
sabin oral	T50.B91-	T50.B92-	T50.B93-	T50.B94-	T50.B95-	T50.B96-
smallpox	T50.B11-	T50.B12-	T50.B13-	T50.B14-	T50.B15-	T50.B16-
TAB	T50.A91-	T50.A92-	T50.A93-	T50.A94-	T50.A95-	T50.A96-
tetanus	T50.A91-	T50.A92-	T50.A93-	T50.A94-	T50.A95-	T50.A96-
typhoid	T50.A91-	T50.A92-	T50.A93-	T50.A94-	T50.A95-	T50.A96-

Substance	Poisoning Accidental (unintentional)	Poisoning Intentional self-harm	Poisoning Assault	Poisoning Undetermined	Adverse effect	Underdosing
Vaccine NEC (continued)						
typhus	T50.A91-	T50.A92-	T50.A93-	T50.A94-	T50.A95-	T50.A96-
viral NEC	T50.B91-	T50.B92-	T50.B93-	T50.B94-	T50.B95-	T50.B96-
yellow fever	T50.B91-	T50.B92-	T50.B93-	T50.B94-	T50.B95-	T50.B96-
Vaccinia immune globulin	T50.Z11-	T50.Z12-	T50.Z13-	T50.Z14-	T50.Z15-	T50.Z16-
Vaginal contraceptives	T49.8X1-	T49.8X2-	T49.8X3-	T49.8X4-	T49.8X5-	T49.8X6-
Valerian						
root	T42.6X1-	T42.6X2-	T42.6X3-	T42.6X4-	T42.6X5-	T42.6X6-
tincture	T42.6X1-	T42.6X2-	T42.6X3-	T42.6X4-	T42.6X5-	T42.6X6-
Valethamate bromide	T44.3X1-	T44.3X2-	T44.3X3-	T44.3X4-	T44.3X5-	T44.3X6-
Valisone	T49.0X1-	T49.0X2-	T49.0X3-	T49.0X4-	T49.0X5-	T49.0X6-
Valium	T42.4X1-	T42.4X2-	T42.4X3-	T42.4X4-	T42.4X5-	T42.4X6-
Valmid	T42.6X1-	T42.6X2-	T42.6X3-	T42.6X4-	T42.6X5-	T42.6X6-
Valnoctamide	T42.6X1-	T42.6X2-	T42.6X3-	T42.6X4-	T42.6X5-	T42.6X6-
Valproate (sodium)	T42.6X1-	T42.6X2-	T42.6X3-	T42.6X4-	T42.6X5-	T42.6X6-
Valproic acid	T42.6X1-	T42.6X2-	T42.6X3-	T42.6X4-	T42.6X5-	T42.6X6-
Valpromide	T42.6X1-	T42.6X2-	T42.6X3-	T42.6X4-	T42.6X5-	T42.6X6-
Vanadium	T56.891-	T56.892-	T56.893-	T56.894-	-	-
Vancomycin	T36.8X1-	T36.8X2-	T36.8X3-	T36.8X4-	T36.8X5-	T36.8X6-
Vapor — *see also Gas*	T59.91X-	T59.92X-	T59.93X-	T59.94X-	-	-
kiln (carbon monoxide)	T58.8X1-	T58.8X2-	T58.8X3-	T58.8X4-	-	-
lead — *see lead*						
specified source NEC	T59.891-	T59.892-	T59.893-	T59.894-	-	-
Vardenafil	T46.7X1-	T46.7X2-	T46.7X3-	T46.7X4-	T46.7X5-	T46.7X6-
Varicose reduction drug	T46.8X1-	T46.8X2-	T46.8X3-	T46.8X4-	T46.8X5-	T46.8X6-
Varnish	T65.4X1-	T65.4X2-	T65.4X3-	T65.4X4-	-	-
cleaner	T52.91X-	T52.92X-	T52.93X-	T52.94X-	-	-
Vaseline	T49.3X1-	T49.3X2-	T49.3X3-	T49.3X4-	T49.3X5-	T49.3X6-
Vasodilan	T46.7X1-	T46.7X2-	T46.7X3-	T46.7X4-	T46.7X5-	T46.7X6-
Vasodilator						
coronary NEC	T46.3X1-	T46.3X2-	T46.3X3-	T46.3X4-	T46.3X5-	T46.3X6-
peripheral NEC	T46.7X1-	T46.7X2-	T46.7X3-	T46.7X4-	T46.7X5-	T46.7X6-
Vasopressin	T38.891-	T38.892-	T38.893-	T38.894-	T38.895-	T38.896-
Vasopressor drugs	T38.891-	T38.892-	T38.893-	T38.894-	T38.895-	T38.896-
Vecuronium bromide	T48.1X1-	T48.1X2-	T48.1X3-	T48.1X4-	T48.1X5-	T48.1X6-
Vegetable extract, astringent	T49.2X1-	T49.2X2-	T49.2X3-	T49.2X4-	T49.2X5-	T49.2X6-
Venlafaxine	T43.211-	T43.212-	T43.213-	T43.214-	T43.215-	T43.216-
Venom, venomous (bite) (sting)	T63.91X-	T63.92X-	T63.93X-	T63.94X-	-	-
amphibian NEC	T63.831-	T63.832-	T63.833-	T63.834-	-	-
animal NEC	T63.891-	T63.892-	T63.893-	T63.894-	-	-
ant	T63.421-	T63.422-	T63.423-	T63.424-	-	-
arthropod NEC	T63.481-	T63.482-	T63.483-	T63.484-	-	-
bee	T63.441-	T63.442-	T63.443-	T63.444-	-	-
centipede	T63.411-	T63.412-	T63.413-	T63.414-	-	-
fish	T63.591-	T63.592-	T63.593-	T63.594-	-	-
frog	T63.811-	T63.812-	T63.813-	T63.814-	-	-
hornet	T63.451-	T63.452-	T63.453-	T63.454-	-	-
insect NEC	T63.481-	T63.482-	T63.483-	T63.484-	-	-
lizard	T63.121-	T63.122-	T63.123-	T63.124-	-	-
marine						
animals	T63.691-	T63.692-	T63.693-	T63.694-	-	-
bluebottle	T63.611-	T63.612-	T63.613-	T63.614-	-	-
jellyfish NEC	T63.621-	T63.622-	T63.623-	T63.624-	-	-
Portuguese Man-o-war	T63.611-	T63.612-	T63.613-	T63.614-	-	-
sea anemone	T63.631-	T63.632-	T63.633-	T63.634-	-	-
specified NEC	T63.691-	T63.692-	T63.693-	T63.694-	-	-
fish	T63.591-	T63.592-	T63.593-	T63.594-	-	-
plants	T63.711-	T63.712-	T63.713-	T63.714-	-	-

Substance	Poisoning Accidental (unintentional)	Poisoning Intentional self-harm	Poisoning Assault	Poisoning Undetermined	Adverse effect	Underdosing
Venom, venomous (bite) (sting) (continued)						
sting ray	T63.511-	T63.512-	T63.513-	T63.514-	-	-
millipede (tropical)	T63.411-	T63.412-	T63.413-	T63.414-	-	-
plant NEC	T63.791-	T63.792-	T63.793-	T63.794-	-	-
marine	T63.711-	T63.712-	T63.713-	T63.714-	-	-
reptile	T63.191-	T63.192-	T63.193-	T63.194-	-	-
gila monster	T63.111-	T63.112-	T63.113-	T63.114-	-	-
lizard NEC	T63.121-	T63.122-	T63.123-	T63.124-	-	-
scorpion	T63.2X1-	T63.2X2-	T63.2X3-	T63.2X4-	-	-
snake	T63.001-	T63.002-	T63.003-	T63.004-	-	-
African NEC	T63.081-	T63.082-	T63.083-	T63.084-	-	-
American (North) (South) NEC	T63.061-	T63.062-	T63.063-	T63.064-	-	-
Asian	T63.081-	T63.082-	T63.083-	T63.084-	-	-
Australian	T63.071-	T63.072-	T63.073-	T63.074-	-	-
cobra	T63.041-	T63.042-	T63.043-	T63.044-	-	-
coral snake	T63.021-	T63.022-	T63.023-	T63.024-	-	-
rattlesnake	T63.011-	T63.012-	T63.013-	T63.014-	-	-
specified NEC	T63.091-	T63.092-	T63.093-	T63.094-	-	-
taipan	T63.031-	T63.032-	T63.033-	T63.034-	-	-
specified NEC	T63.891-	T63.892-	T63.893-	T63.894-	-	-
spider	T63.301-	T63.302-	T63.303-	T63.304-	-	-
black widow	T63.311-	T63.312-	T63.313-	T63.314-	-	-
brown recluse	T63.331-	T63.332-	T63.333-	T63.334-	-	-
specified NEC	T63.391-	T63.392-	T63.393-	T63.394-	-	-
tarantula	T63.321-	T63.322-	T63.323-	T63.324-	-	-
sting ray	T63.511-	T63.512-	T63.513-	T63.514-	-	-
toad	T63.821-	T63.822-	T63.823-	T63.824-	-	-
wasp	T63.461-	T63.462-	T63.463-	T63.464-	-	-
Venous sclerosing drug NEC	T46.8X1-	T46.8X2-	T46.8X3-	T46.8X4-	T46.8X5-	T46.8X6-
Ventolin — *see Albuterol*						
Veramon	T42.3X1-	T42.3X2-	T42.3X3-	T42.3X4-	T42.3X5-	T42.3X6-
Verapamil	T46.1X1-	T46.1X2-	T46.1X3-	T46.1X4-	T46.1X5-	T46.1X6-
Veratrine	T46.5X1-	T46.5X2-	T46.5X3-	T46.5X4-	T46.5X5-	T46.5X6-
Veratrum						
album	T62.2X1-	T62.2X2-	T62.2X3-	T62.2X4-	-	-
alkaloids	T46.5X1-	T46.5X2-	T46.5X3-	T46.5X4-	T46.5X5-	T46.5X6-
viride	T62.2X1-	T62.2X2-	T62.2X3-	T62.2X4-	-	-
Verdigris	T60.3X1-	T60.3X2-	T60.3X3-	T60.3X4-	-	-
Veronal	T42.3X1-	T42.3X2-	T42.3X3-	T42.3X4-	T42.3X5-	T42.3X6-
Veroxil	T37.4X1-	T37.4X2-	T37.4X3-	T37.4X4-	T37.4X5-	T37.4X6-
Versenate	T50.6X1-	T50.6X2-	T50.6X3-	T50.6X4-	T50.6X5-	T50.6X6-
Versidyne	T39.8X1-	T39.8X2-	T39.8X3-	T39.8X4-	T39.8X5-	T39.8X6-
Vetrabutine	T48.0X1-	T48.0X2-	T48.0X3-	T48.0X4-	T48.0X5-	T48.0X6-
Vidarabine	T37.5X1-	T37.5X2-	T37.5X3-	T37.5X4-	T37.5X5-	T37.5X6-
Vienna						
green	T57.0X1-	T57.0X2-	T57.0X3-	T57.0X4-	-	-
insecticide	T60.2X1-	T60.2X2-	T60.2X3-	T60.2X4-	-	-
red	T57.0X1-	T57.0X2-	T57.0X3-	T57.0X4-	-	-
pharmaceutical dye	T50.991-	T50.992-	T50.993-	T50.994-	T50.995-	T50.996-
Vigabatrin	T42.6X1-	T42.6X2-	T42.6X3-	T42.6X4-	T42.6X5-	T42.6X6-
Viloxazine	T43.291-	T43.292-	T43.293-	T43.294-	T43.295-	T43.296-
Viminol	T39.8X1-	T39.8X2-	T39.8X3-	T39.8X4-	T39.8X5-	T39.8X6-
Vinbarbital, vinbarbitone	T42.3X1-	T42.3X2-	T42.3X3-	T42.3X4-	T42.3X5-	T42.3X6-
Vinblastine	T45.1X1-	T45.1X2-	T45.1X3-	T45.1X4-	T45.1X5-	T45.1X6-
Vinburnine	T46.7X1-	T46.7X2-	T46.7X3-	T46.7X4-	T46.7X5-	T46.7X6-
Vincamine	T45.1X1-	T45.1X2-	T45.1X3-	T45.1X4-	T45.1X5-	T45.1X6-
Vincristine	T45.1X1-	T45.1X2-	T45.1X3-	T45.1X4-	T45.1X5-	T45.1X6-
Vindesine	T45.1X1-	T45.1X2-	T45.1X3-	T45.1X4-	T45.1X5-	T45.1X6-

Substance	Poisoning Accidental (unintentional)	Poisoning Intentional self-harm	Poisoning Assault	Poisoning Undetermined	Adverse effect	Underdosing
Vinesthene, vinethene	T41.0X1-	T41.0X2-	T41.0X3-	T41.0X4-	T41.0X5-	T41.0X6-
Vinorelbine tartrate	T45.1X1-	T45.1X2-	T45.1X3-	T45.1X4-	T45.1X5-	T45.1X6-
Vinpocetine	T46.7X1-	T46.7X2-	T46.7X3-	T46.7X4-	T46.7X5-	T46.7X6-
Vinyl						
acetate	T65.891-	T65.892-	T65.893-	T65.894-	-	-
bital	T42.3X1-	T42.3X2-	T42.3X3-	T42.3X4-	T42.3X5-	T42.3X6-
bromide	T65.891-	T65.892-	T65.893-	T65.894-	-	-
chloride	T59.891-	T59.892-	T59.893-	T59.894-	-	-
ether	T41.0X1-	T41.0X2-	T41.0X3-	T41.0X4-	T41.0X5-	T41.0X6-
Vinylbital	T42.3X1-	T42.3X2-	T42.3X3-	T42.3X4-	T42.3X5-	T42.3X6-
Vinylidene chloride	T65.891-	T65.892-	T65.893-	T65.894-	-	-
Vioform	T37.8X1-	T37.8X2-	T37.8X3-	T37.8X4-	T37.8X5-	T37.8X6-
topical	T49.0X1-	T49.0X2-	T49.0X3-	T49.0X4-	T49.0X5-	T49.0X6-
Viomycin	T36.8X1-	T36.8X2-	T36.8X3-	T36.8X4-	T36.8X5-	T36.8X6-
Viosterol	T45.2X1-	T45.2X2-	T45.2X3-	T45.2X4-	T45.2X5-	T45.2X6-
Viper (venom)	T63.091-	T63.092-	T63.093-	T63.094-	-	-
Viprynium	T37.4X1-	T37.4X2-	T37.4X3-	T37.4X4-	T37.4X5-	T37.4X6-
Viquidil	T46.7X1-	T46.7X2-	T46.7X3-	T46.7X4-	T46.7X5-	T46.7X6-
Viral vaccine NEC	T50.B91-	T50.B92-	T50.B93-	T50.B94-	T50.B95-	T50.B96-
Virginiamycin	T36.8X1-	T36.8X2-	T36.8X3-	T36.8X4-	T36.8X5-	T36.8X6-
Virugon	T37.5X1-	T37.5X2-	T37.5X3-	T37.5X4-	T37.5X5-	T37.5X6-
Viscous agent	T50.901-	T50.902-	T50.903-	T50.904-	T50.905-	T50.906-
Visine	T49.5X1-	T49.5X2-	T49.5X3-	T49.5X4-	T49.5X5-	T49.5X6-
Visnadine	T46.3X1-	T46.3X2-	T46.3X3-	T46.3X4-	T46.3X5-	T46.3X6-
Vitamin NEC	T45.2X1-	T45.2X2-	T45.2X3-	T45.2X4-	T45.2X5-	T45.2X6-
A	T45.2X1-	T45.2X2-	T45.2X3-	T45.2X4-	T45.2X5-	T45.2X6-
B NEC	T45.2X1-	T45.2X2-	T45.2X3-	T45.2X4-	T45.2X5-	T45.2X6-
nicotinic acid	T46.7X1-	T46.7X2-	T46.7X3-	T46.7X4-	T46.7X5-	T46.7X6-
B1	T45.2X1-	T45.2X2-	T45.2X3-	T45.2X4-	T45.2X5-	T45.2X6-
B2	T45.2X1-	T45.2X2-	T45.2X3-	T45.2X4-	T45.2X5-	T45.2X6-
B6	T45.2X1-	T45.2X2-	T45.2X3-	T45.2X4-	T45.2X5-	T45.2X6-
B12	T45.2X1-	T45.2X2-	T45.2X3-	T45.2X4-	T45.2X5-	T45.2X6-
B15	T45.2X1-	T45.2X2-	T45.2X3-	T45.2X4-	T45.2X5-	T45.2X6-
C	T45.2X1-	T45.2X2-	T45.2X3-	T45.2X4-	T45.2X5-	T45.2X6-
D	T45.2X1-	T45.2X2-	T45.2X3-	T45.2X4-	T45.2X5-	T45.2X6-
D2	T45.2X1-	T45.2X2-	T45.2X3-	T45.2X4-	T45.2X5-	T45.2X6-
D3	T45.2X1-	T45.2X2-	T45.2X3-	T45.2X4-	T45.2X5-	T45.2X6-
E	T45.2X1-	T45.2X2-	T45.2X3-	T45.2X4-	T45.2X5-	T45.2X6-
E acetate	T45.2X1-	T45.2X2-	T45.2X3-	T45.2X4-	T45.2X5-	T45.2X6-
hematopoietic	T45.8X1-	T45.8X2-	T45.8X3-	T45.8X4-	T45.8X5-	T45.8X6-
K NEC	T45.7X1-	T45.7X2-	T45.7X3-	T45.7X4-	T45.7X5-	T45.7X6-
K1	T45.7X1-	T45.7X2-	T45.7X3-	T45.7X4-	T45.7X5-	T45.7X6-
K2	T45.7X1-	T45.7X2-	T45.7X3-	T45.7X4-	T45.7X5-	T45.7X6-
PP	T45.2X1-	T45.2X2-	T45.2X3-	T45.2X4-	T45.2X5-	T45.2X6-
ulceroprotectant	T47.1X1-	T47.1X2-	T47.1X3-	T47.1X4-	T47.1X5-	T47.1X6-
Vleminckx's solution	T49.4X1-	T49.4X2-	T49.4X3-	T49.4X4-	T49.4X5-	T49.4X6-
Voltaren — *see Diclofenac sodium*						
Warfarin	T45.511-	T45.512-	T45.513-	T45.514-	T45.515-	T45.516-
rodenticide	T60.4X1-	T60.4X2-	T60.4X3-	T60.4X4-	-	-
sodium	T45.511-	T45.512-	T45.513-	T45.514-	T45.515-	T45.516-
Wasp (sting)	T63.461-	T63.462-	T63.463-	T63.464-	-	-
Water						
balance drug	T50.3X1-	T50.3X2-	T50.3X3-	T50.3X4-	T50.3X5-	T50.3X6-
distilled	T50.3X1-	T50.3X2-	T50.3X3-	T50.3X4-	T50.3X5-	T50.3X6-
gas — *see Gas, water*						
incomplete combustion of — *see Carbon, monoxide, fuel, utility*						
hemlock	T62.2X1-	T62.2X2-	T62.2X3-	T62.2X4-	-	-

Substance	Poisoning Accidental (unintentional)	Poisoning Intentional self-harm	Poisoning Assault	Poisoning Undetermined	Adverse effect	Underdosing
Water (continued)						
moccasin (venom)	T63.061-	T63.062-	T63.063-	T63.064-	-	-
purified	T50.3X1-	T50.3X2-	T50.3X3-	T50.3X4-	T50.3X5-	T50.3X6-
Wax (paraffin) (petroleum)	T52.0X1-	T52.0X2-	T52.0X3-	T52.0X4-	-	-
automobile	T65.891-	T65.892-	T65.893-	T65.894-	-	-
floor	T52.0X1-	T52.0X2-	T52.0X3-	T52.0X4-	-	-
Weed killers NEC	T60.3X1-	T60.3X2-	T60.3X3-	T60.3X4-	-	-
Welldorm	T42.6X1-	T42.6X2-	T42.6X3-	T42.6X4-	T42.6X5-	T42.6X6-
White						
arsenic	T57.0X1-	T57.0X2-	T57.0X3-	T57.0X4-	-	-
hellebore	T62.2X1-	T62.2X2-	T62.2X3-	T62.2X4-	-	-
lotion (keratolytic)	T49.4X1-	T49.4X2-	T49.4X3-	T49.4X4-	T49.4X5-	T49.4X6-
spirit	T52.0X1-	T52.0X2-	T52.0X3-	T52.0X4-	-	-
Whitewash	T65.891-	T65.892-	T65.893-	T65.894-	-	-
Whole blood (human)	T45.8X1-	T45.8X2-	T45.8X3-	T45.8X4-	T45.8X5-	T45.8X6-
Wild						
black cherry	T62.2X1-	T62.2X2-	T62.2X3-	T62.2X4-	-	-
poisonous plants NEC	T62.2X1-	T62.2X2-	T62.2X3-	T62.2X4-	-	-
Window cleaning fluid	T65.891-	T65.892-	T65.893-	T65.894-	-	-
Wintergreen (oil)	T49.3X1-	T49.3X2-	T49.3X3-	T49.3X4-	T49.3X5-	T49.3X6-
Wisterine	T62.2X1-	T62.2X2-	T62.2X3-	T62.2X4-	-	-
Witch hazel	T49.2X1-	T49.2X2-	T49.2X3-	T49.2X4-	T49.2X5-	T49.2X6-
Wood alcohol or spirit	T51.1X1-	T51.1X2-	T51.1X3-	T51.1X4-	-	-
Wool fat (hydrous)	T49.3X1-	T49.3X2-	T49.3X3-	T49.3X4-	T49.3X5-	T49.3X6-
Woorali	T48.1X1-	T48.1X2-	T48.1X3-	T48.1X4-	T48.1X5-	T48.1X6-
Wormseed, American	T37.4X1-	T37.4X2-	T37.4X3-	T37.4X4-	T37.4X5-	T37.4X6-
Xamoterol	T44.5X1-	T44.5X2-	T44.5X3-	T44.5X4-	T44.5X5-	T44.5X6-
Xanthine diuretics	T50.2X1-	T50.2X2-	T50.2X3-	T50.2X4-	T50.2X5-	T50.2X6-
Xanthinol nicotinate	T46.7X1-	T46.7X2-	T46.7X3-	T46.7X4-	T46.7X5-	T46.7X6-
Xanthotoxin	T49.3X1-	T49.3X2-	T49.3X3-	T49.3X4-	T49.3X5-	T49.3X6-
Xantinol nicotinate	T46.7X1-	T46.7X2-	T46.7X3-	T46.7X4-	T46.7X5-	T46.7X6-
Xantocillin	T36.0X1-	T36.0X2-	T36.0X3-	T36.0X4-	T36.0X5-	T36.0X6-
Xenon (127Xe) (133Xe)	T50.8X1-	T50.8X2-	T50.8X3-	T50.8X4-	T50.8X5-	T50.8X6-
Xenysalate	T49.4X1-	T49.4X2-	T49.4X3-	T49.4X4-	T49.4X5-	T49.4X6-
Xibornol	T37.8X1-	T37.8X2-	T37.8X3-	T37.8X4-	T37.8X5-	T37.8X6-
Xigris	T45.511-	T45.512-	T45.513-	T45.514-	T45.515-	T45.516-
Xipamide	T50.2X1-	T50.2X2-	T50.2X3-	T50.2X4-	T50.2X5-	T50.2X6-
Xylene (vapor)	T52.2X1-	T52.2X2-	T52.2X3-	T52.2X4-	-	-
Xylocaine (infiltration) (topical)	T41.3X1-	T41.3X2-	T41.3X3-	T41.3X4-	T41.3X5-	T41.3X6-
nerve block (peripheral) (plexus)	T41.3X1-	T41.3X2-	T41.3X3-	T41.3X4-	T41.3X5-	T41.3X6-
spinal	T41.3X1-	T41.3X2-	T41.3X3-	T41.3X4-	T41.3X5-	T41.3X6-
Xylol (vapor)	T52.2X1-	T52.2X2-	T52.2X3-	T52.2X4-	-	-
Xylometazoline	T48.5X1-	T48.5X2-	T48.5X3-	T48.5X4-	T48.5X5-	T48.5X6-
Yeast	T45.2X1-	T45.2X2-	T45.2X3-	T45.2X4-	T45.2X5-	T45.2X6-
dried	T45.2X1-	T45.2X2-	T45.2X3-	T45.2X4-	T45.2X5-	T45.2X6-
Yellow						
fever vaccine	T50.B91-	T50.B92-	T50.B93-	T50.B94-	T50.B95-	T50.B96-
jasmine	T62.2X1-	T62.2X2-	T62.2X3-	T62.2X4-	-	-
phenolphthalein	T47.2X1-	T47.2X2-	T47.2X3-	T47.2X4-	T47.2X5-	T47.2X6-
Yew	T62.2X1-	T62.2X2-	T62.2X3-	T62.2X4-	-	-
Yohimbic acid	T40.991-	T40.992-	T40.993-	T40.994-	T40.995-	T40.996-
Zactane	T39.8X1-	T39.8X2-	T39.8X3-	T39.8X4-	T39.8X5-	T39.8X6-
Zalcitabine	T37.5X1-	T37.5X2-	T37.5X3-	T37.5X4-	T37.5X5-	T37.5X6-
Zaroxolyn	T50.2X1-	T50.2X2-	T50.2X3-	T50.2X4-	T50.2X5-	T50.2X6-
Zephiran (topical)	T49.0X1-	T49.0X2-	T49.0X3-	T49.0X4-	T49.0X5-	T49.0X6-
ophthalmic preparation	T49.5X1-	T49.5X2-	T49.5X3-	T49.5X4-	T49.5X5-	T49.5X6-
Zeranol	T38.7X1-	T38.7X2-	T38.7X3-	T38.7X4-	T38.7X5-	T38.7X6-
Zerone	T51.1X1-	T51.1X2-	T51.1X3-	T51.1X4-	-	-

Substance	Poisoning Accidental (unintentional)	Poisoning Intentional self-harm	Poisoning Assault	Poisoning Undetermined	Adverse effect	Underdosing
Zidovudine	T37.5X1-	T37.5X2-	T37.5X3-	T37.5X4-	T37.5X5-	T37.5X6-
Zimeldine	T43.221-	T43.222-	T43.223-	T43.224-	T43.225-	T43.226-
Zinc (compounds) (fumes) (vapor) NEC	T56.5X1-	T56.5X2-	T56.5X3-	T56.5X4-	-	-
anti-infectives	T49.0X1-	T49.0X2-	T49.0X3-	T49.0X4-	T49.0X5-	T49.0X6-
antivaricose	T46.8X1-	T46.8X2-	T46.8X3-	T46.8X4-	T46.8X5-	T46.8X6-
bacitracin	T49.0X1-	T49.0X2-	T49.0X3-	T49.0X4-	T49.0X5-	T49.0X6-
chloride (mouthwash)	T49.6X1-	T49.6X2-	T49.6X3-	T49.6X4-	T49.6X5-	T49.6X6-
chromate	T56.5X1-	T56.5X2-	T56.5X3-	T56.5X4-	-	-
gelatin	T49.3X1-	T49.3X2-	T49.3X3-	T49.3X4-	T49.3X5-	T49.3X6-
oxide	T49.3X1-	T49.3X2-	T49.3X3-	T49.3X4-	T49.3X5-	T49.3X6-
plaster	T49.3X1-	T49.3X2-	T49.3X3-	T49.3X4-	T49.3X5-	T49.3X6-
peroxide	T49.0X1-	T49.0X2-	T49.0X3-	T49.0X4-	T49.0X5-	T49.0X6-
pesticides	T56.5X1-	T56.5X2-	T56.5X3-	T56.5X4-	-	-
phosphide	T60.4X1-	T60.4X2-	T60.4X3-	T60.4X4-	-	-
pyrithionate	T49.4X1-	T49.4X2-	T49.4X3-	T49.4X4-	T49.4X5-	T49.4X6-
stearate	T49.3X1-	T49.3X2-	T49.3X3-	T49.3X4-	T49.3X5-	T49.3X6-
sulfate	T49.5X1-	T49.5X2-	T49.5X3-	T49.5X4-	T49.5X5-	T49.5X6-
ENT agent	T49.6X1-	T49.6X2-	T49.6X3-	T49.6X4-	T49.6X5-	T49.6X6-
ophthalmic solution	T49.5X1-	T49.5X2-	T49.5X3-	T49.5X4-	T49.5X5-	T49.5X6-
topical NEC	T49.0X1-	T49.0X2-	T49.0X3-	T49.0X4-	T49.0X5-	T49.0X6-
undecylenate	T49.0X1-	T49.0X2-	T49.0X3-	T49.0X4-	T49.0X5-	T49.0X6-
Zineb	T60.0X1-	T60.0X2-	T60.0X3-	T60.0X4-	-	-
Zinostatin	T45.1X1-	T45.1X2-	T45.1X3-	T45.1X4-	T45.1X5-	T45.1X6-
Zipeprol	T48.3X1-	T48.3X2-	T48.3X3-	T48.3X4-	T48.3X5-	T48.3X6-
Zofenopril	T46.4X1-	T46.4X2-	T46.4X3-	T46.4X4-	T46.4X5-	T46.4X6-
Zolpidem	T42.6X1-	T42.6X2-	T42.6X3-	T42.6X4-	T42.6X5-	T42.6X6-
Zomepirac	T39.391-	T39.392-	T39.393-	T39.394-	T39.395-	T39.396-
Zopiclone	T42.6X1-	T42.6X2-	T42.6X3-	T42.6X4-	T42.6X5-	T42.6X6-
Zorubicin	T45.1X1-	T45.1X2-	T45.1X3-	T45.1X4-	T45.1X5-	T45.1X6-
Zotepine	T43.591-	T43.592-	T43.593-	T43.594-	T43.595-	T43.596-
Zovant	T45.511-	T45.512-	T45.513-	T45.514-	T45.515-	T45.516-
Zoxazolamine	T42.8X1-	T42.8X2-	T42.8X3-	T42.8X4-	T42.8X5-	T42.8X6-
Zuclopenthixol	T43.4X1-	T43.4X2-	T43.4X3-	T43.4X4-	T43.4X5-	T43.4X6-
Zygadenus (venenosus)	T62.2X1-	T62.2X2-	T62.2X3-	T62.2X4-	-	-
Zyprexa	T43.591-	T43.592-	T43.593-	T43.594-	T43.595-	T43.596-

Index to External Cause of Injuries

The final section of the Alphabetic Index is the Index to External Cause of Injuries. This section classifies environmental events, circumstances, and conditions as the ***cause of*** injury, poisoning and other adverse effects. The Index to External Cause of Injuries is organized by main terms that describe the accident, circumstance, event, or specific agent causing the injury or other adverse effect.

External cause codes are intended to provide data for injury research and evaluation of injury prevention strategies. These codes capture how the injury or health condition happened (cause), the intent (unintentional or accidental; or intentional, such as suicide or assault), the place where the event occurred, the activity of the patient at the time of the event, and the person's status (e.g., civilian, military).

An external cause code may be used with any code in the range of A00.0 – T88.9, Z00 – Z99, classification that is a health condition due to an external cause. Though they are most applicable to injuries, they are also valid for use with such things as infections or diseases due to an external source, and other health conditions, such as a heart attack that occurs during strenuous physical activity.

Important: An external cause code can never be a principal (**first-listed**) diagnosis.

The selection of the appropriate external cause code is guided by the Alphabetic Index of External Causes and by Inclusion and Exclusion notes in the Tabular List.

A

- **Abandonment (causing exposure to weather conditions) (with intent to injure or kill) NEC** X58
- **Abuse (adult) (child) (mental) (physical) (sexual)** X58
- **Accident (to)** X58
  - aircraft (in transit) (powered) — *see also* Accident, transport, aircraft
    - due to, caused by cataclysm — *see* Forces of nature, by type
  - animal-rider — *see* Accident, transport, animal-rider
  - animal-drawn vehicle — *see* Accident, transport, animal-drawn vehicle occupant
  - automobile — *see* Accident, transport, car occupant
  - bare foot water skiier V94.4
  - boat, boating — *see also* Accident, watercraft
    - striking swimmer
      - powered V94.11
      - unpowered V94.12
  - bus — *see* Accident, transport, bus occupant
  - cable car, not on rails V98.0
    - on rails — *see* Accident, transport, streetcar occupant
  - car — *see* Accident, transport, car occupant
  - caused by, due to
    - animal NEC W64
    - chain hoist W24.0
    - cold (excessive) — *see* Exposure, cold
    - corrosive liquid, substance — *see* Table of Drugs and Chemicals
    - cutting or piercing instrument — *see* Contact, with, by type of instrument
    - drive belt W24.0
    - electric
      - current — *see* Exposure, electric current
      - motor — *see also* Contact, with, by type of machine W31.3
        - current (of) W86.8
    - environmental factor NEC X58
    - explosive material — *see* Explosion
    - fire, flames — *see* Exposure, fire
    - firearm missile — *see* Discharge, firearm by type
    - heat (excessive) — *see* Heat
    - hot — *see* Contact, with, hot
    - ignition — *see* Ignition
    - lifting device W24.0
    - lightning — *see* subcategory T75.0
      - causing fire — *see* Exposure, fire
    - machine, machinery — *see* Contact, with, by type of machine
    - natural factor NEC X58
    - pulley (block) W24.0
    - radiation — *see* Radiation
    - steam X13.1
      - inhalation X13.0
      - pipe X16
    - thunderbolt — *see* subcategory T75.0
      - causing fire — *see* Exposure, fire
    - transmission device W24.1
  - coach — *see* Accident, transport, bus occupant
  - coal car — *see* Accident, transport, industrial vehicle occupant
  - diving — *see also* Fall, into, water
    - with
      - drowning or submersion — *see* Drowning
  - forklift — *see* Accident, transport, industrial vehicle occupant
  - heavy transport vehicle NOS — *see* Accident, transport, truck occupant
  - ice yacht V98.2
  - in
    - medical, surgical procedure
      - as, or due to misadventure — *see* Misadventure

Accident (to) - *continued*

- in - *continued*
  - medical, surgical procedure - *continued*
    - causing an abnormal reaction or later complication without mention of misadventure — *see also* Complication of or following, by type of procedure Y84.9
- land yacht V98.1
- late effect of — *see* W00-X58 with 7th character S
- logging car — *see* Accident, transport, industrial vehicle occupant
- machine, machinery — *see also* Contact, with, by type of machine
  - on board watercraft V93.69
    - explosion — *see* Explosion, in, watercraft
    - fire — *see* Burn, on board watercraft
    - powered craft V93.63
      - ferry boat V93.61
      - fishing boat V93.62
      - jetskis V93.63
      - liner V93.61
      - merchant ship V93.60
      - passenger ship V93.61
      - sailboat V93.64
- mine tram — *see* Accident, transport, industrial vehicle occupant
- mobility scooter (motorized) — *see* Accident, transport, pedestrian, conveyance, specified type NEC
- motor scooter — *see* Accident, transport, motorcyclist
- motor vehicle NOS (traffic) — *see also* Accident, transport V89.2
  - nontraffic V89.0
  - three-wheeled NOS — *see* Accident, transport, three-wheeled motor vehicle occupant
- motorcycle NOS — *see* Accident, transport, motorcyclist
- nonmotor vehicle NOS (nontraffic) — *see also* Accident, transport V89.1
  - traffic NOS V89.3
- nontraffic (victim's mode of transport NOS) V88.9
  - collision (between) V88.7
    - bus and truck V88.5
    - car and:
      - bus V88.3
      - pickup V88.2
      - three-wheeled motor vehicle V88.0
      - train V88.6
      - truck V88.4
      - two-wheeled motor vehicle V88.0
      - van V88.2
    - specified vehicle NEC and:
      - three-wheeled motor vehicle V88.1
      - two-wheeled motor vehicle V88.1
  - known mode of transport — *see* Accident, transport, by type of vehicle
  - noncollision V88.8
- on board watercraft V93.89
  - powered craft V93.83
    - ferry boat V93.81
    - fishing boat V93.82
    - jetskis V93.83
    - liner V93.81
    - merchant ship V93.80
    - passenger ship V93.81
  - unpowered craft V93.88
    - canoe V93.85
    - inflatable V93.86
      - in tow
        - recreational V94.31
        - specified NEC V94.32
    - kayak V93.85
    - sailboat V93.84
    - surf-board V93.88
    - water skis V93.87
    - windsurfer V93.88
- parachutist V97.29
  - entangled in object V97.21
  - injured on landing V97.22

Accident (to) - *continued*

- pedal cycle — *see* Accident, transport, pedal cyclist
- pedestrian (on foot)
  - with
    - another pedestrian W51
      - with fall W03
        - due to ice or snow W00.0
      - on pedestrian conveyance NEC V00.09
    - rider of
      - hoverboard V00.038
      - Segway V00.038
      - standing
        - electric scooter V00.031
        - micro-mobility pedestrian conveyance NEC V00.038
    - roller skater (in-line) V00.01
    - skate boarder V00.02
    - transport vehicle — *see* Accident, transport
  - on pedestrian conveyance — *see* Accident, transport, pedestrian, conveyance
- pick-up truck or van — *see* Accident, transport, pickup truck occupant
- quarry truck — *see* Accident, transport, industrial vehicle occupant
- railway vehicle (any) (in motion) — *see* Accident, transport, railway vehicle occupant
  - due to cataclysm — *see* Forces of nature, by type
- scooter (non-motorized) — *see* Accident, transport, pedestrian, conveyance, scooter
- sequelae of — *see* W00-X58 with 7th character S
- skateboard — *see* Accident, transport, pedestrian, conveyance, skateboard
- ski (ing) — *see* Accident, transport, pedestrian, conveyance
  - lift V98.3
- specified cause NEC X58
- streetcar — *see* Accident, transport, streetcar occupant
- traffic (victim's mode of transport NOS) V87.9
  - collision (between) V87.7
    - bus and truck V87.5
    - car and:
      - bus V87.3
      - pickup V87.2
      - three-wheeled motor vehicle V87.0
      - train V87.6
      - truck V87.4
      - two-wheeled motor vehicle V87.0
      - van V87.2
    - specified vehicle NEC V86.39
      - and
        - three-wheeled motor vehicle V87.1
        - two-wheeled motor vehicle V87.1
      - driver V86.09
      - person on outside V86.29
      - passenger V86.19
      - while boarding or alighting V86.49
  - known mode of transport — *see* Accident, transport, by type of vehicle
  - noncollision V87.8
- transport (involving injury to) V99
  - 18 wheeler — *see* Accident, transport, truck occupant
  - agricultural vehicle occupant (nontraffic) V84.9
    - driver V84.5
    - hanger-on V84.7
    - passenger V84.6
    - traffic V84.3
      - driver V84.0
      - hanger-on V84.2
      - passenger V84.1
    - while boarding or alighting V84.4
  - aircraft NEC V97.89
    - military NEC V97.818
      - with civilian aircraft V97.810
      - civilian injured by V97.811

ACCIDENT - ACCIDENT

- **Accident (to)** - *continued*
  - transport (involving injury to) - *continued*
    - bus occupant - *continued*
      - driver - *continued*
        - collision (with) - *continued*
          - streetcar (traffic) - *continued*
            - nontraffic V76.0
          - three wheeled motor vehicle (traffic) V72.5
            - nontraffic V72.0
          - truck (traffic) V74.5
            - nontraffic V74.0
          - two wheeled motor vehicle (traffic) V72.5
            - nontraffic V72.0
          - van (traffic) V73.5
            - nontraffic V73.0
        - noncollision accident (traffic) V78.5
          - nontraffic V78.0
      - noncollision accident (traffic) V78.9
        - nontraffic V78.3
        - while boarding or alighting V78.4
      - nontraffic V79.3
      - hanger-on
        - collision (with)
          - animal (traffic) V70.7
            - being ridden (traffic) V76.7
              - nontraffic V76.2
            - nontraffic V70.2
          - animal-drawn vehicle (traffic) V76.7
            - nontraffic V76.2
          - bus (traffic) V74.7
            - nontraffic V74.2
          - car (traffic) V73.7
            - nontraffic V73.2
          - pedal cycle (traffic) V71.7
            - nontraffic V71.2
          - pickup truck (traffic) V73.7
            - nontraffic V73.2
          - railway vehicle (traffic) V75.7
            - nontraffic V75.2
          - specified vehicle NEC (traffic) V76.7
            - nontraffic V76.2
          - stationary object (traffic) V77.7
            - nontraffic V77.2
          - streetcar (traffic) V76.7
            - nontraffic V76.2
          - three wheeled motor vehicle (traffic) V72.7
            - nontraffic V72.2
          - truck (traffic) V74.7
            - nontraffic V74.2
          - two wheeled motor vehicle (traffic) V72.7
            - nontraffic V72.2
          - van (traffic) V73.7
            - nontraffic V73.2
        - noncollision accident (traffic) V78.7
          - nontraffic V78.2
      - passenger
        - collision (with)
          - animal (traffic) V70.6
            - being ridden (traffic) V76.6
              - nontraffic V76.1
            - nontraffic V70.1
          - animal-drawn vehicle (traffic) V76.6
            - nontraffic V76.1
          - bus (traffic) V74.6
            - nontraffic V74.1
          - car (traffic) V73.6
            - nontraffic V73.1
          - motor vehicle NOS (traffic) V79.50
            - nontraffic V79.10
            - specified type NEC (traffic) V79.59
              - nontraffic V79.19
          - pedal cycle (traffic) V71.6
            - nontraffic V71.1
          - pickup truck (traffic) V73.6
            - nontraffic V73.1
          - railway vehicle (traffic) V75.6
            - nontraffic V75.1

- **Accident (to)** - *continued*
  - transport (involving injury to) - *continued*
    - bus occupant - *continued*
      - passenger - *continued*
        - collision (with) - *continued*
          - specified vehicle NEC (traffic) V76.6
            - nontraffic V76.1
          - stationary object (traffic) V77.6
            - nontraffic V77.1
          - streetcar (traffic) V76.6
            - nontraffic V76.1
          - three wheeled motor vehicle (traffic) V72.6
            - nontraffic V72.1
          - truck (traffic) V74.6
            - nontraffic V74.1
          - two wheeled motor vehicle (traffic) V72.6
            - nontraffic V72.1
          - van (traffic) V73.6
            - nontraffic V73.1
        - noncollision accident (traffic) V78.6
          - nontraffic V78.1
      - specified type NEC V79.88
        - military vehicle V79.81
    - cable car, not on rails V98.0
      - on rails — *see* Accident, transport, streetcar occupant
    - car occupant V49.9
      - ambulance occupant — *see* Accident, transport, ambulance occupant
      - collision (with)
        - animal (traffic) V40.9
          - being ridden (traffic) V46.9
            - nontraffic V46.3
            - while boarding or alighting V46.4
          - nontraffic V40.3
          - while boarding or alighting V40.4
        - animal-drawn vehicle (traffic) V46.9
          - nontraffic V46.3
          - while boarding or alighting V46.4
        - bus (traffic) V44.9
          - nontraffic V44.3
          - while boarding or alighting V44.4
        - car (traffic) V43.92
          - nontraffic V43.32
          - while boarding or alighting V43.42
        - motor vehicle NOS (traffic) V49.60
          - nontraffic V49.20
          - specified type NEC (traffic) V49.69
            - nontraffic V49.29
        - pedal cycle (traffic) V41.9
          - nontraffic V41.3
          - while boarding or alighting V41.4
        - pickup truck (traffic) V43.93
          - nontraffic V43.33
          - while boarding or alighting V43.43
        - railway vehicle (traffic) V45.9
          - nontraffic V45.3
          - while boarding or alighting V45.4
        - specified vehicle NEC (traffic) V46.9
          - nontraffic V46.3
          - while boarding or alighting V46.4
        - sport utility vehicle (traffic) V43.91
          - nontraffic V43.31
          - while boarding or alighting V43.41
        - stationary object (traffic) V47.9
          - nontraffic V47.3
          - while boarding or alighting V47.4
        - streetcar (traffic) V46.9
          - nontraffic V46.3
          - while boarding or alighting V46.4
        - three wheeled motor vehicle (traffic) V42.9
          - nontraffic V42.3
          - while boarding or alighting V42.4
        - truck (traffic) V44.9
          - nontraffic V44.3
          - while boarding or alighting V44.4
        - two wheeled motor vehicle (traffic) V42.9
          - nontraffic V42.3
          - while boarding or alighting V42.4
        - van (traffic) V43.94

- **Accident (to)** - *continued*
  - transport (involving injury to) - *continued*
    - car occupant - *continued*
      - collision (with) - *continued*
        - van (traffic) - *continued*
          - nontraffic V43.34
          - while boarding or alighting V43.44
      - driver
        - collision (with)
          - animal (traffic) V40.5
            - being ridden (traffic) V46.5
              - nontraffic V46.0
            - nontraffic V40.0
          - animal-drawn vehicle (traffic) V46.5
            - nontraffic V46.0
          - bus (traffic) V44.5
            - nontraffic V44.0
          - car (traffic) V43.52
            - nontraffic V43.02
          - motor vehicle NOS (traffic) V49.40
            - nontraffic V49.00
            - specified type NEC (traffic) V49.49
              - nontraffic V49.09
          - pedal cycle (traffic) V41.5
            - nontraffic V41.0
          - pickup truck (traffic) V43.53
            - nontraffic V43.03
          - railway vehicle (traffic) V45.5
            - nontraffic V45.0
          - specified vehicle NEC (traffic) V46.5
            - nontraffic V46.0
          - sport utility vehicle (traffic) V43.51
            - nontraffic V43.01
          - stationary object (traffic) V47.5
            - nontraffic V47.0
          - streetcar (traffic) V46.5
            - nontraffic V46.0
          - three wheeled motor vehicle (traffic) V42.5
            - nontraffic V42.0
          - truck (traffic) V44.5
            - nontraffic V44.0
          - two wheeled motor vehicle (traffic) V42.5
            - nontraffic V42.0
          - van (traffic) V43.54
            - nontraffic V43.04
        - noncollision accident (traffic) V48.5
          - nontraffic V48.0
      - noncollision accident (traffic) V48.9
        - nontraffic V48.3
        - while boarding or alighting V48.4
      - nontraffic V49.3
      - hanger-on
        - collision (with)
          - animal (traffic) V40.7
            - being ridden (traffic) V46.7
              - nontraffic V46.2
            - nontraffic V40.2
          - animal-drawn vehicle (traffic) V46.7
            - nontraffic V46.2
          - bus (traffic) V44.7
            - nontraffic V44.2
          - car (traffic) V43.72
            - nontraffic V43.22
          - pedal cycle (traffic) V41.7
            - nontraffic V41.2
          - pickup truck (traffic) V43.73
            - nontraffic V43.23
          - railway vehicle (traffic) V45.7
            - nontraffic V45.2
          - specified vehicle NEC (traffic) V46.7
            - nontraffic V46.2
          - sport utility vehicle (traffic) V43.71
            - nontraffic V43.21
          - stationary object (traffic) V47.7
            - nontraffic V47.2
          - streetcar (traffic) V46.7
            - nontraffic V46.2

ACCIDENT - ACCIDENT

- **Accident (to)** - *continued*
  - transport (involving injury to) - *continued*
    - person NEC (unknown way or transportation) - *continued*
      - collision (between) - *continued*
        - bus (with) - *continued*
          - heavy transport vehicle (traffic) V87.5
            - nontraffic V88.5
        - car (with)
          - nontraffic V88.5
          - bus (traffic) V87.3
            - nontraffic V88.3
          - heavy transport vehicle (traffic) V87.4
            - nontraffic V88.4
          - pick-up truck or van (traffic) V87.2
            - nontraffic V88.2
          - train or railway vehicle (traffic) V87.6
            - nontraffic V88.6
          - two-or three-wheeled motor vehicle (traffic) V87.0
            - nontraffic V88.0
        - motor vehicle (traffic) NEC V87.7
          - nontraffic V88.7
        - two-or three-wheeled vehicle (with) (traffic)
          - motor vehicle NEC V87.1
            - nontraffic V88.1
      - nonmotor vehicle (collision) (noncollision) (traffic) V87.9
        - nontraffic V88.9
    - pickup truck occupant V59.9
      - collision (with)
        - animal (traffic) V50.9
          - being ridden (traffic) V56.9
            - nontraffic V56.3
            - while boarding or alighting V56.4
          - nontraffic V50.3
          - while boarding or alighting V50.4
        - animal-drawn vehicle (traffic) V56.9
          - nontraffic V56.3
          - while boarding or alighting V56.4
        - bus (traffic) V54.9
          - nontraffic V54.3
          - while boarding or alighting V54.4
        - car (traffic) V53.9
          - nontraffic V53.3
          - while boarding or alighting V53.4
        - motor vehicle NOS (traffic) V59.60
          - nontraffic V59.20
          - specified type NEC (traffic) V59.69
            - nontraffic V59.29
        - pedal cycle (traffic) V51.9
          - nontraffic V51.3
          - while boarding or alighting V51.4
        - pickup truck (traffic) V53.9
          - nontraffic V53.3
          - while boarding or alighting V53.4
        - railway vehicle (traffic) V55.9
          - nontraffic V55.3
          - while boarding or alighting V55.4
        - specified vehicle NEC (traffic) V56.9
          - nontraffic V56.3
          - while boarding or alighting V56.4
        - stationary object (traffic) V57.9
          - nontraffic V57.3
          - while boarding or alighting V57.4
        - streetcar (traffic) V56.9
          - nontraffic V56.3
          - while boarding or alighting V56.4
        - three wheeled motor vehicle (traffic) V52.9
          - nontraffic V52.3
          - while boarding or alighting V52.4
        - truck (traffic) V54.9
          - nontraffic V54.3
          - while boarding or alighting V54.4
        - two wheeled motor vehicle (traffic) V52.9
          - nontraffic V52.3
          - while boarding or alighting V52.4
        - van (traffic) V53.9
          - nontraffic V53.3

- **Accident (to)** - *continued*
  - transport (involving injury to) - *continued*
    - pickup truck occupant - *continued*
      - collision (with) - *continued*
        - van (traffic) - *continued*
          - while boarding or alighting V53.4
      - driver
        - collision (with)
          - animal (traffic) V50.5
            - being ridden (traffic) V56.5
              - nontraffic V56.0
            - nontraffic V50.0
          - animal-drawn vehicle (traffic) V56.5
            - nontraffic V56.0
          - bus (traffic) V54.5
            - nontraffic V54.0
          - car (traffic) V53.5
            - nontraffic V53.0
          - motor vehicle NOS (traffic) V59.40
            - nontraffic V59.00
            - specified type NEC (traffic) V59.49
              - nontraffic V59.09
          - pedal cycle (traffic) V51.5
            - nontraffic V51.0
          - pickup truck (traffic) V53.5
            - nontraffic V53.0
          - railway vehicle (traffic) V55.5
            - nontraffic V55.0
          - specified vehicle NEC (traffic) V56.5
            - nontraffic V56.0
          - stationary object (traffic) V57.5
            - nontraffic V57.0
          - streetcar (traffic) V56.5
            - nontraffic V56.0
          - three wheeled motor vehicle (traffic) V52.5
            - nontraffic V52.0
          - truck (traffic) V54.5
            - nontraffic V54.0
          - two wheeled motor vehicle (traffic) V52.5
            - nontraffic V52.0
          - van (traffic) V53.5
            - nontraffic V53.0
        - noncollision accident (traffic) V58.5
          - nontraffic V58.0
      - noncollision accident (traffic) V58.9
        - nontraffic V58.3
        - while boarding or alighting V58.4
      - nontraffic V59.3
      - hanger-on
        - collision (with)
          - animal (traffic) V50.7
            - being ridden (traffic) V56.7
              - nontraffic V56.2
            - nontraffic V50.2
          - animal-drawn vehicle (traffic) V56.7
            - nontraffic V56.2
          - bus (traffic) V54.7
            - nontraffic V54.2
          - car (traffic) V53.7
            - nontraffic V53.2
          - pedal cycle (traffic) V51.7
            - nontraffic V51.2
          - pickup truck (traffic) V53.7
            - nontraffic V53.2
          - railway vehicle (traffic) V55.7
            - nontraffic V55.2
          - specified vehicle NEC (traffic) V56.7
            - nontraffic V56.2
          - stationary object (traffic) V57.7
            - nontraffic V57.2
          - streetcar (traffic) V56.7
            - nontraffic V56.2
          - three wheeled motor vehicle (traffic) V52.7
            - nontraffic V52.2
          - truck (traffic) V54.7
            - nontraffic V54.2

- **Accident (to)** - *continued*
  - transport (involving injury to) - *continued*
    - pickup truck occupant - *continued*
      - hanger-on - *continued*
        - collision (with) - *continued*
          - two wheeled motor vehicle (traffic) V52.7
            - nontraffic V52.2
          - van (traffic) V53.7
            - nontraffic V53.2
        - noncollision accident (traffic) V58.7
          - nontraffic V58.2
      - passenger
        - collision (with)
          - animal (traffic) V50.6
            - being ridden (traffic) V56.6
              - nontraffic V56.1
            - nontraffic V50.1
          - animal-drawn vehicle (traffic) V56.6
            - nontraffic V56.1
          - bus (traffic) V54.6
            - nontraffic V54.1
          - car (traffic) V53.6
            - nontraffic V53.1
          - motor vehicle NOS (traffic) V59.50
            - nontraffic V59.10
            - specified type NEC (traffic) V59.59
              - nontraffic V59.19
          - pedal cycle (traffic) V51.6
            - nontraffic V51.1
          - pickup truck (traffic) V53.6
            - nontraffic V53.1
          - railway vehicle (traffic) V55.6
            - nontraffic V55.1
          - specified vehicle NEC (traffic) V56.6
            - nontraffic V56.1
          - stationary object (traffic) V57.6
            - nontraffic V57.1
          - streetcar (traffic) V56.6
            - nontraffic V56.1
          - three wheeled motor vehicle (traffic) V52.6
            - nontraffic V52.1
          - truck (traffic) V54.6
            - nontraffic V54.1
          - two wheeled motor vehicle (traffic) V52.6
            - nontraffic V52.1
          - van (traffic) V53.6
            - nontraffic V53.1
        - noncollision accident (traffic) V58.6
          - nontraffic V58.1
      - specified type NEC V59.88
        - military vehicle V59.81
    - quarry truck — *see* Accident, transport, industrial vehicle occupant
    - race car — *see* Accident, transport, motor vehicle NEC occupant
    - railway vehicle occupant V81.9
      - collision (with) V81.3
        - motor vehicle (non-military) (traffic) V81.1
          - military V81.83
          - nontraffic V81.0
        - rolling stock V81.2
        - specified object NEC V81.3
      - during derailment V81.7
        - with antecedent collision — *see* Accident, transport, railway vehicle occupant, collision
      - explosion V81.81
      - fall (in railway vehicle) V81.5
        - during derailment V81.7
          - with antecedent collision — *see* Accident, transport, railway vehicle occupant, collision
        - from railway vehicle V81.6
          - during derailment V81.7
            - with antecedent collision — *see* Accident, transport, railway vehicle occupant, collision
        - while boarding or alighting V81.4

Accident (to) - *continued*
transport (involving injury to) - *continued*
railway vehicle occupant - *continued*
fire V81.81
object falling onto train V81.82
specified type NEC V81.89
while boarding or alighting V81.4
Segway V00.848
ski lift V98.3
snowmobile occupant (nontraffic) V86.92
driver V86.52
hanger-on V86.72
passenger V86.62
traffic V86.32
driver V86.02
hanger-on V86.22
passenger V86.12
while boarding or alighting V86.42
specified NEC V98.8
sport utility vehicle occupant — *see also* Accident, transport, pickup truck occupant
streetcar occupant V82.9
collision (with) V82.3
motor vehicle (traffic) V82.1
nontraffic V82.0
rolling stock V82.2
during derailment V82.7
with antecedent collision — *see* Accident, transport, streetcar occupant, collision
fall (in streetcar) V82.5
during derailment V82.7
with antecedent collision — *see* Accident, transport, streetcar occupant, collision
from streetcar V82.6
during derailment V82.7
with antecedent collision — *see* Accident, transport, streetcar occupant, collision
while boarding or alighting V82.4
while boarding or alighting V82.4
specified type NEC V82.8
while boarding or alighting V82.4
three-wheeled motor vehicle occupant V39.9
collision (with)
animal (traffic) V30.9
being ridden (traffic) V36.9
nontraffic V36.3
while boarding or alighting V36.4
nontraffic V30.3
while boarding or alighting V30.4
animal-drawn vehicle (traffic) V36.9
nontraffic V36.3
while boarding or alighting V36.4
bus (traffic) V34.9
nontraffic V34.3
while boarding or alighting V34.4
car (traffic) V33.9
nontraffic V33.3
while boarding or alighting V33.4
motor vehicle NOS (traffic) V39.60
nontraffic V39.20
specified type NEC (traffic) V39.69
nontraffic V39.29
pedal cycle (traffic) V31.9
nontraffic V31.3
while boarding or alighting V31.4
pickup truck (traffic) V33.9
nontraffic V33.3
while boarding or alighting V33.4
railway vehicle (traffic) V35.9
nontraffic V35.3
while boarding or alighting V35.4
specified vehicle NEC (traffic) V36.9
nontraffic V36.3
while boarding or alighting V36.4
stationary object (traffic) V37.9
nontraffic V37.3
while boarding or alighting V37.4
streetcar (traffic) V36.9
nontraffic V36.3
while boarding or alighting V36.4

Accident (to) - *continued*
transport (involving injury to) - *continued*
three-wheeled motor vehicle occupant - *continued*
collision (with) - *continued*
three wheeled motor vehicle (traffic) V32.9
nontraffic V32.3
while boarding or alighting V32.4
truck (traffic) V34.9
nontraffic V34.3
while boarding or alighting V34.4
two wheeled motor vehicle (traffic) V32.9
nontraffic V32.3
while boarding or alighting V32.4
van (traffic) V33.9
nontraffic V33.3
while boarding or alighting V33.4
driver
collision (with)
animal (traffic) V30.5
being ridden (traffic) V36.5
nontraffic V36.0
nontraffic V30.0
animal-drawn vehicle (traffic) V36.5
nontraffic V36.0
bus (traffic) V34.5
nontraffic V34.0
car (traffic) V33.5
nontraffic V33.0
motor vehicle NOS (traffic) V39.40
nontraffic V39.00
specified type NEC (traffic) V39.49
nontraffic V39.09
pedal cycle (traffic) V31.5
nontraffic V31.0
pickup truck (traffic) V33.5
nontraffic V33.0
railway vehicle (traffic) V35.5
nontraffic V35.0
specified vehicle NEC (traffic) V36.5
nontraffic V36.0
stationary object (traffic) V37.5
nontraffic V37.0
streetcar (traffic) V36.5
nontraffic V36.0
three wheeled motor vehicle (traffic) V32.5
nontraffic V32.0
truck (traffic) V34.5
nontraffic V34.0
two wheeled motor vehicle (traffic) V32.5
nontraffic V32.0
van (traffic) V33.5
nontraffic V33.0
noncollision accident (traffic) V38.5
nontraffic V38.0
noncollision accident (traffic) V38.9
nontraffic V38.3
while boarding or alighting V38.4
nontraffic V39.3
hanger-on
collision (with)
animal (traffic) V30.7
being ridden (traffic) V36.7
nontraffic V36.2
nontraffic V30.2
animal-drawn vehicle (traffic) V36.7
nontraffic V36.2
bus (traffic) V34.7
nontraffic V34.2
car (traffic) V33.7
nontraffic V33.2
pedal cycle (traffic) V31.7
nontraffic V31.2
pickup truck (traffic) V33.7
nontraffic V33.2
railway vehicle (traffic) V35.7
nontraffic V35.2

Accident (to) - *continued*
transport (involving injury to) - *continued*
three-wheeled motor vehicle occupant - *continued*
hanger-on - *continued*
collision (with) - *continued*
specified vehicle NEC (traffic) V36.7
nontraffic V36.2
stationary object (traffic) V37.7
nontraffic V37.2
streetcar (traffic) V36.7
nontraffic V36.2
three wheeled motor vehicle (traffic) V32.7
nontraffic V32.2
truck (traffic) V34.7
nontraffic V34.2
two wheeled motor vehicle (traffic) V32.7
nontraffic V32.2
van (traffic) V33.7
nontraffic V33.2
noncollision accident (traffic) V38.7
nontraffic V38.2
passenger
collision (with)
animal (traffic) V30.6
being ridden (traffic) V36.6
nontraffic V36.1
nontraffic V30.1
animal-drawn vehicle (traffic) V36.6
nontraffic V36.1
bus (traffic) V34.6
nontraffic V34.1
car (traffic) V33.6
nontraffic V33.1
motor vehicle NOS (traffic) V39.50
nontraffic V39.10
specified type NEC (traffic) V39.59
nontraffic V39.19
pedal cycle (traffic) V31.6
nontraffic V31.1
pickup truck (traffic) V33.6
nontraffic V33.1
railway vehicle (traffic) V35.6
nontraffic V35.1
specified vehicle NEC (traffic) V36.6
nontraffic V36.1
stationary object (traffic) V37.6
nontraffic V37.1
streetcar (traffic) V36.6
nontraffic V36.1
three wheeled motor vehicle (traffic) V32.6
nontraffic V32.1
truck (traffic) V34.6
nontraffic V34.1
two wheeled motor vehicle (traffic) V32.6
nontraffic V32.1
van (traffic) V33.6
nontraffic V33.1
noncollision accident (traffic) V38.6
nontraffic V38.1
specified type NEC V39.89
military vehicle V39.81
tractor (farm) (and trailer) — *see* Accident, transport, agricultural vehicle occupant
tram — *see* Accident, transport, streetcar
in mine or quarry — *see* Accident, transport, industrial vehicle occupant
trolley — *see* Accident, transport, streetcar
in mine or quarry — *see* Accident, transport, industrial vehicle occupant
truck (heavy) occupant V69.9
collision (with)
animal (traffic) V60.9
being ridden (traffic) V66.9

ACCIDENT - ACTIVITY

Activity (involving) (of victim at time of event) - *continued*
- soccer Y93.66
- softball Y93.64
- specified NEC Y93.89
- spectator at an event Y93.82
- sports NEC Y93.79
  - sports played as a team or group NEC Y93.69
  - sports played individually NEC Y93.59
- springboard diving Y93.12
- squash Y93.73
- stationary bike Y93.A1
- step (stepping) exercise (class) Y93.A3
- stepper machine Y93.A1
- stove Y93.G3
- string instrument playing Y93.J3
- surfing Y93.18
  - wind Y93.18
- swimming Y93.11
- tackle football Y93.61
- tap dancing Y93.41
- tennis Y93.73
- tobogganing Y93.23
- touch football Y93.62
- track and field events (non-running) Y93.57
  - running Y93.02
- trampoline Y93.44
- treadmill Y93.A1
- trimming shrubs Y93.H2
- tubing (in calm and turbulent water) Y93.16
  - snow Y93.23
- ultimate frisbee Y93.74
- underwater diving Y93.15
- unpacking in moving to a new residence Y93.E6
- use of stove, oven and microwave oven Y93.G3
- vacuuming Y93.E3
- volleyball (beach) (court) Y93.68
- wake boarding Y93.17
- walking an animal Y93.K1
- walking (on level or elevated terrain) Y93.01
  - an animal Y93.K1
- wall climbing Y93.31
- warm up and cool down exercises Y93.A2
- water NEC Y93.19
  - aerobics Y93.14
  - craft NEC Y93.19
  - exercise Y93.14
  - polo Y93.13
  - skiing Y93.17
  - sliding Y93.18
  - survival training and testing Y93.19
- weeding (garden and lawn) Y93.H2
- wind instrument playing Y93.J4
- windsurfing Y93.18
- wrestling Y93.72
- yoga Y93.42

Adverse effect of drugs — *see* Table of Drugs and Chemicals

Aerosinusitis - — *see* Air, pressure

After-effect, late — *see* Sequelae

Air
- blast in war operations — *see* War operations, air blast
- pressure
  - change, rapid
    - during
      - ascent W94.29
        - while (in) (surfacing from)
          - aircraft W94.23
          - deep water diving W94.21
          - underground W94.22
      - descent W94.39
        - in
          - aircraft W94.31
          - water W94.32
  - high, prolonged W94.0
  - low, prolonged W94.12
    - due to residence or long visit at high altitude W94.11

Alpine sickness W94.11

Altitude sickness W94.11

Anaphylactic shock, anaphylaxis — *see* Table of Drugs and Chemicals

Andes disease W94.11

Arachnidism, arachnoidism X58

Arson (with intent to injure or kill) X97

Asphyxia, asphyxiation
- by
  - food (bone) (seed) — *see* categories T17 and T18
  - gas — *see also* Table of Drugs and Chemicals
    - legal
      - execution — *see* Legal, intervention, gas
      - intervention — *see* Legal, intervention, gas
- from
  - fire — *see also* Exposure, fire
    - in war operations — *see* War operations, fire
  - ignition — *see* Ignition
  - vomitus T17.81
- in war operations — *see* War operations, restriction of airway

Aspiration
- food (any type) (into respiratory tract) (with asphyxia, obstruction respiratory tract, suffocation) — *see* categories T17 and T18
- foreign body — *see* Foreign body, aspiration
- vomitus (with asphyxia, obstruction respiratory tract, suffocation) T17.81

Assassination (attempt) — *see* Assault

Assault (homicidal) (by) (in) Y09
- arson X97
- bite (of human being) Y04.1
- bodily force Y04.8
  - bite Y04.1
  - bumping into Y04.2
  - sexual — *see* subcategories T74.0, T76.0
  - unarmed fight Y04.0
- bomb X96.9
  - antipersonnel X96.0
  - fertilizer X96.3
  - gasoline X96.1
  - letter X96.2
  - petrol X96.1
  - pipe X96.3
  - specified NEC X96.8
- brawl (hand) (fists) (foot) (unarmed) Y04.0
- burning, burns (by fire) NEC X97
  - acid Y08.89
  - caustic, corrosive substance Y08.89
  - chemical from swallowing caustic, corrosive substance — *see* Table of Drugs and Chemicals
  - cigarette (s) X97
  - hot object X98.9
    - fluid NEC X98.2
    - household appliance X98.3
    - specified NEC X98.8
    - steam X98.0
    - tap water X98.1
    - vapors X98.0
  - scalding — *see* Assault, burning
  - steam X98.0
  - vitriol Y08.89
- caustic, corrosive substance (gas) Y08.89
- crashing of
  - aircraft Y08.81
  - motor vehicle Y03.8
    - pushed in front of Y02.0
    - run over Y03.0
    - specified NEC Y03.8
- cutting or piercing instrument X99.9
  - dagger X99.2
  - glass X99.0
  - knife X99.1
  - specified NEC X99.8
  - sword X99.2
- dagger X99.2
- drowning (in) X92.9
  - bathtub X92.0
  - natural water X92.3
  - specified NEC X92.8

Assault (homicidal) (by) (in) - *continued*
- drowning (in) - *continued*
  - swimming pool X92.1
    - following fall X92.2
- dynamite X96.8
- explosive (s) (material) X96.9
- fight (hand) (fists) (foot) (unarmed) Y04.0
  - with weapon — *see* Assault, by type of weapon
- fire X97
- firearm X95.9
  - airgun X95.01
  - handgun X93
  - hunting rifle X94.1
  - larger X94.9
    - specified NEC X94.8
  - machine gun X94.2
  - shotgun X94.0
  - specified NEC X95.8
- gunshot (wound) NEC — *see* Assault, firearm, by type
- incendiary device X97
- injury Y09
  - to child due to criminal abortion attempt NEC Y08.89
- knife X99.1
- late effect of — *see* X92-Y08 with 7th character S
- placing before moving object NEC Y02.8
  - motor vehicle Y02.0
- poisoning — *see* categories T36-T65 with 7th character S
- puncture, any part of body — *see* Assault, cutting or piercing instrument
- pushing
  - before moving object NEC Y02.8
    - motor vehicle Y02.0
    - subway train Y02.1
    - train Y02.1
  - from high place Y01
- rape T74.2-
- scalding — *see* Assault, burning
- sequelae of — *see* X92-Y08 with 7th character S
- sexual (by bodily force) T74.2-
- shooting — *see* Assault, firearm
- specified means NEC Y08.89
- stab, any part of body — *see* Assault, cutting or piercing instrument
- steam X98.0
- striking against
  - other person Y04.2
  - sports equipment Y08.09
    - baseball bat Y08.02
    - hockey stick Y08.01
- struck by
  - sports equipment Y08.09
    - baseball bat Y08.02
    - hockey stick Y08.01
- submersion — *see* Assault, drowning
- violence Y09
- weapon Y09
  - blunt Y00
  - cutting or piercing — *see* Assault, cutting or piercing instrument
  - firearm — *see* Assault, firearm
- wound Y09
  - cutting — *see* Assault, cutting or piercing instrument
  - gunshot — *see* Assault, firearm
  - knife X99.1
  - piercing — *see* Assault, cutting or piercing instrument
  - puncture — *see* Assault, cutting or piercing instrument
  - stab — *see* Assault, cutting or piercing instrument

Attack by mammals NEC W55.89

Avalanche — *see* Landslide

Aviator's disease - — *see* Air, pressure

B

Barotitis, barodontalgia, barosinusitis, barotrauma (otitic) (sinus) - — *see* Air, pressure

C

Complication (delayed) of or following (medical or surgical procedure) - *continued*
- shock therapy Y84.3
- surgical operation NEC — *see also* Complication of or following, by type of operation Y83.9
  - reconstructive NEC Y83.4
    - with
      - anastomosis, bypass or graft Y83.2
      - formation of external stoma Y83.3
  - specified NEC Y83.8
- transfusion — *see also* Table of Drugs and Chemicals
  - procedure Y84.8
- transplant, transplantation (heart) (kidney) (liver) (whole organ, any) Y83.0
  - partial organ Y83.4
- ureterostomy Y83.3
- vaccination — *see also* Table of Drugs and Chemicals
  - procedure Y84.8

Compression
- divers' squeeze - — *see* Air, pressure, change
- trachea by
  - food (lodged in esophagus) — *see* categories T17 and T18
  - vomitus (lodged in esophagus) T17.81-

Conflagration — *see* Exposure, fire, uncontrolled

Constriction (external)
- hair W49.01
- jewelry W49.04
- ring W49.04
- rubber band W49.03
- specified item NEC W49.09
- string W49.02
- thread W49.02

Contact (accidental)
- with
  - abrasive wheel (metalworking) W31.1
  - alligator W58.09
    - bite W58.01
    - crushing W58.03
    - strike W58.02
  - amphibian W62.9
    - frog W62.0
    - toad W62.1
  - animal (nonvenomous) NEC W64
    - marine W56.89
      - bite W56.81
      - dolphin — *see* Contact, with, dolphin
      - fish NEC — *see* Contact, with, fish
      - mammal — *see* Contact, with, mammal, marine
      - orca — *see* Contact, with, orca
      - sea lion — *see* Contact, with, sea lion
      - shark — *see* Contact, with, shark
      - strike W56.82
  - animate mechanical force NEC W64
  - arrow W21.89
    - not thrown, projected or falling W45.8
  - arthropods (nonvenomous) W57
  - axe W27.0
  - band-saw (industrial) W31.2
  - bayonet — *see* Bayonet wound
  - bee (s) X58
  - bench-saw (industrial) W31.2
  - bird W61.99
    - bite W61.91
    - chicken — *see* Contact, with, chicken
    - duck — *see* Contact, with, duck
    - goose — *see* Contact, with, goose
    - macaw — *see* Contact, with, macaw
    - parrot — *see* Contact, with, parrot
    - psittacine — *see* Contact, with, psittacine
    - strike W61.92
    - turkey — *see* Contact, with, turkey
  - blender W29.0
  - boiling water X12
    - stated as undetermined whether accidental or intentional Y27.2
    - suicide (attempt) X77.2
  - bore, earth-drilling or mining (land) (seabed) W31.0

Contact (accidental) - *continued*
- with - *continued*
  - buffalo — *see* Contact, with, hoof stock NEC
  - bull W55.29
    - bite W55.21
    - gored W55.22
    - strike W55.22
  - bumper cars W31.81
  - camel — *see* Contact, with, hoof stock NEC
  - can
    - lid W26.8
    - opener W27.4
      - powered W29.0
  - cat W55.09
    - bite W55.01
    - scratch W55.03
  - caterpillar (venomous) X58
  - centipede (venomous) X58
  - chain
    - hoist W24.0
      - agricultural operations W30.89
    - saw W29.3
  - chicken W61.39
    - peck W61.33
    - strike W61.32
  - chisel W27.0
  - circular saw W31.2
  - cobra X58
  - combine (harvester) W30.0
  - conveyer belt W24.1
  - cooker (hot) X15.8
    - stated as undetermined whether accidental or intentional Y27.3
    - suicide (attempt) X77.3
  - coral X58
  - cotton gin W31.82
  - cow W55.29
    - bite W55.21
    - strike W55.22
  - crane W24.0
    - agricultural operations W30.89
  - crocodile W58.19
    - bite W58.11
    - crushing W58.13
    - strike W58.12
  - dagger W26.1
    - stated as undetermined whether accidental or intentional Y28.2
    - suicide (attempt) X78.2
  - dairy equipment W31.82
  - dart W21.89
    - not thrown, projected or falling W45.8
  - deer — *see* Contact, with, hoof stock NEC
  - derrick W24.0
    - agricultural operations W30.89
      - hay W30.2
  - dog W54.8
    - bite W54.0
    - strike W54.1
  - dolphin W56.09
    - bite W56.01
    - strike W56.02
  - donkey — *see* Contact, with, hoof stock NEC
  - drill (powered) W29.8
    - earth (land) (seabed) W31.0
    - nonpowered W27.8
  - drive belt W24.0
    - agricultural operations W30.89
  - dry ice — *see* Exposure, cold, man-made
  - dryer (clothes) (powered) (spin) W29.2
  - duck W61.69
    - bite W61.61
    - strike W61.62
  - earth (-)
    - drilling machine (industrial) W31.0
    - scraping machine in stationary use W31.83
  - edge of stiff paper W26.2
  - electric
    - beater W29.0
    - blanket X16
    - fan W29.2

Contact (accidental) - *continued*
- with - *continued*
  - electric - *continued*
    - fan - *continued*
      - commercial W31.82
    - knife W29.1
    - mixer W29.0
  - elevator (building) W24.0
    - agricultural operations W30.89
      - grain W30.3
  - engine (s) , hot NEC X17
  - excavating machine W31.0
  - farm machine W30.9
  - feces — *see* Contact, with, by type of animal
  - fer de lance X58
  - fish W56.59
    - bite W56.51
    - shark — *see* Contact, with, shark
    - strike W56.52
  - flying horses W31.81
  - forging (metalworking) machine W31.1
  - fork W27.4
  - forklift (truck) W24.0
    - agricultural operations W30.89
  - frog W62.0
  - garden
    - cultivator (powered) W29.3
      - riding W30.89
    - fork W27.1
  - gas turbine W31.3
  - Gila monster X58
  - giraffe — *see* Contact, with, hoof stock NEC
  - glass (sharp) (broken) W25
    - with subsequent fall W18.02
    - assault X99.0
    - due to fall — *see* Fall, by type
    - stated as undetermined whether accidental or intentional Y28.0
    - suicide (attempt) X78.0
  - goat W55.39
    - bite W55.31
    - strike W55.32
  - goose W61.59
    - bite W61.51
    - strike W61.52
  - hand
    - saw W27.0
    - tool (not powered) NEC W27.8
      - powered W29.8
  - harvester W30.0
  - hay-derrick W30.2
  - heat NEC X19
    - from appliance (electrical) (household) — *see* Contact, with, hot, household appliance
    - heating appliance X16
  - heating
    - appliance (hot) X16
    - pad (electric) X16
  - hedge-trimmer (powered) W29.3
  - hoe W27.1
  - hoist (chain) (shaft) NEC W24.0
    - agricultural W30.89
  - hoof stock NEC W55.39
    - bite W55.31
    - strike W55.32
  - hornet (s) X58
  - horse W55.19
    - bite W55.11
    - strike W55.12
  - hot
    - air X14.1
      - inhalation X14.0
    - cooker X15.8
    - drinks X10.0
    - engine X17
    - fats X10.2
    - fluids NEC X12
      - assault X98.2
      - suicide (attempt) X77.2
      - undetermined whether accidental or intentional Y27.2
    - food X10.1

Contact (accidental) - *continued*
with - *continued*
hot - *continued*
gases X14.1
inhalation X14.0
heating appliance X16
household appliance X15.8
assault X98.3
cooker X15.8
hotplate X15.2
kettle X15.8
light bulb X15.8
object NEC X19
assault X98.8
stated as undetermined whether accidental or intentional Y27.9
suicide (attempt) X77.8
saucepan X15.3
skillet X15.3
stove X15.0
stated as undetermined whether accidental or intentional Y27.3
suicide (attempt) X77.3
toaster X15.1
kettle X15.8
light bulb X15.8
liquid NEC — *see also* Burn X12
drinks X10.0
stated as undetermined whether accidental or intentional Y27.2
suicide (attempt) X77.2
tap water X11.8
stated as undetermined whether accidental or intentional Y27.1
suicide (attempt) X77.1
machinery X17
metal (molten) (liquid) NEC X18
object (not producing fire or flames) NEC X19
oil (cooking) X10.2
pipe X16
plate X15.2
radiator X16
saucepan (glass) (metal) X15.3
skillet X15.3
stove (kitchen) X15.0
substance NEC X19
tap-water X11.8
assault X98.1
heated on stove X12
stated as undetermined whether accidental or intentional Y27.2
suicide (attempt) X77.2
in bathtub X11.0
running X11.1
stated as undetermined whether accidental or intentional Y27.1
suicide (attempt) X77.1
toaster X15.1
tool X17
vapors X13.1
inhalation X13.0
water (tap) X11.8
boiling X12
stated as undetermined whether accidental or intentional Y27.2
suicide (attempt) X77.2
heated on stove X12
stated as undetermined whether accidental or intentional Y27.2
suicide (attempt) X77.2
in bathtub X11.0
running X11.1
stated as undetermined whether accidental or intentional Y27.1
suicide (attempt) X77.1
hotplate X15.2
ice-pick W27.4
insect (nonvenomous) NEC W57
kettle (hot) X15.8
knife W26.0
assault X99.1
electric W29.1
stated as undetermined whether accidental or intentional Y28.1

Contact (accidental) - *continued*
with - *continued*
knife - *continued*
suicide (attempt) X78.1
lathe (metalworking) W31.1
turnings W45.8
woodworking W31.2
lawnmower (powered) (ridden) W28
causing electrocution W86.8
suicide (attempt) X83.1
unpowered W27.1
lift, lifting (devices) W24.0
agricultural operations W30.89
shaft W24.0
liquefied gas — *see* Exposure, cold, man-made
liquid air, hydrogen, nitrogen — *see* Exposure, cold, man-made
lizard (nonvenomous) W59.09
bite W59.01
strike W59.02
llama — *see* Contact, with, hoof stock NEC
macaw W61.19
bite W61.11
strike W61.12
machine, machinery W31.9
abrasive wheel W31.1
agricultural including animal-powered W30.9
combine harvester W30.0
grain storage elevator W30.3
hay derrick W30.2
power take-off device W30.1
reaper W30.0
specified NEC W30.89
thresher W30.0
transport vehicle, stationary W30.81
band saw W31.2
bench saw W31.2
circular saw W31.2
commercial NEC W31.82
drilling, metal (industrial) W31.1
earth-drilling W31.0
earthmoving or scraping W31.89
excavating W31.89
forging machine W31.1
gas turbine W31.3
hot X17
internal combustion engine W31.3
land drill W31.0
lathe W31.1
lifting (devices) W24.0
metal drill W31.1
metalworking (industrial) W31.1
milling, metal W31.1
mining W31.0
molding W31.2
overhead plane W31.2
power press, metal W31.1
prime mover W31.3
printing W31.89
radial saw W31.2
recreational W31.81
roller-coaster W31.81
rolling mill, metal W31.1
sander W31.2
seabed drill W31.0
shaft
hoist W31.0
lift W31.0
specified NEC W31.89
spinning W31.89
steam engine W31.3
transmission W24.1
undercutter W31.0
water driven turbine W31.3
weaving W31.89
woodworking or forming (industrial) W31.2
mammal (feces) (urine) W55.89
bull — *see* Contact, with, bull
cat — *see* Contact, with, cat
cow — *see* Contact, with, cow
goat — *see* Contact, with, goat

Contact (accidental) - *continued*
with - *continued*
mammal (feces) (urine) - *continued*
hoof stock — *see* Contact, with, hoof stock
horse — *see* Contact, with, horse
marine W56.39
dolphin — *see* Contact, with, dolphin
orca — *see* Contact, with, orca
sea lion — *see* Contact, with, sea lion
specified NEC W56.39
bite W56.31
strike W56.32
pig — *see* Contact, with, pig
raccoon — *see* Contact, with, raccoon
rodent — *see* Contact, with, rodent
sheep — *see* Contact, with, sheep
specified NEC W55.89
bite W55.81
strike W55.82
marine
animal W56.89
bite W56.81
dolphin — *see* Contact, with, dolphin
fish NEC — *see* Contact, with, fish
mammal — *see* Contact, with, mammal, marine
orca — *see* Contact, with, orca
sea lion — *see* Contact, with, sea lion
shark — *see* Contact, with, shark
strike W56.82
meat
grinder (domestic) W29.0
industrial W31.82
nonpowered W27.4
slicer (domestic) W29.0
industrial W31.82
merry go round W31.81
metal, hot (liquid) (molten) NEC X18
millipede W57
nail W45.0
gun W29.4
needle (sewing) W27.3
hypodermic W46.0
contaminated W46.1
object (blunt) NEC
hot NEC X19
legal intervention — *see* Legal, intervention, blunt object
sharp NEC W45.8
inflicted by other person NEC W45.8
stated as
intentional homicide (attempt) — *see* Assault, cutting or piercing instrument
legal intervention — *see* Legal, intervention, sharp object
self-inflicted X78.9
orca W56.29
bite W56.21
strike W56.22
overhead plane W31.2
paper (as sharp object) W26.2
paper-cutter W27.5
parrot W61.09
bite W61.01
strike W61.02
pig W55.49
bite W55.41
strike W55.42
pipe, hot X16
pitchfork W27.1
plane (metal) (wood) W27.0
overhead W31.2
plant thorns, spines, sharp leaves or other mechanisms W60
powered
garden cultivator W29.3
household appliance, implement, or machine W29.8
saw (industrial) W31.2
hand W29.8
printing machine W31.89
psittacine bird W61.29
bite W61.21

Contact (accidental) - *continued*
with - *continued*
psittacine bird - *continued*
macaw — *see* Contact, with, macaw
parrot — *see* Contact, with, parrot
strike W61.22
pulley (block) (transmission) W24.0
agricultural operations W30.89
raccoon W55.59
bite W55.51
strike W55.52
radial-saw (industrial) W31.2
radiator (hot) X16
rake W27.1
rattlesnake X58
reaper W30.0
reptile W59.89
lizard — *see* Contact, with, lizard
snake — *see* Contact, with, snake
specified NEC W59.89
bite W59.81
crushing W59.83
strike W59.82
turtle — *see* Contact, with, turtle
rivet gun (powered) W29.4
road scraper — *see* Accident, transport, construction vehicle
rodent (feces) (urine) W53.89
bite W53.81
mouse W53.09
bite W53.01
rat W53.19
bite W53.11
specified NEC W53.89
bite W53.81
squirrel W53.29
bite W53.21
roller coaster W31.81
rope NEC W24.0
agricultural operations W30.89
saliva — *see* Contact, with, by type of animal
sander W29.8
industrial W31.2
saucepan (hot) (glass) (metal) X15.3
saw W27.0
band (industrial) W31.2
bench (industrial) W31.2
chain W29.3
hand W27.0
sawing machine, metal W31.1
scissors W27.2
scorpion X58
screwdriver W27.0
powered W29.8
sea
anemone, cucumber or urchin (spine) X58
lion W56.19
bite W56.11
strike W56.12
serpent — *see* Contact, with, snake, by type
sewing-machine (electric) (powered) W29.2
not powered W27.8
shaft (hoist) (lift) (transmission) NEC W24.0
agricultural W30.89
shark W56.49
bite W56.41
strike W56.42
sharp object (s) W26.9
specified NEC W26.8
shears (hand) W27.2
powered (industrial) W31.1
domestic W29.2
sheep W55.39
bite W55.31
strike W55.32
shovel W27.8
steam — *see* Accident, transport, construction vehicle
snake (nonvenomous) W59.19
bite W59.11

Contact (accidental) - *continued*
with - *continued*
snake (nonvenomous) - *continued*
crushing W59.13
strike W59.12
spade W27.1
spider (venomous) X58
spin-drier W29.2
spinning machine W31.89
splinter W45.8
sports equipment W21.9
staple gun (powered) W29.8
steam X13.1
engine W31.3
inhalation X13.0
pipe X16
shovel W31.89
stove (hot) (kitchen) X15.0
substance, hot NEC X19
molten (metal) X18
sword W26.1
assault X99.2
stated as undetermined whether accidental or intentional Y28.2
suicide (attempt) X78.2
tarantula X58
thresher W30.0
tin can lid W26.8
toad W62.1
toaster (hot) X15.1
tool W27.8
hand (not powered) W27.8
auger W27.0
axe W27.0
can opener W27.4
chisel W27.0
fork W27.4
garden W27.1
handsaw W27.0
hoe W27.1
ice-pick W27.4
kitchen utensil W27.4
manual
lawn mower W27.1
sewing machine W27.8
meat grinder W27.4
needle (sewing) W27.3
hypodermic W46.0
contaminated W46.1
paper cutter W27.5
pitchfork W27.1
rake W27.1
scissors W27.2
screwdriver W27.0
specified NEC W27.8
workbench W27.0
hot X17
powered W29.8
blender W29.0
commercial W31.82
can opener W29.0
commercial W31.82
chainsaw W29.3
clothes dryer W29.2
commercial W31.82
dishwasher W29.2
commercial W31.82
edger W29.3
electric fan W29.2
commercial W31.82
electric knife W29.1
food processor W29.0
commercial W31.82
garbage disposal W29.0
commercial W31.82
garden tool W29.3
hedge trimmer W29.3
ice maker W29.0
commercial W31.82
kitchen appliance W29.0
commercial W31.82
lawn mower W28
meat grinder W29.0
commercial W31.82
mixer W29.0

Contact (accidental) - *continued*
with - *continued*
tool - *continued*
powered - *continued*
mixer - *continued*
commercial W31.82
rototiller W29.3
sewing machine W29.2
commercial W31.82
washing machine W29.2
commercial W31.82
transmission device (belt, cable, chain, gear, pinion, shaft) W24.1
agricultural operations W30.89
turbine (gas) (water-driven) W31.3
turkey W61.49
peck W61.43
strike W61.42
turtle (nonvenomous) W59.29
bite W59.21
strike W59.22
terrestrial W59.89
bite W59.81
crushing W59.83
strike W59.82
under-cutter W31.0
urine — *see* Contact, with, by type of animal
vehicle
agricultural use (transport) — *see* Accident, transport, agricultural vehicle
not on public highway W30.81
industrial use (transport) — *see* Accident, transport, industrial vehicle
not on public highway W31.83
off-road use (transport) — *see* Accident, transport, all-terrain or off-road vehicle
not on public highway W31.83
special construction use (transport) — *see* Accident, transport, construction vehicle
not on public highway W31.83
venomous
animal X58
arthropods X58
lizard X58
marine animal NEC X58
marine plant NEC X58
millipedes (tropical) X58
plant (s) X58
snake X58
spider X58
viper X58
washing-machine (powered) W29.2
wasp X58
weaving-machine W31.89
winch W24.0
agricultural operations W30.89
wire NEC W24.0
agricultural operations W30.89
wood slivers W45.8
yellow jacket X58
zebra — *see* Contact, with, hoof stock NEC
pressure X50.9
stress X50.9
Coup de soleil X32
Crash
aircraft (in transit) (powered) V95.9
balloon V96.01
fixed wing NEC (private) V95.21
commercial V95.31
glider V96.21
hang V96.11
powered V95.11
helicopter V95.01
in war operations — *see* War operations, destruction of aircraft
microlight V95.11
nonpowered V96.9
specified NEC V96.8
powered NEC V95.8

- **Dog bite** W54.0
- **Dragged by transport vehicle NEC** — *see also* Accident, transport V09.9
- **Drinking poison (accidental)** — *see* Table of Drugs and Chemicals
- **Dropped (accidentally) while being carried or supported by other person** W04
- **Drowning (accidental)** W74
  - assault X92.9
  - due to
    - accident (to)
      - machinery — *see* Contact, with, by type of machine
      - watercraft V90.89
        - burning V90.29
          - powered V90.23
            - merchant ship V90.20
            - passenger ship V90.21
            - fishing boat V90.22
            - jetskis V90.23
          - unpowered V90.28
            - canoe V90.25
            - inflatable V90.26
            - kayak V90.25
            - sailboat V90.24
            - water skis V90.27
        - crushed V90.39
          - powered V90.33
            - merchant ship V90.30
            - passenger ship V90.31
            - fishing boat V90.32
            - jetskis V90.33
          - unpowered V90.38
            - canoe V90.35
            - inflatable V90.36
            - kayak V90.35
            - sailboat V90.34
            - water skis V90.37
        - overturning V90.09
          - powered V90.03
            - merchant ship V90.00
            - passenger ship V90.01
            - fishing boat V90.02
            - jetskis V90.03
          - unpowered V90.08
            - canoe V90.05
            - inflatable V90.06
            - kayak V90.05
            - sailboat V90.04
        - sinking V90.19
          - powered V90.13
            - merchant ship V90.10
            - passenger ship V90.11
            - fishing boat V90.12
            - jetskis V90.13
          - unpowered V90.18
            - canoe V90.15
            - inflatable V90.16
            - kayak V90.15
            - sailboat V90.14
        - specified type NEC V90.89
          - powered V90.83
            - merchant ship V90.80
            - passenger ship V90.81
            - fishing boat V90.82
            - jetskis V90.83
          - unpowered V90.88
            - canoe V90.85
            - inflatable V90.86
            - kayak V90.85
            - sailboat V90.84
            - water skis V90.87
    - avalanche — *see* Landslide
    - cataclysmic
      - earth surface movement NEC — *see* Forces of nature, earth movement
      - storm — *see* Forces of nature, cataclysmic storm
    - cloudburst X37.8
    - cyclone X37.1
    - fall overboard (from) V92.09
      - powered craft V92.03
        - ferry boat V92.01
        - liner V92.01
        - merchant ship V92.00

- **Drowning (accidental)** - *continued*
  - due to - *continued*
    - fall overboard (from) - *continued*
      - powered craft - *continued*
        - passenger ship V92.01
        - fishing boat V92.02
        - jetskis V92.03
      - unpowered craft V92.08
        - canoe V92.05
        - inflatable V92.06
        - kayak V92.05
        - sailboat V92.04
        - surf-board V92.08
        - water skis V92.07
        - windsurfer V92.08
      - resulting from
        - accident to watercraft — *see* Drowning, due to, accident to, watercraft
        - being washed overboard (from) V92.29
          - powered craft V92.23
            - ferry boat V92.21
            - liner V92.21
            - merchant ship V92.20
            - passenger ship V92.21
            - fishing boat V92.22
            - jetskis V92.23
          - unpowered craft V92.28
            - canoe V92.25
            - inflatable V92.26
            - kayak V92.25
            - sailboat V92.24
            - surf-board V92.28
            - water skis V92.27
            - windsurfer V92.28
        - motion of watercraft V92.19
          - powered craft V92.13
            - ferry boat V92.11
            - liner V92.11
            - merchant ship V92.10
            - passenger ship V92.11
            - fishing boat V92.12
            - jetskis V92.13
          - unpowered craft
            - canoe V92.15
            - inflatable V92.16
            - kayak V92.15
            - sailboat V92.14
    - hurricane X37.0
    - jumping into water from watercraft (involved in accident) — *see also* Drowning, due to, accident to, watercraft
      - without accident to or on watercraft W16.711
    - tidal wave NEC — *see* Forces of nature, tidal wave
    - torrential rain X37.8
  - following
    - fall
      - into
        - bathtub W16.211
        - bucket W16.221
        - fountain — *see* Drowning, following, fall, into, water, specified NEC
        - quarry — *see* Drowning, following, fall, into, water, specified NEC
        - reservoir — *see* Drowning, following, fall, into, water, specified NEC
        - swimming-pool W16.011
          - striking
            - bottom W16.021
            - wall W16.031
          - stated as undetermined whether accidental or intentional Y21.3
          - suicide (attempt) X71.2
        - water NOS W16.41
          - natural (lake) (open sea) (river) (stream) (pond) W16.111
            - striking
              - bottom W16.121
              - side W16.131
          - specified NEC W16.311
            - striking

- **Drowning (accidental)** - *continued*
  - following - *continued*
    - fall - *continued*
      - into - *continued*
        - water NOS - *continued*
          - specified NEC - *continued*
            - striking - *continued*
              - bottom W16.321
              - wall W16.331
      - overboard NEC — *see* Drowning, due to, fall overboard
    - jump or dive
      - from boat W16.711
        - striking bottom W16.721
      - into
        - fountain — *see* Drowning, following, jump or dive, into, water, specified NEC
        - quarry — *see* Drowning, following, jump or dive, into, water, specified NEC
        - reservoir — *see* Drowning, following, jump or dive, into, water, specified NEC
        - swimming-pool W16.511
          - striking
            - bottom W16.521
            - wall W16.531
          - suicide (attempt) X71.2
        - water NOS W16.91
          - natural (lake) (open sea) (river) (stream) (pond) W16.611
          - specified NEC W16.811
            - striking
              - bottom W16.821
              - wall W16.831
          - striking bottom W16.621
  - homicide (attempt) X92.9
  - in
    - bathtub (accidental) W65
      - assault X92.0
      - following fall W16.211
        - stated as undetermined whether accidental or intentional Y21.1
      - stated as undetermined whether accidental or intentional Y21.0
      - suicide (attempt) X71.0
    - lake — *see* Drowning, in, natural water
    - natural water (lake) (open sea) (river) (stream) (pond) W69
      - assault X92.3
      - following
        - dive or jump W16.611
          - striking bottom W16.621
        - fall W16.111
          - striking
            - bottom W16.121
            - side W16.131
      - stated as undetermined whether accidental or intentional Y21.4
      - suicide (attempt) X71.3
    - quarry — *see* Drowning, in, specified place NEC
    - quenching tank — *see* Drowning, in, specified place NEC
    - reservoir — *see* Drowning, in, specified place NEC
    - river — *see* Drowning, in, natural water
    - sea — *see* Drowning, in, natural water
    - specified place NEC W73
      - assault X92.8
      - following
        - dive or jump W16.811
          - striking
            - bottom W16.821
            - wall W16.831
        - fall W16.311
          - striking
            - bottom W16.321
            - wall W16.331
      - stated as undetermined whether accidental or intentional Y21.8
      - suicide (attempt) X71.8
    - stream — *see* Drowning, in, natural water
    - swimming-pool W67

DOG BITE - DROWNING

- **Exposure (to)** - *continued*
  - mechanical forces NEC - *continued*
    - inanimate NEC W49.9
  - noise W42.9
    - supersonic W42.0
  - noxious substance — *see* Table of Drugs and Chemicals
  - pneumatic jet W49.9
  - prolonged in deep-freeze unit or refrigerator W93.2
  - radiation — *see* Radiation
  - smoke — *see also* Exposure, fire
    - tobacco, second hand Z77.22
  - specified factors NEC X58
  - sunlight X32
    - man-made (sun lamp) W89.8
      - tanning bed W89.1
  - supersonic waves W42.0
  - transmission line (s) , electric W85
  - vibration W49.9
  - waves
    - infrasound W49.9
    - sound W42.9
    - supersonic W42.0
  - weather NEC — *see* Forces of nature
- **External cause status** Y99.9
  - child assisting in compensated work for family Y99.8
  - civilian activity done for financial or other compensation Y99.0
  - civilian activity done for income or pay Y99.0
  - family member assisting in compensated work for other family member Y99.8
  - hobby not done for income Y99.8
  - leisure activity Y99.8
  - military activity Y99.1
  - off-duty activity of military personnel Y99.8
  - recreation or sport not for income or while a student Y99.8
  - specified NEC Y99.8
  - student activity Y99.8
  - volunteer activity Y99.2

F

- **Factors, supplemental**
  - alcohol
    - blood level
      - less than 20mg/100ml Y90.0
      - presence in blood, level not specified Y90.9
      - 20-39mg/100ml Y90.1
      - 40-59mg/100ml Y90.2
      - 60-79mg/100ml Y90.3
      - 80-99mg/100ml Y90.4
      - 100-119mg/100ml Y90.5
      - 120-199mg/100ml Y90.6
      - 200-239mg/100ml Y90.7
      - 240mg/100ml or more Y90.8
    - presence in blood, but level not specified Y90.9
  - environmental-pollution-related condition- see Z57
  - nosocomial condition Y95
  - work-related condition Y99.0
- **Failure**
  - in suture or ligature during surgical procedure Y65.2
  - mechanical, of instrument or apparatus (any) (during any medical or surgical procedure) Y65.8
  - sterile precautions (during medical and surgical care) — *see* Misadventure, failure, sterile precautions, by type of procedure
  - to
    - introduce tube or instrument Y65.4
      - endotracheal tube during anesthesia Y65.3
    - make curve (transport vehicle) NEC — *see* Accident, transport
    - remove tube or instrument Y65.4
- **Fall, falling (accidental)** W19
  - building W20.1
    - burning (uncontrolled fire) X00.3
  - down
- **Fall, falling (accidental)** - *continued*
  - down - *continued*
    - embankment W17.81
    - escalator W10.0
    - hill W17.81
    - ladder W11
    - ramp W10.2
    - stairs, steps W10.9
  - due to
    - bumping against
      - object W18.00
        - sharp glass W18.02
        - specified NEC W18.09
        - sports equipment W18.01
      - person W03
        - due to ice or snow W00.0
        - on pedestrian conveyance — *see* Accident, transport, pedestrian, conveyance
    - collision with another person W03
      - due to ice or snow W00.0
      - involving pedestrian conveyance — *see* Accident, transport, pedestrian, conveyance
    - grocery cart tipping over W17.82
    - ice or snow W00.9
      - from one level to another W00.2
        - on stairs or steps W00.1
      - involving pedestrian conveyance — *see* Accident, transport, pedestrian, conveyance
      - on same level W00.0
    - slipping (on moving sidewalk) W01.0
      - with subsequent striking against object W01.10
        - furniture W01.190
        - sharp object W01.119
          - glass W01.110
          - power tool or machine W01.111
          - specified NEC W01.118
        - specified NEC W01.198
    - striking against
      - object W18.00
        - sharp glass W18.02
        - specified NEC W18.09
        - sports equipment W18.01
      - person W03
        - due to ice or snow W00.0
        - on pedestrian conveyance — *see* Accident, transport, pedestrian, conveyance
  - earth (with asphyxia or suffocation (by pressure)) — *see* Earth, falling
  - from, off, out of
    - aircraft NEC (with accident to aircraft NEC) V97.0
      - while boarding or alighting V97.1
    - balcony W13.0
    - bed W06
    - boat, ship, watercraft NEC (with drowning or submersion) — *see* Drowning, due to, fall overboard
      - with hitting bottom or object V94.0
    - bridge W13.1
    - building W13.9
      - burning (uncontrolled fire) X00.3
    - cavity W17.2
    - chair W07
    - cherry picker W17.89
    - cliff W15
    - dock W17.4
    - embankment W17.81
    - escalator W10.0
    - flagpole W13.8
    - furniture NEC W08
    - grocery cart W17.82
    - haystack W17.89
    - high place NEC W17.89
      - stated as undetermined whether accidental or intentional Y30
    - hole W17.2
    - incline W10.2
    - ladder W11
    - lifting device W17.89
- **Fall, falling (accidental)** - *continued*
  - from, off, out of - *continued*
    - machine, machinery — *see also* Contact, with, by type of machine
      - not in operation W17.89
    - manhole W17.1
    - mobile elevated work platform [MEWP] W17.89
    - motorized mobility scooter W05.2
    - one level to another NEC W17.89
      - intentional, purposeful, suicide (attempt) X80
      - stated as undetermined whether accidental or intentional Y30
    - pit W17.2
    - playground equipment W09.8
      - jungle gym W09.2
      - slide W09.0
      - swing W09.1
    - quarry W17.89
    - railing W13.9
    - ramp W10.2
    - roof W13.2
    - scaffolding W12
    - scooter (nonmotorized) W05.1
      - motorized mobility W05.2
    - sky lift W17.89
    - stairs, steps W10.9
      - curb W10.1
      - due to ice or snow W00.1
      - escalator W10.0
      - incline W10.2
      - ramp W10.2
      - sidewalk curb W10.1
      - specified NEC W10.8
      - standing
        - electric scooter V00.841
        - micro-mobility pedestrian conveyance V00.848
    - stepladder W11
    - storm drain W17.1
    - streetcar NEC V82.6
      - with antecedent collision — *see* Accident, transport, streetcar occupant
      - while boarding or alighting V82.4
    - structure NEC W13.8
      - burning (uncontrolled fire) X00.3
    - table W08
    - toilet W18.11
      - with subsequent striking against object W18.12
    - train NEC V81.6
      - during derailment (without antecedent collision) V81.7
        - with antecedent collision — *see* Accident, transport, railway vehicle occupant
      - while boarding or alighting V81.4
    - transport vehicle after collision — *see* Accident, transport, by type of vehicle, collision
    - tree W14
    - vehicle (in motion) NEC — *see also* Accident, transport V89.9
      - motor NEC — *see also* Accident, transport, occupant, by type of vehicle V87.8
      - stationary W17.89
        - while boarding or alighting — *see* Accident, transport, by type of vehicle, while boarding or alighting
    - viaduct W13.8
    - wall W13.8
    - watercraft — *see also* Drowning, due to, fall overboard
      - with hitting bottom or object V94.0
    - well W17.0
    - wheelchair, non-moving W05.0
      - powered — *see* Accident, transport, pedestrian, conveyance occupant, specified type NEC
    - window W13.4
  - in, on

Incident, adverse - *continued*
device - *continued*
ophthalmic - *continued*
surgical Y77.3
therapeutic Y77.19
orthopedic Y79.8
accessory Y79.2
diagnostic Y79.0
miscellaneous Y79.8
monitoring Y79.0
prosthetic Y79.2
rehabilitative Y79.1
surgical Y79.3
therapeutic Y79.1
otorhinolaryngological Y72.8
accessory Y72.2
diagnostic Y72.0
miscellaneous Y72.8
monitoring Y72.0
prosthetic Y72.2
rehabilitative Y72.1
surgical Y72.3
therapeutic Y72.1
personal use Y74.8
accessory Y74.2
diagnostic Y74.0
miscellaneous Y74.8
monitoring Y74.0
prosthetic Y74.2
rehabilitative Y74.1
surgical Y74.3
therapeutic Y74.1
physical medicine Y80.8
accessory Y80.2
diagnostic Y80.0
miscellaneous Y80.8
monitoring Y80.0
prosthetic Y80.2
rehabilitative Y80.1
surgical Y80.3
therapeutic Y80.1
plastic surgical Y81.8
accessory Y81.2
diagnostic Y81.0
miscellaneous Y81.8
monitoring Y81.0
prosthetic Y81.2
rehabilitative Y81.1
surgical Y81.3
therapeutic Y81.1
radiological Y78.8
accessory Y78.2
diagnostic Y78.0
miscellaneous Y78.8
monitoring Y78.0
prosthetic Y78.2
rehabilitative Y78.1
surgical Y78.3
therapeutic Y78.1
urology Y73.8
accessory Y73.2
diagnostic Y73.0
miscellaneous Y73.8
monitoring Y73.0
prosthetic Y73.2
rehabilitative Y73.1
surgical Y73.3
therapeutic Y73.1
Incineration (accidental) — *see* Exposure, fire
Infanticide — *see* Assault
Infrasound waves (causing injury) W49.9
Ingestion
foreign body (causing injury) (with obstruction) — *see* Foreign body, alimentary canal
poisonous
plant (s) X58
substance NEC — *see* Table of Drugs and Chemicals
Inhalation
excessively cold substance, man-made — *see* Exposure, cold, man-made

Inhalation - *continued*
food (any type) (into respiratory tract) (with asphyxia, obstruction respiratory tract, suffocation) — *see* categories T17 and T18
foreign body — *see* Foreign body, aspiration
gastric contents (with asphyxia, obstruction respiratory passage, suffocation) T17.81-
hot air or gases X14.0
liquid air, hydrogen, nitrogen W93.12
suicide (attempt) X83.2
steam X13.0
assault X98.0
stated as undetermined whether accidental or intentional Y27.0
suicide (attempt) X77.0
toxic gas — *see* Table of Drugs and Chemicals
vomitus (with asphyxia, obstruction respiratory passage, suffocation) T17.81-
Injury, injured (accidental (ly)) NOS X58
by, caused by, from
assault — *see* Assault
law-enforcing agent, police, in course of legal intervention — *see* Legal intervention
suicide (attempt) X83.8
due to, in
civil insurrection — *see* War operations
fight — *see also* Assault, fight Y04.0
war operations — *see* War operations
homicide — *see also* Assault Y09
inflicted (by)
in course of arrest (attempted) , suppression of disturbance, maintenance of order, by law-enforcing agents — *see* Legal intervention
other person
stated as
accidental X58
intentional, homicide (attempt) — *see* Assault
undetermined whether accidental or intentional Y33
purposely (inflicted) by other person (s) — *see* Assault
self-inflicted X83.8
stated as accidental X58
specified cause NEC X58
undetermined whether accidental or intentional Y33
Insolation, effects X30
Insufficient nourishment X58
Interruption of respiration (by)
food (lodged in esophagus) — *see* categories T17 and T18
vomitus (lodged in esophagus) T17.81-
Intervention, legal — *see* Legal intervention
Intoxication
drug — *see* Table of Drugs and Chemicals
poison — *see* Table of Drugs and Chemicals

J

Jammed (accidentally)
between objects (moving) (stationary and moving) W23.0
stationary W23.1
Jumped, jumping
before moving object NEC X81.8
motor vehicle X81.0
subway train X81.1
train X81.1
undetermined whether accidental or intentional Y31
from
boat (into water) voluntarily, without accident (to or on boat) W16.712
with
accident to or on boat — *see* Accident, watercraft
drowning or submersion W16.711
suicide (attempt) X71.3
striking bottom W16.722

Jumped, jumping - *continued*
from - *continued*
boat (into water) voluntarily, without accident (to or on boat) - *continued*
striking bottom - *continued*
causing drowning W16.721
building — *see also* Jumped, from, high place W13.9
burning (uncontrolled fire) X00.5
high place NEC W17.89
suicide (attempt) X80
undetermined whether accidental or intentional Y30
structure — *see also* Jumped, from, high place W13.9
burning (uncontrolled fire) X00.5
into water W16.92
causing drowning W16.91
from, off watercraft — *see* Jumped, from, boat
in
natural body W16.612
causing drowning W16.611
striking bottom W16.622
causing drowning W16.621
specified place NEC W16.812
causing drowning W16.811
striking
bottom W16.822
causing drowning W16.821
wall W16.832
causing drowning W16.831
swimming pool W16.512
causing drowning W16.511
striking
bottom W16.522
causing drowning W16.521
wall W16.532
causing drowning W16.531
suicide (attempt) X71.3

K

Kicked by
animal NEC W55.82
person (s) (accidentally) W50.1
with intent to injure or kill Y04.0
as, or caused by, a crowd or human stampede (with fall) W52
assault Y04.0
homicide (attempt) Y04.0
in
fight Y04.0
legal intervention
injuring
bystander Y35.812
law enforcement personnel Y35.811
suspect Y35.813
unspecified person Y35.819
Kicking
against
object W22.8
sports equipment W21.9
stationary W22.09
sports equipment W21.89
person — *see* Striking against, person
sports equipment W21.9
carpet stretcher with knee X50.3
Killed, killing (accidentally) NOS — *see also* Injury X58
in
action — *see* War operations
brawl, fight (hand) (fists) (foot) Y04.0
by weapon — *see also* Assault
cutting, piercing — *see* Assault, cutting or piercing instrument
firearm — *see* Discharge, firearm, by type, homicide
self
stated as
accident NOS X58
suicide — *see* Suicide
undetermined whether accidental or intentional Y33
Kneeling (prolonged) (static) X50.1

Lying before train, vehicle or other moving object - Misadventure during surgical or medical care

Lying before train, vehicle or other moving object - *continued*
train X81.1
undetermined whether accidental or intentional Y31
Lynching — *see* Assault

M

Malfunction (mechanism or component) (of)
firearm W34.10
airgun W34.110
BB gun W34.110
gas, air or spring-operated gun NEC W34.118
handgun W32.1
hunting rifle W33.12
larger firearm W33.10
specified NEC W33.19
machine gun W33.13
paintball gun W34.111
pellet gun W34.110
shotgun W33.11
specified NEC W34.19
Very pistol [flare] W34.19
handgun — *see* Malfunction, firearm, handgun
Maltreatment — *see* Perpetrator
Mangled (accidentally) NOS X58
Manhandling (in brawl, fight) Y04.0
legal intervention — *see* Legal, intervention, manhandling
Manslaughter (nonaccidental) — *see* Assault
Mauled by animal NEC W55.89
Medical procedure, complication of (delayed or as an abnormal reaction without mention of misadventure) — *see* Complication of or following, by specified type of procedure
due to or as a result of misadventure — *see* Misadventure
Melting (due to fire) — *see also* Exposure, fire
apparel NEC X06.3
clothes, clothing NEC X06.3
nightwear X05
fittings or furniture (burning building) (uncontrolled fire) X00.8
nightwear X05
plastic jewelry X06.1
Mental cruelty X58
Military operations (injuries to military and civilians occuring during peacetime on military property and during routine military exercises and operations) (by) (from) (involving) Y37.90-
air blast Y37.20-
aircraft
destruction — *see* Military operations, destruction of aircraft
airway restriction — *see* Military operations, restriction of airways
asphyxiation — *see* Military operations, restriction of airways
biological weapons Y37.6X-
blast Y37.20-
blast fragments Y37.20-
blast wave Y37.20-
blast wind Y37.20-
bomb Y37.20-
dirty Y37.50-
gasoline Y37.31-
incendiary Y37.31-
petrol Y37.31-
bullet Y37.43-
incendiary Y37.32-
rubber Y37.41-
chemical weapons Y37.7X-
combat
hand to hand (unarmed) combat Y37.44-
using blunt or piercing object Y37.45-
conflagration — *see* Military operations, fire
conventional warfare NEC Y37.49-
depth-charge Y37.01-
destruction of aircraft Y37.10-
due to
air to air missile Y37.11-

Military operations (injuries to military and civilians occuring during peacetime on military property and during routine military exercises and operations) (by) (from) (involving) - *continued*
destruction of aircraft - *continued*
due to - *continued*
collision with other aircraft Y37.12-
detonation (accidental) of onboard munitions and explosives Y37.14-
enemy fire or explosives Y37.11-
explosive placed on aircraft Y37.11-
onboard fire Y37.13-
rocket propelled grenade [RPG] Y37.11-
small arms fire Y37.11-
surface to air missile Y37.11-
specified NEC Y37.19-
detonation (accidental) of
onboard marine weapons Y37.05-
own munitions or munitions launch device Y37.24-
dirty bomb Y37.50-
explosion (of) Y37.20-
aerial bomb Y37.21-
bomb NOS — *see also* Military operations, bomb(s) Y37.20-
own munitions or munitions launch device (accidental) Y37.24-
fragments Y37.20-
grenade Y37.29-
guided missile Y37.22-
improvised explosive device [IED] (person-borne) (roadside) (vehicle-borne) Y37.23-
land mine Y37.29-
marine mine (at sea) (in harbor) Y37.02-
marine weapon Y37.00-
specified NEC Y37.09-
sea-based artillery shell Y37.03-
specified NEC Y37.29-
torpedo Y37.04-
fire Y37.30-
specified NEC Y37.39-
firearms
discharge Y37.43-
pellets Y37.42-
flamethrower Y37.33-
fragments (from) (of)
improvised explosive device [IED] (person-borne) (roadside) (vehicle-borne) Y37.26-
munitions Y37.25-
specified NEC Y37.29-
weapons Y37.27-
friendly fire Y37.92-
hand to hand (unarmed) combat Y37.44-
hot substances — *see* Military operations, fire
incendiary bullet Y37.32-
nuclear weapon (effects of) Y37.50-
acute radiation exposure Y37.54-
blast pressure Y37.51-
direct blast Y37.51-
direct heat Y37.53-
fallout exposure Y37.54-
fireball Y37.53-
indirect blast (struck or crushed by blast debris) (being thrown by blast) Y37.52-
ionizing radiation (immediate exposure) Y37.54-
nuclear radiation Y37.54-
radiation
ionizing (immediate exposure) Y37.54-
nuclear Y37.54-
thermal Y37.53-
specified NEC Y37.59-
secondary effects Y37.54-
thermal radiation Y37.53-
restriction of air (airway)
intentional Y37.46-
unintentional Y37.47-
rubber bullets Y37.41-
shrapnel NOS Y37.29-

Military operations (injuries to military and civilians occuring during peacetime on military property and during routine military exercises and operations) (by) (from) (involving) - *continued*
suffocation — *see* Military operations, restriction of airways
unconventional warfare NEC Y37.7X-
underwater blast NOS Y37.00-
warfare
conventional NEC Y37.49-
unconventional NEC Y37.7X-
weapons
biological weapons Y37.6X-
chemical Y37.7X-
nuclear (effects of) Y37.50-
acute radiation exposure Y37.54-
blast pressure Y37.51-
direct blast Y37.51-
direct heat Y37.53-
fallout exposure Y37.54-
fireball Y37.53-
indirect blast (struck or crushed by blast debris) (being thrown by blast) Y37.52-
radiation
ionizing (immediate exposure) Y37.54-
nuclear Y37.54-
thermal Y37.53-
secondary effects Y37.54-
specified NEC Y37.59-
of mass destruction [WMD] Y37.91-
weapon of mass destruction [WMD] Y37.91-
Misadventure (s) to patient (s) during surgical or medical care Y69
contaminated medical or biological substance (blood, drug, fluid) Y64.9
administered (by) NEC Y64.9
immunization Y64.1
infusion Y64.0
injection Y64.1
specified means NEC Y64.8
transfusion Y64.0
vaccination Y64.1
excessive amount of blood or other fluid during transfusion or infusion Y63.0
failure
in dosage Y63.9
electroshock therapy Y63.4
inappropriate temperature (too hot or too cold) in local application and packing Y63.5
infusion
excessive amount of fluid Y63.0
incorrect dilution of fluid Y63.1
insulin-shock therapy Y63.4
nonadministration of necessary drug or biological substance Y63.6
overdose — *see* Table of Drugs and Chemicals
radiation, in therapy Y63.2
radiation
overdose Y63.2
specified procedure NEC Y63.8
transfusion
excessive amount of blood Y63.0
mechanical, of instrument or apparatus (any) (during any procedure) Y65.8
sterile precautions (during procedure) Y62.9
aspiration of fluid or tissue (by puncture or catheterization, except heart) Y62.6
biopsy (except needle aspiration) Y62.8
needle (aspirating) Y62.6
blood sampling Y62.6
catheterization Y62.6
heart Y62.5
dialysis (kidney) Y62.2
endoscopic examination Y62.4
enema Y62.8
immunization Y62.3
infusion Y62.1
injection Y62.3

LYING BEFORE TRAIN, VEHICLE OR OTHER MOVING OBJECT - MISADVENTURE DURING SURGICAL OR MEDICAL CARE

Misadventure (s) to patient (s) during surgical or medical care - *continued*
failure - *continued*
sterile precautions (during procedure) - *continued*
needle biopsy Y62.6
paracentesis (abdominal) (thoracic) Y62.6
perfusion Y62.2
puncture (lumbar) Y62.6
removal of catheter or packing Y62.8
specified procedure NEC Y62.8
surgical operation Y62.0
transfusion Y62.1
vaccination Y62.3
suture or ligature during surgical procedure Y65.2
to introduce or to remove tube or instrument — *see* Failure, to
hemorrhage — *see* Index to Diseases and Injuries, Complication(s)
inadvertent exposure of patient to radiation Y63.3
inappropriate
operation performed — *see* Inappropriate operation performed
temperature (too hot or too cold) in local application or packing Y63.5
infusion — *see also* Misadventure, by type, infusion Y69
excessive amount of fluid Y63.0
incorrect dilution of fluid Y63.1
wrong fluid Y65.1
mismatched blood in transfusion Y65.0
nonadministration of necessary drug or biological substance Y63.6
overdose — *see* Table of Drugs and Chemicals
radiation (in therapy) Y63.2
perforation — *see* Index to Diseases and Injuries, Complication(s)
performance of inappropriate operation — *see* Inappropriate operation performed
puncture — *see* Index to Diseases and Injuries, Complication(s)
specified type NEC Y65.8
failure
suture or ligature during surgical operation Y65.2
to introduce or to remove tube or instrument — *see* Failure, to
infusion of wrong fluid Y65.1
performance of inappropriate operation — *see* Inappropriate operation performed
transfusion of mismatched blood Y65.0
wrong
fluid in infusion Y65.1
placement of endotracheal tube during anesthetic procedure Y65.3
transfusion — *see* Misadventure, by type, transfusion
excessive amount of blood Y63.0
mismatched blood Y65.0
wrong
drug given in error — *see* Table of Drugs and Chemicals
fluid in infusion Y65.1
placement of endotracheal tube during anesthetic procedure Y65.3
Mismatched blood in transfusion Y65.0
Motion sickness T75.3
Mountain sickness W94.11
Mudslide (of cataclysmic nature) — *see* Landslide
Murder (attempt) — *see* Assault

N

Nail
contact with W45.0
gun W29.4
embedded in skin W45.0
Neglect (criminal) (homicidal intent) X58
Noise (causing injury) (pollution) W42.9
supersonic W42.0
Nonadministration (of)
drug or biological substance (necessary) Y63.6
surgical and medical care Y66
Nosocomial condition Y95

O

Object
falling
from, in, on, hitting
machinery — *see* Contact, with, by type of machine
set in motion by
accidental explosion or rupture of pressure vessel W38
firearm — *see* Discharge, firearm, by type
machine (ry) — *see* Contact, with, by type of machine
Overdose (drug) — *see* Table of Drugs and Chemicals
radiation Y63.2
Overexertion X50.9
from
prolonged static or awkward postures X50.1
repetitive movements X50.3
specified strenuous movements or postures NEC X50.9
strenuous movement or load X50.0
Overexposure (accidental) (to)
cold — *see also* Exposure, cold X31
due to man-made conditions — *see* Exposure, cold, man-made
heat — *see also* Heat X30
radiation — *see* Radiation
radioactivity W88.0
sun (sunburn) X32
weather NEC — *see* Forces of nature
wind NEC — *see* Forces of nature
Overheated — *see* Heat
Overturning (accidental)
machinery — *see* Contact, with, by type of machine
transport vehicle NEC — *see also* Accident, transport V89.9
watercraft (causing drowning, submersion) — *see also* Drowning, due to, accident to, watercraft, overturning
causing injury except drowning or submersion — *see* Accident, watercraft, causing, injury NEC

P

Parachute descent (voluntary) (without accident to aircraft) V97.29
due to accident to aircraft — *see* Accident, transport, aircraft
Pecked by bird W61.99
Perforation during medical or surgical treatment as misadventure — *see* Index to Diseases and Injuries, Complication(s)
Perpetrator, perpetration, of assault, maltreatment and neglect (by) Y07.9
boyfriend Y07.03
brother Y07.410
stepbrother Y07.435
coach Y07.53
cousin
female Y07.491
male Y07.490
daycare provider Y07.519
at-home
adult care Y07.512
childcare Y07.510
care center
adult care Y07.513
childcare Y07.511
family member NEC Y07.499
father Y07.11
adoptive Y07.13
foster Y07.420
stepfather Y07.430
foster father Y07.420
foster mother Y07.421
girl friend Y07.04
healthcare provider Y07.529
mental health Y07.521
Perpetrator, perpetration, of assault, maltreatment and neglect (by) - *continued*
healthcare provider - *continued*
specified NEC Y07.528
husband Y07.01
instructor Y07.53
mother Y07.12
adoptive Y07.14
foster Y07.421
stepmother Y07.433
multiple perpetrators Y07.6
nonfamily member Y07.50
specified NEC Y07.59
nurse Y07.528
occupational therapist Y07.528
partner of parent
female Y07.434
male Y07.432
physical therapist Y07.528
sister Y07.411
speech therapist Y07.528
stepbrother Y07.435
stepfather Y07.430
stepmother Y07.433
stepsister Y07.436
teacher Y07.53
wife Y07.02
Piercing — *see* Contact, with, by type of object or machine
Pinched
between objects (moving) (stationary and moving) W23.0
stationary W23.1
Pinned under machine (ry) — *see* Contact, with, by type of machine
Place of occurrence Y92.9
abandoned house Y92.89
airplane Y92.813
airport Y92.520
ambulatory health services establishment NEC Y92.538
ambulatory surgery center Y92.530
amusement park Y92.831
apartment (co-op) — *see* Place of occurrence, residence, apartment
assembly hall Y92.29
bank Y92.510
barn Y92.71
baseball field Y92.320
basketball court Y92.310
beach Y92.832
boarding house — *see* Place of occurrence, residence, boarding house
boat Y92.814
bowling alley Y92.39
bridge Y92.89
building under construction Y92.61
bus Y92.811
station Y92.521
cafe Y92.511
campsite Y92.833
campus — *see* Place of occurrence, school
canal Y92.89
car Y92.810
casino Y92.59
children's home — *see* Place of occurrence, residence, institutional, orphanage
church Y92.22
cinema Y92.26
clubhouse Y92.29
coal pit Y92.64
college (community) Y92.214
condominium — *see* Place of occurrence, residence, apartment
construction area — *see* Place of occurrence, industrial and construction area
convalescent home — *see* Place of occurrence, residence, institutional, nursing home
court-house Y92.240
cricket ground Y92.328
cultural building Y92.258
art gallery Y92.250
museum Y92.251
music hall Y92.252

MISADVENTURE DURING SURGICAL OR MEDICAL CARE - PLACE OF OCCURRENCE

- **Place of occurrence** - *continued*
  - residence (non-institutional) (private) - *continued*
    - institutional - *continued*
      - specified NEC - *continued*
        - bathroom Y92.192
        - bedroom Y92.193
        - dining room Y92.191
        - driveway Y92.194
        - garage Y92.195
        - garden Y92.197
        - kitchen Y92.190
        - specified NEC Y92.198
        - swimming pool Y92.196
        - yard Y92.197
    - kitchen Y92.000
    - mobile home Y92.029
      - bathroom Y92.022
      - bedroom Y92.023
      - dining room Y92.021
      - driveway Y92.024
      - garage Y92.025
      - garden Y92.027
      - kitchen Y92.020
      - specified NEC Y92.028
      - swimming pool Y92.026
      - yard Y92.027
    - specified place in residence NEC Y92.008
    - specified residence type NEC Y92.099
      - bathroom Y92.091
      - bedroom Y92.092
      - driveway Y92.093
      - garage Y92.094
      - garden Y92.096
      - kitchen Y92.090
      - specified NEC Y92.098
      - swimming pool Y92.095
      - yard Y92.096
  - restaurant Y92.511
  - riding school Y92.39
  - river Y92.828
  - road Y92.410
  - rodeo ring Y92.39
  - rugby field Y92.328
  - same day surgery center Y92.530
  - sand pit Y92.64
  - school (private) (public) (state) Y92.219
    - college Y92.214
    - daycare center Y92.210
    - elementary school Y92.211
    - high school Y92.213
    - kindergarten Y92.211
    - middle school Y92.212
    - specified NEC Y92.218
    - trace school Y92.215
    - university Y92.214
    - vocational school Y92.215
  - sea (shore) Y92.832
  - senior citizen center Y92.29
  - service area
    - airport Y92.520
    - bus station Y92.521
    - gas station Y92.524
    - highway rest stop Y92.523
    - railway station Y92.522
  - shipyard Y92.62
  - shop (commercial) Y92.513
  - sidewalk Y92.480
  - silo Y92.79
  - skating rink (roller) Y92.331
    - ice Y92.330
  - slaughter house Y92.86
  - soccer field Y92.322
  - specified place NEC Y92.89
  - sports area Y92.39
    - athletic
      - court Y92.318
        - basketball Y92.310
        - specified NEC Y92.318
        - squash Y92.311
        - tennis Y92.312
      - field Y92.328
        - baseball Y92.320
        - cricket ground Y92.328
        - football Y92.321

- **Place of occurrence** - *continued*
  - sports area - *continued*
    - athletic - *continued*
      - field - *continued*
        - hockey Y92.328
        - soccer Y92.322
        - specified NEC Y92.328
    - golf course Y92.39
    - gymnasium Y92.39
    - riding school Y92.39
    - skating rink (roller) Y92.331
      - ice Y92.330
    - stadium Y92.39
    - swimming pool Y92.34
  - squash court Y92.311
  - stadium Y92.39
  - steeplechasing course Y92.39
  - store Y92.512
  - stream Y92.828
  - street and highway Y92.410
    - bike path Y92.482
    - freeway Y92.411
    - highway ramp Y92.415
    - interstate highway Y92.411
    - local residential or business street Y92.414
    - motorway Y92.411
    - parkway Y92.412
    - parking lot Y92.481
    - sidewalk Y92.480
    - specified NEC Y92.488
    - state road Y92.413
  - subway car Y92.816
  - supermarket Y92.512
  - swamp Y92.828
  - swimming pool (public) Y92.34
    - private (at) Y92.095
      - boarding house Y92.045
      - military base Y92.136
      - mobile home Y92.026
      - nursing home Y92.125
      - orphanage Y92.115
      - prison Y92.146
      - reform school Y92.156
      - single family residence Y92.016
  - synagogue Y92.22
  - television station Y92.59
  - tennis court Y92.312
  - theater Y92.254
  - trade area Y92.59
    - bank Y92.510
    - cafe Y92.511
    - casino Y92.59
    - garage Y92.59
    - hotel Y92.59
    - market Y92.512
    - office building Y92.59
    - radio station Y92.59
    - restaurant Y92.511
    - shop Y92.513
    - shopping mall Y92.59
    - store Y92.512
    - supermarket Y92.512
    - television station Y92.59
    - warehouse Y92.59
  - trailer park, residential — *see* Place of occurrence, residence, mobile home
  - trailer site NOS Y92.89
  - train Y92.815
    - station Y92.522
  - truck Y92.812
  - tunnel under construction Y92.69
  - urgent (health) care center Y92.532
  - university Y92.214
  - vehicle (transport) Y92.818
    - airplane Y92.813
    - boat Y92.814
    - bus Y92.811
    - car Y92.810
    - specified NEC Y92.818
    - subway car Y92.816
    - train Y92.815
    - truck Y92.812
  - warehouse Y92.59
  - water reservoir Y92.89
  - wilderness area Y92.828

- **Place of occurrence** - *continued*
  - wilderness area - *continued*
    - desert Y92.820
    - forest Y92.821
    - marsh Y92.828
    - mountain Y92.828
    - prairie Y92.828
    - specified NEC Y92.828
    - swamp Y92.828
  - workshop Y92.69
  - yard, private Y92.096
    - boarding house Y92.046
    - single family house Y92.017
    - mobile home Y92.027
  - youth center Y92.29
  - zoo (zoological garden) Y92.834
- **Plumbism** — *see* Table of Drugs and Chemicals, lead
- **Poisoning (accidental) (by)** — *see also* Table of Drugs and Chemicals
  - by plant, thorns, spines, sharp leaves or other mechanisms NEC X58
  - carbon monoxide
    - generated by
      - motor vehicle — *see* Accident, transport
      - watercraft (in transit) (not in transit) V93.89
        - ferry boat V93.81
        - fishing boat V93.82
        - jet skis V93.83
        - liner V93.81
        - merchant ship V93.80
        - passenger ship V93.81
        - powered craft NEC V93.83
  - caused by injection of poisons into skin by plant thorns, spines, sharp leaves X58
    - marine or sea plants (venomous) X58
  - exhaust gas
    - generated by
      - motor vehicle — *see* Accident, transport
      - watercraft (in transit) (not in transit) V93.89
        - ferry boat V93.81
        - fishing boat V93.82
        - jet skis V93.83
        - liner V93.81
        - merchant ship V93.80
        - passenger ship V93.81
        - powered craft NEC V93.83
  - fumes or smoke due to
    - explosion — *see also* Explosion W40.9
    - fire — *see* Exposure, fire
    - ignition — *see* Ignition
  - gas
    - in legal intervention — *see* Legal, intervention, gas
    - legal execution — *see* Legal, intervention, gas
  - in war operations — *see* War operations
  - legal
  - execution — *see* Legal, intervention, gas
    - intervention
      - by gas — *see* Legal, intervention, gas
      - other specified means — *see* Legal, intervention, specified means NEC
- **Powder burn (by) (from)**
  - airgun W34.110
  - BB gun W34.110
  - firearm NEC W34.19
  - gas, air or spring-operated gun NEC W34.118
  - handgun W32.1
  - hunting rifle W33.12
  - larger firearm W33.10
    - specified NEC W33.19
  - machine gun W33.13
  - paintball gun W34.111
  - pellet gun W34.110
  - shotgun W33.11
  - Very pistol [flare] W34.19
- **Premature cessation (of) surgical and medical care** Y66
- **Privation (food) (water)** X58

Procedure (operation)
- correct, on wrong side or body part (wrong side) (wrong site) Y65.53
- intended for another patient done on wrong patient Y65.52
- performed on patient not scheduled for surgery Y65.52
- performed on wrong patient Y65.52
- wrong, performed on correct patient Y65.51

Prolonged
- sitting in transport vehicle — *see* Travel, by type of vehicle
- stay in
  - high altitude as cause of anoxia, barodontalgia, barotitis or hypoxia W94.11
  - weightless environment X52

Pulling, excessive — *see also* Overexertion X50.9

Puncture, puncturing — *see also* Contact, with, by type of object or machine
- by
  - plant thorns, spines, sharp leaves or other mechanisms NEC W60
- during medical or surgical treatment as misadventure — *see* Index to Diseases and Injuries, Complication(s)

Pushed, pushing (accidental) (injury in)
- by other person (s) (accidental) W51
  - with fall W03
    - due to ice or snow W00.0
  - as, or caused by, a crowd or human stampede (with fall) W52
  - before moving object NEC Y02.8
    - motor vehicle Y02.0
    - subway train Y02.1
    - train Y02.1
  - from
    - high place NEC
      - in accidental circumstances W17.89
      - stated as
        - intentional, homicide (attempt) Y01
        - undetermined whether accidental or intentional Y30
    - transport vehicle NEC — *see also* Accident, transport V89.9
      - stated as
        - intentional, homicide (attempt) Y08.89
- overexertion X50.9

R

Radiation (exposure to)
- arc lamps W89.0
- atomic power plant (malfunction) NEC W88.1
- complication of or abnormal reaction to medical radiotherapy Y84.2
- electromagnetic, ionizing W88.0
- gamma rays W88.1
- in
  - war operations (from or following nuclear explosion) — *see* War operations
- inadvertent exposure of patient (receiving test or therapy) Y63.3
- infrared (heaters and lamps) W90.1
  - excessive heat from W92
- ionized, ionizing (particles, artificially accelerated)
  - radioisotopes W88.1
  - specified NEC W88.8
  - x-rays W88.0
- isotopes, radioactive — *see* Radiation, radioactive isotopes
- laser (s) W90.2
  - in war operations — *see* War operations
  - misadventure in medical care Y63.2
- light sources (man-made visible and ultraviolet) W89.9
  - natural X32
  - specified NEC W89.8
  - tanning bed W89.1
  - welding light W89.0
- man-made visible light W89.9
  - specified NEC W89.8
  - tanning bed W89.1

Radiation (exposure to) - *continued*
- man-made visible light - *continued*
  - welding light W89.0
- microwave W90.8
- misadventure in medical or surgical procedure Y63.2
- natural NEC X39.08
  - radon X39.01
- overdose (in medical or surgical procedure) Y63.2
- radar W90.0
- radioactive isotopes (any) W88.1
  - atomic power plant malfunction W88.1
  - misadventure in medical or surgical treatment Y63.2
- radiofrequency W90.0
- radium NEC W88.1
- sun X32
- ultraviolet (light) (man-made) W89.9
  - natural X32
  - specified NEC W89.8
  - tanning bed W89.1
  - welding light W89.0
- welding arc, torch, or light W89.0
  - excessive heat from W92
- x-rays (hard) (soft) W88.0

Range disease W94.11

Rape (attempted) T74.2-

Rat bite W53.11

Reaching (prolonged) (static) X50.1

Reaction, abnormal to medical procedure — *see also* Complication of or following, by type of procedure Y84.9
- with misadventure — *see* Misadventure
- biologicals — *see* Table of Drugs and Chemicals
- drugs — *see* Table of Drugs and Chemicals
- vaccine — *see* Table of Drugs and Chemicals

Recoil
- airgun W34.110
- BB gun W34.110
- firearm NEC W34.19
- gas, air or spring-operated gun NEC W34.118
- handgun W32.1
- hunting rifle W33.12
- larger firearm W33.10
  - specified NEC W33.19
- machine gun W33.13
- paintball gun W34.111
- pellet W34.110
- shotgun W33.11
- Very pistol [flare] W34.19

Reduction in
- atmospheric pressure - — *see* Air, pressure, change

Rock falling on or hitting (accidentally) (person) W20.8
- in cave-in W20.0

Run over (accidentally) (by)
- animal (not being ridden) NEC W55.89
- machinery — *see* Contact, with, by specified type of machine
- transport vehicle NEC — *see also* Accident, transport V09.9
  - intentional homicide (attempt) Y03.0
  - motor NEC V09.20
    - intentional homicide (attempt) Y03.0

Running
- before moving object X81.8
  - motor vehicle X81.0

Running off, away
- animal (being ridden) — *see also* Accident, transport V80.918
  - not being ridden W55.89
- animal-drawn vehicle NEC — *see also* Accident, transport V80.928
- highway, road (way) , street
  - transport vehicle NEC — *see also* Accident, transport V89.9

Rupture pressurized devices — *see* Explosion, by type of device

S

Saturnism — *see* Table of Drugs and Chemicals, lead

Scald, scalding (accidental) (by) (from) (in) X19
- air (hot) X14.1
- gases (hot) X14.1
- homicide (attempt) — *see* Assault, burning, hot object
- inflicted by other person
  - stated as intentional, homicide (attempt) — *see* Assault, burning, hot object
- liquid (boiling) (hot) NEC X12
  - stated as undetermined whether accidental or intentional Y27.2
  - suicide (attempt) X77.2
- local application of externally applied substance in medical or surgical care Y63.5
- metal (molten) (liquid) (hot) NEC X18
- self-inflicted X77.9
- stated as undetermined whether accidental or intentional Y27.8
- steam X13.1
  - assault X98.0
  - stated as undetermined whether accidental or intentional Y27.0
  - suicide (attempt) X77.0
- suicide (attempt) X77.9
- vapor (hot) X13.1
  - assault X98.0
  - stated as undetermined whether accidental or intentional Y27.0
  - suicide (attempt) X77.0

Scratched by
- cat W55.03
- person (s) (accidentally) W50.4
  - with intent to injure or kill Y04.0
  - as, or caused by, a crowd or human stampede (with fall) W52
  - assault Y04.0
  - homicide (attempt) Y04.0
  - in
    - fight Y04.0
    - legal intervention
      - injuring
        - bystander Y35.892
        - law enforcement personnel Y35.891
        - suspect Y35.893
        - unspecified person Y35.899

Seasickness T75.3

Self-harm NEC — *see also* External cause by type, undetermined whether accidental or intentional
- intentional — *see* Suicide
- poisoning NEC — *see* Table of drugs and biologicals, accident

Self-inflicted (injury) NEC — *see also* External cause by type, undetermined whether accidental or intentional
- intentional — *see* Suicide
- poisoning NEC — *see* Table of drugs and biologicals, accident

Sequelae (of)
- accident NEC — *see* W00-X58 with 7th character S
- assault (homicidal) (any means) — *see* X92-Y08 with 7th character S
- homicide, attempt (any means) — *see* X92-Y08 with 7th character S
- injury undetermined whether accidentally or purposely inflicted — *see* Y21-Y33 with 7th character S
- intentional self-harm (classifiable to X71-X83) — *see* X71-X83 with 7th character S
- legal intervention — *see* Y35 with 7th character S
- motor vehicle accident — *see* V00-V99 with 7th character S
- suicide, attempt (any means) — *see* X71-X83 with 7th character S
- transport accident — *see* V00-V99 with 7th character S
- war operations — *see* War operations

Shock
- electric — *see* Exposure, electric current

- **Struck (accidentally) by** - *continued*
  - object - *continued*
    - blunt - *continued*
      - assault Y00
      - suicide (attempt) X79
      - undetermined whether accidental or intentional Y29
    - falling W20.8
      - from, in, on
        - building W20.1
          - burning (uncontrolled fire) X00.4
        - cataclysmic
          - earth surface movement NEC — *see* Landslide
          - storm — *see* Forces of nature, cataclysmic storm
        - cave-in W20.0
        - earthquake X34
        - machine (in operation) — *see* Contact, with, by type of machine
        - structure W20.1
          - burning X00.4
        - transport vehicle (in motion) — *see* Accident, transport, by type of vehicle
        - watercraft V93.49
          - due to
            - accident to craft V91.39
              - powered craft V91.33
                - ferry boat V91.31
                - fishing boat V91.32
                - jetskis V91.33
                - liner V91.31
                - merchant ship V91.30
                - passenger ship V91.31
              - unpowered craft V91.38
                - canoe V91.35
                - inflatable V91.36
                - kayak V91.35
                - sailboat V91.34
                - surf-board V91.38
                - windsurfer V91.38
          - powered craft V93.43
            - ferry boat V93.41
            - fishing boat V93.42
            - jetskis V93.43
            - liner V93.41
            - merchant ship V93.40
            - passenger ship V93.41
          - unpowered craft V93.48
            - sailboat V93.44
            - surf-board V93.48
            - windsurfer V93.48
    - moving NEC W20.8
    - projected W20.8
      - assault Y00
      - in sports W21.9
        - assault Y08.09
        - ball W21.00
          - baseball W21.03
          - basketball W21.05
          - football W21.01
          - golf ball W21.04
          - soccer W21.02
          - softball W21.07
          - specified NEC W21.09
          - volleyball W21.06
        - bat or racquet
          - baseball bat W21.11
            - assault Y08.02
          - golf club W21.13
            - assault Y08.09
          - specified NEC W21.19
            - assault Y08.09
          - tennis racquet W21.12
            - assault Y08.09
        - hockey (ice)
          - field
            - puck W21.221
            - stick W21.211
          - puck W21.220
          - stick W21.210
            - assault Y08.01
        - specified NEC W21.89

- **Struck (accidentally) by** - *continued*
  - object - *continued*
    - set in motion by explosion — *see* Explosion
    - thrown W20.8
      - assault Y00
      - in sports W21.9
        - assault Y08.09
        - ball W21.00
          - baseball W21.03
          - basketball W21.05
          - football W21.01
          - golf ball W21.04
          - soccer W21.02
          - soft ball W21.07
          - specified NEC W21.09
          - volleyball W21.06
        - bat or racquet
          - baseball bat W21.11
            - assault Y08.02
          - golf club W21.13
            - assault Y08.09
          - specified NEC W21.19
            - assault Y08.09
          - tennis racquet W21.12
            - assault Y08.09
        - hockey (ice)
          - field
            - puck W21.221
            - stick W21.211
          - puck W21.220
          - stick W21.210
            - assault Y08.01
        - specified NEC W21.89
  - other person (s) W50.0
    - with
      - blunt object W22.8
        - intentional, homicide (attempt) Y00
        - sports equipment W21.9
        - undetermined whether accidental or intentional Y29
      - fall W03
        - due to ice or snow W00.0
    - as, or caused by, a crowd or human stampede (with fall) W52
    - assault Y04.2
    - homicide (attempt) Y04.2
    - in legal intervention
      - injuring
        - bystander Y35.812
        - law enforcement personnel Y35.811
        - suspect Y35.813
        - unspecified person Y35.819
    - sports equipment W21.9
  - police (on duty) — *see* Legal, intervention, manhandling
    - with blunt object — *see* Legal, intervention, blunt object
  - sports equipment W21.9
    - assault Y08.09
    - ball W21.00
      - baseball W21.03
      - basketball W21.05
      - football W21.01
      - golf ball W21.04
      - soccer W21.02
      - soft ball W21.07
      - specified NEC W21.09
      - volleyball W21.06
    - bat or racquet
      - baseball bat W21.11
        - assault Y08.02
      - golf club W21.13
        - assault Y08.09
      - specified NEC W21.19
      - tennis racquet W21.12
        - assault Y08.09
    - cleats (shoe) W21.31
    - foot wear NEC W21.39
    - football helmet W21.81
    - hockey (ice)
      - field
        - puck W21.221
        - stick W21.211
      - puck W21.220

- **Struck (accidentally) by** - *continued*
  - sports equipment - *continued*
    - hockey (ice) - *continued*
      - stick W21.210
        - assault Y08.01
    - skate blades W21.32
    - specified NEC W21.89
      - assault Y08.09
  - thunderbolt — *see* subcategory T75.0
    - causing fire — *see* Exposure, fire
  - transport vehicle NEC — *see also* Accident, transport V09.9
    - intentional, homicide (attempt) Y03.0
    - motor NEC — *see also* Accident, transport V09.20
      - homicide Y03.0
  - vehicle (transport) NEC — *see* Accident, transport, by type of vehicle
    - stationary (falling from jack, hydraulic lift, ramp) W20.8
- **Stumbling**
  - over
    - animal NEC W01.0
      - with fall W18.09
    - carpet, rug or (small) object W22.8
      - with fall W18.09
    - person W51
      - with fall W03
        - due to ice or snow W00.0
  - without fall W18.40
    - due to
      - specified NEC W18.49
      - stepping from one level to another W18.43
      - stepping into hole or opening W18.42
      - stepping on object W18.41
- **Submersion (accidental)** — *see* Drowning
- **Suffocation (accidental) (by external means) (by pressure) (mechanical)** (*see also* category T71)
  - due to, by
    - avalanche — *see* Landslide
    - explosion — *see* Explosion
    - fire — *see* Exposure, fire
    - food, any type (aspiration) (ingestion) (inhalation) — *see* categories T17 and T18
    - ignition — *see* Ignition
    - landslide — *see* Landslide
    - machine (ry) — *see* Contact, with, by type of machine
    - vomitus (aspiration) (inhalation) T17.81-
  - in
    - burning building X00.8
- **Suicide, suicidal (attempted) (by)** X83.8
  - blunt object X79
  - burning, burns X76
    - hot object X77.9
      - fluid NEC X77.2
      - household appliance X77.3
      - specified NEC X77.8
      - steam X77.0
      - tap water X77.1
      - vapors X77.0
  - caustic substance — *see* Table of Drugs and Chemicals
  - cold, extreme X83.2
  - collision of motor vehicle with
    - motor vehicle X82.0
    - specified NEC X82.8
    - train X82.1
    - tree X82.2
  - crashing of aircraft X83.0
  - cut (any part of body) X78.9
  - cutting or piercing instrument X78.9
    - dagger X78.2
    - glass X78.0
    - knife X78.1
    - specified NEC X78.8
    - sword X78.2
  - drowning (in) X71.9
    - bathtub X71.0
    - natural water X71.3
    - specified NEC X71.8
    - swimming pool X71.1

Suicide, suicidal (attempted) (by) - *continued*
- drowning (in) - *continued*
  - swimming pool - *continued*
    - following fall X71.2
- electrocution X83.1
- explosive (s) (material) X75
- fire, flames X76
- firearm X74.9
  - airgun X74.01
  - handgun X72
  - hunting rifle X73.1
  - larger X73.9
    - specified NEC X73.8
  - machine gun X73.2
  - shotgun X73.0
  - specified NEC X74.8
- hanging X83.8
- hot object — *see* Suicide, burning, hot object
- jumping
  - before moving object X81.8
    - motor vehicle X81.0
    - subway train X81.1
    - train X81.1
  - from high place X80
- late effect of attempt — *see* X71-X83 with 7th character S
- lying before moving object, train, vehicle X81.8
- poisoning — *see* Table of Drugs and Chemicals
- puncture (any part of body) — *see* Suicide, cutting or piercing instrument
- scald — *see* Suicide, burning, hot object
- sequelae of attempt — *see* X71-X83 with 7th character S
- sharp object (any) — *see* Suicide, cutting or piercing instrument
- shooting — *see* Suicide, firearm
- specified means NEC X83.8
- stab (any part of body) — *see* Suicide, cutting or piercing instrument
- steam, hot vapors X77.0
- strangulation X83.8
- submersion — *see* Suicide, drowning
- suffocation X83.8
- wound NEC X83.8

Sunstroke X32

Supersonic waves (causing injury) W42.0

Surgical procedure, complication of (delayed or as an abnormal reaction without mention of misadventure) — *see also* Complication of or following, by type of procedure
- due to or as a result of misadventure — *see* Misadventure

Swallowed, swallowing
- foreign body — *see* Foreign body, alimentary canal
- poison — *see* Table of Drugs and Chemicals
- substance
  - caustic or corrosive — *see* Table of Drugs and Chemicals
  - poisonous — *see* Table of Drugs and Chemicals

T

Tackle in sport W03

Terrorism (involving) Y38.80
- biological weapons Y38.6X-
- chemical weapons Y38.7X-
- conflagration Y38.3X-
- drowning and submersion Y38.89-
- explosion Y38.2X-
  - destruction of aircraft Y38.1X-
  - marine weapons Y38.0X-
- fire Y38.3X-
- firearms Y38.4X-
- hot substances Y38.3X-
- lasers Y38.89-
- nuclear weapons Y38.5X-
- piercing or stabbing instruments Y38.89-
- secondary effects Y38.9X-
- specified method NEC Y38.89-
- suicide bomber Y38.81-

Thirst X58

Threat to breathing
- aspiration — *see* Aspiration
- due to cave-in, falling earth or substance NEC — *see* category T71

Thrown (accidentally)
- against part (any) of or object in transport vehicle (in motion) NEC — *see also* Accident, transport
- from
  - high place, homicide (attempt) Y01
  - machinery — *see* Contact, with, by type of machine
  - transport vehicle NEC — *see also* Accident, transport V89.9
- off — *see* Thrown, from

Thunderbolt — *see* subcategory T75.0
- causing fire — *see* Exposure, fire

Tidal wave (any injury) NEC — *see* Forces of nature, tidal wave

Took
- overdose (drug) — *see* Table of Drugs and Chemicals
- poison — *see* Table of Drugs and Chemicals

Tornado (any injury) X37.1

Torrential rain (any injury) X37.8

Torture X58

Trampled by animal NEC W55.89

Trapped (accidentally)
- between objects (moving) (stationary and moving) — *see* Caught
- by part (any) of
  - motorcycle V29.88
  - pedal cycle V19.88
  - transport vehicle NEC — *see also* Accident, transport V89.9

Travel (effects) (sickness) T75.3

Tree falling on or hitting (accidentally) (person) W20.8

Tripping
- over
  - animal W01.0
    - with fall W01.0
  - carpet, rug or (small) object W22.8
    - with fall W18.09
  - person W51
    - with fall W03
      - due to ice or snow W00.0
- without fall W18.40
  - due to
    - specified NEC W18.49
    - stepping from one level to another W18.43
    - stepping into hole or opening W18.42
    - stepping on object W18.41

Twisted by person (s) (accidentally) W50.2
- with intent to injure or kill Y04.0
- as, or caused by, a crowd or human stampede (with fall) W52
- assault Y04.0
- homicide (attempt) Y04.0
- in
  - fight Y04.0
  - legal intervention — *see* Legal, intervention, manhandling

Twisting (prolonged) (static) X50.1

U

Underdosing of necessary drugs, medicaments or biological substances Y63.6

Undetermined intent (contact) (exposure)
- automobile collision Y32
- blunt object Y29
- drowning (submersion) (in) Y21.9
  - bathtub Y21.0
    - after fall Y21.1
  - natural water (lake) (ocean) (pond) (river) (stream) Y21.4
  - specified place NEC Y21.8
  - swimming pool Y21.2
    - after fall Y21.3
- explosive material Y25
- fall, jump or push from high place Y30
- falling, lying or running before moving object Y31
- fire Y26

Undetermined intent (contact) (exposure) - *continued*
- firearm discharge Y24.9
  - airgun (BB) (pellet) Y24.0
  - handgun (pistol) (revolver) Y22
  - hunting rifle Y23.1
  - larger Y23.9
    - hunting rifle Y23.1
    - machine gun Y23.3
    - military Y23.2
    - shotgun Y23.0
    - specified type NEC Y23.8
  - machine gun Y23.3
  - military Y23.2
  - shotgun Y23.0
  - specified type NEC Y24.8
  - Very pistol Y24.8
- hot object Y27.9
  - fluid NEC Y27.2
  - household appliance Y27.3
  - specified object NEC Y27.8
  - steam Y27.0
  - tap water Y27.1
  - vapor Y27.0
- jump, fall or push from high place Y30
- lying, falling or running before moving object Y31
- motor vehicle crash Y32
- push, fall or jump from high place Y30
- running, falling or lying before moving object Y31
- sharp object Y28.9
  - dagger Y28.2
  - glass Y28.0
  - knife Y28.1
  - specified object NEC Y28.8
  - sword Y28.2
- smoke Y26
- specified event NEC Y33

Use of hand as hammer X50.3

V

Vibration (causing injury) W49.9

Victim (of)
- avalanche — *see* Landslide
- earth movements NEC — *see* Forces of nature, earth movement
- earthquake X34
- flood — *see* Flood
- landslide — *see* Landslide
- lightning — *see* subcategory T75.0
  - causing fire — *see* Exposure, fire
- storm (cataclysmic) NEC — *see* Forces of nature, cataclysmic storm
- volcanic eruption X35

Volcanic eruption (any injury) X35

Vomitus, gastric contents in air passages (with asphyxia, obstruction or suffocation) T17.81-

W

Walked into stationary object (any) W22.09
- furniture W22.03
- lamppost W22.02
- wall W22.01

War operations (injuries to military personnel and civilians during war, civil insurrection and peacekeeping missions) (by) (from) (involving) Y36.90
- after cessation of hostilities Y36.89-
  - explosion (of)
    - bomb placed during war operations Y36.82-
    - mine placed during war operations Y36.81-
  - specified NEC Y36.88-
- air blast Y36.20-
- aircraft
  - destruction — *see* War operations, destruction of aircraft
- airway restriction — *see* War operations, restriction of airways
- asphyxiation — *see* War operations, restriction of airways
- biological weapons Y36.6X-
- blast Y36.20-
- blast fragments Y36.20-

WAR OPERATIONS - WRONG

Chapter 1: Infectious and Parasitic Diseases (A00-B99)

In this chapter, code selection usually is determined by the specific organism involved in the disease process. "Infectious" refers to a disease caused by a microorganism, or capable of being communicated by infection (contagious). "Parasitic" refers to a disease caused by a parasite (e.g., a tick).

In home care, it is rare to receive documentation naming the infection-causing organism, but when the information is available from the physician, it should be used when selecting the diagnosis code. It is acceptable to code a diagnosis in a lab or pathology report provided by a physician (such as a pathologist or radiologist) ***who has interpreted the results***, per Q1 2017 Coding Clinic. As is always the case, the critical data used to assign codes is in the medical record, the assessment, and the Plan of Care documentation. After selecting the correct codes, proper sequencing is the next concern.

Code categories found in this first chapter include infectious conditions related to specific locations or conditions (such as intestinal infectious diseases, tuberculosis and poliomyelitis), viral infections (such as human immunodeficiency virus), bacterial infections (such as leprosy), diseases caused by parasites (zoonotic bacterial and arthropod-borne viral diseases), venereal diseases, mycoses (fungal infections), helminthiases (intestinal parasites or worms), and the late effects of these conditions.

Certain diseases also have been arranged in Chapter 1 of ICD-10-CM within separate subchapters or blocks that group similar conditions together. Examples include: infections with a predominantly sexual mode of transmission (A50-A64), viral hepatitis (B15-B19), and other viral diseases (B25-B34). Some conditions such as streptococcal sore throat and its inclusion terms previously listed in Chapter 1 have been reclassified in ICD-10-CM to Chapter 10: Diseases of the respiratory system.

Many of the codes in Chapter 1 have been expanded to reflect manifestations of the disease with the use of fourth or fifth characters allowing the infectious disease and manifestation to be now captured with one code instead of two.

Example: A01.0 Typhoid fever

Infection due to Salmonella typhi

A01.00, Typhoid fever, unspecified

A01.01, Typhoid meningitis

A01.02, Typhoid fever with heart involvement

A01.03, Typhoid pneumonia

A01.04, Typhoid arthritis

A01.05, Typhoid osteomyelitis

A01.09, Typhoid fever with other complications

The correct code can be found by looking up the term for the condition in the Alphabetic Index and then look at the subterms listed, which will list possible organisms. For example, to find the code for "encephalitis caused by meningococcus, "look up encephalitis with subterm meningococcal, which leads to A39.81.

Remember that sometimes a Chapter 1 code is not the most appropriate choice. The following are a few situations to watch out for:

- If a patient has a **personal or family history of infectious or parasitic disease** reported in this chapter, it may be more appropriate to use a code from the Z code section, such as Z86.19 (Personal history of infectious and parasitic diseases).
- If the patient has **been exposed to an infectious disease** but does not currently have the disease, refer to 'Exposure (to) or Contact, with' in the Alphabetical Index, which leads to Z20.1 (Contact with tuberculosis).
- If the patient is a **carrier or suspected carrier of an infectious disease**, refer to 'Carrier' in the Alphabetical Index, which will generally direct you to a Z22.- code.
- If the organism causing an infection is **resistant to antibiotics (other than methicillin)**, search under 'Resistance' in the Alphabetical Index, which will refer you to a Z16.- code. MRSA is coded with specific codes MRSA codes, and Z16.- codes are not used for MRSA.
- If an **infection is the result of injury or medical treatment**, a code for the injury or medical complication may be reported with a code from this chapter.
- Watch for **combination codes,** especially with pneumonia and influenza under those main terms in the Alphabetical Index. Then, confirm in the Tabular List (Chapter 10: Respiratory Diseases) where the infectious agent is already included in the disease code. For example, Staphylococcus aureus pneumonia is coded with combination code J15.211 (Methicillin susceptible staphylococcus aureus).
- Although not often coded in home health, if reporting an **infectious or parasitic disease in a pregnant patient**, and the condition is complicating the pregnancy, report first a code

from Chapter 15, Pregnancy, Childbirth and the Puerperium, and a code from Chapter 1 as an additional diagnosis.

- For **Zika virus infections**, code only a confirmed diagnosis (A92.5) as documented by the provider. This is an exception to the hospital inpatient guideline. In this context, "confirmation" does not require documentation of the type of test performed; the physician's diagnostic statement that the condition is confirmed is sufficient. If the provider documents "suspected", "possible" or "probable" Zika, do not assign code A92.5. Instead, assign a code(s) explaining the reason for encounter (such as fever, rash, or joint pain) or Z20.828, Contact with and (suspected) exposure to other viral communicable diseases

Multiple Coding and Sequencing

Certain infections are classified in chapters other than Chapter 1 and no organism is identified as part of the infection code. In these instances, it is necessary to use an additional code from Chapter 1 to identify the organism. For example, the following codes are to be used as an additional code to identify the organism: A code from category B95, Streptococcus, Staphylococcus, and Enterococcus, as the cause of the disease classified in other chapters; B96, Other bacterial agents as the cause of diseases classified to other chapters; or B97, Viral agents as the cause of other diseases classified to other chapters. An instructional note will be found at the infection code advising that an additional organism code is required.

For these categories, a code from another chapter is reported first to indicate the condition, and an additional code from Chapter 1 categories B95-B97 is reported to indicate the organism responsible for the condition.

Here are some examples:

- A urinary tract infection due to Escherichia coli (E. coli), site not specified, is reported with code N39.0 for the urinary tract infection, site not specified, from Chapter 14 first followed by (the organism), E. coli (B96.20) from Chapter 1. A note under code N39.0 states "Use additional code to identify organism."
- T87.43 describes an infection of an amputation stump, right lower extremity. If the physician documents the causative organism to be staphylococcus, unspecified, (B95.8), the correct code sequence is T87.43 and then B95.8. If the documentation supports staphylococcus aureus, the correct add-on code is B95.61. If the documentation supports MRSA, the additional code is B95.62. The code from the B95 category should be sequenced right after the code for the condition and never in the primary slot.
- A patient with pulmonary insufficiency as a late effect of tuberculosis is another sequencing exception. This is reported using J98.4 (other pulmonary insufficiency) and an additional code B90.9 (sequelae of respiratory and unspecified tuberculosis).

Always remember that Includes and Excludes notes are crucial, and it is important to follow any other instructions under the code or code category.

Special Issues

HIV

Code only confirmed cases of HIV infection/illness. Human immunodeficiency virus [HIV] disease is only reported if the physician's documentation states that the patient is HIV positive with symptoms, or has an HIV-related illness. If the patient has an HIV-related condition, the principal diagnosis should be B20, Human immunodeficiency virus (HIV), followed by additional diagnosis codes for all related HIV-related conditions. Here are some examples:

- If the patient is being seen for a HIV-related condition, report B20 as the first-listed diagnosis. For example, a patient with Kaposi's sarcoma and HIV/AIDS is reported with B20 as the first-listed diagnosis, and C46.- (Kaposi's sarcoma) as the additional diagnosis.
- If the patient is being seen for a condition unrelated to the HIV, report the other condition as first-listed diagnosis.
- Code Z21 (Asymptomatic human immunodeficiency virus [HIV] infection status) is to be applied when the patient without any documentation of symptoms is listed as being "HIV positive," "known HIV," "HIV test positive," or similar terminology. Do not use this code if "AIDS" is used or is described as having any condition(s) resulting from his/her HIV positive status; use B20 in these cases.
- Patients with inconclusive HIV serology, but no definitive diagnosis or manifestation of the illness, may be assigned code R75, Inconclusive laboratory evidence of human immunodeficiency virus [HIV].
- Patients with any known prior diagnoses of an HIV-related illness should be coded to B20. Once a patient has developed an HIV-related illness, the patient should always be assigned code B20 on every subsequent admission/encounter. Patients previously diagnoses with any HIV illness (B20) should never be assigned to R75 or Z21, Asymptomatic human immunodeficiency virus [HIV] infection status.

- During pregnancy, childbirth or the puerperium, a patient admitted for a health care encounter because of an HIV-related illness should receive a principle diagnosis code of O98.7-, Human immunodeficiency [HIV] disease complicating pregnancy, childbirth and the puerperium, followed by the B20 and the code(s) for the HIV-related illness(es). Codes from Chapter 15, (Pregnancy, Childbirth and the Puerperium) always take sequencing priority.
- Some states and U.S. territories have specific restrictions on the coding of HIV, including Alaska, Arizona, California, Colorado, Connecticut, DC, Delaware, Hawaii, Idaho, Illinois, Iowa, Maryland, Massachusetts, Michigan, Mississippi, Montana, Nevada, New Jersey, New Mexico, North Dakota, Oregon, Puerto Rico, South Carolina, Texas, Utah, Virgin Islands, Washington, West Virginia, Wisconsin and Wyoming. Some of these states restrict the coding of B20 as primary and some prohibit the use of the code. Seek a code for an associated condition in these cases, such as B59, pneumocystosis.

Sepsis, Severe Sepsis and Septic Shock

Sepsis

For a diagnosis of sepsis, assign the appropriate code for the underlying systemic infection. If the type of infection or causal organism is not further specified, assign code A41.9, Sepsis, unspecified organism.

A code from subcategory R65.2, Severe sepsis, should not be assigned unless severe sepsis or an associated acute organ dysfunction is documented. This guideline takes precedence over the fact that acute organ dysfunction is listed under "with" in the alphabetic index listing for "sepsis." [I.C.1.d.1.a]

- **Negative or inconclusive blood cultures** do not preclude a diagnosis of sepsis in patients with clinical evidence of the condition, however, the physician should be queried.
- The term **urosepsis is a nonspecific term and it is not to be considered synonymous with sepsis.** It has no default code in the Alphabetical Index. Should a provider use this term, he/she must be queried for clarification.
- If a patient has sepsis **and** associated acute organ dysfunction or multiple organ dysfunction (MOD), **follow the instructions for coding severe sepsis**.
- If a patient has sepsis and an acute organ dysfunction, but the medical record documentation indicates that the acute organ dysfunction is related to a medical condition other than sepsis, do not assign a code from subcategory R65.2, Severe sepsis. **An acute organ dysfunction must be associated with the sepsis in order to assign the severe sepsis code.** If the documentation is not clear as to whether the acute organ dysfunction is related to the sepsis or another medical condition, query the physician.

Severe sepsis

The coding of severe sepsis requires a minimum of two codes: first a code for the underlying systemic infection, followed by a code from subcategory R65.2, Severe sepsis. If the causal organism is not documented, assign A41.9, Sepsis, unspecified organism, for the infection. Additional code(s) for the associated acute organ dysfunction are also required.

Due to the complex nature of severe sepsis, some cases may require querying the physician prior to assignment of the codes.

Septic shock

Septic shock generally refers to circulatory failure associated with severe sepsis, and therefore, it represents a type of acute organ dysfunction.

For cases of septic shock, the code for the systemic infection should be sequenced first, followed by code R65.21, Severe sepsis with septic shock or code T81.12, Postprocedural septic shock. Any additional codes for the other acute organ dysfunctions should also be assigned. As noted in the sequencing instructions in the Tabular List, the code for the septic shock cannot be assigned as a principal diagnosis.

Sepsis and severe sepsis with a localized infection

If the reason for admission is both sepsis or severe sepsis and a localized infection, such as pneumonia or cellulitis, a code(s) for the underlying systemic infection should be sequenced first, and the code for the localized infection should be assigned as a secondary diagnosis. If the patient has severe sepsis, a code from subcategory R65.2 should also be assigned as a secondary diagnosis. If the patient is admitted with a localized infection, such as pneumonia, and sepsis/severe sepsis doesn't develop until after admission, the localized infection should be assigned first, followed by the appropriate sepsis/severe sepsis codes.

Sepsis due to a post-procedural infection

In cases of sepsis due to post-procedural infection, base the code assignment **on the provider's documentation of the relationship between the infection and the procedure**.

For such cases, the post-procedural infection code, such as T80.2, Infections following infusion, transfusion and therapeutic injection; T81.44, Sepsis following a procedure; T88.0, Infection following immunization; or O86.0-, Infection of obstetrical surgical wound, should be coded first, followed by the code for the specific infection. If the patient has severe sepsis the appropriate code from subcategory R65.2 should also be assigned with the additional code(s) for any acute organ dysfunction.

Sepsis and severe sepsis associated with a noninfectious process (condition)

If sepsis or severe sepsis is documented as associated with a noninfectious condition, such as a burn or serious injury, and this condition meets the definition for principal diagnosis, the code for the noninfectious process is sequenced first, followed by the code for the resulting infection. If severe sepsis is present, a code from subcategory R65.2 should also be assigned with any associated organ dysfunction(s) codes. It is not necessary to assign a code from R65.1, Systemic inflammatory response syndrome (SIRS) of non-infectious origin, for these cases.

MRSA and MSSA

When a patient is diagnoses with an infection that is due to methicillin resistant Staphylococcus aureus (MRSA) or Methicillin susceptible Staphylococcus aureus (MSSA), and that infection has a combination code that includes the causal organism, assign the appropriate combination code for the condition (e.g., A41.02, Sepsis due to MRSA). Do not assign code B95.62, Methicillin resistant Staphylococcus aureus infection, as the cause of diseases classified elsewhere, or Z16.11, Resistance to penicillins, as additional diagnoses. If a patient has a diagnosis of pneumonia due to Methicillin susceptible Staphylococcus aureus, code only the combination code J15.211 without an additional code from B95.61.

When there is documentation of a current infection (e.g., wound infection, stitch abscess, urinary tract infection) due to MRSA, and that infection does not have a combination code that includes the causal organism, assign the appropriate code to identify the condition along with a code from B95.62, Methicillin Resistant Staphylococcus Aureus (MRSA), or B95.61 Methicillin Susceptible Staphylococcus Aureus (MSSA), as the cause of the diseases classified elsewhere for the MRSA or MSSA infection. Do not assign a code from subcategory Z16.11, Resistance to penicillins, along with the B95.62 code.

The condition or state of being colonized or carrying MSSA or MRSA is called colonization or carriage, while an individual person is described as being colonized or being a carrier. Colonization means that MSSA or MRSA is present on or in the body without necessarily causing illness. A positive MRSA colonization test might be documented by the provider as "MRSA positive screen" or "MRSA nasal swab positive."

Assign code Z22.322, Carrier or suspected carrier of Methicillin resistant Staphylococcus aureus, for patients documented as having MRSA colonization. Assign code Z22.321, Carrier or suspected carrier of Methicillin susceptible Staphylococcus aureus, for patients documented as having MSSA colonization. Colonization is not necessarily indicative of a disease process or as the cause of a specific condition the patient may have unless documented as such by the provider. If the patient is stated to have a history of MRSA, use code Z86.14.

If a patient is documented as having both MRSA colonization ***and*** infection, you may assign both code Z22.322, Carrier or suspected carrier of MRSA, and a code for the MRSA infection.

CHAPTER 1: CERTAIN INFECTIOUS AND PARASITIC DISEASES (A00-B99)

INCLUDES diseases generally recognized as communicable or transmissible

Use additional code to identify resistance to antimicrobial drugs (Z16.-)

EXCLUDES 1 certain localized infections - see body system-related chapters

EXCLUDES 2 carrier or suspected carrier of infectious disease (Z22.-)
infectious and parasitic diseases complicating pregnancy, childbirth and the puerperium (O98.-)
infectious and parasitic diseases specific to the perinatal period (P35-P39)
influenza and other acute respiratory infections (J00-J22)

This chapter contains the following blocks:

A00-A09	Intestinal infectious diseases
A15-A19	Tuberculosis
A20-A28	Certain zoonotic bacterial diseases
A30-A49	Other bacterial diseases
A50-A64	Infections with a predominantly sexual mode of transmission
A65-A69	Other spirochetal diseases
A70-A74	Other diseases caused by chlamydiae
A75-A79	Rickettsioses
A80-A89	Viral and prion infections of the central nervous system
A90-A99	Arthropod-borne viral fevers and viral hemorrhagic fevers
B00-B09	Viral infections characterized by skin and mucous membrane lesions
B10	Other human herpesviruses
B15-B19	Viral hepatitis
B20	Human immunodeficiency virus [HIV] disease
B25-B34	Other viral diseases
B35-B49	Mycoses
B50-B64	Protozoal diseases
B65-B83	Helminthiases
B85-B89	Pediculosis, acariasis and other infestations
B90-B94	Sequelae of infectious and parasitic diseases
B95-B97	Bacterial and viral infectious agents
B99	Other infectious diseases

Intestinal infectious diseases (A00-A09)

4 **A00 Cholera**

SP **A00.0 Cholera due to Vibrio cholerae 01, biovar cholerae**
Classical cholera

SP **A00.1 Cholera due to Vibrio cholerae 01, biovar eltor**
Cholera eltor

SP **A00.9 Cholera, unspecified**

4 **A01 Typhoid and paratyphoid fevers**

5 **A01.0 Typhoid fever**
Infection due to Salmonella typhi

SP **A01.00 Typhoid fever, unspecified**

SP **A01.01 Typhoid meningitis**

SP **A01.02 Typhoid fever with heart involvement**
Typhoid endocarditis
Typhoid myocarditis

SP **A01.03 Typhoid pneumonia**

SP **A01.04 Typhoid arthritis**

SP **A01.05 Typhoid osteomyelitis**

SP **A01.09 Typhoid fever with other complications**

SP **A01.1 Paratyphoid fever A**

SP **A01.2 Paratyphoid fever B**

SP **A01.3 Paratyphoid fever C**

SP **A01.4 Paratyphoid fever, unspecified**
Infection due to Salmonella paratyphi NOS

4 **A02 Other salmonella infections**
INCLUDES infection or foodborne intoxication due to any Salmonella species other than S. typhi and S. paratyphi

SP **A02.0 Salmonella enteritis**
Salmonellosis

SP **A02.1 Salmonella sepsis**

5 **A02.2 Localized salmonella infections**

SP **A02.20 Localized salmonella infection, unspecified**

SP **A02.21 Salmonella meningitis**

SP **A02.22 Salmonella pneumonia**

SP **A02.23 Salmonella arthritis**

CODING TIPS ✓ Salmonella arthritis is a form of reactive arthritis. Code A02.23 indicates the arthritis and its cause. Do not assign an additional code for arthritis.

SP **A02.24 Salmonella osteomyelitis**

SP **A02.25 Salmonella pyelonephritis**
Salmonella tubulo-interstitial nephropathy

SP **A02.29 Salmonella with other localized infection**

SP **A02.8 Other specified salmonella infections**

SP **A02.9 Salmonella infection, unspecified**

4 **A03 Shigellosis**

SP **A03.0 Shigellosis due to Shigella dysenteriae**
Group A shigellosis [Shiga-Kruse dysentery]

SP **A03.1 Shigellosis due to Shigella flexneri**
Group B shigellosis

SP **A03.2 Shigellosis due to Shigella boydii**
Group C shigellosis

SP **A03.3 Shigellosis due to Shigella sonnei**
Group D shigellosis

SP **A03.8 Other shigellosis**

SP **A03.9 Shigellosis, unspecified**
Bacillary dysentery NOS

4 **A04 Other bacterial intestinal infections**
EXCLUDES 1 bacterial foodborne intoxications, NEC (A05.-)
tuberculous enteritis (A18.32)

SP **A04.0 Enteropathogenic Escherichia coli infection**

SP **A04.1 Enterotoxigenic Escherichia coli infection**

SP **A04.2 Enteroinvasive Escherichia coli infection**

SP **A04.3 Enterohemorrhagic Escherichia coli infection**

SP **A04.4 Other intestinal Escherichia coli infections**
Escherichia coli enteritis NOS

Chapter 1 | A00 - B99

CODING TIPS✓ This code for E. coli (A04.4) is used when the bacterium causes intestinal infection and is not to be used for other E. coli infections, e.g., UTIs. See B96.2- for other infections caused by E. coli.

SP **A04.5 Campylobacter enteritis**

SP **A04.6 Enteritis due to Yersinia enterocolitica**

EXCLUDES 1 extraintestinal yersiniosis (A28.2)

CODING TIPS✓ Arthropathy associated with Yersinia requires an additional code from M02.-.

5 **A04.7 Enterocolitis due to Clostridium difficile**

Foodborne intoxication by Clostridium difficile

Pseudomembraneous colitis

DEFINITION Clostridium difficile (C. difficile) is an anaerobic gram-positive, spore-forming, toxin-producing bacillus that is transmitted among humans through the fecal–oral route. C. difficile causes antibiotic associated colitis by colonizing the human intestinal tract after the normal gut flora have been altered due to antibiotic therapy. Recurrence is defined by complete abatement of CDI symptoms while on appropriate therapy, followed by subsequent reappearance of diarrhea and other symptoms after treatment has been stopped. Recurrence typically occurs within one week after treatment cessation, however recurrence may occur up to 8 weeks later.

SP **A04.71 Enterocolitis due to Clostridium difficile, recurrent**

CODING TIPS✓ Recurrence is defined by complete abatement of CDI symptoms while on appropriate therapy, followed by subsequent reappearance of diarrhea and other symptoms after treatment has been stopped. Recurrence typically occurs within one week after treatment cessation, however recurrence may occur up to 8 weeks later.

SP **A04.72 Enterocolitis due to Clostridium difficile, not specified as recurrent**

CODING TIPS✓ A04.72 is the default code for C. difficile enteritis. Use this code when there is no documentation of recurrence.

SP **A04.8 Other specified bacterial intestinal infections**

SP **A04.9 Bacterial intestinal infection, unspecified**

Bacterial enteritis NOS

CODING TIPS✓ Report A04.9 if the patient is suffering from diarrhea known to be infectious and bacterial, but only if the condition is otherwise unspecified, i.e., if the specific bacterial agent is unknown.

4 **A05 Other bacterial foodborne intoxications, not elsewhere classified**

EXCLUDES 1 Clostridium difficile foodborne intoxication and infection (A04.7-)
Escherichia coli infection (A04.0-A04.4)
listeriosis (A32.-)
salmonella foodborne intoxication and infection (A02.-)
toxic effect of noxious foodstuffs (T61-T62)

SP **A05.0 Foodborne staphylococcal intoxication**

SP **A05.1 Botulism food poisoning**

Botulism NOS

Classical foodborne intoxication due to Clostridium botulinum

EXCLUDES 1 infant botulism (A48.51)
wound botulism (A48.52)

DEFINITION Muscle-paralyzing disease caused by ingesting the neurotoxins produced by the bacteria Clostridium botulinum.

SP **A05.2 Foodborne Clostridium perfringens [Clostridium welchii] intoxication**

Enteritis necroticans

Pig-bel

SP **A05.3 Foodborne Vibrio parahaemolyticus intoxication**

SP **A05.4 Foodborne Bacillus cereus intoxication**

SP **A05.5 Foodborne Vibrio vulnificus intoxication**

SP **A05.8 Other specified bacterial foodborne intoxications**

SP **A05.9 Bacterial foodborne intoxication, unspecified**

4 **A06 Amebiasis**

INCLUDES infection due to Entamoeba histolytica

EXCLUDES 1 other protozoal intestinal diseases (A07.-)

EXCLUDES 2 acanthamebiasis (B60.1-)
Naegleriasis (B60.2)

SP **A06.0 Acute amebic dysentery**

Acute amebiasis

Intestinal amebiasis NOS

SP **A06.1 Chronic intestinal amebiasis**

SP **A06.2 Amebic nondysenteric colitis**

SP **A06.3 Ameboma of intestine**

Ameboma NOS

SP **A06.4 Amebic liver abscess**

Hepatic amebiasis

SP **A06.5 Amebic lung abscess**

Amebic abscess of lung (and liver)

SP **A06.6 Amebic brain abscess**

Amebic abscess of brain (and liver) (and lung)

CODING TIPS✓ Report A06.6 for an amebic infection of the brain, which may or may not include an infection of the liver and/or lung. Do not report a liver or lung infection separately.

SP **A06.7 Cutaneous amebiasis**

5 **A06.8 Amebic infection of other sites**

SP **A06.81 Amebic cystitis**

SP **A06.82 Other amebic genitourinary infections**

Amebic balanitis

Amebic vesiculitis
Amebic vulvovaginitis

SP A06.89 **Other amebic infections**
Amebic appendicitis
Amebic splenic abscess

SP A06.9 **Amebiasis, unspecified**

4 A07 **Other protozoal intestinal diseases**

SP A07.0 **Balantidiasis**
Balantidial dysentery

SP A07.1 **Giardiasis [lambliasis]**

SP A07.2 **Cryptosporidiosis**

SP A07.3 **Isosporiasis**
Infection due to Isospora belli and Isospora hominis
Intestinal coccidiosis
Isosporosis

SP A07.4 **Cyclosporiasis**

SP A07.8 **Other specified protozoal intestinal diseases**
Intestinal microsporidiosis
Intestinal trichomoniasis
Sarcocystosis
Sarcosporidiosis

SP A07.9 **Protozoal intestinal disease, unspecified**
Flagellate diarrhea
Protozoal colitis
Protozoal diarrhea
Protozoal dysentery

4 A08 **Viral and other specified intestinal infections**
EXCLUDES 1 influenza with involvement of gastrointestinal tract (J09.X3, J10.2, J11.2)

CODING TIPS ✓ Note that an influenza infection that also affects the intestinal tract is reported with J09.x3, J10.2, or J11.2 codes, not A08.

SP A08.0 **Rotaviral enteritis**

5 A08.1 **Acute gastroenteropathy due to Norwalk agent and other small round viruses**

SP A08.11 **Acute gastroenteropathy due to Norwalk agent**
Acute gastroenteropathy due to Norovirus
Acute gastroenteropathy due to Norwalk-like agent

SP A08.19 **Acute gastroenteropathy due to other small round viruses**
Acute gastroenteropathy due to small round virus [SRV] NOS

SP A08.2 **Adenoviral enteritis**

5 A08.3 **Other viral enteritis**

SP A08.31 **Calicivirus enteritis**

SP A08.32 **Astrovirus enteritis**

SP A08.39 **Other viral enteritis**
Coxsackie virus enteritis
Echovirus enteritis
Enterovirus enteritis NEC
Torovirus enteritis

SP A08.4 **Viral intestinal infection, unspecified**
Viral enteritis NOS
Viral gastroenteritis NOS
Viral gastroenteropathy NOS

SP A08.8 **Other specified intestinal infections**

SP A09 **Infectious gastroenteritis and colitis, unspecified**
Infectious colitis NOS
Infectious enteritis NOS
Infectious gastroenteritis NOS
EXCLUDES 1 colitis NOS (K52.9)
diarrhea NOS (R19.7)
enteritis NOS (K52.9)
gastroenteritis NOS (K52.9)
noninfective gastroenteritis and colitis, unspecified (K52.9)

Tuberculosis (A15-A19)

INCLUDES infections due to Mycobacterium tuberculosis and Mycobacterium bovis

EXCLUDES 1 congenital tuberculosis (P37.0)
nonspecific reaction to test for tuberculosis without active tuberculosis (R76.1-)
pneumoconiosis associated with tuberculosis, any type in A15 (J65)
positive PPD (R76.11)
positive tuberculin skin test without active tuberculosis (R76.11)
sequelae of tuberculosis (B90.-)
silicotuberculosis (J65)

CODING TIPS ✓ Codes from A15-A19 should not be assigned to report a positive PPD (Mantoux) test. A positive PPD (Mantoux) skin test without active tuberculosis should be coded to R76.11.

CODING TIPS ✓ These codes are for active TB. See B90 for sequelae of TB and Z86.11 for personal history of TB without residuals.

4 A15 **Respiratory tuberculosis**

SP A15.0 **Tuberculosis of lung**
Tuberculous bronchiectasis
Tuberculous fibrosis of lung
Tuberculous pneumonia
Tuberculous pneumothorax

SP A15.4 **Tuberculosis of intrathoracic lymph nodes**
Tuberculosis of hilar lymph nodes
Tuberculosis of mediastinal lymph nodes
Tuberculosis of tracheobronchial lymph nodes
EXCLUDES 1 tuberculosis specified as primary (A15.7)

SP A15.5 **Tuberculosis of larynx, trachea and bronchus**
Tuberculosis of bronchus
Tuberculosis of glottis
Tuberculosis of larynx
Tuberculosis of trachea

SP A15.6 **Tuberculous pleurisy**
Tuberculosis of pleura Tuberculous empyema
EXCLUDES 1 primary respiratory tuberculosis (A15.7)

SP A15.7 **Primary respiratory tuberculosis**

SP A15.8 **Other respiratory tuberculosis**
Mediastinal tuberculosis
Nasopharyngeal tuberculosis
Tuberculosis of nose
Tuberculosis of sinus [any nasal]

SP A15.9 **Respiratory tuberculosis unspecified**

4 A17 **Tuberculosis of nervous system**

SP A17.0 **Tuberculous meningitis**

Chapter 1

A00 - B99

Tuberculosis of meninges (cerebral)(spinal)
Tuberculous leptomeningitis
EXCLUDES 1 tuberculous meningoencephalitis (A17.82)

SP **A17.1 Meningeal tuberculoma**
Tuberculoma of meninges (cerebral) (spinal)
EXCLUDES 2 tuberculoma of brain and spinal cord (A17.81)

5 **A17.8 Other tuberculosis of nervous system**

SP **A17.81 Tuberculoma of brain and spinal cord**
Tuberculous abscess of brain and spinal cord

SP **A17.82 Tuberculous meningoencephalitis**
Tuberculous myelitis

SP **A17.83 Tuberculous neuritis**
Tuberculous mononeuropathy

SP **A17.89 Other tuberculosis of nervous system**
Tuberculous polyneuropathy

SP **A17.9 Tuberculosis of nervous system, unspecified**

4 **A18 Tuberculosis of other organs**

5 **A18.0 Tuberculosis of bones and joints**

SP **A18.01 Tuberculosis of spine**
Pott's disease or curvature of spine
Tuberculous arthritis
Tuberculous osteomyelitis of spine
Tuberculous spondylitis

SP **A18.02 Tuberculous arthritis of other joints**
Tuberculosis of hip (joint)
Tuberculosis of knee (joint)
CODING TIPS✓ Report A18.02 for a TB infection of the hip or knee joint or bone.

SP **A18.03 Tuberculosis of other bones**
Tuberculous mastoiditis
Tuberculous osteomyelitis
CODING TIPS✓ Report A18.03 for a TB infection of bones, except for hip, knee and spine.

SP **A18.09 Other musculoskeletal tuberculosis**
Tuberculous myositis
Tuberculous synovitis
Tuberculous tenosynovitis

5 **A18.1 Tuberculosis of genitourinary system**

IQ **A18.10 Tuberculosis of genitourinary system, unspecified**

SP **A18.11 Tuberculosis of kidney and ureter**

SP **A18.12 Tuberculosis of bladder**

SP **A18.13 Tuberculosis of other urinary organs**
Tuberculous urethritis

SP **A18.14 Tuberculosis of prostate**

SP **A18.15 Tuberculosis of other male genital organs**

SP **A18.16 Tuberculosis of cervix**

SP **A18.17 Tuberculous female pelvic inflammatory disease**
Tuberculous endometritis
Tuberculous oophoritis and salpingitis

SP **A18.18 Tuberculosis of other female genital organs**
Tuberculous ulceration of vulva

SP **A18.2 Tuberculous peripheral lymphadenopathy**
Tuberculous adenitis
EXCLUDES 2 tuberculosis of bronchial and mediastinal lymph nodes (A15.4)
tuberculosis of mesenteric and retroperitoneal lymph nodes (A18.39)
tuberculous tracheobronchial adenopathy (A15.4)

5 **A18.3 Tuberculosis of intestines, peritoneum and mesenteric glands**

SP **A18.31 Tuberculous peritonitis**
Tuberculous ascites

SP **A18.32 Tuberculous enteritis**
Tuberculosis of anus and rectum
Tuberculosis of intestine (large) (small)

SP **A18.39 Retroperitoneal tuberculosis**
Tuberculosis of mesenteric glands
Tuberculosis of retroperitoneal (lymph glands)

SP **A18.4 Tuberculosis of skin and subcutaneous tissue**
Erythema induratum, tuberculous
Lupus excedens
Lupus vulgaris NOS
Lupus vulgaris of eyelid
Scrofuloderma
Tuberculosis of external ear
EXCLUDES 2 lupus erythematosus (L93.-)
systemic lupus erythematosus (M32.-)

5 **A18.5 Tuberculosis of eye**
EXCLUDES 2 lupus vulgaris of eyelid (A18.4)

SP **A18.50 Tuberculosis of eye, unspecified**

SP **A18.51 Tuberculous episcleritis**

SP **A18.52 Tuberculous keratitis**
Tuberculous interstitial keratitis
Tuberculous keratoconjunctivitis (interstitial) (phlyctenular)

SP **A18.53 Tuberculous chorioretinitis**

SP **A18.54 Tuberculous iridocyclitis**

SP **A18.59 Other tuberculosis of eye**
Tuberculous conjunctivitis

SP **A18.6 Tuberculosis of (inner) (middle) ear**
Tuberculous otitis media
EXCLUDES 2 tuberculosis of external ear (A18.4)
tuberculous mastoiditis (A18.03)

SP **A18.7 Tuberculosis of adrenal glands**
Tuberculous Addison's disease

5 **A18.8 Tuberculosis of other specified organs**

SP **A18.81 Tuberculosis of thyroid gland**

SP **A18.82 Tuberculosis of other endocrine glands**
Tuberculosis of pituitary gland
Tuberculosis of thymus gland

SP **A18.83 Tuberculosis of digestive tract organs, not elsewhere classified**
EXCLUDES 1 tuberculosis of intestine (A18.32)

SP **A18.84 Tuberculosis of heart**
Tuberculous cardiomyopathy
Tuberculous endocarditis

4 4th digit required 5 5th digit required 6 6th digit required 7 7th digit required 7 7th digit placeholder + Additional code Laterality

Tuberculous myocarditis
Tuberculous pericarditis

SP **A18.85 Tuberculosis of spleen**

SP **A18.89 Tuberculosis of other sites**
Tuberculosis of muscle
Tuberculous cerebral arteritis

4 **A19 Miliary tuberculosis**
INCLUDES disseminated tuberculosis
generalized tuberculosis
tuberculous polyserositis

CODING TIPS ✓ Miliary tuberculosis (TB) is the widespread dissemination of Mycobacterium tuberculosis via hematogenous spread. Code A19.8 should be used for miliary TB that is documented as chronic.

SP **A19.0 Acute miliary tuberculosis of a single specified site**

SP **A19.1 Acute miliary tuberculosis of multiple sites**

SP **A19.2 Acute miliary tuberculosis, unspecified**

SP **A19.8 Other miliary tuberculosis**

SP **A19.9 Miliary tuberculosis, unspecified**

Certain zoonotic bacterial diseases (A20-A28)

4 **A20 Plague**
INCLUDES infection due to Yersinia pestis

SP **A20.0 Bubonic plague**
DEFINITION Infection with the Yersinia pestis bacillus, transmitted via flea, tick, and lice bites and by contact with infected persons or materials, causing severe inflammation and death of skin cells.

SP **A20.1 Cellulocutaneous plague**

SP **A20.2 Pneumonic plague**
DEFINITION Rapidly progressive, often fatal plague pneumonia caused by direct inhalation of bacteria with severe cough producing frothy, bloody, mucoid sputum.

SP **A20.3 Plague meningitis**

SP **A20.7 Septicemic plague**
DEFINITION High-density bloodstream infection in acute bubonic plague; may cause death before the appearance of buboes or pulmonary manifestations.

SP **A20.8 Other forms of plague**
Abortive plague
Asymptomatic plague
Pestis minor

SP **A20.9 Plague, unspecified**

4 **A21 Tularemia**
INCLUDES deer-fly fever
infection due to Francisella tularensis
rabbit fever

SP **A21.0 Ulceroglandular tularemia**

SP **A21.1 Oculoglandular tularemia**
Ophthalmic tularemia

SP **A21.2 Pulmonary tularemia**

SP **A21.3 Gastrointestinal tularemia**
Abdominal tularemia

SP **A21.7 Generalized tularemia**

SP **A21.8 Other forms of tularemia**

SP **A21.9 Tularemia, unspecified**

4 **A22 Anthrax**
INCLUDES infection due to Bacillus anthracis

SP **A22.0 Cutaneous anthrax**
Malignant carbuncle
Malignant pustule

SP **A22.1 Pulmonary anthrax**
Inhalation anthrax
Ragpicker's disease
Woolsorter's disease

SP **A22.2 Gastrointestinal anthrax**

SP **A22.7 Anthrax sepsis**

SP **A22.8 Other forms of anthrax**
Anthrax meningitis

SP **A22.9 Anthrax, unspecified**

4 **A23 Brucellosis**
INCLUDES Malta fever
Mediterranean fever
undulant fever

SP **A23.0 Brucellosis due to Brucella melitensis**

SP **A23.1 Brucellosis due to Brucella abortus**

SP **A23.2 Brucellosis due to Brucella suis**

SP **A23.3 Brucellosis due to Brucella canis**

SP **A23.8 Other brucellosis**

SP **A23.9 Brucellosis, unspecified**

4 **A24 Glanders and melioidosis**

SP **A24.0 Glanders**
Infection due to Pseudomonas mallei
Malleus

SP **A24.1 Acute and fulminating melioidosis**
Melioidosis pneumonia
Melioidosis sepsis

SP **A24.2 Subacute and chronic melioidosis**

SP **A24.3 Other melioidosis**

SP **A24.9 Melioidosis, unspecified**
Infection due to Pseudomonas pseudomallei NOS
Whitmore's disease

4 **A25 Rat-bite fevers**

SP **A25.0 Spirillosis**
Sodoku

SP **A25.1 Streptobacillosis**
Epidemic arthritic erythema
Haverhill fever
Streptobacillary rat-bite fever

SP **A25.9 Rat-bite fever, unspecified**

4 **A26 Erysipeloid**

SP **A26.0 Cutaneous erysipeloid**
Erythema migrans

SP **A26.7 Erysipelothrix sepsis**

SP **A26.8 Other forms of erysipeloid**

SP **A26.9 Erysipeloid, unspecified**

4 **A27 Leptospirosis**

SP **A27.0 Leptospirosis icterohemorrhagica**
Leptospiral or spirochetal jaundice (hemorrhagic)
Weil's disease

5 **A27.8 Other forms of leptospirosis**

SP **A27.81 Aseptic meningitis in leptospirosis**

SP **A27.89 Other forms of leptospirosis**

SP **A27.9 Leptospirosis, unspecified**

Chapter 1 A00 - B99

4 **A28 Other zoonotic bacterial diseases, not elsewhere classified**

SP **A28.0 Pasteurellosis**

SP **A28.1 Cat-scratch disease**
Cat-scratch fever

SP **A28.2 Extraintestinal yersiniosis**
EXCLUDES 1 enteritis due to Yersinia enterocolitica (A04.6)
plague (A20.-)

SP **A28.8 Other specified zoonotic bacterial diseases, not elsewhere classified**

IQ **A28.9 Zoonotic bacterial disease, unspecified**

Other bacterial diseases (A30-A49)

4 **A30 Leprosy [Hansen's disease]**
INCLUDES infection due to Mycobacterium leprae
EXCLUDES 1 sequelae of leprosy (B92)
CODING TIPS ✓ Arthropathy associated with leprosy requires an additional code from M01.-.

SP **A30.0 Indeterminate leprosy**
I leprosy

SP **A30.1 Tuberculoid leprosy**
TT leprosy

SP **A30.2 Borderline tuberculoid leprosy**
BT leprosy

SP **A30.3 Borderline leprosy**
BB leprosy

SP **A30.4 Borderline lepromatous leprosy**
BL leprosy

SP **A30.5 Lepromatous leprosy**
LL leprosy

SP **A30.8 Other forms of leprosy**

SP **A30.9 Leprosy, unspecified**

4 **A31 Infection due to other mycobacteria**
EXCLUDES 2 leprosy (A30.-)
tuberculosis (A15-A19)

SP **A31.0 Pulmonary mycobacterial infection**
Infection due to Mycobacterium avium
Infection due to Mycobacterium intracellulare [Battey bacillus]
Infection due to Mycobacterium kansasii

SP **A31.1 Cutaneous mycobacterial infection**
Buruli ulcer
Infection due to Mycobacterium marinum
Infection due to Mycobacterium ulcerans

SP **A31.2 Disseminated mycobacterium avium-intracellulare complex (DMAC)**
MAC sepsis

SP **A31.8 Other mycobacterial infections**

SP **A31.9 Mycobacterial infection, unspecified**
Atypical mycobacterial infection NOS
Mycobacteriosis NOS

4 **A32 Listeriosis**
INCLUDES listerial foodborne infection
EXCLUDES 1 neonatal (disseminated) listeriosis (P37.2)

SP **A32.0 Cutaneous listeriosis**

5 **A32.1 Listerial meningitis and meningoencephalitis**

SP **A32.11 Listerial meningitis**

SP **A32.12 Listerial meningoencephalitis**

SP **A32.7 Listerial sepsis**

5 **A32.8 Other forms of listeriosis**

SP **A32.81 Oculoglandular listeriosis**

SP **A32.82 Listerial endocarditis**

SP **A32.89 Other forms of listeriosis**
Listerial cerebral arteritis

SP **A32.9 Listeriosis, unspecified**

SP **A33 Tetanus neonatorum**

SP **A34 Obstetrical tetanus**

SP **A35 Other tetanus**
Tetanus NOS
EXCLUDES 1 obstetrical tetanus (A34)
tetanus neonatorum (A33)
DEFINITION Potentially fatal disease due to the neurotoxin of Clostridium tetani, entering the body through contaminated wound, burn, or ulcer; causes muscular contractions, hyperreflexia, lockjaw, respiratory spasm, seizures, and paralysis.

4 **A36 Diphtheria**

SP **A36.0 Pharyngeal diphtheria**
Diphtheritic membranous angina
Tonsillar diphtheria
DEFINITION An acute infectious disease usually confined to the upper respiratory tract, caused by toxigenic strains of Corynebacterium diphtheriae, and acquired by contact with an infected person or carrier of the disease.

SP **A36.1 Nasopharyngeal diphtheria**

SP **A36.2 Laryngeal diphtheria**
Diphtheritic laryngotracheitis

SP **A36.3 Cutaneous diphtheria**
EXCLUDES 2 erythrasma (L08.1)

5 **A36.8 Other diphtheria**

SP **A36.81 Diphtheritic cardiomyopathy**
Diphtheritic myocarditis

SP **A36.82 Diphtheritic radiculomyelitis**

SP **A36.83 Diphtheritic polyneuritis**

SP **A36.84 Diphtheritic tubulo-interstitial nephropathy**

SP **A36.85 Diphtheritic cystitis**

SP **A36.86 Diphtheritic conjunctivitis**

SP **A36.89 Other diphtheritic complications**
Diphtheritic peritonitis

SP **A36.9 Diphtheria, unspecified**

4 **A37 Whooping cough**

5 **A37.0 Whooping cough due to Bordetella pertussis**
DEFINITION Infectious disease caused by Bordetella pertussis, marked by inflammation of mucous membranes and cough, ending in a prolonged crowing or whooping respiration.

▲ SP **A37.00 Whooping cough due to Bordetella pertussis without pneumonia**
Paroxysmal cough due to Bordetella pertussis without pneumonia

▲ SP **A37.01 Whooping cough due to Bordetella pertussis with pneumonia**
Paroxysmal cough due to Bordetella pertussis with pneumonia

5 **A37.1 Whooping cough due to Bordetella parapertussis**

SP **A37.10 Whooping cough due to Bordetella parapertussis without pneumonia**

SP **A37.11 Whooping cough due to Bordetella parapertussis with pneumonia**

5 **A37.8 Whooping cough due to other Bordetella species**

SP **A37.80 Whooping cough due to other Bordetella species without pneumonia**

SP **A37.81 Whooping cough due to other Bordetella species with pneumonia**

5 **A37.9 Whooping cough, unspecified species**

SP **A37.90 Whooping cough, unspecified species without pneumonia**

SP **A37.91 Whooping cough, unspecified species with pneumonia**

4 **A38 Scarlet fever**

INCLUDES scarlatina

EXCLUDES 2 streptococcal sore throat (J02.0)

SP **A38.0 Scarlet fever with otitis media**

DEFINITION Infection with group A beta-hemolytic streptococcal bacteria causing sore throat, fever, and rough, bright red "sandpaper" rash over most of the body.

SP **A38.1 Scarlet fever with myocarditis**

SP **A38.8 Scarlet fever with other complications**

SP **A38.9 Scarlet fever, uncomplicated**

Scarlet fever, NOS

4 **A39 Meningococcal infection**

SP **A39.0 Meningococcal meningitis**

DEFINITION Inflammation of the membranes (meninges) around the brain or spinal cord causing fever, headache, stiff neck, muscle aches, and skin rashes.

SP **A39.1 Waterhouse-Friderichsen syndrome**

Meningococcal hemorrhagic adrenalitis
Meningococcic adrenal syndrome

DEFINITION Syndrome associated with meningococcal meningitis, marked by sudden fever, purple skin discoloration, and hemorrhage into the adrenal glands with cardiovascular collapse.

SP **A39.2 Acute meningococcemia**

SP **A39.3 Chronic meningococcemia**

SP **A39.4 Meningococcemia, unspecified**

5 **A39.5 Meningococcal heart disease**

SP **A39.50 Meningococcal carditis, unspecified**

SP **A39.51 Meningococcal endocarditis**

SP **A39.52 Meningococcal myocarditis**

SP **A39.53 Meningococcal pericarditis**

5 **A39.8 Other meningococcal infections**

SP **A39.81 Meningococcal encephalitis**

SP **A39.82 Meningococcal retrobulbar neuritis**

SP **A39.83 Meningococcal arthritis**

SP **A39.84 Postmeningococcal arthritis**

SP **A39.89 Other meningococcal infections**

Meningococcal conjunctivitis

SP **A39.9 Meningococcal infection, unspecified**

Meningococcal disease NOS

4 **A40 Streptococcal sepsis**

Code first:
- postprocedural streptococcal sepsis (T81.4-)
- streptococcal sepsis during labor (O75.3)
- streptococcal sepsis following abortion or ectopic or molar pregnancy (O03-O07, O08.0)
- streptococcal sepsis following immunization (T88.0)
- streptococcal sepsis following infusion, transfusion or therapeutic injection (T80.2-)

EXCLUDES 1 neonatal (P36.0-P36.1)
puerperal sepsis (O85)
sepsis due to Streptococcus, group D (A41.81)

GUIDELINES **Section I.C.1.d.1)(a)(i-iii)**

Negative or inconclusive blood cultures do not preclude a diagnosis of sepsis in patients with clinical evidence of the condition, however, the provider should be queried.

The term urosepsis is a nonspecific term. It is not to be considered synonymous with sepsis. It has no default code in the Alphabetic Index. Should a provider use this term, he/she must be queried for clarification.

If a patient has sepsis and associated acute organ dysfunction or multiple organ dysfunction (MOD), follow the instructions for coding severe sepsis.

GUIDELINES **Section I.C.1.d.1)(a)(iv)**

If a patient has sepsis and an acute organ dysfunction, but the medical record documentation indicates that the acute organ dysfunction is related to a medical condition other than the sepsis, do not assign a code from subcategory R65.2, Severe sepsis. An acute organ dysfunction must be associated with the sepsis in order to assign the severe sepsis code. If the documentation is not clear as to whether an acute organ dysfunction is related to the sepsis or another medical condition, query the provider.

CODING TIPS✓ If sepsis is related to a medical or surgical procedure, the specific complication code is sequenced prior to the A40 or A41 code. If a surgical wound becomes septic, sequence first T81.4-A for the wound infection, followed by T81.44xA. Follow with the appropriate A40-A41 code.

CODING TIPS✓ When sepsis is present with a localized infection, such as UTI or pneumonia, sequence the sepsis and then the localized infection. The causative organism may be identified in the sepsis code, and therefore doesn't need to be repeated with the localized infection, except in the case of combination codes that identify the organism. Use the combination code for the pneumonia, if the localized infection is pneumonia.

CODING TIPS✓ Do not assign a code from A40-A41 to indicate a bacterial infection in conditions classified elsewhere, e.g., a localized infection. Codes classified in A40-A41 are used to indicate systemic infection.

CODING TIPS✓ Sepsis is the systemic inflammatory response to an infection. When assigning a code for sepsis, review clinical documentation to ensure the clinician has provided support for the diagnosis, as well as clearly documented the causative organism. While the organism may be clearly stated in the physician or NPP record, and the coder may use this to assign the correct code, the home health record should support the continued treatment of the unresolved infection and/or systemic response, as well as clearly state the causative organism (when known).

CODING TIPS✓ Severe sepsis is defined as sepsis resulting in organ dysfunction or failure. If sepsis is associated with organ dysfunction or failure, add R65.2 to indicate severe sepsis. Severe sepsis is a complication ordinarily resolved prior to home care, so query the physician or NPP regarding the continued presence of severe sepsis at discharge from the inpatient facility. The organ dysfunction or failure should be added as a third code if organ dysfunction is related to the sepsis. R65.21 indicates the presence of septic shock which is considered organ dysfunction in and of itself.

SP **A40.0 Sepsis due to streptococcus, group A**

SP **A40.1 Sepsis due to streptococcus, group B**

SP **A40.3 Sepsis due to Streptococcus pneumoniae**
Pneumococcal sepsis

SP **A40.8 Other streptococcal sepsis**

SP **A40.9 Streptococcal sepsis, unspecified**

4 **A41 Other sepsis**

Code first:
- postprocedural sepsis (T81.4-)
- sepsis during labor (O75.3)
- sepsis following abortion, ectopic or molar pregnancy (O03-O07, O08.0)
- sepsis following immunization (T88.0)
- sepsis following infusion, transfusion or therapeutic injection (T80.2-)

EXCLUDES 1
- bacteremia NOS (R78.81)
- neonatal (P36.-)
- puerperal sepsis (O85)
- streptococcal sepsis (A40.-)

EXCLUDES 2
- sepsis (due to) (in) actinomycotic (A42.7)
- sepsis (due to) (in) anthrax (A22.7)
- sepsis (due to) (in) candidal (B37.7)
- sepsis (due to) (in) Erysipelothrix (A26.7)
- sepsis (due to) (in) extraintestinal yersiniosis (A28.2)
- sepsis (due to) (in) gonococcal (A54.86)
- sepsis (due to) (in) herpesviral (B00.7)
- sepsis (due to) (in) listerial (A32.7)
- sepsis (due to) (in) melioidosis (A24.1)
- sepsis (due to) (in) meningococcal (A39.2-A39.4)
- sepsis (due to) (in) plague (A20.7)
- sepsis (due to) (in) tularemia (A21.7)
- toxic shock syndrome (A48.3)

GUIDELINES **Section I.C.1.d.1)(a)**
For a diagnosis of sepsis, assign the appropriate code for the underlying systemic infection. If the type of infection or causal organism is not further specified, assign code A41.9, Sepsis, unspecified organism. A code from subcategory R65.2, Severe sepsis, should not be assigned unless severe sepsis or an associated acute organ dysfunction is documented.

GUIDELINES **Section I.C.1.d.1)(b)**
The coding of severe sepsis requires a minimum of two codes: first a code for the underlying systemic infection, followed by a code from subcategory R65.2, Severe sepsis. If the causal organism is not documented, assign code A41.9, Sepsis, unspecified organism, for the infection. Additional code(s) for the associated acute organ dysfunction are also required. Due to the complex nature of severe sepsis, some cases may require querying the provider prior to assignment of the codes.

CODING TIPS✓ If sepsis is related to a medical or surgical procedure, the specific complication code is sequenced prior to the A40 or A41 code. If a surgical wound becomes septic, sequence first T81.4-A for the wound infection, followed by T81.44xA. Follow with the appropriate A40-A41 code.

CODING TIPS✓ When sepsis is present with a localized infection, such as UTI or pneumonia, sequence the sepsis and then the localized infection. The causative organism may be identified in the sepsis code, and therefore doesn't need to be repeated with the localized infection, except in the case of combination codes that identify the organism. Use the combination code for the pneumonia, if the localized infection is pneumonia.

CODING TIPS✓ Sepsis is the systemic inflammatory response to an infection. When assigning a code for sepsis, review clinical documentation to ensure the clinician has provided support for the diagnosis, as well as clearly documented the causative organism. While the organism may be clearly stated in the physician or NPP record, and the coder may use this to assign the correct code, the home health record should support the continued treatment of the unresolved infection and/or systemic response, as well as clearly state the causative organism (when known).

CODING TIPS✓ Do not assign a code from A40-A41 to indicate a bacterial infection in conditions classified elsewhere, e.g., a localized infection. Codes classified in A40-A41 are used to indicate systemic infection.

CODING TIPS✓ Severe sepsis is defined as sepsis resulting in organ dysfunction or failure. If sepsis is associated with organ dysfunction or failure, add R65.2 to indicate severe sepsis. Severe sepsis is a complication ordinarily resolved prior to home care, so query the physician or NPP regarding the continued presence of severe sepsis at discharge from the inpatient facility. The organ dysfunction or failure should be added as a third code if organ dysfunction is related to the sepsis. R65.21 indicates the presence of septic shock which is considered organ dysfunction in and of itself.

5 **A41.0 Sepsis due to Staphylococcus aureus**

SP **A41.01 Sepsis due to Methicillin susceptible Staphylococcus aureus**
MSSA sepsis
Staphylococcus aureus sepsis NOS

CODING TIPS✓ Use this code when the Staph aureus causing the sepsis is not methicillin resistant.

SP **A41.02 Sepsis due to Methicillin resistant Staphylococcus aureus**

GUIDELINES **Section I.C.1.e.1)(a).** When a patient is diagnosed with an infection that is due to methicillin resistant Staphylococcus aureus (MRSA), and that infection has a combination code that includes the causal organism (e.g., sepsis, pneumonia) assign the appropriate combination code for the condition (e.g., code A41.02 ...). Do not assign code B95.62, Methicillin resistant Staphylococcus aureus infection as the cause of diseases classified elsewhere, as an additional code because the combination code includes the type of infection and the MRSA organism.

CODING TIPS✓ Do not assign a Z16 code to indicate Staph aureus resistance to penicillins. Z16 codes may be added for other resistance, such as Vancomycin resistance, or when other bacteria other than Staphylococcus aureus are involved.

SP **A41.1 Sepsis due to other specified staphylococcus**
Coagulase negative staphylococcus sepsis

SP **A41.2 Sepsis due to unspecified staphylococcus**

CODING TIPS✓ Use this code if sepsis is identified as caused by staph without specification as to species.

SP **A41.3 Sepsis due to Hemophilus influenzae**

SP **A41.4 Sepsis due to anaerobes**
EXCLUDES 1 gas gangrene (A48.0)

5 **A41.5 Sepsis due to other Gram-negative organisms**

SP **A41.50 Gram-negative sepsis, unspecified**
Gram-negative sepsis NOS

SP **A41.51 Sepsis due to Escherichia coli [E. coli]**

SP **A41.52 Sepsis due to Pseudomonas**
Pseudomonas aeroginosa

SP **A41.53 Sepsis due to Serratia**

SP **A41.59 Other Gram-negative sepsis**

5 **A41.8 Other specified sepsis**

SP **A41.81 Sepsis due to Enterococcus**

SP **A41.89 Other specified sepsis**

CODING TIPS✓ If a patient is admitted with sepsis due to COVID-19 pneumonia and the sepsis meets the definition of principal diagnosis, then the code for viral sepsis (A41.89) should be assigned as principal diagnosis followed by codes U07.1 and J12.82, as secondary diagnoses.

SP **A41.9 Sepsis, unspecified organism**
Septicemia NOS

CODING TIPS✓ Septicemia is coded to A41.9 when the bacteria has not been identified. A41.9 is also acceptable for sepsis when the bacteria responsible has not been identified. The physician or NPP should be queried.

4 **A42 Actinomycosis**
EXCLUDES 1 actinomycetoma (B47.1)

SP **A42.0 Pulmonary actinomycosis**

SP **A42.1 Abdominal actinomycosis**

SP **A42.2 Cervicofacial actinomycosis**

SP **A42.7 Actinomycotic sepsis**

5 **A42.8 Other forms of actinomycosis**

SP **A42.81 Actinomycotic meningitis**

SP **A42.82 Actinomycotic encephalitis**

SP **A42.89 Other forms of actinomycosis**

SP **A42.9 Actinomycosis, unspecified**

4 **A43 Nocardiosis**

SP **A43.0 Pulmonary nocardiosis**

SP **A43.1 Cutaneous nocardiosis**

SP **A43.8 Other forms of nocardiosis**

SP **A43.9 Nocardiosis, unspecified**

4 **A44 Bartonellosis**

SP **A44.0 Systemic bartonellosis**
Oroya fever

SP **A44.1 Cutaneous and mucocutaneous bartonellosis**
Verruga peruana

SP **A44.8 Other forms of bartonellosis**

SP **A44.9 Bartonellosis, unspecified**

SP **A46 Erysipelas**
EXCLUDES 1 postpartum or puerperal erysipelas (O86.89)

DEFINITION Superficial cellulitis with dermal lymphatic involvement, commonly caused by group A beta-hemolytic streptococci; presents with shiny, raised, indurated, tender lesions with distinct margins, commonly on the legs and face.

4 **A48 Other bacterial diseases, not elsewhere classified**

EXCLUDES 1 actinomycetoma (B47.1)

SP **A48.0 Gas gangrene**
Clostridial cellulitis
Clostridial myonecrosis

CODING TIPS ✓ Gas gangrene is a medical emergency and is not the gangrene routinely coded in home care and hospice, known as dry gangrene. If gas gangrene is documented, there is an assumed relationship between diabetes and gas gangrene and A48.0 is coded after the appropriate code for diabetes with gangrene.

SP **A48.1 Legionnaires' disease**

SP **A48.2 Nonpneumonic Legionnaires' disease [Pontiac fever]**

SP + **A48.3 Toxic shock syndrome**
Use additional code to identify the organism (B95, B96)
EXCLUDES 1 endotoxic shock NOS (R57.8)
sepsis NOS (A41.9)

SP **A48.4 Brazilian purpuric fever**
Systemic Hemophilus aegyptius infection

5 **A48.5 Other specified botulism**
Non-foodborne intoxication due to toxins of Clostridium botulinum [C. botulinum]
EXCLUDES 1 food poisoning due to toxins of Clostridium botulinum (A05.1)

SP **A48.51 Infant botulism**

SP + **A48.52 Wound botulism**
Non-foodborne botulism NOS
Use additional code for associated wound

DEFINITION Wound infection with Clostridium botulinum producing neurological effects of severe hypotonia and paralysis without gastrointestinal symptoms of food poisoning.

SP **A48.8 Other specified bacterial diseases**

4 **A49 Bacterial infection of unspecified site**
EXCLUDES 1 bacterial agents as the cause of diseases classified elsewhere (B95-B96)
chlamydial infection NOS (A74.9)
meningococcal infection NOS (A39.9)
rickettsial infection NOS (A79.9)
spirochetal infection NOS (A69.9)

CODING TIPS ✓ These codes indicate a bacterial infection in an unknown site. Do not use these codes to indicate bacterial infections. See A40-A41 for sepsis or B95 and B96 for causative organisms for localized infections (if a combination code does not apply).

5 **A49.0 Staphylococcal infection, unspecified site**

IQ **A49.01 Methicillin susceptible Staphylococcus aureus infection, unspecified site**
Methicillin susceptible Staphylococcus aureus (MSSA) infection
Staphylococcus aureus infection NOS

IQ **A49.02 Methicillin resistant Staphylococcus aureus infection, unspecified site**
Methicillin resistant Staphylococcus aureus (MRSA) infection

IQ **A49.1 Streptococcal infection, unspecified site**

IQ **A49.2 Hemophilus influenzae infection, unspecified site**

IQ **A49.3 Mycoplasma infection, unspecified site**

IQ **A49.8 Other bacterial infections of unspecified site**

IQ **A49.9 Bacterial infection, unspecified**
EXCLUDES 1 bacteremia NOS (R78.81)

Infections with a predominantly sexual mode of transmission (A50-A64)

EXCLUDES 1 human immunodeficiency virus [HIV] disease (B20)
nonspecific and nongonococcal urethritis (N34.1)
Reiter's disease (M02.3-)

4 **A50 Congenital syphilis**

5 **A50.0 Early congenital syphilis, symptomatic**
Any congenital syphilitic condition specified as early or manifest less than two years after birth.

SP **A50.01 Early congenital syphilitic oculopathy**

SP **A50.02 Early congenital syphilitic osteochondropathy**

SP **A50.03 Early congenital syphilitic pharyngitis**
Early congenital syphilitic laryngitis

SP **A50.04 Early congenital syphilitic pneumonia**

SP **A50.05 Early congenital syphilitic rhinitis**

SP **A50.06 Early cutaneous congenital syphilis**

SP **A50.07 Early mucocutaneous congenital syphilis**

SP **A50.08 Early visceral congenital syphilis**

SP **A50.09 Other early congenital syphilis, symptomatic**

SP **A50.1 Early congenital syphilis, latent**
Congenital syphilis without clinical manifestations, with positive serological reaction and negative spinal fluid test, less than two years after birth.

SP **A50.2 Early congenital syphilis, unspecified**
Congenital syphilis NOS less than two years after birth.

5 **A50.3 Late congenital syphilitic oculopathy**
EXCLUDES 1 Hutchinson's triad (A50.53)

SP **A50.30 Late congenital syphilitic oculopathy, unspecified**

SP **A50.31 Late congenital syphilitic interstitial keratitis**

SP **A50.32 Late congenital syphilitic chorioretinitis**

SP **A50.39 Other late congenital syphilitic oculopathy**

+ 5 **A50.4 Late congenital neurosyphilis [juvenile neurosyphilis]**

Use additional code to identify any associated mental disorder

EXCLUDES 1 Hutchinson's triad (A50.53)

SP + A50.40 **Late congenital neurosyphilis, unspecified**

Juvenile neurosyphilis NOS

SP + A50.41 **Late congenital syphilitic meningitis**

SP + A50.42 **Late congenital syphilitic encephalitis**

SP + A50.43 **Late congenital syphilitic polyneuropathy**

SP + A50.44 **Late congenital syphilitic optic nerve atrophy**

SP + A50.45 **Juvenile general paresis**

Dementia paralytica juvenilis
Juvenile tabetoparetic neurosyphilis

SP + A50.49 **Other late congenital neurosyphilis**

Juvenile tabes dorsalis

5 A50.5 **Other late congenital syphilis, symptomatic**

Any congenital syphilitic condition specified as late or manifest two years or more after birth.

SP A50.51 **Clutton's joints**

SP A50.52 **Hutchinson's teeth**

SP A50.53 **Hutchinson's triad**

SP A50.54 **Late congenital cardiovascular syphilis**

SP A50.55 **Late congenital syphilitic arthropathy**

SP A50.56 **Late congenital syphilitic osteochondropathy**

SP A50.57 **Syphilitic saddle nose**

SP A50.59 **Other late congenital syphilis, symptomatic**

SP A50.6 **Late congenital syphilis, latent**

Congenital syphilis without clinical manifestations, with positive serological reaction and negative spinal fluid test, two years or more after birth.

SP A50.7 **Late congenital syphilis, unspecified**

Congenital syphilis NOS two years or more after birth.

SP A50.9 **Congenital syphilis, unspecified**

4 A51 **Early syphilis**

SP A51.0 **Primary genital syphilis**

Syphilitic chancre NOS

SP A51.1 **Primary anal syphilis**

SP A51.2 **Primary syphilis of other sites**

5 A51.3 **Secondary syphilis of skin and mucous membranes**

SP A51.31 **Condyloma latum**

SP A51.32 **Syphilitic alopecia**

SP A51.39 **Other secondary syphilis of skin**

Syphilitic leukoderma
Syphilitic mucous patch

EXCLUDES 1 late syphilitic leukoderma (A52.79)

5 A51.4 **Other secondary syphilis**

SP A51.41 **Secondary syphilitic meningitis**

SP A51.42 **Secondary syphilitic female pelvic disease**

SP A51.43 **Secondary syphilitic oculopathy**

Secondary syphilitic chorioretinitis
Secondary syphilitic iridocyclitis, iritis
Secondary syphilitic uveitis

SP A51.44 **Secondary syphilitic nephritis**

SP A51.45 **Secondary syphilitic hepatitis**

SP A51.46 **Secondary syphilitic osteopathy**

SP A51.49 **Other secondary syphilitic conditions**

Secondary syphilitic lymphadenopathy
Secondary syphilitic myositis

SP A51.5 **Early syphilis, latent**

Syphilis (acquired) without clinical manifestations, with positive serological reaction and negative spinal fluid test, less than two years after infection.

SP A51.9 **Early syphilis, unspecified**

4 A52 **Late syphilis**

5 A52.0 **Cardiovascular and cerebrovascular syphilis**

SP A52.00 **Cardiovascular syphilis, unspecified**

SP A52.01 **Syphilitic aneurysm of aorta**

SP A52.02 **Syphilitic aortitis**

SP A52.03 **Syphilitic endocarditis**

Syphilitic aortic valve incompetence or stenosis
Syphilitic mitral valve stenosis
Syphilitic pulmonary valve regurgitation

SP A52.04 **Syphilitic cerebral arteritis**

SP A52.05 **Other cerebrovascular syphilis**

Syphilitic cerebral aneurysm (ruptured) (non-ruptured)
Syphilitic cerebral thrombosis

SP A52.06 **Other syphilitic heart involvement**

Syphilitic coronary artery disease
Syphilitic myocarditis
Syphilitic pericarditis

SP A52.09 **Other cardiovascular syphilis**

5 A52.1 **Symptomatic neurosyphilis**

SP A52.10 **Symptomatic neurosyphilis, unspecified**

SP A52.11 **Tabes dorsalis**

Locomotor ataxia (progressive)
Tabetic neurosyphilis

SP A52.12 **Other cerebrospinal syphilis**

SP A52.13 **Late syphilitic meningitis**

SP A52.14 **Late syphilitic encephalitis**

SP A52.15 **Late syphilitic neuropathy**

Late syphilitic acoustic neuritis
Late syphilitic optic (nerve) atrophy
Late syphilitic polyneuropathy
Late syphilitic retrobulbar neuritis

SP A52.16 **Charcôt's arthropathy (tabetic)**

CODING TIPS ✓ Use this code only for Charcot's foot caused by syphillis. Another code is not used to indicate the joint involved, etc. Do not use this code for Charcot's foot caused by other conditions.

SP A52.17 **General paresis**

Dementia paralytica

SP A52.19 **Other symptomatic neurosyphilis**

Syphilitic parkinsonism

SP A52.2 **Asymptomatic neurosyphilis**

SP A52.3 **Neurosyphilis, unspecified**

Gumma (syphilitic)
Syphilis (late)
Syphiloma

5 **A52.7 Other symptomatic late syphilis**

SP **A52.71 Late syphilitic oculopathy**
Late syphilitic chorioretinitis
Late syphilitic episcleritis

SP **A52.72 Syphilis of lung and bronchus**

SP **A52.73 Symptomatic late syphilis of other respiratory organs**

SP **A52.74 Syphilis of liver and other viscera**
Late syphilitic peritonitis

SP **A52.75 Syphilis of kidney and ureter**
Syphilitic glomerular disease

SP **A52.76 Other genitourinary symptomatic late syphilis**
Late syphilitic female pelvic inflammatory disease

SP **A52.77 Syphilis of bone and joint**

SP **A52.78 Syphilis of other musculoskeletal tissue**
Late syphilitic bursitis
Syphilis [stage unspecified] of bursa
Syphilis [stage unspecified] of muscle
Syphilis [stage unspecified] of synovium
Syphilis [stage unspecified] of tendon

SP **A52.79 Other symptomatic late syphilis**
Late syphilitic leukoderma
Syphilis of adrenal gland
Syphilis of pituitary gland
Syphilis of thyroid gland
Syphilitic splenomegaly
EXCLUDES 1 syphilitic leukoderma (secondary) (A51.39)

SP **A52.8 Late syphilis, latent**
Syphilis (acquired) without clinical manifestations, with positive serological reaction and negative spinal fluid test, two years or more after infection

SP **A52.9 Late syphilis, unspecified**

4 **A53 Other and unspecified syphilis**

SP **A53.0 Latent syphilis, unspecified as early or late**
Latent syphilis NOS
Positive serological reaction for syphilis

SP **A53.9 Syphilis, unspecified**
Infection due to Treponema pallidum NOS
Syphilis (acquired) NOS
EXCLUDES 1 syphilis NOS under two years of age (A50.2)

4 **A54 Gonococcal infection**

5 **A54.0 Gonococcal infection of lower genitourinary tract without periurethral or accessory gland abscess**
EXCLUDES 1 gonococcal infection with genitourinary gland abscess (A54.1)
gonococcal infection with periurethral abscess (A54.1)

SP **A54.00 Gonococcal infection of lower genitourinary tract, unspecified**

SP **A54.01 Gonococcal cystitis and urethritis, unspecified**

SP **A54.02 Gonococcal vulvovaginitis, unspecified**

SP **A54.03 Gonococcal cervicitis, unspecified**

SP **A54.09 Other gonococcal infection of lower genitourinary tract**

SP **A54.1 Gonococcal infection of lower genitourinary tract with periurethral and accessory gland abscess**
Gonococcal Bartholin's gland abscess

5 **A54.2 Gonococcal pelviperitonitis and other gonococcal genitourinary infection**

SP **A54.21 Gonococcal infection of kidney and ureter**

SP **A54.22 Gonococcal prostatitis**

SP **A54.23 Gonococcal infection of other male genital organs**
Gonococcal epididymitis
Gonococcal orchitis

SP **A54.24 Gonococcal female pelvic inflammatory disease**
Gonococcal pelviperitonitis
EXCLUDES 1 gonococcal peritonitis (A54.85)

SP **A54.29 Other gonococcal genitourinary infections**

5 **A54.3 Gonococcal infection of eye**

SP **A54.30 Gonococcal infection of eye, unspecified**

SP **A54.31 Gonococcal conjunctivitis**
Ophthalmia neonatorum due to gonococcus

SP **A54.32 Gonococcal iridocyclitis**

SP **A54.33 Gonococcal keratitis**

SP **A54.39 Other gonococcal eye infection**
Gonococcal endophthalmia

5 **A54.4 Gonococcal infection of musculoskeletal system**

SP **A54.40 Gonococcal infection of musculoskeletal system, unspecified**

SP **A54.41 Gonococcal spondylopathy**

SP **A54.42 Gonococcal arthritis**
EXCLUDES 2 gonococcal infection of spine (A54.41)

SP **A54.43 Gonococcal osteomyelitis**
EXCLUDES 2 gonococcal infection of spine (A54.41)

SP **A54.49 Gonococcal infection of other musculoskeletal tissue**
Gonococcal bursitis
Gonococcal myositis
Gonococcal synovitis
Gonococcal tenosynovitis

SP **A54.5 Gonococcal pharyngitis**

SP **A54.6 Gonococcal infection of anus and rectum**

5 **A54.8 Other gonococcal infections**

SP **A54.81 Gonococcal meningitis**

SP **A54.82 Gonococcal brain abscess**

SP **A54.83 Gonococcal heart infection**
Gonococcal endocarditis
Gonococcal myocarditis
Gonococcal pericarditis

SP **A54.84 Gonococcal pneumonia**

SP **A54.85 Gonococcal peritonitis**

EXCLUDES 1 gonococcal pelviperitonitis (A54.24)

SP **A54.86 Gonococcal sepsis**

SP **A54.89 Other gonococcal infections**
Gonococcal keratoderma
Gonococcal lymphadenitis

SP **A54.9 Gonococcal infection, unspecified**

SP **A55 Chlamydial lymphogranuloma (venereum)**
Climatic or tropical bubo
Durand-Nicolas-Favre disease
Esthiomene
Lymphogranuloma inguinale

DEFINITION Sexually transmitted infection by Chlamydia trachomatis, seen in warm climates; presents with primary cutaneous or mucosal lesion at infection site and acute unilateral or bilateral lymphadenopathy.

4 **A56 Other sexually transmitted chlamydial diseases**

INCLUDES sexually transmitted diseases due to Chlamydia trachomatis

EXCLUDES 1 neonatal chlamydial conjunctivitis (P39.1)
neonatal chlamydial pneumonia (P23.1)

EXCLUDES 2 chlamydial lymphogranuloma (A55)
conditions classified to A74.-

5 **A56.0 Chlamydial infection of lower genitourinary tract**

SP **A56.00 Chlamydial infection of lower genitourinary tract, unspecified**

SP **A56.01 Chlamydial cystitis and urethritis**

SP **A56.02 Chlamydial vulvovaginitis**

SP **A56.09 Other chlamydial infection of lower genitourinary tract**
Chlamydial cervicitis

5 **A56.1 Chlamydial infection of pelviperitoneum and other genitourinary organs**

SP **A56.11 Chlamydial female pelvic inflammatory disease**

SP **A56.19 Other chlamydial genitourinary infection**
Chlamydial epididymitis
Chlamydial orchitis

SP **A56.2 Chlamydial infection of genitourinary tract, unspecified**

SP **A56.3 Chlamydial infection of anus and rectum**

SP **A56.4 Chlamydial infection of pharynx**

SP **A56.8 Sexually transmitted chlamydial infection of other sites**

SP **A57 Chancroid**
Ulcus molle

DEFINITION Sexually transmitted disease, characterized by a painful, primary ulcer, usually on the external genitalia.

SP **A58 Granuloma inguinale**
Donovanosis

4 **A59 Trichomoniasis**

EXCLUDES 2 intestinal trichomoniasis (A07.8)

5 **A59.0 Urogenital trichomoniasis**

SP **A59.00 Urogenital trichomoniasis, unspecified**
Fluor (vaginalis) due to Trichomonas
Leukorrhea (vaginalis) due to Trichomonas

SP **A59.01 Trichomonal vulvovaginitis**

DEFINITION Sexually transmitted disease caused by the protozoan Trichomonas vaginalis infecting the vagina and external female genitalia.

SP **A59.02 Trichomonal prostatitis**

SP **A59.03 Trichomonal cystitis and urethritis**

SP **A59.09 Other urogenital trichomoniasis**
Trichomonas cervicitis

SP **A59.8 Trichomoniasis of other sites**

SP **A59.9 Trichomoniasis, unspecified**

4 **A60 Anogenital herpesviral [herpes simplex] infections**

5 **A60.0 Herpesviral infection of genitalia and urogenital tract**

SP **A60.00 Herpesviral infection of urogenital system, unspecified**

SP **A60.01 Herpesviral infection of penis**

SP **A60.02 Herpesviral infection of other male genital organs**

SP **A60.03 Herpesviral cervicitis**

SP **A60.04 Herpesviral vulvovaginitis**
Herpesviral [herpes simplex] ulceration
Herpesviral [herpes simplex] vaginitis
Herpesviral [herpes simplex] vulvitis

SP **A60.09 Herpesviral infection of other urogenital tract**

SP **A60.1 Herpesviral infection of perianal skin and rectum**

SP **A60.9 Anogenital herpesviral infection, unspecified**

4 **A63 Other predominantly sexually transmitted diseases, not elsewhere classified**

EXCLUDES 2 molluscum contagiosum (B08.1)
papilloma of cervix (D26.0)

SP **A63.0 Anogenital (venereal) warts**
Anogenital warts due to (human) papillomavirus [HPV]
Condyloma acuminatum

DEFINITION A wartlike growth on the skin or mucous membrane, in the area of the anus or external genitalia.

SP **A63.8 Other specified predominantly sexually transmitted diseases**

IQ **A64 Unspecified sexually transmitted disease**

Other spirochetal diseases (A65-A69)

EXCLUDES 2 leptospirosis (A27.-)
syphilis (A50-A53)

SP **A65 Nonvenereal syphilis**
Bejel
Endemic syphilis
Njovera

4 **A66 Yaws**

INCLUDES bouba
frambesia (tropica)
pian

SP **A66.0 Initial lesions of yaws**
Chancre of yaws

Frambesia, initial or primary
Initial frambesial ulcer
Mother yaw

SP **A66.1 Multiple papillomata and wet crab yaws**
Frambesioma
Pianoma
Plantar or palmar papilloma of yaws

SP **A66.2 Other early skin lesions of yaws**
Cutaneous yaws, less than five years after infection
Early yaws (cutaneous)(macular)(maculopapular)(micropapular)(papular)
Frambeside of early yaws

SP **A66.3 Hyperkeratosis of yaws**
Ghoul hand
Hyperkeratosis, palmar or plantar (early) (late) due to yaws
Worm-eaten soles

SP **A66.4 Gummata and ulcers of yaws**
Gummatous frambeside
Nodular late yaws (ulcerated)

SP **A66.5 Gangosa**
Rhinopharyngitis mutilans

SP **A66.6 Bone and joint lesions of yaws**
Yaws ganglion
Yaws goundou
Yaws gumma, bone
Yaws gummatous osteitis or periostitis
Yaws hydrarthrosis
Yaws osteitis
Yaws periostitis (hypertrophic)

SP **A66.7 Other manifestations of yaws**
Juxta-articular nodules of yaws
Mucosal yaws

SP **A66.8 Latent yaws**
Yaws without clinical manifestations, with positive serology

SP **A66.9 Yaws, unspecified**

4 **A67 Pinta [carate]**

SP **A67.0 Primary lesions of pinta**
Chancre (primary) of pinta
Papule (primary) of pinta

SP **A67.1 Intermediate lesions of pinta**
Erythematous plaques of pinta
Hyperchromic lesions of pinta
Hyperkeratosis of pinta
Pintids

SP **A67.2 Late lesions of pinta**
Achromic skin lesions of pinta
Cicatricial skin lesions of pinta
Dyschromic skin lesions of pinta

SP **A67.3 Mixed lesions of pinta**
Achromic with hyperchromic skin lesions of pinta [carate]

SP **A67.9 Pinta, unspecified**

4 **A68 Relapsing fevers**
INCLUDES recurrent fever
EXCLUDES 2 Lyme disease (A69.2-)

SP **A68.0 Louse-borne relapsing fever**
Relapsing fever due to Borrelia recurrentis

SP **A68.1 Tick-borne relapsing fever**
Relapsing fever due to any Borrelia species other than Borrelia recurrentis

SP **A68.9 Relapsing fever, unspecified**

4 **A69 Other spirochetal infections**

SP **A69.0 Necrotizing ulcerative stomatitis**
Cancrum oris
Fusospirochetal gangrene
Noma
Stomatitis gangrenosa

SP **A69.1 Other Vincent's infections**
Fusospirochetal pharyngitis
Necrotizing ulcerative (acute) gingivitis
Necrotizing ulcerative (acute) gingivostomatitis
Spirochetal stomatitis
Trench mouth
Vincent's angina
Vincent's gingivitis

5 **A69.2 Lyme disease**
Erythema chronicum migrans due to Borrelia burgdorferi

CODING TIPS✓ A69.2 codes include 5th characters to include the complications of Lyme disease, and no additional codes for the assorted complications are necessary.

DEFINITION Tick-transmitted infection caused by Borrelia burgdorferi, manifesting with erythema chronicum migrans, myalgia, arthritis of the large joints, and nervous and cardiovascular system involvement.

SP **A69.20 Lyme disease, unspecified**

SP **A69.21 Meningitis due to Lyme disease**

SP **A69.22 Other neurologic disorders in Lyme disease**
Cranial neuritis
Meningoencephalitis
Polyneuropathy

SP **A69.23 Arthritis due to Lyme disease**

SP **A69.29 Other conditions associated with Lyme disease**
Myopericarditis due to Lyme disease

SP **A69.8 Other specified spirochetal infections**

SP **A69.9 Spirochetal infection, unspecified**

Other diseases caused by chlamydiae (A70-A74)

EXCLUDES 1 sexually transmitted chlamydial diseases (A55-A56)

SP **A70 Chlamydia psittaci infections**
Ornithosis
Parrot fever
Psittacosis

4 **A71 Trachoma**
EXCLUDES 1 sequelae of trachoma (B94.0)

CODING TIPS✓ When coding category A71, physician or NPP notes may state "granular conjunctivitis" or 'Egyptian ophthalmia." Use B94.0 for sequelae of trachoma.

SP **A71.0 Initial stage of trachoma**
Trachoma dubium

SP **A71.1 Active stage of trachoma**
Granular conjunctivitis (trachomatous)
Trachomatous follicular conjunctivitis
Trachomatous pannus

SP **A71.9 Trachoma, unspecified**

4 **A74 Other diseases caused by chlamydiae**
EXCLUDES 1 neonatal chlamydial conjunctivitis (P39.1)

neonatal chlamydial pneumonia (P23.1)
Reiter's disease (M02.3-)
sexually transmitted chlamydial diseases (A55-A56)

EXCLUDES 2 chlamydial pneumonia (J16.0)

SP **A74.0 Chlamydial conjunctivitis**
Paratrachoma

5 **A74.8 Other chlamydial diseases**

SP **A74.81 Chlamydial peritonitis**

SP **A74.89 Other chlamydial diseases**

SP **A74.9 Chlamydial infection, unspecified**
Chlamydiosis NOS

Rickettsioses (A75-A79)

4 **A75 Typhus fever**

EXCLUDES 1 rickettsiosis due to Ehrlichia sennetsu (A79.81)

SP **A75.0 Epidemic louse-borne typhus fever due to Rickettsia prowazekii**
Classical typhus (fever)
Epidemic (louse-borne) typhus

SP **A75.1 Recrudescent typhus [Brill's disease]**
Brill-Zinsser disease

SP **A75.2 Typhus fever due to Rickettsia typhi**
Murine (flea-borne) typhus

SP **A75.3 Typhus fever due to Rickettsia tsutsugamushi**
Scrub (mite-borne) typhus
Tsutsugamushi fever
Typhus fever due to Orientia Tsutsugamushi (scrub typhus)

SP **A75.9 Typhus fever, unspecified**
Typhus (fever) NOS

4 **A77 Spotted fever [tick-borne rickettsioses]**

SP **A77.0 Spotted fever due to Rickettsia rickettsii**
Rocky Mountain spotted fever
Sao Paulo fever

SP **A77.1 Spotted fever due to Rickettsia conorii**
African tick typhus
Boutonneuse fever
India tick typhus
Kenya tick typhus
Marseilles fever
Mediterranean tick fever

SP **A77.2 Spotted fever due to Rickettsia siberica**
North Asian tick fever
Siberian tick typhus

SP **A77.3 Spotted fever due to Rickettsia australis**
Queensland tick typhus

▲ 5 **A77.4 Ehrlichiosis**

EXCLUDES 1 anaplasmosis [A. phagocytophilum] (A79.82)
rickettsiosis due to Ehrlichia sennetsu (A79.81)

SP **A77.40 Ehrlichiosis, unspecified**

SP **A77.41 Ehrlichiosis chafeensis [E. chafeensis]**

SP **A77.49 Other ehrlichiosis**
Ehrlichiosis due to E. ewingii
Ehrlichiosis due to E. muris euclairensis

SP **A77.8 Other spotted fevers**
Rickettsia 364D/R. philipii (Pacific Coast tick fever)
Spotted fever due to Rickettsia africae (African tick bite fever)
Spotted fever due to Rickettsia parkeri

SP **A77.9 Spotted fever, unspecified**
Tick-borne typhus NOS

SP **A78 Q fever**
Infection due to Coxiella burnetii
Nine Mile fever
Quadrilateral fever

4 **A79 Other rickettsioses**

SP **A79.0 Trench fever**
Quintan fever
Wolhynian fever

SP **A79.1 Rickettsialpox due to Rickettsia akari**
Kew Garden fever
Vesicular rickettsiosis

5 **A79.8 Other specified rickettsioses**

SP **A79.81 Rickettsiosis due to Ehrlichia sennetsu**
Rickettsiosis due to Neorickettsia sennetsu

★ **A79.82 Anaplasmosis [A. phagocytophilum]**
Transfusion transmitted A. phagocytophilum

SP **A79.89 Other specified rickettsioses**

SP **A79.9 Rickettsiosis, unspecified**
Rickettsial infection NOS

Viral and prion infections of the central nervous system (A80-A89)

EXCLUDES 1 postpolio syndrome (G14)
sequelae of poliomyelitis (B91)
sequelae of viral encephalitis (B94.1)

▲ 4 **A80 Acute poliomyelitis**

EXCLUDES 1 acute flaccid myelitis (G04.82)

CODING TIPS✓ Assign a code from category A80 to indicate acute poliomyelitis, not a sequela of polio, or post polio syndrome. A80-codes are used to report acute, active poliomyelitis only. Use B91 for sequelae of polio, or G14 for post polio syndrome, which must be documented by the physician or NPP.

SP **A80.0 Acute paralytic poliomyelitis, vaccine-associated**

SP **A80.1 Acute paralytic poliomyelitis, wild virus, imported**

SP **A80.2 Acute paralytic poliomyelitis, wild virus, indigenous**

5 **A80.3 Acute paralytic poliomyelitis, other and unspecified**

SP **A80.30 Acute paralytic poliomyelitis, unspecified**

SP **A80.39 Other acute paralytic poliomyelitis**

SP **A80.4 Acute nonparalytic poliomyelitis**

SP **A80.9 Acute poliomyelitis, unspecified**

✚ 4 **A81 Atypical virus infections of central nervous system**

INCLUDES diseases of the central nervous system caused by prions

Use additional code to identify:
dementia with behavioral disturbance (F02.81)
dementia without behavioral disturbance (F02.80)

+ 5 A81.0 Creutzfeldt-Jakob disease

DEFINITION Degenerative neural disease caused by a prion (an infectious protein); presents with loss of muscular control, balance, and memory, twitching movements, nervousness and agitation, changes in personality, and dementia.

SP + A81.00 Creutzfeldt-Jakob disease, unspecified

Jakob-Creutzfeldt disease, unspecified

SP + A81.01 Variant Creutzfeldt-Jakob disease

vCJD

DEFINITION Rare, transmissible form of fatal Jakob-Creutzfeldt disease, affecting younger people with a longer duration, causing spongiform degeneration of the brain with unusual psychiatric and sensory symptoms.

SP + A81.09 Other Creutzfeldt-Jakob disease

CJD
Familial Creutzfeldt-Jakob disease
Iatrogenic Creutzfeldt-Jakob disease
Sporadic Creutzfeldt-Jakob disease
Subacute spongiform encephalopathy (with dementia)

SP + A81.1 Subacute sclerosing panencephalitis

Dawson's inclusion body encephalitis
Van Bogaert's sclerosing leukoencephalopathy

SP + A81.2 Progressive multifocal leukoencephalopathy

Multifocal leukoencephalopathy NOS

+ 5 A81.8 Other atypical virus infections of central nervous system

SP + A81.81 Kuru

SP + A81.82 Gerstmann-Sträussler-Scheinker syndrome

GSS syndrome

DEFINITION Extremely rare, inherited, fatal disease of the brain that progresses slowly, causing lack of muscle coordination, unsteady gait, dementia, slurred speech, spasticity, and coma before death.

SP + A81.83 Fatal familial insomnia

FFI

DEFINITION Very rare, inherited brain disease caused by prion protein mutation from soluble to insoluble, resulting in plaques forming in the thalamus, causing insomnia that progresses to dementia, unresponsiveness, and death.

SP + A81.89 Other atypical virus infections of central nervous system

SP + A81.9 Atypical virus infection of central nervous system, unspecified

Prion diseases of the central nervous system NOS

4 A82 Rabies

SP A82.0 Sylvatic rabies

SP A82.1 Urban rabies

SP A82.9 Rabies, unspecified

4 A83 Mosquito-borne viral encephalitis

INCLUDES mosquito-borne viral meningoencephalitis

EXCLUDES 2 Venezuelan equine encephalitis (A92.2)
West Nile fever (A92.3-)
West Nile virus (A92.3-)

SP A83.0 Japanese encephalitis

SP A83.1 Western equine encephalitis

SP A83.2 Eastern equine encephalitis

SP A83.3 St Louis encephalitis

SP A83.4 Australian encephalitis

Kunjin virus disease

SP A83.5 California encephalitis

California meningoencephalitis
La Crosse encephalitis

SP A83.6 Rocio virus disease

SP A83.8 Other mosquito-borne viral encephalitis

SP A83.9 Mosquito-borne viral encephalitis, unspecified

4 A84 Tick-borne viral encephalitis

INCLUDES tick-borne viral meningoencephalitis

SP A84.0 Far Eastern tick-borne encephalitis [Russian spring-summer encephalitis]

SP A84.1 Central European tick-borne encephalitis

5 A84.8 Other tick-borne viral encephalitis

SP A84.81 Powassan virus disease

SP A84.89 Other tick-borne viral encephalitis

Louping ill
Code first:
, if applicable, transfusion related infection (T80.22-)

SP A84.9 Tick-borne viral encephalitis, unspecified

4 A85 Other viral encephalitis, not elsewhere classified

INCLUDES specified viral encephalomyelitis NEC
specified viral meningoencephalitis NEC

EXCLUDES 1 benign myalgic encephalomyelitis (G93.3)
encephalitis due to cytomegalovirus (B25.8)
encephalitis due to herpesvirus NEC (B10.0-)
encephalitis due to herpesvirus [herpes simplex] (B00.4)
encephalitis due to measles virus (B05.0)
encephalitis due to mumps virus (B26.2)
encephalitis due to poliomyelitis virus (A80.-)
encephalitis due to zoster (B02.0)
lymphocytic choriomeningitis (A87.2)

SP A85.0 Enteroviral encephalitis

Enteroviral encephalomyelitis

SP A85.1 Adenoviral encephalitis

Adenoviral meningoencephalitis

SP A85.2 Arthropod-borne viral encephalitis, unspecified

EXCLUDES 1 West nile virus with encephalitis (A92.31)

SP A85.8 Other specified viral encephalitis

Encephalitis lethargica
Von Economo-Cruchet disease

SP A86 **Unspecified viral encephalitis**
Viral encephalomyelitis NOS
Viral meningoencephalitis NOS

4 A87 **Viral meningitis**
EXCLUDES 1 meningitis due to herpesvirus [herpes simplex] (B00.3)
meningitis due to herpesvirus [herpes simplex] (B00.3)
meningitis due to measles virus (B05.1)
meningitis due to mumps virus (B26.1)
meningitis due to poliomyelitis virus (A80.-)
meningitis due to zoster (B02.1)

SP A87.0 **Enteroviral meningitis**
Coxsackievirus meningitis
Echovirus meningitis

SP A87.1 **Adenoviral meningitis**

SP A87.2 **Lymphocytic choriomeningitis**
Lymphocytic meningoencephalitis

SP A87.8 **Other viral meningitis**

SP A87.9 **Viral meningitis, unspecified**

4 A88 **Other viral infections of central nervous system, not elsewhere classified**
EXCLUDES 1 viral encephalitis NOS (A86)
viral meningitis NOS (A87.9)

SP A88.0 **Enteroviral exanthematous fever [Boston exanthem]**

SP A88.1 **Epidemic vertigo**

SP A88.8 **Other specified viral infections of central nervous system**

SP A89 **Unspecified viral infection of central nervous system**

Arthropod-borne viral fevers and viral hemorrhagic fevers (A90-A99)

SP A90 **Dengue fever [classical dengue]**
EXCLUDES 1 dengue hemorrhagic fever (A91)

SP A91 **Dengue hemorrhagic fever**

4 A92 **Other mosquito-borne viral fevers**
EXCLUDES 1 Ross River disease (B33.1)

SP A92.0 **Chikungunya virus disease**
Chikungunya (hemorrhagic) fever

SP A92.1 **O'nyong-nyong fever**

SP A92.2 **Venezuelan equine fever**
Venezuelan equine encephalitis
Venezuelan equine encephalomyelitis virus disease

5 A92.3 **West Nile virus infection**
West Nile fever

SP A92.30 **West Nile virus infection, unspecified**
West Nile fever NOS
West Nile fever without complications
West Nile virus NOS

SP A92.31 **West Nile virus infection with encephalitis**
West Nile encephalitis
West Nile encephalomyelitis

SP + A92.32 **West Nile virus infection with other neurologic manifestation**
Use additional code to specify the neurologic manifestation

SP + A92.39 **West Nile virus infection with other complications**
Use additional code to specify the other conditions

SP A92.4 **Rift Valley fever**

SP A92.5 **Zika virus disease**
Zika virus fever
Zika virus infection
Zika NOS
EXCLUDES 1 congenital Zika virus disease (P35.4)

CODING TIPS✓ Zika virus must be documented by the provider. Suspected or probable Zika should not be coded as Zika. In that case, code the symptoms/signs experienced by the patient.

DEFINITION Disease caused by infection with the Zika virus most commonly presents with fever, rash, joint pain, reddening of the eyes, muscle pain, and headache. Zika viral infection is primarily spread by the bite of infected mosquitoes.

SP A92.8 **Other specified mosquito-borne viral fevers**

SP A92.9 **Mosquito-borne viral fever, unspecified**

4 A93 **Other arthropod-borne viral fevers, not elsewhere classified**

SP A93.0 **Oropouche virus disease**
Oropouche fever

SP A93.1 **Sandfly fever**
Pappataci fever
Phlebotomus fever

SP A93.2 **Colorado tick fever**

SP A93.8 **Other specified arthropod-borne viral fevers**
Piry virus disease
Vesicular stomatitis virus disease [Indiana fever]

SP A94 **Unspecified arthropod-borne viral fever**
Arboviral fever NOS
Arbovirus infection NOS

4 A95 **Yellow fever**

SP A95.0 **Sylvatic yellow fever**
Jungle yellow fever

SP A95.1 **Urban yellow fever**

SP A95.9 **Yellow fever, unspecified**

4 A96 **Arenaviral hemorrhagic fever**

SP A96.0 **Junin hemorrhagic fever**
Argentinian hemorrhagic fever

SP A96.1 **Machupo hemorrhagic fever**
Bolivian hemorrhagic fever

SP A96.2 **Lassa fever**

SP A96.8 **Other arenaviral hemorrhagic fevers**

SP A96.9 **Arenaviral hemorrhagic fever, unspecified**

4 A98 **Other viral hemorrhagic fevers, not elsewhere classified**
EXCLUDES 1 chikungunya hemorrhagic fever (A92.0)
dengue hemorrhagic fever (A91)

SP **A98.0 Crimean-Congo hemorrhagic fever**
Central Asian hemorrhagic fever

SP **A98.1 Omsk hemorrhagic fever**

SP **A98.2 Kyasanur Forest disease**

SP **A98.3 Marburg virus disease**

SP **A98.4 Ebola virus disease**

SP **A98.5 Hemorrhagic fever with renal syndrome**
Epidemic hemorrhagic fever
Korean hemorrhagic fever
Russian hemorrhagic fever
Hantaan virus disease
Hantavirus disease with renal manifestations
Nephropathia epidemica
Songo fever
EXCLUDES 1 hantavirus (cardio)-pulmonary syndrome (B33.4)

SP **A98.8 Other specified viral hemorrhagic fevers**

SP **A99 Unspecified viral hemorrhagic fever**

Viral infections characterized by skin and mucous membrane lesions (B00-B09)

4 **B00 Herpesviral [herpes simplex] infections**
EXCLUDES 1 congenital herpesviral infections (P35.2)
EXCLUDES 2 anogenital herpesviral infection (A60.-)
gammaherpesviral mononucleosis (B27.0-)
herpangina (B08.5)
CODING TIPS ✓ Conditions classified to B00 are due to herpes simplex virus, not those due to herpes zoster virus (such as shingles). Category B02- includes infections due to herpes zoster virus.

SP **B00.0 Eczema herpeticum**
Kaposi's varicelliform eruption
DEFINITION Potentially fatal infection with the herpes simplex virus at the site of an existing skin condition, often atopic dermatitis, causing severe rash, fever, and fatigue.

SP **B00.1 Herpesviral vesicular dermatitis**
Herpes simplex facialis
Herpes simplex labialis
Herpes simplex otitis externa
Vesicular dermatitis of ear
Vesicular dermatitis of lip

SP **B00.2 Herpesviral gingivostomatitis and pharyngotonsillitis**
Herpesviral pharyngitis

SP **B00.3 Herpesviral meningitis**

SP **B00.4 Herpesviral encephalitis**
Herpesviral meningoencephalitis
Simian B disease
EXCLUDES 1 herpesviral encephalitis due to herpesvirus 6 and 7 (B10.01, B10.09)
non-simplex herpesviral encephalitis (B10.0-)

5 **B00.5 Herpesviral ocular disease**

SP **B00.50 Herpesviral ocular disease, unspecified**

SP **B00.51 Herpesviral iridocyclitis**
Herpesviral iritis
Herpesviral uveitis, anterior

SP **B00.52 Herpesviral keratitis**
Herpesviral keratoconjunctivitis

SP **B00.53 Herpesviral conjunctivitis**

SP **B00.59 Other herpesviral disease of eye**
Herpesviral dermatitis of eyelid

SP **B00.7 Disseminated herpesviral disease**
Herpesviral sepsis

5 **B00.8 Other forms of herpesviral infections**

SP **B00.81 Herpesviral hepatitis**

SP **B00.82 Herpes simplex myelitis**

SP **B00.89 Other herpesviral infection**
Herpesviral whitlow
DEFINITION Viral infection that results in a painful, blistery eruption on one of the digits.

SP **B00.9 Herpesviral infection, unspecified**
Herpes simplex infection NOS

4 **B01 Varicella [chickenpox]**

SP **B01.0 Varicella meningitis**

5 **B01.1 Varicella encephalitis, myelitis and encephalomyelitis**
Postchickenpox encephalitis, myelitis and encephalomyelitis

SP **B01.11 Varicella encephalitis and encephalomyelitis**
Postchickenpox encephalitis and encephalomyelitis

SP **B01.12 Varicella myelitis**
Postchickenpox myelitis

SP **B01.2 Varicella pneumonia**

5 **B01.8 Varicella with other complications**

SP **B01.81 Varicella keratitis**

SP **B01.89 Other varicella complications**

SP **B01.9 Varicella without complication**
Varicella NOS

4 **B02 Zoster [herpes zoster]**
INCLUDES shingles
zona

SP **B02.0 Zoster encephalitis**
Zoster meningoencephalitis

SP **B02.1 Zoster meningitis**

5 **B02.2 Zoster with other nervous system involvement**

SP **B02.21 Postherpetic geniculate ganglionitis**

SP **B02.22 Postherpetic trigeminal neuralgia**

SP **B02.23 Postherpetic polyneuropathy**

SP **B02.24 Postherpetic myelitis**
Herpes zoster myelitis

SP **B02.29 Other postherpetic nervous system involvement**
Postherpetic radiculopathy

5 **B02.3 Zoster ocular disease**

SP **B02.30 Zoster ocular disease, unspecified**

SP **B02.31 Zoster conjunctivitis**

SP **B02.32 Zoster iridocyclitis**

SP **B02.33 Zoster keratitis**
Herpes zoster keratoconjunctivitis

SP **B02.34 Zoster scleritis**

SP **B02.39 Other herpes zoster eye disease**
Zoster blepharitis

SP **B02.7 Disseminated zoster**

4 4th digit required 5 5th digit required 6 6th digit required 7 7th digit required 7th digit placeholder + Additional code Laterality

SP **B02.8 Zoster with other complications**
Herpes zoster otitis externa

SP **B02.9 Zoster without complications**
Zoster NOS

IQ **B03 Smallpox**
Note:
In 1980 the 33rd World Health Assembly declared that smallpox had been eradicated.
The classification is maintained for surveillance purposes.

SP **B04 Monkeypox**

4 **B05 Measles**
INCLUDES morbilli
EXCLUDES 1 subacute sclerosing panencephalitis (A81.1)

SP **B05.0 Measles complicated by encephalitis**
Postmeasles encephalitis

SP **B05.1 Measles complicated by meningitis**
Postmeasles meningitis

SP **B05.2 Measles complicated by pneumonia**
Postmeasles pneumonia

SP **B05.3 Measles complicated by otitis media**
Postmeasles otitis media

SP **B05.4 Measles with intestinal complications**

5 **B05.8 Measles with other complications**

SP **B05.81 Measles keratitis and keratoconjunctivitis**

SP **B05.89 Other measles complications**

SP **B05.9 Measles without complication**
Measles NOS

4 **B06 Rubella [German measles]**
EXCLUDES 1 congenital rubella (P35.0)

5 **B06.0 Rubella with neurological complications**

SP **B06.00 Rubella with neurological complication, unspecified**

SP **B06.01 Rubella encephalitis**
Rubella meningoencephalitis

SP **B06.02 Rubella meningitis**

SP **B06.09 Other neurological complications of rubella**

5 **B06.8 Rubella with other complications**

SP **B06.81 Rubella pneumonia**

SP **B06.82 Rubella arthritis**

SP **B06.89 Other rubella complications**

SP **B06.9 Rubella without complication**
Rubella NOS

4 **B07 Viral warts**
INCLUDES verruca simplex
verruca vulgaris
viral warts due to human papillomavirus
EXCLUDES 2 anogenital (venereal) warts (A63.0)
papilloma of bladder (D41.4)
papilloma of cervix (D26.0)
papilloma larynx (D14.1)

SP **B07.0 Plantar wart**
Verruca plantaris
DEFINITION Noncancerous skin growths on the soles of the feet, often under pressure points, caused by the human papilloma virus that enters through tiny cuts or cracks in the skin.

SP **B07.8 Other viral warts**
Common wart
Flat wart
Verruca plana

SP **B07.9 Viral wart, unspecified**

4 **B08 Other viral infections characterized by skin and mucous membrane lesions, not elsewhere classified**
EXCLUDES 1 vesicular stomatitis virus disease (A93.8)

5 **B08.0 Other orthopoxvirus infections**
EXCLUDES 2 monkeypox (B04)

6 **B08.01 Cowpox and vaccinia not from vaccine**

SP **B08.010 Cowpox**

SP **B08.011 Vaccinia not from vaccine**
EXCLUDES 1 vaccinia (from vaccination) (generalized) (T88.1)

SP **B08.02 Orf virus disease**
Contagious pustular dermatitis
Ecthyma contagiosum
DEFINITION Skin disease closely related to smallpox, manifesting with localized, small, red, fluid-filled pustules that scab and heal, providing immunity to smallpox.

SP **B08.03 Pseudocowpox [milker's node]**

SP **B08.04 Paravaccinia, unspecified**

SP **B08.09 Other orthopoxvirus infections**
Orthopoxvirus infection NOS

SP **B08.1 Molluscum contagiosum**

5 **B08.2 Exanthema subitum [sixth disease]**
Roseola infantum

SP **B08.20 Exanthema subitum [sixth disease], unspecified**
Roseola infantum, unspecified
DEFINITION Common childhood herpes viral illness of mild upper respiratory symptoms, swollen glands, high fever lasting 3-7 days ending abruptly, followed by a rash.

SP **B08.21 Exanthema subitum [sixth disease] due to human herpesvirus 6**
Roseola infantum due to human herpesvirus 6

SP **B08.22 Exanthema subitum [sixth disease] due to human herpesvirus 7**
Roseola infantum due to human herpesvirus 7

SP **B08.3 Erythema infectiosum [fifth disease]**
DEFINITION A mild infectious disease occurring mainly in early childhood, marked by a rosy-red rash on the cheeks, often spreading to the trunk and limbs. Fever and arthritis may also be present.

SP **B08.4 Enteroviral vesicular stomatitis with exanthem**
Hand, foot and mouth disease

SP **B08.5 Enteroviral vesicular pharyngitis**
Herpangina

5 **B08.6 Parapoxvirus infections**

SP **B08.60 Parapoxvirus infection, unspecified**

SP **B08.61 Bovine stomatitis**

SP **B08.62 Sealpox**

SP **B08.69 Other parapoxvirus infections**

5 **B08.7 Yatapoxvirus infections**

SP **B08.70 Yatapoxvirus infection, unspecified**

SP **B08.71 Tanapox virus disease**

SP **B08.72 Yaba pox virus disease**
Yaba monkey tumor disease

SP **B08.79 Other yatapoxvirus infections**

SP **B08.8 Other specified viral infections characterized by skin and mucous membrane lesions**
Enteroviral lymphonodular pharyngitis
Foot-and-mouth disease
Poxvirus NEC

SP **B09 Unspecified viral infection characterized by skin and mucous membrane lesions**
Viral enanthema NOS
Viral exanthema NOS

Other human herpesviruses (B10)

4 **B10 Other human herpesviruses**

EXCLUDES 2 cytomegalovirus (B25.9)
Epstein-Barr virus (B27.0-)
herpes NOS (B00.9)
herpes simplex (B00.-)
herpes zoster (B02.-)
human herpesvirus NOS (B00.-)
human herpesvirus 1 and 2 (B00.-)
human herpesvirus 3 (B01.-, B02.-)
human herpesvirus 4 (B27.0-)
human herpesvirus 5 (B25.-)
varicella (B01.-)
zoster (B02.-)

5 **B10.0 Other human herpesvirus encephalitis**

EXCLUDES 2 herpes encephalitis NOS (B00.4)
herpes simplex encephalitis (B00.4)
human herpesvirus encephalitis (B00.4)
simian B herpes virus encephalitis (B00.4)

SP **B10.01 Human herpesvirus 6 encephalitis**

SP **B10.09 Other human herpesvirus encephalitis**
Human herpesvirus 7 encephalitis

5 **B10.8 Other human herpesvirus infection**

SP **B10.81 Human herpesvirus 6 infection**

SP **B10.82 Human herpesvirus 7 infection**

SP **B10.89 Other human herpesvirus infection**
Human herpesvirus 8 infection
Kaposi's sarcoma-associated herpesvirus infection

Viral hepatitis (B15-B19)

EXCLUDES 1 sequelae of viral hepatitis (B94.2)

EXCLUDES 2 cytomegaloviral hepatitis (B25.1)
herpesviral [herpes simplex] hepatitis (B00.81)

CODING TIPS ✓ When viral hepatitis is also documented as a confirmed diagnosis in a patient with any diagnosis classifiable to K74.-, the appropriate code from B15-B19 should also be assigned. The sequencing of the K74.- and the viral hepatitis code is according to focus of care.

4 **B15 Acute hepatitis A**

SP **B15.0 Hepatitis A with hepatic coma**

SP **B15.9 Hepatitis A without hepatic coma**
Hepatitis A (acute)(viral) NOS

4 **B16 Acute hepatitis B**

SP **B16.0 Acute hepatitis B with delta-agent with hepatic coma**

SP **B16.1 Acute hepatitis B with delta-agent without hepatic coma**

SP **B16.2 Acute hepatitis B without delta-agent with hepatic coma**

SP **B16.9 Acute hepatitis B without delta-agent and without hepatic coma**
Hepatitis B (acute) (viral) NOS

4 **B17 Other acute viral hepatitis**

SP **B17.0 Acute delta-(super) infection of hepatitis B carrier**

5 **B17.1 Acute hepatitis C**

SP **B17.10 Acute hepatitis C without hepatic coma**
Acute hepatitis C NOS

SP **B17.11 Acute hepatitis C with hepatic coma**

SP **B17.2 Acute hepatitis E**

SP **B17.8 Other specified acute viral hepatitis**
Hepatitis non-A non-B (acute) (viral) NEC

SP **B17.9 Acute viral hepatitis, unspecified**
Acute hepatitis NOS
Acute infectious hepatitis NOS

4 **B18 Chronic viral hepatitis**

INCLUDES Carrier of viral hepatitis

SP **B18.0 Chronic viral hepatitis B with delta-agent**

SP **B18.1 Chronic viral hepatitis B without delta-agent**
Carrier of viral hepatitis B
Chronic (viral) hepatitis B

SP **B18.2 Chronic viral hepatitis C**
Carrier of viral hepatitis C

SP **B18.8 Other chronic viral hepatitis**
Carrier of other viral hepatitis

SP **B18.9 Chronic viral hepatitis, unspecified**
Carrier of unspecified viral hepatitis

4 **B19 Unspecified viral hepatitis**

SP **B19.0 Unspecified viral hepatitis with hepatic coma**

5 **B19.1 Unspecified viral hepatitis B**

SP **B19.10 Unspecified viral hepatitis B without hepatic coma**
Unspecified viral hepatitis B NOS

SP **B19.11 Unspecified viral hepatitis B with hepatic coma**

5 **B19.2 Unspecified viral hepatitis C**

SP **B19.20 Unspecified viral hepatitis C without hepatic coma**
Viral hepatitis C NOS

SP **B19.21 Unspecified viral hepatitis C with hepatic coma**

SP **B19.9 Unspecified viral hepatitis without hepatic coma**
Viral hepatitis NOS

Human immunodeficiency virus [HIV] disease (B20)

CODING TIPS ✓ B20 is sequenced as primary when the patient is admitted for conditions related to HIV infection. Sequence the conditions caused by the HIV next. If the patient is being admitted for another condition unrelated to HIV, code that condition first and B20 can be used as a secondary code. If the patient has had a HIV related condition in the past, continue to use the B20 code, even if that HIV-related condition is resolved. Z21 is used only for HIV+ patients who have never had a HIV related condition. Some states may have a prohibition against sequencing B20 as primary, or using the code at all. Look for OASIS error code +150 to indicate that state regulations are stricter than HIPAA, disallowing the code for AIDS.

H SP + **B20 Human immunodeficiency virus [HIV] disease**

INCLUDES acquired immune deficiency syndrome [AIDS]
AIDS-related complex [ARC]
HIV infection, symptomatic

Code first:
Human immunodeficiency virus [HIV] disease complicating pregnancy, childbirth and the puerperium, if applicable (O98.7-)

Use additional code(s) to identify all manifestations of HIV infection

EXCLUDES 1 asymptomatic human immunodeficiency virus [HIV] infection status (Z21)
exposure to HIV virus (Z20.6)
inconclusive serologic evidence of HIV (R75)

GUIDELINES **Section I.C.1.a.1)**
Code only confirmed cases of HIV infection/illness: This [guideline] is an exception to the hospital inpatient guideline Section II, H. In this context, "confirmation" does not require documentation of positive serology or culture for HIV; the provider's diagnostic statement that the patient is HIV positive, or has an HIV-related illness is sufficient. B20, Human immunideficiency virus (HIV) disease should be assigned.

GUIDELINES **Section I.C.1.a.2)(a)**
If a patient is admitted for an HIV-related condition, the principal diagnosis should be B20, Human immunodeficiency virus [HIV] disease followed by additional diagnosis codes for all reported HIV-related conditions.

GUIDELINES **Section I.C.1.a.2)(b)**
If a patient with HIV disease is admitted for an unrelated condition (such as a traumatic injury), the code for the unrelated condition (e.g., the nature of injury code) should be the principal diagnosis. Other diagnoses would be B20 followed by additional diagnosis codes for all reported HIV-related conditions.

GUIDELINES **Section I.C.1.a.2)(c)**
Whether the patient is newly diagnosed or has had previous admissions/encounters for HIV conditions is irrelevant to the sequencing decision.

GUIDELINES **Section I.C.1.a.2)(e)**
Patients with inconclusive HIV serology, but no definitive diagnosis or manifestations of the illness, may be assigned code R75, Inconclusive laboratory evidence of human immunodeficiency virus [HIV].

GUIDELINES **Section I.C.1.a.2)(f)**
Patients with any known prior diagnosis of an HIV-related illness should be coded to B20. Once a patient has developed an HIV-related illness, the patient should always be assigned code B20 on every subsequent admission/encounter. Patients previously diagnosed with any HIV illness (B20) should never be assigned to R75 or Z21, Asymptomatic human immunodeficiency virus [HIV] infection status.

Other viral diseases (B25-B34)

4 **B25 Cytomegaloviral disease**

EXCLUDES 1 congenital cytomegalovirus infection (P35.1)
cytomegaloviral mononucleosis (B27.1-)

SP **B25.0 Cytomegaloviral pneumonitis**

SP **B25.1 Cytomegaloviral hepatitis**

SP **B25.2 Cytomegaloviral pancreatitis**

SP **B25.8 Other cytomegaloviral diseases**
Cytomegaloviral encephalitis

SP **B25.9 Cytomegaloviral disease, unspecified**

4 **B26 Mumps**

INCLUDES epidemic parotitis
infectious parotitis

SP **B26.0 Mumps orchitis**

SP **B26.1 Mumps meningitis**

SP **B26.2 Mumps encephalitis**

SP **B26.3 Mumps pancreatitis**

5 **B26.8 Mumps with other complications**

SP **B26.81 Mumps hepatitis**

SP **B26.82 Mumps myocarditis**

SP **B26.83 Mumps nephritis**

SP **B26.84 Mumps polyneuropathy**

SP **B26.85 Mumps arthritis**

SP **B26.89 Other mumps complications**

SP **B26.9 Mumps without complication**
Mumps NOS
Mumps parotitis NOS

4 **B27 Infectious mononucleosis**

INCLUDES glandular fever
monocytic angina
Pfeiffer's disease

5 **B27.0 Gammaherpesviral mononucleosis**
Mononucleosis due to Epstein-Barr virus

SP **B27.00 Gammaherpesviral mononucleosis without complication**

SP **B27.01 Gammaherpesviral mononucleosis with polyneuropathy**

SP **B27.02 Gammaherpesviral mononucleosis with meningitis**

SP **B27.09 Gammaherpesviral mononucleosis with other complications**
Hepatomegaly in gammaherpesviral mononucleosis

5 **B27.1 Cytomegaloviral mononucleosis**

SP **B27.10 Cytomegaloviral mononucleosis without complications**

SP **B27.11 Cytomegaloviral mononucleosis with polyneuropathy**

SP **B27.12 Cytomegaloviral mononucleosis with meningitis**

SP **B27.19 Cytomegaloviral mononucleosis with other complication**
Hepatomegaly in cytomegaloviral mononucleosis

5 **B27.8 Other infectious mononucleosis**

SP **B27.80 Other infectious mononucleosis without complication**

SP **B27.81 Other infectious mononucleosis with polyneuropathy**

SP **B27.82 Other infectious mononucleosis with meningitis**

SP **B27.89 Other infectious mononucleosis with other complication**
Hepatomegaly in other infectious mononucleosis

5 **B27.9 Infectious mononucleosis, unspecified**

SP **B27.90 Infectious mononucleosis, unspecified without complication**

SP **B27.91 Infectious mononucleosis, unspecified with polyneuropathy**

SP **B27.92 Infectious mononucleosis, unspecified with meningitis**

SP **B27.99 Infectious mononucleosis, unspecified with other complication**
Hepatomegaly in unspecified infectious mononucleosis

4 **B30 Viral conjunctivitis**
EXCLUDES 1 herpesviral [herpes simplex] ocular disease (B00.5)
ocular zoster (B02.3)

SP **B30.0 Keratoconjunctivitis due to adenovirus**
Epidemic keratoconjunctivitis
Shipyard eye

SP **B30.1 Conjunctivitis due to adenovirus**
Acute adenoviral follicular conjunctivitis
Swimming-pool conjunctivitis

SP **B30.2 Viral pharyngoconjunctivitis**

SP **B30.3 Acute epidemic hemorrhagic conjunctivitis (enteroviral)**
Conjunctivitis due to coxsackievirus 24
Conjunctivitis due to enterovirus 70
Hemorrhagic conjunctivitis (acute)(epidemic)

SP **B30.8 Other viral conjunctivitis**
Newcastle conjunctivitis

SP **B30.9 Viral conjunctivitis, unspecified**

4 **B33 Other viral diseases, not elsewhere classified**

SP **B33.0 Epidemic myalgia**
Bornholm disease

SP **B33.1 Ross River disease**
Epidemic polyarthritis and exanthema
Ross River fever

5 **B33.2 Viral carditis**
Coxsackie (virus) carditis

SP **B33.20 Viral carditis, unspecified**

SP **B33.21 Viral endocarditis**

SP **B33.22 Viral myocarditis**

SP **B33.23 Viral pericarditis**

SP **B33.24 Viral cardiomyopathy**

SP **B33.3 Retrovirus infections, not elsewhere classified**
Retrovirus infection NOS

SP + **B33.4 Hantavirus (cardio)-pulmonary syndrome [HPS] [HCPS]**
Hantavirus disease with pulmonary manifestations
Sin nombre virus disease
Use additional code to identify any associated acute kidney failure (N17.9)
EXCLUDES 1 hantavirus disease with renal manifestations (A98.5)
hemorrhagic fever with renal manifestations (A98.5)

SP **B33.8 Other specified viral diseases**
EXCLUDES 1 anogenital human papillomavirus infection (A63.0)
viral warts due to human papillomavirus infection (B07)

4 **B34 Viral infection of unspecified site**
EXCLUDES 1 anogenital human papillomavirus infection (A63.0)
cytomegaloviral disease NOS (B25.9)
herpesvirus [herpes simplex] infection NOS (B00.9)
retrovirus infection NOS (B33.3)
viral agents as the cause of diseases classified elsewhere (B97.-)
viral warts due to human papillomavirus infection (B07)

CODING TIPS✓ Avoid using these codes for viral-caused infections. Most viral infections have combination codes.

SP **B34.0 Adenovirus infection, unspecified**

SP **B34.1 Enterovirus infection, unspecified**
Coxsackievirus infection NOS
Echovirus infection NOS

SP **B34.2 Coronavirus infection, unspecified**
EXCLUDES 1 COVID-19 (U07.1)
pneumonia due to SARS-associated coronavirus (J12.81)

CODING TIPS✓ B34.2, although indicating coronavirus, is not appropriate for COVID-19, which is universally respiratory in nature. Do not use B34.2 for COVID-19.

SP **B34.3 Parvovirus infection, unspecified**

SP **B34.4 Papovavirus infection, unspecified**

IQ **B34.8 Other viral infections of unspecified site**

IQ **B34.9 Viral infection, unspecified**
Viremia NOS

Mycoses (B35-B49)

EXCLUDES 2 hypersensitivity pneumonitis due to organic dust (J67.-)
mycosis fungoides (C84.0-)

4 B35 Dermatophytosis
INCLUDES favus
infections due to species of Epidermophyton, Microsporum and Trichophyton
tinea, any type except those in B36.-

SP B35.0 Tinea barbae and tinea capitis
Beard ringworm
Kerion
Scalp ringworm
Sycosis, mycotic
DEFINITION Superficial fungal infections of the skin of bearded parts of the face and neck, and the scalp.

SP B35.1 Tinea unguium
Dermatophytic onychia
Dermatophytosis of nail
Onychomycosis
Ringworm of nails
DEFINITION Fungal infection of the nails, first the surface, lateral and distal edges, and later, the part beneath the nail plate.

SP B35.2 Tinea manuum
Dermatophytosis of hand
Hand ringworm

SP B35.3 Tinea pedis
Athlete's foot
Dermatophytosis of foot
Foot ringworm

SP B35.4 Tinea corporis
Ringworm of the body

SP B35.5 Tinea imbricata
Tokelau
DEFINITION A fungal infection which affects skin with few or no hair follicles, typically seen in humid climates. The early lesion is annular with a circle of scales at the outside boundary.

SP B35.6 Tinea cruris
Dhobi itch
Groin ringworm
Jock itch
DEFINITION Fungal infection of the groin commonly known as jock itch.

SP B35.8 Other dermatophytoses
Disseminated dermatophytosis
Granulomatous dermatophytosis

SP B35.9 Dermatophytosis, unspecified
Ringworm NOS

4 B36 Other superficial mycoses

SP B36.0 Pityriasis versicolor
Tinea flava
Tinea versicolor

SP B36.1 Tinea nigra
Keratomycosis nigricans palmaris
Microsporosis nigra
Pityriasis nigra
DEFINITION A minor fungal infection having dark lesions with the appearance of spattered silver nitrate on the skin.

SP B36.2 White piedra
Tinea blanca
DEFINITION A fungal disease of hair covered skin, marked by pale patches and bald spot where the infection occurred.

SP B36.3 Black piedra

SP B36.8 Other specified superficial mycoses

SP B36.9 Superficial mycosis, unspecified

4 B37 Candidiasis
INCLUDES candidosis
moniliasis
EXCLUDES 1 neonatal candidiasis (P37.5)

SP B37.0 Candidal stomatitis
Oral thrush
DEFINITION Fungal infection located in the mouth.

SP B37.1 Pulmonary candidiasis
Candidal bronchitis
Candidal pneumonia

SP B37.2 Candidiasis of skin and nail
Candidal onychia
Candidal paronychia
EXCLUDES 2 diaper dermatitis (L22)

SP B37.3 Candidiasis of vulva and vagina
Candidal vulvovaginitis
Monilial vulvovaginitis
Vaginal thrush

5 B37.4 Candidiasis of other urogenital sites

SP B37.41 Candidal cystitis and urethritis
CODING TIPS ✓ B37.41 is a combination code that includes both the infection of the urinary tract and candida as the infectious cause. No additional codes should be assigned for urinary infection.

SP B37.42 Candidal balanitis

SP B37.49 Other urogenital candidiasis
Candidal pyelonephritis

SP B37.5 Candidal meningitis

SP B37.6 Candidal endocarditis

SP B37.7 Candidal sepsis
Disseminated candidiasis
Systemic candidiasis

5 B37.8 Candidiasis of other sites

SP B37.81 Candidal esophagitis
DEFINITION Fungal infection of the esophagus, usually occurring in patients with immunocompromised states.

SP B37.82 Candidal enteritis
Candidal proctitis

SP B37.83 Candidal cheilitis

SP B37.84 Candidal otitis externa

SP B37.89 Other sites of candidiasis
Candidal osteomyelitis

SP B37.9 Candidiasis, unspecified
Thrush NOS

4 B38 Coccidioidomycosis

SP B38.0 Acute pulmonary coccidioidomycosis

SP B38.1 Chronic pulmonary coccidioidomycosis

SP B38.2 Pulmonary coccidioidomycosis, unspecified

SP B38.3 Cutaneous coccidioidomycosis

SP B38.4 Coccidioidomycosis meningitis

SP B38.7 Disseminated coccidioidomycosis
Generalized coccidioidomycosis

5 B38.8 Other forms of coccidioidomycosis

SP B38.81 Prostatic coccidioidomycosis

SP B38.89 Other forms of coccidioidomycosis

Chapter 1

A00 - B99

SP **B38.9 Coccidioidomycosis, unspecified**

+ 4 **B39 Histoplasmosis**
Code first:
associated AIDS (B20)
Use additional code for any associated manifestations, such as:
endocarditis (I39)
meningitis (G02)
pericarditis (I32)
retinitis (H32)

CODING TIPS ✓ Histoplasmosis (B39) is usually associated with HIV/AIDS. If so, then B20 (HIV disease) is sequenced prior to using the B39 category code.

SP + **B39.0 Acute pulmonary histoplasmosis capsulati**

SP + **B39.1 Chronic pulmonary histoplasmosis capsulati**

SP + **B39.2 Pulmonary histoplasmosis capsulati, unspecified**

SP + **B39.3 Disseminated histoplasmosis capsulati**
Generalized histoplasmosis capsulati

SP + **B39.4 Histoplasmosis capsulati, unspecified**
American histoplasmosis

SP + **B39.5 Histoplasmosis duboisii**
African histoplasmosis

SP + **B39.9 Histoplasmosis, unspecified**

4 **B40 Blastomycosis**
EXCLUDES 1 Brazilian blastomycosis (B41.-)
keloidal blastomycosis (B48.0)

SP **B40.0 Acute pulmonary blastomycosis**

SP **B40.1 Chronic pulmonary blastomycosis**

SP **B40.2 Pulmonary blastomycosis, unspecified**

SP **B40.3 Cutaneous blastomycosis**

SP **B40.7 Disseminated blastomycosis**
Generalized blastomycosis

5 **B40.8 Other forms of blastomycosis**

SP **B40.81 Blastomycotic meningoencephalitis**
Meningomyelitis due to blastomycosis

SP **B40.89 Other forms of blastomycosis**

SP **B40.9 Blastomycosis, unspecified**

4 **B41 Paracoccidioidomycosis**
INCLUDES Brazilian blastomycosis
Lutz' disease

SP **B41.0 Pulmonary paracoccidioidomycosis**

SP **B41.7 Disseminated paracoccidioidomycosis**
Generalized paracoccidioidomycosis

SP **B41.8 Other forms of paracoccidioidomycosis**

SP **B41.9 Paracoccidioidomycosis, unspecified**

4 **B42 Sporotrichosis**

SP **B42.0 Pulmonary sporotrichosis**

SP **B42.1 Lymphocutaneous sporotrichosis**

SP **B42.7 Disseminated sporotrichosis**
Generalized sporotrichosis

5 **B42.8 Other forms of sporotrichosis**

SP **B42.81 Cerebral sporotrichosis**
Meningitis due to sporotrichosis

SP **B42.82 Sporotrichosis arthritis**

SP **B42.89 Other forms of sporotrichosis**

SP **B42.9 Sporotrichosis, unspecified**

4 **B43 Chromomycosis and pheomycotic abscess**

SP **B43.0 Cutaneous chromomycosis**
Dermatitis verrucosa

SP **B43.1 Pheomycotic brain abscess**
Cerebral chromomycosis

SP **B43.2 Subcutaneous pheomycotic abscess and cyst**

SP **B43.8 Other forms of chromomycosis**

SP **B43.9 Chromomycosis, unspecified**

4 **B44 Aspergillosis**
INCLUDES aspergilloma

SP **B44.0 Invasive pulmonary aspergillosis**

SP **B44.1 Other pulmonary aspergillosis**

SP **B44.2 Tonsillar aspergillosis**

SP **B44.7 Disseminated aspergillosis**
Generalized aspergillosis

5 **B44.8 Other forms of aspergillosis**

SP **B44.81 Allergic bronchopulmonary aspergillosis**

SP **B44.89 Other forms of aspergillosis**

SP **B44.9 Aspergillosis, unspecified**

4 **B45 Cryptococcosis**

SP **B45.0 Pulmonary cryptococcosis**

DEFINITION Yeastlike fungus infection, by cryptococcus neoformans, commonly occurring in the soil, which infects via the lungs and may spread to the brain and meninges.

SP **B45.1 Cerebral cryptococcosis**
Cryptococcal meningitis
Cryptococcosis meningocerebralis

DEFINITION Infection of the brain and/or its surrounding tissues causing hydrocephalus and intracerebral cysts due to infection with cryptococcus fungus.

SP **B45.2 Cutaneous cryptococcosis**

SP **B45.3 Osseous cryptococcosis**

SP **B45.7 Disseminated cryptococcosis**
Generalized cryptococcosis

SP **B45.8 Other forms of cryptococcosis**

SP **B45.9 Cryptococcosis, unspecified**

4 **B46 Zygomycosis**

SP **B46.0 Pulmonary mucormycosis**

SP **B46.1 Rhinocerebral mucormycosis**

SP **B46.2 Gastrointestinal mucormycosis**

SP **B46.3 Cutaneous mucormycosis**
Subcutaneous mucormycosis

SP **B46.4 Disseminated mucormycosis**
Generalized mucormycosis

SP **B46.5 Mucormycosis, unspecified**

SP **B46.8 Other zygomycoses**
Entomophthoromycosis

SP **B46.9 Zygomycosis, unspecified**
Phycomycosis NOS

4 **B47 Mycetoma**

SP **B47.0 Eumycetoma**
Madura foot, mycotic
Maduromycosis

SP **B47.1 Actinomycetoma**

SP **B47.9 Mycetoma, unspecified**
Madura foot NOS

DEFINITION Chronic infection involving the feet, characterized by formation of localized lesions, with swelling and multiple draining sinuses.

4 **B48 Other mycoses, not elsewhere classified**

SP **B48.0 Lobomycosis**
Keloidal blastomycosis
Lobo's disease
DEFINITION A fungal infection of the skin caused by Lobo loboi and characterized by keloidal nodular lesions occurring on the face, ears, and extremities.

SP **B48.1 Rhinosporidiosis**

SP **B48.2 Allescheriasis**
Infection due to Pseudallescheria boydii
EXCLUDES 1 eumycetoma (B47.0)

SP **B48.3 Geotrichosis**
Geotrichum stomatitis

SP **B48.4 Penicillosis**
Talaromycosis

SP **B48.8 Other specified mycoses**
Adiaspiromycosis
Infection of tissue and organs by Alternaria
Infection of tissue and organs by Drechslera
Infection of tissue and organs by Fusarium
Infection of tissue and organs by saprophytic fungi NEC

SP **B49 Unspecified mycosis**
Fungemia NOS

Protozoal diseases (B50-B64)

EXCLUDES 1 amebiasis (A06.-)
other protozoal intestinal diseases (A07.-)

4 **B50 Plasmodium falciparum malaria**
INCLUDES mixed infections of Plasmodium falciparum with any other Plasmodium species

SP **B50.0 Plasmodium falciparum malaria with cerebral complications**
Cerebral malaria NOS

SP **B50.8 Other severe and complicated Plasmodium falciparum malaria**
Severe or complicated Plasmodium falciparum malaria NOS

SP **B50.9 Plasmodium falciparum malaria, unspecified**

4 **B51 Plasmodium vivax malaria**
INCLUDES mixed infections of Plasmodium vivax with other Plasmodium species, except Plasmodium falciparum
EXCLUDES 1 plasmodium vivax with Plasmodium falciparum (B50.-)

SP **B51.0 Plasmodium vivax malaria with rupture of spleen**

SP **B51.8 Plasmodium vivax malaria with other complications**

SP **B51.9 Plasmodium vivax malaria without complication**
Plasmodium vivax malaria NOS

4 **B52 Plasmodium malariae malaria**
INCLUDES mixed infections of Plasmodium malariae with other Plasmodium species, except Plasmodium falciparum and Plasmodium vivax
EXCLUDES 1 Plasmodium falciparum (B50.-)
Plasmodium vivax (B51.-)

SP **B52.0 Plasmodium malariae malaria with nephropathy**

SP **B52.8 Plasmodium malariae malaria with other complications**

SP **B52.9 Plasmodium malariae malaria without complication**
Plasmodium malariae malaria NOS

4 **B53 Other specified malaria**

SP **B53.0 Plasmodium ovale malaria**
EXCLUDES 1 Plasmodium ovale with Plasmodium falciparum (B50.-)
Plasmodium ovale with Plasmodium malariae (B52.-)
Plasmodium ovale with Plasmodium vivax (B51.-)

SP **B53.1 Malaria due to simian plasmodia**
EXCLUDES 1 Malaria due to simian plasmodia with Plasmodium falciparum (B50.-)
Malaria due to simian plasmodia with Plasmodium malariae (B52.-)
Malaria due to simian plasmodia with Plasmodium ovale (B53.0)
Malaria due to simian plasmodia with Plasmodium vivax (B51.-)

SP **B53.8 Other malaria, not elsewhere classified**

SP **B54 Unspecified malaria**

4 **B55 Leishmaniasis**

SP **B55.0 Visceral leishmaniasis**
Kala-azar
Post-kala-azar dermal leishmaniasis

SP **B55.1 Cutaneous leishmaniasis**

SP **B55.2 Mucocutaneous leishmaniasis**

SP **B55.9 Leishmaniasis, unspecified**

4 **B56 African trypanosomiasis**

SP **B56.0 Gambiense trypanosomiasis**
Infection due to Trypanosoma brucei gambiense
West African sleeping sickness

SP **B56.1 Rhodesiense trypanosomiasis**
East African sleeping sickness
Infection due to Trypanosoma brucei rhodesiense

SP **B56.9 African trypanosomiasis, unspecified**
Sleeping sickness NOS

4 **B57 Chagas' disease**
INCLUDES American trypanosomiasis
infection due to Trypanosoma cruzi

SP **B57.0 Acute Chagas' disease with heart involvement**
Acute Chagas' disease with myocarditis

SP **B57.1 Acute Chagas' disease without heart involvement**
Acute Chagas' disease NOS

SP **B57.2 Chagas' disease (chronic) with heart involvement**

American trypanosomiasis NOS
Chagas' disease (chronic) NOS
Chagas' disease (chronic) with myocarditis
Trypanosomiasis NOS

5 **B57.3 Chagas' disease (chronic) with digestive system involvement**

SP **B57.30 Chagas' disease with digestive system involvement, unspecified**

SP **B57.31 Megaesophagus in Chagas' disease**

SP **B57.32 Megacolon in Chagas' disease**

SP **B57.39 Other digestive system involvement in Chagas' disease**

5 **B57.4 Chagas' disease (chronic) with nervous system involvement**

SP **B57.40 Chagas' disease with nervous system involvement, unspecified**

SP **B57.41 Meningitis in Chagas' disease**

SP **B57.42 Meningoencephalitis in Chagas' disease**

SP **B57.49 Other nervous system involvement in Chagas' disease**

SP **B57.5 Chagas' disease (chronic) with other organ involvement**

4 **B58 Toxoplasmosis**

INCLUDES infection due to Toxoplasma gondii

EXCLUDES 1 congenital toxoplasmosis (P37.1)

5 **B58.0 Toxoplasma oculopathy**

SP **B58.00 Toxoplasma oculopathy, unspecified**

SP **B58.01 Toxoplasma chorioretinitis**

SP **B58.09 Other toxoplasma oculopathy**
Toxoplasma uveitis

SP **B58.1 Toxoplasma hepatitis**

SP **B58.2 Toxoplasma meningoencephalitis**

SP **B58.3 Pulmonary toxoplasmosis**

5 **B58.8 Toxoplasmosis with other organ involvement**

SP **B58.81 Toxoplasma myocarditis**

SP **B58.82 Toxoplasma myositis**

SP **B58.83 Toxoplasma tubulo-interstitial nephropathy**
Toxoplasma pyelonephritis

SP **B58.89 Toxoplasmosis with other organ involvement**

SP **B58.9 Toxoplasmosis, unspecified**

SP **B59 Pneumocystosis**
Pneumonia due to Pneumocystis carinii
Pneumonia due to Pneumocystis jiroveci

CODING TIPS ✓ Pneumocystosis is usually associated with HIV/AIDS. If so, then B20 (HIV disease) is sequenced prior to using the B59 category code.

4 **B60 Other protozoal diseases, not elsewhere classified**

EXCLUDES 1 cryptosporidiosis (A07.2)
intestinal microsporidiosis (A07.8)
isosporiasis (A07.3)

5 **B60.0 Babesiosis**

SP **B60.00 Babesiosis, unspecified**
Babesiosis due to unspecified Babesia species
Piroplasmosis, unspecified

SP **B60.01 Babesiosis due to Babesia microti**
Infection due to B. microti

SP **B60.02 Babesiosis due to Babesia duncani**
Infection due to B. duncani and B. duncani-type species

SP **B60.03 Babesiosis due to Babesia divergens**
Babesiosis due to Babesia MO-1
Infection due to B. divergens and B. divergens-like strains

SP **B60.09 Other babesiosis**
Babesiosis due to Babesia KO-1
Babesiosis due to Babesia venatorum
Infection due to other Babesia species
Infection due to other protozoa of the order Piroplasmida
Other piroplasmosis

5 **B60.1 Acanthamebiasis**

SP **B60.10 Acanthamebiasis, unspecified**

SP **B60.11 Meningoencephalitis due to Acanthamoeba (culbertsoni)**

SP **B60.12 Conjunctivitis due to Acanthamoeba**

SP **B60.13 Keratoconjunctivitis due to Acanthamoeba**

SP **B60.19 Other acanthamebic disease**

SP **B60.2 Naegleriasis**
Primary amebic meningoencephalitis

SP **B60.8 Other specified protozoal diseases**
Microsporidiosis

IQ **B64 Unspecified protozoal disease**

Helminthiases (B65-B83)

4 **B65 Schistosomiasis [bilharziasis]**

INCLUDES snail fever

SP **B65.0 Schistosomiasis due to Schistosoma haematobium [urinary schistosomiasis]**

SP **B65.1 Schistosomiasis due to Schistosoma mansoni [intestinal schistosomiasis]**

SP **B65.2 Schistosomiasis due to Schistosoma japonicum**
Asiatic schistosomiasis

SP **B65.3 Cercarial dermatitis**
Swimmer's itch

DEFINITION An itching inflammation of the skin due to penetration of larval forms of schistosomes (parasitic worms), occurring in bathers of infested waters.

SP **B65.8 Other schistosomiasis**
Infection due to Schistosoma intercalatum
Infection due to Schistosoma mattheei
Infection due to Schistosoma mekongi

SP **B65.9 Schistosomiasis, unspecified**

4 **B66 Other fluke infections**

SP **B66.0 Opisthorchiasis**
Infection due to cat liver fluke
Infection due to Opisthorchis (felineus)(viverrini)

SP **B66.1 Clonorchiasis**
Chinese liver fluke disease
Infection due to Clonorchis sinensis
Oriental liver fluke disease

SP **B66.2 Dicroceliasis**
Infection due to Dicrocoelium dendriticum
Lancet fluke infection

SP **B66.3 Fascioliasis**
Infection due to Fasciola gigantica

Infection due to Fasciola hepatica
Infection due to Fasciola indica
Sheep liver fluke disease

SP **B66.4 Paragonimiasis**
Infection due to Paragonimus species
Lung fluke disease
Pulmonary distomiasis

SP **B66.5 Fasciolopsiasis**
Infection due to Fasciolopsis buski
Intestinal distomiasis

SP **B66.8 Other specified fluke infections**
Echinostomiasis
Heterophyiasis
Metagonimiasis
Nanophyetiasis
Watsoniasis

SP **B66.9 Fluke infection, unspecified**

4 **B67 Echinococcosis**
INCLUDES hydatidosis

SP **B67.0 Echinococcus granulosus infection of liver**
DEFINITION A genus of parasitic tapeworm passed from dogs. The larvae form large cysts in the liver, causing serious and sometimes fatal disease.

SP **B67.1 Echinococcus granulosus infection of lung**

SP **B67.2 Echinococcus granulosus infection of bone**

5 **B67.3 Echinococcus granulosus infection, other and multiple sites**

SP **B67.31 Echinococcus granulosus infection, thyroid gland**

SP **B67.32 Echinococcus granulosus infection, multiple sites**

SP **B67.39 Echinococcus granulosus infection, other sites**

IQ **B67.4 Echinococcus granulosus infection, unspecified**
Dog tapeworm (infection)

SP **B67.5 Echinococcus multilocularis infection of liver**

5 **B67.6 Echinococcus multilocularis infection, other and multiple sites**

SP **B67.61 Echinococcus multilocularis infection, multiple sites**

SP **B67.69 Echinococcus multilocularis infection, other sites**

IQ **B67.7 Echinococcus multilocularis infection, unspecified**

SP **B67.8 Echinococcosis, unspecified, of liver**

5 **B67.9 Echinococcosis, other and unspecified**

SP **B67.90 Echinococcosis, unspecified**
Echinococcosis NOS

SP **B67.99 Other echinococcosis**

4 **B68 Taeniasis**
EXCLUDES 1 cysticercosis (B69.-)

SP **B68.0 Taenia solium taeniasis**
Pork tapeworm (infection)

SP **B68.1 Taenia saginata taeniasis**
Beef tapeworm (infection)
Infection due to adult tapeworm Taenia saginata

SP **B68.9 Taeniasis, unspecified**

4 **B69 Cysticercosis**
INCLUDES cysticerciasis infection due to larval form of Taenia solium

SP **B69.0 Cysticercosis of central nervous system**

SP **B69.1 Cysticercosis of eye**

5 **B69.8 Cysticercosis of other sites**

SP **B69.81 Myositis in cysticercosis**

SP **B69.89 Cysticercosis of other sites**

SP **B69.9 Cysticercosis, unspecified**
DEFINITION Infection caused by the pork tapeworm when its larvae enter the body and form cysts.

4 **B70 Diphyllobothriasis and sparganosis**

SP **B70.0 Diphyllobothriasis**
Diphyllobothrium (adult) (latum) (pacificum) infection
Fish tapeworm (infection)
EXCLUDES 2 larval diphyllobothriasis (B70.1)

SP **B70.1 Sparganosis**
Infection due to Sparganum (mansoni) (proliferum)
Infection due to Spirometra larva
Larval diphyllobothriasis
Spirometrosis

4 **B71 Other cestode infections**

SP **B71.0 Hymenolepiasis**
Dwarf tapeworm infection
Rat tapeworm (infection)

SP **B71.1 Dipylidiasis**

SP **B71.8 Other specified cestode infections**
Coenurosis

SP **B71.9 Cestode infection, unspecified**
Tapeworm (infection) NOS

SP **B72 Dracunculiasis**
INCLUDES guinea worm infection
infection due to Dracunculus medinensis

4 **B73 Onchocerciasis**
INCLUDES onchocerca volvulus infection
onchocercosis
river blindness

5 **B73.0 Onchocerciasis with eye disease**

SP **B73.00 Onchocerciasis with eye involvement, unspecified**

SP **B73.01 Onchocerciasis with endophthalmitis**

SP **B73.02 Onchocerciasis with glaucoma**

SP **B73.09 Onchocerciasis with other eye involvement**
Infestation of eyelid due to onchocerciasis

SP **B73.1 Onchocerciasis without eye disease**

▲ 4 **B74 Filariasis**
EXCLUDES 2 onchocerciasis (B73)
tropical (pulmonary) eosinophilia NOS (J82.89)

SP **B74.0 Filariasis due to Wuchereria bancrofti**
Bancroftian elephantiasis
Bancroftian filariasis

SP **B74.1 Filariasis due to Brugia malayi**

SP **B74.2 Filariasis due to Brugia timori**

SP **B74.3 Loiasis**
Calabar swelling
Eyeworm disease of Africa
Loa loa infection

SP **B74.4 Mansonelliasis**
Infection due to Mansonella ozzardi
Infection due to Mansonella perstans
Infection due to Mansonella streptocerca

SP **B74.8 Other filariases**
Dirofilariasis

SP **B74.9 Filariasis, unspecified**

SP **B75 Trichinellosis**
INCLUDES infection due to Trichinella species
trichiniasis

4 **B76 Hookworm diseases**
INCLUDES uncinariasis

SP **B76.0 Ancylostomiasis**
Infection due to Ancylostoma species

SP **B76.1 Necatoriasis**
Infection due to Necator americanus

SP **B76.8 Other hookworm diseases**

SP **B76.9 Hookworm disease, unspecified**
Cutaneous larva migrans NOS

4 **B77 Ascariasis**
INCLUDES ascaridiasis
roundworm infection

SP **B77.0 Ascariasis with intestinal complications**

5 **B77.8 Ascariasis with other complications**

SP **B77.81 Ascariasis pneumonia**

SP **B77.89 Ascariasis with other complications**

SP **B77.9 Ascariasis, unspecified**

4 **B78 Strongyloidiasis**
EXCLUDES 1 trichostrongyliasis (B81.2)

SP **B78.0 Intestinal strongyloidiasis**

SP **B78.1 Cutaneous strongyloidiasis**

SP **B78.7 Disseminated strongyloidiasis**

SP **B78.9 Strongyloidiasis, unspecified**

SP **B79 Trichuriasis**
INCLUDES trichocephaliasis
whipworm (disease) (infection)

SP **B80 Enterobiasis**
INCLUDES oxyuriasis
pinworm infection
threadworm infection

4 **B81 Other intestinal helminthiases, not elsewhere classified**
EXCLUDES 1 angiostrongyliasis due to:
Angiostrongylus cantonensis (B83.2)
Parastrongylus cantonensis (B83.2)

SP **B81.0 Anisakiasis**
Infection due to Anisakis larva

SP **B81.1 Intestinal capillariasis**
Capillariasis NOS
Infection due to Capillaria philippinensis
EXCLUDES 2 hepatic capillariasis (B83.8)

SP **B81.2 Trichostrongyliasis**

SP **B81.3 Intestinal angiostrongyliasis**
Angiostrongyliasis due to:
Angiostrongylus costaricensis
Parastrongylus costaricensis

SP **B81.4 Mixed intestinal helminthiases**
Infection due to intestinal helminths classified to more than one of the categories B65.0-B81.3 and B81.8
Mixed helminthiasis NOS

SP **B81.8 Other specified intestinal helminthiases**
Infection due to Oesophagostomum species [esophagostomiasis]
Infection due to Ternidens diminutus [ternidensiasis]

4 **B82 Unspecified intestinal parasitism**

SP **B82.0 Intestinal helminthiasis, unspecified**

SP **B82.9 Intestinal parasitism, unspecified**

4 **B83 Other helminthiases**
EXCLUDES 1 capillariasis NOS (B81.1)
EXCLUDES 2 intestinal capillariasis (B81.1)

SP **B83.0 Visceral larva migrans**
Toxocariasis

SP **B83.1 Gnathostomiasis**
Wandering swelling

SP **B83.2 Angiostrongyliasis due to Parastrongylus cantonensis**
Eosinophilic meningoencephalitis due to Parastrongylus cantonensis
EXCLUDES 2 intestinal angiostrongyliasis (B81.3)

SP **B83.3 Syngamiasis**
Syngamosis

SP **B83.4 Internal hirudiniasis**
EXCLUDES 2 external hirudiniasis (B88.3)

SP **B83.8 Other specified helminthiases**
Acanthocephaliasis
Gongylonemiasis
Hepatic capillariasis
Metastrongyliasis
Thelaziasis

SP **B83.9 Helminthiasis, unspecified**
Worms NOS
EXCLUDES 1 intestinal helminthiasis NOS (B82.0)

Pediculosis, acariasis and other infestations (B85-B89)

4 **B85 Pediculosis and phthiriasis**

SP **B85.0 Pediculosis due to Pediculus humanus capitis**
Head-louse infestation

SP **B85.1 Pediculosis due to Pediculus humanus corporis**
Body-louse infestation

SP **B85.2 Pediculosis, unspecified**

SP **B85.3 Phthiriasis**
Infestation by crab-louse
Infestation by Phthirus pubis

SP **B85.4 Mixed pediculosis and phthiriasis**
Infestation classifiable to more than one of the categories B85.0-B85.3

SP **B86 Scabies**
Sarcoptic itch

4 **B87 Myiasis**
INCLUDES infestation by larva of flies

SP **B87.0 Cutaneous myiasis**
Creeping myiasis
DEFINITION Infestation by the fly larvae of the genus Oestrus causing inflamed furuncles where the larvae are maturing beneath the skin.

SP **B87.1 Wound myiasis**
Traumatic myiasis

SP **B87.2 Ocular myiasis**

SP **B87.3 Nasopharyngeal myiasis**
Laryngeal myiasis

SP **B87.4 Aural myiasis**

5 **B87.8 Myiasis of other sites**

SP **B87.81 Genitourinary myiasis**

SP **B87.82 Intestinal myiasis**

SP **B87.89 Myiasis of other sites**

SP **B87.9 Myiasis, unspecified**

4 **B88 Other infestations**

SP **B88.0 Other acariasis**
Acarine dermatitis
Dermatitis due to Demodex species
Dermatitis due to Dermanyssus gallinae
Dermatitis due to Liponyssoides sanguineus
Trombiculosis
EXCLUDES 2 scabies (B86)

SP **B88.1 Tungiasis [sandflea infestation]**

SP **B88.2 Other arthropod infestations**
Scarabiasis

SP **B88.3 External hirudiniasis**
Leech infestation NOS
EXCLUDES 2 internal hirudiniasis (B83.4)

SP **B88.8 Other specified infestations**
Ichthyoparasitism due to Vandellia cirrhosa
Linguatulosis
Porocephaliasis

IQ **B88.9 Infestation, unspecified**
Infestation (skin) NOS
Infestation by mites NOS
Skin parasites NOS

IQ **B89 Unspecified parasitic disease**

Sequelae of infectious and parasitic diseases (B90-B94)

Note:
Categories B90-B94 are to be used to indicate conditions in categories A00-B89 as the cause of sequelae, which are themselves classified elsewhere. The 'sequelae' include conditions specified as such; they also include residuals of diseases classifiable to the above categories if there is evidence that the disease itself is no longer present. Codes from these categories are not to be used for chronic infections. Code chronic current infections to active infectious disease as appropriate.
Code first:
condition resulting from (sequela) the infectious or parasitic disease

4 **B90 Sequelae of tuberculosis**

CODING TIPS✓ Conditions classified here are specifically reportable as sequelae or late effects of tuberculosis. The active disease is no longer present. Acute tuberculosis should be coded to A15-A19.

CODING TIPS✓ Do not use B90 to indicate chronic infection. If there are no residuals of a past infection, use Z86.11.

IQ **B90.0 Sequelae of central nervous system tuberculosis**

IQ **B90.1 Sequelae of genitourinary tuberculosis**

IQ **B90.2 Sequelae of tuberculosis of bones and joints**

IQ **B90.8 Sequelae of tuberculosis of other organs**
EXCLUDES 2 sequelae of respiratory tuberculosis (B90.9)

IQ **B90.9 Sequelae of respiratory and unspecified tuberculosis**
Sequelae of tuberculosis NOS

IQ **B91 Sequelae of poliomyelitis**
EXCLUDES 1 postpolio syndrome (G14)

CODING TIPS✓ Conditions classified here are specifically reportable as sequelae of poliomyelitis. Acute poliomyelitis should be coded to A80. When postpolio syndrome is specified, report code G14 rather than B91.

CODING TIPS✓ The general rule is to code the sequela, or residual, first then B91, unless there is a tabular convention that instructs otherwise. If polio has been resolved and there are no residuals, use Z86.12.

IQ **B92 Sequelae of leprosy**

4 **B94 Sequelae of other and unspecified infectious and parasitic diseases**

IQ **B94.0 Sequelae of trachoma**

IQ **B94.1 Sequelae of viral encephalitis**

IQ **B94.2 Sequelae of viral hepatitis**

IQ **B94.8 Sequelae of other specified infectious and parasitic diseases**

CODING TIPS✓ This code is no longer used to indicate sequela of COVID-19 infections. Use U09.9 instead.

▲ IQ **B94.9 Sequelae of unspecified infectious and parasitic disease**
EXCLUDES 2 post COVID-19 condition (U09.9)

Bacterial and viral infectious agents (B95-B97)

Note:
These categories are provided for use as supplementary or additional codes to identify the infectious agent(s) in diseases classified elsewhere.

GUIDELINES **Section I.C.1.b**
Certain infections are classified in chapters other than Chapter 1 and no organism is identified as part of the infection code. In these instances, it is necessary to use an additional code from Chapter 1 to identify the organism. A code from category B95, Streptococcus, Staphylococcus, and Enterococcus as the cause of diseases classified to other chapters, B96, Other bacterial agents as the cause of diseases classified to other chapters, or B97, Viral agents as the cause of diseases classified to other chapters, is to be used as an additional code to identify the organism. An instructional note will be found at the infection code advising that an additional organism code is required.

Section I.C.1.c
Many bacterial infections are resistant to current antibiotics. It is necessary to identify all infections documented as antibiotic resistant. Assign a code from category Z16, Resistance to antimicrobial drugs, following the infection code only if the infection code does not identify drug resistance.

CODING TIPS✓ Conditions classified here are specifically reportable as additional codes to identify infectious agents in diseases classified elsewhere. Do not assign codes from B95-B97 without a code for the underlying disease process first. If the bacteria is unavailable in the documentation, there is no need to add the code.

4 B95 Streptococcus, Staphylococcus, and Enterococcus as the cause of diseases classified elsewhere

CODING TIPS✓ Use B95 codes to identify the organism causing the infection, if known. B95 codes indicate localized streptococcal infections, staphylococcal infections and enterococcal infections (also known as Strep D). These codes are always coded after the code indicating the type of infection from chapters other than chapter 1, such as UTIs and cellulitis, to identify the causative organism. Watch for combination codes. An infectious process, such as pneumonia, is a combination code, and a B95 code is not to be added.

!Q B95.0 Streptococcus, group A, as the cause of diseases classified elsewhere

!Q B95.1 Streptococcus, group B, as the cause of diseases classified elsewhere

!Q B95.2 Enterococcus as the cause of diseases classified elsewhere

!Q B95.3 Streptococcus pneumoniae as the cause of diseases classified elsewhere

!Q B95.4 Other streptococcus as the cause of diseases classified elsewhere

!Q B95.5 Unspecified streptococcus as the cause of diseases classified elsewhere

5 B95.6 Staphylococcus aureus as the cause of diseases classified elsewhere

!Q B95.61 Methicillin susceptible Staphylococcus aureus infection as the cause of diseases classified elsewhere

Methicillin susceptible Staphylococcus aureus (MSSA) infection as the cause of diseases classified elsewhere

Staphylococcus aureus infection NOS as the cause of diseases classified elsewhere

CODING TIPS✓ B95.61 is used when the bacteria is identified as Staphylococcus aureus or MSSA.

!Q B95.62 Methicillin resistant Staphylococcus aureus infection as the cause of diseases classified elsewhere

Methicillin resistant staphylococcus aureus (MRSA) infection as the cause of diseases classified elsewhere

GUIDELINES **Section I.C.1.e.1)**

Selection and sequencing of MRSA codes:

(a) Combination codes for MRSA infection. When a patient is diagnosed with an infection that is due to MRSA, and that infection has a combination code that includes the causal organism (e.g., sepsis, pneumonia) assign the appropriate combination code for the condition (e.g., code A41.02, Sepsis due to Methicillin resistant Staphylococcus aureus or code J15.212, Pneumonia due to Methicillin resistant Staphylococcus aureus). Do not assign code B95.62, Methicillin resistant Staphylococcus aureus infection as the cause of diseases classified elsewhere, as an additional code because the combination code includes the type of infection and the MRSA organism. Do not assign a code from subcategory Z16.11, Resistance to penicillins, as an additional diagnosis.

(b) Other codes for MRSA infection. When there is documentation of a current infection (e.g., wound infection, stitch abscess, urinary tract infection) due to MRSA, and that infection does not have a combination code that includes the causal organism, assign the appropriate code to identify the condition along with code B95.62, Methicillin resistant Staphylococcus aureus infection as the cause of diseases classified elsewhere for the MRSA infection. Do not assign a code from subcategory Z16.11, Resistance to penicillins.

CODING TIPS✓ B95.62 is used when the organism is identified as methicillin-resistant Staph aureus (MRSA). Do not use a Z16 code to indicate resistance to penicillins. Z16 may be added for other resistance, other than penicillins, such as vancomycin.

!Q B95.7 Other staphylococcus as the cause of diseases classified elsewhere

CODING TIPS✓ Use this code when another staph is identified, such as Staphylococcus epidermidis.

!Q B95.8 Unspecified staphylococcus as the cause of diseases classified elsewhere

CODING TIPS✓ Use this code if the organism is identified as "staph" without the species name, such as aureus.

4 B96 Other bacterial agents as the cause of diseases classified elsewhere

CODING TIPS✓ Use B96 codes to identify the organism causing the localized infection, if known. B96 codes indicate other bacterial infections with the exception of streptococcal, staphylococcal, and enterococcal infections. These codes are always coded after the code indicating the type of infection from chapters other than chapter 1, for example, UTIs and cellulitis, to identify the causative organism. Watch for combination codes. An infectious process, such as pneumonia, is a combination code, and a B96 code is not to be added.

IQ **B96.0 Mycoplasma pneumoniae [M. pneumoniae] as the cause of diseases classified elsewhere**
Pleuro-pneumonia-like-organism [PPLO]

IQ **B96.1 Klebsiella pneumoniae [K. pneumoniae] as the cause of diseases classified elsewhere**

5 **B96.2 Escherichia coli [E. coli] as the cause of diseases classified elsewhere**

IQ **B96.20 Unspecified Escherichia coli [E. coli] as the cause of diseases classified elsewhere**
Escherichia coli [E. coli] NOS
CODING TIPS✓ E. coli is the most common bacterial agent identified in UTIs. B96.20 is used when a specific E. coli is not specified by the physician.

IQ **B96.21 Shiga toxin-producing Escherichia coli [E. coli] [STEC] O157 as the cause of diseases classified elsewhere**
E. coli O157:H- (nonmotile) with confirmation of Shiga toxin
E. coli O157 with confirmation of Shiga toxin when H antigen is unknown, or is not H7
O157:H7 Escherichia coli [E.coli] with or without confirmation of Shiga toxin-production
Shiga toxin-producing Escherichia coli [E.coli] O157:H7 with or without confirmation of Shiga toxin-production
STEC O157:H7 with or without confirmation of Shiga toxin-production

IQ **B96.22 Other specified Shiga toxin-producing Escherichia coli [E. coli] [STEC] as the cause of diseases classified elsewhere**
Non-O157 Shiga toxin-producing Escherichia coli [E.coli]
Non-O157 Shiga toxin-producing Escherichia coli [E.coli] with known O group

IQ **B96.23 Unspecified Shiga toxin-producing Escherichia coli [E. coli] [STEC] as the cause of diseases classified elsewhere**
Shiga toxin-producing Escherichia coli [E. coli] with unspecified O group
STEC NOS

IQ **B96.29 Other Escherichia coli [E. coli] as the cause of diseases classified elsewhere**
Non-Shiga toxin-producing E. coli

IQ **B96.3 Hemophilus influenzae [H. influenzae] as the cause of diseases classified elsewhere**
CODING TIPS✓ Hemophilius influenzae (coded to B96.3) is often confused with the influenza virus. H. influenzae is a bacteria.

IQ **B96.4 Proteus (mirabilis) (morganii) as the cause of diseases classified elsewhere**

IQ **B96.5 Pseudomonas (aeruginosa) (mallei) (pseudomallei) as the cause of diseases classified elsewhere**

IQ **B96.6 Bacteroides fragilis [B. fragilis] as the cause of diseases classified elsewhere**

IQ **B96.7 Clostridium perfringens [C. perfringens] as the cause of diseases classified elsewhere**
CODING TIPS✓ Clostridium difficile is coded to A04.7-.

5 **B96.8 Other specified bacterial agents as the cause of diseases classified elsewhere**

IQ **B96.81 Helicobacter pylori [H. pylori] as the cause of diseases classified elsewhere**
DEFINITION Common gastric pathogen causing dyspepsia, gastritis, peptic ulcer disease, gastric adenocarcinoma, and gastric lymphoma.

IQ **B96.82 Vibrio vulnificus as the cause of diseases classified elsewhere**

IQ **B96.89 Other specified bacterial agents as the cause of diseases classified elsewhere**
CODING TIPS✓ Do not use to indicate an unknown bacteria causing a localized infection. If the bacteria is unknown, there is no need to add a code for the bacteria.

4 **B97 Viral agents as the cause of diseases classified elsewhere**
CODING TIPS✓ Most viral conditions use combination codes. Search the index for the specific condition before choosing B97 codes.

IQ **B97.0 Adenovirus as the cause of diseases classified elsewhere**

5 **B97.1 Enterovirus as the cause of diseases classified elsewhere**

IQ **B97.10 Unspecified enterovirus as the cause of diseases classified elsewhere**

IQ **B97.11 Coxsackievirus as the cause of diseases classified elsewhere**

IQ **B97.12 Echovirus as the cause of diseases classified elsewhere**
DEFINITION A group of DNA-containing viruses that affect the tissue linings of the respiratory tract, eyes, intestines, and urinary tract. There are approximately 50 serotypes.

IQ **B97.19 Other enterovirus as the cause of diseases classified elsewhere**

5 **B97.2 Coronavirus as the cause of diseases classified elsewhere**

IQ **B97.21 SARS-associated coronavirus as the cause of diseases classified elsewhere**
EXCLUDES 1 pneumonia due to SARS-associated coronavirus (J12.81)

IQ **B97.29 Other coronavirus as the cause of diseases classified elsewhere**

CODING TIPS✓ Because code B97.29 is not exclusive to the SARS-CoV-2/2019-nCoV virus responsible for the COVID-19 pandemic, it was used only as an interim code until U07.1 was effective. Do not use B97.29 to indicate COVID-19 infections.

5 **B97.3 Retrovirus as the cause of diseases classified elsewhere**

EXCLUDES 1 Human immunodeficiency virus [HIV] disease (B20)

IQ **B97.30 Unspecified retrovirus as the cause of diseases classified elsewhere**

IQ **B97.31 Lentivirus as the cause of diseases classified elsewhere**

IQ **B97.32 Oncovirus as the cause of diseases classified elsewhere**

IQ **B97.33 Human T-cell lymphotrophic virus, type I [HTLV-I] as the cause of diseases classified elsewhere**

IQ **B97.34 Human T-cell lymphotrophic virus, type II [HTLV-II] as the cause of diseases classified elsewhere**

IQ **B97.35 Human immunodeficiency virus, type 2 [HIV 2] as the cause of diseases classified elsewhere**

IQ **B97.39 Other retrovirus as the cause of diseases classified elsewhere**

▲ M IQ **B97.4 *Respiratory syncytial virus as the cause of diseases classified elsewhere***

RSV as the cause of diseases classified elsewhere

Code first related disorders, such as:
- otitis media (H65.-)
- upper respiratory infection (J06.9)

EXCLUDES 1 acute bronchiolitis due to respiratory syncytial virus (RSV) (J21.0)
acute bronchitis due to respiratory syncytial virus (RSV) (J20.5)
respiratory syncytial virus (RSV) pneumonia (J12.1)

IQ **B97.5 Reovirus as the cause of diseases classified elsewhere**

IQ **B97.6 Parvovirus as the cause of diseases classified elsewhere**

IQ **B97.7 Papillomavirus as the cause of diseases classified elsewhere**

5 **B97.8 Other viral agents as the cause of diseases classified elsewhere**

IQ **B97.81 Human metapneumovirus as the cause of diseases classified elsewhere**

IQ **B97.89 Other viral agents as the cause of diseases classified elsewhere**

Other infectious diseases (B99)

4 **B99 Other and unspecified infectious diseases**

CODING TIPS✓ Do not use to indicate an unknown bacteria causing a localized infection. If the bacteria is unknown, there is no need to add a code for the bacteria.

IQ **B99.8 Other infectious disease**

IQ **B99.9 Unspecified infectious disease**

Chapter 1 Scenarios: Certain infectious and parasitic diseases (A00-B99)

Recurrent pneumonia, HIV status

A 65-year-old man is admitted to home health for treatment with intravenous antibiotics for streptococcus pneumoniae pneumonia, which his medical record states is a recurrent diagnosis. His record also indicates that he is HIV positive, lives alone and has very little support, which prompted his physician to order medical social worker services.

Description	Code
Primary: Pneumonia due to Streptococcus pneumoniae	J13
Secondary: Encounter for adjustment and management of vascular access device	Z45.2
Secondary: Asymptomatic human immunodeficiency virus [HIV] infection status	Z21
Secondary: Problems related to living alone	Z60.2
Secondary: Personal history of pneumonia (recurrent)	Z87.01
Secondary: Long term (current) use of antibiotics	Z79.2

The type of pneumonia is specified, prompting the assignment of the specific pneumonia code J13. Though the patient has streptococcus pneumoniae pneumonia that is stated as recurrent and is also HIV positive, Z21 must be assigned to capture the patient's HIV status, not B20 (Human immunodeficiency virus [HIV] disease. Neither streptococcus pneumoniae pneumonia nor the recurrent pneumonia can be assumed to be HIV-related illness, which must be diagnosed by the physician in order to use B20, according to Q1 2019 Coding Clinic guidance. Code Z45.2 can be reported as the principal diagnosis or the first reported secondary diagnosis to be assigned to the Complex Nursing Interventions group in PDGM, according to CMS. The reasoning for looking at the first secondary diagnosis for Z45.2 was to ensure that the complexity of services inherent with a patient who has an IV or is receiving IV therapy was captured for the clinical group assignment under the PDGM in the event that the primary reason for home health services is for IV therapy or management of a patient with an IV line. That will not change in this current grouper even though this is not in accordance with the current coding guidance, according to CMS in an email dated 2/19/20. Additional status codes are assigned to capture that the patient lives alone (Z60.2) and has a history of recurrent pneumonia (Z87.01). The long-term use of IV antibiotics is captured with Z79.2 Note that coding guidelines allow for the assignment of codes between the categories of Z55 and Z65 based on a clinician's documentation.

Streptococcal sepsis, COVID-19

A patient is admitted following hospitalization for streptococcal sepsis with organ dysfunction due to pneumonia (streptococcal), noted to have developed following COVID-19 infection with associated viral pneumonia. Acute renal failure with tubular necrosis, type 1 diabetes mellitus, and chronic kidney disease stage 2 is documented by the provider. The patient will continue oral antibiotics for two weeks.

Description	Code
Primary: Streptococcal sepsis, unspecified	A40.9
Secondary: COVID-19	U07.1
Secondary: Pneumonia due to coronavirus disease 2019	J12.82
Secondary: Pneumonia due to other streptococci	J15.4
Secondary: Severe sepsis without septic shock	R65.20
Secondary: Acute kidney failure with tubular necrosis	N17.0
Secondary: Type 1 diabetes mellitus with diabetic chronic kidney disease	E10.22
Secondary: Chronic kidney disease, stage 2 (mild)	N18.2

This patient experienced a COVID-19 infection that led to sepsis. While the focus of this patient's episode is the infection, coding guidelines for the coding of COVID-19 infections are clear that guidelines for coding sepsis must still be followed and these guidelines require that the code for the systemic infection be listed first, which is streptococcal sepsis. Guidelines for coding of positive COVID-19 cases state that pneumonia associated with COVID-19 is coded to J12.82 and should follow the U07.1 code. This patient also developed complicating streptococcal pneumonia due to COVID-19, so this is listed following the J12.82 code. Guidelines for coding of severe sepsis require that any associated organ failure must be stated by the provider and the code should follow the appropriate R65.2- code. Type 1 diabetics generally use insulin, but do not assign an additional code for insulin use in type 1 diabetics.

Cellulitis with E. coli

A 73-year-old woman comes to home health with a primary diagnosis of cellulitis on her groin that is infected with E.coli and is being treated with oral antibiotics. She also has diabetes and hypertension.

Description	Code
Primary: Cellulitis of groin	L03.314
Secondary: Unspecified Escherichia coli [E. coli] as the cause of diseases classified elsewhere	B96.20
Secondary: Type 2 diabetes mellitus without complications	E11.9
Secondary: Essential (primary) hypertension	I10

E. coli bacteria is the cause of the cellulitis in the patient's groin, which is classified to Chapter 12 (Diseases of Skin and Subcutaneous Tissue). Therefore, the appropriate code to capture the infecting E. coli organism is B96.20. Code B96.20 is sequenced after the disease that it is causing, the cellulitis, in accordance with coding guidelines. As important comorbidities, her diabetes and hypertension are also coded.

Septic shock due to MSSA

A 72-year-old man was admitted to the hospital with acute renal failure due to septic shock, due to Methicillin susceptible Staphylococcus aureus (MSSA). The patient's renal failure is improving, and he was discharged to home health for observation and assessment of the renal condition until the physician determines it has resolved. He received two weeks of IV antibiotics in the hospital to treat the infection, and the home health nurse will administer the remainder of the 8-week course.

Description	Code
Primary: Sepsis due to Methicillin susceptible Staphylococcus aureus	A41.01
Secondary: Severe sepsis with septic shock	R65.21
Secondary: Acute kidney failure, unspecified	N17.9
Secondary: Encounter for adjustment and management of vascular access device	Z45.2
Secondary: Long term (current) use of antibiotics	Z79.2

A single combination code (R65.21) captures both severe sepsis and septic shock. Tabular instruction at R65.21 tells the coder to code first the underlying infection, which is MSSA sepsis in this case. The code for the still-resolving acute renal failure is assigning additionally, in accordance with tabular instruction. Code Z45.2 is assigned for the administration of the IV antibiotics. If the IV is not the primary reason the patient requires home health care, but where there may be some sort of intervention noted on the home health plan of care, then it would be appropriate to report Z45.2 (but not as the principal or first secondary diagnosis), according to CMS.

HIV, cryptosporidiosis

A patient is admitted with an AIDS-related infection specified as Cryptosporidiosis. His symptoms include dehydration and diarrhea.

Description	Code
Primary: HIV	B20
Secondary: Other protozoal intestinal diseases, cryptosporidiosis	A07.2

Cryptosporidiosis is an infection of the small intestine caused by a protozoal organism and is frequently a complication of HIV and AIDS. The ICD-10 guidelines state that if a patient is admitted for an HIV-related condition, the principal diagnosis should be B20, Human immunodeficiency virus (HIV) disease, followed by additional codes for all reported HIV-related conditions. Note that the Coding Clinic issued guidance on the coding of HIV-related illnesses in its Q1 2019 update, saying that B20 should be assigned only when there is a documented diagnosis of AIDS or the patient's illness is documented as related to or resulting from HIV, and that for patients described as "HIV positive" or having known HIV but no HIV-related illnesses, the correct code is Z21 (Asymptomatic human immunodeficiency virus [HIV] infection status. The patient's symptoms of dehydration and diarrhea are not coded additionally as they are integral to the Cryptosporidiosis infection. Note that many states prohibit reporting HIV as a primary diagnosis or reporting it at all. Check with your state's OASIS coordinator to determine the appropriate sequencing of an HIV diagnosis, based on your state's regulations. If prohibited, report the associated condition(s).

Infected abdominal surgical wound, IV antibiotics

A 72-year-old woman recently underwent surgery to remove cancer in her sigmoid colon. The surgery completely eradicated the cancer but the surgical wound developed an intramuscular abscess that's infected with E. coli and the patient was admitted to home health to continue treatment with a wound VAC and IV antibiotics for six weeks. The patient is morbidly obese with a BMI of 35.

Description	Code
Primary: Infection following a procedure, deep incisional surgical site, initial encounter	T81.42xA
Secondary: Unspecified Escherichia coli [E. coli] as the cause of diseases classified elsewhere	B96.20
Secondary: Encounter for adjustment and management of vascular access device	Z45.2
Secondary: Morbid (severe) obesity due to excess calories	E66.01
Secondary: Body mass index (BMI) 35.0-35.9, adult	Z68.35
Secondary: Long term (current) use of antibiotics	Z79.2
Secondary: Personal history of other malignant neoplasm of large intestine	Z85.038

The surgical wound is complicated by an intramuscular abscess, which equates to a deep incisional surgical site, and is appropriately coded to T81.42-, according to the inclusion terms on the code. Because the patient is still undergoing active treatment for the infection, with IV antibiotics and a wound VAC, it is considered active care and thus should take the seventh character "A," according to the Coding Clinic. The infecting organism E. coli is specified and thus is coded following the infection code, in accordance with tabular instruction. Morbid obesity should always be coded when it's documented, according to Q4 2018 Coding Clinic guidance. Therefore, it is coded along with the specified BMI, in accordance with tabular instruction. The patient is receiving IV antibiotic therapy for six weeks and is thus at risk for complications, making the use of Z45.2 and Z79.2 necessary. If the IV is not the primary reason the patient requires home health care, but where there may be some sort of intervention noted on the home health plan of care, then it would be appropriate to report Z45.2 (but not as the principal or first secondary diagnosis), according to CMS. The patient's cancer was said to be eradicated through surgery and thus the personal history code (Z85.038) is assigned, versus a current neoplasm code.

Recurrent Clostridium difficile

A 79-year-old woman was recently hospitalized for severe colitis due to recurrent Clostridium difficile. During her hospitalization she experienced severe diarrhea and acute kidney failure. The kidney failure resolved prior to discharge but the infection is still resolving and she is still experiencing mild to moderate diarrhea. She has comorbidities of chronic diastolic heart failure and hypertension. Following her discharge, she is admitted to home health to continue her recovery. Skilled nursing will provide instruction to her caregiver on the disease process and management of new medications.

Description	Code
Primary: Enterocolitis due to Clostridium difficile, recurrent	A04.71
Secondary: Hypertensive heart disease with heart failure	I11.0
Secondary: Chronic diastolic (congestive) heart failure	I50.32

With the colitis due to Clostridium difficile infection still resolving and the focus of care, it is appropriately coded in the primary position. Since it's noted as recurrent, A04.71 is assigned. Her moderate diarrhea is not coded as it is inherent to the Clostridium difficile infection. There is an assumed relationship between hypertension and heart failure in the ICD-10 classification, unless the physician says they're unrelated to each other. Therefore, the diagnoses are coded as connected with I11.0 and I50.32.

DVT, Sequela of COVID-19

The agency has admitted a 72-year-old male patient who has developed a chronic DVT to the right femoral vein secondary to COVID-19 infection and requires observation, assessment, regarding education related to the condition and use of Xarelto anticoagulant. Physician documentation indicates that the patient's COVID-19 infection has resolved, and patient has chronic atrial fibrillation.

Description	Code
Primary: Chronic embolism and thrombosis of right femoral vein	I82.511
Secondary: Sequelae of other specified infectious and parasitic diseases	B94.8
Secondary: Chronic atrial fibrillation, unspecified	I48.20
Secondary: Long term (current) use of anticoagulants	Z79.01

The physician has specified that this patient's DVT is a sequela of COVID-19, so conventions for coding sequela(e) must be followed, which includes first coding the residual conditions, followed by the code to identify the cause as sequela(e). In this case the DVT of the right femoral is identified as chronic, so the sub-term "chronic" is chosen when searching in the alpha index, leading to I82.511. Guidance from Q3 2021 Coding Clinic, as well as the Centers for Disease Control (CDC) and CMS has indicated to assign B94.8 to indicate conditions as sequela(e) of COVID-19 disease. The atrial fibrillation places the patient at risk for further thrombosis and should be additionally coded, along with Z79.01 to identify the use of the anticoagulant medication.

[illegible]

[illegible]

[illegible]	[illegible]
[illegible]	[illegible]
[illegible]	[illegible]
[illegible]	[illegible]
[illegible]	[illegible]

[illegible]

Chapter 2: Neoplasms (C00- D49)

"Neoplasm" refers to any new, abnormal growth of tissue. The words tumor, fibroid, hyperplasia, mass, or adenoma indicate a neoplasm. However, if documentation states 'mass,' go to 'mass' in the Alphabetic Index. All malignant and most benign neoplasms are classified in this chapter by site (topography) with broad groupings for behavior (malignant, in situ, benign), whether they are functionally active or not. In a few cases, such as malignant melanoma and certain neuroendocrine tumors, the morphology (histologic type) is included in the category and codes. An additional code from Chapter 4, Endocrine, nutritional and metablic diseases, may be used to identify functional activity associated with any neoplasm.

Code selection in this chapter depends on the physician's description of the neoplasm. If there is not enough information to select a code, query the physician.

Types of neoplasms:

- **Malignant neoplasms** (cancers) (C00-C75) grow uncontrollably and may invade healthy surrounding tissues or spread (metastasize) from the point of origin.
- **A primary malignancy** is the area where the tumor first developed in the body.
- **A secondary malignancy** (metastasis) is an area of the body where the first- listed cancer has metastasized.
- **Benign neoplasms** (noncancerous) (D10-D36) do not invade surrounding tissues or metastasize.
- **Carcinoma in situ** (CIS or ca in situ) (D00-D09) is an early form of carcinoma defined by the non-invasion of surrounding tissues. In other words, the neoplastic cells proliferate in their normal habitat, hence the name 'in situ' (Latin for 'in its place'). CIS is considered a precursor or incipient form of cancer that if left untreated long enough may transform into a malignant neoplasm.
- **Uncertain behavior** (D37-D48) describes a neoplasm that is exhibiting characteristics of both malignant and benign neoplasms. Further study is needed to determine the type of neoplasm.
- **Unspecified behavior** (D49) describes a neoplasm when there is not enough information to select the type of neoplasm. This may occur when the physician is waiting for a pathology report before deciding on the nature of the neoplasm. Ask the physician for more information, if possible. Do not code unspecified behavior just because it is unknown whether a cancer is primary or secondary. It is important to code cancers to malignant neoplasms when appropriate.

If the medical record states "**metastatic to**," this refers to the secondary site. The primary neoplasm is metastatic to the secondary site.

If the medical record states "**metastatic from**," this refers to the primary site. A secondary site is metastatic from the primary site.

If the medical record states "**contiguous sites**," this refers to primary neoplasms with overlapping boundaries in which the point of origin (primary site) cannot be determined. Therefore, contiguous sites should be classified to fourth character of 8 (overlapping lesion), unless a combination code is specifically indexed elsewhere. For example, a cancer may involve the skin of cheek and nose, but the physician has not documented which neoplasm is primary. In this case, report C44.80 (unspecified malignant neoplasm of overlapping sites of skin).

For multiple neoplasms of the same site that are not contiguous, such as tumors in different quadrants of the same breast, codes for each site should be assigned.

There are some situations in which a code from Chapter 2 is not the most appropriate. Below are a few situations to watch out for:

- If a patient has a **personal or family history of a condition** reported in this chapter, it may be more appropriate to select from the Z code section, such as Z85.- (personal history of malignant neoplasms), or Z80.9 (family history of malignant neoplasm). Remember that personal history codes are used more often in home health than family history codes.
- **Nonspecific neoplasms** are sometimes reported using codes from other chapters. If the documentation uses words such as "mass," "swelling," or "lump," but offers no definitive diagnosis, refer to that word in the Alphabetic Index in order to find the correct code.

  For example, a breast mass or lump is reported using code N63 from Chapter 14, Diseases of the genitourinary system. An abdominal mass is reported using code R19.00 from Chapter18, Symptoms, signs and abnormal clinical and laboratory findings, not elsewhere classified. Coders should attempt to obtain more specific information before coding lumps or masses as well as the specific location of the mass or lump.
- Although it is not found often in home health, when a **pregnant woman has a malignant**

neoplasm, a code from subcategory O9A.1-, Malignant neoplasm complicating pregnancy, childbirth, and the puerperium, should be sequenced first, followed by the appropriate code from Chapter 2 to indicate the type of neoplasm.

Neoplasms & the alphabetic index

The Alphabetic Index includes a **Neoplasm Table** that can be used to select the correct code. In the left hand column of the table is a list of locations within the body. In the other columns are codes for the types of neoplasms (malignant, benign, uncertain behavior) in that body area. However, **coders should not go directly to the Neoplasm Table unless the only documentation is something like 'lung cancer.'** If the histological term is present in the medical record, first look up the histological term in the alphabetic index. The index will refer you to the table when appropriate.

Consider the following examples of how to use the Index to find a neoplasm code:

- If the documentation states "hyperplasia, adrenal cortex," the Index refers you to E27.8 (other specified disorders of adrenal glands). The Neoplasm Table is not referenced.
- If the documentation states "dysplasia, high grade, focal," of the colon, the Index refers the coder to D12.6, Benign neoplasm of colon, unspecified.

When using the Neoplasm Table, first find the body site, and then refer to the column for malignant, benign, uncertain behavior, or unspecified codes as appropriate. If the neoplasm is malignant, determine whether it is primary, secondary, or cancer in situ. Be sure to refer to the code in the Tabular List to ensure the listed code is correct; do not code using only the Neoplasm Table. If the site is unknown, refer to Neoplasm, unknown site or unspecified, in the Table. There are specific codes for unknown primary malignant, secondary malignant, Ca in situ, benign, uncertain and unspecified behaviors.

Some codes in the Neoplasm Table are grouped under the heading "connective tissue." This includes tissues such as blood vessels, bursa, fascia, ligaments, muscle, peripheral nerves and tendons in a specific body area. Neoplasms of connective tissue have a separate category (C49.-). For example, malignant neoplasm of the abdominal cavity is listed as C76.2 (malignant neoplasm, abdomen). Malignant neoplasm of connective tissue of the abdomen is listed as C49.4 (malignant neoplasm of connective, and other soft tissue, abdomen).

Multiple Coding and Sequencing

It is important to read the Includes and Excludes notes under codes in this chapter, as well as any other instructions under the code or code category. There are many multiple coding and sequencing issues for codes in this chapter.

Important note: Just because a neoplasm is listed as a primary cancer does not mean it should be reported as the primary diagnosis. Sequencing of codes depends on which neoplasm site is the focus of care for that specific episode. If the primary site of the cancer is still present, it is ***usually*** sequenced prior to the secondary site. If the focus of care is the secondary site, the secondary site is listed as the primary diagnosis even though the primary malignancy is still present and the primary site is coded as an additional code.

If a primary site is considered eradicated and there is no further treatment directed to that site and no evidence of any existing primary malignancy, use the appropriate Z85 code for personal history of the primary malignant neoplasm.

If the primary or secondary site is unknown, use C80.1 (primary malignant site unknown) or C79.9 (secondary site is unknown).

If no determination of known primary or secondary sites of malignancy for advanced cancer can be made, use code C80.0, Disseminated malignant neoplasm, unspecified.

Special Coding Issues

Postoperative Treatment

A neoplasm is still considered present if the patient is receiving treatment. That is, if the neoplasm has been excised but the patient is still receiving chemotherapy or radiotherapy, report a code for the cancer, not a Z85 code (personal history of malignant neoplasm).

When the admission/encounter is for a complication resulting from a surgical procedure, designate the complication as the principal or first listed diagnosis if treatment is directed at resolving the complication.

If the neoplasm has been excised, and there is no complication, the code for aftercare following surgery for a neoplasm, Z48.3, is used. This will be followed by the code for the neoplasm if it is unknown that the neoplasm is fully eradicated, or if the neoplasm is still receiving treatment. If the neoplasm is known to be fully eradicated by the surgery, and only routine post-surgical aftercare is needed, then the personal history code is used.

Coding and sequencing of complications

When admission/encounter is for **management of anemia associated with the malignancy,** and the treatment is only for the anemia, the appropriate code for the malignancy is sequenced as the principal or first-listed diagnosis followed by the appropriate code for the anemia (such as code D63.0, Anemia in neoplastic disease).

When the admission/encounter is for management of an anemia associated with an adverse effect of the administration of chemotherapy, immunotherapy or radiation and the only treatment is for the anemia, the anemia code is sequenced first.

When the admission/encounter is for the management of dehydration due to the malignancy and only the dehydration is being treated (intravenous hydration), the dehydration is sequenced first, followed by the code(s) for the malignancy.

Pathological fracture due to a neoplasm

When an encounter is for a pathological fracture due to a neoplasm, and the focus of treatment is the fracture, a code from subcategory M84.5, Pathological fracture in neoplastic disease, should be sequenced first, followed by the code for the neoplasm from Chapter 2.

If the focus of care is the neoplasm with an associated pathological fracture, the neoplasm code should be sequenced first, followed by a code from M84.5 for the pathological fracture.

Patients with long-term use of agents affecting estrogen receptors and estrogen levels

Codes revolving around long-term use of agents affecting estrogen receptors and estrogen levels, such as SERMS, aromatase inhibitors and other agents, are found in the Z79.81- subcategory. The use of long-term prophylactic agents to prevent recurrence of disease raises questions as to when treatment is actually complete. Instructions at the Z79.81 subcategory include: 'Code first, if applicable': malignant neoplasm of breast (C50-) or malignant neoplasm of prostate (C61) and 'Use additional code, if applicable, to identify': estrogen receptor positive status (Z17.0); family history of breast cancer (Z80.3); genetic susceptibility to cancer (Z15.0-); personal history of breast cancer (Z85.3); personal history of prostate cancer (Z85.46) and/or postmenopausal status (Z78.0).

Admissions/Encounters involving chemotherapy, immunotherapy or radiation therapy

If a patient's admission/encounter is solely for the administration of chemotherapy, immunotherapy or radiation therapy, assign a code from Z51.- as the first listed or principal diagnosis. The malignancy for which the therapy is being administered should be assigned as a secondary diagnosis.

Malignant neoplasm associated with a transplanted organ

The incidence of cancer in transplanted organs has increased. A malignant neoplasm of a transplanted organ should be coded as a transplant complication. Assign first the appropriate code from category T86.-. Complications of transplanted organs and tissue, followed by code C80.2, Malignant neoplasm associated with transplanted organ. Use an additional code for the specific malignancy.

Leukemia, multiple myeloma and malignant plasma cell neoplasm

The categories for leukemia and category C90, Multiple myeloma and malignant plasma cell neoplasms, have codes indicating whether or not the leukemia has achieved remission. There are also codes Z85.6, Personal history of leukemia, and Z85.79, Personal history of lymphoid, hematopoietic and related tissues. If the documentation is unclear as to whether the leukemia has achieved remission, the provider should be queried.

CHAPTER 2: NEOPLASMS (C00-D49)

Note:
Functional activity
All neoplasms are classified in this chapter, whether they are functionally active or not. An additional code from Chapter 4 may be used, to identify functional activity associated with any neoplasm.
Morphology [Histology]
Chapter 2 classifies neoplasms primarily by site (topography), with broad groupings for behavior, malignant, in situ, benign, etc. The Table of Neoplasms should be used to identify the correct topography code. In a few cases, such as for malignant melanoma and certain neuroendocrine tumors, the morphology (histologic type) is included in the category and codes.
Primary malignant neoplasms overlapping site boundaries
A primary malignant neoplasm that overlaps two or more contiguous (next to each other) sites should be classified to the subcategory/code .8 ('overlapping lesion'), unless the combination is specifically indexed elsewhere. For multiple neoplasms of the same site that are not contiguous, such as tumors in different quadrants of the same breast, codes for each site should be assigned.
Malignant neoplasm of ectopic tissue
Malignant neoplasms of ectopic tissue are to be coded to the site mentioned, e.g., ectopic pancreatic malignant neoplasms are coded to pancreas, unspecified (C25.9).

GUIDELINES **Section I.C.2**
Chapter 2 of the ICD-10-CM contains the codes for most benign and all malignant neoplasms. Certain benign neoplasms, such as prostatic adenomas, may be found in the specific body system chapters. To properly code a neoplasm it is necessary to determine from the record if the neoplasm is benign, in-situ, malignant, or of uncertain histologic behavior. If malignant, any secondary (metastatic) sites should also be determined.

GUIDELINES **Section I.C.2**
The neoplasm table in the Alphabetic Index should be referenced first. However, if the histological term is documented, that term should be referenced first, rather than going immediately to the Neoplasm Table, in order to determine which column in the Neoplasm Table is appropriate. For example, if the documentation indicates "adenoma," refer to the term in the Alphabetic Index to review the entries under this term and the instructional note to "see also neoplasm, by site, benign." The table provides the proper code based on the type of neoplasm and the site.

This chapter contains the following blocks:

C00-C14	Malignant neoplasms of lip, oral cavity and pharynx
C15-C26	Malignant neoplasms of digestive organs
C30-C39	Malignant neoplasms of respiratory and intrathoracic organs
C40-C41	Malignant neoplasms of bone and articular cartilage
C43-C44	Melanoma and other malignant neoplasms of skin
C45-C49	Malignant neoplasms of mesothelial and soft tissue
C50	Malignant neoplasms of breast
C51-C58	Malignant neoplasms of female genital organs
C60-C63	Malignant neoplasms of male genital organs
C64-C68	Malignant neoplasms of urinary tract
C69-C72	Malignant neoplasms of eye, brain and other parts of central nervous system
C73-C75	Malignant neoplasms of thyroid and other endocrine glands
C7A	Malignant neuroendocrine tumors
C7B	Secondary neuroendocrine tumors
C76-C80	Malignant neoplasms of ill-defined, other secondary and unspecified sites
C81-C96	Malignant neoplasms of lymphoid, hematopoietic and related tissue
D00-D09	In situ neoplasms
D10-D36	Benign neoplasms, except benign neuroendocrine tumors
D3A	Benign neuroendocrine tumors
D37-D48	Neoplasms of uncertain behavior, polycythemia vera and myelodysplastic syndromes
D49	Neoplasms of unspecified behavior

Malignant neoplasms (C00-C96)

Malignant neoplasms, stated or presumed to be primary (of specified sites), and certain specified histologies, except neuroendocrine, and of lymphoid, hematopoietic and related tissue (C00-C75)

Malignant neoplasms of lip, oral cavity and pharynx (C00-C14)

CODING TIPS✓ Codes classifiable to C00-C14 include active cancer. History of cancer to the lip, pharynx, or oral cavity should be coded to Z85.81-.

+ 4 **C00 Malignant neoplasm of lip**
Use additional code to identify:
alcohol abuse and dependence (F10.-)
history of tobacco dependence (Z87.891)
tobacco dependence (F17.-)
tobacco use (Z72.0)

EXCLUDES 1 malignant melanoma of lip (C43.0)
Merkel cell carcinoma of lip (C4A.0)
other and unspecified malignant neoplasm of skin of lip (C44.0-)

CODING TIPS✓ C00 indicates active cancer. See Z85.818 for personal history of primary malignancy of lip, oral cavity and pharynx.

CODING TIPS✓ Area on lip must be specified in documentation to choose an acceptable code.

SP SL + **C00.0 Malignant neoplasm of external upper lip**
Malignant neoplasm of lipstick area of upper lip
Malignant neoplasm of upper lip NOS
Malignant neoplasm of vermilion border of upper lip

SP SL + **C00.1 Malignant neoplasm of external lower lip**
Malignant neoplasm of lower lip NOS
Malignant neoplasm of lipstick area of lower lip
Malignant neoplasm of vermilion border of lower lip

!Q + **C00.2 Malignant neoplasm of external lip, unspecified**
Malignant neoplasm of vermilion border of lip NOS

SP SL + **C00.3 Malignant neoplasm of upper lip, inner aspect**

Malignant neoplasm of buccal aspect of upper lip
Malignant neoplasm of frenulum of upper lip
Malignant neoplasm of mucosa of upper lip
Malignant neoplasm of oral aspect of upper lip

SP SL + C00.4 **Malignant neoplasm of lower lip, inner aspect**
Malignant neoplasm of buccal aspect of lower lip
Malignant neoplasm of frenulum of lower lip
Malignant neoplasm of mucosa of lower lip
Malignant neoplasm of oral aspect of lower lip

IQ + C00.5 **Malignant neoplasm of lip, unspecified, inner aspect**
Malignant neoplasm of buccal aspect of lip, unspecified
Malignant neoplasm of frenulum of lip, unspecified
Malignant neoplasm of mucosa of lip, unspecified
Malignant neoplasm of oral aspect of lip, unspecified

SP + C00.6 **Malignant neoplasm of commissure of lip, unspecified**

SP SL + C00.8 **Malignant neoplasm of overlapping sites of lip**

IQ + C00.9 **Malignant neoplasm of lip, unspecified**

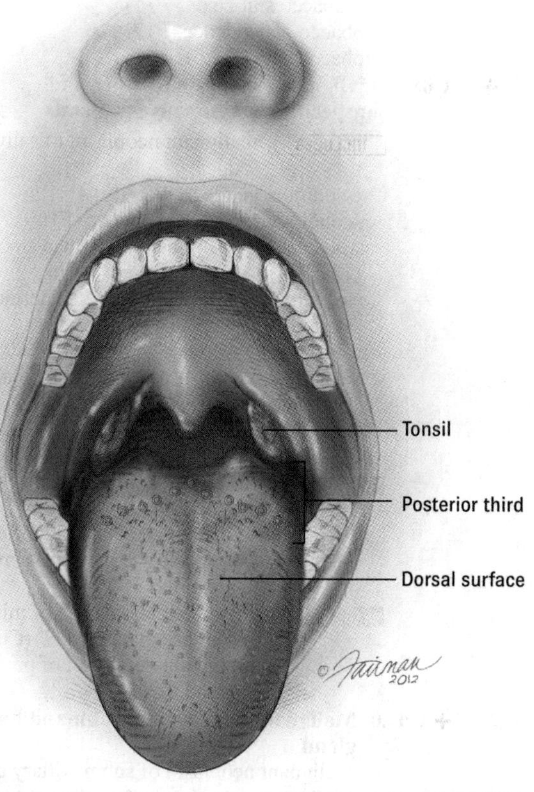

SP SL + C01 **Malignant neoplasm of base of tongue**
Malignant neoplasm of dorsal surface of base of tongue
Malignant neoplasm of fixed part of tongue NOS
Malignant neoplasm of posterior third of tongue
Use additional code to identify:
alcohol abuse and dependence (F10.-)
history of tobacco dependence (Z87.891)
tobacco dependence (F17.-)
tobacco use (Z72.0)

CODING TIPS✓ C01 codes indicate active cancer. See Z85.810 for personal history of primary malignancy of tongue and Z85.818 for tonsils.

+ 4 C02 **Malignant neoplasm of other and unspecified parts of tongue**
Use additional code to identify:
alcohol abuse and dependence (F10.-)
history of tobacco dependence (Z87.891)
tobacco dependence (F17.-)
tobacco use (Z72.0)

CODING TIPS✓ C02 codes indicate active cancer. See Z85.810 for personal history of primary malignancy of tongue and Z85.818 for tonsils.

CODING TIPS✓ Upper or lower gum must be specified in documentation to choose an acceptable code.

SP SL + C02.0 **Malignant neoplasm of dorsal surface of tongue**
Malignant neoplasm of anterior two-thirds of tongue, dorsal surface
EXCLUDES 2 malignant neoplasm of dorsal surface of base of tongue (C01)

SP SL + C02.1 **Malignant neoplasm of border of tongue**
Malignant neoplasm of tip of tongue

SP SL + C02.2 **Malignant neoplasm of ventral surface of tongue**
Malignant neoplasm of anterior two-thirds of tongue, ventral surface
Malignant neoplasm of frenulum linguae

SP SL + C02.3 **Malignant neoplasm of anterior two-thirds of tongue, part unspecified**
Malignant neoplasm of middle third of tongue NOS
Malignant neoplasm of mobile part of tongue NOS

SP SL + C02.4 **Malignant neoplasm of lingual tonsil**
EXCLUDES 2 malignant neoplasm of tonsil NOS (C09.9)

SP SL + C02.8 **Malignant neoplasm of overlapping sites of tongue**
Malignant neoplasm of two or more contiguous sites of tongue

SP SL + C02.9 **Malignant neoplasm of tongue, unspecified**

+ 4 C03 **Malignant neoplasm of gum**
INCLUDES malignant neoplasm of alveolar (ridge) mucosa
malignant neoplasm of gingiva
Use additional code to identify:
alcohol abuse and dependence (F10.-)
history of tobacco dependence (Z87.891)
tobacco dependence (F17.-)
tobacco use (Z72.0)
EXCLUDES 2 malignant odontogenic neoplasms (C41.0-C41.1)

CODING TIPS✓ This category indicates active cancer. See Z85.818 for personal history of primary malignancy of lip, oral cavity and pharynx.

SP + C03.0 **Malignant neoplasm of upper gum**

SP SL + C03.1 **Malignant neoplasm of lower gum**

IQ + C03.9 **Malignant neoplasm of gum, unspecified**

+ 4 C04 **Malignant neoplasm of floor of mouth**
Use additional code to identify:
alcohol abuse and dependence (F10.-)
history of tobacco dependence (Z87.891)
tobacco dependence (F17.-)
tobacco use (Z72.0)

CODING TIPS✓ This category indicates active cancer. See Z85.818 for personal history of primary malignancy of lip, oral cavity and pharynx.

SP SL + C04.0 **Malignant neoplasm of anterior floor of mouth**
Malignant neoplasm of anterior to the premolar-canine junction

SP SL + C04.1 **Malignant neoplasm of lateral floor of mouth**

SP SL + C04.8 **Malignant neoplasm of overlapping sites of floor of mouth**

SP SL + C04.9 **Malignant neoplasm of floor of mouth, unspecified**

+ 4 C05 **Malignant neoplasm of palate**
Use additional code to identify:
alcohol abuse and dependence (F10.-)
history of tobacco dependence (Z87.891)
tobacco dependence (F17.-)
tobacco use (Z72.0)

EXCLUDES 1 Kaposi's sarcoma of palate (C46.2)

CODING TIPS✓ This category indicates active cancer. See Z85.818 for personal history of primary malignancy of lip, oral cavity and pharynx.

SP SL + C05.0 **Malignant neoplasm of hard palate**

SP SL + C05.1 **Malignant neoplasm of soft palate**
EXCLUDES 2 malignant neoplasm of nasopharyngeal surface of soft palate (C11.3)

SP SL + C05.2 **Malignant neoplasm of uvula**

SP SL + C05.8 **Malignant neoplasm of overlapping sites of palate**

SP SL + C05.9 **Malignant neoplasm of palate, unspecified**
Malignant neoplasm of roof of mouth

+ 4 C06 **Malignant neoplasm of other and unspecified parts of mouth**
Use additional code to identify:
alcohol abuse and dependence (F10.-)
history of tobacco dependence (Z87.891)
tobacco dependence (F17.-)
tobacco use (Z72.0)

CODING TIPS✓ This category indicates active cancer. See Z85.818 for personal history of primary malignancy of lip, oral cavity and pharynx.

CODING TIPS✓ Area in mouth should be specified in documentation to choose an acceptable code.

SP SL + C06.0 **Malignant neoplasm of cheek mucosa**
Malignant neoplasm of buccal mucosa NOS
Malignant neoplasm of internal cheek

SP SL + C06.1 **Malignant neoplasm of vestibule of mouth**
Malignant neoplasm of buccal sulcus (upper) (lower)
Malignant neoplasm of labial sulcus (upper) (lower)

SP SL + C06.2 **Malignant neoplasm of retromolar area**

+ 5 C06.8 **Malignant neoplasm of overlapping sites of other and unspecified parts of mouth**

SP SL + C06.80 **Malignant neoplasm of overlapping sites of unspecified parts of mouth**

SP SL + C06.89 **Malignant neoplasm of overlapping sites of other parts of mouth**
'book leaf' neoplasm [ventral surface of tongue and floor of mouth]

IQ SL + C06.9 **Malignant neoplasm of mouth, unspecified**
Malignant neoplasm of minor salivary gland, unspecified site
Malignant neoplasm of oral cavity NOS

SP SL + C07 **Malignant neoplasm of parotid gland**
Use additional code to identify:
alcohol abuse and dependence (F10.-)
exposure to environmental tobacco smoke (Z77.22)
exposure to tobacco smoke in the perinatal period (P96.81)
history of tobacco dependence (Z87.891)
occupational exposure to environmental tobacco smoke (Z57.31)
tobacco dependence (F17.-)
tobacco use (Z72.0)

+ 4 C08 **Malignant neoplasm of other and unspecified major salivary glands**
INCLUDES malignant neoplasm of salivary ducts
Use additional code to identify:
alcohol abuse and dependence (F10.-)
exposure to environmental tobacco smoke (Z77.22)
exposure to tobacco smoke in the perinatal period (P96.81)
history of tobacco dependence (Z87.891)
occupational exposure to environmental tobacco smoke (Z57.31)
tobacco dependence (F17.-)
tobacco use (Z72.0)

EXCLUDES 1 malignant neoplasms of specified minor salivary glands which are classified according to their anatomical location

EXCLUDES 2 malignant neoplasms of minor salivary glands NOS (C06.9)
malignant neoplasm of parotid gland (C07)

SP SL + C08.0 **Malignant neoplasm of submandibular gland**
Malignant neoplasm of submaxillary gland

SP SL + C08.1 **Malignant neoplasm of sublingual gland**

IQ SL + C08.9 **Malignant neoplasm of major salivary gland, unspecified**

Malignant neoplasm of salivary gland (major) NOS

+ 4 C09 Malignant neoplasm of tonsil
Use additional code to identify:
alcohol abuse and dependence (F10.-)
exposure to environmental tobacco smoke (Z77.22)
exposure to tobacco smoke in the perinatal period (P96.81)
history of tobacco dependence (Z87.891)
occupational exposure to environmental tobacco smoke (Z57.31)
tobacco dependence (F17.-)
tobacco use (Z72.0)
EXCLUDES 2 malignant neoplasm of lingual tonsil (C02.4)
malignant neoplasm of pharyngeal tonsil (C11.1)

SP SL + C09.0 Malignant neoplasm of tonsillar fossa

SP SL + C09.1 Malignant neoplasm of tonsillar pillar (anterior) (posterior)

SP SL + C09.8 Malignant neoplasm of overlapping sites of tonsil

SP SL + C09.9 Malignant neoplasm of tonsil, unspecified
Malignant neoplasm of tonsil NOS
Malignant neoplasm of faucial tonsils
Malignant neoplasm of palatine tonsils

+ 4 C10 Malignant neoplasm of oropharynx
Use additional code to identify:
alcohol abuse and dependence (F10.-)
exposure to environmental tobacco smoke (Z77.22)
exposure to tobacco smoke in the perinatal period (P96.81)
history of tobacco dependence (Z87.891)
occupational exposure to environmental tobacco smoke (Z57.31)
tobacco dependence (F17.-)
tobacco use (Z72.0)
EXCLUDES 2 malignant neoplasm of tonsil (C09.-)

SP SL + C10.0 Malignant neoplasm of vallecula

SP SL + C10.1 Malignant neoplasm of anterior surface of epiglottis
Malignant neoplasm of epiglottis, free border [margin]
Malignant neoplasm of glossoepiglottic fold(s)
EXCLUDES 2 malignant neoplasm of epiglottis (suprahyoid portion) NOS (C32.1)

SP SL + C10.2 Malignant neoplasm of lateral wall of oropharynx

SP SL + C10.3 Malignant neoplasm of posterior wall of oropharynx

SP SL + C10.4 Malignant neoplasm of branchial cleft
Malignant neoplasm of branchial cyst [site of neoplasm]

SP SL + C10.8 Malignant neoplasm of overlapping sites of oropharynx
Malignant neoplasm of junctional region of oropharynx

SP SL + C10.9 Malignant neoplasm of oropharynx, unspecified

+ 4 C11 Malignant neoplasm of nasopharynx
Use additional code to identify:
exposure to environmental tobacco smoke (Z77.22)
exposure to tobacco smoke in the perinatal period (P96.81)
history of tobacco dependence (Z87.891)
occupational exposure to environmental tobacco smoke (Z57.31)
tobacco dependence (F17.-)
tobacco use (Z72.0)

SP SL + C11.0 Malignant neoplasm of superior wall of nasopharynx
Malignant neoplasm of roof of nasopharynx

SP SL + C11.1 Malignant neoplasm of posterior wall of nasopharynx
Malignant neoplasm of adenoid
Malignant neoplasm of pharyngeal tonsil

SP SL + C11.2 Malignant neoplasm of lateral wall of nasopharynx
Malignant neoplasm of fossa of Rosenmüller
Malignant neoplasm of opening of auditory tube
Malignant neoplasm of pharyngeal recess

SP SL + C11.3 Malignant neoplasm of anterior wall of nasopharynx
Malignant neoplasm of floor of nasopharynx
Malignant neoplasm of nasopharyngeal (anterior) (posterior) surface of soft palate
Malignant neoplasm of posterior margin of nasal choana
Malignant neoplasm of posterior margin of nasal septum

SP SL + C11.8 Malignant neoplasm of overlapping sites of nasopharynx

SP SL + C11.9 Malignant neoplasm of nasopharynx, unspecified
Malignant neoplasm of nasopharyngeal wall NOS

SP SL + C12 Malignant neoplasm of pyriform sinus
Malignant neoplasm of pyriform fossa
Use additional code to identify:
exposure to environmental tobacco smoke (Z77.22)
exposure to tobacco smoke in the perinatal period (P96.81)
history of tobacco dependence (Z87.891)
occupational exposure to environmental tobacco smoke (Z57.31)
tobacco dependence (F17.-)
tobacco use (Z72.0)

+ 4 C13 Malignant neoplasm of hypopharynx
Use additional code to identify:
exposure to environmental tobacco smoke (Z77.22)
exposure to tobacco smoke in the perinatal period (P96.81)
history of tobacco dependence (Z87.891)
occupational exposure to environmental tobacco smoke (Z57.31)
tobacco dependence (F17.-)
tobacco use (Z72.0)
EXCLUDES 2 malignant neoplasm of pyriform sinus (C12)

SP SL + C13.0 Malignant neoplasm of postcricoid region

SP SL + C13.1 **Malignant neoplasm of aryepiglottic fold, hypopharyngeal aspect**
Malignant neoplasm of aryepiglottic fold, marginal zone
Malignant neoplasm of aryepiglottic fold NOS
Malignant neoplasm of interarytenoid fold, marginal zone
Malignant neoplasm of interarytenoid fold NOS
EXCLUDES 2 malignant neoplasm of aryepiglottic fold or interarytenoid fold, laryngeal aspect (C32.1)

SP SL + C13.2 **Malignant neoplasm of posterior wall of hypopharynx**

SP SL + C13.8 **Malignant neoplasm of overlapping sites of hypopharynx**

SP SL + C13.9 **Malignant neoplasm of hypopharynx, unspecified**
Malignant neoplasm of hypopharyngeal wall NOS

+ 4 C14 **Malignant neoplasm of other and ill-defined sites in the lip, oral cavity and pharynx**
Use additional code to identify:
alcohol abuse and dependence (F10.-)
exposure to environmental tobacco smoke (Z77.22)
exposure to tobacco smoke in the perinatal period (P96.81)
history of tobacco dependence (Z87.891)
occupational exposure to environmental tobacco smoke (Z57.31)
tobacco dependence (F17.-)
tobacco use (Z72.0)
EXCLUDES 1 malignant neoplasm of oral cavity NOS (C06.9)

SP SL + C14.0 **Malignant neoplasm of pharynx, unspecified**

SP SL + C14.2 **Malignant neoplasm of Waldeyer's ring**

SP SL + C14.8 **Malignant neoplasm of overlapping sites of lip, oral cavity and pharynx**
Primary malignant neoplasm of two or more contiguous sites of lip, oral cavity and pharynx
EXCLUDES 1 'book leaf' neoplasm [ventral surface of tongue and floor of mouth] (C06.89)

Malignant neoplasms of digestive organs (C15-C26)

EXCLUDES 1 Kaposi's sarcoma of gastrointestinal sites (C46.4)
EXCLUDES 2 gastrointestinal stromal tumors (C49.A-)
CODING TIPS✓ Codes classifiable to C15-C26 include active cancer. History of cancer to digestive organs should be coded to Z85.0-.

+ 4 C15 **Malignant neoplasm of esophagus**
Use additional code to identify:
alcohol abuse and dependence (F10.-)
CODING TIPS✓ This category indicates active cancer. See Z85.01 for personal history of primary malignancy of esophagus.

SP + C15.3 **Malignant neoplasm of upper third of esophagus**

SP + C15.4 **Malignant neoplasm of middle third of esophagus**

SP + C15.5 **Malignant neoplasm of lower third of esophagus**
EXCLUDES 1 malignant neoplasm of cardio-esophageal junction (C16.0)

SP + C15.8 **Malignant neoplasm of overlapping sites of esophagus**

SP + C15.9 **Malignant neoplasm of esophagus, unspecified**

+ 4 C16 **Malignant neoplasm of stomach**
Use additional code to identify:
alcohol abuse and dependence (F10.-)
EXCLUDES 2 malignant carcinoid tumor of the stomach (C7A.092)
CODING TIPS✓ This category indicates active cancer. See Z85.02 for personal history of primary malignancy of stomach.

SP + C16.0 **Malignant neoplasm of cardia**
Malignant neoplasm of cardiac orifice
Malignant neoplasm of cardio-esophageal junction
Malignant neoplasm of esophagus and stomach
Malignant neoplasm of gastro-esophageal junction

SP + C16.1 **Malignant neoplasm of fundus of stomach**

SP + C16.2 **Malignant neoplasm of body of stomach**

SP + C16.3 **Malignant neoplasm of pyloric antrum**
Malignant neoplasm of gastric antrum

SP + C16.4 **Malignant neoplasm of pylorus**
Malignant neoplasm of prepylorus
Malignant neoplasm of pyloric canal

SP + C16.5 **Malignant neoplasm of lesser curvature of stomach, unspecified**
Malignant neoplasm of lesser curvature of stomach, not classifiable to C16.1-C16.4

SP + C16.6 **Malignant neoplasm of greater curvature of stomach, unspecified**
Malignant neoplasm of greater curvature of stomach, not classifiable to C16.0-C16.4

SP + C16.8 **Malignant neoplasm of overlapping sites of stomach**

SP + C16.9 **Malignant neoplasm of stomach, unspecified**
Gastric cancer NOS

4 C17 **Malignant neoplasm of small intestine**
EXCLUDES 1 malignant carcinoid tumors of the small intestine (C7A.01)
CODING TIPS✓ This category indicates active cancer. See Z85.068 for personal history of primary malignancy of small intestine.

SP C17.0 **Malignant neoplasm of duodenum**

SP C17.1 **Malignant neoplasm of jejunum**

SP C17.2 **Malignant neoplasm of ileum**
EXCLUDES 1 malignant neoplasm of ileocecal valve (C18.0)

SP C17.3 **Meckel's diverticulum, malignant**
EXCLUDES 1 Meckel's diverticulum, congenital (Q43.0)

SP C17.8 **Malignant neoplasm of overlapping sites of small intestine**

SP **C17.9 Malignant neoplasm of small intestine, unspecified**

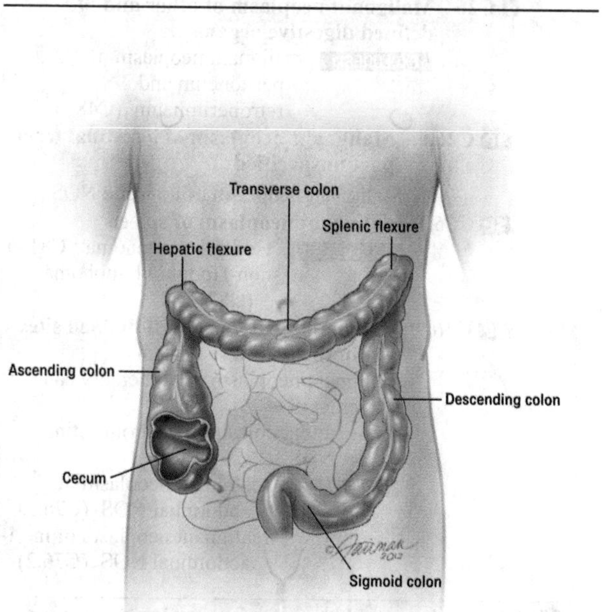

C18 Malignant neoplasm of colon

EXCLUDES 1 malignant carcinoid tumors of the colon (C7A.02-)

CODING TIPS✓ This category indicates active cancer. See Z85.038 for personal history of primary malignancy of large intestine.

SP **C18.0 Malignant neoplasm of cecum**
Malignant neoplasm of ileocecal valve

SP **C18.1 Malignant neoplasm of appendix**

SP **C18.2 Malignant neoplasm of ascending colon**

SP **C18.3 Malignant neoplasm of hepatic flexure**

SP **C18.4 Malignant neoplasm of transverse colon**

SP **C18.5 Malignant neoplasm of splenic flexure**

SP **C18.6 Malignant neoplasm of descending colon**

SP **C18.7 Malignant neoplasm of sigmoid colon**
Malignant neoplasm of sigmoid (flexure)

EXCLUDES 1 malignant neoplasm of rectosigmoid junction (C19)

SP **C18.8 Malignant neoplasm of overlapping sites of colon**

SP **C18.9 Malignant neoplasm of colon, unspecified**
Malignant neoplasm of large intestine NOS

SP **C19 Malignant neoplasm of rectosigmoid junction**
Malignant neoplasm of colon with rectum
Malignant neoplasm of rectosigmoid (colon)

EXCLUDES 1 malignant carcinoid tumors of the colon (C7A.02-)

CODING TIPS✓ This category indicates active cancer. See Z85.048 for personal history of primary malignancy of rectum, rectosigmoid junction and anus.

SP **C20 Malignant neoplasm of rectum**
Malignant neoplasm of rectal ampulla

EXCLUDES 1 malignant carcinoid tumor of the rectum (C7A.026)

CODING TIPS✓ This category indicates active cancer. See Z85.048 for personal history of primary malignancy of rectum, rectosigmoid junction and anus.

C21 Malignant neoplasm of anus and anal canal

EXCLUDES 2 malignant carcinoid tumors of the colon (C7A.02-)
malignant melanoma of anal margin (C43.51)
malignant melanoma of anal skin (C43.51)
malignant melanoma of perianal skin (C43.51)
other and unspecified malignant neoplasm of anal margin (C44.500, C44.510, C44.520, C44.590)
other and unspecified malignant neoplasm of anal skin (C44.500, C44.510, C44.520, C44.590)
other and unspecified malignant neoplasm of perianal skin (C44.500, C44.510, C44.520, C44.590)

CODING TIPS✓ This category indicates active cancer. See Z85.048 for personal history of primary malignancy of rectum, rectosigmoid junction and anus.

SP **C21.0 Malignant neoplasm of anus, unspecified**

SP **C21.1 Malignant neoplasm of anal canal**
Malignant neoplasm of anal sphincter

SP **C21.2 Malignant neoplasm of cloacogenic zone**

SP **C21.8 Malignant neoplasm of overlapping sites of rectum, anus and anal canal**
Malignant neoplasm of anorectal junction
Malignant neoplasm of anorectum
Primary malignant neoplasm of two or more contiguous sites of rectum, anus and anal canal

+ **C22 Malignant neoplasm of liver and intrahepatic bile ducts**
Use additional code to identify:
alcohol abuse and dependence (F10.-)
hepatitis B (B16.-, B18.0-B18.1)
hepatitis C (B17.1-, B18.2)

EXCLUDES 1 malignant neoplasm of biliary tract NOS (C24.9)
secondary malignant neoplasm of liver and intrahepatic bile duct (C78.7)

CODING TIPS✓ This category indicates active cancer. See Z85.05 for personal history of primary malignancy of the liver.

CODING TIPS✓ Primary cancer of the liver (C22) is rare, so look for specific documentation from the physician, such as hepatocellular carcinoma or Kupffer cell sarcoma, before coding primary liver cancer.

H SP + **C22.0 Liver cell carcinoma**
Hepatocellular carcinoma
Hepatoma

SP + **C22.1 Intrahepatic bile duct carcinoma**

Chapter 2 C00-D49

Cholangiocarcinoma
EXCLUDES 1 malignant neoplasm of hepatic duct (C24.0)

H SP + C22.2 **Hepatoblastoma**

H SP + C22.3 **Angiosarcoma of liver**
Kupffer cell sarcoma

H SP + C22.4 **Other sarcomas of liver**

H SP + C22.7 **Other specified carcinomas of liver**

H SP + C22.8 **Malignant neoplasm of liver, primary, unspecified as to type**

SP + C22.9 **Malignant neoplasm of liver, not specified as primary or secondary**

SP C23 **Malignant neoplasm of gallbladder**
CODING TIPS ✓ This category indicates active cancer. See Z85.09 for personal history of primary malignancy of the other digestive organs.

4 C24 **Malignant neoplasm of other and unspecified parts of biliary tract**
EXCLUDES 1 malignant neoplasm of intrahepatic bile duct (C22.1)

SP C24.0 **Malignant neoplasm of extrahepatic bile duct**
Malignant neoplasm of biliary duct or passage NOS
Malignant neoplasm of common bile duct
Malignant neoplasm of cystic duct
Malignant neoplasm of hepatic duct

SP C24.1 **Malignant neoplasm of ampulla of Vater**

SP C24.8 **Malignant neoplasm of overlapping sites of biliary tract**
Malignant neoplasm involving both intrahepatic and extrahepatic bile ducts
Primary malignant neoplasm of two or more contiguous sites of biliary tract

SP C24.9 **Malignant neoplasm of biliary tract, unspecified**

▲ + 4 C25 **Malignant neoplasm of pancreas**
Code also:
if applicable exocrine pancreatic insufficiency (K86.81)
Use additional code to identify:
alcohol abuse and dependence (F10.-)
CODING TIPS ✓ This category indicates active cancer. See Z85.07 for personal history of primary malignancy of the pancreas.

SP + C25.0 **Malignant neoplasm of head of pancreas**

SP + C25.1 **Malignant neoplasm of body of pancreas**

SP + C25.2 **Malignant neoplasm of tail of pancreas**

SP + C25.3 **Malignant neoplasm of pancreatic duct**

SP + C25.4 **Malignant neoplasm of endocrine pancreas**
Malignant neoplasm of islets of Langerhans
Use additional code to identify any functional activity.
CODING TIPS ✓ Use this code when malignant neoplasm of the pancreas has caused diabetes (E08).

SP + C25.7 **Malignant neoplasm of other parts of pancreas**
Malignant neoplasm of neck of pancreas

SP + C25.8 **Malignant neoplasm of overlapping sites of pancreas**

SP + C25.9 **Malignant neoplasm of pancreas, unspecified**

4 C26 **Malignant neoplasm of other and ill-defined digestive organs**
EXCLUDES 1 malignant neoplasm of peritoneum and retroperitoneum (C48.-)

SP C26.0 **Malignant neoplasm of intestinal tract, part unspecified**
Malignant neoplasm of intestine NOS

SP C26.1 **Malignant neoplasm of spleen**
EXCLUDES 1 Hodgkin lymphoma (C81.-)
non-Hodgkin lymphoma (C82-C85)

SP C26.9 **Malignant neoplasm of ill-defined sites within the digestive system**
Malignant neoplasm of alimentary canal or tract NOS
Malignant neoplasm of gastrointestinal tract NOS
EXCLUDES 1 malignant neoplasm of abdominal NOS (C76.2)
malignant neoplasm of intra-abdominal NOS (C76.2)

Malignant neoplasms of respiratory and intrathoracic organs (C30-C39)

INCLUDES malignant neoplasm of middle ear
EXCLUDES 1 mesothelioma (C45.-)

CODING TIPS ✓ Codes classifiable to C30-C39 include active cancer. History of cancer to respiratory system and other intrathoracic organs should be coded using codes from Z85.1- and Z85.2-.

4 C30 **Malignant neoplasm of nasal cavity and middle ear**
CODING TIPS ✓ C30 indicates active cancer. See Z85.22 for personal history of primary malignancy of the nasal cavities, middle ear and accessory sinuses.

SP C30.0 **Malignant neoplasm of nasal cavity**
Malignant neoplasm of cartilage of nose
Malignant neoplasm of nasal concha
Malignant neoplasm of internal nose
Malignant neoplasm of septum of nose
Malignant neoplasm of vestibule of nose
EXCLUDES 1 malignant neoplasm of nasal bone (C41.0)
malignant neoplasm of nose NOS (C76.0)
malignant neoplasm of olfactory bulb (C72.2-)
malignant neoplasm of posterior margin of nasal septum and choana (C11.3)
malignant melanoma of skin of nose (C43.31)
malignant neoplasm of turbinates (C41.0)
other and unspecified malignant neoplasm of skin of nose (C44.301, C44.311, C44.321, C44.391)

SP C30.1 **Malignant neoplasm of middle ear**

Malignant neoplasm of antrum tympanicum
Malignant neoplasm of auditory tube
Malignant neoplasm of eustachian tube
Malignant neoplasm of inner ear
Malignant neoplasm of mastoid air cells
Malignant neoplasm of tympanic cavity

EXCLUDES 1 malignant neoplasm of auricular canal (external) (C43.2-,C44.2-)
malignant neoplasm of bone of ear (meatus) (C41.0)
malignant neoplasm of cartilage of ear (C49.0)
malignant melanoma of skin of (external) ear (C43.2-)
other and unspecified malignant neoplasm of skin of (external) ear (C44.2-)

4 **C31 Malignant neoplasm of accessory sinuses**

CODING TIPS ✓ C31 indicates active cancer. See Z85.22 for personal history of primary malignancy of the nasal cavities, middle ear and accessory sinuses.

SP **C31.0 Malignant neoplasm of maxillary sinus**
Malignant neoplasm of antrum (Highmore) (maxillary)

SP **C31.1 Malignant neoplasm of ethmoidal sinus**

SP **C31.2 Malignant neoplasm of frontal sinus**

SP **C31.3 Malignant neoplasm of sphenoid sinus**

SP **C31.8 Malignant neoplasm of overlapping sites of accessory sinuses**

SP **C31.9 Malignant neoplasm of accessory sinus, unspecified**

+ 4 **C32 Malignant neoplasm of larynx**
Use additional code to identify:
alcohol abuse and dependence (F10.-)
exposure to environmental tobacco smoke (Z77.22)
exposure to tobacco smoke in the perinatal period (P96.81)
history of tobacco dependence (Z87.891)
occupational exposure to environmental tobacco smoke (Z57.31)
tobacco dependence (F17.-)
tobacco use (Z72.0)

CODING TIPS ✓ This code indicates active cancer. See Z85.21 for history of primary malignant neoplasm of larynx.

SP + **C32.0 Malignant neoplasm of glottis**
Malignant neoplasm of intrinsic larynx
Malignant neoplasm of laryngeal commissure (anterior)(posterior)
Malignant neoplasm of vocal cord (true) NOS

SP + **C32.1 Malignant neoplasm of supraglottis**
Malignant neoplasm of aryepiglottic fold or interarytenoid fold, laryngeal aspect
Malignant neoplasm of epiglottis (suprahyoid portion) NOS
Malignant neoplasm of extrinsic larynx
Malignant neoplasm of false vocal cord
Malignant neoplasm of posterior (laryngeal) surface of epiglottis
Malignant neoplasm of ventricular bands

EXCLUDES 2 malignant neoplasm of anterior surface of epiglottis (C10.1)
malignant neoplasm of aryepiglottic fold or interarytenoid fold, hypopharyngeal aspect (C13.1)
malignant neoplasm of aryepiglottic fold or interarytenoid fold, marginal zone (C13.1)
malignant neoplasm of aryepiglottic fold or interarytenoid fold NOS (C13.1)

SP + **C32.2 Malignant neoplasm of subglottis**

SP + **C32.3 Malignant neoplasm of laryngeal cartilage**

SP + **C32.8 Malignant neoplasm of overlapping sites of larynx**

SP + **C32.9 Malignant neoplasm of larynx, unspecified**

SP + **C33 Malignant neoplasm of trachea**
Use additional code to identify:
exposure to environmental tobacco smoke (Z77.22)
exposure to tobacco smoke in the perinatal period (P96.81)
history of tobacco dependence (Z87.891)
occupational exposure to environmental tobacco smoke (Z57.31)
tobacco dependence (F17.-)
tobacco use (Z72.0)

+ 4 **C34 Malignant neoplasm of bronchus and lung**
Use additional code to identify:
exposure to environmental tobacco smoke (Z77.22)
exposure to tobacco smoke in the perinatal period (P96.81)
history of tobacco dependence (Z87.891)
occupational exposure to environmental tobacco smoke (Z57.31)
tobacco dependence (F17.-)
tobacco use (Z72.0)

EXCLUDES 1 Kaposi's sarcoma of lung (C46.5-)
malignant carcinoid tumor of the bronchus and lung (C7A.090)

CODING TIPS ✓ C34 indicates active cancer in the lung. Laterality is important. Unspecified laterality will not be assigned to a Clinical Grouper in PDGM. Query the physician for location of tumors in the lung(s). See Z85.118 for personal history of primary malignancy of the lung and bronchus.

+ 5 **C34.0 Malignant neoplasm of main bronchus**
Malignant neoplasm of carina
Malignant neoplasm of hilus (of lung)

⊟ SP + **C34.00 Malignant neoplasm of unspecified main bronchus**

⊟ SP + **C34.01 Malignant neoplasm of right main bronchus**

⊟ SP + **C34.02 Malignant neoplasm of left main bronchus**

+ 5 **C34.1 Malignant neoplasm of upper lobe, bronchus or lung**

Chapter 2
C00-D49

Laterality IQ + C34.10 **Malignant neoplasm of upper lobe, unspecified bronchus or lung**

Laterality SP + C34.11 **Malignant neoplasm of upper lobe, right bronchus or lung**

Laterality SP + C34.12 **Malignant neoplasm of upper lobe, left bronchus or lung**

SP + C34.2 **Malignant neoplasm of middle lobe, bronchus or lung**

+ 5 C34.3 **Malignant neoplasm of lower lobe, bronchus or lung**

Laterality IQ + C34.30 **Malignant neoplasm of lower lobe, unspecified bronchus or lung**

Laterality SP + C34.31 **Malignant neoplasm of lower lobe, right bronchus or lung**

Laterality SP + C34.32 **Malignant neoplasm of lower lobe, left bronchus or lung**

+ 5 C34.8 **Malignant neoplasm of overlapping sites of bronchus and lung**

Laterality IQ + C34.80 **Malignant neoplasm of overlapping sites of unspecified bronchus and lung**

Laterality SP + C34.81 **Malignant neoplasm of overlapping sites of right bronchus and lung**

Laterality SP + C34.82 **Malignant neoplasm of overlapping sites of left bronchus and lung**

+ 5 C34.9 **Malignant neoplasm of unspecified part of bronchus or lung**

Laterality IQ + C34.90 **Malignant neoplasm of unspecified part of unspecified bronchus or lung**

Lung cancer NOS

Laterality SP + C34.91 **Malignant neoplasm of unspecified part of right bronchus or lung**

Laterality SP + C34.92 **Malignant neoplasm of unspecified part of left bronchus or lung**

SP C37 **Malignant neoplasm of thymus**

EXCLUDES 1 malignant carcinoid tumor of the thymus (C7A.091)

4 C38 **Malignant neoplasm of heart, mediastinum and pleura**

EXCLUDES 1 mesothelioma (C45.-)

SP C38.0 **Malignant neoplasm of heart**

Malignant neoplasm of pericardium

EXCLUDES 1 malignant neoplasm of great vessels (C49.3)

SP C38.1 **Malignant neoplasm of anterior mediastinum**

SP C38.2 **Malignant neoplasm of posterior mediastinum**

SP C38.3 **Malignant neoplasm of mediastinum, part unspecified**

SP C38.4 **Malignant neoplasm of pleura**

SP C38.8 **Malignant neoplasm of overlapping sites of heart, mediastinum and pleura**

+ 4 C39 **Malignant neoplasm of other and ill-defined sites in the respiratory system and intrathoracic organs**

Use additional code to identify:
- exposure to environmental tobacco smoke (Z77.22)
- exposure to tobacco smoke in the perinatal period (P96.81)
- history of tobacco dependence (Z87.891)
- occupational exposure to environmental tobacco smoke (Z57.31)
- tobacco dependence (F17.-)
- tobacco use (Z72.0)

EXCLUDES 1 intrathoracic malignant neoplasm NOS (C76.1)
thoracic malignant neoplasm NOS (C76.1)

IQ + C39.0 **Malignant neoplasm of upper respiratory tract, part unspecified**

IQ + C39.9 **Malignant neoplasm of lower respiratory tract, part unspecified**

Malignant neoplasm of respiratory tract NOS

Malignant neoplasms of bone and articular cartilage (C40-C41)

INCLUDES malignant neoplasm of cartilage (articular) (joint)
malignant neoplasm of periosteum

EXCLUDES 1 malignant neoplasm of bone marrow NOS (C96.9)
malignant neoplasm of synovia (C49.-)

CODING TIPS✓ Codes classifiable to C40-C41 include active cancer. History of cancer to bone or soft tissue should be coded to Z85.83-.

+ 4 C40 **Malignant neoplasm of bone and articular cartilage of limbs**

Use additional code to identify major osseous defect, if applicable (M89.7-)

CODING TIPS✓ If bone cancer is noted in the medical record, confirm with the physician whether the cancer is primary or secondary cancer to the bone. Most commonly, home care agencies care for patients with metastasis to the bone, which is coded C79.51. Category C40 indicates active primary cancer to the bone. See Z85.830 for personal history of primary malignancy of bone.

CODING TIPS✓ Laterality is very important with these codes. Unspecified should not be used and will not be assigned to a Clinical Grouper as primary in PDGM.

+ 5 C40.0 **Malignant neoplasm of scapula and long bones of upper limb**

Laterality IQ + C40.00 **Malignant neoplasm of scapula and long bones of unspecified upper limb**

Laterality SP + C40.01 **Malignant neoplasm of scapula and long bones of right upper limb**

Laterality SP + C40.02 **Malignant neoplasm of scapula and long bones of left upper limb**

+ 5 C40.1 **Malignant neoplasm of short bones of upper limb**

Laterality IQ + C40.10 **Malignant neoplasm of short bones of unspecified upper limb**

Laterality SP + C40.11 **Malignant neoplasm of short bones of right upper limb**

Laterality SP + C40.12 **Malignant neoplasm of short bones of left upper limb**

+ 5 C40.2 **Malignant neoplasm of long bones of lower limb**

Laterality IQ + C40.20 **Malignant neoplasm of long bones of unspecified lower limb**

Laterality SP + C40.21 **Malignant neoplasm of long bones of right lower limb**

Laterality SP + C40.22 **Malignant neoplasm of long bones of left lower limb**

+ 5 C40.3 **Malignant neoplasm of short bones of lower limb**

IQ + C40.30 **Malignant neoplasm of short bones of unspecified lower limb**

SP + C40.31 **Malignant neoplasm of short bones of right lower limb**

SP + C40.32 **Malignant neoplasm of short bones of left lower limb**

+ 5 C40.8 **Malignant neoplasm of overlapping sites of bone and articular cartilage of limb**

IQ + C40.80 **Malignant neoplasm of overlapping sites of bone and articular cartilage of unspecified limb**

SP + C40.81 **Malignant neoplasm of overlapping sites of bone and articular cartilage of right limb**

SP + C40.82 **Malignant neoplasm of overlapping sites of bone and articular cartilage of left limb**

+ 5 C40.9 **Malignant neoplasm of unspecified bones and articular cartilage of limb**

IQ + C40.90 **Malignant neoplasm of unspecified bones and articular cartilage of unspecified limb**

SP + C40.91 **Malignant neoplasm of unspecified bones and articular cartilage of right limb**

SP + C40.92 **Malignant neoplasm of unspecified bones and articular cartilage of left limb**

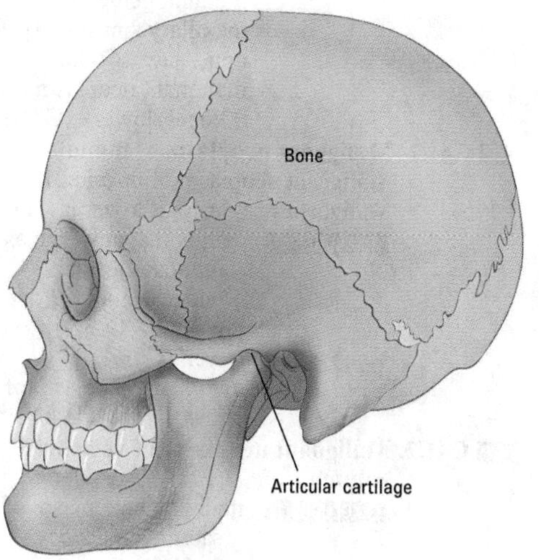

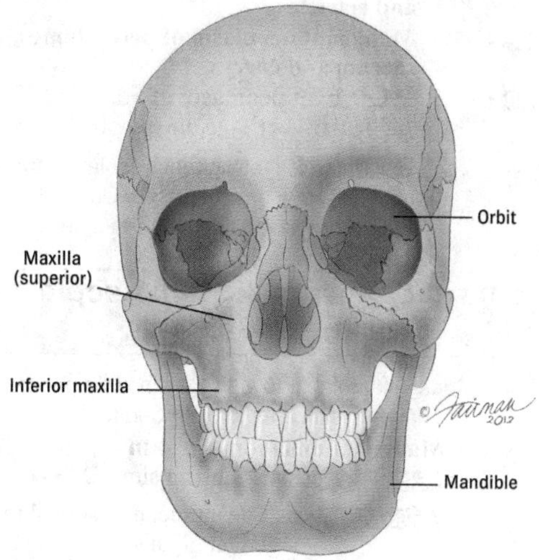

4 C41 **Malignant neoplasm of bone and articular cartilage of other and unspecified sites**

EXCLUDES 1 malignant neoplasm of bones of limbs (C40.-)
malignant neoplasm of cartilage of ear (C49.0)
malignant neoplasm of cartilage of eyelid (C49.0)
malignant neoplasm of cartilage of larynx (C32.3)
malignant neoplasm of cartilage of limbs (C40.-)
malignant neoplasm of cartilage of nose (C30.0)

SP C41.0 **Malignant neoplasm of bones of skull and face**
Malignant neoplasm of maxilla (superior)
Malignant neoplasm of orbital bone

EXCLUDES 2 carcinoma, any type except intraosseous or odontogenic of:
maxillary sinus (C31.0)
upper jaw (C03.0)
malignant neoplasm of jaw bone (lower) (C41.1)

SP **C41.1 Malignant neoplasm of mandible**
Malignant neoplasm of inferior maxilla
Malignant neoplasm of lower jaw bone
EXCLUDES 2 carcinoma, any type except intraosseous or odontogenic of:
jaw NOS (C03.9)
lower (C03.1)
malignant neoplasm of upper jaw bone (C41.0)

SP **C41.2 Malignant neoplasm of vertebral column**
EXCLUDES 1 malignant neoplasm of sacrum and coccyx (C41.4)

SP **C41.3 Malignant neoplasm of ribs, sternum and clavicle**

SP **C41.4 Malignant neoplasm of pelvic bones, sacrum and coccyx**

SP **C41.9 Malignant neoplasm of bone and articular cartilage, unspecified**

CODING TIPS✓ Malignant neoplasm of bone, unspecified is unacceptable. Query the physician for additional information.

Melanoma and other malignant neoplasms of skin (C43-C44)

CODING TIPS✓ Codes classifiable to C43-C44 include active cancer. History of cancer to skin should be coded to Z85.82-.

4 **C43 Malignant melanoma of skin**
EXCLUDES 1 melanoma in situ (D03.-)
EXCLUDES 2 malignant melanoma of skin of genital organs (C51-C52, C60.-, C63.-)
Merkel cell carcinoma (C4A.-)
sites other than skin-code to malignant neoplasm of the site

CODING TIPS✓ Malignant melanoma is rapidly invasive. C43 indicates active cancer. See Z85.820 for personal history of malignant melanoma.

CODING TIPS✓ Laterality is very important with these codes. Unspecified should not be used and will not be assigned to a Clinical Grouper as primary in PDGM.

SP **C43.0 Malignant melanoma of lip**
EXCLUDES 1 malignant neoplasm of vermilion border of lip (C00.0-C00.2)

5 **C43.1 Malignant melanoma of eyelid, including canthus**

⊟ IQ **C43.10 Malignant melanoma of unspecified eyelid, including canthus**

6 **C43.11 Malignant melanoma of right eyelid, including canthus**

⊟ SP **C43.111 Malignant melanoma of right upper eyelid, including canthus**

⊟ SP **C43.112 Malignant melanoma of right lower eyelid, including canthus**

6 **C43.12 Malignant melanoma of left eyelid, including canthus**

⊟ SP **C43.121 Malignant melanoma of left upper eyelid, including canthus**

⊟ SP **C43.122 Malignant melanoma of left lower eyelid, including canthus**

5 **C43.2 Malignant melanoma of ear and external auricular canal**

⊟ IQ **C43.20 Malignant melanoma of unspecified ear and external auricular canal**

⊟ SP **C43.21 Malignant melanoma of right ear and external auricular canal**

⊟ SP **C43.22 Malignant melanoma of left ear and external auricular canal**

5 **C43.3 Malignant melanoma of other and unspecified parts of face**

IQ **C43.30 Malignant melanoma of unspecified part of face**

SP **C43.31 Malignant melanoma of nose**

SP **C43.39 Malignant melanoma of other parts of face**

SP **C43.4 Malignant melanoma of scalp and neck**

5 **C43.5 Malignant melanoma of trunk**
EXCLUDES 2 malignant neoplasm of anus NOS (C21.0)
malignant neoplasm of scrotum (C63.2)

SP **C43.51 Malignant melanoma of anal skin**
Malignant melanoma of anal margin
Malignant melanoma of perianal skin

SP **C43.52 Malignant melanoma of skin of breast**

SP **C43.59 Malignant melanoma of other part of trunk**

5 **C43.6 Malignant melanoma of upper limb, including shoulder**

⊟ IQ **C43.60 Malignant melanoma of unspecified upper limb, including shoulder**

⊟ SP **C43.61 Malignant melanoma of right upper limb, including shoulder**

⊟ SP **C43.62 Malignant melanoma of left upper limb, including shoulder**

5 **C43.7 Malignant melanoma of lower limb, including hip**

⊟ IQ **C43.70 Malignant melanoma of unspecified lower limb, including hip**

⊟ SP **C43.71 Malignant melanoma of right lower limb, including hip**

⊟ SP **C43.72 Malignant melanoma of left lower limb, including hip**

SP **C43.8 Malignant melanoma of overlapping sites of skin**

IQ **C43.9 Malignant melanoma of skin, unspecified**
Malignant melanoma of unspecified site of skin
Melanoma (malignant) NOS

4 **C4A Merkel cell carcinoma**

SP **C4A.0 Merkel cell carcinoma of lip**
EXCLUDES 1 malignant neoplasm of vermilion border of lip (C00.0-C00.2)

5 **C4A.1 Merkel cell carcinoma of eyelid, including canthus**

C4A.10 Merkel cell carcinoma of unspecified eyelid, including canthus

C4A.11 Merkel cell carcinoma of right eyelid, including canthus

C4A.111 Merkel cell carcinoma of right upper eyelid, including canthus

C4A.112 Merkel cell carcinoma of right lower eyelid, including canthus

C4A.12 Merkel cell carcinoma of left eyelid, including canthus

C4A.121 Merkel cell carcinoma of left upper eyelid, including canthus

C4A.122 Merkel cell carcinoma of left lower eyelid, including canthus

C4A.2 Merkel cell carcinoma of ear and external auricular canal

C4A.20 Merkel cell carcinoma of unspecified ear and external auricular canal

C4A.21 Merkel cell carcinoma of right ear and external auricular canal

C4A.22 Merkel cell carcinoma of left ear and external auricular canal

C4A.3 Merkel cell carcinoma of other and unspecified parts of face

C4A.30 Merkel cell carcinoma of unspecified part of face

C4A.31 Merkel cell carcinoma of nose

C4A.39 Merkel cell carcinoma of other parts of face

C4A.4 Merkel cell carcinoma of scalp and neck

C4A.5 Merkel cell carcinoma of trunk

EXCLUDES 2 malignant neoplasm of anus NOS (C21.0)
malignant neoplasm of scrotum (C63.2)

C4A.51 Merkel cell carcinoma of anal skin
Merkel cell carcinoma of anal margin
Merkel cell carcinoma of perianal skin

C4A.52 Merkel cell carcinoma of skin of breast

C4A.59 Merkel cell carcinoma of other part of trunk

C4A.6 Merkel cell carcinoma of upper limb, including shoulder

C4A.60 Merkel cell carcinoma of unspecified upper limb, including shoulder

C4A.61 Merkel cell carcinoma of right upper limb, including shoulder

C4A.62 Merkel cell carcinoma of left upper limb, including shoulder

C4A.7 Merkel cell carcinoma of lower limb, including hip

C4A.70 Merkel cell carcinoma of unspecified lower limb, including hip

C4A.71 Merkel cell carcinoma of right lower limb, including hip

C4A.72 Merkel cell carcinoma of left lower limb, including hip

C4A.8 Merkel cell carcinoma of overlapping sites

C4A.9 Merkel cell carcinoma, unspecified
Merkel cell carcinoma of unspecified site
Merkel cell carcinoma NOS

C44 Other and unspecified malignant neoplasm of skin

INCLUDES malignant neoplasm of sebaceous glands
malignant neoplasm of sweat glands

EXCLUDES 1 Kaposi's sarcoma of skin (C46.0)
malignant melanoma of skin (C43.-)
malignant neoplasm of skin of genital organs (C51-C52, C60.-, C63.2)
Merkel cell carcinoma (C4A.-)

CODING TIPS ✓ C44 is used for squamous cell and basal cell carcinoma of the skin. If malignant melanoma is documented, use C43 instead. See Z85.828 for personal history of skin cancer.

CODING TIPS ✓ Do not code Merkel cell carcinoma to C44. See C4A for Merkel cell carcinoma and Z85.821 for personal history of Merkel cell carcinoma.

CODING TIPS ✓ Metastasis of common sunlight-induced squamous cell carcinoma is unusual. Lesions more likely to metastasize are lesions of the lip or ear.

C44.0 Other and unspecified malignant neoplasm of skin of lip

EXCLUDES 1 malignant neoplasm of lip (C00.-)

C44.00 Unspecified malignant neoplasm of skin of lip

C44.01 Basal cell carcinoma of skin of lip

C44.02 Squamous cell carcinoma of skin of lip

C44.09 Other specified malignant neoplasm of skin of lip

C44.1 Other and unspecified malignant neoplasm of skin of eyelid, including canthus

EXCLUDES 1 connective tissue of eyelid (C49.0)

CODING TIPS ✓ Laterality is very important with these codes. Unspecified should not be used and will not be assigned to a Clinical Grouper as primary in PDGM.

C44.10 Unspecified malignant neoplasm of skin of eyelid, including canthus

C44.101 Unspecified malignant neoplasm of skin of unspecified eyelid, including canthus

C44.102 Unspecified malignant neoplasm of skin of right eyelid, including canthus

CODING TIPS ✓ There was no 7th character table published with codes C44.102- and C44.109-. A 7th character of 1 denotes "upper" and a 7th character of 2 denotes "lower".

C44.109 Unspecified malignant neoplasm of skin of left eyelid, including canthus

Chapter 2 C00-D49

6 C44.11 Basal cell carcinoma of skin of eyelid, including canthus

IQ C44.111 Basal cell carcinoma of skin of unspecified eyelid, including canthus

SP 7 C44.112 Basal cell carcinoma of skin of right eyelid, including canthus

CODING TIPS ✓ There was no 7th character table published with codes C44.112- and C44.119-. A 7th character of 1 denotes "upper" and a 7th character of 2 denotes "lower".

SP 7 C44.119 Basal cell carcinoma of skin of left eyelid, including canthus

6 C44.12 Squamous cell carcinoma of skin of eyelid, including canthus

IQ C44.121 Squamous cell carcinoma of skin of unspecified eyelid, including canthus

SP 7 C44.122 Squamous cell carcinoma of skin of right eyelid, including canthus

CODING TIPS ✓ There was no 7th character table published with codes C44.122- and C44.129-. A 7th character of 1 denotes "upper" and a 7th character of 2 denotes "lower".

SP 7 C44.129 Squamous cell carcinoma of skin of left eyelid, including canthus

6 C44.13 Sebaceous cell carcinoma of skin of eyelid, including canthus

IQ C44.131 Sebaceous cell carcinoma of skin of unspecified eyelid, including canthus

SP 7 C44.132 Sebaceous cell carcinoma of skin of right eyelid, including canthus

CODING TIPS ✓ There was no 7th character table published with codes C44.132- and C44.139-. A 7th character of 1 denotes "upper" and a 7th character of 2 denotes "lower".

SP 7 C44.139 Sebaceous cell carcinoma of skin of left eyelid, including canthus

6 C44.19 Other specified malignant neoplasm of skin of eyelid, including canthus

IQ C44.191 Other specified malignant neoplasm of skin of unspecified eyelid, including canthus

SP 7 C44.192 Other specified malignant neoplasm of skin of right eyelid, including canthus

CODING TIPS ✓ There was no 7th character table published with codes C44.192- and C44.199-. A 7th character of 1 denotes "upper" and a 7th character of 2 denotes "lower".

SP 7 C44.199 Other specified malignant neoplasm of skin of left eyelid, including canthus

5 C44.2 Other and unspecified malignant neoplasm of skin of ear and external auricular canal

EXCLUDES 1 connective tissue of ear (C49.0)

6 C44.20 Unspecified malignant neoplasm of skin of ear and external auricular canal

IQ C44.201 Unspecified malignant neoplasm of skin of unspecified ear and external auricular canal

SP C44.202 Unspecified malignant neoplasm of skin of right ear and external auricular canal

IQ C44.209 Unspecified malignant neoplasm of skin of left ear and external auricular canal

6 C44.21 Basal cell carcinoma of skin of ear and external auricular canal

IQ C44.211 Basal cell carcinoma of skin of unspecified ear and external auricular canal

SP C44.212 Basal cell carcinoma of skin of right ear and external auricular canal

SP C44.219 Basal cell carcinoma of skin of left ear and external auricular canal

6 C44.22 Squamous cell carcinoma of skin of ear and external auricular canal

IQ C44.221 Squamous cell carcinoma of skin of unspecified ear and external auricular canal

SP C44.222 Squamous cell carcinoma of skin of right ear and external auricular canal

SP C44.229 Squamous cell carcinoma of skin of left ear and external auricular canal

6 C44.29 Other specified malignant neoplasm of skin of ear and external auricular canal

IQ C44.291 Other specified malignant neoplasm of skin of unspecified ear and external auricular canal

SP C44.292 Other specified malignant neoplasm of skin of right ear and external auricular canal

SP C44.299 Other specified malignant neoplasm of skin of left ear and external auricular canal

5 C44.3 Other and unspecified malignant neoplasm of skin of other and unspecified parts of face

6 C44.30 Unspecified malignant neoplasm of skin of other and unspecified parts of face

IQ C44.300 Unspecified malignant neoplasm of skin of unspecified part of face

SP C44.301 Unspecified malignant neoplasm of skin of nose

SP C44.309 Unspecified malignant neoplasm of skin of other parts of face

6 C44.31 Basal cell carcinoma of skin of other and unspecified parts of face

IQ C44.310 Basal cell carcinoma of skin of unspecified parts of face

SP C44.311 Basal cell carcinoma of skin of nose

SP C44.319 Basal cell carcinoma of skin of other parts of face

6 C44.32 Squamous cell carcinoma of skin of other and unspecified parts of face

IQ C44.320 Squamous cell carcinoma of skin of unspecified parts of face

Chapter 2

C00-D49

SP C44.321 **Squamous cell carcinoma of skin of nose**

SP C44.329 **Squamous cell carcinoma of skin of other parts of face**

6 C44.39 **Other specified malignant neoplasm of skin of other and unspecified parts of face**

IQ C44.390 **Other specified malignant neoplasm of skin of unspecified parts of face**

SP C44.391 **Other specified malignant neoplasm of skin of nose**

SP C44.399 **Other specified malignant neoplasm of skin of other parts of face**

5 C44.4 **Other and unspecified malignant neoplasm of skin of scalp and neck**

SP C44.40 **Unspecified malignant neoplasm of skin of scalp and neck**

SP C44.41 **Basal cell carcinoma of skin of scalp and neck**

SP C44.42 **Squamous cell carcinoma of skin of scalp and neck**

SP C44.49 **Other specified malignant neoplasm of skin of scalp and neck**

5 C44.5 **Other and unspecified malignant neoplasm of skin of trunk**

EXCLUDES 1 anus NOS (C21.0)
scrotum (C63.2)

6 C44.50 **Unspecified malignant neoplasm of skin of trunk**

SP C44.500 **Unspecified malignant neoplasm of anal skin**
Unspecified malignant neoplasm of anal margin
Unspecified malignant neoplasm of perianal skin

SP C44.501 **Unspecified malignant neoplasm of skin of breast**

SP C44.509 **Unspecified malignant neoplasm of skin of other part of trunk**

6 C44.51 **Basal cell carcinoma of skin of trunk**

SP C44.510 **Basal cell carcinoma of anal skin**
Basal cell carcinoma of anal margin
Basal cell carcinoma of perianal skin

SP C44.511 **Basal cell carcinoma of skin of breast**

SP C44.519 **Basal cell carcinoma of skin of other part of trunk**

6 C44.52 **Squamous cell carcinoma of skin of trunk**

SP C44.520 **Squamous cell carcinoma of anal skin**
Squamous cell carcinoma of anal margin
Squamous cell carcinoma of perianal skin

SP C44.521 **Squamous cell carcinoma of skin of breast**

SP C44.529 **Squamous cell carcinoma of skin of other part of trunk**

6 C44.59 **Other specified malignant neoplasm of skin of trunk**

SP C44.590 **Other specified malignant neoplasm of anal skin**
Other specified malignant neoplasm of anal margin
Other specified malignant neoplasm of perianal skin

SP C44.591 **Other specified malignant neoplasm of skin of breast**

SP C44.599 **Other specified malignant neoplasm of skin of other part of trunk**

5 C44.6 **Other and unspecified malignant neoplasm of skin of upper limb, including shoulder**

6 C44.60 **Unspecified malignant neoplasm of skin of upper limb, including shoulder**

H IQ C44.601 **Unspecified malignant neoplasm of skin of unspecified upper limb, including shoulder**

H SP C44.602 **Unspecified malignant neoplasm of skin of right upper limb, including shoulder**

H SP C44.609 **Unspecified malignant neoplasm of skin of left upper limb, including shoulder**

6 C44.61 **Basal cell carcinoma of skin of upper limb, including shoulder**

H IQ C44.611 **Basal cell carcinoma of skin of unspecified upper limb, including shoulder**

H SP C44.612 **Basal cell carcinoma of skin of right upper limb, including shoulder**

H SP C44.619 **Basal cell carcinoma of skin of left upper limb, including shoulder**

6 C44.62 **Squamous cell carcinoma of skin of upper limb, including shoulder**

H IQ C44.621 **Squamous cell carcinoma of skin of unspecified upper limb, including shoulder**

H SP C44.622 **Squamous cell carcinoma of skin of right upper limb, including shoulder**

H SP C44.629 **Squamous cell carcinoma of skin of left upper limb, including shoulder**

6 C44.69 **Other specified malignant neoplasm of skin of upper limb, including shoulder**

H IQ C44.691 **Other specified malignant neoplasm of skin of unspecified upper limb, including shoulder**

H SP C44.692 **Other specified malignant neoplasm of skin of right upper limb, including shoulder**

H SP C44.699 **Other specified malignant neoplasm of skin of left upper limb, including shoulder**

5 C44.7 **Other and unspecified malignant neoplasm of skin of lower limb, including hip**

6 C44.70 **Unspecified malignant neoplasm of skin of lower limb, including hip**

H IQ C44.701 **Unspecified malignant neoplasm of skin of unspecified lower limb, including hip**

Chapter 2

C00-D49

⊟ SP C44.702 **Unspecified malignant neoplasm of skin of right lower limb, including hip**

⊟ SP C44.709 **Unspecified malignant neoplasm of skin of left lower limb, including hip**

6 C44.71 **Basal cell carcinoma of skin of lower limb, including hip**

⊟ IQ C44.711 **Basal cell carcinoma of skin of unspecified lower limb, including hip**

⊟ SP C44.712 **Basal cell carcinoma of skin of right lower limb, including hip**

⊟ SP C44.719 **Basal cell carcinoma of skin of left lower limb, including hip**

6 C44.72 **Squamous cell carcinoma of skin of lower limb, including hip**

⊟ IQ C44.721 **Squamous cell carcinoma of skin of unspecified lower limb, including hip**

⊟ SP C44.722 **Squamous cell carcinoma of skin of right lower limb, including hip**

⊟ SP C44.729 **Squamous cell carcinoma of skin of left lower limb, including hip**

6 C44.79 **Other specified malignant neoplasm of skin of lower limb, including hip**

⊟ IQ C44.791 **Other specified malignant neoplasm of skin of unspecified lower limb, including hip**

⊟ SP C44.792 **Other specified malignant neoplasm of skin of right lower limb, including hip**

⊟ SP C44.799 **Other specified malignant neoplasm of skin of left lower limb, including hip**

5 C44.8 **Other and unspecified malignant neoplasm of overlapping sites of skin**

SP C44.80 **Unspecified malignant neoplasm of overlapping sites of skin**

SP C44.81 **Basal cell carcinoma of overlapping sites of skin**

SP C44.82 **Squamous cell carcinoma of overlapping sites of skin**

SP C44.89 **Other specified malignant neoplasm of overlapping sites of skin**

5 C44.9 **Other and unspecified malignant neoplasm of skin, unspecified**

IQ C44.90 **Unspecified malignant neoplasm of skin, unspecified**
Malignant neoplasm of unspecified site of skin

IQ C44.91 **Basal cell carcinoma of skin, unspecified**

IQ C44.92 **Squamous cell carcinoma of skin, unspecified**

IQ C44.99 **Other specified malignant neoplasm of skin, unspecified**

Malignant neoplasms of mesothelial and soft tissue (C45-C49)

CODING TIPS ✓ Codes classifiable to C45-C49 include active cancer. History of cancer to soft tissue should be coded to Z85.83-.

4 C45 **Mesothelioma**

SP C45.0 **Mesothelioma of pleura**
EXCLUDES 1 other malignant neoplasm of pleura (C38.4)

SP C45.1 **Mesothelioma of peritoneum**
Mesothelioma of cul-de-sac
Mesothelioma of mesentery
Mesothelioma of mesocolon
Mesothelioma of omentum
Mesothelioma of peritoneum (parietal) (pelvic)
EXCLUDES 1 other malignant neoplasm of soft tissue of peritoneum (C48.-)

SP C45.2 **Mesothelioma of pericardium**
EXCLUDES 1 other malignant neoplasm of pericardium (C38.0)

SP C45.7 **Mesothelioma of other sites**

IQ C45.9 **Mesothelioma, unspecified**

4 C46 **Kaposi's sarcoma**
Code first:
any human immunodeficiency virus [HIV] disease (B20)

CODING TIPS ✓ Kaposi's sarcoma (C46) is usually associated with HIV/AIDS. If so, then B20 is coded prior to using the C46 category code, unless other restrictions apply. (See coding tip at category B20.)

SP C46.0 **Kaposi's sarcoma of skin**

SP C46.1 **Kaposi's sarcoma of soft tissue**
Kaposi's sarcoma of blood vessel
Kaposi's sarcoma of connective tissue
Kaposi's sarcoma of fascia
Kaposi's sarcoma of ligament
Kaposi's sarcoma of lymphatic(s) NEC
Kaposi's sarcoma of muscle
EXCLUDES 2 Kaposi's sarcoma of lymph glands and nodes (C46.3)

SP C46.2 **Kaposi's sarcoma of palate**

SP C46.3 **Kaposi's sarcoma of lymph nodes**

SP C46.4 **Kaposi's sarcoma of gastrointestinal sites**

5 C46.5 **Kaposi's sarcoma of lung**

⊟ IQ C46.50 **Kaposi's sarcoma of unspecified lung**

⊟ SP C46.51 **Kaposi's sarcoma of right lung**

⊟ SP C46.52 **Kaposi's sarcoma of left lung**

SP C46.7 **Kaposi's sarcoma of other sites**

IQ C46.9 **Kaposi's sarcoma, unspecified**
Kaposi's sarcoma of unspecified site

4 C47 **Malignant neoplasm of peripheral nerves and autonomic nervous system**
INCLUDES malignant neoplasm of sympathetic and parasympathetic nerves and ganglia
EXCLUDES 1 Kaposi's sarcoma of soft tissue (C46.1)

SP C47.0 **Malignant neoplasm of peripheral nerves of head, face and neck**
EXCLUDES 1 malignant neoplasm of peripheral nerves of orbit (C69.6-)

5 C47.1 **Malignant neoplasm of peripheral nerves of upper limb, including shoulder**

⊟ IQ **C47.10 Malignant neoplasm of peripheral nerves of unspecified upper limb, including shoulder**

⊟ SP **C47.11 Malignant neoplasm of peripheral nerves of right upper limb, including shoulder**

⊟ SP **C47.12 Malignant neoplasm of peripheral nerves of left upper limb, including shoulder**

5 **C47.2 Malignant neoplasm of peripheral nerves of lower limb, including hip**

⊟ IQ **C47.20 Malignant neoplasm of peripheral nerves of unspecified lower limb, including hip**

⊟ SP **C47.21 Malignant neoplasm of peripheral nerves of right lower limb, including hip**

⊟ SP **C47.22 Malignant neoplasm of peripheral nerves of left lower limb, including hip**

SP **C47.3 Malignant neoplasm of peripheral nerves of thorax**

SP **C47.4 Malignant neoplasm of peripheral nerves of abdomen**

SP **C47.5 Malignant neoplasm of peripheral nerves of pelvis**

SP **C47.6 Malignant neoplasm of peripheral nerves of trunk, unspecified**

Malignant neoplasm of peripheral nerves of unspecified part of trunk

SP **C47.8 Malignant neoplasm of overlapping sites of peripheral nerves and autonomic nervous system**

SP **C47.9 Malignant neoplasm of peripheral nerves and autonomic nervous system, unspecified**

Malignant neoplasm of unspecified site of peripheral nerves and autonomic nervous system

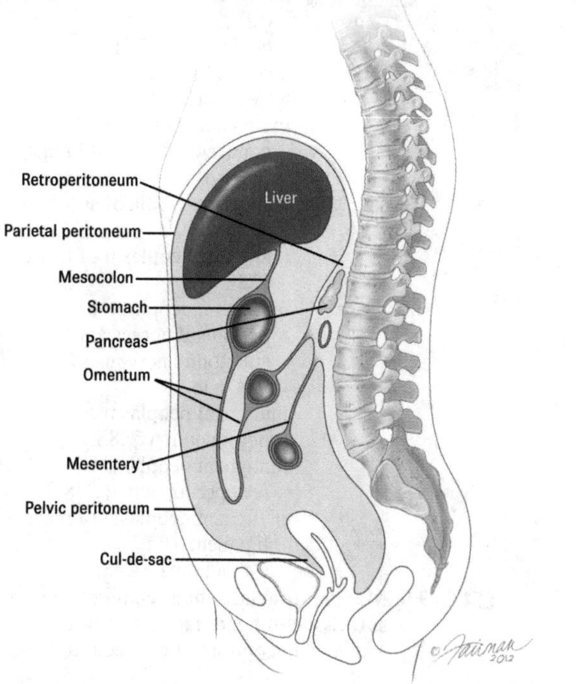

4 **C48 Malignant neoplasm of retroperitoneum and peritoneum**

EXCLUDES 1 Kaposi's sarcoma of connective tissue (C46.1)
mesothelioma (C45.-)

CODING TIPS ✓ This category indicates active cancer. See Z85.09 for personal history of primary malignancy of the other digestive organs.

SP **C48.0 Malignant neoplasm of retroperitoneum**

SP **C48.1 Malignant neoplasm of specified parts of peritoneum**

Malignant neoplasm of cul-de-sac
Malignant neoplasm of mesentery
Malignant neoplasm of mesocolon
Malignant neoplasm of omentum
Malignant neoplasm of parietal peritoneum
Malignant neoplasm of pelvic peritoneum

SP **C48.2 Malignant neoplasm of peritoneum, unspecified**

SP **C48.8 Malignant neoplasm of overlapping sites of retroperitoneum and peritoneum**

4 **C49 Malignant neoplasm of other connective and soft tissue**

INCLUDES malignant neoplasm of blood vessel
malignant neoplasm of bursa
malignant neoplasm of cartilage
malignant neoplasm of fascia
malignant neoplasm of fat
malignant neoplasm of ligament, except uterine
malignant neoplasm of lymphatic vessel
malignant neoplasm of muscle
malignant neoplasm of synovia

Chapter 2 C00-D49

malignant neoplasm of tendon (sheath)

EXCLUDES 1 malignant neoplasm of cartilage (of) :
articular (C40-C41)
larynx (C32.3)
nose (C30.0)
malignant neoplasm of connective tissue of breast (C50.-)

EXCLUDES 2 Kaposi's sarcoma of soft tissue (C46.1)
malignant neoplasm of heart (C38.0)
malignant neoplasm of peripheral nerves and autonomic nervous system (C47.-)
malignant neoplasm of peritoneum (C48.2)
malignant neoplasm of retroperitoneum (C48.0)
malignant neoplasm of uterine ligament (C57.3)
mesothelioma (C45.-)

SP **C49.0 Malignant neoplasm of connective and soft tissue of head, face and neck**
Malignant neoplasm of connective tissue of ear
Malignant neoplasm of connective tissue of eyelid
EXCLUDES 1 connective tissue of orbit (C69.6-)

5 **C49.1 Malignant neoplasm of connective and soft tissue of upper limb, including shoulder**

Laterality IQ **C49.10 Malignant neoplasm of connective and soft tissue of unspecified upper limb, including shoulder**

Laterality SP **C49.11 Malignant neoplasm of connective and soft tissue of right upper limb, including shoulder**

Laterality SP **C49.12 Malignant neoplasm of connective and soft tissue of left upper limb, including shoulder**

5 **C49.2 Malignant neoplasm of connective and soft tissue of lower limb, including hip**

Laterality IQ **C49.20 Malignant neoplasm of connective and soft tissue of unspecified lower limb, including hip**

Laterality SP **C49.21 Malignant neoplasm of connective and soft tissue of right lower limb, including hip**

Laterality SP **C49.22 Malignant neoplasm of connective and soft tissue of left lower limb, including hip**

SP **C49.3 Malignant neoplasm of connective and soft tissue of thorax**
Malignant neoplasm of axilla
Malignant neoplasm of diaphragm
Malignant neoplasm of great vessels
EXCLUDES 1 malignant neoplasm of breast (C50.-)
malignant neoplasm of heart (C38.0)
malignant neoplasm of mediastinum (C38.1-C38.3)
malignant neoplasm of thymus (C37)

SP **C49.4 Malignant neoplasm of connective and soft tissue of abdomen**
Malignant neoplasm of abdominal wall
Malignant neoplasm of hypochondrium

SP **C49.5 Malignant neoplasm of connective and soft tissue of pelvis**
Malignant neoplasm of buttock
Malignant neoplasm of groin
Malignant neoplasm of perineum

SP **C49.6 Malignant neoplasm of connective and soft tissue of trunk, unspecified**
Malignant neoplasm of back NOS

SP **C49.8 Malignant neoplasm of overlapping sites of connective and soft tissue**
Primary malignant neoplasm of two or more contiguous sites of connective and soft tissue

IQ **C49.9 Malignant neoplasm of connective and soft tissue, unspecified**

5 **C49.A Gastrointestinal stromal tumor**

IQ **C49.A0 Gastrointestinal stromal tumor, unspecified site**

SP **C49.A1 Gastrointestinal stromal tumor of esophagus**

SP **C49.A2 Gastrointestinal stromal tumor of stomach**

SP **C49.A3 Gastrointestinal stromal tumor of small intestine**

SP **C49.A4 Gastrointestinal stromal tumor of large intestine**

SP **C49.A5 Gastrointestinal stromal tumor of rectum**

SP **C49.A9 Gastrointestinal stromal tumor of other sites**

Malignant neoplasms of breast (C50)

CODING TIPS✓ Code C50 indicates active cancer. History of cancer to the breast should be coded to Z85.3. Add a Z79.81- code for treatment agents affecting estrogen receptors and estrogen levels.

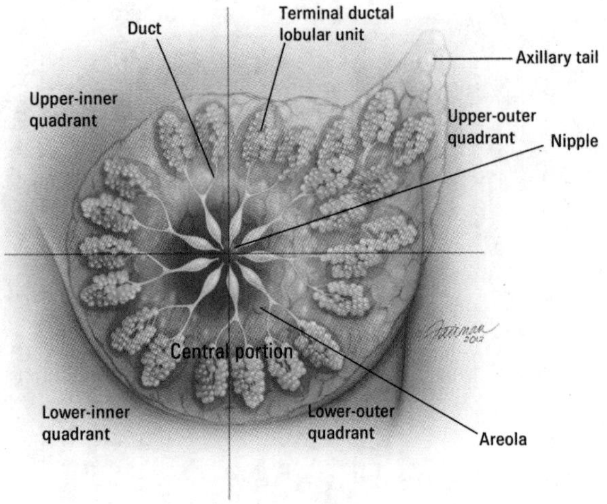

+ 4 **C50 Malignant neoplasm of breast**

INCLUDES connective tissue of breast
Paget's disease of breast
Paget's disease of nipple

Use additional code to identify estrogen receptor status (Z17.0, Z17.1)

EXCLUDES 1 skin of breast (C44.501, C44.511, C44.521, C44.591)

+ 5 C50.0 **Malignant neoplasm of nipple and areola**

+ 6 C50.01 **Malignant neoplasm of nipple and areola, female**

SP + C50.011 **Malignant neoplasm of nipple and areola, right female breast**

SP + C50.012 **Malignant neoplasm of nipple and areola, left female breast**

IQ + C50.019 **Malignant neoplasm of nipple and areola, unspecified female breast**

+ 6 C50.02 **Malignant neoplasm of nipple and areola, male**

SP + C50.021 **Malignant neoplasm of nipple and areola, right male breast**

SP + C50.022 **Malignant neoplasm of nipple and areola, left male breast**

IQ + C50.029 **Malignant neoplasm of nipple and areola, unspecified male breast**

+ 5 C50.1 **Malignant neoplasm of central portion of breast**

+ 6 C50.11 **Malignant neoplasm of central portion of breast, female**

SP + C50.111 **Malignant neoplasm of central portion of right female breast**

SP + C50.112 **Malignant neoplasm of central portion of left female breast**

IQ + C50.119 **Malignant neoplasm of central portion of unspecified female breast**

+ 6 C50.12 **Malignant neoplasm of central portion of breast, male**

SP + C50.121 **Malignant neoplasm of central portion of right male breast**

SP + C50.122 **Malignant neoplasm of central portion of left male breast**

IQ + C50.129 **Malignant neoplasm of central portion of unspecified male breast**

+ 5 C50.2 **Malignant neoplasm of upper-inner quadrant of breast**

+ 6 C50.21 **Malignant neoplasm of upper-inner quadrant of breast, female**

SP + C50.211 **Malignant neoplasm of upper-inner quadrant of right female breast**

SP + C50.212 **Malignant neoplasm of upper-inner quadrant of left female breast**

IQ + C50.219 **Malignant neoplasm of upper-inner quadrant of unspecified female breast**

+ 6 C50.22 **Malignant neoplasm of upper-inner quadrant of breast, male**

SP + C50.221 **Malignant neoplasm of upper-inner quadrant of right male breast**

SP + C50.222 **Malignant neoplasm of upper-inner quadrant of left male breast**

IQ + C50.229 **Malignant neoplasm of upper-inner quadrant of unspecified male breast**

+ 5 C50.3 **Malignant neoplasm of lower-inner quadrant of breast**

+ 6 C50.31 **Malignant neoplasm of lower-inner quadrant of breast, female**

SP + C50.311 **Malignant neoplasm of lower-inner quadrant of right female breast**

SP + C50.312 **Malignant neoplasm of lower-inner quadrant of left female breast**

IQ + C50.319 **Malignant neoplasm of lower-inner quadrant of unspecified female breast**

+ 6 C50.32 **Malignant neoplasm of lower-inner quadrant of breast, male**

SP + C50.321 **Malignant neoplasm of lower-inner quadrant of right male breast**

SP + C50.322 **Malignant neoplasm of lower-inner quadrant of left male breast**

IQ + C50.329 **Malignant neoplasm of lower-inner quadrant of unspecified male breast**

+ 5 C50.4 **Malignant neoplasm of upper-outer quadrant of breast**

+ 6 C50.41 **Malignant neoplasm of upper-outer quadrant of breast, female**

SP + C50.411 **Malignant neoplasm of upper-outer quadrant of right female breast**

SP + C50.412 **Malignant neoplasm of upper-outer quadrant of left female breast**

IQ + C50.419 **Malignant neoplasm of upper-outer quadrant of unspecified female breast**

+ 6 C50.42 **Malignant neoplasm of upper-outer quadrant of breast, male**

SP + C50.421 **Malignant neoplasm of upper-outer quadrant of right male breast**

SP + C50.422 **Malignant neoplasm of upper-outer quadrant of left male breast**

IQ + C50.429 **Malignant neoplasm of upper-outer quadrant of unspecified male breast**

+ 5 C50.5 **Malignant neoplasm of lower-outer quadrant of breast**

+ 6 C50.51 **Malignant neoplasm of lower-outer quadrant of breast, female**

SP + C50.511 **Malignant neoplasm of lower-outer quadrant of right female breast**

SP + C50.512 **Malignant neoplasm of lower-outer quadrant of left female breast**

IQ + C50.519 **Malignant neoplasm of lower-outer quadrant of unspecified female breast**

+ 6 C50.52 **Malignant neoplasm of lower-outer quadrant of breast, male**

⊟ SP + C50.521 **Malignant neoplasm of lower-outer quadrant of right male breast**
⊟ SP + C50.522 **Malignant neoplasm of lower-outer quadrant of left male breast**
⊟ IQ + C50.529 **Malignant neoplasm of lower-outer quadrant of unspecified male breast**

+ 5 C50.6 **Malignant neoplasm of axillary tail of breast**
+ 6 C50.61 **Malignant neoplasm of axillary tail of breast, female**
⊟ SP + C50.611 **Malignant neoplasm of axillary tail of right female breast**
⊟ SP + C50.612 **Malignant neoplasm of axillary tail of left female breast**
⊟ IQ + C50.619 **Malignant neoplasm of axillary tail of unspecified female breast**
+ 6 C50.62 **Malignant neoplasm of axillary tail of breast, male**
⊟ SP + C50.621 **Malignant neoplasm of axillary tail of right male breast**
⊟ SP + C50.622 **Malignant neoplasm of axillary tail of left male breast**
⊟ IQ + C50.629 **Malignant neoplasm of axillary tail of unspecified male breast**

+ 5 C50.8 **Malignant neoplasm of overlapping sites of breast**
+ 6 C50.81 **Malignant neoplasm of overlapping sites of breast, female**
⊟ SP + C50.811 **Malignant neoplasm of overlapping sites of right female breast**
⊟ SP + C50.812 **Malignant neoplasm of overlapping sites of left female breast**
⊟ IQ + C50.819 **Malignant neoplasm of overlapping sites of unspecified female breast**
+ 6 C50.82 **Malignant neoplasm of overlapping sites of breast, male**
⊟ SP + C50.821 **Malignant neoplasm of overlapping sites of right male breast**
⊟ SP + C50.822 **Malignant neoplasm of overlapping sites of left male breast**
⊟ IQ + C50.829 **Malignant neoplasm of overlapping sites of unspecified male breast**

+ 5 C50.9 **Malignant neoplasm of breast of unspecified site**
+ 6 C50.91 **Malignant neoplasm of breast of unspecified site, female**
⊟ SP + C50.911 **Malignant neoplasm of unspecified site of right female breast**
⊟ SP + C50.912 **Malignant neoplasm of unspecified site of left female breast**
⊟ IQ + C50.919 **Malignant neoplasm of unspecified site of unspecified female breast**

CODING TIPS ✓ **Documentation:** If the site is not documented, you **must** query the physician or NPP and specify the site with C50.911 (right breast) or C50.912 (left breast). Use an additional code for estrogen receptor status (Z17.0, Z17.1), when documented.

+ 6 C50.92 **Malignant neoplasm of breast of unspecified site, male**
⊟ SP + C50.921 **Malignant neoplasm of unspecified site of right male breast**
⊟ SP + C50.922 **Malignant neoplasm of unspecified site of left male breast**
⊟ IQ + C50.929 **Malignant neoplasm of unspecified site of unspecified male breast**

Malignant neoplasms of female genital organs (C51-C58)

INCLUDES malignant neoplasm of skin of female genital organs

CODING TIPS ✓ Categories C51-C58 indicate active cancer. See Z85.40-Z85.44 for personal history of primary malignancy of female genital organs and Z85.45-Z85.49 for personal history of primary malignancy of male genital organs.

4 C51 **Malignant neoplasm of vulva**
EXCLUDES 1 carcinoma in situ of vulva (D07.1)
SP C51.0 **Malignant neoplasm of labium majus**
Malignant neoplasm of Bartholin's [greater vestibular] gland
SP C51.1 **Malignant neoplasm of labium minus**
SP C51.2 **Malignant neoplasm of clitoris**
SP C51.8 **Malignant neoplasm of overlapping sites of vulva**
SP C51.9 **Malignant neoplasm of vulva, unspecified**
Malignant neoplasm of external female genitalia NOS
Malignant neoplasm of pudendum

SP C52 **Malignant neoplasm of vagina**
EXCLUDES 1 carcinoma in situ of vagina (D07.2)

4 C53 **Malignant neoplasm of cervix uteri**
EXCLUDES 1 carcinoma in situ of cervix uteri (D06.-)
SP C53.0 **Malignant neoplasm of endocervix**
SP C53.1 **Malignant neoplasm of exocervix**
SP C53.8 **Malignant neoplasm of overlapping sites of cervix uteri**
SP C53.9 **Malignant neoplasm of cervix uteri, unspecified**

4 C54 **Malignant neoplasm of corpus uteri**
SP C54.0 **Malignant neoplasm of isthmus uteri**
Malignant neoplasm of lower uterine segment
SP C54.1 **Malignant neoplasm of endometrium**
SP C54.2 **Malignant neoplasm of myometrium**
SP C54.3 **Malignant neoplasm of fundus uteri**
SP C54.8 **Malignant neoplasm of overlapping sites of corpus uteri**

SP C54.9 **Malignant neoplasm of corpus uteri, unspecified**

SP C55 **Malignant neoplasm of uterus, part unspecified**

+ 4 C56 **Malignant neoplasm of ovary**
Use additional code to identify any functional activity

SP + C56.1 **Malignant neoplasm of right ovary**

SP + C56.2 **Malignant neoplasm of left ovary**

★ + C56.3 **Malignant neoplasm of bilateral ovaries**

IQ + C56.9 **Malignant neoplasm of unspecified ovary**

4 C57 **Malignant neoplasm of other and unspecified female genital organs**

5 C57.0 **Malignant neoplasm of fallopian tube**
Malignant neoplasm of oviduct
Malignant neoplasm of uterine tube

IQ C57.00 **Malignant neoplasm of unspecified fallopian tube**

SP C57.01 **Malignant neoplasm of right fallopian tube**

SP C57.02 **Malignant neoplasm of left fallopian tube**

5 C57.1 **Malignant neoplasm of broad ligament**

IQ C57.10 **Malignant neoplasm of unspecified broad ligament**

SP C57.11 **Malignant neoplasm of right broad ligament**

SP C57.12 **Malignant neoplasm of left broad ligament**

5 C57.2 **Malignant neoplasm of round ligament**

IQ C57.20 **Malignant neoplasm of unspecified round ligament**

SP C57.21 **Malignant neoplasm of right round ligament**

SP C57.22 **Malignant neoplasm of left round ligament**

SP C57.3 **Malignant neoplasm of parametrium**
Malignant neoplasm of uterine ligament NOS

SP C57.4 **Malignant neoplasm of uterine adnexa, unspecified**

SP C57.7 **Malignant neoplasm of other specified female genital organs**
Malignant neoplasm of wolffian body or duct

SP C57.8 **Malignant neoplasm of overlapping sites of female genital organs**
Primary malignant neoplasm of two or more contiguous sites of the female genital organs whose point of origin cannot be determined
Primary tubo-ovarian malignant neoplasm whose point of origin cannot be determined
Primary utero-ovarian malignant neoplasm whose point of origin cannot be determined

IQ C57.9 **Malignant neoplasm of female genital organ, unspecified**
Malignant neoplasm of female genitourinary tract NOS

SP C58 **Malignant neoplasm of placenta**
INCLUDES choriocarcinoma NOS
chorionepithelioma NOS
EXCLUDES 1 chorioadenoma (destruens) (D39.2)
hydatidiform mole NOS (O01.9)
invasive hydatidiform mole (D39.2)
male choriocarcinoma NOS (C62.9-)
malignant hydatidiform mole (D39.2)

Malignant neoplasms of male genital organs (C60-C63)

INCLUDES malignant neoplasm of skin of male genital organs

CODING TIPS✓ Codes classifiable to C60-C63 include active cancer. History of cancer to the male genital organs should be coded to Z85.4-.

4 C60 **Malignant neoplasm of penis**

SP C60.0 **Malignant neoplasm of prepuce**
Malignant neoplasm of foreskin

SP C60.1 **Malignant neoplasm of glans penis**

SP C60.2 **Malignant neoplasm of body of penis**
Malignant neoplasm of corpus cavernosum

SP C60.8 **Malignant neoplasm of overlapping sites of penis**

SP C60.9 **Malignant neoplasm of penis, unspecified**
Malignant neoplasm of skin of penis NOS

SP + C61 **Malignant neoplasm of prostate**
Use additional code to identify:
hormone sensitivity status (Z19.1-Z19.2)
rising PSA following treatment for malignant neoplasm of prostate (R97.21)
EXCLUDES 1 malignant neoplasm of seminal vesicle (C63.7)

+ 4 C62 **Malignant neoplasm of testis**
Use additional code to identify any functional activity

+ 5 C62.0 **Malignant neoplasm of undescended testis**
Malignant neoplasm of ectopic testis
Malignant neoplasm of retained testis

IQ + C62.00 **Malignant neoplasm of unspecified undescended testis**

SP + C62.01 **Malignant neoplasm of undescended right testis**

SP + C62.02 **Malignant neoplasm of undescended left testis**

+ 5 C62.1 **Malignant neoplasm of descended testis**
Malignant neoplasm of scrotal testis

IQ + C62.10 **Malignant neoplasm of unspecified descended testis**

SP + C62.11 **Malignant neoplasm of descended right testis**

SP + C62.12 **Malignant neoplasm of descended left testis**

+ 5 C62.9 **Malignant neoplasm of testis, unspecified whether descended or undescended**

IQ + C62.90 **Malignant neoplasm of unspecified testis, unspecified whether descended or undescended**
Malignant neoplasm of testis NOS

Laterality SP + C62.91 **Malignant neoplasm of right testis, unspecified whether descended or undescended**

Laterality SP + C62.92 **Malignant neoplasm of left testis, unspecified whether descended or undescended**

4 C63 **Malignant neoplasm of other and unspecified male genital organs**

5 C63.0 **Malignant neoplasm of epididymis**

Laterality IQ C63.00 **Malignant neoplasm of unspecified epididymis**

Laterality SP C63.01 **Malignant neoplasm of right epididymis**

Laterality SP C63.02 **Malignant neoplasm of left epididymis**

5 C63.1 **Malignant neoplasm of spermatic cord**

Laterality IQ C63.10 **Malignant neoplasm of unspecified spermatic cord**

Laterality SP C63.11 **Malignant neoplasm of right spermatic cord**

Laterality SP C63.12 **Malignant neoplasm of left spermatic cord**

SP C63.2 **Malignant neoplasm of scrotum**
Malignant neoplasm of skin of scrotum

SP C63.7 **Malignant neoplasm of other specified male genital organs**
Malignant neoplasm of seminal vesicle
Malignant neoplasm of tunica vaginalis

SP C63.8 **Malignant neoplasm of overlapping sites of male genital organs**
Primary malignant neoplasm of two or more contiguous sites of male genital organs whose point of origin cannot be determined

IQ C63.9 **Malignant neoplasm of male genital organ, unspecified**
Malignant neoplasm of male genitourinary tract NOS

Malignant neoplasms of urinary tract (C64-C68)

CODING TIPS ✓ Codes classifiable to C64-C68 include active cancer. History of cancer to the urinary tract should be coded to Z85.5-.

4 C64 **Malignant neoplasm of kidney, except renal pelvis**
EXCLUDES 1 malignant carcinoid tumor of the kidney (C7A.093)
malignant neoplasm of renal calyces (C65.-)
malignant neoplasm of renal pelvis (C65.-)
CODING TIPS ✓ This code indicates active cancer. See Z85.52- for personal history of malignant neoplasm of the kidney.

Laterality SP C64.1 **Malignant neoplasm of right kidney, except renal pelvis**

Laterality SP C64.2 **Malignant neoplasm of left kidney, except renal pelvis**

Laterality IQ C64.9 **Malignant neoplasm of unspecified kidney, except renal pelvis**

4 C65 **Malignant neoplasm of renal pelvis**
INCLUDES malignant neoplasm of pelviureteric junction
malignant neoplasm of renal calyces
CODING TIPS ✓ This code indicates active cancer. See Z85.53 for personal history of the renal pelvis.

Laterality SP C65.1 **Malignant neoplasm of right renal pelvis**

Laterality SP C65.2 **Malignant neoplasm of left renal pelvis**

Laterality IQ C65.9 **Malignant neoplasm of unspecified renal pelvis**

4 C66 **Malignant neoplasm of ureter**
EXCLUDES 1 malignant neoplasm of ureteric orifice of bladder (C67.6)
CODING TIPS ✓ This code indicates active cancer. See Z85.54 for history of primary malignant neoplasm of ureter.

Laterality SP C66.1 **Malignant neoplasm of right ureter**

Laterality SP C66.2 **Malignant neoplasm of left ureter**

Laterality IQ C66.9 **Malignant neoplasm of unspecified ureter**

4 C67 **Malignant neoplasm of bladder**
CODING TIPS ✓ This code indicates active cancer. See Z85.51 for personal history of malignant neoplasm of the bladder.

SP C67.0 **Malignant neoplasm of trigone of bladder**

SP C67.1 **Malignant neoplasm of dome of bladder**

SP C67.2 **Malignant neoplasm of lateral wall of bladder**

SP C67.3 **Malignant neoplasm of anterior wall of bladder**

SP C67.4 **Malignant neoplasm of posterior wall of bladder**

SP C67.5 **Malignant neoplasm of bladder neck**
Malignant neoplasm of internal urethral orifice

SP C67.6 **Malignant neoplasm of ureteric orifice**

SP C67.7 **Malignant neoplasm of urachus**

SP C67.8 **Malignant neoplasm of overlapping sites of bladder**

SP C67.9 **Malignant neoplasm of bladder, unspecified**

4 C68 **Malignant neoplasm of other and unspecified urinary organs**
EXCLUDES 1 malignant neoplasm of female genitourinary tract NOS (C57.9)
malignant neoplasm of male genitourinary tract NOS (C63.9)

SP C68.0 **Malignant neoplasm of urethra**
EXCLUDES 1 malignant neoplasm of urethral orifice of bladder (C67.5)

SP C68.1 **Malignant neoplasm of paraurethral glands**

SP C68.8 **Malignant neoplasm of overlapping sites of urinary organs**
Primary malignant neoplasm of two or more contiguous sites of urinary organs whose point of origin cannot be determined

IQ C68.9 **Malignant neoplasm of urinary organ, unspecified**
Malignant neoplasm of urinary system NOS

Malignant neoplasms of eye, brain and other parts of central nervous system (C69-C72)

CODING TIPS✓ Codes classifiable to C69-C72 include active cancer. History of cancer to eye, brain, or other area of nervous system should be coded to Z85.84-.

4 **C69 Malignant neoplasm of eye and adnexa**
EXCLUDES 1 malignant neoplasm of connective tissue of eyelid (C49.0)
malignant neoplasm of eyelid (skin) (C43.1-, C44.1-)
malignant neoplasm of optic nerve (C72.3-)

CODING TIPS✓ This code indicates active cancer. See Z85.840 for personal history of malignant neoplasm of the eye.

5 **C69.0 Malignant neoplasm of conjunctiva**
IQ **C69.00 Malignant neoplasm of unspecified conjunctiva**
SP **C69.01 Malignant neoplasm of right conjunctiva**
SP **C69.02 Malignant neoplasm of left conjunctiva**
5 **C69.1 Malignant neoplasm of cornea**
IQ **C69.10 Malignant neoplasm of unspecified cornea**
SP **C69.11 Malignant neoplasm of right cornea**
SP **C69.12 Malignant neoplasm of left cornea**
5 **C69.2 Malignant neoplasm of retina**
EXCLUDES 1 dark area on retina (D49.81)
neoplasm of unspecified behavior of retina and choroid (D49.81)
retinal freckle (D49.81)
IQ **C69.20 Malignant neoplasm of unspecified retina**
SP **C69.21 Malignant neoplasm of right retina**
SP **C69.22 Malignant neoplasm of left retina**
5 **C69.3 Malignant neoplasm of choroid**
IQ **C69.30 Malignant neoplasm of unspecified choroid**
SP **C69.31 Malignant neoplasm of right choroid**
SP **C69.32 Malignant neoplasm of left choroid**
5 **C69.4 Malignant neoplasm of ciliary body**
IQ **C69.40 Malignant neoplasm of unspecified ciliary body**
SP **C69.41 Malignant neoplasm of right ciliary body**
SP **C69.42 Malignant neoplasm of left ciliary body**
5 **C69.5 Malignant neoplasm of lacrimal gland and duct**
Malignant neoplasm of lacrimal sac
Malignant neoplasm of nasolacrimal duct
IQ **C69.50 Malignant neoplasm of unspecified lacrimal gland and duct**
SP **C69.51 Malignant neoplasm of right lacrimal gland and duct**
SP **C69.52 Malignant neoplasm of left lacrimal gland and duct**
5 **C69.6 Malignant neoplasm of orbit**
Malignant neoplasm of connective tissue of orbit
Malignant neoplasm of extraocular muscle
Malignant neoplasm of peripheral nerves of orbit
Malignant neoplasm of retrobulbar tissue
Malignant neoplasm of retro-ocular tissue
EXCLUDES 1 malignant neoplasm of orbital bone (C41.0)
IQ **C69.60 Malignant neoplasm of unspecified orbit**
SP **C69.61 Malignant neoplasm of right orbit**
SP **C69.62 Malignant neoplasm of left orbit**
5 **C69.8 Malignant neoplasm of overlapping sites of eye and adnexa**
IQ **C69.80 Malignant neoplasm of overlapping sites of unspecified eye and adnexa**
SP **C69.81 Malignant neoplasm of overlapping sites of right eye and adnexa**
SP **C69.82 Malignant neoplasm of overlapping sites of left eye and adnexa**
5 **C69.9 Malignant neoplasm of unspecified site of eye**
Malignant neoplasm of eyeball
IQ **C69.90 Malignant neoplasm of unspecified site of unspecified eye**
SP **C69.91 Malignant neoplasm of unspecified site of right eye**
SP **C69.92 Malignant neoplasm of unspecified site of left eye**

4 **C70 Malignant neoplasm of meninges**
SP **C70.0 Malignant neoplasm of cerebral meninges**
SP **C70.1 Malignant neoplasm of spinal meninges**
SP **C70.9 Malignant neoplasm of meninges, unspecified**

4 **C71 Malignant neoplasm of brain**
EXCLUDES 1 malignant neoplasm of cranial nerves (C72.2-C72.5)
retrobulbar malignant neoplasm (C69.6-)

CODING TIPS✓ C71 indicates active cancer. See Z85.841 for personal history of malignant neoplasm of the brain. Metastasis to the brain is seen more often than a primary lesion. Metastases to the brain are coded with C79.31.

SP **C71.0 Malignant neoplasm of cerebrum, except lobes and ventricles**
Malignant neoplasm of supratentorial NOS
SP **C71.1 Malignant neoplasm of frontal lobe**
SP **C71.2 Malignant neoplasm of temporal lobe**
SP **C71.3 Malignant neoplasm of parietal lobe**
SP **C71.4 Malignant neoplasm of occipital lobe**
SP **C71.5 Malignant neoplasm of cerebral ventricle**
EXCLUDES 1 malignant neoplasm of fourth cerebral ventricle (C71.7)
SP **C71.6 Malignant neoplasm of cerebellum**
SP **C71.7 Malignant neoplasm of brain stem**
Malignant neoplasm of fourth cerebral ventricle
Infratentorial malignant neoplasm NOS

SP **C71.8 Malignant neoplasm of overlapping sites of brain**

SP **C71.9 Malignant neoplasm of brain, unspecified**

4 **C72 Malignant neoplasm of spinal cord, cranial nerves and other parts of central nervous system**

EXCLUDES 1 malignant neoplasm of meninges (C70.-)
malignant neoplasm of peripheral nerves and autonomic nervous system (C47.-)

CODING TIPS✓ This code indicates active cancer. See Z85.848 for personal history of malignant neoplasm to other parts of the nervous system.

SP **C72.0 Malignant neoplasm of spinal cord**

SP **C72.1 Malignant neoplasm of cauda equina**

5 **C72.2 Malignant neoplasm of olfactory nerve**
Malignant neoplasm of olfactory bulb

Laterality IQ **C72.20 Malignant neoplasm of unspecified olfactory nerve**

Laterality SP **C72.21 Malignant neoplasm of right olfactory nerve**

Laterality SP **C72.22 Malignant neoplasm of left olfactory nerve**

5 **C72.3 Malignant neoplasm of optic nerve**

Laterality IQ **C72.30 Malignant neoplasm of unspecified optic nerve**

Laterality SP **C72.31 Malignant neoplasm of right optic nerve**

Laterality SP **C72.32 Malignant neoplasm of left optic nerve**

5 **C72.4 Malignant neoplasm of acoustic nerve**

Laterality IQ **C72.40 Malignant neoplasm of unspecified acoustic nerve**

Laterality SP **C72.41 Malignant neoplasm of right acoustic nerve**

Laterality SP **C72.42 Malignant neoplasm of left acoustic nerve**

5 **C72.5 Malignant neoplasm of other and unspecified cranial nerves**

IQ **C72.50 Malignant neoplasm of unspecified cranial nerve**
Malignant neoplasm of cranial nerve NOS

SP **C72.59 Malignant neoplasm of other cranial nerves**

SP **C72.9 Malignant neoplasm of central nervous system, unspecified**
Malignant neoplasm of unspecified site of central nervous system
Malignant neoplasm of nervous system NOS

Malignant neoplasms of thyroid and other endocrine glands (C73-C75)

CODING TIPS✓ Codes classifiable to C73-C75 include active cancer. History of cancer to endocrine glands should be coded to Z85.85-.

SP + **C73 Malignant neoplasm of thyroid gland**
Use additional code to identify any functional activity

CODING TIPS✓ Category C73 indicates active cancer. See Z85.850 for personal history of primary malignancy of the thyroid if the thyroid cancer has been eradicated. If the cancer is being treated, code the cancer. If the malignancy is causing abnormal secretion of thyroid hormones, the effects of the thyroid hormones should also be coded.

4 **C74 Malignant neoplasm of adrenal gland**

CODING TIPS✓ This code indicates active cancer. See Z85.858 for personal history of primary history of other endocrine glands if cancer has been eradicated. If cancer is being treated, code the cancer, not the Z code. If the cancer is causing abnormal secretion of hormones, the effects of the hormones should also be coded.

5 **C74.0 Malignant neoplasm of cortex of adrenal gland**

Laterality SP **C74.00 Malignant neoplasm of cortex of unspecified adrenal gland**

Laterality SP **C74.01 Malignant neoplasm of cortex of right adrenal gland**

Laterality SP **C74.02 Malignant neoplasm of cortex of left adrenal gland**

5 **C74.1 Malignant neoplasm of medulla of adrenal gland**

Laterality IQ **C74.10 Malignant neoplasm of medulla of unspecified adrenal gland**

Laterality SP **C74.11 Malignant neoplasm of medulla of right adrenal gland**

Laterality SP **C74.12 Malignant neoplasm of medulla of left adrenal gland**

5 **C74.9 Malignant neoplasm of unspecified part of adrenal gland**

Laterality IQ **C74.90 Malignant neoplasm of unspecified part of unspecified adrenal gland**

Laterality SP **C74.91 Malignant neoplasm of unspecified part of right adrenal gland**

Laterality SP **C74.92 Malignant neoplasm of unspecified part of left adrenal gland**

4 **C75 Malignant neoplasm of other endocrine glands and related structures**

EXCLUDES 1 malignant carcinoid tumors (C7A.0-)
malignant neoplasm of adrenal gland (C74.-)
malignant neoplasm of endocrine pancreas (C25.4)
malignant neoplasm of islets of Langerhans (C25.4)
malignant neoplasm of ovary (C56.-)
malignant neoplasm of testis (C62.-)
malignant neoplasm of thymus (C37)
malignant neoplasm of thyroid gland (C73)
malignant neuroendocrine tumors (C7A.-)

CODING TIPS ✓ This code indicates active cancer. See Z85.858 for personal history of primary history of other endocrine glands if cancer has been eradicated. If cancer is being treated, code the cancer, not the Z code. If the cancer is causing abnormal secretion of hormones, the effects of the hormones should also be coded.

SP **C75.0 Malignant neoplasm of parathyroid gland**

SP **C75.1 Malignant neoplasm of pituitary gland**

SP **C75.2 Malignant neoplasm of craniopharyngeal duct**

SP **C75.3 Malignant neoplasm of pineal gland**

SP **C75.4 Malignant neoplasm of carotid body**

SP **C75.5 Malignant neoplasm of aortic body and other paraganglia**

SP **C75.8 Malignant neoplasm with pluriglandular involvement, unspecified**

SP **C75.9 Malignant neoplasm of endocrine gland, unspecified**

Malignant neuroendocrine tumors (C7A)

CODING TIPS ✓ Codes classifiable to C7A- include primary neuroendocrine tumors, which are considered active malignant carcinoid tumors. A history of any malignant carcinoid tumor (neuroendocrine malignancy) should be coded to the appropriate Z85- code for history of malignant carcinoid tumor of that specific anatomical location.

+ 4 **C7A Malignant neuroendocrine tumors**

Code also:

any associated multiple endocrine neoplasia [MEN] syndromes (E31.2-)

Use additional code to identify any associated endocrine syndrome, such as:

carcinoid syndrome (E34.0)

EXCLUDES 2 malignant pancreatic islet cell tumors (C25.4)

Merkel cell carcinoma (C4A.-)

+ 5 **C7A.0 Malignant carcinoid tumors**

IQ + **C7A.00 Malignant carcinoid tumor of unspecified site**

+ 6 **C7A.01 Malignant carcinoid tumors of the small intestine**

SP + **C7A.010 Malignant carcinoid tumor of the duodenum**

SP + **C7A.011 Malignant carcinoid tumor of the jejunum**

SP + **C7A.012 Malignant carcinoid tumor of the ileum**

SP + **C7A.019 Malignant carcinoid tumor of the small intestine, unspecified portion**

+ 6 **C7A.02 Malignant carcinoid tumors of the appendix, large intestine, and rectum**

SP + **C7A.020 Malignant carcinoid tumor of the appendix**

SP + **C7A.021 Malignant carcinoid tumor of the cecum**

SP + **C7A.022 Malignant carcinoid tumor of the ascending colon**

SP + **C7A.023 Malignant carcinoid tumor of the transverse colon**

SP + **C7A.024 Malignant carcinoid tumor of the descending colon**

SP + **C7A.025 Malignant carcinoid tumor of the sigmoid colon**

SP + **C7A.026 Malignant carcinoid tumor of the rectum**

SP + **C7A.029 Malignant carcinoid tumor of the large intestine, unspecified portion**

Malignant carcinoid tumor of the colon NOS

+ 6 **C7A.09 Malignant carcinoid tumors of other sites**

SP + **C7A.090 Malignant carcinoid tumor of the bronchus and lung**

SP + **C7A.091 Malignant carcinoid tumor of the thymus**

SP + **C7A.092 Malignant carcinoid tumor of the stomach**

SP + **C7A.093 Malignant carcinoid tumor of the kidney**

SP + **C7A.094 Malignant carcinoid tumor of the foregut, unspecified**

SP + **C7A.095 Malignant carcinoid tumor of the midgut, unspecified**

SP + **C7A.096 Malignant carcinoid tumor of the hindgut, unspecified**

SP + **C7A.098 Malignant carcinoid tumors of other sites**

SP + **C7A.1 Malignant poorly differentiated neuroendocrine tumors**

Malignant poorly differentiated neuroendocrine tumor NOS

Malignant poorly differentiated neuroendocrine carcinoma, any site

High grade neuroendocrine carcinoma, any site

SP + **C7A.8 Other malignant neuroendocrine tumors**

Secondary neuroendocrine tumors (C7B)

CODING TIPS ✓ Codes classifiable to C7B- include secondary (metastases) neuroendocrine tumors, which are considered active malignant carcinoid tumors.

+ 4 **C7B Secondary neuroendocrine tumors**

Use additional code to identify any functional activity

+ 5 **C7B.0 Secondary carcinoid tumors**

IQ + **C7B.00 Secondary carcinoid tumors, unspecified site**

SP + **C7B.01 Secondary carcinoid tumors of distant lymph nodes**

SP + **C7B.02 Secondary carcinoid tumors of liver**

SP + **C7B.03 Secondary carcinoid tumors of bone**

SP + **C7B.04 Secondary carcinoid tumors of peritoneum**

Mesentary metastasis of carcinoid tumor

SP + **C7B.09 Secondary carcinoid tumors of other sites**

SP + **C7B.1 Secondary Merkel cell carcinoma**

Merkel cell carcinoma nodal presentation

Merkel cell carcinoma visceral metastatic presentation

SP + **C7B.8 Other secondary neuroendocrine tumors**

Malignant neoplasms of ill-defined, other secondary and unspecified sites (C76-C80)

4 **C76 Malignant neoplasm of other and ill-defined sites**

EXCLUDES 1 malignant neoplasm of female genitourinary tract NOS (C57.9)
malignant neoplasm of male genitourinary tract NOS (C63.9)
malignant neoplasm of lymphoid, hematopoietic and related tissue (C81-C96)
malignant neoplasm of skin (C44.-)
malignant neoplasm of unspecified site NOS (C80.1)

CODING TIPS ✓ Query the physician or NPP before assigning codes from C76. For example, if the documentation indicates cancer of the nose: Is it the nasal passages, skin on the nose, the cartilage of the nose?

SP **C76.0 Malignant neoplasm of head, face and neck**
Malignant neoplasm of cheek NOS
Malignant neoplasm of nose NOS

SP **C76.1 Malignant neoplasm of thorax**
Intrathoracic malignant neoplasm NOS
Malignant neoplasm of axilla NOS
Thoracic malignant neoplasm NOS

SP **C76.2 Malignant neoplasm of abdomen**

SP **C76.3 Malignant neoplasm of pelvis**
Malignant neoplasm of groin NOS
Malignant neoplasm of sites overlapping systems within the pelvis
Rectovaginal (septum) malignant neoplasm
Rectovesical (septum) malignant neoplasm

5 **C76.4 Malignant neoplasm of upper limb**

Laterality IQ **C76.40 Malignant neoplasm of unspecified upper limb**

Laterality SP **C76.41 Malignant neoplasm of right upper limb**

Laterality SP **C76.42 Malignant neoplasm of left upper limb**

5 **C76.5 Malignant neoplasm of lower limb**

Laterality IQ **C76.50 Malignant neoplasm of unspecified lower limb**

Laterality SP **C76.51 Malignant neoplasm of right lower limb**

Laterality SP **C76.52 Malignant neoplasm of left lower limb**

SP **C76.8 Malignant neoplasm of other specified ill-defined sites**
Malignant neoplasm of overlapping ill-defined sites

4 **C77 Secondary and unspecified malignant neoplasm of lymph nodes**

EXCLUDES 1 malignant neoplasm of lymph nodes, specified as primary (C81-C86, C88, C96.-)
mesentary metastasis of carcinoid tumor (C7B.04)
secondary carcinoid tumors of distant lymph nodes (C7B.01)

CODING TIPS ✓ Codes classifiable to C77- include neoplasms specified as secondary or metastatic sites of cancer. Primary neoplasms of lymphatic tissue should not be assigned codes from C77-. See C7B for secondary neuroendocrine tumors, such as carcinoid tumors and Merkel cell carcinoma.

SP **C77.0 Secondary and unspecified malignant neoplasm of lymph nodes of head, face and neck**
Secondary and unspecified malignant neoplasm of supraclavicular lymph nodes

SP **C77.1 Secondary and unspecified malignant neoplasm of intrathoracic lymph nodes**

SP **C77.2 Secondary and unspecified malignant neoplasm of intra-abdominal lymph nodes**

SP **C77.3 Secondary and unspecified malignant neoplasm of axilla and upper limb lymph nodes**
Secondary and unspecified malignant neoplasm of pectoral lymph nodes

SP **C77.4 Secondary and unspecified malignant neoplasm of inguinal and lower limb lymph nodes**

SP **C77.5 Secondary and unspecified malignant neoplasm of intrapelvic lymph nodes**

SP **C77.8 Secondary and unspecified malignant neoplasm of lymph nodes of multiple regions**

IQ **C77.9 Secondary and unspecified malignant neoplasm of lymph node, unspecified**

4 **C78 Secondary malignant neoplasm of respiratory and digestive organs**

EXCLUDES 1 secondary carcinoid tumors of liver (C7B.02)
secondary carcinoid tumors of peritoneum (C7B.04)

EXCLUDES 2 lymph node metastases (C77.0)

CODING TIPS ✓ Codes classifiable to C78- include neoplasms specified as secondary or metastatic sites of cancer. Primary neoplasms should not be assigned codes from C78-. See C7B for secondary neuroendocrine tumors, such as carcinoid tumors and Merkel cell carcinoma.

5 **C78.0 Secondary malignant neoplasm of lung**

Laterality IQ **C78.00 Secondary malignant neoplasm of unspecified lung**

Laterality SP **C78.01 Secondary malignant neoplasm of right lung**

Laterality SP **C78.02 Secondary malignant neoplasm of left lung**

SP **C78.1 Secondary malignant neoplasm of mediastinum**

SP **C78.2 Secondary malignant neoplasm of pleura**

5 **C78.3 Secondary malignant neoplasm of other and unspecified respiratory organs**

IQ C78.30 **Secondary malignant neoplasm of unspecified respiratory organ**

SP C78.39 **Secondary malignant neoplasm of other respiratory organs**

SP C78.4 **Secondary malignant neoplasm of small intestine**

SP C78.5 **Secondary malignant neoplasm of large intestine and rectum**

SP C78.6 **Secondary malignant neoplasm of retroperitoneum and peritoneum**

SP C78.7 **Secondary malignant neoplasm of liver and intrahepatic bile duct**

5 C78.8 **Secondary malignant neoplasm of other and unspecified digestive organs**

IQ C78.80 **Secondary malignant neoplasm of unspecified digestive organ**

SP C78.89 **Secondary malignant neoplasm of other digestive organs**

Code also:
exocrine pancreatic insufficiency (K86.81)

4 C79 **Secondary malignant neoplasm of other and unspecified sites**

EXCLUDES 1 secondary carcinoid tumors (C7B.-)
secondary neuroendocrine tumors (C7B.-)

CODING TIPS✓ Codes classifiable to C79- include neoplasms specified as secondary or metastatic sites of cancer. Primary neoplasms should not be assigned codes from C79-. See C7B for secondary neuroendocrine tumors, such as carcinoid tumors and Merkel cell carcinoma.

5 C79.0 **Secondary malignant neoplasm of kidney and renal pelvis**

⊟ IQ C79.00 **Secondary malignant neoplasm of unspecified kidney and renal pelvis**

⊟ SP C79.01 **Secondary malignant neoplasm of right kidney and renal pelvis**

⊟ SP C79.02 **Secondary malignant neoplasm of left kidney and renal pelvis**

5 C79.1 **Secondary malignant neoplasm of bladder and other and unspecified urinary organs**

IQ C79.10 **Secondary malignant neoplasm of unspecified urinary organs**

SP C79.11 **Secondary malignant neoplasm of bladder**

EXCLUDES 2 lymph node metastases (C77.0)

SP C79.19 **Secondary malignant neoplasm of other urinary organs**

SP C79.2 **Secondary malignant neoplasm of skin**

EXCLUDES 1 secondary Merkel cell carcinoma (C7B.1)

5 C79.3 **Secondary malignant neoplasm of brain and cerebral meninges**

SP C79.31 **Secondary malignant neoplasm of brain**

SP C79.32 **Secondary malignant neoplasm of cerebral meninges**

5 C79.4 **Secondary malignant neoplasm of other and unspecified parts of nervous system**

IQ C79.40 **Secondary malignant neoplasm of unspecified part of nervous system**

SP C79.49 **Secondary malignant neoplasm of other parts of nervous system**

5 C79.5 **Secondary malignant neoplasm of bone and bone marrow**

EXCLUDES 1 secondary carcinoid tumors of bone (C7B.03)

SP C79.51 **Secondary malignant neoplasm of bone**

SP C79.52 **Secondary malignant neoplasm of bone marrow**

5 C79.6 **Secondary malignant neoplasm of ovary**

⊟ IQ C79.60 **Secondary malignant neoplasm of unspecified ovary**

⊟ SP C79.61 **Secondary malignant neoplasm of right ovary**

⊟ SP C79.62 **Secondary malignant neoplasm of left ovary**

★ ⊟ C79.63 **Secondary malignant neoplasm of bilateral ovaries**

5 C79.7 **Secondary malignant neoplasm of adrenal gland**

⊟ IQ C79.70 **Secondary malignant neoplasm of unspecified adrenal gland**

⊟ SP C79.71 **Secondary malignant neoplasm of right adrenal gland**

⊟ SP C79.72 **Secondary malignant neoplasm of left adrenal gland**

5 C79.8 **Secondary malignant neoplasm of other specified sites**

SP C79.81 **Secondary malignant neoplasm of breast**

SP C79.82 **Secondary malignant neoplasm of genital organs**

SP C79.89 **Secondary malignant neoplasm of other specified sites**

IQ C79.9 **Secondary malignant neoplasm of unspecified site**

Metastatic cancer NOS
Metastatic disease NOS

EXCLUDES 1 carcinomatosis NOS (C80.0)
generalized cancer NOS (C80.0)
malignant (primary) neoplasm of unspecified site (C80.1)

CODING TIPS✓ This code should be reported if the physician or NPP documents metastasis but does not indicate the location. Query the physician or NPP prior to using this code.

4 C80 **Malignant neoplasm without specification of site**

EXCLUDES 1 malignant carcinoid tumor of unspecified site (C7A.00)
malignant neoplasm of specified multiple sites- code to each site

SP C80.0 **Disseminated malignant neoplasm, unspecified**

Carcinomatosis NOS
Generalized cancer, unspecified site (primary) (secondary)
Generalized malignancy, unspecified site (primary) (secondary)

Chapter 2 C00-D49

GUIDELINES **Section I.C.2.j**
Code C80.0 is for use only in those cases where the patient has advanced metastatic disease and no known primary or secondary sites are specified. It should not be used in place of assigning codes for the primary site and all known secondary sites.

CODING TIPS✓ This code is used to indicate that the cancer is in multiple locations and no attempt will be made to identify the primary and secondary sites. Advanced metatastic disease may be documented. If there are multiple sites specified, code to each site.

IQ **C80.1 Malignant (primary) neoplasm, unspecified**
Cancer NOS
Cancer unspecified site (primary)
Carcinoma unspecified site (primary)
Malignancy unspecified site (primary)
EXCLUDES 1 secondary malignant neoplasm of unspecified site (C79.9)

GUIDELINES **Section I.C.2.k**
Code C80.1 equates to Cancer, unspecified. This code should only be used when no determination can be made as to the primary site of a malignancy. This code should rarely be used in the inpatient setting.

CODING TIPS✓ When coding a secondary site of the cancer and the primary site is unknown, C80.1 should be added for unknown primary site. A biopsy-proven malignancy for which a primary site cannot be found constitutes 0.5% to 7% of all cancer patients.

IQ + **C80.2 Malignant neoplasm associated with transplanted organ**
Code first:
complication of transplanted organ (T86.-)
Use additional code to identify the specific malignancy

GUIDELINES **Section I.C.2.r**
A malignant neoplasm of a transplanted organ should be coded as a transplant complication. Assign first the appropriate code from category T86.-, Complications of transplanted organs and tissue, followed by code C80.2. Use an additional code for the specific malignancy.

Malignant neoplasms of lymphoid, hematopoietic and related tissue (C81-C96)

EXCLUDES 2 Kaposi's sarcoma of lymph nodes (C46.3)
secondary and unspecified neoplasm of lymph nodes (C77.-)
secondary neoplasm of bone marrow (C79.52)
secondary neoplasm of spleen (C78.89)

CODING TIPS✓ Codes classifiable to C81-C96 include active malignancy of lymphoid, hematopeotic and related tissues. Secondary neoplastic disease of lymph tissue should not be coded using codes from C81-C96.

4 **C81 Hodgkin lymphoma**
EXCLUDES 1 personal history of Hodgkin lymphoma (Z85.71)

5 **C81.0 Nodular lymphocyte predominant Hodgkin lymphoma**
SP **C81.00 Nodular lymphocyte predominant Hodgkin lymphoma, unspecified site**
SP **C81.01 Nodular lymphocyte predominant Hodgkin lymphoma, lymph nodes of head, face, and neck**
SP **C81.02 Nodular lymphocyte predominant Hodgkin lymphoma, intrathoracic lymph nodes**
SP **C81.03 Nodular lymphocyte predominant Hodgkin lymphoma, intra-abdominal lymph nodes**
SP **C81.04 Nodular lymphocyte predominant Hodgkin lymphoma, lymph nodes of axilla and upper limb**
SP **C81.05 Nodular lymphocyte predominant Hodgkin lymphoma, lymph nodes of inguinal region and lower limb**
SP **C81.06 Nodular lymphocyte predominant Hodgkin lymphoma, intrapelvic lymph nodes**
SP **C81.07 Nodular lymphocyte predominant Hodgkin lymphoma, spleen**
SP **C81.08 Nodular lymphocyte predominant Hodgkin lymphoma, lymph nodes of multiple sites**
SP **C81.09 Nodular lymphocyte predominant Hodgkin lymphoma, extranodal and solid organ sites**

5 **C81.1 Nodular sclerosis Hodgkin lymphoma**
Nodular sclerosis classical Hodgkin lymphoma
SP **C81.10 Nodular sclerosis Hodgkin lymphoma, unspecified site**
SP **C81.11 Nodular sclerosis Hodgkin lymphoma, lymph nodes of head, face, and neck**
SP **C81.12 Nodular sclerosis Hodgkin lymphoma, intrathoracic lymph nodes**
SP **C81.13 Nodular sclerosis Hodgkin lymphoma, intra-abdominal lymph nodes**
SP **C81.14 Nodular sclerosis Hodgkin lymphoma, lymph nodes of axilla and upper limb**
SP **C81.15 Nodular sclerosis Hodgkin lymphoma, lymph nodes of inguinal region and lower limb**
SP **C81.16 Nodular sclerosis Hodgkin lymphoma, intrapelvic lymph nodes**
SP **C81.17 Nodular sclerosis Hodgkin lymphoma, spleen**
SP **C81.18 Nodular sclerosis Hodgkin lymphoma, lymph nodes of multiple sites**
SP **C81.19 Nodular sclerosis Hodgkin lymphoma, extranodal and solid organ sites**

5 **C81.2 Mixed cellularity Hodgkin lymphoma**
Mixed cellularity classical Hodgkin lymphoma

Chapter 2
C00-D49

4 4th digit required 5 5th digit required 6 6th digit required 7 7th digit required 7 7th digit placeholder + Additional code Laterality

SP C81.20 Mixed cellularity Hodgkin lymphoma, unspecified site
SP C81.21 Mixed cellularity Hodgkin lymphoma, lymph nodes of head, face, and neck
SP C81.22 Mixed cellularity Hodgkin lymphoma, intrathoracic lymph nodes
SP C81.23 Mixed cellularity Hodgkin lymphoma, intra-abdominal lymph nodes
SP C81.24 Mixed cellularity Hodgkin lymphoma, lymph nodes of axilla and upper limb
SP C81.25 Mixed cellularity Hodgkin lymphoma, lymph nodes of inguinal region and lower limb
SP C81.26 Mixed cellularity Hodgkin lymphoma, intrapelvic lymph nodes
SP C81.27 Mixed cellularity Hodgkin lymphoma, spleen
SP C81.28 Mixed cellularity Hodgkin lymphoma, lymph nodes of multiple sites
SP C81.29 Mixed cellularity Hodgkin lymphoma, extranodal and solid organ sites

5 **C81.3 Lymphocyte depleted Hodgkin lymphoma**
Lymphocyte depleted classical Hodgkin lymphoma

SP C81.30 Lymphocyte depleted Hodgkin lymphoma, unspecified site
SP C81.31 Lymphocyte depleted Hodgkin lymphoma, lymph nodes of head, face, and neck
SP C81.32 Lymphocyte depleted Hodgkin lymphoma, intrathoracic lymph nodes
SP C81.33 Lymphocyte depleted Hodgkin lymphoma, intra-abdominal lymph nodes
SP C81.34 Lymphocyte depleted Hodgkin lymphoma, lymph nodes of axilla and upper limb
SP C81.35 Lymphocyte depleted Hodgkin lymphoma, lymph nodes of inguinal region and lower limb
SP C81.36 Lymphocyte depleted Hodgkin lymphoma, intrapelvic lymph nodes
SP C81.37 Lymphocyte depleted Hodgkin lymphoma, spleen
SP C81.38 Lymphocyte depleted Hodgkin lymphoma, lymph nodes of multiple sites
SP C81.39 Lymphocyte depleted Hodgkin lymphoma, extranodal and solid organ sites

5 **C81.4 Lymphocyte-rich Hodgkin lymphoma**
Lymphocyte-rich classical Hodgkin lymphoma

EXCLUDES 1 nodular lymphocyte predominant Hodgkin lymphoma (C81.0-)

SP C81.40 Lymphocyte-rich Hodgkin lymphoma, unspecified site
SP C81.41 Lymphocyte-rich Hodgkin lymphoma, lymph nodes of head, face, and neck
SP C81.42 Lymphocyte-rich Hodgkin lymphoma, intrathoracic lymph nodes
SP C81.43 Lymphocyte-rich Hodgkin lymphoma, intra-abdominal lymph nodes
SP C81.44 Lymphocyte-rich Hodgkin lymphoma, lymph nodes of axilla and upper limb
SP C81.45 Lymphocyte-rich Hodgkin lymphoma, lymph nodes of inguinal region and lower limb
SP C81.46 Lymphocyte-rich Hodgkin lymphoma, intrapelvic lymph nodes
SP C81.47 Lymphocyte-rich Hodgkin lymphoma, spleen
SP C81.48 Lymphocyte-rich Hodgkin lymphoma, lymph nodes of multiple sites
SP C81.49 Lymphocyte-rich Hodgkin lymphoma, extranodal and solid organ sites

5 **C81.7 Other Hodgkin lymphoma**
Classical Hodgkin lymphoma NOS
Other classical Hodgkin lymphoma

SP C81.70 Other Hodgkin lymphoma, unspecified site
SP C81.71 Other Hodgkin lymphoma, lymph nodes of head, face, and neck
SP C81.72 Other Hodgkin lymphoma, intrathoracic lymph nodes
SP C81.73 Other Hodgkin lymphoma, intra-abdominal lymph nodes
SP C81.74 Other Hodgkin lymphoma, lymph nodes of axilla and upper limb
SP C81.75 Other Hodgkin lymphoma, lymph nodes of inguinal region and lower limb
SP C81.76 Other Hodgkin lymphoma, intrapelvic lymph nodes
SP C81.77 Other Hodgkin lymphoma, spleen
SP C81.78 Other Hodgkin lymphoma, lymph nodes of multiple sites
SP C81.79 Other Hodgkin lymphoma, extranodal and solid organ sites

5 **C81.9 Hodgkin lymphoma, unspecified**

SP C81.90 Hodgkin lymphoma, unspecified, unspecified site
SP C81.91 Hodgkin lymphoma, unspecified, lymph nodes of head, face, and neck
SP C81.92 Hodgkin lymphoma, unspecified, intrathoracic lymph nodes
SP C81.93 Hodgkin lymphoma, unspecified, intra-abdominal lymph nodes
SP C81.94 Hodgkin lymphoma, unspecified, lymph nodes of axilla and upper limb
SP C81.95 Hodgkin lymphoma, unspecified, lymph nodes of inguinal region and lower limb
SP C81.96 Hodgkin lymphoma, unspecified, intrapelvic lymph nodes

SP C81.97 Hodgkin lymphoma, unspecified, spleen

SP C81.98 Hodgkin lymphoma, unspecified, lymph nodes of multiple sites

SP C81.99 Hodgkin lymphoma, unspecified, extranodal and solid organ sites

4 C82 Follicular lymphoma

INCLUDES follicular lymphoma with or without diffuse areas

EXCLUDES 1 mature T/NK-cell lymphomas (C84.-)
personal history of non-Hodgkin lymphoma (Z85.72)

5 C82.0 Follicular lymphoma grade I

SP C82.00 Follicular lymphoma grade I, unspecified site

SP C82.01 Follicular lymphoma grade I, lymph nodes of head, face, and neck

SP C82.02 Follicular lymphoma grade I, intrathoracic lymph nodes

SP C82.03 Follicular lymphoma grade I, intra-abdominal lymph nodes

SP C82.04 Follicular lymphoma grade I, lymph nodes of axilla and upper limb

SP C82.05 Follicular lymphoma grade I, lymph nodes of inguinal region and lower limb

SP C82.06 Follicular lymphoma grade I, intrapelvic lymph nodes

SP C82.07 Follicular lymphoma grade I, spleen

SP C82.08 Follicular lymphoma grade I, lymph nodes of multiple sites

SP C82.09 Follicular lymphoma grade I, extranodal and solid organ sites

5 C82.1 Follicular lymphoma grade II

SP C82.10 Follicular lymphoma grade II, unspecified site

SP C82.11 Follicular lymphoma grade II, lymph nodes of head, face, and neck

SP C82.12 Follicular lymphoma grade II, intrathoracic lymph nodes

SP C82.13 Follicular lymphoma grade II, intra-abdominal lymph nodes

SP C82.14 Follicular lymphoma grade II, lymph nodes of axilla and upper limb

SP C82.15 Follicular lymphoma grade II, lymph nodes of inguinal region and lower limb

SP C82.16 Follicular lymphoma grade II, intrapelvic lymph nodes

SP C82.17 Follicular lymphoma grade II, spleen

SP C82.18 Follicular lymphoma grade II, lymph nodes of multiple sites

SP C82.19 Follicular lymphoma grade II, extranodal and solid organ sites

5 C82.2 Follicular lymphoma grade III, unspecified

SP C82.20 Follicular lymphoma grade III, unspecified, unspecified site

SP C82.21 Follicular lymphoma grade III, unspecified, lymph nodes of head, face, and neck

SP C82.22 Follicular lymphoma grade III, unspecified, intrathoracic lymph nodes

SP C82.23 Follicular lymphoma grade III, unspecified, intra-abdominal lymph nodes

SP C82.24 Follicular lymphoma grade III, unspecified, lymph nodes of axilla and upper limb

SP C82.25 Follicular lymphoma grade III, unspecified, lymph nodes of inguinal region and lower limb

SP C82.26 Follicular lymphoma grade III, unspecified, intrapelvic lymph nodes

SP C82.27 Follicular lymphoma grade III, unspecified, spleen

SP C82.28 Follicular lymphoma grade III, unspecified, lymph nodes of multiple sites

SP C82.29 Follicular lymphoma grade III, unspecified, extranodal and solid organ sites

5 C82.3 Follicular lymphoma grade IIIa

SP C82.30 Follicular lymphoma grade IIIa, unspecified site

SP C82.31 Follicular lymphoma grade IIIa, lymph nodes of head, face, and neck

SP C82.32 Follicular lymphoma grade IIIa, intrathoracic lymph nodes

SP C82.33 Follicular lymphoma grade IIIa, intra-abdominal lymph nodes

SP C82.34 Follicular lymphoma grade IIIa, lymph nodes of axilla and upper limb

SP C82.35 Follicular lymphoma grade IIIa, lymph nodes of inguinal region and lower limb

SP C82.36 Follicular lymphoma grade IIIa, intrapelvic lymph nodes

SP C82.37 Follicular lymphoma grade IIIa, spleen

SP C82.38 Follicular lymphoma grade IIIa, lymph nodes of multiple sites

SP C82.39 Follicular lymphoma grade IIIa, extranodal and solid organ sites

5 C82.4 Follicular lymphoma grade IIIb

SP C82.40 Follicular lymphoma grade IIIb, unspecified site

SP C82.41 Follicular lymphoma grade IIIb, lymph nodes of head, face, and neck

SP C82.42 Follicular lymphoma grade IIIb, intrathoracic lymph nodes

SP C82.43 Follicular lymphoma grade IIIb, intra-abdominal lymph nodes

SP C82.44 Follicular lymphoma grade IIIb, lymph nodes of axilla and upper limb

SP C82.45 Follicular lymphoma grade IIIb, lymph nodes of inguinal region and lower limb

SP C82.46 Follicular lymphoma grade IIIb, intrapelvic lymph nodes

SP C82.47 Follicular lymphoma grade IIIb, spleen

SP C82.48 Follicular lymphoma grade IIIb, lymph nodes of multiple sites

SP C82.49 Follicular lymphoma grade IIIb, extranodal and solid organ sites

5 C82.5 Diffuse follicle center lymphoma
SP C82.50 Diffuse follicle center lymphoma, unspecified site
SP C82.51 Diffuse follicle center lymphoma, lymph nodes of head, face, and neck
SP C82.52 Diffuse follicle center lymphoma, intrathoracic lymph nodes
SP C82.53 Diffuse follicle center lymphoma, intra-abdominal lymph nodes
SP C82.54 Diffuse follicle center lymphoma, lymph nodes of axilla and upper limb
SP C82.55 Diffuse follicle center lymphoma, lymph nodes of inguinal region and lower limb
SP C82.56 Diffuse follicle center lymphoma, intrapelvic lymph nodes
SP C82.57 Diffuse follicle center lymphoma, spleen
SP C82.58 Diffuse follicle center lymphoma, lymph nodes of multiple sites
SP C82.59 Diffuse follicle center lymphoma, extranodal and solid organ sites

5 C82.6 Cutaneous follicle center lymphoma
SP C82.60 Cutaneous follicle center lymphoma, unspecified site
SP C82.61 Cutaneous follicle center lymphoma, lymph nodes of head, face, and neck
SP C82.62 Cutaneous follicle center lymphoma, intrathoracic lymph nodes
SP C82.63 Cutaneous follicle center lymphoma, intra-abdominal lymph nodes
SP C82.64 Cutaneous follicle center lymphoma, lymph nodes of axilla and upper limb
SP C82.65 Cutaneous follicle center lymphoma, lymph nodes of inguinal region and lower limb
SP C82.66 Cutaneous follicle center lymphoma, intrapelvic lymph nodes
SP C82.67 Cutaneous follicle center lymphoma, spleen
SP C82.68 Cutaneous follicle center lymphoma, lymph nodes of multiple sites
SP C82.69 Cutaneous follicle center lymphoma, extranodal and solid organ sites

5 C82.8 Other types of follicular lymphoma
SP C82.80 Other types of follicular lymphoma, unspecified site
SP C82.81 Other types of follicular lymphoma, lymph nodes of head, face, and neck
SP C82.82 Other types of follicular lymphoma, intrathoracic lymph nodes
SP C82.83 Other types of follicular lymphoma, intra-abdominal lymph nodes
SP C82.84 Other types of follicular lymphoma, lymph nodes of axilla and upper limb
SP C82.85 Other types of follicular lymphoma, lymph nodes of inguinal region and lower limb
SP C82.86 Other types of follicular lymphoma, intrapelvic lymph nodes
SP C82.87 Other types of follicular lymphoma, spleen
SP C82.88 Other types of follicular lymphoma, lymph nodes of multiple sites
SP C82.89 Other types of follicular lymphoma, extranodal and solid organ sites

5 C82.9 Follicular lymphoma, unspecified
SP C82.90 Follicular lymphoma, unspecified, unspecified site
SP C82.91 Follicular lymphoma, unspecified, lymph nodes of head, face, and neck
SP C82.92 Follicular lymphoma, unspecified, intrathoracic lymph nodes
SP C82.93 Follicular lymphoma, unspecified, intra-abdominal lymph nodes
SP C82.94 Follicular lymphoma, unspecified, lymph nodes of axilla and upper limb
SP C82.95 Follicular lymphoma, unspecified, lymph nodes of inguinal region and lower limb
SP C82.96 Follicular lymphoma, unspecified, intrapelvic lymph nodes
SP C82.97 Follicular lymphoma, unspecified, spleen
SP C82.98 Follicular lymphoma, unspecified, lymph nodes of multiple sites
SP C82.99 Follicular lymphoma, unspecified, extranodal and solid organ sites

4 C83 Non-follicular lymphoma
EXCLUDES 1 personal history of non-Hodgkin lymphoma (Z85.72)

5 C83.0 Small cell B-cell lymphoma
Lymphoplasmacytic lymphoma
Nodal marginal zone lymphoma
Non-leukemic variant of B-CLL
Splenic marginal zone lymphoma
EXCLUDES 1 chronic lymphocytic leukemia (C91.1)
mature T/NK-cell lymphomas (C84.-)
Waldenström macroglobulinemia (C88.0)

DEFINITION Uncommon, low-grade, slow-growing B-cell non-Hodgkin's lymphoma involving the marginal, patchy area of the lymph node outside the mantle zone; not very responsive to traditional therapy.

SP C83.00 Small cell B-cell lymphoma, unspecified site
SP C83.01 Small cell B-cell lymphoma, lymph nodes of head, face, and neck
SP C83.02 Small cell B-cell lymphoma, intrathoracic lymph nodes
SP C83.03 Small cell B-cell lymphoma, intra-abdominal lymph nodes
SP C83.04 Small cell B-cell lymphoma, lymph nodes of axilla and upper limb
SP C83.05 Small cell B-cell lymphoma, lymph nodes of inguinal region and lower limb
SP C83.06 Small cell B-cell lymphoma, intrapelvic lymph nodes
SP C83.07 Small cell B-cell lymphoma, spleen
SP C83.08 Small cell B-cell lymphoma, lymph nodes of multiple sites
SP C83.09 Small cell B-cell lymphoma, extranodal and solid organ sites

5 **C83.1 Mantle cell lymphoma**
Centrocytic lymphoma
Malignant lymphomatous polyposis

SP **C83.10 Mantle cell lymphoma, unspecified site**

SP **C83.11 Mantle cell lymphoma, lymph nodes of head, face, and neck**

SP **C83.12 Mantle cell lymphoma, intrathoracic lymph nodes**

SP **C83.13 Mantle cell lymphoma, intra-abdominal lymph nodes**

SP **C83.14 Mantle cell lymphoma, lymph nodes of axilla and upper limb**

SP **C83.15 Mantle cell lymphoma, lymph nodes of inguinal region and lower limb**

SP **C83.16 Mantle cell lymphoma, intrapelvic lymph nodes**

SP **C83.17 Mantle cell lymphoma, spleen**

SP **C83.18 Mantle cell lymphoma, lymph nodes of multiple sites**

SP **C83.19 Mantle cell lymphoma, extranodal and solid organ sites**

5 **C83.3 Diffuse large B-cell lymphoma**
Anaplastic diffuse large B-cell lymphoma
CD30-positive diffuse large B-cell lymphoma
Centroblastic diffuse large B-cell lymphoma
Diffuse large B-cell lymphoma, subtype not specified
Immunoblastic diffuse large B-cell lymphoma
Plasmablastic diffuse large B-cell lymphoma
Diffuse large B-cell lymphoma, subtype not specified
T-cell rich diffuse large B-cell lymphoma

EXCLUDES 1 mediastinal (thymic) large B-cell lymphoma (C85.2-)
mature T/NK-cell lymphomas (C84.-)

SP **C83.30 Diffuse large B-cell lymphoma, unspecified site**

SP **C83.31 Diffuse large B-cell lymphoma, lymph nodes of head, face, and neck**

SP **C83.32 Diffuse large B-cell lymphoma, intrathoracic lymph nodes**

SP **C83.33 Diffuse large B-cell lymphoma, intra-abdominal lymph nodes**

SP **C83.34 Diffuse large B-cell lymphoma, lymph nodes of axilla and upper limb**

SP **C83.35 Diffuse large B-cell lymphoma, lymph nodes of inguinal region and lower limb**

SP **C83.36 Diffuse large B-cell lymphoma, intrapelvic lymph nodes**

SP **C83.37 Diffuse large B-cell lymphoma, spleen**

SP **C83.38 Diffuse large B-cell lymphoma, lymph nodes of multiple sites**

SP **C83.39 Diffuse large B-cell lymphoma, extranodal and solid organ sites**

5 **C83.5 Lymphoblastic (diffuse) lymphoma**
B-precursor lymphoma
Lymphoblastic B-cell lymphoma
Lymphoblastic lymphoma NOS
Lymphoblastic T-cell lymphoma
T-precursor lymphoma

SP **C83.50 Lymphoblastic (diffuse) lymphoma, unspecified site**

SP **C83.51 Lymphoblastic (diffuse) lymphoma, lymph nodes of head, face, and neck**

SP **C83.52 Lymphoblastic (diffuse) lymphoma, intrathoracic lymph nodes**

SP **C83.53 Lymphoblastic (diffuse) lymphoma, intra-abdominal lymph nodes**

SP **C83.54 Lymphoblastic (diffuse) lymphoma, lymph nodes of axilla and upper limb**

SP **C83.55 Lymphoblastic (diffuse) lymphoma, lymph nodes of inguinal region and lower limb**

SP **C83.56 Lymphoblastic (diffuse) lymphoma, intrapelvic lymph nodes**

SP **C83.57 Lymphoblastic (diffuse) lymphoma, spleen**

SP **C83.58 Lymphoblastic (diffuse) lymphoma, lymph nodes of multiple sites**

SP **C83.59 Lymphoblastic (diffuse) lymphoma, extranodal and solid organ sites**

5 **C83.7 Burkitt lymphoma**
Atypical Burkitt lymphoma
Burkitt-like lymphoma

EXCLUDES 1 mature B-cell leukemia Burkitt type (C91.A-)

SP **C83.70 Burkitt lymphoma, unspecified site**

SP **C83.71 Burkitt lymphoma, lymph nodes of head, face, and neck**

SP **C83.72 Burkitt lymphoma, intrathoracic lymph nodes**

SP **C83.73 Burkitt lymphoma, intra-abdominal lymph nodes**

SP **C83.74 Burkitt lymphoma, lymph nodes of axilla and upper limb**

SP **C83.75 Burkitt lymphoma, lymph nodes of inguinal region and lower limb**

SP **C83.76 Burkitt lymphoma, intrapelvic lymph nodes**

SP **C83.77 Burkitt lymphoma, spleen**

SP **C83.78 Burkitt lymphoma, lymph nodes of multiple sites**

SP **C83.79 Burkitt lymphoma, extranodal and solid organ sites**

5 **C83.8 Other non-follicular lymphoma**
Intravascular large B-cell lymphoma
Lymphoid granulomatosis
Primary effusion B-cell lymphoma

EXCLUDES 1 mediastinal (thymic) large B-cell lymphoma (C85.2-)
T-cell rich B-cell lymphoma (C83.3-)

SP **C83.80 Other non-follicular lymphoma, unspecified site**

SP **C83.81 Other non-follicular lymphoma, lymph nodes of head, face, and neck**

SP **C83.82 Other non-follicular lymphoma, intrathoracic lymph nodes**

SP **C83.83 Other non-follicular lymphoma, intra-abdominal lymph nodes**

SP **C83.84 Other non-follicular lymphoma, lymph nodes of axilla and upper limb**

SP C83.85 Other non-follicular lymphoma, lymph nodes of inguinal region and lower limb

SP C83.86 Other non-follicular lymphoma, intrapelvic lymph nodes

SP C83.87 Other non-follicular lymphoma, spleen

SP C83.88 Other non-follicular lymphoma, lymph nodes of multiple sites

SP C83.89 Other non-follicular lymphoma, extranodal and solid organ sites

5 C83.9 Non-follicular (diffuse) lymphoma, unspecified

SP C83.90 Non-follicular (diffuse) lymphoma, unspecified, unspecified site

SP C83.91 Non-follicular (diffuse) lymphoma, unspecified, lymph nodes of head, face, and neck

SP C83.92 Non-follicular (diffuse) lymphoma, unspecified, intrathoracic lymph nodes

SP C83.93 Non-follicular (diffuse) lymphoma, unspecified, intra-abdominal lymph nodes

SP C83.94 Non-follicular (diffuse) lymphoma, unspecified, lymph nodes of axilla and upper limb

SP C83.95 Non-follicular (diffuse) lymphoma, unspecified, lymph nodes of inguinal region and lower limb

SP C83.96 Non-follicular (diffuse) lymphoma, unspecified, intrapelvic lymph nodes

SP C83.97 Non-follicular (diffuse) lymphoma, unspecified, spleen

SP C83.98 Non-follicular (diffuse) lymphoma, unspecified, lymph nodes of multiple sites

SP C83.99 Non-follicular (diffuse) lymphoma, unspecified, extranodal and solid organ sites

4 C84 Mature T/NK-cell lymphomas

EXCLUDES 1 personal history of non-Hodgkin lymphoma (Z85.72)

5 C84.0 Mycosis fungoides

EXCLUDES 1 peripheral T-cell lymphoma, not classified (C84.4-)

DEFINITION A rare, progressive form of slow-growing cutaneous T-cell lymphoma associated with a chromosome abnormality that evolves into a generalized, high grade, aggressive systemic form of lymphoma.

SP C84.00 Mycosis fungoides, unspecified site

SP C84.01 Mycosis fungoides, lymph nodes of head, face, and neck

SP C84.02 Mycosis fungoides, intrathoracic lymph nodes

SP C84.03 Mycosis fungoides, intra-abdominal lymph nodes

SP C84.04 Mycosis fungoides, lymph nodes of axilla and upper limb

SP C84.05 Mycosis fungoides, lymph nodes of inguinal region and lower limb

SP C84.06 Mycosis fungoides, intrapelvic lymph nodes

SP C84.07 Mycosis fungoides, spleen

SP C84.08 Mycosis fungoides, lymph nodes of multiple sites

SP C84.09 Mycosis fungoides, extranodal and solid organ sites

5 C84.1 Sézary disease

SP C84.10 Sézary disease, unspecified site

SP C84.11 Sézary disease, lymph nodes of head, face, and neck

SP C84.12 Sézary disease, intrathoracic lymph nodes

SP C84.13 Sézary disease, intra-abdominal lymph nodes

SP C84.14 Sézary disease, lymph nodes of axilla and upper limb

SP C84.15 Sézary disease, lymph nodes of inguinal region and lower limb

SP C84.16 Sézary disease, intrapelvic lymph nodes

SP C84.17 Sézary disease, spleen

SP C84.18 Sézary disease, lymph nodes of multiple sites

SP C84.19 Sézary disease, extranodal and solid organ sites

5 C84.4 Peripheral T-cell lymphoma, not classified

Lennert's lymphoma
Lymphoepithelioid lymphoma
Mature T-cell lymphoma, not elsewhere classified

DEFINITION Aggressive, non-Hodgkin's lymphoma derived from mature neoplastic T-cell lymphocytes that have moved to other tissue, causing site-related symptoms and generalized lymphadenopathy.

SP C84.40 Peripheral T-cell lymphoma, not classified, unspecified site

SP C84.41 Peripheral T-cell lymphoma, not classified, lymph nodes of head, face, and neck

SP C84.42 Peripheral T-cell lymphoma, not classified, intrathoracic lymph nodes

SP C84.43 Peripheral T-cell lymphoma, not classified, intra-abdominal lymph nodes

SP C84.44 Peripheral T-cell lymphoma, not classified, lymph nodes of axilla and upper limb

SP C84.45 Peripheral T-cell lymphoma, not classified, lymph nodes of inguinal region and lower limb

SP C84.46 Peripheral T-cell lymphoma, not classified, intrapelvic lymph nodes

SP C84.47 Peripheral T-cell lymphoma, not classified, spleen

SP C84.48 Peripheral T-cell lymphoma, not classified, lymph nodes of multiple sites

SP C84.49 Peripheral T-cell lymphoma, not classified, extranodal and solid organ sites

5 C84.6 Anaplastic large cell lymphoma, ALK-positive

Anaplastic large cell lymphoma, CD30-positive

SP C84.60 Anaplastic large cell lymphoma, ALK-positive, unspecified site

Chapter 2 C00-D49

SP **C84.61 Anaplastic large cell lymphoma, ALK-positive, lymph nodes of head, face, and neck**
SP **C84.62 Anaplastic large cell lymphoma, ALK-positive, intrathoracic lymph nodes**
SP **C84.63 Anaplastic large cell lymphoma, ALK-positive, intra-abdominal lymph nodes**
SP **C84.64 Anaplastic large cell lymphoma, ALK-positive, lymph nodes of axilla and upper limb**
SP **C84.65 Anaplastic large cell lymphoma, ALK-positive, lymph nodes of inguinal region and lower limb**
SP **C84.66 Anaplastic large cell lymphoma, ALK-positive, intrapelvic lymph nodes**
SP **C84.67 Anaplastic large cell lymphoma, ALK-positive, spleen**
SP **C84.68 Anaplastic large cell lymphoma, ALK-positive, lymph nodes of multiple sites**
SP **C84.69 Anaplastic large cell lymphoma, ALK-positive, extranodal and solid organ sites**

5 **C84.7 Anaplastic large cell lymphoma, ALK-negative**

EXCLUDES 1 primary cutaneous CD30-positive T-cell proliferations (C86.6-)

SP **C84.70 Anaplastic large cell lymphoma, ALK-negative, unspecified site**
SP **C84.71 Anaplastic large cell lymphoma, ALK-negative, lymph nodes of head, face, and neck**
SP **C84.72 Anaplastic large cell lymphoma, ALK-negative, intrathoracic lymph nodes**
SP **C84.73 Anaplastic large cell lymphoma, ALK-negative, intra-abdominal lymph nodes**
SP **C84.74 Anaplastic large cell lymphoma, ALK-negative, lymph nodes of axilla and upper limb**
SP **C84.75 Anaplastic large cell lymphoma, ALK-negative, lymph nodes of inguinal region and lower limb**
SP **C84.76 Anaplastic large cell lymphoma, ALK-negative, intrapelvic lymph nodes**
SP **C84.77 Anaplastic large cell lymphoma, ALK-negative, spleen**
SP **C84.78 Anaplastic large cell lymphoma, ALK-negative, lymph nodes of multiple sites**
SP **C84.79 Anaplastic large cell lymphoma, ALK-negative, extranodal and solid organ sites**
★ + **C84.7A Anaplastic large cell lymphoma, ALK-negative, breast**

Breast implant associated anaplastic large cell lymphoma (BIA-ALCL)

Use additional code to identify:
- breast implant status (Z98.82)
- personal history of breast implant removal (Z98.86)

5 **C84.A Cutaneous T-cell lymphoma, unspecified**

SP **C84.A0 Cutaneous T-cell lymphoma, unspecified, unspecified site**
SP **C84.A1 Cutaneous T-cell lymphoma, unspecified lymph nodes of head, face, and neck**
SP **C84.A2 Cutaneous T-cell lymphoma, unspecified, intrathoracic lymph nodes**
SP **C84.A3 Cutaneous T-cell lymphoma, unspecified, intra-abdominal lymph nodes**
SP **C84.A4 Cutaneous T-cell lymphoma, unspecified, lymph nodes of axilla and upper limb**
SP **C84.A5 Cutaneous T-cell lymphoma, unspecified, lymph nodes of inguinal region and lower limb**
SP **C84.A6 Cutaneous T-cell lymphoma, unspecified, intrapelvic lymph nodes**
SP **C84.A7 Cutaneous T-cell lymphoma, unspecified, spleen**
SP **C84.A8 Cutaneous T-cell lymphoma, unspecified, lymph nodes of multiple sites**
SP **C84.A9 Cutaneous T-cell lymphoma, unspecified, extranodal and solid organ sites**

5 **C84.Z Other mature T/NK-cell lymphomas**

Note:
If T-cell lineage or involvement is mentioned in conjunction with a specific lymphoma, code to the more specific description.

EXCLUDES 1
- angioimmunoblastic T-cell lymphoma (C86.5)
- blastic NK-cell lymphoma (C86.4)
- enteropathy-type T-cell lymphoma (C86.2)
- extranodal NK-cell lymphoma, nasal type (C86.0)
- hepatosplenic T-cell lymphoma (C86.1)
- primary cutaneous CD30-positive T-cell proliferations (C86.6)
- subcutaneous panniculitis-like T-cell lymphoma (C86.3)
- T-cell leukemia (C91.1-)

SP **C84.Z0 Other mature T/NK-cell lymphomas, unspecified site**
SP **C84.Z1 Other mature T/NK-cell lymphomas, lymph nodes of head, face, and neck**
SP **C84.Z2 Other mature T/NK-cell lymphomas, intrathoracic lymph nodes**
SP **C84.Z3 Other mature T/NK-cell lymphomas, intra-abdominal lymph nodes**
SP **C84.Z4 Other mature T/NK-cell lymphomas, lymph nodes of axilla and upper limb**

SP C84.Z5 Other mature T/NK-cell lymphomas, lymph nodes of inguinal region and lower limb

SP C84.Z6 Other mature T/NK-cell lymphomas, intrapelvic lymph nodes

SP C84.Z7 Other mature T/NK-cell lymphomas, spleen

SP C84.Z8 Other mature T/NK-cell lymphomas, lymph nodes of multiple sites

SP C84.Z9 Other mature T/NK-cell lymphomas, extranodal and solid organ sites

5 C84.9 Mature T/NK-cell lymphomas, unspecified

NK/T cell lymphoma NOS

EXCLUDES 1 mature T-cell lymphoma, not elsewhere classified (C84.4-)

SP C84.90 Mature T/NK-cell lymphomas, unspecified, unspecified site

SP C84.91 Mature T/NK-cell lymphomas, unspecified, lymph nodes of head, face, and neck

SP C84.92 Mature T/NK-cell lymphomas, unspecified, intrathoracic lymph nodes

SP C84.93 Mature T/NK-cell lymphomas, unspecified, intra-abdominal lymph nodes

SP C84.94 Mature T/NK-cell lymphomas, unspecified, lymph nodes of axilla and upper limb

SP C84.95 Mature T/NK-cell lymphomas, unspecified, lymph nodes of inguinal region and lower limb

SP C84.96 Mature T/NK-cell lymphomas, unspecified, intrapelvic lymph nodes

SP C84.97 Mature T/NK-cell lymphomas, unspecified, spleen

SP C84.98 Mature T/NK-cell lymphomas, unspecified, lymph nodes of multiple sites

SP C84.99 Mature T/NK-cell lymphomas, unspecified, extranodal and solid organ sites

4 C85 Other specified and unspecified types of non-Hodgkin lymphoma

EXCLUDES 1 other specified types of T/NK-cell lymphoma (C86.-)
personal history of non-Hodgkin lymphoma (Z85.72)

5 C85.1 Unspecified B-cell lymphoma

Note:
If B-cell lineage or involvement is mentioned in conjunction with a specific lymphoma, code to the more specific description.

SP C85.10 Unspecified B-cell lymphoma, unspecified site

SP C85.11 Unspecified B-cell lymphoma, lymph nodes of head, face, and neck

SP C85.12 Unspecified B-cell lymphoma, intrathoracic lymph nodes

SP C85.13 Unspecified B-cell lymphoma, intra-abdominal lymph nodes

SP C85.14 Unspecified B-cell lymphoma, lymph nodes of axilla and upper limb

SP C85.15 Unspecified B-cell lymphoma, lymph nodes of inguinal region and lower limb

SP C85.16 Unspecified B-cell lymphoma, intrapelvic lymph nodes

SP C85.17 Unspecified B-cell lymphoma, spleen

SP C85.18 Unspecified B-cell lymphoma, lymph nodes of multiple sites

SP C85.19 Unspecified B-cell lymphoma, extranodal and solid organ sites

5 C85.2 Mediastinal (thymic) large B-cell lymphoma

SP C85.20 Mediastinal (thymic) large B-cell lymphoma, unspecified site

SP C85.21 Mediastinal (thymic) large B-cell lymphoma, lymph nodes of head, face, and neck

SP C85.22 Mediastinal (thymic) large B-cell lymphoma, intrathoracic lymph nodes

SP C85.23 Mediastinal (thymic) large B-cell lymphoma, intra-abdominal lymph nodes

SP C85.24 Mediastinal (thymic) large B-cell lymphoma, lymph nodes of axilla and upper limb

SP C85.25 Mediastinal (thymic) large B-cell lymphoma, lymph nodes of inguinal region and lower limb

SP C85.26 Mediastinal (thymic) large B-cell lymphoma, intrapelvic lymph nodes

SP C85.27 Mediastinal (thymic) large B-cell lymphoma, spleen

SP C85.28 Mediastinal (thymic) large B-cell lymphoma, lymph nodes of multiple sites

SP C85.29 Mediastinal (thymic) large B-cell lymphoma, extranodal and solid organ sites

5 C85.8 Other specified types of non-Hodgkin lymphoma

SP C85.80 Other specified types of non-Hodgkin lymphoma, unspecified site

SP C85.81 Other specified types of non-Hodgkin lymphoma, lymph nodes of head, face, and neck

SP C85.82 Other specified types of non-Hodgkin lymphoma, intrathoracic lymph nodes

SP C85.83 Other specified types of non-Hodgkin lymphoma, intra-abdominal lymph nodes

SP C85.84 Other specified types of non-Hodgkin lymphoma, lymph nodes of axilla and upper limb

SP C85.85 Other specified types of non-Hodgkin lymphoma, lymph nodes of inguinal region and lower limb

SP C85.86 Other specified types of non-Hodgkin lymphoma, intrapelvic lymph nodes

SP **C85.87 Other specified types of non-Hodgkin lymphoma, spleen**

SP **C85.88 Other specified types of non-Hodgkin lymphoma, lymph nodes of multiple sites**

SP **C85.89 Other specified types of non-Hodgkin lymphoma, extranodal and solid organ sites**

5 **C85.9 Non-Hodgkin lymphoma, unspecified**

Lymphoma NOS
Malignant lymphoma NOS
Non-Hodgkin lymphoma NOS

SP **C85.90 Non-Hodgkin lymphoma, unspecified, unspecified site**

SP **C85.91 Non-Hodgkin lymphoma, unspecified, lymph nodes of head, face, and neck**

SP **C85.92 Non-Hodgkin lymphoma, unspecified, intrathoracic lymph nodes**

SP **C85.93 Non-Hodgkin lymphoma, unspecified, intra-abdominal lymph nodes**

SP **C85.94 Non-Hodgkin lymphoma, unspecified, lymph nodes of axilla and upper limb**

SP **C85.95 Non-Hodgkin lymphoma, unspecified, lymph nodes of inguinal region and lower limb**

SP **C85.96 Non-Hodgkin lymphoma, unspecified, intrapelvic lymph nodes**

SP **C85.97 Non-Hodgkin lymphoma, unspecified, spleen**

SP **C85.98 Non-Hodgkin lymphoma, unspecified, lymph nodes of multiple sites**

SP **C85.99 Non-Hodgkin lymphoma, unspecified, extranodal and solid organ sites**

4 **C86 Other specified types of T/NK-cell lymphoma**

EXCLUDES 1 anaplastic large cell lymphoma, ALK negative (C84.7-)
anaplastic large cell lymphoma, ALK positive (C84.6-)
mature T/NK-cell lymphomas (C84.-)
other specified types of non-Hodgkin lymphoma (C85.8-)

SP **C86.0 Extranodal NK/T-cell lymphoma, nasal type**

SP **C86.1 Hepatosplenic T-cell lymphoma**

Alpha-beta and gamma delta types

SP **C86.2 Enteropathy-type (intestinal) T-cell lymphoma**

Enteropathy associated T-cell lymphoma

SP **C86.3 Subcutaneous panniculitis-like T-cell lymphoma**

SP **C86.4 Blastic NK-cell lymphoma**

Blastic plasmacytoid dendritic cell neoplasm (BPDCN)

SP **C86.5 Angioimmunoblastic T-cell lymphoma**

Angioimmunoblastic lymphadenopathy with dysproteinemia (AILD)

SP **C86.6 Primary cutaneous CD30-positive T-cell proliferations**

Lymphomatoid papulosis
Primary cutaneous anaplastic large cell lymphoma
Primary cutaneous CD30-positive large T-cell lymphoma

4 **C88 Malignant immunoproliferative diseases and certain other B-cell lymphomas**

EXCLUDES 1 B-cell lymphoma, unspecified (C85.1-)
personal history of other malignant neoplasms of lymphoid, hematopoietic and related tissues (Z85.79)

SP **C88.0 Waldenström macroglobulinemia**

Lymphoplasmacytic lymphoma with IgM-production
Macroglobulinemia (idiopathic) (primary)

EXCLUDES 1 small cell B-cell lymphoma (C83.0)

SP **C88.2 Heavy chain disease**

Franklin disease
Gamma heavy chain disease
Mu heavy chain disease

SP **C88.3 Immunoproliferative small intestinal disease**

Alpha heavy chain disease
Mediterranean lymphoma

SP **C88.4 Extranodal marginal zone B-cell lymphoma of mucosa-associated lymphoid tissue [MALT-lymphoma]**

Lymphoma of skin-associated lymphoid tissue [SALT-lymphoma]
Lymphoma of bronchial-associated lymphoid tissue [BALT-lymphoma]

EXCLUDES 1 high malignant (diffuse large B-cell) lymphoma (C83.3-)

SP **C88.8 Other malignant immunoproliferative diseases**

SP **C88.9 Malignant immunoproliferative disease, unspecified**

Immunoproliferative disease NOS

4 **C90 Multiple myeloma and malignant plasma cell neoplasms**

EXCLUDES 1 personal history of other malignant neoplasms of lymphoid, hematopoietic and related tissues (Z85.79)

GUIDELINES **Section I.C.2.n**

The categories for leukemia [C91 - C95], and category C90, Multiple myeloma and malignant plasma cell neoplasms, have codes indicating whether or not the leukemia has achieved remission. There are also codes Z85.6, Personal history of leukemia, and Z85.79, Personal history of other malignant neoplasms of lymphoid, hematopoietic and related tissues. If the documentation is unclear, as to whether the leukemia has achieved remission, the provider should be queried.

CODING TIPS ✓ Terms such as "in remission" and "in relapse" must be specified by the provider in order to indicate assignment of a code specifying these terms. If the provider has not specified one of these terms, select the code for "not having achieved remission."

5 **C90.0 Multiple myeloma**

Kahler's disease

Medullary plasmacytoma
Myelomatosis
Plasma cell myeloma
EXCLUDES 1 solitary myeloma (C90.3-)
solitary plasmactyoma (C90.3-)

SP **C90.00 Multiple myeloma not having achieved remission**
Multiple myeloma with failed remission
Multiple myeloma NOS

SP **C90.01 Multiple myeloma in remission**

SP **C90.02 Multiple myeloma in relapse**

5 **C90.1 Plasma cell leukemia**
Plasmacytic leukemia

SP **C90.10 Plasma cell leukemia not having achieved remission**
Plasma cell leukemia with failed remission
Plasma cell leukemia NOS

SP **C90.11 Plasma cell leukemia in remission**

SP **C90.12 Plasma cell leukemia in relapse**

5 **C90.2 Extramedullary plasmacytoma**

SP **C90.20 Extramedullary plasmacytoma not having achieved remission**
Extramedullary plasmacytoma with failed remission
Extramedullary plasmacytoma NOS

SP **C90.21 Extramedullary plasmacytoma in remission**

SP **C90.22 Extramedullary plasmacytoma in relapse**

5 **C90.3 Solitary plasmacytoma**
Localized malignant plasma cell tumor NOS
Plasmacytoma NOS
Solitary myeloma

SP **C90.30 Solitary plasmacytoma not having achieved remission**
Solitary plasmacytoma with failed remission
Solitary plasmacytoma NOS

SP **C90.31 Solitary plasmacytoma in remission**

SP **C90.32 Solitary plasmacytoma in relapse**

4 **C91 Lymphoid leukemia**
EXCLUDES 1 personal history of leukemia (Z85.6)

CODING TIPS✓ Terms such as "in remission" and "in relapse" must be specified by the provider in order to indicate assignment of a code specifying these terms. If the provider has not specified one of these terms, select the code for "not having achieved remission."

5 **C91.0 Acute lymphoblastic leukemia [ALL]**
Note:
Codes in subcategory C91.0- should only be used for T-cell and B-cell precursor leukemia

SP **C91.00 Acute lymphoblastic leukemia not having achieved remission**
Acute lymphoblastic leukemia with failed remission
Acute lymphoblastic leukemia NOS

SP **C91.01 Acute lymphoblastic leukemia, in remission**

SP **C91.02 Acute lymphoblastic leukemia, in relapse**

5 **C91.1 Chronic lymphocytic leukemia of B-cell type**
Lymphoplasmacytic leukemia
Richter syndrome
EXCLUDES 1 lymphoplasmacytic lymphoma (C83.0-)

SP **C91.10 Chronic lymphocytic leukemia of B-cell type not having achieved remission**
Chronic lymphocytic leukemia of B-cell type with failed remission
Chronic lymphocytic leukemia of B-cell type NOS

SP **C91.11 Chronic lymphocytic leukemia of B-cell type in remission**

SP **C91.12 Chronic lymphocytic leukemia of B-cell type in relapse**

5 **C91.3 Prolymphocytic leukemia of B-cell type**

SP **C91.30 Prolymphocytic leukemia of B-cell type not having achieved remission**
Prolymphocytic leukemia of B-cell type with failed remission
Prolymphocytic leukemia of B-cell type NOS

SP **C91.31 Prolymphocytic leukemia of B-cell type, in remission**

SP **C91.32 Prolymphocytic leukemia of B-cell type, in relapse**

5 **C91.4 Hairy cell leukemia**
Leukemic reticuloendotheliosis

SP **C91.40 Hairy cell leukemia not having achieved remission**
Hairy cell leukemia with failed remission
Hairy cell leukemia NOS

SP **C91.41 Hairy cell leukemia, in remission**

SP **C91.42 Hairy cell leukemia, in relapse**

5 **C91.5 Adult T-cell lymphoma/leukemia (HTLV-1-associated)**
Acute variant of adult T-cell lymphoma/leukemia (HTLV-1-associated)
Chronic variant of adult T-cell lymphoma/leukemia (HTLV-1-associated)
Lymphomatoid variant of adult T-cell lymphoma/leukemia (HTLV-1-associated)
Smouldering variant of adult T-cell lymphoma/leukemia (HTLV-1-associated)

SP **C91.50 Adult T-cell lymphoma/leukemia (HTLV-1-associated) not having achieved remission**
Adult T-cell lymphoma/leukemia (HTLV-1-associated) with failed remission
Adult T-cell lymphoma/leukemia (HTLV-1-associated) NOS

SP **C91.51 Adult T-cell lymphoma/leukemia (HTLV-1-associated), in remission**

SP **C91.52 Adult T-cell lymphoma/leukemia (HTLV-1-associated), in relapse**

5 **C91.6 Prolymphocytic leukemia of T-cell type**

SP **C91.60 Prolymphocytic leukemia of T-cell type not having achieved remission**
Prolymphocytic leukemia of T-cell type with failed remission

Prolymphocytic leukemia of T-cell type NOS

SP **C91.61 Prolymphocytic leukemia of T-cell type, in remission**

SP **C91.62 Prolymphocytic leukemia of T-cell type, in relapse**

5 **C91.A Mature B-cell leukemia Burkitt-type**

EXCLUDES 1 Burkitt lymphoma (C83.7-)

SP **C91.A0 Mature B-cell leukemia Burkitt-type not having achieved remission**

Mature B-cell leukemia Burkitt-type with failed remission

Mature B-cell leukemia Burkitt-type NOS

SP **C91.A1 Mature B-cell leukemia Burkitt-type, in remission**

SP **C91.A2 Mature B-cell leukemia Burkitt-type, in relapse**

5 **C91.Z Other lymphoid leukemia**

T-cell large granular lymphocytic leukemia (associated with rheumatoid arthritis)

SP **C91.Z0 Other lymphoid leukemia not having achieved remission**

Other lymphoid leukemia with failed remission

Other lymphoid leukemia NOS

SP **C91.Z1 Other lymphoid leukemia, in remission**

SP **C91.Z2 Other lymphoid leukemia, in relapse**

5 **C91.9 Lymphoid leukemia, unspecified**

SP **C91.90 Lymphoid leukemia, unspecified not having achieved remission**

Lymphoid leukemia with failed remission

Lymphoid leukemia NOS

SP **C91.91 Lymphoid leukemia, unspecified, in remission**

SP **C91.92 Lymphoid leukemia, unspecified, in relapse**

4 **C92 Myeloid leukemia**

INCLUDES granulocytic leukemia
myelogenous leukemia

EXCLUDES 1 personal history of leukemia (Z85.6)

CODING TIPS✓ Coding these types of cancers in remission or in relapse must be based on physician or NPP documentation or query. Query the physician or NPP to differentiate between leukemia in remission and history of leukemia. History of leukemia is coded to Z85.6. Treatment is different for a patient who has never achieved remission vs. a patient who has achieved remission and then relapsed.

5 **C92.0 Acute myeloblastic leukemia**

Acute myeloblastic leukemia, minimal differentiation

Acute myeloblastic leukemia (with maturation)

Acute myeloblastic leukemia 1/ETO

Acute myeloblastic leukemia M0

Acute myeloblastic leukemia M1

Acute myeloblastic leukemia M2

Acute myeloblastic leukemia with t(8;21)

Acute myeloblastic leukemia (without a FAB classification) NOS

Refractory anemia with excess blasts in transformation [RAEB T]

EXCLUDES 1 acute exacerbation of chronic myeloid leukemia (C92.10)
refractory anemia with excess of blasts not in transformation (D46.2-)

SP **C92.00 Acute myeloblastic leukemia, not having achieved remission**

Acute myeloblastic leukemia with failed remission

Acute myeloblastic leukemia NOS

SP **C92.01 Acute myeloblastic leukemia, in remission**

SP **C92.02 Acute myeloblastic leukemia, in relapse**

5 **C92.1 Chronic myeloid leukemia, BCR/ABL-positive**

Chronic myelogenous leukemia, Philadelphia chromosome (Ph1) positive

Chronic myelogenous leukemia, t(9;22) (q34;q11)

Chronic myelogenous leukemia with crisis of blast cells

EXCLUDES 1 atypical chronic myeloid leukemia BCR/ABL-negative (C92.2-)
chronic myelomonocytic leukemia (C93.1-)
chronic myeloproliferative disease (D47.1)

SP **C92.10 Chronic myeloid leukemia, BCR/ABL-positive, not having achieved remission**

Chronic myeloid leukemia, BCR/ABL-positive with failed remission

Chronic myeloid leukemia, BCR/ABL-positive NOS

SP **C92.11 Chronic myeloid leukemia, BCR/ABL-positive, in remission**

SP **C92.12 Chronic myeloid leukemia, BCR/ABL-positive, in relapse**

5 **C92.2 Atypical chronic myeloid leukemia, BCR/ABL-negative**

SP **C92.20 Atypical chronic myeloid leukemia, BCR/ABL-negative, not having achieved remission**

Atypical chronic myeloid leukemia, BCR/ABL-negative with failed remission

Atypical chronic myeloid leukemia, BCR/ABL-negative NOS

SP **C92.21 Atypical chronic myeloid leukemia, BCR/ABL-negative, in remission**

SP **C92.22 Atypical chronic myeloid leukemia, BCR/ABL-negative, in relapse**

5 **C92.3 Myeloid sarcoma**

A malignant tumor of immature myeloid cells

Chloroma

Granulocytic sarcoma

SP **C92.30 Myeloid sarcoma, not having achieved remission**

Myeloid sarcoma with failed remission

Myeloid sarcoma NOS

SP **C92.31 Myeloid sarcoma, in remission**

SP **C92.32 Myeloid sarcoma, in relapse**

5 **C92.4 Acute promyelocytic leukemia**
AML M3
AML Me with t(15;17) and variants

SP **C92.40 Acute promyelocytic leukemia, not having achieved remission**
Acute promyelocytic leukemia with failed remission
Acute promyelocytic leukemia NOS

SP **C92.41 Acute promyelocytic leukemia, in remission**

SP **C92.42 Acute promyelocytic leukemia, in relapse**

5 **C92.5 Acute myelomonocytic leukemia**
AML M4
AML M4 Eo with inv(16) or t(16;16)

SP **C92.50 Acute myelomonocytic leukemia, not having achieved remission**
Acute myelomonocytic leukemia with failed remission
Acute myelomonocytic leukemia NOS

SP **C92.51 Acute myelomonocytic leukemia, in remission**

SP **C92.52 Acute myelomonocytic leukemia, in relapse**

5 **C92.6 Acute myeloid leukemia with 11q23-abnormality**
Acute myeloid leukemia with variation of MLL-gene

SP **C92.60 Acute myeloid leukemia with 11q23-abnormality not having achieved remission**
Acute myeloid leukemia with 11q23-abnormality with failed remission
Acute myeloid leukemia with 11q23-abnormality NOS

SP **C92.61 Acute myeloid leukemia with 11q23-abnormality in remission**

SP **C92.62 Acute myeloid leukemia with 11q23-abnormality in relapse**

5 **C92.A Acute myeloid leukemia with multilineage dysplasia**
Acute myeloid leukemia with dysplasia of remaining hematopoesis and/or myelodysplastic disease in its history

SP **C92.A0 Acute myeloid leukemia with multilineage dysplasia, not having achieved remission**
Acute myeloid leukemia with multilineage dysplasia with failed remission
Acute myeloid leukemia with multilineage dysplasia NOS

SP **C92.A1 Acute myeloid leukemia with multilineage dysplasia, in remission**

SP **C92.A2 Acute myeloid leukemia with multilineage dysplasia, in relapse**

5 **C92.Z Other myeloid leukemia**

SP **C92.Z0 Other myeloid leukemia not having achieved remission**
Myeloid leukemia NEC with failed remission
Myeloid leukemia NEC

SP **C92.Z1 Other myeloid leukemia, in remission**

SP **C92.Z2 Other myeloid leukemia, in relapse**

5 **C92.9 Myeloid leukemia, unspecified**

SP **C92.90 Myeloid leukemia, unspecified, not having achieved remission**
Myeloid leukemia, unspecified with failed remission
Myeloid leukemia, unspecified NOS

SP **C92.91 Myeloid leukemia, unspecified in remission**

SP **C92.92 Myeloid leukemia, unspecified in relapse**

4 **C93 Monocytic leukemia**
INCLUDES monocytoid leukemia
EXCLUDES 1 personal history of leukemia (Z85.6)
CODING TIPS✓ Coding these types of cancers in remission or in relapse must be based on physician or NPP documentation or query. Query the physician or NPP to differentiate between leukemia in remission and history of leukemia. History of leukemia is coded to Z85.6. Treatment is different for a patient who has never achieved remission vs. a patient who has achieved remission and then relapsed.

5 **C93.0 Acute monoblastic/monocytic leukemia**
AML M5
AML M5a
AML M5b

SP **C93.00 Acute monoblastic/monocytic leukemia, not having achieved remission**
Acute monoblastic/monocytic leukemia with failed remission
Acute monoblastic/monocytic leukemia NOS

SP **C93.01 Acute monoblastic/monocytic leukemia, in remission**

SP **C93.02 Acute monoblastic/monocytic leukemia, in relapse**

5 **C93.1 Chronic myelomonocytic leukemia**
Chronic monocytic leukemia
CMML-1
CMML-2
CMML with eosinophilia
Code also:
, if applicable, eosinophilia (D72.18)

SP **C93.10 Chronic myelomonocytic leukemia not having achieved remission**
Chronic myelomonocytic leukemia with failed remission
Chronic myelomonocytic leukemia NOS

SP **C93.11 Chronic myelomonocytic leukemia, in remission**

SP **C93.12 Chronic myelomonocytic leukemia, in relapse**

5 **C93.3 Juvenile myelomonocytic leukemia**

SP **C93.30 Juvenile myelomonocytic leukemia, not having achieved remission**
Juvenile myelomonocytic leukemia with failed remission
Juvenile myelomonocytic leukemia NOS

SP **C93.31 Juvenile myelomonocytic leukemia, in remission**

SP **C93.32 Juvenile myelomonocytic leukemia, in relapse**

5 **C93.Z Other monocytic leukemia**

SP **C93.Z0 Other monocytic leukemia, not having achieved remission**

Chapter 2

C00-D49

Other monocytic leukemia NOS

SP **C93.Z1 Other monocytic leukemia, in remission**

SP **C93.Z2 Other monocytic leukemia, in relapse**

5 **C93.9 Monocytic leukemia, unspecified**

SP **C93.90 Monocytic leukemia, unspecified, not having achieved remission**

Monocytic leukemia, unspecified with failed remission

Monocytic leukemia, unspecified NOS

SP **C93.91 Monocytic leukemia, unspecified in remission**

SP **C93.92 Monocytic leukemia, unspecified in relapse**

4 **C94 Other leukemias of specified cell type**

EXCLUDES 1 leukemic reticuloendotheliosis (C91.4-)
myelodysplastic syndromes (D46.-)
personal history of leukemia (Z85.6)
plasma cell leukemia (C90.1-)

CODING TIPS✓ Coding these types of cancers in remission or in relapse must be based on physician or NPP documentation or query. Query the physician or NPP to differentiate between leukemia in remission and history of leukemia. History of leukemia is coded to Z85.6. Treatment is different for a patient who has never achieved remission vs. a patient who has achieved remission and then relapsed.

5 **C94.0 Acute erythroid leukemia**

Acute myeloid leukemia M6(a)(b)

Erythroleukemia

SP **C94.00 Acute erythroid leukemia, not having achieved remission**

Acute erythroid leukemia with failed remission

Acute erythroid leukemia NOS

SP **C94.01 Acute erythroid leukemia, in remission**

SP **C94.02 Acute erythroid leukemia, in relapse**

5 **C94.2 Acute megakaryoblastic leukemia**

Acute myeloid leukemia M7

Acute megakaryocytic leukemia

SP **C94.20 Acute megakaryoblastic leukemia not having achieved remission**

Acute megakaryoblastic leukemia with failed remission

Acute megakaryoblastic leukemia NOS

SP **C94.21 Acute megakaryoblastic leukemia, in remission**

SP **C94.22 Acute megakaryoblastic leukemia, in relapse**

5 **C94.3 Mast cell leukemia**

SP **C94.30 Mast cell leukemia not having achieved remission**

Mast cell leukemia with failed remission

Mast cell leukemia NOS

SP **C94.31 Mast cell leukemia, in remission**

SP **C94.32 Mast cell leukemia, in relapse**

5 **C94.4 Acute panmyelosis with myelofibrosis**

Acute myelofibrosis

EXCLUDES 1 myelofibrosis NOS (D75.81)
secondary myelofibrosis NOS (D75.81)

SP **C94.40 Acute panmyelosis with myelofibrosis not having achieved remission**

Acute myelofibrosis NOS

Acute panmyelosis with myelofibrosis with failed remission

Acute panmyelosis NOS

SP **C94.41 Acute panmyelosis with myelofibrosis, in remission**

SP **C94.42 Acute panmyelosis with myelofibrosis, in relapse**

SP **C94.6 Myelodysplastic disease, not classified**

Myeloproliferative disease, not classified

5 **C94.8 Other specified leukemias**

Aggressive NK-cell leukemia

Acute basophilic leukemia

SP **C94.80 Other specified leukemias not having achieved remission**

Other specified leukemia with failed remission

Other specified leukemias NOS

SP **C94.81 Other specified leukemias, in remission**

SP **C94.82 Other specified leukemias, in relapse**

4 **C95 Leukemia of unspecified cell type**

EXCLUDES 1 personal history of leukemia (Z85.6)

CODING TIPS✓ Coding these types of cancers in remission or in relapse must be based on physician or NPP documentation or query. Query the physician or NPP to differentiate between leukemia in remission and history of leukemia. History of leukemia is coded to Z85.6. Treatment is different for a patient who has never achieved remission vs. a patient who has achieved remission and then relapsed.

5 **C95.0 Acute leukemia of unspecified cell type**

Acute bilineal leukemia

Acute mixed lineage leukemia

Biphenotypic acute leukemia

Stem cell leukemia of unclear lineage

EXCLUDES 1 acute exacerbation of unspecified chronic leukemia (C95.10)

SP **C95.00 Acute leukemia of unspecified cell type not having achieved remission**

Acute leukemia of unspecified cell type with failed remission

Acute leukemia NOS

SP **C95.01 Acute leukemia of unspecified cell type, in remission**

SP **C95.02 Acute leukemia of unspecified cell type, in relapse**

5 **C95.1 Chronic leukemia of unspecified cell type**

SP **C95.10 Chronic leukemia of unspecified cell type not having achieved remission**

Chronic leukemia of unspecified cell type with failed remission

Chronic leukemia NOS

Chapter 2

C00-D49

4 4th digit required 5 5th digit required 6 6th digit required 7 7th digit required X 7th digit placeholder ✚ Additional code L Laterality

SP C95.11 Chronic leukemia of unspecified cell type, in remission

SP C95.12 Chronic leukemia of unspecified cell type, in relapse

5 C95.9 Leukemia, unspecified

SP C95.90 Leukemia, unspecified not having achieved remission
Leukemia, unspecified with failed remission
Leukemia NOS

SP C95.91 Leukemia, unspecified, in remission

SP C95.92 Leukemia, unspecified, in relapse

4 C96 Other and unspecified malignant neoplasms of lymphoid, hematopoietic and related tissue
EXCLUDES 1 personal history of other malignant neoplasms of lymphoid, hematopoietic and related tissues (Z85.79)

SP **C96.0 Multifocal and multisystemic (disseminated) Langerhans-cell histiocytosis**
Histiocytosis X, multisystemic
Letterer-Siwe disease
EXCLUDES 1 adult pulmonary Langerhans cell histiocytosis (J84.82)
multifocal and unisystemic Langerhans-cell histiocytosis (C96.5)
unifocal Langerhans-cell histiocytosis (C96.6)

5 **C96.2 Malignant mast cell neoplasm**
EXCLUDES 1 indolent mastocytosis (D47.02)
mast cell leukemia (C94.30)
mastocytosis (congenital) (cutaneous) (Q82.2)

SP C96.20 Malignant mast cell neoplasm, unspecified

SP **C96.21 Aggressive systemic mastocytosis**

SP **C96.22 Mast cell sarcoma**

SP **C96.29 Other malignant mast cell neoplasm**

SP **C96.4 Sarcoma of dendritic cells (accessory cells)**
Follicular dendritic cell sarcoma
Interdigitating dendritic cell sarcoma
Langerhans cell sarcoma

SP **C96.5 Multifocal and unisystemic Langerhans-cell histiocytosis**
Hand-Schüller-Christian disease
Histiocytosis X, multifocal
EXCLUDES 1 multifocal and multisystemic (disseminated) Langerhans-cell histiocytosis (C96.0)
unifocal Langerhans-cell histiocytosis (C96.6)

SP **C96.6 Unifocal Langerhans-cell histiocytosis**
Eosinophilic granuloma
Histiocytosis X, unifocal
Histiocytosis X NOS
Langerhans-cell histiocytosis NOS
EXCLUDES 1 multifocal and multisysemic (disseminated) Langerhans-cell histiocytosis (C96.0)
multifocal and unisystemic Langerhans-cell histiocytosis (C96.5)

SP **C96.A Histiocytic sarcoma**
Malignant histiocytosis

SP **C96.Z Other specified malignant neoplasms of lymphoid, hematopoietic and related tissue**

SP C96.9 Malignant neoplasm of lymphoid, hematopoietic and related tissue, unspecified

In situ neoplasms (D00-D09)

INCLUDES Bowen's disease
erythroplasia
grade III intraepithelial neoplasia
Queyrat's erythroplasia

CODING TIPS ✓ Carcinomas in situ are defined as cancer that has remained in place in the specific location of origin and has not spread or invaded any neighboring tissue. The physician or NPP must state "in situ" or pre-cancerous/pre-malignant lesion in order to indicate the correct assignment of any D00-D09 codes.

4 **D00 Carcinoma in situ of oral cavity, esophagus and stomach**
EXCLUDES 1 melanoma in situ (D03.-)

+ 5 **D00.0 Carcinoma in situ of lip, oral cavity and pharynx**
Use additional code to identify:
exposure to environmental tobacco smoke (Z77.22)
exposure to tobacco smoke in the perinatal period (P96.81)
history of tobacco dependence (Z87.891)
occupational exposure to environmental tobacco smoke (Z57.31)
tobacco dependence (F17.-)
tobacco use (Z72.0)
EXCLUDES 1 carcinoma in situ of aryepiglottic fold or interarytenoid fold, laryngeal aspect (D02.0)
carcinoma in situ of epiglottis NOS (D02.0)
carcinoma in situ of epiglottis suprahyoid portion (D02.0)
carcinoma in situ of skin of lip (D03.0, D04.0)

IQ + D00.00 Carcinoma in situ of oral cavity, unspecified site

SP + **D00.01 Carcinoma in situ of labial mucosa and vermilion border**

SP + **D00.02 Carcinoma in situ of buccal mucosa**

SP + **D00.03 Carcinoma in situ of gingiva and edentulous alveolar ridge**

SP + **D00.04 Carcinoma in situ of soft palate**

SP + **D00.05 Carcinoma in situ of hard palate**

SP + **D00.06 Carcinoma in situ of floor of mouth**

SP + **D00.07 Carcinoma in situ of tongue**

SP + **D00.08 Carcinoma in situ of pharynx**
Carcinoma in situ of aryepiglottic fold NOS
Carcinoma in situ of hypopharyngeal aspect of aryepiglottic fold
Carcinoma in situ of marginal zone of aryepiglottic fold

Chapter 2 C00-D49

SP **D00.1 Carcinoma in situ of esophagus**

SP **D00.2 Carcinoma in situ of stomach**

4 **D01 Carcinoma in situ of other and unspecified digestive organs**

EXCLUDES 1 melanoma in situ (D03.-)

SP **D01.0 Carcinoma in situ of colon**

EXCLUDES 1 carcinoma in situ of rectosigmoid junction (D01.1)

SP **D01.1 Carcinoma in situ of rectosigmoid junction**

SP **D01.2 Carcinoma in situ of rectum**

SP **D01.3 Carcinoma in situ of anus and anal canal**

Anal intraepithelial neoplasia III [AIN III]
Severe dysplasia of anus

EXCLUDES 1 anal intraepithelial neoplasia I and II [AIN I and AIN II] (K62.82)
carcinoma in situ of anal margin (D04.5)
carcinoma in situ of anal skin (D04.5)
carcinoma in situ of perianal skin (D04.5)

5 **D01.4 Carcinoma in situ of other and unspecified parts of intestine**

EXCLUDES 1 carcinoma in situ of ampulla of Vater (D01.5)

IQ **D01.40 Carcinoma in situ of unspecified part of intestine**

SP **D01.49 Carcinoma in situ of other parts of intestine**

SP **D01.5 Carcinoma in situ of liver, gallbladder and bile ducts**

Carcinoma in situ of ampulla of Vater

SP **D01.7 Carcinoma in situ of other specified digestive organs**

Carcinoma in situ of pancreas

IQ **D01.9 Carcinoma in situ of digestive organ, unspecified**

+ 4 **D02 Carcinoma in situ of middle ear and respiratory system**

Use additional code to identify:
exposure to environmental tobacco smoke (Z77.22)
exposure to tobacco smoke in the perinatal period (P96.81)
history of tobacco dependence (Z87.891)
occupational exposure to environmental tobacco smoke (Z57.31)
tobacco dependence (F17.-)
tobacco use (Z72.0)

EXCLUDES 1 melanoma in situ (D03.-)

SP + **D02.0 Carcinoma in situ of larynx**

Carcinoma in situ of aryepiglottic fold or interarytenoid fold, laryngeal aspect
Carcinoma in situ of epiglottis (suprahyoid portion)

EXCLUDES 1 carcinoma in situ of aryepiglottic fold or interarytenoid fold NOS (D00.08)
carcinoma in situ of hypopharyngeal aspect (D00.08)
carcinoma in situ of marginal zone (D00.08)

SP + **D02.1 Carcinoma in situ of trachea**

+ 5 **D02.2 Carcinoma in situ of bronchus and lung**

⊟ IQ + **D02.20 Carcinoma in situ of unspecified bronchus and lung**

⊟ SP + **D02.21 Carcinoma in situ of right bronchus and lung**

⊟ SP + **D02.22 Carcinoma in situ of left bronchus and lung**

SP + **D02.3 Carcinoma in situ of other parts of respiratory system**

Carcinoma in situ of accessory sinuses
Carcinoma in situ of middle ear
Carcinoma in situ of nasal cavities

EXCLUDES 1 carcinoma in situ of ear (external) (skin) (D04.2-)
carcinoma in situ of nose NOS (D09.8)
carcinoma in situ of skin of nose (D04.3)

IQ + **D02.4 Carcinoma in situ of respiratory system, unspecified**

4 **D03 Melanoma in situ**

SP **D03.0 Melanoma in situ of lip**

5 **D03.1 Melanoma in situ of eyelid, including canthus**

⊟ IQ **D03.10 Melanoma in situ of unspecified eyelid, including canthus**

6 **D03.11 Melanoma in situ of right eyelid, including canthus**

⊟ SP **D03.111 Melanoma in situ of right upper eyelid, including canthus**

⊟ SP **D03.112 Melanoma in situ of right lower eyelid, including canthus**

6 **D03.12 Melanoma in situ of left eyelid, including canthus**

⊟ SP **D03.121 Melanoma in situ of left upper eyelid, including canthus**

⊟ SP **D03.122 Melanoma in situ of left lower eyelid, including canthus**

5 **D03.2 Melanoma in situ of ear and external auricular canal**

⊟ IQ **D03.20 Melanoma in situ of unspecified ear and external auricular canal**

⊟ SP **D03.21 Melanoma in situ of right ear and external auricular canal**

⊟ SP **D03.22 Melanoma in situ of left ear and external auricular canal**

5 **D03.3 Melanoma in situ of other and unspecified parts of face**

IQ **D03.30 Melanoma in situ of unspecified part of face**

SP **D03.39 Melanoma in situ of other parts of face**

SP **D03.4 Melanoma in situ of scalp and neck**

5 **D03.5 Melanoma in situ of trunk**

SP **D03.51 Melanoma in situ of anal skin**

Melanoma in situ of anal margin
Melanoma in situ of perianal skin

SP **D03.52 Melanoma in situ of breast (skin) (soft tissue)**

SP **D03.59 Melanoma in situ of other part of trunk**

5 **D03.6 Melanoma in situ of upper limb, including shoulder**

4 4th digit required 5 5th digit required 6 6th digit required 7 7th digit required 7 7th digit placeholder + Additional code ⊟ Laterality

D03.60 Melanoma in situ of unspecified upper limb, including shoulder
D03.61 Melanoma in situ of right upper limb, including shoulder
D03.62 Melanoma in situ of left upper limb, including shoulder
D03.7 Melanoma in situ of lower limb, including hip
D03.70 Melanoma in situ of unspecified lower limb, including hip
D03.71 Melanoma in situ of right lower limb, including hip
D03.72 Melanoma in situ of left lower limb, including hip
D03.8 Melanoma in situ of other sites
Melanoma in situ of scrotum
EXCLUDES 1 carcinoma in situ of scrotum (D07.61)
D03.9 Melanoma in situ, unspecified

D04 Carcinoma in situ of skin
EXCLUDES 1 erythroplasia of Queyrat (penis) NOS (D07.4)
melanoma in situ (D03.-)

D04.0 Carcinoma in situ of skin of lip
EXCLUDES 2 carcinoma in situ of vermilion border of lip (D00.01)
D04.1 Carcinoma in situ of skin of eyelid, including canthus
D04.10 Carcinoma in situ of skin of unspecified eyelid, including canthus
D04.11 Carcinoma in situ of skin of right eyelid, including canthus
D04.111 Carcinoma in situ of skin of right upper eyelid, including canthus
D04.112 Carcinoma in situ of skin of right lower eyelid, including canthus
D04.12 Carcinoma in situ of skin of left eyelid, including canthus
D04.121 Carcinoma in situ of skin of left upper eyelid, including canthus
D04.122 Carcinoma in situ of skin of left lower eyelid, including canthus
D04.2 Carcinoma in situ of skin of ear and external auricular canal
D04.20 Carcinoma in situ of skin of unspecified ear and external auricular canal
D04.21 Carcinoma in situ of skin of right ear and external auricular canal
D04.22 Carcinoma in situ of skin of left ear and external auricular canal
D04.3 Carcinoma in situ of skin of other and unspecified parts of face
D04.30 Carcinoma in situ of skin of unspecified part of face
D04.39 Carcinoma in situ of skin of other parts of face
D04.4 Carcinoma in situ of skin of scalp and neck
D04.5 Carcinoma in situ of skin of trunk
Carcinoma in situ of anal margin
Carcinoma in situ of anal skin
Carcinoma in situ of perianal skin
Carcinoma in situ of skin of breast
EXCLUDES 1 carcinoma in situ of anus NOS (D01.3)
carcinoma in situ of scrotum (D07.61)
carcinoma in situ of skin of genital organs (D07.-)
D04.6 Carcinoma in situ of skin of upper limb, including shoulder
D04.60 Carcinoma in situ of skin of unspecified upper limb, including shoulder
D04.61 Carcinoma in situ of skin of right upper limb, including shoulder
D04.62 Carcinoma in situ of skin of left upper limb, including shoulder
D04.7 Carcinoma in situ of skin of lower limb, including hip
D04.70 Carcinoma in situ of skin of unspecified lower limb, including hip
D04.71 Carcinoma in situ of skin of right lower limb, including hip
D04.72 Carcinoma in situ of skin of left lower limb, including hip
D04.8 Carcinoma in situ of skin of other sites
D04.9 Carcinoma in situ of skin, unspecified

D05 Carcinoma in situ of breast
EXCLUDES 1 carcinoma in situ of skin of breast (D04.5)
melanoma in situ of breast (skin) (D03.5)
Paget's disease of breast or nipple (C50.-)

D05.0 Lobular carcinoma in situ of breast
D05.00 Lobular carcinoma in situ of unspecified breast
D05.01 Lobular carcinoma in situ of right breast
D05.02 Lobular carcinoma in situ of left breast
D05.1 Intraductal carcinoma in situ of breast
D05.10 Intraductal carcinoma in situ of unspecified breast
D05.11 Intraductal carcinoma in situ of right breast
D05.12 Intraductal carcinoma in situ of left breast
D05.8 Other specified type of carcinoma in situ of breast
D05.80 Other specified type of carcinoma in situ of unspecified breast
D05.81 Other specified type of carcinoma in situ of right breast
D05.82 Other specified type of carcinoma in situ of left breast
D05.9 Unspecified type of carcinoma in situ of breast
D05.90 Unspecified type of carcinoma in situ of unspecified breast
D05.91 Unspecified type of carcinoma in situ of right breast
D05.92 Unspecified type of carcinoma in situ of left breast

D06 Carcinoma in situ of cervix uteri
INCLUDES cervical adenocarcinoma in situ

Chapter 2 C00-D49

cervical intraepithelial glandular neoplasia
cervical intraepithelial neoplasia III [CIN III]
severe dysplasia of cervix uteri

EXCLUDES 1 cervical intraepithelial neoplasia II [CIN II] (N87.1)
cytologic evidence of malignancy of cervix without histologic confirmation (R87.614)
high grade squamous intraepithelial lesion (HGSIL) of cervix (R87.613)
melanoma in situ of cervix (D03.5)
moderate cervical dysplasia (N87.1)

CODING TIPS ✓ Class III, or severe dysplasia, is coded to category D06. Mild and moderate dysplasia of the cervix is coded to N87.-

SP **D06.0 Carcinoma in situ of endocervix**

SP **D06.1 Carcinoma in situ of exocervix**

SP **D06.7 Carcinoma in situ of other parts of cervix**

SP **D06.9 Carcinoma in situ of cervix, unspecified**

4 **D07 Carcinoma in situ of other and unspecified genital organs**

EXCLUDES 1 melanoma in situ of trunk (D03.5)

SP **D07.0 Carcinoma in situ of endometrium**

SP **D07.1 Carcinoma in situ of vulva**
Severe dysplasia of vulva
Vulvar intraepithelial neoplasia III [VIN III]

EXCLUDES 1 moderate dysplasia of vulva (N90.1)
vulvar intraepithelial neoplasia II [VIN II] (N90.1)

SP **D07.2 Carcinoma in situ of vagina**
Severe dysplasia of vagina
Vaginal intraepithelial neoplasia III [VAIN III]

EXCLUDES 1 moderate dysplasia of vagina (N89.1)
vaginal intraepithelial neoplasia II [VIN II] (N89.1)

5 **D07.3 Carcinoma in situ of other and unspecified female genital organs**

IQ **D07.30 Carcinoma in situ of unspecified female genital organs**

SP **D07.39 Carcinoma in situ of other female genital organs**

SP **D07.4 Carcinoma in situ of penis**
Erythroplasia of Queyrat NOS

SP **D07.5 Carcinoma in situ of prostate**
Prostatic intraepithelial neoplasia III (PIN III)
Severe dysplasia of prostate

EXCLUDES 1 dysplasia (mild) (moderate) of prostate (N42.3-)
prostatic intraepithelial neoplasia II [PIN II] (N42.3-)

5 **D07.6 Carcinoma in situ of other and unspecified male genital organs**

IQ **D07.60 Carcinoma in situ of unspecified male genital organs**

SP **D07.61 Carcinoma in situ of scrotum**

SP **D07.69 Carcinoma in situ of other male genital organs**

4 **D09 Carcinoma in situ of other and unspecified sites**

EXCLUDES 1 melanoma in situ (D03.-)

SP **D09.0 Carcinoma in situ of bladder**

5 **D09.1 Carcinoma in situ of other and unspecified urinary organs**

IQ **D09.10 Carcinoma in situ of unspecified urinary organ**

SP **D09.19 Carcinoma in situ of other urinary organs**

5 **D09.2 Carcinoma in situ of eye**

EXCLUDES 1 carcinoma in situ of skin of eyelid (D04.1-)

⊟ IQ **D09.20 Carcinoma in situ of unspecified eye**

⊟ SP **D09.21 Carcinoma in situ of right eye**

⊟ SP **D09.22 Carcinoma in situ of left eye**

SP **D09.3 Carcinoma in situ of thyroid and other endocrine glands**

EXCLUDES 1 carcinoma in situ of endocrine pancreas (D01.7)
carcinoma in situ of ovary (D07.39)
carcinoma in situ of testis (D07.69)

SP **D09.8 Carcinoma in situ of other specified sites**

IQ **D09.9 Carcinoma in situ, unspecified**

Benign neoplasms, except benign neuroendocrine tumors (D10-D36)

4 **D10 Benign neoplasm of mouth and pharynx**

SP **D10.0 Benign neoplasm of lip**
Benign neoplasm of lip (frenulum) (inner aspect) (mucosa) (vermilion border)

EXCLUDES 1 benign neoplasm of skin of lip (D22.0, D23.0)

SP **D10.1 Benign neoplasm of tongue**
Benign neoplasm of lingual tonsil

SP **D10.2 Benign neoplasm of floor of mouth**

5 **D10.3 Benign neoplasm of other and unspecified parts of mouth**

IQ **D10.30 Benign neoplasm of unspecified part of mouth**

SP **D10.39 Benign neoplasm of other parts of mouth**
Benign neoplasm of minor salivary gland NOS

EXCLUDES 1 benign odontogenic neoplasms (D16.4-D16.5)
benign neoplasm of mucosa of lip (D10.0)
benign neoplasm of nasopharyngeal surface of soft palate (D10.6)

SP **D10.4 Benign neoplasm of tonsil**

4 4th digit required 5 5th digit required 6 6th digit required 7 7th digit required 7 7th digit placeholder + Additional code ⊟ Laterality

Benign neoplasm of tonsil (faucial) (palatine)
EXCLUDES 1 benign neoplasm of lingual tonsil (D10.1)
benign neoplasm of pharyngeal tonsil (D10.6)
benign neoplasm of tonsillar fossa (D10.5)
benign neoplasm of tonsillar pillars (D10.5)

SP **D10.5 Benign neoplasm of other parts of oropharynx**
Benign neoplasm of epiglottis, anterior aspect
Benign neoplasm of tonsillar fossa
Benign neoplasm of tonsillar pillars
Benign neoplasm of vallecula
EXCLUDES 1 benign neoplasm of epiglottis NOS (D14.1)
benign neoplasm of epiglottis, suprahyoid portion (D14.1)

SP **D10.6 Benign neoplasm of nasopharynx**
Benign neoplasm of pharyngeal tonsil
Benign neoplasm of posterior margin of septum and choanae

SP **D10.7 Benign neoplasm of hypopharynx**

SP **D10.9 Benign neoplasm of pharynx, unspecified**

4 **D11 Benign neoplasm of major salivary glands**
EXCLUDES 1 benign neoplasms of specified minor salivary glands which are classified according to their anatomical location
benign neoplasms of minor salivary glands NOS (D10.39)

SP **D11.0 Benign neoplasm of parotid gland**

SP **D11.7 Benign neoplasm of other major salivary glands**
Benign neoplasm of sublingual salivary gland
Benign neoplasm of submandibular salivary gland

IQ **D11.9 Benign neoplasm of major salivary gland, unspecified**

4 **D12 Benign neoplasm of colon, rectum, anus and anal canal**
EXCLUDES 1 benign carcinoid tumors of the large intestine, and rectum (D3A.02-)
polyp of colon NOS (K63.5)

CODING TIPS✓ Adenomatous polyps are coded to D12. Hyperplastic polyps are coded to K63.5.

SP **D12.0 Benign neoplasm of cecum**
Benign neoplasm of ileocecal valve

SP **D12.1 Benign neoplasm of appendix**
EXCLUDES 1 benign carcinoid tumor of the appendix (D3A.020)

SP **D12.2 Benign neoplasm of ascending colon**

SP **D12.3 Benign neoplasm of transverse colon**
Benign neoplasm of hepatic flexure
Benign neoplasm of splenic flexure

SP **D12.4 Benign neoplasm of descending colon**

SP **D12.5 Benign neoplasm of sigmoid colon**

SP **D12.6 Benign neoplasm of colon, unspecified**
Adenomatosis of colon
Benign neoplasm of large intestine NOS
Polyposis (hereditary) of colon
EXCLUDES 1 inflammatory polyp of colon (K51.4-)

SP **D12.7 Benign neoplasm of rectosigmoid junction**

SP **D12.8 Benign neoplasm of rectum**
EXCLUDES 1 benign carcinoid tumor of the rectum (D3A.026)

SP **D12.9 Benign neoplasm of anus and anal canal**
Benign neoplasm of anus NOS
EXCLUDES 1 benign neoplasm of anal margin (D22.5, D23.5)
benign neoplasm of anal skin (D22.5, D23.5)
benign neoplasm of perianal skin (D22.5, D23.5)

4 **D13 Benign neoplasm of other and ill-defined parts of digestive system**
EXCLUDES 1 benign stromal tumors of digestive system (D21.4)

SP **D13.0 Benign neoplasm of esophagus**

SP **D13.1 Benign neoplasm of stomach**
EXCLUDES 1 benign carcinoid tumor of the stomach (D3A.092)

SP **D13.2 Benign neoplasm of duodenum**
EXCLUDES 1 benign carcinoid tumor of the duodenum (D3A.010)

5 **D13.3 Benign neoplasm of other and unspecified parts of small intestine**
EXCLUDES 1 benign carcinoid tumors of the small intestine (D3A.01-)
benign neoplasm of ileocecal valve (D12.0)

SP **D13.30 Benign neoplasm of unspecified part of small intestine**

SP **D13.39 Benign neoplasm of other parts of small intestine**

SP **D13.4 Benign neoplasm of liver**
Benign neoplasm of intrahepatic bile ducts

SP **D13.5 Benign neoplasm of extrahepatic bile ducts**

SP **D13.6 Benign neoplasm of pancreas**
EXCLUDES 1 benign neoplasm of endocrine pancreas (D13.7)

SP + **D13.7 Benign neoplasm of endocrine pancreas**
Islet cell tumor
Benign neoplasm of islets of Langerhans
Use additional code to identify any functional activity.

SP **D13.9 Benign neoplasm of ill-defined sites within the digestive system**
Benign neoplasm of digestive system NOS
Benign neoplasm of intestine NOS
Benign neoplasm of spleen

4 **D14 Benign neoplasm of middle ear and respiratory system**

SP **D14.0 Benign neoplasm of middle ear, nasal cavity and accessory sinuses**
Benign neoplasm of cartilage of nose
EXCLUDES 1 benign neoplasm of auricular canal (external) (D22.2-, D23.2-)
benign neoplasm of bone of ear (D16.4)

Chapter 2

C00-D49

benign neoplasm of bone of nose (D16.4)
benign neoplasm of cartilage of ear (D21.0)
benign neoplasm of ear (external) (skin) (D22.2-, D23.2-)
benign neoplasm of nose NOS (D36.7)
benign neoplasm of skin of nose (D22.39, D23.39)
benign neoplasm of olfactory bulb (D33.3)
benign neoplasm of posterior margin of septum and choanae (D10.6)
polyp of accessory sinus (J33.8)
polyp of ear (middle) (H74.4)
polyp of nasal (cavity) (J33.-)

SP **D14.1 Benign neoplasm of larynx**
Adenomatous polyp of larynx
Benign neoplasm of epiglottis (suprahyoid portion)
EXCLUDES 1 benign neoplasm of epiglottis, anterior aspect (D10.5)
polyp (nonadenomatous) of vocal cord or larynx (J38.1)

SP **D14.2 Benign neoplasm of trachea**

5 **D14.3 Benign neoplasm of bronchus and lung**
EXCLUDES 1 benign carcinoid tumor of the bronchus and lung (D3A.090)

Laterality !Q **D14.30 Benign neoplasm of unspecified bronchus and lung**

Laterality SP **D14.31 Benign neoplasm of right bronchus and lung**

Laterality SP **D14.32 Benign neoplasm of left bronchus and lung**

!Q **D14.4 Benign neoplasm of respiratory system, unspecified**

4 **D15 Benign neoplasm of other and unspecified intrathoracic organs**
EXCLUDES 1 benign neoplasm of mesothelial tissue (D19.-)

SP **D15.0 Benign neoplasm of thymus**
EXCLUDES 1 benign carcinoid tumor of the thymus (D3A.091)

SP **D15.1 Benign neoplasm of heart**
EXCLUDES 1 benign neoplasm of great vessels (D21.3)

SP **D15.2 Benign neoplasm of mediastinum**

SP **D15.7 Benign neoplasm of other specified intrathoracic organs**

!Q **D15.9 Benign neoplasm of intrathoracic organ, unspecified**

4 **D16 Benign neoplasm of bone and articular cartilage**
EXCLUDES 1 benign neoplasm of connective tissue of ear (D21.0)
benign neoplasm of connective tissue of eyelid (D21.0)
benign neoplasm of connective tissue of larynx (D14.1)
benign neoplasm of connective tissue of nose (D14.0)
benign neoplasm of synovia (D21.-)

5 **D16.0 Benign neoplasm of scapula and long bones of upper limb**

Laterality !Q **D16.00 Benign neoplasm of scapula and long bones of unspecified upper limb**

Laterality SP **D16.01 Benign neoplasm of scapula and long bones of right upper limb**

Laterality SP **D16.02 Benign neoplasm of scapula and long bones of left upper limb**

5 **D16.1 Benign neoplasm of short bones of upper limb**

Laterality !Q **D16.10 Benign neoplasm of short bones of unspecified upper limb**

Laterality SP **D16.11 Benign neoplasm of short bones of right upper limb**

Laterality SP **D16.12 Benign neoplasm of short bones of left upper limb**

5 **D16.2 Benign neoplasm of long bones of lower limb**

Laterality !Q **D16.20 Benign neoplasm of long bones of unspecified lower limb**

Laterality SP **D16.21 Benign neoplasm of long bones of right lower limb**

Laterality SP **D16.22 Benign neoplasm of long bones of left lower limb**

5 **D16.3 Benign neoplasm of short bones of lower limb**

Laterality !Q **D16.30 Benign neoplasm of short bones of unspecified lower limb**

Laterality SP **D16.31 Benign neoplasm of short bones of right lower limb**

Laterality SP **D16.32 Benign neoplasm of short bones of left lower limb**

SP **D16.4 Benign neoplasm of bones of skull and face**
Benign neoplasm of maxilla (superior)
Benign neoplasm of orbital bone
Keratocyst of maxilla
Keratocystic odontogenic tumor of maxilla
EXCLUDES 2 benign neoplasm of lower jaw bone (D16.5)

SP **D16.5 Benign neoplasm of lower jaw bone**
Keratocyst of mandible
Keratocystic odontogenic tumor of mandible

SP **D16.6 Benign neoplasm of vertebral column**
EXCLUDES 1 benign neoplasm of sacrum and coccyx (D16.8)

SP **D16.7 Benign neoplasm of ribs, sternum and clavicle**

SP **D16.8 Benign neoplasm of pelvic bones, sacrum and coccyx**

!Q **D16.9 Benign neoplasm of bone and articular cartilage, unspecified**

4 **D17 Benign lipomatous neoplasm**

SP **D17.0 Benign lipomatous neoplasm of skin and subcutaneous tissue of head, face and neck**

SP **D17.1 Benign lipomatous neoplasm of skin and subcutaneous tissue of trunk**

5 **D17.2 Benign lipomatous neoplasm of skin and subcutaneous tissue of limb**

= IQ **D17.20 Benign lipomatous neoplasm of skin and subcutaneous tissue of unspecified limb**

= SP **D17.21 Benign lipomatous neoplasm of skin and subcutaneous tissue of right arm**

= SP **D17.22 Benign lipomatous neoplasm of skin and subcutaneous tissue of left arm**

= SP **D17.23 Benign lipomatous neoplasm of skin and subcutaneous tissue of right leg**

= SP **D17.24 Benign lipomatous neoplasm of skin and subcutaneous tissue of left leg**

5 **D17.3 Benign lipomatous neoplasm of skin and subcutaneous tissue of other and unspecified sites**

IQ **D17.30 Benign lipomatous neoplasm of skin and subcutaneous tissue of unspecified sites**

SP **D17.39 Benign lipomatous neoplasm of skin and subcutaneous tissue of other sites**

SP **D17.4 Benign lipomatous neoplasm of intrathoracic organs**

SP **D17.5 Benign lipomatous neoplasm of intra-abdominal organs**

EXCLUDES 1 benign lipomatous neoplasm of peritoneum and retroperitoneum (D17.79)

SP **D17.6 Benign lipomatous neoplasm of spermatic cord**

5 **D17.7 Benign lipomatous neoplasm of other sites**

SP **D17.71 Benign lipomatous neoplasm of kidney**

SP **D17.72 Benign lipomatous neoplasm of other genitourinary organ**

SP **D17.79 Benign lipomatous neoplasm of other sites**

Benign lipomatous neoplasm of peritoneum

Benign lipomatous neoplasm of retroperitoneum

IQ **D17.9 Benign lipomatous neoplasm, unspecified**

Lipoma NOS

4 **D18 Hemangioma and lymphangioma, any site**

EXCLUDES 1 benign neoplasm of glomus jugulare (D35.6)
blue or pigmented nevus (D22.-)
nevus NOS (D22.-)
vascular nevus (Q82.5)

5 **D18.0 Hemangioma**

Angioma NOS

Cavernous nevus

IQ **D18.00 Hemangioma unspecified site**

SP **D18.01 Hemangioma of skin and subcutaneous tissue**

SP **D18.02 Hemangioma of intracranial structures**

SP **D18.03 Hemangioma of intra-abdominal structures**

SP **D18.09 Hemangioma of other sites**

SP **D18.1 Lymphangioma, any site**

4 **D19 Benign neoplasm of mesothelial tissue**

SP **D19.0 Benign neoplasm of mesothelial tissue of pleura**

SP **D19.1 Benign neoplasm of mesothelial tissue of peritoneum**

SP **D19.7 Benign neoplasm of mesothelial tissue of other sites**

IQ **D19.9 Benign neoplasm of mesothelial tissue, unspecified**

Benign mesothelioma NOS

4 **D20 Benign neoplasm of soft tissue of retroperitoneum and peritoneum**

EXCLUDES 1 benign lipomatous neoplasm of peritoneum and retroperitoneum (D17.79)
benign neoplasm of mesothelial tissue (D19.-)

SP **D20.0 Benign neoplasm of soft tissue of retroperitoneum**

SP **D20.1 Benign neoplasm of soft tissue of peritoneum**

4 **D21 Other benign neoplasms of connective and other soft tissue**

INCLUDES benign neoplasm of blood vessel
benign neoplasm of bursa
benign neoplasm of cartilage
benign neoplasm of fascia
benign neoplasm of fat
benign neoplasm of ligament, except uterine
benign neoplasm of lymphatic channel
benign neoplasm of muscle
benign neoplasm of synovia
benign neoplasm of tendon (sheath)
benign stromal tumors

EXCLUDES 1 benign neoplasm of articular cartilage (D16.-)
benign neoplasm of cartilage of larynx (D14.1)
benign neoplasm of cartilage of nose (D14.0)
benign neoplasm of connective tissue of breast (D24.-)
benign neoplasm of peripheral nerves and autonomic nervous system (D36.1-)
benign neoplasm of peritoneum (D20.1)
benign neoplasm of retroperitoneum (D20.0)
benign neoplasm of uterine ligament, any (D28.2)
benign neoplasm of vascular tissue (D18.-)
hemangioma (D18.0-)
lipomatous neoplasm (D17.-)
lymphangioma (D18.1)
uterine leiomyoma (D25.-)

SP **D21.0 Benign neoplasm of connective and other soft tissue of head, face and neck**

Benign neoplasm of connective tissue of ear

Benign neoplasm of connective tissue of eyelid

EXCLUDES 1 benign neoplasm of connective tissue of orbit (D31.6-)

Chapter 2

C00-D49

5 D21.1 Benign neoplasm of connective and other soft tissue of upper limb, including shoulder

⊟ IQ D21.10 Benign neoplasm of connective and other soft tissue of unspecified upper limb, including shoulder

⊟ SP D21.11 Benign neoplasm of connective and other soft tissue of right upper limb, including shoulder

⊟ SP D21.12 Benign neoplasm of connective and other soft tissue of left upper limb, including shoulder

5 D21.2 Benign neoplasm of connective and other soft tissue of lower limb, including hip

⊟ IQ D21.20 Benign neoplasm of connective and other soft tissue of unspecified lower limb, including hip

⊟ SP D21.21 Benign neoplasm of connective and other soft tissue of right lower limb, including hip

⊟ SP D21.22 Benign neoplasm of connective and other soft tissue of left lower limb, including hip

SP D21.3 Benign neoplasm of connective and other soft tissue of thorax

Benign neoplasm of axilla
Benign neoplasm of diaphragm
Benign neoplasm of great vessels

EXCLUDES 1 benign neoplasm of heart (D15.1)
benign neoplasm of mediastinum (D15.2)
benign neoplasm of thymus (D15.0)

SP D21.4 Benign neoplasm of connective and other soft tissue of abdomen

Benign stromal tumors of abdomen

SP D21.5 Benign neoplasm of connective and other soft tissue of pelvis

EXCLUDES 1 benign neoplasm of any uterine ligament (D28.2)
uterine leiomyoma (D25.-)

SP D21.6 Benign neoplasm of connective and other soft tissue of trunk, unspecified

Benign neoplasm of connective and other soft tissue of back NOS

IQ D21.9 Benign neoplasm of connective and other soft tissue, unspecified

4 D22 Melanocytic nevi

INCLUDES atypical nevus
blue hairy pigmented nevus
nevus NOS

CODING TIPS ✓ Melanocytic nevi are also known as moles. These benign neoplasms are generally not treated and pose little threat to individuals. Melanocytic nevi are unlikely to impair patient function in any way and do not support a need for medical necessity under the home health benefit.

SP D22.0 Melanocytic nevi of lip

5 D22.1 Melanocytic nevi of eyelid, including canthus

⊟ IQ D22.10 Melanocytic nevi of unspecified eyelid, including canthus

6 D22.11 Melanocytic nevi of right eyelid, including canthus

⊟ SP D22.111 Melanocytic nevi of right upper eyelid, including canthus

⊟ SP D22.112 Melanocytic nevi of right lower eyelid, including canthus

6 D22.12 Melanocytic nevi of left eyelid, including canthus

⊟ SP D22.121 Melanocytic nevi of left upper eyelid, including canthus

⊟ SP D22.122 Melanocytic nevi of left lower eyelid, including canthus

5 D22.2 Melanocytic nevi of ear and external auricular canal

⊟ IQ D22.20 Melanocytic nevi of unspecified ear and external auricular canal

⊟ SP D22.21 Melanocytic nevi of right ear and external auricular canal

⊟ SP D22.22 Melanocytic nevi of left ear and external auricular canal

5 D22.3 Melanocytic nevi of other and unspecified parts of face

IQ D22.30 Melanocytic nevi of unspecified part of face

SP D22.39 Melanocytic nevi of other parts of face

SP D22.4 Melanocytic nevi of scalp and neck

SP D22.5 Melanocytic nevi of trunk

Melanocytic nevi of anal margin
Melanocytic nevi of anal skin
Melanocytic nevi of perianal skin
Melanocytic nevi of skin of breast

5 D22.6 Melanocytic nevi of upper limb, including shoulder

⊟ IQ D22.60 Melanocytic nevi of unspecified upper limb, including shoulder

⊟ SP D22.61 Melanocytic nevi of right upper limb, including shoulder

⊟ SP D22.62 Melanocytic nevi of left upper limb, including shoulder

5 D22.7 Melanocytic nevi of lower limb, including hip

⊟ IQ D22.70 Melanocytic nevi of unspecified lower limb, including hip

⊟ SP D22.71 Melanocytic nevi of right lower limb, including hip

⊟ SP D22.72 Melanocytic nevi of left lower limb, including hip

IQ D22.9 Melanocytic nevi, unspecified

4 D23 Other benign neoplasms of skin

INCLUDES benign neoplasm of hair follicles
benign neoplasm of sebaceous glands
benign neoplasm of sweat glands

EXCLUDES 1 benign lipomatous neoplasms of skin (D17.0-D17.3)

EXCLUDES 2 melanocytic nevi (D22.-)

SP D23.0 Other benign neoplasm of skin of lip

EXCLUDES 1 benign neoplasm of vermilion border of lip (D10.0)

5 D23.1 Other benign neoplasm of skin of eyelid, including canthus

⊟ IQ D23.10 Other benign neoplasm of skin of unspecified eyelid, including canthus

6 **D23.11 Other benign neoplasm of skin of right eyelid, including canthus**

SP D23.111 Other benign neoplasm of skin of right upper eyelid, including canthus

SP D23.112 Other benign neoplasm of skin of right lower eyelid, including canthus

6 **D23.12 Other benign neoplasm of skin of left eyelid, including canthus**

SP D23.121 Other benign neoplasm of skin of left upper eyelid, including canthus

SP D23.122 Other benign neoplasm of skin of left lower eyelid, including canthus

5 **D23.2 Other benign neoplasm of skin of ear and external auricular canal**

IQ D23.20 Other benign neoplasm of skin of unspecified ear and external auricular canal

SP D23.21 Other benign neoplasm of skin of right ear and external auricular canal

SP D23.22 Other benign neoplasm of skin of left ear and external auricular canal

5 **D23.3 Other benign neoplasm of skin of other and unspecified parts of face**

IQ D23.30 Other benign neoplasm of skin of unspecified part of face

SP D23.39 Other benign neoplasm of skin of other parts of face

SP D23.4 Other benign neoplasm of skin of scalp and neck

SP D23.5 Other benign neoplasm of skin of trunk

Other benign neoplasm of anal margin
Other benign neoplasm of anal skin
Other benign neoplasm of perianal skin
Other benign neoplasm of skin of breast

EXCLUDES 1 benign neoplasm of anus NOS (D12.9)

5 **D23.6 Other benign neoplasm of skin of upper limb, including shoulder**

IQ D23.60 Other benign neoplasm of skin of unspecified upper limb, including shoulder

SP D23.61 Other benign neoplasm of skin of right upper limb, including shoulder

SP D23.62 Other benign neoplasm of skin of left upper limb, including shoulder

5 **D23.7 Other benign neoplasm of skin of lower limb, including hip**

IQ D23.70 Other benign neoplasm of skin of unspecified lower limb, including hip

SP D23.71 Other benign neoplasm of skin of right lower limb, including hip

SP D23.72 Other benign neoplasm of skin of left lower limb, including hip

IQ D23.9 Other benign neoplasm of skin, unspecified

4 **D24 Benign neoplasm of breast**

INCLUDES benign neoplasm of connective tissue of breast
benign neoplasm of soft parts of breast
fibroadenoma of breast

EXCLUDES 2 adenofibrosis of breast (N60.2)
benign cyst of breast (N60.-)
benign mammary dysplasia (N60.-)
benign neoplasm of skin of breast (D22.5, D23.5)
fibrocystic disease of breast (N60.-)

SP D24.1 Benign neoplasm of right breast

SP D24.2 Benign neoplasm of left breast

IQ D24.9 Benign neoplasm of unspecified breast

4 **D25 Leiomyoma of uterus**

INCLUDES uterine fibroid
uterine fibromyoma
uterine myoma

SP D25.0 Submucous leiomyoma of uterus

SP D25.1 Intramural leiomyoma of uterus

Interstitial leiomyoma of uterus

SP D25.2 Subserosal leiomyoma of uterus

Subperitoneal leiomyoma of uterus

SP D25.9 Leiomyoma of uterus, unspecified

4 **D26 Other benign neoplasms of uterus**

SP D26.0 Other benign neoplasm of cervix uteri

SP D26.1 Other benign neoplasm of corpus uteri

SP D26.7 Other benign neoplasm of other parts of uterus

SP D26.9 Other benign neoplasm of uterus, unspecified

+ 4 **D27 Benign neoplasm of ovary**

Use additional code to identify any functional activity.

EXCLUDES 2 corpus albicans cyst (N83.2-)
corpus luteum cyst (N83.1-)
endometrial cyst (N80.1)
follicular (atretic) cyst (N83.0-)
graafian follicle cyst (N83.0-)
ovarian cyst NEC (N83.2-)
ovarian retention cyst (N83.2-)

SP + D27.0 Benign neoplasm of right ovary

SP + D27.1 Benign neoplasm of left ovary

IQ + D27.9 Benign neoplasm of unspecified ovary

4 **D28 Benign neoplasm of other and unspecified female genital organs**

INCLUDES adenomatous polyp
benign neoplasm of skin of female genital organs
benign teratoma

EXCLUDES 1 epoophoron cyst (Q50.5)
fimbrial cyst (Q50.4)
Gartner's duct cyst (Q52.4)
parovarian cyst (Q50.5)

SP D28.0 Benign neoplasm of vulva

SP D28.1 Benign neoplasm of vagina

SP D28.2 Benign neoplasm of uterine tubes and ligaments

Benign neoplasm of fallopian tube
Benign neoplasm of uterine ligament (broad) (round)

SP D28.7 Benign neoplasm of other specified female genital organs

IQ D28.9 Benign neoplasm of female genital organ, unspecified

4 **D29 Benign neoplasm of male genital organs**

Chapter 2 C00-D49

INCLUDES benign neoplasm of skin of male genital organs

SP **D29.0 Benign neoplasm of penis**

SP **D29.1 Benign neoplasm of prostate**
EXCLUDES 1 enlarged prostate (N40.-)

+ 5 **D29.2 Benign neoplasm of testis**
Use additional code to identify any functional activity.

Laterality !Q + **D29.20 Benign neoplasm of unspecified testis**

Laterality SP + **D29.21 Benign neoplasm of right testis**

Laterality SP + **D29.22 Benign neoplasm of left testis**

5 **D29.3 Benign neoplasm of epididymis**

Laterality !Q **D29.30 Benign neoplasm of unspecified epididymis**

Laterality SP **D29.31 Benign neoplasm of right epididymis**

Laterality SP **D29.32 Benign neoplasm of left epididymis**

SP **D29.4 Benign neoplasm of scrotum**
Benign neoplasm of skin of scrotum

SP **D29.8 Benign neoplasm of other specified male genital organs**
Benign neoplasm of seminal vesicle
Benign neoplasm of spermatic cord
Benign neoplasm of tunica vaginalis

!Q **D29.9 Benign neoplasm of male genital organ, unspecified**

4 **D30 Benign neoplasm of urinary organs**

5 **D30.0 Benign neoplasm of kidney**
EXCLUDES 1 benign carcinoid tumor of the kidney (D3A.093)
benign neoplasm of renal calyces (D30.1-)
benign neoplasm of renal pelvis (D30.1-)

Laterality !Q **D30.00 Benign neoplasm of unspecified kidney**

Laterality SP **D30.01 Benign neoplasm of right kidney**

Laterality SP **D30.02 Benign neoplasm of left kidney**

5 **D30.1 Benign neoplasm of renal pelvis**

Laterality !Q **D30.10 Benign neoplasm of unspecified renal pelvis**

Laterality SP **D30.11 Benign neoplasm of right renal pelvis**

Laterality SP **D30.12 Benign neoplasm of left renal pelvis**

5 **D30.2 Benign neoplasm of ureter**
EXCLUDES 1 benign neoplasm of ureteric orifice of bladder (D30.3)

Laterality !Q **D30.20 Benign neoplasm of unspecified ureter**

Laterality SP **D30.21 Benign neoplasm of right ureter**

Laterality SP **D30.22 Benign neoplasm of left ureter**

SP **D30.3 Benign neoplasm of bladder**
Benign neoplasm of ureteric orifice of bladder
Benign neoplasm of urethral orifice of bladder

SP **D30.4 Benign neoplasm of urethra**
EXCLUDES 1 benign neoplasm of urethral orifice of bladder (D30.3)

SP **D30.8 Benign neoplasm of other specified urinary organs**
Benign neoplasm of paraurethral glands

!Q **D30.9 Benign neoplasm of urinary organ, unspecified**
Benign neoplasm of urinary system NOS

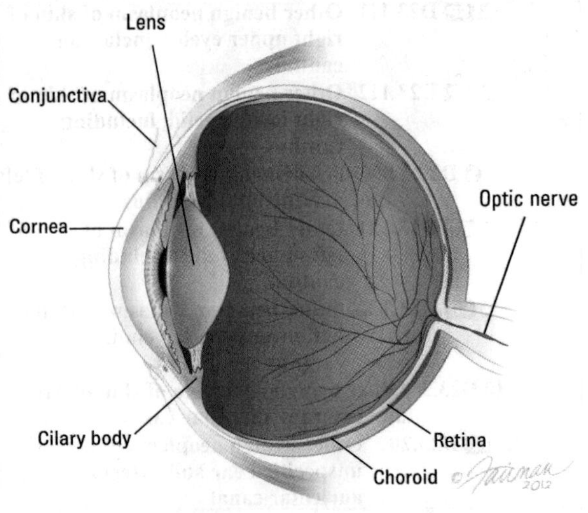

4 **D31 Benign neoplasm of eye and adnexa**
EXCLUDES 1 benign neoplasm of connective tissue of eyelid (D21.0)
benign neoplasm of optic nerve (D33.3)
benign neoplasm of skin of eyelid (D22.1-, D23.1-)

5 **D31.0 Benign neoplasm of conjunctiva**

Laterality !Q **D31.00 Benign neoplasm of unspecified conjunctiva**

Laterality SP **D31.01 Benign neoplasm of right conjunctiva**

Laterality SP **D31.02 Benign neoplasm of left conjunctiva**

5 **D31.1 Benign neoplasm of cornea**

Laterality !Q **D31.10 Benign neoplasm of unspecified cornea**

Laterality SP **D31.11 Benign neoplasm of right cornea**

Laterality SP **D31.12 Benign neoplasm of left cornea**

5 **D31.2 Benign neoplasm of retina**
EXCLUDES 1 dark area on retina (D49.81)
hemangioma of retina (D49.81)
neoplasm of unspecified behavior of retina and choroid (D49.81)
retinal freckle (D49.81)

Laterality !Q **D31.20 Benign neoplasm of unspecified retina**

Laterality SP **D31.21 Benign neoplasm of right retina**

Laterality SP **D31.22 Benign neoplasm of left retina**

5 **D31.3 Benign neoplasm of choroid**

Laterality !Q **D31.30 Benign neoplasm of unspecified choroid**

Laterality SP **D31.31 Benign neoplasm of right choroid**

Laterality SP **D31.32 Benign neoplasm of left choroid**

5 **D31.4 Benign neoplasm of ciliary body**

Laterality !Q **D31.40 Benign neoplasm of unspecified ciliary body**

Laterality SP **D31.41 Benign neoplasm of right ciliary body**

Laterality SP **D31.42 Benign neoplasm of left ciliary body**

5 **D31.5 Benign neoplasm of lacrimal gland and duct**

Benign neoplasm of lacrimal sac
Benign neoplasm of nasolacrimal duct

D31.50 Benign neoplasm of unspecified lacrimal gland and duct

D31.51 Benign neoplasm of right lacrimal gland and duct

D31.52 Benign neoplasm of left lacrimal gland and duct

D31.6 Benign neoplasm of unspecified site of orbit
Benign neoplasm of connective tissue of orbit
Benign neoplasm of extraocular muscle
Benign neoplasm of peripheral nerves of orbit
Benign neoplasm of retrobulbar tissue
Benign neoplasm of retro-ocular tissue
EXCLUDES 1 benign neoplasm of orbital bone (D16.4)

D31.60 Benign neoplasm of unspecified site of unspecified orbit

D31.61 Benign neoplasm of unspecified site of right orbit

D31.62 Benign neoplasm of unspecified site of left orbit

D31.9 Benign neoplasm of unspecified part of eye
Benign neoplasm of eyeball

D31.90 Benign neoplasm of unspecified part of unspecified eye

D31.91 Benign neoplasm of unspecified part of right eye

D31.92 Benign neoplasm of unspecified part of left eye

D32 Benign neoplasm of meninges

D32.0 Benign neoplasm of cerebral meninges

D32.1 Benign neoplasm of spinal meninges

D32.9 Benign neoplasm of meninges, unspecified
Meningioma NOS

D33 Benign neoplasm of brain and other parts of central nervous system
EXCLUDES 1 angioma (D18.0-)
benign neoplasm of meninges (D32.-)
benign neoplasm of peripheral nerves and autonomic nervous system (D36.1-)
hemangioma (D18.0-)
neurofibromatosis (Q85.0-)
retro-ocular benign neoplasm (D31.6-)

CODING TIPS ✓ This code category is used for benign neoplasms of the brain and spinal cord. A personal history of these benign neoplasms is coded to Z86.011.

D33.0 Benign neoplasm of brain, supratentorial
Benign neoplasm of cerebral ventricle
Benign neoplasm of cerebrum
Benign neoplasm of frontal lobe
Benign neoplasm of occipital lobe
Benign neoplasm of parietal lobe
Benign neoplasm of temporal lobe
EXCLUDES 1 benign neoplasm of fourth ventricle (D33.1)

D33.1 Benign neoplasm of brain, infratentorial
Benign neoplasm of brain stem
Benign neoplasm of cerebellum
Benign neoplasm of fourth ventricle

D33.2 Benign neoplasm of brain, unspecified

D33.3 Benign neoplasm of cranial nerves
Benign neoplasm of olfactory bulb

D33.4 Benign neoplasm of spinal cord

D33.7 Benign neoplasm of other specified parts of central nervous system

D33.9 Benign neoplasm of central nervous system, unspecified
Benign neoplasm of nervous system (central) NOS

+ D34 Benign neoplasm of thyroid gland
Use additional code to identify any functional activity

+ D35 Benign neoplasm of other and unspecified endocrine glands
Use additional code to identify any functional activity
EXCLUDES 1 benign neoplasm of endocrine pancreas (D13.7)
benign neoplasm of ovary (D27.-)
benign neoplasm of testis (D29.2.-)
benign neoplasm of thymus (D15.0)

+ D35.0 Benign neoplasm of adrenal gland

+ D35.00 Benign neoplasm of unspecified adrenal gland

+ D35.01 Benign neoplasm of right adrenal gland

+ D35.02 Benign neoplasm of left adrenal gland

+ D35.1 Benign neoplasm of parathyroid gland

+ D35.2 Benign neoplasm of pituitary gland

+ D35.3 Benign neoplasm of craniopharyngeal duct

+ D35.4 Benign neoplasm of pineal gland

+ D35.5 Benign neoplasm of carotid body

+ D35.6 Benign neoplasm of aortic body and other paraganglia
Benign tumor of glomus jugulare

+ D35.7 Benign neoplasm of other specified endocrine glands

+ D35.9 Benign neoplasm of endocrine gland, unspecified
Benign neoplasm of unspecified endocrine gland

D36 Benign neoplasm of other and unspecified sites

D36.0 Benign neoplasm of lymph nodes
EXCLUDES 1 lymphangioma (D18.1)

D36.1 Benign neoplasm of peripheral nerves and autonomic nervous system
EXCLUDES 1 benign neoplasm of peripheral nerves of orbit (D31.6-)
neurofibromatosis (Q85.0-)

D36.10 Benign neoplasm of peripheral nerves and autonomic nervous system, unspecified

Chapter 2 C00-D49

SP D36.11 **Benign neoplasm of peripheral nerves and autonomic nervous system of face, head, and neck**

SP D36.12 **Benign neoplasm of peripheral nerves and autonomic nervous system, upper limb, including shoulder**

SP D36.13 **Benign neoplasm of peripheral nerves and autonomic nervous system of lower limb, including hip**

SP D36.14 **Benign neoplasm of peripheral nerves and autonomic nervous system of thorax**

SP D36.15 **Benign neoplasm of peripheral nerves and autonomic nervous system of abdomen**

SP D36.16 **Benign neoplasm of peripheral nerves and autonomic nervous system of pelvis**

SP D36.17 **Benign neoplasm of peripheral nerves and autonomic nervous system of trunk, unspecified**

SP D36.7 **Benign neoplasm of other specified sites**
Benign neoplasm of back NOS
Benign neoplasm of nose NOS

!Q D36.9 **Benign neoplasm, unspecified site**

Benign neuroendocrine tumors (D3A)

+ 4 D3A **Benign neuroendocrine tumors**
Code also:
any associated multiple endocrine neoplasia [MEN] syndromes (E31.2-)
Use additional code to identify any associated endocrine syndrome, such as:
carcinoid syndrome (E34.0)
EXCLUDES 2 benign pancreatic islet cell tumors (D13.7)

+ 5 D3A.0 **Benign carcinoid tumors**

!Q + D3A.00 **Benign carcinoid tumor of unspecified site**
Carcinoid tumor NOS

+ 6 D3A.01 **Benign carcinoid tumors of the small intestine**

SP + D3A.010 **Benign carcinoid tumor of the duodenum**

SP + D3A.011 **Benign carcinoid tumor of the jejunum**

SP + D3A.012 **Benign carcinoid tumor of the ileum**

SP + D3A.019 **Benign carcinoid tumor of the small intestine, unspecified portion**

+ 6 D3A.02 **Benign carcinoid tumors of the appendix, large intestine, and rectum**

SP + D3A.020 **Benign carcinoid tumor of the appendix**

SP + D3A.021 **Benign carcinoid tumor of the cecum**

SP + D3A.022 **Benign carcinoid tumor of the ascending colon**

SP + D3A.023 **Benign carcinoid tumor of the transverse colon**

SP + D3A.024 **Benign carcinoid tumor of the descending colon**

SP + D3A.025 **Benign carcinoid tumor of the sigmoid colon**

SP + D3A.026 **Benign carcinoid tumor of the rectum**

SP + D3A.029 **Benign carcinoid tumor of the large intestine, unspecified portion**
Benign carcinoid tumor of the colon NOS

+ 6 D3A.09 **Benign carcinoid tumors of other sites**

SP + D3A.090 **Benign carcinoid tumor of the bronchus and lung**

SP + D3A.091 **Benign carcinoid tumor of the thymus**

SP + D3A.092 **Benign carcinoid tumor of the stomach**

SP + D3A.093 **Benign carcinoid tumor of the kidney**

SP + D3A.094 **Benign carcinoid tumor of the foregut, unspecified**

SP + D3A.095 **Benign carcinoid tumor of the midgut, unspecified**

SP + D3A.096 **Benign carcinoid tumor of the hindgut, unspecified**

SP + D3A.098 **Benign carcinoid tumors of other sites**

SP + D3A.8 **Other benign neuroendocrine tumors**
Neuroendocrine tumor NOS

Neoplasms of uncertain behavior, polycythemia vera and myelodysplastic syndromes (D37-D48)

Note:
Categories D37-D44, and D48 classify by site neoplasms of uncertain behavior, i.e., histologic confirmation whether the neoplasm is malignant or benign cannot be made.
EXCLUDES 1 neoplasms of unspecified behavior (D49.-)

CODING TIPS ✓ Codes classifiable to D37-D48 include tumors specifically reported as those of "uncertain behavior." This term is a specific diagnostic statement that must be reported by the physician or NPP in order to support assignment of any code from D37-D48, as these tumors include lesions whose behavior cannot be predicted. The status is currently benign, but the tumor could undergo a malignant transformation. These codes are not to be used when a biopsy has not been performed or results are not available.

4 D37 **Neoplasm of uncertain behavior of oral cavity and digestive organs**
EXCLUDES 1 stromal tumors of uncertain behavior of digestive system (D48.1)

5 D37.0 **Neoplasm of uncertain behavior of lip, oral cavity and pharynx**
EXCLUDES 1 neoplasm of uncertain behavior of aryepiglottic fold or interarytenoid fold, laryngeal aspect (D38.0)
neoplasm of uncertain behavior of epiglottis NOS (D38.0)
neoplasm of uncertain behavior of skin of lip (D48.5)
neoplasm of uncertain behavior of suprahyoid portion of epiglottis (D38.0)

Chapter 2 C00-D49

SP **D37.01 Neoplasm of uncertain behavior of lip**
Neoplasm of uncertain behavior of vermilion border of lip

SP **D37.02 Neoplasm of uncertain behavior of tongue**

6 **D37.03 Neoplasm of uncertain behavior of the major salivary glands**

SP **D37.030 Neoplasm of uncertain behavior of the parotid salivary glands**

SP **D37.031 Neoplasm of uncertain behavior of the sublingual salivary glands**

SP **D37.032 Neoplasm of uncertain behavior of the submandibular salivary glands**

SP **D37.039 Neoplasm of uncertain behavior of the major salivary glands, unspecified**

SP **D37.04 Neoplasm of uncertain behavior of the minor salivary glands**
Neoplasm of uncertain behavior of submucosal salivary glands of lip
Neoplasm of uncertain behavior of submucosal salivary glands of cheek
Neoplasm of uncertain behavior of submucosal salivary glands of hard palate
Neoplasm of uncertain behavior of submucosal salivary glands of soft palate

SP **D37.05 Neoplasm of uncertain behavior of pharynx**
Neoplasm of uncertain behavior of aryepiglottic fold of pharynx NOS
Neoplasm of uncertain behavior of hypopharyngeal aspect of aryepiglottic fold of pharynx
Neoplasm of uncertain behavior of marginal zone of aryepiglottic fold of pharynx

SP **D37.09 Neoplasm of uncertain behavior of other specified sites of the oral cavity**

SP **D37.1 Neoplasm of uncertain behavior of stomach**

SP **D37.2 Neoplasm of uncertain behavior of small intestine**

SP **D37.3 Neoplasm of uncertain behavior of appendix**

SP **D37.4 Neoplasm of uncertain behavior of colon**

SP **D37.5 Neoplasm of uncertain behavior of rectum**
Neoplasm of uncertain behavior of rectosigmoid junction

SP **D37.6 Neoplasm of uncertain behavior of liver, gallbladder and bile ducts**
Neoplasm of uncertain behavior of ampulla of Vater

SP **D37.8 Neoplasm of uncertain behavior of other specified digestive organs**
Neoplasm of uncertain behavior of anal canal
Neoplasm of uncertain behavior of anal sphincter
Neoplasm of uncertain behavior of anus NOS
Neoplasm of uncertain behavior of esophagus
Neoplasm of uncertain behavior of intestine NOS
Neoplasm of uncertain behavior of pancreas
EXCLUDES 1 neoplasm of uncertain behavior of anal margin (D48.5)
neoplasm of uncertain behavior of anal skin (D48.5)
neoplasm of uncertain behavior of perianal skin (D48.5)

IQ **D37.9 Neoplasm of uncertain behavior of digestive organ, unspecified**

4 **D38 Neoplasm of uncertain behavior of middle ear and respiratory and intrathoracic organs**
EXCLUDES 1 neoplasm of uncertain behavior of heart (D48.7)

SP **D38.0 Neoplasm of uncertain behavior of larynx**
Neoplasm of uncertain behavior of aryepiglottic fold or interarytenoid fold, laryngeal aspect
Neoplasm of uncertain behavior of epiglottis (suprahyoid portion)
EXCLUDES 1 neoplasm of uncertain behavior of aryepiglottic fold or interarytenoid fold NOS (D37.05)
neoplasm of uncertain behavior of hypopharyngeal aspect of aryepiglottic fold (D37.05)
neoplasm of uncertain behavior of marginal zone of aryepiglottic fold (D37.05)

SP **D38.1 Neoplasm of uncertain behavior of trachea, bronchus and lung**

SP **D38.2 Neoplasm of uncertain behavior of pleura**

SP **D38.3 Neoplasm of uncertain behavior of mediastinum**

SP **D38.4 Neoplasm of uncertain behavior of thymus**

SP **D38.5 Neoplasm of uncertain behavior of other respiratory organs**
Neoplasm of uncertain behavior of accessory sinuses
Neoplasm of uncertain behavior of cartilage of nose
Neoplasm of uncertain behavior of middle ear
Neoplasm of uncertain behavior of nasal cavities
EXCLUDES 1 neoplasm of uncertain behavior of ear (external) (skin) (D48.5)
neoplasm of uncertain behavior of nose NOS (D48.7)
neoplasm of uncertain behavior of skin of nose (D48.5)

IQ **D38.6 Neoplasm of uncertain behavior of respiratory organ, unspecified**

Chapter 2

C00-D49

4 D39 Neoplasm of uncertain behavior of female genital organs

SP **D39.0 Neoplasm of uncertain behavior of uterus**

+ 5 **D39.1 Neoplasm of uncertain behavior of ovary**

Use additional code to identify any functional activity.

L IQ + **D39.10 Neoplasm of uncertain behavior of unspecified ovary**

L SP + **D39.11 Neoplasm of uncertain behavior of right ovary**

L SP + **D39.12 Neoplasm of uncertain behavior of left ovary**

SP **D39.2 Neoplasm of uncertain behavior of placenta**

Chorioadenoma destruens

Invasive hydatidiform mole

Malignant hydatidiform mole

EXCLUDES 1 hydatidiform mole NOS (O01.9)

SP **D39.8 Neoplasm of uncertain behavior of other specified female genital organs**

Neoplasm of uncertain behavior of skin of female genital organs

IQ **D39.9 Neoplasm of uncertain behavior of female genital organ, unspecified**

4 D40 Neoplasm of uncertain behavior of male genital organs

SP **D40.0 Neoplasm of uncertain behavior of prostate**

5 **D40.1 Neoplasm of uncertain behavior of testis**

L IQ **D40.10 Neoplasm of uncertain behavior of unspecified testis**

L SP **D40.11 Neoplasm of uncertain behavior of right testis**

L SP **D40.12 Neoplasm of uncertain behavior of left testis**

SP **D40.8 Neoplasm of uncertain behavior of other specified male genital organs**

Neoplasm of uncertain behavior of skin of male genital organs

IQ **D40.9 Neoplasm of uncertain behavior of male genital organ, unspecified**

4 D41 Neoplasm of uncertain behavior of urinary organs

5 **D41.0 Neoplasm of uncertain behavior of kidney**

EXCLUDES 1 neoplasm of uncertain behavior of renal pelvis (D41.1-)

L IQ **D41.00 Neoplasm of uncertain behavior of unspecified kidney**

L SP **D41.01 Neoplasm of uncertain behavior of right kidney**

L SP **D41.02 Neoplasm of uncertain behavior of left kidney**

5 **D41.1 Neoplasm of uncertain behavior of renal pelvis**

L IQ **D41.10 Neoplasm of uncertain behavior of unspecified renal pelvis**

L SP **D41.11 Neoplasm of uncertain behavior of right renal pelvis**

L SP **D41.12 Neoplasm of uncertain behavior of left renal pelvis**

5 **D41.2 Neoplasm of uncertain behavior of ureter**

L IQ **D41.20 Neoplasm of uncertain behavior of unspecified ureter**

L SP **D41.21 Neoplasm of uncertain behavior of right ureter**

L SP **D41.22 Neoplasm of uncertain behavior of left ureter**

SP **D41.3 Neoplasm of uncertain behavior of urethra**

SP **D41.4 Neoplasm of uncertain behavior of bladder**

SP **D41.8 Neoplasm of uncertain behavior of other specified urinary organs**

IQ **D41.9 Neoplasm of uncertain behavior of unspecified urinary organ**

4 D42 Neoplasm of uncertain behavior of meninges

SP **D42.0 Neoplasm of uncertain behavior of cerebral meninges**

SP **D42.1 Neoplasm of uncertain behavior of spinal meninges**

SP **D42.9 Neoplasm of uncertain behavior of meninges, unspecified**

4 D43 Neoplasm of uncertain behavior of brain and central nervous system

EXCLUDES 1 neoplasm of uncertain behavior of peripheral nerves and autonomic nervous system (D48.2)

SP **D43.0 Neoplasm of uncertain behavior of brain, supratentorial**

Neoplasm of uncertain behavior of cerebral ventricle

Neoplasm of uncertain behavior of cerebrum

Neoplasm of uncertain behavior of frontal lobe

Neoplasm of uncertain behavior of occipital lobe

Neoplasm of uncertain behavior of parietal lobe

Neoplasm of uncertain behavior of temporal lobe

EXCLUDES 1 neoplasm of uncertain behavior of fourth ventricle (D43.1)

SP **D43.1 Neoplasm of uncertain behavior of brain, infratentorial**

Neoplasm of uncertain behavior of brain stem

Neoplasm of uncertain behavior of cerebellum

Neoplasm of uncertain behavior of fourth ventricle

SP **D43.2 Neoplasm of uncertain behavior of brain, unspecified**

SP **D43.3 Neoplasm of uncertain behavior of cranial nerves**

SP **D43.4 Neoplasm of uncertain behavior of spinal cord**

SP **D43.8 Neoplasm of uncertain behavior of other specified parts of central nervous system**

IQ **D43.9 Neoplasm of uncertain behavior of central nervous system, unspecified**

Neoplasm of uncertain behavior of nervous system (central) NOS

4 D44 Neoplasm of uncertain behavior of endocrine glands

EXCLUDES 1 multiple endocrine adenomatosis (E31.2-)
multiple endocrine neoplasia (E31.2-)
neoplasm of uncertain behavior of endocrine pancreas (D37.8)
neoplasm of uncertain behavior of ovary (D39.1-)
neoplasm of uncertain behavior of testis (D40.1-)
neoplasm of uncertain behavior of thymus (D38.4)

SP **D44.0 Neoplasm of uncertain behavior of thyroid gland**

+ 5 **D44.1 Neoplasm of uncertain behavior of adrenal gland**
Use additional code to identify any functional activity.

IQ + **D44.10 Neoplasm of uncertain behavior of unspecified adrenal gland**

SP + **D44.11 Neoplasm of uncertain behavior of right adrenal gland**

SP + **D44.12 Neoplasm of uncertain behavior of left adrenal gland**

SP **D44.2 Neoplasm of uncertain behavior of parathyroid gland**

SP + **D44.3 Neoplasm of uncertain behavior of pituitary gland**
Use additional code to identify any functional activity.

SP **D44.4 Neoplasm of uncertain behavior of craniopharyngeal duct**

SP **D44.5 Neoplasm of uncertain behavior of pineal gland**

SP **D44.6 Neoplasm of uncertain behavior of carotid body**

SP **D44.7 Neoplasm of uncertain behavior of aortic body and other paraganglia**

IQ **D44.9 Neoplasm of uncertain behavior of unspecified endocrine gland**

SP **D45 Polycythemia vera**
EXCLUDES 1 familial polycythemia (D75.0)
secondary polycythemia (D75.1)

+ 4 **D46 Myelodysplastic syndromes**
Use additional code for adverse effect, if applicable, to identify drug (T36-T50 with fifth or sixth character 5)
EXCLUDES 2 drug-induced aplastic anemia (D61.1)

SP + **D46.0 Refractory anemia without ring sideroblasts, so stated**
Refractory anemia without sideroblasts, without excess of blasts

SP + **D46.1 Refractory anemia with ring sideroblasts**
RARS

+ 5 **D46.2 Refractory anemia with excess of blasts [RAEB]**

SP + **D46.20 Refractory anemia with excess of blasts, unspecified**
RAEB NOS

SP + **D46.21 Refractory anemia with excess of blasts 1**
RAEB 1

SP + **D46.22 Refractory anemia with excess of blasts 2**
RAEB 2

SP + **D46.A Refractory cytopenia with multilineage dysplasia**

SP + **D46.B Refractory cytopenia with multilineage dysplasia and ring sideroblasts**
RCMD RS

SP + **D46.C Myelodysplastic syndrome with isolated del(5q) chromosomal abnormality**
Myelodysplastic syndrome with 5q deletion
5q minus syndrome NOS

SP + **D46.4 Refractory anemia, unspecified**

SP + **D46.Z Other myelodysplastic syndromes**
EXCLUDES 1 chronic myelomonocytic leukemia (C93.1-)

SP + **D46.9 Myelodysplastic syndrome, unspecified**
Myelodysplasia NOS

4 **D47 Other neoplasms of uncertain behavior of lymphoid, hematopoietic and related tissue**

5 **D47.0 Mast cell neoplasms of uncertain behavior**
EXCLUDES 1 congenital cutaneous mastocytosis (Q82.2)
histiocytic neoplasms of uncertain behavior (D47.Z9)
malignant mast cell neoplasm (C96.2-)

SP **D47.01 Cutaneous mastocytosis**
Diffuse cutaneous mastocytosis
Maculopapular cutaneous mastocytosis
Solitary mastocytoma
Telangiectasia macularis eruptiva perstans
Urticaria pigmentosa
EXCLUDES 1 congenital (diffuse) (maculopapular) cutaneous mastocytosis (Q82.2)
congenital urticaria pigmentosa (Q82.2)
extracutaneous mastocytoma (D47.09)

SP **D47.02 Systemic mastocytosis**
Indolent systemic mastocytosis
Isolated bone marrow mastocytosis
Smoldering systemic mastocytosis
Systemic mastocytosis, with an associated hematological non-mast cell lineage disease (SM-AHNMD)
Code also, if applicable, any associated hematological non-mast cell lineage disease, such as:
acute myeloid leukemia (C92.6-, C92.A-)
chronic myelomonocytic leukemia (C93.1-)
essential thrombocytosis (D47.3)
hypereosinophilic syndrome (D72.1)
myelodysplastic syndrome (D46.9)
myeloproliferative syndrome (D47.1)
non-Hodgkin lymphoma (C82-C85)
plasma cell myeloma (C90.0-)
polycythemia vera (D45)
EXCLUDES 1 aggressive systemic mastocytosis (C96.21)

mast cell leukemia (C94.3-)

SP **D47.09 Other mast cell neoplasms of uncertain behavior**
Extracutaneous mastocytoma
Mast cell tumor NOS
Mastocytoma NOS
Mastocytosis NOS

SP **D47.1 Chronic myeloproliferative disease**
Chronic neutrophilic leukemia
Myeloproliferative disease, unspecified
EXCLUDES 1 atypical chronic myeloid leukemia BCR/ABL-negative (C92.2-)
chronic myeloid leukemia BCR/ABL-positive (C92.1-)
myelofibrosis NOS (D75.81)
myelophthisic anemia (D61.82)
myelophthisis (D61.82)
secondary myelofibrosis NOS (D75.81)

SP **D47.2 Monoclonal gammopathy**
Monoclonal gammopathy of undetermined significance [MGUS]

▲ SP **D47.3 Essential (hemorrhagic) thrombocythemia**
Essential thrombocytosis
Idiopathic hemorrhagic thrombocythemia
Primary thrombocytosis
EXCLUDES 2 reactive thrombocytosis (D75.838)
secondary thrombocytosis (D75.838)
thrombocythemia NOS (D75.839)
thrombocytosis NOS (D75.839)

DEFINITION Rare myeloproliferative disorder characterized by uncontrolled over-production of blood platelet precursor cells, leading to splenomegaly, hemorrhaging from the intestines, gums, or nose, and blood vessel thrombosis.

SP **D47.4 Osteomyelofibrosis**
Chronic idiopathic myelofibrosis
Myelofibrosis (idiopathic) (with myeloid metaplasia)
Myelosclerosis (megakaryocytic) with myeloid metaplasia
Secondary myelofibrosis in myeloproliferative disease
EXCLUDES 1 acute myelofibrosis (C94.4-)

5 **D47.Z Other specified neoplasms of uncertain behavior of lymphoid, hematopoietic and related tissue**

IQ **D47.Z1 Post-transplant lymphoproliferative disorder (PTLD)**
Code first:
complications of transplanted organs and tissue (T86.-)

SP **D47.Z2 Castleman disease**
Code also:
, if applicable, human herpesvirus 8 infection (B10.89)

EXCLUDES 2 Kaposi's sarcoma (C46.-)

SP **D47.Z9 Other specified neoplasms of uncertain behavior of lymphoid, hematopoietic and related tissue**
Histiocytic tumors of uncertain behavior

SP **D47.9 Neoplasm of uncertain behavior of lymphoid, hematopoietic and related tissue, unspecified**
Lymphoproliferative disease NOS

4 **D48 Neoplasm of uncertain behavior of other and unspecified sites**
EXCLUDES 1 neurofibromatosis (nonmalignant) (Q85.0-)

SP **D48.0 Neoplasm of uncertain behavior of bone and articular cartilage**
EXCLUDES 1 neoplasm of uncertain behavior of cartilage of ear (D48.1)
neoplasm of uncertain behavior of cartilage of larynx (D38.0)
neoplasm of uncertain behavior of cartilage of nose (D38.5)
neoplasm of uncertain behavior of connective tissue of eyelid (D48.1)
neoplasm of uncertain behavior of synovia (D48.1)

SP **D48.1 Neoplasm of uncertain behavior of connective and other soft tissue**
Neoplasm of uncertain behavior of connective tissue of ear
Neoplasm of uncertain behavior of connective tissue of eyelid
Stromal tumors of uncertain behavior of digestive system
EXCLUDES 1 neoplasm of uncertain behavior of articular cartilage (D48.0)
neoplasm of uncertain behavior of cartilage of larynx (D38.0)
neoplasm of uncertain behavior of cartilage of nose (D38.5)
neoplasm of uncertain behavior of connective tissue of breast (D48.6-)

SP **D48.2 Neoplasm of uncertain behavior of peripheral nerves and autonomic nervous system**
EXCLUDES 1 neoplasm of uncertain behavior of peripheral nerves of orbit (D48.7)

SP **D48.3 Neoplasm of uncertain behavior of retroperitoneum**

SP **D48.4 Neoplasm of uncertain behavior of peritoneum**

SP **D48.5 Neoplasm of uncertain behavior of skin**
Neoplasm of uncertain behavior of anal margin
Neoplasm of uncertain behavior of anal skin
Neoplasm of uncertain behavior of perianal skin

Neoplasm of uncertain behavior of skin of breast

EXCLUDES 1 neoplasm of uncertain behavior of anus NOS (D37.8)
neoplasm of uncertain behavior of skin of genital organs (D39.8, D40.8)
neoplasm of uncertain behavior of vermilion border of lip (D37.0)

5 **D48.6 Neoplasm of uncertain behavior of breast**

Neoplasm of uncertain behavior of connective tissue of breast
Cystosarcoma phyllodes

EXCLUDES 1 neoplasm of uncertain behavior of skin of breast (D48.5)

IQ **D48.60 Neoplasm of uncertain behavior of unspecified breast**

SP **D48.61 Neoplasm of uncertain behavior of right breast**

SP **D48.62 Neoplasm of uncertain behavior of left breast**

SP **D48.7 Neoplasm of uncertain behavior of other specified sites**

Neoplasm of uncertain behavior of eye
Neoplasm of uncertain behavior of heart
Neoplasm of uncertain behavior of peripheral nerves of orbit

EXCLUDES 1 neoplasm of uncertain behavior of connective tissue (D48.1)
neoplasm of uncertain behavior of skin of eyelid (D48.5)

IQ **D48.9 Neoplasm of uncertain behavior, unspecified**

Neoplasms of unspecified behavior (D49)

CODING TIPS✓ Codes classifiable to D49 include tumors that have not been defined as malignant or benign. The term 'mass' should not be interpreted to mean unspecified behavior. The physician or NPP should be queried to determine whether neoplasm codes are applicable.

4 **D49 Neoplasms of unspecified behavior**

Note:
Category D49 classifies by site neoplasms of unspecified morphology and behavior. The term 'mass', unless otherwise stated, is not to be regarded as a neoplastic growth.

INCLUDES 'growth' NOS
neoplasm NOS
new growth NOS
tumor NOS

EXCLUDES 1 neoplasms of uncertain behavior (D37-D44, D48)

SP **D49.0 Neoplasm of unspecified behavior of digestive system**

EXCLUDES 1 neoplasm of unspecified behavior of margin of anus (D49.2)
neoplasm of unspecified behavior of perianal skin (D49.2)
neoplasm of unspecified behavior of skin of anus (D49.2)

SP **D49.1 Neoplasm of unspecified behavior of respiratory system**

SP **D49.2 Neoplasm of unspecified behavior of bone, soft tissue, and skin**

EXCLUDES 1 neoplasm of unspecified behavior of anal canal (D49.0)
neoplasm of unspecified behavior of anus NOS (D49.0)
neoplasm of unspecified behavior of bone marrow (D49.89)
neoplasm of unspecified behavior of cartilage of larynx (D49.1)
neoplasm of unspecified behavior of cartilage of nose (D49.1)
neoplasm of unspecified behavior of connective tissue of breast (D49.3)
neoplasm of unspecified behavior of skin of genital organs (D49.59)
neoplasm of unspecified behavior of vermilion border of lip (D49.0)

SP **D49.3 Neoplasm of unspecified behavior of breast**

EXCLUDES 1 neoplasm of unspecified behavior of skin of breast (D49.2)

SP **D49.4 Neoplasm of unspecified behavior of bladder**

5 **D49.5 Neoplasm of unspecified behavior of other genitourinary organs**

6 **D49.51 Neoplasm of unspecified behavior of kidney**

SP **D49.511 Neoplasm of unspecified behavior of right kidney**

SP **D49.512 Neoplasm of unspecified behavior of left kidney**

IQ **D49.519 Neoplasm of unspecified behavior of unspecified kidney**

SP **D49.59 Neoplasm of unspecified behavior of other genitourinary organ**

SP **D49.6 Neoplasm of unspecified behavior of brain**

EXCLUDES 1 neoplasm of unspecified behavior of cerebral meninges (D49.7)
neoplasm of unspecified behavior of cranial nerves (D49.7)

SP **D49.7 Neoplasm of unspecified behavior of endocrine glands and other parts of nervous system**

EXCLUDES 1 neoplasm of unspecified behavior of peripheral, sympathetic, and parasympathetic nerves and ganglia (D49.2)

Chapter 2
C00-D49

5 D49.8 Neoplasm of unspecified behavior of other specified sites

EXCLUDES 1 neoplasm of unspecified behavior of eyelid (skin) (D49.2)
neoplasm of unspecified behavior of eyelid cartilage (D49.2)
neoplasm of unspecified behavior of great vessels (D49.2)
neoplasm of unspecified behavior of optic nerve (D49.7)

SP D49.81 Neoplasm of unspecified behavior of retina and choroid

Dark area on retina
Retinal freckle

SP D49.89 Neoplasm of unspecified behavior of other specified sites

!Q D49.9 Neoplasm of unspecified behavior of unspecified site

Chapter 2 Scenarios: Neoplasms (C00-D49)

Malignant pericardial effusion, metastatic melanoma

A 79-year-old woman comes to home health for management of malignant pericardial effusion that's causing her symptoms of shortness of breath and fatigue. The cause of the pericardial effusion is documented as metastatic melanoma that began on her forehead and spread to both of her lungs, and her liver. Discharge summary documentation also indicates she has stable hypertensive heart disease and end stage kidney failure, for which she attends hemodialysis three times a week.

Description	Code
Primary: Pericardial effusion (noninflammatory)	I31.3
Secondary: Secondary malignant neoplasm of right lung	C78.01
Secondary: Secondary malignant neoplasm of left lung	C78.02
Secondary: Secondary malignant neoplasm of liver and intrahepatic bile duct	C78.7
Secondary: Malignant melanoma of other parts of face	C43.39
Secondary: Hypertensive heart and chronic kidney disease without heart failure, with stage 5 chronic kidney disease, or end stage renal disease	I13.11
Secondary: End stage renal disease	N18.6
Secondary: Dependence on renal dialysis	Z99.2

Malignant pericardial effusion caused by cancer should be captured first with the I31.3, then the codes for the cancer, according to Q1 2019 Coding Clinic guidance. Thus, I31.3 is assigned first, followed by the codes for each of the secondary sites of the metastatic disease, because the metastatic disease is the cause of the pericardial effusion, as well as the primary site. Her symptoms of shortness of breath and fatigue are not separately coded as they are integral to pericardial effusion and are thus included in I31.3. Additional codes are added to identify her hypertensive heart and chronic kidney disease as these are important to her plan of care and prognosis, and provide important comorbidity adjustment, but these are coded lower as the conditions remain stable. A Z code to identify dependence on dialysis is required when an end stage renal disease patient remains on dialysis.

Paraplegia with bone metastasis and wound care

A 68-year-old diabetic male patient is admitted for wound care to a venous stasis ulcer of the left calf (due to venous insufficiency), which extends to the fat layer. The patient is paraplegic due to untreated bony vertebral metastases from primary prostate cancer for which the patient has also refused treatment. The focus of care will be wound care, but the patient will also receive therapy to improve lower extremity circulation.

Description	Code
Primary: Encounter for change or removal of nonsurgical wound dressing	Z48.00
Secondary: Type 2 diabetes mellitus with diabetic peripheral angiopathy without gangrene	E11.51
Secondary: Venous insufficiency (chronic) (peripheral)	I87.2
Secondary: Non-pressure chronic ulcer of left calf with fat layer exposed	L97.222
Secondary: Paraplegia, unspecified	G82.20
Secondary: Secondary malignant neoplasm of bone	C79.51
Secondary: Malignant neoplasm of prostate	C61

Because the focus of care is wound care, this is coded first. When the focus of care is wound care, first assign Z48.00 if the primary code would otherwise not group to Wounds within the PDGM grouper, such as E11.51. The neoplastic disease has never been treated and is coded as active disease. Because the secondary neoplasm of the bone is resulting in the paraplegia, which is being addressed by home health, this is coded before the primary prostate cancer.

Lung cancer, dressing changes, drain care

Your patient had a pneumonectomy for cancer of the left lower lobe of the lung. He also has a deep tissue injury (DTI) on the right heel, diabetes and congestive heart failure (CHF). He was referred to home health for aftercare, dressing changes, care of a surgical drain, and teaching of oxygen safety since he is receiving oxygen intermittently at 2 liters/minute. The patient will begin chemotherapy in two weeks.

Description	Code
Primary: Aftercare following surgery for neoplasm	Z48.3
Secondary: Malignant neoplasm of lower lobe, left bronchus of lung	C34.32
Secondary: Pressure-induced deep tissue damage of right heel	L89.616
Secondary: Type 2 diabetes mellitus without complications	E11.9
Secondary: Heart failure, unspecified	I50.9
Secondary: Dependence on supplemental oxygen	Z99.81
Secondary: Acquired absence of lung [part of]	Z90.2

If documentation is present that indicates that the lung cancer is eradicated and requires no further treatment, then the cancer will not be reported as an active diagnosis. However, this patient is still under treatment for his lung cancer, so the cancer is coded. The drain care is included in the aftercare code (Z48.3). There is no indication here that the comorbidities are unstable, so they are coded lower than the active lung cancer and pressure ulcer/injury. Note, Z90.2 includes any part of the lung.

Anemia due to neoplasm

A patient is admitted to home care for management of multifactorial anemia including anemia due to a malignant carcinoid tumor of the stomach. His discharge summary also reports acute bleeding gastritis with resulting acute anemia, a history of pernicious anemia, for which the patient's physician administers B12 injections, and diabetes with polyneuropathy.

Description	Code
Primary: Malignant carcinoid tumor of stomach	C7A.092
Secondary: Anemia in neoplastic disease	D63.0
Secondary: Acute gastritis with bleeding	K29.01
Secondary: Acute posthemorrhagic anemia	D62
Secondary: Vitamin B12 deficiency anemia due to intrinsic factor deficiency	D51.0
Secondary: Type 2 diabetes mellitus with diabetic polyneuropathy	E11.42

When the admission/encounter is for management of anemia associated with the malignancy and the treatment is only for anemia, the appropriate code for the malignancy is sequenced as the principal or first-listed diagnosis, followed by the appropriate code for the anemia, according to coding guidelines. The coder will see a "code first" note in the Tabular section under the anemia code. Also, note that carcinoid tumors are not listed in the Neoplasm Table. Reference the Index under "Tumor, carcinoid." In the Tabular List, these are not listed in chronological order. They are found after C75.9 as Malignant neuroendocrine tumors (C7A). *[I.C.2.c.1]*.

When a patient has multifactorial anemia (anemia stated as due to multiple causes), each of the specific anemia types must be coded and the guidelines for each followed. Acute bleeding gastritis, K29.01, does not include the anemia resulting from the loss of blood, so the assignment of D62 is required. Code D51.0 must also be assigned for pernicious anemia and diabetes with polyneuropathy is coded lower as an important comorbid diagnosis that will impact the patient's plan of care.

Cancer and hypertension

Your patient has hypertension due to a secondary aldosterone secreting malignant neoplasm of the brain, which has metastasized from a primary, untreated neoplasm of the lower lobe of the left lung. She has secondary hyperaldosteronism due to the brain tumor and comorbid diastolic congestive heart failure and stage 2 chronic kidney disease.. The focus of care for the patient is the neoplasm.

Description	Code
Primary: Secondary malignant neoplasm of brain	C79.31
Secondary: Other secondary hypertension	I15.8
Secondary: Secondary hyperaldosteronism	E26.1
Secondary: Malignant neoplasm of lower lobe, left bronchus or lung	C34.32
Secondary: Chronic diastolic (congestive) heart failure	I50.32
Secondary: Chronic kidney disease, stage 2 (mild)	N18.2

Sequencing is based on the focus of care for the encounter, which is the brain neoplasm in this case. Per official coding guidelines: "If the reason for the encounter is for treatment of a primary malignancy, assign the malignancy as the principal/first-listed diagnosis." *[I.C.2.l.1].* The secondary hyperaldosteronism must also be coded. This patient's hypertension, heart failure, and chronic kidney disease diagnoses are unrelated so no combination codes are used.

Dehydration due to neoplasm

A patient who has a primary malignant neoplasm of the lower outer quadrant of her right breast was referred to home care for IV hydration due to severe dehydration that is described as a complication of the neoplasm. The dehydration is the focus of care.

Description	Code
Primary: Dehydration	E86.0
Secondary: Malignant neoplasm of lower-outer quadrant of right female breast	C50.511
Secondary: Encounter for adjustment and management of vascular access device	Z45.2

The dehydration is the focus of care and should be coded as the primary diagnosis. The dehydration is sequenced prior to the malignancy. Per official coding guidelines: "When the admission/encounter is for management of dehydration due to the malignancy and only the dehydration is being treated (intravenous rehydration), the dehydration is sequenced first, followed by the code(s) for the malignancy." [*I.C.2.c.3*]. Assign code Z45.2 to capture the IV maintenance. If the IV is not the primary reason the patient requires home health care, but where there may be some sort of intervention noted on the home health plan of care, then it would be appropriate to report Z45.2 (but not as the principal or first secondary diagnosis), according to CMS.

Secondary bone cancer and pathological fracture

A patient has a history of prostate cancer that has metastasized to the right femur where it's caused a pathological fracture. He is admitted to home health for nursing and therapy, which will provide routine care of the pathological right femur fracture, which is the focus of care and is healing normally, as well as observation and assessment, strengthening, transfers and pain management. His dosage of morphine, which he has been taking for his neoplasm-related pain, was increased and has resulted in associated constipation due to the drug, which nursing will monitor.

Description	Code
Primary: Pathological fracture in neoplastic disease, right femur, subsequent encounter with routine healing	M84.551D
Secondary: Secondary malignant neoplasm, bone	C79.51
Secondary: Neoplasm related pain	G89.3
Secondary: Drug induced constipation	K59.03
Secondary: Adverse effect of other opioids, subsequent encounter	T40.2X5D
Secondary: History of prostate cancer	Z85.46

When an encounter is for a pathological fracture due to a neoplasm and the focus of treatment is the fracture, a code from subcategory M84.5- (Pathological fracture in neoplastic disease) should be sequenced first, followed by the code for the neoplasm, according to coding guidelines. That is the case here and thus M84.551D is assigned in the primary position. Note as well as a seventh character is required to describe the timing of the encounter, such as initial, subsequent or sequela. This is expanded further for fractures to include routine or delayed healing, nonunion or malunion. Routine care for a normally healing fracture is the case here, and thus "D" is the appropriate seventh character. Additional codes are assigned for his neoplasm related pain, drug induced constipation, and adverse effect of other opioids (morphine), and history of prostate cancer.

Hodgkin's lymphoma

A 65-year-old man was recently diagnosed with Hodgkin's lymphoma of the lymph nodes of his neck. He is undergoing treatment. He also has hypertension and type 2 diabetes with polyneuropathy and was admitted to home health for teaching on the disease process and management of new medications.

Description	Code
Primary: Hodgkin lymphoma, unspecified, lymph nodes of head, face, and neck	C81.91
Secondary: Type 2 diabetes mellitus with diabetic polyneuropathy	E11.42
Secondary: Essential (primary) hypertension	I10

As the focus of care, the Hodgkin's lymphoma is coded primary. The lymphoma is affecting the lymph nodes of his neck, so the more specific code C81.91 is assigned. The type 2 diabetes with polyneuropathy and hypertension are important comorbidities that should be coded even if they're not the focus of care as they impact the plan of care and E11.42 provides and important low comorbidity adjustment to this episode.

Exacerbated obstructive bronchitis, sessile serrated polyp of the ascending colon

A 78-year-old woman was recently hospitalized for an exacerbation of her chronic obstructive bronchitis. She is admitted to home health to continue her recovery and to teach on and monitor new medications. She also has a sessile serrated polyp of the ascending colon, which her physician wants to monitor but not treat at this time. She also has diabetic polyneuropathy with insulin dependence.

Description	Code
Primary: Chronic obstructive pulmonary disease with (acute) exacerbation	J44.1
Secondary: Benign neoplasm of ascending colon	D12.2
Secondary: Type 2 diabetes mellitus with diabetic polyneuropathy	E11.42
Secondary: Long term (current) use of insulin	Z79.4

The focus of the home health admission is the exacerbated chronic obstructive bronchitis, so that diagnosis is coded primary. The patient also has a sessile serrated polyp of the ascending colon, which is not malignant but can be pre-cancerous and should be coded with D12.2, according to Q2 2018 Coding Clinic guidance. The polyp will require monitoring but isn't the focus of care and thus is coded as a secondary diagnosis. Her diabetic polyneuropathy has the potential to impact her plan of care and is thus also coded. Because she is dependent on insulin but not stated to be a type 1 diabetic, the code for insulin use must be assigned as well.

Aftercare following mastectomy

A 68-year-old female is admitted to home health post-mastectomy of her left breast due to breast cancer of the lower outer quadrant of her left breast. She will begin chemo once the incision is healed. Medical records state she is estrogen receptor positive. The focus of skilled nursing is surgical aftercare and instruction related to the breast cancer.

Description	Code
Primary: Aftercare following surgery for neoplasm	Z48.3
Secondary: Malignant neoplasm of lower-outer quadrant of left female breast	C50.512
Secondary: Estrogen receptor positive status [ER+]	Z17.0
Secondary: Acquired absence of left breast and nipple	Z90.12

The patient is admitted to home health for surgical aftercare following her mastectomy procedure. Her cancer remains under treatment and thus is still coded. Additional Z codes are assigned to capture that she is estrogen receptor positive, which is relevant to her breast cancer diagnosis, and a status code indicating her left breast is now absent following the mastectomy.

Open wounds from lymphoma

A 61-year-old man is admitted to home health following the initial phase of treatment in the hospital for B-cell lymphoma in the lymph nodes of his neck. The lymphoma has caused open wounds on his neck and upper chest, which will require wound care. He also has hypertension, combined chronic end stage systolic and diastolic heart failure, and coronary artery disease. The lymphoma and the open wounds are the focus of care.

Description	Code
Primary: Unspecified B-cell lymphoma, lymph nodes of head, face, and neck	C85.11
Secondary: Atherosclerotic heart disease of native coronary artery without angina pectoris	I25.10
Secondary: Hypertensive heart disease with heart failure	I11.0
Secondary: End stage heart failure	I50.84
Secondary: Chronic combined systolic (congestive) and diastolic (congestive) heart failure	I50.42

Since the open wounds were caused by the lymphoma, no additional code is necessary as the lymphoma code covers both conditions. As the focus of care, it is coded primary. Coronary artery disease and hypertension are relevant comorbidities that will require monitoring and so are also coded. Note the ICD-10 classification does not assume a relationship between hypertension and coronary artery disease, but a relationship between hypertension and heart failure is assumed. When heart failure is stated as "end stage", I50.84 must also be assigned. The "code also" note present at I50.84 allows for discretionary sequencing between I50.84 and the specific type of heart failure (systolic, diastolic, combined).

Malignant ascites, lung cancer

A 70-year-old man is admitted to home health for management of malignant ascites caused by cancer in the upper lobe of his right lung. His medical record indicates that he's been a cigarette smoker for the past 30 years and continues to smoke despite his illness.

Description	Code
Primary: Malignant neoplasm of upper lobe, right bronchus or lung	C34.11
Secondary: Malignant ascites	R18.0
Secondary: Nicotine dependence, cigarettes, uncomplicated	F17.210

Though the focus of care is the malignant ascites, there is a "code first" note at R18.0 that says to code the malignancy first. Thus, C34.11 is coded in the primary position. Note that in PDGM, incorrectly coding R18.0 in the ***primary*** position will cause the claim to be sent back to be re-coded. The fact that the patient is a smoker is coded, in accordance with tabular instruction at C34.11. "Smoker" codes to nicotine dependence in the alphabetic index.

Chapter 3: Diseases of Blood and Blood-Forming Organs and Certain Disorders Involving the Immune Mechanism (D50 –D89)

This chapter includes five primary categories of conditions, including:

- nutritional, hemolytic and aplastic and other forms of anemia, as well as other bone marrow failure syndromes (D50-D64)
- coagulation defects, purpura and other hemorrhagic conditions (D65- D69)
- Other disorders of blood and blood-forming organs (D70-D77)
- Intraoperative and post-procedural complications of the spleen (D78)
- Certain disorders involving the immune mechanism (D80-D89)

The term "blood-forming organs" refers to the spleen, bone marrow and lymph nodes. Codes from this chapter refer to elements within the blood, such as red blood cells (erythrocytes); white blood cells (leukocytes, lymphocytes, neutrophils, eosinophils, monocytes and basophils); and thrombocytes (platelets or clotting cells).

Sometimes a Chapter 3 code isn't the most appropriate choice. Here are a few situations to watch out for:

- If the documentation indicates a **neoplasm or tumor of a blood-forming organ or of the blood**, coders should look up the term (malignancy, tumor, and adenoma) to find the correct code, most likely a code from Chapter 2.
- If a patient has a **personal or family history of a condition** reported in this chapter, it may be appropriate to select from the Z code section, such as Z85.6 (personal history of leukemia) or Z86.2 (personal history of diseases of the blood and blood-forming organs and certain disorders involving the immune mechanism).
- If a condition reported in this chapter is the **result of injury**, a code from Chapter 19 (Injury, poisoning and certain other consequences of external causes) may be reported, such as a contusion of the spleen (S36.02-), along with a code from this chapter.
- **Symptoms related to blood** are sometimes reported using codes from Chapter 18 (Symptoms, signs and laboratory findings, not elsewhere classified), such as precipitous drop in hematocrit (R71.0) or elevated erythrocyte sedimentation rate (R70.0). Every effort should be made to secure a definitive diagnosis.
- Although rarely coded in home health, if reporting diseases of the blood and blood-forming organs in a **pregnant patient**, when the condition is complicating the pregnancy, report first a code from Chapter 15, such as O99.01- (anemia complicating pregnancy) or O46.00- (antepartum hemorrhage with coagulation defect, unspecified) as the first-listed diagnosis, and a code from this chapter as an additional diagnosis.

Multiple Coding and Sequencing

Codes in this chapter can be either primary or additional diagnoses, depending on the focus of care.

It is important to read the Includes and Excludes notes under codes in this chapter, as well as any other instructions under the code or code category. Here are some examples of multiple coding and sequencing issues for codes in this chapter. Code D57.81- (other sickle-cell disorder with crisis) includes the statement "Use additional code for any associated fever (R50.81)." Therefore, D57.81 is coded first followed by the "fever" code. Another example is code D61.82 (myelophthisis), which includes the statement "Code also the underlying disorder, such a malignant neoplasm of breast (C50-); Tuberculosis (A15-)." Therefore, a code for the neoplasm or tuberculosis is sequenced first, followed by the D61.82 code.

Special Coding Issues

Anemia

Anemia (decrease in either red blood cells or hemoglobin) may be caused by other conditions, such as chronic infections (osteomyelitis, hepatitis, infective endocarditis, tuberculosis, chronic urinary tract infection); inflammatory disorders (rheumatoid disease, burns, systemic lupus erythematosus); and cancer and chronic renal failure. Reporting these conditions requires two codes. For example, anemia in chronic kidney disease (D63.1) has a note to code first underlying chronic kidney disease (N18-).

Anemia may also be related to a malignancy or be the result of treatment for a malignancy. In this situation, there is also a "code first underlying neoplasm" note that applies even when the anemia is the focus of care.

Take note of these three situations and their sequencing rules:

- When the admission/encounter is for management of anemia associated with (or caused by) the malignancy, even if the only treatment is for the anemia, the appropriate code for the malignancy is sequenced as the principal or first-listed diagnosis, followed by the appropriate code for the anemia (such as code D63.0, Anemia in neoplastic disease).
- When the admission/encounter is for management of an anemia associated with an adverse effect of the administration of chemotherapy, immunotherapy or radiation and the only treatment is for the anemia, the anemia code is sequenced first.

Detailed and precise terms are vital to accurately coding any anemia diagnosis. If the home health clinician suspects a specific type of anemia, but the physician documentation is vague, the clinician should check with the physician for verification. For example, anemia due to blood loss from a chronic gastric ulcer would code to D50.0 (iron deficiency anemia secondary to blood loss [chronic]) if the anemia is the focus of care, along with code K25.7 (chronic gastric ulcer without hemorrhage or perforation) as a secondary code to describe the source of the blood loss. Pay attention to the note at K25.- to use an additional code to identify alcohol abuse and dependence (F10-). Most of the time, "hemorrhagic disorder" or "coagulation defects" must be specifically diagnosed and documented by the provider in order to assign codes from category D68 (Other coagulation defects). However, for bleeding symptoms associated with a medication as part of anticoagulation therapy, such as hemoptysis, hematuria, hematemesis and/ or hematochezia, assign code D68.32 (Hemorrhagic disorder due to extrinsic circulating anticoagulants), per Q1 2016 Coding Clinic. This is supported by the inclusion term at D68.32 of "Drug-induced hemorrhagic disorder." Sequencing depends on the focus of care.

Note: Assign as many anemia codes as needed to describe the presence of multiple types of anemia.

Neutropenia

Neutropenia is an abnormal decrease of neutrophils in the blood. Neutrophils are the circulating white blood cells essential for phagocytosis and proteolysis that destroy and remove bacteria, cellular debris and other solid particles. Neutrophils can be associated with acute leukemia, infection, rheumatoid arthritis, B12 deficiency and chronic splenomegaly. Symptoms include chills, fever and sores in the throat, stomach or skin.

As with coding from any ICD-10 chapter, the home health agency must determine the principal diagnosis based on the condition that is most relevant to the current plan of care.

The diagnosis may or may not be related to the patient's most recent hospital stay, but must relate to the services the home health agency will be providing.

CHAPTER 3: DISEASES OF THE BLOOD AND BLOOD-FORMING ORGANS AND CERTAIN DISORDERS INVOLVING THE IMMUNE MECHANISM (D50-D89)

EXCLUDES 2 autoimmune disease (systemic) NOS (M35.9)
certain conditions originating in the perinatal period (P00-P96)
complications of pregnancy, childbirth and the puerperium (O00-O9A)
congenital malformations, deformations and chromosomal abnormalities (Q00-Q99)
endocrine, nutritional and metabolic diseases (E00-E88)
human immunodeficiency virus [HIV] disease (B20)
injury, poisoning and certain other consequences of external causes (S00-T88)
neoplasms (C00-D49)
symptoms, signs and abnormal clinical and laboratory findings, not elsewhere classified (R00-R94)

This chapter contains the following blocks:

D50-D53	Nutritional anemias
D55-D59	Hemolytic anemias
D60-D64	Aplastic and other anemias and other bone marrow failure syndromes
D65-D69	Coagulation defects, purpura and other hemorrhagic conditions
D70-D77	Other disorders of blood and blood-forming organs
D78	Intraoperative and postprocedural complications of the spleen
D80-D89	Certain disorders involving the immune mechanism

Nutritional anemias (D50-D53)

4 **D50 Iron deficiency anemia**

INCLUDES asiderotic anemia
hypochromic anemia

ALERT The assignment of iron deficiency anemia to the home health claim does not provide a supportive diagnosis for medical necessity for the administration of B12 injections by the home health agency under the Medicare part A home health benefit. CMS considers the following conditions reasonable and necessary for the administration of B-12 under the home health benefit: pernicious anemia, megaloblastic anemias, macrocytic anemias, fish tapeworm anemia, gastrectomy, malabsorption syndromes such as sprue and idiopathic steatorrhea, surgical and mechanical disorders such as resection of the small intestine, strictures, anastomosis and blind loop syndrome, and posterolateral sclerosis, other neuropathies associated with pernicious anemia, during the acute phase or acute exacerbation of a neuropathy due to malnutrition and alcoholism.

CODING TIPS✓ Do not assign codes from category D50 when the record only reports "iron deficiency" but does not specifically state "iron deficiency anemia" or "anemia due to iron deficiency." Iron deficiency (without anemia) should be coded to E61.1.

SP **D50.0 Iron deficiency anemia secondary to blood loss (chronic)**
Posthemorrhagic anemia (chronic)

EXCLUDES 1 acute posthemorrhagic anemia (D62)
congenital anemia from fetal blood loss (P61.3)

CODING TIPS✓ The term "chronic" is a non-essential modifier in the code title for iron deficiency anemia secondary to blood loss (chronic). When the record specifies posthemorrhagic anemia (not specified as acute), D50.0 should be assigned. No time period is specifically required for the condition.

DEFINITION Iron depletion from sustained RBC loss in long-term bleeding, often from an ulcerous lesion, causing decreased hemoglobin and insufficient tissue oxygenation.

SP **D50.1 Sideropenic dysphagia**
Kelly-Paterson syndrome
Plummer-Vinson syndrome

SP **D50.8 Other iron deficiency anemias**
Iron deficiency anemia due to inadequate dietary iron intake

CODING TIPS✓ Code D50.8 should be used to report anemia due to dietary iron deficiency.

SP **D50.9 Iron deficiency anemia, unspecified**

CODING TIPS✓ When the record specifies only "iron deficiency anemia," with no cause provided, report code D50.9.

DEFINITION Insufficient stores of iron in the body causing decreased hemoglobin and a reduction in red blood cell oxygen carrying capacity.

4 **D51 Vitamin B12 deficiency anemia**

EXCLUDES 1 vitamin B12 deficiency (E53.8)

ALERT The assignment of B12 deficiency anemia alone to the home health claim does not provide a supportive diagnosis for medical necessity for the administration of B12 injections by the home health agency under the Medicare part A home health benefit. CMS considers the following conditions reasonable and necessary for the administration of B12 under the home health benefit: pernicious anemia, megaloblastic anemias, macrocytic anemias, fish tapeworm anemia, gastrectomy, malabsorption syndromes such as sprue and idiopathic steatorrhea, surgical and mechanical disorders such as resection of the small intestine, strictures, anastomosis and blind loop syndrome, and posterolateral sclerosis, other neuropathies associated with pernicious anemia, during the acute phase or acute exacerbation of a neuropathy due to malnutrition and alcoholism.

CODING TIPS✓ Do not assign codes from category D51 when the record reports "B12 deficiency" but does not specifically state "B12 deficiency anemia" or "anemia due to B12 deficiency." B12 deficiency (without anemia) should be coded to E53.8.

SP **D51.0 Vitamin B12 deficiency anemia due to intrinsic factor deficiency**
Addison anemia
Biermer anemia
Pernicious (congenital) anemia
Congenital intrinsic factor deficiency

CODING TIPS✓ When a patient is receiving home health services for the administration of subcutaneous B12 injections, ensure the clinical record contains evidence of an appropriate diagnosis for coverage. Home health coverage for the administration of B12 is limited to specified anemias, such as pernicious, megaloblastic, macrocytic and fish tapeworm (Medicare Benefit Policy Manual, Chapter 7).

CODING TIPS✓ When a patient is receiving home health services for the administration of subcutaneous B12 injections, the clinical record must contain detailed evidence of why the patient is unable to self administer. For example, a patient with rheumatoid arthritis may have impaired ability to manipulate an injectable medication and self inject. It is not appropriate to use vague terms, such as poor vision or poor manual dexterity. The patient is not expected to self-admiinister IM injections.

DEFINITION Anemia due to underlying Vitamin B12 malabsorption caused by inadequate production of intrinsic factor in the gastric mucosa.

SP **D51.1 Vitamin B12 deficiency anemia due to selective vitamin B12 malabsorption with proteinuria**
Imerslund (Gräsbeck) syndrome
Megaloblastic hereditary anemia

SP **D51.2 Transcobalamin II deficiency**

SP **D51.3 Other dietary vitamin B12 deficiency anemia**
Vegan anemia

CODING TIPS✓ Code D51.3 should be used to report anemia due to dietary B12 deficiency. Deficiencies of B Vitamins may result in neuropathies. Look for specific information regarding deficiencies versus anemia.

SP **D51.8 Other vitamin B12 deficiency anemias**

SP **D51.9 Vitamin B12 deficiency anemia, unspecified**

4 **D52 Folate deficiency anemia**
EXCLUDES 1 folate deficiency without anemia (E53.8)

ALERT The assignment of folate deficiency anemia to the home health claim does not provide a supportive diagnosis for medical necessity for the administration of B12 injections by the home health agency under the Medicare part A home health benefit. CMS considers the following conditions reasonable and necessary for the administration of B-12 under the home health benefit: pernicious anemia, megaloblastic anemias, macrocytic anemias, fish tapeworm anemia, gastrectomy, malabsorption syndromes such as sprue and idiopathic steatorrhea, surgical and mechanical disorders such as resection of the small intestine, strictures, anastomosis and blind loop syndrome, and posterolateral sclerosis, other neuropathies associated with pernicious anemia, during the acute phase or acute exacerbation of a neuropathy due to malnutrition and alcoholism.

DEFINITION Lack of folic acid causing large, immature, misshapen red blood cells, called megaloblasts, to form in the bone marrow.

SP **D52.0 Dietary folate deficiency anemia**
Nutritional megaloblastic anemia

CODING TIPS✓ Code D52.0 should be used to report anemia due to dietary folate deficiency.

SP + **D52.1 Drug-induced folate deficiency anemia**
Use additional code for adverse effect, if applicable, to identify drug (T36-T50 with fifth or sixth character 5)

CODING TIPS✓ Code D52.1 indicates folate deficiency anemia due to the effects of a drug. The clinical record should specify the drug and the anemia should be coded as an adverse effect of the drug. A code from T36-T50 should be assigned following D52.1 to identify the drug resulting in anemia.

SP **D52.8 Other folate deficiency anemias**

SP **D52.9 Folate deficiency anemia, unspecified**
Folic acid deficiency anemia NOS

4 **D53 Other nutritional anemias**
INCLUDES megaloblastic anemia unresponsive to vitamin B12 or folate therapy

SP **D53.0 Protein deficiency anemia**
Amino-acid deficiency anemia
Orotaciduric anemia
EXCLUDES 1 Lesch-Nyhan syndrome (E79.1)

SP **D53.1 Other megaloblastic anemias, not elsewhere classified**
Megaloblastic anemia NOS
EXCLUDES 1 Di Guglielmo's disease (C94.0)

SP **D53.2 Scorbutic anemia**
EXCLUDES 1 scurvy (E54)

SP **D53.8 Other specified nutritional anemias**
Anemia associated with deficiency of copper
Anemia associated with deficiency of molybdenum
Anemia associated with deficiency of zinc

EXCLUDES 1 nutritional deficiencies without anemia, such as:
copper deficiency NOS (E61.0)
molybdenum deficiency NOS (E61.5)
zinc deficiency NOS (E60)

SP **D53.9 Nutritional anemia, unspecified**
Simple chronic anemia
EXCLUDES 1 anemia NOS (D64.9)

Hemolytic anemias (D55-D59)

4 **D55 Anemia due to enzyme disorders**
EXCLUDES 1 drug-induced enzyme deficiency anemia (D59.2)

SP **D55.0 Anemia due to glucose-6-phosphate dehydrogenase [G6PD] deficiency**
Favism
G6PD deficiency anemia
EXCLUDES 1 glucose-6-phosphate dehydrogenase (G6PD) deficiency without anemia (D75.A)

SP **D55.1 Anemia due to other disorders of glutathione metabolism**
Anemia (due to) enzyme deficiencies, except G6PD, related to the hexose monophosphate [HMP] shunt pathway
Anemia (due to) hemolytic nonspherocytic (hereditary), type I
DEFINITION Anemia resulting from damage or destruction of RBCs in high numbers due to insufficient glutathione, a tripeptide used by RBCs to protect against oxidative damage.

▲ 5 **D55.2 Anemia due to disorders of glycolytic enzymes**
EXCLUDES 1 disorders of glycolysis not associated with anemia (E74.81-)

★ **D55.21 Anemia due to pyruvate kinase deficiency**
PK deficiency anemia
Pyruvate kinase deficiency anemia

★ **D55.29 Anemia due to other disorders of glycolytic enzymes**
Hexokinase deficiency anemia
Triose-phosphate isomerase deficiency anemia

SP **D55.3 Anemia due to disorders of nucleotide metabolism**

SP **D55.8 Other anemias due to enzyme disorders**

SP **D55.9 Anemia due to enzyme disorder, unspecified**

4 **D56 Thalassemia**
EXCLUDES 1 sickle-cell thalassemia (D57.4-)

SP + **D56.0 Alpha thalassemia**
Alpha thalassemia major
Hemoglobin H Constant Spring
Hemoglobin H disease
Hydrops fetalis due to alpha thalassemia
Severe alpha thalassemia
Triple gene defect alpha thalassemia
Use additional code, if applicable, for hydrops fetalis due to alpha thalassemia (P56.99)
EXCLUDES 1 alpha thalassemia trait or minor (D56.3)
asymptomatic alpha thalassemia (D56.3)
hydrops fetalis due to isoimmunization (P56.0)
hydrops fetalis not due to immune hemolysis (P83.2)
DEFINITION Hemoglobinopathy caused by genetic decrease in alpha globin chain formation needed for normal hemoglobin A (2 alpha and 2 beta chains), forming unstable hemoglobin and leading to RBC breakage.

SP **D56.1 Beta thalassemia**
Beta thalassemia major
Cooley's anemia
Homozygous beta thalassemia
Severe beta thalassemia
Thalassemia intermedia
Thalassemia major
EXCLUDES 1 beta thalassemia minor (D56.3)
beta thalassemia trait (D56.3)
delta-beta thalassemia (D56.2)
hemoglobin E-beta thalassemia (D56.5)
sickle-cell beta thalassemia (D57.4-)
DEFINITION Hemoglobinopathy caused by genetic decrease in beta globin chain formation needed for normal hemoglobin A (2 alpha and 2 beta chains), leaving insoluble alpha chain aggregates that interfere with RBC production, maturation, and membrane function.

SP **D56.2 Delta-beta thalassemia**
Homozygous delta-beta thalassemia
EXCLUDES 1 delta-beta thalassemia minor (D56.3)
delta-beta thalassemia trait (D56.3)

SP **D56.3 Thalassemia minor**
Alpha thalassemia minor
Alpha thalassemia silent carrier
Alpha thalassemia trait
Beta thalassemia minor
Beta thalassemia trait
Delta-beta thalassemia minor
Delta-beta thalassemia trait
Thalassemia trait NOS
EXCLUDES 1 alpha thalassemia (D56.0)
beta thalassemia (D56.1)
delta-beta thalassemia (D56.2)
hemoglobin E-beta thalassemia (D56.5)
sickle-cell trait (D57.3)
DEFINITION Alpha, beta, and delta-beta hemoglobinopathies caused by small gene mutations resulting in mild signs and symptoms of anemia, or asymptomatic trait or silent carrier forms.

SP **D56.4 Hereditary persistence of fetal hemoglobin [HPFH]**

SP **D56.5 Hemoglobin E-beta thalassemia**

EXCLUDES 1 beta thalassemia (D56.1)
beta thalassemia minor (D56.3)
beta thalassemia trait (D56.3)
delta-beta thalassemia (D56.2)
delta-beta thalassemia trait (D56.3)
hemoglobin E disease (D58.2)
other hemoglobinopathies (D58.2)
sickle-cell beta thalassemia (D57.4-)

DEFINITION Hemoglobinopathy caused by variations in beta globin chain formation, producing unstable hemoglobin E and causing microcytic anemia, poor growth, splenomegaly, and heart failure.

SP **D56.8 Other thalassemias**

Dominant thalassemia
Hemoglobin C thalassemia
Mixed thalassemia
Thalassemia with other hemoglobinopathy

EXCLUDES 1 hemoglobin C disease (D58.2)
hemoglobin E disease (D58.2)
other hemoglobinopathies (D58.2)
sickle-cell anemia (D57.-)
sickle-cell thalassemia (D57.4)

SP **D56.9 Thalassemia, unspecified**

Mediterranean anemia (with other hemoglobinopathy)

DEFINITION Inherited blood disease causing disruption in the normal production of hemoglobin and a high rate of red blood cell destruction.

+ 4 **D57 Sickle-cell disorders**

Use additional code for any associated fever (R50.81)

EXCLUDES 1 other hemoglobinopathies (D58.-)

+ 5 **D57.0 Hb-SS disease with crisis**

Sickle-cell disease with crisis
Hb-SS disease with vasoocclusive pain

CODING TIPS ✓ If vaso-occlusive crisis leads to a specific identifiable exacerbation, such as pulmonary infarction, the exacerbation is also coded.

SP + **D57.00 Hb-SS disease with crisis, unspecified**

Hb-SS disease with (painful) crisis NOS
Hb-SS disease with vasoocclusive pain NOS

DEFINITION Hereditary disease in which RBCs contain abnormal hemoglobin S, making them elongated and crescent-shaped. The fragile, sickled cells become blocked in tiny blood vessels and break apart, causing vaso-occlusive pain.

SP + **D57.01 Hb-SS disease with acute chest syndrome**

DEFINITION Life-threatening complication of sickle-cell disease in which blood clots form in the tiny blood vessels of the lungs with repeated episodes of bleeding from the alveoli and hemosiderin buildup.

SP + **D57.02 Hb-SS disease with splenic sequestration**

DEFINITION Life-threatening complication of sickle-cell disease in which sickled cells become trapped in the spleen, causing acute swelling, high fever, intense abdominal pain, jaundice, leukocytosis, and tissue infarction.

SP + **D57.03 Hb-SS disease with cerebral vascular involvement**

Code also:
, if applicable, cerebral infarction (I63.-)

SP + **D57.09 Hb-SS disease with crisis with other specified complication**

Use additional code to identify complications, such as:
cholelithiasis (K80.-)
priapism (N48.32)

SP + **D57.1 Sickle-cell disease without crisis**

Hb-SS disease without crisis
Sickle-cell anemia NOS
Sickle-cell disease NOS
Sickle-cell disorder NOS

DEFINITION Chronic, hereditary disease in which red blood cells contain abnormal hemoglobin S and are stiff and misshapen like a crescent, inhibiting blood flow through small blood vessels.

+ 5 **D57.2 Sickle-cell/Hb-C disease**

Hb-SC disease
Hb-S/Hb-C disease

SP + **D57.20 Sickle-cell/Hb-C disease without crisis**

+ 6 **D57.21 Sickle-cell/Hb-C disease with crisis**

SP + **D57.211 Sickle-cell/Hb-C disease with acute chest syndrome**

SP + **D57.212 Sickle-cell/Hb-C disease with splenic sequestration**

SP + **D57.213 Sickle-cell/Hb-C disease with cerebral vascular involvement**

Code also:
, if applicable, cerebral infarction (I63.-)

SP + **D57.218 Sickle-cell/Hb-C disease with crisis with other specified complication**

Use additional code to identify complications, such as:
cholelithiasis (K80.-)
priapism (N48.32)

SP + **D57.219 Sickle-cell/Hb-C disease with crisis, unspecified**

Sickle-cell/Hb-C disease with crisis NOS
Sickle-cell/Hb-C disease with vasoocclusive pain NOS

IQ + **D57.3 Sickle-cell trait**

Hb-S trait

Heterozygous hemoglobin S

CODING TIPS ✓ When a patient is reported only to have sickle cell "trait" but no sickle cell disease is stated, report only D57.3.

DEFINITION Condition in which a person carries one gene for normal hemoglobin and one for abnormal hemoglobin S that sickles red blood cells, producing only mild anemia or remaining asymptomatic.

+ 5 D57.4 Sickle-cell thalassemia

Sickle-cell beta thalassemia

Thalassemia Hb-S disease

CODING TIPS ✓ Sickle cell thalassemia differs from sickle cell disease in that these patients have a more mild form of sickle cell disease, with some red blood cells containing abnormal hemoglobin (hemoglobin S) and others containing normal hemoglobin (hemoglobin A).

SP + D57.40 Sickle-cell thalassemia without crisis

Microdrepanocytosis

Sickle-cell thalassemia NOS

DEFINITION Inherited form of anemia, occurring mainly among people of Mediterranean descent, caused by faulty synthesis of part of the hemoglobin molecule.

+ 6 D57.41 Sickle-cell thalassemia, unspecified, with crisis

Sickle-cell thalassemia with (painful) crisis NOS

Sickle-cell thalassemia with vasoocclusive pain NOS

SP + D57.411 Sickle-cell thalassemia, unspecified, with acute chest syndrome

SP + D57.412 Sickle-cell thalassemia, unspecified, with splenic sequestration

SP + D57.413 Sickle-cell thalassemia, unspecified, with cerebral vascular involvement

Code also:

, if applicable cerebral infarction (I63.-)

SP + D57.418 Sickle-cell thalassemia, unspecified, with crisis with other specified complication

Use additional code to identify complications, such as:

cholelithiasis (K80.-)

priapism (N48.32)

▲ SP + D57.419 Sickle-cell thalassemia, unspecified, with crisis

Sickle-cell thalassemia with (painful) crisis NOS

Sickle-cell thalassemia with vasoocclusive pain NOS

SP + D57.42 Sickle-cell thalassemia beta zero without crisis

HbS-beta zero without crisis

Sickle-cell beta zero without crisis

DEFINITION HbS-beta zero is clinically similar to sickle cell-SS disease in terms of degree of frequency and severity of acute and chronic complications. The risk of stroke is similar. They both may be managed long term with medications such as hydroxyurea.

+ 6 D57.43 Sickle-cell thalassemia beta zero with crisis

HbS-beta zero with crisis

Sickle-cell beta zero with crisis

DEFINITION HbS-beta zero is clinically similar to sickle cell-SS disease in terms of degree of frequency and severity of acute and chronic complications. The risk of stroke is similar. They both may be managed long term with medications such as hydroxyurea.

SP + D57.431 Sickle-cell thalassemia beta zero with acute chest syndrome

HbS-beta zero with acute chest syndrome

Sickle-cell beta zero with acute chest syndrome

SP + D57.432 Sickle-cell thalassemia beta zero with splenic sequestration

HbS-beta zero with splenic sequestration

Sickle-cell beta zero with splenic sequestration

SP + D57.433 Sickle-cell thalassemia beta zero with cerebral vascular involvement

HbS-beta zero with cerebral vascular involvement

Sickle-cell beta zero with cerebral vascular involvement

Code also:

, if applicable cerebral infarction (I63.-)

SP + D57.438 Sickle-cell thalassemia beta zero with crisis with other specified complication

HbS-beta zero with other specified complication

Sickle-cell beta zero with other specified complication

Use additional code to identify complications, such as:

cholelithiasis (K80.-)

priapism (N48.32)

▲ SP + D57.439 Sickle-cell thalassemia beta zero with crisis, unspecified

HbS-beta zero with other specified complication

Sickle-cell beta zero with crisis unspecified

Sickle-cell thalassemia beta zero with (painful) crisis NOS

Sickle-cell thalassemia beta zero with vasoocclusive pain NOS

SP + D57.44 Sickle-cell thalassemia beta plus without crisis

HbS-beta plus without crisis

Sickle-cell beta plus without crisis

DEFINITION HbS-beta plus is significantly less severe than HbS-beta zero and with little or no anemia. The spectrum and severity of complications is less than HbS-beta zero. It also carries a relative lower risk of stroke.

+ 6 **D57.45 Sickle-cell thalassemia beta plus with crisis**
HbS-beta plus with crisis
Sickle-cell beta plus with crisis
DEFINITION HbS-beta plus is significantly less severe than HbS-beta zero and with little or no anemia. The spectrum and severity of complications is less than HbS-beta zero. It also carries a relative lower risk of stroke.

SP + **D57.451 Sickle-cell thalassemia beta plus with acute chest syndrome**
HbS-beta plus with acute chest syndrome
Sickle-cell beta plus with acute chest syndrome

SP + **D57.452 Sickle-cell thalassemia beta plus with splenic sequestration**
HbS-beta plus with splenic sequestration
Sickle-cell beta plus with splenic sequestration

SP + **D57.453 Sickle-cell thalassemia beta plus with cerebral vascular involvement**
HbS-beta plus with cerebral vascular involvement
Sickle-cell beta plus with cerebral vascular involvement
Code also:
, if applicable cerebral infarction (I63.-)

SP + **D57.458 Sickle-cell thalassemia beta plus with crisis with other specified complication**
HbS-beta plus with crisis with other specified complication
Sickle-cell beta plus with crisis with other specified complication
Use additional code to identify complications, such as:
cholelithiasis (K80.-)
priapism (N48.32)

▲ SP + **D57.459 Sickle-cell thalassemia beta plus with crisis, unspecified**
HbS-beta plus with crisis with unspecified complication
Sickle-cell beta plus with crisis with unspecified complication
Sickle-cell thalassemia beta plus with (painful) crisis NOS
Sickle-cell thalassemia beta plus with vasoocclusive pain NOS

+ 5 **D57.8 Other sickle-cell disorders**
Hb-SD disease
Hb-SE disease

SP + **D57.80 Other sickle-cell disorders without crisis**

+ 6 **D57.81 Other sickle-cell disorders with crisis**

SP + **D57.811 Other sickle-cell disorders with acute chest syndrome**

SP + **D57.812 Other sickle-cell disorders with splenic sequestration**

SP + **D57.813 Other sickle-cell disorders with cerebral vascular involvement**
Code also:
, if applicable: cerebral infarction (I63.-)

SP + **D57.818 Other sickle-cell disorders with crisis with other specified complication**
Use additional code to identify complications, such as:
cholelithiasis (K80.-)
priapism (N48.32)

SP + **D57.819 Other sickle-cell disorders with crisis, unspecified**
Other sickle-cell disorders with crisis NOS
Other sickle-cell disorders with vasooclusive pain NOS

4 **D58 Other hereditary hemolytic anemias**
EXCLUDES 1 hemolytic anemia of the newborn (P55.-)

SP **D58.0 Hereditary spherocytosis**
Acholuric (familial) jaundice
Congenital (spherocytic) hemolytic icterus
Minkowski-Chauffard syndrome
DEFINITION Congenital form of spherocytosis with hemolytic anemia, abnormal fragility of erythrocytes, jaundice, and splenomegaly.

SP **D58.1 Hereditary elliptocytosis**
Elliptocytosis (congenital)
Ovalocytosis (congenital) (hereditary)

SP **D58.2 Other hemoglobinopathies**
Abnormal hemoglobin NOS
Congenital Heinz body anemia
Hb-C disease
Hb-D disease
Hb-E disease
Hemoglobinopathy NOS
Unstable hemoglobin hemolytic disease
EXCLUDES 1 familial polycythemia (D75.0)
Hb-M disease (D74.0)
hemoglobin E-beta thalassemia (D56.5)
hereditary persistence of fetal hemoglobin [HPFH] (D56.4)
high-altitude polycythemia (D75.1)
methemoglobinemia (D74.-)
other hemoglobinopathies with thalassemia (D56.8)

SP **D58.8 Other specified hereditary hemolytic anemias**
Stomatocytosis

SP **D58.9 Hereditary hemolytic anemia, unspecified**

4 **D59 Acquired hemolytic anemia**

SP + **D59.0 Drug-induced autoimmune hemolytic anemia**
Use additional code for adverse effect, if applicable, to identify drug (T36-T50 with fifth or sixth character 5)

4 4th digit required 5 5th digit required 6 6th digit required 7 7th digit required X 7th digit placeholder + Additional code Laterality

CODING TIPS✓ Code D59.0 indicates autoimmune hemolytic anemia due to the effects of a drug. The clinical record should specify the drug, and this should be coded as an adverse effect of the drug causing the anemia. A code from T36-T50 should be assigned following D59.0 to identify the drug resulting in anemia.

5 **D59.1 Other autoimmune hemolytic anemias**
EXCLUDES 2 Evans syndrome (D69.41)
hemolytic disease of newborn (P55.-)
paroxysmal cold hemoglobinuria (D59.6)

SP **D59.10 Autoimmune hemolytic anemia, unspecified**

SP **D59.11 Warm autoimmune hemolytic anemia**
Warm type (primary) (secondary) (symptomatic) autoimmune hemolytic anemia
Warm type autoimmune hemolytic disease

SP **D59.12 Cold autoimmune hemolytic anemia**
Chronic cold hemagglutinin disease
Cold agglutinin disease
Cold agglutinin hemoglobinuria
Cold type (primary) (secondary) (symptomatic) autoimmune hemolytic anemia
Cold type autoimmune hemolytic disease

SP **D59.13 Mixed type autoimmune hemolytic anemia**
Mixed type autoimmune hemolytic disease
Mixed type, cold and warm, (primary) (secondary) (symptomatic) autoimmune hemolytic anemia

SP **D59.19 Other autoimmune hemolytic anemia**

SP + **D59.2 Drug-induced nonautoimmune hemolytic anemia**
Drug-induced enzyme deficiency anemia
Use additional code for adverse effect, if applicable, to identify drug (T36-T50 with fifth or sixth character 5)

CODING TIPS✓ D59.2 indicates non-autoimmune hemolytic anemia due to the effects of a drug. The clinical record should specify the drug, and this should be coded as an adverse effect of the drug causing the anemia. A code from T36-T50 should be assigned following D59.2 to identify the drug resulting in anemia.

SP + **D59.3 Hemolytic-uremic syndrome**
Use additional code to identify associated:
E. coli infection (B96.2-)
Pneumococcal pneumonia (J13)
Shigella dysenteriae (A03.9)

DEFINITION Condition in which platelets become clogged in narrow renal blood vessels, leading to the destruction of red blood cells and kidney failure. Symptoms include severe abdominal pain, diarrhea, nausea, and vomiting.

SP **D59.4 Other nonautoimmune hemolytic anemias**
Mechanical hemolytic anemia
Microangiopathic hemolytic anemia
Toxic hemolytic anemia

SP **D59.5 Paroxysmal nocturnal hemoglobinuria [Marchiafava-Micheli]**
EXCLUDES 1 hemoglobinuria NOS (R82.3)

SP + **D59.6 Hemoglobinuria due to hemolysis from other external causes**
Hemoglobinuria from exertion
March hemoglobinuria
Paroxysmal cold hemoglobinuria
Use additional code (Chapter 20) to identify external cause
EXCLUDES 1 hemoglobinuria NOS (R82.3)

CODING TIPS✓ Hemoglobinuria is a condition where excess hemoglobin is found in high concentrations in the urine. Code D59.6 only when the hemoglobinuria is stated as due to hemolysis related to a specific other cause (the hemolysis of red blood cells due to another specific cause or condition is resulting in the hemoglobinuria). An external cause code (from Chapter 20) may be assigned to identify the external cause.

SP **D59.8 Other acquired hemolytic anemias**

SP **D59.9 Acquired hemolytic anemia, unspecified**
Idiopathic hemolytic anemia, chronic

Aplastic and other anemias and other bone marrow failure syndromes (D60-D64)

4 **D60 Acquired pure red cell aplasia [erythroblastopenia]**
INCLUDES red cell aplasia (acquired) (adult) (with thymoma)
EXCLUDES 1 congenital red cell aplasia (D61.01)

SP **D60.0 Chronic acquired pure red cell aplasia**
DEFINITION Decline of RBC precursor cells in the bone marrow until nearly absent while WBC precursors are present at normal levels; causes normochromic, normoblastic anemia.

SP **D60.1 Transient acquired pure red cell aplasia**

SP **D60.8 Other acquired pure red cell aplasias**

SP **D60.9 Acquired pure red cell aplasia, unspecified**

4 **D61 Other aplastic anemias and other bone marrow failure syndromes**
EXCLUDES 2 neutropenia (D70.-)

5 **D61.0 Constitutional aplastic anemia**

SP **D61.01 Constitutional (pure) red blood cell aplasia**
Blackfan-Diamond syndrome
Congenital (pure) red cell aplasia
Familial hypoplastic anemia
Primary (pure) red cell aplasia
Red cell (pure) aplasia of infants
EXCLUDES 1 acquired red cell aplasia (D60.9)

SP **D61.09 Other constitutional aplastic anemia**
Fanconi's anemia
Pancytopenia with malformations

SP + **D61.1 Drug-induced aplastic anemia**
Use additional code for adverse effect, if applicable, to identify drug (T36-T50 with fifth or sixth character 5)

CODING TIPS ✓ When the clinical record specifies aplastic anemia due to antineoplastic chemotherapy, D61.1 should be assigned, followed by the appropriate code to identify the adverse effect of antineoplastic chemotherapy (T36-T50).

SP **D61.2 Aplastic anemia due to other external agents**
Code first:
, if applicable, toxic effects of substances chiefly nonmedicinal as to source (T51-T65)

SP **D61.3 Idiopathic aplastic anemia**

5 **D61.8 Other specified aplastic anemias and other bone marrow failure syndromes**

6 **D61.81 Pancytopenia**
EXCLUDES 1 pancytopenia (due to) (with) aplastic anemia (D61.9)
pancytopenia (due to) (with) bone marrow infiltration (D61.82)
pancytopenia (due to) (with) congenital (pure) red cell aplasia (D61.01)
pancytopenia (due to) (with) hairy cell leukemia (C91.4-)
pancytopenia (due to) (with) human immunodeficiency virus disease (B20.-)
pancytopenia (due to) (with) leukoerythroblastic anemia (D61.82)
pancytopenia (due to) (with) myeloproliferative disease (D47.1)
EXCLUDES 2 pancytopenia (due to) (with) myelodysplastic syndromes (D46.-)

DEFINITION Decreased count of all elements in the blood: red blood cells, white blood cells, and platelets.

SP **D61.810 Antineoplastic chemotherapy induced pancytopenia**
EXCLUDES 2 aplastic anemia due to antineoplastic chemotherapy (D61.1)

CODING TIPS ✓ This code is reported when pancytopenia results from antineoplastics. Pancytopenia is a reduction of red and white blood cells, as well as platelets.

SP **D61.811 Other drug-induced pancytopenia**
EXCLUDES 2 aplastic anemia due to drugs (D61.1)

SP **D61.818 Other pancytopenia**

SP **D61.82 Myelophthisis**
Leukoerythroblastic anemia
Myelophthisic anemia
Panmyelophthisis
Code also the underlying disorder, such as:
malignant neoplasm of breast (C50.-)
tuberculosis (A15.-)
EXCLUDES 1 idiopathic myelofibrosis (D47.1)
myelofibrosis NOS (D75.81)
myelofibrosis with myeloid metaplasia (D47.4)
primary myelofibrosis (D47.1)
secondary myelofibrosis (D75.81)

DEFINITION Replacement of hemopoietic tissue in the bone marrow by abnormal infiltrates, usually fibrotic tissue or malignant tumors, suppressing bone marrow function.

SP **D61.89 Other specified aplastic anemias and other bone marrow failure syndromes**

SP **D61.9 Aplastic anemia, unspecified**
Hypoplastic anemia NOS
Medullary hypoplasia

SP **D62 Acute posthemorrhagic anemia**
EXCLUDES 1 anemia due to chronic blood loss (D50.0)
blood loss anemia NOS (D50.0)
congenital anemia from fetal blood loss (P61.3)

CODING TIPS ✓ Do not assign D62 when the clinical record documentation specifies only "blood loss," "blood loss anemia" or "chronic blood loss anemia." Code D62 should only be used when posthemorrhagic anemia is specified as acute.

4 **D63 Anemia in chronic diseases classified elsewhere**

IQ **D63.0 Anemia in neoplastic disease**
Code first:
neoplasm (C00-D49)
EXCLUDES 1 aplastic anemia due to antineoplastic chemotherapy (D61.1)
EXCLUDES 2 anemia due to antineoplastic chemotherapy (D64.81)

GUIDELINES **Section 1.C.2.c.1** When admission/encounter is for management of an anemia associated with the malignancy, and the treatment is only for anemia, the appropriate code for the malignancy is sequenced as the principal or first-listed diagnosis followed by the appropriate code for the anemia (such as code D63.0, Anemia in neoplastic disease).

CODING TIPS ✓ When a patient is admitted for anemia due to neoplastic disease (D63.0), a code for the appropriate neoplasm must first be assigned, regardless of whether the focus of care is the neoplastic disease or the anemia. Anemia is assumed related to the neoplastic disease.

IQ **D63.1 Anemia in chronic kidney disease**
Erythropoietin resistant anemia (EPO resistant anemia)
Code first:
underlying chronic kidney disease (CKD) (N18.-)

ALERT Watch out for coverage issues with anemia in chronic kidney disease. The treatment is covered under the dialysis benefit. This type of anemia is a related condition if the terminal diagnosis in hospice is ESRD.

M IQ **D63.8 *Anemia in other chronic diseases classified elsewhere***
Code first underlying disease, such as:
diphyllobothriasis (B70.0)
hookworm disease (B76.0-B76.9)
hypothyroidism (E00.0-E03.9)
malaria (B50.0-B54)
symptomatic late syphilis (A52.79)
tuberculosis (A18.89)

4 **D64 Other anemias**
EXCLUDES 1 refractory anemia (D46.-)
refractory anemia with excess blasts in transformation [RAEB T] (C92.0-)

SP **D64.0 Hereditary sideroblastic anemia**
Sex-linked hypochromic sideroblastic anemia

DEFINITION Group of blood disorders in which the bone marrow's ability to produce normal red blood cells is impaired and sideroblasts, or deformed red blood cells, are present in the bloodstream.

IQ **D64.1 Secondary sideroblastic anemia due to disease**
Code first:
underlying disease

SP + **D64.2 Secondary sideroblastic anemia due to drugs and toxins**
Code first:
poisoning due to drug or toxin, if applicable
(T36-T65 with fifth or sixth character 1-4 or 6)
Use additional code for adverse effect, if applicable, to identify drug (T36-T50 with fifth or sixth character 5)

SP **D64.3 Other sideroblastic anemias**
Sideroblastic anemia NOS
Pyridoxine-responsive sideroblastic anemia NEC

SP **D64.4 Congenital dyserythropoietic anemia**
Dyshematopoietic anemia (congenital)
EXCLUDES 1 Blackfan-Diamond syndrome (D61.01)
Di Guglielmo's disease (C94.0)

CODING TIPS ✓ Congenital dyserythropoletic anemia is defined as a congenital condition resulting in immature red blood cells that are unusually shaped and cannot develop into functional mature cells, leading to a shortage of healthy red blood cells. These patients also frequently have thrombocytopenia, which should be additionally coded if present.

5 **D64.8 Other specified anemias**

▲ SP **D64.81 Anemia due to antineoplastic chemotherapy**
Antineoplastic chemotherapy induced anemia
EXCLUDES 2 anemia in neoplastic disease (D63.0)
aplastic anemia due to antineoplastic chemotherapy (D61.1)

CODING TIPS ✓ Do not assign D64.81 to indicate anemia due to neoplastic disease. Anemia due to neoplastic disease should be coded to D63.0. Anemia is presumed related to neoplasms and to chemotherapy, so both anemias may be coded unless the physician or NPP indicates otherwise.

CODING TIPS ✓ Do not assign D64.81 to indicate aplastic anemia due to antineoplastic chemotherapy. If the diagnostic statements specifically report aplastic anemia due to antineoplastic chemotherapy, assign D61.1.

CODING TIPS ✓ Code D64.81 should be followed in the sequencing by the appropriate T code for adverse effect of antineoplastics. When sequencing, follow the guideline on coding adverse effects.

CODING TIPS ✓ Antineoplastic chemotherapy-induced changes usually are short term, and they do not usually reduce the marrow cells to a point of aplasia.

SP **D64.89 Other specified anemias**
Infantile pseudoleukemia

SP **D64.9 Anemia, unspecified**

CODING TIPS ✓ There are several conditions presumed related to anemia, such as CKD, neoplastic disease and chemotherapy. Reference the index for anemia and the terms 'with' or 'in' prior to using D64.9.

Coagulation defects, purpura and other hemorrhagic conditions (D65-D69)

CODING TIPS ✓ The codes in D65-D69 are used for different kinds of hemophilias. If bleeds are related to anticoagulant drugs, see D68.32.

SP **D65 Disseminated intravascular coagulation [defibrination syndrome]**
Afibrinogenemia, acquired
Consumption coagulopathy
Diffuse or disseminated intravascular coagulation [DIC]
Fibrinolytic hemorrhage, acquired

Fibrinolytic purpura
Purpura fulminans

EXCLUDES 1 disseminated intravascular coagulation (complicating) :
abortion or ectopic or molar pregnancy (O00-O07, O08.1)
in newborn (P60)
pregnancy, childbirth and the puerperium (O45.0, O46.0, O67.0, O72.3)

DEFINITION Bleeding disorder characterized by an abnormal reduction in the elements involved in blood clotting; marked by profuse hemorrhaging in the late stages.

SP D66 Hereditary factor VIII deficiency
Classical hemophilia
Deficiency factor VIII (with functional defect)
Hemophilia NOS
Hemophilia A

EXCLUDES 1 factor VIII deficiency with vascular defect (D68.0)

DEFINITION Most common form of hemophilia, referred to as classic hemophilia or hemophilia A; characterized by profuse bleeding from injuries, as well as bleeding from the joints, muscles, digestive tract, and brain.

SP D67 Hereditary factor IX deficiency
Christmas disease
Factor IX deficiency (with functional defect)
Hemophilia B
Plasma thromboplastin component [PTC] deficiency

DEFINITION A clotting disorder of blood, caused by hereditary deficiency of factor IX.

4 D68 Other coagulation defects

EXCLUDES 1 abnormal coagulation profile (R79.1)
coagulation defects complicating abortion or ectopic or molar pregnancy (O00-O07, O08.1)
coagulation defects complicating pregnancy, childbirth and the puerperium (O45.0, O46.0, O67.0, O72.3)

SP D68.0 Von Willebrand's disease
Angiohemophilia
Factor VIII deficiency with vascular defect
Vascular hemophilia

EXCLUDES 1 capillary fragility (hereditary) (D69.8)
factor VIII deficiency NOS (D66)
factor VIII deficiency with functional defect (D66)

SP D68.1 Hereditary factor XI deficiency
Hemophilia C
Plasma thromboplastin antecedent [PTA] deficiency
Rosenthal's disease

SP D68.2 Hereditary deficiency of other clotting factors
AC globulin deficiency
Congenital afibrinogenemia
Deficiency of factor I [fibrinogen]
Deficiency of factor II [prothrombin]
Deficiency of factor V [labile]
Deficiency of factor VII [stable]
Deficiency of factor X [Stuart-Prower]
Deficiency of factor XII [Hageman]
Deficiency of factor XIII [fibrin stabilizing]
Dysfibrinogenemia (congenital)
Hypoproconvertinemia
Owren's disease
Proaccelerin deficiency

5 D68.3 Hemorrhagic disorder due to circulating anticoagulants

6 D68.31 Hemorrhagic disorder due to intrinsic circulating anticoagulants, antibodies, or inhibitors

SP D68.311 Acquired hemophilia
Autoimmune hemophilia
Autoimmune inhibitors to clotting factors
Secondary hemophilia

SP D68.312 Antiphospholipid antibody with hemorrhagic disorder
Lupus anticoagulant (LAC) with hemorrhagic disorder
Systemic lupus erythematosus [SLE] inhibitor with hemorrhagic disorder

EXCLUDES 1 antiphospholipid antibody, finding without diagnosis (R76.0)
antiphospholipid antibody syndrome (D68.61)
antiphospholipid antibody with hypercoagulable state (D68.61)
lupus anticoagulant (LAC) finding without diagnosis (R76.0)
lupus anticoagulant (LAC) with hypercoagulable state (D68.62)
systemic lupus erythematosus [SLE] inhibitor finding without diagnosis (R76.0)
systemic lupus erythematosus [SLE] inhibitor with hypercoagulable state (D68.62)

SP D68.318 Other hemorrhagic disorder due to intrinsic circulating anticoagulants, antibodies, or inhibitors
Antithromboplastinemia
Antithromboplastinogenemia
Hemorrhagic disorder due to intrinsic increase in antithrombin
Hemorrhagic disorder due to intrinsic increase in anti-VIIIa
Hemorrhagic disorder due to intrinsic increase in anti-IXa
Hemorrhagic disorder due to intrinsic increase in anti-XIa

SP + **D68.32 Hemorrhagic disorder due to extrinsic circulating anticoagulants**
Drug-induced hemorrhagic disorder
Hemorrhagic disorder due to increase in anti-IIa
Hemorrhagic disorder due to increase in anti-Xa
Hyperheparinemia
Use additional code for adverse effect, if applicable, to identify drug (T45.515, T45.525)

CODING TIPS✓ For bleeding such as hemoptysis, hematuria, hematemesis, hematochezia, etc., that is associated with a drug as part of anticoagulation therapy, assign code D68.32.

CODING TIPS✓ When a bleed results as an adverse effect of anticoagulant therapy, such as a gastric bleed, code the bleed, D68.32, and then the adverse effect of the drug or drugs.

SP **D68.4 Acquired coagulation factor deficiency**
Deficiency of coagulation factor due to liver disease
Deficiency of coagulation factor due to vitamin K deficiency
EXCLUDES 1 vitamin K deficiency of newborn (P53)

▲ 5 **D68.5 Primary thrombophilia**
Primary hypercoagulable states
EXCLUDES 1 antiphospholipid syndrome (D68.61)
lupus anticoagulant (D68.62)
secondary activated protein C resistance (D68.69)
secondary antiphospholipid antibody syndrome (D68.69)
secondary lupus anticoagulant with hypercoagulable state (D68.69)
secondary systemic lupus erythematosus [SLE] inhibitor with hypercoagulable state (D68.69)
systemic lupus erythematosus [SLE] inhibitor finding without diagnosis (R76.0)
systemic lupus erythematosus [SLE] inhibitor with hemorrhagic disorder (D68.312)
thrombotic thrombocytopenic purpura (M31.19)

DEFINITION Abnormal development of blood clots in arteries or veins.

SP **D68.51 Activated protein C resistance**
Factor V Leiden mutation

SP **D68.52 Prothrombin gene mutation**

SP **D68.59 Other primary thrombophilia**
Antithrombin III deficiency
Hypercoagulable state NOS
Primary hypercoagulable state NEC
Primary thrombophilia NEC
Protein C deficiency
Protein S deficiency
Thrombophilia NOS

5 **D68.6 Other thrombophilia**
Other hypercoagulable states
EXCLUDES 1 diffuse or disseminated intravascular coagulation [DIC] (D65)
heparin induced thrombocytopenia (HIT) (D75.82)
hyperhomocysteinemia (E72.11)

SP **D68.61 Antiphospholipid syndrome**
Anticardiolipin syndrome
Antiphospholipid antibody syndrome
EXCLUDES 1 anti-phospholipid antibody, finding without diagnosis (R76.0)
anti-phospholipid antibody with hemorrhagic disorder (D68.312)
lupus anticoagulant syndrome (D68.62)

SP **D68.62 Lupus anticoagulant syndrome**
Lupus anticoagulant
Presence of systemic lupus erythematosus [SLE] inhibitor
EXCLUDES 1 anticardiolipin syndrome (D68.61)
antiphospholipid syndrome (D68.61)
lupus anticoagulant (LAC) finding without diagnosis (R76.0)
lupus anticoagulant (LAC) with hemorrhagic disorder (D68.312)

SP **D68.69 Other thrombophilia**
Hypercoagulable states NEC
Secondary hypercoagulable state NOS

SP **D68.8 Other specified coagulation defects**
EXCLUDES 1 hemorrhagic disease of newborn (P53)

SP **D68.9 Coagulation defect, unspecified**

▲ 4 **D69 Purpura and other hemorrhagic conditions**
EXCLUDES 1 benign hypergammaglobulinemic purpura (D89.0)
cryoglobulinemic purpura (D89.1)
essential (hemorrhagic) thrombocythemia (D47.3)
hemorrhagic thrombocythemia (D47.3)
purpura fulminans (D65)
thrombotic thrombocytopenic purpura (M31.19)
Waldenström hypergammaglobulinemic purpura (D89.0)

SP **D69.0 Allergic purpura**
Allergic vasculitis
Nonthrombocytopenic hemorrhagic purpura

Chapter 3
D50-D89

Nonthrombocytopenic idiopathic purpura
Purpura anaphylactoid
Purpura Henoch(-Schönlein)
Purpura rheumatica
Vascular purpura
EXCLUDES 1 thrombocytopenic hemorrhagic purpura (D69.3)

DEFINITION Allergic reaction causing hemorrhaging of the skin and mucous membranes; produces purple discolorations on the skin surface.

SP **D69.1 Qualitative platelet defects**
Bernard-Soulier [giant platelet] syndrome
Glanzmann's disease
Grey platelet syndrome
Thromboasthenia (hemorrhagic) (hereditary)
Thrombocytopathy
EXCLUDES 1 von Willebrand's disease (D68.0)

SP **D69.2 Other nonthrombocytopenic purpura**
Purpura NOS
Purpura simplex
Senile purpura

SP **D69.3 Immune thrombocytopenic purpura**
Hemorrhagic (thrombocytopenic) purpura
Idiopathic thrombocytopenic purpura
Tidal platelet dysgenesis

5 **D69.4 Other primary thrombocytopenia**
EXCLUDES 1 transient neonatal thrombocytopenia (P61.0)
Wiskott-Aldrich syndrome (D82.0)

SP **D69.41 Evans syndrome**

IQ **D69.42 Congenital and hereditary thrombocytopenia purpura**
Congenital thrombocytopenia
Hereditary thrombocytopenia
Code first congential or hereditary disorder, such as:
thrombocytopenia with absent radius (TAR syndrome) (Q87.2)

SP **D69.49 Other primary thrombocytopenia**
Megakaryocytic hypoplasia
Primary thrombocytopenia NOS

5 **D69.5 Secondary thrombocytopenia**
EXCLUDES 1 heparin induced thrombocytopenia (HIT) (D75.82)
transient thrombocytopenia of newborn (P61.0)

DEFINITION Uncommon but life-threatening adverse reaction in which arterial or venous thrombotic complications develop that can lead to pulmonary embolism, amputation, stroke, or acute myocardial infarction.

SP **D69.51 Posttransfusion purpura**
Posttransfusion purpura from whole blood (fresh) or blood products
PTP

SP **D69.59 Other secondary thrombocytopenia**

SP **D69.6 Thrombocytopenia, unspecified**

SP **D69.8 Other specified hemorrhagic conditions**
Capillary fragility (hereditary)
Vascular pseudohemophilia

SP **D69.9 Hemorrhagic condition, unspecified**

Other disorders of blood and blood-forming organs (D70-D77)

+ 4 **D70 Neutropenia**
INCLUDES agranulocytosis
decreased absolute neurophile count (ANC)
Use additional code for any associated:
fever (R50.81)
mucositis (J34.81, K12.3-, K92.81, N76.81)
EXCLUDES 1 neutropenic splenomegaly (D73.81)
transient neonatal neutropenia (P61.5)

SP + **D70.0 Congenital agranulocytosis**
Congenital neutropenia
Infantile genetic agranulocytosis
Kostmann's disease

SP + **D70.1 Agranulocytosis secondary to cancer chemotherapy**
Code also:
underlying neoplasm
Use additional code for adverse effect, if applicable, to identify drug (T45.1X5)

SP + **D70.2 Other drug-induced agranulocytosis**
Use additional code for adverse effect, if applicable, to identify drug (T36-T50 with fifth or sixth character 5)

SP + **D70.3 Neutropenia due to infection**

SP + **D70.4 Cyclic neutropenia**
Cyclic hematopoiesis
Periodic neutropenia

SP + **D70.8 Other neutropenia**

SP + **D70.9 Neutropenia, unspecified**

SP **D71 Functional disorders of polymorphonuclear neutrophils**
Cell membrane receptor complex [CR3] defect
Chronic (childhood) granulomatous disease
Congenital dysphagocytosis
Progressive septic granulomatosis

4 **D72 Other disorders of white blood cells**
EXCLUDES 1 basophilia (D72.824)
immunity disorders (D80-D89)
neutropenia (D70)
preleukemia (syndrome) (D46.9)

SP **D72.0 Genetic anomalies of leukocytes**
Alder (granulation) (granulocyte) anomaly
Alder syndrome
Hereditary leukocytic hypersegmentation
Hereditary leukocytic hyposegmentation
Hereditary leukomelanopathy
May-Hegglin (granulation) (granulocyte) anomaly
May-Hegglin syndrome
Pelger-Huët (granulation) (granulocyte) anomaly
Pelger-Huët syndrome
EXCLUDES 1 Chédiak (-Steinbrinck) -Higashi syndrome (E70.330)

▲ 5 **D72.1 Eosinophilia**
EXCLUDES 2 Löffler's syndrome (J82.89)
pulmonary eosinophilia (J82.-)

SP **D72.10 Eosinophilia, unspecified**

6 **D72.11 Hypereosinophilic syndrome [HES]**

SP **D72.110 Idiopathic hypereosinophilic syndrome [IHES]**

SP **D72.111 Lymphocytic Variant Hypereosinophilic Syndrome [LHES]**
Lymphocyte variant hypereosinophilia
Code also:
, if applicable, any associated lymphocytic neoplastic disorder

SP **D72.118 Other hypereosinophilic syndrome**
Episodic angioedema with eosinophilia
Gleich's syndrome

SP **D72.119 Hypereosinophilic syndrome [HES], unspecified**

SP + **D72.12 Drug rash with eosinophilia and systemic symptoms syndrome**
DRESS syndrome
Use additional code for adverse effect, if applicable, to identify drug (T36-T50 with fifth or sixth character 5)

M **D72.18** ***Eosinophilia in diseases classified elsewhere***
Code first underlying disease, such as:
chronic myelomonocytic leukemia (C93.1-)

SP **D72.19 Other eosinophilia**
Familial eosinophilia
Hereditary eosinophilia

5 **D72.8 Other specified disorders of white blood cells**
EXCLUDES 1 leukemia (C91-C95)

6 **D72.81 Decreased white blood cell count**
EXCLUDES 1 neutropenia (D70.-)

SP **D72.810 Lymphocytopenia**
Decreased lymphocytes

SP **D72.818 Other decreased white blood cell count**
Basophilic leukopenia
Eosinophilic leukopenia
Monocytopenia
Other decreased leukocytes
Plasmacytopenia

SP **D72.819 Decreased white blood cell count, unspecified**
Decreased leukocytes, unspecified
Leukocytopenia, unspecified
Leukopenia
EXCLUDES 1 malignant leukopenia (D70.9)

6 **D72.82 Elevated white blood cell count**
EXCLUDES 1 eosinophilia (D72.1)

SP **D72.820 Lymphocytosis (symptomatic)**
Elevated lymphocytes

SP **D72.821 Monocytosis (symptomatic)**
EXCLUDES 1 infectious mononucleosis (B27.-)

SP **D72.822 Plasmacytosis**

SP **D72.823 Leukemoid reaction**
Basophilic leukemoid reaction
Leukemoid reaction NOS
Lymphocytic leukemoid reaction
Monocytic leukemoid reaction
Myelocytic leukemoid reaction
Neutrophilic leukemoid reaction
DEFINITION A state of circulating blood presenting a clinical picture resembling or indistinguishable from leukemia due to a condition such as infection, bone marrow compromise, liver failure, and inflammatory disorders.

SP **D72.824 Basophilia**
DEFINITION Abnormally increased number of basophils in the blood, which release histamine and serotonin upon stimulation.

SP **D72.825 Bandemia**
Bandemia without diagnosis of specific infection
EXCLUDES 1 confirmed infection - code to infection
leukemia (C91.-, C92.-, C93.-, C94.-, C95.-)
DEFINITION Nonspecific elevated count of immature white blood cells when other white blood cell counts are normal.

SP **D72.828 Other elevated white blood cell count**

SP **D72.829 Elevated white blood cell count, unspecified**
Elevated leukocytes, unspecified
Leukocytosis, unspecified

SP **D72.89 Other specified disorders of white blood cells**
Abnormality of white blood cells NEC

SP **D72.9 Disorder of white blood cells, unspecified**
Abnormal leukocyte differential NOS

4 **D73 Diseases of spleen**

SP **D73.0 Hyposplenism**
Atrophy of spleen
EXCLUDES 1 asplenia (congenital) (Q89.01)
postsurgical absence of spleen (Z90.81)

SP **D73.1 Hypersplenism**
EXCLUDES 1 neutropenic splenomegaly (D73.81)
primary splenic neutropenia (D73.81)
splenitis, splenomegaly in late syphilis (A52.79)
splenitis, splenomegaly in tuberculosis (A18.85)
splenomegaly NOS (R16.1)
splenomegaly congenital (Q89.0)

SP **D73.2 Chronic congestive splenomegaly**

SP **D73.3 Abscess of spleen**

SP **D73.4 Cyst of spleen**

SP **D73.5 Infarction of spleen**
Splenic rupture, nontraumatic
Torsion of spleen

EXCLUDES 1 rupture of spleen due to Plasmodium vivax malaria (B51.0)
traumatic rupture of spleen (S36.03-)

5 **D73.8 Other diseases of spleen**

SP **D73.81 Neutropenic splenomegaly**
Werner-Schultz disease

SP **D73.89 Other diseases of spleen**
Fibrosis of spleen NOS
Perisplenitis
Splenitis NOS

!Q **D73.9 Disease of spleen, unspecified**

4 **D74 Methemoglobinemia**

SP **D74.0 Congenital methemoglobinemia**
Congenital NADH-methemoglobin reductase deficiency
Hemoglobin-M [Hb-M] disease
Methemoglobinemia, hereditary

SP **D74.8 Other methemoglobinemias**
Acquired methemoglobinemia (with sulfhemoglobinemia)
Toxic methemoglobinemia

SP **D74.9 Methemoglobinemia, unspecified**

DEFINITION Presence of a higher than normal level of methemoglobin, a form of hemoglobin that does not bind oxygen, in the blood. When its concentration is elevated in red blood cells, anemia and hypoxia may occur.

4 **D75 Other and unspecified diseases of blood and blood-forming organs**

EXCLUDES 2 acute lymphadenitis (L04.-)
chronic lymphadenitis (I88.1)
enlarged lymph nodes (R59.-)
hypergammaglobulinemia NOS (D89.2)
lymphadenitis NOS (I88.9)
mesenteric lymphadenitis (acute) (chronic) (I88.0)

SP **D75.0 Familial erythrocytosis**
Benign polycythemia
Familial polycythemia
EXCLUDES 1 hereditary ovalocytosis (D58.1)

SP **D75.1 Secondary polycythemia**
Acquired polycythemia
Emotional polycythemia
Erythrocytosis NOS
Hypoxemic polycythemia
Nephrogenous polycythemia
Polycythemia due to erythropoietin
Polycythemia due to fall in plasma volume
Polycythemia due to high altitude
Polycythemia due to stress
Polycythemia NOS
Relative polycythemia
EXCLUDES 1 polycythemia neonatorum (P61.1)
polycythemia vera (D45)

5 **D75.8 Other specified diseases of blood and blood-forming organs**

!Q + **D75.81 Myelofibrosis**
Myelofibrosis NOS
Secondary myelofibrosis NOS
Code first the underlying disorder, such as:
malignant neoplasm of breast (C50.-)
Use additional code, if applicable, for associated therapy-related myelodysplastic syndrome (D46.-)
Use additional code for adverse effect, if applicable, to identify drug (T45.1X5)
EXCLUDES 1 acute myelofibrosis (C94.4-)
idiopathic myelofibrosis (D47.1)
leukoerythroblastic anemia (D61.82)
myelofibrosis with myeloid metaplasia (D47.4)
myelophthisic anemia (D61.82)
myelophthisis (D61.82)
primary myelofibrosis (D47.1)

SP **D75.82 Heparin induced thrombocytopenia (HIT)**

★ 6 **D75.83 Thrombocytosis**
EXCLUDES 2 essential thrombocythemia (D47.3)

★ **D75.838 Other thrombocytosis**
Reactive thrombocytosis
Secondary thrombocytosis
Code also:
underlying condition, if known and applicable

★ **D75.839 Thrombocytosis, unspecified**
Thrombocythemia NOS
Thrombocytosis NOS

SP **D75.89 Other specified diseases of blood and blood-forming organs**

!Q **D75.9 Disease of blood and blood-forming organs, unspecified**

SP **D75.A Glucose-6-phosphate dehydrogenase (G6PD) deficiency without anemia**
EXCLUDES 1 glucose-6-phosphate dehydrogenase (G6PD) deficiency with anemia (D55.0)

4 **D76 Other specified diseases with participation of lymphoreticular and reticulohistiocytic tissue**
EXCLUDES 1 (Abt-) Letterer-Siwe disease (C96.0)
eosinophilic granuloma (C96.6)
Hand-Schüller-Christian disease (C96.5)
histiocytic medullary reticulosis (C96.9)
histiocytic sarcoma (C96.A)
histiocytosis X, multifocal (C96.5)
histiocytosis X, unifocal (C96.6)
Langerhans-cell histiocytosis, multifocal (C96.5)
Langerhans-cell histiocytosis NOS (C96.6)

Langerhans-cell histiocytosis, unifocal (C96.6)
leukemic reticuloendotheliosis (C91.4-)
lipomelanotic reticulosis (I89.8)
malignant histiocytosis (C96.A)
malignant reticulosis (C86.0)
nonlipid reticuloendotheliosis (C96.0)

SP **D76.1 Hemophagocytic lymphohistiocytosis**
Familial hemophagocytic reticulosis
Histiocytoses of mononuclear phagocytes

SP + **D76.2 Hemophagocytic syndrome, infection-associated**
Use additional code to identify infectious agent or disease.

SP **D76.3 Other histiocytosis syndromes**
Reticulohistiocytoma (giant-cell)
Sinus histiocytosis with massive lymphadenopathy
Xanthogranuloma

M IQ **D77** ***Other disorders of blood and blood-forming organs in diseases classified elsewhere***
Code first underlying disease, such as:
amyloidosis (E85.-)
congenital early syphilis (A50.0)
echinococcosis (B67.0-B67.9)
malaria (B50.0-B54)
schistosomiasis [bilharziasis] (B65.0-B65.9)
vitamin C deficiency (E54)
EXCLUDES 1 rupture of spleen due to Plasmodium vivax malaria (B51.0)
splenitis, splenomegaly in late syphilis (A52.79)
splenitis, splenomegaly in tuberculosis (A18.85)

Intraoperative and postprocedural complications of the spleen (D78)

CODING TIPS ✓ Conditions classifiable to D78- are classifiable as intraoperative and postprocedural complications. These conditions should only be assigned when diagnostic statements clearly indicate that the condition is a complication of a procedure.

4 **D78 Intraoperative and postprocedural complications of the spleen**

5 **D78.0 Intraoperative hemorrhage and hematoma of the spleen complicating a procedure**
EXCLUDES 1 intraoperative hemorrhage and hematoma of the spleen due to accidental puncture or laceration during a procedure (D78.1-)

SP **D78.01 Intraoperative hemorrhage and hematoma of the spleen complicating a procedure on the spleen**

SP **D78.02 Intraoperative hemorrhage and hematoma of the spleen complicating other procedure**

5 **D78.1 Accidental puncture and laceration of the spleen during a procedure**

SP **D78.11 Accidental puncture and laceration of the spleen during a procedure on the spleen**

SP **D78.12 Accidental puncture and laceration of the spleen during other procedure**

5 **D78.2 Postprocedural hemorrhage of the spleen following a procedure**

SP **D78.21 Postprocedural hemorrhage of the spleen following a procedure on the spleen**

SP **D78.22 Postprocedural hemorrhage of the spleen following other procedure**

5 **D78.3 Postprocedural hematoma and seroma of the spleen following a procedure**

SP **D78.31 Postprocedural hematoma of the spleen following a procedure on the spleen**

SP **D78.32 Postprocedural hematoma of the spleen following other procedure**

SP **D78.33 Postprocedural seroma of the spleen following a procedure on the spleen**

SP **D78.34 Postprocedural seroma of the spleen following other procedure**

+ 5 **D78.8 Other intraoperative and postprocedural complications of the spleen**
Use additional code, if applicable, to further specify disorder

SP + **D78.81 Other intraoperative complications of the spleen**

SP + **D78.89 Other postprocedural complications of the spleen**

Certain disorders involving the immune mechanism (D80-D89)

INCLUDES defects in the complement system
immunodeficiency disorders, except human immunodeficiency virus [HIV] disease
sarcoidosis

EXCLUDES 1 autoimmune disease (systemic) NOS (M35.9)
functional disorders of polymorphonuclear neutrophils (D71)
human immunodeficiency virus [HIV] disease (B20)

4 **D80 Immunodeficiency with predominantly antibody defects**

SP **D80.0 Hereditary hypogammaglobulinemia**
Autosomal recessive agammaglobulinemia (Swiss type)
X-linked agammaglobulinemia [Bruton] (with growth hormone deficiency)

SP **D80.1 Nonfamilial hypogammaglobulinemia**
Agammaglobulinemia with immunoglobulin-bearing B-lymphocytes
Common variable agammaglobulinemia [CVAgamma]
Hypogammaglobulinemia NOS
DEFINITION Loss of the body's ability to respond to infection because of a lack of immunoglobulins (antibodies) in the blood.

SP **D80.2 Selective deficiency of immunoglobulin A [IgA]**

SP **D80.3 Selective deficiency of immunoglobulin G [IgG] subclasses**

SP **D80.4 Selective deficiency of immunoglobulin M [IgM]**

Chapter 3 D50-D89

SP **D80.5 Immunodeficiency with increased immunoglobulin M [IgM]**

SP **D80.6 Antibody deficiency with near-normal immunoglobulins or with hyperimmunoglobulinemia**

SP **D80.7 Transient hypogammaglobulinemia of infancy**

SP **D80.8 Other immunodeficiencies with predominantly antibody defects**
Kappa light chain deficiency

SP **D80.9 Immunodeficiency with predominantly antibody defects, unspecified**

4 **D81 Combined immunodeficiencies**
EXCLUDES 1 autosomal recessive agammaglobulinemia (Swiss type) (D80.0)

SP **D81.0 Severe combined immunodeficiency [SCID] with reticular dysgenesis**

SP **D81.1 Severe combined immunodeficiency [SCID] with low T- and B-cell numbers**

SP **D81.2 Severe combined immunodeficiency [SCID] with low or normal B-cell numbers**

5 **D81.3 Adenosine deaminase [ADA] deficiency**

SP **D81.30 Adenosine deaminase deficiency, unspecified**
ADA deficiency NOS

SP **D81.31 Severe combined immunodeficiency due to adenosine deaminase deficiency**
ADA deficiency with SCID
Adenosine deaminase [ADA] deficiency with severe combined immunodeficiency
DEFINITION Deficiency of Adenosine Deaminase 1 (DADA1) can result in a severe immunodeficiency while any immunodeficiency in deficiency of adenosine deaminase 2 (DADA2) is mild, if present. DADA1 results from a defect of a gene on chromosome 20, whereas DADA2 results from a gene defect on chromosome 22.

SP **D81.32 Adenosine deaminase 2 deficiency**
ADA2 deficiency
Adenosine deaminase deficiency type 2
Code also, if applicable, any associated manifestations, such as:
polyarteritis nodosa (M30.0)
stroke (I63.-)
DEFINITION Deficiency of Adenosine Deaminase 2 (DADA2), or adenosine deaminase 2 deficiency, is characterized by abnormal inflammation of various tissues, which may be associated with a mottled rash (livedo racemosa), early-onset strokes, other findings of vasculitis (consistent with polyarteritis nodosa), and sometimes immunodeficiency. It is autoinflammatory in nature, and besides the skin and nervous system, may affect the gastrointestinal system or kidneys, and may cause intermittent fevers. It may be associated with hepatosplenomegaly. Onset may be from early childhood to adulthood.

SP **D81.39 Other adenosine deaminase deficiency**
Adenosine deaminase [ADA] deficiency type 1, NOS
Adenosine deaminase [ADA] deficiency type 1, without SCID
Adenosine deaminase [ADA] deficiency type 1, without severe combined immunodeficiency
Partial ADA deficiency (type 1)
Partial adenosine deaminase deficiency (type 1)

SP **D81.4 Nezelof's syndrome**

SP **D81.5 Purine nucleoside phosphorylase [PNP] deficiency**

SP **D81.6 Major histocompatibility complex class I deficiency**
Bare lymphocyte syndrome

SP **D81.7 Major histocompatibility complex class II deficiency**

5 **D81.8 Other combined immunodeficiencies**

6 **D81.81 Biotin-dependent carboxylase deficiency**
Multiple carboxylase deficiency
EXCLUDES 1 biotin-dependent carboxylase deficiency due to dietary deficiency of biotin (E53.8)

SP **D81.810 Biotinidase deficiency**

SP **D81.818 Other biotin-dependent carboxylase deficiency**
Holocarboxylase synthetase deficiency
Other multiple carboxylase deficiency

SP **D81.819 Biotin-dependent carboxylase deficiency, unspecified**
Multiple carboxylase deficiency, unspecified

SP **D81.89 Other combined immunodeficiencies**

SP **D81.9 Combined immunodeficiency, unspecified**
Severe combined immunodeficiency disorder [SCID] NOS

4 **D82 Immunodeficiency associated with other major defects**
EXCLUDES 1 ataxia telangiectasia [Louis-Bar] (G11.3)

SP **D82.0 Wiskott-Aldrich syndrome**
Immunodeficiency with thrombocytopenia and eczema
DEFINITION X-linked immunodeficiency syndrome presenting with eczema, thrombocytopenia, and recurrent pyogenic infection.

SP **D82.1 Di George's syndrome**
Pharyngeal pouch syndrome
Thymic alymphoplasia
Thymic aplasia or hypoplasia with immunodeficiency
DEFINITION Congenital disorder with hypoplasia or aplasia of the thymus and parathyroid glands; associated with congenital heart defects, great vessel anomalies, esophageal atresia, and abnormal facial structure.

SP **D82.2 Immunodeficiency with short-limbed stature**

SP **D82.3 Immunodeficiency following hereditary defective response to Epstein-Barr virus**
X-linked lymphoproliferative disease

SP **D82.4 Hyperimmunoglobulin E [IgE] syndrome**
CODING TIPS✓ Patients with hyperimmunoglobulin E [IgE] syndrome have a lifelong condition characterized by elevated IgE levels, which may also be referred to as "Job syndrome." These patients are highly prone to problematic skin conditions such as eczema, skin lesions and infections (abscesses), sinus infections, and other respiratory infections, which should be additionally coded when present.

SP **D82.8 Immunodeficiency associated with other specified major defects**

SP **D82.9 Immunodeficiency associated with major defect, unspecified**

4 **D83 Common variable immunodeficiency**

SP **D83.0 Common variable immunodeficiency with predominant abnormalities of B-cell numbers and function**

SP **D83.1 Common variable immunodeficiency with predominant immunoregulatory T-cell disorders**

SP **D83.2 Common variable immunodeficiency with autoantibodies to B- or T-cells**

SP **D83.8 Other common variable immunodeficiencies**

SP **D83.9 Common variable immunodeficiency, unspecified**

4 **D84 Other immunodeficiencies**

SP **D84.0 Lymphocyte function antigen-1 [LFA-1] defect**

SP **D84.1 Defects in the complement system**
C1 esterase inhibitor [C1-INH] deficiency

5 **D84.8 Other specified immunodeficiencies**

M IQ **D84.81 *Immunodeficiency due to conditions classified elsewhere***
Code first underlying condition, such as:
chromosomal abnormalities (Q90-Q99)
diabetes mellitus (E08-E13)
malignant neoplasms (C00-C96)
EXCLUDES 1 certain disorders involving the immune mechanism (D80-D83, D84.0, D84.1, D84.9)
human immunodeficiency virus [HIV] disease (B20)

6 **D84.82 Immunodeficiency due to drugs and external causes**
CODING TIPS✓ Multiple codes may be assigned to show immunodeficiency due to multiple causes (e.g., cancer and antineoplastic medication). [AHA: 4Q 2020]

SP + **D84.821 Immunodeficiency due to drugs**
Immunodeficiency due to (current or past) medication
Use additional code for adverse effect if applicable, to identify adverse effect of drug (T36-T50 with fifth or six character 5)
Use additional code, if applicable, for associated long term (current) drug therapy drug or medication such as:
long term (current) drug therapy systemic steroids (Z79.52)
other long term (current) drug therapy (Z79.899)
CODING TIPS✓ An adverse effect code is not assigned when the medication has achieved its intended result in lowering the patient's immune response. If the reduced immune response is not an intended result of the drug, i.e. chemotherapy, then the adverse effect code for the drug is added.

SP + **D84.822 Immunodeficiency due to external causes**
Code also:
, if applicable, radiological procedure and radiotherapy (Y84.2)
Use additional code for external cause such as:
exposure to ionizing radiation (W88)

SP **D84.89 Other immunodeficiencies**

SP **D84.9 Immunodeficiency, unspecified**
Immunocompromised NOS
Immunodeficient NOS
Immunosuppressed NOS

4 **D86 Sarcoidosis**

SP **D86.0 Sarcoidosis of lung**

SP **D86.1 Sarcoidosis of lymph nodes**

SP **D86.2 Sarcoidosis of lung with sarcoidosis of lymph nodes**

SP **D86.3 Sarcoidosis of skin**

5 **D86.8 Sarcoidosis of other sites**

SP **D86.81 Sarcoid meningitis**

SP **D86.82 Multiple cranial nerve palsies in sarcoidosis**

SP **D86.83 Sarcoid iridocyclitis**

SP **D86.84 Sarcoid pyelonephritis**
Tubulo-interstitial nephropathy in sarcoidosis

SP **D86.85 Sarcoid myocarditis**

SP **D86.86 Sarcoid arthropathy**
Polyarthritis in sarcoidosis

SP **D86.87 Sarcoid myositis**

SP **D86.89 Sarcoidosis of other sites**
Hepatic granuloma
Uveoparotid fever [Heerfordt]

SP **D86.9 Sarcoidosis, unspecified**

4 **D89 Other disorders involving the immune mechanism, not elsewhere classified**
EXCLUDES 1 hyperglobulinemia NOS (R77.1)

monoclonal gammopathy (of undetermined significance) (D47.2)

EXCLUDES 2 transplant failure and rejection (T86.-)

SP **D89.0 Polyclonal hypergammaglobulinemia**
Benign hypergammaglobulinemic purpura
Polyclonal gammopathy NOS

SP **D89.1 Cryoglobulinemia**
Cryoglobulinemic purpura
Cryoglobulinemic vasculitis
Essential cryoglobulinemia
Idiopathic cryoglobulinemia
Mixed cryoglobulinemia
Primary cryoglobulinemia
Secondary cryoglobulinemia

SP **D89.2 Hypergammaglobulinemia, unspecified**

SP + **D89.3 Immune reconstitution syndrome**
Immune reconstitution inflammatory syndrome [IRIS]
Use additional code for adverse effect, if applicable, to identify drug (T36-T50 with fifth or sixth character 5)

5 **D89.4 Mast cell activation syndrome and related disorders**

EXCLUDES 1 aggressive systemic mastocytosis (C96.21)
congenital cutaneous mastocytosis (Q82.2)
(non-congenital) cutaneous mastocytosis (D47.01)
(indolent) systemic mastocytosis (D47.02)
malignant mast cell neoplasm (C96.2-)
malignant mastocytoma (C96.29)
mast cell leukemia (C94.3-)
mast cell sarcoma (C96.22)
mastocytoma NOS (D47.09)
other mast cell neoplasms of uncertain behavior (D47.09)
systemic mastocytosis associated with a clonal hematologic non-mast cell lineage disease (SM-AHNMD) (D47.02)

SP **D89.40 Mast cell activation, unspecified**
Mast cell activation disorder, unspecified
Mast cell activation syndrome, NOS

SP **D89.41 Monoclonal mast cell activation syndrome**

SP **D89.42 Idiopathic mast cell activation syndrome**

SP **D89.43 Secondary mast cell activation**
Secondary mast cell activation syndrome
Code also:
underlying etiology, if known

★ + **D89.44 Hereditary alpha tryptasemia**
Use additional code, if applicable, for:
allergy status, other than to drugs and biological substances (Z91.0-)
personal history of anaphylaxis (Z87.892)

SP **D89.49 Other mast cell activation disorder**
Other mast cell activation syndrome

5 **D89.8 Other specified disorders involving the immune mechanism, not elsewhere classified**

+ 6 **D89.81 Graft-versus-host disease**
Code first underlying cause, such as:
complications of transplanted organs and tissue (T86.-)
complications of blood transfusion (T80.89)
Use additional code to identify associated manifestations, such as:
desquamative dermatitis (L30.8)
diarrhea (R19.7)
elevated bilirubin (R17)
hair loss (L65.9)

CODING TIPS✓ Code D89.81 may only be assigned when the provider specifically indicates this condition. Development of complicating disease, such as ESRD or neoplasm in a transplanted organ, should not be assumed to indicate graft versus host disease.

IQ + **D89.810 Acute graft-versus-host disease**

IQ + **D89.811 Chronic graft-versus-host disease**

IQ + **D89.812 Acute on chronic graft-versus-host disease**

IQ + **D89.813 Graft-versus-host disease, unspecified**

SP **D89.82 Autoimmune lymphoproliferative syndrome [ALPS]**

+ 6 **D89.83 Cytokine release syndrome**
Code first underlying cause, such as:
complications following infusion, transfusion and therapeutic injection (T80.89-)
complications of transplanted organs and tissue (T86.-)
Use additional code to identify associated manifestations

DEFINITION Commonly referred to as an infusion reaction, cytokine releast syndrome (CRS) results from the release of cytokines from cells targeted by the antibody as well as immune effector cells. Typical complications of CAR-T therapy, used to treat certain blood cancers, include CRS and/or neurotoxicity, which usually occur in the first few weeks after receiving the cell infusion (when patient is still in hospital). Sometimes, however, such complications occur post-discharge and can be the reason for additional medical encounters (i.e. visit to a physician or ED).

IQ + **D89.831 Cytokine release syndrome, grade 1**

IQ + **D89.832 Cytokine release syndrome, grade 2**

IQ + **D89.833 Cytokine release syndrome, grade 3**

IQ + **D89.834 Cytokine release syndrome, grade 4**

IQ + **D89.835 Cytokine release syndrome, grade 5**

Chapter 3

D50-D89

IQ + **D89.839 Cytokine release syndrome, grade unspecified**

SP **D89.89 Other specified disorders involving the immune mechanism, not elsewhere classified**

EXCLUDES 1 human immunodeficiency virus disease (B20)

SP **D89.9 Disorder involving the immune mechanism, unspecified**

Immune disease NOS

Chapter 3 Scenarios: Diseases of the blood and blood-forming organs and certain disorders involving the immune mechanism (D50-D89)

Hematochezia due to anticoagulant use

A 67-year-old woman takes anticoagulants prophylactically to treat a chronic deep vein thrombosis (DVT) in the soleal vein of her left calf. Recently she began to pass fresh, red blood in her stools. After being evaluated by her physician, it was determined that the bleeding is related to her use of anticoagulants. The patient's anticoagulant dosage has been adjusted but she continues to take the medication. Management of the DVT is the focus of care.

Description	Code
Primary: Chronic embolism and thrombosis of left calf muscular vein	I82.562
Secondary: Melena	K92.1
Secondary: Hemorrhagic disorder due to extrinsic circulating anticoagulants	D68.32
Secondary: Adverse effect of anticoagulants, subsequent encounter	T45.515D

The patient is experiencing bleeding due to her use of anticoagulants, which requires the use of D68.32, according to Q1 2016 Coding Clinic guidance. The condition (bleeding) caused by the drug is coded before the adverse effect code capturing the role of the anticoagulant in causing the bleeding, in accordance with coding guidelines. The chronic DVT is assigned in the primary position as the focus of care. Be sure that the location of the DVT is specified as non-specific codes are unacceptable primary diagnoses in PDGM. Because the location is specified as the soleal vein of her left calf, I82.562 is coded.

Anemia due to throat cancer

A 72-year-old male patient is admitted to home health with anemia secondary to a primary malignant neoplasm of his throat. He has a history of tobacco dependence. The anemia will be the focus of care. He also has a small stage 2 ulcer on his coccyx that is healing and the caregiver is performing dressing changes. Home health will assess the area for complications as it continues to heal and provide supplies.

Description	Code
Primary: Malignant neoplasm of pharynx, unspecified	C14.0
Secondary: Anemia in neoplastic disease	D63.0
Secondary: Pressure ulcer of sacral region, stage 2	L89.152
Secondary: Personal history of nicotine dependence	Z87.891

Even though the anemia is the focus of care, official coding guidelines stipulate that the neoplasm causing the anemia must be sequenced first. The stage 2 sacral ulcer is also coded as it impacts the patient's overall condition and prognosis and provides important comorbidity adjustment, but follows the other diagnoses, as it is stable and healing well. The patient's history of tobacco dependence is coded, in accordance with the instructional note in the Tabular List for category C14.- to use an additional code to identify the status of tobacco use or exposure, if applicable.*[I.C.2.c.1]*

Antineoplastic chemotherapy induced anemia

An 84-year-old woman was admitted to home health for management of antineoplastic chemotherapy-induced anemia resulting from treatment for primary colon cancer. A physical therapist will also be seeing this patient for strengthening due to weakness.

Description	Code
Primary: Anemia due to antineoplastic chemotherapy	D64.81
Secondary: Malignant neoplasm of colon, unspecified	C18.9
Secondary: Adverse effect of antineoplastic and immunosuppressive drugs, subsequent encounter	T45.1x5D

When the admission is for management of anemia associated with an adverse effect of chemotherapy, and the only treatment is for the anemia, the anemia code is sequenced first followed by the appropriate codes for the neoplasm (C18.9) and the adverse effect of chemotherapy (T45.1x5-), according to coding guidelines. The 7th character of "D" will be commonly used in home care, as it indicates subsequent care. The patient's weakness would be inherent to her condition and would, therefore, not require an additional code. *[I.C.2.c.2]*

Anemia and duodenal ulcer

Home health is seeing a patient for anemia. She has a newly diagnosed acute bleeding duodenal ulcer, which is stated to be the cause of her acute anemia. Her medical records also indicate a history of chronic blood loss anemia.

Description	Code
Primary: Acute posthemorrhagic anemia	D62
Secondary: Acute duodenal ulcer with hemorrhage	K26.0

Anemia is the focus of care, so it is listed as the primary diagnosis. The anemia is coded as D62 because the physician has specified the duodenal ulcer and acute blood loss as the cause of the acute anemia, in addition to the patient's diagnosis of chronic blood loss anemia. According to Q3 2019 Coding Clinic guidance, when acute and chronic blood loss anemia are both present, assign only a code for acute blood loss anemia. A combination code is assigned for the duodenal ulcer which indicates the nature of the ulcer (acute), the site of the ulceration (duodenal), and the bleeding.

Anemia due to chronic gastric ulcer

Your patient has anemia due to blood loss from a chronic gastric ulcer. The focus of care is the medical management of the ulcer.

Description	Code
Primary: Chronic gastric ulcer with hemorrhage	K25.4
Secondary: Iron deficiency anemia secondary to blood loss, chronic	D50.0

Any blood loss specified as due to an ulcer is classified as a hemorrhage even though the blood loss may be slow over time as is frequently seen with chronic gastric ulcers. As the focus of care, the ulcer is coded first and the anemia follows it. Anemia due to blood loss is classified as iron deficiency anemia, according to the alphabetic index. Unless the blood loss is specified as acute, it should be coded as chronic based upon the alphabetic index classification of the term since "chronic" is a non-essential modifier to the sub-term "blood loss" under anemia.

Chronic graft vs. host disease

A 65-year-old man is admitted to home health with chronic graft versus host disease that is a complication of a stem cell transplant performed a year ago to treat multiple myeloma. The transplant put his multiple myeloma into remission but he continues to experience diarrhea and desquamative dermatitis, which his doctor diagnosed as manifestations of the chronic graft versus host disease. He'll receive skilled nursing for managing new medications, including multiple new immunosuppressive drugs, and physical therapy for muscle strengthening and stamina.

Description	Code
Primary: Complications of stem cell transplant	T86.5
Secondary: Chronic graft-versus-host disease	D89.811
Secondary: Other specified dermatitis	L30.8
Secondary: Diarrhea, unspecified	R19.7
Secondary: Multiple myeloma in remission	C90.01
Secondary: Other long term (current) drug therapy	Z79.899

Since the graft vs. host disease was documented as a complication of his stem cell transplant, T86.5 is coded first, followed by D89.911, in accordance with tabular instruction. Manifestations of chronic graft versus host disease, such as the desquamative dermatitis and diarrhea in this scenario, are assigned as additional diagnoses, in accordance with tabular instructions. His multiple myeloma is in remission but still present so it is coded with C90.01. Finally, Z79.899 is assigned to capture his use of multiple new immunosuppressive drugs.

Non-traumatic compartment syndrome, hemophilia A

A 53-year-old man is admitted to home health for aftercare following surgery for non-traumatic compartment syndrome in his bicep. Medical record documentation indicates that the patient experienced a spontaneous hemorrhage in the muscle due to hemophilia A, which led to the compartment syndrome. It's also indicated that the surgery completely resolved the non-traumatic compartment syndrome.

Description	Code
Primary: Encounter for other orthopedic aftercare	Z47.89
Secondary: Hereditary factor VIII deficiency	D66

The patient requires surgical aftercare following a procedure on the musculoskeletal system. Since there's no specific code for that nor is there a specific code for surgery to treat non-traumatic compartment syndrome, the best code choice is Z47.89. Hemophilia A will impact his recovery from surgery and requires close monitoring by the nurse. This condition is also known as hereditary factor VIII hemophilia. Note as well that Hemophilia A is listed as a clarifying term at D66. Non-traumatic compartment syndrome is not coded because it is completely resolved.

DVTs, Factor V Leiden mutation

A 47-year-old woman was hospitalized for treatment of acute DVTs in the peroneal veins of both her calves. Blood tests in the hospital revealed a Factor V Leiden mutation, which her physician documented is responsible for her DVTs. The focus of the home health admission are the DVTs. She is now on long-term anticoagulant medication and the nurse will be regularly checking PT/INRs.

Description	Code
Primary: Acute embolism and thrombosis of peroneal vein, bilateral	I82.453
Secondary: Activated protein C resistance	D68.51
Secondary: Encounter for therapeutic drug level monitoring	Z51.81
Secondary: Long term (current) use of anticoagulants	Z79.01

As the focus of care, the DVTs are coded in the primary position. Note, in PDGM, if you assign the code for DVTs of ***unspecified*** distal lower extremity, the claim would be sent back to be recoded. Because the DVTs are specified as affecting the peroneal veins in her calves, I82.452 is appropriately assigned. Her newly diagnosed Factor V Leiden mutation is assigned as the cause of the DVTs, as it is an important condition that will require teaching and monitoring. "Factor V Leiden mutation" is an inclusion term at D68.51. She will be taking long-term anticoagulation therapy and requires blood-level monitoring, thus requiring the assignment of Z51.81 and Z79.01.

Immunodeficiency due to drugs

A 65-year-old male patient with rheumatoid arthritis who has been taking Humira developed cellulitis to his right lower leg. He is sent home from observation with home health for "IV antibiotic therapy due to his high-risk secondary to immunodeficiency due to his current Humira use". Skilled nursing will teach the patient and caregiver administration of the medication/IV and they will administer and provide care for the cellulitis as well as obtain routine lab work.

Description	Code
Primary: Cellulitis of right lower limb	L03.115
Secondary: Immunodeficiency due to drugs	D84.821
Secondary: Other long term (current) drug therapy	Z79.899
Secondary: Rheumatoid arthritis, unspecified	M06.9
Secondary: Encounter for adjustment and management of vascular access device	Z45.2
Secondary: Long term (current) use of antibiotics	Z79.2

The focus of care for this episode will be the care and treatment of this patient's cellulitis, including the treatment of the area infected and teaching/oversight of IV antibiotic administration. The cellulitis is the primary diagnosis for this reason. The patient also has a specific immunodeficiency resulting from his current use of medication to treat RA, so D84.821 is assigned. A "use additional code" note at D84.821 directs the coder to assign an additional code for the drug causing the immunodeficiency, which may either be an adverse effect or long-term use code. Guidance from Q4 2020 Coding Clinic indicates that an adverse effect code is not assigned when the medication has achieved its intended result in lowering the patient's immune response, so Z79.899 is assigned to identify the Humira use. Additional codes to identify rheumatoid arthritis, vascular device (identifying the teaching and care of the IV line) and use of antibiotic medication are also assigned.

Chapter 4: Endocrine, Nutritional and Metabolic Diseases (E00 – E89)

Chapter 4 addresses a variety of conditions, including endocrine, nutritional and metabolic diseases. Home care clinicians will find themselves flipping to these pages often as this chapter contains the codes for diabetes – a common home care diagnosis. Also, codes in Chapter 4 may be used to identify functional activity associated with any neoplasm code from Chapter 2, or by ectopic endocrine tissue. ***Note:*** This chapter excludes transitory endocrine and metabolic disorders specific to newborn (codes P70-P74).

Chapter 4 includes codes for a number of different conditions, including:

- Conditions related to the endocrine glands (thyroid, E00-E07); other disorders of glucose regulation and pancreatic internal secretion (E15-E16); disorders of parathyroid, pituitary, hypothalamus, adrenal glands, ovaries, testes, polyglandular disorders; and other endocrine disorders (E20-E35).
- The largest code group for home health is combination codes related to five categories of diabetes codes. These codes include the type of diabetes mellitus, the body system affected and the complications affecting that body system. These categories include:
  - E08, Diabetes mellitus due to underlying conditions
  - E09, Drug or chemically induced diabetes mellitus
  - E10, Type 1 diabetes mellitus
  - E11, Type 2 diabetes mellitus
  - E13, Other specified diabetes mellitus
- Intraoperative complications of endocrine system (E36)
- Conditions related to nutrition, such as malnutrition (E40-E46); other nutritional deficiencies (E50-E64); and overweight, obesity, and other hyperalimentation (E65-E68).
- Metabolic disorders (E70-E88); Conditions related to metabolism as well as cystic fibrosis, volume depletion, dehydration and fluid overload, and hyperkalemia & hypokalemia.
- Post-procedural endocrine and metabolic complications and disorders, not elsewhere classified (E89).

Sometimes a Chapter 4 code isn't the most appropriate choice. See below a few situations to watch out for:

- If the **documentation indicates a neoplasm or tumor of an endocrine organ,** the term (malignancy, tumor, adenoma) that is used in the medical record should be looked up; it is most likely a code from Chapter 2. When a neoplasm affects an endocrine gland, the hormone levels may be unusually high or low and those conditions are used as additional codes to the neoplasm condition. In these situations, an additional code from Chapter 4 may be used to identify any functional activity associated with the neoplasm code from Chapter 2. The neoplasm is coded first and the functional activity is coded as a secondary code.

  Examples are E05.80 (other thyrotoxicosis without crisis) and E31.2 (multiple endocrine neoplasia syndromes)
- If a patient has a **personal or family history** of a condition reported in this chapter, it may be appropriate to select a code from the Z code section, such as Z86.3- (personal history of endocrine, nutritional and metabolic diseases) or Z83.3 (family history of diabetes mellitus). Remember that personal history is far more important than family history in home health coding.
- When reporting endocrine, nutritional and metabolic diseases in a **pregnant patient,** and the condition is complicating the pregnancy, report first a code from Chapter 15, such as O24.41- (diabetes mellitus in pregnancy) or O24.81- (other pre-existing diabetes mellitus in pregnancy). Pay attention to notes to use an additional code from category E11 to further identify any manifestations. Also assign Z79.4 (long-term (current) use of insulin) or Z79.84 (long-term (current) use of oral hypoglycemic drugs) if the diabetes mellitus is being treated with insulin or oral medications. If the patient is treated with both oral medications and insulin, only assign the code for insulin controlled (Z79.4).

Multiple Coding and Sequencing

In this chapter, you will see many instructions to code first and use additional codes as well as instructions to use codes from other chapters. There are many examples of combination codes related to the etiology/manifestations for diabetes. However, there are also "code first" notes related to poisoning due to drugs or toxins and "add an additional code" notes for multiple coding and sequencing issues for codes in this chapter.

If the note to use an additional code references an adverse effect of a drug, refer to the Table of Drugs and Chemicals, as well as codes T36-T50 in Chapter 19 with a 5th or 6th character of '5' to identify the associated drug.

Important: The subterm "with" or "in" within the Index should be interpreted as a link between diabetes and any of those conditions indented under the word "with" or "in", according to coding conventions.

The classification presumes a causal relationship between the two conditions linked by these terms in the Alphabetic Index or Tabular List. These conditions should be coded as related even in the absence of provider documentation explicitly linking them, unless the documentation clearly states the conditions are unrelated or when another guideline exists that specifically requires a documented linkage between two conditions.

Warning: This convention does not apply to 'not elsewhere classified (NEC)' index entries that cover broad categories of conditions. Rather, you must see specific conditions linked by the terms 'with,' 'due to' or 'associated with' in order to assume a connection based on 'with.' Similarly, coronary artery disease cannot be automatically connected to diabetes and coded with E11.59; dementia cannot be automatically connected to diabetes and coded with E11.49; and blindness cannot be automatically connected to diabetes and coded with E11.39; unless explicitly stated as linked by the physician, according to Q4 2017 Coding Clinic guidance.

Special Coding Issues

Diabetes

The most commonly-used and misused diagnosis codes in this chapter are for **diabetes mellitus.**

Again, it's important to note diabetes mellitus codes are combination codes that include the type of diabetes mellitus, the body system affected, and the complications affecting that body system.

Codes E10- and E11- define the condition as Type 1 or Type 2 diabetes. The 4th and 5th characters are used to indicate the complication, such as E11.29 for Type 2 diabetes mellitus with other diabetic kidney complication. Sometimes a 6th character is used to provide further detail. For example, E11.331 for Type 2 diabetes mellitus with moderate nonproliferative diabetic retinopathy with macular edema.

Usually, the term "diabetes" refers to diabetes mellitus (E11-). If the medical record states only "diabetes," assume that it is Type 2 diabetes mellitus.

Although age is not the sole determining factor, most Type 1 diabetics develop the condition before reaching puberty. For this reason Type 1 diabetes mellitus is also referred to as juvenile diabetes. Type 1 diabetic patients must take daily insulin.

If the documentation in the medical record does not indicate the type of diabetes, but does indicate that the patient uses insulin, assign code E11 (Type 2 diabetes) along with Z79.4 (Long-term (current) use of insulin). Code Z79.4 should ***not*** be assigned if insulin is given temporarily to bring a Type 2 patient's blood sugar under control.

Most Type 2 (formerly called adult onset diabetes or NIDDM) usually is diagnosed in older patients (but not always) and may or may not be treated with insulin. The terms IDDM and NIDDM are archaic and should not be used to determine the type of diabetes.

Take note of the following general rules for coding diabetes mellitus:

- Do not assume that use of terms such as "glycosuria," "glucosuria," "hyperglycemia," or "polyuria" means the patient has diabetes. These are symptoms of diabetes, but may indicate other conditions.
- If the physician documentation indicates that the diabetes is "poorly controlled," "out of control," assign the code for the diabetes mellitus by type with hyperglycemia (EXX.65 code from categories E08-E13). For example, E10.65, Type 1 diabetes mellitus with hyperglycemia; or E11.65, Type 2 diabetes mellitus with hyperglycemia; or any of the other types of diabetes). ***But note,*** diabetes simply referred to as "uncontrolled" could be either hyperglycemia or hypoglycemia. If documentation isn't clear, query the physician, per Q1 2017 Coding Clinic.
- If the physician states the patient has uncontrolled or "out of control" diabetes plus other complications (manifestations) of diabetes, code them all, including the hyperglycemia. For example, medical record documentation states "uncontrolled Type 2 diabetes with diabetic polyneuropathy." You would code E11.42 and E11.65.

- Do not assume that a young diabetic patient has Type 1.
- Do not assume a patient using insulin has Type 1.
- Do not assume that a patient described as insulin dependent has Type 1.
- If the documentation does not state the type of diabetes, the default code is Type 2. Note that 90% to 95% of patients with diabetes have Type 2.
- If the documentation states Type 1.5, and the physician does not provide more specific information confirming either Type 1 or Type 2, assign a code from E13.-.

Use of insulin, oral hypoglycemics, and injectable non-insulin drugs

If the documentation in a medical record does not indicate the type of diabetes but does indicate that the patient uses insulin, code E11-, Type 2 diabetes mellitus, should be assigned. An additional code should be assigned from category Z79 to identify the long-term (current) use of insulin or oral hypoglycemic drugs. If the patient is treated with both oral medications and insulin, only assign the code for insulin controlled (Z79.4).

If the patient is treated with both insulin and an injectable non-insulin antidiabetic drug, assign codes Z79.4, Long-term (current) use of insulin, and Z79.899, Other long term (current) drug therapy. If the patient is treated with both oral hypoglycemic drugs and an injectable non-insulin antidiabetic drug, assign codes Z79.84, Long-term (current) use of oral hypoglycemic drugs, and Z79.899, Other long-term (current) drug therapy. Code Z79.4 should not be assigned if insulin is given temporarily to bring a type 2 patient's blood sugar under control during an encounter.

Complications due to insulin pump malfunction

Underdose of insulin due to insulin pump failure should be assigned with a specific code from subcategory T85.6 (Mechanical complication of other specified internal and external prosthetic devices, implants and grafts), as the principal or first-listed code. It should be followed by code T38.3x6- (Underdosing of insulin and oral hypoglycemic [antidiabetic] drugs). Additional codes for the type of diabetes mellitus and any associated complications due to the underdosing should also be assigned.

Overdose of insulin due to insulin pump failure: The principal or first-listed code for an encounter due to an insulin pump malfunction resulting in an overdose of insulin should also be T85.6-(Mechanical complication of other specified internal and external prosthetic devices, implants and grafts), followed by code T38.3x1- (Poisoning by insulin and oral hypoglycemic [antidiabetic] drugs, accidental (unintentional).

Include as many codes within a particular category as are necessary to describe all of the complications of the diabetes. They should be sequenced based on the reason for a particular encounter. Assign as many codes from Categories E08 – E13 as needed to identify all of the associated conditions that the patient has.

- For example, for a patient who has Type 2 diabetes mellitus **and** diabetic peripheral angiopathy **and** diabetic gastroparesis, report codes E11.5- (Diabetes with diabetic angiopathy) and E11.43 (Diabetes with diabetic gastroparesis).
- If multiple manifestations apply to a specific body system, then sequence them accordingly. For example, for a patient who has diabetic peripheral angiopathy and gangrene, you would assign E11.52.
- Code Z79.4 (long-term [current] use of insulin) also is reported as an additional diagnosis for patients who have Type 2 diabetes, secondary diabetes, or an unspecified type of diabetes who routinely use insulin. However, code Z79.4 is not reported for patients with Type 1 diabetes. Code Z79.84 (oral antidiabetic/hypoglycemic drugs) is also available to report as an additional diagnosis when applicable.

Secondary diabetes mellitus

Codes under categories E08 (Diabetes mellitus due to underlying condition), E09 (Drug or chemical induced diabetes mellitus) and E13 (Other specified diabetes mellitus) all identify secondary diabetes.

Secondary diabetes is always caused by another condition or event (e.g., cystic fibrosis, malignant neoplasm of the pancreas, pancreatectomy, adverse effect of drug or poisoning). Like primary diabetes mellitus, there are combination codes to identify any complications/manifestations due to secondary diabetes.

Assigning and sequencing secondary diabetes codes and its causes

The sequencing of the secondary diabetes codes in relationship to codes for the cause of the diabetes is based on the Tabular instructions for E08, E09 and E13.

Secondary diabetes due to drugs

Secondary diabetes may be caused by an adverse effect of correctly administered medications, poisoning or sequela of a poisoning.

Secondary diabetes due to pancreatectomy

For post pancreatectomy diabetes mellitus (lack of insulin due to the surgical removal of all or part of the pancreas), assign code E89.1 (Postprocedural hypoinsulinemia), then assign a code from category E13, followed by a code from subcategory Z90.41- (Acquired absence of pancreas).

Coding Diabetes after a Pancreas Transplant

After the transplant, diabetes may no longer be an issue, but lingering manifestations may be. Code as you would any patient with diabetic complications. Assign a code from E11 with the appropriate body system to identify any specific manifestations. The patient still has complications associated with the diabetes because the transplant did not resolve the manifestations of diabetes, even though it did resolve the diabetes.

The manifestations require that diabetes be coded as the etiology even if the patient no longer has diabetes. Also code Z94.83, Organ or tissue replaced by transplant, pancreas.

Diabetic Ulcers

Volume 2 (Alphabetic Index) lists diabetic ulcers as a combination code under each of the diabetes mellitus categories. For example: E08.621, Diabetes mellitus due to underlying condition with foot ulcer; and E08.622, Diabetes mellitus due to underlying condition with other skin ulcer. However there is also a notation to use an additional code to identify site of the foot ulcer (L97.4-, L95.5-), and a notation to an use additional code to identify site of the (other) skin ulcer (L97.1-L97.9, L98.41-L98.49)

Malnutrition (E40-E46)

Malnutrition codes are frequently used with hospice patients to further define their terminal status. The physician must document the actual malnutrition diagnoses but clinicians may and should show an associated Body Mass Index (BMI) code from Z68.- that illustrates the extent of the weight loss.

Overweight, Obesity (E65-E68)

Overweight or obesity is coded only if documented by the physician. Even though the coding of overweight/obesity is limited to physician documentation, the BMI is easily calculated and can be determined by a clinician involved in the care of the patient even in the absence of obesity codes. When coding obesity or overweight, the BMI code Z68.- should also be listed as an additional diagnosis.

CHAPTER 4: ENDOCRINE, NUTRITIONAL AND METABOLIC DISEASES (E00-E89)

Note:
All neoplasms, whether functionally active or not, are classified in Chapter 2. Appropriate codes in this chapter (i.e. E05.8, E07.0, E16-E31, E34.-) may be used as additional codes to indicate either functional activity by neoplasms and ectopic endocrine tissue or hyperfunction and hypofunction of endocrine glands associated with neoplasms and other conditions classified elsewhere.

EXCLUDES 1 transitory endocrine and metabolic disorders specific to newborn (P70-P74)

This chapter contains the following blocks:

E00-E07 Disorders of thyroid gland
E08-E13 Diabetes mellitus
E15-E16 Other disorders of glucose regulation and pancreatic internal secretion
E20-E35 Disorders of other endocrine glands
E36 Intraoperative complications of endocrine system
E40-E46 Malnutrition
E50-E64 Other nutritional deficiencies
E65-E68 Overweight, obesity and other hyperalimentation
E70-E88 Metabolic disorders
E89 Postprocedural endocrine and metabolic complications and disorders, not elsewhere classified

Disorders of thyroid gland (E00-E07)

+ 4 **E00 Congenital iodine-deficiency syndrome**
Use additional code (F70-F79) to identify associated intellectual disabilities.
EXCLUDES 1 subclinical iodine-deficiency hypothyroidism (E02)
CODING TIPS ✓ Do not assign a code from E00 to identify any condition that is not reported as "congenital" (present from birth).
DEFINITION Congenital iodine-deficiency syndrome is a congenital disorder often referred to as "cretinism." Congenital iodine-deficiency syndrome results from a thyroid hormone deficiency during fetal development and marked in childhood by dwarfed stature, mental retardation, dystrophy of the bones, and a low basal metabolism.

SP + **E00.0 Congenital iodine-deficiency syndrome, neurological type**
Endemic cretinism, neurological type
DEFINITION Underactive thyroid gland present at birth with inadequate hormone production and slowed metabolic processes. Untreated, it can cause brain damage, mental retardation, and developmental delays.

SP + **E00.1 Congenital iodine-deficiency syndrome, myxedematous type**
Endemic hypothyroid cretinism
Endemic cretinism, myxedematous type

SP + **E00.2 Congenital iodine-deficiency syndrome, mixed type**
Endemic cretinism, mixed type

SP + **E00.9 Congenital iodine-deficiency syndrome, unspecified**
Congenital iodine-deficiency hypothyroidism NOS
Endemic cretinism NOS

4 **E01 Iodine-deficiency related thyroid disorders and allied conditions**
EXCLUDES 1 congenital iodine-deficiency syndrome (E00.-)
subclinical iodine-deficiency hypothyroidism (E02)

SP **E01.0 Iodine-deficiency related diffuse (endemic) goiter**

SP **E01.1 Iodine-deficiency related multinodular (endemic) goiter**
Iodine-deficiency related nodular goiter

SP **E01.2 Iodine-deficiency related (endemic) goiter, unspecified**
Endemic goiter NOS

SP **E01.8 Other iodine-deficiency related thyroid disorders and allied conditions**
Acquired iodine-deficiency hypothyroidism NOS

SP **E02 Subclinical iodine-deficiency hypothyroidism**
DEFINITION Early stage of hypothyroidism marked by increased TSH levels and normal free thyroxin T4 levels; occurs when the body requires additional TSH in order to produce enough thyroxin, and developing into overt hypothyroidism in a few years.

4 **E03 Other hypothyroidism**
EXCLUDES 1 iodine-deficiency related hypothyroidism (E00-E02)
postprocedural hypothyroidism (E89.0)
CODING TIPS ✓ Report E89.0 for patients with hypothyroidism following a thyroidectomy, not other hypothyroidism (E03).

SP **E03.0 Congenital hypothyroidism with diffuse goiter**
Congenital parenchymatous goiter (nontoxic)
Congenital goiter (nontoxic) NOS
EXCLUDES 1 transitory congenital goiter with normal function (P72.0)
DEFINITION Abnormal hormone production or blocked TSH receptors in the fetus causing underactive thyroid with diffuse enlargement at birth, tracheal compression, difficulty breathing, and dysphagia.

SP **E03.1 Congenital hypothyroidism without goiter**
Aplasia of thyroid (with myxedema)
Congenital atrophy of thyroid
Congenital hypothyroidism NOS

SP + **E03.2 Hypothyroidism due to medicaments and other exogenous substances**
Code first:
poisoning due to drug or toxin, if applicable (T36-T65 with fifth or sixth character 1-4 or 6)
Use additional code for adverse effect, if applicable, to identify drug (T36-T50 with fifth or sixth character 5)

CODING TIPS✓ Determine whether the hypothyroidism is due to a poisoning or due to an adverse effect of a medication, such as lithium. Sequencing is determined based on whether the causative factor was a poisoning or an adverse effect. If the physician or NPP uses the term "thyroiditis," see E06.4.

SP **E03.3 Postinfectious hypothyroidism**

DEFINITION Damage to normal thyroid function from a previous infection, resulting in tiredness, weight gain, constipation, cold intolerance, dry skin, slowed mental function, and depression.

SP **E03.4 Atrophy of thyroid (acquired)**

EXCLUDES 1 congenital atrophy of thyroid (E03.1)

DEFINITION Abnormally small thyroid due to tissue degeneration and wasting; the gland becomes nonviable or severely reduced in function.

SP **E03.5 Myxedema coma**

DEFINITION Fully symptomatic hypothyroid disease manifesting with coma in a seriously decompensated state, mostly in the elderly, accompanied by hypothermia, hypoventilation with hypoxia, hypercapnia, hyponatremia, and bradycardia.

SP **E03.8 Other specified hypothyroidism**

SP **E03.9 Hypothyroidism, unspecified**

Myxedema NOS

DEFINITION Failure of the thyroid gland to produce enough hormone to maintain the body's metabolism, causing fatigue, weight gain, muscle aches and cramps, cold intolerance, memory loss, and depression.

4 **E04 Other nontoxic goiter**

EXCLUDES 1 congenital goiter (NOS) (diffuse) (parenchymatous) (E03.0)
iodine-deficiency related goiter (E00-E02)

SP **E04.0 Nontoxic diffuse goiter**

Diffuse (colloid) nontoxic goiter
Simple nontoxic goiter

DEFINITION Generalized, simple, painless thyroid enlargement without impairment of glandular function due to an overload of thyroid-stimulating hormone (TSH) from the pituitary gland.

SP **E04.1 Nontoxic single thyroid nodule**

Colloid nodule (cystic) (thyroid)
Nontoxic uninodular goiter
Thyroid (cystic) nodule NOS

DEFINITION A simple, painless, cyst-like node or singular goiter on the thyroid that is not impairing the normal glandular function.

SP **E04.2 Nontoxic multinodular goiter**

Cystic goiter NOS
Multinodular (cystic) goiter NOS

DEFINITION Multiple hard knobs, or cysts, in the thyroid detected by palpation but not impairing function or causing disease.

SP **E04.8 Other specified nontoxic goiter**

SP **E04.9 Nontoxic goiter, unspecified**

Goiter NOS
Nodular goiter (nontoxic) NOS

4 **E05 Thyrotoxicosis [hyperthyroidism]**

EXCLUDES 1 chronic thyroiditis with transient thyrotoxicosis (E06.2)
neonatal thyrotoxicosis (P72.1)

CODING TIPS✓ Thyrotoxicosis is another term for hyperthyroidism, and these terms may frequently be used interchangeably in clinical records. Unspecified hyperthyroidism should be coded to E05.9-.

CODING TIPS✓ Codes from category E05 are combination codes that indicate the presence or absence of thyrotoxic crisis or storm. A thyrotoxic crisis (also called "thyroid storm") is a condition that may occur among individuals with hyperthyroidism and is marked by tachycardia, fever, and hypertension, which may or may not result in congestive heart failure and/or shock. Thyrotoxic crisis should only be coded when specified by the provider and cannot be assumed based upon other symptoms alone.

5 **E05.0 Thyrotoxicosis with diffuse goiter**

Exophthalmic or toxic goiter NOS
Graves' disease
Toxic diffuse goiter

DEFINITION Thyrotropin receptor antibody production that mimics the pituitary's normal regulatory hormone, overriding it and increasing thyroid hormone production, marked by enlarged thyroid and bulging eyes.

SP **E05.00 Thyrotoxicosis with diffuse goiter without thyrotoxic crisis or storm**

DEFINITION Hyperthyroid conditions with excessive hormone production and speeding up of body functions; increased heart rate and blood pressure, excessive sweating, hand tremors, nervousness and anxiety, insomnia, and weight loss with increased appetite.

SP **E05.01 Thyrotoxicosis with diffuse goiter with thyrotoxic crisis or storm**

DEFINITION Severe, sudden worsening of hyperthyroid conditions from injury, stress, or gland removal that can lead to coma and death, manifesting with tachycardia, arrhythmia, vomiting, high fever, diarrhea, and dehydration.

5 **E05.1 Thyrotoxicosis with toxic single thyroid nodule**

Thyrotoxicosis with toxic uninodular goiter

SP **E05.10 Thyrotoxicosis with toxic single thyroid nodule without thyrotoxic crisis or storm**

SP **E05.11 Thyrotoxicosis with toxic single thyroid nodule with thyrotoxic crisis or storm**

5 **E05.2 Thyrotoxicosis with toxic multinodular goiter**

Toxic nodular goiter NOS

Chapter 4 E00-E89

SP **E05.20 Thyrotoxicosis with toxic multinodular goiter without thyrotoxic crisis or storm**

SP **E05.21 Thyrotoxicosis with toxic multinodular goiter with thyrotoxic crisis or storm**

5 **E05.3 Thyrotoxicosis from ectopic thyroid tissue**

SP **E05.30 Thyrotoxicosis from ectopic thyroid tissue without thyrotoxic crisis or storm**

SP **E05.31 Thyrotoxicosis from ectopic thyroid tissue with thyrotoxic crisis or storm**

5 **E05.4 Thyrotoxicosis factitia**

DEFINITION Thyrotoxicosis factitia is a condition of higher than normal thyroid hormones (T3 and T4) resulting from excess ingestion of thyroid hormone (medication). The condition may be iatrogenic (adverse effect resulting from taking prescription correctly) or due to intentional ingestion of excess medication (poisoning). The cause of the condition should be identified and the coder should follow guidelines for coding of adverse effects and poisoning when assigning a code from E05.4-.

SP **E05.40 Thyrotoxicosis factitia without thyrotoxic crisis or storm**

SP **E05.41 Thyrotoxicosis factitia with thyrotoxic crisis or storm**

5 **E05.8 Other thyrotoxicosis**

Overproduction of thyroid-stimulating hormone

SP **E05.80 Other thyrotoxicosis without thyrotoxic crisis or storm**

SP **E05.81 Other thyrotoxicosis with thyrotoxic crisis or storm**

5 **E05.9 Thyrotoxicosis, unspecified**

Hyperthyroidism NOS

SP **E05.90 Thyrotoxicosis, unspecified without thyrotoxic crisis or storm**

SP **E05.91 Thyrotoxicosis, unspecified with thyrotoxic crisis or storm**

4 **E06 Thyroiditis**

EXCLUDES 1 postpartum thyroiditis (O90.5)

DEFINITION Thyroiditis is a condition marked by inflammation of the thyroid (may or may not be infectious in nature), and should not be confused with hyperthyroidism. Various forms of thyroiditis may result in either hyper- or hypothyroidism.

SP + **E06.0 Acute thyroiditis**

Abscess of thyroid
Pyogenic thyroiditis
Suppurative thyroiditis
Use additional code (B95-B97) to identify infectious agent.

DEFINITION Painful infection of the thyroid gland, often with abscess and pus formation.

SP **E06.1 Subacute thyroiditis**

de Quervain thyroiditis
Giant-cell thyroiditis
Granulomatous thyroiditis
Nonsuppurative thyroiditis
Viral thyroiditis

EXCLUDES 1 autoimmune thyroiditis (E06.3)

DEFINITION Thyroid inflammation often resulting from another disease, such as mumps or flu, presenting with fever, radiating neck pain, and hyperthyroidism symptoms than can last months.

SP **E06.2 Chronic thyroiditis with transient thyrotoxicosis**

EXCLUDES 1 autoimmune thyroiditis (E06.3)

SP **E06.3 Autoimmune thyroiditis**

Hashimoto's thyroiditis
Hashitoxicosis (transient)
Lymphadenoid goiter
Lymphocytic thyroiditis
Struma lymphomatosa

DEFINITION Autoimmune inflammation of the thyroid with lymphocyte infiltration that presents with painless thyroid enlargement and hypothyroid symptoms.

SP + **E06.4 Drug-induced thyroiditis**

Use additional code for adverse effect, if applicable, to identify drug (T36-T50 with fifth or sixth character 5)

CODING TIPS ✓ Drug-induced thyroiditis should only be coded when clinical record documentation clearly indicates thyroiditis (inflammation of the thyroid), resulting from the administration of a specific drug or chemical. The causative drug or chemical should be identified and the coder should follow guidelines for coding of adverse effects and poisoning when assigning E06.4. If the provider documentation states "hypothyroidism, due to drugs or toxins," see E03.2.

DEFINITION Iatrogenic inflammation of the thyroid due to taking certain medications, such as lithium, or an overdose of iodine.

SP **E06.5 Other chronic thyroiditis**

Chronic fibrous thyroiditis
Chronic thyroiditis NOS
Ligneous thyroiditis
Riedel thyroiditis

SP **E06.9 Thyroiditis, unspecified**

DEFINITION Inflammation of the thyroid with noticeable swelling, often on one side, possibly inducing symptoms of hyper- or hypothyroidism, from unspecified causation or acuity.

4 **E07 Other disorders of thyroid**

SP **E07.0 Hypersecretion of calcitonin**

C-cell hyperplasia of thyroid
Hypersecretion of thyrocalcitonin

SP **E07.1 Dyshormogenetic goiter**

Familial dyshormogenetic goiter
Pendred's syndrome

EXCLUDES 1 transitory congenital goiter with normal function (P72.0)

5 **E07.8 Other specified disorders of thyroid**

SP **E07.81 Sick-euthyroid syndrome**

Euthyroid sick-syndrome

Chapter 4 E00-E89

DEFINITION Condition in which thyroid hormone levels are off due to a non-thyroid related problem.

SP **E07.89 Other specified disorders of thyroid**
Abnormality of thyroid-binding globulin
Hemorrhage of thyroid
Infarction of thyroid

IQ **E07.9 Disorder of thyroid, unspecified**

Diabetes mellitus (E08-E13)

GUIDELINES **Section I.C.4.a.1)-3)**
The diabetes mellitus codes are combination codes that include the type of diabetes mellitus, the body system affected, and the complications affecting that body system. As many codes within a particular category as are necessary to describe all of the complications of the disease may be used. They should be sequenced based on the reason for a particular encounter. Assign as many codes from categories E08 – E13 as needed to identify all of the associated conditions that the patient has.

The age of a patient is not the sole determining factor, though most type 1 diabetics develop the condition before reaching puberty. For this reason type 1 diabetes mellitus is also referred to as juvenile diabetes.

If the type of diabetes mellitus is not documented in the medical record the default is E11.-, Type 2 diabetes mellitus.

If the documentation in a medical record does not indicate the type of diabetes but does indicate that the patient uses insulin, code E11, Type 2 diabetes mellitus, should be assigned. An additional code should be assigned from category Z79 to identify the long-term (current) use of insulin or oral hypoglycemic drugs. If the patient is treated with both oral medications and insulin, only the code for long-term (current) use of insulin should be assigned. If the patient is treated with both insulin and an injectable non-insulin antidiabetic drug, assign codes Z79.4, Long-term (current) use of insulin, and Z79.899, Other long term (current) drug therapy. If the patient is treated with both oral hypoglycemic drugs and an injectable non-insulin antidiabetic drug, assign codes Z79.84, Long-term (current) use of oral hypoglycemic drugs, and Z79.899, Other long-term (current) drug therapy. Code Z79.4 should not be assigned if insulin is given temporarily to bring a type 2 patient's blood sugar under control during an encounter.

GUIDELINES **Section I.C.4.a.6)**
Codes under categories E08, Diabetes mellitus due to underlying condition, E09, Drug or chemical induced diabetes mellitus, and E13, Other specified diabetes mellitus, identify complications/manifestations associated with secondary diabetes mellitus. Secondary diabetes is always caused by another condition or event (e.g., cystic fibrosis, malignant neoplasm of pancreas, pancreatectomy, adverse effect of drug, or poisoning).

CODING TIPS✓ When diabetes is treated by a pancreatic transplant or bariatric surgery, and the physician indicates the diabetes is "cured" or "resolved," continue to code any manifestations of diabetes as diabetic. If there are no manifestations of diabetes, do not code diabetes. Assign code Z86.39, Personal history of other endocrine, nutritional and metabolic disease.

CODING TIPS✓ Codes E08-E13 are combination codes that generally do not require a second code to describe the manifestation unless specified by the code specific convention. Specifically, when coding diabetes with an ulcer, diabetic chronic kidney disease, or speciified manifestations that do not belong in a specific subcategory, a second code is required. A second code to identify gastroparesis (K31.84) may be assigned, optionally, when coding diabetic gastroparesis.

CODING TIPS✓ Reference the alphabetical index to review conditions that the classification assumes are related to diabetes. All specified manifestations/complications listed under the word 'with' in the index are presumed related unless the physician or NPP specified a different cause in documentation, or states they're unrelated. The 'with' convention does not apply to "not elsewhere classified (NEC)" index entries that cover broad categories of conditions. Coding professionals should not assume a causal relationship when the diabetic complication is "NEC."

CODING TIPS✓ When a patient is receiving home health services for the administration of insulin, the clinical record must contain detailed evidence of the patient's inability to self administer. For example, a patient with rheumatoid arthritis may have impaired ability to manipulate an injectable medication and self inject. It is not appropriate to use vague terms, such as poor vision or poor manual dexterity.

+ 4 **E08 Diabetes mellitus due to underlying condition**
Code first the underlying condition, such as:
- congenital rubella (P35.0)
- Cushing's syndrome (E24.-)
- cystic fibrosis (E84.-)
- malignant neoplasm (C00-C96)
- malnutrition (E40-E46)
- pancreatitis and other diseases of the pancreas (K85-K86.-)

Use additional code to identify control using:
- insulin (Z79.4)
- oral antidiabetic drugs (Z79.84)
- oral hypoglycemic drugs (Z79.84)

EXCLUDES 1
- drug or chemical induced diabetes mellitus (E09.-)
- gestational diabetes (O24.4-)
- neonatal diabetes mellitus (P70.2)
- postpancreatectomy diabetes mellitus (E13.-)
- postprocedural diabetes mellitus (E13.-)
- secondary diabetes mellitus NEC (E13.-)
- type 1 diabetes mellitus (E10.-)
- type 2 diabetes mellitus (E11.-)

CODING TIPS✓ When coding diabetes mellitus due to an underlying condition, the underlying condition and relationship to diabetes should be specified by the provider.

CODING TIPS✓ If the patient uses an insulin pump, use Z96.41 as an additional code. If there is a complication involving the insulin pump, use a code from T85.6- or T85.7- instead of the Z code.

CODING TIPS✓ Use Z79.4 to indicate the use of insulin, OR use Z79.84 to indicate the use of oral anti-glycemics. Use Z79.84 only when the patient does not also take insulin. Do NOT code both.
Use Z79.899 for non-insulin anti-diabetic medications. Z79.899 may be used with Z79.84 or with Z79.4.

CODING TIPS✓ Reference the alphabetical index to review conditions that the classification assumes are related to diabetes. All specified manifestations/complications listed under the word 'with' in the index are presumed related unless the physician or NPP specifies a different cause in documentation, or states they're unrelated. The "with" convention does not apply to "not elsewhere classified (NEC)" index entries that cover broad categories of conditions. Specific conditions must be linked by the terms "with," "in," "due to" or "associated with." Coding professionals should not assume a causal relationship when the diabetic complication is "NEC."

CODING TIPS✓ E08 codes will never be primary. Common conditions causing diabetes due to underlying condition are listed in the "code first" note. If diabetes is related to a malignant neoplasm of the pancreas, query whether the diabetes is caused by the neoplasm itself (E08); the drugs used to treat the neoplasm (E09); or the removal of part or all of the pancreas (E13).

+ 5 **E08.0 Diabetes mellitus due to underlying condition with hyperosmolarity**

IQ SL + **E08.00 Diabetes mellitus due to underlying condition with hyperosmolarity without nonketotic hyperglycemic-hyperosmolar coma (NKHHC)**

IQ SL + **E08.01 Diabetes mellitus due to underlying condition with hyperosmolarity with coma**

+ 5 **E08.1 Diabetes mellitus due to underlying condition with ketoacidosis**

CODING TIPS✓ Diabetic ketoacidosis is a serious complication of diabetes that occurs when the body produces high levels of blood acids called ketones. This condition is likely resolved before admission to home care, but could be a current diagnosis.

IQ SL + **E08.10 Diabetes mellitus due to underlying condition with ketoacidosis without coma**

IQ SL + **E08.11 Diabetes mellitus due to underlying condition with ketoacidosis with coma**

+ 5 **E08.2 Diabetes mellitus due to underlying condition with kidney complications**

IQ SL + **E08.21 Diabetes mellitus due to underlying condition with diabetic nephropathy**
Diabetes mellitus due to underlying condition with intercapillary glomerulosclerosis
Diabetes mellitus due to underlying condition with intracapillary glomerulonephrosis
Diabetes mellitus due to underlying condition with Kimmelstiel-Wilson disease

IQ SL + **E08.22 Diabetes mellitus due to underlying condition with diabetic chronic kidney disease**
Use additional code to identify stage of chronic kidney disease (N18.1-N18.6)

CODING TIPS✓ Assign an additional code from N18- to indicate the stage of CKD. When diabetic nephropathy and CKD are documented, code diabetic CKD, not nephropathy, because CKD is more specific.

CODING TIPS✓ When diabetes, CKD and hypertension are documented, sequence the appropriate category of diabetes with CKD (E--.22) and the appropriate hypertension code (I12 or I13) prior to N18. The hypertension or the diabetes may be sequenced first depending on the focus of care. Use N18.1-N18.6 or N18.9 to indicate the CKD. These conditions are all considered related unless the physician or NPP indicates they are not related. For example, if the provider documents diabetic CKD, this indicates that hypertension is not related to the CKD.

IQ + **E08.29 Diabetes mellitus due to underlying condition with other diabetic kidney complication**
Renal tubular degeneration in diabetes mellitus due to underlying condition

+ 5 **E08.3 Diabetes mellitus due to underlying condition with ophthalmic complications**

CODING TIPS✓ Diabetic codes indicating specific eye disorders require a 7th character to indicate laterality.

CODING TIPS✓ When a patient has macular edema, the patient also has retinopathy, with the macular edema developing as a complication of the retinopathy. Retinopathy includes three stages: background retinopathy, proliferative retinopathy, and macular edema.

CODING TIPS✓ When coding diabetes with ophthalmic manifestations, review the clinical record and plan of care to ensure that the functional impact of visual impairments is reported. The home health record should clearly report how visual losses impact the function and activities of the patient, including how these conditions impact medication administration, safety, the ability to perform treatments (such as wound care) and other key areas related to the patient's daily living.

+ 6 **E08.31 Diabetes mellitus due to underlying condition with unspecified diabetic retinopathy**

IQ + **E08.311 Diabetes mellitus due to underlying condition with unspecified diabetic retinopathy with macular edema**

!Q $L + E08.319 **Diabetes mellitus due to underlying condition with unspecified diabetic retinopathy without macular edema**

+ 6 E08.32 **Diabetes mellitus due to underlying condition with mild nonproliferative diabetic retinopathy**

Diabetes mellitus due to underlying condition with nonproliferative diabetic retinopathy NOS

One of the following 7th characters is to be assigned to codes in subcategory E08.32 to designate laterality of the disease:
1 right eye
2 left eye
3 bilateral
9 unspecified eye

⊟ !Q + 7 E08.321- **Diabetes mellitus due to underlying condition with mild nonproliferative diabetic retinopathy with macular edema**

⊟ !Q $L + 7 E08.329- **Diabetes mellitus due to underlying condition with mild nonproliferative diabetic retinopathy without macular edema**

+ 6 E08.33 **Diabetes mellitus due to underlying condition with moderate nonproliferative diabetic retinopathy**

One of the following 7th characters is to be assigned to codes in subcategory E08.33 to designate laterality of the disease:
1 right eye
2 left eye
3 bilateral
9 unspecified eye

⊟ !Q + 7 E08.331- **Diabetes mellitus due to underlying condition with moderate nonproliferative diabetic retinopathy with macular edema**

⊟ !Q $L + 7 E08.339- **Diabetes mellitus due to underlying condition with moderate nonproliferative diabetic retinopathy without macular edema**

+ 6 E08.34 **Diabetes mellitus due to underlying condition with severe nonproliferative diabetic retinopathy**

One of the following 7th characters is to be assigned to codes in subcategory E08.34 to designate laterality of the disease:
1 right eye
2 left eye
3 bilateral
9 unspecified eye

⊟ !Q + 7 E08.341- **Diabetes mellitus due to underlying condition with severe nonproliferative diabetic retinopathy with macular edema**

⊟ !Q $L + 7 E08.349- **Diabetes mellitus due to underlying condition with severe nonproliferative diabetic retinopathy without macular edema**

+ 6 E08.35 **Diabetes mellitus due to underlying condition with proliferative diabetic retinopathy**

One of the following 7th characters is to be assigned to codes in subcategory E08.35 to designate laterality of the disease:
1 right eye
2 left eye
3 bilateral
9 unspecified eye

⊟ !Q + 7 E08.351- **Diabetes mellitus due to underlying condition with proliferative diabetic retinopathy with macular edema**

⊟ !Q $L + 7 E08.352- **Diabetes mellitus due to underlying condition with proliferative diabetic retinopathy with traction retinal detachment involving the macula**

⊟ !Q $L + 7 E08.353- **Diabetes mellitus due to underlying condition with proliferative diabetic retinopathy with traction retinal detachment not involving the macula**

⊟ !Q $L + 7 E08.354- **Diabetes mellitus due to underlying condition with proliferative diabetic retinopathy with combined traction retinal detachment and rhegmatogenous retinal detachment**

⊟ !Q $L + 7 E08.355- **Diabetes mellitus due to underlying condition with stable proliferative diabetic retinopathy**

⊟ !Q $L + 7 E08.359- **Diabetes mellitus due to underlying condition with proliferative diabetic retinopathy without macular edema**

!Q $L + E08.36 **Diabetes mellitus due to underlying condition with diabetic cataract**

CODING TIPS ✓ Cataracts are more common in diabetic patients. The classification assumes a relationship between cataracts and diabetes, when the patient has diabetes. Even cataracts specifically described as "cortical, nuclear and posterior subcapsular" and "nuclear sclerotic" should prompt the assignment of E--.36, along with the code for the specific cataract code. (AHA: 2Q 2019)

⊟ !Q $L + E08.37X- 7 **Diabetes mellitus due to underlying condition with diabetic macular edema, resolved following treatment**

One of the following 7th characters is to be assigned to code E08.37 to designate laterality of the disease:
1 right eye
2 left eye
3 bilateral
9 unspecified eye

CODING TIPS✓ The macular edema may be resolved, but the retinopathy remains. This code is like a history code for the macular edema.

IQ SL + **E08.39 Diabetes mellitus due to underlying condition with other diabetic ophthalmic complication**
Use additional code to identify manifestation, such as:
diabetic glaucoma (H40-H42)

CODING TIPS✓ There is no assumed relationship between diabetes and glaucoma. The coder should seek further clarification regarding the relationship between blindness, glaucoma and diabetes before coding as a diabetic manifestation.

+ 5 **E08.4 Diabetes mellitus due to underlying condition with neurological complications**

CODING TIPS✓ Diabetes due to an underlying condition with loss of protective sensation or diabetic peripheral neuropathy should be coded to E08.42.

IQ SH SL + **E08.40 Diabetes mellitus due to underlying condition with diabetic neuropathy, unspecified**

IQ SL + **E08.41 Diabetes mellitus due to underlying condition with diabetic mononeuropathy**

IQ SH SL + **E08.42 Diabetes mellitus due to underlying condition with diabetic polyneuropathy**
Diabetes mellitus due to underlying condition with diabetic neuralgia

CODING TIPS✓ Do not use diabetic polyneuropathy as the etiology of diabetic ulcers. Instead, assign E--.621 or E--.622 followed by the code(s) for the ulcer(s). Assign diabetic polyneuropathy as a comorbidity.

CODING TIPS✓ Diabetic polyneuropathy is the most common type of diabetic neuropathy and causes pain or loss of feeling in the toes, feet, legs, hands and arms.

IQ SL + **E08.43 Diabetes mellitus due to underlying condition with diabetic autonomic (poly)neuropathy**
Diabetes mellitus due to underlying condition with diabetic gastroparesis

CODING TIPS✓ Autonomic neuropathy affects the heart, digestive system and other involuntary functions. This type of neuropathy causes delayed or slowed gastric emptying as well as problems with orthostatic hypotension. This code is not to be used for polyneuropathy of the hands and feet.

CODING TIPS✓ Gastroparesis (K31.84) may be sequenced after this code as an option.

IQ SL + **E08.44 Diabetes mellitus due to underlying condition with diabetic amyotrophy**

CODING TIPS✓ Diabetic amyotrophy is muscle weakness, characterized by weakness followed by wasting of pelvifemoral muscles, either unilaterally or bilaterally, with associated pain.

IQ SL + **E08.49 Diabetes mellitus due to underlying condition with other diabetic neurological complication**

+ 5 **E08.5 Diabetes mellitus due to underlying condition with circulatory complications**

CODING TIPS✓ Peripheral angiopathy includes arterial, venous and capillary conditions. Peripheral angiopathy may be documented as diabetic PVD. There is an assumed relationship between diabetes and PVD and PAD, including peripheral atherosclerosis and venous insufficiency. Diabetic PVD is coded E--.51. Diabetic arteriosclerosis of the peripheral arteries should be coded E--.51 or E--.52 then the appropriate I70.- code. Diabetic venous insufficiency should be coded E--.51 or E--.52 and I87.2 The presence of diabetes and peripheral arterial disease in the record indicates that both diabetes and PVD should be marked in M1028. Venous disease is not included in M1028.

IQ SL + **E08.51 Diabetes mellitus due to underlying condition with diabetic peripheral angiopathy without gangrene**

CODING TIPS✓ Do not use diabetic peripheral angiopathy as the etiology of diabetic ulcers. Assign codes E--.621 or E--.622 instead followed by the code(s) for the ulcer(s). Assign diabetic angiopathy as a comorbidity.

CODING TIPS✓ If the physician or NPP documents diabetes and venous stasis ulcer, the E--.51 code precedes the code for the venous disease and the ulcer. If wound care is the focus of the care, use Z48.00 as the primary code.

IQ SL + **E08.52 Diabetes mellitus due to underlying condition with diabetic peripheral angiopathy with gangrene**
Diabetes mellitus due to underlying condition with diabetic gangrene

IQ SL + **E08.59 Diabetes mellitus due to underlying condition with other circulatory complications**

CODING TIPS✓ Diabetic circulatory complications other than peripheral angiopathy and gangrene, identified as such by the physician or NPP, may be coded to 4th and 5th characters .59. Example: Diabetic CAD or ASHD is documented.

+ 5 **E08.6 Diabetes mellitus due to underlying condition with other specified complications**

+ 6 **E08.61 Diabetes mellitus due to underlying condition with diabetic arthropathy**

IQ SL + **E08.610 Diabetes mellitus due to underlying condition with diabetic neuropathic arthropathy**
Diabetes mellitus due to underlying condition with Charcôt's joints
CODING TIPS✓ Do not add a M14.6 code for Charcot's joint.

IQ SL + **E08.618 Diabetes mellitus due to underlying condition with other diabetic arthropathy**

+ 6 **E08.62 Diabetes mellitus due to underlying condition with skin complications**

IQ SL + **E08.620 Diabetes mellitus due to underlying condition with diabetic dermatitis**
Diabetes mellitus due to underlying condition with diabetic necrobiosis lipoidica

IQ SL + **E08.621 Diabetes mellitus due to underlying condition with foot ulcer**
Use additional code to identify site of ulcer (L97.4-, L97.5-)
CODING TIPS✓ If the patient has had a diabetic foot ulcer in the past, either healed or amputated, also code Z86.31. Ulceration of the foot is assumed related to diabetes unless another cause is indicated.

IQ SL + **E08.622 Diabetes mellitus due to underlying condition with other skin ulcer**
Use additional code to identify site of ulcer (L97.1-L97.9, L98.41-L98.49)
CODING TIPS✓ Diabetes codes with 4th, 5th and 6th characters .622 are used when an ulcer is located on the lower extremity, beginning at the ankle, and not including the foot. Whereas ulcers located on the foot are assumed related to diabetes, ulcers located elsewhere are not assumed related to diabetes and must be confirmed with the provider.

IQ SL + **E08.628 Diabetes mellitus due to underlying condition with other skin complications**

+ 6 **E08.63 Diabetes mellitus due to underlying condition with oral complications**

IQ SL + **E08.630 Diabetes mellitus due to underlying condition with periodontal disease**

IQ SL + **E08.638 Diabetes mellitus due to underlying condition with other oral complications**

+ 6 **E08.64 Diabetes mellitus due to underlying condition with hypoglycemia**

IQ SL + **E08.641 Diabetes mellitus due to underlying condition with hypoglycemia with coma**

IQ SL + **E08.649 Diabetes mellitus due to underlying condition with hypoglycemia without coma**
CODING TIPS✓ The physician or NPP should be queried when the term "uncontrolled" is used to determine whether the patient has hyperglycemia, hypoglycemia or both.
CODING TIPS✓ If encephalopathy is due to hypoglycemia, use G93.41 as an additional code.

IQ SL + **E08.65 Diabetes mellitus due to underlying condition with hyperglycemia**
CODING TIPS✓ Inadequately controlled, poorly controlled and out of control diabetes are coded with hyperglycemia. The physician or NPP should be queried when the term 'uncontrolled' is used to determine whether the patient has hyperglycemia, hypoglycemia, or both. The clinical record should support hyperglycemia. Do not code diabetes with hyperglycemia when ketoacidosis is also documented.

IQ SL + **E08.69 Diabetes mellitus due to underlying condition with other specified complication**
Use additional code to identify complication
CODING TIPS✓ Use this code when the physician or NPP specifies a manifestation of diabetes that does not fit in any of the other subcategories. Follow the diabetes code with the code for the specified condition.
CODING TIPS✓ The classification presumes a cause-and-effect relationship between osteomyelitis and diabetes when no other cause is documented. Osteomyelitis with diabetes is usually associated with ulceration. Use the appropriate code for the osteomyelitis after coding diabetes with other specified manifestation (E--.69). Although not clear when referencing diabetes in the index, it has been confirmed that osteomyelitis is related to all diabetes types.

IQ + **E08.8 Diabetes mellitus due to underlying condition with unspecified complications**
CODING TIPS✓ This code should not be used for unspecified complications. Query the physician or NPP for information regarding suspected manifestations that the classification does not presume related.

IQ SL + **E08.9 Diabetes mellitus due to underlying condition without complications**

CODING TIPS✓ This code is acceptable to use for a diabetic without manifestations. Certain specified conditions are assumed related to diabetes by the classification, if listed indented under the word "with" in the alphabetical index, so the use of .9 as a diabetes 4th character should not be common. Query the physician or NPP for information regarding suspected manifestations when documentation regarding other potential causes is unclear. This code should be used for a diabetic requiring insulin injections only if teaching is the skill, or other comorbidities, unrelated to diabetes, make it unacceptable for the patient to self-inject. If .9 is used as a 4th character, no other diabetes code may be used.

+ 4 E09 Drug or chemical induced diabetes mellitus

Code first:
poisoning due to drug or toxin, if applicable (T36-T65 with fifth or sixth character 1-4 or 6)

Use additional code for adverse effect, if applicable, to identify drug (T36-T50 with fifth or sixth character 5)

Use additional code to identify control using:
insulin (Z79.4)
oral antidiabetic drugs (Z79.84)
oral hypoglycemic drugs (Z79.84)

EXCLUDES 1
diabetes mellitus due to underlying condition (E08.-)
gestational diabetes (O24.4-)
neonatal diabetes mellitus (P70.2)
postpancreatectomy diabetes mellitus (E13.-)
postprocedural diabetes mellitus (E13.-)
secondary diabetes mellitus NEC (E13.-)
type 1 diabetes mellitus (E10.-)
type 2 diabetes mellitus (E11.-)

GUIDELINES **Section I.C.4.a.6(a)**

Codes under categories E08, Diabetes mellitus due to underlying condition, E09, Drug or chemical induced diabetes mellitus, and E13, Other specified diabetes mellitus, identify complications/manifestations associated with secondary diabetes mellitus. Secondary diabetes is always caused by another condition or event (e.g., cystic fibrosis, malignant neoplasm of pancreas, pancreatectomy, adverse effect of drug, or poisoning).

For patients with secondary diabetes mellitus who routinely use insulin or oral hypoglycemic drugs, an additional code from category Z79 should be assigned to identify the long-term (current) use of insulin or oral hypoglycemic drugs. If the patient is treated with both oral medications and insulin, only the code for long-term (current) use of insulin should be assigned ... Code Z79.4 should not be assigned if insulin is given temporarily to bring a secondary diabetic patient's blood sugar under control during an encounter.

GUIDELINES **Section I.C.4.a**

The diabetes mellitus codes are combination codes that include the type of diabetes mellitus, the body system affected, and the complications affecting that body system. As many codes within a particular category as are necessary to describe all of the complications of the disease may be used. They should be sequenced based on the reason for a particular encounter. Assign as many codes from categories E08 – E13 as needed to identify all of the associated conditions that the patient has.

CODING TIPS✓ If the patient uses an insulin pump, use Z96.41 as an additional code. If there is a complication involving the insulin pump, use a code from T85.6- or T85.7- instead of the Z code.

CODING TIPS✓ Use Z79.4 to indicate the use of insulin, OR use Z79.84 to indicate the use of oral anti-glycemics. Use Z79.84 only when the patient does not also take insulin. Do NOT code both.
Use Z79.899 for non-insulin anti-diabetic medications. Z79.899 may be used with Z79.84 or with Z79.4.

CODING TIPS✓ Reference the alphabetical index to review conditions that the classification assumes are related to diabetes. All specified manifestations/complications listed under the word 'with' in the index are presumed related unless the physician or NPP specifies a different cause in documentation, or states they're unrelated. The "with" convention does not apply to "not elsewhere classified (NEC)" index entries that cover broad categories of conditions. Specific conditions must be linked by the terms "with," "in," "due to" or "associated with." Coding professionals should not assume a causal relationship when the diabetic complication is "NEC."

CODING TIPS✓ If diabetes is related to a malignant neoplasm of the pancreas, query whether the diabetes is caused by the neoplasm itself (E08); the drugs used to treat the neoplasm (E09); or the removal of part or all of the pancreas (E13).

+ 5 E09.0 Drug or chemical induced diabetes mellitus with hyperosmolarity

SP SL + E09.00 Drug or chemical induced diabetes mellitus with hyperosmolarity without nonketotic hyperglycemic-hyperosmolar coma (NKHHC)

SP SL + E09.01 Drug or chemical induced diabetes mellitus with hyperosmolarity with coma

+ 5 E09.1 Drug or chemical induced diabetes mellitus with ketoacidosis

CODING TIPS✓ Diabetic ketoacidosis is a serious complication of diabetes that occurs when the body produces high levels of blood acids called ketones. This condition is likely resolved before admission to home care, but could be a current diagnosis.

Chapter 4
E00-E89

SP SL + **E09.10 Drug or chemical induced diabetes mellitus with ketoacidosis without coma**

SP SL + **E09.11 Drug or chemical induced diabetes mellitus with ketoacidosis with coma**

+ 5 **E09.2 Drug or chemical induced diabetes mellitus with kidney complications**

SP SL + **E09.21 Drug or chemical induced diabetes mellitus with diabetic nephropathy**

Drug or chemical induced diabetes mellitus with intercapillary glomerulosclerosis

Drug or chemical induced diabetes mellitus with intracapillary glomerulonephrosis

Drug or chemical induced diabetes mellitus with Kimmelstiel-Wilson disease

SP SL + **E09.22 Drug or chemical induced diabetes mellitus with diabetic chronic kidney disease**

Use additional code to identify stage of chronic kidney disease (N18.1-N18.6)

CODING TIPS✓ When diabetes, CKD and hypertension are documented, sequence the appropriate category of diabetes with CKD (E--.22) and the appropriate hypertension code (I12 or I13) prior to N18. The hypertension or the diabetes may be sequenced first depending on the focus of care. Use N18.1-N18.6 or N18.9 to indicate the CKD. These conditions are all considered related unless the physician or NPP indicates they are not related. For example, if the provider documents diabetic CKD, this indicates that hypertension is not related to the CKD.

CODING TIPS✓ Assign an additional code from N18- to indicate the stage of CKD. When diabetic nephropathy and CKD are documented, code diabetic CKD, not nephropathy, because CKD is more specific.

SP SL + **E09.29 Drug or chemical induced diabetes mellitus with other diabetic kidney complication**

Drug or chemical induced diabetes mellitus with renal tubular degeneration

+ 5 **E09.3 Drug or chemical induced diabetes mellitus with ophthalmic complications**

CODING TIPS✓ Diabetic codes indicating specific eye disorders require a 7th character to indicate laterality.

CODING TIPS✓ When coding diabetes with ophthalmic manifestations, review the clinical record and plan of care to ensure that the functional impact of visual impairments is reported. The home health record should clearly report how visual losses impact the function and activities of the patient, including how these conditions impact medication administration, safety, the ability to perform treatments (such as wound care) and other key areas related to the patient's daily living.

CODING TIPS✓ When a patient has macular edema, the patient also has retinopathy, with the macular edema developing as a complication of the retinopathy. Retinopathy includes three stages: background retinopathy, proliferative retinopathy, and macular edema.

+ 6 **E09.31 Drug or chemical induced diabetes mellitus with unspecified diabetic retinopathy**

SP + **E09.311 Drug or chemical induced diabetes mellitus with unspecified diabetic retinopathy with macular edema**

SP SL + **E09.319 Drug or chemical induced diabetes mellitus with unspecified diabetic retinopathy without macular edema**

+ 6 **E09.32 Drug or chemical induced diabetes mellitus with mild nonproliferative diabetic retinopathy**

Drug or chemical induced diabetes mellitus with nonproliferative diabetic retinopathy NOS

One of the following 7th characters is to be assigned to codes in subcategory E09.32 to designate laterality of the disease:

1	right eye
2	left eye
3	bilateral
9	unspecified eye

L SP + 7 **E09.321- Drug or chemical induced diabetes mellitus with mild nonproliferative diabetic retinopathy with macular edema**

L SP SL + 7 **E09.329- Drug or chemical induced diabetes mellitus with mild nonproliferative diabetic retinopathy without macular edema**

+ 6 **E09.33 Drug or chemical induced diabetes mellitus with moderate nonproliferative diabetic retinopathy**

One of the following 7th characters is to be assigned to codes in subcategory E09.33 to designate laterality of the disease:

1	right eye
2	left eye
3	bilateral
9	unspecified eye

SP + 7 **E09.331-** **Drug or chemical induced diabetes mellitus with moderate nonproliferative diabetic retinopathy with macular edema**

SP SL + 7 **E09.339-** **Drug or chemical induced diabetes mellitus with moderate nonproliferative diabetic retinopathy without macular edema**

+ 6 **E09.34** **Drug or chemical induced diabetes mellitus with severe nonproliferative diabetic retinopathy**

One of the following 7th characters is to be assigned to codes in subcategory E09.34 to designate laterality of the disease:

1 right eye
2 left eye
3 bilateral
9 unspecified eye

SP + 7 **E09.341-** **Drug or chemical induced diabetes mellitus with severe nonproliferative diabetic retinopathy with macular edema**

SP SL + 7 **E09.349-** **Drug or chemical induced diabetes mellitus with severe nonproliferative diabetic retinopathy without macular edema**

+ 6 **E09.35** **Drug or chemical induced diabetes mellitus with proliferative diabetic retinopathy**

One of the following 7th characters is to be assigned to codes in subcategory E09.35 to designate laterality of the disease:

1 right eye
2 left eye
3 bilateral
9 unspecified eye

SP + 7 **E09.351-** **Drug or chemical induced diabetes mellitus with proliferative diabetic retinopathy with macular edema**

SP SL + 7 **E09.352-** **Drug or chemical induced diabetes mellitus with proliferative diabetic retinopathy with traction retinal detachment involving the macula**

SP SL + 7 **E09.353-** **Drug or chemical induced diabetes mellitus with proliferative diabetic retinopathy with traction retinal detachment not involving the macula**

SP SL + 7 **E09.354-** **Drug or chemical induced diabetes mellitus with proliferative diabetic retinopathy with combined traction retinal detachment and rhegmatogenous retinal detachment**

SP SL + 7 **E09.355-** **Drug or chemical induced diabetes mellitus with stable proliferative diabetic retinopathy**

SP SL + 7 **E09.359-** **Drug or chemical induced diabetes mellitus with proliferative diabetic retinopathy without macular edema**

SP SL + **E09.36** **Drug or chemical induced diabetes mellitus with diabetic cataract**

CODING TIPS ✓ Cataracts are more common in diabetic patients. The classification assumes a relationship between cataracts and diabetes, when the patient has diabetes. Even cataracts specifically described as "cortical, nuclear and posterior subcapsular" and "nuclear sclerotic" should prompt the assignment of E--.36, along with the code for the specific cataract code. (AHA: 2Q 2019)

SP SL + **E09.37X-** 7 **Drug or chemical induced diabetes mellitus with diabetic macular edema, resolved following treatment**

One of the following 7th characters is to be assigned to code E09.37 to designate laterality of the disease:

1 right eye
2 left eye
3 bilateral
9 unspecified eye

CODING TIPS ✓ The macular edema may be resolved, but the retinopathy remains. This code is like a history code for the macular edema.

SP SL + **E09.39** **Drug or chemical induced diabetes mellitus with other diabetic ophthalmic complication**

Use additional code to identify manifestation, such as:
diabetic glaucoma (H40-H42)

CODING TIPS ✓ There is no assumed relationship between diabetes and glaucoma. The coder should seek further clarification regarding the relationship between blindness, glaucoma and diabetes before coding as a diabetic manifestation.

+ 5 **E09.4** **Drug or chemical induced diabetes mellitus with neurological complications**

CODING TIPS ✓ Drug or chemical-induced diabetes with loss of protective sensation or diabetic peripheral neuropathy should be coded to E09.42.

SP SH SL + **E09.40** **Drug or chemical induced diabetes mellitus with neurological complications with diabetic neuropathy, unspecified**

SP SL + **E09.41** **Drug or chemical induced diabetes mellitus with neurological complications with diabetic mononeuropathy**

SP SH SL + **E09.42 Drug or chemical induced diabetes mellitus with neurological complications with diabetic polyneuropathy**
Drug or chemical induced diabetes mellitus with diabetic neuralgia

CODING TIPS ✓ Do not use diabetic polyneuropathy as the etiology of diabetic ulcers. Instead, assign E--.621 or E--.622 followed by the code(s) for the ulcer(s). Assign diabetic polyneuropathy as a comorbidity.

CODING TIPS ✓ Diabetic polyneuropathy is the most common type of diabetic neuropathy and causes pain or loss of feeling in the toes, feet, legs, hands and arms.

SP SL + **E09.43 Drug or chemical induced diabetes mellitus with neurological complications with diabetic autonomic (poly)neuropathy**
Drug or chemical induced diabetes mellitus with diabetic gastroparesis

CODING TIPS ✓ Autonomic neuropathy affects the heart, digestive system and other involuntary functions. This type of neuropathy causes delayed or slowed gastric emptying as well as problems with orthostatic hypotension. This code is not to be used for polyneuropathy of the hands and feet.

CODING TIPS ✓ Gastroparesis (K31.84) may be sequenced after this code as an option.

SP SL + **E09.44 Drug or chemical induced diabetes mellitus with neurological complications with diabetic amyotrophy**

CODING TIPS ✓ Diabetic amyotrophy is muscle weakness, characterized by weakness followed by wasting of pelvifemoral muscles, either unilaterally or bilaterally, with associated pain.

SP SL + **E09.49 Drug or chemical induced diabetes mellitus with neurological complications with other diabetic neurological complication**

+ 5 **E09.5 Drug or chemical induced diabetes mellitus with circulatory complications**

CODING TIPS ✓ Peripheral angiopathy includes arterial, venous and capillary conditions. Peripheral angiopathy may be documented as diabetic PVD. There is an assumed relationship between diabetes and PVD and PAD, including peripheral atherosclerosis and venous insufficiency. Diabetic PVD is coded E--.51. Diabetic arteriosclerosis of the peripheral arteries should be coded E--.51 or E--.52 then the appropriate I70.- code. Diabetic venous insufficiency should be coded E--.51 or E--.52 and I87.2 The presence of diabetes and peripheral arterial disease in the record indicates that both diabetes and PVD should be marked in M1028. Venous disease is not included in M1028.

SP SL + **E09.51 Drug or chemical induced diabetes mellitus with diabetic peripheral angiopathy without gangrene**

CODING TIPS ✓ If the physician or NPP documents diabetes and venous stasis ulcer, the E--.51 code precedes the code for the venous disease and the ulcer. If wound care is the focus of the care, use Z48.00 as the primary code.

CODING TIPS ✓ Do not use diabetic peripheral angiopathy as the etiology of diabetic ulcers. Assign codes E--.621 or E--.622 instead followed by the code(s) for the ulcer(s). Assign diabetic angiopathy as a comorbidity.

SP SL + **E09.52 Drug or chemical induced diabetes mellitus with diabetic peripheral angiopathy with gangrene**
Drug or chemical induced diabetes mellitus with diabetic gangrene

SP SL + **E09.59 Drug or chemical induced diabetes mellitus with other circulatory complications**

CODING TIPS ✓ Diabetic circulatory complications other than peripheral angiopathy and gangrene, identified as such by the physician or NPP, may be coded to 4th and 5th characters .59. Example: Diabetic CAD or ASHD is documented.

+ 5 **E09.6 Drug or chemical induced diabetes mellitus with other specified complications**

+ 6 **E09.61 Drug or chemical induced diabetes mellitus with diabetic arthropathy**

SP SL + **E09.610 Drug or chemical induced diabetes mellitus with diabetic neuropathic arthropathy**
Drug or chemical induced diabetes mellitus with Charcôt's joints

CODING TIPS ✓ Do not add a M14.6 code for Charcot's joint.

SP SL + **E09.618 Drug or chemical induced diabetes mellitus with other diabetic arthropathy**

+ 6 **E09.62 Drug or chemical induced diabetes mellitus with skin complications**

SP SL + **E09.620 Drug or chemical induced diabetes mellitus with diabetic dermatitis**
Drug or chemical induced diabetes mellitus with diabetic necrobiosis lipoidica

SP SL + **E09.621 Drug or chemical induced diabetes mellitus with foot ulcer**
Use additional code to identify site of ulcer (L97.4-, L97.5-)

CODING TIPS ✓ If the patient has had a diabetic foot ulcer in the past, either healed or amputated, also code Z86.31. Ulceration of the foot is assumed related to diabetes unless another cause is indicated.

SP SL + **E09.622 Drug or chemical induced diabetes mellitus with other skin ulcer**

Use additional code to identify site of ulcer (L97.1-L97.9, L98.41-L98.49)

CODING TIPS✓ Diabetes codes with 4th, 5th and 6th characters .622 are used when an ulcer is located on the lower extremity, beginning at the ankle, and not including the foot. Whereas ulcers located on the foot are assumed related to diabetes, ulcers located elsewhere are not assumed related to diabetes and must be confirmed with the provider.

SP SL + **E09.628 Drug or chemical induced diabetes mellitus with other skin complications**

+ 6 **E09.63 Drug or chemical induced diabetes mellitus with oral complications**

SP SL + **E09.630 Drug or chemical induced diabetes mellitus with periodontal disease**

SP SL + **E09.638 Drug or chemical induced diabetes mellitus with other oral complications**

+ 6 **E09.64 Drug or chemical induced diabetes mellitus with hypoglycemia**

SP SL + **E09.641 Drug or chemical induced diabetes mellitus with hypoglycemia with coma**

SP SL + **E09.649 Drug or chemical induced diabetes mellitus with hypoglycemia without coma**

CODING TIPS✓ The physician or NPP should be queried when the term "uncontrolled" is used to determine whether the patient has hyperglycemia, hypoglycemia or both.

CODING TIPS✓ If encephalopathy is due to hypoglycemia, use G93.41 as an additional code.

SP SL + **E09.65 Drug or chemical induced diabetes mellitus with hyperglycemia**

CODING TIPS✓ Inadequately controlled, poorly controlled and out of control diabetes are coded with hyperglycemia. The physician or NPP should be queried when the term 'uncontrolled' is used to determine whether the patient has hyperglycemia, hypoglycemia, or both. The clinical record should support hyperglycemia. Do not code diabetes with hyperglycemia when ketoacidosis is also documented.

SP SL + **E09.69 Drug or chemical induced diabetes mellitus with other specified complication**

Use additional code to identify complication

CODING TIPS✓ Use this code when the physician or NPP specifies a manifestation of diabetes that does not fit in any of the other subcategories. Follow the diabetes code with the code for the specified condition.

CODING TIPS✓ The classification presumes a cause-and-effect relationship between osteomyelitis and diabetes when no other cause is documented. Osteomyelitis with diabetes is usually associated with ulceration. Use the appropriate code for the osteomyelitis after coding diabetes with other specified manifestation (E--.69). Although not clear when referencing diabetes in the index, it has been confirmed that osteomyelitis is related to all diabetes types.

IQ + **E09.8 Drug or chemical induced diabetes mellitus with unspecified complications**

CODING TIPS✓ This code should not be used for unspecified complications. Query the physician or NPP for information regarding suspected manifestations that the classification does not presume related.

SP SL + **E09.9 Drug or chemical induced diabetes mellitus without complications**

CODING TIPS✓ This code is acceptable to use for a diabetic without manifestations. Certain specified conditions are assumed related to diabetes by the classification, if listed indented under the word "with" in the alphabetical index, so the use of .9 as a diabetes 4th character should not be common. Query the physician or NPP for information regarding suspected manifestations when documentation regarding other potential causes is unclear. This code should be used for a diabetic requiring insulin injections only if teaching is the skill, or other comorbidities, unrelated to diabetes, make it unacceptable for the patient to self-inject. If .9 is used as a 4th character, no other diabetes code may be used.

4 **E10 Type 1 diabetes mellitus**

INCLUDES
- brittle diabetes (mellitus)
- diabetes (mellitus) due to autoimmune process
- diabetes (mellitus) due to immune mediated pancreatic islet beta-cell destruction
- idiopathic diabetes (mellitus)
- juvenile onset diabetes (mellitus)
- ketosis-prone diabetes (mellitus)

EXCLUDES 1
- diabetes mellitus due to underlying condition (E08.-)
- drug or chemical induced diabetes mellitus (E09.-)
- gestational diabetes (O24.4-)
- hyperglycemia NOS (R73.9)
- neonatal diabetes mellitus (P70.2)
- postpancreatectomy diabetes mellitus (E13.-)
- postprocedural diabetes mellitus (E13.-)
- secondary diabetes mellitus NEC (E13.-)
- type 2 diabetes mellitus (E11.-)

GUIDELINES **Section I.C.4.a.1)**
The age of a patient is not the sole determining factor, though most type 1 diabetics develop the condition before reaching puberty. For this reason type 1 diabetes mellitus is also referred to as juvenile diabetes.

CODING TIPS✓ If the patient uses an insulin pump, use Z96.41 as an additional code. If there is a complication involving the insulin pump, use a code from T85.6- or T85.7- instead of the Z code.

CODING TIPS✓ Reference the alphabetical index to review conditions that the classification assumes are related to diabetes. All specified manifestations/complications listed under the word 'with' in the index are presumed related unless the physician or NPP specifies a different cause in documentation, or states they're unrelated. The "with" convention does not apply to "not elsewhere classified (NEC)" index entries that cover broad categories of conditions. Specific conditions must be linked by the terms "with," "in," "due to" or "associated with." Coding professionals should not assume a causal relationship when the diabetic complication is "NEC."

5 **E10.1 Type 1 diabetes mellitus with ketoacidosis**

CODING TIPS✓ Diabetic ketoacidosis is a serious complication of diabetes that occurs when the body produces high levels of blood acids called ketones. This condition is likely resolved before admission to home care, but could be a current diagnosis.

DEFINITION Diabetic complication characterized by hyperglycemia, hyperketonemia, and metabolic acidosis; often presents with nausea, vomiting, and abdominal pain; may progress to cerebral edema or lead to coma and/or death.

SP SH **E10.10 Type 1 diabetes mellitus with ketoacidosis without coma**

SP SH **E10.11 Type 1 diabetes mellitus with ketoacidosis with coma**

5 **E10.2 Type 1 diabetes mellitus with kidney complications**

SP SH **E10.21 Type 1 diabetes mellitus with diabetic nephropathy**
Type 1 diabetes mellitus with intercapillary glomerulosclerosis
Type 1 diabetes mellitus with intracapillary glomerulonephrosis
Type 1 diabetes mellitus with Kimmelstiel-Wilson disease

SP SH + **E10.22 Type 1 diabetes mellitus with diabetic chronic kidney disease**
Use additional code to identify stage of chronic kidney disease (N18.1-N18.6)

CODING TIPS✓ Assign an additional code from N18- to indicate the stage of CKD. When diabetic nephropathy and CKD are documented, code diabetic CKD, not nephropathy, because CKD is more specific.

CODING TIPS✓ When diabetes, CKD and hypertension are documented, sequence the appropriate category of diabetes with CKD (E--.22) and the appropriate hypertension code (I12 or I13) prior to N18. The hypertension or the diabetes may be sequenced first depending on the focus of care. Use N18.1-N18.6 or N18.9 to indicate the CKD. These conditions are all considered related unless the physician or NPP indicates they are not related. For example, if the provider documents diabetic CKD, this indicates that hypertension is not related to the CKD.

SP SH **E10.29 Type 1 diabetes mellitus with other diabetic kidney complication**
Type 1 diabetes mellitus with renal tubular degeneration

5 **E10.3 Type 1 diabetes mellitus with ophthalmic complications**

CODING TIPS✓ The 7th character codes in this category that are acceptable primary diagnoses in PDGM and contribute to a comorbidity adjustment are those with a 7th character of 1, 2, or 3. Unspecified eye (7th character of 9) is not acceptable as a primary diagnoses in PDGM, nor does it contribute to a comorbidity adjustment.

CODING TIPS✓ Diabetic codes indicating specific eye disorders require a 7th character to indicate laterality.

CODING TIPS✓ When a patient has macular edema, the patient also has retinopathy, with the macular edema developing as a complication of the retinopathy. Retinopathy includes three stages: background retinopathy, proliferative retinopathy, and macular edema.

CODING TIPS✓ When coding diabetes with ophthalmic manifestations, review the clinical record and plan of care to ensure that the functional impact of visual impairments is reported. The home health record should clearly report how visual losses impact the function and activities of the patient, including how these conditions impact medication administration, safety, the ability to perform treatments (such as wound care) and other key areas related to the patient's daily living.

6 **E10.31 Type 1 diabetes mellitus with unspecified diabetic retinopathy**

SP **E10.311 Type 1 diabetes mellitus with unspecified diabetic retinopathy with macular edema**

SP SH **E10.319 Type 1 diabetes mellitus with unspecified diabetic retinopathy without macular edema**

6 **E10.32 Type 1 diabetes mellitus with mild nonproliferative diabetic retinopathy**
Type 1 diabetes mellitus with nonproliferative diabetic retinopathy NOS

4 4th digit required 5 5th digit required 6 6th digit required 7 7th digit required X 7th digit placeholder + Additional code ⊟ Laterality

One of the following 7th characters is to be assigned to codes in subcategory E10.32 to designate laterality of the disease:
1 right eye
2 left eye
3 bilateral
9 unspecified eye

SP 7 E10.321- **Type 1 diabetes mellitus with mild nonproliferative diabetic retinopathy with macular edema**

SP SH 7 E10.329- **Type 1 diabetes mellitus with mild nonproliferative diabetic retinopathy without macular edema**

6 **E10.33 Type 1 diabetes mellitus with moderate nonproliferative diabetic retinopathy**

One of the following 7th characters is to be assigned to codes in subcategory E10.33 to designate laterality of the disease:
1 right eye
2 left eye
3 bilateral
9 unspecified eye

SP 7 E10.331- **Type 1 diabetes mellitus with moderate nonproliferative diabetic retinopathy with macular edema**

SP SH 7 E10.339- **Type 1 diabetes mellitus with moderate nonproliferative diabetic retinopathy without macular edema**

6 **E10.34 Type 1 diabetes mellitus with severe nonproliferative diabetic retinopathy**

One of the following 7th characters is to be assigned to codes in subcategory E10.34 to designate laterality of the disease:
1 right eye
2 left eye
3 bilateral
9 unspecified eye

SP 7 E10.341- **Type 1 diabetes mellitus with severe nonproliferative diabetic retinopathy with macular edema**

SP SH 7 E10.349- **Type 1 diabetes mellitus with severe nonproliferative diabetic retinopathy without macular edema**

6 **E10.35 Type 1 diabetes mellitus with proliferative diabetic retinopathy**

One of the following 7th characters is to be assigned to codes in subcategory E10.35 to designate laterality of the disease:
1 right eye
2 left eye
3 bilateral
9 unspecified eye

SP 7 E10.351- **Type 1 diabetes mellitus with proliferative diabetic retinopathy with macular edema**

SP SH 7 E10.352- **Type 1 diabetes mellitus with proliferative diabetic retinopathy with traction retinal detachment involving the macula**

SP SH 7 E10.353- **Type 1 diabetes mellitus with proliferative diabetic retinopathy with traction retinal detachment not involving the macula**

SP SH 7 E10.354- **Type 1 diabetes mellitus with proliferative diabetic retinopathy with combined traction retinal detachment and rhegmatogenous retinal detachment**

SP SH 7 E10.355- **Type 1 diabetes mellitus with stable proliferative diabetic retinopathy**

SP SH 7 E10.359- **Type 1 diabetes mellitus with proliferative diabetic retinopathy without macular edema**

SP SH **E10.36 Type 1 diabetes mellitus with diabetic cataract**

CODING TIPS✓ Cataracts are more common in diabetic patients. The classification assumes a relationship between cataracts and diabetes, when the patient has diabetes. Even cataracts specifically described as "cortical, nuclear and posterior subcapsular" and "nuclear sclerotic" should prompt the assignment of E--.36, along with the code for the specific cataract code. (AHA: 2Q 2019)

SP SH 7 E10.37X- **Type 1 diabetes mellitus with diabetic macular edema, resolved following treatment**

One of the following 7th characters is to be assigned to code E10.37 to designate laterality of the disease:
1 right eye
2 left eye
3 bilateral
9 unspecified eye

CODING TIPS✓ The macular edema may be resolved, but the retinopathy remains. This code is like a history code for the macular edema.

SP SH + **E10.39 Type 1 diabetes mellitus with other diabetic ophthalmic complication**

Use additional code to identify manifestation, such as:
diabetic glaucoma (H40-H42)

CODING TIPS✓ There is no assumed relationship between diabetes and glaucoma. The coder should seek further clarification regarding the relationship between blindness, glaucoma and diabetes before coding as a diabetic manifestation.

Chapter 4

E00-E89

5 E10.4 Type 1 diabetes mellitus with neurological complications

CODING TIPS✓ Type 1 diabetes with loss of protective sensation or diabetic peripheral neuropathy should be coded to E10.42.

SP SH SL **E10.40 Type 1 diabetes mellitus with diabetic neuropathy, unspecified**

SP SH **E10.41 Type 1 diabetes mellitus with diabetic mononeuropathy**

SP SH SL **E10.42 Type 1 diabetes mellitus with diabetic polyneuropathy**

Type 1 diabetes mellitus with diabetic neuralgia

CODING TIPS✓ Do not use diabetic polyneuropathy as the etiology of diabetic ulcers. Instead, assign E--.621 or E--.622 followed by the code(s) for the ulcer(s). Assign diabetic polyneuropathy as a comorbidity.

CODING TIPS✓ Diabetic polyneuropathy is the most common type of diabetic neuropathy and causes pain or loss of feeling in the toes, feet, legs, hands and arms.

SP SH **E10.43 Type 1 diabetes mellitus with diabetic autonomic (poly)neuropathy**

Type 1 diabetes mellitus with diabetic gastroparesis

CODING TIPS✓ Autonomic neuropathy affects the heart, digestive system and other involuntary functions. This type of neuropathy causes delayed or slowed gastric emptying as well as problems with orthostatic hypotension. This code is not to be used for polyneuropathy of the hands and feet.

CODING TIPS✓ Gastroparesis (K31.84) may be sequenced after this code as an option.

SP SH **E10.44 Type 1 diabetes mellitus with diabetic amyotrophy**

CODING TIPS✓ Diabetic amyotrophy is muscle weakness, characterized by weakness followed by wasting of pelvifemoral muscles, either unilaterally or bilaterally, with associated pain.

SP SH **E10.49 Type 1 diabetes mellitus with other diabetic neurological complication**

5 E10.5 Type 1 diabetes mellitus with circulatory complications

CODING TIPS✓ Peripheral angiopathy includes arterial, venous and capillary conditions. Peripheral angiopathy may be documented as diabetic PVD. There is an assumed relationship between diabetes and PVD and PAD, including peripheral atherosclerosis and venous insufficiency. Diabetic PVD is coded E--.51. Diabetic arteriosclerosis of the peripheral arteries should be coded E--.51 or E--.52 then the appropriate I70.- code. Diabetic venous insufficiency should be coded E--.51 or E--.52 and I87.2 The presence of diabetes and peripheral arterial disease in the record indicates that both diabetes and PVD should be marked in M1028. Venous disease is not included in M1028.

SP SH **E10.51 Type 1 diabetes mellitus with diabetic peripheral angiopathy without gangrene**

CODING TIPS✓ Do not use diabetic peripheral angiopathy as the etiology of diabetic ulcers. Assign codes E--.621 or E--.622 instead followed by the code(s) for the ulcer(s). Assign diabetic angiopathy as a comorbidity.

CODING TIPS✓ If the physician or NPP documents diabetes and venous stasis ulcer, the E--.51 code precedes the code for the venous disease and the ulcer. If wound care is the focus of the care, use Z48.00 as the primary code.

SP SH **E10.52 Type 1 diabetes mellitus with diabetic peripheral angiopathy with gangrene**

Type 1 diabetes mellitus with diabetic gangrene

SP SH **E10.59 Type 1 diabetes mellitus with other circulatory complications**

CODING TIPS✓ Diabetic circulatory complications other than peripheral angiopathy and gangrene, identified as such by the physician or NPP, may be coded to 4th and 5th characters .59. Example: Diabetic CAD or ASHD is documented.

5 E10.6 Type 1 diabetes mellitus with other specified complications

6 E10.61 Type 1 diabetes mellitus with diabetic arthropathy

SP SH **E10.610 Type 1 diabetes mellitus with diabetic neuropathic arthropathy**

Type 1 diabetes mellitus with Charcôt's joints

CODING TIPS✓ Do not add a M14.6 code for Charcot's joint.

SP SH **E10.618 Type 1 diabetes mellitus with other diabetic arthropathy**

6 E10.62 Type 1 diabetes mellitus with skin complications

SP SH **E10.620 Type 1 diabetes mellitus with diabetic dermatitis**

Type 1 diabetes mellitus with diabetic necrobiosis lipoidica

SP SH + **E10.621 Type 1 diabetes mellitus with foot ulcer**

Chapter 4

E00-E89

Use additional code to identify site of ulcer (L97.4-, L97.5-)

CODING TIPS✓ If the patient has had a diabetic foot ulcer in the past, either healed or amputated, also code Z86.31. Ulceration of the foot is assumed related to diabetes unless another cause is indicated.

SP SH + **E10.622 Type 1 diabetes mellitus with other skin ulcer**

Use additional code to identify site of ulcer (L97.1-L97.9, L98.41-L98.49)

CODING TIPS✓ Diabetes codes with 4th, 5th and 6th characters .622 are used when an ulcer is located on the lower extremity, beginning at the ankle, and not including the foot. Whereas ulcers located on the foot are assumed related to diabetes, ulcers located elsewhere are not assumed related to diabetes and must be confirmed with the provider.

SP SH **E10.628 Type 1 diabetes mellitus with other skin complications**

6 **E10.63 Type 1 diabetes mellitus with oral complications**

SP SH **E10.630 Type 1 diabetes mellitus with periodontal disease**

SP SH **E10.638 Type 1 diabetes mellitus with other oral complications**

6 **E10.64 Type 1 diabetes mellitus with hypoglycemia**

SP SH **E10.641 Type 1 diabetes mellitus with hypoglycemia with coma**

SP SH **E10.649 Type 1 diabetes mellitus with hypoglycemia without coma**

CODING TIPS✓ The physician or NPP should be queried when the term "uncontrolled" is used to determine whether the patient has hyperglycemia, hypoglycemia or both.

CODING TIPS✓ If encephalopathy is due to hypoglycemia, use G93.41 as an additional code.

SP SH **E10.65 Type 1 diabetes mellitus with hyperglycemia**

CODING TIPS✓ Inadequately controlled, poorly controlled and out of control diabetes are coded with hyperglycemia. The physician or NPP should be queried when the term 'uncontrolled' is used to determine whether the patient has hyperglycemia, hypoglycemia, or both. The clinical record should support hyperglycemia. Do not code diabetes with hyperglycemia when ketoacidosis is also documented.

SP SH + **E10.69 Type 1 diabetes mellitus with other specified complication**

Use additional code to identify complication

CODING TIPS✓ Use this code when the physician or NPP specifies a manifestation of diabetes that does not fit in any of the other subcategories. Follow the diabetes code with the code for the specified condition.

CODING TIPS✓ The classification presumes a cause-and-effect relationship between osteomyelitis and diabetes when no other cause is documented. Osteomyelitis with diabetes is usually associated with ulceration. Use the appropriate code for the osteomyelitis after coding diabetes with other specified manifestation (E--.69). Although not clear when referencing diabetes in the index, it has been confirmed that osteomyelitis is related to all diabetes types.

IQ **E10.8 Type 1 diabetes mellitus with unspecified complications**

CODING TIPS✓ This code should not be used for unspecified complications. Query the physician or NPP for information regarding suspected manifestations that the classification does not presume related.

SP SH **E10.9 Type 1 diabetes mellitus without complications**

CODING TIPS✓ This code is acceptable to use for a diabetic without manifestations. Certain specified conditions are assumed related to diabetes by the classification, if listed indented under the word "with" in the alphabetical index, so the use of .9 as a diabetes 4th character should not be common. Query the physician or NPP for information regarding suspected manifestations when documentation regarding other potential causes is unclear. This code should be used for a diabetic requiring insulin injections only if teaching is the skill, or other comorbidities, unrelated to diabetes, make it unacceptable for the patient to self-inject. If .9 is used as a 4th character, no other diabetes code may be used.

+ 4 **E11 Type 2 diabetes mellitus**

INCLUDES diabetes (mellitus) due to insulin secretory defect
diabetes NOS
insulin resistant diabetes (mellitus)

Use additional code to identify control using:
insulin (Z79.4)
oral antidiabetic drugs (Z79.84)
oral hypoglycemic drugs (Z79.84)

EXCLUDES 1 diabetes mellitus due to underlying condition (E08.-)
drug or chemical induced diabetes mellitus (E09.-)
gestational diabetes (O24.4-)
neonatal diabetes mellitus (P70.2)
postpancreatectomy diabetes mellitus (E13.-)
postprocedural diabetes mellitus (E13.-)

Chapter 4 E00-E89

secondary diabetes mellitus NEC (E13.-)
type 1 diabetes mellitus (E10.-)

GUIDELINES **Section I.C.4.a.2)-3)**
If the type of diabetes mellitus is not documented in the medical record the default is E11.-, Type 2 diabetes mellitus. If the documentation in a medical record does not indicate the type of diabetes but does indicate that the patient uses insulin, code E11, Type 2 diabetes mellitus, should be assigned.
An additional code should be assigned from category Z79 to identify the long-term (current) use of insulin or oral hypoglycemic drugs. If the patient is treated with both oral medications and insulin, only the code for long-term (current) use of insulin should be assigned ...
Code Z79.4 should not be assigned if insulin is given temporarily to bring a type 2 patient's blood sugar under control during an encounter.

CODING TIPS✓ If the patient uses an insulin pump, use Z96.41 as an additional code. If there is a complication involving the insulin pump, use a code from T85.6- or T85.7- instead of the Z code.

CODING TIPS✓ Use Z79.4 to indicate the use of insulin, OR use Z79.84 to indicate the use of oral anti-glycemics. Use Z79.84 only when the patient does not also take insulin. Do NOT code both.
Use Z79.899 for non-insulin anti-diabetic medications. Z79.899 may be used with Z79.84 or with Z79.4.

CODING TIPS✓ Reference the alphabetical index to review conditions that the classification assumes are related to diabetes. All specified manifestations/complications listed under the word 'with' in the index are presumed related unless the physician or NPP specifies a different cause in documentation, or states they're unrelated. The "with" convention does not apply to "not elsewhere classified (NEC)" index entries that cover broad categories of conditions. Specific conditions must be linked by the terms "with," "in," "due to" or "associated with." Coding professionals should not assume a causal relationship when the diabetic complication is "NEC."

CODING TIPS✓ When clinical record diagnostic statements do not indicate a specific type of diabetes, a code from category E11 (Type 2 diabetes) should be assigned.

+ 5 **E11.0 Type 2 diabetes mellitus with hyperosmolarity**

DEFINITION Metabolic diabetic emergency presenting with altered consciousness varying from confusion or disorientation to coma, with extreme dehydration, and high blood concentrations of sugar and sodium.

SP SH + **E11.00 Type 2 diabetes mellitus with hyperosmolarity without nonketotic hyperglycemic-hyperosmolar coma (NKHHC)**

SP SH + **E11.01 Type 2 diabetes mellitus with hyperosmolarity with coma**

+ 5 **E11.1 Type 2 diabetes mellitus with ketoacidosis**

SP SH + **E11.10 Type 2 diabetes mellitus with ketoacidosis without coma**

CODING TIPS✓ Diabetic ketoacidosis is a serious complication of diabetes that occurs when the body produces high levels of blood acids called ketones. Query the physician or NPP to determine if the condition is resolved prior to home care. Diabetic ketoacidosis is rare in type 2 diabetes, so if the documentation states diabetic ketoacidosis, query the physician or NPP as to type of diabetes.

SP SH + **E11.11 Type 2 diabetes mellitus with ketoacidosis with coma**

+ 5 **E11.2 Type 2 diabetes mellitus with kidney complications**

CODING TIPS✓ Diabetic triopathy refers to the most common types of manifestations of diabetes: nephropathy, retinopathy and neuropathy.

SP SH + **E11.21 Type 2 diabetes mellitus with diabetic nephropathy**
Type 2 diabetes mellitus with intercapillary glomerulosclerosis
Type 2 diabetes mellitus with intracapillary glomerulonephrosis
Type 2 diabetes mellitus with Kimmelstiel-Wilson disease

SP SH + **E11.22 Type 2 diabetes mellitus with diabetic chronic kidney disease**
Use additional code to identify stage of chronic kidney disease (N18.1-N18.6)

CODING TIPS✓ When diabetes, CKD and hypertension are documented, sequence the appropriate category of diabetes with CKD (E--.22) and the appropriate hypertension code (I12 or I13) prior to N18. The hypertension or the diabetes may be sequenced first depending on the focus of care. Use N18.1-N18.6 or N18.9 to indicate the CKD. These conditions are all considered related unless the physician or NPP indicates they are not related. For example, if the provider documents diabetic CKD, this indicates that hypertension is not related to the CKD.

CODING TIPS✓ Assign an additional code from N18- to indicate the stage of CKD. When diabetic nephropathy and CKD are documented, code diabetic CKD, not nephropathy, because CKD is more specific.

SP SH + **E11.29 Type 2 diabetes mellitus with other diabetic kidney complication**
Type 2 diabetes mellitus with renal tubular degeneration

+ 5 **E11.3 Type 2 diabetes mellitus with ophthalmic complications**

CODING TIPS✓ The 7th character codes in this category that are acceptable primary diagnoses in PDGM and contribute to a comorbidity adjustment are those with a 7th character of 1, 2, or 3. Unspecified eye (7th character of 9) is not acceptable as a primary diagnoses in PDGM, nor does it contribute to a comorbidity adjustment.

CODING TIPS✓ Diabetic codes indicating specific eye disorders require a 7th character to indicate laterality.

CODING TIPS✓ Diabetic triopathy refers to the most common types of manifestations of diabetes: nephropathy, retinopathy and neuropathy.

CODING TIPS✓ When coding diabetes with ophthalmic manifestations, review the clinical record and plan of care to ensure that the functional impact of visual impairments is reported. The home health record should clearly report how visual losses impact the function and activities of the patient, including how these conditions impact medication administration, safety, the ability to perform treatments (such as wound care) and other key areas related to the patient's daily living.

CODING TIPS✓ When a patient has macular edema, the patient also has retinopathy, with the macular edema developing as a complication of the retinopathy. Retinopathy includes three stages: background retinopathy, proliferative retinopathy, and macular edema.

+ 6 **E11.31** **Type 2 diabetes mellitus with unspecified diabetic retinopathy**

SP + **E11.311** **Type 2 diabetes mellitus with unspecified diabetic retinopathy with macular edema**

SP SH + **E11.319** **Type 2 diabetes mellitus with unspecified diabetic retinopathy without macular edema**

+ 6 **E11.32** **Type 2 diabetes mellitus with mild nonproliferative diabetic retinopathy**

Type 2 diabetes mellitus with nonproliferative diabetic retinopathy NOS

One of the following 7th characters is to be assigned to codes in subcategory E11.32 to designate laterality of the disease:

1	right eye
2	left eye
3	bilateral
9	unspecified eye

⊟ SP + 7 **E11.321-** **Type 2 diabetes mellitus with mild nonproliferative diabetic retinopathy with macular edema**

⊟ SP SH + 7 **E11.329-** **Type 2 diabetes mellitus with mild nonproliferative diabetic retinopathy without macular edema**

+ 6 **E11.33** **Type 2 diabetes mellitus with moderate nonproliferative diabetic retinopathy**

One of the following 7th characters is to be assigned to codes in subcategory E11.33 to designate laterality of the disease:

1	right eye
2	left eye
3	bilateral
9	unspecified eye

⊟ SP + 7 **E11.331-** **Type 2 diabetes mellitus with moderate nonproliferative diabetic retinopathy with macular edema**

⊟ SP SH + 7 **E11.339-** **Type 2 diabetes mellitus with moderate nonproliferative diabetic retinopathy without macular edema**

+ 6 **E11.34** **Type 2 diabetes mellitus with severe nonproliferative diabetic retinopathy**

One of the following 7th characters is to be assigned to codes in subcategory E11.34 to designate laterality of the disease:

1	right eye
2	left eye
3	bilateral
9	unspecified eye

⊟ SP + 7 **E11.341-** **Type 2 diabetes mellitus with severe nonproliferative diabetic retinopathy with macular edema**

⊟ SP SH + 7 **E11.349-** **Type 2 diabetes mellitus with severe nonproliferative diabetic retinopathy without macular edema**

+ 6 **E11.35** **Type 2 diabetes mellitus with proliferative diabetic retinopathy**

One of the following 7th characters is to be assigned to codes in subcategory E11.35 to designate laterality of the disease:

1	right eye
2	left eye
3	bilateral
9	unspecified eye

⊟ SP + 7 **E11.351-** **Type 2 diabetes mellitus with proliferative diabetic retinopathy with macular edema**

⊟ SP SH + 7 **E11.352-** **Type 2 diabetes mellitus with proliferative diabetic retinopathy with traction retinal detachment involving the macula**

⊟ SP SH + 7 **E11.353-** **Type 2 diabetes mellitus with proliferative diabetic retinopathy with traction retinal detachment not involving the macula**

E11.354- **Type 2 diabetes mellitus with proliferative diabetic retinopathy with combined traction retinal detachment and rhegmatogenous retinal detachment**

E11.355- **Type 2 diabetes mellitus with stable proliferative diabetic retinopathy**

E11.359- **Type 2 diabetes mellitus with proliferative diabetic retinopathy without macular edema**

E11.36 **Type 2 diabetes mellitus with diabetic cataract**

CODING TIPS✓ Cataracts are more common in diabetic patients. The classification assumes a relationship between cataracts and diabetes, when the patient has diabetes. Even cataracts specifically described as "cortical, nuclear and posterior subcapsular" and "nuclear sclerotic" should prompt the assignment of E--.36, along with the code for the specific cataract code. (AHA: 2Q 2019)

E11.37X- **Type 2 diabetes mellitus with diabetic macular edema, resolved following treatment**

One of the following 7th characters is to be assigned to code E11.37 to designate laterality of the disease:

1	right eye
2	left eye
3	bilateral
9	unspecified eye

CODING TIPS✓ The macular edema may be resolved, but the retinopathy remains. This code is like a history code for the macular edema.

E11.39 **Type 2 diabetes mellitus with other diabetic ophthalmic complication**

Use additional code to identify manifestation, such as:
diabetic glaucoma (H40-H42)

CODING TIPS✓ There is no assumed relationship between diabetes and glaucoma. The coder should seek further clarification regarding the relationship between blindness, glaucoma and diabetes before coding as a diabetic manifestation.

E11.4 **Type 2 diabetes mellitus with neurological complications**

CODING TIPS✓ Type 2 or unspecified diabetes with loss of protective sensation or diabetic peripheral neuropathy with loss of protective sensation should be coded to E11.42.

CODING TIPS✓ Diabetic triopathy refers to the most common types of manifestations of diabetes: nephropathy, retinopathy and neuropathy.

E11.40 **Type 2 diabetes mellitus with diabetic neuropathy, unspecified**

E11.41 **Type 2 diabetes mellitus with diabetic mononeuropathy**

E11.42 **Type 2 diabetes mellitus with diabetic polyneuropathy**

Type 2 diabetes mellitus with diabetic neuralgia

CODING TIPS✓ Do not use diabetic polyneuropathy as the etiology of diabetic ulcers. Instead, assign E--.621 or E--.622 followed by the code(s) for the ulcer(s). Assign diabetic polyneuropathy as a comorbidity.

CODING TIPS✓ Diabetic polyneuropathy is the most common type of diabetic neuropathy and causes pain or loss of feeling in the toes, feet, legs, hands and arms.

E11.43 **Type 2 diabetes mellitus with diabetic autonomic (poly)neuropathy**

Type 2 diabetes mellitus with diabetic gastroparesis

CODING TIPS✓ Autonomic neuropathy affects the heart, digestive system and other involuntary functions. This type of neuropathy causes delayed or slowed gastric emptying as well as problems with orthostatic hypotension. This code is not to be used for polyneuropathy of the hands and feet.

CODING TIPS✓ Gastroparesis (K31.84) may be sequenced after this code as an option.

E11.44 **Type 2 diabetes mellitus with diabetic amyotrophy**

CODING TIPS✓ Diabetic amyotrophy is muscle weakness, characterized by weakness followed by wasting of pelvifemoral muscles, either unilaterally or bilaterally, with associated pain.

E11.49 **Type 2 diabetes mellitus with other diabetic neurological complication**

E11.5 **Type 2 diabetes mellitus with circulatory complications**

CODING TIPS✓ Peripheral angiopathy includes arterial, venous and capillary conditions. Peripheral angiopathy may be documented as diabetic PVD. There is an assumed relationship between diabetes and PVD and PAD, including peripheral atherosclerosis and venous insufficiency. Diabetic PVD is coded E--.51. Diabetic arteriosclerosis of the peripheral arteries should be coded E--.51 or E--.52 then the appropriate I70.- code. Diabetic venous insufficiency should be coded E--.51 or E--.52 and I87.2 The presence of diabetes and peripheral arterial disease in the record indicates that both diabetes and PVD should be marked in M1028. Venous disease is not included in M1028.

E11.51 **Type 2 diabetes mellitus with diabetic peripheral angiopathy without gangrene**

CODING TIPS✓ If the physician or NPP documents diabetes and venous stasis ulcer, the E--.51 code precedes the code for the venous disease and the ulcer. If wound care is the focus of the care, use Z48.00 as the primary code.

CODING TIPS✓ Do not use diabetic peripheral angiopathy as the etiology of diabetic ulcers. Assign codes E--.621 or E--.622 instead followed by the code(s) for the ulcer(s). Assign diabetic angiopathy as a comorbidity.

SP SH + **E11.52 Type 2 diabetes mellitus with diabetic peripheral angiopathy with gangrene**
Type 2 diabetes mellitus with diabetic gangrene

SP SH + **E11.59 Type 2 diabetes mellitus with other circulatory complications**

CODING TIPS✓ Diabetic circulatory complications other than peripheral angiopathy and gangrene, identified as such by the physician or NPP, may be coded to 4th and 5th characters .59. Example: Diabetic CAD or ASHD is documented.

+ 5 **E11.6 Type 2 diabetes mellitus with other specified complications**

+ 6 **E11.61 Type 2 diabetes mellitus with diabetic arthropathy**

SP SH + **E11.610 Type 2 diabetes mellitus with diabetic neuropathic arthropathy**
Type 2 diabetes mellitus with Charcôt's joints

CODING TIPS✓ Do not add a M14.6 code for Charcot's joint.

SP SH + **E11.618 Type 2 diabetes mellitus with other diabetic arthropathy**

+ 6 **E11.62 Type 2 diabetes mellitus with skin complications**

SP SH + **E11.620 Type 2 diabetes mellitus with diabetic dermatitis**
Type 2 diabetes mellitus with diabetic necrobiosis lipoidica

SP SH + **E11.621 Type 2 diabetes mellitus with foot ulcer**
Use additional code to identify site of ulcer (L97.4-, L97.5-)

CODING TIPS✓ If the patient has had a diabetic foot ulcer in the past, either healed or amputated, also code Z86.31. Ulceration of the foot is assumed related to diabetes unless another cause is indicated.

SP SH + **E11.622 Type 2 diabetes mellitus with other skin ulcer**
Use additional code to identify site of ulcer (L97.1-L97.9, L98.41-L98.49)

CODING TIPS✓ Diabetes codes with 4th, 5th and 6th characters .622 are used when an ulcer is located on the lower extremity, beginning at the ankle, and not including the foot. Whereas ulcers located on the foot are assumed related to diabetes, ulcers located elsewhere are not assumed related to diabetes and must be confirmed with the provider.

SP SH + **E11.628 Type 2 diabetes mellitus with other skin complications**

+ 6 **E11.63 Type 2 diabetes mellitus with oral complications**

SP SH + **E11.630 Type 2 diabetes mellitus with periodontal disease**

SP SH + **E11.638 Type 2 diabetes mellitus with other oral complications**

+ 6 **E11.64 Type 2 diabetes mellitus with hypoglycemia**

SP SH + **E11.641 Type 2 diabetes mellitus with hypoglycemia with coma**

SP SH + **E11.649 Type 2 diabetes mellitus with hypoglycemia without coma**

CODING TIPS✓ The physician or NPP should be queried when the term "uncontrolled" is used to determine whether the patient has hyperglycemia, hypoglycemia or both.

CODING TIPS✓ If encephalopathy is due to hypoglycemia, use G93.41 as an additional code.

SP SH + **E11.65 Type 2 diabetes mellitus with hyperglycemia**

CODING TIPS✓ Inadequately controlled, poorly controlled and out of control diabetes are coded with hyperglycemia. The physician or NPP should be queried when the term 'uncontrolled' is used to determine whether the patient has hyperglycemia, hypoglycemia, or both. The clinical record should support hyperglycemia. Do not code diabetes with hyperglycemia when ketoacidosis is also documented.

SP SH + **E11.69 Type 2 diabetes mellitus with other specified complication**
Use additional code to identify complication

CODING TIPS✓ Use this code when the physician or NPP specifies a manifestation of diabetes that does not fit in any of the other subcategories. Follow the diabetes code with the code for the specified condition.

CODING TIPS✓ The classification presumes a cause-and-effect relationship between osteomyelitis and diabetes when no other cause is documented. Osteomyelitis with diabetes is usually associated with ulceration. Use the appropriate code for the osteomyelitis after coding diabetes with other specified manifestation (E--.69). Although not clear when referencing diabetes in the index, it has been confirmed that osteomyelitis is related to all diabetes types.

IQ + **E11.8 Type 2 diabetes mellitus with unspecified complications**

CODING TIPS✓ This code should not be used for unspecified complications. Query the physician or NPP for information regarding suspected manifestations that the classification does not presume related.

SP SH + **E11.9 Type 2 diabetes mellitus without complications**

CODING TIPS✓ This code is acceptable to use for a diabetic without manifestations. Certain specified conditions are assumed related to diabetes by the classification, if listed indented under the word "with" in the alphabetical index, so the use of .9 as a diabetes 4th character should not be common. Query the physician or NPP for information regarding suspected manifestations when documentation regarding other potential causes is unclear. This code should be used for a diabetic requiring insulin injections only if teaching is the skill, or other comorbidities, unrelated to diabetes, make it unacceptable for the patient to self-inject. If .9 is used as a 4th character, no other diabetes code may be used.

DEFINITION Underproduction or underutilization of insulin; presents with abnormally high blood sugar (glucose) levels, resulting in impaired carbohydrate and fat metabolism.

+ 4 **E13 Other specified diabetes mellitus**

INCLUDES diabetes mellitus due to genetic defects of beta-cell function
diabetes mellitus due to genetic defects in insulin action
postpancreatectomy diabetes mellitus
postprocedural diabetes mellitus
secondary diabetes mellitus NEC

Use additional code to identify control using:
insulin (Z79.4)
oral antidiabetic drugs (Z79.84)
oral hypoglycemic drugs (Z79.84)

EXCLUDES 1 diabetes (mellitus) due to autoimmune process (E10.-)
diabetes (mellitus) due to immune mediated pancreatic islet beta-cell destruction (E10.-)
diabetes mellitus due to underlying condition (E08.-)
drug or chemical induced diabetes mellitus (E09.-)
gestational diabetes (O24.4-)
neonatal diabetes mellitus (P70.2)
type 1 diabetes mellitus (E10.-)

GUIDELINES **Section I.C.4.a.6(a)**
Codes under categories E08, Diabetes mellitus due to underlying condition, E09, Drug or chemical induced diabetes mellitus, and E13, Other specified diabetes mellitus, identify complications/manifestations associated with secondary diabetes mellitus. Secondary diabetes is always caused by another condition or event (e.g., cystic fibrosis, malignant neoplasm of pancreas, pancreatectomy, adverse effect of drug, or poisoning).
For patients with secondary diabetes mellitus who routinely use insulin or oral hypoglycemic drugs, an additional code from category Z79 should be assigned to identify the long-term (current) use of insulin or oral hypoglycemic drugs. If the patient is treated with both oral medications and insulin, only the code for long-term (current) use of insulin should be assigned ... Code Z79.4 should not be assigned if insulin is given temporarily to bring a secondary diabetic patient's blood sugar under control during an encounter.

GUIDELINES **Section I.C.4.a.6)(b)(i)**
For postpancreatectomy diabetes mellitus (lack of insulin due to the surgical removal of all or part of the pancreas), assign code E89.1, Postprocedural hypoinsulinemia. Assign a code from category E13 and a code from subcategory Z90.41-, Acquired absence of pancreas, as additional codes.

CODING TIPS✓ If the patient uses an insulin pump, use Z96.41 as an additional code. If there is a complication involving the insulin pump, use a code from T85.6- or T85.7- instead of the Z code.

CODING TIPS✓ Use Z79.4 to indicate the use of insulin, OR use Z79.84 to indicate the use of oral anti-glycemics. Use Z79.84 only when the patient does not also take insulin. Do NOT code both.
Use Z79.899 for non-insulin anti-diabetic medications. Z79.899 may be used with Z79.84 or with Z79.4.

CODING TIPS✓ Reference the alphabetical index to review conditions that the classification assumes are related to diabetes. All specified manifestations/complications listed under the word 'with' in the index are presumed related unless the physician or NPP specifies a different cause in documentation, or states they're unrelated. The "with" convention does not apply to "not elsewhere classified (NEC)" index entries that cover broad categories of conditions. Specific conditions must be linked by the terms "with," "in," "due to" or "associated with." Coding professionals should not assume a causal relationship when the diabetic complication is "NEC."

CODING TIPS✓ If diabetes is related to a malignant neoplasm of the pancreas, query whether the diabetes is caused by the neoplasm itself (E08); the drugs used to treat the neoplasm (E09); or the removal of part or all of the pancreas (E13).

CODING TIPS✓ When postpancreatectomy or postprocedural diabetes is specified, the coder should first look in the Alphabetic Index and identify the terms "hypoinsulinemia, postprocedural- E89.1." Review of this code in the tabular index will instruct the coder to use an additional code for acquired absence of pancreas (Z90.41-), diabetes mellitus (postpancreatectomy) (postprocedural) (E13.-), and insulin use (Z79.4).

+ 5 E13.0 Other specified diabetes mellitus with hyperosmolarity

SP SH + E13.00 Other specified diabetes mellitus with hyperosmolarity without nonketotic hyperglycemic-hyperosmolar coma (NKHHC)

EXCLUDES 2 type 2 diabetes mellitus (E11.-)

SP SH + E13.01 Other specified diabetes mellitus with hyperosmolarity with coma

+ 5 E13.1 Other specified diabetes mellitus with ketoacidosis

CODING TIPS✓ Diabetic ketoacidosis is a serious complication of diabetes that occurs when the body produces high levels of blood acids called ketones. This condition is likely resolved before admission to home care, but could be a current diagnosis.

SP SH + E13.10 Other specified diabetes mellitus with ketoacidosis without coma

SP SH + E13.11 Other specified diabetes mellitus with ketoacidosis with coma

+ 5 E13.2 Other specified diabetes mellitus with kidney complications

SP SH + E13.21 Other specified diabetes mellitus with diabetic nephropathy

Other specified diabetes mellitus with intercapillary glomerulosclerosis

Other specified diabetes mellitus with intracapillary glomerulonephrosis

Other specified diabetes mellitus with Kimmelstiel-Wilson disease

SP SH + E13.22 Other specified diabetes mellitus with diabetic chronic kidney disease

Use additional code to identify stage of chronic kidney disease (N18.1-N18.6)

CODING TIPS✓ When diabetes, CKD and hypertension are documented, sequence the appropriate category of diabetes with CKD (E--.22) and the appropriate hypertension code (I12 or I13) prior to N18. The hypertension or the diabetes may be sequenced first depending on the focus of care. Use N18.1-N18.6 or N18.9 to indicate the CKD. These conditions are all considered related unless the physician or NPP indicates they are not related. For example, if the provider documents diabetic CKD, this indicates that hypertension is not related to the CKD.

CODING TIPS✓ Assign an additional code from N18- to indicate the stage of CKD. When diabetic nephropathy and CKD are documented, code diabetic CKD, not nephropathy, because CKD is more specific.

SP SH + E13.29 Other specified diabetes mellitus with other diabetic kidney complication

Other specified diabetes mellitus with renal tubular degeneration

+ 5 E13.3 Other specified diabetes mellitus with ophthalmic complications

CODING TIPS✓ The 7th character codes in this category that are acceptable primary diagnoses in PDGM and contribute to a comorbidity adjustment are those with a 7th character of 1, 2, or 3. Unspecified eye (7th character of 9) is not acceptable as a primary diagnoses in PDGM, nor does it contribute to a comorbidity adjustment.

CODING TIPS✓ Diabetic codes indicating specific eye disorders require a 7th character to indicate laterality.

CODING TIPS✓ When a patient has macular edema, the patient also has retinopathy, with the macular edema developing as a complication of the retinopathy. Retinopathy includes three stages: background retinopathy, proliferative retinopathy, and macular edema.

CODING TIPS✓ When coding diabetes with ophthalmic manifestations, review the clinical record and plan of care to ensure that the functional impact of visual impairments is reported. The home health record should clearly report how visual losses impact the function and activities of the patient, including how these conditions impact medication administration, safety, the ability to perform treatments (such as wound care) and other key areas related to the patient's daily living.

+ 6 E13.31 Other specified diabetes mellitus with unspecified diabetic retinopathy

SP + E13.311 Other specified diabetes mellitus with unspecified diabetic retinopathy with macular edema

SP SH + **E13.319 Other specified diabetes mellitus with unspecified diabetic retinopathy without macular edema**

+ 6 **E13.32 Other specified diabetes mellitus with mild nonproliferative diabetic retinopathy**

Other specified diabetes mellitus with nonproliferative diabetic retinopathy NOS

One of the following 7th characters is to be assigned to codes in subcategory E13.32 to designate laterality of the disease:

1	right eye
2	left eye
3	bilateral
9	unspecified eye

L SP + 7 **E13.321- Other specified diabetes mellitus with mild nonproliferative diabetic retinopathy with macular edema**

L SP SH + 7 **E13.329- Other specified diabetes mellitus with mild nonproliferative diabetic retinopathy without macular edema**

+ 6 **E13.33 Other specified diabetes mellitus with moderate nonproliferative diabetic retinopathy**

One of the following 7th characters is to be assigned to codes in subcategory E13.33 to designate laterality of the disease:

1	right eye
2	left eye
3	bilateral
9	unspecified eye

L SP + 7 **E13.331- Other specified diabetes mellitus with moderate nonproliferative diabetic retinopathy with macular edema**

L SP SH + 7 **E13.339- Other specified diabetes mellitus with moderate nonproliferative diabetic retinopathy without macular edema**

+ 6 **E13.34 Other specified diabetes mellitus with severe nonproliferative diabetic retinopathy**

One of the following 7th characters is to be assigned to codes in subcategory E13.34 to designate laterality of the disease:

1	right eye
2	left eye
3	bilateral
9	unspecified eye

L SP + 7 **E13.341- Other specified diabetes mellitus with severe nonproliferative diabetic retinopathy with macular edema**

L SP SH + 7 **E13.349- Other specified diabetes mellitus with severe nonproliferative diabetic retinopathy without macular edema**

+ 6 **E13.35 Other specified diabetes mellitus with proliferative diabetic retinopathy**

One of the following 7th characters is to be assigned to codes in subcategory E13.35 to designate laterality of the disease:

1	right eye
2	left eye
3	bilateral
9	unspecified eye

L SP + 7 **E13.351- Other specified diabetes mellitus with proliferative diabetic retinopathy with macular edema**

L SP SH + 7 **E13.352- Other specified diabetes mellitus with proliferative diabetic retinopathy with traction retinal detachment involving the macula**

L SP SH + 7 **E13.353- Other specified diabetes mellitus with proliferative diabetic retinopathy with traction retinal detachment not involving the macula**

L SP SH + 7 **E13.354- Other specified diabetes mellitus with proliferative diabetic retinopathy with combined traction retinal detachment and rhegmatogenous retinal detachment**

L SP SH + 7 **E13.355- Other specified diabetes mellitus with stable proliferative diabetic retinopathy**

L SP SH + 7 **E13.359- Other specified diabetes mellitus with proliferative diabetic retinopathy without macular edema**

SP SH + **E13.36 Other specified diabetes mellitus with diabetic cataract**

CODING TIPS✓ Cataracts are more common in diabetic patients. The classification assumes a relationship between cataracts and diabetes, when the patient has diabetes. Even cataracts specifically described as "cortical, nuclear and posterior subcapsular" and "nuclear sclerotic" should prompt the assignment of E--.36, along with the code for the specific cataract code. (AHA: 2Q 2019)

L SP SH + **E13.37X-** X7 **Other specified diabetes mellitus with diabetic macular edema, resolved following treatment**

Chapter 4

E00-E89

One of the following 7th characters is to be assigned to code E13.37 to designate laterality of the disease:
1 right eye
2 left eye
3 bilateral
9 unspecified eye

CODING TIPS✓ The macular edema may be resolved, but the retinopathy remains. This code is like a history code for the macular edema.

SP SH + **E13.39 Other specified diabetes mellitus with other diabetic ophthalmic complication**
Use additional code to identify manifestation, such as:
diabetic glaucoma (H40-H42)

CODING TIPS✓ There is no assumed relationship between diabetes and glaucoma. The coder should seek further clarification regarding the relationship between blindness, glaucoma and diabetes before coding as a diabetic manifestation.

+ 5 **E13.4 Other specified diabetes mellitus with neurological complications**

CODING TIPS✓ Other specified diabetes with loss of protective sensation or diabetic peripheral neuropathy should be coded to E13.42.

!Q SH SL + **E13.40 Other specified diabetes mellitus with diabetic neuropathy, unspecified**

SP SH + **E13.41 Other specified diabetes mellitus with diabetic mononeuropathy**

SP SH SL + **E13.42 Other specified diabetes mellitus with diabetic polyneuropathy**
Other specified diabetes mellitus with diabetic neuralgia

CODING TIPS✓ Do not use diabetic polyneuropathy as the etiology of diabetic ulcers. Instead, assign E--.621 or E--.622 followed by the code(s) for the ulcer(s). Assign diabetic polyneuropathy as a comorbidity.

CODING TIPS✓ Diabetic polyneuropathy is the most common type of diabetic neuropathy and causes pain or loss of feeling in the toes, feet, legs, hands and arms.

SP SH + **E13.43 Other specified diabetes mellitus with diabetic autonomic (poly)neuropathy**
Other specified diabetes mellitus with diabetic gastroparesis

CODING TIPS✓ Autonomic neuropathy affects the heart, digestive system and other involuntary functions. This type of neuropathy causes delayed or slowed gastric emptying as well as problems with orthostatic hypotension. This code is not to be used for polyneuropathy of the hands and feet.

CODING TIPS✓ Gastroparesis (K31.84) may be sequenced after this code as an option.

SP SH + **E13.44 Other specified diabetes mellitus with diabetic amyotrophy**

CODING TIPS✓ Diabetic amyotrophy is muscle weakness, characterized by weakness followed by wasting of pelvifemoral muscles, either unilaterally or bilaterally, with associated pain.

SP SH + **E13.49 Other specified diabetes mellitus with other diabetic neurological complication**

+ 5 **E13.5 Other specified diabetes mellitus with circulatory complications**

CODING TIPS✓ Peripheral angiopathy includes arterial, venous and capillary conditions. Peripheral angiopathy may be documented as diabetic PVD. There is an assumed relationship between diabetes and PVD and PAD, including peripheral atherosclerosis and venous insufficiency. Diabetic PVD is coded E--.51. Diabetic arteriosclerosis of the peripheral arteries should be coded E--.51 or E--.52 then the appropriate I70.- code. Diabetic venous insufficiency should be coded E--.51 or E--.52 and I87.2 The presence of diabetes and peripheral arterial disease in the record indicates that both diabetes and PVD should be marked in M1028. Venous disease is not included in M1028.

SP SH + **E13.51 Other specified diabetes mellitus with diabetic peripheral angiopathy without gangrene**

CODING TIPS✓ Do not use diabetic peripheral angiopathy as the etiology of diabetic ulcers. Assign codes E--.621 or E--.622 instead followed by the code(s) for the ulcer(s). Assign diabetic angiopathy as a comorbidity.

CODING TIPS✓ If the physician or NPP documents diabetes and venous stasis ulcer, the E--.51 code precedes the code for the venous disease and the ulcer. If wound care is the focus of the care, use Z48.00 as the primary code.

SP SH + **E13.52 Other specified diabetes mellitus with diabetic peripheral angiopathy with gangrene**
Other specified diabetes mellitus with diabetic gangrene

SP SH + **E13.59 Other specified diabetes mellitus with other circulatory complications**

CODING TIPS✓ Diabetic circulatory complications other than peripheral angiopathy and gangrene, identified as such by the physician or NPP, may be coded to 4th and 5th characters .59. Example: Diabetic CAD or ASHD is documented.

+ 5 **E13.6 Other specified diabetes mellitus with other specified complications**

+ 6 **E13.61 Other specified diabetes mellitus with diabetic arthropathy**

SP SH + **E13.610 Other specified diabetes mellitus with diabetic neuropathic arthropathy**
Other specified diabetes mellitus with Charcôt's joints
CODING TIPS✓ Do not add a M14.6 code for Charcot's joint.

SP SH + **E13.618 Other specified diabetes mellitus with other diabetic arthropathy**

+ 6 **E13.62 Other specified diabetes mellitus with skin complications**

SP SH + **E13.620 Other specified diabetes mellitus with diabetic dermatitis**
Other specified diabetes mellitus with diabetic necrobiosis lipoidica

SP SH + **E13.621 Other specified diabetes mellitus with foot ulcer**
Use additional code to identify site of ulcer (L97.4-, L97.5-)
CODING TIPS✓ If the patient has had a diabetic foot ulcer in the past, either healed or amputated, also code Z86.31. Ulceration of the foot is assumed related to diabetes unless another cause is indicated.

SP SH + **E13.622 Other specified diabetes mellitus with other skin ulcer**
Use additional code to identify site of ulcer (L97.1-L97.9, L98.41-L98.49)
CODING TIPS✓ Diabetes codes with 4th, 5th and 6th characters .622 are used when an ulcer is located on the lower extremity, beginning at the ankle, and not including the foot. Whereas ulcers located on the foot are assumed related to diabetes, ulcers located elsewhere are not assumed related to diabetes and must be confirmed with the provider.

SP SH + **E13.628 Other specified diabetes mellitus with other skin complications**

+ 6 **E13.63 Other specified diabetes mellitus with oral complications**

SP SH + **E13.630 Other specified diabetes mellitus with periodontal disease**

SP SH + **E13.638 Other specified diabetes mellitus with other oral complications**

+ 6 **E13.64 Other specified diabetes mellitus with hypoglycemia**

SP SH + **E13.641 Other specified diabetes mellitus with hypoglycemia with coma**

SP SH + **E13.649 Other specified diabetes mellitus with hypoglycemia without coma**
CODING TIPS✓ The physician or NPP should be queried when the term "uncontrolled" is used to determine whether the patient has hyperglycemia, hypoglycemia or both.
CODING TIPS✓ If encephalopathy is due to hypoglycemia, use G93.41 as an additional code.

SP SH + **E13.65 Other specified diabetes mellitus with hyperglycemia**
CODING TIPS✓ Inadequately controlled, poorly controlled and out of control diabetes are coded with hyperglycemia. The physician or NPP should be queried when the term 'uncontrolled' is used to determine whether the patient has hyperglycemia, hypoglycemia, or both. The clinical record should support hyperglycemia. Do not code diabetes with hyperglycemia when ketoacidosis is also documented.

SP SH + **E13.69 Other specified diabetes mellitus with other specified complication**
Use additional code to identify complication
CODING TIPS✓ Use this code when the physician or NPP specifies a manifestation of diabetes that does not fit in any of the other subcategories. Follow the diabetes code with the code for the specified condition.
CODING TIPS✓ The classification presumes a cause-and-effect relationship between osteomyelitis and diabetes when no other cause is documented. Osteomyelitis with diabetes is usually associated with ulceration. Use the appropriate code for the osteomyelitis after coding diabetes with other specified manifestation (E--.69). Although not clear when referencing diabetes in the index, it has been confirmed that osteomyelitis is related to all diabetes types.

IQ + **E13.8 Other specified diabetes mellitus with unspecified complications**
CODING TIPS✓ This code should not be used for unspecified complications. Query the physician or NPP for information regarding suspected manifestations that the classification does not presume related.

SP SH + **E13.9 Other specified diabetes mellitus without complications**
CODING TIPS✓ This code is acceptable to use for a diabetic without manifestations. Certain specified conditions are assumed related to diabetes by the classification, if listed indented under the word "with" in the alphabetical index, so the use of .9 as a diabetes 4th character should not be common. Query the physician or NPP for information regarding suspected manifestations when documentation regarding other potential causes is unclear. This code should be used for a diabetic requiring insulin injections only if teaching is the skill, or other comorbidities, unrelated to diabetes, make it unacceptable for the patient to self-inject. If .9 is used as a 4th character, no other diabetes code may be used.

Other disorders of glucose regulation and pancreatic internal secretion (E15-E16)

SP **E15 Nondiabetic hypoglycemic coma**

INCLUDES drug-induced insulin coma in nondiabetic
hyperinsulinism with hypoglycemic coma
hypoglycemic coma NOS

4 **E16 Other disorders of pancreatic internal secretion**

SP + **E16.0 Drug-induced hypoglycemia without coma**

Use additional code for adverse effect, if applicable, to identify drug (T36-T50 with fifth or sixth character 5)

EXCLUDES 1 diabetes with hypoglycemia without coma (E09.649)

CODING TIPS✓ Use this code for drug induced hypoglycemia in someone who is not diabetic.

SP **E16.1 Other hypoglycemia**

Functional hyperinsulinism
Functional nonhyperinsulinemic hypoglycemia
Hyperinsulinism NOS
Hyperplasia of pancreatic islet beta cells NOS

EXCLUDES 1 diabetes with hypoglycemia (E08.649, E10.649, E11.649, E13.649)
hypoglycemia in infant of diabetic mother (P70.1)
neonatal hypoglycemia (P70.4)

CODING TIPS✓ Do not assign E16.1 to report hypoglycemia in a patient with a known diagnosis of diabetes, including post-procedural hypoinsulinemia.

SP **E16.2 Hypoglycemia, unspecified**

EXCLUDES 1 diabetes with hypoglycemia (E08.649, E10.649, E11.649, E13.649)

CODING TIPS✓ Report this code for someone who has hypoglycemia and is not diabetic.

DEFINITION Condition in which blood sugar levels are too low for normal functioning, manifesting as weakness, trembling, hunger, headache, irritability, racing heartbeat, confusion, even convulsions or coma.

SP **E16.3 Increased secretion of glucagon**

Hyperplasia of pancreatic endocrine cells with glucagon excess

SP **E16.4 Increased secretion of gastrin**

Hypergastrinemia
Hyperplasia of pancreatic endocrine cells with gastrin excess
Zollinger-Ellison syndrome

SP **E16.8 Other specified disorders of pancreatic internal secretion**

Increased secretion from endocrine pancreas of growth hormone-releasing hormone
Increased secretion from endocrine pancreas of pancreatic polypeptide
Increased secretion from endocrine pancreas of somatostatin
Increased secretion from endocrine pancreas of vasoactive-intestinal polypeptide

CODING TIPS✓ Do not use E16.8 for steroid induced diabetes. Use E09 instead.

SP **E16.9 Disorder of pancreatic internal secretion, unspecified**

Islet-cell hyperplasia NOS
Pancreatic endocrine cell hyperplasia NOS

Disorders of other endocrine glands (E20-E35)

EXCLUDES 1 galactorrhea (N64.3)
gynecomastia (N62)

4 **E20 Hypoparathyroidism**

EXCLUDES 1 Di George's syndrome (D82.1)
postprocedural hypoparathyroidism (E89.2)
tetany NOS (R29.0)
transitory neonatal hypoparathyroidism (P71.4)

DEFINITION Reduced production of parathyroid hormone causing tingling of the hands, fingers, and mouth, muscle cramps, and possibly convulsions.

SP **E20.0 Idiopathic hypoparathyroidism**

SP **E20.1 Pseudohypoparathyroidism**

CODING TIPS✓ Patients with pseudohypoparathyroidism produce adequate levels of PTH, but are resistant to its effects due to a genetic abnormality. These patients typically exhibit low blood calcium and elevated phosphorus, which are characteristic of hypoparathyroidism and should not be separately coded.

DEFINITION Condition of hypoparathyroidism symptoms manifesting due to an inadequate response to the parathyroid hormone, rather than an insufficient amount of the hormone.

SP **E20.8 Other hypoparathyroidism**

SP **E20.9 Hypoparathyroidism, unspecified**

Parathyroid tetany

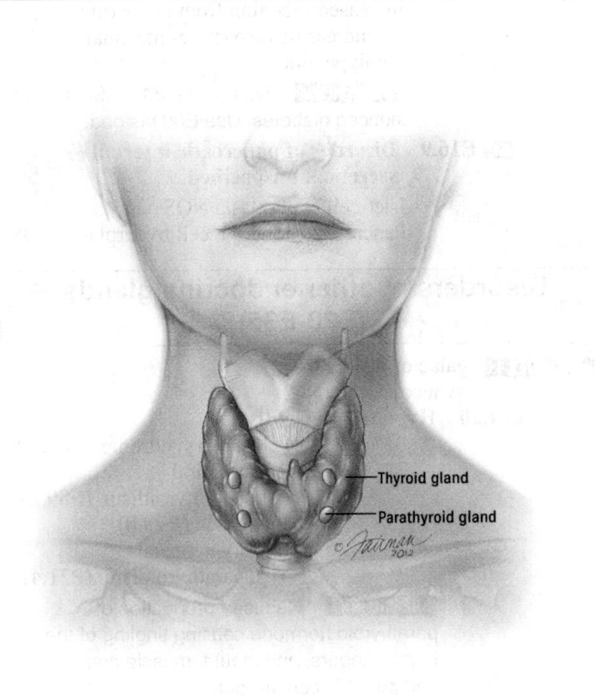

▲ 4 **E21 Hyperparathyroidism and other disorders of parathyroid gland**

EXCLUDES 1 adult osteomalacia (M83.-)
ectopic hyperparathyroidism (E34.2)
hungry bone syndrome (E83.81)
infantile and juvenile osteomalacia (E55.0)

EXCLUDES 2 familial hypocalciuric hypercalcemia (E83.52)

SP **E21.0 Primary hyperparathyroidism**
Hyperplasia of parathyroid
Osteitis fibrosa cystica generalisata [von Recklinghausen's disease of bone]

DEFINITION Excessive production of parathyroid hormone, usually caused by hyperplasia of the gland itself, causing decreased calcium levels in bones.

SP **E21.1 Secondary hyperparathyroidism, not elsewhere classified**

EXCLUDES 1 secondary hyperparathyroidism of renal origin (N25.81)

CODING TIPS ✓ Do not assign E21.1 if the causative mechanism of the diagnosed secondary hyperparathyroid disease is of renal (kidney) origin. E21.1 should only be assigned when the hyperparathyroidism is not reported as primary and has a clear cause reported as not of renal origin.

SP **E21.2 Other hyperparathyroidism**
Tertiary hyperparathyroidism

EXCLUDES 1 familial hypocalciuric hypercalcemia (E83.52)

SP **E21.3 Hyperparathyroidism, unspecified**

SP **E21.4 Other specified disorders of parathyroid gland**

!Q **E21.5 Disorder of parathyroid gland, unspecified**

4 **E22 Hyperfunction of pituitary gland**

EXCLUDES 1 Cushing's syndrome (E24.-)
Nelson's syndrome (E24.1)
overproduction of ACTH not associated with Cushing's disease (E27.0)
overproduction of pituitary ACTH (E24.0)
overproduction of thyroid-stimulating hormone (E05.8-)

SP **E22.0 Acromegaly and pituitary gigantism**
Overproduction of growth hormone

EXCLUDES 1 constitutional gigantism (E34.4)
constitutional tall stature (E34.4)
increased secretion from endocrine pancreas of growth hormone-releasing hormone (E16.8)

DEFINITION Acromegaly: Abnormally large growth of the hands, feet and facial features due to the production of too much growth hormone in adults by the pituitary gland.

SP + **E22.1 Hyperprolactinemia**
Use additional code for adverse effect, if applicable, to identify drug (T36-T50 with fifth or sixth character 5)

SP **E22.2 Syndrome of inappropriate secretion of antidiuretic hormone**

SP **E22.8 Other hyperfunction of pituitary gland**
Central precocious puberty

!Q **E22.9 Hyperfunction of pituitary gland, unspecified**

4 **E23 Hypofunction and other disorders of the pituitary gland**

INCLUDES the listed conditions whether the disorder is in the pituitary or the hypothalamus

EXCLUDES 1 postprocedural hypopituitarism (E89.3)

SP **E23.0 Hypopituitarism**
Fertile eunuch syndrome
Hypogonadotropic hypogonadism
Idiopathic growth hormone deficiency
Isolated deficiency of gonadotropin
Isolated deficiency of growth hormone
Isolated deficiency of pituitary hormone
Kallmann's syndrome
Lorain-Levi short stature
Necrosis of pituitary gland (postpartum)
Panhypopituitarism
Pituitary cachexia
Pituitary insufficiency NOS
Pituitary short stature
Sheehan's syndrome
Simmonds' disease

DEFINITION A type of dwarfism with retention of infantile characteristics, due to undersecretion of growth hormone and gonadotropin deficiency.

SP + **E23.1 Drug-induced hypopituitarism**
Use additional code for adverse effect, if applicable, to identify drug (T36-T50 with fifth or sixth character 5)

!Q **E23.2 Diabetes insipidus**

EXCLUDES 1 nephrogenic diabetes insipidus (N25.1)

CODING TIPS✓ E23.2 is one of the less common kinds of diabetes. It is caused by a malfunction of the pituitary gland. Don't confuse with nephrogenic diabetes insipidus, a problem caused by kidneys (N25.2). Diabetes insipidus is not related to diabetes mellitus.

DEFINITION Insufficient vasopressin production/secretion of antidiuretic hormone (ADH) resulting in intense thirst and excretion of large amounts of urine.

SP **E23.3 Hypothalamic dysfunction, not elsewhere classified**

EXCLUDES 1 Prader-Willi syndrome (Q87.11)
Russell-Silver syndrome (Q87.19)

SP **E23.6 Other disorders of pituitary gland**
Abscess of pituitary
Adiposogenital dystrophy

IQ **E23.7 Disorder of pituitary gland, unspecified**

4 **E24 Cushing's syndrome**

EXCLUDES 1 congenital adrenal hyperplasia (E25.0)

CODING TIPS✓ When Cushing's syndrome is stated as the related cause of diabetes (diabetes due to an underlying condition), assign the appropriate code for Cushing's syndrome (classifiable to E24), followed by a code from E08 to indicate diabetes mellitus due to an underlying condition.

SP **E24.0 Pituitary-dependent Cushing's disease**
Overproduction of pituitary ACTH
Pituitary-dependent hypercorticalism

SP **E24.1 Nelson's syndrome**

SP + **E24.2 Drug-induced Cushing's syndrome**
Use additional code for adverse effect, if applicable, to identify drug (T36-T50 with fifth or sixth character 5)

CODING TIPS✓ Code E24.2 should only be assigned when documentation clearly indicates a relationship between Cushing's syndrome and a drug or chemical as the underlying cause. Assign a code from T36-T50 to indicate the drug and adverse effect.

SP **E24.3 Ectopic ACTH syndrome**

SP **E24.4 Alcohol-induced pseudo-Cushing's syndrome**

SP **E24.8 Other Cushing's syndrome**

SP **E24.9 Cushing's syndrome, unspecified**

DEFINITION Disorder caused by prolonged exposure of body tissues to high levels of cortisol, presenting with upper body obesity, thinning arms and legs, brittle bones, severe fatigue, weakness, high blood pressure, and high blood sugar.

4 **E25 Adrenogenital disorders**

INCLUDES adrenogenital syndromes, virilizing or feminizing, whether acquired or due to adrenal hyperplasia consequent on inborn enzyme defects in hormone synthesis
Female adrenal pseudohermaphroditism
Female heterosexual precocious pseudopuberty
Male isosexual precocious pseudopuberty
Male macrogenitosomia praecox
Male sexual precocity with adrenal hyperplasia
Male virilization (female)

EXCLUDES 1 indeterminate sex and pseudohermaphroditism (Q56)
chromosomal abnormalities (Q90-Q99)

SP **E25.0 Congenital adrenogenital disorders associated with enzyme deficiency**
Congenital adrenal hyperplasia
21-Hydroxylase deficiency
Salt-losing congenital adrenal hyperplasia

SP + **E25.8 Other adrenogenital disorders**
Idiopathic adrenogenital disorder
Use additional code for adverse effect, if applicable, to identify drug (T36-T50 with fifth or sixth character 5)

IQ **E25.9 Adrenogenital disorder, unspecified**
Adrenogenital syndrome NOS

4 **E26 Hyperaldosteronism**

5 **E26.0 Primary hyperaldosteronism**

DEFINITION Excessive aldosterone production; typically presents with loss of potassium, muscular weakness, and elevated blood pressure.

SP **E26.01 Conn's syndrome**
Code also:
adrenal adenoma (D35.0-)

DEFINITION Excess secretion of aldosterone due to an adrenocortical adenoma, causing hypokalemia, alkalosis, muscular weakness, polyuria, polydipsia, and hypertension.

SP **E26.02 Glucocorticoid-remediable aldosteronism**
Familial aldosteronism type I

SP **E26.09 Other primary hyperaldosteronism**
Primary aldosteronism due to adrenal hyperplasia (bilateral)

SP **E26.1 Secondary hyperaldosteronism**

5 **E26.8 Other hyperaldosteronism**

SP **E26.81 Bartter's syndrome**

DEFINITION Group of symptoms caused by the kidneys' inability to reabsorb potassium, also known as urinary potassium wasting; causes renal cell enlargement, alkalosis, hyperaldosteronism, cramping, constipation, urinary frequency, and weakness.

SP **E26.89 Other hyperaldosteronism**

IQ **E26.9 Hyperaldosteronism, unspecified**
Aldosteronism NOS
Hyperaldosteronism NOS

4 **E27 Other disorders of adrenal gland**

SP **E27.0 Other adrenocortical overactivity**

Chapter 4
E00-E89

Overproduction of ACTH, not associated with Cushing's disease
Premature adrenarche
EXCLUDES 1 Cushing's syndrome (E24.-)

SP **E27.1 Primary adrenocortical insufficiency**
Addison's disease
Autoimmune adrenalitis
EXCLUDES 1 Addison only phenotype adrenoleukodystrophy (E71.528)
amyloidosis (E85.-)
tuberculous Addison's disease (A18.7)
Waterhouse-Friderichsen syndrome (A39.1)

SP **E27.2 Addisonian crisis**
Adrenal crisis
Adrenocortical crisis
CODING TIPS✓ Do not assign E27.2 to indicate Addison's disease. Code E27.2 indicates Addisonian crisis, a severe and life-threatening condition that may occur in individuals with Addison's disease or other conditions resulting in severely elevated cortisol levels. Addison's disease in the absence of crisis should be coded to E27.1.
DEFINITION Low levels of the glucocorticoid hormone, cortisol, secreted by the adrenal glands and responsible for regulating blood pressure, cardiovascular function, inflammatory response, insulin effects, and metabolism.

SP + **E27.3 Drug-induced adrenocortical insufficiency**
Use additional code for adverse effect, if applicable, to identify drug (T36-T50 with fifth or sixth character 5)
CODING TIPS✓ Code E27.3 should only be assigned when documentation clearly indicates a relationship between adrenocortical insufficiency and a drug or chemical as the underlying cause. Assign a code from T36-T50 following E27.3 to indicate the drug and adverse effect.

5 **E27.4 Other and unspecified adrenocortical insufficiency**
EXCLUDES 1 adrenoleukodystrophy [Addison-Schilder] (E71.528)
Waterhouse-Friderichsen syndrome (A39.1)

IQ **E27.40 Unspecified adrenocortical insufficiency**
Adrenocortical insufficiency NOS
Hypoaldosteronism

IQ **E27.49 Other adrenocortical insufficiency**
Adrenal hemorrhage
Adrenal infarction

SP **E27.5 Adrenomedullary hyperfunction**
Adrenomedullary hyperplasia
Catecholamine hypersecretion
DEFINITION Overproduction of adrenaline hormones by the adrenal medulla, causing heart disease, high blood pressure, and related problems.

SP **E27.8 Other specified disorders of adrenal gland**
Abnormality of cortisol-binding globulin

IQ **E27.9 Disorder of adrenal gland, unspecified**

4 **E28 Ovarian dysfunction**
EXCLUDES 1 isolated gonadotropin deficiency (E23.0)
postprocedural ovarian failure (E89.4-)

SP + **E28.0 Estrogen excess**
Use additional code for adverse effect, if applicable, to identify drug (T36-T50 with fifth or sixth character 5)

SP + **E28.1 Androgen excess**
Hypersecretion of ovarian androgens
Use additional code for adverse effect, if applicable, to identify drug (T36-T50 with fifth or sixth character 5)

SP **E28.2 Polycystic ovarian syndrome**
Sclerocystic ovary syndrome
Stein-Leventhal syndrome
CODING TIPS✓ Polycystic ovarian syndrome (PCOS) is associated with increased risk for a number of other endocrine disorders, including insulin resistance, hypothyroidism and obesity. When present, these other diagnoses should also be reported.
DEFINITION Syndrome in which the ovaries produce too many androgens, causing ovarian cysts and interfering with the menstrual cycle; results in missed, heavy, or irregular periods, infertility, abdominal discomfort, acne, weight gain, and uterine bleeding.

5 **E28.3 Primary ovarian failure**
EXCLUDES 1 pure gonadal dysgenesis (Q99.1)
Turner's syndrome (Q96.-)

6 **E28.31 Premature menopause**

SP **E28.310 Symptomatic premature menopause**
Symptoms such as flushing, sleeplessness, headache, lack of concentration, associated with premature menopause

SP **E28.319 Asymptomatic premature menopause**
Premature menopause NOS

SP **E28.39 Other primary ovarian failure**
Decreased estrogen
Resistant ovary syndrome

SP **E28.8 Other ovarian dysfunction**
Ovarian hyperfunction NOS
EXCLUDES 1 postprocedural ovarian failure (E89.4-)

IQ **E28.9 Ovarian dysfunction, unspecified**

4 **E29 Testicular dysfunction**
EXCLUDES 1 androgen insensitivity syndrome (E34.5-)
azoospermia or oligospermia NOS (N46.0-N46.1)
isolated gonadotropin deficiency (E23.0)
Klinefelter's syndrome (Q98.0-Q98.1, Q98.4)

SP **E29.0 Testicular hyperfunction**
Hypersecretion of testicular hormones

DEFINITION Excessive testosterone production, often due to an active tumor on the testicle. Commonly presents with increased muscle and bone growth in children and increased secondary sex characteristics.

SP + **E29.1 Testicular hypofunction**
Defective biosynthesis of testicular androgen NOS
5-delta-Reductase deficiency (with male pseudohermaphroditism)
Testicular hypogonadism NOS
Use additional code for adverse effect, if applicable, to identify drug (T36-T50 with fifth or sixth character 5)
EXCLUDES 1 postprocedural testicular hypofunction (E89.5)
DEFINITION Underdevelopment of all the genital tissues with decreased functional activities of the gonads.

SP **E29.8 Other testicular dysfunction**

IQ **E29.9 Testicular dysfunction, unspecified**

4 **E30 Disorders of puberty, not elsewhere classified**

IQ **E30.0 Delayed puberty**
Constitutional delay of puberty
Delayed sexual development

IQ **E30.1 Precocious puberty**
Precocious menstruation
EXCLUDES 1 Albright (-McCune) (-Sternberg) syndrome (Q78.1)
central precocious puberty (E22.8)
congenital adrenal hyperplasia (E25.0)
female heterosexual precocious pseudopuberty (E25.-)
male isosexual precocious pseudopuberty (E25.-)

IQ **E30.8 Other disorders of puberty**
Premature thelarche

IQ **E30.9 Disorder of puberty, unspecified**

4 **E31 Polyglandular dysfunction**
EXCLUDES 1 ataxia telangiectasia [Louis-Bar] (G11.3)
dystrophia myotonica [Steinert] (G71.11)
pseudohypoparathyroidism (E20.1)

SP **E31.0 Autoimmune polyglandular failure**
Schmidt's syndrome
DEFINITION Schmidt's syndrome: hypofunction of more than one endocrine gland in different combinations, including the thyroid, adrenals, gonads, parathyroid, and pancreas; occurs primarily in adult females.

SP **E31.1 Polyglandular hyperfunction**
EXCLUDES 1 multiple endocrine adenomatosis (E31.2-)
multiple endocrine neoplasia (E31.2-)

5 **E31.2 Multiple endocrine neoplasia [MEN] syndromes**
Multiple endocrine adenomatosis
Code also:
any associated malignancies and other conditions associated with the syndromes
CODING TIPS✓ MEN syndromes are distinct, inherited autosomal disorders, which may present in conjunction with endocrine tumors.

SP **E31.20 Multiple endocrine neoplasia [MEN] syndrome, unspecified**
Multiple endocrine adenomatosis NOS
Multiple endocrine neoplasia [MEN] syndrome NOS

SP **E31.21 Multiple endocrine neoplasia [MEN] type I**
Wermer's syndrome
DEFINITION Hyperplasia or tumors of the parathyroid, pancreatic islet cells, and pituitary gland; causes oversecretion of hormones, kidney stones, infertility, and severe peptic ulcers.

SP **E31.22 Multiple endocrine neoplasia [MEN] type IIA**
Sipple's syndrome
DEFINITION Triad of thyroid medullary carcinoma, adrenal gland tumor, and parathyroid hyperplasia.

SP **E31.23 Multiple endocrine neoplasia [MEN] type IIB**

SP **E31.8 Other polyglandular dysfunction**

SP **E31.9 Polyglandular dysfunction, unspecified**

4 **E32 Diseases of thymus**
EXCLUDES 1 aplasia or hypoplasia of thymus with immunodeficiency (D82.1)
myasthenia gravis (G70.0)

IQ **E32.0 Persistent hyperplasia of thymus**
Hypertrophy of thymus

SP **E32.1 Abscess of thymus**

SP **E32.8 Other diseases of thymus**
EXCLUDES 1 aplasia or hypoplasia with immunodeficiency (D82.1)
thymoma (D15.0)

IQ **E32.9 Disease of thymus, unspecified**

4 **E34 Other endocrine disorders**
EXCLUDES 1 pseudohypoparathyroidism (E20.1)

SP **E34.0 Carcinoid syndrome**
Note:
May be used as an additional code to identify functional activity associated with a carcinoid tumor.
CODING TIPS✓ Carcinoid syndrome is a specific syndrome causing a variety of symptoms in patients with advanced stage malignant carcinoid tumors. When coding carcinoid syndrome, the specific type and location of the carcinoid tumor should be identified and additionally coded by assigning the appropriate code(s) from category C7A and/or C7B.

DEFINITION Condition in which cancerous cells secrete hormones into the bloodstream causing chemical imbalances in the body with symptoms of periodic flushing, diarrhea, abdominal pain, and high blood pressure.

SP **E34.1 Other hypersecretion of intestinal hormones**

SP **E34.2 Ectopic hormone secretion, not elsewhere classified**

EXCLUDES 1 ectopic ACTH syndrome (E24.3)

DEFINITION Condition that occurs when a glandular tumor metastasizes, moving from its original location to another area of the body, and continues to secrete hormones.

SP **E34.3 Short stature due to endocrine disorder**

Constitutional short stature
Laron-type short stature

EXCLUDES 1 achondroplastic short stature (Q77.4)
hypochondroplastic short stature (Q77.4)
nutritional short stature (E45)
pituitary short stature (E23.0)
progeria (E34.8)
renal short stature (N25.0)
Russell-Silver syndrome (Q87.19)
short-limbed stature with immunodeficiency (D82.2)
short stature in specific dysmorphic syndromes - code to syndrome - see Alphabetical Index
short stature NOS (R62.52)

SP **E34.4 Constitutional tall stature**

Constitutional gigantism

5 **E34.5 Androgen insensitivity syndrome**

DEFINITION Defects in androgen action causing feminization of external genitalia, abnormal sexual development, infertility, and pseudohermaphroditism in males.

IQ **E34.50 Androgen insensitivity syndrome, unspecified**

Androgen insensitivity NOS

SP **E34.51 Complete androgen insensitivity syndrome**

Complete androgen insensitivity
de Quervain syndrome
Goldberg-Maxwell syndrome

SP **E34.52 Partial androgen insensitivity syndrome**

Partial androgen insensitivity
Reifenstein syndrome

SP **E34.8 Other specified endocrine disorders**

Pineal gland dysfunction
Progeria

EXCLUDES 2 pseudohypoparathyroidism (E20.1)

IQ **E34.9 Endocrine disorder, unspecified**

Endocrine disturbance NOS
Hormone disturbance NOS

M IQ + **E35 *Disorders of endocrine glands in diseases classified elsewhere***

Code first underlying disease, such as:
late congenital syphilis of thymus gland [Dubois disease] (A50.5)

Use additional code, if applicable, to identify:
sequelae of tuberculosis of other organs (B90.8)

EXCLUDES 1 Echinococcus granulosus infection of thyroid gland (B67.3)
meningococcal hemorrhagic adrenalitis (A39.1)
syphilis of endocrine gland (A52.79)
tuberculosis of adrenal gland, except calcification (A18.7)
tuberculosis of endocrine gland NEC (A18.82)
tuberculosis of thyroid gland (A18.81)
Waterhouse-Friderichsen syndrome (A39.1)

Intraoperative complications of endocrine system (E36)

CODING TIPS✓ Codes classifiable to E36 are complication codes (intraoperative complications) and should only be coded when the provider specifically indicates a relationship between the operative procedure and the specific complication. If no relationship between the condition suspected to be a complication and the operative procedure is stated, the provider may be queried to clarify if the condition is classifiable as a complication.

4 **E36 Intraoperative complications of endocrine system**

EXCLUDES 2 postprocedural endocrine and metabolic complications and disorders, not elsewhere classified (E89.-)

5 **E36.0 Intraoperative hemorrhage and hematoma of an endocrine system organ or structure complicating a procedure**

EXCLUDES 1 intraoperative hemorrhage and hematoma of an endocrine system organ or structure due to accidental puncture or laceration during a procedure (E36.1-)

SP **E36.01 Intraoperative hemorrhage and hematoma of an endocrine system organ or structure complicating an endocrine system procedure**

SP **E36.02 Intraoperative hemorrhage and hematoma of an endocrine system organ or structure complicating other procedure**

5 **E36.1 Accidental puncture and laceration of an endocrine system organ or structure during a procedure**

SP **E36.11 Accidental puncture and laceration of an endocrine system organ or structure during an endocrine system procedure**

SP **E36.12 Accidental puncture and laceration of an endocrine system organ or structure during other procedure**

Chapter 4
E00-E89

SP + **E36.8 Other intraoperative complications of endocrine system**
Use additional code, if applicable, to further specify disorder

Malnutrition (E40-E46)

EXCLUDES 1 intestinal malabsorption (K90.-)
sequelae of protein-calorie malnutrition (E64.0)
EXCLUDES 2 nutritional anemias (D50-D53)
starvation (T73.0)

CODING TIPS✓ Malnutrition is defined as insufficient, excessive or imbalanced nutrient consumption. Not all patients experiencing malnutrition will present with inadequate intake or low body weight/BMI. The specific type of malnutrition (such as severe, moderate, Kwashiorkor, etc.) must be indicated by the patient's provider and cannot be assumed. When documentation only states "malnutrition," assign E46.

SP **E40 Kwashiorkor**
Severe malnutrition with nutritional edema with dyspigmentation of skin and hair
EXCLUDES 1 marasmic kwashiorkor (E42)
ALERT Kwashiorkor is a form of severe protein malnutrition that generally affects children living in tropical and subtropical parts of the world during periods of famine or insufficient food supply. It is typically not found in the United States.

SP **E41 Nutritional marasmus**
Severe malnutrition with marasmus
EXCLUDES 1 marasmic kwashiorkor (E42)
DEFINITION Chronic wasting of body tissues, especially in young children, commonly due to prolonged dietary deficiency of protein and calories.

SP **E42 Marasmic kwashiorkor**
Intermediate form severe protein-calorie malnutrition
Severe protein-calorie malnutrition with signs of both kwashiorkor and marasmus

SP **E43 Unspecified severe protein-calorie malnutrition**
Starvation edema
CODING TIPS✓ If the physician/NPP documents emaciation related to malnutrition, assign code E43.

4 **E44 Protein-calorie malnutrition of moderate and mild degree**
SP **E44.0 Moderate protein-calorie malnutrition**
SP **E44.1 Mild protein-calorie malnutrition**

SP **E45 Retarded development following protein-calorie malnutrition**
Nutritional short stature
Nutritional stunting
Physical retardation due to malnutrition

SP **E46 Unspecified protein-calorie malnutrition**
Malnutrition NOS
Protein-calorie imbalance NOS
EXCLUDES 1 nutritional deficiency NOS (E63.9)
ALERT Hospice claims may be rejected for E46 for non-specificity.
CODING TIPS✓ This code should not be reported as primary in hospice due to its non-specific nature. Query the physician or NPP for a more specific code for the malnutrition.

Other nutritional deficiencies (E50-E64)

EXCLUDES 2 nutritional anemias (D50-D53)

CODING TIPS✓ Do not use codes from E50-E64 to indicate anemia due to a nutritional deficiency. When a patient has a specific diagnosis of anemia due to a nutritional deficiency, assign the appropriate specified code from Chapter 3.

4 **E50 Vitamin A deficiency**
EXCLUDES 1 sequelae of vitamin A deficiency (E64.1)

SP **E50.0 Vitamin A deficiency with conjunctival xerosis**
DEFINITION Vitamin A deficiency with dryness of the membrane that lines eyelids and covers the exposed surface of the sclera.

SP **E50.1 Vitamin A deficiency with Bitot's spot and conjunctival xerosis**
Bitot's spot in the young child
DEFINITION Vitamin A deficiency with superficial spots of keratinized epithelium on the conjunctiva, accompanied by dryness.

SP **E50.2 Vitamin A deficiency with corneal xerosis**
SP **E50.3 Vitamin A deficiency with corneal ulceration and xerosis**
SP **E50.4 Vitamin A deficiency with keratomalacia**
DEFINITION Vitamin A deficiency with softening of the corneas that may lead to corneal infection or rupture.

SP **E50.5 Vitamin A deficiency with night blindness**
SP **E50.6 Vitamin A deficiency with xerophthalmic scars of cornea**
SP **E50.7 Other ocular manifestations of vitamin A deficiency**
Xerophthalmia NOS
SP **E50.8 Other manifestations of vitamin A deficiency**
Follicular keratosis
Xeroderma
SP **E50.9 Vitamin A deficiency, unspecified**
Hypovitaminosis A NOS

4 **E51 Thiamine deficiency**
EXCLUDES 1 sequelae of thiamine deficiency (E64.8)

5 **E51.1 Beriberi**
DEFINITION Severe Vitamin B1 (thiamine) deficiency causing nerve, heart, and/or brain abnormalities.

SP **E51.11 Dry beriberi**
Beriberi NOS
Beriberi with polyneuropathy
SP **E51.12 Wet beriberi**
Beriberi with cardiovascular manifestations
Cardiovascular beriberi
Shoshin disease
SP **E51.2 Wernicke's encephalopathy**
SP **E51.8 Other manifestations of thiamine deficiency**
SP **E51.9 Thiamine deficiency, unspecified**

SP **E52 Niacin deficiency [pellagra]**
Niacin (-tryptophan) deficiency

Chapter 4
E00-E89

Nicotinamide deficiency
Pellagra (alcoholic)
EXCLUDES 1 sequelae of niacin deficiency (E64.8)
DEFINITION Niacin and amino acid tryptophan deficiency affecting the skin, digestive tract, and brain.

4 E53 Deficiency of other B group vitamins
EXCLUDES 1 sequelae of vitamin B deficiency (E64.8)

SP E53.0 Riboflavin deficiency
Ariboflavinosis
Vitamin B2 deficiency
DEFINITION Riboflavin deficiency causing dry throat and nasal passages, mouth sores, magenta-colored tongue, and overproduction of oil on the skin.

SP E53.1 Pyridoxine deficiency
Vitamin B6 deficiency
EXCLUDES 1 pyridoxine-responsive sideroblastic anemia (D64.3)

SP E53.8 Deficiency of other specified B group vitamins
Biotin deficiency
Cyanocobalamin deficiency
Folate deficiency
Folic acid deficiency
Pantothenic acid deficiency
Vitamin B12 deficiency
EXCLUDES 1 folate deficiency anemia (D52.-)
vitamin B12 deficiency anemia (D51.-)

SP E53.9 Vitamin B deficiency, unspecified

SP E54 Ascorbic acid deficiency
Deficiency of vitamin C
Scurvy
EXCLUDES 1 scorbutic anemia (D53.2)
sequelae of vitamin C deficiency (E64.2)
DEFINITION Condition known as scurvy caused by deficiency of ascorbic acid (vitamin C) and marked by weakness, anemia, spongy gums, and mucocutaneous hemorrhages.

4 E55 Vitamin D deficiency
EXCLUDES 1 adult osteomalacia (M83.-)
osteoporosis (M80.-)
sequelae of rickets (E64.3)

SP E55.0 Rickets, active
Infantile osteomalacia
Juvenile osteomalacia
EXCLUDES 1 celiac rickets (K90.0)
Crohn's rickets (K50.-)
hereditary vitamin D-dependent rickets (E83.32)
inactive rickets (E64.3)
renal rickets (N25.0)
sequelae of rickets (E64.3)
vitamin D-resistant rickets (E83.31)
DEFINITION Childhood disease caused by a lack of vitamin D, resulting in soft, spongy bones and bone pain as well as skeletal deformities (e.g., bowlegs, scoliosis), distortion of the rib cage, and oddly-shaped skull.

SP E55.9 Vitamin D deficiency, unspecified
Avitaminosis D

4 E56 Other vitamin deficiencies
EXCLUDES 1 sequelae of other vitamin deficiencies (E64.8)

SP E56.0 Deficiency of vitamin E

SP E56.1 Deficiency of vitamin K
EXCLUDES 1 deficiency of coagulation factor due to vitamin K deficiency (D68.4)
vitamin K deficiency of newborn (P53)

SP E56.8 Deficiency of other vitamins

IQ E56.9 Vitamin deficiency, unspecified

SP E58 Dietary calcium deficiency
EXCLUDES 1 disorders of calcium metabolism (E83.5-)
sequelae of calcium deficiency (E64.8)

SP E59 Dietary selenium deficiency
Keshan disease
EXCLUDES 1 sequelae of selenium deficiency (E64.8)

SP E60 Dietary zinc deficiency

+ 4 E61 Deficiency of other nutrient elements
Use additional code for adverse effect, if applicable, to identify drug (T36-T50 with fifth or sixth character 5)
EXCLUDES 1 disorders of mineral metabolism (E83.-)
iodine deficiency related thyroid disorders (E00-E02)
sequelae of malnutrition and other nutritional deficiencies (E64.-)

SP + E61.0 Copper deficiency

SP + E61.1 Iron deficiency
EXCLUDES 1 iron deficiency anemia (D50.-)

SP + E61.2 Magnesium deficiency

SP + E61.3 Manganese deficiency

SP + E61.4 Chromium deficiency

SP + E61.5 Molybdenum deficiency

SP + E61.6 Vanadium deficiency

SP + E61.7 Deficiency of multiple nutrient elements

SP + E61.8 Deficiency of other specified nutrient elements

IQ + E61.9 Deficiency of nutrient element, unspecified

▲ 4 E63 Other nutritional deficiencies
EXCLUDES 2 dehydration (E86.0)
failure to thrive, adult (R62.7)
failure to thrive, child (R62.51)
feeding problems in newborn (P92.-)
sequelae of malnutrition and other nutritional deficiencies (E64.-)

SP E63.0 Essential fatty acid [EFA] deficiency

SP **E63.1 Imbalance of constituents of food intake**

SP **E63.8 Other specified nutritional deficiencies**

IQ **E63.9 Nutritional deficiency, unspecified**

4 **E64 Sequelae of malnutrition and other nutritional deficiencies**

Note:

This category is to be used to indicate conditions in categories E43, E44, E46, E50-E63 as the cause of sequelae, which are themselves classified elsewhere. The 'sequelae' include conditions specified as such; they also include the late effects of diseases classifiable to the above categories if the disease itself is no longer present

Code first:

condition resulting from (sequela) of malnutrition and other nutritional deficiencies

IQ **E64.0 Sequelae of protein-calorie malnutrition**

EXCLUDES 2 retarded development following protein-calorie malnutrition (E45)

IQ **E64.1 Sequelae of vitamin A deficiency**

IQ **E64.2 Sequelae of vitamin C deficiency**

IQ **E64.3 Sequelae of rickets**

IQ **E64.8 Sequelae of other nutritional deficiencies**

IQ **E64.9 Sequelae of unspecified nutritional deficiency**

Overweight, obesity and other hyperalimentation (E65-E68)

SP **E65 Localized adiposity**

Fat pad

+ 4 **E66 Overweight and obesity**

Code first:

obesity complicating pregnancy, childbirth and the puerperium, if applicable (O99.21-)

Use additional code to identify body mass index (BMI), if known (Z68.-)

EXCLUDES 1 adiposogenital dystrophy (E23.6)

lipomatosis NOS (E88.2)

lipomatosis dolorosa [Dercum] (E88.2)

Prader-Willi syndrome (Q87.11)

GUIDELINES **Section I.B.14**

For the Body Mass Index (BMI), depth of non-pressure chronic ulcers, pressure ulcer stage, coma scale, and NIH stroke scale (NIHSS) codes, code assignment may be based on medical record documentation from clinicians who are not the patient's provider (i.e., physician or other qualified healthcare practitioner legally accountable for establishing the patient's diagnosis), since this information is typically documented by other clinicians involved in the care of the patient (e.g., a dietitian often documents the BMI, a nurse often documents the pressure ulcer stages, and an emergency medical technician often documents the coma scale). However, the associated diagnosis (such as overweight, obesity, acute stroke, or pressure ulcer) must be documented by the patient's provider.

CODING TIPS✓ Adult BMI codes are used for people age 20 and over. There are specific BMI codes for ages 2-19 pediatric populations. Code obesity if the physician documents obesity and it is impacting your plan of care.

CODING TIPS✓ When assigning a code for any overweight, obesity or morbid obesity, physician or NPP documentation indicating obesity as a diagnosis is required. The coder may not code obesity without confirmation from the provider. BMI may be calculated based upon nursing documentation (height and weight used to calculate); however, the BMI may only be coded if a physician or NPP-provided diagnosis, such as overweight, obesity or underweight, is coded.

+ 5 **E66.0 Obesity due to excess calories**

DEFINITION Increased body weight with excessive accumulation of fat caused by overeating and/or a sedentary lifestyle.

SP + **E66.01 Morbid (severe) obesity due to excess calories**

EXCLUDES 1 morbid (severe) obesity with alveolar hypoventilation (E66.2)

CODING TIPS✓ Note that the alphabetical index refers to this code for morbid obesity. This code is used when morbid obesity is documented.

SP + **E66.09 Other obesity due to excess calories**

SP + **E66.1 Drug-induced obesity**

Use additional code for adverse effect, if applicable, to identify drug (T36-T50 with fifth or sixth character 5)

CODING TIPS✓ This code should only be assigned when documentation clearly indicates a relationship between obesity and a drug or chemical as the underlying cause. Assign a code from T36-T50 following E66.1 to indicate the drug and adverse effect.

SP + **E66.2 Morbid (severe) obesity with alveolar hypoventilation**

Obesity hypoventilation syndrome (OHS)

Pickwickian syndrome

SP + **E66.3 Overweight**

Chapter 4 E00-E89

SP + **E66.8 Other obesity**

SP + **E66.9 Obesity, unspecified**
Obesity NOS

4 **E67 Other hyperalimentation**
EXCLUDES 1 hyperalimentation NOS (R63.2)
sequelae of hyperalimentation (E68)

SP **E67.0 Hypervitaminosis A**

SP **E67.1 Hypercarotenemia**
DEFINITION Elevated carotene levels in the blood from excessive ingestion of carotenoids or the inability to convert carotenoids to vitamin A; often presents with yellowing of the skin.

SP **E67.2 Megavitamin-B6 syndrome**

SP **E67.3 Hypervitaminosis D**

SP **E67.8 Other specified hyperalimentation**

!Q **E68 Sequelae of hyperalimentation**
Code first:
condition resulting from (sequela) of hyperalimentation

Metabolic disorders (E70-E88)

EXCLUDES 1 androgen insensitivity syndrome (E34.5-)
congenital adrenal hyperplasia (E25.0)
hemolytic anemias attributable to enzyme disorders (D55.-)
Marfan's syndrome (Q87.4)
5-alpha-reductase deficiency (E29.1)

EXCLUDES 2 Ehlers-Danlos syndromes (Q79.6-)

4 **E70 Disorders of aromatic amino-acid metabolism**

SP **E70.0 Classical phenylketonuria**
DEFINITION Inherited metabolic disorder caused by an enzyme deficiency resulting in accumulation of phenylalanine and its metabolites in the blood with excess excretion in the urine; causes mental retardation, seizures, eczema, and abnormal body odor.

SP **E70.1 Other hyperphenylalaninemias**

5 **E70.2 Disorders of tyrosine metabolism**
EXCLUDES 1 transitory tyrosinemia of newborn (P74.5)

SP **E70.20 Disorder of tyrosine metabolism, unspecified**

SP **E70.21 Tyrosinemia**
Hypertyrosinemia

SP **E70.29 Other disorders of tyrosine metabolism**
Alkaptonuria
Ochronosis

5 **E70.3 Albinism**

SP **E70.30 Albinism, unspecified**

6 **E70.31 Ocular albinism**

SP **E70.310 X-linked ocular albinism**

SP **E70.311 Autosomal recessive ocular albinism**

SP **E70.318 Other ocular albinism**

SP **E70.319 Ocular albinism, unspecified**

6 **E70.32 Oculocutaneous albinism**
EXCLUDES 1 Chediak-Higashi syndrome (E70.330)
Hermansky-Pudlak syndrome (E70.331)

SP **E70.320 Tyrosinase negative oculocutaneous albinism**
Albinism I
Oculocutaneous albinism ty-neg

SP **E70.321 Tyrosinase positive oculocutaneous albinism**
Albinism II
Oculocutaneous albinism ty-pos

SP **E70.328 Other oculocutaneous albinism**
Cross syndrome

SP **E70.329 Oculocutaneous albinism, unspecified**

6 **E70.33 Albinism with hematologic abnormality**

SP **E70.330 Chediak-Higashi syndrome**

SP **E70.331 Hermansky-Pudlak syndrome**

SP **E70.338 Other albinism with hematologic abnormality**

SP **E70.339 Albinism with hematologic abnormality, unspecified**

SP **E70.39 Other specified albinism**
Piebaldism

5 **E70.4 Disorders of histidine metabolism**

SP **E70.40 Disorders of histidine metabolism, unspecified**

SP **E70.41 Histidinemia**

SP **E70.49 Other disorders of histidine metabolism**

SP **E70.5 Disorders of tryptophan metabolism**

5 **E70.8 Other disorders of aromatic amino-acid metabolism**

SP **E70.81 Aromatic L-amino acid decarboxylase deficiency**
AADC deficiency
DEFINITION AADC deficiency is a rare disease and usually appears by the age of 3.5 years.

SP **E70.89 Other disorders of aromatic amino-acid metabolism**

SP **E70.9 Disorder of aromatic amino-acid metabolism, unspecified**

4 **E71 Disorders of branched-chain amino-acid metabolism and fatty-acid metabolism**

SP **E71.0 Maple-syrup-urine disease**

5 **E71.1 Other disorders of branched-chain amino-acid metabolism**

6 **E71.11 Branched-chain organic acidurias**

SP **E71.110 Isovaleric acidemia**

SP **E71.111 3-methylglutaconic aciduria**

SP **E71.118 Other branched-chain organic acidurias**

6 **E71.12 Disorders of propionate metabolism**

SP **E71.120 Methylmalonic acidemia**

SP **E71.121 Propionic acidemia**

SP **E71.128 Other disorders of propionate metabolism**

SP **E71.19 Other disorders of branched-chain amino-acid metabolism**
Hyperleucine-isoleucinemia
Hypervalinemia

SP **E71.2 Disorder of branched-chain amino-acid metabolism, unspecified**

5 **E71.3 Disorders of fatty-acid metabolism**
EXCLUDES 1 peroxisomal disorders (E71.5)
Refsum's disease (G60.1)
Schilder's disease (G37.0)
EXCLUDES 2 carnitine deficiency due to inborn error of metabolism (E71.42)

SP **E71.30 Disorder of fatty-acid metabolism, unspecified**

6 **E71.31 Disorders of fatty-acid oxidation**

SP **E71.310 Long chain/very long chain acyl CoA dehydrogenase deficiency**
LCAD
VLCAD

SP **E71.311 Medium chain acyl CoA dehydrogenase deficiency**
MCAD

SP **E71.312 Short chain acyl CoA dehydrogenase deficiency**
SCAD

SP **E71.313 Glutaric aciduria type II**
Glutaric aciduria type II A
Glutaric aciduria type II B
Glutaric aciduria type II C
EXCLUDES 1 glutaric aciduria (type 1) NOS (E72.3)

SP **E71.314 Muscle carnitine palmitoyltransferase deficiency**

SP **E71.318 Other disorders of fatty-acid oxidation**

SP **E71.32 Disorders of ketone metabolism**

SP **E71.39 Other disorders of fatty-acid metabolism**

5 **E71.4 Disorders of carnitine metabolism**
EXCLUDES 1 Muscle carnitine palmitoyltransferase deficiency (E71.314)

SP **E71.40 Disorder of carnitine metabolism, unspecified**

SP **E71.41 Primary carnitine deficiency**

SP **E71.42 Carnitine deficiency due to inborn errors of metabolism**
Code also:
associated inborn error or metabolism

SP **E71.43 Iatrogenic carnitine deficiency**
Carnitine deficiency due to hemodialysis
Carnitine deficiency due to Valproic acid therapy

6 **E71.44 Other secondary carnitine deficiency**

SP **E71.440 Ruvalcaba-Myhre-Smith syndrome**

SP **E71.448 Other secondary carnitine deficiency**

5 **E71.5 Peroxisomal disorders**
EXCLUDES 1 Schilder's disease (G37.0)

SP **E71.50 Peroxisomal disorder, unspecified**

6 **E71.51 Disorders of peroxisome biogenesis**
Group 1 peroxisomal disorders
EXCLUDES 1 Refsum's disease (G60.1)

SP **E71.510 Zellweger syndrome**

SP **E71.511 Neonatal adrenoleukodystrophy**
EXCLUDES 1 X-linked adrenoleukodystrophy (E71.42-)

SP **E71.518 Other disorders of peroxisome biogenesis**

6 **E71.52 X-linked adrenoleukodystrophy**

SP **E71.520 Childhood cerebral X-linked adrenoleukodystrophy**

SP **E71.521 Adolescent X-linked adrenoleukodystrophy**

SP **E71.522 Adrenomyeloneuropathy**

SP **E71.528 Other X-linked adrenoleukodystrophy**
Addison only phenotype adrenoleukodystrophy
Addison-Schilder adrenoleukodystrophy

SP **E71.529 X-linked adrenoleukodystrophy, unspecified type**

SP **E71.53 Other group 2 peroxisomal disorders**

6 **E71.54 Other peroxisomal disorders**

SP **E71.540 Rhizomelic chondrodysplasia punctata**
EXCLUDES 1 chondrodysplasia punctata NOS (Q77.3)

SP **E71.541 Zellweger-like syndrome**

SP **E71.542 Other group 3 peroxisomal disorders**

SP **E71.548 Other peroxisomal disorders**

4 **E72 Other disorders of amino-acid metabolism**
EXCLUDES 1 disorders of:
aromatic amino-acid metabolism (E70.-)
branched-chain amino-acid metabolism (E71.0-E71.2)
fatty-acid metabolism (E71.3)
purine and pyrimidine metabolism (E79.-)
gout (M1A.-, M10.-)

5 **E72.0 Disorders of amino-acid transport**
EXCLUDES 1 disorders of tryptophan metabolism (E70.5)

SP **E72.00 Disorders of amino-acid transport, unspecified**

SP **E72.01 Cystinuria**

SP **E72.02 Hartnup's disease**

SP + **E72.03 Lowe's syndrome**
Use additional code for associated glaucoma (H42)

SP **E72.04 Cystinosis**
Fanconi (-de Toni) (-Debré) syndrome with cystinosis
EXCLUDES 1 Fanconi (-de Toni) (-Debré) syndrome without cystinosis (E72.09)

SP **E72.09 Other disorders of amino-acid transport**
Fanconi (-de Toni) (-Debré) syndrome, unspecified

5 **E72.1 Disorders of sulfur-bearing amino-acid metabolism**
EXCLUDES 1 cystinosis (E72.04)
cystinuria (E72.01)

Chapter 4

E00-E89

transcobalamin II deficiency (D51.2)

SP **E72.10 Disorders of sulfur-bearing amino-acid metabolism, unspecified**

SP **E72.11 Homocystinuria**
Cystathionine synthase deficiency

SP **E72.12 Methylenetetrahydrofolate reductase deficiency**

SP **E72.19 Other disorders of sulfur-bearing amino-acid metabolism**
Cystathioninuria
Methioninemia
Sulfite oxidase deficiency

5 **E72.2 Disorders of urea cycle metabolism**
EXCLUDES 1 disorders of ornithine metabolism (E72.4)

SP **E72.20 Disorder of urea cycle metabolism, unspecified**
Hyperammonemia
EXCLUDES 1 hyperammonemia-hyperornithinemia-homocitrullinemia syndrome E72.4
transient hyperammonemia of newborn (P74.6)

SP **E72.21 Argininemia**

SP **E72.22 Arginosuccinic aciduria**

SP **E72.23 Citrullinemia**

SP **E72.29 Other disorders of urea cycle metabolism**

SP **E72.3 Disorders of lysine and hydroxylysine metabolism**
Glutaric aciduria NOS
Glutaric aciduria (type I)
Hydroxylysinemia
Hyperlysinemia
EXCLUDES 1 glutaric aciduria type II (E71.313)
Refsum's disease (G60.1)
Zellweger syndrome (E71.510)

SP **E72.4 Disorders of ornithine metabolism**
Hyperammonemia-Hyperornithinemia-Homocitrullinemia syndrome
Ornithinemia (types I, II)
Ornithine transcarbamylase deficiency
EXCLUDES 1 hereditary choroidal dystrophy (H31.2-)

5 **E72.5 Disorders of glycine metabolism**

SP **E72.50 Disorder of glycine metabolism, unspecified**

SP **E72.51 Non-ketotic hyperglycinemia**

SP **E72.52 Trimethylaminuria**

SP **E72.53 Primary hyperoxaluria**
Oxalosis
Oxaluria

SP **E72.59 Other disorders of glycine metabolism**
D-glycericacidemia
Hyperhydroxyprolinemia
Hyperprolinemia (types I, II)
Sarcosinemia

5 **E72.8 Other specified disorders of amino-acid metabolism**

SP **E72.81 Disorders of gamma aminobutyric acid metabolism**
4-hydroxybutyric aciduria
Disorders of GABA metabolism
GABA metabolic defect
GABA transaminase deficiency
GABA-T deficiency
Gamma-hydroxybutyric aciduria
SSADHD
Succinic semialdehyde dehydrogenase deficiency

SP **E72.89 Other specified disorders of amino-acid metabolism**
Disorders of beta-amino-acid metabolism
Disorders of gamma-glutamyl cycle

IQ **E72.9 Disorder of amino-acid metabolism, unspecified**

4 **E73 Lactose intolerance**

SP **E73.0 Congenital lactase deficiency**

SP **E73.1 Secondary lactase deficiency**

SP **E73.8 Other lactose intolerance**

SP **E73.9 Lactose intolerance, unspecified**

4 **E74 Other disorders of carbohydrate metabolism**
EXCLUDES 1 diabetes mellitus (E08-E13)
hypoglycemia NOS (E16.2)
increased secretion of glucagon (E16.3)
mucopolysaccharidosis (E76.0-E76.3)

5 **E74.0 Glycogen storage disease**

SP **E74.00 Glycogen storage disease, unspecified**

SP **E74.01 von Gierke disease**
Type I glycogen storage disease

SP **E74.02 Pompe disease**
Cardiac glycogenosis
Type II glycogen storage disease
DEFINITION Pompe disease is also called type II glycogen storage disease and is a congenital disease caused by a metabolic error in which the body deposits an abnormally high amount of glycogen in the kidneys and liver. The disease produces symptoms such as hypoglycemia (low blood sugar) and hyperlipemia (an excess of lipid molecules in the blood, which can lead to problems such as clogged arteries and heart attacks).

SP **E74.03 Cori disease**
Forbes disease
Type III glycogen storage disease

SP **E74.04 McArdle disease**
Type V glycogen storage disease

SP **E74.09 Other glycogen storage disease**
Andersen disease
Hers disease
Tauri disease
Glycogen storage disease, types 0, IV, VI-XI
Liver phosphorylase deficiency
Muscle phosphofructokinase deficiency

5 **E74.1 Disorders of fructose metabolism**
EXCLUDES 1 muscle phosphofructokinase deficiency (E74.09)

SP E74.10 Disorder of fructose metabolism, unspecified

SP E74.11 **Essential fructosuria**
Fructokinase deficiency

SP E74.12 **Hereditary fructose intolerance**
Fructosemia

SP E74.19 **Other disorders of fructose metabolism**
Fructose-1, 6-diphosphatase deficiency

5 E74.2 **Disorders of galactose metabolism**

SP E74.20 Disorders of galactose metabolism, unspecified

SP E74.21 **Galactosemia**

SP E74.29 **Other disorders of galactose metabolism**
Galactokinase deficiency

5 E74.3 **Other disorders of intestinal carbohydrate absorption**
EXCLUDES 2 lactose intolerance (E73.-)

SP E74.31 **Sucrase-isomaltase deficiency**

SP E74.39 **Other disorders of intestinal carbohydrate absorption**
Disorder of intestinal carbohydrate absorption NOS
Glucose-galactose malabsorption
Sucrase deficiency

SP E74.4 **Disorders of pyruvate metabolism and gluconeogenesis**
Deficiency of phosphoenolpyruvate carboxykinase
Deficiency of pyruvate carboxylase
Deficiency of pyruvate dehydrogenase
EXCLUDES 1 disorders of pyruvate metabolism and gluconeogenesis with anemia (D55.-)
Leigh's syndrome (G31.82)

5 E74.8 **Other specified disorders of carbohydrate metabolism**
DEFINITION Excess glucose in the urine with normal levels in the blood, due to renal tubules' inability to reabsorb glucose completely.

6 E74.81 **Disorders of glucose transport, not elsewhere classified**

SP E74.810 **Glucose transporter protein type 1 deficiency**
De Vivo syndrome
Glucose transport defect, blood-brain barrier
Glut1 deficiency
GLUT1 deficiency syndrome 1, infantile onset
GLUT1 deficiency syndrome 2, childhood onset

SP E74.818 **Other disorders of glucose transport**
(Familial) renal glycosuria

SP E74.819 Disorders of glucose transport, unspecified

SP E74.89 **Other specified disorders of carbohydrate metabolism**
Essential pentosuria

IQ E74.9 Disorder of carbohydrate metabolism, unspecified

4 E75 **Disorders of sphingolipid metabolism and other lipid storage disorders**
EXCLUDES 1 mucolipidosis, types I-III (E77.0-E77.1)
Refsum's disease (G60.1)

5 E75.0 **GM2 gangliosidosis**

SP E75.00 GM2 gangliosidosis, unspecified

SP E75.01 **Sandhoff disease**

SP E75.02 **Tay-Sachs disease**

SP E75.09 **Other GM2 gangliosidosis**
Adult GM2 gangliosidosis
Juvenile GM2 gangliosidosis

5 E75.1 Other and unspecified gangliosidosis

SP E75.10 Unspecified gangliosidosis
Gangliosidosis NOS

SP E75.11 **Mucolipidosis IV**

SP E75.19 **Other gangliosidosis**
GM1 gangliosidosis
GM3 gangliosidosis

5 E75.2 **Other sphingolipidosis**
EXCLUDES 1 adrenoleukodystrophy [Addison-Schilder] (E71.528)

SP E75.21 **Fabry (-Anderson) disease**

SP E75.22 **Gaucher disease**

SP E75.23 **Krabbe disease**

▲ 6 E75.24 **Niemann-Pick disease**
Acid sphingomyelinase deficiency (ASMD)

▲ SP E75.240 **Niemann-Pick disease type A**
Acid sphingomyelinase deficiency type A (ASMD type A)
Infantile neurovisceral acid sphingomyelinase deficiency

▲ SP E75.241 **Niemann-Pick disease type B**
Acid sphingomyelinase deficiency type B (ASMD type B)
Chronic visceral acid sphingomyelinase deficiency

SP E75.242 **Niemann-Pick disease type C**

SP E75.243 **Niemann-Pick disease type D**

★ E75.244 **Niemann-Pick disease type A/B**
Acid sphingomyelinase deficiency type A/B (ASMD type A/B)
Chronic neurovisceral acid sphingomyelinase deficiency

SP E75.248 **Other Niemann-Pick disease**

▲ SP E75.249 Niemann-Pick disease, unspecified
Acid sphingomyelinase deficiency (ASMD) NOS

SP E75.25 **Metachromatic leukodystrophy**

SP E75.26 **Sulfatase deficiency**
Multiple sulfatase deficiency (MSD)

SP E75.29 **Other sphingolipidosis**
Farber's syndrome
Sulfatide lipidosis

SP E75.3 Sphingolipidosis, unspecified

SP E75.4 **Neuronal ceroid lipofuscinosis**
Batten disease
Bielschowsky-Jansky disease
Kufs disease
Spielmeyer-Vogt disease

SP E75.5 **Other lipid storage disorders**
Cerebrotendinous cholesterosis [van Bogaert-Scherer-Epstein]
Wolman's disease

SP **E75.6 Lipid storage disorder, unspecified**

4 **E76 Disorders of glycosaminoglycan metabolism**

5 **E76.0 Mucopolysaccharidosis, type I**

SP **E76.01 Hurler's syndrome**

SP **E76.02 Hurler-Scheie syndrome**

SP **E76.03 Scheie's syndrome**

SP **E76.1 Mucopolysaccharidosis, type II**
Hunter's syndrome

5 **E76.2 Other mucopolysaccharidoses**

6 **E76.21 Morquio mucopolysaccharidoses**

SP **E76.210 Morquio A mucopolysaccharidoses**
Classic Morquio syndrome
Morquio syndrome A
Mucopolysaccharidosis, type IVA

SP **E76.211 Morquio B mucopolysaccharidoses**
Morquio-like mucopolysaccharidoses
Morquio-like syndrome
Morquio syndrome B
Mucopolysaccharidosis, type IVB

SP **E76.219 Morquio mucopolysaccharidoses, unspecified**
Morquio syndrome
Mucopolysaccharidosis, type IV

SP **E76.22 Sanfilippo mucopolysaccharidoses**
Mucopolysaccharidosis, type III (A) (B) (C) (D)
Sanfilippo A syndrome
Sanfilippo B syndrome
Sanfilippo C syndrome
Sanfilippo D syndrome

SP **E76.29 Other mucopolysaccharidoses**
beta-Glucuronidase deficiency
Maroteaux-Lamy (mild) (severe) syndrome
Mucopolysaccharidosis, types VI, VII

SP **E76.3 Mucopolysaccharidosis, unspecified**

SP **E76.8 Other disorders of glucosaminoglycan metabolism**

SP **E76.9 Glucosaminoglycan metabolism disorder, unspecified**

4 **E77 Disorders of glycoprotein metabolism**

SP **E77.0 Defects in post-translational modification of lysosomal enzymes**
Mucolipidosis II [I-cell disease]
Mucolipidosis III [pseudo-Hurler polydystrophy]

SP **E77.1 Defects in glycoprotein degradation**
Aspartylglucosaminuria
Fucosidosis
Mannosidosis
Sialidosis [mucolipidosis I]

SP **E77.8 Other disorders of glycoprotein metabolism**

SP **E77.9 Disorder of glycoprotein metabolism, unspecified**

4 **E78 Disorders of lipoprotein metabolism and other lipidemias**
EXCLUDES 1 sphingolipidosis (E75.0-E75.3)

5 **E78.0 Pure hypercholesterolemia**

SP **E78.00 Pure hypercholesterolemia, unspecified**
Fredrickson's hyperlipoproteinemia, type IIa
Hyperbetalipoproteinemia
Low-density-lipoprotein-type [LDL] hyperlipoproteinemia
(Pure) hypercholesterolemia NOS

SP **E78.01 Familial hypercholesterolemia**

SP **E78.1 Pure hyperglyceridemia**
Elevated fasting triglycerides
Endogenous hyperglyceridemia
Fredrickson's hyperlipoproteinemia, type IV
Hyperlipidemia, group B
Hyperprebetalipoproteinemia
Very-low-density-lipoprotein-type [VLDL] hyperlipoproteinemia

SP **E78.2 Mixed hyperlipidemia**
Broad- or floating-betalipoproteinemia
Combined hyperlipidemia NOS
Elevated cholesterol with elevated triglycerides NEC
Fredrickson's hyperlipoproteinemia, type IIb or III
Hyperbetalipoproteinemia with prebetalipoproteinemia
Hypercholesteremia with endogenous hyperglyceridemia
Hyperlipidemia, group C
Tubo-eruptive xanthoma
Xanthoma tuberosum
EXCLUDES 1 cerebrotendinous cholesterosis [van Bogaert-Scherer- Epstein] (E75.5)
familial combined hyperlipidemia (E78.49)

SP **E78.3 Hyperchylomicronemia**
Chylomicron retention disease
Fredrickson's hyperlipoproteinemia, type I or V
Hyperlipidemia, group D
Mixed hyperglyceridemia

5 **E78.4 Other hyperlipidemia**

SP **E78.41 Elevated Lipoprotein(a)**
Elevated Lp(a)

SP **E78.49 Other hyperlipidemia**
Familial combined hyperlipidemia

SP **E78.5 Hyperlipidemia, unspecified**
DEFINITION An excess of lipids or fats in the blood.

SP **E78.6 Lipoprotein deficiency**
Abetalipoproteinemia
Depressed HDL cholesterol
High-density lipoprotein deficiency
Hypoalphalipoproteinemia
Hypobetalipoproteinemia (familial)
Lecithin cholesterol acyltransferase deficiency
Tangier disease

5 **E78.7 Disorders of bile acid and cholesterol metabolism**
EXCLUDES 1 Niemann-Pick disease type C (E75.242)

SP **E78.70 Disorder of bile acid and cholesterol metabolism, unspecified**

SP **E78.71 Barth syndrome**

SP **E78.72 Smith-Lemli-Opitz syndrome**

Chapter 4
E00-E89

SP **E78.79 Other disorders of bile acid and cholesterol metabolism**

5 **E78.8 Other disorders of lipoprotein metabolism**

SP **E78.81 Lipoid dermatoarthritis**

SP **E78.89 Other lipoprotein metabolism disorders**

IQ **E78.9 Disorder of lipoprotein metabolism, unspecified**

4 **E79 Disorders of purine and pyrimidine metabolism**

EXCLUDES 1 Ataxia-telangiectasia (Q87.19)
Bloom's syndrome (Q82.8)
Cockayne's syndrome (Q87.19)
calculus of kidney (N20.0)
combined immunodeficiency disorders (D81.-)
Fanconi's anemia (D61.09)
gout (M1A.-, M10.-)
orotaciduric anemia (D53.0)
progeria (E34.8)
Werner's syndrome (E34.8)
xeroderma pigmentosum (Q82.1)

SP **E79.0 Hyperuricemia without signs of inflammatory arthritis and tophaceous disease**
Asymptomatic hyperuricemia

SP **E79.1 Lesch-Nyhan syndrome**
HGPRT deficiency

SP **E79.2 Myoadenylate deaminase deficiency**

IQ **E79.8 Other disorders of purine and pyrimidine metabolism**
Hereditary xanthinuria

SP **E79.9 Disorder of purine and pyrimidine metabolism, unspecified**

4 **E80 Disorders of porphyrin and bilirubin metabolism**

INCLUDES defects of catalase and peroxidase

SP **E80.0 Hereditary erythropoietic porphyria**
Congenital erythropoietic porphyria
Erythropoietic protoporphyria

SP **E80.1 Porphyria cutanea tarda**

5 **E80.2 Other and unspecified porphyria**

SP **E80.20 Unspecified porphyria**
Porphyria NOS

SP **E80.21 Acute intermittent (hepatic) porphyria**

SP **E80.29 Other porphyria**
Hereditary coproporphyria

SP **E80.3 Defects of catalase and peroxidase**
Acatalasia [Takahara]

SP **E80.4 Gilbert syndrome**

DEFINITION A harmless inborn error of bilirubin metabolism from an abnormal liver enzyme causing a benign elevation of unconjugated bilirubin with no liver damage or hematologic abnormalities.

SP **E80.5 Crigler-Najjar syndrome**

SP **E80.6 Other disorders of bilirubin metabolism**
Dubin-Johnson syndrome
Rotor's syndrome

SP **E80.7 Disorder of bilirubin metabolism, unspecified**

4 **E83 Disorders of mineral metabolism**

EXCLUDES 1 dietary mineral deficiency (E58-E61)
parathyroid disorders (E20-E21)
vitamin D deficiency (E55.-)

5 **E83.0 Disorders of copper metabolism**

SP **E83.00 Disorder of copper metabolism, unspecified**

SP **E83.01 Wilson's disease**
Code also:
associated Kayser Fleischer ring (H18.04-)

SP **E83.09 Other disorders of copper metabolism**
Menkes' (kinky hair) (steely hair) disease

5 **E83.1 Disorders of iron metabolism**

EXCLUDES 1 iron deficiency anemia (D50.-)
sideroblastic anemia (D64.0-D64.3)

SP **E83.10 Disorder of iron metabolism, unspecified**

6 **E83.11 Hemochromatosis**

EXCLUDES 1 GALD (P78.84)
Gestational alloimmune liver disease (P78.84)
Neonatal hemochromatosis (P78.84)

SP **E83.110 Hereditary hemochromatosis**
Bronzed diabetes
Pigmentary cirrhosis (of liver)
Primary (hereditary) hemochromatosis

DEFINITION A genetic problem causing the body to store too much iron, resulting in liver swelling, skin bronzing, and development of diabetes, arthritis, and organ failure.

SP **E83.111 Hemochromatosis due to repeated red blood cell transfusions**
Iron overload due to repeated red blood cell transfusions
Transfusion (red blood cell) associated hemochromatosis

SP **E83.118 Other hemochromatosis**

SP **E83.119 Hemochromatosis, unspecified**

SP + **E83.19 Other disorders of iron metabolism**
Use additional code, if applicable, for idiopathic pulmonary hemosiderosis (J84.03)

SP **E83.2 Disorders of zinc metabolism**
Acrodermatitis enteropathica

5 **E83.3 Disorders of phosphorus metabolism and phosphatases**

EXCLUDES 1 adult osteomalacia (M83.-)
osteoporosis (M80.-)

SP **E83.30 Disorder of phosphorus metabolism, unspecified**

SP **E83.31 Familial hypophosphatemia**
Vitamin D-resistant osteomalacia
Vitamin D-resistant rickets

EXCLUDES 1 vitamin D-deficiency rickets (E55.0)

SP **E83.32 Hereditary vitamin D-dependent rickets (type 1) (type 2)**

25-hydroxyvitamin D 1-alpha-hydroxylase deficiency
Pseudovitamin D deficiency
Vitamin D receptor defect

SP **E83.39 Other disorders of phosphorus metabolism**
Acid phosphatase deficiency
Hypophosphatasia

5 **E83.4 Disorders of magnesium metabolism**

SP **E83.40 Disorders of magnesium metabolism, unspecified**

SP **E83.41 Hypermagnesemia**

SP **E83.42 Hypomagnesemia**

SP **E83.49 Other disorders of magnesium metabolism**

5 **E83.5 Disorders of calcium metabolism**
EXCLUDES 1 chondrocalcinosis (M11.1-M11.2)
hungry bone syndrome (E83.81)
hyperparathyroidism (E21.0-E21.3)

SP **E83.50 Unspecified disorder of calcium metabolism**

SP **E83.51 Hypocalcemia**
DEFINITION Reduced calcium levels in the blood causing hyperactive deep tendon reflexes, Chvostek's sign, muscle and abdominal cramps, and carpopedal spasm.

SP **E83.52 Hypercalcemia**
Familial hypocalciuric hypercalcemia
DEFINITION Excess calcium levels in the blood causing fatigue, muscle weakness, depression, anorexia, nausea, and constipation.

SP **E83.59 Other disorders of calcium metabolism**

5 **E83.8 Other disorders of mineral metabolism**

SP **E83.81 Hungry bone syndrome**
DEFINITION Low levels of calcium due to elevated parathyroid hormone levels or thyrotoxicosis that later return to normal or lower levels after treatment, causing bones to hoard calcium, resulting in increased bone density.

SP **E83.89 Other disorders of mineral metabolism**

IQ **E83.9 Disorder of mineral metabolism, unspecified**

4 **E84 Cystic fibrosis**
INCLUDES mucoviscidosis
Code also:
exocrine pancreatic insufficiency (K86.81)

CODING TIPS ✓ When reporting a E84 code, an additional code should be used to describe the manifestation. Chronic lung disease with bronchiectasis is a common aspect of cystic fibrosis, but is coded separately to provide additional information. An infection, such as pneumonia, should be coded separately. A patient with both pulmonary manifestations and gastrointestinal manifestations is coded with E84.0 and E84.1. Other manifestations (E84.8) include diabetes (E08) and right ventricular hypertrophy (I51.7). [AHA: 1Q 2021]

SP + **E84.0 Cystic fibrosis with pulmonary manifestations**
Use additional code to identify any infectious organism present, such as:
Pseudomonas (B96.5)

5 **E84.1 Cystic fibrosis with intestinal manifestations**

SP **E84.11 Meconium ileus in cystic fibrosis**
EXCLUDES 1 meconium ileus not due to cystic fibrosis (P76.0)

SP **E84.19 Cystic fibrosis with other intestinal manifestations**
Distal intestinal obstruction syndrome

SP **E84.8 Cystic fibrosis with other manifestations**

SP **E84.9 Cystic fibrosis, unspecified**
DEFINITION Defective gene causing overproduction of mucous that builds up in lung passages, resulting in life-threatening respiratory problems.

4 **E85 Amyloidosis**
EXCLUDES 2 Alzheimer's disease (G30.0-)

SP **E85.0 Non-neuropathic heredofamilial amyloidosis**
Hereditary amyloid nephropathy
Code also associated disorders, such as:
autoinflammatory syndromes (M04.-)
EXCLUDES 2 Transthyretin-related (ATTR) familial amyloid cardiomyopathy (E85.4)

SP **E85.1 Neuropathic heredofamilial amyloidosis**
Amyloid polyneuropathy (Portuguese)
Transthyretin-related (ATTR) familial amyloid polyneuropathy

SP **E85.2 Heredofamilial amyloidosis, unspecified**

SP **E85.3 Secondary systemic amyloidosis**
Hemodialysis-associated amyloidosis
DEFINITION Secondary amyloidosis is also known as reactive systemic amyloidosis, in which the deposited protein fibrils are of the AA type caused by a reaction to a chronic infection or other condition, such as osteomyelitis, rheumatoid arthritis, or a noninfectious disease process such as kidney failure with long term hemodialysis.

SP **E85.4 Organ-limited amyloidosis**
Localized amyloidosis
Transthyretin-related (ATTR) familial amyloid cardiomyopathy

5 **E85.8 Other amyloidosis**

SP **E85.81 Light chain (AL) amyloidosis**

SP **E85.82 Wild-type transthyretin-related (ATTR) amyloidosis**
Senile systemic amyloidosis (SSA)

SP **E85.89 Other amyloidosis**

SP **E85.9 Amyloidosis, unspecified**
DEFINITION Abnormal accumulation of amyloid-like proteins in tissues.

+ 4 **E86 Volume depletion**
Use additional code(s) for any associated disorders of electrolyte and acid-base balance (E87.-)
EXCLUDES 1 dehydration of newborn (P74.1)
postprocedural hypovolemic shock (T81.19)
traumatic hypovolemic shock (T79.4)
EXCLUDES 2 hypovolemic shock NOS (R57.1)

SP + **E86.0 Dehydration**
GUIDELINES **Section I.C.2.c.3)**
When the admission/encounter is for management of dehydration due to the malignancy and only the dehydration is being treated (intravenous rehydration), the dehydration is sequenced first, followed by the code(s) for the malignancy.

SP + **E86.1 Hypovolemia**
Depletion of volume of plasma
DEFINITION Abnormal decrease in the total volume of circulating blood with a corresponding loss of sodium electrolytes.

SP + **E86.9 Volume depletion, unspecified**

4 **E87 Other disorders of fluid, electrolyte and acid-base balance**
EXCLUDES 1 diabetes insipidus (E23.2)
electrolyte imbalance associated with hyperemesis gravidarum (O21.1)
electrolyte imbalance following ectopic or molar pregnancy (O08.5)
familial periodic paralysis (G72.3)

SP **E87.0 Hyperosmolality and hypernatremia**
Sodium [Na] excess
Sodium [Na] overload

SP **E87.1 Hypo-osmolality and hyponatremia**
Sodium [Na] deficiency
EXCLUDES 1 syndrome of inappropriate secretion of antidiuretic hormone (E22.2)

▲ SP **E87.2 Acidosis**
Acidosis NOS
Lactic acidosis
Metabolic acidosis
Respiratory acidosis
EXCLUDES 1 diabetic acidosis - see categories E08-E10, E11, E13 with ketoacidosis
DEFINITION An abnormal increase in the acidity of body fluids, caused either by accumulation of acids or by depletion of bicarbonates.

SP **E87.3 Alkalosis**
Alkalosis NOS
Metabolic alkalosis
Respiratory alkalosis

SP **E87.4 Mixed disorder of acid-base balance**

SP **E87.5 Hyperkalemia**
Potassium [K] excess
Potassium [K] overload
DEFINITION An abnormally high concentration of potassium ions in the blood.

SP **E87.6 Hypokalemia**
Potassium [K] deficiency
DEFINITION Low potassium level in the blood causing neuromuscular disorders ranging from weakness to paralysis, electrocardiographic abnormalities, renal disease, and gastrointestinal disorders.

5 **E87.7 Fluid overload**
EXCLUDES 1 edema NOS (R60.9)
fluid retention (R60.9)
DEFINITION High infusion rates or transfusion volumes not processed effectively by the recipient, causing circulatory system overload marked by acute respiratory distress.

SP **E87.70 Fluid overload, unspecified**

SP **E87.71 Transfusion associated circulatory overload**
Fluid overload due to transfusion (blood) (blood components)
TACO

SP **E87.79 Other fluid overload**

SP **E87.8 Other disorders of electrolyte and fluid balance, not elsewhere classified**
Electrolyte imbalance NOS
Hyperchloremia
Hypochloremia

+ 4 **E88 Other and unspecified metabolic disorders**
Use additional codes for associated conditions
EXCLUDES 1 histiocytosis X (chronic) (C96.6)

+ 5 **E88.0 Disorders of plasma-protein metabolism, not elsewhere classified**
EXCLUDES 1 monoclonal gammopathy (of undetermined significance) (D47.2)
polyclonal hypergammaglobulinemia (D89.0)
Waldenström macroglobulinemia (C88.0)
EXCLUDES 2 disorder of lipoprotein metabolism (E78.-)

SP + **E88.01 Alpha-1-antitrypsin deficiency**
AAT deficiency

SP + **E88.02 Plasminogen deficiency**
Dysplasminogenemia
Hypoplasminogenemia
Type 1 plasminogen deficiency
Type 2 plasminogen deficiency
Code also:
, if applicable, ligneous conjunctivitis (H10.51)
Use additional code for associated findings, such as:
hydrocephalus (G91.4)
otitis media (H67.-)

respiratory disorder related to plasminogen deficiency (J99)

SP + E88.09 **Other disorders of plasma-protein metabolism, not elsewhere classified**
Bisalbuminemia

SP + E88.1 **Lipodystrophy, not elsewhere classified**
Lipodystrophy NOS
EXCLUDES 1 Whipple's disease (K90.81)
DEFINITION Defective fat metabolism resulting in abnormal or degenerative subcutaneous fat deposits that appear as lumps or dents under the skin.

SP + E88.2 **Lipomatosis, not elsewhere classified**
Lipomatosis NOS
Lipomatosis (Check) dolorosa [Dercum]

SP + E88.3 **Tumor lysis syndrome**
Tumor lysis syndrome (spontaneous)
Tumor lysis syndrome following antineoplastic drug chemotherapy
Use additional code for adverse effect, if applicable, to identify drug (T45.1X5)

+ 5 E88.4 **Mitochondrial metabolism disorders**
EXCLUDES 1 disorders of pyruvate metabolism (E74.4)
Kearns-Sayre syndrome (H49.81)
Leber's disease (H47.22)
Leigh's encephalopathy (G31.82)
Mitochondrial myopathy, NEC (G71.3)
Reye's syndrome (G93.7)

SP + E88.40 **Mitochondrial metabolism disorder, unspecified**

SP + E88.41 **MELAS syndrome**
Mitochondrial myopathy, encephalopathy, lactic acidosis and stroke-like episodes

SP + E88.42 **MERRF syndrome**
Myoclonic epilepsy associated with ragged-red fibers
Code also:
progressive myoclonic epilepsy (G40.3-)

SP + E88.49 **Other mitochondrial metabolism disorders**

+ 5 E88.8 **Other specified metabolic disorders**

SP + E88.81 **Metabolic syndrome**
Dysmetabolic syndrome X
Use additional codes for associated manifestations, such as:
obesity (E66.-)
CODING TIPS ✓ Metabolic syndrome (also called dysmetabolic syndrome X) involves a cluster of symptoms placing individuals at risk for development of a number of disease processes. Manifestations of metabolic syndrome confirmed by the provider, such as obesity (and BMI as calculated by the clinical record documentation), should additionally be coded following E88.81.

SP + E88.89 **Other specified metabolic disorders**
Launois-Bensaude adenolipomatosis
EXCLUDES 1 adult pulmonary Langerhans cell histiocytosis (J84.82)

IQ + E88.9 **Metabolic disorder, unspecified**

Postprocedural endocrine and metabolic complications and disorders, not elsewhere classified (E89)

CODING TIPS ✓ Conditions classifiable to E89 are classifiable as postprocedural complications. These conditions should only be assigned when diagnostic statements clearly indicate that the condition is a complication of a procedure.

4 E89 **Postprocedural endocrine and metabolic complications and disorders, not elsewhere classified**
EXCLUDES 2 intraoperative complications of endocrine system organ or structure (E36.0-, E36.1-, E36.8)

SP E89.0 **Postprocedural hypothyroidism**
Postirradiation hypothyroidism
Postsurgical hypothyroidism
CODING TIPS ✓ Report E89.0 for patients with hypothyroidism following a thyroidectomy.
DEFINITION Underactive thyroid gland due to surgery or radiation, causing an inadequate production of thyroid hormone and a slowing of metabolic processes.

SP + E89.1 **Postprocedural hypoinsulinemia**
Postpancreatectomy hyperglycemia
Postsurgical hypoinsulinemia
Use additional code, if applicable, to identify:
acquired absence of pancreas (Z90.41-)
diabetes mellitus (postpancreatectomy) (postprocedural) (E13.-)
insulin use (Z79.4)
EXCLUDES 1 transient postprocedural hyperglycemia (R73.9)
transient postprocedural hypoglycemia (E16.2)
GUIDELINES **Section I.C.4.a.6)(b)(i)**
For postpancreatectomy diabetes mellitus (lack of insulin due to the surgical removal of all or part of the pancreas), assign code E89.1, Postprocedural hypoinsulinemia. Assign a code from category E13 and a code from subcategory Z90.41-, Acquired absence of pancreas, as additional codes.
CODING TIPS ✓ Because the pancreas produces insulin, the removal of even a portion of the pancreas can produce diabetic-like symptoms. If manifestations are produced because of the hyperglycemia and lack of insulin, add the codes for manifestations after E89.1 with the appropriate E13 code(s). Also add the acquired absence of pancreas (Z90.41-) and use of insulin (Z79.4).

SP E89.2 **Postprocedural hypoparathyroidism**
Parathyroprival tetany

SP E89.3 **Postprocedural hypopituitarism**
Postirradiation hypopituitarism

5 E89.4 **Postprocedural ovarian failure**

SP E89.40 **Asymptomatic postprocedural ovarian failure**
Postprocedural ovarian failure NOS

Chapter 4
E00-E89

SP **E89.41 Symptomatic postprocedural ovarian failure**
Symptoms such as flushing, sleeplessness, headache, lack of concentration, associated with postprocedural menopause

SP **E89.5 Postprocedural testicular hypofunction**

SP **E89.6 Postprocedural adrenocortical (-medullary) hypofunction**

5 **E89.8 Other postprocedural endocrine and metabolic complications and disorders**

6 **E89.81 Postprocedural hemorrhage of an endocrine system organ or structure following a procedure**

SP **E89.810 Postprocedural hemorrhage of an endocrine system organ or structure following an endocrine system procedure**

SP **E89.811 Postprocedural hemorrhage of an endocrine system organ or structure following other procedure**

6 **E89.82 Postprocedural hematoma and seroma of an endocrine system organ or structure**

SP **E89.820 Postprocedural hematoma of an endocrine system organ or structure following an endocrine system procedure**

SP **E89.821 Postprocedural hematoma of an endocrine system organ or structure following other procedure**

SP **E89.822 Postprocedural seroma of an endocrine system organ or structure following an endocrine system procedure**

SP **E89.823 Postprocedural seroma of an endocrine system organ or structure following other procedure**

SP + **E89.89 Other postprocedural endocrine and metabolic complications and disorders**
Use additional code, if applicable, to further specify disorder

Chapter 4 Scenarios: Endocrine, nutritional and metabolic diseases (E00-E89)

Diabetic hypertension

A 74-year-old man was recently diagnosed with severe hypertension that his physician documented as due to his type 2 diabetes. He also has stage 2 chronic kidney disease, which is also related to the diabetes. The physician confirmed that his additional diagnosis of right heart failure, which predated his diabetes diagnosis, is unrelated to the hypertension. He takes oral hypoglycemic medication. The hypertension is the focus of care.

Description	Code
Primary: Type 2 diabetes mellitus with other circulatory complications	E11.59
Secondary: Hypertension secondary to endocrine disorders	I15.2
Secondary: Type 2 diabetes mellitus with diabetic chronic kidney disease	E11.22
Secondary: Chronic kidney disease, stage 2 (mild)	N18.2
Secondary: Right heart failure, unspecified	I50.810
Secondary: Long term (current) use of oral hypoglycemic drugs	Z79.84

There is no assumed relationship between hypertension and diabetes. However, in this scenario, the physician specifically connected the diagnoses. Thus, it is captured first with E11.59 followed by I15.2. Stage 2 diabetic chronic kidney disease also requires two codes to fully capture the diagnosis: E11.22 and N18.2. While there is normally an assumed relationship between hypertension and heart failure, the physician confirmed the two are unrelated and are thus coded separately, in accordance with coding guidelines.

Diabetic macular edema

A 73-year-old man admitted to home care has just been prescribed insulin for his type 2 diabetes. However, the retinopathy and macular edema from his diabetes is severe enough that it has caused legal blindness. Skilled nursing is ordered for teaching and training regarding insulin and use of insulin syringes with magnifiers.

Description	Code
Primary: Type 2 diabetes with unspecified diabetic retinopathy with macular edema	E11.311
Secondary: Legal blindness	H54.8
Secondary: Long-term (current) use of insulin	Z79.4

There's a "code first" note at H54.8 instructing to assign first the reason for the legal blindness - in this case, that would be the one all-inclusive code for diabetic macular edema, E11.311. The long-term (current) use of insulin should be coded, if it is anticipated that the need for insulin will be ongoing. It should not be used for short-term insulin use.

Diabetes with renal manifestation

A patient is admitted to home health for teaching and training about his diabetes with stage 2 chronic kidney disease. He is not currently taking insulin. The patient's medical record indicates a history of stable chronic systolic heart failure and hypertension.

Description	Code
Primary: Type 2 diabetes mellitus with diabetic chronic kidney disease	E11.22
Secondary: Hypertensive heart and chronic kidney disease with heart failure and stage 1 through stage 4 chronic kidney disease, or unspecified chronic kidney disease	I13.0
Secondary: Chronic systolic (congestive) heart failure	I50.22
Secondary: Chronic kidney disease, stage 2	N18.2

When the type of diabetes is not stated, the default is type 2. There is an assumed relationship in the ICD-10 classification between diabetes and any specific condition listed under "with" in the alphabetic index, and a combination code describes these two conditions: E11.22. Note that E11.22 instructs the coder to use an additional code to identify the stage of chronic kidney disease. Therefore, N18.2 is additionally assigned. The current ICD-10 classification also assumes a relationship between hypertension and chronic kidney disease, as well as hypertension and heart failure, therefore a combination code from category I13.- is assigned and precedes both the heart failure and chronic kidney disease codes.

Amyloidosis with arthropathy

Physical therapy is ordered for a patient who has right shoulder arthropathy due to amyloidosis. Additional diagnoses of "secondary diabetes", polyneuropathy, and gastroparesis are also reported by the physician.

Description	Code
Primary: Organ limited amyloidosis (localized)	E85.4
Secondary: Arthropathy in other specified diseases elsewhere, right shoulder	M14.811
Secondary: Other specified diabetes mellitus with diabetic polyneuropathy	E13.42
Secondary: Other specified diabetes mellitus with diabetic autonomic (poly)neuropathy	E13.43
Secondary: Gastroparesis	K31.84

Amyloidosis can be limited to one organ; e.g., the musculoskeletal system, the heart or the brain. This is an etiology (amyloidosis) and manifestation (arthropathy) pairing. It is evident when searching the alphabetic index for "arthropathy in (due to) "amyloidosis" and you find "E85.4 *[M14.8-]*." Therefore, the etiology (the amyloidosis) must be immediately followed by the manifestation (the arthropathy). Additional codes for the secondary diabetes with manifestations of polyneuropathy and gastroparesis are added as these are important comorbid conditions that impact the patient's rehabilitation prognosis and the comorbidity adjustment for payment. Secondary diabetes, when not further specified is coded to E13.-. Gastroparesis should be assigned using the combination code for diabetes with autonomic (poly)neuropathy. While the assignment of the additional code to identify gastroparesis, K31.84, more specifically, is not required, it may be optionally assigned according to Q1 2016 Coding Clinic guidance.

Type 1 diabetes with neuropathy

A patient is admitted to home care for type 1 diabetes mellitus with neuropathy and with hyperglycemia. She was started on a sliding scale, in addition to her daily insulin, which she is able to administer independently. She also has hypertension, depression and a pressure ulcer/injury of the right buttock (stage 3) that is improving with treatment but still requires dressing changes, which the nurse will be doing twice a week. She also just started taking iron for her anemia. The main reason for admission is diabetic management.

Description	Code
Primary: Type 1 diabetes mellitus with diabetic neuropathy, unspecified	E10.40
Secondary: Type 1 diabetes mellitus with hyperglycemia	E10.65
Secondary: Pressure ulcer of right buttock, stage 3	L89.313
Secondary: Anemia, unspecified	D64.9
Secondary: Essential primary hypertension	I10
Secondary: Depression, unspecified	F32.A

The patient's diabetes is captured with two separate combination codes, one for the diabetic neuropathy, which is not further specified, and one for diabetes with hyperglycemia. The pressure ulcer/injury code is a combination code, which includes the site, stage and laterality. The other relevant co-morbidities, anemia, hypertension and depression, are additionally coded as they have the potential to impact the patient's plan of care. Though she is taking iron for her anemia, it's not specified as iron deficiency anemia and is thus coded as unspecified. Depression that is not specified should be coded to F32.A.

Secondary diabetes with PVD

Your patient has diabetic peripheral vascular disease (PVD), as a result of prolonged use of prednisone for his severe persistent asthma. The focus of care is his diabetes. He continues to take prednisone.

Description	Code
Primary: Drug or chemical induced diabetes mellitus with diabetic peripheral angiopathy without gangrene	E09.51
Secondary: Adverse effect of steroids, subsequent encounter	T38.0X5D
Secondary: Severe persistent asthma, uncomplicated	J45.50
Secondary: Long-term (current) use of systemic steroids	Z79.52

Since the patient took the prednisone, as prescribed, and then developed diabetes (which is considered secondary diabetes), this is coded as an adverse effect. Tabular instruction at category E09.- tells you to use an additional code to identify the drug causing the adverse effect, which is found in the Table of Drugs and Chemicals. The reason the drug was taken in the first place, asthma in this case, should be sequenced next. Note, if an existing diagnosis of diabetes worsens due to steroid use, it is not steroid-induced diabetes. Diabetic PVD should be coded as diabetic peripheral angiopathy, according to Q2 2018 Coding Clinic guidance. The patient's continued use of prednisone is captured with Z79.52.

Diabetes, contracture

A patient is referred for home care with worsening type 2 diabetes, now requiring insulin. She has right hand joint contractures after suffering third-degree burns from contact with boiling water three years ago. Orders include nursing for insulin teaching and administration, and occupational therapy to assist with insulin administration strategies.

Description	Code
Primary: Type 2 diabetes without complications	E11.9
Secondary: Contracture, right hand	M24.541
Secondary: Burn of third degree of right hand, unspecified site, sequela	T23.301S
Secondary: Contact with other hot fluids, sequela	X12.XXXS
Secondary: Long term (current) use of insulin	Z79.4

The code for the sequela condition, the contracture, is sequenced immediately before the sequela form of the etiology injury code, the burn, per coding guidelines. When searching the index for sequelae, burn and corrosion, the code provided is for the sequela condition only, indicating this is not a combination code. The code for the sequela condition or residual (the hand contracture) is found by searching the index at contraction, joint, hand joint, and is then sequenced preceding the sequela form of the etiology injury code to fully capture the fact that the now-healed burn left behind the contracture. In the index at sequelae, burn and corrosion, the direction is to code to injury with the seventh character "S." The letter "S" is added to the sequela code to indicate that the code represents a sequela and not an acute burn. An external cause code is assigned to illustrate how the patient sustained the burn that caused the current contracture (contact with boiling water), which is found by searching the Index to External Cause of Injuries. Notice how the external cause code is only three characters long (X12.-) but requires a 7th character, necessitating the use of placeholder "x" for the fourth, fifth and sixth character positions. The external cause code carries the same seventh character as the injury it's describing, in accordance with coding guidelines. Long-term (current) use of insulin, Z79.4, will be coded because the patient uses insulin and is not a type 1 diabetic.

Cystic fibrosis with pseudomonas pneumonia

A 42-year-old man is admitted to home health following a hospitalization where he was treated with IV antibiotics for a pulmonary exacerbation of his cystic fibrosis with pseudomonas pneumonia. The infection is still resolving and he will continue on oral antibiotics for the next six weeks. His discharge summary also lists secondary diabetes with hyperglycemia due to the cystic fibrosis, for which he takes insulin, polyneuropathy, and vitamin D deficiency.

Description	Code
Primary: Cystic fibrosis with pulmonary manifestations	E84.0
Secondary: Pneumonia due to Pseudomonas	J15.1
Secondary: Diabetes mellitus due to underlying condition with hyperglycemia	E08.65
Secondary: Diabetes mellitus due to underlying condition with diabetic polyneuropathy	E08.42
Secondary: Vitamin D deficiency, unspecified	E55.9
Secondary: Long term (current) use of insulin	Z79.4
Secondary: Long term (current) use of antibiotics	Z79.2

The pseudomonas pneumonia is coded after the cystic fibrosis in accordance with tabular instructions. The code for antibiotic use is assigned as the patient will continue taking antibiotics for several more weeks. Additional codes are added for the diabetes with hyperglycemia and polyneuropathy due to cystic fibrosis, as well as vitamin D deficiency and insulin use. A "code first" note at E08- requires that codes from this category always be assigned after the underlying cause.

Diabetic retinopathy secondary to hereditary hemochromatosis

A 68-year-old man comes to home health with a primary diagnosis of diabetic retinopathy in both eyes. He was diagnosed with hereditary hemochromatosis five years ago and developed diabetes two years later as a result. He is insulin-dependent and also has hypertension and will receive skilled nursing visits for teaching on the disease process.

Description	Code
Primary: Hereditary hemochromatosis	E83.110
Secondary: Diabetes mellitus due to underlying condition with unspecified diabetic retinopathy without macular edema	E08.319
Secondary: Essential (primary) hypertension	I10
Secondary: Long term (current) use of insulin	Z79.4

The patient's diabetic retinopathy resulted from hereditary hemochromatosis and is therefore appropriately coded as a manifestation of diabetes due to any underlying condition, with E08.319. Even though the diabetic retinopathy is the focus of care, because it was caused by hemochromatosis, the underlying condition is coded first, according to tabular instruction. Hypertension is an important comorbidity that should be coded whenever it is present. The patient is insulin dependent but not a type 1 diabetic; therefore, the code for insulin use is required.

Diabetes, obesity

A newly diagnosed diabetic on an oral antidiabetic agent is admitted to home health for observation, assessment and teaching on diabetes. The history and physical notes that she is morbidly obese with a history of hypertension and chronic diastolic heart failure. Her BMI is documented as 56.

Description	Code
Primary: Type 2 diabetes mellitus without complications	E11.9
Secondary: Morbid (severe) obesity due to excess calories	E66.01
Secondary: Hypertensive heart disease with heart failure	I11.0
Secondary: Chronic diastolic (congestive) heart failure	I50.32
Secondary: Body mass index (BMI) 50.0-59.9, adult	Z68.43
Secondary: Long term (current) use of oral hypoglycemic drugs	Z79.84

Since the type of diabetes is not stated, the default is type 2. Morbid obesity should always be coded when it's been documented by the physician, according to Q4 2018 Coding Clinic guidance. If not documented or confirmed, the BMI may be calculated, based on the patient's height and weight, by a non-provider, such as a dietitian or nurse, and may be coded without physician verification. Remember to add the code for use of oral hypoglycemic drugs (Z79.84) per the use additional code note at E11.-. Additional codes for comorbid conditions hypertension and chronic diastolic heart failure are added as these conditions impact the patients overall prognosis and add important comorbidity adjustment to the episode. The ICD-10 classification assumes a relationship between these two conditions, requiring that a combination code be assigned for hypertensive heart disease, I11.0.

Diabetic osteomyelitis, MRSA

A 69-year-old man with diabetes comes to home health with a primary diagnosis of acute osteomyelitis in the bones of his left big toe. The infecting organism is MRSA. He will receive IV antibiotics for several weeks and is dependent on insulin.

Description	Code
Primary: Type 2 diabetes mellitus with other specified complication	E11.69
Secondary: Other acute osteomyelitis, left ankle and foot	M86.172
Secondary: Methicillin resistant Staphylococcus aureus infection as the cause of diseases classified elsewhere	B95.62
Secondary: Encounter for adjustment and management of vascular access device	Z45.2
Secondary: Long term (current) use of antibiotics	Z79.2
Secondary: Long term (current) use of insulin	Z79.4

The patient's osteomyelitis infection can be assumed to be connected to his diabetes as no other cause was given, according to its listing under the subterm "with" in the alphabetic index. Thus, it is coded as diabetic osteomyelitis. The diabetes is coded as type 2 as the type is not specified and type 2 is the default, according to coding guidelines. The code for osteomyelitis is assigned underneath the diabetes code, in accordance with the etiology-manifestation convention. The infecting organism was specified as MRSA, necessitating the use of B95.62. The administration of IV antibiotics is captured with Z45.2 and Z79.2. If the IV is not the primary reason the patient requires home health care, but where there may be some sort of intervention noted on the home health plan of care, then it would be appropriate to report Z45.2 (but not as the principal or first secondary diagnosis), according to CMS. As the patient is not specified to be a type 1 diabetes and is dependent on insulin, code Z79.4 is required to capture this.

Yeast infection, morbid obesity

A 62-year-old woman who is morbidly obese is admitted to home health for medication monitoring, after recently being started on insulin, and physical therapy for a diagnosis of diabetic polyneuropathy. She also requires treatment of a yeast infection in the skin folds of her abdomen. She suffers from severe chafing and irritation from the skin folds constantly rubbing together, which her physician stated led to the yeast infection. Her height is 60 inches and she weighs 502 lbs, which the assessing clinician calculated to 98.

Description	Code
Primary: Type 2 diabetes mellitus with diabetic polyneuropathy	E11.42
Secondary: Erythema intertrigo	L30.4
Secondary: Candidiasis of skin and nail	B37.2
Secondary: Morbid (severe) obesity due to excess calories	E66.01
Secondary: Body mass index (BMI) 70 or greater, adult	Z68.45
Secondary: Long term (current) use of insulin	Z79.4

Diabetic polyneuropathy is captured with the combination code E11.42. As the focus of care, it is coded in the primary position. Codes L30.4 and B37.2 are assigned to capture the irritation in her skin folds from excessive chafing and the resulting yeast infection. Morbid obesity has been diagnosed and must be coded, as it will impact her care and recovery, and because morbid obesity should be coded whenever it has been documented by the physician, according to Q4 2018 Coding Clinic guidance. Her BMI is calculated by the assessing clinician based on her recorded height and weight and coded in accordance with tabular instruction at E66.01. A BMI code can be assigned on the basis of the clinician's documentation, according to coding guidelines. As a type 2 diabetes who uses insulin, an additional code for insulin use, Z79.4, is required.

Severe malnutrition with neoplastic disease

A 38-year-old male patient male patient is admitted with severe malnutrition and anemia due to neoplastic disease including primary liver cancer. He also requires wound care due to a stage 3 pressure wound of the left ankle. His medical record notes that he is wheelchair bound due to C1-C4 complete quadriplegia secondary to a C1 spinal cord injury causing central cord syndrome. The focus of care is malnutrition.

Description	Code
Primary: Unspecified severe protein-calorie malnutrition	E43
Secondary: Malignant neoplasm of liver, primary, unspecified as to type	C22.8
Secondary: Anemia in neoplastic disease	D63.0
Secondary: Pressure ulcer of left ankle, stage 3	L89.523
Secondary: Quadriplegia, C1-C4 complete	G82.51
Secondary: Central cord syndrome at C1 level of cervical spinal cord, sequela	S14.121S
Secondary: Dependence on wheelchair	Z99.3

According to Q1 2020 Coding Clinic guidance, malnutrition is not integral to neoplastic disease and should be coded separately. Because the malnutrition is the focus of care, it is assigned primary. While the patient is also referred for monitoring of anemia due to neoplastic disease, the "code first" note at D63.0 requires that the neoplasm be coded before the anemia. Additional codes are assigned for the wound of the ankle, which requires care, as well as quadriplegia and the cord syndrome with 7th character "S" to indicate that the quadriplegia is a sequela of this and it is not a current condition.

Chapter 5: Mental, Behavioral and Neurodevelopmental Disorders (F01-F99)

When assigning a diagnosis from this chapter, pay close attention to consistency with OASIS data items related to cognitive and behavioral functioning. **Do not choose a mental disorder as a diagnosis unless that diagnosis is confirmed with the physician.** You'll also want to consider whether your agency will be providing psychiatric nursing when using a code from this chapter as primary, or whether you will be training a caregiver to care for a patient with such a condition. Mental disorders are comorbidities that will impact the care, so ordinarily will be coded as secondary even if psychiatric nursing will not be provided.

Chapter 5 includes codes for a number of different conditions including:

- Psychoses with organic and nonorganic causes such as dementia and schizophrenia.
- Neurotic disorders such as anxiety disorders and phobic disorders.
- Personality disorders such as paranoia and antisocial personality disorder.
- Abuse of alcohol and drugs. In this category, the patient has intense desire to obtain increasing amounts of alcohol or drugs to the exclusion of all other activities, but is not dependent.
- Dependence on alcohol and drugs where the patient has a physical need for the alcohol or drug (addiction) and suffers withdrawal symptoms if it is not available.
- Intellectual disabilities where the patient has an IQ of 70 or less.
- Special symptoms or syndromes, not elsewhere classified, including stuttering and anorexia nervosa.

Some conditions in this chapter use the same or similar terms. It is important to check with the physician if there is any doubt as to which code is correct. For example, obsessive-compulsive disorder may be reported using the appropriate code from category F42.- (Obsessive-compulsive disorder) or F60.5 (Obsessive-compulsive personality disorder). Since there is an Excludes 2 note at both of these codes, they can be coded together as long as both diagnoses are verified by the physician. Another example is major depression unspecified, which may be reported using F32.9 (single episode) or F33.9 (recurrent episodes), F41.8 (mixed anxiety and depressive disorder) or F43.21 (Adjustment disorder with depressed mood).

This chapter also includes some codes that are phobias and disorders not due to substance or known physiological condition, such as shyness disorder of childhood/adolescence (F40.10), adult onset fluency disorder (F98.5), sleep disorders unspecified (F51.9), bedwetting (F98.0). Other disorders coded in this chapter are autism disorder (F84.0) and attention deficit hyperactivity disorder (F90.-).

A few situations to watch out for:

- If a patient has a **personal or family history** of a condition reported in this chapter, it may be appropriate to select from the Z code section, such as Z86.59 (Personal history of other mental and behavioral disorders) or Z81.8 (Family history of other mental and behavioral disorders). ***Reminder:*** These are vague codes and would not generally be used in home health or hospice.
- If a condition reported in this chapter is the **result of injury or medical treatment**, a code from Chapter 19 may be reported with a code from this chapter.
- **Symptoms** related to mental disorders are sometimes reported using codes from Chapter 18 such as code R41.81 (Age related cognitive decline or senility NOS) or R54 (Age-related physical debility). Every effort should be made to secure a definitive diagnosis. A symptom code from Chapter 18 may be reported as an additional diagnosis when it describes a significant aspect of the condition but is not an integral part of the condition.
- Although not often recorded in home health, if reporting a **mental disorder in a pregnant patient** when the condition is complicating the pregnancy, report first a code from Chapter 15 category O99.3- (Mental disorders and diseases of the nervous system complicating pregnancy, childbirth and the puerperium) with an additional code from Chapter 5 to describe the mental disease or disorder.

Multiple Coding and Sequencing

Includes and Excludes notes should be followed for codes in this chapter, as well as any other instructions under the code or code category. Some examples of multiple coding and sequencing issues for codes in this chapter include:

Disorders that affect the brain

The majority of codes from categories F01-F09 (Mental disorders due to physiological conditions) are reported **following** a code for the underlying physiological condition. For example, a patient with depressed mood disorder due to cerebrovascular disease would be coded I67.9 (cerebrovascular disease, unspecified) followed by F06.31 (Mood disorder due to known physiological condition with depressive features).

Dementia in Alzheimer's disease

Dementia in Alzheimer's disease is reported with code G30.- (Alzheimer's) as the first diagnosis and F02.80 (Dementia in conditions classified elsewhere without behavioral disturbance) or F02.81 (with behavioral disturbance such as physical or verbal aggression) as the additional diagnosis. When coding F02.81, use Z91.83 (Wandering in diseases classified elsewhere) as an additional diagnosis when appropriate. But remember, wandering can only be coded with the F02.81 to indicate behavior problems even though the patient may not have aggressive, violent or combative behavior. There are many neurological conditions in Chapter 6 that are the underlying etiology for F02.8- so be sure to look at the code first note under F02.

Also, an additional code from F02.8- (Dementia in other diseases classified elsewhere) is required for a patient with Lewy body dementia (G31.83). ***Note***, dementia is inherent to a diagnosis of Alzheimer's disease and the physician does not have to list it separately in order for it to be coded, the Coding Clinic confirmed in its Q1 2017 update.

Note: F03.- (Unspecified dementia) covers many codes, such as senile and presenile dementia. Vascular dementia is coded from category F01 with a 5th character required to identify with or without behavioral disturbance.

Pain disorders related to psychological factors

Assign code F45.41 for pain that is exclusively related to psychological disorders. As indicated by the Excludes 1 note under category G89 (Pain, not elsewhere classified), a code from category G89 should ***not*** be assigned with code F45.41.

Code F45.42 (Pain disorders with related psychological factors) should be used with a code from category G89 (Pain not elsewhere classified) if there is documentation of a psychological component for a patient with acute and chronic pain.

Special Coding Issues

Mental and behavioral disorders due to psychoactive substance use

ICD-10-CM has significantly expanded the coding options related to psychoactive substance use. Codes for psychoactive substance use disorders (codes from subcategories F10.9-, F11.9-, F12.9-, F13.9-, F14.9-, F15.9- and F16.9-) should only be assigned based on provider documentation and when they meet the definition of a reportable diagnosis (see Section III, Reporting Additional Diagnoses). The codes are to be used only when the psychoactive substance use is associated with a physical, mental or behavioral disorder, and such a relationship is documented by the provider, according to coding guidelines.

Selection of codes to indicate "in remission" in categories F10-F19 utilize FXX.11 to indicate abuse in remission, or FXX.21 to indicate dependence in remission. These codes are ***assigned only on the basis of physician documentation that the patient is in remission.***

Take note of the following guidelines when coding these diagnoses:

- Capture mild substance abuse disorder in early or sustained remission as substance abuse in remission. Code moderate or severe substance abuse disorder in early or sustained remission as substance dependence in remission.
- When the physician documentation refers to use, abuse and dependence of the same substance (e.g., alcohol, opioid, cannabis, etc.), only one code should be assigned to identify the pattern of use based on the following hierarchy:
  - If both use and abuse are documented, assign only the code for abuse.
  - If both abuse and dependence are documented, assign only the code for dependence.
  - If use, abuse and dependence are all documented, assign only the code for dependence.
  - If both use and dependence are documented, assign only the code for dependence.
- As with all other diagnoses, the codes for psychoactive substance use should only be assigned ***based on the physician's documentation and when they meet the definition of a reportable diagnosis.*** The definition of other diagnoses is interpreted as additional conditions that affect patient care in terms of requiring:
  - Clinical evaluation, or
  - Therapeutic treatment, or
  - Diagnostic procedures, or extended length of stay, or
  - Increased nursing care and/or monitoring.

The codes are to be used only when the psychoactive substance use is associated with a mental or behavioral disorder, and such a relationship is documented by the physician.

Chapter 5 includes many combination codes that combine the psychoactive substance use with other symptoms such as F10.97 (Alcohol use, unspecified with alcohol-induced persisting dementia) or F10.250 (Alcohol dependence with alcohol induced psychotic disorder with delusions).

CHAPTER 5: MENTAL, BEHAVIORAL AND NEURODEVELOPMENTAL DISORDERS (F01-F99)

INCLUDES disorders of psychological development

EXCLUDES 2 symptoms, signs and abnormal clinical laboratory findings, not elsewhere classified (R00-R99)

CODING TIPS✓ It is important not to code a patient with dementia or other psychiatric disorder unless documented by the physician or NPP. A primary diagnosis of mental disorder may require a psychiatrically trained nurse to provide services. Some services, such as administration of IM medications for treatment of a psychiatric diagnosis, do not require a psychiatrically trained nurse. A mental disorder always impacts the care and should be added as a comorbidity any time the documentation is present.

This chapter contains the following blocks:

F01-F09	Mental disorders due to known physiological conditions
F10-F19	Mental and behavioral disorders due to psychoactive substance use
F20-F29	Schizophrenia, schizotypal, delusional, and other non-mood psychotic disorders
F30-F39	Mood [affective] disorders
F40-F48	Anxiety, dissociative, stress-related, somatoform and other nonpsychotic mental disorders
F50-F59	Behavioral syndromes associated with physiological disturbances and physical factors
F60-F69	Disorders of adult personality and behavior
F70-F79	Intellectual disabilities
F80-F89	Pervasive and specific developmental disorders
F90-F98	Behavioral and emotional disorders with onset usually occurring in childhood and adolescence
F99	Unspecified mental disorder

Mental disorders due to known physiological conditions (F01-F09)

Note:
This block comprises a range of mental disorders grouped together on the basis of their having in common a demonstrable etiology in cerebral disease, brain injury, or other insult leading to cerebral dysfunction. The dysfunction may be primary, as in diseases, injuries, and insults that affect the brain directly and selectively; or secondary, as in systemic diseases and disorders that attack the brain only as one of the multiple organs or systems of the body that are involved.

CODING TIPS✓ Conditions classifiable here are specifically reportable as due to an underlying cause or condition.

4 **F01 Vascular dementia**

Vascular dementia as a result of infarction of the brain due to vascular disease, including hypertensive cerebrovascular disease.

INCLUDES arteriosclerotic dementia

Code first:
the underlying physiological condition or sequelae of cerebrovascular disease.

ALERT F01, F02 and F03 will not be accepted as primary codes in hospice.

5 **F01.5 Vascular dementia**

CODING TIPS✓ Do not assign a code from category F01.5- if the underlying cause is unknown. Assign a code from category F03.9- (Unspecified dementia). (AHA: 2Q 2021)

CODING TIPS✓ It is inappropriate to code vascular dementia as a sequela of unspecified cerebrovascular disease (I69.918), unless the physician documented the dementia as a sequela of cerebrovascular disease. Vascular dementia can be coded with other types of dementia using the F02.8 subcategory.

CODING TIPS✓ Vascular dementia may also be reported as "multi-infarct dementia." In this case it should be coded as a sequelae of cerebrovascular accident (stroke). This type of dementia also may be related to other cerebral vascular disorders including vascular hypertension and cerebral atherosclerosis.

CODING TIPS✓ F01.5 codes may not be sequenced primary in hospice, and do not qualify as a primary diagnosis in PDGM. If related to cerebral infarction, home care and hospice coders should use I69.3-. If the patient has not had a stroke, query the physician or NPP regarding conditions in I65- I67 as causes of vascular dementia.

DEFINITION Major neurocognitive disorder, known previously as dementia, is a decline in mental ability severe enough to interfere with independence and daily life. This term was introduced when the American Psychiatric Association (APA) released the fifth edition of its Diagnostic and Statistical Manual of Mental Disorders (DSM-5).

IQ **F01.50 Vascular dementia without behavioral disturbance**

Major neurocognitive disorder without behavioral disturbance

IQ + **F01.51 Vascular dementia with behavioral disturbance**

Major neurocognitive disorder due to vascular disease, with behavioral disturbance

Major neurocognitive disorder with aggressive behavior

Major neurocognitive disorder with combative behavior

Major neurocognitive disorder with violent behavior

Vascular dementia with aggressive behavior

Vascular dementia with combative behavior

Vascular dementia with violent behavior

Use additional code, if applicable, to identify wandering in vascular dementia (Z91.83)

CODING TIPS✓ Anxiety is not considered a behavior indicated by a 5th character of 1. Anxiety, when documented by the provider, in addition to dementia, should be coded separately.

CODING TIPS✓ Use Z91.83 (Wandering in diseases classified elsewhere) as an additional code when appropriate. Wandering is coded with the 5th digit indicating behavior problems even if the patient does not have aggressive, violent, combative behavior.

4 F02 Dementia in other diseases classified elsewhere

INCLUDES Major neurocognitive disorder in other diseases classified elsewhere

Code first the underlying physiological condition, such as:
- Alzheimer's (G30.-)
- cerebral lipidosis (E75.4)
- Creutzfeldt-Jakob disease (A81.0-)
- dementia with Lewy bodies (G31.83)
- dementia with Parkinsonism (G31.83)
- epilepsy and recurrent seizures (G40.-)
- frontotemporal dementia (G31.09)
- hepatolenticular degeneration (E83.0)
- human immunodeficiency virus [HIV] disease (B20)
- Huntington's disease (G10)
- hypercalcemia (E83.52)
- hypothyroidism, acquired (E00-E03.-)
- intoxications (T36-T65)
- Jakob-Creutzfeldt disease (A81.0-)
- multiple sclerosis (G35)
- neurosyphilis (A52.17)
- niacin deficiency [pellagra] (E52)
- Parkinson's disease (G20)
- Pick's disease (G31.01)
- polyarteritis nodosa (M30.0)
- prion disease (A81.9)
- systemic lupus erythematosus (M32.-)
- traumatic brain injury (S06.-)
- trypanosomiasis (B56.-, B57.-)
- vitamin B deficiency (E53.8)

EXCLUDES 2 dementia in alcohol and psychoactive substance disorders (F10-F19, with .17, .27, .97)
vascular dementia (F01.5-)

5 F02.8 Dementia in other diseases classified elsewhere

CODING TIPS✓ Codes F02.80 and F02.81 are manifestation codes and should be used only to report dementia in an etiology/manifestation pairing. An F02.8- code should never be used alone and inappropriate use of these codes may result in claims edits. Always code the etiology first, followed by the appropriate F02.8- code to specify dementia with or without behavioral disturbance. The provider must document a diagnosis of dementia and the presence of behavioral disturbances.

M IQ SH F02.80 *Dementia in other diseases classified elsewhere without behavioral disturbance*

Dementia in other diseases classified elsewhere NOS
Major neurocognitive disorder in other diseases classified elsewhere

M IQ SH + F02.81 *Dementia in other diseases classified elsewhere with behavioral disturbance*

Dementia in other diseases classified elsewhere with aggressive behavior
Dementia in other diseases classified elsewhere with combative behavior
Dementia in other diseases classified elsewhere with violent behavior
Major neurocognitive disorder in other diseases classified elsewhere with aggressive behavior
Major neurocognitive disorder in other diseases classified elsewhere with combative behavior
Major neurocognitive disorder in other diseases classified elsewhere with violent behavior

Use additional code, if applicable, to identify wandering in dementia in conditions classified elsewhere (Z91.83)

CODING TIPS✓ Anxiety is not considered a behavior indicated by a 5th character of 1. Anxiety, when documented by the provider, in addition to dementia, should be coded separately.

CODING TIPS✓ Use Z91.83 (Wandering in diseases classified elsewhere) as an additional code when appropriate. Wandering is coded with the 5th digit indicating behavior problems even if the patient does not have aggressive, violent, combative behavior.

4 F03 Unspecified dementia

Presenile dementia NOS
Presenile psychosis NOS
Primary degenerative dementia NOS
Senile dementia NOS
Senile dementia depressed or paranoid type
Senile psychosis NOS

EXCLUDES 1 senility NOS (R41.81)

EXCLUDES 2 mild memory disturbance due to known physiological condition (F06.8)
senile dementia with delirium or acute confusional state (F05)

DEFINITION Loss of cognitive and intellectual functions, such as impaired memory, judgment, and intellect, without impaired perception or consciousness.

5 F03.9 Unspecified dementia

CODING TIPS✓ If the physician or NPP documents major neurocognitive disorder without an etiology, use the codes for unspecified dementia.

CODING TIPS✓ Codes F03.90 and F03.91 are to be used for dementia that is not specified as due to another condition, and is reported as unspecified, senile psychosis, senile dementia (may also state depressed or paranoid type), primary degenerative dementia, or presenile dementia/psychosis. Do not confuse these conditions with organic brain disease or senility NOS. Senility NOS should not be coded with an F03.9- code (see excludes 1 notes) as this is less specific. When senile dementia is specified, the appropriate F03.9- code should be used.

CODING TIPS✓ Hospices should NOT assign a code from F03.9- as primary. When only "dementia" is provided as a diagnostic statement, hospices should query the physician or NPP and/or medical director for a more specific diagnosis. Clinical documentation should reflect confirmation of any additional or changed diagnostic statements.

SP SH **F03.90 Unspecified dementia without behavioral disturbance**

Dementia NOS

SP SH + **F03.91 Unspecified dementia with behavioral disturbance**

Unspecified dementia with aggressive behavior

Unspecified dementia with combative behavior

Unspecified dementia with violent behavior

Use additional code, if applicable, to identify wandering in unspecified dementia (Z91.83)

CODING TIPS✓ Anxiety is not considered a behavior indicated by a 5th character of 1. Anxiety, when documented by the provider, in addition to dementia, should be coded separately.

CODING TIPS✓ Use Z91.83 (Wandering in diseases classified elsewhere) as an additional code when appropriate. Wandering is coded with the 5th digit indicating behavior problems even if the patient does not have aggressive, violent, combative behavior.

IQ SH **F04 Amnestic disorder due to known physiological condition**

Korsakov's psychosis or syndrome, nonalcoholic

Code first:

the underlying physiological condition

EXCLUDES 1 amnesia NOS (R41.3)
anterograde amnesia (R41.1)
dissociative amnesia (F44.0)
retrograde amnesia (R41.2)

EXCLUDES 2 alcohol-induced or unspecified Korsakov's syndrome (F10.26, F10.96)
Korsakov's syndrome induced by other psychoactive substances (F13.26, F13.96, F19.16, F19.26, F19.96)

IQ SH **F05 Delirium due to known physiological condition**

Acute or subacute brain syndrome

Acute or subacute confusional state (nonalcoholic)

Acute or subacute infective psychosis

Acute or subacute organic reaction

Acute or subacute psycho-organic syndrome

Delirium of mixed etiology

Delirium superimposed on dementia

Sundowning

Code first:

the underlying physiological condition

EXCLUDES 1 delirium NOS (R41.0)

EXCLUDES 2 delirium tremens alcohol-induced or unspecified (F10.231, F10.921)

CODING TIPS✓ Patients with dementia may also have delirium or sundowning. When appropriate, add F05 when dementia is coded.

4 **F06 Other mental disorders due to known physiological condition**

INCLUDES mental disorders due to endocrine disorder
mental disorders due to exogenous hormone
mental disorders due to exogenous toxic substance
mental disorders due to primary cerebral disease
mental disorders due to somatic illness
mental disorders due to systemic disease affecting the brain

Code first:

the underlying physiological condition

EXCLUDES 1 unspecified dementia (F03)

EXCLUDES 2 delirium due to known physiological condition (F05)
dementia as classified in F01-F02
other mental disorders associated with alcohol and other psychoactive substances (F10-F19)

IQ **F06.0 Psychotic disorder with hallucinations due to known physiological condition**

Organic hallucinatory state (nonalcoholic)

EXCLUDES 2 hallucinations and perceptual disturbance induced by alcohol and other psychoactive substances (F10-F19 with .151, .251, .951)
schizophrenia (F20.-)

IQ SH **F06.1 Catatonic disorder due to known physiological condition**

Catatonia associated with another mental disorder

Catatonia NOS

EXCLUDES 1 catatonic stupor (R40.1)
stupor NOS (R40.1)

EXCLUDES 2 catatonic schizophrenia (F20.2)
dissociative stupor (F44.2)

IQ **F06.2 Psychotic disorder with delusions due to known physiological condition**

Paranoid and paranoid-hallucinatory organic states
Schizophrenia-like psychosis in epilepsy
EXCLUDES 2 alcohol and drug-induced psychotic disorder (F10-F19 with .150, .250, .950)
brief psychotic disorder (F23)
delusional disorder (F22)
schizophrenia (F20.-)

5 F06.3 Mood disorder due to known physiological condition
EXCLUDES 2 mood disorders due to alcohol and other psychoactive substances (F10-F19 with .14, .24, .94)
mood disorders, not due to known physiological condition or unspecified (F30-F39)

IQ F06.30 Mood disorder due to known physiological condition, unspecified

IQ F06.31 Mood disorder due to known physiological condition with depressive features
Depressive disorder due to known physiological condition, with depressive features

IQ F06.32 Mood disorder due to known physiological condition with major depressive-like episode
Depressive disorder due to known physiological condition, with major depressive-like episode

IQ F06.33 Mood disorder due to known physiological condition with manic features
Bipolar and related disorder due to a known physiological condition, with manic features
Bipolar and related disorder due to known physiological condition, with manic- or hypomanic-like episodes

IQ F06.34 Mood disorder due to known physiological condition with mixed features
Bipolar and related disorder due to known physiological condition, with mixed features
Depressive disorder due to known physiological condition, with mixed features

IQ F06.4 Anxiety disorder due to known physiological condition
EXCLUDES 2 anxiety disorders due to alcohol and other psychoactive substances (F10-F19 with .180, .280, .980)
anxiety disorders, not due to known physiological condition or unspecified (F40.-, F41.-)

IQ SH F06.8 Other specified mental disorders due to known physiological condition
Epileptic psychosis NOS
Obsessive-compulsive and related disorder due to a known physiological condition
Organic dissociative disorder
Organic emotionally labile [asthenic] disorder

4 F07 Personality and behavioral disorders due to known physiological condition
Code first:
the underlying physiological condition

IQ F07.0 Personality change due to known physiological condition
Frontal lobe syndrome
Limbic epilepsy personality syndrome
Lobotomy syndrome
Organic personality disorder
Organic pseudopsychopathic personality
Organic pseudoretarded personality
Postleucotomy syndrome
Code first:
underlying physiological condition
EXCLUDES 1 mild cognitive impairment (G31.84)
postconcussional syndrome (F07.81)
postencephalitic syndrome (F07.89)
signs and symptoms involving emotional state (R45.-)
EXCLUDES 2 specific personality disorder (F60.-)

DEFINITION Frontal lobe syndrome: Damage to the frontal lobe of the brain, typically manifesting as apathy, a lack of planning, emotional bluntness, the absence of abstract thought and attention, and judgment changes.

5 F07.8 Other personality and behavioral disorders due to known physiological condition

IQ + F07.81 Postconcussional syndrome
Postcontusional syndrome (encephalopathy)
Post-traumatic brain syndrome, nonpsychotic
Use additional code to identify associated post-traumatic headache, if applicable (G44.3-)
EXCLUDES 1 current concussion (brain) (S06.0-)
postencephalitic syndrome (F07.89)

CODING TIPS ✓ **Documentation:** Post concussion syndrome is a complex disorder resulting from a mild traumatic brain injury and is not associated with the severity of the initial injury. No documented loss of consciousness with the initial injury is necessary for a diagnosis of post concussion syndrome, but the physician or NPP must specify this disorder.

CODING TIPS ✓ Code F07.81 should not be used for the patient who has a current concussion (see the Excludes 1 notes).

DEFINITION Symptoms such as headache, amnesia, and lack of concentration due to a severe blow to the skull.

IQ **F07.89 Other personality and behavioral disorders due to known physiological condition**
Postencephalitic syndrome
Right hemispheric organic affective disorder

IQ **F07.9 Unspecified personality and behavioral disorder due to known physiological condition**
Organic psychosyndrome

IQ **F09 Unspecified mental disorder due to known physiological condition**
Mental disorder NOS due to known physiological condition
Organic brain syndrome NOS
Organic mental disorder NOS
Organic psychosis NOS
Symptomatic psychosis NOS
Code first:
the underlying physiological condition
EXCLUDES 1 psychosis NOS (F29)

Mental and behavioral disorders due to psychoactive substance use (F10-F19)

GUIDELINES **Section I.C.5.b.1)-3)**
Selection of codes for "in remission" for categories F10-F19, Mental and behavioral disorders due to psychoactive substance use (categories F10-F19 with -.21), requires the provider's clinical judgment. The appropriate codes for "in remission" are assigned only on the basis of provider documentation (as defined in the Official Guidelines for Coding and Reporting) unless otherwise instructed by the classification.

Mild substance use disorders in early or sustained remission are classified to the appropriate codes for substance abuse in remission, and moderate or severe substance use disorders in early or sustained remission are classified to the appropriate codes for substance dependence in remission.

When the provider documentation refers to use, abuse and dependence of the same substance (e.g. alcohol, opioid, cannabis, etc.), only one code should be assigned to identify the pattern of use based on the following hierarchy:
- If both use and abuse are documented, assign only the code for abuse
- If both abuse and dependence are documented, assign only the code for dependence
- If use, abuse and dependence are all documented, assign only the code for dependence
- If both use and dependence are documented, assign only the code for dependence.

As with all other unspecified diagnoses, the codes for unspecified psychoactive substance use disorders (F10.9-, F11.9-, F12.9-, F13.9-, F14.9-, F15.9-, F16.9-, F18.9-, F19.9-) should only be assigned based on provider documentation and when they meet the definition of a reportable diagnosis (see Section III, Reporting Additional Diagnoses). The codes are to be used only when the psychoactive substance use is associated with a physical, mental or behavioral disorder, and such a relationship is documented by the provider.

CODING TIPS ✓ Codes for psychoactive substance use are to be used only when the psychoactive substance use is associated with a physical, mental or behavioral disorder, and such a relationship is documented by the physician or NPP. Physical conditions refer only to those conditions included in Chapter 5 and do not refer to pain, digestive disorders, etc.

+ 4 **F10 Alcohol related disorders**
Use additional code for blood alcohol level, if applicable (Y90.-)

CODING TIPS ✓ There are codes for alcohol use, abuse and dependence. Alcoholism is coded to dependence. Use disorder is coded to abuse or dependence depending on the severity.

+ 5 **F10.1 Alcohol abuse**
EXCLUDES 1 alcohol dependence (F10.2-)
alcohol use, unspecified (F10.9-)

SP + **F10.10 Alcohol abuse, uncomplicated**
Alcohol use disorder, mild

IQ + **F10.11 Alcohol abuse, in remission**
Alcohol use disorder, mild, in early remission
Alcohol use disorder, mild, in sustained remission

+ 6 **F10.12 Alcohol abuse with intoxication**

SP + **F10.120 Alcohol abuse with intoxication, uncomplicated**

SP + **F10.121 Alcohol abuse with intoxication delirium**

SP + **F10.129 Alcohol abuse with intoxication, unspecified**

+ 6 **F10.13 Alcohol abuse, with withdrawal**

SP + **F10.130 Alcohol abuse with withdrawal, uncomplicated**

SP + **F10.131 Alcohol abuse with withdrawal delirium**

SP + **F10.132 Alcohol abuse with withdrawal with perceptual disturbance**

SP + **F10.139 Alcohol abuse with withdrawal, unspecified**

SP + **F10.14 Alcohol abuse with alcohol-induced mood disorder**
Alcohol use disorder, mild, with alcohol-induced bipolar or related disorder
Alcohol use disorder, mild, with alcohol-induced depressive disorder

+ 6 **F10.15 Alcohol abuse with alcohol-induced psychotic disorder**

SP + **F10.150 Alcohol abuse with alcohol-induced psychotic disorder with delusions**

SP + **F10.151 Alcohol abuse with alcohol-induced psychotic disorder with hallucinations**

SP + **F10.159 Alcohol abuse with alcohol-induced psychotic disorder, unspecified**

+ 6 **F10.18 Alcohol abuse with other alcohol-induced disorders**

SP + **F10.180 Alcohol abuse with alcohol-induced anxiety disorder**

SP + **F10.181 Alcohol abuse with alcohol-induced sexual dysfunction**

SP + **F10.182 Alcohol abuse with alcohol-induced sleep disorder**

SP + **F10.188 Alcohol abuse with other alcohol-induced disorder**

SP + **F10.19 Alcohol abuse with unspecified alcohol-induced disorder**

+ 5 **F10.2 Alcohol dependence**

EXCLUDES 1 alcohol abuse (F10.1-)
alcohol use, unspecified (F10.9-)

EXCLUDES 2 toxic effect of alcohol (T51.0-)

CODING TIPS✓ Alcoholism is coded to alcohol dependence.

SP + **F10.20 Alcohol dependence, uncomplicated**
Alcohol use disorder, moderate
Alcohol use disorder, severe

SP + **F10.21 Alcohol dependence, in remission**
Alcohol use disorder, moderate, in early remission
Alcohol use disorder, moderate, in sustained remission
Alcohol use disorder, severe, in early remission
Alcohol use disorder, severe, in sustained remission

+ 6 **F10.22 Alcohol dependence with intoxication**
Acute drunkenness (in alcoholism)

EXCLUDES 2 alcohol dependence with withdrawal (F10.23-)

SP + **F10.220 Alcohol dependence with intoxication, uncomplicated**

SP + **F10.221 Alcohol dependence with intoxication delirium**

SP + **F10.229 Alcohol dependence with intoxication, unspecified**

+ 6 **F10.23 Alcohol dependence with withdrawal**

EXCLUDES 2 Alcohol dependence with intoxication (F10.22-)

SP + **F10.230 Alcohol dependence with withdrawal, uncomplicated**

SP + **F10.231 Alcohol dependence with withdrawal delirium**

DEFINITION Delirium occurring when an alcoholic is denied alcohol for a significant period of time.

SP + **F10.232 Alcohol dependence with withdrawal with perceptual disturbance**

SP + **F10.239 Alcohol dependence with withdrawal, unspecified**

SP + **F10.24 Alcohol dependence with alcohol-induced mood disorder**
Alcohol use disorder, moderate, with alcohol-induced bipolar or related disorder
Alcohol use disorder, moderate, with alcohol-induced depressive disorder
Alcohol use disorder, severe, with alcohol-induced bipolar or related disorder
Alcohol use disorder, severe, with alcohol-induced depressive disorder

+ 6 **F10.25 Alcohol dependence with alcohol-induced psychotic disorder**

SP + **F10.250 Alcohol dependence with alcohol-induced psychotic disorder with delusions**

SP + **F10.251 Alcohol dependence with alcohol-induced psychotic disorder with hallucinations**

SP + **F10.259 Alcohol dependence with alcohol-induced psychotic disorder, unspecified**

SP + **F10.26 Alcohol dependence with alcohol-induced persisting amnestic disorder**
Alcohol use disorder, moderate, with alcohol-induced major neurocognitive disorder, amnestic-confabulatory type
Alcohol use disorder, severe, with alcohol-induced major neurocognitive disorder, amnestic-confabulatory type

SP + **F10.27 Alcohol dependence with alcohol-induced persisting dementia**
Alcohol use disorder, moderate, with alcohol-induced major neurocognitive disorder, nonamnestic-confabulatory type
Alcohol use disorder, severe, with alcohol-induced major neurocognitive disorder, nonamnestic-confabulatory type

DEFINITION Lasting state of dementia due to chronic alcoholism.

+ 6 **F10.28 Alcohol dependence with other alcohol-induced disorders**

SP + **F10.280 Alcohol dependence with alcohol-induced anxiety disorder**

SP + **F10.281 Alcohol dependence with alcohol-induced sexual dysfunction**

SP + **F10.282 Alcohol dependence with alcohol-induced sleep disorder**

SP + **F10.288 Alcohol dependence with other alcohol-induced disorder**
Alcohol use disorder, moderate, with alcohol-induced mild neurocognitive disorder
Alcohol use disorder, severe, with alcohol-induced mild neurocognitive disorder

CODING TIPS✓ The physician or NPP must link the physical disorder to the alcoholism to use this code. Only those physical disorders included in Chapter 5 (such as sexual dysfunction and sleep disorder), or mental or behavioral disorders are assigned F10.288. The relationship must be documented by the provider.

SP + **F10.29 Alcohol dependence with unspecified alcohol-induced disorder**

+ 5 **F10.9 Alcohol use, unspecified**

EXCLUDES 1 alcohol abuse (F10.1-)
alcohol dependence (F10.2-)

CODING TIPS✓ The use codes are for use of the alcohol associated with a mental, emotional or physical disorder as documented by the physician or NPP. The use codes are not to be used for the patient who drinks alcohol occasionally or without the additional physician or NPP documentation.

+ 6 **F10.92 Alcohol use, unspecified with intoxication**

SP + **F10.920 Alcohol use, unspecified with intoxication, uncomplicated**

SP + **F10.921 Alcohol use, unspecified with intoxication delirium**

SP + **F10.929 Alcohol use, unspecified with intoxication, unspecified**

+ 6 **F10.93 Alcohol use, unspecified with withdrawal**

SP + **F10.930 Alcohol use, unspecified with withdrawal, uncomplicated**

SP + **F10.931 Alcohol use, unspecified with withdrawal delirium**

SP + **F10.932 Alcohol use, unspecified with withdrawal with perceptual disturbance**

SP + **F10.939 Alcohol use, unspecified with withdrawal, unspecified**

SP + **F10.94 Alcohol use, unspecified with alcohol-induced mood disorder**
Alcohol induced bipolar or related disorder, without use disorder
Alcohol induced depressive disorder, without use disorder

+ 6 **F10.95 Alcohol use, unspecified with alcohol-induced psychotic disorder**

SP + **F10.950 Alcohol use, unspecified with alcohol-induced psychotic disorder with delusions**

SP + **F10.951 Alcohol use, unspecified with alcohol-induced psychotic disorder with hallucinations**

SP + **F10.959 Alcohol use, unspecified with alcohol-induced psychotic disorder, unspecified**
Alcohol-induced psychotic disorder without use disorder

SP + **F10.96 Alcohol use, unspecified with alcohol-induced persisting amnestic disorder**
Alcohol-induced major neurocognitive disorder, amnestic-confabulatory type, without use disorder

SP + **F10.97 Alcohol use, unspecified with alcohol-induced persisting dementia**
Alcohol-induced major neurocognitive disorder, nonamnestic-confabulatory type, without use disorder

+ 6 **F10.98 Alcohol use, unspecified with other alcohol-induced disorders**

SP + **F10.980 Alcohol use, unspecified with alcohol-induced anxiety disorder**
Alcohol induced anxiety disorder, without use disorder

SP + **F10.981 Alcohol use, unspecified with alcohol-induced sexual dysfunction**
Alcohol induced sexual dysfunction, without use disorder

SP + **F10.982 Alcohol use, unspecified with alcohol-induced sleep disorder**
Alcohol induced sleep disorder, without use disorder

DEFINITION Disruption of normal sleep patterns due to the consumption of alcohol.

SP + **F10.988 Alcohol use, unspecified with other alcohol-induced disorder**
Alcohol induced mild neurocognitive disorder, without use disorder

SP + **F10.99 Alcohol use, unspecified with unspecified alcohol-induced disorder**

4 **F11 Opioid related disorders**

5 **F11.1 Opioid abuse**
EXCLUDES 1 opioid dependence (F11.2-)
opioid use, unspecified (F11.9-)

SP **F11.10 Opioid abuse, uncomplicated**
Opioid use disorder, mild

IQ **F11.11 Opioid abuse, in remission**
Opioid use disorder, mild, in early remission
Opioid use disorder, mild, in sustained remission

6 **F11.12 Opioid abuse with intoxication**

SP **F11.120 Opioid abuse with intoxication, uncomplicated**

SP **F11.121 Opioid abuse with intoxication delirium**

SP **F11.122 Opioid abuse with intoxication with perceptual disturbance**

SP **F11.129 Opioid abuse with intoxication, unspecified**

SP **F11.13 Opioid abuse with withdrawal**

SP **F11.14 Opioid abuse with opioid-induced mood disorder**
Opioid use disorder, mild, with opioid-induced depressive disorder

6 **F11.15 Opioid abuse with opioid-induced psychotic disorder**

SP **F11.150 Opioid abuse with opioid-induced psychotic disorder with delusions**

SP **F11.151 Opioid abuse with opioid-induced psychotic disorder with hallucinations**

SP **F11.159 Opioid abuse with opioid-induced psychotic disorder, unspecified**

6 **F11.18 Opioid abuse with other opioid-induced disorder**

SP **F11.181 Opioid abuse with opioid-induced sexual dysfunction**

SP **F11.182 Opioid abuse with opioid-induced sleep disorder**

SP **F11.188 Opioid abuse with other opioid-induced disorder**

SP **F11.19 Opioid abuse with unspecified opioid-induced disorder**

5 **F11.2 Opioid dependence**
EXCLUDES 1 opioid abuse (F11.1-)
opioid use, unspecified (F11.9-)
EXCLUDES 2 opioid poisoning (T40.0-T40.2-)

SP **F11.20 Opioid dependence, uncomplicated**
Opioid use disorder, moderate
Opioid use disorder, severe

Chapter 5

F01-F99

SP **F11.21 Opioid dependence, in remission**
Opioid use disorder, moderate, in early remission
Opioid use disorder, moderate, in sustained remission
Opioid use disorder, severe, in early remission
Opioid use disorder, severe, in sustained remission

6 **F11.22 Opioid dependence with intoxication**
EXCLUDES 1 opioid dependence with withdrawal (F11.23)

SP **F11.220 Opioid dependence with intoxication, uncomplicated**

SP **F11.221 Opioid dependence with intoxication delirium**

SP **F11.222 Opioid dependence with intoxication with perceptual disturbance**

SP **F11.229 Opioid dependence with intoxication, unspecified**

SP **F11.23 Opioid dependence with withdrawal**
EXCLUDES 1 opioid dependence with intoxication (F11.22-)

SP **F11.24 Opioid dependence with opioid-induced mood disorder**
Opioid use disorder, moderate, with opioid induced depressive disorder

6 **F11.25 Opioid dependence with opioid-induced psychotic disorder**

SP **F11.250 Opioid dependence with opioid-induced psychotic disorder with delusions**

SP **F11.251 Opioid dependence with opioid-induced psychotic disorder with hallucinations**

SP **F11.259 Opioid dependence with opioid-induced psychotic disorder, unspecified**

6 **F11.28 Opioid dependence with other opioid-induced disorder**

SP **F11.281 Opioid dependence with opioid-induced sexual dysfunction**

SP **F11.282 Opioid dependence with opioid-induced sleep disorder**

SP **F11.288 Opioid dependence with other opioid-induced disorder**

SP **F11.29 Opioid dependence with unspecified opioid-induced disorder**

5 **F11.9 Opioid use, unspecified**
EXCLUDES 1 opioid abuse (F11.1-)
opioid dependence (F11.2-)

CODING TIPS✓ The use codes are for use of the opioid associated with (causing) a mental, emotional or physical disorder as documented by the physician or NPP. The use codes are not to be used for the patient who uses opioids medicinally or without the additional physician or NPP documentation.

CODING TIPS✓ Use disorder is coded to abuse or dependence depending on the severity. Mild is coded to abuse, and moderate and severe are coded to dependence.

SP **F11.90 Opioid use, unspecified, uncomplicated**

6 **F11.92 Opioid use, unspecified with intoxication**
EXCLUDES 1 opioid use, unspecified with withdrawal (F11.93)

SP **F11.920 Opioid use, unspecified with intoxication, uncomplicated**

SP **F11.921 Opioid use, unspecified with intoxication delirium**
Opioid-induced delirium

SP **F11.922 Opioid use, unspecified with intoxication with perceptual disturbance**

SP **F11.929 Opioid use, unspecified with intoxication, unspecified**

SP **F11.93 Opioid use, unspecified with withdrawal**
EXCLUDES 1 opioid use, unspecified with intoxication (F11.92-)

SP **F11.94 Opioid use, unspecified with opioid-induced mood disorder**
Opioid induced depressive disorder, without use disorder

6 **F11.95 Opioid use, unspecified with opioid-induced psychotic disorder**

SP **F11.950 Opioid use, unspecified with opioid-induced psychotic disorder with delusions**

SP **F11.951 Opioid use, unspecified with opioid-induced psychotic disorder with hallucinations**

SP **F11.959 Opioid use, unspecified with opioid-induced psychotic disorder, unspecified**

6 **F11.98 Opioid use, unspecified with other specified opioid-induced disorder**

SP **F11.981 Opioid use, unspecified with opioid-induced sexual dysfunction**
Opioid induced sexual dysfunction, without use disorder

SP **F11.982 Opioid use, unspecified with opioid-induced sleep disorder**
Opioid induced sleep disorder, without use disorder

SP **F11.988 Opioid use, unspecified with other opioid-induced disorder**
Opioid induced anxiety disorder, without use disorder

SP **F11.99 Opioid use, unspecified with unspecified opioid-induced disorder**

4 **F12 Cannabis related disorders**
INCLUDES marijuana

CODING TIPS✓ Recreational marijuana use or medical use of marijuana should not ordinarily be coded. Do not assign a code for marijuana use without an associated physical, mental or behavioral disorder documented by the provider. Physical disorders include only those in Chapter 5.

5 **F12.1 Cannabis abuse**
EXCLUDES 1 cannabis dependence (F12.2-)

cannabis use, unspecified (F12.9-)

SP **F12.10 Cannabis abuse, uncomplicated**
Cannabis use disorder, mild

IQ **F12.11 Cannabis abuse, in remission**
Cannabis use disorder, mild, in early remission
Cannabis use disorder, mild, in sustained remission

6 **F12.12 Cannabis abuse with intoxication**

SP **F12.120 Cannabis abuse with intoxication, uncomplicated**

SP **F12.121 Cannabis abuse with intoxication delirium**

SP **F12.122 Cannabis abuse with intoxication with perceptual disturbance**

SP **F12.129 Cannabis abuse with intoxication, unspecified**

SP **F12.13 Cannabis abuse with withdrawal**

6 **F12.15 Cannabis abuse with psychotic disorder**

SP **F12.150 Cannabis abuse with psychotic disorder with delusions**

SP **F12.151 Cannabis abuse with psychotic disorder with hallucinations**

SP **F12.159 Cannabis abuse with psychotic disorder, unspecified**

6 **F12.18 Cannabis abuse with other cannabis-induced disorder**

SP **F12.180 Cannabis abuse with cannabis-induced anxiety disorder**

SP **F12.188 Cannabis abuse with other cannabis-induced disorder**
Cannabis use disorder, mild, with cannabis-induced sleep disorder

SP **F12.19 Cannabis abuse with unspecified cannabis-induced disorder**

5 **F12.2 Cannabis dependence**

EXCLUDES 1 cannabis abuse (F12.1-)
cannabis use, unspecified (F12.9-)

EXCLUDES 2 cannabis poisoning (T40.7-)

SP **F12.20 Cannabis dependence, uncomplicated**
Cannabis use disorder, moderate
Cannabis use disorder, severe

SP **F12.21 Cannabis dependence, in remission**
Cannabis use disorder, moderate, in early remission
Cannabis use disorder, moderate, in sustained remission
Cannabis use disorder, severe, in early remission
Cannabis use disorder, severe, in sustained remission

6 **F12.22 Cannabis dependence with intoxication**

SP **F12.220 Cannabis dependence with intoxication, uncomplicated**

SP **F12.221 Cannabis dependence with intoxication delirium**

SP **F12.222 Cannabis dependence with intoxication with perceptual disturbance**

SP **F12.229 Cannabis dependence with intoxication, unspecified**

SP **F12.23 Cannabis dependence with withdrawal**

6 **F12.25 Cannabis dependence with psychotic disorder**

SP **F12.250 Cannabis dependence with psychotic disorder with delusions**

SP **F12.251 Cannabis dependence with psychotic disorder with hallucinations**

SP **F12.259 Cannabis dependence with psychotic disorder, unspecified**

6 **F12.28 Cannabis dependence with other cannabis-induced disorder**

SP **F12.280 Cannabis dependence with cannabis-induced anxiety disorder**

SP **F12.288 Cannabis dependence with other cannabis-induced disorder**
Cannabis use disorder, moderate, with cannabis-induced sleep disorder
Cannabis use disorder, severe, with cannabis-induced sleep disorder

SP **F12.29 Cannabis dependence with unspecified cannabis-induced disorder**

5 **F12.9 Cannabis use, unspecified**

EXCLUDES 1 cannabis abuse (F12.1-)
cannabis dependence (F12.2-)

CODING TIPS ✓ The use codes are for use of the cannibis associated with (causing) a mental, emotional or physical disorder as documented by the physician or NPP.The use codes are not to be used for the patient who uses medical marijuana or uses the marijuana recreationally without the additional physician or NPP documentation.

CODING TIPS ✓ Use disorder is coded to abuse or dependence depending on the severity. Mild is coded to abuse, and moderate and severe are coded to dependence.

SP **F12.90 Cannabis use, unspecified, uncomplicated**

6 **F12.92 Cannabis use, unspecified with intoxication**

SP **F12.920 Cannabis use, unspecified with intoxication, uncomplicated**

SP **F12.921 Cannabis use, unspecified with intoxication delirium**

SP **F12.922 Cannabis use, unspecified with intoxication with perceptual disturbance**

SP **F12.929 Cannabis use, unspecified with intoxication, unspecified**

SP **F12.93 Cannabis use, unspecified with withdrawal**

6 **F12.95 Cannabis use, unspecified with psychotic disorder**

SP **F12.950 Cannabis use, unspecified with psychotic disorder with delusions**

SP **F12.951 Cannabis use, unspecified with psychotic disorder with hallucinations**

SP **F12.959 Cannabis use, unspecified with psychotic disorder, unspecified**
Cannabis induced psychotic disorder, without use disorder

6 **F12.98 Cannabis use, unspecified with other cannabis-induced disorder**

SP **F12.980 Cannabis use, unspecified with anxiety disorder**
Cannabis induced anxiety disorder, without use disorder

SP **F12.988 Cannabis use, unspecified with other cannabis-induced disorder**
Cannabis induced sleep disorder, without use disorder

SP **F12.99 Cannabis use, unspecified with unspecified cannabis-induced disorder**

4 **F13 Sedative, hypnotic, or anxiolytic related disorders**

5 **F13.1 Sedative, hypnotic or anxiolytic-related abuse**
EXCLUDES 1 sedative, hypnotic or anxiolytic-related dependence (F13.2-)
sedative, hypnotic, or anxiolytic use, unspecified (F13.9-)

SP **F13.10 Sedative, hypnotic or anxiolytic abuse, uncomplicated**
Sedative, hypnotic, or anxiolytic use disorder, mild

IQ **F13.11 Sedative, hypnotic or anxiolytic abuse, in remission**
Sedative, hypnotic or anxiolytic use disorder, mild, in early remission
Sedative, hypnotic or anxiolytic use disorder, mild, in sustained remission

6 **F13.12 Sedative, hypnotic or anxiolytic abuse with intoxication**

SP **F13.120 Sedative, hypnotic or anxiolytic abuse with intoxication, uncomplicated**

SP **F13.121 Sedative, hypnotic or anxiolytic abuse with intoxication delirium**

SP **F13.129 Sedative, hypnotic or anxiolytic abuse with intoxication, unspecified**

6 **F13.13 Sedative, hypnotic or anxiolytic abuse with withdrawal**

SP **F13.130 Sedative, hypnotic or anxiolytic abuse with withdrawal, uncomplicated**

SP **F13.131 Sedative, hypnotic or anxiolytic abuse with withdrawal delirium**

SP **F13.132 Sedative, hypnotic or anxiolytic abuse with withdrawal with perceptual disturbance**

SP **F13.139 Sedative, hypnotic or anxiolytic abuse with withdrawal, unspecified**

SP **F13.14 Sedative, hypnotic or anxiolytic abuse with sedative, hypnotic or anxiolytic-induced mood disorder**
Sedative, hypnotic, or anxiolytic use disorder, mild, with sedative, hypnotic, or anxiolytic-induced bipolar or related disorder
Sedative, hypnotic, or anxiolytic use disorder, mild, with sedative, hypnotic, or anxiolytic-induced depressive disorder

6 **F13.15 Sedative, hypnotic or anxiolytic abuse with sedative, hypnotic or anxiolytic-induced psychotic disorder**

SP **F13.150 Sedative, hypnotic or anxiolytic abuse with sedative, hypnotic or anxiolytic-induced psychotic disorder with delusions**

SP **F13.151 Sedative, hypnotic or anxiolytic abuse with sedative, hypnotic or anxiolytic-induced psychotic disorder with hallucinations**

SP **F13.159 Sedative, hypnotic or anxiolytic abuse with sedative, hypnotic or anxiolytic-induced psychotic disorder, unspecified**

6 **F13.18 Sedative, hypnotic or anxiolytic abuse with other sedative, hypnotic or anxiolytic-induced disorders**

SP **F13.180 Sedative, hypnotic or anxiolytic abuse with sedative, hypnotic or anxiolytic-induced anxiety disorder**

SP **F13.181 Sedative, hypnotic or anxiolytic abuse with sedative, hypnotic or anxiolytic-induced sexual dysfunction**

SP **F13.182 Sedative, hypnotic or anxiolytic abuse with sedative, hypnotic or anxiolytic-induced sleep disorder**

SP **F13.188 Sedative, hypnotic or anxiolytic abuse with other sedative, hypnotic or anxiolytic-induced disorder**

SP **F13.19 Sedative, hypnotic or anxiolytic abuse with unspecified sedative, hypnotic or anxiolytic-induced disorder**

5 **F13.2 Sedative, hypnotic or anxiolytic-related dependence**
EXCLUDES 1 sedative, hypnotic or anxiolytic-related abuse (F13.1-)
sedative, hypnotic, or anxiolytic use, unspecified (F13.9-)
EXCLUDES 2 sedative, hypnotic, or anxiolytic poisoning (T42.-)

SP **F13.20 Sedative, hypnotic or anxiolytic dependence, uncomplicated**

SP **F13.21 Sedative, hypnotic or anxiolytic dependence, in remission**
Sedative, hypnotic or anxiolytic use disorder, moderate, in early remission
Sedative, hypnotic or anxiolytic use disorder, moderate, in sustained remission
Sedative, hypnotic or anxiolytic use disorder, severe, in early remission
Sedative, hypnotic or anxiolytic use disorder, severe, in sustained remission

6 **F13.22 Sedative, hypnotic or anxiolytic dependence with intoxication**

EXCLUDES 1 sedative, hypnotic or anxiolytic dependence with withdrawal (F13.23-)

SP **F13.220 Sedative, hypnotic or anxiolytic dependence with intoxication, uncomplicated**

SP **F13.221 Sedative, hypnotic or anxiolytic dependence with intoxication delirium**

SP **F13.229 Sedative, hypnotic or anxiolytic dependence with intoxication, unspecified**

6 **F13.23 Sedative, hypnotic or anxiolytic dependence with withdrawal**

Sedative, hypnotic, or anxiolytic use disorder, moderate

Sedative, hypnotic, or anxiolytic use disorder, severe

EXCLUDES 1 sedative, hypnotic or anxiolytic dependence with intoxication (F13.22-)

DEFINITION Curtailed drug use, resulting in physical or psychological symptoms lasting hours to weeks, commonly featuring headache, anxiety, depression, chills, sweats, and tremors.

SP **F13.230 Sedative, hypnotic or anxiolytic dependence with withdrawal, uncomplicated**

SP **F13.231 Sedative, hypnotic or anxiolytic dependence with withdrawal delirium**

SP **F13.232 Sedative, hypnotic or anxiolytic dependence with withdrawal with perceptual disturbance**

Sedative, hypnotic, or anxiolytic withdrawal with perceptual disturbances

SP **F13.239 Sedative, hypnotic or anxiolytic dependence with withdrawal, unspecified**

Sedative, hypnotic, or anxiolytic withdrawal without perceptual disturbances

SP **F13.24 Sedative, hypnotic or anxiolytic dependence with sedative, hypnotic or anxiolytic-induced mood disorder**

Sedative, hypnotic, or anxiolytic use disorder, moderate, with sedative, hypnotic, or anxiolytic-induced bipolar or related disorder

Sedative, hypnotic, or anxiolytic use disorder, moderate, with sedative, hypnotic, or anxiolytic-induced depressive disorder

Sedative, hypnotic, or anxiolytic use disorder, severe, with sedative, hypnotic, or anxiolytic-induced bipolar or related disorder

Sedative, hypnotic, or anxiolytic use disorder, severe, with sedative, hypnotic, or anxiolytic-induced depressive disorder

6 **F13.25 Sedative, hypnotic or anxiolytic dependence with sedative, hypnotic or anxiolytic-induced psychotic disorder**

SP **F13.250 Sedative, hypnotic or anxiolytic dependence with sedative, hypnotic or anxiolytic-induced psychotic disorder with delusions**

SP **F13.251 Sedative, hypnotic or anxiolytic dependence with sedative, hypnotic or anxiolytic-induced psychotic disorder with hallucinations**

SP **F13.259 Sedative, hypnotic or anxiolytic dependence with sedative, hypnotic or anxiolytic-induced psychotic disorder, unspecified**

SP **F13.26 Sedative, hypnotic or anxiolytic dependence with sedative, hypnotic or anxiolytic-induced persisting amnestic disorder**

SP **F13.27 Sedative, hypnotic or anxiolytic dependence with sedative, hypnotic or anxiolytic-induced persisting dementia**

Sedative, hypnotic, or anxiolytic use disorder, moderate, with sedative, hypnotic, or anxiolytic-induced major neurocognitive disorder

Sedative, hypnotic, or anxiolytic use disorder, severe, with sedative, hypnotic, or anxiolytic-induced major neurocognitive disorder

6 **F13.28 Sedative, hypnotic or anxiolytic dependence with other sedative, hypnotic or anxiolytic-induced disorders**

SP **F13.280 Sedative, hypnotic or anxiolytic dependence with sedative, hypnotic or anxiolytic-induced anxiety disorder**

SP **F13.281 Sedative, hypnotic or anxiolytic dependence with sedative, hypnotic or anxiolytic-induced sexual dysfunction**

SP **F13.282 Sedative, hypnotic or anxiolytic dependence with sedative, hypnotic or anxiolytic-induced sleep disorder**

SP **F13.288 Sedative, hypnotic or anxiolytic dependence with other sedative, hypnotic or anxiolytic-induced disorder**

Sedative, hypnotic, or anxiolytic use disorder, moderate, with sedative, hypnotic, or anxiolytic-induced mild neurocognitive disorder

Sedative, hypnotic, or anxiolytic use disorder, severe, with sedative, hypnotic, or anxiolytic-induced mild neurocognitive disorder

SP **F13.29 Sedative, hypnotic or anxiolytic dependence with unspecified sedative, hypnotic or anxiolytic-induced disorder**

5 **F13.9 Sedative, hypnotic or anxiolytic-related use, unspecified**

EXCLUDES 1 sedative, hypnotic or anxiolytic-related abuse (F13.1-)
sedative, hypnotic or anxiolytic-related dependence (F13.2-)

CODING TIPS✓ The use codes are for use of sedative, hypnotic or anxiolytic when associated with (causing) a mental, emotional or physical disorder as documented by the physician or NPP. The use codes are not to be used for the patient who uses sedatives, hypnotics or anxiolytics without the additional physician or NPP documentation.

CODING TIPS✓ Use disorder is coded to abuse or dependence depending on the severity. Mild is coded to abuse, and moderate and severe are coded to dependence.

SP F13.90 **Sedative, hypnotic, or anxiolytic use, unspecified, uncomplicated**

6 F13.92 **Sedative, hypnotic or anxiolytic use, unspecified with intoxication**

EXCLUDES 1 sedative, hypnotic or anxiolytic use, unspecified with withdrawal (F13.93-)

SP F13.920 **Sedative, hypnotic or anxiolytic use, unspecified with intoxication, uncomplicated**

SP F13.921 **Sedative, hypnotic or anxiolytic use, unspecified with intoxication delirium**

Sedative, hypnotic, or anxiolytic-induced delirium

SP F13.929 **Sedative, hypnotic or anxiolytic use, unspecified with intoxication, unspecified**

6 F13.93 **Sedative, hypnotic or anxiolytic use, unspecified with withdrawal**

EXCLUDES 1 sedative, hypnotic or anxiolytic use, unspecified with intoxication (F13.92-)

SP F13.930 **Sedative, hypnotic or anxiolytic use, unspecified with withdrawal, uncomplicated**

SP F13.931 **Sedative, hypnotic or anxiolytic use, unspecified with withdrawal delirium**

SP F13.932 **Sedative, hypnotic or anxiolytic use, unspecified with withdrawal with perceptual disturbances**

SP F13.939 **Sedative, hypnotic or anxiolytic use, unspecified with withdrawal, unspecified**

SP F13.94 **Sedative, hypnotic or anxiolytic use, unspecified with sedative, hypnotic or anxiolytic-induced mood disorder**

Sedative, hypnotic, or anxiolytic-induced bipolar or related disorder, without use disorder

Sedative, hypnotic, or anxiolytic-induced depressive disorder, without use disorder

6 F13.95 **Sedative, hypnotic or anxiolytic use, unspecified with sedative, hypnotic or anxiolytic-induced psychotic disorder**

SP F13.950 **Sedative, hypnotic or anxiolytic use, unspecified with sedative, hypnotic or anxiolytic-induced psychotic disorder with delusions**

SP F13.951 **Sedative, hypnotic or anxiolytic use, unspecified with sedative, hypnotic or anxiolytic-induced psychotic disorder with hallucinations**

SP F13.959 **Sedative, hypnotic or anxiolytic use, unspecified with sedative, hypnotic or anxiolytic-induced psychotic disorder, unspecified**

Sedative, hypnotic, or anxiolytic-induced psychotic disorder, without use disorder

SP F13.96 **Sedative, hypnotic or anxiolytic use, unspecified with sedative, hypnotic or anxiolytic-induced persisting amnestic disorder**

SP F13.97 **Sedative, hypnotic or anxiolytic use, unspecified with sedative, hypnotic or anxiolytic-induced persisting dementia**

Sedative, hypnotic, or anxiolytic-induced major neurocognitive disorder, without use disorder

6 F13.98 **Sedative, hypnotic or anxiolytic use, unspecified with other sedative, hypnotic or anxiolytic-induced disorders**

SP F13.980 **Sedative, hypnotic or anxiolytic use, unspecified with sedative, hypnotic or anxiolytic-induced anxiety disorder**

Sedative, hypnotic, or anxiolytic-induced anxiety disorder, without use disorder

SP F13.981 **Sedative, hypnotic or anxiolytic use, unspecified with sedative, hypnotic or anxiolytic-induced sexual dysfunction**

Sedative, hypnotic, or anxiolytic-induced sexual dysfunction disorder, without use disorder

SP F13.982 **Sedative, hypnotic or anxiolytic use, unspecified with sedative, hypnotic or anxiolytic-induced sleep disorder**

Sedative, hypnotic, or anxiolytic-induced sleep disorder, without use disorder

SP F13.988 **Sedative, hypnotic or anxiolytic use, unspecified with other sedative, hypnotic or anxiolytic-induced disorder**

Sedative, hypnotic, or anxiolytic-induced mild neurocognitive disorder

SP F13.99 Sedative, hypnotic or anxiolytic use, unspecified with unspecified sedative, hypnotic or anxiolytic-induced disorder

4 **F14 Cocaine related disorders**
EXCLUDES 2 other stimulant-related disorders (F15.-)

5 **F14.1 Cocaine abuse**
EXCLUDES 1 cocaine dependence (F14.2-)
cocaine use, unspecified (F14.9-)

SP **F14.10 Cocaine abuse, uncomplicated**
Cocaine use disorder, mild

IQ **F14.11 Cocaine abuse, in remission**
Cocaine use disorder, mild, in early remission
Cocaine use disorder, mild, in sustained remission

6 **F14.12 Cocaine abuse with intoxication**

SP **F14.120 Cocaine abuse with intoxication, uncomplicated**

SP **F14.121 Cocaine abuse with intoxication with delirium**

SP **F14.122 Cocaine abuse with intoxication with perceptual disturbance**

SP **F14.129 Cocaine abuse with intoxication, unspecified**

SP **F14.13 Cocaine abuse, unspecified with withdrawal**

SP **F14.14 Cocaine abuse with cocaine-induced mood disorder**
Cocaine use disorder, mild, with cocaine-induced bipolar or related disorder
Cocaine use disorder, mild, with cocaine-induced depressive disorder

6 **F14.15 Cocaine abuse with cocaine-induced psychotic disorder**

SP **F14.150 Cocaine abuse with cocaine-induced psychotic disorder with delusions**

SP **F14.151 Cocaine abuse with cocaine-induced psychotic disorder with hallucinations**

SP **F14.159 Cocaine abuse with cocaine-induced psychotic disorder, unspecified**

6 **F14.18 Cocaine abuse with other cocaine-induced disorder**

SP **F14.180 Cocaine abuse with cocaine-induced anxiety disorder**

SP **F14.181 Cocaine abuse with cocaine-induced sexual dysfunction**

SP **F14.182 Cocaine abuse with cocaine-induced sleep disorder**

SP **F14.188 Cocaine abuse with other cocaine-induced disorder**
Cocaine use disorder, mild, with cocaine-induced obsessive compulsive or related disorder

SP **F14.19 Cocaine abuse with unspecified cocaine-induced disorder**

5 **F14.2 Cocaine dependence**
EXCLUDES 1 cocaine abuse (F14.1-)
cocaine use, unspecified (F14.9-)
EXCLUDES 2 cocaine poisoning (T40.5-)

SP **F14.20 Cocaine dependence, uncomplicated**
Cocaine use disorder, moderate
Cocaine use disorder, severe

SP **F14.21 Cocaine dependence, in remission**
Cocaine use disorder, moderate, in early remission
Cocaine use disorder, moderate, in sustained remission
Cocaine use disorder, severe, in early remission
Cocaine use disorder, severe, in sustained remission

6 **F14.22 Cocaine dependence with intoxication**
EXCLUDES 1 cocaine dependence with withdrawal (F14.23)

SP **F14.220 Cocaine dependence with intoxication, uncomplicated**

SP **F14.221 Cocaine dependence with intoxication delirium**

SP **F14.222 Cocaine dependence with intoxication with perceptual disturbance**

SP **F14.229 Cocaine dependence with intoxication, unspecified**

SP **F14.23 Cocaine dependence with withdrawal**
EXCLUDES 1 cocaine dependence with intoxication (F14.22-)

SP **F14.24 Cocaine dependence with cocaine-induced mood disorder**
Cocaine use disorder, moderate, with cocaine-induced bipolar or related disorder
Cocaine use disorder, moderate, with cocaine-induced depressive disorder
Cocaine use disorder, severe, with cocaine-induced bipolar or related disorder
Cocaine use disorder, severe, with cocaine-induced depressive disorder

6 **F14.25 Cocaine dependence with cocaine-induced psychotic disorder**

SP **F14.250 Cocaine dependence with cocaine-induced psychotic disorder with delusions**

SP **F14.251 Cocaine dependence with cocaine-induced psychotic disorder with hallucinations**

SP **F14.259 Cocaine dependence with cocaine-induced psychotic disorder, unspecified**

6 **F14.28 Cocaine dependence with other cocaine-induced disorder**

SP **F14.280 Cocaine dependence with cocaine-induced anxiety disorder**

SP **F14.281 Cocaine dependence with cocaine-induced sexual dysfunction**

SP **F14.282 Cocaine dependence with cocaine-induced sleep disorder**

SP **F14.288 Cocaine dependence with other cocaine-induced disorder**
Cocaine use disorder, moderate, with cocaine-induced obsessive compulsive or related disorder

Cocaine use disorder, severe, with cocaine-induced obsessive compulsive or related disorder

SP **F14.29 Cocaine dependence with unspecified cocaine-induced disorder**

5 **F14.9 Cocaine use, unspecified**

EXCLUDES 1 cocaine abuse (F14.1-)
cocaine dependence (F14.2-)

CODING TIPS✓ The use codes are for use of cocaine when associated with (causing) a mental, emotional or physical disorder as documented by the physician or NPP. The use codes are not to be used for the patient who uses cocaine without the additional physician or NPP documentation.

CODING TIPS✓ Use disorder is coded to abuse or dependence depending on the severity. Mild is coded to abuse, and moderate and severe are coded to dependence.

SP **F14.90 Cocaine use, unspecified, uncomplicated**

6 **F14.92 Cocaine use, unspecified with intoxication**

SP **F14.920 Cocaine use, unspecified with intoxication, uncomplicated**

SP **F14.921 Cocaine use, unspecified with intoxication delirium**

SP **F14.922 Cocaine use, unspecified with intoxication with perceptual disturbance**

SP **F14.929 Cocaine use, unspecified with intoxication, unspecified**

SP **F14.93 Cocaine use, unspecified with withdrawal**

SP **F14.94 Cocaine use, unspecified with cocaine-induced mood disorder**

Cocaine induced bipolar or related disorder, without use disorder
Cocaine induced depressive disorder, without use disorder

6 **F14.95 Cocaine use, unspecified with cocaine-induced psychotic disorder**

SP **F14.950 Cocaine use, unspecified with cocaine-induced psychotic disorder with delusions**

SP **F14.951 Cocaine use, unspecified with cocaine-induced psychotic disorder with hallucinations**

SP **F14.959 Cocaine use, unspecified with cocaine-induced psychotic disorder, unspecified**

Cocaine induced psychotic disorder, without use disorder

6 **F14.98 Cocaine use, unspecified with other specified cocaine-induced disorder**

SP **F14.980 Cocaine use, unspecified with cocaine-induced anxiety disorder**

Cocaine induced anxiety disorder, without use disorder

SP **F14.981 Cocaine use, unspecified with cocaine-induced sexual dysfunction**

Cocaine induced sexual dysfunction, without use disorder

SP **F14.982 Cocaine use, unspecified with cocaine-induced sleep disorder**

Cocaine induced sleep disorder, without use disorder

SP **F14.988 Cocaine use, unspecified with other cocaine-induced disorder**

Cocaine induced obsessive compulsive or related disorder

SP **F14.99 Cocaine use, unspecified with unspecified cocaine-induced disorder**

4 **F15 Other stimulant related disorders**

INCLUDES amphetamine-related disorders
caffeine

EXCLUDES 2 cocaine-related disorders (F14.-)

CODING TIPS✓ Use this category of codes for methamphetamines and "bath salts" abuse and dependence.

5 **F15.1 Other stimulant abuse**

EXCLUDES 1 other stimulant dependence (F15.2-)
other stimulant use, unspecified (F15.9-)

SP **F15.10 Other stimulant abuse, uncomplicated**

Amphetamine type substance use disorder, mild
Other or unspecified stimulant use disorder, mild

IQ **F15.11 Other stimulant abuse, in remission**

Amphetamine type substance use disorder, mild, in early remission
Amphetamine type substance use disorder, mild, in sustained remission
Other or unspecified stimulant use disorder, mild, in early remission
Other or unspecified stimulant use disorder, mild, in sustained remission

6 **F15.12 Other stimulant abuse with intoxication**

SP **F15.120 Other stimulant abuse with intoxication, uncomplicated**

SP **F15.121 Other stimulant abuse with intoxication delirium**

SP **F15.122 Other stimulant abuse with intoxication with perceptual disturbance**

Amphetamine or other stimulant use disorder, mild, with amphetamine or other stimulant intoxication, with perceptual disturbances

SP **F15.129 Other stimulant abuse with intoxication, unspecified**

Amphetamine or other stimulant use disorder, mild, with amphetamine or other stimulant intoxication, without perceptual disturbances

SP **F15.13 Other stimulant abuse with withdrawal**

SP **F15.14 Other stimulant abuse with stimulant-induced mood disorder**

Amphetamine or other stimulant use disorder, mild, with amphetamine or other stimulant induced bipolar or related disorder

Amphetamine or other stimulant use disorder, mild, with amphetamine or other stimulant induced depressive disorder

6 **F15.15 Other stimulant abuse with stimulant-induced psychotic disorder**

SP **F15.150 Other stimulant abuse with stimulant-induced psychotic disorder with delusions**

SP **F15.151 Other stimulant abuse with stimulant-induced psychotic disorder with hallucinations**

SP **F15.159 Other stimulant abuse with stimulant-induced psychotic disorder, unspecified**

6 **F15.18 Other stimulant abuse with other stimulant-induced disorder**

SP **F15.180 Other stimulant abuse with stimulant-induced anxiety disorder**

SP **F15.181 Other stimulant abuse with stimulant-induced sexual dysfunction**

SP **F15.182 Other stimulant abuse with stimulant-induced sleep disorder**

SP **F15.188 Other stimulant abuse with other stimulant-induced disorder**

Amphetamine or other stimulant use disorder, mild, with amphetamine or other stimulant induced obsessive-compulsive or related disorder

SP **F15.19 Other stimulant abuse with unspecified stimulant-induced disorder**

5 **F15.2 Other stimulant dependence**

EXCLUDES 1 other stimulant abuse (F15.1-)
other stimulant use, unspecified (F15.9-)

SP **F15.20 Other stimulant dependence, uncomplicated**

Amphetamine type substance use disorder, moderate

Amphetamine type substance use disorder, severe

Other or unspecified stimulant use disorder, moderate

Other or unspecified stimulant use disorder, severe

SP **F15.21 Other stimulant dependence, in remission**

Amphetamine type substance use disorder, moderate, in early remission

Amphetamine type substance use disorder, moderate, in sustained remission

Amphetamine type substance use disorder, severe, in early remission

Amphetamine type substance use disorder, severe, in sustained remission

Other or unspecified stimulant use disorder, moderate, in early remission

Other or unspecified stimulant use disorder, moderate, in sustained remission

Other or unspecified stimulant use disorder, severe, in early remission

Other or unspecified stimulant use disorder, severe, in sustained remission

6 **F15.22 Other stimulant dependence with intoxication**

EXCLUDES 1 other stimulant dependence with withdrawal (F15.23)

SP **F15.220 Other stimulant dependence with intoxication, uncomplicated**

SP **F15.221 Other stimulant dependence with intoxication delirium**

SP **F15.222 Other stimulant dependence with intoxication with perceptual disturbance**

Amphetamine or other stimulant use disorder, moderate, with amphetamine or other stimulant intoxication, with perceptual disturbances

Amphetamine or other stimulant use disorder, severe, with amphetamine or other stimulant intoxication, with perceptual disturbances

SP **F15.229 Other stimulant dependence with intoxication, unspecified**

Amphetamine or other stimulant use disorder, moderate, with amphetamine or other stimulant intoxication, without perceptual disturbances

Amphetamine or other stimulant use disorder, severe, with amphetamine or other stimulant intoxication, without perceptual disturbances

SP **F15.23 Other stimulant dependence with withdrawal**

Amphetamine or other stimulant withdrawal

EXCLUDES 1 other stimulant dependence with intoxication (F15.22-)

SP **F15.24 Other stimulant dependence with stimulant-induced mood disorder**

Amphetamine or other stimulant use disorder, moderate, with amphetamine or other stimulant-induced bipolar or related disorder

Amphetamine or other stimulant use disorder, moderate, with amphetamine or other stimulant induced depressive disorder

Amphetamine or other stimulant use disorder, severe, with amphetamine or other stimulant-induced bipolar or related disorder

Amphetamine or other stimulant use disorder, severe, with amphetamine or other stimulant-induced depressive disorder

6 **F15.25 Other stimulant dependence with stimulant-induced psychotic disorder**

Chapter 5

F01-F99

SP **F15.250 Other stimulant dependence with stimulant-induced psychotic disorder with delusions**

SP **F15.251 Other stimulant dependence with stimulant-induced psychotic disorder with hallucinations**

SP **F15.259 Other stimulant dependence with stimulant-induced psychotic disorder, unspecified**

6 **F15.28 Other stimulant dependence with other stimulant-induced disorder**

SP **F15.280 Other stimulant dependence with stimulant-induced anxiety disorder**

SP **F15.281 Other stimulant dependence with stimulant-induced sexual dysfunction**

SP **F15.282 Other stimulant dependence with stimulant-induced sleep disorder**

SP **F15.288 Other stimulant dependence with other stimulant-induced disorder**

Amphetamine or other stimulant use disorder, moderate, with amphetamine or other stimulant induced obsessive compulsive or related disorder

Amphetamine or other stimulant use disorder, severe, with amphetamine or other stimulant induced obsessive compulsive or related disorder

SP **F15.29 Other stimulant dependence with unspecified stimulant-induced disorder**

5 **F15.9 Other stimulant use, unspecified**

EXCLUDES 1 other stimulant abuse (F15.1-)
other stimulant dependence (F15.2-)

CODING TIPS✓ The use codes are for use of other stimulants when associated with (causing) a mental, emotional or physical disorder as documented by the physician or NPP. The use codes are not to be used for the patient who uses stimulants without the additional physician or NPP documentation.

CODING TIPS✓ Use disorder is coded to abuse or dependence depending on the severity. Mild is coded to abuse, and moderate and severe are coded to dependence.

SP **F15.90 Other stimulant use, unspecified, uncomplicated**

6 **F15.92 Other stimulant use, unspecified with intoxication**

EXCLUDES 1 other stimulant use, unspecified with withdrawal (F15.93)

SP **F15.920 Other stimulant use, unspecified with intoxication, uncomplicated**

SP **F15.921 Other stimulant use, unspecified with intoxication delirium**

Amphetamine or other stimulant-induced delirium

SP **F15.922 Other stimulant use, unspecified with intoxication with perceptual disturbance**

SP **F15.929 Other stimulant use, unspecified with intoxication, unspecified**

Caffeine intoxication

SP **F15.93 Other stimulant use, unspecified with withdrawal**

Caffeine withdrawal

EXCLUDES 1 other stimulant use, unspecified with intoxication (F15.92-)

SP **F15.94 Other stimulant use, unspecified with stimulant-induced mood disorder**

Amphetamine or other stimulant-induced bipolar or related disorder, without use disorder

Amphetamine or other stimulant-induced depressive disorder, without use disorder

6 **F15.95 Other stimulant use, unspecified with stimulant-induced psychotic disorder**

SP **F15.950 Other stimulant use, unspecified with stimulant-induced psychotic disorder with delusions**

SP **F15.951 Other stimulant use, unspecified with stimulant-induced psychotic disorder with hallucinations**

SP **F15.959 Other stimulant use, unspecified with stimulant-induced psychotic disorder, unspecified**

Amphetamine or other stimulant-induced psychotic disorder, without use disorder

6 **F15.98 Other stimulant use, unspecified with other stimulant-induced disorder**

SP **F15.980 Other stimulant use, unspecified with stimulant-induced anxiety disorder**

Amphetamine or other stimulant-induced anxiety disorder, without use disorder

Caffeine induced anxiety disorder, without use disorder

SP **F15.981 Other stimulant use, unspecified with stimulant-induced sexual dysfunction**

Amphetamine or other stimulant-induced sexual dysfunction, without use disorder

SP **F15.982 Other stimulant use, unspecified with stimulant-induced sleep disorder**

Amphetamine or other stimulant-induced sleep disorder, without use disorder

Caffeine induced sleep disorder, without use disorder

SP **F15.988 Other stimulant use, unspecified with other stimulant-induced disorder**

Amphetamine or other stimulant-induced obsessive compulsive or related disorder, without use disorder

SP **F15.99 Other stimulant use, unspecified with unspecified stimulant-induced disorder**

4 **F16 Hallucinogen related disorders**

INCLUDES ecstasy
PCP
phencyclidine

5 **F16.1 Hallucinogen abuse**

EXCLUDES 1 hallucinogen dependence (F16.2-)
hallucinogen use, unspecified (F16.9-)

SP **F16.10 Hallucinogen abuse, uncomplicated**
Other hallucinogen use disorder, mild
Phencyclidine use disorder, mild

IQ **F16.11 Hallucinogen abuse, in remission**
Other hallucinogen use disorder, mild, in early remission
Other hallucinogen use disorder, mild, in sustained remission
Phencyclidine use disorder, mild, in early remission
Phencyclidine use disorder, mild, in sustained remission

6 **F16.12 Hallucinogen abuse with intoxication**

SP **F16.120 Hallucinogen abuse with intoxication, uncomplicated**

SP **F16.121 Hallucinogen abuse with intoxication with delirium**

SP **F16.122 Hallucinogen abuse with intoxication with perceptual disturbance**

SP **F16.129 Hallucinogen abuse with intoxication, unspecified**

SP **F16.14 Hallucinogen abuse with hallucinogen-induced mood disorder**
Other hallucinogen use disorder, mild, with other hallucinogen induced bipolar or related disorder
Other hallucinogen use disorder, mild, with other hallucinogen induced depressive disorder
Phencyclidine use disorder, mild, with phencyclidine induced bipolar or related disorder
Phencyclidine use disorder, mild, with phencyclidine induced depressive disorder

6 **F16.15 Hallucinogen abuse with hallucinogen-induced psychotic disorder**

SP **F16.150 Hallucinogen abuse with hallucinogen-induced psychotic disorder with delusions**

SP **F16.151 Hallucinogen abuse with hallucinogen-induced psychotic disorder with hallucinations**

SP **F16.159 Hallucinogen abuse with hallucinogen-induced psychotic disorder, unspecified**

6 **F16.18 Hallucinogen abuse with other hallucinogen-induced disorder**

SP **F16.180 Hallucinogen abuse with hallucinogen-induced anxiety disorder**

SP **F16.183 Hallucinogen abuse with hallucinogen persisting perception disorder (flashbacks)**

SP **F16.188 Hallucinogen abuse with other hallucinogen-induced disorder**

SP **F16.19 Hallucinogen abuse with unspecified hallucinogen-induced disorder**

5 **F16.2 Hallucinogen dependence**

EXCLUDES 1 hallucinogen abuse (F16.1-)
hallucinogen use, unspecified (F16.9-)

SP **F16.20 Hallucinogen dependence, uncomplicated**
Other hallucinogen use disorder, moderate
Other hallucinogen use disorder, severe
Phencyclidine use disorder, moderate
Phencyclidine use disorder, severe

SP **F16.21 Hallucinogen dependence, in remission**
Other hallucinogen use disorder, moderate, in early remission
Other hallucinogen use disorder, moderate, in sustained remission
Other hallucinogen use disorder, severe, in early remission
Other hallucinogen use disorder, severe, in sustained remission
Phencyclidine use disorder, moderate, in early remission
Phencyclidine use disorder, moderate, in sustained remission
Phencyclidine use disorder, severe, in early remission
Phencyclidine use disorder, severe, in sustained remission

6 **F16.22 Hallucinogen dependence with intoxication**

SP **F16.220 Hallucinogen dependence with intoxication, uncomplicated**

SP **F16.221 Hallucinogen dependence with intoxication with delirium**

SP **F16.229 Hallucinogen dependence with intoxication, unspecified**

SP **F16.24 Hallucinogen dependence with hallucinogen-induced mood disorder**
Other hallucinogen use disorder, moderate, with other hallucinogen induced bipolar or related disorder
Other hallucinogen use disorder, moderate, with other hallucinogen induced depressive disorder
Other hallucinogen use disorder, severe, with other hallucinogen-induced bipolar or related disorder
Other hallucinogen use disorder, severe, with other hallucinogen-induced depressive disorder
Phencyclidine use disorder, moderate, with phencyclidine induced bipolar or related disorder
Phencyclidine use disorder, moderate, with phencyclidine induced depressive disorder
Phencyclidine use disorder, severe, with phencyclidine induced bipolar or related disorder
Phencyclidine use disorder, severe, with phencyclidine-induced depressive disorder

Chapter 5 F01-F99

6 **F16.25 Hallucinogen dependence with hallucinogen-induced psychotic disorder**

SP **F16.250 Hallucinogen dependence with hallucinogen-induced psychotic disorder with delusions**

SP **F16.251 Hallucinogen dependence with hallucinogen-induced psychotic disorder with hallucinations**

SP **F16.259 Hallucinogen dependence with hallucinogen-induced psychotic disorder, unspecified**

6 **F16.28 Hallucinogen dependence with other hallucinogen-induced disorder**

SP **F16.280 Hallucinogen dependence with hallucinogen-induced anxiety disorder**

SP **F16.283 Hallucinogen dependence with hallucinogen persisting perception disorder (flashbacks)**

SP **F16.288 Hallucinogen dependence with other hallucinogen-induced disorder**

SP **F16.29 Hallucinogen dependence with unspecified hallucinogen-induced disorder**

5 **F16.9 Hallucinogen use, unspecified**

EXCLUDES 1 hallucinogen abuse (F16.1-)
hallucinogen dependence (F16.2-)

CODING TIPS✓ The use codes are for use of hallucinogens when associated with (causing) a mental, emotional or physical disorder as documented by the physician or NPP. The use codes are not to be used for the patient who uses hallucinogens without the additional physician or NPP documentation.

CODING TIPS✓ Use disorder is coded to abuse or dependence depending on the severity. Mild is coded to abuse, and moderate and severe are coded to dependence.

SP **F16.90 Hallucinogen use, unspecified, uncomplicated**

6 **F16.92 Hallucinogen use, unspecified with intoxication**

SP **F16.920 Hallucinogen use, unspecified with intoxication, uncomplicated**

SP **F16.921 Hallucinogen use, unspecified with intoxication with delirium**

Other hallucinogen intoxication delirium

SP **F16.929 Hallucinogen use, unspecified with intoxication, unspecified**

SP **F16.94 Hallucinogen use, unspecified with hallucinogen-induced mood disorder**

Other hallucinogen induced bipolar or related disorder, without use disorder
Other hallucinogen induced depressive disorder, without use disorder
Phencyclidine induced bipolar or related disorder, without use disorder
Phencyclidine induced depressive disorder, without use disorder

6 **F16.95 Hallucinogen use, unspecified with hallucinogen-induced psychotic disorder**

SP **F16.950 Hallucinogen use, unspecified with hallucinogen-induced psychotic disorder with delusions**

SP **F16.951 Hallucinogen use, unspecified with hallucinogen-induced psychotic disorder with hallucinations**

SP **F16.959 Hallucinogen use, unspecified with hallucinogen-induced psychotic disorder, unspecified**

Other hallucinogen induced psychotic disorder, without use disorder
Phencyclidine induced psychotic disorder, without use disorder

6 **F16.98 Hallucinogen use, unspecified with other specified hallucinogen-induced disorder**

SP **F16.980 Hallucinogen use, unspecified with hallucinogen-induced anxiety disorder**

Other hallucinogen-induced anxiety disorder, without use disorder
Phencyclidine induced anxiety disorder, without use disorder

SP **F16.983 Hallucinogen use, unspecified with hallucinogen persisting perception disorder (flashbacks)**

SP **F16.988 Hallucinogen use, unspecified with other hallucinogen-induced disorder**

SP **F16.99 Hallucinogen use, unspecified with unspecified hallucinogen-induced disorder**

4 **F17 Nicotine dependence**

EXCLUDES 1 history of tobacco dependence (Z87.891)
tobacco use NOS (Z72.0)

EXCLUDES 2 tobacco use (smoking) during pregnancy, childbirth and the puerperium (O99.33-)
toxic effect of nicotine (T65.2-)

CODING TIPS✓ Use disorder, regardless of the severity (mild, moderate or severe), is coded to dependence. There is no separate code to indicate abuse.

5 **F17.2 Nicotine dependence**

CODING TIPS✓ Use the appropriate code to specify nicotine product when known. ICD-10 codes provide for greater specificity, allowing the coder to specify dependence on a specific nicotine product.

6 **F17.20 Nicotine dependence, unspecified**

SP **F17.200 Nicotine dependence, unspecified, uncomplicated**

Tobacco use disorder, mild
Tobacco use disorder, moderate
Tobacco use disorder, severe

SP **F17.201 Nicotine dependence, unspecified, in remission**

Tobacco use disorder, mild, in early remission

Tobacco use disorder, mild, in sustained remission
Tobacco use disorder, moderate, in early remission
Tobacco use disorder, moderate, in sustained remission
Tobacco use disorder, severe, in early remission
Tobacco use disorder, severe, in sustained remission

SP **F17.203 Nicotine dependence unspecified, with withdrawal**
Tobacco withdrawal

SP **F17.208 Nicotine dependence, unspecified, with other nicotine-induced disorders**

SP **F17.209 Nicotine dependence, unspecified, with unspecified nicotine-induced disorders**

6 **F17.21 Nicotine dependence, cigarettes**
CODING TIPS✓ If the physician or NPP documents "smoker" and indicates that it is cigarettes, e.g. 2ppd, use a code from F17.21.

SP **F17.210 Nicotine dependence, cigarettes, uncomplicated**
CODING TIPS✓ Assign code U07.0 if the physician indicates a vaping disorder.
CODING TIPS✓ Use this code if the physician or NPP documents "smoker" or tobacco/nicotine dependence and indicates cigarettes.

SP **F17.211 Nicotine dependence, cigarettes, in remission**
Tobacco use disorder, cigarettes, mild, in early remission
Tobacco use disorder, cigarettes, mild, in sustained remission
Tobacco use disorder, cigarettes, moderate, in early remission
Tobacco use disorder, cigarettes, moderate, in sustained remission
Tobacco use disorder, cigarettes, severe, in early remission
Tobacco use disorder, cigarettes, severe, in sustained remission
CODING TIPS✓ The use of the code for remission vs. the code for history (Z87.891) is dependent on the physician or NPP documentation. The ICD-10-CM classifies a history of nicotine dependence differently than other types of drug dependence. Reference the term used by the physician or NPP in the alphabetical index.

SP **F17.213 Nicotine dependence, cigarettes, with withdrawal**

SP **F17.218 Nicotine dependence, cigarettes, with other nicotine-induced disorders**
CODING TIPS✓ The physician or NPP must link the condition to the smoking to use this code.

SP **F17.219 Nicotine dependence, cigarettes, with unspecified nicotine-induced disorders**

6 **F17.22 Nicotine dependence, chewing tobacco**

SP **F17.220 Nicotine dependence, chewing tobacco, uncomplicated**

SP **F17.221 Nicotine dependence, chewing tobacco, in remission**
Tobacco use disorder, chewing tobacco, mild, in early remission
Tobacco use disorder, chewing tobacco, mild, in sustained remission
Tobacco use disorder, chewing tobacco, moderate, in early remission
Tobacco use disorder, chewing tobacco, moderate, in sustained remission
Tobacco use disorder, chewing tobacco, severe, in early remission
Tobacco use disorder, chewing tobacco, severe, in sustained remission

SP **F17.223 Nicotine dependence, chewing tobacco, with withdrawal**

SP **F17.228 Nicotine dependence, chewing tobacco, with other nicotine-induced disorders**

SP **F17.229 Nicotine dependence, chewing tobacco, with unspecified nicotine-induced disorders**

6 **F17.29 Nicotine dependence, other tobacco product**

SP **F17.290 Nicotine dependence, other tobacco product, uncomplicated**
CODING TIPS✓ Assign code U07.0 if the physician indicates a vaping disorder.

SP **F17.291 Nicotine dependence, other tobacco product, in remission**
Tobacco use disorder, other tobacco product, mild, in early remission
Tobacco use disorder, other tobacco product, mild, in sustained remission
Tobacco use disorder, other tobacco product, moderate, in early remission
Tobacco use disorder, other tobacco product, moderate, in sustained remission
Tobacco use disorder, other tobacco product, severe, in early remission
Tobacco use disorder, other tobacco product, severe, in sustained remission

SP **F17.293 Nicotine dependence, other tobacco product, with withdrawal**

SP **F17.298 Nicotine dependence, other tobacco product, with other nicotine-induced disorders**

SP **F17.299 Nicotine dependence, other tobacco product, with unspecified nicotine-induced disorders**

4 **F18 Inhalant related disorders**

INCLUDES volatile solvents

5 **F18.1 Inhalant abuse**

EXCLUDES 1 inhalant dependence (F18.2-)
inhalant use, unspecified (F18.9-)

SP **F18.10 Inhalant abuse, uncomplicated**
Inhalant use disorder, mild

IQ **F18.11 Inhalant abuse, in remission**
Inhalant use disorder, mild, in early remission
Inhalant use disorder, mild, in sustained remission

6 **F18.12 Inhalant abuse with intoxication**

SP **F18.120 Inhalant abuse with intoxication, uncomplicated**

SP **F18.121 Inhalant abuse with intoxication delirium**

SP **F18.129 Inhalant abuse with intoxication, unspecified**

SP **F18.14 Inhalant abuse with inhalant-induced mood disorder**
Inhalant use disorder, mild, with inhalant induced depressive disorder

6 **F18.15 Inhalant abuse with inhalant-induced psychotic disorder**

SP **F18.150 Inhalant abuse with inhalant-induced psychotic disorder with delusions**

SP **F18.151 Inhalant abuse with inhalant-induced psychotic disorder with hallucinations**

SP **F18.159 Inhalant abuse with inhalant-induced psychotic disorder, unspecified**

SP **F18.17 Inhalant abuse with inhalant-induced dementia**
Inhalant use disorder, mild, with inhalant induced major neurocognitive disorder

6 **F18.18 Inhalant abuse with other inhalant-induced disorders**

SP **F18.180 Inhalant abuse with inhalant-induced anxiety disorder**

SP **F18.188 Inhalant abuse with other inhalant-induced disorder**
Inhalant use disorder, mild, with inhalant induced mild neurocognitive disorder

SP **F18.19 Inhalant abuse with unspecified inhalant-induced disorder**

5 **F18.2 Inhalant dependence**

EXCLUDES 1 inhalant abuse (F18.1-)
inhalant use, unspecified (F18.9-)

SP **F18.20 Inhalant dependence, uncomplicated**
Inhalant use disorder, moderate
Inhalant use disorder, severe

SP **F18.21 Inhalant dependence, in remission**
Inhalant use disorder, moderate, in early remission
Inhalant use disorder, moderate, in sustained remission
Inhalant use disorder, severe, in early remission
Inhalant use disorder, severe, in sustained remission

6 **F18.22 Inhalant dependence with intoxication**

SP **F18.220 Inhalant dependence with intoxication, uncomplicated**

SP **F18.221 Inhalant dependence with intoxication delirium**

SP **F18.229 Inhalant dependence with intoxication, unspecified**

SP **F18.24 Inhalant dependence with inhalant-induced mood disorder**
Inhalant use disorder, moderate, with inhalant induced depressive disorder
Inhalant use disorder, severe, with inhalant induced depressive disorder

6 **F18.25 Inhalant dependence with inhalant-induced psychotic disorder**

SP **F18.250 Inhalant dependence with inhalant-induced psychotic disorder with delusions**

SP **F18.251 Inhalant dependence with inhalant-induced psychotic disorder with hallucinations**

SP **F18.259 Inhalant dependence with inhalant-induced psychotic disorder, unspecified**

SP **F18.27 Inhalant dependence with inhalant-induced dementia**
Inhalant use disorder, moderate, with inhalant induced major neurocognitive disorder
Inhalant use disorder, severe, with inhalant induced major neurocognitive disorder

6 **F18.28 Inhalant dependence with other inhalant-induced disorders**

SP **F18.280 Inhalant dependence with inhalant-induced anxiety disorder**

SP **F18.288 Inhalant dependence with other inhalant-induced disorder**
Inhalant use disorder, moderate, with inhalant-induced mild neurocognitive disorder
Inhalant use disorder, severe, with inhalant-induced mild neurocognitive disorder

SP **F18.29 Inhalant dependence with unspecified inhalant-induced disorder**

5 **F18.9 Inhalant use, unspecified**

EXCLUDES 1 inhalant abuse (F18.1-)
inhalant dependence (F18.2-)

CODING TIPS✓ The use codes are for use of inhalants when associated with (causing) a mental, emotional or physical disorder as documented by the physician or NPP. The use codes are not to be used for the patient who uses inhalants without the additional physician or NPP documentation.

CODING TIPS✓ Use disorder is coded to abuse or dependence depending on the severity. Mild is coded to abuse, and moderate and severe are coded to dependence.

SP **F18.90 Inhalant use, unspecified, uncomplicated**

6 **F18.92 Inhalant use, unspecified with intoxication**

SP **F18.920 Inhalant use, unspecified with intoxication, uncomplicated**

SP **F18.921 Inhalant use, unspecified with intoxication with delirium**

SP **F18.929 Inhalant use, unspecified with intoxication, unspecified**

SP **F18.94 Inhalant use, unspecified with inhalant-induced mood disorder**

Inhalant induced depressive disorder

6 **F18.95 Inhalant use, unspecified with inhalant-induced psychotic disorder**

SP **F18.950 Inhalant use, unspecified with inhalant-induced psychotic disorder with delusions**

SP **F18.951 Inhalant use, unspecified with inhalant-induced psychotic disorder with hallucinations**

SP **F18.959 Inhalant use, unspecified with inhalant-induced psychotic disorder, unspecified**

SP **F18.97 Inhalant use, unspecified with inhalant-induced persisting dementia**

Inhalant-induced major neurocognitive disorder

6 **F18.98 Inhalant use, unspecified with other inhalant-induced disorders**

SP **F18.980 Inhalant use, unspecified with inhalant-induced anxiety disorder**

SP **F18.988 Inhalant use, unspecified with other inhalant-induced disorder**

Inhalant-induced mild neurocognitive disorder

SP **F18.99 Inhalant use, unspecified with unspecified inhalant-induced disorder**

4 **F19 Other psychoactive substance related disorders**

INCLUDES polysubstance drug use (indiscriminate drug use)

5 **F19.1 Other psychoactive substance abuse**

EXCLUDES 1 other psychoactive substance dependence (F19.2-)
other psychoactive substance use, unspecified (F19.9-)

SP **F19.10 Other psychoactive substance abuse, uncomplicated**

Other (or unknown) substance use disorder, mild

IQ **F19.11 Other psychoactive substance abuse, in remission**

Other (or unknown) substance use disorder, mild, in early remission

Other (or unknown) substance use disorder, mild, in sustained remission

6 **F19.12 Other psychoactive substance abuse with intoxication**

SP **F19.120 Other psychoactive substance abuse with intoxication, uncomplicated**

SP **F19.121 Other psychoactive substance abuse with intoxication delirium**

SP **F19.122 Other psychoactive substance abuse with intoxication with perceptual disturbances**

SP **F19.129 Other psychoactive substance abuse with intoxication, unspecified**

6 **F19.13 Other psychoactive substance abuse with withdrawal**

SP **F19.130 Other psychoactive substance abuse with withdrawal, uncomplicated**

SP **F19.131 Other psychoactive substance abuse with withdrawal delirium**

SP **F19.132 Other psychoactive substance abuse with withdrawal with perceptual disturbance**

SP **F19.139 Other psychoactive substance abuse with withdrawal, unspecified**

SP **F19.14 Other psychoactive substance abuse with psychoactive substance-induced mood disorder**

Other (or unknown) substance use disorder, mild, with other (or unknown) substance-induced bipolar or related disorder

Other (or unknown) substance use disorder, mild, with other (or unknown) substance-induced depressive disorder

6 **F19.15 Other psychoactive substance abuse with psychoactive substance-induced psychotic disorder**

SP **F19.150 Other psychoactive substance abuse with psychoactive substance-induced psychotic disorder with delusions**

SP **F19.151 Other psychoactive substance abuse with psychoactive substance-induced psychotic disorder with hallucinations**

SP **F19.159 Other psychoactive substance abuse with psychoactive substance-induced psychotic disorder, unspecified**

SP **F19.16 Other psychoactive substance abuse with psychoactive substance-induced persisting amnestic disorder**

SP **F19.17 Other psychoactive substance abuse with psychoactive substance-induced persisting dementia**

Other (or unknown) substance use disorder, mild, with other (or unknown) substance-induced major neurocognitive disorder

6 **F19.18 Other psychoactive substance abuse with other psychoactive substance-induced disorders**

SP **F19.180 Other psychoactive substance abuse with psychoactive substance-induced anxiety disorder**

SP **F19.181 Other psychoactive substance abuse with psychoactive substance-induced sexual dysfunction**

SP **F19.182 Other psychoactive substance abuse with psychoactive substance-induced sleep disorder**

SP **F19.188 Other psychoactive substance abuse with other psychoactive substance-induced disorder**

Other (or unknown) substance use disorder, mild, with other (or unknown) substance induced mild neurocognitive disorder

Other (or unknown) substance use disorder, mild, with other (or unknown) substance induced obsessive-compulsive or related disorder

SP **F19.19 Other psychoactive substance abuse with unspecified psychoactive substance-induced disorder**

5 **F19.2 Other psychoactive substance dependence**

EXCLUDES 1 other psychoactive substance abuse (F19.1-)
other psychoactive substance use, unspecified (F19.9-)

SP **F19.20 Other psychoactive substance dependence, uncomplicated**

Other (or unknown) substance use disorder, moderate

Other (or unknown) substance use disorder, severe

SP **F19.21 Other psychoactive substance dependence, in remission**

Other (or unknown) substance use disorder, moderate, in early remission

Other (or unknown) substance use disorder, moderate, in sustained remission

Other (or unknown) substance use disorder, severe, in early remission

Other (or unknown) substance use disorder, severe, in sustained remission

6 **F19.22 Other psychoactive substance dependence with intoxication**

EXCLUDES 1 other psychoactive substance dependence with withdrawal (F19.23-)

SP **F19.220 Other psychoactive substance dependence with intoxication, uncomplicated**

SP **F19.221 Other psychoactive substance dependence with intoxication delirium**

SP **F19.222 Other psychoactive substance dependence with intoxication with perceptual disturbance**

SP **F19.229 Other psychoactive substance dependence with intoxication, unspecified**

6 **F19.23 Other psychoactive substance dependence with withdrawal**

EXCLUDES 1 other psychoactive substance dependence with intoxication (F19.22-)

SP **F19.230 Other psychoactive substance dependence with withdrawal, uncomplicated**

SP **F19.231 Other psychoactive substance dependence with withdrawal delirium**

SP **F19.232 Other psychoactive substance dependence with withdrawal with perceptual disturbance**

SP **F19.239 Other psychoactive substance dependence with withdrawal, unspecified**

SP **F19.24 Other psychoactive substance dependence with psychoactive substance-induced mood disorder**

Other (or unknown) substance use disorder, moderate, with other (or unknown) substance induced bipolar or related disorder

Other (or unknown) substance use disorder, moderate, with other (or unknown) substance induced depressive disorder

Other (or unknown) substance use disorder, severe, with other (or unknown) substance induced bipolar or related disorder

Other (or unknown) substance use disorder, severe, with other (or unknown) substance induced depressive disorder

6 **F19.25 Other psychoactive substance dependence with psychoactive substance-induced psychotic disorder**

SP **F19.250 Other psychoactive substance dependence with psychoactive substance-induced psychotic disorder with delusions**

SP **F19.251 Other psychoactive substance dependence with psychoactive substance-induced psychotic disorder with hallucinations**

SP **F19.259 Other psychoactive substance dependence with psychoactive substance-induced psychotic disorder, unspecified**

SP **F19.26 Other psychoactive substance dependence with psychoactive substance-induced persisting amnestic disorder**

SP **F19.27 Other psychoactive substance dependence with psychoactive substance-induced persisting dementia**

Other (or unknown) substance use disorder, moderate, with other (or unknown) substance induced major neurocognitive disorder

Other (or unknown) substance use disorder, severe, with other (or unknown) substance induced major neurocognitive disorder

6 **F19.28 Other psychoactive substance dependence with other psychoactive substance-induced disorders**

SP **F19.280 Other psychoactive substance dependence with psychoactive substance-induced anxiety disorder**

SP **F19.281 Other psychoactive substance dependence with psychoactive substance-induced sexual dysfunction**

SP **F19.282 Other psychoactive substance dependence with psychoactive substance-induced sleep disorder**

SP **F19.288 Other psychoactive substance dependence with other psychoactive substance-induced disorder**

Other (or unknown) substance use disorder, moderate, with other (or unknown) substance induced mild neurocognitive disorder

Other (or unknown) substance use disorder, severe, with other (or unknown) substance induced mild neurocognitive disorder

Other (or unknown) substance use disorder, moderate, with other (or unknown) substance induced obsessive compulsive or related disorder

Other (or unknown) substance use disorder, severe, with other (or unknown) substance induced obsessive-compulsive or related disorder

SP **F19.29 Other psychoactive substance dependence with unspecified psychoactive substance-induced disorder**

5 **F19.9 Other psychoactive substance use, unspecified**

EXCLUDES 1 other psychoactive substance abuse (F19.1-)
other psychoactive substance dependence (F19.2-)

CODING TIPS✓ The use codes are for use of psychoactive substances when associated with (causing) a mental, emotional or physical disorder as documented by the physician or NPP. The use codes are not to be used for the patient who uses psychoactive substances without the additional physician or NPP documentation.

CODING TIPS✓ Use disorder is coded to abuse or dependence depending on the severity. Mild is coded to abuse, and moderate and severe are coded to dependence.

SP **F19.90 Other psychoactive substance use, unspecified, uncomplicated**

6 **F19.92 Other psychoactive substance use, unspecified with intoxication**

EXCLUDES 1 other psychoactive substance use, unspecified with withdrawal (F19.93)

SP **F19.920 Other psychoactive substance use, unspecified with intoxication, uncomplicated**

SP **F19.921 Other psychoactive substance use, unspecified with intoxication with delirium**

Other (or unknown) substance-induced delirium

SP **F19.922 Other psychoactive substance use, unspecified with intoxication with perceptual disturbance**

SP **F19.929 Other psychoactive substance use, unspecified with intoxication, unspecified**

6 **F19.93 Other psychoactive substance use, unspecified with withdrawal**

EXCLUDES 1 other psychoactive substance use, unspecified with intoxication (F19.92-)

SP **F19.930 Other psychoactive substance use, unspecified with withdrawal, uncomplicated**

SP **F19.931 Other psychoactive substance use, unspecified with withdrawal delirium**

SP **F19.932 Other psychoactive substance use, unspecified with withdrawal with perceptual disturbance**

SP **F19.939 Other psychoactive substance use, unspecified with withdrawal, unspecified**

SP **F19.94 Other psychoactive substance use, unspecified with psychoactive substance-induced mood disorder**

Other (or unknown) substance-induced bipolar or related disorder, without use disorder

Other (or unknown) substance-induced depressive disorder, without use disorder

6 **F19.95 Other psychoactive substance use, unspecified with psychoactive substance-induced psychotic disorder**

SP **F19.950 Other psychoactive substance use, unspecified with psychoactive substance-induced psychotic disorder with delusions**

SP **F19.951 Other psychoactive substance use, unspecified with psychoactive substance-induced psychotic disorder with hallucinations**

SP **F19.959 Other psychoactive substance use, unspecified with psychoactive substance-induced psychotic disorder, unspecified**

Other or unknown substance-induced psychotic disorder, without use disorder

SP **F19.96 Other psychoactive substance use, unspecified with psychoactive substance-induced persisting amnestic disorder**

SP **F19.97 Other psychoactive substance use, unspecified with psychoactive substance-induced persisting dementia**

Chapter 5

F01-F99

Other (or unknown) substance-induced major neurocognitive disorder, without use disorder

6 **F19.98 Other psychoactive substance use, unspecified with other psychoactive substance-induced disorders**

SP **F19.980 Other psychoactive substance use, unspecified with psychoactive substance-induced anxiety disorder**

Other (or unknown) substance-induced anxiety disorder, without use disorder

SP **F19.981 Other psychoactive substance use, unspecified with psychoactive substance-induced sexual dysfunction**

Other (or unknown) substance-induced sexual dysfunction, without use disorder

SP **F19.982 Other psychoactive substance use, unspecified with psychoactive substance-induced sleep disorder**

Other (or unknown) substance-induced sleep disorder, without use disorder

SP **F19.988 Other psychoactive substance use, unspecified with other psychoactive substance-induced disorder**

Other (or unknown) substance-induced mild neurocognitive disorder, without use disorder

Other (or unknown) substance-induced obsessive-compulsive or related disorder, without use disorder

SP **F19.99 Other psychoactive substance use, unspecified with unspecified psychoactive substance-induced disorder**

Schizophrenia, schizotypal, delusional, and other non-mood psychotic disorders (F20-F29)

4 **F20 Schizophrenia**

EXCLUDES 1 brief psychotic disorder (F23)
cyclic schizophrenia (F25.0)
mood [affective] disorders with psychotic symptoms (F30.2, F31.2, F31.5, F31.64, F32.3, F33.3)
schizoaffective disorder (F25.-)
schizophrenic reaction NOS (F23)

EXCLUDES 2 schizophrenic reaction in:
alcoholism (F10.15-, F10.25-, F10.95-)
brain disease (F06.2)
epilepsy (F06.2)
psychoactive drug use (F11-F19 with .15. .25, .95)
schizotypal disorder (F21)

CODING TIPS✓ Schizophrenia will always impact care so it should be coded. Schizophrenia, as a primary diagnosis, usually requires a psychiatric-trained RN.

SP **F20.0 Paranoid schizophrenia**

Paraphrenic schizophrenia

EXCLUDES 1 involutional paranoid state (F22)
paranoia (F22)

DEFINITION Schizophrenia marked by displays of megalomania, delusions of persecution and/or grandeur, hallucinations, and aggressive behavior.

SP **F20.1 Disorganized schizophrenia**

Hebephrenic schizophrenia
Hebephrenia

SP **F20.2 Catatonic schizophrenia**

Schizophrenic catalepsy
Schizophrenic catatonia
Schizophrenic flexibilitas cerea

EXCLUDES 1 catatonic stupor (R40.1)

SP **F20.3 Undifferentiated schizophrenia**

Atypical schizophrenia

EXCLUDES 1 acute schizophrenia-like psychotic disorder (F23)

EXCLUDES 2 post-schizophrenic depression (F32.89)

SP **F20.5 Residual schizophrenia**

Restzustand (schizophrenic)
Schizophrenic residual state

5 **F20.8 Other schizophrenia**

SP **F20.81 Schizophreniform disorder**

Schizophreniform psychosis NOS

SP **F20.89 Other schizophrenia**

Cenesthopathic schizophrenia
Simple schizophrenia

SP **F20.9 Schizophrenia, unspecified**

SP **F21 Schizotypal disorder**

Borderline schizophrenia
Latent schizophrenia
Latent schizophrenic reaction
Prepsychotic schizophrenia
Prodromal schizophrenia
Pseudoneurotic schizophrenia
Pseudopsychopathic schizophrenia
Schizotypal personality disorder

EXCLUDES 2 Asperger's syndrome (F84.5)
schizoid personality disorder (F60.1)

CODING TIPS✓ Do not use code F21 when schizophrenia or schizoaffective disorder is specified by the provider. Schizotypal disorder is a personality disorder characterized by behaviors that impact interpersonal relationships, affect appearance and often exacerbate depressive and/or anxious symptoms.

SP **F22 Delusional disorders**

Delusional dysmorphophobia
Involutional paranoid state
Paranoia
Paranoia querulans
Paranoid psychosis
Paranoid state
Paraphrenia (late)
Sensitiver Beziehungswahn

EXCLUDES 1 mood [affective] disorders with psychotic symptoms (F30.2, F31.2, F31.5, F31.64, F32.3, F33.3)
paranoid schizophrenia (F20.0)

EXCLUDES 2 paranoid personality disorder (F60.0)
paranoid psychosis, psychogenic (F23)
paranoid reaction (F23)

DEFINITION Paranoia: Extreme, irrational distrust of others.

SP **F23 Brief psychotic disorder**
Paranoid reaction
Psychogenic paranoid psychosis

EXCLUDES 2 mood [affective] disorders with psychotic symptoms (F30.2, F31.2, F31.5, F31.64, F32.3, F33.3)

SP **F24 Shared psychotic disorder**
Folie à deux
Induced paranoid disorder
Induced psychotic disorder

4 **F25 Schizoaffective disorders**

EXCLUDES 1 mood [affective] disorders with psychotic symptoms (F30.2, F31.2, F31.5, F31.64, F32.3, F33.3)
schizophrenia (F20.-)

CODING TIPS ✓ Do not use F25.- codes when schizophrenia is specified by the provider. Schizoaffective disorder is diagnosed in patients who do not meet the criteria for either schizophrenia or bipolar disorder but often demonstrate characteristics of both disorders.

SP **F25.0 Schizoaffective disorder, bipolar type**
Cyclic schizophrenia
Schizoaffective disorder, manic type
Schizoaffective disorder, mixed type
Schizoaffective psychosis, bipolar type

SP **F25.1 Schizoaffective disorder, depressive type**
Schizoaffective psychosis, depressive type

SP **F25.8 Other schizoaffective disorders**

SP **F25.9 Schizoaffective disorder, unspecified**
Schizoaffective psychosis NOS

SP **F28 Other psychotic disorder not due to a substance or known physiological condition**
Chronic hallucinatory psychosis
Other specified schizophrenia spectrum and other psychotic disorder

SP **F29 Unspecified psychosis not due to a substance or known physiological condition**
Psychosis NOS
Unspecified schizophrenia spectrum and other psychotic disorder

EXCLUDES 1 mental disorder NOS (F99)
unspecified mental disorder due to known physiological condition (F09)

Mood [affective] disorders (F30-F39)

4 **F30 Manic episode**

INCLUDES bipolar disorder, single manic episode
mixed affective episode

EXCLUDES 1 bipolar disorder (F31.-)
major depressive disorder, single episode (F32.-)
major depressive disorder, recurrent (F33.-)

5 **F30.1 Manic episode without psychotic symptoms**

SP SH **F30.10 Manic episode without psychotic symptoms, unspecified**

SP SH **F30.11 Manic episode without psychotic symptoms, mild**

SP SH **F30.12 Manic episode without psychotic symptoms, moderate**

SP SH **F30.13 Manic episode, severe, without psychotic symptoms**

SP SH **F30.2 Manic episode, severe with psychotic symptoms**
Manic stupor
Mania with mood-congruent psychotic symptoms
Mania with mood-incongruent psychotic symptoms

SP SH **F30.3 Manic episode in partial remission**

SP SH **F30.4 Manic episode in full remission**

SP SH **F30.8 Other manic episodes**
Hypomania

SP SH **F30.9 Manic episode, unspecified**
Mania NOS

4 **F31 Bipolar disorder**

INCLUDES bipolar I disorder
bipolar type I disorder
manic-depressive illness
manic-depressive psychosis
manic-depressive reaction

EXCLUDES 1 bipolar disorder, single manic episode (F30.-)
major depressive disorder, single episode (F32.-)
major depressive disorder, recurrent (F33.-)

EXCLUDES 2 cyclothymia (F34.0)

CODING TIPS ✓ When assigning a code for bipolar disorder, no additional code for depression or depressive disorder should be assigned if the patient is also reported to have depression and/or depressive symptoms. Individuals with bipolar disorder may have alternating periods of emotional highs and lows reported as cyclothymic features. When cyclothymic features are additionally reported by the provider, cyclothymia (F34.0) should be additionally coded.

SP SH **F31.0 Bipolar disorder, current episode hypomanic**

5 **F31.1 Bipolar disorder, current episode manic without psychotic features**

SP SH **F31.10 Bipolar disorder, current episode manic without psychotic features, unspecified**

SP SH **F31.11 Bipolar disorder, current episode manic without psychotic features, mild**

SP SH **F31.12 Bipolar disorder, current episode manic without psychotic features, moderate**

SP SH **F31.13 Bipolar disorder, current episode manic without psychotic features, severe**

SP SH **F31.2 Bipolar disorder, current episode manic severe with psychotic features**
Bipolar disorder, current episode manic with mood-congruent psychotic symptoms
Bipolar disorder, current episode manic with mood-incongruent psychotic symptoms
Bipolar I disorder, current or most recent episode manic with psychotic features

5 **F31.3 Bipolar disorder, current episode depressed, mild or moderate severity**

SP SH **F31.30 Bipolar disorder, current episode depressed, mild or moderate severity, unspecified**

SP SH **F31.31 Bipolar disorder, current episode depressed, mild**

SP SH **F31.32 Bipolar disorder, current episode depressed, moderate**

SP SH **F31.4 Bipolar disorder, current episode depressed, severe, without psychotic features**

SP SH **F31.5 Bipolar disorder, current episode depressed, severe, with psychotic features**
Bipolar disorder, current episode depressed with mood-incongruent psychotic symptoms
Bipolar disorder, current episode depressed with mood-congruent psychotic symptoms
Bipolar I disorder, current or most recent episode depressed, with psychotic features

5 **F31.6 Bipolar disorder, current episode mixed**

SP SH **F31.60 Bipolar disorder, current episode mixed, unspecified**

SP SH **F31.61 Bipolar disorder, current episode mixed, mild**

SP SH **F31.62 Bipolar disorder, current episode mixed, moderate**

SP SH **F31.63 Bipolar disorder, current episode mixed, severe, without psychotic features**

SP SH **F31.64 Bipolar disorder, current episode mixed, severe, with psychotic features**
Bipolar disorder, current episode mixed with mood-congruent psychotic symptoms
Bipolar disorder, current episode mixed with mood-incongruent psychotic symptoms

5 **F31.7 Bipolar disorder, currently in remission**

SP SH **F31.70 Bipolar disorder, currently in remission, most recent episode unspecified**

SP SH **F31.71 Bipolar disorder, in partial remission, most recent episode hypomanic**

SP SH **F31.72 Bipolar disorder, in full remission, most recent episode hypomanic**

SP SH **F31.73 Bipolar disorder, in partial remission, most recent episode manic**

SP **F31.74 Bipolar disorder, in full remission, most recent episode manic**

SP **F31.75 Bipolar disorder, in partial remission, most recent episode depressed**

SP **F31.76 Bipolar disorder, in full remission, most recent episode depressed**

SP SH **F31.77 Bipolar disorder, in partial remission, most recent episode mixed**

SP SH **F31.78 Bipolar disorder, in full remission, most recent episode mixed**

5 **F31.8 Other bipolar disorders**

SP SH **F31.81 Bipolar II disorder**
Bipolar disorder, type 2

SP SH **F31.89 Other bipolar disorder**
Recurrent manic episodes NOS

SP SH **F31.9 Bipolar disorder, unspecified**
Manic depression

▲ 4 **F32 Depressive episode**

INCLUDES single episode of agitated depression
single episode of depressive reaction
single episode of major depression
single episode of psychogenic depression
single episode of reactive depression
single episode of vital depression

EXCLUDES 1 bipolar disorder (F31.-)
manic episode (F30.-)
recurrent depressive disorder (F33.-)

EXCLUDES 2 adjustment disorder (F43.2)

CODING TIPS✓ A physician or NPP must provide confirmation of the diagnosis of depression to assign this code category, and it should not be assigned based upon the presence of symptoms or use of medications alone.

SP SH **F32.0 Major depressive disorder, single episode, mild**

SP SH **F32.1 Major depressive disorder, single episode, moderate**

SP SH **F32.2 Major depressive disorder, single episode, severe without psychotic features**

SP **F32.3 Major depressive disorder, single episode, severe with psychotic features**
Single episode of major depression with mood-congruent psychotic symptoms
Single episode of major depression with mood-incongruent psychotic symptoms
Single episode of major depression with psychotic symptoms
Single episode of psychogenic depressive psychosis
Single episode of psychotic depression
Single episode of reactive depressive psychosis

SP SH **F32.4 Major depressive disorder, single episode, in partial remission**

SP **F32.5 Major depressive disorder, single episode, in full remission**

5 **F32.8 Other depressive episodes**

SP **F32.81 Premenstrual dysphoric disorder**
EXCLUDES 1 premenstrual tension syndrome (N94.3)
DEFINITION Premenstrual dysphoric disorder (PMDD) is a severe form of premenstrual syndrome (PMS). PMDD is characterized by depression, anxiety, tension and irritability that typically begins after release of the ovum.

SP SH **F32.89 Other specified depressive episodes**
Atypical depression
Post-schizophrenic depression
Single episode of 'masked' depression NOS

▲ SP SH **F32.9 Major depressive disorder, single episode, unspecified**
Major depression NOS
CODING TIPS✓ If the physician or NPP has documented only depression or depressive disorder, the correct code is F32.A. Code F32.9 requires that the physician document major depressive disorder, single episode, but otherwise unspecified as to severity and remission.

★ **F32.A Depression, unspecified**
Depression NOS
Depressive disorder NOS
CODING TIPS✓ If the physician or NPP has documented only depression or depressive disorder, the correct code is F32.A. Code F32.9 requires that the physician document major depressive disorder, single episode, but otherwise unspecified as to severity and remission.

4 **F33 Major depressive disorder, recurrent**
INCLUDES recurrent episodes of depressive reaction
recurrent episodes of endogenous depression
recurrent episodes of major depression
recurrent episodes of psychogenic depression
recurrent episodes of reactive depression
recurrent episodes of seasonal depressive disorder
recurrent episodes of vital depression
EXCLUDES 1 bipolar disorder (F31.-)
manic episode (F30.-)

SP SH **F33.0 Major depressive disorder, recurrent, mild**

SP SH **F33.1 Major depressive disorder, recurrent, moderate**

SP SH **F33.2 Major depressive disorder, recurrent severe without psychotic features**

SP **F33.3 Major depressive disorder, recurrent, severe with psychotic symptoms**
Endogenous depression with psychotic symptoms
Major depressive disorder, recurrent, with psychotic features
Recurrent severe episodes of major depression with mood-congruent psychotic symptoms
Recurrent severe episodes of major depression with mood-incongruent psychotic symptoms
Recurrent severe episodes of major depression with psychotic symptoms
Recurrent severe episodes of psychogenic depressive psychosis
Recurrent severe episodes of psychotic depression
Recurrent severe episodes of reactive depressive psychosis

5 **F33.4 Major depressive disorder, recurrent, in remission**

SP SH **F33.40 Major depressive disorder, recurrent, in remission, unspecified**

SP SH **F33.41 Major depressive disorder, recurrent, in partial remission**

SP **F33.42 Major depressive disorder, recurrent, in full remission**

SP SH **F33.8 Other recurrent depressive disorders**
Recurrent brief depressive episodes

SP SH **F33.9 Major depressive disorder, recurrent, unspecified**
Monopolar depression NOS

4 **F34 Persistent mood [affective] disorders**

SP **F34.0 Cyclothymic disorder**
Affective personality disorder
Cycloid personality
Cyclothymia
Cyclothymic personality
DEFINITION Mild mood swings between elevated mood and mild depression.

SP **F34.1 Dysthymic disorder**
Depressive neurosis
Depressive personality disorder
Dysthymia
Neurotic depression
Persistent anxiety depression
Persistent depressive disorder
EXCLUDES 2 anxiety depression (mild or not persistent) (F41.8)

5 **F34.8 Other persistent mood [affective] disorders**

SP SH **F34.81 Disruptive mood dysregulation disorder**

SP SH **F34.89 Other specified persistent mood disorders**

SP SH **F34.9 Persistent mood [affective] disorder, unspecified**

SP SH **F39 Unspecified mood [affective] disorder**
Affective psychosis NOS

Anxiety, dissociative, stress-related, somatoform and other nonpsychotic mental disorders (F40-F48)

4 **F40 Phobic anxiety disorders**

5 **F40.0 Agoraphobia**

SP **F40.00 Agoraphobia, unspecified**

SP **F40.01 Agoraphobia with panic disorder**
Panic disorder with agoraphobia
EXCLUDES 1 panic disorder without agoraphobia (F41.0)

DEFINITION Fear of open spaces or crowds, traveling, or leaving a safe place, accompanied by panic attacks.

SP **F40.02 Agoraphobia without panic disorder**

5 **F40.1 Social phobias**
Anthropophobia
Social anxiety disorder
Social anxiety disorder of childhood
Social neurosis

DEFINITION Intense fear of appearing in public, especially in situations where one is the center of attention.

IQ **F40.10 Social phobia, unspecified**

SP **F40.11 Social phobia, generalized**

5 **F40.2 Specific (isolated) phobias**
EXCLUDES 2 dysmorphophobia (nondelusional) (F45.22)
nosophobia (F45.22)

6 **F40.21 Animal type phobia**

SP **F40.210 Arachnophobia**
Fear of spiders

SP **F40.218 Other animal type phobia**

6 **F40.22 Natural environment type phobia**

SP **F40.220 Fear of thunderstorms**

SP **F40.228 Other natural environment type phobia**

6 **F40.23 Blood, injection, injury type phobia**

SP **F40.230 Fear of blood**

SP **F40.231 Fear of injections and transfusions**

SP **F40.232 Fear of other medical care**

SP **F40.233 Fear of injury**

6 **F40.24 Situational type phobia**

SP **F40.240 Claustrophobia**

SP **F40.241 Acrophobia**

SP **F40.242 Fear of bridges**

SP **F40.243 Fear of flying**

SP **F40.248 Other situational type phobia**

6 **F40.29 Other specified phobia**

SP **F40.290 Androphobia**
Fear of men

SP **F40.291 Gynephobia**
Fear of women

SP **F40.298 Other specified phobia**

SP **F40.8 Other phobic anxiety disorders**
Phobic anxiety disorder of childhood

IQ **F40.9 Phobic anxiety disorder, unspecified**
Phobia NOS
Phobic state NOS

4 **F41 Other anxiety disorders**
EXCLUDES 2 anxiety in:
acute stress reaction (F43.0)
transient adjustment reaction (F43.2)
neurasthenia (F48.8)
psychophysiologic disorders (F45.-)
separation anxiety (F93.0)

SP **F41.0 Panic disorder [episodic paroxysmal anxiety]**
Panic attack
Panic state
EXCLUDES 1 panic disorder with agoraphobia (F40.01)

DEFINITION Unexplained bouts of intense fear or anxiety, accompanied by physiological symptoms of elevated heart rate, sweating, trembling, dizziness, and dyspnea.

SP **F41.1 Generalized anxiety disorder**
Anxiety neurosis
Anxiety reaction
Anxiety state
Overanxious disorder
EXCLUDES 2 neurasthenia (F48.8)

DEFINITION Persistent, uncontrollable worry about aspects of a person's life; diagnosed when symptoms last longer than six months, with anxiety present on the majority of days in that time.

SP **F41.3 Other mixed anxiety disorders**

SP **F41.8 Other specified anxiety disorders**
Anxiety depression (mild or not persistent)
Anxiety hysteria
Mixed anxiety and depressive disorder

CODING TIPS✓ There is no assumed relationship between depression and anxiety. Do not assume that because the physician or NPP documented depression with anxiety that the two are related. Depression and anxiety should only be coded with F41.8 if the physician or NPP had indicated a relationship or has documented anxiety depression or mixed anxiety and depressive disorder or MADD.[AHA: 1Q 2021]

SP **F41.9 Anxiety disorder, unspecified**
Anxiety NOS

4 **F42 Obsessive-compulsive disorder**
EXCLUDES 2 obsessive-compulsive personality (disorder) (F60.5)
obsessive-compulsive symptoms occurring in depression (F32-F33)
obsessive-compulsive symptoms occurring in schizophrenia (F20.-)

DEFINITION Recurrent obsessions of thought or action that are time-consuming or disruptive to daily life and can produce anxiety or distress.

SP **F42.2 Mixed obsessional thoughts and acts**

SP **F42.3 Hoarding disorder**

CODING TIPS✓ Hoarding disorder must be documented by the physician or NPP. The personal and public health consequences of hoarding can be substantial, putting people at risk for fire, falling (especially elderly people), poor sanitation and health risks.

SP **F42.4 Excoriation (skin-picking) disorder**
EXCLUDES 1 factitial dermatitis (L98.1)
other specified behavioral and emotional disorders with onset usually occurring in early childhood and adolescence (F98.8)

CODING TIPS ✓ Skin picking disorder is defined as recurrent skin picking resulting in skin lesions despite repeated attempts to decrease or stop skin picking. Skin picking also leads to clinically significant distress or disability, and patients with skin picking disorder can have important medical sequelae.

SP **F42.8 Other obsessive-compulsive disorder**
Anancastic neurosis
Obsessive-compulsive neurosis

SP **F42.9 Obsessive-compulsive disorder, unspecified**

4 **F43 Reaction to severe stress, and adjustment disorders**

SP **F43.0 Acute stress reaction**
Acute crisis reaction
Acute reaction to stress
Combat and operational stress reaction
Combat fatigue
Crisis state
Psychic shock

5 **F43.1 Post-traumatic stress disorder (PTSD)**
Traumatic neurosis

CODING TIPS ✓ Post-traumatic stress disorder is coded with F43.1 and combat fatigue is coded to F43.0. History of combat and operations stress reaction is coded to Z86.51.

DEFINITION Chronic stressful response to traumatic events such as combat, rape, physical assault, and natural disasters with sudden, powerful memories (flashbacks) of the event, anxiety, and panic.

SP **F43.10 Post-traumatic stress disorder, unspecified**

SP **F43.11 Post-traumatic stress disorder, acute**

SP **F43.12 Post-traumatic stress disorder, chronic**

5 **F43.2 Adjustment disorders**
Culture shock
Grief reaction
Hospitalism in children

EXCLUDES 2 separation anxiety disorder of childhood (F93.0)

SP **F43.20 Adjustment disorder, unspecified**

SP **F43.21 Adjustment disorder with depressed mood**

CODING TIPS ✓ Complicated bereavement is coded to F43.21. Bereavement (uncomplicated) is coded Z63.4.

DEFINITION Prolonged depressive state as a reaction to an event or change in the patient's life.

SP **F43.22 Adjustment disorder with anxiety**

SP **F43.23 Adjustment disorder with mixed anxiety and depressed mood**

SP **F43.24 Adjustment disorder with disturbance of conduct**

SP **F43.25 Adjustment disorder with mixed disturbance of emotions and conduct**

SP **F43.29 Adjustment disorder with other symptoms**

SP **F43.8 Other reactions to severe stress**
Other specified trauma and stressor-related disorder

IQ **F43.9 Reaction to severe stress, unspecified**
Trauma and stressor-related disorder, NOS

4 **F44 Dissociative and conversion disorders**

INCLUDES conversion hysteria
conversion reaction
hysteria
hysterical psychosis

EXCLUDES 2 malingering [conscious simulation] (Z76.5)

SP **F44.0 Dissociative amnesia**

EXCLUDES 1 amnesia NOS (R41.3)
anterograde amnesia (R41.1)
dissociative amnesia with dissociative fugue (F44.1)
retrograde amnesia (R41.2)

EXCLUDES 2 alcohol-or other psychoactive substance-induced amnestic disorder (F10, F13, F19 with .26, .96)
amnestic disorder due to known physiological condition (F04)
postictal amnesia in epilepsy (G40.-)

DEFINITION Psychological trauma causing temporary forgetting of personal information and inability to perform complex tasks, like driving or cooking.

SP **F44.1 Dissociative fugue**
Dissociative amnesia with dissociative fugue

EXCLUDES 2 postictal fugue in epilepsy (G40.-)

DEFINITION Disorder occurring in response to a severe, recent stressor, in which the patient invents a new personality and becomes unable to remember his/her previous identity, lasting days or months.

SP **F44.2 Dissociative stupor**

EXCLUDES 1 catatonic stupor (R40.1)
stupor NOS (R40.1)

EXCLUDES 2 catatonic disorder due to known physiological condition (F06.1)
depressive stupor (F32, F33)
manic stupor (F30, F31)

SP **F44.4 Conversion disorder with motor symptom or deficit**
Conversion disorder with abnormal movement
Conversion disorder with speech symptoms
Conversion disorder with swallowing symptoms
Conversion disorder with weakness/paralysis
Dissociative motor disorders
Psychogenic aphonia
Psychogenic dysphonia

SP **F44.5 Conversion disorder with seizures or convulsions**
Conversion disorder with attacks or seizures
Dissociative convulsions

SP **F44.6 Conversion disorder with sensory symptom or deficit**
Conversion disorder with anesthesia or sensory loss
Conversion disorder with special sensory symptoms
Dissociative anesthesia and sensory loss
Psychogenic deafness

SP **F44.7 Conversion disorder with mixed symptom presentation**

5 **F44.8 Other dissociative and conversion disorders**

SP **F44.81 Dissociative identity disorder**
Multiple personality disorder

SP **F44.89 Other dissociative and conversion disorders**
Ganser's syndrome
Psychogenic confusion
Psychogenic twilight state
Trance and possession disorders

SP **F44.9 Dissociative and conversion disorder, unspecified**
Dissociative disorder NOS

4 **F45 Somatoform disorders**
EXCLUDES 2 dissociative and conversion disorders (F44.-)
factitious disorders (F68.1-, F68.A)
hair-plucking (F63.3)
lalling (F80.0)
lisping (F80.0)
malingering [conscious simulation] (Z76.5)
nail-biting (F98.8)
psychological or behavioral factors associated with disorders or diseases classified elsewhere (F54)
sexual dysfunction, not due to a substance or known physiological condition (F52.-)
thumb-sucking (F98.8)
tic disorders (in childhood and adolescence) (F95.-)
Tourette's syndrome (F95.2)
trichotillomania (F63.3)

SP **F45.0 Somatization disorder**
Briquet's disorder
Multiple psychosomatic disorder

SP **F45.1 Undifferentiated somatoform disorder**
Somatic symptom disorder
Undifferentiated psychosomatic disorder

5 **F45.2 Hypochondriacal disorders**
EXCLUDES 2 delusional dysmorphophobia (F22)
fixed delusions about bodily functions or shape (F22)

DEFINITION Chronic worry about nonexistent illnesses that one believes one may have.

SP **F45.20 Hypochondriacal disorder, unspecified**

SP **F45.21 Hypochondriasis**
Hypochondriacal neurosis
Illness anxiety disorder

SP **F45.22 Body dysmorphic disorder**
Dysmorphophobia (nondelusional)
Nosophobia

SP **F45.29 Other hypochondriacal disorders**

5 **F45.4 Pain disorders related to psychological factors**
EXCLUDES 1 pain NOS (R52)

SP **F45.41 Pain disorder exclusively related to psychological factors**
Somatoform pain disorder (persistent)

GUIDELINES **Section I.C.5.a**
Assign code F45.41 for pain that is exclusively related to psychological disorders. As indicated by the Excludes 1 note under category G89, a code from category G89 should not be assigned with code F45.41.

CODING TIPS✓ Do not use F45.41 to report somatoform disorder not related to pain, chronic pain syndrome, or psychological factors related to chronic pain disorders (G89.-, F45.42).

SP **F45.42 Pain disorder with related psychological factors**
Code also:
associated acute or chronic pain (G89.-)

GUIDELINES **Section I.C.5.a**
Code F45.42 should be used with a code from category G89, Pain, not elsewhere classified, if there is documentation of a psychological component for a patient with acute or chronic pain.

CODING TIPS✓ When the clinical record specifies that the patient has a pain disorder with related psychological factors, this code should be additionally assigned.

SP **F45.8 Other somatoform disorders**
Psychogenic dysmenorrhea
Psychogenic dysphagia, including 'globus hystericus'
Psychogenic pruritus
Psychogenic torticollis
Somatoform autonomic dysfunction
Teeth grinding
EXCLUDES 1 sleep related teeth grinding (G47.63)

SP **F45.9 Somatoform disorder, unspecified**
Psychosomatic disorder NOS

4 **F48 Other nonpsychotic mental disorders**

SP **F48.1 Depersonalization-derealization syndrome**

SP **F48.2 Pseudobulbar affect**
Involuntary emotional expression disorder
Code first underlying cause, if known, such as:
amyotrophic lateral sclerosis (G12.21)
multiple sclerosis (G35)
sequelae of cerebrovascular disease (I69.-)
sequelae of traumatic intracranial injury (S06.-)

4 4th digit required 5 5th digit required 6 6th digit required 7 7th digit required X 7th digit placeholder + Additional code L Laterality

CODING TIPS ✓ This is an example of a convention in opposition to a guideline. The guideline says to code the residual condition first followed by the sequela. In this case, the convention states to code first the sequelae of traumatic intracranial injury. The convention is followed.

SP **F48.8 Other specified nonpsychotic mental disorders**
Dhat syndrome
Neurasthenia
Occupational neurosis, including writer's cramp
Psychasthenia
Psychasthenic neurosis
Psychogenic syncope

SP **F48.9 Nonpsychotic mental disorder, unspecified**
Neurosis NOS

Behavioral syndromes associated with physiological disturbances and physical factors (F50-F59)

▲ 4 **F50 Eating disorders**
EXCLUDES 1 anorexia NOS (R63.0)
feeding problems of newborn (P92.-)
polyphagia (R63.2)
EXCLUDES 2 feeding difficulties (R63.3)
feeding disorder in infancy or childhood (F98.2-)

5 **F50.0 Anorexia nervosa**
EXCLUDES 1 loss of appetite (R63.0)
psychogenic loss of appetite (F50.89)

CODING TIPS ✓ This code can be assigned only if specified as "anorexia nervosa," which is differentiated from simple anorexia (loss of appetite) due to psychological features, including intense fear of weight gain, body image distortions, and a refusal to maintain normal body weight.

SP **F50.00 Anorexia nervosa, unspecified**

SP **F50.01 Anorexia nervosa, restricting type**

SP **F50.02 Anorexia nervosa, binge eating/purging type**
EXCLUDES 1 bulimia nervosa (F50.2)

SP **F50.2 Bulimia nervosa**
Bulimia NOS
Hyperorexia nervosa
EXCLUDES 1 anorexia nervosa, binge eating/purging type (F50.02)

DEFINITION Repetitive episodes of binge eating followed by excessive measures to avoid gaining weight, such as self-induced vomiting and extreme exercising.

5 **F50.8 Other eating disorders**
EXCLUDES 2 pica of infancy and childhood (F98.3)

SP **F50.81 Binge eating disorder**

SP **F50.82 Avoidant/restrictive food intake disorder**

SP **F50.89 Other specified eating disorder**
Pica in adults
Psychogenic loss of appetite

CODING TIPS ✓ Psychogenic loss of appetite may explain the patient's refusal to eat and be used in addition to, or instead of, malnutrition to better explain the patient's loss of weight and further decline.

DEFINITION This code includes pica in adults. Pica is the urge to eat nonfood substances, such as dirt, paper, paint, and rocks. It also includes the psychogenic loss of appetite characterized by an aversion to food or eating with no pathologic or physiologic explanation.

SP **F50.9 Eating disorder, unspecified**
Atypical anorexia nervosa
Atypical bulimia nervosa
Feeding or eating disorder, unspecified
Other specified feeding disorder

4 **F51 Sleep disorders not due to a substance or known physiological condition**
EXCLUDES 2 organic sleep disorders (G47.-)

5 **F51.0 Insomnia not due to a substance or known physiological condition**
EXCLUDES 2 alcohol related insomnia (F10.182, F10.282, F10.982)
drug-related insomnia (F11.182, F11.282, F11.982, F13.182, F13.282, F13.982, F14.182, F14.282, F14.982, F15.182, F15.282, F15.982, F19.182, F19.282, F19.982)
insomnia NOS (G47.0-)
insomnia due to known physiological condition (G47.0-)
organic insomnia (G47.0-)
sleep deprivation (Z72.820)

SP **F51.01 Primary insomnia**
Idiopathic insomnia

SP **F51.02 Adjustment insomnia**

SP **F51.03 Paradoxical insomnia**

SP **F51.04 Psychophysiologic insomnia**

SP **F51.05 Insomnia due to other mental disorder**
Code also:
associated mental disorder

SP **F51.09 Other insomnia not due to a substance or known physiological condition**

5 **F51.1 Hypersomnia not due to a substance or known physiological condition**
EXCLUDES 2 alcohol related hypersomnia (F10.182, F10.282, F10.982)

Chapter 5

F01-F99

drug-related hypersomnia (F11.182, F11.282, F11.982, F13.182, F13.282, F13.982, F14.182, F14.282, F14.982, F15.182, F15.282, F15.982, F19.182, F19.282, F19.982)
hypersomnia NOS (G47.10)
hypersomnia due to known physiological condition (G47.10)
idiopathic hypersomnia (G47.11, G47.12)
narcolepsy (G47.4-)

SP **F51.11 Primary hypersomnia**

SP **F51.12 Insufficient sleep syndrome**
EXCLUDES 1 sleep deprivation (Z72.820)

SP **F51.13 Hypersomnia due to other mental disorder**
Code also:
associated mental disorder

SP **F51.19 Other hypersomnia not due to a substance or known physiological condition**

SP **F51.3 Sleepwalking [somnambulism]**
Non-rapid eye movement sleep arousal disorders, sleepwalking type

SP **F51.4 Sleep terrors [night terrors]**
Non-rapid eye movement sleep arousal disorders, sleep terror type

SP **F51.5 Nightmare disorder**
Dream anxiety disorder

SP **F51.8 Other sleep disorders not due to a substance or known physiological condition**

SP **F51.9 Sleep disorder not due to a substance or known physiological condition, unspecified**
Emotional sleep disorder NOS

4 **F52 Sexual dysfunction not due to a substance or known physiological condition**
EXCLUDES 2 Dhat syndrome (F48.8)

SP **F52.0 Hypoactive sexual desire disorder**
Lack or loss of sexual desire
Male hypoactive sexual desire disorder
Sexual anhedonia
EXCLUDES 1 decreased libido (R68.82)
DEFINITION Markedly decreased sexual desire.

SP **F52.1 Sexual aversion disorder**
Sexual aversion and lack of sexual enjoyment

5 **F52.2 Sexual arousal disorders**
Failure of genital response

SP **F52.21 Male erectile disorder**
Erectile disorder
Psychogenic impotence
EXCLUDES 1 impotence of organic origin (N52.-)
impotence NOS (N52.-)

SP **F52.22 Female sexual arousal disorder**
Female sexual interest/arousal disorder

5 **F52.3 Orgasmic disorder**
Inhibited orgasm
Psychogenic anorgasmy

SP **F52.31 Female orgasmic disorder**

SP **F52.32 Male orgasmic disorder**
Delayed ejaculation

SP **F52.4 Premature ejaculation**

SP **F52.5 Vaginismus not due to a substance or known physiological condition**
Psychogenic vaginismus
EXCLUDES 2 vaginismus (due to a known physiological condition) (N94.2)

SP **F52.6 Dyspareunia not due to a substance or known physiological condition**
Genito-pelvic pain penetration disorder
Psychogenic dyspareunia
EXCLUDES 2 dyspareunia (due to a known physiological condition) (N94.1-)

SP **F52.8 Other sexual dysfunction not due to a substance or known physiological condition**
Excessive sexual drive
Nymphomania
Satyriasis

SP **F52.9 Unspecified sexual dysfunction not due to a substance or known physiological condition**
Sexual dysfunction NOS

4 **F53 Mental and behavioral disorders associated with the puerperium, not elsewhere classified**
EXCLUDES 1 mood disorders with psychotic features (F30.2, F31.2, F31.5, F31.64, F32.3, F33.3)
postpartum dysphoria (O90.6)
psychosis in schizophrenia, schizotypal, delusional, and other psychotic disorders (F20-F29)

SP **F53.0 Postpartum depression**
Postnatal depression, NOS
Postpartum depression, NOS

SP **F53.1 Puerperal psychosis**
Postpartum psychosis
Puerperal psychosis, NOS

IQ **F54 Psychological and behavioral factors associated with disorders or diseases classified elsewhere**
Psychological factors affecting physical conditions
Code first the associated physical disorder, such as:
asthma (J45.-)
dermatitis (L23-L25)
gastric ulcer (K25.-)
mucous colitis (K58.-)
ulcerative colitis (K51.-)
urticaria (L50.-)
EXCLUDES 2 tension-type headache (G44.2)

CODING TIPS✓ Assign code F54 when a psychological condition causes exacerbation of a specific physical condition, such as asthma or ulcers. This code may not be used alone, and documentation should specify that the psychological condition has caused exacerbation of the physical state. Code the physical condition first, followed by F54.

4 **F55 Abuse of non-psychoactive substances**
EXCLUDES 2 abuse of psychoactive substances (F10-F19)

SP **F55.0 Abuse of antacids**

SP **F55.1 Abuse of herbal or folk remedies**

SP **F55.2 Abuse of laxatives**

SP **F55.3 Abuse of steroids or hormones**

SP **F55.4 Abuse of vitamins**

SP **F55.8 Abuse of other non-psychoactive substances**

SP **F59 Unspecified behavioral syndromes associated with physiological disturbances and physical factors**
Psychogenic physiological dysfunction NOS
CODING TIPS✓ Do not use F59 to report psychosomatic disorder. Psychosomatic disorder has a specific code and should be coded to F45.9.

Disorders of adult personality and behavior (F60-F69)

4 **F60 Specific personality disorders**

SP **F60.0 Paranoid personality disorder**
Expansive paranoid personality (disorder)
Fanatic personality (disorder)
Querulant personality (disorder)
Paranoid personality (disorder)
Sensitive paranoid personality (disorder)
EXCLUDES 2 paranoia (F22)
paranoia querulans (F22)
paranoid psychosis (F22)
paranoid schizophrenia (F20.0)
paranoid state (F22)

SP **F60.1 Schizoid personality disorder**
EXCLUDES 2 Asperger's syndrome (F84.5)
delusional disorder (F22)
schizoid disorder of childhood (F84.5)
schizophrenia (F20.-)
schizotypal disorder (F21)

SP **F60.2 Antisocial personality disorder**
Amoral personality (disorder)
Asocial personality (disorder)
Dissocial personality disorder
Psychopathic personality (disorder)
Sociopathic personality (disorder)
EXCLUDES 1 conduct disorders (F91.-)
EXCLUDES 2 borderline personality disorder (F60.3)

SP **F60.3 Borderline personality disorder**
Aggressive personality (disorder)
Emotionally unstable personality disorder
Explosive personality (disorder)
EXCLUDES 2 antisocial personality disorder (F60.2)
DEFINITION Disorder in which a person is quick to anger, aggressive, abnormally emotional, and argumentative.

SP **F60.4 Histrionic personality disorder**
Hysterical personality (disorder)
Psychoinfantile personality (disorder)

SP **F60.5 Obsessive-compulsive personality disorder**
Anankastic personality (disorder)
Compulsive personality (disorder)
Obsessional personality (disorder)
EXCLUDES 2 obsessive-compulsive disorder (F42.-)

SP **F60.6 Avoidant personality disorder**
Anxious personality disorder

SP **F60.7 Dependent personality disorder**
Asthenic personality (disorder)
Inadequate personality (disorder)
Passive personality (disorder)

5 **F60.8 Other specific personality disorders**

SP **F60.81 Narcissistic personality disorder**

SP **F60.89 Other specific personality disorders**
Eccentric personality disorder
'Haltlose' type personality disorder
Immature personality disorder
Passive-aggressive personality disorder
Psychoneurotic personality disorder
Self-defeating personality disorder

SP **F60.9 Personality disorder, unspecified**
Character disorder NOS
Character neurosis NOS
Pathological personality NOS

4 **F63 Impulse disorders**
EXCLUDES 2 habitual excessive use of alcohol or psychoactive substances (F10-F19)
impulse disorders involving sexual behavior (F65.-)

SP **F63.0 Pathological gambling**
Compulsive gambling
Gambling disorder
EXCLUDES 1 gambling and betting NOS (Z72.6)
EXCLUDES 2 excessive gambling by manic patients (F30, F31)
gambling in antisocial personality disorder (F60.2)

SP **F63.1 Pyromania**
Pathological fire-setting
EXCLUDES 2 fire-setting (by) (in):
adult with antisocial personality disorder (F60.2)
alcohol or psychoactive substance intoxication (F10-F19)
conduct disorders (F91.-)
mental disorders due to known physiological condition (F01-F09)
schizophrenia (F20.-)
DEFINITION Uncontrollable impulse to set fires.

SP **F63.2 Kleptomania**
Pathological stealing

EXCLUDES 1 shoplifting as the reason for observation for suspected mental disorder (Z03.8)

EXCLUDES 2 depressive disorder with stealing (F31-F33)
stealing due to underlying mental condition-code to mental condition
stealing in mental disorders due to known physiological condition (F01-F09)

DEFINITION Irresistible impulse to steal.

SP F63.3 **Trichotillomania**
Hair plucking
EXCLUDES 2 other stereotyped movement disorder (F98.4)

5 F63.8 **Other impulse disorders**

SP F63.81 **Intermittent explosive disorder**

SP F63.89 **Other impulse disorders**

SP F63.9 **Impulse disorder, unspecified**
Impulse control disorder NOS

4 F64 **Gender identity disorders**

SP F64.0 **Transsexualism**
Gender identity disorder in adolescence and adulthood
Gender dysphoria in adolescents and adults

SP + F64.1 **Dual role transvestism**
Use additional code to identify sex reassignment status (Z87.890)
EXCLUDES 1 gender identity disorder in childhood (F64.2)
EXCLUDES 2 fetishistic transvestism (F65.1)

SP F64.2 **Gender identity disorder of childhood**
Gender dysphoria in children
EXCLUDES 1 gender identity disorder in adolescence and adulthood (F64.0)
EXCLUDES 2 sexual maturation disorder (F66)

SP F64.8 **Other gender identity disorders**
Other specified gender dysphoria

SP F64.9 **Gender identity disorder, unspecified**
Gender dysphoria, unspecified
Gender-role disorder NOS

4 F65 **Paraphilias**

SP F65.0 **Fetishism**
Fetishistic disorder

SP F65.1 **Transvestic fetishism**
Fetishistic transvestism
Transvestic disorder

SP F65.2 **Exhibitionism**
Exhibitionistic disorder
DEFINITION Compulsion to expose genitals in public.

SP F65.3 **Voyeurism**
Voyeuristic disorder
DEFINITION Uncontrollable compulsion to covertly observe others who are nude or engaged in sexual activity.

SP F65.4 **Pedophilia**
Pedophilic disorder

5 F65.5 **Sadomasochism**

SP F65.50 **Sadomasochism, unspecified**

SP F65.51 **Sexual masochism**
Sexual masochism disorder
DEFINITION Psychosexual disorder marked by the need to be humiliated or hurt to achieve sexual gratification.

SP F65.52 **Sexual sadism**
Sexual sadism disorder
DEFINITION Psychosexual disorder marked by the need to humiliate or injure others to achieve sexual gratification.

5 F65.8 **Other paraphilias**

SP F65.81 **Frotteurism**
Frotteuristic disorder

SP F65.89 **Other paraphilias**
Necrophilia
Other specified paraphilic disorder
DEFINITION Sexual attraction to corpses.

SP F65.9 **Paraphilia, unspecified**
Paraphilic disorder, unspecified
Sexual deviation NOS

SP F66 **Other sexual disorders**
Sexual maturation disorder
Sexual relationship disorder

4 F68 **Other disorders of adult personality and behavior**

5 F68.1 **Factitious disorder imposed on self**
Compensation neurosis
Elaboration of physical symptoms for psychological reasons
Hospital hopper syndrome
Münchausen's syndrome
Peregrinating patient
EXCLUDES 2 factitial dermatitis (L98.1)
person feigning illness (with obvious motivation) (Z76.5)

SP F68.10 **Factitious disorder imposed on self, unspecified**

SP F68.11 **Factitious disorder imposed on self, with predominantly psychological signs and symptoms**

SP F68.12 **Factitious disorder imposed on self, with predominantly physical signs and symptoms**

SP F68.13 **Factitious disorder imposed on self, with combined psychological and physical signs and symptoms**

SP F68.A **Factitious disorder imposed on another**
Factitious disorder by proxy
Münchausen's by proxy

SP F68.8 **Other specified disorders of adult personality and behavior**

IQ F69 **Unspecified disorder of adult personality and behavior**

Intellectual Disabilities (F70-F79)

Code first:
any associated physical or developmental disorders

EXCLUDES 1 borderline intellectual functioning, IQ above 70 to 84 (R41.83)

CODING TIPS✓ When IQ is specified, use the appropriate code from F70-F79 to specify level of intellectual disability based upon reported IQ. When developmental delays or disorders are additionally noted in a patient with Intellectual disability, these should be coded first.

SP **F70 Mild intellectual disabilities**
IQ level 50-55 to approximately 70
Mild mental subnormality

SP **F71 Moderate intellectual disabilities**
IQ level 35-40 to 50-55
Moderate mental subnormality

SP **F72 Severe intellectual disabilities**
IQ 20-25 to 35-40
Severe mental subnormality

SP **F73 Profound intellectual disabilities**
IQ level below 20-25
Profound mental subnormality

▲ 4 **F78 Other intellectual disabilities**

★ 5 **F78.A Other genetic related intellectual disabilities**

★ **F78.A1 SYNGAP1-related intellectual disability**
Code also, if applicable, any associated:
autism spectrum disorder (F84.0)
autistic disorder (F84.0)
encephalopathy (G93.4-)
epilepsy and recurrent seizures (G40.-)
other pervasive developmental disorders (F84.8)
pervasive developmental disorder, NOS (F84.9)

★ **F78.A9 Other genetic related intellectual disability**
Code also:
, if applicable, any associated disorders

SP **F79 Unspecified intellectual disabilities**
Mental deficiency NOS
Mental subnormality NOS

Pervasive and specific developmental disorders (F80-F89)

CODING TIPS✓ Disorders coded to categories F80-F89 should be specified as related to a developmental origin.

4 **F80 Specific developmental disorders of speech and language**

SP **F80.0 Phonological disorder**
Dyslalia
Functional speech articulation disorder
Lalling
Lisping
Phonological developmental disorder
Speech articulation developmental disorder
Speech-sound disorder
EXCLUDES 1 speech articulation impairment due to aphasia NOS (R47.01)
speech articulation impairment due to apraxia (R48.2)
EXCLUDES 2 speech articulation impairment due to hearing loss (F80.4)
speech articulation impairment due to intellectual disabilities (F70-F79)
speech articulation impairment with expressive language developmental disorder (F80.1)
speech articulation impairment with mixed receptive expressive language developmental disorder (F80.2)

CODING TIPS✓ Lisping, lalling, dyslalia and phonological disorder are classified to the same code, F80.0. Coders should also carefully note the multiple Excludes 1 and 2 notes for this code to ensure any additional speech articulation disorders are correctly coded, when applicable.

SP **F80.1 Expressive language disorder**
Developmental dysphasia or aphasia, expressive type
EXCLUDES 1 mixed receptive-expressive language disorder (F80.2)
dysphasia and aphasia NOS (R47.-)
EXCLUDES 2 acquired aphasia with epilepsy [Landau-Kleffner] (G40.80-)
selective mutism (F94.0)
intellectual disabilities (F70-F79)
pervasive developmental disorders (F84.-)

CODING TIPS✓ Language disorders should not be coded here unless specified as related to a developmental cause.

SP **F80.2 Mixed receptive-expressive language disorder**
Developmental dysphasia or aphasia, receptive type
Developmental Wernicke's aphasia
EXCLUDES 1 central auditory processing disorder (H93.25)
dysphasia or aphasia NOS (R47.-)
expressive language disorder (F80.1)
expressive type dysphasia or aphasia (F80.1)
word deafness (H93.25)
EXCLUDES 2 acquired aphasia with epilepsy [Landau-Kleffner] (G40.80-)
pervasive developmental disorders (F84.-)
selective mutism (F94.0)
intellectual disabilities (F70-F79)

DEFINITION Problems comprehending as well as expressing verbal language.

SP **F80.4 Speech and language development delay due to hearing loss**
Code also:
type of hearing loss (H90.-, H91.-)

Chapter 5 F01-F99

5 **F80.8 Other developmental disorders of speech and language**

SP **F80.81 Childhood onset fluency disorder**
Cluttering NOS
Stuttering NOS
EXCLUDES 1 adult onset fluency disorder (F98.5)
fluency disorder in conditions classified elsewhere (R47.82)
fluency disorder (stuttering) following cerebrovascular disease (I69. with final characters -23)

CODING TIPS ✓ Presently there are three major recognized forms of stuttering: stuttering with onset in early childhood, stuttering with onset after puberty, and fluency disorder subsequent to brain lesion or disease. F80.81 is the specific code for stuttering with onset in childhood.

SP **F80.82 Social pragmatic communication disorder**
EXCLUDES 1 Asperger's syndrome (F84.5)
autistic disorder (F84.0)

SP **F80.89 Other developmental disorders of speech and language**

IQ **F80.9 Developmental disorder of speech and language, unspecified**
Communication disorder NOS
Language disorder NOS

4 **F81 Specific developmental disorders of scholastic skills**

IQ **F81.0 Specific reading disorder**
'Backward reading'
Developmental dyslexia
Specific learning disorder, with impairment in reading
Specific reading retardation
EXCLUDES 1 alexia NOS (R48.0)
dyslexia NOS (R48.0)

IQ **F81.2 Mathematics disorder**
Developmental acalculia
Developmental arithmetical disorder
Developmental Gerstmann's syndrome
Specific learning disorder, with impairment in mathematics
EXCLUDES 1 acalculia NOS (R48.8)
EXCLUDES 2 arithmetical difficulties associated with a reading disorder (F81.0)
arithmetical difficulties associated with a spelling disorder (F81.81)
arithmetical difficulties due to inadequate teaching (Z55.8)

5 **F81.8 Other developmental disorders of scholastic skills**

IQ **F81.81 Disorder of written expression**
Specific learning disorder, with impairment in written expression
Specific spelling disorder

IQ **F81.89 Other developmental disorders of scholastic skills**

IQ **F81.9 Developmental disorder of scholastic skills, unspecified**
Knowledge acquisition disability NOS
Learning disability NOS
Learning disorder NOS

SP **F82 Specific developmental disorder of motor function**
Clumsy child syndrome
Developmental coordination disorder
Developmental dyspraxia
EXCLUDES 1 abnormalities of gait and mobility (R26.-)
lack of coordination (R27.-)
EXCLUDES 2 lack of coordination secondary to intellectual disabilities (F70-F79)

▲ 4 **F84 Pervasive developmental disorders**
Code also:
any associated medical condition and intellectual disabilities

SP **F84.0 Autistic disorder**
Autism spectrum disorder
Infantile autism
Infantile psychosis
Kanner's syndrome
EXCLUDES 1 Asperger's syndrome (F84.5)

DEFINITION Neurological disorder appearing at a young age that impairs social development and communication skills, and resulting in abnormal behavior that varies in degree of severity and ability to function.

SP **F84.2 Rett's syndrome**
EXCLUDES 1 Asperger's syndrome (F84.5)
Autistic disorder (F84.0)
Other childhood disintegrative disorder (F84.3)

SP + **F84.3 Other childhood disintegrative disorder**
Dementia infantilis
Disintegrative psychosis
Heller's syndrome
Symbiotic psychosis
Use additional code to identify any associated neurological condition.
EXCLUDES 1 Asperger's syndrome (F84.5)
Autistic disorder (F84.0)
Rett's syndrome (F84.2)

SP **F84.5 Asperger's syndrome**
Asperger's disorder
Autistic psychopathy
Schizoid disorder of childhood

SP **F84.8 Other pervasive developmental disorders**
Overactive disorder associated with intellectual disabilities and stereotyped movements

IQ **F84.9 Pervasive developmental disorder, unspecified**
Atypical autism

SP **F88 Other disorders of psychological development**
Developmental agnosia
Global developmental delay
Other specified neurodevelopmental disorder

IQ **F89 Unspecified disorder of psychological development**
Developmental disorder NOS
Neurodevelopmental disorder NOS

Behavioral and emotional disorders with onset usually occurring in childhood and adolescence (F90-F98)

Note:
Codes within categories F90-F98 may be used regardless of the age of a patient. These disorders generally have onset within the childhood or adolescent years, but may continue throughout life or not be diagnosed until adulthood

CODING TIPS ✓ Disorders classified to categories F90-F98 are frequently diagnosed in childhood and adolescence. However, a diagnosis may be made at any time during an individual's lifetime and may still be reported here when the diagnosis criteria are applicable.

4 **F90 Attention-deficit hyperactivity disorders**
INCLUDES attention deficit disorder with hyperactivity
attention deficit syndrome with hyperactivity
EXCLUDES 2 anxiety disorders (F40.-, F41.-)
mood [affective] disorders (F30-F39)
pervasive developmental disorders (F84.-)
schizophrenia (F20.-)

SP **F90.0 Attention-deficit hyperactivity disorder, predominantly inattentive type**
Attention-deficit/hyperactivity disorder, predominantly inattentive presentation

SP **F90.1 Attention-deficit hyperactivity disorder, predominantly hyperactive type**
Attention-deficit/hyperactivity disorder, predominantly hyperactive impulsive presentation

SP **F90.2 Attention-deficit hyperactivity disorder, combined type**
Attention-deficit/hyperactivity disorder, combined presentation

SP **F90.8 Attention-deficit hyperactivity disorder, other type**

SP **F90.9 Attention-deficit hyperactivity disorder, unspecified type**
Attention-deficit hyperactivity disorder of childhood or adolescence NOS
Attention-deficit hyperactivity disorder NOS

4 **F91 Conduct disorders**
EXCLUDES 1 antisocial behavior (Z72.81-)
antisocial personality disorder (F60.2)
EXCLUDES 2 conduct problems associated with attention-deficit hyperactivity disorder (F90.-)
mood [affective] disorders (F30-F39)
pervasive developmental disorders (F84.-)
schizophrenia (F20.-)

SP **F91.0 Conduct disorder confined to family context**

SP **F91.1 Conduct disorder, childhood-onset type**
Unsocialized conduct disorder
Conduct disorder, solitary aggressive type
Unsocialized aggressive disorder

SP **F91.2 Conduct disorder, adolescent-onset type**
Socialized conduct disorder
Conduct disorder, group type

SP **F91.3 Oppositional defiant disorder**

SP **F91.8 Other conduct disorders**
Other specified conduct disorder
Other specified disruptive disorder

IQ **F91.9 Conduct disorder, unspecified**
Behavioral disorder NOS
Conduct disorder NOS
Disruptive behavior disorder NOS
Disruptive disorder NOS

4 **F93 Emotional disorders with onset specific to childhood**

SP **F93.0 Separation anxiety disorder of childhood**
EXCLUDES 2 mood [affective] disorders (F30-F39)
nonpsychotic mental disorders (F40-F48)
phobic anxiety disorder of childhood (F40.8)
social phobia (F40.1)

DEFINITION Abnormal anxiety when separated from a parent, guardian, or usual environment.

SP **F93.8 Other childhood emotional disorders**
Identity disorder
EXCLUDES 2 gender identity disorder of childhood (F64.2)

IQ **F93.9 Childhood emotional disorder, unspecified**

4 **F94 Disorders of social functioning with onset specific to childhood and adolescence**

SP **F94.0 Selective mutism**
Elective mutism
EXCLUDES 2 pervasive developmental disorders (F84.-)
schizophrenia (F20.-)
specific developmental disorders of speech and language (F80.-)
transient mutism as part of separation anxiety in young children (F93.0)

SP + **F94.1 Reactive attachment disorder of childhood**
Use additional code to identify any associated failure to thrive or growth retardation
EXCLUDES 1 disinhibited attachment disorder of childhood (F94.2)
normal variation in pattern of selective attachment
EXCLUDES 2 Asperger's syndrome (F84.5)
maltreatment syndromes (T74.-)
sexual or physical abuse in childhood, resulting in psychosocial problems (Z62.81-)

SP **F94.2 Disinhibited attachment disorder of childhood**
Affectionless psychopathy
Institutional syndrome

EXCLUDES 1 reactive attachment disorder of childhood (F94.1)

EXCLUDES 2 Asperger's syndrome (F84.5)
attention-deficit hyperactivity disorders (F90.-)
hospitalism in children (F43.2-)

SP **F94.8 Other childhood disorders of social functioning**

IQ **F94.9 Childhood disorder of social functioning, unspecified**

4 **F95 Tic disorder**

SP **F95.0 Transient tic disorder**
Provisional tic disorder

SP **F95.1 Chronic motor or vocal tic disorder**

SP **F95.2 Tourette's disorder**
Combined vocal and multiple motor tic disorder [de la Tourette]
Tourette's syndrome

SP **F95.8 Other tic disorders**

IQ **F95.9 Tic disorder, unspecified**
Tic NOS

4 **F98 Other behavioral and emotional disorders with onset usually occurring in childhood and adolescence**

EXCLUDES 2 breath-holding spells (R06.89)
gender identity disorder of childhood (F64.2)
Kleine-Levin syndrome (G47.13)
obsessive-compulsive disorder (F42.-)
sleep disorders not due to a substance or known physiological condition (F51.-)

SP **F98.0 Enuresis not due to a substance or known physiological condition**
Enuresis (primary) (secondary) of nonorganic origin
Functional enuresis
Psychogenic enuresis
Urinary incontinence of nonorganic origin

EXCLUDES 1 enuresis NOS (R32)

SP + **F98.1 Encopresis not due to a substance or known physiological condition**
Functional encopresis
Incontinence of feces of nonorganic origin
Psychogenic encopresis
Use additional code to identify the cause of any coexisting constipation.

EXCLUDES 1 encopresis NOS (R15.-)

▲ 5 **F98.2 Other feeding disorders of infancy and childhood**

EXCLUDES 2 anorexia nervosa and other eating disorders (F50.-)
feeding difficulties (R63.3)
feeding problems of newborn (P92.-)
pica of infancy or childhood (F98.3)

SP **F98.21 Rumination disorder of infancy**

SP **F98.29 Other feeding disorders of infancy and early childhood**

SP **F98.3 Pica of infancy and childhood**

DEFINITION Compulsion to eat inedible substances, such as dirt or rocks.

SP **F98.4 Stereotyped movement disorders**
Stereotype/habit disorder

EXCLUDES 1 abnormal involuntary movements (R25.-)

EXCLUDES 2 compulsions in obsessive-compulsive disorder (F42.-)
hair plucking (F63.3)
movement disorders of organic origin (G20-G25)
nail-biting (F98.8)
nose-picking (F98.8)
stereotypies that are part of a broader psychiatric condition (F01-F95)
thumb-sucking (F98.8)
tic disorders (F95.-)
trichotillomania (F63.3)

SP **F98.5 Adult onset fluency disorder**

EXCLUDES 1 childhood onset fluency disorder (F80.81)
dysphasia (R47.02)
fluency disorder in conditions classified elsewhere (R47.82)
fluency disorder (stuttering) following cerebrovascular disease (I69. with final characters -23)
tic disorders (F95.-)

CODING TIPS ✓ This code is used for post-childhood onset of stuttering symptoms secondary to emotional stress or trauma. Do not assign F98.5 to report fluency disorder as a sequela of cerebral vascular disease or another cause or to identify dysphasia.

DEFINITION Normal flow of speech disrupted by repeated sounds or pauses.

SP **F98.8 Other specified behavioral and emotional disorders with onset usually occurring in childhood and adolescence**
Excessive masturbation
Nail-biting
Nose-picking
Thumb-sucking

IQ **F98.9 Unspecified behavioral and emotional disorders with onset usually occurring in childhood and adolescence**

Unspecified mental disorder (F99)

IQ **F99 Mental disorder, not otherwise specified**
Mental illness NOS

EXCLUDES 1 unspecified mental disorder due to known physiological condition (F09)

CODING TIPS ✓ **Documentation:** Use F99 only when the clinical documentation from the provider reports mental illness but does not specify anything further. Whenever possible, query the provider and obtain information specifying the patient's definitive diagnosis.

4 4th digit required 5 5th digit required 6 6th digit required 7 7th digit required 7 7th digit placeholder + Additional code Laterality

Chapter 5 Scenarios: Mental, Behavioral and Neurodevelopmental disorders (F01-F99)

Pancreatitis, alcohol dependence, borderline personality disorder

A 46-year-old woman is admitted to home health for management of acute alcoholic pancreatitis. Her medical record indicates long-term alcohol dependence as well as borderline personality disorder. She will also receive psychiatric care from the agency's certified psych nurse.

Description	Code
Primary: Alcohol induced acute pancreatitis without necrosis or infection	K85.20
Secondary: Alcohol dependence, uncomplicated	F10.20
Secondary: Borderline personality disorder	F60.3

After assigning the primary diagnosis of K85.20 for the acute alcoholic pancreatitis, the code for the patient's alcohol dependence, F10.20, is assigned, in accordance with tabular instruction. In this context, alcoholic pancreatitis is not classified as an alcohol-induced disorder. Therefore, code F10.20 is assigned rather than code F10.288, Alcohol dependence with other alcohol-induced disorder, per Q1 2020 Coding Clinic guidance. The patient will receive psychiatric care from the agency, necessitating the capture of her borderline personality disorder. However, psychiatric diagnoses will always affect the plan of care and should always be coded when they've been diagnosed.

Psychogenic paroxysmal tachycardia

Your patient is diagnosed with recurrent psychogenic paroxysmal atrial tachycardia. The patient has a well documented history of recurrent severe major depression (without psychosis), which is currently exacerbated due to the recent death of her husband. As a result of the recurrent atrial tachycardia, she has developed chronic congestive heart failure and her ejection fraction remains preserved at 65%. Home health will monitor this condition and observe for acute exacerbation.

Description	Code
Primary: Paroxysmal atrial tachycardia	I47.1
Secondary: Psychological and behavioral factors associated with disorders or diseases classified elsewhere	F54
Secondary: Major depressive disorder, recurrent severe without psychotic features	F33.2
Secondary: Chronic diastolic (congestive) heart failure	I50.32

F54 is a manifestation code that requires the underlying disease (I47.1) to be coded first. Additional codes are assigned for the severe recurrent depression and heart failure as these conditions impact the patients prognosis and care plan, as well as my provide important comorbidity adjustment for payment. Heart failure should be coded to diastolic when the ejection fraction is reported as preserved or documentation states "HFpEF" per Q1 2016 Coding Clinic guidance.

Major depression

A patient is admitted for management of a stage 2 right heel pressure ulcer/injury. He also has a history of anemia, which is not currently a problem and will not be addressed in the plan of care. The caregiver said that the patient cries a lot and says he wishes he would die. He is on Prozac. The assessing nurse called the physician, who confirmed a diagnosis of major depression. He increased the dosage of the anti-depressant and requested that the agency continue to monitor the patient's mental status.

Description	Code
Primary: Pressure ulcer, right heel, stage 2	L89.612
Secondary: Major depressive disorder, single episode, unspecified	F32.9

As the focus of care, the stage 2 right heel pressure ulcer is coded in the primary position. Referencing 'Depression, major' in the Index leads to code F32.9. An inclusion term at F32.9 is "Major depression NOS." Since the anemia is not a current problem and will not be addressed in the plan of care, it is not coded here.

Paranoid schizophrenia

Your patient, who has long-term alcoholism, is admitted to home health with a primary diagnosis of paranoid schizophrenia. The skilled nurse will be administering Haldol injections B.I.D., a new treatment for the schizophrenia, and instructing the caregiver how to administer the medication. The patient also has hypertension and atrial fibrillation for which she takes Coumadin.

Description	Code
Primary: Paranoid schizophrenia	F20.0
Secondary: Alcohol dependence, uncomplicated	F10.20
Secondary: Essential (primary) hypertension	I10
Secondary: Unspecified atrial fibrillation	I48.91
Secondary: Other long term (current) drug therapy	Z79.899
Secondary: Long term (current) use of anticoagulants	Z79.01

The home health focus of care is to administer and teach on the Haldol injections to treat the paranoid schizophrenia. Alcoholism codes to alcohol dependence in the alphabetic index. Alcohol dependence and the other co-morbidities of hypertension and atrial fibrillation are relevant to the current plan of care and should therefore be coded. The Z codes for long-term drug therapy, for the Haldol and Coumadin, are added to provide additional information.

Major recurrent depression

Home health nursing is ordered for a patient with a diagnosis of major recurrent depression for medication teaching and monitoring. He has been on two anti-depressants for years and his physician increased the dosage of each. The history and physical notes that the patient consumes an excessive amount of coffee and soda, and caffeine dependence is documented.

Description	Code
Primary: Major depressive disorder, recurrent, unspecified	F33.9
Secondary: Other stimulant dependence, uncomplicated	F15.20
Secondary: Other long-term drug therapy	Z79.899

Use caution when assigning codes from Chapter 5, Mental, behavioral and neurodevelopmental disorders. Make sure a physician has documented, or confirmed, the diagnosis you are coding. Category F33.- (Major depressive disorder, recurrent) is found in the Alphabetic Index under "Disorder" not "Depression." Search under "disorder, depressive, recurrent." A code for long-term (current) drug use (Z79.899) is added to show the focus on medication monitoring. This code is selected since there is not a code specific for psychiatric drugs. While a psychiatric nurse is often required when a psychiatric diagnosis is the first-listed diagnosis, it does not require a psychiatric nurse to teach or monitor medications. A psychiatric nurse is required if the plan of care involves counseling for the psychiatric condition.

Bipolar disorder, alcoholism

A 68-year-old man was recently diagnosed with bipolar disorder and alcoholism after being hospitalized following a severe alcohol binge. In the hospital he was also found to be in the early stages of alcoholic cirrhosis of the liver. He was admitted to home health to monitor new medications for his bipolar as well as counseling from a certified psych nurse. The bipolar is the focus of care.

Description	Code
Primary: Bipolar disorder, unspecified	F31.9
Secondary: Alcoholic cirrhosis of liver without ascites	K70.30
Secondary: Alcohol dependence, uncomplicated	F10.20

The bipolar is the focus of care so it is coded primary. Alcoholism codes to alcohol dependence, according to the alphabetic index. In this context, alcoholic cirrhosis is not classified as an alcohol-induced disorder per Q1 2020 Coding Clinic guidance. Therefore, code F10.20 is assigned rather than code F10.288, Alcohol dependence with other alcohol-induced disorder.

Trichotillomania, hoarding disorder, psych nursing

A 45-year-old woman was recently discharged from an inpatient psych facility where she was diagnosed with severe trichotillomania and hoarding disorder. She will receive counseling and medication management from a certified psych nurse. The nurse will also monitor her hypertension.

Description	Code
Primary: Trichotillomania	F63.3
Secondary: Hoarding disorder	F42.3
Secondary: Essential (primary) hypertension	I10

The patient will receive psych services from a certified psych nurse for her diagnoses of trichotillomania and hoarding disorder. Her hypertension is an important comorbidity that should also be coded.

Bipolar II, panic disorder, alcoholism

A 55-year-old woman is admitted to home health with primary diagnoses of bipolar II disorder. She also has panic disorder. She's been an alcoholic for the past 10 years. She will receive medication management and visits from the agency's certified psych nurse.

Description	Code
Primary: Bipolar II disorder	F31.81
Secondary: Panic disorder [episodic paroxysmal anxiety]	F41.0
Secondary: Alcohol dependence, uncomplicated	F10.20

The patient's bipolar disorder, which was specified as bipolar II, is the focus of care and thus coded primary. Panic disorder is also coded as it will impact her care. Her alcoholism is a relevant comorbidity that will impact her recovery. Alcoholism codes to alcohol dependence, according to the alphabetic index.

Suicide attempt, anxiety with depression

A 69-year-old man with a years-long history of anxiety with depression attempted to commit suicide by taking all of the remaining contents of a bottle of Tylenol he kept in his cupboard. Following acute care in the hospital, he's admitted to home health for care of symptoms related to the overdose, which are severe abdominal pain and diarrhea, as well as management of new medications.

Description	Code
Primary: Poisoning by 4-Aminophenol derivatives, intentional self-harm, subsequent encounter	T39.1x2D
Secondary: Unspecified abdominal pain	R10.9
Secondary: Diarrhea, unspecified	R19.7
Secondary: Other specified anxiety disorders	F41.8
Secondary: Personal history of suicidal behavior	Z91.51

The patient intentionally took too much Tylenol in a suicide attempt, making it an intentional poisoning. Therefore, it is coded first with a T code for the specific drug. The health issues caused by the poisoning, abdominal pain and diarrhea, are coded next, in accordance with coding guidelines. Be sure to follow proper sequencing instructions for poisoning, which require the T code to be sequenced first. The patient's diagnosis of anxiety with depression is an important comorbidity that will require monitoring and so is also coded. Because it is stated as anxiety with depression, it can be coded with the combination code F41.8. A Z code is included to capture the patient's history of suicidal behavior.

Mixed dementia with etiologies

An 82-year-old female patient who has experienced multiple CVAs over the previous 12 months presents for home health speech, physical and occupational therapy with diagnoses of multi-infarct dementia due to the prior CVAs, left hemiplegia due to the most recent CVA, hypertension, and early onset Alzheimer's disease. The dietician was consulted during her recent SNF stay and documented mild malnutrition. The focus of her treatment will be the multi-infarct dementia.

Description	Code
Primary: Other symptoms and signs involving cognitive functions following cerebral infarction	I69.318
Secondary: Vascular dementia without behavioral disturbance	F01.50
Secondary: Hemiplegia and hemiparesis following cerebral infarction affecting left non-dominant side	I69.354
Secondary: Essential (primary) hypertension	I10
Secondary: Alzheimer's disease with early onset	G30.0
Secondary: Dementia in other diseases classified elsewhere without behavioral disturbance	F02.80

Dementia that is diagnosed as "multi-infarct" is coded to vascular dementia based upon classification within the alphabetic index. This is the focus of care so it is listed following the etiology that caused it, which is the prior CVA and the appropriate sequela code is assigned as primary. Additional codes are assigned for hemiplegia as a sequela of the CVAs, hypertension, as well as the early onset Alzheimer's disease with the manifestation of dementia. When multiple specified types of dementia are diagnosed (mixed dementia) all types should be coded. No code is assigned for malnutrition because this was not a diagnostic statement given by her physician or a provider with the ability to diagnose the patient, but rather by the dietician within an evaluation and such a statement may not be used for the purpose of coding per Q1 2020 Coding Clinic guidance.

Chapter 6: Diseases of the Nervous System (G00- G99)

The nervous system is how the body interprets and acts in response to a stimulus (light, heat, sound, or chemicals within the body). The nervous system consists of two parts: the central nervous system and the peripheral nervous system. Chapter 6 includes:

- Inflammatory diseases of the central nervous system (G00-G09) such as meningitis, encephalitis, myelitis and encephalomyelitis;
- Systemic atrophies primarily affecting the central nervous system (G10-G14)
- Extrapyramidal and movement disorders (G20-G26) such as Parkinson's disease (G20), dystonia (G24.9), and other extrapyramidal and movement disorders (G25.8-)
- Other degenerative diseases of the nervous system such as Alzheimer's disease (G30-) and mild cognitive impairment (G31.84)
- Demyelinating diseases of the central nervous system such as multiple sclerosis (G35), subacute necrotizing myelitis of central nervous system (G37.4)
- Episodic and paroxysmal disorder (G40-G47) such as epilepsy and recurrent seizures; migraine and other headache disorders; TIAs; and sleep disorders.
- Nerve, nerve root and plexus disorders (G50-G59)
- Polyneuropathies and other disorder of the peripheral nervous system (G60-G65)
- Diseases of myoneural junction and muscle (G70-G73) such as muscular dystrophy, myopathies
- Cerebral palsy and other paralytic syndromes (G80-G83), including hemiplegia and hemiparesis, paraplegia (G82.20), and other paralytic syndromes
- Other disorders of the nervous system (G89-G99), including pain not elsewhere classified, disorders of the autonomic nervous system, hydrocephalus, other disorders of the brain and spinal cord as well as intraoperative and postoperative complications and disorders of the nervous system not classified elsewhere

To select the correct code, it is important to understand the differences between the central and peripheral nervous systems.

The central nervous system (CNS) consists of the brain and spinal cord. The CNS receives nerve impulses and interprets them.

The peripheral nervous system (PNS) consists of all nerve fibers outside the CNS. Sensory nerves in the PNS send a nerve impulse to the CNS for interpretation following a stimulus.

Conditions of the PNS include: conditions of cranial nerves (trigeminal and facial nerves); disorders of nerve roots (collections of nerves right outside the spinal cord) and plexuses (large interlacing networks of nerves); and myoneural disorders (conditions involving the place where a nerve meets a muscle).

The somatic nervous system (SNS) includes all nerves controlling the muscular system and external sensory receptors. External sense organs (including skin) are receptors. Muscle fibers and gland cells are effectors. The reflex arc is an automatic, involuntary reaction to stimulus. Examples of reflex arcs include balance, the blinking reflex and the stretch reflex.

Conditions of the eye and associated tissues are in chapter categories H00-H59 in Chapter 7, and conditions of the ear and associated tissues are in categories H60-H95 in chapter 8.

A few situations to watch out for:

- If the documentation indicates **a neoplasm or tumor of an organ in the nervous system**, coders should look up the term (malignancy, tumor, adenoma) used to find the correct code. In most cases, a code from Chapter 2 (C000-D49) may be reported with a code from this chapter.
- **Code Parkinson's disease that's caused dementia** with behavioral disturbance with G20 and F02.81.
- You must **assign an additional code from F02.8- (Dementia in other diseases classified elsewhere) for a patient with Lewy body dementia (G31.83).**
- If a patient has a **personal or family history** of a condition reported in this chapter, it may be appropriate to select from the Z code section, such as Z85.841 (personal history of malignant neoplasm of the brain) or Z86.61(personal history of infection of the central nervous system).
- If a condition reported in this chapter is the **result of injury, poisoning and certain other consequences of external causes**, a code from Chapter 19 (S00-T88) may be reported with a code from this chapter.
- **Symptoms** related to the nervous system and sense organs are sometimes reported using codes from Chapter 18 (Symptoms, signs and abnormal clinical factors). Some examples include categories R43- (disturbances of sensation of smell and taste), R23- (symptoms involving skin) and R29- (other

symptoms and signs involving the nervous and musculoskeletal system). Every effort should be made to secure a definitive diagnosis.

- If reporting a **nervous system disease in a pregnant patient** when the condition is complicating the pregnancy, report first a code from Chapter 15 (Pregnancy, childbirth and the puerperium) such as O26.82- (pregnancy related neuritis) or O99.35-(diseases of the nervous system complicating pregnancy, childbirth, and the puerperium), as the first-listed diagnosis, and G40.901 from this chapter as an additional code for epilepsy associated with pregnancy.

Multiple Coding and Sequencing

Many codes in this chapter are related to conditions in other chapters. It is important to read the Includes and Excludes notes under codes in this chapter, as well as any other instructions under the code or code category. Consider this example of multiple coding and sequencing issues for codes in this chapter:

- Meningitis due to listeriosis is reported as A32.11 (listeriosis meningitis) from Chapter 1 as a combination code that includes both the organism and the meningitis. There is an Excludes 1 note under G01 (meningitis in bacterial disease classified elsewhere) that excludes A32.11 from this code.

Special Coding Issues

Dominant/nondominant side

Codes from category G81 (Hemiplegia and hemiparesis) and subcategories G83.1 (Monoplegia of lower limb), G83.2 (Monoplegia of upper limb) and G83.3, (Monoplegia, unspecified) identify whether the dominant or nondominant side is affected. Should the affected side be documented, but not specified as dominant or nondominant, and the classification system does not indicate a default code, code selection is as follows:

- For ambidextrous patients, the default should be dominant.
- If the left side is affected, the default code is nondominant.
- If the right side is affected, the default is dominant.

Coding for Pain

Codes in category G89 (Pain, not elsewhere classified) may be used in conjunction with codes from other categories and chapters to provide more detail about acute and chronic pain and neoplasm-related pain, unless otherwise indicated below.

Take note of the following circumstances:

- If the pain is not specified as acute or chronic, post-thoracotomy, post procedural, or neoplasm related, ***do not*** assign codes from category G89.
- A code from G89 should ***not be assigned*** if the underlying (definitive) diagnosis is known, unless the reason for the encounter is pain control/management and **not** management of the underlying condition.
- Category G89 codes are acceptable as the primary, first-listed, code when pain control or pain management is the reason for the admission/encounter. The underlying cause of the pain (e.g., nerve impingement, severe back pain) should be reported as an additional diagnosis if known.

G89 pain codes may be used in conjunction with site-specific pain codes (including chapter 18 symptom codes) if the category code provides additional information. For example, if the code describes the site of pain, but does not fully describe whether the pain is acute or chronic, then both codes should be assigned.

The sequencing is dependent on the circumstances of the encounter/admission as follows:

- If the encounter is for pain control or pain management, assign the code from category G89 followed by the code identifying the specific site of pain. For example, encounter for pain management for acute neck pain from trauma is assigned to code G89.11 (Acute pain due to trauma), followed by code M54.2 (Cervicalgia) to identify the site of pain.
- When a patient is admitted for the insertion of a neurostimulator for pain control, assign the appropriate pain code as the principal or first-listed diagnosis.
- When an admission/encounter is for a procedure aimed at treating the underlying condition and a neurostimulator is inserted for pain control during the same admission/encounter, a code for the underlying condition should be assigned as the principal diagnosis and the appropriate pain code should be assigned as a secondary diagnosis.

Postoperative pain is based on the physician documentation. The default code for post-thoracotomy and other postoperative pain not specified as acute or chronic would be the code for the acute form. However, routine or expected pain immediately after surgery should not be coded.

Take note of the following circumstances:

- Postoperative pain not associated with a specific postoperative complication is assigned to the appropriate postoperative pain code in G89.
- Postoperative pain associated with a specific postoperative complication (e.g., painful wire sutures, T81.89) is assigned from chapter 19

(Injury, poisoning, and certain other consequences of external causes). If appropriate, use an additional code from G89.18 (acute pain) or G89.28 (chronic pain).

- For pain due to devices, implants or grafts, report code T85.84- (pain due to internal prosthetic devices, implants and grafts, not elsewhere classified). For complication of a device, implant or graft associated with a specific system, assign a code for the specific system device, such as implant and graft (T84-T88) from Chapter 19 (Injury, poisoning and other consequences of external causes) as the first-listed diagnosis. Also, add a code for the pain if it provides additional information. For example, a subsequent encounter for acute pain due to an infection of a right hip prosthesis is reported as T84.51xD (infection of right hip prosthesis) as the primary diagnosis. Use an additional code to identify the infection, and you may assign G89.18 to indicate that acute post-procedural pain has been documented for this patient by the physician as another additional diagnosis.

There is no time frame defining when pain becomes chronic; the physician's documentation should be used to guide use of these codes.

Neoplasm-related pain (G89.3) is assigned to pain documented as being related, associated or due to cancer, primary or secondary malignancy or tumor, whether the pain is acute or chronic.

- This code may be assigned as first-listed when the stated reason for the admission/encounter is documented as pain control/pain management with the underlying neoplasm reported as an additional diagnosis.
- When the reason for the admission/encounter is management of the neoplasm and the pain associated with the neoplasm is also documented, code G89.3 may be assigned as an additional diagnosis. It is not necessary to assign an additional code for the site of the pain.
- Central pain syndrome (G89.0) and chronic pain syndrome (G89.4) are different than the term "chronic pain" and therefore codes should only be used when the physician has specifically documented this condition.

Epilepsy

One specific nervous system diagnosis that shows up in home health coding is epilepsy (G40-). Epilepsy is a chronic disorder of the brain that is characterized by paroxysmal (sudden and unpredictable) and excessive neuronal discharge of the brain, usually accompanied by an alteration in consciousness.

However, although epilepsy often is diagnosed in those with seizures, not every seizure is epilepsy. For example, stroke, metabolic disorders, tumors and brain injuries are other possible causes of seizure not associated with epilepsy. Those 80 years of age or older have a 3% chance of developing epilepsy and an 11% chance of having at least one seizure.

To find the most precise diagnosis code for epilepsy, it is important to understand the kind of seizure suffered by the patient as ICD-10-CM has greatly expanded the number and detail of available codes for epilepsy and seizures (G40-G47), and the correct code requires specific documentation or confirmation with the physician.

There are two major categories of seizures – general and partial:

Generalized seizures: Those in which the focus or starting point of the neuronal discharge in the brain is not localized. In other words, it seems to be all over the brain. Generalized seizures are further categorized as nonconvulsive and convulsive.

Partial seizures: These begin in a specific brain location and may or may not spread (or generalize) throughout the entire brain. With this in mind, the seizure may or may not affect consciousness. If it does not, it is termed a **simple partial** seizure. If it does impair consciousness, it is termed a **complex partial** seizure.

CHAPTER 6: DISEASES OF THE NERVOUS SYSTEM (G00-G99)

EXCLUDES 2 certain conditions originating in the perinatal period (P04-P96)
certain infectious and parasitic diseases (A00-B99)
complications of pregnancy, childbirth and the puerperium (O00-O9A)
congenital malformations, deformations, and chromosomal abnormalities (Q00-Q99)
endocrine, nutritional and metabolic diseases (E00-E88)
injury, poisoning and certain other consequences of external causes (S00-T88)
neoplasms (C00-D49)
symptoms, signs and abnormal clinical and laboratory findings, not elsewhere classified (R00-R94)

This chapter contains the following blocks:

G00-G09	Inflammatory diseases of the central nervous system
G10-G14	Systemic atrophies primarily affecting the central nervous system
G20-G26	Extrapyramidal and movement disorders
G30-G32	Other degenerative diseases of the nervous system
G35-G37	Demyelinating diseases of the central nervous system
G40-G47	Episodic and paroxysmal disorders
G50-G59	Nerve, nerve root and plexus disorders
G60-G65	Polyneuropathies and other disorders of the peripheral nervous system
G70-G73	Diseases of myoneural junction and muscle
G80-G83	Cerebral palsy and other paralytic syndromes
G89-G99	Other disorders of the nervous system

Inflammatory diseases of the central nervous system (G00-G09)

CODING TIPS✓ If the central nervous system infection (CNS) is resolved but has a potential for reoccurence, use Z86.61, personal history of CNS infections. If the CNS infection is resolved, but the patient suffers neurological deficits, code the residual deficit followed by the sequela code G09.

4 **G00 Bacterial meningitis, not elsewhere classified**

INCLUDES bacterial arachnoiditis
bacterial leptomeningitis
bacterial meningitis
bacterial pachymeningitis

EXCLUDES 1 bacterial meningoencephalitis (G04.2)
bacterial meningomyelitis (G04.2)

CODING TIPS✓ Most of these central nervous system infection codes are combination codes and include the bacteria or other organism or are manifestation codes and require that the causative condition be coded first. Follow convention instructions to "code first" or "use additional code."

SP **G00.0 Hemophilus meningitis**
Meningitis due to Hemophilus influenzae

DEFINITION Bacterial infection of the tissues (meninges) surrounding the brain and spinal cord, causing fever, headache, vomiting, malaise, and stiff neck and may progress to confusion, stupor, convulsions, coma, and death.

SP **G00.1 Pneumococcal meningitis**
Meningitis due to Streptococcal pneumoniae

SP + **G00.2 Streptococcal meningitis**
Use additional code to further identify organism (B95.0-B95.5)

SP + **G00.3 Staphylococcal meningitis**
Use additional code to further identify organism (B95.61-B95.8)

SP + **G00.8 Other bacterial meningitis**
Meningitis due to Escherichia coli
Meningitis due to Friedländer's bacillus
Meningitis due to Klebsiella
Use additional code to further identify organism (B96.-)

SP **G00.9 Bacterial meningitis, unspecified**
Meningitis due to gram-negative bacteria, unspecified
Purulent meningitis NOS
Pyogenic meningitis NOS
Suppurative meningitis NOS

M IQ **G01** ***Meningitis in bacterial diseases classified elsewhere***
Code first:
underlying disease

EXCLUDES 1 meningitis (in) :
gonococcal (A54.81)
leptospirosis (A27.81)
listeriosis (A32.11)
Lyme disease (A69.21)
meningococcal (A39.0)
neurosyphilis (A52.13)
tuberculosis (A17.0)
meningoencephalitis and meningomyelitis in bacterial diseases classified elsewhere (G05)

▲ M IQ **G02** ***Meningitis in other infectious and parasitic diseases classified elsewhere***
Code first underlying disease, such as:
African trypanosomiasis (B56.-)
poliovirus infection (A80.-)

EXCLUDES 1 candidal meningitis (B37.5)
coccidioidomycosis meningitis (B38.4)
cryptococcal meningitis (B45.1)
herpesviral [herpes simplex] meningitis (B00.3)
infectious mononucleosis complicated by meningitis (B27.- with fifth character 2)
measles complicated by meningitis (B05.1)
meningoencephalitis and meningomyelitis in other infectious and parasitic diseases classified elsewhere (G05)
mumps meningitis (B26.1)
rubella meningitis (B06.02)

varicella [chickenpox] meningitis (B01.0)
zoster meningitis (B02.1)

4 G03 Meningitis due to other and unspecified causes

INCLUDES arachnoiditis NOS
leptomeningitis NOS
meningitis NOS
pachymeningitis NOS

EXCLUDES 1 meningoencephalitis (G04.-)
meningomyelitis (G04.-)

SP **G03.0 Nonpyogenic meningitis**
Aseptic meningitis
Nonbacterial meningitis

SP **G03.1 Chronic meningitis**

SP **G03.2 Benign recurrent meningitis [Mollaret]**

CODING TIPS✓ Do not confuse chronic meningitis with benign recurrent Mollaret's meningitis. Mollaret's meningitis is a rare disorder characterized by a recurrent, mild, and aseptic inflammation of the meninges due to an unknown cause.

!Q **G03.8 Meningitis due to other specified causes**

!Q **G03.9 Meningitis, unspecified**
Arachnoiditis (spinal) NOS

CODING TIPS✓ Meningitis that is not specified as acute, chronic, or due to a specified cause should be coded to G03.9.

▲ 4 **G04 Encephalitis, myelitis and encephalomyelitis**

INCLUDES acute ascending myelitis
meningoencephalitis
meningomyelitis

EXCLUDES 1 encephalopathy NOS (G93.40)

EXCLUDES 2 acute transverse myelitis (G37.3-)
alcoholic encephalopathy (G31.2)
benign myalgic encephalomyelitis (G93.3)
multiple sclerosis (G35)
subacute necrotizing myelitis (G37.4)
toxic encephalitis (G92.8)
toxic encephalopathy (G92.8)

5 **G04.0 Acute disseminated encephalitis and encephalomyelitis (ADEM)**

EXCLUDES 1 acute necrotizing hemorrhagic encephalopathy (G04.3-)
other noninfectious acute disseminated encephalomyelitis (noninfectious ADEM) (G04.81)

SP **G04.00 Acute disseminated encephalitis and encephalomyelitis, unspecified**

SP **G04.01 Postinfectious acute disseminated encephalitis and encephalomyelitis (postinfectious ADEM)**

EXCLUDES 1 post chickenpox encephalitis (B01.1)
post measles encephalitis (B05.0)
post measles myelitis (B05.1)

SP + **G04.02 Postimmunization acute disseminated encephalitis, myelitis and encephalomyelitis**
Encephalitis, post immunization
Encephalomyelitis, post immunization
Use additional code to identify the vaccine (T50.A-, T50.B-, T50.Z-)

CODING TIPS✓ G04.02 should be assigned for encephalitis, myelitis, and encephalomyelitis caused by the administration of vaccines. Use an additional code from T50.A-, T50.B- or T50.Z- to identify the adverse effect from the specific type of vaccine.

SP SH SL **G04.1 Tropical spastic paraplegia**

SP **G04.2 Bacterial meningoencephalitis and meningomyelitis, not elsewhere classified**

5 **G04.3 Acute necrotizing hemorrhagic encephalopathy**

EXCLUDES 1 acute disseminated encephalitis and encephalomyelitis (G04.0-)

SP **G04.30 Acute necrotizing hemorrhagic encephalopathy, unspecified**

SP **G04.31 Postinfectious acute necrotizing hemorrhagic encephalopathy**

SP + **G04.32 Postimmunization acute necrotizing hemorrhagic encephalopathy**
Use additional code to identify the vaccine (T50.A-, T50.B-, T50.Z-)

SP **G04.39 Other acute necrotizing hemorrhagic encephalopathy**
Code also:
underlying etiology, if applicable

5 **G04.8 Other encephalitis, myelitis and encephalomyelitis**
Code also:
any associated seizure (G40.-, R56.9)

SP **G04.81 Other encephalitis and encephalomyelitis**
Noninfectious acute disseminated encephalomyelitis (noninfectious ADEM)

★ **G04.82 Acute flaccid myelitis**

EXCLUDES 1 transverse myelitis (G37.3)

SP **G04.89 Other myelitis**

5 **G04.9 Encephalitis, myelitis and encephalomyelitis, unspecified**

SP **G04.90 Encephalitis and encephalomyelitis, unspecified**
Ventriculitis (cerebral) NOS

SP **G04.91 Myelitis, unspecified**

▲ 4 **G05 Encephalitis, myelitis and encephalomyelitis in diseases classified elsewhere**
Code first underlying disease, such as:
congenital toxoplasmosis encephalitis, myelitis and encephalomyelitis (P37.1)
cytomegaloviral encephalitis, myelitis and encephalomyelitis (B25.8)
encephalitis, myelitis and encephalomyelitis (in) systemic lupus erythematosus (M32.19)
eosinophilic meningoencephalitis (B83.2)
human immunodeficiency virus [HIV] disease (B20)
poliovirus (A80.-)
suppurative otitis media (H66.01-H66.4)
trichinellosis (B75)

EXCLUDES 1 adenoviral encephalitis, myelitis and encephalomyelitis (A85.1)
encephalitis, myelitis and encephalomyelitis (in) measles (B05.0)
enteroviral encephalitis, myelitis and encephalomyelitis (A85.0)
herpesviral [herpes simplex] encephalitis, myelitis and encephalomyelitis (B00.4)
listerial encephalitis, myelitis and encephalomyelitis (A32.12)
meningococcal encephalitis, myelitis and encephalomyelitis (A39.81)
mumps encephalitis, myelitis and encephalomyelitis (B26.2)
postchickenpox encephalitis, myelitis and encephalomyelitis (B01.1-)
rubella encephalitis, myelitis and encephalomyelitis (B06.01)
toxoplasmosis encephalitis, myelitis and encephalomyelitis (B58.2)
zoster encephalitis, myelitis and encephalomyelitis (B02.0)

M IQ **G05.3** ***Encephalitis and encephalomyelitis in diseases classified elsewhere***
Meningoencephalitis in diseases classified elsewhere

M IQ **G05.4** ***Myelitis in diseases classified elsewhere***
Meningomyelitis in diseases classified elsewhere

+ 4 **G06 Intracranial and intraspinal abscess and granuloma**
Use additional code (B95-B97) to identify infectious agent.

SP + **G06.0 Intracranial abscess and granuloma**
Brain [any part] abscess (embolic)
Cerebellar abscess (embolic)
Cerebral abscess (embolic)
Intracranial epidural abscess or granuloma
Intracranial extradural abscess or granuloma
Intracranial subdural abscess or granuloma
Otogenic abscess (embolic)

EXCLUDES 1 tuberculous intracranial abscess and granuloma (A17.81)

SP + **G06.1 Intraspinal abscess and granuloma**
Abscess (embolic) of spinal cord [any part]
Intraspinal epidural abscess or granuloma
Intraspinal extradural abscess or granuloma
Intraspinal subdural abscess or granuloma

EXCLUDES 1 tuberculous intraspinal abscess and granuloma (A17.81)

SP + **G06.2 Extradural and subdural abscess, unspecified**

M IQ **G07** ***Intracranial and intraspinal abscess and granuloma in diseases classified elsewhere***
Code first underlying disease, such as:
schistosomiasis granuloma of brain (B65.-)

EXCLUDES 1 abscess of brain:
amebic (A06.6)
chromomycotic (B43.1)
gonococcal (A54.82)
tuberculous (A17.81)
tuberculoma of meninges (A17.1)

SP **G08 Intracranial and intraspinal phlebitis and thrombophlebitis**
Septic embolism of intracranial or intraspinal venous sinuses and veins
Septic endophlebitis of intracranial or intraspinal venous sinuses and veins
Septic phlebitis of intracranial or intraspinal venous sinuses and veins
Septic thrombophlebitis of intracranial or intraspinal venous sinuses and veins
Septic thrombosis of intracranial or intraspinal venous sinuses and veins

EXCLUDES 1 intracranial phlebitis and thrombophlebitis complicating:
abortion, ectopic or molar pregnancy (O00-O07, O08.7)
pregnancy, childbirth and the puerperium (O22.5, O87.3)
nonpyogenic intracranial phlebitis and thrombophlebitis (I67.6)

EXCLUDES 2 intracranial phlebitis and thrombophlebitis complicating nonpyogenic intraspinal phlebitis and thrombophlebitis (G95.1)

DEFINITION Inflammation and/or blood clot formation in a large vein or channel for venous blood circulation in the brain or spine.

IQ **G09 Sequelae of inflammatory diseases of central nervous system**
Note:
Category G09 is to be used to indicate conditions whose primary classification is to G00-G08 as the cause of sequelae, themselves classifiable elsewhere. The 'sequelae' include conditions specified as residuals.
Code first:
condition resulting from (sequela) of inflammatory diseases of central nervous system

CODING TIPS✓ Use G09, not the acute infection, to indicate residual effects or sequelae of meningitis, encephalitis or other CNS inflammatory diseases. If an infectious encephalitis, not coded with codes G00-G08, causes residual conditions, see B94.8. Sequence the residual condition followed by the sequela code unless there is a tabular convention that indicates otherwise.

CODING TIPS✓ If the central nervous system infection is resolved but has a potential for reoccurrence, use Z86.61, personal history of CNS infections. If the CNS infection is resolved, but the patient suffers neurological deficits, code the neurological deficit and sequela code G09.

Systemic atrophies primarily affecting the central nervous system (G10-G14)

SP **G10 Huntington's disease**
Huntington's chorea
Huntington's dementia
Code also:
dementia in other diseases classified elsewhere without behavioral disturbance (F02.80)

CODING TIPS✓ Huntington's disease is a progressive neurological disorder that includes mental deterioration and may include dementia as part of its progressive course. When dementia has been diagnosed as related to Huntington's disease, the alpha index instructs to use an additional code (F02-) to identify dementia with or without behavioral disturbance.

DEFINITION A genetic, degenerative disorder of the neurons of the brain, characterized by progressive difficulty with physical and mental tasks until death occurs.

4 **G11 Hereditary ataxia**
EXCLUDES 2 cerebral palsy (G80.-)
hereditary and idiopathic neuropathy (G60.-)
metabolic disorders (E70-E88)

CODING TIPS✓ **Documentation:** When assigning a code from category G11.-, the coder should review the record in full and assign the most specific code. Coders should not, however, assign codes for early vs. late onset or a hereditary vs. congenital condition unless specifically reported as confirmed by the patient's physician in the record.

SP **G11.0 Congenital nonprogressive ataxia**
5 **G11.1 Early-onset cerebellar ataxia**
SP **G11.10 Early-onset cerebellar ataxia, unspecified**
SP **G11.11 Friedreich ataxia**
Autosomal recessive Friedreich ataxia
Friedreich ataxia with retained reflexes
SP **G11.19 Other early-onset cerebellar ataxia**
Early-onset cerebellar ataxia with essential tremor
Early-onset cerebellar ataxia with myoclonus [Hunt's ataxia]
Early-onset cerebellar ataxia with retained tendon reflexes
X-linked recessive spinocerebellar ataxia
SP **G11.2 Late-onset cerebellar ataxia**
SP **G11.3 Cerebellar ataxia with defective DNA repair**
Ataxia telangiectasia [Louis-Bar]
EXCLUDES 2 Cockayne's syndrome (Q87.19)
other disorders of purine and pyrimidine metabolism (E79.-)
xeroderma pigmentosum (Q82.1)
SP **G11.4 Hereditary spastic paraplegia**
DEFINITION Hereditary disorder characterized by lower-limb spasticity and near total loss of joint flexibility while the upper limbs remain unaffected.
SP **G11.8 Other hereditary ataxias**
SP **G11.9 Hereditary ataxia, unspecified**
Hereditary cerebellar ataxia NOS
Hereditary cerebellar degeneration
Hereditary cerebellar disease
Hereditary cerebellar syndrome

4 **G12 Spinal muscular atrophy and related syndromes**
SP **G12.0 Infantile spinal muscular atrophy, type I [Werdnig-Hoffman]**
SP **G12.1 Other inherited spinal muscular atrophy**
Adult form spinal muscular atrophy
Childhood form, type II spinal muscular atrophy
Distal spinal muscular atrophy
Juvenile form, type III spinal muscular atrophy [Kugelberg-Welander]
Progressive bulbar palsy of childhood [Fazio-Londe]
Scapuloperoneal form spinal muscular atrophy
5 **G12.2 Motor neuron disease**
SP **G12.20 Motor neuron disease, unspecified**
H SP **G12.21 Amyotrophic lateral sclerosis**
SP **G12.22 Progressive bulbar palsy**
SP **G12.23 Primary lateral sclerosis**
DEFINITION Primary lateral sclerosis is often mistaken for the more common amyotrophic lateral sclerosis (ALS). However, primary lateral sclerosis progresses more slowly than ALS, and in most cases is not fatal.
SP **G12.24 Familial motor neuron disease**
DEFINITION People with familial MND have the disorder because of a mutation in a gene. Usually at least one other person in the family will have the condition.
SP **G12.25 Progressive spinal muscle atrophy**

Chapter 6 G00-G99

DEFINITION Spinal muscular atrophy is a genetic disorder that affects the control of muscle movement. It is caused by a loss of specialized nerve cells, called motor neurons, in the spinal cord and the part of the brain that is connected to the spinal cord (the brainstem).

SP **G12.29 Other motor neuron disease**

SP **G12.8 Other spinal muscular atrophies and related syndromes**

SP **G12.9 Spinal muscular atrophy, unspecified**

4 **G13 Systemic atrophies primarily affecting central nervous system in diseases classified elsewhere**

M IQ **G13.0 *Paraneoplastic neuromyopathy and neuropathy***

Carcinomatous neuromyopathy
Sensorial paraneoplastic neuropathy [Denny Brown]
Code first:
underlying neoplasm (C00-D49)

M IQ **G13.1 *Other systemic atrophy primarily affecting central nervous system in neoplastic disease***

Paraneoplastic limbic encephalopathy
Code first:
underlying neoplasm (C00-D49)

M IQ **G13.2 *Systemic atrophy primarily affecting the central nervous system in myxedema***

Code first underlying disease, such as:
hypothyroidism (E03.-)
myxedematous congenital iodine deficiency (E00.1)

M IQ **G13.8 *Systemic atrophy primarily affecting central nervous system in other diseases classified elsewhere***

Code first:
underlying disease

SP **G14 Postpolio syndrome**

INCLUDES postpolio myelitic syndrome

EXCLUDES 1 sequelae of poliomyelitis (B91)

CODING TIPS✓ The most common symptoms of postpolio syndrome include slowly progressive muscle weakness, fatigue (both generalized and muscular), and a gradual decrease in the size of muscles (muscle atrophy). Pain from joint degeneration and increasing skeletal deformities such as scoliosis (curvature of the spine) is common and may precede the weakness and muscle atrophy.

CODING TIPS✓ **Documentation:** G14 should be assigned only when the physician specifically reports "post polio syndrome" in the patient's clinical record. Note that this is differentiated from sequelae of poliomyelitis or residual deficits related to resolved poliomyelitis. When the record only specifies residual deficits related to resolved poliomyelitis, but does not specify post polio syndrome, coders should assign B91, Sequelae of poliomyelitis.

Extrapyramidal and movement disorders (G20-G26)

SP SH SL + **G20 Parkinson's disease**

Hemiparkinsonism
Idiopathic Parkinsonism or Parkinson's disease
Paralysis agitans
Parkinsonism or Parkinson's disease NOS
Primary Parkinsonism or Parkinson's disease
Use additional code to identify:
dementia with behavioral disturbance (F02.81)
dementia without behavioral disturbance (F02.80)

EXCLUDES 1 dementia with Parkinsonism (G31.83)

CODING TIPS✓ Do not confuse a patient who has Parkinson's disease with dementia and a patient who has dementia with Parkinsonism. When a patient is reported to have Parkinson's disease and dementia, assign G20 followed by a code from category F02.8-, Dementia in diseases classified elsewhere. By contrast, dementia with Parkinsonism, which is also known as Lewy body dementia or dementia with Lewy bodies, is coded to G31.83, followed by a code from the F02.8- category. G20 cannot be coded with G31.83. If the physician or NPP documents Parkinsons and dementia, but also mentions Parkinsonism or Lewy bodies, the G31.83 code is used instead of G20 along with the code for the dementia (F02.8-).

4 **G21 Secondary parkinsonism**

EXCLUDES 1 dementia with Parkinsonism (G31.83)
Huntington's disease (G10)
Shy-Drager syndrome (G90.3)
syphilitic Parkinsonism (A52.19)

SP + **G21.0 Malignant neuroleptic syndrome**

Use additional code for adverse effect, if applicable, to identify drug (T43.3X5, T43.4X5, T43.505, T43.595)

EXCLUDES 1 neuroleptic induced parkinsonism (G21.11)

5 **G21.1 Other drug-induced secondary parkinsonism**

CODING TIPS✓ When coding drug-induced Parkinsonism, be sure to also assign the appropriate code to identify the drug causing the disorder. Drug-induced Parkinsonism is considered an adverse effect of the drug that caused the condition, and the causative relationship must be stated by the physician or NPP.

SP SH SL + **G21.11 Neuroleptic induced parkinsonism**

Use additional code for adverse effect, if applicable, to identify drug (T43.3X5, T43.4X5, T43.505, T43.595)

EXCLUDES 1 malignant neuroleptic syndrome (G21.0)

SP SH SL + **G21.19 Other drug induced secondary parkinsonism**

Other medication-induced parkinsonism

Use additional code for adverse effect, if applicable, to identify drug (T36-T50 with fifth or sixth character 5)

IQ SH SL **G21.2 Secondary parkinsonism due to other external agents**
Code first:
(T51-T65) to identify external agent

SP SH SL **G21.3 Postencephalitic parkinsonism**

SP SH SL **G21.4 Vascular parkinsonism**

SP SH SL **G21.8 Other secondary parkinsonism**

SP SH SL **G21.9 Secondary parkinsonism, unspecified**

4 **G23 Other degenerative diseases of basal ganglia**
EXCLUDES 2 multi-system degeneration of the autonomic nervous system (G90.3)

SP **G23.0 Hallervorden-Spatz disease**
Pigmentary pallidal degeneration

SP **G23.1 Progressive supranuclear ophthalmoplegia [Steele-Richardson-Olszewski]**
Progressive supranuclear palsy

SP **G23.2 Striatonigral degeneration**

SP **G23.8 Other specified degenerative diseases of basal ganglia**
Calcification of basal ganglia

SP **G23.9 Degenerative disease of basal ganglia, unspecified**

4 **G24 Dystonia**
INCLUDES dyskinesia
EXCLUDES 2 athetoid cerebral palsy (G80.3)

CODING TIPS✓ Dystonias may be specified to congenital or acquired, primary or secondary, and may be anatomically specific. When coding dystonias, the coder should attempt to obtain specific information regarding the origin of the dystonia and the specific type of movement disorder so that the most specific code may be assigned.

+ 5 **G24.0 Drug induced dystonia**
Use additional code for adverse effect, if applicable, to identify drug (T36-T50 with fifth or sixth character 5)

SP + **G24.01 Drug induced subacute dyskinesia**
Drug induced blepharospasm
Drug induced orofacial dyskinesia
Neuroleptic induced tardive dyskinesia
Tardive dyskinesia

CODING TIPS✓ Tardive dyskinesia due to use of medications, also referred to as lingual-facial-buccal dyskinesia, which presents as uncontrollable movements of the mouth, tongue, jaw, and cheeks, should be coded using G24.01 followed by the appropriate code to identify the drug causing the dyskinesia. This effect is commonly found following the use of neuroleptic medications.

DEFINITION Involuntary repetitive movements of facial, buccal, oral, and cervical muscles, induced by long-term use of antipsychotic agent, sometimes persisting after withdrawal of the agent.

SP + **G24.02 Drug induced acute dystonia**
Acute dystonic reaction to drugs
Neuroleptic induced acute dystonia

SP + **G24.09 Other drug induced dystonia**

SP **G24.1 Genetic torsion dystonia**
Dystonia deformans progressiva
Dystonia musculorum deformans
Familial torsion dystonia
Idiopathic familial dystonia
Idiopathic (torsion) dystonia NOS
(Schwalbe-) Ziehen-Oppenheim disease

SP **G24.2 Idiopathic nonfamilial dystonia**

SP **G24.3 Spasmodic torticollis**
EXCLUDES 1 congenital torticollis (Q68.0)
hysterical torticollis (F44.4)
ocular torticollis (R29.891)
psychogenic torticollis (F45.8)
torticollis NOS (M43.6)
traumatic recurrent torticollis (S13.4)

DEFINITION Contractions of the neck muscles causing contortion, pain, and abnormal head posture.

SP **G24.4 Idiopathic orofacial dystonia**
Orofacial dyskinesia
EXCLUDES 1 drug induced orofacial dyskinesia (G24.01)

SP **G24.5 Blepharospasm**
EXCLUDES 1 drug induced blepharospasm (G24.01)

DEFINITION Spasm of the orbicularis oculi muscle, causing uncontrolled winking or blinking.

SP **G24.8 Other dystonia**
Acquired torsion dystonia NOS

IQ **G24.9 Dystonia, unspecified**
Dyskinesia NOS

4 **G25 Other extrapyramidal and movement disorders**
EXCLUDES 2 sleep related movement disorders (G47.6-)

SP **G25.0 Essential tremor**
Familial tremor
EXCLUDES 1 tremor NOS (R25.1)

CODING TIPS✓ Do not assign G25.0 to report unspecified tremors or tremors in a patient with a confirmed diagnosis of Parkinson's disease.

SP + **G25.1 Drug-induced tremor**
Use additional code for adverse effect, if applicable, to identify drug (T36-T50 with fifth or sixth character 5)

SP **G25.2 Other specified forms of tremor**
Intention tremor

SP + **G25.3 Myoclonus**
Drug-induced myoclonus
Palatal myoclonus
Use additional code for adverse effect, if applicable, to identify drug (T36-T50 with fifth or sixth character 5)
EXCLUDES 1 facial myokymia (G51.4)
myoclonic epilepsy (G40.-)

CODING TIPS ✓ Myoclonus is also reported as muscle twitching and is often a symptom of a more specific disease process. When the specific disease process is known, code the underlying disease. If myoclonus is related to the adverse effect of a medication, use an additional code to identify the drug. This code should not be assigned for myoclonic epilepsy or seizures.

DEFINITION Spontaneous contractions of a muscle or group of muscles as a part of a disease process, drug side effect, or abnormal physiological response.

SP + **G25.4 Drug-induced chorea**
Use additional code for adverse effect, if applicable, to identify drug (T36-T50 with fifth or sixth character 5)

SP **G25.5 Other chorea**
Chorea NOS
EXCLUDES 1 chorea NOS with heart involvement (I02.0)
Huntington's chorea (G10)
rheumatic chorea (I02.-)
Sydenham's chorea (I02.-)

5 **G25.6 Drug induced tics and other tics of organic origin**

SP + **G25.61 Drug induced tics**
Use additional code for adverse effect, if applicable, to identify drug (T36-T50 with fifth or sixth character 5)

SP **G25.69 Other tics of organic origin**
EXCLUDES 1 habit spasm (F95.9)
tic NOS (F95.9)
Tourette's syndrome (F95.2)

+ 5 **G25.7 Other and unspecified drug induced movement disorders**
Use additional code for adverse effect, if applicable, to identify drug (T36-T50 with fifth or sixth character 5)

IQ + **G25.70 Drug induced movement disorder, unspecified**

SP + **G25.71 Drug induced akathisia**
Drug induced acathisia
Neuroleptic induced acute akathisia
Tardive akathisia

CODING TIPS ✓ Akathisia is a syndrome characterized by a restless inability to maintain stillness or to "sit still" and is frequently induced by the use of various medications, including antipsychotics. When caused by the effect of a drug, an additional code should be assigned to identify the drug.

SP + **G25.79 Other drug induced movement disorders**

5 **G25.8 Other specified extrapyramidal and movement disorders**

SP **G25.81 Restless legs syndrome**
DEFINITION Irresistible urge to move legs, particularly when sitting or lying down, with leg sensations such as creeping, crawling, itching, tugging, tightening, or pulling alleviated upon movement.

SP **G25.82 Stiff-man syndrome**
DEFINITION Progressive fluctuating rigidity of axial and limb muscles in the absence of any signs of cerebral and/or spinal cord disease.

SP **G25.83 Benign shuddering attacks**

SP **G25.89 Other specified extrapyramidal and movement disorders**

IQ **G25.9 Extrapyramidal and movement disorder, unspecified**

!Q **G26 Extrapyramidal and movement disorders in diseases classified elsewhere**
Code first:
underlying disease

Other degenerative diseases of the nervous system (G30-G32)

+ 4 **G30 Alzheimer's disease**
INCLUDES Alzheimer's dementia senile and presenile forms
Use additional code to identify:
delirium, if applicable (F05)
dementia with behavioral disturbance (F02.81)
dementia without behavioral disturbance (F02.80)
EXCLUDES 1 senile degeneration of brain NEC (G31.1)
senile dementia NOS (F03)
senility NOS (R41.81)

CODING TIPS ✓ **Documentation:** Alzheimer's disease is a particular neurological condition and must be specifically confirmed by a physician or NPP. Early onset Alzheimer's is defined as diagnosis prior to the age of 65; however, the designation of early and late onset must be documented by, or confirmed with, the patient's physician and may not be assumed. Query the provider if the information is not readily available and, if unable to make a determination, assign code G30.9 for Alzheimer's disease, unspecified. Alzheimers is a specific type of dementia, so the provider does not have to specifically mention dementia to be able to code it. The Alzheimers is paired with the F02.8- code as a manifestation of Alzheimer's.

DEFINITION Progressive degenerative disease of the brain of unknown cause with diffuse atrophy throughout the cerebral cortex; it initially presents with slight memory disturbance or personality changes that progressively deteriorate to profound memory loss and dementia.

H SP + **G30.0 Alzheimer's disease with early onset**
CODING TIPS ✓ Early onset Alzheimer's is very uncommon and is diagnosed prior to the age of 65. Coders may not assume a diagnosis of early onset Alzheimer's disease because of the patient's age, but must have confirmed Early Onset Alzheimers with the patient's provider in order to assign the diagnosis appropriately.

H SP + **G30.1 Alzheimer's disease with late onset**

CODING TIPS✓ Late onset Alzheimer's is the most common type and presents with symptoms after the age of 65. Coders may not assume a diagnosis of late onset Alzheimer's disease but must have confirmed evidence of this from the patient's provider to assign the diagnosis appropriately.

H SP + **G30.8 Other Alzheimer's disease**

CODING TIPS✓ This code is used for the familial type of Alzheimer's, which accounts for less than 1% of cases.

H SP + **G30.9 Alzheimer's disease, unspecified**

+ 4 **G31 Other degenerative diseases of nervous system, not elsewhere classified**

Use additional For codes G31.0-G31.83, G31.85-G31.9, use additional code to identify:
dementia with behavioral disturbance (F02.81)
dementia without behavioral disturbance (F02.80)

EXCLUDES 2 Reye's syndrome (G93.7)

+ 5 **G31.0 Frontotemporal dementia**

H SP + **G31.01 Pick's disease**
Primary progressive aphasia
Progressive isolated aphasia

DEFINITION Rare, progressive, degenerative disease of the brain, similar to Alzheimer's disease but with cortical atrophy confined to the frontal and temporal lobes.

SP + **G31.09 Other frontotemporal dementia**
Frontal dementia

H SP + **G31.1 Senile degeneration of brain, not elsewhere classified**

EXCLUDES 1 Alzheimer's disease (G30.-)
senility NOS (R41.81)

SP + **G31.2 Degeneration of nervous system due to alcohol**
Alcoholic cerebellar ataxia
Alcoholic cerebellar degeneration
Alcoholic cerebral degeneration
Alcoholic encephalopathy
Dysfunction of the autonomic nervous system due to alcohol
Code also:
associated alcoholism (F10.-)

CODING TIPS✓ Cerebellar ataxia, encephalopathy, cerebellar degeneration, and autonomic dysfunction/degeneration, when specified as due to alcohol, should be coded to G31.2. Also assign the appropriate F10.- code to identify alcohol dependence/alcoholism, and, when applicable, a code to specify dementia (with or without behavior disturbance) as a manifestation (F02.8-). The dementia in alcohol dependence with alcohol-induced dementia code can be coded with F02.8-.

+ 5 **G31.8 Other specified degenerative diseases of nervous system**

SP + **G31.81 Alpers disease**
Grey-matter degeneration

SP + **G31.82 Leigh's disease**
Subacute necrotizing encephalopathy

SP + **G31.83 Dementia with Lewy bodies**
Dementia with Parkinsonism
Lewy body dementia
Lewy body disease

CODING TIPS✓ Parkinsonism dementia, also known as Lewy body dementia (G31.83), has symptoms similar to Parkinson's disease. However, Parkinson's disease is a distinct condition and is coded to G20. For a patient with Lewy body dementia, assign G31.83 followed by a code from category F02.8-, Dementia in diseases classified elsewhere.

SP + **G31.84 Mild cognitive impairment, so stated**
Mild neurocognitive disorder

EXCLUDES 1 age related cognitive decline (R41.81)
altered mental status (R41.82)
cerebral degeneration (G31.9)
change in mental status (R41.82)
cognitive deficits following (sequelae of) cerebral hemorrhage or infarction (I69.01-, I69.11-, I69.21-, I69.31-, I69.81-, I69.91-)
cognitive impairment due to intracranial or head injury (S06.-)
dementia (F01.-, F02.-, F03)
mild memory disturbance (F06.8)
neurologic neglect syndrome (R41.4)
personality change, nonpsychotic (F68.8)

CODING TIPS✓ To use this code, the physician or NPP must have documented mild cognitive impairment. A patient with mild cognitive impairment does not have dementia. Do not add dementia as an additional code.

DEFINITION Impairment in memory or other specific cognitive function, beyond what is normally seen at a given age, but with function remaining relatively intact in the other cognitive domains.

H SP + **G31.85 Corticobasal degeneration**

SP + **G31.89 Other specified degenerative diseases of nervous system**

IQ + **G31.9 Degenerative disease of nervous system, unspecified**

4 **G32 Other degenerative disorders of nervous system in diseases classified elsewhere**

M IQ **G32.0 *Subacute combined degeneration of spinal cord in diseases classified elsewhere***
Dana-Putnam syndrome

Chapter 6
G00-G99

Sclerosis of spinal cord (combined) (dorsolateral) (posterolateral)
Code first underlying disease, such as:
anemia (D51.9)
dietary (D51.3)
pernicious (D51.0)
vitamin B12 deficiency (E53.8)
EXCLUDES 1 syphilitic combined degeneration of spinal cord (A52.11)

5 **G32.8 Other specified degenerative disorders of nervous system in diseases classified elsewhere**
Code first underlying disease, such as:
amyloidosis cerebral degeneration (E85.-)
cerebral degeneration (due to) hypothyroidism (E00.0-E03.9)
cerebral degeneration (due to) neoplasm (C00-D49)
cerebral degeneration (due to) vitamin B deficiency, except thiamine (E52-E53.-)
EXCLUDES 1 superior hemorrhagic polioencephalitis [Wernicke's encephalopathy] (E51.2)

M IQ **G32.81** ***Cerebellar ataxia in diseases classified elsewhere***
Code first underlying disease, such as:
celiac disease (with gluten ataxia) (K90.0)
cerebellar ataxia (in) neoplastic disease (paraneoplastic cerebellar degeneration) (C00-D49)
non-celiac gluten ataxia (M35.9)
EXCLUDES 1 systemic atrophy primarily affecting the central nervous system in alcoholic cerebellar ataxia (G31.2)
systemic atrophy primarily affecting the central nervous system in myxedema (G13.2)

M IQ **G32.89** ***Other specified degenerative disorders of nervous system in diseases classified elsewhere***
Degenerative encephalopathy in diseases classified elsewhere

Demyelinating diseases of the central nervous system (G35-G37)

SP SH SL **G35 Multiple sclerosis**
Disseminated multiple sclerosis
Generalized multiple sclerosis
Multiple sclerosis NOS
Multiple sclerosis of brain stem
Multiple sclerosis of cord

CODING TIPS✓ Code G35 should be listed primary when the patient is being seen for more than one aspect of the disease. Code associated symptoms of MS from Chapter 18 after code G35 (MS), but only if those symptoms are **not routinely** associated with MS. Conditions associated with MS, such as neuropathy are not symptom codes and should be coded in addition to MS.

4 **G36 Other acute disseminated demyelination**
EXCLUDES 1 postinfectious encephalitis and encephalomyelitis NOS (G04.01)

SP **G36.0 Neuromyelitis optica [Devic]**
Demyelination in optic neuritis
EXCLUDES 1 optic neuritis NOS (H46)

SP **G36.1 Acute and subacute hemorrhagic leukoencephalitis [Hurst]**

SP **G36.8 Other specified acute disseminated demyelination**

SP **G36.9 Acute disseminated demyelination, unspecified**

4 **G37 Other demyelinating diseases of central nervous system**

SP **G37.0 Diffuse sclerosis of central nervous system**
Periaxial encephalitis
Schilder's disease
EXCLUDES 1 X linked adrenoleukodystrophy (E71.52-)

SP **G37.1 Central demyelination of corpus callosum**

SP **G37.2 Central pontine myelinolysis**

▲ SP **G37.3 Acute transverse myelitis in demyelinating disease of central nervous system**
Acute transverse myelitis NOS
Acute transverse myelopathy
EXCLUDES 1 acute flaccid myelitis (G04.82)
multiple sclerosis (G35)
neuromyelitis optica [Devic] (G36.0)

DEFINITION Spinal cord disorder with inflammatory lesions across the entire width of one level; numbness, back pain, weakness, sensory loss, motor and sphincter deficits, loss of bladder and bowel control appear quickly and progress to paraplegia.

SP **G37.4 Subacute necrotizing myelitis of central nervous system**

SP **G37.5 Concentric sclerosis [Balo] of central nervous system**

SP **G37.8 Other specified demyelinating diseases of central nervous system**

SP **G37.9 Demyelinating disease of central nervous system, unspecified**

Episodic and paroxysmal disorders (G40-G47)

4 **G40 Epilepsy and recurrent seizures**

Note:
the following terms are to be considered equivalent to intractable: pharmacoresistant (pharmacologically resistant), treatment resistant, refractory (medically) and poorly controlled

EXCLUDES 1 conversion disorder with seizures (F44.5)
convulsions NOS (R56.9)
post traumatic seizures (R56.1)
seizure (convulsive) NOS (R56.9)
seizure of newborn (P90)

EXCLUDES 2 hippocampal sclerosis (G93.81)
mesial temporal sclerosis (G93.81)
temporal sclerosis (G93.81)
Todd's paralysis (G83.84)

CODING TIPS✓ When coding epileptic syndromes, coders should note that seizure(s)/epileptic disorders noted by the provider as treatment- or medication-resistant, refractory, or poorly controlled should be coded to intractable. Coders should not assign R56.9, Unspecified convulsions, for patients experiencing seizure disorders or recurrent seizures. Recurrent seizures and unspecified seizure disorders, when not reported as intractable, should be coded to G40.909.

5 **G40.0 Localization-related (focal) (partial) idiopathic epilepsy and epileptic syndromes with seizures of localized onset**
Benign childhood epilepsy with centrotemporal EEG spikes
Childhood epilepsy with occipital EEG paroxysms

EXCLUDES 1 adult onset localization-related epilepsy (G40.1-, G40.2-)

6 **G40.00 Localization-related (focal) (partial) idiopathic epilepsy and epileptic syndromes with seizures of localized onset, not intractable**
Localization-related (focal) (partial) idiopathic epilepsy and epileptic syndromes with seizures of localized onset without intractability

SP **G40.001 Localization-related (focal) (partial) idiopathic epilepsy and epileptic syndromes with seizures of localized onset, not intractable, with status epilepticus**

SP **G40.009 Localization-related (focal) (partial) idiopathic epilepsy and epileptic syndromes with seizures of localized onset, not intractable, without status epilepticus**
Localization-related (focal) (partial) idiopathic epilepsy and epileptic syndromes with seizures of localized onset NOS

6 **G40.01 Localization-related (focal) (partial) idiopathic epilepsy and epileptic syndromes with seizures of localized onset, intractable**

SP **G40.011 Localization-related (focal) (partial) idiopathic epilepsy and epileptic syndromes with seizures of localized onset, intractable, with status epilepticus**

SP **G40.019 Localization-related (focal) (partial) idiopathic epilepsy and epileptic syndromes with seizures of localized onset, intractable, without status epilepticus**

5 **G40.1 Localization-related (focal) (partial) symptomatic epilepsy and epileptic syndromes with simple partial seizures**
Attacks without alteration of consciousness
Epilepsia partialis continua [Kozhevnikof]
Simple partial seizures developing into secondarily generalized seizures

6 **G40.10 Localization-related (focal) (partial) symptomatic epilepsy and epileptic syndromes with simple partial seizures, not intractable**
Localization-related (focal) (partial) symptomatic epilepsy and epileptic syndromes with simple partial seizures without intractability

SP **G40.101 Localization-related (focal) (partial) symptomatic epilepsy and epileptic syndromes with simple partial seizures, not intractable, with status epilepticus**

SP **G40.109 Localization-related (focal) (partial) symptomatic epilepsy and epileptic syndromes with simple partial seizures, not intractable, without status epilepticus**
Localization-related (focal) (partial) symptomatic epilepsy and epileptic syndromes with simple partial seizures NOS

6 **G40.11 Localization-related (focal) (partial) symptomatic epilepsy and epileptic syndromes with simple partial seizures, intractable**

SP **G40.111 Localization-related (focal) (partial) symptomatic epilepsy and epileptic syndromes with simple partial seizures, intractable, with status epilepticus**

SP **G40.119 Localization-related (focal) (partial) symptomatic epilepsy and epileptic syndromes with simple partial seizures, intractable, without status epilepticus**

5 **G40.2 Localization-related (focal) (partial) symptomatic epilepsy and epileptic syndromes with complex partial seizures**
Attacks with alteration of consciousness, often with automatisms
Complex partial seizures developing into secondarily generalized seizures

6 **G40.20 Localization-related (focal) (partial) symptomatic epilepsy and epileptic syndromes with complex partial seizures, not intractable**

Localization-related (focal) (partial) symptomatic epilepsy and epileptic syndromes with complex partial seizures without intractability

SP **G40.201 Localization-related (focal) (partial) symptomatic epilepsy and epileptic syndromes with complex partial seizures, not intractable, with status epilepticus**

SP **G40.209 Localization-related (focal) (partial) symptomatic epilepsy and epileptic syndromes with complex partial seizures, not intractable, without status epilepticus**

Localization-related (focal) (partial) symptomatic epilepsy and epileptic syndromes with complex partial seizures NOS

6 **G40.21 Localization-related (focal) (partial) symptomatic epilepsy and epileptic syndromes with complex partial seizures, intractable**

SP **G40.211 Localization-related (focal) (partial) symptomatic epilepsy and epileptic syndromes with complex partial seizures, intractable, with status epilepticus**

SP **G40.219 Localization-related (focal) (partial) symptomatic epilepsy and epileptic syndromes with complex partial seizures, intractable, without status epilepticus**

5 **G40.3 Generalized idiopathic epilepsy and epileptic syndromes**

Code also:

MERRF syndrome, if applicable (E88.42)

6 **G40.30 Generalized idiopathic epilepsy and epileptic syndromes, not intractable**

Generalized idiopathic epilepsy and epileptic syndromes without intractability

SP **G40.301 Generalized idiopathic epilepsy and epileptic syndromes, not intractable, with status epilepticus**

SP **G40.309 Generalized idiopathic epilepsy and epileptic syndromes, not intractable, without status epilepticus**

Generalized idiopathic epilepsy and epileptic syndromes NOS

6 **G40.31 Generalized idiopathic epilepsy and epileptic syndromes, intractable**

SP **G40.311 Generalized idiopathic epilepsy and epileptic syndromes, intractable, with status epilepticus**

SP **G40.319 Generalized idiopathic epilepsy and epileptic syndromes, intractable, without status epilepticus**

5 **G40.A Absence epileptic syndrome**

Childhood absence epilepsy [pyknolepsy]

Juvenile absence epilepsy

Absence epileptic syndrome, NOS

6 **G40.A0 Absence epileptic syndrome, not intractable**

SP **G40.A01 Absence epileptic syndrome, not intractable, with status epilepticus**

SP **G40.A09 Absence epileptic syndrome, not intractable, without status epilepticus**

6 **G40.A1 Absence epileptic syndrome, intractable**

SP **G40.A11 Absence epileptic syndrome, intractable, with status epilepticus**

SP **G40.A19 Absence epileptic syndrome, intractable, without status epilepticus**

5 **G40.B Juvenile myoclonic epilepsy [impulsive petit mal]**

6 **G40.B0 Juvenile myoclonic epilepsy, not intractable**

SP **G40.B01 Juvenile myoclonic epilepsy, not intractable, with status epilepticus**

SP **G40.B09 Juvenile myoclonic epilepsy, not intractable, without status epilepticus**

6 **G40.B1 Juvenile myoclonic epilepsy, intractable**

SP **G40.B11 Juvenile myoclonic epilepsy, intractable, with status epilepticus**

SP **G40.B19 Juvenile myoclonic epilepsy, intractable, without status epilepticus**

5 **G40.4 Other generalized epilepsy and epileptic syndromes**

Epilepsy with grand mal seizures on awakening

Epilepsy with myoclonic absences

Epilepsy with myoclonic-astatic seizures

Grand mal seizure NOS

Nonspecific atonic epileptic seizures

Nonspecific clonic epileptic seizures

Nonspecific myoclonic epileptic seizures

Nonspecific tonic epileptic seizures

Nonspecific tonic-clonic epileptic seizures

Symptomatic early myoclonic encephalopathy

6 **G40.40 Other generalized epilepsy and epileptic syndromes, not intractable**

Other generalized epilepsy and epileptic syndromes without intractability

Other generalized epilepsy and epileptic syndromes NOS

SP **G40.401 Other generalized epilepsy and epileptic syndromes, not intractable, with status epilepticus**

SP **G40.409 Other generalized epilepsy and epileptic syndromes, not intractable, without status epilepticus**

6 **G40.41 Other generalized epilepsy and epileptic syndromes, intractable**

SP **G40.411 Other generalized epilepsy and epileptic syndromes, intractable, with status epilepticus**

SP **G40.419 Other generalized epilepsy and epileptic syndromes, intractable, without status epilepticus**

SP + **G40.42 Cyclin-Dependent Kinase-Like 5 Deficiency Disorder**

CDKL5

Use additional code, if known, to identify associated manifestations, such as:
cortical blindness (H47.61-)
global developmental delay (F88)

DEFINITION Cyclin-Dependent Kinase-Like 5 (CDKL5) Deficiency Disorder is a developmental encephalopathy caused by pathogenic variants in the gene CDKL5. CDKL5 Deficiency Disorder is a unique disorder that presents with early infantile onset refractory epilepsy, hypotonia, developmental intellectual and motor disabilities, and cortical visual impairment 1-6.

+ 5 **G40.5 Epileptic seizures related to external causes**
Epileptic seizures related to alcohol
Epileptic seizures related to drugs
Epileptic seizures related to hormonal changes
Epileptic seizures related to sleep deprivation
Epileptic seizures related to stress
Code also:
, if applicable, associated epilepsy and recurrent seizures (G40.-)
Use additional code for adverse effect, if applicable, to identify drug (T36-T50 with fifth or sixth character 5)

+ 6 **G40.50 Epileptic seizures related to external causes, not intractable**

SP + **G40.501 Epileptic seizures related to external causes, not intractable, with status epilepticus**

SP + **G40.509 Epileptic seizures related to external causes, not intractable, without status epilepticus**
Epileptic seizures related to external causes, NOS

5 **G40.8 Other epilepsy and recurrent seizures**
Epilepsies and epileptic syndromes undetermined as to whether they are focal or generalized
Landau-Kleffner syndrome

6 **G40.80 Other epilepsy**

SP **G40.801 Other epilepsy, not intractable, with status epilepticus**
Other epilepsy without intractability with status epilepticus

SP **G40.802 Other epilepsy, not intractable, without status epilepticus**
Other epilepsy NOS
Other epilepsy without intractability without status epilepticus

SP **G40.803 Other epilepsy, intractable, with status epilepticus**

SP **G40.804 Other epilepsy, intractable, without status epilepticus**

6 **G40.81 Lennox-Gastaut syndrome**

SP **G40.811 Lennox-Gastaut syndrome, not intractable, with status epilepticus**

SP **G40.812 Lennox-Gastaut syndrome, not intractable, without status epilepticus**

SP **G40.813 Lennox-Gastaut syndrome, intractable, with status epilepticus**

SP **G40.814 Lennox-Gastaut syndrome, intractable, without status epilepticus**

6 **G40.82 Epileptic spasms**
Infantile spasms
Salaam attacks
West's syndrome

CODING TIPS✓ Code G40.82 describes infantile spasms, also known as West's syndrome.

SP **G40.821 Epileptic spasms, not intractable, with status epilepticus**

SP **G40.822 Epileptic spasms, not intractable, without status epilepticus**

SP **G40.823 Epileptic spasms, intractable, with status epilepticus**

SP **G40.824 Epileptic spasms, intractable, without status epilepticus**

6 **G40.83 Dravet syndrome**
Polymorphic epilepsy in infancy (PMEI)
Severe myoclonic epilepsy in infancy (SMEI)

SP **G40.833 Dravet syndrome, intractable, with status epilepticus**

SP **G40.834 Dravet syndrome, intractable, without status epilepticus**
Dravet syndrome NOS

SP **G40.89 Other seizures**
EXCLUDES 1 post traumatic seizures (R56.1)
recurrent seizures NOS (G40.909)
seizure NOS (R56.9)

5 **G40.9 Epilepsy, unspecified**

6 **G40.90 Epilepsy, unspecified, not intractable**
Epilepsy, unspecified, without intractability

SP **G40.901 Epilepsy, unspecified, not intractable, with status epilepticus**

SP **G40.909 Epilepsy, unspecified, not intractable, without status epilepticus**
Epilepsy NOS
Epileptic convulsions NOS
Epileptic fits NOS
Epileptic seizures NOS
Recurrent seizures NOS
Seizure disorder NOS

CODING TIPS✓ Recurrent seizures and unspecified seizure disorders, when not identified as intractable, should be reported using this code. Do not assign R56.9, Unspecified convulsions, to report a diagnosis of recurrent seizures or seizure disorder.

6 **G40.91 Epilepsy, unspecified, intractable**
Intractable seizure disorder NOS

SP **G40.911 Epilepsy, unspecified, intractable, with status epilepticus**

SP **G40.919 Epilepsy, unspecified, intractable, without status epilepticus**

+ 4 G43 Migraine

Note:

the following terms are to be considered equivalent to intractable: pharmacoresistant (pharmacologically resistant), treatment resistant, refractory (medically) and poorly controlled

Use additional code for adverse effect, if applicable, to identify drug (T36-T50 with fifth or sixth character 5)

EXCLUDES 1 headache NOS (R51.9)
lower half migraine (G44.00)

EXCLUDES 2 headache syndromes (G44.-)

+ 5 G43.0 Migraine without aura

Common migraine

EXCLUDES 1 chronic migraine without aura (G43.7-)

+ 6 G43.00 Migraine without aura, not intractable

Migraine without aura without mention of refractory migraine

SP + G43.001 Migraine without aura, not intractable, with status migrainosus

SP + G43.009 Migraine without aura, not intractable, without status migrainosus

Migraine without aura NOS

+ 6 G43.01 Migraine without aura, intractable

Migraine without aura with refractory migraine

SP + G43.011 Migraine without aura, intractable, with status migrainosus

SP + G43.019 Migraine without aura, intractable, without status migrainosus

+ 5 G43.1 Migraine with aura

Basilar migraine
Classical migraine
Migraine equivalents
Migraine preceded or accompanied by transient focal neurological phenomena
Migraine triggered seizures
Migraine with acute-onset aura
Migraine with aura without headache (migraine equivalents)
Migraine with prolonged aura
Migraine with typical aura
Retinal migraine

Code also:

any associated seizure (G40.-, R56.9)

EXCLUDES 1 persistent migraine aura (G43.5-, G43.6-)

+ 6 G43.10 Migraine with aura, not intractable

Migraine with aura without mention of refractory migraine

SP + G43.101 Migraine with aura, not intractable, with status migrainosus

SP + G43.109 Migraine with aura, not intractable, without status migrainosus

Migraine with aura NOS

+ 6 G43.11 Migraine with aura, intractable

Migraine with aura with refractory migraine

SP + G43.111 Migraine with aura, intractable, with status migrainosus

SP + G43.119 Migraine with aura, intractable, without status migrainosus

+ 5 G43.4 Hemiplegic migraine

Familial migraine
Sporadic migraine

+ 6 G43.40 Hemiplegic migraine, not intractable

Hemiplegic migraine without refractory migraine

SP + G43.401 Hemiplegic migraine, not intractable, with status migrainosus

SP + G43.409 Hemiplegic migraine, not intractable, without status migrainosus

Hemiplegic migraine NOS

+ 6 G43.41 Hemiplegic migraine, intractable

Hemiplegic migraine with refractory migraine

SP + G43.411 Hemiplegic migraine, intractable, with status migrainosus

SP + G43.419 Hemiplegic migraine, intractable, without status migrainosus

+ 5 G43.5 Persistent migraine aura without cerebral infarction

+ 6 G43.50 Persistent migraine aura without cerebral infarction, not intractable

Persistent migraine aura without cerebral infarction, without refractory migraine

SP + G43.501 Persistent migraine aura without cerebral infarction, not intractable, with status migrainosus

SP + G43.509 Persistent migraine aura without cerebral infarction, not intractable, without status migrainosus

Persistent migraine aura NOS

+ 6 G43.51 Persistent migraine aura without cerebral infarction, intractable

Persistent migraine aura without cerebral infarction, with refractory migraine

SP + G43.511 Persistent migraine aura without cerebral infarction, intractable, with status migrainosus

SP + G43.519 Persistent migraine aura without cerebral infarction, intractable, without status migrainosus

+ 5 G43.6 Persistent migraine aura with cerebral infarction

Code also:

the type of cerebral infarction (I63.-)

+ 6 G43.60 Persistent migraine aura with cerebral infarction, not intractable

Persistent migraine aura with cerebral infarction, without refractory migraine

SP + G43.601 Persistent migraine aura with cerebral infarction, not intractable, with status migrainosus

SP + G43.609 Persistent migraine aura with cerebral infarction, not intractable, without status migrainosus

+ 6 **G43.61 Persistent migraine aura with cerebral infarction, intractable**
Persistent migraine aura with cerebral infarction, with refractory migraine

SP + **G43.611 Persistent migraine aura with cerebral infarction, intractable, with status migrainosus**

SP + **G43.619 Persistent migraine aura with cerebral infarction, intractable, without status migrainosus**

+ 5 **G43.7 Chronic migraine without aura**
Transformed migraine
EXCLUDES 1 migraine without aura (G43.0-)

+ 6 **G43.70 Chronic migraine without aura, not intractable**
Chronic migraine without aura, without refractory migraine

SP + **G43.701 Chronic migraine without aura, not intractable, with status migrainosus**

SP + **G43.709 Chronic migraine without aura, not intractable, without status migrainosus**
Chronic migraine without aura NOS

+ 6 **G43.71 Chronic migraine without aura, intractable**
Chronic migraine without aura, with refractory migraine

SP + **G43.711 Chronic migraine without aura, intractable, with status migrainosus**

SP + **G43.719 Chronic migraine without aura, intractable, without status migrainosus**

+ 5 **G43.A Cyclical vomiting**
EXCLUDES 1 cyclical vomiting syndrome unrelated to migraine (R11.15)

SP + **G43.A0 Cyclical vomiting, in migraine, not intractable**
Cyclical vomiting, without refractory migraine

SP + **G43.A1 Cyclical vomiting, in migraine, intractable**
Cyclical vomiting, with refractory migraine

+ 5 **G43.B Ophthalmoplegic migraine**

SP + **G43.B0 Ophthalmoplegic migraine, not intractable**
Ophthalmoplegic migraine, without refractory migraine

SP + **G43.B1 Ophthalmoplegic migraine, intractable**
Ophthalmoplegic migraine, with refractory migraine

+ 5 **G43.C Periodic headache syndromes in child or adult**

SP + **G43.C0 Periodic headache syndromes in child or adult, not intractable**
Periodic headache syndromes in child or adult, without refractory migraine

SP + **G43.C1 Periodic headache syndromes in child or adult, intractable**
Periodic headache syndromes in child or adult, with refractory migraine

+ 5 **G43.D Abdominal migraine**

SP + **G43.D0 Abdominal migraine, not intractable**
Abdominal migraine, without refractory migraine

SP + **G43.D1 Abdominal migraine, intractable**
Abdominal migraine, with refractory migraine

+ 5 **G43.8 Other migraine**

+ 6 **G43.80 Other migraine, not intractable**
Other migraine, without refractory migraine

SP + **G43.801 Other migraine, not intractable, with status migrainosus**

SP + **G43.809 Other migraine, not intractable, without status migrainosus**

+ 6 **G43.81 Other migraine, intractable**
Other migraine, with refractory migraine

SP + **G43.811 Other migraine, intractable, with status migrainosus**

SP + **G43.819 Other migraine, intractable, without status migrainosus**

+ 6 **G43.82 Menstrual migraine, not intractable**
Menstrual headache, not intractable
Menstrual migraine, without refractory migraine
Menstrually related migraine, not intractable
Pre-menstrual headache, not intractable
Pre-menstrual migraine, not intractable
Pure menstrual migraine, not intractable
Code also:
associated premenstrual tension syndrome (N94.3)

SP + **G43.821 Menstrual migraine, not intractable, with status migrainosus**

SP + **G43.829 Menstrual migraine, not intractable, without status migrainosus**
Menstrual migraine NOS

+ 6 **G43.83 Menstrual migraine, intractable**
Menstrual headache, intractable
Menstrual migraine, with refractory migraine
Menstrually related migraine, intractable
Pre-menstrual headache, intractable
Pre-menstrual migraine, intractable
Pure menstrual migraine, intractable
Code also:
associated premenstrual tension syndrome (N94.3)

SP + **G43.831 Menstrual migraine, intractable, with status migrainosus**

SP + **G43.839 Menstrual migraine, intractable, without status migrainosus**

+ 5 **G43.9 Migraine, unspecified**

+ 6 **G43.90 Migraine, unspecified, not intractable**
Migraine, unspecified, without refractory migraine

SP + **G43.901 Migraine, unspecified, not intractable, with status migrainosus**
Status migrainosus NOS

SP + **G43.909 Migraine, unspecified, not intractable, without status migrainosus**

Chapter 6
G00-G99

Migraine NOS

+ 6 **G43.91 Migraine, unspecified, intractable**
Migraine, unspecified, with refractory migraine

SP + **G43.911 Migraine, unspecified, intractable, with status migrainosus**

SP + **G43.919 Migraine, unspecified, intractable, without status migrainosus**

4 **G44 Other headache syndromes**
EXCLUDES 1 headache NOS (R51.9)
EXCLUDES 2 atypical facial pain (G50.1)
headache due to lumbar puncture (G97.1)
migraines (G43.-)
trigeminal neuralgia (G50.0)

5 **G44.0 Cluster headaches and other trigeminal autonomic cephalgias (TAC)**

6 **G44.00 Cluster headache syndrome, unspecified**
Ciliary neuralgia
Cluster headache NOS
Histamine cephalgia
Lower half migraine
Migrainous neuralgia

SP **G44.001 Cluster headache syndrome, unspecified, intractable**

SP **G44.009 Cluster headache syndrome, unspecified, not intractable**
Cluster headache syndrome NOS

6 **G44.01 Episodic cluster headache**
DEFINITION Distinctive headache marked by excruciating, searing pain that develops quickly without warning on one side and occurs in frequent attacks lasting from 15 minutes to 3 hours, in cyclical patterns of up to 12 weeks, followed by remission periods.

SP **G44.011 Episodic cluster headache, intractable**

SP **G44.019 Episodic cluster headache, not intractable**
Episodic cluster headache NOS

6 **G44.02 Chronic cluster headache**

SP **G44.021 Chronic cluster headache, intractable**

SP **G44.029 Chronic cluster headache, not intractable**
Chronic cluster headache NOS

6 **G44.03 Episodic paroxysmal hemicrania**
Paroxysmal hemicrania NOS
DEFINITION Rare headache with severe throbbing or boring pain in the eye or temple on one side and accompanying autonomic responses; occurring in frequent, daily attacks with relatively long headache-free periods.

SP **G44.031 Episodic paroxysmal hemicrania, intractable**

SP **G44.039 Episodic paroxysmal hemicrania, not intractable**
Episodic paroxysmal hemicrania NOS

6 **G44.04 Chronic paroxysmal hemicrania**

SP **G44.041 Chronic paroxysmal hemicrania, intractable**

SP **G44.049 Chronic paroxysmal hemicrania, not intractable**
Chronic paroxysmal hemicrania NOS

6 **G44.05 Short lasting unilateral neuralgiform headache with conjunctival injection and tearing (SUNCT)**

SP **G44.051 Short lasting unilateral neuralgiform headache with conjunctival injection and tearing (SUNCT), intractable**

SP **G44.059 Short lasting unilateral neuralgiform headache with conjunctival injection and tearing (SUNCT), not intractable**
Short lasting unilateral neuralgiform headache with conjunctival injection and tearing (SUNCT) NOS

6 **G44.09 Other trigeminal autonomic cephalgias (TAC)**

SP **G44.091 Other trigeminal autonomic cephalgias (TAC), intractable**

SP **G44.099 Other trigeminal autonomic cephalgias (TAC), not intractable**

SP **G44.1 Vascular headache, not elsewhere classified**
EXCLUDES 2 cluster headache (G44.0)
complicated headache syndromes (G44.5-)
drug-induced headache (G44.4-)
migraine (G43.-)
other specified headache syndromes (G44.8-)
post-traumatic headache (G44.3-)
tension-type headache (G44.2-)

5 **G44.2 Tension-type headache**

6 **G44.20 Tension-type headache, unspecified**
DEFINITION Common, muscular contraction headaches, that produce a mild to moderate, dull, achy tightening pain over the forehead and sides like a band encircling the head or pain at the back of the neck or base of the skull.

SP **G44.201 Tension-type headache, unspecified, intractable**

SP **G44.209 Tension-type headache, unspecified, not intractable**
Tension headache NOS

6 **G44.21 Episodic tension-type headache**

SP **G44.211 Episodic tension-type headache, intractable**

SP **G44.219 Episodic tension-type headache, not intractable**
Episodic tension-type headache NOS

6 **G44.22 Chronic tension-type headache**

SP **G44.221 Chronic tension-type headache, intractable**

SP **G44.229 Chronic tension-type headache, not intractable**
Chronic tension-type headache NOS

5 G44.3 Post-traumatic headache

6 G44.30 Post-traumatic headache, unspecified

DEFINITION Headache as a result of head trauma or injury, with frequency and severity diminishing over time; symptoms such as insomnia, concentration problems, personality changes, and dizziness often accompany the headache.

SP G44.301 Post-traumatic headache, unspecified, intractable

SP G44.309 Post-traumatic headache, unspecified, not intractable

Post-traumatic headache NOS

6 G44.31 Acute post-traumatic headache

SP G44.311 Acute post-traumatic headache, intractable

SP G44.319 Acute post-traumatic headache, not intractable

Acute post-traumatic headache NOS

6 G44.32 Chronic post-traumatic headache

SP G44.321 Chronic post-traumatic headache, intractable

SP G44.329 Chronic post-traumatic headache, not intractable

Chronic post-traumatic headache NOS

+ 5 G44.4 Drug-induced headache, not elsewhere classified

Medication overuse headache

Use additional code for adverse effect, if applicable, to identify drug (T36-T50 with fifth or sixth character 5)

DEFINITION Most common type of chronic daily headache caused by overuse of migraine-abortive ergot alkaloids and analgesic drugs.

SP + G44.40 Drug-induced headache, not elsewhere classified, not intractable

SP + G44.41 Drug-induced headache, not elsewhere classified, intractable

5 G44.5 Complicated headache syndromes

SP G44.51 Hemicrania continua

SP G44.52 New daily persistent headache (NDPH)

SP G44.53 Primary thunderclap headache

DEFINITION Dramatic, sudden, severe headache coming without warning, peaking within 60 seconds, then fading over several hours; sometimes signaling a potentially life-threatening condition, such as a ruptured cerebral aneurysm or subarachnoid hemorrhage.

SP G44.59 Other complicated headache syndrome

5 G44.8 Other specified headache syndromes

EXCLUDES 2 headache with orthostatic or positional component, not elsewhere classified (R51.0)

SP G44.81 Hypnic headache

DEFINITION Relatively rare headache connected to REM sleep, marked by being awakened with intense throbbing or dull type pain through the head, accompanied by nausea, and lasting about an hour.

SP G44.82 Headache associated with sexual activity

Orgasmic headache

Preorgasmic headache

SP G44.83 Primary cough headache

DEFINITION Headache triggered by bouts of coughing or physically straining movements, such as laughing or sneezing, often described as sharp, stabbing, or splitting on both sides of the head and back of the skull.

SP G44.84 Primary exertional headache

SP G44.85 Primary stabbing headache

★ G44.86 Cervicogenic headache

Code also:
associated cervical spinal condition, if known

SP G44.89 Other headache syndrome

4 G45 Transient cerebral ischemic attacks and related syndromes

EXCLUDES 1 neonatal cerebral ischemia (P91.0)
transient retinal artery occlusion (H34.0-)

SP G45.0 Vertebro-basilar artery syndrome

DEFINITION Obstruction of the vertebral or basilar artery temporarily blocking blood flow to the brain, causing vertigo, diplopia, nystagmus, and muscle weakness.

SP G45.1 Carotid artery syndrome (hemispheric)

SP G45.2 Multiple and bilateral precerebral artery syndromes

SP G45.3 Amaurosis fugax

CODING TIPS✓ Amaurosis fugax is a sudden loss of vision in one eye related to impaired carotid blood flow and impaired retinal blood supply and is generally temporary. Generally such a diagnosis is not appropriate for a home health claim, however if the physician or NPP documented this condition, then the coder may assign the code. The condition may signal pending stroke and should not be confused with blindness. Coders should not code blindness in a patient with this condition.

SP G45.4 Transient global amnesia

EXCLUDES 1 amnesia NOS (R41.3)

SP G45.8 Other transient cerebral ischemic attacks and related syndromes

SP G45.9 Transient cerebral ischemic attack, unspecified

Spasm of cerebral artery

TIA

Transient cerebral ischemia NOS

Chapter 6 G00-G99

CODING TIPS✓ Note that there is no code in ICD-10 to report sequelae of a TIA, as these are considered to be "transient" and should not cause residual effects. If residual effects are noted, the coder should query the physician or NPP to determine if the patient experienced an infarction or stroke. Generally such a diagnosis is not appropriate for a home health claim, however if the physician or NPP documented this condition, then the coder may assign the code. A history of TIA (or CVA) with no residual neurological deficits may be coded to Z86.73, Personal history of transient ischemic attack, and cerebral infarction, without residual deficits.

4 G46 Vascular syndromes of brain in cerebrovascular diseases

Code first:
underlying cerebrovascular disease (I60-I69)

CODING TIPS✓ Conditions classified to G46.- include conditions specific to syndromes occurring as a result of specific types of cerebral vascular disease (I65-I68) and cerebral vascular accidents (CVA). Home health claims generally should not assign codes for acute CVAs (I60-I63) in any circumstance. When a syndrome classifiable to G46.- occurs as a residual of a CVA, assign the appropriate I69 code to indicate sequelae of cerebrovascular disease. These syndromes may be coded as "other sequelae" of CVAs and should then be coded following the appropriate I69 code with the 5th character '9' and 6th character '8,' for example, I69.398.

!Q G46.0 Middle cerebral artery syndrome

!Q G46.1 Anterior cerebral artery syndrome

!Q G46.2 Posterior cerebral artery syndrome

!Q G46.3 Brain stem stroke syndrome

Benedikt syndrome
Claude syndrome
Foville syndrome
Millard-Gubler syndrome
Wallenberg syndrome
Weber syndrome

!Q G46.4 Cerebellar stroke syndrome

!Q G46.5 Pure motor lacunar syndrome

!Q G46.6 Pure sensory lacunar syndrome

!Q G46.7 Other lacunar syndromes

!Q G46.8 Other vascular syndromes of brain in cerebrovascular diseases

4 G47 Sleep disorders

EXCLUDES 2 nightmares (F51.5)
nonorganic sleep disorders (F51.-)
sleep terrors (F51.4)
sleepwalking (F51.3)

5 G47.0 Insomnia

EXCLUDES 2 alcohol related insomnia (F10.182, F10.282, F10.982)
drug-related insomnia (F11.182, F11.282, F11.982, F13.182, F13.282, F13.982, F14.182, F14.282, F14.982, F15.182, F15.282, F15.982, F19.182, F19.282, F19.982)
idiopathic insomnia (F51.01)
insomnia due to a mental disorder (F51.05)
insomnia not due to a substance or known physiological condition (F51.0-)
nonorganic insomnia (F51.0-)
primary insomnia (F51.01)
sleep apnea (G47.3-)

SP G47.00 Insomnia, unspecified

Insomnia NOS

SP G47.01 Insomnia due to medical condition

Code also:
associated medical condition

SP G47.09 Other insomnia

5 G47.1 Hypersomnia

EXCLUDES 2 alcohol-related hypersomnia (F10.182, F10.282, F10.982)
drug-related hypersomnia (F11.182, F11.282, F11.982, F13.182, F13.282, F13.982, F14.182, F14.282, F14.982, F15.182, F15.282, F15.982, F19.182, F19.282, F19.982)
hypersomnia due to a mental disorder (F51.13)
hypersomnia not due to a substance or known physiological condition (F51.1-)
primary hypersomnia (F51.11)
sleep apnea (G47.3-)

SP G47.10 Hypersomnia, unspecified

Hypersomnia NOS

SP G47.11 Idiopathic hypersomnia with long sleep time

Idiopathic hypersomnia NOS

SP G47.12 Idiopathic hypersomnia without long sleep time

SP G47.13 Recurrent hypersomnia

Kleine-Levin syndrome
Menstrual related hypersomnia

SP G47.14 Hypersomnia due to medical condition

Code also:
associated medical condition

SP G47.19 Other hypersomnia

5 G47.2 Circadian rhythm sleep disorders

Disorders of the sleep wake schedule
Inversion of nyctohemeral rhythm
Inversion of sleep rhythm

SP G47.20 Circadian rhythm sleep disorder, unspecified type
Sleep wake schedule disorder NOS

SP G47.21 **Circadian rhythm sleep disorder, delayed sleep phase type**
Delayed sleep phase syndrome

SP G47.22 **Circadian rhythm sleep disorder, advanced sleep phase type**

SP G47.23 **Circadian rhythm sleep disorder, irregular sleep wake type**
Irregular sleep-wake pattern

SP G47.24 **Circadian rhythm sleep disorder, free running type**
Circadian rhythm sleep disorder, non-24-hour sleep-wake type

SP G47.25 **Circadian rhythm sleep disorder, jet lag type**

SP G47.26 **Circadian rhythm sleep disorder, shift work type**

IQ G47.27 **Circadian rhythm sleep disorder in conditions classified elsewhere**
Code first:
underlying condition

SP G47.29 **Other circadian rhythm sleep disorder**

5 G47.3 **Sleep apnea**
Code also:
any associated underlying condition
EXCLUDES 1 apnea NOS (R06.81)
Cheyne-Stokes breathing (R06.3)
pickwickian syndrome (E66.2)
sleep apnea of newborn (P28.3)

SP G47.30 Sleep apnea, unspecified
Sleep apnea NOS

SP G47.31 **Primary central sleep apnea**
Idiopathic central sleep apnea

SP G47.32 **High altitude periodic breathing**

SP G47.33 **Obstructive sleep apnea (adult) (pediatric)**
Obstructive sleep apnea hypopnea
EXCLUDES 1 obstructive sleep apnea of newborn (P28.3)

SP G47.34 **Idiopathic sleep related nonobstructive alveolar hypoventilation**
Sleep related hypoxia

SP G47.35 **Congenital central alveolar hypoventilation syndrome**

IQ G47.36 **Sleep related hypoventilation in conditions classified elsewhere**
Sleep related hypoxemia in conditions classified elsewhere
Code first:
underlying condition

IQ G47.37 **Central sleep apnea in conditions classified elsewhere**
Code first:
underlying condition

SP G47.39 **Other sleep apnea**

5 G47.4 **Narcolepsy and cataplexy**

6 G47.41 **Narcolepsy**

SP G47.411 **Narcolepsy with cataplexy**

SP G47.419 **Narcolepsy without cataplexy**
Narcolepsy NOS

6 G47.42 **Narcolepsy in conditions classified elsewhere**
Code first:
underlying condition

IQ G47.421 **Narcolepsy in conditions classified elsewhere with cataplexy**

IQ G47.429 **Narcolepsy in conditions classified elsewhere without cataplexy**

5 G47.5 **Parasomnia**
EXCLUDES 1 alcohol induced parasomnia (F10.182, F10.282, F10.982)
drug induced parasomnia (F11.182, F11.282, F11.982, F13.182, F13.282, F13.982, F14.182, F14.282, F14.982, F15.182, F15.282, F15.982, F19.182, F19.282, F19.982)
parasomnia not due to a substance or known physiological condition (F51.8)

SP G47.50 Parasomnia, unspecified
Parasomnia NOS

SP G47.51 **Confusional arousals**

SP G47.52 **REM sleep behavior disorder**

SP G47.53 **Recurrent isolated sleep paralysis**

IQ G47.54 **Parasomnia in conditions classified elsewhere**
Code first:
underlying condition

SP G47.59 **Other parasomnia**

5 G47.6 **Sleep related movement disorders**
EXCLUDES 2 restless legs syndrome (G25.81)

SP G47.61 **Periodic limb movement disorder**
DEFINITION Involuntary limb movement or jerking during or just before sleep.

SP G47.62 **Sleep related leg cramps**

SP G47.63 **Sleep related bruxism**
EXCLUDES 1 psychogenic bruxism (F45.8)
DEFINITION Grinding the teeth during sleep.

SP G47.69 **Other sleep related movement disorders**

SP G47.8 **Other sleep disorders**
Other specified sleep-wake disorder

SP G47.9 Sleep disorder, unspecified
Sleep disorder NOS
Unspecified sleep-wake disorder

Nerve, nerve root and plexus disorders (G50-G59)

EXCLUDES 1 current traumatic nerve, nerve root and plexus disorders - see Injury, nerve by body region
neuralgia NOS (M79.2)
neuritis NOS (M79.2)
peripheral neuritis in pregnancy (O26.82-)
radiculitis NOS (M54.1-)

4 G50 **Disorders of trigeminal nerve**

INCLUDES disorders of 5th cranial nerve

SP **G50.0 Trigeminal neuralgia**
Syndrome of paroxysmal facial pain
Tic douloureux

SP **G50.1 Atypical facial pain**

SP **G50.8 Other disorders of trigeminal nerve**

SP **G50.9 Disorder of trigeminal nerve, unspecified**

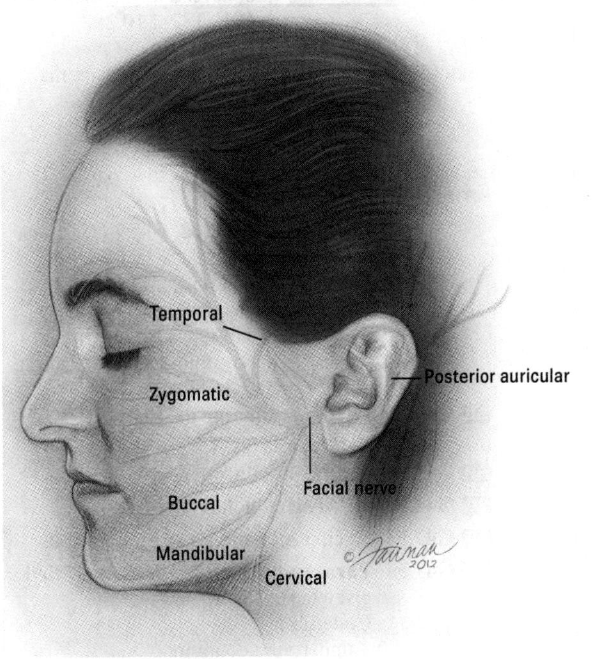

4 **G51 Facial nerve disorders**
INCLUDES disorders of 7th cranial nerve

SP **G51.0 Bell's palsy**
Facial palsy
DEFINITION Temporary, unilateral facial muscle weakness or paralysis resulting from damage or trauma to one of the paired facial nerves.

SP **G51.1 Geniculate ganglionitis**
EXCLUDES 1 postherpetic geniculate ganglionitis (B02.21)
DEFINITION Inflammation of the facial nerve ganglion.

SP **G51.2 Melkersson's syndrome**
Melkersson-Rosenthal syndrome

5 **G51.3 Clonic hemifacial spasm**

SP **G51.31 Clonic hemifacial spasm, right**

SP **G51.32 Clonic hemifacial spasm, left**

SP **G51.33 Clonic hemifacial spasm, bilateral**

SP **G51.39 Clonic hemifacial spasm, unspecified**

SP **G51.4 Facial myokymia**

SP **G51.8 Other disorders of facial nerve**

!Q **G51.9 Disorder of facial nerve, unspecified**

4 **G52 Disorders of other cranial nerves**
EXCLUDES 2 disorders of acoustic [8th] nerve (H93.3)
disorders of optic [2nd] nerve (H46, H47.0)
paralytic strabismus due to nerve palsy (H49.0-H49.2)

SP **G52.0 Disorders of olfactory nerve**
Disorders of 1st cranial nerve

SP **G52.1 Disorders of glossopharyngeal nerve**
Disorder of 9th cranial nerve
Glossopharyngeal neuralgia

SP **G52.2 Disorders of vagus nerve**
Disorders of pneumogastric [10th] nerve

SP **G52.3 Disorders of hypoglossal nerve**
Disorders of 12th cranial nerve

SP **G52.7 Disorders of multiple cranial nerves**
Polyneuritis cranialis

SP **G52.8 Disorders of other specified cranial nerves**

!Q **G52.9 Cranial nerve disorder, unspecified**

M !Q **G53** ***Cranial nerve disorders in diseases classified elsewhere***
Code first underlying disease, such as:
neoplasm (C00-D49)
EXCLUDES 1 multiple cranial nerve palsy in sarcoidosis (D86.82)
multiple cranial nerve palsy in syphilis (A52.15)
postherpetic geniculate ganglionitis (B02.21)
postherpetic trigeminal neuralgia (B02.22)

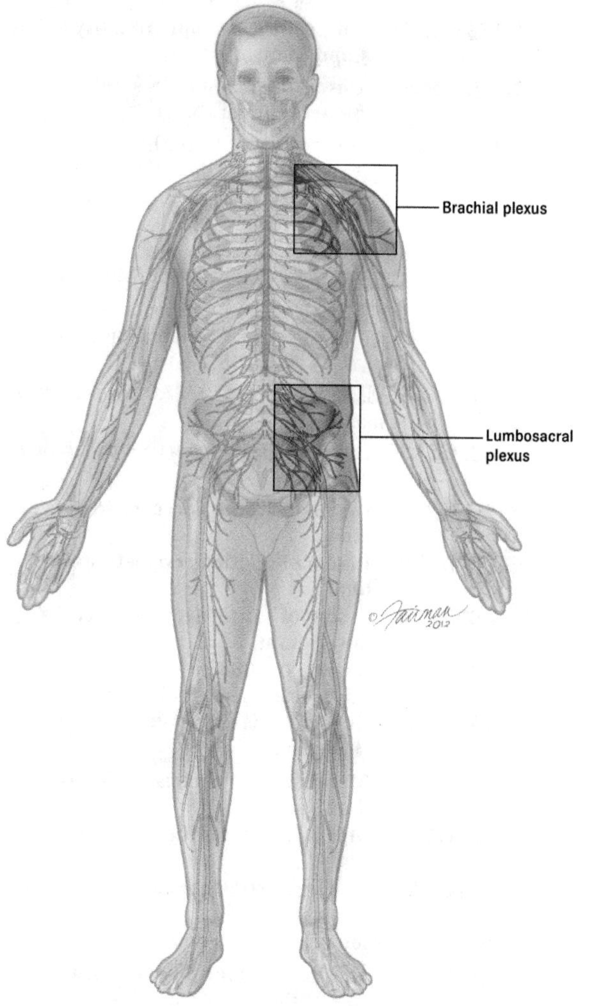

G54 Nerve root and plexus disorders

EXCLUDES 1 current traumatic nerve root and plexus disorders - see nerve injury by body region
intervertebral disc disorders (M50-M51)
neuralgia or neuritis NOS (M79.2)
neuritis or radiculitis brachial NOS (M54.13)
neuritis or radiculitis lumbar NOS (M54.16)
neuritis or radiculitis lumbosacral NOS (M54.17)
neuritis or radiculitis thoracic NOS (M54.14)
radiculitis NOS (M54.10)
radiculopathy NOS (M54.10)
spondylosis (M47.-)

SP **G54.0 Brachial plexus disorders**
Thoracic outlet syndrome

SP **G54.1 Lumbosacral plexus disorders**

SP **G54.2 Cervical root disorders, not elsewhere classified**

SP **G54.3 Thoracic root disorders, not elsewhere classified**

SP **G54.4 Lumbosacral root disorders, not elsewhere classified**

SP **G54.5 Neuralgic amyotrophy**
Parsonage-Aldren-Turner syndrome
Shoulder-girdle neuritis

EXCLUDES 1 neuralgic amyotrophy in diabetes mellitus (E08-E13 with .44)

CODING TIPS ✓ Do not assign code G54.5 for diabetic amyotrophy. Diabetes with amyotrophy should be coded with the appropriate combination code to specify the type of diabetes and the neuralgic amyotrophy manifestation (E08-E13 with 4th and 5th character .44).

SP **G54.6 Phantom limb syndrome with pain**

SP **G54.7 Phantom limb syndrome without pain**
Phantom limb syndrome NOS

SP **G54.8 Other nerve root and plexus disorders**

IQ **G54.9 Nerve root and plexus disorder, unspecified**

▲ M IQ **G55 *Nerve root and plexus compressions in diseases classified elsewhere***

Code first underlying disease, such as:
neoplasm (C00-D49)

EXCLUDES 1 nerve root compression (due to) (in) ankylosing spondylitis (M45.-)
nerve root compression (due to) (in) dorsopathies (M53.-, M54.-)
nerve root compression (due to) (in) intervertebral disc disorders (M50.1.-, M51.1.-)
nerve root compression (due to) (in) spondylopathies (M46.-, M48.-)
nerve root compression (due to) (in) spondylosis (M47.0-, M47.2.-)

G56 Mononeuropathies of upper limb

EXCLUDES 1 current traumatic nerve disorder - see nerve injury by body region

CODING TIPS ✓ Complex regional pain syndromes (CRPS Type I or II or unspecified) are no longer classified and coded to causalgias and mononeuropathies. When CRPS Type I, Type II or unspecified is reported, it should be coded to the appropriate G90.5- code.

G56.0 Carpal tunnel syndrome

DEFINITION Pain, burning, tingling and/or numbness in the fingers and hand, often extending to the elbow, due to compression of the median nerve within the carpal tunnel.

H IQ **G56.00 Carpal tunnel syndrome, unspecified upper limb**

H SP **G56.01 Carpal tunnel syndrome, right upper limb**

H SP **G56.02 Carpal tunnel syndrome, left upper limb**

H SP **G56.03 Carpal tunnel syndrome, bilateral upper limbs**

G56.1 Other lesions of median nerve

Chapter 6
G00-G99

G56.10 Other lesions of median nerve, unspecified upper limb

G56.11 Other lesions of median nerve, right upper limb

G56.12 Other lesions of median nerve, left upper limb

G56.13 Other lesions of median nerve, bilateral upper limbs

G56.2 Lesion of ulnar nerve

Tardy ulnar nerve palsy

G56.20 Lesion of ulnar nerve, unspecified upper limb

G56.21 Lesion of ulnar nerve, right upper limb

G56.22 Lesion of ulnar nerve, left upper limb

G56.23 Lesion of ulnar nerve, bilateral upper limbs

G56.3 Lesion of radial nerve

G56.30 Lesion of radial nerve, unspecified upper limb

G56.31 Lesion of radial nerve, right upper limb

G56.32 Lesion of radial nerve, left upper limb

G56.33 Lesion of radial nerve, bilateral upper limbs

G56.4 Causalgia of upper limb

Complex regional pain syndrome II of upper limb

EXCLUDES 1 complex regional pain syndrome I of lower limb (G90.52-)
complex regional pain syndrome I of upper limb (G90.51-)
complex regional pain syndrome II of lower limb (G57.7-)
reflex sympathetic dystrophy of lower limb (G90.52-)
reflex sympathetic dystrophy of upper limb (G90.51-)

DEFINITION A burning pain in the arm along the course of a peripheral nerve usually associated with skin changes.

G56.40 Causalgia of unspecified upper limb

G56.41 Causalgia of right upper limb

G56.42 Causalgia of left upper limb

G56.43 Causalgia of bilateral upper limbs

G56.8 Other specified mononeuropathies of upper limb

Interdigital neuroma of upper limb

G56.80 Other specified mononeuropathies of unspecified upper limb

G56.81 Other specified mononeuropathies of right upper limb

G56.82 Other specified mononeuropathies of left upper limb

G56.83 Other specified mononeuropathies of bilateral upper limbs

G56.9 Unspecified mononeuropathy of upper limb

G56.90 Unspecified mononeuropathy of unspecified upper limb

G56.91 Unspecified mononeuropathy of right upper limb

G56.92 Unspecified mononeuropathy of left upper limb

G56.93 Unspecified mononeuropathy of bilateral upper limbs

G57 Mononeuropathies of lower limb

EXCLUDES 1 current traumatic nerve disorder - see nerve injury by body region

G57.0 Lesion of sciatic nerve

EXCLUDES 1 sciatica NOS (M54.3-)

EXCLUDES 2 sciatica attributed to intervertebral disc disorder (M51.1.-)

CODING TIPS ✓ Report G57.0- for pyriformis (piriformis) syndrome.

G57.00 Lesion of sciatic nerve, unspecified lower limb

G57.01 Lesion of sciatic nerve, right lower limb

G57.02 Lesion of sciatic nerve, left lower limb

G57.03 Lesion of sciatic nerve, bilateral lower limbs

G57.1 Meralgia paresthetica

Lateral cutaneous nerve of thigh syndrome

G57.10 Meralgia paresthetica, unspecified lower limb

G57.11 Meralgia paresthetica, right lower limb

G57.12 Meralgia paresthetica, left lower limb

G57.13 Meralgia paresthetica, bilateral lower limbs

G57.2 Lesion of femoral nerve

G57.20 Lesion of femoral nerve, unspecified lower limb

G57.21 Lesion of femoral nerve, right lower limb

G57.22 Lesion of femoral nerve, left lower limb

G57.23 Lesion of femoral nerve, bilateral lower limbs

G57.3 Lesion of lateral popliteal nerve

Peroneal nerve palsy

G57.30 Lesion of lateral popliteal nerve, unspecified lower limb

G57.31 Lesion of lateral popliteal nerve, right lower limb

G57.32 Lesion of lateral popliteal nerve, left lower limb

G57.33 Lesion of lateral popliteal nerve, bilateral lower limbs

G57.4 Lesion of medial popliteal nerve

G57.40 Lesion of medial popliteal nerve, unspecified lower limb

G57.41 Lesion of medial popliteal nerve, right lower limb

G57.42 Lesion of medial popliteal nerve, left lower limb

G57.43 Lesion of medial popliteal nerve, bilateral lower limbs

G57.5 Tarsal tunnel syndrome

DEFINITION Pain, burning, tingling, and/or numbness of the sole of the foot, often extending to the ankle, due to compression of the posterior tibial nerve or plantar nerves within the tarsal tunnel.

⊟ IQ **G57.50 Tarsal tunnel syndrome, unspecified lower limb**

⊟ SP **G57.51 Tarsal tunnel syndrome, right lower limb**

⊟ SP **G57.52 Tarsal tunnel syndrome, left lower limb**

⊟ SP **G57.53 Tarsal tunnel syndrome, bilateral lower limbs**

5 **G57.6 Lesion of plantar nerve**

Morton's metatarsalgia

DEFINITION Thickening of tissue that surrounds the digital nerve leading to the toes. Most frequently develops between the third and fourth toes, usually in response to irritation, trauma or excessive pressure.

⊟ IQ **G57.60 Lesion of plantar nerve, unspecified lower limb**

⊟ SP **G57.61 Lesion of plantar nerve, right lower limb**

⊟ SP **G57.62 Lesion of plantar nerve, left lower limb**

⊟ SP **G57.63 Lesion of plantar nerve, bilateral lower limbs**

5 **G57.7 Causalgia of lower limb**

Complex regional pain syndrome II of lower limb

EXCLUDES 1 complex regional pain syndrome I of lower limb (G90.52-)
complex regional pain syndrome I of upper limb (G90.51-)
complex regional pain syndrome II of upper limb (G56.4-)
reflex sympathetic dystrophy of lower limb (G90.52-)
reflex sympathetic dystrophy of upper limb (G90.51-)

⊟ IQ **G57.70 Causalgia of unspecified lower limb**

⊟ SP **G57.71 Causalgia of right lower limb**

⊟ SP **G57.72 Causalgia of left lower limb**

⊟ SP **G57.73 Causalgia of bilateral lower limbs**

5 **G57.8 Other specified mononeuropathies of lower limb**

Interdigital neuroma of lower limb

⊟ IQ **G57.80 Other specified mononeuropathies of unspecified lower limb**

⊟ SP **G57.81 Other specified mononeuropathies of right lower limb**

⊟ SP **G57.82 Other specified mononeuropathies of left lower limb**

⊟ SP **G57.83 Other specified mononeuropathies of bilateral lower limbs**

5 **G57.9 Unspecified mononeuropathy of lower limb**

⊟ IQ **G57.90 Unspecified mononeuropathy of unspecified lower limb**

⊟ SP **G57.91 Unspecified mononeuropathy of right lower limb**

⊟ SP **G57.92 Unspecified mononeuropathy of left lower limb**

⊟ SP **G57.93 Unspecified mononeuropathy of bilateral lower limbs**

4 **G58 Other mononeuropathies**

IQ **G58.0 Intercostal neuropathy**

SP **G58.7 Mononeuritis multiplex**

SP **G58.8 Other specified mononeuropathies**

IQ **G58.9 Mononeuropathy, unspecified**

IQ **G59 Mononeuropathy in diseases classified elsewhere**

Code first:
underlying disease

EXCLUDES 1 diabetic mononeuropathy (E08-E13 with .41)
syphilitic nerve paralysis (A52.19)
syphilitic neuritis (A52.15)
tuberculous mononeuropathy (A17.83)

Polyneuropathies and other disorders of the peripheral nervous system (G60-G65)

EXCLUDES 1 neuralgia NOS (M79.2)
neuritis NOS (M79.2)
peripheral neuritis in pregnancy (O26.82-)
radiculitis NOS (M54.10)

4 **G60 Hereditary and idiopathic neuropathy**

SP **G60.0 Hereditary motor and sensory neuropathy**

Charcot-Marie-Tooth disease
Déjérine-Sottas disease
Hereditary motor and sensory neuropathy, types I-IV
Hypertrophic neuropathy of infancy
Peroneal muscular atrophy (axonal type) (hypertrophic type)
Roussy-Levy syndrome

SP **G60.1 Refsum's disease**

Infantile Refsum disease

SP **G60.2 Neuropathy in association with hereditary ataxia**

SP **G60.3 Idiopathic progressive neuropathy**

SP **G60.8 Other hereditary and idiopathic neuropathies**

Dominantly inherited sensory neuropathy
Morvan's disease
Nelaton's syndrome
Recessively inherited sensory neuropathy

SP **G60.9 Hereditary and idiopathic neuropathy, unspecified**

CODING TIPS ✓ The provider should document hereditary and/or idiopathic neuropathy to assign G60.9. If polyneuropathy is documented without a type or cause, assign G62.9.

4 **G61 Inflammatory polyneuropathy**

CODING TIPS✓ When an inflammatory neuropathy is reported as unresolved, assign the appropriate code from G61.-. If inflammatory neuropathy is documented as resolved but residual neurologic deficits remain as sequelae, assign the appropriate code from category G65.-, Sequelae of inflammatory and toxic polyneuropathies.

SP **G61.0 Guillain-Barre syndrome**
Acute (post-)infective polyneuritis
Miller Fisher Syndrome

CODING TIPS✓ When Guillain-Barre syndrome is reported as unresolved, assign code G61.0. If a Guillain-Barre syndrome is documented as resolved but residual neurologic deficits remain as sequelae, assign code G65.0, Sequelae of Guillain-Barre syndrome (code first the residual defects when coding G65.0). Acute inflammatory demyelinating polyneuropathy is included in this code.

DEFINITION Disorder that causes the body's immune system to attack the nerves; paralysis begins at the feet and progresses upwards through the legs and torso to the arms and face.

SP + **G61.1 Serum neuropathy**
Use additional code for adverse effect, if applicable, to identify serum (T50.-)

5 **G61.8 Other inflammatory polyneuropathies**

SP **G61.81 Chronic inflammatory demyelinating polyneuritis**

SP **G61.82 Multifocal motor neuropathy**
MMN

SP **G61.89 Other inflammatory polyneuropathies**

!Q **G61.9 Inflammatory polyneuropathy, unspecified**

4 **G62 Other and unspecified polyneuropathies**

SP + **G62.0 Drug-induced polyneuropathy**
Use additional code for adverse effect, if applicable, to identify drug (T36-T50 with fifth or sixth character 5)

CODING TIPS✓ Assign G62.0 when the polyneuropathy is specifically reported by the patient's provider as related to the use of a drug. An additional code should be assigned to identify the drug.

SP **G62.1 Alcoholic polyneuropathy**

CODING TIPS✓ This diagnosis indicates that the alcohol was linked to the disorder, so the use, abuse or dependence of alcohol (F10.-) should also be coded, usually with 4th and 5th characters to indicate uncomplicated. Do not include 5th and 6th characters .-88. "Induced disorders" include mental, emotional and physical disorders that are included in Chapter 5 only.

CODING TIPS✓ Assign G62.1 when the patient's provider specifically reports that the polyneuropathy results from alcohol use. The coder should also code any history of, or current use, of alcohol.

DEFINITION Loss of nerve function due to damage from prolonged, excessive alcohol consumption; commonly presents with numbness, weakness, and burning in the feet.

!Q **G62.2 Polyneuropathy due to other toxic agents**
Code first:
(T51-T65) to identify toxic agent

5 **G62.8 Other specified polyneuropathies**

SP **G62.81 Critical illness polyneuropathy**
Acute motor neuropathy

SP + **G62.82 Radiation-induced polyneuropathy**
Use additional external cause code (W88-W90, X39.0-) to identify cause

SP **G62.89 Other specified polyneuropathies**

!Q **G62.9 Polyneuropathy, unspecified**
Neuropathy NOS

CODING TIPS✓ The provider should document hereditary and/or idiopathic neuropathy to assign G60.9. If polyneuropathy is documented without a type or cause, assign G62.9.

▲ M !Q **G63** ***Polyneuropathy in diseases classified elsewhere***
Code first underlying disease, such as:
amyloidosis (E85.-)
endocrine disease, except diabetes (E00-E07, E15-E16, E20-E34)
metabolic diseases (E70-E88)
neoplasm (C00-D49)
nutritional deficiency (E40-E64)

EXCLUDES 1 polyneuropathy (in):
diabetes mellitus (E08-E13 with .42)
diphtheria (A36.83)
infectious mononucleosis complicated by polyneuropathy (B27.0-B27.9 with fifth character 1)
Lyme disease (A69.22)
mumps (B26.84)
postherpetic (B02.23)
rheumatoid arthritis (M05.5-)
scleroderma (M34.83)
systemic lupus erythematosus (M32.19)

CODING TIPS✓ Do not assign code G63 for diabetic polyneuropathy. Diabetes with polyneuropathy should be coded with the appropriate combination code to specify the type of diabetes and the polyneuropathy manifestation.

SP **G64 Other disorders of peripheral nervous system**
Disorder of peripheral nervous system NOS

4 **G65 Sequelae of inflammatory and toxic polyneuropathies**
Code first:
condition resulting from (sequela) of inflammatory and toxic polyneuropathies

SP **G65.0 Sequelae of Guillain-Barré syndrome**

SP **G65.1 Sequelae of other inflammatory polyneuropathy**

SP **G65.2 Sequelae of toxic polyneuropathy**

Chapter 6

G00-G99

4 4th digit required 5 5th digit required 6 6th digit required 7 7th digit required 7 7th digit placeholder + Additional code Laterality

Diseases of myoneural junction and muscle (G70-G73)

4 G70 Myasthenia gravis and other myoneural disorders

EXCLUDES 1 botulism (A05.1, A48.51-A48.52)
transient neonatal myasthenia gravis (P94.0)

5 G70.0 Myasthenia gravis

CODING TIPS✓ When myasthenia gravis is not documented as with or without exacerbation (no exacerbation is specified), assign code G70.00, without (acute) exacerbation.

SP G70.00 Myasthenia gravis without (acute) exacerbation
Myasthenia gravis NOS

SP G70.01 Myasthenia gravis with (acute) exacerbation
Myasthenia gravis in crisis

IQ G70.1 Toxic myoneural disorders
Code first:
(T51-T65) to identify toxic agent

SP IQ G70.2 Congenital and developmental myasthenia

5 G70.8 Other specified myoneural disorders

CODING TIPS✓ Lambert-Eaton myasthenic syndrome (LEMS) is an autoimmune disorder of the neuromuscular junction, the site where nerve cells meet muscle cells and help activate the muscles. The disruption of electrical impulses is associated with antibodies produced as a consequence of this autoimmunity.

SP G70.80 Lambert-Eaton syndrome, unspecified
Lambert-Eaton syndrome NOS

IQ G70.81 Lambert-Eaton syndrome in disease classified elsewhere
Code first:
underlying disease
EXCLUDES 1 Lambert-Eaton syndrome in neoplastic disease (G73.1)

SP G70.89 Other specified myoneural disorders

IQ G70.9 Myoneural disorder, unspecified

4 G71 Primary disorders of muscles

EXCLUDES 2 arthrogryposis multiplex congenita (Q74.3)
metabolic disorders (E70-E88)
myositis (M60.-)

5 G71.0 Muscular dystrophy

SP G71.00 Muscular dystrophy, unspecified

SP G71.01 Duchenne or Becker muscular dystrophy
Autosomal recessive, childhood type, muscular dystrophy resembling Duchenne or Becker muscular dystrophy
Benign [Becker] muscular dystrophy
Severe [Duchenne] muscular dystrophy

SP G71.02 Facioscapulohumeral muscular dystrophy
Scapulohumeral muscular dystrophy

SP G71.09 Other specified muscular dystrophies
Benign scapuloperoneal muscular dystrophy with early contractures [Emery-Dreifuss]
Congenital muscular dystrophy NOS
Congenital muscular dystrophy with specific morphological abnormalities of the muscle fiber
Distal muscular dystrophy
Limb-girdle muscular dystrophy
Ocular muscular dystrophy
Oculopharyngeal muscular dystrophy
Scapuloperoneal muscular dystrophy

5 G71.1 Myotonic disorders

SP G71.11 Myotonic muscular dystrophy
Dystrophia myotonica [Steinert]
Myotonia atrophica
Myotonic dystrophy
Proximal myotonic myopathy (PROMM)
Steinert disease

SP G71.12 Myotonia congenita
Acetazolamide responsive myotonia congenita
Dominant myotonia congenita [Thomsen disease]
Myotonia levior
Recessive myotonia congenita [Becker disease]

SP G71.13 Myotonic chondrodystrophy
Chondrodystrophic myotonia
Congenital myotonic chondrodystrophy
Schwartz-Jampel disease

DEFINITION Muscle disorder of late infancy with distinctive signs: mask-like face with small features, short stature or dwarfism, limited joint mobility, hip dysplasia, and generalized myotonia with hypertrophied diaphragmatic muscles. Death usually occurs due to respiratory compromise.

SP + G71.14 Drug induced myotonia
Use additional code for adverse effect, if applicable, to identify drug (T36-T50 with fifth or sixth character 5)

SP G71.19 Other specified myotonic disorders
Myotonia fluctuans
Myotonia permanens
Neuromyotonia [Isaacs]
Paramyotonia congenita (of von Eulenburg)
Pseudomyotonia
Symptomatic myotonia

5 G71.2 Congenital myopathies

EXCLUDES 2 arthrogryposis multiplex congenita (Q74.3)

SP G71.20 Congenital myopathy, unspecified

SP G71.21 Nemaline myopathy

6 G71.22 Centronuclear myopathy

SP G71.220 X-linked myotubular myopathy
Myotubular (centronuclear) myopathy

SP G71.228 Other centronuclear myopathy
Autosomal centronuclear myopathy

Chapter 6
G00-G99

Autosomal dominant centronuclear myopathy
Autosomal recessive centronuclear myopathy
Centronuclear myopathy, NOS

SP **G71.29 Other congenital myopathy**
Central core disease
Minicore disease
Multicore disease
Multiminicore disease

SP **G71.3 Mitochondrial myopathy, not elsewhere classified**
EXCLUDES 1 Kearns-Sayre syndrome (H49.81)
Leber's disease (H47.21)
Leigh's encephalopathy (G31.82)
mitochondrial metabolism disorders (E88.4.-)
Reye's syndrome (G93.7)

SP **G71.8 Other primary disorders of muscles**

!Q **G71.9 Primary disorder of muscle, unspecified**
Hereditary myopathy NOS

4 **G72 Other and unspecified myopathies**
EXCLUDES 1 arthrogryposis multiplex congenita (Q74.3)
dermatopolymyositis (M33.-)
ischemic infarction of muscle (M62.2-)
myositis (M60.-)
polymyositis (M33.2.-)

SP + **G72.0 Drug-induced myopathy**
Use additional code for adverse effect, if applicable, to identify drug (T36-T50 with fifth or sixth character 5)

SP + **G72.1 Alcoholic myopathy**
Use additional code to identify alcoholism (F10.-)
CODING TIPS✓ This diagnosis indicates that the alcohol was linked to the disorder, so the use, abuse or dependence of alcohol (F10.-) should also be coded, usually with 4th and 5th characters to indicate uncomplicated. Do not include 5th and 6th characters .-88. "Induced disorders" include mental, emotional and physical disorders that are included in Chapter 5 only.

G72.2 Myopathy due to other toxic agents
Code first:
(T51-T65) to identify toxic agent

SP **G72.3 Periodic paralysis**
Familial periodic paralysis
Hyperkalemic periodic paralysis (familial)
Hypokalemic periodic paralysis (familial)
Myotonic periodic paralysis (familial)
Normokalemic paralysis (familial)
Potassium sensitive periodic paralysis
EXCLUDES 1 paramyotonia congenita (of von Eulenburg) (G71.19)

5 **G72.4 Inflammatory and immune myopathies, not elsewhere classified**

SP **G72.41 Inclusion body myositis [IBM]**

SP **G72.49 Other inflammatory and immune myopathies, not elsewhere classified**
Inflammatory myopathy NOS

5 **G72.8 Other specified myopathies**

SP **G72.81 Critical illness myopathy**
Acute necrotizing myopathy
Acute quadriplegic myopathy
Intensive care (ICU) myopathy
Myopathy of critical illness
CODING TIPS✓ Critical illness myopathy typically occurs in the ICU among patients who have been treated with multiple drugs. It commonly occurs in sepsis patients and is responsible for cachexia and weakness.
CODING TIPS✓ This condition may take several weeks to months for a patient to fully recover from, and should be coded in the home health setting when it remains a relevant, current diagnosis for the plan of care.

SP **G72.89 Other specified myopathies**

SP **G72.9 Myopathy, unspecified**

4 **G73 Disorders of myoneural junction and muscle in diseases classified elsewhere**

!Q **G73.1 Lambert-Eaton syndrome in neoplastic disease**
Code first:
underlying neoplasm (C00-D49)
EXCLUDES 1 Lambert-Eaton syndrome not associated with neoplasm (G70.80-G70.81)
CODING TIPS✓ Those with LEMS not associated with malignancy have a benign overall prognosis. Generally the presence of cancer determines the prognosis when the LEMS is associated with a neoplasm.

M !Q ***G73.3 Myasthenic syndromes in other diseases classified elsewhere***
Code first underlying disease, such as:
neoplasm (C00-D49)
thyrotoxicosis (E05.-)

▲ M !Q ***G73.7 Myopathy in diseases classified elsewhere***
Code first underlying disease, such as:
hyperparathyroidism (E21.0, E21.3)
hypoparathyroidism (E20.-)
glycogen storage disease (E74.0)
lipid storage disorders (E75.-)
EXCLUDES 1 myopathy in:
rheumatoid arthritis (M05.32)
sarcoidosis (D86.87)
scleroderma (M34.82)
Sjögren syndrome (M35.03)
systemic lupus erythematosus (M32.19)

Cerebral palsy and other paralytic syndromes (G80-G83)

4 **G80 Cerebral palsy**
EXCLUDES 1 hereditary spastic paraplegia (G11.4)

SP **G80.0 Spastic quadriplegic cerebral palsy**
Congenital spastic paralysis (cerebral)
DEFINITION Palsy presenting with spastic paralysis of all four limbs from early brain damage.

SP **G80.1 Spastic diplegic cerebral palsy**
Spastic cerebral palsy NOS

SP **G80.2 Spastic hemiplegic cerebral palsy**
DEFINITION Palsy affecting the limbs on either the left or the right side (e.g., the right arm and right leg).

SP **G80.3 Athetoid cerebral palsy**
Double athetosis (syndrome)
Dyskinetic cerebral palsy
Dystonic cerebral palsy
Vogt disease
DEFINITION Permanent, nonprogressive, motor disorder caused by brain damage usually occurring shortly before, during, or after birth and characterized by uncontrolled, writhing movements of the hands, feet, arms, or legs.

SP **G80.4 Ataxic cerebral palsy**

SP **G80.8 Other cerebral palsy**
Mixed cerebral palsy syndromes

SP **G80.9 Cerebral palsy, unspecified**
Cerebral palsy NOS

4 **G81 Hemiplegia and hemiparesis**
Note:
This category is to be used only when hemiplegia (complete)(incomplete) is reported without further specification, or is stated to be old or longstanding but of unspecified cause. The category is also for use in multiple coding to identify these types of hemiplegia resulting from any cause.

EXCLUDES 1 congenital cerebral palsy (G80.-)
hemiplegia and hemiparesis due to sequela of cerebrovascular disease (I69.05-, I69.15-, I69.25-, I69.35-, I69.85-, I69.95-)

GUIDELINES **Section I.C.6.a**
Codes from category G81, Hemiplegia and hemiparesis, and subcategories, G83.1, Monoplegia of lower limb, G83.2, Monoplegia of upper limb, and G83.3, Monoplegia, unspecified, identify whether the dominant or nondominant side is affected. Should the affected side be documented, but not specified as dominant or nondominant, and the classification system does not indicate a default, code selection is as follows:
- For ambidextrous patients, the default should be dominant.
- If the left side is affected, the default is non-dominant.
- If the right side is affected, the default is dominant.

CODING TIPS✓ When coding hemiplegia and monoplegia, the dominance rule stated in the guidelines applies. Coders should note that there is no option to code unspecified side since the classification assumes dominant side.

CODING TIPS✓ Hemiparesis refers to one-sided weakness and should be coded with G81.-, not M62.81. Hemiplegia with sequela of stroke is included in the combination code, for example I69.351.

CODING TIPS✓ When paraplegia, hemiplegia, hemiparesis or another paralytic state results from a brain or spinal cord injury, code the paralysis/paresis followed by the code for the brain or spinal injury with the 7th character "S" to report a sequela of the injury.

5 **G81.0 Flaccid hemiplegia**
CODING TIPS✓ Words that describe abnormal muscle tonicity as flaccid (hypotonic) or spastic (hypertonic) point to G81.0 and G81.1, respectively. Documentation of complete versus incomplete must come from the physician.

⊟ IQ **G81.00 Flaccid hemiplegia affecting unspecified side**
⊟ SP SH SL **G81.01 Flaccid hemiplegia affecting right dominant side**
⊟ SP SH SL **G81.02 Flaccid hemiplegia affecting left dominant side**
⊟ SP SH SL **G81.03 Flaccid hemiplegia affecting right nondominant side**
⊟ SP SH SL **G81.04 Flaccid hemiplegia affecting left nondominant side**

5 **G81.1 Spastic hemiplegia**
CODING TIPS✓ Words that describe abnormal muscle tonicity as flaccid (hypotonic) or spastic (hypertonic) point to G81.0 and G81.1, respectively. Documentation of complete versus incomplete must come from the physician.

⊟ IQ **G81.10 Spastic hemiplegia affecting unspecified side**
⊟ SP SH SL **G81.11 Spastic hemiplegia affecting right dominant side**
⊟ SP SH SL **G81.12 Spastic hemiplegia affecting left dominant side**
⊟ SP SH SL **G81.13 Spastic hemiplegia affecting right nondominant side**
⊟ SP SH SL **G81.14 Spastic hemiplegia affecting left nondominant side**

5 **G81.9 Hemiplegia, unspecified**
⊟ IQ **G81.90 Hemiplegia, unspecified affecting unspecified side**
⊟ SP SH SL **G81.91 Hemiplegia, unspecified affecting right dominant side**
⊟ SP SH SL **G81.92 Hemiplegia, unspecified affecting left dominant side**
⊟ SP SH SL **G81.93 Hemiplegia, unspecified affecting right nondominant side**
⊟ SP SH SL **G81.94 Hemiplegia, unspecified affecting left nondominant side**

4 **G82 Paraplegia (paraparesis) and quadriplegia (quadriparesis)**

Chapter 6 G00-G99

Note:
This category is to be used only when the listed conditions are reported without further specification, or are stated to be old or longstanding but of unspecified cause. The category is also for use in multiple coding to identify these conditions resulting from any cause

EXCLUDES 1 congenital cerebral palsy (G80.-)
functional quadriplegia (R53.2)
hysterical paralysis (F44.4)

CODING TIPS ✓ When paraplegia, hemiplegia, hemiparesis or another paralytic state results from a brain or spinal cord injury, code the paralysis/paresis followed by the code for the brain or spinal injury with the 7th character "S" to report a sequela of the injury.

5 G82.2 Paraplegia
Paralysis of both lower limbs NOS
Paraparesis (lower) NOS
Paraplegia (lower) NOS

CODING TIPS ✓ If paraplegia resulted from a spinal cord injury, then code paraplegia followed by the sequela of spinal cord injury code (S14.- with 7th character S for cervical; S24.- with 7th character S for thoracic; S34.- with 7th character S for lumbar). Paraplegia is not likely to result from a CVA. Paraparesis is weakness of both lower limbs without paralysis and is coded with G82.22.

SP SH SL G82.20 Paraplegia, unspecified

ALERT Paraplegia, unspecified, may result in rejected claims in some regions. Query the physician for level of injury and complete/incomplete. "Complete" means that there is complete loss of function below the point of injury. An "incomplete" injury refers to a spinal cord injury in which some feeling or movement is still evident below the point of injury.

SP SH SL G82.21 Paraplegia, complete

SP SH SL G82.22 Paraplegia, incomplete

5 G82.5 Quadriplegia

CODING TIPS ✓ If quadriplegia resulted from a spinal cord injury, then code quadriplegia followed by the sequela of spinal cord injury code (S14.- with 7th character S for cervical; S24.- with 7th character S for thoracic; S34.- with 7th character S for lumbar). If quadriplegia results from a CVA, code the appropriate I69.36- code followed by quadriplegia. Documentation of complete versus incomplete must come from the physician or NPP.

SP SH SL G82.50 Quadriplegia, unspecified

ALERT Quadriplegia, unspecified, may result in rejected claims in some regions. Query the physician for level of injury and complete/incomplete. "Complete" means that there is complete loss of function below the point of injury. An "incomplete" injury refers to a spinal cord injury in which some feeling or movement is still evident below the point of injury.

SP SH SL G82.51 Quadriplegia, C1-C4 complete

SP SH SL G82.52 Quadriplegia, C1-C4 incomplete

SP SH SL G82.53 Quadriplegia, C5-C7 complete

SP SH SL G82.54 Quadriplegia, C5-C7 incomplete

4 G83 Other paralytic syndromes

Note:
This category is to be used only when the listed conditions are reported without further specification, or are stated to be old or longstanding but of unspecified cause. The category is also for use in multiple coding to identify these conditions resulting from any cause.

INCLUDES paralysis (complete) (incomplete), except as in G80-G82

CODING TIPS ✓ When coding hemiplegia and monoplegia, the dominance rule stated in the guidelines applies. Coders should note that there is no option to code unspecified side since the classification assumes dominant side.

CODING TIPS ✓ When paraplegia, hemiplegia, hemiparesis or another paralytic state results from a brain or spinal cord injury, code the paralysis/paresis followed by the code for the brain or spinal injury with the 7th character "S" to report a sequela of the injury.

SP G83.0 Diplegia of upper limbs
Diplegia (upper)
Paralysis of both upper limbs

5 G83.1 Monoplegia of lower limb
Paralysis of lower limb

EXCLUDES 1 monoplegia of lower limbs due to sequela of cerebrovascular disease (I69.04-, I69.14-, I69.24-, I69.34-, I69.84-, I69.94-)

CODING TIPS ✓ If monoplegia is the result of an injury, code the monoplegia and then the injury with 7th character S. If monoplegia is the result of a CVA, then code I69.33- and do not assign a code from G83.-. Unlike the G81 codes where hemiparesis is included, monoparesis is not included in the M83 codes. Weakness of a limb wihout mention of muscle weakness is assigned code R29.898, Other symptoms and signs involving the musculoskeletal system. If muscle weakness is documented, assign M62.81.

Laterality IQ G83.10 Monoplegia of lower limb affecting unspecified side

ALERT Monoplegia not specifying the limb affected may result in a rejected claim.

SP G83.11 **Monoplegia of lower limb affecting right dominant side**

SP G83.12 **Monoplegia of lower limb affecting left dominant side**

SP G83.13 **Monoplegia of lower limb affecting right nondominant side**

SP G83.14 **Monoplegia of lower limb affecting left nondominant side**

5 G83.2 **Monoplegia of upper limb**
Paralysis of upper limb

> **EXCLUDES 1** monoplegia of upper limbs due to sequela of cerebrovascular disease (I69.03-, I69.13-, I69.23-, I69.33-, I69.83-, I69.93-)

CODING TIPS ✓ If monoplegia is the result of an injury, code the monoplegia and then the injury with 7th character S. If monoplegia is the result of a CVA, then code I69.33- and do not assign a code from G83.-. Unlike the G81 codes where hemiparesis is included, monoparesis is not included in the M83 codes. Weakness of a limb wihout mention of muscle weakness is assigned code R29.898, Other symptoms and signs involving the musculoskeletal system. If muscle weakness is documented, assign M62.81.

IQ G83.20 **Monoplegia of upper limb affecting unspecified side**

> **ALERT** Monoplegia not specifying the limb affected may result in a rejected claim.

SP G83.21 **Monoplegia of upper limb affecting right dominant side**

SP G83.22 **Monoplegia of upper limb affecting left dominant side**

SP G83.23 **Monoplegia of upper limb affecting right nondominant side**

SP G83.24 **Monoplegia of upper limb affecting left nondominant side**

5 G83.3 **Monoplegia, unspecified**

> **ALERT** Monoplegia not specifying the limb affected may result in a rejected claim.

IQ G83.30 **Monoplegia, unspecified affecting unspecified side**

SP G83.31 **Monoplegia, unspecified affecting right dominant side**

SP G83.32 **Monoplegia, unspecified affecting left dominant side**

SP G83.33 **Monoplegia, unspecified affecting right nondominant side**

SP G83.34 **Monoplegia, unspecified affecting left nondominant side**

SP G83.4 **Cauda equina syndrome**
Neurogenic bladder due to cauda equina syndrome

> **EXCLUDES 1** cord bladder NOS (G95.89) neurogenic bladder NOS (N31.9)

CODING TIPS ✓ Cauda equina syndrome is a rare condition which is commonly denied for lack of documentation to support the diagnosis.

CODING TIPS ✓ Assign G83.4 only when the provider specifically reports cauda equina syndrome. This code includes neurogenic bladder, and no additional code for neurogenic bladder should be assigned when present.

DEFINITION Emergent condition due to compression of spinal nerve roots causing dull aching pain in the perineum, bladder, and sacrum with associated paresthesia, bladder dysfunction, and/or paralysis.

SP G83.5 **Locked-in state**

CODING TIPS ✓ If the locked-in state results from a CVA, code the appropriate I69.36- code followed by locked-in state.

5 G83.8 **Other specified paralytic syndromes**

> **EXCLUDES 1** paralytic syndromes due to current spinal cord injury- code to spinal cord injury (S14, S24, S34)

SP G83.81 **Brown-Séquard syndrome**

CODING TIPS ✓ Brown-Sequard syndrome results when one side of the spinal cord is damaged. There is loss of movement but preserved sensation on one side of the body, while the other side of the body has loss of sensation but preserved movement.

SP G83.82 **Anterior cord syndrome**

CODING TIPS ✓ Anterior cord syndrome is characterized by damage to the front of the spinal cord. This results in impaired movement, touch, pain, and temperature sensations below the point of injury. In most cases of anterior cord syndrome, some movement can later be recovered.

SP G83.83 **Posterior cord syndrome**

CODING TIPS ✓ Posterior cord syndrome is characterized by damage to the back of the spinal cord. Most patients with posterior cord syndrome maintain good muscle power, pain, and temperature sensation, but experience poor coordination.

SP G83.84 **Todd's paralysis (postepileptic)**

SP G83.89 **Other specified paralytic syndromes**

IQ G83.9 **Paralytic syndrome, unspecified**

> **ALERT** Paralytic syndrome, unspecified may result in a rejected claim. Query the physician for more information.

Other disorders of the nervous system (G89-G99)

▲ 4 G89 **Pain, not elsewhere classified**
Code also:
> related psychological factors associated with pain (F45.42)
> **EXCLUDES 1** generalized pain NOS (R52)

★ New ▲ Revised Px Primary **SP** PDGM Px **SL** Low CoM **SH** High CoM **IQ** Quest. Encounter **H** Hospice non-cancer Dx Unspecified **M** *Manifestation*

pain disorders exclusively related to psychological factors (F45.41)
pain NOS (R52)

EXCLUDES 2 atypical face pain (G50.1)
headache syndromes (G44.-)
localized pain, unspecified type - code to pain by site, such as:
abdomen pain (R10.-)
back pain (M54.9)
breast pain (N64.4)
chest pain (R07.1-R07.9)
ear pain (H92.0-)
eye pain (H57.1)
headache (R51.9)
joint pain (M25.5-)
limb pain (M79.6-)
lumbar region pain (M54.5-)
painful urination (R30.9)
pelvic and perineal pain (R10.2)
shoulder pain (M25.51-)
spine pain (M54.-)
throat pain (R07.0)
tongue pain (K14.6)
tooth pain (K08.8)
renal colic (N23)
migraines (G43.-)
myalgia (M79.1-)
pain from prosthetic devices, implants, and grafts (T82.84, T83.84, T84.84, T85.84-)
phantom limb syndrome with pain (G54.6)
vulvar vestibulitis (N94.810)
vulvodynia (N94.81-)

GUIDELINES **Section I.C.5.a**
Assign code F45.41 for pain that is exclusively related to psychological disorders. As indicated by the Excludes 1 note under category G89, a code from category G89 should not be assigned with code F45.41. Code F45.42, Pain disorders with related psychological factors, should be used with a code from category G89 if there is documentation of a psychological component for a patient with acute or chronic pain.

GUIDELINES **Section I.C.6.b.1)**
Codes in category G89 may be used in conjunction with codes from other categories and chapters to provide more detail about acute or chronic pain and neoplasm-related pain, unless otherwise indicated below. If the pain is not specified as acute or chronic, postthoracotomy, postprocedural, or neoplasm-related, do not assign codes from category G89. A code from category G89 should not be assigned if the underlying (definitive) diagnosis is known, unless the reason for the encounter is pain control/management and not management of the underlying condition.

When an admission or encounter is for a procedure aimed at treating the underlying condition (e.g., spinal fusion, kyphoplasty), a code for the underlying condition (e.g., vertebral fracture, spinal stenosis) should be assigned as the principal diagnosis. No code from category G89 should be assigned.

CODING TIPS✓ **Documentation:** Pain disorders should be coded only when specified by the patient's provider and when the plan of care specifically addresses pain with interventions and goals to address the pain as a focus of care.

SP **G89.0 Central pain syndrome**
Déjérine-Roussy syndrome
Myelopathic pain syndrome
Thalamic pain syndrome (hyperesthetic)

GUIDELINES **Section I.C.6.b.6)**
Central pain syndrome (G89.0) and chronic pain syndrome (G89.4) are different than the term "chronic pain," and therefore codes should only be used when the provider has specifically documented this condition.

CODING TIPS✓ Do not code G89.0 unless the patient's provider specifies central pain syndrome. G89.0 may be appropriate if: 1) Traumatic or brain-related damage to the central nervous system (e.g., damage from stroke, MS, tumors, epilepsy, Parkinson's); 2) The character and extent of the pain is partly related to a variety of causes; 3) Treatment includes pain medications. It also might be appropriate for patients on antidepressants and anticonvulsants.

5 **G89.1 Acute pain, not elsewhere classified**

CODING TIPS✓ When the clinical record specifies that the patient has a pain disorder with related psychological factors, F45.42 should be additionally assigned.

CODING TIPS✓ Do not assign codes from the G89.1 and G89.2 subcategories if the underlying/definitive diagnosis is known, unless the addition of the pain code otherwise adds information as to the pain, i.e., acuity and the cause of the pain - post-surgical or post-traumatic. Use these subcategories as primary only if the reason for home care is encounter for pain control/management, and not treatment for an underlying condition.

SP **G89.11 Acute pain due to trauma**

SP **G89.12 Acute post-thoracotomy pain**
Post-thoracotomy pain NOS

GUIDELINES **Section I.C.6.b.3)(a)-(b)**
The provider's documentation should be used to guide the coding of postoperative pain. The default for post-thoracotomy and other postoperative pain not specified as acute or chronic is the code for the acute form. Routine or expected postoperative pain immediately after surgery should not be coded.

(a) Postoperative pain not associated with a specific postoperative complication is assigned to the appropriate postoperative pain code in category G89.

(b) Postoperative pain associated with specific postoperative complication (such as painful wire sutures) is assigned to the appropriate code(s) found in Chapter 19, Injury, poisoning, and certain other consequences of external causes. If appropriate, use additional code(s) from category G89 to identify acute or chronic pain (G89.18 or G89.28).

SP **G89.18 Other acute postprocedural pain**
Postoperative pain NOS
Postprocedural pain NOS

CODING TIPS✓ **Documentation:** Check the clinical record for documentation that the patient is experiencing a level of pain following a procedure that is indicative of a need for specific focus and attention within the plan of care and is being addressed with specific plan of care interventions and goals.

CODING TIPS✓ G89.18 is the default code for post-operative/post-procedural pain when not specified as acute or chronic. G89.18 should not be coded in all patients who experience pain following a procedure. It is expected that some pain would be experienced following a procedure, and these codes are used for unusual pain.

CODING TIPS✓ If the post-operative pain is associated with a complication (such as a device left in the body), code the complication and the pain. The exception is if the focus of the care is pain management. In that case, the pain code is sequenced as primary.

5 **G89.2 Chronic pain, not elsewhere classified**

EXCLUDES 1 causalgia, lower limb (G57.7-)
causalgia, upper limb (G56.4-)
central pain syndrome (G89.0)
chronic pain syndrome (G89.4)
complex regional pain syndrome II, lower limb (G57.7-)
complex regional pain syndrome II, upper limb (G56.4-)
neoplasm related chronic pain (G89.3)
reflex sympathetic dystrophy (G90.5-)

GUIDELINES **Section I.C.6.b.4)**
Chronic pain is classified to subcategory G89.2. There is no time frame defining when pain becomes chronic pain. The provider's documentation should be used to guide use of these codes.

CODING TIPS✓ When the clinical record specifies that the patient has a pain disorder with related psychological factors, F45.42 should be additionally assigned.

CODING TIPS✓ No specific time frame is required in order to code pain as chronic. Pain must be specified as chronic by the physician or NPP before using these codes. Do not assign codes from the G89.1 and G89.2 subcategories if the underlying/definitive diagnosis is known, unless the addition of the pain code otherwise adds information as to the pain, i.e., acuity and the cause of the pain - post-surgical or post-traumatic. Use these subcategories as primary only if the reason for home care is encounter for pain control/management, and not treatment for an underlying condition.

SP **G89.21 Chronic pain due to trauma**

SP **G89.22 Chronic post-thoracotomy pain**

SP **G89.28 Other chronic postprocedural pain**
Other chronic postoperative pain

CODING TIPS✓ If chronic pain is associated with a postoperative complication, code the complication and then G89.28.

CODING TIPS✓ **Documentation:** Check the clinical record for documentation that the patient is experiencing a level of pain following a procedure that is indicative of a need for specific focus and attention within the plan of care and is being addressed with specific plan of care interventions and goals.

CODING TIPS✓ Post-procedural pain that is not specified as chronic should not be coded to G89.28, Other chronic postprocedural pain. Post operative pain should not be coded in all patients who experience pain following a procedure. It is expected that some pain would be experienced following a procedure.

SP **G89.29 Other chronic pain**

SP **G89.3 Neoplasm related pain (acute) (chronic)**
Cancer associated pain
Pain due to malignancy (primary) (secondary)
Tumor associated pain

GUIDELINES **Section I.C.6.b.5)**
Code G89.3 is assigned to pain documented as being related, associated or due to cancer, primary or secondary malignancy, or tumor. This code is assigned regardless of whether the pain is acute or chronic. This code may be assigned as the principal or first listed code when the stated reason for the admission/encounter is documented as pain control/pain management. The underlying neoplasm should be reported as an additional diagnosis.

When the reason for the admission/encounter is management of the neoplasm and the pain associated with the neoplasm is also documented, code G89.3 may be assigned as an additional diagnosis. It is not necessary to assign an additional code for the site of the pain.

CODING TIPS✓ Use G89.3 for chronic or acute pain, when related to a neoplasm, either benign or malignant. Neoplasm related pain may be assigned as primary if the main reason for home care is admission for pain control. Hospices should not report codes from G89 as primary.

SP **G89.4 Chronic pain syndrome**
Chronic pain associated with significant psychosocial dysfunction

GUIDELINES **Section I.C.6.b.6)**
Central pain syndrome (G89.0) and chronic pain syndrome (G89.4) are different than the term "chronic pain," and therefore codes should only be used when the provider has specifically documented this condition.

CODING TIPS✓ Do not confuse chronic pain syndrome with chronic pain (unspecified). Chronic pain syndrome is a specifically diagnosed condition that must be reported by the patient's provider and includes a cycle of psychological and physical components.

4 **G90 Disorders of autonomic nervous system**
EXCLUDES 1 dysfunction of the autonomic nervous system due to alcohol (G31.2)

5 **G90.0 Idiopathic peripheral autonomic neuropathy**

SP **G90.01 Carotid sinus syncope**
Carotid sinus syndrome

CODING TIPS✓ Carotid sinus syndrome causes a slow heart rate or decreases the blood pressure without slowing the heart rate. Syncope may result from stimulation of the carotid sinus pressure sensors either internally (high blood pressure) or externally (turning the head). This occurs mostly in elderly men.

DEFINITION Exaggerated response to carotid sinus baroreceptor stimulation causing bradycardia, hypotension, and dizziness.

SP **G90.09 Other idiopathic peripheral autonomic neuropathy**
Idiopathic peripheral autonomic neuropathy NOS

CODING TIPS✓ Do not assign G90.09 for polyneuropathy or unspecified peripheral neuropathy. G90.09 is assigned to specify peripheral autonomic neuropathy, a condition that impairs nervous system function between the autonomic nervous system and the brain, resulting in autonomic dysregulation.

SP **G90.1 Familial dysautonomia [Riley-Day]**

SP **G90.2 Horner's syndrome**
Bernard(-Horner) syndrome
Cervical sympathetic dystrophy or paralysis

SP **G90.3 Multi-system degeneration of the autonomic nervous system**
Neurogenic orthostatic hypotension [Shy-Drager]
EXCLUDES 1 orthostatic hypotension NOS (I95.1)

SP + **G90.4 Autonomic dysreflexia**
Use additional code to identify the cause, such as:
fecal impaction (K56.41)
pressure ulcer (pressure area) (L89.-)
urinary tract infection (N39.0)

5 **G90.5 Complex regional pain syndrome I (CRPS I)**
Reflex sympathetic dystrophy
EXCLUDES 1 causalgia of lower limb (G57.7-)
causalgia of upper limb (G56.4-)
complex regional pain syndrome II of lower limb (G57.7-)
complex regional pain syndrome II of upper limb (G56.4-)

SP **G90.50 Complex regional pain syndrome I, unspecified**

6 **G90.51 Complex regional pain syndrome I of upper limb**

⊟ SP **G90.511 Complex regional pain syndrome I of right upper limb**

⊟ SP **G90.512 Complex regional pain syndrome I of left upper limb**

⊟ SP **G90.513 Complex regional pain syndrome I of upper limb, bilateral**

⊟ IQ **G90.519 Complex regional pain syndrome I of unspecified upper limb**

6 **G90.52 Complex regional pain syndrome I of lower limb**

⊟ SP **G90.521 Complex regional pain syndrome I of right lower limb**

⊟ SP **G90.522 Complex regional pain syndrome I of left lower limb**

⊟ SP **G90.523 Complex regional pain syndrome I of lower limb, bilateral**

⊟ IQ **G90.529 Complex regional pain syndrome I of unspecified lower limb**

SP **G90.59 Complex regional pain syndrome I of other specified site**

SP **G90.8 Other disorders of autonomic nervous system**

IQ **G90.9 Disorder of the autonomic nervous system, unspecified**

4 **G91 Hydrocephalus**

INCLUDES acquired hydrocephalus

EXCLUDES 1 Arnold-Chiari syndrome with hydrocephalus (Q07.-)
congenital hydrocephalus (Q03.-)
spina bifida with hydrocephalus (Q05.-)

SP **G91.0 Communicating hydrocephalus**
Secondary normal pressure hydrocephalus

SP **G91.1 Obstructive hydrocephalus**

SP **G91.2 (Idiopathic) normal pressure hydrocephalus**
Normal pressure hydrocephalus NOS

DEFINITION Disruption of normal cerebrospinal fluid circulation and gradual ventricular enlargement without known cause resulting in abnormal gait, cognitive impairment, and urinary incontinence.

SP **G91.3 Post-traumatic hydrocephalus, unspecified**

M IQ ***G91.4 Hydrocephalus in diseases classified elsewhere***
Code first underlying condition, such as:
congenital syphilis (A50.4-)
neoplasm (C00-D49)
plasminogen deficiency (E88.02)

EXCLUDES 1 hydrocephalus due to congenital toxoplasmosis (P37.1)

SP **G91.8 Other hydrocephalus**

IQ **G91.9 Hydrocephalus, unspecified**

▲ 4 **G92 Toxic encephalopathy**

★ 5 **G92.0 Immune effector cell-associated neurotoxicity syndrome**
Code first underlying cause such as:
complications of immune effector cellular therapy (T80.82)
Code also, if applicable:
associated signs and symptoms, such as seizures and cerebral edema
cerebral edema (G93.6)
unspecified convulsions (R56.9)

★ **G92.00 Immune effector cell-associated neurotoxicity syndrome, grade unspecified**
ICANS, grade unspecified

★ **G92.01 Immune effector cell-associated neurotoxicity syndrome, grade 1**
ICANS, grade 1

★ **G92.02 Immune effector cell-associated neurotoxicity syndrome, grade 2**
ICANS, grade 2

★ **G92.03 Immune effector cell-associated neurotoxicity syndrome, grade 3**
ICANS, grade 3

★ **G92.04 Immune effector cell-associated neurotoxicity syndrome, grade 4**
ICANS, grade 4

★ **G92.05 Immune effector cell-associated neurotoxicity syndrome, grade 5**
ICANS, grade 5

★ **G92.8 Other toxic encephalopathy**
Toxic encephalitis
Toxic metabolic encephalopathy
Code first:
poisoning due to drug or toxin, if applicable,
(T36-T65 with fifth or sixth character 1-4 or 6)
Use additional code for adverse effect, if applicable, to identify drug (T36-T50 with fifth or sixth character 5)

★ **G92.9 Unspecified toxic encephalopathy**
Code first:
poisoning due to drug or toxin, if applicable,
(T36-T65 with fifth or sixth character 1-4 or 6)
Use additional code for adverse effect, if applicable, to identify drug (T36-T50 with fifth or sixth character 5)

4 **G93 Other disorders of brain**

SP **G93.0 Cerebral cysts**
Arachnoid cyst
Porencephalic cyst, acquired

EXCLUDES 1 acquired periventricular cysts of newborn (P91.1)
congenital cerebral cysts (Q04.6)

SP **G93.1 Anoxic brain damage, not elsewhere classified**

EXCLUDES 1 cerebral anoxia due to anesthesia during labor and delivery (O74.3)
cerebral anoxia due to anesthesia during the puerperium (O89.2)
neonatal anoxia (P84)

CODING TIPS✓ When the anoxic brain damage is noted as a sequela of an injury and the injury that resulted in the anoxic brain damage is known, a code from Chapter 19, Injury, Poisoning and Certain Other Consequences of External Causes should be additionally assigned (with a 7th character "S").

SP **G93.2 Benign intracranial hypertension**
Pseudotumor

EXCLUDES 1 hypertensive encephalopathy (I67.4)
obstructive hydrocephalus (G91.1)

SP **G93.3 Postviral fatigue syndrome**
Benign myalgic encephalomyelitis

EXCLUDES 1 chronic fatigue syndrome NOS (R53.82)

CODING TIPS✓ Post viral fatigue syndrome has been associated with COVID-19. Do not use the code if the physician documented post-COVID syndrome.

▲ 5 **G93.4 Other and unspecified encephalopathy**

EXCLUDES 1 alcoholic encephalopathy (G31.2)
encephalopathy in diseases classified elsewhere (G94)
hypertensive encephalopathy (I67.4)

EXCLUDES 2 toxic (metabolic) encephalopathy (G92.8)

SP **G93.40 Encephalopathy, unspecified**

SP **G93.41 Metabolic encephalopathy**
Septic encephalopathy
CODING TIPS ✓ Assign G93.41 when encephalopathy is documented related to sepsis. (AHA: 2Q 2017)
DEFINITION Neuropsychiatric disturbances due to metabolic brain disease, commonly caused by hypoxia, ischemia, hypoglycemia, or diseases of other organs.

SP **G93.49 Other encephalopathy**
Encephalopathy NEC
CODING TIPS ✓ Assign G93.49 when encephalopathy is documented related to a CVA or stroke. (AHA: 2Q 2017)

▲ SP **G93.5 Compression of brain**
Arnold-Chiari type 1 compression of brain
Compression of brain (stem)
Herniation of brain (stem)
EXCLUDES 1 traumatic compression of brain (S06.A-)

SP **G93.6 Cerebral edema**
EXCLUDES 1 cerebral edema due to birth injury (P11.0)
traumatic cerebral edema (S06.1-)

SP + **G93.7 Reye's syndrome**
Code first:
poisoning due to salicylates, if applicable (T39.0-, with sixth character 1-4)
Use additional code for adverse effect due to salicylates, if applicable (T39.0-, with sixth character 5)
DEFINITION Rare, acute, sometimes fatal childhood disease with recurrent vomiting, elevated serum transaminase levels and liver changes, then acute brain swelling, consciousness disturbances and seizures.

5 **G93.8 Other specified disorders of brain**

SP **G93.81 Temporal sclerosis**
Hippocampal sclerosis
Mesial temporal sclerosis

IQ **G93.82 Brain death**

SP **G93.89 Other specified disorders of brain**
Postradiation encephalopathy

IQ **G93.9 Disorder of brain, unspecified**

M IQ **G94 *Other disorders of brain in diseases classified elsewhere***
Code first:
underlying disease
EXCLUDES 1 encephalopathy in congenital syphilis (A50.49)
encephalopathy in influenza (J09.X9, J10.81, J11.81)
encephalopathy in syphilis (A52.19)
hydrocephalus in diseases classified elsewhere (G91.4)

4 **G95 Other and unspecified diseases of spinal cord**
EXCLUDES 2 myelitis (G04.-)

SP **G95.0 Syringomyelia and syringobulbia**
DEFINITION Cyst formation within the spinal cord resulting from trauma, hemorrhage, meningitis, tumor, or Chiari 1 malformation. The growing cyst destroys the cord's center, causing neurologic deficits that progress to greater degrees when not treated surgically.

5 **G95.1 Vascular myelopathies**
EXCLUDES 2 intraspinal phlebitis and thrombophlebitis, except non-pyogenic (G08)

SP **G95.11 Acute infarction of spinal cord (embolic) (nonembolic)**
Anoxia of spinal cord
Arterial thrombosis of spinal cord

SP **G95.19 Other vascular myelopathies**
Edema of spinal cord
Hematomyelia
Nonpyogenic intraspinal phlebitis and thrombophlebitis
Subacute necrotic myelopathy

5 **G95.2 Other and unspecified cord compression**

IQ **G95.20 Unspecified cord compression**

SP **G95.29 Other cord compression**

5 **G95.8 Other specified diseases of spinal cord**
EXCLUDES 1 neurogenic bladder NOS (N31.9)
neurogenic bladder due to cauda equina syndrome (G83.4)
neuromuscular dysfunction of bladder without spinal cord lesion (N31.-)

SP **G95.81 Conus medullaris syndrome**

SP **G95.89 Other specified diseases of spinal cord**
Cord bladder NOS
Drug-induced myelopathy
Radiation-induced myelopathy
EXCLUDES 1 myelopathy NOS (G95.9)

IQ **G95.9 Disease of spinal cord, unspecified**
Myelopathy NOS

4 **G96 Other disorders of central nervous system**

5 **G96.0 Cerebrospinal fluid leak**
Code also if applicable:
intracranial hypotension (G96.81-)
EXCLUDES 1 cerebrospinal fluid leak from spinal puncture (G97.0)

SP **G96.00 Cerebrospinal fluid leak, unspecified**
Code also if applicable:
head injury (S00.- to S09.-)

SP **G96.01 Cranial cerebrospinal fluid leak, spontaneous**
Otorrhea due to spontaneous cerebrospinal fluid CSF leak
Rhinorrhea due to spontaneous cerebrospinal fluid CSF leak
Spontaneous cerebrospinal fluid leak from skull base

SP **G96.02 Spinal cerebrospinal fluid leak, spontaneous**
Spontaneous cerebrospinal fluid leak from spine

4 4th digit required 5 5th digit required 6 6th digit required 7 7th digit required 7 7th digit placeholder + Additional code L Laterality

SP **G96.08 Other cranial cerebrospinal fluid leak**
Postoperative cranial cerebrospinal fluid leak
Traumatic cranial cerebrospinal fluid leak
Code also if applicable:
head injury (S00.- to S09.-)

SP **G96.09 Other spinal cerebrospinal fluid leak**
Other spinal CSF leak
Postoperative spinal cerebrospinal fluid leak
Traumatic spinal cerebrospinal fluid leak
Code also if applicable:
head injury (S00.- to S09.-)

5 **G96.1 Disorders of meninges, not elsewhere classified**

SP **G96.11 Dural tear**
Code also:
intracranial hypotension, if applicable (G96.81-)
EXCLUDES 1 accidental puncture or laceration of dura during a procedure (G97.41)

SP **G96.12 Meningeal adhesions (cerebral) (spinal)**

6 **G96.19 Other disorders of meninges, not elsewhere classified**

SP **G96.191 Perineural cyst**
Cervical nerve root cyst
Lumbar nerve root cyst
Sacral nerve root cyst
Tarlov cyst
Thoracic nerve root cyst

SP **G96.198 Other disorders of meninges, not elsewhere classified**

5 **G96.8 Other specified disorders of central nervous system**

6 **G96.81 Intracranial hypotension**
Code also any associated diagnoses, such as:
Brachial amyotrophy (G54.5)
Cerebrospinal fluid leak from spine (G96.02)
Cranial nerve disorders in diseases classified elsewhere (G53)
Nerve root and compressions in diseases classified elsewhere (G55)
Nonpyogenic thrombosis of intracranial venous system (I67.6)
Nontraumatic intracerebral hemorrhage (I61.-)
Nontraumatic subdural hemorrhage (I62.0-)
Other and unspecified cord compression (G95.2-)
Other secondary parkinsonism (G21.8)
Reversible cerebrovascular vasoconstriction syndrome (I67.841)
Spinal cord herniation (G95.89)
Stroke (I63.-)
Syringomyelia (G95.0)

SP **G96.810 Intracranial hypotension, unspecified**

SP **G96.811 Intracranial hypotension, spontaneous**

SP **G96.819 Other intracranial hypotension**

SP **G96.89 Other specified disorders of central nervous system**

IQ **G96.9 Disorder of central nervous system, unspecified**

4 **G97 Intraoperative and postprocedural complications and disorders of nervous system, not elsewhere classified**
EXCLUDES 2 intraoperative and postprocedural cerebrovascular infarction (I97.81-, I97.82-)

CODING TIPS ✓ **Documentation:** Do not assign any code for intraoperative and postprocedural complications and disorders of the nervous system without specific documentation from the patient's provider providing a specific relationship between the complication and the procedure.

SP **G97.0 Cerebrospinal fluid leak from spinal puncture**
Code also any associated diagnoses or complications, such as:
intracranial hypotension following a procedure (G97.83-G97.84)

SP **G97.1 Other reaction to spinal and lumbar puncture**
Headache due to lumbar puncture
Other reaction to spinal dural puncture
Code also:
, if applicable, any associated headache with orthostatic component (R51.0)

SP **G97.2 Intracranial hypotension following ventricular shunting**
Code also:
any associated diagnoses or complications

5 **G97.3 Intraoperative hemorrhage and hematoma of a nervous system organ or structure complicating a procedure**
EXCLUDES 1 intraoperative hemorrhage and hematoma of a nervous system organ or structure due to accidental puncture and laceration during a procedure (G97.4-)

SP **G97.31 Intraoperative hemorrhage and hematoma of a nervous system organ or structure complicating a nervous system procedure**

SP **G97.32 Intraoperative hemorrhage and hematoma of a nervous system organ or structure complicating other procedure**

5 **G97.4 Accidental puncture and laceration of a nervous system organ or structure during a procedure**

SP **G97.41 Accidental puncture or laceration of dura during a procedure**
Incidental (inadvertent) durotomy
Code also:
any associated diagnoses or complications

SP **G97.48 Accidental puncture and laceration of other nervous system organ or structure during a nervous system procedure**

SP **G97.49 Accidental puncture and laceration of other nervous system organ or structure during other procedure**

5 **G97.5 Postprocedural hemorrhage of a nervous system organ or structure following a procedure**

SP **G97.51 Postprocedural hemorrhage of a nervous system organ or structure following a nervous system procedure**

SP **G97.52 Postprocedural hemorrhage of a nervous system organ or structure following other procedure**

5 **G97.6 Postprocedural hematoma and seroma of a nervous system organ or structure following a procedure**

SP **G97.61 Postprocedural hematoma of a nervous system organ or structure following a nervous system procedure**

SP **G97.62 Postprocedural hematoma of a nervous system organ or structure following other procedure**

SP **G97.63 Postprocedural seroma of a nervous system organ or structure following a nervous system procedure**

SP **G97.64 Postprocedural seroma of a nervous system organ or structure following other procedure**

+ 5 **G97.8 Other intraoperative and postprocedural complications and disorders of nervous system**

Use additional code to further specify disorder

SP + **G97.81 Other intraoperative complications of nervous system**

SP + **G97.82 Other postprocedural complications and disorders of nervous system**

SP + **G97.83 Intracranial hypotension following lumbar cerebrospinal fluid shunting**

Code also:
- any associated diagnoses or complications

SP + **G97.84 Intracranial hypotension following other procedure**

Code also, if applicable:
- accidental puncture or laceration of dura during a procedure (G97.41)
- cerebrospinal fluid leak from spinal puncture (G97.0)

4 **G98 Other disorders of nervous system not elsewhere classified**

INCLUDES nervous system disorder NOS

SP **G98.0 Neurogenic arthritis, not elsewhere classified**

Nonsyphilitic neurogenic arthropathy NEC
Nonsyphilitic neurogenic spondylopathy NEC

EXCLUDES 1 spondylopathy (in):
- syringomyelia and syringobulbia (G95.0)
- tabes dorsalis (A52.11)

SP **G98.8 Other disorders of nervous system**

Nervous system disorder NOS

4 **G99 Other disorders of nervous system in diseases classified elsewhere**

M IQ **G99.0** ***Autonomic neuropathy in diseases classified elsewhere***

Code first underlying disease, such as:
- amyloidosis (E85.-)
- gout (M1A.-, M10.-)
- hyperthyroidism (E05.-)

EXCLUDES 1 diabetic autonomic neuropathy (E08-E13 with .43)

CODING TIPS ✓ This neuropathy affects the heart, digestive system and other involuntary functions. This type of neuropathy (G99.0) causes delayed or slowed gastric emptying as well as problems with orthostatic hypotension. This code is not to be used for polyneuropathy of the hands and feet. It is not to be coded as a manifestation of diabetes.

M IQ **G99.2** ***Myelopathy in diseases classified elsewhere***

Code first underlying disease, such as:
- neoplasm (C00-D49)

EXCLUDES 1 myelopathy in:
- intervertebral disease (M50.0-, M51.0-)
- spondylosis (M47.0-, M47.1-)

M IQ **G99.8** ***Other specified disorders of nervous system in diseases classified elsewhere***

Code first underlying disorder, such as:
- amyloidosis (E85.-)
- avitaminosis (E56.9)

EXCLUDES 1 nervous system involvement in:
- cysticercosis (B69.0)
- rubella (B06.0-)
- syphilis (A52.1-)

Chapter 6 Scenarios: Diseases of the nervous system (G00-G99)

Left hip fracture, intractable epilepsy

A 57-year-old woman underwent surgery to repair a fractured left hip sustained during a recent seizure. She has epilepsy that is documented as resistant to treatment. She is admitted to home health to recovery from the fracture and for medication management and occupational therapy.

Description	Code
Primary: Fracture of unspecified part of neck of left femur, subsequent encounter for closed fracture with routine healing	S72.002D
Secondary: Epilepsy, unspecified, intractable, without status epilepticus	G40.919

Though the patient underwent surgery to treat the fracture, a surgical aftercare code is not assigned, in accordance with coding guidelines. Rather, the fracture itself is coded. Since the epilepsy is stated to be resistant to treatment, it is coded as intractable. Be careful to assign the code for the hip fracture that identifies the affected side of the body. Unspecified hip fracture codes are unacceptable primary diagnoses in PDGM.

Neoplasm-related pain, breast cancer, liver mets

A 90-year-old woman is admitted to home health to treat severe pain that is reported as related to breast cancer that has spread to her liver.

Description	Code
Primary: Neoplasm-related pain	G89.3
Secondary: Malignant neoplasm of unspecified site of unspecified female breast	C50.919
Secondary: Secondary malignant neoplasm of liver	C78.7

As the focus of care, the neoplasm-related pain is coded in the primary position. The patient's breast cancer and the mets to the liver are coded in the secondary positions as relevant co-morbidities.

Multiple sclerosis

A 48-year-old woman was admitted to the hospital with intractable pain and muscle spasms. The physician diagnosed it as an exacerbation of multiple sclerosis (MS). Upon admission to home care for physical and occupational therapy, she was found to have continued bouts of spasms, muscle weakness, decreased range of motion in her joints, poor functional mobility and an ataxic gait pattern. The referral further stated the patient has hypertension, chronic diastolic heart failure, neurogenic bladder, and is paraplegic resulting in confinement to the wheelchair.

Description	Code
Primary: Multiple sclerosis	G35
Secondary: Paraplegia, unspecified	G82.20
Secondary: Neurogenic bladder NOS	N31.9
Secondary: Hypertensive heart disease with heart failure	I11.0
Secondary: Chronic diastolic (congestive) heart failure	I50.32

There are no ICD-10 codes that are specifically for therapy. Rather coding guidelines state to code the reason therapy is seeing the patient, which, in this case, would be the multiple sclerosis. G35 is coded primary as this is the focus of care. No additional codes are required for the weakness, spasms, problems with range of motion, gait or functional mobility as these are all integral symptoms to the multiple sclerosis disease process. As such, they should not be additionally coded. Not all MS patients have neurogenic bladder though. Therefore, it should be coded additionally when present with MS. The additional comorbidities of hypertension, chronic diastolic heart failure, and paraplegia, impact the patient's prognosis and may provide important comorbidity adjustment for episodic payment so these are also coded. Paraplegia is not integral to the disease process of MS.

PT for Parkinson's with recent falls

A Parkinson's patient requires physical therapy. The referral notes recent falls and requests that the therapist investigate the increase in falls. The therapist's Plan of Care includes instructing the patient on the signs and symptoms of the disease, strategies to address freezing episodes, stretching of anterior muscles, positioning, strengthening of posterior muscles, fall prevention techniques and gait training. The therapist also performs a home-safety evaluation and modifies the patient's environment as needed to reduce the risk of falls.

Description	Code
Primary: Parkinson's disease	G20
Secondary: Repeated Falls	R29.6
Secondary: History of Falling	Z91.81

There are no therapy codes in ICD-10-CM; coding guidelines state to code the primary reason for therapy. In this scenario, the Parkinson's disease is the primary reason for home health and the focus of care for physical therapy, and is therefore coded as primary. The code R29.6, Repeated falls, is assigned when the patient has had recent falls and the plan of care indicates a need to investigate the cause of recent falls. The Excludes 2 note allows the coder to also code Z91.81, history of falling, with R29.6. The code Z91.81 indicates that a patient has previously fallen in the past and continues to be at risk for future falls.

Hemiplegia affecting non-dominant side

A 70-year-old man suffered a traumatic brain injury with a subdural hematoma following a loss of consciousness, due to a fall down the stairs. He has spastic hemiplegia of the right non-dominant side and dysphagia resulting from the resolved subdural hematoma. He has a PEG tube due to the dysphagia. His family requires teaching on the care of the PEG tube. The patient also has a recurring stage 3 ulcer of the coccyx that the nurse will be providing wound care for. The patient requires PT, OT, and ST to address the residual deficits from the traumatic brain injury and this is the focus of care.

Description	Code
Primary: Spastic hemiplegia affecting right non-dominant side	G81.13
Secondary: Dysphagia, unspecified	R13.10
Secondary: Traumatic subdural hemorrhage with loss of consciousness of unspecified duration, sequela	S06.5x9S
Secondary: Pressure ulcer of sacral region, stage 3	L89.153
Secondary: Encounter for attention to gastrostomy	Z43.1
Secondary: Fall (on) (from) other stairs and steps, sequela	W10.8XXS

Sequence first the residual conditions (non-dominant hemiplegia and dysphagia) resulting from the traumatic brain injury, followed by the injury code with the 7th character "S" (sequela), per coding guidelines. Be sure not to code the symptom, dysphagia, as primary as it is considered a questionable encounter code in PDGM. Assign Z43.1 because the agency will be teaching the family to care for the PEG tube. If the patient/family was independent in the care of the PEG tube, Z93.1 would be assigned instead. The external cause code to report the cause of the accident should also be reported with a 7th character "S," in accordance with coding guidelines.

Epilepsy

A patient is admitted for evaluation and control of his intractable seizures. His video EEGs were consistent with epileptiform discharges of the right temporal lobe origin. Family will be instructed in care and management of epilepsy. Dilantin and Phenobarbital must be adjusted and monitored by home health nurses and venipuncture is ordered for therapeutic/toxicity testing. Diagnosis was partial complex epilepsy localized to the right temporal lobe, with impairment of consciousness.

Description	Code
Primary: Localization related symptomatic epilepsy and epileptic syndromes with complex partial seizures, intractable, without status epilepticus	G40.219
Secondary: Encounter for therapeutic drug monitoring	Z51.81
Secondary: Long-term (current) use of other medications	Z79.899

Partial complex epilepsy references G40.219 when intractable. The venipuncture and medication management are captured with Z51.81 and Z79.899.

Early-onset Alzheimer's disease with wandering

A 60-year-old female with early-onset Alzheimer’s disease is admitted to home care for safety concerns as to a recent onset of agitation and wandering associated with the Alzheimer's disease. She required a replacement of her gastrostomy tube as she pulled it out, and she has a history of dysphagia. She is visibly agitated during clinical interview and her daughter states this has become worse in past few months.

Description	Code
Primary: Alzheimer's disease with early onset	G30.0
Secondary: Dementia in other disease classified elsewhere with behavioral disturbance	F02.81
Secondary: Wandering in diseases classified elsewhere	Z91.83
Secondary: Dysphagia, unspecified	R13.10
Secondary: Encounter for attention to gastrostomy	Z43.1

The patient has a diagnosis of early-onset Alzheimer's dementia. While early onset Alzheimer’s is defined as a diagnosis before the age of 65, you must query the physician to confirm it. Since the diagnosis is confirmed in this case, it is coded with G30.0. The dementia code follows the Alzheimer’s code in accordance with the etiology-manifestation convention and in accordance with Q1 2017 Coding Clinic guidance. Because she is experiencing behavioral disturbance, the dementia code F02.81 is assigned to reflect that. Wandering is coded additionally in accordance with tabular instruction.

Alzheimer's dementia with hypertension

A 72-year-old patient was recently discharged from the hospital where he was treated for uncontrolled hypertension due to inability to take prescribed medications. While there he was diagnosed with late onset Alzheimer's dementia. He is not experiencing behavioral changes, and is now admitted to home care for physical therapy and skilled nursing for safety and medication teaching. The focus of care for the episode will be the Alzheimer's dementia, as this condition is what resulted in the patient's inability to understand and self administer medications safely.

Description	Code
Primary: Alzheimer's disease with late onset	G30.1
Secondary: Dementia in other disease classified elsewhere without behavioral disturbance	F02.80
Secondary: Essential (primary) hypertension	I10
Secondary: Underdosing of other antihypertensive drugs, subsequent encounter	T46.5x6D
Secondary: Patient's unintentional underdosing of medication regimen for other reason	Z91.138

The patient was recently diagnosed with late onset Alzheimer's dementia, so it should be coded with G30.1. An additional code for dementia is also assigned, in accordance with Q1 2017 Coding Clinic guidance. He was treated in the hospital for uncontrolled hypertension, which will require continued monitoring in the home health setting, and thus I10 is assigned to capture that as well. Code T46.5x6D is included to indicate that the patient's uncontrolled hypertension was caused by his inability to take his medication. This code should never be listed primary. Additionally, chapter-specific guidelines instruct the coder to use an additional code to indicate the intent of the patient's non-compliance with his medication regimen and thus Z91.138 is assigned in accordance with this. *[I.C.19.e.5.c]*

Alzheimer's delirium, viral pneumonia

A 56-year-old patient who has had Alzheimer's disease for five years was recently hospitalized with viral pneumonia. She has now been admitted to home care for skilled nursing for continued treatment of the pneumonia. The family says the patient is exhibiting signs of delirium. The nurse queried the physician and confirmed a diagnosis of early onset Alzheimer's with delirium.

Description	Code
Primary: Viral pneumonia, unspecified	J12.9
Secondary: Alzheimer's disease with early onset	G30.0
Secondary: Dementia in other diseases classified elsewhere with behavioral disturbance	F02.81
Secondary: Delirium due to known physiological condition	F05

The patient was diagnosed with Alzheimer's well before the age of 65, and while early onset is defined as a diagnosis before the age of 65, you must query the physician to confirm it, which the nurse did, and thus it is coded with G30.0 As the focus of care, pneumonia is coded primary. The Alzheimer's is coded next because it must be sequenced before the delirium. The dementia code, F02.81, immediately follows the Alzheimer's code as it's part of an etiology/manifestation pairing. Because the patient is experiencing delirium, behavioral disturbance is present and F02.81 is used. The delirium code, F05, follows it.

ALS with tracheostomy care

A 59-year-old man with amyotrophic lateral sclerosis (ALS) recently had a tracheostomy placed to assist in breathing. His family requires reaching on how to care for it. He is wheelchair bound. The tracheostomy is the focus of care.

Description	Code
Primary: Encounter for attention to tracheostomy	Z43.0
Secondary: Amyotrophic lateral sclerosis	G12.21
Secondary: Dependence on wheelchair	Z99.3

The agency will be providing care to the tracheostomy, so a code from Z43.- (Encounter for attention to artificial openings) is appropriate versus a code from Z93.- (Artificial opening status).

Lewy body dementia

A 77-year-old man is admitted to home health for teaching and medication following a recent diagnosis of Lewy body dementia. He has been experiencing agitation and outbursts. Additional comorbidities include congestive heart failure. The Lewy body dementia with outbursts is the focus of care.

Description	Code
Primary: Dementia with Lewy bodies	G31.83
Secondary: Dementia in other diseases classified elsewhere with behavioral disturbance	F02.81
Secondary: Heart failure, unspecified	I50.9

As the primary diagnosis, Lewy body dementia is coded primary. Because the patient is experiencing behavioral disturbance, F02.81 is assigned immediately after. As a comorbidity that will impact his plan of care, his congestive heart failure is coded.

Alcoholic encephalopathy, alcohol-induced diabetes

A 71-year-old man was admitted to home health with a primary diagnosis of alcoholic encephalopathy, which has led to dementia. He also has type 2 diabetes, which his medical record says is the result of heavy drinking, and hypertension. He's been an alcoholic for 37 years and continues to drink heavily.

Description	Code
Primary: Degeneration of nervous system due to alcohol	G31.2
Secondary: Dementia in other diseases classified elsewhere without behavioral disturbance	F02.80
Secondary: Alcohol dependence with alcohol-induced persisting dementia	F10.27
Secondary: Toxic effect of ethanol, accidental (unintentional), subsequent encounter	T51.0x1D
Secondary: Drug or chemical induced diabetes mellitus without complications	E09.9
Secondary: Essential (primary) hypertension	I10

As the focus of care the alcoholic encephalopathy is coded primary. It has caused dementia, so the necessary dementia manifestation code immediately follows it, in accordance with the etiology-manifestation convention. Code F10.27 is coded to capture his continued alcoholism. Alcoholism codes to dependence in the alphabetic index and the more specific code was chosen to show that the alcoholism ultimately led to dementia. His diabetes is an important comorbidity and since it was caused by alcohol use, it must be coded as drug or chemical-induced diabetes, with the code for the toxic effect of alcohol preceding the diabetes code, in accordance with tabular instruction. Hypertension is coded as a relevant comorbidity.

Diabetes with alcoholic neuropathy

A patient is referred for skilled nursing, occupational and physical therapy after being diagnosed with neuropathy due to long-term alcohol dependence, which his physician states is in remission. Prior to these diagnoses, he had been diagnosed with polyneuropathy due to diabetes and PVD. His diabetes is diet controlled.

Description	Code
Primary: Alcoholic polyneuropathy	G62.1
Secondary: Alcohol dependence, in remission	F10.21
Secondary: Type 2 diabetes mellitus with diabetic polyneuropathy	E11.42
Secondary: Type 2 diabetes mellitus with diabetic peripheral angiopathy without gangrene	E11.51

When a diagnosis of alcoholic polyneuropathy is specified, assign G62.1, followed by the appropriate code from category F10, alcohol related disorders. If the provider indicates the patient is not currently drinking, assign the appropriate "in remission" code. If the pattern of alcohol use (dependence or abuse) is not known, assign code F10.988, Alcohol use, unspecified with other alcohol-induced disorder, per Q3 2019 Coding Clinic Guidance. Additional codes for diabetes with polyneuropathy and diabetes with peripheral angiopathy are assigned. Since the provider did not indicate the prior diagnosis of diabetic polyneuropathy was invalid, both may be coded.

Multiple Sclerosis with polyneuropathy

A 52-year-old female patient is referred to home health for physical and occupational therapy due to a decline in functional mobility and self-care. The face-to-face encounter reports that the patient's recent decline is primarily related to an exacerbation of multiple sclerosis with associated polyneuropathy. Comorbid diagnoses listed include diabetes and neurogenic bladder.

Description	Code
Primary: Multiple sclerosis	G35
Secondary: Polyneuropathy in diseases classified elsewhere	G63
Secondary: Type 2 diabetes mellitus without complications	E11.9
Secondary: Neuromuscular dysfunction of bladder, unspecified	N31.9

This patient was referred for therapy services to address a decline in function due to MS and associated polyneuropathy and this is the focus of care, so it is coded as primary. Based upon Q1 2021 Coding Clinic guidance, peripheral/polyneuropathy related to MS should be coded using G63, Polyneuropathy in diseases classified elsewhere, as a manifestation of the MS, when stated as a diagnosis by the provider. While this patient has diabetes, the polyneuropathy is not associated to the diabetes because the provider has clearly indicated a different cause for the condition. Neurogenic bladder also impacts the patient's overall neurological progress and condition and should also be coded.

Chapter 7: Diseases of the Eye and Adnexa (H00-H59)

Chapter 7 includes codes related to conditions of the eye and adnexa, including intraoperative and postprocedural complications and disorders of the eye and adnexa.

Use an external cause code, following the code for the eye condition, if applicable, to identify the cause of the eye condition.

It's important to note that the beginning of this chapter indicates a number of conditions that fall into the Excludes 2 note. In these situations, the conditions are not included in the H00-H59 codes, but may be coded in addition to a code from H00-H59. Refer to the codes in Chapter 7 to determine appropriate sequencing of the codes.

The Excludes 2 note includes the following conditions:

- Certain conditions originating in the perinatal period (P00-P96) located in chapter 16.
- Certain infections and parasitic diseases (A00-B99) located in chapter 1.
- Complications of pregnancy, childbirth and the puerperium (O00–O9A) located in chapter 15.
- Congenital malformations, deformations and chromosomal abnormalities (Q00-Q99) in chapter 17.
- Diabetes mellitus related eye conditions (E09.3-, E10.3-, E11.3-, E13.3-) located in chapter 4.
- Endocrine, nutritional and metabolic diseases (E00-E88) located in chapter 4.
- Injury (trauma) of eye and orbit (S05.-) located in chapter 19.
- Injury, poisoning and certain other consequences of external causes (S00-T88) located in chapter 19.
- Neoplasms (C00-D49) in chapter 2.
- Symptoms, signs and abnormal clinical and laboratory findings (R00-R94) located in chapter 18.
- Syphilis related eye disorders (A50.1, A50.3-, A51.43, A52.71) located in Chapter 1.

Sensory organs

In general, each of the sensory organs has the same basic structure. The sensory organs are composed of sensory receptors, which translate light, mechanical, or chemical stimuli into electrical impulses. Often the tip of the sensory nerve fiber is associated with accessory tissues that amplify the stimulus and increase the sensitivity of the receptor.

Diabetic retinopathy, diabetic glaucoma, and other diabetic vision issues are manifestations of diabetes. In ICD-10-CM, there are combination codes that combine the underlying situation (e.g., diabetes) and the manifestation into one combination code. ***Note:*** Retinopathy due to conditions such as arteriosclerosis and sickle cell disease continue to use the etiology/ manifestation convention in coding.

Conjunctivitis of the eye has more than two dozen different ICD-10-CM codes to sift through. When choosing the appropriate ICD-10-CM code for conjunctivitis, it's important to identify the cause of the inflammation.

Blindness can be found under "blindness" in the Alphabetical Index. The key terms 'low' and 'loss' have a "see blindness notation" but also have references for low vision and loss of vision. Blindness and low vision codes in category H54 have a note to code first any associated underlying cause of the blindness.

Code H54.8 (Legal blindness, as defined in USA) includes a table that gives a classification of severity of visual impairment recommended by a 1972 WHO Study Group on the Prevention of Blindness. The term "low vision" in category H54 comprises categories 1 and 2 of the table, the term blindness is in categories 3, 4, and 5, and the term unqualified visual loss is in category 9. Confirm a low vision diagnosis with the physician to support the use of the code.

If "blindness" or "low vision" of both eyes is documented but the visual impairment category is not documented, assign code H54.3, Unqualified visual loss, both eyes. If "blindness" or "low vision" in one eye is documented but the visual impairment category is not documented, assign a code from H54.6-, Unqualified visual loss, one eye, per coding guidelines.

Glaucoma

Assign as many codes from category H40 (Glaucoma) as needed to identify the type of glaucoma, the affected eye and the glaucoma stage.

When a patient has bilateral glaucoma and both eyes are documented as being the same type and stage, and there is a code for bilateral glaucoma, report only the code for the type of glaucoma, bilateral, with the seventh character for the stage.

When a patient has bilateral glaucoma and both eyes are documented as being the same type and stage, and the classification does not provide a code for bilateral glaucoma (i.e., subcategories H40.10, and H40.20) report only one code for the type of glaucoma with the appropriate seventh character for the stage.

When a patient has bilateral glaucoma and each eye is documented as having a different type or stage, and the classification distinguishes laterality, assign the appropriate code for each eye rather than the code for bilateral glaucoma.

When a patient has bilateral glaucoma and each eye is documented as having a different type, and the classification does not distinguish laterality (i.e. H40.10, and H40.20), assign one code for each type of glaucoma with the appropriate seventh character for the stage.

When a patient has bilateral glaucoma and each eye is documented as having the same type, but different stage, and the classification does not distinguish laterality (i.e. subcategories H40.10, and H40.20), assign a code for the type of glaucoma for each eye.

If a patient is admitted with glaucoma and the stage progresses during the admission, assign the code for the highest stage documented.

Assignment of the seventh character "4" for "indeterminate stage" should be based on the clinical documentation. The seventh character "4" is used for glaucoma in which stage cannot be clinically determined. The seventh character "4" should not be confused with the seventh character "0," unspecified, which should be assigned when there is no documentation regarding the stage of the glaucoma.

As with all coding, watch for notes to code first underlying diseases and add additional codes.

CHAPTER 7: DISEASES OF THE EYE AND ADNEXA (H00-H59)

Note:
Use an external cause code following the code for the eye condition, if applicable, to identify the cause of the eye condition

EXCLUDES 2 certain conditions originating in the perinatal period (P04-P96)
certain infectious and parasitic diseases (A00-B99)
complications of pregnancy, childbirth and the puerperium (O00-O9A)
congenital malformations, deformations, and chromosomal abnormalities (Q00-Q99)
diabetes mellitus related eye conditions (E09.3-, E10.3-, E11.3-, E13.3-)
endocrine, nutritional and metabolic diseases (E00-E88)
injury (trauma) of eye and orbit (S05.-)
injury, poisoning and certain other consequences of external causes (S00-T88)
neoplasms (C00-D49)
symptoms, signs and abnormal clinical and laboratory findings, not elsewhere classified (R00-R94)
syphilis related eye disorders (A50.01, A50.3-, A51.43, A52.71)

This chapter contains the following blocks:

H00-H05	Disorders of eyelid, lacrimal system and orbit
H10-H11	Disorders of conjunctiva
H15-H22	Disorders of sclera, cornea, iris and ciliary body
H25-H28	Disorders of lens
H30-H36	Disorders of choroid and retina
H40-H42	Glaucoma
H43-H44	Disorders of vitreous body and globe
H46-H47	Disorders of optic nerve and visual pathways
H49-H52	Disorders of ocular muscles, binocular movement, accommodation and refraction
H53-H54	Visual disturbances and blindness
H55-H57	Other disorders of eye and adnexa
H59	Intraoperative and postprocedural complications and disorders of eye and adnexa, not elsewhere classified

Disorders of eyelid, lacrimal system and orbit (H00-H05)

EXCLUDES 2 open wound of eyelid (S01.1-)
superficial injury of eyelid (S00.1-, S00.2-)

4 **H00 Hordeolum and chalazion**

5 **H00.0 Hordeolum (externum) (internum) of eyelid**

6 **H00.01 Hordeolum externum**
Hordeolum NOS
Stye
DEFINITION Staph infection of an oil gland in an eyelash follicle.

SP **H00.011 Hordeolum externum right upper eyelid**
SP **H00.012 Hordeolum externum right lower eyelid**
IQ **H00.013 Hordeolum externum right eye, unspecified eyelid**
SP **H00.014 Hordeolum externum left upper eyelid**
SP **H00.015 Hordeolum externum left lower eyelid**
IQ **H00.016 Hordeolum externum left eye, unspecified eyelid**
IQ **H00.019 Hordeolum externum unspecified eye, unspecified eyelid**

6 **H00.02 Hordeolum internum**
Infection of meibomian gland

SP **H00.021 Hordeolum internum right upper eyelid**
SP **H00.022 Hordeolum internum right lower eyelid**
IQ **H00.023 Hordeolum internum right eye, unspecified eyelid**
SP **H00.024 Hordeolum internum left upper eyelid**
SP **H00.025 Hordeolum internum left lower eyelid**
IQ **H00.026 Hordeolum internum left eye, unspecified eyelid**
IQ **H00.029 Hordeolum internum unspecified eye, unspecified eyelid**

6 **H00.03 Abscess of eyelid**
Furuncle of eyelid

SP **H00.031 Abscess of right upper eyelid**
SP **H00.032 Abscess of right lower eyelid**
IQ **H00.033 Abscess of eyelid right eye, unspecified eyelid**
SP **H00.034 Abscess of left upper eyelid**
SP **H00.035 Abscess of left lower eyelid**
IQ **H00.036 Abscess of eyelid left eye, unspecified eyelid**
IQ **H00.039 Abscess of eyelid unspecified eye, unspecified eyelid**

5 **H00.1 Chalazion**
Meibomian (gland) cyst
EXCLUDES 2 infected meibomian gland (H00.02-)
DEFINITION Cyst of the tarsal (eyelid) gland.

SP **H00.11 Chalazion right upper eyelid**
SP **H00.12 Chalazion right lower eyelid**
IQ **H00.13 Chalazion right eye, unspecified eyelid**
SP **H00.14 Chalazion left upper eyelid**
SP **H00.15 Chalazion left lower eyelid**
IQ **H00.16 Chalazion left eye, unspecified eyelid**
IQ **H00.19 Chalazion unspecified eye, unspecified eyelid**

4 **H01 Other inflammation of eyelid**

5 **H01.0 Blepharitis**
EXCLUDES 1 blepharoconjunctivitis (H10.5-)

6 **H01.00 Unspecified blepharitis**
DEFINITION An inflammation of the eyelids or lid margins.

SP **H01.001 Unspecified blepharitis right upper eyelid**
SP **H01.002 Unspecified blepharitis right lower eyelid**
IQ **H01.003 Unspecified blepharitis right eye, unspecified eyelid**

Chapter 7
H00-H59

⊟ SP **H01.004** **Unspecified blepharitis left upper eyelid**
⊟ SP **H01.005** **Unspecified blepharitis left lower eyelid**
⊟ !Q **H01.006** **Unspecified blepharitis left eye, unspecified eyelid**
⊟ !Q **H01.009** **Unspecified blepharitis unspecified eye, unspecified eyelid**
⊟ SP **H01.00A** **Unspecified blepharitis right eye, upper and lower eyelids**
⊟ SP **H01.00B** **Unspecified blepharitis left eye, upper and lower eyelids**

6 **H01.01 Ulcerative blepharitis**
⊟ SP **H01.011** **Ulcerative blepharitis right upper eyelid**
⊟ SP **H01.012** **Ulcerative blepharitis right lower eyelid**
⊟ !Q **H01.013** **Ulcerative blepharitis right eye, unspecified eyelid**
⊟ SP **H01.014** **Ulcerative blepharitis left upper eyelid**
⊟ SP **H01.015** **Ulcerative blepharitis left lower eyelid**
⊟ !Q **H01.016** **Ulcerative blepharitis left eye, unspecified eyelid**
⊟ !Q **H01.019** **Ulcerative blepharitis unspecified eye, unspecified eyelid**
⊟ SP **H01.01A** **Ulcerative blepharitis right eye, upper and lower eyelids**
⊟ SP **H01.01B** **Ulcerative blepharitis left eye, upper and lower eyelids**

6 **H01.02 Squamous blepharitis**
⊟ SP **H01.021** **Squamous blepharitis right upper eyelid**
⊟ SP **H01.022** **Squamous blepharitis right lower eyelid**
⊟ !Q **H01.023** **Squamous blepharitis right eye, unspecified eyelid**
⊟ SP **H01.024** **Squamous blepharitis left upper eyelid**
⊟ SP **H01.025** **Squamous blepharitis left lower eyelid**
⊟ !Q **H01.026** **Squamous blepharitis left eye, unspecified eyelid**
⊟ !Q **H01.029** **Squamous blepharitis unspecified eye, unspecified eyelid**
⊟ SP **H01.02A** **Squamous blepharitis right eye, upper and lower eyelids**
⊟ SP **H01.02B** **Squamous blepharitis left eye, upper and lower eyelids**

5 **H01.1 Noninfectious dermatoses of eyelid**

6 **H01.11 Allergic dermatitis of eyelid**
Contact dermatitis of eyelid
⊟ SP **H01.111** **Allergic dermatitis of right upper eyelid**
⊟ SP **H01.112** **Allergic dermatitis of right lower eyelid**
⊟ !Q **H01.113** **Allergic dermatitis of right eye, unspecified eyelid**
⊟ SP **H01.114** **Allergic dermatitis of left upper eyelid**
⊟ SP **H01.115** **Allergic dermatitis of left lower eyelid**
⊟ !Q **H01.116** **Allergic dermatitis of left eye, unspecified eyelid**
⊟ !Q **H01.119** **Allergic dermatitis of unspecified eye, unspecified eyelid**

6 **H01.12 Discoid lupus erythematosus of eyelid**
⊟ SP **H01.121** **Discoid lupus erythematosus of right upper eyelid**
⊟ SP **H01.122** **Discoid lupus erythematosus of right lower eyelid**
⊟ !Q **H01.123** **Discoid lupus erythematosus of right eye, unspecified eyelid**
⊟ SP **H01.124** **Discoid lupus erythematosus of left upper eyelid**
⊟ SP **H01.125** **Discoid lupus erythematosus of left lower eyelid**
⊟ !Q **H01.126** **Discoid lupus erythematosus of left eye, unspecified eyelid**
⊟ !Q **H01.129** **Discoid lupus erythematosus of unspecified eye, unspecified eyelid**

6 **H01.13 Eczematous dermatitis of eyelid**
⊟ SP **H01.131** **Eczematous dermatitis of right upper eyelid**
⊟ SP **H01.132** **Eczematous dermatitis of right lower eyelid**
⊟ !Q **H01.133** **Eczematous dermatitis of right eye, unspecified eyelid**
⊟ SP **H01.134** **Eczematous dermatitis of left upper eyelid**
⊟ SP **H01.135** **Eczematous dermatitis of left lower eyelid**
⊟ !Q **H01.136** **Eczematous dermatitis of left eye, unspecified eyelid**
⊟ !Q **H01.139** **Eczematous dermatitis of unspecified eye, unspecified eyelid**

6 **H01.14 Xeroderma of eyelid**
⊟ SP **H01.141** **Xeroderma of right upper eyelid**
⊟ SP **H01.142** **Xeroderma of right lower eyelid**
⊟ !Q **H01.143** **Xeroderma of right eye, unspecified eyelid**
⊟ SP **H01.144** **Xeroderma of left upper eyelid**
⊟ SP **H01.145** **Xeroderma of left lower eyelid**
⊟ !Q **H01.146** **Xeroderma of left eye, unspecified eyelid**
⊟ !Q **H01.149** **Xeroderma of unspecified eye, unspecified eyelid**

SP **H01.8 Other specified inflammations of eyelid**

!Q **H01.9 Unspecified inflammation of eyelid**
Inflammation of eyelid NOS

4 **H02 Other disorders of eyelid**
EXCLUDES 1 congenital malformations of eyelid (Q10.0-Q10.3)

5 **H02.0 Entropion and trichiasis of eyelid**

6 **H02.00 Unspecified entropion of eyelid**
DEFINITION Inward curling of the eyelid margin, usually the bottom, so the lashes irritate the surface of the eyeball.
⊟ SP **H02.001** **Unspecified entropion of right upper eyelid**
⊟ SP **H02.002** **Unspecified entropion of right lower eyelid**

4 4th digit required 5 5th digit required 6 6th digit required 7 7th digit required 7 7th digit placeholder + Additional code ⊟ Laterality

- H02.003 Unspecified entropion of right eye, unspecified eyelid
- H02.004 Unspecified entropion of left upper eyelid
- H02.005 Unspecified entropion of left lower eyelid
- H02.006 Unspecified entropion of left eye, unspecified eyelid
- H02.009 Unspecified entropion of unspecified eye, unspecified eyelid

H02.01 Cicatricial entropion of eyelid

- H02.011 Cicatricial entropion of right upper eyelid
- H02.012 Cicatricial entropion of right lower eyelid
- H02.013 Cicatricial entropion of right eye, unspecified eyelid
- H02.014 Cicatricial entropion of left upper eyelid
- H02.015 Cicatricial entropion of left lower eyelid
- H02.016 Cicatricial entropion of left eye, unspecified eyelid
- H02.019 Cicatricial entropion of unspecified eye, unspecified eyelid

H02.02 Mechanical entropion of eyelid

- H02.021 Mechanical entropion of right upper eyelid
- H02.022 Mechanical entropion of right lower eyelid
- H02.023 Mechanical entropion of right eye, unspecified eyelid
- H02.024 Mechanical entropion of left upper eyelid
- H02.025 Mechanical entropion of left lower eyelid
- H02.026 Mechanical entropion of left eye, unspecified eyelid
- H02.029 Mechanical entropion of unspecified eye, unspecified eyelid

H02.03 Senile entropion of eyelid

- H02.031 Senile entropion of right upper eyelid
- H02.032 Senile entropion of right lower eyelid
- H02.033 Senile entropion of right eye, unspecified eyelid
- H02.034 Senile entropion of left upper eyelid
- H02.035 Senile entropion of left lower eyelid
- H02.036 Senile entropion of left eye, unspecified eyelid
- H02.039 Senile entropion of unspecified eye, unspecified eyelid

H02.04 Spastic entropion of eyelid

- H02.041 Spastic entropion of right upper eyelid
- H02.042 Spastic entropion of right lower eyelid
- H02.043 Spastic entropion of right eye, unspecified eyelid
- H02.044 Spastic entropion of left upper eyelid
- H02.045 Spastic entropion of left lower eyelid
- H02.046 Spastic entropion of left eye, unspecified eyelid
- H02.049 Spastic entropion of unspecified eye, unspecified eyelid

H02.05 Trichiasis without entropion

- H02.051 Trichiasis without entropion right upper eyelid
- H02.052 Trichiasis without entropion right lower eyelid
- H02.053 Trichiasis without entropion right eye, unspecified eyelid
- H02.054 Trichiasis without entropion left upper eyelid
- H02.055 Trichiasis without entropion left lower eyelid
- H02.056 Trichiasis without entropion left eye, unspecified eyelid
- H02.059 Trichiasis without entropion unspecified eye, unspecified eyelid

H02.1 Ectropion of eyelid

H02.10 Unspecified ectropion of eyelid

DEFINITION Outward curling of the eyelid away from the eye, usually the lower, exposing the inner surface and causing irritation, dryness, pain and possible conjunctivitis and keratitis.

- H02.101 Unspecified ectropion of right upper eyelid
- H02.102 Unspecified ectropion of right lower eyelid
- H02.103 Unspecified ectropion of right eye, unspecified eyelid
- H02.104 Unspecified ectropion of left upper eyelid
- H02.105 Unspecified ectropion of left lower eyelid
- H02.106 Unspecified ectropion of left eye, unspecified eyelid
- H02.109 Unspecified ectropion of unspecified eye, unspecified eyelid

H02.11 Cicatricial ectropion of eyelid

- H02.111 Cicatricial ectropion of right upper eyelid
- H02.112 Cicatricial ectropion of right lower eyelid
- H02.113 Cicatricial ectropion of right eye, unspecified eyelid
- H02.114 Cicatricial ectropion of left upper eyelid
- H02.115 Cicatricial ectropion of left lower eyelid
- H02.116 Cicatricial ectropion of left eye, unspecified eyelid
- H02.119 Cicatricial ectropion of unspecified eye, unspecified eyelid

H02.12 Mechanical ectropion of eyelid

⊟ SP H02.121 Mechanical ectropion of right upper eyelid
⊟ SP H02.122 Mechanical ectropion of right lower eyelid
⊟ !Q H02.123 Mechanical ectropion of right eye, unspecified eyelid
⊟ SP H02.124 Mechanical ectropion of left upper eyelid
⊟ SP H02.125 Mechanical ectropion of left lower eyelid
⊟ !Q H02.126 Mechanical ectropion of left eye, unspecified eyelid
⊟ !Q H02.129 Mechanical ectropion of unspecified eye, unspecified eyelid

6 H02.13 Senile ectropion of eyelid

⊟ SP H02.131 Senile ectropion of right upper eyelid
⊟ SP H02.132 Senile ectropion of right lower eyelid
⊟ !Q H02.133 Senile ectropion of right eye, unspecified eyelid
⊟ SP H02.134 Senile ectropion of left upper eyelid
⊟ SP H02.135 Senile ectropion of left lower eyelid
⊟ !Q H02.136 Senile ectropion of left eye, unspecified eyelid
⊟ !Q H02.139 Senile ectropion of unspecified eye, unspecified eyelid

6 H02.14 Spastic ectropion of eyelid

⊟ SP H02.141 Spastic ectropion of right upper eyelid
⊟ SP H02.142 Spastic ectropion of right lower eyelid
⊟ !Q H02.143 Spastic ectropion of right eye, unspecified eyelid
⊟ SP H02.144 Spastic ectropion of left upper eyelid
⊟ SP H02.145 Spastic ectropion of left lower eyelid
⊟ !Q H02.146 Spastic ectropion of left eye, unspecified eyelid
⊟ !Q H02.149 Spastic ectropion of unspecified eye, unspecified eyelid

6 H02.15 Paralytic ectropion of eyelid

⊟ SP H02.151 Paralytic ectropion of right upper eyelid
⊟ SP H02.152 Paralytic ectropion of right lower eyelid
⊟ !Q H02.153 Paralytic ectropion of right eye, unspecified eyelid
⊟ SP H02.154 Paralytic ectropion of left upper eyelid
⊟ SP H02.155 Paralytic ectropion of left lower eyelid
⊟ !Q H02.156 Paralytic ectropion of left eye, unspecified eyelid
⊟ !Q H02.159 Paralytic ectropion of unspecified eye, unspecified eyelid

5 H02.2 Lagophthalmos

6 H02.20 Unspecified lagophthalmos

⊟ SP H02.201 Unspecified lagophthalmos right upper eyelid
⊟ SP H02.202 Unspecified lagophthalmos right lower eyelid
⊟ !Q H02.203 Unspecified lagophthalmos right eye, unspecified eyelid
⊟ SP H02.204 Unspecified lagophthalmos left upper eyelid
⊟ SP H02.205 Unspecified lagophthalmos left lower eyelid
⊟ !Q H02.206 Unspecified lagophthalmos left eye, unspecified eyelid
⊟ !Q H02.209 Unspecified lagophthalmos unspecified eye, unspecified eyelid
⊟ SP H02.20A Unspecified lagophthalmos right eye, upper and lower eyelids
⊟ SP H02.20B Unspecified lagophthalmos left eye, upper and lower eyelids
⊟ SP H02.20C Unspecified lagophthalmos, bilateral, upper and lower eyelids

6 H02.21 Cicatricial lagophthalmos

DEFINITION Inability to completely close the eye due to the presence of scar tissue.

⊟ SP H02.211 Cicatricial lagophthalmos right upper eyelid
⊟ SP H02.212 Cicatricial lagophthalmos right lower eyelid
⊟ !Q H02.213 Cicatricial lagophthalmos right eye, unspecified eyelid
⊟ SP H02.214 Cicatricial lagophthalmos left upper eyelid
⊟ SP H02.215 Cicatricial lagophthalmos left lower eyelid
⊟ !Q H02.216 Cicatricial lagophthalmos left eye, unspecified eyelid
⊟ !Q H02.219 Cicatricial lagophthalmos unspecified eye, unspecified eyelid
⊟ SP H02.21A Cicatricial lagophthalmos right eye, upper and lower eyelids
⊟ SP H02.21B Cicatricial lagophthalmos left eye, upper and lower eyelids
⊟ SP H02.21C Cicatricial lagophthalmos, bilateral, upper and lower eyelids

6 H02.22 Mechanical lagophthalmos

⊟ SP H02.221 Mechanical lagophthalmos right upper eyelid
⊟ SP H02.222 Mechanical lagophthalmos right lower eyelid
⊟ !Q H02.223 Mechanical lagophthalmos right eye, unspecified eyelid
⊟ SP H02.224 Mechanical lagophthalmos left upper eyelid
⊟ SP H02.225 Mechanical lagophthalmos left lower eyelid
⊟ !Q H02.226 Mechanical lagophthalmos left eye, unspecified eyelid
⊟ !Q H02.229 Mechanical lagophthalmos unspecified eye, unspecified eyelid
⊟ SP H02.22A Mechanical lagophthalmos right eye, upper and lower eyelids
⊟ SP H02.22B Mechanical lagophthalmos left eye, upper and lower eyelids

SP H02.22C Mechanical lagophthalmos, bilateral, upper and lower eyelids

6 H02.23 Paralytic lagophthalmos

SP H02.231 Paralytic lagophthalmos right upper eyelid

SP H02.232 Paralytic lagophthalmos right lower eyelid

IQ H02.233 Paralytic lagophthalmos right eye, unspecified eyelid

SP H02.234 Paralytic lagophthalmos left upper eyelid

SP H02.235 Paralytic lagophthalmos left lower eyelid

IQ H02.236 Paralytic lagophthalmos left eye, unspecified eyelid

IQ H02.239 Paralytic lagophthalmos unspecified eye, unspecified eyelid

SP H02.23A Paralytic lagophthalmos right eye, upper and lower eyelids

SP H02.23B Paralytic lagophthalmos left eye, upper and lower eyelids

SP H02.23C Paralytic lagophthalmos, bilateral, upper and lower eyelids

5 H02.3 Blepharochalasis

Pseudoptosis

DEFINITION Sagging of the skin of the eyelid. In the upper eyelid, the skin sags over the eye obstructing vision; usually due to changes in elastin and collagen, affecting the skin's elasticity.

IQ H02.30 Blepharochalasis unspecified eye, unspecified eyelid

SP H02.31 Blepharochalasis right upper eyelid

SP H02.32 Blepharochalasis right lower eyelid

IQ H02.33 Blepharochalasis right eye, unspecified eyelid

SP H02.34 Blepharochalasis left upper eyelid

SP H02.35 Blepharochalasis left lower eyelid

IQ H02.36 Blepharochalasis left eye, unspecified eyelid

5 H02.4 Ptosis of eyelid

6 H02.40 Unspecified ptosis of eyelid

SP H02.401 Unspecified ptosis of right eyelid

SP H02.402 Unspecified ptosis of left eyelid

SP H02.403 Unspecified ptosis of bilateral eyelids

IQ H02.409 Unspecified ptosis of unspecified eyelid

6 H02.41 Mechanical ptosis of eyelid

SP H02.411 Mechanical ptosis of right eyelid

SP H02.412 Mechanical ptosis of left eyelid

SP H02.413 Mechanical ptosis of bilateral eyelids

IQ H02.419 Mechanical ptosis of unspecified eyelid

6 H02.42 Myogenic ptosis of eyelid

SP H02.421 Myogenic ptosis of right eyelid

SP H02.422 Myogenic ptosis of left eyelid

SP H02.423 Myogenic ptosis of bilateral eyelids

IQ H02.429 Myogenic ptosis of unspecified eyelid

6 H02.43 Paralytic ptosis of eyelid

Neurogenic ptosis of eyelid

SP H02.431 Paralytic ptosis of right eyelid

SP H02.432 Paralytic ptosis of left eyelid

SP H02.433 Paralytic ptosis of bilateral eyelids

IQ H02.439 Paralytic ptosis unspecified eyelid

5 H02.5 Other disorders affecting eyelid function

EXCLUDES 2 blepharospasm (G24.5)
organic tic (G25.69)
psychogenic tic (F95.-)

6 H02.51 Abnormal innervation syndrome

SP H02.511 Abnormal innervation syndrome right upper eyelid

SP H02.512 Abnormal innervation syndrome right lower eyelid

IQ H02.513 Abnormal innervation syndrome right eye, unspecified eyelid

SP H02.514 Abnormal innervation syndrome left upper eyelid

SP H02.515 Abnormal innervation syndrome left lower eyelid

IQ H02.516 Abnormal innervation syndrome left eye, unspecified eyelid

IQ H02.519 Abnormal innervation syndrome unspecified eye, unspecified eyelid

6 H02.52 Blepharophimosis

Ankyloblepharon

DEFINITION Hereditary disorder in which the palpebral fissures (space between the eyelids) is narrowed, giving the appearance of continually squinting.

SP H02.521 Blepharophimosis right upper eyelid

SP H02.522 Blepharophimosis right lower eyelid

IQ H02.523 Blepharophimosis right eye, unspecified eyelid

SP H02.524 Blepharophimosis left upper eyelid

SP H02.525 Blepharophimosis left lower eyelid

IQ H02.526 Blepharophimosis left eye, unspecified eyelid

IQ H02.529 Blepharophimosis unspecified eye, unspecified lid

6 H02.53 Eyelid retraction

Eyelid lag

SP H02.531 Eyelid retraction right upper eyelid

SP H02.532 Eyelid retraction right lower eyelid

IQ H02.533 Eyelid retraction right eye, unspecified eyelid

SP H02.534 Eyelid retraction left upper eyelid

SP H02.535 Eyelid retraction left lower eyelid

IQ H02.536 Eyelid retraction left eye, unspecified eyelid

IQ H02.539 Eyelid retraction unspecified eye, unspecified lid

SP H02.59 Other disorders affecting eyelid function

Deficient blink reflex

Sensory disorders

5 **H02.6 Xanthelasma of eyelid**

Laterality IQ **H02.60 Xanthelasma of unspecified eye, unspecified eyelid**

Laterality SP **H02.61 Xanthelasma of right upper eyelid**

Laterality SP **H02.62 Xanthelasma of right lower eyelid**

Laterality IQ **H02.63 Xanthelasma of right eye, unspecified eyelid**

Laterality SP **H02.64 Xanthelasma of left upper eyelid**

Laterality SP **H02.65 Xanthelasma of left lower eyelid**

Laterality IQ **H02.66 Xanthelasma of left eye, unspecified eyelid**

5 **H02.7 Other and unspecified degenerative disorders of eyelid and periocular area**

SP **H02.70 Unspecified degenerative disorders of eyelid and periocular area**

6 **H02.71 Chloasma of eyelid and periocular area**

Dyspigmentation of eyelid
Hyperpigmentation of eyelid

Laterality SP **H02.711 Chloasma of right upper eyelid and periocular area**

Laterality SP **H02.712 Chloasma of right lower eyelid and periocular area**

Laterality IQ **H02.713 Chloasma of right eye, unspecified eyelid and periocular area**

Laterality SP **H02.714 Chloasma of left upper eyelid and periocular area**

Laterality SP **H02.715 Chloasma of left lower eyelid and periocular area**

Laterality IQ **H02.716 Chloasma of left eye, unspecified eyelid and periocular area**

Laterality IQ **H02.719 Chloasma of unspecified eye, unspecified eyelid and periocular area**

6 **H02.72 Madarosis of eyelid and periocular area**

Hypotrichosis of eyelid

Laterality SP **H02.721 Madarosis of right upper eyelid and periocular area**

Laterality SP **H02.722 Madarosis of right lower eyelid and periocular area**

Laterality IQ **H02.723 Madarosis of right eye, unspecified eyelid and periocular area**

Laterality SP **H02.724 Madarosis of left upper eyelid and periocular area**

Laterality SP **H02.725 Madarosis of left lower eyelid and periocular area**

Laterality IQ **H02.726 Madarosis of left eye, unspecified eyelid and periocular area**

Laterality IQ **H02.729 Madarosis of unspecified eye, unspecified eyelid and periocular area**

6 **H02.73 Vitiligo of eyelid and periocular area**

Hypopigmentation of eyelid

Laterality SP **H02.731 Vitiligo of right upper eyelid and periocular area**

Laterality SP **H02.732 Vitiligo of right lower eyelid and periocular area**

Laterality IQ **H02.733 Vitiligo of right eye, unspecified eyelid and periocular area**

Laterality SP **H02.734 Vitiligo of left upper eyelid and periocular area**

Laterality SP **H02.735 Vitiligo of left lower eyelid and periocular area**

Laterality IQ **H02.736 Vitiligo of left eye, unspecified eyelid and periocular area**

Laterality IQ **H02.739 Vitiligo of unspecified eye, unspecified eyelid and periocular area**

SP **H02.79 Other degenerative disorders of eyelid and periocular area**

5 **H02.8 Other specified disorders of eyelid**

+ 6 **H02.81 Retained foreign body in eyelid**

Use additional code to identify the type of retained foreign body (Z18.-)

EXCLUDES 1 laceration of eyelid with foreign body (S01.12-)
retained intraocular foreign body (H44.6-, H44.7-)
superficial foreign body of eyelid and periocular area (S00.25-)

Laterality SP + **H02.811 Retained foreign body in right upper eyelid**

Laterality SP + **H02.812 Retained foreign body in right lower eyelid**

Laterality IQ + **H02.813 Retained foreign body in right eye, unspecified eyelid**

Laterality SP + **H02.814 Retained foreign body in left upper eyelid**

Laterality SP + **H02.815 Retained foreign body in left lower eyelid**

Laterality IQ + **H02.816 Retained foreign body in left eye, unspecified eyelid**

Laterality IQ + **H02.819 Retained foreign body in unspecified eye, unspecified eyelid**

6 **H02.82 Cysts of eyelid**

Sebaceous cyst of eyelid

Laterality SP **H02.821 Cysts of right upper eyelid**

Laterality SP **H02.822 Cysts of right lower eyelid**

Laterality IQ **H02.823 Cysts of right eye, unspecified eyelid**

Laterality SP **H02.824 Cysts of left upper eyelid**

Laterality SP **H02.825 Cysts of left lower eyelid**

Laterality IQ **H02.826 Cysts of left eye, unspecified eyelid**

Laterality IQ **H02.829 Cysts of unspecified eye, unspecified eyelid**

6 **H02.83 Dermatochalasis of eyelid**

Laterality SP **H02.831 Dermatochalasis of right upper eyelid**

Laterality SP **H02.832 Dermatochalasis of right lower eyelid**

Laterality IQ **H02.833 Dermatochalasis of right eye, unspecified eyelid**

Laterality SP **H02.834 Dermatochalasis of left upper eyelid**

Laterality SP **H02.835 Dermatochalasis of left lower eyelid**

Laterality IQ **H02.836 Dermatochalasis of left eye, unspecified eyelid**

Laterality IQ **H02.839 Dermatochalasis of unspecified eye, unspecified eyelid**

6 **H02.84 Edema of eyelid**

Chapter 7

H00-H59

Hyperemia of eyelid

H02.841 Edema of right upper eyelid

H02.842 Edema of right lower eyelid

H02.843 Edema of right eye, unspecified eyelid

H02.844 Edema of left upper eyelid

H02.845 Edema of left lower eyelid

H02.846 Edema of left eye, unspecified eyelid

H02.849 Edema of unspecified eye, unspecified eyelid

H02.85 Elephantiasis of eyelid

H02.851 Elephantiasis of right upper eyelid

H02.852 Elephantiasis of right lower eyelid

H02.853 Elephantiasis of right eye, unspecified eyelid

H02.854 Elephantiasis of left upper eyelid

H02.855 Elephantiasis of left lower eyelid

H02.856 Elephantiasis of left eye, unspecified eyelid

H02.859 Elephantiasis of unspecified eye, unspecified eyelid

H02.86 Hypertrichosis of eyelid

H02.861 Hypertrichosis of right upper eyelid

H02.862 Hypertrichosis of right lower eyelid

H02.863 Hypertrichosis of right eye, unspecified eyelid

H02.864 Hypertrichosis of left upper eyelid

H02.865 Hypertrichosis of left lower eyelid

H02.866 Hypertrichosis of left eye, unspecified eyelid

H02.869 Hypertrichosis of unspecified eye, unspecified eyelid

H02.87 Vascular anomalies of eyelid

H02.871 Vascular anomalies of right upper eyelid

H02.872 Vascular anomalies of right lower eyelid

H02.873 Vascular anomalies of right eye, unspecified eyelid

H02.874 Vascular anomalies of left upper eyelid

H02.875 Vascular anomalies of left lower eyelid

H02.876 Vascular anomalies of left eye, unspecified eyelid

H02.879 Vascular anomalies of unspecified eye, unspecified eyelid

H02.88 Meibomian gland dysfunction of eyelid

H02.881 Meibomian gland dysfunction right upper eyelid

H02.882 Meibomian gland dysfunction right lower eyelid

H02.883 Meibomian gland dysfunction of right eye, unspecified eyelid

H02.884 Meibomian gland dysfunction left upper eyelid

H02.885 Meibomian gland dysfunction left lower eyelid

H02.886 Meibomian gland dysfunction of left eye, unspecified eyelid

H02.889 Meibomian gland dysfunction of unspecified eye, unspecified eyelid

H02.88A Meibomian gland dysfunction right eye, upper and lower eyelids

H02.88B Meibomian gland dysfunction left eye, upper and lower eyelids

H02.89 Other specified disorders of eyelid

Hemorrhage of eyelid

H02.9 Unspecified disorder of eyelid

Disorder of eyelid NOS

H04 Disorders of lacrimal system

EXCLUDES 1 congenital malformations of lacrimal system (Q10.4-Q10.6)

H04.0 Dacryoadenitis

H04.00 Unspecified dacryoadenitis

DEFINITION Inflammation of the lacrimal gland.

H04.001 Unspecified dacryoadenitis, right lacrimal gland

H04.002 Unspecified dacryoadenitis, left lacrimal gland

H04.003 Unspecified dacryoadenitis, bilateral lacrimal glands

H04.009 Unspecified dacryoadenitis, unspecified lacrimal gland

H04.01 Acute dacryoadenitis

H04.011 Acute dacryoadenitis, right lacrimal gland

H04.012 Acute dacryoadenitis, left lacrimal gland

H04.013 Acute dacryoadenitis, bilateral lacrimal glands

H04.019 Acute dacryoadenitis, unspecified lacrimal gland

H04.02 Chronic dacryoadenitis

H04.021 Chronic dacryoadenitis, right lacrimal gland

H04.022 Chronic dacryoadenitis, left lacrimal gland

H04.023 Chronic dacryoadenitis, bilateral lacrimal gland

H04.029 Chronic dacryoadenitis, unspecified lacrimal gland

H04.03 Chronic enlargement of lacrimal gland

H04.031 Chronic enlargement of right lacrimal gland

H04.032 Chronic enlargement of left lacrimal gland

H04.033 Chronic enlargement of bilateral lacrimal glands

H04.039 Chronic enlargement of unspecified lacrimal gland

H04.1 Other disorders of lacrimal gland

H04.11 Dacryops

H04.111 Dacryops of right lacrimal gland

H04.112 Dacryops of left lacrimal gland

H04.113 Dacryops of bilateral lacrimal glands

Chapter 7 H00-H59

⊟ IQ **H04.119 Dacryops of unspecified lacrimal gland**

6 **H04.12 Dry eye syndrome**
Tear film insufficiency, NOS

⊟ SP **H04.121 Dry eye syndrome of right lacrimal gland**

⊟ SP **H04.122 Dry eye syndrome of left lacrimal gland**

⊟ SP **H04.123 Dry eye syndrome of bilateral lacrimal glands**

⊟ IQ **H04.129 Dry eye syndrome of unspecified lacrimal gland**

6 **H04.13 Lacrimal cyst**
Lacrimal cystic degeneration

⊟ SP **H04.131 Lacrimal cyst, right lacrimal gland**

⊟ SP **H04.132 Lacrimal cyst, left lacrimal gland**

⊟ SP **H04.133 Lacrimal cyst, bilateral lacrimal glands**

⊟ IQ **H04.139 Lacrimal cyst, unspecified lacrimal gland**

6 **H04.14 Primary lacrimal gland atrophy**

DEFINITION Wasting of the lacrimal glands causing severe dryness with decreased tear production.

⊟ SP **H04.141 Primary lacrimal gland atrophy, right lacrimal gland**

⊟ SP **H04.142 Primary lacrimal gland atrophy, left lacrimal gland**

⊟ SP **H04.143 Primary lacrimal gland atrophy, bilateral lacrimal glands**

⊟ IQ **H04.149 Primary lacrimal gland atrophy, unspecified lacrimal gland**

6 **H04.15 Secondary lacrimal gland atrophy**

⊟ SP **H04.151 Secondary lacrimal gland atrophy, right lacrimal gland**

⊟ SP **H04.152 Secondary lacrimal gland atrophy, left lacrimal gland**

⊟ SP **H04.153 Secondary lacrimal gland atrophy, bilateral lacrimal glands**

⊟ IQ **H04.159 Secondary lacrimal gland atrophy, unspecified lacrimal gland**

6 **H04.16 Lacrimal gland dislocation**

DEFINITION Lacrimal gland separated from the tear ducts, preventing tears from passing normally to the eye.

⊟ SP **H04.161 Lacrimal gland dislocation, right lacrimal gland**

⊟ SP **H04.162 Lacrimal gland dislocation, left lacrimal gland**

⊟ SP **H04.163 Lacrimal gland dislocation, bilateral lacrimal glands**

⊟ IQ **H04.169 Lacrimal gland dislocation, unspecified lacrimal gland**

SP **H04.19 Other specified disorders of lacrimal gland**

5 **H04.2 Epiphora**

6 **H04.20 Unspecified epiphora**

⊟ SP **H04.201 Unspecified epiphora, right side**

⊟ SP **H04.202 Unspecified epiphora, left side**

⊟ SP **H04.203 Unspecified epiphora, bilateral**

⊟ IQ **H04.209 Unspecified epiphora, unspecified side**

6 **H04.21 Epiphora due to excess lacrimation**

⊟ SP **H04.211 Epiphora due to excess lacrimation, right lacrimal gland**

⊟ SP **H04.212 Epiphora due to excess lacrimation, left lacrimal gland**

⊟ SP **H04.213 Epiphora due to excess lacrimation, bilateral lacrimal glands**

⊟ IQ **H04.219 Epiphora due to excess lacrimation, unspecified lacrimal gland**

6 **H04.22 Epiphora due to insufficient drainage**

⊟ SP **H04.221 Epiphora due to insufficient drainage, right side**

⊟ SP **H04.222 Epiphora due to insufficient drainage, left side**

⊟ SP **H04.223 Epiphora due to insufficient drainage, bilateral**

⊟ IQ **H04.229 Epiphora due to insufficient drainage, unspecified side**

5 **H04.3 Acute and unspecified inflammation of lacrimal passages**

EXCLUDES 1 neonatal dacryocystitis (P39.1)

6 **H04.30 Unspecified dacryocystitis**

DEFINITION Inflammation of the lacrimal sac in the eye causing obstruction of the tube draining tears into the nose.

⊟ SP **H04.301 Unspecified dacryocystitis of right lacrimal passage**

⊟ SP **H04.302 Unspecified dacryocystitis of left lacrimal passage**

⊟ SP **H04.303 Unspecified dacryocystitis of bilateral lacrimal passages**

⊟ IQ **H04.309 Unspecified dacryocystitis of unspecified lacrimal passage**

6 **H04.31 Phlegmonous dacryocystitis**

⊟ SP **H04.311 Phlegmonous dacryocystitis of right lacrimal passage**

⊟ SP **H04.312 Phlegmonous dacryocystitis of left lacrimal passage**

⊟ SP **H04.313 Phlegmonous dacryocystitis of bilateral lacrimal passages**

⊟ IQ **H04.319 Phlegmonous dacryocystitis of unspecified lacrimal passage**

6 **H04.32 Acute dacryocystitis**
Acute dacryopericystitis

DEFINITION Sudden, severe inflammation of the tear sac, usually due to blockage of the tear ducts.

⊟ SP **H04.321 Acute dacryocystitis of right lacrimal passage**

⊟ SP **H04.322 Acute dacryocystitis of left lacrimal passage**

⊟ SP **H04.323 Acute dacryocystitis of bilateral lacrimal passages**

⊟ IQ **H04.329 Acute dacryocystitis of unspecified lacrimal passage**

6 **H04.33 Acute lacrimal canaliculitis**

DEFINITION Sudden, severe inflammation of the lacrimal passages or tear ducts.

Chapter 7

H00-H59

7 SP H04.331 Acute lacrimal canaliculitis of right lacrimal passage
7 SP H04.332 Acute lacrimal canaliculitis of left lacrimal passage
7 SP H04.333 Acute lacrimal canaliculitis of bilateral lacrimal passages
7 IQ H04.339 Acute lacrimal canaliculitis of unspecified lacrimal passage

5 H04.4 Chronic inflammation of lacrimal passages
6 H04.41 Chronic dacryocystitis
7 SP H04.411 Chronic dacryocystitis of right lacrimal passage
7 SP H04.412 Chronic dacryocystitis of left lacrimal passage
7 SP H04.413 Chronic dacryocystitis of bilateral lacrimal passages
7 IQ H04.419 Chronic dacryocystitis of unspecified lacrimal passage
6 H04.42 Chronic lacrimal canaliculitis
7 SP H04.421 Chronic lacrimal canaliculitis of right lacrimal passage
7 SP H04.422 Chronic lacrimal canaliculitis of left lacrimal passage
7 SP H04.423 Chronic lacrimal canaliculitis of bilateral lacrimal passages
7 IQ H04.429 Chronic lacrimal canaliculitis of unspecified lacrimal passage
6 H04.43 Chronic lacrimal mucocele

DEFINITION Inflammation of the lacrimal system in which the tear ducts, and then the eyes, become filled with mucous.

7 SP H04.431 Chronic lacrimal mucocele of right lacrimal passage
7 SP H04.432 Chronic lacrimal mucocele of left lacrimal passage
7 SP H04.433 Chronic lacrimal mucocele of bilateral lacrimal passages
7 IQ H04.439 Chronic lacrimal mucocele of unspecified lacrimal passage

5 H04.5 Stenosis and insufficiency of lacrimal passages
6 H04.51 Dacryolith
7 SP H04.511 Dacryolith of right lacrimal passage
7 SP H04.512 Dacryolith of left lacrimal passage
7 SP H04.513 Dacryolith of bilateral lacrimal passages
7 IQ H04.519 Dacryolith of unspecified lacrimal passage
6 H04.52 Eversion of lacrimal punctum

DEFINITION Tear duct exit turned away from the eye, causing tears to flow directly onto the face instead of moistening the eyeball.

7 SP H04.521 Eversion of right lacrimal punctum
7 SP H04.522 Eversion of left lacrimal punctum
7 SP H04.523 Eversion of bilateral lacrimal punctum
7 IQ H04.529 Eversion of unspecified lacrimal punctum
6 H04.53 Neonatal obstruction of nasolacrimal duct

EXCLUDES 1 congenital stenosis and stricture of lacrimal duct (Q10.5)

7 SP H04.531 Neonatal obstruction of right nasolacrimal duct
7 SP H04.532 Neonatal obstruction of left nasolacrimal duct
7 SP H04.533 Neonatal obstruction of bilateral nasolacrimal duct
7 IQ H04.539 Neonatal obstruction of unspecified nasolacrimal duct
6 H04.54 Stenosis of lacrimal canaliculi
7 SP H04.541 Stenosis of right lacrimal canaliculi
7 SP H04.542 Stenosis of left lacrimal canaliculi
7 SP H04.543 Stenosis of bilateral lacrimal canaliculi
7 IQ H04.549 Stenosis of unspecified lacrimal canaliculi
6 H04.55 Acquired stenosis of nasolacrimal duct
7 SP H04.551 Acquired stenosis of right nasolacrimal duct
7 SP H04.552 Acquired stenosis of left nasolacrimal duct
7 SP H04.553 Acquired stenosis of bilateral nasolacrimal duct
7 IQ H04.559 Acquired stenosis of unspecified nasolacrimal duct
6 H04.56 Stenosis of lacrimal punctum
7 SP H04.561 Stenosis of right lacrimal punctum
7 SP H04.562 Stenosis of left lacrimal punctum
7 SP H04.563 Stenosis of bilateral lacrimal punctum
7 IQ H04.569 Stenosis of unspecified lacrimal punctum
6 H04.57 Stenosis of lacrimal sac
7 SP H04.571 Stenosis of right lacrimal sac
7 SP H04.572 Stenosis of left lacrimal sac
7 SP H04.573 Stenosis of bilateral lacrimal sac
7 IQ H04.579 Stenosis of unspecified lacrimal sac

5 H04.6 Other changes of lacrimal passages
6 H04.61 Lacrimal fistula
7 SP H04.611 Lacrimal fistula right lacrimal passage
7 SP H04.612 Lacrimal fistula left lacrimal passage
7 SP H04.613 Lacrimal fistula bilateral lacrimal passages
7 IQ H04.619 Lacrimal fistula unspecified lacrimal passage
SP H04.69 Other changes of lacrimal passages

5 H04.8 Other disorders of lacrimal system
6 H04.81 Granuloma of lacrimal passages
7 SP H04.811 Granuloma of right lacrimal passage
7 SP H04.812 Granuloma of left lacrimal passage
7 SP H04.813 Granuloma of bilateral lacrimal passages
7 IQ H04.819 Granuloma of unspecified lacrimal passage

SP H04.89 Other disorders of lacrimal system

!Q H04.9 Disorder of lacrimal system, unspecified

4 H05 Disorders of orbit
EXCLUDES 1 congenital malformation of orbit (Q10.7)

5 H05.0 Acute inflammation of orbit

SP H05.00 Unspecified acute inflammation of orbit

6 H05.01 Cellulitis of orbit
Abscess of orbit

⊟ SP H05.011 Cellulitis of right orbit
⊟ SP H05.012 Cellulitis of left orbit
⊟ SP H05.013 Cellulitis of bilateral orbits
⊟ !Q H05.019 Cellulitis of unspecified orbit

6 H05.02 Osteomyelitis of orbit

⊟ SP H05.021 Osteomyelitis of right orbit
⊟ SP H05.022 Osteomyelitis of left orbit
⊟ SP H05.023 Osteomyelitis of bilateral orbits
⊟ !Q H05.029 Osteomyelitis of unspecified orbit

6 H05.03 Periostitis of orbit

⊟ SP H05.031 Periostitis of right orbit
⊟ SP H05.032 Periostitis of left orbit
⊟ SP H05.033 Periostitis of bilateral orbits
⊟ !Q H05.039 Periostitis of unspecified orbit

6 H05.04 Tenonitis of orbit

⊟ SP H05.041 Tenonitis of right orbit
⊟ SP H05.042 Tenonitis of left orbit
⊟ SP H05.043 Tenonitis of bilateral orbits
⊟ !Q H05.049 Tenonitis of unspecified orbit

5 H05.1 Chronic inflammatory disorders of orbit

SP H05.10 Unspecified chronic inflammatory disorders of orbit

6 H05.11 Granuloma of orbit
Pseudotumor (inflammatory) of orbit

⊟ SP H05.111 Granuloma of right orbit
⊟ SP H05.112 Granuloma of left orbit
⊟ SP H05.113 Granuloma of bilateral orbits
⊟ !Q H05.119 Granuloma of unspecified orbit

6 H05.12 Orbital myositis
DEFINITION Inflammation of one of the muscles that moves the eyeball.

⊟ SP H05.121 Orbital myositis, right orbit
⊟ SP H05.122 Orbital myositis, left orbit
⊟ SP H05.123 Orbital myositis, bilateral
⊟ !Q H05.129 Orbital myositis, unspecified orbit

5 H05.2 Exophthalmic conditions

SP H05.20 Unspecified exophthalmos

6 H05.21 Displacement (lateral) of globe
DEFINITION Condition in which the eyeball is situated towards the side of the head, away from the nose.

⊟ SP H05.211 Displacement (lateral) of globe, right eye
⊟ SP H05.212 Displacement (lateral) of globe, left eye
⊟ SP H05.213 Displacement (lateral) of globe, bilateral
⊟ !Q H05.219 Displacement (lateral) of globe, unspecified eye

6 H05.22 Edema of orbit
Orbital congestion

⊟ SP H05.221 Edema of right orbit
⊟ SP H05.222 Edema of left orbit
⊟ SP H05.223 Edema of bilateral orbit
⊟ !Q H05.229 Edema of unspecified orbit

6 H05.23 Hemorrhage of orbit

⊟ SP H05.231 Hemorrhage of right orbit
⊟ SP H05.232 Hemorrhage of left orbit
⊟ SP H05.233 Hemorrhage of bilateral orbit
⊟ !Q H05.239 Hemorrhage of unspecified orbit

6 H05.24 Constant exophthalmos

⊟ SP H05.241 Constant exophthalmos, right eye
⊟ SP H05.242 Constant exophthalmos, left eye
⊟ SP H05.243 Constant exophthalmos, bilateral
⊟ !Q H05.249 Constant exophthalmos, unspecified eye

6 H05.25 Intermittent exophthalmos

⊟ SP H05.251 Intermittent exophthalmos, right eye
⊟ SP H05.252 Intermittent exophthalmos, left eye
⊟ SP H05.253 Intermittent exophthalmos, bilateral
⊟ !Q H05.259 Intermittent exophthalmos, unspecified eye

6 H05.26 Pulsating exophthalmos

⊟ SP H05.261 Pulsating exophthalmos, right eye
⊟ SP H05.262 Pulsating exophthalmos, left eye
⊟ SP H05.263 Pulsating exophthalmos, bilateral
⊟ !Q H05.269 Pulsating exophthalmos, unspecified eye

5 H05.3 Deformity of orbit
EXCLUDES 1 congenital deformity of orbit (Q10.7)
hypertelorism (Q75.2)

!Q H05.30 Unspecified deformity of orbit

6 H05.31 Atrophy of orbit

⊟ SP H05.311 Atrophy of right orbit
⊟ SP H05.312 Atrophy of left orbit
⊟ SP H05.313 Atrophy of bilateral orbit
⊟ !Q H05.319 Atrophy of unspecified orbit

6 H05.32 Deformity of orbit due to bone disease
Code also:
associated bone disease

⊟ SP H05.321 Deformity of right orbit due to bone disease
⊟ SP H05.322 Deformity of left orbit due to bone disease
⊟ SP H05.323 Deformity of bilateral orbits due to bone disease
⊟ !Q H05.329 Deformity of unspecified orbit due to bone disease

6 H05.33 Deformity of orbit due to trauma or surgery

⊟ SP H05.331 Deformity of right orbit due to trauma or surgery
⊟ SP H05.332 Deformity of left orbit due to trauma or surgery

4 4th digit required 5 5th digit required 6 6th digit required 7 7th digit required 7 7th digit placeholder ✚ Additional code ⊟ Laterality

SP H05.333 **Deformity of bilateral orbits due to trauma or surgery**

!Q H05.339 **Deformity of unspecified orbit due to trauma or surgery**

6 H05.34 **Enlargement of orbit**

SP H05.341 **Enlargement of right orbit**

SP H05.342 **Enlargement of left orbit**

SP H05.343 **Enlargement of bilateral orbits**

!Q H05.349 **Enlargement of unspecified orbit**

6 H05.35 **Exostosis of orbit**

DEFINITION Abnormal bone growth of the eye socket; can impair vision and prevent the eye from moving properly.

SP H05.351 **Exostosis of right orbit**

SP H05.352 **Exostosis of left orbit**

SP H05.353 **Exostosis of bilateral orbits**

!Q H05.359 **Exostosis of unspecified orbit**

5 H05.4 **Enophthalmos**

6 H05.40 **Unspecified enophthalmos**

DEFINITION Condition in which the eye is recessed abnormally deep within the eye socket.

SP H05.401 **Unspecified enophthalmos, right eye**

SP H05.402 **Unspecified enophthalmos, left eye**

SP H05.403 **Unspecified enophthalmos, bilateral**

!Q H05.409 **Unspecified enophthalmos, unspecified eye**

6 H05.41 **Enophthalmos due to atrophy of orbital tissue**

SP H05.411 **Enophthalmos due to atrophy of orbital tissue, right eye**

SP H05.412 **Enophthalmos due to atrophy of orbital tissue, left eye**

SP H05.413 **Enophthalmos due to atrophy of orbital tissue, bilateral**

!Q H05.419 **Enophthalmos due to atrophy of orbital tissue, unspecified eye**

6 H05.42 **Enophthalmos due to trauma or surgery**

SP H05.421 **Enophthalmos due to trauma or surgery, right eye**

SP H05.422 **Enophthalmos due to trauma or surgery, left eye**

SP H05.423 **Enophthalmos due to trauma or surgery, bilateral**

!Q H05.429 **Enophthalmos due to trauma or surgery, unspecified eye**

+ 5 H05.5 **Retained (old) foreign body following penetrating wound of orbit**

Retrobulbar foreign body

Use additional code to identify the type of retained foreign body (Z18.-)

EXCLUDES 1 current penetrating wound of orbit (S05.4-)

EXCLUDES 2 retained foreign body of eyelid (H02.81-)

retained intraocular foreign body (H44.6-, H44.7-)

!Q + H05.50 **Retained (old) foreign body following penetrating wound of unspecified orbit**

SP + H05.51 **Retained (old) foreign body following penetrating wound of right orbit**

SP + H05.52 **Retained (old) foreign body following penetrating wound of left orbit**

SP + H05.53 **Retained (old) foreign body following penetrating wound of bilateral orbits**

5 H05.8 **Other disorders of orbit**

6 H05.81 **Cyst of orbit**

Encephalocele of orbit

SP H05.811 **Cyst of right orbit**

SP H05.812 **Cyst of left orbit**

SP H05.813 **Cyst of bilateral orbits**

!Q H05.819 **Cyst of unspecified orbit**

6 H05.82 **Myopathy of extraocular muscles**

SP H05.821 **Myopathy of extraocular muscles, right orbit**

SP H05.822 **Myopathy of extraocular muscles, left orbit**

SP H05.823 **Myopathy of extraocular muscles, bilateral**

!Q H05.829 **Myopathy of extraocular muscles, unspecified orbit**

SP H05.89 **Other disorders of orbit**

!Q H05.9 **Unspecified disorder of orbit**

Disorders of conjunctiva (H10-H11)

4 H10 **Conjunctivitis**

EXCLUDES 1 keratoconjunctivitis (H16.2-)

CODING TIPS✓ Consider codes from H10 when an infectious organism is not identified and the documentation only supports a clinical picture of conjunctivitis. If a certain bacterial or viral cause is known, a code from the Infectious and parasitic disease chapter may be more appropriate.

5 H10.0 **Mucopurulent conjunctivitis**

6 H10.01 **Acute follicular conjunctivitis**

SP H10.011 **Acute follicular conjunctivitis, right eye**

SP H10.012 **Acute follicular conjunctivitis, left eye**

SP H10.013 **Acute follicular conjunctivitis, bilateral**

!Q H10.019 **Acute follicular conjunctivitis, unspecified eye**

6 H10.02 **Other mucopurulent conjunctivitis**

CODING TIPS✓ Subcategory H10.02 is commonly referred to as pink eye.

DEFINITION Inflammation of the conjunctiva with the production of mucous and pus.

SP H10.021 **Other mucopurulent conjunctivitis, right eye**

SP H10.022 **Other mucopurulent conjunctivitis, left eye**

SP H10.023 **Other mucopurulent conjunctivitis, bilateral**

!Q H10.029 **Other mucopurulent conjunctivitis, unspecified eye**

5 H10.1 **Acute atopic conjunctivitis**

Chapter 7

H00-H59

Acute papillary conjunctivitis

DEFINITION Sudden, severe case of conjunctivitis caused by allergies.

⊟ IQ **H10.10 Acute atopic conjunctivitis, unspecified eye**

⊟ SP **H10.11 Acute atopic conjunctivitis, right eye**

⊟ SP **H10.12 Acute atopic conjunctivitis, left eye**

⊟ SP **H10.13 Acute atopic conjunctivitis, bilateral**

5 **H10.2 Other acute conjunctivitis**

CODING TIPS✓ Consider subcategory H10.2 when light or noxious chemicals cause conjunctivitis.

6 **H10.21 Acute toxic conjunctivitis**

Acute chemical conjunctivitis

Code first:

(T51-T65) to identify chemical and intent

EXCLUDES 1 burn and corrosion of eye and adnexa (T26.-)

⊟ IQ **H10.211 Acute toxic conjunctivitis, right eye**

⊟ IQ **H10.212 Acute toxic conjunctivitis, left eye**

⊟ IQ **H10.213 Acute toxic conjunctivitis, bilateral**

⊟ IQ **H10.219 Acute toxic conjunctivitis, unspecified eye**

6 **H10.22 Pseudomembranous conjunctivitis**

⊟ SP **H10.221 Pseudomembranous conjunctivitis, right eye**

⊟ SP **H10.222 Pseudomembranous conjunctivitis, left eye**

⊟ SP **H10.223 Pseudomembranous conjunctivitis, bilateral**

⊟ SP **H10.229 Pseudomembranous conjunctivitis, unspecified eye**

6 **H10.23 Serous conjunctivitis, except viral**

EXCLUDES 1 viral conjunctivitis (B30.-)

⊟ SP **H10.231 Serous conjunctivitis, except viral, right eye**

⊟ SP **H10.232 Serous conjunctivitis, except viral, left eye**

⊟ SP **H10.233 Serous conjunctivitis, except viral, bilateral**

⊟ IQ **H10.239 Serous conjunctivitis, except viral, unspecified eye**

5 **H10.3 Unspecified acute conjunctivitis**

EXCLUDES 1 ophthalmia neonatorum NOS (P39.1)

⊟ IQ **H10.30 Unspecified acute conjunctivitis, unspecified eye**

⊟ SP **H10.31 Unspecified acute conjunctivitis, right eye**

⊟ SP **H10.32 Unspecified acute conjunctivitis, left eye**

⊟ SP **H10.33 Unspecified acute conjunctivitis, bilateral**

5 **H10.4 Chronic conjunctivitis**

6 **H10.40 Unspecified chronic conjunctivitis**

⊟ SP **H10.401 Unspecified chronic conjunctivitis, right eye**

⊟ SP **H10.402 Unspecified chronic conjunctivitis, left eye**

⊟ SP **H10.403 Unspecified chronic conjunctivitis, bilateral**

⊟ IQ **H10.409 Unspecified chronic conjunctivitis, unspecified eye**

6 **H10.41 Chronic giant papillary conjunctivitis**

⊟ SP **H10.411 Chronic giant papillary conjunctivitis, right eye**

⊟ SP **H10.412 Chronic giant papillary conjunctivitis, left eye**

⊟ SP **H10.413 Chronic giant papillary conjunctivitis, bilateral**

⊟ IQ **H10.419 Chronic giant papillary conjunctivitis, unspecified eye**

6 **H10.42 Simple chronic conjunctivitis**

⊟ SP **H10.421 Simple chronic conjunctivitis, right eye**

⊟ SP **H10.422 Simple chronic conjunctivitis, left eye**

⊟ SP **H10.423 Simple chronic conjunctivitis, bilateral**

⊟ IQ **H10.429 Simple chronic conjunctivitis, unspecified eye**

6 **H10.43 Chronic follicular conjunctivitis**

⊟ SP **H10.431 Chronic follicular conjunctivitis, right eye**

⊟ SP **H10.432 Chronic follicular conjunctivitis, left eye**

⊟ SP **H10.433 Chronic follicular conjunctivitis, bilateral**

⊟ IQ **H10.439 Chronic follicular conjunctivitis, unspecified eye**

SP **H10.44 Vernal conjunctivitis**

EXCLUDES 1 vernal keratoconjunctivitis with limbar and corneal involvement (H16.26-)

DEFINITION Seasonal inflammation of the conjunctiva due to an allergic reaction to pollen, mold, or another seasonal factor.

SP **H10.45 Other chronic allergic conjunctivitis**

5 **H10.5 Blepharoconjunctivitis**

6 **H10.50 Unspecified blepharoconjunctivitis**

⊟ SP **H10.501 Unspecified blepharoconjunctivitis, right eye**

⊟ SP **H10.502 Unspecified blepharoconjunctivitis, left eye**

⊟ SP **H10.503 Unspecified blepharoconjunctivitis, bilateral**

⊟ IQ **H10.509 Unspecified blepharoconjunctivitis, unspecified eye**

6 **H10.51 Ligneous conjunctivitis**

Code also underlying condition if known, such as:

plasminogen deficiency (E88.02)

⊟ SP **H10.511 Ligneous conjunctivitis, right eye**

⊟ SP **H10.512 Ligneous conjunctivitis, left eye**

⊟ SP **H10.513 Ligneous conjunctivitis, bilateral**

⊟ IQ **H10.519 Ligneous conjunctivitis, unspecified eye**

6 **H10.52 Angular blepharoconjunctivitis**

- H10.521 Angular blepharoconjunctivitis, right eye
- H10.522 Angular blepharoconjunctivitis, left eye
- H10.523 Angular blepharoconjunctivitis, bilateral
- H10.529 Angular blepharoconjunctivitis, unspecified eye

H10.53 Contact blepharoconjunctivitis
- H10.531 Contact blepharoconjunctivitis, right eye
- H10.532 Contact blepharoconjunctivitis, left eye
- H10.533 Contact blepharoconjunctivitis, bilateral
- H10.539 Contact blepharoconjunctivitis, unspecified eye

H10.8 Other conjunctivitis

H10.81 Pingueculitis

EXCLUDES 1 pinguecula (H11.15-)

DEFINITION Yellowish, raised areas of limbal conjunctival tissue, usually seen with chronic sun exposure, that become acutely vascularized, irritated, and inflamed.

- H10.811 Pingueculitis, right eye
- H10.812 Pingueculitis, left eye
- H10.813 Pingueculitis, bilateral
- H10.819 Pingueculitis, unspecified eye

H10.82 Rosacea conjunctivitis

Code first:
underlying rosacea dermatitis (L71.-)

- H10.821 Rosacea conjunctivitis, right eye
- H10.822 Rosacea conjunctivitis, left eye
- H10.823 Rosacea conjunctivitis, bilateral
- H10.829 Rosacea conjunctivitis, unspecified eye

H10.89 Other conjunctivitis

H10.9 Unspecified conjunctivitis

H11 Other disorders of conjunctiva

EXCLUDES 1 keratoconjunctivitis (H16.2-)

H11.0 Pterygium of eye

EXCLUDES 1 pseudopterygium (H11.81-)

H11.00 Unspecified pterygium of eye

DEFINITION Raised, wedge-shaped overgrowth of the conjunctiva onto the cornea of the eye.

- H11.001 Unspecified pterygium of right eye
- H11.002 Unspecified pterygium of left eye
- H11.003 Unspecified pterygium of eye, bilateral
- H11.009 Unspecified pterygium of unspecified eye

H11.01 Amyloid pterygium
- H11.011 Amyloid pterygium of right eye
- H11.012 Amyloid pterygium of left eye
- H11.013 Amyloid pterygium of eye, bilateral
- H11.019 Amyloid pterygium of unspecified eye

H11.02 Central pterygium of eye
- H11.021 Central pterygium of right eye
- H11.022 Central pterygium of left eye
- H11.023 Central pterygium of eye, bilateral
- H11.029 Central pterygium of unspecified eye

H11.03 Double pterygium of eye
- H11.031 Double pterygium of right eye
- H11.032 Double pterygium of left eye
- H11.033 Double pterygium of eye, bilateral
- H11.039 Double pterygium of unspecified eye

H11.04 Peripheral pterygium of eye, stationary
- H11.041 Peripheral pterygium, stationary, right eye
- H11.042 Peripheral pterygium, stationary, left eye
- H11.043 Peripheral pterygium, stationary, bilateral
- H11.049 Peripheral pterygium, stationary, unspecified eye

H11.05 Peripheral pterygium of eye, progressive
- H11.051 Peripheral pterygium, progressive, right eye
- H11.052 Peripheral pterygium, progressive, left eye
- H11.053 Peripheral pterygium, progressive, bilateral
- H11.059 Peripheral pterygium, progressive, unspecified eye

H11.06 Recurrent pterygium of eye
- H11.061 Recurrent pterygium of right eye
- H11.062 Recurrent pterygium of left eye
- H11.063 Recurrent pterygium of eye, bilateral
- H11.069 Recurrent pterygium of unspecified eye

H11.1 Conjunctival degenerations and deposits

EXCLUDES 2 pseudopterygium (H11.81)

H11.10 Unspecified conjunctival degenerations

H11.11 Conjunctival deposits
- H11.111 Conjunctival deposits, right eye
- H11.112 Conjunctival deposits, left eye
- H11.113 Conjunctival deposits, bilateral
- H11.119 Conjunctival deposits, unspecified eye

H11.12 Conjunctival concretions

DEFINITION Yellow-white granules or cysts which form just beneath the conjunctiva, wearing it away and causing the sensation of a foreign body in the eye.

- H11.121 Conjunctival concretions, right eye
- H11.122 Conjunctival concretions, left eye
- H11.123 Conjunctival concretions, bilateral
- H11.129 Conjunctival concretions, unspecified eye

6 **H11.13 Conjunctival pigmentations**
Conjunctival argyrosis [argyria]
L SP **H11.131 Conjunctival pigmentations, right eye**
L SP **H11.132 Conjunctival pigmentations, left eye**
L SP **H11.133 Conjunctival pigmentations, bilateral**
L IQ **H11.139 Conjunctival pigmentations, unspecified eye**
6 **H11.14 Conjunctival xerosis, unspecified**
EXCLUDES 1 xerosis of conjunctiva due to vitamin A deficiency (E50.0, E50.1)
L SP **H11.141 Conjunctival xerosis, unspecified, right eye**
L SP **H11.142 Conjunctival xerosis, unspecified, left eye**
L SP **H11.143 Conjunctival xerosis, unspecified, bilateral**
L IQ **H11.149 Conjunctival xerosis, unspecified, unspecified eye**
6 **H11.15 Pinguecula**
EXCLUDES 1 pingueculitis (H10.81-)
DEFINITION Small, nonmalignant, yellowish growth on the conjunctiva often asymptomatic and requiring no treatment but may cause irritation.
L SP **H11.151 Pinguecula, right eye**
L SP **H11.152 Pinguecula, left eye**
L SP **H11.153 Pinguecula, bilateral**
L IQ **H11.159 Pinguecula, unspecified eye**
5 **H11.2 Conjunctival scars**
6 **H11.21 Conjunctival adhesions and strands (localized)**
L SP **H11.211 Conjunctival adhesions and strands (localized), right eye**
L SP **H11.212 Conjunctival adhesions and strands (localized), left eye**
L SP **H11.213 Conjunctival adhesions and strands (localized), bilateral**
L IQ **H11.219 Conjunctival adhesions and strands (localized), unspecified eye**
6 **H11.22 Conjunctival granuloma**
L SP **H11.221 Conjunctival granuloma, right eye**
L SP **H11.222 Conjunctival granuloma, left eye**
L SP **H11.223 Conjunctival granuloma, bilateral**
L IQ **H11.229 Conjunctival granuloma, unspecified**
6 **H11.23 Symblepharon**
DEFINITION Conjunctiva of the eyelid that has adhered to the eye, sometimes over the cornea, requiring surgical removal.
L SP **H11.231 Symblepharon, right eye**
L SP **H11.232 Symblepharon, left eye**
L SP **H11.233 Symblepharon, bilateral**
L IQ **H11.239 Symblepharon, unspecified eye**
6 **H11.24 Scarring of conjunctiva**
L SP **H11.241 Scarring of conjunctiva, right eye**
L SP **H11.242 Scarring of conjunctiva, left eye**
L SP **H11.243 Scarring of conjunctiva, bilateral**
L IQ **H11.249 Scarring of conjunctiva, unspecified eye**
5 **H11.3 Conjunctival hemorrhage**
Subconjunctival hemorrhage
L IQ **H11.30 Conjunctival hemorrhage, unspecified eye**
L SP **H11.31 Conjunctival hemorrhage, right eye**
L SP **H11.32 Conjunctival hemorrhage, left eye**
L SP **H11.33 Conjunctival hemorrhage, bilateral**
5 **H11.4 Other conjunctival vascular disorders and cysts**
6 **H11.41 Vascular abnormalities of conjunctiva**
Conjunctival aneurysm
L SP **H11.411 Vascular abnormalities of conjunctiva, right eye**
L SP **H11.412 Vascular abnormalities of conjunctiva, left eye**
L SP **H11.413 Vascular abnormalities of conjunctiva, bilateral**
L IQ **H11.419 Vascular abnormalities of conjunctiva, unspecified eye**
6 **H11.42 Conjunctival edema**
L SP **H11.421 Conjunctival edema, right eye**
L SP **H11.422 Conjunctival edema, left eye**
L SP **H11.423 Conjunctival edema, bilateral**
L IQ **H11.429 Conjunctival edema, unspecified eye**
6 **H11.43 Conjunctival hyperemia**
L SP **H11.431 Conjunctival hyperemia, right eye**
L SP **H11.432 Conjunctival hyperemia, left eye**
L SP **H11.433 Conjunctival hyperemia, bilateral**
L IQ **H11.439 Conjunctival hyperemia, unspecified eye**
6 **H11.44 Conjunctival cysts**
L SP **H11.441 Conjunctival cysts, right eye**
L SP **H11.442 Conjunctival cysts, left eye**
L SP **H11.443 Conjunctival cysts, bilateral**
L IQ **H11.449 Conjunctival cysts, unspecified eye**
5 **H11.8 Other specified disorders of conjunctiva**
6 **H11.81 Pseudopterygium of conjunctiva**
L SP **H11.811 Pseudopterygium of conjunctiva, right eye**
L SP **H11.812 Pseudopterygium of conjunctiva, left eye**
L SP **H11.813 Pseudopterygium of conjunctiva, bilateral**
L IQ **H11.819 Pseudopterygium of conjunctiva, unspecified eye**
6 **H11.82 Conjunctivochalasis**
DEFINITION Loosening of the conjunctiva's attachment to the eye, causing wrinkling, dryness, and a tendency to trap particles in the folds, causing chronic inflammation.
L SP **H11.821 Conjunctivochalasis, right eye**
L SP **H11.822 Conjunctivochalasis, left eye**
L SP **H11.823 Conjunctivochalasis, bilateral**

H11.829 Conjunctivochalasis, unspecified eye

H11.89 Other specified disorders of conjunctiva

H11.9 Unspecified disorder of conjunctiva

Disorders of sclera, cornea, iris and ciliary body (H15-H22)

H15 Disorders of sclera

H15.0 Scleritis

H15.00 Unspecified scleritis

H15.001 Unspecified scleritis, right eye

H15.002 Unspecified scleritis, left eye

H15.003 Unspecified scleritis, bilateral

H15.009 Unspecified scleritis, unspecified eye

H15.01 Anterior scleritis

H15.011 Anterior scleritis, right eye

H15.012 Anterior scleritis, left eye

H15.013 Anterior scleritis, bilateral

H15.019 Anterior scleritis, unspecified eye

H15.02 Brawny scleritis

DEFINITION Severe inflammation of the sclera affecting the border between the sclera and the cornea.

H15.021 Brawny scleritis, right eye

H15.022 Brawny scleritis, left eye

H15.023 Brawny scleritis, bilateral

H15.029 Brawny scleritis, unspecified eye

H15.03 Posterior scleritis

Sclerotenonitis

H15.031 Posterior scleritis, right eye

H15.032 Posterior scleritis, left eye

H15.033 Posterior scleritis, bilateral

H15.039 Posterior scleritis, unspecified eye

H15.04 Scleritis with corneal involvement

H15.041 Scleritis with corneal involvement, right eye

H15.042 Scleritis with corneal involvement, left eye

H15.043 Scleritis with corneal involvement, bilateral

H15.049 Scleritis with corneal involvement, unspecified eye

H15.05 Scleromalacia perforans

H15.051 Scleromalacia perforans, right eye

H15.052 Scleromalacia perforans, left eye

H15.053 Scleromalacia perforans, bilateral

H15.059 Scleromalacia perforans, unspecified eye

H15.09 Other scleritis

Scleral abscess

H15.091 Other scleritis, right eye

H15.092 Other scleritis, left eye

H15.093 Other scleritis, bilateral

H15.099 Other scleritis, unspecified eye

H15.1 Episcleritis

H15.10 Unspecified episcleritis

H15.101 Unspecified episcleritis, right eye

H15.102 Unspecified episcleritis, left eye

H15.103 Unspecified episcleritis, bilateral

H15.109 Unspecified episcleritis, unspecified eye

H15.11 Episcleritis periodica fugax

DEFINITION Periodic attacks of inflammation of the sclera; typically of rapid onset and short duration.

H15.111 Episcleritis periodica fugax, right eye

H15.112 Episcleritis periodica fugax, left eye

H15.113 Episcleritis periodica fugax, bilateral

H15.119 Episcleritis periodica fugax, unspecified eye

H15.12 Nodular episcleritis

H15.121 Nodular episcleritis, right eye

H15.122 Nodular episcleritis, left eye

H15.123 Nodular episcleritis, bilateral

H15.129 Nodular episcleritis, unspecified eye

H15.8 Other disorders of sclera

EXCLUDES 2 blue sclera (Q13.5)
degenerative myopia (H44.2-)

H15.81 Equatorial staphyloma

H15.811 Equatorial staphyloma, right eye

H15.812 Equatorial staphyloma, left eye

H15.813 Equatorial staphyloma, bilateral

H15.819 Equatorial staphyloma, unspecified eye

H15.82 Localized anterior staphyloma

H15.821 Localized anterior staphyloma, right eye

H15.822 Localized anterior staphyloma, left eye

H15.823 Localized anterior staphyloma, bilateral

H15.829 Localized anterior staphyloma, unspecified eye

H15.83 Staphyloma posticum

H15.831 Staphyloma posticum, right eye

H15.832 Staphyloma posticum, left eye

H15.833 Staphyloma posticum, bilateral

H15.839 Staphyloma posticum, unspecified eye

H15.84 Scleral ectasia

DEFINITION Contents of the eyeball protrude through an abnormally thin section of the sclera.

H15.841 Scleral ectasia, right eye

H15.842 Scleral ectasia, left eye

H15.843 Scleral ectasia, bilateral

H15.849 Scleral ectasia, unspecified eye

H15.85 Ring staphyloma

H15.851 Ring staphyloma, right eye

H15.852 Ring staphyloma, left eye

H15.853 Ring staphyloma, bilateral

H15.859 Ring staphyloma, unspecified eye

SP H15.89 Other disorders of sclera

!Q H15.9 Unspecified disorder of sclera

4 H16 Keratitis

5 H16.0 Corneal ulcer

6 H16.00 Unspecified corneal ulcer

⊟ SP H16.001 Unspecified corneal ulcer, right eye

⊟ SP H16.002 Unspecified corneal ulcer, left eye

⊟ SP H16.003 Unspecified corneal ulcer, bilateral

⊟ !Q H16.009 Unspecified corneal ulcer, unspecified eye

6 H16.01 Central corneal ulcer

⊟ SP H16.011 Central corneal ulcer, right eye

⊟ SP H16.012 Central corneal ulcer, left eye

⊟ SP H16.013 Central corneal ulcer, bilateral

⊟ !Q H16.019 Central corneal ulcer, unspecified eye

6 H16.02 Ring corneal ulcer

DEFINITION Ring of ulceration encircling the entire edge of the cornea.

⊟ SP H16.021 Ring corneal ulcer, right eye

⊟ SP H16.022 Ring corneal ulcer, left eye

⊟ SP H16.023 Ring corneal ulcer, bilateral

⊟ !Q H16.029 Ring corneal ulcer, unspecified eye

6 H16.03 Corneal ulcer with hypopyon

⊟ SP H16.031 Corneal ulcer with hypopyon, right eye

⊟ SP H16.032 Corneal ulcer with hypopyon, left eye

⊟ SP H16.033 Corneal ulcer with hypopyon, bilateral

⊟ !Q H16.039 Corneal ulcer with hypopyon, unspecified eye

6 H16.04 Marginal corneal ulcer

⊟ SP H16.041 Marginal corneal ulcer, right eye

⊟ SP H16.042 Marginal corneal ulcer, left eye

⊟ SP H16.043 Marginal corneal ulcer, bilateral

⊟ !Q H16.049 Marginal corneal ulcer, unspecified eye

6 H16.05 Mooren's corneal ulcer

⊟ SP H16.051 Mooren's corneal ulcer, right eye

⊟ SP H16.052 Mooren's corneal ulcer, left eye

⊟ SP H16.053 Mooren's corneal ulcer, bilateral

⊟ !Q H16.059 Mooren's corneal ulcer, unspecified eye

6 H16.06 Mycotic corneal ulcer

DEFINITION Corneal ulcer caused by a fungal infection.

⊟ SP H16.061 Mycotic corneal ulcer, right eye

⊟ SP H16.062 Mycotic corneal ulcer, left eye

⊟ SP H16.063 Mycotic corneal ulcer, bilateral

⊟ !Q H16.069 Mycotic corneal ulcer, unspecified eye

6 H16.07 Perforated corneal ulcer

⊟ SP H16.071 Perforated corneal ulcer, right eye

⊟ SP H16.072 Perforated corneal ulcer, left eye

⊟ SP H16.073 Perforated corneal ulcer, bilateral

⊟ !Q H16.079 Perforated corneal ulcer, unspecified eye

5 H16.1 Other and unspecified superficial keratitis without conjunctivitis

6 H16.10 Unspecified superficial keratitis

⊟ SP H16.101 Unspecified superficial keratitis, right eye

⊟ SP H16.102 Unspecified superficial keratitis, left eye

⊟ SP H16.103 Unspecified superficial keratitis, bilateral

⊟ !Q H16.109 Unspecified superficial keratitis, unspecified eye

6 H16.11 Macular keratitis

Areolar keratitis
Nummular keratitis
Stellate keratitis
Striate keratitis

⊟ SP H16.111 Macular keratitis, right eye

⊟ SP H16.112 Macular keratitis, left eye

⊟ SP H16.113 Macular keratitis, bilateral

⊟ !Q H16.119 Macular keratitis, unspecified eye

6 H16.12 Filamentary keratitis

DEFINITION Keratitis with twisted filaments of mucoid material on the surface of the cornea.

⊟ SP H16.121 Filamentary keratitis, right eye

⊟ SP H16.122 Filamentary keratitis, left eye

⊟ SP H16.123 Filamentary keratitis, bilateral

⊟ !Q H16.129 Filamentary keratitis, unspecified eye

6 H16.13 Photokeratitis

Snow blindness
Welders keratitis

DEFINITION Painful, inflamed cornea that develops due to over-exposure to ultraviolet light.

⊟ SP H16.131 Photokeratitis, right eye

⊟ SP H16.132 Photokeratitis, left eye

⊟ SP H16.133 Photokeratitis, bilateral

⊟ !Q H16.139 Photokeratitis, unspecified eye

6 H16.14 Punctate keratitis

⊟ SP H16.141 Punctate keratitis, right eye

⊟ SP H16.142 Punctate keratitis, left eye

⊟ SP H16.143 Punctate keratitis, bilateral

⊟ !Q H16.149 Punctate keratitis, unspecified eye

5 H16.2 Keratoconjunctivitis

DEFINITION Inflammation of both the cornea and the conjunctiva; presents with burning, bloodshot, watery eyes sensitive to bright light, blurred vision, and a sensation of something in the eye.

6 H16.20 Unspecified keratoconjunctivitis

Superficial keratitis with conjunctivitis NOS

⊟ SP H16.201 Unspecified keratoconjunctivitis, right eye

⊟ SP H16.202 Unspecified keratoconjunctivitis, left eye

SP H16.203 Unspecified keratoconjunctivitis, bilateral

IQ H16.209 Unspecified keratoconjunctivitis, unspecified eye

6 H16.21 Exposure keratoconjunctivitis

DEFINITION Dryness and inflammation of the cornea and conjunctiva caused by the failure of the eyelid to completely close during sleep and/or blinking.

SP H16.211 Exposure keratoconjunctivitis, right eye

SP H16.212 Exposure keratoconjunctivitis, left eye

SP H16.213 Exposure keratoconjunctivitis, bilateral

IQ H16.219 Exposure keratoconjunctivitis, unspecified eye

6 H16.22 Keratoconjunctivitis sicca, not specified as Sjögren's

EXCLUDES 1 Sjögren's syndrome (M35.01)

SP H16.221 Keratoconjunctivitis sicca, not specified as Sjögren's, right eye

SP H16.222 Keratoconjunctivitis sicca, not specified as Sjögren's, left eye

SP H16.223 Keratoconjunctivitis sicca, not specified as Sjögren's, bilateral

IQ H16.229 Keratoconjunctivitis sicca, not specified as Sjögren's, unspecified eye

6 H16.23 Neurotrophic keratoconjunctivitis

SP H16.231 Neurotrophic keratoconjunctivitis, right eye

SP H16.232 Neurotrophic keratoconjunctivitis, left eye

SP H16.233 Neurotrophic keratoconjunctivitis, bilateral

IQ H16.239 Neurotrophic keratoconjunctivitis, unspecified eye

6 H16.24 Ophthalmia nodosa

SP H16.241 Ophthalmia nodosa, right eye

SP H16.242 Ophthalmia nodosa, left eye

SP H16.243 Ophthalmia nodosa, bilateral

IQ H16.249 Ophthalmia nodosa, unspecified eye

6 H16.25 Phlyctenular keratoconjunctivitis

SP H16.251 Phlyctenular keratoconjunctivitis, right eye

SP H16.252 Phlyctenular keratoconjunctivitis, left eye

SP H16.253 Phlyctenular keratoconjunctivitis, bilateral

IQ H16.259 Phlyctenular keratoconjunctivitis, unspecified eye

6 H16.26 Vernal keratoconjunctivitis, with limbar and corneal involvement

EXCLUDES 1 vernal conjunctivitis without limbar and corneal involvement (H10.44)

SP H16.261 Vernal keratoconjunctivitis, with limbar and corneal involvement, right eye

SP H16.262 Vernal keratoconjunctivitis, with limbar and corneal involvement, left eye

SP H16.263 Vernal keratoconjunctivitis, with limbar and corneal involvement, bilateral

IQ H16.269 Vernal keratoconjunctivitis, with limbar and corneal involvement, unspecified eye

6 H16.29 Other keratoconjunctivitis

SP H16.291 Other keratoconjunctivitis, right eye

SP H16.292 Other keratoconjunctivitis, left eye

SP H16.293 Other keratoconjunctivitis, bilateral

IQ H16.299 Other keratoconjunctivitis, unspecified eye

5 H16.3 Interstitial and deep keratitis

6 H16.30 Unspecified interstitial keratitis

SP H16.301 Unspecified interstitial keratitis, right eye

SP H16.302 Unspecified interstitial keratitis, left eye

SP H16.303 Unspecified interstitial keratitis, bilateral

IQ H16.309 Unspecified interstitial keratitis, unspecified eye

6 H16.31 Corneal abscess

SP H16.311 Corneal abscess, right eye

SP H16.312 Corneal abscess, left eye

SP H16.313 Corneal abscess, bilateral

IQ H16.319 Corneal abscess, unspecified eye

6 H16.32 Diffuse interstitial keratitis

Cogan's syndrome

DEFINITION Rare disorder characterized by recurrent inflammation of the cornea with episodes of dizziness and hearing loss that can lead to blindness and deafness if left untreated.

SP H16.321 Diffuse interstitial keratitis, right eye

SP H16.322 Diffuse interstitial keratitis, left eye

SP H16.323 Diffuse interstitial keratitis, bilateral

IQ H16.329 Diffuse interstitial keratitis, unspecified eye

6 H16.33 Sclerosing keratitis

SP H16.331 Sclerosing keratitis, right eye

SP H16.332 Sclerosing keratitis, left eye

SP H16.333 Sclerosing keratitis, bilateral

IQ H16.339 Sclerosing keratitis, unspecified eye

6 H16.39 Other interstitial and deep keratitis

SP H16.391 Other interstitial and deep keratitis, right eye

SP H16.392 Other interstitial and deep keratitis, left eye

⊟ SP H16.393 Other interstitial and deep keratitis, bilateral
⊟ IQ H16.399 Other interstitial and deep keratitis, unspecified eye
5 H16.4 Corneal neovascularization
6 H16.40 Unspecified corneal neovascularization
⊟ SP H16.401 Unspecified corneal neovascularization, right eye
⊟ SP H16.402 Unspecified corneal neovascularization, left eye
⊟ SP H16.403 Unspecified corneal neovascularization, bilateral
⊟ IQ H16.409 Unspecified corneal neovascularization, unspecified eye
6 H16.41 Ghost vessels (corneal)
⊟ SP H16.411 Ghost vessels (corneal), right eye
⊟ SP H16.412 Ghost vessels (corneal), left eye
⊟ SP H16.413 Ghost vessels (corneal), bilateral
⊟ IQ H16.419 Ghost vessels (corneal), unspecified eye
6 H16.42 Pannus (corneal)
⊟ SP H16.421 Pannus (corneal), right eye
⊟ SP H16.422 Pannus (corneal), left eye
⊟ SP H16.423 Pannus (corneal), bilateral
⊟ IQ H16.429 Pannus (corneal), unspecified eye
6 H16.43 Localized vascularization of cornea
⊟ SP H16.431 Localized vascularization of cornea, right eye
⊟ SP H16.432 Localized vascularization of cornea, left eye
⊟ SP H16.433 Localized vascularization of cornea, bilateral
⊟ IQ H16.439 Localized vascularization of cornea, unspecified eye
6 H16.44 Deep vascularization of cornea
⊟ SP H16.441 Deep vascularization of cornea, right eye
⊟ SP H16.442 Deep vascularization of cornea, left eye
⊟ SP H16.443 Deep vascularization of cornea, bilateral
⊟ IQ H16.449 Deep vascularization of cornea, unspecified eye
SP H16.8 Other keratitis
SP H16.9 Unspecified keratitis
4 H17 Corneal scars and opacities
5 H17.0 Adherent leukoma
⊟ IQ H17.00 Adherent leukoma, unspecified eye
⊟ SP H17.01 Adherent leukoma, right eye
⊟ SP H17.02 Adherent leukoma, left eye
⊟ SP H17.03 Adherent leukoma, bilateral
5 H17.1 Central corneal opacity
⊟ IQ H17.10 Central corneal opacity, unspecified eye
⊟ SP H17.11 Central corneal opacity, right eye
⊟ SP H17.12 Central corneal opacity, left eye
⊟ SP H17.13 Central corneal opacity, bilateral
5 H17.8 Other corneal scars and opacities
6 H17.81 Minor opacity of cornea
Corneal nebula
⊟ SP H17.811 Minor opacity of cornea, right eye
⊟ SP H17.812 Minor opacity of cornea, left eye
⊟ SP H17.813 Minor opacity of cornea, bilateral
⊟ IQ H17.819 Minor opacity of cornea, unspecified eye
6 H17.82 Peripheral opacity of cornea
⊟ SP H17.821 Peripheral opacity of cornea, right eye
⊟ SP H17.822 Peripheral opacity of cornea, left eye
⊟ SP H17.823 Peripheral opacity of cornea, bilateral
⊟ IQ H17.829 Peripheral opacity of cornea, unspecified eye
SP H17.89 Other corneal scars and opacities
IQ H17.9 Unspecified corneal scar and opacity
4 H18 Other disorders of cornea
5 H18.0 Corneal pigmentations and deposits
6 H18.00 Unspecified corneal deposit
⊟ SP H18.001 Unspecified corneal deposit, right eye
⊟ SP H18.002 Unspecified corneal deposit, left eye
⊟ SP H18.003 Unspecified corneal deposit, bilateral
⊟ IQ H18.009 Unspecified corneal deposit, unspecified eye
6 H18.01 Anterior corneal pigmentations
Staehli's line
⊟ SP H18.011 Anterior corneal pigmentations, right eye
⊟ SP H18.012 Anterior corneal pigmentations, left eye
⊟ SP H18.013 Anterior corneal pigmentations, bilateral
⊟ IQ H18.019 Anterior corneal pigmentations, unspecified eye
6 H18.02 Argentous corneal deposits
⊟ SP H18.021 Argentous corneal deposits, right eye
⊟ SP H18.022 Argentous corneal deposits, left eye
⊟ SP H18.023 Argentous corneal deposits, bilateral
⊟ IQ H18.029 Argentous corneal deposits, unspecified eye
6 H18.03 Corneal deposits in metabolic disorders
Code also:
associated metabolic disorder
⊟ SP H18.031 Corneal deposits in metabolic disorders, right eye
⊟ SP H18.032 Corneal deposits in metabolic disorders, left eye
⊟ SP H18.033 Corneal deposits in metabolic disorders, bilateral
⊟ IQ H18.039 Corneal deposits in metabolic disorders, unspecified eye
6 H18.04 Kayser-Fleischer ring
Code also:
associated Wilson's disease (E83.01)

Chapter 7
H00-H59

4 4th digit required 5 5th digit required 6 6th digit required 7 7th digit required 7 7th digit placeholder + Additional code ⊟ Laterality

DEFINITION Gray-green or brownish ring of copper deposits on the exterior of the cornea that grow slowly inward; often seen with liver disorders.

SP **H18.041 Kayser-Fleischer ring, right eye**

SP **H18.042 Kayser-Fleischer ring, left eye**

SP **H18.043 Kayser-Fleischer ring, bilateral**

IQ **H18.049 Kayser-Fleischer ring, unspecified eye**

6 **H18.05 Posterior corneal pigmentations**
Krukenberg's spindle

SP **H18.051 Posterior corneal pigmentations, right eye**

SP **H18.052 Posterior corneal pigmentations, left eye**

SP **H18.053 Posterior corneal pigmentations, bilateral**

IQ **H18.059 Posterior corneal pigmentations, unspecified eye**

6 **H18.06 Stromal corneal pigmentations**
Hematocornea

SP **H18.061 Stromal corneal pigmentations, right eye**

SP **H18.062 Stromal corneal pigmentations, left eye**

SP **H18.063 Stromal corneal pigmentations, bilateral**

IQ **H18.069 Stromal corneal pigmentations, unspecified eye**

5 **H18.1 Bullous keratopathy**

IQ **H18.10 Bullous keratopathy, unspecified eye**

SP **H18.11 Bullous keratopathy, right eye**

SP **H18.12 Bullous keratopathy, left eye**

SP **H18.13 Bullous keratopathy, bilateral**

5 **H18.2 Other and unspecified corneal edema**

SP **H18.20 Unspecified corneal edema**

6 **H18.21 Corneal edema secondary to contact lens**

EXCLUDES 2 other corneal disorders due to contact lens (H18.82-)

SP **H18.211 Corneal edema secondary to contact lens, right eye**

SP **H18.212 Corneal edema secondary to contact lens, left eye**

SP **H18.213 Corneal edema secondary to contact lens, bilateral**

IQ **H18.219 Corneal edema secondary to contact lens, unspecified eye**

6 **H18.22 Idiopathic corneal edema**

SP **H18.221 Idiopathic corneal edema, right eye**

SP **H18.222 Idiopathic corneal edema, left eye**

SP **H18.223 Idiopathic corneal edema, bilateral**

IQ **H18.229 Idiopathic corneal edema, unspecified eye**

6 **H18.23 Secondary corneal edema**

SP **H18.231 Secondary corneal edema, right eye**

SP **H18.232 Secondary corneal edema, left eye**

SP **H18.233 Secondary corneal edema, bilateral**

IQ **H18.239 Secondary corneal edema, unspecified eye**

5 **H18.3 Changes of corneal membranes**

SP **H18.30 Unspecified corneal membrane change**

6 **H18.31 Folds and rupture in Bowman's membrane**

SP **H18.311 Folds and rupture in Bowman's membrane, right eye**

SP **H18.312 Folds and rupture in Bowman's membrane, left eye**

SP **H18.313 Folds and rupture in Bowman's membrane, bilateral**

IQ **H18.319 Folds and rupture in Bowman's membrane, unspecified eye**

6 **H18.32 Folds in Descemet's membrane**

DEFINITION Fold in the membrane between the innermost layer of the cornea and the stroma (strong, supportive layer), affecting vision and preventing the flow of nutrients out of the cornea.

SP **H18.321 Folds in Descemet's membrane, right eye**

SP **H18.322 Folds in Descemet's membrane, left eye**

SP **H18.323 Folds in Descemet's membrane, bilateral**

IQ **H18.329 Folds in Descemet's membrane, unspecified eye**

6 **H18.33 Rupture in Descemet's membrane**

SP **H18.331 Rupture in Descemet's membrane, right eye**

SP **H18.332 Rupture in Descemet's membrane, left eye**

SP **H18.333 Rupture in Descemet's membrane, bilateral**

IQ **H18.339 Rupture in Descemet's membrane, unspecified eye**

5 **H18.4 Corneal degeneration**

EXCLUDES 1 Mooren's ulcer (H16.0-)
recurrent erosion of cornea (H18.83-)

SP **H18.40 Unspecified corneal degeneration**

6 **H18.41 Arcus senilis**
Senile corneal changes

SP **H18.411 Arcus senilis, right eye**

SP **H18.412 Arcus senilis, left eye**

SP **H18.413 Arcus senilis, bilateral**

IQ **H18.419 Arcus senilis, unspecified eye**

6 **H18.42 Band keratopathy**

DEFINITION Degeneration of the cornea in which calcium deposits are laid in horizontal band-like layers, obscuring the patient's vision.

SP **H18.421 Band keratopathy, right eye**

SP **H18.422 Band keratopathy, left eye**

SP **H18.423 Band keratopathy, bilateral**

IQ **H18.429 Band keratopathy, unspecified eye**

SP **H18.43 Other calcerous corneal degeneration**

6 **H18.44 Keratomalacia**

EXCLUDES 1 keratomalacia due to vitamin A deficiency (E50.4)

- ⊟ SP H18.441 Keratomalacia, right eye
- ⊟ SP H18.442 Keratomalacia, left eye
- ⊟ SP H18.443 Keratomalacia, bilateral
- ⊟ IQ H18.449 Keratomalacia, unspecified eye

6 **H18.45 Nodular corneal degeneration**

- ⊟ SP H18.451 Nodular corneal degeneration, right eye
- ⊟ SP H18.452 Nodular corneal degeneration, left eye
- ⊟ SP H18.453 Nodular corneal degeneration, bilateral
- ⊟ IQ H18.459 Nodular corneal degeneration, unspecified eye

6 **H18.46 Peripheral corneal degeneration**

- ⊟ SP H18.461 Peripheral corneal degeneration, right eye
- ⊟ SP H18.462 Peripheral corneal degeneration, left eye
- ⊟ SP H18.463 Peripheral corneal degeneration, bilateral
- ⊟ IQ H18.469 Peripheral corneal degeneration, unspecified eye

SP **H18.49 Other corneal degeneration**

5 **H18.5 Hereditary corneal dystrophies**

6 **H18.50 Unspecified hereditary corneal dystrophies**

- ⊟ SP H18.501 Unspecified hereditary corneal dystrophies, right eye
- ⊟ SP H18.502 Unspecified hereditary corneal dystrophies, left eye
- ⊟ SP H18.503 Unspecified hereditary corneal dystrophies, bilateral
- ⊟ IQ H18.509 Unspecified hereditary corneal dystrophies, unspecified eye

6 **H18.51 Endothelial corneal dystrophy**

Fuchs' dystrophy

- ⊟ SP H18.511 Endothelial corneal dystrophy, right eye
- ⊟ SP H18.512 Endothelial corneal dystrophy, left eye
- ⊟ SP H18.513 Endothelial corneal dystrophy, bilateral
- ⊟ IQ H18.519 Endothelial corneal dystrophy, unspecified eye

6 **H18.52 Epithelial (juvenile) corneal dystrophy**

DEFINITION Multiple lesions on the outermost layer of the cornea occurring in the early years, which gradually grow together and obscure vision.

- ⊟ SP H18.521 Epithelial (juvenile) corneal dystrophy, right eye
- ⊟ SP H18.522 Epithelial (juvenile) corneal dystrophy, left eye
- ⊟ SP H18.523 Epithelial (juvenile) corneal dystrophy, bilateral
- ⊟ IQ H18.529 Epithelial (juvenile) corneal dystrophy, unspecified eye

6 **H18.53 Granular corneal dystrophy**

- ⊟ SP H18.531 Granular corneal dystrophy, right eye
- ⊟ SP H18.532 Granular corneal dystrophy, left eye
- ⊟ SP H18.533 Granular corneal dystrophy, bilateral
- ⊟ IQ H18.539 Granular corneal dystrophy, unspecified eye

6 **H18.54 Lattice corneal dystrophy**

- ⊟ SP H18.541 Lattice corneal dystrophy, right eye
- ⊟ SP H18.542 Lattice corneal dystrophy, left eye
- ⊟ SP H18.543 Lattice corneal dystrophy, bilateral
- ⊟ IQ H18.549 Lattice corneal dystrophy, unspecified eye

6 **H18.55 Macular corneal dystrophy**

- ⊟ SP H18.551 Macular corneal dystrophy, right eye
- ⊟ SP H18.552 Macular corneal dystrophy, left eye
- ⊟ SP H18.553 Macular corneal dystrophy, bilateral
- ⊟ IQ H18.559 Macular corneal dystrophy, unspecified eye

6 **H18.59 Other hereditary corneal dystrophies**

- ⊟ SP H18.591 Other hereditary corneal dystrophies, right eye
- ⊟ SP H18.592 Other hereditary corneal dystrophies, left eye
- ⊟ SP H18.593 Other hereditary corneal dystrophies, bilateral
- ⊟ IQ H18.599 Other hereditary corneal dystrophies, unspecified eye

5 **H18.6 Keratoconus**

6 **H18.60 Keratoconus, unspecified**

- ⊟ SP H18.601 Keratoconus, unspecified, right eye
- ⊟ SP H18.602 Keratoconus, unspecified, left eye
- ⊟ SP H18.603 Keratoconus, unspecified, bilateral
- ⊟ IQ H18.609 Keratoconus, unspecified, unspecified eye

6 **H18.61 Keratoconus, stable**

- ⊟ SP H18.611 Keratoconus, stable, right eye
- ⊟ SP H18.612 Keratoconus, stable, left eye
- ⊟ SP H18.613 Keratoconus, stable, bilateral
- ⊟ IQ H18.619 Keratoconus, stable, unspecified eye

6 **H18.62 Keratoconus, unstable**

Acute hydrops

- ⊟ SP H18.621 Keratoconus, unstable, right eye
- ⊟ SP H18.622 Keratoconus, unstable, left eye
- ⊟ SP H18.623 Keratoconus, unstable, bilateral
- ⊟ IQ H18.629 Keratoconus, unstable, unspecified eye

5 **H18.7 Other and unspecified corneal deformities**

EXCLUDES 1 congenital malformations of cornea (Q13.3-Q13.4)

IQ **H18.70 Unspecified corneal deformity**

6 **H18.71 Corneal ectasia**

- ⊟ SP H18.711 Corneal ectasia, right eye
- ⊟ SP H18.712 Corneal ectasia, left eye

Chapter 7 H00-H59

4 4th digit required 5 5th digit required 6 6th digit required 7 7th digit required X 7th digit placeholder + Additional code ⊟ Laterality

SP H18.713 Corneal ectasia, bilateral
IQ H18.719 Corneal ectasia, unspecified eye
6 H18.72 Corneal staphyloma
SP H18.721 Corneal staphyloma, right eye
SP H18.722 Corneal staphyloma, left eye
SP H18.723 Corneal staphyloma, bilateral
IQ H18.729 Corneal staphyloma, unspecified eye
6 H18.73 Descemetocele
SP H18.731 Descemetocele, right eye
SP H18.732 Descemetocele, left eye
SP H18.733 Descemetocele, bilateral
IQ H18.739 Descemetocele, unspecified eye
6 H18.79 Other corneal deformities
SP H18.791 Other corneal deformities, right eye
SP H18.792 Other corneal deformities, left eye
SP H18.793 Other corneal deformities, bilateral
IQ H18.799 Other corneal deformities, unspecified eye
5 H18.8 Other specified disorders of cornea
6 H18.81 Anesthesia and hypoesthesia of cornea

DEFINITION Decreased or complete loss of corneal sensitivity to pain and irritation.

SP H18.811 Anesthesia and hypoesthesia of cornea, right eye
SP H18.812 Anesthesia and hypoesthesia of cornea, left eye
SP H18.813 Anesthesia and hypoesthesia of cornea, bilateral
IQ H18.819 Anesthesia and hypoesthesia of cornea, unspecified eye
6 H18.82 Corneal disorder due to contact lens

EXCLUDES 2 corneal edema due to contact lens (H18.21-)

SP H18.821 Corneal disorder due to contact lens, right eye
SP H18.822 Corneal disorder due to contact lens, left eye
SP H18.823 Corneal disorder due to contact lens, bilateral
IQ H18.829 Corneal disorder due to contact lens, unspecified eye
6 H18.83 Recurrent erosion of cornea
SP H18.831 Recurrent erosion of cornea, right eye
SP H18.832 Recurrent erosion of cornea, left eye
SP H18.833 Recurrent erosion of cornea, bilateral
IQ H18.839 Recurrent erosion of cornea, unspecified eye
6 H18.89 Other specified disorders of cornea
SP H18.891 Other specified disorders of cornea, right eye
SP H18.892 Other specified disorders of cornea, left eye
SP H18.893 Other specified disorders of cornea, bilateral
IQ H18.899 Other specified disorders of cornea, unspecified eye
IQ H18.9 Unspecified disorder of cornea
4 H20 Iridocyclitis
5 H20.0 Acute and subacute iridocyclitis

Acute anterior uveitis
Acute cyclitis
Acute iritis
Subacute anterior uveitis
Subacute cyclitis
Subacute iritis

EXCLUDES 1 iridocyclitis, iritis, uveitis (due to) (in) diabetes mellitus (E08-E13 with .39)
iridocyclitis, iritis, uveitis (due to) (in) diphtheria (A36.89)
iridocyclitis, iritis, uveitis (due to) (in) gonococcal (A54.32)
iridocyclitis, iritis, uveitis (due to) (in) herpes (simplex) (B00.51)
iridocyclitis, iritis, uveitis (due to) (in) herpes zoster (B02.32)
iridocyclitis, iritis, uveitis (due to) (in) late congenital syphilis (A50.39)
iridocyclitis, iritis, uveitis (due to) (in) late syphilis (A52.71)
iridocyclitis, iritis, uveitis (due to) (in) sarcoidosis (D86.83)
iridocyclitis, iritis, uveitis (due to) (in) syphilis (A51.43)
iridocyclitis, iritis, uveitis (due to) (in) toxoplasmosis (B58.09)
iridocyclitis, iritis, uveitis (due to) (in) tuberculosis (A18.54)

SP H20.00 Unspecified acute and subacute iridocyclitis
6 H20.01 Primary iridocyclitis
SP H20.011 Primary iridocyclitis, right eye
SP H20.012 Primary iridocyclitis, left eye
SP H20.013 Primary iridocyclitis, bilateral
IQ H20.019 Primary iridocyclitis, unspecified eye
6 H20.02 Recurrent acute iridocyclitis
SP H20.021 Recurrent acute iridocyclitis, right eye
SP H20.022 Recurrent acute iridocyclitis, left eye
SP H20.023 Recurrent acute iridocyclitis, bilateral
IQ H20.029 Recurrent acute iridocyclitis, unspecified eye
6 H20.03 Secondary infectious iridocyclitis
SP H20.031 Secondary infectious iridocyclitis, right eye

Chapter 7

H00-H59

⊟ SP H20.032 Secondary infectious iridocyclitis, left eye
⊟ SP H20.033 Secondary infectious iridocyclitis, bilateral
⊟ IQ H20.039 Secondary infectious iridocyclitis, unspecified eye

6 H20.04 Secondary noninfectious iridocyclitis
⊟ SP H20.041 Secondary noninfectious iridocyclitis, right eye
⊟ SP H20.042 Secondary noninfectious iridocyclitis, left eye
⊟ SP H20.043 Secondary noninfectious iridocyclitis, bilateral
⊟ IQ H20.049 Secondary noninfectious iridocyclitis, unspecified eye

6 H20.05 Hypopyon
DEFINITION Accumulation of pus in the anterior chamber of the eye between the cornea and the iris and lens.
⊟ SP H20.051 Hypopyon, right eye
⊟ SP H20.052 Hypopyon, left eye
⊟ SP H20.053 Hypopyon, bilateral
⊟ IQ H20.059 Hypopyon, unspecified eye

+ 5 H20.1 Chronic iridocyclitis
Use additional code for any associated cataract (H26.21-)
EXCLUDES 2 posterior cyclitis (H30.2-)
⊟ IQ + H20.10 Chronic iridocyclitis, unspecified eye
⊟ SP + H20.11 Chronic iridocyclitis, right eye
⊟ SP + H20.12 Chronic iridocyclitis, left eye
⊟ SP + H20.13 Chronic iridocyclitis, bilateral

5 H20.2 Lens-induced iridocyclitis
⊟ IQ H20.20 Lens-induced iridocyclitis, unspecified eye
⊟ SP H20.21 Lens-induced iridocyclitis, right eye
⊟ SP H20.22 Lens-induced iridocyclitis, left eye
⊟ SP H20.23 Lens-induced iridocyclitis, bilateral

5 H20.8 Other iridocyclitis
EXCLUDES 2 glaucomatocyclitis crises (H40.4-)
posterior cyclitis (H30.2-)
sympathetic uveitis (H44.13-)

6 H20.81 Fuchs' heterochromic cyclitis
⊟ SP H20.811 Fuchs' heterochromic cyclitis, right eye
⊟ SP H20.812 Fuchs' heterochromic cyclitis, left eye
⊟ SP H20.813 Fuchs' heterochromic cyclitis, bilateral
⊟ IQ H20.819 Fuchs' heterochromic cyclitis, unspecified eye

6 H20.82 Vogt-Koyanagi syndrome
⊟ SP H20.821 Vogt-Koyanagi syndrome, right eye
⊟ SP H20.822 Vogt-Koyanagi syndrome, left eye
⊟ SP H20.823 Vogt-Koyanagi syndrome, bilateral
⊟ IQ H20.829 Vogt-Koyanagi syndrome, unspecified eye

SP H20.9 Unspecified iridocyclitis
Uveitis NOS

4 H21 Other disorders of iris and ciliary body
EXCLUDES 2 sympathetic uveitis (H44.1-)

5 H21.0 Hyphema
EXCLUDES 1 traumatic hyphema (S05.1-)
DEFINITION Bleeding in the iris that pools in the bottom of the cornea causing vision to be extremely blurred.
⊟ IQ H21.00 Hyphema, unspecified eye
⊟ SP H21.01 Hyphema, right eye
⊟ SP H21.02 Hyphema, left eye
⊟ SP H21.03 Hyphema, bilateral

5 H21.1 Other vascular disorders of iris and ciliary body
Neovascularization of iris or ciliary body
Rubeosis iridis
Rubeosis of iris

6 H21.1X Other vascular disorders of iris and ciliary body
⊟ SP H21.1X1 Other vascular disorders of iris and ciliary body, right eye
⊟ SP H21.1X2 Other vascular disorders of iris and ciliary body, left eye
⊟ SP H21.1X3 Other vascular disorders of iris and ciliary body, bilateral
⊟ IQ H21.1X9 Other vascular disorders of iris and ciliary body, unspecified eye

5 H21.2 Degeneration of iris and ciliary body

6 H21.21 Degeneration of chamber angle
⊟ SP H21.211 Degeneration of chamber angle, right eye
⊟ SP H21.212 Degeneration of chamber angle, left eye
⊟ SP H21.213 Degeneration of chamber angle, bilateral
⊟ IQ H21.219 Degeneration of chamber angle, unspecified eye

6 H21.22 Degeneration of ciliary body
⊟ SP H21.221 Degeneration of ciliary body, right eye
⊟ SP H21.222 Degeneration of ciliary body, left eye
⊟ SP H21.223 Degeneration of ciliary body, bilateral
⊟ IQ H21.229 Degeneration of ciliary body, unspecified eye

6 H21.23 Degeneration of iris (pigmentary)
Translucency of iris
DEFINITION Fading of the pigmentation (color) of the iris, allowing light to seep in rather than being blocked; presents with light-sensitivity and blurred vision.
⊟ SP H21.231 Degeneration of iris (pigmentary), right eye
⊟ SP H21.232 Degeneration of iris (pigmentary), left eye
⊟ SP H21.233 Degeneration of iris (pigmentary), bilateral
⊟ IQ H21.239 Degeneration of iris (pigmentary), unspecified eye

6 H21.24 Degeneration of pupillary margin
⊟ SP H21.241 Degeneration of pupillary margin, right eye

SP H21.242 Degeneration of pupillary margin, left eye
SP H21.243 Degeneration of pupillary margin, bilateral
IQ H21.249 Degeneration of pupillary margin, unspecified eye
6 H21.25 Iridoschisis
SP H21.251 Iridoschisis, right eye
SP H21.252 Iridoschisis, left eye
SP H21.253 Iridoschisis, bilateral
IQ H21.259 Iridoschisis, unspecified eye
6 H21.26 Iris atrophy (essential) (progressive)
SP H21.261 Iris atrophy (essential) (progressive), right eye
SP H21.262 Iris atrophy (essential) (progressive), left eye
SP H21.263 Iris atrophy (essential) (progressive), bilateral
IQ H21.269 Iris atrophy (essential) (progressive), unspecified eye
6 H21.27 Miotic pupillary cyst
DEFINITION Fluid-filled pockets in the iris at the pupil's edge, causing the iris to contract and interfering with vision when light is less than optimal.
SP H21.271 Miotic pupillary cyst, right eye
SP H21.272 Miotic pupillary cyst, left eye
SP H21.273 Miotic pupillary cyst, bilateral
IQ H21.279 Miotic pupillary cyst, unspecified eye
SP H21.29 Other iris atrophy
5 H21.3 Cyst of iris, ciliary body and anterior chamber
EXCLUDES 2 miotic pupillary cyst (H21.27-)
6 H21.30 Idiopathic cysts of iris, ciliary body or anterior chamber
Cyst of iris, ciliary body or anterior chamber NOS
SP H21.301 Idiopathic cysts of iris, ciliary body or anterior chamber, right eye
SP H21.302 Idiopathic cysts of iris, ciliary body or anterior chamber, left eye
SP H21.303 Idiopathic cysts of iris, ciliary body or anterior chamber, bilateral
IQ H21.309 Idiopathic cysts of iris, ciliary body or anterior chamber, unspecified eye
6 H21.31 Exudative cysts of iris or anterior chamber
SP H21.311 Exudative cysts of iris or anterior chamber, right eye
SP H21.312 Exudative cysts of iris or anterior chamber, left eye
SP H21.313 Exudative cysts of iris or anterior chamber, bilateral
IQ H21.319 Exudative cysts of iris or anterior chamber, unspecified eye
6 H21.32 Implantation cysts of iris, ciliary body or anterior chamber
SP H21.321 Implantation cysts of iris, ciliary body or anterior chamber, right eye
SP H21.322 Implantation cysts of iris, ciliary body or anterior chamber, left eye
SP H21.323 Implantation cysts of iris, ciliary body or anterior chamber, bilateral
IQ H21.329 Implantation cysts of iris, ciliary body or anterior chamber, unspecified eye
6 H21.33 Parasitic cyst of iris, ciliary body or anterior chamber
SP H21.331 Parasitic cyst of iris, ciliary body or anterior chamber, right eye
SP H21.332 Parasitic cyst of iris, ciliary body or anterior chamber, left eye
SP H21.333 Parasitic cyst of iris, ciliary body or anterior chamber, bilateral
IQ H21.339 Parasitic cyst of iris, ciliary body or anterior chamber, unspecified eye
6 H21.34 Primary cyst of pars plana
SP H21.341 Primary cyst of pars plana, right eye
SP H21.342 Primary cyst of pars plana, left eye
SP H21.343 Primary cyst of pars plana, bilateral
IQ H21.349 Primary cyst of pars plana, unspecified eye
6 H21.35 Exudative cyst of pars plana
SP H21.351 Exudative cyst of pars plana, right eye
SP H21.352 Exudative cyst of pars plana, left eye
SP H21.353 Exudative cyst of pars plana, bilateral
IQ H21.359 Exudative cyst of pars plana, unspecified eye
5 H21.4 Pupillary membranes
Iris bombé
Pupillary occlusion
Pupillary seclusion
EXCLUDES 1 congenital pupillary membranes (Q13.8)
IQ H21.40 Pupillary membranes, unspecified eye
SP H21.41 Pupillary membranes, right eye
SP H21.42 Pupillary membranes, left eye
SP H21.43 Pupillary membranes, bilateral
5 H21.5 Other and unspecified adhesions and disruptions of iris and ciliary body
EXCLUDES 1 corectopia (Q13.2)
6 H21.50 Unspecified adhesions of iris
Synechia (iris) NOS
SP H21.501 Unspecified adhesions of iris, right eye
SP H21.502 Unspecified adhesions of iris, left eye
SP H21.503 Unspecified adhesions of iris, bilateral
IQ H21.509 Unspecified adhesions of iris and ciliary body, unspecified eye
6 H21.51 Anterior synechiae (iris)
SP H21.511 Anterior synechiae (iris), right eye
SP H21.512 Anterior synechiae (iris), left eye

Chapter 7
H00-H59

Laterality SP **H21.513 Anterior synechiae (iris), bilateral**

Laterality IQ **H21.519 Anterior synechiae (iris), unspecified eye**

6 **H21.52 Goniosynechiae**

DEFINITION Adhesion of the iris to the posterior surface of the cornea, in the angle of the anterior chamber of the eye.

Laterality SP **H21.521 Goniosynechiae, right eye**

Laterality SP **H21.522 Goniosynechiae, left eye**

Laterality SP **H21.523 Goniosynechiae, bilateral**

Laterality IQ **H21.529 Goniosynechiae, unspecified eye**

6 **H21.53 Iridodialysis**

DEFINITION Separation or loosening of the iris from its root at the ciliary body, usually from trauma or surgical accident.

Laterality SP **H21.531 Iridodialysis, right eye**

Laterality SP **H21.532 Iridodialysis, left eye**

Laterality SP **H21.533 Iridodialysis, bilateral**

Laterality IQ **H21.539 Iridodialysis, unspecified eye**

6 **H21.54 Posterior synechiae (iris)**

DEFINITION Adhesion where the lens and the iris grow together, preventing the iris from dilating and contracting properly.

Laterality SP **H21.541 Posterior synechiae (iris), right eye**

Laterality SP **H21.542 Posterior synechiae (iris), left eye**

Laterality SP **H21.543 Posterior synechiae (iris), bilateral**

Laterality IQ **H21.549 Posterior synechiae (iris), unspecified eye**

6 **H21.55 Recession of chamber angle**

Laterality SP **H21.551 Recession of chamber angle, right eye**

Laterality SP **H21.552 Recession of chamber angle, left eye**

Laterality SP **H21.553 Recession of chamber angle, bilateral**

Laterality IQ **H21.559 Recession of chamber angle, unspecified eye**

6 **H21.56 Pupillary abnormalities**

Deformed pupil
Ectopic pupil
Rupture of sphincter, pupil

EXCLUDES 1 congenital deformity of pupil (Q13.2-)

Laterality SP **H21.561 Pupillary abnormality, right eye**

Laterality SP **H21.562 Pupillary abnormality, left eye**

Laterality SP **H21.563 Pupillary abnormality, bilateral**

Laterality IQ **H21.569 Pupillary abnormality, unspecified eye**

5 **H21.8 Other specified disorders of iris and ciliary body**

SP + **H21.81 Floppy iris syndrome**

Intraoperative floppy iris syndrome (IFIS)

Use additional code for adverse effect, if applicable, to identify drug (T36-T50 with fifth or sixth character 5)

DEFINITION Syndrome occurring in one who has taken alpha-blockers; a dilated iris does not stay dilated, causing potentially injurious surgical complications.

SP **H21.82 Plateau iris syndrome (post-iridectomy) (postprocedural)**

SP **H21.89 Other specified disorders of iris and ciliary body**

IQ **H21.9 Unspecified disorder of iris and ciliary body**

M IQ **H22** ***Disorders of iris and ciliary body in diseases classified elsewhere***

Code first underlying disease, such as:
- gout (M1A.-, M10.-)
- leprosy (A30.-)
- parasitic disease (B89)

Disorders of lens (H25-H28)

4 **H25 Age-related cataract**

Senile cataract

EXCLUDES 2 capsular glaucoma with pseudoexfoliation of lens (H40.1-)

5 **H25.0 Age-related incipient cataract**

6 **H25.01 Cortical age-related cataract**

Laterality SP **H25.011 Cortical age-related cataract, right eye**

Laterality SP **H25.012 Cortical age-related cataract, left eye**

Laterality SP **H25.013 Cortical age-related cataract, bilateral**

Laterality IQ **H25.019 Cortical age-related cataract, unspecified eye**

6 **H25.03 Anterior subcapsular polar age-related cataract**

Laterality SP **H25.031 Anterior subcapsular polar age-related cataract, right eye**

Laterality SP **H25.032 Anterior subcapsular polar age-related cataract, left eye**

Laterality SP **H25.033 Anterior subcapsular polar age-related cataract, bilateral**

Laterality IQ **H25.039 Anterior subcapsular polar age-related cataract, unspecified eye**

6 **H25.04 Posterior subcapsular polar age-related cataract**

Laterality SP **H25.041 Posterior subcapsular polar age-related cataract, right eye**

Laterality SP **H25.042 Posterior subcapsular polar age-related cataract, left eye**

Laterality SP **H25.043 Posterior subcapsular polar age-related cataract, bilateral**

Laterality IQ **H25.049 Posterior subcapsular polar age-related cataract, unspecified eye**

6 **H25.09 Other age-related incipient cataract**

Coronary age-related cataract
Punctate age-related cataract
Water clefts

Laterality SP **H25.091 Other age-related incipient cataract, right eye**

Laterality SP **H25.092 Other age-related incipient cataract, left eye**

Laterality SP **H25.093 Other age-related incipient cataract, bilateral**

Laterality IQ **H25.099 Other age-related incipient cataract, unspecified eye**

Chapter 7 H00-H59

4 4th digit required 5 5th digit required 6 6th digit required 7 7th digit required 7 7th digit placeholder + Additional code Laterality

5 H25.1 Age-related nuclear cataract
Cataracta brunescens
Nuclear sclerosis cataract
IQ H25.10 Age-related nuclear cataract, unspecified eye
SP H25.11 Age-related nuclear cataract, right eye
SP H25.12 Age-related nuclear cataract, left eye
SP H25.13 Age-related nuclear cataract, bilateral
5 H25.2 Age-related cataract, morgagnian type
Age-related hypermature cataract
IQ H25.20 Age-related cataract, morgagnian type, unspecified eye
SP H25.21 Age-related cataract, morgagnian type, right eye
SP H25.22 Age-related cataract, morgagnian type, left eye
SP H25.23 Age-related cataract, morgagnian type, bilateral
5 H25.8 Other age-related cataract
6 H25.81 Combined forms of age-related cataract
SP H25.811 Combined forms of age-related cataract, right eye
SP H25.812 Combined forms of age-related cataract, left eye
SP H25.813 Combined forms of age-related cataract, bilateral
IQ H25.819 Combined forms of age-related cataract, unspecified eye
SP H25.89 Other age-related cataract
SP H25.9 Unspecified age-related cataract

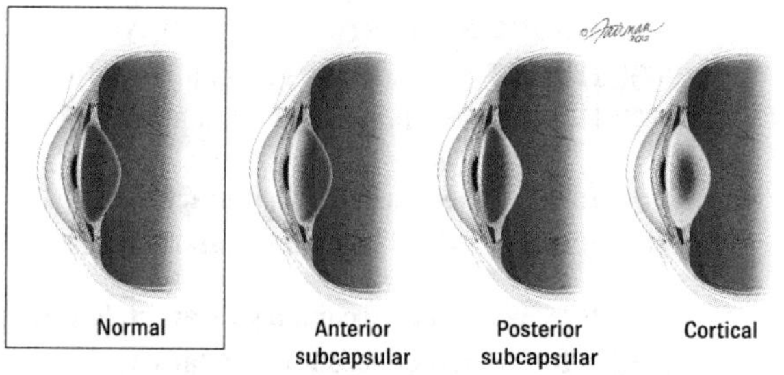

4 H26 Other cataract
EXCLUDES 1 congenital cataract (Q12.0)
DEFINITION Partial or complete clouding on or in the lens or lens capsule of the eye, obscuring vision.
5 H26.0 Infantile and juvenile cataract
6 H26.00 Unspecified infantile and juvenile cataract
SP H26.001 Unspecified infantile and juvenile cataract, right eye
SP H26.002 Unspecified infantile and juvenile cataract, left eye
SP H26.003 Unspecified infantile and juvenile cataract, bilateral
IQ H26.009 Unspecified infantile and juvenile cataract, unspecified eye
6 H26.01 Infantile and juvenile cortical, lamellar, or zonular cataract
SP H26.011 Infantile and juvenile cortical, lamellar, or zonular cataract, right eye
SP H26.012 Infantile and juvenile cortical, lamellar, or zonular cataract, left eye
SP H26.013 Infantile and juvenile cortical, lamellar, or zonular cataract, bilateral
IQ H26.019 Infantile and juvenile cortical, lamellar, or zonular cataract, unspecified eye
6 H26.03 Infantile and juvenile nuclear cataract
SP H26.031 Infantile and juvenile nuclear cataract, right eye
SP H26.032 Infantile and juvenile nuclear cataract, left eye
SP H26.033 Infantile and juvenile nuclear cataract, bilateral
IQ H26.039 Infantile and juvenile nuclear cataract, unspecified eye
6 H26.04 Anterior subcapsular polar infantile and juvenile cataract
SP H26.041 Anterior subcapsular polar infantile and juvenile cataract, right eye
SP H26.042 Anterior subcapsular polar infantile and juvenile cataract, left eye
SP H26.043 Anterior subcapsular polar infantile and juvenile cataract, bilateral
IQ H26.049 Anterior subcapsular polar infantile and juvenile cataract, unspecified eye
6 H26.05 Posterior subcapsular polar infantile and juvenile cataract
SP H26.051 Posterior subcapsular polar infantile and juvenile cataract, right eye
SP H26.052 Posterior subcapsular polar infantile and juvenile cataract, left eye
SP H26.053 Posterior subcapsular polar infantile and juvenile cataract, bilateral
IQ H26.059 Posterior subcapsular polar infantile and juvenile cataract, unspecified eye
6 H26.06 Combined forms of infantile and juvenile cataract
SP H26.061 Combined forms of infantile and juvenile cataract, right eye
SP H26.062 Combined forms of infantile and juvenile cataract, left eye
SP H26.063 Combined forms of infantile and juvenile cataract, bilateral
IQ H26.069 Combined forms of infantile and juvenile cataract, unspecified eye
SP H26.09 Other infantile and juvenile cataract
+ 5 H26.1 Traumatic cataract
Use additional code (Chapter 20) to identify external cause
+ 6 H26.10 Unspecified traumatic cataract
SP + H26.101 Unspecified traumatic cataract, right eye

Chapter 7 H00-H59

H26.102 Unspecified traumatic cataract, left eye
H26.103 Unspecified traumatic cataract, bilateral
H26.109 Unspecified traumatic cataract, unspecified eye
H26.11 Localized traumatic opacities
H26.111 Localized traumatic opacities, right eye
H26.112 Localized traumatic opacities, left eye
H26.113 Localized traumatic opacities, bilateral
H26.119 Localized traumatic opacities, unspecified eye
H26.12 Partially resolved traumatic cataract
H26.121 Partially resolved traumatic cataract, right eye
H26.122 Partially resolved traumatic cataract, left eye
H26.123 Partially resolved traumatic cataract, bilateral
H26.129 Partially resolved traumatic cataract, unspecified eye
H26.13 Total traumatic cataract
H26.131 Total traumatic cataract, right eye
H26.132 Total traumatic cataract, left eye
H26.133 Total traumatic cataract, bilateral
H26.139 Total traumatic cataract, unspecified eye
H26.2 Complicated cataract
H26.20 Unspecified complicated cataract
Cataracta complicata NOS
H26.21 Cataract with neovascularization
Code also associated condition, such as:
chronic iridocyclitis (H20.1-)
H26.211 Cataract with neovascularization, right eye
H26.212 Cataract with neovascularization, left eye
H26.213 Cataract with neovascularization, bilateral
H26.219 Cataract with neovascularization, unspecified eye
H26.22 Cataract secondary to ocular disorders (degenerative) (inflammatory)
Code also:
associated ocular disorder
H26.221 Cataract secondary to ocular disorders (degenerative) (inflammatory), right eye
H26.222 Cataract secondary to ocular disorders (degenerative) (inflammatory), left eye
H26.223 Cataract secondary to ocular disorders (degenerative) (inflammatory), bilateral
H26.229 Cataract secondary to ocular disorders (degenerative) (inflammatory), unspecified eye
H26.23 Glaucomatous flecks (subcapsular)
Code first:
underlying glaucoma (H40-H42)
H26.231 Glaucomatous flecks (subcapsular), right eye
H26.232 Glaucomatous flecks (subcapsular), left eye
H26.233 Glaucomatous flecks (subcapsular), bilateral
H26.239 Glaucomatous flecks (subcapsular), unspecified eye
H26.3 Drug-induced cataract
Toxic cataract
Use additional code for adverse effect, if applicable, to identify drug (T36-T50 with fifth or sixth character 5)
DEFINITION Cataract caused by exposure to a drug or other toxic substance, such as a miotic, antimiotic, corticosteroid, metal, nitro compound, or substituted hydrocarbon.
H26.30 Drug-induced cataract, unspecified eye
H26.31 Drug-induced cataract, right eye
H26.32 Drug-induced cataract, left eye
H26.33 Drug-induced cataract, bilateral
H26.4 Secondary cataract
H26.40 Unspecified secondary cataract
H26.41 Soemmering's ring
DEFINITION Doughnut-shaped remnant of lens behind the pupil, occurring after cataract surgery or secondary to trauma.
H26.411 Soemmering's ring, right eye
H26.412 Soemmering's ring, left eye
H26.413 Soemmering's ring, bilateral
H26.419 Soemmering's ring, unspecified eye
H26.49 Other secondary cataract
H26.491 Other secondary cataract, right eye
H26.492 Other secondary cataract, left eye
H26.493 Other secondary cataract, bilateral
H26.499 Other secondary cataract, unspecified eye
H26.8 Other specified cataract
H26.9 Unspecified cataract
H27 Other disorders of lens
EXCLUDES 1 congenital lens malformations (Q12.-)
mechanical complications of intraocular lens implant (T85.2)
pseudophakia (Z96.1)
H27.0 Aphakia
Acquired absence of lens
Acquired aphakia
Aphakia due to trauma
EXCLUDES 1 cataract extraction status (Z98.4-)
congenital absence of lens (Q12.3)
congenital aphakia (Q12.3)

4th digit required 5th digit required 6th digit required 7th digit required 7th digit placeholder + Additional code Laterality

DEFINITION Absence of the crystalline lens of the eye.

H27.00 Aphakia, unspecified eye
H27.01 Aphakia, right eye
H27.02 Aphakia, left eye
H27.03 Aphakia, bilateral
H27.1 Dislocation of lens
H27.10 Unspecified dislocation of lens
H27.11 Subluxation of lens
H27.111 Subluxation of lens, right eye
H27.112 Subluxation of lens, left eye
H27.113 Subluxation of lens, bilateral
H27.119 Subluxation of lens, unspecified eye
H27.12 Anterior dislocation of lens
H27.121 Anterior dislocation of lens, right eye
H27.122 Anterior dislocation of lens, left eye
H27.123 Anterior dislocation of lens, bilateral
H27.129 Anterior dislocation of lens, unspecified eye
H27.13 Posterior dislocation of lens
H27.131 Posterior dislocation of lens, right eye
H27.132 Posterior dislocation of lens, left eye
H27.133 Posterior dislocation of lens, bilateral
H27.139 Posterior dislocation of lens, unspecified eye
H27.8 Other specified disorders of lens
H27.9 Unspecified disorder of lens
H28 *Cataract in diseases classified elsewhere*

Code first underlying disease, such as:
hypoparathyroidism (E20.-)
myotonia (G71.1-)
myxedema (E03.-)
protein-calorie malnutrition (E40-E46)

EXCLUDES 1 cataract in diabetes mellitus (E08.36, E09.36, E10.36, E11.36, E13.36)

Disorders of choroid and retina (H30-H36)

H30 Chorioretinal inflammation
H30.0 Focal chorioretinal inflammation
Focal chorioretinitis
Focal choroiditis
Focal retinitis
Focal retinochoroiditis
H30.00 Unspecified focal chorioretinal inflammation
Focal chorioretinitis NOS
Focal choroiditis NOS
Focal retinitis NOS
Focal retinochoroiditis NOS
H30.001 Unspecified focal chorioretinal inflammation, right eye
H30.002 Unspecified focal chorioretinal inflammation, left eye
H30.003 Unspecified focal chorioretinal inflammation, bilateral
H30.009 Unspecified focal chorioretinal inflammation, unspecified eye
H30.01 Focal chorioretinal inflammation, juxtapapillary
H30.011 Focal chorioretinal inflammation, juxtapapillary, right eye
H30.012 Focal chorioretinal inflammation, juxtapapillary, left eye
H30.013 Focal chorioretinal inflammation, juxtapapillary, bilateral
H30.019 Focal chorioretinal inflammation, juxtapapillary, unspecified eye
H30.02 Focal chorioretinal inflammation of posterior pole
H30.021 Focal chorioretinal inflammation of posterior pole, right eye
H30.022 Focal chorioretinal inflammation of posterior pole, left eye
H30.023 Focal chorioretinal inflammation of posterior pole, bilateral
H30.029 Focal chorioretinal inflammation of posterior pole, unspecified eye
H30.03 Focal chorioretinal inflammation, peripheral
H30.031 Focal chorioretinal inflammation, peripheral, right eye
H30.032 Focal chorioretinal inflammation, peripheral, left eye
H30.033 Focal chorioretinal inflammation, peripheral, bilateral
H30.039 Focal chorioretinal inflammation, peripheral, unspecified eye
H30.04 Focal chorioretinal inflammation, macular or paramacular
H30.041 Focal chorioretinal inflammation, macular or paramacular, right eye
H30.042 Focal chorioretinal inflammation, macular or paramacular, left eye
H30.043 Focal chorioretinal inflammation, macular or paramacular, bilateral
H30.049 Focal chorioretinal inflammation, macular or paramacular, unspecified eye
H30.1 Disseminated chorioretinal inflammation
Disseminated chorioretinitis
Disseminated choroiditis
Disseminated retinitis
Disseminated retinochoroiditis

EXCLUDES 2 exudative retinopathy (H35.02-)

H30.10 Unspecified disseminated chorioretinal inflammation
Disseminated chorioretinitis NOS
Disseminated choroiditis NOS
Disseminated retinitis NOS
Disseminated retinochoroiditis NOS
H30.101 Unspecified disseminated chorioretinal inflammation, right eye
H30.102 Unspecified disseminated chorioretinal inflammation, left eye

H30.103 Unspecified disseminated chorioretinal inflammation, bilateral
H30.109 Unspecified disseminated chorioretinal inflammation, unspecified eye
H30.11 Disseminated chorioretinal inflammation of posterior pole
H30.111 Disseminated chorioretinal inflammation of posterior pole, right eye
H30.112 Disseminated chorioretinal inflammation of posterior pole, left eye
H30.113 Disseminated chorioretinal inflammation of posterior pole, bilateral
H30.119 Disseminated chorioretinal inflammation of posterior pole, unspecified eye
H30.12 Disseminated chorioretinal inflammation, peripheral
H30.121 Disseminated chorioretinal inflammation, peripheral right eye
H30.122 Disseminated chorioretinal inflammation, peripheral, left eye
H30.123 Disseminated chorioretinal inflammation, peripheral, bilateral
H30.129 Disseminated chorioretinal inflammation, peripheral, unspecified eye
H30.13 Disseminated chorioretinal inflammation, generalized
H30.131 Disseminated chorioretinal inflammation, generalized, right eye
H30.132 Disseminated chorioretinal inflammation, generalized, left eye
H30.133 Disseminated chorioretinal inflammation, generalized, bilateral
H30.139 Disseminated chorioretinal inflammation, generalized, unspecified eye
H30.14 Acute posterior multifocal placoid pigment epitheliopathy
H30.141 Acute posterior multifocal placoid pigment epitheliopathy, right eye
H30.142 Acute posterior multifocal placoid pigment epitheliopathy, left eye
H30.143 Acute posterior multifocal placoid pigment epitheliopathy, bilateral
H30.149 Acute posterior multifocal placoid pigment epitheliopathy, unspecified eye
H30.2 Posterior cyclitis
Pars planitis
DEFINITION Inflammation of the peripheral retina and the ciliary body, the hair-like structures that hold the lens of the eye in place.
H30.20 Posterior cyclitis, unspecified eye
H30.21 Posterior cyclitis, right eye
H30.22 Posterior cyclitis, left eye
H30.23 Posterior cyclitis, bilateral
H30.8 Other chorioretinal inflammations
H30.81 Harada's disease
H30.811 Harada's disease, right eye
H30.812 Harada's disease, left eye
H30.813 Harada's disease, bilateral
H30.819 Harada's disease, unspecified eye
H30.89 Other chorioretinal inflammations
H30.891 Other chorioretinal inflammations, right eye
H30.892 Other chorioretinal inflammations, left eye
H30.893 Other chorioretinal inflammations, bilateral
H30.899 Other chorioretinal inflammations, unspecified eye
H30.9 Unspecified chorioretinal inflammation
Chorioretinitis NOS
Choroiditis NOS
Neuroretinitis NOS
Retinitis NOS
Retinochoroiditis NOS
H30.90 Unspecified chorioretinal inflammation, unspecified eye
H30.91 Unspecified chorioretinal inflammation, right eye
H30.92 Unspecified chorioretinal inflammation, left eye
H30.93 Unspecified chorioretinal inflammation, bilateral
H31 Other disorders of choroid
H31.0 Chorioretinal scars
EXCLUDES 2 postsurgical chorioretinal scars (H59.81-)
H31.00 Unspecified chorioretinal scars
H31.001 Unspecified chorioretinal scars, right eye
H31.002 Unspecified chorioretinal scars, left eye
H31.003 Unspecified chorioretinal scars, bilateral
H31.009 Unspecified chorioretinal scars, unspecified eye
H31.01 Macula scars of posterior pole (postinflammatory) (post-traumatic)
EXCLUDES 1 postprocedural chorioentinal scar (H59.81-)
H31.011 Macula scars of posterior pole (postinflammatory) (post-traumatic), right eye
H31.012 Macula scars of posterior pole (postinflammatory) (post-traumatic), left eye
H31.013 Macula scars of posterior pole (postinflammatory) (post-traumatic), bilateral
H31.019 Macula scars of posterior pole (postinflammatory) (post-traumatic), unspecified eye
H31.02 Solar retinopathy
DEFINITION Scar on the retina resulting from solar radiation.

SP H31.021 Solar retinopathy, right eye
SP H31.022 Solar retinopathy, left eye
SP H31.023 Solar retinopathy, bilateral
!Q H31.029 Solar retinopathy, unspecified eye
6 H31.09 Other chorioretinal scars
SP H31.091 Other chorioretinal scars, right eye
SP H31.092 Other chorioretinal scars, left eye
SP H31.093 Other chorioretinal scars, bilateral
!Q H31.099 Other chorioretinal scars, unspecified eye
5 H31.1 Choroidal degeneration
EXCLUDES 2 angioid streaks of macula (H35.33)
6 H31.10 Unspecified choroidal degeneration
Choroidal sclerosis NOS
SP H31.101 Choroidal degeneration, unspecified, right eye
SP H31.102 Choroidal degeneration, unspecified, left eye
SP H31.103 Choroidal degeneration, unspecified, bilateral
!Q H31.109 Choroidal degeneration, unspecified, unspecified eye
6 H31.11 Age-related choroidal atrophy
SP H31.111 Age-related choroidal atrophy, right eye
SP H31.112 Age-related choroidal atrophy, left eye
SP H31.113 Age-related choroidal atrophy, bilateral
!Q H31.119 Age-related choroidal atrophy, unspecified eye
6 H31.12 Diffuse secondary atrophy of choroid
SP H31.121 Diffuse secondary atrophy of choroid, right eye
SP H31.122 Diffuse secondary atrophy of choroid, left eye
SP H31.123 Diffuse secondary atrophy of choroid, bilateral
!Q H31.129 Diffuse secondary atrophy of choroid, unspecified eye
5 H31.2 Hereditary choroidal dystrophy
EXCLUDES 2 hyperornithinemia (E72.4)
ornithinemia (E72.4)
SP H31.20 Hereditary choroidal dystrophy, unspecified
SP H31.21 Choroideremia
SP H31.22 Choroidal dystrophy (central areolar) (generalized) (peripapillary)
SP H31.23 Gyrate atrophy, choroid
SP H31.29 Other hereditary choroidal dystrophy
5 H31.3 Choroidal hemorrhage and rupture
6 H31.30 Unspecified choroidal hemorrhage
SP H31.301 Unspecified choroidal hemorrhage, right eye
SP H31.302 Unspecified choroidal hemorrhage, left eye
SP H31.303 Unspecified choroidal hemorrhage, bilateral
!Q H31.309 Unspecified choroidal hemorrhage, unspecified eye
6 H31.31 Expulsive choroidal hemorrhage
SP H31.311 Expulsive choroidal hemorrhage, right eye
SP H31.312 Expulsive choroidal hemorrhage, left eye
SP H31.313 Expulsive choroidal hemorrhage, bilateral
!Q H31.319 Expulsive choroidal hemorrhage, unspecified eye
6 H31.32 Choroidal rupture
SP H31.321 Choroidal rupture, right eye
SP H31.322 Choroidal rupture, left eye
SP H31.323 Choroidal rupture, bilateral
!Q H31.329 Choroidal rupture, unspecified eye
5 H31.4 Choroidal detachment
6 H31.40 Unspecified choroidal detachment
SP H31.401 Unspecified choroidal detachment, right eye
SP H31.402 Unspecified choroidal detachment, left eye
SP H31.403 Unspecified choroidal detachment, bilateral
!Q H31.409 Unspecified choroidal detachment, unspecified eye
6 H31.41 Hemorrhagic choroidal detachment
SP H31.411 Hemorrhagic choroidal detachment, right eye
SP H31.412 Hemorrhagic choroidal detachment, left eye
SP H31.413 Hemorrhagic choroidal detachment, bilateral
!Q H31.419 Hemorrhagic choroidal detachment, unspecified eye
6 H31.42 Serous choroidal detachment
SP H31.421 Serous choroidal detachment, right eye
SP H31.422 Serous choroidal detachment, left eye
SP H31.423 Serous choroidal detachment, bilateral
!Q H31.429 Serous choroidal detachment, unspecified eye
SP H31.8 Other specified disorders of choroid
!Q H31.9 Unspecified disorder of choroid
M !Q H32 *Chorioretinal disorders in diseases classified elsewhere*
Code first underlying disease, such as:
congenital toxoplasmosis (P37.1)
histoplasmosis (B39.-)
leprosy (A30.-)
EXCLUDES 1 chorioretinitis (in):
toxoplasmosis (acquired) (B58.01)
tuberculosis (A18.53)
4 H33 Retinal detachments and breaks
EXCLUDES 1 detachment of retinal pigment epithelium (H35.72-, H35.73-)

Chapter 7
H00-H59

DEFINITION Condition in which the retina separates from its underlying layer of cells in the back of the eye, resulting in a decrease in the visual field or blindness.

5 **H33.0 Retinal detachment with retinal break**
Rhegmatogenous retinal detachment
EXCLUDES 1 serous retinal detachment (without retinal break) (H33.2-)

6 **H33.00 Unspecified retinal detachment with retinal break**
SP **H33.001 Unspecified retinal detachment with retinal break, right eye**
SP **H33.002 Unspecified retinal detachment with retinal break, left eye**
SP **H33.003 Unspecified retinal detachment with retinal break, bilateral**
!Q **H33.009 Unspecified retinal detachment with retinal break, unspecified eye**

6 **H33.01 Retinal detachment with single break**
SP **H33.011 Retinal detachment with single break, right eye**
SP **H33.012 Retinal detachment with single break, left eye**
SP **H33.013 Retinal detachment with single break, bilateral**
!Q **H33.019 Retinal detachment with single break, unspecified eye**

6 **H33.02 Retinal detachment with multiple breaks**
SP **H33.021 Retinal detachment with multiple breaks, right eye**
SP **H33.022 Retinal detachment with multiple breaks, left eye**
SP **H33.023 Retinal detachment with multiple breaks, bilateral**
!Q **H33.029 Retinal detachment with multiple breaks, unspecified eye**

6 **H33.03 Retinal detachment with giant retinal tear**
SP **H33.031 Retinal detachment with giant retinal tear, right eye**
SP **H33.032 Retinal detachment with giant retinal tear, left eye**
SP **H33.033 Retinal detachment with giant retinal tear, bilateral**
!Q **H33.039 Retinal detachment with giant retinal tear, unspecified eye**

6 **H33.04 Retinal detachment with retinal dialysis**
SP **H33.041 Retinal detachment with retinal dialysis, right eye**
SP **H33.042 Retinal detachment with retinal dialysis, left eye**
SP **H33.043 Retinal detachment with retinal dialysis, bilateral**
!Q **H33.049 Retinal detachment with retinal dialysis, unspecified eye**

6 **H33.05 Total retinal detachment**
SP **H33.051 Total retinal detachment, right eye**
SP **H33.052 Total retinal detachment, left eye**
SP **H33.053 Total retinal detachment, bilateral**
!Q **H33.059 Total retinal detachment, unspecified eye**

5 **H33.1 Retinoschisis and retinal cysts**
EXCLUDES 1 congenital retinoschisis (Q14.1)
microcystoid degeneration of retina (H35.42-)

6 **H33.10 Unspecified retinoschisis**
SP **H33.101 Unspecified retinoschisis, right eye**
SP **H33.102 Unspecified retinoschisis, left eye**
SP **H33.103 Unspecified retinoschisis, bilateral**
!Q **H33.109 Unspecified retinoschisis, unspecified eye**

6 **H33.11 Cyst of ora serrata**
SP **H33.111 Cyst of ora serrata, right eye**
SP **H33.112 Cyst of ora serrata, left eye**
SP **H33.113 Cyst of ora serrata, bilateral**
!Q **H33.119 Cyst of ora serrata, unspecified eye**

6 **H33.12 Parasitic cyst of retina**
SP **H33.121 Parasitic cyst of retina, right eye**
SP **H33.122 Parasitic cyst of retina, left eye**
SP **H33.123 Parasitic cyst of retina, bilateral**
!Q **H33.129 Parasitic cyst of retina, unspecified eye**

6 **H33.19 Other retinoschisis and retinal cysts**
Pseudocyst of retina
SP **H33.191 Other retinoschisis and retinal cysts, right eye**
SP **H33.192 Other retinoschisis and retinal cysts, left eye**
SP **H33.193 Other retinoschisis and retinal cysts, bilateral**
!Q **H33.199 Other retinoschisis and retinal cysts, unspecified eye**

5 **H33.2 Serous retinal detachment**
Retinal detachment NOS
Retinal detachment without retinal break
EXCLUDES 1 central serous chorioretinopathy (H35.71-)

!Q **H33.20 Serous retinal detachment, unspecified eye**
SP **H33.21 Serous retinal detachment, right eye**
SP **H33.22 Serous retinal detachment, left eye**
SP **H33.23 Serous retinal detachment, bilateral**

5 **H33.3 Retinal breaks without detachment**
EXCLUDES 1 chorioretinal scars after surgery for detachment (H59.81-)
peripheral retinal degeneration without break (H35.4-)

6 **H33.30 Unspecified retinal break**
SP **H33.301 Unspecified retinal break, right eye**
SP **H33.302 Unspecified retinal break, left eye**
SP **H33.303 Unspecified retinal break, bilateral**
!Q **H33.309 Unspecified retinal break, unspecified eye**

6 H33.31 **Horseshoe tear of retina without detachment**
Operculum of retina without detachment

- SP H33.311 **Horseshoe tear of retina without detachment, right eye**
- SP H33.312 **Horseshoe tear of retina without detachment, left eye**
- SP H33.313 **Horseshoe tear of retina without detachment, bilateral**
- IQ H33.319 **Horseshoe tear of retina without detachment, unspecified eye**

6 H33.32 **Round hole of retina without detachment**

- SP H33.321 **Round hole, right eye**
- SP H33.322 **Round hole, left eye**
- SP H33.323 **Round hole, bilateral**
- IQ H33.329 **Round hole, unspecified eye**

6 H33.33 **Multiple defects of retina without detachment**

- SP H33.331 **Multiple defects of retina without detachment, right eye**
- SP H33.332 **Multiple defects of retina without detachment, left eye**
- SP H33.333 **Multiple defects of retina without detachment, bilateral**
- IQ H33.339 **Multiple defects of retina without detachment, unspecified eye**

5 H33.4 **Traction detachment of retina**
Proliferative vitreo-retinopathy with retinal detachment

- IQ H33.40 **Traction detachment of retina, unspecified eye**
- SP H33.41 **Traction detachment of retina, right eye**
- SP H33.42 **Traction detachment of retina, left eye**
- SP H33.43 **Traction detachment of retina, bilateral**

SP H33.8 **Other retinal detachments**

4 H34 **Retinal vascular occlusions**
EXCLUDES 1 amaurosis fugax (G45.3)

5 H34.0 **Transient retinal artery occlusion**

- IQ H34.00 **Transient retinal artery occlusion, unspecified eye**
- SP H34.01 **Transient retinal artery occlusion, right eye**
- SP H34.02 **Transient retinal artery occlusion, left eye**
- SP H34.03 **Transient retinal artery occlusion, bilateral**

5 H34.1 **Central retinal artery occlusion**

- IQ H34.10 **Central retinal artery occlusion, unspecified eye**
- SP H34.11 **Central retinal artery occlusion, right eye**
- SP H34.12 **Central retinal artery occlusion, left eye**
- SP H34.13 **Central retinal artery occlusion, bilateral**

5 H34.2 **Other retinal artery occlusions**

6 H34.21 **Partial retinal artery occlusion**
Hollenhorst's plaque
Retinal microembolism

- SP H34.211 **Partial retinal artery occlusion, right eye**
- SP H34.212 **Partial retinal artery occlusion, left eye**
- SP H34.213 **Partial retinal artery occlusion, bilateral**
- IQ H34.219 **Partial retinal artery occlusion, unspecified eye**

6 H34.23 **Retinal artery branch occlusion**

- SP H34.231 **Retinal artery branch occlusion, right eye**
- SP H34.232 **Retinal artery branch occlusion, left eye**
- SP H34.233 **Retinal artery branch occlusion, bilateral**
- IQ H34.239 **Retinal artery branch occlusion, unspecified eye**

5 H34.8 **Other retinal vascular occlusions**

6 H34.81 **Central retinal vein occlusion**

One of the following 7th characters is to be assigned to codes in subcategory H34.81 to designate the severity of the occlusion:

0	with macular edema
1	with retinal neovascularization
2	stable

- SP 7 H34.811- **Central retinal vein occlusion, right eye**
- SP 7 H34.812- **Central retinal vein occlusion, left eye**
- SP 7 H34.813- **Central retinal vein occlusion, bilateral**
- IQ 7 H34.819- **Central retinal vein occlusion, unspecified eye**

6 H34.82 **Venous engorgement**
Incipient retinal vein occlusion
Partial retinal vein occlusion

- SP H34.821 **Venous engorgement, right eye**
- SP H34.822 **Venous engorgement, left eye**
- SP H34.823 **Venous engorgement, bilateral**
- IQ H34.829 **Venous engorgement, unspecified eye**

6 H34.83 **Tributary (branch) retinal vein occlusion**

One of the following 7th characters is to be assigned to codes in subcategory H34.83 to designate the severity of the occlusion:

0	with macular edema
1	with retinal neovascularization
2	stable

- SP 7 H34.831- **Tributary (branch) retinal vein occlusion, right eye**
- SP 7 H34.832- **Tributary (branch) retinal vein occlusion, left eye**
- SP 7 H34.833- **Tributary (branch) retinal vein occlusion, bilateral**
- IQ 7 H34.839- **Tributary (branch) retinal vein occlusion, unspecified eye**

SP H34.9 **Unspecified retinal vascular occlusion**

4 H35 **Other retinal disorders**

Chapter 7
H00-H59

EXCLUDES 2 diabetic retinal disorders (E08.311-E08.359, E09.311-E09.359, E10.311-E10.359, E11.311-E11.359, E13.311-E13.359)

▲ 5 **H35.0 Background retinopathy and retinal vascular changes**

Code also:

any associated hypertension (I10)

GUIDELINES **Section I.C.9.a.5)**

Subcategory H35.0, Background retinopathy and retinal vascular changes, should be used with a code from category I10-I15, Hypertensive disease to include the systemic hypertension. The sequencing is based on the reason for the encounter.

SP **H35.00 Unspecified background retinopathy**

6 **H35.01 Changes in retinal vascular appearance**

Retinal vascular sheathing

Laterality SP **H35.011 Changes in retinal vascular appearance, right eye**

Laterality SP **H35.012 Changes in retinal vascular appearance, left eye**

Laterality SP **H35.013 Changes in retinal vascular appearance, bilateral**

Laterality IQ **H35.019 Changes in retinal vascular appearance, unspecified eye**

6 **H35.02 Exudative retinopathy**

Coats retinopathy

Laterality SP **H35.021 Exudative retinopathy, right eye**

Laterality SP **H35.022 Exudative retinopathy, left eye**

Laterality SP **H35.023 Exudative retinopathy, bilateral**

Laterality IQ **H35.029 Exudative retinopathy, unspecified eye**

6 **H35.03 Hypertensive retinopathy**

Laterality SP **H35.031 Hypertensive retinopathy, right eye**

Laterality SP **H35.032 Hypertensive retinopathy, left eye**

Laterality SP **H35.033 Hypertensive retinopathy, bilateral**

Laterality IQ **H35.039 Hypertensive retinopathy, specified eye**

6 **H35.04 Retinal micro-aneurysms, unspecified**

Laterality SP **H35.041 Retinal micro-aneurysms, unspecified, right eye**

Laterality SP **H35.042 Retinal micro-aneurysms, unspecified, left eye**

Laterality SP **H35.043 Retinal micro-aneurysms, unspecified, bilateral**

Laterality IQ **H35.049 Retinal micro-aneurysms, unspecified, unspecified eye**

6 **H35.05 Retinal neovascularization, unspecified**

Laterality SP **H35.051 Retinal neovascularization, unspecified, right eye**

Laterality SP **H35.052 Retinal neovascularization, unspecified, left eye**

Laterality SP **H35.053 Retinal neovascularization, unspecified, bilateral**

Laterality IQ **H35.059 Retinal neovascularization, unspecified, unspecified eye**

6 **H35.06 Retinal vasculitis**

Eales disease

Retinal perivasculitis

Laterality SP **H35.061 Retinal vasculitis, right eye**

Laterality SP **H35.062 Retinal vasculitis, left eye**

Laterality SP **H35.063 Retinal vasculitis, bilateral**

Laterality IQ **H35.069 Retinal vasculitis, unspecified eye**

6 **H35.07 Retinal telangiectasis**

Laterality SP **H35.071 Retinal telangiectasis, right eye**

Laterality SP **H35.072 Retinal telangiectasis, left eye**

Laterality SP **H35.073 Retinal telangiectasis, bilateral**

Laterality IQ **H35.079 Retinal telangiectasis, unspecified eye**

SP **H35.09 Other intraretinal microvascular abnormalities**

Retinal varices

5 **H35.1 Retinopathy of prematurity**

6 **H35.10 Retinopathy of prematurity, unspecified**

Retinopathy of prematurity NOS

Laterality SP **H35.101 Retinopathy of prematurity, unspecified, right eye**

Laterality SP **H35.102 Retinopathy of prematurity, unspecified, left eye**

Laterality SP **H35.103 Retinopathy of prematurity, unspecified, bilateral**

Laterality IQ **H35.109 Retinopathy of prematurity, unspecified, unspecified eye**

6 **H35.11 Retinopathy of prematurity, stage 0**

Laterality SP **H35.111 Retinopathy of prematurity, stage 0, right eye**

Laterality SP **H35.112 Retinopathy of prematurity, stage 0, left eye**

Laterality SP **H35.113 Retinopathy of prematurity, stage 0, bilateral**

Laterality IQ **H35.119 Retinopathy of prematurity, stage 0, unspecified eye**

6 **H35.12 Retinopathy of prematurity, stage 1**

Laterality SP **H35.121 Retinopathy of prematurity, stage 1, right eye**

Laterality SP **H35.122 Retinopathy of prematurity, stage 1, left eye**

Laterality SP **H35.123 Retinopathy of prematurity, stage 1, bilateral**

Laterality IQ **H35.129 Retinopathy of prematurity, stage 1, unspecified eye**

6 **H35.13 Retinopathy of prematurity, stage 2**

Laterality SP **H35.131 Retinopathy of prematurity, stage 2, right eye**

Laterality SP **H35.132 Retinopathy of prematurity, stage 2, left eye**

Laterality SP **H35.133 Retinopathy of prematurity, stage 2, bilateral**

Laterality IQ **H35.139 Retinopathy of prematurity, stage 2, unspecified eye**

6 **H35.14 Retinopathy of prematurity, stage 3**

Laterality SP **H35.141 Retinopathy of prematurity, stage 3, right eye**

Laterality SP **H35.142 Retinopathy of prematurity, stage 3, left eye**

Laterality SP **H35.143 Retinopathy of prematurity, stage 3, bilateral**

H35.149 Retinopathy of prematurity, stage 3, unspecified eye

H35.15 Retinopathy of prematurity, stage 4

H35.151 Retinopathy of prematurity, stage 4, right eye

H35.152 Retinopathy of prematurity, stage 4, left eye

H35.153 Retinopathy of prematurity, stage 4, bilateral

H35.159 Retinopathy of prematurity, stage 4, unspecified eye

H35.16 Retinopathy of prematurity, stage 5

H35.161 Retinopathy of prematurity, stage 5, right eye

H35.162 Retinopathy of prematurity, stage 5, left eye

H35.163 Retinopathy of prematurity, stage 5, bilateral

H35.169 Retinopathy of prematurity, stage 5, unspecified eye

H35.17 Retrolental fibroplasia

H35.171 Retrolental fibroplasia, right eye

H35.172 Retrolental fibroplasia, left eye

H35.173 Retrolental fibroplasia, bilateral

H35.179 Retrolental fibroplasia, unspecified eye

H35.2 Other non-diabetic proliferative retinopathy

Proliferative vitreo-retinopathy

EXCLUDES 1 proliferative vitreo-retinopathy with retinal detachment (H33.4-)

H35.20 Other non-diabetic proliferative retinopathy, unspecified eye

H35.21 Other non-diabetic proliferative retinopathy, right eye

H35.22 Other non-diabetic proliferative retinopathy, left eye

H35.23 Other non-diabetic proliferative retinopathy, bilateral

H35.3 Degeneration of macula and posterior pole

H35.30 Unspecified macular degeneration

Age-related macular degeneration

H35.31 Nonexudative age-related macular degeneration

Atrophic age-related macular degeneration

Dry age-related macular degeneration

One of the following 7th characters is to be assigned to codes in subcategory H35.31 to designate the stage of the disease:

0	stage unspecified
1	early dry stage
2	intermediate dry stage
3	advanced atrophic without subfoveal involvement
4	advanced atrophic with subfoveal involvement

H35.311- Nonexudative age-related macular degeneration, right eye

H35.312- Nonexudative age-related macular degeneration, left eye

H35.313- Nonexudative age-related macular degeneration, bilateral

H35.319- Nonexudative age-related macular degeneration, unspecified eye

H35.32 Exudative age-related macular degeneration

Wet age-related macular degeneration

One of the following 7th characters is to be assigned to codes in subcategory H35.32 to designate the stage of the disease:

0	stage unspecified
1	with active choroidal neovascularization
2	with inactive choroidal neovascularization
3	with inactive scar

H35.321- Exudative age-related macular degeneration, right eye

H35.322- Exudative age-related macular degeneration, left eye

H35.323- Exudative age-related macular degeneration, bilateral

H35.329- Exudative age-related macular degeneration, unspecified eye

H35.33 Angioid streaks of macula

H35.34 Macular cyst, hole, or pseudohole

H35.341 Macular cyst, hole, or pseudohole, right eye

H35.342 Macular cyst, hole, or pseudohole, left eye

H35.343 Macular cyst, hole, or pseudohole, bilateral

H35.349 Macular cyst, hole, or pseudohole, unspecified eye

H35.35 Cystoid macular degeneration

EXCLUDES 1 cystoid macular edema following cataract surgery (H59.03-)

H35.351 Cystoid macular degeneration, right eye

H35.352 Cystoid macular degeneration, left eye

H35.353 Cystoid macular degeneration, bilateral

H35.359 Cystoid macular degeneration, unspecified eye

H35.36 Drusen (degenerative) of macula

DEFINITION Small, bright deposits or accumulations of material seen in the retina and/or optic disc that are associated with a variety of eye diseases including macular degeneration, hereditary retinal degeneration, and loss of peripheral vision.

H35.361 Drusen (degenerative) of macula, right eye

H35.362 Drusen (degenerative) of macula, left eye

H35.363 Drusen (degenerative) of macula, bilateral

H35.369 Drusen (degenerative) of macula, unspecified eye

6 **H35.37 Puckering of macula**
L SP **H35.371 Puckering of macula, right eye**
L SP **H35.372 Puckering of macula, left eye**
L SP **H35.373 Puckering of macula, bilateral**
L IQ **H35.379 Puckering of macula, unspecified eye**
+ 6 **H35.38 Toxic maculopathy**
Code first:
poisoning due to drug or toxin, if applicable (T36-T65 with fifth or sixth character 1-4 or 6)
Use additional code for adverse effect, if applicable, to identify drug (T36-T50 with fifth or sixth character 5)
L SP + **H35.381 Toxic maculopathy, right eye**
L SP + **H35.382 Toxic maculopathy, left eye**
L SP + **H35.383 Toxic maculopathy, bilateral**
L IQ + **H35.389 Toxic maculopathy, unspecified eye**
5 **H35.4 Peripheral retinal degeneration**
EXCLUDES 1 hereditary retinal degeneration (dystrophy) (H35.5-)
peripheral retinal degeneration with retinal break (H33.3-)
IQ **H35.40 Unspecified peripheral retinal degeneration**
6 **H35.41 Lattice degeneration of retina**
Palisade degeneration of retina
L SP **H35.411 Lattice degeneration of retina, right eye**
L SP **H35.412 Lattice degeneration of retina, left eye**
L SP **H35.413 Lattice degeneration of retina, bilateral**
L IQ **H35.419 Lattice degeneration of retina, unspecified eye**
6 **H35.42 Microcystoid degeneration of retina**
L SP **H35.421 Microcystoid degeneration of retina, right eye**
L SP **H35.422 Microcystoid degeneration of retina, left eye**
L SP **H35.423 Microcystoid degeneration of retina, bilateral**
L IQ **H35.429 Microcystoid degeneration of retina, unspecified eye**
6 **H35.43 Paving stone degeneration of retina**
L SP **H35.431 Paving stone degeneration of retina, right eye**
L SP **H35.432 Paving stone degeneration of retina, left eye**
L SP **H35.433 Paving stone degeneration of retina, bilateral**
L IQ **H35.439 Paving stone degeneration of retina, unspecified eye**
6 **H35.44 Age-related reticular degeneration of retina**
L SP **H35.441 Age-related reticular degeneration of retina, right eye**
L SP **H35.442 Age-related reticular degeneration of retina, left eye**
L SP **H35.443 Age-related reticular degeneration of retina, bilateral**
L IQ **H35.449 Age-related reticular degeneration of retina, unspecified eye**
6 **H35.45 Secondary pigmentary degeneration**
L SP **H35.451 Secondary pigmentary degeneration, right eye**
L SP **H35.452 Secondary pigmentary degeneration, left eye**
L SP **H35.453 Secondary pigmentary degeneration, bilateral**
L IQ **H35.459 Secondary pigmentary degeneration, unspecified eye**
6 **H35.46 Secondary vitreoretinal degeneration**
L SP **H35.461 Secondary vitreoretinal degeneration, right eye**
L SP **H35.462 Secondary vitreoretinal degeneration, left eye**
L SP **H35.463 Secondary vitreoretinal degeneration, bilateral**
L IQ **H35.469 Secondary vitreoretinal degeneration, unspecified eye**
5 **H35.5 Hereditary retinal dystrophy**
EXCLUDES 1 dystrophies primarily involving Bruch's membrane (H31.1-)
SP **H35.50 Unspecified hereditary retinal dystrophy**
SP **H35.51 Vitreoretinal dystrophy**
SP **H35.52 Pigmentary retinal dystrophy**
Albipunctate retinal dystrophy
Retinitis pigmentosa
Tapetoretinal dystrophy
SP **H35.53 Other dystrophies primarily involving the sensory retina**
Stargardt's disease
DEFINITION Stargardt's disease: genetic condition causing degeneration of the macula, occurring by age 20, with rapid loss of visual acuity and abnormal pigmentation of the macula.
SP **H35.54 Dystrophies primarily involving the retinal pigment epithelium**
Vitelliform retinal dystrophy
5 **H35.6 Retinal hemorrhage**
L IQ **H35.60 Retinal hemorrhage, unspecified eye**
L SP **H35.61 Retinal hemorrhage, right eye**
L SP **H35.62 Retinal hemorrhage, left eye**
L SP **H35.63 Retinal hemorrhage, bilateral**
5 **H35.7 Separation of retinal layers**
EXCLUDES 1 retinal detachment (serous) (H33.2-)
rhegmatogenous retinal detachment (H33.0-)
IQ **H35.70 Unspecified separation of retinal layers**
6 **H35.71 Central serous chorioretinopathy**
DEFINITION Fluid seepage from the choroid into the retina, causing the retinal layers to fill and separate from each other.
L SP **H35.711 Central serous chorioretinopathy, right eye**
L SP **H35.712 Central serous chorioretinopathy, left eye**

H35.713 **Central serous chorioretinopathy, bilateral**

H35.719 **Central serous chorioretinopathy, unspecified eye**

H35.72 **Serous detachment of retinal pigment epithelium**

H35.721 **Serous detachment of retinal pigment epithelium, right eye**

H35.722 **Serous detachment of retinal pigment epithelium, left eye**

H35.723 **Serous detachment of retinal pigment epithelium, bilateral**

H35.729 **Serous detachment of retinal pigment epithelium, unspecified eye**

H35.73 **Hemorrhagic detachment of retinal pigment epithelium**

H35.731 **Hemorrhagic detachment of retinal pigment epithelium, right eye**

H35.732 **Hemorrhagic detachment of retinal pigment epithelium, left eye**

H35.733 **Hemorrhagic detachment of retinal pigment epithelium, bilateral**

H35.739 **Hemorrhagic detachment of retinal pigment epithelium, unspecified eye**

H35.8 **Other specified retinal disorders**

EXCLUDES 2 retinal hemorrhage (H35.6-)

H35.81 **Retinal edema**

Retinal cotton wool spots

H35.82 **Retinal ischemia**

H35.89 **Other specified retinal disorders**

H35.9 **Unspecified retinal disorder**

M **H36** ***Retinal disorders in diseases classified elsewhere***

Code first underlying disease, such as:
- lipid storage disorders (E75.-)
- sickle-cell disorders (D57.-)

EXCLUDES 1 arteriosclerotic retinopathy (H35.0-)
diabetic retinopathy (E08.3-, E09.3-, E10.3-, E11.3-, E13.3-)

Glaucoma (H40-H42)

Glaucoma

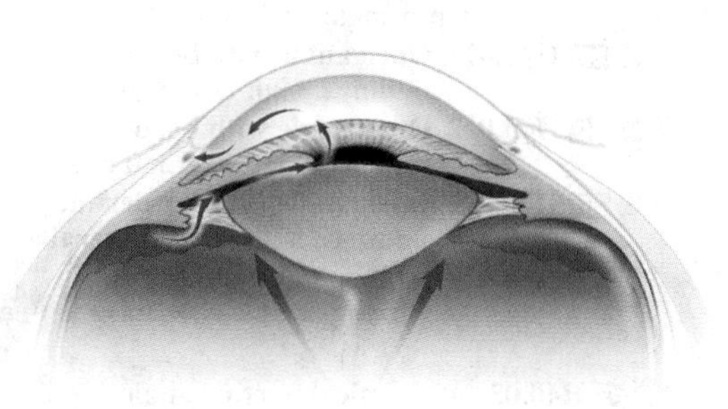

H40 **Glaucoma**

EXCLUDES 1 absolute glaucoma (H44.51-)
congenital glaucoma (Q15.0)
traumatic glaucoma due to birth injury (P15.3)

GUIDELINES **Section I.C.7.a.1)**

Assign as many codes from category H40, Glaucoma, as needed to identify the type of glaucoma, the affected eye, and the glaucoma stage.

GUIDELINES **Section I.C.7.a.2)-3)**

When a patient has bilateral glaucoma and both eyes are documented as being the same type and stage, and there is a code for bilateral glaucoma, report only the code for the type of glaucoma, bilateral, with the seventh character for the stage.

When a patient has bilateral glaucoma and each eye is documented as having a different type or stage, and the classification distinguishes laterality, assign the appropriate code for each eye rather than the code for bilateral glaucoma.

H40.0 **Glaucoma suspect**

DEFINITION Increase in intraocular pressure causing pathologic changes in the optic disk and defects in the field of vision.

H40.00 **Preglaucoma, unspecified**

H40.001 **Preglaucoma, unspecified, right eye**

H40.002 **Preglaucoma, unspecified, left eye**

H40.003 **Preglaucoma, unspecified, bilateral**

H40.009 **Preglaucoma, unspecified, unspecified eye**

H40.01 **Open angle with borderline findings, low risk**

Open angle, low risk

H40.011 **Open angle with borderline findings, low risk, right eye**

H40.012 **Open angle with borderline findings, low risk, left eye**

Chapter 7 H00-H59

Laterality SP H40.013 **Open angle with borderline findings, low risk, bilateral**

Laterality IQ H40.019 **Open angle with borderline findings, low risk, unspecified eye**

6 H40.02 **Open angle with borderline findings, high risk**
Open angle, high risk

Laterality SP H40.021 **Open angle with borderline findings, high risk, right eye**

Laterality SP H40.022 **Open angle with borderline findings, high risk, left eye**

Laterality SP H40.023 **Open angle with borderline findings, high risk, bilateral**

Laterality IQ H40.029 **Open angle with borderline findings, high risk, unspecified eye**

6 H40.03 **Anatomical narrow angle**
Primary angle closure suspect

Laterality SP H40.031 **Anatomical narrow angle, right eye**

Laterality SP H40.032 **Anatomical narrow angle, left eye**

Laterality SP H40.033 **Anatomical narrow angle, bilateral**

Laterality IQ H40.039 **Anatomical narrow angle, unspecified eye**

6 H40.04 **Steroid responder**

Laterality SP H40.041 **Steroid responder, right eye**

Laterality SP H40.042 **Steroid responder, left eye**

Laterality SP H40.043 **Steroid responder, bilateral**

Laterality IQ H40.049 **Steroid responder, unspecified eye**

6 H40.05 **Ocular hypertension**

Laterality SP H40.051 **Ocular hypertension, right eye**

Laterality SP H40.052 **Ocular hypertension, left eye**

Laterality SP H40.053 **Ocular hypertension, bilateral**

Laterality IQ H40.059 **Ocular hypertension, unspecified eye**

6 H40.06 **Primary angle closure without glaucoma damage**

Laterality SP H40.061 **Primary angle closure without glaucoma damage, right eye**

Laterality SP H40.062 **Primary angle closure without glaucoma damage, left eye**

Laterality SP H40.063 **Primary angle closure without glaucoma damage, bilateral**

Laterality IQ H40.069 **Primary angle closure without glaucoma damage, unspecified eye**

5 H40.1 **Open-angle glaucoma**

SP 7th digit placeholder H40.10X- **Unspecified open-angle glaucoma**

One of the following 7th characters is to be assigned to code H40.10 to designate the stage of glaucoma
0 stage unspecified
1 mild stage
2 moderate stage
3 severe stage
4 indeterminate stage

6 H40.11 **Primary open-angle glaucoma**
Chronic simple glaucoma

One of the following 7th characters is to be assigned to each code in subcategory H40.11 to designate the stage of glaucoma
0 stage unspecified
1 mild stage
2 moderate stage
3 severe stage
4 indeterminate stage

Laterality SP 7 H40.111- **Primary open-angle glaucoma, right eye**

Laterality SP 7 H40.112- **Primary open-angle glaucoma, left eye**

Laterality SP 7 H40.113- **Primary open-angle glaucoma, bilateral**

Laterality IQ 7 H40.119- **Primary open-angle glaucoma, unspecified eye**

6 H40.12 **Low-tension glaucoma**

One of the following 7th characters is to be assigned to each code in subcategory H40.12 to designate the stage of glaucoma
0 stage unspecified
1 mild stage
2 moderate stage
3 severe stage
4 indeterminate stage

Laterality SP 7 H40.121- **Low-tension glaucoma, right eye**

Laterality SP 7 H40.122- **Low-tension glaucoma, left eye**

Laterality SP 7 H40.123- **Low-tension glaucoma, bilateral**

Laterality IQ 7 H40.129- **Low-tension glaucoma, unspecified eye**

6 H40.13 **Pigmentary glaucoma**

One of the following 7th characters is to be assigned to each code in subcategory H40.13 to designate the stage of glaucoma
0 stage unspecified
1 mild stage
2 moderate stage
3 severe stage
4 indeterminate stage

DEFINITION Granules of pigment coloring the eye break off and block drainage canals, increasing intraocular pressure.

Laterality SP 7 H40.131- **Pigmentary glaucoma, right eye**

Laterality SP 7 H40.132- **Pigmentary glaucoma, left eye**

Laterality SP 7 H40.133- **Pigmentary glaucoma, bilateral**

Laterality IQ 7 H40.139- **Pigmentary glaucoma, unspecified eye**

6 H40.14 **Capsular glaucoma with pseudoexfoliation of lens**

One of the following 7th characters is to be assigned to each code in subcategory H40.14 to designate the stage of glaucoma
0 stage unspecified
1 mild stage
2 moderate stage
3 severe stage
4 indeterminate stage

SP 7 **H40.141- Capsular glaucoma with pseudoexfoliation of lens, right eye**

SP 7 **H40.142- Capsular glaucoma with pseudoexfoliation of lens, left eye**

SP 7 **H40.143- Capsular glaucoma with pseudoexfoliation of lens, bilateral**

IQ 7 **H40.149- Capsular glaucoma with pseudoexfoliation of lens, unspecified eye**

6 **H40.15 Residual stage of open-angle glaucoma**

SP **H40.151 Residual stage of open-angle glaucoma, right eye**

SP **H40.152 Residual stage of open-angle glaucoma, left eye**

SP **H40.153 Residual stage of open-angle glaucoma, bilateral**

IQ **H40.159 Residual stage of open-angle glaucoma, unspecified eye**

5 **H40.2 Primary angle-closure glaucoma**

EXCLUDES 1 aqueous misdirection (H40.83-)
malignant glaucoma (H40.83-)

SP 7 **H40.20X- Unspecified primary angle-closure glaucoma**

One of the following 7th characters is to be assigned to code H40.20 to designate the stage of glaucoma
0 stage unspecified
1 mild stage
2 moderate stage
3 severe stage
4 indeterminate stage

6 **H40.21 Acute angle-closure glaucoma**
Acute angle-closure glaucoma attack
Acute angle-closure glaucoma crisis

DEFINITION Severe, sudden increase in intraocular pressure due to a blockage of the chamber angle at the junction of the iris and cornea, preventing normal aqueous fluid drainage and causing rapid loss of vision.

SP **H40.211 Acute angle-closure glaucoma, right eye**

SP **H40.212 Acute angle-closure glaucoma, left eye**

SP **H40.213 Acute angle-closure glaucoma, bilateral**

IQ **H40.219 Acute angle-closure glaucoma, unspecified eye**

6 **H40.22 Chronic angle-closure glaucoma**
Chronic primary angle closure glaucoma

One of the following 7th characters is to be assigned to each code in subcategory H40.22 to designate the stage of glaucoma
0 stage unspecified
1 mild stage
2 moderate stage
3 severe stage
4 indeterminate stage

SP 7 **H40.221- Chronic angle-closure glaucoma, right eye**

SP 7 **H40.222- Chronic angle-closure glaucoma, left eye**

SP 7 **H40.223- Chronic angle-closure glaucoma, bilateral**

IQ 7 **H40.229- Chronic angle-closure glaucoma, unspecified eye**

6 **H40.23 Intermittent angle-closure glaucoma**

SP **H40.231 Intermittent angle-closure glaucoma, right eye**

SP **H40.232 Intermittent angle-closure glaucoma, left eye**

SP **H40.233 Intermittent angle-closure glaucoma, bilateral**

IQ **H40.239 Intermittent angle-closure glaucoma, unspecified eye**

6 **H40.24 Residual stage of angle-closure glaucoma**

SP **H40.241 Residual stage of angle-closure glaucoma, right eye**

SP **H40.242 Residual stage of angle-closure glaucoma, left eye**

SP **H40.243 Residual stage of angle-closure glaucoma, bilateral**

IQ **H40.249 Residual stage of angle-closure glaucoma, unspecified eye**

5 **H40.3 Glaucoma secondary to eye trauma**
Code also:
underlying condition

One of the following 7th characters is to be assigned to each code in subcategory H40.3 to designate the stage of glaucoma
0 stage unspecified
1 mild stage
2 moderate stage
3 severe stage
4 indeterminate stage

IQ 7 **H40.30X- Glaucoma secondary to eye trauma, unspecified eye**

SP 7 **H40.31X- Glaucoma secondary to eye trauma, right eye**

SP 7 **H40.32X- Glaucoma secondary to eye trauma, left eye**

SP 7 **H40.33X- Glaucoma secondary to eye trauma, bilateral**

5 **H40.4 Glaucoma secondary to eye inflammation**
Code also:
underlying condition

Chapter 7
H00-H59

One of the following 7th characters is to be assigned to each code in subcategory H40.4 to designate the stage of glaucoma
0   stage unspecified
1   mild stage
2   moderate stage
3   severe stage
4   indeterminate stage

☐ IQ ☑ **H40.40X-** **Glaucoma secondary to eye inflammation, unspecified eye**

☐ SP ☑ **H40.41X-** **Glaucoma secondary to eye inflammation, right eye**

☐ SP ☑ **H40.42X-** **Glaucoma secondary to eye inflammation, left eye**

☐ SP ☑ **H40.43X-** **Glaucoma secondary to eye inflammation, bilateral**

5 **H40.5 Glaucoma secondary to other eye disorders**
Code also:
    underlying eye disorder

One of the following 7th characters is to be assigned to each code in subcategory H40.5 to designate the stage of glaucoma
0   stage unspecified
1   mild stage
2   moderate stage
3   severe stage
4   indeterminate stage

☐ IQ ☑ **H40.50X-** **Glaucoma secondary to other eye disorders, unspecified eye**

☐ SP ☑ **H40.51X-** **Glaucoma secondary to other eye disorders, right eye**

☐ SP ☑ **H40.52X-** **Glaucoma secondary to other eye disorders, left eye**

☐ SP ☑ **H40.53X-** **Glaucoma secondary to other eye disorders, bilateral**

✚ 5 **H40.6 Glaucoma secondary to drugs**
Use additional code for adverse effect, if applicable, to identify drug (T36-T50 with fifth or sixth character 5)

One of the following 7th characters is to be assigned to each code in subcategory H40.6 to designate the stage of glaucoma
0   stage unspecified
1   mild stage
2   moderate stage
3   severe stage
4   indeterminate stage

☐ IQ ✚ ☑ **H40.60X-** **Glaucoma secondary to drugs, unspecified eye**

☐ SP ✚ ☑ **H40.61X-** **Glaucoma secondary to drugs, right eye**

☐ SP ✚ ☑ **H40.62X-** **Glaucoma secondary to drugs, left eye**

☐ SP ✚ ☑ **H40.63X-** **Glaucoma secondary to drugs, bilateral**

5 **H40.8 Other glaucoma**

6 **H40.81 Glaucoma with increased episcleral venous pressure**
DEFINITION   Blood pressure of the veins in the white of the eye increases as the pressure of intraocular fluid increases.

☐ SP **H40.811 Glaucoma with increased episcleral venous pressure, right eye**

☐ SP **H40.812 Glaucoma with increased episcleral venous pressure, left eye**

☐ SP **H40.813 Glaucoma with increased episcleral venous pressure, bilateral**

☐ IQ **H40.819 Glaucoma with increased episcleral venous pressure, unspecified eye**

6 **H40.82 Hypersecretion glaucoma**
DEFINITION   Overproduction of ocular fluid rather than insufficient drainage that causes increased intraocular pressure.

☐ SP **H40.821 Hypersecretion glaucoma, right eye**

☐ SP **H40.822 Hypersecretion glaucoma, left eye**

☐ SP **H40.823 Hypersecretion glaucoma, bilateral**

☐ IQ **H40.829 Hypersecretion glaucoma, unspecified eye**

6 **H40.83 Aqueous misdirection**
Malignant glaucoma

☐ SP **H40.831 Aqueous misdirection, right eye**

☐ SP **H40.832 Aqueous misdirection, left eye**

☐ SP **H40.833 Aqueous misdirection, bilateral**

☐ IQ **H40.839 Aqueous misdirection, unspecified eye**

SP **H40.89 Other specified glaucoma**

SP **H40.9 Unspecified glaucoma**

M IQ **H42** *Glaucoma in diseases classified elsewhere*
Code first underlying condition, such as:
    amyloidosis (E85.-)
    aniridia (Q13.1)
    glaucoma (in) diabetes mellitus (E08.39, E09.39, E10.39, E11.39, E13.39)
    Lowe's syndrome (E72.03)
    Reiger's anomaly (Q13.81)
    specified metabolic disorder (E70-E88)
    EXCLUDES 1   glaucoma (in) onchocerciasis (B73.02)
                   glaucoma (in) syphilis (A52.71)
                   glaucoma (in) tuberculous (A18.59)

Disorders of vitreous body and globe (H43-H44)

4 **H43 Disorders of vitreous body**

5 **H43.0 Vitreous prolapse**
EXCLUDES 1   vitreous syndrome following cataract surgery (H59.0-)
               traumatic vitreous prolapse (S05.2-)

☐ IQ **H43.00 Vitreous prolapse, unspecified eye**

☐ SP **H43.01 Vitreous prolapse, right eye**

☐ SP **H43.02 Vitreous prolapse, left eye**

☐ SP **H43.03 Vitreous prolapse, bilateral**

5 **H43.1 Vitreous hemorrhage**

☐ IQ **H43.10 Vitreous hemorrhage, unspecified eye**

---

4 4th digit required   5 5th digit required   6 6th digit required   7 7th digit required   ☑ 7th digit placeholder   ✚ Additional code   ☐ Laterality

SP **H43.11 Vitreous hemorrhage, right eye**
SP **H43.12 Vitreous hemorrhage, left eye**
SP **H43.13 Vitreous hemorrhage, bilateral**
5 **H43.2 Crystalline deposits in vitreous body**
IQ **H43.20 Crystalline deposits in vitreous body, unspecified eye**
SP **H43.21 Crystalline deposits in vitreous body, right eye**
SP **H43.22 Crystalline deposits in vitreous body, left eye**
SP **H43.23 Crystalline deposits in vitreous body, bilateral**
5 **H43.3 Other vitreous opacities**
6 **H43.31 Vitreous membranes and strands**
SP **H43.311 Vitreous membranes and strands, right eye**
SP **H43.312 Vitreous membranes and strands, left eye**
SP **H43.313 Vitreous membranes and strands, bilateral**
IQ **H43.319 Vitreous membranes and strands, unspecified eye**
6 **H43.39 Other vitreous opacities**
Vitreous floaters
SP **H43.391 Other vitreous opacities, right eye**
SP **H43.392 Other vitreous opacities, left eye**
SP **H43.393 Other vitreous opacities, bilateral**
IQ **H43.399 Other vitreous opacities, unspecified eye**
5 **H43.8 Other disorders of vitreous body**
EXCLUDES 1 proliferative vitreo-retinopathy with retinal detachment (H33.4-)
EXCLUDES 2 vitreous abscess (H44.02-)
6 **H43.81 Vitreous degeneration**
Vitreous detachment
SP **H43.811 Vitreous degeneration, right eye**
SP **H43.812 Vitreous degeneration, left eye**
SP **H43.813 Vitreous degeneration, bilateral**
IQ **H43.819 Vitreous degeneration, unspecified eye**
6 **H43.82 Vitreomacular adhesion**
Vitreomacular traction
SP **H43.821 Vitreomacular adhesion, right eye**
SP **H43.822 Vitreomacular adhesion, left eye**
SP **H43.823 Vitreomacular adhesion, bilateral**
IQ **H43.829 Vitreomacular adhesion, unspecified eye**
SP **H43.89 Other disorders of vitreous body**
IQ **H43.9 Unspecified disorder of vitreous body**

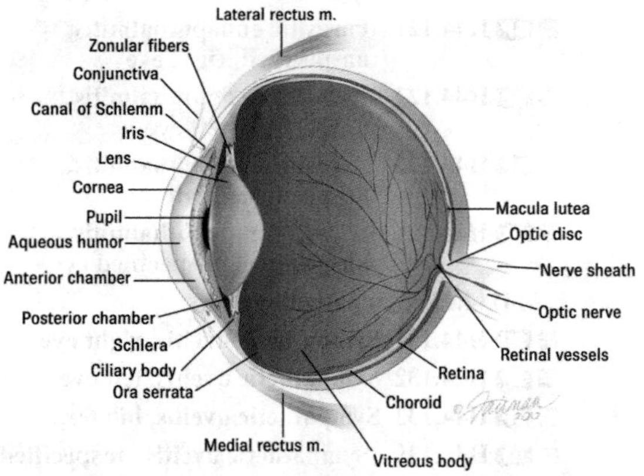

4 **H44 Disorders of globe**
INCLUDES disorders affecting multiple structures of eye
+ 5 **H44.0 Purulent endophthalmitis**
Use additional code to identify organism
EXCLUDES 1 bleb associated endophthalmitis (H59.4-)
+ 6 **H44.00 Unspecified purulent endophthalmitis**
SP + **H44.001 Unspecified purulent endophthalmitis, right eye**
SP + **H44.002 Unspecified purulent endophthalmitis, left eye**
SP + **H44.003 Unspecified purulent endophthalmitis, bilateral**
IQ + **H44.009 Unspecified purulent endophthalmitis, unspecified eye**
+ 6 **H44.01 Panophthalmitis (acute)**
DEFINITION Inflammation affecting all the structures or tissues of the eye.
SP + **H44.011 Panophthalmitis (acute), right eye**
SP + **H44.012 Panophthalmitis (acute), left eye**
SP + **H44.013 Panophthalmitis (acute), bilateral**
IQ + **H44.019 Panophthalmitis (acute), unspecified eye**
+ 6 **H44.02 Vitreous abscess (chronic)**
SP + **H44.021 Vitreous abscess (chronic), right eye**
SP + **H44.022 Vitreous abscess (chronic), left eye**
SP + **H44.023 Vitreous abscess (chronic), bilateral**
IQ + **H44.029 Vitreous abscess (chronic), unspecified eye**
5 **H44.1 Other endophthalmitis**
EXCLUDES 1 bleb associated endophthalmitis (H59.4-)
EXCLUDES 2 ophthalmia nodosa (H16.2-)
6 **H44.11 Panuveitis**
DEFINITION Inflammation of the entire pigmented layer of the eye (uveal tract).
SP **H44.111 Panuveitis, right eye**
SP **H44.112 Panuveitis, left eye**
SP **H44.113 Panuveitis, bilateral**
IQ **H44.119 Panuveitis, unspecified eye**

Chapter 7
H00-H59

6 H44.12 Parasitic endophthalmitis, unspecified
Laterality SP H44.121 Parasitic endophthalmitis, unspecified, right eye
Laterality SP H44.122 Parasitic endophthalmitis, unspecified, left eye
Laterality SP H44.123 Parasitic endophthalmitis, unspecified, bilateral
Laterality !Q H44.129 Parasitic endophthalmitis, unspecified, unspecified eye
6 H44.13 Sympathetic uveitis
Laterality SP H44.131 Sympathetic uveitis, right eye
Laterality SP H44.132 Sympathetic uveitis, left eye
Laterality SP H44.133 Sympathetic uveitis, bilateral
Laterality !Q H44.139 Sympathetic uveitis, unspecified eye
SP H44.19 Other endophthalmitis
5 H44.2 Degenerative myopia
Malignant myopia
Laterality !Q H44.20 Degenerative myopia, unspecified eye
Laterality SP H44.21 Degenerative myopia, right eye
Laterality SP H44.22 Degenerative myopia, left eye
Laterality SP H44.23 Degenerative myopia, bilateral
+ 6 H44.2A Degenerative myopia with choroidal neovascularization
Use additional code for any associated choroid disorders (H31.-)
Laterality SP + H44.2A1 Degenerative myopia with choroidal neovascularization, right eye
Laterality SP + H44.2A2 Degenerative myopia with choroidal neovascularization, left eye
Laterality SP + H44.2A3 Degenerative myopia with choroidal neovascularization, bilateral eye
Laterality !Q + H44.2A9 Degenerative myopia with choroidal neovascularization, unspecified eye
6 H44.2B Degenerative myopia with macular hole
Laterality SP H44.2B1 Degenerative myopia with macular hole, right eye
Laterality SP H44.2B2 Degenerative myopia with macular hole, left eye
Laterality SP H44.2B3 Degenerative myopia with macular hole, bilateral eye
Laterality !Q H44.2B9 Degenerative myopia with macular hole, unspecified eye
+ 6 H44.2C Degenerative myopia with retinal detachment
Use additional code to identify the retinal detachment (H33.-)
Laterality SP + H44.2C1 Degenerative myopia with retinal detachment, right eye
Laterality SP + H44.2C2 Degenerative myopia with retinal detachment, left eye
Laterality SP + H44.2C3 Degenerative myopia with retinal detachment, bilateral eye
Laterality !Q + H44.2C9 Degenerative myopia with retinal detachment, unspecified eye
6 H44.2D Degenerative myopia with foveoschisis
Laterality SP H44.2D1 Degenerative myopia with foveoschisis, right eye
Laterality SP H44.2D2 Degenerative myopia with foveoschisis, left eye
Laterality SP H44.2D3 Degenerative myopia with foveoschisis, bilateral eye
Laterality !Q H44.2D9 Degenerative myopia with foveoschisis, unspecified eye
6 H44.2E Degenerative myopia with other maculopathy
Laterality SP H44.2E1 Degenerative myopia with other maculopathy, right eye
Laterality SP H44.2E2 Degenerative myopia with other maculopathy, left eye
Laterality SP H44.2E3 Degenerative myopia with other maculopathy, bilateral eye
Laterality !Q H44.2E9 Degenerative myopia with other maculopathy, unspecified eye
5 H44.3 Other and unspecified degenerative disorders of globe
!Q H44.30 Unspecified degenerative disorder of globe
6 H44.31 Chalcosis
Laterality SP H44.311 Chalcosis, right eye
Laterality SP H44.312 Chalcosis, left eye
Laterality SP H44.313 Chalcosis, bilateral
Laterality !Q H44.319 Chalcosis, unspecified eye
6 H44.32 Siderosis of eye
Laterality SP H44.321 Siderosis of eye, right eye
Laterality SP H44.322 Siderosis of eye, left eye
Laterality SP H44.323 Siderosis of eye, bilateral
Laterality !Q H44.329 Siderosis of eye, unspecified eye
6 H44.39 Other degenerative disorders of globe
Laterality SP H44.391 Other degenerative disorders of globe, right eye
Laterality SP H44.392 Other degenerative disorders of globe, left eye
Laterality SP H44.393 Other degenerative disorders of globe, bilateral
Laterality !Q H44.399 Other degenerative disorders of globe, unspecified eye
5 H44.4 Hypotony of eye
SP H44.40 Unspecified hypotony of eye
6 H44.41 Flat anterior chamber hypotony of eye
Laterality SP H44.411 Flat anterior chamber hypotony of right eye
Laterality SP H44.412 Flat anterior chamber hypotony of left eye
Laterality SP H44.413 Flat anterior chamber hypotony of eye, bilateral
Laterality !Q H44.419 Flat anterior chamber hypotony of unspecified eye
6 H44.42 Hypotony of eye due to ocular fistula
Laterality SP H44.421 Hypotony of right eye due to ocular fistula
Laterality SP H44.422 Hypotony of left eye due to ocular fistula
Laterality SP H44.423 Hypotony of eye due to ocular fistula, bilateral
Laterality !Q H44.429 Hypotony of unspecified eye due to ocular fistula

4 4th digit required 5 5th digit required 6 6th digit required 7 7th digit required 7 7th digit placeholder + Additional code Laterality

6 H44.43 Hypotony of eye due to other ocular disorders
⊟ SP H44.431 Hypotony of eye due to other ocular disorders, right eye
⊟ SP H44.432 Hypotony of eye due to other ocular disorders, left eye
⊟ SP H44.433 Hypotony of eye due to other ocular disorders, bilateral
⊟ IQ H44.439 Hypotony of eye due to other ocular disorders, unspecified eye
6 H44.44 Primary hypotony of eye
⊟ SP H44.441 Primary hypotony of right eye
⊟ SP H44.442 Primary hypotony of left eye
⊟ SP H44.443 Primary hypotony of eye, bilateral
⊟ IQ H44.449 Primary hypotony of unspecified eye
5 H44.5 Degenerated conditions of globe
IQ H44.50 Unspecified degenerated conditions of globe
6 H44.51 Absolute glaucoma
⊟ SP H44.511 Absolute glaucoma, right eye
⊟ SP H44.512 Absolute glaucoma, left eye
⊟ SP H44.513 Absolute glaucoma, bilateral
⊟ IQ H44.519 Absolute glaucoma, unspecified eye
6 H44.52 Atrophy of globe
Phthisis bulbi
⊟ SP H44.521 Atrophy of globe, right eye
⊟ SP H44.522 Atrophy of globe, left eye
⊟ SP H44.523 Atrophy of globe, bilateral
⊟ IQ H44.529 Atrophy of globe, unspecified eye
6 H44.53 Leucocoria
⊟ SP H44.531 Leucocoria, right eye
⊟ SP H44.532 Leucocoria, left eye
⊟ SP H44.533 Leucocoria, bilateral
⊟ IQ H44.539 Leucocoria, unspecified eye
+ 5 H44.6 Retained (old) intraocular foreign body, magnetic
Use additional code to identify magnetic foreign body (Z18.11)
EXCLUDES 1 current intraocular foreign body (S05.-)
EXCLUDES 2 retained foreign body in eyelid (H02.81-)
retained (old) foreign body following penetrating wound of orbit (H05.5-)
retained (old) intraocular foreign body, nonmagnetic (H44.7-)
+ 6 H44.60 Unspecified retained (old) intraocular foreign body, magnetic
⊟ SP + H44.601 Unspecified retained (old) intraocular foreign body, magnetic, right eye
⊟ SP + H44.602 Unspecified retained (old) intraocular foreign body, magnetic, left eye
⊟ SP + H44.603 Unspecified retained (old) intraocular foreign body, magnetic, bilateral
⊟ IQ + H44.609 Unspecified retained (old) intraocular foreign body, magnetic, unspecified eye
+ 6 H44.61 Retained (old) magnetic foreign body in anterior chamber
⊟ SP + H44.611 Retained (old) magnetic foreign body in anterior chamber, right eye
⊟ SP + H44.612 Retained (old) magnetic foreign body in anterior chamber, left eye
⊟ SP + H44.613 Retained (old) magnetic foreign body in anterior chamber, bilateral
⊟ IQ + H44.619 Retained (old) magnetic foreign body in anterior chamber, unspecified eye
+ 6 H44.62 Retained (old) magnetic foreign body in iris or ciliary body
⊟ SP + H44.621 Retained (old) magnetic foreign body in iris or ciliary body, right eye
⊟ SP + H44.622 Retained (old) magnetic foreign body in iris or ciliary body, left eye
⊟ SP + H44.623 Retained (old) magnetic foreign body in iris or ciliary body, bilateral
⊟ IQ + H44.629 Retained (old) magnetic foreign body in iris or ciliary body, unspecified eye
+ 6 H44.63 Retained (old) magnetic foreign body in lens
⊟ SP + H44.631 Retained (old) magnetic foreign body in lens, right eye
⊟ SP + H44.632 Retained (old) magnetic foreign body in lens, left eye
⊟ SP + H44.633 Retained (old) magnetic foreign body in lens, bilateral
⊟ IQ + H44.639 Retained (old) magnetic foreign body in lens, unspecified eye
+ 6 H44.64 Retained (old) magnetic foreign body in posterior wall of globe
⊟ SP + H44.641 Retained (old) magnetic foreign body in posterior wall of globe, right eye
⊟ SP + H44.642 Retained (old) magnetic foreign body in posterior wall of globe, left eye
⊟ SP + H44.643 Retained (old) magnetic foreign body in posterior wall of globe, bilateral
⊟ IQ + H44.649 Retained (old) magnetic foreign body in posterior wall of globe, unspecified eye
+ 6 H44.65 Retained (old) magnetic foreign body in vitreous body
⊟ SP + H44.651 Retained (old) magnetic foreign body in vitreous body, right eye
⊟ SP + H44.652 Retained (old) magnetic foreign body in vitreous body, left eye
⊟ SP + H44.653 Retained (old) magnetic foreign body in vitreous body, bilateral
⊟ IQ + H44.659 Retained (old) magnetic foreign body in vitreous body, unspecified eye

+ 6 H44.69 Retained (old) intraocular foreign body, magnetic, in other or multiple sites

⊟ SP + H44.691 Retained (old) intraocular foreign body, magnetic, in other or multiple sites, right eye

⊟ SP + H44.692 Retained (old) intraocular foreign body, magnetic, in other or multiple sites, left eye

⊟ SP + H44.693 Retained (old) intraocular foreign body, magnetic, in other or multiple sites, bilateral

⊟ !Q + H44.699 Retained (old) intraocular foreign body, magnetic, in other or multiple sites, unspecified eye

+ 5 H44.7 Retained (old) intraocular foreign body, nonmagnetic

Use additional code to identify nonmagnetic foreign body (Z18.01-Z18.10, Z18.12, Z18.2-Z18.9)

EXCLUDES 1 current intraocular foreign body (S05.-)

EXCLUDES 2 retained foreign body in eyelid (H02.81-)
retained (old) foreign body following penetrating wound of orbit (H05.5-)
retained (old) intraocular foreign body, magnetic (H44.6-)

+ 6 H44.70 Unspecified retained (old) intraocular foreign body, nonmagnetic

⊟ SP + H44.701 Unspecified retained (old) intraocular foreign body, nonmagnetic, right eye

⊟ SP + H44.702 Unspecified retained (old) intraocular foreign body, nonmagnetic, left eye

⊟ SP + H44.703 Unspecified retained (old) intraocular foreign body, nonmagnetic, bilateral

⊟ !Q + H44.709 Unspecified retained (old) intraocular foreign body, nonmagnetic, unspecified eye

Retained (old) intraocular foreign body NOS

+ 6 H44.71 Retained (nonmagnetic) (old) foreign body in anterior chamber

⊟ SP + H44.711 Retained (nonmagnetic) (old) foreign body in anterior chamber, right eye

⊟ SP + H44.712 Retained (nonmagnetic) (old) foreign body in anterior chamber, left eye

⊟ SP + H44.713 Retained (nonmagnetic) (old) foreign body in anterior chamber, bilateral

⊟ !Q + H44.719 Retained (nonmagnetic) (old) foreign body in anterior chamber, unspecified eye

+ 6 H44.72 Retained (nonmagnetic) (old) foreign body in iris or ciliary body

⊟ SP + H44.721 Retained (nonmagnetic) (old) foreign body in iris or ciliary body, right eye

⊟ SP + H44.722 Retained (nonmagnetic) (old) foreign body in iris or ciliary body, left eye

⊟ SP + H44.723 Retained (nonmagnetic) (old) foreign body in iris or ciliary body, bilateral

⊟ SP + H44.729 Retained (nonmagnetic) (old) foreign body in iris or ciliary body, unspecified eye

+ 6 H44.73 Retained (nonmagnetic) (old) foreign body in lens

⊟ SP + H44.731 Retained (nonmagnetic) (old) foreign body in lens, right eye

⊟ SP + H44.732 Retained (nonmagnetic) (old) foreign body in lens, left eye

⊟ SP + H44.733 Retained (nonmagnetic) (old) foreign body in lens, bilateral

⊟ !Q + H44.739 Retained (nonmagnetic) (old) foreign body in lens, unspecified eye

+ 6 H44.74 Retained (nonmagnetic) (old) foreign body in posterior wall of globe

⊟ SP + H44.741 Retained (nonmagnetic) (old) foreign body in posterior wall of globe, right eye

⊟ SP + H44.742 Retained (nonmagnetic) (old) foreign body in posterior wall of globe, left eye

⊟ SP + H44.743 Retained (nonmagnetic) (old) foreign body in posterior wall of globe, bilateral

⊟ !Q + H44.749 Retained (nonmagnetic) (old) foreign body in posterior wall of globe, unspecified eye

+ 6 H44.75 Retained (nonmagnetic) (old) foreign body in vitreous body

⊟ SP + H44.751 Retained (nonmagnetic) (old) foreign body in vitreous body, right eye

⊟ SP + H44.752 Retained (nonmagnetic) (old) foreign body in vitreous body, left eye

⊟ SP + H44.753 Retained (nonmagnetic) (old) foreign body in vitreous body, bilateral

⊟ !Q + H44.759 Retained (nonmagnetic) (old) foreign body in vitreous body, unspecified eye

+ 6 H44.79 Retained (old) intraocular foreign body, nonmagnetic, in other or multiple sites

⊟ SP + H44.791 Retained (old) intraocular foreign body, nonmagnetic, in other or multiple sites, right eye

⊟ SP + H44.792 Retained (old) intraocular foreign body, nonmagnetic, in other or multiple sites, left eye

⊟ SP + H44.793 Retained (old) intraocular foreign body, nonmagnetic, in other or multiple sites, bilateral

⊟ !Q + H44.799 Retained (old) intraocular foreign body, nonmagnetic, in other or multiple sites, unspecified eye

5 H44.8 Other disorders of globe

6 H44.81 Hemophthalmos

Chapter 7 H00-H59

DEFINITION Accumulation of blood within the eyeball that is not due to a current injury.

- H44.811 Hemophthalmos, right eye
- H44.812 Hemophthalmos, left eye
- H44.813 Hemophthalmos, bilateral
- H44.819 Hemophthalmos, unspecified eye
- H44.82 Luxation of globe
- H44.821 Luxation of globe, right eye
- H44.822 Luxation of globe, left eye
- H44.823 Luxation of globe, bilateral
- H44.829 Luxation of globe, unspecified eye
- H44.89 Other disorders of globe
- H44.9 Unspecified disorder of globe

Disorders of optic nerve and visual pathways (H46-H47)

H46 Optic neuritis

EXCLUDES 2 ischemic optic neuropathy (H47.01-)
neuromyelitis optica [Devic] (G36.0)

H46.0 Optic papillitis

DEFINITION Swelling of the optic disc where the optic nerve connects to the retina.

- H46.00 Optic papillitis, unspecified eye
- H46.01 Optic papillitis, right eye
- H46.02 Optic papillitis, left eye
- H46.03 Optic papillitis, bilateral

H46.1 Retrobulbar neuritis

Retrobulbar neuritis NOS

EXCLUDES 1 syphilitic retrobulbar neuritis (A52.15)

DEFINITION Inflammation of the optic nerve directly behind the eye.

- H46.10 Retrobulbar neuritis, unspecified eye
- H46.11 Retrobulbar neuritis, right eye
- H46.12 Retrobulbar neuritis, left eye
- H46.13 Retrobulbar neuritis, bilateral
- H46.2 Nutritional optic neuropathy
- H46.3 Toxic optic neuropathy
  Code first:
  (T51-T65) to identify cause
- H46.8 Other optic neuritis
- H46.9 Unspecified optic neuritis

H47 Other disorders of optic [2nd] nerve and visual pathways

H47.0 Disorders of optic nerve, not elsewhere classified

- H47.01 Ischemic optic neuropathy
- H47.011 Ischemic optic neuropathy, right eye
- H47.012 Ischemic optic neuropathy, left eye
- H47.013 Ischemic optic neuropathy, bilateral
- H47.019 Ischemic optic neuropathy, unspecified eye
- H47.02 Hemorrhage in optic nerve sheath
- H47.021 Hemorrhage in optic nerve sheath, right eye
- H47.022 Hemorrhage in optic nerve sheath, left eye
- H47.023 Hemorrhage in optic nerve sheath, bilateral
- H47.029 Hemorrhage in optic nerve sheath, unspecified eye
- H47.03 Optic nerve hypoplasia
- H47.031 Optic nerve hypoplasia, right eye
- H47.032 Optic nerve hypoplasia, left eye
- H47.033 Optic nerve hypoplasia, bilateral
- H47.039 Optic nerve hypoplasia, unspecified eye
- H47.09 Other disorders of optic nerve, not elsewhere classified
  Compression of optic nerve
- H47.091 Other disorders of optic nerve, not elsewhere classified, right eye
- H47.092 Other disorders of optic nerve, not elsewhere classified, left eye
- H47.093 Other disorders of optic nerve, not elsewhere classified, bilateral
- H47.099 Other disorders of optic nerve, not elsewhere classified, unspecified eye

H47.1 Papilledema

- H47.10 Unspecified papilledema
- H47.11 Papilledema associated with increased intracranial pressure
  DEFINITION Swelling of the optic disk (the part of the retina that connects to the optic nerve) caused by increased intracranial pressure.
- H47.12 Papilledema associated with decreased ocular pressure
- H47.13 Papilledema associated with retinal disorder
- H47.14 Foster-Kennedy syndrome
  DEFINITION Disease that presents with papilledema in one eye and atrophy of the optic nerve of the other; caused by increased intracranial pressure from a tumor.
- H47.141 Foster-Kennedy syndrome, right eye
- H47.142 Foster-Kennedy syndrome, left eye
- H47.143 Foster-Kennedy syndrome, bilateral
- H47.149 Foster-Kennedy syndrome, unspecified eye

H47.2 Optic atrophy

- H47.20 Unspecified optic atrophy
- H47.21 Primary optic atrophy
- H47.211 Primary optic atrophy, right eye
- H47.212 Primary optic atrophy, left eye
- H47.213 Primary optic atrophy, bilateral
- H47.219 Primary optic atrophy, unspecified eye
- H47.22 Hereditary optic atrophy
  Leber's optic atrophy

Chapter 7 H00-H59

New ▲Revised Px Primary SP PDGM Px SL Low CoM SH High CoM IQ Quest. Encounter H Hospice non-cancer Dx Unspecified M Manifestation

6 H47.23 Glaucomatous optic atrophy
- Laterality SP H47.231 **Glaucomatous optic atrophy, right eye**
- Laterality SP H47.232 **Glaucomatous optic atrophy, left eye**
- Laterality SP H47.233 **Glaucomatous optic atrophy, bilateral**
- Laterality IQ H47.239 **Glaucomatous optic atrophy, unspecified eye**

6 H47.29 **Other optic atrophy**
Temporal pallor of optic disc
- Laterality SP H47.291 **Other optic atrophy, right eye**
- Laterality SP H47.292 **Other optic atrophy, left eye**
- Laterality SP H47.293 **Other optic atrophy, bilateral**
- Laterality IQ H47.299 **Other optic atrophy, unspecified eye**

5 H47.3 **Other disorders of optic disc**

6 H47.31 **Coloboma of optic disc**
DEFINITION Congenital defect of the iris in which there is a gap, hole, or cleft that failed to close; may cause ghost images, blurred or decreased visual activity.
- Laterality SP H47.311 **Coloboma of optic disc, right eye**
- Laterality SP H47.312 **Coloboma of optic disc, left eye**
- Laterality SP H47.313 **Coloboma of optic disc, bilateral**
- Laterality IQ H47.319 **Coloboma of optic disc, unspecified eye**

6 H47.32 **Drusen of optic disc**
- Laterality SP H47.321 **Drusen of optic disc, right eye**
- Laterality SP H47.322 **Drusen of optic disc, left eye**
- Laterality SP H47.323 **Drusen of optic disc, bilateral**
- Laterality IQ H47.329 **Drusen of optic disc, unspecified eye**

6 H47.33 **Pseudopapilledema of optic disc**
- Laterality SP H47.331 **Pseudopapilledema of optic disc, right eye**
- Laterality SP H47.332 **Pseudopapilledema of optic disc, left eye**
- Laterality SP H47.333 **Pseudopapilledema of optic disc, bilateral**
- Laterality IQ H47.339 **Pseudopapilledema of optic disc, unspecified eye**

6 H47.39 **Other disorders of optic disc**
- Laterality SP H47.391 **Other disorders of optic disc, right eye**
- Laterality SP H47.392 **Other disorders of optic disc, left eye**
- Laterality SP H47.393 **Other disorders of optic disc, bilateral**
- Laterality IQ H47.399 **Other disorders of optic disc, unspecified eye**

5 H47.4 **Disorders of optic chiasm**
Code also:
underlying condition
- SP H47.41 **Disorders of optic chiasm in (due to) inflammatory disorders**
- SP H47.42 **Disorders of optic chiasm in (due to) neoplasm**
- SP H47.43 **Disorders of optic chiasm in (due to) vascular disorders**
- SP H47.49 **Disorders of optic chiasm in (due to) other disorders**

5 H47.5 **Disorders of other visual pathways**
Disorders of optic tracts, geniculate nuclei and optic radiations
Code also:
underlying condition

6 H47.51 **Disorders of visual pathways in (due to) inflammatory disorders**
- Laterality SP H47.511 **Disorders of visual pathways in (due to) inflammatory disorders, right side**
- Laterality SP H47.512 **Disorders of visual pathways in (due to) inflammatory disorders, left side**
- Laterality IQ H47.519 **Disorders of visual pathways in (due to) inflammatory disorders, unspecified side**

6 H47.52 **Disorders of visual pathways in (due to) neoplasm**
- Laterality SP H47.521 **Disorders of visual pathways in (due to) neoplasm, right side**
- Laterality SP H47.522 **Disorders of visual pathways in (due to) neoplasm, left side**
- Laterality IQ H47.529 **Disorders of visual pathways in (due to) neoplasm, unspecified side**

6 H47.53 **Disorders of visual pathways in (due to) vascular disorders**
- Laterality SP H47.531 **Disorders of visual pathways in (due to) vascular disorders, right side**
- Laterality SP H47.532 **Disorders of visual pathways in (due to) vascular disorders, left side**
- Laterality IQ H47.539 **Disorders of visual pathways in (due to) vascular disorders, unspecified side**

5 H47.6 **Disorders of visual cortex**
Code also:
underlying condition
EXCLUDES 1 injury to visual cortex S04.04-

6 H47.61 **Cortical blindness**
DEFINITION Blindness caused by a defect of the brain and not the eyes.
- Laterality SP H47.611 **Cortical blindness, right side of brain**
- Laterality SP H47.612 **Cortical blindness, left side of brain**
- Laterality IQ H47.619 **Cortical blindness, unspecified side of brain**

6 H47.62 **Disorders of visual cortex in (due to) inflammatory disorders**
- Laterality SP H47.621 **Disorders of visual cortex in (due to) inflammatory disorders, right side of brain**
- Laterality SP H47.622 **Disorders of visual cortex in (due to) inflammatory disorders, left side of brain**
- Laterality IQ H47.629 **Disorders of visual cortex in (due to) inflammatory disorders, unspecified side of brain**

6 H47.63 **Disorders of visual cortex in (due to) neoplasm**
- Laterality SP H47.631 **Disorders of visual cortex in (due to) neoplasm, right side of brain**
- Laterality SP H47.632 **Disorders of visual cortex in (due to) neoplasm, left side of brain**

- H47.639 Disorders of visual cortex in (due to) neoplasm, unspecified side of brain
- H47.64 Disorders of visual cortex in (due to) vascular disorders
- H47.641 Disorders of visual cortex in (due to) vascular disorders, right side of brain
- H47.642 Disorders of visual cortex in (due to) vascular disorders, left side of brain
- H47.649 Disorders of visual cortex in (due to) vascular disorders, unspecified side of brain
- H47.9 Unspecified disorder of visual pathways

Disorders of ocular muscles, binocular movement, accommodation and refraction (H49-H52)

EXCLUDES 2 nystagmus and other irregular eye movements (H55)

- H49 Paralytic strabismus
  - EXCLUDES 2 internal ophthalmoplegia (H52.51-)
  - internuclear ophthalmoplegia (H51.2-)
  - progressive supranuclear ophthalmoplegia (G23.1)
- H49.0 Third [oculomotor] nerve palsy
- H49.00 Third [oculomotor] nerve palsy, unspecified eye
- H49.01 Third [oculomotor] nerve palsy, right eye
- H49.02 Third [oculomotor] nerve palsy, left eye
- H49.03 Third [oculomotor] nerve palsy, bilateral
- H49.1 Fourth [trochlear] nerve palsy
- H49.10 Fourth [trochlear] nerve palsy, unspecified eye
- H49.11 Fourth [trochlear] nerve palsy, right eye
- H49.12 Fourth [trochlear] nerve palsy, left eye
- H49.13 Fourth [trochlear] nerve palsy, bilateral
- H49.2 Sixth [abducent] nerve palsy
- H49.20 Sixth [abducent] nerve palsy, unspecified eye
- H49.21 Sixth [abducent] nerve palsy, right eye
- H49.22 Sixth [abducent] nerve palsy, left eye
- H49.23 Sixth [abducent] nerve palsy, bilateral
- H49.3 Total (external) ophthalmoplegia
  - DEFINITION Paralysis of all of the muscles that move the eye as well as the muscles controlling the diameter of the pupil and shape of the lens.
- H49.30 Total (external) ophthalmoplegia, unspecified eye
- H49.31 Total (external) ophthalmoplegia, right eye
- H49.32 Total (external) ophthalmoplegia, left eye
- H49.33 Total (external) ophthalmoplegia, bilateral
- H49.4 Progressive external ophthalmoplegia
  - EXCLUDES 1 Kearns-Sayre syndrome (H49.81-)
- H49.40 Progressive external ophthalmoplegia, unspecified eye
- H49.41 Progressive external ophthalmoplegia, right eye
- H49.42 Progressive external ophthalmoplegia, left eye
- H49.43 Progressive external ophthalmoplegia, bilateral
- H49.8 Other paralytic strabismus
- + H49.81 Kearns-Sayre syndrome
  - Progressive external ophthalmoplegia with pigmentary retinopathy
  - Use additional code for other manifestation, such as: heart block (I45.9)
- + H49.811 Kearns-Sayre syndrome, right eye
- + H49.812 Kearns-Sayre syndrome, left eye
- + H49.813 Kearns-Sayre syndrome, bilateral
- + H49.819 Kearns-Sayre syndrome, unspecified eye
- H49.88 Other paralytic strabismus
  - External ophthalmoplegia NOS
- H49.881 Other paralytic strabismus, right eye
- H49.882 Other paralytic strabismus, left eye
- H49.883 Other paralytic strabismus, bilateral
- H49.889 Other paralytic strabismus, unspecified eye
- H49.9 Unspecified paralytic strabismus
- H50 Other strabismus
- H50.0 Esotropia
  - Convergent concomitant strabismus
  - EXCLUDES 1 intermittent esotropia (H50.31-, H50.32)
  - DEFINITION Deviation of the visual axis of one or both eyes inward toward that of the other eye.
- H50.00 Unspecified esotropia
- H50.01 Monocular esotropia
- H50.011 Monocular esotropia, right eye
- H50.012 Monocular esotropia, left eye
- H50.02 Monocular esotropia with A pattern
- H50.021 Monocular esotropia with A pattern, right eye
- H50.022 Monocular esotropia with A pattern, left eye
- H50.03 Monocular esotropia with V pattern
- H50.031 Monocular esotropia with V pattern, right eye
- H50.032 Monocular esotropia with V pattern, left eye
- H50.04 Monocular esotropia with other noncomitancies
- H50.041 Monocular esotropia with other noncomitancies, right eye

Chapter 7 H00-H59

SP H50.042 Monocular esotropia with other noncomitancies, left eye
SP H50.05 Alternating esotropia
SP H50.06 Alternating esotropia with A pattern
SP H50.07 Alternating esotropia with V pattern
SP H50.08 Alternating esotropia with other noncomitancies
5 H50.1 Exotropia
Divergent concomitant strabismus
EXCLUDES 1 intermittent exotropia (H50.33-, H50.34)
DEFINITION An abnormal alignment of one or both eyes in which one or both eyes deviate outward.
SP H50.10 Unspecified exotropia
6 H50.11 Monocular exotropia
SP H50.111 Monocular exotropia, right eye
SP H50.112 Monocular exotropia, left eye
6 H50.12 Monocular exotropia with A pattern
SP H50.121 Monocular exotropia with A pattern, right eye
SP H50.122 Monocular exotropia with A pattern, left eye
6 H50.13 Monocular exotropia with V pattern
SP H50.131 Monocular exotropia with V pattern, right eye
SP H50.132 Monocular exotropia with V pattern, left eye
6 H50.14 Monocular exotropia with other noncomitancies
SP H50.141 Monocular exotropia with other noncomitancies, right eye
SP H50.142 Monocular exotropia with other noncomitancies, left eye
SP H50.15 Alternating exotropia
SP H50.16 Alternating exotropia with A pattern
SP H50.17 Alternating exotropia with V pattern
SP H50.18 Alternating exotropia with other noncomitancies
5 H50.2 Vertical strabismus
Hypertropia
SP H50.21 Vertical strabismus, right eye
SP H50.22 Vertical strabismus, left eye
5 H50.3 Intermittent heterotropia
SP H50.30 Unspecified intermittent heterotropia
6 H50.31 Intermittent monocular esotropia
SP H50.311 Intermittent monocular esotropia, right eye
SP H50.312 Intermittent monocular esotropia, left eye
SP H50.32 Intermittent alternating esotropia
6 H50.33 Intermittent monocular exotropia
SP H50.331 Intermittent monocular exotropia, right eye
SP H50.332 Intermittent monocular exotropia, left eye
SP H50.34 Intermittent alternating exotropia
5 H50.4 Other and unspecified heterotropia
SP H50.40 Unspecified heterotropia
6 H50.41 Cyclotropia
SP H50.411 Cyclotropia, right eye
SP H50.412 Cyclotropia, left eye
SP H50.42 Monofixation syndrome
SP H50.43 Accommodative component in esotropia
5 H50.5 Heterophoria
SP H50.50 Unspecified heterophoria
SP H50.51 Esophoria
SP H50.52 Exophoria
SP H50.53 Vertical heterophoria
SP H50.54 Cyclophoria
SP H50.55 Alternating heterophoria
5 H50.6 Mechanical strabismus
SP H50.60 Mechanical strabismus, unspecified
6 H50.61 Brown's sheath syndrome
DEFINITION Condition in which the muscle that moves the eye upward and inward is too short, impairing eye movement.
SP H50.611 Brown's sheath syndrome, right eye
SP H50.612 Brown's sheath syndrome, left eye
SP H50.69 Other mechanical strabismus
Strabismus due to adhesions
Traumatic limitation of duction of eye muscle
5 H50.8 Other specified strabismus
6 H50.81 Duane's syndrome
DEFINITION Congenital eye muscle disorder due to cranial nerve dysfunction that inhibits normal rotation of one or both eyes inward and outward, also causing abnormal inward turning with distant viewing and eye retraction when viewing up close.
SP H50.811 Duane's syndrome, right eye
SP H50.812 Duane's syndrome, left eye
SP H50.89 Other specified strabismus
SP H50.9 Unspecified strabismus
4 H51 Other disorders of binocular movement
SP H51.0 Palsy (spasm) of conjugate gaze
5 H51.1 Convergence insufficiency and excess
SP H51.11 Convergence insufficiency
SP H51.12 Convergence excess
DEFINITION Eyes fail to move in a coordinated fashion when viewing objects up close.
5 H51.2 Internuclear ophthalmoplegia
IQ H51.20 Internuclear ophthalmoplegia, unspecified eye
SP H51.21 Internuclear ophthalmoplegia, right eye
SP H51.22 Internuclear ophthalmoplegia, left eye
SP H51.23 Internuclear ophthalmoplegia, bilateral
SP H51.8 Other specified disorders of binocular movement
IQ H51.9 Unspecified disorder of binocular movement
4 H52 Disorders of refraction and accommodation

4 4th digit required 5 5th digit required 6 6th digit required 7 7th digit required X 7th digit placeholder + Additional code Laterality

5 H52.0 Hypermetropia
- IQ H52.00 Hypermetropia, unspecified eye
- SP H52.01 Hypermetropia, right eye
- SP H52.02 Hypermetropia, left eye
- SP H52.03 Hypermetropia, bilateral

5 H52.1 Myopia
EXCLUDES 1 degenerative myopia (H44.2-)
- IQ H52.10 Myopia, unspecified eye
- SP H52.11 Myopia, right eye
- SP H52.12 Myopia, left eye
- SP H52.13 Myopia, bilateral

5 H52.2 Astigmatism
DEFINITION Condition in which the cornea is not shaped perfectly round, causing light to focus on more than one point of the retina and resulting in blurred vision.

6 H52.20 Unspecified astigmatism
- SP H52.201 Unspecified astigmatism, right eye
- SP H52.202 Unspecified astigmatism, left eye
- SP H52.203 Unspecified astigmatism, bilateral
- IQ H52.209 Unspecified astigmatism, unspecified eye

6 H52.21 Irregular astigmatism
- SP H52.211 Irregular astigmatism, right eye
- SP H52.212 Irregular astigmatism, left eye
- SP H52.213 Irregular astigmatism, bilateral
- IQ H52.219 Irregular astigmatism, unspecified eye

6 H52.22 Regular astigmatism
- SP H52.221 Regular astigmatism, right eye
- SP H52.222 Regular astigmatism, left eye
- SP H52.223 Regular astigmatism, bilateral
- IQ H52.229 Regular astigmatism, unspecified eye

5 H52.3 Anisometropia and aniseikonia

SP H52.31 Anisometropia
DEFINITION Each eye has a different refractive power.

SP H52.32 Aniseikonia
DEFINITION One eye sees an object differently in size and shape than the way the other eye sees it.

SP H52.4 Presbyopia
DEFINITION Lens of the eye loses its elasticity due to age, making it more difficult to focus on near points.

5 H52.5 Disorders of accommodation

6 H52.51 Internal ophthalmoplegia (complete) (total)
- SP H52.511 Internal ophthalmoplegia (complete) (total), right eye
- SP H52.512 Internal ophthalmoplegia (complete) (total), left eye
- SP H52.513 Internal ophthalmoplegia (complete) (total), bilateral
- IQ H52.519 Internal ophthalmoplegia (complete) (total), unspecified eye

6 H52.52 Paresis of accommodation
DEFINITION Paralysis of the ciliary muscles of the eye that results in the loss of visual accommodation.
- SP H52.521 Paresis of accommodation, right eye
- SP H52.522 Paresis of accommodation, left eye
- SP H52.523 Paresis of accommodation, bilateral
- IQ H52.529 Paresis of accommodation, unspecified eye

6 H52.53 Spasm of accommodation
DEFINITION Abnormal, uncontrolled contraction of the ciliary muscle, usually initially presenting as near-sightedness.
- SP H52.531 Spasm of accommodation, right eye
- SP H52.532 Spasm of accommodation, left eye
- SP H52.533 Spasm of accommodation, bilateral
- IQ H52.539 Spasm of accommodation, unspecified eye

SP H52.6 Other disorders of refraction

IQ H52.7 Unspecified disorder of refraction

Visual disturbances and blindness (H53-H54)

4 H53 Visual disturbances

5 H53.0 Amblyopia ex anopsia
EXCLUDES 1 amblyopia due to vitamin A deficiency (E50.5)

6 H53.00 Unspecified amblyopia
- SP H53.001 Unspecified amblyopia, right eye
- SP H53.002 Unspecified amblyopia, left eye
- SP H53.003 Unspecified amblyopia, bilateral
- IQ H53.009 Unspecified amblyopia, unspecified eye

6 H53.01 Deprivation amblyopia
- SP H53.011 Deprivation amblyopia, right eye
- SP H53.012 Deprivation amblyopia, left eye
- SP H53.013 Deprivation amblyopia, bilateral
- IQ H53.019 Deprivation amblyopia, unspecified eye

6 H53.02 Refractive amblyopia
- SP H53.021 Refractive amblyopia, right eye
- SP H53.022 Refractive amblyopia, left eye
- SP H53.023 Refractive amblyopia, bilateral
- IQ H53.029 Refractive amblyopia, unspecified eye

6 H53.03 Strabismic amblyopia
EXCLUDES 1 strabismus (H50.-)
- SP H53.031 Strabismic amblyopia, right eye
- SP H53.032 Strabismic amblyopia, left eye
- SP H53.033 Strabismic amblyopia, bilateral
- IQ H53.039 Strabismic amblyopia, unspecified eye

6 H53.04 Amblyopia suspect
- SP H53.041 Amblyopia suspect, right eye
- SP H53.042 Amblyopia suspect, left eye
- SP H53.043 Amblyopia suspect, bilateral

⊟ IQ **H53.049 Amblyopia suspect, unspecified eye**

5 **H53.1 Subjective visual disturbances**

EXCLUDES 1 subjective visual disturbances due to vitamin A deficiency (E50.5)
visual hallucinations (R44.1)

IQ **H53.10 Unspecified subjective visual disturbances**

SP **H53.11 Day blindness**
Hemeralopia

6 **H53.12 Transient visual loss**
Scintillating scotoma

EXCLUDES 1 amaurosis fugax (G45.3-)
transient retinal artery occlusion (H34.0-)

⊟ SP **H53.121 Transient visual loss, right eye**

⊟ SP **H53.122 Transient visual loss, left eye**

⊟ SP **H53.123 Transient visual loss, bilateral**

⊟ IQ **H53.129 Transient visual loss, unspecified eye**

6 **H53.13 Sudden visual loss**

⊟ SP **H53.131 Sudden visual loss, right eye**

⊟ SP **H53.132 Sudden visual loss, left eye**

⊟ SP **H53.133 Sudden visual loss, bilateral**

⊟ IQ **H53.139 Sudden visual loss, unspecified eye**

6 **H53.14 Visual discomfort**
Asthenopia
Photophobia

⊟ SP **H53.141 Visual discomfort, right eye**

⊟ SP **H53.142 Visual discomfort, left eye**

⊟ SP **H53.143 Visual discomfort, bilateral**

⊟ IQ **H53.149 Visual discomfort, unspecified**

SP **H53.15 Visual distortions of shape and size**
Metamorphopsia

SP **H53.16 Psychophysical visual disturbances**

SP **H53.19 Other subjective visual disturbances**
Visual halos

DEFINITION Photopsia: sparks or flashes in the field of vision, due to retinal irritation.

SP **H53.2 Diplopia**
Double vision

5 **H53.3 Other and unspecified disorders of binocular vision**

IQ **H53.30 Unspecified disorder of binocular vision**

SP **H53.31 Abnormal retinal correspondence**

SP **H53.32 Fusion with defective stereopsis**

SP **H53.33 Simultaneous visual perception without fusion**

DEFINITION Imaging from both eyes reaches the brain and are both processed, but without being merged into a single image; the patient sees two side-by-side images instead of one.

SP **H53.34 Suppression of binocular vision**

5 **H53.4 Visual field defects**

SP **H53.40 Unspecified visual field defects**

6 **H53.41 Scotoma involving central area**
Central scotoma

⊟ SP **H53.411 Scotoma involving central area, right eye**

⊟ SP **H53.412 Scotoma involving central area, left eye**

⊟ SP **H53.413 Scotoma involving central area, bilateral**

⊟ IQ **H53.419 Scotoma involving central area, unspecified eye**

6 **H53.42 Scotoma of blind spot area**
Enlarged blind spot

DEFINITION Blind spot (scotoma) in the central five degrees of the patient's vision.

⊟ SP **H53.421 Scotoma of blind spot area, right eye**

⊟ SP **H53.422 Scotoma of blind spot area, left eye**

⊟ SP **H53.423 Scotoma of blind spot area, bilateral**

⊟ IQ **H53.429 Scotoma of blind spot area, unspecified eye**

6 **H53.43 Sector or arcuate defects**
Arcuate scotoma
Bjerrum scotoma

⊟ SP **H53.431 Sector or arcuate defects, right eye**

⊟ SP **H53.432 Sector or arcuate defects, left eye**

⊟ SP **H53.433 Sector or arcuate defects, bilateral**

⊟ IQ **H53.439 Sector or arcuate defects, unspecified eye**

6 **H53.45 Other localized visual field defect**
Peripheral visual field defect
Ring scotoma NOS
Scotoma NOS

⊟ SP **H53.451 Other localized visual field defect, right eye**

⊟ SP **H53.452 Other localized visual field defect, left eye**

⊟ SP **H53.453 Other localized visual field defect, bilateral**

⊟ IQ **H53.459 Other localized visual field defect, unspecified eye**

6 **H53.46 Homonymous bilateral field defects**
Homonymous hemianopia
Homonymous hemianopsia
Quadrant anopia
Quadrant anopsia

⊟ SP **H53.461 Homonymous bilateral field defects, right side**

⊟ SP **H53.462 Homonymous bilateral field defects, left side**

⊟ IQ **H53.469 Homonymous bilateral field defects, unspecified side**
Homonymous bilateral field defects NOS

SP **H53.47 Heteronymous bilateral field defects**
Heteronymous hemianop(s)ia

6 **H53.48 Generalized contraction of visual field**

⊟ SP **H53.481 Generalized contraction of visual field, right eye**

⊟ SP **H53.482 Generalized contraction of visual field, left eye**

Chapter 7

H00-H59

4 4th digit required 5 5th digit required 6 6th digit required 7 7th digit required X 7th digit placeholder + Additional code ⊟ Laterality

SP H53.483 **Generalized contraction of visual field, bilateral**

IQ H53.489 **Generalized contraction of visual field, unspecified eye**

5 H53.5 **Color vision deficiencies**
Color blindness
EXCLUDES 2 day blindness (H53.11)

IQ H53.50 **Unspecified color vision deficiencies**
Color blindness NOS

SP H53.51 **Achromatopsia**
DEFINITION Nonprogressive, hereditary visual disorder and retinal abnormality causing decreased vision, light sensitivity, nystagmus, and complete color blindness.

SP H53.52 **Acquired color vision deficiency**

SP H53.53 **Deuteranomaly**
Deuteranopia
DEFINITION A deficiency in color perception primarily affecting red-green hues due to deficient pigment sensitive to green wavelengths, a common form of color blindness.

SP H53.54 **Protanomaly**
Protanopia

SP H53.55 **Tritanomaly**
Tritanopia
DEFINITION A deficiency in color perception characterized by an inability to discern blue and yellow due to an absence of blue-sensitive pigment in the retina.

SP H53.59 **Other color vision deficiencies**

5 H53.6 **Night blindness**
EXCLUDES 1 night blindness due to vitamin A deficiency (E50.5)

IQ H53.60 **Unspecified night blindness**

SP H53.61 **Abnormal dark adaptation curve**

SP H53.62 **Acquired night blindness**

SP H53.63 **Congenital night blindness**

SP H53.69 **Other night blindness**

5 H53.7 **Vision sensitivity deficiencies**

SP H53.71 **Glare sensitivity**

SP H53.72 **Impaired contrast sensitivity**

SP H53.8 **Other visual disturbances**

IQ H53.9 **Unspecified visual disturbance**

4 H54 **Blindness and low vision**
Note:
For definition of visual impairment categories see table below
Code first:
any associated underlying cause of the blindness
EXCLUDES 1 amaurosis fugax (G45.3)

GUIDELINES **Section I.C.7.b**
If "blindness" or "low vision" of both eyes is documented but the visual impairment category is not documented, assign code H54.3, Unqualified visual loss, both eyes. If "blindness" or "low vision" in one eye is documented but the visual impairment category is not documented, assign a code from H54.6-, Unqualified visual loss, one eye. If "blindness" or "visual loss" is documented without any information about whether one or both eyes are affected, assign code H54.7, Unspecified visual loss.

CODING TIPS✓ Do not use H54 codes for patients with common refractive errors, e.g. farsightedness, nearsightedness, astigmatism, etc. These codes are to indicate the level of vision for those with other eye conditions such as cataracts, retinopathy, glaucoma, hemianopsia, etc. Blindness should only be coded if documentation supports the code.

5 H54.0 **Blindness, both eyes**
Visual impairment categories 3, 4, 5 in both eyes.
CODING TIPS✓ Do not use H54.0 to indicate blindness in the USA. See H54.3 or H54.8, depending on the physician's documentation.

6 H54.0X **Blindness, both eyes, different category levels**
CODING TIPS✓ The sixth character represents the category of vision in the right eye, and a seventh character represents the category of vision in the left eye.

SP 7 H54.0X3 **Blindness right eye, category 3**

SP 7 H54.0X4 **Blindness right eye, category 4**

SP 7 H54.0X5 **Blindness right eye, category 5**

5 H54.1 **Blindness, one eye, low vision other eye**
Visual impairment categories 3, 4, 5 in one eye, with categories 1 or 2 in the other eye.

SP H54.10 **Blindness, one eye, low vision other eye, unspecified eyes**

6 H54.11 **Blindness, right eye, low vision left eye**
CODING TIPS✓ The sixth character represents the category of vision in the right eye, and a seventh character represents the category of vision in the left eye.

SP 7 H54.113 **Blindness right eye category 3, low vision left eye**

SP 7 H54.114 **Blindness right eye category 4, low vision left eye**

SP 7 H54.115 **Blindness right eye category 5, low vision left eye**

6 H54.12 **Blindness, left eye, low vision right eye**
CODING TIPS✓ The sixth character represents the category of vision in the right eye, and a seventh character represents the category of vision in the left eye.

Chapter 7
H00-H59

H54.121 Low vision right eye category 1, blindness left eye

H54.122 Low vision right eye category 2, blindness left eye

H54.2 Low vision, both eyes
Visual impairment categories 1 or 2 in both eyes.

H54.2X Low vision, both eyes, different category levels
CODING TIPS ✓ The sixth character represents the category of vision in the right eye, and a seventh character represents the category of vision in the left eye.

H54.2X1 Low vision, right eye, category 1

H54.2X2 Low vision, right eye, category 2

H54.3 Unqualified visual loss, both eyes
Visual impairment category 9 in both eyes.
GUIDELINES **Section I.C.7.b**
If "blindness" or "low vision" of both eyes is documented but the visual impairment category is not documented, assign code H54.3, Unqualified visual loss, both eyes.

H54.4 Blindness, one eye
Visual impairment categories 3, 4, 5 in one eye [normal vision in other eye]

H54.40 Blindness, one eye, unspecified eye

H54.41 Blindness, right eye, normal vision left eye
CODING TIPS ✓ The sixth character represents the category of vision in the right eye, and a seventh character represents the category of vision in the left eye.

H54.413 Blindness, right eye, category 3

H54.414 Blindness, right eye, category 4

H54.415 Blindness, right eye, category 5

H54.42 Blindness, left eye, normal vision right eye

H54.42A Blindness, left eye, category 3-5
CODING TIPS ✓ The sixth character represents the category of vision in the right eye, and a seventh character represents the category of vision in the left eye.

H54.5 Low vision, one eye
Visual impairment categories 1 or 2 in one eye [normal vision in other eye].

H54.50 Low vision, one eye, unspecified eye

H54.51 Low vision, right eye, normal vision left eye
CODING TIPS ✓ The sixth character represents the category of vision in the right eye, and a seventh character represents the category of vision in the left eye.

H54.511 Low vision, right eye, category 1-2

H54.52 Low vision, left eye, normal vision right eye

H54.52A Low vision, left eye, category 1-2
CODING TIPS ✓ The sixth character represents the category of vision in the right eye, and a seventh character represents the category of vision in the left eye.

H54.6 Unqualified visual loss, one eye
Visual impairment category 9 in one eye [normal vision in other eye].
GUIDELINES **Section I.C.7.b**
If "blindness" or "low vision" in one eye is documented but the visual impairment category is not documented, assign a code from H54.6-, Unqualified visual loss, one eye.

H54.60 Unqualified visual loss, one eye, unspecified

H54.61 Unqualified visual loss, right eye, normal vision left eye

H54.62 Unqualified visual loss, left eye, normal vision right eye

H54.7 Unspecified visual loss
Visual impairment category 9 NOS
GUIDELINES **Section I.C.7.b**
If "blindness" or "visual loss" is documented without any information about whether one or both eyes are affected, assign code H54.7, Unspecified visual loss.

H54.8 Legal blindness, as defined in USA
Blindness NOS according to USA definition
Note:
The table below gives a classification of severity of visual impairment recommended by a WHO Study Group on the Prevention of Blindness, Geneva, 6-10 November 1972.
The term 'low vision' in category H54 comprises categories 1 and 2 of the table, the term 'blindness' categories 3, 4 and 5, and the term 'unqualified visual loss' category 9.
If the extent of the visual field is taken into account, patients with a field no greater than 10 but greater than 5 around central fixation should be placed in category 3 and patients with a field no greater than 5 around central fixation should be placed in category 4, even if the central acuity is not impaired.

EXCLUDES 1 legal blindness with specification of impairment level (H54.0-H54.7)

Category of visual impairment	Visual acuity with best possible correction	
	Maximum less than:	Minimum equal to or better than:
1	6/18 3/10(0.3) 20/70	6/60 1/10(0.1) 20/200
2	6/60 1/10(0.1) 20/200	3/60 1/20(0.05) 20/400
3	3/60 1/20(0.05) 20/400	1/60(finger counting at one meter) 1/50(0.02) 5/300(20/1200)
4	1/60(finger counting at one meter) 1/50(0.02) 5/300	Light perception
5	No light perception	
9	Undetermined or unspecified	

CODING TIPS✓ Use this code when the provider documents blindness without an indication of eyes involved. If "blindness" or "low vision" of both eyes is documented but the visual impairment category is not documented, assign code H54.3, Unqualified visual loss, both eyes.

Other disorders of eye and adnexa (H55-H57)

4 **H55 Nystagmus and other irregular eye movements**

5 **H55.0 Nystagmus**

SP **H55.00 Unspecified nystagmus**

SP **H55.01 Congenital nystagmus**

SP **H55.02 Latent nystagmus**

DEFINITION Involuntary rapid movement of the eyeball occurring only when one eye is covered.

SP **H55.03 Visual deprivation nystagmus**

SP **H55.04 Dissociated nystagmus**

DEFINITION Involuntary rhythmic movements in both eyes that are dissimilar in direction, extent, and frequency of movement.

SP **H55.09 Other forms of nystagmus**

5 **H55.8 Other irregular eye movements**

SP **H55.81 Deficient saccadic eye movements**

DEFINITION Rapid and involuntary eye movement while changing focus on stationary objects.

SP **H55.82 Deficient smooth pursuit eye movements**

SP **H55.89 Other irregular eye movements**

4 **H57 Other disorders of eye and adnexa**

5 **H57.0 Anomalies of pupillary function**

SP **H57.00 Unspecified anomaly of pupillary function**

SP **H57.01 Argyll Robertson pupil, atypical**

EXCLUDES 1 syphilitic Argyll Robertson pupil (A52.19)

SP **H57.02 Anisocoria**

DEFINITION Pupils of unequal size.

SP **H57.03 Miosis**

DEFINITION Constriction of the pupil.

SP **H57.04 Mydriasis**

6 **H57.05 Tonic pupil**

SP **H57.051 Tonic pupil, right eye**

SP **H57.052 Tonic pupil, left eye**

SP **H57.053 Tonic pupil, bilateral**

IQ **H57.059 Tonic pupil, unspecified eye**

SP **H57.09 Other anomalies of pupillary function**

5 **H57.1 Ocular pain**

IQ **H57.10 Ocular pain, unspecified eye**

SP **H57.11 Ocular pain, right eye**

SP **H57.12 Ocular pain, left eye**

SP **H57.13 Ocular pain, bilateral**

5 **H57.8 Other specified disorders of eye and adnexa**

6 **H57.81 Brow ptosis**

IQ **H57.811 Brow ptosis, right**

IQ **H57.812 Brow ptosis, left**

IQ **H57.813 Brow ptosis, bilateral**

IQ **H57.819 Brow ptosis, unspecified**

SP **H57.89 Other specified disorders of eye and adnexa**

IQ **H57.9 Unspecified disorder of eye and adnexa**

Intraoperative and postprocedural complications and disorders of eye and adnexa, not elsewhere classified (H59)

4 **H59 Intraoperative and postprocedural complications and disorders of eye and adnexa, not elsewhere classified**

EXCLUDES 1 mechanical complication of intraocular lens (T85.2)
mechanical complication of other ocular prosthetic devices, implants and grafts (T85.3)
pseudophakia (Z96.1)
secondary cataracts (H26.4-)

5 **H59.0 Disorders of the eye following cataract surgery**

6 **H59.01 Keratopathy (bullous aphakic) following cataract surgery**

Vitreal corneal syndrome
Vitreous (touch) syndrome

SP **H59.011 Keratopathy (bullous aphakic) following cataract surgery, right eye**

Chapter 7

H00-H59

⊟ SP H59.012 Keratopathy (bullous aphakic) following cataract surgery, left eye

⊟ SP H59.013 Keratopathy (bullous aphakic) following cataract surgery, bilateral

⊟ IQ H59.019 Keratopathy (bullous aphakic) following cataract surgery, unspecified eye

6 H59.02 Cataract (lens) fragments in eye following cataract surgery

⊟ SP H59.021 Cataract (lens) fragments in eye following cataract surgery, right eye

⊟ SP H59.022 Cataract (lens) fragments in eye following cataract surgery, left eye

⊟ SP H59.023 Cataract (lens) fragments in eye following cataract surgery, bilateral

⊟ IQ H59.029 Cataract (lens) fragments in eye following cataract surgery, unspecified eye

6 H59.03 Cystoid macular edema following cataract surgery

⊟ SP H59.031 Cystoid macular edema following cataract surgery, right eye

⊟ SP H59.032 Cystoid macular edema following cataract surgery, left eye

⊟ SP H59.033 Cystoid macular edema following cataract surgery, bilateral

⊟ IQ H59.039 Cystoid macular edema following cataract surgery, unspecified eye

6 H59.09 Other disorders of the eye following cataract surgery

⊟ SP H59.091 Other disorders of the right eye following cataract surgery

⊟ SP H59.092 Other disorders of the left eye following cataract surgery

⊟ SP H59.093 Other disorders of the eye following cataract surgery, bilateral

⊟ IQ H59.099 Other disorders of unspecified eye following cataract surgery

5 H59.1 Intraoperative hemorrhage and hematoma of eye and adnexa complicating a procedure

EXCLUDES 1 intraoperative hemorrhage and hematoma of eye and adnexa due to accidental puncture or laceration during a procedure (H59.2-)

6 H59.11 Intraoperative hemorrhage and hematoma of eye and adnexa complicating an ophthalmic procedure

⊟ SP H59.111 Intraoperative hemorrhage and hematoma of right eye and adnexa complicating an ophthalmic procedure

⊟ SP H59.112 Intraoperative hemorrhage and hematoma of left eye and adnexa complicating an ophthalmic procedure

⊟ SP H59.113 Intraoperative hemorrhage and hematoma of eye and adnexa complicating an ophthalmic procedure, bilateral

⊟ IQ H59.119 Intraoperative hemorrhage and hematoma of unspecified eye and adnexa complicating an ophthalmic procedure

6 H59.12 Intraoperative hemorrhage and hematoma of eye and adnexa complicating other procedure

⊟ SP H59.121 Intraoperative hemorrhage and hematoma of right eye and adnexa complicating other procedure

⊟ SP H59.122 Intraoperative hemorrhage and hematoma of left eye and adnexa complicating other procedure

⊟ SP H59.123 Intraoperative hemorrhage and hematoma of eye and adnexa complicating other procedure, bilateral

⊟ IQ H59.129 Intraoperative hemorrhage and hematoma of unspecified eye and adnexa complicating other procedure

5 H59.2 Accidental puncture and laceration of eye and adnexa during a procedure

6 H59.21 Accidental puncture and laceration of eye and adnexa during an ophthalmic procedure

⊟ SP H59.211 Accidental puncture and laceration of right eye and adnexa during an ophthalmic procedure

⊟ SP H59.212 Accidental puncture and laceration of left eye and adnexa during an ophthalmic procedure

⊟ SP H59.213 Accidental puncture and laceration of eye and adnexa during an ophthalmic procedure, bilateral

⊟ IQ H59.219 Accidental puncture and laceration of unspecified eye and adnexa during an ophthalmic procedure

6 H59.22 Accidental puncture and laceration of eye and adnexa during other procedure

⊟ SP H59.221 Accidental puncture and laceration of right eye and adnexa during other procedure

⊟ SP H59.222 Accidental puncture and laceration of left eye and adnexa during other procedure

⊟ SP H59.223 Accidental puncture and laceration of eye and adnexa during other procedure, bilateral

⊟ IQ H59.229 Accidental puncture and laceration of unspecified eye and adnexa during other procedure

5 H59.3 Postprocedural hemorrhage, hematoma, and seroma of eye and adnexa following a procedure

6 H59.31 Postprocedural hemorrhage of eye and adnexa following an ophthalmic procedure

⊟ SP H59.311 Postprocedural hemorrhage of right eye and adnexa following an ophthalmic procedure

⊟ SP H59.312 Postprocedural hemorrhage of left eye and adnexa following an ophthalmic procedure

SP H59.313 **Postprocedural hemorrhage of eye and adnexa following an ophthalmic procedure, bilateral**

!Q H59.319 **Postprocedural hemorrhage of unspecified eye and adnexa following an ophthalmic procedure**

6 H59.32 **Postprocedural hemorrhage of eye and adnexa following other procedure**

SP H59.321 **Postprocedural hemorrhage of right eye and adnexa following other procedure**

SP H59.322 **Postprocedural hemorrhage of left eye and adnexa following other procedure**

SP H59.323 **Postprocedural hemorrhage of eye and adnexa following other procedure, bilateral**

!Q H59.329 **Postprocedural hemorrhage of unspecified eye and adnexa following other procedure**

6 H59.33 **Postprocedural hematoma of eye and adnexa following an ophthalmic procedure**

SP H59.331 **Postprocedural hematoma of right eye and adnexa following an ophthalmic procedure**

SP H59.332 **Postprocedural hematoma of left eye and adnexa following an ophthalmic procedure**

SP H59.333 **Postprocedural hematoma of eye and adnexa following an ophthalmic procedure, bilateral**

!Q H59.339 **Postprocedural hematoma of unspecified eye and adnexa following an ophthalmic procedure**

6 H59.34 **Postprocedural hematoma of eye and adnexa following other procedure**

SP H59.341 **Postprocedural hematoma of right eye and adnexa following other procedure**

SP H59.342 **Postprocedural hematoma of left eye and adnexa following other procedure**

SP H59.343 **Postprocedural hematoma of eye and adnexa following other procedure, bilateral**

!Q H59.349 **Postprocedural hematoma of unspecified eye and adnexa following other procedure**

6 H59.35 **Postprocedural seroma of eye and adnexa following an ophthalmic procedure**

SP H59.351 **Postprocedural seroma of right eye and adnexa following an ophthalmic procedure**

SP H59.352 **Postprocedural seroma of left eye and adnexa following an ophthalmic procedure**

SP H59.353 **Postprocedural seroma of eye and adnexa following an ophthalmic procedure, bilateral**

!Q H59.359 **Postprocedural seroma of unspecified eye and adnexa following an ophthalmic procedure**

6 H59.36 **Postprocedural seroma of eye and adnexa following other procedure**

SP H59.361 **Postprocedural seroma of right eye and adnexa following other procedure**

SP H59.362 **Postprocedural seroma of left eye and adnexa following other procedure**

SP H59.363 **Postprocedural seroma of eye and adnexa following other procedure, bilateral**

!Q H59.369 **Postprocedural seroma of unspecified eye and adnexa following other procedure**

5 H59.4 **Inflammation (infection) of postprocedural bleb**

Postprocedural blebitis

EXCLUDES 1 filtering (vitreous) bleb after glaucoma surgery status (Z98.83)

SP H59.40 **Inflammation (infection) of postprocedural bleb, unspecified**

SP H59.41 **Inflammation (infection) of postprocedural bleb, stage 1**

SP H59.42 **Inflammation (infection) of postprocedural bleb, stage 2**

SP H59.43 **Inflammation (infection) of postprocedural bleb, stage 3**

Bleb endophthalmitis

5 H59.8 **Other intraoperative and postprocedural complications and disorders of eye and adnexa, not elsewhere classified**

6 H59.81 **Chorioretinal scars after surgery for detachment**

SP H59.811 **Chorioretinal scars after surgery for detachment, right eye**

SP H59.812 **Chorioretinal scars after surgery for detachment, left eye**

SP H59.813 **Chorioretinal scars after surgery for detachment, bilateral**

!Q H59.819 **Chorioretinal scars after surgery for detachment, unspecified eye**

SP H59.88 **Other intraoperative complications of eye and adnexa, not elsewhere classified**

SP H59.89 **Other postprocedural complications and disorders of eye and adnexa, not elsewhere classified**

Chapter 7 Scenarios: Diseases of the eye and adnexa (H00-H59)

Diabetic glaucoma

A 63-year-old woman was recently started on an insulin regimen for her type 2 diabetes. She also has diabetic glaucoma, which has left her legally blind.

Description	Code
Primary: Type 2 diabetes mellitus with other diabetic ophthalmic complication	E11.39
Secondary: Glaucoma in diseases classified elsewhere	H42
Secondary: Legal blindness, as defined in USA	H54.8
Secondary: Long term (current) use of insulin	Z79.4

There is no assumed relationship between diabetes and glaucoma. However, a link has been specified in this scenario. The code for glaucoma caused by diabetes, H42, is a manifestation code and cannot be assigned without a preceding etiology. Therefore, E11.39 must be coded immediately before H42. Note the "code first" note at the H54.- category level, instructing the code to first code the underlying cause of the blindness. Since the patient uses insulin but is not a type 2 diabetic, Z79.4 must be assigned.

Coronary artery bypass graft, glaucoma

An 82-year-old male patient is admitted to home health following surgery for a first-time coronary bypass graft x2 with a history of coronary artery disease. The patient is legally blind due to severe stage open angle glaucoma in both eyes and was recently diagnosed with generalized anxiety disorder. He has a 24-hour caregiver that assists with ADL/IADLs; however, she is not comfortable with managing his surgical site and cardiac status. The physician ordered skilled nursing to assess/monitor the patient's cardiac status and to perform surgical dressing changes.

Description	Code
Primary: Encounter for surgical aftercare following surgery on the circulatory system	Z48.812
Secondary: Atherosclerotic heart disease of native coronary artery without angina pectoris	I25.10
Secondary: Unspecified open-angle glaucoma, severe stage	H40.10x3
Secondary: Legal blindness, as defined in USA	H54.8
Secondary: Generalized anxiety disorder	F41.1
Secondary: Presence of aortocoronary bypass graft	Z95.1

As the focus of care, surgical aftercare is coded primary. The combination code H40.10x3 covers both the type and stage of the patient's glaucoma, which is severe stage unspecified open-angle glaucoma that is occurring in both eyes. "When a patient has bilateral glaucoma and both eyes are documented as being the same type and stage, and the classification does not provide a code for bilateral glaucoma (i.e. subcategories H40.10, and H40.20) report only one code for the type of glaucoma with the appropriate seventh character for the stage," according to coding guidelines. In accordance with tabular instruction, the underlying cause of the blindness (the glaucoma) is coded before the blindness itself. Though the coronary artery bypass graft surgery treats the coronary artery disease, it does not resolve it. Therefore, the condition is still coded.

Senile cataracts

An elderly female patient is admitted to home health for teaching and training for a new diagnosis of type 2 diabetes. She also has comorbid polyneuropathy and atherosclerosis of arteries of the bilateral lower legs. She takes oral medications for her diabetes and her polyneuropathy is impacting her ability to manage obtaining medication and self administering. She also has had cortical senile cataracts in both eyes for years but has not had any surgical intervention for them. The cataracts are unrelated to the patient's diabetes. They impact her ability to accurately manage her medications and disease process. In addition to the neuropathy this is presenting issues with medication self administration and she requires nursing and occupational therapy intervention.

Description	Code
Primary: Type 2 diabetes mellitus with diabetic polyneuropathy	E11.42
Secondary: Type 2 diabetes mellitus with diabetic peripheral angiopathy without gangrene	E11.51
Secondary: Unspecified atherosclerosis of native arteries of extremities, bilateral legs	I70.203
Secondary: Cortical age-related cataract, bilateral	H25.013
Secondary: Long term (current) use of oral hypoglycemic drugs	Z79.84

The patient's cataracts are specified as cortical senile cataracts. In ICD-10 senile cataracts are defined as age-related cataracts. Therefore, H25.013 is the most appropriate code to capture this condition. Though "cataract" appears under the subterm "with" in the alphabetic index "diabetes" listing, they're not related to her diabetes so the "with" convention does not apply and the conditions are coded separately. This patient's diabetic polyneuropathy is significantly impacting her ability to take her medication, so it is listed primary, with the cataract listed as a supportive diagnosis. The ICD-10 classification presumes a relationship between diabetes and atherosclerosis, which is a specific type of peripheral vascular disease.

Diabetic retinopathy, blindness and low vision

A 73-year-old woman has type 2 diabetes that is out of control and has been started on insulin. She has been found to have proliferative diabetic retinopathy in both eyes. The disease had led to macular edema in her left eye. She is now blind in that eye and has low vision in her right eye. The blindness in her left eye is documented as category 3 and the low vision in her right eye is documented as category 2. She also has hypertension. The focus of the admission is skilled nursing care to teach her how to use insulin to better control her diabetes and for occupational therapy for help completing ADLs/IADLs with her vision deficit.

Description	Code
Primary: Type 2 diabetes mellitus with hyperglycemia	E11.65
Secondary: Type 2 diabetes mellitus with proliferative diabetic retinopathy with macular edema, left eye	E11.3512
Secondary: Type 2 diabetes mellitus with proliferative diabetic retinopathy without macular edema, right eye	E11.3591
Secondary: Low vision right eye category 2, blindness left eye category 3	H54.1223
Secondary: Essential (primary) hypertension	I10
Secondary: Long term (current) use of insulin	Z79.4

Since the focus of care is teaching about insulin use and getting the out of control diabetes under better control, diabetes with hyperglycemia is coded in the primary position. Out of control diabetes codes to diabetes with hyperglycemia, according to the alphabetic index. She also has proliferative diabetic retinopathy in both eyes, and it's caused macular edema in her left eye. Two codes are used to capture the condition's different severity in each eye. Code H54.1223 is assigned to indicate that she's blind in her left eye (documented as category 3) and has low vision in her right (documented as category 2). Hypertension is coded as a relevant comorbidity and her use of insulin, as a non-type 1 diabetic, must be captured with Z79.4.

Chapter 8: Diseases of the Ear and Mastoid Process (H60-H95)

Chapter 8 includes codes for diseases of the external ear, middle ear and mastoid, internal ear, other disorders of the ear, and intraoperative and postprocedural complications and disorders of the ear and mastoid process, not elsewhere classified.

There is a note at the beginning of this chapter to use an external cause code following the code for the ear condition, if applicable, to identify the cause of the ear condition. Following the note, there is an Excludes 2 note for chapter 8 codes that defines code categories that are not included in the chapter 8 codes, but could be coded in addition to the chapter 8 code if applicable. These include:

- Certain conditions originating in the perinatal period (P00-P96) located in chapter 16.
- Certain infections and parasitic diseases (A00-B99) located in chapter 1.
- Complications of pregnancy, childbirth and the puerperium (O00 –O9A) located in chapter 15.
- Congenital malformations, deformations and chromosomal abnormalities (Q00-Q99) in chapter 17.
- Endocrine, nutritional and metabolic diseases (E00-E88) in chapter 4.
- Injury, poisoning and certain other consequences of external causes (S00-T88) located in chapter 19.
- Neoplasms (C00-D49) in chapter 2.
- Symptoms, signs and abnormal clinical and laboratory findings (R00-R94) located in chapter 18.

To select the appropriate code, it is important to understand the basic anatomy and physiology of the ear and mastoid process. The ear is divided into three sections: the external, middle and inner ear. The outer and middle ear is strictly involved in hearing and sound wave conduction while the inner ear structures function for both hearing and balance, or equilibrium. The external ear canal leads to the structures inside and is surrounded and protected by cranial bones. The opening of the canal, called the external auditory meatus, opens into the middle ear and lies directly above the mastoid process. The mastoid process is the cone-shaped bony prominence that projects from the undersurface of the temporal bone behind the ear. The tissue structure within the mastoid process also aids the hearing function by promoting conductivity of sound between the external and middle ear.

The external ear is made up of the auricle (pinna), which is the visible portion of the ear and the external auditory canal, which is the tube that leads from the outside environment to the middle portion of the ear and the ear drum. Its main function is to act as the conduit into the auditory receptors located within the ear and to amplify incoming sound waves. The second major function of the external ear is self-cleaning and protection of the tympanic membrane and middle and inner ear structures by providing a physical barrier against moisture, microorganisms, foreign bodies and direct injury.

The middle ear is made up of the tympanic cavity within the temporal bone that is filled with air from the nasopharynx through the auditory tube. It contains three tiny bones called ossicles (malleus, incus and the stirrup) that transmit vibration from the tympanic membrane across the middle ear to the inner ear.

The tympanic membrane functions to transmit sound conducted down the ear canal to the ossicles. Perforations of the ear drum are caused by foreign objects stuck in the ear, waves of external pressure from explosions or a slap to the ear, and infections causing internal pressure.

Damage to the middle ear structures affects the ear's ability to conduct sound to the inner ear and results in conductive hearing loss.

The ossicles transmit and amplify sound. Damage to the middle ear also affects the ear's ability to conduct sound towards the inner ear and results in conductive hearing loss.

The Eustachian tube maintains still air in the middle ear to allow the ossicles to function at optimum level and also serves as a drain to carry mucous or bacterial accumulation out of the middle ear to the throat. The shape and size of the Eustachian tube is different in children than adults. The horizontal orientation of the tube in children results in earaches and infections in the middle ear, especially in children under seven years of age. Obstruction of the tube results in hearing impairment, pain and infections.

The middle ear is comprised of a series of bony labyrinths that are lined with periosteum and filled with fluid. The labyrinthine network is made up of the semicircular canals, the vestibule (responsible for balance and equilibrium) and the cochlea which is embedded in the mastoid (responsible for hearing).

Common infections

Common infections of the ear and mastoid include: **serous otitis media** (fluid in the inner ear as a result of dysfunction of the Eustachian tube**); suppurative otitis media** (infection of the fluid trapped in the middle ear); **mastoiditis** (infection of the air-filled spaces in the mastoid area and even infects the mastoid bone itself); **otitis externa** (infection of the outer auditory canal); and **myringitis** (infection or inflammation of tympanic membrane).

Neoplasms

There also are several possible neoplasms of the ear and mastoid including:

- **Malignant basal cell or squamous cell tumors** of the external ear most commonly in areas exposed to sun, and most commonly found in the elderly and in fair skinned people.
- Benign tumors: **cholesteatomas**, which are most common in middle ear and external ear canal and can eat into the tiny bones of the ossicular chain or erode the bone separating the middle ear cavity from the mastoid area or brain, and cause deafness, nerve destruction, vertigo and infection risk; **acoustic neuromas** are intracranial tumors on vestibulocochlear branch of 8th cranial nerve near the inner ear where the nerve enters the brain. They are also called schwannomas or glomus tumors, which are highly vascularized masses behind the eardrum that can grow into the mastoid or bony wall or wrap around facial nerves, jugular vein, carotid artery and even invade the brain.

Hearing loss

Hearing loss is coded to category H90 in chapter 8 and includes specific codes for

- conductive and sensorineural hearing loss (largest subcategory of hearing loss codes)
- ototoxic hearing loss
- presbycusis
- sudden idiopathic hearing loss
- other hearing loss
- unspecified hearing loss

Other diseases of ear and mastoid

Other diseases and disorders of ear and mastoid include: **non-infective otitis externa**; **acquired stenosis; impacted cerumen, tympanosclerosis** (thickening and hardening of tympanic membrane); **adhesive middle ear disease**; **meniere's disease** (abnormality of inner ear thought to be associated with increased fluid causing swelling and rupture of the membranous labyrinth resulting in unpredictable attacks of vertigo, tinnitus, hearing loss, and/or ear pain/pressure); **vertigo** (many types from severe dizziness/equilibrium dysfunction resulting in a sense that the person or their surroundings are spinning/whirling when there is no motion). ***Important note:*** Most cases of dizziness are not vertigo and are coded as a symptom, while specific types of vertigo are coded from chapter 8 and not as symptoms.

Otosclerosis is a progressive disease causing abnormal growth of bone of the middle ear that can affect all of the ossicles.

Chapter 8 also includes intraoperative and **postprocedural** codes related to hemorrhage and hematoma; accidental puncture and laceration; stenosis of the ear canal; and other complications and disorders of the ear and mastoid process, not elsewhere classified.

Note: Many of the codes in chapter 8 have laterality designations for greater specificity. As in all coding, the specific codes must be documented or confirmed with the physician.

CHAPTER 8: DISEASES OF THE EAR AND MASTOID PROCESS (H60-H95)

Note:
Use an external cause code following the code for the ear condition, if applicable, to identify the cause of the ear condition

EXCLUDES 2 certain conditions originating in the perinatal period (P04-P96)
certain infectious and parasitic diseases (A00-B99)
complications of pregnancy, childbirth and the puerperium (O00-O9A)
congenital malformations, deformations and chromosomal abnormalities (Q00-Q99)
endocrine, nutritional and metabolic diseases (E00-E88)
injury, poisoning and certain other consequences of external causes (S00-T88)
neoplasms (C00-D49)
symptoms, signs and abnormal clinical and laboratory findings, not elsewhere classified (R00-R94)

This chapter contains the following blocks:

H60-H62	Diseases of external ear
H65-H75	Diseases of middle ear and mastoid
H80-H83	Diseases of inner ear
H90-H94	Other disorders of ear
H95	Intraoperative and postprocedural complications and disorders of ear and mastoid process, not elsewhere classified

Diseases of external ear (H60-H62)

4 **H60 Otitis externa**

5 **H60.0 Abscess of external ear**
Boil of external ear
Carbuncle of auricle or external auditory canal
Furuncle of external ear

IQ **H60.00 Abscess of external ear, unspecified ear**

SP **H60.01 Abscess of right external ear**

SP **H60.02 Abscess of left external ear**

SP **H60.03 Abscess of external ear, bilateral**

5 **H60.1 Cellulitis of external ear**
Cellulitis of auricle
Cellulitis of external auditory canal

IQ **H60.10 Cellulitis of external ear, unspecified ear**

SP **H60.11 Cellulitis of right external ear**

SP **H60.12 Cellulitis of left external ear**

SP **H60.13 Cellulitis of external ear, bilateral**

5 **H60.2 Malignant otitis externa**

IQ **H60.20 Malignant otitis externa, unspecified ear**

SP **H60.21 Malignant otitis externa, right ear**

SP **H60.22 Malignant otitis externa, left ear**

SP **H60.23 Malignant otitis externa, bilateral**

5 **H60.3 Other infective otitis externa**

6 **H60.31 Diffuse otitis externa**

SP **H60.311 Diffuse otitis externa, right ear**

SP **H60.312 Diffuse otitis externa, left ear**

SP **H60.313 Diffuse otitis externa, bilateral**

IQ **H60.319 Diffuse otitis externa, unspecified ear**

6 **H60.32 Hemorrhagic otitis externa**

SP **H60.321 Hemorrhagic otitis externa, right ear**

SP **H60.322 Hemorrhagic otitis externa, left ear**

SP **H60.323 Hemorrhagic otitis externa, bilateral**

IQ **H60.329 Hemorrhagic otitis externa, unspecified ear**

6 **H60.33 Swimmer's ear**

SP **H60.331 Swimmer's ear, right ear**

SP **H60.332 Swimmer's ear, left ear**

SP **H60.333 Swimmer's ear, bilateral**

IQ **H60.339 Swimmer's ear, unspecified ear**

6 **H60.39 Other infective otitis externa**

SP **H60.391 Other infective otitis externa, right ear**

SP **H60.392 Other infective otitis externa, left ear**

SP **H60.393 Other infective otitis externa, bilateral**

IQ **H60.399 Other infective otitis externa, unspecified ear**

5 **H60.4 Cholesteatoma of external ear**
Keratosis obturans of external ear (canal)
EXCLUDES 2 cholesteatoma of middle ear (H71.-)
recurrent cholesteatoma of postmastoidectomy cavity (H95.0-)

IQ **H60.40 Cholesteatoma of external ear, unspecified ear**

SP **H60.41 Cholesteatoma of right external ear**

SP **H60.42 Cholesteatoma of left external ear**

SP **H60.43 Cholesteatoma of external ear, bilateral**

5 **H60.5 Acute noninfective otitis externa**

6 **H60.50 Unspecified acute noninfective otitis externa**
Acute otitis externa NOS

SP **H60.501 Unspecified acute noninfective otitis externa, right ear**

SP **H60.502 Unspecified acute noninfective otitis externa, left ear**

SP **H60.503 Unspecified acute noninfective otitis externa, bilateral**

IQ **H60.509 Unspecified acute noninfective otitis externa, unspecified ear**

6 **H60.51 Acute actinic otitis externa**

SP **H60.511 Acute actinic otitis externa, right ear**

SP **H60.512 Acute actinic otitis externa, left ear**

SP **H60.513 Acute actinic otitis externa, bilateral**

IQ **H60.519 Acute actinic otitis externa, unspecified ear**

6 **H60.52 Acute chemical otitis externa**

SP **H60.521 Acute chemical otitis externa, right ear**

SP **H60.522 Acute chemical otitis externa, left ear**

SP H60.523 **Acute chemical otitis externa, bilateral**

IQ H60.529 **Acute chemical otitis externa, unspecified ear**

6 H60.53 **Acute contact otitis externa**

SP H60.531 **Acute contact otitis externa, right ear**

SP H60.532 **Acute contact otitis externa, left ear**

SP H60.533 **Acute contact otitis externa, bilateral**

IQ H60.539 **Acute contact otitis externa, unspecified ear**

6 H60.54 **Acute eczematoid otitis externa**

SP H60.541 **Acute eczematoid otitis externa, right ear**

SP H60.542 **Acute eczematoid otitis externa, left ear**

SP H60.543 **Acute eczematoid otitis externa, bilateral**

IQ H60.549 **Acute eczematoid otitis externa, unspecified ear**

6 H60.55 **Acute reactive otitis externa**

SP H60.551 **Acute reactive otitis externa, right ear**

SP H60.552 **Acute reactive otitis externa, left ear**

SP H60.553 **Acute reactive otitis externa, bilateral**

IQ H60.559 **Acute reactive otitis externa, unspecified ear**

6 H60.59 **Other noninfective acute otitis externa**

SP H60.591 **Other noninfective acute otitis externa, right ear**

SP H60.592 **Other noninfective acute otitis externa, left ear**

SP H60.593 **Other noninfective acute otitis externa, bilateral**

IQ H60.599 **Other noninfective acute otitis externa, unspecified ear**

5 H60.6 **Unspecified chronic otitis externa**

IQ H60.60 **Unspecified chronic otitis externa, unspecified ear**

SP H60.61 **Unspecified chronic otitis externa, right ear**

SP H60.62 **Unspecified chronic otitis externa, left ear**

SP H60.63 **Unspecified chronic otitis externa, bilateral**

5 H60.8 **Other otitis externa**

6 H60.8X **Other otitis externa**

SP H60.8X1 **Other otitis externa, right ear**

SP H60.8X2 **Other otitis externa, left ear**

SP H60.8X3 **Other otitis externa, bilateral**

IQ H60.8X9 **Other otitis externa, unspecified ear**

5 H60.9 **Unspecified otitis externa**

IQ H60.90 **Unspecified otitis externa, unspecified ear**

SP H60.91 **Unspecified otitis externa, right ear**

SP H60.92 **Unspecified otitis externa, left ear**

SP H60.93 **Unspecified otitis externa, bilateral**

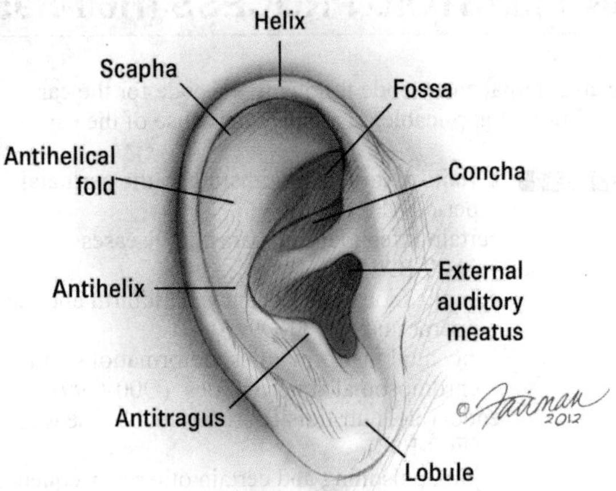

4 H61 **Other disorders of external ear**

5 H61.0 **Chondritis and perichondritis of external ear**
Chondrodermatitis nodularis chronica helicis
Perichondritis of auricle
Perichondritis of pinna
DEFINITION Inflammation of the cartilage of the outer, visible part of the ear.

6 H61.00 **Unspecified perichondritis of external ear**

SP H61.001 **Unspecified perichondritis of right external ear**

SP H61.002 **Unspecified perichondritis of left external ear**

SP H61.003 **Unspecified perichondritis of external ear, bilateral**

IQ H61.009 **Unspecified perichondritis of external ear, unspecified ear**

6 H61.01 **Acute perichondritis of external ear**

SP H61.011 **Acute perichondritis of right external ear**

SP H61.012 **Acute perichondritis of left external ear**

SP H61.013 **Acute perichondritis of external ear, bilateral**

IQ H61.019 **Acute perichondritis of external ear, unspecified ear**

6 H61.02 **Chronic perichondritis of external ear**

SP H61.021 **Chronic perichondritis of right external ear**

SP H61.022 **Chronic perichondritis of left external ear**

SP H61.023 **Chronic perichondritis of external ear, bilateral**

IQ H61.029 **Chronic perichondritis of external ear, unspecified ear**

6 H61.03 **Chondritis of external ear**
Chondritis of auricle
Chondritis of pinna

SP H61.031 **Chondritis of right external ear**

SP H61.032 **Chondritis of left external ear**

Chapter 8
H60-H95

4 4th digit required 5 5th digit required 6 6th digit required 7 7th digit required X 7th digit placeholder + Additional code Laterality

SP H61.033 **Chondritis of external ear, bilateral**
IQ H61.039 **Chondritis of external ear, unspecified ear**

5 H61.1 **Noninfective disorders of pinna**
EXCLUDES 2 cauliflower ear (M95.1-)
gouty tophi of ear (M1A.-)

6 H61.10 **Unspecified noninfective disorders of pinna**
Disorder of pinna NOS
SP H61.101 **Unspecified noninfective disorders of pinna, right ear**
SP H61.102 **Unspecified noninfective disorders of pinna, left ear**
SP H61.103 **Unspecified noninfective disorders of pinna, bilateral**
IQ H61.109 **Unspecified noninfective disorders of pinna, unspecified ear**

6 H61.11 **Acquired deformity of pinna**
Acquired deformity of auricle
EXCLUDES 2 cauliflower ear (M95.1-)
SP H61.111 **Acquired deformity of pinna, right ear**
SP H61.112 **Acquired deformity of pinna, left ear**
SP H61.113 **Acquired deformity of pinna, bilateral**
IQ H61.119 **Acquired deformity of pinna, unspecified ear**

6 H61.12 **Hematoma of pinna**
Hematoma of auricle
DEFINITION Swelling filled with blood on the outer ear.
SP H61.121 **Hematoma of pinna, right ear**
SP H61.122 **Hematoma of pinna, left ear**
SP H61.123 **Hematoma of pinna, bilateral**
IQ H61.129 **Hematoma of pinna, unspecified ear**

6 H61.19 **Other noninfective disorders of pinna**
SP H61.191 **Noninfective disorders of pinna, right ear**
SP H61.192 **Noninfective disorders of pinna, left ear**
SP H61.193 **Noninfective disorders of pinna, bilateral**
IQ H61.199 **Noninfective disorders of pinna, unspecified ear**

5 H61.2 **Impacted cerumen**
Wax in ear
DEFINITION Ear wax blocking the external ear canal.
IQ H61.20 **Impacted cerumen, unspecified ear**
SP H61.21 **Impacted cerumen, right ear**
SP H61.22 **Impacted cerumen, left ear**
SP H61.23 **Impacted cerumen, bilateral**

5 H61.3 **Acquired stenosis of external ear canal**
Collapse of external ear canal
EXCLUDES 1 postprocedural stenosis of external ear canal (H95.81-)

6 H61.30 **Acquired stenosis of external ear canal, unspecified**
SP H61.301 **Acquired stenosis of right external ear canal, unspecified**
SP H61.302 **Acquired stenosis of left external ear canal, unspecified**
SP H61.303 **Acquired stenosis of external ear canal, unspecified, bilateral**
IQ H61.309 **Acquired stenosis of external ear canal, unspecified, unspecified ear**

6 H61.31 **Acquired stenosis of external ear canal secondary to trauma**
SP H61.311 **Acquired stenosis of right external ear canal secondary to trauma**
SP H61.312 **Acquired stenosis of left external ear canal secondary to trauma**
SP H61.313 **Acquired stenosis of external ear canal secondary to trauma, bilateral**
IQ H61.319 **Acquired stenosis of external ear canal secondary to trauma, unspecified ear**

6 H61.32 **Acquired stenosis of external ear canal secondary to inflammation and infection**
SP H61.321 **Acquired stenosis of right external ear canal secondary to inflammation and infection**
SP H61.322 **Acquired stenosis of left external ear canal secondary to inflammation and infection**
SP H61.323 **Acquired stenosis of external ear canal secondary to inflammation and infection, bilateral**
IQ H61.329 **Acquired stenosis of external ear canal secondary to inflammation and infection, unspecified ear**

6 H61.39 **Other acquired stenosis of external ear canal**
SP H61.391 **Other acquired stenosis of right external ear canal**
SP H61.392 **Other acquired stenosis of left external ear canal**
SP H61.393 **Other acquired stenosis of external ear canal, bilateral**
IQ H61.399 **Other acquired stenosis of external ear canal, unspecified ear**

5 H61.8 **Other specified disorders of external ear**

6 H61.81 **Exostosis of external canal**
DEFINITION A bony growth covered with cartilage on the outer ear.
SP H61.811 **Exostosis of right external canal**
SP H61.812 **Exostosis of left external canal**
SP H61.813 **Exostosis of external canal, bilateral**
IQ H61.819 **Exostosis of external canal, unspecified ear**

6 H61.89 **Other specified disorders of external ear**
SP H61.891 **Other specified disorders of right external ear**
SP H61.892 **Other specified disorders of left external ear**
SP H61.893 **Other specified disorders of external ear, bilateral**

IQ H61.899 Other specified disorders of external ear, unspecified ear

5 H61.9 Disorder of external ear, unspecified

IQ H61.90 Disorder of external ear, unspecified, unspecified ear

IQ H61.91 Disorder of right external ear, unspecified

IQ H61.92 Disorder of left external ear, unspecified

IQ H61.93 Disorder of external ear, unspecified, bilateral

4 H62 Disorders of external ear in diseases classified elsewhere

5 H62.4 Otitis externa in other diseases classified elsewhere

Code first underlying disease, such as:
erysipelas (A46)
impetigo (L01.0)

EXCLUDES 1 otitis externa (in):
candidiasis (B37.84)
herpes viral [herpes simplex] (B00.1)
herpes zoster (B02.8)

M IQ H62.40 *Otitis externa in other diseases classified elsewhere, unspecified ear*

M IQ H62.41 *Otitis externa in other diseases classified elsewhere, right ear*

M IQ H62.42 *Otitis externa in other diseases classified elsewhere, left ear*

M IQ H62.43 *Otitis externa in other diseases classified elsewhere, bilateral*

5 H62.8 Other disorders of external ear in diseases classified elsewhere

Code first underlying disease, such as:
gout (M1A.-, M10.-)

6 H62.8X Other disorders of external ear in diseases classified elsewhere

IQ H62.8X1 Other disorders of right external ear in diseases classified elsewhere

IQ H62.8X2 Other disorders of left external ear in diseases classified elsewhere

IQ H62.8X3 Other disorders of external ear in diseases classified elsewhere, bilateral

IQ H62.8X9 Other disorders of external ear in diseases classified elsewhere, unspecified ear

Diseases of middle ear and mastoid (H65-H75)

+ 4 H65 Nonsuppurative otitis media

INCLUDES nonsuppurative otitis media with myringitis

Use additional code for any associated perforated tympanic membrane (H72.-)

Use additional code, if applicable, to identify:
exposure to environmental tobacco smoke (Z77.22)
exposure to tobacco smoke in the perinatal period (P96.81)
history of tobacco dependence (Z87.891)
infectious agent (B95-B97)
occupational exposure to environmental tobacco smoke (Z57.31)
tobacco dependence (F17.-)
tobacco use (Z72.0)

+ 5 H65.0 Acute serous otitis media

Acute and subacute secretory otitis

IQ + H65.00 Acute serous otitis media, unspecified ear

SP + H65.01 Acute serous otitis media, right ear

SP + H65.02 Acute serous otitis media, left ear

SP + H65.03 Acute serous otitis media, bilateral

SP + H65.04 Acute serous otitis media, recurrent, right ear

SP + H65.05 Acute serous otitis media, recurrent, left ear

SP + H65.06 Acute serous otitis media, recurrent, bilateral

IQ + H65.07 Acute serous otitis media, recurrent, unspecified ear

+ 5 H65.1 Other acute nonsuppurative otitis media

EXCLUDES 1 otitic barotrauma (T70.0)
otitis media (acute) NOS (H66.9)

+ 6 H65.11 Acute and subacute allergic otitis media (mucoid) (sanguinous) (serous)

SP + H65.111 Acute and subacute allergic otitis media (mucoid) (sanguinous) (serous), right ear

SP + H65.112 Acute and subacute allergic otitis media (mucoid) (sanguinous) (serous), left ear

SP + H65.113 Acute and subacute allergic otitis media (mucoid) (sanguinous) (serous), bilateral

SP + H65.114 Acute and subacute allergic otitis media (mucoid) (sanguinous) (serous), recurrent, right ear

SP + H65.115 Acute and subacute allergic otitis media (mucoid) (sanguinous) (serous), recurrent, left ear

SP + H65.116 Acute and subacute allergic otitis media (mucoid) (sanguinous) (serous), recurrent, bilateral

IQ + H65.117 Acute and subacute allergic otitis media (mucoid) (sanguinous) (serous), recurrent, unspecified ear

IQ + H65.119 Acute and subacute allergic otitis media (mucoid) (sanguinous) (serous), unspecified ear

+ 6 H65.19 Other acute nonsuppurative otitis media

Acute and subacute mucoid otitis media
Acute and subacute nonsuppurative otitis media NOS
Acute and subacute sanguinous otitis media
Acute and subacute seromucinous otitis media

SP + H65.191 Other acute nonsuppurative otitis media, right ear

SP + H65.192 Other acute nonsuppurative otitis media, left ear

SP + H65.193 Other acute nonsuppurative otitis media, bilateral

SP + H65.194 Other acute nonsuppurative otitis media, recurrent, right ear

SP + H65.195 Other acute nonsuppurative otitis media, recurrent, left ear

SP + H65.196 **Other acute nonsuppurative otitis media, recurrent, bilateral**

IQ + H65.197 **Other acute nonsuppurative otitis media recurrent, unspecified ear**

IQ + H65.199 **Other acute nonsuppurative otitis media, unspecified ear**

+ 5 H65.2 **Chronic serous otitis media**

Chronic tubotympanal catarrh

IQ + H65.20 **Chronic serous otitis media, unspecified ear**

SP + H65.21 **Chronic serous otitis media, right ear**

SP + H65.22 **Chronic serous otitis media, left ear**

SP + H65.23 **Chronic serous otitis media, bilateral**

+ 5 H65.3 **Chronic mucoid otitis media**

Chronic mucinous otitis media
Chronic secretory otitis media
Chronic transudative otitis media
Glue ear

EXCLUDES 1 adhesive middle ear disease (H74.1)

DEFINITION Long-term middle ear infection causing mucous to become trapped in the middle ear.

IQ + H65.30 **Chronic mucoid otitis media, unspecified ear**

SP + H65.31 **Chronic mucoid otitis media, right ear**

SP + H65.32 **Chronic mucoid otitis media, left ear**

SP + H65.33 **Chronic mucoid otitis media, bilateral**

+ 5 H65.4 **Other chronic nonsuppurative otitis media**

+ 6 H65.41 **Chronic allergic otitis media**

SP + H65.411 **Chronic allergic otitis media, right ear**

SP + H65.412 **Chronic allergic otitis media, left ear**

SP + H65.413 **Chronic allergic otitis media, bilateral**

IQ + H65.419 **Chronic allergic otitis media, unspecified ear**

+ 6 H65.49 **Other chronic nonsuppurative otitis media**

Chronic exudative otitis media
Chronic nonsuppurative otitis media NOS
Chronic otitis media with effusion (nonpurulent)
Chronic seromucinous otitis media

SP + H65.491 **Other chronic nonsuppurative otitis media, right ear**

SP + H65.492 **Other chronic nonsuppurative otitis media, left ear**

SP + H65.493 **Other chronic nonsuppurative otitis media, bilateral**

IQ + H65.499 **Other chronic nonsuppurative otitis media, unspecified ear**

+ 5 H65.9 **Unspecified nonsuppurative otitis media**

Allergic otitis media NOS
Catarrhal otitis media NOS
Exudative otitis media NOS
Mucoid otitis media NOS
Otitis media with effusion (nonpurulent) NOS
Secretory otitis media NOS
Seromucinous otitis media NOS
Serous otitis media NOS
Transudative otitis media NOS

IQ + H65.90 **Unspecified nonsuppurative otitis media, unspecified ear**

SP + H65.91 **Unspecified nonsuppurative otitis media, right ear**

SP + H65.92 **Unspecified nonsuppurative otitis media, left ear**

SP + H65.93 **Unspecified nonsuppurative otitis media, bilateral**

+ 4 H66 **Suppurative and unspecified otitis media**

INCLUDES suppurative and unspecified otitis media with myringitis

Use additional code to identify:
- exposure to environmental tobacco smoke (Z77.22)
- exposure to tobacco smoke in the perinatal period (P96.81)
- history of tobacco dependence (Z87.891)
- occupational exposure to environmental tobacco smoke (Z57.31)
- tobacco dependence (F17.-)
- tobacco use (Z72.0)

+ 5 H66.0 **Acute suppurative otitis media**

+ 6 H66.00 **Acute suppurative otitis media without spontaneous rupture of ear drum**

SP + H66.001 **Acute suppurative otitis media without spontaneous rupture of ear drum, right ear**

SP + H66.002 **Acute suppurative otitis media without spontaneous rupture of ear drum, left ear**

SP + H66.003 **Acute suppurative otitis media without spontaneous rupture of ear drum, bilateral**

SP + H66.004 **Acute suppurative otitis media without spontaneous rupture of ear drum, recurrent, right ear**

SP + H66.005 **Acute suppurative otitis media without spontaneous rupture of ear drum, recurrent, left ear**

SP + H66.006 **Acute suppurative otitis media without spontaneous rupture of ear drum, recurrent, bilateral**

IQ + H66.007 **Acute suppurative otitis media without spontaneous rupture of ear drum, recurrent, unspecified ear**

IQ + H66.009 **Acute suppurative otitis media without spontaneous rupture of ear drum, unspecified ear**

+ 6 H66.01 **Acute suppurative otitis media with spontaneous rupture of ear drum**

SP + H66.011 **Acute suppurative otitis media with spontaneous rupture of ear drum, right ear**

SP + H66.012 **Acute suppurative otitis media with spontaneous rupture of ear drum, left ear**

SP + H66.013 **Acute suppurative otitis media with spontaneous rupture of ear drum, bilateral**

Chapter 8

H60-H95

⊟ SP + **H66.014 Acute suppurative otitis media with spontaneous rupture of ear drum, recurrent, right ear**

⊟ SP + **H66.015 Acute suppurative otitis media with spontaneous rupture of ear drum, recurrent, left ear**

⊟ SP + **H66.016 Acute suppurative otitis media with spontaneous rupture of ear drum, recurrent, bilateral**

⊟ !Q + **H66.017 Acute suppurative otitis media with spontaneous rupture of ear drum, recurrent, unspecified ear**

⊟ !Q + **H66.019 Acute suppurative otitis media with spontaneous rupture of ear drum, unspecified ear**

+ 5 **H66.1 Chronic tubotympanic suppurative otitis media**

Benign chronic suppurative otitis media
Chronic tubotympanic disease
Use additional code for any associated perforated tympanic membrane (H72.-)

⊟ !Q + **H66.10 Chronic tubotympanic suppurative otitis media, unspecified**

⊟ SP + **H66.11 Chronic tubotympanic suppurative otitis media, right ear**

⊟ SP + **H66.12 Chronic tubotympanic suppurative otitis media, left ear**

⊟ SP + **H66.13 Chronic tubotympanic suppurative otitis media, bilateral**

+ 5 **H66.2 Chronic atticoantral suppurative otitis media**

Chronic atticoantral disease
Use additional code for any associated perforated tympanic membrane (H72.-)

⊟ !Q + **H66.20 Chronic atticoantral suppurative otitis media, unspecified ear**

⊟ SP + **H66.21 Chronic atticoantral suppurative otitis media, right ear**

⊟ SP + **H66.22 Chronic atticoantral suppurative otitis media, left ear**

⊟ SP + **H66.23 Chronic atticoantral suppurative otitis media, bilateral**

+ 5 **H66.3 Other chronic suppurative otitis media**

Chronic suppurative otitis media NOS
Use additional code for any associated perforated tympanic membrane (H72.-)
EXCLUDES 1 tuberculous otitis media (A18.6)

+ 6 **H66.3X Other chronic suppurative otitis media**

⊟ SP + **H66.3X1 Other chronic suppurative otitis media, right car**

⊟ SP + **H66.3X2 Other chronic suppurative otitis media, left ear**

⊟ SP + **H66.3X3 Other chronic suppurative otitis media, bilateral**

⊟ !Q + **H66.3X9 Other chronic suppurative otitis media, unspecified ear**

+ 5 **H66.4 Suppurative otitis media, unspecified**

Purulent otitis media NOS
Use additional code for any associated perforated tympanic membrane (H72.-)

⊟ !Q + **H66.40 Suppurative otitis media, unspecified, unspecified ear**

⊟ SP + **H66.41 Suppurative otitis media, unspecified, right ear**

⊟ SP + **H66.42 Suppurative otitis media, unspecified, left ear**

⊟ SP + **H66.43 Suppurative otitis media, unspecified, bilateral**

+ 5 **H66.9 Otitis media, unspecified**

Otitis media NOS
Acute otitis media NOS
Chronic otitis media NOS
Use additional code for any associated perforated tympanic membrane (H72.-)

⊟ !Q + **H66.90 Otitis media, unspecified, unspecified ear**

⊟ SP + **H66.91 Otitis media, unspecified, right ear**

⊟ SP + **H66.92 Otitis media, unspecified, left ear**

⊟ SP + **H66.93 Otitis media, unspecified, bilateral**

+ 4 **H67 Otitis media in diseases classified elsewhere**

Code first underlying disease, such as:
plasminogen deficiency (E88.02)
viral disease NEC (B00-B34)
Use additional code for any associated perforated tympanic membrane (H72.-)
EXCLUDES 1 otitis media in:
influenza (J09.X9, J10.83, J11.83)
measles (B05.3)
scarlet fever (A38.0)
tuberculosis (A18.6)

M ⊟ !Q + **H67.1** ***Otitis media in diseases classified elsewhere, right ear***

M ⊟ !Q + **H67.2** ***Otitis media in diseases classified elsewhere, left ear***

M ⊟ !Q + **H67.3** ***Otitis media in diseases classified elsewhere, bilateral***

M ⊟ !Q + **H67.9** ***Otitis media in diseases classified elsewhere, unspecified ear***

4 **H68 Eustachian salpingitis and obstruction**

5 **H68.0 Eustachian salpingitis**

6 **H68.00 Unspecified Eustachian salpingitis**

⊟ SP **H68.001 Unspecified Eustachian salpingitis, right ear**

⊟ SP **H68.002 Unspecified Eustachian salpingitis, left ear**

⊟ SP **H68.003 Unspecified Eustachian salpingitis, bilateral**

⊟ !Q **H68.009 Unspecified Eustachian salpingitis, unspecified ear**

6 **H68.01 Acute Eustachian salpingitis**

⊟ SP **H68.011 Acute Eustachian salpingitis, right ear**

⊟ SP **H68.012 Acute Eustachian salpingitis, left ear**

⊟ SP **H68.013 Acute Eustachian salpingitis, bilateral**

⊟ !Q **H68.019 Acute Eustachian salpingitis, unspecified ear**

6 **H68.02 Chronic Eustachian salpingitis**

⊟ SP **H68.021 Chronic Eustachian salpingitis, right ear**

⊟ SP **H68.022 Chronic Eustachian salpingitis, left ear**

⊟ SP **H68.023 Chronic Eustachian salpingitis, bilateral**

⊟ !Q **H68.029 Chronic Eustachian salpingitis, unspecified ear**

Chapter 8
H60-H95

4 4th digit required 5 5th digit required 6 6th digit required 7 7th digit required 7 7th digit placeholder + Additional code ⊟ Laterality

5 H68.1 **Obstruction of Eustachian tube**
Stenosis of Eustachian tube
Stricture of Eustachian tube

6 H68.10 **Unspecified obstruction of Eustachian tube**

SP H68.101 **Unspecified obstruction of Eustachian tube, right ear**

SP H68.102 **Unspecified obstruction of Eustachian tube, left ear**

SP H68.103 **Unspecified obstruction of Eustachian tube, bilateral**

IQ H68.109 **Unspecified obstruction of Eustachian tube, unspecified ear**

6 H68.11 **Osseous obstruction of Eustachian tube**

SP H68.111 **Osseous obstruction of Eustachian tube, right ear**

SP H68.112 **Osseous obstruction of Eustachian tube, left ear**

SP H68.113 **Osseous obstruction of Eustachian tube, bilateral**

IQ H68.119 **Osseous obstruction of Eustachian tube, unspecified ear**

6 H68.12 **Intrinsic cartilagenous obstruction of Eustachian tube**

SP H68.121 **Intrinsic cartilagenous obstruction of Eustachian tube, right ear**

SP H68.122 **Intrinsic cartilagenous obstruction of Eustachian tube, left ear**

SP H68.123 **Intrinsic cartilagenous obstruction of Eustachian tube, bilateral**

IQ H68.129 **Intrinsic cartilagenous obstruction of Eustachian tube, unspecified ear**

6 H68.13 **Extrinsic cartilagenous obstruction of Eustachian tube**
Compression of Eustachian tube

SP H68.131 **Extrinsic cartilagenous obstruction of Eustachian tube, right ear**

SP H68.132 **Extrinsic cartilagenous obstruction of Eustachian tube, left ear**

SP H68.133 **Extrinsic cartilagenous obstruction of Eustachian tube, bilateral**

IQ H68.139 **Extrinsic cartilagenous obstruction of Eustachian tube, unspecified ear**

4 H69 **Other and unspecified disorders of Eustachian tube**

5 H69.0 **Patulous Eustachian tube**

IQ H69.00 **Patulous Eustachian tube, unspecified ear**

SP H69.01 **Patulous Eustachian tube, right ear**

SP H69.02 **Patulous Eustachian tube, left ear**

SP H69.03 **Patulous Eustachian tube, bilateral**

5 H69.8 **Other specified disorders of Eustachian tube**

IQ H69.80 **Other specified disorders of Eustachian tube, unspecified ear**

SP H69.81 **Other specified disorders of Eustachian tube, right ear**

SP H69.82 **Other specified disorders of Eustachian tube, left ear**

SP H69.83 **Other specified disorders of Eustachian tube, bilateral**

5 H69.9 **Unspecified Eustachian tube disorder**

IQ H69.90 **Unspecified Eustachian tube disorder, unspecified ear**

SP H69.91 **Unspecified Eustachian tube disorder, right ear**

SP H69.92 **Unspecified Eustachian tube disorder, left ear**

SP H69.93 **Unspecified Eustachian tube disorder, bilateral**

4 H70 **Mastoiditis and related conditions**

5 H70.0 **Acute mastoiditis**
Abscess of mastoid
Empyema of mastoid

6 H70.00 **Acute mastoiditis without complications**

SP H70.001 **Acute mastoiditis without complications, right ear**

SP H70.002 **Acute mastoiditis without complications, left ear**

SP H70.003 **Acute mastoiditis without complications, bilateral**

IQ H70.009 **Acute mastoiditis without complications, unspecified ear**

6 H70.01 **Subperiosteal abscess of mastoid**

SP H70.011 **Subperiosteal abscess of mastoid, right ear**

SP H70.012 **Subperiosteal abscess of mastoid, left ear**

SP H70.013 **Subperiosteal abscess of mastoid, bilateral**

IQ H70.019 **Subperiosteal abscess of mastoid, unspecified ear**

6 H70.09 **Acute mastoiditis with other complications**

SP H70.091 **Acute mastoiditis with other complications, right ear**

SP H70.092 **Acute mastoiditis with other complications, left ear**

SP H70.093 **Acute mastoiditis with other complications, bilateral**

IQ H70.099 **Acute mastoiditis with other complications, unspecified ear**

5 H70.1 **Chronic mastoiditis**
Caries of mastoid
Fistula of mastoid
EXCLUDES 1 tuberculous mastoiditis (A18.03)

IQ H70.10 **Chronic mastoiditis, unspecified ear**

SP H70.11 **Chronic mastoiditis, right ear**

SP H70.12 **Chronic mastoiditis, left ear**

SP H70.13 **Chronic mastoiditis, bilateral**

5 H70.2 **Petrositis**
Inflammation of petrous bone

6 H70.20 **Unspecified petrositis**

DEFINITION Inflammation of the dense, hard bone behind the temple protecting the inner ear.

SP H70.201 **Unspecified petrositis, right ear**

H70.202 **Unspecified petrositis, left ear**
H70.203 **Unspecified petrositis, bilateral**
H70.209 **Unspecified petrositis, unspecified ear**
H70.21 **Acute petrositis**
H70.211 **Acute petrositis, right ear**
H70.212 **Acute petrositis, left ear**
H70.213 **Acute petrositis, bilateral**
H70.219 **Acute petrositis, unspecified ear**
H70.22 **Chronic petrositis**
H70.221 **Chronic petrositis, right ear**
H70.222 **Chronic petrositis, left ear**
H70.223 **Chronic petrositis, bilateral**
H70.229 **Chronic petrositis, unspecified ear**
H70.8 **Other mastoiditis and related conditions**
EXCLUDES 1 preauricular sinus and cyst (Q18.1)
sinus, fistula, and cyst of branchial cleft (Q18.0)
H70.81 **Postauricular fistula**
H70.811 **Postauricular fistula, right ear**
H70.812 **Postauricular fistula, left ear**
H70.813 **Postauricular fistula, bilateral**
H70.819 **Postauricular fistula, unspecified ear**
H70.89 **Other mastoiditis and related conditions**
H70.891 **Other mastoiditis and related conditions, right ear**
H70.892 **Other mastoiditis and related conditions, left ear**
H70.893 **Other mastoiditis and related conditions, bilateral**
H70.899 **Other mastoiditis and related conditions, unspecified ear**
H70.9 **Unspecified mastoiditis**
H70.90 **Unspecified mastoiditis, unspecified ear**
H70.91 **Unspecified mastoiditis, right ear**
H70.92 **Unspecified mastoiditis, left ear**
H70.93 **Unspecified mastoiditis, bilateral**
H71 **Cholesteatoma of middle ear**
EXCLUDES 2 cholesteatoma of external ear (H60.4-)
recurrent cholesteatoma of postmastoidectomy cavity (H95.0-)

DEFINITION Cyst-like mass filled with cell debris and cholesterol crystals in the middle ear and/or mastoid process that can damage the ossicles, causing deafness, vertigo, and nerve deterioration.

H71.0 **Cholesteatoma of attic**
H71.00 **Cholesteatoma of attic, unspecified ear**
H71.01 **Cholesteatoma of attic, right ear**
H71.02 **Cholesteatoma of attic, left ear**
H71.03 **Cholesteatoma of attic, bilateral**
H71.1 **Cholesteatoma of tympanum**
H71.10 **Cholesteatoma of tympanum, unspecified ear**
H71.11 **Cholesteatoma of tympanum, right ear**
H71.12 **Cholesteatoma of tympanum, left ear**
H71.13 **Cholesteatoma of tympanum, bilateral**
H71.2 **Cholesteatoma of mastoid**
H71.20 **Cholesteatoma of mastoid, unspecified ear**
H71.21 **Cholesteatoma of mastoid, right ear**
H71.22 **Cholesteatoma of mastoid, left ear**
H71.23 **Cholesteatoma of mastoid, bilateral**
H71.3 **Diffuse cholesteatosis**
H71.30 **Diffuse cholesteatosis, unspecified ear**
H71.31 **Diffuse cholesteatosis, right ear**
H71.32 **Diffuse cholesteatosis, left ear**
H71.33 **Diffuse cholesteatosis, bilateral**
H71.9 **Unspecified cholesteatoma**
H71.90 **Unspecified cholesteatoma, unspecified ear**
H71.91 **Unspecified cholesteatoma, right ear**
H71.92 **Unspecified cholesteatoma, left ear**
H71.93 **Unspecified cholesteatoma, bilateral**
H72 **Perforation of tympanic membrane**
INCLUDES persistent post-traumatic perforation of ear drum
postinflammatory perforation of ear drum
Code first:
any associated otitis media (H65.-, H66.1-, H66.2-, H66.3-, H66.4-, H66.9-, H67.-)
EXCLUDES 1 acute suppurative otitis media with rupture of the tympanic membrane (H66.01-)
traumatic rupture of ear drum (S09.2-)
H72.0 **Central perforation of tympanic membrane**
H72.00 **Central perforation of tympanic membrane, unspecified ear**
H72.01 **Central perforation of tympanic membrane, right ear**
H72.02 **Central perforation of tympanic membrane, left ear**
H72.03 **Central perforation of tympanic membrane, bilateral**
H72.1 **Attic perforation of tympanic membrane**
Perforation of pars flaccida
H72.10 **Attic perforation of tympanic membrane, unspecified ear**
H72.11 **Attic perforation of tympanic membrane, right ear**
H72.12 **Attic perforation of tympanic membrane, left ear**
H72.13 **Attic perforation of tympanic membrane, bilateral**
H72.2 **Other marginal perforations of tympanic membrane**

4th digit required 5th digit required 6th digit required 7th digit required 7th digit placeholder +Additional code Laterality

6 H72.2X Other marginal perforations of tympanic membrane
SP H72.2X1 Other marginal perforations of tympanic membrane, right ear
SP H72.2X2 Other marginal perforations of tympanic membrane, left ear
SP H72.2X3 Other marginal perforations of tympanic membrane, bilateral
IQ H72.2X9 Other marginal perforations of tympanic membrane, unspecified ear
5 H72.8 Other perforations of tympanic membrane
6 H72.81 Multiple perforations of tympanic membrane
SP H72.811 Multiple perforations of tympanic membrane, right ear
SP H72.812 Multiple perforations of tympanic membrane, left ear
SP H72.813 Multiple perforations of tympanic membrane, bilateral
IQ H72.819 Multiple perforations of tympanic membrane, unspecified ear
6 H72.82 Total perforations of tympanic membrane
SP H72.821 Total perforations of tympanic membrane, right ear
SP H72.822 Total perforations of tympanic membrane, left ear
SP H72.823 Total perforations of tympanic membrane, bilateral
IQ H72.829 Total perforations of tympanic membrane, unspecified ear
5 H72.9 Unspecified perforation of tympanic membrane
IQ H72.90 Unspecified perforation of tympanic membrane, unspecified ear
SP H72.91 Unspecified perforation of tympanic membrane, right ear
SP H72.92 Unspecified perforation of tympanic membrane, left ear
SP H72.93 Unspecified perforation of tympanic membrane, bilateral
4 H73 Other disorders of tympanic membrane
5 H73.0 Acute myringitis
EXCLUDES 1 acute myringitis with otitis media (H65, H66)
6 H73.00 Unspecified acute myringitis
Acute tympanitis NOS
SP H73.001 Acute myringitis, right ear
SP H73.002 Acute myringitis, left ear
SP H73.003 Acute myringitis, bilateral
IQ H73.009 Acute myringitis, unspecified ear
6 H73.01 Bullous myringitis
DEFINITION Inflammation of the eardrum caused by a virus and characterized by blood-filled blisters.
SP H73.011 Bullous myringitis, right ear
SP H73.012 Bullous myringitis, left ear
SP H73.013 Bullous myringitis, bilateral
IQ H73.019 Bullous myringitis, unspecified ear
6 H73.09 Other acute myringitis
SP H73.091 Other acute myringitis, right ear
SP H73.092 Other acute myringitis, left ear
SP H73.093 Other acute myringitis, bilateral
IQ H73.099 Other acute myringitis, unspecified ear
5 H73.1 Chronic myringitis
Chronic tympanitis
EXCLUDES 1 chronic myringitis with otitis media (H65, H66)
IQ H73.10 Chronic myringitis, unspecified ear
SP H73.11 Chronic myringitis, right ear
SP H73.12 Chronic myringitis, left ear
SP H73.13 Chronic myringitis, bilateral
5 H73.2 Unspecified myringitis
IQ H73.20 Unspecified myringitis, unspecified ear
SP H73.21 Unspecified myringitis, right ear
SP H73.22 Unspecified myringitis, left ear
SP H73.23 Unspecified myringitis, bilateral
5 H73.8 Other specified disorders of tympanic membrane
6 H73.81 Atrophic flaccid tympanic membrane
DEFINITION Eardrum that has wasted away and lost its tension, resulting in severe hearing loss.
SP H73.811 Atrophic flaccid tympanic membrane, right ear
SP H73.812 Atrophic flaccid tympanic membrane, left ear
SP H73.813 Atrophic flaccid tympanic membrane, bilateral
IQ H73.819 Atrophic flaccid tympanic membrane, unspecified ear
6 H73.82 Atrophic nonflaccid tympanic membrane
SP H73.821 Atrophic nonflaccid tympanic membrane, right ear
SP H73.822 Atrophic nonflaccid tympanic membrane, left ear
SP H73.823 Atrophic nonflaccid tympanic membrane, bilateral
IQ H73.829 Atrophic nonflaccid tympanic membrane, unspecified ear
6 H73.89 Other specified disorders of tympanic membrane
SP H73.891 Other specified disorders of tympanic membrane, right ear
SP H73.892 Other specified disorders of tympanic membrane, left ear
SP H73.893 Other specified disorders of tympanic membrane, bilateral
IQ H73.899 Other specified disorders of tympanic membrane, unspecified ear
5 H73.9 Unspecified disorder of tympanic membrane
IQ H73.90 Unspecified disorder of tympanic membrane, unspecified ear
SP H73.91 Unspecified disorder of tympanic membrane, right ear
SP H73.92 Unspecified disorder of tympanic membrane, left ear

H73.93 Unspecified disorder of tympanic membrane, bilateral

H74 Other disorders of middle ear mastoid
EXCLUDES 2 mastoiditis (H70.-)

H74.0 Tympanosclerosis
DEFINITION Thickening and hardening of the eardrum, reducing its ability to vibrate and transmit sound.

H74.01 Tympanosclerosis, right ear
H74.02 Tympanosclerosis, left ear
H74.03 Tympanosclerosis, bilateral
H74.09 Tympanosclerosis, unspecified ear

H74.1 Adhesive middle ear disease
Adhesive otitis
EXCLUDES 1 glue ear (H65.3-)

H74.11 Adhesive right middle ear disease
H74.12 Adhesive left middle ear disease
H74.13 Adhesive middle ear disease, bilateral
H74.19 Adhesive middle ear disease, unspecified ear

H74.2 Discontinuity and dislocation of ear ossicles

H74.20 Discontinuity and dislocation of ear ossicles, unspecified ear
H74.21 Discontinuity and dislocation of right ear ossicles
H74.22 Discontinuity and dislocation of left ear ossicles
H74.23 Discontinuity and dislocation of ear ossicles, bilateral

H74.3 Other acquired abnormalities of ear ossicles

H74.31 Ankylosis of ear ossicles
H74.311 Ankylosis of ear ossicles, right ear
H74.312 Ankylosis of ear ossicles, left ear
H74.313 Ankylosis of ear ossicles, bilateral
H74.319 Ankylosis of ear ossicles, unspecified ear

H74.32 Partial loss of ear ossicles
H74.321 Partial loss of ear ossicles, right ear
H74.322 Partial loss of ear ossicles, left ear
H74.323 Partial loss of ear ossicles, bilateral
H74.329 Partial loss of ear ossicles, unspecified ear

H74.39 Other acquired abnormalities of ear ossicles
H74.391 Other acquired abnormalities of right ear ossicles
H74.392 Other acquired abnormalities of left ear ossicles
H74.393 Other acquired abnormalities of ear ossicles, bilateral
H74.399 Other acquired abnormalities of ear ossicles, unspecified ear

H74.4 Polyp of middle ear

H74.40 Polyp of middle ear, unspecified ear
H74.41 Polyp of right middle ear
H74.42 Polyp of left middle ear
H74.43 Polyp of middle ear, bilateral

H74.8 Other specified disorders of middle ear and mastoid

H74.8X Other specified disorders of middle ear and mastoid
H74.8X1 Other specified disorders of right middle ear and mastoid
H74.8X2 Other specified disorders of left middle ear and mastoid
H74.8X3 Other specified disorders of middle ear and mastoid, bilateral
H74.8X9 Other specified disorders of middle ear and mastoid, unspecified ear

H74.9 Unspecified disorder of middle ear and mastoid

H74.90 Unspecified disorder of middle ear and mastoid, unspecified ear
H74.91 Unspecified disorder of right middle ear and mastoid
H74.92 Unspecified disorder of left middle ear and mastoid
H74.93 Unspecified disorder of middle ear and mastoid, bilateral

H75 Other disorders of middle ear and mastoid in diseases classified elsewhere
Code first:
underlying disease

H75.0 Mastoiditis in infectious and parasitic diseases classified elsewhere
EXCLUDES 1 mastoiditis (in):
syphilis (A52.77)
tuberculosis (A18.03)

M H75.00 *Mastoiditis in infectious and parasitic diseases classified elsewhere, unspecified ear*
M H75.01 *Mastoiditis in infectious and parasitic diseases classified elsewhere, right ear*
M H75.02 *Mastoiditis in infectious and parasitic diseases classified elsewhere, left ear*
M H75.03 *Mastoiditis in infectious and parasitic diseases classified elsewhere, bilateral*

H75.8 Other specified disorders of middle ear and mastoid in diseases classified elsewhere

H75.80 Other specified disorders of middle ear and mastoid in diseases classified elsewhere, unspecified ear
H75.81 Other specified disorders of right middle ear and mastoid in diseases classified elsewhere
H75.82 Other specified disorders of left middle ear and mastoid in diseases classified elsewhere
H75.83 Other specified disorders of middle ear and mastoid in diseases classified elsewhere, bilateral

Diseases of inner ear (H80-H83)

H80 Otosclerosis
INCLUDES Otospongiosis

H80.0 Otosclerosis involving oval window, nonobliterative

Chapter 8 H60-H95

4th digit required 5th digit required 6th digit required 7th digit required 7th digit placeholder + Additional code Laterality

6 IQ H80.00 Otosclerosis involving oval window, nonobliterative, unspecified ear
6 SP H80.01 Otosclerosis involving oval window, nonobliterative, right ear
6 SP H80.02 Otosclerosis involving oval window, nonobliterative, left ear
6 SP H80.03 Otosclerosis involving oval window, nonobliterative, bilateral
5 H80.1 Otosclerosis involving oval window, obliterative
6 IQ H80.10 Otosclerosis involving oval window, obliterative, unspecified ear
6 SP H80.11 Otosclerosis involving oval window, obliterative, right ear
6 SP H80.12 Otosclerosis involving oval window, obliterative, left ear
6 SP H80.13 Otosclerosis involving oval window, obliterative, bilateral
5 H80.2 Cochlear otosclerosis
Otosclerosis involving otic capsule
Otosclerosis involving round window
DEFINITION Formation of bony tissue in the cochlea, causing hearing loss.
6 IQ H80.20 Cochlear otosclerosis, unspecified ear
6 SP H80.21 Cochlear otosclerosis, right ear
6 SP H80.22 Cochlear otosclerosis, left ear
6 SP H80.23 Cochlear otosclerosis, bilateral
5 H80.8 Other otosclerosis
6 IQ H80.80 Other otosclerosis, unspecified ear
6 SP H80.81 Other otosclerosis, right ear
6 SP H80.82 Other otosclerosis, left ear
6 SP H80.83 Other otosclerosis, bilateral
5 H80.9 Unspecified otosclerosis
6 IQ H80.90 Unspecified otosclerosis, unspecified ear
6 SP H80.91 Unspecified otosclerosis, right ear
6 SP H80.92 Unspecified otosclerosis, left ear
6 SP H80.93 Unspecified otosclerosis, bilateral
4 H81 Disorders of vestibular function
EXCLUDES 1 epidemic vertigo (A88.1)
vertigo NOS (R42)
5 H81.0 Ménière's disease
Labyrinthine hydrops
Ménière's syndrome or vertigo
DEFINITION Disorder of the inner ear causing attacks of vertigo, tinnitus, and progressive hearing loss involving all tones.
6 SP H81.01 Ménière's disease, right ear
6 SP H81.02 Ménière's disease, left ear
6 SP H81.03 Ménière's disease, bilateral
6 IQ H81.09 Ménière's disease, unspecified ear
5 H81.1 Benign paroxysmal vertigo
6 IQ H81.10 Benign paroxysmal vertigo, unspecified ear
6 SP H81.11 Benign paroxysmal vertigo, right ear
6 SP H81.12 Benign paroxysmal vertigo, left ear
6 SP H81.13 Benign paroxysmal vertigo, bilateral
5 H81.2 Vestibular neuronitis
6 IQ H81.20 Vestibular neuronitis, unspecified ear
6 SP H81.21 Vestibular neuronitis, right ear
6 SP H81.22 Vestibular neuronitis, left ear
6 SP H81.23 Vestibular neuronitis, bilateral
5 H81.3 Other peripheral vertigo
6 H81.31 Aural vertigo
7 SP H81.311 Aural vertigo, right ear
7 SP H81.312 Aural vertigo, left ear
7 SP H81.313 Aural vertigo, bilateral
7 IQ H81.319 Aural vertigo, unspecified ear
6 H81.39 Other peripheral vertigo
Lermoyez' syndrome
Otogenic vertigo
Peripheral vertigo NOS
7 SP H81.391 Other peripheral vertigo, right ear
7 SP H81.392 Other peripheral vertigo, left ear
7 SP H81.393 Other peripheral vertigo, bilateral
7 IQ H81.399 Other peripheral vertigo, unspecified ear
SP H81.4 Vertigo of central origin
Central positional nystagmus
5 H81.8 Other disorders of vestibular function
6 H81.8X Other disorders of vestibular function
7 SP H81.8X1 Other disorders of vestibular function, right ear
7 SP H81.8X2 Other disorders of vestibular function, left ear
7 SP H81.8X3 Other disorders of vestibular function, bilateral
7 IQ H81.8X9 Other disorders of vestibular function, unspecified ear
5 H81.9 Unspecified disorder of vestibular function
Vertiginous syndrome NOS
6 IQ H81.90 Unspecified disorder of vestibular function, unspecified ear
6 IQ H81.91 Unspecified disorder of vestibular function, right ear
6 IQ H81.92 Unspecified disorder of vestibular function, left ear
6 IQ H81.93 Unspecified disorder of vestibular function, bilateral
4 H82 Vertiginous syndromes in diseases classified elsewhere
Code first:
underlying disease
EXCLUDES 1 epidemic vertigo (A88.1)
5 IQ H82.1 Vertiginous syndromes in diseases classified elsewhere, right ear
5 IQ H82.2 Vertiginous syndromes in diseases classified elsewhere, left ear
5 IQ H82.3 Vertiginous syndromes in diseases classified elsewhere, bilateral
5 IQ H82.9 Vertiginous syndromes in diseases classified elsewhere, unspecified ear
4 H83 Other diseases of inner ear
5 H83.0 Labyrinthitis
6 SP H83.01 Labyrinthitis, right ear
6 SP H83.02 Labyrinthitis, left ear
6 SP H83.03 Labyrinthitis, bilateral
6 IQ H83.09 Labyrinthitis, unspecified ear

Chapter 8 H60-H95

5 H83.1 Labyrinthine fistula
Laterality SP H83.11 Labyrinthine fistula, right ear
Laterality SP H83.12 Labyrinthine fistula, left ear
Laterality SP H83.13 Labyrinthine fistula, bilateral
Laterality IQ H83.19 Labyrinthine fistula, unspecified ear

5 H83.2 Labyrinthine dysfunction
Labyrinthine hypersensitivity
Labyrinthine hypofunction
Labyrinthine loss of function

6 H83.2X Labyrinthine dysfunction
Laterality SP H83.2X1 Labyrinthine dysfunction, right ear
Laterality SP H83.2X2 Labyrinthine dysfunction, left ear
Laterality SP H83.2X3 Labyrinthine dysfunction, bilateral
Laterality IQ H83.2X9 Labyrinthine dysfunction, unspecified ear

5 H83.3 Noise effects on inner ear
Acoustic trauma of inner ear
Noise-induced hearing loss of inner ear

6 H83.3X Noise effects on inner ear
Laterality SP H83.3X1 Noise effects on right inner ear
Laterality SP H83.3X2 Noise effects on left inner ear
Laterality SP H83.3X3 Noise effects on inner ear, bilateral
Laterality IQ H83.3X9 Noise effects on inner ear, unspecified ear

5 H83.8 Other specified diseases of inner ear

6 H83.8X Other specified diseases of inner ear
Laterality SP H83.8X1 Other specified diseases of right inner ear
Laterality SP H83.8X2 Other specified diseases of left inner ear
Laterality SP H83.8X3 Other specified diseases of inner ear, bilateral
Laterality IQ H83.8X9 Other specified diseases of inner ear, unspecified ear

5 H83.9 Unspecified disease of inner ear
Laterality IQ H83.90 Unspecified disease of inner ear, unspecified ear
Laterality IQ H83.91 Unspecified disease of right inner ear
Laterality IQ H83.92 Unspecified disease of left inner ear
Laterality IQ H83.93 Unspecified disease of inner ear, bilateral

Other disorders of ear (H90-H94)

4 H90 Conductive and sensorineural hearing loss

EXCLUDES 1 deaf nonspeaking NEC (H91.3)
deafness NOS (H91.9-)
hearing loss NOS (H91.9-)
noise-induced hearing loss (H83.3-)
ototoxic hearing loss (H91.0-)
sudden (idiopathic) hearing loss (H91.2-)

SP H90.0 Conductive hearing loss, bilateral

5 H90.1 Conductive hearing loss, unilateral with unrestricted hearing on the contralateral side
Laterality SP H90.11 Conductive hearing loss, unilateral, right ear, with unrestricted hearing on the contralateral side
Laterality SP H90.12 Conductive hearing loss, unilateral, left ear, with unrestricted hearing on the contralateral side

SP H90.2 Conductive hearing loss, unspecified
Conductive deafness NOS

DEFINITION Loss of audio acuity caused by transmission interference of sound waves before they can reach the inner ear and the auditory nerve.

SP H90.3 Sensorineural hearing loss, bilateral

5 H90.4 Sensorineural hearing loss, unilateral with unrestricted hearing on the contralateral side
Laterality SP H90.41 Sensorineural hearing loss, unilateral, right ear, with unrestricted hearing on the contralateral side
Laterality SP H90.42 Sensorineural hearing loss, unilateral, left ear, with unrestricted hearing on the contralateral side

SP H90.5 Unspecified sensorineural hearing loss
Central hearing loss NOS
Congenital deafness NOS
Neural hearing loss NOS
Perceptive hearing loss NOS
Sensorineural deafness NOS
Sensory hearing loss NOS

EXCLUDES 1 abnormal auditory perception (H93.2-)
psychogenic deafness (F44.6)

DEFINITION Sensory-nerve based hearing loss caused by a disorder affecting the VIII cranial nerve, the inner ear sensory perception, or the central processing area of the brain.

SP H90.6 Mixed conductive and sensorineural hearing loss, bilateral

5 H90.7 Mixed conductive and sensorineural hearing loss, unilateral with unrestricted hearing on the contralateral side
Laterality SP H90.71 Mixed conductive and sensorineural hearing loss, unilateral, right ear, with unrestricted hearing on the contralateral side
Laterality SP H90.72 Mixed conductive and sensorineural hearing loss, unilateral, left ear, with unrestricted hearing on the contralateral side

SP H90.8 Mixed conductive and sensorineural hearing loss, unspecified

5 H90.A Conductive and sensorineural hearing loss with restricted hearing on the contralateral side

6 H90.A1 Conductive hearing loss, unilateral, with restricted hearing on the contralateral side
Laterality SP H90.A11 Conductive hearing loss, unilateral, right ear with restricted hearing on the contralateral side
Laterality SP H90.A12 Conductive hearing loss, unilateral, left ear with restricted hearing on the contralateral side

6 H90.A2 Sensorineural hearing loss, unilateral, with restricted hearing on the contralateral side

SP H90.A21 Sensorineural hearing loss, unilateral, right ear, with restricted hearing on the contralateral side

SP H90.A22 Sensorineural hearing loss, unilateral, left ear, with restricted hearing on the contralateral side

6 H90.A3 Mixed conductive and sensorineural hearing loss, unilateral with restricted hearing on the contralateral side

SP H90.A31 Mixed conductive and sensorineural hearing loss, unilateral, right ear with restricted hearing on the contralateral side

SP H90.A32 Mixed conductive and sensorineural hearing loss, unilateral, left ear with restricted hearing on the contralateral side

4 H91 Other and unspecified hearing loss

EXCLUDES 1 abnormal auditory perception (H93.2-)
hearing loss as classified in H90.-
impacted cerumen (H61.2-)
noise-induced hearing loss (H83.3-)
psychogenic deafness (F44.6)
transient ischemic deafness (H93.01-)

+ 5 H91.0 Ototoxic hearing loss

Code first:
poisoning due to drug or toxin, if applicable (T36-T65 with fifth or sixth character 1-4 or 6)
Use additional code for adverse effect, if applicable, to identify drug (T36-T50 with fifth or sixth character 5)

SP + H91.01 Ototoxic hearing loss, right ear

SP + H91.02 Ototoxic hearing loss, left ear

SP + H91.03 Ototoxic hearing loss, bilateral

IQ + H91.09 Ototoxic hearing loss, unspecified ear

5 H91.1 Presbycusis

Presbyacusia

DEFINITION Gradual hearing loss that normally occurs with age.

IQ H91.10 Presbycusis, unspecified ear

SP H91.11 Presbycusis, right ear

SP H91.12 Presbycusis, left ear

SP H91.13 Presbycusis, bilateral

5 H91.2 Sudden idiopathic hearing loss

Sudden hearing loss NOS

IQ H91.20 Sudden idiopathic hearing loss, unspecified ear

SP H91.21 Sudden idiopathic hearing loss, right ear

SP H91.22 Sudden idiopathic hearing loss, left ear

SP H91.23 Sudden idiopathic hearing loss, bilateral

SP H91.3 Deaf nonspeaking, not elsewhere classified

5 H91.8 Other specified hearing loss

6 H91.8X Other specified hearing loss

SP H91.8X1 Other specified hearing loss, right ear

SP H91.8X2 Other specified hearing loss, left ear

SP H91.8X3 Other specified hearing loss, bilateral

IQ H91.8X9 Other specified hearing loss, unspecified ear

5 H91.9 Unspecified hearing loss

Deafness NOS
High frequency deafness
Low frequency deafness

IQ H91.90 Unspecified hearing loss, unspecified ear

SP H91.91 Unspecified hearing loss, right ear

SP H91.92 Unspecified hearing loss, left ear

SP H91.93 Unspecified hearing loss, bilateral

4 H92 Otalgia and effusion of ear

5 H92.0 Otalgia

SP H92.01 Otalgia, right ear

SP H92.02 Otalgia, left ear

SP H92.03 Otalgia, bilateral

IQ H92.09 Otalgia, unspecified ear

5 H92.1 Otorrhea

EXCLUDES 1 leakage of cerebrospinal fluid through ear (G96.0)

DEFINITION Fluid leaking from the ear.

IQ H92.10 Otorrhea, unspecified ear

SP H92.11 Otorrhea, right ear

SP H92.12 Otorrhea, left ear

SP H92.13 Otorrhea, bilateral

5 H92.2 Otorrhagia

EXCLUDES 1 traumatic otorrhagia - code to injury

IQ H92.20 Otorrhagia, unspecified ear

SP H92.21 Otorrhagia, right ear

SP H92.22 Otorrhagia, left ear

SP H92.23 Otorrhagia, bilateral

4 H93 Other disorders of ear, not elsewhere classified

5 H93.0 Degenerative and vascular disorders of ear

EXCLUDES 1 presbycusis (H91.1)

6 H93.01 Transient ischemic deafness

DEFINITION A passing hearing loss that occurs when blood flow to the auditory organs is decreased due to injury or disease.

SP H93.011 Transient ischemic deafness, right ear

SP H93.012 Transient ischemic deafness, left ear

SP H93.013 Transient ischemic deafness, bilateral

IQ H93.019 Transient ischemic deafness, unspecified ear

6 H93.09 Unspecified degenerative and vascular disorders of ear

Laterality SP H93.091 Unspecified degenerative and vascular disorders of right ear
Laterality SP H93.092 Unspecified degenerative and vascular disorders of left ear
Laterality SP H93.093 Unspecified degenerative and vascular disorders of ear, bilateral
Laterality IQ H93.099 Unspecified degenerative and vascular disorders of unspecified ear

5 **H93.1 Tinnitus**
DEFINITION Ringing, hissing, roaring or other sound in the ear in the absence of any apparent stimulus.

Laterality SP H93.11 Tinnitus, right ear
Laterality SP H93.12 Tinnitus, left ear
Laterality SP H93.13 Tinnitus, bilateral
Laterality IQ H93.19 Tinnitus, unspecified ear

5 **H93.A Pulsatile tinnitus**
Laterality SP H93.A1 Pulsatile tinnitus, right ear
Laterality SP H93.A2 Pulsatile tinnitus, left ear
Laterality SP H93.A3 Pulsatile tinnitus, bilateral
Laterality IQ H93.A9 Pulsatile tinnitus, unspecified ear

5 **H93.2 Other abnormal auditory perceptions**
EXCLUDES 2 auditory hallucinations (R44.0)

6 **H93.21 Auditory recruitment**
Laterality SP H93.211 Auditory recruitment, right ear
Laterality SP H93.212 Auditory recruitment, left ear
Laterality SP H93.213 Auditory recruitment, bilateral
Laterality IQ H93.219 Auditory recruitment, unspecified ear

6 **H93.22 Diplacusis**
DEFINITION One sound is heard as two separate sounds at different tones or pitches.

Laterality SP H93.221 Diplacusis, right ear
Laterality SP H93.222 Diplacusis, left ear
Laterality SP H93.223 Diplacusis, bilateral
Laterality IQ H93.229 Diplacusis, unspecified ear

6 **H93.23 Hyperacusis**
DEFINITION Hearing is abnormally heightened; normal sounds seem amplified, even cause ear pain.

Laterality SP H93.231 Hyperacusis, right ear
Laterality SP H93.232 Hyperacusis, left ear
Laterality SP H93.233 Hyperacusis, bilateral
Laterality IQ H93.239 Hyperacusis, unspecified ear

6 **H93.24 Temporary auditory threshold shift**
Laterality SP H93.241 Temporary auditory threshold shift, right ear
Laterality SP H93.242 Temporary auditory threshold shift, left ear
Laterality SP H93.243 Temporary auditory threshold shift, bilateral
Laterality IQ H93.249 Temporary auditory threshold shift, unspecified ear

SP **H93.25 Central auditory processing disorder**
Congenital auditory imperception
Word deafness
EXCLUDES 1 mixed receptive-expressive language disorder (F80.2)

6 **H93.29 Other abnormal auditory perceptions**
Laterality SP H93.291 Other abnormal auditory perceptions, right ear
Laterality SP H93.292 Other abnormal auditory perceptions, left ear
Laterality SP H93.293 Other abnormal auditory perceptions, bilateral
Laterality IQ H93.299 Other abnormal auditory perceptions, unspecified ear

5 **H93.3 Disorders of acoustic nerve**
Disorder of 8th cranial nerve
EXCLUDES 1 acoustic neuroma (D33.3)
syphilitic acoustic neuritis (A52.15)

6 **H93.3X Disorders of acoustic nerve**
Laterality SP H93.3X1 Disorders of right acoustic nerve
Laterality SP H93.3X2 Disorders of left acoustic nerve
Laterality SP H93.3X3 Disorders of bilateral acoustic nerves
Laterality IQ H93.3X9 Disorders of unspecified acoustic nerve

5 **H93.8 Other specified disorders of ear**
6 **H93.8X Other specified disorders of ear**
Laterality SP H93.8X1 Other specified disorders of right ear
Laterality SP H93.8X2 Other specified disorders of left ear
Laterality SP H93.8X3 Other specified disorders of ear, bilateral
Laterality IQ H93.8X9 Other specified disorders of ear, unspecified ear

5 **H93.9 Unspecified disorder of ear**
Laterality IQ H93.90 Unspecified disorder of ear, unspecified ear
Laterality IQ H93.91 Unspecified disorder of right ear
Laterality IQ H93.92 Unspecified disorder of left ear
Laterality IQ H93.93 Unspecified disorder of ear, bilateral

4 **H94 Other disorders of ear in diseases classified elsewhere**
5 **H94.0 Acoustic neuritis in infectious and parasitic diseases classified elsewhere**
Code first underlying disease, such as:
parasitic disease (B65-B89)
EXCLUDES 1 acoustic neuritis (in) :
herpes zoster (B02.29)
syphilis (A52.15)

M Laterality IQ H94.00 *Acoustic neuritis in infectious and parasitic diseases classified elsewhere, unspecified ear*
M Laterality IQ H94.01 *Acoustic neuritis in infectious and parasitic diseases classified elsewhere, right ear*
M Laterality IQ H94.02 *Acoustic neuritis in infectious and parasitic diseases classified elsewhere, left ear*
M Laterality IQ H94.03 *Acoustic neuritis in infectious and parasitic diseases classified elsewhere, bilateral*

Chapter 8
H60-H95

4 4th digit required 5 5th digit required 6 6th digit required 7 7th digit required 7th digit placeholder + Additional code Laterality

5 **H94.8 Other specified disorders of ear in diseases classified elsewhere**
Code first underlying disease, such as:
congenital syphilis (A50.0)
EXCLUDES 1 aural myiasis (B87.4)
syphilitic labyrinthitis (A52.79)

IQ **H94.80 Other specified disorders of ear in diseases classified elsewhere, unspecified ear**

IQ **H94.81 Other specified disorders of right ear in diseases classified elsewhere**

IQ **H94.82 Other specified disorders of left ear in diseases classified elsewhere**

IQ **H94.83 Other specified disorders of ear in diseases classified elsewhere, bilateral**

Intraoperative and postprocedural complications and disorders of ear and mastoid process, not elsewhere classified (H95)

4 **H95 Intraoperative and postprocedural complications and disorders of ear and mastoid process, not elsewhere classified**

5 **H95.0 Recurrent cholesteatoma of postmastoidectomy cavity**

IQ **H95.00 Recurrent cholesteatoma of postmastoidectomy cavity, unspecified ear**

SP **H95.01 Recurrent cholesteatoma of postmastoidectomy cavity, right ear**

SP **H95.02 Recurrent cholesteatoma of postmastoidectomy cavity, left ear**

SP **H95.03 Recurrent cholesteatoma of postmastoidectomy cavity, bilateral ears**

5 **H95.1 Other disorders of ear and mastoid process following mastoidectomy**

6 **H95.11 Chronic inflammation of postmastoidectomy cavity**

SP **H95.111 Chronic inflammation of postmastoidectomy cavity, right ear**

SP **H95.112 Chronic inflammation of postmastoidectomy cavity, left ear**

SP **H95.113 Chronic inflammation of postmastoidectomy cavity, bilateral ears**

IQ **H95.119 Chronic inflammation of postmastoidectomy cavity, unspecified ear**

6 **H95.12 Granulation of postmastoidectomy cavity**

SP **H95.121 Granulation of postmastoidectomy cavity, right ear**

SP **H95.122 Granulation of postmastoidectomy cavity, left ear**

SP **H95.123 Granulation of postmastoidectomy cavity, bilateral ears**

IQ **H95.129 Granulation of postmastoidectomy cavity, unspecified ear**

6 **H95.13 Mucosal cyst of postmastoidectomy cavity**

SP **H95.131 Mucosal cyst of postmastoidectomy cavity, right ear**

SP **H95.132 Mucosal cyst of postmastoidectomy cavity, left ear**

SP **H95.133 Mucosal cyst of postmastoidectomy cavity, bilateral ears**

IQ **H95.139 Mucosal cyst of postmastoidectomy cavity, unspecified ear**

6 **H95.19 Other disorders following mastoidectomy**

SP **H95.191 Other disorders following mastoidectomy, right ear**

SP **H95.192 Other disorders following mastoidectomy, left ear**

SP **H95.193 Other disorders following mastoidectomy, bilateral ears**

IQ **H95.199 Other disorders following mastoidectomy, unspecified ear**

5 **H95.2 Intraoperative hemorrhage and hematoma of ear and mastoid process complicating a procedure**
EXCLUDES 1 intraoperative hemorrhage and hematoma of ear and mastoid process due to accidental puncture or laceration during a procedure (H95.3-)

SP **H95.21 Intraoperative hemorrhage and hematoma of ear and mastoid process complicating a procedure on the ear and mastoid process**

SP **H95.22 Intraoperative hemorrhage and hematoma of ear and mastoid process complicating other procedure**

5 **H95.3 Accidental puncture and laceration of ear and mastoid process during a procedure**

SP **H95.31 Accidental puncture and laceration of the ear and mastoid process during a procedure on the ear and mastoid process**

SP **H95.32 Accidental puncture and laceration of the ear and mastoid process during other procedure**

5 **H95.4 Postprocedural hemorrhage of ear and mastoid process following a procedure**

SP **H95.41 Postprocedural hemorrhage of ear and mastoid process following a procedure on the ear and mastoid process**

SP **H95.42 Postprocedural hemorrhage of ear and mastoid process following other procedure**

5 **H95.5 Postprocedural hematoma and seroma of ear and mastoid process following a procedure**

SP **H95.51 Postprocedural hematoma of ear and mastoid process following a procedure on the ear and mastoid process**

SP **H95.52 Postprocedural hematoma of ear and mastoid process following other procedure**

SP **H95.53 Postprocedural seroma of ear and mastoid process following a procedure on the ear and mastoid process**

SP **H95.54 Postprocedural seroma of ear and mastoid process following other procedure**

5 **H95.8 Other intraoperative and postprocedural complications and disorders of the ear and mastoid process, not elsewhere classified**

EXCLUDES 2 postprocedural complications and disorders following mastoidectomy (H95.0-, H95.1-)

6 **H95.81 Postprocedural stenosis of external ear canal**

Laterality SP **H95.811 Postprocedural stenosis of right external ear canal**

Laterality SP **H95.812 Postprocedural stenosis of left external ear canal**

Laterality SP **H95.813 Postprocedural stenosis of external ear canal, bilateral**

Laterality IQ **H95.819 Postprocedural stenosis of unspecified external ear canal**

SP + **H95.88 Other intraoperative complications and disorders of the ear and mastoid process, not elsewhere classified**

Use additional code, if applicable, to further specify disorder

SP + **H95.89 Other postprocedural complications and disorders of the ear and mastoid process, not elsewhere classified**

Use additional code, if applicable, to further specify disorder

Chapter 8 Scenarios: Diseases of the ear and mastoid process (H60-H95)

Surgical aftercare, vertigo

A 70-year-old man recently underwent joint replacement surgery on his left hip. He had bilateral osteoarthritis in his hips and will have the other hip replaced later on. While in the hospital, he was diagnosed with severe benign paroxysmal positional vertigo. He is admitted to home health for aftercare, including physical and occupational therapy. The home health physical therapist will help him with exercises designed to ease the vertigo symptoms.

Description	Code
Primary: Aftercare following joint replacement surgery	Z47.1
Secondary: Unilateral primary osteoarthritis, right hip	M16.11
Secondary: Benign paroxysmal vertigo, unspecified ear	H81.10
Secondary: Presence of left artificial hip joint	Z96.642

Surgical aftercare is the focus of care, making Z47.1 the appropriate primary code choice. The patient had bilateral osteoarthritis, but since one hip has been replaced, it is resolved on that side. Thus, unilateral hip osteoarthritis is coded instead, in accordance with coding guidelines. The patient's vertigo is specified as benign paroxysmal positional but the ear was not specified, making the correct diagnosis code H81.10. The status code Z96.642 is assigned to identify the joint that was replaced, in accordance with tabular instruction.

Malignant otitis externa, type 1 diabetes

A 68-year-old woman who is a type 1 diabetic comes to home health with a diagnosis of malignant otitis externa in bilateral ears. The record indicates the infecting organism is pseudomonas aeruginosa. She is quadriplegic and unable to self administer the ear drops prescribed. Skilled nursing has been ordered and will provide four planned visits to instruct the caregiver in administration of the drops and prevention of further infection.

Description	Code
Primary: Malignant otitis externa, bilateral	H60.23
Secondary: Pseudomonas (aeruginosa) (mallei) (pseudomallei) as the cause of diseases classified elsewhere	B96.5
Secondary: Type 1 diabetes mellitus without complications	E10.9
Secondary: Quadriplegia, unspecified	G82.50

The infection is the focus of care and is coded primary. The infecting organism immediately follows it. No code for insulin use is assigned because the patient is a type 1 diabetic and insulin dependence is inherent. An additional code for quadriplegia is assigned as this condition impacts her plan of care and provides important comorbidity adjustment.

Ototoxic hearing loss, ankylosing spondylitis

A 66-year-old man with ankylosing spondylitis is suffering from hearing loss in both ears following the completion of treatment with gentamicin for a severe infection which is now resolved. The physician confirms that the hearing loss is a lingering adverse effect of the gentamicin, which was stopped several weeks ago and is no longer in his system. The focus of care is the hearing loss and the patient will receive occupational therapy.

Description	Code
Primary: Ototoxic hearing loss, bilateral	H91.03
Secondary: Adverse effect of aminoglycosides, sequela	T36.5x5S
Secondary: Ankylosing spondylitis of unspecified sites in spine	M45.9

The focus of care is the hearing loss, which is appropriately coded as ototoxic hearing loss, and placed in the primary position. The adverse effect code for the gentamicin is coded following the code for the problem it caused, in accordance with tabular instruction. The seventh character is "S" because the drug is no longer in his system but has left behind a lingering effect. No code for the infection is assigned as it is now resolved. His ankylosing spondylitis is a relevant comorbidity that will impact his recovery and is thus also coded.

Chapter 9: Diseases of the Circulatory System (I00-I99)

Chapter 9 includes the following blocks:

- I00-I02 Acute rheumatic fever
- I05-I09 Chronic rheumatic heart disease
- I10-I16 Hypertensive diseases
- I20-I25 Ischemic heart disease
- I26-I28 Pulmonary heart disease and diseases of pulmonary circulation
- I30-I5A Other forms of heart disease
- I60-I69 Cerebrovascular diseases
- I70-I79 Diseases of arteries, arterioles, and capillaries
- I80-I89 Diseases of veins, lymphatic vessels and lymph nodes, not elsewhere classified.
- I95-I99 Other and unspecified disorders of the circulatory system

Documentation is critically important in coding for conditions in this chapter. Do not try to decipher the condition from the physician's notes. Rather, ask for additional documentation when necessary. Below are some examples of situations and questions to ask when attempting to obtain additional documentation.

Documentation stating **"atrioventricular block"** (I44 category) means occlusion of the chambers within the heart, but more information is needed, such as is the block first or second degree; does it involve the left or right bundle branches (which transmit electricity throughout the heart), or another type of conduction disorder.

Documentation stating **"heart failure"** (I50 category) means that the heart is not able to pump sufficient blood to the body, but more information is needed, such as is it left-sided failure; is it systolic (contraction phase of heartbeat) failure or diastolic (relaxation phase) failure or both; is it congestive heart failure (the blood backs up into the lungs and the tissues of organs and the legs); is it acute, chronic or acute on chronic failure.

Documentation stating **"atherosclerosis"** (I70 category) means hardening of the arteries, but more information is needed, such as is it a native artery or a graft (autologous, nonautologous, biological, nonbiological, or other type) from a bypass surgery; which artery is affected; what side is affected; is there any intermittent claudication, rest pain, ulceration, or gangrene present. ***Note,*** the ICD-10 classification assumes a relationship between atherosclerosis of lower extremities and gangrene, ulceration, rest pain and intermittent claudication.

Circulatory organs and functions tie into nearly all other systems so you will find close linkages to other ICD-10-CM chapters. For instance, the respiratory system carries oxygen to the bloodstream and removes excess carbon dioxide from the body (related codes can be found in Chapter 10, diseases of the respiratory system). Other conditions of the lymphatic system are found throughout the book, depending on the location of the lymph node involved and whether it is a site of a tumor (Chapter 2) or infection (Chapter 1).

Conditions related to the blood or blood-forming organs such as anemias, coagulation deficits, neutropenia, disorders of the spleen are reported using codes from Chapter 3 (Diseases of the Blood and Blood-Forming Organs and Certain Disorders Involving the Immune Mechanism).

As is the case with other ICD-10-CM codes, in certain situations you will need to look beyond this chapter to properly code a case. For example:

- If the documentation indicates **a neoplasm or tumor of an organ in the circulatory system,** look up the term (malignancy, tumor, adenoma) to find the correct code, likely a code from Chapter 2 (C00-D49).
- If a patient has **a personal or family history** of a condition reported in this chapter, it may be appropriate to select from the Z code section, such as Z86.7- (Diseases of circulatory system), or Z82.3 (Family history of stroke).
- If a condition reported in this chapter is the **result of injury, poisoning, or certain other consequences of external causes,** a code from Chapter 19 (S00-T88), may be reported with a code from this chapter.
- **Symptoms, signs and abnormal clinical and laboratory findings** related to the circulatory system are sometimes reported using codes from Chapter 18 (R00-R94) such as R09.89 (Symptoms involving cardiovascular system). Every effort should be made to secure a definitive diagnosis. A symptom code from Chapter 18 may be reported as an additional diagnosis when it describes a significant aspect of the condition but is not an integral part of it.
- Although not often coded in home health, if reporting a circulatory disease in a **pregnant patient** when the condition is complicating the pregnancy, report first a code from Chapter 15 (Pregnancy, childbirth and the puerperium), such as O99.411 (Diseases of the circulatory system complicating pregnancy, first trimester).

A code from Chapter 16, Certain conditions originating in the perinatal period (P00-P96), and codes from Chapter 17, Congenital malformations, deformations, and chromosomal abnormalities (Q00-Q99) are not included in codes in this chapter, but may be used as additional codes to describe the patient's situation.

- Additional disorders and conditions that may be present along with a code within this chapter, but are not included in this chapter include endocrine, nutritional and metabolic diseases (E00-E88) in chapter 4; and systemic connective tissue disorders (M30-M36) in chapter 13. Follow the Tabular directions for sequencing these conditions along with a code from chapter 9.

Multiple Coding and Sequencing

It is important to read the Includes and Excludes notes under codes in this chapter, as well as any other instructions under the code or code category. There are many combination codes in chapter 9, which will decrease the need for multiple codes to be assigned.

If heart disease is caused by an infection, be sure to start your search in the Alphabetical Index under the key term 'pericarditis, inflammation of the pericardium,' and confirm the code in the Tabular List after reading all notes. For example, acute pericarditis due to tuberculosis is reported as A18.84 (tuberculosis of the heart), which includes tuberculosis pericarditis as well as several other cardiac conditions. Code I32 (pericarditis in diseases classified elsewhere) is a manifestation code with an Excludes 1 note for tuberculosis pericarditis so the A18.84 code is the only code needed. However, if a patient has staphylococcal pericarditis, the first listed code would be I30.1 (Infective pericarditis) with an additional code of B95.7 (Other staphylococcus as the cause of diseases classified elsewhere) from Chapter 1. However, if the diagnostic statement or confirmation from the physician indicated the pericarditis was due to methicillin susceptible Staphylococcus aureus, code B95.61 (MSSA infection as the cause of diseases classified elsewhere) would be the choice for the additional code.

Category I50 is used to report **heart failure**. There are multiple types of heart failure, such as left sided, systolic, diastolic, combined systolic and diastolic, and right sided failure that can be unspecified, acute, chronic or acute on chronic.

Code I50.1, left-sided heart failure, includes acute pulmonary edema; no additional code needs to be assigned. Never use I50.1 and I50.9 on the same claim.

Code I50.2 indicates systolic heart failure, which is a decrease in the heart's ability to contract. The heart is unable to pump with enough force to push a sufficient amount of blood into the circulation. Systolic heart failure is coded when the documentation indicates HFrEF, which may also be called heart failure with low ejection fraction, or heart failure with reduced systolic function, or other similar terms meaning systolic heart failure. But remember, do not code systolic failure based on ejection fraction numbers without physician interpretation.

Code I50.3 indicates diastolic heart failure, which occurs when the heart has a problem relaxing. Ventricles are not filling during diastole. All codes for heart failure include any associated pulmonary edema. Diastolic heart failure is coded when the documentation indicates HFpEF, which may also be referred to as heart failure with preserved systolic function, and this condition may also be referred to as diastolic heart failure. Do not code diastolic failure based on ejection fraction numbers without physician interpretation.

Diastolic dysfunction or systolic dysfunction is coded to I51.89 if not related to heart failure. If related to heart failure, then diastolic heart failure or systolic heart failure should be coded.

Category I70 is used to report **atherosclerosis**. Within this category, several codes may be appropriate to assign – both from this category and from other chapters. There is a note to use additional codes with I70 to identify: exposure to environmental tobacco smoke (Z77.22), history of tobacco dependence (Z87.891), occupational exposure to environmental tobacco smoke (Z57.31), tobacco dependence (F17.-) and tobacco use (Z72.0).

Take note of the following circumstances:

- Within specific subcategories of atherosclerosis, there are additional code notes. For example, atherosclerosis of native arteries of the extremities (I70.2-) includes a note to add an additional code, if applicable, to identify chronic total occlusion of artery of an extremity (I70.92). Characters 4, 5 and 6 for I70.- codes identify laterality and additional conditions that may be present such as intermittent claudication, rest pain, presence and location of ulceration, and the presence of gangrene. Codes that indicate ulceration also include a note to add an additional code to identify the severity of any ulcer (L98.49-), if applicable.
- Additional codes in category I70.2 to I70.7 utilize expanded subcategories to identify the atherosclerosis of unspecified type of bypass graft(s)(170.3-); autologous vein bypass graft (I70.4-); nonautologous biological bypass graft(s), (I70.5-); nonbiological bypass graft(s) (I70.6); and other type of bypass graft, (I70.7-) of the extremities.

These are useful terms to know when reviewing documentation related to circulatory disorders:

- Ischemia – decreased blood flow
- Embolism – a clot traveling through the circulatory system
- Infarction – halted blood flow resulting in cellular death
- Occlusion– blockage
- Stenosis – narrowing
- Thrombus – blood clot
- Hemorrhage – heavy or uncontrolled bleeding.

One more pointer: You'll often see the prefixes "epi" and "sub" applied to the anatomical parts. Just remember that "epi" means "upon" and "sub" means "under." Thus, "subarachnoid" means under the arachnoid layer of the meninges.

Special Coding Issues

Hypertension

Hypertensive diseases are organized under one block (I10-I16). Pay attention to the note at the top of the category to use additional codes to identify exposure to environmental tobacco smoke, history of tobacco dependence, occupational exposure to environmental tobacco smoke, tobacco dependence and tobacco use.

The most challenging part of coding for hypertension is establishing its relationship with other conditions. **Remember**, the classification presumes a causal relationship between hypertension and heart involvement and between hypertension and kidney involvement, as the two conditions are linked by the term "with" in the Alphabetic Index. These conditions should be coded as related even in the absence of provider documentation explicitly linking them, unless the documentation clearly states the conditions are unrelated. More specifically:

- **Hypertensive heart disease:** Hypertension with heart conditions classified to I50.-, and I51.4-I51.9, are assigned to a code from category I11 (Hypertensive heart disease) when both conditions are present in the documentation. A cause-and-effect relationship is assumed by the ICD-10 classification system unless the provider states otherwise. If there is uncertainty about the relationship, always query the physician. The hypertensive disease is sequenced first and an additional code is used to identify the specific type(s) of heart disease/failure. If the provider states there is not a relationship between the two conditions, report separate codes for the hypertension and the heart condition in either order based on the impact of each condition on the plan of care.
- **Hypertensive chronic kidney disease:** Report the hypertensive chronic kidney disease (category I12) whether or not a causal relationship is stated in the documentation. Coding Guidelines instruct that you can assume that if both these conditions are present, they are related. You should also report an additional code from category N18 (chronic kidney disease). The classification assumes a relationship between HTN and any condition classifiable to N18 (CKD) and N26. The relationship may be assumed because of the pathology of hypertension, which impacts renal function, often resulting in CKD. However, CKD should not be coded as hypertensive if the physician has specifically documented a different cause. Do not confuse hypertensive chronic kidney disease with renovascular hypertension, a condition in which the kidney dysfunction causes the hypertension. Renovascular hypertension is coded using I15.0.
- **Hypertensive heart and chronic kidney disease (CKD):** Report the hypertensive heart and chronic kidney disease (category I13) when all conditions are present in the documentation. A cause-and-effect relationship is assumed by the ICD-10 classification system unless the provider states otherwise. If there is uncertainty about the relationship, always query the physician. The relationship between the hypertension, heart disease and the chronic kidney disease is presumed by the ICD-10 classification systsem. If heart failure is present, report additional code(s) from category I50 (heart failure) to identify the type(s) of heart failure, and category N18 (chronic kidney disease) to identify the stage of the CKD.

  Example: Patient with CKD stage 3 unspecified, CHF and hypertension is coded as I13.0, I50.9, N18.30.
- **Hypertensive cerebrovascular disease:** An appropriate code from categories I60-I69 (cerebrovascular disease) is assigned first, followed by the appropriate hypertension code from I10-I16.
- **Hypertensiye retinopathy:** Subcategory H35.0 (Background retinopathy and retinal vascular changes) is coded first followed by a code from hypertension category I10 – I16.
- **Hypertension, secondary:** Secondary hypertension is due to an underlying condition. Two codes are required to describe this condition. A code to identify the underlying etiology and a code from category I15, (Secondary hypertension). The actual sequence of the two codes is determined by the reason for admission/encounter.
- **Hypertension transient:** Code R03.0, Elevated blood pressure reading without a diagnosis, is coded unless a patient has an established diagnosis of hypertension.

- **Gestational (pregnancy-induced) hypertension** without significant proteinuria (O13.-), or preeclampsia (O14.-) is coded for transient hypertension associated with pregnancy.
- **Hypertension, controlled** as a diagnosis statement usually refers to an existing state of hypertension under control by therapy. Choose the appropriate code from categories I10-I16 (Hypertensive disease) to describe this situation.
- **Hypertension, uncontrolled** may refer to untreated hypertension or hypertension not responding to current therapeutic regimen. In either case, the appropriate code from categories I10-I16 (Hypertensive disease) is assigned and the terms controlled or uncontrolled do not have any impact on the code assigned. Additional documentation may be included in the medical record to provide this information.
- **Hypertensive Crisis** is assigned with a code from category I16 for documented hypertensive urgency, hypertensive emergency or unspecified hypertensive crisis. Code also any identified hypertensive disease (I10-I15). The sequencing is based on the reason for the encounter.

Atherosclerotic Coronary Artery Disease and Angina

ICD-10-CM has combination codes for atherosclerotic heart disease with angina pectoris: Subcategory I25.11-, Atherosclerotic heart disease of native coronary artery with angina pectoris, and I25.7-, Atherosclerosis of coronary artery bypass graft(s) and coronary artery of transplanted heart with angina pectoris. An additional code for angina pectoris is **not necessary** when using one of these combination codes.

A causal relationship can be assumed in a patient with both atherosclerosis and angina pectoris unless the documentation indicates the angina is due to something other than the atherosclerosis.

If a patient with coronary artery disease is admitted due to an acute myocardial infarction (AMI), the AMI should be sequenced before the coronary artery disease.

CVA

Several conditions, such as a head injury, tumor of the brain or spinal cord, or an infection of the CNS, present with symptoms identical to those found in what a lay person would call "stroke." The symptoms include: weakness, paralysis of facial muscles, clumsiness, paresthesia (numbness), hemiplegia (paralysis in one or both limbs on the same side), loss of sensation, inability to eat or talk, loss of vision or partial vision in one or both eyes, double vision, memory loss, and/or vertigo.

When a physician sees these symptoms, he or she may document the rather generic term "CVA," or "cerebrovascular accident." The acute stage of the condition, reported with codes I60-I63, occurs when brain cells die due to a clot or bleeding in the brain that cuts off the oxygen supply. The acute stage is treated in an inpatient facility, such as with tissue plasminogen activator (t-PA), in order to resolve the clot.

When applicable, use a code from R29.7 to indicate the National Institutes of Health Stroke Scale (NIHSS) score. The NIHSS score can be used as a clinical stroke assessment tool to evaluate and document neurological status in acute stroke patients. The stroke scale is valid for predicting lesion size and can serve as a measure of stroke severity. The NIHSS has been shown to be a predictor of both short and long term outcome of stroke patients.

Sequelae or "late-effects" category I69 includes neurological deficits that persist after the initial onset of conditions classifiable to categories I60-I67. The neurologic deficits caused by cerebrovascular disease may be present from the onset or may arise at any time after the onset of the condition classifiable to I60-I67. You may assign as many of the combination codes in I69 that apply.

Codes from I69 (Sequelae of cerebrovascular disease) that specify hemiplegia, hemiparesis and monoplegia identify whether the dominant or nondominant side is affected. Should the affected side be documented, but not specified as dominant or non-dominant, and the classification system does not indicate a default, code selection is as follows:

- For ambidextrous patients, the default should be dominant.
- If the left side is affected, the default is nondominant.
- If the right side is affected, the default is dominant.

I69 (Sequelae of cerebrovascular disease) codes may be assigned on a health care record **with** codes from I60 – I67, **if** the patient has a current cerebrovascular disease and deficits from an old cerebrovascular disease. However, codes from I69 should not be assigned if the patient does not have neurologic deficits; instead assign Z86.73 (Personal history of TIA and cerebral infarction).

MI

Acute myocardial infarction (AMI) results from a blocked coronary artery that supplies oxygenated blood to a part of the heart's muscle. Interruption of blood and oxygen to the heart muscle causes injury or death of the affected heart muscle tissue. Blockage of a coronary artery that results in a myocardial infarction may be caused by a blood clot due to the rupture of atherosclerotic plaque within arterial walls which causes a blood clot at the site. Other causes of blockage may be mural thrombosis, vegetative endocarditis, or atherosclerotic plaque buildup. A rarer cause of heart attack is spasm of the coronary artery that can prevent blood flow as a result of drug use, such as cocaine.

Types of myocardial infarction:

Transmural infarctions extend through the entire thickness of heart muscle from endocardium to epicardium in the left ventricular wall. These are further classified by site, such as anteriolateral wall or true posterior wall, and are due to complete occlusion of blood supply in the area.

- **STEMI** (ST segment elevation myocardial infarction), the more severe type of MI, occurs when a coronary artery is totally occluded by a blood clot and virtually all the heart muscle dependent on blood supply by that particular artery begins to die. This is a transmural infarction, also known as a Q-wave MI. The ST segment elevation indicates that a large amount of damage to the heart muscle is occurring.

Subendocardial infarctions involve small, multifocal areas of necrosis confined to the inner portion of the wall of the left ventricle, ventricular septum, or papillary muscles and are thought to result from decreased blood supply locally, usually due to narrowing of the vessels.

- **NSTEMI** (non-ST segment elevation myocardial infarction) is a milder form of infarction in which the coronary artery is only partially occluded and only the inner portion of the heart muscle supplied by the coronary artery dies.

The ICD-10-CM codes for type 1 acute myocardial infarction (AMI) identify the site, such as anterolateral wall or true posterior wall. Subcategories I21.0-I21.2 and code I21.3 are used for type 1 ST elevation myocardial infarction (STEMI). Code I21.4, Non-ST elevation (NSTEMI) myocardial infarction, is used for type 1 non ST elevation myocardial infarction (NSTEMI) and nontransmural MIs.

General Guidelines:

- If a type 1 NSTEMI evolves to STEMI, assign the STEMI code.
- If a type 1 STEMI converts to NSTEMI due to thrombolytic therapy, it is still coded as a STEMI.
- If an AMI is documented as nontransmural or subendocardial, but the site is provided, it is still coded as a subendocardial AMI.
- For encounters occurring while the myocardial infarction is equal to, or less than, four weeks old, (including transfers to another acute care setting or a post-acute setting), and the patient requires continued care for the myocardial infarction, you may continue to report codes from category I21.
- For encounters after the four week time frame and the patient is still receiving care related to the myocardial infarction, the appropriate aftercare code should be assigned rather than a code from category I21. For old or healed MIs, not requiring further care, code I25.2 (Old myocardial infarction) may be assigned.
- Code I21.9 is the default for unspecified acute myocardial infarction or unspecified type. Assign I21.3 if only type 1 STEMI or transmural MI without the site is documented.

Subsequent Acute MI:

Assign a code from category I22 when a patient who has suffered a type 1 or unspecified AMI has a new AMI within the 4 week time frame of the initial AMI. Use a code from category I22 with a code from category I21. The sequencing of the I22 and I21 codes depends on the circumstances of the encounter.

Do not assign I22 for subsequent myocardial infarctions other than type 1 or unspecified. For subsequent type 2 AMI assign only assign I21.A1. For subsequent type 4 or type 5 AMI, assign only I21.A9, per coding guidelines.

Other Types of Myocardial Infarction:

There are options for different types of myocardial infarction. Type 1 myocardial infarctions are assigned to codes I21.0-I21.4. Type 2 myocardial infarction (myocardial infarction due to demand ischemia or secondary to ischemic imbalance), is assigned to code I21.A1.

When a type 2 AMI code is described as NSTEMI or STEMI, only assign code I21.A1. Codes I21.01-I21.4 should only be assigned for type 1 AMIs.

Acute myocardial infarctions type 3, 4a, 4b, 4c and 5 are assigned to code I21.A9, Other myocardial infarction type.

CHAPTER 9: DISEASES OF THE CIRCULATORY SYSTEM (I00-I99)

EXCLUDES 2 certain conditions originating in the perinatal period (P04-P96)
certain infectious and parasitic diseases (A00-B99)
complications of pregnancy, childbirth and the puerperium (O00-O9A)
congenital malformations, deformations, and chromosomal abnormalities (Q00-Q99)
endocrine, nutritional and metabolic diseases (E00-E88)
injury, poisoning and certain other consequences of external causes (S00-T88)
neoplasms (C00-D49)
symptoms, signs and abnormal clinical and laboratory findings, not elsewhere classified (R00-R94)
systemic connective tissue disorders (M30-M36)
transient cerebral ischemic attacks and related syndromes (G45.-)

This chapter contains the following blocks:

I00-I02 Acute rheumatic fever
I05-I09 Chronic rheumatic heart diseases
I10-I16 Hypertensive diseases
I20-I25 Ischemic heart diseases
I26-I28 Pulmonary heart disease and diseases of pulmonary circulation
I30-I5A Other forms of heart disease
I60-I69 Cerebrovascular diseases
I70-I79 Diseases of arteries, arterioles and capillaries
I80-I89 Diseases of veins, lymphatic vessels and lymph nodes, not elsewhere classified
I95-I99 Other and unspecified disorders of the circulatory system

Acute rheumatic fever (I00-I02)

SP **I00 Rheumatic fever without heart involvement**
INCLUDES arthritis, rheumatic, acute or subacute
EXCLUDES 1 rheumatic fever with heart involvement (I01.0 -I01.9)
DEFINITION Delayed, febrile, inflammatory disease resulting about 20 days after streptococcal infection; presents with joint pain, migratory arthritis, skin rash on the trunk and proximal extremities, and nosebleeds; can cause cardiac damage.

4 **I01 Rheumatic fever with heart involvement**
EXCLUDES 1 chronic diseases of rheumatic origin (I05-I09) unless rheumatic fever is also present or there is evidence of reactivation or activity of the rheumatic process.
CODING TIPS ✓ Pericarditis, endocarditis, and myocarditis are coded with I01-I02 when specified as rheumatic, or associated with rheumatic fever.

SP **I01.0 Acute rheumatic pericarditis**
Any condition in I00 with pericarditis
Rheumatic pericarditis (acute)
EXCLUDES 1 acute pericarditis not specified as rheumatic (I30.-)

SP **I01.1 Acute rheumatic endocarditis**
Any condition in I00 with endocarditis or valvulitis
Acute rheumatic valvulitis

SP **I01.2 Acute rheumatic myocarditis**
Any condition in I00 with myocarditis

SP **I01.8 Other acute rheumatic heart disease**
Any condition in I00 with other or multiple types of heart involvement
Acute rheumatic pancarditis

SP **I01.9 Acute rheumatic heart disease, unspecified**
Any condition in I00 with unspecified type of heart involvement
Rheumatic carditis, acute
Rheumatic heart disease, active or acute

4 **I02 Rheumatic chorea**
INCLUDES Sydenham's chorea
EXCLUDES 1 chorea NOS (G25.5)
Huntington's chorea (G10)
CODING TIPS ✓ Pericarditis, endocarditis, and myocarditis are coded with I01-I02 when specified as rheumatic, or associated with rheumatic fever.
CODING TIPS ✓ Rheumatic chorea may also be referred to as "St. Vitus dance" and is more frequently diagnosed in children and adolescents.

SP **I02.0 Rheumatic chorea with heart involvement**
Chorea NOS with heart involvement
Rheumatic chorea with heart involvement of any type classifiable under I01.-

SP **I02.9 Rheumatic chorea without heart involvement**
Rheumatic chorea NOS

Chronic rheumatic heart diseases (I05-I09)

CODING TIPS ✓ Category I05 -I09 includes disease of the heart valves. Diseases of the mitral and tricuspid heart valves are considered rheumatic, unless specified by the physician or NPP as nonrheumatic. Aortic and pulmonary heart valve disease is considered nonrheumatic, unless specified as rheumatic. If multiple valves are involved, ICD-10-CM classifies the disease as rheumatic, unless specified by the physician or NPP as non-rheumatic. Pay special attention to includes and excludes 1 notes.

4 **I05 Rheumatic mitral valve diseases**
INCLUDES conditions classifiable to both I05.0 and I05.2-I05.9, whether specified as rheumatic or not
EXCLUDES 1 mitral valve disease specified as nonrheumatic (I34.-)
mitral valve disease with aortic and/or tricuspid valve involvement (I08.-)
CODING TIPS ✓ Mitral valve disease is assumed to be rheumatic unless specified by the physician or NPP as nonrheumatic.

SP **I05.0 Rheumatic mitral stenosis**
Mitral (valve) obstruction (rheumatic)

SP **I05.1 Rheumatic mitral insufficiency**
Rheumatic mitral incompetence
Rheumatic mitral regurgitation

EXCLUDES 1 mitral insufficiency not specified as rheumatic (I34.0)

SP **I05.2 Rheumatic mitral stenosis with insufficiency**
Rheumatic mitral stenosis with incompetence or regurgitation

SP **I05.8 Other rheumatic mitral valve diseases**
Rheumatic mitral (valve) failure

SP **I05.9 Rheumatic mitral valve disease, unspecified**
Rheumatic mitral (valve) disorder (chronic) NOS

4 **I06 Rheumatic aortic valve diseases**
EXCLUDES 1 aortic valve disease not specified as rheumatic (I35.-)
aortic valve disease with mitral and/or tricuspid valve involvement (I08.-)

CODING TIPS✓ Aortic valve disease specified as rheumatic is coded to I06. If not specified as rheumatic, see I35.

SP **I06.0 Rheumatic aortic stenosis**
Rheumatic aortic (valve) obstruction

SP **I06.1 Rheumatic aortic insufficiency**
Rheumatic aortic incompetence
Rheumatic aortic regurgitation

SP **I06.2 Rheumatic aortic stenosis with insufficiency**
Rheumatic aortic stenosis with incompetence or regurgitation

SP **I06.8 Other rheumatic aortic valve diseases**

SP **I06.9 Rheumatic aortic valve disease, unspecified**
Rheumatic aortic (valve) disease NOS

4 **I07 Rheumatic tricuspid valve diseases**
INCLUDES rheumatic tricuspid valve diseases specified as rheumatic or unspecified
EXCLUDES 1 tricuspid valve disease specified as nonrheumatic (I36.-)
tricuspid valve disease with aortic and/or mitral valve involvement (I08.-)

CODING TIPS✓ Tricuspid valve disease is assumed to be rheumatic unless specified as nonrheumatic.

SP **I07.0 Rheumatic tricuspid stenosis**
Tricuspid (valve) stenosis (rheumatic)

SP **I07.1 Rheumatic tricuspid insufficiency**
Tricuspid (valve) insufficiency (rheumatic)

SP **I07.2 Rheumatic tricuspid stenosis and insufficiency**

SP **I07.8 Other rheumatic tricuspid valve diseases**

SP **I07.9 Rheumatic tricuspid valve disease, unspecified**
Rheumatic tricuspid valve disorder NOS

4 **I08 Multiple valve diseases**
INCLUDES multiple valve diseases specified as rheumatic or unspecified
EXCLUDES 1 endocarditis, valve unspecified (I38)
multiple valve disease specified a nonrheumatic (I34.-, I35.-, I36.-, I37.-, I38.-, Q22.-, Q23.-, Q24.8-)
rheumatic valve disease NOS (I09.1)

CODING TIPS✓ Valve disease involving multiple valves is assumed to be rheumatic unless specified as nonrheumatic. Aortic valve disease, by itself, is considered nonrheumatic, unless specified as rheumatic. When aortic valve disease is combined with other heart valves, it is considered rheumatic.

SP **I08.0 Rheumatic disorders of both mitral and aortic valves**
Involvement of both mitral and aortic valves specified as rheumatic or unspecified

CODING TIPS✓ Assign I08.0 for a diagnosis of aortic valve stenosis with mitral valve insufficiency.

SP **I08.1 Rheumatic disorders of both mitral and tricuspid valves**

SP **I08.2 Rheumatic disorders of both aortic and tricuspid valves**

SP **I08.3 Combined rheumatic disorders of mitral, aortic and tricuspid valves**

SP **I08.8 Other rheumatic multiple valve diseases**

CODING TIPS✓ When the clinical record reports rheumatic disease of multiple valves but the descriptions in I08.0, .1, .2 or .3 do not apply, e.g., pulmonary valve along with other specified valves, use I08.8.

SP **I08.9 Rheumatic multiple valve disease, unspecified**

CODING TIPS✓ When the clinical record reports rheumatic disease of multiple valves, but the affected valves are not specified, assign code I08.9.

4 **I09 Other rheumatic heart diseases**

SP **I09.0 Rheumatic myocarditis**
EXCLUDES 1 myocarditis not specified as rheumatic (I51.4)

DEFINITION Chronic inflammation and degeneration of heart muscle due to rheumatic heart disease.

SP **I09.1 Rheumatic diseases of endocardium, valve unspecified**
Rheumatic endocarditis (chronic)
Rheumatic valvulitis (chronic)
EXCLUDES 1 endocarditis, valve unspecified (I38)

SP **I09.2 Chronic rheumatic pericarditis**
Adherent pericardium, rheumatic
Chronic rheumatic mediastinopericarditis
Chronic rheumatic myopericarditis
EXCLUDES 1 chronic pericarditis not specified as rheumatic (I31.-)

5 **I09.8 Other specified rheumatic heart diseases**

SP SH SL + **I09.81 Rheumatic heart failure**
Use additional code to identify type of heart failure (I50.-)

CODING TIPS✓ A diagnosis of heart failure in a patient when documented as related to rheumatic heart disease (severe rheumatic damage to heart valves) is assigned code I09.81 along with a code from I50 to identify the type of heart failure.

DEFINITION Severe rheumatic damage to heart valves causing heart failure.

SP **I09.89 Other specified rheumatic heart diseases**
Rheumatic disease of pulmonary valve

SP **I09.9 Rheumatic heart disease, unspecified**
Rheumatic carditis
EXCLUDES 1 rheumatoid carditis (M05.31)

Hypertensive diseases (I10-I16)

Use additional code to identify:
exposure to environmental tobacco smoke (Z77.22)
history of tobacco dependence (Z87.891)
occupational exposure to environmental tobacco smoke (Z57.31)
tobacco dependence (F17.-)
tobacco use (Z72.0)

EXCLUDES 1 neonatal hypertension (P29.2)
primary pulmonary hypertension (I27.0)

EXCLUDES 2 hypertensive disease complicating pregnancy, childbirth and the puerperium (O10-O11, O13-O16)

GUIDELINES **Section I.C.9.a.**
The classification presumes a causal relationship between hypertension and heart involvement and between hypertension and kidney involvement, as the two conditions are linked by the term “with” in the Alphabetic Index. These conditions should be coded as related even in the absence of provider documentation explicitly linking them, unless the documentation clearly states the conditions are unrelated.
For hypertension and conditions not specifically linked by relational terms such as “with,” “associated with” or “due to” in the classification, provider documentation must link the conditions in order to code them as related.

CODING TIPS✓ Essential hypertension (I10-I13) and pulmonary hypertension (I27) are two different types of hypertension. Essential hypertension, also known as 'high blood pressure' and 'systemic hypertension,' refers to the pressure throughout your body; whereas pulmonary hypertension is high blood pressure that occurs in the arteries in the lungs.

CODING TIPS✓ Arterial, malignant, benign, and unspecified essential hypertension are included in these codes as nonessential modifiers.

SP **I10 Essential (primary) hypertension**
INCLUDES high blood pressure
hypertension (arterial) (benign) (essential) (malignant) (primary) (systemic)
EXCLUDES 1 hypertensive disease complicating pregnancy, childbirth and the puerperium (O10-O11, O13-O16)
EXCLUDES 2 essential (primary) hypertension involving vessels of brain (I60-I69)
essential (primary) hypertension involving vessels of eye (H35.0-)

CODING TIPS✓ Essential hypertension is appropriate when no documentation is present indicating the presence of chronic kidney disease (CKD) or heart disease coded as I51.4-I51.7, I51.89, I51.9 and I50.-. If CKD or heart disease coded as I51.4-I51.7, I51.89, I51.9 and I50 are present, I10 is not the correct hypertension code. I10 is only correct in these circumstances if the physician or NPP documented that the hypertension **was not related** to CKD or the named heart conditions.

4 **I11 Hypertensive heart disease**
INCLUDES any condition in I50.- or I51.4-I51.7, I51.89, I51.9 due to hypertension

GUIDELINES **Section I.C.9.a.1)**
Hypertension with heart conditions classified to I50.- or I51.4-I51.7, I51.89, I51.9, are assigned to a code from category I11, Hypertensive heart disease. Use additional code(s) from category I50, Heart failure, to identify the type(s) of heart failure in those patients with heart failure.

The same heart conditions (I50.-, I51.4-I51.7, I51.89, I51.9) with hypertension are coded separately if the provider has documented they are unrelated to the hypertension. Sequence according to the circumstances of the admission/encounter.

CODING TIPS✓ Heart failure (I50.-) and heart conditions included in I51.4-I51.7, I51.89, I51.9 are assumed related to hypertension. The heart conditions in I51.4-I51.7, I51.89, I51.9 are included in I11 and are not coded separately. The code for the heart failure should be added, when heart failure is present. No other heart conditions are assumed related to hypertension. Takotsubo Syndrome (I51.81) is by definition stress related and therefore should not be coded with I11.9, per CC Q2 2018.

SP SH SL + **I11.0 Hypertensive heart disease with heart failure**
Hypertensive heart failure
Use additional code to identify type of heart failure (I50.-)

SP **I11.9 Hypertensive heart disease without heart failure**
Hypertensive heart disease NOS

4 **I12 Hypertensive chronic kidney disease**
INCLUDES any condition in N18 and N26 - due to hypertension
arteriosclerosis of kidney
arteriosclerotic nephritis (chronic) (interstitial)
hypertensive nephropathy
nephrosclerosis
EXCLUDES 1 hypertension due to kidney disease (I15.0, I15.1)
renovascular hypertension (I15.0)
secondary hypertension (I15.-)
EXCLUDES 2 acute kidney failure (N17.-)

GUIDELINES **Section I.C.9.a.2)**
Assign codes from category I12, Hypertensive chronic kidney disease, when both hypertension and a condition classifiable to category N18, Chronic kidney disease (CKD), are present. CKD should not be coded as hypertensive if the provider indicates the CKD is not related to the hypertension.
The appropriate code from category N18 should be used as a secondary code with a code from category I12 to identify the stage of chronic kidney disease. See Section I.C.14. Chronic kidney disease.
If a patient has hypertensive chronic kidney disease and acute renal failure, the acute renal failure should also be coded. Sequence according to the circumstances of the admission/encounter.

CODING TIPS✓ I12 is coded followed by the appropriate code from N18 to indicate the stage of CKD. If renal sclerosis is documented, use I12.9 and do not code the renal sclerosis as it is considered included in I12.

CODING TIPS✓ When diabetes, CKD and HTN are documented, sequence the appropriate category of diabetes with CKD (E--.22) and the appropriate hypertension code (I12 or I13) prior to N18. Either the hypertension or the diabetes may be sequenced first. Both diabetes and hypertension are coded as related to the CKD, unless the physician has clearly documented that one condition is not related to the CKD. An example of that documentation, is if the physician or NPP states hypertensive CKD or diabetic CKD. If that type of documentation is absent, all three conditions are assumed related.

CODING TIPS✓ The I12 classification assumes a relationship between HTN and any condition classifiable to N18 (CKD) and N26. The classification assumes the relationship because of the pathology of hypertension, which impacts renal function, often resulting in CKD. Do not confuse hypertensive chronic kidney disease with renovascular hypertension, a condition in which the kidney dysfunction causes the hypertension. Renovascular hypertension is coded using I15.0.

H SP SH SL + **I12.0 Hypertensive chronic kidney disease with stage 5 chronic kidney disease or end stage renal disease**
Use additional code to identify the stage of chronic kidney disease (N18.5, N18.6)

SP SH SL + **I12.9 Hypertensive chronic kidney disease with stage 1 through stage 4 chronic kidney disease, or unspecified chronic kidney disease**
Hypertensive chronic kidney disease NOS
Hypertensive renal disease NOS
Use additional code to identify the stage of chronic kidney disease (N18.1-N18.4, N18.9)

4 **I13 Hypertensive heart and chronic kidney disease**
INCLUDES any condition in I11.- with any condition in I12.-
cardiorenal disease
cardiovascular renal disease

GUIDELINES **Section I.C.9.a.3)**
Assign codes from combination category I13, Hypertensive heart and chronic kidney disease, when there is hypertension with both heart and kidney involvement. If heart failure is present, assign an additional code from category I50 to identify the type of heart failure.

The appropriate code from category N18, Chronic kidney disease, should be used as a secondary code with a code from category I13 to identify the stage of chronic kidney disease.

The codes in category I13 are combination codes that include hypertension, heart disease and chronic kidney disease. The Includes note at I13 specifies that the conditions included at I11 and I12 are included together in I13. If a patient has hypertension, heart disease and chronic kidney disease, then a code from I13 should be used, not individual codes for hypertension, heart disease and chronic kidney disease, or codes from I11 or I12. For patients with both acute renal failure and chronic kidney disease, the acute renal failure should also be coded. Sequence according to the circumstances of the admission/encounter.

CODING TIPS✓ Heart failure (I50.-) and conditions included in I51.4-I51.7, I51.89, I51.9 are assumed related to hypertension. CKD is assumed related to hypertension. I13 is a combination code that includes the hypertensive heart disease and the hypertensive chronic kidney disease. Do not code I51.4-I51.7, I51.89, I51.9 in addition to I13 as the conditions are already included. The code for the heart failure should be added, if present. The code for the CKD should be added.

CODING TIPS✓ When diabetes, CKD and HTN are documented, sequence the appropriate category of diabetes with CKD (E--.22) and the appropriate hypertension code (I12 or I13) prior to N18. Either the hypertension or the diabetes may be sequenced first. Both diabetes and hypertension are coded as related to the CKD, unless the physician has clearly documented that one condition is not related to the CKD. An example of that documentation is if the physician or NPP states hypertensive CKD or diabetic CKD. If that type of documentation is absent, all three conditions are assumed related.

SP SH SL + **I13.0 Hypertensive heart and chronic kidney disease with heart failure and stage 1 through stage 4 chronic kidney disease, or unspecified chronic kidney disease**
Use additional code to identify type of heart failure (I50.-)
Use additional code to identify stage of chronic kidney disease (N18.1-N18.4, N18.9)

5 **I13.1 Hypertensive heart and chronic kidney disease without heart failure**

SP SH SL + I13.10 **Hypertensive heart and chronic kidney disease without heart failure, with stage 1 through stage 4 chronic kidney disease, or unspecified chronic kidney disease**

Hypertensive heart disease and hypertensive chronic kidney disease NOS

Use additional code to identify the stage of chronic kidney disease (N18.1-N18.4, N18.9)

SP SH SL + I13.11 **Hypertensive heart and chronic kidney disease without heart failure, with stage 5 chronic kidney disease, or end stage renal disease**

Use additional code to identify the stage of chronic kidney disease (N18.5, N18.6)

SP SH SL + I13.2 **Hypertensive heart and chronic kidney disease with heart failure and with stage 5 chronic kidney disease, or end stage renal disease**

Use additional code to identify type of heart failure (I50.-)

Use additional code to identify the stage of chronic kidney disease (N18.5, N18.6)

4 **I15 Secondary hypertension**

Code also:

underlying condition

EXCLUDES 1 postprocedural hypertension (I97.3)

EXCLUDES 2 secondary hypertension involving vessels of brain (I60-I69)

secondary hypertension involving vessels of eye (H35.0-)

GUIDELINES **Section I.C.9.a.6)**

Secondary hypertension is due to an underlying condition. Two codes are required: one to identify the underlying etiology and one from category I15 to identify the hypertension. Sequencing of codes is determined by the reason for admission/encounter.

CODING TIPS✓ It is more common for hypertension to cause the renal dysfunction, however when hypertension is confirmed caused by the kidney (renal) dysfunction, assign a code from I15.-.

SP **I15.0 Renovascular hypertension**

CODING TIPS✓ Do not confuse hypertensive chronic kidney disease with renovascular hypertension, a condition in which the kidney dysfunction causes the hypertension. When this is the case, the hypertension is secondary to the renal dysfunction and is coded using I15.0. The two conditions may be coded in either order.

SP **I15.1 Hypertension secondary to other renal disorders**

SP **I15.2 Hypertension secondary to endocrine disorders**

CODING TIPS✓ Assign I15.2 when hypertension is specified as due to Cushing's syndrome, primary aldosteronism, acromegaly, hypo/hyperthyroidism, or another specified endocrine disorder. Do not assign a code from I10-I13.0 when hypertension is specified as secondary to one of these causes.

SP **I15.8 Other secondary hypertension**

SP **I15.9 Secondary hypertension, unspecified**

4 **I16 Hypertensive crisis**

Code also:

any identified hypertensive disease (I10-I15)

GUIDELINES **Section I.C.9.a.10)**

Assign a code from category I16, Hypertensive crisis, for documented hypertensive urgency, hypertensive emergency or unspecified hypertensive crisis. Code also any identified hypertensive disease (I10-I15). The sequencing is based on the reason for the encounter.

SP **I16.0 Hypertensive urgency**

CODING TIPS✓ Code hypertensive urgency when documented by the physician or NPP. Hypertensive urgency is a systolic blood pressure greater than 180 or a diastolic pressure greater than 110, without associated progressive organ dysfunction. There may be associated severe headache, shortness of breath, nosebleeds, or severe anxiety.

SP **I16.1 Hypertensive emergency**

CODING TIPS✓ Code hypertensive emergency when documented by the physician or NPP. Hypertensive emergencies occur when blood pressure reaches levels that lead to impending or progressive organ damage. This usually involves blood pressure levels exceeding 180 systolic or 120 diastolic, but it can occur at even lower levels in patients whose blood pressure had not been previously high. Some potential consequences of uncontrolled blood pressure in this range include stroke, loss of consciousness, memory loss, acute myocardial infarction or angina, aortic dissection, damage to the eyes and kidneys, and pulmonary edema.

SP **I16.9 Hypertensive crisis, unspecified**

CODING TIPS✓ Use this code when the physician or NPP documents hypertensive crisis. Hypertensive crisis is when a patient has a systolic blood pressure greater than 180, or a diastolic pressure greater than 110, and it is unknown whether organ damage has occurred.

Ischemic heart diseases (I20-I25)

Code also:

the presence of hypertension (I10-I16)

CODING TIPS✓ Either the hypertension or the condition included in I20-I25 may be sequenced before the other. There is no longer a sequencing rule that applies. Coders should consider the focus of care and the documentation of the physician or NPP.

+ 4 I20 Angina pectoris

Use additional code to identify:
- exposure to environmental tobacco smoke (Z77.22)
- history of tobacco dependence (Z87.891)
- occupational exposure to environmental tobacco smoke (Z57.31)
- tobacco dependence (F17.-)
- tobacco use (Z72.0)

EXCLUDES 1 angina pectoris with atherosclerotic heart disease of native coronary arteries (I25.1-)
atherosclerosis of coronary artery bypass graft (s) and coronary artery of transplanted heart with angina pectoris (I25.7-)
postinfarction angina (I23.7)

GUIDELINES **Section I.C.9.b.** ICD-10-CM has combination codes for atherosclerotic heart disease with angina pectoris. The subcategories for these codes are I25.11, Atherosclerotic heart disease of native coronary artery with angina pectoris and I25.7, Atherosclerosis of coronary artery bypass graft(s) and coronary artery of transplanted heart with angina pectoris.
When using one of these combination codes it is not necessary to use an additional code for angina pectoris. A causal relationship can be assumed in a patient with both atherosclerosis and angina pectoris, unless the documentation indicates the angina is due to something other than the atherosclerosis. If a patient with coronary artery disease is admitted due to an acute myocardial infarction (AMI), the AMI should be sequenced before the coronary artery disease.

CODING TIPS✓ Do not assign a code from I20.- for a patient who also has coronary artery disease (CAD)/atherosclerotic heart disease (ASHD). Angina in a patient with CAD/ASHD should be coded to the appropriate I25.11- code.

SP SH + I20.0 Unstable angina
- Accelerated angina
- Crescendo angina
- De novo effort angina
- Intermediate coronary syndrome
- Preinfarction syndrome
- Worsening effort angina

CODING TIPS✓ Unstable angina is also known as angina at rest.

SP SH + I20.1 Angina pectoris with documented spasm
- Angiospastic angina
- Prinzmetal angina
- Spasm-induced angina
- Variant angina

SP SH + I20.8 Other forms of angina pectoris
- Angina equivalent
- Angina of effort
- Coronary slow flow syndrome
- Stenocardia
- Stable angina

Use additional code(s) for symptoms associated with angina equivalent

SP SH + I20.9 Angina pectoris, unspecified
- Angina NOS
- Anginal syndrome
- Cardiac angina
- Ischemic chest pain

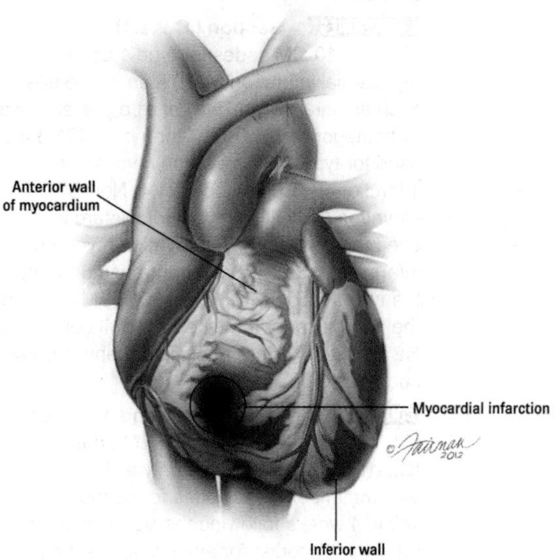

+ 4 I21 Acute myocardial infarction

INCLUDES cardiac infarction
coronary (artery) embolism
coronary (artery) occlusion
coronary (artery) rupture
coronary (artery) thrombosis
infarction of heart, myocardium, or ventricle
myocardial infarction specified as acute or with a stated duration of 4 weeks (28 days) or less from onset

Use additional code, if applicable, to identify:
- exposure to environmental tobacco smoke (Z77.22)
- history of tobacco dependence (Z87.891)
- occupational exposure to environmental tobacco smoke (Z57.31)
- status post administration of tPA (rtPA) in a different facility within the last 24 hours prior to admission to current facility (Z92.82)
- tobacco dependence (F17.-)
- tobacco use (Z72.0)

EXCLUDES 2 old myocardial infarction (I25.2)
postmyocardial infarction syndrome (I24.1)
subsequent type 1 myocardial infarction (I22.-)

GUIDELINES **Section I.C.9.e.4)**
If a subsequent myocardial infarction of one type occurs within 4 weeks of a myocardial infarction of a different type, assign the appropriate codes from category I21 to identify each type. Do not assign a code from I22. Codes from category I22 should only be assigned if both the initial and subsequent myocardial infarctions are type 1 or unspecified.

GUIDELINES **Section I.C.9.e.1)**
The ICD-10-CM codes for type 1 acute myocardial infarction (AMI) identify the site, such as anterolateral wall or true posterior wall. Subcategories I21.0-I21.2 and code I21.3 are used for type 1 ST elevation myocardial infarction (STEMI). Code I21.4, Non-ST elevation (NSTEMI) myocardial infarction, is used for type 1 non ST elevation myocardial infarction (NSTEMI) and nontransmural MIs. If a type 1 NSTEMI evolves to STEMI, assign the STEMI code. If a type 1 STEMI converts to NSTEMI due to thrombolytic therapy, it is still coded as STEMI.

CODING TIPS✓ When assigning any code from I21.- to report STEMI or NSTEMI, note that ICD-10 coding guidelines only allow assignment of these codes for admissions within 4 weeks following the occurrence of the MI. Use I22 codes for any subsequent MI during the same 4 weeks, if both the initial and subsequent MI were Type 1 or unspecified. After 4 weeks, assign I25.2 for the MI.

CODING TIPS✓ I21 codes specify STEMI or ST elevation myocardial infarction. If the physician or NPP has not documented STEMI, but has documented location, use the specific I21 code for that location. STEMI is more common than NSTEMI, and is the default.

+ 5 **I21.0 ST elevation (STEMI) myocardial infarction of anterior wall**
Type 1 ST elevation myocardial infarction of anterior wall

SP + **I21.01 ST elevation (STEMI) myocardial infarction involving left main coronary artery**

SP + **I21.02 ST elevation (STEMI) myocardial infarction involving left anterior descending coronary artery**
ST elevation (STEMI) myocardial infarction involving diagonal coronary artery

SP + **I21.09 ST elevation (STEMI) myocardial infarction involving other coronary artery of anterior wall**
Acute transmural myocardial infarction of anterior wall
Anteroapical transmural (Q wave) infarction (acute)
Anterolateral transmural (Q wave) infarction (acute)
Anteroseptal transmural (Q wave) infarction (acute)
Transmural (Q wave) infarction (acute) (of) anterior (wall) NOS

+ 5 **I21.1 ST elevation (STEMI) myocardial infarction of inferior wall**
Type 1 ST elevation myocardial infarction of inferior wall

SP + **I21.11 ST elevation (STEMI) myocardial infarction involving right coronary artery**
Inferoposterior transmural (Q wave) infarction (acute)

SP + **I21.19 ST elevation (STEMI) myocardial infarction involving other coronary artery of inferior wall**
Acute transmural myocardial infarction of inferior wall
Inferolateral transmural (Q wave) infarction (acute)
Transmural (Q wave) infarction (acute) (of) diaphragmatic wall
Transmural (Q wave) infarction (acute) (of) inferior (wall) NOS
EXCLUDES 2 ST elevation (STEMI) myocardial infarction involving left circumflex coronary artery (I21.21)

+ 5 **I21.2 ST elevation (STEMI) myocardial infarction of other sites**
Type 1 ST elevation myocardial infarction of other sites

SP + **I21.21 ST elevation (STEMI) myocardial infarction involving left circumflex coronary artery**
ST elevation (STEMI) myocardial infarction involving oblique marginal coronary artery

SP + **I21.29 ST elevation (STEMI) myocardial infarction involving other sites**
Acute transmural myocardial infarction of other sites
Apical-lateral transmural (Q wave) infarction (acute)
Basal-lateral transmural (Q wave) infarction (acute)
High lateral transmural (Q wave) infarction (acute)
Lateral (wall) NOS transmural (Q wave) infarction (acute)
Posterior (true) transmural (Q wave) infarction (acute)
Posterobasal transmural (Q wave) infarction (acute)
Posterolateral transmural (Q wave) infarction (acute)
Posteroseptal transmural (Q wave) infarction (acute)
Septal transmural (Q wave) infarction (acute) NOS

SP + **I21.3 ST elevation (STEMI) myocardial infarction of unspecified site**
Acute transmural myocardial infarction of unspecified site
Transmural (Q wave) myocardial infarction NOS
Type 1 ST elevation myocardial infarction of unspecified site
CODING TIPS✓ This code is used for a documented STEMI, but of unspecified location. Do not use this code for MI, NOS. Do not use this code if the physician or NPP has documented Type 2 MI.

SP + I21.4 Non-ST elevation (NSTEMI) myocardial infarction

Acute subendocardial myocardial infarction
Non-Q wave myocardial infarction NOS
Nontransmural myocardial infarction NOS
Type 1 non-ST elevation myocardial infarction

GUIDELINES Section I.C.9.e.1)
Code I21.4, Non-ST elevation (NSTEMI) myocardial infarction, is used for type 1 non ST elevation myocardial infarction (NSTEMI) and nontransmural MIs.

GUIDELINES Section I.C.9.e.3)
If an AMI is documented as nontransmural or subendocardial, but the site is provided, it is still coded as a subendocardial AMI.

SP + I21.9 Acute myocardial infarction, unspecified

Myocardial infarction (acute) NOS

GUIDELINES Section I.C.9.e.2)
Code I21.9, Acute myocardial infarction, unspecified, is the default for unspecified acute myocardial infarction or unspecified type. If only type 1 STEMI or transmural MI without the site is documented, assign code I21.3, ST elevation (STEMI) myocardial infarction of unspecified site.

CODING TIPS✓ This code is used for the initial MI when the physician has not documented the type or location of the infarct.

+ 5 I21.A Other type of myocardial infarction

CODING TIPS✓ There is no code for a subsequent MI of types 2, 3, 4, 5. Continue to use I21.A-, remembering that a code can only be used once on a POC/claim.

SP + I21.A1 Myocardial infarction type 2

Myocardial infarction due to demand ischemia
Myocardial infarction secondary to ischemic imbalance
Code first the underlying cause, such as:
- anemia (D50.0-D64.9)
- chronic obstructive pulmonary disease (J44.-)
- paroxysmal tachycardia (I47.0-I47.9)
- shock (R57.0-R57.9)

GUIDELINES Section I.C.9.e.5)
The ICD-10-CM provides codes for different types of myocardial infarction. Type 1 myocardial infarctions are assigned to codes I21.0-I21.4.
Type 2 myocardial infarction (myocardial infarction due to demand ischemia or secondary to ischemic imbalance) is assigned to code I21.A1, Myocardial infarction type 2 with a code for the underlying cause coded first. Do not assign code I24.8, Other forms of acute ischemic heart disease for the demand ischemia.
Acute myocardial infarctions type 3, 4a, 4b, 4c and 5 are assigned to code I21.A9, Other myocardial infarction type.
The "Code also" and "Code first" notes should be followed related to complications, and for coding of postprocedural myocardial infarctions during or following cardiac surgery.

CODING TIPS✓ When the physician or NPP documents Type 2 MI, assign I21.A1, even if the physician or NPP documents STEMI or NSTEMI. Type 2 MIs are not due to atherosclerotic plaque, but to a problem with supply and demand of oxygen. The documented cause of the problem should be coded first.

SP + I21.A9 Other myocardial infarction type

Myocardial infarction associated with revascularization procedure
Myocardial infarction type 3
Myocardial infarction type 4a
Myocardial infarction type 4b
Myocardial infarction type 4c
Myocardial infarction type 5
Code first:
- , if applicable, postprocedural myocardial infarction following cardiac surgery (I97.190) , or postprocedural myocardial infarction during cardiac surgery (I97.790)

Code also complication, if known and applicable, such as:
- (acute) stent occlusion (T82.897-)
- (acute) stent stenosis (T82.855-)
- (acute) stent thrombosis (T82.867-)
- cardiac arrest due to underlying cardiac condition (I46.2)
- complication of percutaneous coronary intervention (PCI) (I97.89)
- occlusion of coronary artery bypass graft (T82.218-)

+ 4 I22 Subsequent ST elevation (STEMI) and non-ST elevation (NSTEMI) myocardial infarction

INCLUDES acute myocardial infarction occurring within four weeks (28 days) of a previous acute myocardial infarction, regardless of site
cardiac infarction
coronary (artery) embolism

coronary (artery) occlusion
coronary (artery) rupture
coronary (artery) thrombosis
infarction of heart, myocardium, or ventricle
recurrent myocardial infarction
reinfarction of myocardium
rupture of heart, myocardium, or ventricle
subsequent type 1 myocardial infarction

Use additional code, if applicable, to identify:
exposure to environmental tobacco smoke (Z77.22)
history of tobacco dependence (Z87.891)
occupational exposure to environmental tobacco smoke (Z57.31)
status post administration of tPA (rtPA) in a different facility within the last 24 hours prior to admission to current facility (Z92.82)
tobacco dependence (F17.-)
tobacco use (Z72.0)

EXCLUDES 1 subsequent myocardial infarction, type 2 (I21.A1)
subsequent myocardial infarction of other type (type 3) (type 4) (type 5) (I21.A9)

GUIDELINES **Section I.C.9.e.4)**
If a subsequent myocardial infarction of one type occurs within 4 weeks of a myocardial infarction of a different type, assign the appropriate codes from category I21 to identify each type. Do not assign a code from I22. Codes from category I22 should only be assigned if both the initial and subsequent myocardial infarctions are type 1 or unspecified.

GUIDELINES Section I.C.9.e.4)
Do not assign code I22 for subsequent myocardial infarctions other than type 1 or unspecified. For subsequent type 2 AMI assign only code I21.A1. For subsequent type 4 or type 5 AMI, assign only code I21.A9.

CODING TIPS✓ When documentation reports an acute STEMI or NSTEMI occurring within 4 weeks following a prior acute STEMI or NSTEMI, a code from I22.- should be assigned. Codes from I22.- may be assigned for 4 weeks following the occurrence of the initial MI. If the time period since the initial MI (STEMI or NSTEMI) has been less than 4 weeks, then both a code for the initial MI (I21.-) and subsequent MI (I22.-) should be used. If the initial MI (STEMI or NSTEMI) occurred more than 4 weeks ago, then the initial MI cannot be coded as acute. The subsequent MI should be assigned with a code from I21.- to indicate the MI occurring within 4 weeks of admission to home health or hospice. The initial MI is coded as I25.2.

CODING TIPS✓ The term "subsequent" refers to another MI occurring within 4 weeks of the initial MI that was coded with I21, and not the location where the patient has been treated. Code I22 cannot be coded without an I21. If a patient is admitted within 4 weeks of a subsequent MI and the first MI can no longer be coded as acute, code the subsequent MI as I21 and the initial MI as I25.2.

CODING TIPS✓ I22 codes specify subsequent myocardial infarction. Even if the physician or NPP has not documented STEMI, but has documented location, use the specific I22 code for that location. Do not use I22 codes for Types 2, 3, 4, 5 MIs.

SP + **I22.0 Subsequent ST elevation (STEMI) myocardial infarction of anterior wall**
Subsequent acute transmural myocardial infarction of anterior wall
Subsequent transmural (Q wave) infarction (acute)(of) anterior (wall) NOS
Subsequent anteroapical transmural (Q wave) infarction (acute)
Subsequent anterolateral transmural (Q wave) infarction (acute)
Subsequent anteroseptal transmural (Q wave) infarction (acute)

SP + **I22.1 Subsequent ST elevation (STEMI) myocardial infarction of inferior wall**
Subsequent acute transmural myocardial infarction of inferior wall
Subsequent transmural (Q wave) infarction (acute)(of) diaphragmatic wall
Subsequent transmural (Q wave) infarction (acute)(of) inferior (wall) NOS
Subsequent inferolateral transmural (Q wave) infarction (acute)
Subsequent inferoposterior transmural (Q wave) infarction (acute)

SP + **I22.2 Subsequent non-ST elevation (NSTEMI) myocardial infarction**
Subsequent acute subendocardial myocardial infarction
Subsequent non-Q wave myocardial infarction NOS
Subsequent nontransmural myocardial infarction NOS

SP + **I22.8 Subsequent ST elevation (STEMI) myocardial infarction of other sites**
Subsequent acute transmural myocardial infarction of other sites
Subsequent apical-lateral transmural (Q wave) myocardial infarction (acute)
Subsequent basal-lateral transmural (Q wave) myocardial infarction (acute)
Subsequent high lateral transmural (Q wave) myocardial infarction (acute)
Subsequent transmural (Q wave) myocardial infarction (acute)(of) lateral (wall) NOS
Subsequent posterior (true) transmural (Q wave) myocardial infarction (acute)
Subsequent posterobasal transmural (Q wave) myocardial infarction (acute)
Subsequent posterolateral transmural (Q wave) myocardial infarction (acute)
Subsequent posteroseptal transmural (Q wave) myocardial infarction (acute)

Subsequent septal NOS transmural (Q wave) myocardial infarction (acute)

SP + **I22.9 Subsequent ST elevation (STEMI) myocardial infarction of unspecified site**

Subsequent acute myocardial infarction of unspecified site

Subsequent myocardial infarction (acute) NOS

CODING TIPS ✓ This code is used for the subsequent MI when the physician or NPP has not documented the location of the infarct, regardless of whether it is documented as a STEMI. Do not use I22 codes for types 2, 3, 4, 5 MIs.

4 **I23 Certain current complications following ST elevation (STEMI) and non-ST elevation (NSTEMI) myocardial infarction (within the 28 day period)**

CODING TIPS ✓ If a complication occurred after 4 weeks, you can assign a code from I23.-, without a code from I21 or I22. If the complication is post infarction angina and CAD is also present, then code both post infarction angina and CAD with I23.7 and I25.118. If the complication is post infarction angina and it occurs within the 4 weeks, then assign the I23.- code, I21 or I22, I25.118. Post infarction angina is a specific complication of a myocardial infarction and cannot be coded without physician or NPP documentation.

SP **I23.0 Hemopericardium as current complication following acute myocardial infarction**

EXCLUDES 1 hemopericardium not specified as current complication following acute myocardial infarction (I31.2)

CODING TIPS ✓ **Documentation**: Hemopericardium is frequently documented with cardiac wall rupture, including ventricular rupture, following MI, and results in pooling of blood in the pericardial space, leading to tamponade. This life-threatening condition may occur during or shortly after an MI.

SP **I23.1 Atrial septal defect as current complication following acute myocardial infarction**

EXCLUDES 1 acquired atrial septal defect not specified as current complication following acute myocardial infarction (I51.0)

SP **I23.2 Ventricular septal defect as current complication following acute myocardial infarction**

EXCLUDES 1 acquired ventricular septal defect not specified as current complication following acute myocardial infarction (I51.0)

SP **I23.3 Rupture of cardiac wall without hemopericardium as current complication following acute myocardial infarction**

SP **I23.4 Rupture of chordae tendineae as current complication following acute myocardial infarction**

EXCLUDES 1 rupture of chordae tendineae not specified as current complication following acute myocardial infarction (I51.1)

DEFINITION Tear in the fibrous, cord-like tissue connecting the papillary muscles to the valves, holding the valve flaps in place to prevent their eversion.

SP **I23.5 Rupture of papillary muscle as current complication following acute myocardial infarction**

EXCLUDES 1 rupture of papillary muscle not specified as current complication following acute myocardial infarction (I51.2)

SP **I23.6 Thrombosis of atrium, auricular appendage, and ventricle as current complications following acute myocardial infarction**

EXCLUDES 1 thrombosis of atrium, auricular appendage, and ventricle not specified as current complication following acute myocardial infarction (I51.3)

SP **I23.7 Postinfarction angina**

CODING TIPS ✓ If a complication occurred after 4 weeks, you can assign a code from I23.-, without a code from I21 or I22. If the complication is post infarction angina and CAD is also present, then code both post infarction angina and CAD with I23.7 and I25.118. If the complication is post infarction angina and it occurs within the 4 weeks, then assign the I23.- code, I21 or I22, I25.118. Post infarction angina is a specific complication of a myocardial infarction and cannot be coded without physician or NPP documentation.

SP **I23.8 Other current complications following acute myocardial infarction**

▲ 4 **I24 Other acute ischemic heart diseases**

EXCLUDES 1 angina pectoris (I20.-)
transient myocardial ischemia in newborn (P29.4)

EXCLUDES 2 non-ischemic myocardial injury (I5A)

SP SH **I24.0 Acute coronary thrombosis not resulting in myocardial infarction**

Acute coronary (artery) (vein) embolism not resulting in myocardial infarction

Acute coronary (artery) (vein) occlusion not resulting in myocardial infarction

Acute coronary (artery) (vein) thromboembolism not resulting in myocardial infarction

EXCLUDES 1 atherosclerotic heart disease (I25.1-)

SP SH **I24.1 Dressler's syndrome**

Postmyocardial infarction syndrome

EXCLUDES 1 postinfarction angina (I23.7)

Chapter 9

I00-I99

DEFINITION Fever, chest pain, pleuritis, and pericarditis weeks or months after heart injury caused by surgery or myocardial infarction.

SP SH **I24.8 Other forms of acute ischemic heart disease**

EXCLUDES 1 myocardial infarction due to demand ischemia (I21.A1)

SP SH **I24.9 Acute ischemic heart disease, unspecified**

EXCLUDES 1 ischemic heart disease (chronic) NOS (I25.9)

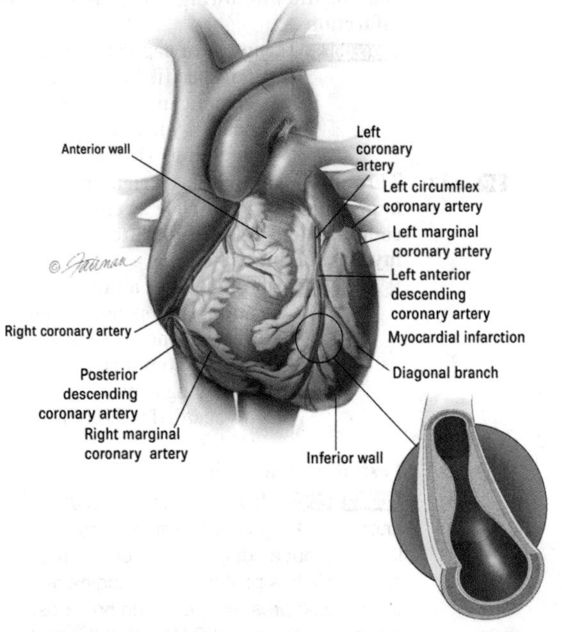

Coronary Artery Disease

▲+4 **I25 Chronic ischemic heart disease**

Use additional code to identify:
- chronic total occlusion of coronary artery (I25.82)
- exposure to environmental tobacco smoke (Z77.22)
- history of tobacco dependence (Z87.891)
- occupational exposure to environmental tobacco smoke (Z57.31)
- tobacco dependence (F17.-)
- tobacco use (Z72.0)

EXCLUDES 2 non-ischemic myocardial injury (I5A)

GUIDELINES **Section I.C.9.b**

ICD-10-CM has combination codes for atherosclerotic heart disease with angina pectoris. The subcategories for these codes are I25.11, Atherosclerotic heart disease of native coronary artery with angina pectoris, and I25.7, Atherosclerosis of coronary artery bypass graft(s) and coronary artery of transplanted heart with angina pectoris.

When using one of these combination codes it is not necessary to use an additional code for angina pectoris. A causal relationship can be assumed in a patient with both atherosclerosis and angina pectoris, unless the documentation indicates the angina is due to something other than the atherosclerosis.

CODING TIPS✓ When angina occurs with atherosclerotic heart disease, the type of angina is included in the code and is not coded separately with I20 codes.

+5 **I25.1 Atherosclerotic heart disease of native coronary artery**

Atherosclerotic cardiovascular disease
Coronary (artery) atheroma
Coronary (artery) atherosclerosis
Coronary (artery) disease
Coronary (artery) sclerosis

Use additional code, if applicable, to identify:
- coronary atherosclerosis due to calcified coronary lesion (I25.84)
- coronary atherosclerosis due to lipid rich plaque (I25.83)

EXCLUDES 2 atheroembolism (I75.-)
atherosclerosis of coronary artery bypass graft (s) and transplanted heart (I25.7-)

CODING TIPS✓ Atherosclerotic heart disease is coded to the native coronary arteries unless there is provider documentation indicating the ASHD of bypass grafts or transplanted hearts.

SP SH+ **I25.10 Atherosclerotic heart disease of native coronary artery without angina pectoris**

Atherosclerotic heart disease NOS

DEFINITION Clogging of coronary arteries with fatty plaque build-up, restricting blood flow and hardening the arteries.

+6 **I25.11 Atherosclerotic heart disease of native coronary artery with angina pectoris**

CODING TIPS✓ When a patient presents with both coronary artery disease (CAD) / atherosclerotic heart disease and angina, a code from I25.11- should be assigned. If the specific type of angina is not specified in the clinical record, assign code I25.119.

SP+ **I25.110 Atherosclerotic heart disease of native coronary artery with unstable angina pectoris**

EXCLUDES 1 unstable angina without atherosclerotic heart disease (I20.0)

CODING TIPS✓ A person with unstable angina is having chest pain at rest and is usually scheduled for an angioplasty or bypass. Unstable angina may be a home health/hospice diagnosis, if the patient is not a surgical candidate.

SP + **I25.111 Atherosclerotic heart disease of native coronary artery with angina pectoris with documented spasm**

EXCLUDES 1 angina pectoris with documented spasm without atherosclerotic heart disease (I20.1)

SP + **I25.118 Atherosclerotic heart disease of native coronary artery with other forms of angina pectoris**

EXCLUDES 1 other forms of angina pectoris without atherosclerotic heart disease (I20.8)

CODING TIPS✓ If a complication occurred after 4 weeks, you can assign a code from I23.-, without a code from I21 or I22. If the complication is post infarction angina and CAD is also present, then code both post infarction angina and CAD with I23.7 and I25.118. If the complication is post infarction angina and it occurs within the 4 weeks, then assign the I23.- code, I21 or I22, I25.118. Post infarction angina is a specific complication of a myocardial infarction and cannot be coded without physician or NPP documentation.

SP + **I25.119 Atherosclerotic heart disease of native coronary artery with unspecified angina pectoris**

Atherosclerotic heart disease with angina NOS

Atherosclerotic heart disease with ischemic chest pain

EXCLUDES 1 unspecified angina pectoris without atherosclerotic heart disease (I20.9)

IQ + **I25.2 Old myocardial infarction**

Healed myocardial infarction

Past myocardial infarction diagnosed by ECG or other investigation, but currently presenting no symptoms

GUIDELINES **Section I.C.9.e.1)**

For old or healed myocardial infarctions not requiring further care, code I25.2 may be assigned.

CODING TIPS✓ Assign code I25.2 (old MI) if a myocardial infarction is specified as: old (greater than 4 weeks after acute attack); healed and not currently presenting with symptoms. You can use this code when a patient has no residual effects of a previous MI, even when its presence shows up on the patient's EKG. If a myocardial infarction older than 4 weeks still requires care, assign Z51.89 and then I25.2. This care cannot be the primary reason for home care.

SP + **I25.3 Aneurysm of heart**

Mural aneurysm

Ventricular aneurysm

+ 5 **I25.4 Coronary artery aneurysm and dissection**

SP + **I25.41 Coronary artery aneurysm**

Coronary arteriovenous fistula, acquired

EXCLUDES 1 congenital coronary (artery) aneurysm (Q24.5)

SP + **I25.42 Coronary artery dissection**

SP + **I25.5 Ischemic cardiomyopathy**

EXCLUDES 2 coronary atherosclerosis (I25.1-, I25.7-)

SP + **I25.6 Silent myocardial ischemia**

+ 5 **I25.7 Atherosclerosis of coronary artery bypass graft(s) and coronary artery of transplanted heart with angina pectoris**

Use additional code, if applicable, to identify:

coronary atherosclerosis due to calcified coronary lesion (I25.84)

coronary atherosclerosis due to lipid rich plaque (I25.83)

EXCLUDES 1 atherosclerosis of bypass graft (s) of transplanted heart without angina pectoris (I25.812)

atherosclerosis of coronary artery bypass graft (s) without angina pectoris (I25.810)

atherosclerosis of native coronary artery of transplanted heart without angina pectoris (I25.811)

CODING TIPS✓ Atherosclerotic heart disease (ASHD) involving the bypass graft (as documented by the physician or NPP) is coded to I25.7. Do not use this code for ASHD for a patient that has had a bypass in the past unless there is specific documentation of the atherosclerosis being present in the bypass graft.

CODING TIPS✓ These codes indicate atherosclerotic plaque in the bypass artery or vein grafts. Restenosis of a stent is coded with a complication code.

+ 6 **I25.70 Atherosclerosis of coronary artery bypass graft(s), unspecified, with angina pectoris**

SP + **I25.700 Atherosclerosis of coronary artery bypass graft(s), unspecified, with unstable angina pectoris**

EXCLUDES 1 unstable angina pectoris without atherosclerosis of coronary artery bypass graft (I20.0)

SP + **I25.701 Atherosclerosis of coronary artery bypass graft(s), unspecified, with angina pectoris with documented spasm**

EXCLUDES 1 angina pectoris with documented spasm without atherosclerosis of coronary artery bypass graft (I20.1)

SP + **I25.708 Atherosclerosis of coronary artery bypass graft(s), unspecified, with other forms of angina pectoris**

EXCLUDES 1 other forms of angina pectoris without atherosclerosis of coronary artery bypass graft (I20.8)

SP + **I25.709 Atherosclerosis of coronary artery bypass graft(s), unspecified, with unspecified angina pectoris**

EXCLUDES 1 unspecified angina pectoris without atherosclerosis of coronary artery bypass graft (I20.9)

+ 6 **I25.71 Atherosclerosis of autologous vein coronary artery bypass graft(s) with angina pectoris**

SP + **I25.710 Atherosclerosis of autologous vein coronary artery bypass graft(s) with unstable angina pectoris**

EXCLUDES 1 unstable angina without atherosclerosis of autologous vein coronary artery bypass graft (s) (I20.0)

EXCLUDES 2 embolism or thrombus of coronary artery bypass graft (s) (T82.8-)

SP + **I25.711 Atherosclerosis of autologous vein coronary artery bypass graft(s) with angina pectoris with documented spasm**

EXCLUDES 1 angina pectoris with documented spasm without atherosclerosis of autologous vein coronary artery bypass graft (s) (I20.1)

SP + **I25.718 Atherosclerosis of autologous vein coronary artery bypass graft(s) with other forms of angina pectoris**

EXCLUDES 1 other forms of angina pectoris without atherosclerosis of autologous vein coronary artery bypass graft (s) (I20.8)

SP + **I25.719 Atherosclerosis of autologous vein coronary artery bypass graft(s) with unspecified angina pectoris**

EXCLUDES 1 unspecified angina pectoris without atherosclerosis of autologous vein coronary artery bypass graft (s) (I20.9)

+ 6 **I25.72 Atherosclerosis of autologous artery coronary artery bypass graft(s) with angina pectoris**

Atherosclerosis of internal mammary artery graft with angina pectoris

SP + **I25.720 Atherosclerosis of autologous artery coronary artery bypass graft(s) with unstable angina pectoris**

EXCLUDES 1 unstable angina without atherosclerosis of autologous artery coronary artery bypass graft (s) (I20.0)

SP + **I25.721 Atherosclerosis of autologous artery coronary artery bypass graft(s) with angina pectoris with documented spasm**

EXCLUDES 1 angina pectoris with documented spasm without atherosclerosis of autologous artery coronary artery bypass graft (s) (I20.1)

SP + **I25.728 Atherosclerosis of autologous artery coronary artery bypass graft(s) with other forms of angina pectoris**

EXCLUDES 1 other forms of angina pectoris without atherosclerosis of autologous artery coronary artery bypass graft (s) (I20.8)

SP + **I25.729 Atherosclerosis of autologous artery coronary artery bypass graft(s) with unspecified angina pectoris**

EXCLUDES 1 unspecified angina pectoris without atherosclerosis of autologous artery coronary artery bypass graft (s) (I20.9)

+ 6 **I25.73 Atherosclerosis of nonautologous biological coronary artery bypass graft(s) with angina pectoris**

SP + **I25.730 Atherosclerosis of nonautologous biological coronary artery bypass graft(s) with unstable angina pectoris**

EXCLUDES 1 unstable angina without atherosclerosis of nonautologous biological coronary artery bypass graft (s) (I20.0)

SP + **I25.731 Atherosclerosis of nonautologous biological coronary artery bypass graft(s) with angina pectoris with documented spasm**

EXCLUDES 1 angina pectoris with documented spasm without atherosclerosis of nonautologous biological coronary artery bypass graft (s) (I20.1)

SP + **I25.738 Atherosclerosis of nonautologous biological coronary artery bypass graft(s) with other forms of angina pectoris**

EXCLUDES 1 other forms of angina pectoris without atherosclerosis of nonautologous biological coronary artery bypass graft (s) (I20.8)

SP + **I25.739 Atherosclerosis of nonautologous biological coronary artery bypass graft(s) with unspecified angina pectoris**

EXCLUDES 1 unspecified angina pectoris without atherosclerosis of nonautologous biological coronary artery bypass graft (s) (I20.9)

+ 6 **I25.75 Atherosclerosis of native coronary artery of transplanted heart with angina pectoris**

EXCLUDES 1 atherosclerosis of native coronary artery of transplanted heart without angina pectoris (I25.811)

SP + **I25.750 Atherosclerosis of native coronary artery of transplanted heart with unstable angina**

SP + **I25.751 Atherosclerosis of native coronary artery of transplanted heart with angina pectoris with documented spasm**

SP + **I25.758 Atherosclerosis of native coronary artery of transplanted heart with other forms of angina pectoris**

SP + **I25.759 Atherosclerosis of native coronary artery of transplanted heart with unspecified angina pectoris**

+ 6 **I25.76 Atherosclerosis of bypass graft of coronary artery of transplanted heart with angina pectoris**

EXCLUDES 1 atherosclerosis of bypass graft of coronary artery of transplanted heart without angina pectoris (I25.812)

SP + **I25.760 Atherosclerosis of bypass graft of coronary artery of transplanted heart with unstable angina**

SP + **I25.761 Atherosclerosis of bypass graft of coronary artery of transplanted heart with angina pectoris with documented spasm**

SP + **I25.768 Atherosclerosis of bypass graft of coronary artery of transplanted heart with other forms of angina pectoris**

SP + **I25.769 Atherosclerosis of bypass graft of coronary artery of transplanted heart with unspecified angina pectoris**

+ 6 **I25.79 Atherosclerosis of other coronary artery bypass graft(s) with angina pectoris**

SP + **I25.790 Atherosclerosis of other coronary artery bypass graft(s) with unstable angina pectoris**

EXCLUDES 1 unstable angina without atherosclerosis of other coronary artery bypass graft (s) (I20.0)

SP + **I25.791 Atherosclerosis of other coronary artery bypass graft(s) with angina pectoris with documented spasm**

EXCLUDES 1 angina pectoris with documented spasm without atherosclerosis of other coronary artery bypass graft (s) (I20.1)

SP + **I25.798 Atherosclerosis of other coronary artery bypass graft(s) with other forms of angina pectoris**

EXCLUDES 1 other forms of angina pectoris without atherosclerosis of other coronary artery bypass graft (s) (I20.8)

SP + **I25.799 Atherosclerosis of other coronary artery bypass graft(s) with unspecified angina pectoris**

EXCLUDES 1 unspecified angina pectoris without atherosclerosis of other coronary artery bypass graft (s) (I20.9)

+ 5 I25.8 Other forms of chronic ischemic heart disease

+ 6 I25.81 Atherosclerosis of other coronary vessels without angina pectoris

Use additional code, if applicable, to identify:
coronary atherosclerosis due to calcified coronary lesion (I25.84)
coronary atherosclerosis due to lipid rich plaque (I25.83)

EXCLUDES 2 atherosclerotic heart disease of native coronary artery without angina pectoris (I25.10)

SP + I25.810 Atherosclerosis of coronary artery bypass graft(s) without angina pectoris

Atherosclerosis of coronary artery bypass graft NOS

EXCLUDES 1 atherosclerosis of coronary bypass graft (s) with angina pectoris (I25.70-I25.73-, I25.79-)

SP + I25.811 Atherosclerosis of native coronary artery of transplanted heart without angina pectoris

Atherosclerosis of native coronary artery of transplanted heart NOS

EXCLUDES 1 atherosclerosis of native coronary artery of transplanted heart with angina pectoris (I25.75-)

SP + I25.812 Atherosclerosis of bypass graft of coronary artery of transplanted heart without angina pectoris

Atherosclerosis of bypass graft of transplanted heart NOS

EXCLUDES 1 atherosclerosis of bypass graft of transplanted heart with angina pectoris (I25.76)

IQ + I25.82 Chronic total occlusion of coronary artery

Complete occlusion of coronary artery
Total occlusion of coronary artery
Code first:
coronary atherosclerosis (I25.1-, I25.7-, I25.81-)

EXCLUDES 1 acute coronary occlusion with myocardial infarction (I21.0-I21.9, I22.-)
acute coronary occlusion without myocardial infarction (I24.0)

IQ + I25.83 Coronary atherosclerosis due to lipid rich plaque

Code first:
coronary atherosclerosis (I25.1-, I25.7-, I25.81-)

IQ + I25.84 Coronary atherosclerosis due to calcified coronary lesion

Coronary atherosclerosis due to severely calcified coronary lesion
Code first:
coronary atherosclerosis (I25.1-, I25.7-, I25.81-)

CODING TIPS✓ Calcified lesions are more difficult to treat with angioplasty and stenting because the calcium deposits may block stents from reaching the desired location and may prevent the stent from fully expanding to the optimal size.

SP + I25.89 Other forms of chronic ischemic heart disease

SP + I25.9 Chronic ischemic heart disease, unspecified

Ischemic heart disease (chronic) NOS

Pulmonary heart disease and diseases of pulmonary circulation (I26-I28)

4 I26 Pulmonary embolism

INCLUDES pulmonary (acute) (artery)(vein) infarction
pulmonary (acute) (artery)(vein) thromboembolism
pulmonary (acute) (artery)(vein) thrombosis

EXCLUDES 2 chronic pulmonary embolism (I27.82)
personal history of pulmonary embolism (Z86.711)
pulmonary embolism complicating abortion, ectopic or molar pregnancy (O00-O07, O08.2)
pulmonary embolism complicating pregnancy, childbirth and the puerperium (O88.-)
pulmonary embolism due to trauma (T79.0, T79.1)
pulmonary embolism due to complications of surgical and medical care (T80.0, T81.7-, T82.8-)
septic (non-pulmonary) arterial embolism (I76)

CODING TIPS✓ Most patients are treated with anticoagulant therapy for an acute embolus for 3-6 months. Do not code chronic pulmonary embolism unless the physician or NPP documents chronic pulmonary embolism (I27.82). Assign Z86.711 for history of pulmonary embolism after 3-6 months if the physician or NPP has not documented chronic pulmonary embolism. Documentation indicating pulmonary embolism, without further information, is assigned I26.99.

5 I26.0 Pulmonary embolism with acute cor pulmonale

CODING TIPS✓ Category I26.0- codes should be assigned only when cor pulmonale is reported as occurring and associated with a pulmonary embolus. Cor pulmonale is a right ventricular dysfunction and failure.

IQ I26.01 Septic pulmonary embolism with acute cor pulmonale

Code first:
underlying infection

CODING TIPS✓ The term septic pulmonary embolism indicates a pulmonary embolus resulting from embolization of infectious particles which enter the lungs in the pulmonary arterial system. This can occur as a result of infectious DVT, periodontal disease, infected venous catheters, endocarditis, or other systemic infections. This code should only be assigned when the embolus is stated as septic and related to an infectious cause. A second code for the underlying/causative infection must be assigned.

SP I26.02 Saddle embolus of pulmonary artery with acute cor pulmonale

SP SL I26.09 Other pulmonary embolism with acute cor pulmonale

Acute cor pulmonale NOS

5 I26.9 Pulmonary embolism without acute cor pulmonale

IQ I26.90 Septic pulmonary embolism without acute cor pulmonale

Code first:
underlying infection

SP I26.92 Saddle embolus of pulmonary artery without acute cor pulmonale

SP SL I26.93 Single subsegmental pulmonary embolism without acute cor pulmonale

Subsegmental pulmonary embolism NOS

DEFINITION Subsegmental PE is defined as PE with no involvement of more proximal pulmonary arteries.

SP SL I26.94 Multiple subsegmental pulmonary emboli without acute cor pulmonale

DEFINITION Subsegmental PE is defined as PE with no involvement of more proximal pulmonary arteries.

SP SL I26.99 Other pulmonary embolism without acute cor pulmonale

Acute pulmonary embolism NOS
Pulmonary embolism NOS

CODING TIPS✓ Documentation indicating pulmonary embolism, without further information, is assigned I26.99.

4 I27 Other pulmonary heart diseases

GUIDELINES **Section I.C.9.a.11)**
Pulmonary hypertension is classified to category I27, Other pulmonary heart diseases. For secondary pulmonary hypertension (I27.1, I27.2-), code also any associated conditions or adverse effects of drugs or toxins. The sequencing is based on the reason for the encounter, except for adverse effects of drugs (See Section I.C.19.e.).

SP I27.0 Primary pulmonary hypertension

Heritable pulmonary arterial hypertension
Idiopathic pulmonary arterial hypertension
Primary group 1 pulmonary hypertension
Primary pulmonary arterial hypertension

EXCLUDES 1 persistent pulmonary hypertension of newborn (P29.30)
pulmonary hypertension NOS (I27.20)
secondary pulmonary arterial hypertension (I27.21)
secondary pulmonary hypertension (I27.29)

SP I27.1 Kyphoscoliotic heart disease

5 I27.2 Other secondary pulmonary hypertension

Code also:
associated underlying condition

EXCLUDES 1 Eisenmenger's syndrome (I27.83)

SP I27.20 Pulmonary hypertension, unspecified

Pulmonary hypertension NOS

SP I27.21 Secondary pulmonary arterial hypertension

(Associated) (drug-induced) (toxin-induced) pulmonary arterial hypertension NOS
(Associated) (drug-induced) (toxin-induced) (secondary) group 1 pulmonary hypertension

Code also associated conditions if applicable, or adverse effects of drugs or toxins, such as:
adverse effect of appetite depressants (T50.5X5)
congenital heart disease (Q20-Q28)
human immunodeficiency virus [HIV] disease (B20)
polymyositis (M33.2-)
portal hypertension (K76.6)
rheumatoid arthritis (M05.-)
schistosomiasis (B65.-)
Sjögren syndrome (M35.0-)
systemic sclerosis (M34.-)

SP I27.22 Pulmonary hypertension due to left heart disease

Group 2 pulmonary hypertension

Code also associated left heart disease, if known, such as:
multiple valve disease (I08.-)
rheumatic mitral valve diseases (I05.-)
rheumatic aortic valve diseases (I06.-)

SP I27.23 Pulmonary hypertension due to lung diseases and hypoxia

Group 3 pulmonary hypertension
Code also associated lung disease, if known, such as:
bronchiectasis (J47.-)
cystic fibrosis with pulmonary manifestations (E84.0)
interstitial lung disease (J84.-)
pleural effusion (J90)
sleep apnea (G47.3-)

SP **I27.24 Chronic thromboembolic pulmonary hypertension**
Group 4 pulmonary hypertension
Code also:
associated pulmonary embolism, if applicable (I26.-, I27.82)

SP **I27.29 Other secondary pulmonary hypertension**
Group 5 pulmonary hypertension
Pulmonary hypertension with unclear multifactorial mechanisms
Pulmonary hypertension due to hematologic disorders
Pulmonary hypertension due to metabolic disorders
Pulmonary hypertension due to other systemic disorders
Code also other associated disorders, if known, such as:
chronic myeloid leukemia (C92.10-C92.22)
essential thrombocythemia (D47.3)
Gaucher disease (E75.22)
hypertensive chronic kidney disease with end stage renal disease (I12.0, I13.11, I13.2)
hyperthyroidism (E05.-)
hypothyroidism (E00-E03)
polycythemia vera (D45)
sarcoidosis (D86.-)

5 **I27.8 Other specified pulmonary heart diseases**

SP **I27.81 Cor pulmonale (chronic)**
Cor pulmonale NOS
EXCLUDES 1 acute cor pulmonale (I26.0-)

SP + **I27.82 Chronic pulmonary embolism**
Use additional code, if applicable, for associated long-term (current) use of anticoagulants (Z79.01)
EXCLUDES 1 personal history of pulmonary embolism (Z86.711)

CODING TIPS Most acute pulmonary emboli do not cause chronic disease. Verify with physician whether chronic disease is being treated or if the patient is being treated prophylactically. Code chronic pulmonary embolism only if the physician has documented the pulmonary embolism as chronic. If treatment persists longer than 3-6 months after the acute pulmonary embolism, query the physician regarding chronicity. If not chronic, code Z86.711 for history of pulmonary embolism.

SP **I27.83 Eisenmenger's syndrome**
Eisenmenger's complex
(Irreversible) Eisenmenger's disease
Pulmonary hypertension with right to left shunt related to congenital heart disease
Code also underlying heart defect, if known, such as:
atrial septal defect (Q21.1)
Eisenmenger's defect (Q21.8)
patent ductus arteriosus (Q25.0)
ventricular septal defect (Q21.0)

SP **I27.89 Other specified pulmonary heart diseases**

SP **I27.9 Pulmonary heart disease, unspecified**
Chronic cardiopulmonary disease

4 **I28 Other diseases of pulmonary vessels**

SP **I28.0 Arteriovenous fistula of pulmonary vessels**
EXCLUDES 1 congenital arteriovenous fistula (Q25.72)

DEFINITION Abnormal passage between the pulmonary arterial and venous systems, which causes unoxygenated blood to enter systemic circulation.

SP **I28.1 Aneurysm of pulmonary artery**
EXCLUDES 1 congenital aneurysm (Q25.79)
congenital arteriovenous aneurysm (Q25.72)

DEFINITION Bulging in one portion of the arterial wall that brings blood to the lungs, forming a pouch or sac with the potential for rupture.

SP **I28.8 Other diseases of pulmonary vessels**
Pulmonary arteritis
Pulmonary endarteritis
Rupture of pulmonary vessels
Stenosis of pulmonary vessels
Stricture of pulmonary vessels

SP **I28.9 Disease of pulmonary vessels, unspecified**

Other forms of heart disease (I30-I5A)

CODING TIPS Pericarditis, endocarditis and myocarditis not specified as rheumatic are coded with these codes when a more specific code (such as meningococcal pericarditis) is not appropriate. Heart valve disease of the mitral and tricuspid valves are assumed rheumatic (I05 and I07), unless specified as nonrheumatic. Heart valve disease of the aortic and pulmonary valves are considered nonrheumatic, unless specified as rheumatic. Valve disease affecting multiple valves is considered rheumatic, unless specified by the physician or NPP as non-rheumatic. Pay special attention to includes and excludes 1 notes.

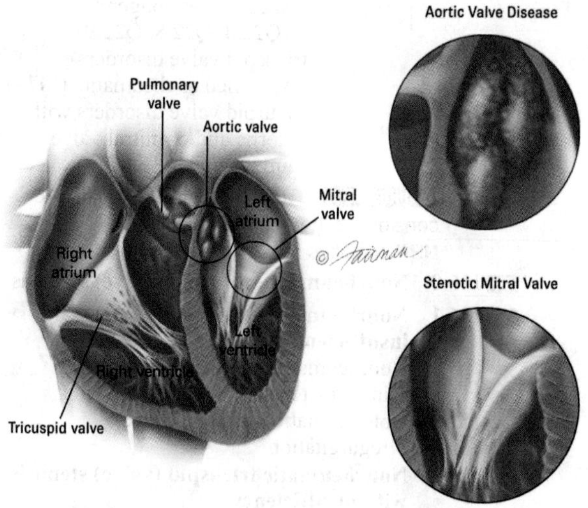

I30 Acute pericarditis
INCLUDES acute mediastinopericarditis
acute myopericarditis
acute pericardial effusion
acute pleuropericarditis
acute pneumopericarditis
EXCLUDES 1 Dressler's syndrome (I24.1)
rheumatic pericarditis (acute) (I01.0)
viral pericarditis due to Coxsakie virus (B33.23)

SP **I30.0 Acute nonspecific idiopathic pericarditis**

SP + **I30.1 Infective pericarditis**
Pneumococcal pericarditis
Pneumopyopericardium
Purulent pericarditis
Pyopericarditis
Pyopericardium
Pyopneumopericardium
Staphylococcal pericarditis
Streptococcal pericarditis
Suppurative pericarditis
Viral pericarditis
Use additional code (B95-B97) to identify infectious agent

SP **I30.8 Other forms of acute pericarditis**

SP **I30.9 Acute pericarditis, unspecified**

I31 Other diseases of pericardium
EXCLUDES 1 diseases of pericardium specified as rheumatic (I09.2)
postcardiotomy syndrome (I97.0)
traumatic injury to pericardium (S26.-)

SP **I31.0 Chronic adhesive pericarditis**
Accretio cordis
Adherent pericardium
Adhesive mediastinopericarditis
DEFINITION Pericardial inflammation with adhesion between the two pericardial layers or between the pericardium and the heart or neighboring structures.

SP **I31.1 Chronic constrictive pericarditis**
Concretio cordis
Pericardial calcification

SP **I31.2 Hemopericardium, not elsewhere classified**
EXCLUDES 1 hemopericardium as current complication following acute myocardial infarction (I23.0)
DEFINITION Bleeding causing the sac around the heart to fill with blood.

SP **I31.3 Pericardial effusion (noninflammatory)**
Chylopericardium
EXCLUDES 1 acute pericardial effusion (I30.9)

IQ **I31.4 Cardiac tamponade**
Code first:
underlying cause
DEFINITION Increased pressure on the heart due to fluid in the pericardial sac, impairing ventricular filling action and causing decreased cardiac output.

SP **I31.8 Other specified diseases of pericardium**
Epicardial plaques
Focal pericardial adhesions

SP **I31.9 Disease of pericardium, unspecified**
Pericarditis (chronic) NOS

M IQ ***I32 Pericarditis in diseases classified elsewhere***
Code first:
underlying disease
EXCLUDES 1 pericarditis (in):
coxsackie (virus) (B33.23)
gonococcal (A54.83)
meningococcal (A39.53)
rheumatoid (arthritis) (M05.31)
syphilitic (A52.06)
systemic lupus erythematosus (M32.12)
tuberculosis (A18.84)
DEFINITION Inflammation of the membranous sac around the heart occurring with another underlying disease process, causing chest pain, coughing, fatigue, and fever.

I33 Acute and subacute endocarditis
EXCLUDES 1 acute rheumatic endocarditis (I01.1)
endocarditis NOS (I38)

SP + **I33.0 Acute and subacute infective endocarditis**
Bacterial endocarditis (acute) (subacute)
Infective endocarditis (acute) (subacute) NOS
Endocarditis lenta (acute) (subacute)
Malignant endocarditis (acute) (subacute)
Purulent endocarditis (acute) (subacute)
Septic endocarditis (acute) (subacute)
Ulcerative endocarditis (acute) (subacute)
Vegetative endocarditis (acute) (subacute)
Use additional code (B95-B97) to identify infectious agent

SP **I33.9 Acute and subacute endocarditis, unspecified**
Acute endocarditis NOS
Acute myoendocarditis NOS
Acute periendocarditis NOS
Subacute endocarditis NOS
Subacute myoendocarditis NOS
Subacute periendocarditis NOS

4 I34 Nonrheumatic mitral valve disorders

EXCLUDES 1 mitral valve disease (I05.9)
mitral valve failure (I05.8)
mitral valve stenosis (I05.0)
mitral valve disorder of unspecified cause with diseases of aortic and/or tricuspid valve (s) (I08.-)
mitral valve disorder of unspecified cause with mitral stenosis or obstruction (I05.0)
mitral valve disorder specified as congenital (Q23.2, Q23.9)
mitral valve disorder specified as rheumatic (I05.-)

CODING TIPS✓ Mitral disorders are considered rheumatic unless the physician or NPP specifies non-rheumatic.

SP I34.0 Nonrheumatic mitral (valve) insufficiency
Nonrheumatic mitral (valve) incompetence NOS
Nonrheumatic mitral (valve) regurgitation NOS

SP I34.1 Nonrheumatic mitral (valve) prolapse
Floppy nonrheumatic mitral valve syndrome
EXCLUDES 1 Marfan's syndrome (Q87.4-)

SP I34.2 Nonrheumatic mitral (valve) stenosis

SP I34.8 Other nonrheumatic mitral valve disorders

SP I34.9 Nonrheumatic mitral valve disorder, unspecified

4 I35 Nonrheumatic aortic valve disorders

EXCLUDES 1 aortic valve disorder of unspecified cause but with diseases of mitral and/or tricuspid valve (s) (I08.-)
aortic valve disorder specified as congenital (Q23.0, Q23.1)
aortic valve disorder specified as rheumatic (I06.-)
hypertrophic subaortic stenosis (I42.1)

CODING TIPS✓ Aortic valve disorders are considered nonrheumatic, unless specified as rheumatic. If aortic valve disease exists with other heart valve disease, consider it rheumatic heart disease, unless specified as nonrheumatic multiple valve disease.

SP I35.0 Nonrheumatic aortic (valve) stenosis

SP I35.1 Nonrheumatic aortic (valve) insufficiency
Nonrheumatic aortic (valve) incompetence NOS
Nonrheumatic aortic (valve) regurgitation NOS

SP I35.2 Nonrheumatic aortic (valve) stenosis with insufficiency

SP I35.8 Other nonrheumatic aortic valve disorders

SP I35.9 Nonrheumatic aortic valve disorder, unspecified

4 I36 Nonrheumatic tricuspid valve disorders

EXCLUDES 1 tricuspid valve disorders of unspecified cause (I07.-)
tricuspid valve disorders specified as congenital (Q22.4, Q22.8, Q22.9)
tricuspid valve disorders specified as rheumatic (I07.-)
tricuspid valve disorders with aortic and/or mitral valve involvement (I08.-)

CODING TIPS✓ Tricuspid valve disorders are considered rheumatic unless the physician or NPP specifies non-rheumatic.

SP I36.0 Nonrheumatic tricuspid (valve) stenosis

SP I36.1 Nonrheumatic tricuspid (valve) insufficiency
Nonrheumatic tricuspid (valve) incompetence
Nonrheumatic tricuspid (valve) regurgitation

SP I36.2 Nonrheumatic tricuspid (valve) stenosis with insufficiency

SP I36.8 Other nonrheumatic tricuspid valve disorders

SP I36.9 Nonrheumatic tricuspid valve disorder, unspecified

4 I37 Nonrheumatic pulmonary valve disorders

EXCLUDES 1 pulmonary valve disorder specified as congenital (Q22.1, Q22.2, Q22.3)
pulmonary valve disorder specified as rheumatic (I09.89)

CODING TIPS✓ Pulmonary valve disorders are considered nonrheumatic unless the physician or NPP specifies rheumatic.

SP I37.0 Nonrheumatic pulmonary valve stenosis

SP I37.1 Nonrheumatic pulmonary valve insufficiency
Nonrheumatic pulmonary valve incompetence
Nonrheumatic pulmonary valve regurgitation

SP I37.2 Nonrheumatic pulmonary valve stenosis with insufficiency

SP I37.8 Other nonrheumatic pulmonary valve disorders

SP I37.9 Nonrheumatic pulmonary valve disorder, unspecified

SP I38 Endocarditis, valve unspecified

INCLUDES endocarditis (chronic) NOS
valvular incompetence NOS
valvular insufficiency NOS
valvular regurgitation NOS
valvular stenosis NOS
valvulitis (chronic) NOS

EXCLUDES 1 congenital insufficiency of cardiac valve NOS (Q24.8)
congenital stenosis of cardiac valve NOS (Q24.8)
endocardial fibroelastosis (I42.4)
endocarditis specified as rheumatic (I09.1)

M IQ I39 *Endocarditis and heart valve disorders in diseases classified elsewhere*
Code first underlying disease, such as:
Q fever (A78)
EXCLUDES 1 endocardial involvement in:

candidiasis (B37.6)
gonococcal infection (A54.83)
Libman-Sacks disease (M32.11)
listerosis (A32.82)
meningococcal infection (A39.51)
rheumatoid arthritis (M05.31)
syphilis (A52.03)
tuberculosis (A18.84)
typhoid fever (A01.02)

CODING TIPS✓ **Documentation:** Assign this code only when the clinical record supports a cause and effect relationship between the underlying disease process and the endocarditis/valve disorder.

CODING TIPS✓ I39 is a manifestation code and may be used only in conjunction with a code to report the causative underlying disease process.

4 **I40 Acute myocarditis**

INCLUDES subacute myocarditis

EXCLUDES 1 acute rheumatic myocarditis (I01.2)

DEFINITION Severe inflammation of heart muscle tissue.

SP + **I40.0 Infective myocarditis**
Septic myocarditis
Use additional code (B95-B97) to identify infectious agent

SP **I40.1 Isolated myocarditis**
Fiedler's myocarditis
Giant cell myocarditis
Idiopathic myocarditis

SP **I40.8 Other acute myocarditis**

SP **I40.9 Acute myocarditis, unspecified**

M IQ **I41** ***Myocarditis in diseases classified elsewhere***

Code first underlying disease, such as:
typhus (A75.0-A75.9)

EXCLUDES 1 myocarditis (in) :
Chagas' disease (chronic) (B57.2)
acute (B57.0)
coxsackie (virus) infection (B33.22)
diphtheritic (A36.81)
gonococcal (A54.83)
influenzal (J09.X9, J10.82, J11.82)
meningococcal (A39.52)
mumps (B26.82)
rheumatoid arthritis (M05.31)
sarcoid (D86.85)
syphilis (A52.06)
toxoplasmosis (B58.81)
tuberculous (A18.84)

CODING TIPS✓ I41 is a manifestation code and may be used only in conjunction with a code to report the causative underlying disease process.

CODING TIPS✓ **Documentation:** Assign this code only when the clinical record supports a cause and effect relationship between the underlying disease process and myocarditis.

4 **I42 Cardiomyopathy**

INCLUDES myocardiopathy

Code first:
pre-existing cardiomyopathy complicating pregnancy and puerperium (O99.4)

EXCLUDES 2 ischemic cardiomyopathy (I25.5)
peripartum cardiomyopathy (O90.3)
ventricular hypertrophy (I51.7)

SP **I42.0 Dilated cardiomyopathy**
Congestive cardiomyopathy

SP **I42.1 Obstructive hypertrophic cardiomyopathy**
Hypertrophic subaortic stenosis (idiopathic)

SP **I42.2 Other hypertrophic cardiomyopathy**
Nonobstructive hypertrophic cardiomyopathy

SP **I42.3 Endomyocardial (eosinophilic) disease**
Endomyocardial (tropical) fibrosis
Löffler's endocarditis

SP **I42.4 Endocardial fibroelastosis**
Congenital cardiomyopathy
Elastomyofibrosis

SP **I42.5 Other restrictive cardiomyopathy**
Constrictive cardiomyopathy NOS

SP **I42.6 Alcoholic cardiomyopathy**
Code also:
presence of alcoholism (F10.-)

CODING TIPS✓ This diagnosis indicates that the alcohol was linked to the disorder, so the use, abuse or dependence of alcohol (F10.-) should also be coded, usually with 4th and 5th characters to indicate uncomplicated. Do not include 5th and 6th characters .-88. "Induced disorders" include mental, emotional and physical disorders that are included in Chapter 5 only.

DEFINITION Dilated disease of the heart muscle due to alcohol abuse.

SP + **I42.7 Cardiomyopathy due to drug and external agent**
Code first:
poisoning due to drug or toxin, if applicable (T36-T65 with fifth or sixth character 1-4 or 6)
Use additional code for adverse effect, if applicable, to identify drug (T36-T50 with fifth or sixth character 5)

SP **I42.8 Other cardiomyopathies**

SP **I42.9 Cardiomyopathy, unspecified**
Cardiomyopathy (primary) (secondary) NOS

M IQ **I43** ***Cardiomyopathy in diseases classified elsewhere***

Code first underlying disease, such as:
amyloidosis (E85.-)
glycogen storage disease (E74.0)
gout (M10.0-)
thyrotoxicosis (E05.0-E05.9-)

EXCLUDES 1 cardiomyopathy (in) :
coxsackie (virus) (B33.24)
diphtheria (A36.81)
sarcoidosis (D86.85)
tuberculosis (A18.84)

CODING TIPS✓ **Documentation:** Assign this code only when the clinical record supports a cause and effect relationship between the underlying disease process and cardiomyopathy.

CODING TIPS✓ I43 is a manifestation code and may be used only in conjunction with a code to report the causative underlying disease process.

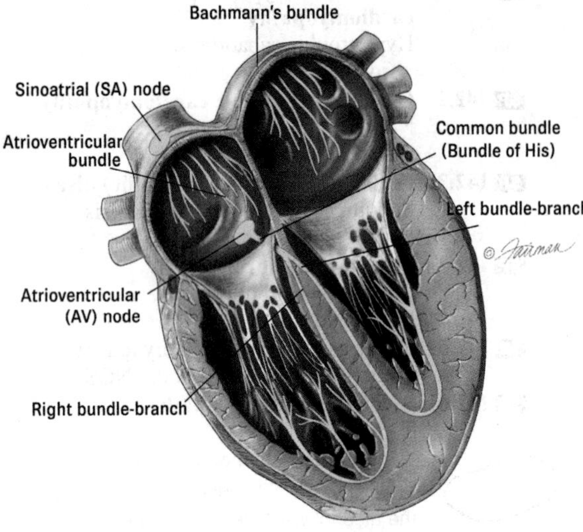

4 I44 Atrioventricular and left bundle-branch block

CODING TIPS✓ When reviewing documentation for heart block, it is important to differentiate heart block degree from heart block type.

SP I44.0 Atrioventricular block, first degree

SP I44.1 Atrioventricular block, second degree
Atrioventricular block, type I and II
Möbitz block, type I and II
Second degree block, type I and II
Wenckebach's block

SP I44.2 Atrioventricular block, complete
Complete heart block NOS
Third degree block

DEFINITION No conduction of electrical impulses occurs between the atria and ventricles, requiring a pacemaker to maintain rhythm.

5 I44.3 Other and unspecified atrioventricular block
Atrioventricular block NOS

SP I44.30 Unspecified atrioventricular block

SP I44.39 Other atrioventricular block

SP I44.4 Left anterior fascicular block

SP I44.5 Left posterior fascicular block

5 I44.6 Other and unspecified fascicular block

SP I44.60 Unspecified fascicular block
Left bundle-branch hemiblock NOS

SP I44.69 Other fascicular block

SP I44.7 Left bundle-branch block, unspecified

4 I45 Other conduction disorders

CODING TIPS✓ When reviewing documentation for heart block, it is important to differentiate heart block degree from heart block type.

SP I45.0 Right fascicular block

5 I45.1 Other and unspecified right bundle-branch block

SP I45.10 Unspecified right bundle-branch block
Right bundle-branch block NOS

SP I45.19 Other right bundle-branch block

SP I45.2 Bifascicular block

SP I45.3 Trifascicular block

SP I45.4 Nonspecific intraventricular block
Bundle-branch block NOS

DEFINITION A condition in which portions of the heart's conduction system are defective and either slow or block the electrical impulses traveling through specialized conduction tissue on the way to the ventricles.

SP I45.5 Other specified heart block
Sinoatrial block
Sinoauricular block
EXCLUDES 1 heart block NOS (I45.9)

SP I45.6 Pre-excitation syndrome
Accelerated atrioventricular conduction
Accessory atrioventricular conduction
Anomalous atrioventricular excitation
Lown-Ganong-Levine syndrome
Pre-excitation atrioventricular conduction
Wolff-Parkinson-White syndrome

5 I45.8 Other specified conduction disorders

SP I45.81 Long QT syndrome

DEFINITION Hereditary defect of the heart's electrical conduction system with an abnormally long gap in the time it takes for the ventricles to contract.

SP I45.89 Other specified conduction disorders
Atrioventricular [AV] dissociation
Interference dissociation
Isorhythmic dissociation
Nonparoxysmal AV nodal tachycardia

CODING TIPS✓ This code is used for short QT syndrome.

SP I45.9 Conduction disorder, unspecified
Heart block NOS
Stokes-Adams syndrome

4 I46 Cardiac arrest
EXCLUDES 2 cardiogenic shock (R57.0)

CODING TIPS✓ Codes from category I46.- should not be assigned to the home health claim. Use Z86.74 for history of cardiac arrest with successful resuscitation on the home health or hospice claim.

IQ I46.2 Cardiac arrest due to underlying cardiac condition
Code first:
underlying cardiac condition

IQ I46.8 Cardiac arrest due to other underlying condition
Code first:
underlying condition

SP I46.9 Cardiac arrest, cause unspecified

4 I47 Paroxysmal tachycardia
Code first tachycardia complicating:
abortion or ectopic or molar pregnancy (O00-O07, O08.8)
obstetric surgery and procedures (O75.4)
EXCLUDES 1 tachycardia NOS (R00.0)
sinoauricular tachycardia NOS (R00.0)
sinus [sinusal] tachycardia NOS (R00.0)

CODING TIPS✓ Do not assign a code from I47.- when only tachycardia is reported in the record and is not specified, or is reported in the record as sinus tachycardia or sinoauricular. When tachycardia is reported as sinus tachycardia or is not specified, report code R00.0 rather than a code from I47.-.

SP I47.0 Re-entry ventricular arrhythmia

SP I47.1 Supraventricular tachycardia
Atrial (paroxysmal) tachycardia
Atrioventricular [AV] (paroxysmal) tachycardia
Atrioventricular re-entrant (nodal) tachycardia [AVNRT] [AVRT]
Junctional (paroxysmal) tachycardia
Nodal (paroxysmal) tachycardia

DEFINITION Abnormally rapid atrial rhythm occurring from time to time, most often in the young.

SP I47.2 Ventricular tachycardia

DEFINITION Potentially lethal rapid heart beat initiating in the ventricles marked by three of more consecutive premature beats.

SP I47.9 Paroxysmal tachycardia, unspecified
Bouveret (-Hoffman) syndrome

4 I48 Atrial fibrillation and flutter

CODING TIPS✓ When assigning a code for atrial fibrillation or flutter, assign the most specific code according to the diagnostic statements given by the patient's provider.

DEFINITION Abnormal heart rhythm that occurs in the atria of the heart.

SP SH I48.0 Paroxysmal atrial fibrillation

CODING TIPS✓ Also known as intermittent atrial fibrillation, paroxysmal atrial fibrillation may spontaneously resolve, only to reappear later.

5 I48.1 Persistent atrial fibrillation
EXCLUDES 1 Permanent atrial fibrillation (I48.21)

CODING TIPS✓ Persistent AF is an abnormal heart rhythm that continues for seven days or longer, or that requires repeat electrical or pharmacological cardioversion. This code may be assigned only with a supportive confirmation diagnosis by the patient's provider. If the provider documents both chronic and persistent AF, assign only a code from category I48.1-, Persistent atrial fibrillation. Persistent atrial fibrillation that is described as chronic, or just persistent, is coded as I48.19. Pay special attention to the terms the physician uses. Persistent is not to be confused with permanent, which is coded as I48.21.

SP SH I48.11 Longstanding persistent atrial fibrillation

DEFINITION Longstanding persistent atrial fibrillation is persistent and continuous lasting longer than one year.

SP SH I48.19 Other persistent atrial fibrillation
Chronic persistent atrial fibrillation
Persistent atrial fibrillation, NOS

5 I48.2 Chronic atrial fibrillation

CODING TIPS✓ Chronic atrial fibrillation is a nonspecific term that could be referring to paroxysmal, persistent, long standing persistent, or permanent atrial fibrillation. If any of these specific terms are used in the diagnostic statement, the specific type should be assigned, and not chronic.

SP SH I48.20 Chronic atrial fibrillation, unspecified
EXCLUDES 1 Chronic persistent atrial fibrillation (I48.19)

CODING TIPS✓ Documentation: Do not assume a diagnosis of chronic atrial fibrillation in a patient who has a long history of atrial fibrillation or has simply had atrial fibrillation for a long period of time. This code may only be assigned with a supportive confirmation diagnosis by the patient's provider. Without such a diagnostic statement, an unspecified code (I48.91) must be assigned.

SP SH I48.21 Permanent atrial fibrillation

CODING TIPS✓ I48.21 is the correct code when permanent atrial fibrillation is documented. Chronic atrial fibrillation without the use of the word 'permanent' is coded I48.20.

SP SH I48.3 Typical atrial flutter
Type I atrial flutter

SP SH I48.4 Atypical atrial flutter
Type II atrial flutter

5 I48.9 Unspecified atrial fibrillation and atrial flutter

SP SH I48.91 Unspecified atrial fibrillation

SP SH I48.92 Unspecified atrial flutter

4 I49 Other cardiac arrhythmias
Code first cardiac arrhythmia complicating:
abortion or ectopic or molar pregnancy (O00-O07, O08.8)
obstetric surgery and procedures (O75.4)
EXCLUDES 1 neonatal dysrhythmia (P29.1-)
sinoatrial bradycardia (R00.1)
sinus bradycardia (R00.1)
vagal bradycardia (R00.1)
EXCLUDES 2 bradycardia NOS (R00.1)

5 I49.0 Ventricular fibrillation and flutter

SP I49.01 Ventricular fibrillation

SP I49.02 Ventricular flutter

SP I49.1 Atrial premature depolarization
Atrial premature beats

SP I49.2 Junctional premature depolarization

SP I49.3 Ventricular premature depolarization

5 I49.4 Other and unspecified premature depolarization

Chapter 9
I00-I99

SP **I49.40 Unspecified premature depolarization**
Premature beats NOS

SP **I49.49 Other premature depolarization**
Ectopic beats
Extrasystoles
Extrasystolic arrhythmias
Premature contractions

SP SH **I49.5 Sick sinus syndrome**
Tachycardia-bradycardia syndrome

SP SH **I49.8 Other specified cardiac arrhythmias**
Brugada syndrome
Coronary sinus rhythm disorder
Ectopic rhythm disorder
Nodal rhythm disorder

SP SH **I49.9 Cardiac arrhythmia, unspecified**
Arrhythmia (cardiac) NOS

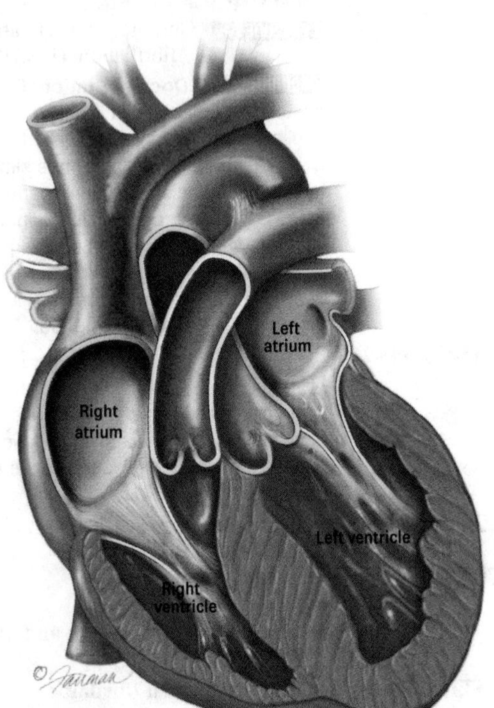

H 4 **I50 Heart failure**
Code first:
heart failure complicating abortion or ectopic or molar pregnancy (O00-O07, O08.8)
heart failure due to hypertension (I11.0)
heart failure due to hypertension with chronic kidney disease (I13.-)
heart failure following surgery (I97.13-)
obstetric surgery and procedures (O75.4)
rheumatic heart failure (I09.81)
EXCLUDES 2 cardiac arrest (I46.-)
neonatal cardiac failure (P29.0)

GUIDELINES **Section I.C.9.a.1)**
Hypertension with heart conditions classified to I50.- or I51.4-I51.7, I51.89, I51.9, are assigned to a code from category I11, Hypertensive heart disease. Use additional code(s) from category I50, Heart failure, to identify the type(s) of heart failure in those patients with heart failure.

The same heart conditions (I50.-, I51.4-I51.7, I51.89, I51.9) with hypertension are coded separately if the provider has documented they are unrelated to the hypertension. Sequence according to the circumstances of the admission/encounter.

CODING TIPS✓ History of heart failure should be coded as chronic heart failure.

CODING TIPS✓ Heart failure includes shortness of breath, pulmonary congestion, and peripheral edema. Pleural effusion may be coded separately with J91.8 if the pleural effusion requires separate treatment.

CODING TIPS✓ When both heart failure and a code from category I11.- will be assigned, the heart failure (I50.-) code should immediately follow the code from category I11.-. When both heart failure and a code from category I13.- will be assigned, the heart failure code (I50.-) and the CKD code (N18.-) should immediately follow the code from I13.- (sequence I50 and N18 depending on which one has the greatest impact on the home health plan of care).

CODING TIPS✓ Decompensated indicates there has been a flare-up or exacerbation of a chronic condition.

CODING TIPS✓ Query the physician or NPP on the type of heart failure (systolic, diastolic, combined systolic and diastolic HF, end stage, right, or CHF) to aid in choosing a more specific 4th character in this category. If the patient has documented CHF and another type of heart failure (systolic, diastolic, end stage or combined) then code just the specific type. If an acute exacerbation of a chronic failure occurs, use 5th character 3 for acute on chronic. An acute heart failure of one type and chronic of another type should be coded separately. Do not code the combined type for these instances.

CODING TIPS✓ The term "congestive" is a non-essential modifier for heart failure codes. When coding heart failure, note the non-essential modifier (congestive) and that no additional code should be used if a patient has both CHF and a more specific form of heart failure, such as diastolic heart failure.

SP SH SL **I50.1 Left ventricular failure, unspecified**
Cardiac asthma
Edema of lung with heart disease NOS
Edema of lung with heart failure
Left heart failure
Pulmonary edema with heart disease NOS
Pulmonary edema with heart failure
EXCLUDES 1 edema of lung without heart disease or heart failure (J81.-)

pulmonary edema without heart disease or failure (J81.-)

CODING TIPS✓ Code I50.1, left-sided heart failure, includes acute pulmonary edema; no additional code needs to be assigned. Never use I50.1 and I50.9 on the same claim.

5 **I50.2 Systolic (congestive) heart failure**
Heart failure with reduced ejection fraction [HFrEF]
Systolic left ventricular heart failure
Code also:
end stage heart failure, if applicable (I50.84)

EXCLUDES 1 combined systolic (congestive) and diastolic (congestive) heart failure (I50.4-)

CODING TIPS✓ Systolic dysfunction documented as linked to heart failure can be coded as systolic heart failure. If the conditions are not linked by the physician or NPP, code them separately with I50.9 and I51.89.

CODING TIPS✓ Systolic heart failure is coded when the documentation indicates HFrEF, which may also be called heart failure with low ejection fraction, or heart failure with reduced systolic function, or other similar terms meaning systolic heart failure. Do not code systolic failure based on ejection fraction numbers without physician or NPP interpretation.

DEFINITION Heart muscle fails to contract with adequate force and not enough oxygen-rich blood is pumped to the body.

SP SH SL **I50.20 Unspecified systolic (congestive) heart failure**

SP SH SL **I50.21 Acute systolic (congestive) heart failure**

SP SH SL **I50.22 Chronic systolic (congestive) heart failure**

SP SH SL **I50.23 Acute on chronic systolic (congestive) heart failure**

CODING TIPS✓ Decompensated indicates there has been a flare-up or exacerbation of a chronic condition.

5 **I50.3 Diastolic (congestive) heart failure**
Diastolic left ventricular heart failure
Heart failure with normal ejection fraction
Heart failure with preserved ejection fraction [HFpEF]
Code also:
end stage heart failure, if applicable (I50.84)

EXCLUDES 1 combined systolic (congestive) and diastolic (congestive) heart failure (I50.4-)

CODING TIPS✓ Diastolic dysfunction documented as linked to heart failure can be coded as diastolic heart failure. If the conditions are not linked by the physician or NPP, code them separately with I50.9 and I51.89.

CODING TIPS✓ Diastolic heart failure is coded when the documentation indicates HFpEF, which may also be referred to as heart failure with preserved systolic function, and this condition may also be referred to as diastolic heart failure. Do not code diastolic failure based on ejection fraction numbers without physician or NPP interpretation.

CODING TIPS✓ All codes for heart failure include any associated pulmonary edema. Pleural effusion may be coded separately with J91.8 if the pleural effusion requires separate treatment.

DEFINITION Heart muscle contracts normally but ventricles fail to relax properly after contraction, resulting in less blood entering the heart.

SP SH SL **I50.30 Unspecified diastolic (congestive) heart failure**

SP SH SL **I50.31 Acute diastolic (congestive) heart failure**

SP SH SL **I50.32 Chronic diastolic (congestive) heart failure**

SP SH SL **I50.33 Acute on chronic diastolic (congestive) heart failure**

CODING TIPS✓ Decompensated indicates there has been a flare-up or exacerbation of a chronic condition.

5 **I50.4 Combined systolic (congestive) and diastolic (congestive) heart failure**
Combined systolic and diastolic left ventricular heart failure
Heart failure with reduced ejection fraction and diastolic dysfunction
Code also:
end stage heart failure, if applicable (I50.84)

DEFINITION Heart fails both to contract and relax properly, resulting in an insufficient amount of blood moving through the circulatory system.

SP SH SL **I50.40 Unspecified combined systolic (congestive) and diastolic (congestive) heart failure**

SP SH SL **I50.41 Acute combined systolic (congestive) and diastolic (congestive) heart failure**

SP SH SL **I50.42 Chronic combined systolic (congestive) and diastolic (congestive) heart failure**

SP SH SL **I50.43 Acute on chronic combined systolic (congestive) and diastolic (congestive) heart failure**

CODING TIPS✓ Decompensated indicates there has been a flare-up or exacerbation of a chronic condition.

5 **I50.8 Other heart failure**

6 **I50.81 Right heart failure**
Right ventricular failure

SP SH SL **I50.810 Right heart failure, unspecified**
Right heart failure without mention of left heart failure
Right ventricular failure NOS

SP SH SL **I50.811 Acute right heart failure**
Acute isolated right heart failure

Acute (isolated) right ventricular failure

SP SH SL **I50.812 Chronic right heart failure**
Chronic isolated right heart failure
Chronic (isolated) right ventricular failure

SP SH SL **I50.813 Acute on chronic right heart failure**
Acute on chronic isolated right heart failure
Acute on chronic (isolated) right ventricular failure
Acute decompensation of chronic (isolated) right ventricular failure
Acute exacerbation of chronic (isolated) right ventricular failure

SP SH SL **I50.814 Right heart failure due to left heart failure**
Right ventricular failure secondary to left ventricular failure
Code also:
the type of left ventricular failure, if known (I50.2-I50.43)
EXCLUDES 1 Right heart failure with but not due to left heart failure (I50.82)

SP SH SL **I50.82 Biventricular heart failure**
Code also:
the type of left ventricular failure as systolic, diastolic, or combined, if known (I50.2-I50.43)

SP SH SL **I50.83 High output heart failure**
CODING TIPS ✓ The term "high output heart failure" is a misnomer because the heart in these conditions is normal, capable of generating high cardiac output. The underlying problem in high output failure is a decrease in the systemic vascular resistance that threatens the arterial blood pressure and causes activation of neurohormones, resulting in an increase in salt and water retention by the kidney. Many high output states are curable conditions, and because they are associated with decreased peripheral vascular resistance, the use of vasodilator therapy for treatment of congestion may aggravate the problem.

SP SH SL **I50.84 End stage heart failure**
Stage D heart failure
Code also:
the type of heart failure as systolic, diastolic, or combined, if known (I50.2-I50.43)
CODING TIPS ✓ Do not code congestive heart failure with end stage heart failure. Code only specific types of heart failure with end stage heart failure.

DEFINITION Patients with end stage heart failure fall into stage D of the ABCD Classification of the American College of Cardiology (ACC)/American Heart Association (AHA), and are characterized by advanced structural heart disease and pronounced symptoms of heart failure at rest or upon minimal physical exertion, despite maximal medical treatment. They frequently develop intolerance to medical therapy and are developing worsening renal function and diuretic resistance according to current guidelines. This patient population has a 1-year mortality rate of approximately 50%, is at highest risk for re-hospitalization and requires special therapeutic interventions such as ventricular assist devices, artificial hearts and heart transplantation or hospice care.

SP SH SL **I50.89 Other heart failure**

SP SH SL **I50.9 Heart failure, unspecified**
Cardiac, heart or myocardial failure NOS
Congestive heart disease
Congestive heart failure NOS
EXCLUDES 2 fluid overload unrelated to congestive heart failure (E87.70)
CODING TIPS ✓ Stage A of the ABCD Classification of the American College of Cardiology (ACC)/American Heart Association (AHA) is the presence of heart failure risk factors but no heart disease and no symptoms. This should not be coded to the regular heart failure codes, but rather to code Z91.89, Other specified personal risk factors, not elsewhere classified. Stage B is where heart disease is present but there are no symptoms; thus there are structural changes in the heart before symptoms occur. Stage C involves structural heart disease, with symptoms.

4 **I51 Complications and ill-defined descriptions of heart disease**
EXCLUDES 1 any condition in I51.4-I51.9 due to hypertension (I11.-)
any condition in I51.4-I51.9 due to hypertension and chronic kidney disease (I13.-)
heart disease specified as rheumatic (I00-I09)

SP **I51.0 Cardiac septal defect, acquired**
Acquired septal atrial defect (old)
Acquired septal auricular defect (old)
Acquired septal ventricular defect (old)
EXCLUDES 1 cardiac septal defect as current complication following acute myocardial infarction (I23.1, I23.2)

SP **I51.1 Rupture of chordae tendineae, not elsewhere classified**

EXCLUDES 1 rupture of chordae tendineae as current complication following acute myocardial infarction (I23.4)

DEFINITION Tear in the fibrous, cord-like tissue connecting the papillary muscles to the valves, holding the valve flaps in place to prevent their eversion.

SP **I51.2 Rupture of papillary muscle, not elsewhere classified**

EXCLUDES 1 rupture of papillary muscle as current complication following acute myocardial infarction (I23.5)

SP SH **I51.3 Intracardiac thrombosis, not elsewhere classified**

Apical thrombosis (old)
Atrial thrombosis (old)
Auricular thrombosis (old)
Mural thrombosis (old)
Ventricular thrombosis (old)

EXCLUDES 1 intracardiac thrombosis as current complication following acute myocardial infarction (I23.6)

SP **I51.4 Myocarditis, unspecified**

Chronic (interstitial) myocarditis
Myocardial fibrosis
Myocarditis NOS

EXCLUDES 1 acute or subacute myocarditis (I40.-)

CODING TIPS✓ If conditions included in I51.4 -I51.7. I51.89, I51.9 are present with hypertension, then do not code them. These conditions are included in codes I11 and I13.

SP **I51.5 Myocardial degeneration**

Fatty degeneration of heart or myocardium
Myocardial disease
Senile degeneration of heart or myocardium

CODING TIPS✓ If conditions included in I51.4 -I51.7. I51.89, I51.9 are present with hypertension, then do not code them. These conditions are included in codes I11 and I13.

DEFINITION Wasting away of the heart muscle.

SP **I51.7 Cardiomegaly**

Cardiac dilatation
Cardiac hypertrophy
Ventricular dilatation

CODING TIPS✓ If conditions included in I51.4 -I51.7. I51.89, I51.9 are present with hypertension, then do not code them. These conditions are included in codes I11 and I13.

5 **I51.8 Other ill-defined heart diseases**

SP **I51.81 Takotsubo syndrome**

Reversible left ventricular dysfunction following sudden emotional stress
Stress induced cardiomyopathy
Takotsubo cardiomyopathy
Transient left ventricular apical ballooning syndrome

CODING TIPS✓ Takotsubo Syndrome (I51.81) is by definition stress related and therefore should not be coded with I11.9, per CC Q2 2018.

DEFINITION Takutosobu Syndrome presents with chest pain and dypsnea and occurs more frequently in postmenopausal females, with a physical or emotional stressor. They may have ST elevation and a troponin elevation, however cardiac catheterization demonstrates normal coronary arteries in more than 80% of cases.

SP SH **I51.89 Other ill-defined heart diseases**

Carditis (acute)(chronic)
Pancarditis (acute)(chronic)

CODING TIPS✓ Diastolic dysfunction or systolic dysfunction is coded to I51.89 if not related to heart failure. If related to heart failure, then diastolic heart failure or systolic heart failure should be coded.

CODING TIPS✓ If conditions included in I51.4 -I51.7. I51.89, I51.9 are present with hypertension, then do not code them. These conditions are included in codes I11 and I13.

SP **I51.9 Heart disease, unspecified**

CODING TIPS✓ This code is assigned for end stage heart disease, but the provider should always be queried for additional information regarding the type of heart disease. For example, end stage heart failure is coded to I51.84.

CODING TIPS✓ If conditions included in I51.4 -I51.7. I51.89, I51.9 are present with hypertension, then do not code them. These conditions are included in codes I11 and I13.

M IQ **I52 *Other heart disorders in diseases classified elsewhere***

Code first underlying disease, such as:
congenital syphilis (A50.5)
mucopolysaccharidosis (E76.3)
schistosomiasis (B65.0-B65.9)

EXCLUDES 1 heart disease (in) :
gonococcal infection (A54.83)
meningococcal infection (A39.50)
rheumatoid arthritis (M05.31)
syphilis (A52.06)

★ **I5A Non-ischemic myocardial injury (non-traumatic)**

Acute (non-ischemic) myocardial injury
Chronic (non-ischemic) myocardial injury

Unspecified (non-ischemic) myocardial injury
Code first the underlying cause, if known and applicable, such as:
- acute kidney failure (N17.-)
- acute myocarditis (I40.-)
- cardiomyopathy (I42.-)
- chronic kidney disease (CKD) (N18.-)
- heart failure (I50.-)
- hypertensive urgency (I16.0)
- nonrheumatic aortic valve disorders (I35.-)
- paroxysmal tachycardia (I47.-)
- pulmonary embolism (I26.-)
- pulmonary hypertension (I27.0, I27.2-)
- sepsis (A41.-)
- takotsubo syndrome (I51.81)

EXCLUDES 1 acute myocardial infarction (I21.-)
injury of heart (S26.-)

EXCLUDES 2 other acute ischemic heart diseases (I24.-)

Cerebrovascular diseases (I60-I69)

Use additional code to identify presence of:
- alcohol abuse and dependence (F10.-)
- exposure to environmental tobacco smoke (Z77.22)
- history of tobacco dependence (Z87.891)
- hypertension (I10-I16)
- occupational exposure to environmental tobacco smoke (Z57.31)
- tobacco dependence (F17.-)
- tobacco use (Z72.0)

EXCLUDES 1 traumatic intracranial hemorrhage (S06.-)

CODING TIPS✓ The hypertensive cerebrovascular disease guideline is based on the instructional note at the I60-I69 block of codes which indicates "use additional code to identify presence of ..." If the physician or NPP documents hypertensive cerebrovascular disease, add the code for hypertension.

CODING TIPS✓ A traumatic head injury and a CVA may both be coded if the two conditions are unrelated.

4 I60 Nontraumatic subarachnoid hemorrhage

EXCLUDES 1 syphilitic ruptured cerebral aneurysm (A52.05)

EXCLUDES 2 sequelae of subarachnoid hemorrhage (I69.0-)

CODING TIPS✓ Codes from category I60.- should ordinarily not be used on the home health or hospice claim because they indicate a continuing cerebrovascular bleed. If documentation indicates an ongoing bleed, the I60.- codes may continue to be reported in home health and hospice. If there is no indication that the bleed continues, I69.0- is used on home health and hospice claims to indicate residual deficits.

CODING TIPS✓ Imaging reports may be utilized to provide greater specificity of the anatomic site as documented by the physician. It is appropriate to utilize the imaging report to determine the location of the stroke or infarction, only if the attending or consulting physician has signed or documented otherwise.

CODING TIPS✓ The use of codes from R29.7 indicate the NIHSS. The NIHSS can be used as a clinical stroke assessment tool to evaluate and document neurological status in acute stroke patients. The stroke scale is valid for predicting lesion size and can serve as a measure of stroke severity. The NIHSS has been shown to be a predictor of both short and long term outcome of stroke patients. The codes are meant for use for acute hospitals only.

5 I60.0 Nontraumatic subarachnoid hemorrhage from carotid siphon and bifurcation

⊟ SP I60.00 Nontraumatic subarachnoid hemorrhage from unspecified carotid siphon and bifurcation

⊟ SP I60.01 Nontraumatic subarachnoid hemorrhage from right carotid siphon and bifurcation

⊟ SP I60.02 Nontraumatic subarachnoid hemorrhage from left carotid siphon and bifurcation

5 I60.1 Nontraumatic subarachnoid hemorrhage from middle cerebral artery

⊟ SP I60.10 Nontraumatic subarachnoid hemorrhage from unspecified middle cerebral artery

⊟ SP I60.11 Nontraumatic subarachnoid hemorrhage from right middle cerebral artery

⊟ SP I60.12 Nontraumatic subarachnoid hemorrhage from left middle cerebral artery

SP I60.2 Nontraumatic subarachnoid hemorrhage from anterior communicating artery

5 I60.3 Nontraumatic subarachnoid hemorrhage from posterior communicating artery

⊟ SP I60.30 Nontraumatic subarachnoid hemorrhage from unspecified posterior communicating artery

⊟ SP I60.31 Nontraumatic subarachnoid hemorrhage from right posterior communicating artery

⊟ SP I60.32 Nontraumatic subarachnoid hemorrhage from left posterior communicating artery

SP I60.4 Nontraumatic subarachnoid hemorrhage from basilar artery

5 I60.5 Nontraumatic subarachnoid hemorrhage from vertebral artery

⊟ SP I60.50 Nontraumatic subarachnoid hemorrhage from unspecified vertebral artery

⊟ SP I60.51 Nontraumatic subarachnoid hemorrhage from right vertebral artery

⊟ SP I60.52 Nontraumatic subarachnoid hemorrhage from left vertebral artery

SP I60.6 Nontraumatic subarachnoid hemorrhage from other intracranial arteries

SP **I60.7 Nontraumatic subarachnoid hemorrhage from unspecified intracranial artery**
Ruptured (congenital) berry aneurysm
Ruptured (congenital) cerebral aneurysm
Subarachnoid hemorrhage (nontraumatic) from cerebral artery NOS
Subarachnoid hemorrhage (nontraumatic) from communicating artery NOS
EXCLUDES 1 berry aneurysm, nonruptured (I67.1)

SP **I60.8 Other nontraumatic subarachnoid hemorrhage**
Meningeal hemorrhage
Rupture of cerebral arteriovenous malformation

SP **I60.9 Nontraumatic subarachnoid hemorrhage, unspecified**

4 **I61 Nontraumatic intracerebral hemorrhage**
EXCLUDES 2 sequelae of intracerebral hemorrhage (I69.1-)

CODING TIPS✓ The use of codes from R29.7 indicate the NIHSS. The NIHSS can be used as a clinical stroke assessment tool to evaluate and document neurological status in acute stroke patients. The stroke scale is valid for predicting lesion size and can serve as a measure of stroke severity. The NIHSS has been shown to be a predictor of both short and long term outcome of stroke patients. The codes are meant for use for acute hospitals only.

CODING TIPS✓ Imaging reports may be utilized to provide greater specificity of the anatomic site as documented by the physician. It is appropriate to utilize the imaging report to determine the location of the stroke or infarction, only if the attending or consulting physician has signed or documented otherwise.

CODING TIPS✓ Codes from category I61.- should ordinarily not be used on the home health or hospice claim because they indicate a continuing cerebrovascular bleed. If documentation indicates an ongoing bleed, the I61.- codes may continue to be reported in home health and hospice. If there is no indication that the bleed continues, I69.1- is used on home health and hospice claims to indicate residual deficits.

SP **I61.0 Nontraumatic intracerebral hemorrhage in hemisphere, subcortical**
Deep intracerebral hemorrhage (nontraumatic)

SP **I61.1 Nontraumatic intracerebral hemorrhage in hemisphere, cortical**
Cerebral lobe hemorrhage (nontraumatic)
Superficial intracerebral hemorrhage (nontraumatic)

SP **I61.2 Nontraumatic intracerebral hemorrhage in hemisphere, unspecified**

SP **I61.3 Nontraumatic intracerebral hemorrhage in brain stem**

SP **I61.4 Nontraumatic intracerebral hemorrhage in cerebellum**

SP **I61.5 Nontraumatic intracerebral hemorrhage, intraventricular**

SP **I61.6 Nontraumatic intracerebral hemorrhage, multiple localized**

SP **I61.8 Other nontraumatic intracerebral hemorrhage**

SP **I61.9 Nontraumatic intracerebral hemorrhage, unspecified**

4 **I62 Other and unspecified nontraumatic intracranial hemorrhage**
EXCLUDES 2 sequelae of intracranial hemorrhage (I69.2)

CODING TIPS✓ Codes from category I62.- should ordinarily not be used on the home health or hospice claim because they indicate a continuing cerebrovascular bleed. If documentation indicates an ongoing bleed, the I62.- codes may continue to be reported in home health and hospice. If there is no indication that the bleed continues, I69.2- is used on home health and hospice claims to indicate residual deficits.

CODING TIPS✓ Imaging reports may be utilized to provide greater specificity of the anatomic site as documented by the physician. It is appropriate to utilize the imaging report to determine the location of the stroke or infarction, only if the attending or consulting physician has signed or documented otherwise.

CODING TIPS✓ The use of codes from R29.7 indicate the NIHSS. The NIHSS can be used as a clinical stroke assessment tool to evaluate and document neurological status in acute stroke patients. The stroke scale is valid for predicting lesion size and can serve as a measure of stroke severity. The NIHSS has been shown to be a predictor of both short and long term outcome of stroke patients. The codes are meant for use for acute hospitals only.

5 **I62.0 Nontraumatic subdural hemorrhage**

SP **I62.00 Nontraumatic subdural hemorrhage, unspecified**

SP **I62.01 Nontraumatic acute subdural hemorrhage**

SP **I62.02 Nontraumatic subacute subdural hemorrhage**

SP **I62.03 Nontraumatic chronic subdural hemorrhage**

SP **I62.1 Nontraumatic extradural hemorrhage**
Nontraumatic epidural hemorrhage

SP **I62.9 Nontraumatic intracranial hemorrhage, unspecified**

+ 4 **I63 Cerebral infarction**
INCLUDES occlusion and stenosis of cerebral and precerebral arteries, resulting in cerebral infarction
Use additional code, if applicable, to identify status post administration of tPA (rtPA) in a different facility within the last 24 hours prior to admission to current facility (Z92.82)
Use additional code, if known, to indicate National Institutes of Health Stroke Scale (NIHSS) score (R29.7-)
EXCLUDES 1 neonatal cerebral infarction (P91.82-)

EXCLUDES 2 sequelae of cerebral infarction (I69.3-)

CODING TIPS✓ The use of codes from R29.7 indicate the NIHSS. The NIHSS can be used as a clinical stroke assessment tool to evaluate and document neurological status in acute stroke patients. The stroke scale is valid for predicting lesion size and can serve as a measure of stroke severity. The NIHSS has been shown to be a predictor of both short and long term outcome of stroke patients. The codes are meant for use for acute hospitals only.

CODING TIPS✓ Imaging reports may be utilized to provide greater specificity of the anatomic site as documented by the physician. It is appropriate to utilize the imaging report to determine the location of the stroke or infarction, only if the attending or consulting physician has signed or documented otherwise.

CODING TIPS✓ Codes from category I63.- should ordinarily not be used on the home health or hospice claim because they indicate a continuing cerebrovascular infarction. If documentation indicates an ongoing infarction, the I63.- codes may continue to be reported in home health and hospice. If there is no indication that the infarction continues, I69.3- is used on home health and hospice claims to indicate residual deficits.

+ 5 I63.0 Cerebral infarction due to thrombosis of precerebral arteries

SP + I63.00 Cerebral infarction due to thrombosis of unspecified precerebral artery

+ 6 I63.01 Cerebral infarction due to thrombosis of vertebral artery

⊟ SP + I63.011 Cerebral infarction due to thrombosis of right vertebral artery

⊟ SP + I63.012 Cerebral infarction due to thrombosis of left vertebral artery

⊟ SP + I63.013 Cerebral infarction due to thrombosis of bilateral vertebral arteries

⊟ SP + I63.019 Cerebral infarction due to thrombosis of unspecified vertebral artery

SP + I63.02 Cerebral infarction due to thrombosis of basilar artery

+ 6 I63.03 Cerebral infarction due to thrombosis of carotid artery

⊟ SP + I63.031 Cerebral infarction due to thrombosis of right carotid artery

⊟ SP + I63.032 Cerebral infarction due to thrombosis of left carotid artery

⊟ SP + I63.033 Cerebral infarction due to thrombosis of bilateral carotid arteries

⊟ SP + I63.039 Cerebral infarction due to thrombosis of unspecified carotid artery

SP + I63.09 Cerebral infarction due to thrombosis of other precerebral artery

+ 5 I63.1 Cerebral infarction due to embolism of precerebral arteries

SP + I63.10 Cerebral infarction due to embolism of unspecified precerebral artery

+ 6 I63.11 Cerebral infarction due to embolism of vertebral artery

⊟ SP + I63.111 Cerebral infarction due to embolism of right vertebral artery

⊟ SP + I63.112 Cerebral infarction due to embolism of left vertebral artery

⊟ SP + I63.113 Cerebral infarction due to embolism of bilateral vertebral arteries

⊟ SP + I63.119 Cerebral infarction due to embolism of unspecified vertebral artery

SP + I63.12 Cerebral infarction due to embolism of basilar artery

+ 6 I63.13 Cerebral infarction due to embolism of carotid artery

⊟ SP + I63.131 Cerebral infarction due to embolism of right carotid artery

⊟ SP + I63.132 Cerebral infarction due to embolism of left carotid artery

⊟ SP + I63.133 Cerebral infarction due to embolism of bilateral carotid arteries

⊟ SP + I63.139 Cerebral infarction due to embolism of unspecified carotid artery

SP + I63.19 Cerebral infarction due to embolism of other precerebral artery

+ 5 I63.2 Cerebral infarction due to unspecified occlusion or stenosis of precerebral arteries

SP + I63.20 Cerebral infarction due to unspecified occlusion or stenosis of unspecified precerebral arteries

+ 6 I63.21 Cerebral infarction due to unspecified occlusion or stenosis of vertebral arteries

⊟ SP + I63.211 Cerebral infarction due to unspecified occlusion or stenosis of right vertebral artery

⊟ SP + I63.212 Cerebral infarction due to unspecified occlusion or stenosis of left vertebral artery

⊟ SP + I63.213 Cerebral infarction due to unspecified occlusion or stenosis of bilateral vertebral arteries

⊟ SP + I63.219 Cerebral infarction due to unspecified occlusion or stenosis of unspecified vertebral artery

SP + I63.22 Cerebral infarction due to unspecified occlusion or stenosis of basilar artery

+ 6 I63.23 Cerebral infarction due to unspecified occlusion or stenosis of carotid arteries

⊟ SP + I63.231 Cerebral infarction due to unspecified occlusion or stenosis of right carotid arteries

⊟ SP + I63.232 Cerebral infarction due to unspecified occlusion or stenosis of left carotid arteries

4 4th digit required   5 5th digit required   6 6th digit required   7 7th digit required   7 7th digit placeholder   + Additional code   ⊟ Laterality

SP + I63.233 Cerebral infarction due to unspecified occlusion or stenosis of bilateral carotid arteries

SP + I63.239 Cerebral infarction due to unspecified occlusion or stenosis of unspecified carotid artery

SP + I63.29 Cerebral infarction due to unspecified occlusion or stenosis of other precerebral arteries

+ 5 I63.3 Cerebral infarction due to thrombosis of cerebral arteries

SP + I63.30 Cerebral infarction due to thrombosis of unspecified cerebral artery

+ 6 I63.31 Cerebral infarction due to thrombosis of middle cerebral artery

SP + I63.311 Cerebral infarction due to thrombosis of right middle cerebral artery

SP + I63.312 Cerebral infarction due to thrombosis of left middle cerebral artery

SP + I63.313 Cerebral infarction due to thrombosis of bilateral middle cerebral arteries

SP + I63.319 Cerebral infarction due to thrombosis of unspecified middle cerebral artery

+ 6 I63.32 Cerebral infarction due to thrombosis of anterior cerebral artery

SP + I63.321 Cerebral infarction due to thrombosis of right anterior cerebral artery

SP + I63.322 Cerebral infarction due to thrombosis of left anterior cerebral artery

SP + I63.323 Cerebral infarction due to thrombosis of bilateral anterior cerebral arteries

SP + I63.329 Cerebral infarction due to thrombosis of unspecified anterior cerebral artery

+ 6 I63.33 Cerebral infarction due to thrombosis of posterior cerebral artery

SP + I63.331 Cerebral infarction due to thrombosis of right posterior cerebral artery

SP + I63.332 Cerebral infarction due to thrombosis of left posterior cerebral artery

SP + I63.333 Cerebral infarction due to thrombosis of bilateral posterior cerebral arteries

SP + I63.339 Cerebral infarction due to thrombosis of unspecified posterior cerebral artery

+ 6 I63.34 Cerebral infarction due to thrombosis of cerebellar artery

SP + I63.341 Cerebral infarction due to thrombosis of right cerebellar artery

SP + I63.342 Cerebral infarction due to thrombosis of left cerebellar artery

SP + I63.343 Cerebral infarction due to thrombosis of bilateral cerebellar arteries

SP + I63.349 Cerebral infarction due to thrombosis of unspecified cerebellar artery

SP + I63.39 Cerebral infarction due to thrombosis of other cerebral artery

+ 5 I63.4 Cerebral infarction due to embolism of cerebral arteries

SP + I63.40 Cerebral infarction due to embolism of unspecified cerebral artery

+ 6 I63.41 Cerebral infarction due to embolism of middle cerebral artery

SP + I63.411 Cerebral infarction due to embolism of right middle cerebral artery

SP + I63.412 Cerebral infarction due to embolism of left middle cerebral artery

SP + I63.413 Cerebral infarction due to embolism of bilateral middle cerebral arteries

SP + I63.419 Cerebral infarction due to embolism of unspecified middle cerebral artery

+ 6 I63.42 Cerebral infarction due to embolism of anterior cerebral artery

SP + I63.421 Cerebral infarction due to embolism of right anterior cerebral artery

SP + I63.422 Cerebral infarction due to embolism of left anterior cerebral artery

SP + I63.423 Cerebral infarction due to embolism of bilateral anterior cerebral arteries

SP + I63.429 Cerebral infarction due to embolism of unspecified anterior cerebral artery

+ 6 I63.43 Cerebral infarction due to embolism of posterior cerebral artery

SP + I63.431 Cerebral infarction due to embolism of right posterior cerebral artery

SP + I63.432 Cerebral infarction due to embolism of left posterior cerebral artery

SP + I63.433 Cerebral infarction due to embolism of bilateral posterior cerebral arteries

SP + I63.439 Cerebral infarction due to embolism of unspecified posterior cerebral artery

+ 6 I63.44 Cerebral infarction due to embolism of cerebellar artery

SP + I63.441 Cerebral infarction due to embolism of right cerebellar artery

SP + I63.442 Cerebral infarction due to embolism of left cerebellar artery

SP + I63.443 Cerebral infarction due to embolism of bilateral cerebellar arteries

SP + I63.449 Cerebral infarction due to embolism of unspecified cerebellar artery

Chapter 9

I00-I99

SP + I63.49 **Cerebral infarction due to embolism of other cerebral artery**

+ 5 I63.5 **Cerebral infarction due to unspecified occlusion or stenosis of cerebral arteries**

SP + I63.50 **Cerebral infarction due to unspecified occlusion or stenosis of unspecified cerebral artery**

+ 6 I63.51 **Cerebral infarction due to unspecified occlusion or stenosis of middle cerebral artery**

⊟ SP + I63.511 **Cerebral infarction due to unspecified occlusion or stenosis of right middle cerebral artery**

⊟ SP + I63.512 **Cerebral infarction due to unspecified occlusion or stenosis of left middle cerebral artery**

⊟ SP + I63.513 **Cerebral infarction due to unspecified occlusion or stenosis of bilateral middle cerebral arteries**

⊟ SP + I63.519 **Cerebral infarction due to unspecified occlusion or stenosis of unspecified middle cerebral artery**

+ 6 I63.52 **Cerebral infarction due to unspecified occlusion or stenosis of anterior cerebral artery**

⊟ SP + I63.521 **Cerebral infarction due to unspecified occlusion or stenosis of right anterior cerebral artery**

⊟ SP + I63.522 **Cerebral infarction due to unspecified occlusion or stenosis of left anterior cerebral artery**

⊟ SP + I63.523 **Cerebral infarction due to unspecified occlusion or stenosis of bilateral anterior cerebral arteries**

⊟ SP + I63.529 **Cerebral infarction due to unspecified occlusion or stenosis of unspecified anterior cerebral artery**

+ 6 I63.53 **Cerebral infarction due to unspecified occlusion or stenosis of posterior cerebral artery**

⊟ SP + I63.531 **Cerebral infarction due to unspecified occlusion or stenosis of right posterior cerebral artery**

⊟ SP + I63.532 **Cerebral infarction due to unspecified occlusion or stenosis of left posterior cerebral artery**

⊟ SP + I63.533 **Cerebral infarction due to unspecified occlusion or stenosis of bilateral posterior cerebral arteries**

⊟ SP + I63.539 **Cerebral infarction due to unspecified occlusion or stenosis of unspecified posterior cerebral artery**

+ 6 I63.54 **Cerebral infarction due to unspecified occlusion or stenosis of cerebellar artery**

⊟ SP + I63.541 **Cerebral infarction due to unspecified occlusion or stenosis of right cerebellar artery**

⊟ SP + I63.542 **Cerebral infarction due to unspecified occlusion or stenosis of left cerebellar artery**

⊟ SP + I63.543 **Cerebral infarction due to unspecified occlusion or stenosis of bilateral cerebellar arteries**

⊟ SP + I63.549 **Cerebral infarction due to unspecified occlusion or stenosis of unspecified cerebellar artery**

SP + I63.59 **Cerebral infarction due to unspecified occlusion or stenosis of other cerebral artery**

SP + I63.6 **Cerebral infarction due to cerebral venous thrombosis, nonpyogenic**

+ 5 I63.8 **Other cerebral infarction**

SP + I63.81 **Other cerebral infarction due to occlusion or stenosis of small artery**
Lacunar infarction

SP + I63.89 **Other cerebral infarction**

SP + I63.9 **Cerebral infarction, unspecified**
Stroke NOS
EXCLUDES 2 transient cerebral ischemic attacks and related syndromes (G45.-)

4 I65 **Occlusion and stenosis of precerebral arteries, not resulting in cerebral infarction**
INCLUDES embolism of precerebral artery
narrowing of precerebral artery
obstruction (complete) (partial) of precerebral artery
thrombosis of precerebral artery
EXCLUDES 1 insufficiency, NOS, of precerebral artery (G45.-)
insufficiency of precerebral arteries causing cerebral infarction (I63.0-I63.2)

CODING TIPS ✓ Codes from categories I65.- and I66.- are used to indicate stenosis and occlusion that do not result in infarction and may be used in the home health setting. Assign the most specific code as appropriate according to diagnostic statements provided by the physician or NPP. If the affected artery is not specified, do not assume a code for an affected location, but rather use an unspecified code. If more than one arterial location is affected and a specific code is available for separate locations, separate codes should be assigned.
Imaging reports may be utilized to provide greater specificity of the anatomic site as documented by the physician or NPP.

5 I65.0 **Occlusion and stenosis of vertebral artery**

⊟ SP I65.01 **Occlusion and stenosis of right vertebral artery**

⊟ SP I65.02 **Occlusion and stenosis of left vertebral artery**

⊟ SP I65.03 **Occlusion and stenosis of bilateral vertebral arteries**

⊟ SP I65.09 **Occlusion and stenosis of unspecified vertebral artery**

SP I65.1 **Occlusion and stenosis of basilar artery**

5 I65.2 **Occlusion and stenosis of carotid artery**

⊟ SP I65.21 **Occlusion and stenosis of right carotid artery**

4 4th digit required | 5 5th digit required | 6 6th digit required | 7 7th digit required | 7 7th digit placeholder | + Additional code | ⊟ Laterality

SP I65.22 **Occlusion and stenosis of left carotid artery**

SP I65.23 **Occlusion and stenosis of bilateral carotid arteries**

CODING TIPS ✓ If the physician or NPP indicates carotid artery disease without occlusion or stenosis, use I77.9 instead. [AHA: 1Q 2021]

SP I65.29 **Occlusion and stenosis of unspecified carotid artery**

SP I65.8 **Occlusion and stenosis of other precerebral arteries**

SP I65.9 **Occlusion and stenosis of unspecified precerebral artery**

Occlusion and stenosis of precerebral artery NOS

4 I66 **Occlusion and stenosis of cerebral arteries, not resulting in cerebral infarction**

INCLUDES embolism of cerebral artery
narrowing of cerebral artery
obstruction (complete) (partial) of cerebral artery
thrombosis of cerebral artery

EXCLUDES 1 Occlusion and stenosis of cerebral artery causing cerebral infarction (I63.3-I63.5)

CODING TIPS ✓ Codes from categories I65.- and I66.- are used to indicate stenosis and occlusion that do not result in infarction and may be used in the home health setting. Assign the most specific code as appropriate according to diagnostic statements provided by the physician or NPP. If the affected artery is not specified, do not assume a code for an affected location, but rather use an unspecified code. If more than one arterial location is affected and a specific code is available for separate locations, separate codes should be assigned.
Imaging reports may be utilized to provide greater specificity of the anatomic site as documented by the physician or NPP.

5 I66.0 **Occlusion and stenosis of middle cerebral artery**

SP I66.01 **Occlusion and stenosis of right middle cerebral artery**

SP I66.02 **Occlusion and stenosis of left middle cerebral artery**

SP I66.03 **Occlusion and stenosis of bilateral middle cerebral arteries**

SP I66.09 **Occlusion and stenosis of unspecified middle cerebral artery**

5 I66.1 **Occlusion and stenosis of anterior cerebral artery**

SP I66.11 **Occlusion and stenosis of right anterior cerebral artery**

SP I66.12 **Occlusion and stenosis of left anterior cerebral artery**

SP I66.13 **Occlusion and stenosis of bilateral anterior cerebral arteries**

SP I66.19 **Occlusion and stenosis of unspecified anterior cerebral artery**

5 I66.2 **Occlusion and stenosis of posterior cerebral artery**

SP I66.21 **Occlusion and stenosis of right posterior cerebral artery**

SP I66.22 **Occlusion and stenosis of left posterior cerebral artery**

SP I66.23 **Occlusion and stenosis of bilateral posterior cerebral arteries**

SP I66.29 **Occlusion and stenosis of unspecified posterior cerebral artery**

SP I66.3 **Occlusion and stenosis of cerebellar arteries**

SP I66.8 **Occlusion and stenosis of other cerebral arteries**

Occlusion and stenosis of perforating arteries

SP I66.9 **Occlusion and stenosis of unspecified cerebral artery**

4 I67 **Other cerebrovascular diseases**

EXCLUDES 2 sequelae of the listed conditions (I69.8)

CODING TIPS ✓ These codes may be used in home health and hospice for various cerebrovascular disease.

SP I67.0 **Dissection of cerebral arteries, nonruptured**

EXCLUDES 1 ruptured cerebral arteries (I60.7)

SP I67.1 **Cerebral aneurysm, nonruptured**

Cerebral aneurysm NOS
Cerebral arteriovenous fistula, acquired
Internal carotid artery aneurysm, intracranial portion
Internal carotid artery aneurysm, NOS

EXCLUDES 1 congenital cerebral aneurysm, nonruptured (Q28.-)
ruptured cerebral aneurysm (I60.7)

SP SH SL I67.2 **Cerebral atherosclerosis**

Atheroma of cerebral and precerebral arteries

SP I67.3 **Progressive vascular leukoencephalopathy**

Binswanger's disease

SP I67.4 **Hypertensive encephalopathy**

EXCLUDES 2 insufficiency, NOS, of precerebral arteries (G45.2)

SP I67.5 **Moyamoya disease**

SP I67.6 **Nonpyogenic thrombosis of intracranial venous system**

Nonpyogenic thrombosis of cerebral vein
Nonpyogenic thrombosis of intracranial venous sinus

EXCLUDES 1 nonpyogenic thrombosis of intracranial venous system causing infarction (I63.6)

SP I67.7 **Cerebral arteritis, not elsewhere classified**

Granulomatous angiitis of the nervous system

EXCLUDES 1 allergic granulomatous angiitis (M30.1)

DEFINITION Inflammation of an artery in the head.

5 I67.8 **Other specified cerebrovascular diseases**

SP SH SL I67.81 **Acute cerebrovascular insufficiency**

Acute cerebrovascular insufficiency unspecified as to location or reversibility

SP SH SL **I67.82 Cerebral ischemia**
Chronic cerebral ischemia

SP **I67.83 Posterior reversible encephalopathy syndrome**
PRES

6 **I67.84 Cerebral vasospasm and vasoconstriction**

SP **I67.841 Reversible cerebrovascular vasoconstriction syndrome**
Call-Fleming syndrome
Code first:
underlying condition, if applicable, such as eclampsia (O15.00-O15.9)

SP **I67.848 Other cerebrovascular vasospasm and vasoconstriction**

6 **I67.85 Hereditary cerebrovascular diseases**

SP **I67.850 Cerebral autosomal dominant arteriopathy with subcortical infarcts and leukoencephalopathy**
CADASIL
Code also any associated diagnoses, such as:
epilepsy (G40.-)
stroke (I63.-)
vascular dementia (F01.-)

SP **I67.858 Other hereditary cerebrovascular disease**

SP SH SL **I67.89 Other cerebrovascular disease**

SP **I67.9 Cerebrovascular disease, unspecified**

CODING TIPS✓ Do not assign I67.9 for sequelae of cerebral vascular accident. Do not assign I67.9 for cerebral atherosclerosis or any other known type of cerebral vascular disorder. If the type of cerebral vascular disease is not specified in the record, query the patient's provider to attempt to obtain a more specific diagnosis.

4 **I68 Cerebrovascular disorders in diseases classified elsewhere**

CODING TIPS✓ These codes may be used in home health and hospice for various cerebrovascular disease.

M IQ **I68.0 *Cerebral amyloid angiopathy***
Code first:
underlying amyloidosis (E85.-)

M IQ **I68.2 *Cerebral arteritis in other diseases classified elsewhere***
Code first:
underlying disease
EXCLUDES 1 cerebral arteritis (in) :
listerosis (A32.89)
systemic lupus erythematosus (M32.19)
syphilis (A52.04)
tuberculosis (A18.89)

M IQ **I68.8 *Other cerebrovascular disorders in diseases classified elsewhere***
Code first:
underlying disease
EXCLUDES 1 syphilitic cerebral aneurysm (A52.05)

H 4 **I69 Sequelae of cerebrovascular disease**

Note:
Category I69 is to be used to indicate conditions in I60-I67 as the cause of sequelae. The 'sequelae' include conditions specified as such or as residuals which may occur at any time after the onset of the causal condition

EXCLUDES 1 personal history of cerebral infarction without residual deficit (Z86.73)
personal history of prolonged reversible ischemic neurologic deficit (PRIND) (Z86.73)
personal history of reversible ischemic neurologcial deficit (RIND) (Z86.73)
sequelae of traumatic intracranial injury (S06.-)

GUIDELINES **Section I.C.9.d.1)**
Category I69 is used to indicate conditions classifiable to categories I60-I67 as the causes of sequela (neurologic deficits), themselves classified elsewhere. These "late effects" include neurologic deficits that persist after initial onset of conditions classifiable to categories I60-I67. The neurologic deficits caused by cerebrovascular disease may be present from the onset or may arise at any time after the onset or may arise at any time after the onset of the condition classifiable to categories I60-I67.

Codes from category I69, Sequelae of cerebrovascular disease, that specify hemiplegia, hemiparesis and monoplegia identify whether the dominant or nondominant side is affected. Should the affected side be documented, but not specified as dominant or nondominant, and the classification system does not indicate a default, code selection is as follows:

- For ambidextrous patients, the default should be dominant.
- If the left side is affected, the default is non-dominant.
- If the right side is affected, the default is dominant.

GUIDELINES **Section I.C.9.d.3)**
Codes from category I69 should not be assigned if the patient does not have neurologic deficits.

CODING TIPS✓ I69 codes are used to indicate neurologic deficits as sequela of acute CVAs, themselves coded as I60-I63.

5 **I69.0 Sequelae of nontraumatic subarachnoid hemorrhage**

CODING TIPS ✓ Use subcategory I69.0, I69.1 or I69.2 for patients who have had a CVA involving a bleed when residual neurological deficits are apparent. If there are no neurological deficits, use Z86.73 instead. The neurologic deficits caused by cerebrovascular disease may be present from the onset or may arise at any time after the onset of the condition. Some I69.- codes are combination codes that include the residual deficit within the code, e.g., I69.-51. Others are combination codes that require additional information in the form of a secondary code to further specify the deficit, e.g., I69.-91.

CODING TIPS ✓ This code is used for residuals from a stroke caused by hemorrhage, not to be confused with a traumatic hemorrhage within or around the brain from an external injury.

IQ **I69.00 Unspecified sequelae of nontraumatic subarachnoid hemorrhage**

6 **I69.01 Cognitive deficits following nontraumatic subarachnoid hemorrhage**

SP SH SL **I69.010 Attention and concentration deficit following nontraumatic subarachnoid hemorrhage**

SP SH SL **I69.011 Memory deficit following nontraumatic subarachnoid hemorrhage**

SP SH SL **I69.012 Visuospatial deficit and spatial neglect following nontraumatic subarachnoid hemorrhage**

SP SH SL **I69.013 Psychomotor deficit following nontraumatic subarachnoid hemorrhage**

SP SH SL **I69.014 Frontal lobe and executive function deficit following nontraumatic subarachnoid hemorrhage**

SP SH SL **I69.015 Cognitive social or emotional deficit following nontraumatic subarachnoid hemorrhage**

SP SH SL **I69.018 Other symptoms and signs involving cognitive functions following nontraumatic subarachnoid hemorrhage**

IQ **I69.019 Unspecified symptoms and signs involving cognitive functions following nontraumatic subarachnoid hemorrhage**

6 **I69.02 Speech and language deficits following nontraumatic subarachnoid hemorrhage**

SP SH SL **I69.020 Aphasia following nontraumatic subarachnoid hemorrhage**

CODING TIPS ✓ Aphasia is the lack of speech, whereas dysphasia is difficulty speaking.

SP SH SL **I69.021 Dysphasia following nontraumatic subarachnoid hemorrhage**

CODING TIPS ✓ Aphasia is the lack of speech, whereas dysphasia is difficulty speaking.

CODING TIPS ✓ Distinguish between dysphasia (difficulty speaking) and dysphagia (difficulty swallowing).

SP SH SL **I69.022 Dysarthria following nontraumatic subarachnoid hemorrhage**

CODING TIPS ✓ Dysarthria is a weakness in the musculature of the mouth and throat causing difficulty with speech.

SP SH SL **I69.023 Fluency disorder following nontraumatic subarachnoid hemorrhage**

Stuttering following nontraumatic subarachnoid hemorrhage

SP SH SL **I69.028 Other speech and language deficits following nontraumatic subarachnoid hemorrhage**

6 **I69.03 Monoplegia of upper limb following nontraumatic subarachnoid hemorrhage**

H SP SH SL **I69.031 Monoplegia of upper limb following nontraumatic subarachnoid hemorrhage affecting right dominant side**

H SP SH SL **I69.032 Monoplegia of upper limb following nontraumatic subarachnoid hemorrhage affecting left dominant side**

H SP SH SL **I69.033 Monoplegia of upper limb following nontraumatic subarachnoid hemorrhage affecting right non-dominant side**

H SP SH SL **I69.034 Monoplegia of upper limb following nontraumatic subarachnoid hemorrhage affecting left non-dominant side**

H IQ **I69.039 Monoplegia of upper limb following nontraumatic subarachnoid hemorrhage affecting unspecified side**

ALERT This code includes unspecified side which may cause the claim to be rejected.

6 **I69.04 Monoplegia of lower limb following nontraumatic subarachnoid hemorrhage**

H SP SH SL **I69.041 Monoplegia of lower limb following nontraumatic subarachnoid hemorrhage affecting right dominant side**

H SP SH SL **I69.042 Monoplegia of lower limb following nontraumatic subarachnoid hemorrhage affecting left dominant side**

H SP SH SL **I69.043 Monoplegia of lower limb following nontraumatic subarachnoid hemorrhage affecting right non-dominant side**

H SP SH SL **I69.044 Monoplegia of lower limb following nontraumatic subarachnoid hemorrhage affecting left non-dominant side**

H IQ **I69.049 Monoplegia of lower limb following nontraumatic subarachnoid hemorrhage affecting unspecified side**

ALERT This code includes unspecified side which may cause the claim to be rejected.

6 **I69.05 Hemiplegia and hemiparesis following nontraumatic subarachnoid hemorrhage**

CODING TIPS✓ Hemiparesis is weakness of one side of the body due to cerebrovascular disease. This is often documented as "left-sided weakness" or "right-sided weakness." Hemiplegia and hemiparesis are represented by the same code and should be coded when one-sided weakness is described as a result of a stroke. When the side affected is documented, but not dominant or nondominant, the coder may choose dominant if the right side is affected and non-dominant if the left side is affected. Best practice is to obtain information from the clinician regarding dominant side.

⊟ SP SH SL **I69.051 Hemiplegia and hemiparesis following nontraumatic subarachnoid hemorrhage affecting right dominant side**

⊟ SP SH SL **I69.052 Hemiplegia and hemiparesis following nontraumatic subarachnoid hemorrhage affecting left dominant side**

⊟ SP SH SL **I69.053 Hemiplegia and hemiparesis following nontraumatic subarachnoid hemorrhage affecting right non-dominant side**

⊟ SP SH SL **I69.054 Hemiplegia and hemiparesis following nontraumatic subarachnoid hemorrhage affecting left non-dominant side**

⊟ IQ **I69.059 Hemiplegia and hemiparesis following nontraumatic subarachnoid hemorrhage affecting unspecified side**

ALERT This code includes unspecified side which may cause the claim to be rejected.

+ 6 **I69.06 Other paralytic syndrome following nontraumatic subarachnoid hemorrhage**

Use additional code to identify type of paralytic syndrome, such as:
- locked-in state (G83.5)
- quadriplegia (G82.5-)

EXCLUDES 1 hemiplegia/hemiparesis following nontraumatic subarachnoid hemorrhage (I69.05-)
monoplegia of lower limb following nontraumatic subarachnoid hemorrhage (I69.04-)
monoplegia of upper limb following nontraumatic subarachnoid hemorrhage (I69.03-)

⊟ SP SH SL + **I69.061 Other paralytic syndrome following nontraumatic subarachnoid hemorrhage affecting right dominant side**

⊟ SP SH SL + **I69.062 Other paralytic syndrome following nontraumatic subarachnoid hemorrhage affecting left dominant side**

⊟ SP SH SL + **I69.063 Other paralytic syndrome following nontraumatic subarachnoid hemorrhage affecting right non-dominant side**

⊟ SP SH SL + **I69.064 Other paralytic syndrome following nontraumatic subarachnoid hemorrhage affecting left non-dominant side**

⊟ SP SH SL + **I69.065 Other paralytic syndrome following nontraumatic subarachnoid hemorrhage, bilateral**

⊟ IQ + **I69.069 Other paralytic syndrome following nontraumatic subarachnoid hemorrhage affecting unspecified side**

6 **I69.09 Other sequelae of nontraumatic subarachnoid hemorrhage**

SP SH SL **I69.090 Apraxia following nontraumatic subarachnoid hemorrhage**

SP SH SL + **I69.091 Dysphagia following nontraumatic subarachnoid hemorrhage**

Use additional code to identify the type of dysphagia, if known (R13.1-)

CODING TIPS✓ Use an additional code from R13.1 to explain the phase of swallowing affected. Avoid coding unspecified dysphagia. Query the physician or NPP regarding phase of dysphagia.

CODING TIPS✓ Distinguish between dysphasia (difficulty speaking) and dysphagia (difficulty swallowing).

SP **I69.092 Facial weakness following nontraumatic subarachnoid hemorrhage**

Facial droop following nontraumatic subarachnoid hemorrhage

SP SH SL **I69.093 Ataxia following nontraumatic subarachnoid hemorrhage**

SP SH SL + **I69.098 Other sequelae following nontraumatic subarachnoid hemorrhage**

Alterations of sensation following nontraumatic subarachnoid hemorrhage

Disturbance of vision following nontraumatic subarachnoid hemorrhage

Use additional code to identify the sequelae

CODING TIPS✓ When generalized muscle weakness, seizures, contractures or other residuals not included in the other sequela codes result from a stroke, assign code I69.398, followed by the code for the specific residual, e.g., M62.81 (muscle weakness), or F48.2 (pseudobulbar affect - also known as involuntary emotional expression disorder).

5 **I69.1 Sequelae of nontraumatic intracerebral hemorrhage**

CODING TIPS✓ Use subcategory I69.0, I69.1 or I69.2 for patients who have had a CVA involving a bleed when residual neurological deficits are apparent. If there are no neurological deficits, use Z86.73 instead. The neurologic deficits caused by cerebrovascular disease may be present from the onset or may arise at any time after the onset of the condition. Some I69.- codes are combination codes that include the residual deficit within the code, e.g., I69.-51. Others are combination codes that require additional information in the form of a secondary code to further specify the deficit, e.g., I69.-91.

CODING TIPS✓ This code is used for residuals from a stroke caused by hemorrhage, not to be confused with a traumatic hemorrhage within or around the brain from an external injury.

SP **I69.10 Unspecified sequelae of nontraumatic intracerebral hemorrhage**

6 **I69.11 Cognitive deficits following nontraumatic intracerebral hemorrhage**

SP SH SL **I69.110 Attention and concentration deficit following nontraumatic intracerebral hemorrhage**

SP SH SL **I69.111 Memory deficit following nontraumatic intracerebral hemorrhage**

SP SH SL **I69.112 Visuospatial deficit and spatial neglect following nontraumatic intracerebral hemorrhage**

SP SH SL **I69.113 Psychomotor deficit following nontraumatic intracerebral hemorrhage**

SP SH SL **I69.114 Frontal lobe and executive function deficit following nontraumatic intracerebral hemorrhage**

SP SH SL **I69.115 Cognitive social or emotional deficit following nontraumatic intracerebral hemorrhage**

SP SH SL **I69.118 Other symptoms and signs involving cognitive functions following nontraumatic intracerebral hemorrhage**

CODING TIPS✓ Use this code to indicate vascular dementia related to a cerebral vascular accident, e.g. I69.--8, F01.50.

IQ **I69.119 Unspecified symptoms and signs involving cognitive functions following nontraumatic intracerebral hemorrhage**

6 **I69.12 Speech and language deficits following nontraumatic intracerebral hemorrhage**

SP SH SL **I69.120 Aphasia following nontraumatic intracerebral hemorrhage**

CODING TIPS✓ Aphasia is the lack of speech, whereas dysphasia is difficulty speaking.

SP SH SL **I69.121 Dysphasia following nontraumatic intracerebral hemorrhage**

CODING TIPS✓ Aphasia is the lack of speech, whereas dysphasia is difficulty speaking.

CODING TIPS✓ Distinguish between dysphasia (difficulty speaking) and dysphagia (difficulty swallowing).

SP SH SL **I69.122 Dysarthria following nontraumatic intracerebral hemorrhage**

CODING TIPS✓ Dysarthria is a weakness in the musculature of the mouth and throat causing difficulty with speech.

SP SH SL **I69.123 Fluency disorder following nontraumatic intracerebral hemorrhage**

Stuttering following nontraumatic intracerebral hemorrhage

SP SH SL **I69.128 Other speech and language deficits following nontraumatic intracerebral hemorrhage**

6 **I69.13 Monoplegia of upper limb following nontraumatic intracerebral hemorrhage**

H SP SH SL **I69.131 Monoplegia of upper limb following nontraumatic intracerebral hemorrhage affecting right dominant side**

H SP SH SL **I69.132 Monoplegia of upper limb following nontraumatic intracerebral hemorrhage affecting left dominant side**

H SP SH SL **I69.133 Monoplegia of upper limb following nontraumatic intracerebral hemorrhage affecting right non-dominant side**

H SP SH SL **I69.134 Monoplegia of upper limb following nontraumatic intracerebral hemorrhage affecting left non-dominant side**

H IQ **I69.139 Monoplegia of upper limb following nontraumatic intracerebral hemorrhage affecting unspecified side**

ALERT This code includes unspecified side which may cause the claim to be rejected.

6 **I69.14 Monoplegia of lower limb following nontraumatic intracerebral hemorrhage**

Chapter 9

I00-I99

I69.141 Monoplegia of lower limb following nontraumatic intracerebral hemorrhage affecting right dominant side (Laterality, SP, SH, SL)

I69.142 Monoplegia of lower limb following nontraumatic intracerebral hemorrhage affecting left dominant side (Laterality, SP, SH, SL)

I69.143 Monoplegia of lower limb following nontraumatic intracerebral hemorrhage affecting right non-dominant side (Laterality, SP, SH, SL)

I69.144 Monoplegia of lower limb following nontraumatic intracerebral hemorrhage affecting left non-dominant side (Laterality, SP, SH, SL)

I69.149 Monoplegia of lower limb following nontraumatic intracerebral hemorrhage affecting unspecified side (Laterality, IQ)

ALERT This code includes unspecified side which may cause the claim to be rejected.

I69.15 Hemiplegia and hemiparesis following nontraumatic intracerebral hemorrhage (6th digit required)

CODING TIPS✓ Hemiparesis is weakness of one side of the body due to cerebrovascular disease. This is often documented as "left-sided weakness" or "right-sided weakness." Hemiplegia and hemiparesis are represented by the same code and should be coded when one-sided weakness is described as a result of a stroke. When the side affected is documented, but not dominant or nondominant, the coder may choose dominant if the right side is affected and non-dominant if the left side is affected. Best practice is to obtain information from the clinician regarding dominant side.

I69.151 Hemiplegia and hemiparesis following nontraumatic intracerebral hemorrhage affecting right dominant side (Laterality, SP, SH, SL)

I69.152 Hemiplegia and hemiparesis following nontraumatic intracerebral hemorrhage affecting left dominant side (Laterality, SP, SH, SL)

I69.153 Hemiplegia and hemiparesis following nontraumatic intracerebral hemorrhage affecting right non-dominant side (Laterality, SP, SH, SL)

I69.154 Hemiplegia and hemiparesis following nontraumatic intracerebral hemorrhage affecting left non-dominant side (Laterality, SP, SH, SL)

I69.159 Hemiplegia and hemiparesis following nontraumatic intracerebral hemorrhage affecting unspecified side (Laterality, IQ)

ALERT This code includes unspecified side which may cause the claim to be rejected.

I69.16 Other paralytic syndrome following nontraumatic intracerebral hemorrhage (Additional code, 6th digit required)

Use additional code to identify type of paralytic syndrome, such as:
- locked-in state (G83.5)
- quadriplegia (G82.5-)

EXCLUDES 1
- hemiplegia/hemiparesis following nontraumatic intracerebral hemorrhage (I69.15-)
- monoplegia of lower limb following nontraumatic intracerebral hemorrhage (I69.14-)
- monoplegia of upper limb following nontraumatic intracerebral hemorrhage (I69.13-)

I69.161 Other paralytic syndrome following nontraumatic intracerebral hemorrhage affecting right dominant side (Laterality, SP, SH, SL, Additional code)

I69.162 Other paralytic syndrome following nontraumatic intracerebral hemorrhage affecting left dominant side (Laterality, SP, SH, SL, Additional code)

I69.163 Other paralytic syndrome following nontraumatic intracerebral hemorrhage affecting right non-dominant side (Laterality, SP, SH, SL, Additional code)

I69.164 Other paralytic syndrome following nontraumatic intracerebral hemorrhage affecting left non-dominant side (Laterality, SP, SH, SL, Additional code)

I69.165 Other paralytic syndrome following nontraumatic intracerebral hemorrhage, bilateral (Laterality, SP, SH, SL, Additional code)

I69.169 Other paralytic syndrome following nontraumatic intracerebral hemorrhage affecting unspecified side (Laterality, IQ, Additional code)

I69.19 Other sequelae of nontraumatic intracerebral hemorrhage (6th digit required)

I69.190 Apraxia following nontraumatic intracerebral hemorrhage (SP, SH, SL)

I69.191 Dysphagia following nontraumatic intracerebral hemorrhage (SP, SH, SL, Additional code)

Use additional code to identify the type of dysphagia, if known (R13.1-)

CODING TIPS✓ Use an additional code from R13.1 to explain the phase of swallowing affected. Avoid coding unspecified dysphagia. Query the physician or NPP regarding phase of dysphagia.

CODING TIPS✓ Distinguish between dysphasia (difficulty speaking) and dysphagia (difficulty swallowing).

I69.192 Facial weakness following nontraumatic intracerebral hemorrhage (SP)

Facial droop following nontraumatic intracerebral hemorrhage

I69.193 Ataxia following nontraumatic intracerebral hemorrhage (SP, SH, SL)

4 4th digit required | 5 5th digit required | 6 6th digit required | 7 7th digit required | 7th digit placeholder | + Additional code | Laterality

SP SH SL + I69.198 **Other sequelae of nontraumatic intracerebral hemorrhage**
Alteration of sensations following nontraumatic intracerebral hemorrhage
Disturbance of vision following nontraumatic intracerebral hemorrhage
Use additional code to identify the sequelae
CODING TIPS✓ When generalized muscle weakness, seizures, contractures or other residuals not included in the other sequela codes result from a stroke, assign code I69.398, followed by the code for the specific residual, e.g., M62.81 (muscle weakness), or F48.2 (pseudobulbar affect - also known as involuntary emotional expression disorder).

5 I69.2 **Sequelae of other nontraumatic intracranial hemorrhage**
CODING TIPS✓ Use subcategory I69.0, I69.1 or I69.2 for patients who have had a CVA involving a bleed when residual neurological deficits are apparent. If there are no neurological deficits, use Z86.73 instead. The neurologic deficits caused by cerebrovascular disease may be present from the onset or may arise at any time after the onset of the condition. Some I69.- codes are combination codes that include the residual deficit within the code, e.g., I69.-51. Others are combination codes that require additional information in the form of a secondary code to further specify the deficit, e.g., I69.-91.
CODING TIPS✓ This code is used for residuals from a stroke caused by hemorrhage, not to be confused with a traumatic hemorrhage within or around the brain from an external injury.

IQ I69.20 **Unspecified sequelae of other nontraumatic intracranial hemorrhage**

6 I69.21 **Cognitive deficits following other nontraumatic intracranial hemorrhage**

SP SH SL I69.210 **Attention and concentration deficit following other nontraumatic intracranial hemorrhage**

SP SH SL I69.211 **Memory deficit following other nontraumatic intracranial hemorrhage**

SP SH SL I69.212 **Visuospatial deficit and spatial neglect following other nontraumatic intracranial hemorrhage**

SP SH SL I69.213 **Psychomotor deficit following other nontraumatic intracranial hemorrhage**

SP SH SL I69.214 **Frontal lobe and executive function deficit following other nontraumatic intracranial hemorrhage**

SP SH SL I69.215 **Cognitive social or emotional deficit following other nontraumatic intracranial hemorrhage**

SP SH SL I69.218 **Other symptoms and signs involving cognitive functions following other nontraumatic intracranial hemorrhage**
CODING TIPS✓ Use this code to indicate vascular dementia related to a cerebral vascular accident, e.g. I69.--8, F01.50.

IQ I69.219 **Unspecified symptoms and signs involving cognitive functions following other nontraumatic intracranial hemorrhage**

6 I69.22 **Speech and language deficits following other nontraumatic intracranial hemorrhage**

SP SH SL I69.220 **Aphasia following other nontraumatic intracranial hemorrhage**
CODING TIPS✓ Aphasia is the lack of speech, whereas dysphasia is difficulty speaking.

SP SH SL I69.221 **Dysphasia following other nontraumatic intracranial hemorrhage**
CODING TIPS✓ Aphasia is the lack of speech, whereas dysphasia is difficulty speaking.
CODING TIPS✓ Distinguish between dysphasia (difficulty speaking) and dysphagia (difficulty swallowing).

SP SH SL I69.222 **Dysarthria following other nontraumatic intracranial hemorrhage**
CODING TIPS✓ Dysarthria is a weakness in the musculature of the mouth and throat causing difficulty with speech.

SP SH SL I69.223 **Fluency disorder following other nontraumatic intracranial hemorrhage**
Stuttering following other nontraumatic intracranial hemorrhage

SP SH SL I69.228 **Other speech and language deficits following other nontraumatic intracranial hemorrhage**

6 I69.23 **Monoplegia of upper limb following other nontraumatic intracranial hemorrhage**

⊟ SP SH SL I69.231 **Monoplegia of upper limb following other nontraumatic intracranial hemorrhage affecting right dominant side**

⊟ SP SH SL I69.232 **Monoplegia of upper limb following other nontraumatic intracranial hemorrhage affecting left dominant side**

⊟ SP SH SL I69.233 **Monoplegia of upper limb following other nontraumatic intracranial hemorrhage affecting right non-dominant side**

Chapter 9
I00-I99

Laterality SP SH SL **I69.234 Monoplegia of upper limb following other nontraumatic intracranial hemorrhage affecting left non-dominant side**

Laterality IQ **I69.239 Monoplegia of upper limb following other nontraumatic intracranial hemorrhage affecting unspecified side**

ALERT This code includes unspecified side which may cause the claim to be rejected.

6th digit required **I69.24 Monoplegia of lower limb following other nontraumatic intracranial hemorrhage**

Laterality SP SH SL **I69.241 Monoplegia of lower limb following other nontraumatic intracranial hemorrhage affecting right dominant side**

Laterality SP SH SL **I69.242 Monoplegia of lower limb following other nontraumatic intracranial hemorrhage affecting left dominant side**

Laterality SP SH SL **I69.243 Monoplegia of lower limb following other nontraumatic intracranial hemorrhage affecting right non-dominant side**

Laterality SP SH SL **I69.244 Monoplegia of lower limb following other nontraumatic intracranial hemorrhage affecting left non-dominant side**

Laterality IQ **I69.249 Monoplegia of lower limb following other nontraumatic intracranial hemorrhage affecting unspecified side**

ALERT This code includes unspecified side which may cause the claim to be rejected.

6th digit required **I69.25 Hemiplegia and hemiparesis following other nontraumatic intracranial hemorrhage**

CODING TIPS✓ Hemiparesis is weakness of one side of the body due to cerebrovascular disease. This is often documented as "left-sided weakness" or "right-sided weakness." Hemiplegia and hemiparesis are represented by the same code and should be coded when one-sided weakness is described as a result of a stroke. When the side affected is documented, but not dominant or nondominant, the coder may choose dominant if the right side is affected and non-dominant if the left side is affected. Best practice is to obtain information from the clinician regarding dominant side.

Laterality SP SH SL **I69.251 Hemiplegia and hemiparesis following other nontraumatic intracranial hemorrhage affecting right dominant side**

Laterality SP SH SL **I69.252 Hemiplegia and hemiparesis following other nontraumatic intracranial hemorrhage affecting left dominant side**

Laterality SP SH SL **I69.253 Hemiplegia and hemiparesis following other nontraumatic intracranial hemorrhage affecting right non-dominant side**

Laterality SP SH SL **I69.254 Hemiplegia and hemiparesis following other nontraumatic intracranial hemorrhage affecting left non-dominant side**

Laterality IQ **I69.259 Hemiplegia and hemiparesis following other nontraumatic intracranial hemorrhage affecting unspecified side**

ALERT This code includes unspecified side which may cause the claim to be rejected.

+ 6th digit required **I69.26 Other paralytic syndrome following other nontraumatic intracranial hemorrhage**

Use additional code to identify type of paralytic syndrome, such as:
- locked-in state (G83.5)
- quadriplegia (G82.5-)

EXCLUDES 1 hemiplegia/hemiparesis following other nontraumatic intracranial hemorrhage (I69.25-)
monoplegia of lower limb following other nontraumatic intracranial hemorrhage (I69.24-)
monoplegia of upper limb following other nontraumatic intracranial hemorrhage (I69.23-)

Laterality SP SH SL + **I69.261 Other paralytic syndrome following other nontraumatic intracranial hemorrhage affecting right dominant side**

Laterality SP SH SL + **I69.262 Other paralytic syndrome following other nontraumatic intracranial hemorrhage affecting left dominant side**

Laterality SP SH SL + **I69.263 Other paralytic syndrome following other nontraumatic intracranial hemorrhage affecting right non-dominant side**

Laterality SP SH SL + **I69.264 Other paralytic syndrome following other nontraumatic intracranial hemorrhage affecting left non-dominant side**

Laterality SP SH SL + **I69.265 Other paralytic syndrome following other nontraumatic intracranial hemorrhage, bilateral**

Laterality IQ + **I69.269 Other paralytic syndrome following other nontraumatic intracranial hemorrhage affecting unspecified side**

6th digit required **I69.29 Other sequelae of other nontraumatic intracranial hemorrhage**

SP SH SL **I69.290 Apraxia following other nontraumatic intracranial hemorrhage**

SP SH SL + **I69.291 Dysphagia following other nontraumatic intracranial hemorrhage**

Use additional code to identify the type of dysphagia, if known (R13.1-)

4th digit required 5th digit required 6th digit required 7th digit required 7th digit placeholder +Additional code Laterality

CODING TIPS✓ Use an additional code from R13.1 to explain the phase of swallowing affected. Avoid coding unspecified dysphagia. Query the physician or NPP regarding phase of dysphagia.

CODING TIPS✓ Distinguish between dysphasia (difficulty speaking) and dysphagia (difficulty swallowing).

SP **I69.292 Facial weakness following other nontraumatic intracranial hemorrhage**
Facial droop following other nontraumatic intracranial hemorrhage

SP SH SL **I69.293 Ataxia following other nontraumatic intracranial hemorrhage**

SP SH SL + **I69.298 Other sequelae of other nontraumatic intracranial hemorrhage**
Alteration of sensation following other nontraumatic intracranial hemorrhage
Disturbance of vision following other nontraumatic intracranial hemorrhage
Use additional code to identify the sequelae

CODING TIPS✓ When generalized muscle weakness, seizures, contractures or other residuals not included in the other sequela codes result from a stroke, assign code I69.398, followed by the code for the specific residual, e.g., M62.81 (muscle weakness), or F48.2 (pseudobulbar affect - also known as involuntary emotional expression disorder).

5 **I69.3 Sequelae of cerebral infarction**
Sequelae of stroke NOS

CODING TIPS✓ Use subcategory I69.3 for all stroke patients when residual neurological deficits are apparent. If there are no neurological deficits, use Z86.73 instead. The neurologic deficits caused by cerebrovascular disease may be present from the onset or may arise at any time after the onset of the condition. Some I69.3 codes are combination codes that include the residual deficit within the code, e.g., I69.351. Others are combination codes that require additional information in the form of a secondary code to further specify the deficit, e.g., I69.391.

IQ **I69.30 Unspecified sequelae of cerebral infarction**

6 **I69.31 Cognitive deficits following cerebral infarction**

SP SH SL **I69.310 Attention and concentration deficit following cerebral infarction**

SP SH SL **I69.311 Memory deficit following cerebral infarction**

SP SH SL **I69.312 Visuospatial deficit and spatial neglect following cerebral infarction**

SP SH SL **I69.313 Psychomotor deficit following cerebral infarction**

SP SH SL **I69.314 Frontal lobe and executive function deficit following cerebral infarction**

SP SH SL **I69.315 Cognitive social or emotional deficit following cerebral infarction**

SP SH SL **I69.318 Other symptoms and signs involving cognitive functions following cerebral infarction**

CODING TIPS✓ Use this code to indicate vascular dementia related to a cerebral vascular accident, e.g. I69.--8, F01.50.

IQ **I69.319 Unspecified symptoms and signs involving cognitive functions following cerebral infarction**

6 **I69.32 Speech and language deficits following cerebral infarction**

SP SH SL **I69.320 Aphasia following cerebral infarction**

CODING TIPS✓ Aphasia is the lack of speech, whereas dysphasia is difficulty speaking.

SP SH SL **I69.321 Dysphasia following cerebral infarction**

CODING TIPS✓ Aphasia is the lack of speech, whereas dysphasia is difficulty speaking.

CODING TIPS✓ Distinguish between dysphasia (difficulty speaking) and dysphagia (difficulty swallowing).

SP SH SL **I69.322 Dysarthria following cerebral infarction**
EXCLUDES 2 transient ischemic attack (TIA) (G45.9)

CODING TIPS✓ Dysarthria is a weakness in the musculature of the mouth and throat causing difficulty with speech.

SP SH SL **I69.323 Fluency disorder following cerebral infarction**
Stuttering following cerebral infarction

SP SH SL **I69.328 Other speech and language deficits following cerebral infarction**

6 **I69.33 Monoplegia of upper limb following cerebral infarction**

CODING TIPS✓ Unlike the I69.35 codes where hemiparesis is included, monoparesis is not included in the I69.33 and I69.34 codes. When monoparesis is documented, use I69.398. Weakness of a limb *without mention of muscle weakness* is assigned code R29.898, Other symptoms and signs involving the musculoskeletal system. If muscle weakness is documented, assign M62.81 as an additional code.

I69.331 Monoplegia of upper limb following cerebral infarction affecting right dominant side

I69.332 Monoplegia of upper limb following cerebral infarction affecting left dominant side

I69.333 Monoplegia of upper limb following cerebral infarction affecting right non-dominant side

I69.334 Monoplegia of upper limb following cerebral infarction affecting left non-dominant side

I69.339 Monoplegia of upper limb following cerebral infarction affecting unspecified side

ALERT This code includes unspecified side which may cause the claim to be rejected.

I69.34 Monoplegia of lower limb following cerebral infarction

CODING TIPS✓ Unlike the I69.35 codes where hemiparesis is included, monoparesis is not included in the I69.33 and I69.34 codes. When monoparesis is documented, use I69.398. Weakness of a limb *without mention of muscle weakness* is assigned code R29.898, Other symptoms and signs involving the musculoskeletal system. If muscle weakness is documented, assign M62.81 as an additional code.

I69.341 Monoplegia of lower limb following cerebral infarction affecting right dominant side

I69.342 Monoplegia of lower limb following cerebral infarction affecting left dominant side

I69.343 Monoplegia of lower limb following cerebral infarction affecting right non-dominant side

I69.344 Monoplegia of lower limb following cerebral infarction affecting left non-dominant side

I69.349 Monoplegia of lower limb following cerebral infarction affecting unspecified side

ALERT This code includes unspecified side which may cause the claim to be rejected.

I69.35 Hemiplegia and hemiparesis following cerebral infarction

CODING TIPS✓ Hemiparesis is weakness of one side of the body due to cerebrovascular disease. This is often documented as "left-sided weakness" or "right-sided weakness." Hemiplegia and hemiparesis are represented by the same code and should be coded when one-sided weakness is described as a result of a stroke. When the side affected is documented, but not dominant or nondominant, the coder may choose dominant if the right side is affected and non-dominant if the left side is affected. Best practice is to obtain information from the clinician regarding dominant side.

I69.351 Hemiplegia and hemiparesis following cerebral infarction affecting right dominant side

EXCLUDES 2 transient ischemic attack (TIA) (G45.9)

I69.352 Hemiplegia and hemiparesis following cerebral infarction affecting left dominant side

I69.353 Hemiplegia and hemiparesis following cerebral infarction affecting right non-dominant side

I69.354 Hemiplegia and hemiparesis following cerebral infarction affecting left non-dominant side

I69.359 Hemiplegia and hemiparesis following cerebral infarction affecting unspecified side

ALERT This code includes unspecified side which may cause the claim to be rejected.

+ I69.36 Other paralytic syndrome following cerebral infarction

Use additional code to identify type of paralytic syndrome, such as:
- locked-in state (G83.5)
- quadriplegia (G82.5-)

EXCLUDES 1 hemiplegia/hemiparesis following cerebral infarction (I69.35-)
monoplegia of lower limb following cerebral infarction (I69.34-)
monoplegia of upper limb following cerebral infarction (I69.33-)

+ I69.361 Other paralytic syndrome following cerebral infarction affecting right dominant side

+ I69.362 Other paralytic syndrome following cerebral infarction affecting left dominant side

+ I69.363 Other paralytic syndrome following cerebral infarction affecting right non-dominant side

+ I69.364 Other paralytic syndrome following cerebral infarction affecting left non-dominant side

+ I69.365 Other paralytic syndrome following cerebral infarction, bilateral

I69.369 Other paralytic syndrome following cerebral infarction affecting unspecified side

I69.39 Other sequelae of cerebral infarction

I69.390 Apraxia following cerebral infarction

I69.391 Dysphagia following cerebral infarction

Use additional code to identify the type of dysphagia, if known (R13.1-)

CODING TIPS ✓ Use an additional code from R13.1 to explain the phase of swallowing affected. Avoid coding unspecified dysphagia. Query the physician or NPP regarding phase of dysphagia.

CODING TIPS ✓ Distinguish between dysphasia (difficulty speaking) and dysphagia (difficulty swallowing).

I69.392 Facial weakness following cerebral infarction

Facial droop following cerebral infarction

I69.393 Ataxia following cerebral infarction

I69.398 Other sequelae of cerebral infarction

Alteration of sensation following cerebral infarction

Disturbance of vision following cerebral infarction

Use additional code to identify the sequelae

CODING TIPS ✓ When generalized muscle weakness, seizures, contractures or other residuals not included in the other sequela codes result from a stroke, assign code I69.398, followed by the code for the specific residual, e.g., M62.81 (muscle weakness), or F48.2 (pseudobulbar affect - also known as involuntary emotional expression disorder).

I69.8 Sequelae of other cerebrovascular diseases

EXCLUDES 1 sequelae of traumatic intracranial injury (S06.-)

I69.80 Unspecified sequelae of other cerebrovascular disease

I69.81 Cognitive deficits following other cerebrovascular disease

I69.810 Attention and concentration deficit following other cerebrovascular disease

I69.811 Memory deficit following other cerebrovascular disease

I69.812 Visuospatial deficit and spatial neglect following other cerebrovascular disease

I69.813 Psychomotor deficit following other cerebrovascular disease

I69.814 Frontal lobe and executive function deficit following other cerebrovascular disease

I69.815 Cognitive social or emotional deficit following other cerebrovascular disease

I69.818 Other symptoms and signs involving cognitive functions following other cerebrovascular disease

I69.819 Unspecified symptoms and signs involving cognitive functions following other cerebrovascular disease

I69.82 Speech and language deficits following other cerebrovascular disease

I69.820 Aphasia following other cerebrovascular disease

I69.821 Dysphasia following other cerebrovascular disease

I69.822 Dysarthria following other cerebrovascular disease

I69.823 Fluency disorder following other cerebrovascular disease

Stuttering following other cerebrovascular disease

I69.828 Other speech and language deficits following other cerebrovascular disease

I69.83 Monoplegia of upper limb following other cerebrovascular disease

I69.831 Monoplegia of upper limb following other cerebrovascular disease affecting right dominant side

I69.832 Monoplegia of upper limb following other cerebrovascular disease affecting left dominant side

I69.833 Monoplegia of upper limb following other cerebrovascular disease affecting right non-dominant side

I69.834 Monoplegia of upper limb following other cerebrovascular disease affecting left non-dominant side

I69.839 Monoplegia of upper limb following other cerebrovascular disease affecting unspecified side

ALERT This code includes unspecified side which may cause the claim to be rejected.

I69.84 Monoplegia of lower limb following other cerebrovascular disease

I69.841 Monoplegia of lower limb following other cerebrovascular disease affecting right dominant side

I69.842 Monoplegia of lower limb following other cerebrovascular disease affecting left dominant side

I69.843 Monoplegia of lower limb following other cerebrovascular disease affecting right non-dominant side

⊟ SP SH SL **I69.844 Monoplegia of lower limb following other cerebrovascular disease affecting left non-dominant side**

⊟ IQ **I69.849 Monoplegia of lower limb following other cerebrovascular disease affecting unspecified side**

ALERT This code includes unspecified side which may cause the claim to be rejected.

6 **I69.85 Hemiplegia and hemiparesis following other cerebrovascular disease**

⊟ SP SH SL **I69.851 Hemiplegia and hemiparesis following other cerebrovascular disease affecting right dominant side**

⊟ SP SH SL **I69.852 Hemiplegia and hemiparesis following other cerebrovascular disease affecting left dominant side**

⊟ SP SH SL **I69.853 Hemiplegia and hemiparesis following other cerebrovascular disease affecting right non-dominant side**

⊟ SP SH SL **I69.854 Hemiplegia and hemiparesis following other cerebrovascular disease affecting left non-dominant side**

⊟ IQ **I69.859 Hemiplegia and hemiparesis following other cerebrovascular disease affecting unspecified side**

ALERT This code includes unspecified side which may cause the claim to be rejected.

+ 6 **I69.86 Other paralytic syndrome following other cerebrovascular disease**

Use additional code to identify type of paralytic syndrome, such as:
locked-in state (G83.5)
quadriplegia (G82.5-)

EXCLUDES 1 hemiplegia/hemiparesis following other cerebrovascular disease (I69.85-)
monoplegia of lower limb following other cerebrovascular disease (I69.84-)
monoplegia of upper limb following other cerebrovascular disease (I69.83-)

⊟ SP SH SL + **I69.861 Other paralytic syndrome following other cerebrovascular disease affecting right dominant side**

⊟ SP SH SL + **I69.862 Other paralytic syndrome following other cerebrovascular disease affecting left dominant side**

⊟ SP SH SL + **I69.863 Other paralytic syndrome following other cerebrovascular disease affecting right non-dominant side**

⊟ SP SH SL + **I69.864 Other paralytic syndrome following other cerebrovascular disease affecting left non-dominant side**

⊟ SP SH SL + **I69.865 Other paralytic syndrome following other cerebrovascular disease, bilateral**

⊟ IQ + **I69.869 Other paralytic syndrome following other cerebrovascular disease affecting unspecified side**

6 **I69.89 Other sequelae of other cerebrovascular disease**

SP SH SL **I69.890 Apraxia following other cerebrovascular disease**

SP SH SL + **I69.891 Dysphagia following other cerebrovascular disease**

Use additional code to identify the type of dysphagia, if known (R13.1-)

SP **I69.892 Facial weakness following other cerebrovascular disease**

Facial droop following other cerebrovascular disease

SP SH SL **I69.893 Ataxia following other cerebrovascular disease**

SP SH SL + **I69.898 Other sequelae of other cerebrovascular disease**

Alteration of sensation following other cerebrovascular disease
Disturbance of vision following other cerebrovascular disease
Use additional code to identify the sequelae

5 **I69.9 Sequelae of unspecified cerebrovascular diseases**

EXCLUDES 1 sequelae of stroke (I69.3)
sequelae of traumatic intracranial injury (S06.-)

CODING TIPS ✓ Do not use this unspecified code for residuals or sequelae of strokes or any other known cerebrovascular diseases. See I69.3-.

IQ **I69.90 Unspecified sequelae of unspecified cerebrovascular disease**

6 **I69.91 Cognitive deficits following unspecified cerebrovascular disease**

SP SH SL **I69.910 Attention and concentration deficit following unspecified cerebrovascular disease**

SP SH SL **I69.911 Memory deficit following unspecified cerebrovascular disease**

SP SH SL **I69.912 Visuospatial deficit and spatial neglect following unspecified cerebrovascular disease**

SP SH SL **I69.913 Psychomotor deficit following unspecified cerebrovascular disease**

SP SH SL **I69.914 Frontal lobe and executive function deficit following unspecified cerebrovascular disease**

SP SH SL **I69.915 Cognitive social or emotional deficit following unspecified cerebrovascular disease**

SP SH SL **I69.918 Other symptoms and signs involving cognitive functions following unspecified cerebrovascular disease**

IQ **I69.919 Unspecified symptoms and signs involving cognitive functions following unspecified cerebrovascular disease**

6 **I69.92 Speech and language deficits following unspecified cerebrovascular disease**

SP SH SL **I69.920 Aphasia following unspecified cerebrovascular disease**

DEFINITION Impaired or complete loss of the ability to communicate with language or symbols resulting from brain damage.

SP SH SL **I69.921 Dysphasia following unspecified cerebrovascular disease**

DEFINITION Impairment in the ability to speak or understand words resulting from brain damage.

SP SH SL **I69.922 Dysarthria following unspecified cerebrovascular disease**

SP SH SL **I69.923 Fluency disorder following unspecified cerebrovascular disease**

Stuttering following unspecified cerebrovascular disease

SP SH SL **I69.928 Other speech and language deficits following unspecified cerebrovascular disease**

6 **I69.93 Monoplegia of upper limb following unspecified cerebrovascular disease**

H SP SH SL **I69.931 Monoplegia of upper limb following unspecified cerebrovascular disease affecting right dominant side**

H SP SH SL **I69.932 Monoplegia of upper limb following unspecified cerebrovascular disease affecting left dominant side**

H SP SH SL **I69.933 Monoplegia of upper limb following unspecified cerebrovascular disease affecting right non-dominant side**

H SP SH SL **I69.934 Monoplegia of upper limb following unspecified cerebrovascular disease affecting left non-dominant side**

H IQ **I69.939 Monoplegia of upper limb following unspecified cerebrovascular disease affecting unspecified side**

6 **I69.94 Monoplegia of lower limb following unspecified cerebrovascular disease**

H SP SH SL **I69.941 Monoplegia of lower limb following unspecified cerebrovascular disease affecting right dominant side**

H SP SH SL **I69.942 Monoplegia of lower limb following unspecified cerebrovascular disease affecting left dominant side**

H SP SH SL **I69.943 Monoplegia of lower limb following unspecified cerebrovascular disease affecting right non-dominant side**

H SP SH SL **I69.944 Monoplegia of lower limb following unspecified cerebrovascular disease affecting left non-dominant side**

H IQ **I69.949 Monoplegia of lower limb following unspecified cerebrovascular disease affecting unspecified side**

6 **I69.95 Hemiplegia and hemiparesis following unspecified cerebrovascular disease**

DEFINITION Paralysis affecting one side of the body.

H SP SH SL **I69.951 Hemiplegia and hemiparesis following unspecified cerebrovascular disease affecting right dominant side**

H SP SH SL **I69.952 Hemiplegia and hemiparesis following unspecified cerebrovascular disease affecting left dominant side**

H SP SH SL **I69.953 Hemiplegia and hemiparesis following unspecified cerebrovascular disease affecting right non-dominant side**

H SP SH SL **I69.954 Hemiplegia and hemiparesis following unspecified cerebrovascular disease affecting left non-dominant side**

H IQ **I69.959 Hemiplegia and hemiparesis following unspecified cerebrovascular disease affecting unspecified side**

+ 6 **I69.96 Other paralytic syndrome following unspecified cerebrovascular disease**

Use additional code to identify type of paralytic syndrome, such as:
locked-in state (G83.5)
quadriplegia (G82.5-)

EXCLUDES 1 hemiplegia/hemiparesis following unspecified cerebrovascular disease (I69.95-)
monoplegia of lower limb following unspecified cerebrovascular disease (I69.94-)
monoplegia of upper limb following unspecified cerebrovascular disease (I69.93-)

H SP SH SL + **I69.961 Other paralytic syndrome following unspecified cerebrovascular disease affecting right dominant side**

H SP SH SL + **I69.962 Other paralytic syndrome following unspecified cerebrovascular disease affecting left dominant side**

Laterality SP SH SL + **I69.963 Other paralytic syndrome following unspecified cerebrovascular disease affecting right non-dominant side**

Laterality SP SH SL + **I69.964 Other paralytic syndrome following unspecified cerebrovascular disease affecting left non-dominant side**

Laterality IQ SH SL + **I69.965 Other paralytic syndrome following unspecified cerebrovascular disease, bilateral**

Laterality IQ + **I69.969 Other paralytic syndrome following unspecified cerebrovascular disease affecting unspecified side**

6 **I69.99 Other sequelae of unspecified cerebrovascular disease**

SP SH SL **I69.990 Apraxia following unspecified cerebrovascular disease**

SP SH SL + **I69.991 Dysphagia following unspecified cerebrovascular disease**

Use additional code to identify the type of dysphagia, if known (R13.1-)

SP **I69.992 Facial weakness following unspecified cerebrovascular disease**

Facial droop following unspecified cerebrovascular disease

SP SH SL **I69.993 Ataxia following unspecified cerebrovascular disease**

DEFINITION Inability to coordinate muscle movement.

SP SH SL + **I69.998 Other sequelae following unspecified cerebrovascular disease**

Alteration in sensation following unspecified cerebrovascular disease
Disturbance of vision following unspecified cerebrovascular disease
Use additional code to identify the sequelae

Diseases of arteries, arterioles and capillaries (I70-I79)

+ 4 **I70 Atherosclerosis**

INCLUDES arteriolosclerosis
arterial degeneration
arteriosclerosis
arteriosclerotic vascular disease
arteriovascular degeneration
atheroma
endarteritis deformans or obliterans
senile arteritis
senile endarteritis
vascular degeneration

Use additional code to identify:
exposure to environmental tobacco smoke (Z77.22)
history of tobacco dependence (Z87.891)
occupational exposure to environmental tobacco smoke (Z57.31)
tobacco dependence (F17.-)
tobacco use (Z72.0)

EXCLUDES 2 arteriosclerotic cardiovascular disease (I25.1-)
arteriosclerotic heart disease (I25.1-)
atheroembolism (I75.-)
cerebral atherosclerosis (I67.2)
coronary atherosclerosis (I25.1-)
mesenteric atherosclerosis (K55.1)
precerebral atherosclerosis (I67.2)
primary pulmonary atherosclerosis (I27.0)

SP + **I70.0 Atherosclerosis of aorta**

DEFINITION Fatty plaque deposits in the aorta that reduce its diameter and elasticity.

SP + **I70.1 Atherosclerosis of renal artery**

Goldblatt's kidney

EXCLUDES 2 atherosclerosis of renal arterioles (I12.-)

CODING TIPS ✓ Atherosclerosis of renal artery may also be reported as renal artery stenosis. When renal artery stenosis is reported as causative of hypertension, an additional code of I15.0, Renovascular hypertension, should be reported.

+ 5 **I70.2 Atherosclerosis of native arteries of the extremities**

Mönckeberg's (medial) sclerosis
Use additional code, if applicable, to identify chronic total occlusion of artery of extremity (I70.92)

EXCLUDES 2 atherosclerosis of bypass graft of extremities (I70.30-I70.79)

CODING TIPS ✓ I70.2 is the correct subcategory for arteriosclerosis of the native arteries of the legs. Peripheral angiopathy may be documented as diabetic PVD. There is an assumed relationship between diabetes and PVD and PAD, including peripheral atherosclerosis. Diabetic arteriosclerosis of the peripheral arteries should be coded E--.51 or E--.52 then the appropriate I70.- code. PAD, PVD on M1028 should be selected.

+ 6 **I70.20 Unspecified atherosclerosis of native arteries of extremities**

Laterality SP + **I70.201 Unspecified atherosclerosis of native arteries of extremities, right leg**

Laterality SP + **I70.202 Unspecified atherosclerosis of native arteries of extremities, left leg**

Laterality SP + **I70.203 Unspecified atherosclerosis of native arteries of extremities, bilateral legs**

Laterality SP + **I70.208 Unspecified atherosclerosis of native arteries of extremities, other extremity**

Laterality IQ + **I70.209 Unspecified atherosclerosis of native arteries of extremities, unspecified extremity**

+ 6 I70.21 Atherosclerosis of native arteries of extremities with intermittent claudication

SP + I70.211 Atherosclerosis of native arteries of extremities with intermittent claudication, right leg

SP + I70.212 Atherosclerosis of native arteries of extremities with intermittent claudication, left leg

SP + I70.213 Atherosclerosis of native arteries of extremities with intermittent claudication, bilateral legs

SP + I70.218 Atherosclerosis of native arteries of extremities with intermittent claudication, other extremity

IQ + I70.219 Atherosclerosis of native arteries of extremities with intermittent claudication, unspecified extremity

+ 6 I70.22 Atherosclerosis of native arteries of extremities with rest pain

INCLUDES any condition classifiable to I70.21-
chronic limb-threatening ischemia NOS of native arteries of extremities
chronic limb-threatening ischemia of native arteries of extremities with rest pain
critical limb ischemia NOS of native arteries of extremities
critical limb ischemia of native arteries of extremities with rest pain

SP + I70.221 Atherosclerosis of native arteries of extremities with rest pain, right leg

SP + I70.222 Atherosclerosis of native arteries of extremities with rest pain, left leg

SP + I70.223 Atherosclerosis of native arteries of extremities with rest pain, bilateral legs

SP + I70.228 Atherosclerosis of native arteries of extremities with rest pain, other extremity

IQ + I70.229 Atherosclerosis of native arteries of extremities with rest pain, unspecified extremity

+ 6 I70.23 Atherosclerosis of native arteries of right leg with ulceration

INCLUDES any condition classifiable to I70.211 and I70.221
chronic limb-threatening ischemia of native arteries of right leg with ulceration
critical limb ischemia of native arteries of right leg with ulceration

Use additional code to identify severity of ulcer (L97.-)

CODING TIPS ✓ When the physician or NPP documents arterial ulcer, query regarding arteriosclerosis.

CODING TIPS ✓ When bilateral ulcers are present or ulcers of multiple specified areas classifiable in a patient with atherosclerosis of the extremities, assign a code for each specific site, taking laterality into account. A second code from category L97.- to specify the severity of the ulcer must be used following each reported site of atherosclerosis to the extremity with ulceration. The ICD-10 classification assumes a relationship between atherosclerosis of lower extremities and gangrene, ulceration, rest pain and intermittent claudication.

SP SH SL + I70.231 Atherosclerosis of native arteries of right leg with ulceration of thigh

SP SH SL + I70.232 Atherosclerosis of native arteries of right leg with ulceration of calf

SP SH SL + I70.233 Atherosclerosis of native arteries of right leg with ulceration of ankle

SP SH SL + I70.234 Atherosclerosis of native arteries of right leg with ulceration of heel and midfoot

Atherosclerosis of native arteries of right leg with ulceration of plantar surface of midfoot

SP SH SL + I70.235 Atherosclerosis of native arteries of right leg with ulceration of other part of foot

Atherosclerosis of native arteries of right leg extremities with ulceration of toe

SP SH SL + I70.238 Atherosclerosis of native arteries of right leg with ulceration of other part of lower leg

IQ + I70.239 Atherosclerosis of native arteries of right leg with ulceration of unspecified site

+ 6 I70.24 Atherosclerosis of native arteries of left leg with ulceration

INCLUDES any condition classifiable to I70.212 and I70.222
chronic limb-threatening ischemia of native arteries of left leg with ulceration
critical limb ischemia of native arteries of left leg with ulceration

Use additional code to identify severity of ulcer (L97.-)

CODING TIPS ✓ When the physician or NPP documents arterial ulcer, query regarding arteriosclerosis.

Chapter 9

I00-I99

CODING TIPS✓ When bilateral ulcers are present or ulcers of multiple specified areas classifiable in a patient with atherosclerosis of the extremities, assign a code for each specific site, taking laterality into account. A second code from category L97.- to specify the severity of the ulcer must be used following each reported site of atherosclerosis to the extremity with ulceration. The ICD-10 classification assumes a relationship between atherosclerosis of lower extremities and gangrene, ulceration, rest pain and intermittent claudication.

Laterality SP SH SL + **I70.241 Atherosclerosis of native arteries of left leg with ulceration of thigh**

Laterality SP SH SL + **I70.242 Atherosclerosis of native arteries of left leg with ulceration of calf**

Laterality SP SH SL + **I70.243 Atherosclerosis of native arteries of left leg with ulceration of ankle**

Laterality SP SH SL + **I70.244 Atherosclerosis of native arteries of left leg with ulceration of heel and midfoot**

Atherosclerosis of native arteries of left leg with ulceration of plantar surface of midfoot

Laterality SP SH SL + **I70.245 Atherosclerosis of native arteries of left leg with ulceration of other part of foot**

Atherosclerosis of native arteries of left leg extremities with ulceration of toe

Laterality SP SH SL + **I70.248 Atherosclerosis of native arteries of left leg with ulceration of other part of lower leg**

Laterality IQ + **I70.249 Atherosclerosis of native arteries of left leg with ulceration of unspecified site**

Laterality SP + **I70.25 Atherosclerosis of native arteries of other extremities with ulceration**

INCLUDES any condition classifiable to I70.218 and I70.228

Use additional code to identify the severity of the ulcer (L98.49-)

CODING TIPS✓ When the physician or NPP documents arterial ulcer, query regarding arteriosclerosis.

CODING TIPS✓ When bilateral ulcers are present or ulcers of multiple specified areas classifiable in a patient with atherosclerosis of the extremities, assign a code for each specific site, taking laterality into account. A second code from category L97.- to specify the severity of the ulcer must be used following each reported site of atherosclerosis to the extremity with ulceration. The ICD-10 classification assumes a relationship between atherosclerosis of lower extremities and gangrene, ulceration, rest pain and intermittent claudication.

+ 6 **I70.26 Atherosclerosis of native arteries of extremities with gangrene**

INCLUDES any condition classifiable to I70.21-, I70.22-, I70.23-, I70.24-, and I70.25-

chronic limb-threatening ischemia of native arteries of extremities with gangrene

critical limb ischemia of native arteries of extremities with gangrene

Use additional code to identify the severity of any ulcer (L97.-, L98.49-), if applicable

CODING TIPS✓ When the clinical record reports atherosclerosis of the lower extremities with ulceration and gangrene, assign a code from I70.26-. Do not code the gangrene separately.

An additional code from category L97.- should be assigned to report the severity of any ulceration.

Laterality SP + **I70.261 Atherosclerosis of native arteries of extremities with gangrene, right leg**

Laterality SP + **I70.262 Atherosclerosis of native arteries of extremities with gangrene, left leg**

Laterality SP + **I70.263 Atherosclerosis of native arteries of extremities with gangrene, bilateral legs**

Laterality SP + **I70.268 Atherosclerosis of native arteries of extremities with gangrene, other extremity**

Laterality IQ + **I70.269 Atherosclerosis of native arteries of extremities with gangrene, unspecified extremity**

+ 6 **I70.29 Other atherosclerosis of native arteries of extremities**

Laterality SP + **I70.291 Other atherosclerosis of native arteries of extremities, right leg**

Laterality SP + **I70.292 Other atherosclerosis of native arteries of extremities, left leg**

Laterality SP + **I70.293 Other atherosclerosis of native arteries of extremities, bilateral legs**

Laterality SP + **I70.298 Other atherosclerosis of native arteries of extremities, other extremity**

Laterality IQ + **I70.299 Other atherosclerosis of native arteries of extremities, unspecified extremity**

+ 5 **I70.3 Atherosclerosis of unspecified type of bypass graft(s) of the extremities**

Use additional code, if applicable, to identify chronic total occlusion of artery of extremity (I70.92)

EXCLUDES 1 embolism or thrombus of bypass graft (s) of extremities (T82.8-)

CODING TIPS✓ M1028 should be marked PAD, PVD on the OASIS.

CODING TIPS ✓ Peripheral angiopathy may be documented as diabetic PVD. There is an assumed relationship between diabetes and PVD and PAD, including peripheral atherosclerosis. Diabetic arteriosclerosis of the peripheral arteries should be coded E--.51 or E--.52 then the appropriate I70.- code.

+ 6 **I70.30 Unspecified atherosclerosis of unspecified type of bypass graft(s) of the extremities**

SP + **I70.301 Unspecified atherosclerosis of unspecified type of bypass graft(s) of the extremities, right leg**

SP + **I70.302 Unspecified atherosclerosis of unspecified type of bypass graft(s) of the extremities, left leg**

SP + **I70.303 Unspecified atherosclerosis of unspecified type of bypass graft(s) of the extremities, bilateral legs**

SP + **I70.308 Unspecified atherosclerosis of unspecified type of bypass graft(s) of the extremities, other extremity**

IQ + **I70.309 Unspecified atherosclerosis of unspecified type of bypass graft(s) of the extremities, unspecified extremity**

+ 6 **I70.31 Atherosclerosis of unspecified type of bypass graft(s) of the extremities with intermittent claudication**

SP + **I70.311 Atherosclerosis of unspecified type of bypass graft(s) of the extremities with intermittent claudication, right leg**

SP + **I70.312 Atherosclerosis of unspecified type of bypass graft(s) of the extremities with intermittent claudication, left leg**

SP + **I70.313 Atherosclerosis of unspecified type of bypass graft(s) of the extremities with intermittent claudication, bilateral legs**

SP + **I70.318 Atherosclerosis of unspecified type of bypass graft(s) of the extremities with intermittent claudication, other extremity**

IQ + **I70.319 Atherosclerosis of unspecified type of bypass graft(s) of the extremities with intermittent claudication, unspecified extremity**

+ 6 **I70.32 Atherosclerosis of unspecified type of bypass graft(s) of the extremities with rest pain**

INCLUDES any condition classifiable to I70.31-
chronic limb-threatening ischemia NOS of unspecified type of bypass graft (s) of the extremities
chronic limb-threatening ischemia of unspecified type of bypass graft (s) of the extremities with rest pain, right leg
critical limb ischemia NOS of unspecified type of bypass graft (s) of the extremities
critical limb ischemia of unspecified type of bypass graft (s) of the extremities with rest pain

SP + **I70.321 Atherosclerosis of unspecified type of bypass graft(s) of the extremities with rest pain, right leg**

SP + **I70.322 Atherosclerosis of unspecified type of bypass graft(s) of the extremities with rest pain, left leg**

SP + **I70.323 Atherosclerosis of unspecified type of bypass graft(s) of the extremities with rest pain, bilateral legs**

SP + **I70.328 Atherosclerosis of unspecified type of bypass graft(s) of the extremities with rest pain, other extremity**

IQ + **I70.329 Atherosclerosis of unspecified type of bypass graft(s) of the extremities with rest pain, unspecified extremity**

+ 6 **I70.33 Atherosclerosis of unspecified type of bypass graft(s) of the right leg with ulceration**

INCLUDES any condition classifiable to I70.311 and I70.321
chronic limb-threatening ischemia of unspecified type of bypass graft (s) of the right leg with ulceration
critical limb ischemia of unspecified type of bypass graft (s) of the right leg with ulceration

Use additional code to identify severity of ulcer (L97.-)

SP SH SL + **I70.331 Atherosclerosis of unspecified type of bypass graft(s) of the right leg with ulceration of thigh**

SP SH SL + **I70.332 Atherosclerosis of unspecified type of bypass graft(s) of the right leg with ulceration of calf**

SP SH SL + **I70.333 Atherosclerosis of unspecified type of bypass graft(s) of the right leg with ulceration of ankle**

SP SH SL + **I70.334 Atherosclerosis of unspecified type of bypass graft(s) of the right leg with ulceration of heel and midfoot**

Atherosclerosis of unspecified type of bypass graft(s) of right leg with ulceration of plantar surface of midfoot

Chapter 9
I00-I99

Laterality SP SH SL + **I70.335 Atherosclerosis of unspecified type of bypass graft(s) of the right leg with ulceration of other part of foot**

Atherosclerosis of unspecified type of bypass graft(s) of the right leg with ulceration of toe

Laterality SP SH SL + **I70.338 Atherosclerosis of unspecified type of bypass graft(s) of the right leg with ulceration of other part of lower leg**

Laterality IQ SH SL + **I70.339 Atherosclerosis of unspecified type of bypass graft(s) of the right leg with ulceration of unspecified site**

+ 6 **I70.34 Atherosclerosis of unspecified type of bypass graft(s) of the left leg with ulceration**

INCLUDES any condition classifiable to I70.312 and I70.322

chronic limb-threatening ischemia of unspecified type of bypass graft (s) of the left leg with ulceration

critical limb ischemia of unspecified type of bypass graft (s) of the left leg with ulceration

Use additional code to identify severity of ulcer (L97.-)

Laterality SP SH SL + **I70.341 Atherosclerosis of unspecified type of bypass graft(s) of the left leg with ulceration of thigh**

Laterality SP SH SL + **I70.342 Atherosclerosis of unspecified type of bypass graft(s) of the left leg with ulceration of calf**

Laterality SP SH SL + **I70.343 Atherosclerosis of unspecified type of bypass graft(s) of the left leg with ulceration of ankle**

Laterality SP SH SL + **I70.344 Atherosclerosis of unspecified type of bypass graft(s) of the left leg with ulceration of heel and midfoot**

Atherosclerosis of unspecified type of bypass graft(s) of left leg with ulceration of plantar surface of midfoot

Laterality SP SH SL + **I70.345 Atherosclerosis of unspecified type of bypass graft(s) of the left leg with ulceration of other part of foot**

Atherosclerosis of unspecified type of bypass graft(s) of the left leg with ulceration of toe

Laterality SP SH SL + **I70.348 Atherosclerosis of unspecified type of bypass graft(s) of the left leg with ulceration of other part of lower leg**

Laterality IQ SH SL + **I70.349 Atherosclerosis of unspecified type of bypass graft(s) of the left leg with ulceration of unspecified site**

Laterality SP + **I70.35 Atherosclerosis of unspecified type of bypass graft(s) of other extremity with ulceration**

INCLUDES any condition classifiable to I70.318 and I70.328

Use additional code to identify severity of ulcer (L98.49-)

+ 6 **I70.36 Atherosclerosis of unspecified type of bypass graft(s) of the extremities with gangrene**

INCLUDES any condition classifiable to I70.31-, I70.32-, I70.33-, I70.34-, I70.35

chronic limb-threatening ischemia of unspecified type of bypass graft (s) of the extremities with gangrene

critical limb ischemia of unspecified type of bypass graft (s) of the extremities with gangrene

Use additional code to identify the severity of any ulcer (L97.-, L98.49-), if applicable

Laterality SP + **I70.361 Atherosclerosis of unspecified type of bypass graft(s) of the extremities with gangrene, right leg**

Laterality SP + **I70.362 Atherosclerosis of unspecified type of bypass graft(s) of the extremities with gangrene, left leg**

Laterality SP + **I70.363 Atherosclerosis of unspecified type of bypass graft(s) of the extremities with gangrene, bilateral legs**

Laterality SP + **I70.368 Atherosclerosis of unspecified type of bypass graft(s) of the extremities with gangrene, other extremity**

Laterality IQ + **I70.369 Atherosclerosis of unspecified type of bypass graft(s) of the extremities with gangrene, unspecified extremity**

+ 6 **I70.39 Other atherosclerosis of unspecified type of bypass graft(s) of the extremities**

Laterality SP + **I70.391 Other atherosclerosis of unspecified type of bypass graft(s) of the extremities, right leg**

Laterality SP + **I70.392 Other atherosclerosis of unspecified type of bypass graft(s) of the extremities, left leg**

Laterality SP + **I70.393 Other atherosclerosis of unspecified type of bypass graft(s) of the extremities, bilateral legs**

Laterality SP + **I70.398 Other atherosclerosis of unspecified type of bypass graft(s) of the extremities, other extremity**

Laterality IQ + **I70.399 Other atherosclerosis of unspecified type of bypass graft(s) of the extremities, unspecified extremity**

+ 5 **I70.4 Atherosclerosis of autologous vein bypass graft(s) of the extremities**

Use additional code, if applicable, to identify chronic total occlusion of artery of extremity (I70.92)

CODING TIPS✓ M1028 should be marked PAD, PVD on the OASIS.

CODING TIPS✓ Peripheral angiopathy may be documented as diabetic PVD. There is an assumed relationship between diabetes and PVD and PAD, including peripheral atherosclerosis. Diabetic arteriosclerosis of the peripheral arteries should be coded E--.51 or E--.52 then the appropriate I70.- code.

+ 6 **I70.40** **Unspecified atherosclerosis of autologous vein bypass graft(s) of the extremities**

SP + **I70.401** **Unspecified atherosclerosis of autologous vein bypass graft(s) of the extremities, right leg**

SP + **I70.402** **Unspecified atherosclerosis of autologous vein bypass graft(s) of the extremities, left leg**

SP + **I70.403** **Unspecified atherosclerosis of autologous vein bypass graft(s) of the extremities, bilateral legs**

SP + **I70.408** **Unspecified atherosclerosis of autologous vein bypass graft(s) of the extremities, other extremity**

IQ + **I70.409** **Unspecified atherosclerosis of autologous vein bypass graft(s) of the extremities, unspecified extremity**

+ 6 **I70.41** **Atherosclerosis of autologous vein bypass graft(s) of the extremities with intermittent claudication**

SP + **I70.411** **Atherosclerosis of autologous vein bypass graft(s) of the extremities with intermittent claudication, right leg**

SP + **I70.412** **Atherosclerosis of autologous vein bypass graft(s) of the extremities with intermittent claudication, left leg**

SP + **I70.413** **Atherosclerosis of autologous vein bypass graft(s) of the extremities with intermittent claudication, bilateral legs**

SP + **I70.418** **Atherosclerosis of autologous vein bypass graft(s) of the extremities with intermittent claudication, other extremity**

IQ + **I70.419** **Atherosclerosis of autologous vein bypass graft(s) of the extremities with intermittent claudication, unspecified extremity**

+ 6 **I70.42** **Atherosclerosis of autologous vein bypass graft(s) of the extremities with rest pain**

INCLUDES any condition classifiable to I70.41-
chronic limb-threatening ischemia NOS of autologous vein bypass graft (s) of the extremities
chronic limb-threatening ischemia of autologous vein bypass graft (s) of the extremities with rest pain
critical limb ischemia NOS of autologous vein bypass graft (s) of the extremities
critical limb ischemia of autologous vein bypass graft (s) of the extremities with rest pain

SP + **I70.421** **Atherosclerosis of autologous vein bypass graft(s) of the extremities with rest pain, right leg**

SP + **I70.422** **Atherosclerosis of autologous vein bypass graft(s) of the extremities with rest pain, left leg**

SP + **I70.423** **Atherosclerosis of autologous vein bypass graft(s) of the extremities with rest pain, bilateral legs**

SP + **I70.428** **Atherosclerosis of autologous vein bypass graft(s) of the extremities with rest pain, other extremity**

IQ + **I70.429** **Atherosclerosis of autologous vein bypass graft(s) of the extremities with rest pain, unspecified extremity**

+ 6 **I70.43** **Atherosclerosis of autologous vein bypass graft(s) of the right leg with ulceration**

INCLUDES any condition classifiable to I70.411 and I70.421
chronic limb-threatening ischemia of autologous vein bypass graft (s) of the right leg with ulceration
critical limb ischemia of autologous vein bypass graft (s) of the right leg with ulceration

Use additional code to identify severity of ulcer (L97.-)

SP SH SL + **I70.431** **Atherosclerosis of autologous vein bypass graft(s) of the right leg with ulceration of thigh**

SP SH SL + **I70.432** **Atherosclerosis of autologous vein bypass graft(s) of the right leg with ulceration of calf**

SP SH SL + **I70.433** **Atherosclerosis of autologous vein bypass graft(s) of the right leg with ulceration of ankle**

SP SH SL + **I70.434** **Atherosclerosis of autologous vein bypass graft(s) of the right leg with ulceration of heel and midfoot**

Atherosclerosis of autologous vein bypass graft(s) of right leg with ulceration of plantar surface of midfoot

SP SH SL + **I70.435** **Atherosclerosis of autologous vein bypass graft(s) of the right leg with ulceration of other part of foot**

Chapter 9

I00-I99

Atherosclerosis of autologous vein bypass graft(s) of right leg with ulceration of toe

SP SH SL + **I70.438 Atherosclerosis of autologous vein bypass graft(s) of the right leg with ulceration of other part of lower leg**

IQ SH SL + **I70.439 Atherosclerosis of autologous vein bypass graft(s) of the right leg with ulceration of unspecified site**

+ 6 **I70.44 Atherosclerosis of autologous vein bypass graft(s) of the left leg with ulceration**

INCLUDES any condition classifiable to I70.412 and I70.422

chronic limb-threatening ischemia of autologous vein bypass graft (s) of the left leg with ulceration

critical limb ischemia of autologous vein bypass graft (s) of the left leg with ulceration

Use additional code to identify severity of ulcer (L97.-)

SP SH SL + **I70.441 Atherosclerosis of autologous vein bypass graft(s) of the left leg with ulceration of thigh**

SP SH SL + **I70.442 Atherosclerosis of autologous vein bypass graft(s) of the left leg with ulceration of calf**

SP SH SL + **I70.443 Atherosclerosis of autologous vein bypass graft(s) of the left leg with ulceration of ankle**

SP SH SL + **I70.444 Atherosclerosis of autologous vein bypass graft(s) of the left leg with ulceration of heel and midfoot**

Atherosclerosis of autologous vein bypass graft(s) of left leg with ulceration of plantar surface of midfoot

SP SH SL + **I70.445 Atherosclerosis of autologous vein bypass graft(s) of the left leg with ulceration of other part of foot**

Atherosclerosis of autologous vein bypass graft(s) of left leg with ulceration of toe

SP SH SL + **I70.448 Atherosclerosis of autologous vein bypass graft(s) of the left leg with ulceration of other part of lower leg**

IQ SH SL + **I70.449 Atherosclerosis of autologous vein bypass graft(s) of the left leg with ulceration of unspecified site**

SP + **I70.45 Atherosclerosis of autologous vein bypass graft(s) of other extremity with ulceration**

INCLUDES any condition classifiable to I70.418, I70.428, and I70.438

Use additional code to identify severity of ulcer (L98.49)

+ 6 **I70.46 Atherosclerosis of autologous vein bypass graft(s) of the extremities with gangrene**

INCLUDES any condition classifiable to I70.41-, I70.42-, and I70.43-, I70.44-, I70.45

chronic limb-threatening ischemia of autologous vein bypass graft (s) of the extremities with gangrene

critical limb ischemia of autologous vein bypass graft (s) of the extremities with gangrene

Use additional code to identify the severity of any ulcer (L97.-, L98.49-), if applicable

SP + **I70.461 Atherosclerosis of autologous vein bypass graft(s) of the extremities with gangrene, right leg**

SP + **I70.462 Atherosclerosis of autologous vein bypass graft(s) of the extremities with gangrene, left leg**

SP + **I70.463 Atherosclerosis of autologous vein bypass graft(s) of the extremities with gangrene, bilateral legs**

SP + **I70.468 Atherosclerosis of autologous vein bypass graft(s) of the extremities with gangrene, other extremity**

IQ + **I70.469 Atherosclerosis of autologous vein bypass graft(s) of the extremities with gangrene, unspecified extremity**

+ 6 **I70.49 Other atherosclerosis of autologous vein bypass graft(s) of the extremities**

SP + **I70.491 Other atherosclerosis of autologous vein bypass graft(s) of the extremities, right leg**

SP + **I70.492 Other atherosclerosis of autologous vein bypass graft(s) of the extremities, left leg**

SP + **I70.493 Other atherosclerosis of autologous vein bypass graft(s) of the extremities, bilateral legs**

SP + **I70.498 Other atherosclerosis of autologous vein bypass graft(s) of the extremities, other extremity**

IQ + **I70.499 Other atherosclerosis of autologous vein bypass graft(s) of the extremities, unspecified extremity**

+ 5 **I70.5 Atherosclerosis of nonautologous biological bypass graft(s) of the extremities**

Use additional code, if applicable, to identify chronic total occlusion of artery of extremity (I70.92)

CODING TIPS ✓ M1028 should be marked PAD, PVD on the OASIS.

CODING TIPS ✓ Peripheral angiopathy may be documented as diabetic PVD. There is an assumed relationship between diabetes and PVD and PAD, including peripheral atherosclerosis. Diabetic arteriosclerosis of the peripheral arteries should be coded E--.51 or E--.52 then the appropriate I70.- code.

+ 6 I70.50 **Unspecified atherosclerosis of nonautologous biological bypass graft(s) of the extremities**

SP + I70.501 **Unspecified atherosclerosis of nonautologous biological bypass graft(s) of the extremities, right leg**

SP + I70.502 **Unspecified atherosclerosis of nonautologous biological bypass graft(s) of the extremities, left leg**

SP + I70.503 **Unspecified atherosclerosis of nonautologous biological bypass graft(s) of the extremities, bilateral legs**

SP + I70.508 **Unspecified atherosclerosis of nonautologous biological bypass graft(s) of the extremities, other extremity**

IQ + I70.509 **Unspecified atherosclerosis of nonautologous biological bypass graft(s) of the extremities, unspecified extremity**

+ 6 I70.51 **Atherosclerosis of nonautologous biological bypass graft(s) of the extremities intermittent claudication**

SP + I70.511 **Atherosclerosis of nonautologous biological bypass graft(s) of the extremities with intermittent claudication, right leg**

SP + I70.512 **Atherosclerosis of nonautologous biological bypass graft(s) of the extremities with intermittent claudication, left leg**

SP + I70.513 **Atherosclerosis of nonautologous biological bypass graft(s) of the extremities with intermittent claudication, bilateral legs**

SP + I70.518 **Atherosclerosis of nonautologous biological bypass graft(s) of the extremities with intermittent claudication, other extremity**

IQ + I70.519 **Atherosclerosis of nonautologous biological bypass graft(s) of the extremities with intermittent claudication, unspecified extremity**

+ 6 I70.52 **Atherosclerosis of nonautologous biological bypass graft(s) of the extremities with rest pain**

INCLUDES any condition classifiable to I70.51-
chronic limb-threatening ischemia NOS of nonautologous biological bypass graft (s) of the extremities
chronic limb-threatening ischemia of nonautologous biological bypass graft (s) of the extremities with rest pain
critical limb ischemia NOS of nonautologous biological bypass graft (s) of the extremities
critical limb ischemia of nonautologous biological bypass graft (s) of the extremities with rest pain

SP + I70.521 **Atherosclerosis of nonautologous biological bypass graft(s) of the extremities with rest pain, right leg**

SP + I70.522 **Atherosclerosis of nonautologous biological bypass graft(s) of the extremities with rest pain, left leg**

SP + I70.523 **Atherosclerosis of nonautologous biological bypass graft(s) of the extremities with rest pain, bilateral legs**

SP + I70.528 **Atherosclerosis of nonautologous biological bypass graft(s) of the extremities with rest pain, other extremity**

IQ + I70.529 **Atherosclerosis of nonautologous biological bypass graft(s) of the extremities with rest pain, unspecified extremity**

+ 6 I70.53 **Atherosclerosis of nonautologous biological bypass graft(s) of the right leg with ulceration**

INCLUDES any condition classifiable to I70.511 and I70.521
chronic limb-threatening ischemia of nonautologous biological bypass graft (s) of the right leg with ulceration
critical limb ischemia of nonautologous biological bypass graft (s) of the right leg with ulceration

Use additional code to identify severity of ulcer (L97.-)

SP SH SL + I70.531 **Atherosclerosis of nonautologous biological bypass graft(s) of the right leg with ulceration of thigh**

SP SH SL + I70.532 **Atherosclerosis of nonautologous biological bypass graft(s) of the right leg with ulceration of calf**

SP SH SL + I70.533 **Atherosclerosis of nonautologous biological bypass graft(s) of the right leg with ulceration of ankle**

SP SH SL + I70.534 **Atherosclerosis of nonautologous biological bypass graft(s) of the right leg with ulceration of heel and midfoot**
Atherosclerosis of nonautologous biological bypass graft(s) of right leg with ulceration of plantar surface of midfoot

SP SH SL + I70.535 **Atherosclerosis of nonautologous biological bypass graft(s) of the right leg with ulceration of other part of foot**
Atherosclerosis of nonautologous biological bypass graft(s) of the right leg with ulceration of toe

Chapter 9 I00-I99

⊟ SP SH SL + **I70.538 Atherosclerosis of nonautologous biological bypass graft(s) of the right leg with ulceration of other part of lower leg**

⊟ IQ SH SL + **I70.539 Atherosclerosis of nonautologous biological bypass graft(s) of the right leg with ulceration of unspecified site**

+ 6 **I70.54 Atherosclerosis of nonautologous biological bypass graft(s) of the left leg with ulceration**

INCLUDES any condition classifiable to I70.512 and I70.522
chronic limb-threatening ischemia of nonautologous biological bypass graft (s) of the left leg with ulceration
critical limb ischemia of nonautologous biological bypass graft (s) of the left leg with ulceration

Use additional code to identify severity of ulcer (L97.-)

⊟ SP SH SL + **I70.541 Atherosclerosis of nonautologous biological bypass graft(s) of the left leg with ulceration of thigh**

⊟ SP SH SL + **I70.542 Atherosclerosis of nonautologous biological bypass graft(s) of the left leg with ulceration of calf**

⊟ SP SH SL + **I70.543 Atherosclerosis of nonautologous biological bypass graft(s) of the left leg with ulceration of ankle**

⊟ SP SH SL + **I70.544 Atherosclerosis of nonautologous biological bypass graft(s) of the left leg with ulceration of heel and midfoot**

Atherosclerosis of nonautologous biological bypass graft(s) of left leg with ulceration of plantar surface of midfoot

⊟ SP SH SL + **I70.545 Atherosclerosis of nonautologous biological bypass graft(s) of the left leg with ulceration of other part of foot**

Atherosclerosis of nonautologous biological bypass graft(s) of the left leg with ulceration of toe

⊟ SP SH SL + **I70.548 Atherosclerosis of nonautologous biological bypass graft(s) of the left leg with ulceration of other part of lower leg**

⊟ IQ SH SL + **I70.549 Atherosclerosis of nonautologous biological bypass graft(s) of the left leg with ulceration of unspecified site**

⊟ SP + **I70.55 Atherosclerosis of nonautologous biological bypass graft(s) of other extremity with ulceration**

INCLUDES any condition classifiable to I70.518, I70.528, and I70.538

Use additional code to identify severity of ulcer (L98.49)

+ 6 **I70.56 Atherosclerosis of nonautologous biological bypass graft(s) of the extremities with gangrene**

INCLUDES any condition classifiable to I70.51-, I70.52-, and I70.53-, I70.54-, I70.55
chronic limb-threatening ischemia of nonautologous biological bypass graft (s) of the extremities with gangrene
critical limb ischemia of nonautologous biological bypass graft (s) of the extremities with gangrene

Use additional code to identify the severity of any ulcer (L97.-, L98.49-), if applicable

⊟ SP + **I70.561 Atherosclerosis of nonautologous biological bypass graft(s) of the extremities with gangrene, right leg**

⊟ SP + **I70.562 Atherosclerosis of nonautologous biological bypass graft(s) of the extremities with gangrene, left leg**

⊟ SP + **I70.563 Atherosclerosis of nonautologous biological bypass graft(s) of the extremities with gangrene, bilateral legs**

⊟ SP + **I70.568 Atherosclerosis of nonautologous biological bypass graft(s) of the extremities with gangrene, other extremity**

⊟ IQ + **I70.569 Atherosclerosis of nonautologous biological bypass graft(s) of the extremities with gangrene, unspecified extremity**

+ 6 **I70.59 Other atherosclerosis of nonautologous biological bypass graft(s) of the extremities**

⊟ SP + **I70.591 Other atherosclerosis of nonautologous biological bypass graft(s) of the extremities, right leg**

⊟ SP + **I70.592 Other atherosclerosis of nonautologous biological bypass graft(s) of the extremities, left leg**

⊟ SP + **I70.593 Other atherosclerosis of nonautologous biological bypass graft(s) of the extremities, bilateral legs**

⊟ SP + **I70.598 Other atherosclerosis of nonautologous biological bypass graft(s) of the extremities, other extremity**

⊟ IQ + **I70.599 Other atherosclerosis of nonautologous biological bypass graft(s) of the extremities, unspecified extremity**

+ 5 **I70.6 Atherosclerosis of nonbiological bypass graft(s) of the extremities**

Use additional code, if applicable, to identify chronic total occlusion of artery of extremity (I70.92)

CODING TIPS ✓ M1028 should be marked PAD, PVD on the OASIS.

CODING TIPS✓ Peripheral angiopathy may be documented as diabetic PVD. There is an assumed relationship between diabetes and PVD and PAD, including peripheral atherosclerosis. Diabetic arteriosclerosis of the peripheral arteries should be coded E--.51 or E--.52 then the appropriate I70.- code.

+ 6 **I70.60 Unspecified atherosclerosis of nonbiological bypass graft(s) of the extremities**

SP + **I70.601 Unspecified atherosclerosis of nonbiological bypass graft(s) of the extremities, right leg**

SP + **I70.602 Unspecified atherosclerosis of nonbiological bypass graft(s) of the extremities, left leg**

SP + **I70.603 Unspecified atherosclerosis of nonbiological bypass graft(s) of the extremities, bilateral legs**

SP + **I70.608 Unspecified atherosclerosis of nonbiological bypass graft(s) of the extremities, other extremity**

IQ + **I70.609 Unspecified atherosclerosis of nonbiological bypass graft(s) of the extremities, unspecified extremity**

+ 6 **I70.61 Atherosclerosis of nonbiological bypass graft(s) of the extremities with intermittent claudication**

SP + **I70.611 Atherosclerosis of nonbiological bypass graft(s) of the extremities with intermittent claudication, right leg**

SP + **I70.612 Atherosclerosis of nonbiological bypass graft(s) of the extremities with intermittent claudication, left leg**

SP + **I70.613 Atherosclerosis of nonbiological bypass graft(s) of the extremities with intermittent claudication, bilateral legs**

SP + **I70.618 Atherosclerosis of nonbiological bypass graft(s) of the extremities with intermittent claudication, other extremity**

IQ + **I70.619 Atherosclerosis of nonbiological bypass graft(s) of the extremities with intermittent claudication, unspecified extremity**

+ 6 **I70.62 Atherosclerosis of nonbiological bypass graft(s) of the extremities with rest pain**

INCLUDES any condition classifiable to I70.61-
chronic limb-threatening ischemia NOS of nonbiological bypass graft (s) of the extremities
chronic limb-threatening ischemia of nonbiological bypass graft (s) of the extremities with rest pain
critical limb ischemia NOS of nonbiological bypass graft (s) of the extremities
critical limb ischemia of nonbiological bypass graft (s) of the extremities with rest pain

SP + **I70.621 Atherosclerosis of nonbiological bypass graft(s) of the extremities with rest pain, right leg**

SP + **I70.622 Atherosclerosis of nonbiological bypass graft(s) of the extremities with rest pain, left leg**

SP + **I70.623 Atherosclerosis of nonbiological bypass graft(s) of the extremities with rest pain, bilateral legs**

SP + **I70.628 Atherosclerosis of nonbiological bypass graft(s) of the extremities with rest pain, other extremity**

IQ + **I70.629 Atherosclerosis of nonbiological bypass graft(s) of the extremities with rest pain, unspecified extremity**

+ 6 **I70.63 Atherosclerosis of nonbiological bypass graft(s) of the right leg with ulceration**

INCLUDES any condition classifiable to I70.611 and I70.621
chronic limb-threatening ischemia of nonbiological bypass graft (s) of the right leg with ulceration
critical limb ischemia of nonbiological bypass graft (s) of the right leg with ulceration

Use additional code to identify severity of ulcer (L97.-)

SP SH SL + **I70.631 Atherosclerosis of nonbiological bypass graft(s) of the right leg with ulceration of thigh**

SP SH SL + **I70.632 Atherosclerosis of nonbiological bypass graft(s) of the right leg with ulceration of calf**

SP SH SL + **I70.633 Atherosclerosis of nonbiological bypass graft(s) of the right leg with ulceration of ankle**

SP SH SL + **I70.634 Atherosclerosis of nonbiological bypass graft(s) of the right leg with ulceration of heel and midfoot**

Atherosclerosis of nonbiological bypass graft(s) of right leg with ulceration of plantar surface of midfoot

SP SH SL + **I70.635 Atherosclerosis of nonbiological bypass graft(s) of the right leg with ulceration of other part of foot**

Atherosclerosis of nonbiological bypass graft(s) of the right leg with ulceration of toe

SP SH SL + **I70.638 Atherosclerosis of nonbiological bypass graft(s) of the right leg with ulceration of other part of lower leg**

⊟ IQ SH SL + I70.639 **Atherosclerosis of nonbiological bypass graft(s) of the right leg with ulceration of unspecified site**

+ 6 I70.64 **Atherosclerosis of nonbiological bypass graft(s) of the left leg with ulceration**

INCLUDES any condition classifiable to I70.612 and I70.622
chronic limb-threatening ischemia of nonbiological bypass graft (s) of the left leg with ulceration
critical limb ischemia of nonbiological bypass graft (s) of the left leg with ulceration

Use additional code to identify severity of ulcer (L97.-)

⊟ SP SH SL + I70.641 **Atherosclerosis of nonbiological bypass graft(s) of the left leg with ulceration of thigh**

⊟ SP SH SL + I70.642 **Atherosclerosis of nonbiological bypass graft(s) of the left leg with ulceration of calf**

⊟ SP SH SL + I70.643 **Atherosclerosis of nonbiological bypass graft(s) of the left leg with ulceration of ankle**

⊟ SP SH SL + I70.644 **Atherosclerosis of nonbiological bypass graft(s) of the left leg with ulceration of heel and midfoot**
Atherosclerosis of nonbiological bypass graft(s) of left leg with ulceration of plantar surface of midfoot

⊟ SP SH SL + I70.645 **Atherosclerosis of nonbiological bypass graft(s) of the left leg with ulceration of other part of foot**
Atherosclerosis of nonbiological bypass graft(s) of the left leg with ulceration of toe

⊟ SP SH SL + I70.648 **Atherosclerosis of nonbiological bypass graft(s) of the left leg with ulceration of other part of lower leg**

⊟ IQ SH SL + I70.649 **Atherosclerosis of nonbiological bypass graft(s) of the left leg with ulceration of unspecified site**

⊟ SP + I70.65 **Atherosclerosis of nonbiological bypass graft(s) of other extremity with ulceration**

INCLUDES any condition classifiable to I70.618 and I70.628

Use additional code to identify severity of ulcer (L98.49)

+ 6 I70.66 **Atherosclerosis of nonbiological bypass graft(s) of the extremities with gangrene**

INCLUDES any condition classifiable to I70.61-, I70.62-, I70.63-, I70.64-, I70.65
chronic limb-threatening ischemia of nonbiological bypass graft (s) of the extremities with gangrene
critical limb ischemia of nonbiological bypass graft (s) of the extremities with gangrene

Use additional code to identify the severity of any ulcer (L97.-, L98.49-), if applicable

⊟ SP + I70.661 **Atherosclerosis of nonbiological bypass graft(s) of the extremities with gangrene, right leg**

⊟ SP + I70.662 **Atherosclerosis of nonbiological bypass graft(s) of the extremities with gangrene, left leg**

⊟ SP + I70.663 **Atherosclerosis of nonbiological bypass graft(s) of the extremities with gangrene, bilateral legs**

⊟ SP + I70.668 **Atherosclerosis of nonbiological bypass graft(s) of the extremities with gangrene, other extremity**

⊟ IQ + I70.669 **Atherosclerosis of nonbiological bypass graft(s) of the extremities with gangrene, unspecified extremity**

+ 6 I70.69 **Other atherosclerosis of nonbiological bypass graft(s) of the extremities**

⊟ SP + I70.691 **Other atherosclerosis of nonbiological bypass graft(s) of the extremities, right leg**

⊟ SP + I70.692 **Other atherosclerosis of nonbiological bypass graft(s) of the extremities, left leg**

⊟ SP + I70.693 **Other atherosclerosis of nonbiological bypass graft(s) of the extremities, bilateral legs**

⊟ SP + I70.698 **Other atherosclerosis of nonbiological bypass graft(s) of the extremities, other extremity**

⊟ IQ + I70.699 **Other atherosclerosis of nonbiological bypass graft(s) of the extremities, unspecified extremity**

+ 5 I70.7 **Atherosclerosis of other type of bypass graft(s) of the extremities**
Use additional code, if applicable, to identify chronic total occlusion of artery of extremity (I70.92)

CODING TIPS✓ M1028 should be marked PAD, PVD on the OASIS.

CODING TIPS✓ Peripheral angiopathy may be documented as diabetic PVD. There is an assumed relationship between diabetes and PVD and PAD, including peripheral atherosclerosis. Diabetic arteriosclerosis of the peripheral arteries should be coded E--.51 or E--.52 then the appropriate I70.- code.

+ 6 I70.70 **Unspecified atherosclerosis of other type of bypass graft(s) of the extremities**

⊟ SP + I70.701 **Unspecified atherosclerosis of other type of bypass graft(s) of the extremities, right leg**

⊟ SP + I70.702 **Unspecified atherosclerosis of other type of bypass graft(s) of the extremities, left leg**

SP + **I70.703 Unspecified atherosclerosis of other type of bypass graft(s) of the extremities, bilateral legs**

SP + **I70.708 Unspecified atherosclerosis of other type of bypass graft(s) of the extremities, other extremity**

IQ + **I70.709 Unspecified atherosclerosis of other type of bypass graft(s) of the extremities, unspecified extremity**

+ 6 **I70.71 Atherosclerosis of other type of bypass graft(s) of the extremities with intermittent claudication**

SP + **I70.711 Atherosclerosis of other type of bypass graft(s) of the extremities with intermittent claudication, right leg**

SP + **I70.712 Atherosclerosis of other type of bypass graft(s) of the extremities with intermittent claudication, left leg**

SP + **I70.713 Atherosclerosis of other type of bypass graft(s) of the extremities with intermittent claudication, bilateral legs**

SP + **I70.718 Atherosclerosis of other type of bypass graft(s) of the extremities with intermittent claudication, other extremity**

IQ + **I70.719 Atherosclerosis of other type of bypass graft(s) of the extremities with intermittent claudication, unspecified extremity**

+ 6 **I70.72 Atherosclerosis of other type of bypass graft(s) of the extremities with rest pain**

INCLUDES any condition classifiable to I70.71-
chronic limb-threatening ischemia NOS of other type of bypass graft (s) of the extremities
chronic limb-threatening ischemia of other type of bypass graft (s) of the extremities with rest pain
critical limb ischemia NOS of other type of bypass graft (s) of the extremities
critical limb ischemia of other type of bypass graft (s) of the extremities with rest pain

SP + **I70.721 Atherosclerosis of other type of bypass graft(s) of the extremities with rest pain, right leg**

SP + **I70.722 Atherosclerosis of other type of bypass graft(s) of the extremities with rest pain, left leg**

SP + **I70.723 Atherosclerosis of other type of bypass graft(s) of the extremities with rest pain, bilateral legs**

SP + **I70.728 Atherosclerosis of other type of bypass graft(s) of the extremities with rest pain, other extremity**

IQ + **I70.729 Atherosclerosis of other type of bypass graft(s) of the extremities with rest pain, unspecified extremity**

+ 6 **I70.73 Atherosclerosis of other type of bypass graft(s) of the right leg with ulceration**

INCLUDES any condition classifiable to I70.711 and I70.721
chronic limb-threatening ischemia of other type of bypass graft (s) of the right leg with ulceration
critical limb ischemia of other type of bypass graft (s) of the right leg with ulceration

Use additional code to identify severity of ulcer (L97.-)

SP SH SL + **I70.731 Atherosclerosis of other type of bypass graft(s) of the right leg with ulceration of thigh**

SP SH SL + **I70.732 Atherosclerosis of other type of bypass graft(s) of the right leg with ulceration of calf**

SP SH SL + **I70.733 Atherosclerosis of other type of bypass graft(s) of the right leg with ulceration of ankle**

SP SH SL + **I70.734 Atherosclerosis of other type of bypass graft(s) of the right leg with ulceration of heel and midfoot**
Atherosclerosis of other type of bypass graft(s) of right leg with ulceration of plantar surface of midfoot

SP SH SL + **I70.735 Atherosclerosis of other type of bypass graft(s) of the right leg with ulceration of other part of foot**
Atherosclerosis of other type of bypass graft(s) of right leg with ulceration of toe

SP SH SL + **I70.738 Atherosclerosis of other type of bypass graft(s) of the right leg with ulceration of other part of lower leg**

IQ SH SL + **I70.739 Atherosclerosis of other type of bypass graft(s) of the right leg with ulceration of unspecified site**

+ 6 **I70.74 Atherosclerosis of other type of bypass graft(s) of the left leg with ulceration**

INCLUDES any condition classifiable to I70.712 and I70.722
chronic limb-threatening ischemia of other type of bypass graft (s) of the left leg with ulceration
critical limb ischemia of other type of bypass graft (s) of the left leg with ulceration

Use additional code to identify severity of ulcer (L97.-)

I70.741 Atherosclerosis of other type of bypass graft(s) of the left leg with ulceration of thigh

I70.742 Atherosclerosis of other type of bypass graft(s) of the left leg with ulceration of calf

I70.743 Atherosclerosis of other type of bypass graft(s) of the left leg with ulceration of ankle

I70.744 Atherosclerosis of other type of bypass graft(s) of the left leg with ulceration of heel and midfoot

Atherosclerosis of other type of bypass graft(s) of left leg with ulceration of plantar surface of midfoot

I70.745 Atherosclerosis of other type of bypass graft(s) of the left leg with ulceration of other part of foot

Atherosclerosis of other type of bypass graft(s) of left leg with ulceration of toe

I70.748 Atherosclerosis of other type of bypass graft(s) of the left leg with ulceration of other part of lower leg

I70.749 Atherosclerosis of other type of bypass graft(s) of the left leg with ulceration of unspecified site

I70.75 Atherosclerosis of other type of bypass graft(s) of other extremity with ulceration

INCLUDES any condition classifiable to I70.718 and I70.728

Use additional code to identify severity of ulcer (L98.49)

I70.76 Atherosclerosis of other type of bypass graft(s) of the extremities with gangrene

INCLUDES any condition classifiable to I70.71-, I70.72-, I70.73-, I70.74-, I70.75

chronic limb-threatening ischemia of other type of bypass graft (s) of the extremities with gangrene

critical limb ischemia of other type of bypass graft (s) of the extremities with gangrene

Use additional code to identify the severity of any ulcer (L97.-, L98.49-), if applicable

I70.761 Atherosclerosis of other type of bypass graft(s) of the extremities with gangrene, right leg

I70.762 Atherosclerosis of other type of bypass graft(s) of the extremities with gangrene, left leg

I70.763 Atherosclerosis of other type of bypass graft(s) of the extremities with gangrene, bilateral legs

I70.768 Atherosclerosis of other type of bypass graft(s) of the extremities with gangrene, other extremity

I70.769 Atherosclerosis of other type of bypass graft(s) of the extremities with gangrene, unspecified extremity

I70.79 Other atherosclerosis of other type of bypass graft(s) of the extremities

I70.791 Other atherosclerosis of other type of bypass graft(s) of the extremities, right leg

I70.792 Other atherosclerosis of other type of bypass graft(s) of the extremities, left leg

I70.793 Other atherosclerosis of other type of bypass graft(s) of the extremities, bilateral legs

I70.798 Other atherosclerosis of other type of bypass graft(s) of the extremities, other extremity

I70.799 Other atherosclerosis of other type of bypass graft(s) of the extremities, unspecified extremity

I70.8 Atherosclerosis of other arteries

CODING TIPS Peripheral angiopathy may be documented as diabetic PVD. There is an assumed relationship between diabetes and PVD and PAD, including peripheral atherosclerosis. Diabetic arteriosclerosis of the peripheral arteries should be coded E--.51 or E--.52 then the appropriate I70.- code.

I70.9 Other and unspecified atherosclerosis

I70.90 Unspecified atherosclerosis

I70.91 Generalized atherosclerosis

CODING TIPS M1028 should be marked PAD, PVD on the OASIS.

I70.92 Chronic total occlusion of artery of the extremities

Complete occlusion of artery of the extremities

Total occlusion of artery of the extremities

Code first:

atherosclerosis of arteries of the extremities (I70.2-, I70.3-, I70.4-, I70.5-, I70.6-, I70.7-)

CODING TIPS M1028 should be marked PAD, PVD on the OASIS.

I71 Aortic aneurysm and dissection

EXCLUDES 1 aortic ectasia (I77.81-)
syphilitic aortic aneurysm (A52.01)
traumatic aortic aneurysm (S25.09, S35.09)

I71.0 Dissection of aorta

I71.00 Dissection of unspecified site of aorta

I71.01 Dissection of thoracic aorta

I71.02 Dissection of abdominal aorta

I71.03 Dissection of thoracoabdominal aorta

I71.1 Thoracic aortic aneurysm, ruptured

I71.2 Thoracic aortic aneurysm, without rupture

I71.3 Abdominal aortic aneurysm, ruptured

SP **I71.4 Abdominal aortic aneurysm, without rupture**

SP **I71.5 Thoracoabdominal aortic aneurysm, ruptured**

SP **I71.6 Thoracoabdominal aortic aneurysm, without rupture**

IQ **I71.8 Aortic aneurysm of unspecified site, ruptured**

Rupture of aorta NOS

IQ **I71.9 Aortic aneurysm of unspecified site, without rupture**

Aneurysm of aorta
Dilatation of aorta
Hyaline necrosis of aorta

4 **I72 Other aneurysm**

INCLUDES aneurysm (cirsoid) (false) (ruptured)

EXCLUDES 2 acquired aneurysm (I77.0)
aneurysm (of) aorta (I71.-)
aneurysm (of) arteriovenous NOS (Q27.3-)
carotid artery dissection (I77.71)
cerebral (nonruptured) aneurysm (I67.1)
coronary aneurysm (I25.4)
coronary artery dissection (I25.42)
dissection of artery NEC (I77.79)
dissection of precerebral artery, congenital (nonruptured) (Q28.1)
heart aneurysm (I25.3)
iliac artery dissection (I77.72)
precerebral artery, congential (nonruptured) (Q28.1)
pulmonary artery aneurysm (I28.1)
renal artery dissection (I77.73)
retinal aneurysm (H35.0)
ruptured cerebral aneurysm (I60.7)
varicose aneurysm (I77.0)
vertebral artery dissection (I77.74)

SP **I72.0 Aneurysm of carotid artery**

Aneurysm of common carotid artery
Aneurysm of external carotid artery
Aneurysm of internal carotid artery, extracranial portion

EXCLUDES 1 aneurysm of internal carotid artery, intracranial portion (I67.1)
aneurysm of internal carotid artery NOS (I67.1)

SP **I72.1 Aneurysm of artery of upper extremity**

SP **I72.2 Aneurysm of renal artery**

SP **I72.3 Aneurysm of iliac artery**

SP **I72.4 Aneurysm of artery of lower extremity**

SP **I72.5 Aneurysm of other precerebral arteries**

Aneurysm of basilar artery (trunk)

EXCLUDES 2 aneurysm of carotid artery (I72.0)
aneurysm of vertebral artery (I72.6)
dissection of carotid artery (I77.71)
dissection of other precerebral arteries (I77.75)
dissection of vertebral artery (I77.74)

SP **I72.6 Aneurysm of vertebral artery**

EXCLUDES 2 dissection of vertebral artery (I77.74)

SP **I72.8 Aneurysm of other specified arteries**

IQ **I72.9 Aneurysm of unspecified site**

4 **I73 Other peripheral vascular diseases**

EXCLUDES 2 chilblains (T69.1)
frostbite (T33-T34)
immersion hand or foot (T69.0-)
spasm of cerebral artery (G45.9)

CODING TIPS ✓ M1028 should be marked PAD, PVD on the OASIS.

5 **I73.0 Raynaud's syndrome**

Raynaud's disease
Raynaud's phenomenon (secondary)

SP **I73.00 Raynaud's syndrome without gangrene**

SP **I73.01 Raynaud's syndrome with gangrene**

DEFINITION Medium-sized blood vessels of the hands and feet become inflamed and blocked by blood clots, causing gangrene of the extremities.

SP **I73.1 Thromboangiitis obliterans [Buerger's disease]**

5 **I73.8 Other specified peripheral vascular diseases**

EXCLUDES 1 diabetic (peripheral) angiopathy (E08-E13 with .51-.52)

SP **I73.81 Erythromelalgia**

DEFINITION Abnormal dilation of extremity blood vessels, especially in the feet, causing a painful, burning sensation, and redness.

SP **I73.89 Other specified peripheral vascular diseases**

Acrocyanosis
Erythrocyanosis
Simple acroparesthesia [Schultze's type]
Vasomotor acroparesthesia [Nothnagel's type]

SP **I73.9 Peripheral vascular disease, unspecified**

Intermittent claudication
Peripheral angiopathy NOS
Spasm of artery

EXCLUDES 1 atherosclerosis of the extremities (I70.2--I70.7-)

CODING TIPS ✓ Do not assign I73.9 when peripheral atherosclerosis is reported in the clinical record. Note, atherosclerosis of the extremities is a more specific diagnosis and should be coded using a code from I70.2- through I70.7-. When PVD is documented in a diabetic, use the appropriate code for diabetic peripheral angiopathy instead, and also assign a code from I70.- if specific information about the diagnosis if available.

CODING TIPS ✓ I73.9 is used for peripheral vascular disease and peripheral arterial disease (angiopathy). If the physician or NPP documents venous disease, I80-I89 should be referenced.

4 I74 Arterial embolism and thrombosis
INCLUDES embolic infarction
embolic occlusion
thrombotic infarction
thrombotic occlusion
Code first:
embolism and thrombosis complicating abortion or ectopic or molar pregnancy (O00-O07, O08.2)
embolism and thrombosis complicating pregnancy, childbirth and the puerperium (O88.-)
EXCLUDES 2 atheroembolism (I75.-)
basilar embolism and thrombosis (I63.0-I63.2, I65.1)
carotid embolism and thrombosis (I63.0-I63.2, I65.2)
cerebral embolism and thrombosis (I63.3-I63.5, I66.-)
coronary embolism and thrombosis (I21-I25)
mesenteric embolism and thrombosis (K55.0-)
ophthalmic embolism and thrombosis (H34.-)
precerebral embolism and thrombosis NOS (I63.0-I63.2, I65.9)
pulmonary embolism and thrombosis (I26.-)
renal embolism and thrombosis (N28.0)
retinal embolism and thrombosis (H34.-)
septic embolism and thrombosis (I76)
vertebral embolism and thrombosis (I63.0-I63.2, I65.0)

5 I74.0 Embolism and thrombosis of abdominal aorta

SP I74.01 Saddle embolus of abdominal aorta

SP I74.09 Other arterial embolism and thrombosis of abdominal aorta
Aortic bifurcation syndrome
Aortoiliac obstruction
Leriche's syndrome

5 I74.1 Embolism and thrombosis of other and unspecified parts of aorta

SP I74.10 Embolism and thrombosis of unspecified parts of aorta

SP I74.11 Embolism and thrombosis of thoracic aorta

SP I74.19 Embolism and thrombosis of other parts of aorta

SP I74.2 Embolism and thrombosis of arteries of the upper extremities

SP I74.3 Embolism and thrombosis of arteries of the lower extremities

IQ I74.4 Embolism and thrombosis of arteries of extremities, unspecified
Peripheral arterial embolism NOS

SP I74.5 Embolism and thrombosis of iliac artery

SP I74.8 Embolism and thrombosis of other arteries

IQ I74.9 Embolism and thrombosis of unspecified artery

4 I75 Atheroembolism
INCLUDES atherothrombotic microembolism
cholesterol embolism

5 I75.0 Atheroembolism of extremities

6 I75.01 Atheroembolism of upper extremity

Laterality SP I75.011 Atheroembolism of right upper extremity

Laterality SP I75.012 Atheroembolism of left upper extremity

Laterality SP I75.013 Atheroembolism of bilateral upper extremities

Laterality IQ I75.019 Atheroembolism of unspecified upper extremity

6 I75.02 Atheroembolism of lower extremity

Laterality SP I75.021 Atheroembolism of right lower extremity

Laterality SP I75.022 Atheroembolism of left lower extremity

Laterality SP I75.023 Atheroembolism of bilateral lower extremities

Laterality IQ I75.029 Atheroembolism of unspecified lower extremity

5 I75.8 Atheroembolism of other sites

SP + I75.81 Atheroembolism of kidney
Use additional code for any associated acute kidney failure and chronic kidney disease (N17.-, N18.-)

SP I75.89 Atheroembolism of other site

IQ + I76 Septic arterial embolism
Code first underlying infection, such as:
infective endocarditis (I33.0)
lung abscess (J85.-)
Use additional code to identify the site of the embolism (I74.-)
EXCLUDES 2 septic pulmonary embolism (I26.01, I26.90)

DEFINITION Dislodged material from a centralized infection lodged in a small arteriole, causing tissue death due to bacteria and lack of blood supply.

4 I77 Other disorders of arteries and arterioles
EXCLUDES 2 collagen (vascular) diseases (M30-M36)
hypersensitivity angiitis (M31.0)
pulmonary artery (I28.-)

SP I77.0 Arteriovenous fistula, acquired
Aneurysmal varix
Arteriovenous aneurysm, acquired
EXCLUDES 1 arteriovenous aneurysm NOS (Q27.3-)
presence of arteriovenous shunt (fistula) for dialysis (Z99.2)
traumatic - see injury of blood vessel by body region

EXCLUDES 2 cerebral (I67.1)
coronary (I25.4)

SP **I77.1 Stricture of artery**
Narrowing of artery

SP **I77.2 Rupture of artery**
Erosion of artery
Fistula of artery
Ulcer of artery
EXCLUDES 1 traumatic rupture of artery - see injury of blood vessel by body region

CODING TIPS✓ Do not assign code I77.2 for a traumatic rupture of the artery. A fistula, ulcer, or arterial erosion would be coded to I77.2.

SP **I77.3 Arterial fibromuscular dysplasia**
Fibromuscular hyperplasia (of) carotid artery
Fibromuscular hyperplasia (of) renal artery

SP **I77.4 Celiac artery compression syndrome**

SP **I77.5 Necrosis of artery**

SP **I77.6 Arteritis, unspecified**
Aortitis NOS
Endarteritis NOS
EXCLUDES 1 arteritis or endarteritis:
aortic arch (M31.4)
cerebral NEC (I67.7)
coronary (I25.89)
deformans (I70.-)
giant cell (M31.5, M31.6)
obliterans (I70.-)
senile (I70.-)

5 **I77.7 Other arterial dissection**
EXCLUDES 2 dissection of aorta (I71.0-)
dissection of coronary artery (I25.42)

IQ **I77.70 Dissection of unspecified artery**

SP **I77.71 Dissection of carotid artery**

SP **I77.72 Dissection of iliac artery**

SP **I77.73 Dissection of renal artery**

SP **I77.74 Dissection of vertebral artery**
EXCLUDES 2 aneurysm of vertebral artery (I72.6)

SP **I77.75 Dissection of other precerebral arteries**
Dissection of basilar artery (trunk)
EXCLUDES 2 aneurysm of carotid artery (I72.0)
aneurysm of other precerebral arteries (I72.5)
aneurysm of vertebral artery (I72.6)
dissection of carotid artery (I77.71)
dissection of vertebral artery (I77.74)

SP **I77.76 Dissection of artery of upper extremity**

SP **I77.77 Dissection of artery of lower extremity**

SP **I77.79 Dissection of other specified artery**

5 **I77.8 Other specified disorders of arteries and arterioles**

6 **I77.81 Aortic ectasia**
Ectasis aorta
EXCLUDES 1 aortic aneurysm and dissection (I71.0-)

SP **I77.810 Thoracic aortic ectasia**

SP **I77.811 Abdominal aortic ectasia**

SP **I77.812 Thoracoabdominal aortic ectasia**

SP **I77.819 Aortic ectasia, unspecified site**

SP **I77.89 Other specified disorders of arteries and arterioles**

IQ **I77.9 Disorder of arteries and arterioles, unspecified**

CODING TIPS✓ This code is used for carotid artery disease when there is no occlusion or stenosis. [AHA: 1Q 2021]

4 **I78 Diseases of capillaries**

SP **I78.0 Hereditary hemorrhagic telangiectasia**
Rendu-Osler-Weber disease

SP **I78.1 Nevus, non-neoplastic**
Araneus nevus
Senile nevus
Spider nevus
Stellar nevus
EXCLUDES 1 nevus NOS (D22.-)
vascular NOS (Q82.5)
EXCLUDES 2 blue nevus (D22.-)
flammeus nevus (Q82.5)
hairy nevus (D22.-)
melanocytic nevus (D22.-)
pigmented nevus (D22.-)
portwine nevus (Q82.5)
sanguineous nevus (Q82.5)
strawberry nevus (Q82.5)
verrucous nevus (Q82.5)

SP **I78.8 Other diseases of capillaries**

IQ **I78.9 Disease of capillaries, unspecified**

4 **I79 Disorders of arteries, arterioles and capillaries in diseases classified elsewhere**

CODING TIPS✓ Codes from category I79.- should be coded only when the arterial disease/dysfunction is specified as due to another primary disease process. The causative disease process should be coded first.

M IQ ***I79.0 Aneurysm of aorta in diseases classified elsewhere***
Code first:
underlying disease
EXCLUDES 1 syphilitic aneurysm (A52.01)

CODING TIPS✓ I79.0 should be coded only when an aortic aneurysm is specified as due to another primary disease process. The causative disease process should be coded first.

M IQ ***I79.1 Aortitis in diseases classified elsewhere***
Code first:
underlying disease
EXCLUDES 1 syphilitic aortitis (A52.02)

M IQ ***I79.8 Other disorders of arteries, arterioles and capillaries in diseases classified elsewhere***
Code first underlying disease, such as:
amyloidosis (E85.-)
EXCLUDES 1 diabetic (peripheral) angiopathy (E08-E13 with .51-.52)

syphilitic endarteritis (A52.09)
tuberculous endarteritis (A18.89)

Diseases of veins, lymphatic vessels and lymph nodes, not elsewhere classified (I80-I89)

4 **I80 Phlebitis and thrombophlebitis**

INCLUDES endophlebitis
inflammation, vein
periphlebitis
suppurative phlebitis

Code first:
phlebitis and thrombophlebitis complicating abortion, ectopic or molar pregnancy (O00-O07, O08.7)
phlebitis and thrombophlebitis complicating pregnancy, childbirth and the puerperium (O22.-, O87.-)

EXCLUDES 1 venous embolism and thrombosis of lower extremities (I82.4-, I82.5-, I82.81-)

5 **I80.0 Phlebitis and thrombophlebitis of superficial vessels of lower extremities**
Phlebitis and thrombophlebitis of femoropopliteal vein

Laterality IQ **I80.00 Phlebitis and thrombophlebitis of superficial vessels of unspecified lower extremity**

Laterality SP **I80.01 Phlebitis and thrombophlebitis of superficial vessels of right lower extremity**

Laterality SP **I80.02 Phlebitis and thrombophlebitis of superficial vessels of left lower extremity**

Laterality SP **I80.03 Phlebitis and thrombophlebitis of superficial vessels of lower extremities, bilateral**

5 **I80.1 Phlebitis and thrombophlebitis of femoral vein**
Phlebitis and thrombophlebitis of common femoral vein
Phlebitis and thrombophlebitis of deep femoral vein

CODING TIPS ✓ Deep vein thrombosis in the proximal deep veins is more significant than deep vein thrombosis in the distal deep veins. Veins of the thigh are the iliac and femoral.

Laterality IQ **I80.10 Phlebitis and thrombophlebitis of unspecified femoral vein**

Laterality SP **I80.11 Phlebitis and thrombophlebitis of right femoral vein**

Laterality SP **I80.12 Phlebitis and thrombophlebitis of left femoral vein**

Laterality SP **I80.13 Phlebitis and thrombophlebitis of femoral vein, bilateral**

5 **I80.2 Phlebitis and thrombophlebitis of other and unspecified deep vessels of lower extremities**

CODING TIPS ✓ Deep vein thrombosis in the proximal deep veins is more significant than deep vein thrombosis in the distal deep veins. Veins of the calf include the peroneal, gastrocnemial, tibial and soleal. Veins of the thigh are the iliac and femoral.

6 **I80.20 Phlebitis and thrombophlebitis of unspecified deep vessels of lower extremities**

Laterality SP **I80.201 Phlebitis and thrombophlebitis of unspecified deep vessels of right lower extremity**

Laterality SP **I80.202 Phlebitis and thrombophlebitis of unspecified deep vessels of left lower extremity**

Laterality SP **I80.203 Phlebitis and thrombophlebitis of unspecified deep vessels of lower extremities, bilateral**

Laterality IQ **I80.209 Phlebitis and thrombophlebitis of unspecified deep vessels of unspecified lower extremity**

6 **I80.21 Phlebitis and thrombophlebitis of iliac vein**
Phlebitis and thrombophlebitis of common iliac vein
Phlebitis and thrombophlebitis of external iliac vein
Phlebitis and thrombophlebitis of internal iliac vein

Laterality SP **I80.211 Phlebitis and thrombophlebitis of right iliac vein**

Laterality SP **I80.212 Phlebitis and thrombophlebitis of left iliac vein**

Laterality SP **I80.213 Phlebitis and thrombophlebitis of iliac vein, bilateral**

Laterality IQ **I80.219 Phlebitis and thrombophlebitis of unspecified iliac vein**

6 **I80.22 Phlebitis and thrombophlebitis of popliteal vein**

Laterality SP **I80.221 Phlebitis and thrombophlebitis of right popliteal vein**

Laterality SP **I80.222 Phlebitis and thrombophlebitis of left popliteal vein**

Laterality SP **I80.223 Phlebitis and thrombophlebitis of popliteal vein, bilateral**

Laterality IQ **I80.229 Phlebitis and thrombophlebitis of unspecified popliteal vein**

6 **I80.23 Phlebitis and thrombophlebitis of tibial vein**
Phlebitis and thrombophlebitis of anterior tibial vein
Phlebitis and thrombophlebitis of posterior tibial vein

Laterality SP **I80.231 Phlebitis and thrombophlebitis of right tibial vein**

Laterality SP **I80.232 Phlebitis and thrombophlebitis of left tibial vein**

Laterality SP **I80.233 Phlebitis and thrombophlebitis of tibial vein, bilateral**

Laterality SP **I80.239 Phlebitis and thrombophlebitis of unspecified tibial vein**

6 **I80.24 Phlebitis and thrombophlebitis of peroneal vein**

Laterality SP **I80.241 Phlebitis and thrombophlebitis of right peroneal vein**

Laterality SP **I80.242 Phlebitis and thrombophlebitis of left peroneal vein**

SP I80.243 **Phlebitis and thrombophlebitis of peroneal vein, bilateral**

I80.249 **Phlebitis and thrombophlebitis of unspecified peroneal vein**

6 I80.25 **Phlebitis and thrombophlebitis of calf muscular vein**
Phlebitis and thrombophlebitis of calf muscular vein, NOS
Phlebitis and thrombophlebitis of gastrocnemial vein
Phlebitis and thrombophlebitis of soleal vein

SP I80.251 **Phlebitis and thrombophlebitis of right calf muscular vein**

SP I80.252 **Phlebitis and thrombophlebitis of left calf muscular vein**

SP I80.253 **Phlebitis and thrombophlebitis of calf muscular vein, bilateral**

I80.259 **Phlebitis and thrombophlebitis of unspecified calf muscular vein**

6 I80.29 **Phlebitis and thrombophlebitis of other deep vessels of lower extremities**

SP I80.291 **Phlebitis and thrombophlebitis of other deep vessels of right lower extremity**

SP I80.292 **Phlebitis and thrombophlebitis of other deep vessels of left lower extremity**

SP I80.293 **Phlebitis and thrombophlebitis of other deep vessels of lower extremity, bilateral**

IQ I80.299 **Phlebitis and thrombophlebitis of other deep vessels of unspecified lower extremity**

SP I80.3 **Phlebitis and thrombophlebitis of lower extremities, unspecified**

SP I80.8 **Phlebitis and thrombophlebitis of other sites**

IQ I80.9 **Phlebitis and thrombophlebitis of unspecified site**

SP I81 **Portal vein thrombosis**
Portal (vein) obstruction

EXCLUDES 2 hepatic vein thrombosis (I82.0)
phlebitis of portal vein (K75.1)

CODING TIPS ✓ Portal vein thrombosis is a specific clinical condition caused by the occlusion/obstruction of the portal vein but does not include occlusion of the hepatic vein, and is relatively common in cirrhosis patients. It often leads to portal hypertension. When this condition occurs, any comorbid hepatic vein thrombosis and/or portal hypertension should also be coded.

4 I82 **Other venous embolism and thrombosis**
Code first venous embolism and thrombosis complicating:
abortion, ectopic or molar pregnancy (O00-O07, O08.7)
pregnancy, childbirth and the puerperium (O22.-, O87.-)

EXCLUDES 2 venous embolism and thrombosis (of) :
cerebral (I63.6, I67.6)
coronary (I21-I25)
intracranial and intraspinal, septic or NOS (G08)
intracranial, nonpyogenic (I67.6)
intraspinal, nonpyogenic (G95.1)
mesenteric (K55.0-)
portal (I81)
pulmonary (I26.-)

SP SL I82.0 **Budd-Chiari syndrome**
Hepatic vein thrombosis

DEFINITION Obstruction or occlusion of the hepatic veins, causing an enlarged liver, abdominal pain/tenderness, intractable ascites, mild jaundice, portal hypertension, and liver failure.

SP SL I82.1 **Thrombophlebitis migrans**

5 I82.2 **Embolism and thrombosis of vena cava and other thoracic veins**

6 I82.21 **Embolism and thrombosis of superior vena cava**

SP SL I82.210 **Acute embolism and thrombosis of superior vena cava**
Embolism and thrombosis of superior vena cava NOS

SP SL I82.211 **Chronic embolism and thrombosis of superior vena cava**

6 I82.22 **Embolism and thrombosis of inferior vena cava**

SP SL I82.220 **Acute embolism and thrombosis of inferior vena cava**
Embolism and thrombosis of inferior vena cava NOS

SP SL I82.221 **Chronic embolism and thrombosis of inferior vena cava**

6 I82.29 **Embolism and thrombosis of other thoracic veins**
Embolism and thrombosis of brachiocephalic (innominate) vein

SP SL I82.290 **Acute embolism and thrombosis of other thoracic veins**

SP SL I82.291 **Chronic embolism and thrombosis of other thoracic veins**

SP SL I82.3 **Embolism and thrombosis of renal vein**

5 I82.4 **Acute embolism and thrombosis of deep veins of lower extremity**

CODING TIPS ✓ Acute embolism and thrombosis codes are used unless the physician or NPP indicates the condition is chronic.

6 I82.40 **Acute embolism and thrombosis of unspecified deep veins of lower extremity**
Deep vein thrombosis NOS
DVT NOS

EXCLUDES 1 acute embolism and thrombosis of unspecified deep veins of distal lower extremity (I82.4Z-)
acute embolism and thrombosis of unspecified deep veins of proximal lower extremity (I82.4Y-)

SP SL I82.401 **Acute embolism and thrombosis of unspecified deep veins of right lower extremity**

Chapter 9

I00-I99

- **I82.402 Acute embolism and thrombosis of unspecified deep veins of left lower extremity**
- **I82.403 Acute embolism and thrombosis of unspecified deep veins of lower extremity, bilateral**
- **I82.409 Acute embolism and thrombosis of unspecified deep veins of unspecified lower extremity**

I82.41 Acute embolism and thrombosis of femoral vein
Acute embolism and thrombosis of common femoral vein
Acute embolism and thrombosis of deep femoral vein

CODING TIPS ✓ Deep vein thrombosis in the proximal deep veins is more significant than deep vein thrombosis in the distal deep veins. Veins of the thigh are the iliac and femoral.

- **I82.411 Acute embolism and thrombosis of right femoral vein**
- **I82.412 Acute embolism and thrombosis of left femoral vein**
- **I82.413 Acute embolism and thrombosis of femoral vein, bilateral**
- **I82.419 Acute embolism and thrombosis of unspecified femoral vein**

I82.42 Acute embolism and thrombosis of iliac vein
Acute embolism and thrombosis of common iliac vein
Acute embolism and thrombosis of external iliac vein
Acute embolism and thrombosis of internal iliac vein

CODING TIPS ✓ Deep vein thrombosis in the proximal deep veins is more significant than deep vein thrombosis in the distal deep veins. Veins of the thigh are the iliac and femoral.

- **I82.421 Acute embolism and thrombosis of right iliac vein**
- **I82.422 Acute embolism and thrombosis of left iliac vein**
- **I82.423 Acute embolism and thrombosis of iliac vein, bilateral**
- **I82.429 Acute embolism and thrombosis of unspecified iliac vein**

I82.43 Acute embolism and thrombosis of popliteal vein

- **I82.431 Acute embolism and thrombosis of right popliteal vein**
- **I82.432 Acute embolism and thrombosis of left popliteal vein**
- **I82.433 Acute embolism and thrombosis of popliteal vein, bilateral**
- **I82.439 Acute embolism and thrombosis of unspecified popliteal vein**

I82.44 Acute embolism and thrombosis of tibial vein
Acute embolism and thrombosis of anterior tibial vein
Acute embolism and thrombosis of posterior tibial vein

CODING TIPS ✓ Deep vein thrombosis in the proximal deep veins is more significant than deep vein thrombosis in the distal deep veins. Veins of the calf include the peroneal, gastrocnemial, tibial and soleal.

- **I82.441 Acute embolism and thrombosis of right tibial vein**
- **I82.442 Acute embolism and thrombosis of left tibial vein**
- **I82.443 Acute embolism and thrombosis of tibial vein, bilateral**
- **I82.449 Acute embolism and thrombosis of unspecified tibial vein**

I82.45 Acute embolism and thrombosis of peroneal vein

CODING TIPS ✓ Deep vein thrombosis in the proximal deep veins is more significant than deep vein thrombosis in the distal deep veins. Veins of the calf include the peroneal, gastrocnemial, tibial and soleal.

- **I82.451 Acute embolism and thrombosis of right peroneal vein**
- **I82.452 Acute embolism and thrombosis of left peroneal vein**
- **I82.453 Acute embolism and thrombosis of peroneal vein, bilateral**
- **I82.459 Acute embolism and thrombosis of unspecified peroneal vein**

I82.46 Acute embolism and thrombosis of calf muscular vein
Acute embolism and thrombosis of calf muscular vein, NOS
Acute embolism and thrombosis of gastrocnemial vein
Acute embolism and thrombosis of soleal vein

CODING TIPS ✓ Deep vein thrombosis in the proximal deep veins is more significant than deep vein thrombosis in the distal deep veins. Veins of the calf include the peroneal, gastrocnemial, tibial and soleal.

- **I82.461 Acute embolism and thrombosis of right calf muscular vein**
- **I82.462 Acute embolism and thrombosis of left calf muscular vein**
- **I82.463 Acute embolism and thrombosis of calf muscular vein, bilateral**
- **I82.469 Acute embolism and thrombosis of unspecified calf muscular vein**

I82.49 Acute embolism and thrombosis of other specified deep vein of lower extremity

- **I82.491 Acute embolism and thrombosis of other specified deep vein of right lower extremity**
- **I82.492 Acute embolism and thrombosis of other specified deep vein of left lower extremity**
- **I82.493 Acute embolism and thrombosis of other specified deep vein of lower extremity, bilateral**
- **I82.499 Acute embolism and thrombosis of other specified deep vein of unspecified lower extremity**

6 **I82.4Y Acute embolism and thrombosis of unspecified deep veins of proximal lower extremity**
Acute embolism and thrombosis of deep vein of thigh NOS
Acute embolism and thrombosis of deep vein of upper leg NOS

SP SL **I82.4Y1 Acute embolism and thrombosis of unspecified deep veins of right proximal lower extremity**

SP SL **I82.4Y2 Acute embolism and thrombosis of unspecified deep veins of left proximal lower extremity**

SP SL **I82.4Y3 Acute embolism and thrombosis of unspecified deep veins of proximal lower extremity, bilateral**

IQ **I82.4Y9 Acute embolism and thrombosis of unspecified deep veins of unspecified proximal lower extremity**

6 **I82.4Z Acute embolism and thrombosis of unspecified deep veins of distal lower extremity**
Acute embolism and thrombosis of deep vein of calf NOS
Acute embolism and thrombosis of deep vein of lower leg NOS

SP SL **I82.4Z1 Acute embolism and thrombosis of unspecified deep veins of right distal lower extremity**

SP SL **I82.4Z2 Acute embolism and thrombosis of unspecified deep veins of left distal lower extremity**

SP SL **I82.4Z3 Acute embolism and thrombosis of unspecified deep veins of distal lower extremity, bilateral**

IQ **I82.4Z9 Acute embolism and thrombosis of unspecified deep veins of unspecified distal lower extremity**

+ 5 **I82.5 Chronic embolism and thrombosis of deep veins of lower extremity**
Use additional code, if applicable, for associated long-term (current) use of anticoagulants (Z79.01)

EXCLUDES 1 personal history of venous embolism and thrombosis (Z86.718)

CODING TIPS✓ These conditions are considered acute, unless the physician or NPP specifies chronic.

+ 6 **I82.50 Chronic embolism and thrombosis of unspecified deep veins of lower extremity**

EXCLUDES 1 chronic embolism and thrombosis of unspecified deep veins of distal lower extremity (I82.5Z-)
chronic embolism and thrombosis of unspecified deep veins of proximal lower extremity (I82.5Y-)

SP SL + **I82.501 Chronic embolism and thrombosis of unspecified deep veins of right lower extremity**

SP SL + **I82.502 Chronic embolism and thrombosis of unspecified deep veins of left lower extremity**

SP SL + **I82.503 Chronic embolism and thrombosis of unspecified deep veins of lower extremity, bilateral**

IQ + **I82.509 Chronic embolism and thrombosis of unspecified deep veins of unspecified lower extremity**

+ 6 **I82.51 Chronic embolism and thrombosis of femoral vein**
Chronic embolism and thrombosis of common femoral vein
Chronic embolism and thrombosis of deep femoral vein

CODING TIPS✓ Deep vein thrombosis in the proximal deep veins is more significant than deep vein thrombosis in the distal deep veins. Veins of the thigh are the iliac and femoral.

SP SL + **I82.511 Chronic embolism and thrombosis of right femoral vein**

SP SL + **I82.512 Chronic embolism and thrombosis of left femoral vein**

SP SL + **I82.513 Chronic embolism and thrombosis of femoral vein, bilateral**

IQ + **I82.519 Chronic embolism and thrombosis of unspecified femoral vein**

+ 6 **I82.52 Chronic embolism and thrombosis of iliac vein**
Chronic embolism and thrombosis of common iliac vein
Chronic embolism and thrombosis of external iliac vein
Chronic embolism and thrombosis of internal iliac vein

CODING TIPS✓ Deep vein thrombosis in the proximal deep veins is more significant than deep vein thrombosis in the distal deep veins. Veins of the thigh are the iliac and femoral.

SP SL + **I82.521 Chronic embolism and thrombosis of right iliac vein**

SP SL + **I82.522 Chronic embolism and thrombosis of left iliac vein**

SP SL + **I82.523 Chronic embolism and thrombosis of iliac vein, bilateral**

IQ + **I82.529 Chronic embolism and thrombosis of unspecified iliac vein**

+ 6 **I82.53 Chronic embolism and thrombosis of popliteal vein**

SP SL + **I82.531 Chronic embolism and thrombosis of right popliteal vein**

SP SL + **I82.532 Chronic embolism and thrombosis of left popliteal vein**

SP SL + **I82.533 Chronic embolism and thrombosis of popliteal vein, bilateral**

IQ + **I82.539 Chronic embolism and thrombosis of unspecified popliteal vein**

Chapter 9
I00-I99

+ 6 **I82.54 Chronic embolism and thrombosis of tibial vein**

Chronic embolism and thrombosis of anterior tibial vein

Chronic embolism and thrombosis of posterior tibial vein

CODING TIPS✓ Deep vein thrombosis in the proximal deep veins is more significant than deep vein thrombosis in the distal deep veins. Veins of the calf include the peroneal, gastrocnemial, tibial and soleal.

⊟ SP SL + **I82.541 Chronic embolism and thrombosis of right tibial vein**

⊟ SP SL + **I82.542 Chronic embolism and thrombosis of left tibial vein**

⊟ SP SL + **I82.543 Chronic embolism and thrombosis of tibial vein, bilateral**

⊟ IQ + **I82.549 Chronic embolism and thrombosis of unspecified tibial vein**

+ 6 **I82.55 Chronic embolism and thrombosis of peroneal vein**

CODING TIPS✓ Deep vein thrombosis in the proximal deep veins is more significant than deep vein thrombosis in the distal deep veins. Veins of the calf include the peroneal, gastrocnemial, tibial and soleal.

⊟ SP SL + **I82.551 Chronic embolism and thrombosis of right peroneal vein**

⊟ SP SL + **I82.552 Chronic embolism and thrombosis of left peroneal vein**

⊟ SP SL + **I82.553 Chronic embolism and thrombosis of peroneal vein, bilateral**

⊟ + **I82.559 Chronic embolism and thrombosis of unspecified peroneal vein**

+ 6 **I82.56 Chronic embolism and thrombosis of calf muscular vein**

Chronic embolism and thrombosis of calf muscular vein NOS

Chronic embolism and thrombosis of gastrocnemial vein

Chronic embolism and thrombosis of soleal vein

CODING TIPS✓ Deep vein thrombosis in the proximal deep veins is more significant than deep vein thrombosis in the distal deep veins. Veins of the calf include the peroneal, gastrocnemial, tibial and soleal.

⊟ SP SL + **I82.561 Chronic embolism and thrombosis of right calf muscular vein**

⊟ SP SL + **I82.562 Chronic embolism and thrombosis of left calf muscular vein**

⊟ SP SL + **I82.563 Chronic embolism and thrombosis of calf muscular vein, bilateral**

⊟ + **I82.569 Chronic embolism and thrombosis of unspecified calf muscular vein**

+ 6 **I82.59 Chronic embolism and thrombosis of other specified deep vein of lower extremity**

⊟ SP SL + **I82.591 Chronic embolism and thrombosis of other specified deep vein of right lower extremity**

⊟ SP SL + **I82.592 Chronic embolism and thrombosis of other specified deep vein of left lower extremity**

⊟ SP SL + **I82.593 Chronic embolism and thrombosis of other specified deep vein of lower extremity, bilateral**

⊟ IQ + **I82.599 Chronic embolism and thrombosis of other specified deep vein of unspecified lower extremity**

+ 6 **I82.5Y Chronic embolism and thrombosis of unspecified deep veins of proximal lower extremity**

Chronic embolism and thrombosis of deep veins of thigh NOS

Chronic embolism and thrombosis of deep veins of upper leg NOS

⊟ SP SL + **I82.5Y1 Chronic embolism and thrombosis of unspecified deep veins of right proximal lower extremity**

⊟ SP SL + **I82.5Y2 Chronic embolism and thrombosis of unspecified deep veins of left proximal lower extremity**

⊟ SP SL + **I82.5Y3 Chronic embolism and thrombosis of unspecified deep veins of proximal lower extremity, bilateral**

⊟ IQ + **I82.5Y9 Chronic embolism and thrombosis of unspecified deep veins of unspecified proximal lower extremity**

+ 6 **I82.5Z Chronic embolism and thrombosis of unspecified deep veins of distal lower extremity**

Chronic embolism and thrombosis of deep veins of calf NOS

Chronic embolism and thrombosis of deep veins of lower leg NOS

⊟ SP SL + **I82.5Z1 Chronic embolism and thrombosis of unspecified deep veins of right distal lower extremity**

⊟ SP SL + **I82.5Z2 Chronic embolism and thrombosis of unspecified deep veins of left distal lower extremity**

⊟ SP SL + **I82.5Z3 Chronic embolism and thrombosis of unspecified deep veins of distal lower extremity, bilateral**

⊟ IQ + **I82.5Z9 Chronic embolism and thrombosis of unspecified deep veins of unspecified distal lower extremity**

5 **I82.6 Acute embolism and thrombosis of veins of upper extremity**

6 **I82.60 Acute embolism and thrombosis of unspecified veins of upper extremity**

⊟ SP SL **I82.601 Acute embolism and thrombosis of unspecified veins of right upper extremity**

⊟ SP SL **I82.602 Acute embolism and thrombosis of unspecified veins of left upper extremity**

SP SL I82.603 Acute embolism and thrombosis of unspecified veins of upper extremity, bilateral

IQ I82.609 Acute embolism and thrombosis of unspecified veins of unspecified upper extremity

6 I82.61 **Acute embolism and thrombosis of superficial veins of upper extremity**
Acute embolism and thrombosis of antecubital vein
Acute embolism and thrombosis of basilic vein
Acute embolism and thrombosis of cephalic vein

SP SL I82.611 **Acute embolism and thrombosis of superficial veins of right upper extremity**

SP SL I82.612 **Acute embolism and thrombosis of superficial veins of left upper extremity**

SP SL I82.613 **Acute embolism and thrombosis of superficial veins of upper extremity, bilateral**

IQ I82.619 Acute embolism and thrombosis of superficial veins of unspecified upper extremity

6 I82.62 **Acute embolism and thrombosis of deep veins of upper extremity**
Acute embolism and thrombosis of brachial vein
Acute embolism and thrombosis of radial vein
Acute embolism and thrombosis of ulnar vein

SP SL I82.621 **Acute embolism and thrombosis of deep veins of right upper extremity**

SP SL I82.622 **Acute embolism and thrombosis of deep veins of left upper extremity**

SP SL I82.623 **Acute embolism and thrombosis of deep veins of upper extremity, bilateral**

IQ I82.629 Acute embolism and thrombosis of deep veins of unspecified upper extremity

+ 5 I82.7 **Chronic embolism and thrombosis of veins of upper extremity**
Use additional code, if applicable, for associated long-term (current) use of anticoagulants (Z79.01)
EXCLUDES 1 personal history of venous embolism and thrombosis (Z86.718)
CODING TIPS These conditions are considered acute, unless the physician or NPP specifies chronic.

+ 6 I82.70 Chronic embolism and thrombosis of unspecified veins of upper extremity

SP SL + I82.701 Chronic embolism and thrombosis of unspecified veins of right upper extremity

SP SL + I82.702 Chronic embolism and thrombosis of unspecified veins of left upper extremity

SP SL + I82.703 Chronic embolism and thrombosis of unspecified veins of upper extremity, bilateral

IQ + I82.709 Chronic embolism and thrombosis of unspecified veins of unspecified upper extremity

+ 6 I82.71 **Chronic embolism and thrombosis of superficial veins of upper extremity**
Chronic embolism and thrombosis of antecubital vein
Chronic embolism and thrombosis of basilic vein
Chronic embolism and thrombosis of cephalic vein

SP SL + I82.711 **Chronic embolism and thrombosis of superficial veins of right upper extremity**

SP SL + I82.712 **Chronic embolism and thrombosis of superficial veins of left upper extremity**

SP SL + I82.713 **Chronic embolism and thrombosis of superficial veins of upper extremity, bilateral**

IQ + I82.719 Chronic embolism and thrombosis of superficial veins of unspecified upper extremity

+ 6 I82.72 **Chronic embolism and thrombosis of deep veins of upper extremity**
Chronic embolism and thrombosis of brachial vein
Chronic embolism and thrombosis of radial vein
Chronic embolism and thrombosis of ulnar vein

SP SL + I82.721 **Chronic embolism and thrombosis of deep veins of right upper extremity**

SP SL + I82.722 **Chronic embolism and thrombosis of deep veins of left upper extremity**

SP SL + I82.723 **Chronic embolism and thrombosis of deep veins of upper extremity, bilateral**

IQ + I82.729 Chronic embolism and thrombosis of deep veins of unspecified upper extremity

5 I82.A **Embolism and thrombosis of axillary vein**

6 I82.A1 **Acute embolism and thrombosis of axillary vein**

SP SL I82.A11 **Acute embolism and thrombosis of right axillary vein**

SP SL I82.A12 **Acute embolism and thrombosis of left axillary vein**

SP SL I82.A13 **Acute embolism and thrombosis of axillary vein, bilateral**

IQ I82.A19 Acute embolism and thrombosis of unspecified axillary vein

6 I82.A2 **Chronic embolism and thrombosis of axillary vein**

SP SL I82.A21 **Chronic embolism and thrombosis of right axillary vein**

SP SL I82.A22 **Chronic embolism and thrombosis of left axillary vein**

SP SL I82.A23 **Chronic embolism and thrombosis of axillary vein, bilateral**

Chapter 9

I00-I99

L IQ **I82.A29 Chronic embolism and thrombosis of unspecified axillary vein**

5 **I82.B Embolism and thrombosis of subclavian vein**

6 **I82.B1 Acute embolism and thrombosis of subclavian vein**

L SP SL **I82.B11 Acute embolism and thrombosis of right subclavian vein**

L SP SL **I82.B12 Acute embolism and thrombosis of left subclavian vein**

L SP SL **I82.B13 Acute embolism and thrombosis of subclavian vein, bilateral**

L IQ **I82.B19 Acute embolism and thrombosis of unspecified subclavian vein**

6 **I82.B2 Chronic embolism and thrombosis of subclavian vein**

L SP SL **I82.B21 Chronic embolism and thrombosis of right subclavian vein**

L SP SL **I82.B22 Chronic embolism and thrombosis of left subclavian vein**

L SP SL **I82.B23 Chronic embolism and thrombosis of subclavian vein, bilateral**

L IQ **I82.B29 Chronic embolism and thrombosis of unspecified subclavian vein**

5 **I82.C Embolism and thrombosis of internal jugular vein**

6 **I82.C1 Acute embolism and thrombosis of internal jugular vein**

L SP SL **I82.C11 Acute embolism and thrombosis of right internal jugular vein**

L SP SL **I82.C12 Acute embolism and thrombosis of left internal jugular vein**

L SP SL **I82.C13 Acute embolism and thrombosis of internal jugular vein, bilateral**

L IQ **I82.C19 Acute embolism and thrombosis of unspecified internal jugular vein**

6 **I82.C2 Chronic embolism and thrombosis of internal jugular vein**

L SP SL **I82.C21 Chronic embolism and thrombosis of right internal jugular vein**

L SP SL **I82.C22 Chronic embolism and thrombosis of left internal jugular vein**

L SP SL **I82.C23 Chronic embolism and thrombosis of internal jugular vein, bilateral**

L IQ **I82.C29 Chronic embolism and thrombosis of unspecified internal jugular vein**

+ 5 **I82.8 Embolism and thrombosis of other specified veins**

Use additional code, if applicable, for associated long-term (current) use of anticoagulants (Z79.01)

+ 6 **I82.81 Embolism and thrombosis of superficial veins of lower extremities**

Embolism and thrombosis of saphenous vein (greater) (lesser)

L SP SL + **I82.811 Embolism and thrombosis of superficial veins of right lower extremity**

L SP SL + **I82.812 Embolism and thrombosis of superficial veins of left lower extremity**

L SP SL + **I82.813 Embolism and thrombosis of superficial veins of lower extremities, bilateral**

L IQ + **I82.819 Embolism and thrombosis of superficial veins of unspecified lower extremity**

+ 6 **I82.89 Embolism and thrombosis of other specified veins**

SP SL + **I82.890 Acute embolism and thrombosis of other specified veins**

SP SL + **I82.891 Chronic embolism and thrombosis of other specified veins**

5 **I82.9 Embolism and thrombosis of unspecified vein**

IQ **I82.90 Acute embolism and thrombosis of unspecified vein**

Embolism of vein NOS

Thrombosis (vein) NOS

IQ **I82.91 Chronic embolism and thrombosis of unspecified vein**

▲ 4 **I83 Varicose veins of lower extremities**

EXCLUDES 2 varicose veins complicating pregnancy (O22.0-)
varicose veins complicating the puerperium (O87.4)

CODING TIPS✓ **Documentation:** When assigning a code from I83.-, coders should assign the most specific code applicable, but cannot assume a specific code. A relationship between a lower extremity wound and varicosity must be stated in the clinical record as a cause and effect relationship by the physician or NPP in order to assign a code from I83.2- or I83.0-. Inflammation should not be assumed to be related to varicosities but should be verified by the provider as related before assigning a code from category I83.1-

+ 5 **I83.0 Varicose veins of lower extremities with ulcer**

Use additional code to identify severity of ulcer (L97.-)

CODING TIPS✓ A stasis ulcer associated with varicose vein is coded to I83.0 or I83.2 (varicose veins of lower extremities). An additional code for the ulcer is required to indicate the severity of the ulcer.

+ 6 **I83.00 Varicose veins of unspecified lower extremity with ulcer**

IQ + **I83.001 Varicose veins of unspecified lower extremity with ulcer of thigh**

IQ + **I83.002 Varicose veins of unspecified lower extremity with ulcer of calf**

IQ + **I83.003 Varicose veins of unspecified lower extremity with ulcer of ankle**

IQ + **I83.004 Varicose veins of unspecified lower extremity with ulcer of heel and midfoot**

Varicose veins of unspecified lower extremity with ulcer of plantar surface of midfoot

IQ + **I83.005 Varicose veins of unspecified lower extremity with ulcer other part of foot**

Varicose veins of unspecified lower extremity with ulcer of toe

IQ + I83.008 **Varicose veins of unspecified lower extremity with ulcer other part of lower leg**

IQ + I83.009 **Varicose veins of unspecified lower extremity with ulcer of unspecified site**

+ 6 I83.01 **Varicose veins of right lower extremity with ulcer**

SP SL + I83.011 **Varicose veins of right lower extremity with ulcer of thigh**

SP SL + I83.012 **Varicose veins of right lower extremity with ulcer of calf**

SP SL + I83.013 **Varicose veins of right lower extremity with ulcer of ankle**

SP SL + I83.014 **Varicose veins of right lower extremity with ulcer of heel and midfoot**

Varicose veins of right lower extremity with ulcer of plantar surface of midfoot

SP SL + I83.015 **Varicose veins of right lower extremity with ulcer other part of foot**

Varicose veins of right lower extremity with ulcer of toe

SP SL + I83.018 **Varicose veins of right lower extremity with ulcer other part of lower leg**

IQ + I83.019 **Varicose veins of right lower extremity with ulcer of unspecified site**

+ 6 I83.02 **Varicose veins of left lower extremity with ulcer**

SP SL + I83.021 **Varicose veins of left lower extremity with ulcer of thigh**

SP SL + I83.022 **Varicose veins of left lower extremity with ulcer of calf**

SP SL + I83.023 **Varicose veins of left lower extremity with ulcer of ankle**

SP SL + I83.024 **Varicose veins of left lower extremity with ulcer of heel and midfoot**

Varicose veins of left lower extremity with ulcer of plantar surface of midfoot

SP SL + I83.025 **Varicose veins of left lower extremity with ulcer other part of foot**

Varicose veins of left lower extremity with ulcer of toe

SP SL + I83.028 **Varicose veins of left lower extremity with ulcer other part of lower leg**

IQ + I83.029 **Varicose veins of left lower extremity with ulcer of unspecified site**

5 I83.1 **Varicose veins of lower extremities with inflammation**

CODING TIPS ✓ **Documentation:** Do not assume inflammation of the lower extremities to be related to varicosities when present. Inflammation present on assessment should be reported to the patient's provider and a cause and effect relationship confirmed in order to assign a code from category I83.1-.

IQ I83.10 **Varicose veins of unspecified lower extremity with inflammation**

SP SL I83.11 **Varicose veins of right lower extremity with inflammation**

SP SL I83.12 **Varicose veins of left lower extremity with inflammation**

+ 5 I83.2 **Varicose veins of lower extremities with both ulcer and inflammation**

Use additional code to identify severity of ulcer (L97.-)

CODING TIPS ✓ If the clinical record reports a confirmed diagnosis of ulcers due to varicosity (condition classifiable to I83.0), as well as inflammation due to varicosity (condition classifiable to I83.1-), then a code from category I83.2- should be reported instead. An additional code is required to indicate the severity of the ulcer.

+ 6 I83.20 **Varicose veins of unspecified lower extremity with both ulcer and inflammation**

IQ + I83.201 **Varicose veins of unspecified lower extremity with both ulcer of thigh and inflammation**

IQ + I83.202 **Varicose veins of unspecified lower extremity with both ulcer of calf and inflammation**

IQ + I83.203 **Varicose veins of unspecified lower extremity with both ulcer of ankle and inflammation**

IQ + I83.204 **Varicose veins of unspecified lower extremity with both ulcer of heel and midfoot and inflammation**

Varicose veins of unspecified lower extremity with both ulcer of plantar surface of midfoot and inflammation

IQ + I83.205 **Varicose veins of unspecified lower extremity with both ulcer other part of foot and inflammation**

Varicose veins of unspecified lower extremity with both ulcer of toe and inflammation

IQ + I83.208 **Varicose veins of unspecified lower extremity with both ulcer of other part of lower extremity and inflammation**

IQ + I83.209 **Varicose veins of unspecified lower extremity with both ulcer of unspecified site and inflammation**

+ 6 I83.21 **Varicose veins of right lower extremity with both ulcer and inflammation**

SP SL + I83.211 **Varicose veins of right lower extremity with both ulcer of thigh and inflammation**

SP SL + I83.212 **Varicose veins of right lower extremity with both ulcer of calf and inflammation**

SP SL + I83.213 **Varicose veins of right lower extremity with both ulcer of ankle and inflammation**

Chapter 9

I00-I99

I83.214 Varicose veins of right lower extremity with both ulcer of heel and midfoot and inflammation
Varicose veins of right lower extremity with both ulcer of plantar surface of midfoot and inflammation

I83.215 Varicose veins of right lower extremity with both ulcer other part of foot and inflammation
Varicose veins of right lower extremity with both ulcer of toe and inflammation

I83.218 Varicose veins of right lower extremity with both ulcer of other part of lower extremity and inflammation

I83.219 Varicose veins of right lower extremity with both ulcer of unspecified site and inflammation

I83.22 Varicose veins of left lower extremity with both ulcer and inflammation

I83.221 Varicose veins of left lower extremity with both ulcer of thigh and inflammation

I83.222 Varicose veins of left lower extremity with both ulcer of calf and inflammation

I83.223 Varicose veins of left lower extremity with both ulcer of ankle and inflammation

I83.224 Varicose veins of left lower extremity with both ulcer of heel and midfoot and inflammation
Varicose veins of left lower extremity with both ulcer of plantar surface of midfoot and inflammation

I83.225 Varicose veins of left lower extremity with both ulcer other part of foot and inflammation
Varicose veins of left lower extremity with both ulcer of toe and inflammation

I83.228 Varicose veins of left lower extremity with both ulcer of other part of lower extremity and inflammation

I83.229 Varicose veins of left lower extremity with both ulcer of unspecified site and inflammation

I83.8 Varicose veins of lower extremities with other complications

I83.81 Varicose veins of lower extremities with pain

I83.811 Varicose veins of right lower extremity with pain

I83.812 Varicose veins of left lower extremity with pain

I83.813 Varicose veins of bilateral lower extremities with pain

I83.819 Varicose veins of unspecified lower extremity with pain

I83.89 Varicose veins of lower extremities with other complications
Varicose veins of lower extremities with edema
Varicose veins of lower extremities with swelling

I83.891 Varicose veins of right lower extremity with other complications

I83.892 Varicose veins of left lower extremity with other complications

I83.893 Varicose veins of bilateral lower extremities with other complications

I83.899 Varicose veins of unspecified lower extremity with other complications

I83.9 Asymptomatic varicose veins of lower extremities
Phlebectasia of lower extremities
Varicose veins of lower extremities
Varix of lower extremities

CODING TIPS✓ Before assigning a code from I83.9-, consider if this diagnosis is the correct one, as I83.9- codes indicate asymptomatic varicosities. Also consider the appropriateness of including I83.9- codes on the home health claim, as these codes indicate a stable and asymptomatic condition that should require little to no intervention.

I83.90 Asymptomatic varicose veins of unspecified lower extremity
Varicose veins NOS

I83.91 Asymptomatic varicose veins of right lower extremity

I83.92 Asymptomatic varicose veins of left lower extremity

I83.93 Asymptomatic varicose veins of bilateral lower extremities

I85 Esophageal varices
Use additional code to identify:
alcohol abuse and dependence (F10.-)

CODING TIPS✓ Esophageal varices are coded to vascular disorders, rather than gastrointestinal disorders, due to the nature of their pathophysiology. Bleeding varices can be life-threatening and cause additional complex cardiovascular complications.

I85.0 Esophageal varices
Idiopathic esophageal varices
Primary esophageal varices

I85.00 Esophageal varices without bleeding
Esophageal varices NOS

CODING TIPS✓ When the clinical record does not specify bleeding or absence of bleeding in a patient with esophageal varices, assign code I85.00, when the varices are not specified as related to any other cause.

I85.01 Esophageal varices with bleeding

I85.1 Secondary esophageal varices
Esophageal varices secondary to alcoholic liver disease
Esophageal varices secondary to cirrhosis of liver
Esophageal varices secondary to schistosomiasis

Esophageal varices secondary to toxic liver disease
Code first:
underlying disease

CODING TIPS ✓ This diagnosis indicates that the alcohol was linked to the disorder, so the use, abuse or dependence of alcohol (F10.-) should also be coded, usually with 4th and 5th characters to indicate uncomplicated. Do not include 5th and 6th characters .-88. "Induced disorders" include mental, emotional and physical disorders that are included in Chapter 5 only.

IQ + **I85.10 Secondary esophageal varices without bleeding**

IQ + **I85.11 Secondary esophageal varices with bleeding**

4 **I86 Varicose veins of other sites**
EXCLUDES 1 varicose veins of unspecified site (I83.9-)
EXCLUDES 2 retinal varices (H35.0-)

SP **I86.0 Sublingual varices**

SP **I86.1 Scrotal varices**
Varicocele

SP **I86.2 Pelvic varices**

SP **I86.3 Vulval varices**
EXCLUDES 1 vulval varices complicating childbirth and the puerperium (O87.8)
vulval varices complicating pregnancy (O22.1-)

SP **I86.4 Gastric varices**

SP **I86.8 Varicose veins of other specified sites**
Varicose ulcer of nasal septum

4 **I87 Other disorders of veins**

5 **I87.0 Postthrombotic syndrome**
Chronic venous hypertension due to deep vein thrombosis
Postphlebitic syndrome
EXCLUDES 1 chronic venous hypertension without deep vein thrombosis (I87.3-)

6 **I87.00 Postthrombotic syndrome without complications**
Asymptomatic Postthrombotic syndrome

SP **I87.001 Postthrombotic syndrome without complications of right lower extremity**

SP **I87.002 Postthrombotic syndrome without complications of left lower extremity**

SP **I87.003 Postthrombotic syndrome without complications of bilateral lower extremity**

IQ **I87.009 Postthrombotic syndrome without complications of unspecified extremity**
Postthrombotic syndrome NOS

+ 6 **I87.01 Postthrombotic syndrome with ulcer**
Use additional code to specify site and severity of ulcer (L97.-)

CODING TIPS ✓ Postphlebitic or postthrombotic syndrome ulcers require that L97 codes be used to identify the location and laterality of the ulcer.

SP + **I87.011 Postthrombotic syndrome with ulcer of right lower extremity**

SP + **I87.012 Postthrombotic syndrome with ulcer of left lower extremity**

SP + **I87.013 Postthrombotic syndrome with ulcer of bilateral lower extremity**

IQ + **I87.019 Postthrombotic syndrome with ulcer of unspecified lower extremity**

6 **I87.02 Postthrombotic syndrome with inflammation**

SP **I87.021 Postthrombotic syndrome with inflammation of right lower extremity**

SP **I87.022 Postthrombotic syndrome with inflammation of left lower extremity**

SP **I87.023 Postthrombotic syndrome with inflammation of bilateral lower extremity**

IQ **I87.029 Postthrombotic syndrome with inflammation of unspecified lower extremity**

+ 6 **I87.03 Postthrombotic syndrome with ulcer and inflammation**
Use additional code to specify site and severity of ulcer (L97.-)

CODING TIPS ✓ Postphlebitic or postthrombotic syndrome ulcers require that L97 codes be used to identify the location and laterality of the ulcer.

SP + **I87.031 Postthrombotic syndrome with ulcer and inflammation of right lower extremity**

SP + **I87.032 Postthrombotic syndrome with ulcer and inflammation of left lower extremity**

SP + **I87.033 Postthrombotic syndrome with ulcer and inflammation of bilateral lower extremity**

IQ + **I87.039 Postthrombotic syndrome with ulcer and inflammation of unspecified lower extremity**

6 **I87.09 Postthrombotic syndrome with other complications**

SP **I87.091 Postthrombotic syndrome with other complications of right lower extremity**

SP **I87.092 Postthrombotic syndrome with other complications of left lower extremity**

SP **I87.093 Postthrombotic syndrome with other complications of bilateral lower extremity**

IQ **I87.099 Postthrombotic syndrome with other complications of unspecified lower extremity**

SP **I87.1 Compression of vein**
Stricture of vein
Vena cava syndrome (inferior) (superior)
EXCLUDES 2 compression of pulmonary vein (I28.8)

SP **I87.2 Venous insufficiency (chronic) (peripheral)**
Stasis dermatitis
EXCLUDES 1 stasis dermatitis with varicose veins of lower extremities (I83.1-, I83.2-)

CODING TIPS✓ Chronic venous insufficiency is considered a peripheral angiopathy and is assumed related to diabetes. Use E--.51 prior to coding I87.2 in the diabetic.

CODING TIPS✓ If the physician or NPP documents only "stasis ulcer" then use I87.2 followed by the ulcer code to indicate severity and laterality. Stasis dermatitis, in the absence of varicosities, is included.

5 **I87.3 Chronic venous hypertension (idiopathic)**
Stasis edema
EXCLUDES 1 chronic venous hypertension due to deep vein thrombosis (I87.0-)
varicose veins of lower extremities (I83.-)

CODING TIPS✓ Chronic venous hypertension is a more severe state of the venous insufficiency. Do not code I87.2 with I87.3.

6 **I87.30 Chronic venous hypertension (idiopathic) without complications**
Asymptomatic chronic venous hypertension (idiopathic)

⊟ SP **I87.301 Chronic venous hypertension (idiopathic) without complications of right lower extremity**

⊟ SP **I87.302 Chronic venous hypertension (idiopathic) without complications of left lower extremity**

⊟ SP **I87.303 Chronic venous hypertension (idiopathic) without complications of bilateral lower extremity**

⊟ IQ **I87.309 Chronic venous hypertension (idiopathic) without complications of unspecified lower extremity**
Chronic venous hypertension NOS

+ 6 **I87.31 Chronic venous hypertension (idiopathic) with ulcer**
Use additional code to specify site and severity of ulcer (L97.-)

CODING TIPS✓ To report an ulcer associated with chronic venous hypertension, report first I87.31 or I87.33 and L97 as an additional diagnosis.

⊟ SP + **I87.311 Chronic venous hypertension (idiopathic) with ulcer of right lower extremity**

⊟ SP + **I87.312 Chronic venous hypertension (idiopathic) with ulcer of left lower extremity**

⊟ SP + **I87.313 Chronic venous hypertension (idiopathic) with ulcer of bilateral lower extremity**

⊟ IQ + **I87.319 Chronic venous hypertension (idiopathic) with ulcer of unspecified lower extremity**

6 **I87.32 Chronic venous hypertension (idiopathic) with inflammation**

⊟ SP **I87.321 Chronic venous hypertension (idiopathic) with inflammation of right lower extremity**

⊟ SP **I87.322 Chronic venous hypertension (idiopathic) with inflammation of left lower extremity**

⊟ SP **I87.323 Chronic venous hypertension (idiopathic) with inflammation of bilateral lower extremity**

⊟ IQ **I87.329 Chronic venous hypertension (idiopathic) with inflammation of unspecified lower extremity**

+ 6 **I87.33 Chronic venous hypertension (idiopathic) with ulcer and inflammation**
Use additional code to specify site and severity of ulcer (L97.-)

CODING TIPS✓ To report an ulcer associated with chronic venous hypertension, report first I87.31 or I87.33 and L97 as an additional diagnosis.

⊟ SP + **I87.331 Chronic venous hypertension (idiopathic) with ulcer and inflammation of right lower extremity**

⊟ SP + **I87.332 Chronic venous hypertension (idiopathic) with ulcer and inflammation of left lower extremity**

⊟ SP + **I87.333 Chronic venous hypertension (idiopathic) with ulcer and inflammation of bilateral lower extremity**

⊟ IQ + **I87.339 Chronic venous hypertension (idiopathic) with ulcer and inflammation of unspecified lower extremity**

6 **I87.39 Chronic venous hypertension (idiopathic) with other complications**

⊟ SP **I87.391 Chronic venous hypertension (idiopathic) with other complications of right lower extremity**

⊟ SP **I87.392 Chronic venous hypertension (idiopathic) with other complications of left lower extremity**

⊟ SP **I87.393 Chronic venous hypertension (idiopathic) with other complications of bilateral lower extremity**

⊟ IQ **I87.399 Chronic venous hypertension (idiopathic) with other complications of unspecified lower extremity**

SP **I87.8 Other specified disorders of veins**
Phlebosclerosis
Venofibrosis

IQ **I87.9 Disorder of vein, unspecified**

4 **I88 Nonspecific lymphadenitis**
EXCLUDES 1 acute lymphadenitis, except mesenteric (L04.-)
enlarged lymph nodes NOS (R59.-)
human immunodeficiency virus [HIV] disease resulting in generalized lymphadenopathy (B20)

SP **I88.0 Nonspecific mesenteric lymphadenitis**
Mesenteric lymphadenitis (acute)(chronic)

SP **I88.1 Chronic lymphadenitis, except mesenteric**
Adenitis
Lymphadenitis
DEFINITION Chronic enlargement of the lymphatic glands.

SP **I88.8 Other nonspecific lymphadenitis**

IQ **I88.9 Nonspecific lymphadenitis, unspecified**
Lymphadenitis NOS

4 **I89 Other noninfective disorders of lymphatic vessels and lymph nodes**
EXCLUDES 1 chylocele, tunica vaginalis (nonfilarial) NOS (N50.89)
enlarged lymph nodes NOS (R59.-)
filarial chylocele (B74.-)
hereditary lymphedema (Q82.0)

SP SL **I89.0 Lymphedema, not elsewhere classified**
Elephantiasis (nonfilarial) NOS
Lymphangiectasis
Obliteration, lymphatic vessel
Praecox lymphedema
Secondary lymphedema
EXCLUDES 1 postmastectomy lymphedema (I97.2)
CODING TIPS✓ Lymphedema is not the same as edema associated with other conditions, such as heart failure, and may not be coded without physician or NPP confirmation.

SP **I89.1 Lymphangitis**
Chronic lymphangitis
Lymphangitis NOS
Subacute lymphangitis
EXCLUDES 1 acute lymphangitis (L03.-)

SP **I89.8 Other specified noninfective disorders of lymphatic vessels and lymph nodes**
Chylocele (nonfilarial)
Chylous ascites
Chylous cyst
Lipomelanotic reticulosis
Lymph node or vessel fistula
Lymph node or vessel infarction
Lymph node or vessel rupture

IQ **I89.9 Noninfective disorder of lymphatic vessels and lymph nodes, unspecified**
Disease of lymphatic vessels NOS

Other and unspecified disorders of the circulatory system (I95-I99)

4 **I95 Hypotension**
EXCLUDES 1 cardiovascular collapse (R57.9)
maternal hypotension syndrome (O26.5-)
nonspecific low blood pressure reading NOS (R03.1)
CODING TIPS✓ A low blood pressure reading in the absence of a diagnosis of hypotension should not be coded to I95.-. A singular low blood pressure reading with no diagnosis of hypotension should be coded to R03.1.

SP **I95.0 Idiopathic hypotension**
CODING TIPS✓ **Documentation:** Idiopathic hypotension requires a confirmed diagnosis by the patient's provider and may not be assumed. Do not assign I95.0 for a patient with hypotension of uncertain cause, with no provider report of idiopathic etiology, and do not assign for a singular low blood pressure reading.

SP **I95.1 Orthostatic hypotension**
Hypotension, postural
EXCLUDES 1 neurogenic orthostatic hypotension [Shy-Drager] (G90.3)
orthostatic hypotension due to drugs (I95.2)
CODING TIPS✓ Do not assign code I95.1 for orthostasis resulting from medication effects. Hypotension secondary to medication/drug effects is coded to I95.2 and is coded as an adverse effect.
DEFINITION Abnormally low blood pressure that occurs when the patient moves to a standing or upright position.

SP + **I95.2 Hypotension due to drugs**
Orthostatic hypotension due to drugs
Use additional code for adverse effect, if applicable, to identify drug (T36-T50 with fifth or sixth character 5)
CODING TIPS✓ A patient can have a diagnosis of hypertension and a problem with hypotension at the same time, especially hypotension related to the anti-hypertensive medications. Continue to code the type of hypertension.
CODING TIPS✓ When hypotension or orthostasis is confirmed and reported in the medical record as resulting from the effects of medications or other drugs, code I95.2 should be assigned. An additional code from category T36-T50 should be assigned to identify the drug.

SP **I95.3 Hypotension of hemodialysis**
Intra-dialytic hypotension

5 **I95.8 Other hypotension**

SP **I95.81 Postprocedural hypotension**

SP **I95.89 Other hypotension**
Chronic hypotension

IQ **I95.9 Hypotension, unspecified**

SP **I96 Gangrene, not elsewhere classified**
Gangrenous cellulitis
EXCLUDES 1 gangrene in atherosclerosis of native arteries of the extremities (I70.26)
gangrene in hernia (K40.1, K40.4, K41.1, K41.4, K42.1, K43.1-, K44.1, K45.1, K46.1)
gangrene in other peripheral vascular diseases (I73.-)
gangrene of certain specified sites - see Alphabetical Index
gas gangrene (A48.0)
pyoderma gangrenosum (L88)
EXCLUDES 2 gangrene in diabetes mellitus (E08-E13 with .52)

Chapter 9
I00-I99

CODING TIPS✓ Gangrene may be documented as gangrenous cellulitis or necrosis, and is also known as dry gangrene.

CODING TIPS✓ Gangrene associated with a pressure ulcer is coded with I96, then assign the L89.- codes for pressure ulcers. Gangrene associated with pressure ulcers is NOT related to diabetes and is not coded as diabetic gangrene. Note the L89 codes instruct to "code first" any associated gangrene at L89.

CODING TIPS✓ Do not use I96 to indicate gangrene in diabetes, atherosclerosis or other vascular disease, pyoderma gangrenosum, gas gangrene, or gangrene in a hernia.

DEFINITION Complication of cell death (necrosis), characterized by tissue decay, which becomes black and malodorous, caused by infection or ischemia, resulting from insufficient blood supply.

4 I97 Intraoperative and postprocedural complications and disorders of circulatory system, not elsewhere classified

EXCLUDES 2 postprocedural shock (T81.1-)

CODING TIPS✓ **Documentation:** Codes in category I97.- are complication codes and require physician or NPP documentation and confirmation of a cause and effect relationship between the procedure and the complicated condition. Documentation in the home health clinical record must also support this relationship. They may be described as "post-status" or "post-op".

SP I97.0 Postcardiotomy syndrome

5 I97.1 Other postprocedural cardiac functional disturbances

EXCLUDES 2 acute pulmonary insufficiency following thoracic surgery (J95.1)
intraoperative cardiac functional disturbances (I97.7-)

6 I97.11 Postprocedural cardiac insufficiency

SP I97.110 Postprocedural cardiac insufficiency following cardiac surgery

SP I97.111 Postprocedural cardiac insufficiency following other surgery

6 I97.12 Postprocedural cardiac arrest

SP I97.120 Postprocedural cardiac arrest following cardiac surgery

SP I97.121 Postprocedural cardiac arrest following other surgery

+ 6 I97.13 Postprocedural heart failure

Use additional code to identify the heart failure (I50.-)

SP + I97.130 Postprocedural heart failure following cardiac surgery

SP + I97.131 Postprocedural heart failure following other surgery

+ 6 I97.19 Other postprocedural cardiac functional disturbances

Use additional code, if applicable, to further specify disorder

SP + I97.190 Other postprocedural cardiac functional disturbances following cardiac surgery

Use additional code, if applicable, for type 4 or type 5 myocardial infarction, to further specify disorder

SP + I97.191 Other postprocedural cardiac functional disturbances following other surgery

SP SL I97.2 Postmastectomy lymphedema syndrome

Elephantiasis due to mastectomy
Obliteration of lymphatic vessels

CODING TIPS✓ Assign code I97.2 only when lymphedema is specifically reported as related to the effects of a mastectomy.

DEFINITION Localized edema in the arm following breast and lymph node removal due to lack of lymph circulation through the chest area.

SP I97.3 Postprocedural hypertension

5 I97.4 Intraoperative hemorrhage and hematoma of a circulatory system organ or structure complicating a procedure

EXCLUDES 1 intraoperative hemorrhage and hematoma of a circulatory system organ or structure due to accidental puncture and laceration during a procedure (I97.5-)

EXCLUDES 2 intraoperative cerebrovascular hemorrhage complicating a procedure (G97.3-)

6 I97.41 Intraoperative hemorrhage and hematoma of a circulatory system organ or structure complicating a circulatory system procedure

SP I97.410 Intraoperative hemorrhage and hematoma of a circulatory system organ or structure complicating a cardiac catheterization

SP I97.411 Intraoperative hemorrhage and hematoma of a circulatory system organ or structure complicating a cardiac bypass

SP I97.418 Intraoperative hemorrhage and hematoma of a circulatory system organ or structure complicating other circulatory system procedure

SP I97.42 Intraoperative hemorrhage and hematoma of a circulatory system organ or structure complicating other procedure

5 I97.5 Accidental puncture and laceration of a circulatory system organ or structure during a procedure

EXCLUDES 2 accidental puncture and laceration of brain during a procedure (G97.4-)

SP I97.51 Accidental puncture and laceration of a circulatory system organ or structure during a circulatory system procedure

SP **I97.52 Accidental puncture and laceration of a circulatory system organ or structure during other procedure**

5 **I97.6 Postprocedural hemorrhage, hematoma and seroma of a circulatory system organ or structure following a procedure**

EXCLUDES 2 postprocedural cerebrovascular hemorrhage complicating a procedure (G97.5-)

6 **I97.61 Postprocedural hemorrhage of a circulatory system organ or structure following a circulatory system procedure**

SP **I97.610 Postprocedural hemorrhage of a circulatory system organ or structure following a cardiac catheterization**

SP **I97.611 Postprocedural hemorrhage of a circulatory system organ or structure following cardiac bypass**

SP **I97.618 Postprocedural hemorrhage of a circulatory system organ or structure following other circulatory system procedure**

6 **I97.62 Postprocedural hemorrhage, hematoma and seroma of a circulatory system organ or structure following other procedure**

SP **I97.620 Postprocedural hemorrhage of a circulatory system organ or structure following other procedure**

SP **I97.621 Postprocedural hematoma of a circulatory system organ or structure following other procedure**

SP **I97.622 Postprocedural seroma of a circulatory system organ or structure following other procedure**

6 **I97.63 Postprocedural hematoma of a circulatory system organ or structure following a circulatory system procedure**

SP **I97.630 Postprocedural hematoma of a circulatory system organ or structure following a cardiac catheterization**

SP **I97.631 Postprocedural hematoma of a circulatory system organ or structure following cardiac bypass**

SP **I97.638 Postprocedural hematoma of a circulatory system organ or structure following other circulatory system procedure**

6 **I97.64 Postprocedural seroma of a circulatory system organ or structure following a circulatory system procedure**

SP **I97.640 Postprocedural seroma of a circulatory system organ or structure following a cardiac catheterization**

SP **I97.641 Postprocedural seroma of a circulatory system organ or structure following cardiac bypass**

SP **I97.648 Postprocedural seroma of a circulatory system organ or structure following other circulatory system procedure**

5 **I97.7 Intraoperative cardiac functional disturbances**

EXCLUDES 2 acute pulmonary insufficiency following thoracic surgery (J95.1)
postprocedural cardiac functional disturbances (I97.1-)

6 **I97.71 Intraoperative cardiac arrest**

CODING TIPS✓ Codes from subcategory I97.71- indicate that the patient experienced cardiac arrest during a surgical procedure. These codes should never be assigned on the home health claim, but history of cardiac arrest with successful resuscitation may be used instead (Z86.74).

SP **I97.710 Intraoperative cardiac arrest during cardiac surgery**

SP **I97.711 Intraoperative cardiac arrest during other surgery**

+ 6 **I97.79 Other intraoperative cardiac functional disturbances**

Use additional code, if applicable, to further specify disorder

SP + **I97.790 Other intraoperative cardiac functional disturbances during cardiac surgery**

SP + **I97.791 Other intraoperative cardiac functional disturbances during other surgery**

+ 5 **I97.8 Other intraoperative and postprocedural complications and disorders of the circulatory system, not elsewhere classified**

Use additional code, if applicable, to further specify disorder

+ 6 **I97.81 Intraoperative cerebrovascular infarction**

CODING TIPS✓ Codes from category I97.81- indicate that the patient experienced a cerebral vascular accident *during* a surgical procedure (either a cardiac- I97.810, or non-cardiac- I97.811 procedure). Home health may assign a code from category I69.- (sequelae of cerebral vascular disease) on the home health claim if residual neurological deficits as a result of the cerebral vascular accident remain.

SP + **I97.810 Intraoperative cerebrovascular infarction during cardiac surgery**

SP + **I97.811 Intraoperative cerebrovascular infarction during other surgery**

+ 6 **I97.82 Postprocedural cerebrovascular infarction**

Chapter 9

I00-I99

CODING TIPS✓ Codes from category I97.82- indicate that the patient experienced a cerebral vascular accident *after* a surgical procedure (either a cardiac- I97.820, or non-cardiac- I97.821 procedure). Home health may assign a code from category I69.- (sequelae of cerebral vascular disease) on the home health claim if residual neurological deficits as a result of the cerebral vascular accident remain.

SP + **I97.820 Postprocedural cerebrovascular infarction following cardiac surgery**

SP + **I97.821 Postprocedural cerebrovascular infarction following other surgery**

SP + **I97.88 Other intraoperative complications of the circulatory system, not elsewhere classified**

SP + **I97.89 Other postprocedural complications and disorders of the circulatory system, not elsewhere classified**

4 **I99 Other and unspecified disorders of circulatory system**

SP **I99.8 Other disorder of circulatory system**

!Q **I99.9 Unspecified disorder of circulatory system**

Chapter 9 Scenarios: Diseases of the circulatory system (I00-I99)

Diabetic ulcer, sick sinus syndrome

A 69-year-old morbidly obese woman with a BMI of 37 comes to home health for wound care to a diabetic foot ulcer on her left heel. The wound has penetrated muscle tissue but there's no mention of necrosis. The documentation also lists a diagnosis of sick sinus syndrome that is controlled with a pacemaker. She is insulin-dependent.

Description	Code
Primary: Type 2 diabetes mellitus with foot ulcer	E11.621
Secondary: Non-pressure chronic ulcer of left heel and midfoot with muscle involvement without evidence of necrosis	L97.425
Secondary: Sick sinus syndrome	I49.5
Secondary: Morbid (severe) obesity due to excess calories	E66.01
Secondary: Presence of cardiac pacemaker	Z95.0
Secondary: Body mass index (BMI) 37.0-37.9, adult	Z68.37
Secondary: Long term (current) use of insulin	Z79.4

Wound care to the diabetic foot ulcer is the focus of care and so it is coded primary. The coding of a diabetic foot ulcer requires two codes – one for the diabetic ulcer and one for the location and severity of the wound. Sick sinus syndrome, even if controlled by a pacemaker, should still be coded, according to Q1 2019 Coding Clinic guidance. Additionally, morbid obesity is always a clinically significant diagnosis and should be coded when it's documented, according to Q4 2018 Coding Clinic guidance. The pacemaker is coded with Z95.0, and an additional status code is assigned to capture the patient's BMI, in accordance with tabular instruction on the obesity code. Finally, since the patient is not a type 1 diabetic, her insulin use must be captured with Z79.4, in accordance with coding guidelines.

Congestive heart failure

Your agency admitted a 70-year-old woman who was discharged from the hospital with acute exacerbation of her chronic congestive heart failure (CHF) with diastolic heart failure. Her Lasix dose was increased and the physician is requesting daily weights for two weeks and urinary output assessment due to her chronic kidney disease. She also has hypertension, dementia and diabetes with polyneuropathy, and is described as pleasantly confused without behavioral disturbances. Her diabetes is reported as diet controlled.

Description	Code
Primary: Hypertensive heart and chronic kidney disease with heart failure and stage 1 through stage 4 chronic kidney disease, or unspecified chronic kidney disease	I13.0
Secondary: Acute on chronic diastolic (congestive) heart failure	I50.33
Secondary: Type 2 diabetes mellitus with diabetic chronic kidney disease	E11.22
Secondary: Chronic kidney disease, unspecified	N18.9
Secondary: Unspecified dementia without behavioral disturbance	F03.90
Secondary: Type 2 diabetes mellitus with diabetic polyneuropathy	E11.42

A cause-and-effect relationship between hypertension, heart failure, diabetes and chronic kidney disease is assumed by the ICD-10 classification system unless the provider states that the conditions are unrelated. CHF and diastolic (or systolic) heart failure diagnoses are combined into one diagnosis and code. In addition, when an acute exacerbation is reported as superimposed upon a chronic condition, the condition should be coded as "acute on chronic." The appropriate code from N18.- for the stage of chronic kidney disease is also assigned in accordance with tabular instruction. No further information or etiology for the dementia is stated, so only F03.90 can be assigned. While the diabetes is well controlled and requires no medication therapy, it must still be coded.

Cerebral vascular accident

A female patient admitted to home health after suffering a CVA with hemiparesis of right side, dysphagia of oral phase and stuttering. Nursing, physical therapy and speech therapy will see the patient. Her co-morbidities of hypertension, diabetes with angiopathy, and well-controlled emphysema are documented. The patient takes insulin and recently has been started on Coumadin. PT/INRs will be monitored. The focus of care is the CVA with hemiparesis.

Description	Code
Primary: Hemiplegia following CVA affecting right dominant side	I69.351
Secondary: Dysphagia following CVA	I69.391
Secondary: Dysphagia oral phase	R13.11
Secondary: Fluency disorder following CVA	I69.323
Secondary: Essential primary hypertension	I10
Secondary: Type 2 diabetes mellitus with angiopathy without gangrene	E11.51
Secondary: Emphysema, unspecified	J43.9
Secondary: Long term (current) use of insulin	Z79.4
Secondary: Encounter for therapeutic drug level monitoring	Z51.81

Even though the documentation does not include whether the right sided CVA is dominant or non-dominant, if the information is not provided, right defaults to dominant, according to official coding guidelines. If the type of diabetes is not specified, it defaults to type 2. Because the patient uses insulin and is not a type 1 diabetic, the code for insulin use is assigned. The patient's emphysema is a relevant comorbidity and is also coded. Code Z79.01 is assigned to capture her Coumadin use. The instructional note on the code for encounter for therapeutic drug monitoring (Z51.81), to also code the condition requiring care, does not include sequencing instructions (code also). The two codes can be in either order. Thus it is sequenced at the bottom of the list.

Exacerbated hypertension, chronic systolic heart failure

A 77-year-old male is admitted to home health with a diagnosis of exacerbated hypertension. He also has chronic systolic heart failure and congestive heart failure (CHF). As a result of his hypertension, he suffered a stroke last year, from which he still suffers some aphasia. Hypertension is the focus of care.

Description	Code
Primary: Hypertensive heart disease with heart failure	I11.0
Secondary: Chronic systolic (congestive) heart failure	I50.22
Secondary: Aphasia following cerebral infarction	I69.320

The patient is having an exacerbation of his hypertension, and since it will be the focus of care, it should be listed as the primary diagnosis. A cause-and-effect relationship between hypertension and heart failure is assumed by the ICD-10 classification system unless the provider states they're unrelated. The patient also has two types of heart failure, chronic systolic heart failure and congestive heart failure. Both types of heart failure should be recognized. However, congestive heart failure is included in the code title for chronic systolic heart failure, and therefore only one heart failure code is needed to complete the diagnostic statement in this scenario. Code a patient with chronic systolic heart failure, who does not also have CHF, with I50.22 because "congestive" is a non-essential modifier. The aphasia resulting from the prior CVA is also coded as this will impact the plan of care and patient progress and may provide important comorbidity adjustment.

Chronic DVT, wound care, morbid obesity

A 57-year-old patient was referred to home health for wound care to a stage 3 pressure ulcer/injury on her right buttock. She is morbidly obese with a documented BMI of 41. She had a Greenfield filter inserted four years ago after she was diagnosed with a chronic DVT of her deep femoral vein on her right side, following a fem-pop bypass due to severe PVD. As a result of her chronic DVT, she is on chronic anticoagulant therapy and the agency will also be obtaining PT/INR levels.

Description	Code
Primary: Pressure ulcer, stage 3, right buttock	L89.313
Secondary: Peripheral vascular disease, unspecified	I73.9
Secondary: Chronic embolism and thrombosis of right femoral vein	I82.511
Secondary: Morbid (severe) obesity due to excess calories	E66.01
Secondary: Body mass index [BMI] 40.0-44.9, adult	Z68.41
Secondary: Encounter for therapeutic drug level monitoring	Z51.81
Secondary: Long term (current) use of anticoagulants	Z79.01

The site, stage and laterality of a pressure ulcer/injury are combined into one code. And, as the focus of care, it is coded primary. The chronic DVT should also be coded, since it may be impacted by the peripheral vascular disease and requires long-term anticoagulant therapy. This DVT code (I82.511) also denotes laterality (i.e. the last character 1 = right, indicates laterality). Morbid obesity is a relevant comorbidity and should always be coded when documented, according to Q4 2018 Coding Clinic guidance. It is coded, along with the BMI code, in accordance with tabular instruction. Monitoring of PT/INR levels is captured by Z51.81 and the long-term anticoagulant use is captured with Z79.01.

Congestive heart failure, hypertensive chronic kidney disease

The patient has congestive heart failure (CHF) and hypertensive chronic kidney disease (CKD) of unspecified stage. The CHF is focus of care.

Description	Code
Primary: Hypertensive heart and chronic kidney disease with heart failure and stage 1 through stage 4 chronic kidney disease, or unspecified chronic kidney disease	I13.0
Secondary: Heart failure, unspecified	I50.9
Secondary: Chronic kidney disease, unspecified	N18.9

A cause-and-effect relationship between hypertension, heart failure and chronic kidney disease is assumed by the ICD-10 classification system unless the provider states they're unrelated. Additional codes for the type of heart failure and stage of chronic kidney disease are assigned in accordance with tabular instruction.

HOME HEALTH CODING SCENARIOS

Hemiplegia after intracerebral hemorrhage, aphasia

The patient is referred for home care after suffering an intracerebral hemorrhage due to uncontrolled hypertension. His deficits include aphasia and left-sided hemiplegia. The patient has a 30-year history of smoking but quit 10 years ago. Nursing, physical therapy, occupational therapy and speech therapy are ordered.

Description	Code
Primary: Hemiplegia following non-traumatic intracerebral hemorrhage affecting left non-dominant side	I69.154
Secondary: Aphasia following non-traumatic intracerebral hemorrhage	I69.120
Secondary: Hypertension	I10
Secondary: Personal history of nicotine dependence	Z87.891

This scenario illustrates how some sequela conditions and the causal illness or injury are combined into one diagnosis code, in this case I69.154 and I69.120. Residual codes are found in the index under the heading "sequelae." Search first for sequelae, hemorrhage, intracerebral, by deficit and then confirm the choice in the tabular. Although the medical record information does not indicate left- or right-hand dominance for the patient, coding guidelines indicate that, when specific information is not available, if the left side of the body is affected, the default code for non-dominant should be used. Tabular instruction at the Hypertensive diseases category level instruct the coder to use an additional code to identify history of tobacco use, which in this case necessitates the addition of Z87.891.

Hypertensive acute systolic heart failure

A 76-year-old woman was admitted to home health with acute systolic heart failure stated in the documentation as secondary to hypertension. She will receive skilled nursing care for management of new medications as well as physical therapy to help increase her stamina in completing ADLs.

Description	Code
Primary: Hypertensive heart disease with heart failure	I11.0
Secondary: Acute systolic (congestive) heart failure	I50.21

The patient's heart failure was caused by her hypertension and is therefore coded as hypertensive heart disease with heart failure. The hypertensive heart disease code is assigned first, in accordance with coding guidelines. An additional code for the specific type of heart failure is also coded, in accordance with tabular instruction.

Secondary hypertension, breast cancer with brain metastasis

A 71-year-old woman comes to home health with uncontrolled hypertension caused by breast cancer in her left breast that has metastasized to her brain. The hypertension is the focus of care.

Description	Code
Primary: Other secondary hypertension	I15.8
Secondary: Secondary malignant neoplasm of brain	C79.31
Secondary: Malignant neoplasm of unspecified site of left female breast	C50.912

The patient's hypertension is caused by the brain neoplasm, so it is coded secondary hypertension. As the focus of care, it is coded first. The brain metastasis is sequenced next as it is causing the hypertension. The original neoplasm is coded as well, as a diagnosis relevant to the plan of care.

Heart attacks

A 75-year-old man suffered a myocardial infarction. Three weeks and four days later, he suffered another myocardial infarction. After treatment in the hospital, which included the placement of stents via an angioplasty, he was admitted to home health one week later. The focus of care is recovery from the myocardial infarction. He also has a diagnosis of coronary artery disease and a history of resolved prostate cancer.

Description	Code
Primary: Acute myocardial infarction, unspecified	I21.9
Secondary: Old myocardial infarction	I25.2
Secondary: Atherosclerotic heart disease of native coronary artery without angina pectoris	I25.10
Secondary: Presence of coronary angioplasty implant and graft	Z95.5
Secondary: Personal history of malignant neoplasm of prostate	Z85.46

Though the patient has had two recent myocardial infarctions, the first one occurred more than four weeks ago, and is thus no longer an acute condition. Therefore it is coded as an old myocardial infarction with I25.2. The second heart attack is coded as an acute myocardial infarction since it is within the four-week acute timeframe. With no further information available about the type and location of the MI, it is most appropriately captured with I21.9. The patient's coronary artery disease is an important comorbidity and thus is coded, as is the status code (Z95.5) indicating he had a stent placed in the hospital. His personal history of resolved prostate cancer is also important to capture, with Z85.46.

Decompensated chronic obstructive bronchitis, aortic valve disease

A 71-year-old woman is admitted to home health with chronic obstructive bronchitis that is acutely decompensated. She also has aortic valve disease and is awaiting valve replacement surgery once her pulmonary disease is stable.

Description	Code
Primary: Chronic obstructive pulmonary disease with (acute) exacerbation	J44.1
Secondary: Nonrheumatic aortic valve disorder, unspecified	I35.9

The focus of care is acutely decompensated chronic obstructive bronchitis, which codes to the J44.- category. Acutely decompensated chronic obstructive bronchitis can be coded as acutely exacerbated COPD, according to the inclusion terms on J44.1. Her aortic valve disease is an important comorbidity that should also be coded. It codes to I35.9, according to the alphabetic index.

Post-infarction angina

A 67-year-old woman suffered a STEMI 30 days ago, she underwent angioplasty and a stent was placed. She has coronary artery disease and still suffers from post-infarction angina. She also has hypertension and stage 2 kidney disease. The post-infarction angina is the focus of care.

Description	Code
Primary: Postinfarction angina	I23.7
Secondary: Atherosclerotic heart disease of native coronary artery with other forms of angina pectoris	I25.118
Secondary: Hypertensive chronic kidney disease with stage 1 through stage 4 chronic kidney disease, or unspecified chronic kidney disease	I12.9
Secondary: Chronic kidney disease, stage 2 (mild)	N18.2
Secondary: Presence of coronary angioplasty implant and graft	Z95.5

The patient's myocardial infarction is no longer considered an acute condition because it occurred longer than 28 days ago. However, the patient is still experiencing symptoms, which have been specified as post-infarction angina. Even though the 28-day acute period has passed, a post-infarction complication can still be assigned, according to Q2 2017 Coding Clinic guidance. The patient has angina and coronary artery disease, which are assumed to be connected and coded with a combination code, according to coding guidelines. The patient's hypertension and chronic kidney disease are assumed to be connected as well, according to coding guidelines, and are captured with combination codes I12.9 and N18.2. The presence of the stent used to treat the myocardial infarction is captured with Z95.5.

Type 2 myocardial infarction

A 74-year-old man is admitted to home health to continue recovery from a heart attack caused by demand ischemia due to a coronary vasospasm. The vasospasm is now under control and recovery from the heart attack will be the focus of care. He also has chronic obstructive asthma, which is currently stable. The physician's H&P states that he smokes a pack of cigarettes a day.

Description	Code
Primary: Angina pectoris with documented spasm	I20.1
Secondary: Myocardial infarction type 2	I21.A1
Secondary: Chronic obstructive pulmonary disease, unspecified	J44.9
Secondary: Nicotine dependence, cigarettes, uncomplicated	F17.210

A myocardial infarction resulting from demand ischemia due to a coronary vasospasm is a Type 2 heart attack. Because the coronary vasospasm is the underlying cause of the MI, it is coded first, according to the code first note at I21.A1. The patient's chronic obstructive asthma is coded as a relevant comorbidity that could impact his recovery. The patient's tobacco use is captured with F17.210 in accordance with tabular instruction.

Heart failure with diastolic dysfunction

A 71-year-old man was recently diagnosed with acute congestive heart failure (CHF) with diastolic dysfunction. He is also a type 2 diabetic with additional diagnoses of polyneuropathy and retinopathy. He uses both insulin and oral antidiabetic medication. The heart failure is the focus of care.

Description	Code
Primary: Acute diastolic (congestive) heart failure	I50.31
Secondary: Type 2 diabetes mellitus with diabetic polyneuropathy	E11.42
Secondary: Type 2 diabetes mellitus with unspecified diabetic retinopathy without macular edema	E11.319
Secondary: Long term (current) use of insulin	Z79.4

A diagnosis of acute congestive heart failure (CHF) with diastolic dysfunction should be coded with I50.31, according to Q1 2017 Coding Clinic guidance. Both the patient's polyneuropathy and retinopathy can be assumed to be connected to the diagnoses diagnosis, according to the alphabetic index. The patient uses both insulin and oral antidiabetic medication, but only insulin use is coded, in accordance with coding guidelines.

Stasis ulcers in diabetes

The patient has diabetes and multiple stasis ulcers on both calves that extend to the fat layer and are caused by venous insufficiency. The patient also has peripheral neuropathy and lymphedema. Oral hypoglycemic medication is used for diabetic control. The wound care is the focus of care.

Description	Code
Primary: Encounter for change or removal of nonsurgical wound dressing	Z48.00
Secondary: Type 2 diabetes mellitus with diabetic peripheral angiopathy without gangrene	E11.51
Secondary: Venous insufficiency (chronic) (peripheral)	I87.2
Secondary: Non-pressure chronic ulcer of left calf with fat layer exposed	L97.222
Secondary: Non-pressure chronic ulcer of right calf with fat layer exposed	L97.212
Secondary: Type 2 diabetes mellitus with diabetic polyneuropathy	E11.42
Secondary: Lymphedema, not elsewhere classified	I89.0
Secondary: Long term (current) use of oral hypoglycemic drugs	Z79.84

Venous insufficiency is a form of peripheral angiopathy and when it occurs in a patient with diabetes, it should be coded as diabetic peripheral angiopathy, according to Coding Clinic guidance. When wound care of a stasis ulcer due to diabetes is the primary focus of care, assign Z48.00 as primary. Z48.00 belongs to the Wounds primary diagnosis group within the PDGM grouper and will assure that the coding for this episode appropriately reflects the care being provided. Additional codes are assigned to identify comorbid diabetic neuropathy and lymphedema as these will impact the healing of the wound and overall plan of care. A code for use of oral hypoglycemic drugs must be assigned.

HOME HEALTH CODING SCENARIOS

Hypertension, diabetic CKD

A patient is referred to home health following multiple medication changes for hypertension. The patient has additional diagnoses listed as ESRD due to diabetic nephropathy on dialysis and diabetic peripheral neuropathy. The patient takes insulin for diabetic control.

Description	Code
Primary: Essential (primary) hypertension	I10
Secondary: Type 2 diabetes mellitus with diabetic chronic kidney disease	E11.22
Secondary: End stage renal disease	N18.6
Secondary: Type 2 diabetes mellitus with diabetic polyneuropathy	E11.42
Secondary: Long term (current) use of insulin	Z79.4

When the patient has diabetes, hypertension and chronic kidney disease (CKD), and the provider documents CKD due to diabetes or diabetic CKD, diabetic nephropathy or other similar terminology, a causal relationship is indicated, and denotes the CKD is not related to the hypertension. In this case, assign a code for diabetic chronic kidney disease. Do not assign a code for hypertensive CKD, as the hypertension would be coded separately per Q3 2019 Coding Clinic Guidance. A code for insulin use must also be assigned.

Central Venous Sinus Thrombosis (CSVT) due to metastatic cancer

An 82-year-old woman is being referred for physical therapy and nursing after an extended hospital and skilled nursing facility stay. She was originally hospitalized for planned lobectomy due to right lower lobe lung cancer, which was not done due to discovery of metastases to brain and cervical lymph nodes. Her hospitalization was complicated by a cerebral venous sinus thrombosis (CVST) caused by pressure on the internal jugular vein due to the cervical metastases. Medical record documentation indicates she has residual right hemiplegia and aphasia. Physical therapy for the hemiplegia is the focus of care.

Description	Code
Primary: Hemiplegia and hemiparesis following cerebral infarction affecting right dominant side	I69.351
Secondary: Aphasia following cerebral infarction	I69.320
Secondary: Secondary and unspecified malignant neoplasm of lymph nodes of head, face and neck	C77.0
Secondary: Malignant neoplasm of lower lobe, right bronchus or lung	C34.31
Secondary: Secondary malignant neoplasm of brain	C79.31

Cerebral venous sinus thrombosis (CVST) is a type of stroke in which the venous channels of the brain become thrombosed, resulting in cerebral infarction in the areas corresponding to the thrombosis. This patient has residual deficits from the infarction (CVA) that are the focus of care and should be coded first for this reason. Sequencing of the neoplastic disease is discretionary, but because the CVST was caused by compression on the internal jugular vein by the cervical lymph node metastases, this is coded next in the scenario. The lung neoplasm and secondary brain neoplasm are also active and are sequenced next.

Atherosclerosis, Critical limb ischemia

A patient with a history of atherosclerosis to the bilateral lower extremities was hospitalized due to critical limb ischemia to both legs, which resulted in an ulcer to the right ankle. During the hospitalization, a femoral-popliteal bypass was performed to the right lower limb and the right ankle ulcer debrided, noting removal of slough with clear fat layer base. The patient has been referred to home health for care of the ankle wound and the nurse will also observe the right leg incision for normal healing.

Description	Code
Primary: Atherosclerosis of native arteries of right leg with ulceration of ankle	I70.233
Secondary: Non-pressure chronic ulcer of right ankle with fat layer exposed	L97.312
Secondary: Encounter for surgical aftercare following surgery on the circulatory system	Z48.812
Secondary: Atherosclerosis of native arteries of extremities with rest pain, left leg	I70.222

The focus of care for this episode is the care of the right ankle ulcer. The etiology of the ulcer must be listed first, and this is critical limb ischemia. When a patient who has atherosclerosis of the lower extremities also has critical limb ischemia, reference arteriosclerosis, with, critical limb ischemia, leg in the alpha index. When such a patient also has an ulcer, follow the next sub-entry under "leg" to the lateral site then with, ulcer. I70.233 includes critical limb ischemia. Guidance issued in Q4 2020 Coding Clinic indicates that critical limb ischemia is a form of atherosclerosis with rest pain. In the absence of ulceration, the condition codes to I70.22-. Because the nurse will also be monitoring the lower extremity bypass site, Z48.812 is also assigned to indicate aftercare.

Orthostatic hypotension, PVCs, bradycardia

A 69-year-old female is referred for skilled nursing for home health following hospitalization for orthostatic hypotension. While hospitalized, it was also determined that the patient was experiencing frequent premature ventricular contractions (PVCs) and intermittent bradycardia, but the cause was not determined. The patient will be following up with cardiology and home health will be observing and assessing to report to the physician.

Description	Code
Primary: Orthostatic hypotension	I95.1
Secondary: Ventricular premature depolarization	I49.3
Secondary: Bradycardia, unspecified	R00.1

The focus of care and reason for admission is orthostatic hypotension, so this should be first assigned. However, nursing will also be monitoring the other cardiovascular abnormalities, PVCs and bradycardia, so these should also be listed. No specific cause is known for the bradycardia, so R00.1 is the most appropriate code. While there is an excludes 1 note at I49 for R00.1, there is an excludes 2 note at R00 indicating that specified arrythmias (I47-I49) may be assigned with codes from R00. Q2 2020 Coding Clinic guidance has specified that these conditions may be assigned together when the excludes 2 conditions are met.

Atherosclerosis, Critical Limb Ischemia

A patient with a history of atherosclerosis of the bilateral lower extremities was hospitalized due to critical limb ischemia of the right foot, which resulted in an ulcer of the right ankle. During the hospitalization, a femoral-popliteal bypass was [illegible] to improve [illegible] the lower limb and the right ankle ulcer [illegible], removal of slough with clear fat layer base. The patient has been referred to home health for care of the ankle wound and the nurse will also observe the right leg incision for normal healing.

Diagnosis	Code
Primary: Atherosclerosis of native arteries of right leg with ulceration of ankle	I70.233
Secondary: Non-pressure chronic ulcer of right ankle with fat layer exposed	L97.312
Secondary: Encounter for other specified aftercare following surgery on the circulatory system	Z48.812
Secondary: Atherosclerosis of native arteries of extremities with rest pain, left leg	I70.222

The focus of care for this episode is the care of the right ankle ulcer. The etiology of the ulcer is atherosclerosis, and [illegible] critical limb ischemia. When a patient who has atherosclerosis of the lower extremity also has critical limb ischemia, [illegible] atherosclerosis [illegible] ICD-10-CM [illegible] Guidance [illegible] OASIS [illegible].

Orthostatic Hypotension, PVCs, Bradycardia

A patient was referred for skilled nursing for home health following hospitalization for orthostatic hypotension. While hospitalized it was also determined that the patient was experiencing premature ventricular contractions (PVCs) and intermittent bradycardia, but the cause was not determined. The patient will be followed by cardiology and home health will be observing and assessing to return to the heart.

Diagnosis	Code
Primary: Orthostatic hypotension	I95.1
Secondary: Ventricular premature depolarization	I49.3
Secondary: Bradycardia, unspecified	R00.1

The focus of care and reason for admission is orthostatic hypotension, so this code is listed first. However, nursing will also be monitoring the PVCs and bradycardia [illegible] R00.1 is the most appropriate code [illegible] I49.3 [illegible] codes [illegible] conditions may be assigned together when the [illegible].

Chapter 10: Diseases of the Respiratory System (J00-J99)

The respiratory system includes the airways (nose and nasal passages, pharynx, larynx, trachea, bronchi, alveoli) and lungs. Also included are structures related to these airways such as the vocal cords, tonsils, adenoids, thorax and diaphragm.

The chapter is divided into the following blocks:

J00-J06	Acute upper respiratory infections
J09-J18	Influenza and pneumonia
J20-J22	Other acute lower respiratory infections
J30-J39	Other diseases of the upper respiratory tract
J40-J47	Chronic lower respiratory diseases
J60-J70	Lung diseases due to external agents
J80-J84	Other respiratory diseases principally affecting the interstitium
J85-J86	Suppurative and necrotic conditions of the lower respiratory tract
J90-J94	Other diseases of the pleura
J95	Intraoperative and post procedural complications and disorders of the respiratory system, NEC
J96-J99	Other diseases of the respiratory system

The airways are divided into the upper and lower airways. The upper airways (and upper respiratory tract) include the nasopharynx (nose), oropharynx (mouth), laryngopharynx and larynx. Their purposes are to warm, filter and humidify inhaled air. They also help make sound and send air to the lower airways.

The lower airways begin with the trachea, which then divides into the right and left mainstream bronchial tubes. The bronchial tubes divide into bronchi that are lined with mucus producing ciliated epithelium, which is one of the lung's major defense systems.

The bronchi then divide into secondary bronchi, tertiary bronchi, terminal bronchioles, respiratory bronchioles, alveolar ducts and, finally, into the alveoli, which are the gas exchange units of the lungs.

The right lung is larger and has three lobes: upper, middle and lower. The left lung is smaller and has only an upper and lower lobe. This leaves room for the heart.

Two systems control breathing: an automatic response and a voluntary response. Patients with diagnosed chronic respiratory diseases have a progressive increase in the mechanical work of breathing and limited respiratory reserve capacities. These factors may lead to symptoms of chronic dyspnea on exertion, wheezing, chronic cough and debilitating functional disabilities that limit exercise and activities of daily living (ADLs). Other respiratory problems that might affect daily life include chronic respiratory inflammation, edema, mucous plugging, hypoxemia, carbon dioxide retention, pulmonary hypertension and pulmonary heart disease.

Codes in this chapter are used to report **pneumonia** (an infection of the lungs). Pneumonia is not a single disease, but refers to many different infections or conditions. Check the documentation for the cause to select the correct code. Pneumonia can be caused by viruses (Category J12.-), bacteria (category J13., J15.-), fungi or organisms called mycoplasma (J15.7), radiation treatment (J70.0), or other causes. Aspiration pneumonia (subcategory J69.0) is caused by the inhalation of substances into the lungs, such as food, vomitus, gastric secretions, milk, oils/essences, etc. Code J18.9 (Pneumonia, organism unspecified) should never be used if the organism or other cause is known.

Some codes are reported for occupational hazards that cause pulmonary problems. Codes in the categories J60-J70 (pneumoconiosis and other lung diseases due to external agents) include conditions involving the aspiration of dust and other substances, such as coal dust (black lung disease at J60) and asbestosis and other mineral fibers (J61), dust containing silica (J62), and other inorganic dusts (J63). Codes from category J67.- (extrinsic allergic alveolitis, pneumonitis due to inhaled organic dust and particles of fungal, actinomycetic or other origin) occur in specific occupations or activities, such as mushroom workers' lung or bird-fanciers' lung.

Other codes found in chapter 10 include: category J98.19 pulmonary collapse (collapsed lung); J98.2, Interstitial emphysema; category J96.-, Respiratory failure (inability of respiratory system to maintain adequate gas exchange); and J95.-Acute pulmonary insufficiency following surgery (problems with the valve between the heart and the artery leading to the lungs).

In certain situations, you'll need to look beyond this chapter to properly code a case. For example:

- If the documentation indicates a **neoplasm or tumor of an organ in the respiratory system,** coders should look up the term (malignancy, tumor, adenoma) to find the correct code in Chapter 2.
- If a patient has a **personal or family history** of a condition reported in this chapter, it may be appropriate to use a code from chapter 21, such as Z87.09 (Diseases of respiratory system); Z85.12 (Personal history of malignant neoplasm of trachea); or Z80.2 (Family history of malignant neoplasm of intrathoracic organs).

- **Symptoms** related to the respiratory system are sometimes reported using codes from Chapter 18 such as code series R09.89 (Symptoms involving respiratory system and other chest symptoms). Every effort should be made to secure a definitive diagnosis. A symptom code from Chapter 18 may be reported as an additional diagnosis when it describes a significant aspect of the condition but is not an integral part of it.
- Although not reported often in home health or hospice, if reporting **a respiratory system disease in a pregnant patient** when the condition is complicating the pregnancy, report a code from Chapter 15 as the first-listed diagnosis and a code from this chapter as an additional diagnosis.

Intraoperative and postoprocedural complications and disorders of respiratory system, not elsewhere classified, are coded from category J95. For example, a complication of a tracheostomy is reported using a code from J95.00-J95.09, such as J95.02 (Infection of the tracheostomy stoma) or J95.03 (Mechanical complication of a tracheostomy). Codes such as infection of a tracheostomy state that additional codes should be reported to indicate the type of infection such as cellulitis of the neck (L03.221) or sepsis (A40, A41-).

Multiple Coding and Sequencing

It is important to read the Includes and Excludes 1 and Excludes 2 notes under codes in this chapter, as well as any other instructions under the code or code category. The following are examples of multiple coding and sequencing issues to keep an eye out for in this chapter.

Because of the higher risk of respiratory conditions related to smoking or smoke exposure, there is a note under the heading of the chapter that states to use an additional code, where applicable, to identify:

- exposure to environmental tobacco smoke (Z77.22)
- exposure to tobacco smoke in the prenatal period (P68.81)
- history of tobacco dependence (Z87.891)
- occupational exposure to environmental tobacco smoke (Z57.31)
- tobacco dependence (F17.-)
- tobacco use (Z72.0)

This note is repeated under codes for disorders of the upper respiratory tract, chronic lower respiratory diseases (i.e., asthma, bronchitis) and interstitial pulmonary diseases.

Many of the conditions listed in Chapter 10 involve infections. For example, a note under the acute sinusitis category (J01) states: "Use additional code (B95-B97) to identify infectious agents." With other codes within chapter 10 there are a variety of other notes to code first or add additional codes for associated conditions and adverse effects.

Some conditions reported with codes in other chapters are reported with manifestations in Chapter 10. For example, cystic fibrosis with pulmonary manifestations (code E84.0 from Chapter 4) is a genetic defect that causes the body to produce abnormally thick, sticky mucus that clogs the airways.

Special Coding Issue

Chronic Obstructive Pulmonary Disease (COPD) and Asthma, emphysema

The codes in categories J44 and J45 distinguish between uncomplicated cases and those in an acute exacerbation. An acute exacerbation is a worsening or a decompensation of a chronic condition. ***An acute exacerbation is not equivalent to an infection superimposed on a chronic condition***, although an exacerbation may be triggered by an infection.

Chronic obstructive pulmonary disease (COPD) (J43-J45) is an irreversible obstruction of the airways. Conditions that fall under the COPD umbrella include chronic obstructive asthma, chronic obstructive bronchitis and emphysema. Code J44.9 is an unspecified code that is reported when a patient has a condition that is classifiable to J44 and there's no information as to whether the condition is exacerbated or occurring with a lower respiratory infection, which would necessitate the coding of J44.1 and J44.0, respectively.

An additional code for the type of asthma should be assigned in a patient with COPD and asthma. For a patient with exacerbated asthma, and a condition classifiable to J44 that's not exacerbated or co-occurring with a lower respiratory infection, you would assign J45.901 along with J44.9. You should not assign an additional code for unspecified asthma in this scenario, but if the asthma is documented as exacerbated, that additional specificity makes the use of an additional asthma code appropriate, according to the Q4 2017 Coding Clinic update.

Assign J43.9 (Emphysema, unspecified) for a patient who has emphysema and acutely exacerbated COPD, according to Q4 2017 Coding Clinic. When it comes to coding COPD, focus on the specificity of the disease, not whether it's exacerbated. If an infection is also present, code it as well and sequence the acute condition first. Conversely, for a diagnosis of exacerbated chronic obstructive bronchitis, the correct code would be J44.1.

Assign a code from J44.0 when a patient has both a condition classifiable to J44 and a diagnosis of a lower respiratory tract infection. An additional code should be assigned to report the infection. If the physician confirms both a diagnosis of a lower respiratory tract infection and exacerbation of chronic obstructive bronchitis, for example, both J44.1, Chronic obstructive pulmonary disease with (acute) exacerbation, and J44.0, Chronic obstructive pulmonary disease with (acute) lower respiratory infection, should be assigned, along with a code for the specific lower respiratory infection. Examples of lower respiratory infections include pneumonia, bronchitis and bronchiolitis. The sequencing of J44.1 and and the lower respiratory infection is discretionary and should be based on the Plan of Care.

Respiratory insufficiency (R06.89) is an integral part of COPD. If the documentation states that the patient has COPD, do not report R06.89 as an additional code.

It is important to locate the diagnosis term in the Alphabetical Index and then review all the notes under the code in the Tabular List to ensure correct code assignment.

Influenza due to certain identified influenza viruses

Code only confirmed cases of influenza due to certain identified influenza viruses (category J09), and due to other identified influenza virus (category J10). In this context, "confirmation" does not require documentation of positive laboratory testing specific for avian or other novel influenza A, or other identified influenza virus. However, coding should be based on the physician's diagnostic statement that the patient has avian influenza, or other novel influenza A, for category J09, or has another particular identified strain influenza, such as H1N1 or H3N2, but not identified as novel or variant, for category J10.

If the physician documents "suspected" or "possible" or "probable" avian influenza, or novel influenza, or other identified influenza, then assign the appropriate influenza code from category J11, Influenza due to unidentified influenza virus. Do not assign a code from category J09, Influenza due to certain identified influenza viruses, or a code from category J10, Influenza due to other identified influenza virus.

Ventilator associated pneumonia

As with all procedural or postprocedural complications, code assignment is based on the physician's documentation of the relationship between the condition and the procedure. Code J95.851, Ventilator associated pneumonia, should be assigned only when the physician has documented ventilator associated pneumonia (VAP). An additional code to identify the organism (e.g., Pseudomonas aeruginosa, code B96.5) should also be assigned. Do not assign an additional code from categories J12-J18 to identify the type of pneumonia.

Code J95.851 should not be assigned in cases where the patient has pneumonia and is on a mechanical ventilator, and the physician has not specifically stated that the pneumonia is ventilator-associated pneumonia. If the documentation is unclear as to whether the patient has pneumonia that is a complication attributable to the mechanical ventilator, query the physician.

If a patient has either aspiration pneumonia or ventilator-associated pneumonia and a condition classifiable to J44, you would not assign J44.0, as neither of the pneumonia diagnoses are considered respiratory infections. For each you'd code J44.9 along with the code for the type of pneumonia, sequenced according to the circumstances of the admission, according to the Q1 2017 Coding Clinic.

CHAPTER 10: DISEASES OF THE RESPIRATORY SYSTEM (J00-J99)

Note:
When a respiratory condition is described as occurring in more than one site and is not specifically indexed, it should be classified to the lower anatomic site (e.g. tracheobronchitis to bronchitis in J40).
Use additional code, where applicable, to identify:
exposure to environmental tobacco smoke (Z77.22)
exposure to tobacco smoke in the perinatal period (P96.81)
history of tobacco dependence (Z87.891)
occupational exposure to environmental tobacco smoke (Z57.31)
tobacco dependence (F17.-)
tobacco use (Z72.0)

EXCLUDES 2 certain conditions originating in the perinatal period (P04-P96)
certain infectious and parasitic diseases (A00-B99)
complications of pregnancy, childbirth and the puerperium (O00-O9A)
congenital malformations, deformations and chromosomal abnormalities (Q00-Q99)
endocrine, nutritional and metabolic diseases (E00-E88)
injury, poisoning and certain other consequences of external causes (S00-T88)
neoplasms (C00-D49)
smoke inhalation (T59.81-)
symptoms, signs and abnormal clinical and laboratory findings, not elsewhere classified (R00-R94)

This chapter contains the following blocks:

J00-J06	Acute upper respiratory infections
J09-J18	Influenza and pneumonia
J20-J22	Other acute lower respiratory infections
J30-J39	Other diseases of upper respiratory tract
J40-J47	Chronic lower respiratory diseases
J60-J70	Lung diseases due to external agents
J80-J84	Other respiratory diseases principally affecting the interstitium
J85-J86	Suppurative and necrotic conditions of the lower respiratory tract
J90-J94	Other diseases of the pleura
J95	Intraoperative and postprocedural complications and disorders of respiratory system, not elsewhere classified
J96-J99	Other diseases of the respiratory system

Acute upper respiratory infections (J00-J06)

EXCLUDES 1 chronic obstructive pulmonary disease with acute lower respiratory infection (J44.0)

CODING TIPS✓ A patient with an upper respiratory infection (J00-J06), such as laryngitis, pharyngitis, sinus infection, etc., who also has a condition classifiable to J44 would not be coded with J44.0. Code J44.0 is only used when the patient with one of those diagnoses also has a lower respiratory infection, such as bronchitis or pneumonia.

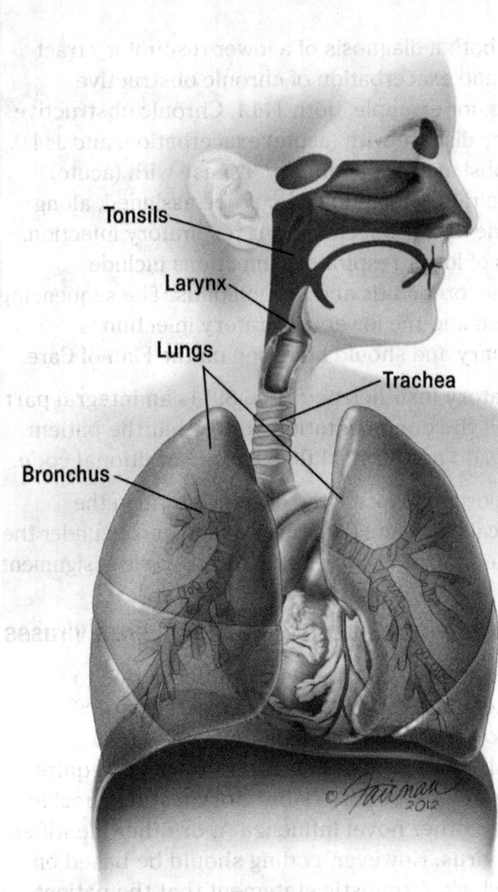

SP J00 Acute nasopharyngitis [common cold]
Acute rhinitis
Coryza (acute)
Infective nasopharyngitis NOS
Infective rhinitis
Nasal catarrh, acute
Nasopharyngitis NOS

EXCLUDES 1 acute pharyngitis (J02.-)
acute sore throat NOS (J02.9)
influenza virus with other respiratory manifestations (J09.X2, J10.1, J11.1)
pharyngitis NOS (J02.9)
rhinitis NOS (J31.0)
sore throat NOS (J02.9)

EXCLUDES 2 allergic rhinitis (J30.1-J30.9)
chronic pharyngitis (J31.2)
chronic rhinitis (J31.0)
chronic sore throat (J31.2)
nasopharyngitis, chronic (J31.1)
vasomotor rhinitis (J30.0)

+4 J01 Acute sinusitis

INCLUDES acute abscess of sinus
acute empyema of sinus
acute infection of sinus
acute inflammation of sinus
acute suppuration of sinus

Use additional code (B95-B97) to identify infectious agent.

EXCLUDES 1 sinusitis NOS (J32.9)

EXCLUDES 2 chronic sinusitis (J32.0-J32.8)

+ 5 J01.0 Acute maxillary sinusitis
Acute antritis

SP + J01.00 Acute maxillary sinusitis, unspecified

SP + J01.01 Acute recurrent maxillary sinusitis

+ 5 J01.1 Acute frontal sinusitis

SP + J01.10 Acute frontal sinusitis, unspecified

SP + J01.11 Acute recurrent frontal sinusitis

+ 5 J01.2 Acute ethmoidal sinusitis

SP + J01.20 Acute ethmoidal sinusitis, unspecified

SP + J01.21 Acute recurrent ethmoidal sinusitis

+ 5 J01.3 Acute sphenoidal sinusitis

SP + J01.30 Acute sphenoidal sinusitis, unspecified

SP + J01.31 Acute recurrent sphenoidal sinusitis

+ 5 J01.4 Acute pansinusitis

SP + J01.40 Acute pansinusitis, unspecified

SP + J01.41 Acute recurrent pansinusitis

+ 5 J01.8 Other acute sinusitis

SP + J01.80 Other acute sinusitis
Acute sinusitis involving more than one sinus but not pansinusitis

SP + J01.81 Other acute recurrent sinusitis
Acute recurrent sinusitis involving more than one sinus but not pansinusitis

+ 5 J01.9 Acute sinusitis, unspecified

SP + J01.90 Acute sinusitis, unspecified

SP + J01.91 Acute recurrent sinusitis, unspecified

4 J02 Acute pharyngitis
INCLUDES acute sore throat
EXCLUDES 1 acute laryngopharyngitis (J06.0)
peritonsillar abscess (J36)
pharyngeal abscess (J39.1)
retropharyngeal abscess (J39.0)
EXCLUDES 2 chronic pharyngitis (J31.2)

SP J02.0 Streptococcal pharyngitis
Septic pharyngitis
Streptococcal sore throat
EXCLUDES 2 scarlet fever (A38.-)

SP + J02.8 Acute pharyngitis due to other specified organisms
Use additional code (B95-B97) to identify infectious agent
EXCLUDES 1 acute pharyngitis due to coxsackie virus (B08.5)
acute pharyngitis due to gonococcus (A54.5)
acute pharyngitis due to herpes [simplex] virus (B00.2)
acute pharyngitis due to infectious mononucleosis (B27.-)
enteroviral vesicular pharyngitis (B08.5)

SP J02.9 Acute pharyngitis, unspecified
Gangrenous pharyngitis (acute)
Infective pharyngitis (acute) NOS
Pharyngitis (acute) NOS
Sore throat (acute) NOS
Suppurative pharyngitis (acute)
Ulcerative pharyngitis (acute)
EXCLUDES 1 influenza virus with other respiratory manifestations (J09.X2, J10.1, J11.1)

4 J03 Acute tonsillitis
EXCLUDES 1 acute sore throat (J02.-)
hypertrophy of tonsils (J35.1)
peritonsillar abscess (J36)
sore throat NOS (J02.9)
streptococcal sore throat (J02.0)
EXCLUDES 2 chronic tonsillitis (J35.0)

5 J03.0 Streptococcal tonsillitis

SP J03.00 Acute streptococcal tonsillitis, unspecified

SP J03.01 Acute recurrent streptococcal tonsillitis

+ 5 J03.8 Acute tonsillitis due to other specified organisms
Use additional code (B95-B97) to identify infectious agent.
EXCLUDES 1 diphtheritic tonsillitis (A36.0)
herpesviral pharyngotonsillitis (B00.2)
streptococcal tonsillitis (J03.0)
tuberculous tonsillitis (A15.8)
Vincent's tonsillitis (A69.1)

SP + J03.80 Acute tonsillitis due to other specified organisms

SP + J03.81 Acute recurrent tonsillitis due to other specified organisms

5 J03.9 Acute tonsillitis, unspecified
Follicular tonsillitis (acute)
Gangrenous tonsillitis (acute)
Infective tonsillitis (acute)
Tonsillitis (acute) NOS
Ulcerative tonsillitis (acute)
EXCLUDES 1 influenza virus with other respiratory manifestations (J09.X2, J10.1, J11.1)

SP J03.90 Acute tonsillitis, unspecified

SP J03.91 Acute recurrent tonsillitis, unspecified

+ 4 J04 Acute laryngitis and tracheitis
Code also influenza, if present, such as:
influenza due to identified novel influenza A virus with other respiratory manifestations (J09.X2)
influenza due to other identified influenza virus with other respiratory manifestations (J10.1)
influenza due to unidentified influenza virus with other respiratory manifestations (J11.1)
Use additional code (B95-B97) to identify infectious agent.
EXCLUDES 1 acute obstructive laryngitis [croup] and epiglottitis (J05.-)
EXCLUDES 2 laryngismus (stridulus) (J38.5)

SP + J04.0 Acute laryngitis

Chapter 10
J00-J99

Edematous laryngitis (acute)
Laryngitis (acute) NOS
Subglottic laryngitis (acute)
Suppurative laryngitis (acute)
Ulcerative laryngitis (acute)
EXCLUDES 1 acute obstructive laryngitis (J05.0)
EXCLUDES 2 chronic laryngitis (J37.0)

+ 5 J04.1 Acute tracheitis
Acute viral tracheitis
Catarrhal tracheitis (acute)
Tracheitis (acute) NOS
EXCLUDES 2 chronic tracheitis (J42)

SP + J04.10 Acute tracheitis without obstruction

SP + J04.11 Acute tracheitis with obstruction

SP + J04.2 Acute laryngotracheitis
Laryngotracheitis NOS
Tracheitis (acute) with laryngitis (acute)
EXCLUDES 1 acute obstructive laryngotracheitis (J05.0)
EXCLUDES 2 chronic laryngotracheitis (J37.1)

CODING TIPS✓ J04.2 is a specific code and should be assigned when the patient is reported as specifically having laryngotracheitis by the physician. This involves inflammation of both the larynx and trachea.

+ 5 J04.3 Supraglottitis, unspecified

CODING TIPS✓ Supraglottitis is a potentially life-threatening inflammation of the supraglottic area of the airway. If airway obstruction is documented, assign J04.31.

SP + J04.30 Supraglottitis, unspecified, without obstruction

SP + J04.31 Supraglottitis, unspecified, with obstruction

▲ + 4 J05 Acute obstructive laryngitis [croup] and epiglottitis
Code also, influenza, if present, such as:
influenza due to identified novel influenza A virus with other respiratory manifestations (J09.X2)
influenza due to other identified influenza virus with other respiratory manifestations (J10.1)
influenza due to unidentified influenza virus with other respiratory manifestations (J11.1)
Use additional code (B95-B97) to identify infectious agent.

SP + J05.0 Acute obstructive laryngitis [croup]
Obstructive laryngitis (acute) NOS
Obstructive laryngotracheitis NOS

+ 5 J05.1 Acute epiglottitis
EXCLUDES 2 epiglottitis, chronic (J37.0)

SP + J05.10 Acute epiglottitis without obstruction
Epiglottitis NOS

SP + J05.11 Acute epiglottitis with obstruction

4 J06 Acute upper respiratory infections of multiple and unspecified sites
EXCLUDES 1 acute respiratory infection NOS (J22)
influenza virus with other respiratory manifestations (J09.X2, J10.1, J11.1)
streptococcal pharyngitis (J02.0)

SP J06.0 Acute laryngopharyngitis

SP + J06.9 Acute upper respiratory infection, unspecified
Upper respiratory disease, acute
Upper respiratory infection NOS
Use additional code (B95-B97) to identify infectious agent, if known, such as: respiratory syncytial virus (RSV) (B97.4)

CODING TIPS✓ When upper respiratory infection and lower respiratory infection are both documented, assign only the code for the lower respiratory infection.

CODING TIPS✓ Assign J06.9 for upper respiratory infection NOS only when a more specific diagnosis to identify the type of infection cannot be identified.

Influenza and pneumonia (J09-J18)

EXCLUDES 2 allergic or eosinophilic pneumonia (J82)
aspiration pneumonia NOS (J69.0)
meconium pneumonia (P24.01)
neonatal aspiration pneumonia (P24.-)
pneumonia due to solids and liquids (J69.-)
congenital pneumonia (P23.9)
lipid pneumonia (J69.1)
rheumatic pneumonia (I00)
ventilator associated pneumonia (J95.851)

CODING TIPS✓ Assign J43.9 with J18.9 for emphysema, COPD and pneumonia. (AHA: 1Q 2019)

CODING TIPS✓ Influenza is not considered a lower respiratory infection for the purposes of coding a condition classifiable to J44 with J44.0. If influenza results in pneumonia, code the condition as J44.0, the influenza with pneumonia combination code and the specific pneumonia. Sequence according to the focus of care.

CODING TIPS✓ Pneumonia should be coded to the specific causative organism using a combination code when a specific code is available. Evaluate all available clinical documentation and assign the most specific code for pneumonia. When the causative organism of bacterial pneumonia is known but no combination code exists, assign J15.8.

CODING TIPS✓ When pneumonia is diagnosed in a patient who also has a condition classifiable to J44, the coder should assign J44.0 and the specific code to indicate the type of pneumonia. Sequence according to the focus of care.

4 J09 Influenza due to certain identified influenza viruses
EXCLUDES 1 influenza A/H1N1 (J10.-)
influenza due to other identified influenza virus (J10.-)
influenza due to unidentified influenza virus (J11.-)
seasonal influenza due to other identified influenza virus (J10.-)
seasonal influenza due to unidentified influenza virus (J11.-)

GUIDELINES **Section I.C.10.c**
Code only confirmed cases of influenza due to certain identified influenza viruses (category J09), and due to other identified influenza virus (category J10).

If the provider records "suspected" or "possible" or "probable" avian influenza, or novel influenza, or other identified influenza, then the appropriate influenza code from category J11, Influenza due to unidentified influenza virus, should be assigned.

CODING TIPS✓ J09 is not used for influenza type A. Influenza due to **novel** influenza A is coded to J09 along with manifestations of other respiratory, gastrointestinal and other manifestations. Use additional codes to identify the manifestations.

5 **J09.X Influenza due to identified novel influenza A virus**
Avian influenza
Bird influenza
Influenza A/H5N1
Influenza of other animal origin, not bird or swine
Swine influenza virus (viruses that normally cause infections in pigs)

SP **J09.X1 Influenza due to identified novel influenza A virus with pneumonia**
Code also, if applicable, associated:
lung abscess (J85.1)
other specified type of pneumonia

SP + **J09.X2 Influenza due to identified novel influenza A virus with other respiratory manifestations**
Influenza due to identified novel influenza A virus NOS
Influenza due to identified novel influenza A virus with laryngitis
Influenza due to identified novel influenza A virus with pharyngitis
Influenza due to identified novel influenza A virus with upper respiratory symptoms
Use additional code, if applicable, for associated:
pleural effusion (J91.8)
sinusitis (J01.-)

SP **J09.X3 Influenza due to identified novel influenza A virus with gastrointestinal manifestations**
Influenza due to identified novel influenza A virus gastroenteritis
EXCLUDES 1 'intestinal flu' [viral gastroenteritis] (A08.-)

SP + **J09.X9 Influenza due to identified novel influenza A virus with other manifestations**
Influenza due to identified novel influenza A virus with encephalopathy
Influenza due to identified novel influenza A virus with myocarditis
Influenza due to identified novel influenza A virus with otitis media
Use additional code to identify manifestation

4 **J10 Influenza due to other identified influenza virus**
INCLUDES influenza A (non-novel)
influenza B
influenza C
EXCLUDES 1 influenza due to avian influenza virus (J09.X-)
influenza due to swine flu (J09.X-)
influenza due to unidentifed influenza virus (J11.-)

GUIDELINES **Section I.C.10.c**
Code only confirmed cases of influenza due to certain identified influenza viruses (category J09), and due to other identified influenza virus (category J10).

If the provider records "suspected" or "possible" or "probable" avian influenza, or novel influenza, or other identified influenza, then the appropriate influenza code from category J11, Influenza due to unidentified influenza virus, should be assigned.

CODING TIPS✓ Influenza due to Type A (not novel) or Type B is coded to J10 along with manifestations of other respiratory, gastrointestinal and other manifestations. Use additional codes to identify the manifestations. If the influenza is identified as influenza A but not documented as novel, use these codes.

5 **J10.0 Influenza due to other identified influenza virus with pneumonia**
Code also:
associated lung abscess, if applicable (J85.1)

SP **J10.00 Influenza due to other identified influenza virus with unspecified type of pneumonia**

SP **J10.01 Influenza due to other identified influenza virus with the same other identified influenza virus pneumonia**

SP **J10.08 Influenza due to other identified influenza virus with other specified pneumonia**
Code also:
other specified type of pneumonia

SP + **J10.1 Influenza due to other identified influenza virus with other respiratory manifestations**
Influenza due to other identified influenza virus NOS
Influenza due to other identified influenza virus with laryngitis
Influenza due to other identified influenza virus with pharyngitis
Influenza due to other identified influenza virus with upper respiratory symptoms
Use additional code for associated pleural effusion, if applicable (J91.8)
Use additional code for associated sinusitis, if applicable (J01.-)

SP **J10.2 Influenza due to other identified influenza virus with gastrointestinal manifestations**
Influenza due to other identified influenza virus gastroenteritis
EXCLUDES 1 'intestinal flu' [viral gastroenteritis] (A08.-)

Chapter 10
J00-J99

5 J10.8 Influenza due to other identified influenza virus with other manifestations

SP J10.81 Influenza due to other identified influenza virus with encephalopathy

SP J10.82 Influenza due to other identified influenza virus with myocarditis

SP + J10.83 Influenza due to other identified influenza virus with otitis media
Use additional code for any associated perforated tympanic membrane (H72.-)

SP + J10.89 Influenza due to other identified influenza virus with other manifestations
Use additional codes to identify the manifestations

4 J11 Influenza due to unidentified influenza virus

CODING TIPS✓ Influenza when the physician or NPP does not specify the influenza virus is coded to J11 along with manifestations of other respiratory, gastrointestinal and other manifestations. Use additional codes to identify the manifestations. Documentation from the physician or NPP would indicate "flu" or "influenza" to use J11.

5 J11.0 Influenza due to unidentified influenza virus with pneumonia
Code also:
associated lung abscess, if applicable (J85.1)

SP J11.00 Influenza due to unidentified influenza virus with unspecified type of pneumonia
Influenza with pneumonia NOS

SP J11.08 Influenza due to unidentified influenza virus with specified pneumonia
Code also:
other specified type of pneumonia

SP + J11.1 Influenza due to unidentified influenza virus with other respiratory manifestations
Influenza NOS
Influenzal laryngitis NOS
Influenzal pharyngitis NOS
Influenza with upper respiratory symptoms NOS
Use additional code for associated pleural effusion, if applicable (J91.8)
Use additional code for associated sinusitis, if applicable (J01.-)

SP J11.2 Influenza due to unidentified influenza virus with gastrointestinal manifestations
Influenza gastroenteritis NOS
EXCLUDES 1 'intestinal flu' [viral gastroenteritis] (A08.-)

5 J11.8 Influenza due to unidentified influenza virus with other manifestations

SP J11.81 Influenza due to unidentified influenza virus with encephalopathy
Influenzal encephalopathy NOS

SP J11.82 Influenza due to unidentified influenza virus with myocarditis
Influenzal myocarditis NOS

SP + J11.83 Influenza due to unidentified influenza virus with otitis media
Influenzal otitis media NOS
Use additional code for any associated perforated tympanic membrane (H72.-)

SP + J11.89 Influenza due to unidentified influenza virus with other manifestations
Use additional codes to identify the manifestations

4 J12 Viral pneumonia, not elsewhere classified
INCLUDES bronchopneumonia due to viruses other than influenza viruses
Code first:
associated influenza, if applicable (J09.X1, J10.0-, J11.0-)
Code also:
associated abscess, if applicable (J85.1)
EXCLUDES 1 aspiration pneumonia due to anesthesia during labor and delivery (O74.0)
aspiration pneumonia due to anesthesia during pregnancy (O29)
aspiration pneumonia due to anesthesia during puerperium (O89.0)
aspiration pneumonia due to solids and liquids (J69.-)
aspiration pneumonia NOS (J69.0)
congenital pneumonia (P23.0)
congenital rubella pneumonitis (P35.0)
interstitial pneumonia NOS (J84.9)
lipid pneumonia (J69.1)
neonatal aspiration pneumonia (P24.-)

SP J12.0 Adenoviral pneumonia

SP J12.1 Respiratory syncytial virus pneumonia
RSV pneumonia

CODING TIPS✓ The description of code J12.1 includes the organism, so no additional code is needed for the organism.

SP J12.2 Parainfluenza virus pneumonia

SP J12.3 Human metapneumovirus pneumonia

5 J12.8 Other viral pneumonia

SP J12.81 Pneumonia due to SARS-associated coronavirus
Severe acute respiratory syndrome NOS

IQ J12.82 Pneumonia due to coronavirus disease 2019
Pneumonia due to 2019 novel coronavirus (SARS-CoV-2)
Pneumonia due to COVID-19
Code first:
COVID-19 (U07.1)

GUIDELINES **Section I.C.1.g.1)(c)(i)**
For a patient with pneumonia confirmed as due to COVID-19, assign codes U07.1, COVID-19, and J12.82, Pneumonia due to coronavirus disease 2019.

CODING TIPS ✓ For pneumonia confirmed as due to COVID-19, assign U07.1 and J12.82.

SP **J12.89 Other viral pneumonia**

CODING TIPS ✓ Do not use this code for pneumonia due to COVID-19. Use J12.82.

SP **J12.9 Viral pneumonia, unspecified**

SP **J13 Pneumonia due to Streptococcus pneumoniae**

Bronchopneumonia due to S. pneumoniae

Code first:

associated influenza, if applicable (J09.X1, ~~J10~~.0-, J11.0-)

Code also:

associated abscess, if applicable (J85.1)

EXCLUDES 1 congenital pneumonia due to S. pneumoniae (P23.6)
lobar pneumonia, unspecified organism (J18.1)
pneumonia due to other streptococci (J15.3-J15.4)

SP **J14 Pneumonia due to Hemophilus influenzae**

Bronchopneumonia due to H. influenzae

Code first:

associated influenza, if applicable (J09.X1, J10.0-, J11.0-)

Code also:

associated abscess, if applicable (J85.1)

EXCLUDES 1 congenital pneumonia due to H. influenzae (P23.6)

4 **J15 Bacterial pneumonia, not elsewhere classified**

INCLUDES bronchopneumonia due to bacteria other than S. pneumoniae and H. influenzae

Code first:

associated influenza, if applicable (J09.X1, J10.0-, J11.0-)

Code also:

associated abscess, if applicable (J85.1)

EXCLUDES 1 chlamydial pneumonia (J16.0)
congenital pneumonia (P23.-)
Legionnaires' disease (A48.1)
spirochetal pneumonia (A69.8)

CODING TIPS ✓ J15 codes are used for bacterial pneumonia when the bacteria is not Streptococcus pneumoniae (J13) or Hemophilus influenzae (J14).

SP **J15.0 Pneumonia due to Klebsiella pneumoniae**

SP **J15.1 Pneumonia due to Pseudomonas**

5 **J15.2 Pneumonia due to staphylococcus**

SP **J15.20 Pneumonia due to staphylococcus, unspecified**

6 **J15.21 Pneumonia due to staphylococcus aureus**

SP **J15.211 Pneumonia due to Methicillin susceptible Staphylococcus aureus**

MSSA pneumonia

Pneumonia due to Staphylococcus aureus NOS

CODING TIPS ✓ J15.211 is used when the organism causing the pneumonia is identified as MSSA-methicillin susceptible Staph aureus, or Staph aureus without information as to resistance.

SP **J15.212 Pneumonia due to Methicillin resistant Staphylococcus aureus**

GUIDELINES **Section I.C.1.e.1)**

When a patient is diagnosed with an infection that is due to methicillin resistant Staphylococcus aureus (MRSA), and that infection has a combination code that includes the causal organism (e.g., sepsis, pneumonia) assign the appropriate combination code for the condition (e.g., code A41.02, Sepsis due to Methicillin resistant Staphylococcus aureus or code J15.212, Pneumonia due to Methicillin resistant Staphylococcus aureus). Do not assign code B95.62, Methicillin resistant Staphylococcus aureus infection as the cause of diseases classified elsewhere, as an additional code because the combination code includes the type of infection and the MRSA organism. Do not assign a code from subcategory Z16.11, Resistance to penicillins, as an additional diagnosis.

CODING TIPS ✓ J15.212 is used when the organism causing the pneumonia is methicillin resistant or MRSA. Do not use Z16 codes unless the organism is resistant to a different antibiotic, such as vancomycin - Z16.21.

SP **J15.29 Pneumonia due to other staphylococcus**

CODING TIPS ✓ When pneumonia is identified as "staph" without information as to species, e.g., aureus, use this code.

SP **J15.3 Pneumonia due to streptococcus, group B**

SP **J15.4 Pneumonia due to other streptococci**

EXCLUDES 1 pneumonia due to streptococcus, group B (J15.3)
pneumonia due to Streptococcus pneumoniae (J13)

SP **J15.5 Pneumonia due to Escherichia coli**

SP **J15.6 Pneumonia due to other Gram-negative bacteria**

Pneumonia due to other aerobic Gram-negative bacteria

Pneumonia due to Serratia marcescens

SP **J15.7 Pneumonia due to Mycoplasma pneumoniae**

SP **J15.8 Pneumonia due to other specified bacteria**

Chapter 10

J00-J99

CODING TIPS ✓ Do not assign code J15.8 for unspecified pneumonia. J15.8 indicates pneumonia with a specified organism for which no combination code exists.

SP **J15.9 Unspecified bacterial pneumonia**

Pneumonia due to gram-positive bacteria

4 **J16 Pneumonia due to other infectious organisms, not elsewhere classified**

Code first:
- associated influenza, if applicable (J09.X1, J10.0-, J11.0-)

Code also:
- associated abscess, if applicable (J85.1)

EXCLUDES 1
- congenital pneumonia (P23.-)
- ornithosis (A70)
- pneumocystosis (B59)
- pneumonia NOS (J18.9)

SP **J16.0 Chlamydial pneumonia**

SP **J16.8 Pneumonia due to other specified infectious organisms**

M IQ **J17 *Pneumonia in diseases classified elsewhere***

Code first underlying disease, such as:
- Q fever (A78)
- rheumatic fever (I00)
- schistosomiasis (B65.0-B65.9)

EXCLUDES 1
- candidial pneumonia (B37.1)
- chlamydial pneumonia (J16.0)
- gonorrheal pneumonia (A54.84)
- histoplasmosis pneumonia (B39.0-B39.2)
- measles pneumonia (B05.2)
- nocardiosis pneumonia (A43.0)
- pneumocystosis (B59)
- pneumonia due to Pneumocystis carinii (B59)
- pneumonia due to Pneumocystis jiroveci (B59)
- pneumonia in actinomycosis (A42.0)
- pneumonia in anthrax (A22.1)
- pneumonia in ascariasis (B77.81)
- pneumonia in aspergillosis (B44.0-B44.1)
- pneumonia in coccidioidomycosis (B38.0-B38.2)
- pneumonia in cytomegalovirus disease (B25.0)
- pneumonia in toxoplasmosis (B58.3)
- rubella pneumonia (B06.81)
- salmonella pneumonia (A02.22)
- spirochetal infection NEC with pneumonia (A69.8)
- tularemia pneumonia (A21.2)
- typhoid fever with pneumonia (A01.03)
- varicella pneumonia (B01.2)
- whooping cough with pneumonia (A37 with fifth-character 1)

4 **J18 Pneumonia, unspecified organism**

Code first:
- associated influenza, if applicable (J09.X1, J10.0-, J11.0-)

EXCLUDES 1
- abscess of lung with pneumonia (J85.1)
- aspiration pneumonia due to anesthesia during labor and delivery (O74.0)
- aspiration pneumonia due to anesthesia during pregnancy (O29)
- aspiration pneumonia due to anesthesia during puerperium (O89.0)
- aspiration pneumonia due to solids and liquids (J69.-)
- aspiration pneumonia NOS (J69.0)
- congenital pneumonia (P23.0)
- drug-induced interstitial lung disorder (J70.2-J70.4)
- interstitial pneumonia NOS (J84.9)
- lipid pneumonia (J69.1)
- neonatal aspiration pneumonia (P24.-)
- pneumonitis due to external agents (J67-J70)
- pneumonitis due to fumes and vapors (J68.0)
- usual interstitial pneumonia (J84.178)

CODING TIPS ✓ Do not use code J18 if the causative agent is known.

SP **J18.0 Bronchopneumonia, unspecified organism**

EXCLUDES 1
- hypostatic bronchopneumonia (J18.2)
- lipid pneumonia (J69.1)

EXCLUDES 2
- acute bronchiolitis (J21.-)
- chronic bronchiolitis (J44.9)

SP **J18.1 Lobar pneumonia, unspecified organism**

SP **J18.2 Hypostatic pneumonia, unspecified organism**

Hypostatic bronchopneumonia
Passive pneumonia

SP **J18.8 Other pneumonia, unspecified organism**

SP **J18.9 Pneumonia, unspecified organism**

CODING TIPS ✓ Assign J43.9 with J18.9 for emphysema, COPD and pneumonia. (AHA: 1Q 2019)

CODING TIPS ✓ Do not assign J18.9 when the causative organism or underlying cause of pneumonia is reported in the clinical record. If the organism or cause of pneumonia is known, a combination code should be assigned. When pneumonia is diagnosed in a patient who also has COPD, the coder should assign J44.0 and the type of pneumonia, and sequence according to the focus of care.

Other acute lower respiratory infections (J20-J22)

EXCLUDES 2
- chronic obstructive pulmonary disease with acute lower respiratory infection (J44.0)

CODING TIPS✓ Assign J43.9 and J20.9 for emphysema, COPD and acute bronchitis when there is no mention of a more specific type of chronic obstructive lung disease, i.e. chronic obstructive bronchitis. (AHA: 1Q 2019)

CODING TIPS✓ The presence of conditions in J20-J22 along with a condition classifiable to J44, require the COPD be coded with J44.0 with the lower respiratory infection code. Sequence according to the focus of care.

CODING TIPS✓ **Documentation:** Be cautious to differentiate the diagnostic differences between bronchitis and bronchiolitis. These are not interchangeable and are not the same disease process. Bronchitis is inflammation of the mucous membranes of the bronchi, while bronchiolitis involves inflammation of the smaller bronchioles which lead directly to the lungs. Bronchiolitis is more commonly diagnosed in children.

4 **J20 Acute bronchitis**

INCLUDES acute and subacute bronchitis (with) bronchospasm
acute and subacute bronchitis (with) tracheitis
acute and subacute bronchitis (with) tracheobronchitis, acute
acute and subacute fibrinous bronchitis
acute and subacute membranous bronchitis
acute and subacute purulent bronchitis
acute and subacute septic bronchitis

EXCLUDES 1 bronchitis NOS (J40)
tracheobronchitis NOS (J40)

EXCLUDES 2 acute bronchitis with bronchiectasis (J47.0)
acute bronchitis with chronic obstructive asthma (J44.0)
acute bronchitis with chronic obstructive pulmonary disease (J44.0)
allergic bronchitis NOS (J45.909-)
bronchitis due to chemicals, fumes and vapors (J68.0)
chronic bronchitis NOS (J42)
chronic mucopurulent bronchitis (J41.1)
chronic obstructive bronchitis (J44.-)
chronic obstructive tracheobronchitis (J44.-)
chronic simple bronchitis (J41.0)
chronic tracheobronchitis (J42)

CODING TIPS✓ If the patient also has a condition classifiable to J44, code J44.0 and the appropriate code from J20, and sequence according to the focus of care. You may not assume that a lower respiratory infection is an exacerbation of the COPD. If exacerbation is documented in a condition classifiable to J44, then add J44.1.

SP **J20.0 Acute bronchitis due to Mycoplasma pneumoniae**

SP **J20.1 Acute bronchitis due to Hemophilus influenzae**

SP **J20.2 Acute bronchitis due to streptococcus**

SP **J20.3 Acute bronchitis due to coxsackievirus**

SP **J20.4 Acute bronchitis due to parainfluenza virus**

SP **J20.5 Acute bronchitis due to respiratory syncytial virus**
Acute bronchitis due to RSV

SP **J20.6 Acute bronchitis due to rhinovirus**

SP **J20.7 Acute bronchitis due to echovirus**

SP **J20.8 Acute bronchitis due to other specified organisms**

CODING TIPS✓ For acute bronchitis confirmed as due to COVID-19, assign U07.1 and J20.8.

SP **J20.9 Acute bronchitis, unspecified**

CODING TIPS✓ Assign J43.9 and J20.9 for emphysema, COPD and acute bronchitis when there is no mention of a more specific type of chronic obstructive lung disease, i.e. chronic obstructive bronchitis. (AHA: 1Q 2019)

4 **J21 Acute bronchiolitis**

INCLUDES acute bronchiolitis with bronchospasm

EXCLUDES 2 respiratory bronchiolitis interstitial lung disease (J84.115)

SP **J21.0 Acute bronchiolitis due to respiratory syncytial virus**
Acute bronchiolitis due to RSV

SP **J21.1 Acute bronchiolitis due to human metapneumovirus**

SP **J21.8 Acute bronchiolitis due to other specified organisms**

SP **J21.9 Acute bronchiolitis, unspecified**
Bronchiolitis (acute)

EXCLUDES 1 chronic bronchiolitis (J44.-)

SP **J22 Unspecified acute lower respiratory infection**
Acute (lower) respiratory (tract) infection NOS

EXCLUDES 1 upper respiratory infection (acute) (J06.9)

CODING TIPS✓ For a lower respiratory infection, not otherwise specified, but confirmed as due to COVID-19, assign U07.1 and J22. If the respiratory infection is not identified as 'lower,' assign J98.8.

CODING TIPS✓ When upper respiratory infection and lower respiratory infection are both documented, assign only the code for the lower respiratory infection.

Other diseases of upper respiratory tract (J30-J39)

4 **J30 Vasomotor and allergic rhinitis**

INCLUDES spasmodic rhinorrhea

EXCLUDES 1 allergic rhinitis with asthma (bronchial) (J45.909)
rhinitis NOS (J31.0)

SP **J30.0 Vasomotor rhinitis**

SP **J30.1 Allergic rhinitis due to pollen**
Allergy NOS due to pollen
Hay fever
Pollinosis

Chapter 10

J00-J99

SP **J30.2 Other seasonal allergic rhinitis**

SP **J30.5 Allergic rhinitis due to food**

5 **J30.8 Other allergic rhinitis**

SP **J30.81 Allergic rhinitis due to animal (cat) (dog) hair and dander**

SP **J30.89 Other allergic rhinitis**
Perennial allergic rhinitis

SP **J30.9 Allergic rhinitis, unspecified**

+ 4 **J31 Chronic rhinitis, nasopharyngitis and pharyngitis**
Use additional code to identify:
exposure to environmental tobacco smoke (Z77.22)
exposure to tobacco smoke in the perinatal period (P96.81)
history of tobacco dependence (Z87.891)
occupational exposure to environmental tobacco smoke (Z57.31)
tobacco dependence (F17.-)
tobacco use (Z72.0)

SP + **J31.0 Chronic rhinitis**
Atrophic rhinitis (chronic)
Granulomatous rhinitis (chronic)
Hypertrophic rhinitis (chronic)
Obstructive rhinitis (chronic)
Ozena
Purulent rhinitis (chronic)
Rhinitis (chronic) NOS
Ulcerative rhinitis (chronic)
EXCLUDES 1 allergic rhinitis (J30.1-J30.9)
vasomotor rhinitis (J30.0)
DEFINITION Long-term inflammation of the nasal mucous membrane, with wasting of the mucous membrane and glands.

SP + **J31.1 Chronic nasopharyngitis**
EXCLUDES 2 acute nasopharyngitis (J00)
DEFINITION Long-term inflammation of the nasal and pharyngeal (throat) mucous membranes.

SP + **J31.2 Chronic pharyngitis**
Chronic sore throat
Atrophic pharyngitis (chronic)
Granular pharyngitis (chronic)
Hypertrophic pharyngitis (chronic)
EXCLUDES 2 acute pharyngitis (J02.9)

+ 4 **J32 Chronic sinusitis**
INCLUDES sinus abscess
sinus empyema
sinus infection
sinus suppuration
Use additional code to identify:
exposure to environmental tobacco smoke (Z77.22)
exposure to tobacco smoke in the perinatal period (P96.81)
history of tobacco dependence (Z87.891)
infectious agent (B95-B97)
occupational exposure to environmental tobacco smoke (Z57.31)
tobacco dependence (F17.-)
tobacco use (Z72.0)
EXCLUDES 2 acute sinusitis (J01.-)

CODING TIPS ✓ Do not assign a code from J32.- when sinusitis is reported as acute or infectious, unless the patient is reported to have both the chronic and acute form of sinusitis. If both forms are reported as confirmed in the medical record, assign separate and specific codes for each.

SP + **J32.0 Chronic maxillary sinusitis**
Antritis (chronic)
Maxillary sinusitis NOS

SP + **J32.1 Chronic frontal sinusitis**
Frontal sinusitis NOS

SP + **J32.2 Chronic ethmoidal sinusitis**
Ethmoidal sinusitis NOS
EXCLUDES 1 Woakes' ethmoiditis (J33.1)

SP + **J32.3 Chronic sphenoidal sinusitis**
Sphenoidal sinusitis NOS

SP + **J32.4 Chronic pansinusitis**
Pansinusitis NOS

SP + **J32.8 Other chronic sinusitis**
Sinusitis (chronic) involving more than one sinus but not pansinusitis

SP + **J32.9 Chronic sinusitis, unspecified**
Sinusitis (chronic) NOS

+ 4 **J33 Nasal polyp**
Use additional code to identify:
exposure to environmental tobacco smoke (Z77.22)
exposure to tobacco smoke in the perinatal period (P96.81)
history of tobacco dependence (Z87.891)
occupational exposure to environmental tobacco smoke (Z57.31)
tobacco dependence (F17.-)
tobacco use (Z72.0)
EXCLUDES 1 adenomatous polyps (D14.0)

SP + **J33.0 Polyp of nasal cavity**
Choanal polyp
Nasopharyngeal polyp

SP + **J33.1 Polypoid sinus degeneration**
Woakes' syndrome or ethmoiditis

SP + **J33.8 Other polyp of sinus**
Accessory polyp of sinus
Ethmoidal polyp of sinus
Maxillary polyp of sinus
Sphenoidal polyp of sinus

SP + **J33.9 Nasal polyp, unspecified**

4 **J34 Other and unspecified disorders of nose and nasal sinuses**
EXCLUDES 2 varicose ulcer of nasal septum (I86.8)

SP **J34.0 Abscess, furuncle and carbuncle of nose**
Cellulitis of nose
Necrosis of nose
Ulceration of nose

SP **J34.1 Cyst and mucocele of nose and nasal sinus**

SP **J34.2 Deviated nasal septum**
Deflection or deviation of septum (nasal) (acquired)
EXCLUDES 1 congenital deviated nasal septum (Q67.4)
DEFINITION Cartilage separating the nostrils is shifted out of position, usually due to an old traumatic injury.

SP **J34.3 Hypertrophy of nasal turbinates**

5 **J34.8 Other specified disorders of nose and nasal sinuses**

SP **J34.81 Nasal mucositis (ulcerative)**
Code also type of associated therapy, such as:
antineoplastic and immunosuppressive drugs (T45.1X-)
radiological procedure and radiotherapy (Y84.2)
EXCLUDES 2 gastrointestinal mucositis (ulcerative) (K92.81)
mucositis (ulcerative) of vagina and vulva (N76.81)
oral mucositis (ulcerative) (K12.3-)

SP **J34.89 Other specified disorders of nose and nasal sinuses**
Perforation of nasal septum NOS
Rhinolith

IQ **J34.9 Unspecified disorder of nose and nasal sinuses**

+ 4 **J35 Chronic diseases of tonsils and adenoids**
Use additional code to identify:
exposure to environmental tobacco smoke (Z77.22)
exposure to tobacco smoke in the perinatal period (P96.81)
history of tobacco dependence (Z87.891)
occupational exposure to environmental tobacco smoke (Z57.31)
tobacco dependence (F17.-)
tobacco use (Z72.0)

+ 5 **J35.0 Chronic tonsillitis and adenoiditis**
EXCLUDES 2 acute tonsillitis (J03.-)

SP + **J35.01 Chronic tonsillitis**

SP + **J35.02 Chronic adenoiditis**

SP + **J35.03 Chronic tonsillitis and adenoiditis**

SP + **J35.1 Hypertrophy of tonsils**
Enlargement of tonsils
EXCLUDES 1 hypertrophy of tonsils with tonsillitis (J35.0-)

SP + **J35.2 Hypertrophy of adenoids**
Enlargement of adenoids
EXCLUDES 1 hypertrophy of adenoids with adenoiditis (J35.0-)

SP + **J35.3 Hypertrophy of tonsils with hypertrophy of adenoids**
EXCLUDES 1 hypertrophy of tonsils and adenoids with tonsillitis and adenoiditis (J35.03)

SP + **J35.8 Other chronic diseases of tonsils and adenoids**
Adenoid vegetations
Amygdalolith
Calculus, tonsil
Cicatrix of tonsil (and adenoid)
Tonsillar tag
Ulcer of tonsil

IQ + **J35.9 Chronic disease of tonsils and adenoids, unspecified**
Disease (chronic) of tonsils and adenoids NOS

SP + **J36 Peritonsillar abscess**
INCLUDES abscess of tonsil
peritonsillar cellulitis
quinsy
Use additional code (B95-B97) to identify infectious agent.
EXCLUDES 1 acute tonsillitis (J03.-)
chronic tonsillitis (J35.0)
retropharyngeal abscess (J39.0)
tonsillitis NOS (J03.9-)

+ 4 **J37 Chronic laryngitis and laryngotracheitis**
Use additional code to identify:
exposure to environmental tobacco smoke (Z77.22)
exposure to tobacco smoke in the perinatal period (P96.81)
history of tobacco dependence (Z87.891)
infectious agent (B95-B97)
occupational exposure to environmental tobacco smoke (Z57.31)
tobacco dependence (F17.-)
tobacco use (Z72.0)

CODING TIPS ✓ Assign a code from J37.- only when the patient's provider specifies laryngitis or laryngotracheitis as "chronic."

SP + **J37.0 Chronic laryngitis**
Catarrhal laryngitis
Hypertrophic laryngitis
Sicca laryngitis
EXCLUDES 2 acute laryngitis (J04.0)
obstructive (acute) laryngitis (J05.0)

SP + **J37.1 Chronic laryngotracheitis**
Laryngitis, chronic, with tracheitis (chronic)
Tracheitis, chronic, with laryngitis
EXCLUDES 1 chronic tracheitis (J42)
EXCLUDES 2 acute laryngotracheitis (J04.2)
acute tracheitis (J04.1)

DEFINITION Long-term inflammation extending past the vocal cords and into the trachea.

+ 4 **J38 Diseases of vocal cords and larynx, not elsewhere classified**
Use additional code to identify:
exposure to environmental tobacco smoke (Z77.22)
exposure to tobacco smoke in the perinatal period (P96.81)
history of tobacco dependence (Z87.891)
occupational exposure to environmental tobacco smoke (Z57.31)
tobacco dependence (F17.-)
tobacco use (Z72.0)
EXCLUDES 1 congenital laryngeal stridor (P28.89)
obstructive laryngitis (acute) (J05.0)
postprocedural subglottic stenosis (J95.5)
stridor (R06.1)
ulcerative laryngitis (J04.0)

+ 5 **J38.0 Paralysis of vocal cords and larynx**
Laryngoplegia
Paralysis of glottis

IQ + **J38.00 Paralysis of vocal cords and larynx, unspecified**

SP + **J38.01 Paralysis of vocal cords and larynx, unilateral**

Chapter 10

J00-J99

SP + **J38.02 Paralysis of vocal cords and larynx, bilateral**

SP + **J38.1 Polyp of vocal cord and larynx**
EXCLUDES 1 adenomatous polyps (D14.1)

SP + **J38.2 Nodules of vocal cords**
Chorditis (fibrinous)(nodosa)(tuberosa)
Singer's nodes
Teacher's nodes

SP + **J38.3 Other diseases of vocal cords**
Abscess of vocal cords
Cellulitis of vocal cords
Granuloma of vocal cords
Leukokeratosis of vocal cords
Leukoplakia of vocal cords

SP + **J38.4 Edema of larynx**
Edema (of) glottis
Subglottic edema
Supraglottic edema
EXCLUDES 1 acute obstructive laryngitis [croup] (J05.0)
edematous laryngitis (J04.0)

SP + **J38.5 Laryngeal spasm**
Laryngismus (stridulus)

SP + **J38.6 Stenosis of larynx**

SP + **J38.7 Other diseases of larynx**
Abscess of larynx
Cellulitis of larynx
Disease of larynx NOS
Necrosis of larynx
Pachyderma of larynx
Perichondritis of larynx
Ulcer of larynx

4 **J39 Other diseases of upper respiratory tract**
EXCLUDES 1 acute respiratory infection NOS (J22)
acute upper respiratory infection (J06.9)
upper respiratory inflammation due to chemicals, gases, fumes or vapors (J68.2)

SP **J39.0 Retropharyngeal and parapharyngeal abscess**
Peripharyngeal abscess
EXCLUDES 1 peritonsillar abscess (J36)

DEFINITION Pus-filled sore at the back of the throat.

SP **J39.1 Other abscess of pharynx**
Cellulitis of pharynx
Nasopharyngeal abscess

CODING TIPS ✓ Do not assign J39.1 for a diagnosis of pharyngitis. Acute pharyngitis should be coded to J02.-

SP **J39.2 Other diseases of pharynx**
Cyst of pharynx
Edema of pharynx
EXCLUDES 2 chronic pharyngitis (J31.2)
ulcerative pharyngitis (J02.9)

SP **J39.3 Upper respiratory tract hypersensitivity reaction, site unspecified**
EXCLUDES 1 hypersensitivity reaction of upper respiratory tract, such as:
extrinsic allergic alveolitis (J67.9)
pneumoconiosis (J60-J67.9)

SP **J39.8 Other specified diseases of upper respiratory tract**

SP **J39.9 Disease of upper respiratory tract, unspecified**

Chronic lower respiratory diseases (J40-J47)

EXCLUDES 1 bronchitis due to chemicals, gases, fumes and vapors (J68.0)
EXCLUDES 2 cystic fibrosis (E84.-)

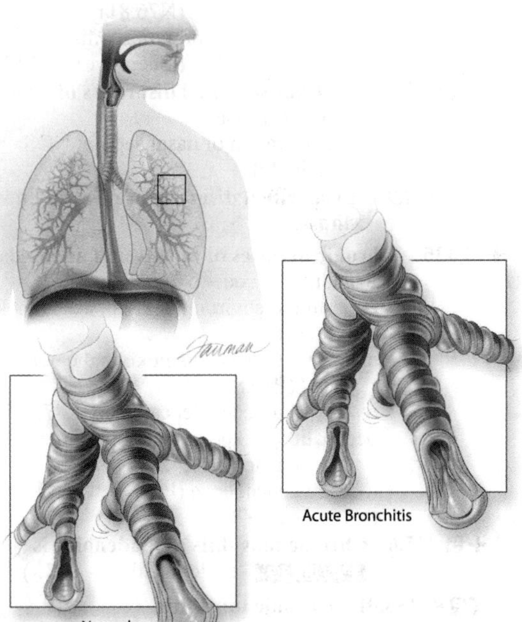

SP + **J40 Bronchitis, not specified as acute or chronic**
Bronchitis NOS
Bronchitis with tracheitis NOS
Catarrhal bronchitis
Tracheobronchitis NOS
Use additional code to identify:
exposure to environmental tobacco smoke (Z77.22)
exposure to tobacco smoke in the perinatal period (P96.81)
history of tobacco dependence (Z87.891)
occupational exposure to environmental tobacco smoke (Z57.31)
tobacco dependence (F17.-)
tobacco use (Z72.0)
EXCLUDES 1 acute bronchitis (J20.-)
allergic bronchitis NOS (J45.909-)
asthmatic bronchitis NOS (J45.9-)
bronchitis due to chemicals, gases, fumes and vapors (J68.0)

CODING TIPS ✓ Do not assign code J40 for chronic, chronic obstructive, or acute bronchitis. J40 should be assigned only when no diagnostic information is available to differentiate the type of bronchitis.

+ 4 J41 Simple and mucopurulent chronic bronchitis

Use additional code to identify:
- exposure to environmental tobacco smoke (Z77.22)
- exposure to tobacco smoke in the perinatal period (P96.81)
- history of tobacco dependence (Z87.891)
- occupational exposure to environmental tobacco smoke (Z57.31)
- tobacco dependence (F17.-)
- tobacco use (Z72.0)

EXCLUDES 1 chronic bronchitis NOS (J42)
chronic obstructive bronchitis (J44.-)

CODING TIPS✓ Chronic bronchitis not specified as "obstructive" should be coded to J41.0-J42. Chronic bronchitis that is specified as obstructive is coded to category J44.-. Chronic indicates cough with mucus most days of the month for at least 3 months out of the year.

SP + J41.0 Simple chronic bronchitis

SP + J41.1 Mucopurulent chronic bronchitis

SP + J41.8 Mixed simple and mucopurulent chronic bronchitis

SP + J42 Unspecified chronic bronchitis

Chronic bronchitis NOS
Chronic tracheitis
Chronic tracheobronchitis

Use additional code to identify:
- exposure to environmental tobacco smoke (Z77.22)
- exposure to tobacco smoke in the perinatal period (P96.81)
- history of tobacco dependence (Z87.891)
- occupational exposure to environmental tobacco smoke (Z57.31)
- tobacco dependence (F17.-)
- tobacco use (Z72.0)

EXCLUDES 1 chronic asthmatic bronchitis (J44.-)
chronic bronchitis with airways obstruction (J44.-)
chronic emphysematous bronchitis (J44.-)
chronic obstructive pulmonary disease NOS (J44.9)
simple and mucopurulent chronic bronchitis (J41.-)

CODING TIPS✓ Chronic bronchitis not specified as "obstructive" should be coded to J41.0-J42. Chronic bronchitis that is specified as obstructive is coded to category J44.-. Chronic indicates cough with mucus most days of the month for at least 3 months out of the year.

+ 4 J43 Emphysema

Use additional code to identify:
- exposure to environmental tobacco smoke (Z77.22)
- history of tobacco dependence (Z87.891)
- occupational exposure to environmental tobacco smoke (Z57.31)
- tobacco dependence (F17.-)
- tobacco use (Z72.0)

EXCLUDES 1 compensatory emphysema (J98.3)
emphysema due to inhalation of chemicals, gases, fumes or vapors (J68.4)
emphysema with chronic (obstructive) bronchitis (J44.-)
emphysematous (obstructive) bronchitis (J44.-)
interstitial emphysema (J98.2)
mediastinal emphysema (J98.2)
neonatal interstitial emphysema (P25.0)
surgical (subcutaneous) emphysema (T81.82)

EXCLUDES 2 traumatic subcutaneous emphysema (T79.7)

CODING TIPS✓ Emphysema and COPD (not documented as a specific chronic obstructive bronchitis, chronic obstructive asthma or emphysematous bronchitis) is coded to J43. Emphysema with documented exacerbated COPD is coded to J43, not J44.

CODING TIPS✓ Do not assign a code from J43.- when the provider's documentation reports emphysema with chronic obstructive bronchitis or emphysematous bronchitis. Emphysema with chronic obstructive bronchitis and emphysematous bronchitis should be coded to J44.- and cannot be coded on the same claim as J43.-.

CODING TIPS✓ Codes in the subclassification J43 include respiratory insufficiency; therefore, do not assign R06.89 as an additional code. However, respiratory failure, if documented, should be coded.

CODING TIPS✓ When a diagnosis supports coding a more specific code for emphysema, such as interstitial emphysema (J98.2), compensatory emphysema (J98.3), or subcutaneous emphysema due to trauma (T79.7), then do not assign J43.-, but assign the more specific code.

SP + J43.0 Unilateral pulmonary emphysema [MacLeod's syndrome]

Swyer-James syndrome
Unilateral emphysema
Unilateral hyperlucent lung
Unilateral pulmonary artery functional hypoplasia
Unilateral transparency of lung

SP + J43.1 Panlobular emphysema

Panacinar emphysema

SP + J43.2 Centrilobular emphysema

SP + J43.8 Other emphysema

SP + J43.9 Emphysema, unspecified

Bullous emphysema (lung)(pulmonary)
Emphysema (lung)(pulmonary) NOS
Emphysematous bleb
Vesicular emphysema (lung)(pulmonary)

CODING TIPS✓ Assign J43.9 and J20.9 for emphysema, COPD and acute bronchitis when there's no mention of chronic bronchitis; assign J43.9 with J18.9 for emphysema, COPD and pneumonia; assign J43.9 with a code from J45 for emphysema, COPD and asthma. (AHA: 1Q 2019)

Chapter 10 J00-J99

DEFINITION Abnormal enlargement of the air sacs in the lungs, which lose their elasticity, making breathing increasingly difficult.

+ 4 J44 Other chronic obstructive pulmonary disease

INCLUDES asthma with chronic obstructive pulmonary disease
chronic asthmatic (obstructive) bronchitis
chronic bronchitis with airway obstruction
chronic bronchitis with emphysema
chronic emphysematous bronchitis
chronic obstructive asthma
chronic obstructive bronchitis
chronic obstructive tracheobronchitis

Code also:
type of asthma, if applicable (J45.-)

Use additional code to identify:
exposure to environmental tobacco smoke (Z77.22)
history of tobacco dependence (Z87.891)
occupational exposure to environmental tobacco smoke (Z57.31)
tobacco dependence (F17.-)
tobacco use (Z72.0)

EXCLUDES 1 bronchiectasis (J47.-)
chronic bronchitis NOS (J42)
chronic simple and mucopurulent bronchitis (J41.-)
chronic tracheitis (J42)
chronic tracheobronchitis (J42)
emphysema without chronic bronchitis (J43.-)

GUIDELINES **Section I.C.10.a**
The codes in categories J44 and J45 distinguish between uncomplicated cases and those in acute exacerbation. An acute exacerbation is a worsening or a decompensation of a chronic condition. An acute exacerbation is not equivalent to an infection superimposed on a chronic condition, though an exacerbation may be triggered by an infection.

CODING TIPS✓ COPD is not the same as chronic bronchitis. COPD is an unspecified term that may encompass multiple components of chronic obstructive pulmonary disease (chronic bronchitis, chronic asthma and emphysema). Code J43.- is used when COPD (unspecified) and emphysema have been documented by the provider.

CODING TIPS✓ If the patient has COPD and asthma and the type of asthma is specified by the physician or NPP, code the J45 for the type of asthma along with the COPD. If the physician or NPP documents that the asthma is exacerbated, but not which type, code J45.901 and the COPD. If the physician or NPP has documented asthma, but not specified the type, or exacerbation, do not code the asthma (J45), if the patient has COPD.

SP SH + J44.0 Chronic obstructive pulmonary disease with (acute) lower respiratory infection

Code also:
* to identify the infection

CODING TIPS✓ Assign a code from J44.0 when a patient has both a condition classifiable to J44 and a diagnosis of a lower respiratory tract infection. Examples of lower respiratory infections include pneumonia, bronchitis and bronchiolitis. An additional code should be assigned to report the infection, and sequence depending on the focus of care.

CODING TIPS✓ If the physician or NPP confirms both a diagnosis of a lower respiratory tract infection and exacerbation of a condition classifiable to J44, both J44.1 and J44.0 should be assigned, along with a code for the specific lower respiratory infection.

SP SH + J44.1 Chronic obstructive pulmonary disease with (acute) exacerbation

Decompensated COPD
Decompensated COPD with (acute) exacerbation

EXCLUDES 2 chronic obstructive pulmonary disease [COPD] with acute bronchitis (J44.0)
lung diseases due to external agents (J60-J70)

CODING TIPS✓ **Documentation:** Do not assign this code unless the physician or NPP has confirmed that the condition is exacerbated. An exacerbation should be documented by the physician or NPP, and changes in treatment and medication regimen do not presume an exacerbation.

CODING TIPS✓ This code is appropriate when the patient has an acute exacerbation of a condition classifiable to J44, or the disease is decompensating. If the disease is **not** decompensating or exacerbated, use J44.9. If there is a lower respiratory infection, use J44.0, not J44.9.

CODING TIPS✓ An acute exacerbation is a worsening or decompensation of a chronic condition. Decompensated indicates there has been a flare-up (acute phase) of a chronic condition. It is not equivalent to an infection superimposed on a chronic condition, so do not assume an exacerbation with an infection. The physician or NPP must indicate an exacerbation, decompensation or flare-up to use this code.

SP SH + J44.9 **Chronic obstructive pulmonary disease, unspecified**

Chronic obstructive airway disease NOS
Chronic obstructive lung disease NOS

EXCLUDES 2 lung diseases due to external agents (J60-J70)

CODING TIPS ✓ If a condition classifiable to J44 is documented with exacerbation or lower respiratory infection, do not assign J44.9, and use the more specific code(s). If any condition is documented that is included in J44 without an exacerbation or lower respiratory infection, use J44.9. Respiratory insufficiency is an integral part of these diseases; therefore, do not assign additional code R06.89. However, respiratory failure, if indicated, is coded as an additional code.

+ 4 J45 **Asthma**

INCLUDES allergic (predominantly) asthma
allergic bronchitis NOS
allergic rhinitis with asthma
atopic asthma
extrinsic allergic asthma
hay fever with asthma
idiosyncratic asthma
intrinsic nonallergic asthma
nonallergic asthma

Use additional code to identify:
eosinophilic asthma (J82.83)
exposure to environmental tobacco smoke (Z77.22)
exposure to tobacco smoke in the perinatal period (P96.81)
history of tobacco dependence (Z87.891)
occupational exposure to environmental tobacco smoke (Z57.31)
tobacco dependence (F17.-)
tobacco use (Z72.0)

EXCLUDES 1 detergent asthma (J69.8)
eosinophilic asthma (J82)
miner's asthma (J60)
wheezing NOS (R06.2)
wood asthma (J67.8)

EXCLUDES 2 asthma with chronic obstructive pulmonary disease (J44.9)
chronic asthmatic (obstructive) bronchitis (J44.9)
chronic obstructive asthma (J44.9)

GUIDELINES **Section I.C.10.a**

The codes in categories J44 and J45 distinguish between uncomplicated cases and those in acute exacerbation. An acute exacerbation is a worsening or a decompensation of a chronic condition. An acute exacerbation is not equivalent to an infection superimposed on a chronic condition, though an exacerbation may be triggered by an infection.

CODING TIPS ✓ Asthma may be referred to as reactive or Reversible Airway Disease in the documentation. Restrictive airway disease is not asthma.

CODING TIPS ✓ Assign J43.9 with a code from J45 for emphysema, COPD and asthma. (AHA: 1Q 2019)

CODING TIPS ✓ The patient can have both asthma and other types of COPD, so when documentation indicates a condition classifiable to J44 and any **specified** type of asthma, or exacerbation of asthma, the asthma should also be coded.

CODING TIPS ✓ Status asthmaticus refers to a patient's failure to respond to therapy administered during an asthmatic episode. It is a life-threatening complication that requires emergency care.

CODING TIPS ✓ Patients are classified as having intermittent or persistent (mild, moderate or severe) asthma depending on the degree of impairment and risk. The severity of asthma is determined based on which of the following factors is the worst: daytime or nocturnal symptoms, rescue SABA use, lung function or exacerbation frequency.

DEFINITION Asthma is also known as reactive airway disease. It is an inflammatory process of the lining of the airways of the lungs and is considered reversible. Patients with asthma typically develop wheezing, shortness of breath and cough. Because the inflammation of the lining of the airways is considered reversible, asthma symptoms are intermittent and cover a spectrum from mild-to-severe disease. Several symptoms overlap in patients with COPD and asthma. A history of wheezing strongly suggests a diagnosis of asthma, whereas chronic cough productive of sputum is more indicative of COPD.

+ 5 J45.2 **Mild intermittent asthma**

SP SH + J45.20 **Mild intermittent asthma, uncomplicated**
Mild intermittent asthma NOS

SP SH + J45.21 **Mild intermittent asthma with (acute) exacerbation**

SP SH + J45.22 **Mild intermittent asthma with status asthmaticus**

+ 5 J45.3 **Mild persistent asthma**

SP SH + J45.30 **Mild persistent asthma, uncomplicated**
Mild persistent asthma NOS

SP SH + J45.31 **Mild persistent asthma with (acute) exacerbation**

SP SH + J45.32 **Mild persistent asthma with status asthmaticus**

+ 5 J45.4 **Moderate persistent asthma**

SP SH + J45.40 **Moderate persistent asthma, uncomplicated**
Moderate persistent asthma NOS

SP SH + J45.41 **Moderate persistent asthma with (acute) exacerbation**

SP SH + J45.42 **Moderate persistent asthma with status asthmaticus**

+ 5 J45.5 **Severe persistent asthma**

SP SH + J45.50 **Severe persistent asthma, uncomplicated**
Severe persistent asthma NOS

SP SH + J45.51 **Severe persistent asthma with (acute) exacerbation**

Chapter 10

J00-J99

SP SH + **J45.52 Severe persistent asthma with status asthmaticus**

+ 5 **J45.9 Other and unspecified asthma**

+ 6 **J45.90 Unspecified asthma**

Asthmatic bronchitis NOS
Childhood asthma NOS
Late onset asthma

SP SH + **J45.901 Unspecified asthma with (acute) exacerbation**

SP SH + **J45.902 Unspecified asthma with status asthmaticus**

SP SH + **J45.909 Unspecified asthma, uncomplicated**

Asthma NOS

EXCLUDES 2 lung diseases due to external agents (J60-J70)

CODING TIPS✓ Do not use this code with J44. Asthma is included in the conditions classifiable to J44, and the asthma code should be added only if asthma is specified or exacerbated.

+ 6 **J45.99 Other asthma**

SP SH + **J45.990 Exercise induced bronchospasm**

SP SH + **J45.991 Cough variant asthma**

SP SH + **J45.998 Other asthma**

+ 4 **J47 Bronchiectasis**

INCLUDES bronchiolectasis

Use additional code to identify:
exposure to environmental tobacco smoke (Z77.22)
exposure to tobacco smoke in the perinatal period (P96.81)
history of tobacco dependence (Z87.891)
occupational exposure to environmental tobacco smoke (Z57.31)
tobacco dependence (F17.-)
tobacco use (Z72.0)

EXCLUDES 1 congenital bronchiectasis (Q33.4)
tuberculous bronchiectasis (current disease) (A15.0)

CODING TIPS✓ Bronchiecstasis is the destruction and dilatation of the airways. Although bronchiecstasis is common with cystic fibrosis, the code for bronchiecstasis should be added to E84.0 as the respiratory manifestation. [AHA: 1Q 2021]

▲ SP SH + **J47.0 Bronchiectasis with acute lower respiratory infection**

Bronchiectasis with acute bronchitis
Code also:
to identify infection, if applicable

SP SH + **J47.1 Bronchiectasis with (acute) exacerbation**

SP SH + **J47.9 Bronchiectasis, uncomplicated**

Bronchiectasis NOS

DEFINITION Destruction and widening of the large airways, often due to recurrent, severe infection or inflammation, or following foreign body obstruction.

Lung diseases due to external agents (J60-J70)

EXCLUDES 2 asthma (J45.-)
malignant neoplasm of bronchus and lung (C34.-)

SP **J60 Coalworker's pneumoconiosis**

Anthracosilicosis
Anthracosis
Black lung disease
Coalworker's lung

EXCLUDES 1 coalworker pneumoconiosis with tuberculosis, any type in A15 (J65)

DEFINITION Silicotic nodules and scar-tissue formation in the lungs due to prolonged inhalation and collection of coal dust particles in the bronchioles.

SP **J61 Pneumoconiosis due to asbestos and other mineral fibers**

Asbestosis

EXCLUDES 1 pleural plaque with asbestosis (J92.0)
pneumoconiosis with tuberculosis, any type in A15 (J65)

DEFINITION Chronic lung disease caused by inhaling asbestos particles over a prolonged period.

4 **J62 Pneumoconiosis due to dust containing silica**

INCLUDES silicotic fibrosis (massive) of lung

EXCLUDES 1 pneumoconiosis with tuberculosis, any type in A15 (J65)

SP **J62.0 Pneumoconiosis due to talc dust**

SP **J62.8 Pneumoconiosis due to other dust containing silica**

Silicosis NOS

4 **J63 Pneumoconiosis due to other inorganic dusts**

EXCLUDES 1 pneumoconiosis with tuberculosis, any type in A15 (J65)

SP **J63.0 Aluminosis (of lung)**

SP **J63.1 Bauxite fibrosis (of lung)**

SP **J63.2 Berylliosis**

SP **J63.3 Graphite fibrosis (of lung)**

SP **J63.4 Siderosis**

SP **J63.5 Stannosis**

SP **J63.6 Pneumoconiosis due to other specified inorganic dusts**

SP **J64 Unspccified pneumoconiosis**

EXCLUDES 1 pneumonoconiosis with tuberculosis, any type in A15 (J65)

SP **J65 Pneumoconiosis associated with tuberculosis**

Any condition in J60-J64 with tuberculosis, any type in A15
Silicotuberculosis

4 **J66 Airway disease due to specific organic dust**

EXCLUDES 2 allergic alveolitis (J67.-)
asbestosis (J61)
bagassosis (J67.1)
farmer's lung (J67.0)
hypersensitivity pneumonitis due to organic dust (J67.-)

4 4th digit required 5 5th digit required 6 6th digit required 7 7th digit required 7th digit placeholder + Additional code Laterality

reactive airways dysfunction syndrome (J68.3)

SP **J66.0 Byssinosis**
Airway disease due to cotton dust

SP **J66.1 Flax-dressers' disease**

SP **J66.2 Cannabinosis**

SP **J66.8 Airway disease due to other specific organic dusts**

4 **J67 Hypersensitivity pneumonitis due to organic dust**
INCLUDES allergic alveolitis and pneumonitis due to inhaled organic dust and particles of fungal, actinomycetic or other origin
EXCLUDES 1 pneumonitis due to inhalation of chemicals, gases, fumes or vapors (J68.0)

SP **J67.0 Farmer's lung**
Harvester's lung
Haymaker's lung
Moldy hay disease
DEFINITION Inflammation of the small, inner air sacs in the lungs, due to an allergic reaction triggered by inhaled organic substances or microorganisms.

SP **J67.1 Bagassosis**
Bagasse disease
Bagasse pneumonitis

SP **J67.2 Bird fancier's lung**
Budgerigar fancier's disease or lung
Pigeon fancier's disease or lung

SP **J67.3 Suberosis**
Corkhandler's disease or lung
Corkworker's disease or lung

SP **J67.4 Maltworker's lung**
Alveolitis due to Aspergillus clavatus

SP **J67.5 Mushroom-worker's lung**

SP **J67.6 Maple-bark-stripper's lung**
Alveolitis due to Cryptostroma corticale
Cryptostromosis

SP **J67.7 Air conditioner and humidifier lung**
Allergic alveolitis due to fungal, thermophilic actinomycetes and other organisms growing in ventilation [air conditioning] systems

SP **J67.8 Hypersensitivity pneumonitis due to other organic dusts**
Cheese-washer's lung
Coffee-worker's lung
Fish-meal worker's lung
Furrier's lung
Sequoiosis

SP **J67.9 Hypersensitivity pneumonitis due to unspecified organic dust**
Allergic alveolitis (extrinsic) NOS
Hypersensitivity pneumonitis NOS

+ 4 **J68 Respiratory conditions due to inhalation of chemicals, gases, fumes and vapors**
Code first:
(T51-T65) to identify cause
Use additional code to identify associated respiratory conditions, such as:
acute respiratory failure (J96.0-)

IQ + **J68.0 Bronchitis and pneumonitis due to chemicals, gases, fumes and vapors**
Chemical bronchitis (acute)

IQ + **J68.1 Pulmonary edema due to chemicals, gases, fumes and vapors**
Chemical pulmonary edema (acute) (chronic)
EXCLUDES 1 pulmonary edema (acute) (chronic) NOS (J81.-)

IQ + **J68.2 Upper respiratory inflammation due to chemicals, gases, fumes and vapors, not elsewhere classified**

IQ + **J68.3 Other acute and subacute respiratory conditions due to chemicals, gases, fumes and vapors**
Reactive airways dysfunction syndrome

IQ + **J68.4 Chronic respiratory conditions due to chemicals, gases, fumes and vapors**
Emphysema (diffuse) (chronic) due to inhalation of chemicals, gases, fumes and vapors
Obliterative bronchiolitis (chronic) (subacute) due to inhalation of chemicals, gases, fumes and vapors
Pulmonary fibrosis (chronic) due to inhalation of chemicals, gases, fumes and vapors
EXCLUDES 1 chronic pulmonary edema due to chemicals, gases, fumes and vapors (J68.1)

IQ + **J68.8 Other respiratory conditions due to chemicals, gases, fumes and vapors**

IQ + **J68.9 Unspecified respiratory condition due to chemicals, gases, fumes and vapors**

4 **J69 Pneumonitis due to solids and liquids**
EXCLUDES 1 neonatal aspiration syndromes (P24.-)
postprocedural pneumonitis (J95.4)
CODING TIPS✓ Aspiration pneumonia is not considered an infection (although it can result in an infection). Code J44.0 is NOT to be used with J69, unless a secondary infection is also documented.

SP **J69.0 Pneumonitis due to inhalation of food and vomit**
Aspiration pneumonia NOS
Aspiration pneumonia (due to) food (regurgitated)
Aspiration pneumonia (due to) gastric secretions
Aspiration pneumonia (due to) milk
Aspiration pneumonia (due to) vomit
Code also:
any associated foreign body in respiratory tract (T17.-)
EXCLUDES 1 chemical pneumonitis due to anesthesia (J95.4)
obstetric aspiration pneumonitis (O74.0)
CODING TIPS✓ When sepsis is documented as related to aspiration pneumonia, code the sepsis, the specified pneumonia, and the pneumonitis due to inhalation of food and vomit. (AHA: 2Q 2020)
CODING TIPS✓ Code J69.0 for aspiration bronchitis that isn't further specified. (AHA: 2Q 2019)

IQ **J69.1 Pneumonitis due to inhalation of oils and essences**
Exogenous lipoid pneumonia

Chapter 10

J00-J99

Lipid pneumonia NOS
Code first:
(T51-T65) to identify substance
EXCLUDES 1 endogenous lipoid pneumonia (J84.89)

IQ **J69.8 Pneumonitis due to inhalation of other solids and liquids**
Pneumonitis due to aspiration of blood
Pneumonitis due to aspiration of detergent
Code first:
(T51-T65) to identify substance

4 **J70 Respiratory conditions due to other external agents**

SP + **J70.0 Acute pulmonary manifestations due to radiation**
Radiation pneumonitis
Use additional code (W88-W90, X39.0-) to identify the external cause

SP + **J70.1 Chronic and other pulmonary manifestations due to radiation**
Fibrosis of lung following radiation
Use additional code (W88-W90, X39.0-) to identify the external cause

SP + **J70.2 Acute drug-induced interstitial lung disorders**
Use additional code for adverse effect, if applicable, to identify drug (T36-T50 with fifth or sixth character 5)
EXCLUDES 1 interstitial pneumonia NOS (J84.9)
lymphoid interstitial pneumonia (J84.2)

SP + **J70.3 Chronic drug-induced interstitial lung disorders**
Use additional code for adverse effect, if applicable, to identify drug (T36-T50 with fifth or sixth character 5)
EXCLUDES 1 interstitial pneumonia NOS (J84.9)
lymphoid interstitial pneumonia (J84.2)

SP + **J70.4 Drug-induced interstitial lung disorders, unspecified**
Use additional code for adverse effect, if applicable, to identify drug (T36-T50 with fifth or sixth character 5)
EXCLUDES 1 interstitial pneumonia NOS (J84.9)
lymphoid interstitial pneumonia (J84.2)

IQ **J70.5 Respiratory conditions due to smoke inhalation**
Code first:
smoke inhalation (T59.81-)
EXCLUDES 2 smoke inhalation due to chemicals, gases, fumes and vapors (J68.9)

IQ **J70.8 Respiratory conditions due to other specified external agents**
Code first:
(T51-T65) to identify the external agent

IQ **J70.9 Respiratory conditions due to unspecified external agent**
Code first:
(T51-T65) to identify the external agent

Other respiratory diseases principally affecting the interstitium (J80-J84)

SP **J80 Acute respiratory distress syndrome**
Acute respiratory distress syndrome in adult or child
Adult hyaline membrane disease
EXCLUDES 1 respiratory distress syndrome in newborn (perinatal) (P22.0)

CODING TIPS ✓ For acute respiratory distress syndrome as due to COVID-19, assign U07.1 and J80.

CODING TIPS ✓ Acute respiratory distress syndrome is a life-threatening condition, which requires acute care treatment. J80 should be assigned as a primary or secondary diagnosis if it is a current condition.

+ 4 **J81 Pulmonary edema**
Use additional code to identify:
exposure to environmental tobacco smoke (Z77.22)
history of tobacco dependence (Z87.891)
occupational exposure to environmental tobacco smoke (Z57.31)
tobacco dependence (F17.-)
tobacco use (Z72.0)
EXCLUDES 1 chemical (acute) pulmonary edema (J68.1)
hypostatic pneumonia (J18.2)
passive pneumonia (J18.2)
pulmonary edema due to external agents (J60-J70)
pulmonary edema with heart disease NOS (I50.1)
pulmonary edema with heart failure (I50.1)

CODING TIPS ✓ Pulmonary congestion is integral to, or routinely associated with, several conditions, such as CHF and pneumonia. Do not use an additional symptom code such as R09.89 when the symptom is routinely associated with the condition.

SP + **J81.0 Acute pulmonary edema**
Acute edema of lung

DEFINITION Sudden, severe accumulation of fluid in the lungs.

SP + **J81.1 Chronic pulmonary edema**
Pulmonary congestion (chronic) (passive)
Pulmonary edema NOS

4 **J82 Pulmonary eosinophilia, not elsewhere classified**
EXCLUDES 2 pulmonary eosinophilia due to aspergillosis (B44.-)
pulmonary eosinophilia due to drugs (J70.2-J70.4)
pulmonary eosinophilia due to specified parasitic infection (B50-B83)
pulmonary eosinophilia due to systemic connective tissue disorders (M30-M36)
pulmonary infiltrate NOS (R91.8)

5 **J82.8 Pulmonary eosinophilia, not elsewhere classified**

SP **J82.81 Chronic eosinophilic pneumonia**
Eosinophilic pneumonia, NOS

SP **J82.82 Acute eosinophilic pneumonia**

IQ **J82.83 Eosinophilic asthma**
Code first asthma, by type, such as:
mild intermittent asthma (J45.2-)
mild persistent asthma (J45.3-)
moderate persistent asthma (J45.4-)
severe persistent asthma (J45.5-)

SP **J82.89 Other pulmonary eosinophilia, not elsewhere classified**
Allergic pneumonia
Löffler's pneumonia
Tropical (pulmonary) eosinophilia NOS

4 **J84 Other interstitial pulmonary diseases**
EXCLUDES 1 drug-induced interstitial lung disorders (J70.2-J70.4)
interstitial emphysema (J98.2)
EXCLUDES 2 lung diseases due to external agents (J60-J70)

5 **J84.0 Alveolar and parieto-alveolar conditions**

SP **J84.01 Alveolar proteinosis**

SP **J84.02 Pulmonary alveolar microlithiasis**

M IQ ***J84.03 Idiopathic pulmonary hemosiderosis***
Essential brown induration of lung
Code first underlying disease, such as:
disorders of iron metabolism (E83.1-)
EXCLUDES 1 acute idiopathic pulmonary hemorrhage in infants [AIPHI] (R04.81)

SP **J84.09 Other alveolar and parieto-alveolar conditions**

5 **J84.1 Other interstitial pulmonary diseases with fibrosis**
EXCLUDES 1 pulmonary fibrosis (chronic) due to inhalation of chemicals, gases, fumes or vapors (J68.4)
pulmonary fibrosis (chronic) following radiation (J70.1)

DEFINITION Formation of fibrous tissue and scarring in the lungs after the lungs have been inflamed for a significant period of time.

SP **J84.10 Pulmonary fibrosis, unspecified**
Capillary fibrosis of lung
Cirrhosis of lung (chronic) NOS
Fibrosis of lung (atrophic) (chronic) (confluent) (massive) (perialveolar) (peribronchial) NOS
Induration of lung (chronic) NOS
Postinflammatory pulmonary fibrosis

6 **J84.11 Idiopathic interstitial pneumonia**
EXCLUDES 1 lymphoid interstitial pneumonia (J84.2)
pneumocystis pneumonia (B59)

SP **J84.111 Idiopathic interstitial pneumonia, not otherwise specified**

SP **J84.112 Idiopathic pulmonary fibrosis**
Cryptogenic fibrosing alveolitis
Idiopathic fibrosing alveolitis

SP **J84.113 Idiopathic non-specific interstitial pneumonitis**
EXCLUDES 1 non-specific interstitial pneumonia NOS, or due to known underlying cause (J84.89)

SP **J84.114 Acute interstitial pneumonitis**
Hamman-Rich syndrome
EXCLUDES 1 pneumocystis pneumonia (B59)

SP **J84.115 Respiratory bronchiolitis interstitial lung disease**

SP **J84.116 Cryptogenic organizing pneumonia**
EXCLUDES 1 organizing pneumonia NOS, or due to known underlying cause (J84.89)

SP **J84.117 Desquamative interstitial pneumonia**

6 **J84.17 Other interstitial pulmonary diseases with fibrosis in diseases classified elsewhere**

M IQ ***J84.170 Interstitial lung disease with progressive fibrotic phenotype in diseases classified elsewhere***
Progressive fibrotic interstitial lung disease
Code first underlying disease, such as:
lung diseases due to external agents (J60-J70)
rheumatoid arthritis (M05.00-M06.9)
sarcoidosis (D86)
systemic connective tissue disorders (M30-M36)

M IQ ***J84.178 Other interstitial pulmonary diseases with fibrosis in diseases classified elsewhere***
Interstitial pneumonia (nonspecific) (usual) due to collagen vascular disease
Interstitial pneumonia (nonspecific) (usual) in diseases classified elsewhere
Organizing pneumonia due to collagen vascular disease
Organizing pneumonia in diseases classified elsewhere
Code first underlying disease, such as:
progressive systemic sclerosis (M34.0)
rheumatoid arthritis (M05.00-M06.9)
systemic lupus erythematosis (M32.0-M32.9)

SP **J84.2 Lymphoid interstitial pneumonia**
Lymphoid interstitial pneumonitis

5 **J84.8 Other specified interstitial pulmonary diseases**
EXCLUDES 1 exogenous lipoid pneumonia (J69.1)
unspecified lipoid pneumonia (J69.1)

SP **J84.81 Lymphangioleiomyomatosis**
Lymphangiomyomatosis

Chapter 10
J00-J99

SP J84.82 **Adult pulmonary Langerhans cell histiocytosis**
Adult PLCH

SP J84.83 **Surfactant mutations of the lung**

6 J84.84 **Other interstitial lung diseases of childhood**

SP J84.841 **Neuroendocrine cell hyperplasia of infancy**

SP J84.842 **Pulmonary interstitial glycogenosis**

SP J84.843 **Alveolar capillary dysplasia with vein misalignment**

SP J84.848 **Other interstitial lung diseases of childhood**

SP + J84.89 **Other specified interstitial pulmonary diseases**
Endogenous lipoid pneumonia
Interstitial pneumonitis
Non-specific interstitial pneumonitis NOS
Organizing pneumonia NOS
Code first, if applicable:
poisoning due to drug or toxin (T51-T65 with fifth or sixth character to indicate intent) , for toxic pneumonopathy
underlying cause of pneumonopathy, if known
Use additional code, for adverse effect, to identify drug (T36-T50 with fifth or sixth character 5), if drug-induced
EXCLUDES 1 cryptogenic organizing pneumonia (J84.116)
idiopathic non-specific interstitial pneumonitis (J84.113)
lipoid pneumonia, exogenous or unspecified (J69.1)
lymphoid interstitial pneumonia (J84.2)

SP J84.9 **Interstitial pulmonary disease, unspecified**
Interstitial pneumonia NOS

Suppurative and necrotic conditions of the lower respiratory tract (J85-J86)

CODING TIPS✓ When the record specifies the causative organism, use an additional code to report the organism specified, following the instructions to "use an additional code."

+ 4 J85 **Abscess of lung and mediastinum**
Use additional code (B95-B97) to identify infectious agent.

SP + J85.0 **Gangrene and necrosis of lung**

SP + J85.1 **Abscess of lung with pneumonia**
Code also:
the type of pneumonia

SP + J85.2 **Abscess of lung without pneumonia**
Abscess of lung NOS

SP + J85.3 **Abscess of mediastinum**

+ 4 J86 **Pyothorax**
Use additional code (B95-B97) to identify infectious agent.
EXCLUDES 1 abscess of lung (J85.-)
pyothorax due to tuberculosis (A15.6)

SP + J86.0 **Pyothorax with fistula**
Bronchocutaneous fistula
Bronchopleural fistula
Hepatopleural fistula
Mediastinal fistula
Pleural fistula
Thoracic fistula
Any condition classifiable to J86.9 with fistula

SP + J86.9 **Pyothorax without fistula**
Abscess of pleura
Abscess of thorax
Empyema (chest) (lung) (pleura)
Fibrinopurulent pleurisy
Purulent pleurisy
Pyopneumothorax
Septic pleurisy
Seropurulent pleurisy
Suppurative pleurisy

Other diseases of the pleura (J90-J94)

SP J90 **Pleural effusion, not elsewhere classified**
Encysted pleurisy
Pleural effusion NOS
Pleurisy with effusion (exudative) (serous)
EXCLUDES 1 chylous (pleural) effusion (J94.0)
malignant pleural effusion (J91.0))
pleurisy NOS (R09.1)
tuberculous pleural effusion (A15.6)

CODING TIPS✓ Pleural effusion indicates excess pleural fluid built up and accumulated in the pleural lining causing respiratory distress. While often treated in the inpatient setting, pleural effusion may also be treated in home health with interventions such as a PleurX drainage catheter and other respiratory interventions. Home health should verify the presence or absence of a diagnosed pleural effusion to clarify a need to report the diagnosis as active.

4 J91 **Pleural effusion in conditions classified elsewhere**
EXCLUDES 2 pleural effusion in heart failure (I50.-)
pleural effusion in systemic lupus erythematosus (M32.13)

IQ J91.0 **Malignant pleural effusion**
Code first:
underlying neoplasm
DEFINITION Dangerous fluid accumulation between the layers of the membrane lining the chest cavity and lungs, most often caused by cancers of the breast, lung, or lymph nodes.

M IQ J91.8 ***Pleural effusion in other conditions classified elsewhere***
Code first underlying disease, such as:
filariasis (B74.0-B74.9)
influenza (J09.X2, J10.1, J11.1)

CODING TIPS✓ Pleural effusion (J91.8) may be used for pleural effusion in systemic lupus erythematosus and pleural effusion in heart failure. The code J91.8 is coded after the condition causing the pleural effusion. Pleural effusion is ordinarily integral to heart failure and is not coded separately. However, if the pleural effusion requires separate treatment, i.e. chest tube for drainage, then add the code for pleural effusion.

4 **J92 Pleural plaque**
INCLUDES pleural thickening

SP **J92.0 Pleural plaque with presence of asbestos**

SP **J92.9 Pleural plaque without asbestos**
Pleural plaque NOS

4 **J93 Pneumothorax and air leak**
EXCLUDES 1 congenital or perinatal pneumothorax (P25.1)
postprocedural air leak (J95.812)
postprocedural pneumothorax (J95.811)
traumatic pneumothorax (S27.0)
tuberculous (current disease) pneumothorax (A15.-)
pyopneumothorax (J86.-)

CODING TIPS✓ Spontaneous pneumothorax may be primary or secondary and thus related to various other conditions. Some causes of secondary pneumothorax include cystic fibrosis, spontaneous rupture of the esophagus, Marfan's syndrome, lymphangioleiomyomatosis, metastatic cancer, primary lung cancer, catamenial, pneumocystis carinii pneumonia, and eosinophilic pneumonia.

SP **J93.0 Spontaneous tension pneumothorax**

5 **J93.1 Other spontaneous pneumothorax**

SP **J93.11 Primary spontaneous pneumothorax**

IQ **J93.12 Secondary spontaneous pneumothorax**
Code first underlying condition, such as:
catamenial pneumothorax due to endometriosis (N80.8)
cystic fibrosis (E84.-)
eosinophilic pneumonia (J82)
lymphangioleiomyomatosis (J84.81)
malignant neoplasm of bronchus and lung (C34.-)
Marfan's syndrome (Q87.4)
pneumonia due to Pneumocystis carinii (B59)
secondary malignant neoplasm of lung (C78.0-)
spontaneous rupture of the esophagus (K22.3)

5 **J93.8 Other pneumothorax and air leak**

SP **J93.81 Chronic pneumothorax**

SP **J93.82 Other air leak**
Persistent air leak

SP **J93.83 Other pneumothorax**
Acute pneumothorax
Spontaneous pneumothorax NOS

SP **J93.9 Pneumothorax, unspecified**
Pneumothorax NOS

4 **J94 Other pleural conditions**
EXCLUDES 1 pleurisy NOS (R09.1)
traumatic hemopneumothorax (S27.2)
traumatic hemothorax (S27.1)
tuberculous pleural conditions (current disease) (A15.-)

SP **J94.0 Chylous effusion**
Chyliform effusion

SP **J94.1 Fibrothorax**

SP **J94.2 Hemothorax**
Hemopneumothorax

SP **J94.8 Other specified pleural conditions**
Hydropneumothorax
Hydrothorax

IQ **J94.9 Pleural condition, unspecified**

Intraoperative and postprocedural complications and disorders of respiratory system, not elsewhere classified (J95)

4 **J95 Intraoperative and postprocedural complications and disorders of respiratory system, not elsewhere classified**
EXCLUDES 2 aspiration pneumonia (J69.-)
emphysema (subcutaneous) resulting from a procedure (T81.82)
hypostatic pneumonia (J18.2)
pulmonary manifestations due to radiation (J70.0-J70.1)

CODING TIPS✓ **Documentation:** Codes in category J95.- are complication codes and require physician or NPP documentation and confirmation of a cause and effect relationship between the procedure and the complicated condition. Documentation in the home health clinical record must also support this relationship. They may be described as "post-status" or "post-op."

5 **J95.0 Tracheostomy complications**
CODING TIPS✓ Do not use Z93.0 or Z43.0 codes when assigning any code from subcategory J95.0-.

IQ **J95.00 Unspecified tracheostomy complication**

SP **J95.01 Hemorrhage from tracheostomy stoma**

SP + **J95.02 Infection of tracheostomy stoma**
Use additional code to identify type of infection, such as:
cellulitis of neck (L03.221)
sepsis (A40, A41.-)

CODING TIPS✓ When coding J95.02, use an additional code to indicate the infection, such as cellulitis, sepsis, or the infectious organism, when the specific information is available.

SP **J95.03 Malfunction of tracheostomy stoma**
Mechanical complication of tracheostomy stoma
Obstruction of tracheostomy airway
Tracheal stenosis due to tracheostomy

Chapter 10 J00-J99

SP **J95.04 Tracheo-esophageal fistula following tracheostomy**

SP **J95.09 Other tracheostomy complication**

CODING TIPS✓ Use this code along with L24.B2 for contact irritant dermatitis related to the respiratory fistula or stoma.

SP **J95.1 Acute pulmonary insufficiency following thoracic surgery**

EXCLUDES 2 Functional disturbances following cardiac surgery (I97.0, I97.1-)

SP **J95.2 Acute pulmonary insufficiency following nonthoracic surgery**

EXCLUDES 2 Functional disturbances following cardiac surgery (I97.0, I97.1-)

SP **J95.3 Chronic pulmonary insufficiency following surgery**

EXCLUDES 2 Functional disturbances following cardiac surgery (I97.0, I97.1-)

SP + **J95.4 Chemical pneumonitis due to anesthesia**

Mendelson's syndrome

Postprocedural aspiration pneumonia

Use additional code for adverse effect, if applicable, to identify drug (T41.- with fifth or sixth character 5)

EXCLUDES 1 aspiration pneumonitis due to anesthesia complicating labor and delivery (O74.0)
aspiration pneumonitis due to anesthesia complicating pregnancy (O29)
aspiration pneumonitis due to anesthesia complicating the puerperium (O89.01)

SP **J95.5 Postprocedural subglottic stenosis**

5 **J95.6 Intraoperative hemorrhage and hematoma of a respiratory system organ or structure complicating a procedure**

EXCLUDES 1 intraoperative hemorrhage and hematoma of a respiratory system organ or structure due to accidental puncture and laceration during procedure (J95.7-)

SP **J95.61 Intraoperative hemorrhage and hematoma of a respiratory system organ or structure complicating a respiratory system procedure**

SP **J95.62 Intraoperative hemorrhage and hematoma of a respiratory system organ or structure complicating other procedure**

5 **J95.7 Accidental puncture and laceration of a respiratory system organ or structure during a procedure**

EXCLUDES 2 postprocedural pneumothorax (J95.811)

SP **J95.71 Accidental puncture and laceration of a respiratory system organ or structure during a respiratory system procedure**

SP **J95.72 Accidental puncture and laceration of a respiratory system organ or structure during other procedure**

5 **J95.8 Other intraoperative and postprocedural complications and disorders of respiratory system, not elsewhere classified**

6 **J95.81 Postprocedural pneumothorax and air leak**

SP **J95.811 Postprocedural pneumothorax**

SP **J95.812 Postprocedural air leak**

6 **J95.82 Postprocedural respiratory failure**

EXCLUDES 1 Respiratory failure in other conditions (J96.-)

SP **J95.821 Acute postprocedural respiratory failure**

Postprocedural respiratory failure NOS

SP **J95.822 Acute and chronic postprocedural respiratory failure**

6 **J95.83 Postprocedural hemorrhage of a respiratory system organ or structure following a procedure**

SP **J95.830 Postprocedural hemorrhage of a respiratory system organ or structure following a respiratory system procedure**

SP **J95.831 Postprocedural hemorrhage of a respiratory system organ or structure following other procedure**

SP **J95.84 Transfusion-related acute lung injury (TRALI)**

6 **J95.85 Complication of respirator [ventilator]**

SP **J95.850 Mechanical complication of respirator**

EXCLUDES 1 encounter for respirator [ventilator] dependence during power failure (Z99.12)

SP + **J95.851 Ventilator associated pneumonia**

Ventilator associated pneumonitis

Use additional code to identify the organism, if known (B95.-, B96.-, B97.-)

EXCLUDES 1 ventilator lung in newborn (P27.8)

CODING TIPS✓ VAP is not considered an infection for the purpose of using J44.0.

SP **J95.859 Other complication of respirator [ventilator]**

6 **J95.86 Postprocedural hematoma and seroma of a respiratory system organ or structure following a procedure**

SP **J95.860 Postprocedural hematoma of a respiratory system organ or structure following a respiratory system procedure**

SP **J95.861 Postprocedural hematoma of a respiratory system organ or structure following other procedure**

SP **J95.862 Postprocedural seroma of a respiratory system organ or structure following a respiratory system procedure**

SP J95.863 **Postprocedural seroma of a respiratory system organ or structure following other procedure**

SP J95.88 **Other intraoperative complications of respiratory system, not elsewhere classified**

SP + J95.89 **Other postprocedural complications and disorders of respiratory system, not elsewhere classified**
Use additional code to identify disorder, such as:
aspiration pneumonia (J69.-)
bacterial or viral pneumonia (J12-J18)
EXCLUDES 2 acute pulmonary insufficiency following thoracic surgery (J95.1)
postprocedural subglottic stenosis (J95.5)

Other diseases of the respiratory system (J96-J99)

4 J96 **Respiratory failure, not elsewhere classified**
EXCLUDES 1 acute respiratory distress syndrome (J80)
cardiorespiratory failure (R09.2)
newborn respiratory distress syndrome (P22.0)
postprocedural respiratory failure (J95.82-)
respiratory arrest (R09.2)
respiratory arrest of newborn (P28.81)
respiratory failure of newborn (P28.5)

CODING TIPS ✓ Respiratory failure can be acute (rapid onset) or chronic (ongoing). Acute respiratory failure can develop quickly and may require emergency treatment. Chronic respiratory failure develops more slowly and lasts longer. If the physician or NPP documents both acute and chronic respiratory failure, report a code from J96.2.

5 J96.0 **Acute respiratory failure**
GUIDELINES **Section I.C.1.g.1)(c)(v)**
For acute respiratory failure due to COVID-19, assign code U07.1, and code J96.0-, Acute respiratory failure.

SP J96.00 **Acute respiratory failure, unspecified whether with hypoxia or hypercapnia**

SP J96.01 **Acute respiratory failure with hypoxia**

SP J96.02 **Acute respiratory failure with hypercapnia**

5 J96.1 **Chronic respiratory failure**

SP J96.10 **Chronic respiratory failure, unspecified whether with hypoxia or hypercapnia**

SP J96.11 **Chronic respiratory failure with hypoxia**

SP J96.12 **Chronic respiratory failure with hypercapnia**

5 J96.2 **Acute and chronic respiratory failure**
Acute on chronic respiratory failure

SP J96.20 **Acute and chronic respiratory failure, unspecified whether with hypoxia or hypercapnia**

SP J96.21 **Acute and chronic respiratory failure with hypoxia**

SP J96.22 **Acute and chronic respiratory failure with hypercapnia**

5 J96.9 **Respiratory failure, unspecified**

SP J96.90 **Respiratory failure, unspecified, unspecified whether with hypoxia or hypercapnia**

SP J96.91 **Respiratory failure, unspecified with hypoxia**

SP J96.92 **Respiratory failure, unspecified with hypercapnia**

+ 4 J98 **Other respiratory disorders**
Use additional code to identify:
exposure to environmental tobacco smoke (Z77.22)
exposure to tobacco smoke in the perinatal period (P96.81)
history of tobacco dependence (Z87.891)
occupational exposure to environmental tobacco smoke (Z57.31)
tobacco dependence (F17.-)
tobacco use (Z72.0)
EXCLUDES 1 newborn apnea (P28.4)
newborn sleep apnea (P28.3)
EXCLUDES 2 apnea NOS (R06.81)
sleep apnea (G47.3-)

+ 5 J98.0 **Diseases of bronchus, not elsewhere classified**

SP + J98.01 **Acute bronchospasm**
EXCLUDES 1 acute bronchiolitis with bronchospasm (J21.-)
acute bronchitis with bronchospasm (J20.-)
asthma (J45.-)
exercise induced bronchospasm (J45.990)
DEFINITION Constriction or contraction of the smooth muscle in the large air passages, severely limiting airflow.

SP + J98.09 **Other diseases of bronchus, not elsewhere classified**
Broncholithiasis
Calcification of bronchus
Stenosis of bronchus
Tracheobronchial collapse
Tracheobronchial dyskinesia
Ulcer of bronchus

+ 5 J98.1 **Pulmonary collapse**
EXCLUDES 1 therapeutic collapse of lung status (Z98.3)

SP + J98.11 **Atelectasis**
EXCLUDES 1 newborn atelectasis
tuberculous atelectasis (current disease) (A15)

SP + J98.19 **Other pulmonary collapse**

SP + J98.2 **Interstitial emphysema**
Mediastinal emphysema
EXCLUDES 1 emphysema NOS (J43.9)

Chapter 10 J00-J99

emphysema in newborn (P25.0)
surgical emphysema (subcutaneous) (T81.82)
traumatic subcutaneous emphysema (T79.7)

SP + **J98.3 Compensatory emphysema**

SP + **J98.4 Other disorders of lung**
Calcification of lung
Cystic lung disease (acquired)
Lung disease NOS
Pulmolithiasis
EXCLUDES 1 acute interstitial pneumonitis (J84.114)
pulmonary insufficiency following surgery (J95.1-J95.2)

+ 5 **J98.5 Diseases of mediastinum, not elsewhere classified**
EXCLUDES 2 abscess of mediastinum (J85.3)

SP + **J98.51 Mediastinitis**
Code first:
underlying condition, if applicable, such as postoperative mediastinitis (T81.-)

SP + **J98.59 Other diseases of mediastinum, not elsewhere classified**
Fibrosis of mediastinum
Hernia of mediastinum
Retraction of mediastinum

SP + **J98.6 Disorders of diaphragm**
Diaphragmatitis
Paralysis of diaphragm
Relaxation of diaphragm
EXCLUDES 1 congenital malformation of diaphragm NEC (Q79.1)
congenital diaphragmatic hernia (Q79.0)
EXCLUDES 2 diaphragmatic hernia (K44.-)

SP + **J98.8 Other specified respiratory disorders**
CODING TIPS ✓ For a respiratory infection confirmed as due to COVID-19, but not otherwise specified, assign U07.1 and J98.8.

IQ + **J98.9 Respiratory disorder, unspecified**
Respiratory disease (chronic) NOS

▲ M IQ **J99 *Respiratory disorders in diseases classified elsewhere***
Code first underlying disease, such as:
amyloidosis (E85.-)
ankylosing spondylitis (M45)
congenital syphilis (A50.5)
cryoglobulinemia (D89.1)
early congenital syphilis (A50.0)
plasminogen deficiency (E88.02)
schistosomiasis (B65.0-B65.9)
EXCLUDES 1 respiratory disorders in:
amebiasis (A06.5)
blastomycosis (B40.0-B40.2)
candidiasis (B37.1)
coccidioidomycosis (B38.0-B38.2)
cystic fibrosis with pulmonary manifestations (E84.0)
dermatomyositis (M33.01, M33.11)
histoplasmosis (B39.0-B39.2)
late syphilis (A52.72, A52.73)
polymyositis (M33.21)
Sjögren syndrome (M35.02)
systemic lupus erythematosus (M32.13)
systemic sclerosis (M34.81)
Wegener's granulomatosis (M31.30-M31.31)

Chapter 10 Scenarios: Diseases of the respiratory system (J00-J99)

Exacerbated COPD with emphysema and acute bronchitis

An 87-year-old man was hospitalized with a severe case of acute bronchitis, which caused an exacerbation of his COPD with emphysema. He is admitted to home health with still-resolving bronchitis, which is the focus of care, and to help get his emphysema back under control. The patient will be taking oral antibiotics for the next three weeks. He smoked cigarettes as a young man but quit several years ago.

Description	Code
Primary: Acute bronchitis, unspecified	J20.9
Secondary: Emphysema, unspecified	J43.9
Secondary: Long term (current) use of antibiotics	Z79.2
Secondary: Personal history of nicotine dependence	Z87.891

Codes J20.9 and J43.9 are assigned for the patient with his acute bronchitis, and exacerbated COPD with emphysema, according to Q1 2019 Coding Clinic guidance. As the focus of care, the acute bronchitis is coded in the primary position. The patient is taking antibiotics for three weeks, prompting the assignment of Z79.2. Since he has a history of tobacco use and a diagnosis from Chapter 10 (J00-J99), Z87.891 is also assigned. There is a chapter-level tabular instruction covering all of Chapter 10, instructing the coder to assign a code if the patient has been exposed to tobacco, or is a current or former user of tobacco.

Chronic obstructive bronchitis with chronic obstructive asthma, hypertension

A 75-year-old male patient is admitted to home care with a primary diagnosis of exacerbated chronic obstructive bronchitis with chronic obstructive mild intermittent asthma also exacerbated. He also has hypertension. His history and physical says that he was a cigarette smoker for several decades but quit 12 years ago.

Description	Code
Primary: Chronic obstructive pulmonary disease with acute exacerbation	J44.1
Secondary: Mild intermittent asthma with (acute) exacerbation	J45.21
Secondary: Hypertension	I10
Secondary: Personal history of nicotine dependence	Z87.891

The patient's exacerbated chronic obstructive bronchitis is captured with J44.1. Because the patient's asthma is specified as mild intermittent asthma, which is also exacerbated, a code should also be assigned to identify the asthma. Hypertension is assigned as a relevant comorbidity. The code for history of tobacco use, required for all codes in Chapter 10 due to chapter-level tabular instruction, is included to capture that the patient is a former smoker.

Emphysema, congestive heart failure, smoker

A 78-year-old female patient is admitted to home health with a primary diagnosis of emphysema. She also has congestive heart failure and the physician documents she is a long-time current cigarette smoker.

Description	Code
Primary: Emphysema, unspecified	J43.9
Secondary: Congestive heart failure, unspecified	I50.9
Secondary: Nicotine dependence, cigarettes, uncomplicated	F17.210

With no other information known about the patient's emphysema, J43.9 is the most appropriate code choice. Congestive heart failure is a relevant comorbidity and is also assigned. Because the patient continues to smoke cigarettes, an additional code is required to report this. The correct code for the cigarette smoking is F17.210, as this is where the alphabetic index leads.

Aftercare of surgery, respiratory issues, GI issues

The patient had gall bladder surgery due to cholecystitis but had an exacerbation of her chronic obstructive bronchitis while in the hospital and additionally developed bacterial pneumonia, which is still being treated with oral antibiotic therapy for 10 days. She also has a gastrostomy that is infected. Her gastrostomy was placed last year because of dysphagia. The focus of care is the exacerbated COPD but she will also receive speech therapy to address the dysphagia.

Description	Code
Primary: Chronic obstructive pulmonary disease with acute exacerbation	J44.1
Secondary: Chronic obstructive pulmonary disease with (acute) lower respiratory infection	J44.0
Secondary: Unspecified bacterial pneumonia	J15.9
Secondary: Gastrostomy infection	K94.22
Secondary: Dysphagia, unspecified	R13.10
Secondary: Encounter for surgical aftercare following surgery on the digestive system	Z48.815

This is a situation in which the patient had surgery, but the aftercare is not the focus of care. Both J44.1 and J44.0 are used as this patient developed an acute lower respiratory tract infection, as well as an exacerbation of her COPD. The Excludes 2 note at J44.1 allows the coder to code both COPD codes. To further specify the lower respiratory tract infection in accordance with tabular instruction, J15.9 (Unspecified bacterial pneumonia) is assigned in this scenario. Code Z43.1 should not be used for the gastrostomy because the gastrostomy is complicated. Dysphagia is coded only if it is a current diagnosis and is addressed by the plan of care, which it is in this case. No code for antibiotic use is assigned because the patient will remain on antibiotics for only 10 days.

Pneumonia, chronic obstructive bronchitis

A patient with chronic obstructive bronchitis is admitted with pneumonia that is still under treatment. The patient's physician confirms that the chronic obstructive bronchitis is acutely exacerbated. Hospitalization records indicate that upon admission the patient was tested for COVID-19 due to known exposure, but tested negative x 2. The pneumonia is the focus of care.

Description	Code
Primary: Pneumonia, unspecified organism	J18.9
Secondary: Chronic obstructive pulmonary disease with (acute) lower respiratory infection	J44.0
Secondary: Chronic obstructive pulmonary disease with (acute) exacerbation	J44.1
Secondary: Contact with and (suspected) exposure to COVID-19	Z20.822

Since the pneumonia is the focus of care, it is coded before both the chronic obstructive bronchitis with lower respiratory infection, and the exacerbated chronic obstructive bronchitis codes. Because the tabular instruction at J44.0 is "code also," either the COPD with lower respiratory infection code, or the code for the infection itself could be sequenced first, depending on the focus of care. The Excludes 2 note at the J44.1 code level directs the coder that chronic obstructive pulmonary disease with a lower respiratory infection is not included in the J44.1 code and, if present, should be coded separately. For cases where there is an actual exposure to someone who is confirmed or suspected (not ruled out) to have COVID-19, and the exposed individual either tests negative or the test results are unknown, assign code Z20.822 per coding guidelines.

Influenza with pneumonia, congestive heart failure

A 92-year-old woman was treated in the hospital with influenza type A that led to a case of klebsiella pneumonia. Upon release from the hospital, she is admitted to home health, but is still taking Tamiflu and antibiotics, as her influenza and pneumonia have not yet completely resolved. She has a long history of chronic systolic congestive heart failure, which is currently stable, but her physician is concerned about the chronic condition decompensating due to the infection the patient is continuing to fight. Other comorbidities include insulin-dependent diabetes and non-dominant left-sided hemiplegia from an old CVA.

Description	Code
Primary: Influenza due to other identified influenza virus with other specified pneumonia	J10.08
Secondary: Pneumonia due to Klebsiella pneumoniae	J15.0
Secondary: Chronic systolic (congestive) heart failure	I50.22
Secondary: Hemiplegia and hemiparesis following cerebral infarction affecting left non-dominant side	I69.354
Secondary: Type 2 diabetes mellitus without complications	E11.9
Secondary: Long term (current) use of insulin	Z79.4

The patient is still being treated for the influenza with pneumonia and it is the focus of are, so it is coded primary. This patient has type A influenza, which is a specific type, but not a novel variant, so a code from category J10 is assigned. Since the type of pneumonia resulting from the influenza is a specified type, but not the same as the influenza type, J10.08 must be used. Her physician is worried that her chronic systolic congestive heart failure may decompensate due to the influenza and pneumonia, and while it is currently stable, it is being closely monitored and thus it is coded directly following the primary diagnosis of influenza with pneumonia. The patient's diabetes and the residual effects of the prior CVA are also listed as these conditions impact prognosis and some may provide important comorbidity adjustment.

MSSA pneumonia

A 71-year-old man was recently hospitalized for treatment of pneumonia, which was caused by staphylococcus aureus bacteria. He improved sufficiently in the hospital and was discharged to home health for continued treatment on a long-term course of oral antibiotic drugs. Three years ago he underwent a kidney transplant and still has stage 2 chronic kidney disease, diabetes with peripheral neuropathy, and hypertension. His diabetes is controlled with oral hypoglycemic medication.

Description	Code
Primary: Pneumonia due to Methicillin susceptible Staphylococcus aureus	J15.211
Secondary: Hypertensive chronic kidney disease with stage 1 through stage 4 chronic kidney disease, or unspecified chronic kidney disease	I12.9
Secondary: Type 2 diabetes mellitus with diabetic chronic kidney disease	E11.22
Secondary: Chronic kidney disease, stage 2 (mild)	N18.2
Secondary: Type 2 diabetes mellitus with diabetic polyneuropathy	E11.42
Secondary: Kidney transplant status	Z94.0
Secondary: Long term (current) use of antibiotics	Z79.2
Secondary: Long term (current) use of oral hypoglycemic drugs	Z79.84

No separate infecting organism code is required in this scenario because it is included in the pneumonia code. Though the patient underwent a kidney transplant, he still has stage 2 chronic kidney disease. Hypertension and chronic kidney disease are assumed to be related and are coded as such, as hypertensive chronic kidney disease, in accordance with coding guidelines. Diabetes and chronic kidney disease are also assumed to be related and E11.22 is assigned to represent this prior to the chronic kidney disease code. The patient is taking oral antibiotics but the course is long-term, making the use of Z79.2 appropriate. An additional code for diabetic polyneuropathy is assigned as this may impact the patient's prognosis and care plan. Coding guidelines require the assignment of an additional code for the use of oral hypoglycemic drugs in type 2 diabetes patients who are using these medications, but not using insulin.

MRSA pneumonia, exacerbated chronic obstructive asthma

A 75-year-old woman is admitted to home health after being hospitalized with MRSA pneumonia, which caused an acute exacerbation of her chronic obstructive asthma. The pneumonia is still resolving and is the focus of care. She will continue taking oral antibiotics for the several weeks.

Description	Code
Primary: Pneumonia due to Methicillin resistant Staphylococcus aureus	J15.212
Secondary: Chronic obstructive pulmonary disease with (acute) lower respiratory infection	J44.0
Secondary: Chronic obstructive pulmonary disease with (acute) exacerbation	J44.1
Secondary: Long term (current) use of antibiotics	Z79.2

As the focus of care, the pneumonia is assigned in the primary position. The code for chronic obstructive asthma with a lower respiratory infection comes next, followed by a code for acutely exacerbated COPD, to show that the pneumonia caused an exacerbation of the chronic condition. An Excludes 2 note on J44.0 allows their assignment of both J44.- codes. Code Z79.2 is assigned to capture continued antibiotics for the next several weeks.

Aspiration pneumonia, Alzheimer's

An 81-year-old woman is admitted following hospitalization to home health with a primary diagnosis of aspiration pneumonia due to choking on an unspecified piece of food during dinner, which was later recovered, but caused infection. She suffers from chronic emphysematous bronchitis and Alzheimer's disease. She will continue on a brief course of oral liquid antibiotics.

Description	Code
Primary: Pneumonitis due to inhalation of food and vomit	J69.0
Secondary: Food in respiratory tract, part unspecified causing asphyxiation, subsequent encounter	T17.920D
Secondary: Chronic obstructive pulmonary disease, unspecified	J44.9
Secondary: Alzheimer's disease, unspecified	G30.9
Secondary: Dementia in other diseases classified elsewhere without behavioral disturbance	F02.80

The primary diagnosis is aspiration pneumonia due to aspirated food, which codes to J69.0. Code J44.9 is assigned to capture her respiratory condition, and not J44.0, as aspiration pneumonia is not considered a respiratory infection that is included under that code, according to Q1 2017 Coding Clinic guidance. See the "code also" note at J69.0 that indicates to add the appropriate code from category T17.- to indicate any associated foreign body in the respiratory tract (with the appropriate 7th character). In this case, the patient choked on a piece of food. A search of "choked, food" in the alphabetic index directs the coder to "see foreign body by site". The term choke is synonymous with asphyxiation. Searching "Foreign body, respiratory tract, causing, asphyxiation, food" directs the coder to T17.920. The 7th character "D" is selected as the condition is not resolved but does not require specific active treatment. Her Alzheimer's disease is an important comorbidity and is thus coded. Dementia is assigned as a manifestation of Alzheimer's disease. While dementia is not specifically stated, it should be coded along with G30.9, according to Q1 2017 Coding Clinic guidance.

Chemical pneumonia

A 57-year-old man is admitted to home health with a primary diagnosis of chemical pneumonia that his physician diagnosed as caused by inhaling excessive smoke from a campfire. He also has type 2 diabetes and PVD and takes oral hypoglycemic medication.

Description	Code
Primary: Toxic effect of smoke, accidental (unintentional), subsequent encounter	T59.811D
Secondary: Bronchitis and pneumonitis due to chemicals, gases, fumes and vapors	J68.0
Secondary: Type 2 diabetes mellitus with diabetic peripheral angiopathy without gangrene	E11.51
Secondary: Exposure to smoke in controlled fire, not in building or structure, subsequent encounter	X03.1xxD
Secondary: Long term (current) use of oral hypoglycemic drugs	Z79.84

The patient's pneumonia was caused by inhaling excessive smoke during a campfire. Because it is caused by fumes, it is chemical pneumonia. Chemical pneumonia codes to J68.0, according to the alphabetic index. The code for the unintentional poisoning from the smoke is assigned before the pneumonia code, in accordance with tabular instruction. The patient's diabetes and PVD, which can be assumed to be connected via the alphabetic index, are also captured together with the combination code E11.51. An external cause code is used to help show how the patient developed chemical pneumonia, from exposure to smoke. Code Z79.84 is assigned to show that he takes oral hypoglycemic medication for his diabetes.

Post COVID organizing pneumonia

A patient is admitted to home health for nursing and therapy after an extended inpatient stay including acute hospitalization, LTACH, and SNF due to exacerbation of COPD and acute on chronic hypoxic respiratory failure. The patient was tested multiple times during her stay for COVID-19 and had no negative tests, but her physician has documented on her discharge paperwork that she have a positive antibody test for COVID-19 with unknown infection date, "now demonstrating post COVID organizing pneumonia." Home health will focus on the COPD exacerbation and overall respiratory issues.

Description	Code
Primary: Chronic obstructive pulmonary disease with (acute) exacerbation	J44.1
Secondary: Other specified interstitial pulmonary diseases	J84.89
Secondary: Post COVID-19 condition, unspecified	U09.9
Secondary: Acute and chronic respiratory failure with hypoxia	J96.21

The focus of care for this episode is the exacerbation of COPD, so this is listed first. The patient was also given a diagnosis of "post COVID organizing pneumonia" and this should be coded as a sequela of COVID-19, per Q1 2021 coding clinic guidance. Effective 10/1/21, the appropriate code for sequela(e) of COVID-19 conditions should be coded by first assigning the code(s) for residual conditions, followed by U09.9. Because this patient has an existing, unresolved condition due to COVID-19, the history of COVID-19 is not sequenced. J96.21 is also listed to indicate the patient has unresolved acute on hypoxic respiratory failure that will be addressed. It should not be assumed that acute respiratory failure has resolved unless so stated by the provider.

Chapter 11: Diseases of the Digestive System (K00- K95)

Chapter 11 includes diseases of the organs of the digestive system: a long, twisting tube stretching from the mouth through the esophagus, stomach, small and large intestines, and ending at the anus. Other areas related to the mouth (teeth, jaws, salivary glands) are also coded in this chapter. Diseases of organs that assist the digestive process (liver, gallbladder, pancreas) are included, as well as diseases of the ducts that carry enzymes and digestive juices from these organs to the intestines (the biliary tract, including the hepatic, cystic and common bile ducts). Finally, this chapter includes conditions affecting the peritoneum (membrane surrounding the organs in the abdominal cavity).

In certain situations you'll need to look beyond this chapter to properly code a case. Here are a few examples of such cases:

- If the documentation indicates a **neoplasm or tumor of an organ in the digestive system**, coders should look up the term (malignancy, tumor, adenoma) to find the correct code, most likely a code from Chapter 2.
- If a patient has a **personal or family history** of a condition reported in this chapter, it may be appropriate to select from chapter 21, the Z code section, such as Z87.11 (Personal history of peptic ulcer disease) or Z87.19 (Personal history of diseases of digestive system), subcategory Z85.0- (Personal history of malignant neoplasm of digestive organs), Z83.79 (Family history of other diseases of digestive system), or Z80.0 (Family history of malignant neoplasm of digestive organs).
- **Symptoms** related to the digestive system are sometimes reported using codes from Chapter 18, such as code series R19.8 (Symptoms involving digestive system and abdomen). Every effort should be made to secure a definitive diagnosis. A symptom code from Chapter 18 may be reported as an additional diagnosis when it describes a significant aspect of the condition but is not an integral part of it.
- Although not coded often in home health, if reporting a **digestive system disease in a pregnant patient** when the condition is complicating the pregnancy, report first a code from Chapter 15, for example O26.61- (Liver and biliary tract disorders in pregnancy), as the first-listed diagnosis and K76.9 (Liver disease unspecified) from this chapter as an additional diagnosis.

Complications of artificial openings of the digestive system are reported using codes from category K94 in this chapter. Each type of ostomy includes specific codes for unspecified complication, hemorrhage, infection (with a note to add an additional code to specify the type of infection), mechanical malfunction and "other" complication. For example, an infection of an esophagostomy is reported using code K94.32 (with an additional code to identify the infection); a mechanical complication of a colostomy is coded as K94.03; a hemorrhage of a gastrostomy is coded as K94.21; and an "other" complication of an enterostomy would be reported as K94.19.

Be aware that if the ostomy is complicated, the complication code is used rather than the Z93.- code for 'status' or the Z43.- code for 'attention to' an artificial opening.

Multiple Coding and Sequencing

Includes and Excludes notes are important to follow, as well as any other instructions under the code or code category. The following are some examples of multiple coding and sequencing issues for codes in this chapter.

- **Peritonitis** is reported using category K65. A note under this code states: use an additional code (B95-B97) if known, to identify infectious agent. Pay close attention to the Excludes 1 note under code K65, since there are many types of peritonitis that are coded using a combination code found in other chapters. Examples include: gonococcal peritonitis (A54.85), neonatal peritonitis (P78.0-P78.1), or aseptic or chemical peritonitis (T81.6-).
- K67 is used as a second diagnosis for disorders of the **peritoneum in infectious diseases** classified elsewhere and includes a note to code first the underlying condition such as helminthiasis (B65.0-B83.9).
- Disorders such as K12.- **(stomatitis and related lesions)** include an extensive note following the category code to use additional codes to identify alcohol abuse and dependence (F10.-) and exposure to tobacco smoke as well as tobacco use, dependence and history of dependence.
- **Oral mucositis** (ulcerative) has notes to add additional codes relative to the cause of the disorder. For example, K12.31 (Mucositis due to antineoplastic therapy) has two instructional notes following the code: use additional code for adverse effect, if applicable, to identify antineoplastic and immunosuppressive drugs (T45.1x5), and use additional code for other neoplastic therapy, such as radiological procedure and radiotherapy (Y84.2).

- Disorders such as **oral thrush (candidiasis)** are not coded in chapter 11. Instead the code is found as a combination code in chapter 1 at B37.0 and provides all of the necessary information with a single code.
- Code K31.84 (**gastroparesis**) includes a note: Code first underlying disease such as anorexia nervosa (F50.0-), scleroderma (M34-) or diabetes mellitus (E08.43, E09.43, E10.43, E11.43, E13.43). However, gastroparesis may be coded alone if the underlying cause is unknown.
- Code K62.81 (**Anal sphincter tear** [healed, old]) includes a note that states: Use additional code for any associated fecal incontinence (R15-).

Special Coding Issues

Ulcers

This chapter includes codes for ulcers (sores or lesions that form in the lining of the stomach or intestinal tract). Code selection depends on the location (stomach, small and large intestine), whether the ulcer is acute, chronic, perforated (lesion extends to entire thickness of organ), hemorrhaging (bleeding), or causing obstruction. Check the physician's documentation carefully in order to report the correct code.

- Category K25.- (stomach ulcer) is used to report a gastric ulcer.
- Category K26.- (duodenal ulcer) is used to report an ulcer involving the duodenum (first section of the small intestine).
- Category K28.- (gastrojejunal ulcer) is used to report an ulcer involving the stomach and jejuneum (second section of the small intestine).
- Category K27.9 (peptic ulcer, site unspecified) is used to report an ulcer in these cases:
  - Ulcer described as gastroduodenal (involving the stomach and duodenum),
  - Ulcer described as a peptic or stress ulcer, or
  - Ulcer is documented as present in digestive tract, but its location is not designated.

Ulcers of the large intestine are reported using codes from either series K51.- (ulcerative colitis), code K63.3 (ulceration of intestine) or code K63.1 (perforation of intestine). If the ulcer is documented as colitis (noninfectious ulcerative colitis), report code K52.9.

Once the location of an ulcer is determined, it's important to recognize the distinguishing factors that most often will lead to the appropriate 4th character. The 4th character denotes whether the ulcer is acute or chronic and whether or not it involves hemorrhage and/or perforation.

Hepatitis

Be careful attaching this diagnosis to your claims. Hepatitis simply means liver inflammation. Do not append a diagnosis of hepatitis because you see elevated liver enzymes on the medical chart because there are two different etiologies for liver inflammation: those due to blockage and those due to infectious or toxic agents.

Hepatitis is due to infectious or toxic agents. Obstructive liver inflammation is not hepatitis. Hepatitis can be caused by alcohol (K70.-), chemical or drug-induced (K71.-), autoimmune (K75.4), or viral (refer to categories B15-B19 in chapter 1), which spans hepatitis A, hepatitis B, hepatitis B with delta and hepatitis C (the most common). Even if an elevated liver enzyme test is present, hepatitis A, B, and C often cannot be differentiated without further lab tests. It is best to use an elevated liver function test diagnosis (code R94.5) until a diagnosis of hepatitis is confirmed. Hepatitis C may be referred to as non-A, non-B or viral.

Once you have a diagnosis, use the patient assessment, coupled with confirmation from the physician, to determine if the hepatitis is: a) chronic or acute, and b) whether it's accompanied by hepatic coma. If newly diagnosed, hepatitis usually is labeled acute since it takes several months to be labeled as chronic. Other diagnosis codes that can be added include those that indicate the mode of transmission, for example, Z20.5 for contact with/exposure to viral hepatitis.

Gastrointestinal Hemorrhage

There are several terms used to describe GI hemorrhage that are linked with the specific area in the GI tract. For example, code K92.2 for GI hemorrhage, unspecified; K29.01 for acute hemorrhagic gastritis; K62.5 for hemorrhage of anus and rectum; K57.- for diverticular disease with hemorrhage; or K25-K28 for peptic ulcer with hemorrhage. The following are some additional terms that describe the presence of GI bleeding:

- Hematemesis, K92.0 (vomiting of blood), indicates acute upper GI hemorrhage;
- Melena, K92.1 (presence of dark-colored blood in the stool), indicates upper or lower GI hemorrhage;
- Occult bleeding (presence of blood in the stool that can be seen only on laboratory exam); and
- Hematochezia/melena (presence of brightly-colored blood in stool), usually indicates blood from the rectum.

Hernias

This chapter also includes codes for hernias in categories K40-K46 (a weakness or defect in the abdominal wall in which the contents of the abdomen protrude into other sites). Check the physician's documentation carefully in order to report the correct code.

Code selection depends first on the location of the hernia: inguinal (into genital area), femoral (into thigh area), umbilical (into area of the navel), hiatal (stomach protruding through the diaphragm), incisional (through an old surgical incision), or ventral (into the front of the abdomen).

Other words describe whether the hernia is obstructing the organs involved. For example, the term "incarcerated" indicates a hernia causing complete obstruction. The term "strangulated" indicates a lack of blood flow to the affected organ due to compression, which can quickly lead to a hernia "with gangrene," in which necrosis or tissue death occurs due to the blocked blood supply and resulting absence of oxygen. You should also know the following terms: unilateral or bilateral (one or both sides, refers to inguinal hernias); recurrent (repaired hernia has reoccurred); reducible, or nonreducible (whether tissue can be put back in its place by manipulation); or sliding (tissue moves into and out of place).

The physician's documentation may include words with the suffix "-cele" or the word "prolapse" (falling, drooping of an organ) to describe hernias. Coders should look up the words used in the documentation to find the correct code since many of the conditions are coded in different body system chapters in ICD-10-CM.

Hernias not related to the digestive system are classified to the system they are associated with. For example, an omphalocele (Q79.2), which is a congenital hernia of the umbilicus, also referred to as an exomphalos, is coded from chapter 17 (Congenital malformations, deformations and chromosomal abnormalities).

Cystocele (herniation of bladder [N81.10]), ureterovaginal prolapse (N81.4), rectocele, prolapse of posterior vaginal wall (N81.6) are other examples of codes found in chapter 14 (Diseases of the genitourinary system) rather than chapter 11.

Constipation

Constipation (Category K59) is the passage of small amounts of hard, dry bowel movements, usually fewer than three times a week. People who are constipated may find it difficult and painful to have a bowel movement. Other symptoms of constipation include feeling bloated, uncomfortable and sluggish.

Constipation codes include:

- Constipation, unspecified (K59.00)
- Slow transit constipation (K59.01)
- Outlet dysfunction constipation (K59.02)
- Drug-induced constipation (K59.03)
- Chronic idiopathic constipation (K59.04)
- Other constipation (K59.09)
- Irritable bowel syndrome with constipation (K58.1)

Diarrhea

Loose, watery stools occurring more than three times in one day is a problem that usually lasts a day or two and resolves on its own. However, prolonged diarrhea can be a sign of other problems and requires use of a more specific code than diarrhea NOS (R19.7), when possible.

Bloody diarrhea is found under Melena (K92.1).

Infectious diarrhea is assigned a code from Chapter 1 when the organism has been identified.

Functional diarrhea is characterized by chronic or recurrent diarrhea not explained by structural or biochemical abnormalities, and is coded with K59.1. This code has an Excludes note: diarrhea, NOS (R19.7); and irritable bowel syndrome with diarrhea (K58.0).

CHAPTER 11: DISEASES OF THE DIGESTIVE SYSTEM (K00-K95)

EXCLUDES 2 certain conditions originating in the perinatal period (P04-P96)
certain infectious and parasitic diseases (A00-B99)
complications of pregnancy, childbirth and the puerperium (O00-O9A)
congenital malformations, deformations and chromosomal abnormalities (Q00-Q99)
endocrine, nutritional and metabolic diseases (E00-E88)
injury, poisoning and certain other consequences of external causes (S00-T88)
neoplasms (C00-D49)
symptoms, signs and abnormal clinical and laboratory findings, not elsewhere classified (R00-R94)

This chapter contains the following blocks:

K00-K14	Diseases of oral cavity and salivary glands
K20-K31	Diseases of esophagus, stomach and duodenum
K35-K38	Diseases of appendix
K40-K46	Hernia
K50-K52	Noninfective enteritis and colitis
K55-K64	Other diseases of intestines
K65-K68	Diseases of peritoneum and retroperitoneum
K70-K77	Diseases of liver
K80-K87	Disorders of gallbladder, biliary tract and pancreas
K90-K95	Other diseases of the digestive system

Diseases of oral cavity and salivary glands (K00-K14)

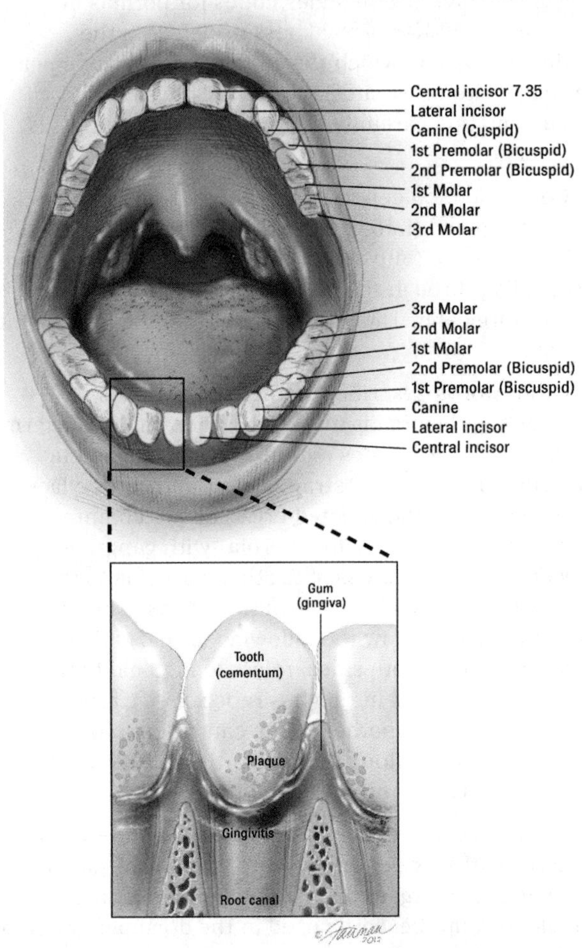

4 K00 Disorders of tooth development and eruption
EXCLUDES 2 embedded and impacted teeth (K01.-)

!Q K00.0 Anodontia
Hypodontia
Oligodontia
EXCLUDES 1 acquired absence of teeth (K08.1-)
DEFINITION Defect in which many or all of the teeth do not develop and are absent from the mouth.

!Q K00.1 Supernumerary teeth
Distomolar
Fourth molar
Mesiodens
Paramolar
Supplementary teeth
EXCLUDES 2 supernumerary roots (K00.2)

!Q K00.2 Abnormalities of size and form of teeth
Concrescence of teeth
Fusion of teeth
Gemination of teeth
Dens evaginatus
Dens in dente
Dens invaginatus

Enamel pearls
Macrodontia
Microdontia
Peg-shaped [conical] teeth
Supernumerary roots
Taurodontism
Tuberculum paramolare
EXCLUDES 1 abnormalities of teeth due to congenital syphilis (A50.5)
tuberculum Carabelli, which is regarded as a normal variation and should not be coded

IQ **K00.3 Mottled teeth**
Dental fluorosis
Mottling of enamel
Nonfluoride enamel opacities
EXCLUDES 2 deposits [accretions] on teeth (K03.6)

IQ **K00.4 Disturbances in tooth formation**
Aplasia and hypoplasia of cementum
Dilaceration of tooth
Enamel hypoplasia (neonatal) (postnatal) (prenatal)
Regional odontodysplasia
Turner's tooth
EXCLUDES 1 Hutchinson's teeth and mulberry molars in congenital syphilis (A50.5)
EXCLUDES 2 mottled teeth (K00.3)

IQ **K00.5 Hereditary disturbances in tooth structure, not elsewhere classified**
Amelogenesis imperfecta
Dentinogenesis imperfecta
Odontogenesis imperfecta
Dentinal dysplasia
Shell teeth

IQ **K00.6 Disturbances in tooth eruption**
Dentia praecox
Natal tooth
Neonatal tooth
Premature eruption of tooth
Premature shedding of primary [deciduous] tooth
Prenatal teeth
Retained [persistent] primary tooth
EXCLUDES 2 embedded and impacted teeth (K01.-)

IQ **K00.7 Teething syndrome**

IQ **K00.8 Other disorders of tooth development**
Color changes during tooth formation
Intrinsic staining of teeth NOS
EXCLUDES 2 posteruptive color changes (K03.7)

IQ **K00.9 Disorder of tooth development, unspecified**
Disorder of odontogenesis NOS

4 **K01 Embedded and impacted teeth**
EXCLUDES 1 abnormal position of fully erupted teeth (M26.3-)

IQ **K01.0 Embedded teeth**

IQ **K01.1 Impacted teeth**

4 **K02 Dental caries**
INCLUDES caries of dentine
dental cavities
early childhood caries
pre-eruptive caries
recurrent caries
(dentino enamel junction)
(enamel) (to the pulp)
tooth decay

IQ **K02.3 Arrested dental caries**
Arrested coronal and root caries

5 **K02.5 Dental caries on pit and fissure surface**
Dental caries on chewing surface of tooth

IQ **K02.51 Dental caries on pit and fissure surface limited to enamel**
White spot lesions [initial caries] on pit and fissure surface of tooth

IQ **K02.52 Dental caries on pit and fissure surface penetrating into dentin**
Primary dental caries, cervical origin

IQ **K02.53 Dental caries on pit and fissure surface penetrating into pulp**

5 **K02.6 Dental caries on smooth surface**

IQ **K02.61 Dental caries on smooth surface limited to enamel**
White spot lesions [initial caries] on smooth surface of tooth

IQ **K02.62 Dental caries on smooth surface penetrating into dentin**

IQ **K02.63 Dental caries on smooth surface penetrating into pulp**

IQ **K02.7 Dental root caries**

IQ **K02.9 Dental caries, unspecified**

4 **K03 Other diseases of hard tissues of teeth**
EXCLUDES 2 bruxism (F45.8)
dental caries (K02.-)
teeth-grinding NOS (F45.8)

IQ **K03.0 Excessive attrition of teeth**
Approximal wear of teeth
Occlusal wear of teeth
DEFINITION Teeth exhibit excessive wear and tear as a result of tooth-to-tooth contact, often due to grinding the teeth.

IQ **K03.1 Abrasion of teeth**
Dentifrice abrasion of teeth
Habitual abrasion of teeth
Occupational abrasion of teeth
Ritual abrasion of teeth
Traditional abrasion of teeth
Wedge defect NOS
DEFINITION Teeth exhibit specific wear and tear as a result of tooth contact with another object.

IQ **K03.2 Erosion of teeth**
Erosion of teeth due to diet
Erosion of teeth due to drugs and medicaments
Erosion of teeth due to persistent vomiting
Erosion of teeth NOS
Idiopathic erosion of teeth
Occupational erosion of teeth

IQ **K03.3 Pathological resorption of teeth**
Internal granuloma of pulp
Resorption of teeth (external)

IQ **K03.4 Hypercementosis**
Cementation hyperplasia

IQ **K03.5 Ankylosis of teeth**
DEFINITION Roots of the teeth grow into and merge with the bone of the jaw; most often occurring during development of baby teeth.

K03.6 Deposits [accretions] on teeth
Betel deposits [accretions] on teeth
Black deposits [accretions] on teeth
Extrinsic staining of teeth NOS
Green deposits [accretions] on teeth
Materia alba deposits [accretions] on teeth
Orange deposits [accretions] on teeth
Staining of teeth NOS
Subgingival dental calculus
Supragingival dental calculus
Tobacco deposits [accretions] on teeth
DEFINITION Calculous deposits or tartar build-up that resists removal by normal brushing and requires professional cleaning.

K03.7 Posteruptive color changes of dental hard tissues
EXCLUDES 2 deposits [accretions] on teeth (K03.6)

K03.8 Other specified diseases of hard tissues of teeth

K03.81 Cracked tooth
EXCLUDES 1 asymptomatic craze lines in enamel - omit code
broken or fractured tooth due to trauma (S02.5)

K03.89 Other specified diseases of hard tissues of teeth

K03.9 Disease of hard tissues of teeth, unspecified

K04 Diseases of pulp and periapical tissues

K04.0 Pulpitis
Acute pulpitis
Chronic (hyperplastic) (ulcerative) pulpitis
DEFINITION Painful inflammation of the soft living tissue containing nerves within the center of the tooth.

K04.01 Reversible pulpitis

K04.02 Irreversible pulpitis

K04.1 Necrosis of pulp
Pulpal gangrene

K04.2 Pulp degeneration
Denticles
Pulpal calcifications
Pulpal stones

K04.3 Abnormal hard tissue formation in pulp
Secondary or irregular dentine

K04.4 Acute apical periodontitis of pulpal origin
Acute apical periodontitis NOS
EXCLUDES 1 acute periodontitis (K05.2-)
DEFINITION Severe inflammation of the periodontal ligament connecting the tooth to the jawbone due to infection or necrosis of the soft, living tissue in the center of the tooth.

K04.5 Chronic apical periodontitis
Apical or periapical granuloma
Apical periodontitis NOS
EXCLUDES 1 chronic periodontitis (K05.3-)

K04.6 Periapical abscess with sinus
Dental abscess with sinus
Dentoalveolar abscess with sinus

K04.7 Periapical abscess without sinus
Dental abscess without sinus
Dentoalveolar abscess without sinus

K04.8 Radicular cyst
Apical (periodontal) cyst
Periapical cyst
Residual radicular cyst
EXCLUDES 2 lateral periodontal cyst (K09.0)

K04.9 Other and unspecified diseases of pulp and periapical tissues

K04.90 Unspecified diseases of pulp and periapical tissues

K04.99 Other diseases of pulp and periapical tissues

+ K05 Gingivitis and periodontal diseases
Use additional code to identify:
alcohol abuse and dependence (F10.-)
exposure to environmental tobacco smoke (Z77.22)
exposure to tobacco smoke in the perinatal period (P96.81)
history of tobacco dependence (Z87.891)
occupational exposure to environmental tobacco smoke (Z57.31)
tobacco dependence (F17.-)
tobacco use (Z72.0)

+ K05.0 Acute gingivitis
EXCLUDES 1 acute necrotizing ulcerative gingivitis (A69.1)
herpesviral [herpes simplex] gingivostomatitis (B00.2)

+ K05.00 Acute gingivitis, plaque induced
Acute gingivitis NOS
Plaque induced gingival disease

+ K05.01 Acute gingivitis, non-plaque induced

+ K05.1 Chronic gingivitis
Desquamative gingivitis (chronic)
Gingivitis (chronic) NOS
Hyperplastic gingivitis (chronic)
Pregnancy associated gingivitis
Simple marginal gingivitis (chronic)
Ulcerative gingivitis (chronic)
Code first:
, if applicable, diseases of the digestive system complicating pregnancy (O99.61-)

+ K05.10 Chronic gingivitis, plaque induced
Chronic gingivitis NOS
Gingivitis NOS

+ K05.11 Chronic gingivitis, non-plaque induced

+ K05.2 Aggressive periodontitis
Acute pericoronitis
EXCLUDES 1 acute apical periodontitis (K04.4)
periapical abscess (K04.7)
periapical abscess with sinus (K04.6)

+ K05.20 Aggressive periodontitis, unspecified
DEFINITION Serious and destructive inflammation and infection of the ligaments and bones supporting the teeth, leading to tooth loss.

+ K05.21 Aggressive periodontitis, localized
Periodontal abscess

+ K05.211 Aggressive periodontitis, localized, slight

Chapter 11
K00-K95

IQ + K05.212 Aggressive periodontitis, localized, moderate

IQ + K05.213 Aggressive periodontitis, localized, severe

IQ + K05.219 Aggressive periodontitis, localized, unspecified severity

+ 6 K05.22 Aggressive periodontitis, generalized

IQ + K05.221 Aggressive periodontitis, generalized, slight

IQ + K05.222 Aggressive periodontitis, generalized, moderate

IQ + K05.223 Aggressive periodontitis, generalized, severe

IQ + K05.229 Aggressive periodontitis, generalized, unspecified severity

+ 5 K05.3 Chronic periodontitis

Chronic pericoronitis
Complex periodontitis
Periodontitis NOS
Simplex periodontitis

EXCLUDES 1 chronic apical periodontitis (K04.5)

IQ + K05.30 Chronic periodontitis, unspecified

+ 6 K05.31 Chronic periodontitis, localized

IQ + K05.311 Chronic periodontitis, localized, slight

IQ + K05.312 Chronic periodontitis, localized, moderate

IQ + K05.313 Chronic periodontitis, localized, severe

IQ + K05.319 Chronic periodontitis, localized, unspecified severity

+ 6 K05.32 Chronic periodontitis, generalized

IQ + K05.321 Chronic periodontitis, generalized, slight

IQ + K05.322 Chronic periodontitis, generalized, moderate

IQ + K05.323 Chronic periodontitis, generalized, severe

IQ + K05.329 Chronic periodontitis, generalized, unspecified severity

IQ + K05.4 Periodontosis

Juvenile periodontosis

IQ + K05.5 Other periodontal diseases

Combined periodontic-endodontic lesion
Narrow gingival width (of periodontal soft tissue)

EXCLUDES 2 leukoplakia of gingiva (K13.21)

IQ + K05.6 Periodontal disease, unspecified

4 K06 Other disorders of gingiva and edentulous alveolar ridge

EXCLUDES 2 acute gingivitis (K05.0)
atrophy of edentulous alveolar ridge (K08.2)
chronic gingivitis (K05.1)
gingivitis NOS (K05.1)

5 K06.0 Gingival recession

Gingival recession (postinfective) (postprocedural)

DEFINITION Gums that have receded, exposing more tooth.

6 K06.01 Gingival recession, localized

IQ K06.010 Localized gingival recession, unspecified

Localized gingival recession, NOS

IQ K06.011 Localized gingival recession, minimal

IQ K06.012 Localized gingival recession, moderate

IQ K06.013 Localized gingival recession, severe

6 K06.02 Gingival recession, generalized

IQ K06.020 Generalized gingival recession, unspecified

Generalized gingival recession, NOS

IQ K06.021 Generalized gingival recession, minimal

IQ K06.022 Generalized gingival recession, moderate

IQ K06.023 Generalized gingival recession, severe

IQ K06.1 Gingival enlargement

Gingival fibromatosis

IQ + K06.2 Gingival and edentulous alveolar ridge lesions associated with trauma

Irritative hyperplasia of edentulous ridge [denture hyperplasia]
Use additional code (Chapter 20) to identify external cause or denture status (Z97.2)

IQ K06.3 Horizontal alveolar bone loss

IQ K06.8 Other specified disorders of gingiva and edentulous alveolar ridge

Fibrous epulis
Flabby alveolar ridge
Giant cell epulis
Peripheral giant cell granuloma of gingiva
Pyogenic granuloma of gingiva
Vertical ridge deficiency

EXCLUDES 2 gingival cyst (K09.0)

IQ K06.9 Disorder of gingiva and edentulous alveolar ridge, unspecified

4 K08 Other disorders of teeth and supporting structures

EXCLUDES 2 dentofacial anomalies [including malocclusion] (M26.-)
disorders of jaw (M27.-)

IQ K08.0 Exfoliation of teeth due to systemic causes

Code also:
underlying systemic condition

5 K08.1 Complete loss of teeth

Acquired loss of teeth, complete

EXCLUDES 1 congenital absence of teeth (K00.0)
exfoliation of teeth due to systemic causes (K08.0)
partial loss of teeth (K08.4-)

6 K08.10 Complete loss of teeth, unspecified cause

IQ K08.101 Complete loss of teeth, unspecified cause, class I

IQ K08.102 Complete loss of teeth, unspecified cause, class II

IQ K08.103 Complete loss of teeth, unspecified cause, class III

IQ K08.104 Complete loss of teeth, unspecified cause, class IV

Chapter 11 K00-K95

IQ **K08.109 Complete loss of teeth, unspecified cause, unspecified class**
Edentulism NOS

6 **K08.11 Complete loss of teeth due to trauma**

IQ **K08.111 Complete loss of teeth due to trauma, class I**

IQ **K08.112 Complete loss of teeth due to trauma, class II**

IQ **K08.113 Complete loss of teeth due to trauma, class III**

IQ **K08.114 Complete loss of teeth due to trauma, class IV**

IQ **K08.119 Complete loss of teeth due to trauma, unspecified class**

6 **K08.12 Complete loss of teeth due to periodontal diseases**

IQ **K08.121 Complete loss of teeth due to periodontal diseases, class I**

IQ **K08.122 Complete loss of teeth due to periodontal diseases, class II**

IQ **K08.123 Complete loss of teeth due to periodontal diseases, class III**

IQ **K08.124 Complete loss of teeth due to periodontal diseases, class IV**

IQ **K08.129 Complete loss of teeth due to periodontal diseases, unspecified class**

6 **K08.13 Complete loss of teeth due to caries**

IQ **K08.131 Complete loss of teeth due to caries, class I**

IQ **K08.132 Complete loss of teeth due to caries, class II**

IQ **K08.133 Complete loss of teeth due to caries, class III**

IQ **K08.134 Complete loss of teeth due to caries, class IV**

IQ **K08.139 Complete loss of teeth due to caries, unspecified class**

6 **K08.19 Complete loss of teeth due to other specified cause**

IQ **K08.191 Complete loss of teeth due to other specified cause, class I**

IQ **K08.192 Complete loss of teeth due to other specified cause, class II**

IQ **K08.193 Complete loss of teeth due to other specified cause, class III**

IQ **K08.194 Complete loss of teeth due to other specified cause, class IV**

IQ **K08.199 Complete loss of teeth due to other specified cause, unspecified class**

5 **K08.2 Atrophy of edentulous alveolar ridge**

IQ **K08.20 Unspecified atrophy of edentulous alveolar ridge**
Atrophy of the mandible NOS
Atrophy of the maxilla NOS

IQ **K08.21 Minimal atrophy of the mandible**
Minimal atrophy of the edentulous mandible

IQ **K08.22 Moderate atrophy of the mandible**
Moderate atrophy of the edentulous mandible

IQ **K08.23 Severe atrophy of the mandible**
Severe atrophy of the edentulous mandible

IQ **K08.24 Minimal atrophy of maxilla**
Minimal atrophy of the edentulous maxilla

IQ **K08.25 Moderate atrophy of the maxilla**
Moderate atrophy of the edentulous maxilla

IQ **K08.26 Severe atrophy of the maxilla**
Severe atrophy of the edentulous maxilla

IQ **K08.3 Retained dental root**
DEFINITION Part or all of the root structure of a tooth remains in the jaw after the tooth is extracted or otherwise lost.

5 **K08.4 Partial loss of teeth**
Acquired loss of teeth, partial
EXCLUDES 1 complete loss of teeth (K08.1-)
congenital absence of teeth (K00.0)
EXCLUDES 2 exfoliation of teeth due to systemic causes (K08.0)

6 **K08.40 Partial loss of teeth, unspecified cause**

IQ **K08.401 Partial loss of teeth, unspecified cause, class I**

IQ **K08.402 Partial loss of teeth, unspecified cause, class II**

IQ **K08.403 Partial loss of teeth, unspecified cause, class III**

IQ **K08.404 Partial loss of teeth, unspecified cause, class IV**

IQ **K08.409 Partial loss of teeth, unspecified cause, unspecified class**
Tooth extraction status NOS

6 **K08.41 Partial loss of teeth due to trauma**

IQ **K08.411 Partial loss of teeth due to trauma, class I**

IQ **K08.412 Partial loss of teeth due to trauma, class II**

IQ **K08.413 Partial loss of teeth due to trauma, class III**

IQ **K08.414 Partial loss of teeth due to trauma, class IV**

IQ **K08.419 Partial loss of teeth due to trauma, unspecified class**

6 **K08.42 Partial loss of teeth due to periodontal diseases**

IQ **K08.421 Partial loss of teeth due to periodontal diseases, class I**

IQ **K08.422 Partial loss of teeth due to periodontal diseases, class II**

IQ **K08.423 Partial loss of teeth due to periodontal diseases, class III**

IQ **K08.424 Partial loss of teeth due to periodontal diseases, class IV**

IQ **K08.429 Partial loss of teeth due to periodontal diseases, unspecified class**

6 **K08.43 Partial loss of teeth due to caries**

IQ **K08.431 Partial loss of teeth due to caries, class I**

IQ **K08.432 Partial loss of teeth due to caries, class II**

IQ **K08.433 Partial loss of teeth due to caries, class III**

Chapter 11
K00-K95

IQ **K08.434 Partial loss of teeth due to caries, class IV**

IQ **K08.439 Partial loss of teeth due to caries, unspecified class**

6 **K08.49 Partial loss of teeth due to other specified cause**

IQ **K08.491 Partial loss of teeth due to other specified cause, class I**

IQ **K08.492 Partial loss of teeth due to other specified cause, class II**

IQ **K08.493 Partial loss of teeth due to other specified cause, class III**

IQ **K08.494 Partial loss of teeth due to other specified cause, class IV**

IQ **K08.499 Partial loss of teeth due to other specified cause, unspecified class**

5 **K08.5 Unsatisfactory restoration of tooth**
Defective bridge, crown, filling
Defective dental restoration
EXCLUDES 1 dental restoration status (Z98.811)
EXCLUDES 2 endosseous dental implant failure (M27.6-)
unsatisfactory endodontic treatment (M27.5-)

IQ **K08.50 Unsatisfactory restoration of tooth, unspecified**
Defective dental restoration NOS

IQ **K08.51 Open restoration margins of tooth**
Dental restoration failure of marginal integrity
Open margin on tooth restoration
Poor gingival margin to tooth restoration

IQ **K08.52 Unrepairable overhanging of dental restorative materials**
Overhanging of tooth restoration

6 **K08.53 Fractured dental restorative material**
EXCLUDES 1 cracked tooth (K03.81)
traumatic fracture of tooth (S02.5)

IQ **K08.530 Fractured dental restorative material without loss of material**

IQ **K08.531 Fractured dental restorative material with loss of material**

IQ **K08.539 Fractured dental restorative material, unspecified**

IQ **K08.54 Contour of existing restoration of tooth biologically incompatible with oral health**
Dental restoration failure of periodontal anatomical integrity
Unacceptable contours of existing restoration of tooth
Unacceptable morphology of existing restoration of tooth

IQ + **K08.55 Allergy to existing dental restorative material**
Use additional code to identify the specific type of allergy

IQ **K08.56 Poor aesthetic of existing restoration of tooth**
Dental restoration aesthetically inadequate or displeasing

IQ **K08.59 Other unsatisfactory restoration of tooth**
Other defective dental restoration

5 **K08.8 Other specified disorders of teeth and supporting structures**

IQ **K08.81 Primary occlusal trauma**

IQ **K08.82 Secondary occlusal trauma**

IQ **K08.89 Other specified disorders of teeth and supporting structures**
Enlargement of alveolar ridge NOS
Insufficient anatomic crown height
Insufficient clinical crown length
Irregular alveolar process
Toothache NOS

IQ **K08.9 Disorder of teeth and supporting structures, unspecified**

4 **K09 Cysts of oral region, not elsewhere classified**
INCLUDES lesions showing histological features both of aneurysmal cyst and of another fibro-osseous lesion
EXCLUDES 2 cysts of jaw (M27.0-, M27.4-)
radicular cyst (K04.8)

IQ **K09.0 Developmental odontogenic cysts**
Dentigerous cyst
Eruption cyst
Follicular cyst
Gingival cyst
Lateral periodontal cyst
Primordial cyst
EXCLUDES 2 keratocysts (D16.4, D16.5)
odontogenic keratocystic tumors (D16.4, D16.5)

IQ **K09.1 Developmental (nonodontogenic) cysts of oral region**
Cyst (of) incisive canal
Cyst (of) palatine of papilla
Globulomaxillary cyst
Median palatal cyst
Nasoalveolar cyst
Nasolabial cyst
Nasopalatine duct cyst

IQ **K09.8 Other cysts of oral region, not elsewhere classified**
Dermoid cyst
Epidermoid cyst
Lymphoepithelial cyst
Epstein's pearl

IQ **K09.9 Cyst of oral region, unspecified**

+ 4 **K11 Diseases of salivary glands**
Use additional code to identify:
alcohol abuse and dependence (F10.-)
exposure to environmental tobacco smoke (Z77.22)
exposure to tobacco smoke in the perinatal period (P96.81)
history of tobacco dependence (Z87.891)
occupational exposure to environmental tobacco smoke (Z57.31)
tobacco dependence (F17.-)
tobacco use (Z72.0)

SP + **K11.0 Atrophy of salivary gland**
DEFINITION Wasting of the saliva glands, resulting in insufficient saliva production.

SP + **K11.1 Hypertrophy of salivary gland**

+ 5 **K11.2 Sialoadenitis**
Parotitis
EXCLUDES 1 epidemic parotitis (B26.-)
mumps (B26.-)

uveoparotid fever [Heerfordt] (D86.89)

SP + **K11.20 Sialoadenitis, unspecified**

SP + **K11.21 Acute sialoadenitis**

EXCLUDES 1 acute recurrent sialoadenitis (K11.22)

SP + **K11.22 Acute recurrent sialoadenitis**

SP + **K11.23 Chronic sialoadenitis**

SP + **K11.3 Abscess of salivary gland**

SP + **K11.4 Fistula of salivary gland**

EXCLUDES 1 congenital fistula of salivary gland (Q38.4)

SP + **K11.5 Sialolithiasis**

Calculus of salivary gland or duct
Stone of salivary gland or duct

SP + **K11.6 Mucocele of salivary gland**

Mucous extravasation cyst of salivary gland
Mucous retention cyst of salivary gland
Ranula

SP + **K11.7 Disturbances of salivary secretion**

Hypoptyalism
Ptyalism
Xerostomia

EXCLUDES 2 dry mouth NOS (R68.2)

▲ SP + **K11.8 Other diseases of salivary glands**

Benign lymphoepithelial lesion of salivary gland
Mikulicz' disease
Necrotizing sialometaplasia
Sialectasia
Stenosis of salivary duct
Stricture of salivary duct

EXCLUDES 1 Sjögren syndrome (M35.0-)

!Q + **K11.9 Disease of salivary gland, unspecified**

Sialoadenopathy NOS

+ 4 **K12 Stomatitis and related lesions**

Use additional code to identify:
alcohol abuse and dependence (F10.-)
exposure to environmental tobacco smoke (Z77.22)
exposure to tobacco smoke in the perinatal period (P96.81)
history of tobacco dependence (Z87.891)
occupational exposure to environmental tobacco smoke (Z57.31)
tobacco dependence (F17.-)
tobacco use (Z72.0)

EXCLUDES 1 cancrum oris (A69.0)
cheilitis (K13.0)
gangrenous stomatitis (A69.0)
herpesviral [herpes simplex] gingivostomatitis (B00.2)
noma (A69.0)

SP + **K12.0 Recurrent oral aphthae**

Aphthous stomatitis (major) (minor)
Bednar's aphthae
Periadenitis mucosa necrotica recurrens
Recurrent aphthous ulcer
Stomatitis herpetiformis

SP + **K12.1 Other forms of stomatitis**

Stomatitis NOS
Denture stomatitis
Ulcerative stomatitis
Vesicular stomatitis

EXCLUDES 1 acute necrotizing ulcerative stomatitis (A69.1)
Vincent's stomatitis (A69.1)

DEFINITION Painful inflammation of the mucosal soft tissues of the mouth, usually from a viral infection that can lead to ulcers or vesicular lesions.

SP + **K12.2 Cellulitis and abscess of mouth**

Cellulitis of mouth (floor)
Submandibular abscess

EXCLUDES 2 abscess of salivary gland (K11.3)
abscess of tongue (K14.0)
periapical abscess (K04.6-K04.7)
periodontal abscess (K05.21)
peritonsillar abscess (J36)

+ 5 **K12.3 Oral mucositis (ulcerative)**

Mucositis (oral) (oropharyneal)

EXCLUDES 2 gastrointestinal mucositis (ulcerative) (K92.81)
mucositis (ulcerative) of vagina and vulva (N76.81)
nasal mucositis (ulcerative) (J34.81)

SP + **K12.30 Oral mucositis (ulcerative), unspecified**

SP + **K12.31 Oral mucositis (ulcerative) due to antineoplastic therapy**

Use additional code for adverse effect, if applicable, to identify antineoplastic and immunosuppressive drugs (T45.1X5)
Use additional code for other antineoplastic therapy, such as: radiological procedure and radiotherapy (Y84.2)

SP + **K12.32 Oral mucositis (ulcerative) due to other drugs**

Use additional code for adverse effect, if applicable, to identify drug (T36-T50 with fifth or sixth character 5)

SP + **K12.33 Oral mucositis (ulcerative) due to radiation**

Use additional external cause code (W88-W90, X39.0-) to identify cause

SP + **K12.39 Other oral mucositis (ulcerative)**

Viral oral mucositis (ulcerative)

+ 4 **K13 Other diseases of lip and oral mucosa**

INCLUDES epithelial disturbances of tongue

Use additional code to identify:
alcohol abuse and dependence (F10.-)
exposure to environmental tobacco smoke (Z77.22)
exposure to tobacco smoke in the perinatal period (P96.81)
history of tobacco dependence (Z87.891)
occupational exposure to environmental tobacco smoke (Z57.31)
tobacco dependence (F17.-)
tobacco use (Z72.0)

EXCLUDES 2 certain disorders of gingiva and edentulous alveolar ridge (K05-K06)
cysts of oral region (K09.-)
diseases of tongue (K14.-)
stomatitis and related lesions (K12.-)

Chapter 11
K00-K95

4 4th digit required 5 5th digit required 6 6th digit required 7 7th digit required X 7th digit placeholder + Additional code ⊟ Laterality

SP + **K13.0 Diseases of lips**
Abscess of lips
Angular cheilitis
Cellulitis of lips
Cheilitis NOS
Cheilodynia
Cheilosis
Exfoliative cheilitis
Fistula of lips
Glandular cheilitis
Hypertrophy of lips
Perlèche NEC
EXCLUDES 1 ariboflavinosis (E53.0)
cheilitis due to radiation-related disorders (L55-L59)
congenital fistula of lips (Q38.0)
congenital hypertrophy of lips (Q18.6)
Perlèche due to candidiasis (B37.83)
Perlèche due to riboflavin deficiency (E53.0)

SP + **K13.1 Cheek and lip biting**

+ 5 **K13.2 Leukoplakia and other disturbances of oral epithelium, including tongue**
EXCLUDES 1 carcinoma in situ of oral epithelium (D00.0-)
hairy leukoplakia (K13.3)

SP + **K13.21 Leukoplakia of oral mucosa, including tongue**
Leukokeratosis of oral mucosa
Leukoplakia of gingiva, lips, tongue
EXCLUDES 1 hairy leukoplakia (K13.3)
leukokeratosis nicotina palati (K13.24)

SP + **K13.22 Minimal keratinized residual ridge mucosa**
Minimal keratinization of alveolar ridge mucosa

SP + **K13.23 Excessive keratinized residual ridge mucosa**
Excessive keratinization of alveolar ridge mucosa

SP + **K13.24 Leukokeratosis nicotina palati**
Smoker's palate

SP + **K13.29 Other disturbances of oral epithelium, including tongue**
Erythroplakia of mouth or tongue
Focal epithelial hyperplasia of mouth or tongue
Leukoedema of mouth or tongue
Other oral epithelium disturbances

SP + **K13.3 Hairy leukoplakia**

SP + **K13.4 Granuloma and granuloma-like lesions of oral mucosa**
Eosinophilic granuloma
Granuloma pyogenicum
Verrucous xanthoma

SP + **K13.5 Oral submucous fibrosis**
Submucous fibrosis of tongue
DEFINITION Build-up of fibrous (scar-like) tissue within the soft tissues of the mouth, causing rigidity and inability to open the mouth.

SP + **K13.6 Irritative hyperplasia of oral mucosa**
EXCLUDES 2 irritative hyperplasia of edentulous ridge [denture hyperplasia] (K06.2)

+ 5 **K13.7 Other and unspecified lesions of oral mucosa**

IQ + **K13.70 Unspecified lesions of oral mucosa**

SP + **K13.79 Other lesions of oral mucosa**
Focal oral mucinosis

+ 4 **K14 Diseases of tongue**
Use additional code to identify:
alcohol abuse and dependence (F10.-)
exposure to environmental tobacco smoke (Z77.22)
history of tobacco dependence (Z87.891)
occupational exposure to environmental tobacco smoke (Z57.31)
tobacco dependence (F17.-)
tobacco use (Z72.0)
EXCLUDES 2 erythroplakia (K13.29)
focal epithelial hyperplasia (K13.29)
leukedema of tongue (K13.29)
leukoplakia of tongue (K13.21)
hairy leukoplakia (K13.3)
macroglossia (congenital) (Q38.2)
submucous fibrosis of tongue (K13.5)

SP + **K14.0 Glossitis**
Abscess of tongue
Ulceration (traumatic) of tongue
EXCLUDES 1 atrophic glossitis (K14.4)
DEFINITION Changes in the appearance of the tongue due to inflammation.

SP + **K14.1 Geographic tongue**
Benign migratory glossitis
Glossitis areata exfoliativa

SP + **K14.2 Median rhomboid glossitis**

SP + **K14.3 Hypertrophy of tongue papillae**
Black hairy tongue
Coated tongue
Hypertrophy of foliate papillae
Lingua villosa nigra

SP + **K14.4 Atrophy of tongue papillae**
Atrophic glossitis

SP + **K14.5 Plicated tongue**
Fissured tongue
Furrowed tongue
Scrotal tongue
EXCLUDES 1 fissured tongue, congenital (Q38.3)

SP + **K14.6 Glossodynia**
Glossopyrosis
Painful tongue
DEFINITION Pain and/or a burning sensation in the tongue.

SP + **K14.8 Other diseases of tongue**
Atrophy of tongue
Crenated tongue
Enlargement of tongue
Glossocele
Glossoptosis
Hypertrophy of tongue

IQ + **K14.9 Disease of tongue, unspecified**
Glossopathy NOS

Chapter 11
K00-K95

Diseases of esophagus, stomach and duodenum (K20-K31)

EXCLUDES 2 hiatus hernia (K44.-)

+ 4 K20 Esophagitis
Use additional code to identify:
alcohol abuse and dependence (F10.-)
EXCLUDES 1 erosion of esophagus (K22.1-)
esophagitis with gastro-esophageal reflux disease (K21.0-)
reflux esophagitis (K21.0-)
ulcerative esophagitis (K22.1-)
EXCLUDES 2 eosinophilic gastritis or gastroenteritis (K52.81)

CODING TIPS ✓ Do not assign a code from K20.- if gastroesophageal reflux is also diagnosed. When a patient has confirmed diagnoses of both gastroesophageal reflux and esophagitis, a code from K21.0 should be assigned.

SP + K20.0 Eosinophilic esophagitis

+ 5 K20.8 Other esophagitis

SP + K20.80 Other esophagitis without bleeding
Abscess of esophagus
Other esophagitis NOS

SP + K20.81 Other esophagitis with bleeding

+ 5 K20.9 Esophagitis, unspecified

SP + K20.90 Esophagitis, unspecified without bleeding
Esophagitis NOS

SP + K20.91 Esophagitis, unspecified with bleeding

4 K21 Gastro-esophageal reflux disease
EXCLUDES 1 newborn esophageal reflux (P78.83)

5 K21.0 Gastro-esophageal reflux disease with esophagitis

DEFINITION Esophageal inflammation due to reflux of gastric acid from the stomach back up into the esophagus.

SP K21.00 Gastro-esophageal reflux disease with esophagitis, without bleeding
Reflux esophagitis

SP K21.01 Gastro-esophageal reflux disease with esophagitis, with bleeding

SP K21.9 Gastro-esophageal reflux disease without esophagitis
Esophageal reflux NOS

DEFINITION A burning sensation, usually centered in the middle of the chest near the breast bone, caused by the reflux of acidic stomach fluids that enter the lower end of the esophagus.

4 K22 Other diseases of esophagus
EXCLUDES 2 esophageal varices (I85.-)

SP K22.0 Achalasia of cardia
Achalasia NOS
Cardiospasm
EXCLUDES 1 congenital cardiospasm (Q39.5)

+ 5 K22.1 Ulcer of esophagus
Barrett's ulcer
Erosion of esophagus
Fungal ulcer of esophagus
Peptic ulcer of esophagus
Ulcer of esophagus due to ingestion of chemicals
Ulcer of esophagus due to ingestion of drugs and medicaments
Ulcerative esophagitis
Code first:
poisoning due to drug or toxin, if applicable (T36-T65 with fifth or sixth character 1-4 or 6)
Use additional code for adverse effect, if applicable, to identify drug (T36-T50 with fifth or sixth character 5)
EXCLUDES 1 Barrett's esophagus (K22.7-)

SP + K22.10 Ulcer of esophagus without bleeding
Ulcer of esophagus NOS

SP + K22.11 Ulcer of esophagus with bleeding
EXCLUDES 2 bleeding esophageal varices (I85.01, I85.11)

SP K22.2 Esophageal obstruction
Compression of esophagus
Constriction of esophagus
Stenosis of esophagus
Stricture of esophagus
EXCLUDES 1 congenital stenosis or stricture of esophagus (Q39.3)

SP K22.3 Perforation of esophagus
Rupture of esophagus
EXCLUDES 1 traumatic perforation of (thoracic) esophagus (S27.8-)

SP K22.4 Dyskinesia of esophagus
Corkscrew esophagus
Diffuse esophageal spasm
Spasm of esophagus
EXCLUDES 1 cardiospasm (K22.0)

DEFINITION Weakened, paralyzed, or uncoordinated movement of esophageal muscles, causing difficulty swallowing.

SP K22.5 Diverticulum of esophagus, acquired
Esophageal pouch, acquired
EXCLUDES 1 diverticulum of esophagus (congenital) (Q39.6)

SP K22.6 Gastro-esophageal laceration-hemorrhage syndrome
Mallory-Weiss syndrome

CODING TIPS ✓ Code K22.6 should be assigned only for patients diagnosed with Mallory-Weiss syndrome or esophageal laceration and bleeding due to Mallory-Weiss tears. When esophageal bleeding is documented as due to esophageal varices, assign a code from I85.-.

DEFINITION Esophagus becomes torn and bleeds near its connection to the stomach due to prolonged vomiting, hiccupping, or other spasmodic activity.

5 K22.7 Barrett's esophagus
Barrett's disease
Barrett's syndrome
EXCLUDES 1 Barrett's ulcer (K22.1)
malignant neoplasm of esophagus (C15.-)

SP **K22.70 Barrett's esophagus without dysplasia**
Barrett's esophagus NOS

6 **K22.71 Barrett's esophagus with dysplasia**

SP **K22.710 Barrett's esophagus with low grade dysplasia**

SP **K22.711 Barrett's esophagus with high grade dysplasia**

SP **K22.719 Barrett's esophagus with dysplasia, unspecified**

▲ 5 **K22.8 Other specified diseases of esophagus**
EXCLUDES 2 esophageal varices (I85.-)
Paterson-Kelly syndrome (D50.1)

★ **K22.81 Esophageal polyp**
EXCLUDES 1 benign neoplasm of esophagus (D13.0)

★ **K22.82 Esophagogastric junction polyp**
EXCLUDES 1 benign neoplasm of stomach (D13.1)

★ **K22.89 Other specified disease of esophagus**
Hemorrhage of esophagus NOS

CODING TIPS✓ Do not assign when esophageal hemorrhage is documented as due to Mallory-Weiss syndrome. When Mallory-Weiss syndrome causes laceration and esophageal hemorrhage, assign code K22.6. Also do not assign for esophageal bleeding due to varices. When esophageal bleeding is documented as due to esophageal varices, assign a code from I85.-.

IQ **K22.9 Disease of esophagus, unspecified**

M IQ **K23** ***Disorders of esophagus in diseases classified elsewhere***
Code first underlying disease, such as:
congenital syphilis (A50.5)
EXCLUDES 1 late syphilis (A52.79)
megaesophagus due to Chagas' disease (B57.31)
tuberculosis (A18.83)

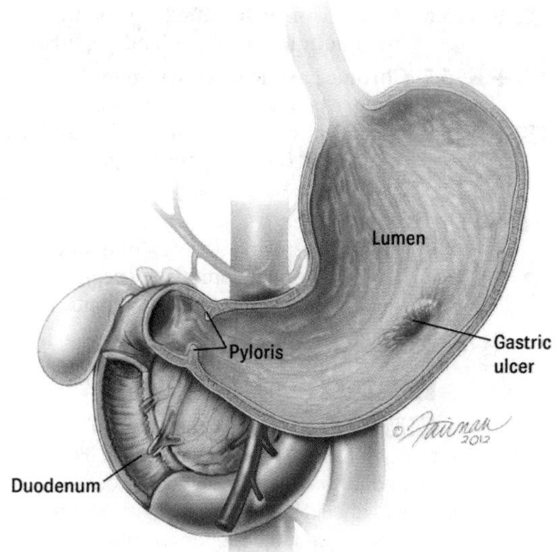

+ 4 **K25 Gastric ulcer**
INCLUDES erosion (acute) of stomach
pylorus ulcer (peptic)
stomach ulcer (peptic)
Use additional code to identify:
alcohol abuse and dependence (F10.-)
EXCLUDES 1 acute gastritis (K29.0-)
peptic ulcer NOS (K27.-)

CODING TIPS✓ When documentation specifies that any gastric, duodenal or peptic ulcer is related to alcohol abuse or dependence, coders should assign an additional code to specify the abuse/dependence as specified. Do not use 5th and 6th digits .88 to indicate alcohol induced disorder with the F10 code as alcohol induced disorders include only mental, emotional and physical disorders in Chapter 5.This is true when assigning code K25, K26 or K27.

CODING TIPS✓ If the physician or NPP documents that the condition is caused or induced by the alcohol, use the appropriate F10 code to indicate the alcohol use, abuse or dependence. Do not use 5th and 6th digits .88 to indicate alcohol induced disorder with the F10 code as alcohol induced disorders include only mental, emotional and physical disorders in Chapter 5.

CODING TIPS✓ Gastric ulcers are often documented as stomach ulcers. Carefully read all documentation in order to code ulcers to the proper anatomic location.

SP + **K25.0 Acute gastric ulcer with hemorrhage**

SP + **K25.1 Acute gastric ulcer with perforation**

SP + **K25.2 Acute gastric ulcer with both hemorrhage and perforation**

SP + **K25.3 Acute gastric ulcer without hemorrhage or perforation**

SP + **K25.4 Chronic or unspecified gastric ulcer with hemorrhage**

Chapter 11

K00-K95

SP + **K25.5 Chronic or unspecified gastric ulcer with perforation**

SP + **K25.6 Chronic or unspecified gastric ulcer with both hemorrhage and perforation**

SP + **K25.7 Chronic gastric ulcer without hemorrhage or perforation**

SP + **K25.9 Gastric ulcer, unspecified as acute or chronic, without hemorrhage or perforation**

+ 4 **K26 Duodenal ulcer**

INCLUDES erosion (acute) of duodenum
duodenum ulcer (peptic)
postpyloric ulcer (peptic)

Use additional code to identify:
alcohol abuse and dependence (F10.-)

EXCLUDES 1 peptic ulcer NOS (K27.-)

CODING TIPS✓ When documentation specifies that any gastric, duodenal or peptic ulcer is related to alcohol abuse or dependence, coders should assign an additional code to specify the abuse/dependence as specified. Do not use 5th and 6th digits .88 to indicate alcohol induced disorder with the F10 code as alcohol induced disorders include only mental, emotional and physical disorders in Chapter 5.This is true when assigning code K25, K26 or K27.

CODING TIPS✓ A peptic ulcer should be coded to K26.- only when specified as duodenal or postpyloric. When documentation reports an ulcer as peptic and does not specify to one of these locations, assign a code from K27.-

SP + **K26.0 Acute duodenal ulcer with hemorrhage**

SP + **K26.1 Acute duodenal ulcer with perforation**

SP + **K26.2 Acute duodenal ulcer with both hemorrhage and perforation**

SP + **K26.3 Acute duodenal ulcer without hemorrhage or perforation**

SP + **K26.4 Chronic or unspecified duodenal ulcer with hemorrhage**

SP + **K26.5 Chronic or unspecified duodenal ulcer with perforation**

SP + **K26.6 Chronic or unspecified duodenal ulcer with both hemorrhage and perforation**

SP + **K26.7 Chronic duodenal ulcer without hemorrhage or perforation**

SP + **K26.9 Duodenal ulcer, unspecified as acute or chronic, without hemorrhage or perforation**

+ 4 **K27 Peptic ulcer, site unspecified**

INCLUDES gastroduodenal ulcer NOS
peptic ulcer NOS

Use additional code to identify:
alcohol abuse and dependence (F10.-)

EXCLUDES 1 peptic ulcer of newborn (P78.82)

CODING TIPS✓ When documentation specifies that any gastric, duodenal or peptic ulcer is related to alcohol abuse or dependence, coders should assign an additional code to specify the abuse/dependence as specified. Do not use 5th and 6th digits .88 to indicate alcohol induced disorder with the F10 code as alcohol induced disorders include only mental, emotional and physical disorders in Chapter 5.This is true when assigning code K25, K26 or K27.

SP + **K27.0 Acute peptic ulcer, site unspecified, with hemorrhage**

SP + **K27.1 Acute peptic ulcer, site unspecified, with perforation**

SP + **K27.2 Acute peptic ulcer, site unspecified, with both hemorrhage and perforation**

SP + **K27.3 Acute peptic ulcer, site unspecified, without hemorrhage or perforation**

SP + **K27.4 Chronic or unspecified peptic ulcer, site unspecified, with hemorrhage**

SP + **K27.5 Chronic or unspecified peptic ulcer, site unspecified, with perforation**

SP + **K27.6 Chronic or unspecified peptic ulcer, site unspecified, with both hemorrhage and perforation**

SP + **K27.7 Chronic peptic ulcer, site unspecified, without hemorrhage or perforation**

SP + **K27.9 Peptic ulcer, site unspecified, unspecified as acute or chronic, without hemorrhage or perforation**

+ 4 **K28 Gastrojejunal ulcer**

INCLUDES anastomotic ulcer (peptic) or erosion
gastrocolic ulcer (peptic) or erosion
gastrointestinal ulcer (peptic) or erosion
gastrojejunal ulcer (peptic) or erosion
jejunal ulcer (peptic) or erosion
marginal ulcer (peptic) or erosion
stomal ulcer (peptic) or erosion

Use additional code to identify:
alcohol abuse and dependence (F10.-)

EXCLUDES 1 primary ulcer of small intestine (K63.3)

SP + **K28.0 Acute gastrojejunal ulcer with hemorrhage**

SP + **K28.1 Acute gastrojejunal ulcer with perforation**

SP + **K28.2 Acute gastrojejunal ulcer with both hemorrhage and perforation**

SP + **K28.3 Acute gastrojejunal ulcer without hemorrhage or perforation**

SP + **K28.4 Chronic or unspecified gastrojejunal ulcer with hemorrhage**

SP + **K28.5 Chronic or unspecified gastrojejunal ulcer with perforation**

SP + **K28.6 Chronic or unspecified gastrojejunal ulcer with both hemorrhage and perforation**

SP + **K28.7 Chronic gastrojejunal ulcer without hemorrhage or perforation**

SP + **K28.9 Gastrojejunal ulcer, unspecified as acute or chronic, without hemorrhage or perforation**

4 **K29 Gastritis and duodenitis**

EXCLUDES 1 eosinophilic gastritis or gastroenteritis (K52.81)
Zollinger-Ellison syndrome (E16.4)

+ 5 **K29.0 Acute gastritis**

Use additional code to identify:
alcohol abuse and dependence (F10.-)

EXCLUDES 1 erosion (acute) of stomach (K25.-)

SP + **K29.00 Acute gastritis without bleeding**

SP + **K29.01 Acute gastritis with bleeding**

+ 5 **K29.2 Alcoholic gastritis**

Use additional code to identify:
alcohol abuse and dependence (F10.-)

SP + **K29.20 Alcoholic gastritis without bleeding**

SP + **K29.21 Alcoholic gastritis with bleeding**

5 **K29.3 Chronic superficial gastritis**

SP **K29.30 Chronic superficial gastritis without bleeding**

SP **K29.31 Chronic superficial gastritis with bleeding**

5 **K29.4 Chronic atrophic gastritis**

Gastric atrophy

SP **K29.40 Chronic atrophic gastritis without bleeding**

SP **K29.41 Chronic atrophic gastritis with bleeding**

5 **K29.5 Unspecified chronic gastritis**

Chronic antral gastritis
Chronic fundal gastritis

SP **K29.50 Unspecified chronic gastritis without bleeding**

SP **K29.51 Unspecified chronic gastritis with bleeding**

5 **K29.6 Other gastritis**

Giant hypertrophic gastritis
Granulomatous gastritis
Ménétrier's disease

SP **K29.60 Other gastritis without bleeding**

SP **K29.61 Other gastritis with bleeding**

5 **K29.7 Gastritis, unspecified**

SP **K29.70 Gastritis, unspecified, without bleeding**

SP **K29.71 Gastritis, unspecified, with bleeding**

5 **K29.8 Duodenitis**

SP **K29.80 Duodenitis without bleeding**

SP **K29.81 Duodenitis with bleeding**

5 **K29.9 Gastroduodenitis, unspecified**

SP **K29.90 Gastroduodenitis, unspecified, without bleeding**

SP **K29.91 Gastroduodenitis, unspecified, with bleeding**

SP **K30 Functional dyspepsia**

Indigestion

EXCLUDES 1 dyspepsia NOS (R10.13)
heartburn (R12)
nervous dyspepsia (F45.8)
neurotic dyspepsia (F45.8)
psychogenic dyspepsia (F45.8)

4 **K31 Other diseases of stomach and duodenum**

INCLUDES functional disorders of stomach

EXCLUDES 2 diabetic gastroparesis (E08.43, E09.43, E10.43, E11.43, E13.43)
diverticulum of duodenum (K57.00-K57.13)

SP **K31.0 Acute dilatation of stomach**

Acute distention of stomach

DEFINITION Distention of the stomach due to excessive gas build-up or bowel obstruction, preventing passage of food.

SP **K31.1 Adult hypertrophic pyloric stenosis**

Pyloric stenosis NOS

EXCLUDES 1 congenital or infantile pyloric stenosis (Q40.0)

SP **K31.2 Hourglass stricture and stenosis of stomach**

EXCLUDES 1 congenital hourglass stomach (Q40.2)
hourglass contraction of stomach (K31.89)

SP **K31.3 Pylorospasm, not elsewhere classified**

EXCLUDES 1 congenital or infantile pylorospasm (Q40.0)
neurotic pylorospasm (F45.8)
psychogenic pylorospasm (F45.8)

SP **K31.4 Gastric diverticulum**

EXCLUDES 1 congenital diverticulum of stomach (Q40.2)

SP **K31.5 Obstruction of duodenum**

Constriction of duodenum
Duodenal ileus (chronic)
Stenosis of duodenum
Stricture of duodenum
Volvulus of duodenum

EXCLUDES 1 congenital stenosis of duodenum (Q41.0)

SP **K31.6 Fistula of stomach and duodenum**

Gastrocolic fistula
Gastrojejunocolic fistula

SP **K31.7 Polyp of stomach and duodenum**

EXCLUDES 1 adenomatous polyp of stomach (D13.1)

5 **K31.8 Other specified diseases of stomach and duodenum**

6 **K31.81 Angiodysplasia of stomach and duodenum**

SP **K31.811 Angiodysplasia of stomach and duodenum with bleeding**

SP **K31.819 Angiodysplasia of stomach and duodenum without bleeding**

Angiodysplasia of stomach and duodenum NOS

SP **K31.82 Dieulafoy lesion (hemorrhagic) of stomach and duodenum**

EXCLUDES 2 Dieulafoy lesion of intestine (K63.81)

DEFINITION Abnormality of arteriole within the digestive tract protruding through a tiny mucosal defect, usually near the gastroesophageal junction, that can cause massive gastrointestinal bleeding.

SP **K31.83 Achlorhydria**

DEFINITION Absence of hydrochloric acid in the stomach's gastric secretions, most often from antibodies against cells producing gastric acid, or a symptom of H. pylori infection, atrophic gastritis, or cancer.

SP **K31.84 Gastroparesis**

Gastroparalysis

Code first underlying disease, if known, such as:

anorexia nervosa (F50.0-)

diabetes mellitus (E08.43, E09.43, E10.43, E11.43, E13.43)

scleroderma (M34.-)

SP **K31.89 Other diseases of stomach and duodenum**

IQ **K31.9 Disease of stomach and duodenum, unspecified**

★ 5 **K31.A Gastric intestinal metaplasia**

★ **K31.A0 Gastric intestinal metaplasia, unspecified**

Gastric intestinal metaplasia indefinite for dysplasia

Gastric intestinal metaplasia NOS

★ 6 **K31.A1 Gastric intestinal metaplasia without dysplasia**

★ **K31.A11 Gastric intestinal metaplasia without dysplasia, involving the antrum**

★ **K31.A12 Gastric intestinal metaplasia without dysplasia, involving the body (corpus)**

★ **K31.A13 Gastric intestinal metaplasia without dysplasia, involving the fundus**

★ **K31.A14 Gastric intestinal metaplasia without dysplasia, involving the cardia**

★ **K31.A15 Gastric intestinal metaplasia without dysplasia, involving multiple sites**

★ **K31.A19 Gastric intestinal metaplasia without dysplasia, unspecified site**

★ 6 **K31.A2 Gastric intestinal metaplasia with dysplasia**

★ **K31.A21 Gastric intestinal metaplasia with low grade dysplasia**

★ **K31.A22 Gastric intestinal metaplasia with high grade dysplasia**

★ **K31.A29 Gastric intestinal metaplasia with dysplasia, unspecified**

Diseases of appendix (K35-K38)

4 **K35 Acute appendicitis**

CODING TIPS ✓ With acute appendicitis, the single most important distinction is between perforation (bacterial contamination of the peritoneal space) and no perforation (no bacterial contamination), rather than the presence or absence of sterile inflammation of the peritoneum. The term peritonitis is used by different surgeons to mean different things.

CODING TIPS ✓ When a patient has had an appendectomy, usually the condition (appendicitis) is resolved. An appendix that is ruptured, however, may have caused peritonitis that may not be resolved. Acute appendicitis progresses from inflammation of the appendix, then gangrene, followed by perforation. Perforation results in contamination of the peritoneal space with enteric bacteria, which can result in abscess formation or generalized bacterial contamination of the peritoneal space (generalized peritonitis). Perforation, the presence of an abscess, and the presence of generalized peritonitis are key characteristics of appendicitis that physicians use to describe the severity of the disease and determine the most appropriate treatment, such as deciding whether or not to perform an appendectomy or drain abscesses (sometimes percutaneously) and determining the duration of antibiotic treatment.

5 **K35.2 Acute appendicitis with generalized peritonitis**

Appendicitis (acute) with generalized (diffuse) peritonitis following rupture or perforation of appendix

SP **K35.20 Acute appendicitis with generalized peritonitis, without abscess**

(Acute) appendicitis with generalized peritonitis NOS

SP **K35.21 Acute appendicitis with generalized peritonitis, with abscess**

5 **K35.3 Acute appendicitis with localized peritonitis**

SP **K35.30 Acute appendicitis with localized peritonitis, without perforation or gangrene**

Acute appendicitis with localized peritonitis NOS

SP **K35.31 Acute appendicitis with localized peritonitis and gangrene, without perforation**

SP **K35.32 Acute appendicitis with perforation and localized peritonitis, without abscess**

(Acute) appendicitis with perforation NOS

Perforated appendix NOS

Ruptured appendix (with localized peritonitis) NOS

SP **K35.33 Acute appendicitis with perforation and localized peritonitis, with abscess**

(Acute) appendicitis with (peritoneal) abscess NOS

Ruptured appendix with localized peritonitis and abscess

5 **K35.8 Other and unspecified acute appendicitis**

SP **K35.80 Unspecified acute appendicitis**

Acute appendicitis NOS

Acute appendicitis without (localized) (generalized) peritonitis

6 **K35.89 Other acute appendicitis**

SP **K35.890 Other acute appendicitis without perforation or gangrene**

SP **K35.891 Other acute appendicitis without perforation, with gangrene**
(Acute) appendicitis with gangrene NOS

SP **K36 Other appendicitis**
Chronic appendicitis
Recurrent appendicitis

SP **K37 Unspecified appendicitis**
EXCLUDES 1 unspecified appendicitis with peritonitis (K35.2-, K35.3-)

4 **K38 Other diseases of appendix**

SP **K38.0 Hyperplasia of appendix**

SP **K38.1 Appendicular concretions**
Fecalith of appendix
Stercolith of appendix

SP **K38.2 Diverticulum of appendix**

SP **K38.3 Fistula of appendix**

SP **K38.8 Other specified diseases of appendix**
Intussusception of appendix

IQ **K38.9 Disease of appendix, unspecified**

Hernia (K40-K46)

Note:
Hernia with both gangrene and obstruction is classified to hernia with gangrene.

INCLUDES acquired hernia
congenital [except diaphragmatic or hiatus] hernia
recurrent hernia

CODING TIPS✓ **Documentation:** Carefully review all documentation when assigning codes for a hernia. It is important to note the various anatomical positions of each type of hernia, as well as the differences between obstructed and non-obstructed hernias. When a hernia is obstructed, gangrene may occur due to the lack of blood flow related to the obstruction. If the hernia has been repaired, assign the appropriate Z code for aftercare.

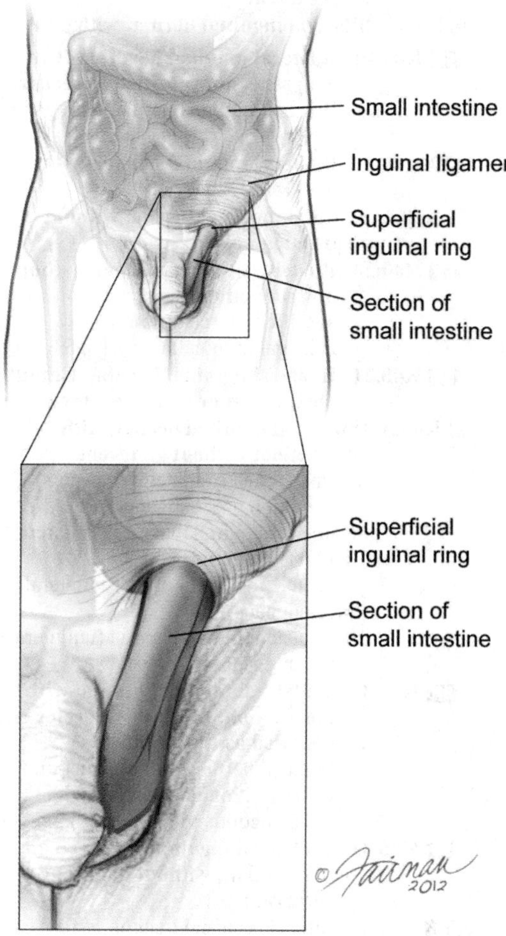

4 **K40 Inguinal hernia**
INCLUDES bubonocele
direct inguinal hernia
double inguinal hernia
indirect inguinal hernia
inguinal hernia NOS
oblique inguinal hernia
scrotal hernia

DEFINITION Weakness in the muscles in the groin area between the abdomen and thigh, allowing part of the intestine to bulge through the muscle wall.

5 **K40.0 Bilateral inguinal hernia, with obstruction, without gangrene**
Inguinal hernia (bilateral) causing obstruction without gangrene
Incarcerated inguinal hernia (bilateral) without gangrene
Irreducible inguinal hernia (bilateral) without gangrene
Strangulated inguinal hernia (bilateral) without gangrene

SP **K40.00 Bilateral inguinal hernia, with obstruction, without gangrene, not specified as recurrent**
Bilateral inguinal hernia, with obstruction, without gangrene NOS

Chapter 11
K00-K95

SP **K40.01 Bilateral inguinal hernia, with obstruction, without gangrene, recurrent**

5 **K40.1 Bilateral inguinal hernia, with gangrene**

SP **K40.10 Bilateral inguinal hernia, with gangrene, not specified as recurrent**
Bilateral inguinal hernia, with gangrene NOS

SP **K40.11 Bilateral inguinal hernia, with gangrene, recurrent**

5 **K40.2 Bilateral inguinal hernia, without obstruction or gangrene**

SP **K40.20 Bilateral inguinal hernia, without obstruction or gangrene, not specified as recurrent**
Bilateral inguinal hernia NOS

SP **K40.21 Bilateral inguinal hernia, without obstruction or gangrene, recurrent**

5 **K40.3 Unilateral inguinal hernia, with obstruction, without gangrene**
Inguinal hernia (unilateral) causing obstruction without gangrene
Incarcerated inguinal hernia (unilateral) without gangrene
Irreducible inguinal hernia (unilateral) without gangrene
Strangulated inguinal hernia (unilateral) without gangrene

SP **K40.30 Unilateral inguinal hernia, with obstruction, without gangrene, not specified as recurrent**
Inguinal hernia, with obstruction NOS
Unilateral inguinal hernia, with obstruction, without gangrene NOS

SP **K40.31 Unilateral inguinal hernia, with obstruction, without gangrene, recurrent**

5 **K40.4 Unilateral inguinal hernia, with gangrene**

SP **K40.40 Unilateral inguinal hernia, with gangrene, not specified as recurrent**
Inguinal hernia with gangrene NOS
Unilateral inguinal hernia with gangrene NOS

SP **K40.41 Unilateral inguinal hernia, with gangrene, recurrent**

5 **K40.9 Unilateral inguinal hernia, without obstruction or gangrene**

SP **K40.90 Unilateral inguinal hernia, without obstruction or gangrene, not specified as recurrent**
Inguinal hernia NOS
Unilateral inguinal hernia NOS

SP **K40.91 Unilateral inguinal hernia, without obstruction or gangrene, recurrent**

4 **K41 Femoral hernia**

5 **K41.0 Bilateral femoral hernia, with obstruction, without gangrene**
Femoral hernia (bilateral) causing obstruction, without gangrene
Incarcerated femoral hernia (bilateral), without gangrene
Irreducible femoral hernia (bilateral), without gangrene
Strangulated femoral hernia (bilateral), without gangrene

SP **K41.00 Bilateral femoral hernia, with obstruction, without gangrene, not specified as recurrent**
Bilateral femoral hernia, with obstruction, without gangrene NOS

SP **K41.01 Bilateral femoral hernia, with obstruction, without gangrene, recurrent**

5 **K41.1 Bilateral femoral hernia, with gangrene**

SP **K41.10 Bilateral femoral hernia, with gangrene, not specified as recurrent**
Bilateral femoral hernia, with gangrene NOS

SP **K41.11 Bilateral femoral hernia, with gangrene, recurrent**

5 **K41.2 Bilateral femoral hernia, without obstruction or gangrene**

SP **K41.20 Bilateral femoral hernia, without obstruction or gangrene, not specified as recurrent**
Bilateral femoral hernia NOS

SP **K41.21 Bilateral femoral hernia, without obstruction or gangrene, recurrent**

5 **K41.3 Unilateral femoral hernia, with obstruction, without gangrene**
Femoral hernia (unilateral) causing obstruction, without gangrene
Incarcerated femoral hernia (unilateral), without gangrene
Irreducible femoral hernia (unilateral), without gangrene
Strangulated femoral hernia (unilateral), without gangrene

SP **K41.30 Unilateral femoral hernia, with obstruction, without gangrene, not specified as recurrent**
Femoral hernia, with obstruction NOS
Unilateral femoral hernia, with obstruction NOS

SP **K41.31 Unilateral femoral hernia, with obstruction, without gangrene, recurrent**

5 **K41.4 Unilateral femoral hernia, with gangrene**

SP **K41.40 Unilateral femoral hernia, with gangrene, not specified as recurrent**
Femoral hernia, with gangrene NOS
Unilateral femoral hernia, with gangrene NOS

SP **K41.41 Unilateral femoral hernia, with gangrene, recurrent**

5 **K41.9 Unilateral femoral hernia, without obstruction or gangrene**

SP **K41.90 Unilateral femoral hernia, without obstruction or gangrene, not specified as recurrent**
Femoral hernia NOS
Unilateral femoral hernia NOS

SP **K41.91 Unilateral femoral hernia, without obstruction or gangrene, recurrent**

4 **K42 Umbilical hernia**
INCLUDES paraumbilical hernia
EXCLUDES 1 omphalocele (Q79.2)

SP **K42.0 Umbilical hernia with obstruction, without gangrene**
Umbilical hernia causing obstruction, without gangrene

Incarcerated umbilical hernia, without gangrene
Irreducible umbilical hernia, without gangrene
Strangulated umbilical hernia, without gangrene

SP **K42.1 Umbilical hernia with gangrene**
Gangrenous umbilical hernia

SP **K42.9 Umbilical hernia without obstruction or gangrene**
Umbilical hernia NOS

4 **K43 Ventral hernia**

SP **K43.0 Incisional hernia with obstruction, without gangrene**
Incisional hernia causing obstruction, without gangrene
Incarcerated incisional hernia, without gangrene
Irreducible incisional hernia, without gangrene
Strangulated incisional hernia, without gangrene

SP **K43.1 Incisional hernia with gangrene**
Gangrenous incisional hernia

SP **K43.2 Incisional hernia without obstruction or gangrene**
Incisional hernia NOS

SP **K43.3 Parastomal hernia with obstruction, without gangrene**
Incarcerated parastomal hernia, without gangrene
Irreducible parastomal hernia, without gangrene
Parastomal hernia causing obstruction, without gangrene
Strangulated parastomal hernia, without gangrene

SP **K43.4 Parastomal hernia with gangrene**
Gangrenous parastomal hernia

SP **K43.5 Parastomal hernia without obstruction or gangrene**
Parastomal hernia NOS

SP **K43.6 Other and unspecified ventral hernia with obstruction, without gangrene**
Epigastric hernia causing obstruction, without gangrene
Hypogastric hernia causing obstruction, without gangrene
Incarcerated epigastric hernia without gangrene
Incarcerated hypogastric hernia without gangrene
Incarcerated midline hernia without gangrene
Incarcerated spigelian hernia without gangrene
Incarcerated subxiphoid hernia without gangrene
Irreducible epigastric hernia without gangrene
Irreducible hypogastric hernia without gangrene
Irreducible midline hernia without gangrene
Irreducible spigelian hernia without gangrene
Irreducible subxiphoid hernia without gangrene
Midline hernia causing obstruction, without gangrene
Spigelian hernia causing obstruction, without gangrene
Strangulated epigastric hernia without gangrene
Strangulated hypogastric hernia without gangrene
Strangulated midline hernia without gangrene
Strangulated spigelian hernia without gangrene
Strangulated subxiphoid hernia without gangrene
Subxiphoid hernia causing obstruction, without gangrene

SP **K43.7 Other and unspecified ventral hernia with gangrene**
Any condition listed under K43.6 specified as gangrenous

SP **K43.9 Ventral hernia without obstruction or gangrene**
Epigastric hernia
Ventral hernia NOS

4 **K44 Diaphragmatic hernia**
INCLUDES hiatus hernia (esophageal) (sliding)
paraesophageal hernia
EXCLUDES 1 congenital diaphragmatic hernia (Q79.0)
congenital hiatus hernia (Q40.1)

SP **K44.0 Diaphragmatic hernia with obstruction, without gangrene**
Diaphragmatic hernia causing obstruction
Incarcerated diaphragmatic hernia
Irreducible diaphragmatic hernia
Strangulated diaphragmatic hernia

SP **K44.1 Diaphragmatic hernia with gangrene**
Gangrenous diaphragmatic hernia

SP **K44.9 Diaphragmatic hernia without obstruction or gangrene**
Diaphragmatic hernia NOS

4 **K45 Other abdominal hernia**
INCLUDES abdominal hernia, specified site NEC
lumbar hernia
obturator hernia
pudendal hernia
retroperitoneal hernia
sciatic hernia

SP **K45.0 Other specified abdominal hernia with obstruction, without gangrene**
Other specified abdominal hernia causing obstruction
Other specified incarcerated abdominal hernia
Other specified irreducible abdominal hernia
Other specified strangulated abdominal hernia

SP **K45.1 Other specified abdominal hernia with gangrene**
Any condition listed under K45 specified as gangrenous

SP **K45.8 Other specified abdominal hernia without obstruction or gangrene**

4 **K46 Unspecified abdominal hernia**

INCLUDES enterocele
epiplocele
hernia NOS
interstitial hernia
intestinal hernia
intra-abdominal hernia
EXCLUDES 1 vaginal enterocele (N81.5)

SP **K46.0 Unspecified abdominal hernia with obstruction, without gangrene**
Unspecified abdominal hernia causing obstruction
Unspecified incarcerated abdominal hernia
Unspecified irreducible abdominal hernia
Unspecified strangulated abdominal hernia

IQ **K46.1 Unspecified abdominal hernia with gangrene**
Any condition listed under K46 specified as gangrenous

IQ **K46.9 Unspecified abdominal hernia without obstruction or gangrene**
Abdominal hernia NOS

Noninfective enteritis and colitis (K50-K52)

INCLUDES noninfective inflammatory bowel disease
EXCLUDES 1 irritable bowel syndrome (K58.-)
megacolon (K59.3-)

CODING TIPS Do not assign a code from K50-K52 when enteritis/colitis is specified as infectious. Infectious colitis requires assignment of a code from Chapter 1, Certain Infectious and Parasitic Diseases.

+4 **K50 Crohn's disease [regional enteritis]**
INCLUDES granulomatous enteritis
Use additional code to identify manifestations, such as:
pyoderma gangrenosum (L88)
EXCLUDES 1 ulcerative colitis (K51.-)

+5 **K50.0 Crohn's disease of small intestine**
Crohn's disease [regional enteritis] of duodenum
Crohn's disease [regional enteritis] of ileum
Crohn's disease [regional enteritis] of jejunum
Regional ileitis
Terminal ileitis
EXCLUDES 1 Crohn's disease of both small and large intestine (K50.8-)

SP + **K50.00 Crohn's disease of small intestine without complications**

+6 **K50.01 Crohn's disease of small intestine with complications**

SP + **K50.011 Crohn's disease of small intestine with rectal bleeding**

SP + **K50.012 Crohn's disease of small intestine with intestinal obstruction**

SP + **K50.013 Crohn's disease of small intestine with fistula**

SP + **K50.014 Crohn's disease of small intestine with abscess**

SP + **K50.018 Crohn's disease of small intestine with other complication**

IQ + **K50.019 Crohn's disease of small intestine with unspecified complications**

+5 **K50.1 Crohn's disease of large intestine**
Crohn's disease [regional enteritis] of colon
Crohn's disease [regional enteritis] of large bowel
Crohn's disease [regional enteritis] of rectum
Granulomatous colitis
Regional colitis
EXCLUDES 1 Crohn's disease of both small and large intestine (K50.8)

SP + **K50.10 Crohn's disease of large intestine without complications**

+6 **K50.11 Crohn's disease of large intestine with complications**

SP + **K50.111 Crohn's disease of large intestine with rectal bleeding**

SP + **K50.112 Crohn's disease of large intestine with intestinal obstruction**

SP + **K50.113 Crohn's disease of large intestine with fistula**

SP + **K50.114 Crohn's disease of large intestine with abscess**

SP + **K50.118 Crohn's disease of large intestine with other complication**

IQ + **K50.119 Crohn's disease of large intestine with unspecified complications**

+5 **K50.8 Crohn's disease of both small and large intestine**

SP + **K50.80 Crohn's disease of both small and large intestine without complications**

+6 **K50.81 Crohn's disease of both small and large intestine with complications**

SP + **K50.811 Crohn's disease of both small and large intestine with rectal bleeding**

SP + **K50.812 Crohn's disease of both small and large intestine with intestinal obstruction**

SP + **K50.813 Crohn's disease of both small and large intestine with fistula**

SP + **K50.814 Crohn's disease of both small and large intestine with abscess**

SP + **K50.818 Crohn's disease of both small and large intestine with other complication**

IQ + **K50.819 Crohn's disease of both small and large intestine with unspecified complications**

+5 **K50.9 Crohn's disease, unspecified**

SP + **K50.90 Crohn's disease, unspecified, without complications**
Crohn's disease NOS
Regional enteritis NOS

+6 **K50.91 Crohn's disease, unspecified, with complications**

SP + **K50.911 Crohn's disease, unspecified, with rectal bleeding**

SP + **K50.912 Crohn's disease, unspecified, with intestinal obstruction**

SP + **K50.913 Crohn's disease, unspecified, with fistula**

SP + **K50.914 Crohn's disease, unspecified, with abscess**

SP + **K50.918 Crohn's disease, unspecified, with other complication**

IQ + **K50.919 Crohn's disease, unspecified, with unspecified complications**

+4 K51 **Ulcerative colitis**
Use additional code to identify manifestations, such as:
pyoderma gangrenosum (L88)
EXCLUDES 1 Crohn's disease [regional enteritis] (K50.-)

+5 K51.0 **Ulcerative (chronic) pancolitis**
Backwash ileitis
SP + K51.00 **Ulcerative (chronic) pancolitis without complications**
Ulcerative (chronic) pancolitis NOS
+6 K51.01 **Ulcerative (chronic) pancolitis with complications**
SP + K51.011 **Ulcerative (chronic) pancolitis with rectal bleeding**
SP + K51.012 **Ulcerative (chronic) pancolitis with intestinal obstruction**
SP + K51.013 **Ulcerative (chronic) pancolitis with fistula**
SP + K51.014 **Ulcerative (chronic) pancolitis with abscess**
SP + K51.018 **Ulcerative (chronic) pancolitis with other complication**
!Q + K51.019 **Ulcerative (chronic) pancolitis with unspecified complications**

+5 K51.2 **Ulcerative (chronic) proctitis**
SP + K51.20 **Ulcerative (chronic) proctitis without complications**
Ulcerative (chronic) proctitis NOS
+6 K51.21 **Ulcerative (chronic) proctitis with complications**
SP + K51.211 **Ulcerative (chronic) proctitis with rectal bleeding**
SP + K51.212 **Ulcerative (chronic) proctitis with intestinal obstruction**
SP + K51.213 **Ulcerative (chronic) proctitis with fistula**
SP + K51.214 **Ulcerative (chronic) proctitis with abscess**
SP + K51.218 **Ulcerative (chronic) proctitis with other complication**
!Q + K51.219 **Ulcerative (chronic) proctitis with unspecified complications**

+5 K51.3 **Ulcerative (chronic) rectosigmoiditis**
SP + K51.30 **Ulcerative (chronic) rectosigmoiditis without complications**
Ulcerative (chronic) rectosigmoiditis NOS
+6 K51.31 **Ulcerative (chronic) rectosigmoiditis with complications**
SP + K51.311 **Ulcerative (chronic) rectosigmoiditis with rectal bleeding**
SP + K51.312 **Ulcerative (chronic) rectosigmoiditis with intestinal obstruction**
SP + K51.313 **Ulcerative (chronic) rectosigmoiditis with fistula**
SP + K51.314 **Ulcerative (chronic) rectosigmoiditis with abscess**
SP + K51.318 **Ulcerative (chronic) rectosigmoiditis with other complication**
!Q + K51.319 **Ulcerative (chronic) rectosigmoiditis with unspecified complications**

+5 K51.4 **Inflammatory polyps of colon**
EXCLUDES 1 adenomatous polyp of colon (D12.6)
polyposis of colon (D12.6)
polyps of colon NOS (K63.5)
SP + K51.40 **Inflammatory polyps of colon without complications**
Inflammatory polyps of colon NOS
+6 K51.41 **Inflammatory polyps of colon with complications**
SP + K51.411 **Inflammatory polyps of colon with rectal bleeding**
SP + K51.412 **Inflammatory polyps of colon with intestinal obstruction**
SP + K51.413 **Inflammatory polyps of colon with fistula**
SP + K51.414 **Inflammatory polyps of colon with abscess**
SP + K51.418 **Inflammatory polyps of colon with other complication**
!Q + K51.419 **Inflammatory polyps of colon with unspecified complications**

+5 K51.5 **Left sided colitis**
Left hemicolitis
SP + K51.50 **Left sided colitis without complications**
Left sided colitis NOS
+6 K51.51 **Left sided colitis with complications**
SP + K51.511 **Left sided colitis with rectal bleeding**
SP + K51.512 **Left sided colitis with intestinal obstruction**
SP + K51.513 **Left sided colitis with fistula**
SP + K51.514 **Left sided colitis with abscess**
SP + K51.518 **Left sided colitis with other complication**
!Q + K51.519 **Left sided colitis with unspecified complications**

+5 K51.8 **Other ulcerative colitis**
SP + K51.80 **Other ulcerative colitis without complications**
DEFINITION Inflammation of the intestinal lining with ulcer formation, causing diarrhea as the colon empties frequently.
+6 K51.81 **Other ulcerative colitis with complications**
SP + K51.811 **Other ulcerative colitis with rectal bleeding**
SP + K51.812 **Other ulcerative colitis with intestinal obstruction**
SP + K51.813 **Other ulcerative colitis with fistula**
SP + K51.814 **Other ulcerative colitis with abscess**
SP + K51.818 **Other ulcerative colitis with other complication**
!Q + K51.819 **Other ulcerative colitis with unspecified complications**

+5 K51.9 **Ulcerative colitis, unspecified**
SP + K51.90 **Ulcerative colitis, unspecified, without complications**
+6 K51.91 **Ulcerative colitis, unspecified, with complications**
SP + K51.911 **Ulcerative colitis, unspecified with rectal bleeding**

Chapter 11 K00-K95

SP + K51.912 **Ulcerative colitis, unspecified with intestinal obstruction**

SP + K51.913 **Ulcerative colitis, unspecified with fistula**

SP + K51.914 **Ulcerative colitis, unspecified with abscess**

SP + K51.918 **Ulcerative colitis, unspecified with other complication**

IQ + K51.919 **Ulcerative colitis, unspecified with unspecified complications**

4 K52 **Other and unspecified noninfective gastroenteritis and colitis**

SP K52.0 **Gastroenteritis and colitis due to radiation**

SP + K52.1 **Toxic gastroenteritis and colitis**
Drug-induced gastroenteritis and colitis
Code first:
(T51-T65) to identify toxic agent
Use additional code for adverse effect, if applicable, to identify drug (T36-T50 with fifth or sixth character 5)

▲ + 5 K52.2 **Allergic and dietetic gastroenteritis and colitis**
Food hypersensitivity gastroenteritis or colitis
Use additional code to identify type of food allergy (Z91.01-, Z91.02-)
EXCLUDES 2 allergic eosinophilic colitis (K52.82)
allergic eosinophilic esophagitis (K20.0)
allergic eosinophilic gastritis (K52.81)
allergic eosinophilic gastroenteritis (K52.81)

SP + K52.21 **Food protein-induced enterocolitis syndrome**
FPIES
Use additional code for hypovolemic shock, if present (R57.1)
DEFINITION A nontypical, non-IgE, food allergy affecting infants and young children with serious gastrointestinal effects that result in profound vomiting, severe diarrhea involving both the large and small intestine, and dehydration as well as severe lethargy and dangerous changes in body temperature and blood pressure. Symptoms may not be immediate or show up on standard allergy tests, but will appear after ingesting a food trigger.

SP + K52.22 **Food protein-induced enteropathy**
DEFINITION A type of food protein intolerance with gastrointestinal manifestations, typically occurring in the pediatric population in the first 6 months of life and most often as intolerance to cow's milk or soy milk protein.

▲ SP + K52.29 **Other allergic and dietetic gastroenteritis and colitis**
Allergic proctocolitis
Food hypersensitivity gastroenteritis or colitis
Food-induced eosinophilic proctocolitis
Food protein-induced proctocolitis
Immediate gastrointestinal hypersensitivity
Milk protein-induced proctocolitis

SP K52.3 **Indeterminate colitis**
Colonic inflammatory bowel disease unclassified (IBDU)
EXCLUDES 1 unspecified colitis (K52.9)

5 K52.8 **Other specified noninfective gastroenteritis and colitis**

SP K52.81 **Eosinophilic gastritis or gastroenteritis**
Eosinophilic enteritis
EXCLUDES 2 eosinophilic esophagitis (K20.0)

▲ SP K52.82 **Eosinophilic colitis**
EXCLUDES 2 allergic proctocolitis (K52.29)
food-induced eosinophilic proctocolitis (K52.29)
food protein-induced enterocolitis syndrome (FPIES) (K52.21)
food protein-induced proctocolitis (K52.29)
milk protein-induced proctocolitis (K52.29)

6 K52.83 **Microscopic colitis**

SP K52.831 **Collagenous colitis**

SP K52.832 **Lymphocytic colitis**

SP K52.838 **Other microscopic colitis**

SP K52.839 **Microscopic colitis, unspecified**

SP K52.89 **Other specified noninfective gastroenteritis and colitis**

SP K52.9 **Noninfective gastroenteritis and colitis, unspecified**
Colitis NOS
Enteritis NOS
Gastroenteritis NOS
Ileitis NOS
Jejunitis NOS
Sigmoiditis NOS
EXCLUDES 1 diarrhea NOS (R19.7)
functional diarrhea (K59.1)
infectious gastroenteritis and colitis NOS (A09)
neonatal diarrhea (noninfective) (P78.3)
psychogenic diarrhea (F45.8)

Other diseases of intestines (K55-K64)

4 K55 **Vascular disorders of intestine**
EXCLUDES 1 necrotizing enterocolitis of newborn (P77.-)

5 K55.0 **Acute vascular disorders of intestine**
Infarction of appendices epiploicae
Mesenteric (artery) (vein) embolism
Mesenteric (artery) (vein) infarction
Mesenteric (artery) (vein) thrombosis

6 K55.01 **Acute (reversible) ischemia of small intestine**

SP K55.011 **Focal (segmental) acute (reversible) ischemia of small intestine**

Chapter 11

K00-K95

4 4th digit required 5 5th digit required 6 6th digit required 7 7th digit required 7 7th digit placeholder + Additional code Laterality

SP **K55.012 Diffuse acute (reversible) ischemia of small intestine**

SP **K55.019 Acute (reversible) ischemia of small intestine, extent unspecified**

6 **K55.02 Acute infarction of small intestine**
Gangrene of small intestine
Necrosis of small intestine

SP **K55.021 Focal (segmental) acute infarction of small intestine**

SP **K55.022 Diffuse acute infarction of small intestine**

SP **K55.029 Acute infarction of small intestine, extent unspecified**

6 **K55.03 Acute (reversible) ischemia of large intestine**
Acute fulminant ischemic colitis
Subacute ischemic colitis

SP **K55.031 Focal (segmental) acute (reversible) ischemia of large intestine**

SP **K55.032 Diffuse acute (reversible) ischemia of large intestine**

SP **K55.039 Acute (reversible) ischemia of large intestine, extent unspecified**

6 **K55.04 Acute infarction of large intestine**
Gangrene of large intestine
Necrosis of large intestine

SP **K55.041 Focal (segmental) acute infarction of large intestine**

SP **K55.042 Diffuse acute infarction of large intestine**

SP **K55.049 Acute infarction of large intestine, extent unspecified**

6 **K55.05 Acute (reversible) ischemia of intestine, part unspecified**

SP **K55.051 Focal (segmental) acute (reversible) ischemia of intestine, part unspecified**

SP **K55.052 Diffuse acute (reversible) ischemia of intestine, part unspecified**

SP **K55.059 Acute (reversible) ischemia of intestine, part and extent unspecified**

6 **K55.06 Acute infarction of intestine, part unspecified**
Acute intestinal infarction
Gangrene of intestine
Necrosis of intestine

SP **K55.061 Focal (segmental) acute infarction of intestine, part unspecified**

SP **K55.062 Diffuse acute infarction of intestine, part unspecified**

SP **K55.069 Acute infarction of intestine, part and extent unspecified**

SP **K55.1 Chronic vascular disorders of intestine**
Chronic ischemic colitis
Chronic ischemic enteritis
Chronic ischemic enterocolitis
Ischemic stricture of intestine
Mesenteric atherosclerosis
Mesenteric vascular insufficiency

5 **K55.2 Angiodysplasia of colon**

SP **K55.20 Angiodysplasia of colon without hemorrhage**

SP **K55.21 Angiodysplasia of colon with hemorrhage**

DEFINITION Dilated intestinal blood vessels with corresponding thinning and weakening of vessel walls and bleeding into the intestinal tract.

5 **K55.3 Necrotizing enterocolitis**

EXCLUDES 1 necrotizing enterocolitis of newborn (P77.-)

EXCLUDES 2 necrotizing enterocolitis due to Clostridium difficile (A04.7-)

CODING TIPS✓ Necrotizing enterocolitis is characterized by damage to the intestine which can be related to inflammation, infection, or ischemia. This leads to necrosis, which may involve just the intestinal lining, or the full thickness, and can cause perforation, and death. Due to its potential severity, necrotizing enterocolitis is considered a medical emergency.

SP **K55.30 Necrotizing enterocolitis, unspecified**
Necrotizing enterocolitis, NOS

SP **K55.31 Stage 1 necrotizing enterocolitis**
Necrotizing enterocolitis without pneumatosis, without perforation

SP **K55.32 Stage 2 necrotizing enterocolitis**
Necrotizing enterocolitis with pneumatosis, without perforation

SP **K55.33 Stage 3 necrotizing enterocolitis**
Necrotizing enterocolitis with perforation
Necrotizing enterocolitis with pneumatosis and perforation

SP **K55.8 Other vascular disorders of intestine**

SP **K55.9 Vascular disorder of intestine, unspecified**
Ischemic colitis
Ischemic enteritis
Ischemic enterocolitis

4 **K56 Paralytic ileus and intestinal obstruction without hernia**

EXCLUDES 1 congenital stricture or stenosis of intestine (Q41-Q42)
cystic fibrosis with meconium ileus (E84.11)
ischemic stricture of intestine (K55.1)
meconium ileus NOS (P76.0)
neonatal intestinal obstructions classifiable to P76.-
obstruction of duodenum (K31.5)
postprocedural intestinal obstruction (K91.3-)

EXCLUDES 2 stenosis of anus or rectum (K62.4)

SP **K56.0 Paralytic ileus**
Paralysis of bowel
Paralysis of colon
Paralysis of intestine

EXCLUDES 1 gallstone ileus (K56.3)
ileus NOS (K56.7)
obstructive ileus NOS (K56.69-)

DEFINITION Blockage in the small or large intestine due to nonfunctioning muscle wall; may occur due to fluid imbalance, nerve damage, decreased blood supply, or toxins.

SP **K56.1 Intussusception**
Intussusception or invagination of bowel
Intussusception or invagination of colon
Intussusception or invagination of intestine
Intussusception or invagination of rectum
EXCLUDES 2 intussusception of appendix (K38.8)

SP **K56.2 Volvulus**
Strangulation of colon or intestine
Torsion of colon or intestine
Twist of colon or intestine
EXCLUDES 2 volvulus of duodenum (K31.5)

DEFINITION Twisting of the intestine, constricting the passageway and cutting off blood supply to the area; presents with sudden, severe abdominal pain, vomiting, and abdominal distention.

SP **K56.3 Gallstone ileus**
Obstruction of intestine by gallstone

5 **K56.4 Other impaction of intestine**

SP **K56.41 Fecal impaction**
EXCLUDES 1 constipation (K59.0-)
incomplete defecation (R15.0)

SP **K56.49 Other impaction of intestine**

5 **K56.5 Intestinal adhesions [bands] with obstruction (postinfection)**
Abdominal hernia due to adhesions with obstruction
Peritoneal adhesions [bands] with intestinal obstruction (postinfection)

CODING TIPS✓ Intestinal obstruction varies in severity, from partial or intermittent obstruction that resolves without intervention to complete obstruction that requires an operation and may lead to intestinal gangrene and perforation. Physicians or NPPs frequently describe intestinal obstruction as partial versus complete. These distinctions are relevant because complete obstruction generally requires an operation and partial obstruction usually does not (especially for the small intestine). These descriptors may differentiate between an aftercare code and a condition that may not yet be resolved.

SP **K56.50 Intestinal adhesions [bands], unspecified as to partial versus complete obstruction**
Intestinal adhesions with obstruction NOS

SP **K56.51 Intestinal adhesions [bands], with partial obstruction**
Intestinal adhesions with incomplete obstruction

SP **K56.52 Intestinal adhesions [bands] with complete obstruction**

5 **K56.6 Other and unspecified intestinal obstruction**

CODING TIPS✓ Intestinal obstruction varies in severity, from partial or intermittent obstruction that resolves without intervention to complete obstruction that requires an operation and may lead to intestinal gangrene and perforation. Physicians or NPPs frequently describe intestinal obstruction as partial versus complete. These distinctions are relevant because complete obstruction generally requires an operation and partial obstruction usually does not (especially for the small intestine). These descriptors may differentiate between an aftercare code and a condition that may not yet be resolved.

6 **K56.60 Unspecified intestinal obstruction**

IQ **K56.600 Partial intestinal obstruction, unspecified as to cause**
Incomplete intestinal obstruction, NOS

IQ **K56.601 Complete intestinal obstruction, unspecified as to cause**

IQ **K56.609 Unspecified intestinal obstruction, unspecified as to partial versus complete obstruction**
Intestinal obstruction NOS

6 **K56.69 Other intestinal obstruction**
Enterostenosis NOS
Obstructive ileus NOS
Occlusion of colon or intestine NOS
Stenosis of colon or intestine NOS
Stricture of colon or intestine NOS
EXCLUDES 1 intestinal obstruction due to specified condition-code to condition

SP **K56.690 Other partial intestinal obstruction**
Other incomplete intestinal obstruction

SP **K56.691 Other complete intestinal obstruction**

SP **K56.699 Other intestinal obstruction unspecified as to partial versus complete obstruction**
Other intestinal obstruction, NEC

SP **K56.7 Ileus, unspecified**
EXCLUDES 1 obstructive ileus (K56.69-)
EXCLUDES 2 intestinal obstruction with hernia (K40-K46)

4 **K57 Diverticular disease of intestine**
Code also:
if applicable peritonitis K65.-
EXCLUDES 1 congenital diverticulum of intestine (Q43.8)
Meckel's diverticulum (Q43.0)
EXCLUDES 2 diverticulum of appendix (K38.2)

CODING TIPS✓ Do not assign a code from K57.- for diverticular conditions reported as congenital. Congenital diverticulum should be coded to the appropriate Q43.- code.

5 **K57.0 Diverticulitis of small intestine with perforation and abscess**

Chapter 11

K00-K95

EXCLUDES 1 diverticulitis of both small and large intestine with perforation and abscess (K57.4-)

SP **K57.00 Diverticulitis of small intestine with perforation and abscess without bleeding**

SP **K57.01 Diverticulitis of small intestine with perforation and abscess with bleeding**

5 **K57.1 Diverticular disease of small intestine without perforation or abscess**

EXCLUDES 1 diverticular disease of both small and large intestine without perforation or abscess (K57.5-)

SP **K57.10 Diverticulosis of small intestine without perforation or abscess without bleeding**

Diverticular disease of small intestine NOS

SP **K57.11 Diverticulosis of small intestine without perforation or abscess with bleeding**

SP **K57.12 Diverticulitis of small intestine without perforation or abscess without bleeding**

SP **K57.13 Diverticulitis of small intestine without perforation or abscess with bleeding**

5 **K57.2 Diverticulitis of large intestine with perforation and abscess**

EXCLUDES 1 diverticulitis of both small and large intestine with perforation and abscess (K57.4-)

SP **K57.20 Diverticulitis of large intestine with perforation and abscess without bleeding**

SP **K57.21 Diverticulitis of large intestine with perforation and abscess with bleeding**

5 **K57.3 Diverticular disease of large intestine without perforation or abscess**

EXCLUDES 1 diverticular disease of both small and large intestine without perforation or abscess (K57.5-)

SP **K57.30 Diverticulosis of large intestine without perforation or abscess without bleeding**

Diverticular disease of colon NOS

SP **K57.31 Diverticulosis of large intestine without perforation or abscess with bleeding**

SP **K57.32 Diverticulitis of large intestine without perforation or abscess without bleeding**

SP **K57.33 Diverticulitis of large intestine without perforation or abscess with bleeding**

5 **K57.4 Diverticulitis of both small and large intestine with perforation and abscess**

SP **K57.40 Diverticulitis of both small and large intestine with perforation and abscess without bleeding**

SP **K57.41 Diverticulitis of both small and large intestine with perforation and abscess with bleeding**

5 **K57.5 Diverticular disease of both small and large intestine without perforation or abscess**

SP **K57.50 Diverticulosis of both small and large intestine without perforation or abscess without bleeding**

Diverticular disease of both small and large intestine NOS

SP **K57.51 Diverticulosis of both small and large intestine without perforation or abscess with bleeding**

SP **K57.52 Diverticulitis of both small and large intestine without perforation or abscess without bleeding**

SP **K57.53 Diverticulitis of both small and large intestine without perforation or abscess with bleeding**

5 **K57.8 Diverticulitis of intestine, part unspecified, with perforation and abscess**

SP **K57.80 Diverticulitis of intestine, part unspecified, with perforation and abscess without bleeding**

SP **K57.81 Diverticulitis of intestine, part unspecified, with perforation and abscess with bleeding**

5 **K57.9 Diverticular disease of intestine, part unspecified, without perforation or abscess**

SP **K57.90 Diverticulosis of intestine, part unspecified, without perforation or abscess without bleeding**

Diverticular disease of intestine NOS

SP **K57.91 Diverticulosis of intestine, part unspecified, without perforation or abscess with bleeding**

SP **K57.92 Diverticulitis of intestine, part unspecified, without perforation or abscess without bleeding**

SP **K57.93 Diverticulitis of intestine, part unspecified, without perforation or abscess with bleeding**

4 **K58 Irritable bowel syndrome**

INCLUDES irritable colon
spastic colon

CODING TIPS✓ Functional gastrointestinal disorders (FGIDs) can affect any part of the gastrointestinal tract; they are disorders of how the GI tract works, not structural or biochemical abnormalities. Irritable bowel syndrome (IBS) is a chronic functional gastrointestinal disorder characterized by abdominal pain or discomfort associated with altered bowel habits. IBS is classified into subtypes based on the predominant alteration in stool form: IBS with constipation (IBS-C), IBS with diarrhea (IBS-D), both (IBS-M for mixed) or neither (IBS-U for unspecified).

DEFINITION Functional disorder of hypersensitive nerves and muscles in the colon, causing cramping, pain, diarrhea, and/or constipation.

SP **K58.0 Irritable bowel syndrome with diarrhea**

Chapter 11

K00-K95

CODING TIPS ✓ Do not assign an additional code for the diarrhea. K58.0 is a combination code and does not require additional coding of the included symptom.

SP **K58.1 Irritable bowel syndrome with constipation**

SP **K58.2 Mixed irritable bowel syndrome**

SP **K58.8 Other irritable bowel syndrome**

SP **K58.9 Irritable bowel syndrome without diarrhea**
Irritable bowel syndrome NOS

4 **K59 Other functional intestinal disorders**
EXCLUDES 1 change in bowel habit NOS (R19.4)
intestinal malabsorption (K90.-)
psychogenic intestinal disorders (F45.8)
EXCLUDES 2 functional disorders of stomach (K31.-)

5 **K59.0 Constipation**
EXCLUDES 1 fecal impaction (K56.41)
incomplete defecation (R15.0)

SP **K59.00 Constipation, unspecified**

SP **K59.01 Slow transit constipation**
DEFINITION Dysfunction of intestinal smooth muscles that move fecal matter, causing slow stool movement.

SP **K59.02 Outlet dysfunction constipation**

SP + **K59.03 Drug induced constipation**
Use additional code for adverse effect, if applicable, to identify drug (T36-T50 with fifth or sixth character 5)

CODING TIPS ✓ Opiate induced constipation is more difficult to manage. Code also the opiate adverse effect.

CODING TIPS ✓ Opioids and other medications affect all segments of the stomach and intestine (particularly the colon) altering nerve input to the GI tract which inhibits movement. Constipation from slowed or absent GI motility requires a long-term bowel program and possible colectomy for chronic constipation resistant to treatment.

SP **K59.04 Chronic idiopathic constipation**
Functional constipation

DEFINITION Chronic idiopathic constipation, also known as functional constipation, is a long-lasting or recurring reduction in stool frequency, usually less than 3 times per week, difficulty passing stools, or both without any underlying illness, medication, or physiological cause, such as hormonal imbalance.

SP **K59.09 Other constipation**
Chronic constipation

SP **K59.1 Functional diarrhea**
EXCLUDES 1 diarrhea NOS (R19.7)
irritable bowel syndrome with diarrhea (K58.0)

CODING TIPS ✓ K59.1, functional diarrhea, is a condition with no detectable organic cause. When the organism is identified, infectious diarrhea must be assigned from code range A00-A09.

SP **K59.2 Neurogenic bowel, not elsewhere classified**
DEFINITION Intestinal dysfunction due to spinal cord damage.

5 **K59.3 Megacolon, not elsewhere classified**
Dilatation of colon
Code first:
, if applicable (T51-T65) to identify toxic agent
EXCLUDES 1 congenital megacolon (aganglionic) (Q43.1)
megacolon (due to) (in) Chagas' disease (B57.32)
megacolon (due to) (in) Clostridium difficile (A04.7-)
megacolon (due to) (in) Hirschsprung's disease (Q43.1)

CODING TIPS ✓ Megacolon is an abnormal dilation of the colon, generally accompanied by reduced peristalsis. Do not assign a code from K59.3- if the cause is known to be due to another condition such as *Clostridium difficile* (A04.7), Hirschsprung's disease (Q43.1), or other congenital or known cause. When the cause is known, code the cause of the megacolon.

DEFINITION Enlargement or dilation of the sigmoid colon.

SP **K59.31 Toxic megacolon**

SP **K59.39 Other megacolon**
Megacolon NOS

DEFINITION A condition in which the large intestine becomes extremely distended and stretched so that it is much larger than usual. This may be an acute, sudden and severe condition due to infection, or a chronic condition due to abnormal growth. Note: Congenital megacolon and that due to exposure to toxins is classified by other codes.

SP **K59.4 Anal spasm**
Proctalgia fugax

5 **K59.8 Other specified functional intestinal disorders**

SP **K59.81 Ogilvie syndrome**
Acute colonic pseudo-obstruction (ACPO)

SP **K59.89 Other specified functional intestinal disorders**
Atony of colon
Pseudo-obstruction (acute) (chronic) of intestine

SP **K59.9 Functional intestinal disorder, unspecified**

4 **K60 Fissure and fistula of anal and rectal regions**
EXCLUDES 1 fissure and fistula of anal and rectal regions with abscess or cellulitis (K61.-)

4 4th digit required 5 5th digit required 6 6th digit required 7 7th digit required 7 7th digit placeholder + Additional code Laterality

EXCLUDES 2 anal sphincter tear (healed) (nontraumatic) (old) (K62.81)

SP **K60.0 Acute anal fissure**

SP **K60.1 Chronic anal fissure**

SP **K60.2 Anal fissure, unspecified**

SP **K60.3 Anal fistula**

DEFINITION An abnormal passage from the anus to the skin.

SP **K60.4 Rectal fistula**

Fistula of rectum to skin

EXCLUDES 1 rectovaginal fistula (N82.3)
vesicorectal fistual (N32.1)

SP **K60.5 Anorectal fistula**

4 **K61 Abscess of anal and rectal regions**

INCLUDES abscess of anal and rectal regions
cellulitis of anal and rectal regions

SP **K61.0 Anal abscess**

Perianal abscess

EXCLUDES 2 intrasphincteric abscess (K61.4)

SP **K61.1 Rectal abscess**

Perirectal abscess

EXCLUDES 1 ischiorectal abscess (K61.39)

SP **K61.2 Anorectal abscess**

5 **K61.3 Ischiorectal abscess**

SP **K61.31 Horseshoe abscess**

SP **K61.39 Other ischiorectal abscess**

Abscess of ischiorectal fossa
Ischiorectal abscess, NOS

SP **K61.4 Intrasphincteric abscess**

Intersphincteric abscess

SP **K61.5 Supralevator abscess**

4 **K62 Other diseases of anus and rectum**

INCLUDES anal canal

EXCLUDES 2 colostomy and enterostomy malfunction (K94.0-, K94.1-)
fecal incontinence (R15.-)
hemorrhoids (K64.-)

SP **K62.0 Anal polyp**

SP **K62.1 Rectal polyp**

EXCLUDES 1 adenomatous polyp (D12.8)

SP **K62.2 Anal prolapse**

Prolapse of anal canal

SP **K62.3 Rectal prolapse**

Prolapse of rectal mucosa

DEFINITION Rectal tissue falls from its usual position, turning itself inside out and protruding from the body in late stages.

SP **K62.4 Stenosis of anus and rectum**

Stricture of anus (sphincter)

SP **K62.5 Hemorrhage of anus and rectum**

EXCLUDES 1 gastrointestinal bleeding NOS (K92.2)
melena (K92.1)
neonatal rectal hemorrhage (P54.2)

SP **K62.6 Ulcer of anus and rectum**

Solitary ulcer of anus and rectum
Stercoral ulcer of anus and rectum

EXCLUDES 1 fissure and fistula of anus and rectum (K60.-)
ulcerative colitis (K51.-)

DEFINITION Open sore in the rectum and/or anus causing pain that worsens during defecation and blood or mucous in the stool.

SP + **K62.7 Radiation proctitis**

Use additional code to identify the type of radiation (W88.-)
or radiation therapy (Y84.2)

CODING TIPS✓ Radiation proctitis includes ulceration of the rectal lining due to the adverse effects of radiation. Assign an additional code from W88.- to identify radiation exposure, or Y84.2 if documentation indicates exposure was an adverse effect or abnormal reaction of a radiological procedure.

5 **K62.8 Other specified diseases of anus and rectum**

EXCLUDES 2 ulcerative proctitis (K51.2)

SP + **K62.81 Anal sphincter tear (healed) (nontraumatic) (old)**

Tear of anus, nontraumatic
Use additional code for any associated fecal incontinence (R15.-)

EXCLUDES 2 anal fissure (K60.-)
anal sphincter tear (healed) (old) complicating delivery (O34.7-)
traumatic tear of anal sphincter (S31.831)

SP **K62.82 Dysplasia of anus**

Anal intraepithelial neoplasia I and II (AIN I and II) (histologically confirmed)
Dysplasia of anus NOS
Mild and moderate dysplasia of anus (histologically confirmed)

EXCLUDES 1 abnormal results from anal cytologic examination without histologic confirmation (R85.61-)
anal intraepithelial neoplasia III (D01.3)
carcinoma in situ of anus (D01.3)
HGSIL of anus (R85.613)
severe dysplasia of anus (D01.3)

SP + **K62.89 Other specified diseases of anus and rectum**

Proctitis NOS
Use additional code for any associated fecal incontinence (R15.-)

IQ **K62.9 Disease of anus and rectum, unspecified**

4 **K63 Other diseases of intestine**

SP **K63.0 Abscess of intestine**

EXCLUDES 1 abscess of intestine with Crohn's disease (K50.014, K50.114, K50.814, K50.914,)
abscess of intestine with diverticular disease (K57.0, K57.2, K57.4, K57.8)

Chapter 11

K00-K95

abscess of intestine with ulcerative colitis (K51.014, K51.214, K51.314, K51.414, K51.514, K51.814, K51.914)

EXCLUDES 2 abscess of anal and rectal regions (K61.-)
abscess of appendix (K35.3-)

SP **K63.1 Perforation of intestine (nontraumatic)**
Perforation (nontraumatic) of rectum
EXCLUDES 1 perforation (nontraumatic) of duodenum (K26.-)
perforation (nontraumatic) of intestine with diverticular disease (K57.0, K57.2, K57.4, K57.8)
EXCLUDES 2 perforation (nontraumatic) of appendix (K35.2-, K35.3-)
DEFINITION Hole in the intestinal wall allowing food and/or fecal matter to leak into the abdominal cavity.

SP **K63.2 Fistula of intestine**
EXCLUDES 1 fistula of duodenum (K31.6)
fistula of intestine with Crohn's disease (K50.013, K50.113, K50.813, K50.913,)
fistula of intestine with ulcerative colitis (K51.013, K51.213, K51.313, K51.413, K51.513, K51.813, K51.913)
EXCLUDES 2 fistula of anal and rectal regions (K60.-)
fistula of appendix (K38.3)
intestinal-genital fistula, female (N82.2-N82.4)
vesicointestinal fistula (N32.1)
DEFINITION Abnormal passageway between loops of the intestine or the intestine and another organ or the abdominal wall.

SP **K63.3 Ulcer of intestine**
Primary ulcer of small intestine
EXCLUDES 1 duodenal ulcer (K26.-)
gastrointestinal ulcer (K28.-)
gastrojejunal ulcer (K28.-)
jejunal ulcer (K28.-)
peptic ulcer, site unspecified (K27.-)
ulcer of intestine with perforation (K63.1)
ulcer of anus or rectum (K62.6)
ulcerative colitis (K51.-)

SP **K63.4 Enteroptosis**

SP **K63.5 Polyp of colon**
EXCLUDES 1 adenomatous polyp of colon (D12.-)
inflammatory polyp of colon (K51.4-)
polyposis of colon (D12.6)
CODING TIPS✓ Most polyps of the colon are coded to D12 because they are considered benign neoplasms. Hyperplastic polyps are coded to K63.5.

5 **K63.8 Other specified diseases of intestine**

SP **K63.81 Dieulafoy lesion of intestine**
EXCLUDES 2 Dieulafoy lesion of stomach and duodenum (K31.82)

SP **K63.89 Other specified diseases of intestine**

IQ **K63.9 Disease of intestine, unspecified**

4 **K64 Hemorrhoids and perianal venous thrombosis**
INCLUDES piles
EXCLUDES 1 hemorrhoids complicating childbirth and the puerperium (O87.2)
hemorrhoids complicating pregnancy (O22.4)

SP **K64.0 First degree hemorrhoids**
Grade/stage I hemorrhoids
Hemorrhoids (bleeding) without prolapse outside of anal canal

SP **K64.1 Second degree hemorrhoids**
Grade/stage II hemorrhoids
Hemorrhoids (bleeding) that prolapse with straining, but retract spontaneously

SP **K64.2 Third degree hemorrhoids**
Grade/stage III hemorrhoids
Hemorrhoids (bleeding) that prolapse with straining and require manual replacement back inside anal canal

SP **K64.3 Fourth degree hemorrhoids**
Grade/stage IV hemorrhoids
Hemorrhoids (bleeding) with prolapsed tissue that cannot be manually replaced

SP **K64.4 Residual hemorrhoidal skin tags**
External hemorrhoids, NOS
Skin tags of anus

SP **K64.5 Perianal venous thrombosis**
External hemorrhoids with thrombosis
Perianal hematoma
Thrombosed hemorrhoids NOS

SP **K64.8 Other hemorrhoids**
Internal hemorrhoids, without mention of degree
Prolapsed hemorrhoids, degree not specified

SP **K64.9 Unspecified hemorrhoids**
Hemorrhoids (bleeding) NOS
Hemorrhoids (bleeding) without mention of degree

Chapter 11

K00-K95

Diseases of peritoneum and retroperitoneum (K65-K68)

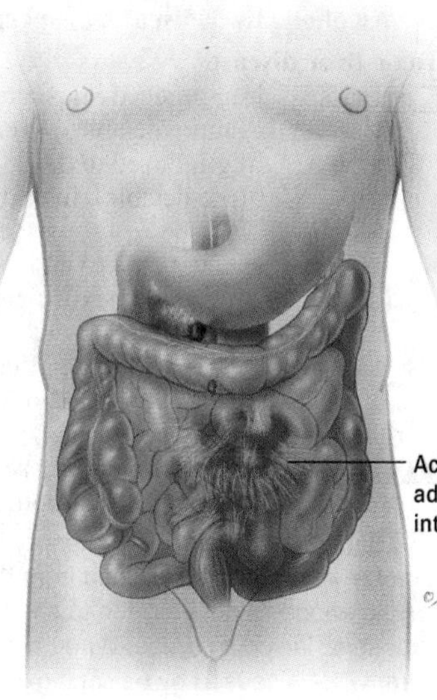

+ 4 **K65 Peritonitis**
Code also:
if applicable diverticular disease of intestine (K57.-)
Use additional code (B95-B97), to identify infectious agent, if known
EXCLUDES 1 acute appendicitis with generalized peritonitis (K35.2-)
aseptic peritonitis (T81.6)
benign paroxysmal peritonitis (E85.0)
chemical peritonitis (T81.6)
gonococcal peritonitis (A54.85)
neonatal peritonitis (P78.0-P78.1)
pelvic peritonitis, female (N73.3-N73.5)
periodic familial peritonitis (E85.0)
peritonitis due to talc or other foreign substance (T81.6)
peritonitis in chlamydia (A74.81)
peritonitis in diphtheria (A36.89)
peritonitis in syphilis (late) (A52.74)
peritonitis in tuberculosis (A18.31)
peritonitis with or following abortion or ectopic or molar pregnancy (O00-O07, O08.0)
peritonitis with or following appendicitis (K35.-)
puerperal peritonitis (O85)
retroperitoneal infections (K68.-)

CODING TIPS✓ When the causative infectious organism is known, always assign an additional code from B95-B97 to identify the infectious agent.

SP + **K65.0 Generalized (acute) peritonitis**
Pelvic peritonitis (acute), male
Subphrenic peritonitis (acute)
Suppurative peritonitis (acute)

SP + **K65.1 Peritoneal abscess**
Abdominopelvic abscess
Abscess (of) omentum
Abscess (of) peritoneum
Mesenteric abscess
Retrocecal abscess
Subdiaphragmatic abscess
Subhepatic abscess
Subphrenic abscess

SP + **K65.2 Spontaneous bacterial peritonitis**
EXCLUDES 1 bacterial peritonitis NOS (K65.9)
CODING TIPS✓ Do not assign K65.2 unless the provider has specifically provided a diagnosis of "spontaneous" bacterial peritonitis. Bacterial peritonitis not specified as spontaneous is classified to K65.9 (Peritonitis NOS).

SP + **K65.3 Choleperitonitis**
Peritonitis due to bile

SP + **K65.4 Sclerosing mesenteritis**
Fat necrosis of peritoneum
(Idiopathic) sclerosing mesenteric fibrosis
Mesenteric lipodystrophy
Mesenteric panniculitis
Retractile mesenteritis
DEFINITION Rare, idiopathic lesions of fat necrosis, fibrosis, and chronic inflammation causing single or multiple lesions, with diffuse thickening of the mesentery.

SP + **K65.8 Other peritonitis**
Chronic proliferative peritonitis
Peritonitis due to urine

SP + **K65.9 Peritonitis, unspecified**
Bacterial peritonitis NOS

4 **K66 Other disorders of peritoneum**
EXCLUDES 2 ascites (R18.-)
peritoneal effusion (chronic) (R18.8)

SP **K66.0 Peritoneal adhesions (postprocedural) (postinfection)**
Adhesions (of) abdominal (wall)
Adhesions (of) diaphragm
Adhesions (of) intestine
Adhesions (of) male pelvis
Adhesions (of) omentum
Adhesions (of) stomach
Adhesive bands
Mesenteric adhesions
EXCLUDES 1 female pelvic adhesions [bands] (N73.6)
peritoneal adhesions with intestinal obstruction (K56.5-)

SP **K66.1 Hemoperitoneum**
EXCLUDES 1 traumatic hemoperitoneum (S36.8-)

SP **K66.8 Other specified disorders of peritoneum**

IQ **K66.9 Disorder of peritoneum, unspecified**

Chapter 11 K00-K95

M IQ **K67** ***Disorders of peritoneum in infectious diseases classified elsewhere***

Code first underlying disease, such as:
congenital syphilis (A50.0)
helminthiasis (B65.0 -B83.9)

EXCLUDES 1 peritonitis in chlamydia (A74.81)
peritonitis in diphtheria (A36.89)
peritonitis in gonococcal (A54.85)
peritonitis in syphilis (late) (A52.74)
peritonitis in tuberculosis (A18.31)

4 **K68 Disorders of retroperitoneum**

5 **K68.1 Retroperitoneal abscess**

SP **K68.11 Postprocedural retroperitoneal abscess**

EXCLUDES 2 infection following procedure (T81.4-)

SP **K68.12 Psoas muscle abscess**

SP **K68.19 Other retroperitoneal abscess**

SP **K68.9 Other disorders of retroperitoneum**

Diseases of liver (K70-K77)

EXCLUDES 1 jaundice NOS (R17)

EXCLUDES 2 hemochromatosis (E83.11-)
Reye's syndrome (G93.7)
viral hepatitis (B15-B19)
Wilson's disease (E83.0)

+ 4 **K70 Alcoholic liver disease**

Use additional code to identify:
alcohol abuse and dependence (F10.-)

CODING TIPS ✓ Codes from category K70.- indicate liver disease resulting from alcohol use. An additional code should be assigned to identify alcohol abuse or dependence. Do not use 5th and 6th digits .88 to indicate alcohol induced disorder with the F10 code as alcohol induced disorders include only mental, emotional and physical disorders in Chapter 5.

SP + **K70.0 Alcoholic fatty liver**

+ 5 **K70.1 Alcoholic hepatitis**

SP + **K70.10 Alcoholic hepatitis without ascites**

SP + **K70.11 Alcoholic hepatitis with ascites**

H SP + **K70.2 Alcoholic fibrosis and sclerosis of liver**

DEFINITION Intermediate stage liver disease in which normal, healthy tissue of the liver is replaced by scar tissue due to long-term, excessive alcohol consumption.

+ 5 **K70.3 Alcoholic cirrhosis of liver**

Alcoholic cirrhosis NOS

DEFINITION Late stage liver disease characterized by inflammation, debilitating scar tissue, and damaged membranes due to long-term, excessive alcohol consumption.

H SP + **K70.30 Alcoholic cirrhosis of liver without ascites**

H SP + **K70.31 Alcoholic cirrhosis of liver with ascites**

+ 5 **K70.4 Alcoholic hepatic failure**

Acute alcoholic hepatic failure
Alcoholic hepatic failure NOS
Chronic alcoholic hepatic failure
Subacute alcoholic hepatic failure

SP + **K70.40 Alcoholic hepatic failure without coma**

H SP + **K70.41 Alcoholic hepatic failure with coma**

SP + **K70.9 Alcoholic liver disease, unspecified**

+ 4 **K71 Toxic liver disease**

INCLUDES drug-induced idiosyncratic (unpredictable) liver disease
drug-induced toxic (predictable) liver disease

Code first:
poisoning due to drug or toxin, if applicable (T36-T65 with fifth or sixth character 1-4 or 6)

Use additional code for adverse effect, if applicable, to identify drug (T36-T50 with fifth or sixth character 5)

EXCLUDES 2 alcoholic liver disease (K70.-)
Budd-Chiari syndrome (I82.0)

CODING TIPS ✓ Codes from category K71.- indicate liver disease resulting from toxicity or toxic damage to the liver due to chemical exposure, including drugs. When a condition from K71.- is caused by poisoning, code first the appropriate T36-T65 code to indicate poisoning. When the condition is diagnosed as an adverse effect, code the appropriate K71.- code followed by the appropriate code from categories T36-T50 to indicate adverse effect.

H SP + **K71.0 Toxic liver disease with cholestasis**

Cholestasis with hepatocyte injury
'Pure' cholestasis

+ 5 **K71.1 Toxic liver disease with hepatic necrosis**

Hepatic failure (acute) (chronic) due to drugs

H SP + **K71.10 Toxic liver disease with hepatic necrosis, without coma**

H SP + **K71.11 Toxic liver disease with hepatic necrosis, with coma**

H SP + **K71.2 Toxic liver disease with acute hepatitis**

H SP + **K71.3 Toxic liver disease with chronic persistent hepatitis**

H SP + **K71.4 Toxic liver disease with chronic lobular hepatitis**

+ 5 **K71.5 Toxic liver disease with chronic active hepatitis**

Toxic liver disease with lupoid hepatitis

H SP + **K71.50 Toxic liver disease with chronic active hepatitis without ascites**

H SP + **K71.51 Toxic liver disease with chronic active hepatitis with ascites**

H SP + **K71.6 Toxic liver disease with hepatitis, not elsewhere classified**

H SP + **K71.7 Toxic liver disease with fibrosis and cirrhosis of liver**

H SP + **K71.8 Toxic liver disease with other disorders of liver**

Toxic liver disease with focal nodular hyperplasia
Toxic liver disease with hepatic granulomas
Toxic liver disease with peliosis hepatis
Toxic liver disease with veno-occlusive disease of liver

H IQ + **K71.9 Toxic liver disease, unspecified**

4 K72 Hepatic failure, not elsewhere classified

INCLUDES fulminant hepatitis NEC, with hepatic failure
hepatic encephalopathy NOS
liver (cell) necrosis with hepatic failure
malignant hepatitis NEC, with hepatic failure
yellow liver atrophy or dystrophy

EXCLUDES 1 alcoholic hepatic failure (K70.4)
hepatic failure with toxic liver disease (K71.1-)
icterus of newborn (P55-P59)
postprocedural hepatic failure (K91.82)

EXCLUDES 2 hepatic failure complicating abortion or ectopic or molar pregnancy (O00-O07, O08.8)
hepatic failure complicating pregnancy, childbirth and the puerperium (O26.6-)
viral hepatitis with hepatic coma (B15-B19)

5 K72.0 Acute and subacute hepatic failure
Acute non-viral hepatitis NOS

SP K72.00 Acute and subacute hepatic failure without coma

CODING TIPS ✓ This code is correct for non-viral acute hepatitis.

H SP K72.01 Acute and subacute hepatic failure with coma

▲ **5 K72.1 Chronic hepatic failure**
End stage liver disease

SP K72.10 Chronic hepatic failure without coma

H SP K72.11 Chronic hepatic failure with coma

5 K72.9 Hepatic failure, unspecified

SP K72.90 Hepatic failure, unspecified without coma

H SP K72.91 Hepatic failure, unspecified with coma
Hepatic coma NOS

4 K73 Chronic hepatitis, not elsewhere classified

EXCLUDES 1 alcoholic hepatitis (chronic) (K70.1-)
drug-induced hepatitis (chronic) (K71.-)
granulomatous hepatitis (chronic) NEC (K75.3)
reactive, nonspecific hepatitis (chronic) (K75.2)
viral hepatitis (chronic) (B15-B19)

CODING TIPS ✓ Do not assign a code from category K73.- when hepatitis is specified as viral or due to a specific cause, such as alcohol use or toxicity.

H SP K73.0 Chronic persistent hepatitis, not elsewhere classified

H SP K73.1 Chronic lobular hepatitis, not elsewhere classified

H SP K73.2 Chronic active hepatitis, not elsewhere classified

H SP K73.8 Other chronic hepatitis, not elsewhere classified

H SP K73.9 Chronic hepatitis, unspecified

4 K74 Fibrosis and cirrhosis of liver
Code also:
, if applicable, viral hepatitis (acute) (chronic) (B15-B19)

EXCLUDES 1 alcoholic cirrhosis (of liver) (K70.3)
alcoholic fibrosis of liver (K70.2)
cardiac sclerosis of liver (K76.1)
cirrhosis (of liver) with toxic liver disease (K71.7)
congenital cirrhosis (of liver) (P78.81)
pigmentary cirrhosis (of liver) (E83.110)

CODING TIPS ✓ When viral hepatitis is also documented as a confirmed diagnosis in a patient with any diagnosis classifiable to K74.-, the appropriate code from B15-B19 should also be assigned. The sequencing of the K74.- and the viral hepatitis code is according to focus of care.

5 K74.0 Hepatic fibrosis
Code first underlying liver disease, such as:
nonalcoholic steatohepatitis (NASH) (K75.81)

IQ K74.00 Hepatic fibrosis, unspecified

IQ K74.01 Hepatic fibrosis, early fibrosis
Hepatic fibrosis, stage F1 or stage F2

IQ K74.02 Hepatic fibrosis, advanced fibrosis
Hepatic fibrosis, stage F3

EXCLUDES 1 cirrhosis of liver (K74.6-)
hepatic fibrosis, stage F4 (K74.6-)

SP K74.1 Hepatic sclerosis

SP K74.2 Hepatic fibrosis with hepatic sclerosis

H SP K74.3 Primary biliary cirrhosis
Chronic nonsuppurative destructive cholangitis
Primary biliary cholangitis

EXCLUDES 2 primary sclerosing cholangitis (K83.01)

DEFINITION Scar tissue formation of the ducts carrying bile from the liver to the small intestine, resulting in bile build-up and liver damage leading to cirrhosis.

H SP K74.4 Secondary biliary cirrhosis

H SP K74.5 Biliary cirrhosis, unspecified

5 K74.6 Other and unspecified cirrhosis of liver

H SP K74.60 Unspecified cirrhosis of liver
Cirrhosis (of liver) NOS

H SP K74.69 Other cirrhosis of liver
Cryptogenic cirrhosis (of liver)
Macronodular cirrhosis (of liver)
Micronodular cirrhosis (of liver)
Mixed type cirrhosis (of liver)
Portal cirrhosis (of liver)
Postnecrotic cirrhosis (of liver)

4 K75 Other inflammatory liver diseases

EXCLUDES 2 toxic liver disease (K71.-)

SP K75.0 Abscess of liver
Cholangitic hepatic abscess

Hematogenic hepatic abscess
Hepatic abscess NOS
Lymphogenic hepatic abscess
Pylephlebitic hepatic abscess
EXCLUDES 1 amebic liver abscess (A06.4)
cholangitis without liver abscess (K83.09)
pylephlebitis without liver abscess (K75.1)
EXCLUDES 2 acute or subacute hepatitis NOS (B17.9)
acute or subacute non-viral hepatitis (K72.0)
chronic hepatitis NEC (K73.8)

SP **K75.1 Phlebitis of portal vein**
Pylephlebitis
EXCLUDES 1 pylephlebitic liver abscess (K75.0)

H SP **K75.2 Nonspecific reactive hepatitis**
EXCLUDES 1 acute or subacute hepatitis (K72.0-)
chronic hepatitis NEC (K73.-)
viral hepatitis (B15-B19)

H SP **K75.3 Granulomatous hepatitis, not elsewhere classified**
EXCLUDES 1 acute or subacute hepatitis (K72.0-)
chronic hepatitis NEC (K73.-)
viral hepatitis (B15-B19)

H SP **K75.4 Autoimmune hepatitis**
Lupoid hepatitis NEC
DEFINITION Continuous inflammation and necrosis of liver cells that progresses to cirrhosis, in association with autoimmune diseases and not infection, alcohol consumption, or toxic exposure.

5 **K75.8 Other specified inflammatory liver diseases**

H SP + **K75.81 Nonalcoholic steatohepatitis (NASH)**
Use additional code, if applicable, hepatic fibrosis (K74.0-)

SP **K75.89 Other specified inflammatory liver diseases**

SP **K75.9 Inflammatory liver disease, unspecified**
Hepatitis NOS
EXCLUDES 1 acute or subacute hepatitis (K72.0-)
chronic hepatitis NEC (K73.-)
viral hepatitis (B15-B19)
CODING TIPS✓ If hepatitis is described as acute and is non-viral, assign code K72.00.
CODING TIPS✓ **Documentation:** When documentation confirms only that a patient has hepatitis but does not provide any further detail, assign K75.9 to indicate hepatitis NOS. Do not assign this code if specific cause/type of hepatitis is specified in diagnostic information.

4 **K76 Other diseases of liver**
EXCLUDES 2 alcoholic liver disease (K70.-)
amyloid degeneration of liver (E85.-)
cystic disease of liver (congenital) (Q44.6)
hepatic vein thrombosis (I82.0)
hepatomegaly NOS (R16.0)
pigmentary cirrhosis (of liver) (E83.110)
portal vein thrombosis (I81)
toxic liver disease (K71.-)

SP **K76.0 Fatty (change of) liver, not elsewhere classified**
Nonalcoholic fatty liver disease (NAFLD)
EXCLUDES 1 nonalcoholic steatohepatitis (NASH) (K75.81)

SP **K76.1 Chronic passive congestion of liver**
Cardiac cirrhosis
Cardiac sclerosis

SP **K76.2 Central hemorrhagic necrosis of liver**
EXCLUDES 1 liver necrosis with hepatic failure (K72.-)

SP **K76.3 Infarction of liver**

H SP **K76.4 Peliosis hepatis**
Hepatic angiomatosis

SP **K76.5 Hepatic veno-occlusive disease**
EXCLUDES 1 Budd-Chiari syndrome (I82.0)

SP + **K76.6 Portal hypertension**
Use additional code for any associated complications, such as:
portal hypertensive gastropathy (K31.89)
DEFINITION Increase in the pressure within the portal vein which carries blood from the digestive organs to the liver, caused by a blockage of blood flow through the liver.

H SP **K76.7 Hepatorenal syndrome**
EXCLUDES 1 hepatorenal syndrome following labor and delivery (O90.4)
postprocedural hepatorenal syndrome (K91.83)

5 **K76.8 Other specified diseases of liver**

H SP **K76.81 Hepatopulmonary syndrome**
Code first underlying liver disease, such as:
alcoholic cirrhosis of liver (K70.3-)
cirrhosis of liver without mention of alcohol (K74.6-)

SP **K76.89 Other specified diseases of liver**
Cyst (simple) of liver
Focal nodular hyperplasia of liver
Hepatoptosis

IQ **K76.9 Liver disease, unspecified**

▲ M IQ **K77** ***Liver disorders in diseases classified elsewhere***
Code first underlying disease, such as:
amyloidosis (E85.-)
congenital syphilis (A50.0, A50.5)
congenital toxoplasmosis (P37.1)
infectious mononucleosis with liver disease (B27.0-B27.9 with .9)
schistosomiasis (B65.0-B65.9)
EXCLUDES 1 alcoholic hepatitis (K70.1-)
alcoholic liver disease (K70.-)
cytomegaloviral hepatitis (B25.1)
herpesviral [herpes simplex] hepatitis (B00.81)

Chapter 11
K00-K95

4 4th digit required 5 5th digit required 6 6th digit required 7 7th digit required 7 7th digit placeholder + Additional code B Laterality

mumps hepatitis (B26.81)
sarcoidosis with liver disease (D86.89)
secondary syphilis with liver disease (A51.45)
syphilis (late) with liver disease (A52.74)
toxoplasmosis (acquired) hepatitis (B58.1)
tuberculosis with liver disease (A18.83)

Disorders of gallbladder, biliary tract and pancreas (K80-K87)

4 **K80 Cholelithiasis**
EXCLUDES 1 retained cholelithiasis following cholecystectomy (K91.86)
CODING TIPS✓ When cholecystitis or cholelithiasis has been diagnosed and treated by surgery, and is resolved by surgery upon home health admission, assign a code for aftercare.

+ 5 **K80.0 Calculus of gallbladder with acute cholecystitis**
Any condition listed in K80.2 with acute cholecystitis
Use additional code if applicable for associated gangrene of gallbladder (K82.A1), or perforation of gallbladder (K82.A2)

SP + **K80.00 Calculus of gallbladder with acute cholecystitis without obstruction**

SP + **K80.01 Calculus of gallbladder with acute cholecystitis with obstruction**

+ 5 **K80.1 Calculus of gallbladder with other cholecystitis**
Use additional code if applicable for associated gangrene of gallbladder (K82.A1), or perforation of gallbladder (K82.A2)

SP + **K80.10 Calculus of gallbladder with chronic cholecystitis without obstruction**
Cholelithiasis with cholecystitis NOS

SP + **K80.11 Calculus of gallbladder with chronic cholecystitis with obstruction**

SP + **K80.12 Calculus of gallbladder with acute and chronic cholecystitis without obstruction**

SP + **K80.13 Calculus of gallbladder with acute and chronic cholecystitis with obstruction**

SP + **K80.18 Calculus of gallbladder with other cholecystitis without obstruction**

SP + **K80.19 Calculus of gallbladder with other cholecystitis with obstruction**

5 **K80.2 Calculus of gallbladder without cholecystitis**
Cholecystolithiasis without cholecystitis
Cholelithiasis (without cholecystitis)
Colic (recurrent) of gallbladder (without cholecystitis)
Gallstone (impacted) of cystic duct (without cholecystitis)
Gallstone (impacted) of gallbladder (without cholecystitis)

SP **K80.20 Calculus of gallbladder without cholecystitis without obstruction**

SP **K80.21 Calculus of gallbladder without cholecystitis with obstruction**

5 **K80.3 Calculus of bile duct with cholangitis**
Any condition listed in K80.5 with cholangitis

SP **K80.30 Calculus of bile duct with cholangitis, unspecified, without obstruction**

SP **K80.31 Calculus of bile duct with cholangitis, unspecified, with obstruction**

SP **K80.32 Calculus of bile duct with acute cholangitis without obstruction**

SP **K80.33 Calculus of bile duct with acute cholangitis with obstruction**

SP **K80.34 Calculus of bile duct with chronic cholangitis without obstruction**

SP **K80.35 Calculus of bile duct with chronic cholangitis with obstruction**

SP **K80.36 Calculus of bile duct with acute and chronic cholangitis without obstruction**

SP **K80.37 Calculus of bile duct with acute and chronic cholangitis with obstruction**

+ 5 **K80.4 Calculus of bile duct with cholecystitis**
Any condition listed in K80.5 with cholecystitis (with cholangitis)
Codes also fistula of bile duct (K83.3)
Use additional code if applicable for associated gangrene of gallbladder (K82.A1), or perforation of gallbladder (K82.A2)

SP + **K80.40 Calculus of bile duct with cholecystitis, unspecified, without obstruction**

SP + **K80.41 Calculus of bile duct with cholecystitis, unspecified, with obstruction**

SP + **K80.42 Calculus of bile duct with acute cholecystitis without obstruction**

SP + **K80.43 Calculus of bile duct with acute cholecystitis with obstruction**

SP + **K80.44 Calculus of bile duct with chronic cholecystitis without obstruction**

SP + **K80.45 Calculus of bile duct with chronic cholecystitis with obstruction**

SP + **K80.46 Calculus of bile duct with acute and chronic cholecystitis without obstruction**

SP + **K80.47 Calculus of bile duct with acute and chronic cholecystitis with obstruction**

5 **K80.5 Calculus of bile duct without cholangitis or cholecystitis**
Choledocholithiasis (without cholangitis or cholecystitis)
Gallstone (impacted) of bile duct NOS (without cholangitis or cholecystitis)
Gallstone (impacted) of common duct (without cholangitis or cholecystitis)
Gallstone (impacted) of hepatic duct (without cholangitis or cholecystitis)
Hepatic cholelithiasis (without cholangitis or cholecystitis)
Hepatic colic (recurrent) (without cholangitis or cholecystitis)

SP **K80.50 Calculus of bile duct without cholangitis or cholecystitis without obstruction**

SP **K80.51 Calculus of bile duct without cholangitis or cholecystitis with obstruction**

+ 5 **K80.6 Calculus of gallbladder and bile duct with cholecystitis**
Use additional code if applicable for associated gangrene of gallbladder (K82.A1), or perforation of gallbladder (K82.A2)

SP + **K80.60 Calculus of gallbladder and bile duct with cholecystitis, unspecified, without obstruction**

SP + **K80.61 Calculus of gallbladder and bile duct with cholecystitis, unspecified, with obstruction**

SP + **K80.62 Calculus of gallbladder and bile duct with acute cholecystitis without obstruction**

SP + **K80.63 Calculus of gallbladder and bile duct with acute cholecystitis with obstruction**

SP + **K80.64 Calculus of gallbladder and bile duct with chronic cholecystitis without obstruction**

SP + **K80.65 Calculus of gallbladder and bile duct with chronic cholecystitis with obstruction**

SP + **K80.66 Calculus of gallbladder and bile duct with acute and chronic cholecystitis without obstruction**

SP + **K80.67 Calculus of gallbladder and bile duct with acute and chronic cholecystitis with obstruction**

5 **K80.7 Calculus of gallbladder and bile duct without cholecystitis**

SP **K80.70 Calculus of gallbladder and bile duct without cholecystitis without obstruction**

SP **K80.71 Calculus of gallbladder and bile duct without cholecystitis with obstruction**

5 **K80.8 Other cholelithiasis**

SP **K80.80 Other cholelithiasis without obstruction**

SP **K80.81 Other cholelithiasis with obstruction**

+ 4 **K81 Cholecystitis**
Use additional code if applicable for associated gangrene of gallbladder (K82.A1), or perforation of gallbladder (K82.A2)
EXCLUDES 1 cholecystitis with cholelithiasis (K80.-)
CODING TIPS ✓ When cholecystitis or cholelithiasis has been diagnosed and treated by surgery, and is resolved by surgery upon home health admission, assign a code for aftercare.

SP + **K81.0 Acute cholecystitis**
Abscess of gallbladder
Angiocholecystitis
Emphysematous (acute) cholecystitis
Empyema of gallbladder
Gangrene of gallbladder
Gangrenous cholecystitis
Suppurative cholecystitis

SP + **K81.1 Chronic cholecystitis**

SP + **K81.2 Acute cholecystitis with chronic cholecystitis**

SP + **K81.9 Cholecystitis, unspecified**

4 **K82 Other diseases of gallbladder**
EXCLUDES 1 nonvisualization of gallbladder (R93.2)
postcholecystectomy syndrome (K91.5)

SP **K82.0 Obstruction of gallbladder**
Occlusion of cystic duct or gallbladder without cholelithiasis
Stenosis of cystic duct or gallbladder without cholelithiasis
Stricture of cystic duct or gallbladder without cholelithiasis
EXCLUDES 1 obstruction of gallbladder with cholelithiasis (K80.-)

SP **K82.1 Hydrops of gallbladder**
Mucocele of gallbladder
DEFINITION Overly full, distended gallbladder due to accumulation of mucous and watery material rather than stone formation.

SP **K82.2 Perforation of gallbladder**
Rupture of cystic duct or gallbladder
EXCLUDES 1 Perforation of gallbladder in cholecystitis (K82.A2)

SP **K82.3 Fistula of gallbladder**
Cholecystocolic fistula
Cholecystoduodenal fistula

SP **K82.4 Cholesterolosis of gallbladder**
Strawberry gallbladder
EXCLUDES 1 cholesterolosis of gallbladder with cholecystitis (K81.-)
cholesterolosis of gallbladder with cholelithiasis (K80.-)
DEFINITION Build-up of cholesterol deposits on the surface of the gallbladder, giving it a 'strawberry' appearance.

SP **K82.8 Other specified diseases of gallbladder**
Adhesions of cystic duct or gallbladder
Atrophy of cystic duct or gallbladder
Cyst of cystic duct or gallbladder
Dyskinesia of cystic duct or gallbladder
Hypertrophy of cystic duct or gallbladder
Nonfunctioning of cystic duct or gallbladder
Ulcer of cystic duct or gallbladder

!Q **K82.9 Disease of gallbladder, unspecified**

5 **K82.A Disorders of gallbladder in diseases classified elsewhere**
Code first:
the type of cholecystitis (K81.-) , or cholelithiasis with cholecystitis (K80.00-K80.19, K80.40-K80.47, K80.60-K80.67)

M IQ **K82.A1** ***Gangrene of gallbladder in cholecystitis***

M IQ **K82.A2** ***Perforation of gallbladder in cholecystitis***

4 **K83 Other diseases of biliary tract**
EXCLUDES 1 postcholecystectomy syndrome (K91.5)
EXCLUDES 2 conditions involving the gallbladder (K81-K82)
conditions involving the cystic duct (K81-K82)

Chapter 11

K00-K95

5 **K83.0 Cholangitis**
EXCLUDES 1 cholangitic liver abscess (K75.0)
cholangitis with choledocholithiasis (K80.3-, K80.4-)
EXCLUDES 2 chronic nonsuppurative destructive cholangitis (K74.3)
primary biliary cholangitis (K74.3)
primary biliary cirrhosis (K74.3)
DEFINITION Infection of the biliary tract; presents with pain in the upper-right abdomen which may grow worse after a fatty meal, fever, nausea, vomiting, flatulence, pale-colored stool, and yellowing of the eyes and skin.

SP **K83.01 Primary sclerosing cholangitis**

SP **K83.09 Other cholangitis**
Ascending cholangitis
Cholangitis NOS
Primary cholangitis
Recurrent cholangitis
Sclerosing cholangitis
Secondary cholangitis
Stenosing cholangitis
Suppurative cholangitis

SP **K83.1 Obstruction of bile duct**
Occlusion of bile duct without cholelithiasis
Stenosis of bile duct without cholelithiasis
Stricture of bile duct without cholelithiasis
EXCLUDES 1 congenital obstruction of bile duct (Q44.3)
obstruction of bile duct with cholelithiasis (K80.-)

SP **K83.2 Perforation of bile duct**
Rupture of bile duct

SP **K83.3 Fistula of bile duct**
Choledochoduodenal fistula

SP **K83.4 Spasm of sphincter of Oddi**

SP **K83.5 Biliary cyst**

SP **K83.8 Other specified diseases of biliary tract**
Adhesions of biliary tract
Atrophy of biliary tract
Hypertrophy of biliary tract
Ulcer of biliary tract

IQ **K83.9 Disease of biliary tract, unspecified**

4 **K85 Acute pancreatitis**
INCLUDES acute (recurrent) pancreatitis
subacute pancreatitis

5 **K85.0 Idiopathic acute pancreatitis**

SP **K85.00 Idiopathic acute pancreatitis without necrosis or infection**

SP **K85.01 Idiopathic acute pancreatitis with uninfected necrosis**

SP **K85.02 Idiopathic acute pancreatitis with infected necrosis**

5 **K85.1 Biliary acute pancreatitis**
Gallstone pancreatitis

SP **K85.10 Biliary acute pancreatitis without necrosis or infection**

SP **K85.11 Biliary acute pancreatitis with uninfected necrosis**

SP **K85.12 Biliary acute pancreatitis with infected necrosis**

5 **K85.2 Alcohol induced acute pancreatitis**
EXCLUDES 2 alcohol induced chronic pancreatitis (K86.0)
CODING TIPS ✓ Assign a code from K85.2- only when physician or NPP documentation clearly confirms acute pancreatitis due to alcohol use. Use the appropriate F10 code to indicate the alcohol use, abuse or dependence. Do not use 5th and 6th digits .88 to indicate alcohol induced disorder with the F10 code as alcohol induced disorders include only mental, emotional and physical disorders in Chapter 5.

SP **K85.20 Alcohol induced acute pancreatitis without necrosis or infection**

SP **K85.21 Alcohol induced acute pancreatitis with uninfected necrosis**

SP **K85.22 Alcohol induced acute pancreatitis with infected necrosis**

+ 5 **K85.3 Drug induced acute pancreatitis**
Use additional code for adverse effect, if applicable, to identify drug (T36-T50 with fifth or sixth character 5)
Use additional code to identify drug abuse and dependence (F11.-F17.-)

SP + **K85.30 Drug induced acute pancreatitis without necrosis or infection**

SP + **K85.31 Drug induced acute pancreatitis with uninfected necrosis**

SP + **K85.32 Drug induced acute pancreatitis with infected necrosis**

5 **K85.8 Other acute pancreatitis**

SP **K85.80 Other acute pancreatitis without necrosis or infection**

SP **K85.81 Other acute pancreatitis with uninfected necrosis**

SP **K85.82 Other acute pancreatitis with infected necrosis**

5 **K85.9 Acute pancreatitis, unspecified**
Pancreatitis NOS

SP **K85.90 Acute pancreatitis without necrosis or infection, unspecified**

SP **K85.91 Acute pancreatitis with uninfected necrosis, unspecified**

SP **K85.92 Acute pancreatitis with infected necrosis, unspecified**

4 **K86 Other diseases of pancreas**
EXCLUDES 2 fibrocystic disease of pancreas (E84.-)
islet cell tumor (of pancreas) (D13.7)
pancreatic steatorrhea (K90.3)

SP + **K86.0 Alcohol-induced chronic pancreatitis**
Code also:
exocrine pancreatic insufficiency (K86.81)
Use additional code to identify:
alcohol abuse and dependence (F10.-)
EXCLUDES 2 alcohol induced acute pancreatitis (K85.2-)

Chapter 11

K00-K95

CODING TIPS✓ Assign code K86.0 only when physician or NPP documentation clearly confirms chronic pancreatitis due to alcohol use. Use the appropriate F10 code to indicate the alcohol use, abuse or dependence. Do not use 5th and 6th digits .88 to indicate alcohol induced disorder with the F10 code as alcohol induced disorders include only mental, emotional and physical disorders in Chapter 5.

SP **K86.1 Other chronic pancreatitis**
Chronic pancreatitis NOS
Infectious chronic pancreatitis
Recurrent chronic pancreatitis
Relapsing chronic pancreatitis
Code also:
exocrine pancreatic insufficiency (K86.81)

SP **K86.2 Cyst of pancreas**

SP **K86.3 Pseudocyst of pancreas**

5 **K86.8 Other specified diseases of pancreas**

SP **K86.81 Exocrine pancreatic insufficiency**
DEFINITION Insufficient pancreatic secretory functioning causes malfunctioning digestion and the malabsorption of fats in particular, which leads to malnutrition, and associated diseases of nutritional deficiencies. It is common in cystic fibrosis patients. Symptoms include chronic diarrhea or passing foul-smelling, voluminous stools, bloating, abdominal pain and cramping, weight loss, and steatorrhea.

SP **K86.89 Other specified diseases of pancreas**
Aseptic pancreatic necrosis, unrelated to acute pancreatitis
Atrophy of pancreas
Calculus of pancreas
Cirrhosis of pancreas
Fibrosis of pancreas
Pancreatic fat necrosis, unrelated to acute pancreatitis
Pancreatic infantilism
Pancreatic necrosis NOS, unrelated to acute pancreatitis

IQ **K86.9 Disease of pancreas, unspecified**

IQ **K87 Disorders of gallbladder, biliary tract and pancreas in diseases classified elsewhere**
Code first:
underlying disease
EXCLUDES 1 cytomegaloviral pancreatitis (B25.2)
mumps pancreatitis (B26.3)
syphilitic gallbladder (A52.74)
syphilitic pancreas (A52.74)
tuberculosis of gallbladder (A18.83)
tuberculosis of pancreas (A18.83)

Other diseases of the digestive system (K90-K95)

4 **K90 Intestinal malabsorption**
EXCLUDES 1 intestinal malabsorption following gastrointestinal surgery (K91.2)

CODING TIPS✓ Do not assign a code from K90.- when malabsorption is reported as post-surgical or post-procedural. Post-procedural / post-surgical complications affecting the gastrointestinal system are coded to category K91.-

SP + **K90.0 Celiac disease**
Celiac disease with steatorrhea
Celiac gluten-sensitive enteropathy
Nontropical sprue
Code also:
exocrine pancreatic insufficiency (K86.81)
Use additional code for associated disorders including:
dermatitis herpetiformis (L13.0)
gluten ataxia (G32.81)
DEFINITION Malabsorption syndrome precipitated by ingestion of gluten with loss of villous projections of the intestinal mucosa; manifests with bulky, frothy diarrhea, abdominal distention, flatulence, weight loss, and vitamin and electrolyte depletion.

SP **K90.1 Tropical sprue**
Sprue NOS
Tropical steatorrhea
DEFINITION A malabsorption syndrome occurring in the tropics and subtropics, marked by inflammation of the mucous tissue of the mouth, diarrhea, and anemia.

SP **K90.2 Blind loop syndrome, not elsewhere classified**
Blind loop syndrome NOS
EXCLUDES 1 congenital blind loop syndrome (Q43.8)
postsurgical blind loop syndrome (K91.2)

SP **K90.3 Pancreatic steatorrhea**
DEFINITION Insufficient pancreatic enzyme excretions causing severe malabsorption and nutrient deficiencies with loose stools containing unabsorbed fat.

5 **K90.4 Other malabsorption due to intolerance**
EXCLUDES 2 celiac gluten-sensitive enteropathy (K90.0)
lactose intolerance (E73.-)

SP **K90.41 Non-celiac gluten sensitivity**
Gluten sensitivity NOS
Non-celiac gluten sensitive enteropathy

SP **K90.49 Malabsorption due to intolerance, not elsewhere classified**
Malabsorption due to intolerance to carbohydrate
Malabsorption due to intolerance to fat
Malabsorption due to intolerance to protein
Malabsorption due to intolerance to starch

5 **K90.8 Other intestinal malabsorption**

SP **K90.81 Whipple's disease**

SP **K90.89 Other intestinal malabsorption**

SP **K90.9 Intestinal malabsorption, unspecified**

4 **K91 Intraoperative and postprocedural complications and disorders of digestive system, not elsewhere classified**

Chapter 11
K00-K95

EXCLUDES 2 complications of artificial opening of digestive system (K94.-)
complications of bariatric procedures (K95.-)
gastrojejunal ulcer (K28.-)
postprocedural (radiation) retroperitoneal abscess (K68.11)
radiation colitis (K52.0)
radiation gastroenteritis (K52.0)
radiation proctitis (K62.7)

CODING TIPS✓ Intestinal obstruction varies in severity, from partial or intermittent obstruction that resolves without intervention (usually involving small intestine) to complete obstruction that requires surgical intervention and may lead to intestinal gangrene and perforation. Physicians and NPPs frequently describe intestinal obstruction as partial versus complete. If the obstruction has been surgically treated without complication, an aftercare code (Z48.815) may be appropriate.

CODING TIPS✓ **Documentation:** Codes in category K91.- are complication codes and require physician or NPP documentation and confirmation of a cause-and-effect relationship between the procedure and the complicated condition. Documentation in the home health clinical record must also support this relationship. Gastrointestinal complications that have been resolved by the time the patient is admitted to home care are coded with aftercare codes, e.g. Z48.815.

SP **K91.0 Vomiting following gastrointestinal surgery**

SP **K91.1 Postgastric surgery syndromes**
Dumping syndrome
Postgastrectomy syndrome
Postvagotomy syndrome

SP **K91.2 Postsurgical malabsorption, not elsewhere classified**
Postsurgical blind loop syndrome
EXCLUDES 1 malabsorption osteomalacia in adults (M83.2)
malabsorption osteoporosis, postsurgical (M80.8-, M81.8)

5 **K91.3 Postprocedural intestinal obstruction**

SP **K91.30 Postprocedural intestinal obstruction, unspecified as to partial versus complete**
Postprocedural intestinal obstruction NOS

SP **K91.31 Postprocedural partial intestinal obstruction**
Postprocedural incomplete intestinal obstruction

SP **K91.32 Postprocedural complete intestinal obstruction**

SP **K91.5 Postcholecystectomy syndrome**

5 **K91.6 Intraoperative hemorrhage and hematoma of a digestive system organ or structure complicating a procedure**
EXCLUDES 1 intraoperative hemorrhage and hematoma of a digestive system organ or structure due to accidental puncture and laceration during a procedure (K91.7-)

SP **K91.61 Intraoperative hemorrhage and hematoma of a digestive system organ or structure complicating a digestive system procedure**

SP **K91.62 Intraoperative hemorrhage and hematoma of a digestive system organ or structure complicating other procedure**

5 **K91.7 Accidental puncture and laceration of a digestive system organ or structure during a procedure**

SP **K91.71 Accidental puncture and laceration of a digestive system organ or structure during a digestive system procedure**

SP **K91.72 Accidental puncture and laceration of a digestive system organ or structure during other procedure**

5 **K91.8 Other intraoperative and postprocedural complications and disorders of digestive system**

SP **K91.81 Other intraoperative complications of digestive system**

SP **K91.82 Postprocedural hepatic failure**

SP **K91.83 Postprocedural hepatorenal syndrome**

6 **K91.84 Postprocedural hemorrhage of a digestive system organ or structure following a procedure**

SP **K91.840 Postprocedural hemorrhage of a digestive system organ or structure following a digestive system procedure**

SP **K91.841 Postprocedural hemorrhage of a digestive system organ or structure following other procedure**

6 **K91.85 Complications of intestinal pouch**

SP **K91.850 Pouchitis**
Inflammation of internal ileoanal pouch

SP **K91.858 Other complications of intestinal pouch**

SP **K91.86 Retained cholelithiasis following cholecystectomy**

6 **K91.87 Postprocedural hematoma and seroma of a digestive system organ or structure following a procedure**

SP **K91.870 Postprocedural hematoma of a digestive system organ or structure following a digestive system procedure**

SP **K91.871 Postprocedural hematoma of a digestive system organ or structure following other procedure**

SP **K91.872 Postprocedural seroma of a digestive system organ or structure following a digestive system procedure**

Chapter 11
K00-K95

SP **K91.873 Postprocedural seroma of a digestive system organ or structure following other procedure**

SP + **K91.89 Other postprocedural complications and disorders of digestive system**
Use additional code, if applicable, to further specify disorder
EXCLUDES 2 postprocedural retroperitoneal abscess (K68.11)

4 **K92 Other diseases of digestive system**
EXCLUDES 1 neonatal gastrointestinal hemorrhage (P54.0-P54.3)
CODING TIPS✓ When gastrointestinal bleeds are related to anti-coagulant or anti-platelet use, also code D68.32 and an additional code to identify the drug.

SP **K92.0 Hematemesis**

SP **K92.1 Melena**
EXCLUDES 1 occult blood in feces (R19.5)

SP **K92.2 Gastrointestinal hemorrhage, unspecified**
Gastric hemorrhage NOS
Intestinal hemorrhage NOS
EXCLUDES 1 acute hemorrhagic gastritis (K29.01)
hemorrhage of anus and rectum (K62.5)
angiodysplasia of stomach with hemorrhage (K31.811)
diverticular disease with hemorrhage (K57.-)
gastritis and duodenitis with hemorrhage (K29.-)
peptic ulcer with hemorrhage (K25-K28)

5 **K92.8 Other specified diseases of the digestive system**

SP **K92.81 Gastrointestinal mucositis (ulcerative)**
Code also type of associated therapy, such as:
antineoplastic and immunosuppressive drugs (T45.1X-)
radiological procedure and radiotherapy (Y84.2)
EXCLUDES 2 mucositis (ulcerative) of vagina and vulva (N76.81)
nasal mucositis (ulcerative) (J34.81)
oral mucositis (ulcerative) (K12.3-)

SP **K92.89 Other specified diseases of the digestive system**

IQ **K92.9 Disease of digestive system, unspecified**

4 **K94 Complications of artificial openings of the digestive system**
CODING TIPS✓ All colostomy, gastrostomy, enterostomy, and esophagostomy complications are coded to category K94.- . This includes excoriation and denuding of the skin surrounding the ostomy, infection of the ostomy site, hemorrhage of the ostomy site, and other complications. No additional code should be used when coding skin complications unless an infection is present, in which case an additional code should be used to specify the infection. When an ostomy complication is present, do not assign a Z code for the ostomy. Z codes indicate routine ostomy care and are not appropriate in the case of a complicated ostomy.

5 **K94.0 Colostomy complications**

IQ **K94.00 Colostomy complication, unspecified**

SP **K94.01 Colostomy hemorrhage**

SP + **K94.02 Colostomy infection**
Use additional code to specify type of infection, such as:
cellulitis of abdominal wall (L03.311)
sepsis (A40.-, A41.-)
CODING TIPS✓ If the patient has cellulitis at the colostomy site, code the infected colostomy followed by cellulitis.

SP **K94.03 Colostomy malfunction**
Mechanical complication of colostomy
CODING TIPS✓ A mechanical complication may include the denuding of the skin around the stoma due to the appliance not fitting a too-small stoma.

SP **K94.09 Other complications of colostomy**
CODING TIPS✓ Use this code along with L24.B1 for contact irritant dermatitis related to the digestive fistula or stoma.

5 **K94.1 Enterostomy complications**

IQ **K94.10 Enterostomy complication, unspecified**

SP **K94.11 Enterostomy hemorrhage**

SP + **K94.12 Enterostomy infection**
Use additional code to specify type of infection, such as:
cellulitis of abdominal wall (L03.311)
sepsis (A40.-, A41.-)
CODING TIPS✓ If the patient has cellulitis at the enterostomy site, code the infected enterostomy followed by cellulitis.

SP **K94.13 Enterostomy malfunction**
Mechanical complication of enterostomy

SP **K94.19 Other complications of enterostomy**
CODING TIPS✓ Use this code along with L24.B1 for contact irritant dermatitis related to the digestive fistula or stoma.

5 **K94.2 Gastrostomy complications**
CODING TIPS✓ Do not use the Z93.1 (status gastrostomy) or Z43.1 (attention to gastrostomy) codes if the gastrostomy is complicated.

IQ **K94.20 Gastrostomy complication, unspecified**

SP **K94.21 Gastrostomy hemorrhage**

SP + **K94.22 Gastrostomy infection**
Use additional code to specify type of infection, such as:
cellulitis of abdominal wall (L03.311)
sepsis (A40.-, A41.-)

CODING TIPS ✓ If the patient has cellulitis at the gastrostomy site, code the infected gastrostomy followed by cellulitis.

SP **K94.23 Gastrostomy malfunction**
Mechanical complication of gastrostomy

SP **K94.29 Other complications of gastrostomy**

CODING TIPS ✓ Use this code along with L24.B1 for contact irritant dermatitis related to the digestive fistula or stoma.

5 **K94.3 Esophagostomy complications**

IQ **K94.30 Esophagostomy complications, unspecified**

SP **K94.31 Esophagostomy hemorrhage**

SP + **K94.32 Esophagostomy infection**
Use additional code to identify the infection

CODING TIPS ✓ If the patient has cellulitis at the esophagostomy site, code the infected esophagostomy followed by cellulitis.

SP **K94.33 Esophagostomy malfunction**
Mechanical complication of esophagostomy

SP **K94.39 Other complications of esophagostomy**

CODING TIPS ✓ Use this code along with L24.B1 for contact irritant dermatitis related to the digestive fistula or stoma.

4 **K95 Complications of bariatric procedures**

CODING TIPS ✓ Do not use Z98.84 for bariatric surgery status if there is a complication.

CODING TIPS ✓ **Documentation:** Codes in category K95.- are complication codes and require physician or NPP documentation and confirmation of a cause and effect relationship between the procedure and the complicated condition. Documentation in the home health clinical record must also support this relationship. Gastrointestinal complications that have been resolved by the time the patient is admitted to home care are coded with aftercare codes, e.g. Z48.815.

5 **K95.0 Complications of gastric band procedure**

SP + **K95.01 Infection due to gastric band procedure**
Use additional code to specify type of infection or organism, such as:
bacterial and viral infectious agents (B95.-, B96.-)
cellulitis of abdominal wall (L03.311)
sepsis (A40.-, A41.-)

SP + **K95.09 Other complications of gastric band procedure**
Use additional code, if applicable, to further specify complication

5 **K95.8 Complications of other bariatric procedure**

EXCLUDES 1 complications of gastric band surgery (K95.0-)

SP + **K95.81 Infection due to other bariatric procedure**
Use additional code to specify type of infection or organism, such as:
bacterial and viral infectious agents (B95.-, B96.-)
cellulitis of abdominal wall (L03.311)
sepsis (A40.-, A41.-)

SP + **K95.89 Other complications of other bariatric procedure**
Use additional code, if applicable, to further specify complication

Chapter 11 Scenarios: Diseases of the digestive system (K00-K95)

Ulcerative colitis with intestinal fistula

A 55-year-old woman is admitted to home health with ulcerative colitis that's caused an intestinal fistula. She also has hypertension and anxiety.

Description	Code
Primary: Ulcerative colitis, unspecified with fistula	K51.913
Secondary: Essential (primary) hypertension	I10
Secondary: Anxiety disorder, unspecified	F41.9

The ulcerative colitis has caused a fistula, necessitating the assignment of K51.913. The patient's hypertension and anxiety are comorbidities that have the potential to impact her care and recovery and thus are coded as secondary diagnoses.

Infection of gastrostomy

A patient with Parkinson's and dysphagia has cellulitis of the abdominal wall extending from an infected gastrostomy site. Documentation confirmed the culture growth of Staphylococcus aureus without mention of MRSA from the gastrostomy site. Home health will focus on the infection. The patient is taking a 3-week course of oral antibiotics.

Description	Code
Primary: Infection of gastrostomy	K94.22
Secondary: Cellulitis of abdominal wall	L03.311
Secondary: Methicillin susceptible Staph aureus infection as the cause of diseases classified elsewhere	B95.61
Secondary: Parkinson's disease	G20
Secondary: Dysphagia, unspecified	R13.10
Secondary: Long term (current) use of antibiotics	Z79.2

Notes at K94.22 instruct coders to use an additional code to identify cellulitis of the abdominal wall (L03.311). The Z code for gastrostomy status should not be used when a complication is present. Additional codes to identify the Parkinson's disease, unspecified dysphagia, and antibiotic use are assigned as they impact the patient's prognosis and care planning and may provide important comorbidity adjustment.

Flare of Crohn's disease

The patient was treated in the hospital for a severe flare of her Crohn's disease of the large intestine, with rectal bleeding. She was placed on new medications for the Crohn's disease in the hospital. Encounter notes indicate that the patient has comorbid COPD that is not exacerbated. Home care is ordered for medical management and education on the new medications.

Description	Code
Primary: Crohn's disease of large intestine with rectal bleeding	K50.111
Secondary: Chronic obstructive pulmonary disease, unspecified	J44.9

A flare of her Crohn's disease is the focus of care and since she is currently experiencing rectal bleeding, the code K50.111 is used. No codes are needed for the management of the new medications, but the COPD is coded due to its impact on the care plan and patient prognosis

Reflux esophagitis

A patient is admitted to home care for medication management and diet teaching for reflux esophagitis without bleeding. Patient also has Type 1 diabetes and is on an insulin sliding scale.

Description	Code
Primary: Gastro-esophageal reflux disease with esophagitis, without bleeding	K21.00
Secondary: Type 1 diabetes mellitus without complications	E10.9

This is a case where a disease is coded, not medication management. Medication management itself is not a skilled service and should not be coded primary. Teaching and diet is aimed at the esophagitis so that disease is the code that should be assigned. Within the ICD-10 code set, GERD has separate codes that include the presence or absence of esophagitis, as well as the presence or absence of bleeding. Type 1 diabetes is defined by the E10.- category. There is not an instructional note to list insulin and an additional code for the use of insulin should not be included when coding type 1 diabetes as these diabetics are assumed to require insulin.

Abdominal abscess following surgery

A 70-year-old male is referred to home health for care of a retroperitoneal abscess described as a complication of surgery for sigmoid colon cancer six months prior. After his initial surgery, he developed pain and was diagnosed with a retroperitoneal abscess and an open incision and drainage was performed, with a drain now present to the area. The patient remains on a three-month course of IV Vancomycin, which the home health agency has been ordered to administer. The history and physical provided reports that he is also diabetic. The record confirms that the colon cancer is eradicated and the surgical wound is healed.

Description	Code
Primary: Postprocedural retroperitoneal abscess	K68.11
Secondary: Type 2 diabetes mellitus without complications	E11.9
Secondary: Encounter for adjustment and management of vascular device	Z45.2
Secondary: Long term (current) use of antibiotics	Z79.2
Secondary: Personal history of other malignant neoplasm of large intestine	Z85.038

In this scenario, the patient has experienced a GI complication following his surgery to remove the neoplasm. The code for a complication specific to any disease process is located in the chapter specific to diseases of that body system within the ICD-10 code set. For that reason, the code for post-procedural retroperitoneal abscess is found within Chapter 11, Diseases of the digestive system.

The history of malignant neoplasm of the large intestine (sigmoid colon) should be included, but is coded using a Z code for personal history, as the cancer has been eliminated/removed and the patient is receiving no further treatment for it. Codes Z45.2 and Z79.2 capture the IV administration. If the IV is not the primary reason the patient requires home health care, but where there may be some sort of intervention noted on the home health plan of care, then it would be appropriate to report Z45.2 (but not as the principal or first secondary diagnosis), according to CMS.

Barrett's esophagus

A patient is admitted to home health for teaching regarding newly diagnosed Barrett's esophagus with low-grade dysplasia. Face-to-face encounter notes from the physician also include comorbid diagnoses of reflux esophagitis without bleeding and chronic emphysematous bronchitis.

Description	Code
Primary: Barrett's esophagus with low grade dysplasia	K22.710
Secondary: Gastro-esophageal reflux disease with esophagitis, without bleeding	K21.00
Secondary: Chronic obstructive pulmonary disease, unspecified	J44.9

There are three separate codes for Barrett's esophagus with dysplasia in ICD-10, depending on the grade of the dysplasia. In this case, K22.710 is the appropriate code choice. Additional codes are assigned for reflux esophagitis and chronic emphysematous bronchitis due to the impact these conditions have on the plan of care. Chronic emphysematous bronchitis is included under category J44.- within the ICD-10-CM classification.

Alcoholic cirrhosis with ascites

A 77-year-old man comes to home health with a diagnosis of alcoholic cirrhosis with ascites. He also has type 2 diabetes with polyneuropathy. The liver disease is the focus of care. He has a diagnosis of alcoholism but the medical record says it is in remission and he is not continuing to drink.

Description	Code
Primary: Alcoholic cirrhosis of liver with ascites	K70.31
Secondary: Alcohol dependence, in remission	F10.21
Secondary: Type 2 diabetes mellitus with diabetic polyneuropathy	E11.42

The alcoholic cirrhosis is the focus of care and is therefore coded primary. Because he also has ascites, the combination code indicating the presence of ascites is assigned. His alcoholism is documented was documented as in remission, making F10.21 the appropriate code. An additional code for diabetes with polyneuropathy is added since this condition has an important impact on the patient's prognosis and care plan and may provide important comorbidity adjustment.

Chronic pancreatitis, exocrine pancreatic insufficiency

A 69-year-old man is admitted to home health for management of chronic pancreatitis, which has caused exocrine pancreatic insufficiency.

Description	Code
Primary: Other chronic pancreatitis	K86.1
Secondary: Exocrine pancreatic insufficiency	K86.81

As the focus of care, chronic pancreatitis is coded in the primary position. Exocrine pancreatic insufficiency is coded next, in accordance with tabular instruction.

Toxic liver injury

A 67-year-old man is admitted to home health with a primary diagnosis of toxic liver disease caused by an unintentional overdose of prescription ibuprofen that he was taking for chronic pain related to hemiplegia of the right non-dominant side following a stroke that occurred last year. He admitted that he had misread the instructions for dosage and had been taking twice the prescribed amount.

Description	Code
Primary: Poisoning by propionic acid derivatives, accidental (unintentional), subsequent encounter	T39.311D
Secondary: Toxic liver disease, unspecified	K71.9
Secondary: Other chronic pain	G89.29
Secondary: Hemiplegia and hemiparesis following cerebral infarction affecting right non-dominant side	I69.353

The patient's toxic liver disease was caused by an unintentional overdose of prescription ibuprofen. Because he did not take the drug as prescribed, it is considered a poisoning. The poisoning code must be assigned before the code for the toxic liver disease, according to tabular instruction. The reasons, chronic pain due to hemiplegia from the prior stroke, the patient was taking the drug are coded immediately after.

HOME HEALTH CODING SCENARIOS

Alcoholic cirrhosis with encephalopathy

An 82-year-old male patient with a history of alcoholic cirrhosis was hospitalized with toxic metabolic encephalopathy, acute hepatic encephalopathy, upper GI bleeding due to esophageal varices with associated acute on chronic blood loss anemia, and gastric varices. He is now referred to home health for skilled nursing follow up, education, and observation/assessment. He has comorbid alcohol dependence, ascites, morbid obesity (BMI 55), and quit smoking cigarettes 25 years ago.

Description	Code
Primary: Acute and subacute hepatic failure without coma	K72.00
Secondary: Other toxic encephalopathy	G92.8
Secondary: Alcoholic cirrhosis of liver with ascites	K70.31
Secondary: Alcohol dependence, uncomplicated	F10.20
Secondary: Esophageal varices with bleeding	I85.01
Secondary: Acute posthemorrhagic anemia	D62
Secondary: Gastric varices	I86.4
Secondary: Personal history of nicotine dependence	Z87.891

This patient was diagnosed with both hepatic encephalopathy and toxic metabolic encephalopathy, neither of which has resolved upon home health admission. These conditions are not excluded from each other and both should be coded when present per guidance from Q1 2021 Coding Clinic. Codes for toxic encephalopathy were updated for FY2022 to include a code for unspecified and other toxic encephalopathy. Because the condition is specified as metabolic, G92.8 is assigned. A combination code identifies that ascites is present with the alcoholic cirrhosis and the code for alcohol dependence should follow this condition. A combination code also identifies that the esophageal varices are the cause of the GI bleeding and no additional code for bleeding is needed. Because the anemia is stated as acute on chronic blood loss, the more specific code identifying acute (D62) is assigned.

Chapter 12: Diseases of the Skin and Subcutaneous Tissue (L00-L99)

Chapter 12 includes conditions of the skin, sweat glands, hair and nails. Among the most common reasons for home health services are the care of skin lesions, surgical wounds and skin ulcers. The ICD-10-CM codes for skin lesions, including ulcers (except vascular ulcers), are found in this chapter. One of the biggest challenges when selecting a code from Chapter 12 is properly defining the type of wound or skin condition. Some common skin conditions, such as boils (carbuncles), rashes, erythema, abscesses (localized collection of pus), sunburns, baldness (alopecia), hives (urticaria), allergic skin reactions, and blisters (bullae) are reported using these codes. Other conditions, such as bed sores (pressure ulcers), cellulitis (acute spreading infection of skin), and acute lymphadenitis are also reported here.

Sometimes, a Chapter 12 code isn't the most appropriate choice. Here are a few situations to watch out for:

- If the documentation indicates **a neoplasm or tumor of the skin or subcutaneous tissues,** coders should look up the term to find the correct code, most likely a code from Chapter 2 (C00-D49). For example, the Alphabetic Index entry for the term "dermatofibrosarcoma" reads "see Neoplasm, skin, malignant," referring the coder to the Neoplasm Table.
- **Venous (stasis) and arterial ulcers** are coded from Chapter 9, Diseases of the Circulatory system. Atherosclerosis of native arteries of the lower extremities are coded within sub-category I70.23, while ulceration associated with various types of bypass grafts are found at I70.3- to I70.73-. Varicose veins of lower extremity with ulcers are coded from category I83 in Chapter 9.
- **Symptoms** related to skin and subcutaneous tissues are reported using codes from either this chapter or Chapter 18. Chapter 12 includes symptom codes, such as itchiness (pruritis, L29.9). Chapter 18 contains the code series R20-R23 (symptoms involving skin and subcutaneous tissue), which include: disturbances of skin sensations; rash and other nonspecific skin eruption; localized swelling; edema; and other skin changes such as cyanosis, flushing, changes in skin texture, etc.

  Every effort should be made to secure a definitive diagnosis. A symptom code from chapters 12 or 18 may be reported as an additional diagnosis when it describes a significant aspect of the condition but is not an integral part of it.
- If a patient has **a personal or family history of a condition of the skin or subcutaneous tissues,** it may be appropriate to select from the V code section, such as Z85.82- (Personal history of malignant neoplasm of skin) or Z87.2 (Personal history of diseases of skin and subcutaneous tissue) or Z84.0 (Family history of skin conditions).
- Although not often found in home care, if reporting a **skin disorder that is complicating pregnancy, childbirth or puerperium**, report a code from Chapter 15, such as O99.71-, as the first-listed diagnosis and a code from this chapter as an additional diagnosis.
- Other code categories that are excluded from chapter 12 include: certain conditions originating in the perinatal period (P00-P96); certain infectious and parasitic diseases (A00-B99); congenital malformations, deformations, and chromosomal abnormalities (Q00-Q99); endocrine, nutritional and metabolic diseases (E00-E88); lipomelanotic reticulosis (I89.8); systemic connective tissue disorders (M30-M36) and viral warts (B07.-).

Multiple Coding and Sequencing

It is very important to read the Includes and Excludes notes under codes in this chapter, as well as any other instructions under the code or code category. Many notes refer to Chapter 1 codes (infections and parasitic conditions). Here are some examples of multiple coding and sequencing issues for codes in this chapter:

A note under classifications L00-L08 (infections of the skin and subcutaneous tissue) states: "Use additional code (B95-B97) to identify infectious agent." The first-listed diagnosis is from chapter 12.

Notes under codes in this chapter may refer to other chapters. For example, a note under the code L97.- non-pressure chronic ulcer of lower limb, not elsewhere classified states: "Code first any associated underlying condition, such as: any associated gangrene (I96). Atherosclerosis of the lower extremities (I70.-), chronic venous hypertension (I87.31-, I87.33-), diabetic ulcers, postphlebitic syndrome (I87.01-, I87.03-), and varicose ulcer (I83.0-, I83.2-)". The code from L97.- is listed following the underlying condition to describe the location and depth of the ulcer.

Important: The L97 "code first" note at means "if present, if applicable." However, if you don't know the underlying etiology you should query the physician, as experts believe auditors will be looking for both codes.

Special Coding Issues

Cellulitis (code series L03.-) literally means inflammation of cells. The condition indicates an acute, spreading infection of the dermis and subcutaneous tissues resulting in pain, erythema, edema and warmth. Cellulitis may spread by invading contiguous tissue or through the lymphatic and circulatory systems. If an organism is specified, report the appropriate code from Chapter 1 (B95-B96) as an additional diagnosis. If the cellulitis is associated with a wound or an ostomy, the wound or complicated ostomy is generally coded first.

Cellulitis resulting from a colostomy, enterostomy, gastrostomy and esophagostomy are reported with code K94.- in chapter 11 (Diseases of the digestive system), and cellulitis associated with stomas of the urinary tract are coded with N99.5- codes found in chapter 14 (Diseases of the genitourinary system). A code for the cellulitis from chapter 12 and a code for the organism from chapter 1 are listed as additional diagnoses following the ostomy complication code if cellulitis is present in addition to the ostomy complication. If cellulitis is present and is the focus of care around an ostomy, the cellulitis by location is listed first.

Cellulitis can occur in many areas of the body and therefore, codes from the appropriate chapters should be assigned. For example, cellulitis of the pharynx is reported using code J39.1 from Chapter 10. Cellulitis of the eyelid is reported using code H00.03- from Chapter 7.

Dermatitis and Eczema

Dermatitis is any inflammation of the skin. Eczema is a type of dermatitis with inflammation, erythema (redness), bumps (papules, vesicles, pustules), scales, and/or scabs. All eczema is dermatitis, but not all dermatitis is eczema.

However, in ICD-10, categories L20-L30, the terms dermatitis and eczema are used synonymously and interchangeably. When the cause of the condition is related to contact with the skin, consider categories L24.- to L25.- for contact dermatitis. Allergic contact dermatitis is coded at L23.3 and is used when dermatitis is caused by contact with metals, adhesives, cosmetics, drugs, dyes, food, plants, animal dander and other agents in contact with the skin. Assign an additional code for adverse effects, if applicable, to identify drug (T36-T50 with fifth or sixth character 5) found in the Table of Drugs and Chemicals, to indicate the drug that caused the dermatitis and verify the code in the Tabular List. When the cause of the dermatitis or eczema is unspecified, consider L23.9, allergic contact dermatitis/eczema.

Irritant contact dermatitis is coded at category L24.-, unspecified contact dermatitis is coded at category L25.-. Specific codes for all of the types of irritants are listed in L23.

There are many other conditions "not elsewhere classified" (NEC) that also fall under this category.

For example, intertriginous dermatitis is found between two skin surfaces that rub against each other, such as under the breasts, between the toes, or in the skin folds of the groin. Consider L25.8, Unspecified dermatitis due to other agents.

When dermatitis is known to be the result of an ingested substance, consider category L27.-. When an internally taken drug or medicine causes dermatitis, select a code depending on whether the dermatitis is generalized (L27.0) or localized (L27.1), and remember to add an additional code for adverse effect, if applicable to identify the drug (T36-T50 with fifth or sixth character 5). When the ingested causative agent is food, use L27.2. If another specified substance taken internally is the cause, use L27.8. If the substance is unspecified but known to have been taken internally, use L27.9.

Ulcers

Just as the plan of care and progress notes support nursing interventions, the ICD-10-CM codes support medical necessity for the wound management services provided. If the code is absent or inaccurate, a red flag will be raised when the claim is reviewed and payment may ultimately be delayed.

Codes from the L97.- are often listed as manifestations of other conditions, such as diabetes, atherosclerosis and postphlebitic syndrome. The L97.- codes are not manifestations in the true sense of the word; however, causal conditions should precede the L97.- codes.

More than one L97.- code (non-pressure ulcer of the lower limb) may be used on a claim/record to capture the total number of ulcer locations, but remember that the same code may **not** be used twice in the same diagnosis list. In ICD-10-CM, the L97.- codes are combination codes including the location, laterality (right, left) and the depth of the ulcer. For example, a non-pressure ulcer of the right calf with fat layer exposed is coded L97.212 as an additional code following a code for the underlying condition. If there is no code available for bilateral and the patient has ulcers on both calves, a code for both the right and left calf would be assigned. For example, if there was a chronic skin ulcer of the right calf with fat exposure (L97.212) and another chronic skin ulcer on the left calf with breakdown limited to the skin (L97.221), both would be coded. If there was the same underlying cause for the ulcers, that code would be listed first followed by the two ulcer codes. Necrosis must be evident in the muscle or bone to use an L97.- code with a sixth character of "3" (corresponding to muscle necrosis) or "4" (corresponding to bone necrosis). If you can't see it, you can't code it.

If an ulcer is caused by inadequate venous circulation in the area, then it's most likely a **stasis ulcer**. ICD -10-CM codes designated for non-pressure chronic ulcers of lower limb, not elsewhere classified are found in Category L97. To select a code, you must distinguish between **pressure ulcers** and other kinds of ulcers. Note that **varicose ulcers** are found under **"varix"** in the Alphabetical Index and direct the coder to lower leg with ulcer category I83.- by location on the leg. But **stasis ulcers without varicose veins** are coded with a code from I87.2 (venous insufficiency), or if the statement indicates **venous hypertension** – found under hypertension, venous, idiopathic in the Alphabetical Index and at I87.33- in the Tabular).

If caused by poor arterial circulation, consider it an arterial ulcer. If the etiology is diabetes, the ulcer most likely will be coded as a diabetic ulcer.

Arterial ulcers occur when arterial blood flow is compromised. Atherosclerosis of the right leg with ulceration of the ankle limited to skin breakdown is coded I70.233 followed by L97.311. An arterial ulcer on the toes with gangrene due to atherosclerosis is coded I70.26- (Atherosclerosis of the extremities with gangrene), L98.499 (Non-pressure chronic ulcer of skin of other sites with unspecified severity). In this case, the gangrene is part of the I70.262 combination code and is not coded separately.

Remember that not all arterial ulcers are caused by atherosclerosis. Inflammatory diseases including vasculitis, lupus and scleroderma can cause arterial ulcers, as can an arterial thrombus and other conditions. Always query the physician to determine the etiology of the ulcer. For example, an ulcer due to Raynaud's syndrome would be captured by coding first the Raynaud's I73.00, followed by the ulcer code L97.823 (Ulcer of left lower leg with necrosis of muscle).

Diabetic ulcers are coded with the appropriate code for the type of diabetes from E08.62-, E09.62-, E10.62-, E11.62-, or E13.62- followed by the appropriate code from L97.-. If the physician documents an ulcer as the result of diabetic neuropathy, code the diabetic ulcer as E08.49, E09.49, E10.49, E11.49 or E13.49 followed by L97.- to show the location and depth of ulcer.

Venous stasis is a type of angiopathy and should be coded as diabetic peripheral angiopathy with E11.51 and I87.2, according to recent Coding Clinic guidance. Remember, when the focus of care is wound care, it is appropriate to first assign Z48.00, Encounter for change or removal of nonsurgical wound dressing. However, if the diabetic ulcer or the venous stasis ulcer is coded first, the Z48.00 code does not need to be primary.

Always confirm the etiology and type of ulcer with the physician.

A **decubitus ulcer** is a **pressure ulcer,** or what is commonly called a "bed sore." Presentations of pressure ulcers range from a deep red coloration of the skin that does not blanche, to a very deep wound extending to and sometimes into the bone. Remember, that stage 1 pressure ulcers of patients who are not Caucasian may present as an area of hyperpigmentation (darker coloration of the natural skin tone) that doesn't blanche, and not as an area of non-blanchable redness.

Code a diagnosis of "pressure injury" the same way you would code a "pressure ulcer" by site and stage. The term "pressure injury" represents a change in termination and not a change in definition, per Q3 2016 Coding Clinic guidance.

Home health agencies may adopt the NPUAP guidelines in their clinical practice and documentation. When discrepancies exist between the NPUAP definitions and the OASIS scoring instructions provided in the Guidance Manual and CMS Q&As, providers should rely on the CMS OASIS instructions, according to CMS.

To view the WOCN's most recent guidance, visit *https://cdn.ymaws.com/www.wocn.org/resource/collection/7406B652-D19C-41C7-906C-0578AABC356B/OASIS-D_Best_Practice_Document__2019_.pdf.* The NPUAP released new pressure ulcer staging definitions in April 2016. *For the NPUAP new definitions visit http://tinyurl.com/gnvnhvg. View schematic artwork reflecting the changes in stages for pressure injury at http://bit.ly/1p0NMaE.*

Codes from category L89, pressure ulcer, are combination codes that identify the site of the pressure ulcer as well as the stage of the ulcer. For example, you list only **one code** for a stage 4 pressure ulcer of the right ankle – L89.514.

The ICD-10-CM classifies pressure ulcers based on severity, which is designated by stages 1 - 4, pressure-induced deep tissue damage, unspecified stage, and unstageable. Assign as many codes from category L89 as needed to identify all the pressure ulcers a patient has, if applicable.

Assignment of the code for unstageable pressure ulcer (L89.xx0) should be based on the clinical documentation. These codes are used for pressure ulcers whose stage cannot be clinically determined (e.g., the pressure ulcer is covered by eschar or has been treated with a skin or muscle graft.) This code should not be confused with codes for unspecified stage.

Assignment of the pressure ulcer stage code should be guided by clinical documentation of the stage or documentation of the terms found in the Alphabetical Index. For clinical terms describing the stage that are not found in the Alphabetical Index and when there is no documentation of the stage, you should query the physician.

No code is assigned if the documentation states the pressure ulcer is completely healed. However, pressure ulcers described as "healing" should be assigned the appropriate pressure ulcer stage code based on the documentation in the medical record. If the documentation does not provide information about the stage of the healing pressure ulcer, assign the appropriate code for unspecified stage (L89.899).

If the documentation is unclear about whether the patient has a current pressure ulcer or if the patient is being treated for a healing pressure ulcer, query the physician.

If a patient is admitted with a pressure ulcer at one stage and it progresses to a worse stage, assign the code for the worse stage reported for that site.

CHAPTER 12: DISEASES OF THE SKIN AND SUBCUTANEOUS TISSUE (L00-L99)

EXCLUDES 2 certain conditions originating in the perinatal period (P04-P96)
certain infectious and parasitic diseases (A00-B99)
complications of pregnancy, childbirth and the puerperium (O00-O9A)
congenital malformations, deformations, and chromosomal abnormalities (Q00-Q99)
endocrine, nutritional and metabolic diseases (E00-E88)
lipomelanotic reticulosis (I89.8)
neoplasms (C00-D49)
symptoms, signs and abnormal clinical and laboratory findings, not elsewhere classified (R00-R94)
systemic connective tissue disorders (M30-M36)
viral warts (B07.-)

This chapter contains the following blocks:

L00-L08	Infections of the skin and subcutaneous tissue
L10-L14	Bullous disorders
L20-L30	Dermatitis and eczema
L40-L45	Papulosquamous disorders
L49-L54	Urticaria and erythema
L55-L59	Radiation-related disorders of the skin and subcutaneous tissue
L60-L75	Disorders of skin appendages
L76	Intraoperative and postprocedural complications of skin and subcutaneous tissue
L80-L99	Other disorders of the skin and subcutaneous tissue

Infections of the skin and subcutaneous tissue (L00-L08)

Use additional code (B95-B97) to identify infectious agent.

EXCLUDES 2 hordeolum (H00.0)
infective dermatitis (L30.3)
local infections of skin classified in Chapter 1
lupus panniculitis (L93.2)
panniculitis NOS (M79.3)
panniculitis of neck and back (M54.0-)
Perlèche NOS (K13.0)
Perlèche due to candidiasis (B37.0)
Perlèche due to riboflavin deficiency (E53.0)
pyogenic granuloma (L98.0)
relapsing panniculitis [Weber-Christian] (M35.6)
viral warts (B07.-)
zoster (B02.-)

SP + **L00 Staphylococcal scalded skin syndrome**
Ritter's disease
Use additional code to identify percentage of skin exfoliation (L49.-)
EXCLUDES 1 bullous impetigo (L01.03)
pemphigus neonatorum (L01.03)
toxic epidermal necrolysis [Lyell] (L51.2)

DEFINITION The breakdown of dermal layer cellular structure by staph bacteria causing large sections of skin to slough off and peel away, leaving raw, exposed areas.

4 **L01 Impetigo**
EXCLUDES 1 impetigo herpetiformis (L40.1)

5 **L01.0 Impetigo**
Impetigo contagiosa
Impetigo vulgaris

DEFINITION Bacterial skin infection in children; small pustules form over a reddish rash and burst, leaving an itchy, yellow crust over the affected area.

SP **L01.00 Impetigo, unspecified**
Impetigo NOS

SP **L01.01 Non-bullous impetigo**

DEFINITION Most common type of impetigo due to staph or strep bacteria, in which tiny blisters form (particularly on the face), burst quickly, and leave a small, wet, weeping spot that crusts over and disappears, leaving a red mark that later heals.

SP **L01.02 Bockhart's impetigo**
Impetigo follicularis
Perifolliculitis NOS
Superficial pustular perifolliculitis

DEFINITION Superficial, pustular folliculitis caused by *S. aureus*; characterized by small, painful, tense, yellowish-white domed pustules in crops around follicular orifices that heal in a few days.

SP **L01.03 Bullous impetigo**
Impetigo neonatorum
Pemphigus neonatorum

DEFINITION Impetigo of longer duration (generally due to *S. aureus*), in which large, clear, fluid-filled blisters form on red sores, become cloudy, then burst and ooze, leaving a large, yellowish, crusty scab.

SP **L01.09 Other impetigo**
Ulcerative impetigo

DEFINITION Ulcerative impetigo: A deeper dermis form of impetigo with small, shallow, purulent ulcers that form under a thick, brownish-black crusted surface infection, surrounded by erythema.

SP **L01.1 Impetiginization of other dermatoses**

DEFINITION Impetigo occurring in an area already experiencing a dermatosis; the infected blisters burst, leaving a weeping wet patch that crusts over, worsening the existing condition.

+ 4 **L02 Cutaneous abscess, furuncle and carbuncle**
Use additional code to identify organism (B95-B96)
EXCLUDES 2 abscess of anus and rectal regions (K61.-)
abscess of female genital organs (external) (N76.4)
abscess of male genital organs (external) (N48.2, N49.-)

CODING TIPS ✓ Abscesses are infected by definition. An aftercare following surgery code is not usually appropriate when an infection is being treated by incision and drainage and/or antibiotics. Continue to code the abscess.

CODING TIPS ✓ Abscesses, carbuncles and furuncles are coded separately from cellulitis (L03). Furuncles are commonly known as boils. Use an additional code to identify the causative organism.

DEFINITION Furuncle: A bacterial infection of a hair follicle characterized by a painful, red, swollen bump filled with fluid, pus, and cellular debris; also called a boil.

DEFINITION Abscess: A pocket of pus that collects within an infected area of skin and is generally red and sore.

DEFINITION Carbuncle: A group of several infected hair follicles, or furuncles, that join together with more than one opening to drain pus, often extending into deeper tissue.

+ 5 **L02.0 Cutaneous abscess, furuncle and carbuncle of face**

EXCLUDES 2 abscess of ear, external (H60.0)
abscess of eyelid (H00.0)
abscess of head [any part, except face] (L02.8)
abscess of lacrimal gland (H04.0)
abscess of lacrimal passages (H04.3)
abscess of mouth (K12.2)
abscess of nose (J34.0)
abscess of orbit (H05.0)
submandibular abscess (K12.2)

SP + **L02.01 Cutaneous abscess of face**

SP + **L02.02 Furuncle of face**
Boil of face
Folliculitis of face

SP + **L02.03 Carbuncle of face**

+ 5 **L02.1 Cutaneous abscess, furuncle and carbuncle of neck**

SP SH SL + **L02.11 Cutaneous abscess of neck**

SP + **L02.12 Furuncle of neck**
Boil of neck
Folliculitis of neck

SP + **L02.13 Carbuncle of neck**

+ 5 **L02.2 Cutaneous abscess, furuncle and carbuncle of trunk**

EXCLUDES 1 non-newborn omphalitis (L08.82)
omphalitis of newborn (P38.-)

EXCLUDES 2 abscess of breast (N61.1)
abscess of buttocks (L02.3)
abscess of female external genital organs (N76.4)
abscess of male external genital organs (N48.2, N49.-)
abscess of hip (L02.4)

+ 6 **L02.21 Cutaneous abscess of trunk**

SP SH SL + **L02.211 Cutaneous abscess of abdominal wall**

SP SH SL + **L02.212 Cutaneous abscess of back [any part, except buttock]**

SP SH SL + **L02.213 Cutaneous abscess of chest wall**

SP SH SL + **L02.214 Cutaneous abscess of groin**

SP SH SL + **L02.215 Cutaneous abscess of perineum**

SP SH SL + **L02.216 Cutaneous abscess of umbilicus**

SP SH SL + **L02.219 Cutaneous abscess of trunk, unspecified**

+ 6 **L02.22 Furuncle of trunk**
Boil of trunk
Folliculitis of trunk

SP + **L02.221 Furuncle of abdominal wall**

SP + **L02.222 Furuncle of back [any part, except buttock]**

SP + **L02.223 Furuncle of chest wall**

SP + **L02.224 Furuncle of groin**

SP + **L02.225 Furuncle of perineum**

SP + **L02.226 Furuncle of umbilicus**

SP + **L02.229 Furuncle of trunk, unspecified**

+ 6 **L02.23 Carbuncle of trunk**

SP + **L02.231 Carbuncle of abdominal wall**

SP + **L02.232 Carbuncle of back [any part, except buttock]**

SP + **L02.233 Carbuncle of chest wall**

SP + **L02.234 Carbuncle of groin**

SP + **L02.235 Carbuncle of perineum**

SP + **L02.236 Carbuncle of umbilicus**

SP + **L02.239 Carbuncle of trunk, unspecified**

+ 5 **L02.3 Cutaneous abscess, furuncle and carbuncle of buttock**

EXCLUDES 1 pilonidal cyst with abscess (L05.01)

SP SH SL + **L02.31 Cutaneous abscess of buttock**
Cutaneous abscess of gluteal region

SP + **L02.32 Furuncle of buttock**
Boil of buttock
Folliculitis of buttock
Furuncle of gluteal region

SP + **L02.33 Carbuncle of buttock**
Carbuncle of gluteal region

+ 5 **L02.4 Cutaneous abscess, furuncle and carbuncle of limb**

EXCLUDES 2 Cutaneous abscess, furuncle and carbuncle of groin (L02.214, L02.224, L02.234)
Cutaneous abscess, furuncle and carbuncle of hand (L02.5-)
Cutaneous abscess, furuncle and carbuncle of foot (L02.6-)

+ 6 **L02.41 Cutaneous abscess of limb**

⊟ SP SH SL + **L02.411 Cutaneous abscess of right axilla**

⊟ SP SH SL + **L02.412 Cutaneous abscess of left axilla**

⊟ SP SH SL + **L02.413 Cutaneous abscess of right upper limb**

⊟ SP SH SL + **L02.414 Cutaneous abscess of left upper limb**

⊟ SP SH SL + **L02.415 Cutaneous abscess of right lower limb**

⊟ SP SH SL + **L02.416 Cutaneous abscess of left lower limb**

⊟ IQ + **L02.419 Cutaneous abscess of limb, unspecified**

+ 6 **L02.42 Furuncle of limb**
Boil of limb
Folliculitis of limb

⊟ SP + **L02.421 Furuncle of right axilla**

Chapter 12

L00-L99

SP + L02.422 Furuncle of left axilla
SP + L02.423 Furuncle of right upper limb
SP + L02.424 Furuncle of left upper limb
SP + L02.425 Furuncle of right lower limb
SP + L02.426 Furuncle of left lower limb
IQ + L02.429 Furuncle of limb, unspecified
+ 6 L02.43 Carbuncle of limb
SP + L02.431 Carbuncle of right axilla
SP + L02.432 Carbuncle of left axilla
SP + L02.433 Carbuncle of right upper limb
SP + L02.434 Carbuncle of left upper limb
SP + L02.435 Carbuncle of right lower limb
SP + L02.436 Carbuncle of left lower limb
IQ + L02.439 Carbuncle of limb, unspecified
+ 5 L02.5 Cutaneous abscess, furuncle and carbuncle of hand
+ 6 L02.51 Cutaneous abscess of hand
SP SH SL + L02.511 Cutaneous abscess of right hand
SP SH SL + L02.512 Cutaneous abscess of left hand
IQ + L02.519 Cutaneous abscess of unspecified hand
+ 6 L02.52 Furuncle hand
Boil of hand
Folliculitis of hand
SP + L02.521 Furuncle right hand
SP + L02.522 Furuncle left hand
IQ + L02.529 Furuncle unspecified hand
+ 6 L02.53 Carbuncle of hand
SP + L02.531 Carbuncle of right hand
SP + L02.532 Carbuncle of left hand
IQ + L02.539 Carbuncle of unspecified hand
+ 5 L02.6 Cutaneous abscess, furuncle and carbuncle of foot
+ 6 L02.61 Cutaneous abscess of foot
SP SH SL + L02.611 Cutaneous abscess of right foot
SP SH SL + L02.612 Cutaneous abscess of left foot
IQ + L02.619 Cutaneous abscess of unspecified foot
+ 6 L02.62 Furuncle of foot
Boil of foot
Folliculitis of foot
SP + L02.621 Furuncle of right foot
SP + L02.622 Furuncle of left foot
IQ + L02.629 Furuncle of unspecified foot
+ 6 L02.63 Carbuncle of foot
SP + L02.631 Carbuncle of right foot
SP + L02.632 Carbuncle of left foot
IQ + L02.639 Carbuncle of unspecified foot
+ 5 L02.8 Cutaneous abscess, furuncle and carbuncle of other sites
+ 6 L02.81 Cutaneous abscess of other sites
SP SH SL + L02.811 Cutaneous abscess of head [any part, except face]
SP SH SL + L02.818 Cutaneous abscess of other sites
+ 6 L02.82 Furuncle of other sites
Boil of other sites
Folliculitis of other sites
SP + L02.821 Furuncle of head [any part, except face]
SP + L02.828 Furuncle of other sites
+ 6 L02.83 Carbuncle of other sites
SP + L02.831 Carbuncle of head [any part, except face]
SP + L02.838 Carbuncle of other sites
+ 5 L02.9 Cutaneous abscess, furuncle and carbuncle, unspecified
IQ + L02.91 Cutaneous abscess, unspecified
IQ + L02.92 Furuncle, unspecified
Boil NOS
Furunculosis NOS
IQ + L02.93 Carbuncle, unspecified
4 L03 Cellulitis and acute lymphangitis
EXCLUDES 2 cellulitis of anal and rectal region (K61.-)
cellulitis of external auditory canal (H60.1)
cellulitis of eyelid (H00.0)
cellulitis of female external genital organs (N76.4)
cellulitis of lacrimal apparatus (H04.3)
cellulitis of male external genital organs (N48.2, N49.-)
cellulitis of mouth (K12.2)
cellulitis of nose (J34.0)
eosinophilic cellulitis [Wells] (L98.3)
febrile neutrophilic dermatosis [Sweet] (L98.2)
lymphangitis (chronic) (subacute) (I89.1)

CODING TIPS✓ L03 includes codes for cellulitis. When diagnostic statements indicate abscess, a code from L02 should be coded.

CODING TIPS✓ Cellulitis usually presents as an abrupt onset of redness, swelling, pain, or heat in the affected area. Unless a diagnosis of cellulitis is documented by the provider, a code from category L03 should not be assigned. If cellulitis is associated with a wound or ostomy, code the wound or complicated ostomy first, followed by the appropriate L03 code for cellulitis.

DEFINITION Cellulitis: A spreading bacterial infection of connective soft tissue extending into deep dermal and subcutaneous layers; produces circumscribed swelling, fever, and swollen lymph nodes.

DEFINITION Acute lymphangitis: A quickly spreading bacterial infection of the lymph vessels appearing as painful, red streaks visible through the skin surface.

5 L03.0 Cellulitis and acute lymphangitis of finger and toe
Infection of nail
Onychia
Paronychia
Perionychia
6 L03.01 Cellulitis of finger
Felon
Whitlow
EXCLUDES 1 herpetic whitlow (B00.89)
SP L03.011 Cellulitis of right finger

Chapter 12 L00-L99

L03.012 Cellulitis of left finger
L03.019 Cellulitis of unspecified finger
L03.02 Acute lymphangitis of finger
Hangnail with lymphangitis of finger
L03.021 Acute lymphangitis of right finger
L03.022 Acute lymphangitis of left finger
L03.029 Acute lymphangitis of unspecified finger
L03.03 Cellulitis of toe
L03.031 Cellulitis of right toe
L03.032 Cellulitis of left toe
L03.039 Cellulitis of unspecified toe
L03.04 Acute lymphangitis of toe
Hangnail with lymphangitis of toe
L03.041 Acute lymphangitis of right toe
L03.042 Acute lymphangitis of left toe
L03.049 Acute lymphangitis of unspecified toe
L03.1 Cellulitis and acute lymphangitis of other parts of limb
L03.11 Cellulitis of other parts of limb
EXCLUDES 2 cellulitis of fingers (L03.01-)
cellulitis of toes (L03.03-)
groin (L03.314)
L03.111 Cellulitis of right axilla
L03.112 Cellulitis of left axilla
L03.113 Cellulitis of right upper limb
L03.114 Cellulitis of left upper limb
L03.115 Cellulitis of right lower limb
L03.116 Cellulitis of left lower limb
L03.119 Cellulitis of unspecified part of limb
L03.12 Acute lymphangitis of other parts of limb
EXCLUDES 2 acute lymphangitis of fingers (L03.2-)
acute lymphangitis of toes (L03.04-)
acute lymphangitis of groin (L03.324)
L03.121 Acute lymphangitis of right axilla
L03.122 Acute lymphangitis of left axilla
L03.123 Acute lymphangitis of right upper limb
L03.124 Acute lymphangitis of left upper limb
L03.125 Acute lymphangitis of right lower limb
L03.126 Acute lymphangitis of left lower limb
L03.129 Acute lymphangitis of unspecified part of limb
L03.2 Cellulitis and acute lymphangitis of face and neck
L03.21 Cellulitis and acute lymphangitis of face
L03.211 Cellulitis of face
EXCLUDES 2 abscess of orbit (H05.01-)
cellulitis of ear (H60.1-)
cellulitis of eyelid (H00.0-)
cellulitis of head (L03.81)
cellulitis of lacrimal apparatus (H04.3)
cellulitis of lip (K13.0)
cellulitis of mouth (K12.2)
cellulitis of nose (internal) (J34.0)
cellulitis of orbit (H05.01-)
cellulitis of scalp (L03.81)
L03.212 Acute lymphangitis of face
L03.213 Periorbital cellulitis
Preseptal cellulitis
L03.22 Cellulitis and acute lymphangitis of neck
L03.221 Cellulitis of neck
L03.222 Acute lymphangitis of neck
L03.3 Cellulitis and acute lymphangitis of trunk
L03.31 Cellulitis of trunk
EXCLUDES 2 cellulitis of anal and rectal regions (K61.-)
cellulitis of breast NOS (N61.0)
cellulitis of female external genital organs (N76.4)
cellulitis of male external genital organs (N48.2, N49.-)
omphalitis of newborn (P38.-)
puerperal cellulitis of breast (O91.2)
L03.311 Cellulitis of abdominal wall
EXCLUDES 2 cellulitis of umbilicus (L03.316)
cellulitis of groin (L03.314)
L03.312 Cellulitis of back [any part except buttock]
L03.313 Cellulitis of chest wall
L03.314 Cellulitis of groin
L03.315 Cellulitis of perineum
L03.316 Cellulitis of umbilicus
L03.317 Cellulitis of buttock
L03.319 Cellulitis of trunk, unspecified
L03.32 Acute lymphangitis of trunk
L03.321 Acute lymphangitis of abdominal wall
L03.322 Acute lymphangitis of back [any part except buttock]
L03.323 Acute lymphangitis of chest wall
L03.324 Acute lymphangitis of groin
L03.325 Acute lymphangitis of perineum
L03.326 Acute lymphangitis of umbilicus
L03.327 Acute lymphangitis of buttock
L03.329 Acute lymphangitis of trunk, unspecified

Chapter 12 L00-L99

4th digit required 5th digit required 6th digit required 7th digit required 7th digit placeholder +Additional code Laterality

5 **L03.8 Cellulitis and acute lymphangitis of other sites**

6 **L03.81 Cellulitis of other sites**

SP SH SL **L03.811 Cellulitis of head [any part, except face]**
Cellulitis of scalp
EXCLUDES 2 cellulitis of face (L03.211)

SP SH SL **L03.818 Cellulitis of other sites**

6 **L03.89 Acute lymphangitis of other sites**

SP SH SL **L03.891 Acute lymphangitis of head [any part, except face]**

SP SH SL **L03.898 Acute lymphangitis of other sites**

5 **L03.9 Cellulitis and acute lymphangitis, unspecified**

!Q **L03.90 Cellulitis, unspecified**

!Q **L03.91 Acute lymphangitis, unspecified**
EXCLUDES 1 lymphangitis NOS (I89.1)

4 **L04 Acute lymphadenitis**
INCLUDES abscess (acute) of lymph nodes, except mesenteric
acute lymphadenitis, except mesenteric
EXCLUDES 1 chronic or subacute lymphadenitis, except mesenteric (I88.1)
enlarged lymph nodes (R59.-)
human immunodeficiency virus [HIV] disease resulting in generalized lymphadenopathy (B20)
lymphadenitis NOS (I88.9)
nonspecific mesenteric lymphadenitis (I88.0)

SP **L04.0 Acute lymphadenitis of face, head and neck**

SP **L04.1 Acute lymphadenitis of trunk**

SP **L04.2 Acute lymphadenitis of upper limb**
Acute lymphadenitis of axilla
Acute lymphadenitis of shoulder

SP **L04.3 Acute lymphadenitis of lower limb**
Acute lymphadenitis of hip
EXCLUDES 2 acute lymphadenitis of groin (L04.1)

SP **L04.8 Acute lymphadenitis of other sites**

!Q **L04.9 Acute lymphadenitis, unspecified**

4 **L05 Pilonidal cyst and sinus**

5 **L05.0 Pilonidal cyst and sinus with abscess**
DEFINITION An abscessed sinus tract draining to the surface and located in the tailbone area, often associated with ingrown hairs.

SP **L05.01 Pilonidal cyst with abscess**
Pilonidal abscess
Pilonidal dimple with abscess
Postanal dimple with abscess
EXCLUDES 2 congenital sacral dimple (Q82.6)
parasacral dimple (Q82.6)

SP **L05.02 Pilonidal sinus with abscess**
Coccygeal fistula with abscess
Coccygeal sinus with abscess
Pilonidal fistula with abscess

5 **L05.9 Pilonidal cyst and sinus without abscess**

SP **L05.91 Pilonidal cyst without abscess**
Pilonidal dimple
Postanal dimple
Pilonidal cyst NOS
EXCLUDES 2 congenital sacral dimple (Q82.6)
parasacral dimple (Q82.6)

SP **L05.92 Pilonidal sinus without abscess**
Coccygeal fistula
Coccygeal sinus without abscess
Pilonidal fistula

4 **L08 Other local infections of skin and subcutaneous tissue**

SP **L08.0 Pyoderma**
Dermatitis gangrenosa
Purulent dermatitis
Septic dermatitis
Suppurative dermatitis
EXCLUDES 1 pyoderma gangrenosum (L88)
pyoderma vegetans (L08.81)
CODING TIPS ✓ Do not assign L08.0 to indicate pyoderma gangrenosum, which is a specific disorder resulting in deep, ulcerative, necrotic ulcers. Pyoderma gangrenosum should be coded to L88 when specified.
DEFINITION A skin condition producing pus.

SP **L08.1 Erythrasma**
DEFINITION Skin infection caused by Corynebacterium minutissimum in which pink-red patches with fine scales and wrinkling appear in perpetually moist skin folds (intergluteal fold, inframammary fold, armpits, groin) and later turn brown and scaly.

5 **L08.8 Other specified local infections of the skin and subcutaneous tissue**

SP **L08.81 Pyoderma vegetans**
EXCLUDES 1 pyoderma gangrenosum (L88)
pyoderma NOS (L08.0)

SP **L08.82 Omphalitis not of newborn**
EXCLUDES 1 omphalitis of newborn (P38.-)

SP **L08.89 Other specified local infections of the skin and subcutaneous tissue**

SP **L08.9 Local infection of the skin and subcutaneous tissue, unspecified**

Bullous disorders (L10-L14)

EXCLUDES 1 benign familial pemphigus [Hailey-Hailey] (Q82.8)
staphylococcal scalded skin syndrome (L00)
toxic epidermal necrolysis [Lyell] (L51.2)

4 **L10 Pemphigus**
EXCLUDES 1 pemphigus neonatorum (L01.03)

SP **L10.0 Pemphigus vulgaris**

SP **L10.1 Pemphigus vegetans**

SP **L10.2 Pemphigus foliaceous**

SP **L10.3 Brazilian pemphigus [fogo selvagem]**

Chapter 12
L00-L99

SP **L10.4 Pemphigus erythematosus**
Senear-Usher syndrome

SP + **L10.5 Drug-induced pemphigus**
Use additional code for adverse effect, if applicable, to identify drug (T36-T50 with fifth or sixth character 5)

CODING TIPS ✓ Code L10.5 should only be assigned when documentation clearly indicates a relationship between pemphigus and a drug or chemical as the underlying cause. Assign a code from T36-T50 following L10.5 to indicate the drug and adverse effect.

5 **L10.8 Other pemphigus**

SP **L10.81 Paraneoplastic pemphigus**

SP **L10.89 Other pemphigus**

SP **L10.9 Pemphigus, unspecified**

4 **L11 Other acantholytic disorders**

SP **L11.0 Acquired keratosis follicularis**
EXCLUDES 1 keratosis follicularis (congenital) [Darier-White] (Q82.8)

SP **L11.1 Transient acantholytic dermatosis [Grover]**

SP **L11.8 Other specified acantholytic disorders**

SP **L11.9 Acantholytic disorder, unspecified**

4 **L12 Pemphigoid**
EXCLUDES 1 herpes gestationis (O26.4-)
impetigo herpetiformis (L40.1)

SP **L12.0 Bullous pemphigoid**

SP **L12.1 Cicatricial pemphigoid**
Benign mucous membrane pemphigoid

SP **L12.2 Chronic bullous disease of childhood**
Juvenile dermatitis herpetiformis

5 **L12.3 Acquired epidermolysis bullosa**
EXCLUDES 1 epidermolysis bullosa (congenital) (Q81.-)

SP **L12.30 Acquired epidermolysis bullosa, unspecified**

SP + **L12.31 Epidermolysis bullosa due to drug**
Use additional code for adverse effect, if applicable, to identify drug (T36-T50 with fifth or sixth character 5)

SP **L12.35 Other acquired epidermolysis bullosa**

SP **L12.8 Other pemphigoid**

SP **L12.9 Pemphigoid, unspecified**

4 **L13 Other bullous disorders**

SP **L13.0 Dermatitis herpetiformis**
Duhring's disease
Hydroa herpetiformis
EXCLUDES 1 juvenile dermatitis herpetiformis (L12.2)
senile dermatitis herpetiformis (L12.0)

DEFINITION Chronic skin disease that can persist indefinitely, characterized by intensely itchy, symmetrical excoriations on the elbows, knees, lower back, buttocks, and shoulders, often accompanied by burning and stinging hours before an eruption.

SP **L13.1 Subcorneal pustular dermatitis**
Sneddon-Wilkinson disease

SP **L13.8 Other specified bullous disorders**

SP **L13.9 Bullous disorder, unspecified**

IQ **L14 Bullous disorders in diseases classified elsewhere**
Code first:
underlying disease

Dermatitis and eczema (L20-L30)

Note:
In this block the terms dermatitis and eczema are used synonymously and interchangeably.

EXCLUDES 2 chronic (childhood) granulomatous disease (D71)
dermatitis gangrenosa (L08.0)
dermatitis herpetiformis (L13.0)
dry skin dermatitis (L85.3)
factitial dermatitis (L98.1)
perioral dermatitis (L71.0)
radiation-related disorders of the skin and subcutaneous tissue (L55-L59)
stasis dermatitis (I87.2)

CODING TIPS ✓ Dermatitis is also referred to as 'rash.'

4 **L20 Atopic dermatitis**

SP **L20.0 Besnier's prurigo**

5 **L20.8 Other atopic dermatitis**
EXCLUDES 2 circumscribed neurodermatitis (L28.0)

SP **L20.81 Atopic neurodermatitis**
Diffuse neurodermatitis

SP **L20.82 Flexural eczema**

SP **L20.83 Infantile (acute) (chronic) eczema**

SP **L20.84 Intrinsic (allergic) eczema**

SP **L20.89 Other atopic dermatitis**

SP **L20.9 Atopic dermatitis, unspecified**

4 **L21 Seborrheic dermatitis**
EXCLUDES 2 infective dermatitis (L30.3)
seborrheic keratosis (L82.-)

SP **L21.0 Seborrhea capitis**
Cradle cap

DEFINITION Inflammatory skin rash on the scalp of infants, characterized by flaky or scaly skin with redness.

SP **L21.1 Seborrheic infantile dermatitis**

SP **L21.8 Other seborrheic dermatitis**

SP **L21.9 Seborrheic dermatitis, unspecified**
Seborrhea NOS

DEFINITION Overactivity of the sebaceous (fat) glands, resulting in an inflammatory skin rash.

SP **L22 Diaper dermatitis**
Diaper erythema
Diaper rash
Psoriasiform diaper rash

4 **L23 Allergic contact dermatitis**
EXCLUDES 1 allergy NOS (T78.40)
contact dermatitis NOS (L25.9)
dermatitis NOS (L30.9)
EXCLUDES 2 dermatitis due to substances taken internally (L27.-)
dermatitis of eyelid (H01.1-)
diaper dermatitis (L22)
eczema of external ear (H60.5-)
irritant contact dermatitis (L24.-)
perioral dermatitis (L71.0)

Chapter 12
L00-L99

radiation-related disorders of the skin and subcutaneous tissue (L55-L59)

CODING TIPS ✓ Do not assign a code from L23 to report a skin reaction or allergy due to drugs or other medications that are ingested (internally). A code from category L27 should be assigned to indicate a skin reaction or allergy due to drugs or other medications ingested internally (with an additional code from T36-T50 assigned to indicate the adverse effect and specific drug).

CODING TIPS ✓ Contact dermatitis indicates that the inflammation of the skin is related to contact with a substance. The specific causative substance that resulted in the condition should be documented and the plan of care should include appropriate interventions for skin care and instruction on prevention of contact with irritants. If the patient had contact with substances and had a non-allergic type reaction, see L24.

DEFINITION Inflammation of the skin upon contact with an allergen, due to hypersensitization.

SP **L23.0 Allergic contact dermatitis due to metals**
Allergic contact dermatitis due to chromium
Allergic contact dermatitis due to nickel

SP **L23.1 Allergic contact dermatitis due to adhesives**

SP **L23.2 Allergic contact dermatitis due to cosmetics**

SP + **L23.3 Allergic contact dermatitis due to drugs in contact with skin**
Use additional code for adverse effect, if applicable, to identify drug (T36-T50 with fifth or sixth character 5)
EXCLUDES 2 dermatitis due to ingested drugs and medicaments (L27.0-L27.1)

SP **L23.4 Allergic contact dermatitis due to dyes**

SP **L23.5 Allergic contact dermatitis due to other chemical products**
Allergic contact dermatitis due to cement
Allergic contact dermatitis due to insecticide
Allergic contact dermatitis due to plastic
Allergic contact dermatitis due to rubber

SP **L23.6 Allergic contact dermatitis due to food in contact with the skin**
EXCLUDES 2 dermatitis due to ingested food (L27.2)

SP **L23.7 Allergic contact dermatitis due to plants, except food**
EXCLUDES 2 allergy NOS due to pollen (J30.1)

5 **L23.8 Allergic contact dermatitis due to other agents**

SP **L23.81 Allergic contact dermatitis due to animal (cat) (dog) dander**
Allergic contact dermatitis due to animal (cat) (dog) hair

SP **L23.89 Allergic contact dermatitis due to other agents**

SP **L23.9 Allergic contact dermatitis, unspecified cause**
Allergic contact eczema NOS

4 **L24 Irritant contact dermatitis**
EXCLUDES 1 allergy NOS (T78.40)
contact dermatitis NOS (L25.9)
dermatitis NOS (L30.9)
EXCLUDES 2 allergic contact dermatitis (L23.-)
dermatitis due to substances taken internally (L27.-)
dermatitis of eyelid (H01.1-)
diaper dermatitis (L22)
eczema of external ear (H60.5-)
perioral dermatitis (L71.0)
radiation-related disorders of the skin and subcutaneous tissue (L55-L59)

CODING TIPS ✓ Contact dermatitis indicates that the inflammation of the skin is related to contact with a substance. The specific causative substance that resulted in the condition should be documented, and the plan of care should include appropriate interventions for skin care and instruction on prevention of contact with irritants.

SP **L24.0 Irritant contact dermatitis due to detergents**

SP **L24.1 Irritant contact dermatitis due to oils and greases**

SP **L24.2 Irritant contact dermatitis due to solvents**
Irritant contact dermatitis due to chlorocompound
Irritant contact dermatitis due to cyclohexane
Irritant contact dermatitis due to ester
Irritant contact dermatitis due to glycol
Irritant contact dermatitis due to hydrocarbon
Irritant contact dermatitis due to ketone

SP **L24.3 Irritant contact dermatitis due to cosmetics**

SP + **L24.4 Irritant contact dermatitis due to drugs in contact with skin**
Use additional code for adverse effect, if applicable, to identify drug (T36-T50 with fifth or sixth character 5)

SP **L24.5 Irritant contact dermatitis due to other chemical products**
Irritant contact dermatitis due to cement
Irritant contact dermatitis due to insecticide
Irritant contact dermatitis due to plastic
Irritant contact dermatitis due to rubber

SP **L24.6 Irritant contact dermatitis due to food in contact with skin**
EXCLUDES 2 dermatitis due to ingested food (L27.2)

SP **L24.7 Irritant contact dermatitis due to plants, except food**
EXCLUDES 2 allergy NOS to pollen (J30.1)

5 **L24.8 Irritant contact dermatitis due to other agents**

SP **L24.81 Irritant contact dermatitis due to metals**
Irritant contact dermatitis due to chromium
Irritant contact dermatitis due to nickel

SP **L24.89 Irritant contact dermatitis due to other agents**
Irritant contact dermatitis due to dyes

SP **L24.9 Irritant contact dermatitis, unspecified cause**
Irritant contact eczema NOS

5 **L24.A Irritant contact dermatitis due to friction or contact with body fluids**
EXCLUDES 1 irritant contact dermatitis related to stoma or fistula (L24.B-)
EXCLUDES 2 erythema intertrigo (L30.4)

L24.A0 Irritant contact dermatitis due to friction or contact with body fluids, unspecified

L24.A1 Irritant contact dermatitis due to saliva

L24.A2 Irritant contact dermatitis due to fecal, urinary or dual incontinence
EXCLUDES 1 diaper dermatitis (L22)

L24.A9 Irritant contact dermatitis due friction or contact with other specified body fluids
Irritant contact dermatitis related to endotracheal tube
Wound fluids, exudate

+ 5 **L24.B Irritant contact dermatitis related to stoma or fistula**
Use additional code to identify any artificial opening status (Z93.-), if applicable, for contact dermatitis related to stoma secretions

+ **L24.B0 Irritant contact dermatitis related to unspecified stoma or fistula**
Irritant contact dermatitis related to fistula NOS
Irritant contact dermatitis related to stoma NOS

+ **L24.B1 Irritant contact dermatitis related to digestive stoma or fistula**
Irritant contact dermatitis related to gastrostomy
Irritant contact dermatitis related to jejunostomy
Irritant contact dermatitis related to saliva or spit fistula

+ **L24.B2 Irritant contact dermatitis related to respiratory stoma or fistula**
Irritant contact dermatitis related to tracheostomy

+ **L24.B3 Irritant contact dermatitis related to fecal or urinary stoma or fistula**
Irritant contact dermatitis related to colostomy
Irritant contact dermatitis related to enterocutaneous fistula
Irritant contact dermatitis related to ileostomy

4 **L25 Unspecified contact dermatitis**
EXCLUDES 1 allergic contact dermatitis (L23.-)
allergy NOS (T78.40)
dermatitis NOS (L30.9)
irritant contact dermatitis (L24.-)
EXCLUDES 2 dermatitis due to ingested substances (L27.-)
dermatitis of eyelid (H01.1-)
eczema of external ear (H60.5-)
perioral dermatitis (L71.0)
radiation-related disorders of the skin and subcutaneous tissue (L55-L59)

CODING TIPS ✓ Contact dermatitis indicates that the inflammation of the skin is related to contact with a substance. The specific causative substance that resulted in the condition should be documented, and the plan of care should include appropriate interventions for skin care and instruction on prevention of contact with irritants.

SP **L25.0 Unspecified contact dermatitis due to cosmetics**

SP + **L25.1 Unspecified contact dermatitis due to drugs in contact with skin**
Use additional code for adverse effect, if applicable, to identify drug (T36-T50 with fifth or sixth character 5)
EXCLUDES 2 dermatitis due to ingested drugs and medicaments (L27.0-L27.1)

SP **L25.2 Unspecified contact dermatitis due to dyes**

SP **L25.3 Unspecified contact dermatitis due to other chemical products**
Unspecified contact dermatitis due to cement
Unspecified contact dermatitis due to insecticide

SP **L25.4 Unspecified contact dermatitis due to food in contact with skin**
EXCLUDES 2 dermatitis due to ingested food (L27.2)

SP **L25.5 Unspecified contact dermatitis due to plants, except food**
EXCLUDES 1 nettle rash (L50.9)
EXCLUDES 2 allergy NOS due to pollen (J30.1)

SP **L25.8 Unspecified contact dermatitis due to other agents**

SP **L25.9 Unspecified contact dermatitis, unspecified cause**
Contact dermatitis (occupational) NOS
Contact eczema (occupational) NOS

SP **L26 Exfoliative dermatitis**
Hebra's pityriasis
EXCLUDES 1 Ritter's disease (L00)

4 **L27 Dermatitis due to substances taken internally**
EXCLUDES 1 allergy NOS (T78.40)
EXCLUDES 2 adverse food reaction, except dermatitis (T78.0-T78.1)
contact dermatitis (L23-L25)
drug photoallergic response (L56.1)
drug phototoxic response (L56.0)
urticaria (L50.-)

SP + **L27.0 Generalized skin eruption due to drugs and medicaments taken internally**
Use additional code for adverse effect, if applicable, to identify drug (T36-T50 with fifth or sixth character 5)

Chapter 12
L00-L99

SP + **L27.1 Localized skin eruption due to drugs and medicaments taken internally**
Use additional code for adverse effect, if applicable, to identify drug (T36-T50 with fifth or sixth character 5)

SP **L27.2 Dermatitis due to ingested food**
EXCLUDES 2 dermatitis due to food in contact with skin (L23.6, L24.6, L25.4)

SP **L27.8 Dermatitis due to other substances taken internally**

SP **L27.9 Dermatitis due to unspecified substance taken internally**

4 **L28 Lichen simplex chronicus and prurigo**

SP **L28.0 Lichen simplex chronicus**
Circumscribed neurodermatitis
Lichen NOS

SP **L28.1 Prurigo nodularis**

SP **L28.2 Other prurigo**
Prurigo NOS
Prurigo Hebra
Prurigo mitis
Urticaria papulosa
DEFINITION Chronic inflammatory skin disease featuring blistering papules and severe itching.

4 **L29 Pruritus**
EXCLUDES 1 neurotic excoriation (L98.1)
psychogenic pruritus (F45.8)
CODING TIPS✓ Do not confuse pruritis with urticaria. Pruritis refers to "itch" or "itching" while urticaria refers to hives. Urticaria should be coded to L50.

SP **L29.0 Pruritus ani**
DEFINITION Severe itching of the perianal region.

SP **L29.1 Pruritus scroti**

SP **L29.2 Pruritus vulvae**

SP **L29.3 Anogenital pruritus, unspecified**

SP **L29.8 Other pruritus**

IQ **L29.9 Pruritus, unspecified**
Itch NOS

4 **L30 Other and unspecified dermatitis**
EXCLUDES 2 contact dermatitis (L23-L25)
dry skin dermatitis (L85.3)
small plaque parapsoriasis (L41.3)
stasis dermatitis (I87.2)

SP **L30.0 Nummular dermatitis**

SP **L30.1 Dyshidrosis [pompholyx]**

SP **L30.2 Cutaneous autosensitization**
Candidid [levurid]
Dermatophytid
Eczematid

SP **L30.3 Infective dermatitis**
Infectious eczematoid dermatitis

SP **L30.4 Erythema intertrigo**
CODING TIPS✓ Consider this code for intertriginous dermatitis for scenarios such as excoriation when two skin surfaces rub together, like between the toes, under the breasts, or between folds of skin.

SP **L30.5 Pityriasis alba**

SP **L30.8 Other specified dermatitis**

SP **L30.9 Dermatitis, unspecified**
Eczema NOS

Papulosquamous disorders (L40-L45)

4 **L40 Psoriasis**

SP **L40.0 Psoriasis vulgaris**
Nummular psoriasis
Plaque psoriasis

SP **L40.1 Generalized pustular psoriasis**
Impetigo herpetiformis
Von Zumbusch's disease

SP **L40.2 Acrodermatitis continua**

SP **L40.3 Pustulosis palmaris et plantaris**

SP **L40.4 Guttate psoriasis**

5 **L40.5 Arthropathic psoriasis**

SP **L40.50 Arthropathic psoriasis, unspecified**

SP **L40.51 Distal interphalangeal psoriatic arthropathy**

SP **L40.52 Psoriatic arthritis mutilans**

SP **L40.53 Psoriatic spondylitis**

SP **L40.54 Psoriatic juvenile arthropathy**

SP **L40.59 Other psoriatic arthropathy**

SP **L40.8 Other psoriasis**
Flexural psoriasis

SP **L40.9 Psoriasis, unspecified**

4 **L41 Parapsoriasis**
EXCLUDES 1 poikiloderma vasculare atrophicans (L94.5)

SP **L41.0 Pityriasis lichenoides et varioliformis acuta**
Mucha-Habermann disease

SP **L41.1 Pityriasis lichenoides chronica**

SP **L41.3 Small plaque parapsoriasis**

SP **L41.4 Large plaque parapsoriasis**

SP **L41.5 Retiform parapsoriasis**

SP **L41.8 Other parapsoriasis**

SP **L41.9 Parapsoriasis, unspecified**

SP **L42 Pityriasis rosea**
DEFINITION Skin that is marked with scaling, pink, oval macules, arranged with the long axes parallel to the cleavage lines of the skin.

4 **L43 Lichen planus**
EXCLUDES 1 lichen planopilaris (L66.1)

SP **L43.0 Hypertrophic lichen planus**

SP **L43.1 Bullous lichen planus**

SP + **L43.2 Lichenoid drug reaction**
Use additional code for adverse effect, if applicable, to identify drug (T36-T50 with fifth or sixth character 5)

SP **L43.3 Subacute (active) lichen planus**
Lichen planus tropicus

SP **L43.8 Other lichen planus**

SP **L43.9 Lichen planus, unspecified**

4 **L44 Other papulosquamous disorders**

SP **L44.0 Pityriasis rubra pilaris**
DEFINITION Rare skin condition of red-orange, scaly patches spreading over the body, thickened palms and soles, and rough, dry plugs within the rash.

SP **L44.1 Lichen nitidus**

SP **L44.2 Lichen striatus**

SP **L44.3 Lichen ruber moniliformis**

SP **L44.4 Infantile papular acrodermatitis [Gianotti-Crosti]**

SP **L44.8 Other specified papulosquamous disorders**

SP **L44.9 Papulosquamous disorder, unspecified**

IQ **L45 Papulosquamous disorders in diseases classified elsewhere**

Code first:
underlying disease.

Urticaria and erythema (L49-L54)

EXCLUDES 1 Lyme disease (A69.2-)
rosacea (L71.-)

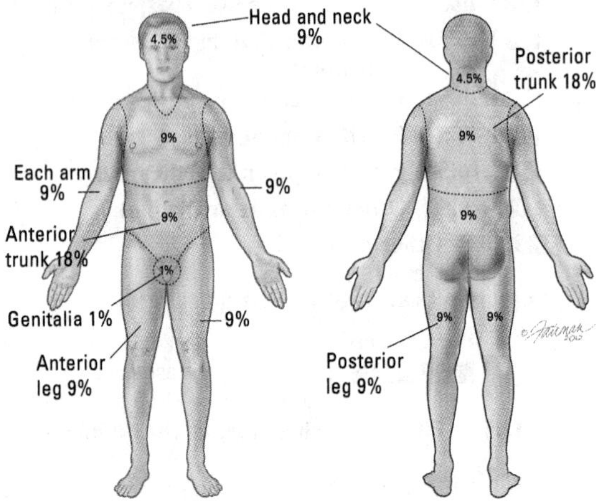

4 **L49 Exfoliation due to erythematous conditions according to extent of body surface involved**

Code first erythematous condition causing exfoliation, such as:
Ritter's disease (L00)
(Staphylococcal) scalded skin syndrome (L00)
Stevens-Johnson syndrome (L51.1)
Stevens-Johnson syndrome-toxic epidermal necrolysis
overlap syndrome (L51.3)
Toxic epidermal necrolysis (L51.2)

CODING TIPS✓ Use the rule of nines to estimate the extent of body surface involved.

IQ **L49.0 Exfoliation due to erythematous condition involving less than 10 percent of body surface**

Exfoliation due to erythematous condition NOS

IQ **L49.1 Exfoliation due to erythematous condition involving 10-19 percent of body surface**

IQ **L49.2 Exfoliation due to erythematous condition involving 20-29 percent of body surface**

IQ **L49.3 Exfoliation due to erythematous condition involving 30-39 percent of body surface**

IQ **L49.4 Exfoliation due to erythematous condition involving 40-49 percent of body surface**

IQ **L49.5 Exfoliation due to erythematous condition involving 50-59 percent of body surface**

IQ **L49.6 Exfoliation due to erythematous condition involving 60-69 percent of body surface**

IQ **L49.7 Exfoliation due to erythematous condition involving 70-79 percent of body surface**

IQ **L49.8 Exfoliation due to erythematous condition involving 80-89 percent of body surface**

IQ **L49.9 Exfoliation due to erythematous condition involving 90 or more percent of body surface**

4 **L50 Urticaria**

EXCLUDES 1 allergic contact dermatitis (L23.-)
angioneurotic edema (T78.3)
giant urticaria (T78.3)
hereditary angio-edema (D84.1)
Quincke's edema (T78.3)
serum urticaria (T80.6-)
solar urticaria (L56.3)
urticaria neonatorum (P83.8)
urticaria papulosa (L28.2)
urticaria pigmentosa (D47.01)

CODING TIPS✓ Do not confuse urticaria with pruritis. Pruritis refers to "itch" or "itching" while urticaria refers to hives. Pruritis should be coded to L29.

SP **L50.0 Allergic urticaria**

DEFINITION The most common form of hives in which smooth, raised, pink or white, itchy welts appear on or beneath the skin as a hypersensitivity response of the immune system to an allergic trigger.

SP **L50.1 Idiopathic urticaria**

DEFINITION The appearance of hives with no known, apparent cause.

SP **L50.2 Urticaria due to cold and heat**

EXCLUDES 2 familial cold urticaria (M04.2)

DEFINITION The appearance of hives in response to external heat or cold that typically fade after moving to a comfortable temperature.

SP **L50.3 Dermatographic urticaria**

DEFINITION The appearance of hives in only one particular area of the body.

SP **L50.4 Vibratory urticaria**

DEFINITION Hives brought on by intense, prolonged vibration, such as that which occurs with the use of heavy mechanical equipment.

SP **L50.5 Cholinergic urticaria**

DEFINITION Hives that occur in response to a rise in body temperature, such as from exercise, stress, or overheating.

SP **L50.6 Contact urticaria**

SP **L50.8 Other urticaria**

Chronic urticaria

Recurrent periodic urticaria

SP L50.9 **Urticaria, unspecified**

+ 4 L51 **Erythema multiforme**

Use additional code for adverse effect, if applicable, to identify drug (T36-T50 with fifth or sixth character 5)

Use additional code to identify associated manifestations, such as:

arthropathy associated with dermatological disorders (M14.8-)
conjunctival edema (H11.42)
conjunctivitis (H10.22-)
corneal scars and opacities (H17.-)
corneal ulcer (H16.0-)
edema of eyelid (H02.84-)
inflammation of eyelid (H01.8)
keratoconjunctivitis sicca (H16.22-)
mechanical lagophthalmos (H02.22-)
stomatitis (K12.-)
symblepharon (H11.23-)

Use additional code to identify percentage of skin exfoliation (L49.-)

EXCLUDES 1 staphylococcal scalded skin syndrome (L00)
Ritter's disease (L00)

SP + L51.0 **Nonbullous erythema multiforme**

SP + L51.1 **Stevens-Johnson syndrome**

SP + L51.2 **Toxic epidermal necrolysis [Lyell]**

SP + L51.3 **Stevens-Johnson syndrome-toxic epidermal necrolysis overlap syndrome**

SJS-TEN overlap syndrome

SP + L51.8 **Other erythema multiforme**

SP + L51.9 **Erythema multiforme, unspecified**

Erythema iris
Erythema multiforme major NOS
Erythema multiforme minor NOS
Herpes iris

DEFINITION Erythema multiforme minor NOS: Acute, localized, self-limiting eruption marked by distinctive, classical target lesions of pink-red blotches with a ring around a pale center.

SP L52 **Erythema nodosum**

EXCLUDES 1 tuberculous erythema nodosum (A18.4)

DEFINITION An inflammatory skin disorder marked by flat, firm, warm, red, tender, or painful nodules about an inch across under the skin that turn purple and fade to brown after several weeks, commonly found on anterior lower legs.

4 L53 **Other erythematous conditions**

EXCLUDES 1 erythema ab igne (L59.0)
erythema due to external agents in contact with skin (L23-L25)
erythema intertrigo (L30.4)

SP + L53.0 **Toxic erythema**

Code first:

poisoning due to drug or toxin, if applicable (T36-T65 with fifth or sixth character 1-4 or 6)

Use additional code for adverse effect, if applicable, to identify drug (T36-T50 with fifth or sixth character 5)

EXCLUDES 1 neonatal erythema toxicum (P83.1)

SP L53.1 **Erythema annulare centrifugum**

SP L53.2 **Erythema marginatum**

SP L53.3 **Other chronic figurate erythema**

SP L53.8 **Other specified erythematous conditions**

IQ L53.9 **Erythematous condition, unspecified**

Erythema NOS
Erythroderma NOS

IQ L54 **Erythema in diseases classified elsewhere**

Code first:

underlying disease.

Radiation-related disorders of the skin and subcutaneous tissue (L55-L59)

4 L55 **Sunburn**

CODING TIPS✓ Sunburns (L55) are differentiated by degree. First degree is erythema; second degree is blistering; and third degree is deep tissue damage.

SP L55.0 **Sunburn of first degree**

SP L55.1 **Sunburn of second degree**

SP L55.2 **Sunburn of third degree**

IQ L55.9 **Sunburn, unspecified**

+ 4 L56 **Other acute skin changes due to ultraviolet radiation**

Use additional code to identify the source of the ultraviolet radiation (W89, X32)

SP + L56.0 **Drug phototoxic response**

Use additional code for adverse effect, if applicable, to identify drug (T36-T50 with fifth or sixth character 5)

SP + L56.1 **Drug photoallergic response**

Use additional code for adverse effect, if applicable, to identify drug (T36-T50 with fifth or sixth character 5)

SP + L56.2 **Photocontact dermatitis [berloque dermatitis]**

SP + L56.3 **Solar urticaria**

SP + L56.4 **Polymorphous light eruption**

SP + L56.5 **Disseminated superficial actinic porokeratosis (DSAP)**

SP + L56.8 **Other specified acute skin changes due to ultraviolet radiation**

SP + L56.9 **Acute skin change due to ultraviolet radiation, unspecified**

+ 4 L57 **Skin changes due to chronic exposure to nonionizing radiation**

Use additional code to identify the source of the ultraviolet radiation (W89), or other nonionizing radiation (W90)

CODING TIPS✓ L57 includes an instruction to use an additional code to identify the source of radiation. According to the guidelines, external cause codes are not required. However, this instruction is a convention, and conventions trump guidelines.

SP + L57.0 **Actinic keratosis**

Keratosis NOS
Senile keratosis
Solar keratosis

SP + L57.1 **Actinic reticuloid**

SP + L57.2 **Cutis rhomboidalis nuchae**

SP + **L57.3 Poikiloderma of Civatte**

SP + **L57.4 Cutis laxa senilis**
Elastosis senilis

SP + **L57.5 Actinic granuloma**

SP + **L57.8 Other skin changes due to chronic exposure to nonionizing radiation**
Farmer's skin
Sailor's skin
Solar dermatitis
DEFINITION Solar dermatitis: Premature aging of the skin and degeneration of the elastic tissue of the dermis due to prolonged exposure to sunlight.

SP + **L57.9 Skin changes due to chronic exposure to nonionizing radiation, unspecified**

+ 4 **L58 Radiodermatitis**
Use additional code to identify the source of the radiation (W88, W90)

SP + **L58.0 Acute radiodermatitis**

SP + **L58.1 Chronic radiodermatitis**

SP + **L58.9 Radiodermatitis, unspecified**

4 **L59 Other disorders of skin and subcutaneous tissue related to radiation**

SP **L59.0 Erythema ab igne [dermatitis ab igne]**

SP **L59.8 Other specified disorders of the skin and subcutaneous tissue related to radiation**

SP **L59.9 Disorder of the skin and subcutaneous tissue related to radiation, unspecified**

Disorders of skin appendages (L60-L75)

EXCLUDES 1 congenital malformations of integument (Q84.-)

4 **L60 Nail disorders**
EXCLUDES 2 clubbing of nails (R68.3)
onychia and paronychia (L03.0-)

SP **L60.0 Ingrowing nail**
CODING TIPS ✓ Care of an ingrown nail (regardless of infection) is generally not complex. Small and superficial wounds, such as caused by an ingrown toenail, generally do not require the skills of a nurse. Simple wound care is generally not covered; however, some conditions can increase the complexity. For example, an infected ingrown toenail in a diabetic may require the skills of a nurse due to the potential for complication.

SP **L60.1 Onycholysis**

SP **L60.2 Onychogryphosis**

IQ **L60.3 Nail dystrophy**

IQ **L60.4 Beau's lines**

IQ **L60.5 Yellow nail syndrome**

SP **L60.8 Other nail disorders**

IQ **L60.9 Nail disorder, unspecified**

M IQ **L62** ***Nail disorders in diseases classified elsewhere***
Code first underlying disease, such as:
pachydermoperiostosis (M89.4-)

4 **L63 Alopecia areata**
DEFINITION Patchy loss of hair on the head or body.

SP **L63.0 Alopecia (capitis) totalis**

SP **L63.1 Alopecia universalis**

SP **L63.2 Ophiasis**

SP **L63.8 Other alopecia areata**

SP **L63.9 Alopecia areata, unspecified**

4 **L64 Androgenic alopecia**
INCLUDES male-pattern baldness

SP + **L64.0 Drug-induced androgenic alopecia**
Use additional code for adverse effect, if applicable, to identify drug (T36-T50 with fifth or sixth character 5)

SP **L64.8 Other androgenic alopecia**

SP **L64.9 Androgenic alopecia, unspecified**

+ 4 **L65 Other nonscarring hair loss**
Use additional code for adverse effect, if applicable, to identify drug (T36-T50 with fifth or sixth character 5)
EXCLUDES 1 trichotillomania (F63.3)

SP + **L65.0 Telogen effluvium**

SP + **L65.1 Anagen effluvium**

SP + **L65.2 Alopecia mucinosa**

SP + **L65.8 Other specified nonscarring hair loss**

IQ + **L65.9 Nonscarring hair loss, unspecified**
Alopecia NOS

4 **L66 Cicatricial alopecia [scarring hair loss]**

SP **L66.0 Pseudopelade**

SP **L66.1 Lichen planopilaris**
Follicular lichen planus

SP **L66.2 Folliculitis decalvans**

SP **L66.3 Perifolliculitis capitis abscedens**

SP **L66.4 Folliculitis ulerythematosa reticulata**

SP **L66.8 Other cicatricial alopecia**

SP **L66.9 Cicatricial alopecia, unspecified**

4 **L67 Hair color and hair shaft abnormalities**
EXCLUDES 1 monilethrix (Q84.1)
pili annulati (Q84.1)
telogen effluvium (L65.0)

SP **L67.0 Trichorrhexis nodosa**

IQ **L67.1 Variations in hair color**
Canities
Greyness, hair (premature)
Heterochromia of hair
Poliosis circumscripta, acquired
Poliosis NOS

IQ **L67.8 Other hair color and hair shaft abnormalities**
Fragilitas crinium

IQ **L67.9 Hair color and hair shaft abnormality, unspecified**

4 **L68 Hypertrichosis**
INCLUDES excess hair
EXCLUDES 1 congenital hypertrichosis (Q84.2)
persistent lanugo (Q84.2)

SP **L68.0 Hirsutism**

SP **L68.1 Acquired hypertrichosis lanuginosa**

SP **L68.2 Localized hypertrichosis**

SP **L68.3 Polytrichia**

SP **L68.8 Other hypertrichosis**

SP **L68.9 Hypertrichosis, unspecified**

4 **L70 Acne**
EXCLUDES 2 acne keloid (L73.0)

SP **L70.0 Acne vulgaris**

SP **L70.1 Acne conglobata**

SP **L70.2 Acne varioliformis**
Acne necrotica miliaris

SP **L70.3 Acne tropica**

SP **L70.4 Infantile acne**

SP **L70.5 Acné excoriée**
Acné excoriée des jeunes filles
Picker's acne

SP **L70.8 Other acne**

SP **L70.9 Acne, unspecified**

+4 **L71 Rosacea**
Use additional code for adverse effect, if applicable, to identify drug (T36-T50 with fifth or sixth character 5)

SP + **L71.0 Perioral dermatitis**

SP + **L71.1 Rhinophyma**

SP + **L71.8 Other rosacea**

SP + **L71.9 Rosacea, unspecified**

4 **L72 Follicular cysts of skin and subcutaneous tissue**

SP **L72.0 Epidermal cyst**

5 **L72.1 Pilar and trichodermal cyst**

SP **L72.11 Pilar cyst**
CODING TIPS✓ Greater than 90% of pilar cysts occur on the scalp. Pilar cysts are the most common cutaneous cyst.

SP **L72.12 Trichodermal cyst**
Trichilemmal (proliferating) cyst

SP **L72.2 Steatocystoma multiplex**

SP **L72.3 Sebaceous cyst**
EXCLUDES 2 pilar cyst (L72.11)
trichilemmal (proliferating) cyst (L72.12)

SP **L72.8 Other follicular cysts of the skin and subcutaneous tissue**

SP **L72.9 Follicular cyst of the skin and subcutaneous tissue, unspecified**

4 **L73 Other follicular disorders**

SP **L73.0 Acne keloid**

SP **L73.1 Pseudofolliculitis barbae**

SP **L73.2 Hidradenitis suppurativa**

SP **L73.8 Other specified follicular disorders**
Sycosis barbae

IQ **L73.9 Follicular disorder, unspecified**

4 **L74 Eccrine sweat disorders**
EXCLUDES 2 generalized hyperhidrosis (R61)

SP **L74.0 Miliaria rubra**
DEFINITION Inflammatory heat rash caused by obstruction of the sweat glands with resultant skin rash of small clusters of red pimples on the skin.

SP **L74.1 Miliaria crystallina**

SP **L74.2 Miliaria profunda**
Miliaria tropicalis

SP **L74.3 Miliaria, unspecified**

SP **L74.4 Anhidrosis**
Hypohidrosis

5 **L74.5 Focal hyperhidrosis**

6 **L74.51 Primary focal hyperhidrosis**

SP **L74.510 Primary focal hyperhidrosis, axilla**

SP **L74.511 Primary focal hyperhidrosis, face**

SP **L74.512 Primary focal hyperhidrosis, palms**

SP **L74.513 Primary focal hyperhidrosis, soles**

SP **L74.519 Primary focal hyperhidrosis, unspecified**

SP **L74.52 Secondary focal hyperhidrosis**
Frey's syndrome

SP **L74.8 Other eccrine sweat disorders**

SP **L74.9 Eccrine sweat disorder, unspecified**
Sweat gland disorder NOS

4 **L75 Apocrine sweat disorders**
EXCLUDES 1 dyshidrosis (L30.1)
hidradenitis suppurativa (L73.2)

SP **L75.0 Bromhidrosis**

SP **L75.1 Chromhidrosis**

SP **L75.2 Apocrine miliaria**
Fox-Fordyce disease

SP **L75.8 Other apocrine sweat disorders**

SP **L75.9 Apocrine sweat disorder, unspecified**

Intraoperative and postprocedural complications of skin and subcutaneous tissue (L76)

CODING TIPS✓ Conditions classifiable to L76 are classifiable as intraoperative and postprocedural complications. These conditions should only be assigned when diagnostic statements clearly indicate that the condition is a complication of a procedure. Complications that are resolved upon admission to home care are coded to Z48.812.

4 **L76 Intraoperative and postprocedural complications of skin and subcutaneous tissue**

5 **L76.0 Intraoperative hemorrhage and hematoma of skin and subcutaneous tissue complicating a procedure**
EXCLUDES 1 intraoperative hemorrhage and hematoma of skin and subcutaneous tissue due to accidental puncture and laceration during a procedure (L76.1-)

SP **L76.01 Intraoperative hemorrhage and hematoma of skin and subcutaneous tissue complicating a dermatologic procedure**

SP **L76.02 Intraoperative hemorrhage and hematoma of skin and subcutaneous tissue complicating other procedure**

5 **L76.1 Accidental puncture and laceration of skin and subcutaneous tissue during a procedure**

SP **L76.11 Accidental puncture and laceration of skin and subcutaneous tissue during a dermatologic procedure**

SP **L76.12 Accidental puncture and laceration of skin and subcutaneous tissue during other procedure**

5 **L76.2 Postprocedural hemorrhage of skin and subcutaneous tissue following a procedure**

SP **L76.21 Postprocedural hemorrhage of skin and subcutaneous tissue following a dermatologic procedure**

SP **L76.22 Postprocedural hemorrhage of skin and subcutaneous tissue following other procedure**

5 **L76.3 Postprocedural hematoma and seroma of skin and subcutaneous tissue following a procedure**

SP **L76.31 Postprocedural hematoma of skin and subcutaneous tissue following a dermatologic procedure**

SP **L76.32 Postprocedural hematoma of skin and subcutaneous tissue following other procedure**

SP **L76.33 Postprocedural seroma of skin and subcutaneous tissue following a dermatologic procedure**

SP **L76.34 Postprocedural seroma of skin and subcutaneous tissue following other procedure**

+ 5 **L76.8 Other intraoperative and postprocedural complications of skin and subcutaneous tissue**
Use additional code, if applicable, to further specify disorder

SP + **L76.81 Other intraoperative complications of skin and subcutaneous tissue**

SP + **L76.82 Other postprocedural complications of skin and subcutaneous tissue**

Other disorders of the skin and subcutaneous tissue (L80-L99)

SP **L80 Vitiligo**
EXCLUDES 2 vitiligo of eyelids (H02.73-)
vitiligo of vulva (N90.89)
DEFINITION White patches devoid of pigmentation appearing on otherwise normal skin.

4 **L81 Other disorders of pigmentation**
EXCLUDES 1 birthmark NOS (Q82.5)
Peutz-Jeghers syndrome (Q85.8)
EXCLUDES 2 nevus - see Alphabetical Index

SP **L81.0 Postinflammatory hyperpigmentation**

SP **L81.1 Chloasma**

IQ **L81.2 Freckles**

IQ **L81.3 Café au lait spots**

SP **L81.4 Other melanin hyperpigmentation**
Lentigo

SP **L81.5 Leukoderma, not elsewhere classified**

SP **L81.6 Other disorders of diminished melanin formation**

SP **L81.7 Pigmented purpuric dermatosis**
Angioma serpiginosum

SP **L81.8 Other specified disorders of pigmentation**
Iron pigmentation
Tattoo pigmentation

IQ **L81.9 Disorder of pigmentation, unspecified**

4 **L82 Seborrheic keratosis**
INCLUDES basal cell papilloma
dermatosis papulosa nigra
Leser-Trélat disease
EXCLUDES 2 seborrheic dermatitis (L21.-)

SP **L82.0 Inflamed seborrheic keratosis**
DEFINITION Noncancerous, barnacle-like skin lesions appearing in areas of long-term sun exposure in the elderly. Growths are irritated, itchy, inflamed, and may even bleed.

SP **L82.1 Other seborrheic keratosis**
Seborrheic keratosis NOS
DEFINITION Noncancerous skin lesion associated with aging and long periods of sun exposure. Growths appear round or oval, slightly elevated, black, brown, or pale in appearance with a crusty or scaly surface.

SP **L83 Acanthosis nigricans**
Confluent and reticulated papillomatosis

SP **L84 Corns and callosities**
Callus
Clavus

4 **L85 Other epidermal thickening**
EXCLUDES 2 hypertrophic disorders of the skin (L91.-)

SP **L85.0 Acquired ichthyosis**
EXCLUDES 1 congenital ichthyosis (Q80.-)

SP **L85.1 Acquired keratosis [keratoderma] palmaris et plantaris**
EXCLUDES 1 inherited keratosis palmaris et plantaris (Q82.8)

SP **L85.2 Keratosis punctata (palmaris et plantaris)**

SP **L85.3 Xerosis cutis**
Dry skin dermatitis

SP **L85.8 Other specified epidermal thickening**
Cutaneous horn

IQ **L85.9 Epidermal thickening, unspecified**

!Q **L86 Keratoderma in diseases classified elsewhere**
Code first underlying disease, such as:
Reiter's disease (M02.3-)
EXCLUDES 1 gonococcal keratoderma (A54.89)
gonococcal keratosis (A54.89)
keratoderma due to vitamin A deficiency (E50.8)
keratosis due to vitamin A deficiency (E50.8)
xeroderma due to vitamin A deficiency (E50.8)

4 **L87 Transepidermal elimination disorders**
EXCLUDES 1 granuloma annulare (perforating) (L92.0)

SP **L87.0 Keratosis follicularis et parafollicularis in cutem penetrans**
Kyrle disease
Hyperkeratosis follicularis penetrans

SP **L87.1 Reactive perforating collagenosis**

SP **L87.2 Elastosis perforans serpiginosa**

SP **L87.8 Other transepidermal elimination disorders**

IQ **L87.9 Transepidermal elimination disorder, unspecified**

SP **L88 Pyoderma gangrenosum**
Phagedenic pyoderma
EXCLUDES 1 dermatitis gangrenosa (L08.0)

4 4th digit required 5 5th digit required 6 6th digit required 7 7th digit required 7 7th digit placeholder + Additional code Laterality

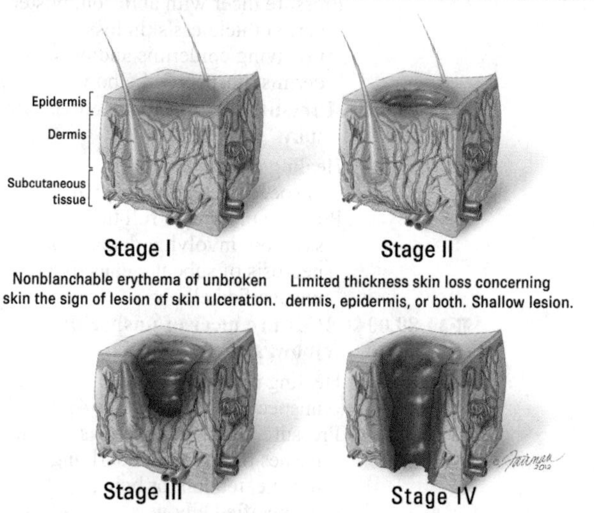

Stage I: Nonblanchable erythema of unbroken skin the sign of lesion of skin ulceration.

Stage II: Limited thickness skin loss concerning dermis, epidermis, or both. Shallow lesion.

Stage III: Total thickness skin loss concerning damage or necrosis of subcutaneous tissue that can expand down to but not underlying fascia. Deep crater-like lesion.

Stage IV: Total thickness skin loss with far-reaching destruction, tissue necrosis.

4 L89 Pressure ulcer

INCLUDES bed sore
decubitus ulcer
plaster ulcer
pressure area
pressure sore

Code first:
any associated gangrene (I96)

EXCLUDES 2 decubitus (trophic) ulcer of cervix (uteri) (N86)
diabetic ulcers (E08.621, E08.622, E09.621, E09.622, E10.621, E10.622, E11.621, E11.622, E13.621, E13.622)
non-pressure chronic ulcer of skin (L97.-)
skin infections (L00-L08)
varicose ulcer (I83.0, I83.2)

GUIDELINES Section I.C.12.a.7)
For pressure-induced deep tissue damage or deep tissue pressure injury, assign only the appropriate code for pressure-induced deep tissue damage (L89.--6).

GUIDELINES Section I.B.14
For the Body Mass Index (BMI), depth of non-pressure chronic ulcers, pressure ulcer stage, coma scale, and NIH stroke scale (NIHSS) codes, code assignment may be based on medical record documentation from clinicians who are not the patient's provider (i.e., physician or other qualified healthcare practitioner legally accountable for establishing the patient's diagnosis), since this information is typically documented by other clinicians involved in the care of the patient (e.g., a dietitian often documents the BMI, a nurse often documents the pressure ulcer stages, and an emergency medical technician often documents the coma scale). However, the associated diagnosis (such as overweight, obesity, acute stroke, or pressure ulcer) must be documented by the patient's provider.

GUIDELINES Section I.C.12.a.1)
Codes in category L89, Pressure ulcer, identify the site and stage of the pressure ulcer. The ICD-10-CM classifies pressure ulcer stages based on severity, which is designated by stages 1-4, deep tissue pressure injury, unspecified stage, and unstageable. Assign as many codes from category L89 as needed to identify all the pressure ulcers the patient has, if applicable.

GUIDELINES Section I.C.12.a.2)
Assignment of the code for unstageable pressure ulcer (L89.--0) should be based on the clinical documentation. These codes are used for pressure ulcers whose stage cannot be clinically determined (e.g., the ulcer is covered by eschar or has been treated with a skin or muscle graft). This code should not be confused with the codes for unspecified stage (L89.--9). When there is no documentation regarding the stage of the pressure ulcer, assign the appropriate code for unspecified stage (L89.--9).

GUIDELINES Section I.C.12.a.4)
No code is assigned if the documentation states that the pressure ulcer is completely healed at the time of admission.

CODING TIPS✓ If a pressure ulcer presents as unstageable and then is debrided so that the stage can be determined, the coder should use the code for the stage. [AHA: 1Q 2021]

CODING TIPS✓ Deep Tissue Pressure Injuries (DTPI) presenting with intact skin or partial thickness skin loss should be marked on the **OASIS** as Deep Tissue Injury, and coded with 6th character 6. DTPI presenting with full thickness loss should be marked on the OASIS as Stage 3 (fatty tissue exposed) or Stage 4 (bone, muscle, ligament, joint capsule), and coded with 6th character 3 or 4 as applicable. *(4/19 CMS Q&As)*

CODING TIPS✓ Although not due to pressure, Kennedy ulcers or terminal ulcers are coded to L89. Kennedy ulcers indicate multi-organ failure and are rarely coded in home care, but may be present in hospice patients.

CODING TIPS✓ Pressure ulcer guidance for the purposes of scoring the OASIS is different than the guidelines regarding coding pressure ulcers. A pressure ulcer covered with a flap or graft is no longer a pressure ulcer according to OASIS, but is coded as an unstageable pressure ulcer. A pressure ulcer covered with a non-removable dressing is unstageable on the OASIS; however, the stage can be coded based on physician or NPP documentation of the stage.

CODING TIPS✓ Closed stage 3 and 4 pressure ulcers are no longer counted on the OASIS as pressure ulcers even though the closed areas are still at risk for further breakdown. If the physician or NPP documents the stage 3 or 4 pressure ulcer as completely healed, do not code the pressure ulcer. Otherwise, the coder should consider whether the pressure ulcer meets the criteria in Section III of the coding guidelines regarding reportable diagnoses.

CODING TIPS✓ Codes in category L89 are combination codes that include a fifth or sixth character indicating the stage. An assessing clinician may mark the OASIS with pressure ulcer/injury based on the characteristics of the wound utilizing WOCN and NPUAP criteria. The physician or NPP must provide confirmation of the diagnosis of pressure ulcer/injury; however, coders may choose the stage based on clinicians' documentation. Home health and hospice coders should never have to use 6th character 9 for unspecified stage.

CODING TIPS✓ Pressure ulcers/injuries on mucous membranes or where the mucosal membrane meets skin, for example at the urethral meatus, are considered mucosal membrane pressure injuries (MMPI). MMPIs are not considered pressure ulcers/injuries for the purpose of OASIS. They cannot be staged because of the different anatomy.

DEFINITION **Deep Tissue Pressure Injury (DTPI)** is defined as intact or non-intact skin with localized area of persistent non-blanchable deep red, maroon, purple discoloration or epidermal separation revealing a dark wound bed or blood filled blister. Pain and temperature change often precede skin color changes. Discoloration may appear differently in darkly pigmented skin. This condition results from intense and/or prolonged pressure and shear forces at the bone-muscle interface. The wound may evolve rapidly to reveal the actual extent of tissue injury, or may resolve without tissue loss.

DEFINITION A pressure-induced ulceration or sore of the skin usually occurring when a patient is confined to bed for long periods of time, due to lack of circulation and oxygenation to the affected tissue.

5 **L89.0 Pressure ulcer of elbow**

6 **L89.00 Pressure ulcer of unspecified elbow**

IQ **L89.000 Pressure ulcer of unspecified elbow, unstageable**

IQ **L89.001 Pressure ulcer of unspecified elbow, stage 1**
- Healing pressure ulcer of unspecified elbow, stage 1
- Pressure pre-ulcer skin changes limited to persistent focal edema, unspecified elbow

IQ **L89.002 Pressure ulcer of unspecified elbow, stage 2**
- Healing pressure ulcer of unspecified elbow, stage 2
- Pressure ulcer with abrasion, blister, partial thickness skin loss involving epidermis and/or dermis, unspecified elbow

IQ **L89.003 Pressure ulcer of unspecified elbow, stage 3**
- Healing pressure ulcer of unspecified elbow, stage 3
- Pressure ulcer with full thickness skin loss involving damage or necrosis of subcutaneous tissue, unspecified elbow

IQ **L89.004 Pressure ulcer of unspecified elbow, stage 4**
- Healing pressure ulcer of unspecified elbow, stage 4
- Pressure ulcer with necrosis of soft tissues through to underlying muscle, tendon, or bone, unspecified elbow

L89.006 Pressure-induced deep tissue damage of unspecified elbow

IQ **L89.009 Pressure ulcer of unspecified elbow, unspecified stage**
- Healing pressure ulcer of elbow NOS
- Healing pressure ulcer of unspecified elbow, unspecified stage

6 **L89.01 Pressure ulcer of right elbow**

⊟ SP SH SL **L89.010 Pressure ulcer of right elbow, unstageable**

⊟ SP **L89.011 Pressure ulcer of right elbow, stage 1**
- Healing pressure ulcer of right elbow, stage 1
- Pressure pre-ulcer skin changes limited to persistent focal edema, right elbow

⊟ SP SH SL **L89.012 Pressure ulcer of right elbow, stage 2**
- Healing pressure ulcer of right elbow, stage 2
- Pressure ulcer with abrasion, blister, partial thickness skin loss involving epidermis and/or dermis, right elbow

⊟ SP SH SL **L89.013 Pressure ulcer of right elbow, stage 3**
- Healing pressure ulcer of right elbow, stage 3
- Pressure ulcer with full thickness skin loss involving damage or necrosis of subcutaneous tissue, right elbow

⊟ SP SH SL **L89.014 Pressure ulcer of right elbow, stage 4**
- Healing pressure ulcer of right elbow, stage 4
- Pressure ulcer with necrosis of soft tissues through to underlying muscle, tendon, or bone, right elbow

⊟ SP SH SL **L89.016 Pressure-induced deep tissue damage of right elbow**

▲ ⊟ IQ **L89.019 Pressure ulcer of right elbow, unspecified stage**

Healing pressure ulcer of right elbow NOS

6 **L89.02 Pressure ulcer of left elbow**

SP SH SL **L89.020 Pressure ulcer of left elbow, unstageable**

SP **L89.021 Pressure ulcer of left elbow, stage 1**

Healing pressure ulcer of left elbow, stage 1

Pressure pre-ulcer skin changes limited to persistent focal edema, left elbow

SP SH SL **L89.022 Pressure ulcer of left elbow, stage 2**

Healing pressure ulcer of left elbow, stage 2

Pressure ulcer with abrasion, blister, partial thickness skin loss involving epidermis and/or dermis, left elbow

SP SH SL **L89.023 Pressure ulcer of left elbow, stage 3**

Healing pressure ulcer of left elbow, stage 3

Pressure ulcer with full thickness skin loss involving damage or necrosis of subcutaneous tissue, left elbow

SP SH SL **L89.024 Pressure ulcer of left elbow, stage 4**

Healing pressure ulcer of left elbow, stage 4

Pressure ulcer with necrosis of soft tissues through to underlying muscle, tendon, or bone, left elbow

SP SH SL **L89.026 Pressure-induced deep tissue damage of left elbow**

▲ IQ **L89.029 Pressure ulcer of left elbow, unspecified stage**

Healing pressure ulcer of left elbow NOS

5 **L89.1 Pressure ulcer of back**

6 **L89.10 Pressure ulcer of unspecified part of back**

IQ **L89.100 Pressure ulcer of unspecified part of back, unstageable**

IQ **L89.101 Pressure ulcer of unspecified part of back, stage 1**

Healing pressure ulcer of unspecified part of back, stage 1

Pressure pre-ulcer skin changes limited to persistent focal edema, unspecified part of back

IQ SH SL **L89.102 Pressure ulcer of unspecified part of back, stage 2**

Healing pressure ulcer of unspecified part of back, stage 2

Pressure ulcer with abrasion, blister, partial thickness skin loss involving epidermis and/or dermis, unspecified part of back

IQ SH SL **L89.103 Pressure ulcer of unspecified part of back, stage 3**

Healing pressure ulcer of unspecified part of back, stage 3

Pressure ulcer with full thickness skin loss involving damage or necrosis of subcutaneous tissue, unspecified part of back

IQ SH SL **L89.104 Pressure ulcer of unspecified part of back, stage 4**

Healing pressure ulcer of unspecified part of back, stage 4

Pressure ulcer with necrosis of soft tissues through to underlying muscle, tendon, or bone, unspecified part of back

L89.106 Pressure-induced deep tissue damage of unspecified part of back

IQ **L89.109 Pressure ulcer of unspecified part of back, unspecified stage**

Healing pressure ulcer of unspecified part of back NOS

Healing pressure ulcer of unspecified part of back, unspecified stage

6 **L89.11 Pressure ulcer of right upper back**

Pressure ulcer of right shoulder blade

SP SH SL **L89.110 Pressure ulcer of right upper back, unstageable**

SP **L89.111 Pressure ulcer of right upper back, stage 1**

Healing pressure ulcer of right upper back, stage 1

Pressure pre-ulcer skin changes limited to persistent focal edema, right upper back

SP SH SL **L89.112 Pressure ulcer of right upper back, stage 2**

Healing pressure ulcer of right upper back, stage 2

Pressure ulcer with abrasion, blister, partial thickness skin loss involving epidermis and/or dermis, right upper back

SP SH SL **L89.113 Pressure ulcer of right upper back, stage 3**

Healing pressure ulcer of right upper back, stage 3

Pressure ulcer with full thickness skin loss involving damage or necrosis of subcutaneous tissue, right upper back

SP SH SL **L89.114 Pressure ulcer of right upper back, stage 4**

Healing pressure ulcer of right upper back, stage 4

Pressure ulcer with necrosis of soft tissues through to underlying muscle, tendon, or bone, right upper back

SP SH SL **L89.116 Pressure-induced deep tissue damage of right upper back**

IQ **L89.119 Pressure ulcer of right upper back, unspecified stage**

Healing pressure ulcer of right upper back NOS

Healing pressure ulcer of right upper back, unspecified stage

6 **L89.12 Pressure ulcer of left upper back**

Pressure ulcer of left shoulder blade

L89.120 Pressure ulcer of left upper back, unstageable

L89.121 Pressure ulcer of left upper back, stage 1
Healing pressure ulcer of left upper back, stage 1
Pressure pre-ulcer skin changes limited to persistent focal edema, left upper back

L89.122 Pressure ulcer of left upper back, stage 2
Healing pressure ulcer of left upper back, stage 2
Pressure ulcer with abrasion, blister, partial thickness skin loss involving epidermis and/or dermis, left upper back

L89.123 Pressure ulcer of left upper back, stage 3
Healing pressure ulcer of left upper back, stage 3
Pressure ulcer with full thickness skin loss involving damage or necrosis of subcutaneous tissue, left upper back

L89.124 Pressure ulcer of left upper back, stage 4
Healing pressure ulcer of left upper back, stage 4
Pressure ulcer with necrosis of soft tissues through to underlying muscle, tendon, or bone, left upper back

L89.126 Pressure-induced deep tissue damage of left upper back

L89.129 Pressure ulcer of left upper back, unspecified stage
Healing pressure ulcer of left upper back NOS
Healing pressure ulcer of left upper back, unspecified stage

L89.13 Pressure ulcer of right lower back

L89.130 Pressure ulcer of right lower back, unstageable

L89.131 Pressure ulcer of right lower back, stage 1
Healing pressure ulcer of right lower back, stage 1
Pressure pre-ulcer skin changes limited to persistent focal edema, right lower back

L89.132 Pressure ulcer of right lower back, stage 2
Healing pressure ulcer of right lower back, stage 2
Pressure ulcer with abrasion, blister, partial thickness skin loss involving epidermis and/or dermis, right lower back

L89.133 Pressure ulcer of right lower back, stage 3
Healing pressure ulcer of right lower back, stage 3
Pressure ulcer with full thickness skin loss involving damage or necrosis of subcutaneous tissue, right lower back

L89.134 Pressure ulcer of right lower back, stage 4
Healing pressure ulcer of right lower back, stage 4
Pressure ulcer with necrosis of soft tissues through to underlying muscle, tendon, or bone, right lower back

L89.136 Pressure-induced deep tissue damage of right lower back

L89.139 Pressure ulcer of right lower back, unspecified stage
Healing pressure ulcer of right lower back NOS
Healing pressure ulcer of right lower back, unspecified stage

L89.14 Pressure ulcer of left lower back

L89.140 Pressure ulcer of left lower back, unstageable

L89.141 Pressure ulcer of left lower back, stage 1
Healing pressure ulcer of left lower back, stage 1
Pressure pre-ulcer skin changes limited to persistent focal edema, left lower back

L89.142 Pressure ulcer of left lower back, stage 2
Healing pressure ulcer of left lower back, stage 2
Pressure ulcer with abrasion, blister, partial thickness skin loss involving epidermis and/or dermis, left lower back

L89.143 Pressure ulcer of left lower back, stage 3
Healing pressure ulcer of left lower back, stage 3
Pressure ulcer with full thickness skin loss involving damage or necrosis of subcutaneous tissue, left lower back

L89.144 Pressure ulcer of left lower back, stage 4
Healing pressure ulcer of left lower back, stage 4
Pressure ulcer with necrosis of soft tissues through to underlying muscle, tendon, or bone, left lower back

L89.146 Pressure-induced deep tissue damage of left lower back

L89.149 Pressure ulcer of left lower back, unspecified stage
Healing pressure ulcer of left lower back NOS
Healing pressure ulcer of left lower back, unspecified stage

L89.15 Pressure ulcer of sacral region
Pressure ulcer of coccyx
Pressure ulcer of tailbone

L89.150 Pressure ulcer of sacral region, unstageable

L89.151 Pressure ulcer of sacral region, stage 1
Healing pressure ulcer of sacral region, stage 1

Pressure pre-ulcer skin changes limited to persistent focal edema, sacral region

SP SH SL **L89.152 Pressure ulcer of sacral region, stage 2**
Healing pressure ulcer of sacral region, stage 2
Pressure ulcer with abrasion, blister, partial thickness skin loss involving epidermis and/or dermis, sacral region

SP SH SL **L89.153 Pressure ulcer of sacral region, stage 3**
Healing pressure ulcer of sacral region, stage 3
Pressure ulcer with full thickness skin loss involving damage or necrosis of subcutaneous tissue, sacral region

SP SH SL **L89.154 Pressure ulcer of sacral region, stage 4**
Healing pressure ulcer of sacral region, stage 4
Pressure ulcer with necrosis of soft tissues through to underlying muscle, tendon, or bone, sacral region

SP SH SL **L89.156 Pressure-induced deep tissue damage of sacral region**

!Q **L89.159 Pressure ulcer of sacral region, unspecified stage**
Healing pressure ulcer of sacral region NOS
Healing pressure ulcer of sacral region, unspecified stage

5 **L89.2 Pressure ulcer of hip**

6 **L89.20 Pressure ulcer of unspecified hip**

!Q **L89.200 Pressure ulcer of unspecified hip, unstageable**

!Q **L89.201 Pressure ulcer of unspecified hip, stage 1**
Healing pressure ulcer of unspecified hip back, stage 1
Pressure pre-ulcer skin changes limited to persistent focal edema, unspecified hip

!Q **L89.202 Pressure ulcer of unspecified hip, stage 2**
Healing pressure ulcer of unspecified hip, stage 2
Pressure ulcer with abrasion, blister, partial thickness skin loss involving epidermis and/or dermis, unspecified hip

!Q **L89.203 Pressure ulcer of unspecified hip, stage 3**
Healing pressure ulcer of unspecified hip, stage 3
Pressure ulcer with full thickness skin loss involving damage or necrosis of subcutaneous tissue, unspecified hip

!Q **L89.204 Pressure ulcer of unspecified hip, stage 4**
Healing pressure ulcer of unspecified hip, stage 4
Pressure ulcer with necrosis of soft tissues through to underlying muscle, tendon, or bone, unspecified hip

L89.206 Pressure-induced deep tissue damage of unspecified hip

!Q **L89.209 Pressure ulcer of unspecified hip, unspecified stage**
Healing pressure ulcer of unspecified hip NOS
Healing pressure ulcer of unspecified hip, unspecified stage

6 **L89.21 Pressure ulcer of right hip**

⇄ SP SH SL **L89.210 Pressure ulcer of right hip, unstageable**

⇄ SP **L89.211 Pressure ulcer of right hip, stage 1**
Healing pressure ulcer of right hip back, stage 1
Pressure pre-ulcer skin changes limited to persistent focal edema, right hip

⇄ SP SH SL **L89.212 Pressure ulcer of right hip, stage 2**
Healing pressure ulcer of right hip, stage 2
Pressure ulcer with abrasion, blister, partial thickness skin loss involving epidermis and/or dermis, right hip

⇄ SP SH SL **L89.213 Pressure ulcer of right hip, stage 3**
Healing pressure ulcer of right hip, stage 3
Pressure ulcer with full thickness skin loss involving damage or necrosis of subcutaneous tissue, right hip

⇄ SP SH SL **L89.214 Pressure ulcer of right hip, stage 4**
Healing pressure ulcer of right hip, stage 4
Pressure ulcer with necrosis of soft tissues through to underlying muscle, tendon, or bone, right hip

⇄ SP SH SL **L89.216 Pressure-induced deep tissue damage of right hip**

⇄ !Q **L89.219 Pressure ulcer of right hip, unspecified stage**
Healing pressure ulcer of right hip NOS
Healing pressure ulcer of right hip, unspecified stage

6 **L89.22 Pressure ulcer of left hip**

⇄ SP SH SL **L89.220 Pressure ulcer of left hip, unstageable**

⇄ SP **L89.221 Pressure ulcer of left hip, stage 1**
Healing pressure ulcer of left hip back, stage 1
Pressure pre-ulcer skin changes limited to persistent focal edema, left hip

⇄ SP SH SL **L89.222 Pressure ulcer of left hip, stage 2**
Healing pressure ulcer of left hip, stage 2
Pressure ulcer with abrasion, blister, partial thickness skin loss involving epidermis and/or dermis, left hip

⇄ SP SH SL **L89.223 Pressure ulcer of left hip, stage 3**
Healing pressure ulcer of left hip, stage 3

Pressure ulcer with full thickness skin loss involving damage or necrosis of subcutaneous tissue, left hip

L89.224 **Pressure ulcer of left hip, stage 4**
Healing pressure ulcer of left hip, stage 4
Pressure ulcer with necrosis of soft tissues through to underlying muscle, tendon, or bone, left hip

L89.226 **Pressure-induced deep tissue damage of left hip**

L89.229 **Pressure ulcer of left hip, unspecified stage**
Healing pressure ulcer of left hip NOS
Healing pressure ulcer of left hip, unspecified stage

L89.3 **Pressure ulcer of buttock**

CODING TIPS ✓ A pressure ulcer/injury described as being on the ischial tuberosity, is considered to be on the buttock.

L89.30 **Pressure ulcer of unspecified buttock**

L89.300 **Pressure ulcer of unspecified buttock, unstageable**

L89.301 **Pressure ulcer of unspecified buttock, stage 1**
Healing pressure ulcer of unspecified buttock, stage 1
Pressure pre-ulcer skin changes limited to persistent focal edema, unspecified buttock

L89.302 **Pressure ulcer of unspecified buttock, stage 2**
Healing pressure ulcer of unspecified buttock, stage 2
Pressure ulcer with abrasion, blister, partial thickness skin loss involving epidermis and/or dermis, unspecified buttock

L89.303 **Pressure ulcer of unspecified buttock, stage 3**
Healing pressure ulcer of unspecified buttock, stage 3
Pressure ulcer with full thickness skin loss involving damage or necrosis of subcutaneous tissue, unspecified buttock

L89.304 **Pressure ulcer of unspecified buttock, stage 4**
Healing pressure ulcer of unspecified buttock, stage 4
Pressure ulcer with necrosis of soft tissues through to underlying muscle, tendon, or bone, unspecified buttock

L89.306 **Pressure-induced deep tissue damage of unspecified buttock**

L89.309 **Pressure ulcer of unspecified buttock, unspecified stage**
Healing pressure ulcer of unspecified buttock NOS
Healing pressure ulcer of unspecified buttock, unspecified stage

L89.31 **Pressure ulcer of right buttock**

L89.310 **Pressure ulcer of right buttock, unstageable**

L89.311 **Pressure ulcer of right buttock, stage 1**
Healing pressure ulcer of right buttock, stage 1
Pressure pre-ulcer skin changes limited to persistent focal edema, right buttock

L89.312 **Pressure ulcer of right buttock, stage 2**
Healing pressure ulcer of right buttock, stage 2
Pressure ulcer with abrasion, blister, partial thickness skin loss involving epidermis and/or dermis, right buttock

L89.313 **Pressure ulcer of right buttock, stage 3**
Healing pressure ulcer of right buttock, stage 3
Pressure ulcer with full thickness skin loss involving damage or necrosis of subcutaneous tissue, right buttock

L89.314 **Pressure ulcer of right buttock, stage 4**
Healing pressure ulcer of right buttock, stage 4
Pressure ulcer with necrosis of soft tissues through to underlying muscle, tendon, or bone, right buttock

L89.316 **Pressure-induced deep tissue damage of right buttock**

L89.319 **Pressure ulcer of right buttock, unspecified stage**
Healing pressure ulcer of right buttock NOS
Healing pressure ulcer of right buttock, unspecified stage

L89.32 **Pressure ulcer of left buttock**

L89.320 **Pressure ulcer of left buttock, unstageable**

L89.321 **Pressure ulcer of left buttock, stage 1**
Healing pressure ulcer of left buttock, stage 1
Pressure pre-ulcer skin changes limited to persistent focal edema, left buttock

L89.322 **Pressure ulcer of left buttock, stage 2**
Healing pressure ulcer of left buttock, stage 2
Pressure ulcer with abrasion, blister, partial thickness skin loss involving epidermis and/or dermis, left buttock

L89.323 **Pressure ulcer of left buttock, stage 3**
Healing pressure ulcer of left buttock, stage 3
Pressure ulcer with full thickness skin loss involving damage or necrosis of subcutaneous tissue, left buttock

SP SH SL **L89.324 Pressure ulcer of left buttock, stage 4**
Healing pressure ulcer of left buttock, stage 4
Pressure ulcer with necrosis of soft tissues through to underlying muscle, tendon, or bone, left buttock

SP SH SL **L89.326 Pressure-induced deep tissue damage of left buttock**

IQ **L89.329 Pressure ulcer of left buttock, unspecified stage**
Healing pressure ulcer of left buttock NOS
Healing pressure ulcer of left buttock, unspecified stage

5 **L89.4 Pressure ulcer of contiguous site of back, buttock and hip**

CODING TIPS✓ When a patient presents with a pressure ulcer/injury that is contiguous to the surface area of the back, buttock, and/or hip, a code from L89.4- should be assigned. The stage of the ulcer/injury should be assigned as the worst stage identifiable (the area of the ulcer which has deteriorated to its worst stage).

IQ **L89.40 Pressure ulcer of contiguous site of back, buttock and hip, unspecified stage**
Healing pressure ulcer of contiguous site of back, buttock and hip NOS
Healing pressure ulcer of contiguous site of back, buttock and hip, unspecified stage

SP **L89.41 Pressure ulcer of contiguous site of back, buttock and hip, stage 1**
Healing pressure ulcer of contiguous site of back, buttock and hip, stage 1
Pressure pre-ulcer skin changes limited to persistent focal edema, contiguous site of back, buttock and hip

SP SH SL **L89.42 Pressure ulcer of contiguous site of back, buttock and hip, stage 2**
Healing pressure ulcer of contiguous site of back, buttock and hip, stage 2
Pressure ulcer with abrasion, blister, partial thickness skin loss involving epidermis and/or dermis, contiguous site of back, buttock and hip

SP SH SL **L89.43 Pressure ulcer of contiguous site of back, buttock and hip, stage 3**
Healing pressure ulcer of contiguous site of back, buttock and hip, stage 3
Pressure ulcer with full thickness skin loss involving damage or necrosis of subcutaneous tissue, contiguous site of back, buttock and hip

SP SH SL **L89.44 Pressure ulcer of contiguous site of back, buttock and hip, stage 4**
Healing pressure ulcer of contiguous site of back, buttock and hip, stage 4
Pressure ulcer with necrosis of soft tissues through to underlying muscle, tendon, or bone, contiguous site of back, buttock and hip

SP SH SL **L89.45 Pressure ulcer of contiguous site of back, buttock and hip, unstageable**

SP SH SL **L89.46 Pressure-induced deep tissue damage of contiguous site of back, buttock and hip**

5 **L89.5 Pressure ulcer of ankle**

6 **L89.50 Pressure ulcer of unspecified ankle**

IQ **L89.500 Pressure ulcer of unspecified ankle, unstageable**

IQ **L89.501 Pressure ulcer of unspecified ankle, stage 1**
Healing pressure ulcer of unspecified ankle, stage 1
Pressure pre-ulcer skin changes limited to persistent focal edema, unspecified ankle

IQ **L89.502 Pressure ulcer of unspecified ankle, stage 2**
Healing pressure ulcer of unspecified ankle, stage 2
Pressure ulcer with abrasion, blister, partial thickness skin loss involving epidermis and/or dermis, unspecified ankle

IQ **L89.503 Pressure ulcer of unspecified ankle, stage 3**
Healing pressure ulcer of unspecified ankle, stage 3
Pressure ulcer with full thickness skin loss involving damage or necrosis of subcutaneous tissue, unspecified ankle

IQ **L89.504 Pressure ulcer of unspecified ankle, stage 4**
Healing pressure ulcer of unspecified ankle, stage 4
Pressure ulcer with necrosis of soft tissues through to underlying muscle, tendon, or bone, unspecified ankle

L89.506 Pressure-induced deep tissue damage of unspecified ankle

IQ **L89.509 Pressure ulcer of unspecified ankle, unspecified stage**
Healing pressure ulcer of unspecified ankle NOS
Healing pressure ulcer of unspecified ankle, unspecified stage

6 **L89.51 Pressure ulcer of right ankle**

SP SH SL **L89.510 Pressure ulcer of right ankle, unstageable**

SP **L89.511 Pressure ulcer of right ankle, stage 1**
Healing pressure ulcer of right ankle, stage 1
Pressure pre-ulcer skin changes limited to persistent focal edema, right ankle

SP SH SL **L89.512 Pressure ulcer of right ankle, stage 2**
Healing pressure ulcer of right ankle, stage 2
Pressure ulcer with abrasion, blister, partial thickness skin loss involving epidermis and/or dermis, right ankle

SP SH SL **L89.513 Pressure ulcer of right ankle, stage 3**

Chapter 12 L00-L99

Healing pressure ulcer of right ankle, stage 3
Pressure ulcer with full thickness skin loss involving damage or necrosis of subcutaneous tissue, right ankle

L89.514 Pressure ulcer of right ankle, stage 4
Healing pressure ulcer of right ankle, stage 4
Pressure ulcer with necrosis of soft tissues through to underlying muscle, tendon, or bone, right ankle

L89.516 Pressure-induced deep tissue damage of right ankle

L89.519 Pressure ulcer of right ankle, unspecified stage
Healing pressure ulcer of right ankle NOS
Healing pressure ulcer of right ankle, unspecified stage

L89.52 Pressure ulcer of left ankle

L89.520 Pressure ulcer of left ankle, unstageable

L89.521 Pressure ulcer of left ankle, stage 1
Healing pressure ulcer of left ankle, stage 1
Pressure pre-ulcer skin changes limited to persistent focal edema, left ankle

L89.522 Pressure ulcer of left ankle, stage 2
Healing pressure ulcer of left ankle, stage 2
Pressure ulcer with abrasion, blister, partial thickness skin loss involving epidermis and/or dermis, left ankle

L89.523 Pressure ulcer of left ankle, stage 3
Healing pressure ulcer of left ankle, stage 3
Pressure ulcer with full thickness skin loss involving damage or necrosis of subcutaneous tissue, left ankle

L89.524 Pressure ulcer of left ankle, stage 4
Healing pressure ulcer of left ankle, stage 4
Pressure ulcer with necrosis of soft tissues through to underlying muscle, tendon, or bone, left ankle

L89.526 Pressure-induced deep tissue damage of left ankle

L89.529 Pressure ulcer of left ankle, unspecified stage
Healing pressure ulcer of left ankle NOS
Healing pressure ulcer of left ankle, unspecified stage

L89.6 Pressure ulcer of heel

L89.60 Pressure ulcer of unspecified heel

L89.600 Pressure ulcer of unspecified heel, unstageable

L89.601 Pressure ulcer of unspecified heel, stage 1
Healing pressure ulcer of unspecified heel, stage 1
Pressure pre-ulcer skin changes limited to persistent focal edema, unspecified heel

L89.602 Pressure ulcer of unspecified heel, stage 2
Healing pressure ulcer of unspecified heel, stage 2
Pressure ulcer with abrasion, blister, partial thickness skin loss involving epidermis and/or dermis, unspecified heel

L89.603 Pressure ulcer of unspecified heel, stage 3
Healing pressure ulcer of unspecified heel, stage 3
Pressure ulcer with full thickness skin loss involving damage or necrosis of subcutaneous tissue, unspecified heel

L89.604 Pressure ulcer of unspecified heel, stage 4
Healing pressure ulcer of unspecified heel, stage 4
Pressure ulcer with necrosis of soft tissues through to underlying muscle, tendon, or bone, unspecified heel

L89.606 Pressure-induced deep tissue damage of unspecified heel

L89.609 Pressure ulcer of unspecified heel, unspecified stage
Healing pressure ulcer of unspecified heel NOS
Healing pressure ulcer of unspecified heel, unspecified stage

L89.61 Pressure ulcer of right heel

L89.610 Pressure ulcer of right heel, unstageable

L89.611 Pressure ulcer of right heel, stage 1
Healing pressure ulcer of right heel, stage 1
Pressure pre-ulcer skin changes limited to persistent focal edema, right heel

L89.612 Pressure ulcer of right heel, stage 2
Healing pressure ulcer of right heel, stage 2
Pressure ulcer with abrasion, blister, partial thickness skin loss involving epidermis and/or dermis, right heel

L89.613 Pressure ulcer of right heel, stage 3
Healing pressure ulcer of right heel, stage 3
Pressure ulcer with full thickness skin loss involving damage or necrosis of subcutaneous tissue, right heel

L89.614 Pressure ulcer of right heel, stage 4

Healing pressure ulcer of right heel, stage 4
Pressure ulcer with necrosis of soft tissues through to underlying muscle, tendon, or bone, right heel

H SP SH SL **L89.616 Pressure-induced deep tissue damage of right heel**

H IQ **L89.619 Pressure ulcer of right heel, unspecified stage**
Healing pressure ulcer of right heel NOS
Healing pressure ulcer of right heel, unspecified stage

6 **L89.62 Pressure ulcer of left heel**

H SP SH SL **L89.620 Pressure ulcer of left heel, unstageable**

H SP **L89.621 Pressure ulcer of left heel, stage 1**
Healing pressure ulcer of left heel, stage 1
Pressure pre-ulcer skin changes limited to persistent focal edema, left heel

H SP SH SL **L89.622 Pressure ulcer of left heel, stage 2**
Healing pressure ulcer of left heel, stage 2
Pressure ulcer with abrasion, blister, partial thickness skin loss involving epidermis and/or dermis, left heel

H SP SH SL **L89.623 Pressure ulcer of left heel, stage 3**
Healing pressure ulcer of left heel, stage 3
Pressure ulcer with full thickness skin loss involving damage or necrosis of subcutaneous tissue, left heel

H SP SH SL **L89.624 Pressure ulcer of left heel, stage 4**
Healing pressure ulcer of left heel, stage 4
Pressure ulcer with necrosis of soft tissues through to underlying muscle, tendon, or bone, left heel

H SP SH SL **L89.626 Pressure-induced deep tissue damage of left heel**

H IQ **L89.629 Pressure ulcer of left heel, unspecified stage**
Healing pressure ulcer of left heel NOS
Healing pressure ulcer of left heel, unspecified stage

5 **L89.8 Pressure ulcer of other site**

CODING TIPS✓ Use this subcategory for pressure ulcers/injuries between the knees, edge of the ear, bridge of the nose and other areas not covered by the other L89 codes. Do not use L89.9.

6 **L89.81 Pressure ulcer of head**
Pressure ulcer of face

SP SH SL **L89.810 Pressure ulcer of head, unstageable**

SP **L89.811 Pressure ulcer of head, stage 1**
Healing pressure ulcer of head, stage 1
Pressure pre-ulcer skin changes limited to persistent focal edema, head

SP SH SL **L89.812 Pressure ulcer of head, stage 2**
Healing pressure ulcer of head, stage 2
Pressure ulcer with abrasion, blister, partial thickness skin loss involving epidermis and/or dermis, head

SP SH SL **L89.813 Pressure ulcer of head, stage 3**
Healing pressure ulcer of head, stage 3
Pressure ulcer with full thickness skin loss involving damage or necrosis of subcutaneous tissue, head

SP SH SL **L89.814 Pressure ulcer of head, stage 4**
Healing pressure ulcer of head, stage 4
Pressure ulcer with necrosis of soft tissues through to underlying muscle, tendon, or bone, head

SP SH SL **L89.816 Pressure-induced deep tissue damage of head**

IQ **L89.819 Pressure ulcer of head, unspecified stage**
Healing pressure ulcer of head NOS
Healing pressure ulcer of head, unspecified stage

6 **L89.89 Pressure ulcer of other site**

SP SH SL **L89.890 Pressure ulcer of other site, unstageable**

SP **L89.891 Pressure ulcer of other site, stage 1**
Healing pressure ulcer of other site, stage 1
Pressure pre-ulcer skin changes limited to persistent focal edema, other site

SP SH SL **L89.892 Pressure ulcer of other site, stage 2**
Healing pressure ulcer of other site, stage 2
Pressure ulcer with abrasion, blister, partial thickness skin loss involving epidermis and/or dermis, other site

SP SH SL **L89.893 Pressure ulcer of other site, stage 3**
Healing pressure ulcer of other site, stage 3
Pressure ulcer with full thickness skin loss involving damage or necrosis of subcutaneous tissue, other site

SP SH SL **L89.894 Pressure ulcer of other site, stage 4**
Healing pressure ulcer of other site, stage 4
Pressure ulcer with necrosis of soft tissues through to underlying muscle, tendon, or bone, other site

SP SH SL **L89.896 Pressure-induced deep tissue damage of other site**

IQ **L89.899 Pressure ulcer of other site, unspecified stage**
Healing pressure ulcer of other site NOS
Healing pressure ulcer of other site, unspecified stage

5 **L89.9 Pressure ulcer of unspecified site**

CODING TIPS✓ Home health and hospice coders should never have to use L89.9- for pressure ulcer of unspecified site.

IQ **L89.90 Pressure ulcer of unspecified site, unspecified stage**
Healing pressure ulcer of unspecified site NOS
Healing pressure ulcer of unspecified site, unspecified stage

IQ **L89.91 Pressure ulcer of unspecified site, stage 1**
Healing pressure ulcer of unspecified site, stage 1
Pressure pre-ulcer skin changes limited to persistent focal edema, unspecified site

IQ **L89.92 Pressure ulcer of unspecified site, stage 2**
Healing pressure ulcer of unspecified site, stage 2
Pressure ulcer with abrasion, blister, partial thickness skin loss involving epidermis and/or dermis, unspecified site

IQ **L89.93 Pressure ulcer of unspecified site, stage 3**
Healing pressure ulcer of unspecified site, stage 3
Pressure ulcer with full thickness skin loss involving damage or necrosis of subcutaneous tissue, unspecified site

IQ **L89.94 Pressure ulcer of unspecified site, stage 4**
Healing pressure ulcer of unspecified site, stage 4
Pressure ulcer with necrosis of soft tissues through to underlying muscle, tendon, or bone, unspecified site

IQ **L89.95 Pressure ulcer of unspecified site, unstageable**

L89.96 Pressure-induced deep tissue damage of unspecified site

4 **L90 Atrophic disorders of skin**

SP **L90.0 Lichen sclerosus et atrophicus**
EXCLUDES 2 lichen sclerosus of external female genital organs (N90.4)
lichen sclerosus of external male genital organs (N48.0)

SP **L90.1 Anetoderma of Schweninger-Buzzi**

SP **L90.2 Anetoderma of Jadassohn-Pellizzari**

SP **L90.3 Atrophoderma of Pasini and Pierini**

SP **L90.4 Acrodermatitis chronica atrophicans**

SP **L90.5 Scar conditions and fibrosis of skin**
Adherent scar (skin)
Cicatrix
Disfigurement of skin due to scar
Fibrosis of skin NOS
Scar NOS
EXCLUDES 2 hypertrophic scar (L91.0)
keloid scar (L91.0)

SP **L90.6 Striae atrophicae**

SP **L90.8 Other atrophic disorders of skin**

IQ **L90.9 Atrophic disorder of skin, unspecified**

4 **L91 Hypertrophic disorders of skin**

SP **L91.0 Hypertrophic scar**
Keloid
Keloid scar
EXCLUDES 2 acne keloid (L73.0)
scar NOS (L90.5)

SP **L91.8 Other hypertrophic disorders of the skin**

IQ **L91.9 Hypertrophic disorder of the skin, unspecified**

4 **L92 Granulomatous disorders of skin and subcutaneous tissue**
EXCLUDES 2 actinic granuloma (L57.5)

SP **L92.0 Granuloma annulare**
Perforating granuloma annulare

SP **L92.1 Necrobiosis lipoidica, not elsewhere classified**
EXCLUDES 1 necrobiosis lipoidica associated with diabetes mellitus (E08-E13 with .620)

SP **L92.2 Granuloma faciale [eosinophilic granuloma of skin]**

SP + **L92.3 Foreign body granuloma of the skin and subcutaneous tissue**
Use additional code to identify the type of retained foreign body (Z18.-)

SP **L92.8 Other granulomatous disorders of the skin and subcutaneous tissue**

SP **L92.9 Granulomatous disorder of the skin and subcutaneous tissue, unspecified**
EXCLUDES 2 umbilical granuloma (P83.81)

+ 4 **L93 Lupus erythematosus**
Use additional code for adverse effect, if applicable, to identify drug (T36-T50 with fifth or sixth character 5)
EXCLUDES 1 lupus exedens (A18.4)
lupus vulgaris (A18.4)
scleroderma (M34.-)
systemic lupus erythematosus (M32.-)

SP + **L93.0 Discoid lupus erythematosus**
Lupus erythematosus NOS

SP + **L93.1 Subacute cutaneous lupus erythematosus**

SP + **L93.2 Other local lupus erythematosus**
Lupus erythematosus profundus
Lupus panniculitis

4 **L94 Other localized connective tissue disorders**
EXCLUDES 1 systemic connective tissue disorders (M30-M36)

SP **L94.0 Localized scleroderma [morphea]**
Circumscribed scleroderma

SP **L94.1 Linear scleroderma**
En coup de sabre lesion

SP **L94.2 Calcinosis cutis**

SP **L94.3 Sclerodactyly**

SP **L94.4 Gottron's papules**

SP **L94.5 Poikiloderma vasculare atrophicans**

SP **L94.6 Ainhum**

SP **L94.8 Other specified localized connective tissue disorders**

IQ **L94.9 Localized connective tissue disorder, unspecified**

4 **L95 Vasculitis limited to skin, not elsewhere classified**

EXCLUDES 1 angioma serpiginosum (L81.7)
Henoch (-Schönlein) purpura (D69.0)
hypersensitivity angiitis (M31.0)
lupus panniculitis (L93.2)
panniculitis NOS (M79.3)
panniculitis of neck and back (M54.0-)
polyarteritis nodosa (M30.0)
relapsing panniculitis (M35.6)
rheumatoid vasculitis (M05.2)
serum sickness (T80.6-)
urticaria (L50.-)
Wegener's granulomatosis (M31.3-)

SP **L95.0 Livedoid vasculitis**
Atrophie blanche (en plaque)

SP **L95.1 Erythema elevatum diutinum**

SP **L95.8 Other vasculitis limited to the skin**

SP **L95.9 Vasculitis limited to the skin, unspecified**

4 **L97 Non-pressure chronic ulcer of lower limb, not elsewhere classified**

INCLUDES chronic ulcer of skin of lower limb NOS
non-healing ulcer of skin
non-infected sinus of skin
trophic ulcer NOS
tropical ulcer NOS
ulcer of skin of lower limb NOS

Code first any associated underlying condition, such as:
any associated gangrene (I96)
atherosclerosis of the lower extremities (I70.23-, I70.24-, I70.33-, I70.34-, I70.43-, I70.44-, I70.53-, I70.54-, I70.63-, I70.64-, I70.73-, I70.74-)
chronic venous hypertension (I87.31-, I87.33-)
diabetic ulcers (E08.621, E08.622, E09.621, E09.622, E10.621, E10.622, E11.621, E11.622, E13.621, E13.622)
postphlebitic syndrome (I87.01-, I87.03-)
postthrombotic syndrome (I87.01-, I87.03-)
varicose ulcer (I83.0-, I83.2-)

EXCLUDES 2 pressure ulcer (pressure area) (L89.-)
skin infections (L00-L08)
specific infections classified to A00-B99

GUIDELINES **Section I.B.14**

For the Body Mass Index (BMI), depth of non-pressure chronic ulcers, pressure ulcer stage, coma scale, and NIH stroke scale (NIHSS) codes, code assignment may be based on medical record documentation from clinicians who are not the patient's provider (i.e., physician or other qualified healthcare practitioner legally accountable for establishing the patient's diagnosis), since this information is typically documented by other clinicians involved in the care of the patient (e.g., a dietitian often documents the BMI, a nurse often documents the pressure ulcer stages, and an emergency medical technician often documents the coma scale). However, the associated diagnosis (such as overweight, obesity, acute stroke, or pressure ulcer) must be documented by the patient's provider.

CODING TIPS ✓ If the ulcer is documented at one severity and after debridement is documented at a worse severity, code the worse severity.

CODING TIPS ✓ When coding any non-pressure chronic ulcer classifiable to L97, first code the underlying cause of the ulcer if known, followed by the appropriate L97 code to identify the ulcer location, site and severity. Gangrene (I96) associated with the ulcer should be coded prior to sequencing of the L97 code. Skin ulceration on the foot in a diabetic is assumed related to the diabetes, unless otherwise specified by the physician or NPP. Skin ulceration on areas other than the foot are not assumed related to diabetes unless documented by the physician or NPP. Diabetic neuropathies and peripheral angiopathies are considered co-morbidities and are not coded as causes of diabetic ulcers.

CODING TIPS ✓ If granulation tissue is documented, the 6th character of L97 should at least be a 2. (Ulcers limited to breakdown of skin do not granulate.) Before assigning 6th character 3, there must be evidence of muscle necrosis, not just muscle exposure. Before assigning 6th character 4, there must be evidence of bone necrosis, not just bone exposure. Sixth characters 5 and 6 may be used if muscle or bone, respectively, is involved, but necrosis cannot be determined. Sixth character 8 may be used if documentation of other structures, such as tendon and bone, are documented. Note, documentation of subcutaneous exposure is coded to fatty layer exposed.

CODING TIPS ✓ L97 codes are specific for location, including laterality and severity (e.g., skin, fat layer exposed, muscle involvement, necrosis of muscle, bone involvement, necrosis of bone, and other specified). The severity of the ulcer may be determined and coded based upon nursing documentation, but the diagnosis of the ulcer must come from the physician.

CODING TIPS✓ More than one L97 code may be used on a claim/record depending on the number of ulcers, cause of the ulcers, location on the lower limb, and severity of the ulcers. The same code may only be used once. Watch out for laterality. Do not choose an unspecified side code. There are no codes for bilateral, so if the condition is bilateral, a code for the right and a code for the left must be used. Two ulcers at the same location, but of different severity, may both be coded.

5 **L97.1 Non-pressure chronic ulcer of thigh**

6 **L97.10 Non-pressure chronic ulcer of unspecified thigh**

IQ **L97.101 Non-pressure chronic ulcer of unspecified thigh limited to breakdown of skin**

IQ **L97.102 Non-pressure chronic ulcer of unspecified thigh with fat layer exposed**

IQ **L97.103 Non-pressure chronic ulcer of unspecified thigh with necrosis of muscle**

IQ **L97.104 Non-pressure chronic ulcer of unspecified thigh with necrosis of bone**

IQ **L97.105 Non-pressure chronic ulcer of unspecified thigh with muscle involvement without evidence of necrosis**

IQ **L97.106 Non-pressure chronic ulcer of unspecified thigh with bone involvement without evidence of necrosis**

IQ **L97.108 Non-pressure chronic ulcer of unspecified thigh with other specified severity**

IQ **L97.109 Non-pressure chronic ulcer of unspecified thigh with unspecified severity**

6 **L97.11 Non-pressure chronic ulcer of right thigh**

⊟ SP SH SL **L97.111 Non-pressure chronic ulcer of right thigh limited to breakdown of skin**

⊟ SP SH SL **L97.112 Non-pressure chronic ulcer of right thigh with fat layer exposed**

⊟ SP SH SL **L97.113 Non-pressure chronic ulcer of right thigh with necrosis of muscle**

⊟ SP SH SL **L97.114 Non-pressure chronic ulcer of right thigh with necrosis of bone**

⊟ SP SH SL **L97.115 Non-pressure chronic ulcer of right thigh with muscle involvement without evidence of necrosis**

⊟ SP SH SL **L97.116 Non-pressure chronic ulcer of right thigh with bone involvement without evidence of necrosis**

⊟ SP SH SL **L97.118 Non-pressure chronic ulcer of right thigh with other specified severity**

⊟ SP SH SL **L97.119 Non-pressure chronic ulcer of right thigh with unspecified severity**

6 **L97.12 Non-pressure chronic ulcer of left thigh**

⊟ SP SH SL **L97.121 Non-pressure chronic ulcer of left thigh limited to breakdown of skin**

⊟ SP SH SL **L97.122 Non-pressure chronic ulcer of left thigh with fat layer exposed**

⊟ SP SH SL **L97.123 Non-pressure chronic ulcer of left thigh with necrosis of muscle**

⊟ SP SH SL **L97.124 Non-pressure chronic ulcer of left thigh with necrosis of bone**

⊟ SP SH SL **L97.125 Non-pressure chronic ulcer of left thigh with muscle involvement without evidence of necrosis**

⊟ SP SH SL **L97.126 Non-pressure chronic ulcer of left thigh with bone involvement without evidence of necrosis**

⊟ SP SH SL **L97.128 Non-pressure chronic ulcer of left thigh with other specified severity**

⊟ SP SH SL **L97.129 Non-pressure chronic ulcer of left thigh with unspecified severity**

5 **L97.2 Non-pressure chronic ulcer of calf**

6 **L97.20 Non-pressure chronic ulcer of unspecified calf**

IQ **L97.201 Non-pressure chronic ulcer of unspecified calf limited to breakdown of skin**

IQ **L97.202 Non-pressure chronic ulcer of unspecified calf with fat layer exposed**

IQ **L97.203 Non-pressure chronic ulcer of unspecified calf with necrosis of muscle**

IQ **L97.204 Non-pressure chronic ulcer of unspecified calf with necrosis of bone**

IQ **L97.205 Non-pressure chronic ulcer of unspecified calf with muscle involvement without evidence of necrosis**

IQ **L97.206 Non-pressure chronic ulcer of unspecified calf with bone involvement without evidence of necrosis**

IQ **L97.208 Non-pressure chronic ulcer of unspecified calf with other specified severity**

IQ **L97.209 Non-pressure chronic ulcer of unspecified calf with unspecified severity**

6 **L97.21 Non-pressure chronic ulcer of right calf**

⊟ SP SH SL **L97.211 Non-pressure chronic ulcer of right calf limited to breakdown of skin**

⊟ SP SH SL **L97.212 Non-pressure chronic ulcer of right calf with fat layer exposed**

⊟ SP SH SL **L97.213 Non-pressure chronic ulcer of right calf with necrosis of muscle**

⊟ SP SH SL **L97.214 Non-pressure chronic ulcer of right calf with necrosis of bone**

⊟ SP SH SL **L97.215 Non-pressure chronic ulcer of right calf with muscle involvement without evidence of necrosis**

⊟ SP SH SL **L97.216 Non-pressure chronic ulcer of right calf with bone involvement without evidence of necrosis**

⊟ SP SH SL **L97.218 Non-pressure chronic ulcer of right calf with other specified severity**

SP SH SL L97.219 Non-pressure chronic ulcer of right calf with unspecified severity

6 L97.22 Non-pressure chronic ulcer of left calf

SP SH SL L97.221 Non-pressure chronic ulcer of left calf limited to breakdown of skin

SP SH SL L97.222 Non-pressure chronic ulcer of left calf with fat layer exposed

SP SH SL L97.223 Non-pressure chronic ulcer of left calf with necrosis of muscle

SP SH SL L97.224 Non-pressure chronic ulcer of left calf with necrosis of bone

SP SH SL L97.225 Non-pressure chronic ulcer of left calf with muscle involvement without evidence of necrosis

SP SH SL L97.226 Non-pressure chronic ulcer of left calf with bone involvement without evidence of necrosis

SP SH SL L97.228 Non-pressure chronic ulcer of left calf with other specified severity

SP SH SL L97.229 Non-pressure chronic ulcer of left calf with unspecified severity

5 L97.3 Non-pressure chronic ulcer of ankle

6 L97.30 Non-pressure chronic ulcer of unspecified ankle

SP L97.301 Non-pressure chronic ulcer of unspecified ankle limited to breakdown of skin

!Q L97.302 Non-pressure chronic ulcer of unspecified ankle with fat layer exposed

!Q L97.303 Non-pressure chronic ulcer of unspecified ankle with necrosis of muscle

!Q L97.304 Non-pressure chronic ulcer of unspecified ankle with necrosis of bone

!Q L97.305 Non-pressure chronic ulcer of unspecified ankle with muscle involvement without evidence of necrosis

!Q L97.306 Non-pressure chronic ulcer of unspecified ankle with bone involvement without evidence of necrosis

!Q L97.308 Non-pressure chronic ulcer of unspecified ankle with other specified severity

!Q L97.309 Non-pressure chronic ulcer of unspecified ankle with unspecified severity

6 L97.31 Non-pressure chronic ulcer of right ankle

SP SH SL L97.311 Non-pressure chronic ulcer of right ankle limited to breakdown of skin

SP SH SL L97.312 Non-pressure chronic ulcer of right ankle with fat layer exposed

SP SH SL L97.313 Non-pressure chronic ulcer of right ankle with necrosis of muscle

SP SH SL L97.314 Non-pressure chronic ulcer of right ankle with necrosis of bone

SP SH SL L97.315 Non-pressure chronic ulcer of right ankle with muscle involvement without evidence of necrosis

SP SH SL L97.316 Non-pressure chronic ulcer of right ankle with bone involvement without evidence of necrosis

SP SH SL L97.318 Non-pressure chronic ulcer of right ankle with other specified severity

SP SH SL L97.319 Non-pressure chronic ulcer of right ankle with unspecified severity

6 L97.32 Non-pressure chronic ulcer of left ankle

SP SH SL L97.321 Non-pressure chronic ulcer of left ankle limited to breakdown of skin

SP SH SL L97.322 Non-pressure chronic ulcer of left ankle with fat layer exposed

SP SH SL L97.323 Non-pressure chronic ulcer of left ankle with necrosis of muscle

SP SH SL L97.324 Non-pressure chronic ulcer of left ankle with necrosis of bone

SP SH SL L97.325 Non-pressure chronic ulcer of left ankle with muscle involvement without evidence of necrosis

SP SH SL L97.326 Non-pressure chronic ulcer of left ankle with bone involvement without evidence of necrosis

SP SH SL L97.328 Non-pressure chronic ulcer of left ankle with other specified severity

SP SH SL L97.329 Non-pressure chronic ulcer of left ankle with unspecified severity

5 L97.4 Non-pressure chronic ulcer of heel and midfoot

Non-pressure chronic ulcer of plantar surface of midfoot

6 L97.40 Non-pressure chronic ulcer of unspecified heel and midfoot

!Q L97.401 Non-pressure chronic ulcer of unspecified heel and midfoot limited to breakdown of skin

!Q L97.402 Non-pressure chronic ulcer of unspecified heel and midfoot with fat layer exposed

!Q L97.403 Non-pressure chronic ulcer of unspecified heel and midfoot with necrosis of muscle

!Q L97.404 Non-pressure chronic ulcer of unspecified heel and midfoot with necrosis of bone

!Q L97.405 Non-pressure chronic ulcer of unspecified heel and midfoot with muscle involvement without evidence of necrosis

!Q L97.406 Non-pressure chronic ulcer of unspecified heel and midfoot with bone involvement without evidence of necrosis

!Q L97.408 Non-pressure chronic ulcer of unspecified heel and midfoot with other specified severity

!Q L97.409 Non-pressure chronic ulcer of unspecified heel and midfoot with unspecified severity

6 L97.41 Non-pressure chronic ulcer of right heel and midfoot

L SP SH SL L97.411 Non-pressure chronic ulcer of right heel and midfoot limited to breakdown of skin

L SP SH SL L97.412 Non-pressure chronic ulcer of right heel and midfoot with fat layer exposed

L SP SH SL L97.413 Non-pressure chronic ulcer of right heel and midfoot with necrosis of muscle

L SP SH SL L97.414 Non-pressure chronic ulcer of right heel and midfoot with necrosis of bone

L SP SH SL L97.415 Non-pressure chronic ulcer of right heel and midfoot with muscle involvement without evidence of necrosis

L SP SH SL L97.416 Non-pressure chronic ulcer of right heel and midfoot with bone involvement without evidence of necrosis

L SP SH SL L97.418 Non-pressure chronic ulcer of right heel and midfoot with other specified severity

L SP SH SL L97.419 Non-pressure chronic ulcer of right heel and midfoot with unspecified severity

6 L97.42 Non-pressure chronic ulcer of left heel and midfoot

L SP SH SL L97.421 Non-pressure chronic ulcer of left heel and midfoot limited to breakdown of skin

L SP SH SL L97.422 Non-pressure chronic ulcer of left heel and midfoot with fat layer exposed

L SP SH SL L97.423 Non-pressure chronic ulcer of left heel and midfoot with necrosis of muscle

L SP SH SL L97.424 Non-pressure chronic ulcer of left heel and midfoot with necrosis of bone

L SP SH SL L97.425 Non-pressure chronic ulcer of left heel and midfoot with muscle involvement without evidence of necrosis

L SP SH SL L97.426 Non-pressure chronic ulcer of left heel and midfoot with bone involvement without evidence of necrosis

L SP SH SL L97.428 Non-pressure chronic ulcer of left heel and midfoot with other specified severity

L SP SH SL L97.429 Non-pressure chronic ulcer of left heel and midfoot with unspecified severity

5 L97.5 Non-pressure chronic ulcer of other part of foot

Non-pressure chronic ulcer of toe

6 L97.50 Non-pressure chronic ulcer of other part of unspecified foot

!Q L97.501 Non-pressure chronic ulcer of other part of unspecified foot limited to breakdown of skin

!Q L97.502 Non-pressure chronic ulcer of other part of unspecified foot with fat layer exposed

!Q L97.503 Non-pressure chronic ulcer of other part of unspecified foot with necrosis of muscle

!Q L97.504 Non-pressure chronic ulcer of other part of unspecified foot with necrosis of bone

!Q L97.505 Non-pressure chronic ulcer of other part of unspecified foot with muscle involvement without evidence of necrosis

!Q L97.506 Non-pressure chronic ulcer of other part of unspecified foot with bone involvement without evidence of necrosis

!Q L97.508 Non-pressure chronic ulcer of other part of unspecified foot with other specified severity

!Q L97.509 Non-pressure chronic ulcer of other part of unspecified foot with unspecified severity

6 L97.51 Non-pressure chronic ulcer of other part of right foot

L SP SH SL L97.511 Non-pressure chronic ulcer of other part of right foot limited to breakdown of skin

L SP SH SL L97.512 Non-pressure chronic ulcer of other part of right foot with fat layer exposed

L SP SH SL L97.513 Non-pressure chronic ulcer of other part of right foot with necrosis of muscle

L SP SH SL L97.514 Non-pressure chronic ulcer of other part of right foot with necrosis of bone

L SP SH SL L97.515 Non-pressure chronic ulcer of other part of right foot with muscle involvement without evidence of necrosis

L SP SH SL L97.516 Non-pressure chronic ulcer of other part of right foot with bone involvement without evidence of necrosis

L SP SH SL L97.518 Non-pressure chronic ulcer of other part of right foot with other specified severity

L SP SH SL L97.519 Non-pressure chronic ulcer of other part of right foot with unspecified severity

6 L97.52 Non-pressure chronic ulcer of other part of left foot

L SP SH SL L97.521 Non-pressure chronic ulcer of other part of left foot limited to breakdown of skin

L SP SH SL L97.522 Non-pressure chronic ulcer of other part of left foot with fat layer exposed

L SP SH SL L97.523 Non-pressure chronic ulcer of other part of left foot with necrosis of muscle

L SP SH SL L97.524 Non-pressure chronic ulcer of other part of left foot with necrosis of bone

L SP SH SL L97.525 Non-pressure chronic ulcer of other part of left foot with muscle involvement without evidence of necrosis

Chapter 12

L00-L99

SP SH SL L97.526 Non-pressure chronic ulcer of other part of left foot with bone involvement without evidence of necrosis

SP SH SL L97.528 Non-pressure chronic ulcer of other part of left foot with other specified severity

SP SH SL L97.529 Non-pressure chronic ulcer of other part of left foot with unspecified severity

5 L97.8 Non-pressure chronic ulcer of other part of lower leg

6 L97.80 Non-pressure chronic ulcer of other part of unspecified lower leg

IQ L97.801 Non-pressure chronic ulcer of other part of unspecified lower leg limited to breakdown of skin

IQ L97.802 Non-pressure chronic ulcer of other part of unspecified lower leg with fat layer exposed

IQ L97.803 Non-pressure chronic ulcer of other part of unspecified lower leg with necrosis of muscle

IQ L97.804 Non-pressure chronic ulcer of other part of unspecified lower leg with necrosis of bone

IQ L97.805 Non-pressure chronic ulcer of other part of unspecified lower leg with muscle involvement without evidence of necrosis

IQ L97.806 Non-pressure chronic ulcer of other part of unspecified lower leg with bone involvement without evidence of necrosis

IQ L97.808 Non-pressure chronic ulcer of other part of unspecified lower leg with other specified severity

IQ L97.809 Non-pressure chronic ulcer of other part of unspecified lower leg with unspecified severity

6 L97.81 Non-pressure chronic ulcer of other part of right lower leg

SP SH SL L97.811 Non-pressure chronic ulcer of other part of right lower leg limited to breakdown of skin

SP SH SL L97.812 Non-pressure chronic ulcer of other part of right lower leg with fat layer exposed

SP SH SL L97.813 Non-pressure chronic ulcer of other part of right lower leg with necrosis of muscle

SP SH SL L97.814 Non-pressure chronic ulcer of other part of right lower leg with necrosis of bone

SP SH SL L97.815 Non-pressure chronic ulcer of other part of right lower leg with muscle involvement without evidence of necrosis

SP SH SL L97.816 Non-pressure chronic ulcer of other part of right lower leg with bone involvement without evidence of necrosis

SP SH SL L97.818 Non-pressure chronic ulcer of other part of right lower leg with other specified severity

SP SH SL L97.819 Non-pressure chronic ulcer of other part of right lower leg with unspecified severity

6 L97.82 Non-pressure chronic ulcer of other part of left lower leg

SP SH SL L97.821 Non-pressure chronic ulcer of other part of left lower leg limited to breakdown of skin

SP SH SL L97.822 Non-pressure chronic ulcer of other part of left lower leg with fat layer exposed

SP SH SL L97.823 Non-pressure chronic ulcer of other part of left lower leg with necrosis of muscle

SP SH SL L97.824 Non-pressure chronic ulcer of other part of left lower leg with necrosis of bone

SP SH SL L97.825 Non-pressure chronic ulcer of other part of left lower leg with muscle involvement without evidence of necrosis

SP SH SL L97.826 Non-pressure chronic ulcer of other part of left lower leg with bone involvement without evidence of necrosis

SP SH SL L97.828 Non-pressure chronic ulcer of other part of left lower leg with other specified severity

SP SH SL L97.829 Non-pressure chronic ulcer of other part of left lower leg with unspecified severity

5 L97.9 Non-pressure chronic ulcer of unspecified part of lower leg

CODING TIPS✓ Coders should not have to use L97.9 as the location of the ulcer should be documented.

6 L97.90 Non-pressure chronic ulcer of unspecified part of unspecified lower leg

IQ L97.901 Non-pressure chronic ulcer of unspecified part of unspecified lower leg limited to breakdown of skin

IQ L97.902 Non-pressure chronic ulcer of unspecified part of unspecified lower leg with fat layer exposed

IQ L97.903 Non-pressure chronic ulcer of unspecified part of unspecified lower leg with necrosis of muscle

IQ L97.904 Non-pressure chronic ulcer of unspecified part of unspecified lower leg with necrosis of bone

IQ L97.905 Non-pressure chronic ulcer of unspecified part of unspecified lower leg with muscle involvement without evidence of necrosis

IQ L97.906 Non-pressure chronic ulcer of unspecified part of unspecified lower leg with bone involvement without evidence of necrosis

IQ L97.908 Non-pressure chronic ulcer of unspecified part of unspecified lower leg with other specified severity

IQ **L97.909 Non-pressure chronic ulcer of unspecified part of unspecified lower leg with unspecified severity**

6 **L97.91 Non-pressure chronic ulcer of unspecified part of right lower leg**

Laterality SP SH SL **L97.911 Non-pressure chronic ulcer of unspecified part of right lower leg limited to breakdown of skin**

Laterality SP SH SL **L97.912 Non-pressure chronic ulcer of unspecified part of right lower leg with fat layer exposed**

Laterality SP SH SL **L97.913 Non-pressure chronic ulcer of unspecified part of right lower leg with necrosis of muscle**

Laterality SP SH SL **L97.914 Non-pressure chronic ulcer of unspecified part of right lower leg with necrosis of bone**

Laterality SP SH SL **L97.915 Non-pressure chronic ulcer of unspecified part of right lower leg with muscle involvement without evidence of necrosis**

Laterality SP SH SL **L97.916 Non-pressure chronic ulcer of unspecified part of right lower leg with bone involvement without evidence of necrosis**

Laterality SP SH SL **L97.918 Non-pressure chronic ulcer of unspecified part of right lower leg with other specified severity**

Laterality SP SH SL **L97.919 Non-pressure chronic ulcer of unspecified part of right lower leg with unspecified severity**

6 **L97.92 Non-pressure chronic ulcer of unspecified part of left lower leg**

Laterality SP SH SL **L97.921 Non-pressure chronic ulcer of unspecified part of left lower leg limited to breakdown of skin**

Laterality SP SH SL **L97.922 Non-pressure chronic ulcer of unspecified part of left lower leg with fat layer exposed**

Laterality SP SH SL **L97.923 Non-pressure chronic ulcer of unspecified part of left lower leg with necrosis of muscle**

Laterality SP SH SL **L97.924 Non-pressure chronic ulcer of unspecified part of left lower leg with necrosis of bone**

Laterality SP SH SL **L97.925 Non-pressure chronic ulcer of unspecified part of left lower leg with muscle involvement without evidence of necrosis**

Laterality SP SH SL **L97.926 Non-pressure chronic ulcer of unspecified part of left lower leg with bone involvement without evidence of necrosis**

Laterality SP SH SL **L97.928 Non-pressure chronic ulcer of unspecified part of left lower leg with other specified severity**

Laterality SP SH SL **L97.929 Non-pressure chronic ulcer of unspecified part of left lower leg with unspecified severity**

4 **L98 Other disorders of skin and subcutaneous tissue, not elsewhere classified**

SP **L98.0 Pyogenic granuloma**

EXCLUDES 2 pyogenic granuloma of gingiva (K06.8)
pyogenic granuloma of maxillary alveolar ridge (K04.5)
pyogenic granuloma of oral mucosa (K13.4)

SP **L98.1 Factitial dermatitis**

Neurotic excoriation

EXCLUDES 1 Excoriation (skin-picking) disorder (F42.4)

CODING TIPS ✓ Factitial dermatitis, L98.1, may also be referred to as neurotic excoriation or dermatitis artefacta and is characterized by deliberate, self-inflicted skin lesions produced as a result of underlying psychological conditions. When specified, any underlying or additional psychological conditions should also be coded. An example of a psychological condition is skin-picking disorder (F42.4).

SP **L98.2 Febrile neutrophilic dermatosis [Sweet]**

SP SH SL **L98.3 Eosinophilic cellulitis [Wells]**

5 **L98.4 Non-pressure chronic ulcer of skin, not elsewhere classified**

Chronic ulcer of skin NOS
Tropical ulcer NOS
Ulcer of skin NOS

EXCLUDES 2 pressure ulcer (pressure area) (L89.-)
gangrene (I96)
skin infections (L00-L08)
specific infections classified to A00-B99
ulcer of lower limb NEC (L97.-)
varicose ulcer (I83.0-I83.93)

CODING TIPS ✓ Do not use L98 to indicate a pressure ulcer/injury. All pressure ulcers/injuries are coded to the L89 category. L98.4 is used for ulcers that are not pressure ulcers/injuries and are not on lower extremities.

6 **L98.41 Non-pressure chronic ulcer of buttock**

SP **L98.411 Non-pressure chronic ulcer of buttock limited to breakdown of skin**

SP **L98.412 Non-pressure chronic ulcer of buttock with fat layer exposed**

SP **L98.413 Non-pressure chronic ulcer of buttock with necrosis of muscle**

SP **L98.414 Non-pressure chronic ulcer of buttock with necrosis of bone**

SP **L98.415 Non-pressure chronic ulcer of buttock with muscle involvement without evidence of necrosis**

SP **L98.416 Non-pressure chronic ulcer of buttock with bone involvement without evidence of necrosis**

SP **L98.418 Non-pressure chronic ulcer of buttock with other specified severity**

SP **L98.419 Non-pressure chronic ulcer of buttock with unspecified severity**

6 **L98.42 Non-pressure chronic ulcer of back**

SP **L98.421 Non-pressure chronic ulcer of back limited to breakdown of skin**

Chapter 12

L00-L99

SP **L98.422 Non-pressure chronic ulcer of back with fat layer exposed**

SP **L98.423 Non-pressure chronic ulcer of back with necrosis of muscle**

SP **L98.424 Non-pressure chronic ulcer of back with necrosis of bone**

SP **L98.425 Non-pressure chronic ulcer of back with muscle involvement without evidence of necrosis**

SP **L98.426 Non-pressure chronic ulcer of back with bone involvement without evidence of necrosis**

SP **L98.428 Non-pressure chronic ulcer of back with other specified severity**

SP **L98.429 Non-pressure chronic ulcer of back with unspecified severity**

6 **L98.49 Non-pressure chronic ulcer of skin of other sites**

Non-pressure chronic ulcer of skin NOS

CODING TIPS✓ Locally advanced, metastatic or recurrent cancer may infiltrate the skin, disrupt its integrity, and cause chronic, poorly healing, and fungating wounds. When an ulcer/wound is the result of cancer, code only the cancer. Query the physician or NPP for metastasis to the skin, e.g. C79.2. Do not use L98.49.

SP **L98.491 Non-pressure chronic ulcer of skin of other sites limited to breakdown of skin**

SP **L98.492 Non-pressure chronic ulcer of skin of other sites with fat layer exposed**

SP **L98.493 Non-pressure chronic ulcer of skin of other sites with necrosis of muscle**

SP **L98.494 Non-pressure chronic ulcer of skin of other sites with necrosis of bone**

SP **L98.495 Non-pressure chronic ulcer of skin of other sites with muscle involvement without evidence of necrosis**

SP **L98.496 Non-pressure chronic ulcer of skin of other sites with bone involvement without evidence of necrosis**

SP **L98.498 Non-pressure chronic ulcer of skin of other sites with other specified severity**

SP **L98.499 Non-pressure chronic ulcer of skin of other sites with unspecified severity**

SP **L98.5 Mucinosis of the skin**

Focal mucinosis

Lichen myxedematosus

Reticular erythematous mucinosis

EXCLUDES 1 focal oral mucinosis (K13.79)
myxedema (E03.9)

SP **L98.6 Other infiltrative disorders of the skin and subcutaneous tissue**

EXCLUDES 1 hyalinosis cutis et mucosae (E78.89)

SP **L98.7 Excessive and redundant skin and subcutaneous tissue**

Loose or sagging skin following bariatric surgery weight loss

Loose or sagging skin following dietary weight loss

Loose or sagging skin, NOS

EXCLUDES 2 acquired excess or redundant skin of eyelid (H02.3-)
congenital excess or redundant skin of eyelid (Q10.3)
skin changes due to chronic exposure to nonionizing radiation (L57.-)

SP **L98.8 Other specified disorders of the skin and subcutaneous tissue**

IQ **L98.9 Disorder of the skin and subcutaneous tissue, unspecified**

▲ M IQ **L99 *Other disorders of skin and subcutaneous tissue in diseases classified elsewhere***

Code first underlying disease, such as:
amyloidosis (E85.-)

EXCLUDES 1 skin disorders in diabetes (E08-E13 with .62-)
skin disorders in gonorrhea (A54.89)
skin disorders in syphilis (A51.31, A52.79)

Chapter 12

L00-L99

Chapter 12 Scenarios: Diseases of the skin and subcutaneous tissue (L00-L99)

Gangrenous pressure ulcer, diabetic neuropathy

A 71-year-old woman is admitted to home health for wound care to a gangrenous stage 3 pressure ulcer to her right heel that's documented as associated with diabetic neuropathy. The diabetes is documented as Type 1.5. She uses both insulin and oral hypoglycemic medication.

Description	Code
Primary: Gangrene, not elsewhere classified	I96
Secondary: Pressure ulcer of right heel, stage 3	L89.613
Secondary: Other specified diabetes mellitus with diabetic polyneuropathy	E13.42
Secondary: Long term (current) use of insulin	Z79.4

A gangrenous pressure ulcer on the heel is not a diabetic ulcer and should not be coded as a diabetic manifestation, according to Q3 2018 Coding Clinic guidance. It is coded as gangrenous pressure ulcer, first with I96 followed by L89.612, in accordance with tabular instruction. The gangrene code must be assigned before the pressure ulcer code, according to a "code first" note at the L89.- category level. Since the diabetes is documented as type 1.5, a diabetes code from the E13.- category is assigned, according to Q3 2018 Coding Clinic guidance. The patient uses both insulin and oral hypoglycemic medication; only the code for insulin use is assigned, in accordance with coding guidelines.

Pressure ulcers/injuries, old spinal stroke

Your new 66-year-old patient was referred for care of a stage 3 pressure ulcer/injury on her right buttock and a stage 2 pressure ulcer/injury on her right hip. Skilled nursing has been ordered for wound care. She also has hypertension and is a paraplegic due to an old spinal stroke

Description	Code
Primary: Pressure ulcer right buttock, stage 3	L89.313
Secondary: Pressure ulcer right hip, stage 2	L89.212
Secondary: Paraplegia	G82.20
Secondary: Essential (primary) hypertension	I10
Secondary: Dependence on wheelchair	Z99.3

ICD-10 provides a great deal of specificity with regard to the pressure ulcers/injuries. For example, take L89.313 and break it down: the L89.3.- root code indicates the buttock, the 5th digit "1" indicates the right side, and the 6th digit "3" indicates the stage of the pressure ulcer/injury. In this scenario, the paraplegia is also reported as due to an old spinal stroke. Only the code for the paraplegia is assigned as there is currently no code for sequela of a spinal stroke, according to Q3 2017 Coding Clinic guidance.

Bilateral pressure ulcers/injuries

A 72-year-old male patient has stage 2 pressure ulcers/injuries on both elbows, for which he will be receiving wound care.

Description	Code
Primary: Pressure ulcer of right elbow, stage 2	L89.012
Secondary: Pressure ulcer of left elbow, stage 2	L89.022

There is no single code to indicate a bilateral pressure ulcer/injury in ICD-10. Thus, both ulcers/injuries are captured by their unique body site codes. No separate code is required for the stage, because the ICD-10 combination code includes the stage.

Venous insufficiency, non-healing stasis ulcer

A 72-year-old man is admitted to home care with diagnoses of venous insufficiency and hypertension. He has skin breakdown on his left heel that does not extend beyond the dermis. The area has been diagnosed by the physician as a stasis ulcer and the ulcer is considered non-healing. Wound care is ordered as well as medication management for his hypertension.

Description	Code
Primary: Venous insufficiency (chronic) (peripheral)	I87.2
Secondary: Non-pressure chronic ulcer of left heel and mid-foot limited to breakdown of skin	L97.421
Secondary: Essential (primary) hypertension	I10

The L97.- codes allow you to identify not only the location, but the severity of the ulcer. In this case, the documentation states the severity is limited to the breakdown of the skin so a 6th character of "1" is appropriate. The L97.421 code includes that the ulcer is non-healing. Hypertension is coded as a relevant comorbidity.

Varicose veins, non-healing stasis ulcer

A 79-year-old woman is admitted to home care for wound care of a non-healing stasis ulcer on her right ankle that has exposed the fat layer. The stasis ulcer is a result of varicose veins.

Description	Code
Primary: Varicose veins of right lower extremity with ulcer of ankle	I83.013
Secondary: Non-pressure chronic ulcer of right ankle with fat layer exposed	L97.312

Tabular instruction under I83.0- tells coders to "use additional code to identify severity of ulcer (L97.-)." In this case, the documentation states the severity includes exposure of the fat layer so L97.312 should be used. The fact that the ulcer is non-healing is captured in the L97.312 code.

HOME HEALTH CODING SCENARIOS

Arterial ulcer

A 75-year-old woman comes to home health after developing an ulcer on her calf, which her physician diagnosed as caused by atherosclerosis. The clinician documents that the ulcer is on her right calf, measures two millimeters in depth and four millimeters in diameter, and that it has gone beyond the skin layers into the patient's fatty tissue. The patient also has hypertension. The nurse also documents that while the patient has never smoked, her husband has been a smoker for 35 years, and continues to smoke. Home health will provide wound care.

Description	Code
Primary: Atherosclerosis of native arteries of right leg, with ulceration of calf	I70.232
Secondary: Non-pressure chronic ulcer of right calf with fat layer exposed	L97.212
Secondary: Essential (primary) hypertension	I10
Secondary: Exposure to environmental tobacco smoke	Z77.22

Diagnosed as an arterial ulcer caused by atherosclerosis, the wound is coded as such. Descriptions of laterality and severity are required in ICD-10, and thus the wound is specified as being on the patient's right calf and extending into the fatty layer of tissue. Hypertension is also coded as a relevant comorbidity. ICD-10 atherosclerosis codes include an instructional note to include, if applicable, whether the patient has any dependence on tobacco. In this case, the patient isn't dependent on tobacco, but is exposed to it, and that should be documented and coded.

Cellulitis

A patient initially sustained a minor laceration injury to her right index finger from the sharp edge of a tin can lid. This injury caused cellulitis and the patient requires treatment with IV antibiotics, as several rounds of oral antibiotics were not successful. The initial wound is still healing but does not require treatment from the agency. The focus of the admission is on the cellulitis.

Description	Code
Primary: Cellulitis of right (index) finger	L03.011
Secondary: Laceration without foreign body right index finger (without damage to nail) subsequent encounter	S61.210D
Secondary: Encounter for adjustment and management of vascular device	Z45.2
Secondary: Long term (current) use of antibiotics	Z79.2
Secondary: Contact with other sharp object(s), not elsewhere classified, subsequent encounter	W26.8XXD

The wound typically is coded before the cellulitis, except when the wound does not require care or is no longer present as in this case. Tabular instructions at S61.- state to "code also any associated wound infection." Note that this instruction is different from a "code first" instruction and does not provide any sequencing direction. If the wound is now closed, then it would not be coded. Because the wound is not receiving active treatment from the agency, the 7th character "D" for subsequent encounter is appropriate. The external cause code is added to help explain how the patient sustained the wound that led to the cellulitis. It carries the same 7th character ("D") as the code it is explaining (S61.210D), in accordance with official coding guidelines. Codes Z45.2 and Z79.2 capture the administration of IV antibiotics. If the IV is not the primary reason the patient requires home health care, but where there may be some sort of intervention noted on the home health plan of care, then it would be appropriate to report Z45.2 (but not as the principal or first secondary diagnosis), according to CMS.

Adverse effect of Lovenox, hives

An 82-year-old man recently was diagnosed with paroxysmal atrial fibrillation and was given injections of Lovenox. The drug was given as directed, but the patient suffered an allergic reaction that caused him to break out in hives. His physician has prescribed new medication and the patient has been admitted to home health for medication management and monitoring. The medical record indicates that at the start of care, the nurse identified a non-blanchable red area on the patient's left heel, which was confirmed with the physician to be due to pressure. A protective dressing was ordered and interventions ordered to the care plan that were initiated at the first visit. Nursing will monitor the area and the caregiver is able to apply the dressing.

Description	Code
Primary: Allergic urticaria	L50.0
Secondary: Adverse effect of anticoagulants, subsequent encounter	T45.515D
Secondary: Paroxysmal atrial fibrillation	I48.0
Secondary: Pressure ulcer of left heel, stage 1	L89.621

The drug was given correctly but the patient experienced a problem anyway. Therefore, the scenario is an adverse effect. The adverse effect of the drug, the hives, is coded first, in accordance with coding guidelines. The code for an adverse effect caused by Lovenox is T45.515-, according to the table of drugs and chemicals. A seventh character of "D" is assigned to indicate the subsequent nature of the encounter. The reason the drug was given is coded after the adverse effect code. The stage 1 pressure ulcer was confirmed with the physician, so it is also coded, but the caregiver is providing all care and nursing is only providing intermittent assessment so this is not the focus of care.

Scar from burn

A 68-year-old female developed an extensive scar on her left forearm after a second degree burn healed. The burn occurred when she accidentally dropped a hot iron. The scar causes her severe pain and difficulty with mobility and completing ADLs/IADLs. She was admitted to home health for nursing care and occupational therapy. She also has peripheral vascular disease and chronic atrial fibrillation, for which she is on long-term anticoagulant therapy.

Description	Code
Primary: Scar conditions and fibrosis of skin	L90.5
Secondary: Burn of second degree of left forearm, sequela	T22.212S
Secondary: Peripheral vascular disease, unspecified	I73.9
Secondary: Chronic atrial fibrillation, unspecified	I48.20
Secondary: Long term (current) use of anticoagulants	Z79.01
Secondary: Contact with other hot household appliances, sequela	X15.8xxS

The burn, though healed, left behind a scar that is causing the patient significant distress. Therefore, the burn is coded with a seventh character "S" to indicate that it is healed but has caused a residual condition, or sequela. The residual condition, the scar, is coded prior to the injury that caused it, in accordance with coding guidelines. As comorbidities that will impact her ability to heal, her peripheral vascular disease and chronic atrial fibrillation are coded as well. Her use of anticoagulant medication carries certain risks and thus should be coded with Z79.01. An external cause code is used to describe how the patient sustained the burn.

Ulcer due to PVD, GERD

An 82-year-old male patient is admitted to home health for wound care to an ulcer of his right lateral plantar foot; the wound is showing bone involvement but there's no evidence of necrosis. The ulcer was caused by PVD. He also has GERD and was recently prescribed new medication for it. The patient complains of pain in his legs with ambulation.

Description	Code
Primary: Peripheral vascular disease, unspecified	I73.9
Secondary: Non-pressure chronic ulcer of other part of right foot with bone involvement without evidence of necrosis	L97.516
Secondary: Gastro-esophageal reflux disease without esophagitis	K21.9

The patient's ulcer has been said to be caused by PVD but there's no mention of atherosclerosis. Thus, I73.9 must be assigned to capture the etiology of the ulcer. The L97.516 code, which specifies that the ulcer is on his right foot and that there is bone involvement but no necrosis, is assigned immediately following. GERD is coded as a relevant comorbidity.

Stasis ulcer

A 76-year-old woman was referred to home health for wound care for an ulcer on her left ankle caused by chronic venous hypertension. Muscle tissue is evident in the wound on her ankle but there's no necrosis.

Description	Code
Primary: Chronic venous hypertension (idiopathic) with ulcer of left lower extremity	I87.312
Secondary: Non-pressure chronic ulcer of left ankle with muscle involvement without evidence of necrosis	L97.325

The wound is the result of chronic venous hypertension and it thus captured first with the combination code I87.312. The L97.325, which specifies that the ulcer is on her left ankle and that muscle tissue is visible but there's no necrosis, is assigned following the code for chronic venous hypertension with ulcer.

Ulcerated laceration, Diabetes

A 45-year-old type 1 diabetic patient lacerated his foot 4 weeks ago when walking barefoot in his home and the wound failed to heal. The patient followed up with his primary physician who ordered home health nursing for wound care to the site, which was also cultured and positive for MSSA. The wound was debrided "with clear exposed subcutaneous tissue" during the physician visit. The physician reports that the patient has the following diagnoses: diabetic foot ulcer of the left foot (non-healing) due to prior laceration, PVD, and coronary atherosclerosis. The patient uses insulin to control his diabetes.

Description	Code
Primary: Type 1 diabetes mellitus with foot ulcer	E10.621
Secondary: Non-pressure chronic ulcer of other part of left foot with fat layer exposed	L97.522
Secondary: Laceration without foreign body, left foot, sequela	S91.312S
Secondary: Methicillin susceptible Staphylococcus aureus infection as the cause of diseases classified elsewhere	B95.61
Secondary: Type 1 diabetes mellitus with diabetic peripheral angiopathy without gangrene	E10.51
Secondary: Atherosclerotic heart disease of native coronary artery without angina pectoris	I25.10

In the case of this patient, the ulcer has developed subsequent to the laceration in the diabetic patient. Guidance from Q1 2021 Coding Clinic indicates that in this type of case, the ulcer is a sequela of the laceration, and codes for both the diabetic ulcer and the laceration should be assigned, with the diabetic ulcer first listed, followed by the laceration, which should be identified as a sequela, with the 7th character 'S'. Because MSSA has been identified in the wound, B95.61 should be listed after the last code identifying this (same) wound to indicate the infection. A relationship is presumed between PVD and diabetes in ICD-10 based upon the "with" convention, so a combination code is assigned for diabetes with peripheral angiopathy (E10.51). No Z79 code is assigned to identify use of insulin because this patient is a type 1 diabetic and insulin use is assumed in these patients with no additional code needed.

Dermatitis due to dual incontinence

A 98-year-old woman is incontinent of urine and feces and was recently found to have excoriation of the skin around genital and buttocks areas caused by contact with urine and feces. She is morbidly obese with a BMI of 41 and the excessive moisture due to the incontinence has resulted in contact dermatitis as well as secondary candidal intertrigo of the skin folds of the buttocks and upper thighs. Skilled nursing will be teaching caregivers appropriate skin and incontinent care, managing healing of the secondary infection, and instructing on appropriate bedding and other products to reduce irritation of the skin.

Description	Code
Primary: Irritant contact dermatitis due to fecal, urinary or dual incontinence	L24.A2
Secondary: Erythema intertrigo	L30.4
Secondary: Candidiasis of skin and nail	B37.2
Secondary: Unspecified urinary incontinence	R32
Secondary: Full incontinence of feces	R15.9
Secondary: Morbid (severe) obesity due to excess calories	E66.01
Secondary: Body mass index [BMI] 40.0-44.9, adult	Z68.41

As the focus of care, dermatitis due to dual incontinence of urine and feces is coded in the primary position. It should be noted that this is a distinct condition and should not be confused with diaper dermatitis, which is excluded (excludes 1) from L24.A- conditions. The patient also has secondary candidal intertrigo which should be coded, as it is a separate condition and will significantly complicate the healing of her skin. Erythema intertrigo (L30.4) is an excludes 2 condition with L24.A- conditions, so these should both be separately coded, including both the code for the erythema intertrigo (L30.4) and secondary candidal infection (B37.2). The patient's obesity will also impact her recovery and should be coded with the current BMI. Her fecal and urine incontinence are coded with R32 and R15.9.

Chapter 13: Diseases of Musculoskeletal System and Connective Tissue (M00-M99)

Note that traumatic fracture codes and pathological fractures codes are ***not*** grouped together in ICD-10. Traumatic fracture codes are found in Chapter 19 (Injury, poisoning and certain other consequences of external causes), while codes for pathological fractures are found in Chapter 13 (Diseases of the Musculoskeletal System and Connective Tissue). This isn't a change from ICD-9, but it is a common mistake for coders to assume that all fractures are found in the same chapter.

"Connective tissue" is material that helps give tissue form and strength, including the structures around joints (cartilage, bursae, and synovial cavity). Chapter 13 includes conditions affecting bones, joints, muscles, ligaments, tendons and connective tissues. The conditions found in this chapter include inflammation, displacement, degeneration, and rupture of these structures.

Pathologic fractures (in which the bone is weakened by a disease, such as cancer or osteoporosis) are reported using codes in this chapter. Traumatic fractures (in which bone is broken by external force or violence), injuries to muscles and tendons, as well as dislocations, are reported using codes from Chapter 19 (Injury, poisoning, and certain other consequences of external causes).

Chapter 13 is divided into 18 blocks of similar conditions, which include:

- M00-M02 **Infectious arthropathies** are arthropathies due to microbiological agents that may result in direct infection of the joint or indirect infection which may be reactive or postinfective arthropathy.
- M04 **Autoinflammatory syndromes**
- M05-M14 **Inflammatory polyarthropathies** include conditions such as: ***rheumatoid arthritis***, an autoimmune disorder that causes chronic inflammation of the joints, particularly those in the hands and feet. It differs from other types of arthritis in that it affects the joint lining causing painful swelling that can eventually result in joint deformity; ***enteropathic arthropathies***, which are diseases of the joints associated or linked to gastrointestinal tract inflammation causing the joints to become inflamed and tender; and ***gout,*** which is a form of inflammatory polyarthropathy and includes acute idiopathic gout or chronic gout (category M1A). Gouty arthritis or crystal arthropathy is a form of arthritis caused by deposits of urate crystals around one or more joints; and villonodular synovitis, a condition that affects joints lined with synovial tissue.
- M15-M19 **Osteoarthritis**
- M20-M25 **Other joint disorders** includes acquired deformities of joints, recurrent dislocations, contractures, pain, stiffness and other joint disorders of upper and lower extremities.
- M26-M27 **Dentofacial anomalies** including malocclusion and other disorders of the jaw.
- M30-M36 **Systemic connective tissue disorders**, which include polyarteritis nodosa, necrotizing vasculopathies, systemic lupus erythematosis, scleroderma and manifestations of diseases classified elswhere
- M40-M43 **Deforming dorsopathies,** such as kyphosis, lordosis, scoliosis, osteochondrosis of spine.
- M45-M49 **Spondylopathies**, which is a degenerative or developmental anomaly of vertebrae, enthesopathy (disorders of ligamentous or muscular attachments of the spine), spondylosis (degenerative arthritis of spine), fatigue fracture of vertebra, collapsed vertebrae, and other disorders of spine.
- M50-M54 **Other dorsopathies**, include spinal disc disorders, radiculopathy, sciatica, lumbago, etc.
- M60-M63 **Disorders of muscles** such as myositis; paralytic calcification and ossification of muscles; non-traumatic separation, rupture and ischemic infarction of muscles; contracture of muscle; muscle wasting & atrophy; rhabdomyolysis, disintegration or destruction of muscle); and disorders of muscles in diseases classified elsewhere.
- M65-M67 **Disorders of synovium and tendon** such as synovitis/tenosynovitis; abscess of tendon sheath; calcific tendinitis; and spontaneous rupture of synovium & tendons;
- M70-M79 **Other soft tissue disorders**, including conditions related to use, overuse & pressure such as bursitis; calcium deposits; fibroblastic disorders; necrotizing fasciitis; non-traumatic rotator cuff tears; bone spurs; rheumatism; myalgia; pain in limbs; and nontraumatic compartment syndrome.
- M80-M85 **Disorders of bone density and structure** such as osteoporosis, pathological fractures, stress fractures; fibrous dysplasia; & bone cysts.
- M86-M90 **Other osteopathies** such as osteomyelitis; osteonecrosis; osteitis deformans (Paget's disease); algoneurodystrophy; disorders

of bone development; osteolysis and osteopathy; major osseous defect, and osteonecrosis in diseases classified elsewhere.

- M91-M94 **Chondropathies** (diseases of the cartilage)
- M95 **Other disorders of the musculoskeletal system and connective tissue**
- M96 **Intraoperative and post procedural complications and disorders** of the musculoskeletal system, not elsewhere classified
- M97 **Periprosthetic fracture around internal prosthetic joint**
- M99 **Biomechanical lesions, not elsewhere classified** such as segmental and somatic dysfunction; subluxation complex (vertebral); and stenosis of neural canal.

As noted by the contents in the blocks, the terminology is considerably different in ICD-10 than ICD-9 so a current medical dictionary will be a useful tool in determining the correct diagnosis. Refer to the term used in the physician's documentation in order to select the correct code. If the documentation is unclear, query the physician.

Sometimes a Chapter 13 code is not the most appropriate choice. The following chapters are all referenced in an Excludes 2 note at the start of the chapter.

- If the documentation indicates a **neoplasm or tumor of the bone, joint or connective tissue**, look up the term (malignancy, tumor, adenoma, or specific name) in the Alphabetical index and verify the correct code in the Tabular List, most likely a code from Chapter 2. The Alpha Index will direct the coder to the neoplasm table and the correct column to use.
- This chapter includes some general **symptom codes**, such as pain in joint (category M25.-), low back pain (M54.5-), and pain in limb (subcategory M79.6-). Symptoms may be reported using codes from Chapter 18, such as difficulty walking (R26.2), symptoms involving nervous and musculoskeletal systems (R29.9-); abnormality of gait (R26.9) and lack of coordination (R27.9). Every effort should be made to secure a definitive diagnosis. A symptom code may be reported as an additional diagnosis when it indicates a significant aspect of the condition, but is not an integral part of it. If the documentation is unclear, query the physician.
- If a patient has a **personal or family history** of a condition reported in this chapter, it may be appropriate to select from the Z code section, such as Z85.830 (Personal history of malignant neoplasm, bone), Z87.311 (Personal history of pathologic fracture), Z87.312 (Personal history of stress fracture), Z82.61 (Family history of arthritis), or Z82.62 (Family history of osteoporosis).

There is an Excludes 2 note at the beginning of chapter 13 that indicates the following situations are not included in Chapter 13 codes, but may be coded in addition, if applicable to the situation. Code selection and sequencing will be determined by finding the code in the Alphabetical Index and verifying it in the Tabular as well as following all instructional notes. Take note of the following conditions **not** included in Chapter 13:

- arthropathic psoriasis (L40.5-)
- certain conditions originating in the perinatal period (P00-P96)
- certain infections and parasitic diseases (A00-B99)
- compartment syndrome (traumatic) (T79.A-)
- complications of pregnancy, childbirth and the puerperium (O00-O9A)
- congenital malformations, deformations, and chromosomal abnormalities (Q00-Q99)
- endocrine, nutritional and metabolic diseases (E00-E88)
- injury, poisoning and certain other consequences of external causes (S00-T88)
- neoplasms (C00-D49)
- symptoms, signs and abnormal clinical and laboratory findings, not elsewhere classified (R00-R94)

General Guidance

Site and laterality

Most of the codes within this chapter have site and laterality designations. The site represents the bone, joint or muscle involved. For some conditions, when more than one bone, joint or muscle is usually involved, such as osteoarthritis, there is a "multiple sites" code available, for example, M15.3, Secondary multiple arthritis. There also are codes to indicate bilateral presence of the condition, such as M16.0, bilateral primary osteoarthritis of hip.

For categories where no multiple site code is provided and more than one bone, joint or muscle is involved, multiple codes should be used to indicate the different sites involved. For example, code both M62.251 and M62.261 for nontraumatic ischemic infarction of muscle right thigh and right lower leg.

Bone versus joint

For certain conditions, the bone may be affected at the upper or lower end (e.g., avascular necrosis of the bone (M87), and osteoporosis (M80, M81). Though the portion of the bone affected may be at the joint, the site designation will be the bone, not the joint. Examples include M87.022, idiopathic avascular necrosis of left humerus; or M80.061D, Subsequent encounter for age related osteoporosis with routine healing of current pathological fracture, right lower leg.

Acute traumatic versus chronic or recurrent musculoskeletal conditions

Many musculoskeletal conditions are a result of previous injury or trauma to a site, or are recurrent conditions. Bone, joint or muscle conditions that are a result of a healed injury or a recurrent condition are usually found in Chapter 13. However, any current acute injury should be coded to the appropriate injury code from Chapter 19. If it is difficult to determine from the documentation in the record which code is best to describe a condition, query the provider.

Coding pathological fractures

Pathological fracture codes are combination codes that include a 7th character to indicate whether the care encounter is initial, subsequent or sequela. The 7th character A is used as long as the patient is receiving active treatment for the fracture. Examples of active treatment are: surgical treatment, emergency department encounter, evaluation and treatment by a new physician. The 7th character D is used for encounters for routine healing after the patient has completed active treatment. The remaining 7th characters, listed under each subcategory in the Tabular List, are to be used for subsequent encounters for treatment of problems associated with the healing, such as delayed healing, malunions, nonunions, and sequelae.

Care for complications of surgical treatment for fracture repairs during the healing or recovery phase should be coded as appropriate complication codes.

Multiple Coding and Sequencing

It is important to read the Includes and Excludes notes under codes in this chapter, as well as any other instructions under the code or code category.

Note, there is an instructional note at the beginning of Chapter 13 that states: use an external cause code following the code for the musculoskeletal condition, if applicable, to identify the cause of the musculoskeletal condition.

Here are some examples of multiple coding and sequencing issues for codes in this chapter:

- **Infectious arthropathies** include pyogenic arthritis (category M00) that include codes for arthritis caused by microbiological organisms of specific joints. Several of the subcategories have an instructional note to add an additional code to identify the bacterial agent. For example, Staphylococcal arthritis, right hip, requires two codes, M00.051 as the first-listed code followed by a code from B95.61-B95.8 to identify the type of staphylococcus involved.
- Codes from category M01, **direct infections of joints** due to infectious and parasitic diseases classified elsewhere, and category M02, postinfective and reactive arthropathies, have a code first note to code the underlying disease that refers to infection codes in chapter 1. The code from chapter 1 is reported as the first-listed code followed by the code from chapter 13.
- Some codes require you to code also any associated conditions, For example, codes from category M07 (**enteropathic arthopathies**) require you to code also any associated enteropathy, such as regional enteritis (Crohn's disease K50- or ulcerative colitis K51-). Also category M08 (juvenile arthritis) instructs to code also any associated underlying conditions as an additional code.
- Code category M63 (**disorders of muscles in diseases classified elsewhere**) requires a code first for the underlying disease from chapter 1.

Throughout Chapter 13, there are many categories that include notes to code first or use an additional code for adverse effect, if applicable, to identify the drug (T36-T50 with fifth or sixth character 5). An example is M81.8 (Drug-induced osteoporosis without current pathological fracture).

Special Coding Issues

Fractures

Spontaneous chronic or pathological fractures are reported using codes from this chapter (subcategory M84.4-), while pathological fractures in neoplastic disease are coded at subcategory M84.5- with a note to code also the underlying neoplasm. Stress fractures are coded to subcategory M84.3, while fatigue fractures of the vertebrae are coded to subcategory M48.4- and collapsed fractures of the vertebra are coded to M48.5-.

All of the pathological, stress, fatigue, and collapsed fractures require the appropriate 7th character to indicate whether the encounter is initial, subsequent or a sequela. There are specific 7th character designations for subsequent encounter for fractures with routine healing, delayed healing, and with nonunion or malunion. **Aftercare codes for healing pathological fractures are not used in ICD-10-CM.**

Traumatic fractures are assigned the appropriate code by site and type of fracture from Chapter 19 (Injury, poisoning and certain other consequences of external causes (S00-S99)).

Report a code from M97 for fractures around a prosthesis that are not complications of the prosthesis, but the result of the same conditions as other fractures, that is, trauma or pathological conditions. Periprosthetic fractures can occur around any prosthesis, but the most common would be the hip, knee, ankle, shoulder, or elbow.

Code T84 includes all of the complications of orthopedic prostheses, implants and grafts. Periprosthetic fractures are not considered complications and can be found in M97. Subcategory T84.0 includes complications of internal prosthetic joints. Most include the joint affected, so there is no need to add Z96.6 for the joint unless the complication code does not indicate the joint. A code from M96.6- or M97.- may provide additional information.

Joint replacements

Continue to assign the injury code for patient who underwent a joint replacement to treat a hip fracture. The aftercare code Z47.1 (Aftercare following joint replacement surgery) is ***not*** *appropriate* in these types of scenarios, according to the Coding Clinic Q3 2016 guidance.

Osteoporosis

Osteoporosis is a systemic condition, meaning that all bones of the musculoskeletal system are affected. Therefore site is not a component of the codes under M81, Osteoporosis without current pathological fracture. The site codes under category M80, Osteoporosis with current pathological fracture, identify the site of the fracture, not the osteoporosis.

Osteoporosis without current pathological fracture, Category M81, is used for patients with osteoporosis who do not currently have a pathological fracture due to osteoporosis, even if they had one in the past. For patients with a history of osteoporosis fractures, status code Z87.310 (Personal history of (healed) osteoporosis fracture) should follow the code from M81.

Category M80, Osteoporosis with current pathological fracture, is for patients who have a current pathological fracture at the time of the encounter. The codes under M80 identify the site of the fracture. A code from M80, not a traumatic fracture code, should be used for any patient with known osteoporosis who suffers a fracture, even if the patient had a minor fall or trauma, if that fall or trauma would not usually break a normal, healthy bone.

Arthropathies (M00-M25)

It is incorrect to code an arthropathy and pain in joint separately because pain is integral to the disease.

ICD-10-CM has greatly expanded the codes for arthropathies addressing them in multiple blocks and including many instructional notes within the code categories. Specific sites and laterality are included in the combination codes.

Osteoarthritis

Osteoarthritis also is referred to as degenerative arthritis or degenerative joint disease. It is the most common form of inflammatory joint disease, caused by deterioration of the cartilage that covers the ends of the bones and typically occurs slowly over a long period of time. As the cartilage deteriorates, it becomes rough and causes irritation of the joint. As deterioration continues, the bone itself becomes exposed and eventually joint movement results in bone rubbing against bone, causing pain and damage to the bone itself. When coding osteoarthritis, differentiate between primary and secondary.

Primary osteoarthritis is without a specific known cause other than the progressive wearing down of the cartilage in the joints and is also referred to as idiopathic osteoarthopathy. Codes by specific site are found at categories M15-M19. Primary arthritis NOS or unspecified osteoarthritis, unspecified site, is coded as M19.90.

Secondary osteoarthritis refers to degenerative disease of the synovial joints that results from some predisposing condition, such as trauma/injury, or the result of congenital or other disease that has adversely altered the articular cartilage and/or subchondral bone of the affected joints. Secondary osteoarthritis codes are found in ICD-10-CM at M19.2- (Secondary osteoarthritis of other joints), or M89.4- in the Tabular defined as Other hypertrophic osteoarthropathy by site.

Code osteoarthritis in a patient's joint as primary osteoarthritis if the type of OA, such as primary, secondary or generalized, is not specified. "When the type of osteoarthritis is not specified, "primary" is the default." For example, you should assign M16.0 (Bilateral primary osteoarthritis of hip) for a patient documented has having bilateral osteoarthritis of the hips, according to Q4 2016 Coding Clinic guidance.

When coding arthritis conditions, you must:

- specify the type of arthritis (rheumatoid, infective/ pyogenic, reactive/Reiter's disease, osteoarthritis,/ degenerative, etc); ***and***
- specify the site – do not use multiple sites code; code each affected site separately. M12.9 is arthropathy unspecified, so it is the best choice if information about the specific type of arthritis is unknown. Traumatic arthropathy (subcategory M12.5-) is an example of a residual effect that occurred because of an injury in the past, but excludes a current injury. Consider this example: The patient fractured her right ankle three years ago and now has arthritis in that ankle (M12.571).

In its early stages, Charcot's arthropathy (M14.60-), also known as neuropathic arthropathy, often is confused with osteoarthritis (OA). Some pain, a prominent and often hemorrhagic effusion, and subluxation and instability of the joint are usually present. Acute joint dislocation sometimes occurs at this stage. Neurogenic arthropathy progresses more rapidly than OA. Arthropathy may not develop until long after onset of the neuropathic condition, but can progress rapidly and lead to complete joint disorganization in a few months.

If the patient has Charcot's joints arthropathy due to diabetes type 2, the correct code would be a combination code E11.610 from chapter 4.

CHAPTER 13: DISEASES OF THE MUSCULOSKELETAL SYSTEM AND CONNECTIVE TISSUE (M00-M99)

Note:
Use an external cause code following the code for the musculoskeletal condition, if applicable, to identify the cause of the musculoskeletal condition

EXCLUDES 2 arthropathic psoriasis (L40.5-)
certain conditions originating in the perinatal period (P04-P96)
certain infectious and parasitic diseases (A00-B99)
compartment syndrome (traumatic) (T79.A-)
complications of pregnancy, childbirth and the puerperium (O00-O9A)
congenital malformations, deformations, and chromosomal abnormalities (Q00-Q99)
endocrine, nutritional and metabolic diseases (E00-E88)
injury, poisoning and certain other consequences of external causes (S00-T88)
neoplasms (C00-D49)
symptoms, signs and abnormal clinical and laboratory findings, not elsewhere classified (R00-R94)

GUIDELINES **Section I.C.13.a**
Most of the codes within Chapter 13 have site and laterality designations. The site represents the bone, joint or the muscle involved. For some conditions where more than one bone, joint or muscle is usually involved, such as osteoarthritis, there is a "multiple sites" code available. For categories where no multiple site code is provided and more than one bone, joint or muscle is involved, multiple codes should be used to indicate the different sites involved.

GUIDELINES **Section I.C.13.a.1)**
For certain conditions, the bone may be affected at the upper or lower end, (e.g., avascular necrosis of bone, M87, Osteoporosis, M80, M81). Though the portion of the bone affected may be at the joint, the site designation will be the bone, not the joint.

GUIDELINES **Section I.C.13.b**
Many musculoskeletal conditions are a result of previous injury or trauma to a site, or are recurrent conditions. Bone, joint or muscle conditions that are the result of a healed injury are usually found in chapter 13. Recurrent bone, joint or muscle conditions are also usually found in chapter 13. Any current, acute injury should be coded to the appropriate injury code from chapter 19. Chronic or recurrent conditions should generally be coded with a code from chapter 13. If it is difficult to determine from the documentation in the record which code is best to describe a condition, query the provider.

This chapter contains the following blocks:

M00-M02	Infectious arthropathies
M04	Autoinflammatory syndromes
M05-M14	Inflammatory polyarthropathies
M15-M19	Osteoarthritis
M20-M25	Other joint disorders
M26-M27	Dentofacial anomalies [including malocclusion] and other disorders of jaw
M30-M36	Systemic connective tissue disorders
M40-M43	Deforming dorsopathies
M45-M49	Spondylopathies
M50-M54	Other dorsopathies
M60-M63	Disorders of muscles
M65-M67	Disorders of synovium and tendon
M70-M79	Other soft tissue disorders
M80-M85	Disorders of bone density and structure
M86-M90	Other osteopathies
M91-M94	Chondropathies
M95	Other disorders of the musculoskeletal system and connective tissue
M96	Intraoperative and postprocedural complications and disorders of musculoskeletal system, not elsewhere classified
M97	Periprosthetic fracture around internal prosthetic joint
M99	Biomechanical lesions, not elsewhere classified

Arthropathies (M00-M25)

INCLUDES Disorders affecting predominantly peripheral (limb) joints

Infectious arthropathies (M00-M02)

Note:
This block comprises arthropathies due to microbiological agents. Distinction is made between the following types of etiological relationship:
a) direct infection of joint, where organisms invade synovial tissue and microbial antigen is present in the joint;
b) indirect infection, which may be of two types: a reactive arthropathy, where microbial infection of the body is established but neither organisms nor antigens can be identified in the joint, and a postinfective arthropathy, where microbial antigen is present but recovery of an organism is inconstant and evidence of local multiplication is lacking.

4 **M00 Pyogenic arthritis**
EXCLUDES 2 infection and inflammatory reaction due to internal joint prosthesis (T84.5-)
CODING TIPS✓ Also known as septic joint or septic arthritis, M00.- may be coded in addition to the infection/inflammation of a joint prosthesis.

+ 5 **M00.0 Staphylococcal arthritis and polyarthritis**
Use additional code (B95.61-B95.8) to identify bacterial agent

IQ + **M00.00 Staphylococcal arthritis, unspecified joint**

+ 6 **M00.01 Staphylococcal arthritis, shoulder**
Laterality SP + **M00.011 Staphylococcal arthritis, right shoulder**
Laterality SP + **M00.012 Staphylococcal arthritis, left shoulder**
Laterality IQ + **M00.019 Staphylococcal arthritis, unspecified shoulder**

+ 6 **M00.02 Staphylococcal arthritis, elbow**
Laterality SP + **M00.021 Staphylococcal arthritis, right elbow**
Laterality SP + **M00.022 Staphylococcal arthritis, left elbow**
Laterality IQ + **M00.029 Staphylococcal arthritis, unspecified elbow**

+ 6 **M00.03 Staphylococcal arthritis, wrist**
Staphylococcal arthritis of carpal bones
Laterality SP + **M00.031 Staphylococcal arthritis, right wrist**
Laterality SP + **M00.032 Staphylococcal arthritis, left wrist**
Laterality IQ + **M00.039 Staphylococcal arthritis, unspecified wrist**

+ 6 **M00.04 Staphylococcal arthritis, hand**

Staphylococcal arthritis of metacarpus and phalanges

SP + **M00.041 Staphylococcal arthritis, right hand**

SP + **M00.042 Staphylococcal arthritis, left hand**

!Q + **M00.049 Staphylococcal arthritis, unspecified hand**

+ 6 **M00.05 Staphylococcal arthritis, hip**

SP + **M00.051 Staphylococcal arthritis, right hip**

SP + **M00.052 Staphylococcal arthritis, left hip**

!Q + **M00.059 Staphylococcal arthritis, unspecified hip**

+ 6 **M00.06 Staphylococcal arthritis, knee**

SP + **M00.061 Staphylococcal arthritis, right knee**

SP + **M00.062 Staphylococcal arthritis, left knee**

!Q + **M00.069 Staphylococcal arthritis, unspecified knee**

+ 6 **M00.07 Staphylococcal arthritis, ankle and foot**

Staphylococcal arthritis, tarsus, metatarsus and phalanges

SP + **M00.071 Staphylococcal arthritis, right ankle and foot**

SP + **M00.072 Staphylococcal arthritis, left ankle and foot**

!Q + **M00.079 Staphylococcal arthritis, unspecified ankle and foot**

SP + **M00.08 Staphylococcal arthritis, vertebrae**

SP + **M00.09 Staphylococcal polyarthritis**

5 **M00.1 Pneumococcal arthritis and polyarthritis**

!Q **M00.10 Pneumococcal arthritis, unspecified joint**

6 **M00.11 Pneumococcal arthritis, shoulder**

SP **M00.111 Pneumococcal arthritis, right shoulder**

SP **M00.112 Pneumococcal arthritis, left shoulder**

!Q **M00.119 Pneumococcal arthritis, unspecified shoulder**

6 **M00.12 Pneumococcal arthritis, elbow**

SP **M00.121 Pneumococcal arthritis, right elbow**

SP **M00.122 Pneumococcal arthritis, left elbow**

!Q **M00.129 Pneumococcal arthritis, unspecified elbow**

6 **M00.13 Pneumococcal arthritis, wrist**

Pneumococcal arthritis of carpal bones

SP **M00.131 Pneumococcal arthritis, right wrist**

SP **M00.132 Pneumococcal arthritis, left wrist**

!Q **M00.139 Pneumococcal arthritis, unspecified wrist**

6 **M00.14 Pneumococcal arthritis, hand**

Pneumococcal arthritis of metacarpus and phalanges

SP **M00.141 Pneumococcal arthritis, right hand**

SP **M00.142 Pneumococcal arthritis, left hand**

!Q **M00.149 Pneumococcal arthritis, unspecified hand**

6 **M00.15 Pneumococcal arthritis, hip**

SP **M00.151 Pneumococcal arthritis, right hip**

SP **M00.152 Pneumococcal arthritis, left hip**

!Q **M00.159 Pneumococcal arthritis, unspecified hip**

6 **M00.16 Pneumococcal arthritis, knee**

SP **M00.161 Pneumococcal arthritis, right knee**

SP **M00.162 Pneumococcal arthritis, left knee**

!Q **M00.169 Pneumococcal arthritis, unspecified knee**

6 **M00.17 Pneumococcal arthritis, ankle and foot**

Pneumococcal arthritis, tarsus, metatarsus and phalanges

SP **M00.171 Pneumococcal arthritis, right ankle and foot**

SP **M00.172 Pneumococcal arthritis, left ankle and foot**

!Q **M00.179 Pneumococcal arthritis, unspecified ankle and foot**

SP **M00.18 Pneumococcal arthritis, vertebrae**

SP **M00.19 Pneumococcal polyarthritis**

+ 5 **M00.2 Other streptococcal arthritis and polyarthritis**

Use additional code (B95.0-B95.2, B95.4-B95.5) to identify bacterial agent

!Q + **M00.20 Other streptococcal arthritis, unspecified joint**

+ 6 **M00.21 Other streptococcal arthritis, shoulder**

SP + **M00.211 Other streptococcal arthritis, right shoulder**

SP + **M00.212 Other streptococcal arthritis, left shoulder**

!Q + **M00.219 Other streptococcal arthritis, unspecified shoulder**

+ 6 **M00.22 Other streptococcal arthritis, elbow**

SP + **M00.221 Other streptococcal arthritis, right elbow**

SP + **M00.222 Other streptococcal arthritis, left elbow**

!Q + **M00.229 Other streptococcal arthritis, unspecified elbow**

+ 6 **M00.23 Other streptococcal arthritis, wrist**

Other streptococcal arthritis of carpal bones

SP + **M00.231 Other streptococcal arthritis, right wrist**

SP + **M00.232 Other streptococcal arthritis, left wrist**

!Q + **M00.239 Other streptococcal arthritis, unspecified wrist**

+ 6 **M00.24 Other streptococcal arthritis, hand**

Other streptococcal arthritis metacarpus and phalanges

SP + **M00.241 Other streptococcal arthritis, right hand**

SP + **M00.242 Other streptococcal arthritis, left hand**

!Q + **M00.249 Other streptococcal arthritis, unspecified hand**

+ 6 **M00.25 Other streptococcal arthritis, hip**

SP + **M00.251 Other streptococcal arthritis, right hip**

Chapter 13

M00-M99

⊟ SP + M00.252 Other streptococcal arthritis, left hip

⊟ IQ + M00.259 Other streptococcal arthritis, unspecified hip

+ 6 M00.26 Other streptococcal arthritis, knee

⊟ SP + M00.261 Other streptococcal arthritis, right knee

⊟ SP + M00.262 Other streptococcal arthritis, left knee

⊟ IQ + M00.269 Other streptococcal arthritis, unspecified knee

+ 6 M00.27 Other streptococcal arthritis, ankle and foot
Other streptococcal arthritis, tarsus, metatarsus and phalanges

⊟ SP + M00.271 Other streptococcal arthritis, right ankle and foot

⊟ SP + M00.272 Other streptococcal arthritis, left ankle and foot

⊟ IQ + M00.279 Other streptococcal arthritis, unspecified ankle and foot

SP + M00.28 Other streptococcal arthritis, vertebrae

SP + M00.29 Other streptococcal polyarthritis

+ 5 M00.8 Arthritis and polyarthritis due to other bacteria
Use additional code (B96) to identify bacteria

IQ + M00.80 Arthritis due to other bacteria, unspecified joint

+ 6 M00.81 Arthritis due to other bacteria, shoulder

⊟ SP + M00.811 Arthritis due to other bacteria, right shoulder

⊟ SP + M00.812 Arthritis due to other bacteria, left shoulder

⊟ IQ + M00.819 Arthritis due to other bacteria, unspecified shoulder

+ 6 M00.82 Arthritis due to other bacteria, elbow

⊟ SP + M00.821 Arthritis due to other bacteria, right elbow

⊟ SP + M00.822 Arthritis due to other bacteria, left elbow

⊟ IQ + M00.829 Arthritis due to other bacteria, unspecified elbow

+ 6 M00.83 Arthritis due to other bacteria, wrist
Arthritis due to other bacteria, carpal bones

⊟ SP + M00.831 Arthritis due to other bacteria, right wrist

⊟ SP + M00.832 Arthritis due to other bacteria, left wrist

⊟ IQ + M00.839 Arthritis due to other bacteria, unspecified wrist

+ 6 M00.84 Arthritis due to other bacteria, hand
Arthritis due to other bacteria, metacarpus and phalanges

⊟ SP + M00.841 Arthritis due to other bacteria, right hand

⊟ SP + M00.842 Arthritis due to other bacteria, left hand

⊟ IQ + M00.849 Arthritis due to other bacteria, unspecified hand

+ 6 M00.85 Arthritis due to other bacteria, hip

⊟ SP + M00.851 Arthritis due to other bacteria, right hip

⊟ SP + M00.852 Arthritis due to other bacteria, left hip

⊟ IQ + M00.859 Arthritis due to other bacteria, unspecified hip

+ 6 M00.86 Arthritis due to other bacteria, knee

⊟ SP + M00.861 Arthritis due to other bacteria, right knee

⊟ SP + M00.862 Arthritis due to other bacteria, left knee

⊟ IQ + M00.869 Arthritis due to other bacteria, unspecified knee

+ 6 M00.87 Arthritis due to other bacteria, ankle and foot
Arthritis due to other bacteria, tarsus, metatarsus, and phalanges

⊟ SP + M00.871 Arthritis due to other bacteria, right ankle and foot

⊟ SP + M00.872 Arthritis due to other bacteria, left ankle and foot

⊟ IQ + M00.879 Arthritis due to other bacteria, unspecified ankle and foot

SP + M00.88 Arthritis due to other bacteria, vertebrae

SP + M00.89 Polyarthritis due to other bacteria

SP M00.9 Pyogenic arthritis, unspecified
Infective arthritis NOS

4 M01 Direct infections of joint in infectious and parasitic diseases classified elsewhere
Code first underlying disease, such as:
- leprosy [Hansen's disease] (A30.-)
- mycoses (B35-B49)
- O'nyong-nyong fever (A92.1)
- paratyphoid fever (A01.1-A01.4)

EXCLUDES 1
- arthropathy in Lyme disease (A69.23)
- gonococcal arthritis (A54.42)
- meningococcal arthritis (A39.83)
- mumps arthritis (B26.85)
- postinfective arthropathy (M02.-)
- postmeningococcal arthritis (A39.84)
- reactive arthritis (M02.3)
- rubella arthritis (B06.82)
- sarcoidosis arthritis (D86.86)
- typhoid fever arthritis (A01.04)
- tuberculosis arthritis (A18.01-A18.02)

5 M01.X Direct infection of joint in infectious and parasitic diseases classified elsewhere

M IQ M01.X0 *Direct infection of unspecified joint in infectious and parasitic diseases classified elsewhere*

6 M01.X1 Direct infection of shoulder joint in infectious and parasitic diseases classified elsewhere

M ⊟ IQ M01.X11 *Direct infection of right shoulder in infectious and parasitic diseases classified elsewhere*

M ⊟ IQ M01.X12 *Direct infection of left shoulder in infectious and parasitic diseases classified elsewhere*

M ⊟ IQ **M01.X19** *Direct infection of unspecified shoulder in infectious and parasitic diseases classified elsewhere*

6 **M01.X2 Direct infection of elbow in infectious and parasitic diseases classified elsewhere**

M ⊟ IQ **M01.X21** *Direct infection of right elbow in infectious and parasitic diseases classified elsewhere*

M ⊟ IQ **M01.X22** *Direct infection of left elbow in infectious and parasitic diseases classified elsewhere*

M ⊟ IQ **M01.X29** *Direct infection of unspecified elbow in infectious and parasitic diseases classified elsewhere*

6 **M01.X3 Direct infection of wrist in infectious and parasitic diseases classified elsewhere**

Direct infection of carpal bones in infectious and parasitic diseases classified elsewhere

M ⊟ IQ **M01.X31** *Direct infection of right wrist in infectious and parasitic diseases classified elsewhere*

M ⊟ IQ **M01.X32** *Direct infection of left wrist in infectious and parasitic diseases classified elsewhere*

M ⊟ IQ **M01.X39** *Direct infection of unspecified wrist in infectious and parasitic diseases classified elsewhere*

6 **M01.X4 Direct infection of hand in infectious and parasitic diseases classified elsewhere**

Direct infection of metacarpus and phalanges in infectious and parasitic diseases classified elsewhere

M ⊟ IQ **M01.X41** *Direct infection of right hand in infectious and parasitic diseases classified elsewhere*

M ⊟ IQ **M01.X42** *Direct infection of left hand in infectious and parasitic diseases classified elsewhere*

M ⊟ IQ **M01.X49** *Direct infection of unspecified hand in infectious and parasitic diseases classified elsewhere*

6 **M01.X5 Direct infection of hip in infectious and parasitic diseases classified elsewhere**

M ⊟ IQ **M01.X51** *Direct infection of right hip in infectious and parasitic diseases classified elsewhere*

M ⊟ IQ **M01.X52** *Direct infection of left hip in infectious and parasitic diseases classified elsewhere*

M ⊟ IQ **M01.X59** *Direct infection of unspecified hip in infectious and parasitic diseases classified elsewhere*

6 **M01.X6 Direct infection of knee in infectious and parasitic diseases classified elsewhere**

M ⊟ IQ **M01.X61** *Direct infection of right knee in infectious and parasitic diseases classified elsewhere*

M ⊟ IQ **M01.X62** *Direct infection of left knee in infectious and parasitic diseases classified elsewhere*

M ⊟ IQ **M01.X69** *Direct infection of unspecified knee in infectious and parasitic diseases classified elsewhere*

6 **M01.X7 Direct infection of ankle and foot in infectious and parasitic diseases classified elsewhere**

Direct infection of tarsus, metatarsus and phalanges in infectious and parasitic diseases classified elsewhere

M ⊟ IQ **M01.X71** *Direct infection of right ankle and foot in infectious and parasitic diseases classified elsewhere*

M ⊟ IQ **M01.X72** *Direct infection of left ankle and foot in infectious and parasitic diseases classified elsewhere*

M ⊟ IQ **M01.X79** *Direct infection of unspecified ankle and foot in infectious and parasitic diseases classified elsewhere*

M IQ **M01.X8** *Direct infection of vertebrae in infectious and parasitic diseases classified elsewhere*

M IQ **M01.X9** *Direct infection of multiple joints in infectious and parasitic diseases classified elsewhere*

4 **M02 Postinfective and reactive arthropathies**

Code first underlying disease, such as:
- congenital syphilis [Clutton's joints] (A50.5)
- enteritis due to Yersinia enterocolitica (A04.6)
- infective endocarditis (I33.0)
- viral hepatitis (B15-B19)

EXCLUDES 1 Behçet's disease (M35.2)
- direct infections of joint in infectious and parasitic diseases classified elsewhere (M01.-)
- postmeningococcal arthritis (A39.84)
- mumps arthritis (B26.85)
- rubella arthritis (B06.82)
- syphilis arthritis (late) (A52.77)
- rheumatic fever (I00)
- tabetic arthropathy [Charcôt's] (A52.16)

CODING TIPS ✓ M02.- codes indicate arthropathy due to another cause. The identified underlying cause should be coded first.

5 **M02.0 Arthropathy following intestinal bypass**

IQ **M02.00** **Arthropathy following intestinal bypass, unspecified site**

6 **M02.01 Arthropathy following intestinal bypass, shoulder**

⊟ IQ **M02.011 Arthropathy following intestinal bypass, right shoulder**

⊟ IQ **M02.012 Arthropathy following intestinal bypass, left shoulder**

⊟ IQ **M02.019** **Arthropathy following intestinal bypass, unspecified shoulder**

6 **M02.02 Arthropathy following intestinal bypass, elbow**
- **M02.021 Arthropathy following intestinal bypass, right elbow**
- **M02.022 Arthropathy following intestinal bypass, left elbow**
- **M02.029 Arthropathy following intestinal bypass, unspecified elbow**

6 **M02.03 Arthropathy following intestinal bypass, wrist**
Arthropathy following intestinal bypass, carpal bones
- **M02.031 Arthropathy following intestinal bypass, right wrist**
- **M02.032 Arthropathy following intestinal bypass, left wrist**
- **M02.039 Arthropathy following intestinal bypass, unspecified wrist**

6 **M02.04 Arthropathy following intestinal bypass, hand**
Arthropathy following intestinal bypass, metacarpals and phalanges
- **M02.041 Arthropathy following intestinal bypass, right hand**
- **M02.042 Arthropathy following intestinal bypass, left hand**
- **M02.049 Arthropathy following intestinal bypass, unspecified hand**

6 **M02.05 Arthropathy following intestinal bypass, hip**
- **M02.051 Arthropathy following intestinal bypass, right hip**
- **M02.052 Arthropathy following intestinal bypass, left hip**
- **M02.059 Arthropathy following intestinal bypass, unspecified hip**

6 **M02.06 Arthropathy following intestinal bypass, knee**
- **M02.061 Arthropathy following intestinal bypass, right knee**
- **M02.062 Arthropathy following intestinal bypass, left knee**
- **M02.069 Arthropathy following intestinal bypass, unspecified knee**

6 **M02.07 Arthropathy following intestinal bypass, ankle and foot**
Arthropathy following intestinal bypass, tarsus, metatarsus and phalanges
- **M02.071 Arthropathy following intestinal bypass, right ankle and foot**
- **M02.072 Arthropathy following intestinal bypass, left ankle and foot**
- **M02.079 Arthropathy following intestinal bypass, unspecified ankle and foot**

M02.08 Arthropathy following intestinal bypass, vertebrae

M02.09 Arthropathy following intestinal bypass, multiple sites

5 **M02.1 Postdysenteric arthropathy**

M02.10 Postdysenteric arthropathy, unspecified site

6 **M02.11 Postdysenteric arthropathy, shoulder**
- **M02.111 Postdysenteric arthropathy, right shoulder**
- **M02.112 Postdysenteric arthropathy, left shoulder**
- **M02.119 Postdysenteric arthropathy, unspecified shoulder**

6 **M02.12 Postdysenteric arthropathy, elbow**
- **M02.121 Postdysenteric arthropathy, right elbow**
- **M02.122 Postdysenteric arthropathy, left elbow**
- **M02.129 Postdysenteric arthropathy, unspecified elbow**

6 **M02.13 Postdysenteric arthropathy, wrist**
Postdysenteric arthropathy, carpal bones
- **M02.131 Postdysenteric arthropathy, right wrist**
- **M02.132 Postdysenteric arthropathy, left wrist**
- **M02.139 Postdysenteric arthropathy, unspecified wrist**

6 **M02.14 Postdysenteric arthropathy, hand**
Postdysenteric arthropathy, metacarpus and phalanges
- **M02.141 Postdysenteric arthropathy, right hand**
- **M02.142 Postdysenteric arthropathy, left hand**
- **M02.149 Postdysenteric arthropathy, unspecified hand**

6 **M02.15 Postdysenteric arthropathy, hip**
- **M02.151 Postdysenteric arthropathy, right hip**
- **M02.152 Postdysenteric arthropathy, left hip**
- **M02.159 Postdysenteric arthropathy, unspecified hip**

6 **M02.16 Postdysenteric arthropathy, knee**
- **M02.161 Postdysenteric arthropathy, right knee**
- **M02.162 Postdysenteric arthropathy, left knee**
- **M02.169 Postdysenteric arthropathy, unspecified knee**

6 **M02.17 Postdysenteric arthropathy, ankle and foot**
Postdysenteric arthropathy, tarsus, metatarsus and phalanges
- **M02.171 Postdysenteric arthropathy, right ankle and foot**
- **M02.172 Postdysenteric arthropathy, left ankle and foot**
- **M02.179 Postdysenteric arthropathy, unspecified ankle and foot**

M02.18 Postdysenteric arthropathy, vertebrae

M02.19 Postdysenteric arthropathy, multiple sites

5 **M02.2 Postimmunization arthropathy**

M02.20 Postimmunization arthropathy, unspecified site

6 **M02.21 Postimmunization arthropathy, shoulder**
- **M02.211 Postimmunization arthropathy, right shoulder**
- **M02.212 Postimmunization arthropathy, left shoulder**

4 4th digit required 5 5th digit required 6 6th digit required 7 7th digit required 7th digit placeholder + Additional code Laterality

M02.219 Postimmunization arthropathy, unspecified shoulder

M02.22 Postimmunization arthropathy, elbow

M02.221 Postimmunization arthropathy, right elbow

M02.222 Postimmunization arthropathy, left elbow

M02.229 Postimmunization arthropathy, unspecified elbow

M02.23 Postimmunization arthropathy, wrist
Postimmunization arthropathy, carpal bones

M02.231 Postimmunization arthropathy, right wrist

M02.232 Postimmunization arthropathy, left wrist

M02.239 Postimmunization arthropathy, unspecified wrist

M02.24 Postimmunization arthropathy, hand
Postimmunization arthropathy, metacarpus and phalanges

M02.241 Postimmunization arthropathy, right hand

M02.242 Postimmunization arthropathy, left hand

M02.249 Postimmunization arthropathy, unspecified hand

M02.25 Postimmunization arthropathy, hip

M02.251 Postimmunization arthropathy, right hip

M02.252 Postimmunization arthropathy, left hip

M02.259 Postimmunization arthropathy, unspecified hip

M02.26 Postimmunization arthropathy, knee

M02.261 Postimmunization arthropathy, right knee

M02.262 Postimmunization arthropathy, left knee

M02.269 Postimmunization arthropathy, unspecified knee

M02.27 Postimmunization arthropathy, ankle and foot
Postimmunization arthropathy, tarsus, metatarsus and phalanges

M02.271 Postimmunization arthropathy, right ankle and foot

M02.272 Postimmunization arthropathy, left ankle and foot

M02.279 Postimmunization arthropathy, unspecified ankle and foot

M02.28 Postimmunization arthropathy, vertebrae

M02.29 Postimmunization arthropathy, multiple sites

M02.3 Reiter's disease
Reactive arthritis

M02.30 Reiter's disease, unspecified site

M02.31 Reiter's disease, shoulder

M02.311 Reiter's disease, right shoulder

M02.312 Reiter's disease, left shoulder

M02.319 Reiter's disease, unspecified shoulder

M02.32 Reiter's disease, elbow

M02.321 Reiter's disease, right elbow

M02.322 Reiter's disease, left elbow

M02.329 Reiter's disease, unspecified elbow

M02.33 Reiter's disease, wrist
Reiter's disease, carpal bones

M02.331 Reiter's disease, right wrist

M02.332 Reiter's disease, left wrist

M02.339 Reiter's disease, unspecified wrist

M02.34 Reiter's disease, hand
Reiter's disease, metacarpus and phalanges

M02.341 Reiter's disease, right hand

M02.342 Reiter's disease, left hand

M02.349 Reiter's disease, unspecified hand

M02.35 Reiter's disease, hip

M02.351 Reiter's disease, right hip

M02.352 Reiter's disease, left hip

M02.359 Reiter's disease, unspecified hip

M02.36 Reiter's disease, knee

M02.361 Reiter's disease, right knee

M02.362 Reiter's disease, left knee

M02.369 Reiter's disease, unspecified knee

M02.37 Reiter's disease, ankle and foot
Reiter's disease, tarsus, metatarsus and phalanges

M02.371 Reiter's disease, right ankle and foot

M02.372 Reiter's disease, left ankle and foot

M02.379 Reiter's disease, unspecified ankle and foot

M02.38 Reiter's disease, vertebrae

M02.39 Reiter's disease, multiple sites

M02.8 Other reactive arthropathies

M02.80 Other reactive arthropathies, unspecified site

M02.81 Other reactive arthropathies, shoulder

M02.811 Other reactive arthropathies, right shoulder

M02.812 Other reactive arthropathies, left shoulder

M02.819 Other reactive arthropathies, unspecified shoulder

M02.82 Other reactive arthropathies, elbow

M02.821 Other reactive arthropathies, right elbow

M02.822 Other reactive arthropathies, left elbow

M02.829 Other reactive arthropathies, unspecified elbow

M02.83 Other reactive arthropathies, wrist
Other reactive arthropathies, carpal bones

M02.831 Other reactive arthropathies, right wrist

M02.832 Other reactive arthropathies, left wrist

M02.839 Other reactive arthropathies, unspecified wrist

M02.84 Other reactive arthropathies, hand

Other reactive arthropathies, metacarpus and phalanges

⊟ IQ **M02.841 Other reactive arthropathies, right hand**

⊟ IQ **M02.842 Other reactive arthropathies, left hand**

⊟ IQ **M02.849 Other reactive arthropathies, unspecified hand**

6 **M02.85 Other reactive arthropathies, hip**

⊟ IQ **M02.851 Other reactive arthropathies, right hip**

⊟ IQ **M02.852 Other reactive arthropathies, left hip**

⊟ IQ **M02.859 Other reactive arthropathies, unspecified hip**

6 **M02.86 Other reactive arthropathies, knee**

⊟ IQ **M02.861 Other reactive arthropathies, right knee**

⊟ IQ **M02.862 Other reactive arthropathies, left knee**

⊟ IQ **M02.869 Other reactive arthropathies, unspecified knee**

6 **M02.87 Other reactive arthropathies, ankle and foot**

Other reactive arthropathies, tarsus, metatarsus and phalanges

⊟ IQ **M02.871 Other reactive arthropathies, right ankle and foot**

⊟ IQ **M02.872 Other reactive arthropathies, left ankle and foot**

⊟ IQ **M02.879 Other reactive arthropathies, unspecified ankle and foot**

IQ **M02.88 Other reactive arthropathies, vertebrae**

IQ **M02.89 Other reactive arthropathies, multiple sites**

IQ **M02.9 Reactive arthropathy, unspecified**

Autoinflammatory syndromes (M04)

4 **M04 Autoinflammatory syndromes**

EXCLUDES 2 Crohn's disease (K50.-)

SP **M04.1 Periodic fever syndromes**

Familial Mediterranean fever
Hyperimmunoglobin D syndrome
Mevalonate kinase deficiency
Tumor necrosis factor receptor associated periodic syndrome [TRAPS]

DEFINITION The disease is characterized by recurrent attacks of fever; intense inflammatory response pain in the abdomen, joints, and chest; and red, swollen skin lesions; it often leads to kidney failure.

SP **M04.2 Cryopyrin-associated periodic syndromes**

Chronic infantile neurological, cutaneous and articular syndrome [CINCA]
Familial cold autoinflammatory syndrome
Familial cold urticaria
Muckle-Wells syndrome
Neonatal onset multisystemic inflammatory disorder [NOMID]

SP **M04.8 Other autoinflammatory syndromes**

Blau syndrome
Deficiency of interleukin 1 receptor antagonist [DIRA]
Majeed syndrome
Periodic fever, aphthous stomatitis, pharyngitis, and adenopathy syndrome [PFAPA]
Pyogenic arthritis, pyoderma gangrenosum, and acne syndrome [PAPA]

IQ **M04.9 Autoinflammatory syndrome, unspecified**

Inflammatory polyarthropathies (M05-M14)

4 **M05 Rheumatoid arthritis with rheumatoid factor**

EXCLUDES 1 rheumatic fever (I00)
juvenile rheumatoid arthritis (M08.-)
rheumatoid arthritis of spine (M45.-)

CODING TIPS✓ Rheumatoid arthritis classified here includes rheumatoid arthritis and associated conditions (see combination codes) that have an identified rheumatoid factor present. Do not assume the presence of rheumatoid factor when a diagnosis of rheumatoid arthritis is noted in the clinical record. Rheumatoid arthritis that is not specified with rheumatoid factor is coded to M06.-. There are many associated conditions that the classification assumes are related to rheumatoid arthritis. Consult the alphabetic index "arthritis, rheumatoid, with."

5 **M05.0 Felty's syndrome**

Rheumatoid arthritis with splenoadenomegaly and leukopenia

DEFINITION Atypical form of rheumatoid arthritis presenting with fever, enlarged spleen, recurring infections, and decreased white cell count.

IQ **M05.00 Felty's syndrome, unspecified site**

6 **M05.01 Felty's syndrome, shoulder**

⊟ SP **M05.011 Felty's syndrome, right shoulder**

⊟ SP **M05.012 Felty's syndrome, left shoulder**

⊟ IQ **M05.019 Felty's syndrome, unspecified shoulder**

6 **M05.02 Felty's syndrome, elbow**

⊟ SP **M05.021 Felty's syndrome, right elbow**

⊟ SP **M05.022 Felty's syndrome, left elbow**

⊟ IQ **M05.029 Felty's syndrome, unspecified elbow**

6 **M05.03 Felty's syndrome, wrist**

Felty's syndrome, carpal bones

⊟ SP **M05.031 Felty's syndrome, right wrist**

⊟ SP **M05.032 Felty's syndrome, left wrist**

⊟ IQ **M05.039 Felty's syndrome, unspecified wrist**

6 **M05.04 Felty's syndrome, hand**

Felty's syndrome, metacarpus and phalanges

⊟ SP **M05.041 Felty's syndrome, right hand**

⊟ SP **M05.042 Felty's syndrome, left hand**

⊟ IQ **M05.049 Felty's syndrome, unspecified hand**

6 **M05.05 Felty's syndrome, hip**

SP M05.051 Felty's syndrome, right hip

SP M05.052 Felty's syndrome, left hip

!Q M05.059 Felty's syndrome, unspecified hip

6 M05.06 Felty's syndrome, knee

SP M05.061 Felty's syndrome, right knee

SP M05.062 Felty's syndrome, left knee

!Q M05.069 Felty's syndrome, unspecified knee

6 M05.07 Felty's syndrome, ankle and foot
Felty's syndrome, tarsus, metatarsus and phalanges

SP M05.071 Felty's syndrome, right ankle and foot

SP M05.072 Felty's syndrome, left ankle and foot

!Q M05.079 Felty's syndrome, unspecified ankle and foot

SP M05.09 Felty's syndrome, multiple sites

5 M05.1 Rheumatoid lung disease with rheumatoid arthritis

!Q M05.10 Rheumatoid lung disease with rheumatoid arthritis of unspecified site

6 M05.11 Rheumatoid lung disease with rheumatoid arthritis of shoulder

SP M05.111 Rheumatoid lung disease with rheumatoid arthritis of right shoulder

SP M05.112 Rheumatoid lung disease with rheumatoid arthritis of left shoulder

!Q M05.119 Rheumatoid lung disease with rheumatoid arthritis of unspecified shoulder

6 M05.12 Rheumatoid lung disease with rheumatoid arthritis of elbow

SP M05.121 Rheumatoid lung disease with rheumatoid arthritis of right elbow

SP M05.122 Rheumatoid lung disease with rheumatoid arthritis of left elbow

!Q M05.129 Rheumatoid lung disease with rheumatoid arthritis of unspecified elbow

6 M05.13 Rheumatoid lung disease with rheumatoid arthritis of wrist
Rheumatoid lung disease with rheumatoid arthritis, carpal bones

SP M05.131 Rheumatoid lung disease with rheumatoid arthritis of right wrist

SP M05.132 Rheumatoid lung disease with rheumatoid arthritis of left wrist

!Q M05.139 Rheumatoid lung disease with rheumatoid arthritis of unspecified wrist

6 M05.14 Rheumatoid lung disease with rheumatoid arthritis of hand
Rheumatoid lung disease with rheumatoid arthritis, metacarpus and phalanges

SP M05.141 Rheumatoid lung disease with rheumatoid arthritis of right hand

SP M05.142 Rheumatoid lung disease with rheumatoid arthritis of left hand

!Q M05.149 Rheumatoid lung disease with rheumatoid arthritis of unspecified hand

6 M05.15 Rheumatoid lung disease with rheumatoid arthritis of hip

SP M05.151 Rheumatoid lung disease with rheumatoid arthritis of right hip

SP M05.152 Rheumatoid lung disease with rheumatoid arthritis of left hip

!Q M05.159 Rheumatoid lung disease with rheumatoid arthritis of unspecified hip

6 M05.16 Rheumatoid lung disease with rheumatoid arthritis of knee

SP M05.161 Rheumatoid lung disease with rheumatoid arthritis of right knee

SP M05.162 Rheumatoid lung disease with rheumatoid arthritis of left knee

!Q M05.169 Rheumatoid lung disease with rheumatoid arthritis of unspecified knee

6 M05.17 Rheumatoid lung disease with rheumatoid arthritis of ankle and foot
Rheumatoid lung disease with rheumatoid arthritis, tarsus, metatarsus and phalanges

SP M05.171 Rheumatoid lung disease with rheumatoid arthritis of right ankle and foot

SP M05.172 Rheumatoid lung disease with rheumatoid arthritis of left ankle and foot

!Q M05.179 Rheumatoid lung disease with rheumatoid arthritis of unspecified ankle and foot

SP M05.19 Rheumatoid lung disease with rheumatoid arthritis of multiple sites

5 M05.2 Rheumatoid vasculitis with rheumatoid arthritis

!Q M05.20 Rheumatoid vasculitis with rheumatoid arthritis of unspecified site

6 M05.21 Rheumatoid vasculitis with rheumatoid arthritis of shoulder

SP M05.211 Rheumatoid vasculitis with rheumatoid arthritis of right shoulder

SP M05.212 Rheumatoid vasculitis with rheumatoid arthritis of left shoulder

!Q M05.219 Rheumatoid vasculitis with rheumatoid arthritis of unspecified shoulder

6 M05.22 Rheumatoid vasculitis with rheumatoid arthritis of elbow

SP M05.221 Rheumatoid vasculitis with rheumatoid arthritis of right elbow

SP M05.222 Rheumatoid vasculitis with rheumatoid arthritis of left elbow

!Q M05.229 Rheumatoid vasculitis with rheumatoid arthritis of unspecified elbow

6 M05.23 Rheumatoid vasculitis with rheumatoid arthritis of wrist

Rheumatoid vasculitis with rheumatoid arthritis, carpal bones

SP M05.231 **Rheumatoid vasculitis with rheumatoid arthritis of right wrist**

SP M05.232 **Rheumatoid vasculitis with rheumatoid arthritis of left wrist**

IQ M05.239 **Rheumatoid vasculitis with rheumatoid arthritis of unspecified wrist**

6 M05.24 **Rheumatoid vasculitis with rheumatoid arthritis of hand**

Rheumatoid vasculitis with rheumatoid arthritis, metacarpus and phalanges

SP M05.241 **Rheumatoid vasculitis with rheumatoid arthritis of right hand**

SP M05.242 **Rheumatoid vasculitis with rheumatoid arthritis of left hand**

IQ M05.249 **Rheumatoid vasculitis with rheumatoid arthritis of unspecified hand**

6 M05.25 **Rheumatoid vasculitis with rheumatoid arthritis of hip**

SP M05.251 **Rheumatoid vasculitis with rheumatoid arthritis of right hip**

SP M05.252 **Rheumatoid vasculitis with rheumatoid arthritis of left hip**

IQ M05.259 **Rheumatoid vasculitis with rheumatoid arthritis of unspecified hip**

6 M05.26 **Rheumatoid vasculitis with rheumatoid arthritis of knee**

SP M05.261 **Rheumatoid vasculitis with rheumatoid arthritis of right knee**

SP M05.262 **Rheumatoid vasculitis with rheumatoid arthritis of left knee**

IQ M05.269 **Rheumatoid vasculitis with rheumatoid arthritis of unspecified knee**

6 M05.27 **Rheumatoid vasculitis with rheumatoid arthritis of ankle and foot**

Rheumatoid vasculitis with rheumatoid arthritis, tarsus, metatarsus and phalanges

SP M05.271 **Rheumatoid vasculitis with rheumatoid arthritis of right ankle and foot**

SP M05.272 **Rheumatoid vasculitis with rheumatoid arthritis of left ankle and foot**

IQ M05.279 **Rheumatoid vasculitis with rheumatoid arthritis of unspecified ankle and foot**

SP M05.29 **Rheumatoid vasculitis with rheumatoid arthritis of multiple sites**

5 M05.3 **Rheumatoid heart disease with rheumatoid arthritis**

Rheumatoid carditis
Rheumatoid endocarditis
Rheumatoid myocarditis
Rheumatoid pericarditis

IQ M05.30 **Rheumatoid heart disease with rheumatoid arthritis of unspecified site**

6 M05.31 **Rheumatoid heart disease with rheumatoid arthritis of shoulder**

SP M05.311 **Rheumatoid heart disease with rheumatoid arthritis of right shoulder**

SP M05.312 **Rheumatoid heart disease with rheumatoid arthritis of left shoulder**

IQ M05.319 **Rheumatoid heart disease with rheumatoid arthritis of unspecified shoulder**

6 M05.32 **Rheumatoid heart disease with rheumatoid arthritis of elbow**

SP M05.321 **Rheumatoid heart disease with rheumatoid arthritis of right elbow**

SP M05.322 **Rheumatoid heart disease with rheumatoid arthritis of left elbow**

IQ M05.329 **Rheumatoid heart disease with rheumatoid arthritis of unspecified elbow**

6 M05.33 **Rheumatoid heart disease with rheumatoid arthritis of wrist**

Rheumatoid heart disease with rheumatoid arthritis, carpal bones

SP M05.331 **Rheumatoid heart disease with rheumatoid arthritis of right wrist**

SP M05.332 **Rheumatoid heart disease with rheumatoid arthritis of left wrist**

IQ M05.339 **Rheumatoid heart disease with rheumatoid arthritis of unspecified wrist**

6 M05.34 **Rheumatoid heart disease with rheumatoid arthritis of hand**

Rheumatoid heart disease with rheumatoid arthritis, metacarpus and phalanges

SP M05.341 **Rheumatoid heart disease with rheumatoid arthritis of right hand**

SP M05.342 **Rheumatoid heart disease with rheumatoid arthritis of left hand**

IQ M05.349 **Rheumatoid heart disease with rheumatoid arthritis of unspecified hand**

6 M05.35 **Rheumatoid heart disease with rheumatoid arthritis of hip**

SP M05.351 **Rheumatoid heart disease with rheumatoid arthritis of right hip**

SP M05.352 **Rheumatoid heart disease with rheumatoid arthritis of left hip**

IQ M05.359 **Rheumatoid heart disease with rheumatoid arthritis of unspecified hip**

6 M05.36 **Rheumatoid heart disease with rheumatoid arthritis of knee**

SP M05.361 **Rheumatoid heart disease with rheumatoid arthritis of right knee**

SP M05.362 **Rheumatoid heart disease with rheumatoid arthritis of left knee**

IQ M05.369 **Rheumatoid heart disease with rheumatoid arthritis of unspecified knee**

6 M05.37 **Rheumatoid heart disease with rheumatoid arthritis of ankle and foot**

Rheumatoid heart disease with rheumatoid arthritis, tarsus, metatarsus and phalanges

M05.371 Rheumatoid heart disease with rheumatoid arthritis of right ankle and foot

M05.372 Rheumatoid heart disease with rheumatoid arthritis of left ankle and foot

M05.379 Rheumatoid heart disease with rheumatoid arthritis of unspecified ankle and foot

M05.39 Rheumatoid heart disease with rheumatoid arthritis of multiple sites

M05.4 Rheumatoid myopathy with rheumatoid arthritis

M05.40 Rheumatoid myopathy with rheumatoid arthritis of unspecified site

M05.41 Rheumatoid myopathy with rheumatoid arthritis of shoulder

M05.411 Rheumatoid myopathy with rheumatoid arthritis of right shoulder

M05.412 Rheumatoid myopathy with rheumatoid arthritis of left shoulder

M05.419 Rheumatoid myopathy with rheumatoid arthritis of unspecified shoulder

M05.42 Rheumatoid myopathy with rheumatoid arthritis of elbow

M05.421 Rheumatoid myopathy with rheumatoid arthritis of right elbow

M05.422 Rheumatoid myopathy with rheumatoid arthritis of left elbow

M05.429 Rheumatoid myopathy with rheumatoid arthritis of unspecified elbow

M05.43 Rheumatoid myopathy with rheumatoid arthritis of wrist
Rheumatoid myopathy with rheumatoid arthritis, carpal bones

M05.431 Rheumatoid myopathy with rheumatoid arthritis of right wrist

M05.432 Rheumatoid myopathy with rheumatoid arthritis of left wrist

M05.439 Rheumatoid myopathy with rheumatoid arthritis of unspecified wrist

M05.44 Rheumatoid myopathy with rheumatoid arthritis of hand
Rheumatoid myopathy with rheumatoid arthritis, metacarpus and phalanges

M05.441 Rheumatoid myopathy with rheumatoid arthritis of right hand

M05.442 Rheumatoid myopathy with rheumatoid arthritis of left hand

M05.449 Rheumatoid myopathy with rheumatoid arthritis of unspecified hand

M05.45 Rheumatoid myopathy with rheumatoid arthritis of hip

M05.451 Rheumatoid myopathy with rheumatoid arthritis of right hip

M05.452 Rheumatoid myopathy with rheumatoid arthritis of left hip

M05.459 Rheumatoid myopathy with rheumatoid arthritis of unspecified hip

M05.46 Rheumatoid myopathy with rheumatoid arthritis of knee

M05.461 Rheumatoid myopathy with rheumatoid arthritis of right knee

M05.462 Rheumatoid myopathy with rheumatoid arthritis of left knee

M05.469 Rheumatoid myopathy with rheumatoid arthritis of unspecified knee

M05.47 Rheumatoid myopathy with rheumatoid arthritis of ankle and foot
Rheumatoid myopathy with rheumatoid arthritis, tarsus, metatarsus and phalanges

M05.471 Rheumatoid myopathy with rheumatoid arthritis of right ankle and foot

M05.472 Rheumatoid myopathy with rheumatoid arthritis of left ankle and foot

M05.479 Rheumatoid myopathy with rheumatoid arthritis of unspecified ankle and foot

M05.49 Rheumatoid myopathy with rheumatoid arthritis of multiple sites

M05.5 Rheumatoid polyneuropathy with rheumatoid arthritis

M05.50 Rheumatoid polyneuropathy with rheumatoid arthritis of unspecified site

M05.51 Rheumatoid polyneuropathy with rheumatoid arthritis of shoulder

M05.511 Rheumatoid polyneuropathy with rheumatoid arthritis of right shoulder

M05.512 Rheumatoid polyneuropathy with rheumatoid arthritis of left shoulder

M05.519 Rheumatoid polyneuropathy with rheumatoid arthritis of unspecified shoulder

M05.52 Rheumatoid polyneuropathy with rheumatoid arthritis of elbow

M05.521 Rheumatoid polyneuropathy with rheumatoid arthritis of right elbow

M05.522 Rheumatoid polyneuropathy with rheumatoid arthritis of left elbow

M05.529 Rheumatoid polyneuropathy with rheumatoid arthritis of unspecified elbow

M05.53 Rheumatoid polyneuropathy with rheumatoid arthritis of wrist
Rheumatoid polyneuropathy with rheumatoid arthritis, carpal bones

M05.531 Rheumatoid polyneuropathy with rheumatoid arthritis of right wrist

M05.532 Rheumatoid polyneuropathy with rheumatoid arthritis of left wrist

M05.539 Rheumatoid polyneuropathy with rheumatoid arthritis of unspecified wrist

6 **M05.54 Rheumatoid polyneuropathy with rheumatoid arthritis of hand**
Rheumatoid polyneuropathy with rheumatoid arthritis, metacarpus and phalanges

Laterality SP **M05.541 Rheumatoid polyneuropathy with rheumatoid arthritis of right hand**

Laterality SP **M05.542 Rheumatoid polyneuropathy with rheumatoid arthritis of left hand**

Laterality IQ **M05.549 Rheumatoid polyneuropathy with rheumatoid arthritis of unspecified hand**

6 **M05.55 Rheumatoid polyneuropathy with rheumatoid arthritis of hip**

Laterality SP **M05.551 Rheumatoid polyneuropathy with rheumatoid arthritis of right hip**

Laterality SP **M05.552 Rheumatoid polyneuropathy with rheumatoid arthritis of left hip**

Laterality IQ **M05.559 Rheumatoid polyneuropathy with rheumatoid arthritis of unspecified hip**

6 **M05.56 Rheumatoid polyneuropathy with rheumatoid arthritis of knee**

Laterality SP **M05.561 Rheumatoid polyneuropathy with rheumatoid arthritis of right knee**

Laterality SP **M05.562 Rheumatoid polyneuropathy with rheumatoid arthritis of left knee**

Laterality IQ **M05.569 Rheumatoid polyneuropathy with rheumatoid arthritis of unspecified knee**

6 **M05.57 Rheumatoid polyneuropathy with rheumatoid arthritis of ankle and foot**
Rheumatoid polyneuropathy with rheumatoid arthritis, tarsus, metatarsus and phalanges

Laterality SP **M05.571 Rheumatoid polyneuropathy with rheumatoid arthritis of right ankle and foot**

Laterality SP **M05.572 Rheumatoid polyneuropathy with rheumatoid arthritis of left ankle and foot**

Laterality IQ **M05.579 Rheumatoid polyneuropathy with rheumatoid arthritis of unspecified ankle and foot**

SP **M05.59 Rheumatoid polyneuropathy with rheumatoid arthritis of multiple sites**

5 **M05.6 Rheumatoid arthritis with involvement of other organs and systems**

SP **M05.60 Rheumatoid arthritis of unspecified site with involvement of other organs and systems**

6 **M05.61 Rheumatoid arthritis of shoulder with involvement of other organs and systems**

Laterality SP **M05.611 Rheumatoid arthritis of right shoulder with involvement of other organs and systems**

Laterality SP **M05.612 Rheumatoid arthritis of left shoulder with involvement of other organs and systems**

Laterality IQ **M05.619 Rheumatoid arthritis of unspecified shoulder with involvement of other organs and systems**

6 **M05.62 Rheumatoid arthritis of elbow with involvement of other organs and systems**

Laterality SP **M05.621 Rheumatoid arthritis of right elbow with involvement of other organs and systems**

Laterality SP **M05.622 Rheumatoid arthritis of left elbow with involvement of other organs and systems**

Laterality IQ **M05.629 Rheumatoid arthritis of unspecified elbow with involvement of other organs and systems**

6 **M05.63 Rheumatoid arthritis of wrist with involvement of other organs and systems**
Rheumatoid arthritis of carpal bones with involvement of other organs and systems

Laterality SP **M05.631 Rheumatoid arthritis of right wrist with involvement of other organs and systems**

Laterality SP **M05.632 Rheumatoid arthritis of left wrist with involvement of other organs and systems**

Laterality IQ **M05.639 Rheumatoid arthritis of unspecified wrist with involvement of other organs and systems**

6 **M05.64 Rheumatoid arthritis of hand with involvement of other organs and systems**
Rheumatoid arthritis of metacarpus and phalanges with involvement of other organs and systems

Laterality SP **M05.641 Rheumatoid arthritis of right hand with involvement of other organs and systems**

Laterality SP **M05.642 Rheumatoid arthritis of left hand with involvement of other organs and systems**

Laterality IQ **M05.649 Rheumatoid arthritis of unspecified hand with involvement of other organs and systems**

6 **M05.65 Rheumatoid arthritis of hip with involvement of other organs and systems**

Laterality SP **M05.651 Rheumatoid arthritis of right hip with involvement of other organs and systems**

Laterality SP **M05.652 Rheumatoid arthritis of left hip with involvement of other organs and systems**

Laterality IQ **M05.659 Rheumatoid arthritis of unspecified hip with involvement of other organs and systems**

6 **M05.66 Rheumatoid arthritis of knee with involvement of other organs and systems**

Laterality SP **M05.661 Rheumatoid arthritis of right knee with involvement of other organs and systems**

Laterality SP **M05.662 Rheumatoid arthritis of left knee with involvement of other organs and systems**

Laterality IQ **M05.669 Rheumatoid arthritis of unspecified knee with involvement of other organs and systems**

6 **M05.67 Rheumatoid arthritis of ankle and foot with involvement of other organs and systems**
Rheumatoid arthritis of tarsus, metatarsus and phalanges with involvement of other organs and systems

SP **M05.671 Rheumatoid arthritis of right ankle and foot with involvement of other organs and systems**

SP **M05.672 Rheumatoid arthritis of left ankle and foot with involvement of other organs and systems**

IQ **M05.679 Rheumatoid arthritis of unspecified ankle and foot with involvement of other organs and systems**

SP **M05.69 Rheumatoid arthritis of multiple sites with involvement of other organs and systems**

5 **M05.7 Rheumatoid arthritis with rheumatoid factor without organ or systems involvement**

SP **M05.70 Rheumatoid arthritis with rheumatoid factor of unspecified site without organ or systems involvement**

6 **M05.71 Rheumatoid arthritis with rheumatoid factor of shoulder without organ or systems involvement**

SP **M05.711 Rheumatoid arthritis with rheumatoid factor of right shoulder without organ or systems involvement**

SP **M05.712 Rheumatoid arthritis with rheumatoid factor of left shoulder without organ or systems involvement**

IQ **M05.719 Rheumatoid arthritis with rheumatoid factor of unspecified shoulder without organ or systems involvement**

6 **M05.72 Rheumatoid arthritis with rheumatoid factor of elbow without organ or systems involvement**

SP **M05.721 Rheumatoid arthritis with rheumatoid factor of right elbow without organ or systems involvement**

SP **M05.722 Rheumatoid arthritis with rheumatoid factor of left elbow without organ or systems involvement**

IQ **M05.729 Rheumatoid arthritis with rheumatoid factor of unspecified elbow without organ or systems involvement**

6 **M05.73 Rheumatoid arthritis with rheumatoid factor of wrist without organ or systems involvement**

SP **M05.731 Rheumatoid arthritis with rheumatoid factor of right wrist without organ or systems involvement**

SP **M05.732 Rheumatoid arthritis with rheumatoid factor of left wrist without organ or systems involvement**

IQ **M05.739 Rheumatoid arthritis with rheumatoid factor of unspecified wrist without organ or systems involvement**

6 **M05.74 Rheumatoid arthritis with rheumatoid factor of hand without organ or systems involvement**

SP **M05.741 Rheumatoid arthritis with rheumatoid factor of right hand without organ or systems involvement**

SP **M05.742 Rheumatoid arthritis with rheumatoid factor of left hand without organ or systems involvement**

IQ **M05.749 Rheumatoid arthritis with rheumatoid factor of unspecified hand without organ or systems involvement**

6 **M05.75 Rheumatoid arthritis with rheumatoid factor of hip without organ or systems involvement**

SP **M05.751 Rheumatoid arthritis with rheumatoid factor of right hip without organ or systems involvement**

SP **M05.752 Rheumatoid arthritis with rheumatoid factor of left hip without organ or systems involvement**

IQ **M05.759 Rheumatoid arthritis with rheumatoid factor of unspecified hip without organ or systems involvement**

6 **M05.76 Rheumatoid arthritis with rheumatoid factor of knee without organ or systems involvement**

SP **M05.761 Rheumatoid arthritis with rheumatoid factor of right knee without organ or systems involvement**

SP **M05.762 Rheumatoid arthritis with rheumatoid factor of left knee without organ or systems involvement**

IQ **M05.769 Rheumatoid arthritis with rheumatoid factor of unspecified knee without organ or systems involvement**

6 **M05.77 Rheumatoid arthritis with rheumatoid factor of ankle and foot without organ or systems involvement**

SP **M05.771 Rheumatoid arthritis with rheumatoid factor of right ankle and foot without organ or systems involvement**

SP **M05.772 Rheumatoid arthritis with rheumatoid factor of left ankle and foot without organ or systems involvement**

M05.779 Rheumatoid arthritis with rheumatoid factor of unspecified ankle and foot without organ or systems involvement

SP M05.79 Rheumatoid arthritis with rheumatoid factor of multiple sites without organ or systems involvement

SP M05.7A Rheumatoid arthritis with rheumatoid factor of other specified site without organ or systems involvement

5 M05.8 Other rheumatoid arthritis with rheumatoid factor

IQ M05.80 Other rheumatoid arthritis with rheumatoid factor of unspecified site

6 M05.81 Other rheumatoid arthritis with rheumatoid factor of shoulder

SP M05.811 Other rheumatoid arthritis with rheumatoid factor of right shoulder

SP M05.812 Other rheumatoid arthritis with rheumatoid factor of left shoulder

IQ M05.819 Other rheumatoid arthritis with rheumatoid factor of unspecified shoulder

6 M05.82 Other rheumatoid arthritis with rheumatoid factor of elbow

SP M05.821 Other rheumatoid arthritis with rheumatoid factor of right elbow

SP M05.822 Other rheumatoid arthritis with rheumatoid factor of left elbow

IQ M05.829 Other rheumatoid arthritis with rheumatoid factor of unspecified elbow

6 M05.83 Other rheumatoid arthritis with rheumatoid factor of wrist

SP M05.831 Other rheumatoid arthritis with rheumatoid factor of right wrist

SP M05.832 Other rheumatoid arthritis with rheumatoid factor of left wrist

IQ M05.839 Other rheumatoid arthritis with rheumatoid factor of unspecified wrist

6 M05.84 Other rheumatoid arthritis with rheumatoid factor of hand

SP M05.841 Other rheumatoid arthritis with rheumatoid factor of right hand

SP M05.842 Other rheumatoid arthritis with rheumatoid factor of left hand

IQ M05.849 Other rheumatoid arthritis with rheumatoid factor of unspecified hand

6 M05.85 Other rheumatoid arthritis with rheumatoid factor of hip

SP M05.851 Other rheumatoid arthritis with rheumatoid factor of right hip

SP M05.852 Other rheumatoid arthritis with rheumatoid factor of left hip

IQ M05.859 Other rheumatoid arthritis with rheumatoid factor of unspecified hip

6 M05.86 Other rheumatoid arthritis with rheumatoid factor of knee

SP M05.861 Other rheumatoid arthritis with rheumatoid factor of right knee

SP M05.862 Other rheumatoid arthritis with rheumatoid factor of left knee

IQ M05.869 Other rheumatoid arthritis with rheumatoid factor of unspecified knee

6 M05.87 Other rheumatoid arthritis with rheumatoid factor of ankle and foot

SP M05.871 Other rheumatoid arthritis with rheumatoid factor of right ankle and foot

SP M05.872 Other rheumatoid arthritis with rheumatoid factor of left ankle and foot

IQ M05.879 Other rheumatoid arthritis with rheumatoid factor of unspecified ankle and foot

SP M05.89 Other rheumatoid arthritis with rheumatoid factor of multiple sites

SP M05.8A Other rheumatoid arthritis with rheumatoid factor of other specified site

IQ M05.9 Rheumatoid arthritis with rheumatoid factor, unspecified

4 M06 Other rheumatoid arthritis

5 M06.0 Rheumatoid arthritis without rheumatoid factor

IQ M06.00 Rheumatoid arthritis without rheumatoid factor, unspecified site

6 M06.01 Rheumatoid arthritis without rheumatoid factor, shoulder

SP M06.011 Rheumatoid arthritis without rheumatoid factor, right shoulder

SP M06.012 Rheumatoid arthritis without rheumatoid factor, left shoulder

IQ M06.019 Rheumatoid arthritis without rheumatoid factor, unspecified shoulder

6 M06.02 Rheumatoid arthritis without rheumatoid factor, elbow

SP M06.021 Rheumatoid arthritis without rheumatoid factor, right elbow

SP M06.022 Rheumatoid arthritis without rheumatoid factor, left elbow

IQ M06.029 Rheumatoid arthritis without rheumatoid factor, unspecified elbow

6 M06.03 Rheumatoid arthritis without rheumatoid factor, wrist

SP M06.031 Rheumatoid arthritis without rheumatoid factor, right wrist

SP M06.032 Rheumatoid arthritis without rheumatoid factor, left wrist

IQ M06.039 Rheumatoid arthritis without rheumatoid factor, unspecified wrist

6 M06.04 Rheumatoid arthritis without rheumatoid factor, hand

SP M06.041 Rheumatoid arthritis without rheumatoid factor, right hand

SP M06.042 Rheumatoid arthritis without rheumatoid factor, left hand

IQ M06.049 Rheumatoid arthritis without rheumatoid factor, unspecified hand

6 M06.05 Rheumatoid arthritis without rheumatoid factor, hip

SP M06.051 Rheumatoid arthritis without rheumatoid factor, right hip

SP M06.052 Rheumatoid arthritis without rheumatoid factor, left hip

IQ M06.059 Rheumatoid arthritis without rheumatoid factor, unspecified hip

6 M06.06 Rheumatoid arthritis without rheumatoid factor, knee

SP M06.061 Rheumatoid arthritis without rheumatoid factor, right knee

SP M06.062 Rheumatoid arthritis without rheumatoid factor, left knee

IQ M06.069 Rheumatoid arthritis without rheumatoid factor, unspecified knee

6 M06.07 Rheumatoid arthritis without rheumatoid factor, ankle and foot

SP M06.071 Rheumatoid arthritis without rheumatoid factor, right ankle and foot

SP M06.072 Rheumatoid arthritis without rheumatoid factor, left ankle and foot

IQ M06.079 Rheumatoid arthritis without rheumatoid factor, unspecified ankle and foot

SP M06.08 Rheumatoid arthritis without rheumatoid factor, vertebrae

SP M06.09 Rheumatoid arthritis without rheumatoid factor, multiple sites

SP M06.0A Rheumatoid arthritis without rheumatoid factor, other specified site

SP M06.1 Adult-onset Still's disease

EXCLUDES 1 Still's disease NOS (M08.2-)

5 M06.2 Rheumatoid bursitis

IQ M06.20 Rheumatoid bursitis, unspecified site

6 M06.21 Rheumatoid bursitis, shoulder

SP M06.211 Rheumatoid bursitis, right shoulder

SP M06.212 Rheumatoid bursitis, left shoulder

IQ M06.219 Rheumatoid bursitis, unspecified shoulder

6 M06.22 Rheumatoid bursitis, elbow

SP M06.221 Rheumatoid bursitis, right elbow

SP M06.222 Rheumatoid bursitis, left elbow

IQ M06.229 Rheumatoid bursitis, unspecified elbow

6 M06.23 Rheumatoid bursitis, wrist

SP M06.231 Rheumatoid bursitis, right wrist

SP M06.232 Rheumatoid bursitis, left wrist

IQ M06.239 Rheumatoid bursitis, unspecified wrist

6 M06.24 Rheumatoid bursitis, hand

SP M06.241 Rheumatoid bursitis, right hand

SP M06.242 Rheumatoid bursitis, left hand

IQ M06.249 Rheumatoid bursitis, unspecified hand

6 M06.25 Rheumatoid bursitis, hip

SP M06.251 Rheumatoid bursitis, right hip

SP M06.252 Rheumatoid bursitis, left hip

IQ M06.259 Rheumatoid bursitis, unspecified hip

6 M06.26 Rheumatoid bursitis, knee

SP M06.261 Rheumatoid bursitis, right knee

SP M06.262 Rheumatoid bursitis, left knee

IQ M06.269 Rheumatoid bursitis, unspecified knee

6 M06.27 Rheumatoid bursitis, ankle and foot

SP M06.271 Rheumatoid bursitis, right ankle and foot

SP M06.272 Rheumatoid bursitis, left ankle and foot

IQ M06.279 Rheumatoid bursitis, unspecified ankle and foot

SP M06.28 Rheumatoid bursitis, vertebrae

SP M06.29 Rheumatoid bursitis, multiple sites

5 M06.3 Rheumatoid nodule

IQ M06.30 Rheumatoid nodule, unspecified site

6 M06.31 Rheumatoid nodule, shoulder

SP M06.311 Rheumatoid nodule, right shoulder

SP M06.312 Rheumatoid nodule, left shoulder

IQ M06.319 Rheumatoid nodule, unspecified shoulder

6 M06.32 Rheumatoid nodule, elbow

SP M06.321 Rheumatoid nodule, right elbow

SP M06.322 Rheumatoid nodule, left elbow

IQ M06.329 Rheumatoid nodule, unspecified elbow

6 M06.33 Rheumatoid nodule, wrist

SP M06.331 Rheumatoid nodule, right wrist

SP M06.332 Rheumatoid nodule, left wrist

IQ M06.339 Rheumatoid nodule, unspecified wrist

6 M06.34 Rheumatoid nodule, hand

SP M06.341 Rheumatoid nodule, right hand

SP M06.342 Rheumatoid nodule, left hand

IQ M06.349 Rheumatoid nodule, unspecified hand

6 M06.35 Rheumatoid nodule, hip

SP M06.351 Rheumatoid nodule, right hip

SP M06.352 Rheumatoid nodule, left hip

IQ M06.359 Rheumatoid nodule, unspecified hip

6 M06.36 Rheumatoid nodule, knee

SP M06.361 Rheumatoid nodule, right knee

SP M06.362 Rheumatoid nodule, left knee

IQ M06.369 Rheumatoid nodule, unspecified knee

6 M06.37 Rheumatoid nodule, ankle and foot

SP M06.371 Rheumatoid nodule, right ankle and foot

SP M06.372 Rheumatoid nodule, left ankle and foot

IQ M06.379 Rheumatoid nodule, unspecified ankle and foot

SP M06.38 Rheumatoid nodule, vertebrae

SP M06.39 Rheumatoid nodule, multiple sites

SP M06.4 Inflammatory polyarthropathy

EXCLUDES 1 polyarthritis NOS (M13.0)

5 **M06.8 Other specified rheumatoid arthritis**

IQ **M06.80 Other specified rheumatoid arthritis, unspecified site**

6 **M06.81 Other specified rheumatoid arthritis, shoulder**

Laterality SP **M06.811 Other specified rheumatoid arthritis, right shoulder**

Laterality SP **M06.812 Other specified rheumatoid arthritis, left shoulder**

Laterality IQ **M06.819 Other specified rheumatoid arthritis, unspecified shoulder**

6 **M06.82 Other specified rheumatoid arthritis, elbow**

Laterality SP **M06.821 Other specified rheumatoid arthritis, right elbow**

Laterality SP **M06.822 Other specified rheumatoid arthritis, left elbow**

Laterality IQ **M06.829 Other specified rheumatoid arthritis, unspecified elbow**

6 **M06.83 Other specified rheumatoid arthritis, wrist**

Laterality SP **M06.831 Other specified rheumatoid arthritis, right wrist**

Laterality SP **M06.832 Other specified rheumatoid arthritis, left wrist**

Laterality IQ **M06.839 Other specified rheumatoid arthritis, unspecified wrist**

6 **M06.84 Other specified rheumatoid arthritis, hand**

Laterality SP **M06.841 Other specified rheumatoid arthritis, right hand**

Laterality SP **M06.842 Other specified rheumatoid arthritis, left hand**

Laterality IQ **M06.849 Other specified rheumatoid arthritis, unspecified hand**

6 **M06.85 Other specified rheumatoid arthritis, hip**

Laterality SP **M06.851 Other specified rheumatoid arthritis, right hip**

Laterality SP **M06.852 Other specified rheumatoid arthritis, left hip**

Laterality IQ **M06.859 Other specified rheumatoid arthritis, unspecified hip**

6 **M06.86 Other specified rheumatoid arthritis, knee**

Laterality SP **M06.861 Other specified rheumatoid arthritis, right knee**

Laterality SP **M06.862 Other specified rheumatoid arthritis, left knee**

Laterality IQ **M06.869 Other specified rheumatoid arthritis, unspecified knee**

6 **M06.87 Other specified rheumatoid arthritis, ankle and foot**

Laterality SP **M06.871 Other specified rheumatoid arthritis, right ankle and foot**

Laterality SP **M06.872 Other specified rheumatoid arthritis, left ankle and foot**

Laterality IQ **M06.879 Other specified rheumatoid arthritis, unspecified ankle and foot**

SP **M06.88 Other specified rheumatoid arthritis, vertebrae**

SP **M06.89 Other specified rheumatoid arthritis, multiple sites**

SP **M06.8A Other specified rheumatoid arthritis, other specified site**

IQ **M06.9 Rheumatoid arthritis, unspecified**

4 **M07 Enteropathic arthropathies**

Code also associated enteropathy, such as:
- regional enteritis [Crohn's disease] (K50.-)
- ulcerative colitis (K51.-)

EXCLUDES 1 psoriatic arthropathies (L40.5-)

5 **M07.6 Enteropathic arthropathies**

IQ **M07.60 Enteropathic arthropathies, unspecified site**

6 **M07.61 Enteropathic arthropathies, shoulder**

Laterality SP **M07.611 Enteropathic arthropathies, right shoulder**

Laterality SP **M07.612 Enteropathic arthropathies, left shoulder**

Laterality IQ **M07.619 Enteropathic arthropathies, unspecified shoulder**

6 **M07.62 Enteropathic arthropathies, elbow**

Laterality SP **M07.621 Enteropathic arthropathies, right elbow**

Laterality SP **M07.622 Enteropathic arthropathies, left elbow**

Laterality IQ **M07.629 Enteropathic arthropathies, unspecified elbow**

6 **M07.63 Enteropathic arthropathies, wrist**

Laterality SP **M07.631 Enteropathic arthropathies, right wrist**

Laterality SP **M07.632 Enteropathic arthropathies, left wrist**

Laterality IQ **M07.639 Enteropathic arthropathies, unspecified wrist**

6 **M07.64 Enteropathic arthropathies, hand**

Laterality SP **M07.641 Enteropathic arthropathies, right hand**

Laterality SP **M07.642 Enteropathic arthropathies, left hand**

Laterality IQ **M07.649 Enteropathic arthropathies, unspecified hand**

6 **M07.65 Enteropathic arthropathies, hip**

Laterality SP **M07.651 Enteropathic arthropathies, right hip**

Laterality SP **M07.652 Enteropathic arthropathies, left hip**

Laterality IQ **M07.659 Enteropathic arthropathies, unspecified hip**

6 **M07.66 Enteropathic arthropathies, knee**

Laterality SP **M07.661 Enteropathic arthropathies, right knee**

Laterality SP **M07.662 Enteropathic arthropathies, left knee**

Laterality IQ **M07.669 Enteropathic arthropathies, unspecified knee**

6 **M07.67 Enteropathic arthropathies, ankle and foot**

Laterality SP **M07.671 Enteropathic arthropathies, right ankle and foot**

Laterality SP **M07.672 Enteropathic arthropathies, left ankle and foot**

Laterality IQ **M07.679 Enteropathic arthropathies, unspecified ankle and foot**

SP **M07.68 Enteropathic arthropathies, vertebrae**

SP **M07.69 Enteropathic arthropathies, multiple sites**

4 **M08 Juvenile arthritis**

Code also any associated underlying condition, such as:
regional enteritis [Crohn's disease] (K50.-)
ulcerative colitis (K51.-)

EXCLUDES 1 arthropathy in Whipple's disease (M14.8)
Felty's syndrome (M05.0)
juvenile dermatomyositis (M33.0-)
psoriatic juvenile arthropathy (L40.54)

CODING TIPS✓ Juvenile arthritis generally indicates arthritic conditions that have developed in individuals under 16 years of age. Autoimmune disorders are often the cause of these conditions, and all available records should be carefully reviewed to assign the most specific diagnosis and identify any underlying conditions.

5 **M08.0 Unspecified juvenile rheumatoid arthritis**

Juvenile rheumatoid arthritis with or without rheumatoid factor

IQ **M08.00 Unspecified juvenile rheumatoid arthritis of unspecified site**

6 **M08.01 Unspecified juvenile rheumatoid arthritis, shoulder**

SP **M08.011 Unspecified juvenile rheumatoid arthritis, right shoulder**

SP **M08.012 Unspecified juvenile rheumatoid arthritis, left shoulder**

IQ **M08.019 Unspecified juvenile rheumatoid arthritis, unspecified shoulder**

6 **M08.02 Unspecified juvenile rheumatoid arthritis of elbow**

SP **M08.021 Unspecified juvenile rheumatoid arthritis, right elbow**

SP **M08.022 Unspecified juvenile rheumatoid arthritis, left elbow**

IQ **M08.029 Unspecified juvenile rheumatoid arthritis, unspecified elbow**

6 **M08.03 Unspecified juvenile rheumatoid arthritis, wrist**

SP **M08.031 Unspecified juvenile rheumatoid arthritis, right wrist**

SP **M08.032 Unspecified juvenile rheumatoid arthritis, left wrist**

IQ **M08.039 Unspecified juvenile rheumatoid arthritis, unspecified wrist**

6 **M08.04 Unspecified juvenile rheumatoid arthritis, hand**

SP **M08.041 Unspecified juvenile rheumatoid arthritis, right hand**

SP **M08.042 Unspecified juvenile rheumatoid arthritis, left hand**

IQ **M08.049 Unspecified juvenile rheumatoid arthritis, unspecified hand**

6 **M08.05 Unspecified juvenile rheumatoid arthritis, hip**

SP **M08.051 Unspecified juvenile rheumatoid arthritis, right hip**

SP **M08.052 Unspecified juvenile rheumatoid arthritis, left hip**

IQ **M08.059 Unspecified juvenile rheumatoid arthritis, unspecified hip**

6 **M08.06 Unspecified juvenile rheumatoid arthritis, knee**

SP **M08.061 Unspecified juvenile rheumatoid arthritis, right knee**

SP **M08.062 Unspecified juvenile rheumatoid arthritis, left knee**

IQ **M08.069 Unspecified juvenile rheumatoid arthritis, unspecified knee**

6 **M08.07 Unspecified juvenile rheumatoid arthritis, ankle and foot**

SP **M08.071 Unspecified juvenile rheumatoid arthritis, right ankle and foot**

SP **M08.072 Unspecified juvenile rheumatoid arthritis, left ankle and foot**

IQ **M08.079 Unspecified juvenile rheumatoid arthritis, unspecified ankle and foot**

SP **M08.08 Unspecified juvenile rheumatoid arthritis, vertebrae**

SP **M08.09 Unspecified juvenile rheumatoid arthritis, multiple sites**

SP **M08.0A Unspecified juvenile rheumatoid arthritis, other specified site**

SP **M08.1 Juvenile ankylosing spondylitis**

EXCLUDES 1 ankylosing spondylitis in adults (M45.0-)

5 **M08.2 Juvenile rheumatoid arthritis with systemic onset**

Still's disease NOS

EXCLUDES 1 adult-onset Still's disease (M06.1-)

IQ **M08.20 Juvenile rheumatoid arthritis with systemic onset, unspecified site**

6 **M08.21 Juvenile rheumatoid arthritis with systemic onset, shoulder**

SP **M08.211 Juvenile rheumatoid arthritis with systemic onset, right shoulder**

SP **M08.212 Juvenile rheumatoid arthritis with systemic onset, left shoulder**

IQ **M08.219 Juvenile rheumatoid arthritis with systemic onset, unspecified shoulder**

6 **M08.22 Juvenile rheumatoid arthritis with systemic onset, elbow**

SP **M08.221 Juvenile rheumatoid arthritis with systemic onset, right elbow**

SP **M08.222 Juvenile rheumatoid arthritis with systemic onset, left elbow**

IQ **M08.229 Juvenile rheumatoid arthritis with systemic onset, unspecified elbow**

6 **M08.23 Juvenile rheumatoid arthritis with systemic onset, wrist**

SP **M08.231 Juvenile rheumatoid arthritis with systemic onset, right wrist**

SP **M08.232 Juvenile rheumatoid arthritis with systemic onset, left wrist**

IQ **M08.239 Juvenile rheumatoid arthritis with systemic onset, unspecified wrist**

Chapter 13 M00-M99

6 **M08.24 Juvenile rheumatoid arthritis with systemic onset, hand**

Laterality SP **M08.241 Juvenile rheumatoid arthritis with systemic onset, right hand**

Laterality SP **M08.242 Juvenile rheumatoid arthritis with systemic onset, left hand**

Laterality IQ **M08.249 Juvenile rheumatoid arthritis with systemic onset, unspecified hand**

6 **M08.25 Juvenile rheumatoid arthritis with systemic onset, hip**

Laterality SP **M08.251 Juvenile rheumatoid arthritis with systemic onset, right hip**

Laterality SP **M08.252 Juvenile rheumatoid arthritis with systemic onset, left hip**

Laterality IQ **M08.259 Juvenile rheumatoid arthritis with systemic onset, unspecified hip**

6 **M08.26 Juvenile rheumatoid arthritis with systemic onset, knee**

Laterality SP **M08.261 Juvenile rheumatoid arthritis with systemic onset, right knee**

Laterality SP **M08.262 Juvenile rheumatoid arthritis with systemic onset, left knee**

Laterality IQ **M08.269 Juvenile rheumatoid arthritis with systemic onset, unspecified knee**

6 **M08.27 Juvenile rheumatoid arthritis with systemic onset, ankle and foot**

Laterality SP **M08.271 Juvenile rheumatoid arthritis with systemic onset, right ankle and foot**

Laterality SP **M08.272 Juvenile rheumatoid arthritis with systemic onset, left ankle and foot**

Laterality IQ **M08.279 Juvenile rheumatoid arthritis with systemic onset, unspecified ankle and foot**

SP **M08.28 Juvenile rheumatoid arthritis with systemic onset, vertebrae**

SP **M08.29 Juvenile rheumatoid arthritis with systemic onset, multiple sites**

SP **M08.2A Juvenile rheumatoid arthritis with systemic onset, other specified site**

SP **M08.3 Juvenile rheumatoid polyarthritis (seronegative)**

5 **M08.4 Pauciarticular juvenile rheumatoid arthritis**

IQ **M08.40 Pauciarticular juvenile rheumatoid arthritis, unspecified site**

6 **M08.41 Pauciarticular juvenile rheumatoid arthritis, shoulder**

Laterality SP **M08.411 Pauciarticular juvenile rheumatoid arthritis, right shoulder**

Laterality SP **M08.412 Pauciarticular juvenile rheumatoid arthritis, left shoulder**

Laterality IQ **M08.419 Pauciarticular juvenile rheumatoid arthritis, unspecified shoulder**

6 **M08.42 Pauciarticular juvenile rheumatoid arthritis, elbow**

Laterality SP **M08.421 Pauciarticular juvenile rheumatoid arthritis, right elbow**

Laterality SP **M08.422 Pauciarticular juvenile rheumatoid arthritis, left elbow**

Laterality IQ **M08.429 Pauciarticular juvenile rheumatoid arthritis, unspecified elbow**

6 **M08.43 Pauciarticular juvenile rheumatoid arthritis, wrist**

Laterality SP **M08.431 Pauciarticular juvenile rheumatoid arthritis, right wrist**

Laterality SP **M08.432 Pauciarticular juvenile rheumatoid arthritis, left wrist**

Laterality IQ **M08.439 Pauciarticular juvenile rheumatoid arthritis, unspecified wrist**

6 **M08.44 Pauciarticular juvenile rheumatoid arthritis, hand**

Laterality SP **M08.441 Pauciarticular juvenile rheumatoid arthritis, right hand**

Laterality SP **M08.442 Pauciarticular juvenile rheumatoid arthritis, left hand**

Laterality IQ **M08.449 Pauciarticular juvenile rheumatoid arthritis, unspecified hand**

6 **M08.45 Pauciarticular juvenile rheumatoid arthritis, hip**

Laterality SP **M08.451 Pauciarticular juvenile rheumatoid arthritis, right hip**

Laterality SP **M08.452 Pauciarticular juvenile rheumatoid arthritis, left hip**

Laterality IQ **M08.459 Pauciarticular juvenile rheumatoid arthritis, unspecified hip**

6 **M08.46 Pauciarticular juvenile rheumatoid arthritis, knee**

Laterality SP **M08.461 Pauciarticular juvenile rheumatoid arthritis, right knee**

Laterality SP **M08.462 Pauciarticular juvenile rheumatoid arthritis, left knee**

Laterality IQ **M08.469 Pauciarticular juvenile rheumatoid arthritis, unspecified knee**

6 **M08.47 Pauciarticular juvenile rheumatoid arthritis, ankle and foot**

Laterality SP **M08.471 Pauciarticular juvenile rheumatoid arthritis, right ankle and foot**

Laterality SP **M08.472 Pauciarticular juvenile rheumatoid arthritis, left ankle and foot**

Laterality IQ **M08.479 Pauciarticular juvenile rheumatoid arthritis, unspecified ankle and foot**

SP **M08.48 Pauciarticular juvenile rheumatoid arthritis, vertebrae**

SP **M08.4A Pauciarticular juvenile rheumatoid arthritis, other specified site**

5 **M08.8 Other juvenile arthritis**

IQ **M08.80 Other juvenile arthritis, unspecified site**

6 **M08.81 Other juvenile arthritis, shoulder**

Laterality SP **M08.811 Other juvenile arthritis, right shoulder**

Laterality SP **M08.812 Other juvenile arthritis, left shoulder**

Laterality IQ **M08.819 Other juvenile arthritis, unspecified shoulder**

6 **M08.82 Other juvenile arthritis, elbow**

SP M08.821 Other juvenile arthritis, right elbow

SP M08.822 Other juvenile arthritis, left elbow

IQ M08.829 Other juvenile arthritis, unspecified elbow

6 M08.83 Other juvenile arthritis, wrist

SP M08.831 Other juvenile arthritis, right wrist

SP M08.832 Other juvenile arthritis, left wrist

IQ M08.839 Other juvenile arthritis, unspecified wrist

6 M08.84 Other juvenile arthritis, hand

SP M08.841 Other juvenile arthritis, right hand

SP M08.842 Other juvenile arthritis, left hand

IQ M08.849 Other juvenile arthritis, unspecified hand

6 M08.85 Other juvenile arthritis, hip

SP M08.851 Other juvenile arthritis, right hip

SP M08.852 Other juvenile arthritis, left hip

IQ M08.859 Other juvenile arthritis, unspecified hip

6 M08.86 Other juvenile arthritis, knee

SP M08.861 Other juvenile arthritis, right knee

SP M08.862 Other juvenile arthritis, left knee

IQ M08.869 Other juvenile arthritis, unspecified knee

6 M08.87 Other juvenile arthritis, ankle and foot

SP M08.871 Other juvenile arthritis, right ankle and foot

SP M08.872 Other juvenile arthritis, left ankle and foot

IQ M08.879 Other juvenile arthritis, unspecified ankle and foot

SP M08.88 Other juvenile arthritis, other specified site

Other juvenile arthritis, vertebrae

SP M08.89 Other juvenile arthritis, multiple sites

5 M08.9 Juvenile arthritis, unspecified

EXCLUDES 1 juvenile rheumatoid arthritis, unspecified (M08.0-)

IQ M08.90 Juvenile arthritis, unspecified, unspecified site

6 M08.91 Juvenile arthritis, unspecified, shoulder

SP M08.911 Juvenile arthritis, unspecified, right shoulder

SP M08.912 Juvenile arthritis, unspecified, left shoulder

IQ M08.919 Juvenile arthritis, unspecified, unspecified shoulder

6 M08.92 Juvenile arthritis, unspecified, elbow

SP M08.921 Juvenile arthritis, unspecified, right elbow

SP M08.922 Juvenile arthritis, unspecified, left elbow

IQ M08.929 Juvenile arthritis, unspecified, unspecified elbow

6 M08.93 Juvenile arthritis, unspecified, wrist

SP M08.931 Juvenile arthritis, unspecified, right wrist

SP M08.932 Juvenile arthritis, unspecified, left wrist

IQ M08.939 Juvenile arthritis, unspecified, unspecified wrist

6 M08.94 Juvenile arthritis, unspecified, hand

SP M08.941 Juvenile arthritis, unspecified, right hand

SP M08.942 Juvenile arthritis, unspecified, left hand

IQ M08.949 Juvenile arthritis, unspecified, unspecified hand

6 M08.95 Juvenile arthritis, unspecified, hip

SP M08.951 Juvenile arthritis, unspecified, right hip

SP M08.952 Juvenile arthritis, unspecified, left hip

IQ M08.959 Juvenile arthritis, unspecified, unspecified hip

6 M08.96 Juvenile arthritis, unspecified, knee

SP M08.961 Juvenile arthritis, unspecified, right knee

SP M08.962 Juvenile arthritis, unspecified, left knee

IQ M08.969 Juvenile arthritis, unspecified, unspecified knee

6 M08.97 Juvenile arthritis, unspecified, ankle and foot

SP M08.971 Juvenile arthritis, unspecified, right ankle and foot

SP M08.972 Juvenile arthritis, unspecified, left ankle and foot

IQ M08.979 Juvenile arthritis, unspecified, unspecified ankle and foot

SP M08.98 Juvenile arthritis, unspecified, vertebrae

SP M08.99 Juvenile arthritis, unspecified, multiple sites

SP M08.9A Juvenile arthritis, unspecified, other specified site

+ 4 M1A Chronic gout

Use additional code to identify:

Autonomic neuropathy in diseases classified elsewhere (G99.0)

Calculus of urinary tract in diseases classified elsewhere (N22)

Cardiomyopathy in diseases classified elsewhere (I43)

Disorders of external ear in diseases classified elsewhere (H61.1-, H62.8-)

Disorders of iris and ciliary body in diseases classified elsewhere (H22)

Glomerular disorders in diseases classified elsewhere (N08)

EXCLUDES 1 gout NOS (M10.-)

EXCLUDES 2 acute gout (M10.-)

The appropriate 7th character is to be added to each code from category M1A

0 without tophus (tophi)

1 with tophus (tophi)

Chapter 13

M00-M99

CODING TIPS✓ Do not assign a code from category M1A.- unless the physician or NPP has specifically provided a diagnosis of "chronic" gout.

M1A.0 Idiopathic chronic gout
Chronic gouty bursitis
Primary chronic gout

M1A.00X- Idiopathic chronic gout, unspecified site

M1A.01 Idiopathic chronic gout, shoulder

M1A.011- Idiopathic chronic gout, right shoulder

M1A.012- Idiopathic chronic gout, left shoulder

M1A.019- Idiopathic chronic gout, unspecified shoulder

M1A.02 Idiopathic chronic gout, elbow

M1A.021- Idiopathic chronic gout, right elbow

M1A.022- Idiopathic chronic gout, left elbow

M1A.029- Idiopathic chronic gout, unspecified elbow

M1A.03 Idiopathic chronic gout, wrist

M1A.031- Idiopathic chronic gout, right wrist

M1A.032- Idiopathic chronic gout, left wrist

M1A.039- Idiopathic chronic gout, unspecified wrist

M1A.04 Idiopathic chronic gout, hand

M1A.041- Idiopathic chronic gout, right hand

M1A.042- Idiopathic chronic gout, left hand

M1A.049- Idiopathic chronic gout, unspecified hand

M1A.05 Idiopathic chronic gout, hip

M1A.051- Idiopathic chronic gout, right hip

M1A.052- Idiopathic chronic gout, left hip

M1A.059- Idiopathic chronic gout, unspecified hip

M1A.06 Idiopathic chronic gout, knee

M1A.061- Idiopathic chronic gout, right knee

M1A.062- Idiopathic chronic gout, left knee

M1A.069- Idiopathic chronic gout, unspecified knee

M1A.07 Idiopathic chronic gout, ankle and foot

M1A.071- Idiopathic chronic gout, right ankle and foot

M1A.072- Idiopathic chronic gout, left ankle and foot

M1A.079- Idiopathic chronic gout, unspecified ankle and foot

M1A.08X- Idiopathic chronic gout, vertebrae

M1A.09X- Idiopathic chronic gout, multiple sites

M1A.1 Lead-induced chronic gout
Code first:
toxic effects of lead and its compounds (T56.0-)

M1A.10X- Lead-induced chronic gout, unspecified site

M1A.11 Lead-induced chronic gout, shoulder

M1A.111- Lead-induced chronic gout, right shoulder

M1A.112- Lead-induced chronic gout, left shoulder

M1A.119- Lead-induced chronic gout, unspecified shoulder

M1A.12 Lead-induced chronic gout, elbow

M1A.121- Lead-induced chronic gout, right elbow

M1A.122- Lead-induced chronic gout, left elbow

M1A.129- Lead-induced chronic gout, unspecified elbow

M1A.13 Lead-induced chronic gout, wrist

M1A.131- Lead-induced chronic gout, right wrist

M1A.132- Lead-induced chronic gout, left wrist

M1A.139- Lead-induced chronic gout, unspecified wrist

M1A.14 Lead-induced chronic gout, hand

M1A.141- Lead-induced chronic gout, right hand

M1A.142- Lead-induced chronic gout, left hand

M1A.149- Lead-induced chronic gout, unspecified hand

M1A.15 Lead-induced chronic gout, hip

M1A.151- Lead-induced chronic gout, right hip

M1A.152- Lead-induced chronic gout, left hip

M1A.159- Lead-induced chronic gout, unspecified hip

M1A.16 Lead-induced chronic gout, knee

M1A.161- Lead-induced chronic gout, right knee

M1A.162- Lead-induced chronic gout, left knee

M1A.169- Lead-induced chronic gout, unspecified knee

M1A.17 Lead-induced chronic gout, ankle and foot

M1A.171- Lead-induced chronic gout, right ankle and foot

M1A.172- Lead-induced chronic gout, left ankle and foot

M1A.179- Lead-induced chronic gout, unspecified ankle and foot

M1A.18X- Lead-induced chronic gout, vertebrae

M1A.19X- Lead-induced chronic gout, multiple sites

M1A.2 Drug-induced chronic gout
Use additional code for adverse effect, if applicable, to identify drug (T36-T50 with fifth or sixth character 5)

M1A.20X- Drug-induced chronic gout, unspecified site

M1A.21 Drug-induced chronic gout, shoulder

M1A.211- Drug-induced chronic gout, right shoulder

4th digit required 5th digit required 6th digit required 7th digit required 7th digit placeholder +Additional code Laterality

SP + 7 M1A.212- Drug-induced chronic gout, left shoulder
IQ + 7 M1A.219- Drug-induced chronic gout, unspecified shoulder
+ 6 M1A.22 Drug-induced chronic gout, elbow
SP + 7 M1A.221- Drug-induced chronic gout, right elbow
SP + 7 M1A.222- Drug-induced chronic gout, left elbow
IQ + 7 M1A.229- Drug-induced chronic gout, unspecified elbow
+ 6 M1A.23 Drug-induced chronic gout, wrist
SP + 7 M1A.231- Drug-induced chronic gout, right wrist
SP + 7 M1A.232- Drug-induced chronic gout, left wrist
IQ + 7 M1A.239- Drug-induced chronic gout, unspecified wrist
+ 6 M1A.24 Drug-induced chronic gout, hand
SP + 7 M1A.241- Drug-induced chronic gout, right hand
SP + 7 M1A.242- Drug-induced chronic gout, left hand
IQ + 7 M1A.249- Drug-induced chronic gout, unspecified hand
+ 6 M1A.25 Drug-induced chronic gout, hip
SP + 7 M1A.251- Drug-induced chronic gout, right hip
SP + 7 M1A.252- Drug-induced chronic gout, left hip
IQ + 7 M1A.259- Drug-induced chronic gout, unspecified hip
+ 6 M1A.26 Drug-induced chronic gout, knee
SP + 7 M1A.261- Drug-induced chronic gout, right knee
SP + 7 M1A.262- Drug-induced chronic gout, left knee
IQ + 7 M1A.269- Drug-induced chronic gout, unspecified knee
+ 6 M1A.27 Drug-induced chronic gout, ankle and foot
SP + 7 M1A.271- Drug-induced chronic gout, right ankle and foot
SP + 7 M1A.272- Drug-induced chronic gout, left ankle and foot
IQ + 7 M1A.279- Drug-induced chronic gout, unspecified ankle and foot
SP + 7 M1A.28X- Drug-induced chronic gout, vertebrae
SP + 7 M1A.29X- Drug-induced chronic gout, multiple sites
+ 5 M1A.3 Chronic gout due to renal impairment
Code first:
associated renal disease
IQ + 7 M1A.30X- Chronic gout due to renal impairment, unspecified site
+ 6 M1A.31 Chronic gout due to renal impairment, shoulder
+ 7 M1A.311- Chronic gout due to renal impairment, right shoulder
+ 7 M1A.312- Chronic gout due to renal impairment, left shoulder
IQ + 7 M1A.319- Chronic gout due to renal impairment, unspecified shoulder
+ 6 M1A.32 Chronic gout due to renal impairment, elbow
+ 7 M1A.321- Chronic gout due to renal impairment, right elbow
+ 7 M1A.322- Chronic gout due to renal impairment, left elbow
IQ + 7 M1A.329- Chronic gout due to renal impairment, unspecified elbow
+ 6 M1A.33 Chronic gout due to renal impairment, wrist
+ 7 M1A.331- Chronic gout due to renal impairment, right wrist
+ 7 M1A.332- Chronic gout due to renal impairment, left wrist
IQ + 7 M1A.339- Chronic gout due to renal impairment, unspecified wrist
+ 6 M1A.34 Chronic gout due to renal impairment, hand
+ 7 M1A.341- Chronic gout due to renal impairment, right hand
+ 7 M1A.342- Chronic gout due to renal impairment, left hand
IQ + 7 M1A.349- Chronic gout due to renal impairment, unspecified hand
+ 6 M1A.35 Chronic gout due to renal impairment, hip
+ 7 M1A.351- Chronic gout due to renal impairment, right hip
+ 7 M1A.352- Chronic gout due to renal impairment, left hip
IQ + 7 M1A.359- Chronic gout due to renal impairment, unspecified hip
+ 6 M1A.36 Chronic gout due to renal impairment, knee
+ 7 M1A.361- Chronic gout due to renal impairment, right knee
+ 7 M1A.362- Chronic gout due to renal impairment, left knee
IQ + 7 M1A.369- Chronic gout due to renal impairment, unspecified knee
+ 6 M1A.37 Chronic gout due to renal impairment, ankle and foot
+ 7 M1A.371- Chronic gout due to renal impairment, right ankle and foot
+ 7 M1A.372- Chronic gout due to renal impairment, left ankle and foot
IQ + 7 M1A.379- Chronic gout due to renal impairment, unspecified ankle and foot
+ 7 M1A.38X- Chronic gout due to renal impairment, vertebrae
+ 7 M1A.39X- Chronic gout due to renal impairment, multiple sites
+ 5 M1A.4 Other secondary chronic gout
Code first:
associated condition
IQ + 7 M1A.40X- Other secondary chronic gout, unspecified site
+ 6 M1A.41 Other secondary chronic gout, shoulder
+ 7 M1A.411- Other secondary chronic gout, right shoulder
+ 7 M1A.412- Other secondary chronic gout, left shoulder
IQ + 7 M1A.419- Other secondary chronic gout, unspecified shoulder

Chapter 13

M00-M99

+ 6 **M1A.42 Other secondary chronic gout, elbow**

⊟ + 7 **M1A.421- Other secondary chronic gout, right elbow**

⊟ + 7 **M1A.422- Other secondary chronic gout, left elbow**

⊟ IQ + 7 **M1A.429- Other secondary chronic gout, unspecified elbow**

+ 6 **M1A.43 Other secondary chronic gout, wrist**

⊟ + 7 **M1A.431- Other secondary chronic gout, right wrist**

⊟ + 7 **M1A.432- Other secondary chronic gout, left wrist**

⊟ IQ + 7 **M1A.439- Other secondary chronic gout, unspecified wrist**

+ 6 **M1A.44 Other secondary chronic gout, hand**

⊟ + 7 **M1A.441- Other secondary chronic gout, right hand**

⊟ + 7 **M1A.442- Other secondary chronic gout, left hand**

⊟ IQ + 7 **M1A.449- Other secondary chronic gout, unspecified hand**

+ 6 **M1A.45 Other secondary chronic gout, hip**

⊟ + 7 **M1A.451- Other secondary chronic gout, right hip**

⊟ + 7 **M1A.452- Other secondary chronic gout, left hip**

⊟ IQ + 7 **M1A.459- Other secondary chronic gout, unspecified hip**

+ 6 **M1A.46 Other secondary chronic gout, knee**

⊟ + 7 **M1A.461- Other secondary chronic gout, right knee**

⊟ + 7 **M1A.462- Other secondary chronic gout, left knee**

⊟ IQ + 7 **M1A.469- Other secondary chronic gout, unspecified knee**

+ 6 **M1A.47 Other secondary chronic gout, ankle and foot**

⊟ + 7 **M1A.471- Other secondary chronic gout, right ankle and foot**

⊟ + 7 **M1A.472- Other secondary chronic gout, left ankle and foot**

⊟ IQ + 7 **M1A.479- Other secondary chronic gout, unspecified ankle and foot**

+ 7 **M1A.48X- Other secondary chronic gout, vertebrae**

+ 7 **M1A.49X- Other secondary chronic gout, multiple sites**

SP + 7 **M1A.9XX- Chronic gout, unspecified**

+ 4 **M10 Gout**

Acute gout
Gout attack
Gout flare
Podagra
Use additional code to identify:
- Autonomic neuropathy in diseases classified elsewhere (G99.0)
- Calculus of urinary tract in diseases classified elsewhere (N22)
- Cardiomyopathy in diseases classified elsewhere (I43)
- Disorders of external ear in diseases classified elsewhere (H61.1-, H62.8-)
- Disorders of iris and ciliary body in diseases classified elsewhere (H22)
- Glomerular disorders in diseases classified elsewhere (N08)

EXCLUDES 2 chronic gout (M1A.-)

+ 5 **M10.0 Idiopathic gout**

Gouty bursitis
Primary gout

IQ + **M10.00 Idiopathic gout, unspecified site**

+ 6 **M10.01 Idiopathic gout, shoulder**

⊟ SP + **M10.011 Idiopathic gout, right shoulder**

⊟ SP + **M10.012 Idiopathic gout, left shoulder**

⊟ IQ + **M10.019 Idiopathic gout, unspecified shoulder**

+ 6 **M10.02 Idiopathic gout, elbow**

⊟ SP + **M10.021 Idiopathic gout, right elbow**

⊟ SP + **M10.022 Idiopathic gout, left elbow**

⊟ IQ + **M10.029 Idiopathic gout, unspecified elbow**

+ 6 **M10.03 Idiopathic gout, wrist**

⊟ SP + **M10.031 Idiopathic gout, right wrist**

⊟ SP + **M10.032 Idiopathic gout, left wrist**

⊟ IQ + **M10.039 Idiopathic gout, unspecified wrist**

+ 6 **M10.04 Idiopathic gout, hand**

⊟ SP + **M10.041 Idiopathic gout, right hand**

⊟ SP + **M10.042 Idiopathic gout, left hand**

⊟ IQ + **M10.049 Idiopathic gout, unspecified hand**

+ 6 **M10.05 Idiopathic gout, hip**

⊟ SP + **M10.051 Idiopathic gout, right hip**

⊟ SP + **M10.052 Idiopathic gout, left hip**

⊟ IQ + **M10.059 Idiopathic gout, unspecified hip**

+ 6 **M10.06 Idiopathic gout, knee**

⊟ SP + **M10.061 Idiopathic gout, right knee**

⊟ SP + **M10.062 Idiopathic gout, left knee**

⊟ IQ + **M10.069 Idiopathic gout, unspecified knee**

+ 6 **M10.07 Idiopathic gout, ankle and foot**

⊟ SP + **M10.071 Idiopathic gout, right ankle and foot**

⊟ SP + **M10.072 Idiopathic gout, left ankle and foot**

⊟ IQ + **M10.079 Idiopathic gout, unspecified ankle and foot**

SP + **M10.08 Idiopathic gout, vertebrae**

SP + **M10.09 Idiopathic gout, multiple sites**

+ 5 **M10.1 Lead-induced gout**

Code first:
- toxic effects of lead and its compounds (T56.0-)

IQ + **M10.10 Lead-induced gout, unspecified site**

+ 6 **M10.11 Lead-induced gout, shoulder**

⊟ IQ + **M10.111 Lead-induced gout, right shoulder**

⊟ IQ + **M10.112 Lead-induced gout, left shoulder**

⊟ IQ + **M10.119 Lead-induced gout, unspecified shoulder**

+ 6 **M10.12 Lead-induced gout, elbow**

⊟ IQ + **M10.121 Lead-induced gout, right elbow**

⊟ IQ + **M10.122 Lead-induced gout, left elbow**

⊟ IQ + **M10.129 Lead-induced gout, unspecified elbow**

+ 6 **M10.13 Lead-induced gout, wrist**

⊟ IQ + **M10.131 Lead-induced gout, right wrist**

⊟ IQ + **M10.132 Lead-induced gout, left wrist**

H IQ + M10.139 Lead-induced gout, unspecified wrist

+ 6 M10.14 Lead-induced gout, hand

H IQ + M10.141 Lead-induced gout, right hand

H IQ + M10.142 Lead-induced gout, left hand

H IQ + M10.149 Lead-induced gout, unspecified hand

+ 6 M10.15 Lead-induced gout, hip

H IQ + M10.151 Lead-induced gout, right hip

H IQ + M10.152 Lead-induced gout, left hip

H IQ + M10.159 Lead-induced gout, unspecified hip

+ 6 M10.16 Lead-induced gout, knee

H IQ + M10.161 Lead-induced gout, right knee

H IQ + M10.162 Lead-induced gout, left knee

H IQ + M10.169 Lead-induced gout, unspecified knee

+ 6 M10.17 Lead-induced gout, ankle and foot

H IQ + M10.171 Lead-induced gout, right ankle and foot

H IQ + M10.172 Lead-induced gout, left ankle and foot

H IQ + M10.179 Lead-induced gout, unspecified ankle and foot

IQ + M10.18 Lead-induced gout, vertebrae

IQ + M10.19 Lead-induced gout, multiple sites

+ 5 M10.2 Drug-induced gout

Use additional code for adverse effect, if applicable, to identify drug (T36-T50 with fifth or sixth character 5)

IQ + M10.20 Drug-induced gout, unspecified site

+ 6 M10.21 Drug-induced gout, shoulder

H SP + M10.211 Drug-induced gout, right shoulder

H SP + M10.212 Drug-induced gout, left shoulder

H IQ + M10.219 Drug-induced gout, unspecified shoulder

+ 6 M10.22 Drug-induced gout, elbow

H SP + M10.221 Drug-induced gout, right elbow

H SP + M10.222 Drug-induced gout, left elbow

H IQ + M10.229 Drug-induced gout, unspecified elbow

+ 6 M10.23 Drug-induced gout, wrist

H SP + M10.231 Drug-induced gout, right wrist

H SP + M10.232 Drug-induced gout, left wrist

H IQ + M10.239 Drug-induced gout, unspecified wrist

+ 6 M10.24 Drug-induced gout, hand

H SP + M10.241 Drug-induced gout, right hand

H SP + M10.242 Drug-induced gout, left hand

H IQ + M10.249 Drug-induced gout, unspecified hand

+ 6 M10.25 Drug-induced gout, hip

H SP + M10.251 Drug-induced gout, right hip

H SP + M10.252 Drug-induced gout, left hip

H IQ + M10.259 Drug-induced gout, unspecified hip

+ 6 M10.26 Drug-induced gout, knee

H SP + M10.261 Drug-induced gout, right knee

H SP + M10.262 Drug-induced gout, left knee

H IQ + M10.269 Drug-induced gout, unspecified knee

+ 6 M10.27 Drug-induced gout, ankle and foot

H SP + M10.271 Drug-induced gout, right ankle and foot

H SP + M10.272 Drug-induced gout, left ankle and foot

H IQ + M10.279 Drug-induced gout, unspecified ankle and foot

SP + M10.28 Drug-induced gout, vertebrae

SP + M10.29 Drug-induced gout, multiple sites

+ 5 M10.3 Gout due to renal impairment

Code first:

associated renal disease

IQ + M10.30 Gout due to renal impairment, unspecified site

+ 6 M10.31 Gout due to renal impairment, shoulder

H IQ + M10.311 Gout due to renal impairment, right shoulder

H IQ + M10.312 Gout due to renal impairment, left shoulder

H IQ + M10.319 Gout due to renal impairment, unspecified shoulder

+ 6 M10.32 Gout due to renal impairment, elbow

H IQ + M10.321 Gout due to renal impairment, right elbow

H IQ + M10.322 Gout due to renal impairment, left elbow

H IQ + M10.329 Gout due to renal impairment, unspecified elbow

+ 6 M10.33 Gout due to renal impairment, wrist

H IQ + M10.331 Gout due to renal impairment, right wrist

H IQ + M10.332 Gout due to renal impairment, left wrist

H IQ + M10.339 Gout due to renal impairment, unspecified wrist

+ 6 M10.34 Gout due to renal impairment, hand

H IQ + M10.341 Gout due to renal impairment, right hand

H IQ + M10.342 Gout due to renal impairment, left hand

H IQ + M10.349 Gout due to renal impairment, unspecified hand

+ 6 M10.35 Gout due to renal impairment, hip

H IQ + M10.351 Gout due to renal impairment, right hip

H IQ + M10.352 Gout due to renal impairment, left hip

H IQ + M10.359 Gout due to renal impairment, unspecified hip

+ 6 M10.36 Gout due to renal impairment, knee

H IQ + M10.361 Gout due to renal impairment, right knee

H IQ + M10.362 Gout due to renal impairment, left knee

H IQ + M10.369 Gout due to renal impairment, unspecified knee

+ 6 M10.37 Gout due to renal impairment, ankle and foot

H IQ + M10.371 Gout due to renal impairment, right ankle and foot

H IQ + M10.372 Gout due to renal impairment, left ankle and foot

⊟ IQ + M10.379 **Gout due to renal impairment, unspecified ankle and foot**

IQ + M10.38 **Gout due to renal impairment, vertebrae**

IQ + M10.39 **Gout due to renal impairment, multiple sites**

+ 5 M10.4 **Other secondary gout**

Code first:

associated condition

IQ + M10.40 **Other secondary gout, unspecified site**

+ 6 M10.41 **Other secondary gout, shoulder**

⊟ IQ + M10.411 **Other secondary gout, right shoulder**

⊟ IQ + M10.412 **Other secondary gout, left shoulder**

⊟ IQ + M10.419 **Other secondary gout, unspecified shoulder**

+ 6 M10.42 **Other secondary gout, elbow**

⊟ IQ + M10.421 **Other secondary gout, right elbow**

⊟ IQ + M10.422 **Other secondary gout, left elbow**

⊟ IQ + M10.429 **Other secondary gout, unspecified elbow**

+ 6 M10.43 **Other secondary gout, wrist**

⊟ IQ + M10.431 **Other secondary gout, right wrist**

⊟ IQ + M10.432 **Other secondary gout, left wrist**

⊟ IQ + M10.439 **Other secondary gout, unspecified wrist**

+ 6 M10.44 **Other secondary gout, hand**

⊟ IQ + M10.441 **Other secondary gout, right hand**

⊟ IQ + M10.442 **Other secondary gout, left hand**

⊟ IQ + M10.449 **Other secondary gout, unspecified hand**

+ 6 M10.45 **Other secondary gout, hip**

⊟ IQ + M10.451 **Other secondary gout, right hip**

⊟ IQ + M10.452 **Other secondary gout, left hip**

⊟ IQ + M10.459 **Other secondary gout, unspecified hip**

+ 6 M10.46 **Other secondary gout, knee**

⊟ IQ + M10.461 **Other secondary gout, right knee**

⊟ IQ + M10.462 **Other secondary gout, left knee**

⊟ IQ + M10.469 **Other secondary gout, unspecified knee**

+ 6 M10.47 **Other secondary gout, ankle and foot**

⊟ IQ + M10.471 **Other secondary gout, right ankle and foot**

⊟ IQ + M10.472 **Other secondary gout, left ankle and foot**

⊟ IQ + M10.479 **Other secondary gout, unspecified ankle and foot**

IQ + M10.48 **Other secondary gout, vertebrae**

IQ + M10.49 **Other secondary gout, multiple sites**

SP + M10.9 **Gout, unspecified**

Gout NOS

4 M11 **Other crystal arthropathies**

5 M11.0 **Hydroxyapatite deposition disease**

IQ M11.00 **Hydroxyapatite deposition disease, unspecified site**

6 M11.01 **Hydroxyapatite deposition disease, shoulder**

⊟ SP M11.011 **Hydroxyapatite deposition disease, right shoulder**

⊟ SP M11.012 **Hydroxyapatite deposition disease, left shoulder**

⊟ IQ M11.019 **Hydroxyapatite deposition disease, unspecified shoulder**

6 M11.02 **Hydroxyapatite deposition disease, elbow**

⊟ SP M11.021 **Hydroxyapatite deposition disease, right elbow**

⊟ SP M11.022 **Hydroxyapatite deposition disease, left elbow**

⊟ IQ M11.029 **Hydroxyapatite deposition disease, unspecified elbow**

6 M11.03 **Hydroxyapatite deposition disease, wrist**

⊟ SP M11.031 **Hydroxyapatite deposition disease, right wrist**

⊟ SP M11.032 **Hydroxyapatite deposition disease, left wrist**

⊟ IQ M11.039 **Hydroxyapatite deposition disease, unspecified wrist**

6 M11.04 **Hydroxyapatite deposition disease, hand**

⊟ SP M11.041 **Hydroxyapatite deposition disease, right hand**

⊟ SP M11.042 **Hydroxyapatite deposition disease, left hand**

⊟ IQ M11.049 **Hydroxyapatite deposition disease, unspecified hand**

6 M11.05 **Hydroxyapatite deposition disease, hip**

⊟ SP M11.051 **Hydroxyapatite deposition disease, right hip**

⊟ SP M11.052 **Hydroxyapatite deposition disease, left hip**

⊟ IQ M11.059 **Hydroxyapatite deposition disease, unspecified hip**

6 M11.06 **Hydroxyapatite deposition disease, knee**

⊟ SP M11.061 **Hydroxyapatite deposition disease, right knee**

⊟ SP M11.062 **Hydroxyapatite deposition disease, left knee**

⊟ IQ M11.069 **Hydroxyapatite deposition disease, unspecified knee**

6 M11.07 **Hydroxyapatite deposition disease, ankle and foot**

⊟ SP M11.071 **Hydroxyapatite deposition disease, right ankle and foot**

⊟ SP M11.072 **Hydroxyapatite deposition disease, left ankle and foot**

⊟ IQ M11.079 **Hydroxyapatite deposition disease, unspecified ankle and foot**

SP M11.08 **Hydroxyapatite deposition disease, vertebrae**

SP M11.09 **Hydroxyapatite deposition disease, multiple sites**

5 M11.1 **Familial chondrocalcinosis**

IQ M11.10 **Familial chondrocalcinosis, unspecified site**

6 M11.11 **Familial chondrocalcinosis, shoulder**

⊟ SP M11.111 **Familial chondrocalcinosis, right shoulder**

SP M11.112 Familial chondrocalcinosis, left shoulder
IQ M11.119 Familial chondrocalcinosis, unspecified shoulder
6 M11.12 Familial chondrocalcinosis, elbow
IQ M11.121 Familial chondrocalcinosis, right elbow
SP M11.122 Familial chondrocalcinosis, left elbow
IQ M11.129 Familial chondrocalcinosis, unspecified elbow
6 M11.13 Familial chondrocalcinosis, wrist
SP M11.131 Familial chondrocalcinosis, right wrist
SP M11.132 Familial chondrocalcinosis, left wrist
IQ M11.139 Familial chondrocalcinosis, unspecified wrist
6 M11.14 Familial chondrocalcinosis, hand
SP M11.141 Familial chondrocalcinosis, right hand
SP M11.142 Familial chondrocalcinosis, left hand
IQ M11.149 Familial chondrocalcinosis, unspecified hand
6 M11.15 Familial chondrocalcinosis, hip
SP M11.151 Familial chondrocalcinosis, right hip
SP M11.152 Familial chondrocalcinosis, left hip
IQ M11.159 Familial chondrocalcinosis, unspecified hip
6 M11.16 Familial chondrocalcinosis, knee
SP M11.161 Familial chondrocalcinosis, right knee
SP M11.162 Familial chondrocalcinosis, left knee
IQ M11.169 Familial chondrocalcinosis, unspecified knee
6 M11.17 Familial chondrocalcinosis, ankle and foot
SP M11.171 Familial chondrocalcinosis, right ankle and foot
SP M11.172 Familial chondrocalcinosis, left ankle and foot
IQ M11.179 Familial chondrocalcinosis, unspecified ankle and foot
SP M11.18 Familial chondrocalcinosis, vertebrae
SP M11.19 Familial chondrocalcinosis, multiple sites
5 M11.2 Other chondrocalcinosis
Chondrocalcinosis NOS
IQ M11.20 Other chondrocalcinosis, unspecified site
6 M11.21 Other chondrocalcinosis, shoulder
SP M11.211 Other chondrocalcinosis, right shoulder
SP M11.212 Other chondrocalcinosis, left shoulder
IQ M11.219 Other chondrocalcinosis, unspecified shoulder
6 M11.22 Other chondrocalcinosis, elbow
SP M11.221 Other chondrocalcinosis, right elbow
SP M11.222 Other chondrocalcinosis, left elbow
IQ M11.229 Other chondrocalcinosis, unspecified elbow
6 M11.23 Other chondrocalcinosis, wrist
SP M11.231 Other chondrocalcinosis, right wrist
SP M11.232 Other chondrocalcinosis, left wrist
IQ M11.239 Other chondrocalcinosis, unspecified wrist
6 M11.24 Other chondrocalcinosis, hand
SP M11.241 Other chondrocalcinosis, right hand
SP M11.242 Other chondrocalcinosis, left hand
IQ M11.249 Other chondrocalcinosis, unspecified hand
6 M11.25 Other chondrocalcinosis, hip
SP M11.251 Other chondrocalcinosis, right hip
SP M11.252 Other chondrocalcinosis, left hip
IQ M11.259 Other chondrocalcinosis, unspecified hip
6 M11.26 Other chondrocalcinosis, knee
SP M11.261 Other chondrocalcinosis, right knee
SP M11.262 Other chondrocalcinosis, left knee
IQ M11.269 Other chondrocalcinosis, unspecified knee
6 M11.27 Other chondrocalcinosis, ankle and foot
SP M11.271 Other chondrocalcinosis, right ankle and foot
SP M11.272 Other chondrocalcinosis, left ankle and foot
IQ M11.279 Other chondrocalcinosis, unspecified ankle and foot
SP M11.28 Other chondrocalcinosis, vertebrae
SP M11.29 Other chondrocalcinosis, multiple sites
5 M11.8 Other specified crystal arthropathies
IQ M11.80 Other specified crystal arthropathies, unspecified site
6 M11.81 Other specified crystal arthropathies, shoulder
SP M11.811 Other specified crystal arthropathies, right shoulder
SP M11.812 Other specified crystal arthropathies, left shoulder
IQ M11.819 Other specified crystal arthropathies, unspecified shoulder
6 M11.82 Other specified crystal arthropathies, elbow
SP M11.821 Other specified crystal arthropathies, right elbow
SP M11.822 Other specified crystal arthropathies, left elbow
IQ M11.829 Other specified crystal arthropathies, unspecified elbow
6 M11.83 Other specified crystal arthropathies, wrist
SP M11.831 Other specified crystal arthropathies, right wrist
SP M11.832 Other specified crystal arthropathies, left wrist

Chapter 13
M00-M99

Laterality IQ **M11.839 Other specified crystal arthropathies, unspecified wrist**

6 **M11.84 Other specified crystal arthropathies, hand**

Laterality SP **M11.841 Other specified crystal arthropathies, right hand**

Laterality SP **M11.842 Other specified crystal arthropathies, left hand**

Laterality IQ **M11.849 Other specified crystal arthropathies, unspecified hand**

6 **M11.85 Other specified crystal arthropathies, hip**

Laterality SP **M11.851 Other specified crystal arthropathies, right hip**

Laterality SP **M11.852 Other specified crystal arthropathies, left hip**

Laterality IQ **M11.859 Other specified crystal arthropathies, unspecified hip**

6 **M11.86 Other specified crystal arthropathies, knee**

Laterality SP **M11.861 Other specified crystal arthropathies, right knee**

Laterality SP **M11.862 Other specified crystal arthropathies, left knee**

Laterality IQ **M11.869 Other specified crystal arthropathies, unspecified knee**

6 **M11.87 Other specified crystal arthropathies, ankle and foot**

Laterality SP **M11.871 Other specified crystal arthropathies, right ankle and foot**

Laterality SP **M11.872 Other specified crystal arthropathies, left ankle and foot**

Laterality IQ **M11.879 Other specified crystal arthropathies, unspecified ankle and foot**

SP **M11.88 Other specified crystal arthropathies, vertebrae**

SP **M11.89 Other specified crystal arthropathies, multiple sites**

IQ **M11.9 Crystal arthropathy, unspecified**

4 **M12 Other and unspecified arthropathy**

EXCLUDES 1 arthrosis (M15-M19)
cricoarytenoid arthropathy (J38.7)

5 **M12.0 Chronic postrheumatic arthropathy [Jaccoud]**

IQ **M12.00 Chronic postrheumatic arthropathy [Jaccoud], unspecified site**

6 **M12.01 Chronic postrheumatic arthropathy [Jaccoud], shoulder**

Laterality SP **M12.011 Chronic postrheumatic arthropathy [Jaccoud], right shoulder**

Laterality SP **M12.012 Chronic postrheumatic arthropathy [Jaccoud], left shoulder**

Laterality IQ **M12.019 Chronic postrheumatic arthropathy [Jaccoud], unspecified shoulder**

6 **M12.02 Chronic postrheumatic arthropathy [Jaccoud], elbow**

Laterality SP **M12.021 Chronic postrheumatic arthropathy [Jaccoud], right elbow**

Laterality SP **M12.022 Chronic postrheumatic arthropathy [Jaccoud], left elbow**

Laterality IQ **M12.029 Chronic postrheumatic arthropathy [Jaccoud], unspecified elbow**

6 **M12.03 Chronic postrheumatic arthropathy [Jaccoud], wrist**

Laterality SP **M12.031 Chronic postrheumatic arthropathy [Jaccoud], right wrist**

Laterality SP **M12.032 Chronic postrheumatic arthropathy [Jaccoud], left wrist**

Laterality IQ **M12.039 Chronic postrheumatic arthropathy [Jaccoud], unspecified wrist**

6 **M12.04 Chronic postrheumatic arthropathy [Jaccoud], hand**

Laterality SP **M12.041 Chronic postrheumatic arthropathy [Jaccoud], right hand**

Laterality SP **M12.042 Chronic postrheumatic arthropathy [Jaccoud], left hand**

Laterality IQ **M12.049 Chronic postrheumatic arthropathy [Jaccoud], unspecified hand**

6 **M12.05 Chronic postrheumatic arthropathy [Jaccoud], hip**

Laterality SP **M12.051 Chronic postrheumatic arthropathy [Jaccoud], right hip**

Laterality SP **M12.052 Chronic postrheumatic arthropathy [Jaccoud], left hip**

Laterality IQ **M12.059 Chronic postrheumatic arthropathy [Jaccoud], unspecified hip**

6 **M12.06 Chronic postrheumatic arthropathy [Jaccoud], knee**

Laterality SP **M12.061 Chronic postrheumatic arthropathy [Jaccoud], right knee**

Laterality SP **M12.062 Chronic postrheumatic arthropathy [Jaccoud], left knee**

Laterality IQ **M12.069 Chronic postrheumatic arthropathy [Jaccoud], unspecified knee**

6 **M12.07 Chronic postrheumatic arthropathy [Jaccoud], ankle and foot**

Laterality SP **M12.071 Chronic postrheumatic arthropathy [Jaccoud], right ankle and foot**

Laterality SP **M12.072 Chronic postrheumatic arthropathy [Jaccoud], left ankle and foot**

Laterality IQ **M12.079 Chronic postrheumatic arthropathy [Jaccoud], unspecified ankle and foot**

SP **M12.08 Chronic postrheumatic arthropathy [Jaccoud], other specified site**
Chronic postrheumatic arthropathy [Jaccoud], vertebrae

SP **M12.09 Chronic postrheumatic arthropathy [Jaccoud], multiple sites**

5 **M12.1 Kaschin-Beck disease**
Osteochondroarthrosis deformans endemica

IQ **M12.10 Kaschin-Beck disease, unspecified site**

6 **M12.11 Kaschin-Beck disease, shoulder**

Laterality SP **M12.111 Kaschin-Beck disease, right shoulder**

Laterality SP **M12.112 Kaschin-Beck disease, left shoulder**

M12.119 Kaschin-Beck disease, unspecified shoulder
M12.12 Kaschin-Beck disease, elbow
M12.121 Kaschin-Beck disease, right elbow
M12.122 Kaschin-Beck disease, left elbow
M12.129 Kaschin-Beck disease, unspecified elbow
M12.13 Kaschin-Beck disease, wrist
M12.131 Kaschin-Beck disease, right wrist
M12.132 Kaschin-Beck disease, left wrist
M12.139 Kaschin-Beck disease, unspecified wrist
M12.14 Kaschin-Beck disease, hand
M12.141 Kaschin-Beck disease, right hand
M12.142 Kaschin-Beck disease, left hand
M12.149 Kaschin-Beck disease, unspecified hand
M12.15 Kaschin-Beck disease, hip
M12.151 Kaschin-Beck disease, right hip
M12.152 Kaschin-Beck disease, left hip
M12.159 Kaschin-Beck disease, unspecified hip
M12.16 Kaschin-Beck disease, knee
M12.161 Kaschin-Beck disease, right knee
M12.162 Kaschin-Beck disease, left knee
M12.169 Kaschin-Beck disease, unspecified knee
M12.17 Kaschin-Beck disease, ankle and foot
M12.171 Kaschin-Beck disease, right ankle and foot
M12.172 Kaschin-Beck disease, left ankle and foot
M12.179 Kaschin-Beck disease, unspecified ankle and foot
SP M12.18 Kaschin-Beck disease, vertebrae
SP M12.19 Kaschin-Beck disease, multiple sites
M12.2 Villonodular synovitis (pigmented)
IQ M12.20 Villonodular synovitis (pigmented), unspecified site
M12.21 Villonodular synovitis (pigmented), shoulder
M12.211 Villonodular synovitis (pigmented), right shoulder
M12.212 Villonodular synovitis (pigmented), left shoulder
M12.219 Villonodular synovitis (pigmented), unspecified shoulder
M12.22 Villonodular synovitis (pigmented), elbow
M12.221 Villonodular synovitis (pigmented), right elbow
M12.222 Villonodular synovitis (pigmented), left elbow
M12.229 Villonodular synovitis (pigmented), unspecified elbow
M12.23 Villonodular synovitis (pigmented), wrist
M12.231 Villonodular synovitis (pigmented), right wrist
M12.232 Villonodular synovitis (pigmented), left wrist
M12.239 Villonodular synovitis (pigmented), unspecified wrist
M12.24 Villonodular synovitis (pigmented), hand
M12.241 Villonodular synovitis (pigmented), right hand
M12.242 Villonodular synovitis (pigmented), left hand
M12.249 Villonodular synovitis (pigmented), unspecified hand
M12.25 Villonodular synovitis (pigmented), hip
M12.251 Villonodular synovitis (pigmented), right hip
M12.252 Villonodular synovitis (pigmented), left hip
M12.259 Villonodular synovitis (pigmented), unspecified hip
M12.26 Villonodular synovitis (pigmented), knee
M12.261 Villonodular synovitis (pigmented), right knee
M12.262 Villonodular synovitis (pigmented), left knee
M12.269 Villonodular synovitis (pigmented), unspecified knee
M12.27 Villonodular synovitis (pigmented), ankle and foot
M12.271 Villonodular synovitis (pigmented), right ankle and foot
M12.272 Villonodular synovitis (pigmented), left ankle and foot
M12.279 Villonodular synovitis (pigmented), unspecified ankle and foot
SP M12.28 Villonodular synovitis (pigmented), other specified site
Villonodular synovitis (pigmented), vertebrae
SP M12.29 Villonodular synovitis (pigmented), multiple sites
M12.3 Palindromic rheumatism
IQ M12.30 Palindromic rheumatism, unspecified site
M12.31 Palindromic rheumatism, shoulder
M12.311 Palindromic rheumatism, right shoulder
M12.312 Palindromic rheumatism, left shoulder
M12.319 Palindromic rheumatism, unspecified shoulder
M12.32 Palindromic rheumatism, elbow
M12.321 Palindromic rheumatism, right elbow
M12.322 Palindromic rheumatism, left elbow
M12.329 Palindromic rheumatism, unspecified elbow
M12.33 Palindromic rheumatism, wrist
M12.331 Palindromic rheumatism, right wrist
M12.332 Palindromic rheumatism, left wrist
M12.339 Palindromic rheumatism, unspecified wrist

6 **M12.34 Palindromic rheumatism, hand**
L SP **M12.341 Palindromic rheumatism, right hand**
L SP **M12.342 Palindromic rheumatism, left hand**
L IQ **M12.349 Palindromic rheumatism, unspecified hand**
6 **M12.35 Palindromic rheumatism, hip**
L SP **M12.351 Palindromic rheumatism, right hip**
L SP **M12.352 Palindromic rheumatism, left hip**
L IQ **M12.359 Palindromic rheumatism, unspecified hip**
6 **M12.36 Palindromic rheumatism, knee**
L SP **M12.361 Palindromic rheumatism, right knee**
L SP **M12.362 Palindromic rheumatism, left knee**
L IQ **M12.369 Palindromic rheumatism, unspecified knee**
6 **M12.37 Palindromic rheumatism, ankle and foot**
L SP **M12.371 Palindromic rheumatism, right ankle and foot**
L SP **M12.372 Palindromic rheumatism, left ankle and foot**
L IQ **M12.379 Palindromic rheumatism, unspecified ankle and foot**
SP **M12.38 Palindromic rheumatism, other specified site**
Palindromic rheumatism, vertebrae
SP **M12.39 Palindromic rheumatism, multiple sites**
5 **M12.4 Intermittent hydrarthrosis**
IQ **M12.40 Intermittent hydrarthrosis, unspecified site**
6 **M12.41 Intermittent hydrarthrosis, shoulder**
L SP **M12.411 Intermittent hydrarthrosis, right shoulder**
L SP **M12.412 Intermittent hydrarthrosis, left shoulder**
L IQ **M12.419 Intermittent hydrarthrosis, unspecified shoulder**
6 **M12.42 Intermittent hydrarthrosis, elbow**
L SP **M12.421 Intermittent hydrarthrosis, right elbow**
L SP **M12.422 Intermittent hydrarthrosis, left elbow**
L IQ **M12.429 Intermittent hydrarthrosis, unspecified elbow**
6 **M12.43 Intermittent hydrarthrosis, wrist**
L SP **M12.431 Intermittent hydrarthrosis, right wrist**
L SP **M12.432 Intermittent hydrarthrosis, left wrist**
L IQ **M12.439 Intermittent hydrarthrosis, unspecified wrist**
6 **M12.44 Intermittent hydrarthrosis, hand**
L SP **M12.441 Intermittent hydrarthrosis, right hand**
L SP **M12.442 Intermittent hydrarthrosis, left hand**
L IQ **M12.449 Intermittent hydrarthrosis, unspecified hand**
6 **M12.45 Intermittent hydrarthrosis, hip**
L SP **M12.451 Intermittent hydrarthrosis, right hip**
L SP **M12.452 Intermittent hydrarthrosis, left hip**
L IQ **M12.459 Intermittent hydrarthrosis, unspecified hip**
6 **M12.46 Intermittent hydrarthrosis, knee**
L SP **M12.461 Intermittent hydrarthrosis, right knee**
L SP **M12.462 Intermittent hydrarthrosis, left knee**
L IQ **M12.469 Intermittent hydrarthrosis, unspecified knee**
6 **M12.47 Intermittent hydrarthrosis, ankle and foot**
L SP **M12.471 Intermittent hydrarthrosis, right ankle and foot**
L SP **M12.472 Intermittent hydrarthrosis, left ankle and foot**
L IQ **M12.479 Intermittent hydrarthrosis, unspecified ankle and foot**
SP **M12.48 Intermittent hydrarthrosis, other site**
SP **M12.49 Intermittent hydrarthrosis, multiple sites**
5 **M12.5 Traumatic arthropathy**
EXCLUDES 1 current injury-see Alphabetic Index
post-traumatic osteoarthritis of first carpometacarpal joint (M18.2-M18.3)
post-traumatic osteoarthritis of hip (M16.4-M16.5)
post-traumatic osteoarthritis of knee (M17.2-M17.3)
post-traumatic osteoarthritis NOS (M19.1-)
post-traumatic osteoarthritis of other single joints (M19.1-)

CODING TIPS✓ Report the injury that caused the traumatic arthropathy using a code from Chapter 19 (Injury, Poisoning and Certain Other Consequences of External Causes). If the injury requires a 7th character, use "S" for sequela.

IQ **M12.50 Traumatic arthropathy, unspecified site**
6 **M12.51 Traumatic arthropathy, shoulder**
L SP **M12.511 Traumatic arthropathy, right shoulder**
L SP **M12.512 Traumatic arthropathy, left shoulder**
L IQ **M12.519 Traumatic arthropathy, unspecified shoulder**
6 **M12.52 Traumatic arthropathy, elbow**
L SP **M12.521 Traumatic arthropathy, right elbow**
L SP **M12.522 Traumatic arthropathy, left elbow**
L IQ **M12.529 Traumatic arthropathy, unspecified elbow**
6 **M12.53 Traumatic arthropathy, wrist**
L SP **M12.531 Traumatic arthropathy, right wrist**
L SP **M12.532 Traumatic arthropathy, left wrist**

IQ M12.539 Traumatic arthropathy, unspecified wrist

6 M12.54 Traumatic arthropathy, hand

SP M12.541 Traumatic arthropathy, right hand

SP M12.542 Traumatic arthropathy, left hand

IQ M12.549 Traumatic arthropathy, unspecified hand

6 M12.55 Traumatic arthropathy, hip

SP M12.551 Traumatic arthropathy, right hip

SP M12.552 Traumatic arthropathy, left hip

IQ M12.559 Traumatic arthropathy, unspecified hip

6 M12.56 Traumatic arthropathy, knee

SP M12.561 Traumatic arthropathy, right knee

SP M12.562 Traumatic arthropathy, left knee

IQ M12.569 Traumatic arthropathy, unspecified knee

6 M12.57 Traumatic arthropathy, ankle and foot

SP M12.571 Traumatic arthropathy, right ankle and foot

SP M12.572 Traumatic arthropathy, left ankle and foot

IQ M12.579 Traumatic arthropathy, unspecified ankle and foot

SP M12.58 Traumatic arthropathy, other specified site
Traumatic arthropathy, vertebrae

SP M12.59 Traumatic arthropathy, multiple sites

5 M12.8 Other specific arthropathies, not elsewhere classified
Transient arthropathy

IQ M12.80 Other specific arthropathies, not elsewhere classified, unspecified site

6 M12.81 Other specific arthropathies, not elsewhere classified, shoulder

SP M12.811 Other specific arthropathies, not elsewhere classified, right shoulder

SP M12.812 Other specific arthropathies, not elsewhere classified, left shoulder

IQ M12.819 Other specific arthropathies, not elsewhere classified, unspecified shoulder

6 M12.82 Other specific arthropathies, not elsewhere classified, elbow

SP M12.821 Other specific arthropathies, not elsewhere classified, right elbow

SP M12.822 Other specific arthropathies, not elsewhere classified, left elbow

IQ M12.829 Other specific arthropathies, not elsewhere classified, unspecified elbow

6 M12.83 Other specific arthropathies, not elsewhere classified, wrist

SP M12.831 Other specific arthropathies, not elsewhere classified, right wrist

SP M12.832 Other specific arthropathies, not elsewhere classified, left wrist

IQ M12.839 Other specific arthropathies, not elsewhere classified, unspecified wrist

6 M12.84 Other specific arthropathies, not elsewhere classified, hand

SP M12.841 Other specific arthropathies, not elsewhere classified, right hand

SP M12.842 Other specific arthropathies, not elsewhere classified, left hand

IQ M12.849 Other specific arthropathies, not elsewhere classified, unspecified hand

6 M12.85 Other specific arthropathies, not elsewhere classified, hip

SP M12.851 Other specific arthropathies, not elsewhere classified, right hip

SP M12.852 Other specific arthropathies, not elsewhere classified, left hip

IQ M12.859 Other specific arthropathies, not elsewhere classified, unspecified hip

6 M12.86 Other specific arthropathies, not elsewhere classified, knee

SP M12.861 Other specific arthropathies, not elsewhere classified, right knee

SP M12.862 Other specific arthropathies, not elsewhere classified, left knee

IQ M12.869 Other specific arthropathies, not elsewhere classified, unspecified knee

6 M12.87 Other specific arthropathies, not elsewhere classified, ankle and foot

SP M12.871 Other specific arthropathies, not elsewhere classified, right ankle and foot

SP M12.872 Other specific arthropathies, not elsewhere classified, left ankle and foot

IQ M12.879 Other specific arthropathies, not elsewhere classified, unspecified ankle and foot

SP M12.88 Other specific arthropathies, not elsewhere classified, other specified site
Other specific arthropathies, not elsewhere classified, vertebrae

SP M12.89 Other specific arthropathies, not elsewhere classified, multiple sites

SP M12.9 Arthropathy, unspecified

CODING TIPS ✓ This code should **not** be used in home care, unless the physician or NPP specifically documents arthropathy. Arthritis should be coded to osteoarthritis, unless the physician or NPP has specifically stated another type.

4 M13 Other arthritis

EXCLUDES 1 arthrosis (M15-M19)
osteoarthritis (M15-M19)

SP M13.0 Polyarthritis, unspecified

5 M13.1 Monoarthritis, not elsewhere classified

IQ M13.10 Monoarthritis, not elsewhere classified, unspecified site

6 M13.11 Monoarthritis, not elsewhere classified, shoulder

SP M13.111 Monoarthritis, not elsewhere classified, right shoulder

SP M13.112 Monoarthritis, not elsewhere classified, left shoulder

Chapter 13

M00-M99

M13.119 Monoarthritis, not elsewhere classified, unspecified shoulder

M13.12 Monoarthritis, not elsewhere classified, elbow

M13.121 Monoarthritis, not elsewhere classified, right elbow

M13.122 Monoarthritis, not elsewhere classified, left elbow

M13.129 Monoarthritis, not elsewhere classified, unspecified elbow

M13.13 Monoarthritis, not elsewhere classified, wrist

M13.131 Monoarthritis, not elsewhere classified, right wrist

M13.132 Monoarthritis, not elsewhere classified, left wrist

M13.139 Monoarthritis, not elsewhere classified, unspecified wrist

M13.14 Monoarthritis, not elsewhere classified, hand

M13.141 Monoarthritis, not elsewhere classified, right hand

M13.142 Monoarthritis, not elsewhere classified, left hand

M13.149 Monoarthritis, not elsewhere classified, unspecified hand

M13.15 Monoarthritis, not elsewhere classified, hip

M13.151 Monoarthritis, not elsewhere classified, right hip

M13.152 Monoarthritis, not elsewhere classified, left hip

M13.159 Monoarthritis, not elsewhere classified, unspecified hip

M13.16 Monoarthritis, not elsewhere classified, knee

M13.161 Monoarthritis, not elsewhere classified, right knee

M13.162 Monoarthritis, not elsewhere classified, left knee

M13.169 Monoarthritis, not elsewhere classified, unspecified knee

M13.17 Monoarthritis, not elsewhere classified, ankle and foot

M13.171 Monoarthritis, not elsewhere classified, right ankle and foot

M13.172 Monoarthritis, not elsewhere classified, left ankle and foot

M13.179 Monoarthritis, not elsewhere classified, unspecified ankle and foot

M13.8 Other specified arthritis

Allergic arthritis

EXCLUDES 1 osteoarthritis (M15-M19)

M13.80 Other specified arthritis, unspecified site

M13.81 Other specified arthritis, shoulder

M13.811 Other specified arthritis, right shoulder

M13.812 Other specified arthritis, left shoulder

M13.819 Other specified arthritis, unspecified shoulder

M13.82 Other specified arthritis, elbow

M13.821 Other specified arthritis, right elbow

M13.822 Other specified arthritis, left elbow

M13.829 Other specified arthritis, unspecified elbow

M13.83 Other specified arthritis, wrist

M13.831 Other specified arthritis, right wrist

M13.832 Other specified arthritis, left wrist

M13.839 Other specified arthritis, unspecified wrist

M13.84 Other specified arthritis, hand

M13.841 Other specified arthritis, right hand

M13.842 Other specified arthritis, left hand

M13.849 Other specified arthritis, unspecified hand

M13.85 Other specified arthritis, hip

M13.851 Other specified arthritis, right hip

M13.852 Other specified arthritis, left hip

M13.859 Other specified arthritis, unspecified hip

M13.86 Other specified arthritis, knee

M13.861 Other specified arthritis, right knee

M13.862 Other specified arthritis, left knee

M13.869 Other specified arthritis, unspecified knee

M13.87 Other specified arthritis, ankle and foot

M13.871 Other specified arthritis, right ankle and foot

M13.872 Other specified arthritis, left ankle and foot

M13.879 Other specified arthritis, unspecified ankle and foot

M13.88 Other specified arthritis, other site

M13.89 Other specified arthritis, multiple sites

M14 Arthropathies in other diseases classified elsewhere

EXCLUDES 1 arthropathy in:
- diabetes mellitus (E08-E13 with .61-)
- hematological disorders (M36.2-M36.3)
- hypersensitivity reactions (M36.4)
- neoplastic disease (M36.1)
- neurosyphillis (A52.16)
- sarcoidosis (D86.86)
- enteropathic arthropathies (M07.-)
- juvenile psoriatic arthropathy (L40.54)
- lipoid dermatoarthritis (E78.81)

M14.6 Charcôt's joint

Neuropathic arthropathy

EXCLUDES 1 Charcôt's joint in diabetes mellitus (E08-E13 with .610)
Charcôt's joint in tabes dorsalis (A52.16)

CODING TIPS✓ Do not assign a code from M14.6- to report Charcot arthropathy in diabetes or syphilis. Charcot's joint in diabetes mellitus should be coded to the appropriate combination code from E08-E13 indicating the manifestation.

M14.60 Charcôt's joint, unspecified site

M14.61 Charcôt's joint, shoulder

M14.611 Charcôt's joint, right shoulder

M14.612 Charcôt's joint, left shoulder

M14.619 Charcôt's joint, unspecified shoulder

M14.62 Charcôt's joint, elbow

M14.621 Charcôt's joint, right elbow

M14.622 Charcôt's joint, left elbow

M14.629 Charcôt's joint, unspecified elbow

M14.63 Charcôt's joint, wrist

M14.631 Charcôt's joint, right wrist

M14.632 Charcôt's joint, left wrist

M14.639 Charcôt's joint, unspecified wrist

M14.64 Charcôt's joint, hand

M14.641 Charcôt's joint, right hand

M14.642 Charcôt's joint, left hand

M14.649 Charcôt's joint, unspecified hand

M14.65 Charcôt's joint, hip

M14.651 Charcôt's joint, right hip

M14.652 Charcôt's joint, left hip

M14.659 Charcôt's joint, unspecified hip

M14.66 Charcôt's joint, knee

M14.661 Charcôt's joint, right knee

M14.662 Charcôt's joint, left knee

M14.669 Charcôt's joint, unspecified knee

M14.67 Charcôt's joint, ankle and foot

M14.671 Charcôt's joint, right ankle and foot

M14.672 Charcôt's joint, left ankle and foot

M14.679 Charcôt's joint, unspecified ankle and foot

M14.68 Charcôt's joint, vertebrae

M14.69 Charcôt's joint, multiple sites

M14.8 Arthropathies in other specified diseases classified elsewhere

Code first underlying disease, such as:
- amyloidosis (E85.-)
- erythema multiforme (L51.-)
- erythema nodosum (L52)
- hemochromatosis (E83.11-)
- hyperparathyroidism (E21.-)
- hypothyroidism (E00-E03)
- sickle-cell disorders (D57.-)
- thyrotoxicosis [hyperthyroidism] (E05.-)
- Whipple's disease (K90.81)

M14.80 ***Arthropathies in other specified diseases classified elsewhere, unspecified site***

M14.81 Arthropathies in other specified diseases classified elsewhere, shoulder

M14.811 ***Arthropathies in other specified diseases classified elsewhere, right shoulder***

M14.812 ***Arthropathies in other specified diseases classified elsewhere, left shoulder***

M14.819 ***Arthropathies in other specified diseases classified elsewhere, unspecified shoulder***

M14.82 Arthropathies in other specified diseases classified elsewhere, elbow

M14.821 ***Arthropathies in other specified diseases classified elsewhere, right elbow***

M14.822 ***Arthropathies in other specified diseases classified elsewhere, left elbow***

M14.829 ***Arthropathies in other specified diseases classified elsewhere, unspecified elbow***

M14.83 Arthropathies in other specified diseases classified elsewhere, wrist

M14.831 ***Arthropathies in other specified diseases classified elsewhere, right wrist***

M14.832 ***Arthropathies in other specified diseases classified elsewhere, left wrist***

M14.839 ***Arthropathies in other specified diseases classified elsewhere, unspecified wrist***

M14.84 Arthropathies in other specified diseases classified elsewhere, hand

M14.841 ***Arthropathies in other specified diseases classified elsewhere, right hand***

M14.842 ***Arthropathies in other specified diseases classified elsewhere, left hand***

M14.849 ***Arthropathies in other specified diseases classified elsewhere, unspecified hand***

M14.85 Arthropathies in other specified diseases classified elsewhere, hip

M14.851 ***Arthropathies in other specified diseases classified elsewhere, right hip***

M14.852 ***Arthropathies in other specified diseases classified elsewhere, left hip***

M14.859 ***Arthropathies in other specified diseases classified elsewhere, unspecified hip***

M14.86 Arthropathies in other specified diseases classified elsewhere, knee

M14.861 ***Arthropathies in other specified diseases classified elsewhere, right knee***

M14.862 ***Arthropathies in other specified diseases classified elsewhere, left knee***

M14.869 ***Arthropathies in other specified diseases classified elsewhere, unspecified knee***

Chapter 13

M00-M99

6 **M14.87 Arthropathies in other specified diseases classified elsewhere, ankle and foot**

M ⊟ IQ **M14.871** ***Arthropathies in other specified diseases classified elsewhere, right ankle and foot***

M ⊟ IQ **M14.872** ***Arthropathies in other specified diseases classified elsewhere, left ankle and foot***

M ⊟ IQ **M14.879** ***Arthropathies in other specified diseases classified elsewhere, unspecified ankle and foot***

M IQ **M14.88** ***Arthropathies in other specified diseases classified elsewhere, vertebrae***

M IQ **M14.89** ***Arthropathies in other specified diseases classified elsewhere, multiple sites***

Osteoarthritis (M15-M19)

EXCLUDES 2 osteoarthritis of spine (M47.-)

ALERT Laterality is important. Most of the osteoarthritis codes may be subject to review if laterality is not coded. Query for additional information to avoid assigning a last digit of 9.

CODING TIPS✓ Osteoarthritis/degenerative joint disease (Categories M15-M19) is the most common type of arthritis in the elderly, and is the default if the physician or NPP documents arthritis. If the arthritis is in the spine, refer to Category M47. When coding osteoarthritis, review the medical records to determine whether the OA is localized or generalized; primary or secondary. Bilateral osteoarthritis of the same site is considered localized. Osteoarthritis, when the joint is known, is considered primary by default. If the joints affected are unknown, primary is not assumed. Generalized OA affects multiple joints (M15). Primary osteoarthritis is caused by aging. Secondary OA is caused by other conditions such as obesity.

CODING TIPS✓ Documented arthritis defaults to osteoarthritis, and osteoarthritis defaults to primary, when the joints are known, and when otherwise not noted to be secondary or due to some other cause.

4 **M15 Polyosteoarthritis**

INCLUDES arthritis of multiple sites

EXCLUDES 1 bilateral involvement of single joint (M16-M19)

SP **M15.0 Primary generalized (osteo)arthritis**

SP **M15.1 Heberden's nodes (with arthropathy)**
Interphalangeal distal osteoarthritis

SP **M15.2 Bouchard's nodes (with arthropathy)**
Juxtaphalangeal distal osteoarthritis

SP **M15.3 Secondary multiple arthritis**
Post-traumatic polyosteoarthritis

SP **M15.4 Erosive (osteo)arthritis**

SP **M15.8 Other polyosteoarthritis**

SP **M15.9 Polyosteoarthritis, unspecified**
Generalized osteoarthritis NOS

4 **M16 Osteoarthritis of hip**

SP **M16.0 Bilateral primary osteoarthritis of hip**

5 **M16.1 Unilateral primary osteoarthritis of hip**
Primary osteoarthritis of hip NOS

⊟ IQ **M16.10 Unilateral primary osteoarthritis, unspecified hip**

⊟ SP **M16.11 Unilateral primary osteoarthritis, right hip**

⊟ SP **M16.12 Unilateral primary osteoarthritis, left hip**

SP **M16.2 Bilateral osteoarthritis resulting from hip dysplasia**

5 **M16.3 Unilateral osteoarthritis resulting from hip dysplasia**
Dysplastic osteoarthritis of hip NOS

⊟ IQ **M16.30 Unilateral osteoarthritis resulting from hip dysplasia, unspecified hip**

⊟ SP **M16.31 Unilateral osteoarthritis resulting from hip dysplasia, right hip**

⊟ SP **M16.32 Unilateral osteoarthritis resulting from hip dysplasia, left hip**

SP **M16.4 Bilateral post-traumatic osteoarthritis of hip**

5 **M16.5 Unilateral post-traumatic osteoarthritis of hip**
Post-traumatic osteoarthritis of hip NOS

⊟ IQ **M16.50 Unilateral post-traumatic osteoarthritis, unspecified hip**

⊟ SP **M16.51 Unilateral post-traumatic osteoarthritis, right hip**

⊟ SP **M16.52 Unilateral post-traumatic osteoarthritis, left hip**

SP **M16.6 Other bilateral secondary osteoarthritis of hip**

SP **M16.7 Other unilateral secondary osteoarthritis of hip**
Secondary osteoarthritis of hip NOS

IQ **M16.9 Osteoarthritis of hip, unspecified**

4 **M17 Osteoarthritis of knee**

SP **M17.0 Bilateral primary osteoarthritis of knee**

5 **M17.1 Unilateral primary osteoarthritis of knee**
Primary osteoarthritis of knee NOS

⊟ IQ **M17.10 Unilateral primary osteoarthritis, unspecified knee**

⊟ SP **M17.11 Unilateral primary osteoarthritis, right knee**

⊟ SP **M17.12 Unilateral primary osteoarthritis, left knee**

SP **M17.2 Bilateral post-traumatic osteoarthritis of knee**

5 **M17.3 Unilateral post-traumatic osteoarthritis of knee**
Post-traumatic osteoarthritis of knee NOS

⊟ IQ **M17.30 Unilateral post-traumatic osteoarthritis, unspecified knee**

⊟ SP **M17.31 Unilateral post-traumatic osteoarthritis, right knee**

⊟ SP **M17.32 Unilateral post-traumatic osteoarthritis, left knee**

SP **M17.4 Other bilateral secondary osteoarthritis of knee**

SP **M17.5 Other unilateral secondary osteoarthritis of knee**
Secondary osteoarthritis of knee NOS

IQ **M17.9 Osteoarthritis of knee, unspecified**

4 **M18 Osteoarthritis of first carpometacarpal joint**

SP **M18.0 Bilateral primary osteoarthritis of first carpometacarpal joints**

5 **M18.1 Unilateral primary osteoarthritis of first carpometacarpal joint**
Primary osteoarthritis of first carpometacarpal joint NOS

M18.10 Unilateral primary osteoarthritis of first carpometacarpal joint, unspecified hand

M18.11 Unilateral primary osteoarthritis of first carpometacarpal joint, right hand

M18.12 Unilateral primary osteoarthritis of first carpometacarpal joint, left hand

M18.2 Bilateral post-traumatic osteoarthritis of first carpometacarpal joints

M18.3 Unilateral post-traumatic osteoarthritis of first carpometacarpal joint
Post-traumatic osteoarthritis of first carpometacarpal joint NOS

M18.30 Unilateral post-traumatic osteoarthritis of first carpometacarpal joint, unspecified hand

M18.31 Unilateral post-traumatic osteoarthritis of first carpometacarpal joint, right hand

M18.32 Unilateral post-traumatic osteoarthritis of first carpometacarpal joint, left hand

M18.4 Other bilateral secondary osteoarthritis of first carpometacarpal joints

M18.5 Other unilateral secondary osteoarthritis of first carpometacarpal joint
Secondary osteoarthritis of first carpometacarpal joint NOS

M18.50 Other unilateral secondary osteoarthritis of first carpometacarpal joint, unspecified hand

M18.51 Other unilateral secondary osteoarthritis of first carpometacarpal joint, right hand

M18.52 Other unilateral secondary osteoarthritis of first carpometacarpal joint, left hand

M18.9 Osteoarthritis of first carpometacarpal joint, unspecified

M19 Other and unspecified osteoarthritis
EXCLUDES 1 polyarthritis (M15.-)
EXCLUDES 2 arthrosis of spine (M47.-)
hallux rigidus (M20.2)
osteoarthritis of spine (M47.-)

M19.0 Primary osteoarthritis of other joints
ALERT Laterality is important. Osteoarthritis not specifying the joint affected may result in medical claim rejection. Query for additional information to avoid assigning a last digit 9.

M19.01 Primary osteoarthritis, shoulder

M19.011 Primary osteoarthritis, right shoulder

M19.012 Primary osteoarthritis, left shoulder

M19.019 Primary osteoarthritis, unspecified shoulder

M19.02 Primary osteoarthritis, elbow

M19.021 Primary osteoarthritis, right elbow

M19.022 Primary osteoarthritis, left elbow

M19.029 Primary osteoarthritis, unspecified elbow

M19.03 Primary osteoarthritis, wrist

M19.031 Primary osteoarthritis, right wrist

M19.032 Primary osteoarthritis, left wrist

M19.039 Primary osteoarthritis, unspecified wrist

M19.04 Primary osteoarthritis, hand
EXCLUDES 2 primary osteoarthritis of first carpometacarpal joint (M18.0-, M18.1-)

M19.041 Primary osteoarthritis, right hand

M19.042 Primary osteoarthritis, left hand

M19.049 Primary osteoarthritis, unspecified hand

M19.07 Primary osteoarthritis ankle and foot

M19.071 Primary osteoarthritis, right ankle and foot

M19.072 Primary osteoarthritis, left ankle and foot

M19.079 Primary osteoarthritis, unspecified ankle and foot

M19.09 Primary osteoarthritis, other specified site
CODING TIPS✓ The site of the osteoarthritis must be documented to assign M19.09.

M19.1 Post-traumatic osteoarthritis of other joints

M19.11 Post-traumatic osteoarthritis, shoulder

M19.111 Post-traumatic osteoarthritis, right shoulder

M19.112 Post-traumatic osteoarthritis, left shoulder

M19.119 Post-traumatic osteoarthritis, unspecified shoulder

M19.12 Post-traumatic osteoarthritis, elbow

M19.121 Post-traumatic osteoarthritis, right elbow

M19.122 Post-traumatic osteoarthritis, left elbow

M19.129 Post-traumatic osteoarthritis, unspecified elbow

M19.13 Post-traumatic osteoarthritis, wrist

M19.131 Post-traumatic osteoarthritis, right wrist

M19.132 Post-traumatic osteoarthritis, left wrist

M19.139 Post-traumatic osteoarthritis, unspecified wrist

M19.14 Post-traumatic osteoarthritis, hand
EXCLUDES 2 post-traumatic osteoarthritis of first carpometacarpal joint (M18.2-, M18.3-)

M19.141 Post-traumatic osteoarthritis, right hand

M19.142 Post-traumatic osteoarthritis, left hand

M19.149 Post-traumatic osteoarthritis, unspecified hand

M19.17 Post-traumatic osteoarthritis, ankle and foot

M19.171 Post-traumatic osteoarthritis, right ankle and foot

M19.172 Post-traumatic osteoarthritis, left ankle and foot

M19.179 Post-traumatic osteoarthritis, unspecified ankle and foot

M19.19 Post-traumatic osteoarthritis, other specified site

M19.2 Secondary osteoarthritis of other joints

M19.21 Secondary osteoarthritis, shoulder

M19.211 Secondary osteoarthritis, right shoulder

M19.212 Secondary osteoarthritis, left shoulder

M19.219 Secondary osteoarthritis, unspecified shoulder

M19.22 Secondary osteoarthritis, elbow

M19.221 Secondary osteoarthritis, right elbow

M19.222 Secondary osteoarthritis, left elbow

M19.229 Secondary osteoarthritis, unspecified elbow

M19.23 Secondary osteoarthritis, wrist

M19.231 Secondary osteoarthritis, right wrist

M19.232 Secondary osteoarthritis, left wrist

M19.239 Secondary osteoarthritis, unspecified wrist

M19.24 Secondary osteoarthritis, hand

M19.241 Secondary osteoarthritis, right hand

M19.242 Secondary osteoarthritis, left hand

M19.249 Secondary osteoarthritis, unspecified hand

M19.27 Secondary osteoarthritis, ankle and foot

M19.271 Secondary osteoarthritis, right ankle and foot

M19.272 Secondary osteoarthritis, left ankle and foot

M19.279 Secondary osteoarthritis, unspecified ankle and foot

M19.29 Secondary osteoarthritis, other specified site

M19.9 Osteoarthritis, unspecified site

ALERT Osteoarthritis not specifying the joint affected may result in a medical claim rejection. Query for additional information to avoid assigning a last digit 9.

CODING TIPS✓ If the site is known, do not use M19.90 and M19.91 codes. Primary is not the default when the joints are unknown.

M19.90 Unspecified osteoarthritis, unspecified site

Arthrosis NOS
Arthritis NOS
Osteoarthritis NOS

CODING TIPS✓ Avoid using M19.90. M19.90 is assigned when no information is available regarding the osteoarthritis.

M19.91 Primary osteoarthritis, unspecified site

Primary osteoarthritis NOS

CODING TIPS✓ Avoid using M19.91. This code is appropriate only when the physician or NPP documents "primary osteoarthritis" without naming joints affected.

M19.92 Post-traumatic osteoarthritis, unspecified site

Post-traumatic osteoarthritis NOS

M19.93 Secondary osteoarthritis, unspecified site

Secondary osteoarthritis NOS

Other joint disorders (M20-M25)

EXCLUDES 2 joints of the spine (M40-M54)

M20 Acquired deformities of fingers and toes

EXCLUDES 1 acquired absence of fingers and toes (Z89.-)
congenital absence of fingers and toes (Q71.3-, Q72.3-)
congenital deformities and malformations of fingers and toes (Q66.-, Q68-Q70, Q74.-)

CODING TIPS✓ Acquired deformities are different than congenital deformities. If the deformity was present at birth or considered congenital, refer to the Q codes.

M20.0 Deformity of finger(s)

EXCLUDES 1 clubbing of fingers (R68.3)
palmar fascial fibromatosis [Dupuytren] (M72.0)
trigger finger (M65.3)

M20.00 Unspecified deformity of finger(s)

M20.001 Unspecified deformity of right finger(s)

M20.002 Unspecified deformity of left finger(s)

M20.009 Unspecified deformity of unspecified finger(s)

M20.01 Mallet finger

M20.011 Mallet finger of right finger(s)

M20.012 Mallet finger of left finger(s)

M20.019 Mallet finger of unspecified finger(s)

M20.02 Boutonnière deformity

M20.021 Boutonnière deformity of right finger(s)

M20.022 Boutonnière deformity of left finger(s)

M20.029 Boutonnière deformity of unspecified finger(s)

M20.03 Swan-neck deformity

M20.031 Swan-neck deformity of right finger(s)

M20.032 Swan-neck deformity of left finger(s)

M20.039 Swan-neck deformity of unspecified finger(s)

M20.09 Other deformity of finger(s)

M20.091 Other deformity of right finger(s)

M20.092 Other deformity of left finger(s)

4th digit required 5th digit required 6th digit required 7th digit required 7th digit placeholder +Additional code Laterality

M20.099 Other deformity of finger(s), unspecified finger(s)

M20.1 Hallux valgus (acquired)
EXCLUDES 2 bunion (M21.6-)

M20.10 Hallux valgus (acquired), unspecified foot

M20.11 Hallux valgus (acquired), right foot

M20.12 Hallux valgus (acquired), left foot

M20.2 Hallux rigidus
DEFINITION Inflexible, stiff great toe, with limited motion at the metatarsophalangeal joint.

M20.20 Hallux rigidus, unspecified foot

M20.21 Hallux rigidus, right foot

M20.22 Hallux rigidus, left foot

M20.3 Hallux varus (acquired)
DEFINITION Displaced joint of the big toe which is pointed away from the rest of the toes.

M20.30 Hallux varus (acquired), unspecified foot

M20.31 Hallux varus (acquired), right foot

M20.32 Hallux varus (acquired), left foot

M20.4 Other hammer toe(s) (acquired)

M20.40 Other hammer toe(s) (acquired), unspecified foot

M20.41 Other hammer toe(s) (acquired), right foot

M20.42 Other hammer toe(s) (acquired), left foot

M20.5 Other deformities of toe(s) (acquired)

M20.5X Other deformities of toe(s) (acquired)

M20.5X1 Other deformities of toe(s) (acquired), right foot

M20.5X2 Other deformities of toe(s) (acquired), left foot

M20.5X9 Other deformities of toe(s) (acquired), unspecified foot

M20.6 Acquired deformities of toe(s), unspecified

M20.60 Acquired deformities of toe(s), unspecified, unspecified foot

M20.61 Acquired deformities of toe(s), unspecified, right foot

M20.62 Acquired deformities of toe(s), unspecified, left foot

M21 Other acquired deformities of limbs
EXCLUDES 1 acquired absence of limb (Z89.-)
congenital absence of limbs (Q71-Q73)
congenital deformities and malformations of limbs (Q65-Q66, Q68-Q74)
EXCLUDES 2 acquired deformities of fingers or toes (M20.-)
coxa plana (M91.2)

M21.0 Valgus deformity, not elsewhere classified
EXCLUDES 1 metatarsus valgus (Q66.6)
talipes calcaneovalgus (Q66.4-)

M21.00 Valgus deformity, not elsewhere classified, unspecified site

M21.02 Valgus deformity, not elsewhere classified, elbow
Cubitus valgus

M21.021 Valgus deformity, not elsewhere classified, right elbow

M21.022 Valgus deformity, not elsewhere classified, left elbow

M21.029 Valgus deformity, not elsewhere classified, unspecified elbow

M21.05 Valgus deformity, not elsewhere classified, hip

M21.051 Valgus deformity, not elsewhere classified, right hip

M21.052 Valgus deformity, not elsewhere classified, left hip

M21.059 Valgus deformity, not elsewhere classified, unspecified hip

M21.06 Valgus deformity, not elsewhere classified, knee
Genu valgum
Knock knee
DEFINITION Deformity in which the knees are angled abnormally close together with the ankles apart when standing erect with the legs straightened.

M21.061 Valgus deformity, not elsewhere classified, right knee

M21.062 Valgus deformity, not elsewhere classified, left knee

M21.069 Valgus deformity, not elsewhere classified, unspecified knee

M21.07 Valgus deformity, not elsewhere classified, ankle

M21.071 Valgus deformity, not elsewhere classified, right ankle

M21.072 Valgus deformity, not elsewhere classified, left ankle

M21.079 Valgus deformity, not elsewhere classified, unspecified ankle

M21.1 Varus deformity, not elsewhere classified
EXCLUDES 1 metatarsus varus (Q66.22-)
tibia vara (M92.51-)

M21.10 Varus deformity, not elsewhere classified, unspecified site

M21.12 Varus deformity, not elsewhere classified, elbow
Cubitus varus, elbow

M21.121 Varus deformity, not elsewhere classified, right elbow

M21.122 Varus deformity, not elsewhere classified, left elbow

M21.129 Varus deformity, not elsewhere classified, unspecified elbow

M21.15 Varus deformity, not elsewhere classified, hip

M21.151 Varus deformity, not elsewhere classified, right hip

M21.152 Varus deformity, not elsewhere classified, left hip

M21.159 Varus deformity, not elsewhere classified, unspecified

M21.16 Varus deformity, not elsewhere classified, knee

Chapter 13
M00-M99

Bow leg
Genu varum

M21.161 Varus deformity, not elsewhere classified, right knee

M21.162 Varus deformity, not elsewhere classified, left knee

M21.169 Varus deformity, not elsewhere classified, unspecified knee

M21.17 Varus deformity, not elsewhere classified, ankle

DEFINITION Inward angulation of the tibia and fibula on the talus generally due to trauma or overpull by the tibialis posterior and anterior tendons.

M21.171 Varus deformity, not elsewhere classified, right ankle

M21.172 Varus deformity, not elsewhere classified, left ankle

M21.179 Varus deformity, not elsewhere classified, unspecified ankle

M21.2 Flexion deformity

M21.20 Flexion deformity, unspecified site

M21.21 Flexion deformity, shoulder

M21.211 Flexion deformity, right shoulder

M21.212 Flexion deformity, left shoulder

M21.219 Flexion deformity, unspecified shoulder

M21.22 Flexion deformity, elbow

M21.221 Flexion deformity, right elbow

M21.222 Flexion deformity, left elbow

M21.229 Flexion deformity, unspecified elbow

M21.23 Flexion deformity, wrist

M21.231 Flexion deformity, right wrist

M21.232 Flexion deformity, left wrist

M21.239 Flexion deformity, unspecified wrist

M21.24 Flexion deformity, finger joints

M21.241 Flexion deformity, right finger joints

M21.242 Flexion deformity, left finger joints

M21.249 Flexion deformity, unspecified finger joints

M21.25 Flexion deformity, hip

M21.251 Flexion deformity, right hip

M21.252 Flexion deformity, left hip

M21.259 Flexion deformity, unspecified hip

M21.26 Flexion deformity, knee

M21.261 Flexion deformity, right knee

M21.262 Flexion deformity, left knee

M21.269 Flexion deformity, unspecified knee

M21.27 Flexion deformity, ankle and toes

M21.271 Flexion deformity, right ankle and toes

M21.272 Flexion deformity, left ankle and toes

M21.279 Flexion deformity, unspecified ankle and toes

M21.3 Wrist or foot drop (acquired)

M21.33 Wrist drop (acquired)

M21.331 Wrist drop, right wrist

M21.332 Wrist drop, left wrist

M21.339 Wrist drop, unspecified wrist

M21.37 Foot drop (acquired)

M21.371 Foot drop, right foot

M21.372 Foot drop, left foot

M21.379 Foot drop, unspecified foot

M21.4 Flat foot [pes planus] (acquired)

EXCLUDES 1 congenital pes planus (Q66.5-)

M21.40 Flat foot [pes planus] (acquired), unspecified foot

M21.41 Flat foot [pes planus] (acquired), right foot

M21.42 Flat foot [pes planus] (acquired), left foot

M21.5 Acquired clawhand, clubhand, clawfoot and clubfoot

EXCLUDES 1 clubfoot, not specified as acquired (Q66.89)

M21.51 Acquired clawhand

M21.511 Acquired clawhand, right hand

M21.512 Acquired clawhand, left hand

M21.519 Acquired clawhand, unspecified hand

M21.52 Acquired clubhand

M21.521 Acquired clubhand, right hand

M21.522 Acquired clubhand, left hand

M21.529 Acquired clubhand, unspecified hand

M21.53 Acquired clawfoot

M21.531 Acquired clawfoot, right foot

M21.532 Acquired clawfoot, left foot

M21.539 Acquired clawfoot, unspecified foot

M21.54 Acquired clubfoot

M21.541 Acquired clubfoot, right foot

M21.542 Acquired clubfoot, left foot

M21.549 Acquired clubfoot, unspecified foot

M21.6 Other acquired deformities of foot

EXCLUDES 2 deformities of toe (acquired) (M20.1-M20.6-)

M21.61 Bunion

M21.611 Bunion of right foot

M21.612 Bunion of left foot

M21.619 Bunion of unspecified foot

M21.62 Bunionette

M21.621 Bunionette of right foot

M21.622 Bunionette of left foot

M21.629 Bunionette of unspecified foot

M21.6X Other acquired deformities of foot

M21.6X1 Other acquired deformities of right foot

M21.6X2 Other acquired deformities of left foot

M21.6X9 Other acquired deformities of unspecified foot

M21.7 Unequal limb length (acquired)

4th digit required 5th digit required 6th digit required 7th digit required 7th digit placeholder + Additional code Laterality

Note:
The site used should correspond to the shorter limb

CODING TIPS✓ Acquired unequal limb length is usually due to an injury. Consider adding the injury with 7th character S.

IQ **M21.70 Unequal limb length (acquired), unspecified site**

6 **M21.72 Unequal limb length (acquired), humerus**

SP **M21.721 Unequal limb length (acquired), right humerus**

SP **M21.722 Unequal limb length (acquired), left humerus**

IQ **M21.729 Unequal limb length (acquired), unspecified humerus**

6 **M21.73 Unequal limb length (acquired), ulna and radius**

SP **M21.731 Unequal limb length (acquired), right ulna**

SP **M21.732 Unequal limb length (acquired), left ulna**

SP **M21.733 Unequal limb length (acquired), right radius**

SP **M21.734 Unequal limb length (acquired), left radius**

IQ **M21.739 Unequal limb length (acquired), unspecified ulna and radius**

6 **M21.75 Unequal limb length (acquired), femur**

SP **M21.751 Unequal limb length (acquired), right femur**

SP **M21.752 Unequal limb length (acquired), left femur**

IQ **M21.759 Unequal limb length (acquired), unspecified femur**

6 **M21.76 Unequal limb length (acquired), tibia and fibula**

SP **M21.761 Unequal limb length (acquired), right tibia**

SP **M21.762 Unequal limb length (acquired), left tibia**

SP **M21.763 Unequal limb length (acquired), right fibula**

SP **M21.764 Unequal limb length (acquired), left fibula**

IQ **M21.769 Unequal limb length (acquired), unspecified tibia and fibula**

5 **M21.8 Other specified acquired deformities of limbs**

EXCLUDES 2 coxa plana (M91.2)

IQ **M21.80 Other specified acquired deformities of unspecified limb**

6 **M21.82 Other specified acquired deformities of upper arm**

SP **M21.821 Other specified acquired deformities of right upper arm**

SP **M21.822 Other specified acquired deformities of left upper arm**

IQ **M21.829 Other specified acquired deformities of unspecified upper arm**

6 **M21.83 Other specified acquired deformities of forearm**

SP **M21.831 Other specified acquired deformities of right forearm**

SP **M21.832 Other specified acquired deformities of left forearm**

IQ **M21.839 Other specified acquired deformities of unspecified forearm**

6 **M21.85 Other specified acquired deformities of thigh**

SP **M21.851 Other specified acquired deformities of right thigh**

SP **M21.852 Other specified acquired deformities of left thigh**

IQ **M21.859 Other specified acquired deformities of unspecified thigh**

6 **M21.86 Other specified acquired deformities of lower leg**

SP **M21.861 Other specified acquired deformities of right lower leg**

SP **M21.862 Other specified acquired deformities of left lower leg**

IQ **M21.869 Other specified acquired deformities of unspecified lower leg**

5 **M21.9 Unspecified acquired deformity of limb and hand**

IQ **M21.90 Unspecified acquired deformity of unspecified limb**

6 **M21.92 Unspecified acquired deformity of upper arm**

SP **M21.921 Unspecified acquired deformity of right upper arm**

SP **M21.922 Unspecified acquired deformity of left upper arm**

IQ **M21.929 Unspecified acquired deformity of unspecified upper arm**

6 **M21.93 Unspecified acquired deformity of forearm**

SP **M21.931 Unspecified acquired deformity of right forearm**

SP **M21.932 Unspecified acquired deformity of left forearm**

IQ **M21.939 Unspecified acquired deformity of unspecified forearm**

6 **M21.94 Unspecified acquired deformity of hand**

SP **M21.941 Unspecified acquired deformity of hand, right hand**

SP **M21.942 Unspecified acquired deformity of hand, left hand**

IQ **M21.949 Unspecified acquired deformity of hand, unspecified hand**

6 **M21.95 Unspecified acquired deformity of thigh**

SP **M21.951 Unspecified acquired deformity of right thigh**

SP **M21.952 Unspecified acquired deformity of left thigh**

IQ **M21.959 Unspecified acquired deformity of unspecified thigh**

6 **M21.96 Unspecified acquired deformity of lower leg**

SP **M21.961 Unspecified acquired deformity of right lower leg**

SP **M21.962 Unspecified acquired deformity of left lower leg**

☐ !Q M21.969   **Unspecified acquired deformity of unspecified lower leg**

☐ M22   **Disorder of patella**
> EXCLUDES 2   traumatic dislocation of patella (S83.0-)

☐ M22.0 **Recurrent dislocation of patella**

☐ !Q M22.00   **Recurrent dislocation of patella, unspecified knee**

☐ SP M22.01   **Recurrent dislocation of patella, right knee**

☐ SP M22.02   **Recurrent dislocation of patella, left knee**

☐ M22.1 **Recurrent subluxation of patella**
Incomplete dislocation of patella

☐ !Q M22.10   **Recurrent subluxation of patella, unspecified knee**

☐ SP M22.11   **Recurrent subluxation of patella, right knee**

☐ SP M22.12   **Recurrent subluxation of patella, left knee**

☐ M22.2 **Patellofemoral disorders**

☐ M22.2X **Patellofemoral disorders**

☐ SP M22.2X1 **Patellofemoral disorders, right knee**

☐ SP M22.2X2 **Patellofemoral disorders, left knee**

☐ !Q M22.2X9   **Patellofemoral disorders, unspecified knee**

☐ M22.3 **Other derangements of patella**

☐ M22.3X **Other derangements of patella**

☐ SP M22.3X1 **Other derangements of patella, right knee**

☐ SP M22.3X2 **Other derangements of patella, left knee**

☐ !Q M22.3X9   **Other derangements of patella, unspecified knee**

☐ M22.4 **Chondromalacia patellae**
> CODING TIPS ✓   Chondromalacia patellae (CMP) is also referred to as "runner's knee."

☐ !Q M22.40   **Chondromalacia patellae, unspecified knee**

☐ SP M22.41   **Chondromalacia patellae, right knee**

☐ SP M22.42   **Chondromalacia patellae, left knee**

☐ M22.8 **Other disorders of patella**

☐ M22.8X **Other disorders of patella**

☐ SP M22.8X1 **Other disorders of patella, right knee**

☐ SP M22.8X2 **Other disorders of patella, left knee**

☐ !Q M22.8X9   **Other disorders of patella, unspecified knee**

☐ M22.9 **Unspecified disorder of patella**

☐ !Q M22.90   **Unspecified disorder of patella, unspecified knee**

☐ SP M22.91   **Unspecified disorder of patella, right knee**

☐ SP M22.92   **Unspecified disorder of patella, left knee**

☐ M23   **Internal derangement of knee**
> EXCLUDES 1   ankylosis (M24.66)
deformity of knee (M21.-)
osteochondritis dissecans (M93.2)

> EXCLUDES 2   current injury - see injury of knee and lower leg (S80-S89)
recurrent dislocation or subluxation of joints (M24.4)
recurrent dislocation or subluxation of patella (M22.0-M22.1)

> CODING TIPS ✓   Categories M23 and M24 are used for patients who have old injuries. New injuries are coded with codes from Chapter 19.

☐ M23.0 **Cystic meniscus**

☐ M23.00   **Cystic meniscus, unspecified meniscus**
Cystic meniscus, unspecified lateral meniscus
Cystic meniscus, unspecified medial meniscus

☐ SP M23.000   **Cystic meniscus, unspecified lateral meniscus, right knee**

☐ SP M23.001   **Cystic meniscus, unspecified lateral meniscus, left knee**

☐ !Q M23.002   **Cystic meniscus, unspecified lateral meniscus, unspecified knee**

☐ SP M23.003   **Cystic meniscus, unspecified medial meniscus, right knee**

☐ SP M23.004   **Cystic meniscus, unspecified medial meniscus, left knee**

☐ !Q M23.005   **Cystic meniscus, unspecified medial meniscus, unspecified knee**

☐ SP M23.006   **Cystic meniscus, unspecified meniscus, right knee**

☐ SP M23.007   **Cystic meniscus, unspecified meniscus, left knee**

☐ !Q M23.009   **Cystic meniscus, unspecified meniscus, unspecified knee**

☐ M23.01   **Cystic meniscus, anterior horn of medial meniscus**

☐ SP M23.011 **Cystic meniscus, anterior horn of medial meniscus, right knee**

☐ SP M23.012 **Cystic meniscus, anterior horn of medial meniscus, left knee**

☐ !Q M23.019   **Cystic meniscus, anterior horn of medial meniscus, unspecified knee**

☐ M23.02   **Cystic meniscus, posterior horn of medial meniscus**

☐ SP M23.021 **Cystic meniscus, posterior horn of medial meniscus, right knee**

☐ SP M23.022 **Cystic meniscus, posterior horn of medial meniscus, left knee**

☐ !Q M23.029   **Cystic meniscus, posterior horn of medial meniscus, unspecified knee**

☐ M23.03   **Cystic meniscus, other medial meniscus**

☐ SP M23.031 **Cystic meniscus, other medial meniscus, right knee**

☐ SP M23.032 **Cystic meniscus, other medial meniscus, left knee**

☐ !Q M23.039   **Cystic meniscus, other medial meniscus, unspecified knee**

☐ M23.04   **Cystic meniscus, anterior horn of lateral meniscus**

☐4th digit required   ☐5th digit required   ☐6th digit required   ☐7th digit required   ☐7th digit placeholder   ✚Additional code   ☐Laterality

SP M23.041 Cystic meniscus, anterior horn of lateral meniscus, right knee
SP M23.042 Cystic meniscus, anterior horn of lateral meniscus, left knee
IQ M23.049 Cystic meniscus, anterior horn of lateral meniscus, unspecified knee

6 M23.05 Cystic meniscus, posterior horn of lateral meniscus
SP M23.051 Cystic meniscus, posterior horn of lateral meniscus, right knee
SP M23.052 Cystic meniscus, posterior horn of lateral meniscus, left knee
IQ M23.059 Cystic meniscus, posterior horn of lateral meniscus, unspecified knee

6 M23.06 Cystic meniscus, other lateral meniscus
SP M23.061 Cystic meniscus, other lateral meniscus, right knee
SP M23.062 Cystic meniscus, other lateral meniscus, left knee
IQ M23.069 Cystic meniscus, other lateral meniscus, unspecified knee

5 M23.2 Derangement of meniscus due to old tear or injury
Old bucket-handle tear

6 M23.20 Derangement of unspecified meniscus due to old tear or injury
Derangement of unspecified lateral meniscus due to old tear or injury
Derangement of unspecified medial meniscus due to old tear or injury
SP M23.200 Derangement of unspecified lateral meniscus due to old tear or injury, right knee
SP M23.201 Derangement of unspecified lateral meniscus due to old tear or injury, left knee
IQ M23.202 Derangement of unspecified lateral meniscus due to old tear or injury, unspecified knee
SP M23.203 Derangement of unspecified medial meniscus due to old tear or injury, right knee
SP M23.204 Derangement of unspecified medial meniscus due to old tear or injury, left knee
IQ M23.205 Derangement of unspecified medial meniscus due to old tear or injury, unspecified knee
SP M23.206 Derangement of unspecified meniscus due to old tear or injury, right knee
SP M23.207 Derangement of unspecified meniscus due to old tear or injury, left knee
IQ M23.209 Derangement of unspecified meniscus due to old tear or injury, unspecified knee

6 M23.21 Derangement of anterior horn of medial meniscus due to old tear or injury
SP M23.211 Derangement of anterior horn of medial meniscus due to old tear or injury, right knee
SP M23.212 Derangement of anterior horn of medial meniscus due to old tear or injury, left knee
IQ M23.219 Derangement of anterior horn of medial meniscus due to old tear or injury, unspecified knee

6 M23.22 Derangement of posterior horn of medial meniscus due to old tear or injury
SP M23.221 Derangement of posterior horn of medial meniscus due to old tear or injury, right knee
SP M23.222 Derangement of posterior horn of medial meniscus due to old tear or injury, left knee
IQ M23.229 Derangement of posterior horn of medial meniscus due to old tear or injury, unspecified knee

6 M23.23 Derangement of other medial meniscus due to old tear or injury
SP M23.231 Derangement of other medial meniscus due to old tear or injury, right knee
SP M23.232 Derangement of other medial meniscus due to old tear or injury, left knee
IQ M23.239 Derangement of other medial meniscus due to old tear or injury, unspecified knee

6 M23.24 Derangement of anterior horn of lateral meniscus due to old tear or injury
SP M23.241 Derangement of anterior horn of lateral meniscus due to old tear or injury, right knee
SP M23.242 Derangement of anterior horn of lateral meniscus due to old tear or injury, left knee
IQ M23.249 Derangement of anterior horn of lateral meniscus due to old tear or injury, unspecified knee

6 M23.25 Derangement of posterior horn of lateral meniscus due to old tear or injury
SP M23.251 Derangement of posterior horn of lateral meniscus due to old tear or injury, right knee
SP M23.252 Derangement of posterior horn of lateral meniscus due to old tear or injury, left knee
IQ M23.259 Derangement of posterior horn of lateral meniscus due to old tear or injury, unspecified knee

6 M23.26 Derangement of other lateral meniscus due to old tear or injury
SP M23.261 Derangement of other lateral meniscus due to old tear or injury, right knee
SP M23.262 Derangement of other lateral meniscus due to old tear or injury, left knee
IQ M23.269 Derangement of other lateral meniscus due to old tear or injury, unspecified knee

5 M23.3 Other meniscus derangements
Degenerate meniscus
Detached meniscus
Retained meniscus

6 M23.30 Other meniscus derangements, unspecified meniscus
Other meniscus derangements, unspecified lateral meniscus
Other meniscus derangements, unspecified medial meniscus

Laterality SP M23.300 Other meniscus derangements, unspecified lateral meniscus, right knee

Laterality SP M23.301 Other meniscus derangements, unspecified lateral meniscus, left knee

Laterality IQ M23.302 Other meniscus derangements, unspecified lateral meniscus, unspecified knee

Laterality SP M23.303 Other meniscus derangements, unspecified medial meniscus, right knee

Laterality SP M23.304 Other meniscus derangements, unspecified medial meniscus, left knee

Laterality IQ M23.305 Other meniscus derangements, unspecified medial meniscus, unspecified knee

Laterality SP M23.306 Other meniscus derangements, unspecified meniscus, right knee

Laterality SP M23.307 Other meniscus derangements, unspecified meniscus, left knee

Laterality IQ M23.309 Other meniscus derangements, unspecified meniscus, unspecified knee

6 M23.31 Other meniscus derangements, anterior horn of medial meniscus

Laterality SP M23.311 Other meniscus derangements, anterior horn of medial meniscus, right knee

Laterality SP M23.312 Other meniscus derangements, anterior horn of medial meniscus, left knee

Laterality IQ M23.319 Other meniscus derangements, anterior horn of medial meniscus, unspecified knee

6 M23.32 Other meniscus derangements, posterior horn of medial meniscus

Laterality SP M23.321 Other meniscus derangements, posterior horn of medial meniscus, right knee

Laterality SP M23.322 Other meniscus derangements, posterior horn of medial meniscus, left knee

Laterality IQ M23.329 Other meniscus derangements, posterior horn of medial meniscus, unspecified knee

6 M23.33 Other meniscus derangements, other medial meniscus

Laterality SP M23.331 Other meniscus derangements, other medial meniscus, right knee

Laterality SP M23.332 Other meniscus derangements, other medial meniscus, left knee

Laterality IQ M23.339 Other meniscus derangements, other medial meniscus, unspecified knee

6 M23.34 Other meniscus derangements, anterior horn of lateral meniscus

Laterality SP M23.341 Other meniscus derangements, anterior horn of lateral meniscus, right knee

Laterality SP M23.342 Other meniscus derangements, anterior horn of lateral meniscus, left knee

Laterality IQ M23.349 Other meniscus derangements, anterior horn of lateral meniscus, unspecified knee

6 M23.35 Other meniscus derangements, posterior horn of lateral meniscus

Laterality SP M23.351 Other meniscus derangements, posterior horn of lateral meniscus, right knee

Laterality SP M23.352 Other meniscus derangements, posterior horn of lateral meniscus, left knee

Laterality IQ M23.359 Other meniscus derangements, posterior horn of lateral meniscus, unspecified knee

6 M23.36 Other meniscus derangements, other lateral meniscus

Laterality SP M23.361 Other meniscus derangements, other lateral meniscus, right knee

Laterality SP M23.362 Other meniscus derangements, other lateral meniscus, left knee

Laterality IQ M23.369 Other meniscus derangements, other lateral meniscus, unspecified knee

5 M23.4 Loose body in knee

Laterality IQ M23.40 Loose body in knee, unspecified knee

Laterality SP M23.41 Loose body in knee, right knee

Laterality SP M23.42 Loose body in knee, left knee

5 M23.5 Chronic instability of knee

Laterality IQ M23.50 Chronic instability of knee, unspecified knee

Laterality SP M23.51 Chronic instability of knee, right knee

Laterality SP M23.52 Chronic instability of knee, left knee

5 M23.6 Other spontaneous disruption of ligament(s) of knee

6 M23.60 Other spontaneous disruption of unspecified ligament of knee

Laterality SP M23.601 Other spontaneous disruption of unspecified ligament of right knee

Laterality SP M23.602 Other spontaneous disruption of unspecified ligament of left knee

Laterality IQ M23.609 Other spontaneous disruption of unspecified ligament of unspecified knee

6 M23.61 Other spontaneous disruption of anterior cruciate ligament of knee

Laterality SP M23.611 Other spontaneous disruption of anterior cruciate ligament of right knee

Laterality SP M23.612 Other spontaneous disruption of anterior cruciate ligament of left knee

Laterality IQ M23.619 Other spontaneous disruption of anterior cruciate ligament of unspecified knee

6 M23.62 Other spontaneous disruption of posterior cruciate ligament of knee

⊟ SP M23.621 Other spontaneous disruption of posterior cruciate ligament of right knee

⊟ SP M23.622 Other spontaneous disruption of posterior cruciate ligament of left knee

⊟ IQ M23.629 Other spontaneous disruption of posterior cruciate ligament of unspecified knee

6 M23.63 Other spontaneous disruption of medial collateral ligament of knee

⊟ SP M23.631 Other spontaneous disruption of medial collateral ligament of right knee

⊟ SP M23.632 Other spontaneous disruption of medial collateral ligament of left knee

⊟ IQ M23.639 Other spontaneous disruption of medial collateral ligament of unspecified knee

6 M23.64 Other spontaneous disruption of lateral collateral ligament of knee

⊟ SP M23.641 Other spontaneous disruption of lateral collateral ligament of right knee

⊟ SP M23.642 Other spontaneous disruption of lateral collateral ligament of left knee

⊟ IQ M23.649 Other spontaneous disruption of lateral collateral ligament of unspecified knee

6 M23.67 Other spontaneous disruption of capsular ligament of knee

⊟ SP M23.671 Other spontaneous disruption of capsular ligament of right knee

⊟ SP M23.672 Other spontaneous disruption of capsular ligament of left knee

⊟ IQ M23.679 Other spontaneous disruption of capsular ligament of unspecified knee

5 M23.8 Other internal derangements of knee
Laxity of ligament of knee
Snapping knee

6 M23.8X Other internal derangements of knee

⊟ SP M23.8X1 Other internal derangements of right knee

⊟ SP M23.8X2 Other internal derangements of left knee

⊟ IQ M23.8X9 Other internal derangements of unspecified knee

5 M23.9 Unspecified internal derangement of knee

⊟ IQ M23.90 Unspecified internal derangement of unspecified knee

⊟ IQ M23.91 Unspecified internal derangement of right knee

⊟ IQ M23.92 Unspecified internal derangement of left knee

4 M24 Other specific joint derangements
EXCLUDES 1 current injury - see injury of joint by body region
EXCLUDES 2 ganglion (M67.4)
snapping knee (M23.8-)
temporomandibular joint disorders (M26.6-)

CODING TIPS ✓ Categories M23 and M24 are used for patients who have old injuries. New injuries are coded with codes from Chapter 19.

5 M24.0 Loose body in joint
EXCLUDES 2 loose body in knee (M23.4)

IQ M24.00 Loose body in unspecified joint

6 M24.01 Loose body in shoulder

⊟ SP M24.011 Loose body in right shoulder

⊟ SP M24.012 Loose body in left shoulder

⊟ IQ M24.019 Loose body in unspecified shoulder

6 M24.02 Loose body in elbow

⊟ SP M24.021 Loose body in right elbow

⊟ SP M24.022 Loose body in left elbow

⊟ IQ M24.029 Loose body in unspecified elbow

6 M24.03 Loose body in wrist

⊟ SP M24.031 Loose body in right wrist

⊟ SP M24.032 Loose body in left wrist

⊟ IQ M24.039 Loose body in unspecified wrist

6 M24.04 Loose body in finger joints

⊟ SP M24.041 Loose body in right finger joint(s)

⊟ SP M24.042 Loose body in left finger joint(s)

⊟ IQ M24.049 Loose body in unspecified finger joint(s)

6 M24.05 Loose body in hip

⊟ SP M24.051 Loose body in right hip

⊟ SP M24.052 Loose body in left hip

⊟ IQ M24.059 Loose body in unspecified hip

6 M24.07 Loose body in ankle and toe joints

⊟ SP M24.071 Loose body in right ankle

⊟ SP M24.072 Loose body in left ankle

⊟ IQ M24.073 Loose body in unspecified ankle

⊟ SP M24.074 Loose body in right toe joint(s)

⊟ SP M24.075 Loose body in left toe joint(s)

⊟ IQ M24.076 Loose body in unspecified toe joints

SP M24.08 Loose body, other site

5 M24.1 Other articular cartilage disorders
EXCLUDES 2 chondrocalcinosis (M11.1, M11.2-)
internal derangement of knee (M23.-)
metastatic calcification (E83.5)
ochronosis (E70.2)

IQ M24.10 Other articular cartilage disorders, unspecified site

6 M24.11 Other articular cartilage disorders, shoulder

⊟ SP M24.111 Other articular cartilage disorders, right shoulder

⊟ SP M24.112 Other articular cartilage disorders, left shoulder

⊟ IQ M24.119 Other articular cartilage disorders, unspecified shoulder

6 M24.12 Other articular cartilage disorders, elbow

⊟ SP M24.121 Other articular cartilage disorders, right elbow

⊟ SP M24.122 Other articular cartilage disorders, left elbow

M24.129 Other articular cartilage disorders, unspecified elbow

M24.13 Other articular cartilage disorders, wrist

M24.131 Other articular cartilage disorders, right wrist

M24.132 Other articular cartilage disorders, left wrist

M24.139 Other articular cartilage disorders, unspecified wrist

M24.14 Other articular cartilage disorders, hand

M24.141 Other articular cartilage disorders, right hand

M24.142 Other articular cartilage disorders, left hand

M24.149 Other articular cartilage disorders, unspecified hand

M24.15 Other articular cartilage disorders, hip

M24.151 Other articular cartilage disorders, right hip

M24.152 Other articular cartilage disorders, left hip

M24.159 Other articular cartilage disorders, unspecified hip

M24.17 Other articular cartilage disorders, ankle and foot

M24.171 Other articular cartilage disorders, right ankle

M24.172 Other articular cartilage disorders, left ankle

M24.173 Other articular cartilage disorders, unspecified ankle

M24.174 Other articular cartilage disorders, right foot

M24.175 Other articular cartilage disorders, left foot

M24.176 Other articular cartilage disorders, unspecified foot

M24.19 Other articular cartilage disorders, other specified site

M24.2 Disorder of ligament

Instability secondary to old ligament injury
Ligamentous laxity NOS

EXCLUDES 1 familial ligamentous laxity (M35.7)

EXCLUDES 2 internal derangement of knee (M23.5-M23.8X9)

M24.20 Disorder of ligament, unspecified site

M24.21 Disorder of ligament, shoulder

M24.211 Disorder of ligament, right shoulder

M24.212 Disorder of ligament, left shoulder

M24.219 Disorder of ligament, unspecified shoulder

M24.22 Disorder of ligament, elbow

M24.221 Disorder of ligament, right elbow

M24.222 Disorder of ligament, left elbow

M24.229 Disorder of ligament, unspecified elbow

M24.23 Disorder of ligament, wrist

M24.231 Disorder of ligament, right wrist

M24.232 Disorder of ligament, left wrist

M24.239 Disorder of ligament, unspecified wrist

M24.24 Disorder of ligament, hand

M24.241 Disorder of ligament, right hand

M24.242 Disorder of ligament, left hand

M24.249 Disorder of ligament, unspecified hand

M24.25 Disorder of ligament, hip

M24.251 Disorder of ligament, right hip

M24.252 Disorder of ligament, left hip

M24.259 Disorder of ligament, unspecified hip

M24.27 Disorder of ligament, ankle and foot

M24.271 Disorder of ligament, right ankle

M24.272 Disorder of ligament, left ankle

M24.273 Disorder of ligament, unspecified ankle

M24.274 Disorder of ligament, right foot

M24.275 Disorder of ligament, left foot

M24.276 Disorder of ligament, unspecified foot

M24.28 Disorder of ligament, vertebrae

M24.29 Disorder of ligament, other specified site

M24.3 Pathological dislocation of joint, not elsewhere classified

EXCLUDES 1 congenital dislocation or displacement of joint- see congenital malformations and deformations of the musculoskeletal system (Q65-Q79)
current injury - see injury of joints and ligaments by body region
recurrent dislocation of joint (M24.4-)

M24.30 Pathological dislocation of unspecified joint, not elsewhere classified

M24.31 Pathological dislocation of shoulder, not elsewhere classified

M24.311 Pathological dislocation of right shoulder, not elsewhere classified

M24.312 Pathological dislocation of left shoulder, not elsewhere classified

M24.319 Pathological dislocation of unspecified shoulder, not elsewhere classified

M24.32 Pathological dislocation of elbow, not elsewhere classified

M24.321 Pathological dislocation of right elbow, not elsewhere classified

M24.322 Pathological dislocation of left elbow, not elsewhere classified

M24.329 Pathological dislocation of unspecified elbow, not elsewhere classified

M24.33 Pathological dislocation of wrist, not elsewhere classified

M24.331 Pathological dislocation of right wrist, not elsewhere classified

M24.332 Pathological dislocation of left wrist, not elsewhere classified

IQ M24.339 Pathological dislocation of unspecified wrist, not elsewhere classified

6 M24.34 Pathological dislocation of hand, not elsewhere classified

SP M24.341 Pathological dislocation of right hand, not elsewhere classified

SP M24.342 Pathological dislocation of left hand, not elsewhere classified

IQ M24.349 Pathological dislocation of unspecified hand, not elsewhere classified

6 M24.35 Pathological dislocation of hip, not elsewhere classified

SP M24.351 Pathological dislocation of right hip, not elsewhere classified

SP M24.352 Pathological dislocation of left hip, not elsewhere classified

IQ M24.359 Pathological dislocation of unspecified hip, not elsewhere classified

6 M24.36 Pathological dislocation of knee, not elsewhere classified

SP M24.361 Pathological dislocation of right knee, not elsewhere classified

SP M24.362 Pathological dislocation of left knee, not elsewhere classified

IQ M24.369 Pathological dislocation of unspecified knee, not elsewhere classified

6 M24.37 Pathological dislocation of ankle and foot, not elsewhere classified

SP M24.371 Pathological dislocation of right ankle, not elsewhere classified

SP M24.372 Pathological dislocation of left ankle, not elsewhere classified

IQ M24.373 Pathological dislocation of unspecified ankle, not elsewhere classified

SP M24.374 Pathological dislocation of right foot, not elsewhere classified

SP M24.375 Pathological dislocation of left foot, not elsewhere classified

IQ M24.376 Pathological dislocation of unspecified foot, not elsewhere classified

SP M24.39 Pathological dislocation of other specified joint, not elsewhere classified

5 M24.4 Recurrent dislocation of joint

Recurrent subluxation of joint

EXCLUDES 2 recurrent dislocation of patella (M22.0-M22.1)
recurrent vertebral dislocation (M43.3-, M43.4, M43.5-)

IQ M24.40 Recurrent dislocation, unspecified joint

6 M24.41 Recurrent dislocation, shoulder

SP M24.411 Recurrent dislocation, right shoulder

SP M24.412 Recurrent dislocation, left shoulder

IQ M24.419 Recurrent dislocation, unspecified shoulder

6 M24.42 Recurrent dislocation, elbow

SP M24.421 Recurrent dislocation, right elbow

SP M24.422 Recurrent dislocation, left elbow

IQ M24.429 Recurrent dislocation, unspecified elbow

6 M24.43 Recurrent dislocation, wrist

SP M24.431 Recurrent dislocation, right wrist

SP M24.432 Recurrent dislocation, left wrist

IQ M24.439 Recurrent dislocation, unspecified wrist

6 M24.44 Recurrent dislocation, hand and finger(s)

SP M24.441 Recurrent dislocation, right hand

SP M24.442 Recurrent dislocation, left hand

IQ M24.443 Recurrent dislocation, unspecified hand

SP M24.444 Recurrent dislocation, right finger

SP M24.445 Recurrent dislocation, left finger

IQ M24.446 Recurrent dislocation, unspecified finger

6 M24.45 Recurrent dislocation, hip

SP M24.451 Recurrent dislocation, right hip

SP M24.452 Recurrent dislocation, left hip

IQ M24.459 Recurrent dislocation, unspecified hip

6 M24.46 Recurrent dislocation, knee

SP M24.461 Recurrent dislocation, right knee

SP M24.462 Recurrent dislocation, left knee

IQ M24.469 Recurrent dislocation, unspecified knee

6 M24.47 Recurrent dislocation, ankle, foot and toes

SP M24.471 Recurrent dislocation, right ankle

SP M24.472 Recurrent dislocation, left ankle

IQ M24.473 Recurrent dislocation, unspecified ankle

SP M24.474 Recurrent dislocation, right foot

SP M24.475 Recurrent dislocation, left foot

IQ M24.476 Recurrent dislocation, unspecified foot

SP M24.477 Recurrent dislocation, right toe(s)

SP M24.478 Recurrent dislocation, left toe(s)

IQ M24.479 Recurrent dislocation, unspecified toe(s)

SP M24.49 Recurrent dislocation, other specified joint

5 M24.5 Contracture of joint

EXCLUDES 1 contracture of muscle without contracture of joint (M62.4-)
contracture of tendon (sheath) without contracture of joint (M62.4-)
Dupuytren's contracture (M72.0)

EXCLUDES 2 acquired deformities of limbs (M20-M21)

IQ M24.50 Contracture, unspecified joint

6 M24.51 Contracture, shoulder

SP M24.511 Contracture, right shoulder

SP M24.512 Contracture, left shoulder

M24.519 Contracture, unspecified shoulder
M24.52 Contracture, elbow
M24.521 Contracture, right elbow
M24.522 Contracture, left elbow
M24.529 Contracture, unspecified elbow
M24.53 Contracture, wrist
M24.531 Contracture, right wrist
M24.532 Contracture, left wrist
M24.539 Contracture, unspecified wrist
M24.54 Contracture, hand
M24.541 Contracture, right hand
M24.542 Contracture, left hand
M24.549 Contracture, unspecified hand
M24.55 Contracture, hip
M24.551 Contracture, right hip
M24.552 Contracture, left hip
M24.559 Contracture, unspecified hip
M24.56 Contracture, knee
M24.561 Contracture, right knee
M24.562 Contracture, left knee
M24.569 Contracture, unspecified knee
M24.57 Contracture, ankle and foot
M24.571 Contracture, right ankle
M24.572 Contracture, left ankle
M24.573 Contracture, unspecified ankle
M24.574 Contracture, right foot
M24.575 Contracture, left foot
M24.576 Contracture, unspecified foot
M24.59 Contracture, other specified joint
M24.6 Ankylosis of joint
EXCLUDES 1 stiffness of joint without ankylosis (M25.6-)
EXCLUDES 2 spine (M43.2-)
M24.60 Ankylosis, unspecified joint
M24.61 Ankylosis, shoulder
M24.611 Ankylosis, right shoulder
M24.612 Ankylosis, left shoulder
M24.619 Ankylosis, unspecified shoulder
M24.62 Ankylosis, elbow
M24.621 Ankylosis, right elbow
M24.622 Ankylosis, left elbow
M24.629 Ankylosis, unspecified elbow
M24.63 Ankylosis, wrist
M24.631 Ankylosis, right wrist
M24.632 Ankylosis, left wrist
M24.639 Ankylosis, unspecified wrist
M24.64 Ankylosis, hand
M24.641 Ankylosis, right hand
M24.642 Ankylosis, left hand
M24.649 Ankylosis, unspecified hand
M24.65 Ankylosis, hip
M24.651 Ankylosis, right hip
M24.652 Ankylosis, left hip
M24.659 Ankylosis, unspecified hip
M24.66 Ankylosis, knee
M24.661 Ankylosis, right knee
M24.662 Ankylosis, left knee
M24.669 Ankylosis, unspecified knee
M24.67 Ankylosis, ankle and foot
M24.671 Ankylosis, right ankle
M24.672 Ankylosis, left ankle
M24.673 Ankylosis, unspecified ankle
M24.674 Ankylosis, right foot
M24.675 Ankylosis, left foot
M24.676 Ankylosis, unspecified foot
M24.69 Ankylosis, other specified joint
M24.7 Protrusio acetabuli
M24.8 Other specific joint derangements, not elsewhere classified
EXCLUDES 2 iliotibial band syndrome (M76.3)
M24.80 Other specific joint derangements of unspecified joint, not elsewhere classified
M24.81 Other specific joint derangements of shoulder, not elsewhere classified
M24.811 Other specific joint derangements of right shoulder, not elsewhere classified
M24.812 Other specific joint derangements of left shoulder, not elsewhere classified
M24.819 Other specific joint derangements of unspecified shoulder, not elsewhere classified
M24.82 Other specific joint derangements of elbow, not elsewhere classified
M24.821 Other specific joint derangements of right elbow, not elsewhere classified
M24.822 Other specific joint derangements of left elbow, not elsewhere classified
M24.829 Other specific joint derangements of unspecified elbow, not elsewhere classified
M24.83 Other specific joint derangements of wrist, not elsewhere classified
M24.831 Other specific joint derangements of right wrist, not elsewhere classified
M24.832 Other specific joint derangements of left wrist, not elsewhere classified
M24.839 Other specific joint derangements of unspecified wrist, not elsewhere classified
M24.84 Other specific joint derangements of hand, not elsewhere classified
M24.841 Other specific joint derangements of right hand, not elsewhere classified
M24.842 Other specific joint derangements of left hand, not elsewhere classified
M24.849 Other specific joint derangements of unspecified hand, not elsewhere classified
M24.85 Other specific joint derangements of hip, not elsewhere classified

4th digit required 5th digit required 6th digit required 7th digit required 7th digit placeholder +Additional code Laterality

Irritable hip

⊟ SP **M24.851 Other specific joint derangements of right hip, not elsewhere classified**

⊟ SP **M24.852 Other specific joint derangements of left hip, not elsewhere classified**

⊟ IQ **M24.859 Other specific joint derangements of unspecified hip, not elsewhere classified**

6 **M24.87 Other specific joint derangements of ankle and foot, not elsewhere classified**

⊟ SP **M24.871 Other specific joint derangements of right ankle, not elsewhere classified**

⊟ SP **M24.872 Other specific joint derangements of left ankle, not elsewhere classified**

⊟ IQ **M24.873 Other specific joint derangements of unspecified ankle, not elsewhere classified**

⊟ SP **M24.874 Other specific joint derangements of right foot, not elsewhere classified**

⊟ SP **M24.875 Other specific joint derangements left foot, not elsewhere classified**

⊟ IQ **M24.876 Other specific joint derangements of unspecified foot, not elsewhere classified**

SP **M24.89 Other specific joint derangement of other specified joint, not elsewhere classified**

IQ **M24.9 Joint derangement, unspecified**

4 **M25 Other joint disorder, not elsewhere classified**

EXCLUDES 2 abnormality of gait and mobility (R26.-)
acquired deformities of limb (M20-M21)
calcification of bursa (M71.4-)
calcification of shoulder (joint) (M75.3)
calcification of tendon (M65.2-)
difficulty in walking (R26.2)
temporomandibular joint disorder (M26.6-)

5 **M25.0 Hemarthrosis**

EXCLUDES 1 current injury - see injury of joint by body region
hemophilic arthropathy (M36.2)

IQ **M25.00 Hemarthrosis, unspecified joint**

6 **M25.01 Hemarthrosis, shoulder**

⊟ SP **M25.011 Hemarthrosis, right shoulder**

⊟ SP **M25.012 Hemarthrosis, left shoulder**

⊟ IQ **M25.019 Hemarthrosis, unspecified shoulder**

6 **M25.02 Hemarthrosis, elbow**

⊟ SP **M25.021 Hemarthrosis, right elbow**

⊟ SP **M25.022 Hemarthrosis, left elbow**

⊟ IQ **M25.029 Hemarthrosis, unspecified elbow**

6 **M25.03 Hemarthrosis, wrist**

⊟ SP **M25.031 Hemarthrosis, right wrist**

⊟ SP **M25.032 Hemarthrosis, left wrist**

⊟ IQ **M25.039 Hemarthrosis, unspecified wrist**

6 **M25.04 Hemarthrosis, hand**

⊟ SP **M25.041 Hemarthrosis, right hand**

⊟ SP **M25.042 Hemarthrosis, left hand**

⊟ IQ **M25.049 Hemarthrosis, unspecified hand**

6 **M25.05 Hemarthrosis, hip**

⊟ SP **M25.051 Hemarthrosis, right hip**

⊟ SP **M25.052 Hemarthrosis, left hip**

⊟ IQ **M25.059 Hemarthrosis, unspecified hip**

6 **M25.06 Hemarthrosis, knee**

⊟ SP **M25.061 Hemarthrosis, right knee**

⊟ SP **M25.062 Hemarthrosis, left knee**

⊟ IQ **M25.069 Hemarthrosis, unspecified knee**

6 **M25.07 Hemarthrosis, ankle and foot**

⊟ SP **M25.071 Hemarthrosis, right ankle**

⊟ SP **M25.072 Hemarthrosis, left ankle**

⊟ IQ **M25.073 Hemarthrosis, unspecified ankle**

⊟ SP **M25.074 Hemarthrosis, right foot**

⊟ SP **M25.075 Hemarthrosis, left foot**

⊟ IQ **M25.076 Hemarthrosis, unspecified foot**

SP **M25.08 Hemarthrosis, other specified site**
Hemarthrosis, vertebrae

5 **M25.1 Fistula of joint**

IQ **M25.10 Fistula, unspecified joint**

6 **M25.11 Fistula, shoulder**

⊟ SP **M25.111 Fistula, right shoulder**

⊟ SP **M25.112 Fistula, left shoulder**

⊟ IQ **M25.119 Fistula, unspecified shoulder**

6 **M25.12 Fistula, elbow**

⊟ SP **M25.121 Fistula, right elbow**

⊟ SP **M25.122 Fistula, left elbow**

⊟ IQ **M25.129 Fistula, unspecified elbow**

6 **M25.13 Fistula, wrist**

⊟ SP **M25.131 Fistula, right wrist**

⊟ SP **M25.132 Fistula, left wrist**

⊟ IQ **M25.139 Fistula, unspecified wrist**

6 **M25.14 Fistula, hand**

⊟ SP **M25.141 Fistula, right hand**

⊟ SP **M25.142 Fistula, left hand**

⊟ IQ **M25.149 Fistula, unspecified hand**

6 **M25.15 Fistula, hip**

⊟ SP **M25.151 Fistula, right hip**

⊟ SP **M25.152 Fistula, left hip**

⊟ IQ **M25.159 Fistula, unspecified hip**

6 **M25.16 Fistula, knee**

⊟ SP **M25.161 Fistula, right knee**

⊟ SP **M25.162 Fistula, left knee**

⊟ IQ **M25.169 Fistula, unspecified knee**

6 **M25.17 Fistula, ankle and foot**

⊟ SP **M25.171 Fistula, right ankle**

⊟ SP **M25.172 Fistula, left ankle**

⊟ IQ **M25.173 Fistula, unspecified ankle**

⊟ SP **M25.174 Fistula, right foot**

⊟ SP **M25.175 Fistula, left foot**

⊟ IQ **M25.176 Fistula, unspecified foot**

SP **M25.18 Fistula, other specified site**

Fistula, vertebrae

5 **M25.2 Flail joint**

IQ **M25.20 Flail joint, unspecified joint**

6 **M25.21 Flail joint, shoulder**

Laterality SP **M25.211 Flail joint, right shoulder**

Laterality SP **M25.212 Flail joint, left shoulder**

Laterality IQ **M25.219 Flail joint, unspecified shoulder**

6 **M25.22 Flail joint, elbow**

Laterality SP **M25.221 Flail joint, right elbow**

Laterality SP **M25.222 Flail joint, left elbow**

Laterality IQ **M25.229 Flail joint, unspecified elbow**

6 **M25.23 Flail joint, wrist**

Laterality SP **M25.231 Flail joint, right wrist**

Laterality SP **M25.232 Flail joint, left wrist**

Laterality IQ **M25.239 Flail joint, unspecified wrist**

6 **M25.24 Flail joint, hand**

Laterality SP **M25.241 Flail joint, right hand**

Laterality SP **M25.242 Flail joint, left hand**

Laterality IQ **M25.249 Flail joint, unspecified hand**

6 **M25.25 Flail joint, hip**

Laterality SP **M25.251 Flail joint, right hip**

Laterality SP **M25.252 Flail joint, left hip**

Laterality IQ **M25.259 Flail joint, unspecified hip**

6 **M25.26 Flail joint, knee**

Laterality SP **M25.261 Flail joint, right knee**

Laterality SP **M25.262 Flail joint, left knee**

Laterality IQ **M25.269 Flail joint, unspecified knee**

6 **M25.27 Flail joint, ankle and foot**

Laterality SP **M25.271 Flail joint, right ankle and foot**

Laterality SP **M25.272 Flail joint, left ankle and foot**

Laterality IQ **M25.279 Flail joint, unspecified ankle and foot**

SP **M25.28 Flail joint, other site**

5 **M25.3 Other instability of joint**

EXCLUDES 1 instability of joint secondary to old ligament injury (M24.2-)
instability of joint secondary to removal of joint prosthesis (M96.8-)

EXCLUDES 2 spinal instabilities (M53.2-)

IQ **M25.30 Other instability, unspecified joint**

6 **M25.31 Other instability, shoulder**

Laterality SP **M25.311 Other instability, right shoulder**

Laterality SP **M25.312 Other instability, left shoulder**

Laterality IQ **M25.319 Other instability, unspecified shoulder**

6 **M25.32 Other instability, elbow**

Laterality SP **M25.321 Other instability, right elbow**

Laterality SP **M25.322 Other instability, left elbow**

Laterality IQ **M25.329 Other instability, unspecified elbow**

6 **M25.33 Other instability, wrist**

Laterality SP **M25.331 Other instability, right wrist**

Laterality SP **M25.332 Other instability, left wrist**

Laterality IQ **M25.339 Other instability, unspecified wrist**

6 **M25.34 Other instability, hand**

Laterality SP **M25.341 Other instability, right hand**

Laterality SP **M25.342 Other instability, left hand**

Laterality IQ **M25.349 Other instability, unspecified hand**

6 **M25.35 Other instability, hip**

Laterality SP **M25.351 Other instability, right hip**

Laterality SP **M25.352 Other instability, left hip**

Laterality IQ **M25.359 Other instability, unspecified hip**

6 **M25.36 Other instability, knee**

Laterality SP **M25.361 Other instability, right knee**

Laterality SP **M25.362 Other instability, left knee**

Laterality IQ **M25.369 Other instability, unspecified knee**

6 **M25.37 Other instability, ankle and foot**

Laterality SP **M25.371 Other instability, right ankle**

Laterality SP **M25.372 Other instability, left ankle**

Laterality IQ **M25.373 Other instability, unspecified ankle**

Laterality SP **M25.374 Other instability, right foot**

Laterality SP **M25.375 Other instability, left foot**

Laterality IQ **M25.376 Other instability, unspecified foot**

IQ **M25.39 Other instability, other specified joint**

5 **M25.4 Effusion of joint**

EXCLUDES 1 hydrarthrosis in yaws (A66.6)
intermittent hydrarthrosis (M12.4-)
other infective (teno) synovitis (M65.1-)

IQ **M25.40 Effusion, unspecified joint**

6 **M25.41 Effusion, shoulder**

Laterality SP **M25.411 Effusion, right shoulder**

Laterality SP **M25.412 Effusion, left shoulder**

Laterality IQ **M25.419 Effusion, unspecified shoulder**

6 **M25.42 Effusion, elbow**

Laterality SP **M25.421 Effusion, right elbow**

Laterality SP **M25.422 Effusion, left elbow**

Laterality IQ **M25.429 Effusion, unspecified elbow**

6 **M25.43 Effusion, wrist**

Laterality SP **M25.431 Effusion, right wrist**

Laterality SP **M25.432 Effusion, left wrist**

Laterality IQ **M25.439 Effusion, unspecified wrist**

6 **M25.44 Effusion, hand**

Laterality SP **M25.441 Effusion, right hand**

Laterality SP **M25.442 Effusion, left hand**

Laterality IQ **M25.449 Effusion, unspecified hand**

6 **M25.45 Effusion, hip**

Laterality SP **M25.451 Effusion, right hip**

Laterality SP **M25.452 Effusion, left hip**

Laterality IQ **M25.459 Effusion, unspecified hip**

6 **M25.46 Effusion, knee**

Laterality SP **M25.461 Effusion, right knee**

Laterality SP **M25.462 Effusion, left knee**

Laterality IQ **M25.469 Effusion, unspecified knee**

6 **M25.47 Effusion, ankle and foot**

Laterality SP **M25.471 Effusion, right ankle**

Laterality SP **M25.472 Effusion, left ankle**

IQ M25.473 Effusion, unspecified ankle
SP M25.474 Effusion, right foot
SP M25.475 Effusion, left foot
IQ M25.476 Effusion, unspecified foot
SP M25.48 Effusion, other site
5 M25.5 Pain in joint
EXCLUDES 2 pain in hand (M79.64-)
pain in fingers (M79.64-)
pain in foot (M79.67-)
pain in limb (M79.6-)
pain in toes (M79.67-)
CODING TIPS ✓ These codes should be used when 1) the cause of the pain is unknown; 2) the pain is a sequela of an injury; or 3) in conjunction with a G89 code. Do not use these codes with conditions like arthritis.
IQ M25.50 Pain in unspecified joint
6 M25.51 Pain in shoulder
IQ M25.511 Pain in right shoulder
IQ M25.512 Pain in left shoulder
IQ M25.519 Pain in unspecified shoulder
6 M25.52 Pain in elbow
IQ M25.521 Pain in right elbow
IQ M25.522 Pain in left elbow
IQ M25.529 Pain in unspecified elbow
6 M25.53 Pain in wrist
IQ M25.531 Pain in right wrist
IQ M25.532 Pain in left wrist
IQ M25.539 Pain in unspecified wrist
6 M25.54 Pain in joints of hand
IQ M25.541 Pain in joints of right hand
IQ M25.542 Pain in joints of left hand
IQ M25.549 Pain in joints of unspecified hand
Pain in joints of hand NOS
6 M25.55 Pain in hip
IQ M25.551 Pain in right hip
IQ M25.552 Pain in left hip
IQ M25.559 Pain in unspecified hip
6 M25.56 Pain in knee
IQ M25.561 Pain in right knee
IQ M25.562 Pain in left knee
IQ M25.569 Pain in unspecified knee
6 M25.57 Pain in ankle and joints of foot
IQ M25.571 Pain in right ankle and joints of right foot
IQ M25.572 Pain in left ankle and joints of left foot
IQ M25.579 Pain in unspecified ankle and joints of unspecified foot
IQ M25.59 Pain in other specified joint
5 M25.6 Stiffness of joint, not elsewhere classified
EXCLUDES 1 ankylosis of joint (M24.6-)
contracture of joint (M24.5-)
CODING TIPS ✓ These codes should be used when 1) the cause of the stiffness is unknown; 2) the stiffness is a sequela of an injury. Do not use these codes with conditions like arthritis.
IQ M25.60 Stiffness of unspecified joint, not elsewhere classified
6 M25.61 Stiffness of shoulder, not elsewhere classified
IQ M25.611 Stiffness of right shoulder, not elsewhere classified
IQ M25.612 Stiffness of left shoulder, not elsewhere classified
IQ M25.619 Stiffness of unspecified shoulder, not elsewhere classified
6 M25.62 Stiffness of elbow, not elsewhere classified
IQ M25.621 Stiffness of right elbow, not elsewhere classified
IQ M25.622 Stiffness of left elbow, not elsewhere classified
IQ M25.629 Stiffness of unspecified elbow, not elsewhere classified
6 M25.63 Stiffness of wrist, not elsewhere classified
IQ M25.631 Stiffness of right wrist, not elsewhere classified
IQ M25.632 Stiffness of left wrist, not elsewhere classified
IQ M25.639 Stiffness of unspecified wrist, not elsewhere classified
6 M25.64 Stiffness of hand, not elsewhere classified
IQ M25.641 Stiffness of right hand, not elsewhere classified
IQ M25.642 Stiffness of left hand, not elsewhere classified
IQ M25.649 Stiffness of unspecified hand, not elsewhere classified
6 M25.65 Stiffness of hip, not elsewhere classified
IQ M25.651 Stiffness of right hip, not elsewhere classified
IQ M25.652 Stiffness of left hip, not elsewhere classified
IQ M25.659 Stiffness of unspecified hip, not elsewhere classified
6 M25.66 Stiffness of knee, not elsewhere classified
IQ M25.661 Stiffness of right knee, not elsewhere classified
IQ M25.662 Stiffness of left knee, not elsewhere classified
IQ M25.669 Stiffness of unspecified knee, not elsewhere classified
6 M25.67 Stiffness of ankle and foot, not elsewhere classified
IQ M25.671 Stiffness of right ankle, not elsewhere classified
IQ M25.672 Stiffness of left ankle, not elsewhere classified
IQ M25.673 Stiffness of unspecified ankle, not elsewhere classified
IQ M25.674 Stiffness of right foot, not elsewhere classified
IQ M25.675 Stiffness of left foot, not elsewhere classified
IQ M25.676 Stiffness of unspecified foot, not elsewhere classified
IQ M25.69 Stiffness of other specified joint, not elsewhere classified

5 M25.7 Osteophyte
IQ M25.70 Osteophyte, unspecified joint
6 M25.71 Osteophyte, shoulder
SP M25.711 Osteophyte, right shoulder
SP M25.712 Osteophyte, left shoulder
IQ M25.719 Osteophyte, unspecified shoulder
6 M25.72 Osteophyte, elbow
SP M25.721 Osteophyte, right elbow
SP M25.722 Osteophyte, left elbow
IQ M25.729 Osteophyte, unspecified elbow
6 M25.73 Osteophyte, wrist
SP M25.731 Osteophyte, right wrist
SP M25.732 Osteophyte, left wrist
IQ M25.739 Osteophyte, unspecified wrist
6 M25.74 Osteophyte, hand
SP M25.741 Osteophyte, right hand
SP M25.742 Osteophyte, left hand
IQ M25.749 Osteophyte, unspecified hand
6 M25.75 Osteophyte, hip
SP M25.751 Osteophyte, right hip
SP M25.752 Osteophyte, left hip
IQ M25.759 Osteophyte, unspecified hip
6 M25.76 Osteophyte, knee
SP M25.761 Osteophyte, right knee
SP M25.762 Osteophyte, left knee
IQ M25.769 Osteophyte, unspecified knee
6 M25.77 Osteophyte, ankle and foot
SP M25.771 Osteophyte, right ankle
SP M25.772 Osteophyte, left ankle
IQ M25.773 Osteophyte, unspecified ankle
SP M25.774 Osteophyte, right foot
SP M25.775 Osteophyte, left foot
IQ M25.776 Osteophyte, unspecified foot
SP M25.78 Osteophyte, vertebrae
5 M25.8 Other specified joint disorders
IQ M25.80 Other specified joint disorders, unspecified joint
6 M25.81 Other specified joint disorders, shoulder
SP M25.811 Other specified joint disorders, right shoulder
SP M25.812 Other specified joint disorders, left shoulder
IQ M25.819 Other specified joint disorders, unspecified shoulder
6 M25.82 Other specified joint disorders, elbow
SP M25.821 Other specified joint disorders, right elbow
SP M25.822 Other specified joint disorders, left elbow
IQ M25.829 Other specified joint disorders, unspecified elbow
6 M25.83 Other specified joint disorders, wrist
SP M25.831 Other specified joint disorders, right wrist
SP M25.832 Other specified joint disorders, left wrist
IQ M25.839 Other specified joint disorders, unspecified wrist
6 M25.84 Other specified joint disorders, hand
SP M25.841 Other specified joint disorders, right hand
SP M25.842 Other specified joint disorders, left hand
IQ M25.849 Other specified joint disorders, unspecified hand
6 M25.85 Other specified joint disorders, hip
SP M25.851 Other specified joint disorders, right hip
SP M25.852 Other specified joint disorders, left hip
IQ M25.859 Other specified joint disorders, unspecified hip
6 M25.86 Other specified joint disorders, knee
SP M25.861 Other specified joint disorders, right knee
SP M25.862 Other specified joint disorders, left knee
IQ M25.869 Other specified joint disorders, unspecified knee
6 M25.87 Other specified joint disorders, ankle and foot
SP M25.871 Other specified joint disorders, right ankle and foot
SP M25.872 Other specified joint disorders, left ankle and foot
IQ M25.879 Other specified joint disorders, unspecified ankle and foot
IQ M25.9 Joint disorder, unspecified

Dentofacial anomalies [including malocclusion] and other disorders of jaw (M26-M27)

EXCLUDES 1 hemifacial atrophy or hypertrophy (Q67.4)
unilateral condylar hyperplasia or hypoplasia (M27.8)

4 M26 Dentofacial anomalies [including malocclusion]
5 M26.0 Major anomalies of jaw size
EXCLUDES 1 acromegaly (E22.0)
Robin's syndrome (Q87.0)
IQ M26.00 Unspecified anomaly of jaw size
IQ M26.01 Maxillary hyperplasia
IQ M26.02 Maxillary hypoplasia
IQ M26.03 Mandibular hyperplasia
IQ M26.04 Mandibular hypoplasia
IQ M26.05 Macrogenia
DEFINITION Abnormally large chin.
IQ M26.06 Microgenia
IQ M26.07 Excessive tuberosity of jaw
Entire maxillary tuberosity
IQ M26.09 Other specified anomalies of jaw size
5 M26.1 Anomalies of jaw-cranial base relationship
IQ M26.10 Unspecified anomaly of jaw-cranial base relationship
IQ M26.11 Maxillary asymmetry
IQ M26.12 Other jaw asymmetry

IQ **M26.19 Other specified anomalies of jaw-cranial base relationship**

5 **M26.2 Anomalies of dental arch relationship**

IQ **M26.20 Unspecified anomaly of dental arch relationship**

6 **M26.21 Malocclusion, Angle's class**

IQ **M26.211 Malocclusion, Angle's class I**
Neutro-occlusion

IQ **M26.212 Malocclusion, Angle's class II**
Disto-occlusion Division I
Disto-occlusion Division II

IQ **M26.213 Malocclusion, Angle's class III**
Mesio-occlusion

IQ **M26.219 Malocclusion, Angle's class, unspecified**

6 **M26.22 Open occlusal relationship**

IQ **M26.220 Open anterior occlusal relationship**
Anterior open bite

IQ **M26.221 Open posterior occlusal relationship**
Posterior open bite

IQ **M26.23 Excessive horizontal overlap**
Excessive horizontal overjet

IQ **M26.24 Reverse articulation**
Crossbite (anterior) (posterior)

IQ **M26.25 Anomalies of interarch distance**

IQ **M26.29 Other anomalies of dental arch relationship**
Midline deviation of dental arch
Overbite (excessive) deep
Overbite (excessive) horizontal
Overbite (excessive) vertical
Posterior lingual occlusion of mandibular teeth

5 **M26.3 Anomalies of tooth position of fully erupted tooth or teeth**
EXCLUDES 2 embedded and impacted teeth (K01.-)

IQ **M26.30 Unspecified anomaly of tooth position of fully erupted tooth or teeth**
Abnormal spacing of fully erupted tooth or teeth NOS
Displacement of fully erupted tooth or teeth NOS
Transposition of fully erupted tooth or teeth NOS

IQ **M26.31 Crowding of fully erupted teeth**

IQ **M26.32 Excessive spacing of fully erupted teeth**
Diastema of fully erupted tooth or teeth NOS

IQ **M26.33 Horizontal displacement of fully erupted tooth or teeth**
Tipped tooth or teeth
Tipping of fully erupted tooth

IQ **M26.34 Vertical displacement of fully erupted tooth or teeth**
Extruded tooth
Infraeruption of tooth or teeth
Supraeruption of tooth or teeth

IQ **M26.35 Rotation of fully erupted tooth or teeth**

IQ **M26.36 Insufficient interocclusal distance of fully erupted teeth (ridge)**
Lack of adequate intermaxillary vertical dimension of fully erupted teeth

IQ **M26.37 Excessive interocclusal distance of fully erupted teeth**
Excessive intermaxillary vertical dimension of fully erupted teeth
Loss of occlusal vertical dimension of fully erupted teeth

IQ **M26.39 Other anomalies of tooth position of fully erupted tooth or teeth**

IQ **M26.4 Malocclusion, unspecified**

5 **M26.5 Dentofacial functional abnormalities**
EXCLUDES 1 bruxism (F45.8)
teeth-grinding NOS (F45.8)

IQ **M26.50 Dentofacial functional abnormalities, unspecified**

IQ **M26.51 Abnormal jaw closure**

IQ **M26.52 Limited mandibular range of motion**

IQ **M26.53 Deviation in opening and closing of the mandible**

IQ **M26.54 Insufficient anterior guidance**
Insufficient anterior occlusal guidance

IQ **M26.55 Centric occlusion maximum intercuspation discrepancy**
EXCLUDES 1 centric occlusion NOS (M26.59)

IQ **M26.56 Non-working side interference**
Balancing side interference

IQ **M26.57 Lack of posterior occlusal support**

IQ **M26.59 Other dentofacial functional abnormalities**
Centric occlusion (of teeth) NOS
Malocclusion due to abnormal swallowing
Malocclusion due to mouth breathing
Malocclusion due to tongue, lip or finger habits

5 **M26.6 Temporomandibular joint disorders**
EXCLUDES 2 current temporomandibular joint dislocation (S03.0)
current temporomandibular joint sprain (S03.4)

6 **M26.60 Temporomandibular joint disorder, unspecified**

H IQ **M26.601 Right temporomandibular joint disorder, unspecified**

H IQ **M26.602 Left temporomandibular joint disorder, unspecified**

H IQ **M26.603 Bilateral temporomandibular joint disorder, unspecified**

H IQ **M26.609 Unspecified temporomandibular joint disorder, unspecified side**
Temporomandibular joint disorder NOS

6 **M26.61 Adhesions and ankylosis of temporomandibular joint**

H IQ **M26.611 Adhesions and ankylosis of right temporomandibular joint**

H IQ **M26.612 Adhesions and ankylosis of left temporomandibular joint**

H IQ **M26.613 Adhesions and ankylosis of bilateral temporomandibular joint**

H IQ **M26.619 Adhesions and ankylosis of temporomandibular joint, unspecified side**

Chapter 13

M00-M99

6 **M26.62 Arthralgia of temporomandibular joint**
⊟ IQ **M26.621 Arthralgia of right temporomandibular joint**
⊟ IQ **M26.622 Arthralgia of left temporomandibular joint**
⊟ IQ **M26.623 Arthralgia of bilateral temporomandibular joint**
⊟ IQ **M26.629 Arthralgia of temporomandibular joint, unspecified side**
6 **M26.63 Articular disc disorder of temporomandibular joint**
⊟ IQ **M26.631 Articular disc disorder of right temporomandibular joint**
⊟ IQ **M26.632 Articular disc disorder of left temporomandibular joint**
⊟ IQ **M26.633 Articular disc disorder of bilateral temporomandibular joint**
⊟ IQ **M26.639 Articular disc disorder of temporomandibular joint, unspecified side**
6 **M26.64 Arthritis of temporomandibular joint**
⊟ SP **M26.641 Arthritis of right temporomandibular joint**
⊟ SP **M26.642 Arthritis of left temporomandibular joint**
⊟ SP **M26.643 Arthritis of bilateral temporomandibular joint**
⊟ IQ **M26.649 Arthritis of unspecified temporomandibular joint**
6 **M26.65 Arthropathy of temporomandibular joint**
⊟ SP **M26.651 Arthropathy of right temporomandibular joint**
⊟ SP **M26.652 Arthropathy of left temporomandibular joint**
⊟ SP **M26.653 Arthropathy of bilateral temporomandibular joint**
⊟ IQ **M26.659 Arthropathy of unspecified temporomandibular joint**
IQ **M26.69 Other specified disorders of temporomandibular joint**
5 **M26.7 Dental alveolar anomalies**
IQ **M26.70 Unspecified alveolar anomaly**
IQ **M26.71 Alveolar maxillary hyperplasia**
IQ **M26.72 Alveolar mandibular hyperplasia**
IQ **M26.73 Alveolar maxillary hypoplasia**
IQ **M26.74 Alveolar mandibular hypoplasia**
IQ **M26.79 Other specified alveolar anomalies**
5 **M26.8 Other dentofacial anomalies**
IQ **M26.81 Anterior soft tissue impingement**
Anterior soft tissue impingement on teeth
IQ **M26.82 Posterior soft tissue impingement**
Posterior soft tissue impingement on teeth
IQ **M26.89 Other dentofacial anomalies**
IQ **M26.9 Dentofacial anomaly, unspecified**
4 **M27 Other diseases of jaws**
IQ **M27.0 Developmental disorders of jaws**
Latent bone cyst of jaw
Stafne's cyst
Torus mandibularis
Torus palatinus
IQ **M27.1 Giant cell granuloma, central**
Giant cell granuloma NOS
EXCLUDES 1 peripheral giant cell granuloma (K06.8)
SP + **M27.2 Inflammatory conditions of jaws**
Osteitis of jaw(s)
Osteomyelitis (neonatal) jaw(s)
Osteoradionecrosis jaw(s)
Periostitis jaw(s)
Sequestrum of jaw bone
Use additional code (W88-W90, X39.0) to identify radiation, if radiation-induced
EXCLUDES 2 osteonecrosis of jaw due to drug (M87.180)
IQ **M27.3 Alveolitis of jaws**
Alveolar osteitis
Dry socket
DEFINITION Inflammation of the tooth sockets.
5 **M27.4 Other and unspecified cysts of jaw**
EXCLUDES 1 cysts of oral region (K09.-)
latent bone cyst of jaw (M27.0)
Stafne's cyst (M27.0)
IQ **M27.40 Unspecified cyst of jaw**
Cyst of jaw NOS
IQ **M27.49 Other cysts of jaw**
Aneurysmal cyst of jaw
Hemorrhagic cyst of jaw
Traumatic cyst of jaw
5 **M27.5 Periradicular pathology associated with previous endodontic treatment**
IQ **M27.51 Perforation of root canal space due to endodontic treatment**
IQ **M27.52 Endodontic overfill**
IQ **M27.53 Endodontic underfill**
IQ **M27.59 Other periradicular pathology associated with previous endodontic treatment**
5 **M27.6 Endosseous dental implant failure**
IQ **M27.61 Osseointegration failure of dental implant**
Hemorrhagic complications of dental implant placement
Iatrogenic osseointegration failure of dental implant
Osseointegration failure of dental implant due to complications of systemic disease
Osseointegration failure of dental implant due to poor bone quality
Pre-integration failure of dental implant NOS
Pre-osseointegration failure of dental implant
IQ **M27.62 Post-osseointegration biological failure of dental implant**
Failure of dental implant due to lack of attached gingiva
Failure of dental implant due to occlusal trauma (caused by poor prosthetic design)
Failure of dental implant due to parafunctional habits

Failure of dental implant due to periodontal infection (peri-implantitis)
Failure of dental implant due to poor oral hygiene
Iatrogenic post-osseointegration failure of dental implant
Post-osseointegration failure of dental implant due to complications of systemic disease

IQ **M27.63 Post-osseointegration mechanical failure of dental implant**
Failure of dental prosthesis causing loss of dental implant
Fracture of dental implant
EXCLUDES 2 cracked tooth (K03.81)
fractured dental restorative material with loss of material (K08.531)
fractured dental restorative material without loss of material (K08.530)
fractured tooth (S02.5)

IQ **M27.69 Other endosseous dental implant failure**
Dental implant failure NOS

IQ **M27.8 Other specified diseases of jaws**
Cherubism
Exostosis
Fibrous dysplasia
Unilateral condylar hyperplasia
Unilateral condylar hypoplasia
EXCLUDES 1 jaw pain (R68.84)

IQ **M27.9 Disease of jaws, unspecified**

Systemic connective tissue disorders (M30-M36)

INCLUDES autoimmune disease NOS
collagen (vascular) disease NOS
systemic autoimmune disease
systemic collagen (vascular) disease
EXCLUDES 1 autoimmune disease, single organ or single cell-type -code to relevant condition category

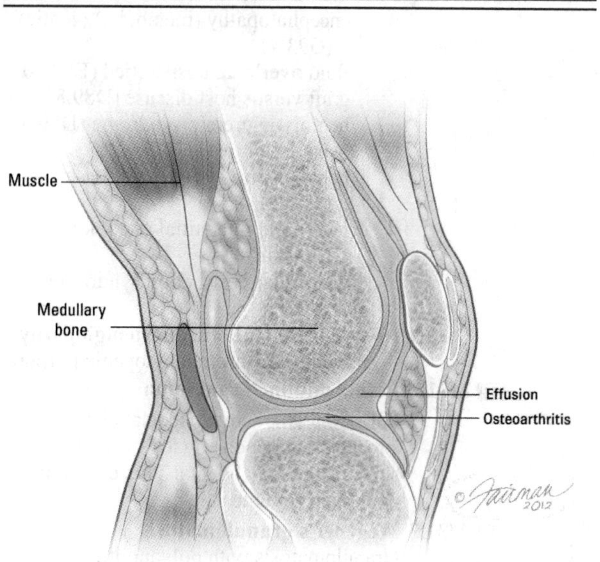

4 **M30 Polyarteritis nodosa and related conditions**
EXCLUDES 1 microscopic polyarteritis (M31.7)

SP **M30.0 Polyarteritis nodosa**
DEFINITION The body's immune system mistakenly attacks small and medium-sized blood vessels, resulting in tissue death.

SP **M30.1 Polyarteritis with lung involvement [Churg-Strauss]**
Allergic granulomatous angiitis
Eosinophilic granulomatosis with polyangiitis [EGPA]

SP **M30.2 Juvenile polyarteritis**

SP **M30.3 Mucocutaneous lymph node syndrome [Kawasaki]**

SP **M30.8 Other conditions related to polyarteritis nodosa**
Polyangiitis overlap syndrome

4 **M31 Other necrotizing vasculopathies**

SP **M31.0 Hypersensitivity angiitis**
Goodpasture's syndrome

▲ 5 **M31.1 Thrombotic microangiopathy**

★ **M31.10 Thrombotic microangiopathy, unspecified**

★ **M31.11 Hematopoietic stem cell transplantation-associated thrombotic microangiopathy [HSCT-TMA]**
Transplant-associated thrombotic microangiopathy [TA-TMA]
Code first if applicable:
complications of bone marrow transplant (T86.0-)
complications of stem cell transplant (T86.5)
Use additional code to identify specific organ dysfunction, such as:
acute kidney failure (N17.-)
acute respiratory distress syndrome (J80)
capillary leak syndrome (I78.8)
diffuse alveolar hemorrhage (R04.89)

encephalopathy (metabolic) (septic) (G93.41)
fluid overload, unspecified (E87.70)
graft versus host disease (D89.81-)
hemolytic uremic syndrome (D59.3)
hepatic failure (K72.-)
hepatic veno-occlusive disease (K76.5)
idiopathic interstitial pneumonia (J84.11-)
sinusoidal obstruction syndrome (K76.5)

★ **M31.19 Other thrombotic microangiopathy**
Thrombotic thrombocytopenic purpura

SP **M31.2 Lethal midline granuloma**
DEFINITION Tumor associated with infection that appears in the nose or sinuses that may be fatal if not diagnosed and treated in time.

5 **M31.3 Wegener's granulomatosis**
Granulomatosis with polyangiitis
Necrotizing respiratory granulomatosis

SP **M31.30 Wegener's granulomatosis without renal involvement**
Wegener's granulomatosis NOS

SP **M31.31 Wegener's granulomatosis with renal involvement**

SP **M31.4 Aortic arch syndrome [Takayasu]**

SP **M31.5 Giant cell arteritis with polymyalgia rheumatica**

SP **M31.6 Other giant cell arteritis**

SP **M31.7 Microscopic polyangiitis**
Microscopic polyarteritis
EXCLUDES 1 polyarteritis nodosa (M30.0)

SP **M31.8 Other specified necrotizing vasculopathies**
Hypocomplementemic vasculitis
Septic vasculitis

SP **M31.9 Necrotizing vasculopathy, unspecified**

4 **M32 Systemic lupus erythematosus (SLE)**
EXCLUDES 1 lupus erythematosus (discoid) (NOS) (L93.0)
CODING TIPS✓ Do not assign a code from category M32.- unless lupus is specified as systemic.

SP + **M32.0 Drug-induced systemic lupus erythematosus**
Use additional code for adverse effect, if applicable, to identify drug (T36-T50 with fifth or sixth character 5)
CODING TIPS✓ Assign code M32.0 only when documentation clearly confirms that the systemic lupus diagnosis is secondary to the effects of a drug. An additional code from categories T36-T50 should be used to identify the drug.

5 **M32.1 Systemic lupus erythematosus with organ or system involvement**

SP **M32.10 Systemic lupus erythematosus, organ or system involvement unspecified**

SP **M32.11 Endocarditis in systemic lupus erythematosus**
Libman-Sacks disease

SP **M32.12 Pericarditis in systemic lupus erythematosus**
Lupus pericarditis

SP **M32.13 Lung involvement in systemic lupus erythematosus**
Pleural effusion due to systemic lupus erythematosus

SP **M32.14 Glomerular disease in systemic lupus erythematosus**
Lupus renal disease NOS

SP **M32.15 Tubulo-interstitial nephropathy in systemic lupus erythematosus**

SP **M32.19 Other organ or system involvement in systemic lupus erythematosus**

SP **M32.8 Other forms of systemic lupus erythematosus**

SP **M32.9 Systemic lupus erythematosus, unspecified**
SLE NOS
Systemic lupus erythematosus NOS
Systemic lupus erythematosus without organ involvement

4 **M33 Dermatopolymyositis**

5 **M33.0 Juvenile dermatomyositis**

SP **M33.00 Juvenile dermatomyositis, organ involvement unspecified**

SP **M33.01 Juvenile dermatomyositis with respiratory involvement**

SP **M33.02 Juvenile dermatomyositis with myopathy**

SP **M33.03 Juvenile dermatomyositis without myopathy**

SP **M33.09 Juvenile dermatomyositis with other organ involvement**

5 **M33.1 Other dermatomyositis**
Adult dermatomyositis

SP **M33.10 Other dermatomyositis, organ involvement unspecified**

SP **M33.11 Other dermatomyositis with respiratory involvement**

SP **M33.12 Other dermatomyositis with myopathy**

SP **M33.13 Other dermatomyositis without myopathy**
Dermatomyositis NOS

SP **M33.19 Other dermatomyositis with other organ involvement**

5 **M33.2 Polymyositis**

SP **M33.20 Polymyositis, organ involvement unspecified**

SP **M33.21 Polymyositis with respiratory involvement**

SP **M33.22 Polymyositis with myopathy**

SP **M33.29 Polymyositis with other organ involvement**

5 **M33.9 Dermatopolymyositis, unspecified**

SP **M33.90 Dermatopolymyositis, unspecified, organ involvement unspecified**

SP **M33.91 Dermatopolymyositis, unspecified with respiratory involvement**

SP **M33.92 Dermatopolymyositis, unspecified with myopathy**

SP **M33.93 Dermatopolymyositis, unspecified without myopathy**

SP **M33.99 Dermatopolymyositis, unspecified with other organ involvement**

4 **M34 Systemic sclerosis [scleroderma]**

EXCLUDES 1 circumscribed scleroderma (L94.0)
neonatal scleroderma (P83.88)

SP **M34.0 Progressive systemic sclerosis**

SP **M34.1 CR(E)ST syndrome**
Combination of calcinosis, Raynaud's phenomenon, esophageal dysfunction, sclerodactyly, telangiectasia

SP + **M34.2 Systemic sclerosis induced by drug and chemical**
Code first:
poisoning due to drug or toxin, if applicable (T36-T65 with fifth or sixth character 1-4 or 6)
Use additional code for adverse effect, if applicable, to identify drug (T36-T50 with fifth or sixth character 5)

5 **M34.8 Other forms of systemic sclerosis**

▲ SP **M34.81 Systemic sclerosis with lung involvement**
Code also if applicable:
other interstitial pulmonary diseases (J84.89)
secondary pulmonary arterial hypertension (I27.21)

SP **M34.82 Systemic sclerosis with myopathy**

SP **M34.83 Systemic sclerosis with polyneuropathy**

SP **M34.89 Other systemic sclerosis**

SP **M34.9 Systemic sclerosis, unspecified**

4 **M35 Other systemic involvement of connective tissue**
EXCLUDES 1 reactive perforating collagenosis (L87.1)

▲ + 5 **M35.0 Sjögren syndrome**
Sicca syndrome
Use additional code to identify associated manifestations
EXCLUDES 1 dry mouth, unspecified (R68.2)

▲ SP + **M35.00 Sjögren syndrome, unspecified**

▲ SP + **M35.01 Sjögren syndrome with keratoconjunctivitis**

▲ SP + **M35.02 Sjögren syndrome with lung involvement**

▲ SP + **M35.03 Sjögren syndrome with myopathy**

▲ SP + **M35.04 Sjögren syndrome with tubulo-interstitial nephropathy**
Renal tubular acidosis in sicca syndrome

★ + **M35.05 Sjögren syndrome with inflammatory arthritis**

★ + **M35.06 Sjögren syndrome with peripheral nervous system involvement**

★ + **M35.07 Sjögren syndrome with central nervous system involvement**

★ + **M35.08 Sjögren syndrome with gastrointestinal involvement**

★ + **M35.0A Sjögren syndrome with glomerular disease**

★ + **M35.0B Sjögren syndrome with vasculitis**

★ + **M35.0C Sjögren syndrome with dental involvement**

▲ SP + **M35.09 Sjögren syndrome with other organ involvement**

SP **M35.1 Other overlap syndromes**
Mixed connective tissue disease
EXCLUDES 1 polyangiitis overlap syndrome (M30.8)

SP **M35.2 Behçet's disease**
DEFINITION Relapsing inflammatory disorder with recurring painful sores of the mouth, skin, and genitals, swollen joints, severe uveitis, retinal vasculitis, optic atrophy, and digestive system involvement.

SP **M35.3 Polymyalgia rheumatica**
EXCLUDES 1 polymyalgia rheumatica with giant cell arteritis (M31.5)

SP **M35.4 Diffuse (eosinophilic) fasciitis**

SP **M35.5 Multifocal fibrosclerosis**

SP **M35.6 Relapsing panniculitis [Weber-Christian]**
EXCLUDES 1 lupus panniculitis (L93.2)
panniculitis NOS (M79.3-)

▲ SP **M35.7 Hypermobility syndrome**
Familial ligamentous laxity
EXCLUDES 1 ligamentous laxity, NOS (M24.2-)
EXCLUDES 2 Ehlers-Danlos syndromes (Q79.6-)

5 **M35.8 Other specified systemic involvement of connective tissue**

▲ SP + **M35.81 Multisystem inflammatory syndrome**
MIS-A
MIS-C
Multisystem inflammatory syndrome in adults
Multisystem inflammatory syndrome in children
Pediatric inflammatory multisystem syndrome
PIMS
Code first:
, if applicable, COVID-19 (U07.1)
Code also any associated complications such as:
acute hepatic failure (K72.0-)
acute kidney failure (N17.-)
acute myocarditis (I40.-)
acute respiratory distress syndrome (J80)
cardiac arrhythmia (I47-I49.-)
pneumonia due to COVID-19 (J12.82)
severe sepsis (R65.2-)
viral cardiomyopathy (B33.24)
viral pericarditis (B33.23)
Use additional code, if applicable, for:
exposure to COVID-19 or SARS-CoV-2 infection (Z20.822)
personal history of COVID-19 (Z86.16)
post COVID-19 condition (U09.9)
DEFINITION Multisystem inflammatory syndrome is a serious, systemic, hyperinflammatory syndrome associated with a previous or current COVID-19 (SARS-CoV-2) infection, predominantly seen in children, and presenting with clinical features similar to sepsis or toxic shock syndrome.

SP **M35.89 Other specified systemic involvement of connective tissue**

Chapter 13
M00-M99

IQ **M35.9 Systemic involvement of connective tissue, unspecified**
Autoimmune disease (systemic) NOS
Collagen (vascular) disease NOS

4 **M36 Systemic disorders of connective tissue in diseases classified elsewhere**
EXCLUDES 2 arthropathies in diseases classified elsewhere (M14.-)

M IQ **M36.0 *Dermato(poly)myositis in neoplastic disease***
Code first:
underlying neoplasm (C00-D49)

M IQ **M36.1 *Arthropathy in neoplastic disease***
Code first underlying neoplasm, such as:
leukemia (C91-C95)
malignant histiocytosis (C96.A)
multiple myeloma (C90.0)

M IQ **M36.2 *Hemophilic arthropathy***
Hemarthrosis in hemophilic arthropathy
Code first underlying disease, such as:
factor VIII deficiency (D66)
with vascular defect (D68.0)
factor IX deficiency (D67)
hemophilia (classical) (D66)
hemophilia B (D67)
hemophilia C (D68.1)

M IQ **M36.3 *Arthropathy in other blood disorders***

M IQ **M36.4 *Arthropathy in hypersensitivity reactions classified elsewhere***
Code first underlying disease, such as:
Henoch (-Schönlein) purpura (D69.0)
serum sickness (T80.6-)

M IQ **M36.8 *Systemic disorders of connective tissue in other diseases classified elsewhere***
Code first underlying disease, such as:
alkaptonuria (E70.2)
hypogammaglobulinemia (D80.-)
ochronosis (E70.2)

Dorsopathies (M40-M54)

Deforming dorsopathies (M40-M43)

▲ 4 **M40 Kyphosis and lordosis**
Code first:
underlying disease
EXCLUDES 1 congenital kyphosis and lordosis (Q76.4)
kyphoscoliosis (M41.-)
postprocedural kyphosis and lordosis (M96.-)

5 **M40.0 Postural kyphosis**
EXCLUDES 1 osteochondrosis of spine (M42.-)

IQ **M40.00 Postural kyphosis, site unspecified**
SP **M40.03 Postural kyphosis, cervicothoracic region**
SP **M40.04 Postural kyphosis, thoracic region**
SP **M40.05 Postural kyphosis, thoracolumbar region**

5 **M40.1 Other secondary kyphosis**
IQ **M40.10 Other secondary kyphosis, site unspecified**
SP **M40.12 Other secondary kyphosis, cervical region**
SP **M40.13 Other secondary kyphosis, cervicothoracic region**
SP **M40.14 Other secondary kyphosis, thoracic region**
SP **M40.15 Other secondary kyphosis, thoracolumbar region**

5 **M40.2 Other and unspecified kyphosis**
6 **M40.20 Unspecified kyphosis**
SP **M40.202 Unspecified kyphosis, cervical region**
SP **M40.203 Unspecified kyphosis, cervicothoracic region**
SP **M40.204 Unspecified kyphosis, thoracic region**
SP **M40.205 Unspecified kyphosis, thoracolumbar region**
IQ **M40.209 Unspecified kyphosis, site unspecified**
6 **M40.29 Other kyphosis**
SP **M40.292 Other kyphosis, cervical region**
SP **M40.293 Other kyphosis, cervicothoracic region**
SP **M40.294 Other kyphosis, thoracic region**
SP **M40.295 Other kyphosis, thoracolumbar region**
IQ **M40.299 Other kyphosis, site unspecified**

5 **M40.3 Flatback syndrome**
IQ **M40.30 Flatback syndrome, site unspecified**
SP **M40.35 Flatback syndrome, thoracolumbar region**
SP **M40.36 Flatback syndrome, lumbar region**
SP **M40.37 Flatback syndrome, lumbosacral region**

5 **M40.4 Postural lordosis**
Acquired lordosis
IQ **M40.40 Postural lordosis, site unspecified**
SP **M40.45 Postural lordosis, thoracolumbar region**
SP **M40.46 Postural lordosis, lumbar region**
SP **M40.47 Postural lordosis, lumbosacral region**

5 **M40.5 Lordosis, unspecified**
IQ **M40.50 Lordosis, unspecified, site unspecified**
SP **M40.55 Lordosis, unspecified, thoracolumbar region**
SP **M40.56 Lordosis, unspecified, lumbar region**
SP **M40.57 Lordosis, unspecified, lumbosacral region**

▲ 4 **M41 Scoliosis**
INCLUDES kyphoscoliosis
EXCLUDES 1 congenital scoliosis NOS (Q67.5)
congenital scoliosis due to bony malformation (Q76.3)
postural congenital scoliosis (Q67.5)
kyphoscoliotic heart disease (I27.1)
EXCLUDES 2 postprocedural scoliosis (M96.-)

CODING TIPS✓ The correct aftercare code to use for surgeries for treatment of scoliosis is Z47.82.

5 **M41.0 Infantile idiopathic scoliosis**

IQ **M41.00 Infantile idiopathic scoliosis, site unspecified**

SP **M41.02 Infantile idiopathic scoliosis, cervical region**

SP **M41.03 Infantile idiopathic scoliosis, cervicothoracic region**

SP **M41.04 Infantile idiopathic scoliosis, thoracic region**

SP **M41.05 Infantile idiopathic scoliosis, thoracolumbar region**

SP **M41.06 Infantile idiopathic scoliosis, lumbar region**

SP **M41.07 Infantile idiopathic scoliosis, lumbosacral region**

SP **M41.08 Infantile idiopathic scoliosis, sacral and sacrococcygeal region**

5 **M41.1 Juvenile and adolescent idiopathic scoliosis**

6 **M41.11 Juvenile idiopathic scoliosis**

SP **M41.112 Juvenile idiopathic scoliosis, cervical region**

SP **M41.113 Juvenile idiopathic scoliosis, cervicothoracic region**

SP **M41.114 Juvenile idiopathic scoliosis, thoracic region**

SP **M41.115 Juvenile idiopathic scoliosis, thoracolumbar region**

SP **M41.116 Juvenile idiopathic scoliosis, lumbar region**

SP **M41.117 Juvenile idiopathic scoliosis, lumbosacral region**

IQ **M41.119 Juvenile idiopathic scoliosis, site unspecified**

6 **M41.12 Adolescent scoliosis**

SP **M41.122 Adolescent idiopathic scoliosis, cervical region**

SP **M41.123 Adolescent idiopathic scoliosis, cervicothoracic region**

SP **M41.124 Adolescent idiopathic scoliosis, thoracic region**

SP **M41.125 Adolescent idiopathic scoliosis, thoracolumbar region**

SP **M41.126 Adolescent idiopathic scoliosis, lumbar region**

SP **M41.127 Adolescent idiopathic scoliosis, lumbosacral region**

IQ **M41.129 Adolescent idiopathic scoliosis, site unspecified**

5 **M41.2 Other idiopathic scoliosis**

SP **M41.20 Other idiopathic scoliosis, site unspecified**

SP **M41.22 Other idiopathic scoliosis, cervical region**

SP **M41.23 Other idiopathic scoliosis, cervicothoracic region**

SP **M41.24 Other idiopathic scoliosis, thoracic region**

SP **M41.25 Other idiopathic scoliosis, thoracolumbar region**

SP **M41.26 Other idiopathic scoliosis, lumbar region**

SP **M41.27 Other idiopathic scoliosis, lumbosacral region**

5 **M41.3 Thoracogenic scoliosis**

IQ **M41.30 Thoracogenic scoliosis, site unspecified**

SP **M41.34 Thoracogenic scoliosis, thoracic region**

SP **M41.35 Thoracogenic scoliosis, thoracolumbar region**

5 **M41.4 Neuromuscular scoliosis**

Scoliosis secondary to cerebral palsy, Friedreich's ataxia, poliomyelitis and other neuromuscular disorders

Code also:
underlying condition

IQ **M41.40 Neuromuscular scoliosis, site unspecified**

SP **M41.41 Neuromuscular scoliosis, occipito-atlanto-axial region**

SP **M41.42 Neuromuscular scoliosis, cervical region**

SP **M41.43 Neuromuscular scoliosis, cervicothoracic region**

SP **M41.44 Neuromuscular scoliosis, thoracic region**

SP **M41.45 Neuromuscular scoliosis, thoracolumbar region**

SP **M41.46 Neuromuscular scoliosis, lumbar region**

SP **M41.47 Neuromuscular scoliosis, lumbosacral region**

▲ 5 **M41.5 Other secondary scoliosis**

Code first:
underlying disease

IQ **M41.50 Other secondary scoliosis, site unspecified**

SP **M41.52 Other secondary scoliosis, cervical region**

SP **M41.53 Other secondary scoliosis, cervicothoracic region**

SP **M41.54 Other secondary scoliosis, thoracic region**

SP **M41.55 Other secondary scoliosis, thoracolumbar region**

SP **M41.56 Other secondary scoliosis, lumbar region**

SP **M41.57 Other secondary scoliosis, lumbosacral region**

5 **M41.8 Other forms of scoliosis**

IQ **M41.80 Other forms of scoliosis, site unspecified**

SP **M41.82 Other forms of scoliosis, cervical region**

SP **M41.83 Other forms of scoliosis, cervicothoracic region**

SP **M41.84 Other forms of scoliosis, thoracic region**

SP **M41.85 Other forms of scoliosis, thoracolumbar region**

SP **M41.86 Other forms of scoliosis, lumbar region**

SP **M41.87 Other forms of scoliosis, lumbosacral region**

SP **M41.9 Scoliosis, unspecified**

4 **M42 Spinal osteochondrosis**

5 **M42.0 Juvenile osteochondrosis of spine**

Calvé's disease
Scheuermann's disease
EXCLUDES 1 postural kyphosis (M40.0)

!Q **M42.00 Juvenile osteochondrosis of spine, site unspecified**

SP **M42.01 Juvenile osteochondrosis of spine, occipito-atlanto-axial region**

SP **M42.02 Juvenile osteochondrosis of spine, cervical region**

SP **M42.03 Juvenile osteochondrosis of spine, cervicothoracic region**

SP **M42.04 Juvenile osteochondrosis of spine, thoracic region**

SP **M42.05 Juvenile osteochondrosis of spine, thoracolumbar region**

SP **M42.06 Juvenile osteochondrosis of spine, lumbar region**

SP **M42.07 Juvenile osteochondrosis of spine, lumbosacral region**

SP **M42.08 Juvenile osteochondrosis of spine, sacral and sacrococcygeal region**

SP **M42.09 Juvenile osteochondrosis of spine, multiple sites in spine**

5 **M42.1 Adult osteochondrosis of spine**

!Q **M42.10 Adult osteochondrosis of spine, site unspecified**

SP **M42.11 Adult osteochondrosis of spine, occipito-atlanto-axial region**

SP **M42.12 Adult osteochondrosis of spine, cervical region**

SP **M42.13 Adult osteochondrosis of spine, cervicothoracic region**

SP **M42.14 Adult osteochondrosis of spine, thoracic region**

SP **M42.15 Adult osteochondrosis of spine, thoracolumbar region**

SP **M42.16 Adult osteochondrosis of spine, lumbar region**

SP **M42.17 Adult osteochondrosis of spine, lumbosacral region**

SP **M42.18 Adult osteochondrosis of spine, sacral and sacrococcygeal region**

SP **M42.19 Adult osteochondrosis of spine, multiple sites in spine**

SP **M42.9 Spinal osteochondrosis, unspecified**

4 **M43 Other deforming dorsopathies**

EXCLUDES 1 congenital spondylolysis and spondylolisthesis (Q76.2)
hemivertebra (Q76.3-Q76.4)
Klippel-Feil syndrome (Q76.1)
lumbarization and sacralization (Q76.4)
platyspondylisis (Q76.4)
spina bifida occulta (Q76.0)
spinal curvature in osteoporosis (M80.-)
spinal curvature in Paget's disease of bone [osteitis deformans] (M88.-)

5 **M43.0 Spondylolysis**

EXCLUDES 1 congenital spondylolysis (Q76.2)
spondylolisthesis (M43.1)

DEFINITION A defect of the pars interarticularis segment of vertebral bone that connects the facet joints, causing stress fracture and predisposing to slippage; occurs most commonly in the lumbar region (specifically L5) during adolescence.

!Q **M43.00 Spondylolysis, site unspecified**

SP **M43.01 Spondylolysis, occipito-atlanto-axial region**

SP **M43.02 Spondylolysis, cervical region**

SP **M43.03 Spondylolysis, cervicothoracic region**

SP **M43.04 Spondylolysis, thoracic region**

SP **M43.05 Spondylolysis, thoracolumbar region**

SP **M43.06 Spondylolysis, lumbar region**

SP **M43.07 Spondylolysis, lumbosacral region**

SP **M43.08 Spondylolysis, sacral and sacrococcygeal region**

SP **M43.09 Spondylolysis, multiple sites in spine**

5 **M43.1 Spondylolisthesis**

EXCLUDES 1 acute traumatic of lumbosacral region (S33.1)
acute traumatic of sites other than lumbosacral- code to Fracture, vertebra, by region
congenital spondylolisthesis (Q76.2)

DEFINITION An acquired condition in which one vertebra slips forward over the one below it, often from degenerative aging or a small fracture in the piece of bone (pars interarticularis) connecting the facet joint above to the one below.

!Q **M43.10 Spondylolisthesis, site unspecified**

SP **M43.11 Spondylolisthesis, occipito-atlanto-axial region**

SP **M43.12 Spondylolisthesis, cervical region**

SP **M43.13 Spondylolisthesis, cervicothoracic region**

SP **M43.14 Spondylolisthesis, thoracic region**

SP **M43.15 Spondylolisthesis, thoracolumbar region**

SP **M43.16 Spondylolisthesis, lumbar region**

SP **M43.17 Spondylolisthesis, lumbosacral region**

SP **M43.18 Spondylolisthesis, sacral and sacrococcygeal region**

SP **M43.19 Spondylolisthesis, multiple sites in spine**

5 **M43.2 Fusion of spine**

Ankylosis of spinal joint

EXCLUDES 1 ankylosing spondylitis (M45.0-)
congenital fusion of spine (Q76.4)

EXCLUDES 2 arthrodesis status (Z98.1)
pseudoarthrosis after fusion or arthrodesis (M96.0)

CODING TIPS✓ Ankylosis of the joint is caused by arthritis, traumatic injury or infection. The joint will assume the least painful position and become permanently fixed. A surgical fusion is coded Z98.1. Surgical fusions are never coded with M43.

IQ **M43.20 Fusion of spine, site unspecified**

SP **M43.21 Fusion of spine, occipito-atlanto-axial region**

SP **M43.22 Fusion of spine, cervical region**

SP **M43.23 Fusion of spine, cervicothoracic region**

SP **M43.24 Fusion of spine, thoracic region**

SP **M43.25 Fusion of spine, thoracolumbar region**

SP **M43.26 Fusion of spine, lumbar region**

SP **M43.27 Fusion of spine, lumbosacral region**

SP **M43.28 Fusion of spine, sacral and sacrococcygeal region**

SP **M43.3 Recurrent atlantoaxial dislocation with myelopathy**

SP **M43.4 Other recurrent atlantoaxial dislocation**

5 **M43.5 Other recurrent vertebral dislocation**

EXCLUDES 1 biomechanical lesions NEC (M99.-)

6 **M43.5X Other recurrent vertebral dislocation**

SP **M43.5X2 Other recurrent vertebral dislocation, cervical region**

SP **M43.5X3 Other recurrent vertebral dislocation, cervicothoracic region**

SP **M43.5X4 Other recurrent vertebral dislocation, thoracic region**

SP **M43.5X5 Other recurrent vertebral dislocation, thoracolumbar region**

SP **M43.5X6 Other recurrent vertebral dislocation, lumbar region**

SP **M43.5X7 Other recurrent vertebral dislocation, lumbosacral region**

SP **M43.5X8 Other recurrent vertebral dislocation, sacral and sacrococcygeal region**

IQ **M43.5X9 Other recurrent vertebral dislocation, site unspecified**

SP **M43.6 Torticollis**

EXCLUDES 1 congenital (sternomastoid) torticollis (Q68.0)
current injury - see Injury, of spine, by body region
ocular torticollis (R29.891)
psychogenic torticollis (F45.8)
spasmodic torticollis (G24.3)
torticollis due to birth injury (P15.2)

DEFINITION Contraction of the neck muscles causing limited neck motion and head positioned to one side.

5 **M43.8 Other specified deforming dorsopathies**

EXCLUDES 2 kyphosis and lordosis (M40.-)
scoliosis (M41.-)

6 **M43.8X Other specified deforming dorsopathies**

SP **M43.8X1 Other specified deforming dorsopathies, occipito-atlanto-axial region**

SP **M43.8X2 Other specified deforming dorsopathies, cervical region**

SP **M43.8X3 Other specified deforming dorsopathies, cervicothoracic region**

SP **M43.8X4 Other specified deforming dorsopathies, thoracic region**

SP **M43.8X5 Other specified deforming dorsopathies, thoracolumbar region**

SP **M43.8X6 Other specified deforming dorsopathies, lumbar region**

SP **M43.8X7 Other specified deforming dorsopathies, lumbosacral region**

SP **M43.8X8 Other specified deforming dorsopathies, sacral and sacrococcygeal region**

IQ **M43.8X9 Other specified deforming dorsopathies, site unspecified**

IQ **M43.9 Deforming dorsopathy, unspecified**

Curvature of spine NOS

Spondylopathies (M45-M49)

4 **M45 Ankylosing spondylitis**

Rheumatoid arthritis of spine

EXCLUDES 1 arthropathy in Reiter's disease (M02.3-)
juvenile (ankylosing) spondylitis (M08.1)

EXCLUDES 2 Behçet's disease (M35.2)

DEFINITION Autoimmune arthritis causing chronic inflammation of the spine and sacroiliac joints, eventually leading to spinal fusion from calcification of ligaments and discs that progresses up the spine, possibly affecting other organs.

SP **M45.0 Ankylosing spondylitis of multiple sites in spine**

SP **M45.1 Ankylosing spondylitis of occipito-atlanto-axial region**

SP **M45.2 Ankylosing spondylitis of cervical region**

SP **M45.3 Ankylosing spondylitis of cervicothoracic region**

SP **M45.4 Ankylosing spondylitis of thoracic region**

SP **M45.5 Ankylosing spondylitis of thoracolumbar region**

SP **M45.6 Ankylosing spondylitis lumbar region**

SP **M45.7 Ankylosing spondylitis of lumbosacral region**

SP **M45.8 Ankylosing spondylitis sacral and sacrococcygeal region**

IQ **M45.9 Ankylosing spondylitis of unspecified sites in spine**

★ 5 **M45.A Non-radiographic axial spondyloarthritis**

★ **M45.A0 Non-radiographic axial spondyloarthritis of unspecified sites in spine**

★ **M45.A1 Non-radiographic axial spondyloarthritis of occipito-atlanto-axial region**

★ **M45.A2 Non-radiographic axial spondyloarthritis of cervical region**

★ **M45.A3 Non-radiographic axial spondyloarthritis of cervicothoracic region**

★ **M45.A4 Non-radiographic axial spondyloarthritis of thoracic region**

★ **M45.A5 Non-radiographic axial spondyloarthritis of thoracolumbar region**

★ **M45.A6 Non-radiographic axial spondyloarthritis of lumbar region**

★ **M45.A7 Non-radiographic axial spondyloarthritis of lumbosacral region**

★ **M45.A8 Non-radiographic axial spondyloarthritis of sacral and sacrococcygeal region**

★ **M45.AB Non-radiographic axial spondyloarthritis of multiple sites in spine**

4 **M46 Other inflammatory spondylopathies**

5 **M46.0 Spinal enthesopathy**

Disorder of ligamentous or muscular attachments of spine

!Q **M46.00 Spinal enthesopathy, site unspecified**

SP **M46.01 Spinal enthesopathy, occipito-atlanto-axial region**

SP **M46.02 Spinal enthesopathy, cervical region**

SP **M46.03 Spinal enthesopathy, cervicothoracic region**

SP **M46.04 Spinal enthesopathy, thoracic region**

SP **M46.05 Spinal enthesopathy, thoracolumbar region**

SP **M46.06 Spinal enthesopathy, lumbar region**

SP **M46.07 Spinal enthesopathy, lumbosacral region**

SP **M46.08 Spinal enthesopathy, sacral and sacrococcygeal region**

SP **M46.09 Spinal enthesopathy, multiple sites in spine**

SP **M46.1 Sacroiliitis, not elsewhere classified**

CODING TIPS✓ DJD of the sacroiliac joint is coded to M46.1 until a future code can be created.

5 **M46.2 Osteomyelitis of vertebra**

!Q **M46.20 Osteomyelitis of vertebra, site unspecified**

SP **M46.21 Osteomyelitis of vertebra, occipito-atlanto-axial region**

SP **M46.22 Osteomyelitis of vertebra, cervical region**

SP **M46.23 Osteomyelitis of vertebra, cervicothoracic region**

SP **M46.24 Osteomyelitis of vertebra, thoracic region**

SP **M46.25 Osteomyelitis of vertebra, thoracolumbar region**

SP **M46.26 Osteomyelitis of vertebra, lumbar region**

SP **M46.27 Osteomyelitis of vertebra, lumbosacral region**

SP **M46.28 Osteomyelitis of vertebra, sacral and sacrococcygeal region**

+ 5 **M46.3 Infection of intervertebral disc (pyogenic)**

Use additional code (B95-B97) to identify infectious agent.

!Q + **M46.30 Infection of intervertebral disc (pyogenic), site unspecified**

SP + **M46.31 Infection of intervertebral disc (pyogenic), occipito-atlanto-axial region**

SP + **M46.32 Infection of intervertebral disc (pyogenic), cervical region**

SP + **M46.33 Infection of intervertebral disc (pyogenic), cervicothoracic region**

SP + **M46.34 Infection of intervertebral disc (pyogenic), thoracic region**

SP + **M46.35 Infection of intervertebral disc (pyogenic), thoracolumbar region**

SP + **M46.36 Infection of intervertebral disc (pyogenic), lumbar region**

SP + **M46.37 Infection of intervertebral disc (pyogenic), lumbosacral region**

SP + **M46.38 Infection of intervertebral disc (pyogenic), sacral and sacrococcygeal region**

SP + **M46.39 Infection of intervertebral disc (pyogenic), multiple sites in spine**

5 **M46.4 Discitis, unspecified**

!Q **M46.40 Discitis, unspecified, site unspecified**

SP **M46.41 Discitis, unspecified, occipito-atlanto-axial region**

SP **M46.42 Discitis, unspecified, cervical region**

SP **M46.43 Discitis, unspecified, cervicothoracic region**

SP **M46.44 Discitis, unspecified, thoracic region**

SP **M46.45 Discitis, unspecified, thoracolumbar region**

SP **M46.46 Discitis, unspecified, lumbar region**

SP **M46.47 Discitis, unspecified, lumbosacral region**

SP **M46.48 Discitis, unspecified, sacral and sacrococcygeal region**

SP **M46.49 Discitis, unspecified, multiple sites in spine**

5 **M46.5 Other infective spondylopathies**

!Q **M46.50 Other infective spondylopathies, site unspecified**

SP **M46.51 Other infective spondylopathies, occipito-atlanto-axial region**

SP **M46.52 Other infective spondylopathies, cervical region**

SP **M46.53 Other infective spondylopathies, cervicothoracic region**

SP **M46.54 Other infective spondylopathies, thoracic region**

SP **M46.55 Other infective spondylopathies, thoracolumbar region**

SP **M46.56 Other infective spondylopathies, lumbar region**

SP **M46.57 Other infective spondylopathies, lumbosacral region**

SP **M46.58 Other infective spondylopathies, sacral and sacrococcygeal region**

SP **M46.59 Other infective spondylopathies, multiple sites in spine**

5 **M46.8 Other specified inflammatory spondylopathies**

IQ **M46.80 Other specified inflammatory spondylopathies, site unspecified**

SP **M46.81 Other specified inflammatory spondylopathies, occipito-atlanto-axial region**

SP **M46.82 Other specified inflammatory spondylopathies, cervical region**

SP **M46.83 Other specified inflammatory spondylopathies, cervicothoracic region**

SP **M46.84 Other specified inflammatory spondylopathies, thoracic region**

SP **M46.85 Other specified inflammatory spondylopathies, thoracolumbar region**

SP **M46.86 Other specified inflammatory spondylopathies, lumbar region**

SP **M46.87 Other specified inflammatory spondylopathies, lumbosacral region**

SP **M46.88 Other specified inflammatory spondylopathies, sacral and sacrococcygeal region**

SP **M46.89 Other specified inflammatory spondylopathies, multiple sites in spine**

5 **M46.9 Unspecified inflammatory spondylopathy**

IQ **M46.90 Unspecified inflammatory spondylopathy, site unspecified**

SP **M46.91 Unspecified inflammatory spondylopathy, occipito-atlanto-axial region**

SP **M46.92 Unspecified inflammatory spondylopathy, cervical region**

SP **M46.93 Unspecified inflammatory spondylopathy, cervicothoracic region**

SP **M46.94 Unspecified inflammatory spondylopathy, thoracic region**

SP **M46.95 Unspecified inflammatory spondylopathy, thoracolumbar region**

SP **M46.96 Unspecified inflammatory spondylopathy, lumbar region**

SP **M46.97 Unspecified inflammatory spondylopathy, lumbosacral region**

SP **M46.98 Unspecified inflammatory spondylopathy, sacral and sacrococcygeal region**

SP **M46.99 Unspecified inflammatory spondylopathy, multiple sites in spine**

4 **M47 Spondylosis**

INCLUDES arthrosis or osteoarthritis of spine
degeneration of facet joints

CODING TIPS✓ OA of spine is coded M47.-. OA of the spine causing weakness, spasticity, clumsiness, altered tonus, but generally no pain, should be coded M47.1-. OA of the spine causing pain, numbness and weakness is coded as M47.2. Query the provider for more specificity when clinical documentation includes those symptoms.

5 **M47.0 Anterior spinal and vertebral artery compression syndromes**

6 **M47.01 Anterior spinal artery compression syndromes**

SP **M47.011 Anterior spinal artery compression syndromes, occipito-atlanto-axial region**

SP **M47.012 Anterior spinal artery compression syndromes, cervical region**

SP **M47.013 Anterior spinal artery compression syndromes, cervicothoracic region**

SP **M47.014 Anterior spinal artery compression syndromes, thoracic region**

SP **M47.015 Anterior spinal artery compression syndromes, thoracolumbar region**

SP **M47.016 Anterior spinal artery compression syndromes, lumbar region**

IQ **M47.019 Anterior spinal artery compression syndromes, site unspecified**

6 **M47.02 Vertebral artery compression syndromes**

SP **M47.021 Vertebral artery compression syndromes, occipito-atlanto-axial region**

SP **M47.022 Vertebral artery compression syndromes, cervical region**

IQ **M47.029 Vertebral artery compression syndromes, site unspecified**

5 **M47.1 Other spondylosis with myelopathy**

Spondylogenic compression of spinal cord

EXCLUDES 1 vertebral subluxation (M43.3-M43.5X9)

CODING TIPS✓ Myelopathy refers to weakness, spasticity, clumsiness, altered tonus, hyperreflexia and pathological reflexes, but generally no pain.

IQ **M47.10 Other spondylosis with myelopathy, site unspecified**

SP **M47.11 Other spondylosis with myelopathy, occipito-atlanto-axial region**

SP **M47.12 Other spondylosis with myelopathy, cervical region**

SP **M47.13 Other spondylosis with myelopathy, cervicothoracic region**

SP **M47.14 Other spondylosis with myelopathy, thoracic region**

SP **M47.15 Other spondylosis with myelopathy, thoracolumbar region**

SP **M47.16 Other spondylosis with myelopathy, lumbar region**

5 **M47.2 Other spondylosis with radiculopathy**

CODING TIPS✓ Radiculopathy refers to symptoms of pain, numbness and weakness in a pattern consistent with the distribution of a particular nerve root.

IQ **M47.20 Other spondylosis with radiculopathy, site unspecified**

SP **M47.21 Other spondylosis with radiculopathy, occipito-atlanto-axial region**

Chapter 13

M00-M99

SP **M47.22 Other spondylosis with radiculopathy, cervical region**

SP **M47.23 Other spondylosis with radiculopathy, cervicothoracic region**

SP **M47.24 Other spondylosis with radiculopathy, thoracic region**

SP **M47.25 Other spondylosis with radiculopathy, thoracolumbar region**

SP **M47.26 Other spondylosis with radiculopathy, lumbar region**

SP **M47.27 Other spondylosis with radiculopathy, lumbosacral region**

SP **M47.28 Other spondylosis with radiculopathy, sacral and sacrococcygeal region**

5 **M47.8 Other spondylosis**

6 **M47.81 Spondylosis without myelopathy or radiculopathy**

SP **M47.811 Spondylosis without myelopathy or radiculopathy, occipito-atlanto-axial region**

SP **M47.812 Spondylosis without myelopathy or radiculopathy, cervical region**

SP **M47.813 Spondylosis without myelopathy or radiculopathy, cervicothoracic region**

SP **M47.814 Spondylosis without myelopathy or radiculopathy, thoracic region**

SP **M47.815 Spondylosis without myelopathy or radiculopathy, thoracolumbar region**

SP **M47.816 Spondylosis without myelopathy or radiculopathy, lumbar region**

SP **M47.817 Spondylosis without myelopathy or radiculopathy, lumbosacral region**

SP **M47.818 Spondylosis without myelopathy or radiculopathy, sacral and sacrococcygeal region**

IQ **M47.819 Spondylosis without myelopathy or radiculopathy, site unspecified**

6 **M47.89 Other spondylosis**

SP **M47.891 Other spondylosis, occipito-atlanto-axial region**

SP **M47.892 Other spondylosis, cervical region**

SP **M47.893 Other spondylosis, cervicothoracic region**

SP **M47.894 Other spondylosis, thoracic region**

SP **M47.895 Other spondylosis, thoracolumbar region**

SP **M47.896 Other spondylosis, lumbar region**

SP **M47.897 Other spondylosis, lumbosacral region**

SP **M47.898 Other spondylosis, sacral and sacrococcygeal region**

IQ **M47.899 Other spondylosis, site unspecified**

IQ **M47.9 Spondylosis, unspecified**

4 **M48 Other spondylopathies**

5 **M48.0 Spinal stenosis**

Caudal stenosis

CODING TIPS ✓ To determine if spinal stenosis has been resolved by surgery, look for physician or NPP documentation regarding decompression or release.

IQ **M48.00 Spinal stenosis, site unspecified**

SP **M48.01 Spinal stenosis, occipito-atlanto-axial region**

SP **M48.02 Spinal stenosis, cervical region**

SP **M48.03 Spinal stenosis, cervicothoracic region**

SP **M48.04 Spinal stenosis, thoracic region**

SP **M48.05 Spinal stenosis, thoracolumbar region**

6 **M48.06 Spinal stenosis, lumbar region**

DEFINITION Neurogenic claudication may present in one or both legs and usually presents as some combination of discomfort, pain, numbness and weakness in the calves, buttocks, and/or thighs.

SP **M48.061 Spinal stenosis, lumbar region without neurogenic claudication**

Spinal stenosis, lumbar region NOS

SP **M48.062 Spinal stenosis, lumbar region with neurogenic claudication**

SP **M48.07 Spinal stenosis, lumbosacral region**

SP **M48.08 Spinal stenosis, sacral and sacrococcygeal region**

5 **M48.1 Ankylosing hyperostosis [Forestier]**

Diffuse idiopathic skeletal hyperostosis [DISH]

SP **M48.10 Ankylosing hyperostosis [Forestier], site unspecified**

SP **M48.11 Ankylosing hyperostosis [Forestier], occipito-atlanto-axial region**

SP **M48.12 Ankylosing hyperostosis [Forestier], cervical region**

SP **M48.13 Ankylosing hyperostosis [Forestier], cervicothoracic region**

SP **M48.14 Ankylosing hyperostosis [Forestier], thoracic region**

SP **M48.15 Ankylosing hyperostosis [Forestier], thoracolumbar region**

SP **M48.16 Ankylosing hyperostosis [Forestier], lumbar region**

SP **M48.17 Ankylosing hyperostosis [Forestier], lumbosacral region**

SP **M48.18 Ankylosing hyperostosis [Forestier], sacral and sacrococcygeal region**

SP **M48.19 Ankylosing hyperostosis [Forestier], multiple sites in spine**

5 **M48.2 Kissing spine**

IQ **M48.20 Kissing spine, site unspecified**

SP **M48.21 Kissing spine, occipito-atlanto-axial region**

SP **M48.22 Kissing spine, cervical region**

SP **M48.23 Kissing spine, cervicothoracic region**

SP **M48.24 Kissing spine, thoracic region**

SP **M48.25 Kissing spine, thoracolumbar region**

SP **M48.26 Kissing spine, lumbar region**

SP **M48.27 Kissing spine, lumbosacral region**

5 **M48.3 Traumatic spondylopathy**

IQ **M48.30 Traumatic spondylopathy, site unspecified**

SP **M48.31 Traumatic spondylopathy, occipito-atlanto-axial region**

SP **M48.32 Traumatic spondylopathy, cervical region**

SP **M48.33 Traumatic spondylopathy, cervicothoracic region**

SP **M48.34 Traumatic spondylopathy, thoracic region**

SP **M48.35 Traumatic spondylopathy, thoracolumbar region**

SP **M48.36 Traumatic spondylopathy, lumbar region**

SP **M48.37 Traumatic spondylopathy, lumbosacral region**

SP **M48.38 Traumatic spondylopathy, sacral and sacrococcygeal region**

5 **M48.4 Fatigue fracture of vertebra**

Stress fracture of vertebra

EXCLUDES 1 pathological fracture NOS (M84.4-)
pathological fracture of vertebra due to neoplasm (M84.58)
pathological fracture of vertebra due to other diagnosis (M84.68)
pathological fracture of vertebra due to osteoporosis (M80.-)
traumatic fracture of vertebrae (S12.0-S12.3-, S22.0-, S32.0-)

The appropriate 7th character is to be added to each code from subcategory M48.4:

A	initial encounter for fracture
D	subsequent encounter for fracture with routine healing
G	subsequent encounter for fracture with delayed healing
S	sequela of fracture

CODING TIPS ✓ Fractures repaired by joint replacements are NOT coded with Z47.1. Fractures repaired by any other orthopedic surgery are NOT coded with Z47.89. Z codes are not appropriate for fractures of any kind. Code the fracture with 7th character D for fractures undergoing surgical repair.

!Q 7 **M48.40X- Fatigue fracture of vertebra, site unspecified**

SP 7 **M48.41X- Fatigue fracture of vertebra, occipito-atlanto-axial region**

SP 7 **M48.42X- Fatigue fracture of vertebra, cervical region**

SP 7 **M48.43X- Fatigue fracture of vertebra, cervicothoracic region**

SP 7 **M48.44X- Fatigue fracture of vertebra, thoracic region**

SP 7 **M48.45X- Fatigue fracture of vertebra, thoracolumbar region**

SP 7 **M48.46X- Fatigue fracture of vertebra, lumbar region**

SP 7 **M48.47X- Fatigue fracture of vertebra, lumbosacral region**

SP 7 **M48.48X- Fatigue fracture of vertebra, sacral and sacrococcygeal region**

5 **M48.5 Collapsed vertebra, not elsewhere classified**

Collapsed vertebra NOS
Compression fracture of vertebra NOS
Wedging of vertebra NOS

EXCLUDES 1 current injury - see Injury of spine, by body region
fatigue fracture of vertebra (M48.4)
pathological fracture of vertebra due to neoplasm (M84.58)
pathological fracture of vertebra due to other diagnosis (M84.68)
pathological fracture of vertebra due to osteoporosis (M80.-)
pathological fracture NOS (M84.4-)
stress fracture of vertebra (M48.4-)
traumatic fracture of vertebra (S12.-, S22.-, S32.-)

The appropriate 7th character is to be added to each code from subcategory M48.5:

A	initial encounter for fracture
D	subsequent encounter for fracture with routine healing
G	subsequent encounter for fracture with delayed healing
S	sequela of fracture

CODING TIPS ✓ Fractures repaired by joint replacements are NOT coded with Z47.1. Fractures repaired by any other orthopedic surgery are NOT coded with Z47.89. Z codes are not appropriate for fractures of any kind. Code the fracture with 7th character D for fractures undergoing surgical repair.

!Q 7 **M48.50X- Collapsed vertebra, not elsewhere classified, site unspecified**

SP 7 **M48.51X- Collapsed vertebra, not elsewhere classified, occipito-atlanto-axial region**

SP 7 **M48.52X- Collapsed vertebra, not elsewhere classified, cervical region**

SP 7 **M48.53X- Collapsed vertebra, not elsewhere classified, cervicothoracic region**

SP 7 **M48.54X- Collapsed vertebra, not elsewhere classified, thoracic region**

SP 7 **M48.55X- Collapsed vertebra, not elsewhere classified, thoracolumbar region**

SP 7 **M48.56X- Collapsed vertebra, not elsewhere classified, lumbar region**

SP 7 **M48.57X- Collapsed vertebra, not elsewhere classified, lumbosacral region**

SP 7 **M48.58X- Collapsed vertebra, not elsewhere classified, sacral and sacrococcygeal region**

5 **M48.8 Other specified spondylopathies**

Ossification of posterior longitudinal ligament

6 **M48.8X Other specified spondylopathies**

SP **M48.8X1 Other specified spondylopathies, occipito-atlanto-axial region**

SP **M48.8X2 Other specified spondylopathies, cervical region**

SP **M48.8X3 Other specified spondylopathies, cervicothoracic region**

SP **M48.8X4 Other specified spondylopathies, thoracic region**

SP **M48.8X5 Other specified spondylopathies, thoracolumbar region**

SP **M48.8X6 Other specified spondylopathies, lumbar region**

SP **M48.8X7 Other specified spondylopathies, lumbosacral region**

SP **M48.8X8 Other specified spondylopathies, sacral and sacrococcygeal region**

!Q **M48.8X9 Other specified spondylopathies, site unspecified**

SP **M48.9 Spondylopathy, unspecified**

4 **M49 Spondylopathies in diseases classified elsewhere**

INCLUDES curvature of spine in diseases classified elsewhere
deformity of spine in diseases classified elsewhere
kyphosis in diseases classified elsewhere
scoliosis in diseases classified elsewhere
spondylopathy in diseases classified elsewhere

Code first underlying disease, such as:
brucellosis (A23.-)
Charcot-Marie-Tooth disease (G60.0)
enterobacterial infections (A01-A04)
osteitis fibrosa cystica (E21.0)

EXCLUDES 1 curvature of spine in tuberculosis [Pott's] (A18.01)
enteropathic arthropathies (M07.-)
gonococcal spondylitis (A54.41)
neuropathic [tabes dorsalis] spondylitis (A52.11)
neuropathic spondylopathy in syringomyelia (G95.0)
neuropathic spondylopathy in tabes dorsalis (A52.11)
nonsyphilitic neuropathic spondylopathy NEC (G98.0)
spondylitis in syphilis (acquired) (A52.77)
tuberculous spondylitis (A18.01)
typhoid fever spondylitis (A01.05)

5 **M49.8 Spondylopathy in diseases classified elsewhere**

CODING TIPS ✓ M49.8- codes indicate spondylopathy due to an underlying condition. The underlying condition should be identified and coded first.

M !Q **M49.80** ***Spondylopathy in diseases classified elsewhere, site unspecified***

M !Q **M49.81** ***Spondylopathy in diseases classified elsewhere, occipito-atlanto-axial region***

M !Q **M49.82** ***Spondylopathy in diseases classified elsewhere, cervical region***

M !Q **M49.83** ***Spondylopathy in diseases classified elsewhere, cervicothoracic region***

M !Q **M49.84** ***Spondylopathy in diseases classified elsewhere, thoracic region***

M !Q **M49.85** ***Spondylopathy in diseases classified elsewhere, thoracolumbar region***

M !Q **M49.86** ***Spondylopathy in diseases classified elsewhere, lumbar region***

M !Q **M49.87** ***Spondylopathy in diseases classified elsewhere, lumbosacral region***

M !Q **M49.88** ***Spondylopathy in diseases classified elsewhere, sacral and sacrococcygeal region***

M !Q **M49.89** ***Spondylopathy in diseases classified elsewhere, multiple sites in spine***

Other dorsopathies (M50-M54)

EXCLUDES 1 current injury - see injury of spine by body region
discitis NOS (M46.4-)

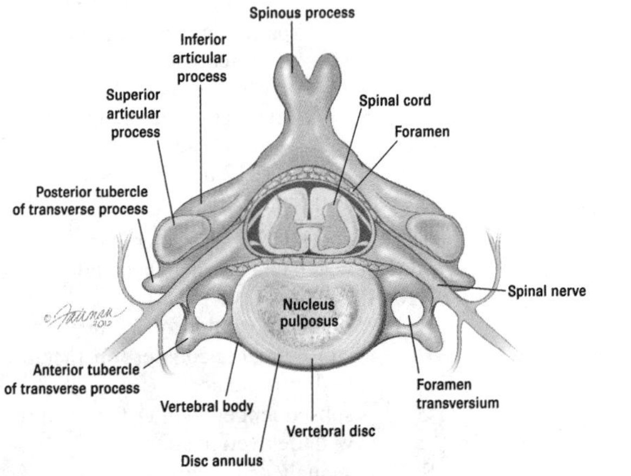

4 **M50 Cervical disc disorders**

Note:
code to the most superior level of disorder

INCLUDES cervicothoracic disc disorders with cervicalgia
cervicothoracic disc disorders

CODING TIPS ✓ If the patient has a disc disorder at more than one region, code to the highest level of each region. Note the excludes 2 note at M51.

5 **M50.0 Cervical disc disorder with myelopathy**

CODING TIPS ✓ Myelopathy refers to weakness, spasticity, clumsiness, altered tonus, hyperreflexia and pathological reflexes, but generally no pain.

SP **M50.00 Cervical disc disorder with myelopathy, unspecified cervical region**

SP **M50.01 Cervical disc disorder with myelopathy, high cervical region**
C2-C3 disc disorder with myelopathy
C3-C4 disc disorder with myelopathy

6 **M50.02 Cervical disc disorder with myelopathy, mid-cervical region**

!Q **M50.020 Cervical disc disorder with myelopathy, mid-cervical region, unspecified level**

SP **M50.021 Cervical disc disorder at C4-C5 level with myelopathy**
C4-C5 disc disorder with myelopathy

SP **M50.022 Cervical disc disorder at C5-C6 level with myelopathy**
C5-C6 disc disorder with myelopathy

SP **M50.023 Cervical disc disorder at C6-C7 level with myelopathy**
C6-C7 disc disorder with myelopathy

SP **M50.03 Cervical disc disorder with myelopathy, cervicothoracic region**
C7-T1 disc disorder with myelopathy

5 **M50.1 Cervical disc disorder with radiculopathy**

EXCLUDES 2 brachial radiculitis NOS (M54.13)

CODING TIPS✓ Radiculopathy refers to symptoms of pain, numbness and weakness in a pattern consistent with the distribution of a particular nerve root.

!Q **M50.10 Cervical disc disorder with radiculopathy, unspecified cervical region**

SP **M50.11 Cervical disc disorder with radiculopathy, high cervical region**
C2-C3 disc disorder with radiculopathy
C3 radiculopathy due to disc disorder
C3-C4 disc disorder with radiculopathy
C4 radiculopathy due to disc disorder

6 **M50.12 Cervical disc disorder with radiculopathy, mid-cervical region**

!Q **M50.120 Mid-cervical disc disorder, unspecified level**

SP **M50.121 Cervical disc disorder at C4-C5 level with radiculopathy**
C4-C5 disc disorder with radiculopathy
C5 radiculopathy due to disc disorder

SP **M50.122 Cervical disc disorder at C5-C6 level with radiculopathy**
C5-C6 disc disorder with radiculopathy
C6 radiculopathy due to disc disorder

SP **M50.123 Cervical disc disorder at C6-C7 level with radiculopathy**
C6-C7 disc disorder with radiculopathy
C7 radiculopathy due to disc disorder

SP **M50.13 Cervical disc disorder with radiculopathy, cervicothoracic region**
C7-T1 disc disorder with radiculopathy
C8 radiculopathy due to disc disorder

5 **M50.2 Other cervical disc displacement**

!Q **M50.20 Other cervical disc displacement, unspecified cervical region**

SP **M50.21 Other cervical disc displacement, high cervical region**
Other C2-C3 cervical disc displacement
Other C3-C4 cervical disc displacement

6 **M50.22 Other cervical disc displacement, mid-cervical region**

!Q **M50.220 Other cervical disc displacement, mid-cervical region, unspecified level**

SP **M50.221 Other cervical disc displacement at C4-C5 level**
Other C4-C5 cervical disc displacement

SP **M50.222 Other cervical disc displacement at C5-C6 level**
Other C5-C6 cervical disc displacement

SP **M50.223 Other cervical disc displacement at C6-C7 level**
Other C6-C7 cervical disc displacement

SP **M50.23 Other cervical disc displacement, cervicothoracic region**
Other C7-T1 cervical disc displacement

5 **M50.3 Other cervical disc degeneration**

!Q **M50.30 Other cervical disc degeneration, unspecified cervical region**

SP **M50.31 Other cervical disc degeneration, high cervical region**
Other C2-C3 cervical disc degeneration
Other C3-C4 cervical disc degeneration

6 **M50.32 Other cervical disc degeneration, mid-cervical region**

!Q **M50.320 Other cervical disc degeneration, mid-cervical region, unspecified level**

SP **M50.321 Other cervical disc degeneration at C4-C5 level**
Other C4-C5 cervical disc degeneration

SP **M50.322 Other cervical disc degeneration at C5-C6 level**
Other C5-C6 cervical disc degeneration

SP **M50.323 Other cervical disc degeneration at C6-C7 level**
Other C6-C7 cervical disc degeneration

SP **M50.33 Other cervical disc degeneration, cervicothoracic region**
Other C7-T1 cervical disc degeneration

5 **M50.8 Other cervical disc disorders**

!Q **M50.80 Other cervical disc disorders, unspecified cervical region**

SP **M50.81 Other cervical disc disorders, high cervical region**
Other C2-C3 cervical disc disorders
Other C3-C4 cervical disc disorders

6 **M50.82 Other cervical disc disorders, mid-cervical region**

!Q **M50.820 Other cervical disc disorders, mid-cervical region, unspecified level**

SP **M50.821 Other cervical disc disorders at C4-C5 level**
Other C4-C5 cervical disc disorders

SP **M50.822 Other cervical disc disorders at C5-C6 level**
Other C5-C6 cervical disc disorders

Chapter 13

M00-M99

SP **M50.823 Other cervical disc disorders at C6-C7 level**
Other C6-C7 cervical disc disorders

SP **M50.83 Other cervical disc disorders, cervicothoracic region**
Other C7-T1 cervical disc disorders

5 **M50.9 Cervical disc disorder, unspecified**

IQ **M50.90 Cervical disc disorder, unspecified, unspecified cervical region**

SP **M50.91 Cervical disc disorder, unspecified, high cervical region**
C2-C3 cervical disc disorder, unspecified
C3-C4 cervical disc disorder, unspecified

6 **M50.92 Cervical disc disorder, unspecified, mid-cervical region**

IQ **M50.920 Unspecified cervical disc disorder, mid-cervical region, unspecified level**

SP **M50.921 Unspecified cervical disc disorder at C4-C5 level**
Unspecified C4-C5 cervical disc disorder

SP **M50.922 Unspecified cervical disc disorder at C5-C6 level**
Unspecified C5-C6 cervical disc disorder

SP **M50.923 Unspecified cervical disc disorder at C6-C7 level**
Unspecified C6-C7 cervical disc disorder

SP **M50.93 Cervical disc disorder, unspecified, cervicothoracic region**
C7-T1 cervical disc disorder, unspecified

4 **M51 Thoracic, thoracolumbar, and lumbosacral intervertebral disc disorders**

EXCLUDES 2 cervical and cervicothoracic disc disorders (M50.-)
sacral and sacrococcygeal disorders (M53.3)

CODING TIPS✓ If the patient has a disc disorder at more than one region, code to the highest level of each region. Note the excludes 2 note at M51.

5 **M51.0 Thoracic, thoracolumbar and lumbosacral intervertebral disc disorders with myelopathy**

CODING TIPS✓ Myelopathy refers to weakness, spasticity, clumsiness, altered tonus, hyperreflexia and pathological reflexes, but generally no pain.

SP **M51.04 Intervertebral disc disorders with myelopathy, thoracic region**

SP **M51.05 Intervertebral disc disorders with myelopathy, thoracolumbar region**

SP **M51.06 Intervertebral disc disorders with myelopathy, lumbar region**

5 **M51.1 Thoracic, thoracolumbar and lumbosacral intervertebral disc disorders with radiculopathy**
Sciatica due to intervertebral disc disorder

EXCLUDES 1 lumbar radiculitis NOS (M54.16)
sciatica NOS (M54.3)

CODING TIPS✓ Radiculopathy refers to symptoms of pain, numbness and weakness in a pattern consistent with the distribution of a particular nerve root.

SP **M51.14 Intervertebral disc disorders with radiculopathy, thoracic region**

SP **M51.15 Intervertebral disc disorders with radiculopathy, thoracolumbar region**

SP **M51.16 Intervertebral disc disorders with radiculopathy, lumbar region**

SP **M51.17 Intervertebral disc disorders with radiculopathy, lumbosacral region**

5 **M51.2 Other thoracic, thoracolumbar and lumbosacral intervertebral disc displacement**
Lumbago due to displacement of intervertebral disc

SP **M51.24 Other intervertebral disc displacement, thoracic region**

SP **M51.25 Other intervertebral disc displacement, thoracolumbar region**

SP **M51.26 Other intervertebral disc displacement, lumbar region**

SP **M51.27 Other intervertebral disc displacement, lumbosacral region**

5 **M51.3 Other thoracic, thoracolumbar and lumbosacral intervertebral disc degeneration**

SP **M51.34 Other intervertebral disc degeneration, thoracic region**

SP **M51.35 Other intervertebral disc degeneration, thoracolumbar region**

SP **M51.36 Other intervertebral disc degeneration, lumbar region**

SP **M51.37 Other intervertebral disc degeneration, lumbosacral region**

5 **M51.4 Schmorl's nodes**

SP **M51.44 Schmorl's nodes, thoracic region**

SP **M51.45 Schmorl's nodes, thoracolumbar region**

SP **M51.46 Schmorl's nodes, lumbar region**

SP **M51.47 Schmorl's nodes, lumbosacral region**

5 **M51.8 Other thoracic, thoracolumbar and lumbosacral intervertebral disc disorders**

SP **M51.84 Other intervertebral disc disorders, thoracic region**

SP **M51.85 Other intervertebral disc disorders, thoracolumbar region**

SP **M51.86 Other intervertebral disc disorders, lumbar region**

SP **M51.87 Other intervertebral disc disorders, lumbosacral region**

SP **M51.9 Unspecified thoracic, thoracolumbar and lumbosacral intervertebral disc disorder**

4 **M53 Other and unspecified dorsopathies, not elsewhere classified**

SP **M53.0 Cervicocranial syndrome**
Posterior cervical sympathetic syndrome

SP **M53.1 Cervicobrachial syndrome**

EXCLUDES 2 cervical disc disorder (M50.-)
thoracic outlet syndrome (G54.0)

5 **M53.2 Spinal instabilities**

6 **M53.2X Spinal instabilities**

SP **M53.2X1 Spinal instabilities, occipito-atlanto-axial region**

SP **M53.2X2 Spinal instabilities, cervical region**

SP **M53.2X3 Spinal instabilities, cervicothoracic region**

SP **M53.2X4 Spinal instabilities, thoracic region**

SP **M53.2X5 Spinal instabilities, thoracolumbar region**

SP **M53.2X6 Spinal instabilities, lumbar region**

SP **M53.2X7 Spinal instabilities, lumbosacral region**

SP **M53.2X8 Spinal instabilities, sacral and sacrococcygeal region**

!Q **M53.2X9 Spinal instabilities, site unspecified**

SP **M53.3 Sacrococcygeal disorders, not elsewhere classified**

Coccygodynia

5 **M53.8 Other specified dorsopathies**

!Q **M53.80 Other specified dorsopathies, site unspecified**

SP **M53.81 Other specified dorsopathies, occipito-atlanto-axial region**

SP **M53.82 Other specified dorsopathies, cervical region**

SP **M53.83 Other specified dorsopathies, cervicothoracic region**

SP **M53.84 Other specified dorsopathies, thoracic region**

SP **M53.85 Other specified dorsopathies, thoracolumbar region**

SP **M53.86 Other specified dorsopathies, lumbar region**

SP **M53.87 Other specified dorsopathies, lumbosacral region**

SP **M53.88 Other specified dorsopathies, sacral and sacrococcygeal region**

!Q **M53.9 Dorsopathy, unspecified**

4 **M54 Dorsalgia**

EXCLUDES 1 psychogenic dorsalgia (F45.41)

5 **M54.0 Panniculitis affecting regions of neck and back**

EXCLUDES 1 lupus panniculitis (L93.2)
panniculitis NOS (M79.3)
relapsing [Weber-Christian] panniculitis (M35.6)

!Q **M54.00 Panniculitis affecting regions of neck and back, site unspecified**

SP **M54.01 Panniculitis affecting regions of neck and back, occipito-atlanto-axial region**

SP **M54.02 Panniculitis affecting regions of neck and back, cervical region**

SP **M54.03 Panniculitis affecting regions of neck and back, cervicothoracic region**

SP **M54.04 Panniculitis affecting regions of neck and back, thoracic region**

SP **M54.05 Panniculitis affecting regions of neck and back, thoracolumbar region**

SP **M54.06 Panniculitis affecting regions of neck and back, lumbar region**

SP **M54.07 Panniculitis affecting regions of neck and back, lumbosacral region**

SP **M54.08 Panniculitis affecting regions of neck and back, sacral and sacrococcygeal region**

SP **M54.09 Panniculitis affecting regions, neck and back, multiple sites in spine**

5 **M54.1 Radiculopathy**

Brachial neuritis or radiculitis NOS
Lumbar neuritis or radiculitis NOS
Lumbosacral neuritis or radiculitis NOS
Thoracic neuritis or radiculitis NOS
Radiculitis NOS

EXCLUDES 1 neuralgia and neuritis NOS (M79.2)
radiculopathy with cervical disc disorder (M50.1)
radiculopathy with lumbar and other intervertebral disc disorder (M51.1-)
radiculopathy with spondylosis (M47.2-)

CODING TIPS✓ Radiculopathy associated with a certain disc disorder should not be coded to M54.1. Note the excludes 1 note.

!Q **M54.10 Radiculopathy, site unspecified**

SP **M54.11 Radiculopathy, occipito-atlanto-axial region**

SP **M54.12 Radiculopathy, cervical region**

SP **M54.13 Radiculopathy, cervicothoracic region**

SP **M54.14 Radiculopathy, thoracic region**

SP **M54.15 Radiculopathy, thoracolumbar region**

SP **M54.16 Radiculopathy, lumbar region**

SP **M54.17 Radiculopathy, lumbosacral region**

SP **M54.18 Radiculopathy, sacral and sacrococcygeal region**

SP **M54.2 Cervicalgia**

EXCLUDES 1 cervicalgia due to intervertebral cervical disc disorder (M50.-)

CODING TIPS✓ Cervicalgia associated with a certain disc disorder should not be coded to M54.2. Note the excludes 1 note.

5 **M54.3 Sciatica**

EXCLUDES 1 lesion of sciatic nerve (G57.0)
sciatica due to intervertebral disc disorder (M51.1-)
sciatica with lumbago (M54.4-)

CODING TIPS✓ Sciatica associated with a certain disc disorder should not be coded to M54.3. Note the excludes 1 note.

DEFINITION Severe pain in the sciatic nerve running down the lower back through the leg; usually resulting from nerve compression or pinching.

H !Q **M54.30 Sciatica, unspecified side**

H SP **M54.31 Sciatica, right side**

H SP **M54.32 Sciatica, left side**

5 **M54.4 Lumbago with sciatica**

EXCLUDES 1 lumbago with sciatica due to intervertebral disc disorder (M51.1-)

Chapter 13

M00-M99

CODING TIPS✓ Lumbago associated with a certain disc disorder should not be coded with this code. Note the excludes 1 note.

M54.40 Lumbago with sciatica, unspecified side

M54.41 Lumbago with sciatica, right side

M54.42 Lumbago with sciatica, left side

M54.5 Low back pain

EXCLUDES 1 low back strain (S39.012)
lumbago due to intervertebral disc displacement (M51.2-)
lumbago with sciatica (M54.4-)

CODING TIPS✓ Lumbago associated with a certain disc disorder should not be coded with this code. Note the excludes 1 note.

M54.50 Low back pain, unspecified

Loin pain
Lumbago NOS

M54.51 Vertebrogenic low back pain

Low back vertebral endplate pain

M54.59 Other low back pain

M54.6 Pain in thoracic spine

EXCLUDES 1 pain in thoracic spine due to intervertebral disc disorder (M51.-)

M54.8 Other dorsalgia

EXCLUDES 1 dorsalgia in thoracic region (M54.6)
low back pain (M54.5-)

M54.81 Occipital neuralgia

M54.89 Other dorsalgia

M54.9 Dorsalgia, unspecified

Backache NOS
Back pain NOS

Soft tissue disorders (M60-M79)

Disorders of muscles (M60-M63)

EXCLUDES 1 dermatopolymyositis (M33.-)
muscular dystrophies and myopathies (G71-G72)
myopathy in amyloidosis (E85.-)
myopathy in polyarteritis nodosa (M30.0)
myopathy in rheumatoid arthritis (M05.32)
myopathy in scleroderma (M34.-)
myopathy in Sjögren's syndrome (M35.03)
myopathy in systemic lupus erythematosus (M32.-)

M60 Myositis

EXCLUDES 2 inclusion body myositis [IBM] (G72.41)

CODING TIPS✓ **Documentation:** Myositis indicates inflammation of the muscles. This may be caused by inflammatory disorders/autoimmune conditions, infection, or injury. Review all clinical documentation carefully to identify any cause and assign the most specific code for the condition.

CODING TIPS✓ Category M60.- does not include inflammatory myositis specified as inclusion body myositis (IBM), a chronic progressive neurologic condition leading to inflammation and weakness of the muscle. IBM should be coded to G72.41.

M60.0 Infective myositis

Tropical pyomyositis
Use additional code (B95-B97) to identify infectious agent

M60.00 Infective myositis, unspecified site

M60.000 Infective myositis, unspecified right arm

Infective myositis, right upper limb NOS

M60.001 Infective myositis, unspecified left arm

Infective myositis, left upper limb NOS

M60.002 Infective myositis, unspecified arm

Infective myositis, upper limb NOS

M60.003 Infective myositis, unspecified right leg

Infective myositis, right lower limb NOS

M60.004 Infective myositis, unspecified left leg

Infective myositis, left lower limb NOS

M60.005 Infective myositis, unspecified leg

Infective myositis, lower limb NOS

M60.009 Infective myositis, unspecified site

M60.01 Infective myositis, shoulder

M60.011 Infective myositis, right shoulder

M60.012 Infective myositis, left shoulder

M60.019 Infective myositis, unspecified shoulder

M60.02 Infective myositis, upper arm

M60.021 Infective myositis, right upper arm

M60.022 Infective myositis, left upper arm

M60.029 Infective myositis, unspecified upper arm

M60.03 Infective myositis, forearm

M60.031 Infective myositis, right forearm

M60.032 Infective myositis, left forearm

M60.039 Infective myositis, unspecified forearm

M60.04 Infective myositis, hand and fingers

M60.041 Infective myositis, right hand

M60.042 Infective myositis, left hand

M60.043 Infective myositis, unspecified hand

M60.044 Infective myositis, right finger(s)

M60.045 Infective myositis, left finger(s)

M60.046 Infective myositis, unspecified finger(s)

M60.05 Infective myositis, thigh

M60.051 Infective myositis, right thigh

M60.052 Infective myositis, left thigh

IQ + M60.059 Infective myositis, unspecified thigh
+ 6 M60.06 Infective myositis, lower leg
SP + M60.061 Infective myositis, right lower leg
SP + M60.062 Infective myositis, left lower leg
IQ + M60.069 Infective myositis, unspecified lower leg
+ 6 M60.07 Infective myositis, ankle, foot and toes
SP + M60.070 Infective myositis, right ankle
SP + M60.071 Infective myositis, left ankle
IQ + M60.072 Infective myositis, unspecified ankle
SP + M60.073 Infective myositis, right foot
SP + M60.074 Infective myositis, left foot
IQ + M60.075 Infective myositis, unspecified foot
SP + M60.076 Infective myositis, right toe(s)
SP + M60.077 Infective myositis, left toe(s)
IQ + M60.078 Infective myositis, unspecified toe(s)
SP + M60.08 Infective myositis, other site
SP + M60.09 Infective myositis, multiple sites
5 M60.1 Interstitial myositis
IQ M60.10 Interstitial myositis of unspecified site
6 M60.11 Interstitial myositis, shoulder
SP M60.111 Interstitial myositis, right shoulder
SP M60.112 Interstitial myositis, left shoulder
IQ M60.119 Interstitial myositis, unspecified shoulder
6 M60.12 Interstitial myositis, upper arm
SP M60.121 Interstitial myositis, right upper arm
SP M60.122 Interstitial myositis, left upper arm
IQ M60.129 Interstitial myositis, unspecified upper arm
6 M60.13 Interstitial myositis, forearm
SP M60.131 Interstitial myositis, right forearm
IQ M60.132 Interstitial myositis, left forearm
IQ M60.139 Interstitial myositis, unspecified forearm
6 M60.14 Interstitial myositis, hand
SP M60.141 Interstitial myositis, right hand
SP M60.142 Interstitial myositis, left hand
IQ M60.149 Interstitial myositis, unspecified hand
6 M60.15 Interstitial myositis, thigh
SP M60.151 Interstitial myositis, right thigh
SP M60.152 Interstitial myositis, left thigh
IQ M60.159 Interstitial myositis, unspecified thigh
6 M60.16 Interstitial myositis, lower leg
SP M60.161 Interstitial myositis, right lower leg
SP M60.162 Interstitial myositis, left lower leg
IQ M60.169 Interstitial myositis, unspecified lower leg
6 M60.17 Interstitial myositis, ankle and foot
SP M60.171 Interstitial myositis, right ankle and foot
SP M60.172 Interstitial myositis, left ankle and foot
IQ M60.179 Interstitial myositis, unspecified ankle and foot
SP M60.18 Interstitial myositis, other site
SP M60.19 Interstitial myositis, multiple sites
+ 5 M60.2 Foreign body granuloma of soft tissue, not elsewhere classified
Use additional code to identify the type of retained foreign body (Z18.-)
EXCLUDES 1 foreign body granuloma of skin and subcutaneous tissue (L92.3)
IQ + M60.20 Foreign body granuloma of soft tissue, not elsewhere classified, unspecified site
+ 6 M60.21 Foreign body granuloma of soft tissue, not elsewhere classified, shoulder
SP + M60.211 Foreign body granuloma of soft tissue, not elsewhere classified, right shoulder
SP + M60.212 Foreign body granuloma of soft tissue, not elsewhere classified, left shoulder
IQ + M60.219 Foreign body granuloma of soft tissue, not elsewhere classified, unspecified shoulder
+ 6 M60.22 Foreign body granuloma of soft tissue, not elsewhere classified, upper arm
SP + M60.221 Foreign body granuloma of soft tissue, not elsewhere classified, right upper arm
SP + M60.222 Foreign body granuloma of soft tissue, not elsewhere classified, left upper arm
IQ + M60.229 Foreign body granuloma of soft tissue, not elsewhere classified, unspecified upper arm
+ 6 M60.23 Foreign body granuloma of soft tissue, not elsewhere classified, forearm
SP + M60.231 Foreign body granuloma of soft tissue, not elsewhere classified, right forearm
SP + M60.232 Foreign body granuloma of soft tissue, not elsewhere classified, left forearm
IQ + M60.239 Foreign body granuloma of soft tissue, not elsewhere classified, unspecified forearm
+ 6 M60.24 Foreign body granuloma of soft tissue, not elsewhere classified, hand
SP + M60.241 Foreign body granuloma of soft tissue, not elsewhere classified, right hand
SP + M60.242 Foreign body granuloma of soft tissue, not elsewhere classified, left hand
IQ + M60.249 Foreign body granuloma of soft tissue, not elsewhere classified, unspecified hand

+ 6 **M60.25** Foreign body granuloma of soft tissue, not elsewhere classified, thigh

L SP + **M60.251** Foreign body granuloma of soft tissue, not elsewhere classified, right thigh

L SP + **M60.252** Foreign body granuloma of soft tissue, not elsewhere classified, left thigh

L !Q + **M60.259** Foreign body granuloma of soft tissue, not elsewhere classified, unspecified thigh

+ 6 **M60.26** Foreign body granuloma of soft tissue, not elsewhere classified, lower leg

L SP + **M60.261** Foreign body granuloma of soft tissue, not elsewhere classified, right lower leg

L SP + **M60.262** Foreign body granuloma of soft tissue, not elsewhere classified, left lower leg

L !Q + **M60.269** Foreign body granuloma of soft tissue, not elsewhere classified, unspecified lower leg

+ 6 **M60.27** Foreign body granuloma of soft tissue, not elsewhere classified, ankle and foot

L SP + **M60.271** Foreign body granuloma of soft tissue, not elsewhere classified, right ankle and foot

L SP + **M60.272** Foreign body granuloma of soft tissue, not elsewhere classified, left ankle and foot

L !Q + **M60.279** Foreign body granuloma of soft tissue, not elsewhere classified, unspecified ankle and foot

SP + **M60.28** Foreign body granuloma of soft tissue, not elsewhere classified, other site

5 **M60.8** Other myositis

!Q **M60.80** Other myositis, unspecified site

6 **M60.81** Other myositis shoulder

L SP **M60.811** Other myositis, right shoulder

L SP **M60.812** Other myositis, left shoulder

L !Q **M60.819** Other myositis, unspecified shoulder

6 **M60.82** Other myositis, upper arm

L SP **M60.821** Other myositis, right upper arm

L SP **M60.822** Other myositis, left upper arm

L !Q **M60.829** Other myositis, unspecified upper arm

6 **M60.83** Other myositis, forearm

L SP **M60.831** Other myositis, right forearm

L SP **M60.832** Other myositis, left forearm

L !Q **M60.839** Other myositis, unspecified forearm

6 **M60.84** Other myositis, hand

L SP **M60.841** Other myositis, right hand

L SP **M60.842** Other myositis, left hand

L !Q **M60.849** Other myositis, unspecified hand

6 **M60.85** Other myositis, thigh

L SP **M60.851** Other myositis, right thigh

L SP **M60.852** Other myositis, left thigh

L !Q **M60.859** Other myositis, unspecified thigh

6 **M60.86** Other myositis, lower leg

L SP **M60.861** Other myositis, right lower leg

L SP **M60.862** Other myositis, left lower leg

L !Q **M60.869** Other myositis, unspecified lower leg

6 **M60.87** Other myositis, ankle and foot

L SP **M60.871** Other myositis, right ankle and foot

L SP **M60.872** Other myositis, left ankle and foot

L !Q **M60.879** Other myositis, unspecified ankle and foot

SP **M60.88** Other myositis, other site

SP **M60.89** Other myositis, multiple sites

!Q **M60.9** Myositis, unspecified

4 **M61** Calcification and ossification of muscle

5 **M61.0** Myositis ossificans traumatica

!Q **M61.00** Myositis ossificans traumatica, unspecified site

6 **M61.01** Myositis ossificans traumatica, shoulder

L SP **M61.011** Myositis ossificans traumatica, right shoulder

L SP **M61.012** Myositis ossificans traumatica, left shoulder

L !Q **M61.019** Myositis ossificans traumatica, unspecified shoulder

6 **M61.02** Myositis ossificans traumatica, upper arm

L SP **M61.021** Myositis ossificans traumatica, right upper arm

L SP **M61.022** Myositis ossificans traumatica, left upper arm

L !Q **M61.029** Myositis ossificans traumatica, unspecified upper arm

6 **M61.03** Myositis ossificans traumatica, forearm

L SP **M61.031** Myositis ossificans traumatica, right forearm

L SP **M61.032** Myositis ossificans traumatica, left forearm

L !Q **M61.039** Myositis ossificans traumatica, unspecified forearm

6 **M61.04** Myositis ossificans traumatica, hand

L SP **M61.041** Myositis ossificans traumatica, right hand

L SP **M61.042** Myositis ossificans traumatica, left hand

L !Q **M61.049** Myositis ossificans traumatica, unspecified hand

6 **M61.05** Myositis ossificans traumatica, thigh

L SP **M61.051** Myositis ossificans traumatica, right thigh

L SP **M61.052** Myositis ossificans traumatica, left thigh

L !Q **M61.059** Myositis ossificans traumatica, unspecified thigh

6 **M61.06** Myositis ossificans traumatica, lower leg

L SP **M61.061** Myositis ossificans traumatica, right lower leg

L SP **M61.062** Myositis ossificans traumatica, left lower leg

L !Q **M61.069** Myositis ossificans traumatica, unspecified lower leg

4 4th digit required 5 5th digit required 6 6th digit required 7 7th digit required 7 7th digit placeholder + Additional code L Laterality

6 M61.07 Myositis ossificans traumatica, ankle and foot
⊟ SP M61.071 Myositis ossificans traumatica, right ankle and foot
⊟ SP M61.072 Myositis ossificans traumatica, left ankle and foot
⊟ IQ M61.079 Myositis ossificans traumatica, unspecified ankle and foot
SP M61.08 Myositis ossificans traumatica, other site
SP M61.09 Myositis ossificans traumatica, multiple sites
5 M61.1 Myositis ossificans progressiva
Fibrodysplasia ossificans progressiva
IQ M61.10 Myositis ossificans progressiva, unspecified site
6 M61.11 Myositis ossificans progressiva, shoulder
⊟ SP M61.111 Myositis ossificans progressiva, right shoulder
⊟ SP M61.112 Myositis ossificans progressiva, left shoulder
⊟ IQ M61.119 Myositis ossificans progressiva, unspecified shoulder
6 M61.12 Myositis ossificans progressiva, upper arm
⊟ SP M61.121 Myositis ossificans progressiva, right upper arm
⊟ SP M61.122 Myositis ossificans progressiva, left upper arm
⊟ IQ M61.129 Myositis ossificans progressiva, unspecified arm
6 M61.13 Myositis ossificans progressiva, forearm
⊟ SP M61.131 Myositis ossificans progressiva, right forearm
⊟ SP M61.132 Myositis ossificans progressiva, left forearm
⊟ IQ M61.139 Myositis ossificans progressiva, unspecified forearm
6 M61.14 Myositis ossificans progressiva, hand and finger(s)
⊟ SP M61.141 Myositis ossificans progressiva, right hand
⊟ SP M61.142 Myositis ossificans progressiva, left hand
⊟ IQ M61.143 Myositis ossificans progressiva, unspecified hand
⊟ SP M61.144 Myositis ossificans progressiva, right finger(s)
⊟ SP M61.145 Myositis ossificans progressiva, left finger(s)
⊟ IQ M61.146 Myositis ossificans progressiva, unspecified finger(s)
6 M61.15 Myositis ossificans progressiva, thigh
⊟ SP M61.151 Myositis ossificans progressiva, right thigh
⊟ SP M61.152 Myositis ossificans progressiva, left thigh
⊟ IQ M61.159 Myositis ossificans progressiva, unspecified thigh
6 M61.16 Myositis ossificans progressiva, lower leg
⊟ SP M61.161 Myositis ossificans progressiva, right lower leg
⊟ SP M61.162 Myositis ossificans progressiva, left lower leg
⊟ IQ M61.169 Myositis ossificans progressiva, unspecified lower leg
6 M61.17 Myositis ossificans progressiva, ankle, foot and toe(s)
⊟ SP M61.171 Myositis ossificans progressiva, right ankle
⊟ SP M61.172 Myositis ossificans progressiva, left ankle
⊟ IQ M61.173 Myositis ossificans progressiva, unspecified ankle
⊟ SP M61.174 Myositis ossificans progressiva, right foot
⊟ SP M61.175 Myositis ossificans progressiva, left foot
⊟ IQ M61.176 Myositis ossificans progressiva, unspecified foot
⊟ SP M61.177 Myositis ossificans progressiva, right toe(s)
⊟ SP M61.178 Myositis ossificans progressiva, left toe(s)
⊟ IQ M61.179 Myositis ossificans progressiva, unspecified toe(s)
SP M61.18 Myositis ossificans progressiva, other site
SP M61.19 Myositis ossificans progressiva, multiple sites
5 M61.2 Paralytic calcification and ossification of muscle
Myositis ossificans associated with quadriplegia or paraplegia
IQ M61.20 Paralytic calcification and ossification of muscle, unspecified site
6 M61.21 Paralytic calcification and ossification of muscle, shoulder
⊟ SP M61.211 Paralytic calcification and ossification of muscle, right shoulder
⊟ SP M61.212 Paralytic calcification and ossification of muscle, left shoulder
⊟ IQ M61.219 Paralytic calcification and ossification of muscle, unspecified shoulder
6 M61.22 Paralytic calcification and ossification of muscle, upper arm
⊟ SP M61.221 Paralytic calcification and ossification of muscle, right upper arm
⊟ SP M61.222 Paralytic calcification and ossification of muscle, left upper arm
⊟ IQ M61.229 Paralytic calcification and ossification of muscle, unspecified upper arm
6 M61.23 Paralytic calcification and ossification of muscle, forearm
⊟ SP M61.231 Paralytic calcification and ossification of muscle, right forearm
⊟ SP M61.232 Paralytic calcification and ossification of muscle, left forearm
⊟ IQ M61.239 Paralytic calcification and ossification of muscle, unspecified forearm

6 **M61.24 Paralytic calcification and ossification of muscle, hand**

Laterality SP **M61.241 Paralytic calcification and ossification of muscle, right hand**

Laterality SP **M61.242 Paralytic calcification and ossification of muscle, left hand**

Laterality IQ **M61.249 Paralytic calcification and ossification of muscle, unspecified hand**

6 **M61.25 Paralytic calcification and ossification of muscle, thigh**

Laterality SP **M61.251 Paralytic calcification and ossification of muscle, right thigh**

Laterality SP **M61.252 Paralytic calcification and ossification of muscle, left thigh**

Laterality IQ **M61.259 Paralytic calcification and ossification of muscle, unspecified thigh**

6 **M61.26 Paralytic calcification and ossification of muscle, lower leg**

Laterality SP **M61.261 Paralytic calcification and ossification of muscle, right lower leg**

Laterality SP **M61.262 Paralytic calcification and ossification of muscle, left lower leg**

Laterality IQ **M61.269 Paralytic calcification and ossification of muscle, unspecified lower leg**

6 **M61.27 Paralytic calcification and ossification of muscle, ankle and foot**

Laterality SP **M61.271 Paralytic calcification and ossification of muscle, right ankle and foot**

Laterality SP **M61.272 Paralytic calcification and ossification of muscle, left ankle and foot**

Laterality IQ **M61.279 Paralytic calcification and ossification of muscle, unspecified ankle and foot**

SP **M61.28 Paralytic calcification and ossification of muscle, other site**

SP **M61.29 Paralytic calcification and ossification of muscle, multiple sites**

5 **M61.3 Calcification and ossification of muscles associated with burns**

Myositis ossificans associated with burns

IQ **M61.30 Calcification and ossification of muscles associated with burns, unspecified site**

6 **M61.31 Calcification and ossification of muscles associated with burns, shoulder**

Laterality SP **M61.311 Calcification and ossification of muscles associated with burns, right shoulder**

Laterality SP **M61.312 Calcification and ossification of muscles associated with burns, left shoulder**

Laterality IQ **M61.319 Calcification and ossification of muscles associated with burns, unspecified shoulder**

6 **M61.32 Calcification and ossification of muscles associated with burns, upper arm**

Laterality SP **M61.321 Calcification and ossification of muscles associated with burns, right upper arm**

Laterality SP **M61.322 Calcification and ossification of muscles associated with burns, left upper arm**

Laterality IQ **M61.329 Calcification and ossification of muscles associated with burns, unspecified upper arm**

6 **M61.33 Calcification and ossification of muscles associated with burns, forearm**

Laterality SP **M61.331 Calcification and ossification of muscles associated with burns, right forearm**

Laterality SP **M61.332 Calcification and ossification of muscles associated with burns, left forearm**

Laterality IQ **M61.339 Calcification and ossification of muscles associated with burns, unspecified forearm**

6 **M61.34 Calcification and ossification of muscles associated with burns, hand**

Laterality SP **M61.341 Calcification and ossification of muscles associated with burns, right hand**

Laterality SP **M61.342 Calcification and ossification of muscles associated with burns, left hand**

Laterality IQ **M61.349 Calcification and ossification of muscles associated with burns, unspecified hand**

6 **M61.35 Calcification and ossification of muscles associated with burns, thigh**

Laterality SP **M61.351 Calcification and ossification of muscles associated with burns, right thigh**

Laterality SP **M61.352 Calcification and ossification of muscles associated with burns, left thigh**

Laterality IQ **M61.359 Calcification and ossification of muscles associated with burns, unspecified thigh**

6 **M61.36 Calcification and ossification of muscles associated with burns, lower leg**

Laterality SP **M61.361 Calcification and ossification of muscles associated with burns, right lower leg**

Laterality SP **M61.362 Calcification and ossification of muscles associated with burns, left lower leg**

Laterality IQ **M61.369 Calcification and ossification of muscles associated with burns, unspecified lower leg**

6 **M61.37 Calcification and ossification of muscles associated with burns, ankle and foot**

Laterality SP **M61.371 Calcification and ossification of muscles associated with burns, right ankle and foot**

Laterality SP **M61.372 Calcification and ossification of muscles associated with burns, left ankle and foot**

Laterality IQ **M61.379 Calcification and ossification of muscles associated with burns, unspecified ankle and foot**

SP **M61.38 Calcification and ossification of muscles associated with burns, other site**

SP **M61.39 Calcification and ossification of muscles associated with burns, multiple sites**

5 **M61.4 Other calcification of muscle**

EXCLUDES 1 calcific tendinitis NOS (M65.2-)
calcific tendinitis of shoulder (M75.3)

!Q **M61.40 Other calcification of muscle, unspecified site**

6 **M61.41 Other calcification of muscle, shoulder**

⊟ SP **M61.411 Other calcification of muscle, right shoulder**

⊟ SP **M61.412 Other calcification of muscle, left shoulder**

⊟ !Q **M61.419 Other calcification of muscle, unspecified shoulder**

6 **M61.42 Other calcification of muscle, upper arm**

⊟ SP **M61.421 Other calcification of muscle, right upper arm**

⊟ SP **M61.422 Other calcification of muscle, left upper arm**

⊟ !Q **M61.429 Other calcification of muscle, unspecified upper arm**

6 **M61.43 Other calcification of muscle, forearm**

⊟ SP **M61.431 Other calcification of muscle, right forearm**

⊟ SP **M61.432 Other calcification of muscle, left forearm**

⊟ !Q **M61.439 Other calcification of muscle, unspecified forearm**

6 **M61.44 Other calcification of muscle, hand**

⊟ SP **M61.441 Other calcification of muscle, right hand**

⊟ SP **M61.442 Other calcification of muscle, left hand**

⊟ !Q **M61.449 Other calcification of muscle, unspecified hand**

6 **M61.45 Other calcification of muscle, thigh**

⊟ SP **M61.451 Other calcification of muscle, right thigh**

⊟ SP **M61.452 Other calcification of muscle, left thigh**

⊟ !Q **M61.459 Other calcification of muscle, unspecified thigh**

6 **M61.46 Other calcification of muscle, lower leg**

⊟ SP **M61.461 Other calcification of muscle, right lower leg**

⊟ SP **M61.462 Other calcification of muscle, left lower leg**

⊟ !Q **M61.469 Other calcification of muscle, unspecified lower leg**

6 **M61.47 Other calcification of muscle, ankle and foot**

⊟ SP **M61.471 Other calcification of muscle, right ankle and foot**

⊟ SP **M61.472 Other calcification of muscle, left ankle and foot**

⊟ !Q **M61.479 Other calcification of muscle, unspecified ankle and foot**

SP **M61.48 Other calcification of muscle, other site**

SP **M61.49 Other calcification of muscle, multiple sites**

5 **M61.5 Other ossification of muscle**

!Q **M61.50 Other ossification of muscle, unspecified site**

6 **M61.51 Other ossification of muscle, shoulder**

⊟ SP **M61.511 Other ossification of muscle, right shoulder**

⊟ SP **M61.512 Other ossification of muscle, left shoulder**

⊟ !Q **M61.519 Other ossification of muscle, unspecified shoulder**

6 **M61.52 Other ossification of muscle, upper arm**

⊟ SP **M61.521 Other ossification of muscle, right upper arm**

⊟ SP **M61.522 Other ossification of muscle, left upper arm**

⊟ !Q **M61.529 Other ossification of muscle, unspecified upper arm**

6 **M61.53 Other ossification of muscle, forearm**

⊟ SP **M61.531 Other ossification of muscle, right forearm**

⊟ SP **M61.532 Other ossification of muscle, left forearm**

⊟ !Q **M61.539 Other ossification of muscle, unspecified forearm**

6 **M61.54 Other ossification of muscle, hand**

⊟ SP **M61.541 Other ossification of muscle, right hand**

⊟ SP **M61.542 Other ossification of muscle, left hand**

⊟ !Q **M61.549 Other ossification of muscle, unspecified hand**

6 **M61.55 Other ossification of muscle, thigh**

⊟ SP **M61.551 Other ossification of muscle, right thigh**

⊟ SP **M61.552 Other ossification of muscle, left thigh**

⊟ !Q **M61.559 Other ossification of muscle, unspecified thigh**

6 **M61.56 Other ossification of muscle, lower leg**

⊟ SP **M61.561 Other ossification of muscle, right lower leg**

⊟ SP **M61.562 Other ossification of muscle, left lower leg**

⊟ !Q **M61.569 Other ossification of muscle, unspecified lower leg**

6 **M61.57 Other ossification of muscle, ankle and foot**

⊟ SP **M61.571 Other ossification of muscle, right ankle and foot**

⊟ SP **M61.572 Other ossification of muscle, left ankle and foot**

⊟ !Q **M61.579 Other ossification of muscle, unspecified ankle and foot**

SP **M61.58 Other ossification of muscle, other site**

SP **M61.59 Other ossification of muscle, multiple sites**

IQ **M61.9 Calcification and ossification of muscle, unspecified**

4 **M62 Other disorders of muscle**

EXCLUDES 1 alcoholic myopathy (G72.1)
cramp and spasm (R25.2)
drug-induced myopathy (G72.0)
myalgia (M79.1-)
stiff-man syndrome (G25.82)

EXCLUDES 2 nontraumatic hematoma of muscle (M79.81)

5 **M62.0 Separation of muscle (nontraumatic)**

Diastasis of muscle

EXCLUDES 1 diastasis recti complicating pregnancy, labor and delivery (O71.8)
traumatic separation of muscle- see strain of muscle by body region

CODING TIPS✓ Codes classified in M62.0- through M62.28 indicate muscle separation, rupture and ischemia of a non-traumatic origin. When a traumatic muscle injury is reported, do not assign a code from M62.0- through M62.28, but instead assign a code from Chapter 19, Injury, Poisoning and Certain Other Consequences of External Causes.

IQ **M62.00 Separation of muscle (nontraumatic), unspecified site**

6 **M62.01 Separation of muscle (nontraumatic), shoulder**

⊟ SP **M62.011 Separation of muscle (nontraumatic), right shoulder**

⊟ SP **M62.012 Separation of muscle (nontraumatic), left shoulder**

⊟ IQ **M62.019 Separation of muscle (nontraumatic), unspecified shoulder**

6 **M62.02 Separation of muscle (nontraumatic), upper arm**

⊟ SP **M62.021 Separation of muscle (nontraumatic), right upper arm**

⊟ SP **M62.022 Separation of muscle (nontraumatic), left upper arm**

⊟ IQ **M62.029 Separation of muscle (nontraumatic), unspecified upper arm**

6 **M62.03 Separation of muscle (nontraumatic), forearm**

⊟ SP **M62.031 Separation of muscle (nontraumatic), right forearm**

⊟ SP **M62.032 Separation of muscle (nontraumatic), left forearm**

⊟ IQ **M62.039 Separation of muscle (nontraumatic), unspecified forearm**

6 **M62.04 Separation of muscle (nontraumatic), hand**

⊟ SP **M62.041 Separation of muscle (nontraumatic), right hand**

⊟ SP **M62.042 Separation of muscle (nontraumatic), left hand**

⊟ IQ **M62.049 Separation of muscle (nontraumatic), unspecified hand**

6 **M62.05 Separation of muscle (nontraumatic), thigh**

⊟ SP **M62.051 Separation of muscle (nontraumatic), right thigh**

⊟ SP **M62.052 Separation of muscle (nontraumatic), left thigh**

⊟ IQ **M62.059 Separation of muscle (nontraumatic), unspecified thigh**

6 **M62.06 Separation of muscle (nontraumatic), lower leg**

⊟ SP **M62.061 Separation of muscle (nontraumatic), right lower leg**

⊟ SP **M62.062 Separation of muscle (nontraumatic), left lower leg**

⊟ IQ **M62.069 Separation of muscle (nontraumatic), unspecified lower leg**

6 **M62.07 Separation of muscle (nontraumatic), ankle and foot**

⊟ SP **M62.071 Separation of muscle (nontraumatic), right ankle and foot**

⊟ SP **M62.072 Separation of muscle (nontraumatic), left ankle and foot**

⊟ IQ **M62.079 Separation of muscle (nontraumatic), unspecified ankle and foot**

SP **M62.08 Separation of muscle (nontraumatic), other site**

5 **M62.1 Other rupture of muscle (nontraumatic)**

EXCLUDES 1 traumatic rupture of muscle - see strain of muscle by body region

EXCLUDES 2 rupture of tendon (M66.-)

CODING TIPS✓ Codes classified in M62.0- through M62.28 indicate muscle separation, rupture and ischemia of a non-traumatic origin. When a traumatic muscle injury is reported, do not assign a code from M62.0- through M62.28, but instead assign a code from Chapter 19, Injury, Poisoning and Certain Other Consequences of External Causes.

IQ **M62.10 Other rupture of muscle (nontraumatic), unspecified site**

6 **M62.11 Other rupture of muscle (nontraumatic), shoulder**

⊟ SP **M62.111 Other rupture of muscle (nontraumatic), right shoulder**

⊟ SP **M62.112 Other rupture of muscle (nontraumatic), left shoulder**

⊟ IQ **M62.119 Other rupture of muscle (nontraumatic), unspecified shoulder**

6 **M62.12 Other rupture of muscle (nontraumatic), upper arm**

⊟ SP **M62.121 Other rupture of muscle (nontraumatic), right upper arm**

⊟ SP **M62.122 Other rupture of muscle (nontraumatic), left upper arm**

⊟ IQ **M62.129 Other rupture of muscle (nontraumatic), unspecified upper arm**

6 **M62.13 Other rupture of muscle (nontraumatic), forearm**

⊟ SP **M62.131 Other rupture of muscle (nontraumatic), right forearm**

SP M62.132 Other rupture of muscle (nontraumatic), left forearm

IQ M62.139 Other rupture of muscle (nontraumatic), unspecified forearm

6 M62.14 Other rupture of muscle (nontraumatic), hand

SP M62.141 Other rupture of muscle (nontraumatic), right hand

SP M62.142 Other rupture of muscle (nontraumatic), left hand

IQ M62.149 Other rupture of muscle (nontraumatic), unspecified hand

6 M62.15 Other rupture of muscle (nontraumatic), thigh

SP M62.151 Other rupture of muscle (nontraumatic), right thigh

SP M62.152 Other rupture of muscle (nontraumatic), left thigh

IQ M62.159 Other rupture of muscle (nontraumatic), unspecified thigh

6 M62.16 Other rupture of muscle (nontraumatic), lower leg

SP M62.161 Other rupture of muscle (nontraumatic), right lower leg

SP M62.162 Other rupture of muscle (nontraumatic), left lower leg

IQ M62.169 Other rupture of muscle (nontraumatic), unspecified lower leg

6 M62.17 Other rupture of muscle (nontraumatic), ankle and foot

SP M62.171 Other rupture of muscle (nontraumatic), right ankle and foot

SP M62.172 Other rupture of muscle (nontraumatic), left ankle and foot

IQ M62.179 Other rupture of muscle (nontraumatic), unspecified ankle and foot

SP M62.18 Other rupture of muscle (nontraumatic), other site

5 M62.2 Nontraumatic ischemic infarction of muscle

EXCLUDES 1 compartment syndrome (traumatic) (T79.A-)
nontraumatic compartment syndrome (M79.A-)
traumatic ischemia of muscle (T79.6)
rhabdomyolysis (M62.82)
Volkmann's ischemic contracture (T79.6)

CODING TIPS✓ Codes classified in M62.0- through M62.28 indicate muscle separation, rupture and ischemia of a non-traumatic origin. When a traumatic muscle injury is reported, do not assign a code from M62.0- through M62.28, but instead assign a code from Chapter 19, Injury, Poisoning and Certain Other Consequences of External Causes.

IQ M62.20 Nontraumatic ischemic infarction of muscle, unspecified site

6 M62.21 Nontraumatic ischemic infarction of muscle, shoulder

SP M62.211 Nontraumatic ischemic infarction of muscle, right shoulder

SP M62.212 Nontraumatic ischemic infarction of muscle, left shoulder

IQ M62.219 Nontraumatic ischemic infarction of muscle, unspecified shoulder

6 M62.22 Nontraumatic ischemic infarction of muscle, upper arm

SP M62.221 Nontraumatic ischemic infarction of muscle, right upper arm

SP M62.222 Nontraumatic ischemic infarction of muscle, left upper arm

IQ M62.229 Nontraumatic ischemic infarction of muscle, unspecified upper arm

6 M62.23 Nontraumatic ischemic infarction of muscle, forearm

SP M62.231 Nontraumatic ischemic infarction of muscle, right forearm

SP M62.232 Nontraumatic ischemic infarction of muscle, left forearm

IQ M62.239 Nontraumatic ischemic infarction of muscle, unspecified forearm

6 M62.24 Nontraumatic ischemic infarction of muscle, hand

SP M62.241 Nontraumatic ischemic infarction of muscle, right hand

SP M62.242 Nontraumatic ischemic infarction of muscle, left hand

IQ M62.249 Nontraumatic ischemic infarction of muscle, unspecified hand

6 M62.25 Nontraumatic ischemic infarction of muscle, thigh

SP M62.251 Nontraumatic ischemic infarction of muscle, right thigh

SP M62.252 Nontraumatic ischemic infarction of muscle, left thigh

IQ M62.259 Nontraumatic ischemic infarction of muscle, unspecified thigh

6 M62.26 Nontraumatic ischemic infarction of muscle, lower leg

SP M62.261 Nontraumatic ischemic infarction of muscle, right lower leg

SP M62.262 Nontraumatic ischemic infarction of muscle, left lower leg

IQ M62.269 Nontraumatic ischemic infarction of muscle, unspecified lower leg

6 M62.27 Nontraumatic ischemic infarction of muscle, ankle and foot

SP M62.271 Nontraumatic ischemic infarction of muscle, right ankle and foot

SP M62.272 Nontraumatic ischemic infarction of muscle, left ankle and foot

IQ M62.279 Nontraumatic ischemic infarction of muscle, unspecified ankle and foot

SP M62.28 Nontraumatic ischemic infarction of muscle, other site

SP M62.3 Immobility syndrome (paraplegic)

CODING TIPS✓ Do not assign M62.3 for paraplegia that is due to a neurologic condition or injury. M62.3 indicates paraplegia of a non-neurologic origin. Do not use this code when the condition is due to an injury or other neurologic condition.

M62.4 Contracture of muscle
Contracture of tendon (sheath)
EXCLUDES 1 contracture of joint (M24.5-)

M62.40 Contracture of muscle, unspecified site

M62.41 Contracture of muscle, shoulder
M62.411 Contracture of muscle, right shoulder
M62.412 Contracture of muscle, left shoulder
M62.419 Contracture of muscle, unspecified shoulder

M62.42 Contracture of muscle, upper arm
M62.421 Contracture of muscle, right upper arm
M62.422 Contracture of muscle, left upper arm
M62.429 Contracture of muscle, unspecified upper arm

M62.43 Contracture of muscle, forearm
M62.431 Contracture of muscle, right forearm
M62.432 Contracture of muscle, left forearm
M62.439 Contracture of muscle, unspecified forearm

M62.44 Contracture of muscle, hand
M62.441 Contracture of muscle, right hand
M62.442 Contracture of muscle, left hand
M62.449 Contracture of muscle, unspecified hand

M62.45 Contracture of muscle, thigh
M62.451 Contracture of muscle, right thigh
M62.452 Contracture of muscle, left thigh
M62.459 Contracture of muscle, unspecified thigh

M62.46 Contracture of muscle, lower leg
M62.461 Contracture of muscle, right lower leg
M62.462 Contracture of muscle, left lower leg
M62.469 Contracture of muscle, unspecified lower leg

M62.47 Contracture of muscle, ankle and foot
M62.471 Contracture of muscle, right ankle and foot
M62.472 Contracture of muscle, left ankle and foot
M62.479 Contracture of muscle, unspecified ankle and foot

M62.48 Contracture of muscle, other site

M62.49 Contracture of muscle, multiple sites

M62.5 Muscle wasting and atrophy, not elsewhere classified
Disuse atrophy NEC
EXCLUDES 1 neuralgic amyotrophy (G54.5)
progressive muscular atrophy (G12.21)
sarcopenia (M62.84)
EXCLUDES 2 pelvic muscle wasting (N81.84)

CODING TIPS✓ Muscle wasting and atrophy has been suggested by CMS as an alternative to muscle weakness when documentation from the physician or NPP supports muscle atrophy.

M62.50 Muscle wasting and atrophy, not elsewhere classified, unspecified site

M62.51 Muscle wasting and atrophy, not elsewhere classified, shoulder
M62.511 Muscle wasting and atrophy, not elsewhere classified, right shoulder
M62.512 Muscle wasting and atrophy, not elsewhere classified, left shoulder
M62.519 Muscle wasting and atrophy, not elsewhere classified, unspecified shoulder

M62.52 Muscle wasting and atrophy, not elsewhere classified, upper arm
M62.521 Muscle wasting and atrophy, not elsewhere classified, right upper arm
M62.522 Muscle wasting and atrophy, not elsewhere classified, left upper arm
M62.529 Muscle wasting and atrophy, not elsewhere classified, unspecified upper arm

M62.53 Muscle wasting and atrophy, not elsewhere classified, forearm
M62.531 Muscle wasting and atrophy, not elsewhere classified, right forearm
M62.532 Muscle wasting and atrophy, not elsewhere classified, left forearm
M62.539 Muscle wasting and atrophy, not elsewhere classified, unspecified forearm

M62.54 Muscle wasting and atrophy, not elsewhere classified, hand
M62.541 Muscle wasting and atrophy, not elsewhere classified, right hand
M62.542 Muscle wasting and atrophy, not elsewhere classified, left hand
M62.549 Muscle wasting and atrophy, not elsewhere classified, unspecified hand

M62.55 Muscle wasting and atrophy, not elsewhere classified, thigh
M62.551 Muscle wasting and atrophy, not elsewhere classified, right thigh
M62.552 Muscle wasting and atrophy, not elsewhere classified, left thigh
M62.559 Muscle wasting and atrophy, not elsewhere classified, unspecified thigh

M62.56 Muscle wasting and atrophy, not elsewhere classified, lower leg
M62.561 Muscle wasting and atrophy, not elsewhere classified, right lower leg

4th digit required 5th digit required 6th digit required 7th digit required 7th digit placeholder +Additional code Laterality

M62.562 Muscle wasting and atrophy, not elsewhere classified, left lower leg

M62.569 Muscle wasting and atrophy, not elsewhere classified, unspecified lower leg

M62.57 Muscle wasting and atrophy, not elsewhere classified, ankle and foot

M62.571 Muscle wasting and atrophy, not elsewhere classified, right ankle and foot

M62.572 Muscle wasting and atrophy, not elsewhere classified, left ankle and foot

M62.579 Muscle wasting and atrophy, not elsewhere classified, unspecified ankle and foot

M62.58 Muscle wasting and atrophy, not elsewhere classified, other site

M62.59 Muscle wasting and atrophy, not elsewhere classified, multiple sites

M62.8 Other specified disorders of muscle

EXCLUDES 2 nontraumatic hematoma of muscle (M79.81)

M62.81 Muscle weakness (generalized)

EXCLUDES 1 muscle weakness in sarcopenia (M62.84)

CODING TIPS ✓ Use M62.81 for true muscle weakness. Muscle weakness may be the result of musculoskeletal disorders, neuromuscular disease or degenerative disease otherwise unidentified. If muscle weakness is part of a condition, do not use the code. Unilateral weakness associated with stroke, brain disorders or injury is coded to hemiplegia/hemiparesis, not M62.81. Muscle group measurements are not required, but measurable muscle weakness must be documented.

M62.82 Rhabdomyolysis

EXCLUDES 1 traumatic rhabdomyolysis (T79.6)

M62.83 Muscle spasm

M62.830 Muscle spasm of back

M62.831 Muscle spasm of calf

Charley-horse

M62.838 Other muscle spasm

M62.84 Sarcopenia

Age-related sarcopenia

Code first underlying disease, if applicable, such as:
- disorders of myoneural junction and muscle disease in diseases classified elsewhere (G73.-)
- other and unspecified myopathies (G72.-)
- primary disorders of muscles (G71.-)

CODING TIPS ✓ Patients with sarcopenia typically experience mobility limitations and other functional issues such as an inability to carry out activities of daily living. Low grip strength and slow gait speed are strongly correlated with decreased ability to recover from serious injury, falls, disability, hospital and nursing home admissions, and increased mortality. Conditions which may be associated with sarcopenia include hip fracture, bed rest with immobilization, chronic obstructive pulmonary disease, diabetes mellitus Type 2, stroke, Parkinson's disease and congestive heart failure. While all people lose muscle mass and strength as they age, some older adults may have accelerated loss of muscle and may develop sarcopenia without having any of these conditions.

M62.89 Other specified disorders of muscle

Muscle (sheath) hernia

ALERT Beware of choosing this code as primary because the code for muscle weakness (M62.81) no longer works as primary in PDGM. Physician or NPP documentation must support the code used. Codes that include "other" are appropriate for use when the information in the medical record provides detail for which a specific code does not exist.

M62.9 Disorder of muscle, unspecified

M63 Disorders of muscle in diseases classified elsewhere

Code first underlying disease, such as:
- leprosy (A30.-)
- neoplasm (C49.-, C79.89, D21.-, D48.1)
- schistosomiasis (B65.-)
- trichinellosis (B75)

EXCLUDES 1 myopathy in cysticercosis (B69.81)
myopathy in endocrine diseases (G73.7)
myopathy in metabolic diseases (G73.7)
myopathy in sarcoidosis (D86.87)
myopathy in secondary syphilis (A51.49)
myopathy in syphilis (late) (A52.78)
myopathy in toxoplasmosis (B58.82)
myopathy in tuberculosis (A18.09)

M63.8 Disorders of muscle in diseases classified elsewhere

M63.80 ***Disorders of muscle in diseases classified elsewhere, unspecified site***

M63.81 Disorders of muscle in diseases classified elsewhere, shoulder

M63.811 ***Disorders of muscle in diseases classified elsewhere, right shoulder***

Chapter 13

M00-M99

M ⊟ IQ M63.812 *Disorders of muscle in diseases classified elsewhere, left shoulder*

M ⊟ IQ M63.819 *Disorders of muscle in diseases classified elsewhere, unspecified shoulder*

6 **M63.82 Disorders of muscle in diseases classified elsewhere, upper arm**

M ⊟ IQ M63.821 *Disorders of muscle in diseases classified elsewhere, right upper arm*

M ⊟ IQ M63.822 *Disorders of muscle in diseases classified elsewhere, left upper arm*

M ⊟ IQ M63.829 *Disorders of muscle in diseases classified elsewhere, unspecified upper arm*

6 **M63.83 Disorders of muscle in diseases classified elsewhere, forearm**

M ⊟ IQ M63.831 *Disorders of muscle in diseases classified elsewhere, right forearm*

M ⊟ IQ M63.832 *Disorders of muscle in diseases classified elsewhere, left forearm*

M ⊟ IQ M63.839 *Disorders of muscle in diseases classified elsewhere, unspecified forearm*

6 **M63.84 Disorders of muscle in diseases classified elsewhere, hand**

M ⊟ IQ M63.841 *Disorders of muscle in diseases classified elsewhere, right hand*

M ⊟ IQ M63.842 *Disorders of muscle in diseases classified elsewhere, left hand*

M ⊟ IQ M63.849 *Disorders of muscle in diseases classified elsewhere, unspecified hand*

6 **M63.85 Disorders of muscle in diseases classified elsewhere, thigh**

M ⊟ IQ M63.851 *Disorders of muscle in diseases classified elsewhere, right thigh*

M ⊟ IQ M63.852 *Disorders of muscle in diseases classified elsewhere, left thigh*

M ⊟ IQ M63.859 *Disorders of muscle in diseases classified elsewhere, unspecified thigh*

6 **M63.86 Disorders of muscle in diseases classified elsewhere, lower leg**

M ⊟ IQ M63.861 *Disorders of muscle in diseases classified elsewhere, right lower leg*

M ⊟ IQ M63.862 *Disorders of muscle in diseases classified elsewhere, left lower leg*

M ⊟ IQ M63.869 *Disorders of muscle in diseases classified elsewhere, unspecified lower leg*

6 **M63.87 Disorders of muscle in diseases classified elsewhere, ankle and foot**

M ⊟ IQ M63.871 *Disorders of muscle in diseases classified elsewhere, right ankle and foot*

M ⊟ IQ M63.872 *Disorders of muscle in diseases classified elsewhere, left ankle and foot*

M ⊟ IQ M63.879 *Disorders of muscle in diseases classified elsewhere, unspecified ankle and foot*

M IQ M63.88 *Disorders of muscle in diseases classified elsewhere, other site*

M IQ M63.89 *Disorders of muscle in diseases classified elsewhere, multiple sites*

Disorders of synovium and tendon (M65-M67)

4 **M65 Synovitis and tenosynovitis**

EXCLUDES 1 chronic crepitant synovitis of hand and wrist (M70.0-)
current injury - see injury of ligament or tendon by body region
soft tissue disorders related to use, overuse and pressure (M70.-)

+ 5 **M65.0 Abscess of tendon sheath**

Use additional code (B95-B96) to identify bacterial agent.

IQ + M65.00 **Abscess of tendon sheath, unspecified site**

+ 6 **M65.01 Abscess of tendon sheath, shoulder**

⊟ SP + M65.011 **Abscess of tendon sheath, right shoulder**

⊟ SP + M65.012 **Abscess of tendon sheath, left shoulder**

⊟ IQ + M65.019 **Abscess of tendon sheath, unspecified shoulder**

+ 6 **M65.02 Abscess of tendon sheath, upper arm**

⊟ SP + M65.021 **Abscess of tendon sheath, right upper arm**

⊟ SP + M65.022 **Abscess of tendon sheath, left upper arm**

⊟ IQ + M65.029 **Abscess of tendon sheath, unspecified upper arm**

+ 6 **M65.03 Abscess of tendon sheath, forearm**

⊟ SP + M65.031 **Abscess of tendon sheath, right forearm**

⊟ SP + M65.032 **Abscess of tendon sheath, left forearm**

⊟ IQ + M65.039 **Abscess of tendon sheath, unspecified forearm**

+ 6 **M65.04 Abscess of tendon sheath, hand**

⊟ SP + M65.041 **Abscess of tendon sheath, right hand**

⊟ SP + M65.042 **Abscess of tendon sheath, left hand**

⊟ IQ + M65.049 **Abscess of tendon sheath, unspecified hand**

+ 6 **M65.05 Abscess of tendon sheath, thigh**

⊟ SP + M65.051 **Abscess of tendon sheath, right thigh**

⊟ SP + M65.052 **Abscess of tendon sheath, left thigh**

⊟ IQ + M65.059 **Abscess of tendon sheath, unspecified thigh**

+ 6 **M65.06 Abscess of tendon sheath, lower leg**

⊟ SP + M65.061 **Abscess of tendon sheath, right lower leg**

⊟ SP + M65.062 **Abscess of tendon sheath, left lower leg**

⊟ IQ + M65.069 **Abscess of tendon sheath, unspecified lower leg**

+ 6 **M65.07 Abscess of tendon sheath, ankle and foot**
SP + **M65.071 Abscess of tendon sheath, right ankle and foot**
SP + **M65.072 Abscess of tendon sheath, left ankle and foot**
IQ + **M65.079 Abscess of tendon sheath, unspecified ankle and foot**
SP + **M65.08 Abscess of tendon sheath, other site**
5 **M65.1 Other infective (teno)synovitis**
IQ **M65.10 Other infective (teno)synovitis, unspecified site**
6 **M65.11 Other infective (teno)synovitis, shoulder**
SP **M65.111 Other infective (teno)synovitis, right shoulder**
SP **M65.112 Other infective (teno)synovitis, left shoulder**
IQ **M65.119 Other infective (teno)synovitis, unspecified shoulder**
6 **M65.12 Other infective (teno)synovitis, elbow**
SP **M65.121 Other infective (teno)synovitis, right elbow**
SP **M65.122 Other infective (teno)synovitis, left elbow**
IQ **M65.129 Other infective (teno)synovitis, unspecified elbow**
6 **M65.13 Other infective (teno)synovitis, wrist**
SP **M65.131 Other infective (teno)synovitis, right wrist**
SP **M65.132 Other infective (teno)synovitis, left wrist**
IQ **M65.139 Other infective (teno)synovitis, unspecified wrist**
6 **M65.14 Other infective (teno)synovitis, hand**
SP **M65.141 Other infective (teno)synovitis, right hand**
SP **M65.142 Other infective (teno)synovitis, left hand**
IQ **M65.149 Other infective (teno)synovitis, unspecified hand**
6 **M65.15 Other infective (teno)synovitis, hip**
SP **M65.151 Other infective (teno)synovitis, right hip**
SP **M65.152 Other infective (teno)synovitis, left hip**
IQ **M65.159 Other infective (teno)synovitis, unspecified hip**
6 **M65.16 Other infective (teno)synovitis, knee**
SP **M65.161 Other infective (teno)synovitis, right knee**
SP **M65.162 Other infective (teno)synovitis, left knee**
IQ **M65.169 Other infective (teno)synovitis, unspecified knee**
6 **M65.17 Other infective (teno)synovitis, ankle and foot**
SP **M65.171 Other infective (teno)synovitis, right ankle and foot**
SP **M65.172 Other infective (teno)synovitis, left ankle and foot**
IQ **M65.179 Other infective (teno)synovitis, unspecified ankle and foot**
SP **M65.18 Other infective (teno)synovitis, other site**
SP **M65.19 Other infective (teno)synovitis, multiple sites**
5 **M65.2 Calcific tendinitis**
EXCLUDES 1 tendinitis as classified in M75-M77
calcified tendinitis of shoulder (M75.3)
IQ **M65.20 Calcific tendinitis, unspecified site**
6 **M65.22 Calcific tendinitis, upper arm**
SP **M65.221 Calcific tendinitis, right upper arm**
SP **M65.222 Calcific tendinitis, left upper arm**
IQ **M65.229 Calcific tendinitis, unspecified upper arm**
6 **M65.23 Calcific tendinitis, forearm**
SP **M65.231 Calcific tendinitis, right forearm**
SP **M65.232 Calcific tendinitis, left forearm**
IQ **M65.239 Calcific tendinitis, unspecified forearm**
6 **M65.24 Calcific tendinitis, hand**
SP **M65.241 Calcific tendinitis, right hand**
SP **M65.242 Calcific tendinitis, left hand**
IQ **M65.249 Calcific tendinitis, unspecified hand**
6 **M65.25 Calcific tendinitis, thigh**
SP **M65.251 Calcific tendinitis, right thigh**
SP **M65.252 Calcific tendinitis, left thigh**
IQ **M65.259 Calcific tendinitis, unspecified thigh**
6 **M65.26 Calcific tendinitis, lower leg**
SP **M65.261 Calcific tendinitis, right lower leg**
SP **M65.262 Calcific tendinitis, left lower leg**
IQ **M65.269 Calcific tendinitis, unspecified lower leg**
6 **M65.27 Calcific tendinitis, ankle and foot**
SP **M65.271 Calcific tendinitis, right ankle and foot**
SP **M65.272 Calcific tendinitis, left ankle and foot**
IQ **M65.279 Calcific tendinitis, unspecified ankle and foot**
SP **M65.28 Calcific tendinitis, other site**
SP **M65.29 Calcific tendinitis, multiple sites**
5 **M65.3 Trigger finger**
Nodular tendinous disease
IQ **M65.30 Trigger finger, unspecified finger**
6 **M65.31 Trigger thumb**
SP **M65.311 Trigger thumb, right thumb**
SP **M65.312 Trigger thumb, left thumb**
IQ **M65.319 Trigger thumb, unspecified thumb**
6 **M65.32 Trigger finger, index finger**
SP **M65.321 Trigger finger, right index finger**
SP **M65.322 Trigger finger, left index finger**
IQ **M65.329 Trigger finger, unspecified index finger**
6 **M65.33 Trigger finger, middle finger**
SP **M65.331 Trigger finger, right middle finger**
SP **M65.332 Trigger finger, left middle finger**

Chapter 13
M00-M99

⊟ IQ M65.339 Trigger finger, unspecified middle finger

6 M65.34 Trigger finger, ring finger

⊟ SP M65.341 Trigger finger, right ring finger

⊟ SP M65.342 Trigger finger, left ring finger

⊟ IQ M65.349 Trigger finger, unspecified ring finger

6 M65.35 Trigger finger, little finger

⊟ SP M65.351 Trigger finger, right little finger

⊟ SP M65.352 Trigger finger, left little finger

⊟ IQ M65.359 Trigger finger, unspecified little finger

SP M65.4 Radial styloid tenosynovitis [de Quervain]

5 M65.8 Other synovitis and tenosynovitis

IQ M65.80 Other synovitis and tenosynovitis, unspecified site

6 M65.81 Other synovitis and tenosynovitis, shoulder

⊟ SP M65.811 Other synovitis and tenosynovitis, right shoulder

⊟ SP M65.812 Other synovitis and tenosynovitis, left shoulder

⊟ IQ M65.819 Other synovitis and tenosynovitis, unspecified shoulder

6 M65.82 Other synovitis and tenosynovitis, upper arm

⊟ SP M65.821 Other synovitis and tenosynovitis, right upper arm

⊟ SP M65.822 Other synovitis and tenosynovitis, left upper arm

⊟ IQ M65.829 Other synovitis and tenosynovitis, unspecified upper arm

6 M65.83 Other synovitis and tenosynovitis, forearm

⊟ SP M65.831 Other synovitis and tenosynovitis, right forearm

⊟ SP M65.832 Other synovitis and tenosynovitis, left forearm

⊟ IQ M65.839 Other synovitis and tenosynovitis, unspecified forearm

6 M65.84 Other synovitis and tenosynovitis, hand

⊟ SP M65.841 Other synovitis and tenosynovitis, right hand

⊟ SP M65.842 Other synovitis and tenosynovitis, left hand

⊟ IQ M65.849 Other synovitis and tenosynovitis, unspecified hand

6 M65.85 Other synovitis and tenosynovitis, thigh

⊟ SP M65.851 Other synovitis and tenosynovitis, right thigh

⊟ SP M65.852 Other synovitis and tenosynovitis, left thigh

⊟ IQ M65.859 Other synovitis and tenosynovitis, unspecified thigh

6 M65.86 Other synovitis and tenosynovitis, lower leg

⊟ SP M65.861 Other synovitis and tenosynovitis, right lower leg

⊟ SP M65.862 Other synovitis and tenosynovitis, left lower leg

⊟ IQ M65.869 Other synovitis and tenosynovitis, unspecified lower leg

6 M65.87 Other synovitis and tenosynovitis, ankle and foot

⊟ SP M65.871 Other synovitis and tenosynovitis, right ankle and foot

⊟ SP M65.872 Other synovitis and tenosynovitis, left ankle and foot

⊟ IQ M65.879 Other synovitis and tenosynovitis, unspecified ankle and foot

SP M65.88 Other synovitis and tenosynovitis, other site

SP M65.89 Other synovitis and tenosynovitis, multiple sites

IQ M65.9 Synovitis and tenosynovitis, unspecified

4 M66 Spontaneous rupture of synovium and tendon

INCLUDES rupture that occurs when a normal force is applied to tissues that are inferred to have less than normal strength

EXCLUDES 2 rotator cuff syndrome (M75.1-)
rupture where an abnormal force is applied to normal tissue - see injury of tendon by body region

SP M66.0 Rupture of popliteal cyst

5 M66.1 Rupture of synovium

Rupture of synovial cyst

EXCLUDES 2 rupture of popliteal cyst (M66.0)

IQ M66.10 Rupture of synovium, unspecified joint

6 M66.11 Rupture of synovium, shoulder

⊟ SP M66.111 Rupture of synovium, right shoulder

⊟ SP M66.112 Rupture of synovium, left shoulder

⊟ IQ M66.119 Rupture of synovium, unspecified shoulder

6 M66.12 Rupture of synovium, elbow

⊟ SP M66.121 Rupture of synovium, right elbow

⊟ SP M66.122 Rupture of synovium, left elbow

⊟ IQ M66.129 Rupture of synovium, unspecified elbow

6 M66.13 Rupture of synovium, wrist

⊟ SP M66.131 Rupture of synovium, right wrist

⊟ SP M66.132 Rupture of synovium, left wrist

⊟ IQ M66.139 Rupture of synovium, unspecified wrist

6 M66.14 Rupture of synovium, hand and fingers

⊟ SP M66.141 Rupture of synovium, right hand

⊟ SP M66.142 Rupture of synovium, left hand

⊟ IQ M66.143 Rupture of synovium, unspecified hand

⊟ SP M66.144 Rupture of synovium, right finger(s)

⊟ SP M66.145 Rupture of synovium, left finger(s)

IQ M66.146 Rupture of synovium, unspecified finger(s)

6 M66.15 Rupture of synovium, hip

SP M66.151 Rupture of synovium, right hip

SP M66.152 Rupture of synovium, left hip

IQ M66.159 Rupture of synovium, unspecified hip

6 M66.17 Rupture of synovium, ankle, foot and toes

SP M66.171 Rupture of synovium, right ankle

SP M66.172 Rupture of synovium, left ankle

IQ M66.173 Rupture of synovium, unspecified ankle

SP M66.174 Rupture of synovium, right foot

SP M66.175 Rupture of synovium, left foot

IQ M66.176 Rupture of synovium, unspecified foot

SP M66.177 Rupture of synovium, right toe(s)

SP M66.178 Rupture of synovium, left toe(s)

IQ M66.179 Rupture of synovium, unspecified toe(s)

SP M66.18 Rupture of synovium, other site

5 M66.2 Spontaneous rupture of extensor tendons

IQ M66.20 Spontaneous rupture of extensor tendons, unspecified site

6 M66.21 Spontaneous rupture of extensor tendons, shoulder

SP M66.211 Spontaneous rupture of extensor tendons, right shoulder

SP M66.212 Spontaneous rupture of extensor tendons, left shoulder

IQ M66.219 Spontaneous rupture of extensor tendons, unspecified shoulder

6 M66.22 Spontaneous rupture of extensor tendons, upper arm

SP M66.221 Spontaneous rupture of extensor tendons, right upper arm

SP M66.222 Spontaneous rupture of extensor tendons, left upper arm

IQ M66.229 Spontaneous rupture of extensor tendons, unspecified upper arm

6 M66.23 Spontaneous rupture of extensor tendons, forearm

SP M66.231 Spontaneous rupture of extensor tendons, right forearm

SP M66.232 Spontaneous rupture of extensor tendons, left forearm

IQ M66.239 Spontaneous rupture of extensor tendons, unspecified forearm

6 M66.24 Spontaneous rupture of extensor tendons, hand

SP M66.241 Spontaneous rupture of extensor tendons, right hand

SP M66.242 Spontaneous rupture of extensor tendons, left hand

IQ M66.249 Spontaneous rupture of extensor tendons, unspecified hand

6 M66.25 Spontaneous rupture of extensor tendons, thigh

SP M66.251 Spontaneous rupture of extensor tendons, right thigh

SP M66.252 Spontaneous rupture of extensor tendons, left thigh

IQ M66.259 Spontaneous rupture of extensor tendons, unspecified thigh

6 M66.26 Spontaneous rupture of extensor tendons, lower leg

SP M66.261 Spontaneous rupture of extensor tendons, right lower leg

SP M66.262 Spontaneous rupture of extensor tendons, left lower leg

IQ M66.269 Spontaneous rupture of extensor tendons, unspecified lower leg

6 M66.27 Spontaneous rupture of extensor tendons, ankle and foot

SP M66.271 Spontaneous rupture of extensor tendons, right ankle and foot

SP M66.272 Spontaneous rupture of extensor tendons, left ankle and foot

IQ M66.279 Spontaneous rupture of extensor tendons, unspecified ankle and foot

SP M66.28 Spontaneous rupture of extensor tendons, other site

SP M66.29 Spontaneous rupture of extensor tendons, multiple sites

5 M66.3 Spontaneous rupture of flexor tendons

IQ M66.30 Spontaneous rupture of flexor tendons, unspecified site

6 M66.31 Spontaneous rupture of flexor tendons, shoulder

SP M66.311 Spontaneous rupture of flexor tendons, right shoulder

SP M66.312 Spontaneous rupture of flexor tendons, left shoulder

IQ M66.319 Spontaneous rupture of flexor tendons, unspecified shoulder

6 M66.32 Spontaneous rupture of flexor tendons, upper arm

SP M66.321 Spontaneous rupture of flexor tendons, right upper arm

SP M66.322 Spontaneous rupture of flexor tendons, left upper arm

IQ M66.329 Spontaneous rupture of flexor tendons, unspecified upper arm

6 M66.33 Spontaneous rupture of flexor tendons, forearm

SP M66.331 Spontaneous rupture of flexor tendons, right forearm

SP M66.332 Spontaneous rupture of flexor tendons, left forearm

IQ M66.339 Spontaneous rupture of flexor tendons, unspecified forearm

6 M66.34 Spontaneous rupture of flexor tendons, hand

SP M66.341 Spontaneous rupture of flexor tendons, right hand

SP M66.342 Spontaneous rupture of flexor tendons, left hand

IQ M66.349 Spontaneous rupture of flexor tendons, unspecified hand

6 M66.35 Spontaneous rupture of flexor tendons, thigh

SP M66.351 Spontaneous rupture of flexor tendons, right thigh

SP M66.352 Spontaneous rupture of flexor tendons, left thigh

IQ M66.359 Spontaneous rupture of flexor tendons, unspecified thigh

6 M66.36 Spontaneous rupture of flexor tendons, lower leg

Laterality SP M66.361 Spontaneous rupture of flexor tendons, right lower leg

Laterality SP M66.362 Spontaneous rupture of flexor tendons, left lower leg

Laterality IQ M66.369 Spontaneous rupture of flexor tendons, unspecified lower leg

6 M66.37 Spontaneous rupture of flexor tendons, ankle and foot

Laterality SP M66.371 Spontaneous rupture of flexor tendons, right ankle and foot

Laterality SP M66.372 Spontaneous rupture of flexor tendons, left ankle and foot

Laterality IQ M66.379 Spontaneous rupture of flexor tendons, unspecified ankle and foot

SP M66.38 Spontaneous rupture of flexor tendons, other site

SP M66.39 Spontaneous rupture of flexor tendons, multiple sites

5 M66.8 Spontaneous rupture of other tendons

IQ M66.80 Spontaneous rupture of other tendons, unspecified site

6 M66.81 Spontaneous rupture of other tendons, shoulder

Laterality SP M66.811 Spontaneous rupture of other tendons, right shoulder

Laterality SP M66.812 Spontaneous rupture of other tendons, left shoulder

Laterality IQ M66.819 Spontaneous rupture of other tendons, unspecified shoulder

6 M66.82 Spontaneous rupture of other tendons, upper arm

Laterality SP M66.821 Spontaneous rupture of other tendons, right upper arm

Laterality SP M66.822 Spontaneous rupture of other tendons, left upper arm

Laterality IQ M66.829 Spontaneous rupture of other tendons, unspecified upper arm

6 M66.83 Spontaneous rupture of other tendons, forearm

Laterality SP M66.831 Spontaneous rupture of other tendons, right forearm

Laterality SP M66.832 Spontaneous rupture of other tendons, left forearm

Laterality IQ M66.839 Spontaneous rupture of other tendons, unspecified forearm

6 M66.84 Spontaneous rupture of other tendons, hand

Laterality SP M66.841 Spontaneous rupture of other tendons, right hand

Laterality SP M66.842 Spontaneous rupture of other tendons, left hand

Laterality IQ M66.849 Spontaneous rupture of other tendons, unspecified hand

6 M66.85 Spontaneous rupture of other tendons, thigh

Laterality SP M66.851 Spontaneous rupture of other tendons, right thigh

Laterality SP M66.852 Spontaneous rupture of other tendons, left thigh

Laterality IQ M66.859 Spontaneous rupture of other tendons, unspecified thigh

6 M66.86 Spontaneous rupture of other tendons, lower leg

Laterality SP M66.861 Spontaneous rupture of other tendons, right lower leg

Laterality SP M66.862 Spontaneous rupture of other tendons, left lower leg

Laterality IQ M66.869 Spontaneous rupture of other tendons, unspecified lower leg

6 M66.87 Spontaneous rupture of other tendons, ankle and foot

Laterality SP M66.871 Spontaneous rupture of other tendons, right ankle and foot

Laterality SP M66.872 Spontaneous rupture of other tendons, left ankle and foot

Laterality IQ M66.879 Spontaneous rupture of other tendons, unspecified ankle and foot

SP M66.88 Spontaneous rupture of other tendons, other sites

SP M66.89 Spontaneous rupture of other tendons, multiple sites

IQ M66.9 Spontaneous rupture of unspecified tendon

Rupture at musculotendinous junction, nontraumatic

4 M67 Other disorders of synovium and tendon

EXCLUDES 1 palmar fascial fibromatosis [Dupuytren] (M72.0)
tendinitis NOS (M77.9-)
xanthomatosis localized to tendons (E78.2)

5 M67.0 Short Achilles tendon (acquired)

Laterality IQ M67.00 Short Achilles tendon (acquired), unspecified ankle

Laterality SP M67.01 Short Achilles tendon (acquired), right ankle

Laterality SP M67.02 Short Achilles tendon (acquired), left ankle

5 M67.2 Synovial hypertrophy, not elsewhere classified

EXCLUDES 1 villonodular synovitis (pigmented) (M12.2-)

IQ M67.20 Synovial hypertrophy, not elsewhere classified, unspecified site

6 M67.21 Synovial hypertrophy, not elsewhere classified, shoulder

Laterality SP M67.211 Synovial hypertrophy, not elsewhere classified, right shoulder

Laterality SP M67.212 Synovial hypertrophy, not elsewhere classified, left shoulder

Laterality IQ M67.219 Synovial hypertrophy, not elsewhere classified, unspecified shoulder

6 M67.22 Synovial hypertrophy, not elsewhere classified, upper arm

Laterality SP M67.221 Synovial hypertrophy, not elsewhere classified, right upper arm

Laterality SP M67.222 Synovial hypertrophy, not elsewhere classified, left upper arm

Laterality IQ M67.229 Synovial hypertrophy, not elsewhere classified, unspecified upper arm

6 M67.23 Synovial hypertrophy, not elsewhere classified, forearm

Laterality SP M67.231 Synovial hypertrophy, not elsewhere classified, right forearm

M67.232 Synovial hypertrophy, not elsewhere classified, left forearm
M67.239 Synovial hypertrophy, not elsewhere classified, unspecified forearm
M67.24 Synovial hypertrophy, not elsewhere classified, hand
M67.241 Synovial hypertrophy, not elsewhere classified, right hand
M67.242 Synovial hypertrophy, not elsewhere classified, left hand
M67.249 Synovial hypertrophy, not elsewhere classified, unspecified hand
M67.25 Synovial hypertrophy, not elsewhere classified, thigh
M67.251 Synovial hypertrophy, not elsewhere classified, right thigh
M67.252 Synovial hypertrophy, not elsewhere classified, left thigh
M67.259 Synovial hypertrophy, not elsewhere classified, unspecified thigh
M67.26 Synovial hypertrophy, not elsewhere classified, lower leg
M67.261 Synovial hypertrophy, not elsewhere classified, right lower leg
M67.262 Synovial hypertrophy, not elsewhere classified, left lower leg
M67.269 Synovial hypertrophy, not elsewhere classified, unspecified lower leg
M67.27 Synovial hypertrophy, not elsewhere classified, ankle and foot
M67.271 Synovial hypertrophy, not elsewhere classified, right ankle and foot
M67.272 Synovial hypertrophy, not elsewhere classified, left ankle and foot
M67.279 Synovial hypertrophy, not elsewhere classified, unspecified ankle and foot
M67.28 Synovial hypertrophy, not elsewhere classified, other site
M67.29 Synovial hypertrophy, not elsewhere classified, multiple sites
M67.3 Transient synovitis
Toxic synovitis
EXCLUDES 1 palindromic rheumatism (M12.3-)
M67.30 Transient synovitis, unspecified site
M67.31 Transient synovitis, shoulder
M67.311 Transient synovitis, right shoulder
M67.312 Transient synovitis, left shoulder
M67.319 Transient synovitis, unspecified shoulder
M67.32 Transient synovitis, elbow
M67.321 Transient synovitis, right elbow
M67.322 Transient synovitis, left elbow
M67.329 Transient synovitis, unspecified elbow
M67.33 Transient synovitis, wrist
M67.331 Transient synovitis, right wrist
M67.332 Transient synovitis, left wrist
M67.339 Transient synovitis, unspecified wrist
M67.34 Transient synovitis, hand
M67.341 Transient synovitis, right hand
M67.342 Transient synovitis, left hand
M67.349 Transient synovitis, unspecified hand
M67.35 Transient synovitis, hip
M67.351 Transient synovitis, right hip
M67.352 Transient synovitis, left hip
M67.359 Transient synovitis, unspecified hip
M67.36 Transient synovitis, knee
M67.361 Transient synovitis, right knee
M67.362 Transient synovitis, left knee
M67.369 Transient synovitis, unspecified knee
M67.37 Transient synovitis, ankle and foot
M67.371 Transient synovitis, right ankle and foot
M67.372 Transient synovitis, left ankle and foot
M67.379 Transient synovitis, unspecified ankle and foot
M67.38 Transient synovitis, other site
M67.39 Transient synovitis, multiple sites
M67.4 Ganglion
Ganglion of joint or tendon (sheath)
EXCLUDES 1 ganglion in yaws (A66.6)
EXCLUDES 2 cyst of bursa (M71.2-M71.3)
cyst of synovium (M71.2-M71.3)
M67.40 Ganglion, unspecified site
M67.41 Ganglion, shoulder
M67.411 Ganglion, right shoulder
M67.412 Ganglion, left shoulder
M67.419 Ganglion, unspecified shoulder
M67.42 Ganglion, elbow
M67.421 Ganglion, right elbow
M67.422 Ganglion, left elbow
M67.429 Ganglion, unspecified elbow
M67.43 Ganglion, wrist
M67.431 Ganglion, right wrist
M67.432 Ganglion, left wrist
M67.439 Ganglion, unspecified wrist
M67.44 Ganglion, hand
M67.441 Ganglion, right hand
M67.442 Ganglion, left hand
M67.449 Ganglion, unspecified hand
M67.45 Ganglion, hip
M67.451 Ganglion, right hip
M67.452 Ganglion, left hip
M67.459 Ganglion, unspecified hip
M67.46 Ganglion, knee
M67.461 Ganglion, right knee
M67.462 Ganglion, left knee

M67.469 Ganglion, unspecified knee
M67.47 Ganglion, ankle and foot
M67.471 Ganglion, right ankle and foot
M67.472 Ganglion, left ankle and foot
M67.479 Ganglion, unspecified ankle and foot
M67.48 Ganglion, other site
M67.49 Ganglion, multiple sites
M67.5 Plica syndrome
Plica knee
M67.50 Plica syndrome, unspecified knee
M67.51 Plica syndrome, right knee
M67.52 Plica syndrome, left knee
M67.8 Other specified disorders of synovium and tendon
M67.80 Other specified disorders of synovium and tendon, unspecified site
M67.81 Other specified disorders of synovium and tendon, shoulder
M67.811 Other specified disorders of synovium, right shoulder
M67.812 Other specified disorders of synovium, left shoulder
M67.813 Other specified disorders of tendon, right shoulder
M67.814 Other specified disorders of tendon, left shoulder
M67.819 Other specified disorders of synovium and tendon, unspecified shoulder
M67.82 Other specified disorders of synovium and tendon, elbow
M67.821 Other specified disorders of synovium, right elbow
M67.822 Other specified disorders of synovium, left elbow
M67.823 Other specified disorders of tendon, right elbow
M67.824 Other specified disorders of tendon, left elbow
M67.829 Other specified disorders of synovium and tendon, unspecified elbow
M67.83 Other specified disorders of synovium and tendon, wrist
M67.831 Other specified disorders of synovium, right wrist
M67.832 Other specified disorders of synovium, left wrist
M67.833 Other specified disorders of tendon, right wrist
M67.834 Other specified disorders of tendon, left wrist
M67.839 Other specified disorders of synovium and tendon, unspecified wrist
M67.84 Other specified disorders of synovium and tendon, hand
M67.841 Other specified disorders of synovium, right hand
M67.842 Other specified disorders of synovium, left hand
M67.843 Other specified disorders of tendon, right hand
M67.844 Other specified disorders of tendon, left hand
M67.849 Other specified disorders of synovium and tendon, unspecified hand
M67.85 Other specified disorders of synovium and tendon, hip
M67.851 Other specified disorders of synovium, right hip
M67.852 Other specified disorders of synovium, left hip
M67.853 Other specified disorders of tendon, right hip
M67.854 Other specified disorders of tendon, left hip
M67.859 Other specified disorders of synovium and tendon, unspecified hip
M67.86 Other specified disorders of synovium and tendon, knee
M67.861 Other specified disorders of synovium, right knee
M67.862 Other specified disorders of synovium, left knee
M67.863 Other specified disorders of tendon, right knee
M67.864 Other specified disorders of tendon, left knee
M67.869 Other specified disorders of synovium and tendon, unspecified knee
M67.87 Other specified disorders of synovium and tendon, ankle and foot
M67.871 Other specified disorders of synovium, right ankle and foot
M67.872 Other specified disorders of synovium, left ankle and foot
M67.873 Other specified disorders of tendon, right ankle and foot
M67.874 Other specified disorders of tendon, left ankle and foot
M67.879 Other specified disorders of synovium and tendon, unspecified ankle and foot
M67.88 Other specified disorders of synovium and tendon, other site
M67.89 Other specified disorders of synovium and tendon, multiple sites
M67.9 Unspecified disorder of synovium and tendon
M67.90 Unspecified disorder of synovium and tendon, unspecified site
M67.91 Unspecified disorder of synovium and tendon, shoulder
M67.911 Unspecified disorder of synovium and tendon, right shoulder
M67.912 Unspecified disorder of synovium and tendon, left shoulder
M67.919 Unspecified disorder of synovium and tendon, unspecified shoulder
M67.92 Unspecified disorder of synovium and tendon, upper arm
M67.921 Unspecified disorder of synovium and tendon, right upper arm
M67.922 Unspecified disorder of synovium and tendon, left upper arm

4th digit required 5th digit required 6th digit required 7th digit required 7th digit placeholder +Additional code Laterality

M67.929 Unspecified disorder of synovium and tendon, unspecified upper arm

M67.93 Unspecified disorder of synovium and tendon, forearm

M67.931 Unspecified disorder of synovium and tendon, right forearm

M67.932 Unspecified disorder of synovium and tendon, left forearm

M67.939 Unspecified disorder of synovium and tendon, unspecified forearm

M67.94 Unspecified disorder of synovium and tendon, hand

M67.941 Unspecified disorder of synovium and tendon, right hand

M67.942 Unspecified disorder of synovium and tendon, left hand

M67.949 Unspecified disorder of synovium and tendon, unspecified hand

M67.95 Unspecified disorder of synovium and tendon, thigh

M67.951 Unspecified disorder of synovium and tendon, right thigh

M67.952 Unspecified disorder of synovium and tendon, left thigh

M67.959 Unspecified disorder of synovium and tendon, unspecified thigh

M67.96 Unspecified disorder of synovium and tendon, lower leg

M67.961 Unspecified disorder of synovium and tendon, right lower leg

M67.962 Unspecified disorder of synovium and tendon, left lower leg

M67.969 Unspecified disorder of synovium and tendon, unspecified lower leg

M67.97 Unspecified disorder of synovium and tendon, ankle and foot

M67.971 Unspecified disorder of synovium and tendon, right ankle and foot

M67.972 Unspecified disorder of synovium and tendon, left ankle and foot

M67.979 Unspecified disorder of synovium and tendon, unspecified ankle and foot

M67.98 Unspecified disorder of synovium and tendon, other site

M67.99 Unspecified disorder of synovium and tendon, multiple sites

Other soft tissue disorders (M70-M79)

+ **M70 Soft tissue disorders related to use, overuse and pressure**

INCLUDES soft tissue disorders of occupational origin

Use additional external cause code to identify activity causing disorder (Y93.-)

EXCLUDES 1 bursitis NOS (M71.9-)

EXCLUDES 2 bursitis of shoulder (M75.5)
enthesopathies (M76-M77)
pressure ulcer (pressure area) (L89.-)

+ **M70.0 Crepitant synovitis (acute) (chronic) of hand and wrist**

+ M70.03 Crepitant synovitis (acute) (chronic), wrist

+ M70.031 Crepitant synovitis (acute) (chronic), right wrist

+ M70.032 Crepitant synovitis (acute) (chronic), left wrist

+ M70.039 Crepitant synovitis (acute) (chronic), unspecified wrist

+ M70.04 Crepitant synovitis (acute) (chronic), hand

+ M70.041 Crepitant synovitis (acute) (chronic), right hand

+ M70.042 Crepitant synovitis (acute) (chronic), left hand

+ M70.049 Crepitant synovitis (acute) (chronic), unspecified hand

+ **M70.1 Bursitis of hand**

+ M70.10 Bursitis, unspecified hand

+ M70.11 Bursitis, right hand

+ M70.12 Bursitis, left hand

+ **M70.2 Olecranon bursitis**

+ M70.20 Olecranon bursitis, unspecified elbow

+ M70.21 Olecranon bursitis, right elbow

+ M70.22 Olecranon bursitis, left elbow

+ **M70.3 Other bursitis of elbow**

+ M70.30 Other bursitis of elbow, unspecified elbow

+ M70.31 Other bursitis of elbow, right elbow

+ M70.32 Other bursitis of elbow, left elbow

+ **M70.4 Prepatellar bursitis**

+ M70.40 Prepatellar bursitis, unspecified knee

+ M70.41 Prepatellar bursitis, right knee

+ M70.42 Prepatellar bursitis, left knee

+ **M70.5 Other bursitis of knee**

+ M70.50 Other bursitis of knee, unspecified knee

+ M70.51 Other bursitis of knee, right knee

+ M70.52 Other bursitis of knee, left knee

+ **M70.6 Trochanteric bursitis**
Trochanteric tendinitis

+ M70.60 Trochanteric bursitis, unspecified hip

+ M70.61 Trochanteric bursitis, right hip

+ M70.62 Trochanteric bursitis, left hip

+ **M70.7 Other bursitis of hip**
Ischial bursitis

+ M70.70 Other bursitis of hip, unspecified hip

+ M70.71 Other bursitis of hip, right hip

+ M70.72 Other bursitis of hip, left hip

+ **M70.8 Other soft tissue disorders related to use, overuse and pressure**

+ M70.80 Other soft tissue disorders related to use, overuse and pressure of unspecified site

+ M70.81 Other soft tissue disorders related to use, overuse and pressure of shoulder

Chapter 13

M00-M99

- ⊟ SP + M70.811 Other soft tissue disorders related to use, overuse and pressure, right shoulder
- ⊟ SP + M70.812 Other soft tissue disorders related to use, overuse and pressure, left shoulder
- ⊟ IQ + M70.819 Other soft tissue disorders related to use, overuse and pressure, unspecified shoulder
- + 6 M70.82 Other soft tissue disorders related to use, overuse and pressure of upper arm
- ⊟ SP + M70.821 Other soft tissue disorders related to use, overuse and pressure, right upper arm
- ⊟ SP + M70.822 Other soft tissue disorders related to use, overuse and pressure, left upper arm
- ⊟ IQ + M70.829 Other soft tissue disorders related to use, overuse and pressure, unspecified upper arms
- + 6 M70.83 Other soft tissue disorders related to use, overuse and pressure of forearm
- ⊟ SP + M70.831 Other soft tissue disorders related to use, overuse and pressure, right forearm
- ⊟ SP + M70.832 Other soft tissue disorders related to use, overuse and pressure, left forearm
- ⊟ IQ + M70.839 Other soft tissue disorders related to use, overuse and pressure, unspecified forearm
- + 6 M70.84 Other soft tissue disorders related to use, overuse and pressure of hand
- ⊟ SP + M70.841 Other soft tissue disorders related to use, overuse and pressure, right hand
- ⊟ SP + M70.842 Other soft tissue disorders related to use, overuse and pressure, left hand
- ⊟ IQ + M70.849 Other soft tissue disorders related to use, overuse and pressure, unspecified hand
- + 6 M70.85 Other soft tissue disorders related to use, overuse and pressure of thigh
- ⊟ SP + M70.851 Other soft tissue disorders related to use, overuse and pressure, right thigh
- ⊟ SP + M70.852 Other soft tissue disorders related to use, overuse and pressure, left thigh
- ⊟ IQ + M70.859 Other soft tissue disorders related to use, overuse and pressure, unspecified thigh
- + 6 M70.86 Other soft tissue disorders related to use, overuse and pressure lower leg
- ⊟ SP + M70.861 Other soft tissue disorders related to use, overuse and pressure, right lower leg
- ⊟ SP + M70.862 Other soft tissue disorders related to use, overuse and pressure, left lower leg
- ⊟ IQ + M70.869 Other soft tissue disorders related to use, overuse and pressure, unspecified leg
- + 6 M70.87 Other soft tissue disorders related to use, overuse and pressure of ankle and foot
- ⊟ SP + M70.871 Other soft tissue disorders related to use, overuse and pressure, right ankle and foot
- ⊟ SP + M70.872 Other soft tissue disorders related to use, overuse and pressure, left ankle and foot
- ⊟ IQ + M70.879 Other soft tissue disorders related to use, overuse and pressure, unspecified ankle and foot
- SP + M70.88 Other soft tissue disorders related to use, overuse and pressure other site
- SP + M70.89 Other soft tissue disorders related to use, overuse and pressure multiple sites
- + 5 M70.9 Unspecified soft tissue disorder related to use, overuse and pressure
- IQ + M70.90 Unspecified soft tissue disorder related to use, overuse and pressure of unspecified site
- + 6 M70.91 Unspecified soft tissue disorder related to use, overuse and pressure of shoulder
- ⊟ SP + M70.911 Unspecified soft tissue disorder related to use, overuse and pressure, right shoulder
- ⊟ SP + M70.912 Unspecified soft tissue disorder related to use, overuse and pressure, left shoulder
- ⊟ IQ + M70.919 Unspecified soft tissue disorder related to use, overuse and pressure, unspecified shoulder
- + 6 M70.92 Unspecified soft tissue disorder related to use, overuse and pressure of upper arm
- ⊟ SP + M70.921 Unspecified soft tissue disorder related to use, overuse and pressure, right upper arm
- ⊟ SP + M70.922 Unspecified soft tissue disorder related to use, overuse and pressure, left upper arm
- ⊟ IQ + M70.929 Unspecified soft tissue disorder related to use, overuse and pressure, unspecified upper arm
- + 6 M70.93 Unspecified soft tissue disorder related to use, overuse and pressure of forearm
- ⊟ SP + M70.931 Unspecified soft tissue disorder related to use, overuse and pressure, right forearm
- ⊟ SP + M70.932 Unspecified soft tissue disorder related to use, overuse and pressure, left forearm
- ⊟ IQ + M70.939 Unspecified soft tissue disorder related to use, overuse and pressure, unspecified forearm
- + 6 M70.94 Unspecified soft tissue disorder related to use, overuse and pressure of hand
- ⊟ SP + M70.941 Unspecified soft tissue disorder related to use, overuse and pressure, right hand
- ⊟ SP + M70.942 Unspecified soft tissue disorder related to use, overuse and pressure, left hand

M70.949 Unspecified soft tissue disorder related to use, overuse and pressure, unspecified hand

M70.95 Unspecified soft tissue disorder related to use, overuse and pressure of thigh

M70.951 Unspecified soft tissue disorder related to use, overuse and pressure, right thigh

M70.952 Unspecified soft tissue disorder related to use, overuse and pressure, left thigh

M70.959 Unspecified soft tissue disorder related to use, overuse and pressure, unspecified thigh

M70.96 Unspecified soft tissue disorder related to use, overuse and pressure lower leg

M70.961 Unspecified soft tissue disorder related to use, overuse and pressure, right lower leg

M70.962 Unspecified soft tissue disorder related to use, overuse and pressure, left lower leg

M70.969 Unspecified soft tissue disorder related to use, overuse and pressure, unspecified lower leg

M70.97 Unspecified soft tissue disorder related to use, overuse and pressure of ankle and foot

M70.971 Unspecified soft tissue disorder related to use, overuse and pressure, right ankle and foot

M70.972 Unspecified soft tissue disorder related to use, overuse and pressure, left ankle and foot

M70.979 Unspecified soft tissue disorder related to use, overuse and pressure, unspecified ankle and foot

SP M70.98 Unspecified soft tissue disorder related to use, overuse and pressure other

SP M70.99 Unspecified soft tissue disorder related to use, overuse and pressure multiple sites

4 M71 Other bursopathies

EXCLUDES 1 bunion (M20.1)
bursitis related to use, overuse or pressure (M70.-)
enthesopathies (M76-M77)

5 M71.0 Abscess of bursa

Use additional code (B95.-, B96.-) to identify causative organism

M71.00 Abscess of bursa, unspecified site

6 M71.01 Abscess of bursa, shoulder

M71.011 Abscess of bursa, right shoulder

M71.012 Abscess of bursa, left shoulder

M71.019 Abscess of bursa, unspecified shoulder

6 M71.02 Abscess of bursa, elbow

M71.021 Abscess of bursa, right elbow

M71.022 Abscess of bursa, left elbow

M71.029 Abscess of bursa, unspecified elbow

6 M71.03 Abscess of bursa, wrist

M71.031 Abscess of bursa, right wrist

M71.032 Abscess of bursa, left wrist

M71.039 Abscess of bursa, unspecified wrist

6 M71.04 Abscess of bursa, hand

M71.041 Abscess of bursa, right hand

M71.042 Abscess of bursa, left hand

M71.049 Abscess of bursa, unspecified hand

6 M71.05 Abscess of bursa, hip

M71.051 Abscess of bursa, right hip

M71.052 Abscess of bursa, left hip

M71.059 Abscess of bursa, unspecified hip

6 M71.06 Abscess of bursa, knee

M71.061 Abscess of bursa, right knee

M71.062 Abscess of bursa, left knee

M71.069 Abscess of bursa, unspecified knee

6 M71.07 Abscess of bursa, ankle and foot

M71.071 Abscess of bursa, right ankle and foot

M71.072 Abscess of bursa, left ankle and foot

M71.079 Abscess of bursa, unspecified ankle and foot

SP M71.08 Abscess of bursa, other site

SP M71.09 Abscess of bursa, multiple sites

5 M71.1 Other infective bursitis

Use additional code (B95.-, B96.-) to identify causative organism

M71.10 Other infective bursitis, unspecified site

6 M71.11 Other infective bursitis, shoulder

M71.111 Other infective bursitis, right shoulder

M71.112 Other infective bursitis, left shoulder

M71.119 Other infective bursitis, unspecified shoulder

6 M71.12 Other infective bursitis, elbow

M71.121 Other infective bursitis, right elbow

M71.122 Other infective bursitis, left elbow

M71.129 Other infective bursitis, unspecified elbow

6 M71.13 Other infective bursitis, wrist

M71.131 Other infective bursitis, right wrist

M71.132 Other infective bursitis, left wrist

M71.139 Other infective bursitis, unspecified wrist

6 M71.14 Other infective bursitis, hand

M71.141 Other infective bursitis, right hand

M71.142 Other infective bursitis, left hand

M71.149 Other infective bursitis, unspecified hand

6 M71.15 Other infective bursitis, hip

Chapter 13

M00-M99

M71.151 Other infective bursitis, right hip
M71.152 Other infective bursitis, left hip
M71.159 Other infective bursitis, unspecified hip
M71.16 Other infective bursitis, knee
M71.161 Other infective bursitis, right knee
M71.162 Other infective bursitis, left knee
M71.169 Other infective bursitis, unspecified knee
M71.17 Other infective bursitis, ankle and foot
M71.171 Other infective bursitis, right ankle and foot
M71.172 Other infective bursitis, left ankle and foot
M71.179 Other infective bursitis, unspecified ankle and foot
M71.18 Other infective bursitis, other site
M71.19 Other infective bursitis, multiple sites
M71.2 Synovial cyst of popliteal space [Baker]
EXCLUDES 1 synovial cyst of popliteal space with rupture (M66.0)
DEFINITION Collection of synovial fluid that has escaped from the knee joint or bursa and has formed a synovial-lined sac behind the knee.
M71.20 Synovial cyst of popliteal space [Baker], unspecified knee
M71.21 Synovial cyst of popliteal space [Baker], right knee
M71.22 Synovial cyst of popliteal space [Baker], left knee
M71.3 Other bursal cyst
Synovial cyst NOS
EXCLUDES 1 synovial cyst with rupture (M66.1-)
M71.30 Other bursal cyst, unspecified site
M71.31 Other bursal cyst, shoulder
M71.311 Other bursal cyst, right shoulder
M71.312 Other bursal cyst, left shoulder
M71.319 Other bursal cyst, unspecified shoulder
M71.32 Other bursal cyst, elbow
M71.321 Other bursal cyst, right elbow
M71.322 Other bursal cyst, left elbow
M71.329 Other bursal cyst, unspecified elbow
M71.33 Other bursal cyst, wrist
M71.331 Other bursal cyst, right wrist
M71.332 Other bursal cyst, left wrist
M71.339 Other bursal cyst, unspecified wrist
M71.34 Other bursal cyst, hand
M71.341 Other bursal cyst, right hand
M71.342 Other bursal cyst, left hand
M71.349 Other bursal cyst, unspecified hand
M71.35 Other bursal cyst, hip
M71.351 Other bursal cyst, right hip
M71.352 Other bursal cyst, left hip
M71.359 Other bursal cyst, unspecified hip
M71.37 Other bursal cyst, ankle and foot
M71.371 Other bursal cyst, right ankle and foot
M71.372 Other bursal cyst, left ankle and foot
M71.379 Other bursal cyst, unspecified ankle and foot
M71.38 Other bursal cyst, other site
M71.39 Other bursal cyst, multiple sites
M71.4 Calcium deposit in bursa
EXCLUDES 2 calcium deposit in bursa of shoulder (M75.3)
M71.40 Calcium deposit in bursa, unspecified site
M71.42 Calcium deposit in bursa, elbow
M71.421 Calcium deposit in bursa, right elbow
M71.422 Calcium deposit in bursa, left elbow
M71.429 Calcium deposit in bursa, unspecified elbow
M71.43 Calcium deposit in bursa, wrist
M71.431 Calcium deposit in bursa, right wrist
M71.432 Calcium deposit in bursa, left wrist
M71.439 Calcium deposit in bursa, unspecified wrist
M71.44 Calcium deposit in bursa, hand
M71.441 Calcium deposit in bursa, right hand
M71.442 Calcium deposit in bursa, left hand
M71.449 Calcium deposit in bursa, unspecified hand
M71.45 Calcium deposit in bursa, hip
M71.451 Calcium deposit in bursa, right hip
M71.452 Calcium deposit in bursa, left hip
M71.459 Calcium deposit in bursa, unspecified hip
M71.46 Calcium deposit in bursa, knee
M71.461 Calcium deposit in bursa, right knee
M71.462 Calcium deposit in bursa, left knee
M71.469 Calcium deposit in bursa, unspecified knee
M71.47 Calcium deposit in bursa, ankle and foot
M71.471 Calcium deposit in bursa, right ankle and foot
M71.472 Calcium deposit in bursa, left ankle and foot
M71.479 Calcium deposit in bursa, unspecified ankle and foot
M71.48 Calcium deposit in bursa, other site
M71.49 Calcium deposit in bursa, multiple sites
M71.5 Other bursitis, not elsewhere classified
EXCLUDES 1 bursitis NOS (M71.9-)

EXCLUDES 2 bursitis of shoulder (M75.5)
bursitis of tibial collateral [Pellegrini-Stieda] (M76.4-)

IQ M71.50 Other bursitis, not elsewhere classified, unspecified site
6 M71.52 Other bursitis, not elsewhere classified, elbow
SP M71.521 Other bursitis, not elsewhere classified, right elbow
SP M71.522 Other bursitis, not elsewhere classified, left elbow
IQ M71.529 Other bursitis, not elsewhere classified, unspecified elbow
6 M71.53 Other bursitis, not elsewhere classified, wrist
SP M71.531 Other bursitis, not elsewhere classified, right wrist
SP M71.532 Other bursitis, not elsewhere classified, left wrist
IQ M71.539 Other bursitis, not elsewhere classified, unspecified wrist
6 M71.54 Other bursitis, not elsewhere classified, hand
SP M71.541 Other bursitis, not elsewhere classified, right hand
SP M71.542 Other bursitis, not elsewhere classified, left hand
IQ M71.549 Other bursitis, not elsewhere classified, unspecified hand
6 M71.55 Other bursitis, not elsewhere classified, hip
SP M71.551 Other bursitis, not elsewhere classified, right hip
SP M71.552 Other bursitis, not elsewhere classified, left hip
IQ M71.559 Other bursitis, not elsewhere classified, unspecified hip
6 M71.56 Other bursitis, not elsewhere classified, knee
SP M71.561 Other bursitis, not elsewhere classified, right knee
SP M71.562 Other bursitis, not elsewhere classified, left knee
IQ M71.569 Other bursitis, not elsewhere classified, unspecified knee
6 M71.57 Other bursitis, not elsewhere classified, ankle and foot
SP M71.571 Other bursitis, not elsewhere classified, right ankle and foot
SP M71.572 Other bursitis, not elsewhere classified, left ankle and foot
IQ M71.579 Other bursitis, not elsewhere classified, unspecified ankle and foot
SP M71.58 Other bursitis, not elsewhere classified, other site
5 M71.8 Other specified bursopathies
IQ M71.80 Other specified bursopathies, unspecified site
6 M71.81 Other specified bursopathies, shoulder
SP M71.811 Other specified bursopathies, right shoulder
SP M71.812 Other specified bursopathies, left shoulder
IQ M71.819 Other specified bursopathies, unspecified shoulder
6 M71.82 Other specified bursopathies, elbow
SP M71.821 Other specified bursopathies, right elbow
SP M71.822 Other specified bursopathies, left elbow
IQ M71.829 Other specified bursopathies, unspecified elbow
6 M71.83 Other specified bursopathies, wrist
SP M71.831 Other specified bursopathies, right wrist
SP M71.832 Other specified bursopathies, left wrist
IQ M71.839 Other specified bursopathies, unspecified wrist
6 M71.84 Other specified bursopathies, hand
SP M71.841 Other specified bursopathies, right hand
SP M71.842 Other specified bursopathies, left hand
IQ M71.849 Other specified bursopathies, unspecified hand
6 M71.85 Other specified bursopathies, hip
SP M71.851 Other specified bursopathies, right hip
SP M71.852 Other specified bursopathies, left hip
IQ M71.859 Other specified bursopathies, unspecified hip
6 M71.86 Other specified bursopathies, knee
SP M71.861 Other specified bursopathies, right knee
SP M71.862 Other specified bursopathies, left knee
IQ M71.869 Other specified bursopathies, unspecified knee
6 M71.87 Other specified bursopathies, ankle and foot
SP M71.871 Other specified bursopathies, right ankle and foot
SP M71.872 Other specified bursopathies, left ankle and foot
IQ M71.879 Other specified bursopathies, unspecified ankle and foot
SP M71.88 Other specified bursopathies, other site
SP M71.89 Other specified bursopathies, multiple sites
IQ M71.9 Bursopathy, unspecified
Bursitis NOS

4 M72 Fibroblastic disorders
EXCLUDES 2 retroperitoneal fibromatosis (D48.3)

SP M72.0 Palmar fascial fibromatosis [Dupuytren]
SP M72.1 Knuckle pads
SP M72.2 Plantar fascial fibromatosis
Plantar fasciitis
SP M72.4 Pseudosarcomatous fibromatosis
Nodular fasciitis
SP + M72.6 Necrotizing fasciitis
Use additional code (B95.-, B96.-) to identify causative organism
SP + M72.8 Other fibroblastic disorders
Abscess of fascia

Fasciitis NEC
Other infective fasciitis
Use additional code to (B95.-, B96.-) identify causative organism
EXCLUDES 1 diffuse (eosinophilic) fasciitis (M35.4)
necrotizing fasciitis (M72.6)
nodular fasciitis (M72.4)
perirenal fasciitis NOS (N13.5)
perirenal fasciitis with infection (N13.6)
plantar fasciitis (M72.2)

IQ **M72.9 Fibroblastic disorder, unspecified**
Fasciitis NOS
Fibromatosis NOS

4 **M75 Shoulder lesions**
EXCLUDES 2 shoulder-hand syndrome (M89.0-)

5 **M75.0 Adhesive capsulitis of shoulder**
Frozen shoulder
Periarthritis of shoulder

L IQ **M75.00 Adhesive capsulitis of unspecified shoulder**

L SP **M75.01 Adhesive capsulitis of right shoulder**

L SP **M75.02 Adhesive capsulitis of left shoulder**

5 **M75.1 Rotator cuff tear or rupture, not specified as traumatic**
Rotator cuff syndrome
Supraspinatus tear or rupture, not specified as traumatic
Supraspinatus syndrome
EXCLUDES 1 tear of rotator cuff, traumatic (S46.01-)

6 **M75.10 Unspecified rotator cuff tear or rupture, not specified as traumatic**

L IQ **M75.100 Unspecified rotator cuff tear or rupture of unspecified shoulder, not specified as traumatic**

L SP **M75.101 Unspecified rotator cuff tear or rupture of right shoulder, not specified as traumatic**

L SP **M75.102 Unspecified rotator cuff tear or rupture of left shoulder, not specified as traumatic**

6 **M75.11 Incomplete rotator cuff tear or rupture not specified as traumatic**

CODING TIPS ✓ A partial tear of the rotator cuff is an area of damage to the rotator cuff tendons, where the tear does not go all the way through the tendons. Note that a complete tear is coded to M75.12. A traumatic tear is coded to S46.01-.

L IQ **M75.110 Incomplete rotator cuff tear or rupture of unspecified shoulder, not specified as traumatic**

L SP **M75.111 Incomplete rotator cuff tear or rupture of right shoulder, not specified as traumatic**

L SP **M75.112 Incomplete rotator cuff tear or rupture of left shoulder, not specified as traumatic**

6 **M75.12 Complete rotator cuff tear or rupture not specified as traumatic**

L IQ **M75.120 Complete rotator cuff tear or rupture of unspecified shoulder, not specified as traumatic**

L SP **M75.121 Complete rotator cuff tear or rupture of right shoulder, not specified as traumatic**

L SP **M75.122 Complete rotator cuff tear or rupture of left shoulder, not specified as traumatic**

5 **M75.2 Bicipital tendinitis**

L IQ **M75.20 Bicipital tendinitis, unspecified shoulder**

L SP **M75.21 Bicipital tendinitis, right shoulder**

L SP **M75.22 Bicipital tendinitis, left shoulder**

5 **M75.3 Calcific tendinitis of shoulder**
Calcified bursa of shoulder

L IQ **M75.30 Calcific tendinitis of unspecified shoulder**

L SP **M75.31 Calcific tendinitis of right shoulder**

L SP **M75.32 Calcific tendinitis of left shoulder**

5 **M75.4 Impingement syndrome of shoulder**

L IQ **M75.40 Impingement syndrome of unspecified shoulder**

L SP **M75.41 Impingement syndrome of right shoulder**

L SP **M75.42 Impingement syndrome of left shoulder**

5 **M75.5 Bursitis of shoulder**

L IQ **M75.50 Bursitis of unspecified shoulder**

L SP **M75.51 Bursitis of right shoulder**

L SP **M75.52 Bursitis of left shoulder**

5 **M75.8 Other shoulder lesions**

L IQ **M75.80 Other shoulder lesions, unspecified shoulder**

L SP **M75.81 Other shoulder lesions, right shoulder**

L SP **M75.82 Other shoulder lesions, left shoulder**

5 **M75.9 Shoulder lesion, unspecified**

L IQ **M75.90 Shoulder lesion, unspecified, unspecified shoulder**

L SP **M75.91 Shoulder lesion, unspecified, right shoulder**

L SP **M75.92 Shoulder lesion, unspecified, left shoulder**

4 **M76 Enthesopathies, lower limb, excluding foot**
EXCLUDES 2 bursitis due to use, overuse and pressure (M70.-)
enthesopathies of ankle and foot (M77.5-)

5 **M76.0 Gluteal tendinitis**

L IQ **M76.00 Gluteal tendinitis, unspecified hip**

L SP **M76.01 Gluteal tendinitis, right hip**

L SP **M76.02 Gluteal tendinitis, left hip**

5 **M76.1 Psoas tendinitis**

L IQ **M76.10 Psoas tendinitis, unspecified hip**

L SP **M76.11 Psoas tendinitis, right hip**

L SP **M76.12 Psoas tendinitis, left hip**

5 **M76.2 Iliac crest spur**

L IQ **M76.20 Iliac crest spur, unspecified hip**

L SP **M76.21 Iliac crest spur, right hip**

L SP **M76.22 Iliac crest spur, left hip**

M76.3 Iliotibial band syndrome

M76.30 Iliotibial band syndrome, unspecified leg

M76.31 Iliotibial band syndrome, right leg

M76.32 Iliotibial band syndrome, left leg

M76.4 Tibial collateral bursitis [Pellegrini-Stieda]

M76.40 Tibial collateral bursitis [Pellegrini-Stieda], unspecified leg

M76.41 Tibial collateral bursitis [Pellegrini-Stieda], right leg

M76.42 Tibial collateral bursitis [Pellegrini-Stieda], left leg

M76.5 Patellar tendinitis

M76.50 Patellar tendinitis, unspecified knee

M76.51 Patellar tendinitis, right knee

M76.52 Patellar tendinitis, left knee

M76.6 Achilles tendinitis

Achilles bursitis

M76.60 Achilles tendinitis, unspecified leg

M76.61 Achilles tendinitis, right leg

M76.62 Achilles tendinitis, left leg

M76.7 Peroneal tendinitis

M76.70 Peroneal tendinitis, unspecified leg

M76.71 Peroneal tendinitis, right leg

M76.72 Peroneal tendinitis, left leg

M76.8 Other specified enthesopathies of lower limb, excluding foot

M76.81 Anterior tibial syndrome

M76.811 Anterior tibial syndrome, right leg

M76.812 Anterior tibial syndrome, left leg

M76.819 Anterior tibial syndrome, unspecified leg

M76.82 Posterior tibial tendinitis

M76.821 Posterior tibial tendinitis, right leg

M76.822 Posterior tibial tendinitis, left leg

M76.829 Posterior tibial tendinitis, unspecified leg

M76.89 Other specified enthesopathies of lower limb, excluding foot

M76.891 Other specified enthesopathies of right lower limb, excluding foot

M76.892 Other specified enthesopathies of left lower limb, excluding foot

M76.899 Other specified enthesopathies of unspecified lower limb, excluding foot

M76.9 Unspecified enthesopathy, lower limb, excluding foot

M77 Other enthesopathies

EXCLUDES 1 bursitis NOS (M71.9-)

EXCLUDES 2 bursitis due to use, overuse and pressure (M70.-)
osteophyte (M25.7)
spinal enthesopathy (M46.0-)

M77.0 Medial epicondylitis

M77.00 Medial epicondylitis, unspecified elbow

M77.01 Medial epicondylitis, right elbow

M77.02 Medial epicondylitis, left elbow

M77.1 Lateral epicondylitis

Tennis elbow

DEFINITION A painful inflammation of the tendons that anchor the extensor carpi radialis brevis muscle to the outer aspect of the humerus at the elbow.

M77.10 Lateral epicondylitis, unspecified elbow

M77.11 Lateral epicondylitis, right elbow

M77.12 Lateral epicondylitis, left elbow

M77.2 Periarthritis of wrist

M77.20 Periarthritis, unspecified wrist

M77.21 Periarthritis, right wrist

M77.22 Periarthritis, left wrist

M77.3 Calcaneal spur

M77.30 Calcaneal spur, unspecified foot

M77.31 Calcaneal spur, right foot

M77.32 Calcaneal spur, left foot

M77.4 Metatarsalgia

EXCLUDES 1 Morton's metatarsalgia (G57.6)

M77.40 Metatarsalgia, unspecified foot

M77.41 Metatarsalgia, right foot

M77.42 Metatarsalgia, left foot

M77.5 Other enthesopathy of foot and ankle

M77.50 Other enthesopathy of unspecified foot and ankle

M77.51 Other enthesopathy of right foot and ankle

M77.52 Other enthesopathy of left foot and ankle

M77.8 Other enthesopathies, not elsewhere classified

M77.9 Enthesopathy, unspecified

Bone spur NOS
Capsulitis NOS
Periarthritis NOS
Tendinitis NOS

M79 Other and unspecified soft tissue disorders, not elsewhere classified

EXCLUDES 1 psychogenic rheumatism (F45.8)
soft tissue pain, psychogenic (F45.41)

M79.0 Rheumatism, unspecified

EXCLUDES 1 fibromyalgia (M79.7)
palindromic rheumatism (M12.3-)

M79.1 Myalgia

Myofascial pain syndrome

EXCLUDES 1 fibromyalgia (M79.7)
myositis (M60.-)

M79.10 Myalgia, unspecified site

M79.11 Myalgia of mastication muscle

M79.12 Myalgia of auxiliary muscles, head and neck

M79.18 Myalgia, other site

M79.2 Neuralgia and neuritis, unspecified

EXCLUDES 1 brachial radiculitis NOS (M54.1)
lumbosacral radiculitis NOS (M54.1)
mononeuropathies (G56-G58)

Chapter 13

M00-M99

★ New ▲ Revised Px Primary SP PDGM Px SL Low CoM SH High CoM IQ Quest. Encounter H Hospice non-cancer Dx Unspecified M *Manifestation*

radiculitis NOS (M54.1)
sciatica (M54.3-M54.4)

SP **M79.3 Panniculitis, unspecified**

EXCLUDES 1 lupus panniculitis (L93.2)
neck and back panniculitis (M54.0-)
relapsing [Weber-Christian] panniculitis (M35.6)

SP **M79.4 Hypertrophy of (infrapatellar) fat pad**

SP **M79.5 Residual foreign body in soft tissue**

EXCLUDES 1 foreign body granuloma of skin and subcutaneous tissue (L92.3)
foreign body granuloma of soft tissue (M60.2-)

5 **M79.6 Pain in limb, hand, foot, fingers and toes**

EXCLUDES 2 pain in joint (M25.5-)

CODING TIPS ✓ These codes should be used when 1) the cause of the pain is unknown; 2) the pain is a sequela of an injury; or 3) in conjunction with a G89 code. Do not use these codes with conditions where this type is integral.

6 **M79.60 Pain in limb, unspecified**

⊟ IQ **M79.601 Pain in right arm**
Pain in right upper limb NOS

⊟ IQ **M79.602 Pain in left arm**
Pain in left upper limb NOS

⊟ IQ **M79.603 Pain in arm, unspecified**
Pain in upper limb NOS

⊟ IQ **M79.604 Pain in right leg**
Pain in right lower limb NOS

⊟ IQ **M79.605 Pain in left leg**
Pain in left lower limb NOS

⊟ IQ **M79.606 Pain in leg, unspecified**
Pain in lower limb NOS

⊟ IQ **M79.609 Pain in unspecified limb**
Pain in limb NOS

6 **M79.62 Pain in upper arm**
Pain in axillary region

⊟ IQ **M79.621 Pain in right upper arm**

⊟ IQ **M79.622 Pain in left upper arm**

⊟ IQ **M79.629 Pain in unspecified upper arm**

6 **M79.63 Pain in forearm**

⊟ IQ **M79.631 Pain in right forearm**

⊟ IQ **M79.632 Pain in left forearm**

⊟ IQ **M79.639 Pain in unspecified forearm**

6 **M79.64 Pain in hand and fingers**

⊟ IQ **M79.641 Pain in right hand**

⊟ IQ **M79.642 Pain in left hand**

⊟ IQ **M79.643 Pain in unspecified hand**

⊟ IQ **M79.644 Pain in right finger(s)**

⊟ IQ **M79.645 Pain in left finger(s)**

⊟ IQ **M79.646 Pain in unspecified finger(s)**

6 **M79.65 Pain in thigh**

⊟ IQ **M79.651 Pain in right thigh**

⊟ IQ **M79.652 Pain in left thigh**

⊟ IQ **M79.659 Pain in unspecified thigh**

6 **M79.66 Pain in lower leg**

⊟ IQ **M79.661 Pain in right lower leg**

⊟ IQ **M79.662 Pain in left lower leg**

⊟ IQ **M79.669 Pain in unspecified lower leg**

6 **M79.67 Pain in foot and toes**

⊟ IQ **M79.671 Pain in right foot**

⊟ IQ **M79.672 Pain in left foot**

⊟ IQ **M79.673 Pain in unspecified foot**

⊟ IQ **M79.674 Pain in right toe(s)**

⊟ IQ **M79.675 Pain in left toe(s)**

⊟ IQ **M79.676 Pain in unspecified toe(s)**

SP **M79.7 Fibromyalgia**
Fibromyositis
Fibrositis
Myofibrositis

5 **M79.A Nontraumatic compartment syndrome**
Code first:
, if applicable, associated postprocedural complication

EXCLUDES 1 compartment syndrome NOS (T79.A-)
fibromyalgia (M79.7)
nontraumatic ischemic infarction of muscle (M62.2-)
traumatic compartment syndrome (T79.A-)

6 **M79.A1 Nontraumatic compartment syndrome of upper extremity**
Nontraumatic compartment syndrome of shoulder, arm, forearm, wrist, hand, and fingers

⊟ SP **M79.A11 Nontraumatic compartment syndrome of right upper extremity**

⊟ SP **M79.A12 Nontraumatic compartment syndrome of left upper extremity**

⊟ IQ **M79.A19 Nontraumatic compartment syndrome of unspecified upper extremity**

6 **M79.A2 Nontraumatic compartment syndrome of lower extremity**
Nontraumatic compartment syndrome of hip, buttock, thigh, leg, foot, and toes

⊟ SP **M79.A21 Nontraumatic compartment syndrome of right lower extremity**

⊟ SP **M79.A22 Nontraumatic compartment syndrome of left lower extremity**

⊟ IQ **M79.A29 Nontraumatic compartment syndrome of unspecified lower extremity**

SP **M79.A3 Nontraumatic compartment syndrome of abdomen**

SP **M79.A9 Nontraumatic compartment syndrome of other sites**

5 **M79.8 Other specified soft tissue disorders**

SP **M79.81 Nontraumatic hematoma of soft tissue**
Nontraumatic hematoma of muscle
Nontraumatic seroma of muscle and soft tissue

DEFINITION A spontaneous, nontraumatic localized collection of partially clotted blood within a soft tissue such as muscle.

SP **M79.89 Other specified soft tissue disorders**
Polyalgia

IQ **M79.9 Soft tissue disorder, unspecified**

Osteopathies and chondropathies (M80-M94)

Disorders of bone density and structure (M80-M85)

+ 4 M80 Osteoporosis with current pathological fracture

INCLUDES osteoporosis with current fragility fracture

Use additional code to identify major osseous defect, if applicable (M89.7-)

EXCLUDES 1 collapsed vertebra NOS (M48.5)
pathological fracture NOS (M84.4)
wedging of vertebra NOS (M48.5)

EXCLUDES 2 personal history of (healed) osteoporosis fracture (Z87.310)

The appropriate 7th character is to be added to each code from category M80:

A	initial encounter for fracture
D	subsequent encounter for fracture with routine healing
G	subsequent encounter for fracture with delayed healing
K	subsequent encounter for fracture with nonunion
P	subsequent encounter for fracture with malunion
S	sequela

GUIDELINES **Section I.C.13.c**

Coding of Pathologic Fractures: 7th character D is to be used for encounters after the patient has completed active treatment for the fracture and is receiving routine care for the fracture during the healing or recovery phase. The other 7th characters, listed under each subcategory in the Tabular List, are to be used for subsequent encounters for treatment of problems associated with the healing, such as malunions, nonunions, and sequelae.

Care for complications of surgical treatment for fracture repairs during the healing or recovery phase should be coded with the appropriate complication codes.

GUIDELINES **Section I.C.13.d.2)**

Category M80, Osteoporosis with current pathological fracture, is for patients who have a current pathologic fracture at the time of an encounter. The codes under M80 identify the site of the fracture. A code from category M80, not a traumatic fracture code, should be used for any patient with known osteoporosis who suffers a fracture, even if the patient had a minor fall or trauma, if that fall or trauma would not usually break a normal, healthy bone.

GUIDELINES **Section I.C.13.a.1)**

For certain conditions, the bone may be affected at the upper or lower end, (e.g., avascular necrosis of bone, M87, Osteoporosis, M80, M81). Though the portion of the bone affected may be at the joint, the site designation will be the bone, not the joint.

CODING TIPS✓ Fractures repaired by joint replacements are NOT coded with Z47.1. Fractures repaired by any other orthopedic surgery are NOT coded with Z47.89. Z codes are not appropriate for fractures of any kind. Code the fracture with 7th character D for fractures undergoing surgical repair.

CODING TIPS✓ When a patient with osteoporosis is noted to have an active fracture, use the osteoporosis fracture codes, unless the physician or NPP has identified the fracture as a trauma fracture. Age-related osteoporosis includes post-menopausal and senile osteoporosis, as well as unspecified. Age-related osteoporosis is the default if the type of osteoporosis is not identified. Code Z87.310 is assigned for an osteoporosis fracture that has healed.

+ 5 M80.0 Age-related osteoporosis with current pathological fracture

Involutional osteoporosis with current pathological fracture
Osteoporosis NOS with current pathological fracture
Postmenopausal osteoporosis with current pathological fracture
Senile osteoporosis with current pathological fracture

IQ + 7 M80.00X- Age-related osteoporosis with current pathological fracture, unspecified site

CODING TIPS✓ Do NOT use this code for osteoporosis fractures of the rib and pelvis. See M80.0A-.

+ 6 M80.01 Age-related osteoporosis with current pathological fracture, shoulder

H SP + 7 M80.011- Age-related osteoporosis with current pathological fracture, right shoulder

H SP + 7 M80.012- Age-related osteoporosis with current pathological fracture, left shoulder

H IQ + 7 M80.019- Age-related osteoporosis with current pathological fracture, unspecified shoulder

+ 6 M80.02 Age-related osteoporosis with current pathological fracture, humerus

H SP + 7 M80.021- Age-related osteoporosis with current pathological fracture, right humerus

H SP + 7 M80.022- Age-related osteoporosis with current pathological fracture, left humerus

H IQ + 7 M80.029- Age-related osteoporosis with current pathological fracture, unspecified humerus

+ 6 **M80.03 Age-related osteoporosis with current pathological fracture, forearm**
Age-related osteoporosis with current pathological fracture of wrist

⊟ SP + 7 **M80.031- Age-related osteoporosis with current pathological fracture, right forearm**

⊟ SP + 7 **M80.032- Age-related osteoporosis with current pathological fracture, left forearm**

⊟ !Q + 7 **M80.039- Age-related osteoporosis with current pathological fracture, unspecified forearm**

+ 6 **M80.04 Age-related osteoporosis with current pathological fracture, hand**

⊟ SP + 7 **M80.041- Age-related osteoporosis with current pathological fracture, right hand**

⊟ SP + 7 **M80.042- Age-related osteoporosis with current pathological fracture, left hand**

⊟ !Q + 7 **M80.049- Age-related osteoporosis with current pathological fracture, unspecified hand**

+ 6 **M80.05 Age-related osteoporosis with current pathological fracture, femur**
Age-related osteoporosis with current pathological fracture of hip

⊟ SP + 7 **M80.051- Age-related osteoporosis with current pathological fracture, right femur**

⊟ SP + 7 **M80.052- Age-related osteoporosis with current pathological fracture, left femur**

⊟ !Q + 7 **M80.059- Age-related osteoporosis with current pathological fracture, unspecified femur**

+ 6 **M80.06 Age-related osteoporosis with current pathological fracture, lower leg**

⊟ SP + 7 **M80.061- Age-related osteoporosis with current pathological fracture, right lower leg**

⊟ SP + 7 **M80.062- Age-related osteoporosis with current pathological fracture, left lower leg**

⊟ !Q + 7 **M80.069- Age-related osteoporosis with current pathological fracture, unspecified lower leg**

+ 6 **M80.07 Age-related osteoporosis with current pathological fracture, ankle and foot**

⊟ SP + 7 **M80.071- Age-related osteoporosis with current pathological fracture, right ankle and foot**

⊟ SP + 7 **M80.072- Age-related osteoporosis with current pathological fracture, left ankle and foot**

⊟ !Q + 7 **M80.079- Age-related osteoporosis with current pathological fracture, unspecified ankle and foot**

SP + X **M80.08X- Age-related osteoporosis with current pathological fracture, vertebra(e)**

SP + X **M80.0AX- Age-related osteoporosis with current pathological fracture, other site**

CODING TIPS✓ Assign this code for osteoporosis fractures of sites other than those listed in other codes in M80.0, such as ribs and pubic bone.

+ 5 **M80.8 Other osteoporosis with current pathological fracture**
Drug-induced osteoporosis with current pathological fracture
Idiopathic osteoporosis with current pathological fracture
Osteoporosis of disuse with current pathological fracture
Postoophorectomy osteoporosis with current pathological fracture
Postsurgical malabsorption osteoporosis with current pathological fracture
Post-traumatic osteoporosis with current pathological fracture
Use additional code for adverse effect, if applicable, to identify drug (T36-T50 with fifth or sixth character 5)

!Q + X **M80.80X- Other osteoporosis with current pathological fracture, unspecified site**

+ 6 **M80.81 Other osteoporosis with pathological fracture, shoulder**

⊟ SP + 7 **M80.811- Other osteoporosis with current pathological fracture, right shoulder**

⊟ SP + 7 **M80.812- Other osteoporosis with current pathological fracture, left shoulder**

⊟ !Q + 7 **M80.819- Other osteoporosis with current pathological fracture, unspecified shoulder**

+ 6 **M80.82 Other osteoporosis with current pathological fracture, humerus**

⊟ SP + 7 **M80.821- Other osteoporosis with current pathological fracture, right humerus**

⊟ SP + 7 **M80.822- Other osteoporosis with current pathological fracture, left humerus**

⊟ !Q + 7 **M80.829- Other osteoporosis with current pathological fracture, unspecified humerus**

+ 6 **M80.83 Other osteoporosis with current pathological fracture, forearm**
Other osteoporosis with current pathological fracture of wrist

⊟ SP + 7 **M80.831- Other osteoporosis with current pathological fracture, right forearm**

⊟ SP + 7 **M80.832- Other osteoporosis with current pathological fracture, left forearm**

⊟ !Q + 7 **M80.839- Other osteoporosis with current pathological fracture, unspecified forearm**

+ 6 **M80.84 Other osteoporosis with current pathological fracture, hand**

⊟ SP + 7 **M80.841- Other osteoporosis with current pathological fracture, right hand**

⊟ SP + 7 **M80.842- Other osteoporosis with current pathological fracture, left hand**

4 4th digit required 5 5th digit required 6 6th digit required 7 7th digit required X 7th digit placeholder + Additional code ⊟ Laterality

IQ + 7 **M80.849- Other osteoporosis with current pathological fracture, unspecified hand**

+ 6 **M80.85 Other osteoporosis with current pathological fracture, femur**
Other osteoporosis with current pathological fracture of hip

SP + 7 **M80.851- Other osteoporosis with current pathological fracture, right femur**

SP + 7 **M80.852- Other osteoporosis with current pathological fracture, left femur**

IQ + 7 **M80.859- Other osteoporosis with current pathological fracture, unspecified femur**

+ 6 **M80.86 Other osteoporosis with current pathological fracture, lower leg**

SP + 7 **M80.861- Other osteoporosis with current pathological fracture, right lower leg**

SP + 7 **M80.862- Other osteoporosis with current pathological fracture, left lower leg**

IQ + 7 **M80.869- Other osteoporosis with current pathological fracture, unspecified lower leg**

+ 6 **M80.87 Other osteoporosis with current pathological fracture, ankle and foot**

SP + 7 **M80.871- Other osteoporosis with current pathological fracture, right ankle and foot**

SP + 7 **M80.872- Other osteoporosis with current pathological fracture, left ankle and foot**

IQ + 7 **M80.879- Other osteoporosis with current pathological fracture, unspecified ankle and foot**

SP + 7 **M80.88X- Other osteoporosis with current pathological fracture, vertebra(e)**

SP + 7 **M80.8AX- Other osteoporosis with current pathological fracture, other site**

CODING TIPS✓ Assign this code for osteoporosis fractures of sites other than those listed in other codes in M80.8, such as ribs and pubic bone, when the type of osteoporosis is specified as other than senile, age-related, or post-menopausal.

+ 4 **M81 Osteoporosis without current pathological fracture**
Use additional code to identify:
major osseous defect, if applicable (M89.7-)
personal history of (healed) osteoporosis fracture, if applicable (Z87.310)

EXCLUDES 1 osteoporosis with current pathological fracture (M80.-)
Sudeck's atrophy (M89.0)

GUIDELINES **Section I.C.13.a.1)**
For certain conditions, the bone may be affected at the upper or lower end, (e.g., avascular necrosis of bone, M87, Osteoporosis, M80, M81). Though the portion of the bone affected may be at the joint, the site designation will be the bone, not the joint.

GUIDELINES **Section I.C.13.d.1)**
Category M81, Osteoporosis without current pathological fracture, is for use for patients with osteoporosis who do not currently have a pathologic fracture due to the osteoporosis, even if they have had a fracture in the past. For patients with a history of osteoporosis fractures, status code Z87.310, Personal history of (healed) osteoporosis fracture, should follow the code from M81.

CODING TIPS✓ M81 is coded for patients with osteoporosis with no current fracture. Osteoporosis is not site-specific since it's considered a systemic condition.

SP + **M81.0 Age-related osteoporosis without current pathological fracture**
Involutional osteoporosis without current pathological fracture
Osteoporosis NOS
Postmenopausal osteoporosis without current pathological fracture
Senile osteoporosis without current pathological fracture

SP + **M81.6 Localized osteoporosis [Lequesne]**
EXCLUDES 1 Sudeck's atrophy (M89.0)

SP + **M81.8 Other osteoporosis without current pathological fracture**
Drug-induced osteoporosis without current pathological fracture
Idiopathic osteoporosis without current pathological fracture
Osteoporosis of disuse without current pathological fracture
Postoophorectomy osteoporosis without current pathological fracture
Postsurgical malabsorption osteoporosis without current pathological fracture
Post-traumatic osteoporosis without current pathological fracture
Use additional code for adverse effect, if applicable, to identify drug (T36-T50 with fifth or sixth character 5)

4 **M83 Adult osteomalacia**
EXCLUDES 1 infantile and juvenile osteomalacia (E55.0)
renal osteodystrophy (N25.0)
rickets (active) (E55.0)
rickets (active) sequelae (E64.3)
vitamin D-resistant osteomalacia (E83.3)
vitamin D-resistant rickets (active) (E83.3)

DEFINITION Deficient levels of calcium in the bone, resulting in bone softening.

SP **M83.0 Puerperal osteomalacia**

SP **M83.1 Senile osteomalacia**

SP **M83.2 Adult osteomalacia due to malabsorption**
Postsurgical malabsorption osteomalacia in adults

SP **M83.3 Adult osteomalacia due to malnutrition**

SP **M83.4 Aluminum bone disease**

SP + **M83.5 Other drug-induced osteomalacia in adults**

Use additional code for adverse effect, if applicable, to identify drug (T36-T50 with fifth or sixth character 5)

SP **M83.8 Other adult osteomalacia**

SP **M83.9 Adult osteomalacia, unspecified**

4 **M84 Disorder of continuity of bone**

EXCLUDES 2 traumatic fracture of bone-see fracture, by site

GUIDELINES **Section I.C.13.c**

Coding of Pathologic Fractures: 7th character D is to be used for encounters after the patient has completed active treatment for the fracture and is receiving routine care for the fracture during the healing or recovery phase. The other 7th characters, listed under each subcategory in the Tabular List, are to be used for subsequent encounters for treatment of problems associated with the healing, such as malunions, nonunions, and sequelae.

Care for complications of surgical treatment for fracture repairs during the healing or recovery phase should be coded with the appropriate complication codes.

+ 5 **M84.3 Stress fracture**

Fatigue fracture
March fracture
Stress fracture NOS
Stress reaction

Use additional external cause code(s) to identify the cause of the stress fracture

EXCLUDES 1 pathological fracture NOS (M84.4.-)
pathological fracture due to osteoporosis (M80.-)
traumatic fracture (S12.-, S22.-, S32.-, S42.-, S52.-, S62.-, S72.-, S82.-, S92.-)

EXCLUDES 2 personal history of (healed) stress (fatigue) fracture (Z87.312)
stress fracture of vertebra (M48.4-)

The appropriate 7th character is to be added to each code from subcategory M84.3:

A	initial encounter for fracture
D	subsequent encounter for fracture with routine healing
G	subsequent encounter for fracture with delayed healing
K	subsequent encounter for fracture with nonunion
P	subsequent encounter for fracture with malunion
S	sequela

CODING TIPS✓ Fractures repaired by joint replacements are NOT coded with Z47.1. Fractures repaired by any other orthopedic surgery are NOT coded with Z47.89. Z codes are not appropriate for fractures of any kind. Code the fracture with 7th character D for fractures undergoing surgical repair.

CODING TIPS✓ Stress fractures are coded with M84.3. History of healed stress fracture is coded to Z87.312.

DEFINITION Small, hairline crack(s) in the surface of a bone due to overuse or activity that applies a repetitive force to a particular area, most commonly occurring in the lower legs and feet.

IQ + 7 **M84.30X- Stress fracture, unspecified site**

+ 6 **M84.31 Stress fracture, shoulder**

L SP + 7 **M84.311- Stress fracture, right shoulder**

L SP + 7 **M84.312- Stress fracture, left shoulder**

L IQ + 7 **M84.319- Stress fracture, unspecified shoulder**

+ 6 **M84.32 Stress fracture, humerus**

L SP + 7 **M84.321- Stress fracture, right humerus**

L SP + 7 **M84.322- Stress fracture, left humerus**

L IQ + 7 **M84.329- Stress fracture, unspecified humerus**

+ 6 **M84.33 Stress fracture, ulna and radius**

L SP + 7 **M84.331- Stress fracture, right ulna**

L SP + 7 **M84.332- Stress fracture, left ulna**

L SP + 7 **M84.333- Stress fracture, right radius**

L SP + 7 **M84.334- Stress fracture, left radius**

L IQ + 7 **M84.339- Stress fracture, unspecified ulna and radius**

+ 6 **M84.34 Stress fracture, hand and fingers**

L SP + 7 **M84.341- Stress fracture, right hand**

L SP + 7 **M84.342- Stress fracture, left hand**

L IQ + 7 **M84.343- Stress fracture, unspecified hand**

L SP + 7 **M84.344- Stress fracture, right finger(s)**

L SP + 7 **M84.345- Stress fracture, left finger(s)**

L IQ + 7 **M84.346- Stress fracture, unspecified finger(s)**

+ 6 **M84.35 Stress fracture, pelvis and femur**

Stress fracture, hip

L SP + 7 **M84.350- Stress fracture, pelvis**

L SP + 7 **M84.351- Stress fracture, right femur**

L SP + 7 **M84.352- Stress fracture, left femur**

L IQ + 7 **M84.353- Stress fracture, unspecified femur**

L IQ + 7 **M84.359- Stress fracture, hip, unspecified**

+ 6 **M84.36 Stress fracture, tibia and fibula**

L SP + 7 **M84.361- Stress fracture, right tibia**

L SP + 7 **M84.362- Stress fracture, left tibia**

L SP + 7 **M84.363- Stress fracture, right fibula**

L SP + 7 **M84.364- Stress fracture, left fibula**

L IQ + 7 **M84.369- Stress fracture, unspecified tibia and fibula**

+ 6 **M84.37 Stress fracture, ankle, foot and toes**

L SP + 7 **M84.371- Stress fracture, right ankle**

L SP + 7 **M84.372- Stress fracture, left ankle**

L IQ + 7 **M84.373- Stress fracture, unspecified ankle**

L SP + 7 **M84.374- Stress fracture, right foot**

L SP + 7 **M84.375- Stress fracture, left foot**

L IQ + 7 **M84.376- Stress fracture, unspecified foot**

SP + 7 **M84.377- Stress fracture, right toe(s)**

SP + 7 **M84.378- Stress fracture, left toe(s)**

!Q + 7 **M84.379- Stress fracture, unspecified toe(s)**

SP + 7 **M84.38X- Stress fracture, other site**

EXCLUDES 2 stress fracture of vertebra (M48.4-)

5 **M84.4 Pathological fracture, not elsewhere classified**

Chronic fracture

Pathological fracture NOS

EXCLUDES 1 collapsed vertebra NEC (M48.5)
pathological fracture in neoplastic disease (M84.5-)
pathological fracture in osteoporosis (M80.-)
pathological fracture in other disease (M84.6-)
stress fracture (M84.3-)
traumatic fracture (S12.-, S22.-, S32.-, S42.-, S52.-, S62.-, S72.-, S82.-, S92.-)

EXCLUDES 2 personal history of (healed) pathological fracture (Z87.311)

The appropriate 7th character is to be added to each code from subcategory M84.4:

A	initial encounter for fracture
D	subsequent encounter for fracture with routine healing
G	subsequent encounter for fracture with delayed healing
K	subsequent encounter for fracture with nonunion
P	subsequent encounter for fracture with malunion
S	sequela

CODING TIPS✓ Fractures repaired by joint replacements are NOT coded with Z47.1. Fractures repaired by any other orthopedic surgery are NOT coded with Z47.89. Z codes are not appropriate for fractures of any kind. Code the fracture with 7th character D for fractures undergoing surgical repair.

CODING TIPS✓ Spontaneous fractures occur without external blunt trauma and are almost always considered pathologic. Compression fractures are considered pathologic fractures. If the patient falls and has a compression fracture or unusual fracture, ask the physician or NPP whether it is considered trauma or pathologic. Pathologic fractures due to osteoporosis (M80) and due to neoplasm (M84.5) are not coded here. Pathologic fractures may be coded with 7th character D or S. Aftercare codes are not used in ICD-10 for fractures.

CODING TIPS✓ Watch out for laterality. Do not choose unspecified. Use Z87.311 for history of healed pathological fracture. Collapsed vertebra or compression fracture of the vertebra is coded to M48.5 when no other cause is identified.

DEFINITION A break resulting from widespread lesions or disease process that destroys normal bone mass, causing the weakened bone to break spontaneously without obvious external force.

!Q 7 **M84.40X- Pathological fracture, unspecified site**

6 **M84.41 Pathological fracture, shoulder**

SP 7 **M84.411- Pathological fracture, right shoulder**

SP 7 **M84.412- Pathological fracture, left shoulder**

!Q 7 **M84.419- Pathological fracture, unspecified shoulder**

6 **M84.42 Pathological fracture, humerus**

SP 7 **M84.421- Pathological fracture, right humerus**

SP 7 **M84.422- Pathological fracture, left humerus**

!Q 7 **M84.429- Pathological fracture, unspecified humerus**

6 **M84.43 Pathological fracture, ulna and radius**

SP 7 **M84.431- Pathological fracture, right ulna**

SP 7 **M84.432- Pathological fracture, left ulna**

SP 7 **M84.433- Pathological fracture, right radius**

SP 7 **M84.434- Pathological fracture, left radius**

!Q 7 **M84.439- Pathological fracture, unspecified ulna and radius**

6 **M84.44 Pathological fracture, hand and fingers**

SP 7 **M84.441- Pathological fracture, right hand**

SP 7 **M84.442- Pathological fracture, left hand**

!Q 7 **M84.443- Pathological fracture, unspecified hand**

SP 7 **M84.444- Pathological fracture, right finger(s)**

SP 7 **M84.445- Pathological fracture, left finger(s)**

!Q 7 **M84.446- Pathological fracture, unspecified finger(s)**

6 **M84.45 Pathological fracture, femur and pelvis**

SP 7 **M84.451- Pathological fracture, right femur**

SP 7 **M84.452- Pathological fracture, left femur**

!Q 7 **M84.453- Pathological fracture, unspecified femur**

SP 7 **M84.454- Pathological fracture, pelvis**

!Q 7 **M84.459- Pathological fracture, hip, unspecified**

6 **M84.46 Pathological fracture, tibia and fibula**

SP 7 **M84.461- Pathological fracture, right tibia**

SP 7 **M84.462- Pathological fracture, left tibia**

M84.463- Pathological fracture, right fibula

M84.464- Pathological fracture, left fibula

M84.469- Pathological fracture, unspecified tibia and fibula

M84.47 Pathological fracture, ankle, foot and toes

M84.471- Pathological fracture, right ankle

M84.472- Pathological fracture, left ankle

M84.473- Pathological fracture, unspecified ankle

M84.474- Pathological fracture, right foot

M84.475- Pathological fracture, left foot

M84.476- Pathological fracture, unspecified foot

M84.477- Pathological fracture, right toe(s)

M84.478- Pathological fracture, left toe(s)

M84.479- Pathological fracture, unspecified toe(s)

M84.48X- Pathological fracture, other site

M84.5 Pathological fracture in neoplastic disease

Code also:
underlying neoplasm

The appropriate 7th character is to be added to each code from subcategory M84.5:

A	initial encounter for fracture
D	subsequent encounter for fracture with routine healing
G	subsequent encounter for fracture with delayed healing
K	subsequent encounter for fracture with nonunion
P	subsequent encounter for fracture with malunion
S	sequela

GUIDELINES **Section I.C.2.l.6)**
When an encounter is for a pathological fracture due to a neoplasm, and the focus of treatment is the fracture, a code from subcategory M84.5, Pathological fracture in neoplastic disease, should be sequenced first, followed by the code for the neoplasm. If the focus of treatment is the neoplasm with an associated pathological fracture, the neoplasm code should be sequenced first, followed by a code from M84.5 for the pathological fracture.

CODING TIPS✓ Fractures repaired by joint replacements are NOT coded with Z47.1. Fractures repaired by any other orthopedic surgery are NOT coded with Z47.89. Z codes are not appropriate for fractures of any kind. Code the fracture with 7th character D for fractures undergoing surgical repair.

CODING TIPS✓ M84.5 indicates pathological fractures related to a neoplasm, most likely a primary or secondary neoplasm to the bone. A fracture in a bone with a primary or secondary neoplasm is assumed a neoplastic fracture by the classification. The neoplasm is also coded and sequenced depending on the focus of care.

DEFINITION A break resulting from metastatic invasion or tumor growth that destroys normal bone mass, resulting in fracture without obvious trauma to the bone.

M84.50X- Pathological fracture in neoplastic disease, unspecified site

M84.51 Pathological fracture in neoplastic disease, shoulder

M84.511- Pathological fracture in neoplastic disease, right shoulder

M84.512- Pathological fracture in neoplastic disease, left shoulder

M84.519- Pathological fracture in neoplastic disease, unspecified shoulder

M84.52 Pathological fracture in neoplastic disease, humerus

M84.521- Pathological fracture in neoplastic disease, right humerus

M84.522- Pathological fracture in neoplastic disease, left humerus

M84.529- Pathological fracture in neoplastic disease, unspecified humerus

M84.53 Pathological fracture in neoplastic disease, ulna and radius

M84.531- Pathological fracture in neoplastic disease, right ulna

M84.532- Pathological fracture in neoplastic disease, left ulna

M84.533- Pathological fracture in neoplastic disease, right radius

M84.534- Pathological fracture in neoplastic disease, left radius

M84.539- Pathological fracture in neoplastic disease, unspecified ulna and radius

M84.54 Pathological fracture in neoplastic disease, hand

M84.541- Pathological fracture in neoplastic disease, right hand

M84.542- Pathological fracture in neoplastic disease, left hand

M84.549- Pathological fracture in neoplastic disease, unspecified hand

M84.55 Pathological fracture in neoplastic disease, pelvis and femur

M84.550- Pathological fracture in neoplastic disease, pelvis

M84.551- Pathological fracture in neoplastic disease, right femur

M84.552- Pathological fracture in neoplastic disease, left femur

M84.553- Pathological fracture in neoplastic disease, unspecified femur

M84.559- Pathological fracture in neoplastic disease, hip, unspecified

M84.56 Pathological fracture in neoplastic disease, tibia and fibula

M84.561- Pathological fracture in neoplastic disease, right tibia

M84.562- Pathological fracture in neoplastic disease, left tibia

M84.563- Pathological fracture in neoplastic disease, right fibula

M84.564- Pathological fracture in neoplastic disease, left fibula

M84.569- Pathological fracture in neoplastic disease, unspecified tibia and fibula

M84.57 Pathological fracture in neoplastic disease, ankle and foot

M84.571- Pathological fracture in neoplastic disease, right ankle

M84.572- Pathological fracture in neoplastic disease, left ankle

M84.573- Pathological fracture in neoplastic disease, unspecified ankle

M84.574- Pathological fracture in neoplastic disease, right foot

M84.575- Pathological fracture in neoplastic disease, left foot

M84.576- Pathological fracture in neoplastic disease, unspecified foot

M84.58X- Pathological fracture in neoplastic disease, other specified site
Pathological fracture in neoplastic disease, vertebrae

M84.6 Pathological fracture in other disease
Code also:
underlying condition
EXCLUDES 1 pathological fracture in osteoporosis (M80.-)

The appropriate 7th character is to be added to each code from subcategory M84.6:

A	initial encounter for fracture
D	subsequent encounter for fracture with routine healing
G	subsequent encounter for fracture with delayed healing
K	subsequent encounter for fracture with nonunion
P	subsequent encounter for fracture with malunion
S	sequela

CODING TIPS✓ Fractures repaired by joint replacements are NOT coded with Z47.1. Fractures repaired by any other orthopedic surgery are NOT coded with Z47.89. Z codes are not appropriate for fractures of any kind. Code the fracture with 7th character D for fractures undergoing surgical repair.

M84.60X- Pathological fracture in other disease, unspecified site

M84.61 Pathological fracture in other disease, shoulder

M84.611- Pathological fracture in other disease, right shoulder

M84.612- Pathological fracture in other disease, left shoulder

M84.619- Pathological fracture in other disease, unspecified shoulder

M84.62 Pathological fracture in other disease, humerus

M84.621- Pathological fracture in other disease, right humerus

M84.622- Pathological fracture in other disease, left humerus

M84.629- Pathological fracture in other disease, unspecified humerus

M84.63 Pathological fracture in other disease, ulna and radius

M84.631- Pathological fracture in other disease, right ulna

M84.632- Pathological fracture in other disease, left ulna

M84.633- Pathological fracture in other disease, right radius

M84.634- Pathological fracture in other disease, left radius

M84.639- Pathological fracture in other disease, unspecified ulna and radius

M84.64 Pathological fracture in other disease, hand

M84.641- Pathological fracture in other disease, right hand

M84.642- Pathological fracture in other disease, left hand

M84.649- Pathological fracture in other disease, unspecified hand

M84.65 Pathological fracture in other disease, pelvis and femur

M84.650- Pathological fracture in other disease, pelvis

M84.651- Pathological fracture in other disease, right femur

M84.652- Pathological fracture in other disease, left femur

M84.653- Pathological fracture in other disease, unspecified femur

M84.659- Pathological fracture in other disease, hip, unspecified

M84.66 Pathological fracture in other disease, tibia and fibula

M84.661- Pathological fracture in other disease, right tibia

M84.662- Pathological fracture in other disease, left tibia

M84.663- Pathological fracture in other disease, right fibula

M84.664- Pathological fracture in other disease, left fibula

M84.669- Pathological fracture in other disease, unspecified tibia and fibula

M84.67 Pathological fracture in other disease, ankle and foot

M84.671- Pathological fracture in other disease, right ankle

M84.672- Pathological fracture in other disease, left ankle

⊟ IQ 7 M84.673- Pathological fracture in other disease, unspecified ankle

⊟ SP 7 M84.674- Pathological fracture in other disease, right foot

⊟ SP 7 M84.675- Pathological fracture in other disease, left foot

⊟ IQ 7 M84.676- Pathological fracture in other disease, unspecified foot

SP 7 M84.68X- Pathological fracture in other disease, other site

5 M84.7 Nontraumatic fracture, not elsewhere classified

CODING TIPS ✓ Fractures repaired by joint replacements are NOT coded with Z47.1. Fractures repaired by any other orthopedic surgery are NOT coded with Z47.89. Z codes are not appropriate for fractures of any kind. Code the fracture with 7th character D for fractures undergoing surgical repair.

6 M84.75 Atypical femoral fracture

The appropriate 7th character is to be added to each code from M84.75:
- A initial encounter for fracture
- D subsequent encounter for fracture with routine healing
- G subsequent encounter for fracture with delayed healing
- K subsequent encounter for fracture with nonunion
- P subsequent encounter for fracture with malunion
- S sequela

IQ 7 M84.750- Atypical femoral fracture, unspecified

⊟ SP 7 M84.751- Incomplete atypical femoral fracture, right leg

⊟ SP 7 M84.752- Incomplete atypical femoral fracture, left leg

⊟ IQ 7 M84.753- Incomplete atypical femoral fracture, unspecified leg

⊟ SP 7 M84.754- Complete transverse atypical femoral fracture, right leg

⊟ SP 7 M84.755- Complete transverse atypical femoral fracture, left leg

⊟ IQ 7 M84.756- Complete transverse atypical femoral fracture, unspecified leg

⊟ SP 7 M84.757- Complete oblique atypical femoral fracture, right leg

⊟ SP 7 M84.758- Complete oblique atypical femoral fracture, left leg

⊟ IQ 7 M84.759- Complete oblique atypical femoral fracture, unspecified leg

5 M84.8 Other disorders of continuity of bone

IQ M84.80 Other disorders of continuity of bone, unspecified site

6 M84.81 Other disorders of continuity of bone, shoulder

⊟ SP M84.811 Other disorders of continuity of bone, right shoulder

⊟ SP M84.812 Other disorders of continuity of bone, left shoulder

⊟ IQ M84.819 Other disorders of continuity of bone, unspecified shoulder

6 M84.82 Other disorders of continuity of bone, humerus

⊟ SP M84.821 Other disorders of continuity of bone, right humerus

⊟ SP M84.822 Other disorders of continuity of bone, left humerus

⊟ IQ M84.829 Other disorders of continuity of bone, unspecified humerus

6 M84.83 Other disorders of continuity of bone, ulna and radius

⊟ SP M84.831 Other disorders of continuity of bone, right ulna

⊟ SP M84.832 Other disorders of continuity of bone, left ulna

⊟ SP M84.833 Other disorders of continuity of bone, right radius

⊟ SP M84.834 Other disorders of continuity of bone, left radius

⊟ IQ M84.839 Other disorders of continuity of bone, unspecified ulna and radius

6 M84.84 Other disorders of continuity of bone, hand

⊟ SP M84.841 Other disorders of continuity of bone, right hand

⊟ SP M84.842 Other disorders of continuity of bone, left hand

⊟ IQ M84.849 Other disorders of continuity of bone, unspecified hand

6 M84.85 Other disorders of continuity of bone, pelvic region and thigh

⊟ SP M84.851 Other disorders of continuity of bone, right pelvic region and thigh

⊟ SP M84.852 Other disorders of continuity of bone, left pelvic region and thigh

⊟ IQ M84.859 Other disorders of continuity of bone, unspecified pelvic region and thigh

6 M84.86 Other disorders of continuity of bone, tibia and fibula

⊟ SP M84.861 Other disorders of continuity of bone, right tibia

⊟ SP M84.862 Other disorders of continuity of bone, left tibia

⊟ SP M84.863 Other disorders of continuity of bone, right fibula

⊟ SP M84.864 Other disorders of continuity of bone, left fibula

⊟ IQ M84.869 Other disorders of continuity of bone, unspecified tibia and fibula

6 M84.87 Other disorders of continuity of bone, ankle and foot

⊟ SP M84.871 Other disorders of continuity of bone, right ankle and foot

⊟ SP M84.872 Other disorders of continuity of bone, left ankle and foot

⊟ IQ M84.879 Other disorders of continuity of bone, unspecified ankle and foot

SP M84.88 Other disorders of continuity of bone, other site

IQ M84.9 Disorder of continuity of bone, unspecified

4 M85 Other disorders of bone density and structure

EXCLUDES 1 osteogenesis imperfecta (Q78.0)
osteopetrosis (Q78.2)

osteopoikilosis (Q78.8)
polyostotic fibrous dysplasia (Q78.1)

5 **M85.0 Fibrous dysplasia (monostotic)**
EXCLUDES 2 fibrous dysplasia of jaw (M27.8)

IQ **M85.00 Fibrous dysplasia (monostotic), unspecified site**

6 **M85.01 Fibrous dysplasia (monostotic), shoulder**

SP **M85.011 Fibrous dysplasia (monostotic), right shoulder**

SP **M85.012 Fibrous dysplasia (monostotic), left shoulder**

IQ **M85.019 Fibrous dysplasia (monostotic), unspecified shoulder**

6 **M85.02 Fibrous dysplasia (monostotic), upper arm**

SP **M85.021 Fibrous dysplasia (monostotic), right upper arm**

SP **M85.022 Fibrous dysplasia (monostotic), left upper arm**

IQ **M85.029 Fibrous dysplasia (monostotic), unspecified upper arm**

6 **M85.03 Fibrous dysplasia (monostotic), forearm**

SP **M85.031 Fibrous dysplasia (monostotic), right forearm**

SP **M85.032 Fibrous dysplasia (monostotic), left forearm**

IQ **M85.039 Fibrous dysplasia (monostotic), unspecified forearm**

6 **M85.04 Fibrous dysplasia (monostotic), hand**

SP **M85.041 Fibrous dysplasia (monostotic), right hand**

SP **M85.042 Fibrous dysplasia (monostotic), left hand**

IQ **M85.049 Fibrous dysplasia (monostotic), unspecified hand**

6 **M85.05 Fibrous dysplasia (monostotic), thigh**

SP **M85.051 Fibrous dysplasia (monostotic), right thigh**

SP **M85.052 Fibrous dysplasia (monostotic), left thigh**

IQ **M85.059 Fibrous dysplasia (monostotic), unspecified thigh**

6 **M85.06 Fibrous dysplasia (monostotic), lower leg**

SP **M85.061 Fibrous dysplasia (monostotic), right lower leg**

SP **M85.062 Fibrous dysplasia (monostotic), left lower leg**

IQ **M85.069 Fibrous dysplasia (monostotic), unspecified lower leg**

6 **M85.07 Fibrous dysplasia (monostotic), ankle and foot**

SP **M85.071 Fibrous dysplasia (monostotic), right ankle and foot**

SP **M85.072 Fibrous dysplasia (monostotic), left ankle and foot**

IQ **M85.079 Fibrous dysplasia (monostotic), unspecified ankle and foot**

SP **M85.08 Fibrous dysplasia (monostotic), other site**

SP **M85.09 Fibrous dysplasia (monostotic), multiple sites**

5 **M85.1 Skeletal fluorosis**

IQ **M85.10 Skeletal fluorosis, unspecified site**

6 **M85.11 Skeletal fluorosis, shoulder**

SP **M85.111 Skeletal fluorosis, right shoulder**

SP **M85.112 Skeletal fluorosis, left shoulder**

IQ **M85.119 Skeletal fluorosis, unspecified shoulder**

6 **M85.12 Skeletal fluorosis, upper arm**

SP **M85.121 Skeletal fluorosis, right upper arm**

SP **M85.122 Skeletal fluorosis, left upper arm**

IQ **M85.129 Skeletal fluorosis, unspecified upper arm**

6 **M85.13 Skeletal fluorosis, forearm**

SP **M85.131 Skeletal fluorosis, right forearm**

SP **M85.132 Skeletal fluorosis, left forearm**

IQ **M85.139 Skeletal fluorosis, unspecified forearm**

6 **M85.14 Skeletal fluorosis, hand**

SP **M85.141 Skeletal fluorosis, right hand**

SP **M85.142 Skeletal fluorosis, left hand**

IQ **M85.149 Skeletal fluorosis, unspecified hand**

6 **M85.15 Skeletal fluorosis, thigh**

SP **M85.151 Skeletal fluorosis, right thigh**

SP **M85.152 Skeletal fluorosis, left thigh**

IQ **M85.159 Skeletal fluorosis, unspecified thigh**

6 **M85.16 Skeletal fluorosis, lower leg**

SP **M85.161 Skeletal fluorosis, right lower leg**

SP **M85.162 Skeletal fluorosis, left lower leg**

IQ **M85.169 Skeletal fluorosis, unspecified lower leg**

6 **M85.17 Skeletal fluorosis, ankle and foot**

SP **M85.171 Skeletal fluorosis, right ankle and foot**

SP **M85.172 Skeletal fluorosis, left ankle and foot**

IQ **M85.179 Skeletal fluorosis, unspecified ankle and foot**

SP **M85.18 Skeletal fluorosis, other site**

SP **M85.19 Skeletal fluorosis, multiple sites**

IQ **M85.2 Hyperostosis of skull**

5 **M85.3 Osteitis condensans**

IQ **M85.30 Osteitis condensans, unspecified site**

6 **M85.31 Osteitis condensans, shoulder**

SP **M85.311 Osteitis condensans, right shoulder**

SP **M85.312 Osteitis condensans, left shoulder**

IQ **M85.319 Osteitis condensans, unspecified shoulder**

6 **M85.32 Osteitis condensans, upper arm**

SP **M85.321 Osteitis condensans, right upper arm**

SP **M85.322 Osteitis condensans, left upper arm**

IQ **M85.329 Osteitis condensans, unspecified upper arm**

6 **M85.33 Osteitis condensans, forearm**

SP **M85.331 Osteitis condensans, right forearm**

Chapter 13

M00-M99

M85.332 Osteitis condensans, left forearm
M85.339 Osteitis condensans, unspecified forearm
M85.34 Osteitis condensans, hand
M85.341 Osteitis condensans, right hand
M85.342 Osteitis condensans, left hand
M85.349 Osteitis condensans, unspecified hand
M85.35 Osteitis condensans, thigh
M85.351 Osteitis condensans, right thigh
M85.352 Osteitis condensans, left thigh
M85.359 Osteitis condensans, unspecified thigh
M85.36 Osteitis condensans, lower leg
M85.361 Osteitis condensans, right lower leg
M85.362 Osteitis condensans, left lower leg
M85.369 Osteitis condensans, unspecified lower leg
M85.37 Osteitis condensans, ankle and foot
M85.371 Osteitis condensans, right ankle and foot
M85.372 Osteitis condensans, left ankle and foot
M85.379 Osteitis condensans, unspecified ankle and foot
M85.38 Osteitis condensans, other site
M85.39 Osteitis condensans, multiple sites
M85.4 Solitary bone cyst
EXCLUDES 2 solitary cyst of jaw (M27.4)
M85.40 Solitary bone cyst, unspecified site
M85.41 Solitary bone cyst, shoulder
M85.411 Solitary bone cyst, right shoulder
M85.412 Solitary bone cyst, left shoulder
M85.419 Solitary bone cyst, unspecified shoulder
M85.42 Solitary bone cyst, humerus
M85.421 Solitary bone cyst, right humerus
M85.422 Solitary bone cyst, left humerus
M85.429 Solitary bone cyst, unspecified humerus
M85.43 Solitary bone cyst, ulna and radius
M85.431 Solitary bone cyst, right ulna and radius
M85.432 Solitary bone cyst, left ulna and radius
M85.439 Solitary bone cyst, unspecified ulna and radius
M85.44 Solitary bone cyst, hand
M85.441 Solitary bone cyst, right hand
M85.442 Solitary bone cyst, left hand
M85.449 Solitary bone cyst, unspecified hand
M85.45 Solitary bone cyst, pelvis
M85.451 Solitary bone cyst, right pelvis
M85.452 Solitary bone cyst, left pelvis
M85.459 Solitary bone cyst, unspecified pelvis
M85.46 Solitary bone cyst, tibia and fibula
M85.461 Solitary bone cyst, right tibia and fibula
M85.462 Solitary bone cyst, left tibia and fibula
M85.469 Solitary bone cyst, unspecified tibia and fibula
M85.47 Solitary bone cyst, ankle and foot
M85.471 Solitary bone cyst, right ankle and foot
M85.472 Solitary bone cyst, left ankle and foot
M85.479 Solitary bone cyst, unspecified ankle and foot
M85.48 Solitary bone cyst, other site
M85.5 Aneurysmal bone cyst
EXCLUDES 2 aneurysmal cyst of jaw (M27.4)
M85.50 Aneurysmal bone cyst, unspecified site
M85.51 Aneurysmal bone cyst, shoulder
M85.511 Aneurysmal bone cyst, right shoulder
M85.512 Aneurysmal bone cyst, left shoulder
M85.519 Aneurysmal bone cyst, unspecified shoulder
M85.52 Aneurysmal bone cyst, upper arm
M85.521 Aneurysmal bone cyst, right upper arm
M85.522 Aneurysmal bone cyst, left upper arm
M85.529 Aneurysmal bone cyst, unspecified upper arm
M85.53 Aneurysmal bone cyst, forearm
M85.531 Aneurysmal bone cyst, right forearm
M85.532 Aneurysmal bone cyst, left forearm
M85.539 Aneurysmal bone cyst, unspecified forearm
M85.54 Aneurysmal bone cyst, hand
M85.541 Aneurysmal bone cyst, right hand
M85.542 Aneurysmal bone cyst, left hand
M85.549 Aneurysmal bone cyst, unspecified hand
M85.55 Aneurysmal bone cyst, thigh
M85.551 Aneurysmal bone cyst, right thigh
M85.552 Aneurysmal bone cyst, left thigh
M85.559 Aneurysmal bone cyst, unspecified thigh
M85.56 Aneurysmal bone cyst, lower leg
M85.561 Aneurysmal bone cyst, right lower leg
M85.562 Aneurysmal bone cyst, left lower leg
M85.569 Aneurysmal bone cyst, unspecified lower leg
M85.57 Aneurysmal bone cyst, ankle and foot
M85.571 Aneurysmal bone cyst, right ankle and foot
M85.572 Aneurysmal bone cyst, left ankle and foot

6 IQ M85.579 Aneurysmal bone cyst, unspecified ankle and foot

SP M85.58 Aneurysmal bone cyst, other site

SP M85.59 Aneurysmal bone cyst, multiple sites

5 M85.6 Other cyst of bone

EXCLUDES 1 cyst of jaw NEC (M27.4)
osteitis fibrosa cystica generalisata [von Recklinghausen's disease of bone] (E21.0)

IQ M85.60 Other cyst of bone, unspecified site

6 M85.61 Other cyst of bone, shoulder

6 SP M85.611 Other cyst of bone, right shoulder

6 SP M85.612 Other cyst of bone, left shoulder

6 IQ M85.619 Other cyst of bone, unspecified shoulder

6 M85.62 Other cyst of bone, upper arm

6 SP M85.621 Other cyst of bone, right upper arm

6 SP M85.622 Other cyst of bone, left upper arm

6 IQ M85.629 Other cyst of bone, unspecified upper arm

6 M85.63 Other cyst of bone, forearm

6 SP M85.631 Other cyst of bone, right forearm

6 SP M85.632 Other cyst of bone, left forearm

6 IQ M85.639 Other cyst of bone, unspecified forearm

6 M85.64 Other cyst of bone, hand

6 SP M85.641 Other cyst of bone, right hand

6 SP M85.642 Other cyst of bone, left hand

6 IQ M85.649 Other cyst of bone, unspecified hand

6 M85.65 Other cyst of bone, thigh

6 SP M85.651 Other cyst of bone, right thigh

6 SP M85.652 Other cyst of bone, left thigh

6 IQ M85.659 Other cyst of bone, unspecified thigh

6 M85.66 Other cyst of bone, lower leg

6 SP M85.661 Other cyst of bone, right lower leg

6 SP M85.662 Other cyst of bone, left lower leg

6 IQ M85.669 Other cyst of bone, unspecified lower leg

6 M85.67 Other cyst of bone, ankle and foot

6 SP M85.671 Other cyst of bone, right ankle and foot

6 SP M85.672 Other cyst of bone, left ankle and foot

6 IQ M85.679 Other cyst of bone, unspecified ankle and foot

SP M85.68 Other cyst of bone, other site

SP M85.69 Other cyst of bone, multiple sites

5 M85.8 Other specified disorders of bone density and structure

Hyperostosis of bones, except skull
Osteosclerosis, acquired

EXCLUDES 1 diffuse idiopathic skeletal hyperostosis [DISH] (M48.1)
osteosclerosis congenita (Q77.4)
osteosclerosis fragilitas (generalista) (Q78.2)
osteosclerosis myelofibrosis (D75.81)

IQ M85.80 Other specified disorders of bone density and structure, unspecified site

6 M85.81 Other specified disorders of bone density and structure, shoulder

6 SP M85.811 Other specified disorders of bone density and structure, right shoulder

6 SP M85.812 Other specified disorders of bone density and structure, left shoulder

6 IQ M85.819 Other specified disorders of bone density and structure, unspecified shoulder

6 M85.82 Other specified disorders of bone density and structure, upper arm

6 SP M85.821 Other specified disorders of bone density and structure, right upper arm

6 SP M85.822 Other specified disorders of bone density and structure, left upper arm

6 IQ M85.829 Other specified disorders of bone density and structure, unspecified upper arm

6 M85.83 Other specified disorders of bone density and structure, forearm

6 SP M85.831 Other specified disorders of bone density and structure, right forearm

6 SP M85.832 Other specified disorders of bone density and structure, left forearm

6 IQ M85.839 Other specified disorders of bone density and structure, unspecified forearm

6 M85.84 Other specified disorders of bone density and structure, hand

6 SP M85.841 Other specified disorders of bone density and structure, right hand

6 SP M85.842 Other specified disorders of bone density and structure, left hand

6 IQ M85.849 Other specified disorders of bone density and structure, unspecified hand

6 M85.85 Other specified disorders of bone density and structure, thigh

6 SP M85.851 Other specified disorders of bone density and structure, right thigh

6 SP M85.852 Other specified disorders of bone density and structure, left thigh

6 IQ M85.859 Other specified disorders of bone density and structure, unspecified thigh

6 M85.86 Other specified disorders of bone density and structure, lower leg

6 SP M85.861 Other specified disorders of bone density and structure, right lower leg

6 SP M85.862 Other specified disorders of bone density and structure, left lower leg

6 IQ M85.869 Other specified disorders of bone density and structure, unspecified lower leg

6 **M85.87 Other specified disorders of bone density and structure, ankle and foot**

Laterality SP **M85.871 Other specified disorders of bone density and structure, right ankle and foot**

Laterality SP **M85.872 Other specified disorders of bone density and structure, left ankle and foot**

Laterality IQ **M85.879 Other specified disorders of bone density and structure, unspecified ankle and foot**

SP **M85.88 Other specified disorders of bone density and structure, other site**

SP **M85.89 Other specified disorders of bone density and structure, multiple sites**

IQ **M85.9 Disorder of bone density and structure, unspecified**

Other osteopathies (M86-M90)

EXCLUDES 1 postprocedural osteopathies (M96.-)

+ 4 **M86 Osteomyelitis**

Use additional code (B95-B97) to identify infectious agent

Use additional code to identify major osseous defect, if applicable (M89.7-)

EXCLUDES 1 osteomyelitis due to:
- echinococcus (B67.2)
- gonococcus (A54.43)
- salmonella (A02.24)

EXCLUDES 2 ostemyelitis of:
- orbit (H05.0-)
- petrous bone (H70.2-)
- vertebra (M46.2-)

CODING TIPS✓ Osteomyelitis commonly occurs in diabetic patients. When osteomyelitis occurs in a diabetic patient and the physician or NPP has not clearly stated they are unrelated, the appropriate code from E08-E13 should be assigned with 4th and 5th characters of .69 followed by the appropriate code for osteomyelitis. When the osteomyelitis does not involve the lower extremity, look carefully for a different cause other than diabetes.

CODING TIPS✓ Codes classified to M86.- do not include osteomyelitis of the orbit, petrous bone, or vertebrae. Look for other causes of the osteomyelitis in the record, besides diabetes.

+ 5 **M86.0 Acute hematogenous osteomyelitis**

IQ + **M86.00 Acute hematogenous osteomyelitis, unspecified site**

+ 6 **M86.01 Acute hematogenous osteomyelitis, shoulder**

Laterality SP + **M86.011 Acute hematogenous osteomyelitis, right shoulder**

Laterality SP + **M86.012 Acute hematogenous osteomyelitis, left shoulder**

Laterality IQ + **M86.019 Acute hematogenous osteomyelitis, unspecified shoulder**

+ 6 **M86.02 Acute hematogenous osteomyelitis, humerus**

Laterality SP + **M86.021 Acute hematogenous osteomyelitis, right humerus**

Laterality SP + **M86.022 Acute hematogenous osteomyelitis, left humerus**

Laterality IQ + **M86.029 Acute hematogenous osteomyelitis, unspecified humerus**

+ 6 **M86.03 Acute hematogenous osteomyelitis, radius and ulna**

Laterality SP + **M86.031 Acute hematogenous osteomyelitis, right radius and ulna**

Laterality SP + **M86.032 Acute hematogenous osteomyelitis, left radius and ulna**

Laterality IQ + **M86.039 Acute hematogenous osteomyelitis, unspecified radius and ulna**

+ 6 **M86.04 Acute hematogenous osteomyelitis, hand**

Laterality SP + **M86.041 Acute hematogenous osteomyelitis, right hand**

Laterality SP + **M86.042 Acute hematogenous osteomyelitis, left hand**

Laterality IQ + **M86.049 Acute hematogenous osteomyelitis, unspecified hand**

+ 6 **M86.05 Acute hematogenous osteomyelitis, femur**

Laterality SP + **M86.051 Acute hematogenous osteomyelitis, right femur**

Laterality SP + **M86.052 Acute hematogenous osteomyelitis, left femur**

Laterality IQ + **M86.059 Acute hematogenous osteomyelitis, unspecified femur**

+ 6 **M86.06 Acute hematogenous osteomyelitis, tibia and fibula**

Laterality SP + **M86.061 Acute hematogenous osteomyelitis, right tibia and fibula**

Laterality SP + **M86.062 Acute hematogenous osteomyelitis, left tibia and fibula**

Laterality IQ + **M86.069 Acute hematogenous osteomyelitis, unspecified tibia and fibula**

+ 6 **M86.07 Acute hematogenous osteomyelitis, ankle and foot**

Laterality SP + **M86.071 Acute hematogenous osteomyelitis, right ankle and foot**

Laterality SP + **M86.072 Acute hematogenous osteomyelitis, left ankle and foot**

Laterality IQ + **M86.079 Acute hematogenous osteomyelitis, unspecified ankle and foot**

SP + **M86.08 Acute hematogenous osteomyelitis, other sites**

SP + **M86.09 Acute hematogenous osteomyelitis, multiple sites**

+ 5 **M86.1 Other acute osteomyelitis**

IQ + **M86.10 Other acute osteomyelitis, unspecified site**

+ 6 **M86.11 Other acute osteomyelitis, shoulder**

Laterality SP + **M86.111 Other acute osteomyelitis, right shoulder**

Laterality SP + **M86.112 Other acute osteomyelitis, left shoulder**

Laterality IQ + **M86.119 Other acute osteomyelitis, unspecified shoulder**

+ 6 **M86.12 Other acute osteomyelitis, humerus**

Laterality SP + **M86.121 Other acute osteomyelitis, right humerus**

SP + M86.122 Other acute osteomyelitis, left humerus

IQ + M86.129 Other acute osteomyelitis, unspecified humerus

+ 6 M86.13 Other acute osteomyelitis, radius and ulna

SP + M86.131 Other acute osteomyelitis, right radius and ulna

SP + M86.132 Other acute osteomyelitis, left radius and ulna

IQ + M86.139 Other acute osteomyelitis, unspecified radius and ulna

+ 6 M86.14 Other acute osteomyelitis, hand

SP + M86.141 Other acute osteomyelitis, right hand

SP + M86.142 Other acute osteomyelitis, left hand

IQ + M86.149 Other acute osteomyelitis, unspecified hand

+ 6 M86.15 Other acute osteomyelitis, femur

SP + M86.151 Other acute osteomyelitis, right femur

SP + M86.152 Other acute osteomyelitis, left femur

IQ + M86.159 Other acute osteomyelitis, unspecified femur

+ 6 M86.16 Other acute osteomyelitis, tibia and fibula

SP + M86.161 Other acute osteomyelitis, right tibia and fibula

SP + M86.162 Other acute osteomyelitis, left tibia and fibula

IQ + M86.169 Other acute osteomyelitis, unspecified tibia and fibula

+ 6 M86.17 Other acute osteomyelitis, ankle and foot

SP + M86.171 Other acute osteomyelitis, right ankle and foot

SP + M86.172 Other acute osteomyelitis, left ankle and foot

IQ + M86.179 Other acute osteomyelitis, unspecified ankle and foot

SP + M86.18 Other acute osteomyelitis, other site

SP + M86.19 Other acute osteomyelitis, multiple sites

+ 5 M86.2 Subacute osteomyelitis

IQ + M86.20 Subacute osteomyelitis, unspecified site

+ 6 M86.21 Subacute osteomyelitis, shoulder

SP + M86.211 Subacute osteomyelitis, right shoulder

SP + M86.212 Subacute osteomyelitis, left shoulder

IQ + M86.219 Subacute osteomyelitis, unspecified shoulder

+ 6 M86.22 Subacute osteomyelitis, humerus

SP + M86.221 Subacute osteomyelitis, right humerus

SP + M86.222 Subacute osteomyelitis, left humerus

IQ + M86.229 Subacute osteomyelitis, unspecified humerus

+ 6 M86.23 Subacute osteomyelitis, radius and ulna

SP + M86.231 Subacute osteomyelitis, right radius and ulna

SP + M86.232 Subacute osteomyelitis, left radius and ulna

IQ + M86.239 Subacute osteomyelitis, unspecified radius and ulna

+ 6 M86.24 Subacute osteomyelitis, hand

SP + M86.241 Subacute osteomyelitis, right hand

SP + M86.242 Subacute osteomyelitis, left hand

IQ + M86.249 Subacute osteomyelitis, unspecified hand

+ 6 M86.25 Subacute osteomyelitis, femur

SP + M86.251 Subacute osteomyelitis, right femur

SP + M86.252 Subacute osteomyelitis, left femur

IQ + M86.259 Subacute osteomyelitis, unspecified femur

+ 6 M86.26 Subacute osteomyelitis, tibia and fibula

SP + M86.261 Subacute osteomyelitis, right tibia and fibula

SP + M86.262 Subacute osteomyelitis, left tibia and fibula

IQ + M86.269 Subacute osteomyelitis, unspecified tibia and fibula

+ 6 M86.27 Subacute osteomyelitis, ankle and foot

SP + M86.271 Subacute osteomyelitis, right ankle and foot

SP + M86.272 Subacute osteomyelitis, left ankle and foot

IQ + M86.279 Subacute osteomyelitis, unspecified ankle and foot

SP + M86.28 Subacute osteomyelitis, other site

SP + M86.29 Subacute osteomyelitis, multiple sites

+ 5 M86.3 Chronic multifocal osteomyelitis

IQ + M86.30 Chronic multifocal osteomyelitis, unspecified site

+ 6 M86.31 Chronic multifocal osteomyelitis, shoulder

SP + M86.311 Chronic multifocal osteomyelitis, right shoulder

SP + M86.312 Chronic multifocal osteomyelitis, left shoulder

IQ + M86.319 Chronic multifocal osteomyelitis, unspecified shoulder

+ 6 M86.32 Chronic multifocal osteomyelitis, humerus

SP + M86.321 Chronic multifocal osteomyelitis, right humerus

SP + M86.322 Chronic multifocal osteomyelitis, left humerus

IQ + M86.329 Chronic multifocal osteomyelitis, unspecified humerus

+ 6 M86.33 Chronic multifocal osteomyelitis, radius and ulna

SP + M86.331 Chronic multifocal osteomyelitis, right radius and ulna

SP + M86.332 Chronic multifocal osteomyelitis, left radius and ulna

IQ + M86.339 Chronic multifocal osteomyelitis, unspecified radius and ulna

+ 6 M86.34 Chronic multifocal osteomyelitis, hand

M86.341 Chronic multifocal osteomyelitis, right hand
M86.342 Chronic multifocal osteomyelitis, left hand
M86.349 Chronic multifocal osteomyelitis, unspecified hand
M86.35 Chronic multifocal osteomyelitis, femur
M86.351 Chronic multifocal osteomyelitis, right femur
M86.352 Chronic multifocal osteomyelitis, left femur
M86.359 Chronic multifocal osteomyelitis, unspecified femur
M86.36 Chronic multifocal osteomyelitis, tibia and fibula
M86.361 Chronic multifocal osteomyelitis, right tibia and fibula
M86.362 Chronic multifocal osteomyelitis, left tibia and fibula
M86.369 Chronic multifocal osteomyelitis, unspecified tibia and fibula
M86.37 Chronic multifocal osteomyelitis, ankle and foot
M86.371 Chronic multifocal osteomyelitis, right ankle and foot
M86.372 Chronic multifocal osteomyelitis, left ankle and foot
M86.379 Chronic multifocal osteomyelitis, unspecified ankle and foot
M86.38 Chronic multifocal osteomyelitis, other site
M86.39 Chronic multifocal osteomyelitis, multiple sites
M86.4 Chronic osteomyelitis with draining sinus
M86.40 Chronic osteomyelitis with draining sinus, unspecified site
M86.41 Chronic osteomyelitis with draining sinus, shoulder
M86.411 Chronic osteomyelitis with draining sinus, right shoulder
M86.412 Chronic osteomyelitis with draining sinus, left shoulder
M86.419 Chronic osteomyelitis with draining sinus, unspecified shoulder
M86.42 Chronic osteomyelitis with draining sinus, humerus
M86.421 Chronic osteomyelitis with draining sinus, right humerus
M86.422 Chronic osteomyelitis with draining sinus, left humerus
M86.429 Chronic osteomyelitis with draining sinus, unspecified humerus
M86.43 Chronic osteomyelitis with draining sinus, radius and ulna
M86.431 Chronic osteomyelitis with draining sinus, right radius and ulna
M86.432 Chronic osteomyelitis with draining sinus, left radius and ulna
M86.439 Chronic osteomyelitis with draining sinus, unspecified radius and ulna
M86.44 Chronic osteomyelitis with draining sinus, hand
M86.441 Chronic osteomyelitis with draining sinus, right hand
M86.442 Chronic osteomyelitis with draining sinus, left hand
M86.449 Chronic osteomyelitis with draining sinus, unspecified hand
M86.45 Chronic osteomyelitis with draining sinus, femur
M86.451 Chronic osteomyelitis with draining sinus, right femur
M86.452 Chronic osteomyelitis with draining sinus, left femur
M86.459 Chronic osteomyelitis with draining sinus, unspecified femur
M86.46 Chronic osteomyelitis with draining sinus, tibia and fibula
M86.461 Chronic osteomyelitis with draining sinus, right tibia and fibula
M86.462 Chronic osteomyelitis with draining sinus, left tibia and fibula
M86.469 Chronic osteomyelitis with draining sinus, unspecified tibia and fibula
M86.47 Chronic osteomyelitis with draining sinus, ankle and foot
M86.471 Chronic osteomyelitis with draining sinus, right ankle and foot
M86.472 Chronic osteomyelitis with draining sinus, left ankle and foot
M86.479 Chronic osteomyelitis with draining sinus, unspecified ankle and foot
M86.48 Chronic osteomyelitis with draining sinus, other site
M86.49 Chronic osteomyelitis with draining sinus, multiple sites
M86.5 Other chronic hematogenous osteomyelitis
M86.50 Other chronic hematogenous osteomyelitis, unspecified site
M86.51 Other chronic hematogenous osteomyelitis, shoulder
M86.511 Other chronic hematogenous osteomyelitis, right shoulder
M86.512 Other chronic hematogenous osteomyelitis, left shoulder
M86.519 Other chronic hematogenous osteomyelitis, unspecified shoulder
M86.52 Other chronic hematogenous osteomyelitis, humerus
M86.521 Other chronic hematogenous osteomyelitis, right humerus
M86.522 Other chronic hematogenous osteomyelitis, left humerus
M86.529 Other chronic hematogenous osteomyelitis, unspecified humerus
M86.53 Other chronic hematogenous osteomyelitis, radius and ulna

4th digit required | 5th digit required | 6th digit required | 7th digit required | 7th digit placeholder | + Additional code | Laterality

SP + M86.531 Other chronic hematogenous osteomyelitis, right radius and ulna
SP + M86.532 Other chronic hematogenous osteomyelitis, left radius and ulna
IQ + M86.539 Other chronic hematogenous osteomyelitis, unspecified radius and ulna
+ 6 M86.54 Other chronic hematogenous osteomyelitis, hand
SP + M86.541 Other chronic hematogenous osteomyelitis, right hand
SP + M86.542 Other chronic hematogenous osteomyelitis, left hand
IQ + M86.549 Other chronic hematogenous osteomyelitis, unspecified hand
+ 6 M86.55 Other chronic hematogenous osteomyelitis, femur
SP + M86.551 Other chronic hematogenous osteomyelitis, right femur
SP + M86.552 Other chronic hematogenous osteomyelitis, left femur
IQ + M86.559 Other chronic hematogenous osteomyelitis, unspecified femur
+ 6 M86.56 Other chronic hematogenous osteomyelitis, tibia and fibula
SP + M86.561 Other chronic hematogenous osteomyelitis, right tibia and fibula
SP + M86.562 Other chronic hematogenous osteomyelitis, left tibia and fibula
IQ + M86.569 Other chronic hematogenous osteomyelitis, unspecified tibia and fibula
+ 6 M86.57 Other chronic hematogenous osteomyelitis, ankle and foot
SP + M86.571 Other chronic hematogenous osteomyelitis, right ankle and foot
SP + M86.572 Other chronic hematogenous osteomyelitis, left ankle and foot
IQ + M86.579 Other chronic hematogenous osteomyelitis, unspecified ankle and foot
SP + M86.58 Other chronic hematogenous osteomyelitis, other site
SP + M86.59 Other chronic hematogenous osteomyelitis, multiple sites
+ 5 M86.6 Other chronic osteomyelitis
IQ + M86.60 Other chronic osteomyelitis, unspecified site
+ 6 M86.61 Other chronic osteomyelitis, shoulder
SP + M86.611 Other chronic osteomyelitis, right shoulder
SP + M86.612 Other chronic osteomyelitis, left shoulder
IQ + M86.619 Other chronic osteomyelitis, unspecified shoulder
+ 6 M86.62 Other chronic osteomyelitis, humerus
SP + M86.621 Other chronic osteomyelitis, right humerus
SP + M86.622 Other chronic osteomyelitis, left humerus
IQ + M86.629 Other chronic osteomyelitis, unspecified humerus
+ 6 M86.63 Other chronic osteomyelitis, radius and ulna
SP + M86.631 Other chronic osteomyelitis, right radius and ulna
SP + M86.632 Other chronic osteomyelitis, left radius and ulna
IQ + M86.639 Other chronic osteomyelitis, unspecified radius and ulna
+ 6 M86.64 Other chronic osteomyelitis, hand
SP + M86.641 Other chronic osteomyelitis, right hand
SP + M86.642 Other chronic osteomyelitis, left hand
IQ + M86.649 Other chronic osteomyelitis, unspecified hand
+ 6 M86.65 Other chronic osteomyelitis, thigh
SP + M86.651 Other chronic osteomyelitis, right thigh
SP + M86.652 Other chronic osteomyelitis, left thigh
IQ + M86.659 Other chronic osteomyelitis, unspecified thigh
+ 6 M86.66 Other chronic osteomyelitis, tibia and fibula
SP + M86.661 Other chronic osteomyelitis, right tibia and fibula
SP + M86.662 Other chronic osteomyelitis, left tibia and fibula
IQ + M86.669 Other chronic osteomyelitis, unspecified tibia and fibula
+ 6 M86.67 Other chronic osteomyelitis, ankle and foot
SP + M86.671 Other chronic osteomyelitis, right ankle and foot
SP + M86.672 Other chronic osteomyelitis, left ankle and foot
IQ + M86.679 Other chronic osteomyelitis, unspecified ankle and foot
SP + M86.68 Other chronic osteomyelitis, other site
SP + M86.69 Other chronic osteomyelitis, multiple sites
+ 5 M86.8 Other osteomyelitis
Brodie's abscess
+ 6 M86.8X Other osteomyelitis
SP + M86.8X0 Other osteomyelitis, multiple sites
SP + M86.8X1 Other osteomyelitis, shoulder
SP + M86.8X2 Other osteomyelitis, upper arm
SP + M86.8X3 Other osteomyelitis, forearm
SP + M86.8X4 Other osteomyelitis, hand
SP + M86.8X5 Other osteomyelitis, thigh
SP + M86.8X6 Other osteomyelitis, lower leg
SP + M86.8X7 Other osteomyelitis, ankle and foot
SP + M86.8X8 Other osteomyelitis, other site
SP + M86.8X9 Other osteomyelitis, unspecified sites
IQ + M86.9 Osteomyelitis, unspecified
Infection of bone NOS
Periostitis without osteomyelitis
+ 4 M87 Osteonecrosis
INCLUDES avascular necrosis of bone
Use additional code to identify major osseous defect, if applicable (M89.7-)

EXCLUDES 1 juvenile osteonecrosis (M91-M92)
osteochondropathies (M90-M93)

GUIDELINES **Section I.C.13.a.1)**
For certain conditions, the bone may be affected at the upper or lower end, (e.g., avascular necrosis of bone, M87, Osteoporosis, M80, M81). Though the portion of the bone affected may be at the joint, the site designation will be the bone, not the joint.

CODING TIPS✓ **Documentation:** Osteonecrosis also may be termed avascular necrosis or aseptic necrosis of the bone. The condition indicates a necrosis of bone due to impaired blood supply and may be related to trauma, use of drugs or another cause. Review documentation carefully to determine if a causative condition is known.

DEFINITION The death of bone tissue from an interruption of its blood supply.

+ 5 M87.0 Idiopathic aseptic necrosis of bone

DEFINITION The death of bone tissue from ischemia of unknown cause.

!Q + M87.00 Idiopathic aseptic necrosis of unspecified bone

+ 6 M87.01 Idiopathic aseptic necrosis of shoulder
Idiopathic aseptic necrosis of clavicle and scapula

L !Q + M87.011 Idiopathic aseptic necrosis of right shoulder
L SP + M87.012 Idiopathic aseptic necrosis of left shoulder
L !Q + M87.019 Idiopathic aseptic necrosis of unspecified shoulder

+ 6 M87.02 Idiopathic aseptic necrosis of humerus

L SP + M87.021 Idiopathic aseptic necrosis of right humerus
L SP + M87.022 Idiopathic aseptic necrosis of left humerus
L !Q + M87.029 Idiopathic aseptic necrosis of unspecified humerus

+ 6 M87.03 Idiopathic aseptic necrosis of radius, ulna and carpus

L SP + M87.031 Idiopathic aseptic necrosis of right radius
L SP + M87.032 Idiopathic aseptic necrosis of left radius
L !Q + M87.033 Idiopathic aseptic necrosis of unspecified radius
L SP + M87.034 Idiopathic aseptic necrosis of right ulna
L SP + M87.035 Idiopathic aseptic necrosis of left ulna
L !Q + M87.036 Idiopathic aseptic necrosis of unspecified ulna
L SP + M87.037 Idiopathic aseptic necrosis of right carpus
L SP + M87.038 Idiopathic aseptic necrosis of left carpus
L !Q + M87.039 Idiopathic aseptic necrosis of unspecified carpus

+ 6 M87.04 Idiopathic aseptic necrosis of hand and fingers
Idiopathic aseptic necrosis of metacarpals and phalanges of hands

L SP + M87.041 Idiopathic aseptic necrosis of right hand
L SP + M87.042 Idiopathic aseptic necrosis of left hand
L !Q + M87.043 Idiopathic aseptic necrosis of unspecified hand
L SP + M87.044 Idiopathic aseptic necrosis of right finger(s)
L SP + M87.045 Idiopathic aseptic necrosis of left finger(s)
L !Q + M87.046 Idiopathic aseptic necrosis of unspecified finger(s)

+ 6 M87.05 Idiopathic aseptic necrosis of pelvis and femur

L SP + M87.050 Idiopathic aseptic necrosis of pelvis
L SP + M87.051 Idiopathic aseptic necrosis of right femur
L SP + M87.052 Idiopathic aseptic necrosis of left femur
L !Q + M87.059 Idiopathic aseptic necrosis of unspecified femur
Idiopathic aseptic necrosis of hip NOS

+ 6 M87.06 Idiopathic aseptic necrosis of tibia and fibula

L SP + M87.061 Idiopathic aseptic necrosis of right tibia
L SP + M87.062 Idiopathic aseptic necrosis of left tibia
L !Q + M87.063 Idiopathic aseptic necrosis of unspecified tibia
L SP + M87.064 Idiopathic aseptic necrosis of right fibula
L SP + M87.065 Idiopathic aseptic necrosis of left fibula
L !Q + M87.066 Idiopathic aseptic necrosis of unspecified fibula

+ 6 M87.07 Idiopathic aseptic necrosis of ankle, foot and toes
Idiopathic aseptic necrosis of metatarsus, tarsus, and phalanges of toes

L SP + M87.071 Idiopathic aseptic necrosis of right ankle
L SP + M87.072 Idiopathic aseptic necrosis of left ankle
L !Q + M87.073 Idiopathic aseptic necrosis of unspecified ankle
L SP + M87.074 Idiopathic aseptic necrosis of right foot
L SP + M87.075 Idiopathic aseptic necrosis of left foot
L !Q + M87.076 Idiopathic aseptic necrosis of unspecified foot
L SP + M87.077 Idiopathic aseptic necrosis of right toe(s)
L SP + M87.078 Idiopathic aseptic necrosis of left toe(s)
L !Q + M87.079 Idiopathic aseptic necrosis of unspecified toe(s)

SP + M87.08 Idiopathic aseptic necrosis of bone, other site
SP + M87.09 Idiopathic aseptic necrosis of bone, multiple sites

+ 5 **M87.1 Osteonecrosis due to drugs**
Use additional code for adverse effect, if applicable, to identify drug (T36-T50 with fifth or sixth character 5)

IQ + **M87.10** Osteonecrosis due to drugs, unspecified bone

+ 6 **M87.11 Osteonecrosis due to drugs, shoulder**

SP + **M87.111** Osteonecrosis due to drugs, right shoulder

SP + **M87.112** Osteonecrosis due to drugs, left shoulder

IQ + **M87.119** Osteonecrosis due to drugs, unspecified shoulder

+ 6 **M87.12 Osteonecrosis due to drugs, humerus**

SP + **M87.121** Osteonecrosis due to drugs, right humerus

SP + **M87.122** Osteonecrosis due to drugs, left humerus

IQ + **M87.129** Osteonecrosis due to drugs, unspecified humerus

+ 6 **M87.13 Osteonecrosis due to drugs of radius, ulna and carpus**

SP + **M87.131** Osteonecrosis due to drugs of right radius

SP + **M87.132** Osteonecrosis due to drugs of left radius

IQ + **M87.133** Osteonecrosis due to drugs of unspecified radius

SP + **M87.134** Osteonecrosis due to drugs of right ulna

SP + **M87.135** Osteonecrosis due to drugs of left ulna

IQ + **M87.136** Osteonecrosis due to drugs of unspecified ulna

SP + **M87.137** Osteonecrosis due to drugs of right carpus

SP + **M87.138** Osteonecrosis due to drugs of left carpus

IQ + **M87.139** Osteonecrosis due to drugs of unspecified carpus

+ 6 **M87.14 Osteonecrosis due to drugs, hand and fingers**

SP + **M87.141** Osteonecrosis due to drugs, right hand

SP + **M87.142** Osteonecrosis due to drugs, left hand

IQ + **M87.143** Osteonecrosis due to drugs, unspecified hand

SP + **M87.144** Osteonecrosis due to drugs, right finger(s)

SP + **M87.145** Osteonecrosis due to drugs, left finger(s)

IQ + **M87.146** Osteonecrosis due to drugs, unspecified finger(s)

+ 6 **M87.15 Osteonecrosis due to drugs, pelvis and femur**

SP + **M87.150** Osteonecrosis due to drugs, pelvis

SP + **M87.151** Osteonecrosis due to drugs, right femur

SP + **M87.152** Osteonecrosis due to drugs, left femur

IQ + **M87.159** Osteonecrosis due to drugs, unspecified femur

+ 6 **M87.16 Osteonecrosis due to drugs, tibia and fibula**

SP + **M87.161** Osteonecrosis due to drugs, right tibia

SP + **M87.162** Osteonecrosis due to drugs, left tibia

IQ + **M87.163** Osteonecrosis due to drugs, unspecified tibia

SP + **M87.164** Osteonecrosis due to drugs, right fibula

SP + **M87.165** Osteonecrosis due to drugs, left fibula

IQ + **M87.166** Osteonecrosis due to drugs, unspecified fibula

+ 6 **M87.17 Osteonecrosis due to drugs, ankle, foot and toes**

SP + **M87.171** Osteonecrosis due to drugs, right ankle

SP + **M87.172** Osteonecrosis due to drugs, left ankle

IQ + **M87.173** Osteonecrosis due to drugs, unspecified ankle

SP + **M87.174** Osteonecrosis due to drugs, right foot

SP + **M87.175** Osteonecrosis due to drugs, left foot

IQ + **M87.176** Osteonecrosis due to drugs, unspecified foot

SP + **M87.177** Osteonecrosis due to drugs, right toe(s)

SP + **M87.178** Osteonecrosis due to drugs, left toe(s)

IQ + **M87.179** Osteonecrosis due to drugs, unspecified toe(s)

+ 6 **M87.18 Osteonecrosis due to drugs, other site**

SP + **M87.180** Osteonecrosis due to drugs, jaw

SP + **M87.188** Osteonecrosis due to drugs, other site

SP + **M87.19** Osteonecrosis due to drugs, multiple sites

+ 5 **M87.2 Osteonecrosis due to previous trauma**

IQ + **M87.20** Osteonecrosis due to previous trauma, unspecified bone

+ 6 **M87.21 Osteonecrosis due to previous trauma, shoulder**

SP + **M87.211** Osteonecrosis due to previous trauma, right shoulder

SP + **M87.212** Osteonecrosis due to previous trauma, left shoulder

IQ + **M87.219** Osteonecrosis due to previous trauma, unspecified shoulder

+ 6 **M87.22 Osteonecrosis due to previous trauma, humerus**

SP + **M87.221** Osteonecrosis due to previous trauma, right humerus

SP + **M87.222** Osteonecrosis due to previous trauma, left humerus

IQ + **M87.229** Osteonecrosis due to previous trauma, unspecified humerus

+ 6 **M87.23 Osteonecrosis due to previous trauma of radius, ulna and carpus**

SP + **M87.231** Osteonecrosis due to previous trauma of right radius

SP + **M87.232** Osteonecrosis due to previous trauma of left radius

IQ + **M87.233** Osteonecrosis due to previous trauma of unspecified radius

⊟ SP + M87.234 Osteonecrosis due to previous trauma of right ulna

⊟ SP + M87.235 Osteonecrosis due to previous trauma of left ulna

⊟ !Q + M87.236 Osteonecrosis due to previous trauma of unspecified ulna

⊟ SP + M87.237 Osteonecrosis due to previous trauma of right carpus

⊟ SP + M87.238 Osteonecrosis due to previous trauma of left carpus

⊟ !Q + M87.239 Osteonecrosis due to previous trauma of unspecified carpus

+ 6 M87.24 Osteonecrosis due to previous trauma, hand and fingers

⊟ SP + M87.241 Osteonecrosis due to previous trauma, right hand

⊟ SP + M87.242 Osteonecrosis due to previous trauma, left hand

⊟ !Q + M87.243 Osteonecrosis due to previous trauma, unspecified hand

⊟ SP + M87.244 Osteonecrosis due to previous trauma, right finger(s)

⊟ SP + M87.245 Osteonecrosis due to previous trauma, left finger(s)

⊟ !Q + M87.246 Osteonecrosis due to previous trauma, unspecified finger(s)

+ 6 M87.25 Osteonecrosis due to previous trauma, pelvis and femur

⊟ SP + M87.250 Osteonecrosis due to previous trauma, pelvis

⊟ SP + M87.251 Osteonecrosis due to previous trauma, right femur

⊟ SP + M87.252 Osteonecrosis due to previous trauma, left femur

⊟ !Q + M87.256 Osteonecrosis due to previous trauma, unspecified femur

+ 6 M87.26 Osteonecrosis due to previous trauma, tibia and fibula

⊟ SP + M87.261 Osteonecrosis due to previous trauma, right tibia

⊟ SP + M87.262 Osteonecrosis due to previous trauma, left tibia

⊟ !Q + M87.263 Osteonecrosis due to previous trauma, unspecified tibia

⊟ SP + M87.264 Osteonecrosis due to previous trauma, right fibula

⊟ SP + M87.265 Osteonecrosis due to previous trauma, left fibula

⊟ !Q + M87.266 Osteonecrosis due to previous trauma, unspecified fibula

+ 6 M87.27 Osteonecrosis due to previous trauma, ankle, foot and toes

⊟ SP + M87.271 Osteonecrosis due to previous trauma, right ankle

⊟ SP + M87.272 Osteonecrosis due to previous trauma, left ankle

⊟ !Q + M87.273 Osteonecrosis due to previous trauma, unspecified ankle

⊟ SP + M87.274 Osteonecrosis due to previous trauma, right foot

⊟ SP + M87.275 Osteonecrosis due to previous trauma, left foot

⊟ !Q + M87.276 Osteonecrosis due to previous trauma, unspecified foot

⊟ SP + M87.277 Osteonecrosis due to previous trauma, right toe(s)

⊟ SP + M87.278 Osteonecrosis due to previous trauma, left toe(s)

⊟ !Q + M87.279 Osteonecrosis due to previous trauma, unspecified toe(s)

SP + M87.28 Osteonecrosis due to previous trauma, other site

SP + M87.29 Osteonecrosis due to previous trauma, multiple sites

+ 5 M87.3 Other secondary osteonecrosis

!Q + M87.30 Other secondary osteonecrosis, unspecified bone

+ 6 M87.31 Other secondary osteonecrosis, shoulder

⊟ SP + M87.311 Other secondary osteonecrosis, right shoulder

⊟ SP + M87.312 Other secondary osteonecrosis, left shoulder

⊟ !Q + M87.319 Other secondary osteonecrosis, unspecified shoulder

+ 6 M87.32 Other secondary osteonecrosis, humerus

⊟ SP + M87.321 Other secondary osteonecrosis, right humerus

⊟ SP + M87.322 Other secondary osteonecrosis, left humerus

⊟ !Q + M87.329 Other secondary osteonecrosis, unspecified humerus

+ 6 M87.33 Other secondary osteonecrosis of radius, ulna and carpus

⊟ SP + M87.331 Other secondary osteonecrosis of right radius

⊟ SP + M87.332 Other secondary osteonecrosis of left radius

⊟ !Q + M87.333 Other secondary osteonecrosis of unspecified radius

⊟ SP + M87.334 Other secondary osteonecrosis of right ulna

⊟ SP + M87.335 Other secondary osteonecrosis of left ulna

⊟ !Q + M87.336 Other secondary osteonecrosis of unspecified ulna

⊟ SP + M87.337 Other secondary osteonecrosis of right carpus

⊟ SP + M87.338 Other secondary osteonecrosis of left carpus

⊟ !Q + M87.339 Other secondary osteonecrosis of unspecified carpus

+ 6 M87.34 Other secondary osteonecrosis, hand and fingers

⊟ SP + M87.341 Other secondary osteonecrosis, right hand

⊟ SP + M87.342 Other secondary osteonecrosis, left hand

⊟ !Q + M87.343 Other secondary osteonecrosis, unspecified hand

⊟ SP + M87.344 Other secondary osteonecrosis, right finger(s)

⊟ SP + M87.345 Other secondary osteonecrosis, left finger(s)

⊟ !Q + M87.346 Other secondary osteonecrosis, unspecified finger(s)

+ 6 M87.35 Other secondary osteonecrosis, pelvis and femur

⊟ SP + M87.350 Other secondary osteonecrosis, pelvis

SP + M87.351 Other secondary osteonecrosis, right femur
SP + M87.352 Other secondary osteonecrosis, left femur
IQ + M87.353 Other secondary osteonecrosis, unspecified femur
+ 6 M87.36 Other secondary osteonecrosis, tibia and fibula
SP + M87.361 Other secondary osteonecrosis, right tibia
SP + M87.362 Other secondary osteonecrosis, left tibia
IQ + M87.363 Other secondary osteonecrosis, unspecified tibia
SP + M87.364 Other secondary osteonecrosis, right fibula
SP + M87.365 Other secondary osteonecrosis, left fibula
IQ + M87.366 Other secondary osteonecrosis, unspecified fibula
+ 6 M87.37 Other secondary osteonecrosis, ankle and foot
SP + M87.371 Other secondary osteonecrosis, right ankle
SP + M87.372 Other secondary osteonecrosis, left ankle
IQ + M87.373 Other secondary osteonecrosis, unspecified ankle
SP + M87.374 Other secondary osteonecrosis, right foot
SP + M87.375 Other secondary osteonecrosis, left foot
IQ + M87.376 Other secondary osteonecrosis, unspecified foot
SP + M87.377 Other secondary osteonecrosis, right toe(s)
SP + M87.378 Other secondary osteonecrosis, left toe(s)
IQ + M87.379 Other secondary osteonecrosis, unspecified toe(s)
SP + M87.38 Other secondary osteonecrosis, other site
SP + M87.39 Other secondary osteonecrosis, multiple sites
+ 5 M87.8 Other osteonecrosis
IQ + M87.80 Other osteonecrosis, unspecified bone
+ 6 M87.81 Other osteonecrosis, shoulder
SP + M87.811 Other osteonecrosis, right shoulder
SP + M87.812 Other osteonecrosis, left shoulder
IQ + M87.819 Other osteonecrosis, unspecified shoulder
+ 6 M87.82 Other osteonecrosis, humerus
SP + M87.821 Other osteonecrosis, right humerus
SP + M87.822 Other osteonecrosis, left humerus
IQ + M87.829 Other osteonecrosis, unspecified humerus
+ 6 M87.83 Other osteonecrosis of radius, ulna and carpus
SP + M87.831 Other osteonecrosis of right radius
SP + M87.832 Other osteonecrosis of left radius
IQ + M87.833 Other osteonecrosis of unspecified radius
SP + M87.834 Other osteonecrosis of right ulna
SP + M87.835 Other osteonecrosis of left ulna
IQ + M87.836 Other osteonecrosis of unspecified ulna
SP + M87.837 Other osteonecrosis of right carpus
SP + M87.838 Other osteonecrosis of left carpus
IQ + M87.839 Other osteonecrosis of unspecified carpus
+ 6 M87.84 Other osteonecrosis, hand and fingers
SP + M87.841 Other osteonecrosis, right hand
SP + M87.842 Other osteonecrosis, left hand
IQ + M87.843 Other osteonecrosis, unspecified hand
SP + M87.844 Other osteonecrosis, right finger(s)
SP + M87.845 Other osteonecrosis, left finger(s)
IQ + M87.849 Other osteonecrosis, unspecified finger(s)
+ 6 M87.85 Other osteonecrosis, pelvis and femur
SP + M87.850 Other osteonecrosis, pelvis
SP + M87.851 Other osteonecrosis, right femur
SP + M87.852 Other osteonecrosis, left femur
IQ + M87.859 Other osteonecrosis, unspecified femur
+ 6 M87.86 Other osteonecrosis, tibia and fibula
SP + M87.861 Other osteonecrosis, right tibia
SP + M87.862 Other osteonecrosis, left tibia
IQ + M87.863 Other osteonecrosis, unspecified tibia
SP + M87.864 Other osteonecrosis, right fibula
SP + M87.865 Other osteonecrosis, left fibula
IQ + M87.869 Other osteonecrosis, unspecified fibula
+ 6 M87.87 Other osteonecrosis, ankle, foot and toes
SP + M87.871 Other osteonecrosis, right ankle
SP + M87.872 Other osteonecrosis, left ankle
IQ + M87.873 Other osteonecrosis, unspecified ankle
SP + M87.874 Other osteonecrosis, right foot
SP + M87.875 Other osteonecrosis, left foot
IQ + M87.876 Other osteonecrosis, unspecified foot
SP + M87.877 Other osteonecrosis, right toe(s)
SP + M87.878 Other osteonecrosis, left toe(s)
IQ + M87.879 Other osteonecrosis, unspecified toe(s)
SP + M87.88 Other osteonecrosis, other site
SP + M87.89 Other osteonecrosis, multiple sites
IQ + M87.9 Osteonecrosis, unspecified
Necrosis of bone NOS
4 M88 Osteitis deformans [Paget's disease of bone]
EXCLUDES 1 osteitis deformans in neoplastic disease (M90.6)

DEFINITION A bone disorder characterized by cycles of bone loss followed by excessive attempts at repair; results in painful, deformed, enlarged bones of porous tissue prone to fractures and arthritic affected joints.

SP **M88.0 Osteitis deformans of skull**

DEFINITION Excessive breakdown and rebuilding of bone tissue in the skull, resulting in an enlarged head with abnormally remodeled skull bones that may press on nerves causing headache, vertigo, tinnitus, or hearing loss.

SP **M88.1 Osteitis deformans of vertebrae**

DEFINITION Excessive breakdown and rebuilding of the vertebrae with bone material that is less dense, resulting in an abnormally remodeled, thickened spine prone to fracture that may compress nerve roots causing pain, numbness, and tingling in arms or legs.

5 **M88.8 Osteitis deformans of other bones**

6 **M88.81 Osteitis deformans of shoulder**

⊟ SP **M88.811 Osteitis deformans of right shoulder**

⊟ SP **M88.812 Osteitis deformans of left shoulder**

⊟ IQ **M88.819 Osteitis deformans of unspecified shoulder**

6 **M88.82 Osteitis deformans of upper arm**

⊟ SP **M88.821 Osteitis deformans of right upper arm**

⊟ SP **M88.822 Osteitis deformans of left upper arm**

⊟ IQ **M88.829 Osteitis deformans of unspecified upper arm**

6 **M88.83 Osteitis deformans of forearm**

⊟ SP **M88.831 Osteitis deformans of right forearm**

⊟ SP **M88.832 Osteitis deformans of left forearm**

⊟ IQ **M88.839 Osteitis deformans of unspecified forearm**

6 **M88.84 Osteitis deformans of hand**

⊟ SP **M88.841 Osteitis deformans of right hand**

⊟ SP **M88.842 Osteitis deformans of left hand**

⊟ IQ **M88.849 Osteitis deformans of unspecified hand**

6 **M88.85 Osteitis deformans of thigh**

⊟ SP **M88.851 Osteitis deformans of right thigh**

⊟ SP **M88.852 Osteitis deformans of left thigh**

⊟ IQ **M88.859 Osteitis deformans of unspecified thigh**

6 **M88.86 Osteitis deformans of lower leg**

⊟ SP **M88.861 Osteitis deformans of right lower leg**

⊟ SP **M88.862 Osteitis deformans of left lower leg**

⊟ IQ **M88.869 Osteitis deformans of unspecified lower leg**

6 **M88.87 Osteitis deformans of ankle and foot**

⊟ SP **M88.871 Osteitis deformans of right ankle and foot**

⊟ SP **M88.872 Osteitis deformans of left ankle and foot**

⊟ IQ **M88.879 Osteitis deformans of unspecified ankle and foot**

SP **M88.88 Osteitis deformans of other bones**

EXCLUDES 2 osteitis deformans of skull (M88.0)
osteitis deformans of vertebrae (M88.1)

SP **M88.89 Osteitis deformans of multiple sites**

IQ **M88.9 Osteitis deformans of unspecified bone**

4 **M89 Other disorders of bone**

5 **M89.0 Algoneurodystrophy**

Shoulder-hand syndrome
Sudeck's atrophy

EXCLUDES 1 causalgia, lower limb (G57.7-)
causalgia, upper limb (G56.4-)
complex regional pain syndrome II, lower limb (G57.7-)
complex regional pain syndrome II, upper limb (G56.4-)
reflex sympathetic dystrophy (G90.5-)

DEFINITION Acute wasting away of bone(s) following relatively minor injury; presents with severe burning pain in the affected extremity, trophic changes in bone, and vasomotor disturbances without specific nerve injury.

IQ **M89.00 Algoneurodystrophy, unspecified site**

6 **M89.01 Algoneurodystrophy, shoulder**

⊟ SP **M89.011 Algoneurodystrophy, right shoulder**

⊟ SP **M89.012 Algoneurodystrophy, left shoulder**

⊟ IQ **M89.019 Algoneurodystrophy, unspecified shoulder**

6 **M89.02 Algoneurodystrophy, upper arm**

⊟ SP **M89.021 Algoneurodystrophy, right upper arm**

⊟ SP **M89.022 Algoneurodystrophy, left upper arm**

⊟ IQ **M89.029 Algoneurodystrophy, unspecified upper arm**

6 **M89.03 Algoneurodystrophy, forearm**

⊟ SP **M89.031 Algoneurodystrophy, right forearm**

⊟ SP **M89.032 Algoneurodystrophy, left forearm**

⊟ IQ **M89.039 Algoneurodystrophy, unspecified forearm**

6 **M89.04 Algoneurodystrophy, hand**

⊟ SP **M89.041 Algoneurodystrophy, right hand**

⊟ SP **M89.042 Algoneurodystrophy, left hand**

⊟ IQ **M89.049 Algoneurodystrophy, unspecified hand**

6 **M89.05 Algoneurodystrophy, thigh**

⊟ SP **M89.051 Algoneurodystrophy, right thigh**

⊟ SP **M89.052 Algoneurodystrophy, left thigh**

⊟ IQ **M89.059 Algoneurodystrophy, unspecified thigh**

6 **M89.06 Algoneurodystrophy, lower leg**

M89.061 Algoneurodystrophy, right lower leg
M89.062 Algoneurodystrophy, left lower leg
M89.069 Algoneurodystrophy, unspecified lower leg
M89.07 Algoneurodystrophy, ankle and foot
M89.071 Algoneurodystrophy, right ankle and foot
M89.072 Algoneurodystrophy, left ankle and foot
M89.079 Algoneurodystrophy, unspecified ankle and foot
M89.08 Algoneurodystrophy, other site
M89.09 Algoneurodystrophy, multiple sites
M89.1 Physeal arrest
Arrest of growth plate
Epiphyseal arrest
Growth plate arrest
M89.12 Physeal arrest, humerus
M89.121 Complete physeal arrest, right proximal humerus
M89.122 Complete physeal arrest, left proximal humerus
M89.123 Partial physeal arrest, right proximal humerus
M89.124 Partial physeal arrest, left proximal humerus
M89.125 Complete physeal arrest, right distal humerus
M89.126 Complete physeal arrest, left distal humerus
M89.127 Partial physeal arrest, right distal humerus
M89.128 Partial physeal arrest, left distal humerus
M89.129 Physeal arrest, humerus, unspecified
M89.13 Physeal arrest, forearm
M89.131 Complete physeal arrest, right distal radius
M89.132 Complete physeal arrest, left distal radius
M89.133 Partial physeal arrest, right distal radius
M89.134 Partial physeal arrest, left distal radius
M89.138 Other physeal arrest of forearm
M89.139 Physeal arrest, forearm, unspecified
M89.15 Physeal arrest, femur
M89.151 Complete physeal arrest, right proximal femur
M89.152 Complete physeal arrest, left proximal femur
M89.153 Partial physeal arrest, right proximal femur
M89.154 Partial physeal arrest, left proximal femur
M89.155 Complete physeal arrest, right distal femur
M89.156 Complete physeal arrest, left distal femur
M89.157 Partial physeal arrest, right distal femur
M89.158 Partial physeal arrest, left distal femur
M89.159 Physeal arrest, femur, unspecified
M89.16 Physeal arrest, lower leg
M89.160 Complete physeal arrest, right proximal tibia
M89.161 Complete physeal arrest, left proximal tibia
M89.162 Partial physeal arrest, right proximal tibia
M89.163 Partial physeal arrest, left proximal tibia
M89.164 Complete physeal arrest, right distal tibia
M89.165 Complete physeal arrest, left distal tibia
M89.166 Partial physeal arrest, right distal tibia
M89.167 Partial physeal arrest, left distal tibia
M89.168 Other physeal arrest of lower leg
M89.169 Physeal arrest, lower leg, unspecified
M89.18 Physeal arrest, other site
M89.2 Other disorders of bone development and growth
M89.20 Other disorders of bone development and growth, unspecified site
M89.21 Other disorders of bone development and growth, shoulder
M89.211 Other disorders of bone development and growth, right shoulder
M89.212 Other disorders of bone development and growth, left shoulder
M89.219 Other disorders of bone development and growth, unspecified shoulder
M89.22 Other disorders of bone development and growth, humerus
M89.221 Other disorders of bone development and growth, right humerus
M89.222 Other disorders of bone development and growth, left humerus
M89.229 Other disorders of bone development and growth, unspecified humerus
M89.23 Other disorders of bone development and growth, ulna and radius
M89.231 Other disorders of bone development and growth, right ulna
M89.232 Other disorders of bone development and growth, left ulna
M89.233 Other disorders of bone development and growth, right radius
M89.234 Other disorders of bone development and growth, left radius

M89.239 Other disorders of bone development and growth, unspecified ulna and radius

M89.24 Other disorders of bone development and growth, hand

M89.241 Other disorders of bone development and growth, right hand

M89.242 Other disorders of bone development and growth, left hand

M89.249 Other disorders of bone development and growth, unspecified hand

M89.25 Other disorders of bone development and growth, femur

M89.251 Other disorders of bone development and growth, right femur

M89.252 Other disorders of bone development and growth, left femur

M89.259 Other disorders of bone development and growth, unspecified femur

M89.26 Other disorders of bone development and growth, tibia and fibula

M89.261 Other disorders of bone development and growth, right tibia

M89.262 Other disorders of bone development and growth, left tibia

M89.263 Other disorders of bone development and growth, right fibula

M89.264 Other disorders of bone development and growth, left fibula

M89.269 Other disorders of bone development and growth, unspecified lower leg

M89.27 Other disorders of bone development and growth, ankle and foot

M89.271 Other disorders of bone development and growth, right ankle and foot

M89.272 Other disorders of bone development and growth, left ankle and foot

M89.279 Other disorders of bone development and growth, unspecified ankle and foot

M89.28 Other disorders of bone development and growth, other site

M89.29 Other disorders of bone development and growth, multiple sites

M89.3 Hypertrophy of bone

M89.30 Hypertrophy of bone, unspecified site

M89.31 Hypertrophy of bone, shoulder

M89.311 Hypertrophy of bone, right shoulder

M89.312 Hypertrophy of bone, left shoulder

M89.319 Hypertrophy of bone, unspecified shoulder

M89.32 Hypertrophy of bone, humerus

M89.321 Hypertrophy of bone, right humerus

M89.322 Hypertrophy of bone, left humerus

M89.329 Hypertrophy of bone, unspecified humerus

M89.33 Hypertrophy of bone, ulna and radius

M89.331 Hypertrophy of bone, right ulna

M89.332 Hypertrophy of bone, left ulna

M89.333 Hypertrophy of bone, right radius

M89.334 Hypertrophy of bone, left radius

M89.339 Hypertrophy of bone, unspecified ulna and radius

M89.34 Hypertrophy of bone, hand

M89.341 Hypertrophy of bone, right hand

M89.342 Hypertrophy of bone, left hand

M89.349 Hypertrophy of bone, unspecified hand

M89.35 Hypertrophy of bone, femur

M89.351 Hypertrophy of bone, right femur

M89.352 Hypertrophy of bone, left femur

M89.359 Hypertrophy of bone, unspecified femur

M89.36 Hypertrophy of bone, tibia and fibula

M89.361 Hypertrophy of bone, right tibia

M89.362 Hypertrophy of bone, left tibia

M89.363 Hypertrophy of bone, right fibula

M89.364 Hypertrophy of bone, left fibula

M89.369 Hypertrophy of bone, unspecified tibia and fibula

M89.37 Hypertrophy of bone, ankle and foot

M89.371 Hypertrophy of bone, right ankle and foot

M89.372 Hypertrophy of bone, left ankle and foot

M89.379 Hypertrophy of bone, unspecified ankle and foot

M89.38 Hypertrophy of bone, other site

M89.39 Hypertrophy of bone, multiple sites

M89.4 Other hypertrophic osteoarthropathy
Marie-Bamberger disease
Pachydermoperiostosis

M89.40 Other hypertrophic osteoarthropathy, unspecified site

M89.41 Other hypertrophic osteoarthropathy, shoulder

M89.411 Other hypertrophic osteoarthropathy, right shoulder

M89.412 Other hypertrophic osteoarthropathy, left shoulder

M89.419 Other hypertrophic osteoarthropathy, unspecified shoulder

M89.42 Other hypertrophic osteoarthropathy, upper arm

M89.421 Other hypertrophic osteoarthropathy, right upper arm

M89.422 Other hypertrophic osteoarthropathy, left upper arm

4th digit required 5th digit required 6th digit required 7th digit required 7th digit placeholder +Additional code Laterality

M89.429 Other hypertrophic osteoarthropathy, unspecified upper arm

M89.43 Other hypertrophic osteoarthropathy, forearm

M89.431 Other hypertrophic osteoarthropathy, right forearm

M89.432 Other hypertrophic osteoarthropathy, left forearm

M89.439 Other hypertrophic osteoarthropathy, unspecified forearm

M89.44 Other hypertrophic osteoarthropathy, hand

M89.441 Other hypertrophic osteoarthropathy, right hand

M89.442 Other hypertrophic osteoarthropathy, left hand

M89.449 Other hypertrophic osteoarthropathy, unspecified hand

M89.45 Other hypertrophic osteoarthropathy, thigh

M89.451 Other hypertrophic osteoarthropathy, right thigh

M89.452 Other hypertrophic osteoarthropathy, left thigh

M89.459 Other hypertrophic osteoarthropathy, unspecified thigh

M89.46 Other hypertrophic osteoarthropathy, lower leg

M89.461 Other hypertrophic osteoarthropathy, right lower leg

M89.462 Other hypertrophic osteoarthropathy, left lower leg

M89.469 Other hypertrophic osteoarthropathy, unspecified lower leg

M89.47 Other hypertrophic osteoarthropathy, ankle and foot

M89.471 Other hypertrophic osteoarthropathy, right ankle and foot

M89.472 Other hypertrophic osteoarthropathy, left ankle and foot

M89.479 Other hypertrophic osteoarthropathy, unspecified ankle and foot

M89.48 Other hypertrophic osteoarthropathy, other site

M89.49 Other hypertrophic osteoarthropathy, multiple sites

+ M89.5 Osteolysis

Use additional code to identify major osseous defect, if applicable (M89.7-)

EXCLUDES 2 periprosthetic osteolysis of internal prosthetic joint (T84.05-)

+ M89.50 Osteolysis, unspecified site

+ M89.51 Osteolysis, shoulder

+ M89.511 Osteolysis, right shoulder

+ M89.512 Osteolysis, left shoulder

+ M89.519 Osteolysis, unspecified shoulder

+ M89.52 Osteolysis, upper arm

+ M89.521 Osteolysis, right upper arm

+ M89.522 Osteolysis, left upper arm

+ M89.529 Osteolysis, unspecified upper arm

+ M89.53 Osteolysis, forearm

+ M89.531 Osteolysis, right forearm

+ M89.532 Osteolysis, left forearm

+ M89.539 Osteolysis, unspecified forearm

+ M89.54 Osteolysis, hand

+ M89.541 Osteolysis, right hand

+ M89.542 Osteolysis, left hand

+ M89.549 Osteolysis, unspecified hand

+ M89.55 Osteolysis, thigh

+ M89.551 Osteolysis, right thigh

+ M89.552 Osteolysis, left thigh

+ M89.559 Osteolysis, unspecified thigh

+ M89.56 Osteolysis, lower leg

+ M89.561 Osteolysis, right lower leg

+ M89.562 Osteolysis, left lower leg

+ M89.569 Osteolysis, unspecified lower leg

+ M89.57 Osteolysis, ankle and foot

+ M89.571 Osteolysis, right ankle and foot

+ M89.572 Osteolysis, left ankle and foot

+ M89.579 Osteolysis, unspecified ankle and foot

+ M89.58 Osteolysis, other site

+ M89.59 Osteolysis, multiple sites

+ M89.6 Osteopathy after poliomyelitis

Use additional code (B91) to identify previous poliomyelitis

EXCLUDES 1 postpolio syndrome (G14)

+ M89.60 Osteopathy after poliomyelitis, unspecified site

CODING TIPS✓ Osteopathy caused by polio will be coded as a sequela of polio with code B91 as an additional code.

+ M89.61 Osteopathy after poliomyelitis, shoulder

+ M89.611 Osteopathy after poliomyelitis, right shoulder

+ M89.612 Osteopathy after poliomyelitis, left shoulder

+ M89.619 Osteopathy after poliomyelitis, unspecified shoulder

+ M89.62 Osteopathy after poliomyelitis, upper arm

+ M89.621 Osteopathy after poliomyelitis, right upper arm

+ M89.622 Osteopathy after poliomyelitis, left upper arm

+ M89.629 Osteopathy after poliomyelitis, unspecified upper arm

+ M89.63 Osteopathy after poliomyelitis, forearm

+ M89.631 Osteopathy after poliomyelitis, right forearm

+ M89.632 Osteopathy after poliomyelitis, left forearm

+ M89.639 Osteopathy after poliomyelitis, unspecified forearm

+ M89.64 Osteopathy after poliomyelitis, hand

Chapter 13

M00-M99

M89.641 Osteopathy after poliomyelitis, right hand
M89.642 Osteopathy after poliomyelitis, left hand
M89.649 Osteopathy after poliomyelitis, unspecified hand
M89.65 Osteopathy after poliomyelitis, thigh
M89.651 Osteopathy after poliomyelitis, right thigh
M89.652 Osteopathy after poliomyelitis, left thigh
M89.659 Osteopathy after poliomyelitis, unspecified thigh
M89.66 Osteopathy after poliomyelitis, lower leg
M89.661 Osteopathy after poliomyelitis, right lower leg
M89.662 Osteopathy after poliomyelitis, left lower leg
M89.669 Osteopathy after poliomyelitis, unspecified lower leg
M89.67 Osteopathy after poliomyelitis, ankle and foot
M89.671 Osteopathy after poliomyelitis, right ankle and foot
M89.672 Osteopathy after poliomyelitis, left ankle and foot
M89.679 Osteopathy after poliomyelitis, unspecified ankle and foot
M89.68 Osteopathy after poliomyelitis, other site
M89.69 Osteopathy after poliomyelitis, multiple sites
M89.7 Major osseous defect

Code first underlying disease, if known, such as:
- aseptic necrosis of bone (M87.-)
- malignant neoplasm of bone (C40.-)
- osteolysis (M89.5)
- osteomyelitis (M86.-)
- osteonecrosis (M87.-)
- osteoporosis (M80.-, M81.-)
- periprosthetic osteolysis (T84.05-)

M89.70 Major osseous defect, unspecified site
M89.71 Major osseous defect, shoulder region

Major osseous defect clavicle or scapula

M89.711 Major osseous defect, right shoulder region
M89.712 Major osseous defect, left shoulder region
M89.719 Major osseous defect, unspecified shoulder region
M89.72 Major osseous defect, humerus
M89.721 Major osseous defect, right humerus
M89.722 Major osseous defect, left humerus
M89.729 Major osseous defect, unspecified humerus
M89.73 Major osseous defect, forearm

Major osseous defect of radius and ulna

M89.731 Major osseous defect, right forearm
M89.732 Major osseous defect, left forearm
M89.739 Major osseous defect, unspecified forearm
M89.74 Major osseous defect, hand

Major osseous defect of carpus, fingers, metacarpus

M89.741 Major osseous defect, right hand
M89.742 Major osseous defect, left hand
M89.749 Major osseous defect, unspecified hand
M89.75 Major osseous defect, pelvic region and thigh

Major osseous defect of femur and pelvis

M89.751 Major osseous defect, right pelvic region and thigh
M89.752 Major osseous defect, left pelvic region and thigh
M89.759 Major osseous defect, unspecified pelvic region and thigh
M89.76 Major osseous defect, lower leg

Major osseous defect of fibula and tibia

M89.761 Major osseous defect, right lower leg
M89.762 Major osseous defect, left lower leg
M89.769 Major osseous defect, unspecified lower leg
M89.77 Major osseous defect, ankle and foot

Major osseous defect of metatarsus, tarsus, toes

M89.771 Major osseous defect, right ankle and foot
M89.772 Major osseous defect, left ankle and foot
M89.779 Major osseous defect, unspecified ankle and foot
M89.78 Major osseous defect, other site
M89.79 Major osseous defect, multiple sites
M89.8 Other specified disorders of bone

Infantile cortical hyperostoses
Post-traumatic subperiosteal ossification

M89.8X Other specified disorders of bone
M89.8X0 Other specified disorders of bone, multiple sites
M89.8X1 Other specified disorders of bone, shoulder
M89.8X2 Other specified disorders of bone, upper arm
M89.8X3 Other specified disorders of bone, forearm
M89.8X4 Other specified disorders of bone, hand
M89.8X5 Other specified disorders of bone, thigh
M89.8X6 Other specified disorders of bone, lower leg
M89.8X7 Other specified disorders of bone, ankle and foot
M89.8X8 Other specified disorders of bone, other site
M89.8X9 Other specified disorders of bone, unspecified site

4th digit required | 5th digit required | 6th digit required | 7th digit required | 7th digit placeholder | + Additional code | Laterality

IQ **M89.9** **Disorder of bone, unspecified**

4 **M90 Osteopathies in diseases classified elsewhere**

EXCLUDES 1 osteochondritis, osteomyelitis, and osteopathy (in):
cryptococcosis (B45.3)
diabetes mellitus (E08-E13 with .69-)
gonococcal (A54.43)
neurogenic syphilis (A52.11)
renal osteodystrophy (N25.0)
salmonellosis (A02.24)
secondary syphilis (A51.46)
syphilis (late) (A52.77)

5 **M90.5 Osteonecrosis in diseases classified elsewhere**

Code first underlying disease, such as:
caisson disease (T70.3)
hemoglobinopathy (D50-D64)

M IQ **M90.50** ***Osteonecrosis in diseases classified elsewhere, unspecified site***

6 **M90.51 Osteonecrosis in diseases classified elsewhere, shoulder**

M H IQ **M90.511** ***Osteonecrosis in diseases classified elsewhere, right shoulder***

M H IQ **M90.512** ***Osteonecrosis in diseases classified elsewhere, left shoulder***

M H IQ **M90.519** ***Osteonecrosis in diseases classified elsewhere, unspecified shoulder***

6 **M90.52 Osteonecrosis in diseases classified elsewhere, upper arm**

M H IQ **M90.521** ***Osteonecrosis in diseases classified elsewhere, right upper arm***

M H IQ **M90.522** ***Osteonecrosis in diseases classified elsewhere, left upper arm***

M H IQ **M90.529** ***Osteonecrosis in diseases classified elsewhere, unspecified upper arm***

6 **M90.53 Osteonecrosis in diseases classified elsewhere, forearm**

M H IQ **M90.531** ***Osteonecrosis in diseases classified elsewhere, right forearm***

M H IQ **M90.532** ***Osteonecrosis in diseases classified elsewhere, left forearm***

M H IQ **M90.539** ***Osteonecrosis in diseases classified elsewhere, unspecified forearm***

6 **M90.54 Osteonecrosis in diseases classified elsewhere, hand**

M H IQ **M90.541** ***Osteonecrosis in diseases classified elsewhere, right hand***

M H IQ **M90.542** ***Osteonecrosis in diseases classified elsewhere, left hand***

M H IQ **M90.549** ***Osteonecrosis in diseases classified elsewhere, unspecified hand***

6 **M90.55 Osteonecrosis in diseases classified elsewhere, thigh**

M H IQ **M90.551** ***Osteonecrosis in diseases classified elsewhere, right thigh***

M H IQ **M90.552** ***Osteonecrosis in diseases classified elsewhere, left thigh***

M H IQ **M90.559** ***Osteonecrosis in diseases classified elsewhere, unspecified thigh***

6 **M90.56 Osteonecrosis in diseases classified elsewhere, lower leg**

M H IQ **M90.561** ***Osteonecrosis in diseases classified elsewhere, right lower leg***

M H IQ **M90.562** ***Osteonecrosis in diseases classified elsewhere, left lower leg***

M H IQ **M90.569** ***Osteonecrosis in diseases classified elsewhere, unspecified lower leg***

6 **M90.57 Osteonecrosis in diseases classified elsewhere, ankle and foot**

M H IQ **M90.571** ***Osteonecrosis in diseases classified elsewhere, right ankle and foot***

M H IQ **M90.572** ***Osteonecrosis in diseases classified elsewhere, left ankle and foot***

M H IQ **M90.579** ***Osteonecrosis in diseases classified elsewhere, unspecified ankle and foot***

M IQ **M90.58** ***Osteonecrosis in diseases classified elsewhere, other site***

M IQ **M90.59** ***Osteonecrosis in diseases classified elsewhere, multiple sites***

5 **M90.6 Osteitis deformans in neoplastic diseases**

Osteitis deformans in malignant neoplasm of bone
Code first:
the neoplasm (C40.-, C41.-)

EXCLUDES 1 osteitis deformans [Paget's disease of bone] (M88.-)

DEFINITION Excessive breakdown with abnormal reformation of bone tissue in the presence of a malignant neoplasm of the bone; results in painful, deformed bones prone to pathological fractures.

M IQ **M90.60** ***Osteitis deformans in neoplastic diseases, unspecified site***

6 **M90.61 Osteitis deformans in neoplastic diseases, shoulder**

M H IQ **M90.611** ***Osteitis deformans in neoplastic diseases, right shoulder***

M H IQ **M90.612** ***Osteitis deformans in neoplastic diseases, left shoulder***

M H IQ **M90.619** ***Osteitis deformans in neoplastic diseases, unspecified shoulder***

6 **M90.62 Osteitis deformans in neoplastic diseases, upper arm**

M H IQ **M90.621** ***Osteitis deformans in neoplastic diseases, right upper arm***

M H IQ **M90.622** ***Osteitis deformans in neoplastic diseases, left upper arm***

M H IQ **M90.629** ***Osteitis deformans in neoplastic diseases, unspecified upper arm***

6 **M90.63 Osteitis deformans in neoplastic diseases, forearm**

M H IQ **M90.631** ***Osteitis deformans in neoplastic diseases, right forearm***

M H IQ **M90.632** ***Osteitis deformans in neoplastic diseases, left forearm***

Chapter 13

M00-M99

M ⊟ IQ **M90.639** *Osteitis deformans in neoplastic diseases, unspecified forearm*

6 **M90.64 Osteitis deformans in neoplastic diseases, hand**

M ⊟ IQ **M90.641** *Osteitis deformans in neoplastic diseases, right hand*

M ⊟ IQ **M90.642** *Osteitis deformans in neoplastic diseases, left hand*

M ⊟ IQ **M90.649** *Osteitis deformans in neoplastic diseases, unspecified hand*

6 **M90.65 Osteitis deformans in neoplastic diseases, thigh**

M ⊟ IQ **M90.651** *Osteitis deformans in neoplastic diseases, right thigh*

M ⊟ IQ **M90.652** *Osteitis deformans in neoplastic diseases, left thigh*

M ⊟ IQ **M90.659** *Osteitis deformans in neoplastic diseases, unspecified thigh*

6 **M90.66 Osteitis deformans in neoplastic diseases, lower leg**

M ⊟ IQ **M90.661** *Osteitis deformans in neoplastic diseases, right lower leg*

M ⊟ IQ **M90.662** *Osteitis deformans in neoplastic diseases, left lower leg*

M ⊟ IQ **M90.669** *Osteitis deformans in neoplastic diseases, unspecified lower leg*

6 **M90.67 Osteitis deformans in neoplastic diseases, ankle and foot**

M ⊟ IQ **M90.671** *Osteitis deformans in neoplastic diseases, right ankle and foot*

M ⊟ IQ **M90.672** *Osteitis deformans in neoplastic diseases, left ankle and foot*

M ⊟ IQ **M90.679** *Osteitis deformans in neoplastic diseases, unspecified ankle and foot*

M IQ **M90.68** *Osteitis deformans in neoplastic diseases, other site*

M IQ **M90.69** *Osteitis deformans in neoplastic diseases, multiple sites*

5 **M90.8 Osteopathy in diseases classified elsewhere**

Code first underlying disease, such as:
- rickets (E55.0)
- vitamin-D-resistant rickets (E83.3)

CODING TIPS ✓ The addition of this code is not necessary for diabetic osteomyelitis. If diabetic osteomyelitis is confirmed, use the appropriate diabetes category (E08-E13) with 4th and 5th digits .69 followed by the osteomyelitis. Query the physician or NPP if acute or chronic is not documented.

M IQ **M90.80** *Osteopathy in diseases classified elsewhere, unspecified site*

6 **M90.81 Osteopathy in diseases classified elsewhere, shoulder**

M ⊟ IQ **M90.811** *Osteopathy in diseases classified elsewhere, right shoulder*

M ⊟ IQ **M90.812** *Osteopathy in diseases classified elsewhere, left shoulder*

M ⊟ IQ **M90.819** *Osteopathy in diseases classified elsewhere, unspecified shoulder*

6 **M90.82 Osteopathy in diseases classified elsewhere, upper arm**

M ⊟ IQ **M90.821** *Osteopathy in diseases classified elsewhere, right upper arm*

M ⊟ IQ **M90.822** *Osteopathy in diseases classified elsewhere, left upper arm*

M ⊟ IQ **M90.829** *Osteopathy in diseases classified elsewhere, unspecified upper arm*

6 **M90.83 Osteopathy in diseases classified elsewhere, forearm**

M ⊟ IQ **M90.831** *Osteopathy in diseases classified elsewhere, right forearm*

M ⊟ IQ **M90.832** *Osteopathy in diseases classified elsewhere, left forearm*

M ⊟ IQ **M90.839** *Osteopathy in diseases classified elsewhere, unspecified forearm*

6 **M90.84 Osteopathy in diseases classified elsewhere, hand**

M ⊟ IQ **M90.841** *Osteopathy in diseases classified elsewhere, right hand*

M ⊟ IQ **M90.842** *Osteopathy in diseases classified elsewhere, left hand*

M ⊟ IQ **M90.849** *Osteopathy in diseases classified elsewhere, unspecified hand*

6 **M90.85 Osteopathy in diseases classified elsewhere, thigh**

M ⊟ IQ **M90.851** *Osteopathy in diseases classified elsewhere, right thigh*

M ⊟ IQ **M90.852** *Osteopathy in diseases classified elsewhere, left thigh*

M ⊟ IQ **M90.859** *Osteopathy in diseases classified elsewhere, unspecified thigh*

6 **M90.86 Osteopathy in diseases classified elsewhere, lower leg**

M ⊟ IQ **M90.861** *Osteopathy in diseases classified elsewhere, right lower leg*

M ⊟ IQ **M90.862** *Osteopathy in diseases classified elsewhere, left lower leg*

M ⊟ IQ **M90.869** *Osteopathy in diseases classified elsewhere, unspecified lower leg*

6 **M90.87 Osteopathy in diseases classified elsewhere, ankle and foot**

M ⊟ IQ **M90.871** *Osteopathy in diseases classified elsewhere, right ankle and foot*

M ⊟ IQ **M90.872** *Osteopathy in diseases classified elsewhere, left ankle and foot*

M ⊟ IQ **M90.879** *Osteopathy in diseases classified elsewhere, unspecified ankle and foot*

M IQ **M90.88** *Osteopathy in diseases classified elsewhere, other site*

M IQ **M90.89** *Osteopathy in diseases classified elsewhere, multiple sites*

Chondropathies (M91-M94)

EXCLUDES 1 postprocedural chondropathies (M96.-)

4 **M91 Juvenile osteochondrosis of hip and pelvis**

EXCLUDES 1 slipped upper femoral epiphysis (nontraumatic) (M93.0)

SP **M91.0 Juvenile osteochondrosis of pelvis**

Osteochondrosis (juvenile) of acetabulum
Osteochondrosis (juvenile) of iliac crest [Buchanan]
Osteochondrosis (juvenile) of ischiopubic synchondrosis [van Neck]

Osteochondrosis (juvenile) of symphysis pubis [Pierson]

5 **M91.1 Juvenile osteochondrosis of head of femur [Legg-Calvé-Perthes]**

DEFINITION Disruption of blood supply to the femoral head epiphysis in children, resulting in death of bone; occurs most commonly in boys age 4-8.

IQ **M91.10 Juvenile osteochondrosis of head of femur [Legg-Calvé-Perthes], unspecified leg**

SP **M91.11 Juvenile osteochondrosis of head of femur [Legg-Calvé-Perthes], right leg**

SP **M91.12 Juvenile osteochondrosis of head of femur [Legg-Calvé-Perthes], left leg**

5 **M91.2 Coxa plana**

Hip deformity due to previous juvenile osteochondrosis

DEFINITION Residual effect of Legg-Calve-Perthes in which the necrotic bone of the normally rounded femoral head is flattened due to gradual bone replacement; secondary deformity of the acetabulum occurs with growth.

IQ **M91.20 Coxa plana, unspecified hip**

SP **M91.21 Coxa plana, right hip**

SP **M91.22 Coxa plana, left hip**

5 **M91.3 Pseudocoxalgia**

IQ **M91.30 Pseudocoxalgia, unspecified hip**

SP **M91.31 Pseudocoxalgia, right hip**

SP **M91.32 Pseudocoxalgia, left hip**

5 **M91.4 Coxa magna**

DEFINITION Residual effect of Legg-Calve-Perthes in which the femoral head is enlarged, becoming broad and overgrown due to the gradual bone replacement process.

IQ **M91.40 Coxa magna, unspecified hip**

SP **M91.41 Coxa magna, right hip**

SP **M91.42 Coxa magna, left hip**

5 **M91.8 Other juvenile osteochondrosis of hip and pelvis**

Juvenile osteochondrosis after reduction of congenital dislocation of hip

IQ **M91.80 Other juvenile osteochondrosis of hip and pelvis, unspecified leg**

SP **M91.81 Other juvenile osteochondrosis of hip and pelvis, right leg**

SP **M91.82 Other juvenile osteochondrosis of hip and pelvis, left leg**

5 **M91.9 Juvenile osteochondrosis of hip and pelvis, unspecified**

IQ **M91.90 Juvenile osteochondrosis of hip and pelvis, unspecified, unspecified leg**

SP **M91.91 Juvenile osteochondrosis of hip and pelvis, unspecified, right leg**

SP **M91.92 Juvenile osteochondrosis of hip and pelvis, unspecified, left leg**

4 **M92 Other juvenile osteochondrosis**

DEFINITION Condition of unknown etiology affecting the developing growth plate and ossification centers in children where increased stress occurs; genetics, repeated trauma, mechanical factors, hormone imbalances, and vascular abnormalities may be a factor.

5 **M92.0 Juvenile osteochondrosis of humerus**

Osteochondrosis (juvenile) of capitulum of humerus [Panner]

Osteochondrosis (juvenile) of head of humerus [Haas]

IQ **M92.00 Juvenile osteochondrosis of humerus, unspecified arm**

SP **M92.01 Juvenile osteochondrosis of humerus, right arm**

SP **M92.02 Juvenile osteochondrosis of humerus, left arm**

5 **M92.1 Juvenile osteochondrosis of radius and ulna**

Osteochondrosis (juvenile) of lower ulna [Burns]

Osteochondrosis (juvenile) of radial head [Brailsford]

IQ **M92.10 Juvenile osteochondrosis of radius and ulna, unspecified arm**

SP **M92.11 Juvenile osteochondrosis of radius and ulna, right arm**

SP **M92.12 Juvenile osteochondrosis of radius and ulna, left arm**

5 **M92.2 Juvenile osteochondrosis, hand**

6 **M92.20 Unspecified juvenile osteochondrosis, hand**

SP **M92.201 Unspecified juvenile osteochondrosis, right hand**

SP **M92.202 Unspecified juvenile osteochondrosis, left hand**

IQ **M92.209 Unspecified juvenile osteochondrosis, unspecified hand**

6 **M92.21 Osteochondrosis (juvenile) of carpal lunate [Kienböck]**

SP **M92.211 Osteochondrosis (juvenile) of carpal lunate [Kienböck], right hand**

SP **M92.212 Osteochondrosis (juvenile) of carpal lunate [Kienböck], left hand**

IQ **M92.219 Osteochondrosis (juvenile) of carpal lunate [Kienböck], unspecified hand**

6 **M92.22 Osteochondrosis (juvenile) of metacarpal heads [Mauclaire]**

SP **M92.221 Osteochondrosis (juvenile) of metacarpal heads [Mauclaire], right hand**

SP **M92.222 Osteochondrosis (juvenile) of metacarpal heads [Mauclaire], left hand**

IQ **M92.229 Osteochondrosis (juvenile) of metacarpal heads [Mauclaire], unspecified hand**

6 **M92.29 Other juvenile osteochondrosis, hand**

SP **M92.291 Other juvenile osteochondrosis, right hand**

⊟ SP M92.292 **Other juvenile osteochondrosis, left hand**

⊟ IQ M92.299 **Other juvenile osteochondrosis, unspecified hand**

5 M92.3 **Other juvenile osteochondrosis, upper limb**

⊟ IQ M92.30 **Other juvenile osteochondrosis, unspecified upper limb**

⊟ SP M92.31 **Other juvenile osteochondrosis, right upper limb**

⊟ SP M92.32 **Other juvenile osteochondrosis, left upper limb**

5 M92.4 **Juvenile osteochondrosis of patella**
Osteochondrosis (juvenile) of primary patellar center [Köhler]
Osteochondrosis (juvenile) of secondary patellar centre [Sinding Larsen]

⊟ IQ M92.40 **Juvenile osteochondrosis of patella, unspecified knee**

⊟ SP M92.41 **Juvenile osteochondrosis of patella, right knee**

⊟ SP M92.42 **Juvenile osteochondrosis of patella, left knee**

5 M92.5 **Juvenile osteochondrosis of tibia and fibula**

6 M92.50 **Unspecified juvenile osteochondrosis of tibia and fibula**

⊟ SP M92.501 **Unspecified juvenile osteochondrosis, right leg**

⊟ SP M92.502 **Unspecified juvenile osteochondrosis, left leg**

⊟ SP M92.503 **Unspecified juvenile osteochondrosis, bilateral leg**

⊟ IQ M92.509 **Unspecified juvenile osteochondrosis, unspecified leg**

6 M92.51 **Juvenile osteochondrosis of proximal tibia**
Blount disease
Tibia vara

⊟ SP M92.511 **Juvenile osteochondrosis of proximal tibia, right leg**

⊟ SP M92.512 **Juvenile osteochondrosis of proximal tibia, left leg**

⊟ SP M92.513 **Juvenile osteochondrosis of proximal tibia, bilateral**

⊟ IQ M92.519 **Juvenile osteochondrosis of proximal tibia, unspecified leg**

6 M92.52 **Juvenile osteochondrosis of tibia tubercle**
Osgood-Schlatter disease

⊟ SP M92.521 **Juvenile osteochondrosis of tibia tubercle, right leg**

⊟ SP M92.522 **Juvenile osteochondrosis of tibia tubercle, left leg**

⊟ SP M92.523 **Juvenile osteochondrosis of tibia tubercle, bilateral**

⊟ IQ M92.529 **Juvenile osteochondrosis of tibia tubercle, unspecified leg**

6 M92.59 **Other juvenile osteochondrosis of tibia and fibula**

⊟ SP M92.591 **Other juvenile osteochondrosis of tibia and fibula, right leg**

⊟ SP M92.592 **Other juvenile osteochondrosis of tibia and fibula, left leg**

⊟ SP M92.593 **Other juvenile osteochondrosis of tibia and fibula, bilateral**

⊟ IQ M92.599 **Other juvenile osteochondrosis of tibia and fibula, unspecified leg**

5 M92.6 **Juvenile osteochondrosis of tarsus**
Osteochondrosis (juvenile) of calcaneum [Sever]
Osteochondrosis (juvenile) of os tibiale externum [Haglund]
Osteochondrosis (juvenile) of talus [Diaz]
Osteochondrosis (juvenile) of tarsal navicular [Köhler]

⊟ IQ M92.60 **Juvenile osteochondrosis of tarsus, unspecified ankle**

⊟ SP M92.61 **Juvenile osteochondrosis of tarsus, right ankle**

⊟ SP M92.62 **Juvenile osteochondrosis of tarsus, left ankle**

5 M92.7 **Juvenile osteochondrosis of metatarsus**
Osteochondrosis (juvenile) of fifth metatarsus [Iselin]
Osteochondrosis (juvenile) of second metatarsus [Freiberg]

⊟ IQ M92.70 **Juvenile osteochondrosis of metatarsus, unspecified foot**

⊟ SP M92.71 **Juvenile osteochondrosis of metatarsus, right foot**

⊟ SP M92.72 **Juvenile osteochondrosis of metatarsus, left foot**

SP M92.8 **Other specified juvenile osteochondrosis**
Calcaneal apophysitis

IQ M92.9 **Juvenile osteochondrosis, unspecified**
Juvenile apophysitis NOS
Juvenile epiphysitis NOS
Juvenile osteochondritis NOS
Juvenile osteochondrosis NOS

4 M93 **Other osteochondropathies**
EXCLUDES 2 osteochondrosis of spine (M42.-)

+ 5 M93.0 **Slipped upper femoral epiphysis (nontraumatic)**
Use additional code for associated chondrolysis (M94.3)
DEFINITION Nontraumatic slippage of the femoral head of the epiphysis occurring in adolescence.

+ 6 M93.00 **Unspecified slipped upper femoral epiphysis (nontraumatic)**

⊟ SP + M93.001 **Unspecified slipped upper femoral epiphysis (nontraumatic), right hip**

⊟ SP + M93.002 **Unspecified slipped upper femoral epiphysis (nontraumatic), left hip**

⊟ IQ + M93.003 **Unspecified slipped upper femoral epiphysis (nontraumatic), unspecified hip**

+ 6 M93.01 **Acute slipped upper femoral epiphysis (nontraumatic)**

⊟ SP + M93.011 **Acute slipped upper femoral epiphysis (nontraumatic), right hip**

⊟ SP + M93.012 **Acute slipped upper femoral epiphysis (nontraumatic), left hip**

⊟ IQ + M93.013 **Acute slipped upper femoral epiphysis (nontraumatic), unspecified hip**

4 4th digit required 5 5th digit required 6 6th digit required 7 7th digit required 7 7th digit placeholder + Additional code ⊟ Laterality

+ 6 **M93.02 Chronic slipped upper femoral epiphysis (nontraumatic)**
SP + **M93.021 Chronic slipped upper femoral epiphysis (nontraumatic), right hip**
SP + **M93.022 Chronic slipped upper femoral epiphysis (nontraumatic), left hip**
IQ + **M93.023 Chronic slipped upper femoral epiphysis (nontraumatic), unspecified hip**
+ 6 **M93.03 Acute on chronic slipped upper femoral epiphysis (nontraumatic)**
SP + **M93.031 Acute on chronic slipped upper femoral epiphysis (nontraumatic), right hip**
SP + **M93.032 Acute on chronic slipped upper femoral epiphysis (nontraumatic), left hip**
IQ + **M93.033 Acute on chronic slipped upper femoral epiphysis (nontraumatic), unspecified hip**
SP **M93.1 Kienböck's disease of adults**
Adult osteochondrosis of carpal lunates
DEFINITION Idiopathic disruption of blood supply to the carpal lunate bone in adults, resulting in death of the bone tissue.
5 **M93.2 Osteochondritis dissecans**
DEFINITION Joint condition in which a piece of cartilage and thin, underlying bone detaches from the bone's end; occurs most often in boys age 10-20 after a joint injury, and commonly affecting the knee.
IQ **M93.20 Osteochondritis dissecans of unspecified site**
6 **M93.21 Osteochondritis dissecans of shoulder**
SP **M93.211 Osteochondritis dissecans, right shoulder**
SP **M93.212 Osteochondritis dissecans, left shoulder**
IQ **M93.219 Osteochondritis dissecans, unspecified shoulder**
6 **M93.22 Osteochondritis dissecans of elbow**
SP **M93.221 Osteochondritis dissecans, right elbow**
SP **M93.222 Osteochondritis dissecans, left elbow**
IQ **M93.229 Osteochondritis dissecans, unspecified elbow**
6 **M93.23 Osteochondritis dissecans of wrist**
SP **M93.231 Osteochondritis dissecans, right wrist**
SP **M93.232 Osteochondritis dissecans, left wrist**
IQ **M93.239 Osteochondritis dissecans, unspecified wrist**
6 **M93.24 Osteochondritis dissecans of joints of hand**
SP **M93.241 Osteochondritis dissecans, joints of right hand**
SP **M93.242 Osteochondritis dissecans, joints of left hand**
IQ **M93.249 Osteochondritis dissecans, joints of unspecified hand**
6 **M93.25 Osteochondritis dissecans of hip**
SP **M93.251 Osteochondritis dissecans, right hip**
SP **M93.252 Osteochondritis dissecans, left hip**
IQ **M93.259 Osteochondritis dissecans, unspecified hip**
6 **M93.26 Osteochondritis dissecans knee**
SP **M93.261 Osteochondritis dissecans, right knee**
SP **M93.262 Osteochondritis dissecans, left knee**
IQ **M93.269 Osteochondritis dissecans, unspecified knee**
6 **M93.27 Osteochondritis dissecans of ankle and joints of foot**
SP **M93.271 Osteochondritis dissecans, right ankle and joints of right foot**
SP **M93.272 Osteochondritis dissecans, left ankle and joints of left foot**
IQ **M93.279 Osteochondritis dissecans, unspecified ankle and joints of foot**
SP **M93.28 Osteochondritis dissecans other site**
SP **M93.29 Osteochondritis dissecans multiple sites**
5 **M93.8 Other specified osteochondropathies**
DEFINITION Other conditions affecting bone and cartilage at any age, noted by abnormal endochondral ossification.
IQ **M93.80 Other specified osteochondropathies of unspecified site**
6 **M93.81 Other specified osteochondropathies of shoulder**
SP **M93.811 Other specified osteochondropathies, right shoulder**
SP **M93.812 Other specified osteochondropathies, left shoulder**
IQ **M93.819 Other specified osteochondropathies, unspecified shoulder**
6 **M93.82 Other specified osteochondropathies of upper arm**
SP **M93.821 Other specified osteochondropathies, right upper arm**
SP **M93.822 Other specified osteochondropathies, left upper arm**
IQ **M93.829 Other specified osteochondropathies, unspecified upper arm**
6 **M93.83 Other specified osteochondropathies of forearm**
SP **M93.831 Other specified osteochondropathies, right forearm**
SP **M93.832 Other specified osteochondropathies, left forearm**
IQ **M93.839 Other specified osteochondropathies, unspecified forearm**
6 **M93.84 Other specified osteochondropathies of hand**
SP **M93.841 Other specified osteochondropathies, right hand**

M93.842 Other specified osteochondropathies, left hand

M93.849 Other specified osteochondropathies, unspecified hand

M93.85 Other specified osteochondropathies of thigh

M93.851 Other specified osteochondropathies, right thigh

M93.852 Other specified osteochondropathies, left thigh

M93.859 Other specified osteochondropathies, unspecified thigh

M93.86 Other specified osteochondropathies lower leg

M93.861 Other specified osteochondropathies, right lower leg

M93.862 Other specified osteochondropathies, left lower leg

M93.869 Other specified osteochondropathies, unspecified lower leg

M93.87 Other specified osteochondropathies of ankle and foot

M93.871 Other specified osteochondropathies, right ankle and foot

M93.872 Other specified osteochondropathies, left ankle and foot

M93.879 Other specified osteochondropathies, unspecified ankle and foot

M93.88 Other specified osteochondropathies other

M93.89 Other specified osteochondropathies multiple sites

M93.9 Osteochondropathy, unspecified

Apophysitis NOS
Epiphysitis NOS
Osteochondritis NOS
Osteochondrosis NOS

M93.90 Osteochondropathy, unspecified of unspecified site

M93.91 Osteochondropathy, unspecified of shoulder

M93.911 Osteochondropathy, unspecified, right shoulder

M93.912 Osteochondropathy, unspecified, left shoulder

M93.919 Osteochondropathy, unspecified, unspecified shoulder

M93.92 Osteochondropathy, unspecified of upper arm

M93.921 Osteochondropathy, unspecified, right upper arm

M93.922 Osteochondropathy, unspecified, left upper arm

M93.929 Osteochondropathy, unspecified, unspecified upper arm

M93.93 Osteochondropathy, unspecified of forearm

M93.931 Osteochondropathy, unspecified, right forearm

M93.932 Osteochondropathy, unspecified, left forearm

M93.939 Osteochondropathy, unspecified, unspecified forearm

M93.94 Osteochondropathy, unspecified of hand

M93.941 Osteochondropathy, unspecified, right hand

M93.942 Osteochondropathy, unspecified, left hand

M93.949 Osteochondropathy, unspecified, unspecified hand

M93.95 Osteochondropathy, unspecified of thigh

M93.951 Osteochondropathy, unspecified, right thigh

M93.952 Osteochondropathy, unspecified, left thigh

M93.959 Osteochondropathy, unspecified, unspecified thigh

M93.96 Osteochondropathy, unspecified lower leg

M93.961 Osteochondropathy, unspecified, right lower leg

M93.962 Osteochondropathy, unspecified, left lower leg

M93.969 Osteochondropathy, unspecified, unspecified lower leg

M93.97 Osteochondropathy, unspecified of ankle and foot

M93.971 Osteochondropathy, unspecified, right ankle and foot

M93.972 Osteochondropathy, unspecified, left ankle and foot

M93.979 Osteochondropathy, unspecified, unspecified ankle and foot

M93.98 Osteochondropathy, unspecified other

M93.99 Osteochondropathy, unspecified multiple sites

M94 Other disorders of cartilage

M94.0 Chondrocostal junction syndrome [Tietze]

Costochondritis

M94.1 Relapsing polychondritis

M94.2 Chondromalacia

EXCLUDES 1 chondromalacia patellae (M22.4)

DEFINITION Joint cartilage softens and degenerates, causing tenderness, pain, and a grinding sensation.

M94.20 Chondromalacia, unspecified site

M94.21 Chondromalacia, shoulder

M94.211 Chondromalacia, right shoulder

M94.212 Chondromalacia, left shoulder

M94.219 Chondromalacia, unspecified shoulder

M94.22 Chondromalacia, elbow

M94.221 Chondromalacia, right elbow

M94.222 Chondromalacia, left elbow

- **M94.229 Chondromalacia, unspecified elbow**
- **M94.23 Chondromalacia, wrist**
- **M94.231 Chondromalacia, right wrist**
- **M94.232 Chondromalacia, left wrist**
- **M94.239 Chondromalacia, unspecified wrist**
- **M94.24 Chondromalacia, joints of hand**
- **M94.241 Chondromalacia, joints of right hand**
- **M94.242 Chondromalacia, joints of left hand**
- **M94.249 Chondromalacia, joints of unspecified hand**
- **M94.25 Chondromalacia, hip**
- **M94.251 Chondromalacia, right hip**
- **M94.252 Chondromalacia, left hip**
- **M94.259 Chondromalacia, unspecified hip**
- **M94.26 Chondromalacia, knee**

CODING TIPS Do not assign M94.26- for chondromalacia patellae (also called "runner's knee" or CMP). Chondromalacia patellae is an inflammation of the underside of the patella and is coded to M22.4.

- **M94.261 Chondromalacia, right knee**
- **M94.262 Chondromalacia, left knee**
- **M94.269 Chondromalacia, unspecified knee**
- **M94.27 Chondromalacia, ankle and joints of foot**
- **M94.271 Chondromalacia, right ankle and joints of right foot**
- **M94.272 Chondromalacia, left ankle and joints of left foot**
- **M94.279 Chondromalacia, unspecified ankle and joints of foot**
- **M94.28 Chondromalacia, other site**
- **M94.29 Chondromalacia, multiple sites**
- **M94.3 Chondrolysis**

Code first:
any associated slipped upper femoral epiphysis (nontraumatic) (M93.0-)

DEFINITION Sudden, severe damage to joint cartilage causing rapid death of normal cartilage cells and abrupt loss of the joint's cartilage layer.

- **M94.35 Chondrolysis, hip**
- **M94.351 Chondrolysis, right hip**
- **M94.352 Chondrolysis, left hip**
- **M94.359 Chondrolysis, unspecified hip**
- **M94.8 Other specified disorders of cartilage**
- **M94.8X Other specified disorders of cartilage**
- **M94.8X0 Other specified disorders of cartilage, multiple sites**
- **M94.8X1 Other specified disorders of cartilage, shoulder**
- **M94.8X2 Other specified disorders of cartilage, upper arm**
- **M94.8X3 Other specified disorders of cartilage, forearm**
- **M94.8X4 Other specified disorders of cartilage, hand**
- **M94.8X5 Other specified disorders of cartilage, thigh**
- **M94.8X6 Other specified disorders of cartilage, lower leg**
- **M94.8X7 Other specified disorders of cartilage, ankle and foot**
- **M94.8X8 Other specified disorders of cartilage, other site**
- **M94.8X9 Other specified disorders of cartilage, unspecified sites**
- **M94.9 Disorder of cartilage, unspecified**

Other disorders of the musculoskeletal system and connective tissue (M95)

- **M95 Other acquired deformities of musculoskeletal system and connective tissue**

EXCLUDES 2 acquired absence of limbs and organs (Z89-Z90)
acquired deformities of limbs (M20-M21)
congenital malformations and deformations of the musculoskeletal system (Q65-Q79)
deforming dorsopathies (M40-M43)
dentofacial anomalies [including malocclusion] (M26.-)
postprocedural musculoskeletal disorders (M96.-)

- **M95.0 Acquired deformity of nose**

EXCLUDES 2 deviated nasal septum (J34.2)

- **M95.1 Cauliflower ear**

EXCLUDES 2 other acquired deformities of ear (H61.1)

- **M95.10 Cauliflower ear, unspecified ear**
- **M95.11 Cauliflower ear, right ear**
- **M95.12 Cauliflower ear, left ear**
- **M95.2 Other acquired deformity of head**
- **M95.3 Acquired deformity of neck**
- **M95.4 Acquired deformity of chest and rib**
- **M95.5 Acquired deformity of pelvis**

EXCLUDES 1 maternal care for known or suspected disproportion (O33.-)

- **M95.8 Other specified acquired deformities of musculoskeletal system**
- **M95.9 Acquired deformity of musculoskeletal system, unspecified**

Intraoperative and postprocedural complications and disorders of musculoskeletal system, not elsewhere classified (M96)

- **M96 Intraoperative and postprocedural complications and disorders of musculoskeletal system, not elsewhere classified**

EXCLUDES 2 arthropathy following intestinal bypass (M02.0-)
complications of internal orthopedic prosthetic devices, implants and grafts (T84.-)
disorders associated with osteoporosis (M80)
periprosthetic fracture around internal prosthetic joint (M97.-)
presence of functional implants and other devices (Z96-Z97)

CODING TIPS✓ These conditions may be used in addition to complication codes found in the T chapter.

CODING TIPS✓ **Documentation:** Codes in category M96.- are complication codes and require physician or NPP documentation and confirmation of a cause and effect relationship between the procedure and the complicated condition. Documentation in the home health clinical record must also support this relationship.

SP **M96.0 Pseudarthrosis after fusion or arthrodesis**

SP **M96.1 Postlaminectomy syndrome, not elsewhere classified**

SP **M96.2 Postradiation kyphosis**

SP **M96.3 Postlaminectomy kyphosis**

SP **M96.4 Postsurgical lordosis**

SP **M96.5 Postradiation scoliosis**

5 **M96.6 Fracture of bone following insertion of orthopedic implant, joint prosthesis, or bone plate**

Intraoperative fracture of bone during insertion of orthopedic implant, joint prosthesis, or bone plate

EXCLUDES 2 complication of internal orthopedic devices, implants or grafts (T84.-)

6 **M96.62 Fracture of humerus following insertion of orthopedic implant, joint prosthesis, or bone plate**

⊟ SP **M96.621 Fracture of humerus following insertion of orthopedic implant, joint prosthesis, or bone plate, right arm**

⊟ SP **M96.622 Fracture of humerus following insertion of orthopedic implant, joint prosthesis, or bone plate, left arm**

⊟ IQ **M96.629 Fracture of humerus following insertion of orthopedic implant, joint prosthesis, or bone plate, unspecified arm**

6 **M96.63 Fracture of radius or ulna following insertion of orthopedic implant, joint prosthesis, or bone plate**

⊟ SP **M96.631 Fracture of radius or ulna following insertion of orthopedic implant, joint prosthesis, or bone plate, right arm**

⊟ SP **M96.632 Fracture of radius or ulna following insertion of orthopedic implant, joint prosthesis, or bone plate, left arm**

⊟ IQ **M96.639 Fracture of radius or ulna following insertion of orthopedic implant, joint prosthesis, or bone plate, unspecified arm**

SP **M96.65 Fracture of pelvis following insertion of orthopedic implant, joint prosthesis, or bone plate**

6 **M96.66 Fracture of femur following insertion of orthopedic implant, joint prosthesis, or bone plate**

⊟ SP **M96.661 Fracture of femur following insertion of orthopedic implant, joint prosthesis, or bone plate, right leg**

⊟ SP **M96.662 Fracture of femur following insertion of orthopedic implant, joint prosthesis, or bone plate, left leg**

⊟ IQ **M96.669 Fracture of femur following insertion of orthopedic implant, joint prosthesis, or bone plate, unspecified leg**

6 **M96.67 Fracture of tibia or fibula following insertion of orthopedic implant, joint prosthesis, or bone plate**

⊟ SP **M96.671 Fracture of tibia or fibula following insertion of orthopedic implant, joint prosthesis, or bone plate, right leg**

⊟ SP **M96.672 Fracture of tibia or fibula following insertion of orthopedic implant, joint prosthesis, or bone plate, left leg**

⊟ IQ **M96.679 Fracture of tibia or fibula following insertion of orthopedic implant, joint prosthesis, or bone plate, unspecified leg**

SP **M96.69 Fracture of other bone following insertion of orthopedic implant, joint prosthesis, or bone plate**

5 **M96.8 Other intraoperative and postprocedural complications and disorders of musculoskeletal system, not elsewhere classified**

6 **M96.81 Intraoperative hemorrhage and hematoma of a musculoskeletal structure complicating a procedure**

EXCLUDES 1 intraoperative hemorrhage and hematoma of a musculoskeletal structure due to accidental puncture and laceration during a procedure (M96.82-)

SP **M96.810 Intraoperative hemorrhage and hematoma of a musculoskeletal structure complicating a musculoskeletal system procedure**

SP **M96.811 Intraoperative hemorrhage and hematoma of a musculoskeletal structure complicating other procedure**

6 **M96.82 Accidental puncture and laceration of a musculoskeletal structure during a procedure**

SP **M96.820 Accidental puncture and laceration of a musculoskeletal structure during a musculoskeletal system procedure**

SP **M96.821 Accidental puncture and laceration of a musculoskeletal structure during other procedure**

6 **M96.83 Postprocedural hemorrhage of a musculoskeletal structure following a procedure**

SP **M96.830 Postprocedural hemorrhage of a musculoskeletal structure following a musculoskeletal system procedure**

SP **M96.831 Postprocedural hemorrhage of a musculoskeletal structure following other procedure**

6 **M96.84 Postprocedural hematoma and seroma of a musculoskeletal structure following a procedure**

SP **M96.840 Postprocedural hematoma of a musculoskeletal structure following a musculoskeletal system procedure**

SP **M96.841 Postprocedural hematoma of a musculoskeletal structure following other procedure**

SP **M96.842 Postprocedural seroma of a musculoskeletal structure following a musculoskeletal system procedure**

SP **M96.843 Postprocedural seroma of a musculoskeletal structure following other procedure**

SP + **M96.89 Other intraoperative and postprocedural complications and disorders of the musculoskeletal system**

Instability of joint secondary to removal of joint prosthesis

Use additional code, if applicable, to further specify disorder

CODING TIPS ✓ Traumatic injury codes should not be assigned for injuries that occur during, or as a result of, a medical intervention. If the patient has rib fractures as the result of chest compressions, use this code and do not code the rib fractures. Add a Y code to indicate the situation resulting in the injury. [AHA: 1Q 2021]

Periprosthetic fracture around internal prosthetic joint (M97)

4 **M97 Periprosthetic fracture around internal prosthetic joint**

EXCLUDES 2 fracture of bone following insertion of orthopedic implant, joint prosthesis or bone plate (M96.6-)

breakage (fracture) of prosthetic joint (T84.01-)

The appropriate 7th character is to be added to each code from category M97

- A initial encounter
- D subsequent encounter
- S sequela

CODING TIPS ✓ Fractures around a prosthesis are not complications of the prosthesis, but the result of the same conditions as other fractures, that is, trauma or pathological conditions. Periprosthetic fractures can occur around any prosthesis, but the most common is the hip, knee, ankle, shoulder, or elbow. The type of fracture, whether traumatic or pathologic, should also be coded.

5 **M97.0 Periprosthetic fracture around internal prosthetic hip joint**

SP **M97.01X- Periprosthetic fracture around internal prosthetic right hip joint**

SP **M97.02X- Periprosthetic fracture around internal prosthetic left hip joint**

5 **M97.1 Periprosthetic fracture around internal prosthetic knee joint**

SP **M97.11X- Periprosthetic fracture around internal prosthetic right knee joint**

SP **M97.12X- Periprosthetic fracture around internal prosthetic left knee joint**

5 **M97.2 Periprosthetic fracture around internal prosthetic ankle joint**

SP **M97.21X- Periprosthetic fracture around internal prosthetic right ankle joint**

SP **M97.22X- Periprosthetic fracture around internal prosthetic left ankle joint**

5 **M97.3 Periprosthetic fracture around internal prosthetic shoulder joint**

SP **M97.31X- Periprosthetic fracture around internal prosthetic right shoulder joint**

SP **M97.32X- Periprosthetic fracture around internal prosthetic left shoulder joint**

5 **M97.4 Periprosthetic fracture around internal prosthetic elbow joint**

SP **M97.41X- Periprosthetic fracture around internal prosthetic right elbow joint**

SP **M97.42X- Periprosthetic fracture around internal prosthetic left elbow joint**

SP + **M97.8XX- Periprosthetic fracture around other internal prosthetic joint**

Periprosthetic fracture around internal prosthetic finger joint

Periprosthetic fracture around internal prosthetic spinal joint

Periprosthetic fracture around internal prosthetic toe joint

Periprosthetic fracture around internal prosthetic wrist joint

Use additional code to identify the joint (Z96.6-)

IQ **M97.9XX- Periprosthetic fracture around unspecified internal prosthetic joint**

Biomechanical lesions, not elsewhere classified (M99)

4 **M99 Biomechanical lesions, not elsewhere classified**

Note:

This category should not be used if the condition can be classified elsewhere.

5 **M99.0 Segmental and somatic dysfunction**

SP M99.00 Segmental and somatic dysfunction of head region
SP M99.01 Segmental and somatic dysfunction of cervical region
SP M99.02 Segmental and somatic dysfunction of thoracic region
SP M99.03 Segmental and somatic dysfunction of lumbar region
SP M99.04 Segmental and somatic dysfunction of sacral region
SP M99.05 Segmental and somatic dysfunction of pelvic region
SP M99.06 Segmental and somatic dysfunction of lower extremity
SP M99.07 Segmental and somatic dysfunction of upper extremity
SP M99.08 Segmental and somatic dysfunction of rib cage
SP M99.09 Segmental and somatic dysfunction of abdomen and other regions

5 M99.1 Subluxation complex (vertebral)
SP M99.10 Subluxation complex (vertebral) of head region
SP M99.11 Subluxation complex (vertebral) of cervical region
SP M99.12 Subluxation complex (vertebral) of thoracic region
SP M99.13 Subluxation complex (vertebral) of lumbar region
SP M99.14 Subluxation complex (vertebral) of sacral region
SP M99.15 Subluxation complex (vertebral) of pelvic region
SP M99.16 Subluxation complex (vertebral) of lower extremity
SP M99.17 Subluxation complex (vertebral) of upper extremity
SP M99.18 Subluxation complex (vertebral) of rib cage
SP M99.19 Subluxation complex (vertebral) of abdomen and other regions

5 M99.2 Subluxation stenosis of neural canal
SP M99.20 Subluxation stenosis of neural canal of head region
SP M99.21 Subluxation stenosis of neural canal of cervical region
SP M99.22 Subluxation stenosis of neural canal of thoracic region
SP M99.23 Subluxation stenosis of neural canal of lumbar region
SP M99.24 Subluxation stenosis of neural canal of sacral region
SP M99.25 Subluxation stenosis of neural canal of pelvic region
SP M99.26 Subluxation stenosis of neural canal of lower extremity
SP M99.27 Subluxation stenosis of neural canal of upper extremity
SP M99.28 Subluxation stenosis of neural canal of rib cage
SP M99.29 Subluxation stenosis of neural canal of abdomen and other regions

5 M99.3 Osseous stenosis of neural canal
SP M99.30 Osseous stenosis of neural canal of head region
SP M99.31 Osseous stenosis of neural canal of cervical region
SP M99.32 Osseous stenosis of neural canal of thoracic region
SP M99.33 Osseous stenosis of neural canal of lumbar region
SP M99.34 Osseous stenosis of neural canal of sacral region
SP M99.35 Osseous stenosis of neural canal of pelvic region
SP M99.36 Osseous stenosis of neural canal of lower extremity
SP M99.37 Osseous stenosis of neural canal of upper extremity
SP M99.38 Osseous stenosis of neural canal of rib cage
SP M99.39 Osseous stenosis of neural canal of abdomen and other regions

5 M99.4 Connective tissue stenosis of neural canal
SP M99.40 Connective tissue stenosis of neural canal of head region
SP M99.41 Connective tissue stenosis of neural canal of cervical region
SP M99.42 Connective tissue stenosis of neural canal of thoracic region
SP M99.43 Connective tissue stenosis of neural canal of lumbar region
SP M99.44 Connective tissue stenosis of neural canal of sacral region
SP M99.45 Connective tissue stenosis of neural canal of pelvic region
SP M99.46 Connective tissue stenosis of neural canal of lower extremity
SP M99.47 Connective tissue stenosis of neural canal of upper extremity
SP M99.48 Connective tissue stenosis of neural canal of rib cage
SP M99.49 Connective tissue stenosis of neural canal of abdomen and other regions

5 M99.5 Intervertebral disc stenosis of neural canal
SP M99.50 Intervertebral disc stenosis of neural canal of head region
SP M99.51 Intervertebral disc stenosis of neural canal of cervical region
SP M99.52 Intervertebral disc stenosis of neural canal of thoracic region
SP M99.53 Intervertebral disc stenosis of neural canal of lumbar region
SP M99.54 Intervertebral disc stenosis of neural canal of sacral region
SP M99.55 Intervertebral disc stenosis of neural canal of pelvic region
SP M99.56 Intervertebral disc stenosis of neural canal of lower extremity
SP M99.57 Intervertebral disc stenosis of neural canal of upper extremity
SP M99.58 Intervertebral disc stenosis of neural canal of rib cage
SP M99.59 Intervertebral disc stenosis of neural canal of abdomen and other regions

5 M99.6 Osseous and subluxation stenosis of intervertebral foramina
SP M99.60 Osseous and subluxation stenosis of intervertebral foramina of head region
SP M99.61 Osseous and subluxation stenosis of intervertebral foramina of cervical region

SP M99.62 Osseous and subluxation stenosis of intervertebral foramina of thoracic region
SP M99.63 Osseous and subluxation stenosis of intervertebral foramina of lumbar region
SP M99.64 Osseous and subluxation stenosis of intervertebral foramina of sacral region
SP M99.65 Osseous and subluxation stenosis of intervertebral foramina of pelvic region
SP M99.66 Osseous and subluxation stenosis of intervertebral foramina of lower extremity
SP M99.67 Osseous and subluxation stenosis of intervertebral foramina of upper extremity
SP M99.68 Osseous and subluxation stenosis of intervertebral foramina of rib cage
SP M99.69 Osseous and subluxation stenosis of intervertebral foramina of abdomen and other regions

5 M99.7 Connective tissue and disc stenosis of intervertebral foramina

SP M99.70 Connective tissue and disc stenosis of intervertebral foramina of head region
SP M99.71 Connective tissue and disc stenosis of intervertebral foramina of cervical region
SP M99.72 Connective tissue and disc stenosis of intervertebral foramina of thoracic region
SP M99.73 Connective tissue and disc stenosis of intervertebral foramina of lumbar region
SP M99.74 Connective tissue and disc stenosis of intervertebral foramina of sacral region
SP M99.75 Connective tissue and disc stenosis of intervertebral foramina of pelvic region
SP M99.76 Connective tissue and disc stenosis of intervertebral foramina of lower extremity
SP M99.77 Connective tissue and disc stenosis of intervertebral foramina of upper extremity
SP M99.78 Connective tissue and disc stenosis of intervertebral foramina of rib cage
SP M99.79 Connective tissue and disc stenosis of intervertebral foramina of abdomen and other regions

5 M99.8 Other biomechanical lesions

SP M99.80 Other biomechanical lesions of head region
SP M99.81 Other biomechanical lesions of cervical region
SP M99.82 Other biomechanical lesions of thoracic region
SP M99.83 Other biomechanical lesions of lumbar region
SP M99.84 Other biomechanical lesions of sacral region
SP M99.85 Other biomechanical lesions of pelvic region
SP M99.86 Other biomechanical lesions of lower extremity
SP M99.87 Other biomechanical lesions of upper extremity
SP M99.88 Other biomechanical lesions of rib cage
SP M99.89 Other biomechanical lesions of abdomen and other regions

IQ M99.9 Biomechanical lesion, unspecified

Chapter 13 Scenarios: Diseases of the musculoskeletal system and connective tissue (M00-M99)

Osteoporosis and pathologic fracture

An elderly gentleman is admitted for home care after undergoing surgery for a pathological fracture of the left femur. Physical therapy is ordered for muscle strengthening and gait training. Skilled nursing is ordered for surgical wound assessment. Medical documentation includes hypertension, heart failure and osteoporosis.

Description	Code
Primary: Age-related osteoporosis with current pathological fracture, left femur	M80.052D
Secondary: Hypertensive heart disease with heart failure	I11.0
Secondary: Heart failure, unspecified	I50.9

A code from category M80.-, not a traumatic fracture code, should be used for any patient with known osteoporosis who suffers a fracture, even if the patient had a minor fall or trauma, if that fall or trauma would not usually break a normal, healthy bone, according to coding guidelines. The M80.0- subcategory indicates age-related osteoporosis with current pathologic fracture. The fifth digit "5" indicates femur, the sixth digit "2" indicates the left side and the seventh character "D" indicates subsequent care. Osteoporosis that is not otherwise specified codes to age-related osteoporosis within the ICD-10 classification system. Additional codes are assigned for hypertension and heart failure comorbidities due to the impact of these conditions on the patient's prognosis and care plan and they may provide important comorbidity adjustment for PDGM.

Pathologic fracture, bone cancer

A 75-year-old male patient has brain cancer that has metastasized to his bones. As a result, he has suffered a pathologic fracture to his right femur, which was treated surgically in the hospital. The focus of the home health admission is the fracture aftercare, which is routine.

Description	Code
Primary: Pathologic fracture in neoplastic disease, right femur, subsequent encounter with routine healing	M84.551D
Secondary: Secondary malignant neoplasm of bone	C79.51
Secondary: Malignant neoplasm of brain, unspecified	C71.9

As the focus of care, the pathological fracture caused by the bone metastasis is coded in the primary position. When an encounter is for a pathological fracture due to a neoplasm, and the focus of treatment is the fracture, a code from subcategory M84.5- (Pathological fracture in neoplastic disease) should be sequenced first followed by the code for the neoplasm, according to coding guidelines. As the reason for the pathological fracture, the secondary malignant neoplasm in the bones is coded before the primary malignant neoplasm in the brain. The care is routine, so the appropriate seventh character is D, which specifies that the case is a subsequent encounter for fracture with routine healing. The underlying neoplasms also are coded, as required by the note in the tabular.

Multiple therapies and fracture

Your patient sustained a pathological fracture of her left femur when rolling over in bed. She has a diagnosis of senile osteoporosis. Skilled nursing and physical and occupational therapy are ordered. She has a history of vertebral pathologic fracture one year ago, and COPD.

Description	Code
Primary: Age-related osteoporosis with current pathologic fracture of left femur, subsequent encounter with routine healing	M80.052D
Secondary: Chronic obstructive pulmonary disease, unspecified	J44.9
Secondary: Personal history of (healed) osteoporosis fracture	Z87.310

The combination code M80.052D covers both the patient's osteoporosis and pathological fracture of her left femur. The seventh character "D" identifies the subsequent nature of the encounter. Her personal history of a healed pathological fracture is relevant to this case and is thus coded. Senile osteoporosis is coded as age-related osteoporosis, according to the alphabetic index. An additional code is assigned to identify the patient's COPD due to the impact this condition has on the patient's rehabilitation and care plan.

Spinal stenosis

The home health agency received a referral for a home care assessment for a patient recently discharged from the hospital after an acute exacerbation of chronic systolic heart failure following suspected COVID-19 exposure. The patient has acute back pain in the lumbar area, diagnosed as spinal stenosis of the lumbar region with neurogenic claudication, and has a history of COPD. The focus for home care is the spinal stenosis/back pain. The nursing staff is to assess her response to pain medications and new cardiac medications. Physical therapy will provide therapeutic exercises and training, and occupational therapy will provide ADL training, adaptive equipment, and motor/sensory treatment. COVID-19 is noted as suspected but testing was negative.

Description	Code
Primary: Spinal stenosis, lumbar region with neurogenic claudication	M48.062
Secondary: Acute on chronic systolic (congestive) heart failure	I50.23
Secondary: Chronic obstructive pulmonary disease, unspecified	J44.9
Secondary: Contact with and (suspected) exposure to COVID-19	Z20.822

The combination code M48.062 covers both the spinal stenosis of the lumbar region and the neurogenic claudication. It is not acceptable to code spinal stenosis of an ***unspecified*** location as primary under PDGM. Back pain is integral to spinal stenosis and thus no additional code is required to capture it. Code I50.23 is assigned for the heart failure as ICD-10-CM coding guidelines require that a single acute on chronic code be assigned when an acute exacerbation of a chronic condition is present. COPD is not exacerbated but should be coded due to the impact of this condition on the patient's prognosis and plan of care. Because the patient was only suspected for COVID-19, but did not test positive, Z20.822 is assigned based upon the most recent guidelines for this condition.

Ankle arthritis

A 73-year-old man was admitted for physical therapy for difficulty in ambulating. Per the medical record, the patient sustained a left ankle fracture four years ago, and now has arthritis in the joint as a result. Due to the pain, the patient has fallen several times in recent weeks.

Description	Code
Primary: Traumatic arthropathy, left ankle and foot	M12.572
Secondary: Other fracture of left lower leg, sequela	S82.892S
Secondary: History of falling	Z91.81

Traumatic arthropathy is coded as it is a residual effect that occurred because of an injury in the past. The now-resolved ankle fracture, which is the reason for the traumatic arthritis, is coded immediately following the arthritis code, in accordance with coding guidelines. It includes the seventh character "S" to indicate that it is not an active condition but rather has left behind a residual, or sequela. The history of falling code (Z91.81) is used when a patient has fallen in the past and is at risk for future falls.

Rheumatoid arthritis, monthly infusions

A 67-year-old man receives home health care for monthly infusions of Actemra to treat his severe rheumatoid arthritis (RA) of both hands. He is positive for rheumatoid factor. He is frequently monitored for potential side effects and complications from the long-term use of Actemra.

Description	Code
Primary: Rheumatoid arthritis with rheumatoid factor of right hand without organ or systems involvement	M05.741
Secondary: Rheumatoid arthritis with rheumatoid factor of left hand without organ or systems involvement	M05.742
Secondary: Encounter for adjustment and management of vascular access device	Z45.2
Secondary: Other long term (current) drug therapy	Z79.899

Two codes are assigned to capture the rheumatoid arthritis being present in both hands, since a bilateral code is not available. Code Z45.2 is assigned to capture the care of the vascular device used to deliver the infusion. If the IV is not the primary reason the patient requires home health care, but where there may be some sort of intervention noted on the home health plan of care, then it would be appropriate to report Z45.2 (but not as the principal or first secondary diagnosis), according to CMS. Additionally, Z79.899 is assigned to capture the patient's long-term use of Actemra in the absence of a more specific code from Z79.-. Note that it is not acceptable to code unspecified rheumatoid arthritis as the primary reason for home health in PDGM.

Traumatic arthritis, stroke sequela

A 67-year-old woman suffered a stroke last year, in which she lost consciousness, fell and broke her left wrist. After the stroke, she continues to suffer from right dominant side hemiplegia, aphasia and dysphagia. Additionally, she has traumatic arthritis in her left wrist as a result of the now-healed fracture. She has orders for physical, occupational and speech therapy to continue her recovery from the stroke sequela. The hemiplegia is the focus of care.

Description	Code
Primary: Hemiplegia and hemiparesis following cerebral infarction affecting right dominant side	I69.351
Secondary: Aphasia following cerebral infarction	I69.320
Secondary: Dysphagia following cerebral infarction	I69.391
Secondary: Dysphagia, unspecified	R13.10
Secondary: Traumatic arthropathy, left wrist	M12.532
Secondary: Fracture of unspecified carpal bone, left wrist, sequela	S62.102S

Though it is a therapy-only case, there is no need to assign a rehab code in ICD-10. The conditions requiring therapy will suffice. As the focus of care, the right dominant side hemiplegia is coded primary. An additional code for dysphagia is assigned, in accordance with tabular instructions at I69.391. The patient's arthritis has been specified as traumatic arthritis, resulting from an old healed wrist fracture. Though the fracture is healed, it left the patient with arthritis. Therefore, the code for the fracture is assigned immediately following the residual it caused (the traumatic arthritis) with the seventh character "S" to indicate that it's no longer an active condition but a sequela.

Nephritis due to lupus

A 60-year-old woman comes to home health for nephritis secondary to systemic lupus erythematosus. Physician encounter notes indicate the nephritis has led to stage 2 chronic kidney disease and the patient also has diabetes with polyneuropathy. She will receive skilled nursing for management of medications, including an increased dosage of systemic steroids, which she has taken for the last year. The nephritis is the focus of care.

Description	Code
Primary: Glomerular disease in systemic lupus erythematosus	M32.14
Secondary: Chronic kidney disease, stage 2 (mild)	N18.2
Secondary: Type 2 diabetes mellitus with diabetic polyneuropathy	E11.42
Secondary: Long term (current) use of systemic steroids	Z79.52

The patient's nephritis is documented as being caused by systemic lupus erythematosus. Thus it is appropriate to code it with the combination code M32.14. As the focus of care, it is coded in the primary position. Since the combination code covers both conditions, an additional code for the lupus is not necessary. Lupus nephritis most commonly results in chronic kidney disease and when this is documented by the provider it should be coded following with the appropriate code to identify the stage of the chronic kidney disease. While this patient is diabetic, the chronic kidney disease is not assumed to be related to the diabetes because another cause is specified by the patient's physician. A code for the diabetic polyneuropathy is also assigned due to the impact this condition has on the patient's care plan.The patient has taken systemic steroids over a long period of time, which carries certain risks and thus must be captured with Z79.52.

Sequelae of rickets

A 70-year-old man is admitted to home health for physical therapy due to cervical scoliosis resulting from childhood rickets. He also has advanced degenerative changes in both of his knees.

Description	Code
Primary: Spondylopathy in diseases classified elsewhere, cervical region	M49.82
Secondary: Sequelae of rickets	E64.3
Secondary: Bilateral primary osteoarthritis of knee	M17.0

In this scenario, the sequelae code is coded after the code that identifies the residual condition, scoliosis (M49.82), due to a specific note at E64.3 that directs the coder to "code first" the condition resulting from (sequela) of malnutrition and other nutrition deficiencies. This is a variation from the convention for sequela(e) coding and when noted for specific codes, should be followed. Advanced degenerative changes in the knee joints is coded as osteoarthritis, according to Q2 2018 Coding Clinic guidance. The osteoarthritis will impact his recovery and thus should also be coded. Also, you can code a patient's osteoarthritis as primary osteoarthritis if the type isn't specified, according to Q4 2016 Coding Clinic guidance.

Chronic idiopathic gout

A 67-year-old man is admitted to home health for skilled nursing, managing new medications, and physical and occupational therapy to address trouble with ADLs/IADLs due to a primary diagnosis of chronic idiopathic gout that affects both of his elbows. He also has a diagnosis of hypertension for which he was recently prescribed new medication.

Description	Code
Primary: Idiopathic chronic gout, right elbow, without tophus (tophi)	M1A.0210
Secondary: Idiopathic chronic gout, left elbow, without tophus (tophi)	M1A.0220
Secondary: Essential (primary) hypertension	I10

The patient's gout is specified as chronic idiopathic gout of both elbows. Because no bilateral code is available, two codes (one for the right and one for the left) are used. It's imperative to know the specific joint affected by the gout, as codes for gout in an unspecified location and laterality are not acceptable as primary diagnoses in PDGM. His hypertension will require monitoring and thus should also be coded.

Pseudogout

A 70-year-old man is experiencing a severe flare of pseudogout in bilateral ankles. He was admitted to home health for management of medications, including prednisone, and physical therapy.

Description	Code
Primary: Other chondrocalcinosis, right ankle and foot	M11.271
Secondary: Other chondrocalcinosis, left ankle and foot	M11.272
Secondary: Long term (current) use of systemic steroids	Z79.52

Pseudogout is classified under chondrocalcinosis. Because there is not a code that captures chondrocalcinosis in both ankles, two codes are used for the right and left ankles. The specific joint and side of the body must be documented in order to code pseudogout as a primary diagnosis in home health. Note, codes for pseudogout in an unspecified location or that don't specify the left or right side of the body are not acceptable as primary diagnoses in PDGM. Taking the systemic steroid drug prednisone comes with certain risks, so it should be captured with Z79.52.

Pathological periprosthetic fracture

An 84-year-old woman with a left knee prosthesis was walking in her home when she felt a sharp pain in her left lower leg and heard a snap sound. She was admitted to the hospital where a fracture of the tibia, around the left knee prosthesis, was discovered. The hospitalist diagnosed the fracture as a pathological periprosthetic fracture and ordered home health for skilled nursing, physical and occupational therapy with a focus on care to and recovery from the fracture. She also has diagnoses of hypertension and depression.

Description	Code
Primary: Pathological fracture, left tibia, subsequent encounter for fracture with routine healing	M84.462D
Secondary: Periprosthetic fracture around internal prosthetic left knee joint, subsequent encounter	M97.12xD
Secondary: Essential (primary) hypertension	I10
Secondary: Depression, unspecified	F32.A

The fracture was diagnosed as a pathological periprosthetic fracture around the left knee prosthesis. Therefore, the pathologic fracture is sequenced first, followed by the periprosthetic fracture code, in accordance with Q4 2016 Coding Clinic guidance. The patient's hypertension and depression are important comorbidities that will impact her ability to recover and are thus coded as secondary diagnoses. Depression that is not specified should be coded to F32.A.

Impending pathologic fracture in neoplastic disease

A 68-year-old female with recently diagnosed left lower lobe lung cancer presented to the hospital with severe right upper leg pain and a secondary neoplasm of the right femur was identified with significant osteolysis and impending fracture. A prophylactic right hip replacement was done due to the impending neoplastic fracture. The inpatient physician's encounter notes also report that the patient has comorbid primary osteoarthritis of the bilateral hips and COPD.

Description	Code
Primary: Aftercare following joint replacement surgery	Z47.1
Secondary: Secondary malignant neoplasm of bone	C79.51
Secondary: Malignant neoplasm of lower lobe, left bronchus or lung	C34.32
Secondary: Chronic obstructive pulmonary disease, unspecified	J44.9
Secondary: Unilateral primary osteoarthritis, left hip	M16.12
Secondary: Presence of right artificial hip joint	Z96.641

While this patient did have a surgical hip replacement, there was no actual fracture to the femur, it was only considered impending due to the bone condition with the identified lesion. Coding guidelines state that "impending" conditions that did not actually occur should only be coded if there is a specific alphabetic index entry for the main or subterm(s) "impending" or "threatened." If there is not, then the existing underlying condition(s), in this case the neoplastic disease, should be coded. Additional codes are assigned for COPD and arthritis of the hip due to the impact of these conditions. While the physician stated that the patient had arthritis of the bilateral hips, the joint to the right hip was removed with the placement of the prosthesis, so only the left hip arthritis is coded. Addition of a code to identify joint replaced is required, so Z96.641 is assigned.

Multisystem Inflammatory Syndrome, history of COVID

A 76-year-old female was hospitalized 2 months ago due to COVID-19 with associated pneumonia, then admitted to home health. The patient was then re-hospitalized due to decline in status and diagnosed with Multisystem Inflammatory Syndrome (MIS) and acute renal failure. Physician documentation upon discharge from the hospital indicates MIS, acute renal failure, history of COVID-19/resolved, COPD, and CKD stage 4.

Description	Code
Primary: Multisystem inflammatory syndrome	M35.81
Secondary: Acute kidney failure, unspecified	N17.9
Secondary: Chronic obstructive pulmonary disease, unspecified	J44.9
Secondary: Chronic kidney disease, stage 4 (severe)	N18.4
Secondary: Personal history of COVID-19	Z86.16

While this patient did have an infection with COVID-19 two months ago, it cannot be assumed that Multisystem inflammatory syndrome (MIS) is a sequela of the condition unless specified by the provider. Per Q1 2021 Coding Clinic guidance, if an individual with a history of COVID-19 develops MIS and the provider does not indicate the MIS is due to the previous COVID-19 infection, assign codes M35.81, Multisystem inflammatory syndrome, and Z86.16, Personal history of COVID-19. The acute renal failure is unresolved, so this is also coded along with CKD stage 4. COPD is a comorbid condition that will impact the patient's progress and plan of care, so this is also sequenced.

Chapter 14: Diseases of the Genitourinary System (N00-N99)

Chapter 14 includes codes arranged in the following blocks:

- Glomerular diseases such as nephritic syndrome, hematuria and hereditary nephropathy (N00-N08);
- Renal tubulo-interstitial diseases and disorders such as hereditary nephritis and chronic pylonephritis, hydronephrosis, and vesicoureteral-reflux nephropathy (N10-N16);
- Acute kidney failure and chronic kidney disease (N17-N19);
- Urolithiasis (N20-N23);
- Other disorders of kidney and ureter including nephrogenic diabetes insipidus, secondary hyperparathyroidism of renal origin, contracted (small) kidney, ischemia and infarction of kidney, and acquired cyst of kidney (N25-N29);
- Other disorders of urinary system including cystitis, neuromuscular dysfunction of the bladder, overactive bladder, uretheral stricture, UTI and urinary incontinence (N30-N39);
- Diseases of male genital organs including enlarged prostate, inflammatory diseases of prostate, hydrocele & spermatocele, noninflammatory disorders of testes, orchitis & epididymitis, male infertility, inflammatory disorders of penis, priaprism, inflammatory disorders of male genitalia, and erectile dysfunction (N40-N53);
- Disorders of breast including benign mammary dysplasia, cystic mastopathy, fibroadenosis of breast & mammary ducts, other inflammatory disorders of breast – hypertrophy & hypoplasia, fat necrosis of breast, other signs and symptoms in breast, and deformity & disproportion of reconstructed breast (N60-N65);
- Inflammatory diseases of female pelvic organs including salpingitis & oophoritis, inflammatory disease of uterus and cervix, pelvic inflammatory diseases and other inflammation of vagina and vulva (N70-N77);
- Noninflammatory disorders of female genital tract including endometriosis, female genital prolapses, urethrocele, cystocele, and rectocele, genital prolapsed, fistulas involving female genital tract, atrophy & polyps genital organs, cervical and vaginal disorders, female genital mutilation status, abnormal uterine & vaginal bleeding, menopausal and perimenopausal disorders and female infertility (N80-N98); and
- Intraoperative and postprocedural complications and disorders of genitourinary system such as uretheral strictures, adhesions, complications of urinary tract stomas, hemorrhage, and accidental puncture and lacerations (N99).

This chapter also includes a number of codes for symptoms, such as N95 for those related to menopausal and perimenopausal disorders and N64.4 for mastodynia (breast pain). Codes in category N92 for conditions related to menstrual periods (unusually heavy [menorrhagia], unusually light [oligomenorrhea], painful [dysmenorrhea], or no periods at all [amenorrhea]). Every effort should be made to secure a definitive diagnosis.

Home health and hospice coding will deal mostly with these areas of Chapter 14:

- Chronic kidney failure (N18.-)
- Urinary incontinence (N39.3, N39.4-)
- Cystitis (N30.-) and Urinary tract infection (N39.0)
- Problems with prostate (N40.- , N41.-, N42.-)

Symptoms related to the genitourinary system are sometimes reported using codes from Chapter 18, symptoms, signs and abnormal clinical and laboratory findings, not elsewhere classified. More specifically, using codes in subcategory R39.- (symptoms involving urinary system) and R82.-(nonspecific findings on examination of urine). Every effort should be made to secure a definitive diagnosis. A symptom code from Chapter 18 may be reported as an additional diagnosis when it describes a significant aspect of the condition but is not an integral part of it.

Other situations when codes outside of Chapter 14 are needed include:

- If the documentation indicates a **neoplasm or tumor of an organ in the genitourinary system**, look up the term (malignancy, tumor, adenoma) to find the correct code, most likely a code from C00 – D49 in Chapter 2.
- If a patient has a **personal or family history** of a condition reported in this chapter, it may be more appropriate to select from the Z code section, such as Z87.448 (Personal history disorder of urinary system), Z85.40 and Z85.45 (Personal history of malignant neoplasm of female and male genital organs), or Z80.4 (Family history of malignant neoplasm of genital organs).
- If a condition reported in this chapter is the result of **injury, poisoning and certain other consequences** of external causes, a code from

Chapter 14

N00 - N99

Chapter 19 may be reported with or instead of a code from this chapter.

- Additional codes in the following categories may be coded in addition to or instead of codes from chapter 14. Refer to the Alphabetical List for the code and follow the notes, if applicable, at the appropriate code. They are:
  - Certain conditions originating in the perinatal period (P00-P96)
  - Complications of pregnancy, childbirth or the puerperium (O00-O9A)
  - Congenital malformations, deformations and chromosomal abnormalities (Q00-O99)
  - Certain infectious and parasitic diseases (A00-B99)
  - Endocrine, nutritional and metabolic diseases (E00-E88)

Multiple Coding and Sequencing

It is important to read the Includes and Excludes notes under codes in this chapter, as well as any other instructions under the code or code category. Below are some examples of multiple coding and sequencing issues for codes in this chapter.

Codes N40.1 (Benign prostatic hyperplasia with lower urinary tract symptoms) and N40.3 (Nodular prostate with lower urinary tract symptoms) include a note that states: "Use additional code(s) for associated symptoms when specified." The note lists symptoms such as incomplete bladder emptying, nocturia, straining on urination, urinary frequency, hesitancy, incontinence, obstruction, retention, urgency and weak urinary stream from Chapter 18, including signs and symptoms involving the genitourinary system (R30-R39), as well as codes N13.8 and N39.4- from this chapter.

Special Coding Issues

There are many more specific combination codes in ICD-10 CM that reduce the need for multiple codes related to genitourinary conditions. Therefore, all codes must be referenced in the Alphabetical Index and then verified in the Tabular list to ensure the correct code is selected.

The Kidneys

The kidneys are responsible for removing waste from the body, regulating electrolyte balance and blood pressure, and stimulating red blood cell production. Although inflammation, scarring, or a decrease in membrane surface area lowers the rate of glomerular filtration, the kidney so effectively compensates that people rarely know they have lost kidney function until only 10% to 20% remains. High blood pressure and anemia may develop with increasing frequency after loss of 30% to 50% kidney function, but these signs develop so gradually they often produce no symptoms.

Because of their intimate relationship with such a large portion of the circulating blood, up to 25% of diseases of the kidney, or any disturbance in the kidney's delicate mechanism, can adversely influence blood pressure, and in turn, may alter kidney function.

Chronic Kidney Disease (CKD)

There are two notes found at N18, Chronic kidney disease. First is a code first note to assign any associated disease, such as:

- diabetic chronic kidney disease (E08.22. E09.22, E10.22, E11.22, E13.22)
- hypertensive chronic kidney disease (I12.-, I13.-)

There is also a note to use an additional code to identify kidney transplant status, such as Z94.0, if applicable.

Stages of chronic kidney disease (CKD)

Chronic kidney disease is classified according to severity. The severity of CKD is designated by stages 1 – 5. Stage 2, code N18.2, equates to mild CKD; stage 3, code N18.3-, equates to moderate CKD; stage 4, N18.4, equates to severe CKD. Also note, CKD stage 3 (moderate) should be further specified as unspecified (N18.30), stage 3a (N18.31) or stage 3b (N18.32). Code N18.6, End stage renal disease (ESRD), is assigned when the provider has documented end-stage-renal disease (ESRD) or chronic kidney disease requiring long-term dialysis. If both a stage of CKD and ESRD are documented, assign code N18.6 only.

When both hypertension and a condition classifiable to category N18, Chronic kidney disease (CKD), are present, assign codes from category I12, Hypertensive chronic kidney disease. CKD should not be coded as hypertensive if the physician has specifically documented a different cause. The appropriate code from category N18 should be used as a secondary code with a code from category I12 to identify the stage of chronic kidney disease.

Abnormal lab findings are not coded and reported unless the provider indicates clinical significance. Therefore, it would be inappropriate to assign a stage for CKD based solely on glomerular filtration rate (GFR). If that information is not available, the coder may select N18.9 for unspecified CKD, or N18.6, if the patient is undergoing dialysis.

If CKD, hypertension and heart disease are all present, it may be appropriate to report a code from Category I13.- (**hypertensive heart and chronic kidney disease**). A code from N18.- (CKD) is reported as an additional code. The classification assumes a relationship between HTN and any condition classifiable to N18 (CKD) and N26. The relationship may be assumed because of the pathology of hypertension, which impacts renal function, often resulting in CKD. Do not confuse hypertensive chronic kidney disease with renovascular hypertension, a condition in which the kidney dysfunction causes the hypertension. Renovascular hypertension is coded using I15.0.

Chronic kidney disease and kidney transplant status

Patients who have undergone a kidney transplant may still have some form of CKD because the kidney transplant may not fully restore kidney function. Therefore, the presence of CKD alone does not constitute a transplant complication. Assign the appropriate N18 code for the patient's stage of CKD and code Z94.0, kidney transplant status. If a transplant complication, such as failure or rejection or other transplant complication is documented, refer to section I.C.19.g of the Official Coding Guidelines for information on coding complications of a kidney transplant. If the documentation is unclear as to whether the patient has a complication of the transplant, query the physician.

Chronic kidney disease with other complications

Patients with CKD may also suffer from other serious conditions, most commonly diabetes mellitus and hypertension. The sequencing of the CKD code in relationship to codes for other contributing conditions is based on conventions in the Tabular List.

Kidney failure is the inability of the kidneys to excrete waste products and occurs for various reasons. It may be acute (N17.-) or chronic (N18.9) in nature. Causes include surgery or trauma, pregnancy, various medical conditions, nephrotoxins, and irreversible conditions that diminish nephron function.

Acute kidney failure (N17.-) most often is due to reduced blood volume or perfusion of the kidney. Causes include infections, severe dehydration, vascular disease, and damage to renal tissues. Factors outside the kidney, such as obstruction, stones, prostatic hypertrophy and tumors also may cause acute kidney failure. Depending on the cause, severity, and medical treatment, 30% to 60% of acute kidney failure patients will recover.

Note: Code N08 (Glomerular disorders in diseases classified elsewhere) is a manifestation code that is assigned when there is not specific information about the kidney disease provided. The code first note at N08 lists the most common causes of glomerulonephritis, nephritis and nephropathy.

Diabetic nephropathy is coded using a code from the most appropriate diabetes category (E08-E13) with a 4th and 5th character of XXX.21. One of the diabetic category codes with 4th and 5th characters, XXX.22 is used when the diagnosis is diabetic chronic kidney disease and requires a second additional code from N18 to identify the stage of the chronic kidney disease (stage 1, 2, 3, 4, 5, or ESRD). ESRD is not technically a stage but used for any patient with CKD who requires chronic dialysis. If both a specific stage of CKD and dialysis are documented for a patient, only N18.6 is assigned.

Acquired renal cysts are classified to N28.1, while a congenital cyst of the kidney is coded Q61.- from chapter 17.

Infections

E. coli is the most common disease-causing organism for urinary system infections, but other organisms including Staphylococcus may be the culprit. When the organism is known, an additional code from B95-B97, infection in diseases classified elsewhere, is added to identify the infectious agent.

Cystitis

Category N30.-, or inflammation of the bladder, usually resulting from a urinary tract infection may also involve other associated organs, such as the kidney, prostate or urethra. Cystitis is more common in women than men. Nonetheless, the diagnosis must be documented by the physician before being coded. Sexual intercourse, trauma or poor hygiene allows bacteria to enter the bladder — typically a sterile vesicle. Urinary frequency, urgency, difficulty and pain just above the pubic area are all symptoms of urinary tract infections. There are a number of combination codes within the N30.- category to describe cystitis as acute, chronic, interstitial, with or without hematuria or other conditions present for greater specificity.

Pyelonephritis, an inflammation of the kidney and renal pelvis, is a more severe condition, which occurs when the invading organisms reach the renal pelvis and kidney tissue. When coded to N12, this condition is also referred to as tubule-interstitial nephritis, not specified as acute or chronic. If the documentation states acute tubulo-interstitial nephritis or acute pyelonephritis, the appropriate code is N10. If the documentation states chronic pyelonephritis or chronic tubule-interstitial nephritis, the appropriate code is N11.-. An additional code is added from B95-B97 to identify the infectious agent, when known, in each of these situations.

Chapter 14

N00 - N99

Urinary tract infection

Category N39.0, Urinary tract infection site not specified, also has a note to use an additional code (B95-B97) to identify the infectious agent.

A urinary tract infection occurring in a patient with a urinary catheter is **not assumed** to be a complication of the catheter. Therefore, code N39.0 and code Z46.6 (fitting and adjustment of urinary device) can be assigned unless the physician documentation supports the infection was caused by the catheter.

If the infection is caused by the catheter, assign a code from T83.51- (infection and inflammatory reaction due to urinary catheter). When T83.51- is used, do not use the Z46.6 code for catheter care. Follow the T83.51- code with an additional code for the specified infection, such as UTI (N39.0 plus an additional code from B95-B97).

Other Issues

The urethra differs in men and women. The female urethra is about 9.5 cm long and the male urethra is about 20 cm long. In men, it serves the dual purpose of conveying sperm and discharging urine from the bladder. The female urethra performs only the latter function.

Neurogenic bladder or neuromuscular dysfunction of bladder, unspecified normally is coded N31.9. There is a note at the N31 category to use an additional code to identify any associated urinary incontinence (N39.3-, N39.4-). Another code for neurogenic bladder, G83.4 (Neurogenic bladder due to cauda equina syndrome) is from Chapter 6, Diseases of the nervous system, but it should not be used unless it is documented or verified with the physician. Improper use of neurogenic bladder codes is a red flag and typically leads to denials. Rarely will a neurogenic bladder be accurately coded at G83.4.

Hyperplasia (benign) of the prostate is coded to N40.- in ICD-10. Prostate growth involves hormones, occurs in different types of tissue (e.g., muscular, glandular), and affects men differently. As a result of these differences, treatment varies in each case. There is no cure for BPH and once prostate growth starts, it often continues unless medical therapy is started.

The prostate can grow in two different ways. In one type of growth, cells multiply around the urethra and squeeze it, much like squeezing a straw. The second type of growth is middle-lobe prostate growth in which cells grow into the urethra and the bladder outlet area. This type of growth typically requires surgery. Hyperplasia, or enlarged prostate, causes a number of symptoms, such as hematuria from straining, a weak urine stream and dribbling. When an enlarged prostrate has associated lower urinary tract symptoms, assign code N40.1 first followed by codes to identify the lower urinary tract symptoms (LUTS).

CHAPTER 14: DISEASES OF THE GENITOURINARY SYSTEM (N00-N99)

EXCLUDES 2 certain conditions originating in the perinatal period (P04-P96)
certain infectious and parasitic diseases (A00-B99)
complications of pregnancy, childbirth and the puerperium (O00-O9A)
congenital malformations, deformations and chromosomal abnormalities (Q00-Q99)
endocrine, nutritional and metabolic diseases (E00-E88)
injury, poisoning and certain other consequences of external causes (S00-T88)
neoplasms (C00-D49)
symptoms, signs and abnormal clinical and laboratory findings, not elsewhere classified (R00-R94)

This chapter contains the following blocks:

N00-N08	Glomerular diseases
N10-N16	Renal tubulo-interstitial diseases
N17-N19	Acute kidney failure and chronic kidney disease
N20-N23	Urolithiasis
N25-N29	Other disorders of kidney and ureter
N30-N39	Other diseases of the urinary system
N40-N53	Diseases of male genital organs
N60-N65	Disorders of breast
N70-N77	Inflammatory diseases of female pelvic organs
N80-N98	Noninflammatory disorders of female genital tract
N99	Intraoperative and postprocedural complications and disorders of genitourinary system, not elsewhere classified

Glomerular diseases (N00-N08)

Code also:
any associated kidney failure (N17-N19) .

EXCLUDES 1 hypertensive chronic kidney disease (I12.-)

4 **N00 Acute nephritic syndrome**

INCLUDES acute glomerular disease
acute glomerulonephritis
acute nephritis

EXCLUDES 1 acute tubulo-interstitial nephritis (N10)
nephritic syndrome NOS (N05.-)

SP **N00.0 Acute nephritic syndrome with minor glomerular abnormality**
Acute nephritic syndrome with minimal change lesion

SP **N00.1 Acute nephritic syndrome with focal and segmental glomerular lesions**
Acute nephritic syndrome with focal and segmental hyalinosis
Acute nephritic syndrome with focal and segmental sclerosis
Acute nephritic syndrome with focal glomerulonephritis

SP **N00.2 Acute nephritic syndrome with diffuse membranous glomerulonephritis**

SP **N00.3 Acute nephritic syndrome with diffuse mesangial proliferative glomerulonephritis**

SP **N00.4 Acute nephritic syndrome with diffuse endocapillary proliferative glomerulonephritis**

SP **N00.5 Acute nephritic syndrome with diffuse mesangiocapillary glomerulonephritis**
Acute nephritic syndrome with membranoproliferative glomerulonephritis, types 1 and 3, or NOS

EXCLUDES 1 Acute nephritic syndrome with C3 glomerulonephritis (N00.A)
Acute nephritic syndrome with C3 glomerulopathy (N00.A)

SP **N00.6 Acute nephritic syndrome with dense deposit disease**
Acute nephritic syndrome with C3 glomerulopathy with dense deposit disease
Acute nephritic syndrome with membranoproliferative glomerulonephritis, type 2

SP **N00.7 Acute nephritic syndrome with diffuse crescentic glomerulonephritis**
Acute nephritic syndrome with extracapillary glomerulonephritis

SP **N00.8 Acute nephritic syndrome with other morphologic changes**
Acute nephritic syndrome with proliferative glomerulonephritis NOS

IQ **N00.9 Acute nephritic syndrome with unspecified morphologic changes**

SP **N00.A Acute nephritic syndrome with C3 glomerulonephritis**
Acute nephritic syndrome with C3 glomerulopathy, NOS

EXCLUDES 1 Acute nephritic syndrome (with C3 glomerulopathy) with dense deposit disease (N00.6)

4 **N01 Rapidly progressive nephritic syndrome**

INCLUDES rapidly progressive glomerular disease
rapidly progressive glomerulonephritis
rapidly progressive nephritis

EXCLUDES 1 nephritic syndrome NOS (N05.-)

SP **N01.0 Rapidly progressive nephritic syndrome with minor glomerular abnormality**
Rapidly progressive nephritic syndrome with minimal change lesion

SP **N01.1 Rapidly progressive nephritic syndrome with focal and segmental glomerular lesions**
Rapidly progressive nephritic syndrome with focal and segmental hyalinosis
Rapidly progressive nephritic syndrome with focal and segmental sclerosis
Rapidly progressive nephritic syndrome with focal glomerulonephritis

SP **N01.2 Rapidly progressive nephritic syndrome with diffuse membranous glomerulonephritis**

SP **N01.3 Rapidly progressive nephritic syndrome with diffuse mesangial proliferative glomerulonephritis**

SP **N01.4 Rapidly progressive nephritic syndrome with diffuse endocapillary proliferative glomerulonephritis**

Chapter 14
N00-N99

SP **N01.5 Rapidly progressive nephritic syndrome with diffuse mesangiocapillary glomerulonephritis**
Rapidly progressive nephritic syndrome with membranoproliferative glomerulonephritis, types 1 and 3, or NOS
EXCLUDES 1 Rapidly progressive nephritic syndrome with C3 glomerulonephritis (N01.A)
Rapidly progressive nephritic syndrome with C3 glomerulopathy (N01.A)

SP **N01.6 Rapidly progressive nephritic syndrome with dense deposit disease**
Rapidly progressive nephritic syndrome with C3 glomerulopathy with dense deposit disease
Rapidly progressive nephritic syndrome with membranoproliferative glomerulonephritis, type 2

SP **N01.7 Rapidly progressive nephritic syndrome with diffuse crescentic glomerulonephritis**
Rapidly progressive nephritic syndrome with extracapillary glomerulonephritis

SP **N01.8 Rapidly progressive nephritic syndrome with other morphologic changes**
Rapidly progressive nephritic syndrome with proliferative glomerulonephritis NOS

IQ **N01.9 Rapidly progressive nephritic syndrome with unspecified morphologic changes**

SP **N01.A Rapidly progressive nephritic syndrome with C3 glomerulonephritis**
Rapidly progressive nephritic syndrome with C3 glomerulopathy, NOS
EXCLUDES 1 Rapidly progressive nephritic syndrome (with C3 glomerulopathy) with dense deposit disease (N01.6)

4 **N02 Recurrent and persistent hematuria**
EXCLUDES 1 acute cystitis with hematuria (N30.01)
hematuria NOS (R31.9)
hematuria not associated with specified morphologic lesions (R31.-)

SP **N02.0 Recurrent and persistent hematuria with minor glomerular abnormality**
Recurrent and persistent hematuria with minimal change lesion

SP **N02.1 Recurrent and persistent hematuria with focal and segmental glomerular lesions**
Recurrent and persistent hematuria with focal and segmental hyalinosis
Recurrent and persistent hematuria with focal and segmental sclerosis
Recurrent and persistent hematuria with focal glomerulonephritis

SP **N02.2 Recurrent and persistent hematuria with diffuse membranous glomerulonephritis**

SP **N02.3 Recurrent and persistent hematuria with diffuse mesangial proliferative glomerulonephritis**

SP **N02.4 Recurrent and persistent hematuria with diffuse endocapillary proliferative glomerulonephritis**

SP **N02.5 Recurrent and persistent hematuria with diffuse mesangiocapillary glomerulonephritis**
Recurrent and persistent hematuria with membranoproliferative glomerulonephritis, types 1 and 3, or NOS
EXCLUDES 1 Recurrent and persistent hematuria with C3 glomerulonephritis (N02.A)
Recurrent and persistent hematuria with C3 glomerulopathy (N02.A)

SP **N02.6 Recurrent and persistent hematuria with dense deposit disease**
Recurrent and persistent hematuria with C3 glomerulopathy with dense deposit disease
Recurrent and persistent hematuria with membranoproliferative glomerulonephritis, type 2

SP **N02.7 Recurrent and persistent hematuria with diffuse crescentic glomerulonephritis**
Recurrent and persistent hematuria with extracapillary glomerulonephritis

SP **N02.8 Recurrent and persistent hematuria with other morphologic changes**
Recurrent and persistent hematuria with proliferative glomerulonephritis NOS

IQ **N02.9 Recurrent and persistent hematuria with unspecified morphologic changes**

SP SH **N02.A Recurrent and persistent hematuria with C3 glomerulonephritis**
Recurrent and persistent hematuria with C3 glomerulopathy
EXCLUDES 1 Recurrent and persistent hematuria (with C3 glomerulopathy) with dense deposit disease (N02.6)

4 **N03 Chronic nephritic syndrome**
INCLUDES chronic glomerular disease
chronic glomerulonephritis
chronic nephritis
EXCLUDES 1 chronic tubulo-interstitial nephritis (N11.-)
diffuse sclerosing glomerulonephritis (N05.8-)
nephritic syndrome NOS (N05.-)

SP **N03.0 Chronic nephritic syndrome with minor glomerular abnormality**
Chronic nephritic syndrome with minimal change lesion

SP **N03.1 Chronic nephritic syndrome with focal and segmental glomerular lesions**
Chronic nephritic syndrome with focal and segmental hyalinosis
Chronic nephritic syndrome with focal and segmental sclerosis

Chapter 14

N00-N99

Chronic nephritic syndrome with focal glomerulonephritis

SP **N03.2 Chronic nephritic syndrome with diffuse membranous glomerulonephritis**

SP **N03.3 Chronic nephritic syndrome with diffuse mesangial proliferative glomerulonephritis**

SP **N03.4 Chronic nephritic syndrome with diffuse endocapillary proliferative glomerulonephritis**

SP **N03.5 Chronic nephritic syndrome with diffuse mesangiocapillary glomerulonephritis**

Chronic nephritic syndrome with membranoproliferative glomerulonephritis, types 1 and 3, or NOS

EXCLUDES 1 Chronic nephritic syndrome with C3 glomerulonephritis (N03.A)
Chronic nephritic syndrome with C3 glomerulopathy (N03.A)

SP **N03.6 Chronic nephritic syndrome with dense deposit disease**

Chronic nephritic syndrome with C3 glomerulopathy with dense deposit disease

Chronic nephritic syndrome with membranoproliferative glomerulonephritis, type 2

SP **N03.7 Chronic nephritic syndrome with diffuse crescentic glomerulonephritis**

Chronic nephritic syndrome with extracapillary glomerulonephritis

SP **N03.8 Chronic nephritic syndrome with other morphologic changes**

Chronic nephritic syndrome with proliferative glomerulonephritis NOS

IQ **N03.9 Chronic nephritic syndrome with unspecified morphologic changes**

SP SH **N03.A Chronic nephritic syndrome with C3 glomerulonephritis**

Chronic nephritic syndrome with C3 glomerulopathy

EXCLUDES 1 Chronic nephritic syndrome (with C3 glomerulopathy) with dense deposit disease (N03.6)

4 **N04 Nephrotic syndrome**

INCLUDES congenital nephrotic syndrome
lipoid nephrosis

SP **N04.0 Nephrotic syndrome with minor glomerular abnormality**

Nephrotic syndrome with minimal change lesion

SP **N04.1 Nephrotic syndrome with focal and segmental glomerular lesions**

Nephrotic syndrome with focal and segmental hyalinosis

Nephrotic syndrome with focal and segmental sclerosis

Nephrotic syndrome with focal glomerulonephritis

SP **N04.2 Nephrotic syndrome with diffuse membranous glomerulonephritis**

SP **N04.3 Nephrotic syndrome with diffuse mesangial proliferative glomerulonephritis**

SP **N04.4 Nephrotic syndrome with diffuse endocapillary proliferative glomerulonephritis**

SP **N04.5 Nephrotic syndrome with diffuse mesangiocapillary glomerulonephritis**

Nephrotic syndrome with membranoproliferative glomerulonephritis, types 1 and 3, or NOS

EXCLUDES 1 Nephrotic syndrome with C3 glomerulonephritis (N04.A)
Nephrotic syndrome with C3 glomerulopathy (N04.A)

SP **N04.6 Nephrotic syndrome with dense deposit disease**

Nephrotic syndrome with C3 glomerulopathy with dense deposit disease

Nephrotic syndrome with membranoproliferative glomerulonephritis, type 2

SP **N04.7 Nephrotic syndrome with diffuse crescentic glomerulonephritis**

Nephrotic syndrome with extracapillary glomerulonephritis

SP **N04.8 Nephrotic syndrome with other morphologic changes**

Nephrotic syndrome with proliferative glomerulonephritis NOS

IQ **N04.9 Nephrotic syndrome with unspecified morphologic changes**

SP SH **N04.A Nephrotic syndrome with C3 glomerulonephritis**

Nephrotic syndrome with C3 glomerulopathy

EXCLUDES 1 Nephrotic syndrome (with C3 glomerulopathy) with dense deposit disease (N04.6)

4 **N05 Unspecified nephritic syndrome**

INCLUDES glomerular disease NOS
glomerulonephritis NOS
nephritis NOS
nephropathy NOS and renal disease NOS with morphological lesion specified in .0-.8

EXCLUDES 1 nephropathy NOS with no stated morphological lesion (N28.9)
renal disease NOS with no stated morphological lesion (N28.9)
tubulo-interstitial nephritis NOS (N12)

SP **N05.0 Unspecified nephritic syndrome with minor glomerular abnormality**

Unspecified nephritic syndrome with minimal change lesion

SP **N05.1 Unspecified nephritic syndrome with focal and segmental glomerular lesions**

Unspecified nephritic syndrome with focal and segmental hyalinosis

Unspecified nephritic syndrome with focal and segmental sclerosis

Unspecified nephritic syndrome with focal glomerulonephritis

Chapter 14

N00-N99

SP **N05.2 Unspecified nephritic syndrome with diffuse membranous glomerulonephritis**

SP **N05.3 Unspecified nephritic syndrome with diffuse mesangial proliferative glomerulonephritis**

SP **N05.4 Unspecified nephritic syndrome with diffuse endocapillary proliferative glomerulonephritis**

SP **N05.5 Unspecified nephritic syndrome with diffuse mesangiocapillary glomerulonephritis**

Unspecified nephritic syndrome with membranoproliferative glomerulonephritis, types 1 and 3, or NOS

EXCLUDES 1 Unspecified nephritic syndrome with C3 glomerulonephritis (N05.A)
Unspecified nephritic syndrome with C3 glomerulopathy (N05.A)

SP **N05.6 Unspecified nephritic syndrome with dense deposit disease**

Unspecified nephritic syndrome with C3 glomerulopathy with dense deposit disease

Unspecified nephritic syndrome with membranoproliferative glomerulonephritis, type 2

SP **N05.7 Unspecified nephritic syndrome with diffuse crescentic glomerulonephritis**

Unspecified nephritic syndrome with extracapillary glomerulonephritis

SP **N05.8 Unspecified nephritic syndrome with other morphologic changes**

Unspecified nephritic syndrome with proliferative glomerulonephritis NOS

IQ **N05.9 Unspecified nephritic syndrome with unspecified morphologic changes**

SP SH **N05.A Unspecified nephritic syndrome with C3 glomerulonephritis**

Unspecified nephritic syndrome with C3 glomerulopathy

EXCLUDES 1 Unspecified nephritic syndrome (with C3 glomerulopathy) with dense deposit disease (N05.6)

4 **N06 Isolated proteinuria with specified morphological lesion**

EXCLUDES 1 Proteinuria not associated with specific morphologic lesions (R80.0)

SP **N06.0 Isolated proteinuria with minor glomerular abnormality**

Isolated proteinuria with minimal change lesion

SP **N06.1 Isolated proteinuria with focal and segmental glomerular lesions**

Isolated proteinuria with focal and segmental hyalinosis

Isolated proteinuria with focal and segmental sclerosis

Isolated proteinuria with focal glomerulonephritis

SP **N06.2 Isolated proteinuria with diffuse membranous glomerulonephritis**

SP **N06.3 Isolated proteinuria with diffuse mesangial proliferative glomerulonephritis**

SP **N06.4 Isolated proteinuria with diffuse endocapillary proliferative glomerulonephritis**

SP **N06.5 Isolated proteinuria with diffuse mesangiocapillary glomerulonephritis**

Isolated proteinuria with membranoproliferative glomerulonephritis, types 1 and 3, or NOS

EXCLUDES 1 Isolated proteinuria with C3 glomerulonephritis (N06.A)
Isolated proteinuria with C3 glomerulopathy (N06.A)

SP **N06.6 Isolated proteinuria with dense deposit disease**

Isolated proteinuria with C3 glomerulopathy with dense deposit disease

Isolated proteinuria with membranoproliferative glomerulonephritis, type 2

SP **N06.7 Isolated proteinuria with diffuse crescentic glomerulonephritis**

Isolated proteinuria with extracapillary glomerulonephritis

SP **N06.8 Isolated proteinuria with other morphologic lesion**

Isolated proteinuria with proliferative glomerulonephritis NOS

IQ **N06.9 Isolated proteinuria with unspecified morphologic lesion**

SP SH **N06.A Isolated proteinuria with C3 glomerulonephritis**

Isolated proteinuria with C3 glomerulopathy

EXCLUDES 1 Isolated proteinuria (with C3 glomerulopathy) with dense deposit disease (N06.6)

4 **N07 Hereditary nephropathy, not elsewhere classified**

EXCLUDES 2 Alport's syndrome (Q87.81-)
hereditary amyloid nephropathy (E85.-)
nail patella syndrome (Q87.2)
non-neuropathic heredofamilial amyloidosis (E85.-)

SP **N07.0 Hereditary nephropathy, not elsewhere classified with minor glomerular abnormality**

Hereditary nephropathy, not elsewhere classified with minimal change lesion

SP **N07.1 Hereditary nephropathy, not elsewhere classified with focal and segmental glomerular lesions**

Hereditary nephropathy, not elsewhere classified with focal and segmental hyalinosis

Hereditary nephropathy, not elsewhere classified with focal and segmental sclerosis

Hereditary nephropathy, not elsewhere classified with focal glomerulonephritis

Chapter 14

N00-N99

SP **N07.2 Hereditary nephropathy, not elsewhere classified with diffuse membranous glomerulonephritis**

SP **N07.3 Hereditary nephropathy, not elsewhere classified with diffuse mesangial proliferative glomerulonephritis**

SP **N07.4 Hereditary nephropathy, not elsewhere classified with diffuse endocapillary proliferative glomerulonephritis**

SP **N07.5 Hereditary nephropathy, not elsewhere classified with diffuse mesangiocapillary glomerulonephritis**

Hereditary nephropathy, not elsewhere classified with membranoproliferative glomerulonephritis, types 1 and 3, or NOS

EXCLUDES 1 Hereditary nephropathy, not elsewhere classified with C3 glomerulonephritis (N07.A)
Hereditary nephropathy, not elsewhere classified with C3 glomerulopathy (N07.A)

SP **N07.6 Hereditary nephropathy, not elsewhere classified with dense deposit disease**

Hereditary nephropathy, not elsewhere classified with C3 glomerulopathy with dense deposit disease
Hereditary nephropathy, not elsewhere classified with membranoproliferative glomerulonephritis, type 2

SP **N07.7 Hereditary nephropathy, not elsewhere classified with diffuse crescentic glomerulonephritis**

Hereditary nephropathy, not elsewhere classified with extracapillary glomerulonephritis

SP **N07.8 Hereditary nephropathy, not elsewhere classified with other morphologic lesions**

Hereditary nephropathy, not elsewhere classified with proliferative glomerulonephritis NOS

IQ **N07.9 Hereditary nephropathy, not elsewhere classified with unspecified morphologic lesions**

SP SH **N07.A Hereditary nephropathy, not elsewhere classified with C3 glomerulonephritis**

Hereditary nephropathy, not elsewhere classified with C3 glomerulopathy

EXCLUDES 1 Hereditary nephropathy, not elsewhere classified (with C3 glomerulopathy) with dense deposit disease (N07.6)

M IQ **N08** ***Glomerular disorders in diseases classified elsewhere***

Glomerulonephritis
Nephritis
Nephropathy

Code first underlying disease, such as:
amyloidosis (E85.-)
congenital syphilis (A50.5)
cryoglobulinemia (D89.1)
disseminated intravascular coagulation (D65)
gout (M1A.-, M10.-)
microscopic polyangiitis (M31.7)
multiple myeloma (C90.0-)
sepsis (A40.0-A41.9)
sickle-cell disease (D57.0-D57.8)

EXCLUDES 1 glomerulonephritis, nephritis and nephropathy (in) :
antiglomerular basement membrane disease (M31.0)
diabetes (E08-E13 with .21)
gonococcal (A54.21)
Goodpasture's syndrome (M31.0)
hemolytic-uremic syndrome (D59.3)
lupus (M32.14)
mumps (B26.83)
syphilis (A52.75)
systemic lupus erythematosus (M32.14)
Wegener's granulomatosis (M31.31)
pyelonephritis in diseases classified elsewhere (N16)
renal tubulo-interstitial disorders classified elsewhere (N16)

CODING TIPS✓ Do not assign code N08 for a patient diagnosed with diabetic nephropathy. For a patient diagnosed with diabetic nephropathy, choose and assign the appropriate combination code to specify the manifestation from categories E08-E13 with 4th and 5th characters .21.

Renal tubulo-interstitial diseases (N10-N16)

INCLUDES pyelonephritis

EXCLUDES 1 pyeloureteritis cystica (N28.85)

CODING TIPS✓ If the urinary tract infection is resolved, or if the patient has recurrent infections, consider the use of Z87.440.

SP + **N10 Acute pyelonephritis**

Acute infectious interstitial nephritis
Acute pyelitis
Acute tubulo-interstitial nephritis
Hemoglobin nephrosis
Myoglobin nephrosis
Use additional code (B95-B97), to identify infectious agent.

+ 4 **N11 Chronic tubulo-interstitial nephritis**

INCLUDES chronic infectious interstitial nephritis
chronic pyelitis
chronic pyelonephritis

Use additional code (B95-B97), to identify infectious agent.

SP SH + **N11.0 Nonobstructive reflux-associated chronic pyelonephritis**

Pyelonephritis (chronic) associated with (vesicoureteral) reflux

EXCLUDES 1 vesicoureteral reflux NOS (N13.70)

SP SH + **N11.1 Chronic obstructive pyelonephritis**
Pyelonephritis (chronic) associated with anomaly of pelviureteric junction
Pyelonephritis (chronic) associated with anomaly of pyeloureteric junction
Pyelonephritis (chronic) associated with crossing of vessel
Pyelonephritis (chronic) associated with kinking of ureter
Pyelonephritis (chronic) associated with obstruction of ureter
Pyelonephritis (chronic) associated with stricture of pelviureteric junction
Pyelonephritis (chronic) associated with stricture of ureter
EXCLUDES 1 calculous pyelonephritis (N20.9)
obstructive uropathy (N13.-)

SP SH + **N11.8 Other chronic tubulo-interstitial nephritis**
Nonobstructive chronic pyelonephritis NOS

SP + **N11.9 Chronic tubulo-interstitial nephritis, unspecified**
Chronic interstitial nephritis NOS
Chronic pyelitis NOS
Chronic pyelonephritis NOS

SP **N12 Tubulo-interstitial nephritis, not specified as acute or chronic**
Interstitial nephritis NOS
Pyelitis NOS
Pyelonephritis NOS
EXCLUDES 1 calculous pyelonephritis (N20.9)

CODING TIPS ✓ A patient with unspecified pyelonephritis and urinary calculus unspecified is coded as N12 and N20 in either order.

4 **N13 Obstructive and reflux uropathy**
EXCLUDES 2 calculus of kidney and ureter without hydronephrosis (N20.-)
congenital obstructive defects of renal pelvis and ureter (Q62.0-Q62.3)
hydronephrosis with ureteropelvic junction obstruction (Q62.11)
obstructive pyelonephritis (N11.1)

SP **N13.0 Hydronephrosis with ureteropelvic junction obstruction**
Hydronephrosis due to acquired occlusion of ureteropelvic junction
EXCLUDES 2 Hydronephrosis with ureteropelvic junction obstruction due to calculus (N13.2)

SP **N13.1 Hydronephrosis with ureteral stricture, not elsewhere classified**
EXCLUDES 1 Hydronephrosis with ureteral stricture with infection (N13.6)

SP SH **N13.2 Hydronephrosis with renal and ureteral calculous obstruction**
EXCLUDES 1 Hydronephrosis with renal and ureteral calculous obstruction with infection (N13.6)

5 **N13.3 Other and unspecified hydronephrosis**
EXCLUDES 1 hydronephrosis with infection (N13.6)

SP **N13.30 Unspecified hydronephrosis**

SP **N13.39 Other hydronephrosis**

SP **N13.4 Hydroureter**
EXCLUDES 1 congenital hydroureter (Q62.3-)
hydroureter with infection (N13.6)
vesicoureteral-reflux with hydroureter (N13.73-)

SP **N13.5 Crossing vessel and stricture of ureter without hydronephrosis**
Kinking and stricture of ureter without hydronephrosis
EXCLUDES 1 Crossing vessel and stricture of ureter without hydronephrosis with infection (N13.6)

SP + **N13.6 Pyonephrosis**
Conditions in N13.0-N13.5 with infection
Obstructive uropathy with infection
Use additional code (B95-B97), to identify infectious agent.

5 **N13.7 Vesicoureteral-reflux**
EXCLUDES 1 reflux-associated pyelonephritis (N11.0)

SP **N13.70 Vesicoureteral-reflux, unspecified**
Vesicoureteral-reflux NOS

DEFINITION Abnormal retrograde flow of urine from bladder back into the ureter and kidney; may cause progressive, long-term damage.

SP **N13.71 Vesicoureteral-reflux without reflux nephropathy**

6 **N13.72 Vesicoureteral-reflux with reflux nephropathy without hydroureter**

SP **N13.721 Vesicoureteral-reflux with reflux nephropathy without hydroureter, unilateral**

SP **N13.722 Vesicoureteral-reflux with reflux nephropathy without hydroureter, bilateral**

!Q **N13.729 Vesicoureteral-reflux with reflux nephropathy without hydroureter, unspecified**

6 **N13.73 Vesicoureteral-reflux with reflux nephropathy with hydroureter**

SP **N13.731 Vesicoureteral-reflux with reflux nephropathy with hydroureter, unilateral**

SP **N13.732 Vesicoureteral-reflux with reflux nephropathy with hydroureter, bilateral**

!Q **N13.739 Vesicoureteral-reflux with reflux nephropathy with hydroureter, unspecified**

SP **N13.8 Other obstructive and reflux uropathy**

Chapter 14
N00-N99

Urinary tract obstruction due to specified cause
Code first, if applicable, any causal condition, such as:
enlarged prostate (N40.1)

SP **N13.9 Obstructive and reflux uropathy, unspecified**
Urinary tract obstruction NOS

+ 4 **N14 Drug- and heavy-metal-induced tubulo-interstitial and tubular conditions**
Code first:
poisoning due to drug or toxin, if applicable (T36-T65 with fifth or sixth character 1-4 or 6)
Use additional code for adverse effect, if applicable, to identify drug (T36-T50 with fifth or sixth character 5)

CODING TIPS ✓ Conditions classified to N14.- indicate nephropathy due to drugs, metals, or other toxic exposure. When one of these conditions has been specifically reported, first assign the appropriate code from T36-T65 when the condition is due to a poisoning. Or, to indicate adverse effect, assign a second code from T36-T50 following the appropriate N14.- code.

SP + **N14.0 Analgesic nephropathy**
SP + **N14.1 Nephropathy induced by other drugs, medicaments and biological substances**
SP + **N14.2 Nephropathy induced by unspecified drug, medicament or biological substance**
SP + **N14.3 Nephropathy induced by heavy metals**
SP + **N14.4 Toxic nephropathy, not elsewhere classified**

4 **N15 Other renal tubulo-interstitial diseases**
SP **N15.0 Balkan nephropathy**
Balkan endemic nephropathy
SP **N15.1 Renal and perinephric abscess**
SP **N15.8 Other specified renal tubulo-interstitial diseases**
SP **N15.9 Renal tubulo-interstitial disease, unspecified**
Infection of kidney NOS
EXCLUDES 1 urinary tract infection NOS (N39.0)

▲ M IQ **N16 *Renal tubulo-interstitial disorders in diseases classified elsewhere***
Pyelonephritis
Tubulo-interstitial nephritis
Code first underlying disease, such as:
brucellosis (A23.0-A23.9)
cryoglobulinemia (D89.1)
glycogen storage disease (E74.0)
leukemia (C91-C95)
lymphoma (C81.0-C85.9, C96.0-C96.9)
multiple myeloma (C90.0-)
sepsis (A40.0-A41.9)
Wilson's disease (E83.0)
EXCLUDES 1 diphtheritic pyelonephritis and tubulo-interstitial nephritis (A36.84)
pyelonephritis and tubulo-interstitial nephritis in candidiasis (B37.49)
pyelonephritis and tubulo-interstitial nephritis in cystinosis (E72.04)
pyelonephritis and tubulo-interstitial nephritis in salmonella infection (A02.25)
pyelonephritis and tubulo-interstitial nephritis in sarcoidosis (D86.84)
pyelonephritis and tubulo-interstitial nephritis in Sjogren syndrome (M35.04)
pyelonephritis and tubulo-interstitial nephritis in systemic lupus erythematosus (M32.15)
pyelonephritis and tubulo-interstitial nephritis in toxoplasmosis (B58.83)
renal tubular degeneration in diabetes (E08-E13 with .29)
syphilitic pyelonephritis and tubulo-interstitial nephritis (A52.75)

Acute kidney failure and chronic kidney disease (N17-N19)

EXCLUDES 2 congenital renal failure (P96.0)
drug- and heavy-metal-induced tubulo-interstitial and tubular conditions (N14.-)
extrarenal uremia (R39.2)
hemolytic-uremic syndrome (D59.3)
hepatorenal syndrome (K76.7)
postpartum hepatorenal syndrome (O90.4)
posttraumatic renal failure (T79.5)
prerenal uremia (R39.2)
renal failure complicating abortion or ectopic or molar pregnancy (O00-O07, O08.4)
renal failure following labor and delivery (O90.4)
renal failure postprocedural (N99.0)

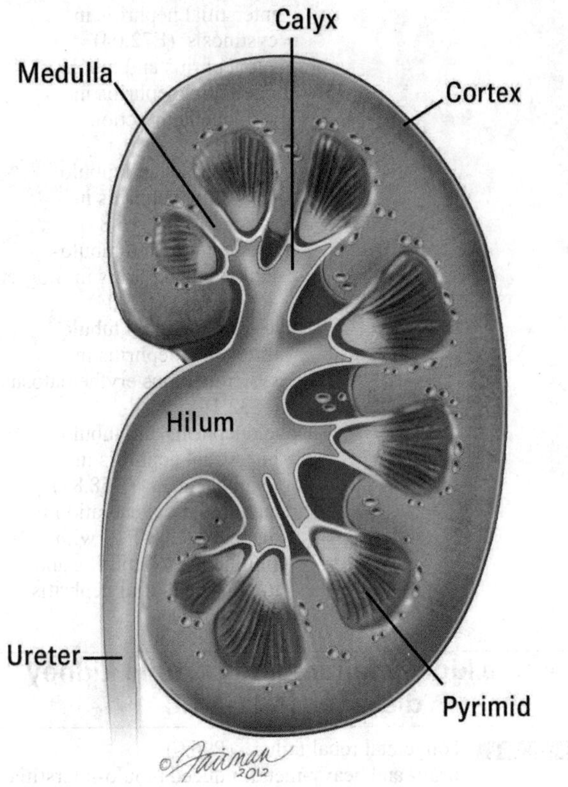

N17 Acute kidney failure
Code also:
associated underlying condition
EXCLUDES 1 posttraumatic renal failure (T79.5)
GUIDELINES **Section I.C.9.a.2)**
If a patient has hypertensive chronic kidney disease and acute renal failure, the acute renal failure should also be coded. Sequence according to the circumstances of the admission/encounter.
CODING TIPS✓ When acute renal failure and chronic renal failure are both documented, both must be coded. Sequencing may be according to importance of care.

H SP **N17.0 Acute kidney failure with tubular necrosis**
Acute tubular necrosis
Renal tubular necrosis
Tubular necrosis NOS

H SP **N17.1 Acute kidney failure with acute cortical necrosis**
Acute cortical necrosis
Cortical necrosis NOS
Renal cortical necrosis

H SP **N17.2 Acute kidney failure with medullary necrosis**
Medullary [papillary] necrosis NOS
Acute medullary [papillary] necrosis
Renal medullary [papillary] necrosis

H SP **N17.8 Other acute kidney failure**

H SP **N17.9 Acute kidney failure, unspecified**
Acute kidney injury (nontraumatic)

EXCLUDES 2 traumatic kidney injury (S37.0-)

+ **N18 Chronic kidney disease (CKD)**
Code first any associated:
diabetic chronic kidney disease (E08.22, E09.22, E10.22, E11.22, E13.22)
hypertensive chronic kidney disease (I12.-, I13.-)
Use additional code to identify kidney transplant status, if applicable, (Z94.0)
GUIDELINES **Section I.C.14.a.3)**
Patients with CKD may also suffer from other serious conditions, most commonly diabetes mellitus and hypertension. The sequencing of the CKD code in relationship to codes for other contributing conditions is based on the conventions in the Tabular List.
CODING TIPS✓ Diabetes and hypertension are assumed related to chronic kidney disease unless the physician documents that they are unrelated. Examples of documentation may be hypertensive CKD or diabetic CKD.
CODING TIPS✓ The stage of CKD may not be coded based on lab data such as glomerular filtration rates (GFR).
CODING TIPS✓ Chronic kidney disease (CKD) is assumed related to hypertension and diabetes. Hypertension (I12 or I13) is sequenced prior to chronic kidney disease (CKD) if both are present. Any associated diabetes also must be sequenced prior to the CKD. Diabetic CKD and hypertension is coded either E11.22, I12.9, N18.9 or I12.9, E11.22, N18.9. If documentation indicates that the patient also has heart disease related to hypertension, the hypertension code will be from the I13 category.
CODING TIPS✓ The presence of CKD alone after a kidney transplant doesn't necessarily mean the transplant is complicated. Patients who have undergone a kidney transplant may still have some form of CKD because the kidney transplant may not fully restore kidney function. Assign the appropriate N18 code (chronic kidney disease) to indicate the stage of CKD, and code Z94.0 (kidney organ or tissue replaced by transplant), if a transplant complication is not documented.

SP SH + **N18.1 Chronic kidney disease, stage 1**

SP SH + **N18.2 Chronic kidney disease, stage 2 (mild)**

+ **N18.3 Chronic kidney disease, stage 3 (moderate)**
CODING TIPS✓ Kidney disease is usually asymptomatic just prior to kidney failure and the need for kidney replacement therapy. Stage 3 has been given more specificity to capture more stage 3 detail. Stage 3a is based on an eGFR of 45-59. Stage 3b is based on an eGFR of 30-44. Determination of the correct code must be based on physician or NPP documentation and not lab data.

SP SH + **N18.30 Chronic kidney disease, stage 3 unspecified**

SP SH + **N18.31 Chronic kidney disease, stage 3a**

SP SH + **N18.32 Chronic kidney disease, stage 3b**

SP SH + **N18.4 Chronic kidney disease, stage 4 (severe)**

!Q SH + **N18.5 Chronic kidney disease, stage 5**

EXCLUDES 1 chronic kidney disease, stage 5 requiring chronic dialysis (N18.6)

H !Q SH + **N18.6 End stage renal disease**

Chronic kidney disease requiring chronic dialysis

Use additional code to identify dialysis status (Z99.2)

ALERT ESRD is not appropriate for assignment to the primary diagnosis in home care. ESRD and related care to the dialysis catheter is the responsibility of the dialysis center.

CODING TIPS✓ All CKD patients requiring dialysis are coded as N18.6, even if the physician or NPP documents a different stage. Do not code ESRD as primary in home health. Add the appropriate Z99.2 or Z91.15 if on dialysis. If the patient with ESRD is not on dialysis, then the code for palliative care may be appropriate (Z51.5).

CODING TIPS✓ If ESRD is documented along with another stage of CKD, code only N18.6.

!Q + **N18.9 Chronic kidney disease, unspecified**

Chronic renal disease
Chronic renal failure NOS
Chronic renal insufficiency
Chronic uremia NOS
Diffuse sclerosing glomerulonephritis NOS

H !Q **N19 Unspecified kidney failure**

Uremia NOS

EXCLUDES 1 acute kidney failure (N17.-)
chronic kidney disease (N18.-)
chronic uremia (N18.9)
extrarenal uremia (R39.2)
prerenal uremia (R39.2)
renal insufficiency (acute) (N28.9)
uremia of newborn (P96.0)

Urolithiasis (N20-N23)

4 **N20 Calculus of kidney and ureter**

Calculous pyelonephritis

EXCLUDES 1 nephrocalcinosis (E83.5)
that with hydronephrosis (N13.2)

CODING TIPS✓ If the renal calculi is resolved, or if the patient has recurrent kidney stones, consider the use of Z87.442.

CODING TIPS✓ A patient with unspecified pyelonephritis and urinary calculus unspecified is coded as N12 and N20 in either order.

SP SH **N20.0 Calculus of kidney**

Nephrolithiasis NOS
Renal calculus
Renal stone
Staghorn calculus
Stone in kidney

SP **N20.1 Calculus of ureter**

Calculus of the ureteropelvic junction
Ureteric stone

SP SH **N20.2 Calculus of kidney with calculus of ureter**

!Q **N20.9 Urinary calculus, unspecified**

4 **N21 Calculus of lower urinary tract**

INCLUDES calculus of lower urinary tract with cystitis and urethritis

SP **N21.0 Calculus in bladder**

Calculus in diverticulum of bladder
Urinary bladder stone

EXCLUDES 2 staghorn calculus (N20.0)

DEFINITION An abnormal concretion of mineral salts, occurring in the bladder.

SP **N21.1 Calculus in urethra**

EXCLUDES 2 calculus of prostate (N42.0)

SP **N21.8 Other lower urinary tract calculus**

!Q **N21.9 Calculus of lower urinary tract, unspecified**

EXCLUDES 1 calculus of urinary tract NOS (N20.9)

M !Q **N22** ***Calculus of urinary tract in diseases classified elsewhere***

Code first underlying disease, such as:
gout (M1A.-, M10.-)
schistosomiasis (B65.0-B65.9)

SP **N23 Unspecified renal colic**

Other disorders of kidney and ureter (N25-N29)

EXCLUDES 2 disorders of kidney and ureter with urolithiasis (N20-N23)

4 **N25 Disorders resulting from impaired renal tubular function**

SP **N25.0 Renal osteodystrophy**

Azotemic osteodystrophy
Phosphate-losing tubular disorders
Renal rickets
Renal short stature

EXCLUDES 2 metabolic disorders classifiable to E70-E88

SP SH **N25.1 Nephrogenic diabetes insipidus**

EXCLUDES 1 diabetes insipidus NOS (E23.2)

5 **N25.8 Other disorders resulting from impaired renal tubular function**

SP **N25.81 Secondary hyperparathyroidism of renal origin**

EXCLUDES 1 secondary hyperparathyroidism, non-renal (E21.1)

EXCLUDES 2 metabolic disorders classifiable to E70-E88

SP **N25.89 Other disorders resulting from impaired renal tubular function**

Hypokalemic nephropathy
Lightwood-Albright syndrome
Renal tubular acidosis NOS

!Q **N25.9 Disorder resulting from impaired renal tubular function, unspecified**

4 **N26 Unspecified contracted kidney**

EXCLUDES 1 contracted kidney due to hypertension (I12.-)
diffuse sclerosing glomerulonephritis (N05.8.-)

Chapter 14 N00-N99

hypertensive nephrosclerosis (arteriolar) (arteriosclerotic) (I12.-)
small kidney of unknown cause (N27.-)

CODING TIPS✓ When a condition classifiable to N26.-is present with a diagnosis of hypertension, I12.9 should be assigned, unless the provider documents secondary hypertension. N26 is included in I12.

SP **N26.1 Atrophy of kidney (terminal)**

SP **N26.2 Page kidney**

!Q **N26.9 Renal sclerosis, unspecified**

4 **N27 Small kidney of unknown cause**

INCLUDES oligonephronia

SP **N27.0 Small kidney, unilateral**

SP **N27.1 Small kidney, bilateral**

!Q **N27.9 Small kidney, unspecified**

4 **N28 Other disorders of kidney and ureter, not elsewhere classified**

SP **N28.0 Ischemia and infarction of kidney**

Renal artery embolism
Renal artery obstruction
Renal artery occlusion
Renal artery thrombosis
Renal infarct

EXCLUDES 1 atherosclerosis of renal artery (extrarenal part) (I70.1)
congenital stenosis of renal artery (Q27.1)
Goldblatt's kidney (I70.1)

SP **N28.1 Cyst of kidney, acquired**

Cyst (multiple) (solitary) of kidney (acquired)

EXCLUDES 1 cystic kidney disease (congenital) (Q61.-)

CODING TIPS✓ N28.1 is coded only for acquired renal cysts. If the medical record does not indicate acquired or congenital, ICD-10 assumes the cyst is congenital (Q61). Carefully review documentation provided to ensure the cysts are in the kidney when assigning this code. Cysts noted to be present in the ureters are not classified here.

5 **N28.8 Other specified disorders of kidney and ureter**

EXCLUDES 1 hydroureter (N13.4)
ureteric stricture with hydronephrosis (N13.1)
ureteric stricture without hydronephrosis (N13.5)

SP **N28.81 Hypertrophy of kidney**

SP **N28.82 Megaloureter**

SP **N28.83 Nephroptosis**

SP **N28.84 Pyelitis cystica**

SP **N28.85 Pyeloureteritis cystica**

DEFINITION Infection of the renal pelvis and ureter with development of small cysts in the kidney and ureter.

SP **N28.86 Ureteritis cystica**

SP **N28.89 Other specified disorders of kidney and ureter**

!Q **N28.9 Disorder of kidney and ureter, unspecified**

Nephropathy NOS
Renal disease (acute) NOS
Renal insufficiency (acute)

EXCLUDES 1 chronic renal insufficiency (N18.9)
unspecified nephritic syndrome (N05.-)

M !Q SH **N29 *Other disorders of kidney and ureter in diseases classified elsewhere***

Code first underlying disease, such as:
amyloidosis (E85.-)
nephrocalcinosis (E83.5)
schistosomiasis (B65.0-B65.9)

EXCLUDES 1 disorders of kidney and ureter in:
cystinosis (E72.0)
gonorrhea (A54.21)
syphilis (A52.75)
tuberculosis (A18.11)

Other diseases of the urinary system (N30-N39)

EXCLUDES 2 urinary infection (complicating) :
abortion or ectopic or molar pregnancy (O00-O07, O08.8)
pregnancy, childbirth and the puerperium (O23.-, O75.3, O86.2-)

+ 4 **N30 Cystitis**

Use additional code to identify infectious agent (B95-B97)

EXCLUDES 1 prostatocystitis (N41.3)

CODING TIPS✓ If the urinary tract infection is resolved, or if the patient has recurrent infections, consider the use of Z87.440.

CODING TIPS✓ Gross hematuria means that the blood in the urine can be seen with the naked eye. If hematuria is related to anticoagulant/antiplatelets, also code D68.32 and the T code for the drug.

CODING TIPS✓ Cystitis indicates inflammation and/or infection localized to the bladder. When a urinary tract infection is specified as cystitis, assign the appropriate N30.- code. Also assign a code for the causative organism, when known. An unspecified urinary tract infection should be coded to N39.0.

+ 5 **N30.0 Acute cystitis**

EXCLUDES 1 irradiation cystitis (N30.4-)
trigonitis (N30.3-)

SP + **N30.00 Acute cystitis without hematuria**

SP + **N30.01 Acute cystitis with hematuria**

+ 5 **N30.1 Interstitial cystitis (chronic)**

SP + **N30.10 Interstitial cystitis (chronic) without hematuria**

SP + **N30.11 Interstitial cystitis (chronic) with hematuria**

+ 5 **N30.2 Other chronic cystitis**

SP + **N30.20 Other chronic cystitis without hematuria**

SP + **N30.21 Other chronic cystitis with hematuria**

+ 5 **N30.3 Trigonitis**

Urethrotrigonitis

DEFINITION Inflammation of the mouth of the bladder where it drains into the urethra.

SP + **N30.30 Trigonitis without hematuria**

SP + **N30.31 Trigonitis with hematuria**

+ 5 **N30.4 Irradiation cystitis**

SP + **N30.40 Irradiation cystitis without hematuria**

SP + **N30.41 Irradiation cystitis with hematuria**

+ 5 **N30.8 Other cystitis**

Abscess of bladder

SP + **N30.80 Other cystitis without hematuria**

SP + **N30.81 Other cystitis with hematuria**

DEFINITION Bullous (cystic) cystitis: Inflammation of the bladder with formation of cysts on the interior bladder wall.

+ 5 **N30.9 Cystitis, unspecified**

SP + **N30.90 Cystitis, unspecified without hematuria**

SP + **N30.91 Cystitis, unspecified with hematuria**

+ 4 **N31 Neuromuscular dysfunction of bladder, not elsewhere classified**

Use additional code to identify any associated urinary incontinence (N39.3-N39.4-)

EXCLUDES 1 cord bladder NOS (G95.89)
neurogenic bladder due to cauda equina syndrome (G83.4)
neuromuscular dysfunction due to spinal cord lesion (G95.89)

SP SH + **N31.0 Uninhibited neuropathic bladder, not elsewhere classified**

SP SH + **N31.1 Reflex neuropathic bladder, not elsewhere classified**

SP + **N31.2 Flaccid neuropathic bladder, not elsewhere classified**

Atonic (motor) (sensory) neuropathic bladder
Autonomous neuropathic bladder
Nonreflex neuropathic bladder

SP + **N31.8 Other neuromuscular dysfunction of bladder**

SP SH + **N31.9 Neuromuscular dysfunction of bladder, unspecified**

Neurogenic bladder dysfunction NOS

4 **N32 Other disorders of bladder**

EXCLUDES 2 calculus of bladder (N21.0)
cystocele (N81.1-)
hernia or prolapse of bladder, female (N81.1-)

SP **N32.0 Bladder-neck obstruction**

Bladder-neck stenosis (acquired)

EXCLUDES 1 congenital bladder-neck obstruction (Q64.3-)

DEFINITION Blockage in the opening between the bladder and the urethra, causing bladder distention and decreased urine output.

SP **N32.1 Vesicointestinal fistula**

Vesicorectal fistula

DEFINITION Abnormal passage between the bladder and the intestines.

SP **N32.2 Vesical fistula, not elsewhere classified**

EXCLUDES 1 fistula between bladder and female genital tract (N82.0-N82.1)

SP **N32.3 Diverticulum of bladder**

EXCLUDES 1 congenital diverticulum of bladder (Q64.6)
diverticulitis of bladder (N30.8-)

5 **N32.8 Other specified disorders of bladder**

SP **N32.81 Overactive bladder**

Detrusor muscle hyperactivity

EXCLUDES 1 frequent urination due to specified bladder condition- code to condition

SP **N32.89 Other specified disorders of bladder**

Bladder hemorrhage
Bladder hypertrophy
Calcified bladder
Contracted bladder

IQ **N32.9 Bladder disorder, unspecified**

M IQ ***N33 Bladder disorders in diseases classified elsewhere***

Code first underlying disease, such as:
schistosomiasis (B65.0-B65.9)

EXCLUDES 1 bladder disorder in syphilis (A52.76)
bladder disorder in tuberculosis (A18.12)
candidal cystitis (B37.41)
chlamydial cystitis (A56.01)
cystitis in gonorrhea (A54.01)
cystitis in neurogenic bladder (N31.-)
diphtheritic cystitis (A36.85)
syphilitic cystitis (A52.76)
trichomonal cystitis (A59.03)

+ 4 **N34 Urethritis and urethral syndrome**

Use additional code (B95-B97), to identify infectious agent.

EXCLUDES 2 Reiter's disease (M02.3-)
urethritis in diseases with a predominantly sexual mode of transmission (A50-A64)
urethrotrigonitis (N30.3-)

SP + **N34.0 Urethral abscess**

Abscess (of) Cowper's gland
Abscess (of) Littré's gland
Abscess (of) urethral (gland)
Periurethral abscess

EXCLUDES 1 urethral caruncle (N36.2)

SP + **N34.1 Nonspecific urethritis**

Nongonococcal urethritis
Nonvenereal urethritis

SP + **N34.2 Other urethritis**

Meatitis, urethral
Postmenopausal urethritis
Ulcer of urethra (meatus)
Urethritis NOS

SP + **N34.3 Urethral syndrome, unspecified**

4 **N35 Urethral stricture**

EXCLUDES 1 congenital urethral stricture (Q64.3-)
postprocedural urethral stricture (N99.1-)

5 **N35.0 Post-traumatic urethral stricture**

Urethral stricture due to injury

Chapter 14

N00-N99

EXCLUDES 1 postprocedural urethral stricture (N99.1-)

6 **N35.01 Post-traumatic urethral stricture, male**

SP **N35.010 Post-traumatic urethral stricture, male, meatal**

SP **N35.011 Post-traumatic bulbous urethral stricture**

SP **N35.012 Post-traumatic membranous urethral stricture**

SP **N35.013 Post-traumatic anterior urethral stricture**

SP **N35.014 Post-traumatic urethral stricture, male, unspecified**

SP **N35.016 Post-traumatic urethral stricture, male, overlapping sites**

6 **N35.02 Post-traumatic urethral stricture, female**

SP **N35.021 Urethral stricture due to childbirth**

SP **N35.028 Other post-traumatic urethral stricture, female**

5 **N35.1 Postinfective urethral stricture, not elsewhere classified**

EXCLUDES 1 urethral stricture associated with schistosomiasis (B65.-, N29)
gonococcal urethral stricture (A54.01)
syphilitic urethral stricture (A52.76)

6 **N35.11 Postinfective urethral stricture, not elsewhere classified, male**

SP **N35.111 Postinfective urethral stricture, not elsewhere classified, male, meatal**

SP **N35.112 Postinfective bulbous urethral stricture, not elsewhere classified, male**

SP **N35.113 Postinfective membranous urethral stricture, not elsewhere classified, male**

SP **N35.114 Postinfective anterior urethral stricture, not elsewhere classified, male**

SP **N35.116 Postinfective urethral stricture, not elsewhere classified, male, overlapping sites**

SP **N35.119 Postinfective urethral stricture, not elsewhere classified, male, unspecified**

SP **N35.12 Postinfective urethral stricture, not elsewhere classified, female**

5 **N35.8 Other urethral stricture**

EXCLUDES 1 postprocedural urethral stricture (N99.1-)

6 **N35.81 Other urethral stricture, male**

SP **N35.811 Other urethral stricture, male, meatal**

SP **N35.812 Other urethral bulbous stricture, male**

SP **N35.813 Other membranous urethral stricture, male**

SP **N35.814 Other anterior urethral stricture, male**

SP **N35.816 Other urethral stricture, male, overlapping sites**

SP **N35.819 Other urethral stricture, male, unspecified site**

SP **N35.82 Other urethral stricture, female**

5 **N35.9 Urethral stricture, unspecified**

6 **N35.91 Urethral stricture, unspecified, male**

SP **N35.911 Unspecified urethral stricture, male, meatal**

SP **N35.912 Unspecified bulbous urethral stricture, male**

SP **N35.913 Unspecified membranous urethral stricture, male**

SP **N35.914 Unspecified anterior urethral stricture, male**

SP **N35.916 Unspecified urethral stricture, male, overlapping sites**

SP **N35.919 Unspecified urethral stricture, male, unspecified site**
Pinhole meatus NOS
Urethral stricture NOS

SP **N35.92 Unspecified urethral stricture, female**

4 **N36 Other disorders of urethra**

SP **N36.0 Urethral fistula**
Urethroperineal fistula
Urethrorectal fistula
Urinary fistula NOS

EXCLUDES 1 urethroscrotal fistula (N50.89)
urethrovaginal fistula (N82.1)
urethrovesicovaginal fistula (N82.1)

DEFINITION An abnormal passage communicating with the urethra.

SP **N36.1 Urethral diverticulum**

DEFINITION Sac-like out-pouching of the urethral wall.

SP **N36.2 Urethral caruncle**

DEFINITION A fleshy outgrowth in the urethra that may be normal or abnormal, often growing from mucous membranes.

+ 5 **N36.4 Urethral functional and muscular disorders**
Use additional code to identify associated urinary stress incontinence (N39.3)

SP + **N36.41 Hypermobility of urethra**

SP + **N36.42 Intrinsic sphincter deficiency (ISD)**

SP + **N36.43 Combined hypermobility of urethra and intrinsic sphincter deficiency**

SP + **N36.44 Muscular disorders of urethra**
Bladder sphincter dyssynergy

SP **N36.5 Urethral false passage**

SP **N36.8 Other specified disorders of urethra**

EXCLUDES 1 congenital urethrocele (Q64.7)
female urethrocele (N81.0)

IQ **N36.9 Urethral disorder, unspecified**

M IQ **N37** ***Urethral disorders in diseases classified elsewhere***
Code first:
underlying disease

EXCLUDES 1 urethritis (in):
candidal infection (B37.41)
chlamydial (A56.01)

gonorrhea (A54.01)
syphilis (A52.76)
trichomonal infection (A59.03)
tuberculosis (A18.13)

4 N39 Other disorders of urinary system

EXCLUDES 2 hematuria NOS (R31.-)
recurrent or persistent hematuria (N02.-)
recurrent or persistent hematuria with specified morphological lesion (N02.-)
proteinuria NOS (R80.-)

SP SH + N39.0 Urinary tract infection, site not specified

Use additional code (B95-B97), to identify infectious agent.

EXCLUDES 1 candidiasis of urinary tract (B37.4-)
neonatal urinary tract infection (P39.3)
pyuria (R82.81)
urinary tract infection of specified site, such as:
cystitis (N30.-)
urethritis (N34.-)

CODING TIPS✓ Bacteriuria is a condition where there are bacteria present in a microscopic examination of the urine. Do not code bacteriuria as a UTI. See R82.7.

CODING TIPS✓ The urinary tract includes the kidneys, ureters, bladder and urethra. Infection involving the bladder is coded with category N30. Infection of the kidney should be coded N15.9 (unless specific information is available). Urethritis is coded with category N34. Infection involving the ureter(s) should be coded with N28.86. Query for specific information.

CODING TIPS✓ If UTI is not a confirmed diagnosis, report a symptom code (e.g., codes in R30-R39 series) instead of this code.

CODING TIPS✓ Code N39.0 is appropriate only when the site of the UTI is unspecified. Remember to use additional code (B95-B97) to identify infectious agent. If the urinary tract infection is resolved, or if the patient has recurrent infections, consider the use of Z87.440.

SP N39.3 Stress incontinence (female) (male)

Code also:
any associated overactive bladder (N32.81)

EXCLUDES 1 mixed incontinence (N39.46)

DEFINITION Involuntary loss of bladder control during physical movements, such as coughing, sneezing, or other strenuous activity.

5 N39.4 Other specified urinary incontinence

Code also:
any associated overactive bladder (N32.81)

EXCLUDES 1 enuresis NOS (R32)
functional urinary incontinence (R39.81)
urinary incontinence associated with cognitive impairment (R39.81)
urinary incontinence NOS (R32)
urinary incontinence of nonorganic origin (F98.0)

SP N39.41 Urge incontinence

EXCLUDES 1 mixed incontinence (N39.46)

DEFINITION Inability to control urination after the urge to urinate.

SP N39.42 Incontinence without sensory awareness

Insensible (urinary) incontinence

IQ N39.43 Post-void dribbling

▲ IQ N39.44 Nocturnal enuresis

EXCLUDES 2 nocturnal polyuria (R35.81)

IQ N39.45 Continuous leakage

SP N39.46 Mixed incontinence

Urge and stress incontinence

6 N39.49 Other specified urinary incontinence

SP N39.490 Overflow incontinence

DEFINITION Urinary incontinence due to pressure of retained urine in the bladder, after the bladder has contracted to its limits, with dribbling urine.

SP N39.491 Coital incontinence

SP N39.492 Postural (urinary) incontinence

SP N39.498 Other specified urinary incontinence

Reflex incontinence
Total incontinence

SP N39.8 Other specified disorders of urinary system

IQ N39.9 Disorder of urinary system, unspecified

Diseases of male genital organs (N40-N53)

4 N40 Benign prostatic hyperplasia

INCLUDES adenofibromatous hypertrophy of prostate
benign hypertrophy of the prostate
benign prostatic hypertrophy
BPH
enlarged prostate
nodular prostate
polyp of prostate

EXCLUDES 1 benign neoplasms of prostate (adenoma, benign) (fibroadenoma) (fibroma) (myoma) (D29.1)

EXCLUDES 2 malignant neoplasm of prostate (C61)

CODING TIPS✓ Enlarged prostate disorders no longer include the benign neoplasms of the prostate. Benign tumors of the prostate are coded to D29.1, not N40.

Chapter 14 N00-N99

CODING TIPS✓ Although hyperplasia (increase in number of cells) and hypertrophy (increase in size of cells) are not synonymous, benign prostatic hyperplasia and benign prostatic hypertrophy are classified to the same code. When a patient diagnosed with a condition classifiable to N40.- also has lower urinary tract symptoms present – such as obstruction, incontinence, hesitancy, frequency, urgency or other included conditions – assign code N40.1 and the associated symptoms.

SP **N40.0 Benign prostatic hyperplasia without lower urinary tract symptoms**
Enlarged prostate without LUTS
Enlarged prostate NOS

SP SH + **N40.1 Benign prostatic hyperplasia with lower urinary tract symptoms**
Enlarged prostate with LUTS
Use additional code for associated symptoms, when specified:
- incomplete bladder emptying (R39.14)
- nocturia (R35.1)
- straining on urination (R39.16)
- urinary frequency (R35.0)
- urinary hesitancy (R39.11)
- urinary incontinence (N39.4-)
- urinary obstruction (N13.8)
- urinary retention (R33.8)
- urinary urgency (R39.15)
- weak urinary stream (R39.12)

SP **N40.2 Nodular prostate without lower urinary tract symptoms**
Nodular prostate without LUTS

SP + **N40.3 Nodular prostate with lower urinary tract symptoms**
Use additional code for associated symptoms, when specified:
- incomplete bladder emptying (R39.14)
- nocturia (R35.1)
- straining on urination (R39.16)
- urinary frequency (R35.0)
- urinary hesitancy (R39.11)
- urinary incontinence (N39.4-)
- urinary obstruction (N13.8)
- urinary retention (R33.8)
- urinary urgency (R39.15)
- weak urinary stream (R39.12)

+ 4 **N41 Inflammatory diseases of prostate**
Use additional code (B95-B97), to identify infectious agent.

SP + **N41.0 Acute prostatitis**

SP + **N41.1 Chronic prostatitis**

SP + **N41.2 Abscess of prostate**

SP + **N41.3 Prostatocystitis**

SP + **N41.4 Granulomatous prostatitis**

SP + **N41.8 Other inflammatory diseases of prostate**

IQ + **N41.9 Inflammatory disease of prostate, unspecified**
Prostatitis NOS

4 **N42 Other and unspecified disorders of prostate**

SP **N42.0 Calculus of prostate**
Prostatic stone

SP **N42.1 Congestion and hemorrhage of prostate**
EXCLUDES 1 enlarged prostate (N40.-)
hematuria (R31.-)
hyperplasia of prostate (N40.-)
inflammatory diseases of prostate (N41.-)

5 **N42.3 Dysplasia of prostate**

SP **N42.30 Unspecified dysplasia of prostate**

SP **N42.31 Prostatic intraepithelial neoplasia**
PIN
Prostatic intraepithelial neoplasia I (PIN I)
Prostatic intraepithelial neoplasia II (PIN II)
EXCLUDES 1 prostatic intraepithelial neoplasia III (PIN III) (D07.5)

SP **N42.32 Atypical small acinar proliferation of prostate**

SP **N42.39 Other dysplasia of prostate**

5 **N42.8 Other specified disorders of prostate**

SP **N42.81 Prostatodynia syndrome**
Painful prostate syndrome

SP **N42.82 Prostatosis syndrome**

SP **N42.83 Cyst of prostate**

SP **N42.89 Other specified disorders of prostate**

IQ **N42.9 Disorder of prostate, unspecified**

4 **N43 Hydrocele and spermatocele**
INCLUDES hydrocele of spermatic cord, testis or tunica vaginalis
EXCLUDES 1 congenital hydrocele (P83.5)

CODING TIPS✓ Conditions classifiable to N43.- indicate cysts of fluid that develop near the head of the epididymis (spermatocele), or surrounding the testicle (hydrocele). They are often painless but may cause discomfort due to pressure on surrounding areas. When a hydrocele is reported as infected, assign N43.1 with an additional code for the causative organism, if known.

SP **N43.0 Encysted hydrocele**

SP + **N43.1 Infected hydrocele**
Use additional code (B95-B97), to identify infectious agent

SP **N43.2 Other hydrocele**

IQ **N43.3 Hydrocele, unspecified**

DEFINITION Collection of serous fluid on the tunica vaginalis, spermatic cord, or testicle from acute local injury, infection, radiotherapy, or gradual fluid accumulation.

5 **N43.4 Spermatocele of epididymis**
Spermatic cyst

DEFINITION Cyst on the epididymis containing sperm.

IQ **N43.40 Spermatocele of epididymis, unspecified**

SP **N43.41 Spermatocele of epididymis, single**

SP **N43.42 Spermatocele of epididymis, multiple**

4 **N44 Noninflammatory disorders of testis**

5 **N44.0 Torsion of testis**

SP **N44.00 Torsion of testis, unspecified**

DEFINITION Testicle becomes twisted inside the scrotum, cutting off the blood supply.

SP **N44.01 Extravaginal torsion of spermatic cord**

SP **N44.02 Intravaginal torsion of spermatic cord**
Torsion of spermatic cord NOS

SP **N44.03 Torsion of appendix testis**

SP **N44.04 Torsion of appendix epididymis**

SP **N44.1 Cyst of tunica albuginea testis**

SP **N44.2 Benign cyst of testis**

SP **N44.8 Other noninflammatory disorders of the testis**

+ 4 **N45 Orchitis and epididymitis**
Use additional code (B95-B97), to identify infectious agent.

CODING TIPS ✓ When coding conditions classifiable to N45.-, review documentation to identify the causative organism(s) if known, and assign an additional code.

SP + **N45.1 Epididymitis**

SP + **N45.2 Orchitis**

SP + **N45.3 Epididymo-orchitis**

SP + **N45.4 Abscess of epididymis or testis**

4 **N46 Male infertility**
EXCLUDES 1 vasectomy status (Z98.52)

5 **N46.0 Azoospermia**
Absolute male infertility
Male infertility due to germinal (cell) aplasia
Male infertility due to spermatogenic arrest (complete)

IQ **N46.01 Organic azoospermia**
Azoospermia NOS

6 **N46.02 Azoospermia due to extratesticular causes**
Code also:
associated cause

IQ **N46.021 Azoospermia due to drug therapy**

IQ **N46.022 Azoospermia due to infection**

IQ **N46.023 Azoospermia due to obstruction of efferent ducts**

IQ **N46.024 Azoospermia due to radiation**

IQ **N46.025 Azoospermia due to systemic disease**

IQ **N46.029 Azoospermia due to other extratesticular causes**

5 **N46.1 Oligospermia**
Male infertility due to germinal cell desquamation
Male infertility due to hypospermatogenesis
Male infertility due to incomplete spermatogenic arrest

DEFINITION Insufficient spermatozoa in the semen.

IQ **N46.11 Organic oligospermia**
Oligospermia NOS

6 **N46.12 Oligospermia due to extratesticular causes**
Code also:
associated cause

IQ **N46.121 Oligospermia due to drug therapy**

IQ **N46.122 Oligospermia due to infection**

IQ **N46.123 Oligospermia due to obstruction of efferent ducts**

IQ **N46.124 Oligospermia due to radiation**

IQ **N46.125 Oligospermia due to systemic disease**

IQ **N46.129 Oligospermia due to other extratesticular causes**

IQ **N46.8 Other male infertility**

IQ **N46.9 Male infertility, unspecified**

4 **N47 Disorders of prepuce**

SP **N47.0 Adherent prepuce, newborn**

SP **N47.1 Phimosis**

SP **N47.2 Paraphimosis**

SP **N47.3 Deficient foreskin**

SP **N47.4 Benign cyst of prepuce**

SP **N47.5 Adhesions of prepuce and glans penis**

SP + **N47.6 Balanoposthitis**
Use additional code (B95-B97), to identify infectious agent.
EXCLUDES 1 balanitis (N48.1)

DEFINITION Inflammation of the head of the penis and foreskin.

SP + **N47.7 Other inflammatory diseases of prepuce**
Use additional code (B95-B97), to identify infectious agent.

SP **N47.8 Other disorders of prepuce**

4 **N48 Other disorders of penis**

SP **N48.0 Leukoplakia of penis**
Balanitis xerotica obliterans
Kraurosis of penis
Lichen sclerosus of external male genital organs
EXCLUDES 1 carcinoma in situ of penis (D07.4)

DEFINITION Chronic skin condition of the penis causing atrophic, white, patches on the foreskin and glans with hardened, indurated tissue near the meatus.

SP + **N48.1 Balanitis**
Use additional code (B95-B97), to identify infectious agent
EXCLUDES 1 amebic balanitis (A06.8)
balanitis xerotica obliterans (N48.0)
candidal balanitis (B37.42)
gonococcal balanitis (A54.23)
herpesviral [herpes simplex] balanitis (A60.01)

DEFINITION Inflammation of the glans penis (the head of the penis).

+ 5 **N48.2 Other inflammatory disorders of penis**
Use additional code (B95-B97), to identify infectious agent.
EXCLUDES 1 balanitis (N48.1)
balanitis xerotica obliterans (N48.0)
balanoposthitis (N47.6)

SP + **N48.21 Abscess of corpus cavernosum and penis**

SP + **N48.22 Cellulitis of corpus cavernosum and penis**

SP + **N48.29 Other inflammatory disorders of penis**

5 **N48.3 Priapism**

Chapter 14 N00-N99

Painful erection
Code first:
underlying cause

IQ **N48.30 Priapism, unspecified**

IQ **N48.31 Priapism due to trauma**

IQ **N48.32 Priapism due to disease classified elsewhere**

IQ **N48.33 Priapism, drug-induced**

IQ **N48.39 Other priapism**

SP **N48.5 Ulcer of penis**

SP **N48.6 Induration penis plastica**
Peyronie's disease
Plastic induration of penis

5 **N48.8 Other specified disorders of penis**

SP **N48.81 Thrombosis of superficial vein of penis**

SP **N48.82 Acquired torsion of penis**
Acquired torsion of penis NOS
EXCLUDES 1 congenital torsion of penis (Q55.63)

SP **N48.83 Acquired buried penis**
EXCLUDES 1 congenital hidden penis (Q55.64)

SP **N48.89 Other specified disorders of penis**

IQ **N48.9 Disorder of penis, unspecified**

+ 4 **N49 Inflammatory disorders of male genital organs, not elsewhere classified**
Use additional code (B95-B97), to identify infectious agent
EXCLUDES 1 inflammation of penis (N48.1, N48.2-)
orchitis and epididymitis (N45.-)

SP + **N49.0 Inflammatory disorders of seminal vesicle**
Vesiculitis NOS

SP + **N49.1 Inflammatory disorders of spermatic cord, tunica vaginalis and vas deferens**
Vasitis

SP + **N49.2 Inflammatory disorders of scrotum**

SP + **N49.3 Fournier gangrene**
CODING TIPS✓ Fournier gangrene is not assumed related to diabetes.
CODING TIPS✓ Fournier gangrene is a specific condition typically occurring in males, which includes a necrotizing or gangrenous infection of the perineal region often including a mix of aerobic and anaerobic bacteria. An additional code should be assigned to identify causative organism(s). Females diagnosed with Fournier's gangrene should be coded to N76.89.
DEFINITION Necrosis affecting the perineal, genital, or perianal regions, characterized by black and malodorous tissue decay caused by infection or ischemia.

SP + **N49.8 Inflammatory disorders of other specified male genital organs**
Inflammation of multiple sites in male genital organs

IQ + **N49.9 Inflammatory disorder of unspecified male genital organ**
Abscess of unspecified male genital organ
Boil of unspecified male genital organ
Carbuncle of unspecified male genital organ
Cellulitis of unspecified male genital organ

4 **N50 Other and unspecified disorders of male genital organs**
EXCLUDES 2 torsion of testis (N44.0-)

SP **N50.0 Atrophy of testis**

SP **N50.1 Vascular disorders of male genital organs**
Hematocele, NOS, of male genital organs
Hemorrhage of male genital organs
Thrombosis of male genital organs

SP **N50.3 Cyst of epididymis**

5 **N50.8 Other specified disorders of male genital organs**
DEFINITION Chylocele: A cyst-like lesion resulting from the escape of chyle (milky fluid consisting of lymph and emulsified fat) into the tunica vaginalis of the testes.

6 **N50.81 Testicular pain**

⊟ SP **N50.811 Right testicular pain**

⊟ SP **N50.812 Left testicular pain**

⊟ IQ **N50.819 Testicular pain, unspecified**

SP **N50.82 Scrotal pain**

SP **N50.89 Other specified disorders of the male genital organs**
Atrophy of scrotum, seminal vesicle, spermatic cord, tunica vaginalis and vas deferens
Chylocele, tunica vaginalis (nonfilarial) NOS
Edema of scrotum, seminal vesicle, spermatic cord, tunica vaginalis and vas deferens
Hypertrophy of scrotum, seminal vesicle, spermatic cord, tunica vaginalis and vas deferens
Stricture of spermatic cord, tunica vaginalis, and vas deferens
Ulcer of scrotum, seminal vesicle, spermatic cord, testis, tunica vaginalis and vas deferens
Urethroscrotal fistula

IQ **N50.9 Disorder of male genital organs, unspecified**

M IQ **N51** ***Disorders of male genital organs in diseases classified elsewhere***
Code first underlying disease, such as:
filariasis (B74.0-B74.9)
EXCLUDES 1 amebic balanitis (A06.8)
candidal balanitis (B37.42)
gonococcal balanitis (A54.23)
gonococcal prostatitis (A54.22)
herpesviral [herpes simplex] balanitis (A60.01)
trichomonal prostatitis (A59.02)
tuberculous prostatitis (A18.14)

4 **N52 Male erectile dysfunction**
EXCLUDES 1 psychogenic impotence (F52.21)

5 **N52.0 Vasculogenic erectile dysfunction**

SP **N52.01 Erectile dysfunction due to arterial insufficiency**

SP **N52.02 Corporo-venous occlusive erectile dysfunction**

SP **N52.03 Combined arterial insufficiency and corporo-venous occlusive erectile dysfunction**

IQ **N52.1 Erectile dysfunction due to diseases classified elsewhere**
Code first:
underlying disease

SP **N52.2 Drug-induced erectile dysfunction**

5 **N52.3 Postprocedural erectile dysfunction**

SP **N52.31 Erectile dysfunction following radical prostatectomy**

SP **N52.32 Erectile dysfunction following radical cystectomy**

SP **N52.33 Erectile dysfunction following urethral surgery**

SP **N52.34 Erectile dysfunction following simple prostatectomy**

SP **N52.35 Erectile dysfunction following radiation therapy**

SP **N52.36 Erectile dysfunction following interstitial seed therapy**

SP **N52.37 Erectile dysfunction following prostate ablative therapy**
Erectile dysfunction following cryotherapy
Erectile dysfunction following other prostate ablative therapies
Erectile dysfunction following ultrasound ablative therapies

SP **N52.39 Other and unspecified postprocedural erectile dysfunction**

SP **N52.8 Other male erectile dysfunction**

SP **N52.9 Male erectile dysfunction, unspecified**
Impotence NOS

4 **N53 Other male sexual dysfunction**
EXCLUDES 1 psychogenic sexual dysfunction (F52.-)

5 **N53.1 Ejaculatory dysfunction**
EXCLUDES 1 premature ejaculation (F52.4)

SP **N53.11 Retarded ejaculation**

SP **N53.12 Painful ejaculation**

SP **N53.13 Anejaculatory orgasm**

SP **N53.14 Retrograde ejaculation**

SP **N53.19 Other ejaculatory dysfunction**
Ejaculatory dysfunction NOS

SP **N53.8 Other male sexual dysfunction**

IQ **N53.9 Unspecified male sexual dysfunction**

Disorders of breast (N60-N65)

EXCLUDES 1 disorders of breast associated with childbirth (O91-O92)

CODING TIPS✓ Code malignancies of the breast to Category C50.

4 **N60 Benign mammary dysplasia**
INCLUDES fibrocystic mastopathy

5 **N60.0 Solitary cyst of breast**
Cyst of breast

SP **N60.01 Solitary cyst of right breast**

SP **N60.02 Solitary cyst of left breast**

IQ **N60.09 Solitary cyst of unspecified breast**

5 **N60.1 Diffuse cystic mastopathy**
Cystic breast
Fibrocystic disease of breast
EXCLUDES 1 diffuse cystic mastopathy with epithelial proliferation (N60.3-)

SP **N60.11 Diffuse cystic mastopathy of right breast**

SP **N60.12 Diffuse cystic mastopathy of left breast**

IQ **N60.19 Diffuse cystic mastopathy of unspecified breast**

5 **N60.2 Fibroadenosis of breast**
Adenofibrosis of breast
EXCLUDES 2 fibroadenoma of breast (D24.-)

SP **N60.21 Fibroadenosis of right breast**

SP **N60.22 Fibroadenosis of left breast**

IQ **N60.29 Fibroadenosis of unspecified breast**

5 **N60.3 Fibrosclerosis of breast**
Cystic mastopathy with epithelial proliferation

SP **N60.31 Fibrosclerosis of right breast**

SP **N60.32 Fibrosclerosis of left breast**

IQ **N60.39 Fibrosclerosis of unspecified breast**

5 **N60.4 Mammary duct ectasia**
DEFINITION Dilated milk duct filled with fluid; becomes inflamed and clogged with a thick, sticky substance, causing discharge and tenderness.

SP **N60.41 Mammary duct ectasia of right breast**

SP **N60.42 Mammary duct ectasia of left breast**

IQ **N60.49 Mammary duct ectasia of unspecified breast**

5 **N60.8 Other benign mammary dysplasias**

SP **N60.81 Other benign mammary dysplasias of right breast**

SP **N60.82 Other benign mammary dysplasias of left breast**

IQ **N60.89 Other benign mammary dysplasias of unspecified breast**

5 **N60.9 Unspecified benign mammary dysplasia**

SP **N60.91 Unspecified benign mammary dysplasia of right breast**

SP **N60.92 Unspecified benign mammary dysplasia of left breast**

IQ **N60.99 Unspecified benign mammary dysplasia of unspecified breast**

4 **N61 Inflammatory disorders of breast**
EXCLUDES 1 inflammatory carcinoma of breast (C50.9)
inflammatory disorder of breast associated with childbirth (O91.-)
neonatal infective mastitis (P39.0)
thrombophlebitis of breast [Mondor's disease] (I80.8)

CODING TIPS✓ Do not assign a code from N61.- for patients who also have inflammatory breast cancer.

SP **N61.0 Mastitis without abscess**
Infective mastitis (acute) (nonpuerperal) (subacute)

Chapter 14
N00-N99

Mastitis (acute) (nonpuerperal) (subacute) NOS
Cellulitis (acute) (nonpuerperal) (subacute) of breast NOS
Cellulitis (acute) (nonpuerperal) (subacute) of nipple NOS

SP **N61.1 Abscess of the breast and nipple**
Abscess (acute) (chronic) (nonpuerperal) of areola
Abscess (acute) (chronic) (nonpuerperal) of breast
Carbuncle of breast
Mastitis with abscess

5 **N61.2 Granulomatous mastitis**

IQ **N61.20 Granulomatous mastitis, unspecified breast**

L SP **N61.21 Granulomatous mastitis, right breast**

L SP **N61.22 Granulomatous mastitis, left breast**

L SP **N61.23 Granulomatous mastitis, bilateral breast**

SP **N62 Hypertrophy of breast**
Gynecomastia
Hypertrophy of breast NOS
Massive pubertal hypertrophy of breast
EXCLUDES 1 breast engorgement of newborn (P83.4)
disproportion of reconstructed breast (N65.1)

DEFINITION Abnormal largeness of the breast.

4 **N63 Unspecified lump in breast**
Nodule(s) NOS in breast

CODING TIPS ✓ These codes are for abnormal nodules or lumps in the breast that are not identified as a neoplasm or tumor.

IQ **N63.0 Unspecified lump in unspecified breast**

5 **N63.1 Unspecified lump in the right breast**

L SP **N63.10 Unspecified lump in the right breast, unspecified quadrant**

L SP **N63.11 Unspecified lump in the right breast, upper outer quadrant**

L SP **N63.12 Unspecified lump in the right breast, upper inner quadrant**

L SP **N63.13 Unspecified lump in the right breast, lower outer quadrant**

L SP **N63.14 Unspecified lump in the right breast, lower inner quadrant**

L SP **N63.15 Unspecified lump in the right breast, overlapping quadrants**

5 **N63.2 Unspecified lump in the left breast**

L SP **N63.20 Unspecified lump in the left breast, unspecified quadrant**

L SP **N63.21 Unspecified lump in the left breast, upper outer quadrant**

L SP **N63.22 Unspecified lump in the left breast, upper inner quadrant**

L SP **N63.23 Unspecified lump in the left breast, lower outer quadrant**

L SP **N63.24 Unspecified lump in the left breast, lower inner quadrant**

L SP **N63.25 Unspecified lump in the left breast, overlapping quadrants**

5 **N63.3 Unspecified lump in axillary tail**

L SP **N63.31 Unspecified lump in axillary tail of the right breast**

L SP **N63.32 Unspecified lump in axillary tail of the left breast**

5 **N63.4 Unspecified lump in breast, subareolar**

L SP **N63.41 Unspecified lump in right breast, subareolar**

L SP **N63.42 Unspecified lump in left breast, subareolar**

4 **N64 Other disorders of breast**
EXCLUDES 2 mechanical complication of breast prosthesis and implant (T85.4-)

SP **N64.0 Fissure and fistula of nipple**

SP **N64.1 Fat necrosis of breast**
Fat necrosis (segmental) of breast
Code first:
breast necrosis due to breast graft (T85.898)

SP **N64.2 Atrophy of breast**

SP **N64.3 Galactorrhea not associated with childbirth**

DEFINITION Inappropriate discharge of milk from the breast.

SP **N64.4 Mastodynia**

5 **N64.5 Other signs and symptoms in breast**
EXCLUDES 2 abnormal findings on diagnostic imaging of breast (R92.-)

SP **N64.51 Induration of breast**

SP **N64.52 Nipple discharge**
EXCLUDES 1 abnormal findings in nipple discharge (R89.-)

SP **N64.53 Retraction of nipple**

SP **N64.59 Other signs and symptoms in breast**

5 **N64.8 Other specified disorders of breast**

SP **N64.81 Ptosis of breast**
EXCLUDES 1 ptosis of native breast in relation to reconstructed breast (N65.1)

DEFINITION Falling, drooping, or sagging of the breast tissue which can occur naturally, or following pregnancy or weight gain and loss.

SP **N64.82 Hypoplasia of breast**
Micromastia
EXCLUDES 1 congenital absence of breast (Q83.0)
hypoplasia of native breast in relation to reconstructed breast (N65.1)

SP **N64.89 Other specified disorders of breast**
Galactocele
Subinvolution of breast (postlactational)

IQ **N64.9 Disorder of breast, unspecified**

4 **N65 Deformity and disproportion of reconstructed breast**

SP **N65.0 Deformity of reconstructed breast**
Contour irregularity in reconstructed breast
Excess tissue in reconstructed breast
Misshapen reconstructed breast

Chapter 14
N00-N99

SP N65.1 **Disproportion of reconstructed breast**
Breast asymmetry between native breast and reconstructed breast
Disproportion between native breast and reconstructed breast

Inflammatory diseases of female pelvic organs (N70-N77)

EXCLUDES 1 inflammatory diseases of female pelvic organs complicating:
abortion or ectopic or molar pregnancy (O00-O07, O08.0)
pregnancy, childbirth and the puerperium (O23.-, O75.3, O85, O86.-)

+ 4 N70 **Salpingitis and oophoritis**
INCLUDES abscess (of) fallopian tube
abscess (of) ovary
pyosalpinx
salpingo-oophoritis
tubo-ovarian abscess
tubo-ovarian inflammatory disease
Use additional code (B95-B97), to identify infectious agent
EXCLUDES 1 gonococcal infection (A54.24)
tuberculous infection (A18.17)
CODING TIPS ✓ When coding a condition classifiable to N70.-, review documentation to identify the causative organism(s) if known, and assign an additional code.

+ 5 N70.0 **Acute salpingitis and oophoritis**
SP + N70.01 **Acute salpingitis**
SP + N70.02 **Acute oophoritis**
SP + N70.03 **Acute salpingitis and oophoritis**
+ 5 N70.1 **Chronic salpingitis and oophoritis**
Hydrosalpinx
SP + N70.11 **Chronic salpingitis**
SP + N70.12 **Chronic oophoritis**
SP + N70.13 **Chronic salpingitis and oophoritis**
+ 5 N70.9 **Salpingitis and oophoritis, unspecified**
DEFINITION Inflammation of appendages of the uterus (adnexa uteri).
SP + N70.91 **Salpingitis, unspecified**
SP + N70.92 **Oophoritis, unspecified**
SP + N70.93 **Salpingitis and oophoritis, unspecified**

+ 4 N71 **Inflammatory disease of uterus, except cervix**
INCLUDES endo (myo) metritis
metritis
myometritis
pyometra
uterine abscess
Use additional code (B95-B97), to identify infectious agent
EXCLUDES 1 hyperplastic endometritis (N85.0-)
infection of uterus following delivery (O85, O86.-)
SP + N71.0 **Acute inflammatory disease of uterus**
SP + N71.1 **Chronic inflammatory disease of uterus**
IQ + N71.9 **Inflammatory disease of uterus, unspecified**

SP + N72 **Inflammatory disease of cervix uteri**
INCLUDES cervicitis
(with or without erosion or ectropion)
endocervicitis
(with or without erosion or ectropion)
exocervicitis
(with or without erosion or ectropion)
Use additional code (B95-B97), to identify infectious agent
EXCLUDES 1 erosion and ectropion of cervix without cervicitis (N86)

+ 4 N73 **Other female pelvic inflammatory diseases**
Use additional code (B95-B97), to identify infectious agent.
SP + N73.0 **Acute parametritis and pelvic cellulitis**
Abscess of broad ligament
Abscess of parametrium
Pelvic cellulitis, female
SP + N73.1 **Chronic parametritis and pelvic cellulitis**
Any condition in N73.0 specified as chronic
EXCLUDES 1 tuberculous parametritis and pelvic cellultis (A18.17)
SP + N73.2 **Unspecified parametritis and pelvic cellulitis**
Any condition in N73.0 unspecified whether acute or chronic
SP + N73.3 **Female acute pelvic peritonitis**
SP + N73.4 **Female chronic pelvic peritonitis**
EXCLUDES 1 tuberculous pelvic (female) peritonitis (A18.17)
SP + N73.5 **Female pelvic peritonitis, unspecified**
SP + N73.6 **Female pelvic peritoneal adhesions (postinfective)**
EXCLUDES 2 postprocedural pelvic peritoneal adhesions (N99.4)
SP + N73.8 **Other specified female pelvic inflammatory diseases**
IQ + N73.9 **Female pelvic inflammatory disease, unspecified**
Female pelvic infection or inflammation NOS

IQ N74 **Female pelvic inflammatory disorders in diseases classified elsewhere**
Code first:
underlying disease
EXCLUDES 1 chlamydial cervicitis (A56.02)
chlamydial pelvic inflammatory disease (A56.11)
gonococcal cervicitis (A54.03)
gonococcal pelvic inflammatory disease (A54.24)
herpesviral [herpes simplex] cervicitis (A60.03)
herpesviral [herpes simplex] pelvic inflammatory disease (A60.09)
syphilitic cervicitis (A52.76)
syphilitic pelvic inflammatory disease (A52.76)
trichomonal cervicitis (A59.09)
tuberculous cervicitis (A18.16)

Chapter 14
N00-N99

tuberculous pelvic inflammatory disease (A18.17)

4 **N75 Diseases of Bartholin's gland**

SP **N75.0 Cyst of Bartholin's gland**

SP **N75.1 Abscess of Bartholin's gland**

SP **N75.8 Other diseases of Bartholin's gland**
Bartholinitis

IQ **N75.9 Disease of Bartholin's gland, unspecified**

+ 4 **N76 Other inflammation of vagina and vulva**
Use additional code (B95-B97), to identify infectious agent
EXCLUDES 2 senile (atrophic) vaginitis (N95.2)
vulvar vestibulitis (N94.810)

SP + **N76.0 Acute vaginitis**
Acute vulvovaginitis
Vaginitis NOS
Vulvovaginitis NOS

SP + **N76.1 Subacute and chronic vaginitis**
Chronic vulvovaginitis
Subacute vulvovaginitis

SP + **N76.2 Acute vulvitis**
Vulvitis NOS

SP + **N76.3 Subacute and chronic vulvitis**

SP + **N76.4 Abscess of vulva**
Furuncle of vulva

SP + **N76.5 Ulceration of vagina**

SP + **N76.6 Ulceration of vulva**

+ 5 **N76.8 Other specified inflammation of vagina and vulva**

SP + **N76.81 Mucositis (ulcerative) of vagina and vulva**
Code also type of associated therapy, such as:
antineoplastic and immunosuppressive drugs (T45.1X-)
radiological procedure and radiotherapy (Y84.2)
EXCLUDES 2 gastrointestinal mucositis (ulcerative) (K92.81)
nasal mucositis (ulcerative) (J34.81)
oral mucositis (ulcerative) (K12.3-)

SP + **N76.89 Other specified inflammation of vagina and vulva**

4 **N77 Vulvovaginal ulceration and inflammation in diseases classified elsewhere**

M IQ **N77.0 *Ulceration of vulva in diseases classified elsewhere***
Code first underlying disease, such as:
Behçet's disease (M35.2)
EXCLUDES 1 ulceration of vulva in gonococcal infection (A54.02)
ulceration of vulva in herpesviral [herpes simplex] infection (A60.04)
ulceration of vulva in syphilis (A51.0)
ulceration of vulva in tuberculosis (A18.18)

M IQ **N77.1 *Vaginitis, vulvitis and vulvovaginitis in diseases classified elsewhere***
Code first underlying disease, such as:
pinworm (B80)
EXCLUDES 1 candidal vulvovaginitis (B37.3)
chlamydial vulvovaginitis (A56.02)
gonococcal vulvovaginitis (A54.02)
herpesviral [herpes simplex] vulvovaginitis (A60.04)
trichomonal vulvovaginitis (A59.01)
tuberculous vulvovaginitis (A18.18)
vulvovaginitis in early syphilis (A51.0)
vulvovaginitis in late syphilis (A52.76)

Noninflammatory disorders of female genital tract (N80-N98)

4 **N80 Endometriosis**
DEFINITION Tissue that lines the uterus growing outside the uterus in the pelvis, abdomen, and on other organs; causes pain and infertility.

SP **N80.0 Endometriosis of uterus**
Adenomyosis
EXCLUDES 1 stromal endometriosis (D39.0)

SP **N80.1 Endometriosis of ovary**

SP **N80.2 Endometriosis of fallopian tube**

SP **N80.3 Endometriosis of pelvic peritoneum**

SP **N80.4 Endometriosis of rectovaginal septum and vagina**

SP **N80.5 Endometriosis of intestine**

SP **N80.6 Endometriosis in cutaneous scar**

SP **N80.8 Other endometriosis**
Endometriosis of thorax

SP **N80.9 Endometriosis, unspecified**

4 **N81 Female genital prolapse**
EXCLUDES 1 genital prolapse complicating pregnancy, labor or delivery (O34.5-)
prolapse and hernia of ovary and fallopian tube (N83.4-)
prolapse of vaginal vault after hysterectomy (N99.3)

SP **N81.0 Urethrocele**
EXCLUDES 1 urethrocele with cystocele (N81.1-)
urethrocele with prolapse of uterus (N81.2-N81.4)

5 **N81.1 Cystocele**
Cystocele with urethrocele
Cystourethrocele
EXCLUDES 1 cystocele with prolapse of uterus (N81.2-N81.4)

SP **N81.10 Cystocele, unspecified**
Prolapse of (anterior) vaginal wall NOS

SP **N81.11 Cystocele, midline**

SP **N81.12 Cystocele, lateral**

Paravaginal cystocele

DEFINITION Bladder bulges through the side wall of the vagina.

SP **N81.2 Incomplete uterovaginal prolapse**
First degree uterine prolapse
Prolapse of cervix NOS
Second degree uterine prolapse
EXCLUDES 1 cervical stump prolapse (N81.85)

SP **N81.3 Complete uterovaginal prolapse**
Procidentia (uteri) NOS
Third degree uterine prolapse

SP **N81.4 Uterovaginal prolapse, unspecified**
Prolapse of uterus NOS

SP **N81.5 Vaginal enterocele**
EXCLUDES 1 enterocele with prolapse of uterus (N81.2-N81.4)

SP + **N81.6 Rectocele**
Prolapse of posterior vaginal wall
Use additional code for any associated fecal incontinence, if applicable (R15.-)
EXCLUDES 2 perineocele (N81.81)
rectal prolapse (K62.3)
rectocele with prolapse of uterus (N81.2-N81.4)

5 **N81.8 Other female genital prolapse**

SP **N81.81 Perineocele**

SP **N81.82 Incompetence or weakening of pubocervical tissue**

SP **N81.83 Incompetence or weakening of rectovaginal tissue**

SP **N81.84 Pelvic muscle wasting**
Disuse atrophy of pelvic muscles and anal sphincter

SP **N81.85 Cervical stump prolapse**
CODING TIPS ✓ A cervical stump prolapse, N81.85, occurs when the cervix falls into the vaginal vault following a supracervical hysterectomy.

SP **N81.89 Other female genital prolapse**
Deficient perineum
Old laceration of muscles of pelvic floor

SP **N81.9 Female genital prolapse, unspecified**

4 **N82 Fistulae involving female genital tract**
EXCLUDES 1 vesicointestinal fistulae (N32.1)

SP **N82.0 Vesicovaginal fistula**

SP **N82.1 Other female urinary-genital tract fistulae**
Cervicovesical fistula
Ureterovaginal fistula
Urethrovaginal fistula
Uteroureteric fistula
Uterovesical fistula

SP **N82.2 Fistula of vagina to small intestine**

SP **N82.3 Fistula of vagina to large intestine**
Rectovaginal fistula

SP **N82.4 Other female intestinal-genital tract fistulae**
Intestinouterine fistula

SP **N82.5 Female genital tract-skin fistulae**
Uterus to abdominal wall fistula
Vaginoperineal fistula

SP **N82.8 Other female genital tract fistulae**

IQ **N82.9 Female genital tract fistula, unspecified**

4 **N83 Noninflammatory disorders of ovary, fallopian tube and broad ligament**
EXCLUDES 2 hydrosalpinx (N70.1-)

5 **N83.0 Follicular cyst of ovary**
Cyst of graafian follicle
Hemorrhagic follicular cyst (of ovary)
DEFINITION Fluid-filled sac on the ovary caused by larger than normal growth of a follicle that does not rupture to release the egg.

H IQ **N83.00 Follicular cyst of ovary, unspecified side**

H SP **N83.01 Follicular cyst of right ovary**

H SP **N83.02 Follicular cyst of left ovary**

5 **N83.1 Corpus luteum cyst**
Hemorrhagic corpus luteum cyst

H IQ **N83.10 Corpus luteum cyst of ovary, unspecified side**

H SP **N83.11 Corpus luteum cyst of right ovary**

H SP **N83.12 Corpus luteum cyst of left ovary**

5 **N83.2 Other and unspecified ovarian cysts**
EXCLUDES 1 developmental ovarian cyst (Q50.1)
neoplastic ovarian cyst (D27.-)
polycystic ovarian syndrome (E28.2)
Stein-Leventhal syndrome (E28.2)

6 **N83.20 Unspecified ovarian cysts**

H SP **N83.201 Unspecified ovarian cyst, right side**

H SP **N83.202 Unspecified ovarian cyst, left side**

H IQ **N83.209 Unspecified ovarian cyst, unspecified side**
Ovarian cyst, NOS

6 **N83.29 Other ovarian cysts**
Retention cyst of ovary
Simple cyst of ovary

H SP **N83.291 Other ovarian cyst, right side**

H SP **N83.292 Other ovarian cyst, left side**

H IQ **N83.299 Other ovarian cyst, unspecified side**

5 **N83.3 Acquired atrophy of ovary and fallopian tube**

6 **N83.31 Acquired atrophy of ovary**

H SP **N83.311 Acquired atrophy of right ovary**

H SP **N83.312 Acquired atrophy of left ovary**

H IQ **N83.319 Acquired atrophy of ovary, unspecified side**
Acquired atrophy of ovary, NOS

6 **N83.32 Acquired atrophy of fallopian tube**

H SP **N83.321 Acquired atrophy of right fallopian tube**

H SP **N83.322 Acquired atrophy of left fallopian tube**

H IQ **N83.329 Acquired atrophy of fallopian tube, unspecified side**
Acquired atrophy of fallopian tube, NOS

6 **N83.33 Acquired atrophy of ovary and fallopian tube**

Chapter 14

N00-N99

N83.331 Acquired atrophy of right ovary and fallopian tube

N83.332 Acquired atrophy of left ovary and fallopian tube

N83.339 Acquired atrophy of ovary and fallopian tube, unspecified side
Acquired atrophy of ovary and fallopian tube, NOS

N83.4 Prolapse and hernia of ovary and fallopian tube

N83.40 Prolapse and hernia of ovary and fallopian tube, unspecified side
Prolapse and hernia of ovary and fallopian tube, NOS

N83.41 Prolapse and hernia of right ovary and fallopian tube

N83.42 Prolapse and hernia of left ovary and fallopian tube

N83.5 Torsion of ovary, ovarian pedicle and fallopian tube
Torsion of accessory tube

N83.51 Torsion of ovary and ovarian pedicle

N83.511 Torsion of right ovary and ovarian pedicle

N83.512 Torsion of left ovary and ovarian pedicle

N83.519 Torsion of ovary and ovarian pedicle, unspecified side
Torsion of ovary and ovarian pedicle, NOS

N83.52 Torsion of fallopian tube
Torsion of hydatid of Morgagni

N83.521 Torsion of right fallopian tube

N83.522 Torsion of left fallopian tube

N83.529 Torsion of fallopian tube, unspecified side
Torsion of fallopian tube, NOS

N83.53 Torsion of ovary, ovarian pedicle and fallopian tube

N83.6 Hematosalpinx
EXCLUDES 1 hematosalpinx (with) (in):
hematocolpos (N89.7)
hematometra (N85.7)
tubal pregnancy (O00.1-)

N83.7 Hematoma of broad ligament

N83.8 Other noninflammatory disorders of ovary, fallopian tube and broad ligament
Broad ligament laceration syndrome [Allen-Masters]

N83.9 Noninflammatory disorder of ovary, fallopian tube and broad ligament, unspecified

N84 Polyp of female genital tract
EXCLUDES 1 adenomatous polyp (D28.-)
placental polyp (O90.89)

N84.0 Polyp of corpus uteri
Polyp of endometrium
Polyp of uterus NOS
EXCLUDES 1 polypoid endometrial hyperplasia (N85.0-)

N84.1 Polyp of cervix uteri
Mucous polyp of cervix

N84.2 Polyp of vagina

N84.3 Polyp of vulva
Polyp of labia

N84.8 Polyp of other parts of female genital tract

N84.9 Polyp of female genital tract, unspecified

N85 Other noninflammatory disorders of uterus, except cervix
EXCLUDES 1 endometriosis (N80.-)
inflammatory diseases of uterus (N71.-)
noninflammatory disorders of cervix, except malposition (N86-N88)
polyp of corpus uteri (N84.0)
uterine prolapse (N81.-)

N85.0 Endometrial hyperplasia
DEFINITION Overgrowth of cells lining the uterus.

N85.00 Endometrial hyperplasia, unspecified
Hyperplasia (adenomatous) (cystic) (glandular) of endometrium
Hyperplastic endometritis

N85.01 Benign endometrial hyperplasia
Endometrial hyperplasia (complex) (simple) without atypia

N85.02 Endometrial intraepithelial neoplasia [EIN]
Endometrial hyperplasia with atypia
EXCLUDES 1 malignant neoplasm of endometrium (with endometrial intraepithelial neoplasia [EIN]) (C54.1)

N85.2 Hypertrophy of uterus
Bulky or enlarged uterus
EXCLUDES 1 puerperal hypertrophy of uterus (O90.89)

N85.3 Subinvolution of uterus
EXCLUDES 1 puerperal subinvolution of uterus (O90.89)

N85.4 Malposition of uterus
Anteversion of uterus
Retroflexion of uterus
Retroversion of uterus
EXCLUDES 1 malposition of uterus complicating pregnancy, labor or delivery (O34.5-, O65.5)

N85.5 Inversion of uterus
EXCLUDES 1 current obstetric trauma (O71.2)
postpartum inversion of uterus (O71.2)

N85.6 Intrauterine synechiae

N85.7 Hematometra
Hematosalpinx with hematometra
EXCLUDES 1 hematometra with hematocolpos (N89.7)
DEFINITION Blood accumulated in the uterus.

N85.8 Other specified noninflammatory disorders of uterus
Atrophy of uterus, acquired
Fibrosis of uterus NOS

N85.9 Noninflammatory disorder of uterus, unspecified

4th digit required · 5th digit required · 6th digit required · 7th digit required · 7th digit placeholder · + Additional code · Laterality

Disorder of uterus NOS

SP **N86 Erosion and ectropion of cervix uteri**
Decubitus (trophic) ulcer of cervix
Eversion of cervix
EXCLUDES 1 erosion and ectropion of cervix with cervicitis (N72)

4 **N87 Dysplasia of cervix uteri**
EXCLUDES 1 abnormal results from cervical cytologic examination without histologic confirmation (R87.61-)
carcinoma in situ of cervix uteri (D06.-)
cervical intraepithelial neoplasia III [CIN III] (D06.-)
HGSIL of cervix (R87.613)
severe dysplasia of cervix uteri (D06.-)

CODING TIPS ✓ Mild and moderate dysplasia of the cervix is coded to this category. Class III is coded to D06.

SP **N87.0 Mild cervical dysplasia**
Cervical intraepithelial neoplasia I [CIN I]

SP **N87.1 Moderate cervical dysplasia**
Cervical intraepithelial neoplasia II [CIN II]

SP **N87.9 Dysplasia of cervix uteri, unspecified**
Anaplasia of cervix
Cervical atypism
Cervical dysplasia NOS

4 **N88 Other noninflammatory disorders of cervix uteri**
EXCLUDES 2 inflammatory disease of cervix (N72)
polyp of cervix (N84.1)

SP **N88.0 Leukoplakia of cervix uteri**

SP **N88.1 Old laceration of cervix uteri**
Adhesions of cervix
EXCLUDES 1 current obstetric trauma (O71.3)

SP **N88.2 Stricture and stenosis of cervix uteri**
EXCLUDES 1 stricture and stenosis of cervix uteri complicating labor (O65.5)

SP **N88.3 Incompetence of cervix uteri**
Investigation and management of (suspected) cervical incompetence in a nonpregnant woman
EXCLUDES 1 cervical incompetence complicating pregnancy (O34.3-)

SP **N88.4 Hypertrophic elongation of cervix uteri**

SP **N88.8 Other specified noninflammatory disorders of cervix uteri**
EXCLUDES 1 current obstetric trauma (O71.3)

IQ **N88.9 Noninflammatory disorder of cervix uteri, unspecified**

4 **N89 Other noninflammatory disorders of vagina**
EXCLUDES 1 abnormal results from vaginal cytologic examination without histologic confirmation (R87.62-)
carcinoma in situ of vagina (D07.2)
HGSIL of vagina (R87.623)
inflammation of vagina (N76.-)
senile (atrophic) vaginitis (N95.2)
severe dysplasia of vagina (D07.2)
trichomonal leukorrhea (A59.00)
vaginal intraepithelial neoplasia [VAIN], grade III (D07.2)

SP **N89.0 Mild vaginal dysplasia**
Vaginal intraepithelial neoplasia [VAIN], grade I

SP **N89.1 Moderate vaginal dysplasia**
Vaginal intraepithelial neoplasia [VAIN], grade II

SP **N89.3 Dysplasia of vagina, unspecified**

SP **N89.4 Leukoplakia of vagina**
DEFINITION White plaque on the mucosal surface of the vagina that develops into thickened, rough-textured grayish white lesions.

SP **N89.5 Stricture and atresia of vagina**
Vaginal adhesions
Vaginal stenosis
EXCLUDES 1 congenital atresia or stricture (Q52.4)
postprocedural adhesions of vagina (N99.2)

SP **N89.6 Tight hymenal ring**
Rigid hymen
Tight introitus
EXCLUDES 1 imperforate hymen (Q52.3)

SP **N89.7 Hematocolpos**
Hematocolpos with hematometra or hematosalpinx

SP **N89.8 Other specified noninflammatory disorders of vagina**
Leukorrhea NOS
Old vaginal laceration
Pessary ulcer of vagina
EXCLUDES 1 current obstetric trauma (O70.-, O71.4, O71.7-O71.8)
old laceration involving muscles of pelvic floor (N81.8)

IQ **N89.9 Noninflammatory disorder of vagina, unspecified**

4 **N90 Other noninflammatory disorders of vulva and perineum**
EXCLUDES 1 anogenital (venereal) warts (A63.0)
carcinoma in situ of vulva (D07.1)
condyloma acuminatum (A63.0)
current obstetric trauma (O70.-, O71.7-O71.8)
inflammation of vulva (N76.-)
severe dysplasia of vulva (D07.1)
vulvar intraepithelial neoplasm III [VIN III] (D07.1)

SP **N90.0 Mild vulvar dysplasia**
Vulvar intraepithelial neoplasia [VIN], grade I

SP **N90.1 Moderate vulvar dysplasia**

Chapter 14
N00-N99

Vulvar intraepithelial neoplasia [VIN], grade II

SP **N90.3 Dysplasia of vulva, unspecified**

SP **N90.4 Leukoplakia of vulva**
Dystrophy of vulva
Kraurosis of vulva
Lichen sclerosus of external female genital organs

SP **N90.5 Atrophy of vulva**
Stenosis of vulva

5 **N90.6 Hypertrophy of vulva**

SP **N90.60 Unspecified hypertrophy of vulva**
Unspecified hypertrophy of labia

SP **N90.61 Childhood asymmetric labium majus enlargement**
CALME

SP **N90.69 Other specified hypertrophy of vulva**
Other specified hypertrophy of labia

SP **N90.7 Vulvar cyst**

5 **N90.8 Other specified noninflammatory disorders of vulva and perineum**

6 **N90.81 Female genital mutilation status**
Female genital cutting status

SP **N90.810 Female genital mutilation status, unspecified**
Female genital cutting status, unspecified
Female genital mutilation status NOS

SP **N90.811 Female genital mutilation Type I status**
Clitorectomy status
Female genital cutting Type I status

SP **N90.812 Female genital mutilation Type II status**
Clitorectomy with excision of labia minora status
Female genital cutting Type II status

SP **N90.813 Female genital mutilation Type III status**
Female genital cutting Type III status
Infibulation status

SP **N90.818 Other female genital mutilation status**
Female genital cutting Type IV status
Female genital mutilation Type IV status
Other female genital cutting status

SP **N90.89 Other specified noninflammatory disorders of vulva and perineum**
Adhesions of vulva
Hypertrophy of clitoris

!Q **N90.9 Noninflammatory disorder of vulva and perineum, unspecified**

4 **N91 Absent, scanty and rare menstruation**
EXCLUDES 1 ovarian dysfunction (E28.-)

SP **N91.0 Primary amenorrhea**

SP **N91.1 Secondary amenorrhea**

!Q **N91.2 Amenorrhea, unspecified**

SP **N91.3 Primary oligomenorrhea**

SP **N91.4 Secondary oligomenorrhea**

!Q **N91.5 Oligomenorrhea, unspecified**
Hypomenorrhea NOS

4 **N92 Excessive, frequent and irregular menstruation**
EXCLUDES 1 postmenopausal bleeding (N95.0)
precocious puberty (menstruation) (E30.1)

!Q **N92.0 Excessive and frequent menstruation with regular cycle**
Heavy periods NOS
Menorrhagia NOS
Polymenorrhea

!Q **N92.1 Excessive and frequent menstruation with irregular cycle**
Irregular intermenstrual bleeding
Irregular, shortened intervals between menstrual bleeding
Menometrorrhagia
Metrorrhagia

!Q **N92.2 Excessive menstruation at puberty**
Excessive bleeding associated with onset of menstrual periods
Pubertal menorrhagia
Puberty bleeding

!Q **N92.3 Ovulation bleeding**
Regular intermenstrual bleeding

SP **N92.4 Excessive bleeding in the premenopausal period**
Climacteric menorrhagia or metrorrhagia
Menopausal menorrhagia or metrorrhagia
Perimenopausal bleeding
Perimenopausal menorrhagia or metrorrhagia
Preclimacteric menorrhagia or metrorrhagia
Premenopausal menorrhagia or metrorrhagia

SP **N92.5 Other specified irregular menstruation**

!Q **N92.6 Irregular menstruation, unspecified**
Irregular bleeding NOS
Irregular periods NOS
EXCLUDES 1 irregular menstruation with:
lengthened intervals or scanty bleeding (N91.3-N91.5)
shortened intervals or excessive bleeding (N92.1)

4 **N93 Other abnormal uterine and vaginal bleeding**
EXCLUDES 1 neonatal vaginal hemorrhage (P54.6)
precocious puberty (menstruation) (E30.1)
pseudomenses (P54.6)

SP **N93.0 Postcoital and contact bleeding**
DEFINITION Bleeding after sexual intercourse.

SP **N93.1 Pre-pubertal vaginal bleeding**

SP **N93.8 Other specified abnormal uterine and vaginal bleeding**
Dysfunctional or functional uterine or vaginal bleeding NOS

!Q **N93.9 Abnormal uterine and vaginal bleeding, unspecified**

4 **N94 Pain and other conditions associated with female genital organs and menstrual cycle**

SP **N94.0 Mittelschmerz**

4 4th digit required 5 5th digit required 6 6th digit required 7 7th digit required 7 7th digit placeholder + Additional code Laterality

DEFINITION Pain accompanying ovulation, usually occurring midway between menstruation periods.

5 **N94.1 Dyspareunia**

EXCLUDES 1 psychogenic dyspareunia (F52.6)

DEFINITION Pain during sexual intercourse.

SP **N94.10 Unspecified dyspareunia**

SP **N94.11 Superficial (introital) dyspareunia**

SP **N94.12 Deep dyspareunia**

SP **N94.19 Other specified dyspareunia**

SP **N94.2 Vaginismus**

EXCLUDES 1 psychogenic vaginismus (F52.5)

DEFINITION Severe, painful spasms of the vaginal muscles that prevent sexual intercourse.

SP **N94.3 Premenstrual tension syndrome**

Code also:

associated menstrual migraine (G43.82-, G43.83-)

EXCLUDES 1 Premenstrual dysphoric disorder (F32.81)

SP **N94.4 Primary dysmenorrhea**

SP **N94.5 Secondary dysmenorrhea**

SP **N94.6 Dysmenorrhea, unspecified**

EXCLUDES 1 psychogenic dysmenorrhea (F45.8)

5 **N94.8 Other specified conditions associated with female genital organs and menstrual cycle**

6 **N94.81 Vulvodynia**

SP **N94.810 Vulvar vestibulitis**

DEFINITION Pain, tenderness, and redness in the vestibule area of the female external genitalia of unknown cause.

SP **N94.818 Other vulvodynia**

SP **N94.819 Vulvodynia, unspecified**

Vulvodynia NOS

SP **N94.89 Other specified conditions associated with female genital organs and menstrual cycle**

IQ **N94.9 Unspecified condition associated with female genital organs and menstrual cycle**

4 **N95 Menopausal and other perimenopausal disorders**

Menopausal and other perimenopausal disorders due to naturally occurring (age-related) menopause and perimenopause

EXCLUDES 1 excessive bleeding in the premenopausal period (N92.4)

menopausal and perimenopausal disorders due to artificial or premature menopause (E89.4-, E28.31-)

premature menopause (E28.31-)

EXCLUDES 2 postmenopausal osteoporosis (M81.0-)

postmenopausal osteoporosis with current pathological fracture (M80.0-)

postmenopausal urethritis (N34.2)

SP **N95.0 Postmenopausal bleeding**

SP + **N95.1 Menopausal and female climacteric states**

Symptoms such as flushing, sleeplessness, headache, lack of concentration, associated with natural (age-related) menopause

Use additional code for associated symptoms

EXCLUDES 1 asymptomatic menopausal state (Z78.0)

symptoms associated with artificial menopause (E89.41)

symptoms associated with premature menopause (E28.310)

SP **N95.2 Postmenopausal atrophic vaginitis**

Senile (atrophic) vaginitis

DEFINITION Thinning of vaginal epithelium due to decreased estrogen levels.

SP **N95.8 Other specified menopausal and perimenopausal disorders**

IQ **N95.9 Unspecified menopausal and perimenopausal disorder**

SP **N96 Recurrent pregnancy loss**

Investigation or care in a nonpregnant woman with history of recurrent pregnancy loss

EXCLUDES 1 recurrent pregancy loss with current pregnancy (O26.2-)

▲ 4 **N97 Female infertility**

INCLUDES inability to achieve a pregnancy

sterility, female NOS

EXCLUDES 2 female infertility associated with:

hypopituitarism (E23.0)

Stein-Leventhal syndrome (E28.2)

incompetence of cervix uteri (N88.3)

SP **N97.0 Female infertility associated with anovulation**

SP **N97.1 Female infertility of tubal origin**

Female infertility associated with congenital anomaly of tube

Female infertility due to tubal block

Female infertility due to tubal occlusion

Female infertility due to tubal stenosis

SP **N97.2 Female infertility of uterine origin**

Female infertility associated with congenital anomaly of uterus

Female infertility due to nonimplantation of ovum

SP **N97.8 Female infertility of other origin**

IQ **N97.9 Female infertility, unspecified**

4 **N98 Complications associated with artificial fertilization**

SP **N98.0 Infection associated with artificial insemination**

SP **N98.1 Hyperstimulation of ovaries**

Hyperstimulation of ovaries NOS

Chapter 14

N00-N99

Hyperstimulation of ovaries associated with induced ovulation

SP **N98.2 Complications of attempted introduction of fertilized ovum following in vitro fertilization**

SP **N98.3 Complications of attempted introduction of embryo in embryo transfer**

SP **N98.8 Other complications associated with artificial fertilization**

IQ **N98.9 Complication associated with artificial fertilization, unspecified**

Intraoperative and postprocedural complications and disorders of genitourinary system, not elsewhere classified (N99)

4 **N99 Intraoperative and postprocedural complications and disorders of genitourinary system, not elsewhere classified**

EXCLUDES 2 irradiation cystitis (N30.4-)
postoophorectomy osteoporosis with current pathological fracture (M80.8-)
postoophorectomy osteoporosis without current pathological fracture (M81.8)

CODING TIPS✓ **Documentation:** Codes in category N99.- are complication codes and require physician or NPP documentation and confirmation of a cause and effect relationship between any specified procedure and the complicated condition. Documentation in the home health clinical record must also support this relationship. If the complication has been resolved, the aftercare code may be appropriate (Z48.816).

SP + **N99.0 Postprocedural (acute) (chronic) kidney failure**
Use additional code to type of kidney disease

5 **N99.1 Postprocedural urethral stricture**
Postcatheterization urethral stricture

6 **N99.11 Postprocedural urethral stricture, male**

SP **N99.110 Postprocedural urethral stricture, male, meatal**

SP **N99.111 Postprocedural bulbous urethral stricture, male**

SP **N99.112 Postprocedural membranous urethral stricture, male**

SP **N99.113 Postprocedural anterior bulbous urethral stricture, male**

SP **N99.114 Postprocedural urethral stricture, male, unspecified**

SP **N99.115 Postprocedural fossa navicularis urethral stricture**

SP **N99.116 Postprocedural urethral stricture, male, overlapping sites**

SP **N99.12 Postprocedural urethral stricture, female**

SP **N99.2 Postprocedural adhesions of vagina**

SP **N99.3 Prolapse of vaginal vault after hysterectomy**

SP **N99.4 Postprocedural pelvic peritoneal adhesions**

EXCLUDES 2 pelvic peritoneal adhesions NOS (N73.6)
postinfective pelvic peritoneal adhesions (N73.6)

5 **N99.5 Complications of stoma of urinary tract**

EXCLUDES 2 mechanical complication of urinary catheter (T83.0-)

CODING TIPS✓ All cystostomy and other urinary stoma complications (including ileoconduit, urostomy and nephrostomy) are coded to N99.51-N99.53. This includes excoriation and denuding of the skin surrounding the ostomy, infection of the ostomy site, hemorrhage of the ostomy site and other complications. Code L24.B3 may be added if irritant contact dermatitis is documented related to fecal or urine around the fistula or stoma. When an ostomy complication is present, do not assign a Z code for the ostomy. Z codes indicate routine ostomy care, which is not appropriate in the case of a complicated ostomy.

6 **N99.51 Complication of cystostomy**

SP **N99.510 Cystostomy hemorrhage**

SP **N99.511 Cystostomy infection**

CODING TIPS✓ Code the cystostomy infection first, followed by cellulitis (if documented), followed by the bacteria causing the infection, if known.

SP **N99.512 Cystostomy malfunction**

SP **N99.518 Other cystostomy complication**

6 **N99.52 Complication of incontinent external stoma of urinary tract**

SP **N99.520 Hemorrhage of incontinent external stoma of urinary tract**

SP **N99.521 Infection of incontinent external stoma of urinary tract**

SP **N99.522 Malfunction of incontinent external stoma of urinary tract**

SP **N99.523 Herniation of incontinent stoma of urinary tract**

SP **N99.524 Stenosis of incontinent stoma of urinary tract**

SP **N99.528 Other complication of incontinent external stoma of urinary tract**

6 **N99.53 Complication of continent stoma of urinary tract**

SP **N99.530 Hemorrhage of continent stoma of urinary tract**

SP **N99.531 Infection of continent stoma of urinary tract**

SP **N99.532 Malfunction of continent stoma of urinary tract**

SP **N99.533 Herniation of continent stoma of urinary tract**

SP **N99.534 Stenosis of continent stoma of urinary tract**

SP **N99.538 Other complication of continent stoma of urinary tract**

5 N99.6 **Intraoperative hemorrhage and hematoma of a genitourinary system organ or structure complicating a procedure**

EXCLUDES 1 intraoperative hemorrhage and hematoma of a genitourinary system organ or structure due to accidental puncture or laceration during a procedure (N99.7-)

SP N99.61 **Intraoperative hemorrhage and hematoma of a genitourinary system organ or structure complicating a genitourinary system procedure**

SP N99.62 **Intraoperative hemorrhage and hematoma of a genitourinary system organ or structure complicating other procedure**

5 N99.7 **Accidental puncture and laceration of a genitourinary system organ or structure during a procedure**

SP N99.71 **Accidental puncture and laceration of a genitourinary system organ or structure during a genitourinary system procedure**

SP N99.72 **Accidental puncture and laceration of a genitourinary system organ or structure during other procedure**

5 N99.8 **Other intraoperative and postprocedural complications and disorders of genitourinary system**

SP N99.81 **Other intraoperative complications of genitourinary system**

6 N99.82 **Postprocedural hemorrhage of a genitourinary system organ or structure following a procedure**

SP N99.820 **Postprocedural hemorrhage of a genitourinary system organ or structure following a genitourinary system procedure**

SP N99.821 **Postprocedural hemorrhage of a genitourinary system organ or structure following other procedure**

SP N99.83 **Residual ovary syndrome**

6 N99.84 **Postprocedural hematoma and seroma of a genitourinary system organ or structure following a procedure**

SP N99.840 **Postprocedural hematoma of a genitourinary system organ or structure following a genitourinary system procedure**

SP N99.841 **Postprocedural hematoma of a genitourinary system organ or structure following other procedure**

SP N99.842 **Postprocedural seroma of a genitourinary system organ or structure following a genitourinary system procedure**

SP N99.843 **Postprocedural seroma of a genitourinary system organ or structure following other procedure**

SP N99.85 **Post endometrial ablation syndrome**

SP N99.89 **Other postprocedural complications and disorders of genitourinary system**

Chapter 14 Scenarios: Diseases of the genitourinary system (N00-N99)

Sickle cell nephropathy

A 51-year-old woman is admitted to home health with a primary diagnosis of sickle cell nephropathy.

Description	Code
Primary: Other sickle-cell disorders without crisis	D57.80
Secondary: Glomerular disorders in diseases classified elsewhere	N08

Sickle cell nephropathy is coded first with a code from the D57.- category (Other sickle-cell disorders without crisis) followed immediately by N08, according to the alphabetic index. Note that the way the codes are listed in the index specifies that they are an unbreakable etiology-manifestation pair, meaning that the N08 code must always immediately follow the D57.- code, according to coding guidelines.

UTI, catheter care, functional incontinence

A 72-year-old woman who is incontinent of urine is referred to home health with a urinary tract infection (UTI). She had a suprapubic catheter placed while she was in the hospital in hopes that it would be less likely than a Foley to cause UTIs. The patient also had a stroke four years ago that left her with residual conditions of left-sided hemiplegia (left side dominant) and aphasia. There is no indication that the stroke is the cause of her incontinence, except that she cannot get to the toilet in time due to her decreased mobility. Documentation in the chart offers no indication that the UTI is secondary to the indwelling catheter, and calls to the physician's office seeking clarification were not returned. The plan of care will focus on treatment of the UTI, as well as teaching care of the new suprapubic catheter.

Description	Code
Primary: Urinary tract infection, site not specified	N39.0
Secondary: Encounter for attention to cystostomy	Z43.5
Secondary: Functional urinary incontinence	R39.81
Secondary: Hemiplegia and hemiparesis following cerebral infarction affecting left dominant side	I69.352
Secondary: Aphasia following cerebral infarction	I69.320

N39.0 has a "Use additional code" note for the infectious agent to be included if known. No organism is listed here so none can be coded. The UTI cannot be assumed to be a complication of the catheter unless the physician has said that it is. Since that is not the case, it is not coded as a complication. Functional urinary incontinence, R39.81, is used to clarify the cause of the incontinence, distinguishing it from a medical condition. Code Z43.5 (Encounter for attention to cystostomy) is used for the catheter care because the agency is changing and caring for a patient's suprapubic catheter and the code captures "attention to" which communicates the provision of more comprehensive care such as assessing, cleaning and teaching, versus simply changing the catheter.

Multiple sclerosis, neurogenic bladder, history of UTI

A 50-year-old woman, diagnosed with multiple sclerosis for the past 20 years, has decreased visual acuity and some impaired mobility, balance and fine motor control, all of which have been relatively stable for six months. She requires home care for the management of her neurogenic bladder, which is causing urinary retention and incontinence without awareness and is managed with a chronic Foley catheter. She has had several UTIs. A nurse visits every four weeks to change the catheter, perform other care associated with the Foley catheter, monitor for signs of urinary tract infection and perform management of the neurogenic bladder.

Description	Code
Primary: Neurogenic bladder NOS	N31.9
Secondary: Multiple sclerosis	G35
Secondary: Incontinence without sensory awareness	N39.42
Secondary: Fitting and adjustment of urinary devices	Z46.6
Secondary: Personal history of urinary (tract) infection	Z87.440

Code N31.9 (neurogenic bladder) is the principal diagnosis code because it represents the most acute condition, which requires the most intensive services. Instruction at N31.- states to use an additional code for urinary incontinence. Assign G35, multiple sclerosis, if the patient is being seen for more than one aspect of this chronic condition. In this case, the neurogenic bladder is the focus of care. History of UTIs (Z87.440) is also assigned.

Diabetic kidney disease

A 67-year-old female patient is admitted to home health with a new diagnosis of chronic kidney disease stage 2. The patient also has a history of diabetes, hypertension and recently diagnosed anemia. The focus of care is the newly diagnosed kidney disease.

Description	Code
Primary: Type 2 diabetes mellitus with diabetic chronic kidney disease	E11.22
Secondary: Hypertensive chronic kidney disease with stage 1 through stage 4 chronic kidney disease, or unspecified chronic kidney disease	I12.9
Secondary: Chronic kidney disease stage 2	N18.2
Secondary: Anemia in chronic kidney disease	D63.1

Even though the kidney disease is the main reason for admission, manifestation sequencing rules take precedence, so the underlying etiology must be listed primary. Many ICD-10 diabetes codes are combination codes and do not require an additional code. However, diabetes with kidney disease has an instruction in the Tabular to "use additional code" to identify the stage of kidney disease. ICD-10-CM assumes a relationship between diabetes and hypertension, so I12.9 is assigned and precedes N18.2 since the physician did not specifically indicate that the chronic kidney disease is due to the diabetes. In the absence of any other stated cause, a relationship is also assumed between anemia and chronic kidney disease, so D63.1 must be assigned.

Congestive heart failure, hypertension, chronic kidney disease

A patient is admitted to home health after being hospitalized for congestive heart failure with shortness of breath, chest pain and acute renal failure. The patient's comorbidities include hypertension and stage 3a chronic kidney disease (CKD). The patient continues to have edema, but other acute symptoms, as well as the acute renal failure, are resolved upon admission to home care. Skilled nursing is ordered to teach on the disease process and monitor symptoms.

Description	Code
Primary: Hypertensive heart and chronic kidney disease with heart failure and stage 1 through stage 4 chronic kidney disease, or unspecified chronic kidney disease	I13.0
Secondary: Heart failure, unspecified	I50.9
Secondary: Chronic kidney disease, stage 3a	N18.31

A cause-and-effect relationship between hypertension, heart failure and chronic kidney disease is assumed by the ICD-10 classification system unless the provider states otherwise. The heart failure is not specified as systolic or diastolic, and therefore would be unspecified. An additional code from N18.- is assigned for the stage of chronic kidney disease in accordance with tabular instruction. The edema is not coded as it is a symptom of the congestive heart failure.

CKD with kidney transplant

A patient was admitted to home health for skilled nursing care following a successful kidney transplant. He still has stage 3b chronic kidney disease (CKD). Discharge encounter notes indicate that the patient also has early stage Parkinson's disease.

Description	Code
Primary: Aftercare following kidney transplant	Z48.22
Secondary: Chronic kidney disease, stage 3b	N18.32
Secondary: Parkinson's disease	G20

Patients who have undergone a kidney transplant may still have some form of CKD because the kidney transplant may not fully restore kidney function. Therefore, the presence of CKD alone does not constitute a transplant complication, and would not be coded as such, according to coding guidelines. Assign the appropriate N18.- code for the patient's stage of CKD. Code Z94.0 (Kidney transplant status) is not required here because the aftercare code already identifies the patient's transplanted organ. *[I.C.14.a.2]* An additional code to identify the patient's Parkinson's disease is assigned due to the impact this condition has on the patient's care planning and need for resource utilization.

HOME HEALTH CODING SCENARIOS

Benign prostatic hyperplasia

An 85-year-old man is admitted to home health with benign prostatic hyperplasia (BPH) to address debilitating symptoms of urinary overflow incontinence and nocturia. He will receive skilled nursing and occupational therapy. He also has hypertension and chronic heart failure with reduced ejection fraction.

Description	Code
Primary: Benign prostatic hyperplasia with lower urinary tract symptoms	N40.1
Secondary: Overflow incontinence	N39.490
Secondary: Nocturia	R35.1
Secondary: Hypertensive heart disease with heart failure	I11.0
Secondary: Chronic systolic (congestive) heart failure	I50.22

Even though incontinence and nocturia are symptoms of an enlarged prostate, or benign prostatic hyperplasia (BPH), and would not normally be additionally coded, they are in this scenario because tabular instructions call for it. Be sure to follow tabular instructions that state to assign the symptom codes after the BPH code. Hypertension and heart failure have an assumed relationship within the ICD-10-CM classification and a combination code is assigned for hypertensive heart disease with heart failure to identify this. Heart failure with reduced ejection fraction should be coded I50.2-, based upon coding guidelines and the "with" convention. The term "reduced ejection fraction" falls under the subterm "heart" below the main term "failure" in the alphabetic index.

Cellulitis around cystostomy site

A 71-year-old woman has a cystostomy in place due to paraplegia. Recently the site around the opening became irritated and her physician diagnosed cellulitis due to group B streptococcus bacteria. She was prescribed a 10-day course of antibiotics and will receive skilled nursing visits to monitor the infection until it resolves. She is wheelchair bound.

Description	Code
Primary: Cystostomy infection	N99.511
Secondary: Cellulitis of groin	L03.314
Secondary: Streptococcus, group B, as the cause of diseases classified elsewhere	B95.1
Secondary: Paraplegia, unspecified	G82.20
Secondary: Dependence on wheelchair	Z99.3

The infection is affecting the skin around the stoma and should thus be coded as a complication of the stoma, with N99.511. Codes for the cellulitis and the group B streptococcus bacteria are added to further describe the infection, in accordance with tabular instruction. The patient's paraplegia and wheelchair dependence are coded as relevant comorbidity factors that will impact the patient's recovery. Long-term antibiotic use is not coded as she is only taking antibiotics for 10 days.

Urethral stricture of overlapping sites

A 75-year-old man comes to home health with a primary diagnosis of a urethral stricture affecting the membranous and bulbous areas. He requires Foley care and teaching. There is no documented cause stated for the urethral stricture in the medical record. He also has diabetic polyneuropathy and hypertension. He takes oral hypoglycemic medication for his diabetes.

Description	Code
Primary: Unspecified urethral stricture, male, overlapping sites	N35.916
Secondary: Encounter for fitting and adjustment of urinary device	Z46.6
Secondary: Type 2 diabetes mellitus with diabetic polyneuropathy	E11.42
Secondary: Essential (primary) hypertension	I10
Secondary: Long term (current) use of oral hypoglycemic drugs	Z79.84

The patient has a primary diagnosis of a urethral stricture affecting overlapping sites that has no documented etiology, which is appropriately coded with N35.916. The care and teaching for the Foley catheter is coded with Z46.6. The patient's diabetic polyneuropathy and hypertension have the potential to impact his care and recovery and are coded as secondary diagnoses as well. His use of oral hypoglycemic medication is captured with Z79.84.

Chapter 15: Pregnancy, Childbirth and the Puerperium (O00-O9A)

Codes from Chapter 15 are reported for ectopic pregnancies (the implantation of a fertilized egg outside the uterus) and molar pregnancies (abnormal products of conception), abortions (including miscarriages), and pregnancy complications. Complications of pregnancy may occur during the antepartum period (before delivery), intrapartum period (during labor and delivery), or puerperium (postpartum period of six weeks following delivery).

The pregnancy codes found here include problems and symptoms related to both the mother and the fetus. The conditions in the mother may have been present before she became pregnant, or developed during the pregnancy or postpartum period. Complication codes in this chapter are reported when the maternal or fetal conditions are affecting management of the pregnancy, or are requiring diagnostic tests, additional observation, special care, or termination of the pregnancy. If it is unclear whether the condition is affecting the management, query the physician.

Codes from this chapter are used only on the mother's medical record, never on the newborn's record. To report complications for a newborn or a fetus during delivery, see Chapter 16 (perinatal period) and Chapter 17 (congenital anomalies).

The principal diagnosis code assignment should correspond to the complication of pregnancy that was the reason for the patient encounter. Conditions usually classified in other chapters of ICD-10-CM are reclassified in Chapter 15 when they are related to or are aggravated by the pregnancy, childbirth, or by the puerperium.

Hypertension, for example, is classified in category O10.- during pregnancy, delivery, and the puerperium.

The majority of codes in Chapter 15 have a final character indicating the trimester of pregnancy. The timeframe for trimesters are:

- 1st trimester – less than 14 weeks 0 days
- 2nd trimester – 14 weeks 0 days to less than 28 weeks 0 days
- 3rd trimester – 28 weeks 0 days until delivery

If the trimester is not a component of a code, it is because the condition always occurs in a specific trimester, or the concept of trimester of pregnancy is not applicable. Certain codes have characters for only certain trimesters because the condition does not occur in all trimesters, but it may occur in more than one.

Assignment of the final character for trimester should be based on the provider's (physician's) documentation of the trimester (or number of weeks) for the current admission/encounter. This applies to the assignment of trimester for pre-existing conditions as well as those that develop during or are due to pregnancy. The provider's documentation of the number of weeks may be used to assign the appropriate code identifying the trimester.

Whenever delivery occurs during the current admission, and there is an "in childbirth" option for the obstetric complication being coded, the "in childbirth" code should be assigned.

Each category that includes codes for trimester has a code for "unspecified trimester." The "unspecified trimester" code should rarely be used, such as when the documentation in the record is insufficient to determine the trimester and it is not possible to obtain clarification.

Chapter 15 codes have sequencing priority over codes from other chapters. An additional code from category Z3A, weeks of gestation, is used with codes from this chapter to identify specific weeks of pregnancy following any complications of pregnancy, childbirth and the puerperium. An outcome of delivery code, Z37.0-Z37.9, should be included on every maternal record when a delivery has occurred.

Maternity and postpartum care is a specialty in home care. OASIS is not involved with these patients if the care is provided for maternity reasons. Should the pregnancy be incidental to the home care encounter, then code Z33.1, Pregnant state incidental, should be used in place of any Chapter 15 codes. It is the physician's responsibility to state that the condition being treated is not affecting the pregnancy.

The circumstances of the encounter govern the selection of the principal diagnosis.

In episodes when no delivery occurs, the principal diagnosis should correspond to the principal complication of the pregnancy that necessitated the encounter. When more than one complication is being treated or monitored, any of the complication codes may be sequenced first.

Codes from category O35 (Maternal care for known or suspected fetal abnormality and damage), and category O36 (Maternal care for other fetal problems), are assigned only when the fetal condition is actually responsible for modifying the management of the mother, i.e., by requiring diagnostic studies, additional observation, special care, or termination of pregnancy. The fact that the fetal condition exists does not justify assigning a code from this series to the mother's record.

In cases when surgery is performed on the fetus, a diagnosis code from category O35, Maternal care for known or suspected fetal abnormality and damage, should be assigned to identify the fetal condition.

No code from Chapter 16, the perinatal codes, should be used on the mother's record to identify fetal conditions. Surgery performed in utero on a fetus is still to be coded as an obstetric encounter.

The postpartum period begins immediately after delivery and continues for six weeks following delivery. The peripartum period is defined as the last month of pregnancy to five months postpartum. A postpartum complication is any complication occurring within the six-week period. (NOTE: Chapter 15 codes also may be used to describe pregnancy-related complications of the mother after the six-week period, should the physician document that a condition is pregnancy related). It is acceptable to use codes specifically for the puerperium with codes complicating pregnancy and childbirth if a condition arises postpartum during the delivery encounter.

Code O94, Sequelae of complication of pregnancy, childbirth, and the puerperium, is used when an initial complication of a pregnancy develops a sequelae requiring treatment at a future date. This code may be used at any time after the initial postpartum period. This code, like all sequela codes, is to be sequenced following the code describing the sequelae of the complication.

Sometimes a Chapter 15 code is not the most appropriate choice. Here are a few situations to watch out for:

- If the documentation indicates **a neoplasm or tumor of an organ**, coders should look up the term (malignancy, tumor, adenoma) used in the medical record to find the correct code, most likely a code from Chapter 2. A code from Chapter 15 is reported (such as subcategory O9A.1- Malignant neoplasm complicating pregnancy, childbirth and the puerperium) as the first- listed diagnosis with an additional code (C00-C96) to identify the neoplasm.
- If a patient has a **personal history of a condition that may complicate the pregnancy in the future but is not currently a complication,** use a code from the Z code section. Examples are Z22.330 (Carrier or suspected carrier of Group B streptococcus), or Z87.51 (Personal history of pre-term labor. However, use code O09.21- (Supervision of pregnancy with history of pre-term labor) if the patient is currently pregnant. If a code from Chapter 15 also is being reported, the Z code is reported as an additional diagnosis.

General Rules for OB Cases

7th Character for Fetus Identification

Where applicable, a 7th character is to be assigned for certain categories (such as O31, O32, O33.3- O33.7, O35, O40, O41, O60.1, O60.2, O64, and O69) to identify the fetus for which the complication code applies. In some of these code categories, there are specific codes for each option. In other code subcategories, coders will need to refer to the 7th character boxes for the definition of the 7th character options.

Assign 7th character "0":

- For single gestations
- When the documentation in the record is insufficient to determine the fetus affected and it is not possible to obtain clarification.
- When it is not possible to clinically determine which fetus is affected.

Selection of OB Principal or First-Listed Diagnosis

For **routine outpatient prenatal visits** when no complications are present, a code from category Z34, Encounter for supervision of normal pregnancy, should be used as a first-listed diagnosis. These codes should not be used in conjunction with Chapter 15 codes, according to the coding guidelines.

For routine prenatal outpatient visits for patients with high-risk pregnancies, a code from category O09 (Supervision of high risk pregnancy) should be used as the first-listed diagnosis. Secondary Chapter 15 codes may be used in conjunction with these codes, if appropriate.

In episodes when no delivery occurs, the principal diagnosis should correspond to the principal complication of the pregnancy which necessitated the encounter. Should more than one complication exist, all of which are treated or monitored, any of the complications codes may be sequenced first.

When an obstetric patient is admitted and delivers during that admission, the condition that prompted the admission should be sequenced as the principal diagnosis. If multiple conditions prompted the admission, sequence the one most related to the delivery as the principal diagnosis. A code for any complication of the delivery should be assigned as an additional diagnosis. In cases of cesarean delivery, the selection of the principal diagnosis should be the condition established after study that was responsible for the patient's admission. If the patient was admitted with a condition that resulted in the performance of the cesarean procedure, then that condition should be selected as the principal diagnosis. If the reason for the admission/encounter was unrelated to the condition resulting in the cesarean delivery, the condition related to the reason for the admission/encounter should be selected as the principal diagnosis.

A code from category Z37, Outcome of delivery, should be included on every maternal record when a delivery has occurred. These codes are not to be used on subsequent records or on the newborn record.

Pre-existing Conditions versus Conditions due to pregnancy

Certain categories in Chapter 15 distinguish between conditions of the mother that existed prior to the pregnancy (pre-existing) and those that are a direct result of pregnancy. When assigning codes from Chapter 15, it is important to assess if a condition was pre-existing prior to pregnancy or developed during or due to pregnancy in order to assign the correct code.

Categories that do not distinguish between pre-existing and pregnancy-related conditions may be used for either.

Pre-existing hypertension in pregnancy

Category O10 (pre-existing hypertension complicating pregnancy, childbirth and the puerperium) includes codes for hypertensive heart and hypertensive chronic kidney disease. When assigning one of the O10 codes that includes hypertensive heart disease or hypertensive chronic kidney disease, it is necessary to add a secondary code from the appropriate hypertension category to specify the type of heart failure or chronic kidney disease.

Multiple Coding and Sequencing

Codes from this chapter almost always are reported as the first-listed diagnosis. Exceptions are category O94 (Sequelae of pregnancy, childbirth and the puerperium), which requires coding first the condition resulting from (sequel) of complication of pregnancy, childbirth and the puerperium, and some Z codes designated as primary only in the Tabular List.

Most complication codes include notes instructing the coder to report an additional code to provide more information as to the nature of the complication. The following are some examples of coding for complications during pregnancy, delivery and the postpartum periods:

- During pregnancy, childbirth or the puerperium, a patient admitted because of an **HIV-related illness** should receive a principal diagnosis from subcategory O98.7-, Human immunodeficiency [HIV] disease complicating pregnancy, childbirth and the puerperium, followed by the code(s) for the HIV-related illness(es). Patients with asymptomatic HIV infection status admitted during pregnancy, childbirth and the puerperium should be assigned codes O98.7- and Z21, Asymptomatic human immunodeficiency virus [HIV] infection status.
- **Diabetes mellitus** is a significant complicating factor in pregnancy. Pregnant women who are diabetic should be assigned a code from category O24, Diabetes mellitus in pregnancy, childbirth and the puerperium, first, followed by the appropriate code(s) (E08-E13) from chapter 4. Code Z79.4, Long-term (current) use of insulin, or code Z79.84, Long-term (current) use of oral hypoglycemic drugs, should also be assigned if the diabetes mellitus is being treated with insulin or oral medications. If the patient is treated with both oral medications and insulin, only the code for insulin-controlled should be assigned, per the Chapter 15 coding guidelines. Remember, these are chapter specific guidelines and therefore only apply to Chapter 15 codes.
- **Gestational (pregnancy induced) diabetes** can occur during the second and third trimester of pregnancy in women who were not diabetic prior to pregnancy. Gestational diabetes can cause complications in the pregnancy similar to those of pre-existing diabetes mellitus. It also puts the woman at greater risk of developing diabetes after the pregnancy. Codes for gestational diabetes are in subcategory O24.4, Gestational diabetes mellitus. No other code from category O24, Diabetes mellitus in pregnancy, childbirth, and the puerperium should be used with a code from O24.4.

The codes under subcategory O24.4 include diet controlled, insulin controlled, and controlled by oral hypoglycemic drugs. If a patient with gestational diabetes is treated with both diet and insulin, only assign the code for insulin-controlled. If a patient with gestational diabetes is treated with both diet and oral hypoglycemic medications, only assign the code for "controlled by oral hypoglycemic drugs." Code Z79.4 or code Z79.84 should not be assigned with codes from subcategory O24.4.

An abnormal glucose tolerance in pregnancy is assigned a code from subcategory O99.81, Abnormal glucose complicating pregnancy, childbirth and the puerperium.

Sepsis and septic shock complicating abortion, pregnancy, childbirth and the puerperium

When assigning a chapter 15 code for sepsis complicating abortion, pregnancy, childbirth, and the puerperium, a code for the specific type of infection should be assigned as an additional diagnosis. If

Chapter 15

O00 - O9A

severe sepsis is present, a code from subcategory R65.2, Severe sepsis, and code(s) for associated organ dysfunction(s) should also be assigned as additional diagnoses.

Code O85, Puerperal sepsis, should be assigned with a secondary code to identify the causal organism (e.g., for a bacterial infection, assign a code from category B95-B96, bacterial infections in conditions classified elsewhere). A code from category A40, streptococcal sepsis, or A41, other sepsis, should not be used for puerperal sepsis. If applicable, use additional codes to identify severe sepsis (R65.2-) and any associated acute organ dysfunction.

Pregnancy-related Cardiomyopathy

Pregnancy associated cardiomyopathy, code O90.3, is unique in that it may be diagnosed in the third trimester of pregnancy but may continue to progress months after the delivery. For this reason, it is referred to as peripartum cardiomyopathy. Code O90.3 is only for use when the cardiomyopathy develops as a result of pregnancy in a woman who did not have pre-existing heart disease.

Alcohol and tobacco use during pregnancy, childbirth and the puerperium

Codes under subcategory O99.31, Alcohol use complicating pregnancy, childbirth and the puerperium, should be assigned for any pregnancy case when a mother uses alcohol during the pregnancy or postpartum. A secondary code from category F10, alcohol related disorders, should also be assigned to identify manifestations of alcohol use.

Codes under subcategory O99.33, Tobacco use disorder complicating pregnancy, childbirth, and the puerperium, should be assigned for any pregnancy case when a mother used any type of tobacco product during the pregnancy or postpartum. A secondary code from F17, nicotine dependence, should also be assigned to identify the type of nicotine dependence.

Poisoning, toxic effects, adverse effects and underdosing in a pregnant patient

A code from subcategory O9A.2, Injury, poisoning and certain other consequences of external causes complicating pregnancy, childbirth, and the puerperium, should be sequenced first, followed by the appropriate injury, poisoning, toxic effect, adverse effect, or underdosing code, and then the additional code(s) that specifies the condition caused by the poisoning, toxic effect, adverse effect or underdosing.

Abuse in a Pregnant Patient

For suspected or confirmed cases of abuse of a pregnant patient, a code(s) from subcategories O9A.3, Physical abuse complicating pregnancy, childbirth, and the puerperium, O9A.4, Sexual abuse complicating pregnancy, childbirth, and the puerperium, and O9A.5, Psychological abuse complicating pregnancy, childbirth, and the puerperium, should be sequenced first, followed by the appropriate codes (if applicable) to identify any associated current injury due to physical abuse, sexual abuse, and the perpetrator of abuse. Refer to chapter 19 for codes related to current injuries and Y07- for codes to describe the perpetrator of abuse.

CHAPTER 15: PREGNANCY, CHILDBIRTH AND THE PUERPERIUM (O00-O9A)

Note:
CODES FROM THIS CHAPTER ARE FOR USE ONLY ON MATERNAL RECORDS, NEVER ON NEWBORN RECORDS
Codes from this chapter are for use for conditions related to or aggravated by the pregnancy, childbirth, or by the puerperium (maternal causes or obstetric causes)
Trimesters are counted from the first day of the last menstrual period. They are defined as follows:
1st trimester- less than 14 weeks 0 days
2nd trimester- 14 weeks 0 days to less than 28 weeks 0 days
3rd trimester- 28 weeks 0 days until delivery
Use additional code from category Z3A, Weeks of gestation, to identify the specific week of the pregnancy, if known.

EXCLUDES 1 supervision of normal pregnancy (Z34.-)

EXCLUDES 2 mental and behavioral disorders associated with the puerperium (F53.-)
obstetrical tetanus (A34)
postpartum necrosis of pituitary gland (E23.0)
puerperal osteomalacia (M83.0)

GUIDELINES **Section I.C.15.a.1)**
Obstetric cases require codes from chapter 15, codes in the range O00-O9A, Pregnancy, Childbirth, and the Puerperium. Chapter 15 codes have sequencing priority over codes from other chapters. Additional codes from other chapters may be used in conjunction with chapter 15 codes to further specify conditions. Should the provider document that the pregnancy is incidental to the encounter, then code Z33.1, Pregnant state, incidental, should be used in place of any chapter 15 codes. It is the provider's responsibility to state that the condition being treated is not affecting the pregnancy.

GUIDELINES **Section I.C.15.a.2)**
Chapter 15 codes are to be used only on the maternal record, never on the record of the newborn.

GUIDELINES **Section I.C.15.c**
When assigning codes from Chapter 15, it is important to assess if a condition was pre-existing prior to pregnancy or developed during or due to the pregnancy in order to assign the correct code. Categories that do not distinguish between pre-existing and pregnancy related conditions may be used for either. It is acceptable to use codes specifically for the puerperium with codes complicating pregnancy and childbirth if a condition arises postpartum during the delivery encounter.

This chapter contains the following blocks:

O00-O08	Pregnancy with abortive outcome
O09	Supervision of high risk pregnancy
O10-O16	Edema, proteinuria and hypertensive disorders in pregnancy, childbirth and the puerperium
O20-O29	Other maternal disorders predominantly related to pregnancy
O30-O48	Maternal care related to the fetus and amniotic cavity and possible delivery problems
O60-O77	Complications of labor and delivery
O80-O82	Encounter for delivery
O85-O92	Complications predominantly related to the puerperium
O94-O9A	Other obstetric conditions, not elsewhere classified

Pregnancy with abortive outcome (O00-O08)

EXCLUDES 1 continuing pregnancy in multiple gestation after abortion of one fetus or more (O31.1-, O31.3-)

+4 **O00 Ectopic pregnancy**
INCLUDES ruptured ectopic pregnancy
Use additional code from category O08 to identify any associated complication

+5 **O00.0 Abdominal pregnancy**
EXCLUDES 1 maternal care for viable fetus in abdominal pregnancy (O36.7-)

SP + **O00.00 Abdominal pregnancy without intrauterine pregnancy**
Abdominal pregnancy NOS

SP + **O00.01 Abdominal pregnancy with intrauterine pregnancy**

+5 **O00.1 Tubal pregnancy**
Fallopian pregnancy
Rupture of (fallopian) tube due to pregnancy
Tubal abortion
DEFINITION Fertilized egg implants itself within the fallopian tube where the embryo grows and may rupture the tube.

+6 **O00.10 Tubal pregnancy without intrauterine pregnancy**
Tubal pregnancy NOS

SP + **O00.101 Right tubal pregnancy without intrauterine pregnancy**

SP + **O00.102 Left tubal pregnancy without intrauterine pregnancy**

SP + **O00.109 Unspecified tubal pregnancy without intrauterine pregnancy**

+6 **O00.11 Tubal pregnancy with intrauterine pregnancy**

SP + **O00.111 Right tubal pregnancy with intrauterine pregnancy**

SP + **O00.112 Left tubal pregnancy with intrauterine pregnancy**

SP + **O00.119 Unspecified tubal pregnancy with intrauterine pregnancy**

+5 **O00.2 Ovarian pregnancy**

+6 **O00.20 Ovarian pregnancy without intrauterine pregnancy**
Ovarian pregnancy NOS

SP + **O00.201 Right ovarian pregnancy without intrauterine pregnancy**

SP + **O00.202 Left ovarian pregnancy without intrauterine pregnancy**

SP + **O00.209 Unspecified ovarian pregnancy without intrauterine pregnancy**

+6 **O00.21 Ovarian pregnancy with intrauterine pregnancy**

SP + **O00.211 Right ovarian pregnancy with intrauterine pregnancy**

SP + **O00.212 Left ovarian pregnancy with intrauterine pregnancy**

SP + **O00.219 Unspecified ovarian pregnancy with intrauterine pregnancy**

+5 **O00.8 Other ectopic pregnancy**
Cervical pregnancy
Cornual pregnancy
Intraligamentous pregnancy
Mural pregnancy

SP + **O00.80 Other ectopic pregnancy without intrauterine pregnancy**
Other ectopic pregnancy NOS

SP + **O00.81 Other ectopic pregnancy with intrauterine pregnancy**

Chapter 15 O00-O9A

+ 5 O00.9 Ectopic pregnancy, unspecified

SP + O00.90 Unspecified ectopic pregnancy without intrauterine pregnancy
Ectopic pregnancy NOS

SP + O00.91 Unspecified ectopic pregnancy with intrauterine pregnancy

+ 4 O01 Hydatidiform mole
Use additional code from category O08 to identify any associated complication.
EXCLUDES 1 chorioadenoma (destruens) (D39.2)
malignant hydatidiform mole (D39.2)

SP + O01.0 Classical hydatidiform mole
Complete hydatidiform mole

SP + O01.1 Incomplete and partial hydatidiform mole

SP + O01.9 Hydatidiform mole, unspecified
Trophoblastic disease NOS
Vesicular mole NOS

+ 4 O02 Other abnormal products of conception
Use additional code from category O08 to identify any associated complication.
EXCLUDES 1 papyraceous fetus (O31.0-)

SP + O02.0 Blighted ovum and nonhydatidiform mole
Carneous mole
Fleshy mole
Intrauterine mole NOS
Molar pregnancy NEC
Pathological ovum

SP + O02.1 Missed abortion
Early fetal death, before completion of 20 weeks of gestation, with retention of dead fetus
EXCLUDES 1 failed induced abortion (O07.-)
fetal death (intrauterine) (late) (O36.4)
missed abortion with blighted ovum (O02.0)
missed abortion with hydatidiform mole (O01.-)
missed abortion with nonhydatidiform (O02.0)
missed abortion with other abnormal products of conception (O02.8-)
missed delivery (O36.4)
stillbirth (P95)

+ 5 O02.8 Other specified abnormal products of conception
EXCLUDES 1 abnormal products of conception with blighted ovum (O02.0)
abnormal products of conception with hydatidiform mole (O01.-)
abnormal products of conception with nonhydatidiform mole (O02.0)

SP + O02.81 Inappropriate change in quantitative human chorionic gonadotropin (hCG) in early pregnancy
Biochemical pregnancy
Chemical pregnancy
Inappropriate level of quantitative human chorionic gonadotropin (hCG) for gestational age in early pregnancy

SP + O02.89 Other abnormal products of conception

SP + O02.9 Abnormal product of conception, unspecified

4 O03 Spontaneous abortion
Note:
Incomplete abortion includes retained products of conception following spontaneous abortion
INCLUDES miscarriage

SP O03.0 Genital tract and pelvic infection following incomplete spontaneous abortion
Endometritis following incomplete spontaneous abortion
Oophoritis following incomplete spontaneous abortion
Parametritis following incomplete spontaneous abortion
Pelvic peritonitis following incomplete spontaneous abortion
Salpingitis following incomplete spontaneous abortion
Salpingo-oophoritis following incomplete spontaneous abortion
EXCLUDES 1 sepsis following incomplete spontaneous abortion (O03.37)
urinary tract infection following incomplete spontaneous abortion (O03.38)

SP O03.1 Delayed or excessive hemorrhage following incomplete spontaneous abortion
Afibrinogenemia following incomplete spontaneous abortion
Defibrination syndrome following incomplete spontaneous abortion
Hemolysis following incomplete spontaneous abortion
Intravascular coagulation following incomplete spontaneous abortion

SP O03.2 Embolism following incomplete spontaneous abortion
Air embolism following incomplete spontaneous abortion
Amniotic fluid embolism following incomplete spontaneous abortion
Blood-clot embolism following incomplete spontaneous abortion
Embolism NOS following incomplete spontaneous abortion
Fat embolism following incomplete spontaneous abortion
Pulmonary embolism following incomplete spontaneous abortion
Pyemic embolism following incomplete spontaneous abortion
Septic or septicopyemic embolism following incomplete spontaneous abortion
Soap embolism following incomplete spontaneous abortion

5 O03.3 Other and unspecified complications following incomplete spontaneous abortion

SP O03.30 Unspecified complication following incomplete spontaneous abortion

SP O03.31 Shock following incomplete spontaneous abortion
Circulatory collapse following incomplete spontaneous abortion
Shock (postprocedural) following incomplete spontaneous abortion
EXCLUDES 1 shock due to infection following incomplete spontaneous abortion (O03.37)

SP O03.32 Renal failure following incomplete spontaneous abortion
Kidney failure (acute) following incomplete spontaneous abortion
Oliguria following incomplete spontaneous abortion
Renal shutdown following incomplete spontaneous abortion
Renal tubular necrosis following incomplete spontaneous abortion
Uremia following incomplete spontaneous abortion

SP O03.33 Metabolic disorder following incomplete spontaneous abortion

SP O03.34 Damage to pelvic organs following incomplete spontaneous abortion
Laceration, perforation, tear or chemical damage of bladder following incomplete spontaneous abortion
Laceration, perforation, tear or chemical damage of bowel following incomplete spontaneous abortion
Laceration, perforation, tear or chemical damage of broad ligament following incomplete spontaneous abortion
Laceration, perforation, tear or chemical damage of cervix following incomplete spontaneous abortion
Laceration, perforation, tear or chemical damage of periurethral tissue following incomplete spontaneous abortion
Laceration, perforation, tear or chemical damage of uterus following incomplete spontaneous abortion
Laceration, perforation, tear or chemical damage of vagina following incomplete spontaneous abortion

SP O03.35 Other venous complications following incomplete spontaneous abortion

SP O03.36 Cardiac arrest following incomplete spontaneous abortion

SP + O03.37 Sepsis following incomplete spontaneous abortion
Use additional code to identify infectious agent (B95-B97)
Use additional code to identify severe sepsis, if applicable (R65.2-)
EXCLUDES 1 septic or septicopyemic embolism following incomplete spontaneous abortion (O03.2)

SP O03.38 Urinary tract infection following incomplete spontaneous abortion
Cystitis following incomplete spontaneous abortion

SP O03.39 Incomplete spontaneous abortion with other complications

SP O03.4 Incomplete spontaneous abortion without complication

SP O03.5 Genital tract and pelvic infection following complete or unspecified spontaneous abortion
Endometritis following complete or unspecified spontaneous abortion
Oophoritis following complete or unspecified spontaneous abortion
Parametritis following complete or unspecified spontaneous abortion
Pelvic peritonitis following complete or unspecified spontaneous abortion
Salpingitis following complete or unspecified spontaneous abortion
Salpingo-oophoritis following complete or unspecified spontaneous abortion
EXCLUDES 1 sepsis following complete or unspecified spontaneous abortion (O03.87)
urinary tract infection following complete or unspecified spontaneous abortion (O03.88)

SP O03.6 Delayed or excessive hemorrhage following complete or unspecified spontaneous abortion
Afibrinogenemia following complete or unspecified spontaneous abortion
Defibrination syndrome following complete or unspecified spontaneous abortion
Hemolysis following complete or unspecified spontaneous abortion
Intravascular coagulation following complete or unspecified spontaneous abortion

SP O03.7 Embolism following complete or unspecified spontaneous abortion
Air embolism following complete or unspecified spontaneous abortion
Amniotic fluid embolism following complete or unspecified spontaneous abortion
Blood-clot embolism following complete or unspecified spontaneous abortion
Embolism NOS following complete or unspecified spontaneous abortion
Fat embolism following complete or unspecified spontaneous abortion
Pulmonary embolism following complete or unspecified spontaneous abortion
Pyemic embolism following complete or unspecified spontaneous abortion
Septic or septicopyemic embolism following complete or unspecified spontaneous abortion

Chapter 15 O00-O9A

Soap embolism following complete or unspecified spontaneous abortion

5 O03.8 Other and unspecified complications following complete or unspecified spontaneous abortion

SP O03.80 Unspecified complication following complete or unspecified spontaneous abortion

SP O03.81 Shock following complete or unspecified spontaneous abortion

Circulatory collapse following complete or unspecified spontaneous abortion

Shock (postprocedural) following complete or unspecified spontaneous abortion

EXCLUDES 1 shock due to infection following complete or unspecified spontaneous abortion (O03.87)

SP O03.82 Renal failure following complete or unspecified spontaneous abortion

Kidney failure (acute) following complete or unspecified spontaneous abortion

Oliguria following complete or unspecified spontaneous abortion

Renal shutdown following complete or unspecified spontaneous abortion

Renal tubular necrosis following complete or unspecified spontaneous abortion

Uremia following complete or unspecified spontaneous abortion

SP O03.83 Metabolic disorder following complete or unspecified spontaneous abortion

SP O03.84 Damage to pelvic organs following complete or unspecified spontaneous abortion

Laceration, perforation, tear or chemical damage of bladder following complete or unspecified spontaneous abortion

Laceration, perforation, tear or chemical damage of bowel following complete or unspecified spontaneous abortion

Laceration, perforation, tear or chemical damage of broad ligament following complete or unspecified spontaneous abortion

Laceration, perforation, tear or chemical damage of cervix following complete or unspecified spontaneous abortion

Laceration, perforation, tear or chemical damage of periurethral tissue following complete or unspecified spontaneous abortion

Laceration, perforation, tear or chemical damage of uterus following complete or unspecified spontaneous abortion

Laceration, perforation, tear or chemical damage of vagina following complete or unspecified spontaneous abortion

SP O03.85 Other venous complications following complete or unspecified spontaneous abortion

SP O03.86 Cardiac arrest following complete or unspecified spontaneous abortion

SP + O03.87 Sepsis following complete or unspecified spontaneous abortion

Use additional code to identify infectious agent (B95-B97)

Use additional code to identify severe sepsis, if applicable (R65.2-)

EXCLUDES 1 septic or septicopyemic embolism following complete or unspecified spontaneous abortion (O03.7)

SP O03.88 Urinary tract infection following complete or unspecified spontaneous abortion

Cystitis following complete or unspecified spontaneous abortion

SP O03.89 Complete or unspecified spontaneous abortion with other complications

SP O03.9 Complete or unspecified spontaneous abortion without complication

Miscarriage NOS

Spontaneous abortion NOS

4 O04 Complications following (induced) termination of pregnancy

INCLUDES complications following (induced) termination of pregnancy

EXCLUDES 1 encounter for elective termination of pregnancy, uncomplicated (Z33.2)

failed attempted termination of pregnancy (O07.-)

SP O04.5 Genital tract and pelvic infection following (induced) termination of pregnancy

Endometritis following (induced) termination of pregnancy

Oophoritis following (induced) termination of pregnancy

Parametritis following (induced) termination of pregnancy

Pelvic peritonitis following (induced) termination of pregnancy

Salpingitis following (induced) termination of pregnancy

Salpingo-oophoritis following (induced) termination of pregnancy

EXCLUDES 1 sepsis following (induced) termination of pregnancy (O04.87)

urinary tract infection following (induced) termination of pregnancy (O04.88)

SP O04.6 Delayed or excessive hemorrhage following (induced) termination of pregnancy

Chapter 15

O00-O9A

Afibrinogenemia following (induced) termination of pregnancy
Defibrination syndrome following (induced) termination of pregnancy
Hemolysis following (induced) termination of pregnancy
Intravascular coagulation following (induced) termination of pregnancy

SP **O04.7 Embolism following (induced) termination of pregnancy**
Air embolism following (induced) termination of pregnancy
Amniotic fluid embolism following (induced) termination of pregnancy
Blood-clot embolism following (induced) termination of pregnancy
Embolism NOS following (induced) termination of pregnancy
Fat embolism following (induced) termination of pregnancy
Pulmonary embolism following (induced) termination of pregnancy
Pyemic embolism following (induced) termination of pregnancy
Septic or septicopyemic embolism following (induced) termination of pregnancy
Soap embolism following (induced) termination of pregnancy

5 **O04.8 (Induced) termination of pregnancy with other and unspecified complications**

SP **O04.80 (Induced) termination of pregnancy with unspecified complications**

SP **O04.81 Shock following (induced) termination of pregnancy**
Circulatory collapse following (induced) termination of pregnancy
Shock (postprocedural) following (induced) termination of pregnancy
EXCLUDES 1 shock due to infection following (induced) termination of pregnancy (O04.87)

SP **O04.82 Renal failure following (induced) termination of pregnancy**
Kidney failure (acute) following (induced) termination of pregnancy
Oliguria following (induced) termination of pregnancy
Renal shutdown following (induced) termination of pregnancy
Renal tubular necrosis following (induced) termination of pregnancy
Uremia following (induced) termination of pregnancy

SP **O04.83 Metabolic disorder following (induced) termination of pregnancy**

SP **O04.84 Damage to pelvic organs following (induced) termination of pregnancy**
Laceration, perforation, tear or chemical damage of bladder following (induced) termination of pregnancy
Laceration, perforation, tear or chemical damage of bowel following (induced) termination of pregnancy
Laceration, perforation, tear or chemical damage of broad ligament following (induced) termination of pregnancy
Laceration, perforation, tear or chemical damage of cervix following (induced) termination of pregnancy
Laceration, perforation, tear or chemical damage of periurethral tissue following (induced) termination of pregnancy
Laceration, perforation, tear or chemical damage of uterus following (induced) termination of pregnancy
Laceration, perforation, tear or chemical damage of vagina following (induced) termination of pregnancy

SP **O04.85 Other venous complications following (induced) termination of pregnancy**

SP **O04.86 Cardiac arrest following (induced) termination of pregnancy**

SP + **O04.87 Sepsis following (induced) termination of pregnancy**
Use additional code to identify infectious agent (B95-B97)
Use additional code to identify severe sepsis, if applicable (R65.2-)
EXCLUDES 1 septic or septicopyemic embolism following (induced) termination of pregnancy (O04.7)

SP **O04.88 Urinary tract infection following (induced) termination of pregnancy**
Cystitis following (induced) termination of pregnancy

SP **O04.89 (Induced) termination of pregnancy with other complications**

4 **O07 Failed attempted termination of pregnancy**
INCLUDES failure of attempted induction of termination of pregnancy
incomplete elective abortion
EXCLUDES 1 incomplete spontaneous abortion (O03.0-)

SP **O07.0 Genital tract and pelvic infection following failed attempted termination of pregnancy**
Endometritis following failed attempted termination of pregnancy
Oophoritis following failed attempted termination of pregnancy
Parametritis following failed attempted termination of pregnancy
Pelvic peritonitis following failed attempted termination of pregnancy
Salpingitis following failed attempted termination of pregnancy
Salpingo-oophoritis following failed attempted termination of pregnancy
EXCLUDES 1 sepsis following failed attempted termination of pregnancy (O07.37)
urinary tract infection following failed attempted termination of pregnancy (O07.38)

SP **O07.1 Delayed or excessive hemorrhage following failed attempted termination of pregnancy**

Chapter 15 O00-O9A

Afibrinogenemia following failed attempted termination of pregnancy
Defibrination syndrome following failed attempted termination of pregnancy
Hemolysis following failed attempted termination of pregnancy
Intravascular coagulation following failed attempted termination of pregnancy

SP **O07.2 Embolism following failed attempted termination of pregnancy**
Air embolism following failed attempted termination of pregnancy
Amniotic fluid embolism following failed attempted termination of pregnancy
Blood-clot embolism following failed attempted termination of pregnancy
Embolism NOS following failed attempted termination of pregnancy
Fat embolism following failed attempted termination of pregnancy
Pulmonary embolism following failed attempted termination of pregnancy
Pyemic embolism following failed attempted termination of pregnancy
Septic or septicopyemic embolism following failed attempted termination of pregnancy
Soap embolism following failed attempted termination of pregnancy

5 **O07.3 Failed attempted termination of pregnancy with other and unspecified complications**

SP **O07.30 Failed attempted termination of pregnancy with unspecified complications**

SP **O07.31 Shock following failed attempted termination of pregnancy**
Circulatory collapse following failed attempted termination of pregnancy
Shock (postprocedural) following failed attempted termination of pregnancy
EXCLUDES 1 shock due to infection following failed attempted termination of pregnancy (O07.37)

SP **O07.32 Renal failure following failed attempted termination of pregnancy**
Kidney failure (acute) following failed attempted termination of pregnancy
Oliguria following failed attempted termination of pregnancy
Renal shutdown following failed attempted termination of pregnancy
Renal tubular necrosis following failed attempted termination of pregnancy
Uremia following failed attempted termination of pregnancy

SP **O07.33 Metabolic disorder following failed attempted termination of pregnancy**

SP **O07.34 Damage to pelvic organs following failed attempted termination of pregnancy**
Laceration, perforation, tear or chemical damage of bladder following failed attempted termination of pregnancy
Laceration, perforation, tear or chemical damage of bowel following failed attempted termination of pregnancy
Laceration, perforation, tear or chemical damage of broad ligament following failed attempted termination of pregnancy
Laceration, perforation, tear or chemical damage of cervix following failed attempted termination of pregnancy
Laceration, perforation, tear or chemical damage of periurethral tissue following failed attempted termination of pregnancy
Laceration, perforation, tear or chemical damage of uterus following failed attempted termination of pregnancy
Laceration, perforation, tear or chemical damage of vagina following failed attempted termination of pregnancy

SP **O07.35 Other venous complications following failed attempted termination of pregnancy**

SP **O07.36 Cardiac arrest following failed attempted termination of pregnancy**

SP + **O07.37 Sepsis following failed attempted termination of pregnancy**
Use additional code (B95-B97), to identify infectious agent
Use additional code (R65.2-) to identify severe sepsis, if applicable
EXCLUDES 1 septic or septicopyemic embolism following failed attempted termination of pregnancy (O07.2)

SP **O07.38 Urinary tract infection following failed attempted termination of pregnancy**
Cystitis following failed attempted termination of pregnancy

SP **O07.39 Failed attempted termination of pregnancy with other complications**

SP **O07.4 Failed attempted termination of pregnancy without complication**

4 **O08 Complications following ectopic and molar pregnancy**
This category is for use with categories O00-O02 to identify any associated complications

SP **O08.0 Genital tract and pelvic infection following ectopic and molar pregnancy**
Endometritis following ectopic and molar pregnancy
Oophoritis following ectopic and molar pregnancy
Parametritis following ectopic and molar pregnancy
Pelvic peritonitis following ectopic and molar pregnancy
Salpingitis following ectopic and molar pregnancy
Salpingo-oophoritis following ectopic and molar pregnancy

EXCLUDES 1 sepsis following ectopic and molar pregnancy (O08.82)
urinary tract infection (O08.83)

SP **O08.1 Delayed or excessive hemorrhage following ectopic and molar pregnancy**
Afibrinogenemia following ectopic and molar pregnancy
Defibrination syndrome following ectopic and molar pregnancy
Hemolysis following ectopic and molar pregnancy
Intravascular coagulation following ectopic and molar pregnancy
EXCLUDES 1 delayed or excessive hemorrhage due to incomplete abortion (O03.1)

SP **O08.2 Embolism following ectopic and molar pregnancy**
Air embolism following ectopic and molar pregnancy
Amniotic fluid embolism following ectopic and molar pregnancy
Blood-clot embolism following ectopic and molar pregnancy
Embolism NOS following ectopic and molar pregnancy
Fat embolism following ectopic and molar pregnancy
Pulmonary embolism following ectopic and molar pregnancy
Pyemic embolism following ectopic and molar pregnancy
Septic or septicopyemic embolism following ectopic and molar pregnancy
Soap embolism following ectopic and molar pregnancy

SP **O08.3 Shock following ectopic and molar pregnancy**
Circulatory collapse following ectopic and molar pregnancy
Shock (postprocedural) following ectopic and molar pregnancy
EXCLUDES 1 shock due to infection following ectopic and molar pregnancy (O08.82)

SP **O08.4 Renal failure following ectopic and molar pregnancy**
Kidney failure (acute) following ectopic and molar pregnancy
Oliguria following ectopic and molar pregnancy
Renal shutdown following ectopic and molar pregnancy
Renal tubular necrosis following ectopic and molar pregnancy
Uremia following ectopic and molar pregnancy

SP **O08.5 Metabolic disorders following an ectopic and molar pregnancy**

SP **O08.6 Damage to pelvic organs and tissues following an ectopic and molar pregnancy**
Laceration, perforation, tear or chemical damage of bladder following an ectopic and molar pregnancy
Laceration, perforation, tear or chemical damage of bowel following an ectopic and molar pregnancy
Laceration, perforation, tear or chemical damage of broad ligament following an ectopic and molar pregnancy
Laceration, perforation, tear or chemical damage of cervix following an ectopic and molar pregnancy
Laceration, perforation, tear or chemical damage of periurethral tissue following an ectopic and molar pregnancy
Laceration, perforation, tear or chemical damage of uterus following an ectopic and molar pregnancy
Laceration, perforation, tear or chemical damage of vagina following an ectopic and molar pregnancy

SP **O08.7 Other venous complications following an ectopic and molar pregnancy**

5 **O08.8 Other complications following an ectopic and molar pregnancy**

SP **O08.81 Cardiac arrest following an ectopic and molar pregnancy**

SP + **O08.82 Sepsis following ectopic and molar pregnancy**
Use additional code (B95-B97), to identify infectious agent
Use additional code (R65.2-) to identify severe sepsis, if applicable
EXCLUDES 1 septic or septicopyemic embolism following ectopic and molar pregnancy (O08.2)

SP **O08.83 Urinary tract infection following an ectopic and molar pregnancy**
Cystitis following an ectopic and molar pregnancy

SP **O08.89 Other complications following an ectopic and molar pregnancy**

SP **O08.9 Unspecified complication following an ectopic and molar pregnancy**

Supervision of high risk pregnancy (O09)

4 **O09 Supervision of high risk pregnancy**

5 **O09.0 Supervision of pregnancy with history of infertility**

IQ **O09.00 Supervision of pregnancy with history of infertility, unspecified trimester**

SP **O09.01 Supervision of pregnancy with history of infertility, first trimester**

SP **O09.02 Supervision of pregnancy with history of infertility, second trimester**

SP **O09.03 Supervision of pregnancy with history of infertility, third trimester**

5 **O09.1 Supervision of pregnancy with history of ectopic pregnancy**

IQ **O09.10 Supervision of pregnancy with history of ectopic pregnancy, unspecified trimester**

SP **O09.11 Supervision of pregnancy with history of ectopic pregnancy, first trimester**

SP **O09.12 Supervision of pregnancy with history of ectopic pregnancy, second trimester**

Chapter 15

O00-O9A

★ New ▲Revised Px Primary SP PDGM Px SL Low CoM SH High CoM IQ Quest. Encounter H Hospice non-cancer Dx Unspecified M Manifestation

SP **O09.13 Supervision of pregnancy with history of ectopic pregnancy, third trimester**

5 **O09.A Supervision of pregnancy with history of molar pregnancy**

DEFINITION An abnormal product of conception that occurs when the cells proliferate out of control, creating a growth or mass of cell clusters that causes the body to continue producing hormones as if in pregnancy, even though there is no fetus developing. This gives a false positive pregnancy result. Molar pregnancies have the potential of developing into a cancerous growth, called choriocarinoma if left untreated.

IQ **O09.A0 Supervision of pregnancy with history of molar pregnancy, unspecified trimester**

SP **O09.A1 Supervision of pregnancy with history of molar pregnancy, first trimester**

SP **O09.A2 Supervision of pregnancy with history of molar pregnancy, second trimester**

SP **O09.A3 Supervision of pregnancy with history of molar pregnancy, third trimester**

5 **O09.2 Supervision of pregnancy with other poor reproductive or obstetric history**

EXCLUDES 2 pregnancy care for patient with history of recurrent pregnancy loss (O26.2-)

6 **O09.21 Supervision of pregnancy with history of pre-term labor**

SP **O09.211 Supervision of pregnancy with history of pre-term labor, first trimester**

SP **O09.212 Supervision of pregnancy with history of pre-term labor, second trimester**

SP **O09.213 Supervision of pregnancy with history of pre-term labor, third trimester**

IQ **O09.219 Supervision of pregnancy with history of pre-term labor, unspecified trimester**

6 **O09.29 Supervision of pregnancy with other poor reproductive or obstetric history**

Supervision of pregnancy with history of neonatal death

Supervision of pregnancy with history of stillbirth

SP **O09.291 Supervision of pregnancy with other poor reproductive or obstetric history, first trimester**

SP **O09.292 Supervision of pregnancy with other poor reproductive or obstetric history, second trimester**

SP **O09.293 Supervision of pregnancy with other poor reproductive or obstetric history, third trimester**

IQ **O09.299 Supervision of pregnancy with other poor reproductive or obstetric history, unspecified trimester**

5 **O09.3 Supervision of pregnancy with insufficient antenatal care**

Supervision of concealed pregnancy

Supervision of hidden pregnancy

IQ **O09.30 Supervision of pregnancy with insufficient antenatal care, unspecified trimester**

SP **O09.31 Supervision of pregnancy with insufficient antenatal care, first trimester**

SP **O09.32 Supervision of pregnancy with insufficient antenatal care, second trimester**

SP **O09.33 Supervision of pregnancy with insufficient antenatal care, third trimester**

5 **O09.4 Supervision of pregnancy with grand multiparity**

IQ **O09.40 Supervision of pregnancy with grand multiparity, unspecified trimester**

SP **O09.41 Supervision of pregnancy with grand multiparity, first trimester**

SP **O09.42 Supervision of pregnancy with grand multiparity, second trimester**

SP **O09.43 Supervision of pregnancy with grand multiparity, third trimester**

5 **O09.5 Supervision of elderly primigravida and multigravida**

Pregnancy for a female 35 years and older at expected date of delivery

6 **O09.51 Supervision of elderly primigravida**

SP **O09.511 Supervision of elderly primigravida, first trimester**

SP **O09.512 Supervision of elderly primigravida, second trimester**

SP **O09.513 Supervision of elderly primigravida, third trimester**

IQ **O09.519 Supervision of elderly primigravida, unspecified trimester**

6 **O09.52 Supervision of elderly multigravida**

SP **O09.521 Supervision of elderly multigravida, first trimester**

SP **O09.522 Supervision of elderly multigravida, second trimester**

SP **O09.523 Supervision of elderly multigravida, third trimester**

IQ **O09.529 Supervision of elderly multigravida, unspecified trimester**

5 **O09.6 Supervision of young primigravida and multigravida**

Supervision of pregnancy for a female less than 16 years old at expected date of delivery

6 **O09.61 Supervision of young primigravida**

SP **O09.611 Supervision of young primigravida, first trimester**

SP **O09.612 Supervision of young primigravida, second trimester**

SP **O09.613 Supervision of young primigravida, third trimester**

IQ **O09.619 Supervision of young primigravida, unspecified trimester**

6 **O09.62 Supervision of young multigravida**

Chapter 15

O00-O9A

4 4th digit required 5 5th digit required 6 6th digit required 7 7th digit required 7th digit placeholder + Additional code Laterality

SP **O09.621 Supervision of young multigravida, first trimester**

SP **O09.622 Supervision of young multigravida, second trimester**

SP **O09.623 Supervision of young multigravida, third trimester**

IQ **O09.629 Supervision of young multigravida, unspecified trimester**

5 **O09.7 Supervision of high risk pregnancy due to social problems**

IQ **O09.70 Supervision of high risk pregnancy due to social problems, unspecified trimester**

IQ **O09.71 Supervision of high risk pregnancy due to social problems, first trimester**

IQ **O09.72 Supervision of high risk pregnancy due to social problems, second trimester**

IQ **O09.73 Supervision of high risk pregnancy due to social problems, third trimester**

5 **O09.8 Supervision of other high risk pregnancies**

6 **O09.81 Supervision of pregnancy resulting from assisted reproductive technology**

Supervision of pregnancy resulting from in-vitro fertilization

EXCLUDES 2 gestational carrier status (Z33.3)

SP **O09.811 Supervision of pregnancy resulting from assisted reproductive technology, first trimester**

SP **O09.812 Supervision of pregnancy resulting from assisted reproductive technology, second trimester**

SP **O09.813 Supervision of pregnancy resulting from assisted reproductive technology, third trimester**

IQ **O09.819 Supervision of pregnancy resulting from assisted reproductive technology, unspecified trimester**

6 **O09.82 Supervision of pregnancy with history of in utero procedure during previous pregnancy**

SP **O09.821 Supervision of pregnancy with history of in utero procedure during previous pregnancy, first trimester**

SP **O09.822 Supervision of pregnancy with history of in utero procedure during previous pregnancy, second trimester**

SP **O09.823 Supervision of pregnancy with history of in utero procedure during previous pregnancy, third trimester**

IQ **O09.829 Supervision of pregnancy with history of in utero procedure during previous pregnancy, unspecified trimester**

EXCLUDES 1 supervision of pregnancy affected by in utero procedure during current pregnancy (O35.7)

6 **O09.89 Supervision of other high risk pregnancies**

SP **O09.891 Supervision of other high risk pregnancies, first trimester**

SP **O09.892 Supervision of other high risk pregnancies, second trimester**

SP **O09.893 Supervision of other high risk pregnancies, third trimester**

IQ **O09.899 Supervision of other high risk pregnancies, unspecified trimester**

5 **O09.9 Supervision of high risk pregnancy, unspecified**

IQ **O09.90 Supervision of high risk pregnancy, unspecified, unspecified trimester**

SP **O09.91 Supervision of high risk pregnancy, unspecified, first trimester**

SP **O09.92 Supervision of high risk pregnancy, unspecified, second trimester**

SP **O09.93 Supervision of high risk pregnancy, unspecified, third trimester**

Edema, proteinuria and hypertensive disorders in pregnancy, childbirth and the puerperium (O10-O16)

4 **O10 Pre-existing hypertension complicating pregnancy, childbirth and the puerperium**

INCLUDES pre-existing hypertension with pre-existing proteinuria complicating pregnancy, childbirth and the puerperium

EXCLUDES 2 pre-existing hypertension with superimposed pre-eclampsia complicating pregnancy, childbirth and the puerperium (O11.-)

GUIDELINES **Section I.C.15.d**

Category O10 includes codes for hypertensive heart and hypertensive chronic kidney disease. When assigning one of the O10 codes that includes hypertensive heart disease or hypertensive chronic kidney disease, it is necessary to add a secondary code from the appropriate hypertension category to specify the type of heart failure or chronic kidney disease.

5 **O10.0 Pre-existing essential hypertension complicating pregnancy, childbirth and the puerperium**

Any condition in I10 specified as a reason for obstetric care during pregnancy, childbirth or the puerperium

6 **O10.01 Pre-existing essential hypertension complicating pregnancy,**

SP **O10.011 Pre-existing essential hypertension complicating pregnancy, first trimester**

SP **O10.012 Pre-existing essential hypertension complicating pregnancy, second trimester**

Chapter 15

O00-O9A

SP **O10.013 Pre-existing essential hypertension complicating pregnancy, third trimester**

!Q **O10.019 Pre-existing essential hypertension complicating pregnancy, unspecified trimester**

SP **O10.02 Pre-existing essential hypertension complicating childbirth**

SP **O10.03 Pre-existing essential hypertension complicating the puerperium**

+ 5 **O10.1 Pre-existing hypertensive heart disease complicating pregnancy, childbirth and the puerperium**

Any condition in I11 specified as a reason for obstetric care during pregnancy, childbirth or the puerperium

Use additional code from I11 to identify the type of hypertensive heart disease

+ 6 **O10.11 Pre-existing hypertensive heart disease complicating pregnancy**

SP + **O10.111 Pre-existing hypertensive heart disease complicating pregnancy, first trimester**

SP + **O10.112 Pre-existing hypertensive heart disease complicating pregnancy, second trimester**

SP + **O10.113 Pre-existing hypertensive heart disease complicating pregnancy, third trimester**

!Q + **O10.119 Pre-existing hypertensive heart disease complicating pregnancy, unspecified trimester**

SP + **O10.12 Pre-existing hypertensive heart disease complicating childbirth**

SP + **O10.13 Pre-existing hypertensive heart disease complicating the puerperium**

+ 5 **O10.2 Pre-existing hypertensive chronic kidney disease complicating pregnancy, childbirth and the puerperium**

Any condition in I12 specified as a reason for obstetric care during pregnancy, childbirth or the puerperium

Use additional code from I12 to identify the type of hypertensive chronic kidney disease

+ 6 **O10.21 Pre-existing hypertensive chronic kidney disease complicating pregnancy**

SP + **O10.211 Pre-existing hypertensive chronic kidney disease complicating pregnancy, first trimester**

SP + **O10.212 Pre-existing hypertensive chronic kidney disease complicating pregnancy, second trimester**

SP + **O10.213 Pre-existing hypertensive chronic kidney disease complicating pregnancy, third trimester**

!Q + **O10.219 Pre-existing hypertensive chronic kidney disease complicating pregnancy, unspecified trimester**

SP + **O10.22 Pre-existing hypertensive chronic kidney disease complicating childbirth**

SP + **O10.23 Pre-existing hypertensive chronic kidney disease complicating the puerperium**

+ 5 **O10.3 Pre-existing hypertensive heart and chronic kidney disease complicating pregnancy, childbirth and the puerperium**

Any condition in I13 specified as a reason for obstetric care during pregnancy, childbirth or the puerperium

Use additional code from I13 to identify the type of hypertensive heart and chronic kidney disease

+ 6 **O10.31 Pre-existing hypertensive heart and chronic kidney disease complicating pregnancy**

SP + **O10.311 Pre-existing hypertensive heart and chronic kidney disease complicating pregnancy, first trimester**

SP + **O10.312 Pre-existing hypertensive heart and chronic kidney disease complicating pregnancy, second trimester**

SP + **O10.313 Pre-existing hypertensive heart and chronic kidney disease complicating pregnancy, third trimester**

!Q + **O10.319 Pre-existing hypertensive heart and chronic kidney disease complicating pregnancy, unspecified trimester**

SP + **O10.32 Pre-existing hypertensive heart and chronic kidney disease complicating childbirth**

SP + **O10.33 Pre-existing hypertensive heart and chronic kidney disease complicating the puerperium**

+ 5 **O10.4 Pre-existing secondary hypertension complicating pregnancy, childbirth and the puerperium**

Any condition in I15 specified as a reason for obstetric care during pregnancy, childbirth or the puerperium

Use additional code from I15 to identify the type of secondary hypertension

+ 6 **O10.41 Pre-existing secondary hypertension complicating pregnancy**

SP + **O10.411 Pre-existing secondary hypertension complicating pregnancy, first trimester**

SP + **O10.412 Pre-existing secondary hypertension complicating pregnancy, second trimester**

SP + **O10.413 Pre-existing secondary hypertension complicating pregnancy, third trimester**

!Q + **O10.419 Pre-existing secondary hypertension complicating pregnancy, unspecified trimester**

SP + **O10.42 Pre-existing secondary hypertension complicating childbirth**

SP + **O10.43 Pre-existing secondary hypertension complicating the puerperium**

5 **O10.9 Unspecified pre-existing hypertension complicating pregnancy, childbirth and the puerperium**

6 **O10.91 Unspecified pre-existing hypertension complicating pregnancy**

Chapter 15

O00-O9A

SP O10.911 **Unspecified pre-existing hypertension complicating pregnancy, first trimester**

SP O10.912 **Unspecified pre-existing hypertension complicating pregnancy, second trimester**

SP O10.913 **Unspecified pre-existing hypertension complicating pregnancy, third trimester**

IQ O10.919 **Unspecified pre-existing hypertension complicating pregnancy, unspecified trimester**

SP O10.92 **Unspecified pre-existing hypertension complicating childbirth**

SP O10.93 **Unspecified pre-existing hypertension complicating the puerperium**

+ 4 O11 **Pre-existing hypertension with pre-eclampsia**

INCLUDES conditions in O10 complicated by pre-eclampsia
pre-eclampsia superimposed pre-existing hypertension

Use additional code from O10 to identify the type of hypertension

SP + O11.1 **Pre-existing hypertension with pre-eclampsia, first trimester**

SP + O11.2 **Pre-existing hypertension with pre-eclampsia, second trimester**

SP + O11.3 **Pre-existing hypertension with pre-eclampsia, third trimester**

SP + O11.4 **Pre-existing hypertension with pre-eclampsia, complicating childbirth**

SP + O11.5 **Pre-existing hypertension with pre-eclampsia, complicating the puerperium**

IQ + O11.9 **Pre-existing hypertension with pre-eclampsia, unspecified trimester**

4 O12 **Gestational [pregnancy-induced] edema and proteinuria without hypertension**

5 O12.0 **Gestational edema**

IQ O12.00 **Gestational edema, unspecified trimester**

SP O12.01 **Gestational edema, first trimester**

SP O12.02 **Gestational edema, second trimester**

SP O12.03 **Gestational edema, third trimester**

SP O12.04 **Gestational edema, complicating childbirth**

SP O12.05 **Gestational edema, complicating the puerperium**

5 O12.1 **Gestational proteinuria**

IQ O12.10 **Gestational proteinuria, unspecified trimester**

SP O12.11 **Gestational proteinuria, first trimester**

SP O12.12 **Gestational proteinuria, second trimester**

SP O12.13 **Gestational proteinuria, third trimester**

SP O12.14 **Gestational proteinuria, complicating childbirth**

SP O12.15 **Gestational proteinuria, complicating the puerperium**

5 O12.2 **Gestational edema with proteinuria**

IQ O12.20 **Gestational edema with proteinuria, unspecified trimester**

SP O12.21 **Gestational edema with proteinuria, first trimester**

SP O12.22 **Gestational edema with proteinuria, second trimester**

SP O12.23 **Gestational edema with proteinuria, third trimester**

SP O12.24 **Gestational edema with proteinuria, complicating childbirth**

SP O12.25 **Gestational edema with proteinuria, complicating the puerperium**

4 O13 **Gestational [pregnancy-induced] hypertension without significant proteinuria**

INCLUDES gestational hypertension NOS
transient hypertension of pregnancy

GUIDELINES **Section I.9.a.7)**

Unless patient has an established diagnosis of hypertension, assign code O13.-, Gestational [pregnancy-induced] hypertension without significant proteinuria, or O14.-, Pre-eclampsia, for transient hypertension of pregnancy.

SP O13.1 **Gestational [pregnancy-induced] hypertension without significant proteinuria, first trimester**

SP O13.2 **Gestational [pregnancy-induced] hypertension without significant proteinuria, second trimester**

SP O13.3 **Gestational [pregnancy-induced] hypertension without significant proteinuria, third trimester**

SP O13.4 **Gestational [pregnancy-induced] hypertension without significant proteinuria, complicating childbirth**

SP O13.5 **Gestational [pregnancy-induced] hypertension without significant proteinuria, complicating the puerperium**

IQ O13.9 **Gestational [pregnancy-induced] hypertension without significant proteinuria, unspecified trimester**

4 O14 **Pre-eclampsia**

EXCLUDES 1 pre-existing hypertension with pre-eclampsia (O11)

GUIDELINES **Section I.9.a.7)**

Unless patient has an established diagnosis of hypertension, assign code O13.-, Gestational [pregnancy-induced] hypertension without significant proteinuria, or O14.-, Pre-eclampsia, for transient hypertension of pregnancy.

5 O14.0 **Mild to moderate pre-eclampsia**

DEFINITION Hypertension (BP >140/90 mmHg) after the 20th week of gestation and up to 6 weeks postpartum, with proteinuria.

IQ O14.00 **Mild to moderate pre-eclampsia, unspecified trimester**

SP O14.02 **Mild to moderate pre-eclampsia, second trimester**

SP O14.03 **Mild to moderate pre-eclampsia, third trimester**

SP O14.04 **Mild to moderate pre-eclampsia, complicating childbirth**

SP O14.05 **Mild to moderate pre-eclampsia, complicating the puerperium**

5 O14.1 **Severe pre-eclampsia**

Chapter 15 O00-O9A

EXCLUDES 1 HELLP syndrome (O14.2-)

DEFINITION Severe hypertension (BP >160/110 mmHg) after the 20th week of gestation and up to 6 weeks postpartum, with proteinuria, and additional symptoms such as pulmonary edema, upper abdominal pain, severe headaches, and blurred vision.

SP **O14.10 Severe pre-eclampsia, unspecified trimester**

SP **O14.12 Severe pre-eclampsia, second trimester**

SP **O14.13 Severe pre-eclampsia, third trimester**

SP **O14.14 Severe pre-eclampsia complicating childbirth**

SP **O14.15 Severe pre-eclampsia, complicating the puerperium**

5 **O14.2 HELLP syndrome**

Severe pre-eclampsia with hemolysis, elevated liver enzymes and low platelet count (HELLP)

DEFINITION Severe pre-eclampsia with hemolysis, elevated liver enzymes and low platelet count (HELLP).

!Q **O14.20 HELLP syndrome (HELLP), unspecified trimester**

SP **O14.22 HELLP syndrome (HELLP), second trimester**

SP **O14.23 HELLP syndrome (HELLP), third trimester**

SP **O14.24 HELLP syndrome, complicating childbirth**

SP **O14.25 HELLP syndrome, complicating the puerperium**

5 **O14.9 Unspecified pre-eclampsia**

!Q **O14.90 Unspecified pre-eclampsia, unspecified trimester**

SP **O14.92 Unspecified pre-eclampsia, second trimester**

SP **O14.93 Unspecified pre-eclampsia, third trimester**

SP **O14.94 Unspecified pre-eclampsia, complicating childbirth**

SP **O14.95 Unspecified pre-eclampsia, complicating the puerperium**

4 **O15 Eclampsia**

INCLUDES convulsions following conditions in O10-O14 and O16

5 **O15.0 Eclampsia complicating pregnancy**

SP **O15.00 Eclampsia complicating pregnancy, unspecified trimester**

SP **O15.02 Eclampsia complicating pregnancy, second trimester**

SP **O15.03 Eclampsia complicating pregnancy, third trimester**

SP **O15.1 Eclampsia complicating labor**

SP **O15.2 Eclampsia complicating the puerperium**

!Q **O15.9 Eclampsia, unspecified as to time period**

Eclampsia NOS

4 **O16 Unspecified maternal hypertension**

SP **O16.1 Unspecified maternal hypertension, first trimester**

SP **O16.2 Unspecified maternal hypertension, second trimester**

SP **O16.3 Unspecified maternal hypertension, third trimester**

SP **O16.4 Unspecified maternal hypertension, complicating childbirth**

SP **O16.5 Unspecified maternal hypertension, complicating the puerperium**

!Q **O16.9 Unspecified maternal hypertension, unspecified trimester**

Other maternal disorders predominantly related to pregnancy (O20-O29)

EXCLUDES 2 maternal care related to the fetus and amniotic cavity and possible delivery problems (O30-O48)
maternal diseases classifiable elsewhere but complicating pregnancy, labor and delivery, and the puerperium (O98-O99)

4 **O20 Hemorrhage in early pregnancy**

INCLUDES hemorrhage before completion of 20 weeks gestation

EXCLUDES 1 pregnancy with abortive outcome (O00-O08)

SP **O20.0 Threatened abortion**

Hemorrhage specified as due to threatened abortion

SP **O20.8 Other hemorrhage in early pregnancy**

SP **O20.9 Hemorrhage in early pregnancy, unspecified**

4 **O21 Excessive vomiting in pregnancy**

SP **O21.0 Mild hyperemesis gravidarum**

Hyperemesis gravidarum, mild or unspecified, starting before the end of the 20th week of gestation

SP **O21.1 Hyperemesis gravidarum with metabolic disturbance**

Hyperemesis gravidarum, starting before the end of the 20th week of gestation, with metabolic disturbance such as carbohydrate depletion

Hyperemesis gravidarum, starting before the end of the 20th week of gestation, with metabolic disturbance such as dehydration

Hyperemesis gravidarum, starting before the end of the 20th week of gestation, with metabolic disturbance such as electrolyte imbalance

SP **O21.2 Late vomiting of pregnancy**

Excessive vomiting starting after 20 completed weeks of gestation

SP + **O21.8 Other vomiting complicating pregnancy**

Vomiting due to diseases classified elsewhere, complicating pregnancy

Use additional code, to identify cause.

SP **O21.9 Vomiting of pregnancy, unspecified**

4 **O22 Venous complications and hemorrhoids in pregnancy**

EXCLUDES 1 venous complications of:
abortion NOS (O03.9)
ectopic or molar pregnancy (O08.7)
failed attempted abortion (O07.35)
induced abortion (O04.85)

Chapter 15 O00-O9A

spontaneous abortion (O03.89)

EXCLUDES 2 obstetric pulmonary embolism (O88.-)
venous complications and hemorrhoids of childbirth and the puerperium (O87.-)

5 **O22.0 Varicose veins of lower extremity in pregnancy**
Varicose veins NOS in pregnancy

IQ **O22.00 Varicose veins of lower extremity in pregnancy, unspecified trimester**

SP **O22.01 Varicose veins of lower extremity in pregnancy, first trimester**

SP **O22.02 Varicose veins of lower extremity in pregnancy, second trimester**

SP **O22.03 Varicose veins of lower extremity in pregnancy, third trimester**

5 **O22.1 Genital varices in pregnancy**
Perineal varices in pregnancy
Vaginal varices in pregnancy
Vulval varices in pregnancy

IQ **O22.10 Genital varices in pregnancy, unspecified trimester**

SP **O22.11 Genital varices in pregnancy, first trimester**

SP **O22.12 Genital varices in pregnancy, second trimester**

SP **O22.13 Genital varices in pregnancy, third trimester**

+ 5 **O22.2 Superficial thrombophlebitis in pregnancy**
Phlebitis in pregnancy NOS
Thrombophlebitis of legs in pregnancy
Thrombosis in pregnancy NOS
Use additional code to identify the superficial thrombophlebitis (I80.0-)

IQ + **O22.20 Superficial thrombophlebitis in pregnancy, unspecified trimester**

SP + **O22.21 Superficial thrombophlebitis in pregnancy, first trimester**

SP + **O22.22 Superficial thrombophlebitis in pregnancy, second trimester**

SP + **O22.23 Superficial thrombophlebitis in pregnancy, third trimester**

+ 5 **O22.3 Deep phlebothrombosis in pregnancy**
Deep vein thrombosis, antepartum
Use additional code to identify the deep vein thrombosis (I82.4-, I82.5-, I82.62-, I82.72-)
Use additional code, if applicable, for associated long-term (current) use of anticoagulants (Z79.01)

IQ + **O22.30 Deep phlebothrombosis in pregnancy, unspecified trimester**

SP + **O22.31 Deep phlebothrombosis in pregnancy, first trimester**

SP + **O22.32 Deep phlebothrombosis in pregnancy, second trimester**

SP + **O22.33 Deep phlebothrombosis in pregnancy, third trimester**

5 **O22.4 Hemorrhoids in pregnancy**

IQ **O22.40 Hemorrhoids in pregnancy, unspecified trimester**

SP **O22.41 Hemorrhoids in pregnancy, first trimester**

SP **O22.42 Hemorrhoids in pregnancy, second trimester**

SP **O22.43 Hemorrhoids in pregnancy, third trimester**

5 **O22.5 Cerebral venous thrombosis in pregnancy**
Cerebrovenous sinus thrombosis in pregnancy

IQ **O22.50 Cerebral venous thrombosis in pregnancy, unspecified trimester**

SP **O22.51 Cerebral venous thrombosis in pregnancy, first trimester**

SP **O22.52 Cerebral venous thrombosis in pregnancy, second trimester**

SP **O22.53 Cerebral venous thrombosis in pregnancy, third trimester**

5 **O22.8 Other venous complications in pregnancy**

6 **O22.8X Other venous complications in pregnancy**

SP **O22.8X1 Other venous complications in pregnancy, first trimester**

SP **O22.8X2 Other venous complications in pregnancy, second trimester**

SP **O22.8X3 Other venous complications in pregnancy, third trimester**

IQ **O22.8X9 Other venous complications in pregnancy, unspecified trimester**

5 **O22.9 Venous complication in pregnancy, unspecified**
Gestational phlebitis NOS
Gestational phlebopathy NOS
Gestational thrombosis NOS

IQ **O22.90 Venous complication in pregnancy, unspecified, unspecified trimester**

SP **O22.91 Venous complication in pregnancy, unspecified, first trimester**

SP **O22.92 Venous complication in pregnancy, unspecified, second trimester**

SP **O22.93 Venous complication in pregnancy, unspecified, third trimester**

+ 4 **O23 Infections of genitourinary tract in pregnancy**
Use additional code to identify organism (B95.-, B96.-)

EXCLUDES 2 gonococcal infections complicating pregnancy, childbirth and the puerperium (O98.2)
infections with a predominantly sexual mode of transmission NOS complicating pregnancy, childbirth and the puerperium (O98.3)
syphilis complicating pregnancy, childbirth and the puerperium (O98.1)
tuberculosis of genitourinary system complicating pregnancy, childbirth and the puerperium (O98.0)
venereal disease NOS complicating pregnancy, childbirth and the puerperium (O98.3)

+ 5 **O23.0 Infections of kidney in pregnancy**
Pyelonephritis in pregnancy

IQ + **O23.00 Infections of kidney in pregnancy, unspecified trimester**

SP + O23.01 **Infections of kidney in pregnancy, first trimester**

SP + O23.02 **Infections of kidney in pregnancy, second trimester**

SP + O23.03 **Infections of kidney in pregnancy, third trimester**

+ 5 O23.1 **Infections of bladder in pregnancy**

!Q + O23.10 **Infections of bladder in pregnancy, unspecified trimester**

SP + O23.11 **Infections of bladder in pregnancy, first trimester**

SP + O23.12 **Infections of bladder in pregnancy, second trimester**

SP + O23.13 **Infections of bladder in pregnancy, third trimester**

+ 5 O23.2 **Infections of urethra in pregnancy**

!Q + O23.20 **Infections of urethra in pregnancy, unspecified trimester**

SP + O23.21 **Infections of urethra in pregnancy, first trimester**

SP + O23.22 **Infections of urethra in pregnancy, second trimester**

SP + O23.23 **Infections of urethra in pregnancy, third trimester**

+ 5 O23.3 **Infections of other parts of urinary tract in pregnancy**

!Q + O23.30 **Infections of other parts of urinary tract in pregnancy, unspecified trimester**

SP + O23.31 **Infections of other parts of urinary tract in pregnancy, first trimester**

SP + O23.32 **Infections of other parts of urinary tract in pregnancy, second trimester**

SP + O23.33 **Infections of other parts of urinary tract in pregnancy, third trimester**

+ 5 O23.4 **Unspecified infection of urinary tract in pregnancy**

!Q + O23.40 **Unspecified infection of urinary tract in pregnancy, unspecified trimester**

SP + O23.41 **Unspecified infection of urinary tract in pregnancy, first trimester**

SP + O23.42 **Unspecified infection of urinary tract in pregnancy, second trimester**

SP + O23.43 **Unspecified infection of urinary tract in pregnancy, third trimester**

+ 5 O23.5 **Infections of the genital tract in pregnancy**

+ 6 O23.51 **Infection of cervix in pregnancy**

SP + O23.511 **Infections of cervix in pregnancy, first trimester**

SP + O23.512 **Infections of cervix in pregnancy, second trimester**

SP + O23.513 **Infections of cervix in pregnancy, third trimester**

!Q + O23.519 **Infections of cervix in pregnancy, unspecified trimester**

+ 6 O23.52 **Salpingo-oophoritis in pregnancy**
Oophoritis in pregnancy
Salpingitis in pregnancy

SP + O23.521 **Salpingo-oophoritis in pregnancy, first trimester**

SP + O23.522 **Salpingo-oophoritis in pregnancy, second trimester**

SP + O23.523 **Salpingo-oophoritis in pregnancy, third trimester**

!Q + O23.529 **Salpingo-oophoritis in pregnancy, unspecified trimester**

+ 6 O23.59 **Infection of other part of genital tract in pregnancy**

SP + O23.591 **Infection of other part of genital tract in pregnancy, first trimester**

SP + O23.592 **Infection of other part of genital tract in pregnancy, second trimester**

SP + O23.593 **Infection of other part of genital tract in pregnancy, third trimester**

!Q + O23.599 **Infection of other part of genital tract in pregnancy, unspecified trimester**

+ 5 O23.9 **Unspecified genitourinary tract infection in pregnancy**
Genitourinary tract infection in pregnancy NOS

!Q + O23.90 **Unspecified genitourinary tract infection in pregnancy, unspecified trimester**

SP + O23.91 **Unspecified genitourinary tract infection in pregnancy, first trimester**

SP + O23.92 **Unspecified genitourinary tract infection in pregnancy, second trimester**

SP + O23.93 **Unspecified genitourinary tract infection in pregnancy, third trimester**

4 O24 **Diabetes mellitus in pregnancy, childbirth, and the puerperium**

GUIDELINES **Section I.C.15.g-h**

Diabetes mellitus is a significant complicating factor in pregnancy. Pregnant women who are diabetic should be assigned a code from category O24, Diabetes mellitus in pregnancy, childbirth, and the puerperium, first, followed by the appropriate diabetes code(s) (E08-E13) from Chapter 4.

An additional code should be assigned from category Z79 to identify the long-term (current) use of insulin or oral hypoglycemic drugs. If the patient is treated with both oral medications and insulin, only the code for long-term (current) use of insulin should be assigned ...

Code Z79.4 should not be assigned if insulin is given temporarily to bring a type 2 patient's blood sugar under control during an encounter.

+ 5 O24.0 **Pre-existing type 1 diabetes mellitus, in pregnancy, childbirth and the puerperium**
Juvenile onset diabetes mellitus, in pregnancy, childbirth and the puerperium
Ketosis-prone diabetes mellitus in pregnancy, childbirth and the puerperium
Use additional code from category E10 to further identify any manifestations

+ 6 O24.01 **Pre-existing type 1 diabetes mellitus, in pregnancy**

SP + O24.011 **Pre-existing type 1 diabetes mellitus, in pregnancy, first trimester**

SP + O24.012 **Pre-existing type 1 diabetes mellitus, in pregnancy, second trimester**

Chapter 15
O00-O9A

4 4th digit required 5 5th digit required 6 6th digit required 7 7th digit required 7th digit placeholder + Additional code Laterality

SP + **O24.013 Pre-existing type 1 diabetes mellitus, in pregnancy, third trimester**

IQ + **O24.019 Pre-existing type 1 diabetes mellitus, in pregnancy, unspecified trimester**

SP + **O24.02 Pre-existing type 1 diabetes mellitus, in childbirth**

SP + **O24.03 Pre-existing type 1 diabetes mellitus, in the puerperium**

+ 5 **O24.1 Pre-existing type 2 diabetes mellitus, in pregnancy, childbirth and the puerperium**

Insulin-resistant diabetes mellitus in pregnancy, childbirth and the puerperium

Use additional code (for):

from category E11 to further identify any manifestations

long-term (current) use of insulin (Z79.4)

+ 6 **O24.11 Pre-existing type 2 diabetes mellitus, in pregnancy**

SP + **O24.111 Pre-existing type 2 diabetes mellitus, in pregnancy, first trimester**

SP + **O24.112 Pre-existing type 2 diabetes mellitus, in pregnancy, second trimester**

SP + **O24.113 Pre-existing type 2 diabetes mellitus, in pregnancy, third trimester**

IQ + **O24.119 Pre-existing type 2 diabetes mellitus, in pregnancy, unspecified trimester**

SP + **O24.12 Pre-existing type 2 diabetes mellitus, in childbirth**

SP + **O24.13 Pre-existing type 2 diabetes mellitus, in the puerperium**

+ 5 **O24.3 Unspecified pre-existing diabetes mellitus in pregnancy, childbirth and the puerperium**

Use additional code (for):

from category E11 to further identify any manifestation

long-term (current) use of insulin (Z79.4)

+ 6 **O24.31 Unspecified pre-existing diabetes mellitus in pregnancy**

SP + **O24.311 Unspecified pre-existing diabetes mellitus in pregnancy, first trimester**

SP + **O24.312 Unspecified pre-existing diabetes mellitus in pregnancy, second trimester**

SP + **O24.313 Unspecified pre-existing diabetes mellitus in pregnancy, third trimester**

IQ + **O24.319 Unspecified pre-existing diabetes mellitus in pregnancy, unspecified trimester**

SP + **O24.32 Unspecified pre-existing diabetes mellitus in childbirth**

SP + **O24.33 Unspecified pre-existing diabetes mellitus in the puerperium**

5 **O24.4 Gestational diabetes mellitus**

Diabetes mellitus arising in pregnancy

Gestational diabetes mellitus NOS

GUIDELINES **Section I.C.15.i**

Gestational (pregnancy induced) diabetes can occur during the second and third trimester of pregnancy in women who were not diabetic prior to pregnancy. Gestational diabetes can cause complications in the pregnancy similar to those of pre-existing diabetes mellitus. It also puts the woman at greater risk of developing diabetes after the pregnancy. Codes for gestational diabetes are in subcategory O24.4, Gestational diabetes mellitus. No other code from category O24, Diabetes mellitus in pregnancy, childbirth, and the puerperium, should be used with a code from O24.4. The codes under subcategory O24.4 include diet controlled, insulin controlled, and controlled by oral hypoglycemic drugs. If a patient with gestational diabetes is treated with both diet and insulin, only the code for insulin-controlled is required. If a patient with gestational diabetes is treated with both diet and oral hypoglycemic medications, only the code for "controlled by oral hypoglycemic drugs" is required. An abnormal glucose tolerance in pregnancy is assigned a code from subcategory O99.81, Abnormal glucose complicating pregnancy, childbirth, and the puerperium.

CODING TIPS✓ Do not use O24.4 if diabetes persists after the puerperium. Use E08 -E13 code.

6 **O24.41 Gestational diabetes mellitus in pregnancy**

SP **O24.410 Gestational diabetes mellitus in pregnancy, diet controlled**

SP **O24.414 Gestational diabetes mellitus in pregnancy, insulin controlled**

SP **O24.415 Gestational diabetes mellitus in pregnancy, controlled by oral hypoglycemic drugs**

Gestational diabetes mellitus in pregnancy, controlled by oral antidiabetic drugs

SP **O24.419 Gestational diabetes mellitus in pregnancy, unspecified control**

6 **O24.42 Gestational diabetes mellitus in childbirth**

SP **O24.420 Gestational diabetes mellitus in childbirth, diet controlled**

SP **O24.424 Gestational diabetes mellitus in childbirth, insulin controlled**

SP **O24.425 Gestational diabetes mellitus in childbirth, controlled by oral hypoglycemic drugs**

Gestational diabetes mellitus in childbirth, controlled by oral antidiabetic drugs

SP **O24.429 Gestational diabetes mellitus in childbirth, unspecified control**

6 **O24.43 Gestational diabetes mellitus in the puerperium**

SP **O24.430 Gestational diabetes mellitus in the puerperium, diet controlled**

SP **O24.434 Gestational diabetes mellitus in the puerperium, insulin controlled**

SP O24.435 **Gestational diabetes mellitus in puerperium, controlled by oral hypoglycemic drugs**
Gestational diabetes mellitus in puerperium, controlled by oral antidiabetic drugs

SP O24.439 **Gestational diabetes mellitus in the puerperium, unspecified control**

+ 5 O24.8 **Other pre-existing diabetes mellitus in pregnancy, childbirth, and the puerperium**
Use additional code (for):
from categories E08, E09 and E13 to further identify any manifestation
long-term (current) use of insulin (Z79.4)

CODING TIPS ✓ Use this code for the obstetric patient who had pre-existing diabetes before pregnancy. Use an additional code for the type of diabetes, E08-E13.

+ 6 O24.81 **Other pre-existing diabetes mellitus in pregnancy**

SP + O24.811 **Other pre-existing diabetes mellitus in pregnancy, first trimester**

SP + O24.812 **Other pre-existing diabetes mellitus in pregnancy, second trimester**

SP + O24.813 **Other pre-existing diabetes mellitus in pregnancy, third trimester**

IQ + O24.819 **Other pre-existing diabetes mellitus in pregnancy, unspecified trimester**

SP + O24.82 **Other pre-existing diabetes mellitus in childbirth**

SP + O24.83 **Other pre-existing diabetes mellitus in the puerperium**

+ 5 O24.9 **Unspecified diabetes mellitus in pregnancy, childbirth and the puerperium**
Use additional code for long-term (current) use of insulin (Z79.4)

+ 6 O24.91 **Unspecified diabetes mellitus in pregnancy**

SP + O24.911 **Unspecified diabetes mellitus in pregnancy, first trimester**

SP + O24.912 **Unspecified diabetes mellitus in pregnancy, second trimester**

SP + O24.913 **Unspecified diabetes mellitus in pregnancy, third trimester**

IQ + O24.919 **Unspecified diabetes mellitus in pregnancy, unspecified trimester**

SP + O24.92 **Unspecified diabetes mellitus in childbirth**

SP + O24.93 **Unspecified diabetes mellitus in the puerperium**

4 O25 **Malnutrition in pregnancy, childbirth and the puerperium**

5 O25.1 **Malnutrition in pregnancy**

IQ O25.10 **Malnutrition in pregnancy, unspecified trimester**

SP O25.11 **Malnutrition in pregnancy, first trimester**

SP O25.12 **Malnutrition in pregnancy, second trimester**

SP O25.13 **Malnutrition in pregnancy, third trimester**

SP O25.2 **Malnutrition in childbirth**

SP O25.3 **Malnutrition in the puerperium**

4 O26 **Maternal care for other conditions predominantly related to pregnancy**

5 O26.0 **Excessive weight gain in pregnancy**
EXCLUDES 2 gestational edema (O12.0, O12.2)

IQ O26.00 **Excessive weight gain in pregnancy, unspecified trimester**

SP O26.01 **Excessive weight gain in pregnancy, first trimester**

SP O26.02 **Excessive weight gain in pregnancy, second trimester**

SP O26.03 **Excessive weight gain in pregnancy, third trimester**

5 O26.1 **Low weight gain in pregnancy**

IQ O26.10 **Low weight gain in pregnancy, unspecified trimester**

SP O26.11 **Low weight gain in pregnancy, first trimester**

SP O26.12 **Low weight gain in pregnancy, second trimester**

SP O26.13 **Low weight gain in pregnancy, third trimester**

5 O26.2 **Pregnancy care for patient with recurrent pregnancy loss**

IQ O26.20 **Pregnancy care for patient with recurrent pregnancy loss, unspecified trimester**

SP O26.21 **Pregnancy care for patient with recurrent pregnancy loss, first trimester**

SP O26.22 **Pregnancy care for patient with recurrent pregnancy loss, second trimester**

SP O26.23 **Pregnancy care for patient with recurrent pregnancy loss, third trimester**

5 O26.3 **Retained intrauterine contraceptive device in pregnancy**

IQ O26.30 **Retained intrauterine contraceptive device in pregnancy, unspecified trimester**

SP O26.31 **Retained intrauterine contraceptive device in pregnancy, first trimester**

SP O26.32 **Retained intrauterine contraceptive device in pregnancy, second trimester**

SP O26.33 **Retained intrauterine contraceptive device in pregnancy, third trimester**

5 O26.4 **Herpes gestationis**

IQ O26.40 **Herpes gestationis, unspecified trimester**

SP O26.41 **Herpes gestationis, first trimester**

SP O26.42 **Herpes gestationis, second trimester**

SP O26.43 **Herpes gestationis, third trimester**

5 O26.5 **Maternal hypotension syndrome**
Supine hypotensive syndrome

IQ O26.50 **Maternal hypotension syndrome, unspecified trimester**

SP O26.51 **Maternal hypotension syndrome, first trimester**

SP **O26.52 Maternal hypotension syndrome, second trimester**

SP **O26.53 Maternal hypotension syndrome, third trimester**

+ 5 **O26.6 Liver and biliary tract disorders in pregnancy, childbirth and the puerperium**

Use additional code to identify the specific disorder

EXCLUDES 2 hepatorenal syndrome following labor and delivery (O90.4)

+ 6 **O26.61 Liver and biliary tract disorders in pregnancy**

SP + **O26.611 Liver and biliary tract disorders in pregnancy, first trimester**

!Q + **O26.612 Liver and biliary tract disorders in pregnancy, second trimester**

SP + **O26.613 Liver and biliary tract disorders in pregnancy, third trimester**

!Q + **O26.619 Liver and biliary tract disorders in pregnancy, unspecified trimester**

SP + **O26.62 Liver and biliary tract disorders in childbirth**

SP + **O26.63 Liver and biliary tract disorders in the puerperium**

5 **O26.7 Subluxation of symphysis (pubis) in pregnancy, childbirth and the puerperium**

EXCLUDES 1 traumatic separation of symphysis (pubis) during childbirth (O71.6)

6 **O26.71 Subluxation of symphysis (pubis) in pregnancy**

SP **O26.711 Subluxation of symphysis (pubis) in pregnancy, first trimester**

SP **O26.712 Subluxation of symphysis (pubis) in pregnancy, second trimester**

SP **O26.713 Subluxation of symphysis (pubis) in pregnancy, third trimester**

!Q **O26.719 Subluxation of symphysis (pubis) in pregnancy, unspecified trimester**

SP **O26.72 Subluxation of symphysis (pubis) in childbirth**

SP **O26.73 Subluxation of symphysis (pubis) in the puerperium**

5 **O26.8 Other specified pregnancy related conditions**

6 **O26.81 Pregnancy related exhaustion and fatigue**

SP **O26.811 Pregnancy related exhaustion and fatigue, first trimester**

SP **O26.812 Pregnancy related exhaustion and fatigue, second trimester**

SP **O26.813 Pregnancy related exhaustion and fatigue, third trimester**

!Q **O26.819 Pregnancy related exhaustion and fatigue, unspecified trimester**

6 **O26.82 Pregnancy related peripheral neuritis**

SP **O26.821 Pregnancy related peripheral neuritis, first trimester**

SP **O26.822 Pregnancy related peripheral neuritis, second trimester**

SP **O26.823 Pregnancy related peripheral neuritis, third trimester**

!Q **O26.829 Pregnancy related peripheral neuritis, unspecified trimester**

+ 6 **O26.83 Pregnancy related renal disease**

Use additional code to identify the specific disorder

SP + **O26.831 Pregnancy related renal disease, first trimester**

SP + **O26.832 Pregnancy related renal disease, second trimester**

SP + **O26.833 Pregnancy related renal disease, third trimester**

!Q + **O26.839 Pregnancy related renal disease, unspecified trimester**

6 **O26.84 Uterine size-date discrepancy complicating pregnancy**

EXCLUDES 1 encounter for suspected problem with fetal growth ruled out (Z03.74)

SP **O26.841 Uterine size-date discrepancy, first trimester**

SP **O26.842 Uterine size-date discrepancy, second trimester**

SP **O26.843 Uterine size-date discrepancy, third trimester**

!Q **O26.849 Uterine size-date discrepancy, unspecified trimester**

6 **O26.85 Spotting complicating pregnancy**

SP **O26.851 Spotting complicating pregnancy, first trimester**

SP **O26.852 Spotting complicating pregnancy, second trimester**

SP **O26.853 Spotting complicating pregnancy, third trimester**

!Q **O26.859 Spotting complicating pregnancy, unspecified trimester**

SP **O26.86 Pruritic urticarial papules and plaques of pregnancy (PUPPP)**

Polymorphic eruption of pregnancy

6 **O26.87 Cervical shortening**

EXCLUDES 1 encounter for suspected cervical shortening ruled out (Z03.75)

SP **O26.872 Cervical shortening, second trimester**

DEFINITION Sonographic evidence of a cervix shortened to 2.5 cm or less in the second trimester; a warning of impending premature birth in women with a prior history of early delivery.

SP **O26.873 Cervical shortening, third trimester**

!Q **O26.879 Cervical shortening, unspecified trimester**

6 **O26.89 Other specified pregnancy related conditions**

SP **O26.891 Other specified pregnancy related conditions, first trimester**

SP **O26.892 Other specified pregnancy related conditions, second trimester**

SP **O26.893 Other specified pregnancy related conditions, third trimester**

!Q **O26.899 Other specified pregnancy related conditions, unspecified trimester**

Chapter 15

O00-O9A

5 **O26.9 Pregnancy related conditions, unspecified**

IQ **O26.90 Pregnancy related conditions, unspecified, unspecified trimester**

IQ **O26.91 Pregnancy related conditions, unspecified, first trimester**

IQ **O26.92 Pregnancy related conditions, unspecified, second trimester**

IQ **O26.93 Pregnancy related conditions, unspecified, third trimester**

4 **O28 Abnormal findings on antenatal screening of mother**

EXCLUDES 1 diagnostic findings classified elsewhere - see Alphabetical Index

IQ **O28.0 Abnormal hematological finding on antenatal screening of mother**

IQ **O28.1 Abnormal biochemical finding on antenatal screening of mother**

IQ **O28.2 Abnormal cytological finding on antenatal screening of mother**

IQ **O28.3 Abnormal ultrasonic finding on antenatal screening of mother**

IQ **O28.4 Abnormal radiological finding on antenatal screening of mother**

IQ **O28.5 Abnormal chromosomal and genetic finding on antenatal screening of mother**

IQ **O28.8 Other abnormal findings on antenatal screening of mother**

IQ **O28.9 Unspecified abnormal findings on antenatal screening of mother**

+ 4 **O29 Complications of anesthesia during pregnancy**

INCLUDES maternal complications arising from the administration of a general, regional or local anesthetic, analgesic or other sedation during pregnancy

Use additional code, if necessary, to identify the complication

EXCLUDES 2 complications of anesthesia during labor and delivery (O74.-)
complications of anesthesia during the puerperium (O89.-)

+ 5 **O29.0 Pulmonary complications of anesthesia during pregnancy**

+ 6 **O29.01 Aspiration pneumonitis due to anesthesia during pregnancy**

Inhalation of stomach contents or secretions NOS due to anesthesia during pregnancy

Mendelson's syndrome due to anesthesia during pregnancy

SP + **O29.011 Aspiration pneumonitis due to anesthesia during pregnancy, first trimester**

SP + **O29.012 Aspiration pneumonitis due to anesthesia during pregnancy, second trimester**

SP + **O29.013 Aspiration pneumonitis due to anesthesia during pregnancy, third trimester**

IQ + **O29.019 Aspiration pneumonitis due to anesthesia during pregnancy, unspecified trimester**

+ 6 **O29.02 Pressure collapse of lung due to anesthesia during pregnancy**

SP + **O29.021 Pressure collapse of lung due to anesthesia during pregnancy, first trimester**

SP + **O29.022 Pressure collapse of lung due to anesthesia during pregnancy, second trimester**

SP + **O29.023 Pressure collapse of lung due to anesthesia during pregnancy, third trimester**

IQ + **O29.029 Pressure collapse of lung due to anesthesia during pregnancy, unspecified trimester**

+ 6 **O29.09 Other pulmonary complications of anesthesia during pregnancy**

SP + **O29.091 Other pulmonary complications of anesthesia during pregnancy, first trimester**

SP + **O29.092 Other pulmonary complications of anesthesia during pregnancy, second trimester**

SP + **O29.093 Other pulmonary complications of anesthesia during pregnancy, third trimester**

IQ + **O29.099 Other pulmonary complications of anesthesia during pregnancy, unspecified trimester**

+ 5 **O29.1 Cardiac complications of anesthesia during pregnancy**

+ 6 **O29.11 Cardiac arrest due to anesthesia during pregnancy**

SP + **O29.111 Cardiac arrest due to anesthesia during pregnancy, first trimester**

SP + **O29.112 Cardiac arrest due to anesthesia during pregnancy, second trimester**

SP + **O29.113 Cardiac arrest due to anesthesia during pregnancy, third trimester**

IQ + **O29.119 Cardiac arrest due to anesthesia during pregnancy, unspecified trimester**

+ 6 **O29.12 Cardiac failure due to anesthesia during pregnancy**

SP + **O29.121 Cardiac failure due to anesthesia during pregnancy, first trimester**

SP + **O29.122 Cardiac failure due to anesthesia during pregnancy, second trimester**

SP + **O29.123 Cardiac failure due to anesthesia during pregnancy, third trimester**

IQ + **O29.129 Cardiac failure due to anesthesia during pregnancy, unspecified trimester**

+ 6 **O29.19 Other cardiac complications of anesthesia during pregnancy**

SP + **O29.191 Other cardiac complications of anesthesia during pregnancy, first trimester**

SP + **O29.192 Other cardiac complications of anesthesia during pregnancy, second trimester**

SP + **O29.193 Other cardiac complications of anesthesia during pregnancy, third trimester**

IQ + **O29.199 Other cardiac complications of anesthesia during pregnancy, unspecified trimester**

+ 5 O29.2 Central nervous system complications of anesthesia during pregnancy

+ 6 O29.21 Cerebral anoxia due to anesthesia during pregnancy

SP + O29.211 Cerebral anoxia due to anesthesia during pregnancy, first trimester

SP + O29.212 Cerebral anoxia due to anesthesia during pregnancy, second trimester

SP + O29.213 Cerebral anoxia due to anesthesia during pregnancy, third trimester

!Q + O29.219 Cerebral anoxia due to anesthesia during pregnancy, unspecified trimester

+ 6 O29.29 Other central nervous system complications of anesthesia during pregnancy

SP + O29.291 Other central nervous system complications of anesthesia during pregnancy, first trimester

SP + O29.292 Other central nervous system complications of anesthesia during pregnancy, second trimester

SP + O29.293 Other central nervous system complications of anesthesia during pregnancy, third trimester

!Q + O29.299 Other central nervous system complications of anesthesia during pregnancy, unspecified trimester

+ 5 O29.3 Toxic reaction to local anesthesia during pregnancy

+ 6 O29.3X Toxic reaction to local anesthesia during pregnancy

SP + O29.3X1 Toxic reaction to local anesthesia during pregnancy, first trimester

SP + O29.3X2 Toxic reaction to local anesthesia during pregnancy, second trimester

SP + O29.3X3 Toxic reaction to local anesthesia during pregnancy, third trimester

!Q + O29.3X9 Toxic reaction to local anesthesia during pregnancy, unspecified trimester

+ 5 O29.4 Spinal and epidural anesthesia induced headache during pregnancy

!Q + O29.40 Spinal and epidural anesthesia induced headache during pregnancy, unspecified trimester

SP + O29.41 Spinal and epidural anesthesia induced headache during pregnancy, first trimester

SP + O29.42 Spinal and epidural anesthesia induced headache during pregnancy, second trimester

SP + O29.43 Spinal and epidural anesthesia induced headache during pregnancy, third trimester

+ 5 O29.5 Other complications of spinal and epidural anesthesia during pregnancy

+ 6 O29.5X Other complications of spinal and epidural anesthesia during pregnancy

SP + O29.5X1 Other complications of spinal and epidural anesthesia during pregnancy, first trimester

SP + O29.5X2 Other complications of spinal and epidural anesthesia during pregnancy, second trimester

SP + O29.5X3 Other complications of spinal and epidural anesthesia during pregnancy, third trimester

!Q + O29.5X9 Other complications of spinal and epidural anesthesia during pregnancy, unspecified trimester

+ 5 O29.6 Failed or difficult intubation for anesthesia during pregnancy

!Q + O29.60 Failed or difficult intubation for anesthesia during pregnancy, unspecified trimester

SP + O29.61 Failed or difficult intubation for anesthesia during pregnancy, first trimester

SP + O29.62 Failed or difficult intubation for anesthesia during pregnancy, second trimester

SP + O29.63 Failed or difficult intubation for anesthesia during pregnancy, third trimester

+ 5 O29.8 Other complications of anesthesia during pregnancy

+ 6 O29.8X Other complications of anesthesia during pregnancy

SP + O29.8X1 Other complications of anesthesia during pregnancy, first trimester

SP + O29.8X2 Other complications of anesthesia during pregnancy, second trimester

SP + O29.8X3 Other complications of anesthesia during pregnancy, third trimester

!Q + O29.8X9 Other complications of anesthesia during pregnancy, unspecified trimester

+ 5 O29.9 Unspecified complication of anesthesia during pregnancy

!Q + O29.90 Unspecified complication of anesthesia during pregnancy, unspecified trimester

!Q + O29.91 Unspecified complication of anesthesia during pregnancy, first trimester

!Q + O29.92 Unspecified complication of anesthesia during pregnancy, second trimester

!Q + O29.93 Unspecified complication of anesthesia during pregnancy, third trimester

Maternal care related to the fetus and amniotic cavity and possible delivery problems (O30-O48)

4 O30 Multiple gestation

Code also:

any complications specific to multiple gestation

5 O30.0 Twin pregnancy

6 O30.00 Twin pregnancy, unspecified number of placenta and unspecified number of amniotic sacs

IQ **O30.001 Twin pregnancy, unspecified number of placenta and unspecified number of amniotic sacs, first trimester**

IQ **O30.002 Twin pregnancy, unspecified number of placenta and unspecified number of amniotic sacs, second trimester**

IQ **O30.003 Twin pregnancy, unspecified number of placenta and unspecified number of amniotic sacs, third trimester**

IQ **O30.009 Twin pregnancy, unspecified number of placenta and unspecified number of amniotic sacs, unspecified trimester**

6 **O30.01 Twin pregnancy, monochorionic/monoamniotic**

Twin pregnancy, one placenta, one amniotic sac

EXCLUDES 1 conjoined twins (O30.02-)

IQ **O30.011 Twin pregnancy, monochorionic/monoamniotic, first trimester**

IQ **O30.012 Twin pregnancy, monochorionic/monoamniotic, second trimester**

IQ **O30.013 Twin pregnancy, monochorionic/monoamniotic, third trimester**

IQ **O30.019 Twin pregnancy, monochorionic/monoamniotic, unspecified trimester**

6 **O30.02 Conjoined twin pregnancy**

SP **O30.021 Conjoined twin pregnancy, first trimester**

SP **O30.022 Conjoined twin pregnancy, second trimester**

SP **O30.023 Conjoined twin pregnancy, third trimester**

IQ **O30.029 Conjoined twin pregnancy, unspecified trimester**

6 **O30.03 Twin pregnancy, monochorionic/diamniotic**

Twin pregnancy, one placenta, two amniotic sacs

IQ **O30.031 Twin pregnancy, monochorionic/diamniotic, first trimester**

IQ **O30.032 Twin pregnancy, monochorionic/diamniotic, second trimester**

IQ **O30.033 Twin pregnancy, monochorionic/diamniotic, third trimester**

IQ **O30.039 Twin pregnancy, monochorionic/diamniotic, unspecified trimester**

6 **O30.04 Twin pregnancy, dichorionic/diamniotic**

Twin pregnancy, two placentae, two amniotic sacs

IQ **O30.041 Twin pregnancy, dichorionic/diamniotic, first trimester**

IQ **O30.042 Twin pregnancy, dichorionic/diamniotic, second trimester**

IQ **O30.043 Twin pregnancy, dichorionic/diamniotic, third trimester**

IQ **O30.049 Twin pregnancy, dichorionic/diamniotic, unspecified trimester**

6 **O30.09 Twin pregnancy, unable to determine number of placenta and number of amniotic sacs**

IQ **O30.091 Twin pregnancy, unable to determine number of placenta and number of amniotic sacs, first trimester**

IQ **O30.092 Twin pregnancy, unable to determine number of placenta and number of amniotic sacs, second trimester**

IQ **O30.093 Twin pregnancy, unable to determine number of placenta and number of amniotic sacs, third trimester**

IQ **O30.099 Twin pregnancy, unable to determine number of placenta and number of amniotic sacs, unspecified trimester**

5 **O30.1 Triplet pregnancy**

6 **O30.10 Triplet pregnancy, unspecified number of placenta and unspecified number of amniotic sacs**

IQ **O30.101 Triplet pregnancy, unspecified number of placenta and unspecified number of amniotic sacs, first trimester**

IQ **O30.102 Triplet pregnancy, unspecified number of placenta and unspecified number of amniotic sacs, second trimester**

IQ **O30.103 Triplet pregnancy, unspecified number of placenta and unspecified number of amniotic sacs, third trimester**

IQ **O30.109 Triplet pregnancy, unspecified number of placenta and unspecified number of amniotic sacs, unspecified trimester**

6 **O30.11 Triplet pregnancy with two or more monochorionic fetuses**

IQ **O30.111 Triplet pregnancy with two or more monochorionic fetuses, first trimester**

IQ **O30.112 Triplet pregnancy with two or more monochorionic fetuses, second trimester**

IQ **O30.113 Triplet pregnancy with two or more monochorionic fetuses, third trimester**

IQ **O30.119 Triplet pregnancy with two or more monochorionic fetuses, unspecified trimester**

6 **O30.12 Triplet pregnancy with two or more monoamniotic fetuses**

IQ **O30.121 Triplet pregnancy with two or more monoamniotic fetuses, first trimester**

IQ O30.122 Triplet pregnancy with two or more monoamniotic fetuses, second trimester

IQ O30.123 Triplet pregnancy with two or more monoamniotic fetuses, third trimester

IQ O30.129 Triplet pregnancy with two or more monoamniotic fetuses, unspecified trimester

6 O30.13 Triplet pregnancy, trichorionic/triamniotic

IQ O30.131 Triplet pregnancy, trichorionic/triamniotic, first trimester

IQ O30.132 Triplet pregnancy, trichorionic/triamniotic, second trimester

IQ O30.133 Triplet pregnancy, trichorionic/triamniotic, third trimester

IQ O30.139 Triplet pregnancy, trichorionic/triamniotic, unspecified trimester

6 O30.19 Triplet pregnancy, unable to determine number of placenta and number of amniotic sacs

IQ O30.191 Triplet pregnancy, unable to determine number of placenta and number of amniotic sacs, first trimester

IQ O30.192 Triplet pregnancy, unable to determine number of placenta and number of amniotic sacs, second trimester

IQ O30.193 Triplet pregnancy, unable to determine number of placenta and number of amniotic sacs, third trimester

IQ O30.199 Triplet pregnancy, unable to determine number of placenta and number of amniotic sacs, unspecified trimester

5 O30.2 Quadruplet pregnancy

6 O30.20 Quadruplet pregnancy, unspecified number of placenta and unspecified number of amniotic sacs

IQ O30.201 Quadruplet pregnancy, unspecified number of placenta and unspecified number of amniotic sacs, first trimester

IQ O30.202 Quadruplet pregnancy, unspecified number of placenta and unspecified number of amniotic sacs, second trimester

IQ O30.203 Quadruplet pregnancy, unspecified number of placenta and unspecified number of amniotic sacs, third trimester

IQ O30.209 Quadruplet pregnancy, unspecified number of placenta and unspecified number of amniotic sacs, unspecified trimester

6 O30.21 Quadruplet pregnancy with two or more monochorionic fetuses

IQ O30.211 Quadruplet pregnancy with two or more monochorionic fetuses, first trimester

IQ O30.212 Quadruplet pregnancy with two or more monochorionic fetuses, second trimester

IQ O30.213 Quadruplet pregnancy with two or more monochorionic fetuses, third trimester

IQ O30.219 Quadruplet pregnancy with two or more monochorionic fetuses, unspecified trimester

6 O30.22 Quadruplet pregnancy with two or more monoamniotic fetuses

IQ O30.221 Quadruplet pregnancy with two or more monoamniotic fetuses, first trimester

IQ O30.222 Quadruplet pregnancy with two or more monoamniotic fetuses, second trimester

IQ O30.223 Quadruplet pregnancy with two or more monoamniotic fetuses, third trimester

IQ O30.229 Quadruplet pregnancy with two or more monoamniotic fetuses, unspecified trimester

6 O30.23 Quadruplet pregnancy, quadrachorionic/quadra-amniotic

IQ O30.231 Quadruplet pregnancy, quadrachorionic/quadra-amniotic, first trimester

IQ O30.232 Quadruplet pregnancy, quadrachorionic/quadra-amniotic, second trimester

IQ O30.233 Quadruplet pregnancy, quadrachorionic/quadra-amniotic, third trimester

IQ O30.239 Quadruplet pregnancy, quadrachorionic/quadra-amniotic, unspecified trimester

6 O30.29 Quadruplet pregnancy, unable to determine number of placenta and number of amniotic sacs

IQ O30.291 Quadruplet pregnancy, unable to determine number of placenta and number of amniotic sacs, first trimester

IQ O30.292 Quadruplet pregnancy, unable to determine number of placenta and number of amniotic sacs, second trimester

IQ O30.293 Quadruplet pregnancy, unable to determine number of placenta and number of amniotic sacs, third trimester

IQ O30.299 Quadruplet pregnancy, unable to determine number of placenta and number of amniotic sacs, unspecified trimester

5 O30.8 Other specified multiple gestation
Multiple gestation pregnancy greater then quadruplets

6 O30.80 Other specified multiple gestation, unspecified number of placenta and unspecified number of amniotic sacs

IQ **O30.801 Other specified multiple gestation, unspecified number of placenta and unspecified number of amniotic sacs, first trimester**

IQ **O30.802 Other specified multiple gestation, unspecified number of placenta and unspecified number of amniotic sacs, second trimester**

IQ **O30.803 Other specified multiple gestation, unspecified number of placenta and unspecified number of amniotic sacs, third trimester**

IQ **O30.809 Other specified multiple gestation, unspecified number of placenta and unspecified number of amniotic sacs, unspecified trimester**

6 **O30.81 Other specified multiple gestation with two or more monochorionic fetuses**

IQ **O30.811 Other specified multiple gestation with two or more monochorionic fetuses, first trimester**

IQ **O30.812 Other specified multiple gestation with two or more monochorionic fetuses, second trimester**

IQ **O30.813 Other specified multiple gestation with two or more monochorionic fetuses, third trimester**

IQ **O30.819 Other specified multiple gestation with two or more monochorionic fetuses, unspecified trimester**

6 **O30.82 Other specified multiple gestation with two or more monoamniotic fetuses**

IQ **O30.821 Other specified multiple gestation with two or more monoamniotic fetuses, first trimester**

IQ **O30.822 Other specified multiple gestation with two or more monoamniotic fetuses, second trimester**

IQ **O30.823 Other specified multiple gestation with two or more monoamniotic fetuses, third trimester**

IQ **O30.829 Other specified multiple gestation with two or more monoamniotic fetuses, unspecified trimester**

6 **O30.83 Other specified multiple gestation, number of chorions and amnions are both equal to the number of fetuses**

Pentachorionic, penta-amniotic pregnancy (quintuplets)
Hexachorionic, hexa-amniotic pregnancy (sextuplets)
Heptachorionic, hepta-amniotic pregnancy (septuplets)

IQ **O30.831 Other specified multiple gestation, number of chorions and amnions are both equal to the number of fetuses, first trimester**

IQ **O30.832 Other specified multiple gestation, number of chorions and amnions are both equal to the number of fetuses, second trimester**

IQ **O30.833 Other specified multiple gestation, number of chorions and amnions are both equal to the number of fetuses, third trimester**

IQ **O30.839 Other specified multiple gestation, number of chorions and amnions are both equal to the number of fetuses, unspecified trimester**

6 **O30.89 Other specified multiple gestation, unable to determine number of placenta and number of amniotic sacs**

IQ **O30.891 Other specified multiple gestation, unable to determine number of placenta and number of amniotic sacs, first trimester**

IQ **O30.892 Other specified multiple gestation, unable to determine number of placenta and number of amniotic sacs, second trimester**

IQ **O30.893 Other specified multiple gestation, unable to determine number of placenta and number of amniotic sacs, third trimester**

IQ **O30.899 Other specified multiple gestation, unable to determine number of placenta and number of amniotic sacs, unspecified trimester**

5 **O30.9 Multiple gestation, unspecified**

Multiple pregnancy NOS

IQ **O30.90 Multiple gestation, unspecified, unspecified trimester**

IQ **O30.91 Multiple gestation, unspecified, first trimester**

IQ **O30.92 Multiple gestation, unspecified, second trimester**

IQ **O30.93 Multiple gestation, unspecified, third trimester**

4 **O31 Complications specific to multiple gestation**

EXCLUDES 2 delayed delivery of second twin, triplet, etc. (O63.2)
malpresentation of one fetus or more (O32.9)
placental transfusion syndromes (O43.0-)

One of the following 7th characters is to be assigned to each code under category O31. 7th character 0 is for single gestations and multiple gestations where the fetus is unspecified. 7th characters 1 through 9 are for cases of multiple gestations to identify the fetus for which the code applies. The appropriate code from category O30, Multiple gestation, must also be assigned when assigning a code from category O31 that has a 7th character of 1 through 9.

0 not applicable or unspecified
1 fetus 1
2 fetus 2
3 fetus 3
4 fetus 4
5 fetus 5
9 other fetus

5 **O31.0 Papyraceous fetus**

Chapter 15
O00-O9A

Fetus compressus

IQ 7 **O31.00X- Papyraceous fetus, unspecified trimester**

IQ 7 **O31.01X- Papyraceous fetus, first trimester**

IQ 7 **O31.02X- Papyraceous fetus, second trimester**

IQ 7 **O31.03X- Papyraceous fetus, third trimester**

5 **O31.1 Continuing pregnancy after spontaneous abortion of one fetus or more**

IQ 7 **O31.10X- Continuing pregnancy after spontaneous abortion of one fetus or more, unspecified trimester**

IQ 7 **O31.11X- Continuing pregnancy after spontaneous abortion of one fetus or more, first trimester**

IQ 7 **O31.12X- Continuing pregnancy after spontaneous abortion of one fetus or more, second trimester**

IQ 7 **O31.13X- Continuing pregnancy after spontaneous abortion of one fetus or more, third trimester**

5 **O31.2 Continuing pregnancy after intrauterine death of one fetus or more**

IQ 7 **O31.20X- Continuing pregnancy after intrauterine death of one fetus or more, unspecified trimester**

IQ 7 **O31.21X- Continuing pregnancy after intrauterine death of one fetus or more, first trimester**

IQ 7 **O31.22X- Continuing pregnancy after intrauterine death of one fetus or more, second trimester**

IQ 7 **O31.23X- Continuing pregnancy after intrauterine death of one fetus or more, third trimester**

5 **O31.3 Continuing pregnancy after elective fetal reduction of one fetus or more**

Continuing pregnancy after selective termination of one fetus or more

IQ 7 **O31.30X- Continuing pregnancy after elective fetal reduction of one fetus or more, unspecified trimester**

IQ 7 **O31.31X- Continuing pregnancy after elective fetal reduction of one fetus or more, first trimester**

IQ 7 **O31.32X- Continuing pregnancy after elective fetal reduction of one fetus or more, second trimester**

IQ 7 **O31.33X- Continuing pregnancy after elective fetal reduction of one fetus or more, third trimester**

5 **O31.8 Other complications specific to multiple gestation**

6 **O31.8X Other complications specific to multiple gestation**

IQ 7 **O31.8X1- Other complications specific to multiple gestation, first trimester**

IQ 7 **O31.8X2- Other complications specific to multiple gestation, second trimester**

IQ 7 **O31.8X3- Other complications specific to multiple gestation, third trimester**

IQ 7 **O31.8X9- Other complications specific to multiple gestation, unspecified trimester**

4 **O32 Maternal care for malpresentation of fetus**

INCLUDES the listed conditions as a reason for observation, hospitalization or other obstetric care of the mother, or for cesarean delivery before onset of labor

EXCLUDES 1 malpresentation of fetus with obstructed labor (O64.-)

One of the following 7th characters is to be assigned to each code under category O32. 7th character 0 is for single gestations and multiple gestations where the fetus is unspecified. 7th characters 1 through 9 are for cases of multiple gestations to identify the fetus for which the code applies. The appropriate code from category O30, Multiple gestation, must also be assigned when assigning a code from category O32 that has a 7th character of 1 through 9.

0 not applicable or unspecified
1 fetus 1
2 fetus 2
3 fetus 3
4 fetus 4
5 fetus 5
9 other fetus

IQ 7 **O32.0XX- Maternal care for unstable lie**

IQ 7 **O32.1XX- Maternal care for breech presentation**

Maternal care for buttocks presentation
Maternal care for complete breech
Maternal care for frank breech

EXCLUDES 1 footling presentation (O32.8)
incomplete breech (O32.8)

IQ 7 **O32.2XX- Maternal care for transverse and oblique lie**

Maternal care for oblique presentation
Maternal care for transverse presentation

IQ 7 **O32.3XX- Maternal care for face, brow and chin presentation**

IQ 7 **O32.4XX- Maternal care for high head at term**

Maternal care for failure of head to enter pelvic brim

IQ 7 **O32.6XX- Maternal care for compound presentation**

IQ 7 **O32.8XX- Maternal care for other malpresentation of fetus**

Maternal care for footling presentation
Maternal care for incomplete breech

IQ 7 **O32.9XX- Maternal care for malpresentation of fetus, unspecified**

4 **O33 Maternal care for disproportion**

Chapter 15 O00-O9A

INCLUDES the listed conditions as a reason for observation, hospitalization or other obstetric care of the mother, or for cesarean delivery before onset of labor

EXCLUDES 1 disproportion with obstructed labor (O65-O66)

!Q **O33.0 Maternal care for disproportion due to deformity of maternal pelvic bones**
Maternal care for disproportion due to pelvic deformity causing disproportion NOS

!Q **O33.1 Maternal care for disproportion due to generally contracted pelvis**
Maternal care for disproportion due to contracted pelvis NOS causing disproportion

!Q **O33.2 Maternal care for disproportion due to inlet contraction of pelvis**
Maternal care for disproportion due to inlet contraction (pelvis) causing disproportion

!Q 7 **O33.3XX- Maternal care for disproportion due to outlet contraction of pelvis**
Maternal care for disproportion due to mid-cavity contraction (pelvis)
Maternal care for disproportion due to outlet contraction (pelvis)

One of the following 7th characters is to be assigned to code O33.3. 7th character 0 is for single gestations and multiple gestations where the fetus is unspecified. 7th characters 1 through 9 are for cases of multiple gestations to identify the fetus for which the code applies. The appropriate code from category O30, Multiple gestation, must also be assigned when assigning code O33.3 with a 7th character of 1 through 9.

0	not applicable or unspecified
1	fetus 1
2	fetus 2
3	fetus 3
4	fetus 4
5	fetus 5
9	other fetus

!Q 7 **O33.4XX- Maternal care for disproportion of mixed maternal and fetal origin**

One of the following 7th characters is to be assigned to code O33.4. 7th character 0 is for single gestations and multiple gestations where the fetus is unspecified. 7th characters 1 through 9 are for cases of multiple gestations to identify the fetus for which the code applies. The appropriate code from category O30, Multiple gestation, must also be assigned when assigning code O33.4 with a 7th character of 1 through 9.

0	not applicable or unspecified
1	fetus 1
2	fetus 2
3	fetus 3
4	fetus 4
5	fetus 5
9	other fetus

!Q 7 **O33.5XX- Maternal care for disproportion due to unusually large fetus**
Maternal care for disproportion due to disproportion of fetal origin with normally formed fetus
Maternal care for disproportion due to fetal disproportion NOS

One of the following 7th characters is to be assigned to code O33.5. 7th character 0 is for single gestations and multiple gestations where the fetus is unspecified. 7th characters 1 through 9 are for cases of multiple gestations to identify the fetus for which the code applies. The appropriate code from category O30, Multiple gestation, must also be assigned when assigning code O33.5 with a 7th character of 1 through 9.

0	not applicable or unspecified
1	fetus 1
2	fetus 2
3	fetus 3
4	fetus 4
5	fetus 5
9	other fetus

!Q 7 **O33.6XX- Maternal care for disproportion due to hydrocephalic fetus**

One of the following 7th characters is to be assigned to code O33.6. 7th character 0 is for single gestations and multiple gestations where the fetus is unspecified. 7th characters 1 through 9 are for cases of multiple gestations to identify the fetus for which the code applies. The appropriate code from category O30, Multiple gestation, must also be assigned when assigning code O33.6 with a 7th character of 1 through 9.

0	not applicable or unspecified
1	fetus 1
2	fetus 2
3	fetus 3
4	fetus 4
5	fetus 5
9	other fetus

!Q 7 **O33.7XX- Maternal care for disproportion due to other fetal deformities**

Maternal care for disproportion due to fetal ascites
Maternal care for disproportion due to fetal hydrops
Maternal care for disproportion due to fetal meningomyelocele
Maternal care for disproportion due to fetal sacral teratoma
Maternal care for disproportion due to fetal tumor

EXCLUDES 1 obstructed labor due to other fetal deformities (O66.3)

One of the following 7th characters is to be assigned to code O33.7. 7th character 0 is for single gestations and multiple gestations where the fetus is unspecified. 7th characters 1 through 9 are for cases of multiple gestations to identify the fetus for which the code applies. The appropriate code from category O30, Multiple gestation, must also be assigned when assigning code O33.7 with a 7th character of 1 through 9.

0	not applicable or unspecified
1	fetus 1
2	fetus 2
3	fetus 3
4	fetus 4
5	fetus 5
9	other fetus

!Q **O33.8 Maternal care for disproportion of other origin**

!Q **O33.9 Maternal care for disproportion, unspecified**

Maternal care for disproportion due to cephalopelvic disproportion NOS
Maternal care for disproportion due to fetopelvic disproportion NOS

+ 4 **O34 Maternal care for abnormality of pelvic organs**

INCLUDES the listed conditions as a reason for hospitalization or other obstetric care of the mother, or for cesarean delivery before onset of labor

Code first:
any associated obstructed labor (O65.5)
Use additional code for specific condition

+ 5 **O34.0 Maternal care for congenital malformation of uterus**

Maternal care for double uterus
Maternal care for uterus bicornis

!Q + **O34.00 Maternal care for unspecified congenital malformation of uterus, unspecified trimester**

!Q + **O34.01 Maternal care for unspecified congenital malformation of uterus, first trimester**

!Q + **O34.02 Maternal care for unspecified congenital malformation of uterus, second trimester**

!Q + **O34.03 Maternal care for unspecified congenital malformation of uterus, third trimester**

+ 5 **O34.1 Maternal care for benign tumor of corpus uteri**

EXCLUDES 2 maternal care for benign tumor of cervix (O34.4-)
maternal care for malignant neoplasm of uterus (O9A.1-)

!Q + **O34.10 Maternal care for benign tumor of corpus uteri, unspecified trimester**

!Q + **O34.11 Maternal care for benign tumor of corpus uteri, first trimester**

!Q + **O34.12 Maternal care for benign tumor of corpus uteri, second trimester**

!Q + **O34.13 Maternal care for benign tumor of corpus uteri, third trimester**

+ 5 **O34.2 Maternal care due to uterine scar from previous surgery**

+ 6 **O34.21 Maternal care for scar from previous cesarean delivery**

!Q + **O34.211 Maternal care for low transverse scar from previous cesarean delivery**

!Q + **O34.212 Maternal care for vertical scar from previous cesarean delivery**

Maternal care for classical scar from previous cesarean delivery

!Q + **O34.218 Maternal care for other type scar from previous cesarean delivery**

Mid-transverse T incision

!Q + **O34.219 Maternal care for unspecified type scar from previous cesarean delivery**

!Q + **O34.22 Maternal care for cesarean scar defect (isthmocele)**

!Q + **O34.29 Maternal care due to uterine scar from other previous surgery**

Maternal care due to uterine scar from other transmural uterine incision

+ 5 **O34.3 Maternal care for cervical incompetence**

Maternal care for cerclage with or without cervical incompetence
Maternal care for Shirodkar suture with or without cervical incompetence

Chapter 15
O00-O9A

O34.30 Maternal care for cervical incompetence, unspecified trimester

O34.31 Maternal care for cervical incompetence, first trimester

O34.32 Maternal care for cervical incompetence, second trimester

O34.33 Maternal care for cervical incompetence, third trimester

O34.4 Maternal care for other abnormalities of cervix

O34.40 Maternal care for other abnormalities of cervix, unspecified trimester

O34.41 Maternal care for other abnormalities of cervix, first trimester

O34.42 Maternal care for other abnormalities of cervix, second trimester

O34.43 Maternal care for other abnormalities of cervix, third trimester

O34.5 Maternal care for other abnormalities of gravid uterus

O34.51 Maternal care for incarceration of gravid uterus

O34.511 Maternal care for incarceration of gravid uterus, first trimester

O34.512 Maternal care for incarceration of gravid uterus, second trimester

O34.513 Maternal care for incarceration of gravid uterus, third trimester

O34.519 Maternal care for incarceration of gravid uterus, unspecified trimester

O34.52 Maternal care for prolapse of gravid uterus

O34.521 Maternal care for prolapse of gravid uterus, first trimester

O34.522 Maternal care for prolapse of gravid uterus, second trimester

O34.523 Maternal care for prolapse of gravid uterus, third trimester

O34.529 Maternal care for prolapse of gravid uterus, unspecified trimester

O34.53 Maternal care for retroversion of gravid uterus

O34.531 Maternal care for retroversion of gravid uterus, first trimester

O34.532 Maternal care for retroversion of gravid uterus, second trimester

O34.533 Maternal care for retroversion of gravid uterus, third trimester

O34.539 Maternal care for retroversion of gravid uterus, unspecified trimester

O34.59 Maternal care for other abnormalities of gravid uterus

O34.591 Maternal care for other abnormalities of gravid uterus, first trimester

O34.592 Maternal care for other abnormalities of gravid uterus, second trimester

O34.593 Maternal care for other abnormalities of gravid uterus, third trimester

O34.599 Maternal care for other abnormalities of gravid uterus, unspecified trimester

O34.6 Maternal care for abnormality of vagina

EXCLUDES 2 maternal care for vaginal varices in pregnancy (O22.1-)

O34.60 Maternal care for abnormality of vagina, unspecified trimester

O34.61 Maternal care for abnormality of vagina, first trimester

O34.62 Maternal care for abnormality of vagina, second trimester

O34.63 Maternal care for abnormality of vagina, third trimester

O34.7 Maternal care for abnormality of vulva and perineum

EXCLUDES 2 maternal care for perineal and vulval varices in pregnancy (O22.1-)

O34.70 Maternal care for abnormality of vulva and perineum, unspecified trimester

O34.71 Maternal care for abnormality of vulva and perineum, first trimester

O34.72 Maternal care for abnormality of vulva and perineum, second trimester

O34.73 Maternal care for abnormality of vulva and perineum, third trimester

O34.8 Maternal care for other abnormalities of pelvic organs

O34.80 Maternal care for other abnormalities of pelvic organs, unspecified trimester

O34.81 Maternal care for other abnormalities of pelvic organs, first trimester

O34.82 Maternal care for other abnormalities of pelvic organs, second trimester

O34.83 Maternal care for other abnormalities of pelvic organs, third trimester

O34.9 Maternal care for abnormality of pelvic organ, unspecified

O34.90 Maternal care for abnormality of pelvic organ, unspecified, unspecified trimester

O34.91 Maternal care for abnormality of pelvic organ, unspecified, first trimester

O34.92 Maternal care for abnormality of pelvic organ, unspecified, second trimester

O34.93 Maternal care for abnormality of pelvic organ, unspecified, third trimester

O35 Maternal care for known or suspected fetal abnormality and damage

Chapter 15 O00-O9A

INCLUDES the listed conditions in the fetus as a reason for hospitalization or other obstetric care to the mother, or for termination of pregnancy

Code also:
any associated maternal condition

EXCLUDES 1 encounter for suspected maternal and fetal conditions ruled out (Z03.7-)

One of the following 7th characters is to be assigned to each code under category O35. 7th character 0 is for single gestations and multiple gestations where the fetus is unspecified. 7th characters 1 through 9 are for cases of multiple gestations to identify the fetus for which the code applies. The appropriate code from category O30, Multiple gestation, must also be assigned when assigning a code from category O35 that has a 7th character of 1 through 9.

0 not applicable or unspecified
1 fetus 1
2 fetus 2
3 fetus 3
4 fetus 4
5 fetus 5
9 other fetus

IQ 7 O35.0XX- **Maternal care for (suspected) central nervous system malformation in fetus**
Maternal care for fetal anencephaly
Maternal care for fetal hydrocephalus
Maternal care for fetal spina bifida
EXCLUDES 2 chromosomal abnormality in fetus (O35.1)

IQ 7 O35.1XX- **Maternal care for (suspected) chromosomal abnormality in fetus**

IQ 7 O35.2XX- **Maternal care for (suspected) hereditary disease in fetus**
EXCLUDES 2 chromosomal abnormality in fetus (O35.1)

IQ 7 O35.3XX- **Maternal care for (suspected) damage to fetus from viral disease in mother**
Maternal care for damage to fetus from maternal cytomegalovirus infection
Maternal care for damage to fetus from maternal rubella

IQ 7 O35.4XX- **Maternal care for (suspected) damage to fetus from alcohol**

IQ 7 O35.5XX- **Maternal care for (suspected) damage to fetus by drugs**
Maternal care for damage to fetus from drug addiction

IQ 7 O35.6XX- **Maternal care for (suspected) damage to fetus by radiation**

IQ 7 O35.7XX- **Maternal care for (suspected) damage to fetus by other medical procedures**
Maternal care for damage to fetus by amniocentesis
Maternal care for damage to fetus by biopsy procedures
Maternal care for damage to fetus by hematological investigation
Maternal care for damage to fetus by intrauterine contraceptive device
Maternal care for damage to fetus by intrauterine surgery

IQ 7 O35.8XX- **Maternal care for other (suspected) fetal abnormality and damage**
Maternal care for damage to fetus from maternal listeriosis
Maternal care for damage to fetus from maternal toxoplasmosis

IQ 7 O35.9XX- **Maternal care for (suspected) fetal abnormality and damage, unspecified**

4 O36 **Maternal care for other fetal problems**

INCLUDES the listed conditions in the fetus as a reason for hospitalization or other obstetric care of the mother, or for termination of pregnancy

EXCLUDES 1 encounter for suspected maternal and fetal conditions ruled out (Z03.7-)
placental transfusion syndromes (O43.0-)

EXCLUDES 2 labor and delivery complicated by fetal stress (O77.-)

One of the following 7th characters is to be assigned to each code under category O36. 7th character 0 is for single gestations and multiple gestations where the fetus is unspecified. 7th characters 1 through 9 are for cases of multiple gestations to identify the fetus for which the code applies. The appropriate code from category O30, Multiple gestation, must also be assigned when assigning a code from category O36 that has a 7th character of 1 through 9.

0 not applicable or unspecified
1 fetus 1
2 fetus 2
3 fetus 3
4 fetus 4
5 fetus 5
9 other fetus

CODING TIPS ✓ It is common to have abnormalities of the fetal heart rate or rhythm during the antepartum period, including fetal tachycardia, fetal bradycardia, decelerations of the fetal heart rate and loss of variability. Abnormalities during antenatal tests such as non-stress tests (NSTs) and contraction stress tests (CSTs) are also reported.

5 O36.0 **Maternal care for rhesus isoimmunization**
Maternal care for Rh incompatibility (with hydrops fetalis)

6 O36.01 **Maternal care for anti-D [Rh] antibodies**

IQ 7 O36.011- **Maternal care for anti-D [Rh] antibodies, first trimester**

IQ 7 O36.012- **Maternal care for anti-D [Rh] antibodies, second trimester**

!Q 7 **O36.013- Maternal care for anti-D [Rh] antibodies, third trimester**

!Q 7 **O36.019- Maternal care for anti-D [Rh] antibodies, unspecified trimester**

6 **O36.09 Maternal care for other rhesus isoimmunization**

!Q 7 **O36.091- Maternal care for other rhesus isoimmunization, first trimester**

!Q 7 **O36.092- Maternal care for other rhesus isoimmunization, second trimester**

!Q 7 **O36.093- Maternal care for other rhesus isoimmunization, third trimester**

!Q 7 **O36.099- Maternal care for other rhesus isoimmunization, unspecified trimester**

5 **O36.1 Maternal care for other isoimmunization**

Maternal care for ABO isoimmunization

6 **O36.11 Maternal care for Anti-A sensitization**

Maternal care for isoimmunization NOS (with hydrops fetalis)

!Q 7 **O36.111- Maternal care for Anti-A sensitization, first trimester**

!Q 7 **O36.112- Maternal care for Anti-A sensitization, second trimester**

!Q 7 **O36.113- Maternal care for Anti-A sensitization, third trimester**

!Q 7 **O36.119- Maternal care for Anti-A sensitization, unspecified trimester**

6 **O36.19 Maternal care for other isoimmunization**

Maternal care for Anti-B sensitization

!Q 7 **O36.191- Maternal care for other isoimmunization, first trimester**

!Q 7 **O36.192- Maternal care for other isoimmunization, second trimester**

!Q 7 **O36.193- Maternal care for other isoimmunization, third trimester**

!Q 7 **O36.199- Maternal care for other isoimmunization, unspecified trimester**

5 **O36.2 Maternal care for hydrops fetalis**

Maternal care for hydrops fetalis NOS

Maternal care for hydrops fetalis not associated with isoimmunization

EXCLUDES 1 hydrops fetalis associated with ABO isoimmunization (O36.1-)
hydrops fetalis associated with rhesus isoimmunization (O36.0-)

!Q 7 **O36.20X- Maternal care for hydrops fetalis, unspecified trimester**

!Q 7 **O36.21X- Maternal care for hydrops fetalis, first trimester**

!Q 7 **O36.22X- Maternal care for hydrops fetalis, second trimester**

!Q 7 **O36.23X- Maternal care for hydrops fetalis, third trimester**

!Q 7 **O36.4XX- Maternal care for intrauterine death**

Maternal care for intrauterine fetal death NOS

Maternal care for intrauterine fetal death after completion of 20 weeks of gestation

Maternal care for late fetal death

Maternal care for missed delivery

EXCLUDES 1 missed abortion (O02.1)
stillbirth (P95)

5 **O36.5 Maternal care for known or suspected poor fetal growth**

6 **O36.51 Maternal care for known or suspected placental insufficiency**

!Q 7 **O36.511- Maternal care for known or suspected placental insufficiency, first trimester**

!Q 7 **O36.512- Maternal care for known or suspected placental insufficiency, second trimester**

!Q 7 **O36.513- Maternal care for known or suspected placental insufficiency, third trimester**

!Q 7 **O36.519- Maternal care for known or suspected placental insufficiency, unspecified trimester**

6 **O36.59 Maternal care for other known or suspected poor fetal growth**

Maternal care for known or suspected light-for-dates NOS

Maternal care for known or suspected small-for-dates NOS

!Q 7 **O36.591- Maternal care for other known or suspected poor fetal growth, first trimester**

!Q 7 **O36.592- Maternal care for other known or suspected poor fetal growth, second trimester**

!Q 7 **O36.593- Maternal care for other known or suspected poor fetal growth, third trimester**

!Q 7 **O36.599- Maternal care for other known or suspected poor fetal growth, unspecified trimester**

5 **O36.6 Maternal care for excessive fetal growth**

Maternal care for known or suspected large-for-dates

!Q 7 **O36.60X- Maternal care for excessive fetal growth, unspecified trimester**

!Q 7 **O36.61X- Maternal care for excessive fetal growth, first trimester**

!Q 7 **O36.62X- Maternal care for excessive fetal growth, second trimester**

!Q 7 **O36.63X- Maternal care for excessive fetal growth, third trimester**

5 **O36.7 Maternal care for viable fetus in abdominal pregnancy**

!Q 7 **O36.70X- Maternal care for viable fetus in abdominal pregnancy, unspecified trimester**

IQ 7 **O36.71X- Maternal care for viable fetus in abdominal pregnancy, first trimester**

IQ 7 **O36.72X- Maternal care for viable fetus in abdominal pregnancy, second trimester**

IQ 7 **O36.73X- Maternal care for viable fetus in abdominal pregnancy, third trimester**

5 **O36.8 Maternal care for other specified fetal problems**

IQ 7 **O36.80X- Pregnancy with inconclusive fetal viability**

Encounter to determine fetal viability of pregnancy

6 **O36.81 Decreased fetal movements**

IQ 7 **O36.812- Decreased fetal movements, second trimester**

IQ 7 **O36.813- Decreased fetal movements, third trimester**

IQ 7 **O36.819- Decreased fetal movements, unspecified trimester**

6 **O36.82 Fetal anemia and thrombocytopenia**

IQ 7 **O36.821- Fetal anemia and thrombocytopenia, first trimester**

IQ 7 **O36.822- Fetal anemia and thrombocytopenia, second trimester**

IQ 7 **O36.823- Fetal anemia and thrombocytopenia, third trimester**

IQ 7 **O36.829- Fetal anemia and thrombocytopenia, unspecified trimester**

6 **O36.83 Maternal care for abnormalities of the fetal heart rate or rhythm**

Maternal care for depressed fetal heart rate tones
Maternal care for fetal bradycardia
Maternal care for fetal heart rate abnormal variability
Maternal care for fetal heart rate decelerations
Maternal care for fetal heart rate irregularity
Maternal care for fetal tachycardia
Maternal care for non-reassuring fetal heart rate or rhythm

IQ 7 **O36.831- Maternal care for abnormalities of the fetal heart rate or rhythm, first trimester**

IQ 7 **O36.832- Maternal care for abnormalities of the fetal heart rate or rhythm, second trimester**

IQ 7 **O36.833- Maternal care for abnormalities of the fetal heart rate or rhythm, third trimester**

IQ 7 **O36.839- Maternal care for abnormalities of the fetal heart rate or rhythm, unspecified trimester**

6 **O36.89 Maternal care for other specified fetal problems**

IQ 7 **O36.891- Maternal care for other specified fetal problems, first trimester**

IQ 7 **O36.892- Maternal care for other specified fetal problems, second trimester**

IQ 7 **O36.893- Maternal care for other specified fetal problems, third trimester**

IQ 7 **O36.899- Maternal care for other specified fetal problems, unspecified trimester**

5 **O36.9 Maternal care for fetal problem, unspecified**

IQ 7 **O36.90X- Maternal care for fetal problem, unspecified, unspecified trimester**

IQ 7 **O36.91X- Maternal care for fetal problem, unspecified, first trimester**

IQ 7 **O36.92X- Maternal care for fetal problem, unspecified, second trimester**

IQ 7 **O36.93X- Maternal care for fetal problem, unspecified, third trimester**

4 **O40 Polyhydramnios**

INCLUDES hydramnios

EXCLUDES 1 encounter for suspected maternal and fetal conditions ruled out (Z03.7-)

One of the following 7th characters is to be assigned to each code under category O40. 7th character 0 is for single gestations and multiple gestations where the fetus is unspecified. 7th characters 1 through 9 are for cases of multiple gestations to identify the fetus for which the code applies. The appropriate code from category O30, Multiple gestation, must also be assigned when assigning a code from category O40 that has a 7th character of 1 through 9.

0	not applicable or unspecified
1	fetus 1
2	fetus 2
3	fetus 3
4	fetus 4
5	fetus 5
9	other fetus

SP IQ 7 **O40.1XX- Polyhydramnios, first trimester**

SP 7 **O40.2XX- Polyhydramnios, second trimester**

SP 7 **O40.3XX- Polyhydramnios, third trimester**

IQ 7 **O40.9XX- Polyhydramnios, unspecified trimester**

4 **O41 Other disorders of amniotic fluid and membranes**

EXCLUDES 1 encounter for suspected maternal and fetal conditions ruled out (Z03.7-)

Chapter 15

O00-O9A

One of the following 7th characters is to be assigned to each code under category O41. 7th character 0 is for single gestations and multiple gestations where the fetus is unspecified. 7th characters 1 through 9 are for cases of multiple gestations to identify the fetus for which the code applies. The appropriate code from category O30, Multiple gestation, must also be assigned when assigning a code from category O41 that has a 7th character of 1 through 9.

0 not applicable or unspecified
1 fetus 1
2 fetus 2
3 fetus 3
4 fetus 4
5 fetus 5
9 other fetus

5 **O41.0 Oligohydramnios**
Oligohydramnios without rupture of membranes

!Q 7 **O41.00X- Oligohydramnios, unspecified trimester**

SP 7 **O41.01X- Oligohydramnios, first trimester**

SP 7 **O41.02X- Oligohydramnios, second trimester**

SP 7 **O41.03X- Oligohydramnios, third trimester**

5 **O41.1 Infection of amniotic sac and membranes**

6 **O41.10 Infection of amniotic sac and membranes, unspecified**

!Q 7 **O41.101- Infection of amniotic sac and membranes, unspecified, first trimester**

!Q 7 **O41.102- Infection of amniotic sac and membranes, unspecified, second trimester**

!Q 7 **O41.103- Infection of amniotic sac and membranes, unspecified, third trimester**

!Q 7 **O41.109- Infection of amniotic sac and membranes, unspecified, unspecified trimester**

6 **O41.12 Chorioamnionitis**

SP 7 **O41.121- Chorioamnionitis, first trimester**

SP 7 **O41.122- Chorioamnionitis, second trimester**

SP 7 **O41.123- Chorioamnionitis, third trimester**

!Q 7 **O41.129- Chorioamnionitis, unspecified trimester**

6 **O41.14 Placentitis**

SP 7 **O41.141- Placentitis, first trimester**

SP 7 **O41.142- Placentitis, second trimester**

SP 7 **O41.143- Placentitis, third trimester**

!Q 7 **O41.149- Placentitis, unspecified trimester**

5 **O41.8 Other specified disorders of amniotic fluid and membranes**

6 **O41.8X Other specified disorders of amniotic fluid and membranes**

SP 7 **O41.8X1- Other specified disorders of amniotic fluid and membranes, first trimester**

SP 7 **O41.8X2- Other specified disorders of amniotic fluid and membranes, second trimester**

SP 7 **O41.8X3- Other specified disorders of amniotic fluid and membranes, third trimester**

!Q 7 **O41.8X9- Other specified disorders of amniotic fluid and membranes, unspecified trimester**

5 **O41.9 Disorder of amniotic fluid and membranes, unspecified**

!Q 7 **O41.90X- Disorder of amniotic fluid and membranes, unspecified, unspecified trimester**

!Q 7 **O41.91X- Disorder of amniotic fluid and membranes, unspecified, first trimester**

!Q 7 **O41.92X- Disorder of amniotic fluid and membranes, unspecified, second trimester**

!Q 7 **O41.93X- Disorder of amniotic fluid and membranes, unspecified, third trimester**

4 **O42 Premature rupture of membranes**

5 **O42.0 Premature rupture of membranes, onset of labor within 24 hours of rupture**

!Q **O42.00 Premature rupture of membranes, onset of labor within 24 hours of rupture, unspecified weeks of gestation**

6 **O42.01 Preterm premature rupture of membranes, onset of labor within 24 hours of rupture**
Premature rupture of membranes before 37 completed weeks of gestation

SP **O42.011 Preterm premature rupture of membranes, onset of labor within 24 hours of rupture, first trimester**

SP **O42.012 Preterm premature rupture of membranes, onset of labor within 24 hours of rupture, second trimester**

SP **O42.013 Preterm premature rupture of membranes, onset of labor within 24 hours of rupture, third trimester**

!Q **O42.019 Preterm premature rupture of membranes, onset of labor within 24 hours of rupture, unspecified trimester**

SP **O42.02 Full-term premature rupture of membranes, onset of labor within 24 hours of rupture**
Premature rupture of membranes at or after 37 completed weeks of gestation, onset of labor within 24 hours of rupture

5 **O42.1 Premature rupture of membranes, onset of labor more than 24 hours following rupture**

!Q **O42.10 Premature rupture of membranes, onset of labor more than 24 hours following rupture, unspecified weeks of gestation**

6 **O42.11 Preterm premature rupture of membranes, onset of labor more than 24 hours following rupture**
Premature rupture of membranes before 37 completed weeks of gestation

SP **O42.111 Preterm premature rupture of membranes, onset of labor more than 24 hours following rupture, first trimester**

SP **O42.112 Preterm premature rupture of membranes, onset of labor more than 24 hours following rupture, second trimester**

SP **O42.113 Preterm premature rupture of membranes, onset of labor more than 24 hours following rupture, third trimester**

!Q **O42.119 Preterm premature rupture of membranes, onset of labor more than 24 hours following rupture, unspecified trimester**

SP **O42.12 Full-term premature rupture of membranes, onset of labor more than 24 hours following rupture**
Premature rupture of membranes at or after 37 completed weeks of gestation, onset of labor more than 24 hours following rupture

5 **O42.9 Premature rupture of membranes, unspecified as to length of time between rupture and onset of labor**

!Q **O42.90 Premature rupture of membranes, unspecified as to length of time between rupture and onset of labor, unspecified weeks of gestation**

6 **O42.91 Preterm premature rupture of membranes, unspecified as to length of time between rupture and onset of labor**
Premature rupture of membranes before 37 completed weeks of gestation

SP **O42.911 Preterm premature rupture of membranes, unspecified as to length of time between rupture and onset of labor, first trimester**

SP **O42.912 Preterm premature rupture of membranes, unspecified as to length of time between rupture and onset of labor, second trimester**

SP **O42.913 Preterm premature rupture of membranes, unspecified as to length of time between rupture and onset of labor, third trimester**

!Q **O42.919 Preterm premature rupture of membranes, unspecified as to length of time between rupture and onset of labor, unspecified trimester**

SP **O42.92 Full-term premature rupture of membranes, unspecified as to length of time between rupture and onset of labor**
Premature rupture of membranes at or after 37 completed weeks of gestation, unspecified as to length of time between rupture and onset of labor

4 **O43 Placental disorders**

EXCLUDES 2 maternal care for poor fetal growth due to placental insufficiency (O36.5-)
placenta previa (O44.-)
placental polyp (O90.89)
placentitis (O41.14-)
premature separation of placenta [abruptio placentae] (O45.-)

5 **O43.0 Placental transfusion syndromes**

6 **O43.01 Fetomaternal placental transfusion syndrome**
Maternofetal placental transfusion syndrome

SP **O43.011 Fetomaternal placental transfusion syndrome, first trimester**

SP **O43.012 Fetomaternal placental transfusion syndrome, second trimester**

SP **O43.013 Fetomaternal placental transfusion syndrome, third trimester**

!Q **O43.019 Fetomaternal placental transfusion syndrome, unspecified trimester**

6 **O43.02 Fetus-to-fetus placental transfusion syndrome**

SP **O43.021 Fetus-to-fetus placental transfusion syndrome, first trimester**

SP **O43.022 Fetus-to-fetus placental transfusion syndrome, second trimester**

SP **O43.023 Fetus-to-fetus placental transfusion syndrome, third trimester**

!Q **O43.029 Fetus-to-fetus placental transfusion syndrome, unspecified trimester**

5 **O43.1 Malformation of placenta**

6 **O43.10 Malformation of placenta, unspecified**
Abnormal placenta NOS

!Q **O43.101 Malformation of placenta, unspecified, first trimester**

!Q **O43.102 Malformation of placenta, unspecified, second trimester**

!Q **O43.103 Malformation of placenta, unspecified, third trimester**

!Q **O43.109 Malformation of placenta, unspecified, unspecified trimester**

6 **O43.11 Circumvallate placenta**

SP **O43.111 Circumvallate placenta, first trimester**

SP **O43.112 Circumvallate placenta, second trimester**

Chapter 15

O00-O9A

SP **O43.113 Circumvallate placenta, third trimester**
!Q **O43.119 Circumvallate placenta, unspecified trimester**
6 **O43.12 Velamentous insertion of umbilical cord**
SP **O43.121 Velamentous insertion of umbilical cord, first trimester**
SP **O43.122 Velamentous insertion of umbilical cord, second trimester**
SP **O43.123 Velamentous insertion of umbilical cord, third trimester**
!Q **O43.129 Velamentous insertion of umbilical cord, unspecified trimester**
6 **O43.19 Other malformation of placenta**
SP **O43.191 Other malformation of placenta, first trimester**
SP **O43.192 Other malformation of placenta, second trimester**
SP **O43.193 Other malformation of placenta, third trimester**
!Q **O43.199 Other malformation of placenta, unspecified trimester**
5 **O43.2 Morbidly adherent placenta**
Code also:
associated third stage postpartum hemorrhage, if applicable (O72.0)
EXCLUDES 1 retained placenta (O73.-)
6 **O43.21 Placenta accreta**
SP **O43.211 Placenta accreta, first trimester**
SP **O43.212 Placenta accreta, second trimester**
SP **O43.213 Placenta accreta, third trimester**
!Q **O43.219 Placenta accreta, unspecified trimester**
6 **O43.22 Placenta increta**
SP **O43.221 Placenta increta, first trimester**
SP **O43.222 Placenta increta, second trimester**
SP **O43.223 Placenta increta, third trimester**
!Q **O43.229 Placenta increta, unspecified trimester**
6 **O43.23 Placenta percreta**
SP **O43.231 Placenta percreta, first trimester**
SP **O43.232 Placenta percreta, second trimester**
SP **O43.233 Placenta percreta, third trimester**
!Q **O43.239 Placenta percreta, unspecified trimester**
5 **O43.8 Other placental disorders**
6 **O43.81 Placental infarction**
SP **O43.811 Placental infarction, first trimester**
SP **O43.812 Placental infarction, second trimester**
SP **O43.813 Placental infarction, third trimester**
!Q **O43.819 Placental infarction, unspecified trimester**
6 **O43.89 Other placental disorders**
Placental dysfunction
SP **O43.891 Other placental disorders, first trimester**
SP **O43.892 Other placental disorders, second trimester**
SP **O43.893 Other placental disorders, third trimester**
!Q **O43.899 Other placental disorders, unspecified trimester**
5 **O43.9 Unspecified placental disorder**
!Q **O43.90 Unspecified placental disorder, unspecified trimester**
!Q **O43.91 Unspecified placental disorder, first trimester**
!Q **O43.92 Unspecified placental disorder, second trimester**
!Q **O43.93 Unspecified placental disorder, third trimester**
4 **O44 Placenta previa**
5 **O44.0 Complete placenta previa NOS or without hemorrhage**
Placenta previa NOS
!Q **O44.00 Complete placenta previa NOS or without hemorrhage, unspecified trimester**
SP **O44.01 Complete placenta previa NOS or without hemorrhage, first trimester**
SP **O44.02 Complete placenta previa NOS or without hemorrhage, second trimester**
SP **O44.03 Complete placenta previa NOS or without hemorrhage, third trimester**
5 **O44.1 Complete placenta previa with hemorrhage**
EXCLUDES 1 labor and delivery complicated by hemorrhage from vasa previa (O69.4)
!Q **O44.10 Complete placenta previa with hemorrhage, unspecified trimester**
SP **O44.11 Complete placenta previa with hemorrhage, first trimester**
SP **O44.12 Complete placenta previa with hemorrhage, second trimester**
SP **O44.13 Complete placenta previa with hemorrhage, third trimester**
5 **O44.2 Partial placenta previa without hemorrhage**
Marginal placenta previa, NOS or without hemorrhage
!Q **O44.20 Partial placenta previa NOS or without hemorrhage, unspecified trimester**
SP **O44.21 Partial placenta previa NOS or without hemorrhage, first trimester**
SP **O44.22 Partial placenta previa NOS or without hemorrhage, second trimester**
SP **O44.23 Partial placenta previa NOS or without hemorrhage, third trimester**
5 **O44.3 Partial placenta previa with hemorrhage**
Marginal placenta previa with hemorrhage
!Q **O44.30 Partial placenta previa with hemorrhage, unspecified trimester**
SP **O44.31 Partial placenta previa with hemorrhage, first trimester**
SP **O44.32 Partial placenta previa with hemorrhage, second trimester**

SP O44.33 **Partial placenta previa with hemorrhage, third trimester**

5 O44.4 **Low lying placenta NOS or without hemorrhage**
INCLUDES Low implantation of placenta NOS or without hemorrhage

!Q O44.40 **Low lying placenta NOS or without hemorrhage, unspecified trimester**

SP O44.41 **Low lying placenta NOS or without hemorrhage, first trimester**

SP O44.42 **Low lying placenta NOS or without hemorrhage, second trimester**

SP O44.43 **Low lying placenta NOS or without hemorrhage, third trimester**

5 O44.5 **Low lying placenta with hemorrhage**
Low implantation of placenta with hemorrhage

!Q O44.50 **Low lying placenta with hemorrhage, unspecified trimester**

SP O44.51 **Low lying placenta with hemorrhage, first trimester**

SP O44.52 **Low lying placenta with hemorrhage, second trimester**

SP O44.53 **Low lying placenta with hemorrhage, third trimester**

4 O45 **Premature separation of placenta [abruptio placentae]**

5 O45.0 **Premature separation of placenta with coagulation defect**

6 O45.00 **Premature separation of placenta with coagulation defect, unspecified**

!Q O45.001 **Premature separation of placenta with coagulation defect, unspecified, first trimester**

SP O45.002 **Premature separation of placenta with coagulation defect, unspecified, second trimester**

SP O45.003 **Premature separation of placenta with coagulation defect, unspecified, third trimester**

!Q O45.009 **Premature separation of placenta with coagulation defect, unspecified, unspecified trimester**

6 O45.01 **Premature separation of placenta with afibrinogenemia**
Premature separation of placenta with hypofibrinogenemia

SP O45.011 **Premature separation of placenta with afibrinogenemia, first trimester**

SP O45.012 **Premature separation of placenta with afibrinogenemia, second trimester**

SP O45.013 **Premature separation of placenta with afibrinogenemia, third trimester**

!Q O45.019 **Premature separation of placenta with afibrinogenemia, unspecified trimester**

6 O45.02 **Premature separation of placenta with disseminated intravascular coagulation**

SP O45.021 **Premature separation of placenta with disseminated intravascular coagulation, first trimester**

SP O45.022 **Premature separation of placenta with disseminated intravascular coagulation, second trimester**

SP O45.023 **Premature separation of placenta with disseminated intravascular coagulation, third trimester**

!Q O45.029 **Premature separation of placenta with disseminated intravascular coagulation, unspecified trimester**

6 O45.09 **Premature separation of placenta with other coagulation defect**

SP O45.091 **Premature separation of placenta with other coagulation defect, first trimester**

SP O45.092 **Premature separation of placenta with other coagulation defect, second trimester**

SP O45.093 **Premature separation of placenta with other coagulation defect, third trimester**

!Q O45.099 **Premature separation of placenta with other coagulation defect, unspecified trimester**

5 O45.8 **Other premature separation of placenta**

6 O45.8X **Other premature separation of placenta**

SP O45.8X1 **Other premature separation of placenta, first trimester**

SP O45.8X2 **Other premature separation of placenta, second trimester**

SP O45.8X3 **Other premature separation of placenta, third trimester**

!Q O45.8X9 **Other premature separation of placenta, unspecified trimester**

5 O45.9 **Premature separation of placenta, unspecified**
Abruptio placentae NOS

!Q O45.90 **Premature separation of placenta, unspecified, unspecified trimester**

SP O45.91 **Premature separation of placenta, unspecified, first trimester**

SP O45.92 **Premature separation of placenta, unspecified, second trimester**

SP O45.93 **Premature separation of placenta, unspecified, third trimester**

4 O46 **Antepartum hemorrhage, not elsewhere classified**
EXCLUDES 1 hemorrhage in early pregnancy (O20.-)
intrapartum hemorrhage NEC (O67.-)
placenta previa (O44.-)
premature separation of placenta [abruptio placentae] (O45.-)

5 O46.0 **Antepartum hemorrhage with coagulation defect**

6 O46.00 **Antepartum hemorrhage with coagulation defect, unspecified**

SP O46.001 **Antepartum hemorrhage with coagulation defect, unspecified, first trimester**

SP O46.002 **Antepartum hemorrhage with coagulation defect, unspecified, second trimester**

Chapter 15 O00-O9A

SP **O46.003 Antepartum hemorrhage with coagulation defect, unspecified, third trimester**

IQ **O46.009 Antepartum hemorrhage with coagulation defect, unspecified, unspecified trimester**

6 **O46.01 Antepartum hemorrhage with afibrinogenemia**
Antepartum hemorrhage with hypofibrinogenemia

SP **O46.011 Antepartum hemorrhage with afibrinogenemia, first trimester**

SP **O46.012 Antepartum hemorrhage with afibrinogenemia, second trimester**

SP **O46.013 Antepartum hemorrhage with afibrinogenemia, third trimester**

IQ **O46.019 Antepartum hemorrhage with afibrinogenemia, unspecified trimester**

6 **O46.02 Antepartum hemorrhage with disseminated intravascular coagulation**

SP **O46.021 Antepartum hemorrhage with disseminated intravascular coagulation, first trimester**

SP **O46.022 Antepartum hemorrhage with disseminated intravascular coagulation, second trimester**

SP **O46.023 Antepartum hemorrhage with disseminated intravascular coagulation, third trimester**

IQ **O46.029 Antepartum hemorrhage with disseminated intravascular coagulation, unspecified trimester**

6 **O46.09 Antepartum hemorrhage with other coagulation defect**

SP **O46.091 Antepartum hemorrhage with other coagulation defect, first trimester**

SP **O46.092 Antepartum hemorrhage with other coagulation defect, second trimester**

SP **O46.093 Antepartum hemorrhage with other coagulation defect, third trimester**

IQ **O46.099 Antepartum hemorrhage with other coagulation defect, unspecified trimester**

5 **O46.8 Other antepartum hemorrhage**

6 **O46.8X Other antepartum hemorrhage**

SP **O46.8X1 Other antepartum hemorrhage, first trimester**

SP **O46.8X2 Other antepartum hemorrhage, second trimester**

SP **O46.8X3 Other antepartum hemorrhage, third trimester**

IQ **O46.8X9 Other antepartum hemorrhage, unspecified trimester**

5 **O46.9 Antepartum hemorrhage, unspecified**

IQ **O46.90 Antepartum hemorrhage, unspecified, unspecified trimester**

SP **O46.91 Antepartum hemorrhage, unspecified, first trimester**

SP **O46.92 Antepartum hemorrhage, unspecified, second trimester**

SP **O46.93 Antepartum hemorrhage, unspecified, third trimester**

4 **O47 False labor**
INCLUDES Braxton Hicks contractions
threatened labor
EXCLUDES 1 preterm labor (O60.-)

5 **O47.0 False labor before 37 completed weeks of gestation**

IQ **O47.00 False labor before 37 completed weeks of gestation, unspecified trimester**

SP **O47.02 False labor before 37 completed weeks of gestation, second trimester**

SP **O47.03 False labor before 37 completed weeks of gestation, third trimester**

SP **O47.1 False labor at or after 37 completed weeks of gestation**

IQ **O47.9 False labor, unspecified**

4 **O48 Late pregnancy**

SP **O48.0 Post-term pregnancy**
Pregnancy over 40 completed weeks to 42 completed weeks gestation

SP **O48.1 Prolonged pregnancy**
Pregnancy which has advanced beyond 42 completed weeks gestation

Complications of labor and delivery (O60-O77)

4 **O60 Preterm labor**
INCLUDES onset (spontaneous) of labor before 37 completed weeks of gestation
EXCLUDES 1 false labor (O47.0-)
threatened labor NOS (O47.0-)

5 **O60.0 Preterm labor without delivery**

IQ **O60.00 Preterm labor without delivery, unspecified trimester**

SP **O60.02 Preterm labor without delivery, second trimester**

SP **O60.03 Preterm labor without delivery, third trimester**

5 **O60.1 Preterm labor with preterm delivery**

One of the following 7th characters is to be assigned to each code under subcategory O60.1. 7th character 0 is for single gestations and multiple gestations where the fetus is unspecified. 7th characters 1 through 9 are for cases of multiple gestations to identify the fetus for which the code applies. The appropriate code from category O30, Multiple gestation, must also be assigned when assigning a code from subcategory O60.1 that has a 7th character of 1 through 9.

0	not applicable or unspecified
1	fetus 1
2	fetus 2
3	fetus 3
4	fetus 4
5	fetus 5
9	other fetus

IQ 7 **O60.10X- Preterm labor with preterm delivery, unspecified trimester**
Preterm labor with delivery NOS

Chapter 15

O00-O9A

4 4th digit required 5 5th digit required 6 6th digit required 7 7th digit required 7th digit placeholder + Additional code Laterality

SP 7 **O60.12X- Preterm labor second trimester with preterm delivery second trimester**

SP 7 **O60.13X- Preterm labor second trimester with preterm delivery third trimester**

SP 7 **O60.14X- Preterm labor third trimester with preterm delivery third trimester**

5 **O60.2 Term delivery with preterm labor**

One of the following 7th characters is to be assigned to each code under subcategory O60.2. 7th character 0 is for single gestations and multiple gestations where the fetus is unspecified. 7th characters 1 through 9 are for cases of multiple gestations to identify the fetus for which the code applies. The appropriate code from category O30, Multiple gestation, must also be assigned when assigning a code from subcategory O60.2 that has a 7th character of 1 through 9.

0 not applicable or unspecified
1 fetus 1
2 fetus 2
3 fetus 3
4 fetus 4
5 fetus 5
9 other fetus

IQ 7 **O60.20X- Term delivery with preterm labor, unspecified trimester**

SP 7 **O60.22X- Term delivery with preterm labor, second trimester**

SP 7 **O60.23X- Term delivery with preterm labor, third trimester**

4 **O61 Failed induction of labor**

IQ **O61.0 Failed medical induction of labor**
Failed induction (of labor) by oxytocin
Failed induction (of labor) by prostaglandins

IQ **O61.1 Failed instrumental induction of labor**
Failed mechanical induction (of labor)
Failed surgical induction (of labor)

IQ **O61.8 Other failed induction of labor**

IQ **O61.9 Failed induction of labor, unspecified**

4 **O62 Abnormalities of forces of labor**

IQ **O62.0 Primary inadequate contractions**
Failure of cervical dilatation
Primary hypotonic uterine dysfunction
Uterine inertia during latent phase of labor

IQ **O62.1 Secondary uterine inertia**
Arrested active phase of labor
Secondary hypotonic uterine dysfunction

IQ **O62.2 Other uterine inertia**
Atony of uterus without hemorrhage
Atony of uterus NOS
Desultory labor
Hypotonic uterine dysfunction NOS
Irregular labor
Poor contractions
Slow slope active phase of labor
Uterine inertia NOS

EXCLUDES 1 atony of uterus with hemorrhage (postpartum) (O72.1)
postpartum atony of uterus without hemorrhage (O75.89)

IQ **O62.3 Precipitate labor**

DEFINITION Labor occurring quickly, with rapid expulsion of the fetus.

IQ **O62.4 Hypertonic, incoordinate, and prolonged uterine contractions**
Cervical spasm
Contraction ring dystocia
Dyscoordinate labor
Hour-glass contraction of uterus
Hypertonic uterine dysfunction
Incoordinate uterine action
Tetanic contractions
Uterine dystocia NOS
Uterine spasm

EXCLUDES 1 dystocia (fetal) (maternal) NOS (O66.9)

IQ **O62.8 Other abnormalities of forces of labor**

IQ **O62.9 Abnormality of forces of labor, unspecified**

4 **O63 Long labor**

IQ **O63.0 Prolonged first stage (of labor)**

IQ **O63.1 Prolonged second stage (of labor)**

IQ **O63.2 Delayed delivery of second twin, triplet, etc.**

IQ **O63.9 Long labor, unspecified**
Prolonged labor NOS

4 **O64 Obstructed labor due to malposition and malpresentation of fetus**

One of the following 7th characters is to be assigned to each code under category O64. 7th character 0 is for single gestations and multiple gestations where the fetus is unspecified. 7th characters 1 through 9 are for cases of multiple gestations to identify the fetus for which the code applies. The appropriate code from category O30, Multiple gestation, must also be assigned when assigning a code from category O64 that has a 7th character of 1 through 9.

0 not applicable or unspecified
1 fetus 1
2 fetus 2
3 fetus 3
4 fetus 4
5 fetus 5
9 other fetus

IQ 7 **O64.0XX- Obstructed labor due to incomplete rotation of fetal head**
Deep transverse arrest
Obstructed labor due to persistent occipitoiliac (position)
Obstructed labor due to persistent occipitoposterior (position)
Obstructed labor due to persistent occipitosacral (position)
Obstructed labor due to persistent occipitotransverse (position)

IQ 7 **O64.1XX- Obstructed labor due to breech presentation**
Obstructed labor due to buttocks presentation
Obstructed labor due to complete breech presentation

Chapter 15
O00-O9A

Obstructed labor due to frank breech presentation

!Q ☑ O64.2XX- Obstructed labor due to face presentation

Obstructed labor due to chin presentation

!Q ☑ O64.3XX- Obstructed labor due to brow presentation

!Q ☑ O64.4XX- Obstructed labor due to shoulder presentation

Prolapsed arm

EXCLUDES 1 impacted shoulders (O66.0)
shoulder dystocia (O66.0)

!Q ☑ O64.5XX- Obstructed labor due to compound presentation

!Q ☑ O64.8XX- Obstructed labor due to other malposition and malpresentation

Obstructed labor due to footling presentation

Obstructed labor due to incomplete breech presentation

!Q ☑ O64.9XX- Obstructed labor due to malposition and malpresentation, unspecified

4 O65 Obstructed labor due to maternal pelvic abnormality

!Q O65.0 Obstructed labor due to deformed pelvis

!Q O65.1 Obstructed labor due to generally contracted pelvis

!Q O65.2 Obstructed labor due to pelvic inlet contraction

!Q O65.3 Obstructed labor due to pelvic outlet and mid-cavity contraction

!Q O65.4 Obstructed labor due to fetopelvic disproportion, unspecified

EXCLUDES 1 dystocia due to abnormality of fetus (O66.2-O66.3)

!Q + O65.5 Obstructed labor due to abnormality of maternal pelvic organs

Obstructed labor due to conditions listed in O34.-

Use additional code to identify abnormality of pelvic organs O34.-

!Q O65.8 Obstructed labor due to other maternal pelvic abnormalities

!Q O65.9 Obstructed labor due to maternal pelvic abnormality, unspecified

4 O66 Other obstructed labor

!Q O66.0 Obstructed labor due to shoulder dystocia

Impacted shoulders

DEFINITION Shoulders of the fetus become caught in the pelvis during delivery.

!Q O66.1 Obstructed labor due to locked twins

!Q O66.2 Obstructed labor due to unusually large fetus

!Q + O66.3 Obstructed labor due to other abnormalities of fetus

Dystocia due to fetal ascites
Dystocia due to fetal hydrops
Dystocia due to fetal meningomyelocele
Dystocia due to fetal sacral teratoma
Dystocia due to fetal tumor
Dystocia due to hydrocephalic fetus

Use additional code to identify cause of obstruction

5 O66.4 Failed trial of labor

!Q O66.40 Failed trial of labor, unspecified

!Q O66.41 Failed attempted vaginal birth after previous cesarean delivery

Code first:
rupture of uterus, if applicable (O71.0-, O71.1)

!Q O66.5 Attempted application of vacuum extractor and forceps

Attempted application of vacuum or forceps, with subsequent delivery by forceps or cesarean delivery

!Q O66.6 Obstructed labor due to other multiple fetuses

!Q + O66.8 Other specified obstructed labor

Use additional code to identify cause of obstruction

!Q O66.9 Obstructed labor, unspecified

Dystocia NOS
Fetal dystocia NOS
Maternal dystocia NOS

4 O67 Labor and delivery complicated by intrapartum hemorrhage, not elsewhere classified

EXCLUDES 1 antepartum hemorrhage NEC (O46.-)
placenta previa (O44.-)
premature separation of placenta [abruptio placentae] (O45.-)

EXCLUDES 2 postpartum hemorrhage (O72.-)

SP O67.0 Intrapartum hemorrhage with coagulation defect

Intrapartum hemorrhage (excessive) associated with afibrinogenemia
Intrapartum hemorrhage (excessive) associated with disseminated intravascular coagulation
Intrapartum hemorrhage (excessive) associated with hyperfibrinolysis
Intrapartum hemorrhage (excessive) associated with hypofibrinogenemia

SP O67.8 Other intrapartum hemorrhage

Excessive intrapartum hemorrhage

SP O67.9 Intrapartum hemorrhage, unspecified

SP O68 Labor and delivery complicated by abnormality of fetal acid-base balance

Fetal acidemia complicating labor and delivery
Fetal acidosis complicating labor and delivery
Fetal alkalosis complicating labor and delivery
Fetal metabolic acidemia complicating labor and delivery

EXCLUDES 1 fetal stress NOS (O77.9)
labor and delivery complicated by electrocardiographic evidence of fetal stress (O77.8)
labor and delivery complicated by ultrasonic evidence of fetal stress (O77.8)

EXCLUDES 2 abnormality in fetal heart rate or rhythm (O76)

labor and delivery complicated by meconium in amniotic fluid (O77.0)

4 O69 **Labor and delivery complicated by umbilical cord complications**

One of the following 7th characters is to be assigned to each code under category O69. 7th character 0 is for single gestations and multiple gestations where the fetus is unspecified. 7th characters 1 through 9 are for cases of multiple gestations to identify the fetus for which the code applies. The appropriate code from category O30, Multiple gestation, must also be assigned when assigning a code from category O69 that has a 7th character of 1 through 9.

0	not applicable or unspecified
1	fetus 1
2	fetus 2
3	fetus 3
4	fetus 4
5	fetus 5
9	other fetus

!Q 7 O69.0XX- **Labor and delivery complicated by prolapse of cord**

!Q 7 O69.1XX- **Labor and delivery complicated by cord around neck, with compression**

EXCLUDES 1 labor and delivery complicated by cord around neck, without compression (O69.81)

!Q 7 O69.2XX- **Labor and delivery complicated by other cord entanglement, with compression**

Labor and delivery complicated by compression of cord NOS

Labor and delivery complicated by entanglement of cords of twins in monoamniotic sac

Labor and delivery complicated by knot in cord

EXCLUDES 1 labor and delivery complicated by other cord entanglement, without compression (O69.82)

!Q 7 O69.3XX- **Labor and delivery complicated by short cord**

!Q 7 O69.4XX- **Labor and delivery complicated by vasa previa**

Labor and delivery complicated by hemorrhage from vasa previa

!Q 7 O69.5XX- **Labor and delivery complicated by vascular lesion of cord**

Labor and delivery complicated by cord bruising

Labor and delivery complicated by cord hematoma

Labor and delivery complicated by thrombosis of umbilical vessels

5 O69.8 **Labor and delivery complicated by other cord complications**

!Q 7 O69.81X- **Labor and delivery complicated by cord around neck, without compression**

!Q 7 O69.82X- **Labor and delivery complicated by other cord entanglement, without compression**

!Q 7 O69.89X- **Labor and delivery complicated by other cord complications**

SP !Q 7 O69.9XX- **Labor and delivery complicated by cord complication, unspecified**

4 O70 **Perineal laceration during delivery**

INCLUDES episiotomy extended by laceration

EXCLUDES 1 obstetric high vaginal laceration alone (O71.4)

SP O70.0 **First degree perineal laceration during delivery**

Perineal laceration, rupture or tear involving fourchette during delivery

Perineal laceration, rupture or tear involving labia during delivery

Perineal laceration, rupture or tear involving skin during delivery

Perineal laceration, rupture or tear involving vagina during delivery

Perineal laceration, rupture or tear involving vulva during delivery

Slight perineal laceration, rupture or tear during delivery

SP O70.1 **Second degree perineal laceration during delivery**

Perineal laceration, rupture or tear during delivery as in O70.0, also involving pelvic floor

Perineal laceration, rupture or tear during delivery as in O70.0, also involving perineal muscles

Perineal laceration, rupture or tear during delivery as in O70.0, also involving vaginal muscles

EXCLUDES 1 perineal laceration involving anal sphincter (O70.2)

5 O70.2 **Third degree perineal laceration during delivery**

Perineal laceration, rupture or tear during delivery as in O70.1, also involving anal sphincter

Perineal laceration, rupture or tear during delivery as in O70.1, also involving rectovaginal septum

Perineal laceration, rupture or tear during delivery as in O70.1, also involving sphincter NOS

EXCLUDES 1 anal sphincter tear during delivery without third degree perineal laceration (O70.4)

perineal laceration involving anal or rectal mucosa (O70.3)

SP O70.20 **Third degree perineal laceration during delivery, unspecified**

SP O70.21 **Third degree perineal laceration during delivery, IIIa**

Third degree perineal laceration during delivery with less than 50% of external anal sphincter (EAS) thickness torn

Chapter 15

O00-O9A

SP **O70.22 Third degree perineal laceration during delivery, IIIb**
Third degree perineal laceration during delivery with more than 50% external anal sphincter (EAS) thickness torn

SP **O70.23 Third degree perineal laceration during delivery, IIIc**
Third degree perineal laceration during delivery with both external anal sphincter (EAS) and internal anal sphincter (IAS) torn

SP **O70.3 Fourth degree perineal laceration during delivery**
Perineal laceration, rupture or tear during delivery as in O70.2, also involving anal mucosa
Perineal laceration, rupture or tear during delivery as in O70.2, also involving rectal mucosa

SP **O70.4 Anal sphincter tear complicating delivery, not associated with third degree laceration**
EXCLUDES 1 anal sphincter tear with third degree perineal laceration (O70.2)

SP **O70.9 Perineal laceration during delivery, unspecified**

4 **O71 Other obstetric trauma**
INCLUDES obstetric damage from instruments

5 **O71.0 Rupture of uterus (spontaneous) before onset of labor**
EXCLUDES 1 disruption of (current) cesarean delivery wound (O90.0)
laceration of uterus, NEC (O71.81)

IQ **O71.00 Rupture of uterus before onset of labor, unspecified trimester**

SP **O71.02 Rupture of uterus before onset of labor, second trimester**

SP **O71.03 Rupture of uterus before onset of labor, third trimester**

SP **O71.1 Rupture of uterus during labor**
Rupture of uterus not stated as occurring before onset of labor
EXCLUDES 1 disruption of cesarean delivery wound (O90.0)
laceration of uterus, NEC (O71.81)

SP **O71.2 Postpartum inversion of uterus**

SP **O71.3 Obstetric laceration of cervix**
Annular detachment of cervix

SP **O71.4 Obstetric high vaginal laceration alone**
Laceration of vaginal wall without perineal laceration
EXCLUDES 1 obstetric high vaginal laceration with perineal laceration (O70.-)

SP **O71.5 Other obstetric injury to pelvic organs**
Obstetric injury to bladder
Obstetric injury to urethra
EXCLUDES 2 obstetric periurethral trauma (O71.82)

SP **O71.6 Obstetric damage to pelvic joints and ligaments**
Obstetric avulsion of inner symphyseal cartilage
Obstetric damage to coccyx
Obstetric traumatic separation of symphysis (pubis)

SP **O71.7 Obstetric hematoma of pelvis**
Obstetric hematoma of perineum
Obstetric hematoma of vagina
Obstetric hematoma of vulva

5 **O71.8 Other specified obstetric trauma**

SP **O71.81 Laceration of uterus, not elsewhere classified**

SP **O71.82 Other specified trauma to perineum and vulva**
Obstetric periurethral trauma

SP **O71.89 Other specified obstetric trauma**

IQ **O71.9 Obstetric trauma, unspecified**

4 **O72 Postpartum hemorrhage**
INCLUDES hemorrhage after delivery of fetus or infant

SP **O72.0 Third-stage hemorrhage**
Hemorrhage associated with retained, trapped or adherent placenta
Retained placenta NOS
Code also:
type of adherent placenta (O43.2-)

SP **O72.1 Other immediate postpartum hemorrhage**
Hemorrhage following delivery of placenta
Postpartum hemorrhage (atonic) NOS
Uterine atony with hemorrhage
EXCLUDES 1 uterine atony NOS (O62.2)
uterine atony without hemorrhage (O62.2)
postpartum atony of uterus without hemorrhage (O75.89)

SP **O72.2 Delayed and secondary postpartum hemorrhage**
Hemorrhage associated with retained portions of placenta or membranes after the first 24 hours following delivery of placenta
Retained products of conception NOS, following delivery

SP **O72.3 Postpartum coagulation defects**
Postpartum afibrinogenemia
Postpartum fibrinolysis

4 **O73 Retained placenta and membranes, without hemorrhage**
EXCLUDES 1 placenta accreta (O43.21-)
placenta increta (O43.22-)
placenta percreta (O43.23-)

SP **O73.0 Retained placenta without hemorrhage**
Adherent placenta, without hemorrhage
Trapped placenta without hemorrhage

SP **O73.1 Retained portions of placenta and membranes, without hemorrhage**
Retained products of conception following delivery, without hemorrhage

+ 4 **O74 Complications of anesthesia during labor and delivery**
INCLUDES maternal complications arising from the administration of a general, regional or local anesthetic, analgesic or other sedation during labor and delivery

Chapter 15

O00-O9A

Use additional code, if applicable, to identify specific complication

SP + O74.0 **Aspiration pneumonitis due to anesthesia during labor and delivery**
Inhalation of stomach contents or secretions NOS due to anesthesia during labor and delivery
Mendelson's syndrome due to anesthesia during labor and delivery

SP + O74.1 **Other pulmonary complications of anesthesia during labor and delivery**

SP + O74.2 **Cardiac complications of anesthesia during labor and delivery**

SP + O74.3 **Central nervous system complications of anesthesia during labor and delivery**

SP + O74.4 **Toxic reaction to local anesthesia during labor and delivery**

SP + O74.5 **Spinal and epidural anesthesia-induced headache during labor and delivery**

SP + O74.6 **Other complications of spinal and epidural anesthesia during labor and delivery**

SP + O74.7 **Failed or difficult intubation for anesthesia during labor and delivery**

SP + O74.8 **Other complications of anesthesia during labor and delivery**

IQ + O74.9 **Complication of anesthesia during labor and delivery, unspecified**

4 O75 **Other complications of labor and delivery, not elsewhere classified**
EXCLUDES 2 puerperal (postpartum) infection (O86.-)
puerperal (postpartum) sepsis (O85)

SP O75.0 **Maternal distress during labor and delivery**

SP O75.1 **Shock during or following labor and delivery**
Obstetric shock following labor and delivery

SP O75.2 **Pyrexia during labor, not elsewhere classified**

SP + O75.3 **Other infection during labor**
Sepsis during labor
Use additional code (B95-B97), to identify infectious agent

SP + O75.4 **Other complications of obstetric surgery and procedures**
Cardiac arrest following obstetric surgery or procedures
Cardiac failure following obstetric surgery or procedures
Cerebral anoxia following obstetric surgery or procedures
Pulmonary edema following obstetric surgery or procedures
Use additional code to identify specific complication
EXCLUDES 2 complications of anesthesia during labor and delivery (O74.-)
disruption of obstetrical (surgical) wound (O90.0-O90.1)
hematoma of obstetrical (surgical) wound (O90.2)
infection of obstetrical (surgical) wound (O86.0-)

SP O75.5 **Delayed delivery after artificial rupture of membranes**

5 O75.8 **Other specified complications of labor and delivery**

SP O75.81 **Maternal exhaustion complicating labor and delivery**

IQ O75.82 **Onset (spontaneous) of labor after 37 completed weeks of gestation but before 39 completed weeks gestation, with delivery by (planned) cesarean section**
Delivery by (planned) cesarean section occurring after 37 completed weeks of gestation but before 39 completed weeks gestation due to (spontaneous) onset of labor
Code first to specify reason for planned cesarean section such as:
cephalopelvic disproportion (normally formed fetus) (O33.9)
previous cesarean delivery (O34.21)

SP O75.89 **Other specified complications of labor and delivery**

IQ O75.9 **Complication of labor and delivery, unspecified**

SP O76 **Abnormality in fetal heart rate and rhythm complicating labor and delivery**
Depressed fetal heart rate tones complicating labor and delivery
Fetal bradycardia complicating labor and delivery
Fetal heart rate decelerations complicating labor and delivery
Fetal heart rate irregularity complicating labor and delivery
Fetal heart rate abnormal variability complicating labor and delivery
Fetal tachycardia complicating labor and delivery
Non-reassuring fetal heart rate or rhythm complicating labor and delivery
EXCLUDES 1 fetal stress NOS (O77.9)
labor and delivery complicated by electrocardiographic evidence of fetal stress (O77.8)
labor and delivery complicated by ultrasonic evidence of fetal stress (O77.8)
EXCLUDES 2 fetal metabolic acidemia (O68)
other fetal stress (O77.0-O77.1)

4 O77 **Other fetal stress complicating labor and delivery**

SP O77.0 **Labor and delivery complicated by meconium in amniotic fluid**

SP O77.1 **Fetal stress in labor or delivery due to drug administration**

SP O77.8 **Labor and delivery complicated by other evidence of fetal stress**
Labor and delivery complicated by electrocardiographic evidence of fetal stress
Labor and delivery complicated by ultrasonic evidence of fetal stress
EXCLUDES 1 abnormality of fetal acid-base balance (O68)
abnormality in fetal heart rate or rhythm (O76)

Chapter 15

O00-O9A

fetal metabolic acidemia (O68)

IQ O77.9 Labor and delivery complicated by fetal stress, unspecified

EXCLUDES 1 abnormality of fetal acid-base balance (O68)
abnormality in fetal heart rate or rhythm (O76)
fetal metabolic acidemia (O68)

Encounter for delivery (O80-O82)

IQ + O80 Encounter for full-term uncomplicated delivery
Delivery requiring minimal or no assistance, with or without episiotomy, without fetal manipulation [e.g., rotation version] or instrumentation [forceps] of a spontaneous, cephalic, vaginal, full-term, single, live-born infant. This code is for use as a single diagnosis code and is not to be used with any other code from chapter 15.
Use additional code to indicate outcome of delivery (Z37.0)

IQ + O82 Encounter for cesarean delivery without indication
Use additional code to indicate outcome of delivery (Z37.0)

Complications predominantly related to the puerperium (O85-O92)

EXCLUDES 2 mental and behavioral disorders associated with the puerperium (F53.-)
obstetrical tetanus (A34)
puerperal osteomalacia (M83.0)

GUIDELINES **Section I.C.15.a.2)**
Chapter 15 codes are to be used only on the maternal record, never on the record of the newborn.

SP + O85 Puerperal sepsis
Postpartum sepsis
Puerperal peritonitis
Puerperal pyemia
Use additional code (B95-B97), to identify infectious agent
Use additional code (R65.2-) to identify severe sepsis, if applicable
EXCLUDES 1 fever of unknown origin following delivery (O86.4)
genital tract infection following delivery (O86.1-)
obstetric pyemic and septic embolism (O88.3-)
puerperal septic thrombophlebitis (O86.81)
urinary tract infection following delivery (O86.2-)
EXCLUDES 2 sepsis during labor (O75.3)

+ 4 O86 Other puerperal infections
Use additional code (B95-B97), to identify infectious agent
EXCLUDES 2 infection during labor (O75.3)
obstetrical tetanus (A34)

GUIDELINES **Section I.C.1.d.5)(b-c)**
For infections following a procedure, a code from T81.40, to T81.43 Infection following a procedure, or a code from O86.00 to O86.03, Infection of obstetric surgical wound, that identifies the site of the infection should be coded first, if known. Assign an additional code for sepsis following a procedure (T81.44) or sepsis following an obstetrical procedure (O86.04). Use an additional code to identify the infectious agent. If the patient has severe sepsis, the appropriate code from subcategory R65.2 should also be assigned with the additional code(s) for any acute organ dysfunction.

If a postprocedural infection has resulted in postprocedural septic shock, assign the codes indicated above for sepsis due to a postprocedural infection, followed by code T81.12-, Postprocedural septic shock. Do not assign code R65.21, Severe sepsis with septic shock. Additional code(s) should be assigned for any acute organ dysfunction.

+ 5 O86.0 Infection of obstetric surgical wound
Infected cesarean delivery wound following delivery
Infected perineal repair following delivery
EXCLUDES 1 complications of procedures, not elsewhere classified (T81.4-)
postprocedural fever NOS (R50.82)
postprocedural retroperitoneal abscess (K68.11)

SP + O86.00 Infection of obstetric surgical wound, unspecified

SP + O86.01 Infection of obstetric surgical wound, superficial incisional site
Subcutaneous abscess following an obstetrical procedure
Stitch abscess following an obstetrical procedure

SP + O86.02 Infection of obstetric surgical wound, deep incisional site
Intramuscular abscess following an obstetrical procedure
Sub-fascial abscess following an obstetrical procedure

SP + O86.03 Infection of obstetric surgical wound, organ and space site
Intraabdominal abscess following an obstetrical procedure
Subphrenic abscess following an obstetrical procedure

SP + O86.04 Sepsis following an obstetrical procedure
Use additional code to identify the sepsis

SP + O86.09 Infection of obstetric surgical wound, other surgical site

+ 5 O86.1 Other infection of genital tract following delivery

SP + O86.11 Cervicitis following delivery

SP + O86.12 Endometritis following delivery

SP + O86.13 Vaginitis following delivery

Chapter 15 O00-O9A

4 4th digit required 5 5th digit required 6 6th digit required 7 7th digit required 7th digit placeholder + Additional code Laterality

SP + **O86.19 Other infection of genital tract following delivery**

+ 5 **O86.2 Urinary tract infection following delivery**

SP + **O86.20 Urinary tract infection following delivery, unspecified**

Puerperal urinary tract infection NOS

SP + **O86.21 Infection of kidney following delivery**

SP + **O86.22 Infection of bladder following delivery**

Infection of urethra following delivery

SP + **O86.29 Other urinary tract infection following delivery**

SP + **O86.4 Pyrexia of unknown origin following delivery**

Puerperal infection NOS following delivery

Puerperal pyrexia NOS following delivery

EXCLUDES 2 pyrexia during labor (O75.2)

+ 5 **O86.8 Other specified puerperal infections**

SP + **O86.81 Puerperal septic thrombophlebitis**

SP + **O86.89 Other specified puerperal infections**

4 **O87 Venous complications and hemorrhoids in the puerperium**

INCLUDES venous complications in labor, delivery and the puerperium

EXCLUDES 2 obstetric embolism (O88.-)
puerperal septic thrombophlebitis (O86.81)
venous complications in pregnancy (O22.-)

SP **O87.0 Superficial thrombophlebitis in the puerperium**

Puerperal phlebitis NOS

Puerperal thrombosis NOS

SP + **O87.1 Deep phlebothrombosis in the puerperium**

Deep vein thrombosis, postpartum

Pelvic thrombophlebitis, postpartum

Use additional code to identify the deep vein thrombosis (I82.4-, I82.5-, I82.62-, I82.72-)

Use additional code, if applicable, for associated long-term (current) use of anticoagulants (Z79.01)

SP **O87.2 Hemorrhoids in the puerperium**

SP **O87.3 Cerebral venous thrombosis in the puerperium**

Cerebrovenous sinus thrombosis in the puerperium

SP **O87.4 Varicose veins of lower extremity in the puerperium**

SP **O87.8 Other venous complications in the puerperium**

Genital varices in the puerperium

SP **O87.9 Venous complication in the puerperium, unspecified**

Puerperal phlebopathy NOS

4 **O88 Obstetric embolism**

EXCLUDES 1 embolism complicating abortion NOS (O03.2)
embolism complicating ectopic or molar pregnancy (O08.2)
embolism complicating failed attempted abortion (O07.2)
embolism complicating induced abortion (O04.7)
embolism complicating spontaneous abortion (O03.2, O03.7)

5 **O88.0 Obstetric air embolism**

6 **O88.01 Obstetric air embolism in pregnancy**

SP **O88.011 Air embolism in pregnancy, first trimester**

SP **O88.012 Air embolism in pregnancy, second trimester**

SP **O88.013 Air embolism in pregnancy, third trimester**

SP **O88.019 Air embolism in pregnancy, unspecified trimester**

SP **O88.02 Air embolism in childbirth**

SP **O88.03 Air embolism in the puerperium**

5 **O88.1 Amniotic fluid embolism**

Anaphylactoid syndrome in pregnancy

6 **O88.11 Amniotic fluid embolism in pregnancy**

SP **O88.111 Amniotic fluid embolism in pregnancy, first trimester**

SP **O88.112 Amniotic fluid embolism in pregnancy, second trimester**

SP **O88.113 Amniotic fluid embolism in pregnancy, third trimester**

SP **O88.119 Amniotic fluid embolism in pregnancy, unspecified trimester**

SP **O88.12 Amniotic fluid embolism in childbirth**

SP **O88.13 Amniotic fluid embolism in the puerperium**

5 **O88.2 Obstetric thromboembolism**

6 **O88.21 Thromboembolism in pregnancy**

Obstetric (pulmonary) embolism NOS

SP **O88.211 Thromboembolism in pregnancy, first trimester**

SP **O88.212 Thromboembolism in pregnancy, second trimester**

SP **O88.213 Thromboembolism in pregnancy, third trimester**

SP **O88.219 Thromboembolism in pregnancy, unspecified trimester**

SP **O88.22 Thromboembolism in childbirth**

SP **O88.23 Thromboembolism in the puerperium**

Puerperal (pulmonary) embolism NOS

5 **O88.3 Obstetric pyemic and septic embolism**

6 **O88.31 Pyemic and septic embolism in pregnancy**

SP **O88.311 Pyemic and septic embolism in pregnancy, first trimester**

SP **O88.312 Pyemic and septic embolism in pregnancy, second trimester**

SP **O88.313 Pyemic and septic embolism in pregnancy, third trimester**

SP **O88.319 Pyemic and septic embolism in pregnancy, unspecified trimester**

SP **O88.32 Pyemic and septic embolism in childbirth**

SP **O88.33 Pyemic and septic embolism in the puerperium**

5 **O88.8 Other obstetric embolism**

Obstetric fat embolism

Chapter 15

O00-O9A

6 O88.81 **Other embolism in pregnancy**

SP O88.811 **Other embolism in pregnancy, first trimester**

SP O88.812 **Other embolism in pregnancy, second trimester**

SP O88.813 **Other embolism in pregnancy, third trimester**

SP O88.819 **Other embolism in pregnancy, unspecified trimester**

SP O88.82 **Other embolism in childbirth**

SP O88.83 **Other embolism in the puerperium**

+ 4 O89 **Complications of anesthesia during the puerperium**

INCLUDES maternal complications arising from the administration of a general, regional or local anesthetic, analgesic or other sedation during the puerperium

Use additional code, if applicable, to identify specific complication

+ 5 O89.0 **Pulmonary complications of anesthesia during the puerperium**

SP + O89.01 **Aspiration pneumonitis due to anesthesia during the puerperium**

Inhalation of stomach contents or secretions NOS due to anesthesia during the puerperium

Mendelson's syndrome due to anesthesia during the puerperium

SP + O89.09 **Other pulmonary complications of anesthesia during the puerperium**

SP + O89.1 **Cardiac complications of anesthesia during the puerperium**

SP + O89.2 **Central nervous system complications of anesthesia during the puerperium**

SP + O89.3 **Toxic reaction to local anesthesia during the puerperium**

SP + O89.4 **Spinal and epidural anesthesia-induced headache during the puerperium**

SP + O89.5 **Other complications of spinal and epidural anesthesia during the puerperium**

SP + O89.6 **Failed or difficult intubation for anesthesia during the puerperium**

SP + O89.8 **Other complications of anesthesia during the puerperium**

SP + O89.9 **Complication of anesthesia during the puerperium, unspecified**

4 O90 **Complications of the puerperium, not elsewhere classified**

SP O90.0 **Disruption of cesarean delivery wound**

Dehiscence of cesarean delivery wound

EXCLUDES 1 rupture of uterus (spontaneous) before onset of labor (O71.0-)
rupture of uterus during labor (O71.1)

SP O90.1 **Disruption of perineal obstetric wound**

Disruption of wound of episiotomy

Disruption of wound of perineal laceration

Secondary perineal tear

SP O90.2 **Hematoma of obstetric wound**

SP O90.3 **Peripartum cardiomyopathy**

Conditions in I42.- arising during pregnancy and the puerperium

EXCLUDES 1 pre-existing heart disease complicating pregnancy and the puerperium (O99.4-)

GUIDELINES **Section I.C.15.o.5)**

Pregnancy associated cardiomyopathy, code O90.3, is unique in that it may be diagnosed in the third trimester of pregnancy but may continue to progress months after delivery. For this reason, it is referred to as peripartum cardiomyopathy. Code O90.3 is only for use when the cardiomyopathy develops as a result of pregnancy in a woman who did not have pre-existing heart disease.

SP O90.4 **Postpartum acute kidney failure**

Hepatorenal syndrome following labor and delivery

SP O90.5 **Postpartum thyroiditis**

SP O90.6 **Postpartum mood disturbance**

Postpartum blues

Postpartum dysphoria

Postpartum sadness

EXCLUDES 1 postpartum depression (F53.0)
puerperal psychosis (F53.1)

5 O90.8 **Other complications of the puerperium, not elsewhere classified**

SP O90.81 **Anemia of the puerperium**

Postpartum anemia NOS

EXCLUDES 1 pre-existing anemia complicating the puerperium (O99.03)

CODING TIPS ✓ Use O90.81 for diagnosed anemia complicating the postpartum period. Use O99.01 for anemia complicating pregnancy. Use O99.03 for pre-existing anemia complicating the puerperium.

SP O90.89 **Other complications of the puerperium, not elsewhere classified**

Placental polyp

SP O90.9 **Complication of the puerperium, unspecified**

+ 4 O91 **Infections of breast associated with pregnancy, the puerperium and lactation**

Use additional code to identify infection

+ 5 O91.0 **Infection of nipple associated with pregnancy, the puerperium and lactation**

+ 6 O91.01 **Infection of nipple associated with pregnancy**

Gestational abscess of nipple

SP + O91.011 **Infection of nipple associated with pregnancy, first trimester**

SP + O91.012 **Infection of nipple associated with pregnancy, second trimester**

SP + O91.013 **Infection of nipple associated with pregnancy, third trimester**

SP + O91.019 **Infection of nipple associated with pregnancy, unspecified trimester**

SP + O91.02 **Infection of nipple associated with the puerperium**

Puerperal abscess of nipple

SP + O91.03 **Infection of nipple associated with lactation**

Abscess of nipple associated with lactation

+ 5 O91.1 **Abscess of breast associated with pregnancy, the puerperium and lactation**

+ 6 O91.11 **Abscess of breast associated with pregnancy**
Gestational mammary abscess
Gestational purulent mastitis
Gestational subareolar abscess

SP + O91.111 **Abscess of breast associated with pregnancy, first trimester**

SP + O91.112 **Abscess of breast associated with pregnancy, second trimester**

SP + O91.113 **Abscess of breast associated with pregnancy, third trimester**

SP + O91.119 **Abscess of breast associated with pregnancy, unspecified trimester**

SP + O91.12 **Abscess of breast associated with the puerperium**
Puerperal mammary abscess
Puerperal purulent mastitis
Puerperal subareolar abscess

SP + O91.13 **Abscess of breast associated with lactation**
Mammary abscess associated with lactation
Purulent mastitis associated with lactation
Subareolar abscess associated with lactation

+ 5 O91.2 **Nonpurulent mastitis associated with pregnancy, the puerperium and lactation**

+ 6 O91.21 **Nonpurulent mastitis associated with pregnancy**
Gestational interstitial mastitis
Gestational lymphangitis of breast
Gestational mastitis NOS
Gestational parenchymatous mastitis

SP + O91.211 **Nonpurulent mastitis associated with pregnancy, first trimester**

SP + O91.212 **Nonpurulent mastitis associated with pregnancy, second trimester**

SP + O91.213 **Nonpurulent mastitis associated with pregnancy, third trimester**

!Q + O91.219 **Nonpurulent mastitis associated with pregnancy, unspecified trimester**

SP + O91.22 **Nonpurulent mastitis associated with the puerperium**
Puerperal interstitial mastitis
Puerperal lymphangitis of breast
Puerperal mastitis NOS
Puerperal parenchymatous mastitis

SP + O91.23 **Nonpurulent mastitis associated with lactation**
Interstitial mastitis associated with lactation
Lymphangitis of breast associated with lactation
Mastitis NOS associated with lactation
Parenchymatous mastitis associated with lactation

4 O92 **Other disorders of breast and disorders of lactation associated with pregnancy and the puerperium**

5 O92.0 **Retracted nipple associated with pregnancy, the puerperium, and lactation**

6 O92.01 **Retracted nipple associated with pregnancy**

SP O92.011 **Retracted nipple associated with pregnancy, first trimester**

SP O92.012 **Retracted nipple associated with pregnancy, second trimester**

SP O92.013 **Retracted nipple associated with pregnancy, third trimester**

!Q O92.019 **Retracted nipple associated with pregnancy, unspecified trimester**

SP O92.02 **Retracted nipple associated with the puerperium**

SP O92.03 **Retracted nipple associated with lactation**

5 O92.1 **Cracked nipple associated with pregnancy, the puerperium, and lactation**
Fissure of nipple, gestational or puerperal

6 O92.11 **Cracked nipple associated with pregnancy**

SP O92.111 **Cracked nipple associated with pregnancy, first trimester**

SP O92.112 **Cracked nipple associated with pregnancy, second trimester**

SP O92.113 **Cracked nipple associated with pregnancy, third trimester**

!Q O92.119 **Cracked nipple associated with pregnancy, unspecified trimester**

SP O92.12 **Cracked nipple associated with the puerperium**

SP O92.13 **Cracked nipple associated with lactation**

5 O92.2 **Other and unspecified disorders of breast associated with pregnancy and the puerperium**

!Q O92.20 **Unspecified disorder of breast associated with pregnancy and the puerperium**

SP O92.29 **Other disorders of breast associated with pregnancy and the puerperium**

SP O92.3 **Agalactia**
Primary agalactia
EXCLUDES 1 Elective agalactia (O92.5)
Secondary agalactia (O92.5)
Therapeutic agalactia (O92.5)

SP O92.4 **Hypogalactia**

SP O92.5 **Suppressed lactation**
Elective agalactia
Secondary agalactia
Therapeutic agalactia
EXCLUDES 1 primary agalactia (O92.3)

SP O92.6 **Galactorrhea**

5 O92.7 **Other and unspecified disorders of lactation**

!Q O92.70 **Unspecified disorders of lactation**

SP O92.79 **Other disorders of lactation**
Puerperal galactocele

Chapter 15 O00-O9A

Other obstetric conditions, not elsewhere classified (O94-O9A)

IQ **O94 Sequelae of complication of pregnancy, childbirth, and the puerperium**
Note:
This category is to be used to indicate conditions in O00-O77.-, O85-O94 and O98-O9A.- as the cause of late effects. The sequelae include conditions specified as such, or as late effects, which may occur at any time after the puerperium
Code first:
condition resulting from (sequela) of complication of pregnancy, childbirth, and the puerperium
GUIDELINES **Section I.C.15.p.1)-3)**
Code O94 is for use in those cases when an initial complication of a pregnancy develops a sequelae requiring care or treatment at a future date. This code may be used at any time after the initial postpartum period. This code, like all sequela codes, is to be sequenced following the code describing the sequelae of the complication.

+ 4 **O98 Maternal infectious and parasitic diseases classifiable elsewhere but complicating pregnancy, childbirth and the puerperium**
INCLUDES the listed conditions when complicating the pregnant state, when aggravated by the pregnancy, or as a reason for obstetric care
Use additional code (Chapter 1), to identify specific infectious or parasitic disease
EXCLUDES 2 herpes gestationis (O26.4-)
infectious carrier state (O99.82-, O99.83-)
obstetrical tetanus (A34)
puerperal infection (O86.-)
puerperal sepsis (O85)
when the reason for maternal care is that the disease is known or suspected to have affected the fetus (O35-O36)

+ 5 **O98.0 Tuberculosis complicating pregnancy, childbirth and the puerperium**
Conditions in A15-A19
+ 6 **O98.01 Tuberculosis complicating pregnancy**
SP + **O98.011 Tuberculosis complicating pregnancy, first trimester**
SP + **O98.012 Tuberculosis complicating pregnancy, second trimester**
SP + **O98.013 Tuberculosis complicating pregnancy, third trimester**
IQ + **O98.019 Tuberculosis complicating pregnancy, unspecified trimester**
SP + **O98.02 Tuberculosis complicating childbirth**
SP + **O98.03 Tuberculosis complicating the puerperium**
+ 5 **O98.1 Syphilis complicating pregnancy, childbirth and the puerperium**
Conditions in A50-A53
+ 6 **O98.11 Syphilis complicating pregnancy**
SP + **O98.111 Syphilis complicating pregnancy, first trimester**
SP + **O98.112 Syphilis complicating pregnancy, second trimester**
SP + **O98.113 Syphilis complicating pregnancy, third trimester**
IQ + **O98.119 Syphilis complicating pregnancy, unspecified trimester**
SP + **O98.12 Syphilis complicating childbirth**
SP + **O98.13 Syphilis complicating the puerperium**
+ 5 **O98.2 Gonorrhea complicating pregnancy, childbirth and the puerperium**
Conditions in A54.-
+ 6 **O98.21 Gonorrhea complicating pregnancy**
SP + **O98.211 Gonorrhea complicating pregnancy, first trimester**
SP + **O98.212 Gonorrhea complicating pregnancy, second trimester**
SP + **O98.213 Gonorrhea complicating pregnancy, third trimester**
IQ + **O98.219 Gonorrhea complicating pregnancy, unspecified trimester**
SP + **O98.22 Gonorrhea complicating childbirth**
SP + **O98.23 Gonorrhea complicating the puerperium**
+ 5 **O98.3 Other infections with a predominantly sexual mode of transmission complicating pregnancy, childbirth and the puerperium**
Conditions in A55-A64
+ 6 **O98.31 Other infections with a predominantly sexual mode of transmission complicating pregnancy**
SP + **O98.311 Other infections with a predominantly sexual mode of transmission complicating pregnancy, first trimester**
SP + **O98.312 Other infections with a predominantly sexual mode of transmission complicating pregnancy, second trimester**
SP + **O98.313 Other infections with a predominantly sexual mode of transmission complicating pregnancy, third trimester**
IQ + **O98.319 Other infections with a predominantly sexual mode of transmission complicating pregnancy, unspecified trimester**
SP + **O98.32 Other infections with a predominantly sexual mode of transmission complicating childbirth**
SP + **O98.33 Other infections with a predominantly sexual mode of transmission complicating the puerperium**
+ 5 **O98.4 Viral hepatitis complicating pregnancy, childbirth and the puerperium**
Conditions in B15-B19
+ 6 **O98.41 Viral hepatitis complicating pregnancy**
SP + **O98.411 Viral hepatitis complicating pregnancy, first trimester**
SP + **O98.412 Viral hepatitis complicating pregnancy, second trimester**
SP + **O98.413 Viral hepatitis complicating pregnancy, third trimester**

IQ + **O98.419 Viral hepatitis complicating pregnancy, unspecified trimester**

SP + **O98.42 Viral hepatitis complicating childbirth**

SP + **O98.43 Viral hepatitis complicating the puerperium**

+ 5 **O98.5 Other viral diseases complicating pregnancy, childbirth and the puerperium**

Conditions in A80-B09, B25-B34, R87.81-, R87.82-

EXCLUDES 1 human immunodeficiency virus [HIV] disease complicating pregnancy, childbirth and the puerperium (O98.7-)

GUIDELINES **Section I.C.15.s**

During pregnancy, childbirth or the puerperium, when COVID-19 is the reason for admission/encounter , code O98.5-, Other viral diseases complicating pregnancy, childbirth and the puerperium, should be sequenced as the principal/first-listed diagnosis, and code U07.1, COVID-19, and the appropriate codes for associated manifestation(s) should be assigned as additional diagnoses. Codes from Chapter 15 always take sequencing priority.

If the reason for admission/encounter is unrelated to COVID-19 but the patient tests positive for COVID-19 during the admission/encounter, the appropriate code for the reason for admission/encounter should be sequenced as the principal/first-listed diagnosis, and codes O98.5- and U07.1, as well as the appropriate codes for associated COVID-19 manifestations, should be assigned as additional diagnoses.

+ 6 **O98.51 Other viral diseases complicating pregnancy**

SP + **O98.511 Other viral diseases complicating pregnancy, first trimester**

SP + **O98.512 Other viral diseases complicating pregnancy, second trimester**

SP + **O98.513 Other viral diseases complicating pregnancy, third trimester**

IQ + **O98.519 Other viral diseases complicating pregnancy, unspecified trimester**

SP + **O98.52 Other viral diseases complicating childbirth**

SP + **O98.53 Other viral diseases complicating the puerperium**

+ 5 **O98.6 Protozoal diseases complicating pregnancy, childbirth and the puerperium**

Conditions in B50-B64

+ 6 **O98.61 Protozoal diseases complicating pregnancy**

SP + **O98.611 Protozoal diseases complicating pregnancy, first trimester**

SP + **O98.612 Protozoal diseases complicating pregnancy, second trimester**

SP + **O98.613 Protozoal diseases complicating pregnancy, third trimester**

IQ + **O98.619 Protozoal diseases complicating pregnancy, unspecified trimester**

SP + **O98.62 Protozoal diseases complicating childbirth**

SP + **O98.63 Protozoal diseases complicating the puerperium**

+ 5 **O98.7 Human immunodeficiency virus [HIV] disease complicating pregnancy, childbirth and the puerperium**

Use additional code to identify the type of HIV disease:

Acquired immune deficiency syndrome (AIDS) (B20)

Asymptomatic HIV status (Z21)

HIV positive NOS (Z21)

Symptomatic HIV disease (B20)

GUIDELINES **Section I.C.1.a.2)(g)**

During pregnancy, childbirth or the puerperium, a patient admitted (or presenting for a health care encounter) because of an HIV-related illness should receive a principal diagnosis code of O98.7-, followed by B20 and the code(s) for the HIV-related illness(es). Codes from Chapter 15 always take sequencing priority.

Patients with asymptomatic HIV infection status admitted (or presenting for a health care encounter) during pregnancy, childbirth, or the puerperium should receive codes of O98.7- and Z21.

+ 6 **O98.71 Human immunodeficiency virus [HIV] disease complicating pregnancy**

SP + **O98.711 Human immunodeficiency virus [HIV] disease complicating pregnancy, first trimester**

SP + **O98.712 Human immunodeficiency virus [HIV] disease complicating pregnancy, second trimester**

SP + **O98.713 Human immunodeficiency virus [HIV] disease complicating pregnancy, third trimester**

IQ + **O98.719 Human immunodeficiency virus [HIV] disease complicating pregnancy, unspecified trimester**

SP + **O98.72 Human immunodeficiency virus [HIV] disease complicating childbirth**

SP + **O98.73 Human immunodeficiency virus [HIV] disease complicating the puerperium**

+ 5 **O98.8 Other maternal infectious and parasitic diseases complicating pregnancy, childbirth and the puerperium**

+ 6 **O98.81 Other maternal infectious and parasitic diseases complicating pregnancy**

SP + **O98.811 Other maternal infectious and parasitic diseases complicating pregnancy, first trimester**

SP + **O98.812 Other maternal infectious and parasitic diseases complicating pregnancy, second trimester**

SP + **O98.813 Other maternal infectious and parasitic diseases complicating pregnancy, third trimester**

Chapter 15

O00-O9A

IQ + O98.819 **Other maternal infectious and parasitic diseases complicating pregnancy, unspecified trimester**

SP + O98.82 **Other maternal infectious and parasitic diseases complicating childbirth**

SP + O98.83 **Other maternal infectious and parasitic diseases complicating the puerperium**

+ 5 O98.9 **Unspecified maternal infectious and parasitic disease complicating pregnancy, childbirth and the puerperium**

+ 6 O98.91 **Unspecified maternal infectious and parasitic disease complicating pregnancy**

IQ + O98.911 **Unspecified maternal infectious and parasitic disease complicating pregnancy, first trimester**

IQ + O98.912 **Unspecified maternal infectious and parasitic disease complicating pregnancy, second trimester**

IQ + O98.913 **Unspecified maternal infectious and parasitic disease complicating pregnancy, third trimester**

IQ + O98.919 **Unspecified maternal infectious and parasitic disease complicating pregnancy, unspecified trimester**

IQ + O98.92 **Unspecified maternal infectious and parasitic disease complicating childbirth**

IQ + O98.93 **Unspecified maternal infectious and parasitic disease complicating the puerperium**

+ 4 O99 **Other maternal diseases classifiable elsewhere but complicating pregnancy, childbirth and the puerperium**

INCLUDES conditions which complicate the pregnant state, are aggravated by the pregnancy or are a main reason for obstetric care

Use additional code to identify specific condition

EXCLUDES 2 when the reason for maternal care is that the condition is known or suspected to have affected the fetus (O35-O36)

+ 5 O99.0 **Anemia complicating pregnancy, childbirth and the puerperium**

Conditions in D50-D64

EXCLUDES 1 anemia arising in the puerperium (O90.81)
postpartum anemia NOS (O90.81)

+ 6 O99.01 **Anemia complicating pregnancy**

CODING TIPS ✓ Use O90.81 for diagnosed anemia complicating the postpartum period. Use O99.01 for anemia complicating pregnancy. Use O99.03 for pre-existing anemia complicating the puerperium.

SP + O99.011 **Anemia complicating pregnancy, first trimester**

SP + O99.012 **Anemia complicating pregnancy, second trimester**

SP + O99.013 **Anemia complicating pregnancy, third trimester**

IQ + O99.019 **Anemia complicating pregnancy, unspecified trimester**

SP + O99.02 **Anemia complicating childbirth**

SP + O99.03 **Anemia complicating the puerperium**

EXCLUDES 1 postpartum anemia not pre-existing prior to delivery (O90.81)

CODING TIPS ✓ Use O90.81 for diagnosed anemia complicating the postpartum period. Use O99.01 for anemia complicating pregnancy. Use O99.03 for pre-existing anemia complicating the puerperium.

+ 5 O99.1 **Other diseases of the blood and blood-forming organs and certain disorders involving the immune mechanism complicating pregnancy, childbirth and the puerperium**

Conditions in D65-D89

EXCLUDES 1 hemorrhage with coagulation defects (O45.-, O46.0-, O67.0, O72.3)

+ 6 O99.11 **Other diseases of the blood and blood-forming organs and certain disorders involving the immune mechanism complicating pregnancy**

SP + O99.111 **Other diseases of the blood and blood-forming organs and certain disorders involving the immune mechanism complicating pregnancy, first trimester**

SP + O99.112 **Other diseases of the blood and blood-forming organs and certain disorders involving the immune mechanism complicating pregnancy, second trimester**

SP + O99.113 **Other diseases of the blood and blood-forming organs and certain disorders involving the immune mechanism complicating pregnancy, third trimester**

IQ + O99.119 **Other diseases of the blood and blood-forming organs and certain disorders involving the immune mechanism complicating pregnancy, unspecified trimester**

SP + O99.12 **Other diseases of the blood and blood-forming organs and certain disorders involving the immune mechanism complicating childbirth**

SP + O99.13 **Other diseases of the blood and blood-forming organs and certain disorders involving the immune mechanism complicating the puerperium**

+ 5 O99.2 **Endocrine, nutritional and metabolic diseases complicating pregnancy, childbirth and the puerperium**

Conditions in E00-E89

EXCLUDES 2 diabetes mellitus (O24.-)
malnutrition (O25.-)

postpartum thyroiditis (O90.5)

+ 6 **O99.21 Obesity complicating pregnancy, childbirth, and the puerperium**
Use additional code to identify the type of obesity (E66.-)

IQ + **O99.210 Obesity complicating pregnancy, unspecified trimester**

SP + **O99.211 Obesity complicating pregnancy, first trimester**

SP + **O99.212 Obesity complicating pregnancy, second trimester**

SP + **O99.213 Obesity complicating pregnancy, third trimester**

SP + **O99.214 Obesity complicating childbirth**

SP + **O99.215 Obesity complicating the puerperium**

+ 6 **O99.28 Other endocrine, nutritional and metabolic diseases complicating pregnancy, childbirth and the puerperium**

IQ + **O99.280 Endocrine, nutritional and metabolic diseases complicating pregnancy, unspecified trimester**

SP + **O99.281 Endocrine, nutritional and metabolic diseases complicating pregnancy, first trimester**

SP + **O99.282 Endocrine, nutritional and metabolic diseases complicating pregnancy, second trimester**

SP + **O99.283 Endocrine, nutritional and metabolic diseases complicating pregnancy, third trimester**

SP + **O99.284 Endocrine, nutritional and metabolic diseases complicating childbirth**

SP + **O99.285 Endocrine, nutritional and metabolic diseases complicating the puerperium**

+ 5 **O99.3 Mental disorders and diseases of the nervous system complicating pregnancy, childbirth and the puerperium**

+ 6 **O99.31 Alcohol use complicating pregnancy, childbirth, and the puerperium**
Use additional code(s) from F10 to identify manifestations of the alcohol use

IQ + **O99.310 Alcohol use complicating pregnancy, unspecified trimester**

SP + **O99.311 Alcohol use complicating pregnancy, first trimester**

SP + **O99.312 Alcohol use complicating pregnancy, second trimester**

SP + **O99.313 Alcohol use complicating pregnancy, third trimester**

SP + **O99.314 Alcohol use complicating childbirth**

SP + **O99.315 Alcohol use complicating the puerperium**

+ 6 **O99.32 Drug use complicating pregnancy, childbirth, and the puerperium**
Use additional code(s) from F11-F16 and F18-F19 to identify manifestations of the drug use

IQ + **O99.320 Drug use complicating pregnancy, unspecified trimester**

SP + **O99.321 Drug use complicating pregnancy, first trimester**

SP + **O99.322 Drug use complicating pregnancy, second trimester**

SP + **O99.323 Drug use complicating pregnancy, third trimester**

SP + **O99.324 Drug use complicating childbirth**

SP + **O99.325 Drug use complicating the puerperium**

+ 6 **O99.33 Tobacco use disorder complicating pregnancy, childbirth, and the puerperium**
Smoking complicating pregnancy, childbirth, and the puerperium
Use additional code from category F17 to identify type of tobacco nicotine dependence

IQ + **O99.330 Smoking (tobacco) complicating pregnancy, unspecified trimester**

SP + **O99.331 Smoking (tobacco) complicating pregnancy, first trimester**

SP + **O99.332 Smoking (tobacco) complicating pregnancy, second trimester**

SP + **O99.333 Smoking (tobacco) complicating pregnancy, third trimester**

SP + **O99.334 Smoking (tobacco) complicating childbirth**

SP + **O99.335 Smoking (tobacco) complicating the puerperium**

+ 6 **O99.34 Other mental disorders complicating pregnancy, childbirth, and the puerperium**
Conditions in F01-F09, F20-F52 and F54-F99

EXCLUDES 2 postpartum mood disturbance (O90.6)
postnatal psychosis (F53.1)
puerperal psychosis (F53.1)

IQ + **O99.340 Other mental disorders complicating pregnancy, unspecified trimester**

SP + **O99.341 Other mental disorders complicating pregnancy, first trimester**

SP + **O99.342 Other mental disorders complicating pregnancy, second trimester**

SP + **O99.343 Other mental disorders complicating pregnancy, third trimester**

SP + **O99.344 Other mental disorders complicating childbirth**

SP + **O99.345 Other mental disorders complicating the puerperium**

+ 6 **O99.35 Diseases of the nervous system complicating pregnancy, childbirth, and the puerperium**
Conditions in G00-G99

EXCLUDES 2 pregnancy related peripheral neuritis (O26.8-)

IQ + **O99.350 Diseases of the nervous system complicating pregnancy, unspecified trimester**

SP + **O99.351 Diseases of the nervous system complicating pregnancy, first trimester**

SP + **O99.352 Diseases of the nervous system complicating pregnancy, second trimester**

SP + **O99.353 Diseases of the nervous system complicating pregnancy, third trimester**

SP + **O99.354 Diseases of the nervous system complicating childbirth**

SP + **O99.355 Diseases of the nervous system complicating the puerperium**

+ 5 **O99.4 Diseases of the circulatory system complicating pregnancy, childbirth and the puerperium**

Conditions in I00-I99

EXCLUDES 1 peripartum cardiomyopathy (O90.3)

EXCLUDES 2 hypertensive disorders (O10-O16)
obstetric embolism (O88.-)
venous complications and cerebrovenous sinus thrombosis in labor, childbirth and the puerperium (O87.-)
venous complications and cerebrovenous sinus thrombosis in pregnancy (O22.-)

+ 6 **O99.41 Diseases of the circulatory system complicating pregnancy**

SP + **O99.411 Diseases of the circulatory system complicating pregnancy, first trimester**

SP + **O99.412 Diseases of the circulatory system complicating pregnancy, second trimester**

SP + **O99.413 Diseases of the circulatory system complicating pregnancy, third trimester**

IQ + **O99.419 Diseases of the circulatory system complicating pregnancy, unspecified trimester**

SP + **O99.42 Diseases of the circulatory system complicating childbirth**

SP + **O99.43 Diseases of the circulatory system complicating the puerperium**

+ 5 **O99.5 Diseases of the respiratory system complicating pregnancy, childbirth and the puerperium**

Conditions in J00-J99

+ 6 **O99.51 Diseases of the respiratory system complicating pregnancy**

SP + **O99.511 Diseases of the respiratory system complicating pregnancy, first trimester**

SP + **O99.512 Diseases of the respiratory system complicating pregnancy, second trimester**

SP + **O99.513 Diseases of the respiratory system complicating pregnancy, third trimester**

IQ + **O99.519 Diseases of the respiratory system complicating pregnancy, unspecified trimester**

SP + **O99.52 Diseases of the respiratory system complicating childbirth**

SP + **O99.53 Diseases of the respiratory system complicating the puerperium**

+ 5 **O99.6 Diseases of the digestive system complicating pregnancy, childbirth and the puerperium**

Conditions in K00-K93

EXCLUDES 2 hemorrhoids in pregnancy (O22.4-)
liver and biliary tract disorders in pregnancy, childbirth and the puerperium (O26.6-)

+ 6 **O99.61 Diseases of the digestive system complicating pregnancy**

SP + **O99.611 Diseases of the digestive system complicating pregnancy, first trimester**

SP + **O99.612 Diseases of the digestive system complicating pregnancy, second trimester**

SP + **O99.613 Diseases of the digestive system complicating pregnancy, third trimester**

IQ + **O99.619 Diseases of the digestive system complicating pregnancy, unspecified trimester**

SP + **O99.62 Diseases of the digestive system complicating childbirth**

SP + **O99.63 Diseases of the digestive system complicating the puerperium**

+ 5 **O99.7 Diseases of the skin and subcutaneous tissue complicating pregnancy, childbirth and the puerperium**

Conditions in L00-L99

EXCLUDES 2 herpes gestationis (O26.4)
pruritic urticarial papules and plaques of pregnancy (PUPPP) (O26.86)

+ 6 **O99.71 Diseases of the skin and subcutaneous tissue complicating pregnancy**

SP + **O99.711 Diseases of the skin and subcutaneous tissue complicating pregnancy, first trimester**

SP + **O99.712 Diseases of the skin and subcutaneous tissue complicating pregnancy, second trimester**

SP + **O99.713 Diseases of the skin and subcutaneous tissue complicating pregnancy, third trimester**

IQ + **O99.719 Diseases of the skin and subcutaneous tissue complicating pregnancy, unspecified trimester**

SP + **O99.72 Diseases of the skin and subcutaneous tissue complicating childbirth**

SP + **O99.73 Diseases of the skin and subcutaneous tissue complicating the puerperium**

+ 5 **O99.8 Other specified diseases and conditions complicating pregnancy, childbirth and the puerperium**

Conditions in D00-D48, H00-H95, M00-N99, and Q00-Q99

Use additional code to identify condition

EXCLUDES 2 genitourinary infections in pregnancy (O23.-)
infection of genitourinary tract following delivery (O86.1-O86.4)
malignant neoplasm complicating pregnancy, childbirth and the puerperium (O9A.1-)
maternal care for known or suspected abnormality of maternal pelvic organs (O34.-)
postpartum acute kidney failure (O90.4)
traumatic injuries in pregnancy (O9A.2-)

+ 6 **O99.81 Abnormal glucose complicating pregnancy, childbirth and the puerperium**
EXCLUDES 1 gestational diabetes (O24.4-)

SP + **O99.810 Abnormal glucose complicating pregnancy**

SP + **O99.814 Abnormal glucose complicating childbirth**

SP + **O99.815 Abnormal glucose complicating the puerperium**

+ 6 **O99.82 Streptococcus B carrier state complicating pregnancy, childbirth and the puerperium**
EXCLUDES 1 Carrier of streptococcus group B (GBS) in a nonpregnant woman (Z22.330)

SP + **O99.820 Streptococcus B carrier state complicating pregnancy**

SP + **O99.824 Streptococcus B carrier state complicating childbirth**

SP + **O99.825 Streptococcus B carrier state complicating the puerperium**

+ 6 **O99.83 Other infection carrier state complicating pregnancy, childbirth and the puerperium**
Use additional code to identify the carrier state (Z22.-)

SP + **O99.830 Other infection carrier state complicating pregnancy**

SP + **O99.834 Other infection carrier state complicating childbirth**

SP + **O99.835 Other infection carrier state complicating the puerperium**

+ 6 **O99.84 Bariatric surgery status complicating pregnancy, childbirth and the puerperium**
Gastric banding status complicating pregnancy, childbirth and the puerperium
Gastric bypass status for obesity complicating pregnancy, childbirth and the puerperium
Obesity surgery status complicating pregnancy, childbirth and the puerperium

IQ + **O99.840 Bariatric surgery status complicating pregnancy, unspecified trimester**

SP + **O99.841 Bariatric surgery status complicating pregnancy, first trimester**

SP + **O99.842 Bariatric surgery status complicating pregnancy, second trimester**

SP + **O99.843 Bariatric surgery status complicating pregnancy, third trimester**

SP + **O99.844 Bariatric surgery status complicating childbirth**

SP + **O99.845 Bariatric surgery status complicating the puerperium**

+ 6 **O99.89 Other specified diseases and conditions complicating pregnancy, childbirth and the puerperium**

SP + **O99.891 Other specified diseases and conditions complicating pregnancy**

SP + **O99.892 Other specified diseases and conditions complicating childbirth**

SP + **O99.893 Other specified diseases and conditions complicating puerperium**

4 **O9A Maternal malignant neoplasms, traumatic injuries and abuse classifiable elsewhere but complicating pregnancy, childbirth and the puerperium**

+ 5 **O9A.1 Malignant neoplasm complicating pregnancy, childbirth and the puerperium**
Conditions in C00-C96
Use additional code to identify neoplasm
EXCLUDES 2 maternal care for benign tumor of corpus uteri (O34.1-)
maternal care for benign tumor of cervix (O34.4-)

+ 6 **O9A.11 Malignant neoplasm complicating pregnancy**

SP + **O9A.111 Malignant neoplasm complicating pregnancy, first trimester**

SP + **O9A.112 Malignant neoplasm complicating pregnancy, second trimester**

SP + **O9A.113 Malignant neoplasm complicating pregnancy, third trimester**

IQ + **O9A.119 Malignant neoplasm complicating pregnancy, unspecified trimester**

SP + **O9A.12 Malignant neoplasm complicating childbirth**

SP + **O9A.13 Malignant neoplasm complicating the puerperium**

+ 5 **O9A.2 Injury, poisoning and certain other consequences of external causes complicating pregnancy, childbirth and the puerperium**
Conditions in S00-T88, except T74 and T76
Use additional code(s) to identify the injury or poisoning
EXCLUDES 2 physical, sexual and psychological abuse complicating pregnancy, childbirth and the puerperium (O9A.3-, O9A.4-, O9A.5-)

Chapter 15
O00-O9A

+ 6 O9A.21 Injury, poisoning and certain other consequences of external causes complicating pregnancy

SP + O9A.211 Injury, poisoning and certain other consequences of external causes complicating pregnancy, first trimester

SP + O9A.212 Injury, poisoning and certain other consequences of external causes complicating pregnancy, second trimester

SP + O9A.213 Injury, poisoning and certain other consequences of external causes complicating pregnancy, third trimester

IQ + O9A.219 Injury, poisoning and certain other consequences of external causes complicating pregnancy, unspecified trimester

SP + O9A.22 Injury, poisoning and certain other consequences of external causes complicating childbirth

SP + O9A.23 Injury, poisoning and certain other consequences of external causes complicating the puerperium

+ 5 O9A.3 Physical abuse complicating pregnancy, childbirth and the puerperium

Conditions in T74.11 or T76.11

Use additional code (if applicable):

to identify any associated current injury due to physical abuse

to identify the perpetrator of abuse (Y07.-)

EXCLUDES 2 sexual abuse complicating pregnancy, childbirth and the puerperium (O9A.4)

GUIDELINES **Section I.C.15.r**

For suspected or confirmed cases of abuse of a pregnant patient, a code(s) from subcategories O9A.3, O9A.4, and O9A.5, should be sequenced first, followed by the appropriate codes (if applicable) to identify any associated current injury due to physical abuse, sexual abuse, and the perpetrator of abuse.

+ 6 O9A.31 Physical abuse complicating pregnancy

SP + O9A.311 Physical abuse complicating pregnancy, first trimester

SP + O9A.312 Physical abuse complicating pregnancy, second trimester

SP + O9A.313 Physical abuse complicating pregnancy, third trimester

IQ + O9A.319 Physical abuse complicating pregnancy, unspecified trimester

SP + O9A.32 Physical abuse complicating childbirth

SP + O9A.33 Physical abuse complicating the puerperium

+ 5 O9A.4 Sexual abuse complicating pregnancy, childbirth and the puerperium

Conditions in T74.21 or T76.21

Use additional code (if applicable):

to identify any associated current injury due to sexual abuse

to identify the perpetrator of abuse (Y07.-)

+ 6 O9A.41 Sexual abuse complicating pregnancy

SP + O9A.411 Sexual abuse complicating pregnancy, first trimester

SP + O9A.412 Sexual abuse complicating pregnancy, second trimester

SP + O9A.413 Sexual abuse complicating pregnancy, third trimester

IQ + O9A.419 Sexual abuse complicating pregnancy, unspecified trimester

SP + O9A.42 Sexual abuse complicating childbirth

SP + O9A.43 Sexual abuse complicating the puerperium

+ 5 O9A.5 Psychological abuse complicating pregnancy, childbirth and the puerperium

Conditions in T74.31 or T76.31

Use additional code to identify the perpetrator of abuse (Y07.-)

+ 6 O9A.51 Psychological abuse complicating pregnancy

SP + O9A.511 Psychological abuse complicating pregnancy, first trimester

SP + O9A.512 Psychological abuse complicating pregnancy, second trimester

SP + O9A.513 Psychological abuse complicating pregnancy, third trimester

IQ + O9A.519 Psychological abuse complicating pregnancy, unspecified trimester

SP + O9A.52 Psychological abuse complicating childbirth

SP + O9A.53 Psychological abuse complicating the puerperium

Chapter 16: Certain Conditions Originating in the Perinatal Period (P00-P96)

The codes in this chapter are for conditions that have their origin in the fetal or perinatal period (before birth and through the first 28 days after birth) even if morbidity occurs later. If a condition originates in the perinatal period and continues throughout life, the perinatal code should continue to be used, regardless of the age of the patient.

Codes from this chapter ***are used on newborn records only, never on maternal records***. Codes from chapter 15, the obstetric chapter, are never permitted on the newborn record.

When coding the birth episode in a newborn record, assign a code from category Z38, Liveborn infants according to place of birth and type of delivery, as the principal diagnosis. A code from category Z38 is assigned only once, to a newborn at the time of birth. If a newborn is transferred to another institution, a code from category Z38 should not be used at the receiving hospital.

All clinically significant conditions noted during the routine newborn examination should be coded. A condition is clinically significant if it requires any of the following: clinical evaluation; therapeutic treatment; diagnostic procedures; extended length of hospital stay, increased nursing care and/or monitoring; or if the condition has implications for future health care needs. Codes should be assigned for conditions that have been specified by the provider as having implications for future health care needs.

Codes from other chapters may be used with codes from Chapter 16 if the codes from the other chapters provide more detail. If the reason for the encounter is a perinatal condition, the code from chapter 16 should be sequenced first.

If a newborn has **a condition that may be either due to the birth process or community-acquired** and the documentation does not indicate whether it is congenital or community-acquired, the default code choice is due to the birth process, and the code from Chapter 16 should be used.

If the condition is community-acquired, a code from Chapter 16 should not be assigned. For example, a newborn may have an injured shoulder. Unless otherwise specified, assume that the condition is related to the delivery and report a code P03.1, (Newborn affected by other malpresentation, malposition and disproportion during labor and delivery) as the first-listed diagnosis.

Special Coding Issues

Newborn affected by maternal factors and by complications of pregnancy, labor, and delivery

Codes P00-P04 are used when the listed maternal conditions are specified as the cause of confirmed morbidity or potential morbidity which have their origin in the perinatal period. Several of these codes have a note to code first any current condition in the newborn.

Just because the mother had a medical condition or experienced some complication of pregnancy, labor or delivery does not mean the mother's condition affected the newborn. For example, the mother may have had hypertension (category O10-O11, O13-O16) listed on her chart. If the condition affected the newborn, then code P00.0 (Newborn affected by maternal hypertensive disorders) should be reported on the newborn's chart. If the mother's condition did not affect the fetus, code P00.0 is not reported.

Expanded codes reference specific types of complications. Read the notes under each code carefully to determine the specific code to use.

Prematurity and Fetal Growth Retardation

Providers utilize different criteria in determining prematurity. A code for prematurity should not be assigned unless it is documented. Assignment of codes in categories P05, Disorders of newborn related to slow fetal growth and fetal malnutrition, and P07, Disorders of newborn related to short gestation and low birth weight, not elsewhere classified, should be based on the recorded birth weight and estimated gestational age. Codes from category P05 should not be assigned with codes from subcategory P07.0 or P07.1.

When both birth weight and gestational age are available, two codes from category P07 should be assigned, with the code for birth weight sequenced before the code for gestational age.

Codes from category P07, Disorders of newborn related to short gestation and low birth weight, not elsewhere classified, are for use for a child or adult who was premature or had a low birth weight as a newborn and this is affecting the patient's current health status.

Bacterial Sepsis of Newborn

Category P36, Bacterial sepsis of newborn, includes congenital sepsis. If a perinate is documented as having sepsis without documentation of congenital or community acquired, the default is congenital and a code from category P36 should be assigned. If the P36 code includes the causal organism, an additional code from category B95, Streptococcus, Staphylococcus, and Enterococcus as the cause of diseases classified elsewhere, or B96, Other bacterial agents as the cause of disease classified elsewhere, should not be assigned. If the P36 code does not include the causal organism, assign an additional code from category B96. If applicable, use additional codes to identify severe sepsis (R65.2-) and any associated acute organ dysfunction.

CHAPTER 16: CERTAIN CONDITIONS ORIGINATING IN THE PERINATAL PERIOD (P00-P96)

Note:
Codes from this chapter are for use on newborn records only, never on maternal records

INCLUDES conditions that have their origin in the fetal or perinatal period (before birth through the first 28 days after birth) even if morbidity occurs later

EXCLUDES 2 congenital malformations, deformations and chromosomal abnormalities (Q00-Q99)
endocrine, nutritional and metabolic diseases (E00-E88)
injury, poisoning and certain other consequences of external causes (S00-T88)
neoplasms (C00-D49)
tetanus neonatorum (A33)

ALERT Sometimes payer policy conflicts with official guidelines, rules and conventions, and other official guidance. When a payer refuses to pay based on code(s) used in compliance with that guidance, take the following steps: 1) Determine whether the denial or rejection is truly a coding dispute and not a different coverage or payment issue; 2) Remind the payer that following official guidelines and conventions is required by HIPAA code set standards and provide the official guidance in question. If a payer does have a policy that clearly conflicts with official coding rules or guidelines, every effort should be made to resolve the issue with the payer; 3) If the payer refuses to change its policy, obtain the payer requirements in writing. If the payer refuses to provide their policy in writing, document all discussions, including dates and names of individuals involved; 4) Conform to the payer's policy if the payer continues to deny or reject the claim; 5) Keep a permanent file of the documentation obtained regarding payer coding policies. It may be come in handy in the event of an audit.

This chapter contains the following blocks:

P00-P04	Newborn affected by maternal factors and by complications of pregnancy, labor, and delivery
P05-P08	Disorders of newborn related to length of gestation and fetal growth
P09	Abnormal findings on neonatal screening
P10-P15	Birth trauma
P19-P29	Respiratory and cardiovascular disorders specific to the perinatal period
P35-P39	Infections specific to the perinatal period
P50-P61	Hemorrhagic and hematological disorders of newborn
P70-P74	Transitory endocrine and metabolic disorders specific to newborn
P76-P78	Digestive system disorders of newborn
P80-P83	Conditions involving the integument and temperature regulation of newborn
P84	Other problems with newborn
P90-P96	Other disorders originating in the perinatal period

Newborn affected by maternal factors and by complications of pregnancy, labor, and delivery (P00-P04)

Note:
These codes are for use when the listed maternal conditions are specified as the cause of confirmed morbidity or potential morbidity which have their origin in the perinatal period (before birth through the first 28 days after birth).

4 **P00 Newborn affected by maternal conditions that may be unrelated to present pregnancy**
Code first:
any current condition in newborn
EXCLUDES 2 encounter for observation of newborn for suspected diseases and conditions ruled out (Z05.-)
newborn affected by maternal complications of pregnancy (P01.-)
newborn affected by maternal endocrine and metabolic disorders (P70-P74)
newborn affected by noxious substances transmitted via placenta or breast milk (P04.-)

SP **P00.0 Newborn affected by maternal hypertensive disorders**
Newborn affected by maternal conditions classifiable to O10-O11, O13-O16

SP **P00.1 Newborn affected by maternal renal and urinary tract diseases**
Newborn affected by maternal conditions classifiable to N00-N39

▲ SP **P00.2 Newborn affected by maternal infectious and parasitic diseases**
Newborn affected by maternal infectious disease classifiable to A00-B99, J09 and J10
EXCLUDES 1 maternal genital tract or other localized infections (P00.8)
EXCLUDES 2 infections specific to the perinatal period (P35-P39)
newborn affected by (positive) maternal group B streptococcus (GBS) colonization (P00.82)

SP **P00.3 Newborn affected by other maternal circulatory and respiratory diseases**
Newborn affected by maternal conditions classifiable to I00-I99, J00-J99, Q20-Q34 and not included in P00.0, P00.2

SP **P00.4 Newborn affected by maternal nutritional disorders**
Newborn affected by maternal disorders classifiable to E40-E64
Maternal malnutrition NOS

SP **P00.5 Newborn affected by maternal injury**
Newborn affected by maternal conditions classifiable to O9A.2-

SP **P00.6 Newborn affected by surgical procedure on mother**
Newborn affected by amniocentesis
EXCLUDES 1 Cesarean delivery for present delivery (P03.4)
damage to placenta from amniocentesis, Cesarean delivery or surgical induction (P02.1)
previous surgery to uterus or pelvic organs (P03.89)
EXCLUDES 2 newborn affected by complication of (fetal) intrauterine procedure (P96.5)

Chapter 16
P00-P96

SP **P00.7 Newborn affected by other medical procedures on mother, not elsewhere classified**
Newborn affected by radiation to mother
EXCLUDES 1 damage to placenta from amniocentesis, cesarean delivery or surgical induction (P02.1)
newborn affected by other complications of labor and delivery (P03.-)

5 **P00.8 Newborn affected by other maternal conditions**

SP **P00.81 Newborn affected by periodontal disease in mother**

★ **P00.82 Newborn affected by (positive) maternal group B streptococcus (GBS) colonization**
Contact with positive maternal group B streptococcus

▲ SP + **P00.89 Newborn affected by other maternal conditions**
Newborn affected by conditions classifiable to T80-T88
Newborn affected by maternal genital tract or other localized infections
Newborn affected by maternal systemic lupus erythematosus
Use additional code to identify infectious agent, if known
Excludes 2: newborn affected by positive maternal group B streptococcus (GBS) colonization (P00.82)

IQ **P00.9 Newborn affected by unspecified maternal condition**

4 **P01 Newborn affected by maternal complications of pregnancy**
Code first:
any current condition in newborn
EXCLUDES 2 encounter for observation of newborn for suspected diseases and conditions ruled out (Z05.-)

SP **P01.0 Newborn affected by incompetent cervix**

SP **P01.1 Newborn affected by premature rupture of membranes**

SP **P01.2 Newborn affected by oligohydramnios**
EXCLUDES 1 oligohydramnios due to premature rupture of membranes (P01.1)
DEFINITION Inadequate amount of amniotic fluid in the womb affecting the fetus.

SP **P01.3 Newborn affected by polyhydramnios**
Newborn affected by hydramnios
DEFINITION Excessive amount of amniotic fluid in the womb affecting the fetus.

SP **P01.4 Newborn affected by ectopic pregnancy**
Newborn affected by abdominal pregnancy

SP **P01.5 Newborn affected by multiple pregnancy**
Newborn affected by triplet (pregnancy)
Newborn affected by twin (pregnancy)

SP **P01.6 Newborn affected by maternal death**

SP **P01.7 Newborn affected by malpresentation before labor**
Newborn affected by breech presentation before labor
Newborn affected by external version before labor
Newborn affected by face presentation before labor
Newborn affected by transverse lie before labor
Newborn affected by unstable lie before labor

SP **P01.8 Newborn affected by other maternal complications of pregnancy**

SP **P01.9 Newborn affected by maternal complication of pregnancy, unspecified**

4 **P02 Newborn affected by complications of placenta, cord and membranes**
Code first:
any current condition in newborn
EXCLUDES 2 encounter for observation of newborn for suspected diseases and conditions ruled out (Z05.-)

SP **P02.0 Newborn affected by placenta previa**

SP **P02.1 Newborn affected by other forms of placental separation and hemorrhage**
Newborn affected by abruptio placenta
Newborn affected by accidental hemorrhage
Newborn affected by antepartum hemorrhage
Newborn affected by damage to placenta from amniocentesis, cesarean delivery or surgical induction
Newborn affected by maternal blood loss
Newborn affected by premature separation of placenta

5 **P02.2 Newborn affected by other and unspecified morphological and functional abnormalities of placenta**

SP **P02.20 Newborn affected by unspecified morphological and functional abnormalities of placenta**

SP **P02.29 Newborn affected by other morphological and functional abnormalities of placenta**
Newborn affected by placental dysfunction
Newborn affected by placental infarction
Newborn affected by placental insufficiency

SP **P02.3 Newborn affected by placental transfusion syndromes**
Newborn affected by placental and cord abnormalities resulting in twin-to-twin or other transplacental transfusion

SP **P02.4 Newborn affected by prolapsed cord**

SP **P02.5 Newborn affected by other compression of umbilical cord**
Newborn affected by umbilical cord (tightly) around neck
Newborn affected by entanglement of umbilical cord
Newborn affected by knot in umbilical cord

Chapter 16

P00-P96

5 **P02.6 Newborn affected by other and unspecified conditions of umbilical cord**

SP **P02.60 Newborn affected by unspecified conditions of umbilical cord**

SP **P02.69 Newborn affected by other conditions of umbilical cord**
Newborn affected by short umbilical cord
Newborn affected by vasa previa
EXCLUDES 1 newborn affected by single umbilical artery (Q27.0)

5 **P02.7 Newborn affected by chorioamnionitis**

SP **P02.70 Newborn affected by fetal inflammatory response syndrome**
Newborn affected by FIRS

SP **P02.78 Newborn affected by other conditions from chorioamnionitis**
Newborn affected by amnionitis
Newborn affected by membranitis
Newborn affected by placentitis

SP **P02.8 Newborn affected by other abnormalities of membranes**

SP **P02.9 Newborn affected by abnormality of membranes, unspecified**

4 **P03 Newborn affected by other complications of labor and delivery**
Code first:
any current condition in newborn
EXCLUDES 2 encounter for observation of newborn for suspected diseases and conditions ruled out (Z05.-)

SP **P03.0 Newborn affected by breech delivery and extraction**

SP **P03.1 Newborn affected by other malpresentation, malposition and disproportion during labor and delivery**
Newborn affected by contracted pelvis
Newborn affected by conditions classifiable to O64-O66
Newborn affected by persistent occipitoposterior
Newborn affected by transverse lie

SP **P03.2 Newborn affected by forceps delivery**

SP **P03.3 Newborn affected by delivery by vacuum extractor [ventouse]**

SP **P03.4 Newborn affected by Cesarean delivery**

SP **P03.5 Newborn affected by precipitate delivery**
Newborn affected by rapid second stage
DEFINITION Fetus affected by labor occurring quickly, with rapid expulsion.

SP **P03.6 Newborn affected by abnormal uterine contractions**
Newborn affected by conditions classifiable to O62.-, except O62.3
Newborn affected by hypertonic labor
Newborn affected by uterine inertia

5 **P03.8 Newborn affected by other specified complications of labor and delivery**

6 **P03.81 Newborn affected by abnormality in fetal (intrauterine) heart rate or rhythm**
EXCLUDES 1 neonatal cardiac dysrhythmia (P29.1-)

SP **P03.810 Newborn affected by abnormality in fetal (intrauterine) heart rate or rhythm before the onset of labor**

SP **P03.811 Newborn affected by abnormality in fetal (intrauterine) heart rate or rhythm during labor**

SP **P03.819 Newborn affected by abnormality in fetal (intrauterine) heart rate or rhythm, unspecified as to time of onset**

SP **P03.82 Meconium passage during delivery**
EXCLUDES 1 meconium aspiration (P24.00, P24.01)
meconium staining (P96.83)

SP **P03.89 Newborn affected by other specified complications of labor and delivery**
Newborn affected by abnormality of maternal soft tissues
Newborn affected by conditions classifiable to O60-O75 and by procedures used in labor and delivery not included in P02.- and P03.0-P03.6
Newborn affected by induction of labor

IQ **P03.9 Newborn affected by complication of labor and delivery, unspecified**

▲ 4 **P04 Newborn affected by noxious substances transmitted via placenta or breast milk**
INCLUDES nonteratogenic effects of substances transmitted via placenta
Code first:
any current condition in newborn, if applicable
EXCLUDES 2 congenital malformations (Q00-Q99)
encounter for observation of newborn for suspected diseases and conditions ruled out (Z05.-)
neonatal jaundice from excessive hemolysis due to drugs or toxins transmitted from mother (P58.4)
newborn in contact with and (suspected) exposures hazardous to health not transmitted via placenta or breast milk (Z77.-)

SP **P04.0 Newborn affected by maternal anesthesia and analgesia in pregnancy, labor and delivery**
Newborn affected by reactions and intoxications from maternal opiates and tranquilizers administered for procedures during pregnancy or labor and delivery
EXCLUDES 2 newborn affected by other maternal medication (P04.1-)

5 **P04.1 Newborn affected by other maternal medication**
Code first:
withdrawal symptoms from maternal use of drugs of addiction, if applicable (P96.1)
EXCLUDES 1 dysmorphism due to warfarin (Q86.2)

Chapter 16 P00-P96

fetal hydantoin syndrome (Q86.1)
EXCLUDES 2 maternal anesthesia and analgesia in pregnancy, labor and delivery (P04.0)
maternal use of drugs of addiction (P04.4-)

SP **P04.11 Newborn affected by maternal antineoplastic chemotherapy**

SP **P04.12 Newborn affected by maternal cytotoxic drugs**

SP **P04.13 Newborn affected by maternal use of anticonvulsants**

SP **P04.14 Newborn affected by maternal use of opiates**

SP **P04.15 Newborn affected by maternal use of antidepressants**

SP **P04.16 Newborn affected by maternal use of amphetamines**

SP **P04.17 Newborn affected by maternal use of sedative-hypnotics**

SP **P04.1A Newborn affected by maternal use of anxiolytics**

SP **P04.18 Newborn affected by other maternal medication**

SP **P04.19 Newborn affected by maternal use of unspecified medication**

SP **P04.2 Newborn affected by maternal use of tobacco**
Newborn affected by exposure in utero to tobacco smoke
EXCLUDES 2 newborn exposure to environmental tobacco smoke (P96.81)

SP **P04.3 Newborn affected by maternal use of alcohol**
EXCLUDES 1 fetal alcohol syndrome (Q86.0)

5 **P04.4 Newborn affected by maternal use of drugs of addiction**

SP **P04.40 Newborn affected by maternal use of unspecified drugs of addiction**

SP **P04.41 Newborn affected by maternal use of cocaine**

SP **P04.42 Newborn affected by maternal use of hallucinogens**
EXCLUDES 2 newborn affected by other maternal medication (P04.1-)

SP **P04.49 Newborn affected by maternal use of other drugs of addiction**
EXCLUDES 2 newborn affected by maternal anesthesia and analgesia (P04.0)
withdrawal symptoms from maternal use of drugs of addiction (P96.1)

SP **P04.5 Newborn affected by maternal use of nutritional chemical substances**

SP **P04.6 Newborn affected by maternal exposure to environmental chemical substances**

5 **P04.8 Newborn affected by other maternal noxious substances**

SP **P04.81 Newborn affected by maternal use of cannabis**

SP **P04.89 Newborn affected by other maternal noxious substances**

IQ **P04.9 Newborn affected by maternal noxious substance, unspecified**

Disorders of newborn related to length of gestation and fetal growth (P05-P08)

4 **P05 Disorders of newborn related to slow fetal growth and fetal malnutrition**

5 **P05.0 Newborn light for gestational age**
Newborn light-for-dates
Weight below but length above 10th percentile for gestational age

IQ **P05.00 Newborn light for gestational age, unspecified weight**

SP **P05.01 Newborn light for gestational age, less than 500 grams**

SP **P05.02 Newborn light for gestational age, 500-749 grams**

SP **P05.03 Newborn light for gestational age, 750-999 grams**

SP **P05.04 Newborn light for gestational age, 1000-1249 grams**

SP **P05.05 Newborn light for gestational age, 1250-1499 grams**

SP **P05.06 Newborn light for gestational age, 1500-1749 grams**

SP **P05.07 Newborn light for gestational age, 1750-1999 grams**

SP **P05.08 Newborn light for gestational age, 2000-2499 grams**

SP **P05.09 Newborn light for gestational age, 2500 grams and over**
Newborn light for gestational age, other

5 **P05.1 Newborn small for gestational age**
Newborn small-and-light-for-dates
Newborn small-for-dates
Weight and length below 10th percentile for gestational age

IQ **P05.10 Newborn small for gestational age, unspecified weight**

SP **P05.11 Newborn small for gestational age, less than 500 grams**

SP **P05.12 Newborn small for gestational age, 500-749 grams**

SP **P05.13 Newborn small for gestational age, 750-999 grams**

SP **P05.14 Newborn small for gestational age, 1000-1249 grams**

SP **P05.15 Newborn small for gestational age, 1250-1499 grams**

SP **P05.16 Newborn small for gestational age, 1500-1749 grams**

SP **P05.17 Newborn small for gestational age, 1750-1999 grams**

SP **P05.18 Newborn small for gestational age, 2000-2499 grams**

SP **P05.19 Newborn small for gestational age, other**
Newborn small for gestational age, 2500 grams and over

SP **P05.2 Newborn affected by fetal (intrauterine) malnutrition not light or small for gestational age**
Infant, not light or small for gestational age, showing signs of fetal malnutrition, such as dry, peeling skin and loss of subcutaneous tissue

Chapter 16
P00-P96

4 4th digit required 5 5th digit required 6 6th digit required 7 7th digit required X 7th digit placeholder + Additional code L Laterality

EXCLUDES 1 newborn affected by fetal malnutrition with light for gestational age (P05.0-)
newborn affected by fetal malnutrition with small for gestational age (P05.1-)

SP **P05.9 Newborn affected by slow intrauterine growth, unspecified**
Newborn affected by fetal growth retardation NOS

4 **P07 Disorders of newborn related to short gestation and low birth weight, not elsewhere classified**
Note:
When both birth weight and gestational age of the newborn are available, both should be coded with birth weight sequenced before gestational age
INCLUDES the listed conditions, without further specification, as the cause of morbidity or additional care, in newborn

5 **P07.0 Extremely low birth weight newborn**
Newborn birth weight 999 g. or less
EXCLUDES 1 low birth weight due to slow fetal growth and fetal malnutrition (P05.-)

!Q **P07.00 Extremely low birth weight newborn, unspecified weight**

SP **P07.01 Extremely low birth weight newborn, less than 500 grams**

SP **P07.02 Extremely low birth weight newborn, 500-749 grams**

SP **P07.03 Extremely low birth weight newborn, 750-999 grams**

5 **P07.1 Other low birth weight newborn**
Newborn birth weight 1000-2499 g.
EXCLUDES 1 low birth weight due to slow fetal growth and fetal malnutrition (P05.-)

!Q **P07.10 Other low birth weight newborn, unspecified weight**

SP **P07.14 Other low birth weight newborn, 1000-1249 grams**

SP **P07.15 Other low birth weight newborn, 1250-1499 grams**

SP **P07.16 Other low birth weight newborn, 1500-1749 grams**

SP **P07.17 Other low birth weight newborn, 1750-1999 grams**

SP **P07.18 Other low birth weight newborn, 2000-2499 grams**

5 **P07.2 Extreme immaturity of newborn**
Less than 28 completed weeks (less than 196 completed days) of gestation.

!Q **P07.20 Extreme immaturity of newborn, unspecified weeks of gestation**
Gestational age less than 28 completed weeks NOS

SP **P07.21 Extreme immaturity of newborn, gestational age less than 23 completed weeks**
Extreme immaturity of newborn, gestational age less than 23 weeks, 0 days

SP **P07.22 Extreme immaturity of newborn, gestational age 23 completed weeks**
Extreme immaturity of newborn, gestational age 23 weeks, 0 days through 23 weeks, 6 days

SP **P07.23 Extreme immaturity of newborn, gestational age 24 completed weeks**
Extreme immaturity of newborn, gestational age 24 weeks, 0 days through 24 weeks, 6 days

SP **P07.24 Extreme immaturity of newborn, gestational age 25 completed weeks**
Extreme immaturity of newborn, gestational age 25 weeks, 0 days through 25 weeks, 6 days

SP **P07.25 Extreme immaturity of newborn, gestational age 26 completed weeks**
Extreme immaturity of newborn, gestational age 26 weeks, 0 days through 26 weeks, 6 days

SP **P07.26 Extreme immaturity of newborn, gestational age 27 completed weeks**
Extreme immaturity of newborn, gestational age 27 weeks, 0 days through 27 weeks, 6 days

5 **P07.3 Preterm [premature] newborn [other]**
28 completed weeks or more but less than 37 completed weeks (196 completed days but less than 259 completed days) of gestation.
Prematurity NOS

!Q **P07.30 Preterm newborn, unspecified weeks of gestation**

SP **P07.31 Preterm newborn, gestational age 28 completed weeks**
Preterm newborn, gestational age 28 weeks, 0 days through 28 weeks, 6 days

SP **P07.32 Preterm newborn, gestational age 29 completed weeks**
Preterm newborn, gestational age 29 weeks, 0 days through 29 weeks, 6 days

SP **P07.33 Preterm newborn, gestational age 30 completed weeks**
Preterm newborn, gestational age 30 weeks, 0 days through 30 weeks, 6 days

SP **P07.34 Preterm newborn, gestational age 31 completed weeks**
Preterm newborn, gestational age 31 weeks, 0 days through 31 weeks, 6 days

SP **P07.35 Preterm newborn, gestational age 32 completed weeks**
Preterm newborn, gestational age 32 weeks, 0 days through 32 weeks, 6 days

SP **P07.36 Preterm newborn, gestational age 33 completed weeks**
Preterm newborn, gestational age 33 weeks, 0 days through 33 weeks, 6 days

SP **P07.37 Preterm newborn, gestational age 34 completed weeks**
Preterm newborn, gestational age 34 weeks, 0 days through 34 weeks, 6 days

SP **P07.38 Preterm newborn, gestational age 35 completed weeks**

Preterm newborn, gestational age 35 weeks, 0 days through 35 weeks, 6 days

SP **P07.39 Preterm newborn, gestational age 36 completed weeks**
Preterm newborn, gestational age 36 weeks, 0 days through 36 weeks, 6 days

4 **P08 Disorders of newborn related to long gestation and high birth weight**
Note:
When both birth weight and gestational age of the newborn are available, priority of assignment should be given to birth weight
INCLUDES the listed conditions, without further specification, as causes of morbidity or additional care, in newborn

SP **P08.0 Exceptionally large newborn baby**
Usually implies a birth weight of 4500 g. or more
EXCLUDES 1 syndrome of infant of diabetic mother (P70.1)
syndrome of infant of mother with gestational diabetes (P70.0)

SP **P08.1 Other heavy for gestational age newborn**
Other newborn heavy- or large-for-dates regardless of period of gestation
Usually implies a birth weight of 4000 g. to 4499 g.
EXCLUDES 1 newborn with a birth weight of 4500 or more (P08.0)
syndrome of infant of diabetic mother (P70.1)
syndrome of infant of mother with gestational diabetes (P70.0)

5 **P08.2 Late newborn, not heavy for gestational age**

SP **P08.21 Post-term newborn**
Newborn with gestation period over 40 completed weeks to 42 completed weeks

SP **P08.22 Prolonged gestation of newborn**
Newborn with gestation period over 42 completed weeks (294 days or more), not heavy- or large-for-dates.
Postmaturity NOS

Abnormal findings on neonatal screening (P09)

▲ 4 **P09 Abnormal findings on neonatal screening**
INCLUDES Abnormal findings on state mandated newborn screens
Failed newborn screening
EXCLUDES 2 nonspecific serologic evidence of human immunodeficiency virus [HIV] (R75)

★ **P09.1 Abnormal findings on neonatal screening for inborn errors of metabolism**

★ **P09.2 Abnormal findings on neonatal screening for congenital endocrine disease**
Abnormal findings on neonatal screening for congenital adrenal hyperplasia
Abnormal findings on neonatal screening for hypothyroidism screen

★ **P09.3 Abnormal findings on neonatal screening for congenital hematologic disorders**
Abnormal findings for hemoglobinothies screen
Abnormal findings on red cell membrane defects screen
Abnormal findings on sickle cell screen

★ **P09.4 Abnormal findings on neonatal screening for cystic fibrosis**

★ **P09.5 Abnormal findings on neonatal screening for critical congenital heart disease**
Neonatal congenital heart disease screening failure

★ **P09.6 Abnormal findings on neonatal screening for neonatal hearing loss**
EXCLUDES 2 encounter for hearing examination following failed hearing screening (Z01.110)

★ **P09.8 Other abnormal findings on neonatal screening**

★ **P09.9 Abnormal findings on neonatal screening, unspecified**

Birth trauma (P10-P15)

4 **P10 Intracranial laceration and hemorrhage due to birth injury**
EXCLUDES 1 intracranial hemorrhage of newborn NOS (P52.9)
intracranial hemorrhage of newborn due to anoxia or hypoxia (P52.-)
nontraumatic intracranial hemorrhage of newborn (P52.-)

SP **P10.0 Subdural hemorrhage due to birth injury**
Subdural hematoma (localized) due to birth injury
EXCLUDES 1 subdural hemorrhage accompanying tentorial tear (P10.4)

SP **P10.1 Cerebral hemorrhage due to birth injury**

SP **P10.2 Intraventricular hemorrhage due to birth injury**

SP **P10.3 Subarachnoid hemorrhage due to birth injury**

SP **P10.4 Tentorial tear due to birth injury**

SP **P10.8 Other intracranial lacerations and hemorrhages due to birth injury**

IQ **P10.9 Unspecified intracranial laceration and hemorrhage due to birth injury**

4 **P11 Other birth injuries to central nervous system**

SP **P11.0 Cerebral edema due to birth injury**

SP **P11.1 Other specified brain damage due to birth injury**

IQ **P11.2 Unspecified brain damage due to birth injury**

SP **P11.3 Birth injury to facial nerve**
Facial palsy due to birth injury

DEFINITION Facial muscle weakness or paralysis resulting from damage or trauma to one of the paired facial nerves.

SP **P11.4 Birth injury to other cranial nerves**

SP **P11.5 Birth injury to spine and spinal cord**
Fracture of spine due to birth injury

IQ **P11.9 Birth injury to central nervous system, unspecified**

4 **P12 Birth injury to scalp**

SP **P12.0 Cephalhematoma due to birth injury**

SP **P12.1 Chignon (from vacuum extraction) due to birth injury**

SP **P12.2 Epicranial subaponeurotic hemorrhage due to birth injury**
Subgaleal hemorrhage

SP **P12.3 Bruising of scalp due to birth injury**

SP **P12.4 Injury of scalp of newborn due to monitoring equipment**
Sampling incision of scalp of newborn
Scalp clip (electrode) injury of newborn

5 **P12.8 Other birth injuries to scalp**

SP **P12.81 Caput succedaneum**

SP **P12.89 Other birth injuries to scalp**

IQ **P12.9 Birth injury to scalp, unspecified**

4 **P13 Birth injury to skeleton**
EXCLUDES 2 birth injury to spine (P11.5)

SP **P13.0 Fracture of skull due to birth injury**

SP **P13.1 Other birth injuries to skull**
EXCLUDES 1 cephalhematoma (P12.0)

SP **P13.2 Birth injury to femur**

SP **P13.3 Birth injury to other long bones**

SP **P13.4 Fracture of clavicle due to birth injury**

SP **P13.8 Birth injuries to other parts of skeleton**

IQ **P13.9 Birth injury to skeleton, unspecified**

4 **P14 Birth injury to peripheral nervous system**

SP **P14.0 Erb's paralysis due to birth injury**

SP **P14.1 Klumpke's paralysis due to birth injury**

SP **P14.2 Phrenic nerve paralysis due to birth injury**

SP **P14.3 Other brachial plexus birth injuries**

SP **P14.8 Birth injuries to other parts of peripheral nervous system**

IQ **P14.9 Birth injury to peripheral nervous system, unspecified**

4 **P15 Other birth injuries**

SP **P15.0 Birth injury to liver**
Rupture of liver due to birth injury

SP **P15.1 Birth injury to spleen**
Rupture of spleen due to birth injury

SP **P15.2 Sternomastoid injury due to birth injury**

SP **P15.3 Birth injury to eye**
Subconjunctival hemorrhage due to birth injury
Traumatic glaucoma due to birth injury

SP **P15.4 Birth injury to face**
Facial congestion due to birth injury

SP **P15.5 Birth injury to external genitalia**

SP **P15.6 Subcutaneous fat necrosis due to birth injury**

SP **P15.8 Other specified birth injuries**

IQ **P15.9 Birth injury, unspecified**

Respiratory and cardiovascular disorders specific to the perinatal period (P19-P29)

4 **P19 Metabolic acidemia in newborn**
INCLUDES metabolic acidemia in newborn

SP **P19.0 Metabolic acidemia in newborn first noted before onset of labor**

SP **P19.1 Metabolic acidemia in newborn first noted during labor**

SP **P19.2 Metabolic acidemia noted at birth**

SP **P19.9 Metabolic acidemia, unspecified**

4 **P22 Respiratory distress of newborn**

SP **P22.0 Respiratory distress syndrome of newborn**
Cardiorespiratory distress syndrome of newborn
Hyaline membrane disease
Idiopathic respiratory distress syndrome [IRDS or RDS] of newborn
Pulmonary hypoperfusion syndrome
Respiratory distress syndrome, type I
EXCLUDES 2 respiratory arrest of newborn (P28.81)
respiratory failure of newborn NOS (P28.5)

SP **P22.1 Transient tachypnea of newborn**
Idiopathic tachypnea of newborn
Respiratory distress syndrome, type II
Wet lung syndrome
DEFINITION Rapid breathing of a newborn.

SP **P22.8 Other respiratory distress of newborn**
EXCLUDES 1 respiratory arrest of newborn (P28.81)
respiratory failure of newborn NOS (P28.5)

SP **P22.9 Respiratory distress of newborn, unspecified**
EXCLUDES 1 respiratory arrest of newborn (P28.81)
respiratory failure of newborn NOS (P28.5)

4 **P23 Congenital pneumonia**
INCLUDES infective pneumonia acquired in utero or during birth
EXCLUDES 1 neonatal pneumonia resulting from aspiration (P24.-)

SP + **P23.0 Congenital pneumonia due to viral agent**
Use additional code (B97) to identify organism
EXCLUDES 1 congenital rubella pneumonitis (P35.0)

SP **P23.1 Congenital pneumonia due to Chlamydia**

SP **P23.2 Congenital pneumonia due to staphylococcus**

SP **P23.3 Congenital pneumonia due to streptococcus, group B**

SP **P23.4 Congenital pneumonia due to Escherichia coli**

SP **P23.5 Congenital pneumonia due to Pseudomonas**

SP + **P23.6 Congenital pneumonia due to other bacterial agents**
Congenital pneumonia due to Hemophilus influenzae

Congenital pneumonia due to Klebsiella pneumoniae
Congenital pneumonia due to Mycoplasma
Congenital pneumonia due to Streptococcus, except group B
Use additional code (B95-B96) to identify organism

SP **P23.8 Congenital pneumonia due to other organisms**

IQ **P23.9 Congenital pneumonia, unspecified**

4 **P24 Neonatal aspiration**

INCLUDES aspiration in utero and during delivery

5 **P24.0 Meconium aspiration**

EXCLUDES 1 meconium passage (without aspiration) during delivery (P03.82)
meconium staining (P96.83)

SP **P24.00 Meconium aspiration without respiratory symptoms**
Meconium aspiration NOS

SP + **P24.01 Meconium aspiration with respiratory symptoms**
Meconium aspiration pneumonia
Meconium aspiration pneumonitis
Meconium aspiration syndrome NOS
Use additional code to identify any secondary pulmonary hypertension, if applicable (I27.2-)

5 **P24.1 Neonatal aspiration of (clear) amniotic fluid and mucus**
Neonatal aspiration of liquor (amnii)

SP **P24.10 Neonatal aspiration of (clear) amniotic fluid and mucus without respiratory symptoms**
Neonatal aspiration of amniotic fluid and mucus NOS

SP + **P24.11 Neonatal aspiration of (clear) amniotic fluid and mucus with respiratory symptoms**
Neonatal aspiration of amniotic fluid and mucus with pneumonia
Neonatal aspiration of amniotic fluid and mucus with pneumonitis
Use additional code to identify any secondary pulmonary hypertension, if applicable (I27.2-)

5 **P24.2 Neonatal aspiration of blood**

SP **P24.20 Neonatal aspiration of blood without respiratory symptoms**
Neonatal aspiration of blood NOS

SP + **P24.21 Neonatal aspiration of blood with respiratory symptoms**
Neonatal aspiration of blood with pneumonia
Neonatal aspiration of blood with pneumonitis
Use additional code to identify any secondary pulmonary hypertension, if applicable (I27.2-)

5 **P24.3 Neonatal aspiration of milk and regurgitated food**
Neonatal aspiration of stomach contents

SP **P24.30 Neonatal aspiration of milk and regurgitated food without respiratory symptoms**
Neonatal aspiration of milk and regurgitated food NOS

SP + **P24.31 Neonatal aspiration of milk and regurgitated food with respiratory symptoms**
Neonatal aspiration of milk and regurgitated food with pneumonia
Neonatal aspiration of milk and regurgitated food with pneumonitis
Use additional code to identify any secondary pulmonary hypertension, if applicable (I27.2-)

5 **P24.8 Other neonatal aspiration**

SP **P24.80 Other neonatal aspiration without respiratory symptoms**
Neonatal aspiration NEC

SP + **P24.81 Other neonatal aspiration with respiratory symptoms**
Neonatal aspiration pneumonia NEC
Neonatal aspiration with pneumonitis NEC
Neonatal aspiration with pneumonia NOS
Neonatal aspiration with pneumonitis NOS
Use additional code to identify any secondary pulmonary hypertension, if applicable (I27.2-)

SP **P24.9 Neonatal aspiration, unspecified**

4 **P25 Interstitial emphysema and related conditions originating in the perinatal period**

SP **P25.0 Interstitial emphysema originating in the perinatal period**

SP **P25.1 Pneumothorax originating in the perinatal period**

SP **P25.2 Pneumomediastinum originating in the perinatal period**

SP **P25.3 Pneumopericardium originating in the perinatal period**

SP **P25.8 Other conditions related to interstitial emphysema originating in the perinatal period**

4 **P26 Pulmonary hemorrhage originating in the perinatal period**

EXCLUDES 1 acute idiopathic hemorrhage in infants over 28 days old (R04.81)

SP **P26.0 Tracheobronchial hemorrhage originating in the perinatal period**

SP **P26.1 Massive pulmonary hemorrhage originating in the perinatal period**

SP **P26.8 Other pulmonary hemorrhages originating in the perinatal period**

SP **P26.9 Unspecified pulmonary hemorrhage originating in the perinatal period**

4 **P27 Chronic respiratory disease originating in the perinatal period**

EXCLUDES 2 respiratory distress of newborn (P22.0-P22.9)

SP **P27.0 Wilson-Mikity syndrome**
Pulmonary dysmaturity

SP **P27.1 Bronchopulmonary dysplasia originating in the perinatal period**

SP **P27.8 Other chronic respiratory diseases originating in the perinatal period**
Congenital pulmonary fibrosis
Ventilator lung in newborn

Chapter 16

P00-P96

IQ **P27.9 Unspecified chronic respiratory disease originating in the perinatal period**

4 **P28 Other respiratory conditions originating in the perinatal period**

EXCLUDES 1 congenital malformations of the respiratory system (Q30-Q34)

SP **P28.0 Primary atelectasis of newborn**

Primary failure to expand terminal respiratory units

Pulmonary hypoplasia associated with short gestation

Pulmonary immaturity NOS

5 **P28.1 Other and unspecified atelectasis of newborn**

SP **P28.10 Unspecified atelectasis of newborn**

Atelectasis of newborn NOS

SP **P28.11 Resorption atelectasis without respiratory distress syndrome**

EXCLUDES 1 resorption atelectasis with respiratory distress syndrome (P22.0)

SP **P28.19 Other atelectasis of newborn**

Partial atelectasis of newborn

Secondary atelectasis of newborn

SP **P28.2 Cyanotic attacks of newborn**

EXCLUDES 1 apnea of newborn (P28.3-P28.4)

DEFINITION A newborn with normal skin tone suddenly turns blue due to a lack of oxygen for a certain period of time before returning to normal color.

SP **P28.3 Primary sleep apnea of newborn**

Central sleep apnea of newborn

Obstructive sleep apnea of newborn

Sleep apnea of newborn NOS

SP **P28.4 Other apnea of newborn**

Apnea of prematurity

Obstructive apnea of newborn

EXCLUDES 1 obstructive sleep apnea of newborn (P28.3)

SP **P28.5 Respiratory failure of newborn**

EXCLUDES 1 respiratory arrest of newborn (P28.81)

respiratory distress of newborn (P22.0-)

5 **P28.8 Other specified respiratory conditions of newborn**

SP **P28.81 Respiratory arrest of newborn**

SP **P28.89 Other specified respiratory conditions of newborn**

Congenital laryngeal stridor

Sniffles in newborn

Snuffles in newborn

EXCLUDES 1 early congenital syphilitic rhinitis (A50.05)

IQ **P28.9 Respiratory condition of newborn, unspecified**

Respiratory depression in newborn

▲ 4 **P29 Cardiovascular disorders originating in the perinatal period**

EXCLUDES 2 congenital malformations of the circulatory system (Q20-Q28)

SP **P29.0 Neonatal cardiac failure**

5 **P29.1 Neonatal cardiac dysrhythmia**

SP **P29.11 Neonatal tachycardia**

SP **P29.12 Neonatal bradycardia**

DEFINITION Abnormally slow newborn heartbeat.

SP **P29.2 Neonatal hypertension**

5 **P29.3 Persistent fetal circulation**

IQ **P29.30 Pulmonary hypertension of newborn**

Persistent pulmonary hypertension of newborn

IQ **P29.38 Other persistent fetal circulation**

Delayed closure of ductus arteriosus

SP **P29.4 Transient myocardial ischemia in newborn**

5 **P29.8 Other cardiovascular disorders originating in the perinatal period**

SP **P29.81 Cardiac arrest of newborn**

SP **P29.89 Other cardiovascular disorders originating in the perinatal period**

IQ **P29.9 Cardiovascular disorder originating in the perinatal period, unspecified**

Infections specific to the perinatal period (P35-P39)

Infections acquired in utero, during birth via the umbilicus, or during the first 28 days after birth

EXCLUDES 2 asymptomatic human immunodeficiency virus [HIV] infection status (Z21)

congenital gonococcal infection (A54.-)

congenital pneumonia (P23.-)

congenital syphilis (A50.-)

human immunodeficiency virus [HIV] disease (B20)

infant botulism (A48.51)

infectious diseases not specific to the perinatal period (A00-B99, J09, J10.-)

intestinal infectious disease (A00-A09)

laboratory evidence of human immunodeficiency virus [HIV] (R75)

tetanus neonatorum (A33)

4 **P35 Congenital viral diseases**

INCLUDES infections acquired in utero or during birth

SP **P35.0 Congenital rubella syndrome**

Congenital rubella pneumonitis

SP **P35.1 Congenital cytomegalovirus infection**

SP **P35.2 Congenital herpesviral [herpes simplex] infection**

SP **P35.3 Congenital viral hepatitis**

SP + **P35.4 Congenital Zika virus disease**

Use additional code to identify manifestations of congenital Zika virus disease

SP **P35.8 Other congenital viral diseases**

Congenital varicella [chickenpox]

IQ **P35.9 Congenital viral disease, unspecified**

+ 4 **P36 Bacterial sepsis of newborn**

INCLUDES congenital sepsis

Use additional code(s), if applicable, to identify severe sepsis (R65.2-) and associated acute organ dysfunction(s)

SP + **P36.0 Sepsis of newborn due to streptococcus, group B**

+ 5 **P36.1 Sepsis of newborn due to other and unspecified streptococci**

Chapter 16

P00-P96

SP + P36.10 **Sepsis of newborn due to unspecified streptococci**

SP + P36.19 **Sepsis of newborn due to other streptococci**

SP + P36.2 **Sepsis of newborn due to Staphylococcus aureus**

+ 5 P36.3 **Sepsis of newborn due to other and unspecified staphylococci**

SP + P36.30 **Sepsis of newborn due to unspecified staphylococci**

SP + P36.39 **Sepsis of newborn due to other staphylococci**

SP + P36.4 **Sepsis of newborn due to Escherichia coli**

SP + P36.5 **Sepsis of newborn due to anaerobes**

SP + P36.8 **Other bacterial sepsis of newborn**
Use additional code from category B96 to identify organism

SP + P36.9 **Bacterial sepsis of newborn, unspecified**

4 P37 **Other congenital infectious and parasitic diseases**
EXCLUDES 2 congenital syphilis (A50.-)
infectious neonatal diarrhea (A00-A09)
necrotizing enterocolitis in newborn (P77.-)
noninfectious neonatal diarrhea (P78.3)
ophthalmia neonatorum due to gonococcus (A54.31)
tetanus neonatorum (A33)

SP P37.0 **Congenital tuberculosis**

SP P37.1 **Congenital toxoplasmosis**
Hydrocephalus due to congenital toxoplasmosis

SP P37.2 **Neonatal (disseminated) listeriosis**

SP P37.3 **Congenital falciparum malaria**

SP P37.4 **Other congenital malaria**

SP P37.5 **Neonatal candidiasis**

SP P37.8 **Other specified congenital infectious and parasitic diseases**

IQ P37.9 **Congenital infectious or parasitic disease, unspecified**

4 P38 **Omphalitis of newborn**
EXCLUDES 1 omphalitis not of newborn (L08.82)
tetanus omphalitis (A33)
umbilical hemorrhage of newborn (P51.-)

SP P38.1 **Omphalitis with mild hemorrhage**

SP P38.9 **Omphalitis without hemorrhage**
Omphalitis of newborn NOS

+ 4 P39 **Other infections specific to the perinatal period**
Use additional code to identify organism or specific infection

SP + P39.0 **Neonatal infective mastitis**
EXCLUDES 1 breast engorgement of newborn (P83.4)
noninfective mastitis of newborn (P83.4)
DEFINITION Inflammation of the breast in a newborn.

SP + P39.1 **Neonatal conjunctivitis and dacryocystitis**
Neonatal chlamydial conjunctivitis
Ophthalmia neonatorum NOS
EXCLUDES 1 gonococcal conjunctivitis (A54.31)

SP + P39.2 **Intra-amniotic infection affecting newborn, not elsewhere classified**

SP + P39.3 **Neonatal urinary tract infection**

SP + P39.4 **Neonatal skin infection**
Neonatal pyoderma
EXCLUDES 1 pemphigus neonatorum (L00)
staphylococcal scalded skin syndrome (L00)

SP + P39.8 **Other specified infections specific to the perinatal period**

IQ + P39.9 **Infection specific to the perinatal period, unspecified**

Hemorrhagic and hematological disorders of newborn (P50-P61)

EXCLUDES 1 congenital stenosis and stricture of bile ducts (Q44.3)
Crigler-Najjar syndrome (E80.5)
Dubin-Johnson syndrome (E80.6)
Gilbert syndrome (E80.4)
hereditary hemolytic anemias (D55-D58)

4 P50 **Newborn affected by intrauterine (fetal) blood loss**
EXCLUDES 1 congenital anemia from intrauterine (fetal) blood loss (P61.3)

SP P50.0 **Newborn affected by intrauterine (fetal) blood loss from vasa previa**

SP P50.1 **Newborn affected by intrauterine (fetal) blood loss from ruptured cord**

SP P50.2 **Newborn affected by intrauterine (fetal) blood loss from placenta**

SP P50.3 **Newborn affected by hemorrhage into co-twin**

SP P50.4 **Newborn affected by hemorrhage into maternal circulation**

SP P50.5 **Newborn affected by intrauterine (fetal) blood loss from cut end of co-twin's cord**

SP P50.8 **Newborn affected by other intrauterine (fetal) blood loss**

SP P50.9 **Newborn affected by intrauterine (fetal) blood loss, unspecified**
Newborn affected by fetal hemorrhage NOS

4 P51 **Umbilical hemorrhage of newborn**
EXCLUDES 1 omphalitis with mild hemorrhage (P38.1)
umbilical hemorrhage from cut end of co-twins cord (P50.5)

SP P51.0 **Massive umbilical hemorrhage of newborn**

SP P51.8 **Other umbilical hemorrhages of newborn**
Slipped umbilical ligature NOS

SP P51.9 **Umbilical hemorrhage of newborn, unspecified**

4 P52 **Intracranial nontraumatic hemorrhage of newborn**
INCLUDES intracranial hemorrhage due to anoxia or hypoxia
EXCLUDES 1 intracranial hemorrhage due to birth injury (P10.-)

Chapter 16
P00-P96

intracranial hemorrhage due to other injury (S06.-)

SP **P52.0 Intraventricular (nontraumatic) hemorrhage, grade 1, of newborn**
Subependymal hemorrhage (without intraventricular extension)
Bleeding into germinal matrix

SP **P52.1 Intraventricular (nontraumatic) hemorrhage, grade 2, of newborn**
Subependymal hemorrhage with intraventricular extension
Bleeding into ventricle

5 **P52.2 Intraventricular (nontraumatic) hemorrhage, grade 3 and grade 4, of newborn**

SP **P52.21 Intraventricular (nontraumatic) hemorrhage, grade 3, of newborn**
Subependymal hemorrhage with intraventricular extension with enlargement of ventricle

SP **P52.22 Intraventricular (nontraumatic) hemorrhage, grade 4, of newborn**
Bleeding into cerebral cortex
Subependymal hemorrhage with intracerebral extension

!Q **P52.3 Unspecified intraventricular (nontraumatic) hemorrhage of newborn**

SP **P52.4 Intracerebral (nontraumatic) hemorrhage of newborn**

SP **P52.5 Subarachnoid (nontraumatic) hemorrhage of newborn**

SP **P52.6 Cerebellar (nontraumatic) and posterior fossa hemorrhage of newborn**

SP **P52.8 Other intracranial (nontraumatic) hemorrhages of newborn**

!Q **P52.9 Intracranial (nontraumatic) hemorrhage of newborn, unspecified**

SP **P53 Hemorrhagic disease of newborn**
Vitamin K deficiency of newborn

4 **P54 Other neonatal hemorrhages**
EXCLUDES 1 newborn affected by (intrauterine) blood loss (P50.-)
pulmonary hemorrhage originating in the perinatal period (P26.-)

SP **P54.0 Neonatal hematemesis**
EXCLUDES 1 neonatal hematemesis due to swallowed maternal blood (P78.2)

SP **P54.1 Neonatal melena**
EXCLUDES 1 neonatal melena due to swallowed maternal blood (P78.2)

SP **P54.2 Neonatal rectal hemorrhage**

SP **P54.3 Other neonatal gastrointestinal hemorrhage**

SP **P54.4 Neonatal adrenal hemorrhage**

SP **P54.5 Neonatal cutaneous hemorrhage**
Neonatal bruising
Neonatal ecchymoses
Neonatal petechiae
Neonatal superficial hematomata
EXCLUDES 2 bruising of scalp due to birth injury (P12.3)
cephalhematoma due to birth injury (P12.0)

DEFINITION Minute red spots on the surface of the skin, due to escape of a small amount of blood from the vessels.

SP **P54.6 Neonatal vaginal hemorrhage**
Neonatal pseudomenses

SP **P54.8 Other specified neonatal hemorrhages**

!Q **P54.9 Neonatal hemorrhage, unspecified**

4 **P55 Hemolytic disease of newborn**

SP **P55.0 Rh isoimmunization of newborn**

SP **P55.1 ABO isoimmunization of newborn**

SP **P55.8 Other hemolytic diseases of newborn**

!Q **P55.9 Hemolytic disease of newborn, unspecified**

4 **P56 Hydrops fetalis due to hemolytic disease**
EXCLUDES 1 hydrops fetalis NOS (P83.2)

SP **P56.0 Hydrops fetalis due to isoimmunization**

5 **P56.9 Hydrops fetalis due to other and unspecified hemolytic disease**

!Q **P56.90 Hydrops fetalis due to unspecified hemolytic disease**

SP **P56.99 Hydrops fetalis due to other hemolytic disease**

4 **P57 Kernicterus**

SP **P57.0 Kernicterus due to isoimmunization**

DEFINITION Encephalopathy due to severe jaundice caused by destruction of the infant's red blood cells by the mother's immune system. Excess bilirubin crosses the blood-brain barrier and accumulates toxically in the brain.

SP **P57.8 Other specified kernicterus**
EXCLUDES 1 Crigler-Najjar syndrome (E80.5)

SP **P57.9 Kernicterus, unspecified**

4 **P58 Neonatal jaundice due to other excessive hemolysis**
EXCLUDES 1 jaundice due to isoimmunization (P55-P57)

SP **P58.0 Neonatal jaundice due to bruising**

SP **P58.1 Neonatal jaundice due to bleeding**

SP **P58.2 Neonatal jaundice due to infection**

SP **P58.3 Neonatal jaundice due to polycythemia**

+ 5 **P58.4 Neonatal jaundice due to drugs or toxins transmitted from mother or given to newborn**
Code first:
poisoning due to drug or toxin, if applicable (T36-T65 with fifth or sixth character 1-4 or 6)
Use additional code for adverse effect, if applicable, to identify drug (T36-T50 with fifth or sixth character 5)

SP + **P58.41 Neonatal jaundice due to drugs or toxins transmitted from mother**

SP + **P58.42 Neonatal jaundice due to drugs or toxins given to newborn**

SP **P58.5 Neonatal jaundice due to swallowed maternal blood**

SP **P58.8 Neonatal jaundice due to other specified excessive hemolysis**

SP **P58.9 Neonatal jaundice due to excessive hemolysis, unspecified**

Chapter 16 P00-P96

4 **P59 Neonatal jaundice from other and unspecified causes**
EXCLUDES 1 jaundice due to inborn errors of metabolism (E70-E88)
kernicterus (P57.-)

SP **P59.0 Neonatal jaundice associated with preterm delivery**
Hyperbilirubinemia of prematurity
Jaundice due to delayed conjugation associated with preterm delivery

SP **P59.1 Inspissated bile syndrome**

5 **P59.2 Neonatal jaundice from other and unspecified hepatocellular damage**
EXCLUDES 1 congenital viral hepatitis (P35.3)

SP **P59.20 Neonatal jaundice from unspecified hepatocellular damage**

SP **P59.29 Neonatal jaundice from other hepatocellular damage**
Neonatal giant cell hepatitis
Neonatal (idiopathic) hepatitis

SP **P59.3 Neonatal jaundice from breast milk inhibitor**

SP **P59.8 Neonatal jaundice from other specified causes**

SP **P59.9 Neonatal jaundice, unspecified**
Neonatal physiological jaundice (intense)(prolonged) NOS

SP **P60 Disseminated intravascular coagulation of newborn**
Defibrination syndrome of newborn

4 **P61 Other perinatal hematological disorders**
EXCLUDES 1 transient hypogammaglobulinemia of infancy (D80.7)

SP **P61.0 Transient neonatal thrombocytopenia**
Neonatal thrombocytopenia due to exchange transfusion
Neonatal thrombocytopenia due to idiopathic maternal thrombocytopenia
Neonatal thrombocytopenia due to isoimmunization

SP **P61.1 Polycythemia neonatorum**
DEFINITION Abnormally increased number of red blood cells in the neonate's bloodstream.

SP **P61.2 Anemia of prematurity**

SP **P61.3 Congenital anemia from fetal blood loss**

SP **P61.4 Other congenital anemias, not elsewhere classified**
Congenital anemia NOS

SP **P61.5 Transient neonatal neutropenia**
EXCLUDES 1 congenital neutropenia (nontransient) (D70.0)

SP **P61.6 Other transient neonatal disorders of coagulation**

SP **P61.8 Other specified perinatal hematological disorders**

IQ **P61.9 Perinatal hematological disorder, unspecified**

Transitory endocrine and metabolic disorders specific to newborn (P70-P74)

INCLUDES transitory endocrine and metabolic disturbances caused by the infant's response to maternal endocrine and metabolic factors, or its adjustment to extrauterine environment

4 **P70 Transitory disorders of carbohydrate metabolism specific to newborn**

SP **P70.0 Syndrome of infant of mother with gestational diabetes**
Newborn (with hypoglycemia) affected by maternal gestational diabetes
EXCLUDES 1 newborn (with hypoglycemia) affected by maternal (pre-existing) diabetes mellitus (P70.1)
syndrome of infant of a diabetic mother (P70.1)

SP **P70.1 Syndrome of infant of a diabetic mother**
Newborn (with hypoglycemia) affected by maternal (pre-existing) diabetes mellitus
EXCLUDES 1 newborn (with hypoglycemia) affected by maternal gestational diabetes (P70.0)
syndrome of infant of mother with gestational diabetes (P70.0)

SP **P70.2 Neonatal diabetes mellitus**

SP **P70.3 Iatrogenic neonatal hypoglycemia**

SP **P70.4 Other neonatal hypoglycemia**
Transitory neonatal hypoglycemia

SP **P70.8 Other transitory disorders of carbohydrate metabolism of newborn**

SP **P70.9 Transitory disorder of carbohydrate metabolism of newborn, unspecified**

4 **P71 Transitory neonatal disorders of calcium and magnesium metabolism**

SP **P71.0 Cow's milk hypocalcemia in newborn**

SP **P71.1 Other neonatal hypocalcemia**
EXCLUDES 1 neonatal hypoparathyroidism (P71.4)

SP **P71.2 Neonatal hypomagnesemia**

SP **P71.3 Neonatal tetany without calcium or magnesium deficiency**
Neonatal tetany NOS

SP **P71.4 Transitory neonatal hypoparathyroidism**

SP **P71.8 Other transitory neonatal disorders of calcium and magnesium metabolism**

SP **P71.9 Transitory neonatal disorder of calcium and magnesium metabolism, unspecified**

4 **P72 Other transitory neonatal endocrine disorders**
EXCLUDES 1 congenital hypothyroidism with or without goiter (E03.0-E03.1)
dyshormogenetic goiter (E07.1)
Pendred's syndrome (E07.1)

SP **P72.0 Neonatal goiter, not elsewhere classified**
Transitory congenital goiter with normal functioning

SP **P72.1 Transitory neonatal hyperthyroidism**

Chapter 16
P00-P96

4 4th digit required 5 5th digit required 6 6th digit required 7 7th digit required 7th digit placeholder + Additional code Laterality

Neonatal thyrotoxicosis
DEFINITION Abnormally high levels of thyroid hormone in the neonate.

SP P72.2 Other transitory neonatal disorders of thyroid function, not elsewhere classified
Transitory neonatal hypothyroidism

SP P72.8 Other specified transitory neonatal endocrine disorders

IQ P72.9 Transitory neonatal endocrine disorder, unspecified

4 P74 Other transitory neonatal electrolyte and metabolic disturbances

SP P74.0 Late metabolic acidosis of newborn
EXCLUDES 1 (fetal) metabolic acidosis of newborn (P19)
DEFINITION Imbalance in the acid to alkaline ratio in the blood, most often affecting premature infants in the 2nd and 3rd week of life.

SP P74.1 Dehydration of newborn

5 P74.2 Disturbances of sodium balance of newborn

SP P74.21 Hypernatremia of newborn

SP P74.22 Hyponatremia of newborn

5 P74.3 Disturbances of potassium balance of newborn

SP P74.31 Hyperkalemia of newborn

SP P74.32 Hypokalemia of newborn

5 P74.4 Other transitory electrolyte disturbances of newborn

SP P74.41 Alkalosis of newborn
Hyperbicarbonatemia

6 P74.42 Disturbances of chlorine balance of newborn

SP P74.421 Hyperchloremia of newborn
Hyperchloremic metabolic acidosis
EXCLUDES 2 late metabolic acidosis of the newborn (P74.0)

SP P74.422 Hypochloremia of newborn

SP P74.49 Other transitory electrolyte disturbance of newborn

SP P74.5 Transitory tyrosinemia of newborn

SP P74.6 Transitory hyperammonemia of newborn

SP P74.8 Other transitory metabolic disturbances of newborn
Amino-acid metabolic disorders described as transitory

IQ P74.9 Transitory metabolic disturbance of newborn, unspecified

Digestive system disorders of newborn (P76-P78)

4 P76 Other intestinal obstruction of newborn

SP P76.0 Meconium plug syndrome
Meconium ileus NOS
EXCLUDES 1 meconium ileus in cystic fibrosis (E84.11)
DEFINITION Dark green feces that normally comprises a newborn's first bowel movement does not pass through the bowel, causing blockage of the intestine.

SP P76.1 Transitory ileus of newborn
EXCLUDES 1 Hirschsprung's disease (Q43.1)

SP P76.2 Intestinal obstruction due to inspissated milk

SP P76.8 Other specified intestinal obstruction of newborn
EXCLUDES 1 intestinal obstruction classifiable to K56.-

IQ P76.9 Intestinal obstruction of newborn, unspecified

4 P77 Necrotizing enterocolitis of newborn

SP P77.1 Stage 1 necrotizing enterocolitis in newborn
Necrotizing enterocolitis without pneumatosis, without perforation

SP P77.2 Stage 2 necrotizing enterocolitis in newborn
Necrotizing enterocolitis with pneumatosis, without perforation

SP P77.3 Stage 3 necrotizing enterocolitis in newborn
Necrotizing enterocolitis with perforation
Necrotizing enterocolitis with pneumatosis and perforation

IQ P77.9 Necrotizing enterocolitis in newborn, unspecified
Necrotizing enterocolitis in newborn, NOS

4 P78 Other perinatal digestive system disorders
EXCLUDES 1 cystic fibrosis (E84.0-E84.9)
neonatal gastrointestinal hemorrhages (P54.0-P54.3)

SP P78.0 Perinatal intestinal perforation
Meconium peritonitis

SP P78.1 Other neonatal peritonitis
Neonatal peritonitis NOS

SP P78.2 Neonatal hematemesis and melena due to swallowed maternal blood

SP P78.3 Noninfective neonatal diarrhea
Neonatal diarrhea NOS

5 P78.8 Other specified perinatal digestive system disorders

SP P78.81 Congenital cirrhosis (of liver)

SP P78.82 Peptic ulcer of newborn

SP P78.83 Newborn esophageal reflux
Neonatal esophageal reflux

SP P78.84 Gestational alloimmune liver disease
GALD
Neonatal hemochromatosis
EXCLUDES 1 hemochromatosis (E83.11-)

SP P78.89 Other specified perinatal digestive system disorders

SP P78.9 Perinatal digestive system disorder, unspecified

Conditions involving the integument and temperature regulation of newborn (P80-P83)

4 P80 Hypothermia of newborn

SP P80.0 Cold injury syndrome
Severe and usually chronic hypothermia associated with a pink flushed appearance, edema and neurological and biochemical abnormalities.
EXCLUDES 1 mild hypothermia of newborn (P80.8)

SP **P80.8 Other hypothermia of newborn**
Mild hypothermia of newborn

SP **P80.9 Hypothermia of newborn, unspecified**

4 **P81 Other disturbances of temperature regulation of newborn**

SP **P81.0 Environmental hyperthermia of newborn**

SP **P81.8 Other specified disturbances of temperature regulation of newborn**

SP **P81.9 Disturbance of temperature regulation of newborn, unspecified**
Fever of newborn NOS

4 **P83 Other conditions of integument specific to newborn**
EXCLUDES 1 congenital malformations of skin and integument (Q80-Q84)
hydrops fetalis due to hemolytic disease (P56.-)
neonatal skin infection (P39.4)
staphylococcal scalded skin syndrome (L00)
EXCLUDES 2 cradle cap (L21.0)
diaper [napkin] dermatitis (L22)

SP **P83.0 Sclerema neonatorum**

SP **P83.1 Neonatal erythema toxicum**

SP **P83.2 Hydrops fetalis not due to hemolytic disease**
Hydrops fetalis NOS

5 **P83.3 Other and unspecified edema specific to newborn**

SP **P83.30 Unspecified edema specific to newborn**

SP **P83.39 Other edema specific to newborn**

SP **P83.4 Breast engorgement of newborn**
Noninfective mastitis of newborn

SP **P83.5 Congenital hydrocele**

SP **P83.6 Umbilical polyp of newborn**

5 **P83.8 Other specified conditions of integument specific to newborn**

SP **P83.81 Umbilical granuloma**
EXCLUDES 2 Granulomatous disorder of the skin and subcutaneous tissue, unspecified (L92.9)

SP **P83.88 Other specified conditions of integument specific to newborn**
Bronze baby syndrome
Neonatal scleroderma
Urticaria neonatorum

IQ **P83.9 Condition of the integument specific to newborn, unspecified**

Other problems with newborn (P84)

SP **P84 Other problems with newborn**
Acidemia of newborn
Acidosis of newborn
Anoxia of newborn NOS
Asphyxia of newborn NOS
Hypercapnia of newborn
Hypoxemia of newborn
Hypoxia of newborn NOS
Mixed metabolic and respiratory acidosis of newborn
EXCLUDES 1 intracranial hemorrhage due to anoxia or hypoxia (P52.-)
hypoxic ischemic encephalopathy [HIE] (P91.6-)
late metabolic acidosis of newborn (P74.0)

Other disorders originating in the perinatal period (P90-P96)

SP **P90 Convulsions of newborn**
EXCLUDES 1 benign myoclonic epilepsy in infancy (G40.3-)
benign neonatal convulsions (familial) (G40.3-)

4 **P91 Other disturbances of cerebral status of newborn**

SP **P91.0 Neonatal cerebral ischemia**
EXCLUDES 1 Neonatal cerebral infarction (P91.82-)

SP **P91.1 Acquired periventricular cysts of newborn**

SP **P91.2 Neonatal cerebral leukomalacia**
Periventricular leukomalacia

SP **P91.3 Neonatal cerebral irritability**

SP **P91.4 Neonatal cerebral depression**

SP **P91.5 Neonatal coma**

5 **P91.6 Hypoxic ischemic encephalopathy [HIE]**
EXCLUDES 1 Neonatal cerebral depression (P91.4)
Neonatal cerebral irritability (P91.3)
Neonatal coma (P91.5)

SP **P91.60 Hypoxic ischemic encephalopathy [HIE], unspecified**

SP **P91.61 Mild hypoxic ischemic encephalopathy [HIE]**

SP **P91.62 Moderate hypoxic ischemic encephalopathy [HIE]**

SP **P91.63 Severe hypoxic ischemic encephalopathy [HIE]**

5 **P91.8 Other specified disturbances of cerebral status of newborn**

6 **P91.81 Neonatal encephalopathy**

IQ **P91.811 Neonatal encephalopathy in diseases classified elsewhere**
Code first underlying condition, if known, such as:
congenital cirrhosis (of liver) (P78.81)
intracranial nontraumatic hemorrhage of newborn (P52.-)
kernicterus (P57.-)

SP **P91.819 Neonatal encephalopathy, unspecified**

6 **P91.82 Neonatal cerebral infarction**
Neonatal stroke
Perinatal arterial ischemic stroke
Perinatal cerebral infarction
EXCLUDES 1 cerebral infarction (I63.-)
EXCLUDES 2 intracranial hemorrhage of newborn (P52.-)

SP **P91.821 Neonatal cerebral infarction, right side of brain**

H SP **P91.822 Neonatal cerebral infarction, left side of brain**

H SP **P91.823 Neonatal cerebral infarction, bilateral**

H SP **P91.829 Neonatal cerebral infarction, unspecified side**

SP **P91.88 Other specified disturbances of cerebral status of newborn**

IQ **P91.9 Disturbance of cerebral status of newborn, unspecified**

▲ 4 **P92 Feeding problems of newborn**

EXCLUDES 1 eating disorders (F50.-)

EXCLUDES 2 feeding problems in child over 28 days old (R63.3)

5 **P92.0 Vomiting of newborn**

EXCLUDES 1 vomiting of child over 28 days old (R11.-)

SP **P92.01 Bilious vomiting of newborn**

EXCLUDES 1 bilious vomiting in child over 28 days old (R11.14)

SP **P92.09 Other vomiting of newborn**

EXCLUDES 1 regurgitation of food in newborn (P92.1)

SP **P92.1 Regurgitation and rumination of newborn**

SP **P92.2 Slow feeding of newborn**

SP **P92.3 Underfeeding of newborn**

SP **P92.4 Overfeeding of newborn**

SP **P92.5 Neonatal difficulty in feeding at breast**

SP **P92.6 Failure to thrive in newborn**

EXCLUDES 1 failure to thrive in child over 28 days old (R62.51)

SP **P92.8 Other feeding problems of newborn**

IQ **P92.9 Feeding problem of newborn, unspecified**

4 **P93 Reactions and intoxications due to drugs administered to newborn**

INCLUDES reactions and intoxications due to drugs administered to fetus affecting newborn

EXCLUDES 1 jaundice due to drugs or toxins transmitted from mother or given to newborn (P58.4-)
reactions and intoxications from maternal opiates, tranquilizers and other medication (P04.0-P04.1, P04.4-)
withdrawal symptoms from maternal use of drugs of addiction (P96.1)
withdrawal symptoms from therapeutic use of drugs in newborn (P96.2)

SP **P93.0 Grey baby syndrome**

Grey syndrome from chloramphenicol administration in newborn

SP + **P93.8 Other reactions and intoxications due to drugs administered to newborn**

Use additional code for adverse effect, if applicable, to identify drug (T36-T50 with fifth or sixth character 5)

4 **P94 Disorders of muscle tone of newborn**

SP **P94.0 Transient neonatal myasthenia gravis**

EXCLUDES 1 myasthenia gravis (G70.0)

SP **P94.1 Congenital hypertonia**

SP **P94.2 Congenital hypotonia**

Floppy baby syndrome, unspecified

SP **P94.8 Other disorders of muscle tone of newborn**

IQ **P94.9 Disorder of muscle tone of newborn, unspecified**

IQ **P95 Stillbirth**

Deadborn fetus NOS
Fetal death of unspecified cause
Stillbirth NOS

EXCLUDES 1 maternal care for intrauterine death (O36.4)
missed abortion (O02.1)
outcome of delivery, stillbirth (Z37.1, Z37.3, Z37.4, Z37.7)

4 **P96 Other conditions originating in the perinatal period**

SP **P96.0 Congenital renal failure**

Uremia of newborn

SP **P96.1 Neonatal withdrawal symptoms from maternal use of drugs of addiction**

Drug withdrawal syndrome in infant of dependent mother
Neonatal abstinence syndrome

EXCLUDES 1 reactions and intoxications from maternal opiates and tranquilizers administered during labor and delivery (P04.0)

SP **P96.2 Withdrawal symptoms from therapeutic use of drugs in newborn**

SP **P96.3 Wide cranial sutures of newborn**

Neonatal craniotabes

SP **P96.5 Complication to newborn due to (fetal) intrauterine procedure**

EXCLUDES 2 newborn affected by amniocentesis (P00.6)

5 **P96.8 Other specified conditions originating in the perinatal period**

SP **P96.81 Exposure to (parental) (environmental) tobacco smoke in the perinatal period**

EXCLUDES 2 newborn affected by in utero exposure to tobacco (P04.2)
exposure to environmental tobacco smoke after the perinatal period (Z77.22)

SP **P96.82 Delayed separation of umbilical cord**

IQ **P96.83 Meconium staining**

EXCLUDES 1 meconium aspiration (P24.00, P24.01)
meconium passage during delivery (P03.82)

SP + **P96.89 Other specified conditions originating in the perinatal period**

Use additional code to specify condition

IQ **P96.9 Condition originating in the perinatal period, unspecified**

Congenital debility NOS

Chapter 17: Congenital Malformations, Deformations and Chromosomal Abnormalities (Q00-Q99)

"Congenital" indicates a condition that is present at birth. A congenital anomaly may be caused by an inherited abnormality (such as webbed fingers or syndactyly), or due to environmental factors (such as fetal alcohol syndrome). Chapter 17 includes codes for congenital conditions related to problems inherited from parents as well as environmental causes. Chapter 16 includes congenital conditions related to environmental problems or injuries occurring during birth.

Codes for these conditions are located in the Alphabetic Index under the terms "anomaly", malformations, deformity/deformations or abnormal chromosomal.

Assign appropriate codes from this chapter when a malformation/deformation or chromosomal abnormality is documented. The diagnosis may be principal/first-listed or a secondary diagnosis.

Codes in this chapter most often are reported for pediatric patients, but may be listed throughout the patient's life. Some anomalies are present at birth but do not become apparent until later in life, e.g., arteriovenous malformations in the brain. Whenever the condition is diagnosed during the patient's lifetime, it is appropriate to assign a code from code range Q00-Q99.

If a congenital malformation or deformity has been corrected, a personal history code should be used to **identify the history of the malformation or deformity. Note,** codes from this chapter are not for use on maternal records.

Multiple Coding and Sequencing

It is important to read the Includes and Excludes notes under codes in this chapter, as well as any other instructions under the code or code category. The following are examples of multiple coding and sequencing issues for codes in this chapter:

- When a congenital anomaly does not have a unique code assignment, assign additional codes for any manifestation that may be present. An example is the use of code Q79.1 (Other congenital malformations of diaphragm) for a patient with congenital absence of diaphragm. Report the associated respiratory conditions as additional diagnoses to provide more information.
- When the code assignment specifically identifies the malformation, deformity or chromosomal abnormality, manifestations that are an inherent component of the anomaly should not be coded separately. An example is code Q21.3 (Tetralogy of Fallot). The individual cardiac conditions associated with this anomaly such as ventricular septal defect with pulmonary stenosis or atresia, dextroposition of aorta, and hypertrophy of right ventricle, are not reported separately. However, additional codes should be assigned for manifestations that are not an inherent component of the condition.

  When a malformation, deformation or chromosomal abnormality does not have a unique code assignment, assign additional codes for any manifestations that may be present,
- For the birth admission, the appropriate code from category Z38, Liveborn infants, according to place of birth and type of delivery, should be sequenced as the principal diagnosis, followed by any congenital anomaly codes (Q00-Q99) as additional diagnoses.

Special Coding Issues – Congenital or Acquired

Coders should be cautious when selecting codes from this chapter. Some conditions can be either congenital or acquired (developed after birth). The Alphabetical Index in ICD-10 shows acquired and congenital as subentries under the main term.

Defect
    Circulation I99.9
        congenital Q28.9

A congenital circulation defect is reported using code Q28.9; an acquired defect is reported using code I99.9. If not specified as acquired or congenital, query the physician or report as acquired.

The Alphabetic Index sometimes indicates an acquired condition using parentheses as a nonessential modifier. For example, the index for cyst of kidney reads:

Cyst
    Kidney (acquired) N28.1
        congenital Q61.00

Congenital cysts are reported using code Q61.00; acquired cysts are reported using code N28.1. If not specified as acquired or congenital, query the physician or report as acquired.

Coders often make mistakes when referencing the Alphabetic Index for the status codes for absent body parts, such as amputation status codes. Many entries under the term "absence" include two choices – one for the congenital absence of the body part and one for the acquired absence. Acquired absence is usually the result of surgical removal. Reference: 'Absence, lung.' The first code listed is Q33.3 for the congenital absence of the lung. The second code listed is Z90.2 for the acquired absence of lung, i.e., surgical removal.

CHAPTER 17: CONGENITAL MALFORMATIONS, DEFORMATIONS AND CHROMOSOMAL ABNORMALITIES (Q00-Q99)

Note:
Codes from this chapter are not for use on maternal records

EXCLUDES 2 inborn errors of metabolism (E70-E88)

ALERT Sometimes payer policy conflicts with official guidelines, rules and conventions, and other official guidance. When a payer refuses to pay based on code(s) used in compliance with that guidance, take the following steps: 1) Determine whether the denial or rejection is truly a coding dispute and not a different coverage or payment issue; 2) Remind the payer that following official guidelines and conventions is required by HIPAA code set standards and provide the official guidance in question. If a payer does have a policy that clearly conflicts with official coding rules or guidelines, every effort should be made to resolve the issue with the payer; 3) If the payer refuses to change its policy, obtain the payer requirements in writing. If the payer refuses to provide their policy in writing, document all discussions, including dates and names of individuals involved; 4) Conform to the payer's policy if the payer continues to deny or reject the claim; 5) Keep a permanent file of the documentation obtained regarding payer coding policies. It may be come in handy in the event of an audit.

GUIDELINES **Section I.C.17**

Codes from Chapter 17 may be used throughout the life of the patient. If a congenital malformation or deformity has been corrected, a personal history code should be used to identify the history of the malformation or deformity. Although present at birth, a malformation/deformation/or chromosomal abnormality may not be identified until later in life. Whenever the condition is diagnosed by the provider, it is appropriate to assign a code from codes Q00-Q99. For the birth admission, the appropriate code from category Z38, Liveborn infants, according to place of birth and type of delivery, should be sequenced as the principal diagnosis, followed by any congenital anomaly codes, Q00- Q99.

This chapter contains the following blocks:

Q00-Q07	Congenital malformations of the nervous system
Q10-Q18	Congenital malformations of eye, ear, face and neck
Q20-Q28	Congenital malformations of the circulatory system
Q30-Q34	Congenital malformations of the respiratory system
Q35-Q37	Cleft lip and cleft palate
Q38-Q45	Other congenital malformations of the digestive system
Q50-Q56	Congenital malformations of genital organs
Q60-Q64	Congenital malformations of the urinary system
Q65-Q79	Congenital malformations and deformations of the musculoskeletal system
Q80-Q89	Other congenital malformations
Q90-Q99	Chromosomal abnormalities, not elsewhere classified

Congenital malformations of the nervous system (Q00-Q07)

4 Q00 Anencephaly and similar malformations

IQ Q00.0 Anencephaly
Acephaly
Acrania
Amyelencephaly
Hemianencephaly
Hemicephaly

IQ Q00.1 Craniorachischisis

IQ Q00.2 Iniencephaly

DEFINITION Neural tube birth defect in which the fetal head is severely bent backwards, the neck is usually absent, and other severe birth defects are present.

4 Q01 Encephalocele

INCLUDES Arnold-Chiari syndrome, type III
encephalocystocele
encephalomyelocele
hydroencephalocele
hydromeningocele, cranial
meningocele, cerebral
meningoencephalocele

EXCLUDES 1 Meckel-Gruber syndrome (Q61.9)

IQ Q01.0 Frontal encephalocele

IQ Q01.1 Nasofrontal encephalocele

IQ Q01.2 Occipital encephalocele

IQ Q01.8 Encephalocele of other sites

IQ Q01.9 Encephalocele, unspecified

IQ Q02 Microcephaly

INCLUDES hydromicrocephaly
micrencephalon

Code first:
, if applicable, congenital Zika virus disease

EXCLUDES 1 Meckel-Gruber syndrome (Q61.9)

DEFINITION Abnormal smallness of the head.

4 Q03 Congenital hydrocephalus

INCLUDES hydrocephalus in newborn

EXCLUDES 1 Arnold-Chiari syndrome, type II (Q07.0-)
acquired hydrocephalus (G91.-)
hydrocephalus due to congenital toxoplasmosis (P37.1)
hydrocephalus with spina bifida (Q05.0-Q05.4)

CODING TIPS✓ Use Z98.2 as a secondary code to indicate a cerebrospinal fluid drainage shunt.

IQ Q03.0 Malformations of aqueduct of Sylvius
Anomaly of aqueduct of Sylvius
Obstruction of aqueduct of Sylvius, congenital
Stenosis of aqueduct of Sylvius

IQ Q03.1 Atresia of foramina of Magendie and Luschka
Dandy-Walker syndrome

IQ Q03.8 Other congenital hydrocephalus

IQ Q03.9 Congenital hydrocephalus, unspecified

4 Q04 Other congenital malformations of brain

EXCLUDES 1 cyclopia (Q87.0)
macrocephaly (Q75.3)

IQ Q04.0 Congenital malformations of corpus callosum
Agenesis of corpus callosum

IQ Q04.1 Arhinencephaly

IQ Q04.2 Holoprosencephaly

IQ Q04.3 Other reduction deformities of brain
Absence of part of brain
Agenesis of part of brain

Agyria
Aplasia of part of brain
Hydranencephaly
Hypoplasia of part of brain
Lissencephaly
Microgyria
Pachygyria
EXCLUDES 1 congenital malformations of corpus callosum (Q04.0)

IQ **Q04.4 Septo-optic dysplasia of brain**

IQ **Q04.5 Megalencephaly**

IQ **Q04.6 Congenital cerebral cysts**
Porencephaly
Schizencephaly
EXCLUDES 1 acquired porencephalic cyst (G93.0)

IQ **Q04.8 Other specified congenital malformations of brain**
Arnold-Chiari syndrome, type IV
Macrogyria

IQ **Q04.9 Congenital malformation of brain, unspecified**
Congenital anomaly NOS of brain
Congenital deformity NOS of brain
Congenital disease or lesion NOS of brain
Multiple anomalies NOS of brain, congenital

+ 4 **Q05 Spina bifida**
INCLUDES hydromeningocele (spinal)
meningocele (spinal)
meningomyelocele
myelocele
myelomeningocele
rachischisis
spina bifida (aperta) (cystica)
syringomyelocele
Use additional code for any associated paraplegia (paraparesis) (G82.2-)
EXCLUDES 1 Arnold-Chiari syndrome, type II (Q07.0-)
spina bifida occulta (Q76.0)
CODING TIPS ✓ Use Z98.2 as a secondary code to indicate a cerebrospinal fluid drainage shunt.

SP + **Q05.0 Cervical spina bifida with hydrocephalus**

SP + **Q05.1 Thoracic spina bifida with hydrocephalus**
Dorsal spina bifida with hydrocephalus
Thoracolumbar spina bifida with hydrocephalus

SP + **Q05.2 Lumbar spina bifida with hydrocephalus**
Lumbosacral spina bifida with hydrocephalus

SP + **Q05.3 Sacral spina bifida with hydrocephalus**

SP + **Q05.4 Unspecified spina bifida with hydrocephalus**

SP + **Q05.5 Cervical spina bifida without hydrocephalus**

SP + **Q05.6 Thoracic spina bifida without hydrocephalus**
Dorsal spina bifida NOS
Thoracolumbar spina bifida NOS

SP + **Q05.7 Lumbar spina bifida without hydrocephalus**
Lumbosacral spina bifida NOS

SP + **Q05.8 Sacral spina bifida without hydrocephalus**

SP + **Q05.9 Spina bifida, unspecified**

4 **Q06 Other congenital malformations of spinal cord**

IQ **Q06.0 Amyelia**

IQ **Q06.1 Hypoplasia and dysplasia of spinal cord**
Atelomyelia
Myelatelia
Myelodysplasia of spinal cord

IQ **Q06.2 Diastematomyelia**

IQ **Q06.3 Other congenital cauda equina malformations**

IQ **Q06.4 Hydromyelia**
Hydrorachis

IQ **Q06.8 Other specified congenital malformations of spinal cord**

IQ **Q06.9 Congenital malformation of spinal cord, unspecified**
Congenital anomaly NOS of spinal cord
Congenital deformity NOS of spinal cord
Congenital disease or lesion NOS of spinal cord

4 **Q07 Other congenital malformations of nervous system**
EXCLUDES 2 congenital central alveolar hypoventilation syndrome (G47.35)
familial dysautonomia [Riley-Day] (G90.1)
neurofibromatosis (nonmalignant) (Q85.0-)
CODING TIPS ✓ Chiari malformation, also referred to as Arnold-Chiari malformation, is an anomaly where cerebellar tissue extends into the spinal canal. The most common form, type IV, includes spina bifida and hydrocephalus. Type IV is an anomaly where cerebellar hypoplasia is present.

5 **Q07.0 Arnold-Chiari syndrome**
Arnold-Chiari syndrome, type II
EXCLUDES 1 Arnold-Chiari syndrome, type III (Q01.-)
Arnold-Chiari syndrome, type IV (Q04.8)

SP **Q07.00 Arnold-Chiari syndrome without spina bifida or hydrocephalus**

SP **Q07.01 Arnold-Chiari syndrome with spina bifida**

SP **Q07.02 Arnold-Chiari syndrome with hydrocephalus**

SP **Q07.03 Arnold-Chiari syndrome with spina bifida and hydrocephalus**

SP **Q07.8 Other specified congenital malformations of nervous system**
Agenesis of nerve
Displacement of brachial plexus
Jaw-winking syndrome
Marcus Gunn's syndrome

IQ **Q07.9 Congenital malformation of nervous system, unspecified**
Congenital anomaly NOS of nervous system
Congenital deformity NOS of nervous system
Congenital disease or lesion NOS of nervous system

Congenital malformations of eye, ear, face and neck (Q10-Q18)

EXCLUDES 2 cleft lip and cleft palate (Q35-Q37)
congenital malformation of cervical spine (Q05.0, Q05.5, Q67.5, Q76.0-Q76.4)
congenital malformation of larynx (Q31.-)
congenital malformation of lip NEC (Q38.0)
congenital malformation of nose (Q30.-)
congenital malformation of parathyroid gland (Q89.2)
congenital malformation of thyroid gland (Q89.2)

4 **Q10 Congenital malformations of eyelid, lacrimal apparatus and orbit**
EXCLUDES 1 cryptophthalmos NOS (Q11.2)
cryptophthalmos syndrome (Q87.0)

IQ **Q10.0 Congenital ptosis**
DEFINITION Congenital drooping of the upper eyelid.

IQ **Q10.1 Congenital ectropion**

IQ **Q10.2 Congenital entropion**

IQ **Q10.3 Other congenital malformations of eyelid**
Ablepharon
Blepharophimosis, congenital
Coloboma of eyelid
Congenital absence or agenesis of cilia
Congenital absence or agenesis of eyelid
Congenital accessory eyelid
Congenital accessory eye muscle
Congenital malformation of eyelid NOS

IQ **Q10.4 Absence and agenesis of lacrimal apparatus**
Congenital absence of punctum lacrimale

IQ **Q10.5 Congenital stenosis and stricture of lacrimal duct**

IQ **Q10.6 Other congenital malformations of lacrimal apparatus**
Congenital malformation of lacrimal apparatus NOS

IQ **Q10.7 Congenital malformation of orbit**

4 **Q11 Anophthalmos, microphthalmos and macrophthalmos**

IQ **Q11.0 Cystic eyeball**

IQ **Q11.1 Other anophthalmos**
Anophthalmos NOS
Agenesis of eye
Aplasia of eye

IQ **Q11.2 Microphthalmos**
Cryptophthalmos NOS
Dysplasia of eye
Hypoplasia of eye
Rudimentary eye
EXCLUDES 1 cryptophthalmos syndrome (Q87.0)
DEFINITION Abnormal smallness in all dimensions of one or both eyes.

IQ **Q11.3 Macrophthalmos**
EXCLUDES 1 macrophthalmos in congenital glaucoma (Q15.0)

4 **Q12 Congenital lens malformations**

IQ **Q12.0 Congenital cataract**

IQ **Q12.1 Congenital displaced lens**

IQ **Q12.2 Coloboma of lens**

IQ **Q12.3 Congenital aphakia**

IQ **Q12.4 Spherophakia**

IQ **Q12.8 Other congenital lens malformations**
Microphakia

IQ **Q12.9 Congenital lens malformation, unspecified**

4 **Q13 Congenital malformations of anterior segment of eye**

IQ **Q13.0 Coloboma of iris**
Coloboma NOS

IQ + **Q13.1 Absence of iris**
Aniridia
Use additional code for associated glaucoma (H42)

IQ **Q13.2 Other congenital malformations of iris**
Anisocoria, congenital
Atresia of pupil
Congenital malformation of iris NOS
Corectopia

IQ **Q13.3 Congenital corneal opacity**

IQ **Q13.4 Other congenital corneal malformations**
Congenital malformation of cornea NOS
Microcornea
Peter's anomaly

IQ **Q13.5 Blue sclera**

5 **Q13.8 Other congenital malformations of anterior segment of eye**

IQ + **Q13.81 Rieger's anomaly**
Use additional code for associated glaucoma (H42)

IQ **Q13.89 Other congenital malformations of anterior segment of eye**

IQ **Q13.9 Congenital malformation of anterior segment of eye, unspecified**

4 **Q14 Congenital malformations of posterior segment of eye**
EXCLUDES 2 optic nerve hypoplasia (H47.03-)

IQ **Q14.0 Congenital malformation of vitreous humor**
Congenital vitreous opacity

IQ **Q14.1 Congenital malformation of retina**
Congenital retinal aneurysm

IQ **Q14.2 Congenital malformation of optic disc**
Coloboma of optic disc

IQ **Q14.3 Congenital malformation of choroid**

IQ **Q14.8 Other congenital malformations of posterior segment of eye**
Coloboma of the fundus

IQ **Q14.9 Congenital malformation of posterior segment of eye, unspecified**

4 **Q15 Other congenital malformations of eye**
EXCLUDES 1 congenital nystagmus (H55.01)
ocular albinism (E70.31-)
optic nerve hypoplasia (H47.03-)
retinitis pigmentosa (H35.52)

IQ **Q15.0 Congenital glaucoma**
Axenfeld's anomaly
Buphthalmos
Glaucoma of childhood
Glaucoma of newborn
Hydrophthalmos
Keratoglobus, congenital, with glaucoma
Macrocornea with glaucoma

Macrophthalmos in congenital glaucoma
Megalocornea with glaucoma

DEFINITION Disease of infancy, marked by an increase of intraocular fluid, elevated eye pressure, and enlargement of the eyeball.

!Q **Q15.8 Other specified congenital malformations of eye**

!Q **Q15.9 Congenital malformation of eye, unspecified**
Congenital anomaly of eye
Congenital deformity of eye

4 **Q16 Congenital malformations of ear causing impairment of hearing**
EXCLUDES 1 congenital deafness (H90.-)

!Q **Q16.0 Congenital absence of (ear) auricle**

!Q **Q16.1 Congenital absence, atresia and stricture of auditory canal (external)**
Congenital atresia or stricture of osseous meatus

!Q **Q16.2 Absence of eustachian tube**

!Q **Q16.3 Congenital malformation of ear ossicles**
Congenital fusion of ear ossicles

!Q **Q16.4 Other congenital malformations of middle ear**
Congenital malformation of middle ear NOS

!Q **Q16.5 Congenital malformation of inner ear**
Congenital anomaly of membranous labyrinth
Congenital anomaly of organ of Corti

!Q **Q16.9 Congenital malformation of ear causing impairment of hearing, unspecified**
Congenital absence of ear NOS

4 **Q17 Other congenital malformations of ear**
EXCLUDES 1 congenital malformations of ear with impairment of hearing (Q16.0-Q16.9)
preauricular sinus (Q18.1)

!Q **Q17.0 Accessory auricle**
Accessory tragus
Polyotia
Preauricular appendage or tag
Supernumerary ear
Supernumerary lobule

!Q **Q17.1 Macrotia**
DEFINITION Excessive enlargement of the auricle (outer portion of ear).

!Q **Q17.2 Microtia**

!Q **Q17.3 Other misshapen ear**
Pointed ear

!Q **Q17.4 Misplaced ear**
Low-set ears
EXCLUDES 1 cervical auricle (Q18.2)

!Q **Q17.5 Prominent ear**
Bat ear

!Q **Q17.8 Other specified congenital malformations of ear**
Congenital absence of lobe of ear

!Q **Q17.9 Congenital malformation of ear, unspecified**
Congenital anomaly of ear NOS

4 **Q18 Other congenital malformations of face and neck**
EXCLUDES 1 cleft lip and cleft palate (Q35-Q37)
conditions classified to Q67.0-Q67.4
congenital malformations of skull and face bones (Q75.-)
cyclopia (Q87.0)
dentofacial anomalies [including malocclusion] (M26.-)
malformation syndromes affecting facial appearance (Q87.0)
persistent thyroglossal duct (Q89.2)

!Q **Q18.0 Sinus, fistula and cyst of branchial cleft**
Branchial vestige

!Q **Q18.1 Preauricular sinus and cyst**
Fistula of auricle, congenital
Cervicoaural fistula

!Q **Q18.2 Other branchial cleft malformations**
Branchial cleft malformation NOS
Cervical auricle
Otocephaly

!Q **Q18.3 Webbing of neck**
Pterygium colli
DEFINITION A thick flap of skin extending from the side of the neck to the shoulder, often in concert with other birth defects.

!Q **Q18.4 Macrostomia**
DEFINITION Abnormally large mouth.

!Q **Q18.5 Microstomia**
DEFINITION Abnormally small mouth.

!Q **Q18.6 Macrocheilia**
Hypertrophy of lip, congenital
DEFINITION Abnormally large lips.

!Q **Q18.7 Microcheilia**

!Q **Q18.8 Other specified congenital malformations of face and neck**
Medial cyst of face and neck
Medial fistula of face and neck
Medial sinus of face and neck

!Q **Q18.9 Congenital malformation of face and neck, unspecified**
Congenital anomaly NOS of face and neck

Congenital malformations of the circulatory system (Q20-Q28)

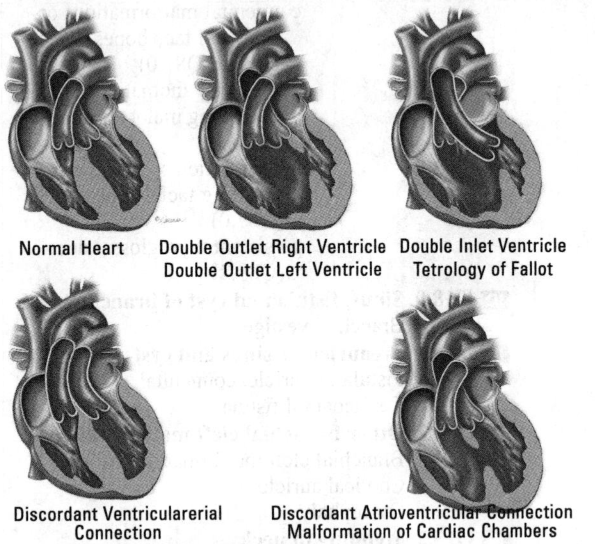

4 Q20 Congenital malformations of cardiac chambers and connections
EXCLUDES 1 dextrocardia with situs inversus (Q89.3)
mirror-image atrial arrangement with situs inversus (Q89.3)

SP Q20.0 Common arterial trunk
Persistent truncus arteriosus
EXCLUDES 1 aortic septal defect (Q21.4)
DEFINITION Congenital anomaly in which there is abnormal communication between the ascending aorta and pulmonary artery, near the semilunar valve.

SP Q20.1 Double outlet right ventricle
Taussig-Bing syndrome

SP Q20.2 Double outlet left ventricle

SP Q20.3 Discordant ventriculoarterial connection
Dextrotransposition of aorta
Transposition of great vessels (complete)

SP Q20.4 Double inlet ventricle
Common ventricle
Cor triloculare biatriatum
Single ventricle
DEFINITION No septum or membrane is present dividing the right ventricle from the left ventricle.

SP Q20.5 Discordant atrioventricular connection
Corrected transposition
Levotransposition
Ventricular inversion

SP Q20.6 Isomerism of atrial appendages
Isomerism of atrial appendages with asplenia or polysplenia

SP Q20.8 Other congenital malformations of cardiac chambers and connections
Cor binoculare

IQ Q20.9 Congenital malformation of cardiac chambers and connections, unspecified

4 Q21 Congenital malformations of cardiac septa
EXCLUDES 1 acquired cardiac septal defect (I51.0)

SP Q21.0 Ventricular septal defect
Roger's disease

SP Q21.1 Atrial septal defect
Coronary sinus defect
Patent or persistent foramen ovale
Patent or persistent ostium secundum defect (type II)
Patent or persistent sinus venosus defect

SP Q21.2 Atrioventricular septal defect
Common atrioventricular canal
Endocardial cushion defect
Ostium primum atrial septal defect (type I)

SP Q21.3 Tetralogy of Fallot
Ventricular septal defect with pulmonary stenosis or atresia, dextroposition of aorta and hypertrophy of right ventricle.

SP Q21.4 Aortopulmonary septal defect
Aortic septal defect
Aortopulmonary window

SP Q21.8 Other congenital malformations of cardiac septa
Eisenmenger's defect
Pentalogy of Fallot
Code also, if applicable:
Eisenmenger's complex (I27.83)
Eisenmenger's syndrome (I27.83)

IQ Q21.9 Congenital malformation of cardiac septum, unspecified
Septal (heart) defect NOS

4 Q22 Congenital malformations of pulmonary and tricuspid valves

SP Q22.0 Pulmonary valve atresia
DEFINITION Congenital absence of a normal valvular opening into the pulmonary artery.

SP Q22.1 Congenital pulmonary valve stenosis

SP Q22.2 Congenital pulmonary valve insufficiency
Congenital pulmonary valve regurgitation

SP Q22.3 Other congenital malformations of pulmonary valve
Congenital malformation of pulmonary valve NOS
Supernumerary cusps of pulmonary valve

SP Q22.4 Congenital tricuspid stenosis
Congenital tricuspid atresia
DEFINITION Abnormal narrowing of the valve that prevents blood from flowing back into the right atrium from the right ventricle.

SP Q22.5 Ebstein's anomaly

SP Q22.6 Hypoplastic right heart syndrome

SP Q22.8 Other congenital malformations of tricuspid valve

SP Q22.9 Congenital malformation of tricuspid valve, unspecified

4 Q23 Congenital malformations of aortic and mitral valves

SP Q23.0 Congenital stenosis of aortic valve
Congenital aortic atresia
Congenital aortic stenosis NOS
EXCLUDES 1 congenital stenosis of aortic valve in hypoplastic left heart syndrome (Q23.4)
congenital subaortic stenosis (Q24.4)
supravalvular aortic stenosis (congenital) (Q25.3)

4 4th digit required 5 5th digit required 6 6th digit required 7 7th digit required X 7th digit placeholder + Additional code = Laterality

SP Q23.1 Congenital insufficiency of aortic valve
Bicuspid aortic valve
Congenital aortic insufficiency

SP Q23.2 Congenital mitral stenosis
Congenital mitral atresia

SP Q23.3 Congenital mitral insufficiency

SP Q23.4 Hypoplastic left heart syndrome

SP Q23.8 Other congenital malformations of aortic and mitral valves

!Q Q23.9 Congenital malformation of aortic and mitral valves, unspecified

4 Q24 Other congenital malformations of heart
EXCLUDES 1 endocardial fibroelastosis (I42.4)

SP Q24.0 Dextrocardia
EXCLUDES 1 dextrocardia with situs inversus (Q89.3)
isomerism of atrial appendages (with asplenia or polysplenia) (Q20.6)
mirror-image atrial arrangement with situs inversus (Q89.3)

SP Q24.1 Levocardia

SP Q24.2 Cor triatriatum
DEFINITION The heart has three atrial chambers with the left atrium divided into two segments.

SP Q24.3 Pulmonary infundibular stenosis
Subvalvular pulmonic stenosis

SP Q24.4 Congenital subaortic stenosis

SP Q24.5 Malformation of coronary vessels
Congenital coronary (artery) aneurysm

SP Q24.6 Congenital heart block

SP Q24.8 Other specified congenital malformations of heart
Congenital diverticulum of left ventricle
Congenital malformation of myocardium
Congenital malformation of pericardium
Malposition of heart
Uhl's disease

!Q Q24.9 Congenital malformation of heart, unspecified
Congenital anomaly of heart
Congenital disease of heart

4 Q25 Congenital malformations of great arteries
CODING TIPS✓ If the condition has been corrected or is no longer a problem, then code Z87.74, Personal history of (corrected) congenital malformations of heart and circulatory system.

SP Q25.0 Patent ductus arteriosus
Patent ductus Botallo
Persistent ductus arteriosus

SP Q25.1 Coarctation of aorta
Coarctation of aorta (preductal) (postductal)
Stenosis of aorta

5 Q25.2 Atresia of aorta

SP Q25.21 Interruption of aortic arch
Atresia of aortic arch

SP Q25.29 Other atresia of aorta
Atresia of aorta

SP Q25.3 Supravalvular aortic stenosis
EXCLUDES 1 congenital aortic stenosis NOS (Q23.0)
congenital stenosis of aortic valve (Q23.0)

5 Q25.4 Other congenital malformations of aorta
EXCLUDES 1 hypoplasia of aorta in hypoplastic left heart syndrome (Q23.4)

!Q Q25.40 Congenital malformation of aorta unspecified

SP Q25.41 Absence and aplasia of aorta

SP Q25.42 Hypoplasia of aorta

SP Q25.43 Congenital aneurysm of aorta
Congenital aneurysm of aortic root
Congenital aneurysm of aortic sinus

SP Q25.44 Congenital dilation of aorta

SP Q25.45 Double aortic arch
Vascular ring of aorta

SP Q25.46 Tortuous aortic arch
Persistent convolutions of aortic arch

SP Q25.47 Right aortic arch
Persistent right aortic arch

SP Q25.48 Anomalous origin of subclavian artery

SP Q25.49 Other congenital malformations of aorta
Aortic arch
Bovine arch

SP Q25.5 Atresia of pulmonary artery

SP Q25.6 Stenosis of pulmonary artery
Supravalvular pulmonary stenosis

5 Q25.7 Other congenital malformations of pulmonary artery

SP Q25.71 Coarctation of pulmonary artery

SP Q25.72 Congenital pulmonary arteriovenous malformation
Congenital pulmonary arteriovenous aneurysm

SP Q25.79 Other congenital malformations of pulmonary artery
Aberrant pulmonary artery
Agenesis of pulmonary artery
Congenital aneurysm of pulmonary artery
Congenital anomaly of pulmonary artery
Hypoplasia of pulmonary artery

SP Q25.8 Other congenital malformations of other great arteries

!Q Q25.9 Congenital malformation of great arteries, unspecified

4 Q26 Congenital malformations of great veins

SP Q26.0 Congenital stenosis of vena cava
Congenital stenosis of vena cava (inferior)(superior)

SP Q26.1 Persistent left superior vena cava

SP Q26.2 Total anomalous pulmonary venous connection
Total anomalous pulmonary venous return [TAPVR], subdiaphragmatic
Total anomalous pulmonary venous return [TAPVR], supradiaphragmatic

SP Q26.3 Partial anomalous pulmonary venous connection
Partial anomalous pulmonary venous return

Chapter 17 Q00-Q99

SP **Q26.4 Anomalous pulmonary venous connection, unspecified**

SP **Q26.5 Anomalous portal venous connection**

SP **Q26.6 Portal vein-hepatic artery fistula**

SP **Q26.8 Other congenital malformations of great veins**
Absence of vena cava (inferior) (superior)
Azygos continuation of inferior vena cava
Persistent left posterior cardinal vein
Scimitar syndrome

SP **Q26.9 Congenital malformation of great vein, unspecified**
Congenital anomaly of vena cava (inferior) (superior) NOS

4 **Q27 Other congenital malformations of peripheral vascular system**
EXCLUDES 2 anomalies of cerebral and precerebral vessels (Q28.0-Q28.3)
anomalies of coronary vessels (Q24.5)
anomalies of pulmonary artery (Q25.5-Q25.7)
congenital retinal aneurysm (Q14.1)
hemangioma and lymphangioma (D18.-)

SP **Q27.0 Congenital absence and hypoplasia of umbilical artery**
Single umbilical artery

SP **Q27.1 Congenital renal artery stenosis**

SP **Q27.2 Other congenital malformations of renal artery**
Congenital malformation of renal artery NOS
Multiple renal arteries

5 **Q27.3 Arteriovenous malformation (peripheral)**
Arteriovenous aneurysm
EXCLUDES 1 acquired arteriovenous aneurysm (I77.0)
EXCLUDES 2 arteriovenous malformation of cerebral vessels (Q28.2)
arteriovenous malformation of precerebral vessels (Q28.0)

IQ **Q27.30 Arteriovenous malformation, site unspecified**

SP **Q27.31 Arteriovenous malformation of vessel of upper limb**

SP **Q27.32 Arteriovenous malformation of vessel of lower limb**

SP **Q27.33 Arteriovenous malformation of digestive system vessel**

SP **Q27.34 Arteriovenous malformation of renal vessel**

SP **Q27.39 Arteriovenous malformation, other site**

SP **Q27.4 Congenital phlebectasia**

SP **Q27.8 Other specified congenital malformations of peripheral vascular system**
Absence of peripheral vascular system
Atresia of peripheral vascular system
Congenital aneurysm (peripheral)
Congenital stricture, artery
Congenital varix
EXCLUDES 1 arteriovenous malformation (Q27.3-)

IQ **Q27.9 Congenital malformation of peripheral vascular system, unspecified**
Anomaly of artery or vein NOS

4 **Q28 Other congenital malformations of circulatory system**
EXCLUDES 1 congenital aneurysm NOS (Q27.8)
congenital coronary aneurysm (Q24.5)
ruptured cerebral arteriovenous malformation (I60.8)
ruptured malformation of precerebral vessels (I72.0)
EXCLUDES 2 congenital peripheral aneurysm (Q27.8)
congenital pulmonary aneurysm (Q25.79)
congenital retinal aneurysm (Q14.1)

SP **Q28.0 Arteriovenous malformation of precerebral vessels**
Congenital arteriovenous precerebral aneurysm (nonruptured)

SP **Q28.1 Other malformations of precerebral vessels**
Congenital malformation of precerebral vessels NOS
Congenital precerebral aneurysm (nonruptured)

SP **Q28.2 Arteriovenous malformation of cerebral vessels**
Arteriovenous malformation of brain NOS
Congenital arteriovenous cerebral aneurysm (nonruptured)

SP **Q28.3 Other malformations of cerebral vessels**
Congenital cerebral aneurysm (nonruptured)
Congenital malformation of cerebral vessels NOS
Developmental venous anomaly

SP **Q28.8 Other specified congenital malformations of circulatory system**
Congenital aneurysm, specified site NEC
Spinal vessel anomaly

IQ **Q28.9 Congenital malformation of circulatory system, unspecified**

Congenital malformations of the respiratory system (Q30-Q34)

4 **Q30 Congenital malformations of nose**
EXCLUDES 1 congenital deviation of nasal septum (Q67.4)

SP **Q30.0 Choanal atresia**
Atresia of nares (anterior) (posterior)
Congenital stenosis of nares (anterior) (posterior)
DEFINITION Fetal nasal airways are obstructed by membranous or bony tissue; infant is unable to breathe and nurse simultaneously.

SP **Q30.1 Agenesis and underdevelopment of nose**
Congenital absent of nose

SP **Q30.2 Fissured, notched and cleft nose**

SP **Q30.3 Congenital perforated nasal septum**

SP **Q30.8 Other congenital malformations of nose**
Accessory nose
Congenital anomaly of nasal sinus wall

IQ **Q30.9 Congenital malformation of nose, unspecified**

4 **Q31 Congenital malformations of larynx**
EXCLUDES 1 congenital laryngeal stridor NOS (P28.89)

SP **Q31.0 Web of larynx**
Glottic web of larynx
Subglottic web of larynx
Web of larynx NOS

SP **Q31.1 Congenital subglottic stenosis**

SP **Q31.2 Laryngeal hypoplasia**

SP **Q31.3 Laryngocele**

SP **Q31.5 Congenital laryngomalacia**

SP **Q31.8 Other congenital malformations of larynx**
Absence of larynx
Agenesis of larynx
Atresia of larynx
Congenital cleft thyroid cartilage
Congenital fissure of epiglottis
Congenital stenosis of larynx NEC
Posterior cleft of cricoid cartilage

IQ **Q31.9 Congenital malformation of larynx, unspecified**

4 **Q32 Congenital malformations of trachea and bronchus**
EXCLUDES 1 congenital bronchiectasis (Q33.4)

SP **Q32.0 Congenital tracheomalacia**

SP **Q32.1 Other congenital malformations of trachea**
Atresia of trachea
Congenital anomaly of tracheal cartilage
Congenital dilatation of trachea
Congenital malformation of trachea
Congenital stenosis of trachea
Congenital tracheocele

SP **Q32.2 Congenital bronchomalacia**

SP **Q32.3 Congenital stenosis of bronchus**

SP **Q32.4 Other congenital malformations of bronchus**
Absence of bronchus
Agenesis of bronchus
Atresia of bronchus
Congenital diverticulum of bronchus
Congenital malformation of bronchus NOS

4 **Q33 Congenital malformations of lung**

SP **Q33.0 Congenital cystic lung**
Congenital cystic lung disease
Congenital honeycomb lung
Congenital polycystic lung disease
EXCLUDES 1 cystic fibrosis (E84.0)
cystic lung disease, acquired or unspecified (J98.4)

SP **Q33.1 Accessory lobe of lung**
Azygos lobe (fissured), lung

SP **Q33.2 Sequestration of lung**

SP **Q33.3 Agenesis of lung**
Congenital absence of lung (lobe)

SP **Q33.4 Congenital bronchiectasis**

SP **Q33.5 Ectopic tissue in lung**

SP **Q33.6 Congenital hypoplasia and dysplasia of lung**
EXCLUDES 1 pulmonary hypoplasia associated with short gestation (P28.0)

SP **Q33.8 Other congenital malformations of lung**

IQ **Q33.9 Congenital malformation of lung, unspecified**

4 **Q34 Other congenital malformations of respiratory system**
EXCLUDES 2 congenital central alveolar hypoventilation syndrome (G47.35)

SP **Q34.0 Anomaly of pleura**

SP **Q34.1 Congenital cyst of mediastinum**

SP **Q34.8 Other specified congenital malformations of respiratory system**
Atresia of nasopharynx

IQ **Q34.9 Congenital malformation of respiratory system, unspecified**
Congenital absence of respiratory system
Congenital anomaly of respiratory system NOS

Cleft lip and cleft palate (Q35-Q37)

Use additional code to identify associated malformation of the nose (Q30.2)
EXCLUDES 2 Robin's syndrome (Q87.0)

4 **Q35 Cleft palate**
INCLUDES fissure of palate
palatoschisis
EXCLUDES 1 cleft palate with cleft lip (Q37.-)

IQ **Q35.1 Cleft hard palate**

IQ **Q35.3 Cleft soft palate**

IQ **Q35.5 Cleft hard palate with cleft soft palate**

IQ **Q35.7 Cleft uvula**

IQ **Q35.9 Cleft palate, unspecified**
Cleft palate NOS
DEFINITION A congenital fissure in the roof of the mouth, resulting from incomplete fusion of the palate during embryonic development.

4 **Q36 Cleft lip**
INCLUDES cheiloschisis
congenital fissure of lip
harelip
labium leporinum
EXCLUDES 1 cleft lip with cleft palate (Q37.-)
CODING TIPS✓ If the cleft palate/cleft lip has been corrected, use Z87.730, Personal history of (corrected) congenital malformations of cleft lip and palate.

SP **Q36.0 Cleft lip, bilateral**

SP **Q36.1 Cleft lip, median**

IQ **Q36.9 Cleft lip, unilateral**
Cleft lip NOS

4 **Q37 Cleft palate with cleft lip**
INCLUDES cheilopalatoschisis
CODING TIPS✓ If the cleft palate/cleft lip has been corrected, use Z87.730, Personal history of (corrected) congenital malformations of cleft lip and palate.

SP **Q37.0 Cleft hard palate with bilateral cleft lip**

SP **Q37.1 Cleft hard palate with unilateral cleft lip**
Cleft hard palate with cleft lip NOS

SP **Q37.2 Cleft soft palate with bilateral cleft lip**

SP **Q37.3 Cleft soft palate with unilateral cleft lip**
Cleft soft palate with cleft lip NOS

SP **Q37.4 Cleft hard and soft palate with bilateral cleft lip**

SP **Q37.5 Cleft hard and soft palate with unilateral cleft lip**
Cleft hard and soft palate with cleft lip NOS

SP **Q37.8 Unspecified cleft palate with bilateral cleft lip**

IQ **Q37.9 Unspecified cleft palate with unilateral cleft lip**
Cleft palate with cleft lip NOS

Other congenital malformations of the digestive system (Q38-Q45)

4 **Q38 Other congenital malformations of tongue, mouth and pharynx**
EXCLUDES 1 dentofacial anomalies (M26.-)
macrostomia (Q18.4)
microstomia (Q18.5)

SP **Q38.0 Congenital malformations of lips, not elsewhere classified**
Congenital fistula of lip
Congenital malformation of lip NOS
Van der Woude's syndrome
EXCLUDES 1 cleft lip (Q36.-)
cleft lip with cleft palate (Q37.-)
macrocheilia (Q18.6)
microcheilia (Q18.7)

SP **Q38.1 Ankyloglossia**
Tongue tie

SP **Q38.2 Macroglossia**
Congenital hypertrophy of tongue
DEFINITION Congenital enlargement of the tongue.

SP **Q38.3 Other congenital malformations of tongue**
Aglossia
Bifid tongue
Congenital adhesion of tongue
Congenital fissure of tongue
Congenital malformation of tongue NOS
Double tongue
Hypoglossia
Hypoplasia of tongue
Microglossia

SP **Q38.4 Congenital malformations of salivary glands and ducts**
Atresia of salivary glands and ducts
Congenital absence of salivary glands and ducts
Congenital accessory salivary glands and ducts
Congenital fistula of salivary gland
DEFINITION Congenital salivary gland fistula: Abnormal passage communicating with a salivary gland and present at birth.

SP **Q38.5 Congenital malformations of palate, not elsewhere classified**
Congenital absence of uvula
Congenital malformation of palate NOS
Congenital high arched palate
EXCLUDES 1 cleft palate (Q35.-)
cleft palate with cleft lip (Q37.-)

SP **Q38.6 Other congenital malformations of mouth**
Congenital malformation of mouth NOS

SP **Q38.7 Congenital pharyngeal pouch**
Congenital diverticulum of pharynx
EXCLUDES 1 pharyngeal pouch syndrome (D82.1)

SP **Q38.8 Other congenital malformations of pharynx**
Congenital malformation of pharynx NOS
Imperforate pharynx

4 **Q39 Congenital malformations of esophagus**

SP **Q39.0 Atresia of esophagus without fistula**
Atresia of esophagus NOS

SP **Q39.1 Atresia of esophagus with tracheo-esophageal fistula**
Atresia of esophagus with broncho-esophageal fistula
CODING TIPS ✓ Code Q39.1 is used for a congenital tracheoesophageal fistula (TE fistula). A fistula as a complication of a tracheostomy is coded J95.04.

SP **Q39.2 Congenital tracheo-esophageal fistula without atresia**
Congenital tracheo-esophageal fistula NOS

SP **Q39.3 Congenital stenosis and stricture of esophagus**

SP **Q39.4 Esophageal web**

SP **Q39.5 Congenital dilatation of esophagus**
Congenital cardiospasm

SP **Q39.6 Congenital diverticulum of esophagus**
Congenital esophageal pouch

SP **Q39.8 Other congenital malformations of esophagus**
Congenital absence of esophagus
Congenital displacement of esophagus
Congenital duplication of esophagus

IQ **Q39.9 Congenital malformation of esophagus, unspecified**

4 **Q40 Other congenital malformations of upper alimentary tract**

SP **Q40.0 Congenital hypertrophic pyloric stenosis**
Congenital or infantile constriction
Congenital or infantile hypertrophy
Congenital or infantile spasm
Congenital or infantile stenosis
Congenital or infantile stricture
DEFINITION Congenital narrowing and partial obstruction of the gastric outlet due to muscular hypertrophy and mucosal edema of the ring-like muscle at the lower end of the stomach (pyloric orifice) in newborns.

SP **Q40.1 Congenital hiatus hernia**
Congenital displacement of cardia through esophageal hiatus
EXCLUDES 1 congenital diaphragmatic hernia (Q79.0)

SP **Q40.2 Other specified congenital malformations of stomach**
Congenital displacement of stomach
Congenital diverticulum of stomach
Congenital hourglass stomach

Congenital duplication of stomach
Megalogastria
Microgastria

IQ **Q40.3 Congenital malformation of stomach, unspecified**

SP **Q40.8 Other specified congenital malformations of upper alimentary tract**

IQ **Q40.9 Congenital malformation of upper alimentary tract, unspecified**
Congenital anomaly of upper alimentary tract
Congenital deformity of upper alimentary tract

4 **Q41 Congenital absence, atresia and stenosis of small intestine**
INCLUDES congenital obstruction, occlusion or stricture of small intestine or intestine NOS
EXCLUDES 1 cystic fibrosis with intestinal manifestation (E84.11)
meconium ileus NOS (without cystic fibrosis) (P76.0)

SP **Q41.0 Congenital absence, atresia and stenosis of duodenum**

SP **Q41.1 Congenital absence, atresia and stenosis of jejunum**
Apple peel syndrome
Imperforate jejunum

SP **Q41.2 Congenital absence, atresia and stenosis of ileum**

SP **Q41.8 Congenital absence, atresia and stenosis of other specified parts of small intestine**

SP **Q41.9 Congenital absence, atresia and stenosis of small intestine, part unspecified**
Congenital absence, atresia and stenosis of intestine NOS

4 **Q42 Congenital absence, atresia and stenosis of large intestine**
INCLUDES congenital obstruction, occlusion and stricture of large intestine

SP **Q42.0 Congenital absence, atresia and stenosis of rectum with fistula**

SP **Q42.1 Congenital absence, atresia and stenosis of rectum without fistula**
Imperforate rectum

SP **Q42.2 Congenital absence, atresia and stenosis of anus with fistula**

SP **Q42.3 Congenital absence, atresia and stenosis of anus without fistula**
Imperforate anus

SP **Q42.8 Congenital absence, atresia and stenosis of other parts of large intestine**

SP **Q42.9 Congenital absence, atresia and stenosis of large intestine, part unspecified**

4 **Q43 Other congenital malformations of intestine**

SP **Q43.0 Meckel's diverticulum (displaced) (hypertrophic)**
Persistent omphalomesenteric duct
Persistent vitelline duct

SP **Q43.1 Hirschsprung's disease**
Aganglionosis
Congenital (aganglionic) megacolon

SP **Q43.2 Other congenital functional disorders of colon**
Congenital dilatation of colon

SP **Q43.3 Congenital malformations of intestinal fixation**
Congenital omental, anomalous adhesions [bands]
Congenital peritoneal adhesions [bands]
Incomplete rotation of cecum and colon
Insufficient rotation of cecum and colon
Jackson's membrane
Malrotation of colon
Rotation failure of cecum and colon
Universal mesentery

SP **Q43.4 Duplication of intestine**

SP **Q43.5 Ectopic anus**

SP **Q43.6 Congenital fistula of rectum and anus**
EXCLUDES 1 congenital fistula of anus with absence, atresia and stenosis (Q42.2)
congenital fistula of rectum with absence, atresia and stenosis (Q42.0)
congenital rectovaginal fistula (Q52.2)
congenital urethrorectal fistula (Q64.73)
pilonidal fistula or sinus (L05.-)

SP **Q43.7 Persistent cloaca**
Cloaca NOS

SP **Q43.8 Other specified congenital malformations of intestine**
Congenital blind loop syndrome
Congenital diverticulitis, colon
Congenital diverticulum, intestine
Dolichocolon
Megaloappendix
Megaloduodenum
Microcolon
Transposition of appendix
Transposition of colon
Transposition of intestine

IQ **Q43.9 Congenital malformation of intestine, unspecified**

4 **Q44 Congenital malformations of gallbladder, bile ducts and liver**

SP **Q44.0 Agenesis, aplasia and hypoplasia of gallbladder**
Congenital absence of gallbladder

SP **Q44.1 Other congenital malformations of gallbladder**
Congenital malformation of gallbladder NOS
Intrahepatic gallbladder

SP **Q44.2 Atresia of bile ducts**

SP **Q44.3 Congenital stenosis and stricture of bile ducts**

SP **Q44.4 Choledochal cyst**

SP **Q44.5 Other congenital malformations of bile ducts**
Accessory hepatic duct
Biliary duct duplication
Congenital malformation of bile duct NOS
Cystic duct duplication

SP **Q44.6 Cystic disease of liver**
Fibrocystic disease of liver

SP **Q44.7 Other congenital malformations of liver**
Accessory liver
Alagille's syndrome
Congenital absence of liver
Congenital hepatomegaly
Congenital malformation of liver NOS

4 **Q45 Other congenital malformations of digestive system**
EXCLUDES 2 congenital diaphragmatic hernia (Q79.0)
congenital hiatus hernia (Q40.1)

SP **Q45.0 Agenesis, aplasia and hypoplasia of pancreas**
Congenital absence of pancreas

SP **Q45.1 Annular pancreas**

SP **Q45.2 Congenital pancreatic cyst**

SP **Q45.3 Other congenital malformations of pancreas and pancreatic duct**
Accessory pancreas
Congenital malformation of pancreas or pancreatic duct NOS
EXCLUDES 1 congenital diabetes mellitus (E10.-)
cystic fibrosis (E84.0-E84.9)
fibrocystic disease of pancreas (E84.-)
neonatal diabetes mellitus (P70.2)

SP **Q45.8 Other specified congenital malformations of digestive system**
Absence (complete) (partial) of alimentary tract NOS
Duplication of digestive system
Malposition, congenital of digestive system

IQ **Q45.9 Congenital malformation of digestive system, unspecified**
Congenital anomaly of digestive system
Congenital deformity of digestive system

Congenital malformations of genital organs (Q50-Q56)

EXCLUDES 1 androgen insensitivity syndrome (E34.5-)
syndromes associated with anomalies in the number and form of chromosomes (Q90-Q99)

4 **Q50 Congenital malformations of ovaries, fallopian tubes and broad ligaments**

5 **Q50.0 Congenital absence of ovary**
EXCLUDES 1 Turner's syndrome (Q96.-)

SP **Q50.01 Congenital absence of ovary, unilateral**

SP **Q50.02 Congenital absence of ovary, bilateral**

SP **Q50.1 Developmental ovarian cyst**

SP **Q50.2 Congenital torsion of ovary**

5 **Q50.3 Other congenital malformations of ovary**

SP **Q50.31 Accessory ovary**

SP **Q50.32 Ovarian streak**
46, XX with streak gonads

SP **Q50.39 Other congenital malformation of ovary**
Congenital malformation of ovary NOS

SP **Q50.4 Embryonic cyst of fallopian tube**
Fimbrial cyst

SP **Q50.5 Embryonic cyst of broad ligament**
Epoophoron cyst
Parovarian cyst

SP **Q50.6 Other congenital malformations of fallopian tube and broad ligament**
Absence of fallopian tube and broad ligament
Accessory fallopian tube and broad ligament
Atresia of fallopian tube and broad ligament
Congenital malformation of fallopian tube or broad ligament NOS

4 **Q51 Congenital malformations of uterus and cervix**

SP **Q51.0 Agenesis and aplasia of uterus**
Congenital absence of uterus

5 **Q51.1 Doubling of uterus with doubling of cervix and vagina**

SP **Q51.10 Doubling of uterus with doubling of cervix and vagina without obstruction**
Doubling of uterus with doubling of cervix and vagina NOS

SP **Q51.11 Doubling of uterus with doubling of cervix and vagina with obstruction**

5 **Q51.2 Other doubling of uterus**
Doubling of uterus NOS
Septate uterus

SP **Q51.21 Complete doubling of uterus**
Complete septate uterus

SP **Q51.22 Partial doubling of uterus**
Partial septate uterus

SP **Q51.28 Other and unspecified doubling of uterus**
Septate uterus NOS

SP **Q51.3 Bicornate uterus**
Bicornate uterus, complete or partial

SP **Q51.4 Unicornate uterus**
Unicornate uterus with or without a separate uterine horn
Uterus with only one functioning horn

SP **Q51.5 Agenesis and aplasia of cervix**
Congenital absence of cervix

SP **Q51.6 Embryonic cyst of cervix**

SP **Q51.7 Congenital fistulae between uterus and digestive and urinary tracts**

5 **Q51.8 Other congenital malformations of uterus and cervix**

6 **Q51.81 Other congenital malformations of uterus**

SP **Q51.810 Arcuate uterus**
Arcuatus uterus

SP **Q51.811 Hypoplasia of uterus**

SP **Q51.818 Other congenital malformations of uterus**
Müllerian anomaly of uterus NEC

6 **Q51.82 Other congenital malformations of cervix**

SP **Q51.820 Cervical duplication**

SP **Q51.821 Hypoplasia of cervix**

SP **Q51.828 Other congenital malformations of cervix**

IQ **Q51.9 Congenital malformation of uterus and cervix, unspecified**

4 Q52 **Other congenital malformations of female genitalia**

SP Q52.0 **Congenital absence of vagina**
Vaginal agenesis, total or partial

5 Q52.1 **Doubling of vagina**
EXCLUDES 1 doubling of vagina with doubling of uterus and cervix (Q51.1-)

SP Q52.10 **Doubling of vagina, unspecified**
Septate vagina NOS

SP Q52.11 **Transverse vaginal septum**

6 Q52.12 **Longitudinal vaginal septum**

SP Q52.120 **Longitudinal vaginal septum, nonobstructing**

SP Q52.121 **Longitudinal vaginal septum, obstructing, right side**

SP Q52.122 **Longitudinal vaginal septum, obstructing, left side**

SP Q52.123 **Longitudinal vaginal septum, microperforate, right side**

SP Q52.124 **Longitudinal vaginal septum, microperforate, left side**

SP Q52.129 **Other and unspecified longitudinal vaginal septum**

SP Q52.2 **Congenital rectovaginal fistula**
EXCLUDES 1 cloaca (Q43.7)

SP Q52.3 **Imperforate hymen**

SP Q52.4 **Other congenital malformations of vagina**
Canal of Nuck cyst, congenital
Congenital malformation of vagina NOS
Embryonic vaginal cyst
Gartner's duct cyst

SP Q52.5 **Fusion of labia**

SP Q52.6 **Congenital malformation of clitoris**

5 Q52.7 **Other and unspecified congenital malformations of vulva**

IQ Q52.70 **Unspecified congenital malformations of vulva**
Congenital malformation of vulva NOS

SP Q52.71 **Congenital absence of vulva**

SP Q52.79 **Other congenital malformations of vulva**
Congenital cyst of vulva

SP Q52.8 **Other specified congenital malformations of female genitalia**

IQ Q52.9 **Congenital malformation of female genitalia, unspecified**

4 Q53 **Undescended and ectopic testicle**

5 Q53.0 **Ectopic testis**

IQ Q53.00 **Ectopic testis, unspecified**

SP Q53.01 **Ectopic testis, unilateral**

SP Q53.02 **Ectopic testes, bilateral**

5 Q53.1 **Undescended testicle, unilateral**

IQ Q53.10 **Unspecified undescended testicle, unilateral**

6 Q53.11 **Abdominal testis, unilateral**

SP Q53.111 **Unilateral intraabdominal testis**

SP Q53.112 **Unilateral inguinal testis**

SP Q53.12 **Ectopic perineal testis, unilateral**

SP Q53.13 **Unilateral high scrotal testis**

5 Q53.2 **Undescended testicle, bilateral**

SP Q53.20 **Undescended testicle, unspecified, bilateral**

6 Q53.21 **Abdominal testis, bilateral**

SP Q53.211 **Bilateral intraabdominal testes**

SP Q53.212 **Bilateral inguinal testes**

SP Q53.22 **Ectopic perineal testis, bilateral**

SP Q53.23 **Bilateral high scrotal testes**

IQ Q53.9 **Undescended testicle, unspecified**
Cryptorchism NOS

4 Q54 **Hypospadias**
EXCLUDES 1 epispadias (Q64.0)

CODING TIPS ✓ Use category Q54 when hypospadias is still present. If the condition has been corrected, then code Z87.710, Personal history of hypospadias.

SP Q54.0 **Hypospadias, balanic**
Hypospadias, coronal
Hypospadias, glandular

SP Q54.1 **Hypospadias, penile**

SP Q54.2 **Hypospadias, penoscrotal**

SP Q54.3 **Hypospadias, perineal**

SP Q54.4 **Congenital chordee**
Chordee without hypospadias

DEFINITION Abnormal downward or upward bowing of the penis, due to a congenital anomaly.

SP Q54.8 **Other hypospadias**
Hypospadias with intersex state

SP Q54.9 **Hypospadias, unspecified**

4 Q55 **Other congenital malformations of male genital organs**
EXCLUDES 1 congenital hydrocele (P83.5)
hypospadias (Q54.-)

SP Q55.0 **Absence and aplasia of testis**
Monorchism

SP Q55.1 **Hypoplasia of testis and scrotum**
Fusion of testes

5 Q55.2 **Other and unspecified congenital malformations of testis and scrotum**

IQ Q55.20 **Unspecified congenital malformations of testis and scrotum**
Congenital malformation of testis or scrotum NOS

SP Q55.21 **Polyorchism**

SP Q55.22 **Retractile testis**

SP Q55.23 **Scrotal transposition**

SP Q55.29 **Other congenital malformations of testis and scrotum**

SP Q55.3 **Atresia of vas deferens**
Code first:
any associated cystic fibrosis (E84.-)

SP Q55.4 **Other congenital malformations of vas deferens, epididymis, seminal vesicles and prostate**
Absence or aplasia of prostate
Absence or aplasia of spermatic cord
Congenital malformation of vas deferens, epididymis, seminal vesicles or prostate NOS

SP Q55.5 **Congenital absence and aplasia of penis**

5 Q55.6 **Other congenital malformations of penis**

SP Q55.61 **Curvature of penis (lateral)**

SP Q55.62 **Hypoplasia of penis**

Micropenis

SP **Q55.63 Congenital torsion of penis**
EXCLUDES 1 acquired torsion of penis (N48.82)

SP **Q55.64 Hidden penis**
Buried penis
Concealed penis
EXCLUDES 1 acquired buried penis (N48.83)

SP **Q55.69 Other congenital malformation of penis**
Congenital malformation of penis NOS

SP **Q55.7 Congenital vasocutaneous fistula**

SP **Q55.8 Other specified congenital malformations of male genital organs**

!Q **Q55.9 Congenital malformation of male genital organ, unspecified**
Congenital anomaly of male genital organ
Congenital deformity of male genital organ

4 **Q56 Indeterminate sex and pseudohermaphroditism**
EXCLUDES 1 46,XX true hermaphrodite (Q99.1)
androgen insensitivity syndrome (E34.5-)
chimera 46,XX/46,XY true hermaphrodite (Q99.0)
female pseudohermaphroditism with adrenocortical disorder (E25.-)
pseudohermaphroditism with specified chromosomal anomaly (Q96-Q99)
pure gonadal dysgenesis (Q99.1)

SP **Q56.0 Hermaphroditism, not elsewhere classified**
Ovotestis

SP **Q56.1 Male pseudohermaphroditism, not elsewhere classified**
46, XY with streak gonads
Male pseudohermaphroditism NOS

SP **Q56.2 Female pseudohermaphroditism, not elsewhere classified**
Female pseudohermaphroditism NOS

SP **Q56.3 Pseudohermaphroditism, unspecified**

SP **Q56.4 Indeterminate sex, unspecified**
Ambiguous genitalia

Congenital malformations of the urinary system (Q60-Q64)

4 **Q60 Renal agenesis and other reduction defects of kidney**
INCLUDES congenital absence of kidney
congenital atrophy of kidney
infantile atrophy of kidney

SP **Q60.0 Renal agenesis, unilateral**

SP **Q60.1 Renal agenesis, bilateral**

!Q **Q60.2 Renal agenesis, unspecified**

SP **Q60.3 Renal hypoplasia, unilateral**

SP **Q60.4 Renal hypoplasia, bilateral**

!Q **Q60.5 Renal hypoplasia, unspecified**

SP **Q60.6 Potter's syndrome**

4 **Q61 Cystic kidney disease**
EXCLUDES 1 acquired cyst of kidney (N28.1)
Potter's syndrome (Q60.6)

5 **Q61.0 Congenital renal cyst**

SP **Q61.00 Congenital renal cyst, unspecified**
Cyst of kidney NOS (congenital)

SP **Q61.01 Congenital single renal cyst**

SP **Q61.02 Congenital multiple renal cysts**

5 **Q61.1 Polycystic kidney, infantile type**
Polycystic kidney, autosomal recessive

SP **Q61.11 Cystic dilatation of collecting ducts**

SP **Q61.19 Other polycystic kidney, infantile type**

SP **Q61.2 Polycystic kidney, adult type**
Polycystic kidney, autosomal dominant

SP **Q61.3 Polycystic kidney, unspecified**

SP **Q61.4 Renal dysplasia**
Multicystic dysplastic kidney
Multicystic kidney (development)
Multicystic kidney disease
Multicystic renal dysplasia
EXCLUDES 1 polycystic kidney disease (Q61.11-Q61.3)

SP **Q61.5 Medullary cystic kidney**
Nephronophthisis
Sponge kidney NOS

SP **Q61.8 Other cystic kidney diseases**
Fibrocystic kidney
Fibrocystic renal degeneration or disease

!Q **Q61.9 Cystic kidney disease, unspecified**
Meckel-Gruber syndrome

4 **Q62 Congenital obstructive defects of renal pelvis and congenital malformations of ureter**

SP **Q62.0 Congenital hydronephrosis**

5 **Q62.1 Congenital occlusion of ureter**
Atresia and stenosis of ureter

SP **Q62.10 Congenital occlusion of ureter, unspecified**

SP **Q62.11 Congenital occlusion of ureteropelvic junction**

SP **Q62.12 Congenital occlusion of ureterovesical orifice**

SP **Q62.2 Congenital megaureter**
Congenital dilatation of ureter

5 **Q62.3 Other obstructive defects of renal pelvis and ureter**

SP **Q62.31 Congenital ureterocele, orthotopic**

SP **Q62.32 Cecoureterocele**
Ectopic ureterocele

SP **Q62.39 Other obstructive defects of renal pelvis and ureter**
Ureteropelvic junction obstruction NOS

SP **Q62.4 Agenesis of ureter**
Congenital absence ureter

SP **Q62.5 Duplication of ureter**
Accessory ureter
Double ureter

5 **Q62.6 Malposition of ureter**

SP **Q62.60 Malposition of ureter, unspecified**

SP **Q62.61 Deviation of ureter**

SP **Q62.62 Displacement of ureter**

SP **Q62.63 Anomalous implantation of ureter**
Ectopia of ureter
Ectopic ureter

SP **Q62.69 Other malposition of ureter**

SP **Q62.7 Congenital vesico-uretero-renal reflux**

SP **Q62.8 Other congenital malformations of ureter**
Anomaly of ureter NOS

4 **Q63 Other congenital malformations of kidney**
EXCLUDES 1 congenital nephrotic syndrome (N04.-)

SP **Q63.0 Accessory kidney**

SP **Q63.1 Lobulated, fused and horseshoe kidney**

SP **Q63.2 Ectopic kidney**
Congenital displaced kidney
Malrotation of kidney

SP **Q63.3 Hyperplastic and giant kidney**
Compensatory hypertrophy of kidney

SP **Q63.8 Other specified congenital malformations of kidney**
Congenital renal calculi

IQ **Q63.9 Congenital malformation of kidney, unspecified**

4 **Q64 Other congenital malformations of urinary system**

SP **Q64.0 Epispadias**
EXCLUDES 1 hypospadias (Q54.-)
DEFINITION A rare, congenital defect in which the urethra typically opens on the upper penile surface in boys, although, the urethral opening may also be positioned in the abdomen.

5 **Q64.1 Exstrophy of urinary bladder**

SP **Q64.10 Exstrophy of urinary bladder, unspecified**
Ectopia vesicae

SP **Q64.11 Supravesical fissure of urinary bladder**

SP **Q64.12 Cloacal exstrophy of urinary bladder**

SP **Q64.19 Other exstrophy of urinary bladder**
Extroversion of bladder

SP **Q64.2 Congenital posterior urethral valves**

5 **Q64.3 Other atresia and stenosis of urethra and bladder neck**

SP **Q64.31 Congenital bladder neck obstruction**
Congenital obstruction of vesicourethral orifice

SP **Q64.32 Congenital stricture of urethra**

SP **Q64.33 Congenital stricture of urinary meatus**

SP **Q64.39 Other atresia and stenosis of urethra and bladder neck**
Atresia and stenosis of urethra and bladder neck NOS

SP **Q64.4 Malformation of urachus**
Cyst of urachus
Patent urachus
Prolapse of urachus

SP **Q64.5 Congenital absence of bladder and urethra**

SP **Q64.6 Congenital diverticulum of bladder**

5 **Q64.7 Other and unspecified congenital malformations of bladder and urethra**
EXCLUDES 1 congenital prolapse of bladder (mucosa) (Q79.4)

IQ **Q64.70 Unspecified congenital malformation of bladder and urethra**
Malformation of bladder or urethra NOS

SP **Q64.71 Congenital prolapse of urethra**

SP **Q64.72 Congenital prolapse of urinary meatus**

SP **Q64.73 Congenital urethrorectal fistula**

SP **Q64.74 Double urethra**

SP **Q64.75 Double urinary meatus**

SP **Q64.79 Other congenital malformations of bladder and urethra**

SP **Q64.8 Other specified congenital malformations of urinary system**

IQ **Q64.9 Congenital malformation of urinary system, unspecified**
Congenital anomaly NOS of urinary system
Congenital deformity NOS of urinary system

Congenital malformations and deformations of the musculoskeletal system (Q65-Q79)

4 **Q65 Congenital deformities of hip**
EXCLUDES 1 clicking hip (R29.4)

5 **Q65.0 Congenital dislocation of hip, unilateral**

IQ **Q65.00 Congenital dislocation of unspecified hip, unilateral**

SP **Q65.01 Congenital dislocation of right hip, unilateral**

SP **Q65.02 Congenital dislocation of left hip, unilateral**

SP **Q65.1 Congenital dislocation of hip, bilateral**

IQ **Q65.2 Congenital dislocation of hip, unspecified**

5 **Q65.3 Congenital partial dislocation of hip, unilateral**

IQ **Q65.30 Congenital partial dislocation of unspecified hip, unilateral**

SP **Q65.31 Congenital partial dislocation of right hip, unilateral**

SP **Q65.32 Congenital partial dislocation of left hip, unilateral**

SP **Q65.4 Congenital partial dislocation of hip, bilateral**

IQ **Q65.5 Congenital partial dislocation of hip, unspecified**

SP **Q65.6 Congenital unstable hip**
Congenital dislocatable hip

5 **Q65.8 Other congenital deformities of hip**

SP **Q65.81 Congenital coxa valga**

SP **Q65.82 Congenital coxa vara**

SP **Q65.89 Other specified congenital deformities of hip**
Anteversion of femoral neck
Congenital acetabular dysplasia

IQ **Q65.9 Congenital deformity of hip, unspecified**

4 **Q66 Congenital deformities of feet**
EXCLUDES 1 reduction defects of feet (Q72.-)
valgus deformities (acquired) (M21.0-)
varus deformities (acquired) (M21.1-)

5 **Q66.0 Congenital talipes equinovarus**

- **Q66.00 Congenital talipes equinovarus, unspecified foot**
- SP **Q66.01 Congenital talipes equinovarus, right foot**
- SP **Q66.02 Congenital talipes equinovarus, left foot**

5 **Q66.1 Congenital talipes calcaneovarus**

- **Q66.10 Congenital talipes calcaneovarus, unspecified foot**
- SP **Q66.11 Congenital talipes calcaneovarus, right foot**
- SP **Q66.12 Congenital talipes calcaneovarus, left foot**

5 **Q66.2 Congenital metatarsus (primus) varus**

6 **Q66.21 Congenital metatarsus primus varus**

- SP **Q66.211 Congenital metatarsus primus varus, right foot**
- SP **Q66.212 Congenital metatarsus primus varus, left foot**
- **Q66.219 Congenital metatarsus primus varus, unspecified foot**

6 **Q66.22 Congenital metatarsus adductus**
Congenital metatarsus varus

- SP **Q66.221 Congenital metatarsus adductus, right foot**
- SP **Q66.222 Congenital metatarsus adductus, left foot**
- SP **Q66.229 Congenital metatarsus adductus, unspecified foot**

5 **Q66.3 Other congenital varus deformities of feet**
Hallux varus, congenital

- **Q66.30 Other congenital varus deformities of feet, unspecified foot**
- SP **Q66.31 Other congenital varus deformities of feet, right foot**
- SP **Q66.32 Other congenital varus deformities of feet, left foot**

5 **Q66.4 Congenital talipes calcaneovalgus**

- **Q66.40 Congenital talipes calcaneovalgus, unspecified foot**
- SP **Q66.41 Congenital talipes calcaneovalgus, right foot**
- SP **Q66.42 Congenital talipes calcaneovalgus, left foot**

5 **Q66.5 Congenital pes planus**
Congenital flat foot
Congenital rigid flat foot
Congenital spastic (everted) flat foot
EXCLUDES 1 pes planus, acquired (M21.4)

- IQ **Q66.50 Congenital pes planus, unspecified foot**
- SP **Q66.51 Congenital pes planus, right foot**
- SP **Q66.52 Congenital pes planus, left foot**

SP **Q66.6 Other congenital valgus deformities of feet**
Congenital metatarsus valgus

5 **Q66.7 Congenital pes cavus**

- **Q66.70 Congenital pes cavus, unspecified foot**
- SP **Q66.71 Congenital pes cavus, right foot**
- SP **Q66.72 Congenital pes cavus, left foot**

5 **Q66.8 Other congenital deformities of feet**

- IQ **Q66.80 Congenital vertical talus deformity, unspecified foot**
- SP **Q66.81 Congenital vertical talus deformity, right foot**
- SP **Q66.82 Congenital vertical talus deformity, left foot**
- SP **Q66.89 Other specified congenital deformities of feet**
  Congenital asymmetric talipes
  Congenital clubfoot NOS
  Congenital talipes NOS
  Congenital tarsal coalition
  Hammer toe, congenital

5 **Q66.9 Congenital deformity of feet, unspecified**

- **Q66.90 Congenital deformity of feet, unspecified, unspecified foot**
- **Q66.91 Congenital deformity of feet, unspecified, right foot**
- **Q66.92 Congenital deformity of feet, unspecified, left foot**

4 **Q67 Congenital musculoskeletal deformities of head, face, spine and chest**
EXCLUDES 1 congenital malformation syndromes classified to Q87.-
Potter's syndrome (Q60.6)

SP **Q67.0 Congenital facial asymmetry**

SP **Q67.1 Congenital compression facies**

SP **Q67.2 Dolichocephaly**

SP **Q67.3 Plagiocephaly**

SP **Q67.4 Other congenital deformities of skull, face and jaw**
Congenital depressions in skull
Congenital hemifacial atrophy or hypertrophy
Deviation of nasal septum, congenital
Squashed or bent nose, congenital
EXCLUDES 1 dentofacial anomalies [including malocclusion] (M26.-)
syphilitic saddle nose (A50.5)

SP **Q67.5 Congenital deformity of spine**
Congenital postural scoliosis
Congenital scoliosis NOS
EXCLUDES 1 infantile idiopathic scoliosis (M41.0)
scoliosis due to congenital bony malformation (Q76.3)

SP **Q67.6 Pectus excavatum**
Congenital funnel chest

SP **Q67.7 Pectus carinatum**
Congenital pigeon chest
DEFINITION A protrusion deformity of the chest wall in which the sternum and ribs are prominent, due to obstruction of infantile respiration or to rickets.

SP **Q67.8 Other congenital deformities of chest**
Congenital deformity of chest wall NOS

4 **Q68 Other congenital musculoskeletal deformities**
EXCLUDES 1 reduction defects of limb (s) (Q71-Q73)

EXCLUDES 2 congenital myotonic chondrodystrophy (G71.13)

SP **Q68.0 Congenital deformity of sternocleidomastoid muscle**
Congenital contracture of sternocleidomastoid (muscle)
Congenital (sternomastoid) torticollis
Sternomastoid tumor (congenital)

SP **Q68.1 Congenital deformity of finger(s) and hand**
Congenital clubfinger
Spade-like hand (congenital)

SP **Q68.2 Congenital deformity of knee**
Congenital dislocation of knee
Congenital genu recurvatum

SP **Q68.3 Congenital bowing of femur**
EXCLUDES 1 anteversion of femur (neck) (Q65.89)

SP **Q68.4 Congenital bowing of tibia and fibula**

IQ **Q68.5 Congenital bowing of long bones of leg, unspecified**

SP **Q68.6 Discoid meniscus**

SP **Q68.8 Other specified congenital musculoskeletal deformities**
Congenital deformity of clavicle
Congenital deformity of elbow
Congenital deformity of forearm
Congenital deformity of scapula
Congenital deformity of wrist
Congenital dislocation of elbow
Congenital dislocation of shoulder
Congenital dislocation of wrist

4 **Q69 Polydactyly**

SP **Q69.0 Accessory finger(s)**

SP **Q69.1 Accessory thumb(s)**

SP **Q69.2 Accessory toe(s)**
Accessory hallux

IQ **Q69.9 Polydactyly, unspecified**
Supernumerary digit(s) NOS
DEFINITION An extra number of digits on a hand or foot.

4 **Q70 Syndactyly**

5 **Q70.0 Fused fingers**
Complex syndactyly of fingers with synostosis

6 IQ **Q70.00 Fused fingers, unspecified hand**

6 SP **Q70.01 Fused fingers, right hand**

6 SP **Q70.02 Fused fingers, left hand**

6 SP **Q70.03 Fused fingers, bilateral**

5 **Q70.1 Webbed fingers**
Simple syndactyly of fingers without synostosis

6 IQ **Q70.10 Webbed fingers, unspecified hand**

6 SP **Q70.11 Webbed fingers, right hand**

6 SP **Q70.12 Webbed fingers, left hand**

6 SP **Q70.13 Webbed fingers, bilateral**

5 **Q70.2 Fused toes**
Complex syndactyly of toes with synostosis

6 IQ **Q70.20 Fused toes, unspecified foot**

6 SP **Q70.21 Fused toes, right foot**

6 SP **Q70.22 Fused toes, left foot**

6 SP **Q70.23 Fused toes, bilateral**

5 **Q70.3 Webbed toes**
Simple syndactyly of toes without synostosis

6 IQ **Q70.30 Webbed toes, unspecified foot**

6 IQ **Q70.31 Webbed toes, right foot**

6 SP **Q70.32 Webbed toes, left foot**

6 SP **Q70.33 Webbed toes, bilateral**

SP **Q70.4 Polysyndactyly, unspecified**
EXCLUDES 1 specified syndactyly of hand and feet - code to specified conditions (Q70.0- -Q70.3-)

SP **Q70.9 Syndactyly, unspecified**
Symphalangy NOS
DEFINITION Partial or total webbing connecting two or more fingers or toes; may involve skin/soft tissue only or include fusion of bone.

4 **Q71 Reduction defects of upper limb**

5 **Q71.0 Congenital complete absence of upper limb**

6 IQ **Q71.00 Congenital complete absence of unspecified upper limb**

6 SP **Q71.01 Congenital complete absence of right upper limb**

6 SP **Q71.02 Congenital complete absence of left upper limb**

6 SP **Q71.03 Congenital complete absence of upper limb, bilateral**

5 **Q71.1 Congenital absence of upper arm and forearm with hand present**

6 IQ **Q71.10 Congenital absence of unspecified upper arm and forearm with hand present**

6 SP **Q71.11 Congenital absence of right upper arm and forearm with hand present**

6 SP **Q71.12 Congenital absence of left upper arm and forearm with hand present**

6 SP **Q71.13 Congenital absence of upper arm and forearm with hand present, bilateral**

5 **Q71.2 Congenital absence of both forearm and hand**

6 IQ **Q71.20 Congenital absence of both forearm and hand, unspecified upper limb**

6 SP **Q71.21 Congenital absence of both forearm and hand, right upper limb**

6 SP **Q71.22 Congenital absence of both forearm and hand, left upper limb**

6 SP **Q71.23 Congenital absence of both forearm and hand, bilateral**

5 **Q71.3 Congenital absence of hand and finger**

6 IQ **Q71.30 Congenital absence of unspecified hand and finger**

6 SP **Q71.31 Congenital absence of right hand and finger**

6 SP **Q71.32 Congenital absence of left hand and finger**

6 SP **Q71.33 Congenital absence of hand and finger, bilateral**

5 **Q71.4 Longitudinal reduction defect of radius**
Clubhand (congenital)
Radial clubhand

6 IQ **Q71.40 Longitudinal reduction defect of unspecified radius**

Chapter 17 Q00-Q99

Q71.41 Longitudinal reduction defect of right radius
Q71.42 Longitudinal reduction defect of left radius
Q71.43 Longitudinal reduction defect of radius, bilateral
Q71.5 Longitudinal reduction defect of ulna
Q71.50 Longitudinal reduction defect of unspecified ulna
Q71.51 Longitudinal reduction defect of right ulna
Q71.52 Longitudinal reduction defect of left ulna
Q71.53 Longitudinal reduction defect of ulna, bilateral
Q71.6 Lobster-claw hand
Q71.60 Lobster-claw hand, unspecified hand
Q71.61 Lobster-claw right hand
Q71.62 Lobster-claw left hand
Q71.63 Lobster-claw hand, bilateral
Q71.8 Other reduction defects of upper limb
Q71.81 Congenital shortening of upper limb
Q71.811 Congenital shortening of right upper limb
Q71.812 Congenital shortening of left upper limb
Q71.813 Congenital shortening of upper limb, bilateral
Q71.819 Congenital shortening of unspecified upper limb
Q71.89 Other reduction defects of upper limb
Q71.891 Other reduction defects of right upper limb
Q71.892 Other reduction defects of left upper limb
Q71.893 Other reduction defects of upper limb, bilateral
Q71.899 Other reduction defects of unspecified upper limb
Q71.9 Unspecified reduction defect of upper limb
Q71.90 Unspecified reduction defect of unspecified upper limb
Q71.91 Unspecified reduction defect of right upper limb
Q71.92 Unspecified reduction defect of left upper limb
Q71.93 Unspecified reduction defect of upper limb, bilateral
Q72 Reduction defects of lower limb
Q72.0 Congenital complete absence of lower limb
Q72.00 Congenital complete absence of unspecified lower limb
Q72.01 Congenital complete absence of right lower limb
Q72.02 Congenital complete absence of left lower limb
Q72.03 Congenital complete absence of lower limb, bilateral
Q72.1 Congenital absence of thigh and lower leg with foot present
Q72.10 Congenital absence of unspecified thigh and lower leg with foot present
Q72.11 Congenital absence of right thigh and lower leg with foot present
Q72.12 Congenital absence of left thigh and lower leg with foot present
Q72.13 Congenital absence of thigh and lower leg with foot present, bilateral
Q72.2 Congenital absence of both lower leg and foot
Q72.20 Congenital absence of both lower leg and foot, unspecified lower limb
Q72.21 Congenital absence of both lower leg and foot, right lower limb
Q72.22 Congenital absence of both lower leg and foot, left lower limb
Q72.23 Congenital absence of both lower leg and foot, bilateral
Q72.3 Congenital absence of foot and toe(s)
Q72.30 Congenital absence of unspecified foot and toe(s)
Q72.31 Congenital absence of right foot and toe(s)
Q72.32 Congenital absence of left foot and toe(s)
Q72.33 Congenital absence of foot and toe(s), bilateral
Q72.4 Longitudinal reduction defect of femur
Proximal femoral focal deficiency
Q72.40 Longitudinal reduction defect of unspecified femur
Q72.41 Longitudinal reduction defect of right femur
Q72.42 Longitudinal reduction defect of left femur
Q72.43 Longitudinal reduction defect of femur, bilateral
Q72.5 Longitudinal reduction defect of tibia
Q72.50 Longitudinal reduction defect of unspecified tibia
Q72.51 Longitudinal reduction defect of right tibia
Q72.52 Longitudinal reduction defect of left tibia
Q72.53 Longitudinal reduction defect of tibia, bilateral
Q72.6 Longitudinal reduction defect of fibula
Q72.60 Longitudinal reduction defect of unspecified fibula
Q72.61 Longitudinal reduction defect of right fibula
Q72.62 Longitudinal reduction defect of left fibula
Q72.63 Longitudinal reduction defect of fibula, bilateral
Q72.7 Split foot
Q72.70 Split foot, unspecified lower limb
Q72.71 Split foot, right lower limb
Q72.72 Split foot, left lower limb
Q72.73 Split foot, bilateral
Q72.8 Other reduction defects of lower limb
Q72.81 Congenital shortening of lower limb
Q72.811 Congenital shortening of right lower limb

H SP Q72.812 Congenital shortening of left lower limb
H SP Q72.813 Congenital shortening of lower limb, bilateral
H IQ Q72.819 Congenital shortening of unspecified lower limb
6 Q72.89 Other reduction defects of lower limb
H SP Q72.891 Other reduction defects of right lower limb
H SP Q72.892 Other reduction defects of left lower limb
H SP Q72.893 Other reduction defects of lower limb, bilateral
H IQ Q72.899 Other reduction defects of unspecified lower limb
5 Q72.9 Unspecified reduction defect of lower limb
H IQ Q72.90 Unspecified reduction defect of unspecified lower limb
H SP Q72.91 Unspecified reduction defect of right lower limb
H SP Q72.92 Unspecified reduction defect of left lower limb
H SP Q72.93 Unspecified reduction defect of lower limb, bilateral

4 Q73 Reduction defects of unspecified limb
IQ Q73.0 Congenital absence of unspecified limb(s)
Amelia NOS
IQ Q73.1 Phocomelia, unspecified limb(s)
Phocomelia NOS
IQ Q73.8 Other reduction defects of unspecified limb(s)
Longitudinal reduction deformity of unspecified limb(s)
Ectromelia of limb NOS
Hemimelia of limb NOS
Reduction defect of limb NOS

4 Q74 Other congenital malformations of limb(s)
EXCLUDES 1 polydactyly (Q69.-)
reduction defect of limb (Q71-Q73)
syndactyly (Q70.-)
SP Q74.0 Other congenital malformations of upper limb(s), including shoulder girdle
Accessory carpal bones
Cleidocranial dysostosis
Congenital pseudarthrosis of clavicle
Macrodactylia (fingers)
Madelung's deformity
Radioulnar synostosis
Sprengel's deformity
Triphalangeal thumb
SP Q74.1 Congenital malformation of knee
Congenital absence of patella
Congenital dislocation of patella
Congenital genu valgum
Congenital genu varum
Rudimentary patella
EXCLUDES 1 congenital dislocation of knee (Q68.2)
congenital genu recurvatum (Q68.2)
nail patella syndrome (Q87.2)
SP Q74.2 Other congenital malformations of lower limb(s), including pelvic girdle
Congenital fusion of sacroiliac joint
Congenital malformation of ankle joint
Congenital malformation of sacroiliac joint
EXCLUDES 1 anteversion of femur (neck) (Q65.89)
SP Q74.3 Arthrogryposis multiplex congenita
SP Q74.8 Other specified congenital malformations of limb(s)
IQ Q74.9 Unspecified congenital malformation of limb(s)
Congenital anomaly of limb(s) NOS

4 Q75 Other congenital malformations of skull and face bones
EXCLUDES 1 congenital malformation of face NOS (Q18.-)
congenital malformation syndromes classified to Q87.-
dentofacial anomalies [including malocclusion] (M26.-)
musculoskeletal deformities of head and face (Q67.0-Q67.4)
skull defects associated with congenital anomalies of brain such as:
anencephaly (Q00.0)
encephalocele (Q01.-)
hydrocephalus (Q03.-)
microcephaly (Q02)
SP Q75.0 Craniosynostosis
Acrocephaly
Imperfect fusion of skull
Oxycephaly
Trigonocephaly
SP Q75.1 Craniofacial dysostosis
Crouzon's disease
SP Q75.2 Hypertelorism
SP Q75.3 Macrocephaly
SP Q75.4 Mandibulofacial dysostosis
Franceschetti syndrome
Treacher Collins syndrome
SP Q75.5 Oculomandibular dysostosis
SP Q75.8 Other specified congenital malformations of skull and face bones
Absence of skull bone, congenital
Congenital deformity of forehead
Platybasia
IQ Q75.9 Congenital malformation of skull and face bones, unspecified
Congenital anomaly of face bones NOS
Congenital anomaly of skull NOS

4 Q76 Congenital malformations of spine and bony thorax
EXCLUDES 1 congenital musculoskeletal deformities of spine and chest (Q67.5-Q67.8)
SP Q76.0 Spina bifida occulta
EXCLUDES 1 meningocele (spinal) (Q05.-)
spina bifida (aperta) (cystica) (Q05.-)
SP Q76.1 Klippel-Feil syndrome
Cervical fusion syndrome
SP Q76.2 Congenital spondylolisthesis
Congenital spondylolysis

Chapter 17

Q00-Q99

EXCLUDES 1 spondylolisthesis (acquired) (M43.1-)
spondylolysis (acquired) (M43.0-)

SP **Q76.3 Congenital scoliosis due to congenital bony malformation**
Hemivertebra fusion or failure of segmentation with scoliosis

5 **Q76.4 Other congenital malformations of spine, not associated with scoliosis**

6 **Q76.41 Congenital kyphosis**

SP **Q76.411 Congenital kyphosis, occipito-atlanto-axial region**

SP **Q76.412 Congenital kyphosis, cervical region**

SP **Q76.413 Congenital kyphosis, cervicothoracic region**

SP **Q76.414 Congenital kyphosis, thoracic region**

SP **Q76.415 Congenital kyphosis, thoracolumbar region**

!Q **Q76.419 Congenital kyphosis, unspecified region**

6 **Q76.42 Congenital lordosis**

SP **Q76.425 Congenital lordosis, thoracolumbar region**

SP **Q76.426 Congenital lordosis, lumbar region**

SP **Q76.427 Congenital lordosis, lumbosacral region**

SP **Q76.428 Congenital lordosis, sacral and sacrococcygeal region**

!Q **Q76.429 Congenital lordosis, unspecified region**

SP **Q76.49 Other congenital malformations of spine, not associated with scoliosis**
Congenital absence of vertebra NOS
Congenital fusion of spine NOS
Congenital malformation of lumbosacral (joint) (region) NOS
Congenital malformation of spine NOS
Hemivertebra NOS
Malformation of spine NOS
Platyspondylisis NOS
Supernumerary vertebra NOS

SP **Q76.5 Cervical rib**
Supernumerary rib in cervical region

SP **Q76.6 Other congenital malformations of ribs**
Accessory rib
Congenital absence of rib
Congenital fusion of ribs
Congenital malformation of ribs NOS
EXCLUDES 1 short rib syndrome (Q77.2)

SP **Q76.7 Congenital malformation of sternum**
Congenital absence of sternum
Sternum bifidum

SP **Q76.8 Other congenital malformations of bony thorax**

!Q **Q76.9 Congenital malformation of bony thorax, unspecified**

4 **Q77 Osteochondrodysplasia with defects of growth of tubular bones and spine**
EXCLUDES 1 mucopolysaccharidosis (E76.0-E76.3)
EXCLUDES 2 congenital myotonic chondrodystrophy (G71.13)

SP **Q77.0 Achondrogenesis**
Hypochondrogenesis

SP **Q77.1 Thanatophoric short stature**

SP **Q77.2 Short rib syndrome**
Asphyxiating thoracic dysplasia [Jeune]

SP **Q77.3 Chondrodysplasia punctata**
EXCLUDES 1 Rhizomelic chondrodysplasia punctata (E71.43)

SP **Q77.4 Achondroplasia**
Hypochondroplasia
Osteosclerosis congenita

SP **Q77.5 Diastrophic dysplasia**

SP **Q77.6 Chondroectodermal dysplasia**
Ellis-van Creveld syndrome

SP **Q77.7 Spondyloepiphyseal dysplasia**

SP **Q77.8 Other osteochondrodysplasia with defects of growth of tubular bones and spine**

SP **Q77.9 Osteochondrodysplasia with defects of growth of tubular bones and spine, unspecified**

4 **Q78 Other osteochondrodysplasias**
EXCLUDES 2 congenital myotonic chondrodystrophy (G71.13)

SP **Q78.0 Osteogenesis imperfecta**
Fragilitas ossium
Osteopsathyrosis

SP **Q78.1 Polyostotic fibrous dysplasia**
Albright(-McCune)(-Sternberg) syndrome
DEFINITION Genetic bone disorder causing multiple areas of normal bone to be replaced by bands of abnormal fibrous tissue, causing pain, fractures, and deformity.

SP **Q78.2 Osteopetrosis**
Albers-Schönberg syndrome
Osteosclerosis NOS

SP **Q78.3 Progressive diaphyseal dysplasia**
Camurati-Engelmann syndrome

SP **Q78.4 Enchondromatosis**
Maffucci's syndrome
Ollier's disease

SP **Q78.5 Metaphyseal dysplasia**
Pyle's syndrome

SP **Q78.6 Multiple congenital exostoses**
Diaphyseal aclasis

SP **Q78.8 Other specified osteochondrodysplasias**
Osteopoikilosis

!Q **Q78.9 Osteochondrodysplasia, unspecified**
Chondrodystrophy NOS
Osteodystrophy NOS

4 **Q79 Congenital malformations of musculoskeletal system, not elsewhere classified**
EXCLUDES 2 congenital (sternomastoid) torticollis (Q68.0)

SP **Q79.0 Congenital diaphragmatic hernia**
EXCLUDES 1 congenital hiatus hernia (Q40.1)

SP **Q79.1 Other congenital malformations of diaphragm**
Absence of diaphragm
Congenital malformation of diaphragm NOS
Eventration of diaphragm

SP **Q79.2 Exomphalos**
Omphalocele

EXCLUDES 1 umbilical hernia (K42.-)

SP **Q79.3 Gastroschisis**

SP **Q79.4 Prune belly syndrome**
Congenital prolapse of bladder mucosa
Eagle-Barrett syndrome

5 **Q79.5 Other congenital malformations of abdominal wall**
EXCLUDES 1 umbilical hernia (K42.-)

SP **Q79.51 Congenital hernia of bladder**

SP **Q79.59 Other congenital malformations of abdominal wall**

5 **Q79.6 Ehlers-Danlos syndromes**
DEFINITION Ehlers-Danlos syndromes are a clinically and genetically heterogeneous group of heritable connective tissue disorders characterized by articular hypermobility, skin hyperextensibility or laxity, and tissue fragility affecting virtually every organ system: skin, ligaments, joints, bone, muscle, blood vessels and various organs.

SP **Q79.60 Ehlers-Danlos syndrome, unspecified**

SP **Q79.61 Classical Ehlers-Danlos syndrome**
Classical EDS (cEDS)

SP **Q79.62 Hypermobile Ehlers-Danlos syndrome**
Hypermobile EDS (hEDS)

SP **Q79.63 Vascular Ehlers-Danlos syndrome**
Vascular EDS (vEDS)

SP **Q79.69 Other Ehlers-Danlos syndromes**

SP **Q79.8 Other congenital malformations of musculoskeletal system**
Absence of muscle
Absence of tendon
Accessory muscle
Amyotrophia congenita
Congenital constricting bands
Congenital shortening of tendon
Poland syndrome

IQ **Q79.9 Congenital malformation of musculoskeletal system, unspecified**
Congenital anomaly of musculoskeletal system NOS
Congenital deformity of musculoskeletal system NOS

Other congenital malformations (Q80-Q89)

4 **Q80 Congenital ichthyosis**
EXCLUDES 1 Refsum's disease (G60.1)

IQ **Q80.0 Ichthyosis vulgaris**

IQ **Q80.1 X-linked ichthyosis**

IQ **Q80.2 Lamellar ichthyosis**
Collodion baby

IQ **Q80.3 Congenital bullous ichthyosiform erythroderma**

IQ **Q80.4 Harlequin fetus**

IQ **Q80.8 Other congenital ichthyosis**

IQ **Q80.9 Congenital ichthyosis, unspecified**

4 **Q81 Epidermolysis bullosa**

SP **Q81.0 Epidermolysis bullosa simplex**
EXCLUDES 1 Cockayne's syndrome (Q87.19)

SP **Q81.1 Epidermolysis bullosa letalis**
Herlitz' syndrome

SP **Q81.2 Epidermolysis bullosa dystrophica**

SP **Q81.8 Other epidermolysis bullosa**

IQ **Q81.9 Epidermolysis bullosa, unspecified**

4 **Q82 Other congenital malformations of skin**
EXCLUDES 1 acrodermatitis enteropathica (E83.2)
congenital erythropoietic porphyria (E80.0)
pilonidal cyst or sinus (L05.-)
Sturge-Weber (-Dimitri) syndrome (Q85.8)

SP **Q82.0 Hereditary lymphedema**

SP **Q82.1 Xeroderma pigmentosum**

SP **Q82.2 Congenital cutaneous mastocytosis**
Congenital diffuse cutaneous mastocytosis
Congenital maculopapular cutaneous mastocytosis
Congenital urticaria pigmentosa
EXCLUDES 1 cutaneous mastocytosis NOS (D47.01)
diffuse cutaneous mastocytosis (with onset after newborn period) (D47.01)
malignant mastocytosis (C96.2-)
systemic mastocytosis (D47.02)
urticaria pigmentosa (non-congenital) (with onset after newborn period) (D47.01)

SP **Q82.3 Incontinentia pigmenti**

SP **Q82.4 Ectodermal dysplasia (anhidrotic)**
EXCLUDES 1 Ellis-van Creveld syndrome (Q77.6)

SP **Q82.5 Congenital non-neoplastic nevus**
Birthmark NOS
Flammeus Nevus
Portwine Nevus
Sanguineous Nevus
Strawberry Nevus
Vascular Nevus NOS
Verrucous Nevus
EXCLUDES 2 Café au lait spots (L81.3)
lentigo (L81.4)
nevus NOS (D22.-)
araneus nevus (I78.1)
melanocytic nevus (D22.-)
pigmented nevus (D22.-)
spider nevus (I78.1)
stellar nevus (I78.1)

SP **Q82.6 Congenital sacral dimple**
Parasacral dimple
EXCLUDES 2 pilonidal cyst with abscess (L05.01)
pilonidal cyst without abscess (L05.91)

SP **Q82.8 Other specified congenital malformations of skin**
Abnormal palmar creases
Accessory skin tags
Benign familial pemphigus [Hailey-Hailey]
Congenital poikiloderma
Cutis laxa (hyperelastica)

Dermatoglyphic anomalies
Inherited keratosis palmaris et plantaris
Keratosis follicularis [Darier-White]
EXCLUDES 1 Ehlers-Danlos syndromes (Q79.6-)

IQ **Q82.9 Congenital malformation of skin, unspecified**

4 **Q83 Congenital malformations of breast**
EXCLUDES 2 absence of pectoral muscle (Q79.8)
hypoplasia of breast (N64.82)
micromastia (N64.82)

SP **Q83.0 Congenital absence of breast with absent nipple**

SP **Q83.1 Accessory breast**
Supernumerary breast

SP **Q83.2 Absent nipple**

SP **Q83.3 Accessory nipple**
Supernumerary nipple

SP **Q83.8 Other congenital malformations of breast**

IQ **Q83.9 Congenital malformation of breast, unspecified**

4 **Q84 Other congenital malformations of integument**

SP **Q84.0 Congenital alopecia**
Congenital atrichosis

IQ **Q84.1 Congenital morphological disturbances of hair, not elsewhere classified**
Beaded hair
Monilethrix
Pili annulati
EXCLUDES 1 Menkes' kinky hair syndrome (E83.0)

IQ **Q84.2 Other congenital malformations of hair**
Congenital hypertrichosis
Congenital malformation of hair NOS
Persistent lanugo

IQ **Q84.3 Anonychia**
EXCLUDES 1 nail patella syndrome (Q87.2)

IQ **Q84.4 Congenital leukonychia**

IQ **Q84.5 Enlarged and hypertrophic nails**
Congenital onychauxis
Pachyonychia

IQ **Q84.6 Other congenital malformations of nails**
Congenital clubnail
Congenital koilonychia
Congenital malformation of nail NOS

SP **Q84.8 Other specified congenital malformations of integument**
Aplasia cutis congenita

IQ **Q84.9 Congenital malformation of integument, unspecified**
Congenital anomaly of integument NOS
Congenital deformity of integument NOS

4 **Q85 Phakomatoses, not elsewhere classified**
EXCLUDES 1 ataxia telangiectasia [Louis-Bar] (G11.3)
familial dysautonomia [Riley-Day] (G90.1)

5 **Q85.0 Neurofibromatosis (nonmalignant)**

SP **Q85.00 Neurofibromatosis, unspecified**

SP **Q85.01 Neurofibromatosis, type 1**
Von Recklinghausen disease

SP **Q85.02 Neurofibromatosis, type 2**
Acoustic neurofibromatosis

SP **Q85.03 Schwannomatosis**
DEFINITION A rare type of neurofibromatosis causing tumors on nerve sheaths of spinal, peripheral, and cranial nerves - except the eighth (vestibular) cranial nerve.

SP **Q85.09 Other neurofibromatosis**

SP **Q85.1 Tuberous sclerosis**
Bourneville's disease
Epiloia

SP **Q85.8 Other phakomatoses, not elsewhere classified**
Peutz-Jeghers Syndrome
Sturge-Weber(-Dimitri) syndrome
von Hippel-Lindau syndrome
EXCLUDES 1 Meckel-Gruber syndrome (Q61.9)

SP **Q85.9 Phakomatosis, unspecified**
Hamartosis NOS

4 **Q86 Congenital malformation syndromes due to known exogenous causes, not elsewhere classified**
EXCLUDES 2 iodine-deficiency-related hypothyroidism (E00-E02)
nonteratogenic effects of substances transmitted via placenta or breast milk (P04.-)

SP **Q86.0 Fetal alcohol syndrome (dysmorphic)**

SP **Q86.1 Fetal hydantoin syndrome**
Meadow's syndrome

SP **Q86.2 Dysmorphism due to warfarin**

SP **Q86.8 Other congenital malformation syndromes due to known exogenous causes**

+ 4 **Q87 Other specified congenital malformation syndromes affecting multiple systems**
Use additional code(s) to identify all associated manifestations

SP + **Q87.0 Congenital malformation syndromes predominantly affecting facial appearance**
Acrocephalopolysyndactyly
Acrocephalosyndactyly [Apert]
Cryptophthalmos syndrome
Cyclopia
Goldenhar syndrome
Moebius syndrome
Oro-facial-digital syndrome
Robin syndrome
Whistling face

+ 5 **Q87.1 Congenital malformation syndromes predominantly associated with short stature**
EXCLUDES 1 Ellis-van Creveld syndrome (Q77.6)
Smith-Lemli-Opitz syndrome (E78.72)

SP + **Q87.11 Prader-Willi syndrome**

SP + **Q87.19 Other congenital malformation syndromes predominantly associated with short stature**
Aarskog syndrome
Cockayne syndrome
De Lange syndrome
Dubowitz syndrome
Noonan syndrome

Robinow-Silverman-Smith syndrome
Russell-Silver syndrome
Seckel syndrome

SP + Q87.2 **Congenital malformation syndromes predominantly involving limbs**
Holt-Oram syndrome
Klippel-Trenaunay-Weber syndrome
Nail patella syndrome
Rubinstein-Taybi syndrome
Sirenomelia syndrome
Thrombocytopenia with absent radius [TAR] syndrome
VATER syndrome

SP + Q87.3 **Congenital malformation syndromes involving early overgrowth**
Beckwith-Wiedemann syndrome
Sotos syndrome
Weaver syndrome

+ 5 Q87.4 **Marfan's syndrome**

SP + Q87.40 **Marfan's syndrome, unspecified**

+ 6 Q87.41 **Marfan's syndrome with cardiovascular manifestations**

SP + Q87.410 **Marfan's syndrome with aortic dilation**

SP + Q87.418 **Marfan's syndrome with other cardiovascular manifestations**

SP + Q87.42 **Marfan's syndrome with ocular manifestations**

SP + Q87.43 **Marfan's syndrome with skeletal manifestation**

SP + Q87.5 **Other congenital malformation syndromes with other skeletal changes**

+ 5 Q87.8 **Other specified congenital malformation syndromes, not elsewhere classified**
EXCLUDES 1 Zellweger syndrome (E71.510)

SP + Q87.81 **Alport syndrome**
Use additional code to identify stage of chronic kidney disease (N18.1-N18.6)

SP + Q87.82 **Arterial tortuosity syndrome**

SP + Q87.89 **Other specified congenital malformation syndromes, not elsewhere classified**
Laurence-Moon (-Bardet)-Biedl syndrome

4 Q89 **Other congenital malformations, not elsewhere classified**

5 Q89.0 **Congenital absence and malformations of spleen**
EXCLUDES 1 isomerism of atrial appendages (with asplenia or polysplenia) (Q20.6)

SP Q89.01 **Asplenia (congenital)**

SP Q89.09 **Congenital malformations of spleen**
Congenital splenomegaly

SP Q89.1 **Congenital malformations of adrenal gland**
EXCLUDES 1 adrenogenital disorders (E25.-)
congenital adrenal hyperplasia (E25.0)

SP Q89.2 **Congenital malformations of other endocrine glands**
Congenital malformation of parathyroid or thyroid gland
Persistent thyroglossal duct
Thyroglossal cyst
EXCLUDES 1 congenital goiter (E03.0)
congenital hypothyroidism (E03.1)

SP Q89.3 **Situs inversus**
Dextrocardia with situs inversus
Mirror-image atrial arrangement with situs inversus
Situs inversus or transversus abdominalis
Situs inversus or transversus thoracis
Transposition of abdominal viscera
Transposition of thoracic viscera
EXCLUDES 1 dextrocardia NOS (Q24.0)
DEFINITION Congenital disorder in which the position of all major organs in the chest and abdomen are reversed horizontally.

SP Q89.4 **Conjoined twins**
Craniopagus
Dicephaly
Pygopagus
Thoracopagus

SP Q89.7 **Multiple congenital malformations, not elsewhere classified**
Multiple congenital anomalies NOS
Multiple congenital deformities NOS
EXCLUDES 1 congenital malformation syndromes affecting multiple systems (Q87.-)

SP + Q89.8 **Other specified congenital malformations**
Use additional code(s) to identify all associated manifestations

IQ Q89.9 **Congenital malformation, unspecified**
Congenital anomaly NOS
Congenital deformity NOS

Chromosomal abnormalities, not elsewhere classified (Q90-Q99)

EXCLUDES 2 mitochondrial metabolic disorders (E88.4-)

+ 4 Q90 **Down syndrome**
Use additional code(s) to identify any associated physical conditions and degree of intellectual disabilities (F70-F79)

SP + Q90.0 **Trisomy 21, nonmosaicism (meiotic nondisjunction)**

SP + Q90.1 **Trisomy 21, mosaicism (mitotic nondisjunction)**

SP + Q90.2 **Trisomy 21, translocation**

SP + Q90.9 **Down syndrome, unspecified**
Trisomy 21 NOS

4 Q91 **Trisomy 18 and Trisomy 13**

SP Q91.0 **Trisomy 18, nonmosaicism (meiotic nondisjunction)**

SP Q91.1 **Trisomy 18, mosaicism (mitotic nondisjunction)**

SP Q91.2 **Trisomy 18, translocation**

SP Q91.3 **Trisomy 18, unspecified**

SP Q91.4 **Trisomy 13, nonmosaicism (meiotic nondisjunction)**

SP Q91.5 **Trisomy 13, mosaicism (mitotic nondisjunction)**

SP Q91.6 **Trisomy 13, translocation**

SP Q91.7 **Trisomy 13, unspecified**

4 Q92 **Other trisomies and partial trisomies of the autosomes, not elsewhere classified**

INCLUDES unbalanced translocations and insertions

EXCLUDES 1 trisomies of chromosomes 13, 18, 21 (Q90-Q91)

SP **Q92.0 Whole chromosome trisomy, nonmosaicism (meiotic nondisjunction)**

SP **Q92.1 Whole chromosome trisomy, mosaicism (mitotic nondisjunction)**

SP **Q92.2 Partial trisomy**
Less than whole arm duplicated
Whole arm or more duplicated
EXCLUDES 1 partial trisomy due to unbalanced translocation (Q92.5)

SP **Q92.5 Duplications with other complex rearrangements**
Partial trisomy due to unbalanced translocations
Code also:
any associated deletions due to unbalanced translocations, inversions and insertions (Q93.7)

5 **Q92.6 Marker chromosomes**
Trisomies due to dicentrics
Trisomies due to extra rings
Trisomies due to isochromosomes
Individual with marker heterochromatin

SP **Q92.61 Marker chromosomes in normal individual**

SP **Q92.62 Marker chromosomes in abnormal individual**

SP **Q92.7 Triploidy and polyploidy**

SP **Q92.8 Other specified trisomies and partial trisomies of autosomes**
Duplications identified by fluorescence in situ hybridization (FISH)
Duplications identified by in situ hybridization (ISH)
Duplications seen only at prometaphase

!Q **Q92.9 Trisomy and partial trisomy of autosomes, unspecified**

4 **Q93 Monosomies and deletions from the autosomes, not elsewhere classified**

SP **Q93.0 Whole chromosome monosomy, nonmosaicism (meiotic nondisjunction)**

SP **Q93.1 Whole chromosome monosomy, mosaicism (mitotic nondisjunction)**

SP **Q93.2 Chromosome replaced with ring, dicentric or isochromosome**

SP **Q93.3 Deletion of short arm of chromosome 4**
Wolff-Hirschorn syndrome

SP **Q93.4 Deletion of short arm of chromosome 5**
Cri-du-chat syndrome

5 **Q93.5 Other deletions of part of a chromosome**

SP **Q93.51 Angelman syndrome**

SP **Q93.59 Other deletions of part of a chromosome**

SP **Q93.7 Deletions with other complex rearrangements**
Deletions due to unbalanced translocations, inversions and insertions
Code also:
any associated duplications due to unbalanced translocations, inversions and insertions (Q92.5)

5 **Q93.8 Other deletions from the autosomes**

SP **Q93.81 Velo-cardio-facial syndrome**
Deletion 22q11.2

SP **Q93.82 Williams syndrome**

SP **Q93.88 Other microdeletions**
Miller-Dieker syndrome
Smith-Magenis syndrome

SP **Q93.89 Other deletions from the autosomes**
Deletions identified by fluorescence in situ hybridization (FISH)
Deletions identified by in situ hybridization (ISH)
Deletions seen only at prometaphase

!Q **Q93.9 Deletion from autosomes, unspecified**

4 **Q95 Balanced rearrangements and structural markers, not elsewhere classified**
INCLUDES Robertsonian and balanced reciprocal translocations and insertions

SP **Q95.0 Balanced translocation and insertion in normal individual**

SP **Q95.1 Chromosome inversion in normal individual**

SP **Q95.2 Balanced autosomal rearrangement in abnormal individual**

SP **Q95.3 Balanced sex/autosomal rearrangement in abnormal individual**

SP **Q95.5 Individual with autosomal fragile site**

SP **Q95.8 Other balanced rearrangements and structural markers**

SP **Q95.9 Balanced rearrangement and structural marker, unspecified**

4 **Q96 Turner's syndrome**
EXCLUDES 1 Noonan syndrome (Q87.19)

SP **Q96.0 Karyotype 45, X**

SP **Q96.1 Karyotype 46, X iso (Xq)**
Karyotype 46, isochromosome Xq

SP **Q96.2 Karyotype 46, X with abnormal sex chromosome, except iso (Xq)**
Karyotype 46, X with abnormal sex chromosome, except isochromosome Xq

SP **Q96.3 Mosaicism, 45, X/46, XX or XY**

SP **Q96.4 Mosaicism, 45, X/other cell line(s) with abnormal sex chromosome**

SP **Q96.8 Other variants of Turner's syndrome**

SP **Q96.9 Turner's syndrome, unspecified**

4 **Q97 Other sex chromosome abnormalities, female phenotype, not elsewhere classified**
EXCLUDES 1 Turner's syndrome (Q96.-)

SP **Q97.0 Karyotype 47, XXX**

SP **Q97.1 Female with more than three X chromosomes**

SP **Q97.2 Mosaicism, lines with various numbers of X chromosomes**

SP **Q97.3 Female with 46, XY karyotype**

SP **Q97.8 Other specified sex chromosome abnormalities, female phenotype**

SP **Q97.9 Sex chromosome abnormality, female phenotype, unspecified**

4 **Q98 Other sex chromosome abnormalities, male phenotype, not elsewhere classified**

SP **Q98.0 Klinefelter syndrome karyotype 47, XXY**

SP **Q98.1 Klinefelter syndrome, male with more than two X chromosomes**

SP **Q98.3 Other male with 46, XX karyotype**

SP **Q98.4 Klinefelter syndrome, unspecified**

SP **Q98.5 Karyotype 47, XYY**

SP **Q98.6 Male with structurally abnormal sex chromosome**

SP **Q98.7 Male with sex chromosome mosaicism**

SP **Q98.8 Other specified sex chromosome abnormalities, male phenotype**

SP **Q98.9 Sex chromosome abnormality, male phenotype, unspecified**

4 **Q99 Other chromosome abnormalities, not elsewhere classified**

SP **Q99.0 Chimera 46, XX/46, XY**
Chimera 46, XX/46, XY true hermaphrodite

SP **Q99.1 46, XX true hermaphrodite**
46, XX with streak gonads
46, XY with streak gonads
Pure gonadal dysgenesis

SP **Q99.2 Fragile X chromosome**
Fragile X syndrome

SP **Q99.8 Other specified chromosome abnormalities**

IQ **Q99.9 Chromosomal abnormality, unspecified**

Chapter 17 Scenarios: Congenital malformations, deformations and chromosomal abnormalities (Q00-Q99)

Open heart surgery, Marfan syndrome

A 65-year-old man underwent open heart surgery to replace his aortic root as well as his aortic valve. The surgery resolved aortic dilation associated with Marfan syndrome. He was admitted to home health for routine surgical aftercare.

Description	Code
Primary: Encounter for surgical aftercare following surgery on the circulatory system	Z48.812
Secondary: Marfan's syndrome, unspecified	Q87.40

Routine surgical aftercare following cardiac surgery is coded with Z48.812. Note that aftercare codes should only be used routine care. The open heart surgery resolved the aortic dilation but did not resolve the Marfan syndrome, which is a congenital condition that can cause a variety of manifestations. Thus, Q87.40 is assigned to capture it.

Pressure ulcers/injuries, spina bifida

A 21-year-old woman who was born with spina bifida is admitted to home health for wound care to a stage 3 pressure ulcer/injury on her right buttock and a stage 2 pressure ulcer/injury on her sacrum. She is confined to a wheelchair due to paraplegia of the bilateral lower limbs.

Description	Code
Primary: Pressure ulcer of right buttock, stage 3	L89.313
Secondary: Pressure ulcer of sacral region, stage 2	L89.152
Secondary: Spina bifida, unspecified	Q05.9
Secondary: Paraplegia, unspecified	G82.20
Secondary: Dependence on wheelchair	Z99.3

As the focus of care, the pressure ulcers/injuries are coded primary. Her spina bifida, paraplegia, and wheelchair dependence are also coded as it will impact her care. Note that while some conditions are considered integral to spina bifida, there is a "use additional code" note for all codes within category Q05 that directs the coder to add the additional code for any associated paraplegia (G82.2-). "Use additional code" notes dictate sequencing, meaning the code must immediately follow the code from category Q05.

Tetralogy of Fallot

A 28-year-old man is admitted for aftercare following surgery to replace his pulmonary valve with a prosthetic one. He was diagnosed with Tetralogy of Fallot as a baby, which necessitated the valve replacement. He has had numerous heart surgeries over the years. He also has a history of melanoma, requiring the removal of several moles and is frequently monitored for recurrence.

Description	Code
Primary: Encounter for surgical aftercare following surgery on the circulatory system	Z48.812
Secondary: Tetralogy of Fallot	Q21.3
Secondary: Presence of prosthetic heart valve	Z95.2
Secondary: Personal history of malignant melanoma of skin	Z85.820

Surgical aftercare is the focus of care, making Z48.812 the appropriate primary diagnosis code. The surgical procedure treats an aspect of the heart condition, Tetralogy of Fallot, but does not cure it. Thus, it is still coded. Tetralogy of Fallot is a congenital condition and as such may be assigned throughout the life of the patient, according to coding guidelines. Code Z95.2 is assigned to indicate the presence of a prosthetic heart valve. An additional code is assigned to capture his history of malignant melanoma and need for frequent monitoring.

Chapter 18: Symptoms, Signs and Abnormal Clinical and Laboratory Findings, not Elsewhere Classified (R00-R99)

Chapter 18 includes symptoms, signs, abnormal results of clinical or other investigative procedures, and ill-defined conditions where no diagnosis classifiable elsewhere is recorded. Signs and symptoms that point rather definitively to a given diagnosis have been assigned to a category in other chapters within ICD-10-CM. In general, categories in this chapter include the less well-defined conditions and symptoms that, without the necessary study of the case to establish a final diagnosis, point perhaps equally to two or more diseases or to two or more systems of the body. Practically all categories in the chapter should be designated "not otherwise specified," "unknown etiology" or "transient." The Alphabetical Index should be consulted to determine which signs and symptoms are to be allocated here and which to other chapters. The residual subcategories numbered .8 are generally provided for other relevant symptoms that cannot be allocated elsewhere in the classification.

In the Patient Driven Groupings Model (PDGM) payment system, the majority of common home health symptom codes carry a questionable encounter designation.

Using a questionable encounter code as a primary diagnosis could result in claims getting kicked back, payment delays and potential red flags for auditors.

CMS states that "the majority of the R codes (codes that describe signs and symptoms, as opposed to diagnoses) are not appropriate as principal diagnosis codes for grouping home health periods into clinical groups" under PDGM.

To avoid these issues, take steps to identify which symptom codes your agency uses and work to gather more detailed information that will lead to more specific, acceptable codes instead.

The conditions and signs or symptoms included in categories R00-R99 of this chapter consist of:

- cases for which no more specific diagnosis can be made even after all the facts bearing on the case have been investigated;
- signs or symptoms existing at the time of initial encounter that proved to be transient and whose causes could not be determined;
- provisional diagnosis in a patient who failed to return for further investigation or care;
- cases referred elsewhere for investigation or treatment before the diagnosis was made;
- cases in which a more precise diagnosis was not available for any other reason;
- certain symptoms, for which supplementary information is provided, that represent important problems in medical care in their own right.

There is an Excludes 2 note at the beginning of this chapter for conditions, signs or symptoms that may be coded in addition to a code from Chapter 18, but are not included as part of the codes that are available in this chapter such as abnormal findings on antenatal screening of the mother (O28.-), certain conditions originating in the perinatal period (P00-P96), signs and symptoms classified in the body system chapters, and signs and symptoms of the breast (N63, N64.5).

The chapter is organized into blocks that correspond to signs and symptoms involving specific body systems such as circulatory, digestive, skin and subcutaneous tissue, nervous and musculoskeletal, genitourinary, cognitive perception/emotional state/behavior, and speech and voice; general signs and symptoms; abnormal findings on examination of blood, urine, other body fluids, substances and tissues; abnormal findings on diagnostic imaging and in functional studies; abnormal tumor markers; and ill-defined and unknown cause of mortality.

A "symptom" is any subjective evidence of disease, or a patient's condition, as reported by the patient. A "sign" is an indication of a problem that is observed by the physician or the clinician. For example, a patient may report a **symptom** by stating that he/she is feeling dizzy. A physician may report a **sign**, such as fever or irregular heartbeat.

More thorough examination may be needed to determine the cause of the symptom or sign (a definitive diagnosis). Coders should not assume a condition is present based on documentation of symptoms. If the documentation lists symptoms but no definitive diagnosis, query the doctor for a definitive diagnosis.

Many codes have an Excludes 1 note that lists more definitive diagnoses. If any of these conditions are documented, do not report the symptom code. For example, category R22, (Localized superficial swelling, mass or lump of skin) includes this note: "Excludes 1: abnormal findings on diagnostic imaging (R90-R93), edema (R60.-), enlarged lymph nodes (R59.-), localized adiposity (E65), and swelling of joint (M25.4-).

Sometimes, a Chapter 18 code is not the most appropriate choice. **Symptom codes also are found in other chapters.** Here are a few situations to watch out for:

- A breast mass or lump is reported using code N63 (lump or mass in breast) from Chapter 14.
- An itch is reported using code Subcategory L29.9 (pruritus and related conditions) from Chapter 12.
- Pain in the eye is reported using code H57.1- (pain in or around the eye) from Chapter 7.

Multiple Coding and Sequencing

It is important to read the Includes and Excludes notes under codes in this chapter, as well as any other instructions under the code or code category. Below are some examples of multiple coding and sequencing issues for codes in this chapter.

A symptom code is not reported if the symptom is an integral part of the condition. For example, congestive heart failure and edema would be reported using only a code from the I50.- category (heart failure) because the edema is an integral part of the heart failure.

A symptom code is reported as an additional diagnosis when it describes a significant aspect of the condition but is not an integral part of it. Code N40.1 Benign prostatic hyperplasia with lower urinary tract symptoms has a note that reads: "Use additional codes to identify symptoms," and lists subcategory N39.4- (Urinary incontinence), code N13.8 (Urinary obstruction) plus several codes from subcategories R33.-, R35.- or R39.- to report the urinary symptoms present.

Category R50 (Fever of other and unknown origin) includes R50.81, fever in conditions classified elsewhere, with a note stating to code first the underlying condition when fever is present – such as with leukemia, neutropenia and sickle-cell disease. Fever is not an integral part of these conditions; therefore, it is reported as an additional diagnosis when present. There are many symptom codes for fever in certain situations: R50.2 (drug induced); R50.82 (postprocedural); R50.83 postvaccination; R50.84 (Febrile nonhemolytic transfusion reaction); and R50.9, (unspecified). However, there are dozens of codes, especially in Chapter 1, for specific diseases in which fever is an integral symptom and a code from category R50 is not used.

Special Coding Issues

Symptoms as reasons for receiving home care

Neither coding nor OASIS instructions prevent an agency from reporting a symptom when a related definitive diagnosis has not been established (confirmed by the provider). However, every effort should be made to establish/confirm a definitive diagnosis. As previously noted, "the majority of the R codes (codes that describe signs and symptoms, as opposed to diagnoses) are not appropriate as **principal** diagnosis codes for grouping home health periods into clinical groups" under PDGM, according to CMS. Codes for signs and symptoms may be reported in addition to a related definitive diagnosis when the sign or symptom is not routinely associated with that diagnosis, such as the various signs and symptoms associated with complex syndromes. The definitive diagnosis should be sequenced before the symptom code.

Signs or symptoms that are associated routinely with a disease process should not be assigned as additional codes, unless otherwise instructed by the classification.

Gait training

For patients needing gait training, the correct principal diagnosis code usually is the illness, especially if there is a disease code indicating gait problem as part of the illness. For example, **abnormality of gait and mobility** (R26.-) is integral to a patient with hemiplegia due to a CVA, lower back pain, or when using aftercare following joint replacement (Z47.1) of the lower extremity. If the therapist or physician documents "abnormal gait" or "unsteady gait," attempt to obtain the definitive diagnosis or a more specific description of the abnormal gait problem, such as R26.0 (Ataxic gait), R26.1 (Paralytic gait), R26.81 (Unsteadiness on feet gait), R26.89 (Other abnormalities of gait and mobility) or R26.9 (Unspecified abnormalities of gait and mobility).

Clinicians should investigate the cause of the gait abnormality. If the gait abnormality is integral to the condition causing the abnormal gait, then code the condition and not the abnormal gait.

Repeated falls (R29.6) is for use for encounters when a patient has recently fallen or has a tendency to fall and the reason for the fall is being investigated. There is an Excludes 2 note at this code to indicate at risk of or history of falling (Z91.81) is not included in this code, but may be coded as either a first-listed or additional code with R29.6.

Combination codes – ICD-10-CM contains a number of combination codes that identify both the definitive diagnosis and common symptoms of that diagnosis. When using one of these combination codes, an additional code should not be assigned for the symptom. The physician must identify a cause-and-effect relationship, if one exists. For example, in some elderly patients with incontinence, the incontinence may be attributed to one of several diseases or conditions.

Gangrene is a complication of necrosis (i.e., cell death) characterized by the decay of body tissues, which become black and malodorous. It is usually the result of critically insufficient blood supply (e.g., peripheral vascular disease) and often is associated with diabetes and long-term smoking. In ICD-10-CM, gangrene is included in multiple combination codes when it is present with another diagnosis or condition. A separate code for gangrene has been reassigned to I96 in Chapter 9, Diseases of the circulatory system and is no longer within the Symptoms chapter. Refer to the Alphabetical Index for the correct combination code based on the diagnostic statement.

Coma scale codes (R40.2-) can be used in conjunction with traumatic brain injury codes, acute cerebrovascular disease or sequelae of cerebrovascular disease codes. These codes are primarily for use by trauma registries, but they may be used in any setting where this information is collected. The coma scale codes should be sequenced after the diagnosis code(s).

These codes, one from each subcategory, are needed to complete the scale. The 7th character indicates when the scale was recorded and should match on all three codes. At a minimum, report the initial score documented on presentation at your facility. This may be a score from the emergency medical technician (EMT) or in the emergency department. If desired, a facility may choose to capture multiple coma scale scores.

Functional quadriplegia (R53.2) is the lack of ability to use one's limbs or ambulate due to extreme debility. It is not associated with neurologic deficit or injury, and code R53.2 should not be used for cases of neurologic quadriplegia. It should be assigned only if functional quadriplegia is specifically documented in the medical record.

SIRS due to non-infectious process – The systemic inflammatory response syndrome (SIRS) can develop as a result of certain non-infectious disease processes, such as trauma, malignant neoplasm or pancreatitis. When SIRS is documented with a noninfectious condition, and no subsequent infection is documented, the code for the underlying condition, such as an injury, should be assigned followed by code R65.10, Systemic inflammatory response syndrome (SIRS) of non-infectious origin without acute organ dysfunction, or code R65.11, Systemic inflammatory response syndrome (SIRS) of non-infectious origin with acute organ dysfunction. If an associated acute organ dysfunction is documented, the appropriate code(s) for the specific type of organ dysfunction(s) should be assigned in addition to code R65.11. If acute organ dysfunction is documented, but it cannot be determined if the acute organ dysfunction is associated with SIRS or due to another condition (e.g., directly due to the trauma), the provider should be queried.

Death NOS – Code R99, Ill-defined and unknown cause of mortality, is only for use in the very limited circumstance when a patient who has already died is brought into an emergency department or other health care facility and is pronounced dead upon arrival. It does not represent the discharge disposition of death.

A patient's **National Institutes of Health Stroke Scale** (NIHSS) score can be reported with the new **R29.7-** codes. The NIHSS score can be used as a clinical stroke assessment tool to evaluate and document neurological status in acute stroke patients. The stroke scale is valid for predicting lesion size and can serve as a measure of stroke severity.

The NIHSS has been shown to be a predictor of both short and long term outcome of stroke patients. Additionally, the stroke scale serves as a data collection tool for planning patient care and provides a common language for information exchanges among healthcare providers. The scale is designed to be a simple, valid and reliable tool that can be administered at the bedside consistently by physicians, nurses or therapists.

The NIH stroke scale (NIHSS) codes (R29.7- -) can be used in conjunction with acute stroke codes (I63) to identify the patient's neurological status and the severity of the stroke. The stroke scale codes should be sequenced after the acute stroke diagnosis code(s). At a minimum, report the initial score documented. If desired, a facility may choose to capture multiple stroke scale scores, per coding guidelines.

For coma scale and NIHSS codes, code assignment may be based on medical record documentation from clinicians who are not the patient's provider such as an emergency medical technician. However, the associated diagnosis (such as acute stroke) must be documented by patient's provider.

CHAPTER 18: SYMPTOMS, SIGNS AND ABNORMAL CLINICAL AND LABORATORY FINDINGS, NOT ELSEWHERE CLASSIFIED (R00-R99)

Note:
This chapter includes symptoms, signs, abnormal results of clinical or other investigative procedures, and ill-defined conditions regarding which no diagnosis classifiable elsewhere is recorded.
Signs and symptoms that point rather definitely to a given diagnosis have been assigned to a category in other chapters of the classification. In general, categories in this chapter include the less well-defined conditions and symptoms that, without the necessary study of the case to establish a final diagnosis, point perhaps equally to two or more diseases or to two or more systems of the body. Practically all categories in the chapter could be designated 'not otherwise specified', 'unknown etiology' or 'transient'. The Alphabetical Index should be consulted to determine which symptoms and signs are to be allocated here and which to other chapters. The residual subcategories, numbered .8, are generally provided for other relevant symptoms that cannot be allocated elsewhere in the classification.
The conditions and signs or symptoms included in categories R00-R94 consist of:
(a) cases for which no more specific diagnosis can be made even after all the facts bearing on the case have been investigated;
(b) signs or symptoms existing at the time of initial encounter that proved to be transient and whose causes could not be determined;
(c) provisional diagnosis in a patient who failed to return for further investigation or care;
(d) cases referred elsewhere for investigation or treatment before the diagnosis was made;
(e) cases in which a more precise diagnosis was not available for any other reason;
(f) certain symptoms, for which supplementary information is provided, that represent important problems in medical care in their own right.

EXCLUDES 2 abnormal findings on antenatal screening of mother (O28.-)
certain conditions originating in the perinatal period (P04-P96)
signs and symptoms classified in the body system chapters
signs and symptoms of breast (N63, N64.5)

GUIDELINES **Section I.C.18.a-c**

Codes that describe symptoms and signs are acceptable for reporting purposes when a related definitive diagnosis has not been established (confirmed) by the provider.

Codes for signs and symptoms may be reported in addition to a related definitive diagnosis when the sign or symptom is not routinely associated with that diagnosis, such as the various signs and symptoms associated with complex syndromes. The definitive diagnosis code should be sequenced before the symptom code. Signs or symptoms that are associated routinely with a disease process should not be assigned as additional codes, unless otherwise instructed by the classification.

ICD-10-CM contains a number of combination codes that identify both the definitive diagnosis and common symptoms of that diagnosis. When using one of these combination codes, an additional code should not be assigned for the symptom.

CODING TIPS✓ The R codes, except for dysphagia codes, are not allowed as primary in PDGM. They are allowed as secondary codes when not routinely associated with the definitive diagnosis. Symptom/sign diagnoses should be coded if there is no definitive diagnosis or the symptom/sign is not routinely associated with the definitive diagnosis, e.g. hemoptysis with pneumonia.

This chapter contains the following blocks:

R00-R09	Symptoms and signs involving the circulatory and respiratory systems
R10-R19	Symptoms and signs involving the digestive system and abdomen
R20-R23	Symptoms and signs involving the skin and subcutaneous tissue
R25-R29	Symptoms and signs involving the nervous and musculoskeletal systems
R30-R39	Symptoms and signs involving the genitourinary system
R40-R46	Symptoms and signs involving cognition, perception, emotional state and behavior
R47-R49	Symptoms and signs involving speech and voice
R50-R69	General symptoms and signs
R70-R79	Abnormal findings on examination of blood, without diagnosis
R80-R82	Abnormal findings on examination of urine, without diagnosis
R83-R89	Abnormal findings on examination of other body fluids, substances and tissues, without diagnosis
R90-R94	Abnormal findings on diagnostic imaging and in function studies, without diagnosis
R97	Abnormal tumor markers
R99	Ill-defined and unknown cause of mortality

Symptoms and signs involving the circulatory and respiratory systems (R00-R09)

4 **R00 Abnormalities of heart beat**
EXCLUDES 1 abnormalities originating in the perinatal period (P29.1-)
EXCLUDES 2 specified arrhythmias (I47-I49)

IQ **R00.0 Tachycardia, unspecified**
Rapid heart beat
Sinoauricular tachycardia NOS
Sinus [sinusal] tachycardia NOS
EXCLUDES 1 neonatal tachycardia (P29.11)
paroxysmal tachycardia (I47.-)

CODING TIPS✓ Tachycardia that is not specified as due to a specific arrhythmia or any particular cause is coded here. When the record reports "sinus tachycardia," assign code R00.0. Sinus tachycardia indicates a high heart rate with an impulse that continues to originate from the SA node.

IQ SH + **R00.1 Bradycardia, unspecified**
Sinoatrial bradycardia
Sinus bradycardia
Slow heart beat
Vagal bradycardia
Use additional code for adverse effect, if applicable, to identify drug (T36-T50 with fifth or sixth character 5)
EXCLUDES 1 neonatal bradycardia (P29.12)

IQ **R00.2 Palpitations**
Awareness of heart beat
DEFINITION Sensation of feeling the heart beat.

IQ **R00.8 Other abnormalities of heart beat**

IQ **R00.9 Unspecified abnormalities of heart beat**

4 **R01 Cardiac murmurs and other cardiac sounds**
EXCLUDES 1 cardiac murmurs and sounds originating in the perinatal period (P29.8)

IQ **R01.0 Benign and innocent cardiac murmurs**
Functional cardiac murmur

IQ **R01.1 Cardiac murmur, unspecified**
Cardiac bruit NOS
Heart murmur NOS
Systolic murmur NOS

IQ **R01.2 Other cardiac sounds**
Cardiac dullness, increased or decreased
Precordial friction

4 **R03 Abnormal blood-pressure reading, without diagnosis**

IQ **R03.0 Elevated blood-pressure reading, without diagnosis of hypertension**
Note:
This category is to be used to record an episode of elevated blood pressure in a patient in whom no formal diagnosis of hypertension has been made, or as an isolated incidental finding.

GUIDELINES **Section I.C.9.a.7)**
Assign code R03.0, Elevated blood pressure reading without diagnosis of hypertension, unless patient has an established diagnosis of hypertension. Assign code O13.-, Gestational [pregnancy-induced] hypertension without significant proteinuria, or O14.-, Pre-eclampsia, for transient hypertension of pregnancy.

CODING TIPS✓ Do not assign this code for a patient with a diagnosis of hypertension (I10-I13).

IQ **R03.1 Nonspecific low blood-pressure reading**
EXCLUDES 1 hypotension (I95.-)
maternal hypotension syndrome (O26.5-)
neurogenic orthostatic hypotension (G90.3)

CODING TIPS✓ Assign code R03.1 when a patient has a low blood pressure reading but has not been diagnosed with hypotension or orthostasis.

4 **R04 Hemorrhage from respiratory passages**
CODING TIPS✓ If these bleeds are the result of an adverse effect of anticoagulant, add D68.32 and the T code for anticoagulant from the Table of Drugs and Chemicals.

IQ **R04.0 Epistaxis**
Hemorrhage from nose
Nosebleed

IQ **R04.1 Hemorrhage from throat**
EXCLUDES 2 hemoptysis (R04.2)

IQ **R04.2 Hemoptysis**
Blood-stained sputum
Cough with hemorrhage
DEFINITION Coughing up blood or bloody mucous.

5 **R04.8 Hemorrhage from other sites in respiratory passages**

IQ **R04.81 Acute idiopathic pulmonary hemorrhage in infants**
AIPHI
Acute idiopathic hemorrhage in infants over 28 days old
EXCLUDES 1 perinatal pulmonary hemorrhage (P26.-)
von Willebrand's disease (D68.0)

IQ **R04.89 Hemorrhage from other sites in respiratory passages**
Pulmonary hemorrhage NOS

IQ **R04.9 Hemorrhage from respiratory passages, unspecified**

▲4 **R05 Cough**
EXCLUDES 1 paroxysmal cough due to Bordetella pertussis (A37.0-)
smoker's cough (J41.0)
EXCLUDES 2 cough with hemorrhage (R04.2)

★ **R05.1 Acute cough**
DEFINITION Cough of less than 3 weeks duration in adults is defined as acute cough (Chung and Pavord, 2008). Acute cough is most associated with upper respiratory infections.

★ **R05.2 Subacute cough**
DEFINITION Subacute cough may be related to URTI and typically resolve after the infection clears. Subacute cough also may be caused by post-infectious cough, pertussis, infection with Mycoplasma or Chlamydia, and – similarly to acute cough – exacerbations of other diseases such as asthma or COPD (Chung and Pavord, 2008). The defining difference between subacute and acute in adults is the duration of the cough, subacute being longer, lasting from three to eight weeks. In children, a cough is defined as chronic beginning at 8 weeks duration (Chang et al, 2017).

★ **R05.3 Chronic cough**
Persistent cough
Refractory cough
Unexplained cough
DEFINITION Chronic cough is a cough that persists despite guideline-based treatment of underlying etiologies.

★ **R05.4 Cough syncope**
Code first:
syncope and collapse (R55)
DEFINITION Some of the more severe symptoms of chronic cough include syncope, incontinence, vomiting, and sleep deprivation. (Irwin, 2006)

★ **R05.8 Other specified cough**

★ **R05.9 Cough, unspecified**

4 **R06 Abnormalities of breathing**
EXCLUDES 1 acute respiratory distress syndrome (J80)
respiratory arrest (R09.2)

Chapter 18

R00-R99

respiratory arrest of newborn (P28.81)
respiratory distress syndrome of newborn (P22.-)
respiratory failure (J96.-)
respiratory failure of newborn (P28.5)

CODING TIPS✓ Do not assign a code from R06.- as an additional code when the respiratory symptom is routinely associated with another disease process also coded, such as COPD, bronchitis, asthma, or another condition known to be the cause of the presenting symptom. The more specific condition should be coded.

5 **R06.0 Dyspnea**
EXCLUDES 1 tachypnea NOS (R06.82)
transient tachypnea of newborn (P22.1)

IQ **R06.00 Dyspnea, unspecified**

IQ **R06.01 Orthopnea**
DEFINITION Difficulty breathing while lying down, necessitating sleeping propped up or in a chair.

IQ **R06.02 Shortness of breath**

IQ **R06.03 Acute respiratory distress**

IQ **R06.09 Other forms of dyspnea**

IQ **R06.1 Stridor**
EXCLUDES 1 congenital laryngeal stridor (P28.89)
laryngismus (stridulus) (J38.5)
DEFINITION A whistling sound when breathing, usually heard on inspiration, indicating obstruction of the trachea or larynx.

IQ **R06.2 Wheezing**
EXCLUDES 1 Asthma (J45.-)

IQ **R06.3 Periodic breathing**
Cheyne-Stokes breathing

IQ **R06.4 Hyperventilation**
EXCLUDES 1 psychogenic hyperventilation (F45.8)

IQ **R06.5 Mouth breathing**
EXCLUDES 2 dry mouth NOS (R68.2)

IQ **R06.6 Hiccough**
EXCLUDES 1 psychogenic hiccough (F45.8)
DEFINITION Sharp sound of inhalation, with spasm of the glottis and diaphragm.

IQ **R06.7 Sneezing**

5 **R06.8 Other abnormalities of breathing**

IQ **R06.81 Apnea, not elsewhere classified**
Apnea NOS
EXCLUDES 1 apnea (of) newborn (P28.4)
sleep apnea (G47.3-)
sleep apnea of newborn (primary) (P28.3)
DEFINITION Temporary cessation of breathing.

IQ **R06.82 Tachypnea, not elsewhere classified**
Tachypnea NOS
EXCLUDES 1 transitory tachypnea of newborn (P22.1)
DEFINITION Rapid breathing.

IQ **R06.83 Snoring**

IQ **R06.89 Other abnormalities of breathing**
Breath-holding (spells)
Sighing
CODING TIPS✓ Respiratory **insufficiency** is part of COPD and therefore is not coded separately. Respiratory **failure** is coded in addition to COPD when documented. Respiratory failure is often confused with respiratory arrest. Respiratory failure means not enough oxygen is getting into the blood and there is a carbon dioxide buildup.

IQ **R06.9 Unspecified abnormalities of breathing**

4 **R07 Pain in throat and chest**
EXCLUDES 1 epidemic myalgia (B33.0)
EXCLUDES 2 jaw pain R68.84
pain in breast (N64.4)
CODING TIPS✓ Do not assign a code from R07.- for a patient with angina. Chest pain due to angina should be coded to the appropriate I20.- or I25.- code

IQ **R07.0 Pain in throat**
EXCLUDES 1 chronic sore throat (J31.2)
sore throat (acute) NOS (J02.9)
EXCLUDES 2 dysphagia (R13.1-)
pain in neck (M54.2)

IQ **R07.1 Chest pain on breathing**
Painful respiration

IQ **R07.2 Precordial pain**

5 **R07.8 Other chest pain**

IQ **R07.81 Pleurodynia**
Pleurodynia NOS
EXCLUDES 1 epidemic pleurodynia (B33.0)

IQ **R07.82 Intercostal pain**

IQ **R07.89 Other chest pain**
Anterior chest-wall pain NOS

IQ **R07.9 Chest pain, unspecified**

4 **R09 Other symptoms and signs involving the circulatory and respiratory system**
EXCLUDES 1 acute respiratory distress syndrome (J80)
respiratory arrest of newborn (P28.81)
respiratory distress syndrome of newborn (P22.0)
respiratory failure (J96.-)
respiratory failure of newborn (P28.5)

5 **R09.0 Asphyxia and hypoxemia**
EXCLUDES 1 asphyxia due to carbon monoxide (T58.-)
asphyxia due to foreign body in respiratory tract (T17.-)
birth (intrauterine) asphyxia (P84)
hyperventilation (R06.4)
traumatic asphyxia (T71.-)
EXCLUDES 2 hypercapnia (R06.89)

IQ **R09.01 Asphyxia**

DEFINITION Extreme decrease in the amount of oxygen in the body, accompanied by an increase of carbon dioxide, leading to loss of consciousness or death.

IQ **R09.02 Hypoxemia**

DEFINITION Abnormally low levels of oxygen in arterial blood.

IQ **R09.1 Pleurisy**

EXCLUDES 1 pleurisy with effusion (J90)

IQ **R09.2 Respiratory arrest**

Cardiorespiratory failure

EXCLUDES 1 cardiac arrest (I46.-)
respiratory arrest of newborn (P28.81)
respiratory distress of newborn (P22.0)
respiratory failure (J96.-)
respiratory failure of newborn (P28.5)
respiratory insufficiency (R06.89)
respiratory insufficiency of newborn (P28.5)

IQ **R09.3 Abnormal sputum**

Abnormal amount of sputum
Abnormal color of sputum
Abnormal odor of sputum
Excessive sputum

EXCLUDES 1 blood-stained sputum (R04.2)

5 **R09.8 Other specified symptoms and signs involving the circulatory and respiratory systems**

IQ **R09.81 Nasal congestion**

IQ **R09.82 Postnasal drip**

IQ **R09.89 Other specified symptoms and signs involving the circulatory and respiratory systems**

Bruit (arterial)
Abnormal chest percussion
Feeling of foreign body in throat
Friction sounds in chest
Chest tympany
Choking sensation
Rales
Weak pulse

EXCLUDES 2 foreign body in throat (T17.2-)
wheezing (R06.2)

CODING TIPS ✓ Pulmonary congestion is integral to, or routinely associated with, several conditions, such as CHF and pneumonia. Do not use an additional symptom code such as R09.89 when the symptom is routinely associated with the condition.

Symptoms and signs involving the digestive system and abdomen (R10-R19)

EXCLUDES 2 congenital or infantile pylorospasm (Q40.0)
gastrointestinal hemorrhage (K92.0-K92.2)
intestinal obstruction (K56.-)
newborn gastrointestinal hemorrhage (P54.0-P54.3)
newborn intestinal obstruction (P76.-)
pylorospasm (K31.3)
signs and symptoms involving the urinary system (R30-R39)
symptoms referable to female genital organs (N94.-)
symptoms referable to male genital organs (N48-N50)

4 **R10 Abdominal and pelvic pain**

EXCLUDES 1 renal colic (N23)

EXCLUDES 2 dorsalgia (M54.-)
flatulence and related conditions (R14.-)

IQ **R10.0 Acute abdomen**

Severe abdominal pain (generalized) (with abdominal rigidity)

EXCLUDES 1 abdominal rigidity NOS (R19.3)
generalized abdominal pain NOS (R10.84)
localized abdominal pain (R10.1-R10.3-)

5 **R10.1 Pain localized to upper abdomen**

IQ **R10.10 Upper abdominal pain, unspecified**

H IQ **R10.11 Right upper quadrant pain**

H IQ **R10.12 Left upper quadrant pain**

IQ **R10.13 Epigastric pain**

Dyspepsia

EXCLUDES 1 functional dyspepsia (K30)

IQ **R10.2 Pelvic and perineal pain**

EXCLUDES 1 vulvodynia (N94.81)

5 **R10.3 Pain localized to other parts of lower abdomen**

IQ **R10.30 Lower abdominal pain, unspecified**

H IQ **R10.31 Right lower quadrant pain**

H IQ **R10.32 Left lower quadrant pain**

IQ **R10.33 Periumbilical pain**

5 **R10.8 Other abdominal pain**

6 **R10.81 Abdominal tenderness**

Abdominal tenderness NOS

H IQ **R10.811 Right upper quadrant abdominal tenderness**

H IQ **R10.812 Left upper quadrant abdominal tenderness**

H IQ **R10.813 Right lower quadrant abdominal tenderness**

H IQ **R10.814 Left lower quadrant abdominal tenderness**

IQ **R10.815 Periumbilic abdominal tenderness**

IQ **R10.816 Epigastric abdominal tenderness**

IQ **R10.817 Generalized abdominal tenderness**

IQ **R10.819 Abdominal tenderness, unspecified site**

6 **R10.82 Rebound abdominal tenderness**

H IQ **R10.821 Right upper quadrant rebound abdominal tenderness**

H IQ **R10.822 Left upper quadrant rebound abdominal tenderness**

H IQ **R10.823 Right lower quadrant rebound abdominal tenderness**

H IQ **R10.824 Left lower quadrant rebound abdominal tenderness**

IQ **R10.825 Periumbilic rebound abdominal tenderness**

Chapter 18
R00-R99

IQ **R10.826 Epigastric rebound abdominal tenderness**

IQ **R10.827 Generalized rebound abdominal tenderness**

IQ **R10.829 Rebound abdominal tenderness, unspecified site**

IQ **R10.83 Colic**
Colic NOS
Infantile colic
EXCLUDES 1 colic in adult and child over 12 months old (R10.84)

IQ **R10.84 Generalized abdominal pain**
EXCLUDES 1 generalized abdominal pain associated with acute abdomen (R10.0)

IQ **R10.9 Unspecified abdominal pain**

4 **R11 Nausea and vomiting**
EXCLUDES 1 cyclical vomiting associated with migraine (G43.A-)
excessive vomiting in pregnancy (O21.-)
hematemesis (K92.0)
neonatal hematemesis (P54.0)
newborn vomiting (P92.0-)
psychogenic vomiting (F50.89)
vomiting associated with bulimia nervosa (F50.2)
vomiting following gastrointestinal surgery (K91.0)

IQ **R11.0 Nausea**
Nausea NOS
Nausea without vomiting

5 **R11.1 Vomiting**

IQ **R11.10 Vomiting, unspecified**
Vomiting NOS

IQ **R11.11 Vomiting without nausea**

IQ **R11.12 Projectile vomiting**

IQ **R11.13 Vomiting of fecal matter**

IQ **R11.14 Bilious vomiting**
Bilious emesis

IQ **R11.15 Cyclical vomiting syndrome unrelated to migraine**
Cyclic vomiting syndrome NOS
Persistent vomiting
EXCLUDES 1 cyclical vomiting in migraine (G43.A-)
EXCLUDES 2 bulimia nervosa (F50.2)
diabetes mellitus due to underlying condition (E08.-)

IQ **R11.2 Nausea with vomiting, unspecified**
Persistent nausea with vomiting NOS

IQ **R12 Heartburn**
EXCLUDES 1 dyspepsia NOS (R10.13)
functional dyspepsia (K30)

4 **R13 Aphagia and dysphagia**

IQ **R13.0 Aphagia**
Inability to swallow
EXCLUDES 1 psychogenic aphagia (F50.9)

5 **R13.1 Dysphagia**
Code first:
, if applicable, dysphagia following cerebrovascular disease (I69. with final characters -91)
EXCLUDES 1 psychogenic dysphagia (F45.8)

CODING TIPS✓ The R codes, except for dysphagia codes, are not allowed as primary in PDGM. They are allowed as secondary codes when not routinely associated with the definitive diagnosis. Symptom/sign diagnoses should be coded if there is no definitive diagnosis or the symptom/sign is not routinely associated with the definitive diagnosis, e.g. hemoptysis with pneumonia.

CODING TIPS✓ The results from tests such as the video fluoroscopic swallowing study, video endoscopic swallowing study, barium-contrast esophagogram or an upper endoscopy or manometry may identify the swallowing stage affected.

CODING TIPS✓ Assign a code from R13.1- following a code from I69.- when dysphagia is reported as a sequela of cerebral vascular disease to report the specified level of dysphagia.

DEFINITION Difficulty in swallowing.

SP **R13.10 Dysphagia, unspecified**
Difficulty in swallowing NOS

SP **R13.11 Dysphagia, oral phase**

SP **R13.12 Dysphagia, oropharyngeal phase**

SP **R13.13 Dysphagia, pharyngeal phase**

SP **R13.14 Dysphagia, pharyngoesophageal phase**

SP **R13.19 Other dysphagia**
Cervical dysphagia
Neurogenic dysphagia

4 **R14 Flatulence and related conditions**
EXCLUDES 1 psychogenic aerophagy (F45.8)

IQ **R14.0 Abdominal distension (gaseous)**
Bloating
Tympanites (abdominal) (intestinal)

IQ **R14.1 Gas pain**

IQ **R14.2 Eructation**

IQ **R14.3 Flatulence**

4 **R15 Fecal incontinence**
INCLUDES encopresis NOS
EXCLUDES 1 fecal incontinence of nonorganic origin (F98.1)

IQ **R15.0 Incomplete defecation**
EXCLUDES 1 constipation (K59.0-)
fecal impaction (K56.41)

IQ **R15.1 Fecal smearing**
Fecal soiling

IQ **R15.2 Fecal urgency**

IQ **R15.9 Full incontinence of feces**
Fecal incontinence NOS

4 **R16 Hepatomegaly and splenomegaly, not elsewhere classified**

IQ **R16.0 Hepatomegaly, not elsewhere classified**
Hepatomegaly NOS

IQ **R16.1 Splenomegaly, not elsewhere classified**
Splenomegaly NOS

Chapter 18

R00-R99

IQ **R16.2 Hepatomegaly with splenomegaly, not elsewhere classified**
Hepatosplenomegaly NOS

IQ **R17 Unspecified jaundice**
EXCLUDES 1 neonatal jaundice (P55, P57-P59)

4 **R18 Ascites**
INCLUDES fluid in peritoneal cavity
EXCLUDES 1 ascites in alcoholic cirrhosis (K70.31)
ascites in alcoholic hepatitis (K70.11)
ascites in toxic liver disease with chronic active hepatitis (K71.51)

IQ **R18.0 Malignant ascites**
Code first malignancy, such as:
malignant neoplasm of ovary (C56.-)
secondary malignant neoplasm of retroperitoneum and peritoneum (C78.6)
DEFINITION Abnormal accumulation of fluid containing cancer cells in the peritoneal cavity, usually from metastatic spread of a malignancy.

IQ **R18.8 Other ascites**
Ascites NOS
Peritoneal effusion (chronic)

4 **R19 Other symptoms and signs involving the digestive system and abdomen**
EXCLUDES 1 acute abdomen (R10.0)

5 **R19.0 Intra-abdominal and pelvic swelling, mass and lump**
EXCLUDES 1 abdominal distension (gaseous) (R14.-)
ascites (R18.-)
CODING TIPS ✓ A mass should not be coded for an area that has been clearly identified as a neoplasm. If a mass has been biopsied and reported as a neoplasm, code the appropriate neoplasm code.

IQ **R19.00 Intra-abdominal and pelvic swelling, mass and lump, unspecified site**

H IQ **R19.01 Right upper quadrant abdominal swelling, mass and lump**

H IQ **R19.02 Left upper quadrant abdominal swelling, mass and lump**

H IQ **R19.03 Right lower quadrant abdominal swelling, mass and lump**

H IQ **R19.04 Left lower quadrant abdominal swelling, mass and lump**

IQ **R19.05 Periumbilic swelling, mass or lump**
Diffuse or generalized umbilical swelling or mass

IQ **R19.06 Epigastric swelling, mass or lump**

IQ **R19.07 Generalized intra-abdominal and pelvic swelling, mass and lump**
Diffuse or generalized intra-abdominal swelling or mass NOS
Diffuse or generalized pelvic swelling or mass NOS

IQ **R19.09 Other intra-abdominal and pelvic swelling, mass and lump**

5 **R19.1 Abnormal bowel sounds**

IQ **R19.11 Absent bowel sounds**

IQ **R19.12 Hyperactive bowel sounds**

IQ **R19.15 Other abnormal bowel sounds**
Abnormal bowel sounds NOS

IQ **R19.2 Visible peristalsis**
Hyperperistalsis

5 **R19.3 Abdominal rigidity**
EXCLUDES 1 abdominal rigidity with severe abdominal pain (R10.0)

IQ **R19.30 Abdominal rigidity, unspecified site**

H IQ **R19.31 Right upper quadrant abdominal rigidity**

H IQ **R19.32 Left upper quadrant abdominal rigidity**

H IQ **R19.33 Right lower quadrant abdominal rigidity**

H IQ **R19.34 Left lower quadrant abdominal rigidity**

IQ **R19.35 Periumbilic abdominal rigidity**

IQ **R19.36 Epigastric abdominal rigidity**

IQ **R19.37 Generalized abdominal rigidity**

IQ **R19.4 Change in bowel habit**
EXCLUDES 1 constipation (K59.0-)
functional diarrhea (K59.1)

IQ **R19.5 Other fecal abnormalities**
Abnormal stool color
Bulky stools
Mucus in stools
Occult blood in feces
Occult blood in stools
EXCLUDES 1 melena (K92.1)
neonatal melena (P54.1)

IQ **R19.6 Halitosis**

IQ **R19.7 Diarrhea, unspecified**
Diarrhea NOS
EXCLUDES 1 functional diarrhea (K59.1)
neonatal diarrhea (P78.3)
psychogenic diarrhea (F45.8)

IQ **R19.8 Other specified symptoms and signs involving the digestive system and abdomen**

Symptoms and signs involving the skin and subcutaneous tissue (R20-R23)

EXCLUDES 2 symptoms relating to breast (N64.4-N64.5)

4 **R20 Disturbances of skin sensation**
EXCLUDES 1 dissociative anesthesia and sensory loss (F44.6)
psychogenic disturbances (F45.8)

IQ **R20.0 Anesthesia of skin**

IQ **R20.1 Hypoesthesia of skin**

IQ **R20.2 Paresthesia of skin**
Formication
Pins and needles
Tingling skin
EXCLUDES 1 acroparesthesia (I73.8)

IQ **R20.3 Hyperesthesia**

IQ **R20.8 Other disturbances of skin sensation**

IQ **R20.9 Unspecified disturbances of skin sensation**

IQ **R21 Rash and other nonspecific skin eruption**
INCLUDES rash NOS

Chapter 18

R00-R99

EXCLUDES 1 specified type of rash- code to condition
vesicular eruption (R23.8)

R22 Localized swelling, mass and lump of skin and subcutaneous tissue

INCLUDES subcutaneous nodules (localized) (superficial)

EXCLUDES 1 abnormal findings on diagnostic imaging (R90-R93)
edema (R60.-)
enlarged lymph nodes (R59.-)
localized adiposity (E65)
swelling of joint (M25.4-)

R22.0 Localized swelling, mass and lump, head

R22.1 Localized swelling, mass and lump, neck

R22.2 Localized swelling, mass and lump, trunk

EXCLUDES 1 intra-abdominal or pelvic mass and lump (R19.0-)
intra-abdominal or pelvic swelling (R19.0-)

EXCLUDES 2 breast mass and lump (N63)

R22.3 Localized swelling, mass and lump, upper limb

R22.30 Localized swelling, mass and lump, unspecified upper limb

R22.31 Localized swelling, mass and lump, right upper limb

R22.32 Localized swelling, mass and lump, left upper limb

R22.33 Localized swelling, mass and lump, upper limb, bilateral

R22.4 Localized swelling, mass and lump, lower limb

R22.40 Localized swelling, mass and lump, unspecified lower limb

R22.41 Localized swelling, mass and lump, right lower limb

R22.42 Localized swelling, mass and lump, left lower limb

R22.43 Localized swelling, mass and lump, lower limb, bilateral

R22.9 Localized swelling, mass and lump, unspecified

R23 Other skin changes

R23.0 Cyanosis

EXCLUDES 1 acrocyanosis (I73.8)
cyanotic attacks of newborn (P28.2)

DEFINITION Bluish tint of the skin from lack of oxygen.

R23.1 Pallor

Clammy skin

DEFINITION Excessive paleness of the skin, especially the face.

R23.2 Flushing

Excessive blushing
Code first:
, if applicable, menopausal and female climacteric states (N95.1)

R23.3 Spontaneous ecchymoses

Petechiae

EXCLUDES 1 ecchymoses of newborn (P54.5)
purpura (D69.-)

DEFINITION Minute red spots on the skin, due to escape of a small amount of blood from the vessels.

R23.4 Changes in skin texture

Desquamation of skin
Induration of skin
Scaling of skin

EXCLUDES 1 epidermal thickening NOS (L85.9)

R23.8 Other skin changes

CODING TIPS✓ When vesicular ulcerations (weeping ulcers) occur to the lower extremities as a result of edema (such as due to CHF or other edema producing conditions), assign R23.8 to indicate the resulting open vesicular (blister) ulceration. Do not assign this code to indicate other ulcerations such as due to friction or unspecified ulcers.

CODING TIPS✓ Because this code may be assigned to report blistering due to edema, it is important that clear assessment of the patient's patterns of edema are present in the clinical record. The plan of care should include interventions to address the patient's edema, as well as the resulting ulcers.

R23.9 Unspecified skin changes

Symptoms and signs involving the nervous and musculoskeletal systems (R25-R29)

R25 Abnormal involuntary movements

EXCLUDES 1 specific movement disorders (G20-G26)
stereotyped movement disorders (F98.4)
tic disorders (F95.-)

R25.0 Abnormal head movements

R25.1 Tremor, unspecified

EXCLUDES 1 chorea NOS (G25.5)
essential tremor (G25.0)
hysterical tremor (F44.4)
intention tremor (G25.2)

R25.2 Cramp and spasm

EXCLUDES 2 carpopedal spasm (R29.0)
charley-horse (M62.831)
infantile spasms (G40.4-)
muscle spasm of back (M62.830)
muscle spasm of calf (M62.831)

R25.3 Fasciculation

Twitching NOS

R25.8 Other abnormal involuntary movements

R25.9 Unspecified abnormal involuntary movements

R26 Abnormalities of gait and mobility

EXCLUDES 1 ataxia NOS (R27.0)
hereditary ataxia (G11.-)
locomotor (syphilitic) ataxia (A52.11)
immobility syndrome (paraplegic) (M62.3)

Chapter 18 R00-R99

4th digit required 5th digit required 6th digit required 7th digit required 7th digit placeholder +Additional code Laterality

CODING TIPS✓ Clinicians should investigate the cause of the gait abnormality when documented by the physician or NPP. Note the exclusions under R26. Consider M62.81 or M23 when the focus is on progressive muscle strengthening or limitations of motion (respectively) for affecting activities of daily living. Use R27, lack of coordination, if equilibrium or nonequilibrium tests show considerable muscle weakness, limitations of movement (LOMs) and balance problems.

CODING TIPS✓ Code gait issues based on physician or NPP documentation, not therapy documentation. Even if documented by the physician or NPP, symptom codes should not be used when the symptom is routinely associated with the condition. For example, do not code difficulty walking (R26.2) for a diagnosis of arthritis. If the gait issue is the result of Parkinsons, then use Parkinsons, not abnormality of gait.The rules specifiying the restricted use of symptom coding apply to therapy "codes." Report the code for the type of gait that is documented by the physician when the symptom is not routinely associated with the condition.

IQ **R26.0 Ataxic gait**
Staggering gait
CODING TIPS✓ Ataxia involves all four limbs and is coded to R27.

IQ **R26.1 Paralytic gait**
Spastic gait

IQ **R26.2 Difficulty in walking, not elsewhere classified**
EXCLUDES 1 falling (R29.6)
unsteadiness on feet (R26.81)

5 **R26.8 Other abnormalities of gait and mobility**

IQ **R26.81 Unsteadiness on feet**

IQ **R26.89 Other abnormalities of gait and mobility**

IQ **R26.9 Unspecified abnormalities of gait and mobility**
CODING TIPS✓ Keep in mind when assigning R26.9 that if the cause of the gait abnormality is known, the code for the underlying cause of the gait abnormality should be assigned. It is not appropriate to assign the code for a symptom when a more specific condition has been identified.

4 **R27 Other lack of coordination**
EXCLUDES 1 ataxic gait (R26.0)
hereditary ataxia (G11.-)
vertigo NOS (R42)

CODING TIPS✓ Category R27 includes problems related to equilibrium (vestibular/balance coordination) and nonequilibrium (nonvestibular coordination) issues. This results from neurological conditions or can indirectly result from orthopedic corrective treatment.

IQ **R27.0 Ataxia, unspecified**
EXCLUDES 1 ataxia following cerebrovascular disease (I69. with final characters -93)

DEFINITION Distortion or impairment of voluntary movement.

IQ **R27.8 Other lack of coordination**

IQ **R27.9 Unspecified lack of coordination**

4 **R29 Other symptoms and signs involving the nervous and musculoskeletal systems**

IQ **R29.0 Tetany**
Carpopedal spasm
EXCLUDES 1 hysterical tetany (F44.5)
neonatal tetany (P71.3)
parathyroid tetany (E20.9)
post-thyroidectomy tetany (E89.2)

IQ **R29.1 Meningismus**

IQ **R29.2 Abnormal reflex**
EXCLUDES 2 abnormal pupillary reflex (H57.0)
hyperactive gag reflex (J39.2)
vasovagal reaction or syncope (R55)

IQ **R29.3 Abnormal posture**

IQ **R29.4 Clicking hip**
EXCLUDES 1 congenital deformities of hip (Q65.-)

IQ **R29.5 Transient paralysis**
Code first:
any associated spinal cord injury (S14.0, S14.1-, S24.0, S24.1-, S34.0-, S34.1-)
EXCLUDES 1 transient ischemic attack (G45.9)

IQ **R29.6 Repeated falls**
Falling
Tendency to fall
EXCLUDES 2 at risk for falling (Z91.81)
history of falling (Z91.81)

GUIDELINES **Section I.C.18.d**
Code R29.6, Repeated falls, is for use for encounters when a patient has recently fallen and the reason for the fall is being investigated. Code Z91.81, History of falling, is for use when a patient has fallen in the past and is at risk for future falls. When appropriate, both codes R29.6 and Z91.81 may be assigned together.

CODING TIPS✓ Code R29.6 indicates that a patient has been experiencing recent falls. When home health will be assessing the patient's pattern of falls and home safety, as well as addressing methods to reduce the falls, this code may be assigned to provide additional information.

5 **R29.7 National Institutes of Health Stroke Scale (NIHSS) score**
Code first:
the type of cerebral infarction (I63.-)

CODING TIPS✓ The NIHSS is used as a clinical stroke assessment tool to evaluate and document neurological status in acute stroke patients and is used for inpatient admissions only. The stroke scale is valid for predicting lesion size and can serve as a measure of stroke severity. The NIHSS has been shown to be a predictor of both short and long term outcome of stroke patients. The stroke scale also serves as a data collection tool for planning patient care and provides a common language for information exchanges among healthcare providers. The scale is designed to be a simple, valid, and reliable tool that can be administered at the bedside consistently by physicians, nurses or therapists.

6 **R29.70 NIHSS score 0-9**

IQ **R29.700 NIHSS score 0**

IQ **R29.701 NIHSS score 1**

IQ **R29.702 NIHSS score 2**

IQ **R29.703 NIHSS score 3**

IQ **R29.704 NIHSS score 4**

IQ **R29.705 NIHSS score 5**

IQ **R29.706 NIHSS score 6**

IQ **R29.707 NIHSS score 7**

IQ **R29.708 NIHSS score 8**

IQ **R29.709 NIHSS score 9**

6 **R29.71 NIHSS score 10-19**

IQ **R29.710 NIHSS score 10**

IQ **R29.711 NIHSS score 11**

IQ **R29.712 NIHSS score 12**

IQ **R29.713 NIHSS score 13**

IQ **R29.714 NIHSS score 14**

IQ **R29.715 NIHSS score 15**

IQ **R29.716 NIHSS score 16**

IQ **R29.717 NIHSS score 17**

IQ **R29.718 NIHSS score 18**

IQ **R29.719 NIHSS score 19**

6 **R29.72 NIHSS score 20-29**

IQ **R29.720 NIHSS score 20**

IQ **R29.721 NIHSS score 21**

IQ **R29.722 NIHSS score 22**

IQ **R29.723 NIHSS score 23**

IQ **R29.724 NIHSS score 24**

IQ **R29.725 NIHSS score 25**

IQ **R29.726 NIHSS score 26**

IQ **R29.727 NIHSS score 27**

IQ **R29.728 NIHSS score 28**

IQ **R29.729 NIHSS score 29**

6 **R29.73 NIHSS score 30-39**

IQ **R29.730 NIHSS score 30**

IQ **R29.731 NIHSS score 31**

IQ **R29.732 NIHSS score 32**

IQ **R29.733 NIHSS score 33**

IQ **R29.734 NIHSS score 34**

IQ **R29.735 NIHSS score 35**

IQ **R29.736 NIHSS score 36**

IQ **R29.737 NIHSS score 37**

IQ **R29.738 NIHSS score 38**

IQ **R29.739 NIHSS score 39**

6 **R29.74 NIHSS score 40-42**

IQ **R29.740 NIHSS score 40**

IQ **R29.741 NIHSS score 41**

IQ **R29.742 NIHSS score 42**

5 **R29.8 Other symptoms and signs involving the nervous and musculoskeletal systems**

6 **R29.81 Other symptoms and signs involving the nervous system**

IQ **R29.810 Facial weakness**

Facial droop

EXCLUDES 1 Bell's palsy (G51.0)
facial weakness following cerebrovascular disease (I69. with final characters -92)

IQ **R29.818 Other symptoms and signs involving the nervous system**

CODING TIPS✓ R29.818 is a nonspecific code, so be sure that documentation supports its use.

6 **R29.89 Other symptoms and signs involving the musculoskeletal system**

EXCLUDES 2 pain in limb (M79.6-)

IQ **R29.890 Loss of height**

EXCLUDES 1 osteoporosis (M80-M81)

IQ **R29.891 Ocular torticollis**

EXCLUDES 1 congenital (sternomastoid) torticollis Q68.0
psychogenic torticollis (F45.8)
spasmodic torticollis (G24.3)
torticollis due to birth injury (P15.8)
torticollis NOS M43.6

IQ **R29.898 Other symptoms and signs involving the musculoskeletal system**

5 **R29.9 Unspecified symptoms and signs involving the nervous and musculoskeletal systems**

IQ **R29.90 Unspecified symptoms and signs involving the nervous system**

IQ **R29.91 Unspecified symptoms and signs involving the musculoskeletal system**

Symptoms and signs involving the genitourinary system (R30-R39)

4 **R30 Pain associated with micturition**

EXCLUDES 1 psychogenic pain associated with micturition (F45.8)

IQ **R30.0 Dysuria**

Strangury

IQ **R30.1 Vesical tenesmus**

IQ **R30.9 Painful micturition, unspecified**

Painful urination NOS

4 **R31 Hematuria**
EXCLUDES 1 hematuria included with underlying conditions, such as:
acute cystitis with hematuria (N30.01)
recurrent and persistent hematuria in glomerular diseases (N02.-)

IQ **R31.0 Gross hematuria**
CODING TIPS✓ Gross hematuria means that the blood in the urine can be seen with the naked eye. If hematuria is related to anticoagulant/antiplatelets, also code D68.32 and the T code for the drug.

IQ **R31.1 Benign essential microscopic hematuria**

5 **R31.2 Other microscopic hematuria**

IQ **R31.21 Asymptomatic microscopic hematuria**
AMH

IQ **R31.29 Other microscopic hematuria**

IQ **R31.9 Hematuria, unspecified**
DEFINITION Presence of blood in the urine.

IQ **R32 Unspecified urinary incontinence**
Enuresis NOS
EXCLUDES 1 functional urinary incontinence (R39.81)
nonorganic enuresis (F98.0)
stress incontinence and other specified urinary incontinence (N39.3-N39.4-)
urinary incontinence associated with cognitive impairment (R39.81)

4 **R33 Retention of urine**
EXCLUDES 1 psychogenic retention of urine (F45.8)

IQ + **R33.0 Drug induced retention of urine**
Use additional code for adverse effect, if applicable, to identify drug (T36-T50 with fifth or sixth character 5)

IQ **R33.8 Other retention of urine**
Code first, if applicable, any causal condition, such as:
enlarged prostate (N40.1)

IQ **R33.9 Retention of urine, unspecified**

IQ **R34 Anuria and oliguria**
EXCLUDES 1 anuria and oliguria complicating abortion or ectopic or molar pregnancy (O00-O07, O08.4)
anuria and oliguria complicating pregnancy (O26.83-)
anuria and oliguria complicating the puerperium (O90.4)

4 **R35 Polyuria**
Code first, if applicable, any causal condition, such as:
enlarged prostate (N40.1)
EXCLUDES 1 psychogenic polyuria (F45.8)

IQ **R35.0 Frequency of micturition**

IQ **R35.1 Nocturia**

▲ 5 **R35.8 Other polyuria**

★ **R35.81 Nocturnal polyuria**
EXCLUDES 2 nocturnal enuresis (N39.44)

★ **R35.89 Other polyuria**
Polyuria NOS

4 **R36 Urethral discharge**

IQ **R36.0 Urethral discharge without blood**

IQ **R36.1 Hematospermia**

IQ **R36.9 Urethral discharge, unspecified**
Penile discharge NOS
Urethrorrhea

IQ **R37 Sexual dysfunction, unspecified**

4 **R39 Other and unspecified symptoms and signs involving the genitourinary system**

IQ **R39.0 Extravasation of urine**

5 **R39.1 Other difficulties with micturition**
Code first, if applicable, any causal condition, such as:
enlarged prostate (N40.1)

IQ **R39.11 Hesitancy of micturition**
DEFINITION Difficulty starting urination.

IQ **R39.12 Poor urinary stream**
Weak urinary steam

IQ **R39.13 Splitting of urinary stream**

IQ **R39.14 Feeling of incomplete bladder emptying**

IQ **R39.15 Urgency of urination**
EXCLUDES 1 urge incontinence (N39.41, N39.46)

IQ **R39.16 Straining to void**

6 **R39.19 Other difficulties with micturition**

IQ **R39.191 Need to immediately re-void**

IQ **R39.192 Position dependent micturition**
CODING TIPS✓ Having to take specific positions to be able to micturate spontaneously or to improve bladder emptying (for example, leaning forwards or backwards on the toilet seat or voiding in the semi-standing position) is called position-dependent micturition.

IQ **R39.198 Other difficulties with micturition**

IQ **R39.2 Extrarenal uremia**
Prerenal uremia
EXCLUDES 1 uremia NOS (N19)

5 **R39.8 Other symptoms and signs involving the genitourinary system**

IQ **R39.81 Functional urinary incontinence**
Urinary incontinence due to cognitive impairment, or severe physical disability or immobility
EXCLUDES 1 stress incontinence and other specified urinary incontinence (N39.3-N39.4-)
urinary incontinence NOS (R32)
DEFINITION Leaking urine due to cognitive impairment or physical disability leading to the inability for volitional control over bladder function.

IQ **R39.82 Chronic bladder pain**

Chapter 18
R00-R99

IQ **R39.83 Unilateral non-palpable testicle**

IQ **R39.84 Bilateral non-palpable testicles**

IQ **R39.89 Other symptoms and signs involving the genitourinary system**

IQ **R39.9 Unspecified symptoms and signs involving the genitourinary system**

Symptoms and signs involving cognition, perception, emotional state and behavior (R40-R46)

EXCLUDES 2 symptoms and signs constituting part of a pattern of mental disorder (F01-F99)

4 **R40 Somnolence, stupor and coma**

EXCLUDES 1 neonatal coma (P91.5)
somnolence, stupor and coma in diabetes (E08-E13)
somnolence, stupor and coma in hepatic failure (K72.-)
somnolence, stupor and coma in hypoglycemia (nondiabetic) (E15)

IQ **R40.0 Somnolence**
Drowsiness
EXCLUDES 1 coma (R40.2-)

IQ **R40.1 Stupor**
Catatonic stupor
Semicoma
EXCLUDES 1 catatonic schizophrenia (F20.2)
coma (R40.2-)
depressive stupor (F31-F33)
dissociative stupor (F44.2)
manic stupor (F30.2)

H 5 **R40.2 Coma**
Note:
One code from each subcategory, R40.21-R40.23, is required to complete the coma scale
Code first any associated:
fracture of skull (S02.-)
intracranial injury (S06.-)

GUIDELINES **Section I.B.14**
For the Body Mass Index (BMI), depth of non-pressure chronic ulcers, pressure ulcer stage, coma scale, and NIH stroke scale (NIHSS) codes, code assignment may be based on medical record documentation from clinicians who are not the patient's provider (i.e., physician or other qualified healthcare practitioner legally accountable for establishing the patient's diagnosis), since this information is typically documented by other clinicians involved in the care of the patient (e.g., a dietitian often documents the BMI, a nurse often documents the pressure ulcer stages, and an emergency medical technician often documents the coma scale). However, the associated diagnosis (such as overweight, obesity, acute stroke, or pressure ulcer) must be documented by the patient's provider.

CODING TIPS✓ Documentation from other than the physician or NPP is appropriate for coding of the Glasgow Coma Scale. It would be appropriate to use the pre-hospital report containing the EMT's documentation and other non-physician documentation to determine the Glasgow coma score.

CODING TIPS✓ If the provider's documentation clearly shows that the ratings are specific scores or numeric values for the Glasgow scale, rather than description, i.e., eyes open to pain, it would be appropriate to report codes from R40.21, R40.22 and R40.23.

CODING TIPS✓ Coma takes at least 3 codes unless the Glasgow Coma Scale total score is available. A 7th character is needed to indicate when the scale was performed.

IQ **R40.20 Unspecified coma**
Coma NOS
Unconsciousness NOS

6 **R40.21 Coma scale, eyes open**

The following appropriate 7th character is to be added to subcategory R40.21-:
0 unspecified time
1 in the field [EMT or ambulance]
2 at arrival to emergency department
3 at hospital admission
4 24 hours or more after hospital admission

IQ 7 **R40.211- Coma scale, eyes open, never**
Coma scale eye opening score of 1

IQ 7 **R40.212- Coma scale, eyes open, to pain**
Coma scale eye opening score of 2

IQ 7 **R40.213- Coma scale, eyes open, to sound**
Coma scale eye opening score of 3

IQ 7 **R40.214- Coma scale, eyes open, spontaneous**
Coma scale eye opening score of 4

6 **R40.22 Coma scale, best verbal response**

The following appropriate 7th character is to be added to subcategory R40.22-:
0 unspecified time
1 in the field [EMT or ambulance]
2 at arrival to emergency department
3 at hospital admission
4 24 hours or more after hospital admission

IQ 7 **R40.221- Coma scale, best verbal response, none**
Coma scale verbal score of 1

IQ 7 **R40.222- Coma scale, best verbal response, incomprehensible words**
Coma scale verbal score of 2
Incomprehensible sounds (2-5 years of age)

Moans/grunts to pain; restless (< 2 years old)

R40.223- Coma scale, best verbal response, inappropriate words

Coma scale verbal score of 3
Inappropriate crying or screaming (< 2 years of age)
Screaming (2-5 years of age)

R40.224- Coma scale, best verbal response, confused conversation

Coma scale verbal score of 4
Inappropriate words (2-5 years of age)
Irritable cries (< 2 years of age)

R40.225- Coma scale, best verbal response, oriented

Coma scale verbal score of 5
Cooing or babbling or crying appropriately (< 2 years of age)
Uses appropriate words (2- 5 years of age)

R40.23 Coma scale, best motor response

The following appropriate 7th character is to be added to subcategory R40.23-:

0	unspecified time
1	in the field [EMT or ambulance]
2	at arrival to emergency department
3	at hospital admission
4	24 hours or more after hospital admission

R40.231- Coma scale, best motor response, none

Coma scale motor score of 1

R40.232- Coma scale, best motor response, extension

Abnormal extensor posturing to pain or noxious stimuli (< 2 years of age)
Coma scale motor score of 2
Extensor posturing to pain or noxious stimuli (2-5 years of age)

R40.233- Coma scale, best motor response, abnormal flexion

Abnormal flexure posturing to pain or noxious stimuli (2-5 years of age)
Coma scale motor score of 3
Flexion/decorticate posturing (< 2 years of age)

R40.234- Coma scale, best motor response, flexion withdrawal

Coma scale motor score of 4
Withdraws from pain or noxious stimuli (2-5 years of age)

R40.235- Coma scale, best motor response, localizes pain

Coma scale motor score of 5
Localizes pain (2-5 years of age)
Withdraws to touch (< 2 years of age)

R40.236- Coma scale, best motor response, obeys commands

Coma scale motor score of 6
Normal or spontaneous movement (< 2 years of age)
Obeys commands (2-5 years of age)

R40.24 Glasgow coma scale, total score

Note:
Assign a code from subcategory R40.24, when only the total coma score is documented

The following appropriate 7th character is to be added to subcategory R40.24-:

0	unspecified time
1	in the field [EMT or ambulance]
2	at arrival to emergency department
3	at hospital admission
4	24 hours or more after hospital admission

CODING TIPS ✓ If the total score is documented, do not code the individual scores for the Glasgow Coma Scale.

R40.241- Glasgow coma scale score 13-15

R40.242- Glasgow coma scale score 9-12

R40.243- Glasgow coma scale score 3-8

R40.244- Other coma, without documented Glasgow coma scale score, or with partial score reported

R40.3 Persistent vegetative state

CODING TIPS ✓ Assign code R40.3 only when the patient's provider has specifically confirmed persistent vegetative state (PVS). Also note that PVS differs from coma.

R40.4 Transient alteration of awareness

CODING TIPS ✓ Code R40.4 for transient alteration of awareness that is not associated with delirium or with another identified condition. It may be prevalent for those at the end of life.

R41 Other symptoms and signs involving cognitive functions and awareness

EXCLUDES 1 dissociative [conversion] disorders (F44.-)
mild cognitive impairment, so stated (G31.84)

R41.0 Disorientation, unspecified

Confusion NOS
Delirium NOS

R41.1 Anterograde amnesia

R41.2 Retrograde amnesia

R41.3 Other amnesia

Amnesia NOS
Memory loss NOS

EXCLUDES 1 amnestic disorder due to known physiologic condition (F04)
amnestic syndrome due to psychoactive substance use (F10-F19 with 5th character .6)

Chapter 18

R00-R99

mild memory disturbance due to known physiological condition (F06.8)
transient global amnesia (G45.4)

IQ R41.4 Neurologic neglect syndrome
Asomatognosia
Hemi-akinesia
Hemi-inattention
Hemispatial neglect
Left-sided neglect
Sensory neglect
Visuospatial neglect
EXCLUDES 1 visuospatial deficit (R41.842)
CODING TIPS ✓ If neurologic neglect syndrome is related to a stroke, use the sequela code for the visuospatial neglect, for example I69.312.

5 R41.8 Other symptoms and signs involving cognitive functions and awareness

IQ R41.81 Age-related cognitive decline
Senility NOS

IQ R41.82 Altered mental status, unspecified
Change in mental status NOS
EXCLUDES 1 altered level of consciousness (R40.-)
altered mental status due to known condition - code to condition
delirium NOS (R41.0)
CODING TIPS ✓ Code R41.82 is used for an altered mental status such as an acute onset of confusion with unknown cause. If altered mental status is due to another condition, code that condition instead.

IQ R41.83 Borderline intellectual functioning
IQ level 71 to 84
EXCLUDES 1 intellectual disabilities (F70-F79)
CODING TIPS ✓ Do not assign R41.83 when intellectual disability is specified. Intellectual disabilities are coded to categories F70-F79.

6 R41.84 Other specified cognitive deficit
EXCLUDES 1 cognitive deficits as sequelae of cerebrovascular disease (I69.01-, I69.11-, I69.21-, I69.31-, I69.81-, I69.91-)
CODING TIPS ✓ The R41.84 codes were created to identify cognitive deficits related to a traumatic brain injury (TBI) and other neurological conditions. They describe cognitive impairments such as problems with memory, concentration, attention, communication and executive function. They are intended to be used as supplementary codes when the cause of the deficit is known as well as before a more specific diagnosis is made. R41.84 codes are not to be used for sequelae of cerebral infarction/strokes. For sequelae of strokes, reference I69.-1 for specific codes, for example I69.311 (Memory deficit following cerebral infarction).

IQ R41.840 Attention and concentration deficit
EXCLUDES 1 attention-deficit hyperactivity disorders (F90.-)

IQ R41.841 Cognitive communication deficit

IQ R41.842 Visuospatial deficit

IQ R41.843 Psychomotor deficit

IQ R41.844 Frontal lobe and executive function deficit

IQ R41.89 Other symptoms and signs involving cognitive functions and awareness
Anosognosia

IQ R41.9 Unspecified symptoms and signs involving cognitive functions and awareness
Unspecified neurocognitive disorder

IQ R42 Dizziness and giddiness
Light-headedness
Vertigo NOS
EXCLUDES 1 vertiginous syndromes (H81.-)
vertigo from infrasound (T75.23)

4 R43 Disturbances of smell and taste

IQ R43.0 Anosmia

IQ R43.1 Parosmia

IQ R43.2 Parageusia

IQ R43.8 Other disturbances of smell and taste
Mixed disturbance of smell and taste

IQ R43.9 Unspecified disturbances of smell and taste

4 R44 Other symptoms and signs involving general sensations and perceptions
EXCLUDES 1 alcoholic hallucinations (F10.151, F10.251, F10.951)
hallucinations in drug psychosis (F11-F19 with fifth to sixth characters 51)
hallucinations in mood disorders with psychotic symptoms (F30.2, F31.5, F32.3, F33.3)
hallucinations in schizophrenia, schizotypal and delusional disorders (F20-F29)
EXCLUDES 2 disturbances of skin sensation (R20.-)

IQ R44.0 Auditory hallucinations

IQ R44.1 Visual hallucinations

IQ **R44.2 Other hallucinations**

IQ **R44.3 Hallucinations, unspecified**

IQ **R44.8 Other symptoms and signs involving general sensations and perceptions**

IQ **R44.9 Unspecified symptoms and signs involving general sensations and perceptions**

4 **R45 Symptoms and signs involving emotional state**

IQ **R45.0 Nervousness**
Nervous tension

IQ **R45.1 Restlessness and agitation**

IQ **R45.2 Unhappiness**

IQ **R45.3 Demoralization and apathy**
EXCLUDES 1 anhedonia (R45.84)

IQ **R45.4 Irritability and anger**

IQ **R45.5 Hostility**

IQ **R45.6 Violent behavior**

IQ **R45.7 State of emotional shock and stress, unspecified**

5 **R45.8 Other symptoms and signs involving emotional state**

IQ **R45.81 Low self-esteem**

IQ **R45.82 Worries**

IQ **R45.83 Excessive crying of child, adolescent or adult**
EXCLUDES 1 excessive crying of infant (baby) R68.11

IQ **R45.84 Anhedonia**
CODING TIPS✓ R45.84 is a nonspecific code used to describe a decreased desire to engage in activities, often with decreased motivation. Anhedonia is frequently identified as a symptom of psychiatric conditions such as depression. Report a more specific code when the cause of anhedonia is known.

6 **R45.85 Homicidal and suicidal ideations**
EXCLUDES 1 suicide attempt (T14.91)

IQ **R45.850 Homicidal ideations**

IQ **R45.851 Suicidal ideations**

IQ **R45.86 Emotional lability**

IQ **R45.87 Impulsiveness**

★ **R45.88 Nonsuicidal self-harm**
Nonsuicidal self-injury
Nonsuicidal self-mutilation
Self-inflicted injury without suicidal intent
Code also:
injury, if known

IQ **R45.89 Other symptoms and signs involving emotional state**

4 **R46 Symptoms and signs involving appearance and behavior**
EXCLUDES 1 appearance and behavior in schizophrenia, schizotypal and delusional disorders (F20-F29)
mental and behavioral disorders (F01-F99)

IQ **R46.0 Very low level of personal hygiene**

IQ **R46.1 Bizarre personal appearance**

IQ **R46.2 Strange and inexplicable behavior**

IQ **R46.3 Overactivity**

IQ **R46.4 Slowness and poor responsiveness**
EXCLUDES 1 stupor (R40.1)

IQ **R46.5 Suspiciousness and marked evasiveness**

IQ **R46.6 Undue concern and preoccupation with stressful events**

IQ **R46.7 Verbosity and circumstantial detail obscuring reason for contact**

5 **R46.8 Other symptoms and signs involving appearance and behavior**

IQ **R46.81 Obsessive-compulsive behavior**
EXCLUDES 1 obsessive-compulsive disorder (F42.-)

IQ **R46.89 Other symptoms and signs involving appearance and behavior**

Symptoms and signs involving speech and voice (R47-R49)

4 **R47 Speech disturbances, not elsewhere classified**
EXCLUDES 1 autism (F84.0)
cluttering (F80.81)
specific developmental disorders of speech and language (F80.-)
stuttering (F80.81)

5 **R47.0 Dysphasia and aphasia**
CODING TIPS✓ Do not use R47.0 codes for sequela of cerebral infarctions or stroke. Use, for example, I69.32 instead for these sequelae. Do not confuse dysphasia with dysphagia (difficulty in swallowing), which is another possible sequela of a stroke.

IQ **R47.01 Aphasia**
EXCLUDES 1 aphasia following cerebrovascular disease (I69. with final characters -20)
progressive isolated aphasia (G31.01)
DEFINITION The inability to speak, write, or understand spoken or written language.

IQ **R47.02 Dysphasia**
EXCLUDES 1 dysphasia following cerebrovascular disease (I69. with final characters -21)

IQ **R47.1 Dysarthria and anarthria**
EXCLUDES 1 dysarthria following cerebrovascular disease (I69. with final characters -22)

5 **R47.8 Other speech disturbances**
EXCLUDES 1 dysarthria following cerebrovascular disease (I69. with final characters -28)

IQ **R47.81 Slurred speech**

IQ **R47.82 Fluency disorder in conditions classified elsewhere**
Stuttering in conditions classified elsewhere
Code first underlying disease or condition, such as:
Parkinson's disease (G20)

Chapter 18 R00-R99

EXCLUDES 1 adult onset fluency disorder (F98.5)
childhood onset fluency disorder (F80.81)
fluency disorder (stuttering) following cerebrovascular disease (I69. with final characters -23)

IQ **R47.89 Other speech disturbances**

IQ **R47.9 Unspecified speech disturbances**

4 **R48 Dyslexia and other symbolic dysfunctions, not elsewhere classified**

EXCLUDES 1 specific developmental disorders of scholastic skills (F81.-)

IQ **R48.0 Dyslexia and alexia**

IQ **R48.1 Agnosia**

Astereognosia (astereognosis)
Autotopagnosia

EXCLUDES 1 visual object agnosia (R48.3)

IQ **R48.2 Apraxia**

EXCLUDES 1 apraxia following cerebrovascular disease (I69. with final characters -90)

IQ **R48.3 Visual agnosia**

Prosopagnosia
Simultanagnosia (asimultagnosia)

IQ **R48.8 Other symbolic dysfunctions**

Acalculia
Agraphia

IQ **R48.9 Unspecified symbolic dysfunctions**

4 **R49 Voice and resonance disorders**

EXCLUDES 1 psychogenic voice and resonance disorders (F44.4)

CODING TIPS ✓ Do not use R49 codes for sequelae of cerebral infarctions or stroke. Use, for example, I69.32 instead for these sequelae.

IQ **R49.0 Dysphonia**

Hoarseness

IQ **R49.1 Aphonia**

Loss of voice

DEFINITION Inability to produce vocal sounds.

5 **R49.2 Hypernasality and hyponasality**

IQ **R49.21 Hypernasality**

IQ **R49.22 Hyponasality**

IQ **R49.8 Other voice and resonance disorders**

IQ **R49.9 Unspecified voice and resonance disorder**

Change in voice NOS
Resonance disorder NOS

General symptoms and signs (R50-R69)

4 **R50 Fever of other and unknown origin**

EXCLUDES 1 chills without fever (R68.83)
febrile convulsions (R56.0-)
fever of unknown origin during labor (O75.2)
fever of unknown origin in newborn (P81.9)
hypothermia due to illness (R68.0)
malignant hyperthermia due to anesthesia (T88.3)
puerperal pyrexia NOS (O86.4)

IQ + **R50.2 Drug induced fever**

Use additional code for adverse effect, if applicable, to identify drug (T36-T50 with fifth or sixth character 5)

EXCLUDES 1 postvaccination (postimmunization) fever (R50.83)

5 **R50.8 Other specified fever**

IQ **R50.81 Fever presenting with conditions classified elsewhere**

Code first underlying condition when associated fever is present, such as with:
leukemia (C91-C95)
neutropenia (D70.-)
sickle-cell disease (D57.-)

IQ **R50.82 Postprocedural fever**

EXCLUDES 1 postprocedural infection (T81.4-)
posttransfusion fever (R50.84)
postvaccination (postimmunization) fever (R50.83)

IQ **R50.83 Postvaccination fever**

Postimmunization fever

IQ **R50.84 Febrile nonhemolytic transfusion reaction**

FNHTR
Posttransfusion fever

IQ **R50.9 Fever, unspecified**

Fever NOS
Fever of unknown origin [FUO]
Fever with chills
Fever with rigors
Hyperpyrexia NOS
Persistent fever
Pyrexia NOS

CODING TIPS ✓ When an infection causing a fever has been diagnosed, do not assign R50.9, but instead code the causative infectious disease specifically.

4 **R51 Headache**

EXCLUDES 2 atypical face pain (G50.1)
migraine and other headache syndromes (G43-G44)
trigeminal neuralgia (G50.0)

IQ **R51.0 Headache with orthostatic component, not elsewhere classified**

Headache with positional component, not elsewhere classified

DEFINITION Orthostatic headache is a medical condition in which a person develops a headache while vertical and the headache is relieved when horizontal.

IQ **R51.9 Headache, unspecified**

Facial pain NOS

▲ IQ **R52 Pain, unspecified**

Acute pain NOS
Generalized pain NOS
Pain NOS

EXCLUDES 1 acute and chronic pain, not elsewhere classified (G89.-)

localized pain, unspecified type - code to pain by site, such as:
abdomen pain (R10.-)
back pain (M54.9)
breast pain (N64.4)
chest pain (R07.1-R07.9)
ear pain (H92.0-)
eye pain (H57.1)
headache (R51.9)
joint pain (M25.5-)
limb pain (M79.6-)
lumbar region pain (M54.5-)
pelvic and perineal pain (R10.2)
shoulder pain (M25.51-)
spine pain (M54.-)
throat pain (R07.0)
tongue pain (K14.6)
tooth pain (K08.8)
renal colic (N23)
pain disorders exclusively related to psychological factors (F45.41)

CODING TIPS✓ R52 should not be coded to identify pain when the underlying cause of pain is known. Code the specific cause of the pain when a diagnosis is present for the cause, such as osteoarthritis. Pay special attention to the Excludes 1 note.

4 **R53 Malaise and fatigue**

IQ **R53.0 Neoplastic (malignant) related fatigue**
Code first:
associated neoplasm

IQ **R53.1 Weakness**
Asthenia NOS
EXCLUDES 1 age-related weakness (R54)
muscle weakness (generalized) (M62.81)
sarcopenia (M62.84)
senile asthenia (R54)

CODING TIPS✓ Do not assign R53.1 to indicate muscle weakness or weakness resulting as a sequela of a cerebral vascular accident. Muscle weakness (generalized) is coded to M62.81.

CODING TIPS✓ Not to be confused with generalized muscle weakness, R53.1 is also known as general weakness. The condition may include excessive tiredness, lacking energy, listlessness, and/or sleepiness. Generally used for patients with cardiorespiratory diseases. May be part of many different illnesses, including the flu, pneumonia, congestive heart failure (CHF) and arteriosclerotic heart disease (ASHD). If weakness is routinely associated with the condition, weakness is not coded additionally.

IQ **R53.2 Functional quadriplegia**
Complete immobility due to severe physical disability or frailty
EXCLUDES 1 frailty NOS (R54)
hysterical paralysis (F44.4)
immobility syndrome (M62.3)
neurologic quadriplegia (G82.5-)
quadriplegia (G82.50)

CODING TIPS✓ Functional quadriplegia refers to the inability to move due to another condition (such as severe contractures or arthritis), resulting in the patient being quadriplegia-like. Do not use code R53.2 for quadriplegia or in addition to quadriplegia. Code only if documented by the physician.

DEFINITION Inability to move due to non-neurological condition, such as severe spasticity, arthritis, or severe muscle contracture.

5 **R53.8 Other malaise and fatigue**
EXCLUDES 1 combat exhaustion and fatigue (F43.0)
congenital debility (P96.9)
exhaustion and fatigue due to excessive exertion (T73.3)
exhaustion and fatigue due to exposure (T73.2)
exhaustion and fatigue due to heat (T67.-)
exhaustion and fatigue due to pregnancy (O26.8-)
exhaustion and fatigue due to recurrent depressive episode (F33)
exhaustion and fatigue due to senile debility (R54)

IQ **R53.81 Other malaise**
Chronic debility
Debility NOS
General physical deterioration
Malaise NOS
Nervous debility
EXCLUDES 1 age-related physical debility (R54)

ALERT This diagnosis is prohibited from use as a terminal diagnosis in hospice.

CODING TIPS✓ Note that debility is a non-specific condition characterized by weight loss, functional decline, malnutrition and multiple chronic conditions. Coding a non-specific diagnosis such as this should be avoided if possible. If the diagnosis causing the debility is known, code that condition.

IQ **R53.82 Chronic fatigue, unspecified**
Chronic fatigue syndrome NOS
EXCLUDES 1 postviral fatigue syndrome (G93.3)

IQ **R53.83 Other fatigue**
Fatigue NOS
Lack of energy
Lethargy
Tiredness
EXCLUDES 2 exhaustion and fatigue due to depressive episode (F32.-)

IQ **R54 Age-related physical debility**
Frailty
Old age
Senescence
Senile asthenia
Senile debility

Chapter 18 R00-R99

EXCLUDES 1 age-related cognitive decline (R41.81)
sarcopenia (M62.84)
senile psychosis (F03)
senility NOS (R41.81)

CODING TIPS ✓ Note that debility is a non-specific condition characterized by weight loss, functional decline, malnutrition and multiple chronic conditions. Coding a non-specific diagnosis such as this should be avoided if possible. If the diagnosis causing the debility is known, code that condition.

!Q **R55 Syncope and collapse**
Blackout
Fainting
Vasovagal attack

EXCLUDES 1 cardiogenic shock (R57.0)
carotid sinus syncope (G90.01)
heat syncope (T67.1)
neurocirculatory asthenia (F45.8)
neurogenic orthostatic hypotension (G90.3)
orthostatic hypotension (I95.1)
postprocedural shock (T81.1-)
psychogenic syncope (F48.8)
shock NOS (R57.9)
shock complicating or following abortion or ectopic or molar pregnancy (O00-O07, O08.3)
shock complicating or following labor and delivery (O75.1)
Stokes-Adams attack (I45.9)
unconsciousness NOS (R40.2-)

DEFINITION Fainting and collapse due to a lack of blood flow to the brain.

4 **R56 Convulsions, not elsewhere classified**

EXCLUDES 1 dissociative convulsions and seizures (F44.5)
epileptic convulsions and seizures (G40.-)
newborn convulsions and seizures (P90)

5 **R56.0 Febrile convulsions**

DEFINITION A convulsion accompanying high fever, characterized by loss of consciousness with stiffness and jerking of the limbs. The skin may become pale or turn blue. Once the jerking subsides, the child goes limp and then normal color and consciousness return.

!Q **R56.00 Simple febrile convulsions**
Febrile convulsion NOS
Febrile seizure NOS

CODING TIPS ✓ Febrile seizures, code R56.00, affect 3%-5% of all children. Fever triggers these seizures.

!Q **R56.01 Complex febrile convulsions**
Atypical febrile seizure
Complex febrile seizure
Complicated febrile seizure

EXCLUDES 1 status epilepticus (G40.901)

!Q **R56.1 Post traumatic seizures**

EXCLUDES 1 post traumatic epilepsy (G40.-)

!Q **R56.9 Unspecified convulsions**
Convulsion disorder
Fit NOS
Recurrent convulsions
Seizure(s) (convulsive) NOS

CODING TIPS ✓ Do not assign R56.9 when a patient has had recurrent seizures or a seizure disorder. When recurrent seizures or seizure disorder are present, report the appropriate code from category G40.-. This code is assigned for non-epileptic pseudoseizures. [AHA: 1Q 2021]

▲ 4 **R57 Shock, not elsewhere classified**

EXCLUDES 1 anaphylactic shock NOS (T78.2)
anaphylactic reaction or shock due to adverse food reaction (T78.0-)
anaphylactic shock due to adverse effect of correct drug or medicament properly administered (T88.6)
anaphylactic shock due to serum (T80.5-)
electric shock (T75.4)
obstetric shock (O75.1)
postprocedural shock (T81.1-)
psychic shock (F43.0)
shock complicating or following ectopic or molar pregnancy (O00-O07, O08.3)
shock due to anesthesia (T88.2)
shock due to lightning (T75.01)
traumatic shock (T79.4)
toxic shock syndrome (A48.3)

!Q **R57.0 Cardiogenic shock**

EXCLUDES 2 septic shock (R65.21)

!Q **R57.1 Hypovolemic shock**

!Q **R57.8 Other shock**

!Q **R57.9 Shock, unspecified**
Failure of peripheral circulation NOS

!Q **R58 Hemorrhage, not elsewhere classified**
Hemorrhage NOS

EXCLUDES 1 hemorrhage included with underlying conditions, such as:
acute duodenal ulcer with hemorrhage (K26.0)
acute gastritis with bleeding (K29.01)
ulcerative enterocolitis with rectal bleeding (K51.01)

4 **R59 Enlarged lymph nodes**

INCLUDES swollen glands

EXCLUDES 1 lymphadenitis NOS (I88.9)
acute lymphadenitis (L04.-)
chronic lymphadenitis (I88.1)
mesenteric (acute) (chronic) lymphadenitis (I88.0)

!Q **R59.0 Localized enlarged lymph nodes**

!Q **R59.1 Generalized enlarged lymph nodes**
Lymphadenopathy NOS

!Q **R59.9 Enlarged lymph nodes, unspecified**

4 **R60 Edema, not elsewhere classified**

EXCLUDES 1 angioneurotic edema (T78.3)
ascites (R18.-)
cerebral edema (G93.6)
cerebral edema due to birth injury (P11.0)
edema of larynx (J38.4)
edema of nasopharynx (J39.2)
edema of pharynx (J39.2)
gestational edema (O12.0-)
hereditary edema (Q82.0)
hydrops fetalis NOS (P83.2)
hydrothorax (J94.8)
newborn edema (P83.3)
pulmonary edema (J81.-)

CODING TIPS✓ Report R60 only when the cause of the edema is unknown, as it is usually integral to another condition where you would not report this symptom code. Never code edema in addition to CHF.

!Q **R60.0 Localized edema**

CODING TIPS✓ Do not report R60.0 in a patient with heart failure or any other known cause for the edema.

!Q **R60.1 Generalized edema**

EXCLUDES 2 nutritional edema (E40-E46)

!Q **R60.9 Edema, unspecified**

Fluid retention NOS

!Q **R61 Generalized hyperhidrosis**

Excessive sweating
Night sweats
Secondary hyperhidrosis
Code first:
, if applicable, menopausal and female climacteric states (N95.1)

EXCLUDES 1 focal (primary) (secondary) hyperhidrosis (L74.5-)
Frey's syndrome (L74.52)
localized (primary) (secondary) hyperhidrosis (L74.5-)

4 **R62 Lack of expected normal physiological development in childhood and adults**

EXCLUDES 1 delayed puberty (E30.0)
gonadal dysgenesis (Q99.1)
hypopituitarism (E23.0)

!Q **R62.0 Delayed milestone in childhood**

Delayed attainment of expected physiological developmental stage
Late talker
Late walker

5 **R62.5 Other and unspecified lack of expected normal physiological development in childhood**

EXCLUDES 1 HIV disease resulting in failure to thrive (B20)
physical retardation due to malnutrition (E45)

!Q **R62.50 Unspecified lack of expected normal physiological development in childhood**

Infantilism NOS

!Q **R62.51 Failure to thrive (child)**

Failure to gain weight

EXCLUDES 1 failure to thrive in child under 28 days old (P92.6)

!Q **R62.52 Short stature (child)**

Lack of growth
Physical retardation
Short stature NOS

EXCLUDES 1 short stature due to endocrine disorder (E34.3)

!Q **R62.59 Other lack of expected normal physiological development in childhood**

!Q **R62.7 Adult failure to thrive**

ALERT This diagnosis is prohibited from use as a primary terminal diagnosis.

CODING TIPS✓ When coding failure to thrive, identify the conditions leading to the patient's failure to thrive and code these underlying conditions first.

4 **R63 Symptoms and signs concerning food and fluid intake**

EXCLUDES 1 bulimia NOS (F50.2)

!Q **R63.0 Anorexia**

Loss of appetite

EXCLUDES 1 anorexia nervosa (F50.0-)
loss of appetite of nonorganic origin (F50.89)

CODING TIPS✓ Anorexia indicates a loss of appetite or intake resulting from appetite loss. Note that anorexia nervosa, which is coded to F50.0-, differs from anorexia coded to R63.0 in that anorexia nervosa includes a psychological component of body image disturbance.

!Q **R63.1 Polydipsia**

Excessive thirst

!Q **R63.2 Polyphagia**

Excessive eating
Hyperalimentation NOS

▲ 5 **R63.3 Feeding difficulties**

EXCLUDES 2 eating disorders (F50.-)
feeding problems of newborn (P92.-)
infant feeding disorder of nonorganic origin (F98.2-)

★ **R63.30 Feeding difficulties, unspecified**

★ **R63.31 Pediatric feeding disorder, acute**

Pediatric feeding dysfunction, acute
Code also, if applicable, associated conditions such as:
aspiration pneumonia (J69.0)
dysphagia (R13.1-)
gastro-esophageal reflux disease (K21.-)
malnutrition (E40-E46)

★ **R63.32 Pediatric feeding disorder, chronic**

Pediatric feeding dysfunction, chronic
Code also, if applicable, associated conditions such as:
aspiration pneumonia (J69.0)
dysphagia (R13.1-)
gastro-esophageal reflux disease (K21.-)
malnutrition (E40-E46)

★ **R63.39 Other feeding difficulties**

Feeding problem (elderly) (infant) NOS
Picky eater

!Q **R63.4 Abnormal weight loss**

CODING TIPS✓ Code also for BMI (Z68) with code R63.4. The Z68 codes are for adults 20 years of age and older.

IQ **R63.5 Abnormal weight gain**

EXCLUDES 1 excessive weight gain in pregnancy (O26.0-)
obesity (E66.-)

IQ + **R63.6 Underweight**

Use additional code to identify body mass index (BMI), if known (Z68.-)

EXCLUDES 1 abnormal weight loss (R63.4)
anorexia nervosa (F50.0-)
malnutrition (E40-E46)

IQ **R63.8 Other symptoms and signs concerning food and fluid intake**

IQ **R64 Cachexia**

Wasting syndrome

Code first:
underlying condition, if known

EXCLUDES 1 abnormal weight loss (R63.4)
nutritional marasmus (E41)

CODING TIPS✓ Emaciation related to malnutrition is assigned E43, and not R64.

4 **R65 Symptoms and signs specifically associated with systemic inflammation and infection**

GUIDELINES **Section I.C.1.d.6)**

Only one code from category R65, Symptoms and signs specifically associated with systemic inflammation and infection, should be assigned. Therefore, when a non-infectious condition leads to an infection resulting in severe sepsis, assign the appropriate code from subcategory R65.2, Severe sepsis. Do not additionally assign a code from subcategory R65.1, Systemic inflammatory response syndrome (SIRS) of noninfectious origin.

5 **R65.1 Systemic inflammatory response syndrome (SIRS) of non-infectious origin**

Code first underlying condition, such as:
heatstroke (T67.0-)
injury and trauma (S00-T88)

EXCLUDES 1 sepsis- code to infection
severe sepsis (R65.2)

CODING TIPS✓ R65.1 codes are used for systemic inflammatory response syndrome (SIRS) of non-infectious origin. Some physicians or NPPs will document "sepsis," but not indicate an infectious process, for example, "due to a pulmonary embolism." Sepsis implies an infection, so the physician should be queried. SIRS is an overreaction to the inflammatory process that triggers changes throughout the body.

IQ **R65.10 Systemic inflammatory response syndrome (SIRS) of non-infectious origin without acute organ dysfunction**

Systemic inflammatory response syndrome (SIRS) NOS

IQ + **R65.11 Systemic inflammatory response syndrome (SIRS) of non-infectious origin with acute organ dysfunction**

Use additional code to identify specific acute organ dysfunction, such as:
acute kidney failure (N17.-)
acute respiratory failure (J96.0-)
critical illness myopathy (G72.81)
critical illness polyneuropathy (G62.81)
disseminated intravascular coagulopathy [DIC] (D65)
encephalopathy (metabolic) (septic) (G93.41)
hepatic failure (K72.0-)

GUIDELINES **Section I.C.18.g**

The systemic inflammatory response syndrome (SIRS) can develop as a result of certain non-infectious disease processes, such as trauma, malignant neoplasm, or pancreatitis. When SIRS is documented with a noninfectious condition, and no subsequent infection is documented, the code for the underlying condition, such as an injury, should be assigned, followed by code R65.10, Systemic inflammatory response syndrome (SIRS) of non-infectious origin without acute organ dysfunction, or code R65.11, Systemic inflammatory response syndrome (SIRS) of non-infectious origin with acute organ dysfunction. If an associated acute organ dysfunction is documented, the appropriate code(s) for the specific type of organ dysfunction(s) should be assigned in addition to code R65.11. If acute organ dysfunction is documented, but it cannot be determined if the acute organ dysfunction is associated with SIRS or due to another condition (e.g., directly due to the trauma), the provider should be queried.

+ 5 **R65.2 Severe sepsis**

Infection with associated acute organ dysfunction
Sepsis with acute organ dysfunction
Sepsis with multiple organ dysfunction
Systemic inflammatory response syndrome due to infectious process with acute organ dysfunction

Code first underlying infection, such as:
infection following a procedure (T81.4-)
infections following infusion, transfusion and therapeutic injection (T80.2-)
puerperal sepsis (O85)
sepsis following complete or unspecified spontaneous abortion (O03.87)
sepsis following ectopic and molar pregnancy (O08.82)
sepsis following incomplete spontaneous abortion (O03.37)
sepsis following (induced) termination of pregnancy (O04.87)
sepsis NOS (A41.9)

Use additional code to identify specific acute organ dysfunction, such as:
acute kidney failure (N17.-)
acute respiratory failure (J96.0-)
critical illness myopathy (G72.81)
critical illness polyneuropathy (G62.81)

disseminated intravascular coagulopathy [DIC] (D65)
encephalopathy (metabolic) (septic) (G93.41)
hepatic failure (K72.0-)

GUIDELINES **Section I.C.1.d.4)**
If the reason for admission is both sepsis or severe sepsis and a localized infection, such as pneumonia or cellulitis, a code(s) for the underlying systemic infection should be assigned first and the code for the localized infection should be assigned as a secondary diagnosis. If the patient has severe sepsis, a code from subcategory R65.2 should also be assigned as a secondary diagnosis. If the patient is admitted with a localized infection, such as pneumonia, and sepsis/severe sepsis doesn't develop until after admission, the localized infection should be assigned first, followed by the appropriate sepsis/severe sepsis codes.

GUIDELINES **Section I.C.1.d.1)(a)(iv)**
If a patient has sepsis and an acute organ dysfunction, but the medical record documentation indicates that the acute organ dysfunction is related to a medical condition other than the sepsis, do not assign a code from subcategory R65.2, Severe sepsis. An acute organ dysfunction must be associated with the sepsis in order to assign the severe sepsis code. If the documentation is not clear as to whether an acute organ dysfunction is related to the sepsis or another medical condition, query the provider.

GUIDELINES **Section I.C.1.d.1)(b)**
The coding of severe sepsis requires a minimum of two codes: first a code for the underlying systemic infection, followed by a code from subcategory R65.2, Severe sepsis. If the causal organism is not documented, assign code A41.9, Sepsis, unspecified organism, for the infection. Additional code(s) for the associated acute organ dysfunction are also required. Due to the complex nature of severe sepsis, some cases may require querying the provider prior to assignment of the codes.

CODING TIPS✓ When severe sepsis is present in a patient (sepsis with the additional presence of organ dysfunction, hypotension, or hypoperfusion), a code from R65.2- must be assigned in addition to the code identifying the underlying infection. An additional code(s) also should be assigned to identify all organ dysfunction present.

IQ + **R65.20 Severe sepsis without septic shock**
Severe sepsis NOS

GUIDELINES **Section I.C.1.d.5)(b-c)**
For infections following a procedure, a code from T81.40, to T81.43 Infection following a procedure, or a code from O86.00 to O86.03, Infection of obstetric surgical wound, that identifies the site of the infection should be coded first, if known. Assign an additional code for sepsis following a procedure (T81.44) or sepsis following an obstetrical procedure (O86.04). Use an additional code to identify the infectious agent. If the patient has severe sepsis, the appropriate code from subcategory R65.2 should also be assigned with the additional code(s) for any acute organ dysfunction.

If a postprocedural infection has resulted in postprocedural septic shock, assign the codes indicated above for sepsis due to a postprocedural infection, followed by code T81.12-, Postprocedural septic shock. Do not assign code R65.21, Severe sepsis with septic shock. Additional code(s) should be assigned for any acute organ dysfunction.

IQ + **R65.21 Severe sepsis with septic shock**

GUIDELINES **Section I.C.1.d.2)(a)**
Septic shock generally refers to circulatory failure associated with severe sepsis, and therefore, it represents a type of acute organ dysfunction. For cases of septic shock, the code for the systemic infection should be sequenced first, followed by code R65.21, Severe sepsis with septic shock or code T81.12, Postprocedural septic shock. Any additional codes for the other acute organ dysfunctions should also be assigned. As noted in the sequencing instructions in the Tabular List, the code for septic shock cannot be assigned as a principal diagnosis.

4 **R68 Other general symptoms and signs**

IQ **R68.0 Hypothermia, not associated with low environmental temperature**

EXCLUDES 1 hypothermia NOS (accidental) (T68)
hypothermia due to anesthesia (T88.51)
hypothermia due to low environmental temperature (T68)
newborn hypothermia (P80.-)

5 **R68.1 Nonspecific symptoms peculiar to infancy**

EXCLUDES 1 colic, infantile (R10.83)
neonatal cerebral irritability (P91.3)
teething syndrome (K00.7)

IQ **R68.11 Excessive crying of infant (baby)**

Chapter 18

R00-R99

EXCLUDES 1 excessive crying of child, adolescent, or adult (R45.83)

IQ **R68.12 Fussy infant (baby)**
Irritable infant

IQ + **R68.13 Apparent life threatening event in infant (ALTE)**
Apparent life threatening event in newborn
Brief resolved unexplained event (BRUE)
Code first:
confirmed diagnosis, if known
Use additional code(s) for associated signs and symptoms if no confirmed diagnosis established, or if signs and symptoms are not associated routinely with confirmed diagnosis, or provide additional information for cause of ALTE

IQ **R68.19 Other nonspecific symptoms peculiar to infancy**

▲ IQ **R68.2 Dry mouth, unspecified**
EXCLUDES 1 dry mouth due to dehydration (E86.0)
dry mouth due to Sjögren syndrome (M35.0-)
salivary gland hyposecretion (K11.7)

IQ **R68.3 Clubbing of fingers**
Clubbing of nails
EXCLUDES 1 congenital clubfinger (Q68.1)

5 **R68.8 Other general symptoms and signs**

IQ **R68.81 Early satiety**

IQ **R68.82 Decreased libido**
Decreased sexual desire

IQ **R68.83 Chills (without fever)**
Chills NOS
EXCLUDES 1 chills with fever (R50.9)

IQ **R68.84 Jaw pain**
Mandibular pain
Maxilla pain
EXCLUDES 1 temporomandibular joint arthralgia (M26.62-)
CODING TIPS✓ Jaw pain may be a symptom of myocardial infarction. If the condition causing the pain is known, such as a jaw disorder, then, for example, use a M26.62 code instead.

IQ **R68.89 Other general symptoms and signs**

IQ **R69 Illness, unspecified**
Unknown and unspecified cases of morbidity
CODING TIPS✓ R69 indicates unknown illness of unknown origin and should not be assigned on a home health claim.

Abnormal findings on examination of blood, without diagnosis (R70-R79)

EXCLUDES 2 abnormal findings on antenatal screening of mother (O28.-)
abnormalities of lipids (E78.-)
abnormalities of platelets and thrombocytes (D69.-)
abnormalities of white blood cells classified elsewhere (D70-D72)
coagulation hemorrhagic disorders (D65-D68)
diagnostic abnormal findings classified elsewhere - see Alphabetical Index
hemorrhagic and hematological disorders of newborn (P50-P61)

4 **R70 Elevated erythrocyte sedimentation rate and abnormality of plasma viscosity**

IQ **R70.0 Elevated erythrocyte sedimentation rate**

IQ **R70.1 Abnormal plasma viscosity**

4 **R71 Abnormality of red blood cells**
EXCLUDES 1 anemias (D50-D64)
anemia of premature infant (P61.2)
benign (familial) polycythemia (D75.0)
congenital anemias (P61.2-P61.4)
newborn anemia due to isoimmunization (P55.-)
polycythemia neonatorum (P61.1)
polycythemia NOS (D75.1)
polycythemia vera (D45)
secondary polycythemia (D75.1)

IQ **R71.0 Precipitous drop in hematocrit**
Drop (precipitous) in hemoglobin
Drop in hematocrit

IQ **R71.8 Other abnormality of red blood cells**
Abnormal red-cell morphology NOS
Abnormal red-cell volume NOS
Anisocytosis
Poikilocytosis

4 **R73 Elevated blood glucose level**
EXCLUDES 1 diabetes mellitus (E08-E13)
diabetes mellitus in pregnancy, childbirth and the puerperium (O24.-)
neonatal disorders (P70.0-P70.2)
postsurgical hypoinsulinemia (E89.1)

5 **R73.0 Abnormal glucose**
EXCLUDES 1 abnormal glucose in pregnancy (O99.81-)
diabetes mellitus (E08-E13)
dysmetabolic syndrome X (E88.81)
gestational diabetes (O24.4-)
glycosuria (R81)
hypoglycemia (E16.2)

IQ **R73.01 Impaired fasting glucose**
Elevated fasting glucose

IQ **R73.02 Impaired glucose tolerance (oral)**
Elevated glucose tolerance

IQ **R73.03 Prediabetes**
Latent diabetes
CODING TIPS✓ Prediabetes is defined as having an impaired fasting glucose (IFG): fasting blood glucose of 100-125 mg/dL, impaired glucose tolerance (IGT): blood glucose of 140-199 mg/dL 2 hours after a 75 g oral glucose tolerance test (OGTT) or a hemoglobin A1c value of 5.7%-6.4%.

DEFINITION An elevated blood sugar level that is higher than normal, but not high enough to be diagnosed as type 2 diabetes. When left untreated, prediabetes progresses to type 2 diabetes in less than 10 years. For many people, prediabetes has no signs or symptoms.

IQ **R73.09 Other abnormal glucose**
Abnormal glucose NOS
Abnormal non-fasting glucose tolerance

IQ **R73.9 Hyperglycemia, unspecified**

CODING TIPS ✓ Hyperglycemia should be coded to R73.9 only when not associated with diabetes mellitus or any form of post-procedural hyperinsulinemia. R73.9 indicates hyperglycemia that is of an unspecified origin.

4 **R74 Abnormal serum enzyme levels**

5 **R74.0 Nonspecific elevation of levels of transaminase and lactic acid dehydrogenase [LDH]**

IQ **R74.01 Elevation of levels of liver transaminase levels**
Elevation of levels of alanine transaminase (ALT)
Elevation of levels of aspartate transaminase (AST)

IQ **R74.02 Elevation of levels of lactic acid dehydrogenase [LDH]**

IQ **R74.8 Abnormal levels of other serum enzymes**
Abnormal level of acid phosphatase
Abnormal level of alkaline phosphatase
Abnormal level of amylase
Abnormal level of lipase [triacylglycerol lipase]

IQ **R74.9 Abnormal serum enzyme level, unspecified**

IQ **R75 Inconclusive laboratory evidence of human immunodeficiency virus [HIV]**
Nonconclusive HIV-test finding in infants

EXCLUDES 1 asymptomatic human immunodeficiency virus [HIV] infection status (Z21)
human immunodeficiency virus [HIV] disease (B20)

GUIDELINES **Section I.C.1.a.2)(f)**
Patients with any known prior diagnosis of an HIV-related illness should be coded to B20. Once a patient has developed an HIV-related illness, the patient should always be assigned code B20 on every subsequent admission/encounter. Patients previously diagnosed with any HIV illness (B20) should never be assigned to R75 or Z21, Asymptomatic human immunodeficiency virus [HIV] infection status.

GUIDELINES **Section I.C.1.a.2)(e)**
Patients with inconclusive HIV serology, but no definitive diagnosis or manifestations of the illness, may be assigned code R75, Inconclusive laboratory evidence of human immunodeficiency virus [HIV].

4 **R76 Other abnormal immunological findings in serum**

IQ **R76.0 Raised antibody titer**

EXCLUDES 1 isoimmunization in pregnancy (O36.0-O36.1)
isoimmunization affecting newborn (P55.-)

5 **R76.1 Nonspecific reaction to test for tuberculosis**

IQ **R76.11 Nonspecific reaction to tuberculin skin test without active tuberculosis**
Abnormal result of Mantoux test
PPD positive
Tuberculin (skin test) positive
Tuberculin (skin test) reactor

EXCLUDES 1 nonspecific reaction to cell mediated immunity measurement of gamma interferon antigen response without active tuberculosis (R76.12)

IQ **R76.12 Nonspecific reaction to cell mediated immunity measurement of gamma interferon antigen response without active tuberculosis**
Nonspecific reaction to QuantiFERON-TB test (QFT) without active tuberculosis

EXCLUDES 1 nonspecific reaction to tuberculin skin test without active tuberculosis (R76.11)
positive tuberculin skin test (R76.11)

IQ **R76.8 Other specified abnormal immunological findings in serum**
Raised level of immunoglobulins NOS

IQ **R76.9 Abnormal immunological finding in serum, unspecified**

4 **R77 Other abnormalities of plasma proteins**

EXCLUDES 1 disorders of plasma-protein metabolism (E88.0-)

IQ **R77.0 Abnormality of albumin**

IQ **R77.1 Abnormality of globulin**
Hyperglobulinemia NOS

IQ **R77.2 Abnormality of alphafetoprotein**

IQ **R77.8 Other specified abnormalities of plasma proteins**

IQ **R77.9 Abnormality of plasma protein, unspecified**

+ 4 **R78 Findings of drugs and other substances, not normally found in blood**
Use additional code to identify the any retained foreign body, if applicable (Z18.-)

EXCLUDES 1 mental or behavioral disorders due to psychoactive substance use (F10-F19)

IQ + **R78.0 Finding of alcohol in blood**
Use additional external cause code (Y90.-), for detail regarding alcohol level.

IQ + **R78.1 Finding of opiate drug in blood**

IQ + **R78.2 Finding of cocaine in blood**

IQ + **R78.3 Finding of hallucinogen in blood**

IQ + **R78.4 Finding of other drugs of addictive potential in blood**

IQ + **R78.5 Finding of other psychotropic drug in blood**

IQ + **R78.6 Finding of steroid agent in blood**

Chapter 18

R00-R99

+ 5 R78.7 Finding of abnormal level of heavy metals in blood

IQ + R78.71 Abnormal lead level in blood

EXCLUDES 1 lead poisoning (T56.0-)

IQ + R78.79 Finding of abnormal level of heavy metals in blood

+ 5 R78.8 Finding of other specified substances, not normally found in blood

IQ + R78.81 Bacteremia

EXCLUDES 1 sepsis-code to specified infection

CODING TIPS ✓ Do not assign code R78.81 to indicate the presence of sepsis. Bacteremia only indicates the presence of bacteria identified in the bloodstream, not the infectious process. Do not assign R78.81 with any code identifying sepsis. Sepsis should be coded to the appropriate code identifying the specific type of sepsis present.

DEFINITION The presence of small numbers of bacteria in the bloodstream, usually as a temporary condition, and without causing symptoms.

IQ + R78.89 Finding of other specified substances, not normally found in blood

Finding of abnormal level of lithium in blood

CODING TIPS ✓ Code R78.89 indicates that the patient has elevated non-therapeutic levels of a drug found in the blood on testing, but has no adverse effects of the drug. If the clinical record indicates poisoning or adverse effect, reference the Table of Drugs and Chemicals for the correct code, including drug and intent.

IQ + R78.9 Finding of unspecified substance, not normally found in blood

+ 4 R79 Other abnormal findings of blood chemistry

Use additional code to identify any retained foreign body, if applicable (Z18.-)

EXCLUDES 1 asymptomatic hyperuricemia (E79.0)
hyperglycemia NOS (R73.9)
hypoglycemia NOS (E16.2)
neonatal hypoglycemia (P70.3-P70.4)
specific findings indicating disorder of amino-acid metabolism (E70-E72)
specific findings indicating disorder of carbohydrate metabolism (E73-E74)
specific findings indicating disorder of lipid metabolism (E75.-)

IQ + R79.0 Abnormal level of blood mineral

Abnormal blood level of cobalt
Abnormal blood level of copper
Abnormal blood level of iron
Abnormal blood level of magnesium
Abnormal blood level of mineral NEC
Abnormal blood level of zinc

EXCLUDES 1 abnormal level of lithium (R78.89)
disorders of mineral metabolism (E83.-)
neonatal hypomagnesemia (P71.2)
nutritional mineral deficiency (E58-E61)

IQ + R79.1 Abnormal coagulation profile

Abnormal or prolonged bleeding time
Abnormal or prolonged coagulation time
Abnormal or prolonged partial thromboplastin time [PTT]
Abnormal or prolonged prothrombin time [PT]

EXCLUDES 1 coagulation defects (D68.-)

EXCLUDES 2 abnormality of fluid, electrolyte or acid-base balance (E86-E87)

CODING TIPS ✓ This code is not for those on Coumadin or other blood thinners for prophylactic purposes. Use Z51.81 and Z79.01 instead. If a bleed has occurred because of anticoagulants/antiplatelets, code the bleed and D68.32 and the T code for the drug.

+ 5 R79.8 Other specified abnormal findings of blood chemistry

IQ + R79.81 Abnormal blood-gas level

DEFINITION Abnormal oxygen or carbon dioxide level in the blood.

IQ + R79.82 Elevated C-reactive protein (CRP)

★ + R79.83 Abnormal findings of blood amino-acid level

Homocysteinemia

EXCLUDES 1 disorders of amino-acid metabolism (E70-E72)

IQ + R79.89 Other specified abnormal findings of blood chemistry

IQ + R79.9 Abnormal finding of blood chemistry, unspecified

Abnormal findings on examination of urine, without diagnosis (R80-R82)

EXCLUDES 1 abnormal findings on antenatal screening of mother (O28.-)
diagnostic abnormal findings classified elsewhere - see Alphabetical Index
specific findings indicating disorder of amino-acid metabolism (E70-E72)
specific findings indicating disorder of carbohydrate metabolism (E73-E74)

4 R80 Proteinuria

EXCLUDES 1 gestational proteinuria (O12.1-)

IQ R80.0 Isolated proteinuria

Idiopathic proteinuria

EXCLUDES 1 isolated proteinuria with specific morphological lesion (N06.-)

IQ R80.1 Persistent proteinuria, unspecified

IQ R80.2 Orthostatic proteinuria, unspecified

Postural proteinuria

IQ R80.3 Bence Jones proteinuria

IQ R80.8 Other proteinuria

IQ R80.9 Proteinuria, unspecified

4 4th digit required 5 5th digit required 6 6th digit required 7 7th digit required 7 7th digit placeholder + Additional code ⊟ Laterality

Albuminuria NOS

IQ **R81 Glycosuria**

EXCLUDES 1 renal glycosuria (E74.818)

+ 4 **R82 Other and unspecified abnormal findings in urine**

INCLUDES chromoabnormalities in urine

Use additional code to identify any retained foreign body, if applicable (Z18.-)

EXCLUDES 2 hematuria (R31.-)

IQ + **R82.0 Chyluria**

EXCLUDES 1 filarial chyluria (B74.-)

IQ + **R82.1 Myoglobinuria**

IQ + **R82.2 Biliuria**

IQ + **R82.3 Hemoglobinuria**

EXCLUDES 1 hemoglobinuria due to hemolysis from external causes NEC (D59.6)
hemoglobinuria due to paroxysmal nocturnal [Marchiafava-Micheli] (D59.5)

IQ + **R82.4 Acetonuria**

Ketonuria

IQ + **R82.5 Elevated urine levels of drugs, medicaments and biological substances**

Elevated urine levels of catecholamines
Elevated urine levels of indoleacetic acid
Elevated urine levels of 17-ketosteroids
Elevated urine levels of steroids

IQ + **R82.6 Abnormal urine levels of substances chiefly nonmedicinal as to source**

Abnormal urine level of heavy metals

+ 5 **R82.7 Abnormal findings on microbiological examination of urine**

EXCLUDES 1 colonization status (Z22.-)

CODING TIPS ✓ Bacteriuria is a condition where there are bacteria present in a microscopic examination of the urine. It is not definitive evidence of a UTI.

IQ + **R82.71 Bacteriuria**

DEFINITION The presence of bacteria identified in the urine. It affects more women than men and commonly occurs asymptomatically.

IQ + **R82.79 Other abnormal findings on microbiological examination of urine**

Positive culture findings of urine

+ 5 **R82.8 Abnormal findings on cytological and histological examination of urine**

+ **R82.81 Pyuria**

Sterile pyuria

+ **R82.89 Other abnormal findings on cytological and histological examination of urine**

+ 5 **R82.9 Other and unspecified abnormal findings in urine**

IQ + **R82.90 Unspecified abnormal findings in urine**

IQ + **R82.91 Other chromoabnormalities of urine**

Chromoconversion (dipstick)
Idiopathic dipstick converts positive for blood with no cellular forms in sediment

EXCLUDES 1 hemoglobinuria (R82.3)
myoglobinuria (R82.1)

+ 6 **R82.99 Other abnormal findings in urine**

IQ + **R82.991 Hypocitraturia**

IQ + **R82.992 Hyperoxaluria**

EXCLUDES 1 Primary hyperoxaluria (E72.53)

IQ + **R82.993 Hyperuricosuria**

IQ + **R82.994 Hypercalciuria**

Idiopathic hypercalciuria

IQ + **R82.998 Other abnormal findings in urine**

Cells and casts in urine
Crystalluria
Melanuria

Abnormal findings on examination of other body fluids, substances and tissues, without diagnosis (R83-R89)

EXCLUDES 1 abnormal findings on antenatal screening of mother (O28.-)
diagnostic abnormal findings classified elsewhere - see Alphabetical Index

EXCLUDES 2 abnormal findings on examination of blood, without diagnosis (R70-R79)
abnormal findings on examination of urine, without diagnosis (R80-R82)
abnormal tumor markers (R97.-)

4 **R83 Abnormal findings in cerebrospinal fluid**

IQ **R83.0 Abnormal level of enzymes in cerebrospinal fluid**

IQ **R83.1 Abnormal level of hormones in cerebrospinal fluid**

IQ **R83.2 Abnormal level of other drugs, medicaments and biological substances in cerebrospinal fluid**

IQ **R83.3 Abnormal level of substances chiefly nonmedicinal as to source in cerebrospinal fluid**

IQ **R83.4 Abnormal immunological findings in cerebrospinal fluid**

IQ **R83.5 Abnormal microbiological findings in cerebrospinal fluid**

Positive culture findings in cerebrospinal fluid

EXCLUDES 1 colonization status (Z22.-)

IQ **R83.6 Abnormal cytological findings in cerebrospinal fluid**

IQ **R83.8 Other abnormal findings in cerebrospinal fluid**

Abnormal chromosomal findings in cerebrospinal fluid

IQ **R83.9 Unspecified abnormal finding in cerebrospinal fluid**

4 **R84 Abnormal findings in specimens from respiratory organs and thorax**

INCLUDES abnormal findings in bronchial washings
abnormal findings in nasal secretions
abnormal findings in pleural fluid
abnormal findings in sputum
abnormal findings in throat scrapings

EXCLUDES 1 blood-stained sputum (R04.2)

IQ **R84.0 Abnormal level of enzymes in specimens from respiratory organs and thorax**

Chapter 18 R00-R99

IQ **R84.1 Abnormal level of hormones in specimens from respiratory organs and thorax**

IQ **R84.2 Abnormal level of other drugs, medicaments and biological substances in specimens from respiratory organs and thorax**

IQ **R84.3 Abnormal level of substances chiefly nonmedicinal as to source in specimens from respiratory organs and thorax**

IQ **R84.4 Abnormal immunological findings in specimens from respiratory organs and thorax**

IQ **R84.5 Abnormal microbiological findings in specimens from respiratory organs and thorax**

Positive culture findings in specimens from respiratory organs and thorax

EXCLUDES 1 colonization status (Z22.-)

IQ **R84.6 Abnormal cytological findings in specimens from respiratory organs and thorax**

IQ **R84.7 Abnormal histological findings in specimens from respiratory organs and thorax**

IQ **R84.8 Other abnormal findings in specimens from respiratory organs and thorax**

Abnormal chromosomal findings in specimens from respiratory organs and thorax

IQ **R84.9 Unspecified abnormal finding in specimens from respiratory organs and thorax**

4 **R85 Abnormal findings in specimens from digestive organs and abdominal cavity**

INCLUDES abnormal findings in peritoneal fluid

abnormal findings in saliva

EXCLUDES 1 cloudy peritoneal dialysis effluent (R88.0)

fecal abnormalities (R19.5)

IQ **R85.0 Abnormal level of enzymes in specimens from digestive organs and abdominal cavity**

IQ **R85.1 Abnormal level of hormones in specimens from digestive organs and abdominal cavity**

IQ **R85.2 Abnormal level of other drugs, medicaments and biological substances in specimens from digestive organs and abdominal cavity**

IQ **R85.3 Abnormal level of substances chiefly nonmedicinal as to source in specimens from digestive organs and abdominal cavity**

IQ **R85.4 Abnormal immunological findings in specimens from digestive organs and abdominal cavity**

IQ **R85.5 Abnormal microbiological findings in specimens from digestive organs and abdominal cavity**

Positive culture findings in specimens from digestive organs and abdominal cavity

EXCLUDES 1 colonization status (Z22.-)

5 **R85.6 Abnormal cytological findings in specimens from digestive organs and abdominal cavity**

6 **R85.61 Abnormal cytologic smear of anus**

EXCLUDES 1 abnormal cytological findings in specimens from other digestive organs and abdominal cavity (R85.69)

carcinoma in situ of anus (histologically confirmed) (D01.3)

anal intraepithelial neoplasia I [AIN I] (K62.82)

anal intraepithelial neoplasia II [AIN II] (K62.82)

anal intraepithelial neoplasia III [AIN III] (D01.3)

dysplasia (mild) (moderate) of anus (histologically confirmed) (K62.82)

severe dysplasia of anus (histologically confirmed) (D01.3)

EXCLUDES 2 anal high risk human papillomavirus (HPV) DNA test positive (R85.81)

anal low risk human papillomavirus (HPV) DNA test positive (R85.82)

IQ **R85.610 Atypical squamous cells of undetermined significance on cytologic smear of anus (ASC-US)**

IQ **R85.611 Atypical squamous cells cannot exclude high grade squamous intraepithelial lesion on cytologic smear of anus (ASC-H)**

IQ **R85.612 Low grade squamous intraepithelial lesion on cytologic smear of anus (LGSIL)**

IQ **R85.613 High grade squamous intraepithelial lesion on cytologic smear of anus (HGSIL)**

IQ **R85.614 Cytologic evidence of malignancy on smear of anus**

IQ **R85.615 Unsatisfactory cytologic smear of anus**

Inadequate sample of cytologic smear of anus

IQ **R85.616 Satisfactory anal smear but lacking transformation zone**

IQ **R85.618 Other abnormal cytological findings on specimens from anus**

IQ **R85.619 Unspecified abnormal cytological findings in specimens from anus**

Abnormal anal cytology NOS

Atypical glandular cells of anus NOS

IQ **R85.69 Abnormal cytological findings in specimens from other digestive organs and abdominal cavity**

IQ **R85.7 Abnormal histological findings in specimens from digestive organs and abdominal cavity**

Chapter 18

R00-R99

5 **R85.8 Other abnormal findings in specimens from digestive organs and abdominal cavity**

IQ **R85.81 Anal high risk human papillomavirus (HPV) DNA test positive**

EXCLUDES 1 anogenital warts due to human papillomavirus (HPV) (A63.0)
condyloma acuminatum (A63.0)

IQ + **R85.82 Anal low risk human papillomavirus (HPV) DNA test positive**

Use additional code for associated human papillomavirus (B97.7)

IQ **R85.89 Other abnormal findings in specimens from digestive organs and abdominal cavity**

Abnormal chromosomal findings in specimens from digestive organs and abdominal cavity

IQ **R85.9 Unspecified abnormal finding in specimens from digestive organs and abdominal cavity**

4 **R86 Abnormal findings in specimens from male genital organs**

INCLUDES abnormal findings in prostatic secretions
abnormal findings in semen, seminal fluid
abnormal spermatozoa

EXCLUDES 1 azoospermia (N46.0-)
oligospermia (N46.1-)

IQ **R86.0 Abnormal level of enzymes in specimens from male genital organs**

IQ **R86.1 Abnormal level of hormones in specimens from male genital organs**

IQ **R86.2 Abnormal level of other drugs, medicaments and biological substances in specimens from male genital organs**

IQ **R86.3 Abnormal level of substances chiefly nonmedicinal as to source in specimens from male genital organs**

IQ **R86.4 Abnormal immunological findings in specimens from male genital organs**

IQ **R86.5 Abnormal microbiological findings in specimens from male genital organs**

Positive culture findings in specimens from male genital organs

EXCLUDES 1 colonization status (Z22.-)

IQ **R86.6 Abnormal cytological findings in specimens from male genital organs**

IQ **R86.7 Abnormal histological findings in specimens from male genital organs**

IQ **R86.8 Other abnormal findings in specimens from male genital organs**

Abnormal chromosomal findings in specimens from male genital organs

IQ **R86.9 Unspecified abnormal finding in specimens from male genital organs**

4 **R87 Abnormal findings in specimens from female genital organs**

INCLUDES abnormal findings in secretion and smears from cervix uteri
abnormal findings in secretion and smears from vagina
abnormal findings in secretion and smears from vulva

IQ **R87.0 Abnormal level of enzymes in specimens from female genital organs**

IQ **R87.1 Abnormal level of hormones in specimens from female genital organs**

IQ **R87.2 Abnormal level of other drugs, medicaments and biological substances in specimens from female genital organs**

IQ **R87.3 Abnormal level of substances chiefly nonmedicinal as to source in specimens from female genital organs**

IQ **R87.4 Abnormal immunological findings in specimens from female genital organs**

IQ **R87.5 Abnormal microbiological findings in specimens from female genital organs**

Positive culture findings in specimens from female genital organs

EXCLUDES 1 colonization status (Z22.-)

5 **R87.6 Abnormal cytological findings in specimens from female genital organs**

6 **R87.61 Abnormal cytological findings in specimens from cervix uteri**

EXCLUDES 1 abnormal cytological findings in specimens from other female genital organs (R87.69)
abnormal cytological findings in specimens from vagina (R87.62-)
carcinoma in situ of cervix uteri (histologically confirmed) (D06.-)
cervical intraepithelial neoplasia I [CIN I] (N87.0)
cervical intraepithelial neoplasia II [CIN II] (N87.1)
cervical intraepithelial neoplasia III [CIN III] (D06.-)
dysplasia (mild) (moderate) of cervix uteri (histologically confirmed) (N87.-)
severe dysplasia of cervix uteri (histologically confirmed) (D06.-)

EXCLUDES 2 cervical high risk human papillomavirus (HPV) DNA test positive (R87.810)
cervical low risk human papillomavirus (HPV) DNA test positive (R87.820)

IQ **R87.610 Atypical squamous cells of undetermined significance on cytologic smear of cervix (ASC-US)**

IQ **R87.611 Atypical squamous cells cannot exclude high grade squamous intraepithelial lesion on cytologic smear of cervix (ASC-H)**

IQ **R87.612 Low grade squamous intraepithelial lesion on cytologic smear of cervix (LGSIL)**

Chapter 18

R00-R99

IQ **R87.613 High grade squamous intraepithelial lesion on cytologic smear of cervix (HGSIL)**

IQ **R87.614 Cytologic evidence of malignancy on smear of cervix**

IQ **R87.615 Unsatisfactory cytologic smear of cervix**
Inadequate sample of cytologic smear of cervix

IQ **R87.616 Satisfactory cervical smear but lacking transformation zone**

IQ **R87.618 Other abnormal cytological findings on specimens from cervix uteri**

IQ **R87.619 Unspecified abnormal cytological findings in specimens from cervix uteri**
Abnormal cervical cytology NOS
Abnormal Papanicolaou smear of cervix NOS
Abnormal thin preparation smear of cervix NOS
Atypical endocervial cells of cervix NOS
Atypical endometrial cells of cervix NOS
Atypical glandular cells of cervix NOS

+ 6 **R87.62 Abnormal cytological findings in specimens from vagina**
Use additional code to identify acquired absence of uterus and cervix, if applicable (Z90.71-)

EXCLUDES 1 abnormal cytological findings in specimens from cervix uteri (R87.61-)
abnormal cytological findings in specimens from other female genital organs (R87.69)
carcinoma in situ of vagina (histologically confirmed) (D07.2)
vaginal intraepithelial neoplasia I [VAIN I] (N89.0)
vaginal intraepithelial neoplasia II [VAIN II] (N89.1)
vaginal intraepithelial neoplasia III [VAIN III] (D07.2)
dysplasia (mild) (moderate) of vagina (histologically confirmed) (N89.-)
severe dysplasia of vagina (histologically confirmed) (D07.2)

EXCLUDES 2 vaginal high risk human papillomavirus (HPV) DNA test positive (R87.811)
vaginal low risk human papillomavirus (HPV) DNA test positive (R87.821)

IQ + **R87.620 Atypical squamous cells of undetermined significance on cytologic smear of vagina (ASC-US)**

IQ + **R87.621 Atypical squamous cells cannot exclude high grade squamous intraepithelial lesion on cytologic smear of vagina (ASC-H)**

IQ + **R87.622 Low grade squamous intraepithelial lesion on cytologic smear of vagina (LGSIL)**

IQ + **R87.623 High grade squamous intraepithelial lesion on cytologic smear of vagina (HGSIL)**

IQ + **R87.624 Cytologic evidence of malignancy on smear of vagina**

IQ + **R87.625 Unsatisfactory cytologic smear of vagina**
Inadequate sample of cytologic smear of vagina

IQ + **R87.628 Other abnormal cytological findings on specimens from vagina**

IQ + **R87.629 Unspecified abnormal cytological findings in specimens from vagina**
Abnormal Papanicolaou smear of vagina NOS
Abnormal thin preparation smear of vagina NOS
Abnormal vaginal cytology NOS
Atypical endocervical cells of vagina NOS
Atypical endometrial cells of vagina NOS
Atypical glandular cells of vagina NOS

IQ **R87.69 Abnormal cytological findings in specimens from other female genital organs**
Abnormal cytological findings in specimens from female genital organs NOS

EXCLUDES 1 dysplasia of vulva (histologically confirmed) (N90.0-N90.3)

IQ **R87.7 Abnormal histological findings in specimens from female genital organs**

EXCLUDES 1 carcinoma in situ (histologically confirmed) of female genital organs (D06-D07.3)
cervical intraepithelial neoplasia I [CIN I] (N87.0)
cervical intraepithelial neoplasia II [CIN II] (N87.1)
cervical intraepithelial neoplasia III [CIN III] (D06.-)

Chapter 18

R00-R99

dysplasia (mild) (moderate) of cervix uteri (histologically confirmed) (N87.-)
dysplasia (mild) (moderate) of vagina (histologically confirmed) (N89.-)
vaginal intraepithelial neoplasia I [VAIN I] (N89.0)
vaginal intraepithelial neoplasia II [VAIN II] (N89.1)
vaginal intraepithelial neoplasia III [VAIN III] (D07.2)
severe dysplasia of cervix uteri (histologically confirmed) (D06.-)
severe dysplasia of vagina (histologically confirmed) (D07.2)

5 **R87.8 Other abnormal findings in specimens from female genital organs**

6 **R87.81 High risk human papillomavirus (HPV) DNA test positive from female genital organs**

EXCLUDES 1 anogenital warts due to human papillomavirus (HPV) (A63.0)
condyloma acuminatum (A63.0)

IQ **R87.810 Cervical high risk human papillomavirus (HPV) DNA test positive**

IQ **R87.811 Vaginal high risk human papillomavirus (HPV) DNA test positive**

+ 6 **R87.82 Low risk human papillomavirus (HPV) DNA test positive from female genital organs**
Use additional code for associated human papillomavirus (B97.7)

IQ + **R87.820 Cervical low risk human papillomavirus (HPV) DNA test positive**

IQ + **R87.821 Vaginal low risk human papillomavirus (HPV) DNA test positive**

IQ **R87.89 Other abnormal findings in specimens from female genital organs**
Abnormal chromosomal findings in specimens from female genital organs

IQ **R87.9 Unspecified abnormal finding in specimens from female genital organs**

4 **R88 Abnormal findings in other body fluids and substances**

IQ **R88.0 Cloudy (hemodialysis) (peritoneal) dialysis effluent**

IQ **R88.8 Abnormal findings in other body fluids and substances**

4 **R89 Abnormal findings in specimens from other organs, systems and tissues**

INCLUDES abnormal findings in nipple discharge
abnormal findings in synovial fluid
abnormal findings in wound secretions

IQ **R89.0 Abnormal level of enzymes in specimens from other organs, systems and tissues**

IQ **R89.1 Abnormal level of hormones in specimens from other organs, systems and tissues**

IQ **R89.2 Abnormal level of other drugs, medicaments and biological substances in specimens from other organs, systems and tissues**

IQ **R89.3 Abnormal level of substances chiefly nonmedicinal as to source in specimens from other organs, systems and tissues**

IQ **R89.4 Abnormal immunological findings in specimens from other organs, systems and tissues**

IQ **R89.5 Abnormal microbiological findings in specimens from other organs, systems and tissues**
Positive culture findings in specimens from other organs, systems and tissues
EXCLUDES 1 colonization status (Z22.-)

IQ **R89.6 Abnormal cytological findings in specimens from other organs, systems and tissues**

IQ **R89.7 Abnormal histological findings in specimens from other organs, systems and tissues**

IQ **R89.8 Other abnormal findings in specimens from other organs, systems and tissues**
Abnormal chromosomal findings in specimens from other organs, systems and tissues

IQ **R89.9 Unspecified abnormal finding in specimens from other organs, systems and tissues**

Abnormal findings on diagnostic imaging and in function studies, without diagnosis (R90-R94)

INCLUDES nonspecific abnormal findings on diagnostic imaging by computerized axial tomography [CAT scan]
nonspecific abnormal findings on diagnostic imaging by magnetic resonance imaging [MRI][NMR]
nonspecific abnormal findings on diagnostic imaging by positron emission tomography [PET scan]
nonspecific abnormal findings on diagnostic imaging by thermography
nonspecific abnormal findings on diagnostic imaging by ultrasound [echogram]
nonspecific abnormal findings on diagnostic imaging by X-ray examination

EXCLUDES 1 abnormal findings on antenatal screening of mother (O28.-)
diagnostic abnormal findings classified elsewhere - see Alphabetical Index

4 **R90 Abnormal findings on diagnostic imaging of central nervous system**

IQ **R90.0 Intracranial space-occupying lesion found on diagnostic imaging of central nervous system**

Chapter 18 R00-R99

5 **R90.8 Other abnormal findings on diagnostic imaging of central nervous system**

IQ **R90.81 Abnormal echoencephalogram**

IQ **R90.82 White matter disease, unspecified**

IQ **R90.89 Other abnormal findings on diagnostic imaging of central nervous system**

Other cerebrovascular abnormality found on diagnostic imaging of central nervous system

4 **R91 Abnormal findings on diagnostic imaging of lung**

IQ **R91.1 Solitary pulmonary nodule**

Coin lesion lung

Solitary pulmonary nodule, subsegmental branch of the bronchial tree

IQ **R91.8 Other nonspecific abnormal finding of lung field**

Lung mass NOS found on diagnostic imaging of lung

Pulmonary infiltrate NOS

Shadow, lung

4 **R92 Abnormal and inconclusive findings on diagnostic imaging of breast**

IQ **R92.0 Mammographic microcalcification found on diagnostic imaging of breast**

EXCLUDES 2 mammographic calcification (calculus) found on diagnostic imaging of breast (R92.1)

IQ **R92.1 Mammographic calcification found on diagnostic imaging of breast**

Mammographic calculus found on diagnostic imaging of breast

IQ **R92.2 Inconclusive mammogram**

Dense breasts NOS

Inconclusive mammogram NEC

Inconclusive mammography due to dense breasts

Inconclusive mammography NEC

IQ **R92.8 Other abnormal and inconclusive findings on diagnostic imaging of breast**

4 **R93 Abnormal findings on diagnostic imaging of other body structures**

IQ **R93.0 Abnormal findings on diagnostic imaging of skull and head, not elsewhere classified**

EXCLUDES 1 intracranial space-occupying lesion found on diagnostic imaging (R90.0)

IQ **R93.1 Abnormal findings on diagnostic imaging of heart and coronary circulation**

Abnormal echocardiogram NOS

Abnormal heart shadow

IQ **R93.2 Abnormal findings on diagnostic imaging of liver and biliary tract**

Nonvisualization of gallbladder

IQ **R93.3 Abnormal findings on diagnostic imaging of other parts of digestive tract**

5 **R93.4 Abnormal findings on diagnostic imaging of urinary organs**

EXCLUDES 2 hypertrophy of kidney (N28.81)

IQ **R93.41 Abnormal radiologic findings on diagnostic imaging of renal pelvis, ureter, or bladder**

Filling defect of bladder found on diagnostic imaging

Filling defect of renal pelvis found on diagnostic imaging

Filling defect of ureter found on diagnostic imaging

6 **R93.42 Abnormal radiologic findings on diagnostic imaging of kidney**

Laterality IQ **R93.421 Abnormal radiologic findings on diagnostic imaging of right kidney**

Laterality IQ **R93.422 Abnormal radiologic findings on diagnostic imaging of left kidney**

Laterality IQ **R93.429 Abnormal radiologic findings on diagnostic imaging of unspecified kidney**

IQ **R93.49 Abnormal radiologic findings on diagnostic imaging of other urinary organs**

IQ **R93.5 Abnormal findings on diagnostic imaging of other abdominal regions, including retroperitoneum**

IQ **R93.6 Abnormal findings on diagnostic imaging of limbs**

EXCLUDES 2 abnormal finding in skin and subcutaneous tissue (R93.8-)

IQ **R93.7 Abnormal findings on diagnostic imaging of other parts of musculoskeletal system**

EXCLUDES 2 abnormal findings on diagnostic imaging of skull (R93.0)

5 **R93.8 Abnormal findings on diagnostic imaging of other specified body structures**

6 **R93.81 Abnormal radiologic findings on diagnostic imaging of testis**

Laterality IQ **R93.811 Abnormal radiologic findings on diagnostic imaging of right testicle**

Laterality IQ **R93.812 Abnormal radiologic findings on diagnostic imaging of left testicle**

Laterality IQ **R93.813 Abnormal radiologic findings on diagnostic imaging of testicles, bilateral**

Laterality IQ **R93.819 Abnormal radiologic findings on diagnostic imaging of unspecified testicle**

IQ **R93.89 Abnormal findings on diagnostic imaging of other specified body structures**

Abnormal finding by radioisotope localization of placenta

Abnormal radiological finding in skin and subcutaneous tissue

Mediastinal shift

IQ **R93.9 Diagnostic imaging inconclusive due to excess body fat of patient**

4 **R94 Abnormal results of function studies**

INCLUDES abnormal results of radionuclide [radioisotope] uptake studies

abnormal results of scintigraphy

5 **R94.0 Abnormal results of function studies of central nervous system**

IQ **R94.01 Abnormal electroencephalogram [EEG]**

IQ **R94.02 Abnormal brain scan**

IQ **R94.09 Abnormal results of other function studies of central nervous system**

Chapter 18

R00-R99

5 **R94.1 Abnormal results of function studies of peripheral nervous system and special senses**

6 **R94.11 Abnormal results of function studies of eye**

IQ **R94.110 Abnormal electro-oculogram [EOG]**

IQ **R94.111 Abnormal electroretinogram [ERG]**
Abnormal retinal function study

IQ **R94.112 Abnormal visually evoked potential [VEP]**

IQ **R94.113 Abnormal oculomotor study**

IQ **R94.118 Abnormal results of other function studies of eye**

6 **R94.12 Abnormal results of function studies of ear and other special senses**

IQ **R94.120 Abnormal auditory function study**

IQ **R94.121 Abnormal vestibular function study**

IQ **R94.128 Abnormal results of other function studies of ear and other special senses**

6 **R94.13 Abnormal results of function studies of peripheral nervous system**

IQ **R94.130 Abnormal response to nerve stimulation, unspecified**

IQ **R94.131 Abnormal electromyogram [EMG]**
EXCLUDES 1 electromyogram of eye (R94.113)

IQ **R94.138 Abnormal results of other function studies of peripheral nervous system**

IQ **R94.2 Abnormal results of pulmonary function studies**
Reduced ventilatory capacity
Reduced vital capacity

5 **R94.3 Abnormal results of cardiovascular function studies**

IQ **R94.30 Abnormal result of cardiovascular function study, unspecified**

IQ **R94.31 Abnormal electrocardiogram [ECG] [EKG]**
EXCLUDES 1 long QT syndrome (I45.81)

IQ **R94.39 Abnormal result of other cardiovascular function study**
Abnormal electrophysiological intracardiac studies
Abnormal phonocardiogram
Abnormal vectorcardiogram

IQ **R94.4 Abnormal results of kidney function studies**
Abnormal renal function test

IQ **R94.5 Abnormal results of liver function studies**

IQ **R94.6 Abnormal results of thyroid function studies**

IQ **R94.7 Abnormal results of other endocrine function studies**
EXCLUDES 2 abnormal glucose (R73.0-)

IQ **R94.8 Abnormal results of function studies of other organs and systems**
Abnormal basal metabolic rate [BMR]
Abnormal bladder function test
Abnormal splenic function test

Abnormal tumor markers (R97)

4 **R97 Abnormal tumor markers**
Elevated tumor associated antigens [TAA]
Elevated tumor specific antigens [TSA]

IQ **R97.0 Elevated carcinoembryonic antigen [CEA]**

IQ **R97.1 Elevated cancer antigen 125 [CA 125]**

5 **R97.2 Elevated prostate specific antigen [PSA]**

IQ **R97.20 Elevated prostate specific antigen [PSA]**
DEFINITION Elevated levels of prostate specific antigen (PSA) in the bloodstream can indicate prostate cancer, or precursor conditions that can develop into prostate cancer.

IQ **R97.21 Rising PSA following treatment for malignant neoplasm of prostate**

IQ **R97.8 Other abnormal tumor markers**

Ill-defined and unknown cause of mortality (R99)

H IQ **R99 Ill-defined and unknown cause of mortality**
Death (unexplained) NOS
Unspecified cause of mortality
CODING TIPS ✓ Code R99 indicates that a patient has expired. This code should never be assigned on a home health claim.

Chapter 18 Scenarios: Symptoms, signs and abnormal clinical and laboratory findings, not elsewhere classified (R00-R99)

Gait abnormality, orthostatic hypotension

A patient is admitted for gait abnormality documented by the physician as unsteadiness on feet. The patient has experienced repeated falls. It was determined that the unsteadiness is due to the patient's severe orthostatic hypotension. The patient will receive physical and occupational therapy to address the gait as well as safety concerns in the home.

Description	Code
Primary: Orthostatic hypotension	I95.1
Secondary: Unsteadiness on feet	R26.81
Secondary: History of falling	Z91.81

It is imperative to determine the underlying diagnosis behind a patient's symptoms as most symptom codes are not acceptable as primary diagnoses in the PDGM system. In this case, because orthostatic hypotension was determined to be the underlying diagnosis and the focus of the admission, it is assigned first. You may code symptoms when a more definitive diagnosis is known but the symptom is not integral to the condition and provides important additional information.The history of falling code (Z91.81) is used when a patient has fallen in the past and is at risk for future falls.

Gastrostomy care, Alzheimer's

An elderly male patient with severe late-onset Alzheimer's with dementia and a seizure disorder had a bout of aspiration pneumonia, resulting from dysphagia, that required hospitalization. The patient is confined to bed and dependent on his caregivers for all aspects of his care. Before his admission to home health, the pneumonia resolved but the patient has a gastrostomy tube with continuous tube feedings due to the dysphagia. The home health nurse will visit three times a week to educate his wife on tube feedings, make sure his nutritional needs are met, and assess for risks of further aspiration. The focus of care is the care and teaching of the g-tube.

Description	Code
Primary: Encounter for attention to gastrostomy	Z43.1
Secondary: Dysphagia, unspecified	R13.10
Secondary: Alzheimer's disease with late onset	G30.1
Secondary: Dementia in other diseases classified elsewhere without behavioral disturbance	F02.80
Secondary: Epilepsy, unspecified, not intractable, without status epilepticus	G40.909
Secondary: Personal history of pneumonia (recurrent)	Z87.01

In this case, since the focus of care is the g-tube, Z43.1 is assigned primary. The Alzheimer's disease has been specified as late-onset and is thus coded that way. The code for dementia follows the Alzheimer's code in accordance with the etiology-manifestation convention and the Q1 2017 Coding Clinic guidance. Though the pneumonia is resolved, the patient is at risk for future aspiration, thus Z87.01 is assigned.

Dysphagia, stroke sequelae

A patient is referred to home care for skilled nursing and speech-language therapy for treatment of dysphagia and dysarthria, which resulted from a stroke. Nursing is teaching on medications and diet. The patient also has a history of multiple sclerosis.

Description	Code
Primary: Dysphagia following cerebral infarction	I69.391
Secondary: Dysphagia, unspecified	R13.10
Secondary: Dysarthria following cerebral infarction	I69.322
Secondary: Multiple sclerosis	G35

The patient's dysphagia and dysarthria are stroke sequela. While the dysphagia and dysarthria due to the prior stroke are symptoms, they are also sequela of the stroke, so a sequela code is assigned to identify these conditions. Code I69.391 requires the assignment of an additional code to identify the type of dysphagia (based upon the "use additional code" note), so both the sequela code and a code from Chapter 18 are used to fully describe this condition. An additional code is assigned for this patient's multiple sclerosis as this condition impacts prognosis and care planning and may provide important comorbidity adjustment.

Chronic Afib, unspecified nausea, atypical chest pain

A 94-year-old female patient is admitted to home health for teaching on new medications prescribed for chronic atrial fibrillation and hypertension. Lately, she's also been experiencing nausea without vomiting, atypical chest pain, and epigastric pain. Radiology suggests possible gastric outlet obstruction or gastric volvulus.

Description	Code
Primary: Chronic atrial fibrillation, unspecified	I48.20
Secondary: Essential (primary) hypertension	I10
Secondary: Nausea without vomiting	R11.0
Secondary: Anterior chest-wall pain NOS	R07.89
Secondary: Epigastric pain	R10.13

The patient is admitted for teaching on new medications for chronic Afib and hypertension; thus they are assigned as primary and first secondary diagnosis. Her additional symptoms of nausea, chest pain and epigastric pain are not associated by the physician with her definitive diagnoses, and so they are coded separately. The physician's differential diagnoses may not be used until confirmed. Remember, most symptom codes are not acceptable as primary diagnoses in PDGM.

HOME HEALTH CODING SCENARIOS

Exacerbated CAD with angina, fall with hip pain

A 93-year-old female is admitted to home health with exacerbated coronary artery disease with angina. She's also complaining of left hip pain after tripping over a root in her yard and landing on her left side. The physician documents a possible subtle fracture and sends her home with an order for a home health skilled nursing and physical therapy. Her history includes chronic obstructive tracheobronchitis, resolved breast cancer and a past right hip replacement. Her left hip x-ray was inconclusive.

Description	Code
Primary: Atherosclerotic heart disease of native coronary artery with unspecified angina pectoris	I25.119
Secondary: Pain in left hip	M25.552
Secondary: Chronic obstructive pulmonary disease, unspecified	J44.9
Secondary: Personal history of malignant neoplasm of breast	Z85.3
Secondary: Presence of right artificial hip joint	Z96.641
Secondary: Fall on same level from slipping, tripping and stumbling without subsequent striking against object, subsequent encounter	W01.0xxD

As the focus of care, CAD with angina is coded in the primary position. Although the physician suspects a hip fracture, testing so far is inconclusive and, therefore, only her symptoms can be coded. Note that most symptom codes are not acceptable primary diagnoses in the PDGM system.

Generalized anxiety disorder, syncope

A 93-year-old woman was hospitalized after fainting during a bingo game at the senior center. While in the hospital she was diagnosed with generalized anxiety disorder and was later admitted to home health for teaching on the condition, new medications prescribed to manage her symptoms and to monitor her for continued fainting episodes. She has mild hypertension and congestive heart failure, but these conditions are currently stable on medication.

Description	Code
Primary: Generalized anxiety disorder	F41.1
Secondary: Syncope and collapse	R55
Secondary: Hypertensive heart disease with heart failure	I11.0
Secondary: Heart failure, unspecified	I50.9

Generalized anxiety disorder is the focus of care and is thus coded primary. Since her syncope symptoms will be monitored, the symptom code is also assigned. Hypertension and heart failure are additionally coded as these conditions impact the patient's prognosis and care planning, as well as may provide important comorbidity adjustment. Remember, most symptom codes are unacceptable as primary diagnoses in PDGM.

Crohn's, seizures

A 70-year-old man with a prior history of dementia suffered three seizures in two days and was hospitalized for investigate the cause. There is no diagnosis of epilepsy or any other reason given for the seizures. While in the hospital, he also suffered a flare of his Crohn's disease. He is admitted to home health with new medication for the Crohn's flare and to manage the seizure symptoms, for which no cause has been found.

Description	Code
Primary: Crohn's disease, unspecified, without complications	K50.90
Secondary: Unspecified convulsions	R56.9
Secondary: Unspecified dementia without behavioral disturbance	F03.90

As the focus of care, Crohn's is coded primary. Without an underlying diagnosis for the seizures, you must assign a symptom code. Remember, most symptom codes are unacceptable as primary diagnoses in PDGM. An additional code is assigned for the patient's diagnosis of dementia due to the impact of this diagnosis on the patient's prognosis and care plan.

Heart failure exacerbation, epistaxis from anticoagulant

A 70-year-old man is experiencing an acute exacerbation of chronic systolic heart failure. He also takes Coumadin for paroxysmal atrial fibrillation and began experiencing nosebleeds as an adverse effect from long-term use of the anticoagulant. He is still taking Coumadin.

Description	Code
Primary: Acute on chronic systolic (congestive) heart failure	I50.23
Secondary: Epistaxis	R04.0
Secondary: Adverse effect of anticoagulants, subsequent encounter	T45.515D
Secondary: Paroxysmal atrial fibrillation	I48.0
Secondary: Long term (current) use of anticoagulants	Z79.01

The acute heart failure exacerbation is the focus of care and is thus coded primary. Epistaxis, being caused by anticoagulant medication, is coded before the adverse effect of the drug code, in accordance with coding guidelines. The reason for the drug that caused the adverse effect, the paroxysmal atrial fibrillation, is assigned next. The patient's continued use of Coumadin is captured with Z79.01. Remember that most symptom codes cannot be a coded as the primary reason for home health under PDGM.

Nausea and vomiting from ibuprofen, rheumatoid arthritis

A 71-year-old woman is admitted to home health after being hospitalized for severe nausea and vomiting. It was determined that she took several 800-mg tablets of ibuprofen to manage joint pain caused by rheumatoid arthritis. The ibuprofen tablets had originally been prescribed for her daughter, with whom she lives. The patient thought they were the same as the over-the-counter Advil, which are 200-mg, she normally takes. She also suffers from mild hypertension.

Description	Code
Primary: Poisoning by propionic acid derivatives, accidental (unintentional), subsequent encounter	T39.311D
Secondary: Nausea with vomiting, unspecified	R11.2
Secondary: Rheumatoid arthritis, unspecified	M06.9
Secondary: Essential (primary) hypertension	I10

The patient took a medication that was prescribed for someone else and believed she was taking a smaller dose than what she actually was. Therefore, this scenario is a poisoning and the T code for the drug is coded before what it caused, the nausea and vomiting. The reason the patient was taking the ibuprofen, rheumatoid arthritis, is also coded. Since no further detail is provided, the unspecified code M06.9, must be used. Note that without more detail about which joints are affected and whether the diagnosis is seropositive, etc., a more specific rheumatoid arthritis code cannot be assigned. Her hypertension will require monitoring and thus it is coded.

Respiratory symptoms, COVID-19 ruled out

A 67-year-old female with a history of COPD presented to her physician's office with cough, persistent fever and shortness of breath. She reports that her sister was diagnosed with COVID-19 two-weeks ago and that she has had no contact since. Her physician's encounter notes report suspicion of COVID-19, however a PCR test for COVID-19 was negative. A chest X-ray was also inconclusive for all findings. Prophylactic oral antibiotic therapy was ordered for ten days, but no official cause of the fever was determined. Home health has been ordered to provide observation of her overall respiratory condition and instruct the patient in better managing her COPD to prevent complications.

Description	Code
Primary: Chronic obstructive pulmonary disease, unspecified	J44.9
Secondary: Fever, unspecified	R50.9
Secondary: Contact with and (suspected) exposure to COVID-19	Z20.822

This patient presented for vague respiratory symptoms with fever and COVID-19 was ruled out. The physician has indicated that home health should focus on COPD and general respiratory assessment, so COPD is coded first, followed by a symptom code for the unspecified fever, since no cause was identified. Z20.822 is additionally coded since the patient had a known COVID-19 exposure, despite testing negative for the virus.

Chapter 19: Injury, Poisoning and Certain Other Consequences of External Causes (S00-T88)

Chapter 19 includes injuries, organized by body part or site beginning with the head and concluding with the ankle and foot, rather than by categories of injury. Other blocks within this chapter include effects of foreign body entering through natural orifice; burns and corrosions; frostbite; poisoning by, adverse effect of and under-dosing of drugs, medicaments and biological substances; toxic effects of substances chiefly non-medicinal as to source; other and unspecified effects of external causes; certain early complications of trauma; and complications of surgical and medical care, not elsewhere classified.

This chapter is the largest in the ICD-10-CM manual and encompasses the S and T alpha characters. The S-section is used for coding different types of injuries related to single body regions and the T-section covers injuries to unspecified body regions as well as poisoning and certain other consequences of external causes.

Secondary code(s) from Chapter 20, External causes of morbidity, are used to indicate the cause of injury. Codes within the T section that include the external cause do not require an additional external cause code.

A note at the beginning of the chapter indicates an additional code should be used to identify any retained foreign body, if applicable (Z18.-)

Chapter 19 has an Excludes 1 note indicating that this chapter specifically excludes birth trauma, found in Chapter 16 (P10-P15) and obstetrical trauma found in Chapter 15 (O70-O71).

Application of 7th Characters

Most categories in Chapter 19 have a 7th character requirement for each applicable code. With the exception of fractures, most categories have one of three 7th character values: A for initial encounter; D for subsequent encounter; and S for sequela. Categories for traumatic fractures have additional 7th character values. In general, focus on whether the patient is ***still receiving active treatment*** for the condition described by the code title when you choose a seventh character that corresponds to either an "initial" or "subsequent" encounter, according to the Coding Clinic. Note, the physician must determine whether the patient is receiving active treatment or ongoing care for the condition.

More specifically:

- 7th character "A", initial encounter, is used while the patient is receiving active treatment for the condition. Examples of active treatment are: surgical treatment, emergency department encounter, and evaluation and treatment by a new physician. It doesn't matter if your agency isn't the first provider to see the patient for the condition, as long as your agency is providing active treatment for it, the seventh character "A" is what you should assign.

  Specifically, antibiotic therapy for infected post-operative wounds as well as wound vac treatment for trauma wounds or dehisced wounds are both examples of active treatment that should be coded with an "A," regardless of setting.
- 7th character "D", subsequent encounter, is used for encounters after the patient has received active treatment of the condition and is receiving routine care for the condition during the healing or recovery phase. Examples of subsequent care are: cast change or removal, removal of external or internal fixation device, medication adjustment, routine aftercare and fracture care with the exception of when the patient delays seeking treatment and it results in a malunion or nonunion, and follow up visits following treatment of the injury or condition. ***The aftercare Z codes should not be used for aftercare for conditions such as injuries or poisonings, where the 7th characters are provided to identify subsequent care.*** For example, for aftercare of an injury, assign the original injury code with the 7th character "D" (subsequent encounter). **Also note**, you will continue to assign the injury code for patient who underwent a joint replacement to treat a hip fracture. The aftercare code Z47.1 (Aftercare following joint replacement surgery) is ***not*** *appropriate* in these types of scenarios, according to Coding Clinic Q3 2016 guidance.
- 7th character "S", sequela, is used for complications or conditions that arise as a direct result of an injury, such as scar formation and skin contractures after a burn, traumatic arthritis and quadriplegia after a spinal cord injury. The scars are sequelae of the burn, traumatic arthritis and quadriplegia after a spinal cord injury. When using a 7th character "S", it is necessary to use both the injury code that precipitated the sequela and the code for the sequela itself. The "S" is added only to the injury code, not the sequela code. The 7th character "S" identifies the injury responsible for the sequela. The specific type of sequela (e.g., scar) is sequenced first, followed by the injury code.

Note: 7th characters D and S do not apply to codes in category S06 with 6th character 7 - death due to brain injury prior to regaining consciousness, or 8 - death due to other cause prior to regaining consciousness.

In general, scenarios involving complications in which the agency is providing continuing treatment, such as for infected and dehisced wounds, are the most appropriate for considering the assignment of an initial encounter seventh character.

Situations that aren't truly complicated, like routine fracture healing, routine aftercare or when a patient experiences a complication in the hospital that resolves prior to the home health admission, don't meet these criteria and shouldn't be coded as initial encounters.

Nevertheless, be aware that every code choice must be supportable and defensible.

Coding of Injuries

Codes for traumatic wounds are classified in different ways, which may overlap. Consider:

- Wounds may be open (e.g., lacerations, punctures, animal bites, fractures), superficial (e.g., insect bites, splinters, abrasions, skin tears), or open/internal (e.g., intracranial hematoma, organ rupture, fractures).
- Wounds may be described as with or without an opening into a cavity. Example: S31.604D, Subsequent encounter for care of an unspecified open wound of abdominal wall, left lower quadrant with penetration into peritoneal cavity.
- Wounds may be described as complicated or without mention of complication. A wound is considered complicated if there is delayed healing, presence of a foreign body in the wound, or an infection.

A common error made by new coders is reporting a code for an open wound (trauma) injury for surgical wound complications or other wounds, including ulcers, because the referral information referred to "**an open wound**" of a particular location rather than the type of wound.

Almost all amputations are the result of other medical conditions rather than accidents and are not coded with codes from Chapter 19 unless there are complications of the post-surgical amputation stump, such as dehiscence (T87.81), infection (T87.4-), necrosis (T85.5-) or neuroma (T87.3-).

When coding injuries, assign separate codes for each injury unless a combination code is provided, in which case the combination code is assigned. Code T07, unspecified multiple injuries, should **not** be used in the inpatient setting unless information for a more specific code is not available. Traumatic injury codes (S00-T14.9) are **not** to be used for normal, healing surgical wounds or to identify complications of surgical wounds. The code for the most serious injury, as determined by the provider and the focus of treatment, is sequenced first.

- Superficial injuries, such as abrasions or contusions, are not coded when associated with more severe injuries of the same site.
- When a primary injury results in damage to peripheral nerves or blood vessels, the primary injury is sequenced first with additional code(s) for injuries to the nerves and spinal cord (such as category S04), and/or injury to blood vessels (such as category S15). When the primary injury is to the blood vessels or nerves, that injury should be sequenced first.

Coding of Traumatic Fractures

The principles of multiple coding of injuries should be followed in coding fractures. Fractures of specific sites are coded individually by site in accordance with both the provisions within categories S02, S12, S22, S32, S42, S49, S52, S59, S62, S72, S79, S82, S89, S92 and the level of detail furnished by the medical record content. Multiple fractures are sequenced in accordance with the severity of the fracture.

Fracture codes require a great amount of specificity in order to code them accurately. Information that may be found in fracture codes includes the type of fracture (open or closed), specific anatomical site, whether the fracture is displaced or not, laterality, and healing status (i.e., routine healing versus delayed healing, nonunion or malunion). Laterality and identification of encounter type (initial, subsequent or sequela) are significant components of the code expansion.

A fracture not indicated as open or closed should be coded as closed. A fracture not indicated as displaced or not displaced should be coded as displaced.

More specific guidelines for traumatic fractures include:

- Traumatic fractures are coded using the appropriate 7th character for initial encounter (i.e., A, B, C) while receiving active treatment for the fracture. Examples of active treatment for the fracture are: surgical treatment, emergency department encounter, and evaluation and treatment by a new physician. The appropriate 7th character for initial encounter should also be assigned for a patient who delayed seeking treatment for the fracture or non-union. **Home health and hospice never use the 7th characters A, B or C when coding fractures.**
- In home health and hospice, fractures are coded using the appropriate 7th character for subsequent care for encounters after the patient has completed active treatment of the fracture and is receiving routine care for the fracture during the healing or recovery phase. Examples of fracture aftercare are: cast change or removal, removal of external or

Chapter 19

S00 - T88

internal fixation device, medication adjustment, and follow-up visits following fracture treatment.

- Care for complications of surgical treatment for fracture repairs during the healing or recovery phase should be coded with the appropriate complication codes.
- Care of complications of fractures, such as malunion and nonunion, should be reported with the appropriate 7th character for subsequent care with nonunion (i.e., K, M, N) or subsequent care with malunion (i.e., P, Q, R).
- Some fracture categories provide for 7th character extensions to designate the type of open fracture based on the Gustilo open fracture classification. Refer to the shaded box of 7th character extension definitions at the top of category S52, (fracture of upper end of ulna) for a listing of all 7th character extension codes as an example. ***Coders must pay special attention to the list of appropriate 7th character codes at the top of each category of fracture in Chapter 19 to select the most appropriate code.***

Some situations related to fractures are coded from chapters other than chapter 19 such as the following:

- A code from category M80 should be used for any patient with known osteoporosis who suffers a fracture, even if the patient had a minor fall or trauma, if that fall or trauma would not usually break a normal, healthy bone. (Refer to M80, Osteoporosis with current pathological fracture in Chapter 13, Diseases of Musculoskeletal System.)
- Refer to Chapter 13, Diseases of the Musculoskeletal System and Connective Tissue for codes related to stress fractures (M84.3-), pathological fractures (M84.5-) or collapsed vertebrae (M48.5-).
- The aftercare Z codes should **not** be used for aftercare for traumatic fractures. For aftercare of a traumatic fracture, assign the original (acute) fracture code with the appropriate 7th character.

Coding of Burns and Corrosions

ICD-10-CM makes a distinction between burns and corrosions. The burn codes are for thermal burns, except sunburns, that come from a heat source, such as a fire or hot appliance. The burn codes are also for burns resulting from electricity and radiation. Corrosions are burns due to chemicals. The guidelines are the same for burns and corrosions.

Current burns (T20-T25) are classified by depth, extent and by agent (X code). Burns are classified as first degree (erythema), second degree (blistering), and third degree (full-thickness involvement). Burns of the eye and internal organs (T26-T28) are classified by site, but not by degree.

Sequencing of burn and related condition codes

- Sequence first the code that reflects the highest degree of burn when more than one burn is present.
- When the reason for the admission or encounter is for treatment of multiple external burns, sequence first the code that reflects the burn of the highest degree.
- When the patient has both internal and external burns, the circumstances of admission govern the selection of the principal or first-listed diagnosis.
- When a patient is admitted for burn injuries and other related conditions, such as smoke inhalation and/or respiratory failure, the circumstances of admission govern the selection of the principal or first-listed diagnosis.
- Classify **burns of the same local site** (three character category level, T20-T28) but of different degrees to the subcategory identifying the highest degree recorded in the diagnosis.
- **Non-healing burns** are coded as acute burns.
- **Necrosis of burned skin** should be coded as a non-healing burn.
- For any documented **infected burn site**, use an additional code for the infection.
- Burns treated with **skin grafts** should be coded with the trauma codes for burns; and when applicable you can also code aftercare for transplant if you're also caring for the donor site (Z48.298).

Burns and corrosions Classified According to Extent of Body Surface Involved

Assign codes from category T31, Burns classified according to the extent of body surface involved, or T32, Corrosions classified to the extent of body surface involved, when the site of the burn is not specified or when there is a need for additional data. It is advisable to use category T31 as additional coding, when needed, to provide data for evaluating burn mortality, such as that needed by burn units. It also is advisable to use category T31 as an additional code for reporting purposes when there is mention of a third-degree burn involving 20% or more of the body surface.

Categories T31 and T32 are based on the classic "rule of nines" in estimating body surface: head and neck are assigned 9%, each arm 9%, each leg 18%, the anterior and posterior trunk 18% each, and genitalia 1%. Providers may change these percentage assignments where necessary to accommodate infants and children who have proportionately larger heads than adults, and adults who have large buttocks, thighs or abdomen that involve burns.

Coding sequela of burns

Encounters **for treatment of sequela** (late effects) of burns (i.e., scars or joint contractures) should be coded with the 7th character "S".

When appropriate, **both a code for a current burn or corrosion** with a 7th character of "D" and a burn or corrosion code with a 7th character "S" may be assigned on the same record (when both a current burn and a sequel of an old burn exist). Burns and corrosions do not heal at the same rate and a current healing wound may still exist with sequela of a healed burn or corrosion.

An **external cause code** should be used with burns and corrosions to identify the source and intent of the burn, as well as the place where it occurred.

Adverse Effects, Poisoning, Underdosing and Toxic Effects

Codes in categories T36-T65 are combination codes that include the substance that was taken as well as the intent. No additional external cause code is required for poisoning, toxic effects, adverse effects and underdosing codes.

- Do not code directly from the Table of Drugs and Chemicals. Always refer back to the Tabular List to confirm the correct code.
- Use as many codes as necessary to describe completely all drugs, medicinal or biological substances.
- If the same code would describe the causative agent for more than one adverse reaction, poisoning, toxic effect or underdosing, assign the code only once.
- If two or more drugs, medicinal or biological substances are reported, code each individually unless a combination code is listed in the Table of Drugs and Chemicals.

The occurrence of drug toxicity is classified in ICD-10-CM as follows:

Adverse Effect

When coding an adverse effect (hypersensitivity, reaction) of a drug that has been correctly prescribed and properly administered, assign the appropriate code for the nature of the adverse effect followed by the appropriate code for the adverse effect of the drug (T36-T50). The code for the drug should have a 5th or 6th character "5" (e.g., T36.0X5-). Examples of the nature of an adverse effect are tachycardia, delirium, gastrointestinal hemorrhaging, vomiting, hypokalemia, hepatitis, renal failure or respiratory failure.

Poisoning

When coding a poisoning or reaction to the improper use of a medication (e.g., overdose, wrong substance given or taken in error, wrong route of administration), first assign the appropriate code from categories T36-T50, followed by additional code(s) for all manifestations of the poisoning. The poisoning codes have an associated intent as their 5th or 6th character (accidental, intentional self-harm, assault, and undetermined). When no intent of poisoning is indicated, code to accidental. Undetermined intent is only used when there is specific documentation in the record that the intent of the poisoning cannot be determined.

If there is also a diagnosis of abuse or dependence of the substance, the abuse or dependence is assigned as an additional code.

Examples of poisoning include:

- **Error** was made in drug prescription or in the administration of the drug by provider, nurse, patient or other person.
- If an **overdose of a drug** was intentionally taken or administered and resulted in drug toxicity, it would be coded as a poisoning.
- **Nonprescription drug or medicinal agent taken in combination with a correctly prescribed** and properly administered drug, any drug toxicity or other reaction resulting from the interaction of the two drugs would be classified as a poisoning.
- When a reaction results from the **interaction of drug(s) and alcohol,** this would be classified as a poisoning.

Underdosing

Underdosing refers to taking less of a medication than is prescribed by the provider or as instructed by the manufacturer whether inadvertently or deliberately. For underdosing, a code from categories T36-T50 with a fifth or sixth character of "6" is used.

Use an additional code for underdosing intent such as patient's non-compliance with medical treatment and regimen (Z91.12-, Z91.13- or Z91.14) or failure in dosage during surgical and medical care (Y63.6-Y63.9). Reminder, the physician needs to confirm this occurrence.

Codes for underdosing should never be assigned as principal or first-listed codes. If a patient has a relapse or exacerbation of the medical condition for which the drug is prescribed because of the reduction in dose, then the medical condition itself should be coded.

Toxic Effects

A toxic effect is classified when a harmful substance is ingested or comes in contact with a person. Codes for the toxic effect of substances that are chiefly nonmedicinal as a source (T51-T65) include a 7th character to indicate the intention.

There are multiple notes at the top of this block of codes. One states to use an additional code for all associated manifestations of toxic effect, such as respiratory conditions due to external agents (J60-J70), personal history of foreign body fully removed (Z87.821) and to identify any retained foreign body, if applicable (Z18.-). The second instructional note states: when no intent is indicated, code to accidental. Undetermined intent is only for use when there is specific documentation in the record that the intent of the toxic effect cannot be determined.

Adult and child abuse, neglect and other maltreatment

Sequence first the appropriate code from categories T74.- (Adult and child abuse, neglect and other maltreatment, confirmed) or T76.- (Adult and child abuse, neglect and other maltreatment, unspecified) for any abuse, neglect and other maltreatment, followed by any accompanying mental health or injury code(s).

If the documentation in the medical record states abuse or neglect, it is coded as confirmed (T74.-). An external cause code from the assault section (X92-Y08) for the cause of any physical injuries and a perpetrator code (Y07) also should be added if the perpetrator of the abuse is known for cases of confirmed abuse or neglect.

If **suspected abuse and neglect** is documented in the medical record, the abuse or neglect is coded as suspected (T76.-) without an external cause or perpetrator code reported.

Complications of care

Code assignment for complications of care is ***based on the provider's documentation of the relationship between the condition and the care or procedure.*** This guideline applies to any complication of care, regardless of the chapter the code is located in. There must be a cause-and-effect relationship between the care provided and the condition, and an indication in the documentation that it is a complication. ***Reminder: Not all conditions that occur during or following medical care or surgery are classified as complications.***

Pain due to medical devices

Pain associated with devices, implants or grafts left in a surgical site is assigned to the appropriate code(s) found in Chapter 19. Specific codes for pain due to medical devices are found in the T code section of ICD-10-CM, according to type of device.

Use additional code(s) from category G89 to identify acute or chronic pain due to the presence of a device, implant or graft (G89.18 or G89.28). Example: a subsequent encounter for a painful hip prosthesis is coded T84.84xD. Additional pain codes are located in multiple body system chapters.

Transplant complications

Codes under category T86, Complications of transplanted organs and tissues, are used for both complications and rejection of transplanted organs. A transplant complication code is only assigned if the complication affects the function of the transplanted organ. Two codes are required to fully describe a transplant complication: the appropriate code from category T86 and a secondary code that identifies the complication.

Pre-existing conditions or conditions that develop after the transplant are not coded as complications unless they affect the function of the transplanted organs.

Patients who have undergone kidney transplant may still have some form of chronic kidney disease (CKD) because the kidney transplant may not fully restore kidney function. A code from T86.1- should be assigned for documented complications of a kidney transplant, such as a transplant failure or rejection or other transplant complication. A code from T86.1- should not be assigned for post kidney transplant patients who have chronic kidney disease (CKD) unless a transplant complication such as transplant failure or rejection is documented. If the documentation is unclear as to whether the patient has a complication of the transplant, query the provider.

Conditions that affect the function of the transplanted kidney, other than CKD, should be assigned a code from T86.1-, Complications of kidney transplant, and a secondary code that identifies the complication. For patients with CKD following a kidney transplant, but who do not have complications such as failure or rejection, refer to codes in category N18 for CKD stages.

Complication codes that include external cause

As with certain other T codes, some of the complications of care codes have the external cause included in the code. These combination codes include the nature of the complication as well as the type of procedure that caused the complication. No external cause code indicating the type of procedure is necessary for these codes.

Complications of care codes within body system chapters

Intraoperative and postprocedural complication codes are found within body system chapters with codes specific to the organs and structures to that body system. These codes should be sequenced first, followed by a code(s) for the specific complication, if applicable.

Codes for personal or family history of conditions that have been resolved related to injuries such as traumatic fractures, and other consequences are found in chapter 21, Factors influencing health status and contact with health services, rather than in Chapter 19. Some examples include: Z87.81, Personal history of healed traumatic fracture; and Personal history of abuse or neglect (childhood Z62.81- or adult Z91.41-).

Codes for complications of surgical and medical care not elsewhere classified include:

- **Complications following infusion, transfusion and therapeutic injection (e.g., T80.212-, Local infection due to central venous catheter)**
- **ABO, Rh and non-ABO incompatibility reactions due to transfusions of blood and blood products. Anaphylactic reaction due to serum, administration of blood and blood products, vaccine, and other serum (T80.3-T80.89).**
- **Complications of procedures, not elsewhere classified such as postprocedural shock (T81.1-T81.19); disruption of wound (T81.30-T81.33); infection following a procedure (T81.4-), with an additional code to identify infection and an additional code from R65.2- to identify severe sepsis, if applicable; and complications of foreign body accidentally left in the body (T81.5-, T81.6-)**
- Complications of cardiac and vascular prosthetic devices, implants and grafts (T82.-)
- Complications of genitourinary prosthetic devices, implants and grafts (T83.-), which includes complications of urinary catheters, cystostomy catheters, other urinary devices and implants, and complications related to prosthetic devices, implants and grafts of the genitourinary tract.
- Complications of internal orthopedic prosthetic devices, implants and grafts. (T84.-).
- Complications of other internal prosthetic devices, implants and grafts. (T85.-)
- Complications of transplanted organs and tissues (T86.-).
- Complications peculiar to reattachment and amputation (T87.-)
- Other complications of surgical and medical care, not elsewhere classified (T88.-).

Complications involving stoma may be reported elsewhere. For example, a tracheostomy complication is reported using a code from J95.0- in Chapter 10. A complication of an esophagostomy, colostomy or enterostomy is reported using a code from K94.- from Chapter 11.

Special Coding Issues

Wounds

Many wounds in the Medicare home care population are the intentional result of medical treatment. Coding surgical wounds and medical amputations using Chapter 19 open wound codes is a mistake because those codes are reserved for injuries (from accidents or violence). Medically-caused wounds should not be coded from Chapter 19, unless they are complicated. Even then, they should never be coded as open wounds. If there is a complication of a surgery, a code from Chapter 19 will be used instead of the Z code for aftercare. The term "complication" should be referenced in the Volume 2 Alphabetic Index. Once the term "complication" is found, reference the type of complication, such as infection or mechanical, to find the correct code.

Superficial injuries

Skin tears or partial thickness wounds are typically superficial, and may only require first aid and therefore the care is not considered skilled. In ICD-10-CM, the coder would reference "tear" in the Alphabetic Index. The term "tear" indicates to code laceration. Laceration indicates a trauma wound. The real question with coding of a skin tear is not how to code it, but whether to code it at all. Care for skin tears is typically not covered by Medicare because the wound care is simple. In that case the skin tear is not coded. If the skin tear is complicated in some way – the tear no longer has a flap and is infected or there is an underlying condition that is complicating the wound's healing – then you may consider coding the skin tear as a laceration. Coding the laceration as primary will place the claim into the wound grouper so ensure the skin tear is really the focus of care, that skilled care is being provided, and that documentation supports the coding. Most often the care of the skin tear is incidental to other skilled care and would be coded as a secondary diagnosis. Lacerations do not provide any comorbidity adjustment. Consult your specific MAC's instructions for coding skin tears that require skilled care.

Infection/complication coding

Occasionally, a post-surgical infection or other surgical complication code may be appropriate. OASIS requires that home care clinicians use the WOCN guidelines to indicate the status of the surgical wound. "Not healing" includes signs and symptoms of infection and delayed healing. If there are signs and symptoms of infection, do not use the aftercare code for that surgery. The aftercare code is indicated only for routine, uncomplicated care. Subcategory T81.4- codes are commonly used for a post-surgical infection; however, some post-operative infections have more

Chapter 19

S00 - T88

specific codes, such as infected amputation, which is coded with T87.4-. Reference the Alphabetic Index to find the most specific code.

The T81.4- subcategory allows coders to report the depth of the infection. There are codes to specify whether the surgical wound infection is affecting the superficial incision surgical site (T81.41-), the deep incisional surgical site (T81.42-) or the organ and space surgical site (T81.43-). Other surgical site and unspecified options are also available (T81.49- and T81.40-). Each of these codes requires a seventh character: "A," "D" or "S." Also, make note of the inclusion terms at each code, such as "subcutaneous abscess following a procedure," to help guide the appropriate code choice.

When a patient is admitted to home care primarily for **surgical wound assessment and treatment**, the presence of a surgical drain is not a complication; it is a normal part of care for some surgical wounds. Care of surgical drains is included in the aftercare code for routine surgical care. If care includes removal or changing of the surgical drain, use Z48.03.

What counts as a wound?

A **lesion** is a broad term used to describe an area of pathologically altered tissue. Sores, ulcers, rashes, crusts, edema, trauma wounds, etc. are all considered lesions.

The **port-a-cath or mediport site** is considered a surgical wound as long as it is present, even if healed over. Implanted infusion devices or venous access devices are considered surgical wounds, and it does not matter whether the device is accessed with any particular frequency. Only **central venous catheters** are considered surgical wounds. Care of the uncomplicated venous or arterial line is coded Z45.2, Adjustment and management of a vascular catheter. Subsequent encounter to care for a bloodstream infection due to central venous catheter is coded T80.211D. Local infection at the exit or insertion site due to central venous catheter is coded with T80.212D, but central line associated infections (including PICC lines) are coded to T80.218D.

Extravasation or infiltration of a vesicant agent into surrounding tissue is a more serious complication of IV therapy and is coded to T80.810 if related to the administration of vesicant antineoplastic chemotherapy or T80.818 if there is extravasation of another vesicant agent.

CHAPTER 19: INJURY, POISONING AND CERTAIN OTHER CONSEQUENCES OF EXTERNAL CAUSES (S00-T88)

Note:
Use secondary code(s) from Chapter 20, External causes of morbidity, to indicate cause of injury. Codes within the T section that include the external cause do not require an additional external cause code
The chapter uses the S-section for coding different types of injuries related to single body regions and the T-section to cover injuries to unspecified body regions as well as poisoning and certain other consequences of external causes.
Use additional code to identify any retained foreign body, if applicable (Z18.-)

EXCLUDES 1 birth trauma (P10-P15)
obstetric trauma (O70-O71)

GUIDELINES **Section I.C.19.a**
Most categories in chapter 19 have a 7th character requirement for each applicable code ... While the patient may be seen by a new or different provider over the course of treatment for an injury, assignment of the 7th character is based on whether the patient is undergoing active treatment and not whether the provider is seeing the patient for the first time ... 7th character "D" subsequent encounter is used for encounters after the patient has completed active treatment of the condition and is receiving routine care for the condition during the healing or recovery phase.

The aftercare Z codes should not be used for aftercare for conditions such as injuries or poisonings, where 7th characters are provided to identify subsequent care. For example, for aftercare of an injury, assign the acute injury code with the 7th character "D" (subsequent encounter).

7th character "S", sequela, is for use for complications or conditions that arise as a direct result of a condition, such as scar formation after a burn. The scars are sequelae of the burn. When using 7th character "S", it is necessary to use both the injury code that precipitated the sequela and the code for the sequela itself. The "S" is added only to the injury code, not the sequela code. The 7th character "S" identifies the injury responsible for the sequela. The specific type of sequela (e.g. scar) is sequenced first, followed by the injury code.

CODING TIPS✓ 7th character A is acceptable in home health and hospice when active treatment is provided, such as antibiotics for an infected wound or a wound vac for a dehisced wound. D is used when the complication or injury is now healing. Think of D as aftercare. S is used for sequela of the injury or complication. Sequela is a residual deficit or condition produced as a result of the injury or complication after the original injury or complication has healed.

This chapter contains the following blocks:

S00-S09	Injuries to the head
S10-S19	Injuries to the neck
S20-S29	Injuries to the thorax
S30-S39	Injuries to the abdomen, lower back, lumbar spine, pelvis and external genitals
S40-S49	Injuries to the shoulder and upper arm
S50-S59	Injuries to the elbow and forearm
S60-S69	Injuries to the wrist, hand and fingers
S70-S79	Injuries to the hip and thigh
S80-S89	Injuries to the knee and lower leg
S90-S99	Injuries to the ankle and foot
T07	Injuries involving multiple body regions
T14	Injury of unspecified body region
T15-T19	Effects of foreign body entering through natural orifice
T20-T25	Burns and corrosions of external body surface, specified by site
T26-T28	Burns and corrosions confined to eye and internal organs
T30-T32	Burns and corrosions of multiple and unspecified body regions
T33-T34	Frostbite
T36-T50	Poisoning by, adverse effect of and underdosing of drugs, medicaments and biological substances
T51-T65	Toxic effects of substances chiefly nonmedicinal as to source
T66-T78	Other and unspecified effects of external causes
T79	Certain early complications of trauma
T80-T88	Complications of surgical and medical care, not elsewhere classified

Injuries to the head (S00-S09)

INCLUDES injuries of ear
injuries of eye
injuries of face [any part]
injuries of gum
injuries of jaw
injuries of oral cavity
injuries of palate
injuries of periocular area
injuries of scalp
injuries of temporomandibular joint area
injuries of tongue
injuries of tooth

Code also:
for any associated infection

EXCLUDES 2 burns and corrosions (T20-T32)
effects of foreign body in ear (T16)
effects of foreign body in larynx (T17.3)
effects of foreign body in mouth NOS (T18.0)
effects of foreign body in nose (T17.0-T17.1)
effects of foreign body in pharynx (T17.2)
effects of foreign body on external eye (T15.-)
frostbite (T33-T34)
insect bite or sting, venomous (T63.4)

GUIDELINES **Section I.C.19.c.2)**
Multiple fractures are sequenced in accordance with the severity of the fracture.

GUIDELINES **Section I.C.19.b.1)-2)**
When coding injuries, assign separate codes for each injury unless a combination code is provided, in which case the combination code is assigned ... Traumatic injury codes (S00-T14.9) are not to be used for normal, healing surgical wounds or to identify complications of surgical wounds. The code for the most serious injury, as determined by the provider and the focus of treatment, is sequenced first.

1) Superficial injuries such as abrasions or contusions are not coded when associated with more severe injuries of the same site.

2) When a primary injury results in minor damage to peripheral nerves or blood vessels, the primary injury is sequenced first with additional code(s) for injuries to nerves and spinal cord (such as category S04), and/or injury to blood vessels (such as category S15). When the primary injury is to the blood vessels or nerves, that injury should be sequenced first.

Chapter 19
S00-T88

GUIDELINES **Section I.C.19.c**

Coding of Traumatic Fractures: The principles of multiple coding of injuries should be followed in coding fractures. Fractures of specified sites are coded individually by site in accordance with both the provisions within categories S02, S12, S22, S32, S42, S49, S52, S59, S62, S72, S79, S82, S89, S92 and the level of detail furnished by medical record content. A fracture not indicated as open or closed should be coded to closed. A fracture not indicated whether displaced or not displaced should be coded to displaced.

CODING TIPS✓ 7th character A is acceptable in home health and hospice when active treatment is provided, such as antibiotics for an infected wound or a wound vac for a dehisced wound. D is used when the complication or injury is now healing. Think of D as aftercare. S is used for sequela of the injury or complication. Sequela is a residual deficit or condition produced as a result of the injury or complication after the original injury or complication has healed.

4 **S00 Superficial injury of head**

EXCLUDES 1 diffuse cerebral contusion (S06.2-)
focal cerebral contusion (S06.3-)
injury of eye and orbit (S05.-)
open wound of head (S01.-)

The appropriate 7th character is to be added to each code from category S00
A initial encounter
D subsequent encounter
S sequela

5 **S00.0 Superficial injury of scalp**

IQ 7 **S00.00X- Unspecified superficial injury of scalp**

IQ 7 **S00.01X- Abrasion of scalp**

IQ 7 **S00.02X- Blister (nonthermal) of scalp**

IQ 7 **S00.03X- Contusion of scalp**
Bruise of scalp
Hematoma of scalp

IQ 7 **S00.04X- External constriction of part of scalp**

IQ 7 **S00.05X- Superficial foreign body of scalp**
Splinter in the scalp

IQ 7 **S00.06X- Insect bite (nonvenomous) of scalp**

IQ 7 **S00.07X- Other superficial bite of scalp**
EXCLUDES 1 open bite of scalp (S01.05)

▲ 5 **S00.1 Contusion of eyelid and periocular area**
Black eye
EXCLUDES 2 contusion of eyeball and orbital tissues (S05.1-)

H IQ 7 **S00.10X- Contusion of unspecified eyelid and periocular area**

H IQ 7 **S00.11X- Contusion of right eyelid and periocular area**

H IQ 7 **S00.12X- Contusion of left eyelid and periocular area**

5 **S00.2 Other and unspecified superficial injuries of eyelid and periocular area**
EXCLUDES 2 superficial injury of conjunctiva and cornea (S05.0-)

6 **S00.20 Unspecified superficial injury of eyelid and periocular area**

H IQ 7 **S00.201- Unspecified superficial injury of right eyelid and periocular area**

H IQ 7 **S00.202- Unspecified superficial injury of left eyelid and periocular area**

H IQ 7 **S00.209- Unspecified superficial injury of unspecified eyelid and periocular area**

6 **S00.21 Abrasion of eyelid and periocular area**

H IQ 7 **S00.211- Abrasion of right eyelid and periocular area**

H IQ 7 **S00.212- Abrasion of left eyelid and periocular area**

H IQ 7 **S00.219- Abrasion of unspecified eyelid and periocular area**

6 **S00.22 Blister (nonthermal) of eyelid and periocular area**

H IQ 7 **S00.221- Blister (nonthermal) of right eyelid and periocular area**

H IQ 7 **S00.222- Blister (nonthermal) of left eyelid and periocular area**

H IQ 7 **S00.229- Blister (nonthermal) of unspecified eyelid and periocular area**

6 **S00.24 External constriction of eyelid and periocular area**

H IQ 7 **S00.241- External constriction of right eyelid and periocular area**

H IQ 7 **S00.242- External constriction of left eyelid and periocular area**

H IQ 7 **S00.249- External constriction of unspecified eyelid and periocular area**

6 **S00.25 Superficial foreign body of eyelid and periocular area**
Splinter of eyelid and periocular area
EXCLUDES 2 retained foreign body in eyelid (H02.81-)

H IQ 7 **S00.251- Superficial foreign body of right eyelid and periocular area**

H IQ 7 **S00.252- Superficial foreign body of left eyelid and periocular area**

H IQ 7 **S00.259- Superficial foreign body of unspecified eyelid and periocular area**

6 **S00.26 Insect bite (nonvenomous) of eyelid and periocular area**

H IQ 7 **S00.261- Insect bite (nonvenomous) of right eyelid and periocular area**

H IQ 7 **S00.262- Insect bite (nonvenomous) of left eyelid and periocular area**

H IQ 7 **S00.269- Insect bite (nonvenomous) of unspecified eyelid and periocular area**

6 **S00.27 Other superficial bite of eyelid and periocular area**
EXCLUDES 1 open bite of eyelid and periocular area (S01.15)

H IQ 7 **S00.271- Other superficial bite of right eyelid and periocular area**

H IQ 7 **S00.272- Other superficial bite of left eyelid and periocular area**

H IQ 7 **S00.279- Other superficial bite of unspecified eyelid and periocular area**

S00.3 Superficial injury of nose

S00.30X- Unspecified superficial injury of nose

S00.31X- Abrasion of nose

S00.32X- Blister (nonthermal) of nose

S00.33X- Contusion of nose
Bruise of nose
Hematoma of nose

S00.34X- External constriction of nose

S00.35X- Superficial foreign body of nose
Splinter in the nose

S00.36X- Insect bite (nonvenomous) of nose

S00.37X- Other superficial bite of nose
EXCLUDES 1 open bite of nose (S01.25)

S00.4 Superficial injury of ear

S00.40 Unspecified superficial injury of ear

S00.401- Unspecified superficial injury of right ear

S00.402- Unspecified superficial injury of left ear

S00.409- Unspecified superficial injury of unspecified ear

S00.41 Abrasion of ear

S00.411- Abrasion of right ear

S00.412- Abrasion of left ear

S00.419- Abrasion of unspecified ear

S00.42 Blister (nonthermal) of ear

S00.421- Blister (nonthermal) of right ear

S00.422- Blister (nonthermal) of left ear

S00.429- Blister (nonthermal) of unspecified ear

S00.43 Contusion of ear
Bruise of ear
Hematoma of ear

S00.431- Contusion of right ear

S00.432- Contusion of left ear

S00.439- Contusion of unspecified ear

S00.44 External constriction of ear

S00.441- External constriction of right ear

S00.442- External constriction of left ear

S00.449- External constriction of unspecified ear

S00.45 Superficial foreign body of ear
Splinter in the ear

S00.451- Superficial foreign body of right ear

S00.452- Superficial foreign body of left ear

S00.459- Superficial foreign body of unspecified ear

S00.46 Insect bite (nonvenomous) of ear

S00.461- Insect bite (nonvenomous) of right ear

S00.462- Insect bite (nonvenomous) of left ear

S00.469- Insect bite (nonvenomous) of unspecified ear

S00.47 Other superficial bite of ear
EXCLUDES 1 open bite of ear (S01.35)

S00.471- Other superficial bite of right ear

S00.472- Other superficial bite of left ear

S00.479- Other superficial bite of unspecified ear

S00.5 Superficial injury of lip and oral cavity

S00.50 Unspecified superficial injury of lip and oral cavity

S00.501- Unspecified superficial injury of lip

S00.502- Unspecified superficial injury of oral cavity

S00.51 Abrasion of lip and oral cavity

S00.511- Abrasion of lip

S00.512- Abrasion of oral cavity

S00.52 Blister (nonthermal) of lip and oral cavity

S00.521- Blister (nonthermal) of lip

S00.522- Blister (nonthermal) of oral cavity

S00.53 Contusion of lip and oral cavity

S00.531- Contusion of lip
Bruise of lip
Hematoma of lip

S00.532- Contusion of oral cavity
Bruise of oral cavity
Hematoma of oral cavity

S00.54 External constriction of lip and oral cavity

S00.541- External constriction of lip

S00.542- External constriction of oral cavity

S00.55 Superficial foreign body of lip and oral cavity

S00.551- Superficial foreign body of lip
Splinter of lip and oral cavity

S00.552- Superficial foreign body of oral cavity
Splinter of lip and oral cavity

S00.56 Insect bite (nonvenomous) of lip and oral cavity

S00.561- Insect bite (nonvenomous) of lip

S00.562- Insect bite (nonvenomous) of oral cavity

S00.57 Other superficial bite of lip and oral cavity

S00.571- Other superficial bite of lip
EXCLUDES 1 open bite of lip (S01.551)

S00.572- Other superficial bite of oral cavity
EXCLUDES 1 open bite of oral cavity (S01.552)

S00.8 Superficial injury of other parts of head
Superficial injuries of face [any part]

S00.80X- Unspecified superficial injury of other part of head

S00.81X- Abrasion of other part of head

S00.82X- Blister (nonthermal) of other part of head

S00.83X- Contusion of other part of head
Bruise of other part of head
Hematoma of other part of head

S00.84X- External constriction of other part of head

S00.85X- Superficial foreign body of other part of head

Splinter in other part of head

IQ 7 S00.86X- **Insect bite (nonvenomous) of other part of head**

IQ 7 S00.87X- **Other superficial bite of other part of head**

EXCLUDES 1 open bite of other part of head (S01.85)

5 S00.9 **Superficial injury of unspecified part of head**

IQ 7 S00.90X- **Unspecified superficial injury of unspecified part of head**

IQ 7 S00.91X- **Abrasion of unspecified part of head**

IQ 7 S00.92X- **Blister (nonthermal) of unspecified part of head**

IQ 7 S00.93X- **Contusion of unspecified part of head**

Bruise of head
Hematoma of head

IQ 7 S00.94X- **External constriction of unspecified part of head**

IQ 7 S00.95X- **Superficial foreign body of unspecified part of head**

Splinter of head

IQ 7 S00.96X- **Insect bite (nonvenomous) of unspecified part of head**

IQ 7 S00.97X- **Other superficial bite of unspecified part of head**

EXCLUDES 1 open bite of head (S01.95)

4 S01 **Open wound of head**

Code also any associated:
- injury of cranial nerve (S04.-)
- injury of muscle and tendon of head (S09.1-)
- intracranial injury (S06.-)
- wound infection

EXCLUDES 1 open skull fracture (S02.- with 7th character B)

EXCLUDES 2 injury of eye and orbit (S05.-)
traumatic amputation of part of head (S08.-)

The appropriate 7th character is to be added to each code from category S01
- A initial encounter
- D subsequent encounter
- S sequela

CODING TIPS✓ Open wound codes are used for wounds caused by trauma. Do not assign a code for "open wound" unless the etiology of the wound is related to trauma. Do not use Z codes for any aspect of care of a trauma wound, e.g. no Z code for dressing changes, drain care, or suture removal.

CODING TIPS✓ No aftercare code applies. The 7th character "D" is the default for home care and hospice when providing aftercare for a healing or resolving condition; "A" is used for active treatment such as antibiotics or more than routine wound care; "S" may be used to indicate a residual condition after the original injury has healed.

▲ 5 S01.0 **Open wound of scalp**

EXCLUDES 1 avulsion of scalp (S08.0-)

SP 7 S01.00X- **Unspecified open wound of scalp**

SP 7 S01.01X- **Laceration without foreign body of scalp**

SP 7 S01.02X- **Laceration with foreign body of scalp**

SP 7 S01.03X- **Puncture wound without foreign body of scalp**

SP 7 S01.04X- **Puncture wound with foreign body of scalp**

SP 7 S01.05X- **Open bite of scalp**

Bite of scalp NOS

EXCLUDES 1 superficial bite of scalp (S00.06, S00.07-)

5 S01.1 **Open wound of eyelid and periocular area**

Open wound of eyelid and periocular area with or without involvement of lacrimal passages

6 S01.10 **Unspecified open wound of eyelid and periocular area**

H SP 7 S01.101- **Unspecified open wound of right eyelid and periocular area**

H SP 7 S01.102- **Unspecified open wound of left eyelid and periocular area**

H IQ 7 S01.109- **Unspecified open wound of unspecified eyelid and periocular area**

6 S01.11 **Laceration without foreign body of eyelid and periocular area**

H SP 7 S01.111- **Laceration without foreign body of right eyelid and periocular area**

H SP 7 S01.112- **Laceration without foreign body of left eyelid and periocular area**

H IQ 7 S01.119- **Laceration without foreign body of unspecified eyelid and periocular area**

6 S01.12 **Laceration with foreign body of eyelid and periocular area**

H SP 7 S01.121- **Laceration with foreign body of right eyelid and periocular area**

H SP 7 S01.122- **Laceration with foreign body of left eyelid and periocular area**

H IQ 7 S01.129- **Laceration with foreign body of unspecified eyelid and periocular area**

6 S01.13 **Puncture wound without foreign body of eyelid and periocular area**

H SP 7 S01.131- **Puncture wound without foreign body of right eyelid and periocular area**

H SP 7 S01.132- **Puncture wound without foreign body of left eyelid and periocular area**

H IQ 7 S01.139- **Puncture wound without foreign body of unspecified eyelid and periocular area**

6 S01.14 **Puncture wound with foreign body of eyelid and periocular area**

H SP 7 S01.141- **Puncture wound with foreign body of right eyelid and periocular area**

H SP 7 S01.142- **Puncture wound with foreign body of left eyelid and periocular area**

S01.149- **Puncture wound with foreign body of unspecified eyelid and periocular area**

S01.15 **Open bite of eyelid and periocular area**
Bite of eyelid and periocular area NOS
EXCLUDES 1 superficial bite of eyelid and periocular area (S00.26, S00.27)

S01.151- **Open bite of right eyelid and periocular area**

S01.152- **Open bite of left eyelid and periocular area**

S01.159- **Open bite of unspecified eyelid and periocular area**

S01.2 **Open wound of nose**

S01.20X- **Unspecified open wound of nose**

S01.21X- **Laceration without foreign body of nose**

S01.22X- **Laceration with foreign body of nose**

S01.23X- **Puncture wound without foreign body of nose**

S01.24X- **Puncture wound with foreign body of nose**

S01.25X- **Open bite of nose**
Bite of nose NOS
EXCLUDES 1 superficial bite of nose (S00.36, S00.37)

S01.3 **Open wound of ear**

S01.30 **Unspecified open wound of ear**

S01.301- **Unspecified open wound of right ear**

S01.302- **Unspecified open wound of left ear**

S01.309- **Unspecified open wound of unspecified ear**

S01.31 **Laceration without foreign body of ear**

S01.311- **Laceration without foreign body of right ear**

S01.312- **Laceration without foreign body of left ear**

S01.319- **Laceration without foreign body of unspecified ear**

S01.32 **Laceration with foreign body of ear**

S01.321- **Laceration with foreign body of right ear**

S01.322- **Laceration with foreign body of left ear**

S01.329- **Laceration with foreign body of unspecified ear**

S01.33 **Puncture wound without foreign body of ear**

S01.331- **Puncture wound without foreign body of right ear**

S01.332- **Puncture wound without foreign body of left ear**

S01.339- **Puncture wound without foreign body of unspecified ear**

S01.34 **Puncture wound with foreign body of ear**

S01.341- **Puncture wound with foreign body of right ear**

S01.342- **Puncture wound with foreign body of left ear**

S01.349- **Puncture wound with foreign body of unspecified ear**

S01.35 **Open bite of ear**
Bite of ear NOS
EXCLUDES 1 superficial bite of ear (S00.46, S00.47)

S01.351- **Open bite of right ear**

S01.352- **Open bite of left ear**

S01.359- **Open bite of unspecified ear**

S01.4 **Open wound of cheek and temporomandibular area**

S01.40 **Unspecified open wound of cheek and temporomandibular area**

S01.401- **Unspecified open wound of right cheek and temporomandibular area**

S01.402- **Unspecified open wound of left cheek and temporomandibular area**

S01.409- **Unspecified open wound of unspecified cheek and temporomandibular area**

S01.41 **Laceration without foreign body of cheek and temporomandibular area**

S01.411- **Laceration without foreign body of right cheek and temporomandibular area**

S01.412- **Laceration without foreign body of left cheek and temporomandibular area**

S01.419- **Laceration without foreign body of unspecified cheek and temporomandibular area**

S01.42 **Laceration with foreign body of cheek and temporomandibular area**

S01.421- **Laceration with foreign body of right cheek and temporomandibular area**

S01.422- **Laceration with foreign body of left cheek and temporomandibular area**

S01.429- **Laceration with foreign body of unspecified cheek and temporomandibular area**

S01.43 **Puncture wound without foreign body of cheek and temporomandibular area**

S01.431- **Puncture wound without foreign body of right cheek and temporomandibular area**

S01.432- **Puncture wound without foreign body of left cheek and temporomandibular area**

S01.439- **Puncture wound without foreign body of unspecified cheek and temporomandibular area**

S01.44 **Puncture wound with foreign body of cheek and temporomandibular area**

S01.441- **Puncture wound with foreign body of right cheek and temporomandibular area**

S01.442- **Puncture wound with foreign body of left cheek and temporomandibular area**

S01.449- **Puncture wound with foreign body of unspecified cheek and temporomandibular area**

S01.45 **Open bite of cheek and temporomandibular area**
Bite of cheek and temporomandibular area NOS
EXCLUDES 2 superficial bite of cheek and temporomandibular area (S00.86, S00.87)

S01.451- **Open bite of right cheek and temporomandibular area**

S01.452- **Open bite of left cheek and temporomandibular area**

S01.459- **Open bite of unspecified cheek and temporomandibular area**

S01.5 **Open wound of lip and oral cavity**
EXCLUDES 2 tooth dislocation (S03.2)
tooth fracture (S02.5)

S01.50 **Unspecified open wound of lip and oral cavity**

S01.501- **Unspecified open wound of lip**

S01.502- **Unspecified open wound of oral cavity**

S01.51 **Laceration of lip and oral cavity without foreign body**

S01.511- **Laceration without foreign body of lip**

S01.512- **Laceration without foreign body of oral cavity**

S01.52 **Laceration of lip and oral cavity with foreign body**

S01.521- **Laceration with foreign body of lip**

S01.522- **Laceration with foreign body of oral cavity**

S01.53 **Puncture wound of lip and oral cavity without foreign body**

S01.531- **Puncture wound without foreign body of lip**

S01.532- **Puncture wound without foreign body of oral cavity**

S01.54 **Puncture wound of lip and oral cavity with foreign body**

S01.541- **Puncture wound with foreign body of lip**

S01.542- **Puncture wound with foreign body of oral cavity**

S01.55 **Open bite of lip and oral cavity**

S01.551- **Open bite of lip**
Bite of lip NOS
EXCLUDES 1 superficial bite of lip (S00.571)

S01.552- **Open bite of oral cavity**
Bite of oral cavity NOS
EXCLUDES 1 superficial bite of oral cavity (S00.572)

S01.8 **Open wound of other parts of head**

S01.80X- **Unspecified open wound of other part of head**

S01.81X- **Laceration without foreign body of other part of head**

S01.82X- **Laceration with foreign body of other part of head**

S01.83X- **Puncture wound without foreign body of other part of head**

S01.84X- **Puncture wound with foreign body of other part of head**

S01.85X- **Open bite of other part of head**
Bite of other part of head NOS
EXCLUDES 1 superficial bite of other part of head (S00.87)

S01.9 **Open wound of unspecified part of head**

S01.90X- **Unspecified open wound of unspecified part of head**

S01.91X- **Laceration without foreign body of unspecified part of head**

S01.92X- **Laceration with foreign body of unspecified part of head**

S01.93X- **Puncture wound without foreign body of unspecified part of head**

S01.94X- **Puncture wound with foreign body of unspecified part of head**

S01.95X- **Open bite of unspecified part of head**
Bite of head NOS
EXCLUDES 1 superficial bite of head NOS (S00.97)

S02 **Fracture of skull and facial bones**
Note:
A fracture not indicated as open or closed should be coded to closed
Code also:
any associated intracranial injury (S06.-)

The appropriate 7th character is to be added to each code from category S02

A	initial encounter for closed fracture
B	initial encounter for open fracture
D	subsequent encounter for fracture with routine healing
G	subsequent encounter for fracture with delayed healing
K	subsequent encounter for fracture with nonunion
S	sequela

CODING TIPS ✓ Fractures are not coded with aftercare codes. Displaced and closed are default choices when documentation is absent. "D" is the 7th character for home care and hospice unless the physician or NPP has documented delayed healing, nonunion or malunion. A sequela is a condition left after the fracture has healed.

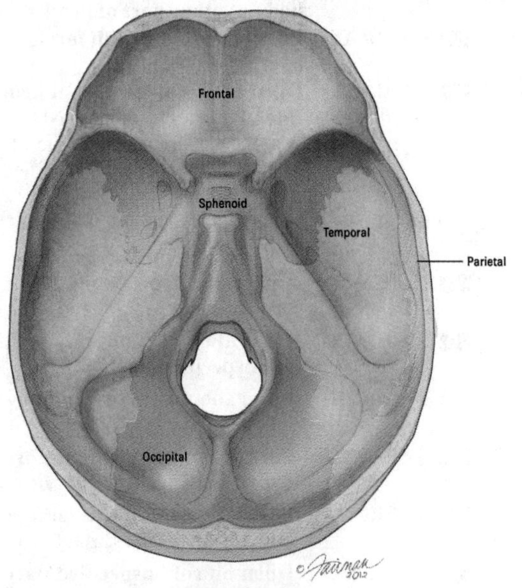

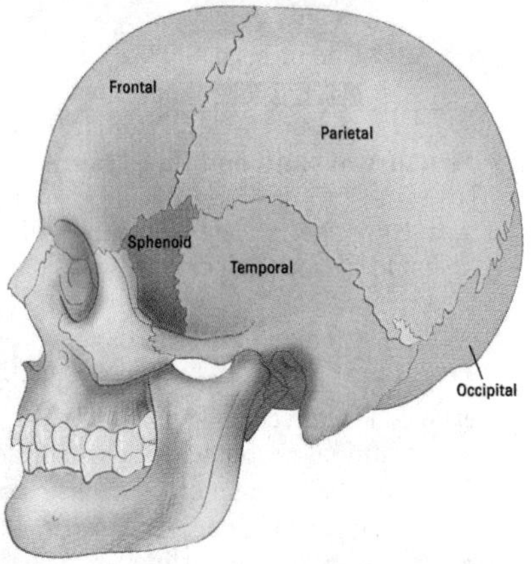

SP 7 S02.0XX- **Fracture of vault of skull**
Fracture of frontal bone
Fracture of parietal bone

5 S02.1 **Fracture of base of skull**
EXCLUDES 2 lateral orbital wall (S02.84-)
medial orbital wall (S02.83-)
orbital floor (S02.3-)

6 S02.10 **Unspecified fracture of base of skull**

Laterality SP 7 S02.101- **Fracture of base of skull, right side**

Laterality SP 7 S02.102- **Fracture of base of skull, left side**

Laterality !Q 7 S02.109- **Fracture of base of skull, unspecified side**

6 S02.11 **Fracture of occiput**

!Q 7 S02.110- **Type I occipital condyle fracture, unspecified side**

!Q 7 S02.111- **Type II occipital condyle fracture, unspecified side**

!Q 7 S02.112- **Type III occipital condyle fracture, unspecified side**

SP 7 S02.113- **Unspecified occipital condyle fracture**

!Q 7 S02.118- **Other fracture of occiput, unspecified side**

SP 7 S02.119- **Unspecified fracture of occiput**

Laterality SP 7 S02.11A- **Type I occipital condyle fracture, right side**

Laterality SP 7 S02.11B- **Type I occipital condyle fracture, left side**

Laterality SP 7 S02.11C- **Type II occipital condyle fracture, right side**

Laterality SP 7 S02.11D- **Type II occipital condyle fracture, left side**

Laterality SP 7 S02.11E- **Type III occipital condyle fracture, right side**

Laterality SP 7 S02.11F- **Type III occipital condyle fracture, left side**

Laterality SP 7 S02.11G- **Other fracture of occiput, right side**

Laterality SP 7 S02.11H- **Other fracture of occiput, left side**

6 S02.12 **Fracture of orbital roof**
CODING TIPS✓ Orbital fractures may be defined in terms of anatomic location, including isolated fractures of the orbital floor, medial wall, temporal wall, and roof. These fractures are commonly seen with midfacial trauma.

Laterality SP 7 S02.121- **Fracture of orbital roof, right side**

Laterality SP 7 S02.122- **Fracture of orbital roof, left side**

Laterality 7 S02.129- **Fracture of orbital roof, unspecified side**

SP 7 S02.19X- **Other fracture of base of skull**
Fracture of anterior fossa of base of skull
Fracture of ethmoid sinus
Fracture of frontal sinus
Fracture of middle fossa of base of skull
Fracture of posterior fossa of base of skull
Fracture of sphenoid
Fracture of temporal bone

SP 7 S02.2XX- **Fracture of nasal bones**

5 S02.3 **Fracture of orbital floor**
Fracture of inferior orbital wall
EXCLUDES 1 orbit NOS (S02.85)
EXCLUDES 2 lateral orbital wall (S02.84-)
medial orbital wall (S02.83-)
orbital roof (S02.1-)

Laterality !Q 7 S02.30X- **Fracture of orbital floor, unspecified side**

Laterality SP 7 S02.31X- **Fracture of orbital floor, right side**

Laterality SP 7 S02.32X- **Fracture of orbital floor, left side**

5 S02.4 **Fracture of malar, maxillary and zygoma bones**
Fracture of superior maxilla
Fracture of upper jaw (bone)
Fracture of zygomatic process of temporal bone

6 S02.40 **Fracture of malar, maxillary and zygoma bones, unspecified**

Laterality !Q 7 S02.400- **Malar fracture, unspecified side**

Laterality !Q 7 S02.401- **Maxillary fracture, unspecified side**

Laterality !Q 7 S02.402- **Zygomatic fracture, unspecified side**

4 4th digit required 5 5th digit required 6 6th digit required 7 7th digit required 7 7th digit placeholder + Additional code Laterality

SP 7 **S02.40A- Malar fracture, right side**
SP 7 **S02.40B- Malar fracture, left side**
SP 7 **S02.40C- Maxillary fracture, right side**
SP 7 **S02.40D- Maxillary fracture, left side**
SP 7 **S02.40E- Zygomatic fracture, right side**
SP 7 **S02.40F- Zygomatic fracture, left side**
6 **S02.41 LeFort fracture**
SP 7 **S02.411- LeFort I fracture**
SP 7 **S02.412- LeFort II fracture**
SP 7 **S02.413- LeFort III fracture**
SP 7 **S02.42X- Fracture of alveolus of maxilla**
!Q 7 **S02.5XX- Fracture of tooth (traumatic)**
Broken tooth
EXCLUDES 1 cracked tooth (nontraumatic) (K03.81)
5 **S02.6 Fracture of mandible**
Fracture of lower jaw (bone)
6 **S02.60 Fracture of mandible, unspecified**
!Q 7 **S02.600- Fracture of unspecified part of body of mandible, unspecified side**
SP 7 **S02.601- Fracture of unspecified part of body of right mandible**
SP 7 **S02.602- Fracture of unspecified part of body of left mandible**
SP 7 **S02.609- Fracture of mandible, unspecified**
6 **S02.61 Fracture of condylar process of mandible**
!Q 7 **S02.610- Fracture of condylar process of mandible, unspecified side**
SP 7 **S02.611- Fracture of condylar process of right mandible**
SP 7 **S02.612- Fracture of condylar process of left mandible**
6 **S02.62 Fracture of subcondylar process of mandible**
!Q 7 **S02.620- Fracture of subcondylar process of mandible, unspecified side**
SP 7 **S02.621- Fracture of subcondylar process of right mandible**
SP 7 **S02.622- Fracture of subcondylar process of left mandible**
6 **S02.63 Fracture of coronoid process of mandible**
!Q 7 **S02.630- Fracture of coronoid process of mandible, unspecified side**
SP 7 **S02.631- Fracture of coronoid process of right mandible**
SP 7 **S02.632- Fracture of coronoid process of left mandible**
6 **S02.64 Fracture of ramus of mandible**
!Q 7 **S02.640- Fracture of ramus of mandible, unspecified side**
SP 7 **S02.641- Fracture of ramus of right mandible**
SP 7 **S02.642- Fracture of ramus of left mandible**
6 **S02.65 Fracture of angle of mandible**
!Q 7 **S02.650- Fracture of angle of mandible, unspecified side**
SP 7 **S02.651- Fracture of angle of right mandible**
SP 7 **S02.652- Fracture of angle of left mandible**
SP 7 **S02.66X- Fracture of symphysis of mandible**
6 **S02.67 Fracture of alveolus of mandible**
!Q 7 **S02.670- Fracture of alveolus of mandible, unspecified side**
SP 7 **S02.671- Fracture of alveolus of right mandible**
SP 7 **S02.672- Fracture of alveolus of left mandible**
SP 7 **S02.69X- Fracture of mandible of other specified site**
5 **S02.8 Fractures of other specified skull and facial bones**
Fracture of palate
EXCLUDES 2 fracture of orbital floor (S02.3-)
fracture of orbital roof (S02.12-)
!Q 7 **S02.80X- Fracture of other specified skull and facial bones, unspecified side**
SP 7 **S02.81X- Fracture of other specified skull and facial bones, right side**
SP 7 **S02.82X- Fracture of other specified skull and facial bones, left side**
6 **S02.83 Fracture of medial orbital wall**
EXCLUDES 2 orbital floor (S02.3-)
orbital roof (S02.12-)
CODING TIPS✓ Orbital fractures may be defined in terms of anatomic location, including isolated fractures of the orbital floor, medial wall, temporal wall, and roof. These fractures are commonly seen with midfacial trauma.
SP 7 **S02.831- Fracture of medial orbital wall, right side**
SP 7 **S02.832- Fracture of medial orbital wall, left side**
7 **S02.839- Fracture of medial orbital wall, unspecified side**
6 **S02.84 Fracture of lateral orbital wall**
EXCLUDES 2 orbital floor (S02.3-)
orbital roof (S02.12-)
CODING TIPS✓ Orbital fractures may be defined in terms of anatomic location, including isolated fractures of the orbital floor, medial wall, temporal wall, and roof. These fractures are commonly seen with midfacial trauma.
SP 7 **S02.841- Fracture of lateral orbital wall, right side**
SP 7 **S02.842- Fracture of lateral orbital wall, left side**
7 **S02.849- Fracture of lateral orbital wall, unspecified side**
7 **S02.85X- Fracture of orbit, unspecified**
Fracture of orbit NOS
Fracture of orbit wall NOS
EXCLUDES 1 lateral orbital wall (S02.84-)
medial orbital wall (S02.83-)
orbital floor (S02.3-)
orbital roof (S02.12-)

Chapter 19
S00-T88

CODING TIPS ✓ Orbital fractures may be defined in terms of anatomic location, including isolated fractures of the orbital floor, medial wall, temporal wall, and roof. These fractures are commonly seen with midfacial trauma.

5 **S02.9 Fracture of unspecified skull and facial bones**

SP 7 **S02.91X- Unspecified fracture of skull**

SP 7 **S02.92X- Unspecified fracture of facial bones**

4 **S03 Dislocation and sprain of joints and ligaments of head**

INCLUDES avulsion of joint (capsule) or ligament of head
laceration of cartilage, joint (capsule) or ligament of head
sprain of cartilage, joint (capsule) or ligament of head
traumatic hemarthrosis of joint or ligament of head
traumatic rupture of joint or ligament of head
traumatic subluxation of joint or ligament of head
traumatic tear of joint or ligament of head

Code also:
any associated open wound

EXCLUDES 2 Strain of muscle or tendon of head (S09.1)

The appropriate 7th character is to be added to each code from category S03
A initial encounter
D subsequent encounter
S sequela

5 **S03.0 Dislocation of jaw**
Dislocation of jaw (cartilage) (meniscus)
Dislocation of mandible
Dislocation of temporomandibular (joint)

L IQ 7 **S03.00X- Dislocation of jaw, unspecified side**

L SP 7 **S03.01X- Dislocation of jaw, right side**

L SP 7 **S03.02X- Dislocation of jaw, left side**

L SP 7 **S03.03X- Dislocation of jaw, bilateral**

SP 7 **S03.1XX- Dislocation of septal cartilage of nose**

IQ 7 **S03.2XX- Dislocation of tooth**

5 **S03.4 Sprain of jaw**
Sprain of temporomandibular (joint) (ligament)

L IQ 7 **S03.40X- Sprain of jaw, unspecified side**

L SP 7 **S03.41X- Sprain of jaw, right side**

L SP 7 **S03.42X- Sprain of jaw, left side**

L SP 7 **S03.43X- Sprain of jaw, bilateral**

SP 7 **S03.8XX- Sprain of joints and ligaments of other parts of head**

SP 7 **S03.9XX- Sprain of joints and ligaments of unspecified parts of head**

4 **S04 Injury of cranial nerve**

The selection of side should be based on the side of the body being affected

Code first:
any associated intracranial injury (S06.-)

Code also any associated:
open wound of head (S01.-)
skull fracture (S02.-)

The appropriate 7th character is to be added to each code from category S04
A initial encounter
D subsequent encounter
S sequela

+ 5 **S04.0 Injury of optic nerve and pathways**
Use additional code to identify any visual field defect or blindness (H53.4-, H54.-)

+ 6 **S04.01 Injury of optic nerve**
Injury of 2nd cranial nerve

L SP + 7 **S04.011- Injury of optic nerve, right eye**

L SP + 7 **S04.012- Injury of optic nerve, left eye**

L IQ + 7 **S04.019- Injury of optic nerve, unspecified eye**
Injury of optic nerve NOS

SP + 7 **S04.02X- Injury of optic chiasm**

+ 6 **S04.03 Injury of optic tract and pathways**
Injury of optic radiation

L SP + 7 **S04.031- Injury of optic tract and pathways, right side**

L SP + 7 **S04.032- Injury of optic tract and pathways, left side**

L IQ + 7 **S04.039- Injury of optic tract and pathways, unspecified side**
Injury of optic tract and pathways NOS

+ 6 **S04.04 Injury of visual cortex**

L SP + 7 **S04.041- Injury of visual cortex, right side**

L SP + 7 **S04.042- Injury of visual cortex, left side**

L IQ + 7 **S04.049- Injury of visual cortex, unspecified side**
Injury of visual cortex NOS

5 **S04.1 Injury of oculomotor nerve**
Injury of 3rd cranial nerve

L IQ 7 **S04.10X- Injury of oculomotor nerve, unspecified side**

L SP 7 **S04.11X- Injury of oculomotor nerve, right side**

L SP 7 **S04.12X- Injury of oculomotor nerve, left side**

5 **S04.2 Injury of trochlear nerve**
Injury of 4th cranial nerve

L IQ 7 **S04.20X- Injury of trochlear nerve, unspecified side**

L SP 7 **S04.21X- Injury of trochlear nerve, right side**

L SP 7 **S04.22X- Injury of trochlear nerve, left side**

5 **S04.3 Injury of trigeminal nerve**
Injury of 5th cranial nerve

L IQ 7 **S04.30X- Injury of trigeminal nerve, unspecified side**

L SP 7 **S04.31X- Injury of trigeminal nerve, right side**

L SP 7 **S04.32X- Injury of trigeminal nerve, left side**

5 **S04.4 Injury of abducent nerve**
Injury of 6th cranial nerve

Chapter 19

S00-T88

IQ 7 **S04.40X- Injury of abducent nerve, unspecified side**
SP 7 **S04.41X- Injury of abducent nerve, right side**
SP 7 **S04.42X- Injury of abducent nerve, left side**

5 **S04.5 Injury of facial nerve**
Injury of 7th cranial nerve
IQ 7 **S04.50X- Injury of facial nerve, unspecified side**
SP 7 **S04.51X- Injury of facial nerve, right side**
SP 7 **S04.52X- Injury of facial nerve, left side**

5 **S04.6 Injury of acoustic nerve**
Injury of auditory nerve
Injury of 8th cranial nerve
IQ 7 **S04.60X- Injury of acoustic nerve, unspecified side**
SP 7 **S04.61X- Injury of acoustic nerve, right side**
SP 7 **S04.62X- Injury of acoustic nerve, left side**

5 **S04.7 Injury of accessory nerve**
Injury of 11th cranial nerve
IQ 7 **S04.70X- Injury of accessory nerve, unspecified side**
SP 7 **S04.71X- Injury of accessory nerve, right side**
SP 7 **S04.72X- Injury of accessory nerve, left side**

5 **S04.8 Injury of other cranial nerves**

6 **S04.81 Injury of olfactory [1st] nerve**
SP 7 **S04.811- Injury of olfactory [1st] nerve, right side**
SP 7 **S04.812- Injury of olfactory [1st] nerve, left side**
IQ 7 **S04.819- Injury of olfactory [1st] nerve, unspecified side**

6 **S04.89 Injury of other cranial nerves**
Injury of vagus [10th] nerve
SP 7 **S04.891- Injury of other cranial nerves, right side**
SP 7 **S04.892- Injury of other cranial nerves, left side**
IQ 7 **S04.899- Injury of other cranial nerves, unspecified side**

IQ 7 **S04.9XX- Injury of unspecified cranial nerve**

4 **S05 Injury of eye and orbit**
INCLUDES open wound of eye and orbit
EXCLUDES 2 2nd cranial [optic] nerve injury (S04.0-)
3rd cranial [oculomotor] nerve injury (S04.1-)
open wound of eyelid and periocular area (S01.1-)
orbital bone fracture (S02.1-, S02.3-, S02.8-)
superficial injury of eyelid (S00.1-S00.2)

The appropriate 7th character is to be added to each code from category S05
A initial encounter
D subsequent encounter
S sequela

5 **S05.0 Injury of conjunctiva and corneal abrasion without foreign body**
EXCLUDES 1 foreign body in conjunctival sac (T15.1)
foreign body in cornea (T15.0)
IQ 7 **S05.00X- Injury of conjunctiva and corneal abrasion without foreign body, unspecified eye**
IQ 7 **S05.01X- Injury of conjunctiva and corneal abrasion without foreign body, right eye**
IQ 7 **S05.02X- Injury of conjunctiva and corneal abrasion without foreign body, left eye**

5 **S05.1 Contusion of eyeball and orbital tissues**
Traumatic hyphema
EXCLUDES 2 black eye NOS (S00.1)
contusion of eyelid and periocular area (S00.1)
IQ 7 **S05.10X- Contusion of eyeball and orbital tissues, unspecified eye**
IQ 7 **S05.11X- Contusion of eyeball and orbital tissues, right eye**
IQ 7 **S05.12X- Contusion of eyeball and orbital tissues, left eye**

5 **S05.2 Ocular laceration and rupture with prolapse or loss of intraocular tissue**
IQ 7 **S05.20X- Ocular laceration and rupture with prolapse or loss of intraocular tissue, unspecified eye**
SP 7 **S05.21X- Ocular laceration and rupture with prolapse or loss of intraocular tissue, right eye**
SP 7 **S05.22X- Ocular laceration and rupture with prolapse or loss of intraocular tissue, left eye**

5 **S05.3 Ocular laceration without prolapse or loss of intraocular tissue**
Laceration of eye NOS
IQ 7 **S05.30X- Ocular laceration without prolapse or loss of intraocular tissue, unspecified eye**
SP 7 **S05.31X- Ocular laceration without prolapse or loss of intraocular tissue, right eye**
SP 7 **S05.32X- Ocular laceration without prolapse or loss of intraocular tissue, left eye**

5 **S05.4 Penetrating wound of orbit with or without foreign body**
EXCLUDES 2 retained (old) foreign body following penetrating wound in orbit (H05.5-)
IQ 7 **S05.40X- Penetrating wound of orbit with or without foreign body, unspecified eye**
SP 7 **S05.41X- Penetrating wound of orbit with or without foreign body, right eye**
SP 7 **S05.42X- Penetrating wound of orbit with or without foreign body, left eye**

5 **S05.5 Penetrating wound with foreign body of eyeball**
EXCLUDES 2 retained (old) intraocular foreign body (H44.6-, H44.7)
IQ 7 **S05.50X- Penetrating wound with foreign body of unspecified eyeball**
SP 7 **S05.51X- Penetrating wound with foreign body of right eyeball**

S05.52X- **Penetrating wound with foreign body of left eyeball**

S05.6 **Penetrating wound without foreign body of eyeball**
Ocular penetration NOS

S05.60X- **Penetrating wound without foreign body of unspecified eyeball**

S05.61X- **Penetrating wound without foreign body of right eyeball**

S05.62X- **Penetrating wound without foreign body of left eyeball**

S05.7 **Avulsion of eye**
Traumatic enucleation

S05.70X- **Avulsion of unspecified eye**

S05.71X- **Avulsion of right eye**

S05.72X- **Avulsion of left eye**

S05.8 **Other injuries of eye and orbit**
Lacrimal duct injury

S05.8X **Other injuries of eye and orbit**

S05.8X1- **Other injuries of right eye and orbit**

S05.8X2- **Other injuries of left eye and orbit**

S05.8X9- **Other injuries of unspecified eye and orbit**

S05.9 **Unspecified injury of eye and orbit**
Injury of eye NOS

S05.90X- **Unspecified injury of unspecified eye and orbit**

S05.91X- **Unspecified injury of right eye and orbit**

S05.92X- **Unspecified injury of left eye and orbit**

S06 **Intracranial injury**
Note:
7th characters D and S do not apply to codes in category S06 with 6th character 7 - death due to brain injury prior to regaining consciousness, or 8 - death due to other cause prior to regaining consciousness.

INCLUDES traumatic brain injury

Code also any associated:
open wound of head (S01.-)
skull fracture (S02.-)

EXCLUDES 1 head injury NOS (S09.90)

The appropriate 7th character is to be added to each code from category S06
A initial encounter
D subsequent encounter
S sequela

CODING TIPS✓ Intracranial injuries are caused by trauma, not strokes. To determine whether the intracranial injury with 7th character "D" or "S" should be used, look at the plan of care (POC) and the length of time since the head injury. Is the POC directed at the head injury or the residuals of the head injury?

CODING TIPS✓ When coding sequelae of a traumatic brain injury, the guideline indicates to first list the residual condition(s), followed by the specific traumatic brain injury diagnosed, using the appropriate code from category S06 with the seventh character "S" to indicate sequelae. In some cases with traumatic brain injury, there is a tabular convention that indicates to code the intracranial injury first and then the residual, e.g. R40.2-. A convention always overrules a conflicting guideline.

S06.0 **Concussion**
Commotio cerebri

EXCLUDES 1 concussion with other intracranial injuries classified in subcategories S06.1- to S06.6- , S06.81- and S06.82- code to specified intracranial injury

CODING TIPS✓ Loss of consciousness (LOC) of more than 30 minutes should not be classified as a concussion or mild traumatic brain injury. Query the physician or NPP if documentation indicates longer than 30 minutes LOC.

S06.0X **Concussion**

S06.0X0- **Concussion without loss of consciousness**

S06.0X1- **Concussion with loss of consciousness of 30 minutes or less**

S06.0X9- **Concussion with loss of consciousness of unspecified duration**
Concussion NOS

S06.1 **Traumatic cerebral edema**
Diffuse traumatic cerebral edema
Focal traumatic cerebral edema

S06.1X **Traumatic cerebral edema**

S06.1X0- **Traumatic cerebral edema without loss of consciousness**

S06.1X1- **Traumatic cerebral edema with loss of consciousness of 30 minutes or less**

S06.1X2- **Traumatic cerebral edema with loss of consciousness of 31 minutes to 59 minutes**

S06.1X3- **Traumatic cerebral edema with loss of consciousness of 1 hour to 5 hours 59 minutes**

S06.1X4- **Traumatic cerebral edema with loss of consciousness of 6 hours to 24 hours**

S06.1X5- **Traumatic cerebral edema with loss of consciousness greater than 24 hours with return to pre-existing conscious level**

S06.1X6- **Traumatic cerebral edema with loss of consciousness greater than 24 hours without return to pre-existing conscious level with patient surviving**

Chapter 19
S00-T88

IQ 7 **S06.1X7- Traumatic cerebral edema with loss of consciousness of any duration with death due to brain injury prior to regaining consciousness**

IQ 7 **S06.1X8- Traumatic cerebral edema with loss of consciousness of any duration with death due to other cause prior to regaining consciousness**

SP 7 **S06.1X9- Traumatic cerebral edema with loss of consciousness of unspecified duration**

Traumatic cerebral edema NOS

▲ + 5 **S06.2 Diffuse traumatic brain injury**

Diffuse axonal brain injury

Use additional code, if applicable, for traumatic brain compression or herniation (S06.A-)

EXCLUDES 1 traumatic diffuse cerebral edema (S06.1X-)

+ 6 **S06.2X Diffuse traumatic brain injury**

SP + 7 **S06.2X0- Diffuse traumatic brain injury without loss of consciousness**

SP + 7 **S06.2X1- Diffuse traumatic brain injury with loss of consciousness of 30 minutes or less**

SP + 7 **S06.2X2- Diffuse traumatic brain injury with loss of consciousness of 31 minutes to 59 minutes**

SP + 7 **S06.2X3- Diffuse traumatic brain injury with loss of consciousness of 1 hour to 5 hours 59 minutes**

SP + 7 **S06.2X4- Diffuse traumatic brain injury with loss of consciousness of 6 hours to 24 hours**

SP + 7 **S06.2X5- Diffuse traumatic brain injury with loss of consciousness greater than 24 hours with return to pre-existing conscious levels**

SP + 7 **S06.2X6- Diffuse traumatic brain injury with loss of consciousness greater than 24 hours without return to pre-existing conscious level with patient surviving**

IQ + 7 **S06.2X7- Diffuse traumatic brain injury with loss of consciousness of any duration with death due to brain injury prior to regaining consciousness**

IQ + 7 **S06.2X8- Diffuse traumatic brain injury with loss of consciousness of any duration with death due to other cause prior to regaining consciousness**

SP + 7 **S06.2X9- Diffuse traumatic brain injury with loss of consciousness of unspecified duration**

Diffuse traumatic brain injury NOS

▲ + 5 **S06.3 Focal traumatic brain injury**

Use additional code, if applicable, for traumatic brain compression or herniation (S06.A-)

EXCLUDES 1 any condition classifiable to S06.4-S06.6

EXCLUDES 2 focal cerebral edema (S06.1)

+ 6 **S06.30 Unspecified focal traumatic brain injury**

SP + 7 **S06.300- Unspecified focal traumatic brain injury without loss of consciousness**

SP + 7 **S06.301- Unspecified focal traumatic brain injury with loss of consciousness of 30 minutes or less**

SP + 7 **S06.302- Unspecified focal traumatic brain injury with loss of consciousness of 31 minutes to 59 minutes**

SP + 7 **S06.303- Unspecified focal traumatic brain injury with loss of consciousness of 1 hour to 5 hours 59 minutes**

SP + 7 **S06.304- Unspecified focal traumatic brain injury with loss of consciousness of 6 hours to 24 hours**

SP + 7 **S06.305- Unspecified focal traumatic brain injury with loss of consciousness greater than 24 hours with return to pre-existing conscious level**

SP + 7 **S06.306- Unspecified focal traumatic brain injury with loss of consciousness greater than 24 hours without return to pre-existing conscious level with patient surviving**

IQ + 7 **S06.307- Unspecified focal traumatic brain injury with loss of consciousness of any duration with death due to brain injury prior to regaining consciousness**

IQ + 7 **S06.308- Unspecified focal traumatic brain injury with loss of consciousness of any duration with death due to other cause prior to regaining consciousness**

SP + 7 **S06.309- Unspecified focal traumatic brain injury with loss of consciousness of unspecified duration**

Unspecified focal traumatic brain injury NOS

+ 6 **S06.31 Contusion and laceration of right cerebrum**

H SP + 7 **S06.310- Contusion and laceration of right cerebrum without loss of consciousness**

H SP + 7 **S06.311- Contusion and laceration of right cerebrum with loss of consciousness of 30 minutes or less**

H SP + 7 **S06.312- Contusion and laceration of right cerebrum with loss of consciousness of 31 minutes to 59 minutes**

H SP + 7 **S06.313- Contusion and laceration of right cerebrum with loss of consciousness of 1 hour to 5 hours 59 minutes**

⊟ SP + 7 **S06.314- Contusion and laceration of right cerebrum with loss of consciousness of 6 hours to 24 hours**

⊟ SP + 7 **S06.315- Contusion and laceration of right cerebrum with loss of consciousness greater than 24 hours with return to pre-existing conscious level**

⊟ SP + 7 **S06.316- Contusion and laceration of right cerebrum with loss of consciousness greater than 24 hours without return to pre-existing conscious level with patient surviving**

⊟ !Q + 7 **S06.317- Contusion and laceration of right cerebrum with loss of consciousness of any duration with death due to brain injury prior to regaining consciousness**

⊟ !Q + 7 **S06.318- Contusion and laceration of right cerebrum with loss of consciousness of any duration with death due to other cause prior to regaining consciousness**

⊟ SP + 7 **S06.319- Contusion and laceration of right cerebrum with loss of consciousness of unspecified duration**

Contusion and laceration of right cerebrum NOS

+ 6 **S06.32 Contusion and laceration of left cerebrum**

⊟ SP + 7 **S06.320- Contusion and laceration of left cerebrum without loss of consciousness**

⊟ SP + 7 **S06.321- Contusion and laceration of left cerebrum with loss of consciousness of 30 minutes or less**

⊟ SP + 7 **S06.322- Contusion and laceration of left cerebrum with loss of consciousness of 31 minutes to 59 minutes**

⊟ SP + 7 **S06.323- Contusion and laceration of left cerebrum with loss of consciousness of 1 hour to 5 hours 59 minutes**

⊟ SP + 7 **S06.324- Contusion and laceration of left cerebrum with loss of consciousness of 6 hours to 24 hours**

⊟ SP + 7 **S06.325- Contusion and laceration of left cerebrum with loss of consciousness greater than 24 hours with return to pre-existing conscious level**

⊟ SP + 7 **S06.326- Contusion and laceration of left cerebrum with loss of consciousness greater than 24 hours without return to pre-existing conscious level with patient surviving**

⊟ !Q + 7 **S06.327- Contusion and laceration of left cerebrum with loss of consciousness of any duration with death due to brain injury prior to regaining consciousness**

⊟ !Q + 7 **S06.328- Contusion and laceration of left cerebrum with loss of consciousness of any duration with death due to other cause prior to regaining consciousness**

⊟ SP + 7 **S06.329- Contusion and laceration of left cerebrum with loss of consciousness of unspecified duration**

Contusion and laceration of left cerebrum NOS

+ 6 **S06.33 Contusion and laceration of cerebrum, unspecified**

SP + 7 **S06.330- Contusion and laceration of cerebrum, unspecified, without loss of consciousness**

SP + 7 **S06.331- Contusion and laceration of cerebrum, unspecified, with loss of consciousness of 30 minutes or less**

SP + 7 **S06.332- Contusion and laceration of cerebrum, unspecified, with loss of consciousness of 31 minutes to 59 minutes**

SP + 7 **S06.333- Contusion and laceration of cerebrum, unspecified, with loss of consciousness of 1 hour to 5 hours 59 minutes**

SP + 7 **S06.334- Contusion and laceration of cerebrum, unspecified, with loss of consciousness of 6 hours to 24 hours**

SP + 7 **S06.335- Contusion and laceration of cerebrum, unspecified, with loss of consciousness greater than 24 hours with return to pre-existing conscious level**

SP + 7 **S06.336- Contusion and laceration of cerebrum, unspecified, with loss of consciousness greater than 24 hours without return to pre-existing conscious level with patient surviving**

!Q + 7 **S06.337- Contusion and laceration of cerebrum, unspecified, with loss of consciousness of any duration with death due to brain injury prior to regaining consciousness**

!Q + 7 **S06.338- Contusion and laceration of cerebrum, unspecified, with loss of consciousness of any duration with death due to other cause prior to regaining consciousness**

SP + 7 **S06.339- Contusion and laceration of cerebrum, unspecified, with loss of consciousness of unspecified duration**

Contusion and laceration of cerebrum NOS

+ 6 **S06.34 Traumatic hemorrhage of right cerebrum**

Traumatic intracerebral hemorrhage and hematoma of right cerebrum

⊟ SP + 7 **S06.340- Traumatic hemorrhage of right cerebrum without loss of consciousness**

Chapter 19

S00-T88

SP + 7 **S06.341- Traumatic hemorrhage of right cerebrum with loss of consciousness of 30 minutes or less**

SP + 7 **S06.342- Traumatic hemorrhage of right cerebrum with loss of consciousness of 31 minutes to 59 minutes**

SP + 7 **S06.343- Traumatic hemorrhage of right cerebrum with loss of consciousness of 1 hours to 5 hours 59 minutes**

SP + 7 **S06.344- Traumatic hemorrhage of right cerebrum with loss of consciousness of 6 hours to 24 hours**

SP + 7 **S06.345- Traumatic hemorrhage of right cerebrum with loss of consciousness greater than 24 hours with return to pre-existing conscious level**

SP IQ + 7 **S06.346- Traumatic hemorrhage of right cerebrum with loss of consciousness greater than 24 hours without return to pre-existing conscious level with patient surviving**

IQ + 7 **S06.347- Traumatic hemorrhage of right cerebrum with loss of consciousness of any duration with death due to brain injury prior to regaining consciousness**

IQ + 7 **S06.348- Traumatic hemorrhage of right cerebrum with loss of consciousness of any duration with death due to other cause prior to regaining consciousness**

SP + 7 **S06.349- Traumatic hemorrhage of right cerebrum with loss of consciousness of unspecified duration**

Traumatic hemorrhage of right cerebrum NOS

+ 6 **S06.35 Traumatic hemorrhage of left cerebrum**

Traumatic intracerebral hemorrhage and hematoma of left cerebrum

SP + 7 **S06.350- Traumatic hemorrhage of left cerebrum without loss of consciousness**

SP + 7 **S06.351- Traumatic hemorrhage of left cerebrum with loss of consciousness of 30 minutes or less**

SP + 7 **S06.352- Traumatic hemorrhage of left cerebrum with loss of consciousness of 31 minutes to 59 minutes**

SP + 7 **S06.353- Traumatic hemorrhage of left cerebrum with loss of consciousness of 1 hours to 5 hours 59 minutes**

SP + 7 **S06.354- Traumatic hemorrhage of left cerebrum with loss of consciousness of 6 hours to 24 hours**

SP + 7 **S06.355- Traumatic hemorrhage of left cerebrum with loss of consciousness greater than 24 hours with return to pre-existing conscious level**

SP + 7 **S06.356- Traumatic hemorrhage of left cerebrum with loss of consciousness greater than 24 hours without return to pre-existing conscious level with patient surviving**

IQ + 7 **S06.357- Traumatic hemorrhage of left cerebrum with loss of consciousness of any duration with death due to brain injury prior to regaining consciousness**

IQ + 7 **S06.358- Traumatic hemorrhage of left cerebrum with loss of consciousness of any duration with death due to other cause prior to regaining consciousness**

SP + 7 **S06.359- Traumatic hemorrhage of left cerebrum with loss of consciousness of unspecified duration**

Traumatic hemorrhage of left cerebrum NOS

+ 6 **S06.36 Traumatic hemorrhage of cerebrum, unspecified**

Traumatic intracerebral hemorrhage and hematoma, unspecified

SP + 7 **S06.360- Traumatic hemorrhage of cerebrum, unspecified, without loss of consciousness**

SP + 7 **S06.361- Traumatic hemorrhage of cerebrum, unspecified, with loss of consciousness of 30 minutes or less**

SP + 7 **S06.362- Traumatic hemorrhage of cerebrum, unspecified, with loss of consciousness of 31 minutes to 59 minutes**

SP + 7 **S06.363- Traumatic hemorrhage of cerebrum, unspecified, with loss of consciousness of 1 hours to 5 hours 59 minutes**

SP + 7 **S06.364- Traumatic hemorrhage of cerebrum, unspecified, with loss of consciousness of 6 hours to 24 hours**

SP + 7 **S06.365- Traumatic hemorrhage of cerebrum, unspecified, with loss of consciousness greater than 24 hours with return to pre-existing conscious level**

SP + 7 **S06.366- Traumatic hemorrhage of cerebrum, unspecified, with loss of consciousness greater than 24 hours without return to pre-existing conscious level with patient surviving**

IQ + 7 **S06.367- Traumatic hemorrhage of cerebrum, unspecified, with loss of consciousness of any duration with death due to brain injury prior to regaining consciousness**

Chapter 19

S00-T88

!Q + 7 **S06.368- Traumatic hemorrhage of cerebrum, unspecified, with loss of consciousness of any duration with death due to other cause prior to regaining consciousness**

SP + 7 **S06.369- Traumatic hemorrhage of cerebrum, unspecified, with loss of consciousness of unspecified duration**
Traumatic hemorrhage of cerebrum NOS

+ 6 **S06.37 Contusion, laceration, and hemorrhage of cerebellum**

SP + 7 **S06.370- Contusion, laceration, and hemorrhage of cerebellum without loss of consciousness**

SP + 7 **S06.371- Contusion, laceration, and hemorrhage of cerebellum with loss of consciousness of 30 minutes or less**

SP + 7 **S06.372- Contusion, laceration, and hemorrhage of cerebellum with loss of consciousness of 31 minutes to 59 minutes**

SP + 7 **S06.373- Contusion, laceration, and hemorrhage of cerebellum with loss of consciousness of 1 hour to 5 hours 59 minutes**

SP + 7 **S06.374- Contusion, laceration, and hemorrhage of cerebellum with loss of consciousness of 6 hours to 24 hours**

SP + 7 **S06.375- Contusion, laceration, and hemorrhage of cerebellum with loss of consciousness greater than 24 hours with return to pre-existing conscious level**

SP + 7 **S06.376- Contusion, laceration, and hemorrhage of cerebellum with loss of consciousness greater than 24 hours without return to pre-existing conscious level with patient surviving**

!Q + 7 **S06.377- Contusion, laceration, and hemorrhage of cerebellum with loss of consciousness of any duration with death due to brain injury prior to regaining consciousness**

!Q + 7 **S06.378- Contusion, laceration, and hemorrhage of cerebellum with loss of consciousness of any duration with death due to other cause prior to regaining consciousness**

SP + 7 **S06.379- Contusion, laceration, and hemorrhage of cerebellum with loss of consciousness of unspecified duration**
Contusion, laceration, and hemorrhage of cerebellum NOS

+ 6 **S06.38 Contusion, laceration, and hemorrhage of brainstem**

SP + 7 **S06.380- Contusion, laceration, and hemorrhage of brainstem without loss of consciousness**

SP + 7 **S06.381- Contusion, laceration, and hemorrhage of brainstem with loss of consciousness of 30 minutes or less**

SP + 7 **S06.382- Contusion, laceration, and hemorrhage of brainstem with loss of consciousness of 31 minutes to 59 minutes**

SP + 7 **S06.383- Contusion, laceration, and hemorrhage of brainstem with loss of consciousness of 1 hour to 5 hours 59 minutes**

SP + 7 **S06.384- Contusion, laceration, and hemorrhage of brainstem with loss of consciousness of 6 hours to 24 hours**

SP + 7 **S06.385- Contusion, laceration, and hemorrhage of brainstem with loss of consciousness greater than 24 hours with return to pre-existing conscious level**

SP + 7 **S06.386- Contusion, laceration, and hemorrhage of brainstem with loss of consciousness greater than 24 hours without return to pre-existing conscious level with patient surviving**

!Q + 7 **S06.387- Contusion, laceration, and hemorrhage of brainstem with loss of consciousness of any duration with death due to brain injury prior to regaining consciousness**

!Q + 7 **S06.388- Contusion, laceration, and hemorrhage of brainstem with loss of consciousness of any duration with death due to other cause prior to regaining consciousness**

SP + 7 **S06.389- Contusion, laceration, and hemorrhage of brainstem with loss of consciousness of unspecified duration**
Contusion, laceration, and hemorrhage of brainstem NOS

5 **S06.4 Epidural hemorrhage**
Extradural hemorrhage NOS
Extradural hemorrhage (traumatic)

6 **S06.4X Epidural hemorrhage**

SP 7 **S06.4X0- Epidural hemorrhage without loss of consciousness**

SP 7 **S06.4X1- Epidural hemorrhage with loss of consciousness of 30 minutes or less**

SP 7 **S06.4X2- Epidural hemorrhage with loss of consciousness of 31 minutes to 59 minutes**

SP 7 **S06.4X3- Epidural hemorrhage with loss of consciousness of 1 hour to 5 hours 59 minutes**

SP 7 **S06.4X4- Epidural hemorrhage with loss of consciousness of 6 hours to 24 hours**

SP 7 **S06.4X5- Epidural hemorrhage with loss of consciousness greater than 24 hours with return to pre-existing conscious level**

SP 7 **S06.4X6- Epidural hemorrhage with loss of consciousness greater than 24 hours without return to pre-existing conscious level with patient surviving**

!Q 7 **S06.4X7- Epidural hemorrhage with loss of consciousness of any duration with death due to brain injury prior to regaining consciousness**

!Q 7 **S06.4X8- Epidural hemorrhage with loss of consciousness of any duration with death due to other causes prior to regaining consciousness**

SP 7 **S06.4X9- Epidural hemorrhage with loss of consciousness of unspecified duration**

Epidural hemorrhage NOS

▲ + 5 **S06.5 Traumatic subdural hemorrhage**

Use additional code, if applicable, for traumatic brain compression or herniation (S06.A-)

\+ 6 **S06.5X Traumatic subdural hemorrhage**

SP + 7 **S06.5X0- Traumatic subdural hemorrhage without loss of consciousness**

SP + 7 **S06.5X1- Traumatic subdural hemorrhage with loss of consciousness of 30 minutes or less**

SP + 7 **S06.5X2- Traumatic subdural hemorrhage with loss of consciousness of 31 minutes to 59 minutes**

SP + 7 **S06.5X3- Traumatic subdural hemorrhage with loss of consciousness of 1 hour to 5 hours 59 minutes**

SP + 7 **S06.5X4- Traumatic subdural hemorrhage with loss of consciousness of 6 hours to 24 hours**

SP + 7 **S06.5X5- Traumatic subdural hemorrhage with loss of consciousness greater than 24 hours with return to pre-existing conscious level**

SP + 7 **S06.5X6- Traumatic subdural hemorrhage with loss of consciousness greater than 24 hours without return to pre-existing conscious level with patient surviving**

!Q + 7 **S06.5X7- Traumatic subdural hemorrhage with loss of consciousness of any duration with death due to brain injury before regaining consciousness**

!Q + 7 **S06.5X8- Traumatic subdural hemorrhage with loss of consciousness of any duration with death due to other cause before regaining consciousness**

SP + 7 **S06.5X9- Traumatic subdural hemorrhage with loss of consciousness of unspecified duration**

Traumatic subdural hemorrhage NOS

▲ + 5 **S06.6 Traumatic subarachnoid hemorrhage**

Use additional code, if applicable, for traumatic brain compression or herniation (S06.A-)

\+ 6 **S06.6X Traumatic subarachnoid hemorrhage**

SP + 7 **S06.6X0- Traumatic subarachnoid hemorrhage without loss of consciousness**

SP + 7 **S06.6X1- Traumatic subarachnoid hemorrhage with loss of consciousness of 30 minutes or less**

SP + 7 **S06.6X2- Traumatic subarachnoid hemorrhage with loss of consciousness of 31 minutes to 59 minutes**

SP + 7 **S06.6X3- Traumatic subarachnoid hemorrhage with loss of consciousness of 1 hour to 5 hours 59 minutes**

SP + 7 **S06.6X4- Traumatic subarachnoid hemorrhage with loss of consciousness of 6 hours to 24 hours**

SP + 7 **S06.6X5- Traumatic subarachnoid hemorrhage with loss of consciousness greater than 24 hours with return to pre-existing conscious level**

SP + 7 **S06.6X6- Traumatic subarachnoid hemorrhage with loss of consciousness greater than 24 hours without return to pre-existing conscious level with patient surviving**

!Q + 7 **S06.6X7- Traumatic subarachnoid hemorrhage with loss of consciousness of any duration with death due to brain injury prior to regaining consciousness**

!Q + 7 **S06.6X8- Traumatic subarachnoid hemorrhage with loss of consciousness of any duration with death due to other cause prior to regaining consciousness**

SP + 7 **S06.6X9- Traumatic subarachnoid hemorrhage with loss of consciousness of unspecified duration**

Traumatic subarachnoid hemorrhage NOS

5 **S06.8 Other specified intracranial injuries**

6 **S06.81 Injury of right internal carotid artery, intracranial portion, not elsewhere classified**

H SP 7 **S06.810- Injury of right internal carotid artery, intracranial portion, not elsewhere classified without loss of consciousness**

H SP 7 **S06.811- Injury of right internal carotid artery, intracranial portion, not elsewhere classified with loss of consciousness of 30 minutes or less**

H SP 7 **S06.812- Injury of right internal carotid artery, intracranial portion, not elsewhere classified with loss of consciousness of 31 minutes to 59 minutes**

H SP 7 **S06.813- Injury of right internal carotid artery, intracranial portion, not elsewhere classified with loss of consciousness of 1 hour to 5 hours 59 minutes**

S06.814- Injury of right internal carotid artery, intracranial portion, not elsewhere classified with loss of consciousness of 6 hours to 24 hours

S06.815- Injury of right internal carotid artery, intracranial portion, not elsewhere classified with loss of consciousness greater than 24 hours with return to pre-existing conscious level

S06.816- Injury of right internal carotid artery, intracranial portion, not elsewhere classified with loss of consciousness greater than 24 hours without return to pre-existing conscious level with patient surviving

S06.817- Injury of right internal carotid artery, intracranial portion, not elsewhere classified with loss of consciousness of any duration with death due to brain injury prior to regaining consciousness

S06.818- Injury of right internal carotid artery, intracranial portion, not elsewhere classified with loss of consciousness of any duration with death due to other cause prior to regaining consciousness

S06.819- Injury of right internal carotid artery, intracranial portion, not elsewhere classified with loss of consciousness of unspecified duration

Injury of right internal carotid artery, intracranial portion, not elsewhere classified NOS

S06.82 Injury of left internal carotid artery, intracranial portion, not elsewhere classified

S06.820- Injury of left internal carotid artery, intracranial portion, not elsewhere classified without loss of consciousness

S06.821- Injury of left internal carotid artery, intracranial portion, not elsewhere classified with loss of consciousness of 30 minutes or less

S06.822- Injury of left internal carotid artery, intracranial portion, not elsewhere classified with loss of consciousness of 31 minutes to 59 minutes

S06.823- Injury of left internal carotid artery, intracranial portion, not elsewhere classified with loss of consciousness of 1 hour to 5 hours 59 minutes

S06.824- Injury of left internal carotid artery, intracranial portion, not elsewhere classified with loss of consciousness of 6 hours to 24 hours

S06.825- Injury of left internal carotid artery, intracranial portion, not elsewhere classified with loss of consciousness greater than 24 hours with return to pre-existing conscious level

S06.826- Injury of left internal carotid artery, intracranial portion, not elsewhere classified with loss of consciousness greater than 24 hours without return to pre-existing conscious level with patient surviving

S06.827- Injury of left internal carotid artery, intracranial portion, not elsewhere classified with loss of consciousness of any duration with death due to brain injury prior to regaining consciousness

S06.828- Injury of left internal carotid artery, intracranial portion, not elsewhere classified with loss of consciousness of any duration with death due to other cause prior to regaining consciousness

S06.829- Injury of left internal carotid artery, intracranial portion, not elsewhere classified with loss of consciousness of unspecified duration

Injury of left internal carotid artery, intracranial portion, not elsewhere classified NOS

S06.89 Other specified intracranial injury

EXCLUDES 1 concussion (S06.0X-)

S06.890- Other specified intracranial injury without loss of consciousness

S06.891- Other specified intracranial injury with loss of consciousness of 30 minutes or less

S06.892- Other specified intracranial injury with loss of consciousness of 31 minutes to 59 minutes

S06.893- Other specified intracranial injury with loss of consciousness of 1 hour to 5 hours 59 minutes

S06.894- Other specified intracranial injury with loss of consciousness of 6 hours to 24 hours

S06.895- Other specified intracranial injury with loss of consciousness greater than 24 hours with return to pre-existing conscious level

S06.896- Other specified intracranial injury with loss of consciousness greater than 24 hours without return to pre-existing conscious level with patient surviving

S06.897- Other specified intracranial injury with loss of consciousness of any duration with death due to brain injury prior to regaining consciousness

IQ 7 **S06.898- Other specified intracranial injury with loss of consciousness of any duration with death due to other cause prior to regaining consciousness**

SP 7 **S06.899- Other specified intracranial injury with loss of consciousness of unspecified duration**

5 **S06.9 Unspecified intracranial injury**

Brain injury NOS
Head injury NOS with loss of consciousness
Traumatic brain injury NOS

EXCLUDES 1 conditions classifiable to S06.0- to S06.8-code to specified intracranial injury
head injury NOS (S09.90)

6 **S06.9X Unspecified intracranial injury**

IQ 7 **S06.9X0- Unspecified intracranial injury without loss of consciousness**

IQ 7 **S06.9X1- Unspecified intracranial injury with loss of consciousness of 30 minutes or less**

IQ 7 **S06.9X2- Unspecified intracranial injury with loss of consciousness of 31 minutes to 59 minutes**

IQ 7 **S06.9X3- Unspecified intracranial injury with loss of consciousness of 1 hour to 5 hours 59 minutes**

IQ 7 **S06.9X4- Unspecified intracranial injury with loss of consciousness of 6 hours to 24 hours**

IQ 7 **S06.9X5- Unspecified intracranial injury with loss of consciousness greater than 24 hours with return to pre-existing conscious level**

IQ 7 **S06.9X6- Unspecified intracranial injury with loss of consciousness greater than 24 hours without return to pre-existing conscious level with patient surviving**

IQ 7 **S06.9X7- Unspecified intracranial injury with loss of consciousness of any duration with death due to brain injury prior to regaining consciousness**

IQ 7 **S06.9X8- Unspecified intracranial injury with loss of consciousness of any duration with death due to other cause prior to regaining consciousness**

IQ 7 **S06.9X9- Unspecified intracranial injury with loss of consciousness of unspecified duration**

★ 5 **S06.A Traumatic brain compression and herniation**

Traumatic cerebral compression
Code first the underlying traumatic brain injury, such as:
diffuse traumatic brain injury (S06.2-)
focal traumatic brain injury (S06.3-)
traumatic subdural hemorrhage (S06.5-)
traumatic subarachnoid hemorrhage (S06.6-)

★ 7 **S06.A0X- Traumatic brain compression without herniation**

Traumatic brain compression NOS
Traumatic cerebral compression NOS

★ 7 **S06.A1X- Traumatic brain compression with herniation**

Traumatic brain herniation
Traumatic brainstem compression with herniation
Traumatic cerebellar compression with herniation
Traumatic cerebral compression with herniation

+ 4 **S07 Crushing injury of head**

Use additional code for all associated injuries, such as:
intracranial injuries (S06.-)
skull fractures (S02.-)

The appropriate 7th character is to be added to each code from category S07

A	initial encounter
D	subsequent encounter
S	sequela

SP + 7 **S07.0XX- Crushing injury of face**

SP + 7 **S07.1XX- Crushing injury of skull**

SP + 7 **S07.8XX- Crushing injury of other parts of head**

SP + 7 **S07.9XX- Crushing injury of head, part unspecified**

4 **S08 Avulsion and traumatic amputation of part of head**

An amputation not identified as partial or complete should be coded to complete

The appropriate 7th character is to be added to each code from category S08

A	initial encounter
D	subsequent encounter
S	sequela

SP 7 **S08.0XX- Avulsion of scalp**

5 **S08.1 Traumatic amputation of ear**

6 **S08.11 Complete traumatic amputation of ear**

SP 7 **S08.111- Complete traumatic amputation of right ear**

SP 7 **S08.112- Complete traumatic amputation of left ear**

IQ 7 **S08.119- Complete traumatic amputation of unspecified ear**

6 **S08.12 Partial traumatic amputation of ear**

SP 7 **S08.121- Partial traumatic amputation of right ear**

SP 7 **S08.122- Partial traumatic amputation of left ear**

IQ 7 **S08.129- Partial traumatic amputation of unspecified ear**

5 **S08.8 Traumatic amputation of other parts of head**

6 **S08.81 Traumatic amputation of nose**

SP 7 **S08.811- Complete traumatic amputation of nose**

SP 7 **S08.812- Partial traumatic amputation of nose**

SP 7 **S08.89X- Traumatic amputation of other parts of head**

Chapter 19
S00-T88

4 **S09 Other and unspecified injuries of head**

The appropriate 7th character is to be added to each code from category S09
A initial encounter
D subsequent encounter
S sequela

SP 7 **S09.0XX- Injury of blood vessels of head, not elsewhere classified**
EXCLUDES 1 injury of cerebral blood vessels (S06.-)
injury of precerebral blood vessels (S15.-)

5 **S09.1 Injury of muscle and tendon of head**
Code also:
any associated open wound (S01.-)
EXCLUDES 2 sprain to joints and ligament of head (S03.9)

IQ 7 **S09.10X- Unspecified injury of muscle and tendon of head**
Injury of muscle and tendon of head NOS

IQ 7 **S09.11X- Strain of muscle and tendon of head**

SP 7 **S09.12X- Laceration of muscle and tendon of head**

IQ 7 **S09.19X- Other specified injury of muscle and tendon of head**

5 **S09.2 Traumatic rupture of ear drum**
EXCLUDES 1 traumatic rupture of ear drum due to blast injury (S09.31-)

Laterality IQ 7 **S09.20X- Traumatic rupture of unspecified ear drum**

Laterality SP 7 **S09.21X- Traumatic rupture of right ear drum**

Laterality SP 7 **S09.22X- Traumatic rupture of left ear drum**

5 **S09.3 Other specified and unspecified injury of middle and inner ear**
EXCLUDES 1 injury to ear NOS (S09.91-)
EXCLUDES 2 injury to external ear (S00.4-, S01.3-, S08.1-)

6 **S09.30 Unspecified injury of middle and inner ear**

Laterality IQ 7 **S09.301- Unspecified injury of right middle and inner ear**

Laterality IQ 7 **S09.302- Unspecified injury of left middle and inner ear**

Laterality IQ 7 **S09.309- Unspecified injury of unspecified middle and inner ear**

6 **S09.31 Primary blast injury of ear**
Blast injury of ear NOS

Laterality SP 7 **S09.311- Primary blast injury of right ear**

Laterality SP 7 **S09.312- Primary blast injury of left ear**

Laterality SP 7 **S09.313- Primary blast injury of ear, bilateral**

Laterality IQ 7 **S09.319- Primary blast injury of unspecified ear**

6 **S09.39 Other specified injury of middle and inner ear**
Secondary blast injury to ear

Laterality SP 7 **S09.391- Other specified injury of right middle and inner ear**

Laterality SP 7 **S09.392- Other specified injury of left middle and inner ear**

Laterality IQ 7 **S09.399- Other specified injury of unspecified middle and inner ear**

SP 7 **S09.8XX- Other specified injuries of head**

5 **S09.9 Unspecified injury of face and head**

IQ 7 **S09.90X- Unspecified injury of head**
Head injury NOS
EXCLUDES 1 brain injury NOS (S06.9-)
head injury NOS with loss of consciousness (S06.9-)
intracranial injury NOS (S06.9-)

IQ 7 **S09.91X- Unspecified injury of ear**
Injury of ear NOS

IQ 7 **S09.92X- Unspecified injury of nose**
Injury of nose NOS

IQ 7 **S09.93X- Unspecified injury of face**
Injury of face NOS

Injuries to the neck (S10-S19)

INCLUDES injuries of nape
injuries of supraclavicular region
injuries of throat

EXCLUDES 2 burns and corrosions (T20-T32)
effects of foreign body in esophagus (T18.1)
effects of foreign body in larynx (T17.3)
effects of foreign body in pharynx (T17.2)
effects of foreign body in trachea (T17.4)
frostbite (T33-T34)
insect bite or sting, venomous (T63.4)

GUIDELINES **Section I.C.19.c.2)**
Multiple fractures are sequenced in accordance with the severity of the fracture.

GUIDELINES **Section I.C.19.b.1)-2)**
When coding injuries, assign separate codes for each injury unless a combination code is provided, in which case the combination code is assigned ... Traumatic injury codes (S00-T14.9) are not to be used for normal, healing surgical wounds or to identify complications of surgical wounds. The code for the most serious injury, as determined by the provider and the focus of treatment, is sequenced first.

1) Superficial injuries such as abrasions or contusions are not coded when associated with more severe injuries of the same site.

2) When a primary injury results in minor damage to peripheral nerves or blood vessels, the primary injury is sequenced first with additional code(s) for injuries to nerves and spinal cord (such as category S04), and/or injury to blood vessels (such as category S15). When the primary injury is to the blood vessels or nerves, that injury should be sequenced first.

GUIDELINES **Section I.C.19.c**
Coding of Traumatic Fractures: The principles of multiple coding of injuries should be followed in coding fractures. Fractures of specified sites are coded individually by site in accordance with both the provisions within categories S02, S12, S22, S32, S42, S49, S52, S59, S62, S72, S79, S82, S89, S92 and the level of detail furnished by medical record content. A fracture not indicated as open or closed should be coded to closed. A fracture not indicated whether displaced or not displaced should be coded to displaced.

CODING TIPS✓ 7th character A is acceptable in home health and hospice when active treatment is provided, such as antibiotics for an infected wound or a wound vac for a dehisced wound. D is used when the complication or injury is now healing. Think of D as aftercare. S is used for sequela of the injury or complication. Sequela is a residual deficit or condition produced as a result of the injury or complication after the original injury or complication has healed.

4 **S10 Superficial injury of neck**

The appropriate 7th character is to be added to each code from category S10
A initial encounter
D subsequent encounter
S sequela

IQ 7 **S10.0XX- Contusion of throat**
Contusion of cervical esophagus
Contusion of larynx
Contusion of pharynx
Contusion of trachea

5 **S10.1 Other and unspecified superficial injuries of throat**

IQ 7 **S10.10X- Unspecified superficial injuries of throat**

IQ 7 **S10.11X- Abrasion of throat**

IQ 7 **S10.12X- Blister (nonthermal) of throat**

IQ 7 **S10.14X- External constriction of part of throat**

IQ 7 **S10.15X- Superficial foreign body of throat**
Splinter in the throat

IQ 7 **S10.16X- Insect bite (nonvenomous) of throat**

IQ 7 **S10.17X- Other superficial bite of throat**
EXCLUDES 1 open bite of throat (S11.85)

5 **S10.8 Superficial injury of other specified parts of neck**

IQ 7 **S10.80X- Unspecified superficial injury of other specified part of neck**

IQ 7 **S10.81X- Abrasion of other specified part of neck**

IQ 7 **S10.82X- Blister (nonthermal) of other specified part of neck**

IQ 7 **S10.83X- Contusion of other specified part of neck**

IQ 7 **S10.84X- External constriction of other specified part of neck**

IQ 7 **S10.85X- Superficial foreign body of other specified part of neck**
Splinter in other specified part of neck

IQ 7 **S10.86X- Insect bite of other specified part of neck**

IQ 7 **S10.87X- Other superficial bite of other specified part of neck**
EXCLUDES 1 open bite of other specified parts of neck (S11.85)

5 **S10.9 Superficial injury of unspecified part of neck**

IQ 7 **S10.90X- Unspecified superficial injury of unspecified part of neck**

IQ 7 **S10.91X- Abrasion of unspecified part of neck**

IQ 7 **S10.92X- Blister (nonthermal) of unspecified part of neck**

IQ 7 **S10.93X- Contusion of unspecified part of neck**

IQ 7 **S10.94X- External constriction of unspecified part of neck**

IQ 7 **S10.95X- Superficial foreign body of unspecified part of neck**

IQ 7 **S10.96X- Insect bite of unspecified part of neck**

IQ 7 **S10.97X- Other superficial bite of unspecified part of neck**

4 **S11 Open wound of neck**
Code also any associated:
spinal cord injury (S14.0, S14.1-)
wound infection
EXCLUDES 2 open fracture of vertebra (S12.- with 7th character B)

The appropriate 7th character is to be added to each code from category S11
A initial encounter
D subsequent encounter
S sequela

CODING TIPS✓ Open wound codes are used for wounds caused by trauma. Do not assign a code for "open wound" unless the etiology of the wound is related to trauma. Do not use Z codes for any aspect of care of a trauma wound, e.g. no Z code for dressing changes, drain care, or suture removal.

CODING TIPS✓ No aftercare code applies. The 7th character "D" is the default for home care and hospice when providing aftercare for a healing or resolving condition; "A" is used for active treatment such as antibiotics or more than routine wound care; "S" may be used to indicate a residual condition after the original injury has healed.

5 **S11.0 Open wound of larynx and trachea**

6 **S11.01 Open wound of larynx**
EXCLUDES 2 open wound of vocal cord (S11.03)

SP 7 **S11.011- Laceration without foreign body of larynx**

SP 7 **S11.012- Laceration with foreign body of larynx**

SP 7 **S11.013- Puncture wound without foreign body of larynx**

SP 7 **S11.014- Puncture wound with foreign body of larynx**

SP 7 **S11.015- Open bite of larynx**
Bite of larynx NOS

SP 7 **S11.019- Unspecified open wound of larynx**

6 **S11.02 Open wound of trachea**
Open wound of cervical trachea

Chapter 19

S00-T88

★New ▲Revised Px Primary SP PDGM Px SL Low CoM SH High CoM IQ Quest. Encounter H Hospice non-cancer Dx Unspecified M *Manifestation*

Open wound of trachea NOS
EXCLUDES 2 open wound of thoracic trachea (S27.5-)

SP 7 **S11.021- Laceration without foreign body of trachea**
SP 7 **S11.022- Laceration with foreign body of trachea**
SP 7 **S11.023- Puncture wound without foreign body of trachea**
SP 7 **S11.024- Puncture wound with foreign body of trachea**
SP 7 **S11.025- Open bite of trachea**
Bite of trachea NOS
SP 7 **S11.029- Unspecified open wound of trachea**

6 **S11.03 Open wound of vocal cord**
SP 7 **S11.031- Laceration without foreign body of vocal cord**
SP 7 **S11.032- Laceration with foreign body of vocal cord**
SP 7 **S11.033- Puncture wound without foreign body of vocal cord**
SP 7 **S11.034- Puncture wound with foreign body of vocal cord**
SP 7 **S11.035- Open bite of vocal cord**
Bite of vocal cord NOS
SP 7 **S11.039- Unspecified open wound of vocal cord**

5 **S11.1 Open wound of thyroid gland**
SP 7 **S11.10X- Unspecified open wound of thyroid gland**
SP 7 **S11.11X- Laceration without foreign body of thyroid gland**
SP 7 **S11.12X- Laceration with foreign body of thyroid gland**
SP 7 **S11.13X- Puncture wound without foreign body of thyroid gland**
SP 7 **S11.14X- Puncture wound with foreign body of thyroid gland**
SP 7 **S11.15X- Open bite of thyroid gland**
Bite of thyroid gland NOS

5 **S11.2 Open wound of pharynx and cervical esophagus**
EXCLUDES 1 open wound of esophagus NOS (S27.8-)
SP 7 **S11.20X- Unspecified open wound of pharynx and cervical esophagus**
SP 7 **S11.21X- Laceration without foreign body of pharynx and cervical esophagus**
SP 7 **S11.22X- Laceration with foreign body of pharynx and cervical esophagus**
SP 7 **S11.23X- Puncture wound without foreign body of pharynx and cervical esophagus**
SP 7 **S11.24X- Puncture wound with foreign body of pharynx and cervical esophagus**
SP 7 **S11.25X- Open bite of pharynx and cervical esophagus**
Bite of pharynx and cervical esophagus NOS

5 **S11.8 Open wound of other specified parts of neck**
SP 7 **S11.80X- Unspecified open wound of other specified part of neck**
SP 7 **S11.81X- Laceration without foreign body of other specified part of neck**
SP 7 **S11.82X- Laceration with foreign body of other specified part of neck**
SP 7 **S11.83X- Puncture wound without foreign body of other specified part of neck**
SP 7 **S11.84X- Puncture wound with foreign body of other specified part of neck**
SP 7 **S11.85X- Open bite of other specified part of neck**
Bite of other specified part of neck NOS
EXCLUDES 1 superficial bite of other specified part of neck (S10.87)
SP 7 **S11.89X- Other open wound of other specified part of neck**

5 **S11.9 Open wound of unspecified part of neck**
SP 7 **S11.90X- Unspecified open wound of unspecified part of neck**
SP 7 **S11.91X- Laceration without foreign body of unspecified part of neck**
SP 7 **S11.92X- Laceration with foreign body of unspecified part of neck**
!Q 7 **S11.93X- Puncture wound without foreign body of unspecified part of neck**
!Q 7 **S11.94X- Puncture wound with foreign body of unspecified part of neck**
!Q 7 **S11.95X- Open bite of unspecified part of neck**
Bite of neck NOS
EXCLUDES 1 superficial bite of neck (S10.97)

4 **S12 Fracture of cervical vertebra and other parts of neck**
Note:
A fracture not indicated as displaced or nondisplaced should be coded to displaced
A fracture not indicated as open or closed should be coded to closed
INCLUDES fracture of cervical neural arch
fracture of cervical spine
fracture of cervical spinous process
fracture of cervical transverse process
fracture of cervical vertebral arch
fracture of neck
Code first:
any associated cervical spinal cord injury (S14.0, S14.1-)

The appropriate 7th character is to be added to all codes from subcategories S12.0-S12.6

A	initial encounter for closed fracture
B	initial encounter for open fracture
D	subsequent encounter for fracture with routine healing
G	subsequent encounter for fracture with delayed healing
K	subsequent encounter for fracture with nonunion
S	sequela

Chapter 19
S00-T88

CODING TIPS✓ Fractures repaired by joint replacements are NOT coded with Z47.1. Fractures repaired by any other orthopedic surgery are NOT coded with Z47.89. Z codes are not appropriate for fractures of any kind. Code the fracture with 7th character D for fractures undergoing surgical repair.

CODING TIPS✓ A fracture not indicated as displaced or nondisplaced should be coded to displaced. A fracture not indicated as open or closed should be coded to closed.

CODING TIPS✓ 'D' is the 7th character for home care and hospice unless the physician or NPP has documented delayed healing, nonunion or malunion. A sequela is a condition left after the fracture has healed. The Gustilo open fracture classification must be used for open fractures. The default 7th character for open fractures is E.

5 **S12.0 Fracture of first cervical vertebra**
Atlas

6 **S12.00 Unspecified fracture of first cervical vertebra**

SP 7 **S12.000- Unspecified displaced fracture of first cervical vertebra**

SP 7 **S12.001- Unspecified nondisplaced fracture of first cervical vertebra**

SP 7 **S12.01X- Stable burst fracture of first cervical vertebra**

SP 7 **S12.02X- Unstable burst fracture of first cervical vertebra**

6 **S12.03 Posterior arch fracture of first cervical vertebra**

SP 7 **S12.030- Displaced posterior arch fracture of first cervical vertebra**

SP 7 **S12.031- Nondisplaced posterior arch fracture of first cervical vertebra**

6 **S12.04 Lateral mass fracture of first cervical vertebra**

SP 7 **S12.040- Displaced lateral mass fracture of first cervical vertebra**

SP 7 **S12.041- Nondisplaced lateral mass fracture of first cervical vertebra**

6 **S12.09 Other fracture of first cervical vertebra**

SP 7 **S12.090- Other displaced fracture of first cervical vertebra**

SP 7 **S12.091- Other nondisplaced fracture of first cervical vertebra**

5 **S12.1 Fracture of second cervical vertebra**
Axis

6 **S12.10 Unspecified fracture of second cervical vertebra**

SP 7 **S12.100- Unspecified displaced fracture of second cervical vertebra**

SP 7 **S12.101- Unspecified nondisplaced fracture of second cervical vertebra**

6 **S12.11 Type II dens fracture**

SP 7 **S12.110- Anterior displaced Type II dens fracture**

SP 7 **S12.111- Posterior displaced Type II dens fracture**

SP 7 **S12.112- Nondisplaced Type II dens fracture**

6 **S12.12 Other dens fracture**

SP 7 **S12.120- Other displaced dens fracture**

SP 7 **S12.121- Other nondisplaced dens fracture**

6 **S12.13 Unspecified traumatic spondylolisthesis of second cervical vertebra**

SP 7 **S12.130- Unspecified traumatic displaced spondylolisthesis of second cervical vertebra**

SP 7 **S12.131- Unspecified traumatic nondisplaced spondylolisthesis of second cervical vertebra**

SP 7 **S12.14X- Type III traumatic spondylolisthesis of second cervical vertebra**

6 **S12.15 Other traumatic spondylolisthesis of second cervical vertebra**

SP 7 **S12.150- Other traumatic displaced spondylolisthesis of second cervical vertebra**

SP 7 **S12.151- Other traumatic nondisplaced spondylolisthesis of second cervical vertebra**

6 **S12.19 Other fracture of second cervical vertebra**

SP 7 **S12.190- Other displaced fracture of second cervical vertebra**

SP 7 **S12.191- Other nondisplaced fracture of second cervical vertebra**

5 **S12.2 Fracture of third cervical vertebra**

6 **S12.20 Unspecified fracture of third cervical vertebra**

SP 7 **S12.200- Unspecified displaced fracture of third cervical vertebra**

SP 7 **S12.201- Unspecified nondisplaced fracture of third cervical vertebra**

6 **S12.23 Unspecified traumatic spondylolisthesis of third cervical vertebra**

SP 7 **S12.230- Unspecified traumatic displaced spondylolisthesis of third cervical vertebra**

SP 7 **S12.231- Unspecified traumatic nondisplaced spondylolisthesis of third cervical vertebra**

SP 7 **S12.24X- Type III traumatic spondylolisthesis of third cervical vertebra**

6 **S12.25 Other traumatic spondylolisthesis of third cervical vertebra**

SP 7 **S12.250- Other traumatic displaced spondylolisthesis of third cervical vertebra**

SP 7 **S12.251- Other traumatic nondisplaced spondylolisthesis of third cervical vertebra**

6 **S12.29 Other fracture of third cervical vertebra**

SP 7 **S12.290- Other displaced fracture of third cervical vertebra**

SP 7 **S12.291- Other nondisplaced fracture of third cervical vertebra**

5 **S12.3 Fracture of fourth cervical vertebra**

6 S12.30 Unspecified fracture of fourth cervical vertebra

SP 7 S12.300- Unspecified displaced fracture of fourth cervical vertebra

SP 7 S12.301- Unspecified nondisplaced fracture of fourth cervical vertebra

6 S12.33 Unspecified traumatic spondylolisthesis of fourth cervical vertebra

SP 7 S12.330- Unspecified traumatic displaced spondylolisthesis of fourth cervical vertebra

SP 7 S12.331- Unspecified traumatic nondisplaced spondylolisthesis of fourth cervical vertebra

SP 7 S12.34X- Type III traumatic spondylolisthesis of fourth cervical vertebra

6 S12.35 Other traumatic spondylolisthesis of fourth cervical vertebra

SP 7 S12.350- Other traumatic displaced spondylolisthesis of fourth cervical vertebra

SP 7 S12.351- Other traumatic nondisplaced spondylolisthesis of fourth cervical vertebra

6 S12.39 Other fracture of fourth cervical vertebra

SP 7 S12.390- Other displaced fracture of fourth cervical vertebra

SP 7 S12.391- Other nondisplaced fracture of fourth cervical vertebra

5 S12.4 Fracture of fifth cervical vertebra

6 S12.40 Unspecified fracture of fifth cervical vertebra

SP 7 S12.400- Unspecified displaced fracture of fifth cervical vertebra

SP 7 S12.401- Unspecified nondisplaced fracture of fifth cervical vertebra

6 S12.43 Unspecified traumatic spondylolisthesis of fifth cervical vertebra

SP 7 S12.430- Unspecified traumatic displaced spondylolisthesis of fifth cervical vertebra

SP 7 S12.431- Unspecified traumatic nondisplaced spondylolisthesis of fifth cervical vertebra

SP 7 S12.44X- Type III traumatic spondylolisthesis of fifth cervical vertebra

6 S12.45 Other traumatic spondylolisthesis of fifth cervical vertebra

SP 7 S12.450- Other traumatic displaced spondylolisthesis of fifth cervical vertebra

SP 7 S12.451- Other traumatic nondisplaced spondylolisthesis of fifth cervical vertebra

6 S12.49 Other fracture of fifth cervical vertebra

SP 7 S12.490- Other displaced fracture of fifth cervical vertebra

SP 7 S12.491- Other nondisplaced fracture of fifth cervical vertebra

5 S12.5 Fracture of sixth cervical vertebra

6 S12.50 Unspecified fracture of sixth cervical vertebra

SP 7 S12.500- Unspecified displaced fracture of sixth cervical vertebra

SP 7 S12.501- Unspecified nondisplaced fracture of sixth cervical vertebra

6 S12.53 Unspecified traumatic spondylolisthesis of sixth cervical vertebra

SP 7 S12.530- Unspecified traumatic displaced spondylolisthesis of sixth cervical vertebra

SP 7 S12.531- Unspecified traumatic nondisplaced spondylolisthesis of sixth cervical vertebra

SP 7 S12.54X- Type III traumatic spondylolisthesis of sixth cervical vertebra

6 S12.55 Other traumatic spondylolisthesis of sixth cervical vertebra

SP 7 S12.550- Other traumatic displaced spondylolisthesis of sixth cervical vertebra

SP 7 S12.551- Other traumatic nondisplaced spondylolisthesis of sixth cervical vertebra

6 S12.59 Other fracture of sixth cervical vertebra

SP 7 S12.590- Other displaced fracture of sixth cervical vertebra

SP 7 S12.591- Other nondisplaced fracture of sixth cervical vertebra

5 S12.6 Fracture of seventh cervical vertebra

6 S12.60 Unspecified fracture of seventh cervical vertebra

SP 7 S12.600- Unspecified displaced fracture of seventh cervical vertebra

SP 7 S12.601- Unspecified nondisplaced fracture of seventh cervical vertebra

6 S12.63 Unspecified traumatic spondylolisthesis of seventh cervical vertebra

SP 7 S12.630- Unspecified traumatic displaced spondylolisthesis of seventh cervical vertebra

SP 7 S12.631- Unspecified traumatic nondisplaced spondylolisthesis of seventh cervical vertebra

SP 7 S12.64X- Type III traumatic spondylolisthesis of seventh cervical vertebra

6 S12.65 Other traumatic spondylolisthesis of seventh cervical vertebra

SP 7 S12.650- Other traumatic displaced spondylolisthesis of seventh cervical vertebra

SP 7 S12.651- Other traumatic nondisplaced spondylolisthesis of seventh cervical vertebra

6 S12.69 Other fracture of seventh cervical vertebra

SP 7 **S12.690- Other displaced fracture of seventh cervical vertebra**

SP 7 **S12.691- Other nondisplaced fracture of seventh cervical vertebra**

SP 7 **S12.8XX- Fracture of other parts of neck**
Hyoid bone
Larynx
Thyroid cartilage
Trachea

The appropriate 7th character is to be added to code S12.8
A initial encounter
D subsequent encounter
S sequela

SP 7 **S12.9XX- Fracture of neck, unspecified**
Fracture of neck NOS
Fracture of cervical spine NOS
Fracture of cervical vertebra NOS

The appropriate 7th character is to be added to code S12.9
A initial encounter
D subsequent encounter
S sequela

4 **S13 Dislocation and sprain of joints and ligaments at neck level**
INCLUDES avulsion of joint or ligament at neck level
laceration of cartilage, joint or ligament at neck level
sprain of cartilage, joint or ligament at neck level
traumatic hemarthrosis of joint or ligament at neck level
traumatic rupture of joint or ligament at neck level
traumatic subluxation of joint or ligament at neck level
traumatic tear of joint or ligament at neck level

Code also:
any associated open wound

EXCLUDES 2 strain of muscle or tendon at neck level (S16.1)

The appropriate 7th character is to be added to each code from category S13
A initial encounter
D subsequent encounter
S sequela

SP 7 **S13.0XX- Traumatic rupture of cervical intervertebral disc**
EXCLUDES 1 rupture or displacement (nontraumatic) of cervical intervertebral disc NOS (M50.-)

5 **S13.1 Subluxation and dislocation of cervical vertebrae**
Code also any associated:
open wound of neck (S11.-)
spinal cord injury (S14.1-)
EXCLUDES 2 fracture of cervical vertebrae (S12.0-S12.3-)

6 **S13.10 Subluxation and dislocation of unspecified cervical vertebrae**

SP 7 **S13.100- Subluxation of unspecified cervical vertebrae**

SP 7 **S13.101- Dislocation of unspecified cervical vertebrae**

6 **S13.11 Subluxation and dislocation of C0/C1 cervical vertebrae**
Subluxation and dislocation of atlantooccipital joint
Subluxation and dislocation of atloidooccipital joint
Subluxation and dislocation of occipitoatloid joint

SP 7 **S13.110- Subluxation of C0/C1 cervical vertebrae**

SP 7 **S13.111- Dislocation of C0/C1 cervical vertebrae**

6 **S13.12 Subluxation and dislocation of C1/C2 cervical vertebrae**
Subluxation and dislocation of atlantoaxial joint

SP 7 **S13.120- Subluxation of C1/C2 cervical vertebrae**

SP 7 **S13.121- Dislocation of C1/C2 cervical vertebrae**

6 **S13.13 Subluxation and dislocation of C2/C3 cervical vertebrae**

SP 7 **S13.130- Subluxation of C2/C3 cervical vertebrae**

SP 7 **S13.131- Dislocation of C2/C3 cervical vertebrae**

6 **S13.14 Subluxation and dislocation of C3/C4 cervical vertebrae**

SP 7 **S13.140- Subluxation of C3/C4 cervical vertebrae**

SP 7 **S13.141- Dislocation of C3/C4 cervical vertebrae**

6 **S13.15 Subluxation and dislocation of C4/C5 cervical vertebrae**

SP 7 **S13.150- Subluxation of C4/C5 cervical vertebrae**

SP 7 **S13.151- Dislocation of C4/C5 cervical vertebrae**

6 **S13.16 Subluxation and dislocation of C5/C6 cervical vertebrae**

SP 7 **S13.160- Subluxation of C5/C6 cervical vertebrae**

SP 7 **S13.161- Dislocation of C5/C6 cervical vertebrae**

6 **S13.17 Subluxation and dislocation of C6/C7 cervical vertebrae**

SP 7 **S13.170- Subluxation of C6/C7 cervical vertebrae**

SP 7 **S13.171- Dislocation of C6/C7 cervical vertebrae**

6 **S13.18 Subluxation and dislocation of C7/T1 cervical vertebrae**

SP 7 **S13.180- Subluxation of C7/T1 cervical vertebrae**

SP 7 **S13.181- Dislocation of C7/T1 cervical vertebrae**

5 **S13.2 Dislocation of other and unspecified parts of neck**

SP 7 **S13.20X- Dislocation of unspecified parts of neck**

SP 7 **S13.29X- Dislocation of other parts of neck**

SP 7 **S13.4XX- Sprain of ligaments of cervical spine**
Sprain of anterior longitudinal (ligament), cervical

Chapter 19

S00-T88

★ New ▲ Revised Px Primary SP PDGM Px SL Low CoM SH High CoM IQ Quest. Encounter H Hospice non-cancer Dx Unspecified M *Manifestation*

Sprain of atlanto-axial (joints)
Sprain of atlanto-occipital (joints)
Whiplash injury of cervical spine

SP 7 **S13.5XX- Sprain of thyroid region**
Sprain of cricoarytenoid (joint) (ligament)
Sprain of cricothyroid (joint) (ligament)
Sprain of thyroid cartilage

SP 7 **S13.8XX- Sprain of joints and ligaments of other parts of neck**

SP 7 **S13.9XX- Sprain of joints and ligaments of unspecified parts of neck**

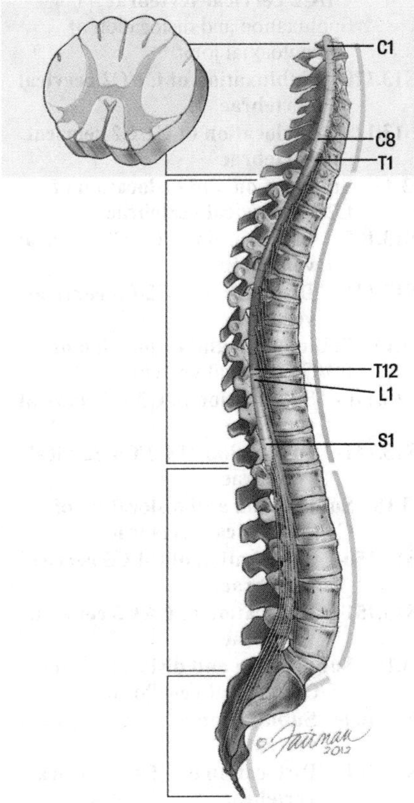

4 **S14 Injury of nerves and spinal cord at neck level**
Note:
Code to highest level of cervical cord injury
Code also any associated:
fracture of cervical vertebra (S12.0--S12.6.-)
open wound of neck (S11.-)
transient paralysis (R29.5)

The appropriate 7th character is to be added to each code from category S14

A	initial encounter
D	subsequent encounter
S	sequela

CODING TIPS ✓ When coding sequelae of a cervical spinal cord injury, first list the residual condition(s), followed by the specific spinal cord injury diagnosed using the appropriate code from this category with the seventh character "S" to indicate sequelae. If there are multiple levels of injury, code only the highest injury in each section of the spine (cervical, thoracic, and lumbar).

SP 7 **S14.0XX- Concussion and edema of cervical spinal cord**

5 **S14.1 Other and unspecified injuries of cervical spinal cord**

6 **S14.10 Unspecified injury of cervical spinal cord**

IQ 7 **S14.101- Unspecified injury at C1 level of cervical spinal cord**

IQ 7 **S14.102- Unspecified injury at C2 level of cervical spinal cord**

IQ 7 **S14.103- Unspecified injury at C3 level of cervical spinal cord**

IQ 7 **S14.104- Unspecified injury at C4 level of cervical spinal cord**

IQ 7 **S14.105- Unspecified injury at C5 level of cervical spinal cord**

IQ 7 **S14.106- Unspecified injury at C6 level of cervical spinal cord**

IQ 7 **S14.107- Unspecified injury at C7 level of cervical spinal cord**

IQ 7 **S14.108- Unspecified injury at C8 level of cervical spinal cord**

IQ 7 **S14.109- Unspecified injury at unspecified level of cervical spinal cord**
Injury of cervical spinal cord NOS

6 **S14.11 Complete lesion of cervical spinal cord**

SP 7 **S14.111- Complete lesion at C1 level of cervical spinal cord**

SP 7 **S14.112- Complete lesion at C2 level of cervical spinal cord**

SP 7 **S14.113- Complete lesion at C3 level of cervical spinal cord**

SP 7 **S14.114- Complete lesion at C4 level of cervical spinal cord**

SP 7 **S14.115- Complete lesion at C5 level of cervical spinal cord**

SP 7 **S14.116- Complete lesion at C6 level of cervical spinal cord**

SP 7 **S14.117- Complete lesion at C7 level of cervical spinal cord**

SP 7 **S14.118- Complete lesion at C8 level of cervical spinal cord**

IQ 7 **S14.119- Complete lesion at unspecified level of cervical spinal cord**

6 **S14.12 Central cord syndrome of cervical spinal cord**

SP 7 **S14.121- Central cord syndrome at C1 level of cervical spinal cord**

SP 7 **S14.122- Central cord syndrome at C2 level of cervical spinal cord**

SP 7 **S14.123- Central cord syndrome at C3 level of cervical spinal cord**

SP 7 **S14.124- Central cord syndrome at C4 level of cervical spinal cord**

SP 7 **S14.125- Central cord syndrome at C5 level of cervical spinal cord**
SP 7 **S14.126- Central cord syndrome at C6 level of cervical spinal cord**
SP 7 **S14.127- Central cord syndrome at C7 level of cervical spinal cord**
SP 7 **S14.128- Central cord syndrome at C8 level of cervical spinal cord**
!Q 7 **S14.129- Central cord syndrome at unspecified level of cervical spinal cord**

6 **S14.13 Anterior cord syndrome of cervical spinal cord**
SP 7 **S14.131- Anterior cord syndrome at C1 level of cervical spinal cord**
SP 7 **S14.132- Anterior cord syndrome at C2 level of cervical spinal cord**
SP 7 **S14.133- Anterior cord syndrome at C3 level of cervical spinal cord**
SP 7 **S14.134- Anterior cord syndrome at C4 level of cervical spinal cord**
SP 7 **S14.135- Anterior cord syndrome at C5 level of cervical spinal cord**
SP 7 **S14.136- Anterior cord syndrome at C6 level of cervical spinal cord**
SP 7 **S14.137- Anterior cord syndrome at C7 level of cervical spinal cord**
SP 7 **S14.138- Anterior cord syndrome at C8 level of cervical spinal cord**
!Q 7 **S14.139- Anterior cord syndrome at unspecified level of cervical spinal cord**

6 **S14.14 Brown-Séquard syndrome of cervical spinal cord**
SP 7 **S14.141- Brown-Séquard syndrome at C1 level of cervical spinal cord**
SP 7 **S14.142- Brown-Séquard syndrome at C2 level of cervical spinal cord**
SP 7 **S14.143- Brown-Séquard syndrome at C3 level of cervical spinal cord**
SP 7 **S14.144- Brown-Séquard syndrome at C4 level of cervical spinal cord**
SP 7 **S14.145- Brown-Séquard syndrome at C5 level of cervical spinal cord**
SP 7 **S14.146- Brown-Séquard syndrome at C6 level of cervical spinal cord**
SP 7 **S14.147- Brown-Séquard syndrome at C7 level of cervical spinal cord**
SP 7 **S14.148- Brown-Séquard syndrome at C8 level of cervical spinal cord**
!Q 7 **S14.149- Brown-Séquard syndrome at unspecified level of cervical spinal cord**

6 **S14.15 Other incomplete lesions of cervical spinal cord**
Incomplete lesion of cervical spinal cord NOS
Posterior cord syndrome of cervical spinal cord
SP 7 **S14.151- Other incomplete lesion at C1 level of cervical spinal cord**
SP 7 **S14.152- Other incomplete lesion at C2 level of cervical spinal cord**
SP 7 **S14.153- Other incomplete lesion at C3 level of cervical spinal cord**
SP 7 **S14.154- Other incomplete lesion at C4 level of cervical spinal cord**
SP 7 **S14.155- Other incomplete lesion at C5 level of cervical spinal cord**
SP 7 **S14.156- Other incomplete lesion at C6 level of cervical spinal cord**
SP 7 **S14.157- Other incomplete lesion at C7 level of cervical spinal cord**
SP 7 **S14.158- Other incomplete lesion at C8 level of cervical spinal cord**
!Q 7 **S14.159- Other incomplete lesion at unspecified level of cervical spinal cord**

SP 7 **S14.2XX- Injury of nerve root of cervical spine**
SP 7 **S14.3XX- Injury of brachial plexus**
SP 7 **S14.4XX- Injury of peripheral nerves of neck**
SP 7 **S14.5XX- Injury of cervical sympathetic nerves**
SP 7 **S14.8XX- Injury of other specified nerves of neck**
!Q 7 **S14.9XX- Injury of unspecified nerves of neck**

4 **S15 Injury of blood vessels at neck level**
Code also:
any associated open wound (S11.-)

The appropriate 7th character is to be added to each code from category S15
A initial encounter
D subsequent encounter
S sequela

5 **S15.0 Injury of carotid artery of neck**
Injury of carotid artery (common) (external) (internal, extracranial portion)
Injury of carotid artery NOS
EXCLUDES 1 injury of internal carotid artery, intracranial portion (S06.8)

6 **S15.00 Unspecified injury of carotid artery**
H !Q 7 **S15.001- Unspecified injury of right carotid artery**
H !Q 7 **S15.002- Unspecified injury of left carotid artery**
H !Q 7 **S15.009- Unspecified injury of unspecified carotid artery**

6 **S15.01 Minor laceration of carotid artery**
Incomplete transection of carotid artery
Laceration of carotid artery NOS
Superficial laceration of carotid artery
H SP 7 **S15.011- Minor laceration of right carotid artery**
H SP 7 **S15.012- Minor laceration of left carotid artery**
H SP !Q 7 **S15.019- Minor laceration of unspecified carotid artery**

6 **S15.02 Major laceration of carotid artery**
Complete transection of carotid artery
Traumatic rupture of carotid artery
H SP 7 **S15.021- Major laceration of right carotid artery**
H SP 7 **S15.022- Major laceration of left carotid artery**
H SP !Q 7 **S15.029- Major laceration of unspecified carotid artery**

6 **S15.09 Other specified injury of carotid artery**

Chapter 19
S00-T88

S15.091- Other specified injury of right carotid artery
S15.092- Other specified injury of left carotid artery
S15.099- Other specified injury of unspecified carotid artery

S15.1 Injury of vertebral artery
S15.10 Unspecified injury of vertebral artery
S15.101- Unspecified injury of right vertebral artery
S15.102- Unspecified injury of left vertebral artery
S15.109- Unspecified injury of unspecified vertebral artery
S15.11 Minor laceration of vertebral artery
Incomplete transection of vertebral artery
Laceration of vertebral artery NOS
Superficial laceration of vertebral artery
S15.111- Minor laceration of right vertebral artery
S15.112- Minor laceration of left vertebral artery
S15.119- Minor laceration of unspecified vertebral artery
S15.12 Major laceration of vertebral artery
Complete transection of vertebral artery
Traumatic rupture of vertebral artery
S15.121- Major laceration of right vertebral artery
S15.122- Major laceration of left vertebral artery
S15.129- Major laceration of unspecified vertebral artery
S15.19 Other specified injury of vertebral artery
S15.191- Other specified injury of right vertebral artery
S15.192- Other specified injury of left vertebral artery
S15.199- Other specified injury of unspecified vertebral artery

S15.2 Injury of external jugular vein
S15.20 Unspecified injury of external jugular vein
S15.201- Unspecified injury of right external jugular vein
S15.202- Unspecified injury of left external jugular vein
S15.209- Unspecified injury of unspecified external jugular vein
S15.21 Minor laceration of external jugular vein
Incomplete transection of external jugular vein
Laceration of external jugular vein NOS
Superficial laceration of external jugular vein
S15.211- Minor laceration of right external jugular vein
S15.212- Minor laceration of left external jugular vein
S15.219- Minor laceration of unspecified external jugular vein
S15.22 Major laceration of external jugular vein
Complete transection of external jugular vein
Traumatic rupture of external jugular vein
S15.221- Major laceration of right external jugular vein
S15.222- Major laceration of left external jugular vein
S15.229- Major laceration of unspecified external jugular vein
S15.29 Other specified injury of external jugular vein
S15.291- Other specified injury of right external jugular vein
S15.292- Other specified injury of left external jugular vein
S15.299- Other specified injury of unspecified external jugular vein

S15.3 Injury of internal jugular vein
S15.30 Unspecified injury of internal jugular vein
S15.301- Unspecified injury of right internal jugular vein
S15.302- Unspecified injury of left internal jugular vein
S15.309- Unspecified injury of unspecified internal jugular vein
S15.31 Minor laceration of internal jugular vein
Incomplete transection of internal jugular vein
Laceration of internal jugular vein NOS
Superficial laceration of internal jugular vein
S15.311- Minor laceration of right internal jugular vein
S15.312- Minor laceration of left internal jugular vein
S15.319- Minor laceration of unspecified internal jugular vein
S15.32 Major laceration of internal jugular vein
Complete transection of internal jugular vein
Traumatic rupture of internal jugular vein
S15.321- Major laceration of right internal jugular vein
S15.322- Major laceration of left internal jugular vein
S15.329- Major laceration of unspecified internal jugular vein
S15.39 Other specified injury of internal jugular vein
S15.391- Other specified injury of right internal jugular vein

H SP 7 **S15.392- Other specified injury of left internal jugular vein**

H IQ 7 **S15.399- Other specified injury of unspecified internal jugular vein**

SP 7 **S15.8XX- Injury of other specified blood vessels at neck level**

IQ 7 **S15.9XX- Injury of unspecified blood vessel at neck level**

4 **S16 Injury of muscle, fascia and tendon at neck level**

Code also:
any associated open wound (S11.-)

EXCLUDES 2 sprain of joint or ligament at neck level (S13.9)

The appropriate 7th character is to be added to each code from category S16
A initial encounter
D subsequent encounter
S sequela

SP 7 **S16.1XX- Strain of muscle, fascia and tendon at neck level**

SP 7 **S16.2XX- Laceration of muscle, fascia and tendon at neck level**

IQ 7 **S16.8XX- Other specified injury of muscle, fascia and tendon at neck level**

IQ 7 **S16.9XX- Unspecified injury of muscle, fascia and tendon at neck level**

+ 4 **S17 Crushing injury of neck**

Use additional code for all associated injuries, such as:
injury of blood vessels (S15.-)
open wound of neck (S11.-)
spinal cord injury (S14.0, S14.1-)
vertebral fracture (S12.0--S12.3-)

The appropriate 7th character is to be added to each code from category S17
A initial encounter
D subsequent encounter
S sequela

SP + 7 **S17.0XX- Crushing injury of larynx and trachea**

SP + 7 **S17.8XX- Crushing injury of other specified parts of neck**

IQ + 7 **S17.9XX- Crushing injury of neck, part unspecified**

4 **S19 Other specified and unspecified injuries of neck**

The appropriate 7th character is to be added to each code from category S19
A initial encounter
D subsequent encounter
S sequela

5 **S19.8 Other specified injuries of neck**

SP 7 **S19.80X- Other specified injuries of unspecified part of neck**

SP 7 **S19.81X- Other specified injuries of larynx**

SP 7 **S19.82X- Other specified injuries of cervical trachea**

EXCLUDES 2 other specified injury of thoracic trachea (S27.5-)

SP 7 **S19.83X- Other specified injuries of vocal cord**

SP 7 **S19.84X- Other specified injuries of thyroid gland**

SP 7 **S19.85X- Other specified injuries of pharynx and cervical esophagus**

SP 7 **S19.89X- Other specified injuries of other specified part of neck**

IQ 7 **S19.9XX- Unspecified injury of neck**

Injuries to the thorax (S20-S29)

INCLUDES
injuries of breast
injuries of chest (wall)
injuries of interscapular area

EXCLUDES 2
burns and corrosions (T20-T32)
effects of foreign body in bronchus (T17.5)
effects of foreign body in esophagus (T18.1)
effects of foreign body in lung (T17.8)
effects of foreign body in trachea (T17.4)
frostbite (T33-T34)
injuries of axilla
injuries of clavicle
injuries of scapular region
injuries of shoulder
insect bite or sting, venomous (T63.4)

GUIDELINES **Section I.C.19.c.2)**

Multiple fractures are sequenced in accordance with the severity of the fracture.

GUIDELINES **Section I.C.19.b.1)-2)**

When coding injuries, assign separate codes for each injury unless a combination code is provided, in which case the combination code is assigned ... Traumatic injury codes (S00-T14.9) are not to be used for normal, healing surgical wounds or to identify complications of surgical wounds. The code for the most serious injury, as determined by the provider and the focus of treatment, is sequenced first.

1) Superficial injuries such as abrasions or contusions are not coded when associated with more severe injuries of the same site.

2) When a primary injury results in minor damage to peripheral nerves or blood vessels, the primary injury is sequenced first with additional code(s) for injuries to nerves and spinal cord (such as category S04), and/or injury to blood vessels (such as category S15). When the primary injury is to the blood vessels or nerves, that injury should be sequenced first.

GUIDELINES **Section I.C.19.c**

Coding of Traumatic Fractures: The principles of multiple coding of injuries should be followed in coding fractures. Fractures of specified sites are coded individually by site in accordance with both the provisions within categories S02, S12, S22, S32, S42, S49, S52, S59, S62, S72, S79, S82, S89, S92 and the level of detail furnished by medical record content. A fracture not indicated as open or closed should be coded to closed. A fracture not indicated whether displaced or not displaced should be coded to displaced.

CODING TIPS ✓ 7th character A is acceptable in home health and hospice when active treatment is provided, such as antibiotics for an infected wound or a wound vac for a dehisced wound. D is used when the complication or injury is now healing. Think of D as aftercare. S is used for sequela of the injury or complication. Sequela is a residual deficit or condition produced as a result of the injury or complication after the original injury or complication has healed.

S20 Superficial injury of thorax

The appropriate 7th character is to be added to each code from category S20
A initial encounter
D subsequent encounter
S sequela

S20.0 Contusion of breast
S20.00X- Contusion of breast, unspecified breast
S20.01X- Contusion of right breast
S20.02X- Contusion of left breast

S20.1 Other and unspecified superficial injuries of breast

S20.10 Unspecified superficial injuries of breast
S20.101- Unspecified superficial injuries of breast, right breast
S20.102- Unspecified superficial injuries of breast, left breast
S20.109- Unspecified superficial injuries of breast, unspecified breast

S20.11 Abrasion of breast
S20.111- Abrasion of breast, right breast
S20.112- Abrasion of breast, left breast
S20.119- Abrasion of breast, unspecified breast

S20.12 Blister (nonthermal) of breast
S20.121- Blister (nonthermal) of breast, right breast
S20.122- Blister (nonthermal) of breast, left breast
S20.129- Blister (nonthermal) of breast, unspecified breast

S20.14 External constriction of part of breast
S20.141- External constriction of part of breast, right breast
S20.142- External constriction of part of breast, left breast
S20.149- External constriction of part of breast, unspecified breast

S20.15 Superficial foreign body of breast
Splinter in the breast
S20.151- Superficial foreign body of breast, right breast
S20.152- Superficial foreign body of breast, left breast
S20.159- Superficial foreign body of breast, unspecified breast

S20.16 Insect bite (nonvenomous) of breast
S20.161- Insect bite (nonvenomous) of breast, right breast
S20.162- Insect bite (nonvenomous) of breast, left breast
S20.169- Insect bite (nonvenomous) of breast, unspecified breast

S20.17 Other superficial bite of breast
EXCLUDES 1 open bite of breast (S21.05-)
S20.171- Other superficial bite of breast, right breast
S20.172- Other superficial bite of breast, left breast
S20.179- Other superficial bite of breast, unspecified breast

S20.2 Contusion of thorax
S20.20X- Contusion of thorax, unspecified

S20.21 Contusion of front wall of thorax
S20.211- Contusion of right front wall of thorax
S20.212- Contusion of left front wall of thorax
S20.213- Contusion of bilateral front wall of thorax
S20.214- Contusion of middle front wall of thorax
S20.219- Contusion of unspecified front wall of thorax

S20.22 Contusion of back wall of thorax
S20.221- Contusion of right back wall of thorax
S20.222- Contusion of left back wall of thorax
S20.223- Contusion of bilateral back wall of thorax
S20.224- Contusion of middle back wall of thorax
S20.229- Contusion of unspecified back wall of thorax

S20.3 Other and unspecified superficial injuries of front wall of thorax

S20.30 Unspecified superficial injuries of front wall of thorax
S20.301- Unspecified superficial injuries of right front wall of thorax
S20.302- Unspecified superficial injuries of left front wall of thorax
S20.303- Unspecified superficial injuries of bilateral front wall of thorax
S20.304- Unspecified superficial injuries of middle front wall of thorax
S20.309- Unspecified superficial injuries of unspecified front wall of thorax

S20.31 Abrasion of front wall of thorax
S20.311- Abrasion of right front wall of thorax
S20.312- Abrasion of left front wall of thorax
S20.313- Abrasion of bilateral front wall of thorax
S20.314- Abrasion of middle front wall of thorax
S20.319- Abrasion of unspecified front wall of thorax

S20.32 Blister (nonthermal) of front wall of thorax
S20.321- Blister (nonthermal) of right front wall of thorax
S20.322- Blister (nonthermal) of left front wall of thorax
S20.323- Blister (nonthermal) of bilateral front wall of thorax
S20.324- Blister (nonthermal) of middle front wall of thorax
S20.329- Blister (nonthermal) of unspecified front wall of thorax

Chapter 19 S00-T88

4th digit required | 5th digit required | 6th digit required | 7th digit required | 7th digit placeholder | + Additional code | Laterality

S20.34 External constriction of front wall of thorax

S20.341- External constriction of right front wall of thorax

S20.342- External constriction of left front wall of thorax

S20.343- External constriction of bilateral front wall of thorax

S20.344- External constriction of middle front wall of thorax

S20.349- External constriction of unspecified front wall of thorax

S20.35 Superficial foreign body of front wall of thorax

Splinter in front wall of thorax

S20.351- Superficial foreign body of right front wall of thorax

S20.352- Superficial foreign body of left front wall of thorax

S20.353- Superficial foreign body of bilateral front wall of thorax

S20.354- Superficial foreign body of middle front wall of thorax

S20.359- Superficial foreign body of unspecified front wall of thorax

S20.36 Insect bite (nonvenomous) of front wall of thorax

S20.361- Insect bite (nonvenomous) of right front wall of thorax

S20.362- Insect bite (nonvenomous) of left front wall of thorax

S20.363- Insect bite (nonvenomous) of bilateral front wall of thorax

S20.364- Insect bite (nonvenomous) of middle front wall of thorax

S20.369- Insect bite (nonvenomous) of unspecified front wall of thorax

S20.37 Other superficial bite of front wall of thorax

EXCLUDES 1 open bite of front wall of thorax (S21.14)

S20.371- Other superficial bite of right front wall of thorax

S20.372- Other superficial bite of left front wall of thorax

S20.373- Other superficial bite of bilateral front wall of thorax

S20.374- Other superficial bite of middle front wall of thorax

S20.379- Other superficial bite of unspecified front wall of thorax

S20.4 Other and unspecified superficial injuries of back wall of thorax

S20.40 Unspecified superficial injuries of back wall of thorax

S20.401- Unspecified superficial injuries of right back wall of thorax

S20.402- Unspecified superficial injuries of left back wall of thorax

S20.409- Unspecified superficial injuries of unspecified back wall of thorax

S20.41 Abrasion of back wall of thorax

S20.411- Abrasion of right back wall of thorax

S20.412- Abrasion of left back wall of thorax

S20.419- Abrasion of unspecified back wall of thorax

S20.42 Blister (nonthermal) of back wall of thorax

S20.421- Blister (nonthermal) of right back wall of thorax

S20.422- Blister (nonthermal) of left back wall of thorax

S20.429- Blister (nonthermal) of unspecified back wall of thorax

S20.44 External constriction of back wall of thorax

S20.441- External constriction of right back wall of thorax

S20.442- External constriction of left back wall of thorax

S20.449- External constriction of unspecified back wall of thorax

S20.45 Superficial foreign body of back wall of thorax

Splinter of back wall of thorax

S20.451- Superficial foreign body of right back wall of thorax

S20.452- Superficial foreign body of left back wall of thorax

S20.459- Superficial foreign body of unspecified back wall of thorax

S20.46 Insect bite (nonvenomous) of back wall of thorax

S20.461- Insect bite (nonvenomous) of right back wall of thorax

S20.462- Insect bite (nonvenomous) of left back wall of thorax

S20.469- Insect bite (nonvenomous) of unspecified back wall of thorax

S20.47 Other superficial bite of back wall of thorax

EXCLUDES 1 open bite of back wall of thorax (S21.24)

S20.471- Other superficial bite of right back wall of thorax

S20.472- Other superficial bite of left back wall of thorax

S20.479- Other superficial bite of unspecified back wall of thorax

S20.9 Superficial injury of unspecified parts of thorax

EXCLUDES 1 contusion of thorax NOS (S20.20)

S20.90X- Unspecified superficial injury of unspecified parts of thorax

Superficial injury of thoracic wall NOS

S20.91X- Abrasion of unspecified parts of thorax

S20.92X- Blister (nonthermal) of unspecified parts of thorax

S20.94X- External constriction of unspecified parts of thorax

S20.95X- Superficial foreign body of unspecified parts of thorax

Splinter in thorax NOS

S20.96X- Insect bite (nonvenomous) of unspecified parts of thorax

!Q 7 **S20.97X- Other superficial bite of unspecified parts of thorax**

EXCLUDES 1 open bite of thorax NOS (S21.95)

4 **S21 Open wound of thorax**

Code also any associated injury, such as:
injury of heart (S26.-)
injury of intrathoracic organs (S27.-)
rib fracture (S22.3-, S22.4-)
spinal cord injury (S24.0-, S24.1-)
traumatic hemopneumothorax (S27.3)
traumatic hemothorax (S27.1)
traumatic pneumothorax (S27.0)
wound infection

EXCLUDES 1 traumatic amputation (partial) of thorax (S28.1)

The appropriate 7th character is to be added to each code from category S21

A	initial encounter
D	subsequent encounter
S	sequela

CODING TIPS✓ Open wound codes are used for wounds caused by trauma. Do not assign a code for "open wound" unless the etiology of the wound is related to trauma. Do not use Z codes for any aspect of care of a trauma wound, e.g. no Z code for dressing changes, drain care, or suture removal.

CODING TIPS✓ No aftercare code applies. The 7th character "D" is the default for home care and hospice when providing aftercare for a healing or resolving condition; "A" is used for active treatment such as antibiotics or more than routine wound care; "S" may be used to indicate a residual condition after the original injury has healed.

5 **S21.0 Open wound of breast**

6 **S21.00 Unspecified open wound of breast**

⊟ SP 7 **S21.001- Unspecified open wound of right breast**

⊟ SP 7 **S21.002- Unspecified open wound of left breast**

⊟ !Q 7 **S21.009- Unspecified open wound of unspecified breast**

6 **S21.01 Laceration without foreign body of breast**

⊟ SP 7 **S21.011- Laceration without foreign body of right breast**

⊟ SP 7 **S21.012- Laceration without foreign body of left breast**

⊟ !Q 7 **S21.019- Laceration without foreign body of unspecified breast**

6 **S21.02 Laceration with foreign body of breast**

⊟ SP 7 **S21.021- Laceration with foreign body of right breast**

⊟ SP 7 **S21.022- Laceration with foreign body of left breast**

⊟ !Q 7 **S21.029- Laceration with foreign body of unspecified breast**

6 **S21.03 Puncture wound without foreign body of breast**

⊟ SP 7 **S21.031- Puncture wound without foreign body of right breast**

⊟ SP 7 **S21.032- Puncture wound without foreign body of left breast**

⊟ !Q 7 **S21.039- Puncture wound without foreign body of unspecified breast**

6 **S21.04 Puncture wound with foreign body of breast**

⊟ SP 7 **S21.041- Puncture wound with foreign body of right breast**

⊟ SP 7 **S21.042- Puncture wound with foreign body of left breast**

⊟ !Q 7 **S21.049- Puncture wound with foreign body of unspecified breast**

6 **S21.05 Open bite of breast**

Bite of breast NOS

EXCLUDES 1 superficial bite of breast (S20.17)

⊟ SP 7 **S21.051- Open bite of right breast**

⊟ SP 7 **S21.052- Open bite of left breast**

⊟ !Q 7 **S21.059- Open bite of unspecified breast**

5 **S21.1 Open wound of front wall of thorax without penetration into thoracic cavity**

Open wound of chest without penetration into thoracic cavity

6 **S21.10 Unspecified open wound of front wall of thorax without penetration into thoracic cavity**

⊟ SP 7 **S21.101- Unspecified open wound of right front wall of thorax without penetration into thoracic cavity**

⊟ SP 7 **S21.102- Unspecified open wound of left front wall of thorax without penetration into thoracic cavity**

⊟ SP 7 **S21.109- Unspecified open wound of unspecified front wall of thorax without penetration into thoracic cavity**

6 **S21.11 Laceration without foreign body of front wall of thorax without penetration into thoracic cavity**

⊟ SP 7 **S21.111- Laceration without foreign body of right front wall of thorax without penetration into thoracic cavity**

⊟ SP 7 **S21.112- Laceration without foreign body of left front wall of thorax without penetration into thoracic cavity**

⊟ SP 7 **S21.119- Laceration without foreign body of unspecified front wall of thorax without penetration into thoracic cavity**

6 **S21.12 Laceration with foreign body of front wall of thorax without penetration into thoracic cavity**

⊟ SP 7 **S21.121- Laceration with foreign body of right front wall of thorax without penetration into thoracic cavity**

⊟ SP 7 **S21.122- Laceration with foreign body of left front wall of thorax without penetration into thoracic cavity**

⊟ SP 7 **S21.129- Laceration with foreign body of unspecified front wall of thorax without penetration into thoracic cavity**

6 **S21.13 Puncture wound without foreign body of front wall of thorax without penetration into thoracic cavity**

SP 7 **S21.131- Puncture wound without foreign body of right front wall of thorax without penetration into thoracic cavity**

SP 7 **S21.132- Puncture wound without foreign body of left front wall of thorax without penetration into thoracic cavity**

IQ 7 **S21.139- Puncture wound without foreign body of unspecified front wall of thorax without penetration into thoracic cavity**

6 **S21.14 Puncture wound with foreign body of front wall of thorax without penetration into thoracic cavity**

SP 7 **S21.141- Puncture wound with foreign body of right front wall of thorax without penetration into thoracic cavity**

SP 7 **S21.142- Puncture wound with foreign body of left front wall of thorax without penetration into thoracic cavity**

IQ 7 **S21.149- Puncture wound with foreign body of unspecified front wall of thorax without penetration into thoracic cavity**

6 **S21.15 Open bite of front wall of thorax without penetration into thoracic cavity**

Bite of front wall of thorax NOS

EXCLUDES 1 superficial bite of front wall of thorax (S20.37)

SP 7 **S21.151- Open bite of right front wall of thorax without penetration into thoracic cavity**

SP 7 **S21.152- Open bite of left front wall of thorax without penetration into thoracic cavity**

IQ 7 **S21.159- Open bite of unspecified front wall of thorax without penetration into thoracic cavity**

5 **S21.2 Open wound of back wall of thorax without penetration into thoracic cavity**

6 **S21.20 Unspecified open wound of back wall of thorax without penetration into thoracic cavity**

SP 7 **S21.201- Unspecified open wound of right back wall of thorax without penetration into thoracic cavity**

SP 7 **S21.202- Unspecified open wound of left back wall of thorax without penetration into thoracic cavity**

SP 7 **S21.209- Unspecified open wound of unspecified back wall of thorax without penetration into thoracic cavity**

6 **S21.21 Laceration without foreign body of back wall of thorax without penetration into thoracic cavity**

SP 7 **S21.211- Laceration without foreign body of right back wall of thorax without penetration into thoracic cavity**

SP 7 **S21.212- Laceration without foreign body of left back wall of thorax without penetration into thoracic cavity**

SP 7 **S21.219- Laceration without foreign body of unspecified back wall of thorax without penetration into thoracic cavity**

6 **S21.22 Laceration with foreign body of back wall of thorax without penetration into thoracic cavity**

SP 7 **S21.221- Laceration with foreign body of right back wall of thorax without penetration into thoracic cavity**

SP 7 **S21.222- Laceration with foreign body of left back wall of thorax without penetration into thoracic cavity**

SP 7 **S21.229- Laceration with foreign body of unspecified back wall of thorax without penetration into thoracic cavity**

6 **S21.23 Puncture wound without foreign body of back wall of thorax without penetration into thoracic cavity**

SP 7 **S21.231- Puncture wound without foreign body of right back wall of thorax without penetration into thoracic cavity**

SP 7 **S21.232- Puncture wound without foreign body of left back wall of thorax without penetration into thoracic cavity**

IQ 7 **S21.239- Puncture wound without foreign body of unspecified back wall of thorax without penetration into thoracic cavity**

6 **S21.24 Puncture wound with foreign body of back wall of thorax without penetration into thoracic cavity**

SP 7 **S21.241- Puncture wound with foreign body of right back wall of thorax without penetration into thoracic cavity**

SP 7 **S21.242- Puncture wound with foreign body of left back wall of thorax without penetration into thoracic cavity**

IQ 7 **S21.249- Puncture wound with foreign body of unspecified back wall of thorax without penetration into thoracic cavity**

6 **S21.25 Open bite of back wall of thorax without penetration into thoracic cavity**

Bite of back wall of thorax NOS

EXCLUDES 1 superficial bite of back wall of thorax (S20.47)

SP 7 **S21.251- Open bite of right back wall of thorax without penetration into thoracic cavity**

SP 7 **S21.252- Open bite of left back wall of thorax without penetration into thoracic cavity**

S21.259- Open bite of unspecified back wall of thorax without penetration into thoracic cavity

S21.3 Open wound of front wall of thorax with penetration into thoracic cavity
Open wound of chest with penetration into thoracic cavity

S21.30 Unspecified open wound of front wall of thorax with penetration into thoracic cavity
S21.301- Unspecified open wound of right front wall of thorax with penetration into thoracic cavity
S21.302- Unspecified open wound of left front wall of thorax with penetration into thoracic cavity
S21.309- Unspecified open wound of unspecified front wall of thorax with penetration into thoracic cavity

S21.31 Laceration without foreign body of front wall of thorax with penetration into thoracic cavity
S21.311- Laceration without foreign body of right front wall of thorax with penetration into thoracic cavity
S21.312- Laceration without foreign body of left front wall of thorax with penetration into thoracic cavity
S21.319- Laceration without foreign body of unspecified front wall of thorax with penetration into thoracic cavity

S21.32 Laceration with foreign body of front wall of thorax with penetration into thoracic cavity
S21.321- Laceration with foreign body of right front wall of thorax with penetration into thoracic cavity
S21.322- Laceration with foreign body of left front wall of thorax with penetration into thoracic cavity
S21.329- Laceration with foreign body of unspecified front wall of thorax with penetration into thoracic cavity

S21.33 Puncture wound without foreign body of front wall of thorax with penetration into thoracic cavity
S21.331- Puncture wound without foreign body of right front wall of thorax with penetration into thoracic cavity
S21.332- Puncture wound without foreign body of left front wall of thorax with penetration into thoracic cavity
S21.339- Puncture wound without foreign body of unspecified front wall of thorax with penetration into thoracic cavity

S21.34 Puncture wound with foreign body of front wall of thorax with penetration into thoracic cavity
S21.341- Puncture wound with foreign body of right front wall of thorax with penetration into thoracic cavity
S21.342- Puncture wound with foreign body of left front wall of thorax with penetration into thoracic cavity
S21.349- Puncture wound with foreign body of unspecified front wall of thorax with penetration into thoracic cavity

S21.35 Open bite of front wall of thorax with penetration into thoracic cavity
EXCLUDES 1 superficial bite of front wall of thorax (S20.37)
S21.351- Open bite of right front wall of thorax with penetration into thoracic cavity
S21.352- Open bite of left front wall of thorax with penetration into thoracic cavity
S21.359- Open bite of unspecified front wall of thorax with penetration into thoracic cavity

S21.4 Open wound of back wall of thorax with penetration into thoracic cavity

S21.40 Unspecified open wound of back wall of thorax with penetration into thoracic cavity
S21.401- Unspecified open wound of right back wall of thorax with penetration into thoracic cavity
S21.402- Unspecified open wound of left back wall of thorax with penetration into thoracic cavity
S21.409- Unspecified open wound of unspecified back wall of thorax with penetration into thoracic cavity

S21.41 Laceration without foreign body of back wall of thorax with penetration into thoracic cavity
S21.411- Laceration without foreign body of right back wall of thorax with penetration into thoracic cavity
S21.412- Laceration without foreign body of left back wall of thorax with penetration into thoracic cavity
S21.419- Laceration without foreign body of unspecified back wall of thorax with penetration into thoracic cavity

S21.42 Laceration with foreign body of back wall of thorax with penetration into thoracic cavity
S21.421- Laceration with foreign body of right back wall of thorax with penetration into thoracic cavity
S21.422- Laceration with foreign body of left back wall of thorax with penetration into thoracic cavity
S21.429- Laceration with foreign body of unspecified back wall of thorax with penetration into thoracic cavity

S21.43 Puncture wound without foreign body of back wall of thorax with penetration into thoracic cavity

SP 7 **S21.431- Puncture wound without foreign body of right back wall of thorax with penetration into thoracic cavity**

SP 7 **S21.432- Puncture wound without foreign body of left back wall of thorax with penetration into thoracic cavity**

IQ 7 **S21.439- Puncture wound without foreign body of unspecified back wall of thorax with penetration into thoracic cavity**

6 **S21.44 Puncture wound with foreign body of back wall of thorax with penetration into thoracic cavity**

SP 7 **S21.441- Puncture wound with foreign body of right back wall of thorax with penetration into thoracic cavity**

SP 7 **S21.442- Puncture wound with foreign body of left back wall of thorax with penetration into thoracic cavity**

IQ 7 **S21.449- Puncture wound with foreign body of unspecified back wall of thorax with penetration into thoracic cavity**

6 **S21.45 Open bite of back wall of thorax with penetration into thoracic cavity**

Bite of back wall of thorax NOS

EXCLUDES 1 superficial bite of back wall of thorax (S20.47)

SP 7 **S21.451- Open bite of right back wall of thorax with penetration into thoracic cavity**

SP 7 **S21.452- Open bite of left back wall of thorax with penetration into thoracic cavity**

IQ 7 **S21.459- Open bite of unspecified back wall of thorax with penetration into thoracic cavity**

5 **S21.9 Open wound of unspecified part of thorax**

Open wound of thoracic wall NOS

SP 7 **S21.90X- Unspecified open wound of unspecified part of thorax**

SP 7 **S21.91X- Laceration without foreign body of unspecified part of thorax**

SP 7 **S21.92X- Laceration with foreign body of unspecified part of thorax**

IQ 7 **S21.93X- Puncture wound without foreign body of unspecified part of thorax**

IQ 7 **S21.94X- Puncture wound with foreign body of unspecified part of thorax**

IQ 7 **S21.95X- Open bite of unspecified part of thorax**

EXCLUDES 1 superficial bite of thorax (S20.97)

4 **S22 Fracture of rib(s), sternum and thoracic spine**

Note:

A fracture not indicated as displaced or nondisplaced should be coded to displaced

A fracture not indicated as open or closed should be coded to closed

INCLUDES fracture of thoracic neural arch

fracture of thoracic spinous process

fracture of thoracic transverse process

fracture of thoracic vertebra

fracture of thoracic vertebral arch

Code first any associated:

injury of intrathoracic organ (S27.-)

spinal cord injury (S24.0-, S24.1-)

EXCLUDES 1 transection of thorax (S28.1)

EXCLUDES 2 fracture of clavicle (S42.0-)

fracture of scapula (S42.1-)

The appropriate 7th character is to be added to each code from category S22

A	initial encounter for closed fracture
B	initial encounter for open fracture
D	subsequent encounter for fracture with routine healing
G	subsequent encounter for fracture with delayed healing
K	subsequent encounter for fracture with nonunion
S	sequela

CODING TIPS ✓ Fractures repaired by joint replacements are NOT coded with Z47.1. Fractures repaired by any other orthopedic surgery are NOT coded with Z47.89. Z codes are not appropriate for fractures of any kind. Code the fracture with 7th character D for fractures undergoing surgical repair.

CODING TIPS ✓ A fracture not indicated as displaced or nondisplaced should be coded to displaced. A fracture not indicated as open or closed should be coded to closed.

CODING TIPS ✓ 'D' is the 7th character for home care and hospice unless the physician or NPP has documented delayed healing, nonunion or malunion. A sequela is a condition left after the fracture has healed. The Gustilo open fracture classification must be used for open fractures. The default 7th character for open fractures is E.

5 **S22.0 Fracture of thoracic vertebra**

6 **S22.00 Fracture of unspecified thoracic vertebra**

SP 7 **S22.000- Wedge compression fracture of unspecified thoracic vertebra**

SP 7 **S22.001- Stable burst fracture of unspecified thoracic vertebra**

SP 7 **S22.002- Unstable burst fracture of unspecified thoracic vertebra**

SP 7 **S22.008- Other fracture of unspecified thoracic vertebra**

SP 7 **S22.009- Unspecified fracture of unspecified thoracic vertebra**

6 **S22.01 Fracture of first thoracic vertebra**

SP 7 **S22.010- Wedge compression fracture of first thoracic vertebra**

SP 7 **S22.011- Stable burst fracture of first thoracic vertebra**

SP 7 **S22.012- Unstable burst fracture of first thoracic vertebra**

SP 7 **S22.018- Other fracture of first thoracic vertebra**

SP 7 **S22.019- Unspecified fracture of first thoracic vertebra**

6 **S22.02 Fracture of second thoracic vertebra**

SP 7 **S22.020- Wedge compression fracture of second thoracic vertebra**

SP 7 **S22.021- Stable burst fracture of second thoracic vertebra**

SP 7 **S22.022- Unstable burst fracture of second thoracic vertebra**

SP 7 **S22.028- Other fracture of second thoracic vertebra**

SP 7 **S22.029- Unspecified fracture of second thoracic vertebra**

6 **S22.03 Fracture of third thoracic vertebra**

SP 7 **S22.030- Wedge compression fracture of third thoracic vertebra**

SP 7 **S22.031- Stable burst fracture of third thoracic vertebra**

SP 7 **S22.032- Unstable burst fracture of third thoracic vertebra**

SP 7 **S22.038- Other fracture of third thoracic vertebra**

SP 7 **S22.039- Unspecified fracture of third thoracic vertebra**

6 **S22.04 Fracture of fourth thoracic vertebra**

SP 7 **S22.040- Wedge compression fracture of fourth thoracic vertebra**

SP 7 **S22.041- Stable burst fracture of fourth thoracic vertebra**

SP 7 **S22.042- Unstable burst fracture of fourth thoracic vertebra**

SP 7 **S22.048- Other fracture of fourth thoracic vertebra**

SP 7 **S22.049- Unspecified fracture of fourth thoracic vertebra**

6 **S22.05 Fracture of T5-T6 vertebra**

SP 7 **S22.050- Wedge compression fracture of T5-T6 vertebra**

SP 7 **S22.051- Stable burst fracture of T5-T6 vertebra**

SP 7 **S22.052- Unstable burst fracture of T5-T6 vertebra**

SP 7 **S22.058- Other fracture of T5-T6 vertebra**

SP 7 **S22.059- Unspecified fracture of T5-T6 vertebra**

6 **S22.06 Fracture of T7-T8 vertebra**

SP 7 **S22.060- Wedge compression fracture of T7-T8 vertebra**

SP 7 **S22.061- Stable burst fracture of T7-T8 vertebra**

SP 7 **S22.062- Unstable burst fracture of T7-T8 vertebra**

SP 7 **S22.068- Other fracture of T7-T8 thoracic vertebra**

SP 7 **S22.069- Unspecified fracture of T7-T8 vertebra**

6 **S22.07 Fracture of T9-T10 vertebra**

SP 7 **S22.070- Wedge compression fracture of T9-T10 vertebra**

SP 7 **S22.071- Stable burst fracture of T9-T10 vertebra**

SP 7 **S22.072- Unstable burst fracture of T9-T10 vertebra**

SP 7 **S22.078- Other fracture of T9-T10 vertebra**

SP 7 **S22.079- Unspecified fracture of T9-T10 vertebra**

6 **S22.08 Fracture of T11-T12 vertebra**

SP 7 **S22.080- Wedge compression fracture of T11-T12 vertebra**

SP 7 **S22.081- Stable burst fracture of T11-T12 vertebra**

SP 7 **S22.082- Unstable burst fracture of T11-T12 vertebra**

SP 7 **S22.088- Other fracture of T11-T12 vertebra**

SP 7 **S22.089- Unspecified fracture of T11-T12 vertebra**

5 **S22.2 Fracture of sternum**

SP 7 **S22.20X- Unspecified fracture of sternum**

SP 7 **S22.21X- Fracture of manubrium**

SP 7 **S22.22X- Fracture of body of sternum**

SP 7 **S22.23X- Sternal manubrial dissociation**

SP 7 **S22.24X- Fracture of xiphoid process**

5 **S22.3 Fracture of one rib**

SP 7 **S22.31X- Fracture of one rib, right side**

SP 7 **S22.32X- Fracture of one rib, left side**

IQ 7 **S22.39X- Fracture of one rib, unspecified side**

5 **S22.4 Multiple fractures of ribs**

Fractures of two or more ribs

EXCLUDES 1 flail chest (S22.5-)

SP 7 **S22.41X- Multiple fractures of ribs, right side**

SP 7 **S22.42X- Multiple fractures of ribs, left side**

SP 7 **S22.43X- Multiple fractures of ribs, bilateral**

IQ 7 **S22.49X- Multiple fractures of ribs, unspecified side**

SP 7 **S22.5XX- Flail chest**

SP 7 **S22.9XX- Fracture of bony thorax, part unspecified**

4 **S23 Dislocation and sprain of joints and ligaments of thorax**

INCLUDES avulsion of joint or ligament of thorax
laceration of cartilage, joint or ligament of thorax
sprain of cartilage, joint or ligament of thorax
traumatic hemarthrosis of joint or ligament of thorax
traumatic rupture of joint or ligament of thorax
traumatic subluxation of joint or ligament of thorax
traumatic tear of joint or ligament of thorax

Code also:
any associated open wound

EXCLUDES 2 dislocation, sprain of sternoclavicular joint (S43.2, S43.6)
strain of muscle or tendon of thorax (S29.01-)

The appropriate 7th character is to be added to each code from category S23
A initial encounter
D subsequent encounter
S sequela

SP 7 **S23.0XX- Traumatic rupture of thoracic intervertebral disc**
EXCLUDES 1 rupture or displacement (nontraumatic) of thoracic intervertebral disc NOS (M51.- with fifth character 4)

5 **S23.1 Subluxation and dislocation of thoracic vertebra**
Code also any associated:
open wound of thorax (S21.-)
spinal cord injury (S24.0-, S24.1-)
EXCLUDES 2 fracture of thoracic vertebrae (S22.0-)

6 **S23.10 Subluxation and dislocation of unspecified thoracic vertebra**
IQ 7 **S23.100- Subluxation of unspecified thoracic vertebra**
IQ 7 **S23.101- Dislocation of unspecified thoracic vertebra**

6 **S23.11 Subluxation and dislocation of T1/T2 thoracic vertebra**
SP 7 **S23.110- Subluxation of T1/T2 thoracic vertebra**
SP 7 **S23.111- Dislocation of T1/T2 thoracic vertebra**

6 **S23.12 Subluxation and dislocation of T2/T3-T3/T4 thoracic vertebra**
SP 7 **S23.120- Subluxation of T2/T3 thoracic vertebra**
SP 7 **S23.121- Dislocation of T2/T3 thoracic vertebra**
SP 7 **S23.122- Subluxation of T3/T4 thoracic vertebra**
SP 7 **S23.123- Dislocation of T3/T4 thoracic vertebra**

6 **S23.13 Subluxation and dislocation of T4/T5-T5/T6 thoracic vertebra**
SP 7 **S23.130- Subluxation of T4/T5 thoracic vertebra**
SP 7 **S23.131- Dislocation of T4/T5 thoracic vertebra**
SP 7 **S23.132- Subluxation of T5/T6 thoracic vertebra**
SP 7 **S23.133- Dislocation of T5/T6 thoracic vertebra**

6 **S23.14 Subluxation and dislocation of T6/T7-T7/T8 thoracic vertebra**
SP 7 **S23.140- Subluxation of T6/T7 thoracic vertebra**
SP 7 **S23.141- Dislocation of T6/T7 thoracic vertebra**
SP 7 **S23.142- Subluxation of T7/T8 thoracic vertebra**
SP 7 **S23.143- Dislocation of T7/T8 thoracic vertebra**

6 **S23.15 Subluxation and dislocation of T8/T9-T9/T10 thoracic vertebra**
SP 7 **S23.150- Subluxation of T8/T9 thoracic vertebra**
SP 7 **S23.151- Dislocation of T8/T9 thoracic vertebra**
SP 7 **S23.152- Subluxation of T9/T10 thoracic vertebra**
SP 7 **S23.153- Dislocation of T9/T10 thoracic vertebra**

6 **S23.16 Subluxation and dislocation of T10/T11-T11/T12 thoracic vertebra**
SP 7 **S23.160- Subluxation of T10/T11 thoracic vertebra**
SP 7 **S23.161- Dislocation of T10/T11 thoracic vertebra**
SP 7 **S23.162- Subluxation of T11/T12 thoracic vertebra**
SP 7 **S23.163- Dislocation of T11/T12 thoracic vertebra**

6 **S23.17 Subluxation and dislocation of T12/L1 thoracic vertebra**
SP 7 **S23.170- Subluxation of T12/L1 thoracic vertebra**
SP 7 **S23.171- Dislocation of T12/L1 thoracic vertebra**

5 **S23.2 Dislocation of other and unspecified parts of thorax**
IQ 7 **S23.20X- Dislocation of unspecified part of thorax**
IQ 7 **S23.29X- Dislocation of other parts of thorax**

SP 7 **S23.3XX- Sprain of ligaments of thoracic spine**

5 **S23.4 Sprain of ribs and sternum**
SP 7 **S23.41X- Sprain of ribs**
6 **S23.42 Sprain of sternum**
SP 7 **S23.420- Sprain of sternoclavicular (joint) (ligament)**
SP 7 **S23.421- Sprain of chondrosternal joint**
SP 7 **S23.428- Other sprain of sternum**
SP 7 **S23.429- Unspecified sprain of sternum**

SP 7 **S23.8XX- Sprain of other specified parts of thorax**
SP 7 **S23.9XX- Sprain of unspecified parts of thorax**

4 **S24 Injury of nerves and spinal cord at thorax level**
Note:
Code to highest level of thoracic spinal cord injury
Injuries to the spinal cord (S24.0 and S24.1) refer to the cord level and not bone level injury, and can affect nerve roots at and below the level given.
Code also any associated:
fracture of thoracic vertebra (S22.0-)
open wound of thorax (S21.-)
transient paralysis (R29.5)
EXCLUDES 2 injury of brachial plexus (S14.3)

The appropriate 7th character is to be added to each code from category S24
A initial encounter
D subsequent encounter
S sequela

Chapter 19
S00-T88

CODING TIPS ✓ When coding sequelae of a cervical spinal cord injury, first list the residual condition(s), followed by the specific spinal cord injury diagnosed using the appropriate code from this category with the seventh character "S" to indicate sequelae. If there are multiple levels of injury, code only the highest injury in each section of the spine (cervical, thoracic, and lumbar).

SP 7 **S24.0XX- Concussion and edema of thoracic spinal cord**

5 **S24.1 Other and unspecified injuries of thoracic spinal cord**

6 **S24.10 Unspecified injury of thoracic spinal cord**

!Q 7 **S24.101- Unspecified injury at T1 level of thoracic spinal cord**

!Q 7 **S24.102- Unspecified injury at T2-T6 level of thoracic spinal cord**

!Q 7 **S24.103- Unspecified injury at T7-T10 level of thoracic spinal cord**

!Q 7 **S24.104- Unspecified injury at T11-T12 level of thoracic spinal cord**

!Q 7 **S24.109- Unspecified injury at unspecified level of thoracic spinal cord**
Injury of thoracic spinal cord NOS

6 **S24.11 Complete lesion of thoracic spinal cord**

SP 7 **S24.111- Complete lesion at T1 level of thoracic spinal cord**

SP 7 **S24.112- Complete lesion at T2-T6 level of thoracic spinal cord**

SP 7 **S24.113- Complete lesion at T7-T10 level of thoracic spinal cord**

SP 7 **S24.114- Complete lesion at T11-T12 level of thoracic spinal cord**

!Q 7 **S24.119- Complete lesion at unspecified level of thoracic spinal cord**

6 **S24.13 Anterior cord syndrome of thoracic spinal cord**

SP 7 **S24.131- Anterior cord syndrome at T1 level of thoracic spinal cord**

SP 7 **S24.132- Anterior cord syndrome at T2-T6 level of thoracic spinal cord**

SP 7 **S24.133- Anterior cord syndrome at T7-T10 level of thoracic spinal cord**

SP 7 **S24.134- Anterior cord syndrome at T11-T12 level of thoracic spinal cord**

!Q 7 **S24.139- Anterior cord syndrome at unspecified level of thoracic spinal cord**

6 **S24.14 Brown-Séquard syndrome of thoracic spinal cord**

SP 7 **S24.141- Brown-Séquard syndrome at T1 level of thoracic spinal cord**

SP 7 **S24.142- Brown-Séquard syndrome at T2-T6 level of thoracic spinal cord**

SP 7 **S24.143- Brown-Séquard syndrome at T7-T10 level of thoracic spinal cord**

SP 7 **S24.144- Brown-Séquard syndrome at T11-T12 level of thoracic spinal cord**

!Q 7 **S24.149- Brown-Séquard syndrome at unspecified level of thoracic spinal cord**

6 **S24.15 Other incomplete lesions of thoracic spinal cord**
Incomplete lesion of thoracic spinal cord NOS
Posterior cord syndrome of thoracic spinal cord

SP 7 **S24.151- Other incomplete lesion at T1 level of thoracic spinal cord**

SP 7 **S24.152- Other incomplete lesion at T2-T6 level of thoracic spinal cord**

SP 7 **S24.153- Other incomplete lesion at T7-T10 level of thoracic spinal cord**

SP 7 **S24.154- Other incomplete lesion at T11-T12 level of thoracic spinal cord**

!Q 7 **S24.159- Other incomplete lesion at unspecified level of thoracic spinal cord**

SP 7 **S24.2XX- Injury of nerve root of thoracic spine**

SP 7 **S24.3XX- Injury of peripheral nerves of thorax**

SP 7 **S24.4XX- Injury of thoracic sympathetic nervous system**
Injury of cardiac plexus
Injury of esophageal plexus
Injury of pulmonary plexus
Injury of stellate ganglion
Injury of thoracic sympathetic ganglion

SP 7 **S24.8XX- Injury of other specified nerves of thorax**

!Q 7 **S24.9XX- Injury of unspecified nerve of thorax**

4 **S25 Injury of blood vessels of thorax**
Code also:
any associated open wound (S21.-)

The appropriate 7th character is to be added to each code from category S25

A	initial encounter
D	subsequent encounter
S	sequela

5 **S25.0 Injury of thoracic aorta**
Injury of aorta NOS

!Q 7 **S25.00X- Unspecified injury of thoracic aorta**

SP 7 **S25.01X- Minor laceration of thoracic aorta**
Incomplete transection of thoracic aorta
Laceration of thoracic aorta NOS
Superficial laceration of thoracic aorta

SP 7 **S25.02X- Major laceration of thoracic aorta**
Complete transection of thoracic aorta
Traumatic rupture of thoracic aorta

SP 7 **S25.09X- Other specified injury of thoracic aorta**

5 **S25.1 Injury of innominate or subclavian artery**

6 **S25.10 Unspecified injury of innominate or subclavian artery**

⊟ !Q 7 **S25.101- Unspecified injury of right innominate or subclavian artery**

⊟ !Q 7 **S25.102- Unspecified injury of left innominate or subclavian artery**

Chapter 19
S00-T88

4 4th digit required 5 5th digit required 6 6th digit required 7 7th digit required 7 7th digit placeholder + Additional code ⊟ Laterality

S25.109- **Unspecified injury of unspecified innominate or subclavian artery**

S25.11 **Minor laceration of innominate or subclavian artery**
Incomplete transection of innominate or subclavian artery
Laceration of innominate or subclavian artery NOS
Superficial laceration of innominate or subclavian artery

S25.111- **Minor laceration of right innominate or subclavian artery**

S25.112- **Minor laceration of left innominate or subclavian artery**

S25.119- **Minor laceration of unspecified innominate or subclavian artery**

S25.12 **Major laceration of innominate or subclavian artery**
Complete transection of innominate or subclavian artery
Traumatic rupture of innominate or subclavian artery

S25.121- **Major laceration of right innominate or subclavian artery**

S25.122- **Major laceration of left innominate or subclavian artery**

S25.129- **Major laceration of unspecified innominate or subclavian artery**

S25.19 **Other specified injury of innominate or subclavian artery**

S25.191- **Other specified injury of right innominate or subclavian artery**

S25.192- **Other specified injury of left innominate or subclavian artery**

S25.199- **Other specified injury of unspecified innominate or subclavian artery**

S25.2 **Injury of superior vena cava**
Injury of vena cava NOS

S25.20X- **Unspecified injury of superior vena cava**

S25.21X- **Minor laceration of superior vena cava**
Incomplete transection of superior vena cava
Laceration of superior vena cava NOS
Superficial laceration of superior vena cava

S25.22X- **Major laceration of superior vena cava**
Complete transection of superior vena cava
Traumatic rupture of superior vena cava

S25.29X- **Other specified injury of superior vena cava**

S25.3 **Injury of innominate or subclavian vein**

S25.30 **Unspecified injury of innominate or subclavian vein**

S25.301- **Unspecified injury of right innominate or subclavian vein**

S25.302- **Unspecified injury of left innominate or subclavian vein**

S25.309- **Unspecified injury of unspecified innominate or subclavian vein**

S25.31 **Minor laceration of innominate or subclavian vein**
Incomplete transection of innominate or subclavian vein
Laceration of innominate or subclavian vein NOS
Superficial laceration of innominate or subclavian vein

S25.311- **Minor laceration of right innominate or subclavian vein**

S25.312- **Minor laceration of left innominate or subclavian vein**

S25.319- **Minor laceration of unspecified innominate or subclavian vein**

S25.32 **Major laceration of innominate or subclavian vein**
Complete transection of innominate or subclavian vein
Traumatic rupture of innominate or subclavian vein

S25.321- **Major laceration of right innominate or subclavian vein**

S25.322- **Major laceration of left innominate or subclavian vein**

S25.329- **Major laceration of unspecified innominate or subclavian vein**

S25.39 **Other specified injury of innominate or subclavian vein**

S25.391- **Other specified injury of right innominate or subclavian vein**

S25.392- **Other specified injury of left innominate or subclavian vein**

S25.399- **Other specified injury of unspecified innominate or subclavian vein**

S25.4 **Injury of pulmonary blood vessels**

S25.40 **Unspecified injury of pulmonary blood vessels**

S25.401- **Unspecified injury of right pulmonary blood vessels**

S25.402- **Unspecified injury of left pulmonary blood vessels**

S25.409- **Unspecified injury of unspecified pulmonary blood vessels**

S25.41 **Minor laceration of pulmonary blood vessels**
Incomplete transection of pulmonary blood vessels
Laceration of pulmonary blood vessels NOS
Superficial laceration of pulmonary blood vessels

S25.411- **Minor laceration of right pulmonary blood vessels**

S25.412- **Minor laceration of left pulmonary blood vessels**

S25.419- **Minor laceration of unspecified pulmonary blood vessels**

S25.42 **Major laceration of pulmonary blood vessels**
Complete transection of pulmonary blood vessels
blood vessels

Chapter 19 S00-T88

Traumatic rupture of pulmonary blood vessels

⊟ SP 7 **S25.421-** **Major laceration of right pulmonary blood vessels**

⊟ SP 7 **S25.422-** **Major laceration of left pulmonary blood vessels**

⊟ !Q 7 **S25.429-** Major laceration of unspecified pulmonary blood vessels

6 **S25.49** Other specified injury of pulmonary blood vessels

⊟ SP 7 **S25.491-** **Other specified injury of right pulmonary blood vessels**

⊟ SP 7 **S25.492-** **Other specified injury of left pulmonary blood vessels**

⊟ !Q 7 **S25.499-** Other specified injury of unspecified pulmonary blood vessels

5 **S25.5** Injury of intercostal blood vessels

6 **S25.50** Unspecified injury of intercostal blood vessels

⊟ !Q 7 **S25.501-** Unspecified injury of intercostal blood vessels, right side

⊟ !Q 7 **S25.502-** Unspecified injury of intercostal blood vessels, left side

⊟ !Q 7 **S25.509-** Unspecified injury of intercostal blood vessels, unspecified side

6 **S25.51** Laceration of intercostal blood vessels

⊟ SP 7 **S25.511-** **Laceration of intercostal blood vessels, right side**

⊟ SP 7 **S25.512-** **Laceration of intercostal blood vessels, left side**

⊟ SP !Q 7 **S25.519-** Laceration of intercostal blood vessels, unspecified side

6 **S25.59** Other specified injury of intercostal blood vessels

⊟ SP 7 **S25.591-** **Other specified injury of intercostal blood vessels, right side**

⊟ SP 7 **S25.592-** **Other specified injury of intercostal blood vessels, left side**

⊟ !Q 7 **S25.599-** Other specified injury of intercostal blood vessels, unspecified side

5 **S25.8** Injury of other blood vessels of thorax
Injury of azygos vein
Injury of mammary artery or vein

6 **S25.80** Unspecified injury of other blood vessels of thorax

⊟ !Q 7 **S25.801-** Unspecified injury of other blood vessels of thorax, right side

⊟ !Q 7 **S25.802-** Unspecified injury of other blood vessels of thorax, left side

⊟ !Q 7 **S25.809-** Unspecified injury of other blood vessels of thorax, unspecified side

6 **S25.81** Laceration of other blood vessels of thorax

⊟ SP 7 **S25.811-** **Laceration of other blood vessels of thorax, right side**

⊟ SP 7 **S25.812-** **Laceration of other blood vessels of thorax, left side**

⊟ !Q 7 **S25.819-** Laceration of other blood vessels of thorax, unspecified side

6 **S25.89** **Other specified injury of other blood vessels of thorax**

⊟ SP 7 **S25.891-** **Other specified injury of other blood vessels of thorax, right side**

⊟ SP 7 **S25.892-** **Other specified injury of other blood vessels of thorax, left side**

⊟ !Q 7 **S25.899-** Other specified injury of other blood vessels of thorax, unspecified side

5 **S25.9** Injury of unspecified blood vessel of thorax

!Q ☑ **S25.90X-** Unspecified injury of unspecified blood vessel of thorax

!Q ☑ **S25.91X-** Laceration of unspecified blood vessel of thorax

!Q ☑ **S25.99X-** Other specified injury of unspecified blood vessel of thorax

4 **S26** **Injury of heart**
Code also any associated:
open wound of thorax (S21.-)
traumatic hemopneumothorax (S27.2)
traumatic hemothorax (S27.1)
traumatic pneumothorax (S27.0)

The appropriate 7th character is to be added to each code from category S26
A   initial encounter
D   subsequent encounter
S   sequela

5 **S26.0** Injury of heart with hemopericardium

!Q ☑ **S26.00X-** Unspecified injury of heart with hemopericardium

SP ☑ **S26.01X-** Contusion of heart with hemopericardium

6 **S26.02** Laceration of heart with hemopericardium

SP 7 **S26.020-** **Mild laceration of heart with hemopericardium**
Laceration of heart without penetration of heart chamber

SP 7 **S26.021-** **Moderate laceration of heart with hemopericardium**
Laceration of heart with penetration of heart chamber

SP 7 **S26.022-** **Major laceration of heart with hemopericardium**
Laceration of heart with penetration of multiple heart chambers

SP ☑ **S26.09X-** Other injury of heart with hemopericardium

5 **S26.1** Injury of heart without hemopericardium

!Q ☑ **S26.10X-** Unspecified injury of heart without hemopericardium

SP ☑ **S26.11X-** Contusion of heart without hemopericardium

SP ☑ **S26.12X-** Laceration of heart without hemopericardium

SP ☑ **S26.19X-** Other injury of heart without hemopericardium

5 **S26.9** Injury of heart, unspecified with or without hemopericardium

!Q ☑ **S26.90X-** Unspecified injury of heart, unspecified with or without hemopericardium

---

4 4th digit required   5 5th digit required   6 6th digit required   7 7th digit required   ☑ 7th digit placeholder   ✚ Additional code   ⊟ Laterality

SP 7 **S26.91X- Contusion of heart, unspecified with or without hemopericardium**

SP 7 **S26.92X- Laceration of heart, unspecified with or without hemopericardium**
Laceration of heart NOS

SP 7 **S26.99X- Other injury of heart, unspecified with or without hemopericardium**

4 **S27 Injury of other and unspecified intrathoracic organs**
Code also:
any associated open wound of thorax (S21.-)
EXCLUDES 2 injury of cervical esophagus (S10-S19)
injury of trachea (cervical) (S10-S19)

The appropriate 7th character is to be added to each code from category S27
A initial encounter
D subsequent encounter
S sequela

SP 7 **S27.0XX- Traumatic pneumothorax**
EXCLUDES 1 spontaneous pneumothorax (J93.-)
CODING TIPS✓ Do not assign S27.0- to indicate a pneumothorax that is not specifically identified as due to trauma. Chapter 19 codes are for those diagnoses due to injury and trauma. S27.0- indicates pneumothorax resulting from traumatic origin. Nontraumatic (spontaneous or unspecified pneumothorax) should be coded to J93.-.

SP 7 **S27.1XX- Traumatic hemothorax**

SP 7 **S27.2XX- Traumatic hemopneumothorax**

5 **S27.3 Other and unspecified injuries of lung**

6 **S27.30 Unspecified injury of lung**

!Q 7 **S27.301- Unspecified injury of lung, unilateral**

!Q 7 **S27.302- Unspecified injury of lung, bilateral**

!Q 7 **S27.309- Unspecified injury of lung, unspecified**

6 **S27.31 Primary blast injury of lung**
Blast injury of lung NOS

SP 7 **S27.311- Primary blast injury of lung, unilateral**

SP 7 **S27.312- Primary blast injury of lung, bilateral**

SP 7 **S27.319- Primary blast injury of lung, unspecified**

6 **S27.32 Contusion of lung**

SP 7 **S27.321- Contusion of lung, unilateral**

SP 7 **S27.322- Contusion of lung, bilateral**

SP 7 **S27.329- Contusion of lung, unspecified**

6 **S27.33 Laceration of lung**

SP 7 **S27.331- Laceration of lung, unilateral**

SP 7 **S27.332- Laceration of lung, bilateral**

!Q 7 **S27.339- Laceration of lung, unspecified**

6 **S27.39 Other injuries of lung**
Secondary blast injury of lung

SP 7 **S27.391- Other injuries of lung, unilateral**

SP 7 **S27.392- Other injuries of lung, bilateral**

!Q 7 **S27.399- Other injuries of lung, unspecified**

5 **S27.4 Injury of bronchus**

6 **S27.40 Unspecified injury of bronchus**

!Q 7 **S27.401- Unspecified injury of bronchus, unilateral**

!Q 7 **S27.402- Unspecified injury of bronchus, bilateral**

!Q 7 **S27.409- Unspecified injury of bronchus, unspecified**

6 **S27.41 Primary blast injury of bronchus**
Blast injury of bronchus NOS

SP 7 **S27.411- Primary blast injury of bronchus, unilateral**

SP 7 **S27.412- Primary blast injury of bronchus, bilateral**

!Q 7 **S27.419- Primary blast injury of bronchus, unspecified**

6 **S27.42 Contusion of bronchus**

SP 7 **S27.421- Contusion of bronchus, unilateral**

SP 7 **S27.422- Contusion of bronchus, bilateral**

!Q 7 **S27.429- Contusion of bronchus, unspecified**

6 **S27.43 Laceration of bronchus**

SP 7 **S27.431- Laceration of bronchus, unilateral**

SP 7 **S27.432- Laceration of bronchus, bilateral**

!Q 7 **S27.439- Laceration of bronchus, unspecified**

6 **S27.49 Other injury of bronchus**
Secondary blast injury of bronchus

SP 7 **S27.491- Other injury of bronchus, unilateral**

SP 7 **S27.492- Other injury of bronchus, bilateral**

!Q 7 **S27.499- Other injury of bronchus, unspecified**

5 **S27.5 Injury of thoracic trachea**

!Q 7 **S27.50X- Unspecified injury of thoracic trachea**

SP 7 **S27.51X- Primary blast injury of thoracic trachea**
Blast injury of thoracic trachea NOS

SP 7 **S27.52X- Contusion of thoracic trachea**

SP 7 **S27.53X- Laceration of thoracic trachea**

SP 7 **S27.59X- Other injury of thoracic trachea**
Secondary blast injury of thoracic trachea

5 **S27.6 Injury of pleura**

!Q 7 **S27.60X- Unspecified injury of pleura**

SP 7 **S27.63X- Laceration of pleura**

SP 7 **S27.69X- Other injury of pleura**

5 **S27.8 Injury of other specified intrathoracic organs**

6 **S27.80 Injury of diaphragm**

SP 7 **S27.802- Contusion of diaphragm**

SP 7 **S27.803- Laceration of diaphragm**

SP 7 **S27.808- Other injury of diaphragm**

!Q 7 **S27.809- Unspecified injury of diaphragm**

6 **S27.81 Injury of esophagus (thoracic part)**

SP 7 **S27.812- Contusion of esophagus (thoracic part)**

SP 7 **S27.813- Laceration of esophagus (thoracic part)**

SP 7 **S27.818- Other injury of esophagus (thoracic part)**

IQ 7 **S27.819- Unspecified injury of esophagus (thoracic part)**

6 **S27.89 Injury of other specified intrathoracic organs**

Injury of lymphatic thoracic duct
Injury of thymus gland

SP 7 **S27.892- Contusion of other specified intrathoracic organs**

SP 7 **S27.893- Laceration of other specified intrathoracic organs**

SP 7 **S27.898- Other injury of other specified intrathoracic organs**

IQ 7 **S27.899- Unspecified injury of other specified intrathoracic organs**

IQ X **S27.9XX- Injury of unspecified intrathoracic organ**

4 **S28 Crushing injury of thorax, and traumatic amputation of part of thorax**

The appropriate 7th character is to be added to each code from category S28
A initial encounter
D subsequent encounter
S sequela

SP + X **S28.0XX- Crushed chest**

Use additional code for all associated injuries

EXCLUDES 1 flail chest (S22.5)

SP X **S28.1XX- Traumatic amputation (partial) of part of thorax, except breast**

5 **S28.2 Traumatic amputation of breast**

6 **S28.21 Complete traumatic amputation of breast**

Traumatic amputation of breast NOS

L SP 7 **S28.211- Complete traumatic amputation of right breast**

L SP 7 **S28.212- Complete traumatic amputation of left breast**

L IQ 7 **S28.219- Complete traumatic amputation of unspecified breast**

6 **S28.22 Partial traumatic amputation of breast**

L SP 7 **S28.221- Partial traumatic amputation of right breast**

L SP 7 **S28.222- Partial traumatic amputation of left breast**

L IQ 7 **S28.229- Partial traumatic amputation of unspecified breast**

4 **S29 Other and unspecified injuries of thorax**

Code also:
any associated open wound (S21.-)

The appropriate 7th character is to be added to each code from category S29
A initial encounter
D subsequent encounter
S sequela

5 **S29.0 Injury of muscle and tendon at thorax level**

6 **S29.00 Unspecified injury of muscle and tendon of thorax**

IQ 7 **S29.001- Unspecified injury of muscle and tendon of front wall of thorax**

IQ 7 **S29.002- Unspecified injury of muscle and tendon of back wall of thorax**

IQ 7 **S29.009- Unspecified injury of muscle and tendon of unspecified wall of thorax**

6 **S29.01 Strain of muscle and tendon of thorax**

SP 7 **S29.011- Strain of muscle and tendon of front wall of thorax**

SP 7 **S29.012- Strain of muscle and tendon of back wall of thorax**

SP 7 **S29.019- Strain of muscle and tendon of unspecified wall of thorax**

6 **S29.02 Laceration of muscle and tendon of thorax**

SP 7 **S29.021- Laceration of muscle and tendon of front wall of thorax**

SP 7 **S29.022- Laceration of muscle and tendon of back wall of thorax**

IQ 7 **S29.029- Laceration of muscle and tendon of unspecified wall of thorax**

6 **S29.09 Other injury of muscle and tendon of thorax**

SP 7 **S29.091- Other injury of muscle and tendon of front wall of thorax**

SP 7 **S29.092- Other injury of muscle and tendon of back wall of thorax**

IQ 7 **S29.099- Other injury of muscle and tendon of unspecified wall of thorax**

SP X **S29.8XX- Other specified injuries of thorax**

IQ X **S29.9XX- Unspecified injury of thorax**

Injuries to the abdomen, lower back, lumbar spine, pelvis and external genitals (S30-S39)

INCLUDES injuries to the abdominal wall
injuries to the anus
injuries to the buttock
injuries to the external genitalia
injuries to the flank
injuries to the groin

EXCLUDES 2 burns and corrosions (T20-T32)
effects of foreign body in anus and rectum (T18.5)
effects of foreign body in genitourinary tract (T19.-)
effects of foreign body in stomach, small intestine and colon (T18.2-T18.4)
frostbite (T33-T34)
insect bite or sting, venomous (T63.4)

GUIDELINES **Section I.C.19.c.2)**

Multiple fractures are sequenced in accordance with the severity of the fracture.

Chapter 19

S00-T88

4 4th digit required 5 5th digit required 6 6th digit required 7 7th digit required X 7th digit placeholder + Additional code L Laterality

GUIDELINES **Section I.C.19.b.1)-2)**

When coding injuries, assign separate codes for each injury unless a combination code is provided, in which case the combination code is assigned ... Traumatic injury codes (S00-T14.9) are not to be used for normal, healing surgical wounds or to identify complications of surgical wounds. The code for the most serious injury, as determined by the provider and the focus of treatment, is sequenced first.

1) Superficial injuries such as abrasions or contusions are not coded when associated with more severe injuries of the same site.

2) When a primary injury results in minor damage to peripheral nerves or blood vessels, the primary injury is sequenced first with additional code(s) for injuries to nerves and spinal cord (such as category S04), and/or injury to blood vessels (such as category S15). When the primary injury is to the blood vessels or nerves, that injury should be sequenced first.

GUIDELINES **Section I.C.19.c**

Coding of Traumatic Fractures: The principles of multiple coding of injuries should be followed in coding fractures. Fractures of specified sites are coded individually by site in accordance with both the provisions within categories S02, S12, S22, S32, S42, S49, S52, S59, S62, S72, S79, S82, S89, S92 and the level of detail furnished by medical record content. A fracture not indicated as open or closed should be coded to closed. A fracture not indicated whether displaced or not displaced should be coded to displaced.

CODING TIPS✓ 7th character A is acceptable in home health and hospice when active treatment is provided, such as antibiotics for an infected wound or a wound vac for a dehisced wound. D is used when the complication or injury is now healing. Think of D as aftercare. S is used for sequela of the injury or complication. Sequela is a residual deficit or condition produced as a result of the injury or complication after the original injury or complication has healed.

4 **S30 Superficial injury of abdomen, lower back, pelvis and external genitals**

EXCLUDES 2 superficial injury of hip (S70.-)

The appropriate 7th character is to be added to each code from category S30
A initial encounter
D subsequent encounter
S sequela

SP 7 **S30.0XX- Contusion of lower back and pelvis**
Contusion of buttock

SP 7 **S30.1XX- Contusion of abdominal wall**
Contusion of flank
Contusion of groin

5 **S30.2 Contusion of external genital organs**

6 **S30.20 Contusion of unspecified external genital organ**

SP 7 **S30.201- Contusion of unspecified external genital organ, male**

SP IQ 7 **S30.202- Contusion of unspecified external genital organ, female**

SP 7 **S30.21X- Contusion of penis**

SP 7 **S30.22X- Contusion of scrotum and testes**

SP 7 **S30.23X- Contusion of vagina and vulva**

SP 7 **S30.3XX- Contusion of anus**

5 **S30.8 Other superficial injuries of abdomen, lower back, pelvis and external genitals**

6 **S30.81 Abrasion of abdomen, lower back, pelvis and external genitals**

IQ 7 **S30.810- Abrasion of lower back and pelvis**

IQ 7 **S30.811- Abrasion of abdominal wall**

IQ 7 **S30.812- Abrasion of penis**

IQ 7 **S30.813- Abrasion of scrotum and testes**

IQ 7 **S30.814- Abrasion of vagina and vulva**

IQ 7 **S30.815- Abrasion of unspecified external genital organs, male**

IQ 7 **S30.816- Abrasion of unspecified external genital organs, female**

IQ 7 **S30.817- Abrasion of anus**

6 **S30.82 Blister (nonthermal) of abdomen, lower back, pelvis and external genitals**

IQ 7 **S30.820- Blister (nonthermal) of lower back and pelvis**

IQ 7 **S30.821- Blister (nonthermal) of abdominal wall**

IQ 7 **S30.822- Blister (nonthermal) of penis**

IQ 7 **S30.823- Blister (nonthermal) of scrotum and testes**

IQ 7 **S30.824- Blister (nonthermal) of vagina and vulva**

IQ 7 **S30.825- Blister (nonthermal) of unspecified external genital organs, male**

IQ 7 **S30.826- Blister (nonthermal) of unspecified external genital organs, female**

IQ 7 **S30.827- Blister (nonthermal) of anus**

6 **S30.84 External constriction of abdomen, lower back, pelvis and external genitals**

IQ 7 **S30.840- External constriction of lower back and pelvis**

IQ 7 **S30.841- External constriction of abdominal wall**

IQ + 7 **S30.842- External constriction of penis**
Hair tourniquet syndrome of penis
Use additional cause code to identify the constricting item (W49.0-)

IQ 7 **S30.843- External constriction of scrotum and testes**

IQ 7 **S30.844- External constriction of vagina and vulva**

IQ 7 **S30.845- External constriction of unspecified external genital organs, male**

IQ 7 **S30.846- External constriction of unspecified external genital organs, female**

6 **S30.85 Superficial foreign body of abdomen, lower back, pelvis and external genitals**
Splinter in the abdomen, lower back, pelvis and external genitals

IQ 7 **S30.850- Superficial foreign body of lower back and pelvis**

IQ 7 **S30.851- Superficial foreign body of abdominal wall**

Chapter 19

S00-T88

IQ 7 **S30.852- Superficial foreign body of penis**

IQ 7 **S30.853- Superficial foreign body of scrotum and testes**

IQ 7 **S30.854- Superficial foreign body of vagina and vulva**

IQ 7 **S30.855- Superficial foreign body of unspecified external genital organs, male**

IQ 7 **S30.856- Superficial foreign body of unspecified external genital organs, female**

IQ 7 **S30.857- Superficial foreign body of anus**

6 **S30.86 Insect bite (nonvenomous) of abdomen, lower back, pelvis and external genitals**

IQ 7 **S30.860- Insect bite (nonvenomous) of lower back and pelvis**

IQ 7 **S30.861- Insect bite (nonvenomous) of abdominal wall**

IQ 7 **S30.862- Insect bite (nonvenomous) of penis**

IQ 7 **S30.863- Insect bite (nonvenomous) of scrotum and testes**

IQ 7 **S30.864- Insect bite (nonvenomous) of vagina and vulva**

IQ 7 **S30.865- Insect bite (nonvenomous) of unspecified external genital organs, male**

IQ 7 **S30.866- Insect bite (nonvenomous) of unspecified external genital organs, female**

IQ 7 **S30.867- Insect bite (nonvenomous) of anus**

6 **S30.87 Other superficial bite of abdomen, lower back, pelvis and external genitals**

EXCLUDES 1 open bite of abdomen, lower back, pelvis and external genitals (S31.05, S31.15, S31.25, S31.35, S31.45, S31.55)

IQ 7 **S30.870- Other superficial bite of lower back and pelvis**

IQ 7 **S30.871- Other superficial bite of abdominal wall**

IQ 7 **S30.872- Other superficial bite of penis**

IQ 7 **S30.873- Other superficial bite of scrotum and testes**

IQ 7 **S30.874- Other superficial bite of vagina and vulva**

IQ 7 **S30.875- Other superficial bite of unspecified external genital organs, male**

IQ 7 **S30.876- Other superficial bite of unspecified external genital organs, female**

IQ 7 **S30.877- Other superficial bite of anus**

5 **S30.9 Unspecified superficial injury of abdomen, lower back, pelvis and external genitals**

IQ 7 **S30.91X- Unspecified superficial injury of lower back and pelvis**

IQ 7 **S30.92X- Unspecified superficial injury of abdominal wall**

IQ 7 **S30.93X- Unspecified superficial injury of penis**

IQ 7 **S30.94X- Unspecified superficial injury of scrotum and testes**

IQ 7 **S30.95X- Unspecified superficial injury of vagina and vulva**

IQ 7 **S30.96X- Unspecified superficial injury of unspecified external genital organs, male**

IQ 7 **S30.97X- Unspecified superficial injury of unspecified external genital organs, female**

IQ 7 **S30.98X- Unspecified superficial injury of anus**

4 **S31 Open wound of abdomen, lower back, pelvis and external genitals**

Code also any associated:
spinal cord injury (S24.0, S24.1-, S34.0-, S34.1-)
wound infection

EXCLUDES 1 traumatic amputation of part of abdomen, lower back and pelvis (S38.2-, S38.3)

EXCLUDES 2 open wound of hip (S71.00-S71.02)
open fracture of pelvis (S32.1--S32.9 with 7th character B)

The appropriate 7th character is to be added to each code from category S31
A initial encounter
D subsequent encounter
S sequela

CODING TIPS✓ Open wound codes are used for wounds caused by trauma. Do not assign a code for "open wound" unless the etiology of the wound is related to trauma. Do not use Z codes for any aspect of care of a trauma wound, e.g. no Z code for dressing changes, drain care, or suture removal.

CODING TIPS✓ No aftercare code applies, including those indicating dressing changes, drain care, or suture removal. 7th character 'D' is the default for home care and hospice when providing aftercare for a healing or resolving condition; 'A' is used for active treatment such as antibiotics or more than routine wound care; 'S' may be used to indicate a residual condition after the original injury has healed.

5 **S31.0 Open wound of lower back and pelvis**

6 **S31.00 Unspecified open wound of lower back and pelvis**

SP 7 **S31.000- Unspecified open wound of lower back and pelvis without penetration into retroperitoneum**

Unspecified open wound of lower back and pelvis NOS

SP 7 **S31.001- Unspecified open wound of lower back and pelvis with penetration into retroperitoneum**

6 **S31.01 Laceration without foreign body of lower back and pelvis**

Chapter 19 S00-T88

4 4th digit required 5 5th digit required 6 6th digit required 7 7th digit required 7 7th digit placeholder + Additional code Laterality

SP 7 **S31.010- Laceration without foreign body of lower back and pelvis without penetration into retroperitoneum**
Laceration without foreign body of lower back and pelvis NOS

SP 7 **S31.011- Laceration without foreign body of lower back and pelvis with penetration into retroperitoneum**

6 **S31.02 Laceration with foreign body of lower back and pelvis**

SP 7 **S31.020- Laceration with foreign body of lower back and pelvis without penetration into retroperitoneum**
Laceration with foreign body of lower back and pelvis NOS

SP 7 **S31.021- Laceration with foreign body of lower back and pelvis with penetration into retroperitoneum**

6 **S31.03 Puncture wound without foreign body of lower back and pelvis**

SP 7 **S31.030- Puncture wound without foreign body of lower back and pelvis without penetration into retroperitoneum**
Puncture wound without foreign body of lower back and pelvis NOS

SP 7 **S31.031- Puncture wound without foreign body of lower back and pelvis with penetration into retroperitoneum**

6 **S31.04 Puncture wound with foreign body of lower back and pelvis**

SP 7 **S31.040- Puncture wound with foreign body of lower back and pelvis without penetration into retroperitoneum**
Puncture wound with foreign body of lower back and pelvis NOS

SP 7 **S31.041- Puncture wound with foreign body of lower back and pelvis with penetration into retroperitoneum**

6 **S31.05 Open bite of lower back and pelvis**
Bite of lower back and pelvis NOS
EXCLUDES 1 superficial bite of lower back and pelvis (S30.860, S30.870)

SP 7 **S31.050- Open bite of lower back and pelvis without penetration into retroperitoneum**
Open bite of lower back and pelvis NOS

SP 7 **S31.051- Open bite of lower back and pelvis with penetration into retroperitoneum**

5 **S31.1 Open wound of abdominal wall without penetration into peritoneal cavity**
Open wound of abdominal wall NOS
EXCLUDES 2 open wound of abdominal wall with penetration into peritoneal cavity (S31.6-)

6 **S31.10 Unspecified open wound of abdominal wall without penetration into peritoneal cavity**

H SP 7 **S31.100- Unspecified open wound of abdominal wall, right upper quadrant without penetration into peritoneal cavity**

H SP 7 **S31.101- Unspecified open wound of abdominal wall, left upper quadrant without penetration into peritoneal cavity**

H SP 7 **S31.102- Unspecified open wound of abdominal wall, epigastric region without penetration into peritoneal cavity**

H SP 7 **S31.103- Unspecified open wound of abdominal wall, right lower quadrant without penetration into peritoneal cavity**

H SP 7 **S31.104- Unspecified open wound of abdominal wall, left lower quadrant without penetration into peritoneal cavity**

H SP 7 **S31.105- Unspecified open wound of abdominal wall, periumbilic region without penetration into peritoneal cavity**

H SP 7 **S31.109- Unspecified open wound of abdominal wall, unspecified quadrant without penetration into peritoneal cavity**
Unspecified open wound of abdominal wall NOS

6 **S31.11 Laceration without foreign body of abdominal wall without penetration into peritoneal cavity**

H SP 7 **S31.110- Laceration without foreign body of abdominal wall, right upper quadrant without penetration into peritoneal cavity**

H SP 7 **S31.111- Laceration without foreign body of abdominal wall, left upper quadrant without penetration into peritoneal cavity**

H SP 7 **S31.112- Laceration without foreign body of abdominal wall, epigastric region without penetration into peritoneal cavity**

H SP 7 **S31.113- Laceration without foreign body of abdominal wall, right lower quadrant without penetration into peritoneal cavity**

H SP 7 **S31.114- Laceration without foreign body of abdominal wall, left lower quadrant without penetration into peritoneal cavity**

H SP 7 **S31.115- Laceration without foreign body of abdominal wall, periumbilic region without penetration into peritoneal cavity**

H SP 7 **S31.119- Laceration without foreign body of abdominal wall, unspecified quadrant without penetration into peritoneal cavity**

6 **S31.12 Laceration with foreign body of abdominal wall without penetration into peritoneal cavity**

H SP 7 **S31.120- Laceration of abdominal wall with foreign body, right upper quadrant without penetration into peritoneal cavity**

H SP 7 **S31.121- Laceration of abdominal wall with foreign body, left upper quadrant without penetration into peritoneal cavity**

S31.122- Laceration of abdominal wall with foreign body, epigastric region without penetration into peritoneal cavity

S31.123- Laceration of abdominal wall with foreign body, right lower quadrant without penetration into peritoneal cavity

S31.124- Laceration of abdominal wall with foreign body, left lower quadrant without penetration into peritoneal cavity

S31.125- Laceration of abdominal wall with foreign body, periumbilic region without penetration into peritoneal cavity

S31.129- Laceration of abdominal wall with foreign body, unspecified quadrant without penetration into peritoneal cavity

S31.13 Puncture wound of abdominal wall without foreign body without penetration into peritoneal cavity

S31.130- Puncture wound of abdominal wall without foreign body, right upper quadrant without penetration into peritoneal cavity

S31.131- Puncture wound of abdominal wall without foreign body, left upper quadrant without penetration into peritoneal cavity

S31.132- Puncture wound of abdominal wall without foreign body, epigastric region without penetration into peritoneal cavity

S31.133- Puncture wound of abdominal wall without foreign body, right lower quadrant without penetration into peritoneal cavity

S31.134- Puncture wound of abdominal wall without foreign body, left lower quadrant without penetration into peritoneal cavity

S31.135- Puncture wound of abdominal wall without foreign body, periumbilic region without penetration into peritoneal cavity

S31.139- Puncture wound of abdominal wall without foreign body, unspecified quadrant without penetration into peritoneal cavity

S31.14 Puncture wound of abdominal wall with foreign body without penetration into peritoneal cavity

S31.140- Puncture wound of abdominal wall with foreign body, right upper quadrant without penetration into peritoneal cavity

S31.141- Puncture wound of abdominal wall with foreign body, left upper quadrant without penetration into peritoneal cavity

S31.142- Puncture wound of abdominal wall with foreign body, epigastric region without penetration into peritoneal cavity

S31.143- Puncture wound of abdominal wall with foreign body, right lower quadrant without penetration into peritoneal cavity

S31.144- Puncture wound of abdominal wall with foreign body, left lower quadrant without penetration into peritoneal cavity

S31.145- Puncture wound of abdominal wall with foreign body, periumbilic region without penetration into peritoneal cavity

S31.149- Puncture wound of abdominal wall with foreign body, unspecified quadrant without penetration into peritoneal cavity

S31.15 Open bite of abdominal wall without penetration into peritoneal cavity

Bite of abdominal wall NOS

EXCLUDES 1 superficial bite of abdominal wall (S30.871)

S31.150- Open bite of abdominal wall, right upper quadrant without penetration into peritoneal cavity

S31.151- Open bite of abdominal wall, left upper quadrant without penetration into peritoneal cavity

S31.152- Open bite of abdominal wall, epigastric region without penetration into peritoneal cavity

S31.153- Open bite of abdominal wall, right lower quadrant without penetration into peritoneal cavity

S31.154- Open bite of abdominal wall, left lower quadrant without penetration into peritoneal cavity

S31.155- Open bite of abdominal wall, periumbilic region without penetration into peritoneal cavity

S31.159- Open bite of abdominal wall, unspecified quadrant without penetration into peritoneal cavity

S31.2 Open wound of penis

S31.20X- Unspecified open wound of penis

S31.21X- Laceration without foreign body of penis

S31.22X- Laceration with foreign body of penis

S31.23X- Puncture wound without foreign body of penis

S31.24X- Puncture wound with foreign body of penis

S31.25X- Open bite of penis

Bite of penis NOS

EXCLUDES 1 superficial bite of penis (S30.862, S30.872)

S31.3 Open wound of scrotum and testes

S31.30X- Unspecified open wound of scrotum and testes

S31.31X- Laceration without foreign body of scrotum and testes

S31.32X- Laceration with foreign body of scrotum and testes

Chapter 19

S00-T88

4th digit required 5th digit required 6th digit required 7th digit required 7th digit placeholder + Additional code Laterality

SP 7 **S31.33X- Puncture wound without foreign body of scrotum and testes**

SP 7 **S31.34X- Puncture wound with foreign body of scrotum and testes**

SP 7 **S31.35X- Open bite of scrotum and testes**

Bite of scrotum and testes NOS

EXCLUDES 1 superficial bite of scrotum and testes (S30.863, S30.873)

5 **S31.4 Open wound of vagina and vulva**

EXCLUDES 1 injury to vagina and vulva during delivery (O70.-, O71.4)

SP 7 **S31.40X- Unspecified open wound of vagina and vulva**

SP 7 **S31.41X- Laceration without foreign body of vagina and vulva**

SP 7 **S31.42X- Laceration with foreign body of vagina and vulva**

SP 7 **S31.43X- Puncture wound without foreign body of vagina and vulva**

SP 7 **S31.44X- Puncture wound with foreign body of vagina and vulva**

SP 7 **S31.45X- Open bite of vagina and vulva**

Bite of vagina and vulva NOS

EXCLUDES 1 superficial bite of vagina and vulva (S30.864, S30.874)

5 **S31.5 Open wound of unspecified external genital organs**

EXCLUDES 1 traumatic amputation of external genital organs (S38.21, S38.22)

6 **S31.50 Unspecified open wound of unspecified external genital organs**

IQ 7 **S31.501- Unspecified open wound of unspecified external genital organs, male**

IQ 7 **S31.502- Unspecified open wound of unspecified external genital organs, female**

6 **S31.51 Laceration without foreign body of unspecified external genital organs**

IQ 7 **S31.511- Laceration without foreign body of unspecified external genital organs, male**

IQ 7 **S31.512- Laceration without foreign body of unspecified external genital organs, female**

6 **S31.52 Laceration with foreign body of unspecified external genital organs**

IQ 7 **S31.521- Laceration with foreign body of unspecified external genital organs, male**

IQ 7 **S31.522- Laceration with foreign body of unspecified external genital organs, female**

6 **S31.53 Puncture wound without foreign body of unspecified external genital organs**

IQ 7 **S31.531- Puncture wound without foreign body of unspecified external genital organs, male**

IQ 7 **S31.532- Puncture wound without foreign body of unspecified external genital organs, female**

6 **S31.54 Puncture wound with foreign body of unspecified external genital organs**

IQ 7 **S31.541- Puncture wound with foreign body of unspecified external genital organs, male**

IQ 7 **S31.542- Puncture wound with foreign body of unspecified external genital organs, female**

6 **S31.55 Open bite of unspecified external genital organs**

Bite of unspecified external genital organs NOS

EXCLUDES 1 superficial bite of unspecified external genital organs (S30.865, S30.866, S30.875, S30.876)

IQ 7 **S31.551- Open bite of unspecified external genital organs, male**

IQ 7 **S31.552- Open bite of unspecified external genital organs, female**

5 **S31.6 Open wound of abdominal wall with penetration into peritoneal cavity**

6 **S31.60 Unspecified open wound of abdominal wall with penetration into peritoneal cavity**

H SP 7 **S31.600- Unspecified open wound of abdominal wall, right upper quadrant with penetration into peritoneal cavity**

H SP 7 **S31.601- Unspecified open wound of abdominal wall, left upper quadrant with penetration into peritoneal cavity**

H SP 7 **S31.602- Unspecified open wound of abdominal wall, epigastric region with penetration into peritoneal cavity**

H SP 7 **S31.603- Unspecified open wound of abdominal wall, right lower quadrant with penetration into peritoneal cavity**

H SP 7 **S31.604- Unspecified open wound of abdominal wall, left lower quadrant with penetration into peritoneal cavity**

H SP 7 **S31.605- Unspecified open wound of abdominal wall, periumbilic region with penetration into peritoneal cavity**

H SP 7 **S31.609- Unspecified open wound of abdominal wall, unspecified quadrant with penetration into peritoneal cavity**

6 **S31.61 Laceration without foreign body of abdominal wall with penetration into peritoneal cavity**

H SP 7 **S31.610- Laceration without foreign body of abdominal wall, right upper quadrant with penetration into peritoneal cavity**

H SP 7 **S31.611- Laceration without foreign body of abdominal wall, left upper quadrant with penetration into peritoneal cavity**

S31.612- Laceration without foreign body of abdominal wall, epigastric region with penetration into peritoneal cavity

S31.613- Laceration without foreign body of abdominal wall, right lower quadrant with penetration into peritoneal cavity

S31.614- Laceration without foreign body of abdominal wall, left lower quadrant with penetration into peritoneal cavity

S31.615- Laceration without foreign body of abdominal wall, periumbilic region with penetration into peritoneal cavity

S31.619- Laceration without foreign body of abdominal wall, unspecified quadrant with penetration into peritoneal cavity

S31.62 Laceration with foreign body of abdominal wall with penetration into peritoneal cavity

S31.620- Laceration with foreign body of abdominal wall, right upper quadrant with penetration into peritoneal cavity

S31.621- Laceration with foreign body of abdominal wall, left upper quadrant with penetration into peritoneal cavity

S31.622- Laceration with foreign body of abdominal wall, epigastric region with penetration into peritoneal cavity

S31.623- Laceration with foreign body of abdominal wall, right lower quadrant with penetration into peritoneal cavity

S31.624- Laceration with foreign body of abdominal wall, left lower quadrant with penetration into peritoneal cavity

S31.625- Laceration with foreign body of abdominal wall, periumbilic region with penetration into peritoneal cavity

S31.629- Laceration with foreign body of abdominal wall, unspecified quadrant with penetration into peritoneal cavity

S31.63 Puncture wound without foreign body of abdominal wall with penetration into peritoneal cavity

S31.630- Puncture wound without foreign body of abdominal wall, right upper quadrant with penetration into peritoneal cavity

S31.631- Puncture wound without foreign body of abdominal wall, left upper quadrant with penetration into peritoneal cavity

S31.632- Puncture wound without foreign body of abdominal wall, epigastric region with penetration into peritoneal cavity

S31.633- Puncture wound without foreign body of abdominal wall, right lower quadrant with penetration into peritoneal cavity

S31.634- Puncture wound without foreign body of abdominal wall, left lower quadrant with penetration into peritoneal cavity

S31.635- Puncture wound without foreign body of abdominal wall, periumbilic region with penetration into peritoneal cavity

S31.639- Puncture wound without foreign body of abdominal wall, unspecified quadrant with penetration into peritoneal cavity

S31.64 Puncture wound with foreign body of abdominal wall with penetration into peritoneal cavity

S31.640- Puncture wound with foreign body of abdominal wall, right upper quadrant with penetration into peritoneal cavity

S31.641- Puncture wound with foreign body of abdominal wall, left upper quadrant with penetration into peritoneal cavity

S31.642- Puncture wound with foreign body of abdominal wall, epigastric region with penetration into peritoneal cavity

S31.643- Puncture wound with foreign body of abdominal wall, right lower quadrant with penetration into peritoneal cavity

S31.644- Puncture wound with foreign body of abdominal wall, left lower quadrant with penetration into peritoneal cavity

S31.645- Puncture wound with foreign body of abdominal wall, periumbilic region with penetration into peritoneal cavity

S31.649- Puncture wound with foreign body of abdominal wall, unspecified quadrant with penetration into peritoneal cavity

S31.65 Open bite of abdominal wall with penetration into peritoneal cavity

EXCLUDES 1 superficial bite of abdominal wall (S30.861, S30.871)

S31.650- Open bite of abdominal wall, right upper quadrant with penetration into peritoneal cavity

S31.651- Open bite of abdominal wall, left upper quadrant with penetration into peritoneal cavity

S31.652- Open bite of abdominal wall, epigastric region with penetration into peritoneal cavity

S31.653- Open bite of abdominal wall, right lower quadrant with penetration into peritoneal cavity

S31.654- Open bite of abdominal wall, left lower quadrant with penetration into peritoneal cavity

☰ SP 7 **S31.655-** Open bite of abdominal wall, periumbilic region with penetration into peritoneal cavity

☰ IQ 7 **S31.659-** Open bite of abdominal wall, unspecified quadrant with penetration into peritoneal cavity

5 **S31.8 Open wound of other parts of abdomen, lower back and pelvis**

6 **S31.80   Open wound of unspecified buttock**

IQ 7 **S31.801-** Laceration without foreign body of unspecified buttock

IQ 7 **S31.802-** Laceration with foreign body of unspecified buttock

IQ 7 **S31.803-** Puncture wound without foreign body of unspecified buttock

IQ 7 **S31.804-** Puncture wound with foreign body of unspecified buttock

IQ 7 **S31.805-** Open bite of unspecified buttock
Bite of buttock NOS
EXCLUDES 1 superficial bite of buttock (S30.870)

IQ 7 **S31.809-** Unspecified open wound of unspecified buttock

6 **S31.81   Open wound of right buttock**

☰ SP 7 **S31.811-** Laceration without foreign body of right buttock

☰ SP 7 **S31.812-** Laceration with foreign body of right buttock

☰ SP 7 **S31.813-** Puncture wound without foreign body of right buttock

☰ SP 7 **S31.814-** Puncture wound with foreign body of right buttock

☰ SP 7 **S31.815-** Open bite of right buttock
Bite of right buttock NOS
EXCLUDES 1 superficial bite of buttock (S30.870)

☰ SP 7 **S31.819-** Unspecified open wound of right buttock

6 **S31.82   Open wound of left buttock**

☰ SP 7 **S31.821-** Laceration without foreign body of left buttock

☰ SP 7 **S31.822-** Laceration with foreign body of left buttock

☰ SP 7 **S31.823-** Puncture wound without foreign body of left buttock

☰ SP 7 **S31.824-** Puncture wound with foreign body of left buttock

☰ SP 7 **S31.825-** Open bite of left buttock
Bite of left buttock NOS
EXCLUDES 1 superficial bite of buttock (S30.870)

☰ SP 7 **S31.829-** Unspecified open wound of left buttock

6 **S31.83   Open wound of anus**

SP 7 **S31.831-** Laceration without foreign body of anus

SP 7 **S31.832-** Laceration with foreign body of anus

SP 7 **S31.833-** Puncture wound without foreign body of anus

SP 7 **S31.834-** Puncture wound with foreign body of anus

SP 7 **S31.835-** Open bite of anus
Bite of anus NOS
EXCLUDES 1 superficial bite of anus (S30.877)

SP 7 **S31.839-** Unspecified open wound of anus

4 **S32   Fracture of lumbar spine and pelvis**
Note:
A fracture not indicated as displaced or nondisplaced should be coded to displaced
A fracture not indicated as opened or closed should be coded to closed
INCLUDES fracture of lumbosacral neural arch
fracture of lumbosacral spinous process
fracture of lumbosacral transverse process
fracture of lumbosacral vertebra
fracture of lumbosacral vertebral arch

Code first:
any associated spinal cord and spinal nerve injury (S34.-)
EXCLUDES 1 transection of abdomen (S38.3)
EXCLUDES 2 fracture of hip NOS (S72.0-)

The appropriate 7th character is to be added to each code from category S32
A   initial encounter for closed fracture
B   initial encounter for open fracture
D   subsequent encounter for fracture with routine healing
G   subsequent encounter for fracture with delayed healing
K   subsequent encounter for fracture with nonunion
S   sequela

CODING TIPS ✓ Fractures repaired by joint replacements are NOT coded with Z47.1. Fractures repaired by any other orthopedic surgery are NOT coded with Z47.89. Z codes are not appropriate for fractures of any kind. Code the fracture with 7th character D for fractures undergoing surgical repair.

CODING TIPS ✓ 'D' is the 7th character for home care and hospice unless the physician or NPP has documented delayed healing, nonunion or malunion. A sequela is a condition left after the fracture has healed. The Gustilo open fracture classification must be used for open fractures. The default 7th character for open fractures is E.

CODING TIPS ✓ A fracture not indicated as displaced or nondisplaced should be coded to displaced. A fracture not indicated as open or closed should be coded to closed.

5 **S32.0 Fracture of lumbar vertebra**
Fracture of lumbar spine NOS

6 **S32.00   Fracture of unspecified lumbar vertebra**

SP 7 **S32.000-** Wedge compression fracture of unspecified lumbar vertebra

SP 7 **S32.001-** Stable burst fracture of unspecified lumbar vertebra

SP 7 **S32.002-** Unstable burst fracture of unspecified lumbar vertebra

★ New ▲ Revised Px Primary SP PDGM Px SL Low CoM SH High CoM IQ Quest. Encounter H Hospice non-cancer Dx Unspecified M Manifestation

DecisionHealth's FY 2022 Complete Home Health ICD-10-CM Diagnosis Coding Manual   1527

Chapter 19

S00-T88

SP 7 S32.008- Other fracture of unspecified lumbar vertebra

SP 7 S32.009- Unspecified fracture of unspecified lumbar vertebra

6 S32.01 Fracture of first lumbar vertebra

SP 7 S32.010- Wedge compression fracture of first lumbar vertebra

SP 7 S32.011- Stable burst fracture of first lumbar vertebra

SP 7 S32.012- Unstable burst fracture of first lumbar vertebra

SP 7 S32.018- Other fracture of first lumbar vertebra

SP 7 S32.019- Unspecified fracture of first lumbar vertebra

6 S32.02 Fracture of second lumbar vertebra

SP 7 S32.020- Wedge compression fracture of second lumbar vertebra

SP 7 S32.021- Stable burst fracture of second lumbar vertebra

SP 7 S32.022- Unstable burst fracture of second lumbar vertebra

SP 7 S32.028- Other fracture of second lumbar vertebra

SP 7 S32.029- Unspecified fracture of second lumbar vertebra

6 S32.03 Fracture of third lumbar vertebra

SP 7 S32.030- Wedge compression fracture of third lumbar vertebra

SP 7 S32.031- Stable burst fracture of third lumbar vertebra

SP 7 S32.032- Unstable burst fracture of third lumbar vertebra

SP 7 S32.038- Other fracture of third lumbar vertebra

SP 7 S32.039- Unspecified fracture of third lumbar vertebra

6 S32.04 Fracture of fourth lumbar vertebra

SP 7 S32.040- Wedge compression fracture of fourth lumbar vertebra

SP 7 S32.041- Stable burst fracture of fourth lumbar vertebra

SP 7 S32.042- Unstable burst fracture of fourth lumbar vertebra

SP 7 S32.048- Other fracture of fourth lumbar vertebra

SP 7 S32.049- Unspecified fracture of fourth lumbar vertebra

6 S32.05 Fracture of fifth lumbar vertebra

SP 7 S32.050- Wedge compression fracture of fifth lumbar vertebra

SP 7 S32.051- Stable burst fracture of fifth lumbar vertebra

SP 7 S32.052- Unstable burst fracture of fifth lumbar vertebra

SP 7 S32.058- Other fracture of fifth lumbar vertebra

SP 7 S32.059- Unspecified fracture of fifth lumbar vertebra

5 S32.1 Fracture of sacrum

For vertical fractures, code to most medial fracture extension

Use two codes if both a vertical and transverse fracture are present

Code also:

any associated fracture of pelvic ring (S32.8-)

SP X S32.10X- Unspecified fracture of sacrum

6 S32.11 Zone I fracture of sacrum

Vertical sacral ala fracture of sacrum

SP 7 S32.110- Nondisplaced Zone I fracture of sacrum

SP 7 S32.111- Minimally displaced Zone I fracture of sacrum

SP 7 S32.112- Severely displaced Zone I fracture of sacrum

SP 7 S32.119- Unspecified Zone I fracture of sacrum

6 S32.12 Zone II fracture of sacrum

Vertical foraminal region fracture of sacrum

SP 7 S32.120- Nondisplaced Zone II fracture of sacrum

SP 7 S32.121- Minimally displaced Zone II fracture of sacrum

SP 7 S32.122- Severely displaced Zone II fracture of sacrum

SP 7 S32.129- Unspecified Zone II fracture of sacrum

6 S32.13 Zone III fracture of sacrum

Vertical fracture into spinal canal region of sacrum

SP 7 S32.130- Nondisplaced Zone III fracture of sacrum

SP 7 S32.131- Minimally displaced Zone III fracture of sacrum

SP 7 S32.132- Severely displaced Zone III fracture of sacrum

SP 7 S32.139- Unspecified Zone III fracture of sacrum

SP X S32.14X- Type 1 fracture of sacrum

Transverse flexion fracture of sacrum without displacement

SP X S32.15X- Type 2 fracture of sacrum

Transverse flexion fracture of sacrum with posterior displacement

SP X S32.16X- Type 3 fracture of sacrum

Transverse extension fracture of sacrum with anterior displacement

SP X S32.17X- Type 4 fracture of sacrum

Transverse segmental comminution of upper sacrum

SP X S32.19X- Other fracture of sacrum

SP X S32.2XX- Fracture of coccyx

5 S32.3 Fracture of ilium

EXCLUDES 1 fracture of ilium with associated disruption of pelvic ring (S32.8-)

6 S32.30 Unspecified fracture of ilium

L SP 7 S32.301- Unspecified fracture of right ilium

L SP 7 S32.302- Unspecified fracture of left ilium

L !Q 7 S32.309- Unspecified fracture of unspecified ilium

6 S32.31 Avulsion fracture of ilium

Chapter 19

S00-T88

SP 7 S32.311- Displaced avulsion fracture of right ilium
SP 7 S32.312- Displaced avulsion fracture of left ilium
!Q 7 S32.313- Displaced avulsion fracture of unspecified ilium
SP 7 S32.314- Nondisplaced avulsion fracture of right ilium
SP 7 S32.315- Nondisplaced avulsion fracture of left ilium
!Q 7 S32.316- Nondisplaced avulsion fracture of unspecified ilium
6 S32.39 Other fracture of ilium
SP 7 S32.391- Other fracture of right ilium
SP 7 S32.392- Other fracture of left ilium
!Q 7 S32.399- Other fracture of unspecified ilium
5 S32.4 Fracture of acetabulum
Code also:
any associated fracture of pelvic ring (S32.8-)
6 S32.40 Unspecified fracture of acetabulum
SP 7 S32.401- Unspecified fracture of right acetabulum
SP 7 S32.402- Unspecified fracture of left acetabulum
!Q 7 S32.409- Unspecified fracture of unspecified acetabulum
6 S32.41 Fracture of anterior wall of acetabulum
SP 7 S32.411- Displaced fracture of anterior wall of right acetabulum
SP 7 S32.412- Displaced fracture of anterior wall of left acetabulum
!Q 7 S32.413- Displaced fracture of anterior wall of unspecified acetabulum
SP 7 S32.414- Nondisplaced fracture of anterior wall of right acetabulum
SP 7 S32.415- Nondisplaced fracture of anterior wall of left acetabulum
SP !Q 7 S32.416- Nondisplaced fracture of anterior wall of unspecified acetabulum
6 S32.42 Fracture of posterior wall of acetabulum
SP 7 S32.421- Displaced fracture of posterior wall of right acetabulum
SP 7 S32.422- Displaced fracture of posterior wall of left acetabulum
!Q 7 S32.423- Displaced fracture of posterior wall of unspecified acetabulum
SP 7 S32.424- Nondisplaced fracture of posterior wall of right acetabulum
SP 7 S32.425- Nondisplaced fracture of posterior wall of left acetabulum
!Q 7 S32.426- Nondisplaced fracture of posterior wall of unspecified acetabulum
6 S32.43 Fracture of anterior column [iliopubic] of acetabulum
SP 7 S32.431- Displaced fracture of anterior column [iliopubic] of right acetabulum
SP 7 S32.432- Displaced fracture of anterior column [iliopubic] of left acetabulum
!Q 7 S32.433- Displaced fracture of anterior column [iliopubic] of unspecified acetabulum
SP 7 S32.434- Nondisplaced fracture of anterior column [iliopubic] of right acetabulum
SP 7 S32.435- Nondisplaced fracture of anterior column [iliopubic] of left acetabulum
!Q 7 S32.436- Nondisplaced fracture of anterior column [iliopubic] of unspecified acetabulum
6 S32.44 Fracture of posterior column [ilioischial] of acetabulum
SP 7 S32.441- Displaced fracture of posterior column [ilioischial] of right acetabulum
SP 7 S32.442- Displaced fracture of posterior column [ilioischial] of left acetabulum
!Q 7 S32.443- Displaced fracture of posterior column [ilioischial] of unspecified acetabulum
SP 7 S32.444- Nondisplaced fracture of posterior column [ilioischial] of right acetabulum
SP 7 S32.445- Nondisplaced fracture of posterior column [ilioischial] of left acetabulum
!Q 7 S32.446- Nondisplaced fracture of posterior column [ilioischial] of unspecified acetabulum
6 S32.45 Transverse fracture of acetabulum
SP 7 S32.451- Displaced transverse fracture of right acetabulum
SP 7 S32.452- Displaced transverse fracture of left acetabulum
!Q 7 S32.453- Displaced transverse fracture of unspecified acetabulum
SP 7 S32.454- Nondisplaced transverse fracture of right acetabulum
SP 7 S32.455- Nondisplaced transverse fracture of left acetabulum
!Q 7 S32.456- Nondisplaced transverse fracture of unspecified acetabulum
6 S32.46 Associated transverse-posterior fracture of acetabulum
SP 7 S32.461- Displaced associated transverse-posterior fracture of right acetabulum
SP 7 S32.462- Displaced associated transverse-posterior fracture of left acetabulum
!Q 7 S32.463- Displaced associated transverse-posterior fracture of unspecified acetabulum
SP 7 S32.464- Nondisplaced associated transverse-posterior fracture of right acetabulum
SP 7 S32.465- Nondisplaced associated transverse-posterior fracture of left acetabulum

S32.466- Nondisplaced associated transverse-posterior fracture of unspecified acetabulum

S32.47 Fracture of medial wall of acetabulum

S32.471- Displaced fracture of medial wall of right acetabulum

S32.472- Displaced fracture of medial wall of left acetabulum

S32.473- Displaced fracture of medial wall of unspecified acetabulum

S32.474- Nondisplaced fracture of medial wall of right acetabulum

S32.475- Nondisplaced fracture of medial wall of left acetabulum

S32.476- Nondisplaced fracture of medial wall of unspecified acetabulum

S32.48 Dome fracture of acetabulum

S32.481- Displaced dome fracture of right acetabulum

S32.482- Displaced dome fracture of left acetabulum

S32.483- Displaced dome fracture of unspecified acetabulum

S32.484- Nondisplaced dome fracture of right acetabulum

S32.485- Nondisplaced dome fracture of left acetabulum

S32.486- Nondisplaced dome fracture of unspecified acetabulum

S32.49 Other specified fracture of acetabulum

S32.491- Other specified fracture of right acetabulum

S32.492- Other specified fracture of left acetabulum

S32.499- Other specified fracture of unspecified acetabulum

S32.5 Fracture of pubis

EXCLUDES 1 fracture of pubis with associated disruption of pelvic ring (S32.8-)

S32.50 Unspecified fracture of pubis

S32.501- Unspecified fracture of right pubis

S32.502- Unspecified fracture of left pubis

S32.509- Unspecified fracture of unspecified pubis

S32.51 Fracture of superior rim of pubis

S32.511- Fracture of superior rim of right pubis

S32.512- Fracture of superior rim of left pubis

S32.519- Fracture of superior rim of unspecified pubis

S32.59 Other specified fracture of pubis

S32.591- Other specified fracture of right pubis

S32.592- Other specified fracture of left pubis

S32.599- Other specified fracture of unspecified pubis

S32.6 Fracture of ischium

EXCLUDES 1 fracture of ischium with associated disruption of pelvic ring (S32.8-)

S32.60 Unspecified fracture of ischium

S32.601- Unspecified fracture of right ischium

S32.602- Unspecified fracture of left ischium

S32.609- Unspecified fracture of unspecified ischium

S32.61 Avulsion fracture of ischium

S32.611- Displaced avulsion fracture of right ischium

S32.612- Displaced avulsion fracture of left ischium

S32.613- Displaced avulsion fracture of unspecified ischium

S32.614- Nondisplaced avulsion fracture of right ischium

S32.615- Nondisplaced avulsion fracture of left ischium

S32.616- Nondisplaced avulsion fracture of unspecified ischium

S32.69 Other specified fracture of ischium

S32.691- Other specified fracture of right ischium

S32.692- Other specified fracture of left ischium

S32.699- Other specified fracture of unspecified ischium

S32.8 Fracture of other parts of pelvis

Code also any associated:
fracture of acetabulum (S32.4-)
sacral fracture (S32.1-)

S32.81 Multiple fractures of pelvis with disruption of pelvic ring

Multiple pelvic fractures with disruption of pelvic circle

S32.810- Multiple fractures of pelvis with stable disruption of pelvic ring

S32.811- Multiple fractures of pelvis with unstable disruption of pelvic ring

S32.82X- Multiple fractures of pelvis without disruption of pelvic ring

Multiple pelvic fractures without disruption of pelvic circle

S32.89X- Fracture of other parts of pelvis

S32.9XX- Fracture of unspecified parts of lumbosacral spine and pelvis

Fracture of lumbosacral spine NOS
Fracture of pelvis NOS

S33 Dislocation and sprain of joints and ligaments of lumbar spine and pelvis

INCLUDES avulsion of joint or ligament of lumbar spine and pelvis
laceration of cartilage, joint or ligament of lumbar spine and pelvis
sprain of cartilage, joint or ligament of lumbar spine and pelvis
traumatic hemarthrosis of joint or ligament of lumbar spine and pelvis

Chapter 19 S00-T88

4th digit required 5th digit required 6th digit required 7th digit required 7th digit placeholder + Additional code Laterality

traumatic rupture of joint or ligament of lumbar spine and pelvis
traumatic subluxation of joint or ligament of lumbar spine and pelvis
traumatic tear of joint or ligament of lumbar spine and pelvis

Code also:
any associated open wound

EXCLUDES 1 nontraumatic rupture or displacement of lumbar intervertebral disc NOS (M51.-)
obstetric damage to pelvic joints and ligaments (O71.6)

EXCLUDES 2 dislocation and sprain of joints and ligaments of hip (S73.-)
strain of muscle of lower back and pelvis (S39.01-)

The appropriate 7th character is to be added to each code from category S33
A initial encounter
D subsequent encounter
S sequela

SP 7 **S33.0XX- Traumatic rupture of lumbar intervertebral disc**
EXCLUDES 1 rupture or displacement (nontraumatic) of lumbar intervertebral disc NOS (M51.- with fifth character 6)

5 **S33.1 Subluxation and dislocation of lumbar vertebra**
Code also any associated:
open wound of abdomen, lower back and pelvis (S31)
spinal cord injury (S24.0, S24.1-, S34.0-, S34.1-)
EXCLUDES 2 fracture of lumbar vertebrae (S32.0-)

6 **S33.10 Subluxation and dislocation of unspecified lumbar vertebra**

IQ 7 **S33.100- Subluxation of unspecified lumbar vertebra**

IQ 7 **S33.101- Dislocation of unspecified lumbar vertebra**

6 **S33.11 Subluxation and dislocation of L1/L2 lumbar vertebra**

SP 7 **S33.110- Subluxation of L1/L2 lumbar vertebra**

SP 7 **S33.111- Dislocation of L1/L2 lumbar vertebra**

6 **S33.12 Subluxation and dislocation of L2/L3 lumbar vertebra**

SP 7 **S33.120- Subluxation of L2/L3 lumbar vertebra**

SP 7 **S33.121- Dislocation of L2/L3 lumbar vertebra**

6 **S33.13 Subluxation and dislocation of L3/L4 lumbar vertebra**

SP 7 **S33.130- Subluxation of L3/L4 lumbar vertebra**

SP 7 **S33.131- Dislocation of L3/L4 lumbar vertebra**

6 **S33.14 Subluxation and dislocation of L4/L5 lumbar vertebra**

SP 7 **S33.140- Subluxation of L4/L5 lumbar vertebra**

SP 7 **S33.141- Dislocation of L4/L5 lumbar vertebra**

SP 7 **S33.2XX- Dislocation of sacroiliac and sacrococcygeal joint**

5 **S33.3 Dislocation of other and unspecified parts of lumbar spine and pelvis**

IQ 7 **S33.30X- Dislocation of unspecified parts of lumbar spine and pelvis**

SP 7 **S33.39X- Dislocation of other parts of lumbar spine and pelvis**

SP 7 **S33.4XX- Traumatic rupture of symphysis pubis**

SP 7 **S33.5XX- Sprain of ligaments of lumbar spine**

SP 7 **S33.6XX- Sprain of sacroiliac joint**

SP 7 **S33.8XX- Sprain of other parts of lumbar spine and pelvis**

SP 7 **S33.9XX- Sprain of unspecified parts of lumbar spine and pelvis**

4 **S34 Injury of lumbar and sacral spinal cord and nerves at abdomen, lower back and pelvis level**
Note:
Code to highest level of lumbar cord injury
Injuries to the spinal cord (S34.0 and S34.1) refer to the cord level and not bone level injury, and can affect nerve roots at and below the level given.
Code also any associated:
fracture of vertebra (S22.0-, S32.0-)
open wound of abdomen, lower back and pelvis (S31.-)
transient paralysis (R29.5)

The appropriate 7th character is to be added to each code from category S34
A initial encounter
D subsequent encounter
S sequela

CODING TIPS ✓ When coding sequelae of a cervical spinal cord injury, first list the residual condition(s), followed by the specific spinal cord injury diagnosed using the appropriate code from this category with the seventh character "S" to indicate sequelae. If there are multiple levels of injury, code only the highest injury in each section of the spine (cervical, thoracic, and lumbar).

5 **S34.0 Concussion and edema of lumbar and sacral spinal cord**

SP 7 **S34.01X- Concussion and edema of lumbar spinal cord**

SP 7 **S34.02X- Concussion and edema of sacral spinal cord**
Concussion and edema of conus medullaris

5 **S34.1 Other and unspecified injury of lumbar and sacral spinal cord**

6 **S34.10 Unspecified injury to lumbar spinal cord**

IQ 7 **S34.101- Unspecified injury to L1 level of lumbar spinal cord**
Unspecified injury to lumbar spinal cord level 1

Chapter 19

S00-T88

IQ 7 S34.102- **Unspecified injury to L2 level of lumbar spinal cord**
Unspecified injury to lumbar spinal cord level 2

IQ 7 S34.103- **Unspecified injury to L3 level of lumbar spinal cord**
Unspecified injury to lumbar spinal cord level 3

IQ 7 S34.104- **Unspecified injury to L4 level of lumbar spinal cord**
Unspecified injury to lumbar spinal cord level 4

IQ 7 S34.105- **Unspecified injury to L5 level of lumbar spinal cord**
Unspecified injury to lumbar spinal cord level 5

IQ 7 S34.109- **Unspecified injury to unspecified level of lumbar spinal cord**

6 **S34.11 Complete lesion of lumbar spinal cord**

SP 7 S34.111- **Complete lesion of L1 level of lumbar spinal cord**
Complete lesion of lumbar spinal cord level 1

SP 7 S34.112- **Complete lesion of L2 level of lumbar spinal cord**
Complete lesion of lumbar spinal cord level 2

SP 7 S34.113- **Complete lesion of L3 level of lumbar spinal cord**
Complete lesion of lumbar spinal cord level 3

SP 7 S34.114- **Complete lesion of L4 level of lumbar spinal cord**
Complete lesion of lumbar spinal cord level 4

SP 7 S34.115- **Complete lesion of L5 level of lumbar spinal cord**
Complete lesion of lumbar spinal cord level 5

IQ 7 S34.119- **Complete lesion of unspecified level of lumbar spinal cord**

6 **S34.12 Incomplete lesion of lumbar spinal cord**

SP 7 S34.121- **Incomplete lesion of L1 level of lumbar spinal cord**
Incomplete lesion of lumbar spinal cord level 1

SP 7 S34.122- **Incomplete lesion of L2 level of lumbar spinal cord**
Incomplete lesion of lumbar spinal cord level 2

SP 7 S34.123- **Incomplete lesion of L3 level of lumbar spinal cord**
Incomplete lesion of lumbar spinal cord level 3

SP 7 S34.124- **Incomplete lesion of L4 level of lumbar spinal cord**
Incomplete lesion of lumbar spinal cord level 4

SP 7 S34.125- **Incomplete lesion of L5 level of lumbar spinal cord**
Incomplete lesion of lumbar spinal cord level 5

IQ 7 S34.129- **Incomplete lesion of unspecified level of lumbar spinal cord**

6 **S34.13 Other and unspecified injury to sacral spinal cord**
Other injury to conus medullaris

SP 7 S34.131- **Complete lesion of sacral spinal cord**
Complete lesion of conus medullaris

SP 7 S34.132- **Incomplete lesion of sacral spinal cord**
Incomplete lesion of conus medullaris

IQ 7 S34.139- **Unspecified injury to sacral spinal cord**
Unspecified injury of conus medullaris

5 **S34.2 Injury of nerve root of lumbar and sacral spine**

SP 7 S34.21X- **Injury of nerve root of lumbar spine**

SP 7 S34.22X- **Injury of nerve root of sacral spine**

SP 7 S34.3XX- **Injury of cauda equina**

SP 7 S34.4XX- **Injury of lumbosacral plexus**

SP 7 S34.5XX- **Injury of lumbar, sacral and pelvic sympathetic nerves**
Injury of celiac ganglion or plexus
Injury of hypogastric plexus
Injury of mesenteric plexus (inferior) (superior)
Injury of splanchnic nerve

SP 7 S34.6XX- **Injury of peripheral nerve(s) at abdomen, lower back and pelvis level**

SP 7 S34.8XX- **Injury of other nerves at abdomen, lower back and pelvis level**

IQ 7 S34.9XX- **Injury of unspecified nerves at abdomen, lower back and pelvis level**

4 **S35 Injury of blood vessels at abdomen, lower back and pelvis level**
Code also:
any associated open wound (S31.-)

The appropriate 7th character is to be added to each code from category S35
A initial encounter
D subsequent encounter
S sequela

5 **S35.0 Injury of abdominal aorta**
EXCLUDES 1 injury of aorta NOS (S25.0)

IQ 7 S35.00X- **Unspecified injury of abdominal aorta**

SP 7 S35.01X- **Minor laceration of abdominal aorta**
Incomplete transection of abdominal aorta
Laceration of abdominal aorta NOS
Superficial laceration of abdominal aorta

SP 7 S35.02X- **Major laceration of abdominal aorta**
Complete transection of abdominal aorta
Traumatic rupture of abdominal aorta

SP 7 S35.09X- **Other injury of abdominal aorta**

5 **S35.1 Injury of inferior vena cava**
Injury of hepatic vein

Chapter 19
S00-T88

4 4th digit required 5 5th digit required 6 6th digit required 7 7th digit required 7 7th digit placeholder + Additional code Laterality

EXCLUDES 1 injury of vena cava NOS (S25.2)

IQ 7 **S35.10X- Unspecified injury of inferior vena cava**

SP 7 **S35.11X- Minor laceration of inferior vena cava**
Incomplete transection of inferior vena cava
Laceration of inferior vena cava NOS
Superficial laceration of inferior vena cava

SP 7 **S35.12X- Major laceration of inferior vena cava**
Complete transection of inferior vena cava
Traumatic rupture of inferior vena cava

SP 7 **S35.19X- Other injury of inferior vena cava**

5 **S35.2 Injury of celiac or mesenteric artery and branches**

6 **S35.21 Injury of celiac artery**

SP 7 **S35.211- Minor laceration of celiac artery**
Incomplete transection of celiac artery
Laceration of celiac artery NOS
Superficial laceration of celiac artery

SP 7 **S35.212- Major laceration of celiac artery**
Complete transection of celiac artery
Traumatic rupture of celiac artery

SP 7 **S35.218- Other injury of celiac artery**

IQ 7 **S35.219- Unspecified injury of celiac artery**

6 **S35.22 Injury of superior mesenteric artery**

SP 7 **S35.221- Minor laceration of superior mesenteric artery**
Incomplete transection of superior mesenteric artery
Laceration of superior mesenteric artery NOS
Superficial laceration of superior mesenteric artery

SP 7 **S35.222- Major laceration of superior mesenteric artery**
Complete transection of superior mesenteric artery
Traumatic rupture of superior mesenteric artery

SP 7 **S35.228- Other injury of superior mesenteric artery**

IQ 7 **S35.229- Unspecified injury of superior mesenteric artery**

6 **S35.23 Injury of inferior mesenteric artery**

SP 7 **S35.231- Minor laceration of inferior mesenteric artery**
Incomplete transection of inferior mesenteric artery
Laceration of inferior mesenteric artery NOS
Superficial laceration of inferior mesenteric artery

SP 7 **S35.232- Major laceration of inferior mesenteric artery**
Complete transection of inferior mesenteric artery
Traumatic rupture of inferior mesenteric artery

SP 7 **S35.238- Other injury of inferior mesenteric artery**

IQ 7 **S35.239- Unspecified injury of inferior mesenteric artery**

6 **S35.29 Injury of branches of celiac and mesenteric artery**
Injury of gastric artery
Injury of gastroduodenal artery
Injury of hepatic artery
Injury of splenic artery

SP 7 **S35.291- Minor laceration of branches of celiac and mesenteric artery**
Incomplete transection of branches of celiac and mesenteric artery
Laceration of branches of celiac and mesenteric artery NOS
Superficial laceration of branches of celiac and mesenteric artery

SP 7 **S35.292- Major laceration of branches of celiac and mesenteric artery**
Complete transection of branches of celiac and mesenteric artery
Traumatic rupture of branches of celiac and mesenteric artery

SP 7 **S35.298- Other injury of branches of celiac and mesenteric artery**

IQ 7 **S35.299- Unspecified injury of branches of celiac and mesenteric artery**

5 **S35.3 Injury of portal or splenic vein and branches**

6 **S35.31 Injury of portal vein**

SP 7 **S35.311- Laceration of portal vein**

SP 7 **S35.318- Other specified injury of portal vein**

IQ 7 **S35.319- Unspecified injury of portal vein**

6 **S35.32 Injury of splenic vein**

SP 7 **S35.321- Laceration of splenic vein**

SP 7 **S35.328- Other specified injury of splenic vein**

IQ 7 **S35.329- Unspecified injury of splenic vein**

6 **S35.33 Injury of superior mesenteric vein**

SP 7 **S35.331- Laceration of superior mesenteric vein**

SP 7 **S35.338- Other specified injury of superior mesenteric vein**

IQ 7 **S35.339- Unspecified injury of superior mesenteric vein**

6 **S35.34 Injury of inferior mesenteric vein**

SP 7 **S35.341- Laceration of inferior mesenteric vein**

SP 7 **S35.348- Other specified injury of inferior mesenteric vein**

IQ 7 **S35.349- Unspecified injury of inferior mesenteric vein**

5 **S35.4 Injury of renal blood vessels**

6 **S35.40 Unspecified injury of renal blood vessel**

IQ 7 **S35.401- Unspecified injury of right renal artery**

IQ 7 **S35.402- Unspecified injury of left renal artery**

Chapter 19 S00-T88

🚫 !Q 7 **S35.403-** **Unspecified injury of unspecified renal artery**

🚫 !Q 7 **S35.404-** **Unspecified injury of right renal vein**

🚫 !Q 7 **S35.405-** **Unspecified injury of left renal vein**

🚫 !Q 7 **S35.406-** **Unspecified injury of unspecified renal vein**

6 **S35.41**   Laceration of renal blood vessel

🚫 SP 7 **S35.411-**   Laceration of right renal artery

🚫 SP 7 **S35.412-**   Laceration of left renal artery

🚫 !Q 7 **S35.413-**   **Laceration of unspecified renal artery**

🚫 SP 7 **S35.414-**   Laceration of right renal vein

🚫 SP 7 **S35.415-**   Laceration of left renal vein

🚫 !Q 7 **S35.416-**   **Laceration of unspecified renal vein**

6 **S35.49**   Other specified injury of renal blood vessel

🚫 SP 7 **S35.491-**   **Other specified injury of right renal artery**

🚫 SP 7 **S35.492-**   **Other specified injury of left renal artery**

🚫 !Q 7 **S35.493-**   **Other specified injury of unspecified renal artery**

🚫 SP 7 **S35.494-**   **Other specified injury of right renal vein**

🚫 SP 7 **S35.495-**   **Other specified injury of left renal vein**

🚫 !Q 7 **S35.496-**   **Other specified injury of unspecified renal vein**

5 **S35.5** Injury of iliac blood vessels

!Q ✓ **S35.50X-**   **Injury of unspecified iliac blood vessel(s)**

6 **S35.51**   Injury of iliac artery or vein
Injury of hypogastric artery or vein

🚫 SP 7 **S35.511-**   **Injury of right iliac artery**

🚫 SP 7 **S35.512-**   **Injury of left iliac artery**

🚫 !Q 7 **S35.513-**   **Injury of unspecified iliac artery**

🚫 SP 7 **S35.514-**   **Injury of right iliac vein**

🚫 SP 7 **S35.515-**   **Injury of left iliac vein**

🚫 !Q 7 **S35.516-**   **Injury of unspecified iliac vein**

6 **S35.53**   Injury of uterine artery or vein

🚫 SP 7 **S35.531-**   **Injury of right uterine artery**

🚫 SP 7 **S35.532-**   **Injury of left uterine artery**

🚫 !Q 7 **S35.533-**   **Injury of unspecified uterine artery**

🚫 SP 7 **S35.534-**   **Injury of right uterine vein**

🚫 SP 7 **S35.535-**   **Injury of left uterine vein**

🚫 !Q 7 **S35.536-**   **Injury of unspecified uterine vein**

SP ✓ **S35.59X-**   Injury of other iliac blood vessels

5 **S35.8** Injury of other blood vessels at abdomen, lower back and pelvis level
Injury of ovarian artery or vein

6 **S35.8X** Injury of other blood vessels at abdomen, lower back and pelvis level

SP 7 **S35.8X1-**   Laceration of other blood vessels at abdomen, lower back and pelvis level

SP 7 **S35.8X8-**   Other specified injury of other blood vessels at abdomen, lower back and pelvis level

!Q 7 **S35.8X9-**   **Unspecified injury of other blood vessels at abdomen, lower back and pelvis level**

5 **S35.9**   Injury of unspecified blood vessel at abdomen, lower back and pelvis level

!Q ✓ **S35.90X-**   **Unspecified injury of unspecified blood vessel at abdomen, lower back and pelvis level**

!Q ✓ **S35.91X-**   **Laceration of unspecified blood vessel at abdomen, lower back and pelvis level**

!Q ✓ **S35.99X-**   **Other specified injury of unspecified blood vessel at abdomen, lower back and pelvis level**

4 **S36**   **Injury of intra-abdominal organs**
Code also:
   any associated open wound (S31.-)

The appropriate 7th character is to be added to each code from category S36
A   initial encounter
D   subsequent encounter
S   sequela

CODING TIPS ✓   Codes from category S36 do not include injury to intra-abdominal organs resulting from intraoperative complications. When intraoperative complications occur, the appropriate complication code from the disease-specific chapter should be assigned (intraoperative and post-procedural complications), as well as any T codes indicating further information on the complication.

5 **S36.0** Injury of spleen

!Q ✓ **S36.00X-**   **Unspecified injury of spleen**

6 **S36.02**   Contusion of spleen

SP 7 **S36.020-**   **Minor contusion of spleen**
Contusion of spleen less than 2 cm

SP 7 **S36.021-**   **Major contusion of spleen**
Contusion of spleen greater than 2 cm

!Q 7 **S36.029-**   **Unspecified contusion of spleen**

6 **S36.03**   Laceration of spleen

SP 7 **S36.030-**   **Superficial (capsular) laceration of spleen**
Laceration of spleen less than 1 cm
Minor laceration of spleen

SP 7 **S36.031-**   **Moderate laceration of spleen**
Laceration of spleen 1 to 3 cm

SP 7 **S36.032-**   **Major laceration of spleen**
Avulsion of spleen
Laceration of spleen greater than 3 cm
Massive laceration of spleen
Multiple moderate lacerations of spleen
Stellate laceration of spleen

!Q 7 **S36.039-**   **Unspecified laceration of spleen**

SP ✓ **S36.09X-**   Other injury of spleen

5 **S36.1**   Injury of liver and gallbladder and bile duct

4 4th digit required   5 5th digit required   6 6th digit required   7 7th digit required   ✓ 7th digit placeholder   ➕ Additional code   🚫 Laterality

1534   *DecisionHealth's* FY 2022 Complete Home Health ICD-10-CM Diagnosis Coding Manual

Chapter 19

S00-T88

6 S36.11 Injury of liver

SP 7 S36.112- Contusion of liver

SP 7 S36.113- Laceration of liver, unspecified degree

SP 7 S36.114- Minor laceration of liver
Laceration involving capsule only, or, without significant involvement of hepatic parenchyma [i.e., less than 1 cm deep]

SP 7 S36.115- Moderate laceration of liver
Laceration involving parenchyma but without major disruption of parenchyma [i.e., less than 10 cm long and less than 3 cm deep]

SP 7 S36.116- Major laceration of liver
Laceration with significant disruption of hepatic parenchyma [i.e., greater than 10 cm long and 3 cm deep]
Multiple moderate lacerations, with or without hematoma
Stellate laceration of liver

SP 7 S36.118- Other injury of liver

IQ 7 S36.119- Unspecified injury of liver

6 S36.12 Injury of gallbladder

SP 7 S36.122- Contusion of gallbladder

SP 7 S36.123- Laceration of gallbladder

SP 7 S36.128- Other injury of gallbladder

IQ 7 S36.129- Unspecified injury of gallbladder

SP 7 S36.13X- Injury of bile duct

5 S36.2 Injury of pancreas

6 S36.20 Unspecified injury of pancreas

IQ 7 S36.200- Unspecified injury of head of pancreas

IQ 7 S36.201- Unspecified injury of body of pancreas

IQ 7 S36.202- Unspecified injury of tail of pancreas

IQ 7 S36.209- Unspecified injury of unspecified part of pancreas

6 S36.22 Contusion of pancreas

SP 7 S36.220- Contusion of head of pancreas

SP 7 S36.221- Contusion of body of pancreas

SP 7 S36.222- Contusion of tail of pancreas

IQ 7 S36.229- Contusion of unspecified part of pancreas

6 S36.23 Laceration of pancreas, unspecified degree

SP 7 S36.230- Laceration of head of pancreas, unspecified degree

SP 7 S36.231- Laceration of body of pancreas, unspecified degree

SP 7 S36.232- Laceration of tail of pancreas, unspecified degree

IQ 7 S36.239- Laceration of unspecified part of pancreas, unspecified degree

6 S36.24 Minor laceration of pancreas

SP 7 S36.240- Minor laceration of head of pancreas

SP 7 S36.241- Minor laceration of body of pancreas

SP 7 S36.242- Minor laceration of tail of pancreas

IQ 7 S36.249- Minor laceration of unspecified part of pancreas

6 S36.25 Moderate laceration of pancreas

SP 7 S36.250- Moderate laceration of head of pancreas

SP 7 S36.251- Moderate laceration of body of pancreas

SP 7 S36.252- Moderate laceration of tail of pancreas

IQ 7 S36.259- Moderate laceration of unspecified part of pancreas

6 S36.26 Major laceration of pancreas

SP 7 S36.260- Major laceration of head of pancreas

SP 7 S36.261- Major laceration of body of pancreas

SP 7 S36.262- Major laceration of tail of pancreas

IQ 7 S36.269- Major laceration of unspecified part of pancreas

6 S36.29 Other injury of pancreas

SP 7 S36.290- Other injury of head of pancreas

SP 7 S36.291- Other injury of body of pancreas

SP 7 S36.292- Other injury of tail of pancreas

SP IQ 7 S36.299- Other injury of unspecified part of pancreas

5 S36.3 Injury of stomach

IQ 7 S36.30X- Unspecified injury of stomach

SP 7 S36.32X- Contusion of stomach

SP 7 S36.33X- Laceration of stomach

SP 7 S36.39X- Other injury of stomach

5 S36.4 Injury of small intestine

6 S36.40 Unspecified injury of small intestine

IQ 7 S36.400- Unspecified injury of duodenum

IQ 7 S36.408- Unspecified injury of other part of small intestine

IQ 7 S36.409- Unspecified injury of unspecified part of small intestine

6 S36.41 Primary blast injury of small intestine
Blast injury of small intestine NOS

SP 7 S36.410- Primary blast injury of duodenum

SP 7 S36.418- Primary blast injury of other part of small intestine

IQ 7 S36.419- Primary blast injury of unspecified part of small intestine

6 S36.42 Contusion of small intestine

SP 7 S36.420- Contusion of duodenum

SP 7 S36.428- Contusion of other part of small intestine

IQ 7 S36.429- Contusion of unspecified part of small intestine

6 S36.43 Laceration of small intestine

SP 7 S36.430- Laceration of duodenum

SP 7 S36.438- Laceration of other part of small intestine

Chapter 19

S00-T88

!Q 7 S36.439- Laceration of unspecified part of small intestine

6 S36.49 Other injury of small intestine

SP 7 S36.490- Other injury of duodenum

SP 7 S36.498- Other injury of other part of small intestine

!Q 7 S36.499- Other injury of unspecified part of small intestine

5 S36.5 Injury of colon

EXCLUDES 2 injury of rectum (S36.6-)

6 S36.50 Unspecified injury of colon

!Q 7 S36.500- Unspecified injury of ascending [right] colon

!Q 7 S36.501- Unspecified injury of transverse colon

!Q 7 S36.502- Unspecified injury of descending [left] colon

!Q 7 S36.503- Unspecified injury of sigmoid colon

!Q 7 S36.508- Unspecified injury of other part of colon

!Q 7 S36.509- Unspecified injury of unspecified part of colon

6 S36.51 Primary blast injury of colon

Blast injury of colon NOS

SP 7 S36.510- Primary blast injury of ascending [right] colon

SP 7 S36.511- Primary blast injury of transverse colon

SP 7 S36.512- Primary blast injury of descending [left] colon

SP 7 S36.513- Primary blast injury of sigmoid colon

SP 7 S36.518- Primary blast injury of other part of colon

!Q 7 S36.519- Primary blast injury of unspecified part of colon

6 S36.52 Contusion of colon

SP 7 S36.520- Contusion of ascending [right] colon

SP 7 S36.521- Contusion of transverse colon

SP 7 S36.522- Contusion of descending [left] colon

SP 7 S36.523- Contusion of sigmoid colon

SP 7 S36.528- Contusion of other part of colon

!Q 7 S36.529- Contusion of unspecified part of colon

6 S36.53 Laceration of colon

SP 7 S36.530- Laceration of ascending [right] colon

SP 7 S36.531- Laceration of transverse colon

SP 7 S36.532- Laceration of descending [left] colon

SP 7 S36.533- Laceration of sigmoid colon

SP 7 S36.538- Laceration of other part of colon

!Q 7 S36.539- Laceration of unspecified part of colon

6 S36.59 Other injury of colon

Secondary blast injury of colon

SP 7 S36.590- Other injury of ascending [right] colon

SP 7 S36.591- Other injury of transverse colon

SP 7 S36.592- Other injury of descending [left] colon

SP 7 S36.593- Other injury of sigmoid colon

SP 7 S36.598- Other injury of other part of colon

!Q 7 S36.599- Other injury of unspecified part of colon

5 S36.6 Injury of rectum

!Q X S36.60X- Unspecified injury of rectum

SP X S36.61X- Primary blast injury of rectum

Blast injury of rectum NOS

SP X S36.62X- Contusion of rectum

SP X S36.63X- Laceration of rectum

SP X S36.69X- Other injury of rectum

Secondary blast injury of rectum

5 S36.8 Injury of other intra-abdominal organs

SP X S36.81X- Injury of peritoneum

6 S36.89 Injury of other intra-abdominal organs

Injury of retroperitoneum

SP 7 S36.892- Contusion of other intra-abdominal organs

SP 7 S36.893- Laceration of other intra-abdominal organs

SP 7 S36.898- Other injury of other intra-abdominal organs

!Q 7 S36.899- Unspecified injury of other intra-abdominal organs

5 S36.9 Injury of unspecified intra-abdominal organ

!Q X S36.90X- Unspecified injury of unspecified intra-abdominal organ

!Q X S36.92X- Contusion of unspecified intra-abdominal organ

!Q X S36.93X- Laceration of unspecified intra-abdominal organ

!Q X S36.99X- Other injury of unspecified intra-abdominal organ

4 S37 Injury of urinary and pelvic organs

Code also:

any associated open wound (S31.-)

EXCLUDES 1 obstetric trauma to pelvic organs (O71.-)

EXCLUDES 2 injury of peritoneum (S36.81)
injury of retroperitoneum (S36.89-)

The appropriate 7th character is to be added to each code from category S37
A initial encounter
D subsequent encounter
S sequela

CODING TIPS ✓ Codes from category S37 do not include injury to urinary and pelvic organs resulting from intraoperative complications. When intraoperative complications occur, the appropriate complication code from the disease-specific chapter should be assigned (intraoperative and post-procedural complications), as well as any T codes indicating further information on the complication.

5 S37.0 Injury of kidney

EXCLUDES 2 acute kidney injury (nontraumatic) (N17.9)

Chapter 19 S00-T88

6 S37.00 Unspecified injury of kidney
H IQ 7 S37.001- Unspecified injury of right kidney
H IQ 7 S37.002- Unspecified injury of left kidney
H IQ 7 S37.009- Unspecified injury of unspecified kidney
6 S37.01 Minor contusion of kidney
Contusion of kidney less than 2 cm
Contusion of kidney NOS
H SP 7 S37.011- Minor contusion of right kidney
H SP 7 S37.012- Minor contusion of left kidney
H SP 7 S37.019- Minor contusion of unspecified kidney
6 S37.02 Major contusion of kidney
Contusion of kidney greater than 2 cm
H SP 7 S37.021- Major contusion of right kidney
H SP 7 S37.022- Major contusion of left kidney
H IQ 7 S37.029- Major contusion of unspecified kidney
6 S37.03 Laceration of kidney, unspecified degree
H SP 7 S37.031- Laceration of right kidney, unspecified degree
H SP 7 S37.032- Laceration of left kidney, unspecified degree
H IQ 7 S37.039- Laceration of unspecified kidney, unspecified degree
6 S37.04 Minor laceration of kidney
Laceration of kidney less than 1 cm
H SP 7 S37.041- Minor laceration of right kidney
H SP 7 S37.042- Minor laceration of left kidney
H IQ 7 S37.049- Minor laceration of unspecified kidney
6 S37.05 Moderate laceration of kidney
Laceration of kidney 1 to 3 cm
H SP 7 S37.051- Moderate laceration of right kidney
H SP 7 S37.052- Moderate laceration of left kidney
H IQ 7 S37.059- Moderate laceration of unspecified kidney
6 S37.06 Major laceration of kidney
Avulsion of kidney
Laceration of kidney greater than 3 cm
Massive laceration of kidney
Multiple moderate lacerations of kidney
Stellate laceration of kidney
H SP 7 S37.061- Major laceration of right kidney
H SP 7 S37.062- Major laceration of left kidney
H SP 7 S37.069- Major laceration of unspecified kidney
6 S37.09 Other injury of kidney
H SP 7 S37.091- Other injury of right kidney
H SP 7 S37.092- Other injury of left kidney
H IQ 7 S37.099- Other injury of unspecified kidney
5 S37.1 Injury of ureter
IQ 7 S37.10X- Unspecified injury of ureter
SP 7 S37.12X- Contusion of ureter
SP 7 S37.13X- Laceration of ureter
SP 7 S37.19X- Other injury of ureter

5 S37.2 Injury of bladder
IQ 7 S37.20X- Unspecified injury of bladder
SP 7 S37.22X- Contusion of bladder
SP 7 S37.23X- Laceration of bladder
SP 7 S37.29X- Other injury of bladder
5 S37.3 Injury of urethra
IQ 7 S37.30X- Unspecified injury of urethra
SP 7 S37.32X- Contusion of urethra
SP 7 S37.33X- Laceration of urethra
SP 7 S37.39X- Other injury of urethra
5 S37.4 Injury of ovary
6 S37.40 Unspecified injury of ovary
IQ 7 S37.401- Unspecified injury of ovary, unilateral
IQ 7 S37.402- Unspecified injury of ovary, bilateral
IQ 7 S37.409- Unspecified injury of ovary, unspecified
6 S37.42 Contusion of ovary
SP 7 S37.421- Contusion of ovary, unilateral
SP 7 S37.422- Contusion of ovary, bilateral
IQ 7 S37.429- Contusion of ovary, unspecified
6 S37.43 Laceration of ovary
SP 7 S37.431- Laceration of ovary, unilateral
SP 7 S37.432- Laceration of ovary, bilateral
IQ 7 S37.439- Laceration of ovary, unspecified
6 S37.49 Other injury of ovary
SP 7 S37.491- Other injury of ovary, unilateral
SP 7 S37.492- Other injury of ovary, bilateral
IQ 7 S37.499- Other injury of ovary, unspecified
5 S37.5 Injury of fallopian tube
6 S37.50 Unspecified injury of fallopian tube
IQ 7 S37.501- Unspecified injury of fallopian tube, unilateral
IQ 7 S37.502- Unspecified injury of fallopian tube, bilateral
IQ 7 S37.509- Unspecified injury of fallopian tube, unspecified
6 S37.51 Primary blast injury of fallopian tube
Blast injury of fallopian tube NOS
SP 7 S37.511- Primary blast injury of fallopian tube, unilateral
SP 7 S37.512- Primary blast injury of fallopian tube, bilateral
IQ 7 S37.519- Primary blast injury of fallopian tube, unspecified
6 S37.52 Contusion of fallopian tube
SP 7 S37.521- Contusion of fallopian tube, unilateral
SP 7 S37.522- Contusion of fallopian tube, bilateral
IQ 7 S37.529- Contusion of fallopian tube, unspecified
6 S37.53 Laceration of fallopian tube
SP 7 S37.531- Laceration of fallopian tube, unilateral
SP 7 S37.532- Laceration of fallopian tube, bilateral

IQ 7 S37.539- **Laceration of fallopian tube, unspecified**

6 S37.59 **Other injury of fallopian tube**
Secondary blast injury of fallopian tube

SP 7 S37.591- **Other injury of fallopian tube, unilateral**

SP 7 S37.592- **Other injury of fallopian tube, bilateral**

IQ 7 S37.599- **Other injury of fallopian tube, unspecified**

5 S37.6 **Injury of uterus**
EXCLUDES 1 injury to gravid uterus (O9A.2-)
injury to uterus during delivery (O71.-)

IQ 7 S37.60X- **Unspecified injury of uterus**

SP 7 S37.62X- **Contusion of uterus**

SP 7 S37.63X- **Laceration of uterus**

SP 7 S37.69X- **Other injury of uterus**

5 S37.8 **Injury of other urinary and pelvic organs**

6 S37.81 **Injury of adrenal gland**

SP 7 S37.812- **Contusion of adrenal gland**

SP 7 S37.813- **Laceration of adrenal gland**

SP 7 S37.818- **Other injury of adrenal gland**

IQ 7 S37.819- **Unspecified injury of adrenal gland**

6 S37.82 **Injury of prostate**

SP 7 S37.822- **Contusion of prostate**

SP 7 S37.823- **Laceration of prostate**

SP 7 S37.828- **Other injury of prostate**

IQ 7 S37.829- **Unspecified injury of prostate**

6 S37.89 **Injury of other urinary and pelvic organ**

SP 7 S37.892- **Contusion of other urinary and pelvic organ**

SP 7 S37.893- **Laceration of other urinary and pelvic organ**

SP 7 S37.898- **Other injury of other urinary and pelvic organ**

IQ 7 S37.899- **Unspecified injury of other urinary and pelvic organ**

5 S37.9 **Injury of unspecified urinary and pelvic organ**

IQ 7 S37.90X- **Unspecified injury of unspecified urinary and pelvic organ**

IQ 7 S37.92X- **Contusion of unspecified urinary and pelvic organ**

IQ 7 S37.93X- **Laceration of unspecified urinary and pelvic organ**

IQ 7 S37.99X- **Other injury of unspecified urinary and pelvic organ**

4 S38 **Crushing injury and traumatic amputation of abdomen, lower back, pelvis and external genitals**
An amputation not identified as partial or complete should be coded to complete

The appropriate 7th character is to be added to each code from category S38
A initial encounter
D subsequent encounter
S sequela

CODING TIPS ✓ Use these codes only when the amputation was due to trauma. There is no need for adding Z89 with traumatic amputations. See Z47.81 for care of amputations not due to trauma.

+ 5 S38.0 **Crushing injury of external genital organs**
Use additional code for any associated injuries

+ 6 S38.00 **Crushing injury of unspecified external genital organs**

IQ + 7 S38.001- **Crushing injury of unspecified external genital organs, male**

IQ + 7 S38.002- **Crushing injury of unspecified external genital organs, female**

SP + 7 S38.01X- **Crushing injury of penis**

SP + 7 S38.02X- **Crushing injury of scrotum and testis**

SP + 7 S38.03X- **Crushing injury of vulva**

SP + 7 S38.1XX- **Crushing injury of abdomen, lower back, and pelvis**
Use additional code for all associated injuries, such as:
fracture of thoracic or lumbar spine and pelvis (S22.0-, S32.-)
injury to intra-abdominal organs (S36.-)
injury to urinary and pelvic organs (S37.-)
open wound of abdominal wall (S31.-)
spinal cord injury (S34.0, S34.1-)
EXCLUDES 2 crushing injury of external genital organs (S38.0-)

5 S38.2 **Traumatic amputation of external genital organs**

6 S38.21 **Traumatic amputation of female external genital organs**
Traumatic amputation of clitoris
Traumatic amputation of labium (majus) (minus)
Traumatic amputation of vulva

SP 7 S38.211- **Complete traumatic amputation of female external genital organs**

SP 7 S38.212- **Partial traumatic amputation of female external genital organs**

6 S38.22 **Traumatic amputation of penis**

SP 7 S38.221- **Complete traumatic amputation of penis**

SP 7 S38.222- **Partial traumatic amputation of penis**

6 S38.23 **Traumatic amputation of scrotum and testis**

SP 7 S38.231- **Complete traumatic amputation of scrotum and testis**

SP 7 S38.232- **Partial traumatic amputation of scrotum and testis**

SP 7 S38.3XX- **Transection (partial) of abdomen**

4 S39 **Other and unspecified injuries of abdomen, lower back, pelvis and external genitals**
Code also:
any associated open wound (S31.-)
EXCLUDES 2 sprain of joints and ligaments of lumbar spine and pelvis (S33.-)

Chapter 19

S00-T88

The appropriate 7th character is to be added to each code from category S39
A initial encounter
D subsequent encounter
S sequela

5 **S39.0 Injury of muscle, fascia and tendon of abdomen, lower back and pelvis**

6 **S39.00 Unspecified injury of muscle, fascia and tendon of abdomen, lower back and pelvis**

IQ 7 **S39.001- Unspecified injury of muscle, fascia and tendon of abdomen**

IQ 7 **S39.002- Unspecified injury of muscle, fascia and tendon of lower back**

IQ 7 **S39.003- Unspecified injury of muscle, fascia and tendon of pelvis**

6 **S39.01 Strain of muscle, fascia and tendon of abdomen, lower back and pelvis**

SP 7 **S39.011- Strain of muscle, fascia and tendon of abdomen**

SP 7 **S39.012- Strain of muscle, fascia and tendon of lower back**

SP 7 **S39.013- Strain of muscle, fascia and tendon of pelvis**

6 **S39.02 Laceration of muscle, fascia and tendon of abdomen, lower back and pelvis**

SP 7 **S39.021- Laceration of muscle, fascia and tendon of abdomen**

SP 7 **S39.022- Laceration of muscle, fascia and tendon of lower back**

SP 7 **S39.023- Laceration of muscle, fascia and tendon of pelvis**

6 **S39.09 Other injury of muscle, fascia and tendon of abdomen, lower back and pelvis**

SP 7 **S39.091- Other injury of muscle, fascia and tendon of abdomen**

SP 7 **S39.092- Other injury of muscle, fascia and tendon of lower back**

SP 7 **S39.093- Other injury of muscle, fascia and tendon of pelvis**

5 **S39.8 Other specified injuries of abdomen, lower back, pelvis and external genitals**

SP 7 **S39.81X- Other specified injuries of abdomen**

SP 7 **S39.82X- Other specified injuries of lower back**

SP 7 **S39.83X- Other specified injuries of pelvis**

6 **S39.84 Other specified injuries of external genitals**

SP 7 **S39.840- Fracture of corpus cavernosum penis**

SP 7 **S39.848- Other specified injuries of external genitals**

5 **S39.9 Unspecified injury of abdomen, lower back, pelvis and external genitals**

IQ 7 **S39.91X- Unspecified injury of abdomen**

IQ 7 **S39.92X- Unspecified injury of lower back**

IQ 7 **S39.93X- Unspecified injury of pelvis**

IQ 7 **S39.94X- Unspecified injury of external genitals**

Injuries to the shoulder and upper arm (S40-S49)

INCLUDES injuries of axilla
injuries of scapular region

EXCLUDES 2 burns and corrosions (T20-T32)
frostbite (T33-T34)
injuries of elbow (S50-S59)
insect bite or sting, venomous (T63.4)

GUIDELINES **Section I.C.19.c.2)**
Multiple fractures are sequenced in accordance with the severity of the fracture.

GUIDELINES **Section I.C.19.b.1)-2)**
When coding injuries, assign separate codes for each injury unless a combination code is provided, in which case the combination code is assigned ... Traumatic injury codes (S00-T14.9) are not to be used for normal, healing surgical wounds or to identify complications of surgical wounds. The code for the most serious injury, as determined by the provider and the focus of treatment, is sequenced first.

1) Superficial injuries such as abrasions or contusions are not coded when associated with more severe injuries of the same site.

2) When a primary injury results in minor damage to peripheral nerves or blood vessels, the primary injury is sequenced first with additional code(s) for injuries to nerves and spinal cord (such as category S04), and/or injury to blood vessels (such as category S15). When the primary injury is to the blood vessels or nerves, that injury should be sequenced first.

GUIDELINES **Section I.C.19.c**
Coding of Traumatic Fractures: The principles of multiple coding of injuries should be followed in coding fractures. Fractures of specified sites are coded individually by site in accordance with both the provisions within categories S02, S12, S22, S32, S42, S49, S52, S59, S62, S72, S79, S82, S89, S92 and the level of detail furnished by medical record content. A fracture not indicated as open or closed should be coded to closed. A fracture not indicated whether displaced or not displaced should be coded to displaced.

CODING TIPS ✓ 7th character A is acceptable in home health and hospice when active treatment is provided, such as antibiotics for an infected wound or a wound vac for a dehisced wound. D is used when the complication or injury is now healing. Think of D as aftercare. S is used for sequela of the injury or complication. Sequela is a residual deficit or condition produced as a result of the injury or complication after the original injury or complication has healed.

4 **S40 Superficial injury of shoulder and upper arm**

The appropriate 7th character is to be added to each code from category S40
A initial encounter
D subsequent encounter
S sequela

5 **S40.0 Contusion of shoulder and upper arm**

6 **S40.01 Contusion of shoulder**

⊟ IQ 7 **S40.011- Contusion of right shoulder**

⊟ IQ 7 **S40.012- Contusion of left shoulder**

⊟ IQ 7 **S40.019- Contusion of unspecified shoulder**

6 S40.02 Contusion of upper arm
- S40.021- Contusion of right upper arm
- S40.022- Contusion of left upper arm
- S40.029- Contusion of unspecified upper arm

5 S40.2 Other superficial injuries of shoulder

6 S40.21 Abrasion of shoulder
- S40.211- Abrasion of right shoulder
- S40.212- Abrasion of left shoulder
- S40.219- Abrasion of unspecified shoulder

6 S40.22 Blister (nonthermal) of shoulder
- S40.221- Blister (nonthermal) of right shoulder
- S40.222- Blister (nonthermal) of left shoulder
- S40.229- Blister (nonthermal) of unspecified shoulder

6 S40.24 External constriction of shoulder
- S40.241- External constriction of right shoulder
- S40.242- External constriction of left shoulder
- S40.249- External constriction of unspecified shoulder

6 S40.25 Superficial foreign body of shoulder
Splinter in the shoulder
- S40.251- Superficial foreign body of right shoulder
- S40.252- Superficial foreign body of left shoulder
- S40.259- Superficial foreign body of unspecified shoulder

6 S40.26 Insect bite (nonvenomous) of shoulder
- S40.261- Insect bite (nonvenomous) of right shoulder
- S40.262- Insect bite (nonvenomous) of left shoulder
- S40.269- Insect bite (nonvenomous) of unspecified shoulder

6 S40.27 Other superficial bite of shoulder
EXCLUDES 1 open bite of shoulder (S41.05)
- S40.271- Other superficial bite of right shoulder
- S40.272- Other superficial bite of left shoulder
- S40.279- Other superficial bite of unspecified shoulder

5 S40.8 Other superficial injuries of upper arm

6 S40.81 Abrasion of upper arm
- S40.811- Abrasion of right upper arm
- S40.812- Abrasion of left upper arm
- S40.819- Abrasion of unspecified upper arm

6 S40.82 Blister (nonthermal) of upper arm
- S40.821- Blister (nonthermal) of right upper arm
- S40.822- Blister (nonthermal) of left upper arm
- S40.829- Blister (nonthermal) of unspecified upper arm

6 S40.84 External constriction of upper arm
- S40.841- External constriction of right upper arm
- S40.842- External constriction of left upper arm
- S40.849- External constriction of unspecified upper arm

6 S40.85 Superficial foreign body of upper arm
Splinter in the upper arm
- S40.851- Superficial foreign body of right upper arm
- S40.852- Superficial foreign body of left upper arm
- S40.859- Superficial foreign body of unspecified upper arm

6 S40.86 Insect bite (nonvenomous) of upper arm
- S40.861- Insect bite (nonvenomous) of right upper arm
- S40.862- Insect bite (nonvenomous) of left upper arm
- S40.869- Insect bite (nonvenomous) of unspecified upper arm

6 S40.87 Other superficial bite of upper arm
EXCLUDES 1 open bite of upper arm (S41.14)
EXCLUDES 2 other superficial bite of shoulder (S40.27-)
- S40.871- Other superficial bite of right upper arm
- S40.872- Other superficial bite of left upper arm
- S40.879- Other superficial bite of unspecified upper arm

5 S40.9 Unspecified superficial injury of shoulder and upper arm

6 S40.91 Unspecified superficial injury of shoulder
- S40.911- Unspecified superficial injury of right shoulder
- S40.912- Unspecified superficial injury of left shoulder
- S40.919- Unspecified superficial injury of unspecified shoulder

6 S40.92 Unspecified superficial injury of upper arm
- S40.921- Unspecified superficial injury of right upper arm
- S40.922- Unspecified superficial injury of left upper arm
- S40.929- Unspecified superficial injury of unspecified upper arm

4 S41 Open wound of shoulder and upper arm
Code also:
any associated wound infection
EXCLUDES 1 traumatic amputation of shoulder and upper arm (S48.-)
EXCLUDES 2 open fracture of shoulder and upper arm (S42.- with 7th character B or C)

Chapter 19 S00-T88

The appropriate 7th character is to be added to each code from category S41
A initial encounter
D subsequent encounter
S sequela

CODING TIPS ✓ Open wound codes indicate a wound resulting from a traumatic origin. Do not assign a code for "open wound" unless the etiology of the wound is related to trauma.

CODING TIPS ✓ No aftercare code applies, including those indicating dressing changes, drain care, or suture removal. 7th character 'D' is the default for home care and hospice when providing aftercare for a healing or resolving condition; 'A' is used for active treatment such as antibiotics or more than routine wound care; 'S' may be used to indicate a residual condition after the original injury has healed.

5 **S41.0 Open wound of shoulder**
6 **S41.00 Unspecified open wound of shoulder**
SP 7 **S41.001- Unspecified open wound of right shoulder**
SP 7 **S41.002- Unspecified open wound of left shoulder**
IQ 7 **S41.009- Unspecified open wound of unspecified shoulder**
6 **S41.01 Laceration without foreign body of shoulder**
SP 7 **S41.011- Laceration without foreign body of right shoulder**
SP 7 **S41.012- Laceration without foreign body of left shoulder**
IQ 7 **S41.019- Laceration without foreign body of unspecified shoulder**
6 **S41.02 Laceration with foreign body of shoulder**
SP 7 **S41.021- Laceration with foreign body of right shoulder**
SP 7 **S41.022- Laceration with foreign body of left shoulder**
IQ 7 **S41.029- Laceration with foreign body of unspecified shoulder**
6 **S41.03 Puncture wound without foreign body of shoulder**
SP 7 **S41.031- Puncture wound without foreign body of right shoulder**
SP 7 **S41.032- Puncture wound without foreign body of left shoulder**
IQ 7 **S41.039- Puncture wound without foreign body of unspecified shoulder**
6 **S41.04 Puncture wound with foreign body of shoulder**
SP 7 **S41.041- Puncture wound with foreign body of right shoulder**
SP 7 **S41.042- Puncture wound with foreign body of left shoulder**
IQ 7 **S41.049- Puncture wound with foreign body of unspecified shoulder**
6 **S41.05 Open bite of shoulder**
Bite of shoulder NOS
EXCLUDES 1 superficial bite of shoulder (S40.27)
SP 7 **S41.051- Open bite of right shoulder**
SP 7 **S41.052- Open bite of left shoulder**
IQ 7 **S41.059- Open bite of unspecified shoulder**

5 **S41.1 Open wound of upper arm**
6 **S41.10 Unspecified open wound of upper arm**
SP 7 **S41.101- Unspecified open wound of right upper arm**
SP 7 **S41.102- Unspecified open wound of left upper arm**
IQ 7 **S41.109- Unspecified open wound of unspecified upper arm**
6 **S41.11 Laceration without foreign body of upper arm**
SP 7 **S41.111- Laceration without foreign body of right upper arm**
SP 7 **S41.112- Laceration without foreign body of left upper arm**
IQ 7 **S41.119- Laceration without foreign body of unspecified upper arm**
6 **S41.12 Laceration with foreign body of upper arm**
SP 7 **S41.121- Laceration with foreign body of right upper arm**
SP 7 **S41.122- Laceration with foreign body of left upper arm**
IQ 7 **S41.129- Laceration with foreign body of unspecified upper arm**
6 **S41.13 Puncture wound without foreign body of upper arm**
SP 7 **S41.131- Puncture wound without foreign body of right upper arm**
SP 7 **S41.132- Puncture wound without foreign body of left upper arm**
IQ 7 **S41.139- Puncture wound without foreign body of unspecified upper arm**
6 **S41.14 Puncture wound with foreign body of upper arm**
SP 7 **S41.141- Puncture wound with foreign body of right upper arm**
SP 7 **S41.142- Puncture wound with foreign body of left upper arm**
IQ 7 **S41.149- Puncture wound with foreign body of unspecified upper arm**
6 **S41.15 Open bite of upper arm**
Bite of upper arm NOS
EXCLUDES 1 superficial bite of upper arm (S40.87)
SP 7 **S41.151- Open bite of right upper arm**
SP 7 **S41.152- Open bite of left upper arm**
IQ 7 **S41.159- Open bite of unspecified upper arm**

4 **S42 Fracture of shoulder and upper arm**
Note:
A fracture not indicated as displaced or nondisplaced should be coded to displaced
A fracture not indicated as open or closed should be coded to closed
EXCLUDES 1 traumatic amputation of shoulder and upper arm (S48.-)

The appropriate 7th character is to be added to all codes from category S42

A	initial encounter for closed fracture
B	initial encounter for open fracture
D	subsequent encounter for fracture with routine healing
G	subsequent encounter for fracture with delayed healing
K	subsequent encounter for fracture with nonunion
P	subsequent encounter for fracture with malunion
S	sequela

CODING TIPS✓ Fractures repaired by joint replacements are NOT coded with Z47.1. Fractures repaired by any other orthopedic surgery are NOT coded with Z47.89. Z codes are not appropriate for fractures of any kind. Code the fracture with 7th character D for fractures undergoing surgical repair.

CODING TIPS✓ 'D' is the 7th character for home care and hospice unless the physician or NPP has documented delayed healing, nonunion or malunion. A sequela is a condition left after the fracture has healed. The Gustilo open fracture classification must be used for open fractures. The default 7th character for open fractures is E.

CODING TIPS✓ A fracture not indicated as displaced or nondisplaced should be coded to displaced. A fracture not indicated as open or closed should be coded to closed.

5 **S42.0 Fracture of clavicle**

6 **S42.00 Fracture of unspecified part of clavicle**

⊟ SP 7 **S42.001- Fracture of unspecified part of right clavicle**

⊟ SP 7 **S42.002- Fracture of unspecified part of left clavicle**

⊟ IQ 7 **S42.009- Fracture of unspecified part of unspecified clavicle**

6 **S42.01 Fracture of sternal end of clavicle**

⊟ SP 7 **S42.011- Anterior displaced fracture of sternal end of right clavicle**

⊟ SP 7 **S42.012- Anterior displaced fracture of sternal end of left clavicle**

⊟ IQ 7 **S42.013- Anterior displaced fracture of sternal end of unspecified clavicle**

Displaced fracture of sternal end of clavicle NOS

⊟ SP 7 **S42.014- Posterior displaced fracture of sternal end of right clavicle**

⊟ SP 7 **S42.015- Posterior displaced fracture of sternal end of left clavicle**

⊟ IQ 7 **S42.016- Posterior displaced fracture of sternal end of unspecified clavicle**

⊟ SP 7 **S42.017- Nondisplaced fracture of sternal end of right clavicle**

⊟ SP 7 **S42.018- Nondisplaced fracture of sternal end of left clavicle**

⊟ IQ 7 **S42.019- Nondisplaced fracture of sternal end of unspecified clavicle**

6 **S42.02 Fracture of shaft of clavicle**

⊟ SP 7 **S42.021- Displaced fracture of shaft of right clavicle**

⊟ SP 7 **S42.022- Displaced fracture of shaft of left clavicle**

⊟ SP IQ 7 **S42.023- Displaced fracture of shaft of unspecified clavicle**

⊟ SP 7 **S42.024- Nondisplaced fracture of shaft of right clavicle**

⊟ SP 7 **S42.025- Nondisplaced fracture of shaft of left clavicle**

⊟ IQ 7 **S42.026- Nondisplaced fracture of shaft of unspecified clavicle**

6 **S42.03 Fracture of lateral end of clavicle**

Fracture of acromial end of clavicle

⊟ SP 7 **S42.031- Displaced fracture of lateral end of right clavicle**

⊟ SP 7 **S42.032- Displaced fracture of lateral end of left clavicle**

⊟ IQ 7 **S42.033- Displaced fracture of lateral end of unspecified clavicle**

⊟ SP 7 **S42.034- Nondisplaced fracture of lateral end of right clavicle**

⊟ SP 7 **S42.035- Nondisplaced fracture of lateral end of left clavicle**

⊟ IQ 7 **S42.036- Nondisplaced fracture of lateral end of unspecified clavicle**

5 **S42.1 Fracture of scapula**

6 **S42.10 Fracture of unspecified part of scapula**

⊟ SP 7 **S42.101- Fracture of unspecified part of scapula, right shoulder**

⊟ SP 7 **S42.102- Fracture of unspecified part of scapula, left shoulder**

⊟ IQ 7 **S42.109- Fracture of unspecified part of scapula, unspecified shoulder**

6 **S42.11 Fracture of body of scapula**

⊟ SP 7 **S42.111- Displaced fracture of body of scapula, right shoulder**

⊟ SP 7 **S42.112- Displaced fracture of body of scapula, left shoulder**

⊟ IQ 7 **S42.113- Displaced fracture of body of scapula, unspecified shoulder**

⊟ SP 7 **S42.114- Nondisplaced fracture of body of scapula, right shoulder**

⊟ SP 7 **S42.115- Nondisplaced fracture of body of scapula, left shoulder**

⊟ IQ 7 **S42.116- Nondisplaced fracture of body of scapula, unspecified shoulder**

6 **S42.12 Fracture of acromial process**

⊟ SP 7 **S42.121- Displaced fracture of acromial process, right shoulder**

⊟ SP 7 **S42.122- Displaced fracture of acromial process, left shoulder**

⊟ IQ 7 **S42.123- Displaced fracture of acromial process, unspecified shoulder**

⊟ SP 7 **S42.124- Nondisplaced fracture of acromial process, right shoulder**

⊟ SP 7 **S42.125- Nondisplaced fracture of acromial process, left shoulder**

⊟ IQ 7 **S42.126- Nondisplaced fracture of acromial process, unspecified shoulder**

6 **S42.13 Fracture of coracoid process**

SP 7 S42.131- Displaced fracture of coracoid process, right shoulder
SP 7 S42.132- Displaced fracture of coracoid process, left shoulder
!Q 7 S42.133- Displaced fracture of coracoid process, unspecified shoulder
SP 7 S42.134- Nondisplaced fracture of coracoid process, right shoulder
SP 7 S42.135- Nondisplaced fracture of coracoid process, left shoulder
!Q 7 S42.136- Nondisplaced fracture of coracoid process, unspecified shoulder

6 S42.14 Fracture of glenoid cavity of scapula

SP 7 S42.141- Displaced fracture of glenoid cavity of scapula, right shoulder
SP 7 S42.142- Displaced fracture of glenoid cavity of scapula, left shoulder
!Q 7 S42.143- Displaced fracture of glenoid cavity of scapula, unspecified shoulder
SP 7 S42.144- Nondisplaced fracture of glenoid cavity of scapula, right shoulder
SP 7 S42.145- Nondisplaced fracture of glenoid cavity of scapula, left shoulder
!Q 7 S42.146- Nondisplaced fracture of glenoid cavity of scapula, unspecified shoulder

6 S42.15 Fracture of neck of scapula

SP 7 S42.151- Displaced fracture of neck of scapula, right shoulder
SP 7 S42.152- Displaced fracture of neck of scapula, left shoulder
!Q 7 S42.153- Displaced fracture of neck of scapula, unspecified shoulder
SP 7 S42.154- Nondisplaced fracture of neck of scapula, right shoulder
SP 7 S42.155- Nondisplaced fracture of neck of scapula, left shoulder
!Q 7 S42.156- Nondisplaced fracture of neck of scapula, unspecified shoulder

6 S42.19 Fracture of other part of scapula

SP 7 S42.191- Fracture of other part of scapula, right shoulder
SP 7 S42.192- Fracture of other part of scapula, left shoulder
!Q 7 S42.199- Fracture of other part of scapula, unspecified shoulder

5 S42.2 Fracture of upper end of humerus

Fracture of proximal end of humerus

EXCLUDES 2 fracture of shaft of humerus (S42.3-)
physeal fracture of upper end of humerus (S49.0-)

6 S42.20 Unspecified fracture of upper end of humerus

SP 7 S42.201- Unspecified fracture of upper end of right humerus
SP 7 S42.202- Unspecified fracture of upper end of left humerus
!Q 7 S42.209- Unspecified fracture of upper end of unspecified humerus

6 S42.21 Unspecified fracture of surgical neck of humerus

Fracture of neck of humerus NOS

SP 7 S42.211- Unspecified displaced fracture of surgical neck of right humerus
SP 7 S42.212- Unspecified displaced fracture of surgical neck of left humerus
!Q 7 S42.213- Unspecified displaced fracture of surgical neck of unspecified humerus
SP 7 S42.214- Unspecified nondisplaced fracture of surgical neck of right humerus
SP 7 S42.215- Unspecified nondisplaced fracture of surgical neck of left humerus
!Q 7 S42.216- Unspecified nondisplaced fracture of surgical neck of unspecified humerus

6 S42.22 2-part fracture of surgical neck of humerus

SP 7 S42.221- 2-part displaced fracture of surgical neck of right humerus
SP 7 S42.222- 2-part displaced fracture of surgical neck of left humerus
!Q 7 S42.223- 2-part displaced fracture of surgical neck of unspecified humerus
SP 7 S42.224- 2-part nondisplaced fracture of surgical neck of right humerus
SP 7 S42.225- 2-part nondisplaced fracture of surgical neck of left humerus
!Q 7 S42.226- 2-part nondisplaced fracture of surgical neck of unspecified humerus

6 S42.23 3-part fracture of surgical neck of humerus

SP 7 S42.231- 3-part fracture of surgical neck of right humerus
SP 7 S42.232- 3-part fracture of surgical neck of left humerus
!Q 7 S42.239- 3-part fracture of surgical neck of unspecified humerus

6 S42.24 4-part fracture of surgical neck of humerus

SP 7 S42.241- 4-part fracture of surgical neck of right humerus
SP 7 S42.242- 4-part fracture of surgical neck of left humerus
!Q 7 S42.249- 4-part fracture of surgical neck of unspecified humerus

6 S42.25 Fracture of greater tuberosity of humerus

SP 7 S42.251- Displaced fracture of greater tuberosity of right humerus
SP 7 S42.252- Displaced fracture of greater tuberosity of left humerus
!Q 7 S42.253- Displaced fracture of greater tuberosity of unspecified humerus
SP 7 S42.254- Nondisplaced fracture of greater tuberosity of right humerus
SP 7 S42.255- Nondisplaced fracture of greater tuberosity of left humerus
!Q 7 S42.256- Nondisplaced fracture of greater tuberosity of unspecified humerus

6 S42.26 Fracture of lesser tuberosity of humerus

Laterality SP 7 S42.261- Displaced fracture of lesser tuberosity of right humerus

Laterality SP 7 S42.262- Displaced fracture of lesser tuberosity of left humerus

Laterality IQ 7 S42.263- Displaced fracture of lesser tuberosity of unspecified humerus

Laterality SP 7 S42.264- Nondisplaced fracture of lesser tuberosity of right humerus

Laterality SP 7 S42.265- Nondisplaced fracture of lesser tuberosity of left humerus

Laterality IQ 7 S42.266- Nondisplaced fracture of lesser tuberosity of unspecified humerus

6 S42.27 Torus fracture of upper end of humerus

The appropriate 7th character is to be added to all codes in subcategory S42.27

A	initial encounter for closed fracture
D	subsequent encounter for fracture with routine healing
G	subsequent encounter for fracture with delayed healing
K	subsequent encounter for fracture with nonunion
P	subsequent encounter for fracture with malunion
S	sequela

Laterality SP 7 S42.271- Torus fracture of upper end of right humerus

Laterality SP 7 S42.272- Torus fracture of upper end of left humerus

Laterality IQ 7 S42.279- Torus fracture of upper end of unspecified humerus

6 S42.29 Other fracture of upper end of humerus

Fracture of anatomical neck of humerus

Fracture of articular head of humerus

Laterality SP 7 S42.291- Other displaced fracture of upper end of right humerus

Laterality SP 7 S42.292- Other displaced fracture of upper end of left humerus

Laterality IQ 7 S42.293- Other displaced fracture of upper end of unspecified humerus

Laterality SP 7 S42.294- Other nondisplaced fracture of upper end of right humerus

Laterality SP 7 S42.295- Other nondisplaced fracture of upper end of left humerus

Laterality IQ 7 S42.296- Other nondisplaced fracture of upper end of unspecified humerus

5 S42.3 Fracture of shaft of humerus

Fracture of humerus NOS

Fracture of upper arm NOS

EXCLUDES 2 physeal fractures of upper end of humerus (S49.0-)
physeal fractures of lower end of humerus (S49.1-)

6 S42.30 Unspecified fracture of shaft of humerus

Laterality SP 7 S42.301- Unspecified fracture of shaft of humerus, right arm

Laterality SP 7 S42.302- Unspecified fracture of shaft of humerus, left arm

Laterality IQ 7 S42.309- Unspecified fracture of shaft of humerus, unspecified arm

6 S42.31 Greenstick fracture of shaft of humerus

The appropriate 7th character is to be added to all codes in subcategory S42.31

A	initial encounter for closed fracture
D	subsequent encounter for fracture with routine healing
G	subsequent encounter for fracture with delayed healing
K	subsequent encounter for fracture with nonunion
P	subsequent encounter for fracture with malunion
S	sequela

Laterality SP 7 S42.311- Greenstick fracture of shaft of humerus, right arm

Laterality SP 7 S42.312- Greenstick fracture of shaft of humerus, left arm

Laterality IQ 7 S42.319- Greenstick fracture of shaft of humerus, unspecified arm

6 S42.32 Transverse fracture of shaft of humerus

Laterality SP 7 S42.321- Displaced transverse fracture of shaft of humerus, right arm

Laterality SP 7 S42.322- Displaced transverse fracture of shaft of humerus, left arm

Laterality IQ 7 S42.323- Displaced transverse fracture of shaft of humerus, unspecified arm

Laterality SP 7 S42.324- Nondisplaced transverse fracture of shaft of humerus, right arm

Laterality SP 7 S42.325- Nondisplaced transverse fracture of shaft of humerus, left arm

Laterality IQ 7 S42.326- Nondisplaced transverse fracture of shaft of humerus, unspecified arm

6 S42.33 Oblique fracture of shaft of humerus

Laterality SP 7 S42.331- Displaced oblique fracture of shaft of humerus, right arm

Laterality SP 7 S42.332- Displaced oblique fracture of shaft of humerus, left arm

Laterality IQ 7 S42.333- Displaced oblique fracture of shaft of humerus, unspecified arm

Laterality SP 7 S42.334- Nondisplaced oblique fracture of shaft of humerus, right arm

Laterality SP 7 S42.335- Nondisplaced oblique fracture of shaft of humerus, left arm

Laterality IQ 7 S42.336- Nondisplaced oblique fracture of shaft of humerus, unspecified arm

6 S42.34 Spiral fracture of shaft of humerus

Laterality SP 7 S42.341- Displaced spiral fracture of shaft of humerus, right arm

Laterality SP 7 S42.342- Displaced spiral fracture of shaft of humerus, left arm

IQ 7 S42.343- Displaced spiral fracture of shaft of humerus, unspecified arm

SP 7 S42.344- Nondisplaced spiral fracture of shaft of humerus, right arm

SP 7 S42.345- Nondisplaced spiral fracture of shaft of humerus, left arm

IQ 7 S42.346- Nondisplaced spiral fracture of shaft of humerus, unspecified arm

6 S42.35 Comminuted fracture of shaft of humerus

SP 7 S42.351- Displaced comminuted fracture of shaft of humerus, right arm

SP 7 S42.352- Displaced comminuted fracture of shaft of humerus, left arm

IQ 7 S42.353- Displaced comminuted fracture of shaft of humerus, unspecified arm

SP 7 S42.354- Nondisplaced comminuted fracture of shaft of humerus, right arm

SP 7 S42.355- Nondisplaced comminuted fracture of shaft of humerus, left arm

IQ 7 S42.356- Nondisplaced comminuted fracture of shaft of humerus, unspecified arm

6 S42.36 Segmental fracture of shaft of humerus

SP 7 S42.361- Displaced segmental fracture of shaft of humerus, right arm

SP 7 S42.362- Displaced segmental fracture of shaft of humerus, left arm

IQ 7 S42.363- Displaced segmental fracture of shaft of humerus, unspecified arm

SP 7 S42.364- Nondisplaced segmental fracture of shaft of humerus, right arm

SP 7 S42.365- Nondisplaced segmental fracture of shaft of humerus, left arm

IQ 7 S42.366- Nondisplaced segmental fracture of shaft of humerus, unspecified arm

6 S42.39 Other fracture of shaft of humerus

SP 7 S42.391- Other fracture of shaft of right humerus

SP 7 S42.392- Other fracture of shaft of left humerus

IQ 7 S42.399- Other fracture of shaft of unspecified humerus

5 S42.4 Fracture of lower end of humerus

Fracture of distal end of humerus

EXCLUDES 2 fracture of shaft of humerus (S42.3-)
physeal fracture of lower end of humerus (S49.1-)

6 S42.40 Unspecified fracture of lower end of humerus

Fracture of elbow NOS

SP 7 S42.401- Unspecified fracture of lower end of right humerus

SP 7 S42.402- Unspecified fracture of lower end of left humerus

IQ 7 S42.409- Unspecified fracture of lower end of unspecified humerus

6 S42.41 Simple supracondylar fracture without intercondylar fracture of humerus

SP 7 S42.411- Displaced simple supracondylar fracture without intercondylar fracture of right humerus

SP 7 S42.412- Displaced simple supracondylar fracture without intercondylar fracture of left humerus

IQ 7 S42.413- Displaced simple supracondylar fracture without intercondylar fracture of unspecified humerus

SP 7 S42.414- Nondisplaced simple supracondylar fracture without intercondylar fracture of right humerus

SP 7 S42.415- Nondisplaced simple supracondylar fracture without intercondylar fracture of left humerus

IQ 7 S42.416- Nondisplaced simple supracondylar fracture without intercondylar fracture of unspecified humerus

6 S42.42 Comminuted supracondylar fracture without intercondylar fracture of humerus

SP 7 S42.421- Displaced comminuted supracondylar fracture without intercondylar fracture of right humerus

SP 7 S42.422- Displaced comminuted supracondylar fracture without intercondylar fracture of left humerus

IQ 7 S42.423- Displaced comminuted supracondylar fracture without intercondylar fracture of unspecified humerus

SP 7 S42.424- Nondisplaced comminuted supracondylar fracture without intercondylar fracture of right humerus

SP 7 S42.425- Nondisplaced comminuted supracondylar fracture without intercondylar fracture of left humerus

IQ 7 S42.426- Nondisplaced comminuted supracondylar fracture without intercondylar fracture of unspecified humerus

6 S42.43 Fracture (avulsion) of lateral epicondyle of humerus

SP 7 S42.431- Displaced fracture (avulsion) of lateral epicondyle of right humerus

SP 7 S42.432- Displaced fracture (avulsion) of lateral epicondyle of left humerus

IQ 7 S42.433- Displaced fracture (avulsion) of lateral epicondyle of unspecified humerus

SP 7 S42.434- Nondisplaced fracture (avulsion) of lateral epicondyle of right humerus

SP 7 S42.435- Nondisplaced fracture (avulsion) of lateral epicondyle of left humerus

S42.436- Nondisplaced fracture (avulsion) of lateral epicondyle of unspecified humerus

S42.44 Fracture (avulsion) of medial epicondyle of humerus

S42.441- Displaced fracture (avulsion) of medial epicondyle of right humerus

S42.442- Displaced fracture (avulsion) of medial epicondyle of left humerus

S42.443- Displaced fracture (avulsion) of medial epicondyle of unspecified humerus

S42.444- Nondisplaced fracture (avulsion) of medial epicondyle of right humerus

S42.445- Nondisplaced fracture (avulsion) of medial epicondyle of left humerus

S42.446- Nondisplaced fracture (avulsion) of medial epicondyle of unspecified humerus

S42.447- Incarcerated fracture (avulsion) of medial epicondyle of right humerus

S42.448- Incarcerated fracture (avulsion) of medial epicondyle of left humerus

S42.449- Incarcerated fracture (avulsion) of medial epicondyle of unspecified humerus

S42.45 Fracture of lateral condyle of humerus

Fracture of capitellum of humerus

S42.451- Displaced fracture of lateral condyle of right humerus

S42.452- Displaced fracture of lateral condyle of left humerus

S42.453- Displaced fracture of lateral condyle of unspecified humerus

S42.454- Nondisplaced fracture of lateral condyle of right humerus

S42.455- Nondisplaced fracture of lateral condyle of left humerus

S42.456- Nondisplaced fracture of lateral condyle of unspecified humerus

S42.46 Fracture of medial condyle of humerus

Trochlea fracture of humerus

S42.461- Displaced fracture of medial condyle of right humerus

S42.462- Displaced fracture of medial condyle of left humerus

S42.463- Displaced fracture of medial condyle of unspecified humerus

S42.464- Nondisplaced fracture of medial condyle of right humerus

S42.465- Nondisplaced fracture of medial condyle of left humerus

S42.466- Nondisplaced fracture of medial condyle of unspecified humerus

S42.47 Transcondylar fracture of humerus

S42.471- Displaced transcondylar fracture of right humerus

S42.472- Displaced transcondylar fracture of left humerus

S42.473- Displaced transcondylar fracture of unspecified humerus

S42.474- Nondisplaced transcondylar fracture of right humerus

S42.475- Nondisplaced transcondylar fracture of left humerus

S42.476- Nondisplaced transcondylar fracture of unspecified humerus

S42.48 Torus fracture of lower end of humerus

The appropriate 7th character is to be added to all codes in subcategory S42.48

A initial encounter for closed fracture
D subsequent encounter for fracture with routine healing
G subsequent encounter for fracture with delayed healing
K subsequent encounter for fracture with nonunion
P subsequent encounter for fracture with malunion
S sequela

S42.481- Torus fracture of lower end of right humerus

S42.482- Torus fracture of lower end of left humerus

S42.489- Torus fracture of lower end of unspecified humerus

S42.49 Other fracture of lower end of humerus

S42.491- Other displaced fracture of lower end of right humerus

S42.492- Other displaced fracture of lower end of left humerus

S42.493- Other displaced fracture of lower end of unspecified humerus

S42.494- Other nondisplaced fracture of lower end of right humerus

S42.495- Other nondisplaced fracture of lower end of left humerus

S42.496- Other nondisplaced fracture of lower end of unspecified humerus

S42.9 Fracture of shoulder girdle, part unspecified

Fracture of shoulder NOS

S42.90X- Fracture of unspecified shoulder girdle, part unspecified

S42.91X- Fracture of right shoulder girdle, part unspecified

S42.92X- Fracture of left shoulder girdle, part unspecified

S43 Dislocation and sprain of joints and ligaments of shoulder girdle

INCLUDES avulsion of joint or ligament of shoulder girdle
laceration of cartilage, joint or ligament of shoulder girdle
sprain of cartilage, joint or ligament of shoulder girdle
traumatic hemarthrosis of joint or ligament of shoulder girdle

4th digit required | 5th digit required | 6th digit required | 7th digit required | 7th digit placeholder | +Additional code | Laterality

traumatic rupture of joint or ligament of shoulder girdle
traumatic subluxation of joint or ligament of shoulder girdle
traumatic tear of joint or ligament of shoulder girdle

Code also:
any associated open wound

EXCLUDES 2 strain of muscle, fascia and tendon of shoulder and upper arm (S46.-)

The appropriate 7th character is to be added to each code from category S43
A initial encounter
D subsequent encounter
S sequela

5 **S43.0 Subluxation and dislocation of shoulder joint**
Dislocation of glenohumeral joint
Subluxation of glenohumeral joint

6 **S43.00 Unspecified subluxation and dislocation of shoulder joint**
Dislocation of humerus NOS
Subluxation of humerus NOS

SP 7 **S43.001- Unspecified subluxation of right shoulder joint**
SP 7 **S43.002- Unspecified subluxation of left shoulder joint**
IQ 7 **S43.003- Unspecified subluxation of unspecified shoulder joint**
SP 7 **S43.004- Unspecified dislocation of right shoulder joint**
SP 7 **S43.005- Unspecified dislocation of left shoulder joint**
IQ 7 **S43.006- Unspecified dislocation of unspecified shoulder joint**

6 **S43.01 Anterior subluxation and dislocation of humerus**
SP 7 **S43.011- Anterior subluxation of right humerus**
SP 7 **S43.012- Anterior subluxation of left humerus**
IQ 7 **S43.013- Anterior subluxation of unspecified humerus**
SP 7 **S43.014- Anterior dislocation of right humerus**
SP 7 **S43.015- Anterior dislocation of left humerus**
IQ 7 **S43.016- Anterior dislocation of unspecified humerus**

6 **S43.02 Posterior subluxation and dislocation of humerus**
SP 7 **S43.021- Posterior subluxation of right humerus**
SP 7 **S43.022- Posterior subluxation of left humerus**
IQ 7 **S43.023- Posterior subluxation of unspecified humerus**
SP 7 **S43.024- Posterior dislocation of right humerus**
SP 7 **S43.025- Posterior dislocation of left humerus**
IQ 7 **S43.026- Posterior dislocation of unspecified humerus**

6 **S43.03 Inferior subluxation and dislocation of humerus**
SP 7 **S43.031- Inferior subluxation of right humerus**
SP 7 **S43.032- Inferior subluxation of left humerus**
IQ 7 **S43.033- Inferior subluxation of unspecified humerus**
SP 7 **S43.034- Inferior dislocation of right humerus**
SP 7 **S43.035- Inferior dislocation of left humerus**
IQ 7 **S43.036- Inferior dislocation of unspecified humerus**

6 **S43.08 Other subluxation and dislocation of shoulder joint**
SP 7 **S43.081- Other subluxation of right shoulder joint**
SP 7 **S43.082- Other subluxation of left shoulder joint**
IQ 7 **S43.083- Other subluxation of unspecified shoulder joint**
SP 7 **S43.084- Other dislocation of right shoulder joint**
SP 7 **S43.085- Other dislocation of left shoulder joint**
IQ 7 **S43.086- Other dislocation of unspecified shoulder joint**

5 **S43.1 Subluxation and dislocation of acromioclavicular joint**

6 **S43.10 Unspecified dislocation of acromioclavicular joint**
SP 7 **S43.101- Unspecified dislocation of right acromioclavicular joint**
SP 7 **S43.102- Unspecified dislocation of left acromioclavicular joint**
IQ 7 **S43.109- Unspecified dislocation of unspecified acromioclavicular joint**

6 **S43.11 Subluxation of acromioclavicular joint**
SP 7 **S43.111- Subluxation of right acromioclavicular joint**
SP 7 **S43.112- Subluxation of left acromioclavicular joint**
IQ 7 **S43.119- Subluxation of unspecified acromioclavicular joint**

6 **S43.12 Dislocation of acromioclavicular joint, 100%-200% displacement**
SP 7 **S43.121- Dislocation of right acromioclavicular joint, 100%-200% displacement**
SP 7 **S43.122- Dislocation of left acromioclavicular joint, 100%-200% displacement**
IQ 7 **S43.129- Dislocation of unspecified acromioclavicular joint, 100%-200% displacement**

6 **S43.13 Dislocation of acromioclavicular joint, greater than 200% displacement**
SP 7 **S43.131- Dislocation of right acromioclavicular joint, greater than 200% displacement**

Chapter 19 S00-T88

☐ SP 7 **S43.132-** Dislocation of left acromioclavicular joint, greater than 200% displacement

☐ IQ 7 **S43.139-** Dislocation of unspecified acromioclavicular joint, greater than 200% displacement

6 **S43.14** Inferior dislocation of acromioclavicular joint

☐ SP 7 **S43.141-** Inferior dislocation of right acromioclavicular joint

☐ SP 7 **S43.142-** Inferior dislocation of left acromioclavicular joint

☐ IQ 7 **S43.149-** Inferior dislocation of unspecified acromioclavicular joint

6 **S43.15** Posterior dislocation of acromioclavicular joint

☐ SP 7 **S43.151-** Posterior dislocation of right acromioclavicular joint

☐ SP 7 **S43.152-** Posterior dislocation of left acromioclavicular joint

☐ IQ 7 **S43.159-** Posterior dislocation of unspecified acromioclavicular joint

5 **S43.2** Subluxation and dislocation of sternoclavicular joint

6 **S43.20** Unspecified subluxation and dislocation of sternoclavicular joint

☐ SP 7 **S43.201-** Unspecified subluxation of right sternoclavicular joint

☐ SP 7 **S43.202-** Unspecified subluxation of left sternoclavicular joint

☐ IQ 7 **S43.203-** Unspecified subluxation of unspecified sternoclavicular joint

☐ SP 7 **S43.204-** Unspecified dislocation of right sternoclavicular joint

☐ SP 7 **S43.205-** Unspecified dislocation of left sternoclavicular joint

☐ IQ 7 **S43.206-** Unspecified dislocation of unspecified sternoclavicular joint

6 **S43.21** Anterior subluxation and dislocation of sternoclavicular joint

☐ SP 7 **S43.211-** Anterior subluxation of right sternoclavicular joint

☐ SP 7 **S43.212-** Anterior subluxation of left sternoclavicular joint

☐ IQ 7 **S43.213-** Anterior subluxation of unspecified sternoclavicular joint

☐ SP 7 **S43.214-** Anterior dislocation of right sternoclavicular joint

☐ SP 7 **S43.215-** Anterior dislocation of left sternoclavicular joint

☐ IQ 7 **S43.216-** Anterior dislocation of unspecified sternoclavicular joint

6 **S43.22** Posterior subluxation and dislocation of sternoclavicular joint

☐ SP 7 **S43.221-** Posterior subluxation of right sternoclavicular joint

☐ SP 7 **S43.222-** Posterior subluxation of left sternoclavicular joint

☐ IQ 7 **S43.223-** Posterior subluxation of unspecified sternoclavicular joint

☐ SP 7 **S43.224-** Posterior dislocation of right sternoclavicular joint

☐ SP 7 **S43.225-** Posterior dislocation of left sternoclavicular joint

☐ IQ 7 **S43.226-** Posterior dislocation of unspecified sternoclavicular joint

5 **S43.3** Subluxation and dislocation of other and unspecified parts of shoulder girdle

6 **S43.30** Subluxation and dislocation of unspecified parts of shoulder girdle

Dislocation of shoulder girdle NOS
Subluxation of shoulder girdle NOS

☐ SP 7 **S43.301-** Subluxation of unspecified parts of right shoulder girdle

☐ SP 7 **S43.302-** Subluxation of unspecified parts of left shoulder girdle

☐ IQ 7 **S43.303-** Subluxation of unspecified parts of unspecified shoulder girdle

☐ SP 7 **S43.304-** Dislocation of unspecified parts of right shoulder girdle

☐ SP 7 **S43.305-** Dislocation of unspecified parts of left shoulder girdle

☐ IQ 7 **S43.306-** Dislocation of unspecified parts of unspecified shoulder girdle

6 **S43.31** Subluxation and dislocation of scapula

☐ SP 7 **S43.311-** Subluxation of right scapula

☐ SP 7 **S43.312-** Subluxation of left scapula

☐ IQ 7 **S43.313-** Subluxation of unspecified scapula

☐ SP 7 **S43.314-** Dislocation of right scapula

☐ SP 7 **S43.315-** Dislocation of left scapula

☐ IQ 7 **S43.316-** Dislocation of unspecified scapula

6 **S43.39** Subluxation and dislocation of other parts of shoulder girdle

☐ SP 7 **S43.391-** Subluxation of other parts of right shoulder girdle

☐ SP 7 **S43.392-** Subluxation of other parts of left shoulder girdle

☐ IQ 7 **S43.393-** Subluxation of other parts of unspecified shoulder girdle

☐ SP 7 **S43.394-** Dislocation of other parts of right shoulder girdle

☐ SP 7 **S43.395-** Dislocation of other parts of left shoulder girdle

☐ IQ 7 **S43.396-** Dislocation of other parts of unspecified shoulder girdle

5 **S43.4** Sprain of shoulder joint

6 **S43.40** Unspecified sprain of shoulder joint

☐ SP 7 **S43.401-** Unspecified sprain of right shoulder joint

☐ SP 7 **S43.402-** Unspecified sprain of left shoulder joint

☐ IQ 7 **S43.409-** Unspecified sprain of unspecified shoulder joint

6 **S43.41** Sprain of coracohumeral (ligament)

☐ SP 7 **S43.411-** Sprain of right coracohumeral (ligament)

☐4 4th digit required   ☐5 5th digit required   ☐6 6th digit required   ☐7 7th digit required   ⑦ 7th digit placeholder   ✚ Additional code   ☐ Laterality

SP 7 **S43.412- Sprain of left coracohumeral (ligament)**

IQ 7 **S43.419- Sprain of unspecified coracohumeral (ligament)**

6 **S43.42 Sprain of rotator cuff capsule**

EXCLUDES 1 rotator cuff syndrome (complete) (incomplete), not specified as traumatic (M75.1-)

EXCLUDES 2 injury of tendon of rotator cuff (S46.0-)

SP 7 **S43.421- Sprain of right rotator cuff capsule**

SP 7 **S43.422- Sprain of left rotator cuff capsule**

IQ 7 **S43.429- Sprain of unspecified rotator cuff capsule**

6 **S43.43 Superior glenoid labrum lesion**

SLAP lesion

SP 7 **S43.431- Superior glenoid labrum lesion of right shoulder**

SP 7 **S43.432- Superior glenoid labrum lesion of left shoulder**

IQ 7 **S43.439- Superior glenoid labrum lesion of unspecified shoulder**

6 **S43.49 Other sprain of shoulder joint**

SP 7 **S43.491- Other sprain of right shoulder joint**

SP 7 **S43.492- Other sprain of left shoulder joint**

IQ 7 **S43.499- Other sprain of unspecified shoulder joint**

5 **S43.5 Sprain of acromioclavicular joint**

Sprain of acromioclavicular ligament

IQ 7 **S43.50X- Sprain of unspecified acromioclavicular joint**

SP 7 **S43.51X- Sprain of right acromioclavicular joint**

SP 7 **S43.52X- Sprain of left acromioclavicular joint**

5 **S43.6 Sprain of sternoclavicular joint**

IQ 7 **S43.60X- Sprain of unspecified sternoclavicular joint**

SP 7 **S43.61X- Sprain of right sternoclavicular joint**

SP 7 **S43.62X- Sprain of left sternoclavicular joint**

5 **S43.8 Sprain of other specified parts of shoulder girdle**

IQ 7 **S43.80X- Sprain of other specified parts of unspecified shoulder girdle**

SP 7 **S43.81X- Sprain of other specified parts of right shoulder girdle**

SP 7 **S43.82X- Sprain of other specified parts of left shoulder girdle**

5 **S43.9 Sprain of unspecified parts of shoulder girdle**

IQ 7 **S43.90X- Sprain of unspecified parts of unspecified shoulder girdle**

Sprain of shoulder girdle NOS

SP 7 **S43.91X- Sprain of unspecified parts of right shoulder girdle**

SP 7 **S43.92X- Sprain of unspecified parts of left shoulder girdle**

4 **S44 Injury of nerves at shoulder and upper arm level**

Code also:

any associated open wound (S41.-)

EXCLUDES 2 injury of brachial plexus (S14.3-)

The appropriate 7th character is to be added to each code from category S44

A	initial encounter
D	subsequent encounter
S	sequela

5 **S44.0 Injury of ulnar nerve at upper arm level**

EXCLUDES 1 ulnar nerve NOS (S54.0)

IQ 7 **S44.00X- Injury of ulnar nerve at upper arm level, unspecified arm**

SP 7 **S44.01X- Injury of ulnar nerve at upper arm level, right arm**

SP 7 **S44.02X- Injury of ulnar nerve at upper arm level, left arm**

5 **S44.1 Injury of median nerve at upper arm level**

EXCLUDES 1 median nerve NOS (S54.1)

IQ 7 **S44.10X- Injury of median nerve at upper arm level, unspecified arm**

SP 7 **S44.11X- Injury of median nerve at upper arm level, right arm**

SP 7 **S44.12X- Injury of median nerve at upper arm level, left arm**

5 **S44.2 Injury of radial nerve at upper arm level**

EXCLUDES 1 radial nerve NOS (S54.2)

IQ 7 **S44.20X- Injury of radial nerve at upper arm level, unspecified arm**

SP 7 **S44.21X- Injury of radial nerve at upper arm level, right arm**

SP 7 **S44.22X- Injury of radial nerve at upper arm level, left arm**

5 **S44.3 Injury of axillary nerve**

IQ 7 **S44.30X- Injury of axillary nerve, unspecified arm**

SP 7 **S44.31X- Injury of axillary nerve, right arm**

SP 7 **S44.32X- Injury of axillary nerve, left arm**

5 **S44.4 Injury of musculocutaneous nerve**

IQ 7 **S44.40X- Injury of musculocutaneous nerve, unspecified arm**

SP 7 **S44.41X- Injury of musculocutaneous nerve, right arm**

SP 7 **S44.42X- Injury of musculocutaneous nerve, left arm**

5 **S44.5 Injury of cutaneous sensory nerve at shoulder and upper arm level**

IQ 7 **S44.50X- Injury of cutaneous sensory nerve at shoulder and upper arm level, unspecified arm**

SP 7 **S44.51X- Injury of cutaneous sensory nerve at shoulder and upper arm level, right arm**

SP 7 **S44.52X- Injury of cutaneous sensory nerve at shoulder and upper arm level, left arm**

5 **S44.8 Injury of other nerves at shoulder and upper arm level**

6 **S44.8X Injury of other nerves at shoulder and upper arm level**

Chapter 19 S00-T88

S44.8X1- Injury of other nerves at shoulder and upper arm level, right arm

S44.8X2- Injury of other nerves at shoulder and upper arm level, left arm

S44.8X9- Injury of other nerves at shoulder and upper arm level, unspecified arm

S44.9 Injury of unspecified nerve at shoulder and upper arm level

S44.90X- Injury of unspecified nerve at shoulder and upper arm level, unspecified arm

S44.91X- Injury of unspecified nerve at shoulder and upper arm level, right arm

S44.92X- Injury of unspecified nerve at shoulder and upper arm level, left arm

S45 Injury of blood vessels at shoulder and upper arm level

Code also:

any associated open wound (S41.-)

EXCLUDES 2 injury of subclavian artery (S25.1)

injury of subclavian vein (S25.3)

The appropriate 7th character is to be added to each code from category S45

A initial encounter

D subsequent encounter

S sequela

S45.0 Injury of axillary artery

S45.00 Unspecified injury of axillary artery

S45.001- Unspecified injury of axillary artery, right side

S45.002- Unspecified injury of axillary artery, left side

S45.009- Unspecified injury of axillary artery, unspecified side

S45.01 Laceration of axillary artery

S45.011- Laceration of axillary artery, right side

S45.012- Laceration of axillary artery, left side

S45.019- Laceration of axillary artery, unspecified side

S45.09 Other specified injury of axillary artery

S45.091- Other specified injury of axillary artery, right side

S45.092- Other specified injury of axillary artery, left side

S45.099- Other specified injury of axillary artery, unspecified side

S45.1 Injury of brachial artery

S45.10 Unspecified injury of brachial artery

S45.101- Unspecified injury of brachial artery, right side

S45.102- Unspecified injury of brachial artery, left side

S45.109- Unspecified injury of brachial artery, unspecified side

S45.11 Laceration of brachial artery

S45.111- Laceration of brachial artery, right side

S45.112- Laceration of brachial artery, left side

S45.119- Laceration of brachial artery, unspecified side

S45.19 Other specified injury of brachial artery

S45.191- Other specified injury of brachial artery, right side

S45.192- Other specified injury of brachial artery, left side

S45.199- Other specified injury of brachial artery, unspecified side

S45.2 Injury of axillary or brachial vein

S45.20 Unspecified injury of axillary or brachial vein

S45.201- Unspecified injury of axillary or brachial vein, right side

S45.202- Unspecified injury of axillary or brachial vein, left side

S45.209- Unspecified injury of axillary or brachial vein, unspecified side

S45.21 Laceration of axillary or brachial vein

S45.211- Laceration of axillary or brachial vein, right side

S45.212- Laceration of axillary or brachial vein, left side

S45.219- Laceration of axillary or brachial vein, unspecified side

S45.29 Other specified injury of axillary or brachial vein

S45.291- Other specified injury of axillary or brachial vein, right side

S45.292- Other specified injury of axillary or brachial vein, left side

S45.299- Other specified injury of axillary or brachial vein, unspecified side

S45.3 Injury of superficial vein at shoulder and upper arm level

S45.30 Unspecified injury of superficial vein at shoulder and upper arm level

S45.301- Unspecified injury of superficial vein at shoulder and upper arm level, right arm

S45.302- Unspecified injury of superficial vein at shoulder and upper arm level, left arm

S45.309- Unspecified injury of superficial vein at shoulder and upper arm level, unspecified arm

S45.31 Laceration of superficial vein at shoulder and upper arm level

S45.311- Laceration of superficial vein at shoulder and upper arm level, right arm

S45.312- Laceration of superficial vein at shoulder and upper arm level, left arm

Chapter 19

S00-T88

S45.319- Laceration of superficial vein at shoulder and upper arm level, unspecified arm

S45.39 Other specified injury of superficial vein at shoulder and upper arm level

S45.391- Other specified injury of superficial vein at shoulder and upper arm level, right arm

S45.392- Other specified injury of superficial vein at shoulder and upper arm level, left arm

S45.399- Other specified injury of superficial vein at shoulder and upper arm level, unspecified arm

S45.8 Injury of other specified blood vessels at shoulder and upper arm level

S45.80 Unspecified injury of other specified blood vessels at shoulder and upper arm level

S45.801- Unspecified injury of other specified blood vessels at shoulder and upper arm level, right arm

S45.802- Unspecified injury of other specified blood vessels at shoulder and upper arm level, left arm

S45.809- Unspecified injury of other specified blood vessels at shoulder and upper arm level, unspecified arm

S45.81 Laceration of other specified blood vessels at shoulder and upper arm level

S45.811- Laceration of other specified blood vessels at shoulder and upper arm level, right arm

S45.812- Laceration of other specified blood vessels at shoulder and upper arm level, left arm

S45.819- Laceration of other specified blood vessels at shoulder and upper arm level, unspecified arm

S45.89 Other specified injury of other specified blood vessels at shoulder and upper arm level

S45.891- Other specified injury of other specified blood vessels at shoulder and upper arm level, right arm

S45.892- Other specified injury of other specified blood vessels at shoulder and upper arm level, left arm

S45.899- Other specified injury of other specified blood vessels at shoulder and upper arm level, unspecified arm

S45.9 Injury of unspecified blood vessel at shoulder and upper arm level

S45.90 Unspecified injury of unspecified blood vessel at shoulder and upper arm level

S45.901- Unspecified injury of unspecified blood vessel at shoulder and upper arm level, right arm

S45.902- Unspecified injury of unspecified blood vessel at shoulder and upper arm level, left arm

S45.909- Unspecified injury of unspecified blood vessel at shoulder and upper arm level, unspecified arm

S45.91 Laceration of unspecified blood vessel at shoulder and upper arm level

S45.911- Laceration of unspecified blood vessel at shoulder and upper arm level, right arm

S45.912- Laceration of unspecified blood vessel at shoulder and upper arm level, left arm

S45.919- Laceration of unspecified blood vessel at shoulder and upper arm level, unspecified arm

S45.99 Other specified injury of unspecified blood vessel at shoulder and upper arm level

S45.991- Other specified injury of unspecified blood vessel at shoulder and upper arm level, right arm

S45.992- Other specified injury of unspecified blood vessel at shoulder and upper arm level, left arm

S45.999- Other specified injury of unspecified blood vessel at shoulder and upper arm level, unspecified arm

S46 Injury of muscle, fascia and tendon at shoulder and upper arm level

Code also:

any associated open wound (S41.-)

EXCLUDES 2 injury of muscle, fascia and tendon at elbow (S56.-)

sprain of joints and ligaments of shoulder girdle (S43.9)

The appropriate 7th character is to be added to each code from category S46

A initial encounter
D subsequent encounter
S sequela

S46.0 Injury of muscle(s) and tendon(s) of the rotator cuff of shoulder

S46.00 Unspecified injury of muscle(s) and tendon(s) of the rotator cuff of shoulder

S46.001- Unspecified injury of muscle(s) and tendon(s) of the rotator cuff of right shoulder

S46.002- Unspecified injury of muscle(s) and tendon(s) of the rotator cuff of left shoulder

Chapter 19

S00-T88

Laterality IQ 7 S46.009- Unspecified injury of muscle(s) and tendon(s) of the rotator cuff of unspecified shoulder

6 S46.01 Strain of muscle(s) and tendon(s) of the rotator cuff of shoulder

Laterality SP 7 S46.011- Strain of muscle(s) and tendon(s) of the rotator cuff of right shoulder

Laterality SP 7 S46.012- Strain of muscle(s) and tendon(s) of the rotator cuff of left shoulder

Laterality IQ 7 S46.019- Strain of muscle(s) and tendon(s) of the rotator cuff of unspecified shoulder

6 S46.02 Laceration of muscle(s) and tendon(s) of the rotator cuff of shoulder

Laterality SP 7 S46.021- Laceration of muscle(s) and tendon(s) of the rotator cuff of right shoulder

Laterality SP 7 S46.022- Laceration of muscle(s) and tendon(s) of the rotator cuff of left shoulder

Laterality IQ 7 S46.029- Laceration of muscle(s) and tendon(s) of the rotator cuff of unspecified shoulder

6 S46.09 Other injury of muscle(s) and tendon(s) of the rotator cuff of shoulder

Laterality SP 7 S46.091- Other injury of muscle(s) and tendon(s) of the rotator cuff of right shoulder

Laterality SP 7 S46.092- Other injury of muscle(s) and tendon(s) of the rotator cuff of left shoulder

Laterality IQ 7 S46.099- Other injury of muscle(s) and tendon(s) of the rotator cuff of unspecified shoulder

5 S46.1 Injury of muscle, fascia and tendon of long head of biceps

6 S46.10 Unspecified injury of muscle, fascia and tendon of long head of biceps

Laterality IQ 7 S46.101- Unspecified injury of muscle, fascia and tendon of long head of biceps, right arm

Laterality IQ 7 S46.102- Unspecified injury of muscle, fascia and tendon of long head of biceps, left arm

Laterality IQ 7 S46.109- Unspecified injury of muscle, fascia and tendon of long head of biceps, unspecified arm

6 S46.11 Strain of muscle, fascia and tendon of long head of biceps

Laterality SP 7 S46.111- Strain of muscle, fascia and tendon of long head of biceps, right arm

Laterality SP 7 S46.112- Strain of muscle, fascia and tendon of long head of biceps, left arm

Laterality IQ 7 S46.119- Strain of muscle, fascia and tendon of long head of biceps, unspecified arm

6 S46.12 Laceration of muscle, fascia and tendon of long head of biceps

Laterality SP 7 S46.121- Laceration of muscle, fascia and tendon of long head of biceps, right arm

Laterality SP 7 S46.122- Laceration of muscle, fascia and tendon of long head of biceps, left arm

Laterality IQ 7 S46.129- Laceration of muscle, fascia and tendon of long head of biceps, unspecified arm

6 S46.19 Other injury of muscle, fascia and tendon of long head of biceps

Laterality SP 7 S46.191- Other injury of muscle, fascia and tendon of long head of biceps, right arm

Laterality SP 7 S46.192- Other injury of muscle, fascia and tendon of long head of biceps, left arm

Laterality IQ 7 S46.199- Other injury of muscle, fascia and tendon of long head of biceps, unspecified arm

5 S46.2 Injury of muscle, fascia and tendon of other parts of biceps

6 S46.20 Unspecified injury of muscle, fascia and tendon of other parts of biceps

Laterality IQ 7 S46.201- Unspecified injury of muscle, fascia and tendon of other parts of biceps, right arm

Laterality IQ 7 S46.202- Unspecified injury of muscle, fascia and tendon of other parts of biceps, left arm

Laterality IQ 7 S46.209- Unspecified injury of muscle, fascia and tendon of other parts of biceps, unspecified arm

6 S46.21 Strain of muscle, fascia and tendon of other parts of biceps

Laterality SP 7 S46.211- Strain of muscle, fascia and tendon of other parts of biceps, right arm

Laterality SP 7 S46.212- Strain of muscle, fascia and tendon of other parts of biceps, left arm

Laterality IQ 7 S46.219- Strain of muscle, fascia and tendon of other parts of biceps, unspecified arm

6 S46.22 Laceration of muscle, fascia and tendon of other parts of biceps

Laterality SP 7 S46.221- Laceration of muscle, fascia and tendon of other parts of biceps, right arm

Laterality SP 7 S46.222- Laceration of muscle, fascia and tendon of other parts of biceps, left arm

Laterality IQ 7 S46.229- Laceration of muscle, fascia and tendon of other parts of biceps, unspecified arm

6 S46.29 Other injury of muscle, fascia and tendon of other parts of biceps

Laterality SP 7 S46.291- Other injury of muscle, fascia and tendon of other parts of biceps, right arm

Laterality SP 7 S46.292- Other injury of muscle, fascia and tendon of other parts of biceps, left arm

Laterality IQ 7 S46.299- Other injury of muscle, fascia and tendon of other parts of biceps, unspecified arm

5 S46.3 Injury of muscle, fascia and tendon of triceps

6 S46.30 Unspecified injury of muscle, fascia and tendon of triceps

Chapter 19

S00-T88

IQ 7 S46.301- Unspecified injury of muscle, fascia and tendon of triceps, right arm

IQ 7 S46.302- Unspecified injury of muscle, fascia and tendon of triceps, left arm

IQ 7 S46.309- Unspecified injury of muscle, fascia and tendon of triceps, unspecified arm

6 S46.31 Strain of muscle, fascia and tendon of triceps

SP 7 S46.311- Strain of muscle, fascia and tendon of triceps, right arm

SP 7 S46.312- Strain of muscle, fascia and tendon of triceps, left arm

IQ 7 S46.319- Strain of muscle, fascia and tendon of triceps, unspecified arm

6 S46.32 Laceration of muscle, fascia and tendon of triceps

SP 7 S46.321- Laceration of muscle, fascia and tendon of triceps, right arm

SP 7 S46.322- Laceration of muscle, fascia and tendon of triceps, left arm

IQ 7 S46.329- Laceration of muscle, fascia and tendon of triceps, unspecified arm

6 S46.39 Other injury of muscle, fascia and tendon of triceps

SP 7 S46.391- Other injury of muscle, fascia and tendon of triceps, right arm

SP 7 S46.392- Other injury of muscle, fascia and tendon of triceps, left arm

IQ 7 S46.399- Other injury of muscle, fascia and tendon of triceps, unspecified arm

5 S46.8 Injury of other muscles, fascia and tendons at shoulder and upper arm level

6 S46.80 Unspecified injury of other muscles, fascia and tendons at shoulder and upper arm level

IQ 7 S46.801- Unspecified injury of other muscles, fascia and tendons at shoulder and upper arm level, right arm

IQ 7 S46.802- Unspecified injury of other muscles, fascia and tendons at shoulder and upper arm level, left arm

IQ 7 S46.809- Unspecified injury of other muscles, fascia and tendons at shoulder and upper arm level, unspecified arm

6 S46.81 Strain of other muscles, fascia and tendons at shoulder and upper arm level

SP 7 S46.811- Strain of other muscles, fascia and tendons at shoulder and upper arm level, right arm

SP 7 S46.812- Strain of other muscles, fascia and tendons at shoulder and upper arm level, left arm

IQ 7 S46.819- Strain of other muscles, fascia and tendons at shoulder and upper arm level, unspecified arm

6 S46.82 Laceration of other muscles, fascia and tendons at shoulder and upper arm level

SP 7 S46.821- Laceration of other muscles, fascia and tendons at shoulder and upper arm level, right arm

SP 7 S46.822- Laceration of other muscles, fascia and tendons at shoulder and upper arm level, left arm

IQ 7 S46.829- Laceration of other muscles, fascia and tendons at shoulder and upper arm level, unspecified arm

6 S46.89 Other injury of other muscles, fascia and tendons at shoulder and upper arm level

SP 7 S46.891- Other injury of other muscles, fascia and tendons at shoulder and upper arm level, right arm

SP 7 S46.892- Other injury of other muscles, fascia and tendons at shoulder and upper arm level, left arm

IQ 7 S46.899- Other injury of other muscles, fascia and tendons at shoulder and upper arm level, unspecified arm

5 S46.9 Injury of unspecified muscle, fascia and tendon at shoulder and upper arm level

6 S46.90 Unspecified injury of unspecified muscle, fascia and tendon at shoulder and upper arm level

IQ 7 S46.901- Unspecified injury of unspecified muscle, fascia and tendon at shoulder and upper arm level, right arm

IQ 7 S46.902- Unspecified injury of unspecified muscle, fascia and tendon at shoulder and upper arm level, left arm

IQ 7 S46.909- Unspecified injury of unspecified muscle, fascia and tendon at shoulder and upper arm level, unspecified arm

6 S46.91 Strain of unspecified muscle, fascia and tendon at shoulder and upper arm level

SP 7 S46.911- Strain of unspecified muscle, fascia and tendon at shoulder and upper arm level, right arm

SP 7 S46.912- Strain of unspecified muscle, fascia and tendon at shoulder and upper arm level, left arm

IQ 7 S46.919- Strain of unspecified muscle, fascia and tendon at shoulder and upper arm level, unspecified arm

6 S46.92 Laceration of unspecified muscle, fascia and tendon at shoulder and upper arm level

SP 7 S46.921- Laceration of unspecified muscle, fascia and tendon at shoulder and upper arm level, right arm

S46.922- Laceration of unspecified muscle, fascia and tendon at shoulder and upper arm level, left arm

S46.929- Laceration of unspecified muscle, fascia and tendon at shoulder and upper arm level, unspecified arm

S46.99 Other injury of unspecified muscle, fascia and tendon at shoulder and upper arm level

S46.991- Other injury of unspecified muscle, fascia and tendon at shoulder and upper arm level, right arm

S46.992- Other injury of unspecified muscle, fascia and tendon at shoulder and upper arm level, left arm

S46.999- Other injury of unspecified muscle, fascia and tendon at shoulder and upper arm level, unspecified arm

S47 Crushing injury of shoulder and upper arm

Use additional code for all associated injuries

EXCLUDES 2 crushing injury of elbow (S57.0-)

The appropriate 7th character is to be added to each code from category S47
- A initial encounter
- D subsequent encounter
- S sequela

S47.1XX- Crushing injury of right shoulder and upper arm

S47.2XX- Crushing injury of left shoulder and upper arm

S47.9XX- Crushing injury of shoulder and upper arm, unspecified arm

S48 Traumatic amputation of shoulder and upper arm

An amputation not identified as partial or complete should be coded to complete

EXCLUDES 1 traumatic amputation at elbow level (S58.0)

The appropriate 7th character is to be added to each code from category S48
- A initial encounter
- D subsequent encounter
- S sequela

CODING TIPS ✓ Use these codes only when the amputation was due to trauma. There is no need for adding Z89 with traumatic amputations. See Z47.81 for care of amputations not due to trauma.

S48.0 Traumatic amputation at shoulder joint

S48.01 Complete traumatic amputation at shoulder joint

S48.011- Complete traumatic amputation at right shoulder joint

S48.012- Complete traumatic amputation at left shoulder joint

S48.019- Complete traumatic amputation at unspecified shoulder joint

S48.02 Partial traumatic amputation at shoulder joint

S48.021- Partial traumatic amputation at right shoulder joint

S48.022- Partial traumatic amputation at left shoulder joint

S48.029- Partial traumatic amputation at unspecified shoulder joint

S48.1 Traumatic amputation at level between shoulder and elbow

S48.11 Complete traumatic amputation at level between shoulder and elbow

S48.111- Complete traumatic amputation at level between right shoulder and elbow

S48.112- Complete traumatic amputation at level between left shoulder and elbow

S48.119- Complete traumatic amputation at level between unspecified shoulder and elbow

S48.12 Partial traumatic amputation at level between shoulder and elbow

S48.121- Partial traumatic amputation at level between right shoulder and elbow

S48.122- Partial traumatic amputation at level between left shoulder and elbow

S48.129- Partial traumatic amputation at level between unspecified shoulder and elbow

S48.9 Traumatic amputation of shoulder and upper arm, level unspecified

S48.91 Complete traumatic amputation of shoulder and upper arm, level unspecified

S48.911- Complete traumatic amputation of right shoulder and upper arm, level unspecified

S48.912- Complete traumatic amputation of left shoulder and upper arm, level unspecified

S48.919- Complete traumatic amputation of unspecified shoulder and upper arm, level unspecified

S48.92 Partial traumatic amputation of shoulder and upper arm, level unspecified

S48.921- Partial traumatic amputation of right shoulder and upper arm, level unspecified

S48.922- Partial traumatic amputation of left shoulder and upper arm, level unspecified

S48.929- Partial traumatic amputation of unspecified shoulder and upper arm, level unspecified

S49 Other and unspecified injuries of shoulder and upper arm

Chapter 19

S00-T88

4 4th digit required 5 5th digit required 6 6th digit required 7 7th digit required 7th digit placeholder + Additional code Laterality

The appropriate 7th character is to be added to each code from subcategories S49.0 and S49.1

A	initial encounter for closed fracture
D	subsequent encounter for fracture with routine healing
G	subsequent encounter for fracture with delayed healing
K	subsequent encounter for fracture with nonunion
P	subsequent encounter for fracture with malunion
S	sequela

5 **S49.0 Physeal fracture of upper end of humerus**

6 **S49.00 Unspecified physeal fracture of upper end of humerus**

SP 7 **S49.001- Unspecified physeal fracture of upper end of humerus, right arm**

SP 7 **S49.002- Unspecified physeal fracture of upper end of humerus, left arm**

!Q 7 **S49.009- Unspecified physeal fracture of upper end of humerus, unspecified arm**

6 **S49.01 Salter-Harris Type I physeal fracture of upper end of humerus**

SP 7 **S49.011- Salter-Harris Type I physeal fracture of upper end of humerus, right arm**

SP 7 **S49.012- Salter-Harris Type I physeal fracture of upper end of humerus, left arm**

!Q 7 **S49.019- Salter-Harris Type I physeal fracture of upper end of humerus, unspecified arm**

6 **S49.02 Salter-Harris Type II physeal fracture of upper end of humerus**

SP 7 **S49.021- Salter-Harris Type II physeal fracture of upper end of humerus, right arm**

SP 7 **S49.022- Salter-Harris Type II physeal fracture of upper end of humerus, left arm**

!Q 7 **S49.029- Salter-Harris Type II physeal fracture of upper end of humerus, unspecified arm**

6 **S49.03 Salter-Harris Type III physeal fracture of upper end of humerus**

SP 7 **S49.031- Salter-Harris Type III physeal fracture of upper end of humerus, right arm**

SP 7 **S49.032- Salter-Harris Type III physeal fracture of upper end of humerus, left arm**

!Q 7 **S49.039- Salter-Harris Type III physeal fracture of upper end of humerus, unspecified arm**

6 **S49.04 Salter-Harris Type IV physeal fracture of upper end of humerus**

SP 7 **S49.041- Salter-Harris Type IV physeal fracture of upper end of humerus, right arm**

SP 7 **S49.042- Salter-Harris Type IV physeal fracture of upper end of humerus, left arm**

!Q 7 **S49.049- Salter-Harris Type IV physeal fracture of upper end of humerus, unspecified arm**

6 **S49.09 Other physeal fracture of upper end of humerus**

SP 7 **S49.091- Other physeal fracture of upper end of humerus, right arm**

SP 7 **S49.092- Other physeal fracture of upper end of humerus, left arm**

!Q 7 **S49.099- Other physeal fracture of upper end of humerus, unspecified arm**

5 **S49.1 Physeal fracture of lower end of humerus**

6 **S49.10 Unspecified physeal fracture of lower end of humerus**

SP 7 **S49.101- Unspecified physeal fracture of lower end of humerus, right arm**

SP 7 **S49.102- Unspecified physeal fracture of lower end of humerus, left arm**

!Q 7 **S49.109- Unspecified physeal fracture of lower end of humerus, unspecified arm**

6 **S49.11 Salter-Harris Type I physeal fracture of lower end of humerus**

SP 7 **S49.111- Salter-Harris Type I physeal fracture of lower end of humerus, right arm**

SP 7 **S49.112- Salter-Harris Type I physeal fracture of lower end of humerus, left arm**

!Q 7 **S49.119- Salter-Harris Type I physeal fracture of lower end of humerus, unspecified arm**

6 **S49.12 Salter-Harris Type II physeal fracture of lower end of humerus**

SP 7 **S49.121- Salter-Harris Type II physeal fracture of lower end of humerus, right arm**

SP 7 **S49.122- Salter-Harris Type II physeal fracture of lower end of humerus, left arm**

!Q 7 **S49.129- Salter-Harris Type II physeal fracture of lower end of humerus, unspecified arm**

6 **S49.13 Salter-Harris Type III physeal fracture of lower end of humerus**

SP 7 **S49.131- Salter-Harris Type III physeal fracture of lower end of humerus, right arm**

SP 7 **S49.132- Salter-Harris Type III physeal fracture of lower end of humerus, left arm**

!Q 7 **S49.139- Salter-Harris Type III physeal fracture of lower end of humerus, unspecified arm**

6 **S49.14 Salter-Harris Type IV physeal fracture of lower end of humerus**

SP 7 **S49.141- Salter-Harris Type IV physeal fracture of lower end of humerus, right arm**

SP 7 **S49.142- Salter-Harris Type IV physeal fracture of lower end of humerus, left arm**

S49.149- Salter-Harris Type IV physeal fracture of lower end of humerus, unspecified arm

S49.19 Other physeal fracture of lower end of humerus

S49.191- Other physeal fracture of lower end of humerus, right arm

S49.192- Other physeal fracture of lower end of humerus, left arm

S49.199- Other physeal fracture of lower end of humerus, unspecified arm

S49.8 Other specified injuries of shoulder and upper arm

The appropriate 7th character is to be added to each code in subcategory S49.8
A initial encounter
D subsequent encounter
S sequela

S49.80X- Other specified injuries of shoulder and upper arm, unspecified arm

S49.81X- Other specified injuries of right shoulder and upper arm

S49.82X- Other specified injuries of left shoulder and upper arm

S49.9 Unspecified injury of shoulder and upper arm

The appropriate 7th character is to be added to each code in subcategory S49.9
A initial encounter
D subsequent encounter
S sequela

S49.90X- Unspecified injury of shoulder and upper arm, unspecified arm

S49.91X- Unspecified injury of right shoulder and upper arm

S49.92X- Unspecified injury of left shoulder and upper arm

Injuries to the elbow and forearm (S50-S59)

EXCLUDES 2 burns and corrosions (T20-T32)
frostbite (T33-T34)
injuries of wrist and hand (S60-S69)
insect bite or sting, venomous (T63.4)

GUIDELINES **Section I.C.19.c.2)**
Multiple fractures are sequenced in accordance with the severity of the fracture.

GUIDELINES **Section I.C.19.b.1)-2)**
When coding injuries, assign separate codes for each injury unless a combination code is provided, in which case the combination code is assigned ... Traumatic injury codes (S00-T14.9) are not to be used for normal, healing surgical wounds or to identify complications of surgical wounds. The code for the most serious injury, as determined by the provider and the focus of treatment, is sequenced first.

1) Superficial injuries such as abrasions or contusions are not coded when associated with more severe injuries of the same site.

2) When a primary injury results in minor damage to peripheral nerves or blood vessels, the primary injury is sequenced first with additional code(s) for injuries to nerves and spinal cord (such as category S04), and/or injury to blood vessels (such as category S15). When the primary injury is to the blood vessels or nerves, that injury should be sequenced first.

GUIDELINES **Section I.C.19.c**
Coding of Traumatic Fractures: The principles of multiple coding of injuries should be followed in coding fractures. Fractures of specified sites are coded individually by site in accordance with both the provisions within categories S02, S12, S22, S32, S42, S49, S52, S59, S62, S72, S79, S82, S89, S92 and the level of detail furnished by medical record content. A fracture not indicated as open or closed should be coded to closed. A fracture not indicated whether displaced or not displaced should be coded to displaced.

CODING TIPS✓ 7th character A is acceptable in home health and hospice when active treatment is provided, such as antibiotics for an infected wound or a wound vac for a dehisced wound. D is used when the complication or injury is now healing. Think of D as aftercare. S is used for sequela of the injury or complication. Sequela is a residual deficit or condition produced as a result of the injury or complication after the original injury or complication has healed.

S50 Superficial injury of elbow and forearm
EXCLUDES 2 superficial injury of wrist and hand (S60.-)

The appropriate 7th character is to be added to each code from category S50
A initial encounter
D subsequent encounter
S sequela

S50.0 Contusion of elbow

S50.00X- Contusion of unspecified elbow

S50.01X- Contusion of right elbow

S50.02X- Contusion of left elbow

S50.1 Contusion of forearm

S50.10X- Contusion of unspecified forearm

S50.11X- Contusion of right forearm

S50.12X- Contusion of left forearm

S50.3 Other superficial injuries of elbow

S50.31 Abrasion of elbow

S50.311- Abrasion of right elbow

S50.312- Abrasion of left elbow

S50.319- Abrasion of unspecified elbow

S50.32 Blister (nonthermal) of elbow

S50.321- Blister (nonthermal) of right elbow

Chapter 19

S00-T88

4th digit required 5th digit required 6th digit required 7th digit required 7th digit placeholder +Additional code Laterality

S50.322- Blister (nonthermal) of left elbow
S50.329- Blister (nonthermal) of unspecified elbow

S50.34 External constriction of elbow
S50.341- External constriction of right elbow
S50.342- External constriction of left elbow
S50.349- External constriction of unspecified elbow

S50.35 Superficial foreign body of elbow
Splinter in the elbow
S50.351- Superficial foreign body of right elbow
S50.352- Superficial foreign body of left elbow
S50.359- Superficial foreign body of unspecified elbow

S50.36 Insect bite (nonvenomous) of elbow
S50.361- Insect bite (nonvenomous) of right elbow
S50.362- Insect bite (nonvenomous) of left elbow
S50.369- Insect bite (nonvenomous) of unspecified elbow

S50.37 Other superficial bite of elbow
EXCLUDES 1 open bite of elbow (S51.04)
S50.371- Other superficial bite of right elbow
S50.372- Other superficial bite of left elbow
S50.379- Other superficial bite of unspecified elbow

S50.8 Other superficial injuries of forearm

S50.81 Abrasion of forearm
S50.811- Abrasion of right forearm
S50.812- Abrasion of left forearm
S50.819- Abrasion of unspecified forearm

S50.82 Blister (nonthermal) of forearm
S50.821- Blister (nonthermal) of right forearm
S50.822- Blister (nonthermal) of left forearm
S50.829- Blister (nonthermal) of unspecified forearm

S50.84 External constriction of forearm
S50.841- External constriction of right forearm
S50.842- External constriction of left forearm
S50.849- External constriction of unspecified forearm

S50.85 Superficial foreign body of forearm
Splinter in the forearm
S50.851- Superficial foreign body of right forearm
S50.852- Superficial foreign body of left forearm
S50.859- Superficial foreign body of unspecified forearm

S50.86 Insect bite (nonvenomous) of forearm
S50.861- Insect bite (nonvenomous) of right forearm
S50.862- Insect bite (nonvenomous) of left forearm
S50.869- Insect bite (nonvenomous) of unspecified forearm

S50.87 Other superficial bite of forearm
EXCLUDES 1 open bite of forearm (S51.84)
S50.871- Other superficial bite of right forearm
S50.872- Other superficial bite of left forearm
S50.879- Other superficial bite of unspecified forearm

S50.9 Unspecified superficial injury of elbow and forearm

S50.90 Unspecified superficial injury of elbow
S50.901- Unspecified superficial injury of right elbow
S50.902- Unspecified superficial injury of left elbow
S50.909- Unspecified superficial injury of unspecified elbow

S50.91 Unspecified superficial injury of forearm
S50.911- Unspecified superficial injury of right forearm
S50.912- Unspecified superficial injury of left forearm
S50.919- Unspecified superficial injury of unspecified forearm

S51 Open wound of elbow and forearm
Code also:
any associated wound infection
EXCLUDES 1 open fracture of elbow and forearm (S52.- with open fracture 7th character)
traumatic amputation of elbow and forearm (S58.-)
EXCLUDES 2 open wound of wrist and hand (S61.-)

The appropriate 7th character is to be added to each code from category S51
A initial encounter
D subsequent encounter
S sequela

CODING TIPS✓ No aftercare code applies, including those indicating dressing changes, drain care, or suture removal. 7th character 'D' is the default for home care and hospice when providing aftercare for a healing or resolving condition; 'A' is used for active treatment such as antibiotics or more than routine wound care; 'S' may be used to indicate a residual condition after the original injury has healed.

CODING TIPS✓ Open wound codes indicate a wound resulting from a traumatic origin. Do not assign a code for "open wound" unless the etiology of the wound is related to trauma.

S51.0 Open wound of elbow
S51.00 Unspecified open wound of elbow

Chapter 19 S00-T88

S51.001- Unspecified open wound of right elbow
S51.002- Unspecified open wound of left elbow
S51.009- Unspecified open wound of unspecified elbow
Open wound of elbow NOS

S51.01 Laceration without foreign body of elbow
S51.011- Laceration without foreign body of right elbow
S51.012- Laceration without foreign body of left elbow
S51.019- Laceration without foreign body of unspecified elbow

S51.02 Laceration with foreign body of elbow
S51.021- Laceration with foreign body of right elbow
S51.022- Laceration with foreign body of left elbow
S51.029- Laceration with foreign body of unspecified elbow

S51.03 Puncture wound without foreign body of elbow
S51.031- Puncture wound without foreign body of right elbow
S51.032- Puncture wound without foreign body of left elbow
S51.039- Puncture wound without foreign body of unspecified elbow

S51.04 Puncture wound with foreign body of elbow
S51.041- Puncture wound with foreign body of right elbow
S51.042- Puncture wound with foreign body of left elbow
S51.049- Puncture wound with foreign body of unspecified elbow

S51.05 Open bite of elbow
Bite of elbow NOS
EXCLUDES 1 superficial bite of elbow (S50.36, S50.37)
S51.051- Open bite, right elbow
S51.052- Open bite, left elbow
S51.059- Open bite, unspecified elbow

S51.8 Open wound of forearm
EXCLUDES 2 open wound of elbow (S51.0-)

S51.80 Unspecified open wound of forearm
S51.801- Unspecified open wound of right forearm
S51.802- Unspecified open wound of left forearm
S51.809- Unspecified open wound of unspecified forearm
Open wound of forearm NOS

S51.81 Laceration without foreign body of forearm
S51.811- Laceration without foreign body of right forearm
S51.812- Laceration without foreign body of left forearm
S51.819- Laceration without foreign body of unspecified forearm

S51.82 Laceration with foreign body of forearm
S51.821- Laceration with foreign body of right forearm
S51.822- Laceration with foreign body of left forearm
S51.829- Laceration with foreign body of unspecified forearm

S51.83 Puncture wound without foreign body of forearm
S51.831- Puncture wound without foreign body of right forearm
S51.832- Puncture wound without foreign body of left forearm
S51.839- Puncture wound without foreign body of unspecified forearm

S51.84 Puncture wound with foreign body of forearm
S51.841- Puncture wound with foreign body of right forearm
S51.842- Puncture wound with foreign body of left forearm
S51.849- Puncture wound with foreign body of unspecified forearm

S51.85 Open bite of forearm
Bite of forearm NOS
EXCLUDES 1 superficial bite of forearm (S50.86, S50.87)
S51.851- Open bite of right forearm
S51.852- Open bite of left forearm
S51.859- Open bite of unspecified forearm

Chapter 19

S00-T88

4 4th digit required 5 5th digit required 6 6th digit required 7 7th digit required 7th digit placeholder + Additional code Laterality

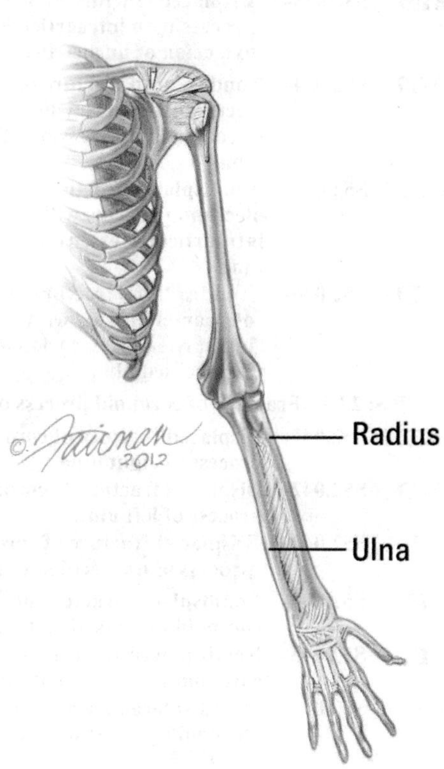

4 S52 Fracture of forearm

Note:

A fracture not indicated as displaced or nondisplaced should be coded to displaced

A fracture not indicated as open or closed should be coded to closed

The open fracture designations are based on the Gustilo open fracture classification

EXCLUDES 1 traumatic amputation of forearm (S58.-)

EXCLUDES 2 fracture at wrist and hand level (S62.-)

The appropriate 7th character is to be added to all codes from category S52

A	initial encounter for closed fracture
B	initial encounter for open fracture type I or II
C	initial encounter for open fracture type IIIA, IIIB, or IIIC
D	subsequent encounter for closed fracture with routine healing
E	subsequent encounter for open fracture type I or II with routine healing
F	subsequent encounter for open fracture type IIIA, IIIB, or IIIC with routine healing
G	subsequent encounter for closed fracture with delayed healing
H	subsequent encounter for open fracture type I or II with delayed healing
J	subsequent encounter for open fracture type IIIA, IIIB, or IIIC with delayed healing
K	subsequent encounter for closed fracture with nonunion
M	subsequent encounter for open fracture type I or II with nonunion
N	subsequent encounter for open fracture type IIIA, IIIB, or IIIC with nonunion
P	subsequent encounter for closed fracture with malunion
Q	subsequent encounter for open fracture type I or II with malunion
R	subsequent encounter for open fracture type IIIA, IIIB, or IIIC with malunion
S	sequela

CODING TIPS✓ Fractures repaired by joint replacements are NOT coded with Z47.1. Fractures repaired by any other orthopedic surgery are NOT coded with Z47.89. Z codes are not appropriate for fractures of any kind. Code the fracture with 7th character D for fractures undergoing surgical repair.

CODING TIPS✓ "D" is the 7th character for home care and hospice unless the physician or NPP has documented delayed healing, nonunion or malunion. A sequela is a condition left after the fracture has healed.

CODING TIPS✓ A fracture not indicated as displaced or nondisplaced should be coded to displaced. A fracture not indicated as open or closed should be coded to closed. The open fracture designations are based on the Gustilo open fracture classification. The 7th characters E, H, M and Q are the default for the Gustilo classification when no information is available. Always query the physician or NPP.

5 S52.0 Fracture of upper end of ulna

Fracture of proximal end of ulna

EXCLUDES 2 fracture of elbow NOS (S42.40-)

fractures of shaft of ulna (S52.2-)

Chapter 19

S00-T88

6 **S52.00 Unspecified fracture of upper end of ulna**

Laterality SP 7 **S52.001- Unspecified fracture of upper end of right ulna**

Laterality SP 7 **S52.002- Unspecified fracture of upper end of left ulna**

Laterality IQ 7 **S52.009- Unspecified fracture of upper end of unspecified ulna**

6 **S52.01 Torus fracture of upper end of ulna**

The appropriate 7th character is to be added to all codes in subcategory S52.01

- A initial encounter for closed fracture
- D subsequent encounter for fracture with routine healing
- G subsequent encounter for fracture with delayed healing
- K subsequent encounter for fracture with nonunion
- P subsequent encounter for fracture with malunion
- S sequela

CODING TIPS✓ Open fractures do not occur with torus fractures and greenstick fractures, therefore the 7th characters for open fractures are not available.

Laterality SP 7 **S52.011- Torus fracture of upper end of right ulna**

Laterality SP 7 **S52.012- Torus fracture of upper end of left ulna**

Laterality IQ 7 **S52.019- Torus fracture of upper end of unspecified ulna**

6 **S52.02 Fracture of olecranon process without intraarticular extension of ulna**

Laterality SP 7 **S52.021- Displaced fracture of olecranon process without intraarticular extension of right ulna**

Laterality SP 7 **S52.022- Displaced fracture of olecranon process without intraarticular extension of left ulna**

Laterality IQ 7 **S52.023- Displaced fracture of olecranon process without intraarticular extension of unspecified ulna**

Laterality SP 7 **S52.024- Nondisplaced fracture of olecranon process without intraarticular extension of right ulna**

Laterality SP 7 **S52.025- Nondisplaced fracture of olecranon process without intraarticular extension of left ulna**

Laterality IQ 7 **S52.026- Nondisplaced fracture of olecranon process without intraarticular extension of unspecified ulna**

6 **S52.03 Fracture of olecranon process with intraarticular extension of ulna**

Laterality SP 7 **S52.031- Displaced fracture of olecranon process with intraarticular extension of right ulna**

Laterality SP 7 **S52.032- Displaced fracture of olecranon process with intraarticular extension of left ulna**

Laterality IQ 7 **S52.033- Displaced fracture of olecranon process with intraarticular extension of unspecified ulna**

Laterality SP 7 **S52.034- Nondisplaced fracture of olecranon process with intraarticular extension of right ulna**

Laterality SP 7 **S52.035- Nondisplaced fracture of olecranon process with intraarticular extension of left ulna**

Laterality IQ 7 **S52.036- Nondisplaced fracture of olecranon process with intraarticular extension of unspecified ulna**

6 **S52.04 Fracture of coronoid process of ulna**

Laterality SP 7 **S52.041- Displaced fracture of coronoid process of right ulna**

Laterality SP 7 **S52.042- Displaced fracture of coronoid process of left ulna**

Laterality IQ 7 **S52.043- Displaced fracture of coronoid process of unspecified ulna**

Laterality SP 7 **S52.044- Nondisplaced fracture of coronoid process of right ulna**

Laterality SP 7 **S52.045- Nondisplaced fracture of coronoid process of left ulna**

Laterality IQ 7 **S52.046- Nondisplaced fracture of coronoid process of unspecified ulna**

6 **S52.09 Other fracture of upper end of ulna**

Laterality SP 7 **S52.091- Other fracture of upper end of right ulna**

Laterality SP 7 **S52.092- Other fracture of upper end of left ulna**

Laterality IQ 7 **S52.099- Other fracture of upper end of unspecified ulna**

5 **S52.1 Fracture of upper end of radius**

Fracture of proximal end of radius

EXCLUDES 2 physeal fractures of upper end of radius (S59.2-)
fracture of shaft of radius (S52.3-)

6 **S52.10 Unspecified fracture of upper end of radius**

Laterality SP 7 **S52.101- Unspecified fracture of upper end of right radius**

Laterality SP 7 **S52.102- Unspecified fracture of upper end of left radius**

Laterality IQ 7 **S52.109- Unspecified fracture of upper end of unspecified radius**

6 **S52.11 Torus fracture of upper end of radius**

The appropriate 7th character is to be added to all codes in subcategory S52.11
A initial encounter for closed fracture
D subsequent encounter for fracture with routine healing
G subsequent encounter for fracture with delayed healing
K subsequent encounter for fracture with nonunion
P subsequent encounter for fracture with malunion
S sequela

CODING TIPS✓ Open fractures do not occur with torus fractures and greenstick fractures, therefore the 7th characters for open fractures are not available.

SP 7 **S52.111- Torus fracture of upper end of right radius**
SP 7 **S52.112- Torus fracture of upper end of left radius**
!Q 7 **S52.119- Torus fracture of upper end of unspecified radius**

6 **S52.12 Fracture of head of radius**
SP 7 **S52.121- Displaced fracture of head of right radius**
SP 7 **S52.122- Displaced fracture of head of left radius**
!Q 7 **S52.123- Displaced fracture of head of unspecified radius**
SP 7 **S52.124- Nondisplaced fracture of head of right radius**
SP 7 **S52.125- Nondisplaced fracture of head of left radius**
!Q 7 **S52.126- Nondisplaced fracture of head of unspecified radius**

6 **S52.13 Fracture of neck of radius**
SP 7 **S52.131- Displaced fracture of neck of right radius**
SP 7 **S52.132- Displaced fracture of neck of left radius**
!Q 7 **S52.133- Displaced fracture of neck of unspecified radius**
SP 7 **S52.134- Nondisplaced fracture of neck of right radius**
SP 7 **S52.135- Nondisplaced fracture of neck of left radius**
!Q 7 **S52.136- Nondisplaced fracture of neck of unspecified radius**

6 **S52.18 Other fracture of upper end of radius**
SP 7 **S52.181- Other fracture of upper end of right radius**
SP 7 **S52.182- Other fracture of upper end of left radius**
!Q 7 **S52.189- Other fracture of upper end of unspecified radius**

5 **S52.2 Fracture of shaft of ulna**

6 **S52.20 Unspecified fracture of shaft of ulna**
Fracture of ulna NOS
SP 7 **S52.201- Unspecified fracture of shaft of right ulna**
SP 7 **S52.202- Unspecified fracture of shaft of left ulna**
!Q 7 **S52.209- Unspecified fracture of shaft of unspecified ulna**

6 **S52.21 Greenstick fracture of shaft of ulna**

The appropriate 7th character is to be added to all codes in subcategory S52.21
A initial encounter for closed fracture
D subsequent encounter for fracture with routine healing
G subsequent encounter for fracture with delayed healing
K subsequent encounter for fracture with nonunion
P subsequent encounter for fracture with malunion
S sequela

CODING TIPS✓ Open fractures do not occur with torus fractures and greenstick fractures, therefore the 7th characters for open fractures are not available.

SP 7 **S52.211- Greenstick fracture of shaft of right ulna**
SP 7 **S52.212- Greenstick fracture of shaft of left ulna**
!Q 7 **S52.219- Greenstick fracture of shaft of unspecified ulna**

6 **S52.22 Transverse fracture of shaft of ulna**
SP 7 **S52.221- Displaced transverse fracture of shaft of right ulna**
SP 7 **S52.222- Displaced transverse fracture of shaft of left ulna**
!Q 7 **S52.223- Displaced transverse fracture of shaft of unspecified ulna**
SP 7 **S52.224- Nondisplaced transverse fracture of shaft of right ulna**
SP 7 **S52.225- Nondisplaced transverse fracture of shaft of left ulna**
!Q 7 **S52.226- Nondisplaced transverse fracture of shaft of unspecified ulna**

6 **S52.23 Oblique fracture of shaft of ulna**
SP 7 **S52.231- Displaced oblique fracture of shaft of right ulna**
SP 7 **S52.232- Displaced oblique fracture of shaft of left ulna**
!Q 7 **S52.233- Displaced oblique fracture of shaft of unspecified ulna**
SP 7 **S52.234- Nondisplaced oblique fracture of shaft of right ulna**
SP 7 **S52.235- Nondisplaced oblique fracture of shaft of left ulna**
!Q 7 **S52.236- Nondisplaced oblique fracture of shaft of unspecified ulna**

6 **S52.24 Spiral fracture of shaft of ulna**
SP !Q 7 **S52.241- Displaced spiral fracture of shaft of ulna, right arm**
SP 7 **S52.242- Displaced spiral fracture of shaft of ulna, left arm**
!Q 7 **S52.243- Displaced spiral fracture of shaft of ulna, unspecified arm**

S52.244- Nondisplaced spiral fracture of shaft of ulna, right arm
S52.245- Nondisplaced spiral fracture of shaft of ulna, left arm
S52.246- Nondisplaced spiral fracture of shaft of ulna, unspecified arm

S52.25 Comminuted fracture of shaft of ulna
S52.251- Displaced comminuted fracture of shaft of ulna, right arm
S52.252- Displaced comminuted fracture of shaft of ulna, left arm
S52.253- Displaced comminuted fracture of shaft of ulna, unspecified arm
S52.254- Nondisplaced comminuted fracture of shaft of ulna, right arm
S52.255- Nondisplaced comminuted fracture of shaft of ulna, left arm
S52.256- Nondisplaced comminuted fracture of shaft of ulna, unspecified arm

S52.26 Segmental fracture of shaft of ulna
S52.261- Displaced segmental fracture of shaft of ulna, right arm
S52.262- Displaced segmental fracture of shaft of ulna, left arm
S52.263- Displaced segmental fracture of shaft of ulna, unspecified arm
S52.264- Nondisplaced segmental fracture of shaft of ulna, right arm
S52.265- Nondisplaced segmental fracture of shaft of ulna, left arm
S52.266- Nondisplaced segmental fracture of shaft of ulna, unspecified arm

S52.27 Monteggia's fracture of ulna
Fracture of upper shaft of ulna with dislocation of radial head
S52.271- Monteggia's fracture of right ulna
S52.272- Monteggia's fracture of left ulna
S52.279- Monteggia's fracture of unspecified ulna

S52.28 Bent bone of ulna
S52.281- Bent bone of right ulna
S52.282- Bent bone of left ulna
S52.283- Bent bone of unspecified ulna

S52.29 Other fracture of shaft of ulna
S52.291- Other fracture of shaft of right ulna
S52.292- Other fracture of shaft of left ulna
S52.299- Other fracture of shaft of unspecified ulna

S52.3 Fracture of shaft of radius
S52.30 Unspecified fracture of shaft of radius
S52.301- Unspecified fracture of shaft of right radius
S52.302- Unspecified fracture of shaft of left radius
S52.309- Unspecified fracture of shaft of unspecified radius

S52.31 Greenstick fracture of shaft of radius

The appropriate 7th character is to be added to all codes in subcategory S52.31

A	initial encounter for closed fracture
D	subsequent encounter for fracture with routine healing
G	subsequent encounter for fracture with delayed healing
K	subsequent encounter for fracture with nonunion
P	subsequent encounter for fracture with malunion
S	sequela

CODING TIPS ✓ Open fractures do not occur with torus fractures and greenstick fractures, therefore the 7th characters for open fractures are not available.

S52.311- Greenstick fracture of shaft of radius, right arm
S52.312- Greenstick fracture of shaft of radius, left arm
S52.319- Greenstick fracture of shaft of radius, unspecified arm

S52.32 Transverse fracture of shaft of radius
S52.321- Displaced transverse fracture of shaft of right radius
S52.322- Displaced transverse fracture of shaft of left radius
S52.323- Displaced transverse fracture of shaft of unspecified radius
S52.324- Nondisplaced transverse fracture of shaft of right radius
S52.325- Nondisplaced transverse fracture of shaft of left radius
S52.326- Nondisplaced transverse fracture of shaft of unspecified radius

S52.33 Oblique fracture of shaft of radius
S52.331- Displaced oblique fracture of shaft of right radius
S52.332- Displaced oblique fracture of shaft of left radius
S52.333- Displaced oblique fracture of shaft of unspecified radius
S52.334- Nondisplaced oblique fracture of shaft of right radius
S52.335- Nondisplaced oblique fracture of shaft of left radius
S52.336- Nondisplaced oblique fracture of shaft of unspecified radius

S52.34 Spiral fracture of shaft of radius
S52.341- Displaced spiral fracture of shaft of radius, right arm
S52.342- Displaced spiral fracture of shaft of radius, left arm
S52.343- Displaced spiral fracture of shaft of radius, unspecified arm
S52.344- Nondisplaced spiral fracture of shaft of radius, right arm
S52.345- Nondisplaced spiral fracture of shaft of radius, left arm

Chapter 19
S00-T88

IQ 7 **S52.346-** **Nondisplaced spiral fracture of shaft of radius, unspecified arm**

6 **S52.35** **Comminuted fracture of shaft of radius**

SP 7 **S52.351-** **Displaced comminuted fracture of shaft of radius, right arm**

SP 7 **S52.352-** **Displaced comminuted fracture of shaft of radius, left arm**

IQ 7 **S52.353-** **Displaced comminuted fracture of shaft of radius, unspecified arm**

SP 7 **S52.354-** **Nondisplaced comminuted fracture of shaft of radius, right arm**

SP 7 **S52.355-** **Nondisplaced comminuted fracture of shaft of radius, left arm**

IQ 7 **S52.356-** **Nondisplaced comminuted fracture of shaft of radius, unspecified arm**

6 **S52.36** **Segmental fracture of shaft of radius**

SP 7 **S52.361-** **Displaced segmental fracture of shaft of radius, right arm**

SP 7 **S52.362-** **Displaced segmental fracture of shaft of radius, left arm**

IQ 7 **S52.363-** **Displaced segmental fracture of shaft of radius, unspecified arm**

SP 7 **S52.364-** **Nondisplaced segmental fracture of shaft of radius, right arm**

SP 7 **S52.365-** **Nondisplaced segmental fracture of shaft of radius, left arm**

IQ 7 **S52.366-** **Nondisplaced segmental fracture of shaft of radius, unspecified arm**

6 **S52.37** **Galeazzi's fracture**

Fracture of lower shaft of radius with radioulnar joint dislocation

SP 7 **S52.371-** **Galeazzi's fracture of right radius**

SP 7 **S52.372-** **Galeazzi's fracture of left radius**

IQ 7 **S52.379-** **Galeazzi's fracture of unspecified radius**

6 **S52.38** **Bent bone of radius**

SP 7 **S52.381-** **Bent bone of right radius**

SP 7 **S52.382-** **Bent bone of left radius**

SP IQ 7 **S52.389-** **Bent bone of unspecified radius**

6 **S52.39** **Other fracture of shaft of radius**

SP 7 **S52.391-** **Other fracture of shaft of radius, right arm**

SP 7 **S52.392-** **Other fracture of shaft of radius, left arm**

IQ 7 **S52.399-** **Other fracture of shaft of radius, unspecified arm**

5 **S52.5** **Fracture of lower end of radius**

Fracture of distal end of radius

EXCLUDES 2 physeal fractures of lower end of radius (S59.2-)

6 **S52.50** **Unspecified fracture of the lower end of radius**

SP 7 **S52.501-** **Unspecified fracture of the lower end of right radius**

SP 7 **S52.502-** **Unspecified fracture of the lower end of left radius**

IQ 7 **S52.509-** **Unspecified fracture of the lower end of unspecified radius**

6 **S52.51** **Fracture of radial styloid process**

SP 7 **S52.511-** **Displaced fracture of right radial styloid process**

SP 7 **S52.512-** **Displaced fracture of left radial styloid process**

IQ 7 **S52.513-** **Displaced fracture of unspecified radial styloid process**

SP 7 **S52.514-** **Nondisplaced fracture of right radial styloid process**

SP 7 **S52.515-** **Nondisplaced fracture of left radial styloid process**

IQ 7 **S52.516-** **Nondisplaced fracture of unspecified radial styloid process**

6 **S52.52** **Torus fracture of lower end of radius**

The appropriate 7th character is to be added to all codes in subcategory S52.52

A	initial encounter for closed fracture
D	subsequent encounter for fracture with routine healing
G	subsequent encounter for fracture with delayed healing
K	subsequent encounter for fracture with nonunion
P	subsequent encounter for fracture with malunion
S	sequela

CODING TIPS✓ Open fractures do not occur with torus fractures and greenstick fractures, therefore the 7th characters for open fractures are not available.

SP 7 **S52.521-** **Torus fracture of lower end of right radius**

SP 7 **S52.522-** **Torus fracture of lower end of left radius**

IQ 7 **S52.529-** **Torus fracture of lower end of unspecified radius**

6 **S52.53** **Colles' fracture**

DEFINITION Break in the lower end of the radius with posterior displacement of the wrist, often caused by breaking a fall with an extended, outstretched hand.

SP 7 **S52.531-** **Colles' fracture of right radius**

SP 7 **S52.532-** **Colles' fracture of left radius**

IQ 7 **S52.539-** **Colles' fracture of unspecified radius**

6 **S52.54** **Smith's fracture**

DEFINITION Break in the lower end of the radius with palmar displacement of the wrist; a reverse Colles' fracture.

SP 7 **S52.541-** **Smith's fracture of right radius**

SP 7 **S52.542-** **Smith's fracture of left radius**

IQ 7 **S52.549-** **Smith's fracture of unspecified radius**

6 **S52.55** **Other extraarticular fracture of lower end of radius**

SP 7 **S52.551-** **Other extraarticular fracture of lower end of right radius**

SP 7 **S52.552-** **Other extraarticular fracture of lower end of left radius**

Chapter 19

S00-T88

S52.559- **Other extraarticular fracture of lower end of unspecified radius**

S52.56 **Barton's fracture**

S52.561- **Barton's fracture of right radius**

S52.562- **Barton's fracture of left radius**

S52.569- **Barton's fracture of unspecified radius**

S52.57 **Other intraarticular fracture of lower end of radius**

S52.571- **Other intraarticular fracture of lower end of right radius**

S52.572- **Other intraarticular fracture of lower end of left radius**

S52.579- **Other intraarticular fracture of lower end of unspecified radius**

S52.59 **Other fractures of lower end of radius**

S52.591- **Other fractures of lower end of right radius**

S52.592- **Other fractures of lower end of left radius**

S52.599- **Other fractures of lower end of unspecified radius**

S52.6 **Fracture of lower end of ulna**

S52.60 **Unspecified fracture of lower end of ulna**

S52.601- **Unspecified fracture of lower end of right ulna**

S52.602- **Unspecified fracture of lower end of left ulna**

S52.609- **Unspecified fracture of lower end of unspecified ulna**

S52.61 **Fracture of ulna styloid process**

S52.611- **Displaced fracture of right ulna styloid process**

S52.612- **Displaced fracture of left ulna styloid process**

S52.613- **Displaced fracture of unspecified ulna styloid process**

S52.614- **Nondisplaced fracture of right ulna styloid process**

S52.615- **Nondisplaced fracture of left ulna styloid process**

S52.616- **Nondisplaced fracture of unspecified ulna styloid process**

S52.62 **Torus fracture of lower end of ulna**

The appropriate 7th character is to be added to all codes in subcategory S52.62

A	initial encounter for closed fracture
D	subsequent encounter for fracture with routine healing
G	subsequent encounter for fracture with delayed healing
K	subsequent encounter for fracture with nonunion
P	subsequent encounter for fracture with malunion
S	sequela

S52.621- **Torus fracture of lower end of right ulna**

S52.622- **Torus fracture of lower end of left ulna**

S52.629- **Torus fracture of lower end of unspecified ulna**

S52.69 **Other fracture of lower end of ulna**

S52.691- **Other fracture of lower end of right ulna**

S52.692- **Other fracture of lower end of left ulna**

S52.699- **Other fracture of lower end of unspecified ulna**

S52.9 **Unspecified fracture of forearm**

S52.90X- **Unspecified fracture of unspecified forearm**

S52.91X- **Unspecified fracture of right forearm**

S52.92X- **Unspecified fracture of left forearm**

S53 **Dislocation and sprain of joints and ligaments of elbow**

INCLUDES avulsion of joint or ligament of elbow
laceration of cartilage, joint or ligament of elbow
sprain of cartilage, joint or ligament of elbow
traumatic hemarthrosis of joint or ligament of elbow
traumatic rupture of joint or ligament of elbow
traumatic subluxation of joint or ligament of elbow
traumatic tear of joint or ligament of elbow

Code also:
any associated open wound

EXCLUDES 2 strain of muscle, fascia and tendon at forearm level (S56.-)

The appropriate 7th character is to be added to each code from category S53

A	initial encounter
D	subsequent encounter
S	sequela

S53.0 **Subluxation and dislocation of radial head**
Dislocation of radiohumeral joint
Subluxation of radiohumeral joint

EXCLUDES 1 Monteggia's fracture-dislocation (S52.27-)

S53.00 **Unspecified subluxation and dislocation of radial head**

S53.001- **Unspecified subluxation of right radial head**

S53.002- **Unspecified subluxation of left radial head**

S53.003- **Unspecified subluxation of unspecified radial head**

S53.004- **Unspecified dislocation of right radial head**

S53.005- **Unspecified dislocation of left radial head**

S53.006- **Unspecified dislocation of unspecified radial head**

S53.01 **Anterior subluxation and dislocation of radial head**

Chapter 19

S00-T88

4th digit required 5th digit required 6th digit required 7th digit required 7th digit placeholder + Additional code Laterality

Anteriomedial subluxation and dislocation of radial head

H SP 7 S53.011- **Anterior subluxation of right radial head**

H SP 7 S53.012- **Anterior subluxation of left radial head**

H IQ 7 S53.013- **Anterior subluxation of unspecified radial head**

H SP 7 S53.014- **Anterior dislocation of right radial head**

H SP 7 S53.015- **Anterior dislocation of left radial head**

H IQ 7 S53.016- **Anterior dislocation of unspecified radial head**

6 S53.02 **Posterior subluxation and dislocation of radial head**

Posteriolateral subluxation and dislocation of radial head

H SP 7 S53.021- **Posterior subluxation of right radial head**

H SP 7 S53.022- **Posterior subluxation of left radial head**

H IQ 7 S53.023- **Posterior subluxation of unspecified radial head**

H SP 7 S53.024- **Posterior dislocation of right radial head**

H SP 7 S53.025- **Posterior dislocation of left radial head**

H IQ 7 S53.026- **Posterior dislocation of unspecified radial head**

6 S53.03 **Nursemaid's elbow**

H SP 7 S53.031- **Nursemaid's elbow, right elbow**

H SP 7 S53.032- **Nursemaid's elbow, left elbow**

H IQ 7 S53.033- **Nursemaid's elbow, unspecified elbow**

6 S53.09 **Other subluxation and dislocation of radial head**

H SP 7 S53.091- **Other subluxation of right radial head**

H SP 7 S53.092- **Other subluxation of left radial head**

H IQ 7 S53.093- **Other subluxation of unspecified radial head**

H SP 7 S53.094- **Other dislocation of right radial head**

H SP 7 S53.095- **Other dislocation of left radial head**

H IQ 7 S53.096- **Other dislocation of unspecified radial head**

5 S53.1 **Subluxation and dislocation of ulnohumeral joint**

Subluxation and dislocation of elbow NOS

EXCLUDES 1 dislocation of radial head alone (S53.0-)

6 S53.10 **Unspecified subluxation and dislocation of ulnohumeral joint**

H SP 7 S53.101- **Unspecified subluxation of right ulnohumeral joint**

H SP 7 S53.102- **Unspecified subluxation of left ulnohumeral joint**

H IQ 7 S53.103- **Unspecified subluxation of unspecified ulnohumeral joint**

H SP 7 S53.104- **Unspecified dislocation of right ulnohumeral joint**

H SP 7 S53.105- **Unspecified dislocation of left ulnohumeral joint**

H IQ 7 S53.106- **Unspecified dislocation of unspecified ulnohumeral joint**

6 S53.11 **Anterior subluxation and dislocation of ulnohumeral joint**

H SP 7 S53.111- **Anterior subluxation of right ulnohumeral joint**

H SP 7 S53.112- **Anterior subluxation of left ulnohumeral joint**

H IQ 7 S53.113- **Anterior subluxation of unspecified ulnohumeral joint**

H SP 7 S53.114- **Anterior dislocation of right ulnohumeral joint**

H SP 7 S53.115- **Anterior dislocation of left ulnohumeral joint**

H IQ 7 S53.116- **Anterior dislocation of unspecified ulnohumeral joint**

6 S53.12 **Posterior subluxation and dislocation of ulnohumeral joint**

H SP 7 S53.121- **Posterior subluxation of right ulnohumeral joint**

H SP 7 S53.122- **Posterior subluxation of left ulnohumeral joint**

H IQ 7 S53.123- **Posterior subluxation of unspecified ulnohumeral joint**

H SP 7 S53.124- **Posterior dislocation of right ulnohumeral joint**

H SP 7 S53.125- **Posterior dislocation of left ulnohumeral joint**

H IQ 7 S53.126- **Posterior dislocation of unspecified ulnohumeral joint**

6 S53.13 **Medial subluxation and dislocation of ulnohumeral joint**

H SP 7 S53.131- **Medial subluxation of right ulnohumeral joint**

H SP 7 S53.132- **Medial subluxation of left ulnohumeral joint**

H IQ 7 S53.133- **Medial subluxation of unspecified ulnohumeral joint**

H SP 7 S53.134- **Medial dislocation of right ulnohumeral joint**

H SP 7 S53.135- **Medial dislocation of left ulnohumeral joint**

H IQ 7 S53.136- **Medial dislocation of unspecified ulnohumeral joint**

6 S53.14 **Lateral subluxation and dislocation of ulnohumeral joint**

H SP 7 S53.141- **Lateral subluxation of right ulnohumeral joint**

H SP 7 S53.142- **Lateral subluxation of left ulnohumeral joint**

H IQ 7 S53.143- **Lateral subluxation of unspecified ulnohumeral joint**

H SP 7 S53.144- **Lateral dislocation of right ulnohumeral joint**

H SP 7 S53.145- **Lateral dislocation of left ulnohumeral joint**

H IQ 7 S53.146- **Lateral dislocation of unspecified ulnohumeral joint**

6 S53.19 **Other subluxation and dislocation of ulnohumeral joint**

H SP 7 S53.191- **Other subluxation of right ulnohumeral joint**

H SP 7 S53.192- **Other subluxation of left ulnohumeral joint**

⊟ IQ 7 **S53.193- Other subluxation of unspecified ulnohumeral joint**

⊟ SP 7 **S53.194- Other dislocation of right ulnohumeral joint**

⊟ SP 7 **S53.195- Other dislocation of left ulnohumeral joint**

⊟ IQ 7 **S53.196- Other dislocation of unspecified ulnohumeral joint**

5 **S53.2 Traumatic rupture of radial collateral ligament**

EXCLUDES 1 sprain of radial collateral ligament NOS (S53.43-)

⊟ IQ 7 **S53.20X- Traumatic rupture of unspecified radial collateral ligament**

⊟ SP 7 **S53.21X- Traumatic rupture of right radial collateral ligament**

⊟ SP 7 **S53.22X- Traumatic rupture of left radial collateral ligament**

5 **S53.3 Traumatic rupture of ulnar collateral ligament**

EXCLUDES 1 sprain of ulnar collateral ligament (S53.44-)

⊟ IQ 7 **S53.30X- Traumatic rupture of unspecified ulnar collateral ligament**

⊟ SP 7 **S53.31X- Traumatic rupture of right ulnar collateral ligament**

⊟ SP 7 **S53.32X- Traumatic rupture of left ulnar collateral ligament**

5 **S53.4 Sprain of elbow**

EXCLUDES 2 traumatic rupture of radial collateral ligament (S53.2-)
traumatic rupture of ulnar collateral ligament (S53.3-)

6 **S53.40 Unspecified sprain of elbow**

⊟ SP 7 **S53.401- Unspecified sprain of right elbow**

⊟ SP 7 **S53.402- Unspecified sprain of left elbow**

⊟ IQ 7 **S53.409- Unspecified sprain of unspecified elbow**

Sprain of elbow NOS

6 **S53.41 Radiohumeral (joint) sprain**

⊟ SP 7 **S53.411- Radiohumeral (joint) sprain of right elbow**

⊟ SP 7 **S53.412- Radiohumeral (joint) sprain of left elbow**

⊟ IQ 7 **S53.419- Radiohumeral (joint) sprain of unspecified elbow**

6 **S53.42 Ulnohumeral (joint) sprain**

⊟ SP 7 **S53.421- Ulnohumeral (joint) sprain of right elbow**

⊟ SP 7 **S53.422- Ulnohumeral (joint) sprain of left elbow**

⊟ IQ 7 **S53.429- Ulnohumeral (joint) sprain of unspecified elbow**

6 **S53.43 Radial collateral ligament sprain**

⊟ SP 7 **S53.431- Radial collateral ligament sprain of right elbow**

⊟ SP 7 **S53.432- Radial collateral ligament sprain of left elbow**

⊟ IQ 7 **S53.439- Radial collateral ligament sprain of unspecified elbow**

6 **S53.44 Ulnar collateral ligament sprain**

⊟ SP 7 **S53.441- Ulnar collateral ligament sprain of right elbow**

⊟ SP 7 **S53.442- Ulnar collateral ligament sprain of left elbow**

⊟ IQ 7 **S53.449- Ulnar collateral ligament sprain of unspecified elbow**

6 **S53.49 Other sprain of elbow**

⊟ SP 7 **S53.491- Other sprain of right elbow**

⊟ SP 7 **S53.492- Other sprain of left elbow**

⊟ IQ 7 **S53.499- Other sprain of unspecified elbow**

4 **S54 Injury of nerves at forearm level**

Code also:
any associated open wound (S51.-)

EXCLUDES 2 injury of nerves at wrist and hand level (S64.-)

The appropriate 7th character is to be added to each code from category S54

A	initial encounter
D	subsequent encounter
S	sequela

5 **S54.0 Injury of ulnar nerve at forearm level**

Injury of ulnar nerve NOS

⊟ IQ 7 **S54.00X- Injury of ulnar nerve at forearm level, unspecified arm**

⊟ SP 7 **S54.01X- Injury of ulnar nerve at forearm level, right arm**

⊟ SP 7 **S54.02X- Injury of ulnar nerve at forearm level, left arm**

5 **S54.1 Injury of median nerve at forearm level**

Injury of median nerve NOS

⊟ IQ 7 **S54.10X- Injury of median nerve at forearm level, unspecified arm**

⊟ SP 7 **S54.11X- Injury of median nerve at forearm level, right arm**

⊟ SP 7 **S54.12X- Injury of median nerve at forearm level, left arm**

5 **S54.2 Injury of radial nerve at forearm level**

Injury of radial nerve NOS

⊟ IQ 7 **S54.20X- Injury of radial nerve at forearm level, unspecified arm**

⊟ SP 7 **S54.21X- Injury of radial nerve at forearm level, right arm**

⊟ SP 7 **S54.22X- Injury of radial nerve at forearm level, left arm**

5 **S54.3 Injury of cutaneous sensory nerve at forearm level**

⊟ IQ 7 **S54.30X- Injury of cutaneous sensory nerve at forearm level, unspecified arm**

⊟ SP 7 **S54.31X- Injury of cutaneous sensory nerve at forearm level, right arm**

⊟ SP 7 **S54.32X- Injury of cutaneous sensory nerve at forearm level, left arm**

5 **S54.8 Injury of other nerves at forearm level**

6 **S54.8X Injury of other nerves at forearm level**

⊟ SP 7 **S54.8X1- Injury of other nerves at forearm level, right arm**

⊟ SP 7 **S54.8X2- Injury of other nerves at forearm level, left arm**

⊟ IQ 7 **S54.8X9- Injury of other nerves at forearm level, unspecified arm**

5 **S54.9 Injury of unspecified nerve at forearm level**

4 4th digit required 5 5th digit required 6 6th digit required 7 7th digit required 7 7th digit placeholder + Additional code ⊟ Laterality

S54.90X- Injury of unspecified nerve at forearm level, unspecified arm

S54.91X- Injury of unspecified nerve at forearm level, right arm

S54.92X- Injury of unspecified nerve at forearm level, left arm

4 S55 Injury of blood vessels at forearm level

Code also:

any associated open wound (S51.-)

EXCLUDES 2 injury of blood vessels at wrist and hand level (S65.-)

injury of brachial vessels (S45.1-S45.2)

The appropriate 7th character is to be added to each code from category S55

A initial encounter

D subsequent encounter

S sequela

5 S55.0 Injury of ulnar artery at forearm level

6 S55.00 Unspecified injury of ulnar artery at forearm level

IQ 7 S55.001- Unspecified injury of ulnar artery at forearm level, right arm

IQ 7 S55.002- Unspecified injury of ulnar artery at forearm level, left arm

IQ 7 S55.009- Unspecified injury of ulnar artery at forearm level, unspecified arm

6 S55.01 Laceration of ulnar artery at forearm level

SP 7 S55.011- Laceration of ulnar artery at forearm level, right arm

SP 7 S55.012- Laceration of ulnar artery at forearm level, left arm

IQ 7 S55.019- Laceration of ulnar artery at forearm level, unspecified arm

6 S55.09 Other specified injury of ulnar artery at forearm level

SP 7 S55.091- Other specified injury of ulnar artery at forearm level, right arm

SP 7 S55.092- Other specified injury of ulnar artery at forearm level, left arm

IQ 7 S55.099- Other specified injury of ulnar artery at forearm level, unspecified arm

5 S55.1 Injury of radial artery at forearm level

6 S55.10 Unspecified injury of radial artery at forearm level

IQ 7 S55.101- Unspecified injury of radial artery at forearm level, right arm

IQ 7 S55.102- Unspecified injury of radial artery at forearm level, left arm

IQ 7 S55.109- Unspecified injury of radial artery at forearm level, unspecified arm

6 S55.11 Laceration of radial artery at forearm level

SP 7 S55.111- Laceration of radial artery at forearm level, right arm

SP 7 S55.112- Laceration of radial artery at forearm level, left arm

IQ 7 S55.119- Laceration of radial artery at forearm level, unspecified arm

6 S55.19 Other specified injury of radial artery at forearm level

SP 7 S55.191- Other specified injury of radial artery at forearm level, right arm

SP 7 S55.192- Other specified injury of radial artery at forearm level, left arm

IQ 7 S55.199- Other specified injury of radial artery at forearm level, unspecified arm

5 S55.2 Injury of vein at forearm level

6 S55.20 Unspecified injury of vein at forearm level

IQ 7 S55.201- Unspecified injury of vein at forearm level, right arm

IQ 7 S55.202- Unspecified injury of vein at forearm level, left arm

IQ 7 S55.209- Unspecified injury of vein at forearm level, unspecified arm

6 S55.21 Laceration of vein at forearm level

SP 7 S55.211- Laceration of vein at forearm level, right arm

SP 7 S55.212- Laceration of vein at forearm level, left arm

IQ 7 S55.219- Laceration of vein at forearm level, unspecified arm

6 S55.29 Other specified injury of vein at forearm level

SP 7 S55.291- Other specified injury of vein at forearm level, right arm

SP 7 S55.292- Other specified injury of vein at forearm level, left arm

IQ 7 S55.299- Other specified injury of vein at forearm level, unspecified arm

5 S55.8 Injury of other blood vessels at forearm level

6 S55.80 Unspecified injury of other blood vessels at forearm level

IQ 7 S55.801- Unspecified injury of other blood vessels at forearm level, right arm

IQ 7 S55.802- Unspecified injury of other blood vessels at forearm level, left arm

IQ 7 S55.809- Unspecified injury of other blood vessels at forearm level, unspecified arm

6 S55.81 Laceration of other blood vessels at forearm level

SP 7 S55.811- Laceration of other blood vessels at forearm level, right arm

SP 7 S55.812- Laceration of other blood vessels at forearm level, left arm

IQ 7 S55.819- Laceration of other blood vessels at forearm level, unspecified arm

6 S55.89 Other specified injury of other blood vessels at forearm level

SP 7 S55.891- Other specified injury of other blood vessels at forearm level, right arm

S55.892- Other specified injury of other blood vessels at forearm level, left arm

S55.899- Other specified injury of other blood vessels at forearm level, unspecified arm

S55.9 Injury of unspecified blood vessel at forearm level

S55.90 Unspecified injury of unspecified blood vessel at forearm level

S55.901- Unspecified injury of unspecified blood vessel at forearm level, right arm

S55.902- Unspecified injury of unspecified blood vessel at forearm level, left arm

S55.909- Unspecified injury of unspecified blood vessel at forearm level, unspecified arm

S55.91 Laceration of unspecified blood vessel at forearm level

S55.911- Laceration of unspecified blood vessel at forearm level, right arm

S55.912- Laceration of unspecified blood vessel at forearm level, left arm

S55.919- Laceration of unspecified blood vessel at forearm level, unspecified arm

S55.99 Other specified injury of unspecified blood vessel at forearm level

S55.991- Other specified injury of unspecified blood vessel at forearm level, right arm

S55.992- Other specified injury of unspecified blood vessel at forearm level, left arm

S55.999- Other specified injury of unspecified blood vessel at forearm level, unspecified arm

S56 Injury of muscle, fascia and tendon at forearm level

Code also:
any associated open wound (S51.-)

EXCLUDES 2 injury of muscle, fascia and tendon at or below wrist (S66.-)
sprain of joints and ligaments of elbow (S53.4-)

The appropriate 7th character is to be added to each code from category S56
A initial encounter
D subsequent encounter
S sequela

S56.0 Injury of flexor muscle, fascia and tendon of thumb at forearm level

S56.00 Unspecified injury of flexor muscle, fascia and tendon of thumb at forearm level

S56.001- Unspecified injury of flexor muscle, fascia and tendon of right thumb at forearm level

S56.002- Unspecified injury of flexor muscle, fascia and tendon of left thumb at forearm level

S56.009- Unspecified injury of flexor muscle, fascia and tendon of unspecified thumb at forearm level

S56.01 Strain of flexor muscle, fascia and tendon of thumb at forearm level

S56.011- Strain of flexor muscle, fascia and tendon of right thumb at forearm level

S56.012- Strain of flexor muscle, fascia and tendon of left thumb at forearm level

S56.019- Strain of flexor muscle, fascia and tendon of unspecified thumb at forearm level

S56.02 Laceration of flexor muscle, fascia and tendon of thumb at forearm level

S56.021- Laceration of flexor muscle, fascia and tendon of right thumb at forearm level

S56.022- Laceration of flexor muscle, fascia and tendon of left thumb at forearm level

S56.029- Laceration of flexor muscle, fascia and tendon of unspecified thumb at forearm level

S56.09 Other injury of flexor muscle, fascia and tendon of thumb at forearm level

S56.091- Other injury of flexor muscle, fascia and tendon of right thumb at forearm level

S56.092- Other injury of flexor muscle, fascia and tendon of left thumb at forearm level

S56.099- Other injury of flexor muscle, fascia and tendon of unspecified thumb at forearm level

S56.1 Injury of flexor muscle, fascia and tendon of other and unspecified finger at forearm level

S56.10 Unspecified injury of flexor muscle, fascia and tendon of other and unspecified finger at forearm level

S56.101- Unspecified injury of flexor muscle, fascia and tendon of right index finger at forearm level

S56.102- Unspecified injury of flexor muscle, fascia and tendon of left index finger at forearm level

S56.103- Unspecified injury of flexor muscle, fascia and tendon of right middle finger at forearm level

S56.104- Unspecified injury of flexor muscle, fascia and tendon of left middle finger at forearm level

S56.105- Unspecified injury of flexor muscle, fascia and tendon of right ring finger at forearm level

Chapter 19

S00-T88

IQ 7 S56.106- Unspecified injury of flexor muscle, fascia and tendon of left ring finger at forearm level

IQ 7 S56.107- Unspecified injury of flexor muscle, fascia and tendon of right little finger at forearm level

IQ 7 S56.108- Unspecified injury of flexor muscle, fascia and tendon of left little finger at forearm level

IQ 7 S56.109- Unspecified injury of flexor muscle, fascia and tendon of unspecified finger at forearm level

6 S56.11 Strain of flexor muscle, fascia and tendon of other and unspecified finger at forearm level

SP 7 S56.111- Strain of flexor muscle, fascia and tendon of right index finger at forearm level

SP 7 S56.112- Strain of flexor muscle, fascia and tendon of left index finger at forearm level

SP 7 S56.113- Strain of flexor muscle, fascia and tendon of right middle finger at forearm level

SP 7 S56.114- Strain of flexor muscle, fascia and tendon of left middle finger at forearm level

SP 7 S56.115- Strain of flexor muscle, fascia and tendon of right ring finger at forearm level

SP 7 S56.116- Strain of flexor muscle, fascia and tendon of left ring finger at forearm level

SP 7 S56.117- Strain of flexor muscle, fascia and tendon of right little finger at forearm level

SP 7 S56.118- Strain of flexor muscle, fascia and tendon of left little finger at forearm level

IQ 7 S56.119- Strain of flexor muscle, fascia and tendon of finger of unspecified finger at forearm level

6 S56.12 Laceration of flexor muscle, fascia and tendon of other and unspecified finger at forearm level

SP 7 S56.121- Laceration of flexor muscle, fascia and tendon of right index finger at forearm level

SP 7 S56.122- Laceration of flexor muscle, fascia and tendon of left index finger at forearm level

SP 7 S56.123- Laceration of flexor muscle, fascia and tendon of right middle finger at forearm level

SP 7 S56.124- Laceration of flexor muscle, fascia and tendon of left middle finger at forearm level

SP 7 S56.125- Laceration of flexor muscle, fascia and tendon of right ring finger at forearm level

SP 7 S56.126- Laceration of flexor muscle, fascia and tendon of left ring finger at forearm level

SP 7 S56.127- Laceration of flexor muscle, fascia and tendon of right little finger at forearm level

SP 7 S56.128- Laceration of flexor muscle, fascia and tendon of left little finger at forearm level

IQ 7 S56.129- Laceration of flexor muscle, fascia and tendon of unspecified finger at forearm level

6 S56.19 Other injury of flexor muscle, fascia and tendon of other and unspecified finger at forearm level

SP 7 S56.191- Other injury of flexor muscle, fascia and tendon of right index finger at forearm level

SP 7 S56.192- Other injury of flexor muscle, fascia and tendon of left index finger at forearm level

SP 7 S56.193- Other injury of flexor muscle, fascia and tendon of right middle finger at forearm level

SP 7 S56.194- Other injury of flexor muscle, fascia and tendon of left middle finger at forearm level

SP 7 S56.195- Other injury of flexor muscle, fascia and tendon of right ring finger at forearm level

SP 7 S56.196- Other injury of flexor muscle, fascia and tendon of left ring finger at forearm level

SP 7 S56.197- Other injury of flexor muscle, fascia and tendon of right little finger at forearm level

SP 7 S56.198- Other injury of flexor muscle, fascia and tendon of left little finger at forearm level

IQ 7 S56.199- Other injury of flexor muscle, fascia and tendon of unspecified finger at forearm level

5 S56.2 Injury of other flexor muscle, fascia and tendon at forearm level

6 S56.20 Unspecified injury of other flexor muscle, fascia and tendon at forearm level

IQ 7 S56.201- Unspecified injury of other flexor muscle, fascia and tendon at forearm level, right arm

IQ 7 S56.202- Unspecified injury of other flexor muscle, fascia and tendon at forearm level, left arm

IQ 7 S56.209- Unspecified injury of other flexor muscle, fascia and tendon at forearm level, unspecified arm

6 S56.21 Strain of other flexor muscle, fascia and tendon at forearm level

SP 7 S56.211- Strain of other flexor muscle, fascia and tendon at forearm level, right arm

SP 7 S56.212- Strain of other flexor muscle, fascia and tendon at forearm level, left arm

IQ 7 S56.219- Strain of other flexor muscle, fascia and tendon at forearm level, unspecified arm

6 S56.22 Laceration of other flexor muscle, fascia and tendon at forearm level

Chapter 19

S00-T88

- S56.221- Laceration of other flexor muscle, fascia and tendon at forearm level, right arm
- S56.222- Laceration of other flexor muscle, fascia and tendon at forearm level, left arm
- S56.229- Laceration of other flexor muscle, fascia and tendon at forearm level, unspecified arm

S56.29 Other injury of other flexor muscle, fascia and tendon at forearm level

- S56.291- Other injury of other flexor muscle, fascia and tendon at forearm level, right arm
- S56.292- Other injury of other flexor muscle, fascia and tendon at forearm level, left arm
- S56.299- Other injury of other flexor muscle, fascia and tendon at forearm level, unspecified arm

S56.3 Injury of extensor or abductor muscles, fascia and tendons of thumb at forearm level

S56.30 Unspecified injury of extensor or abductor muscles, fascia and tendons of thumb at forearm level

- S56.301- Unspecified injury of extensor or abductor muscles, fascia and tendons of right thumb at forearm level
- S56.302- Unspecified injury of extensor or abductor muscles, fascia and tendons of left thumb at forearm level
- S56.309- Unspecified injury of extensor or abductor muscles, fascia and tendons of unspecified thumb at forearm level

S56.31 Strain of extensor or abductor muscles, fascia and tendons of thumb at forearm level

- S56.311- Strain of extensor or abductor muscles, fascia and tendons of right thumb at forearm level
- S56.312- Strain of extensor or abductor muscles, fascia and tendons of left thumb at forearm level
- S56.319- Strain of extensor or abductor muscles, fascia and tendons of unspecified thumb at forearm level

S56.32 Laceration of extensor or abductor muscles, fascia and tendons of thumb at forearm level

- S56.321- Laceration of extensor or abductor muscles, fascia and tendons of right thumb at forearm level
- S56.322- Laceration of extensor or abductor muscles, fascia and tendons of left thumb at forearm level
- S56.329- Laceration of extensor or abductor muscles, fascia and tendons of unspecified thumb at forearm level

S56.39 Other injury of extensor or abductor muscles, fascia and tendons of thumb at forearm level

- S56.391- Other injury of extensor or abductor muscles, fascia and tendons of right thumb at forearm level
- S56.392- Other injury of extensor or abductor muscles, fascia and tendons of left thumb at forearm level
- S56.399- Other injury of extensor or abductor muscles, fascia and tendons of unspecified thumb at forearm level

S56.4 Injury of extensor muscle, fascia and tendon of other and unspecified finger at forearm level

S56.40 Unspecified injury of extensor muscle, fascia and tendon of other and unspecified finger at forearm level

- S56.401- Unspecified injury of extensor muscle, fascia and tendon of right index finger at forearm level
- S56.402- Unspecified injury of extensor muscle, fascia and tendon of left index finger at forearm level
- S56.403- Unspecified injury of extensor muscle, fascia and tendon of right middle finger at forearm level
- S56.404- Unspecified injury of extensor muscle, fascia and tendon of left middle finger at forearm level
- S56.405- Unspecified injury of extensor muscle, fascia and tendon of right ring finger at forearm level
- S56.406- Unspecified injury of extensor muscle, fascia and tendon of left ring finger at forearm level
- S56.407- Unspecified injury of extensor muscle, fascia and tendon of right little finger at forearm level
- S56.408- Unspecified injury of extensor muscle, fascia and tendon of left little finger at forearm level
- S56.409- Unspecified injury of extensor muscle, fascia and tendon of unspecified finger at forearm level

S56.41 Strain of extensor muscle, fascia and tendon of other and unspecified finger at forearm level

- S56.411- Strain of extensor muscle, fascia and tendon of right index finger at forearm level
- S56.412- Strain of extensor muscle, fascia and tendon of left index finger at forearm level
- S56.413- Strain of extensor muscle, fascia and tendon of right middle finger at forearm level

Chapter 19

S00-T88

4th digit required 5th digit required 6th digit required 7th digit required 7th digit placeholder + Additional code Laterality

S56.414- Strain of extensor muscle, fascia and tendon of left middle finger at forearm level

S56.415- Strain of extensor muscle, fascia and tendon of right ring finger at forearm level

S56.416- Strain of extensor muscle, fascia and tendon of left ring finger at forearm level

S56.417- Strain of extensor muscle, fascia and tendon of right little finger at forearm level

S56.418- Strain of extensor muscle, fascia and tendon of left little finger at forearm level

S56.419- Strain of extensor muscle, fascia and tendon of finger, unspecified finger at forearm level

S56.42 Laceration of extensor muscle, fascia and tendon of other and unspecified finger at forearm level

S56.421- Laceration of extensor muscle, fascia and tendon of right index finger at forearm level

S56.422- Laceration of extensor muscle, fascia and tendon of left index finger at forearm level

S56.423- Laceration of extensor muscle, fascia and tendon of right middle finger at forearm level

S56.424- Laceration of extensor muscle, fascia and tendon of left middle finger at forearm level

S56.425- Laceration of extensor muscle, fascia and tendon of right ring finger at forearm level

S56.426- Laceration of extensor muscle, fascia and tendon of left ring finger at forearm level

S56.427- Laceration of extensor muscle, fascia and tendon of right little finger at forearm level

S56.428- Laceration of extensor muscle, fascia and tendon of left little finger at forearm level

S56.429- Laceration of extensor muscle, fascia and tendon of unspecified finger at forearm level

S56.49 Other injury of extensor muscle, fascia and tendon of other and unspecified finger at forearm level

S56.491- Other injury of extensor muscle, fascia and tendon of right index finger at forearm level

S56.492- Other injury of extensor muscle, fascia and tendon of left index finger at forearm level

S56.493- Other injury of extensor muscle, fascia and tendon of right middle finger at forearm level

S56.494- Other injury of extensor muscle, fascia and tendon of left middle finger at forearm level

S56.495- Other injury of extensor muscle, fascia and tendon of right ring finger at forearm level

S56.496- Other injury of extensor muscle, fascia and tendon of left ring finger at forearm level

S56.497- Other injury of extensor muscle, fascia and tendon of right little finger at forearm level

S56.498- Other injury of extensor muscle, fascia and tendon of left little finger at forearm level

S56.499- Other injury of extensor muscle, fascia and tendon of unspecified finger at forearm level

S56.5 Injury of other extensor muscle, fascia and tendon at forearm level

S56.50 Unspecified injury of other extensor muscle, fascia and tendon at forearm level

S56.501- Unspecified injury of other extensor muscle, fascia and tendon at forearm level, right arm

S56.502- Unspecified injury of other extensor muscle, fascia and tendon at forearm level, left arm

S56.509- Unspecified injury of other extensor muscle, fascia and tendon at forearm level, unspecified arm

S56.51 Strain of other extensor muscle, fascia and tendon at forearm level

S56.511- Strain of other extensor muscle, fascia and tendon at forearm level, right arm

S56.512- Strain of other extensor muscle, fascia and tendon at forearm level, left arm

S56.519- Strain of other extensor muscle, fascia and tendon at forearm level, unspecified arm

S56.52 Laceration of other extensor muscle, fascia and tendon at forearm level

S56.521- Laceration of other extensor muscle, fascia and tendon at forearm level, right arm

S56.522- Laceration of other extensor muscle, fascia and tendon at forearm level, left arm

S56.529- Laceration of other extensor muscle, fascia and tendon at forearm level, unspecified arm

S56.59 Other injury of other extensor muscle, fascia and tendon at forearm level

S56.591- Other injury of other extensor muscle, fascia and tendon at forearm level, right arm

S56.592- Other injury of other extensor muscle, fascia and tendon at forearm level, left arm

S56.599- Other injury of other extensor muscle, fascia and tendon at forearm level, unspecified arm

S56.8 Injury of other muscles, fascia and tendons at forearm level

S56.80 Unspecified injury of other muscles, fascia and tendons at forearm level

S56.801- Unspecified injury of other muscles, fascia and tendons at forearm level, right arm

S56.802- Unspecified injury of other muscles, fascia and tendons at forearm level, left arm

S56.809- Unspecified injury of other muscles, fascia and tendons at forearm level, unspecified arm

S56.81 Strain of other muscles, fascia and tendons at forearm level

S56.811- Strain of other muscles, fascia and tendons at forearm level, right arm

S56.812- Strain of other muscles, fascia and tendons at forearm level, left arm

S56.819- Strain of other muscles, fascia and tendons at forearm level, unspecified arm

S56.82 Laceration of other muscles, fascia and tendons at forearm level

S56.821- Laceration of other muscles, fascia and tendons at forearm level, right arm

S56.822- Laceration of other muscles, fascia and tendons at forearm level, left arm

S56.829- Laceration of other muscles, fascia and tendons at forearm level, unspecified arm

S56.89 Other injury of other muscles, fascia and tendons at forearm level

S56.891- Other injury of other muscles, fascia and tendons at forearm level, right arm

S56.892- Other injury of other muscles, fascia and tendons at forearm level, left arm

S56.899- Other injury of other muscles, fascia and tendons at forearm level, unspecified arm

S56.9 Injury of unspecified muscles, fascia and tendons at forearm level

S56.90 Unspecified injury of unspecified muscles, fascia and tendons at forearm level

S56.901- Unspecified injury of unspecified muscles, fascia and tendons at forearm level, right arm

S56.902- Unspecified injury of unspecified muscles, fascia and tendons at forearm level, left arm

S56.909- Unspecified injury of unspecified muscles, fascia and tendons at forearm level, unspecified arm

S56.91 Strain of unspecified muscles, fascia and tendons at forearm level

S56.911- Strain of unspecified muscles, fascia and tendons at forearm level, right arm

S56.912- Strain of unspecified muscles, fascia and tendons at forearm level, left arm

S56.919- Strain of unspecified muscles, fascia and tendons at forearm level, unspecified arm

S56.92 Laceration of unspecified muscles, fascia and tendons at forearm level

S56.921- Laceration of unspecified muscles, fascia and tendons at forearm level, right arm

S56.922- Laceration of unspecified muscles, fascia and tendons at forearm level, left arm

S56.929- Laceration of unspecified muscles, fascia and tendons at forearm level, unspecified arm

S56.99 Other injury of unspecified muscles, fascia and tendons at forearm level

S56.991- Other injury of unspecified muscles, fascia and tendons at forearm level, right arm

S56.992- Other injury of unspecified muscles, fascia and tendons at forearm level, left arm

S56.999- Other injury of unspecified muscles, fascia and tendons at forearm level, unspecified arm

+ S57 Crushing injury of elbow and forearm

Use additional code(s) for all associated injuries

EXCLUDES 2 crushing injury of wrist and hand (S67.-)

The appropriate 7th character is to be added to each code from category S57
A initial encounter
D subsequent encounter
S sequela

+ S57.0 Crushing injury of elbow

+ S57.00X- Crushing injury of unspecified elbow

+ S57.01X- Crushing injury of right elbow

+ S57.02X- Crushing injury of left elbow

+ S57.8 Crushing injury of forearm

+ S57.80X- Crushing injury of unspecified forearm

+ S57.81X- Crushing injury of right forearm

+ S57.82X- Crushing injury of left forearm

S58 Traumatic amputation of elbow and forearm

An amputation not identified as partial or complete should be coded to complete

EXCLUDES 1 traumatic amputation of wrist and hand (S68.-)

The appropriate 7th character is to be added to each code from category S58
A initial encounter
D subsequent encounter
S sequela

Chapter 19

S00-T88

4th digit required 5th digit required 6th digit required 7th digit required 7th digit placeholder +Additional code Laterality

CODING TIPS ✓ Use these codes only when the amputation was due to trauma. There is no need for adding Z89 with traumatic amputations. See Z47.81 for care of amputations not due to trauma.

5 **S58.0 Traumatic amputation at elbow level**

6 **S58.01 Complete traumatic amputation at elbow level**

SP 7 **S58.011- Complete traumatic amputation at elbow level, right arm**

SP 7 **S58.012- Complete traumatic amputation at elbow level, left arm**

IQ 7 **S58.019- Complete traumatic amputation at elbow level, unspecified arm**

6 **S58.02 Partial traumatic amputation at elbow level**

SP 7 **S58.021- Partial traumatic amputation at elbow level, right arm**

SP 7 **S58.022- Partial traumatic amputation at elbow level, left arm**

IQ 7 **S58.029- Partial traumatic amputation at elbow level, unspecified arm**

5 **S58.1 Traumatic amputation at level between elbow and wrist**

6 **S58.11 Complete traumatic amputation at level between elbow and wrist**

SP 7 **S58.111- Complete traumatic amputation at level between elbow and wrist, right arm**

SP 7 **S58.112- Complete traumatic amputation at level between elbow and wrist, left arm**

IQ 7 **S58.119- Complete traumatic amputation at level between elbow and wrist, unspecified arm**

6 **S58.12 Partial traumatic amputation at level between elbow and wrist**

SP 7 **S58.121- Partial traumatic amputation at level between elbow and wrist, right arm**

SP 7 **S58.122- Partial traumatic amputation at level between elbow and wrist, left arm**

SP IQ 7 **S58.129- Partial traumatic amputation at level between elbow and wrist, unspecified arm**

5 **S58.9 Traumatic amputation of forearm, level unspecified**

EXCLUDES 1 traumatic amputation of wrist (S68.-)

6 **S58.91 Complete traumatic amputation of forearm, level unspecified**

SP 7 **S58.911- Complete traumatic amputation of right forearm, level unspecified**

SP 7 **S58.912- Complete traumatic amputation of left forearm, level unspecified**

IQ 7 **S58.919- Complete traumatic amputation of unspecified forearm, level unspecified**

6 **S58.92 Partial traumatic amputation of forearm, level unspecified**

SP 7 **S58.921- Partial traumatic amputation of right forearm, level unspecified**

SP 7 **S58.922- Partial traumatic amputation of left forearm, level unspecified**

IQ 7 **S58.929- Partial traumatic amputation of unspecified forearm, level unspecified**

4 **S59 Other and unspecified injuries of elbow and forearm**

EXCLUDES 2 other and unspecified injuries of wrist and hand (S69.-)

The appropriate 7th character is to be added to each code from subcategories S59.0, S59.1, and S59.2

- A initial encounter for closed fracture
- D subsequent encounter for fracture with routine healing
- G subsequent encounter for fracture with delayed healing
- K subsequent encounter for fracture with nonunion
- P subsequent encounter for fracture with malunion
- S sequela

5 **S59.0 Physeal fracture of lower end of ulna**

6 **S59.00 Unspecified physeal fracture of lower end of ulna**

SP 7 **S59.001- Unspecified physeal fracture of lower end of ulna, right arm**

SP 7 **S59.002- Unspecified physeal fracture of lower end of ulna, left arm**

IQ 7 **S59.009- Unspecified physeal fracture of lower end of ulna, unspecified arm**

6 **S59.01 Salter-Harris Type I physeal fracture of lower end of ulna**

SP 7 **S59.011- Salter-Harris Type I physeal fracture of lower end of ulna, right arm**

SP 7 **S59.012- Salter-Harris Type I physeal fracture of lower end of ulna, left arm**

IQ 7 **S59.019- Salter-Harris Type I physeal fracture of lower end of ulna, unspecified arm**

6 **S59.02 Salter-Harris Type II physeal fracture of lower end of ulna**

SP 7 **S59.021- Salter-Harris Type II physeal fracture of lower end of ulna, right arm**

SP 7 **S59.022- Salter-Harris Type II physeal fracture of lower end of ulna, left arm**

IQ 7 **S59.029- Salter-Harris Type II physeal fracture of lower end of ulna, unspecified arm**

6 **S59.03 Salter-Harris Type III physeal fracture of lower end of ulna**

SP 7 **S59.031- Salter-Harris Type III physeal fracture of lower end of ulna, right arm**

SP 7 **S59.032- Salter-Harris Type III physeal fracture of lower end of ulna, left arm**

IQ 7 **S59.039- Salter-Harris Type III physeal fracture of lower end of ulna, unspecified arm**

6 **S59.04 Salter-Harris Type IV physeal fracture of lower end of ulna**

Chapter 19

S00-T88

Laterality SP 7 S59.041- Salter-Harris Type IV physeal fracture of lower end of ulna, right arm

Laterality SP 7 S59.042- Salter-Harris Type IV physeal fracture of lower end of ulna, left arm

Laterality IQ 7 S59.049- Salter-Harris Type IV physeal fracture of lower end of ulna, unspecified arm

6 S59.09 Other physeal fracture of lower end of ulna

Laterality SP 7 S59.091- Other physeal fracture of lower end of ulna, right arm

Laterality SP 7 S59.092- Other physeal fracture of lower end of ulna, left arm

Laterality IQ 7 S59.099- Other physeal fracture of lower end of ulna, unspecified arm

5 S59.1 Physeal fracture of upper end of radius

6 S59.10 Unspecified physeal fracture of upper end of radius

Laterality SP 7 S59.101- Unspecified physeal fracture of upper end of radius, right arm

Laterality SP 7 S59.102- Unspecified physeal fracture of upper end of radius, left arm

Laterality SP IQ 7 S59.109- Unspecified physeal fracture of upper end of radius, unspecified arm

6 S59.11 Salter-Harris Type I physeal fracture of upper end of radius

Laterality SP 7 S59.111- Salter-Harris Type I physeal fracture of upper end of radius, right arm

Laterality SP 7 S59.112- Salter-Harris Type I physeal fracture of upper end of radius, left arm

Laterality IQ 7 S59.119- Salter-Harris Type I physeal fracture of upper end of radius, unspecified arm

6 S59.12 Salter-Harris Type II physeal fracture of upper end of radius

Laterality SP 7 S59.121- Salter-Harris Type II physeal fracture of upper end of radius, right arm

Laterality SP 7 S59.122- Salter-Harris Type II physeal fracture of upper end of radius, left arm

Laterality IQ 7 S59.129- Salter-Harris Type II physeal fracture of upper end of radius, unspecified arm

6 S59.13 Salter-Harris Type III physeal fracture of upper end of radius

Laterality SP 7 S59.131- Salter-Harris Type III physeal fracture of upper end of radius, right arm

Laterality SP 7 S59.132- Salter-Harris Type III physeal fracture of upper end of radius, left arm

Laterality IQ 7 S59.139- Salter-Harris Type III physeal fracture of upper end of radius, unspecified arm

6 S59.14 Salter-Harris Type IV physeal fracture of upper end of radius

Laterality SP 7 S59.141- Salter-Harris Type IV physeal fracture of upper end of radius, right arm

Laterality SP 7 S59.142- Salter-Harris Type IV physeal fracture of upper end of radius, left arm

Laterality IQ 7 S59.149- Salter-Harris Type IV physeal fracture of upper end of radius, unspecified arm

6 S59.19 Other physeal fracture of upper end of radius

Laterality SP 7 S59.191- Other physeal fracture of upper end of radius, right arm

Laterality SP 7 S59.192- Other physeal fracture of upper end of radius, left arm

Laterality IQ 7 S59.199- Other physeal fracture of upper end of radius, unspecified arm

5 S59.2 Physeal fracture of lower end of radius

6 S59.20 Unspecified physeal fracture of lower end of radius

Laterality SP 7 S59.201- Unspecified physeal fracture of lower end of radius, right arm

Laterality SP 7 S59.202- Unspecified physeal fracture of lower end of radius, left arm

Laterality IQ 7 S59.209- Unspecified physeal fracture of lower end of radius, unspecified arm

6 S59.21 Salter-Harris Type I physeal fracture of lower end of radius

Laterality SP 7 S59.211- Salter-Harris Type I physeal fracture of lower end of radius, right arm

Laterality SP 7 S59.212- Salter-Harris Type I physeal fracture of lower end of radius, left arm

Laterality IQ 7 S59.219- Salter-Harris Type I physeal fracture of lower end of radius, unspecified arm

6 S59.22 Salter-Harris Type II physeal fracture of lower end of radius

Laterality SP 7 S59.221- Salter-Harris Type II physeal fracture of lower end of radius, right arm

Laterality SP 7 S59.222- Salter-Harris Type II physeal fracture of lower end of radius, left arm

Laterality IQ 7 S59.229- Salter-Harris Type II physeal fracture of lower end of radius, unspecified arm

6 S59.23 Salter-Harris Type III physeal fracture of lower end of radius

Laterality SP 7 S59.231- Salter-Harris Type III physeal fracture of lower end of radius, right arm

Laterality SP 7 S59.232- Salter-Harris Type III physeal fracture of lower end of radius, left arm

Laterality IQ 7 S59.239- Salter-Harris Type III physeal fracture of lower end of radius, unspecified arm

6 S59.24 Salter-Harris Type IV physeal fracture of lower end of radius

Laterality SP 7 S59.241- Salter-Harris Type IV physeal fracture of lower end of radius, right arm

Laterality SP 7 S59.242- Salter-Harris Type IV physeal fracture of lower end of radius, left arm

IQ 7 S59.249- **Salter-Harris Type IV physeal fracture of lower end of radius, unspecified arm**

6 S59.29 **Other physeal fracture of lower end of radius**

SP 7 S59.291- **Other physeal fracture of lower end of radius, right arm**

SP 7 S59.292- **Other physeal fracture of lower end of radius, left arm**

IQ 7 S59.299- **Other physeal fracture of lower end of radius, unspecified arm**

5 S59.8 **Other specified injuries of elbow and forearm**

The appropriate 7th character is to be added to each code in subcategory S59.8
A initial encounter
D subsequent encounter
S sequela

6 S59.80 **Other specified injuries of elbow**

SP 7 S59.801- **Other specified injuries of right elbow**

SP 7 S59.802- **Other specified injuries of left elbow**

IQ 7 S59.809- **Other specified injuries of unspecified elbow**

6 S59.81 **Other specified injuries of forearm**

SP 7 S59.811- **Other specified injuries right forearm**

SP 7 S59.812- **Other specified injuries left forearm**

IQ 7 S59.819- **Other specified injuries unspecified forearm**

5 S59.9 **Unspecified injury of elbow and forearm**

The appropriate 7th character is to be added to each code in subcategory S59.9
A initial encounter
D subsequent encounter
S sequela

6 S59.90 **Unspecified injury of elbow**

IQ 7 S59.901- **Unspecified injury of right elbow**

IQ 7 S59.902- **Unspecified injury of left elbow**

IQ 7 S59.909- **Unspecified injury of unspecified elbow**

6 S59.91 **Unspecified injury of forearm**

IQ 7 S59.911- **Unspecified injury of right forearm**

IQ 7 S59.912- **Unspecified injury of left forearm**

IQ 7 S59.919- **Unspecified injury of unspecified forearm**

Injuries to the wrist, hand and fingers (S60-S69)

EXCLUDES 2 burns and corrosions (T20-T32)
frostbite (T33-T34)
insect bite or sting, venomous (T63.4)

GUIDELINES **Section I.C.19.c.2)**
Multiple fractures are sequenced in accordance with the severity of the fracture.

GUIDELINES **Section I.C.19.b.1)-2)**
When coding injuries, assign separate codes for each injury unless a combination code is provided, in which case the combination code is assigned ... Traumatic injury codes (S00-T14.9) are not to be used for normal, healing surgical wounds or to identify complications of surgical wounds. The code for the most serious injury, as determined by the provider and the focus of treatment, is sequenced first.

1) Superficial injuries such as abrasions or contusions are not coded when associated with more severe injuries of the same site.

2) When a primary injury results in minor damage to peripheral nerves or blood vessels, the primary injury is sequenced first with additional code(s) for injuries to nerves and spinal cord (such as category S04), and/or injury to blood vessels (such as category S15). When the primary injury is to the blood vessels or nerves, that injury should be sequenced first.

GUIDELINES **Section I.C.19.c**
Coding of Traumatic Fractures: The principles of multiple coding of injuries should be followed in coding fractures. Fractures of specified sites are coded individually by site in accordance with both the provisions within categories S02, S12, S22, S32, S42, S49, S52, S59, S62, S72, S79, S82, S89, S92 and the level of detail furnished by medical record content. A fracture not indicated as open or closed should be coded to closed. A fracture not indicated whether displaced or not displaced should be coded to displaced.

CODING TIPS ✓ 7th character A is acceptable in home health and hospice when active treatment is provided, such as antibiotics for an infected wound or a wound vac for a dehisced wound. D is used when the complication or injury is now healing. Think of D as aftercare. S is used for sequela of the injury or complication. Sequela is a residual deficit or condition produced as a result of the injury or complication after the original injury or complication has healed.

4 S60 **Superficial injury of wrist, hand and fingers**

The appropriate 7th character is to be added to each code from category S60
A initial encounter
D subsequent encounter
S sequela

5 S60.0 **Contusion of finger without damage to nail**

EXCLUDES 1 contusion involving nail (matrix) (S60.1)

IQ 7 S60.00X- **Contusion of unspecified finger without damage to nail**
Contusion of finger(s) NOS

6 S60.01 **Contusion of thumb without damage to nail**

IQ 7 S60.011- **Contusion of right thumb without damage to nail**

IQ 7 S60.012- **Contusion of left thumb without damage to nail**

IQ 7 S60.019- **Contusion of unspecified thumb without damage to nail**

6 S60.02 **Contusion of index finger without damage to nail**

IQ 7 S60.021- **Contusion of right index finger without damage to nail**

Chapter 19

S00-T88

S60.022- Contusion of left index finger without damage to nail
S60.029- Contusion of unspecified index finger without damage to nail
S60.03 Contusion of middle finger without damage to nail
S60.031- Contusion of right middle finger without damage to nail
S60.032- Contusion of left middle finger without damage to nail
S60.039- Contusion of unspecified middle finger without damage to nail
S60.04 Contusion of ring finger without damage to nail
S60.041- Contusion of right ring finger without damage to nail
S60.042- Contusion of left ring finger without damage to nail
S60.049- Contusion of unspecified ring finger without damage to nail
S60.05 Contusion of little finger without damage to nail
S60.051- Contusion of right little finger without damage to nail
S60.052- Contusion of left little finger without damage to nail
S60.059- Contusion of unspecified little finger without damage to nail
S60.1 Contusion of finger with damage to nail
S60.10X- Contusion of unspecified finger with damage to nail
S60.11 Contusion of thumb with damage to nail
S60.111- Contusion of right thumb with damage to nail
S60.112- Contusion of left thumb with damage to nail
S60.119- Contusion of unspecified thumb with damage to nail
S60.12 Contusion of index finger with damage to nail
S60.121- Contusion of right index finger with damage to nail
S60.122- Contusion of left index finger with damage to nail
S60.129- Contusion of unspecified index finger with damage to nail
S60.13 Contusion of middle finger with damage to nail
S60.131- Contusion of right middle finger with damage to nail
S60.132- Contusion of left middle finger with damage to nail
S60.139- Contusion of unspecified middle finger with damage to nail
S60.14 Contusion of ring finger with damage to nail
S60.141- Contusion of right ring finger with damage to nail
S60.142- Contusion of left ring finger with damage to nail
S60.149- Contusion of unspecified ring finger with damage to nail
S60.15 Contusion of little finger with damage to nail
S60.151- Contusion of right little finger with damage to nail
S60.152- Contusion of left little finger with damage to nail
S60.159- Contusion of unspecified little finger with damage to nail
S60.2 Contusion of wrist and hand
EXCLUDES 2 contusion of fingers (S60.0-, S60.1-)
S60.21 Contusion of wrist
S60.211- Contusion of right wrist
S60.212- Contusion of left wrist
S60.219- Contusion of unspecified wrist
S60.22 Contusion of hand
S60.221- Contusion of right hand
S60.222- Contusion of left hand
S60.229- Contusion of unspecified hand
S60.3 Other superficial injuries of thumb
S60.31 Abrasion of thumb
S60.311- Abrasion of right thumb
S60.312- Abrasion of left thumb
S60.319- Abrasion of unspecified thumb
S60.32 Blister (nonthermal) of thumb
S60.321- Blister (nonthermal) of right thumb
S60.322- Blister (nonthermal) of left thumb
S60.329- Blister (nonthermal) of unspecified thumb
+ **S60.34** External constriction of thumb
Hair tourniquet syndrome of thumb
Use additional cause code to identify the constricting item (W49.0-)
+ **S60.341-** External constriction of right thumb
+ **S60.342-** External constriction of left thumb
+ **S60.349-** External constriction of unspecified thumb
S60.35 Superficial foreign body of thumb
Splinter in the thumb
S60.351- Superficial foreign body of right thumb
S60.352- Superficial foreign body of left thumb
S60.359- Superficial foreign body of unspecified thumb
S60.36 Insect bite (nonvenomous) of thumb
S60.361- Insect bite (nonvenomous) of right thumb
S60.362- Insect bite (nonvenomous) of left thumb
S60.369- Insect bite (nonvenomous) of unspecified thumb
S60.37 Other superficial bite of thumb
EXCLUDES 1 open bite of thumb (S61.05-, S61.15-)
S60.371- Other superficial bite of right thumb
S60.372- Other superficial bite of left thumb
S60.379- Other superficial bite of unspecified thumb

4th digit required | 5th digit required | 6th digit required | 7th digit required | 7th digit placeholder | + Additional code | Laterality

6 S60.39 **Other superficial injuries of thumb**

- 7 S60.391- **Other superficial injuries of right thumb**
- 7 S60.392- **Other superficial injuries of left thumb**
- 7 S60.399- **Other superficial injuries of unspecified thumb**

5 S60.4 **Other superficial injuries of other fingers**

6 S60.41 **Abrasion of fingers**

- 7 S60.410- **Abrasion of right index finger**
- 7 S60.411- **Abrasion of left index finger**
- 7 S60.412- **Abrasion of right middle finger**
- 7 S60.413- **Abrasion of left middle finger**
- 7 S60.414- **Abrasion of right ring finger**
- 7 S60.415- **Abrasion of left ring finger**
- 7 S60.416- **Abrasion of right little finger**
- 7 S60.417- **Abrasion of left little finger**
- 7 S60.418- **Abrasion of other finger**
  Abrasion of specified finger with unspecified laterality
- 7 S60.419- **Abrasion of unspecified finger**

6 S60.42 **Blister (nonthermal) of fingers**

- 7 S60.420- **Blister (nonthermal) of right index finger**
- 7 S60.421- **Blister (nonthermal) of left index finger**
- 7 S60.422- **Blister (nonthermal) of right middle finger**
- 7 S60.423- **Blister (nonthermal) of left middle finger**
- 7 S60.424- **Blister (nonthermal) of right ring finger**
- 7 S60.425- **Blister (nonthermal) of left ring finger**
- 7 S60.426- **Blister (nonthermal) of right little finger**
- 7 S60.427- **Blister (nonthermal) of left little finger**
- 7 S60.428- **Blister (nonthermal) of other finger**
  Blister (nonthermal) of specified finger with unspecified laterality
- 7 S60.429- **Blister (nonthermal) of unspecified finger**

+ 6 S60.44 **External constriction of fingers**
Hair tourniquet syndrome of finger
Use additional cause code to identify the constricting item (W49.0-)

- + 7 S60.440- **External constriction of right index finger**
- + 7 S60.441- **External constriction of left index finger**
- + 7 S60.442- **External constriction of right middle finger**
- + 7 S60.443- **External constriction of left middle finger**
- + 7 S60.444- **External constriction of right ring finger**
- + 7 S60.445- **External constriction of left ring finger**
- + 7 S60.446- **External constriction of right little finger**
- + 7 S60.447- **External constriction of left little finger**
- + 7 S60.448- **External constriction of other finger**
  External constriction of specified finger with unspecified laterality
- + 7 S60.449- **External constriction of unspecified finger**

6 S60.45 **Superficial foreign body of fingers**
Splinter in the finger(s)

- 7 S60.450- **Superficial foreign body of right index finger**
- 7 S60.451- **Superficial foreign body of left index finger**
- 7 S60.452- **Superficial foreign body of right middle finger**
- 7 S60.453- **Superficial foreign body of left middle finger**
- 7 S60.454- **Superficial foreign body of right ring finger**
- 7 S60.455- **Superficial foreign body of left ring finger**
- 7 S60.456- **Superficial foreign body of right little finger**
- 7 S60.457- **Superficial foreign body of left little finger**
- 7 S60.458- **Superficial foreign body of other finger**
  Superficial foreign body of specified finger with unspecified laterality
- 7 S60.459- **Superficial foreign body of unspecified finger**

6 S60.46 **Insect bite (nonvenomous) of fingers**

- 7 S60.460- **Insect bite (nonvenomous) of right index finger**
- 7 S60.461- **Insect bite (nonvenomous) of left index finger**
- 7 S60.462- **Insect bite (nonvenomous) of right middle finger**
- 7 S60.463- **Insect bite (nonvenomous) of left middle finger**
- 7 S60.464- **Insect bite (nonvenomous) of right ring finger**
- 7 S60.465- **Insect bite (nonvenomous) of left ring finger**
- 7 S60.466- **Insect bite (nonvenomous) of right little finger**
- 7 S60.467- **Insect bite (nonvenomous) of left little finger**
- 7 S60.468- **Insect bite (nonvenomous) of other finger**
  Insect bite (nonvenomous) of specified finger with unspecified laterality
- 7 S60.469- **Insect bite (nonvenomous) of unspecified finger**

6 S60.47 **Other superficial bite of fingers**
EXCLUDES 1 open bite of fingers (S61.25-, S61.35-)

- 7 S60.470- **Other superficial bite of right index finger**
- 7 S60.471- **Other superficial bite of left index finger**
- 7 S60.472- **Other superficial bite of right middle finger**
- 7 S60.473- **Other superficial bite of left middle finger**

Chapter 19 S00-T88

S60.474- Other superficial bite of right ring finger
S60.475- Other superficial bite of left ring finger
S60.476- Other superficial bite of right little finger
S60.477- Other superficial bite of left little finger
S60.478- Other superficial bite of other finger
Other superficial bite of specified finger with unspecified laterality
S60.479- Other superficial bite of unspecified finger

S60.5 Other superficial injuries of hand
EXCLUDES 2 superficial injuries of fingers (S60.3-, S60.4-)

S60.51 Abrasion of hand
S60.511- Abrasion of right hand
S60.512- Abrasion of left hand
S60.519- Abrasion of unspecified hand

S60.52 Blister (nonthermal) of hand
S60.521- Blister (nonthermal) of right hand
S60.522- Blister (nonthermal) of left hand
S60.529- Blister (nonthermal) of unspecified hand

S60.54 External constriction of hand
S60.541- External constriction of right hand
S60.542- External constriction of left hand
S60.549- External constriction of unspecified hand

S60.55 Superficial foreign body of hand
Splinter in the hand
S60.551- Superficial foreign body of right hand
S60.552- Superficial foreign body of left hand
S60.559- Superficial foreign body of unspecified hand

S60.56 Insect bite (nonvenomous) of hand
S60.561- Insect bite (nonvenomous) of right hand
S60.562- Insect bite (nonvenomous) of left hand
S60.569- Insect bite (nonvenomous) of unspecified hand

S60.57 Other superficial bite of hand
EXCLUDES 1 open bite of hand (S61.45-)
S60.571- Other superficial bite of hand of right hand
S60.572- Other superficial bite of hand of left hand
S60.579- Other superficial bite of hand of unspecified hand

S60.8 Other superficial injuries of wrist

S60.81 Abrasion of wrist
S60.811- Abrasion of right wrist
S60.812- Abrasion of left wrist
S60.819- Abrasion of unspecified wrist

S60.82 Blister (nonthermal) of wrist
S60.821- Blister (nonthermal) of right wrist
S60.822- Blister (nonthermal) of left wrist
S60.829- Blister (nonthermal) of unspecified wrist

S60.84 External constriction of wrist
S60.841- External constriction of right wrist
S60.842- External constriction of left wrist
S60.849- External constriction of unspecified wrist

S60.85 Superficial foreign body of wrist
Splinter in the wrist
S60.851- Superficial foreign body of right wrist
S60.852- Superficial foreign body of left wrist
S60.859- Superficial foreign body of unspecified wrist

S60.86 Insect bite (nonvenomous) of wrist
S60.861- Insect bite (nonvenomous) of right wrist
S60.862- Insect bite (nonvenomous) of left wrist
S60.869- Insect bite (nonvenomous) of unspecified wrist

S60.87 Other superficial bite of wrist
EXCLUDES 1 open bite of wrist (S61.55)
S60.871- Other superficial bite of right wrist
S60.872- Other superficial bite of left wrist
S60.879- Other superficial bite of unspecified wrist

S60.9 Unspecified superficial injury of wrist, hand and fingers

S60.91 Unspecified superficial injury of wrist
S60.911- Unspecified superficial injury of right wrist
S60.912- Unspecified superficial injury of left wrist
S60.919- Unspecified superficial injury of unspecified wrist

S60.92 Unspecified superficial injury of hand
S60.921- Unspecified superficial injury of right hand
S60.922- Unspecified superficial injury of left hand
S60.929- Unspecified superficial injury of unspecified hand

S60.93 Unspecified superficial injury of thumb
S60.931- Unspecified superficial injury of right thumb
S60.932- Unspecified superficial injury of left thumb
S60.939- Unspecified superficial injury of unspecified thumb

S60.94 Unspecified superficial injury of other fingers

S60.940- Unspecified superficial injury of right index finger

S60.941- Unspecified superficial injury of left index finger

S60.942- Unspecified superficial injury of right middle finger

S60.943- Unspecified superficial injury of left middle finger

S60.944- Unspecified superficial injury of right ring finger

S60.945- Unspecified superficial injury of left ring finger

S60.946- Unspecified superficial injury of right little finger

S60.947- Unspecified superficial injury of left little finger

S60.948- Unspecified superficial injury of other finger
Unspecified superficial injury of specified finger with unspecified laterality

S60.949- Unspecified superficial injury of unspecified finger

S61 Open wound of wrist, hand and fingers
Code also:
any associated wound infection
EXCLUDES 1 open fracture of wrist, hand and finger (S62.- with 7th character B)
traumatic amputation of wrist and hand (S68.-)

The appropriate 7th character is to be added to each code from category S61
A initial encounter
D subsequent encounter
S sequela

CODING TIPS✓ Open wound codes indicate a wound resulting from a traumatic origin. Do not assign a code for "open wound" unless the etiology of the wound is related to trauma.

CODING TIPS✓ No aftercare code applies, including those indicating dressing changes, drain care, or suture removal. 7th character 'D' is the default for home care and hospice when providing aftercare for a healing or resolving condition; 'A' is used for active treatment such as antibiotics or more than routine wound care; 'S' may be used to indicate a residual condition after the original injury has healed.

S61.0 Open wound of thumb without damage to nail
EXCLUDES 1 open wound of thumb with damage to nail (S61.1-)

S61.00 Unspecified open wound of thumb without damage to nail

S61.001- Unspecified open wound of right thumb without damage to nail

S61.002- Unspecified open wound of left thumb without damage to nail

S61.009- Unspecified open wound of unspecified thumb without damage to nail

S61.01 Laceration without foreign body of thumb without damage to nail

S61.011- Laceration without foreign body of right thumb without damage to nail

S61.012- Laceration without foreign body of left thumb without damage to nail

S61.019- Laceration without foreign body of unspecified thumb without damage to nail

S61.02 Laceration with foreign body of thumb without damage to nail

S61.021- Laceration with foreign body of right thumb without damage to nail

S61.022- Laceration with foreign body of left thumb without damage to nail

S61.029- Laceration with foreign body of unspecified thumb without damage to nail

S61.03 Puncture wound without foreign body of thumb without damage to nail

S61.031- Puncture wound without foreign body of right thumb without damage to nail

S61.032- Puncture wound without foreign body of left thumb without damage to nail

S61.039- Puncture wound without foreign body of unspecified thumb without damage to nail

S61.04 Puncture wound with foreign body of thumb without damage to nail

S61.041- Puncture wound with foreign body of right thumb without damage to nail

S61.042- Puncture wound with foreign body of left thumb without damage to nail

S61.049- Puncture wound with foreign body of unspecified thumb without damage to nail

S61.05 Open bite of thumb without damage to nail
Bite of thumb NOS
EXCLUDES 1 superficial bite of thumb (S60.36-, S60.37-)

S61.051- Open bite of right thumb without damage to nail

S61.052- Open bite of left thumb without damage to nail

S61.059- Open bite of unspecified thumb without damage to nail

S61.1 Open wound of thumb with damage to nail

S61.10 Unspecified open wound of thumb with damage to nail

S61.101- Unspecified open wound of right thumb with damage to nail

S61.102- Unspecified open wound of left thumb with damage to nail

S61.109- Unspecified open wound of unspecified thumb with damage to nail

6 **S61.11 Laceration without foreign body of thumb with damage to nail**

Laterality SP 7 **S61.111- Laceration without foreign body of right thumb with damage to nail**

Laterality SP 7 **S61.112- Laceration without foreign body of left thumb with damage to nail**

Laterality !Q 7 **S61.119- Laceration without foreign body of unspecified thumb with damage to nail**

6 **S61.12 Laceration with foreign body of thumb with damage to nail**

Laterality SP 7 **S61.121- Laceration with foreign body of right thumb with damage to nail**

Laterality SP 7 **S61.122- Laceration with foreign body of left thumb with damage to nail**

Laterality !Q 7 **S61.129- Laceration with foreign body of unspecified thumb with damage to nail**

6 **S61.13 Puncture wound without foreign body of thumb with damage to nail**

Laterality SP 7 **S61.131- Puncture wound without foreign body of right thumb with damage to nail**

Laterality SP 7 **S61.132- Puncture wound without foreign body of left thumb with damage to nail**

Laterality !Q 7 **S61.139- Puncture wound without foreign body of unspecified thumb with damage to nail**

6 **S61.14 Puncture wound with foreign body of thumb with damage to nail**

Laterality SP 7 **S61.141- Puncture wound with foreign body of right thumb with damage to nail**

Laterality SP 7 **S61.142- Puncture wound with foreign body of left thumb with damage to nail**

Laterality !Q 7 **S61.149- Puncture wound with foreign body of unspecified thumb with damage to nail**

6 **S61.15 Open bite of thumb with damage to nail**

Bite of thumb with damage to nail NOS

EXCLUDES 1 superficial bite of thumb (S60.36-, S60.37-)

Laterality SP 7 **S61.151- Open bite of right thumb with damage to nail**

Laterality SP 7 **S61.152- Open bite of left thumb with damage to nail**

Laterality !Q 7 **S61.159- Open bite of unspecified thumb with damage to nail**

5 **S61.2 Open wound of other finger without damage to nail**

EXCLUDES 1 open wound of finger involving nail (matrix) (S61.3-)

EXCLUDES 2 open wound of thumb without damage to nail (S61.0-)

6 **S61.20 Unspecified open wound of other finger without damage to nail**

Laterality SP 7 **S61.200- Unspecified open wound of right index finger without damage to nail**

Laterality SP 7 **S61.201- Unspecified open wound of left index finger without damage to nail**

Laterality SP 7 **S61.202- Unspecified open wound of right middle finger without damage to nail**

Laterality SP 7 **S61.203- Unspecified open wound of left middle finger without damage to nail**

Laterality SP 7 **S61.204- Unspecified open wound of right ring finger without damage to nail**

Laterality SP 7 **S61.205- Unspecified open wound of left ring finger without damage to nail**

Laterality SP 7 **S61.206- Unspecified open wound of right little finger without damage to nail**

Laterality SP 7 **S61.207- Unspecified open wound of left little finger without damage to nail**

Laterality SP 7 **S61.208- Unspecified open wound of other finger without damage to nail**

Unspecified open wound of specified finger with unspecified laterality without damage to nail

Laterality !Q 7 **S61.209- Unspecified open wound of unspecified finger without damage to nail**

6 **S61.21 Laceration without foreign body of finger without damage to nail**

Laterality SP 7 **S61.210- Laceration without foreign body of right index finger without damage to nail**

Laterality SP 7 **S61.211- Laceration without foreign body of left index finger without damage to nail**

Laterality SP 7 **S61.212- Laceration without foreign body of right middle finger without damage to nail**

Laterality SP 7 **S61.213- Laceration without foreign body of left middle finger without damage to nail**

Laterality SP 7 **S61.214- Laceration without foreign body of right ring finger without damage to nail**

Laterality SP 7 **S61.215- Laceration without foreign body of left ring finger without damage to nail**

Laterality SP 7 **S61.216- Laceration without foreign body of right little finger without damage to nail**

Laterality SP 7 **S61.217- Laceration without foreign body of left little finger without damage to nail**

Laterality SP 7 **S61.218- Laceration without foreign body of other finger without damage to nail**

Laceration without foreign body of specified finger with unspecified laterality without damage to nail

Laterality !Q 7 **S61.219- Laceration without foreign body of unspecified finger without damage to nail**

6 **S61.22 Laceration with foreign body of finger without damage to nail**

Chapter 19

S00-T88

4 4th digit required | 5 5th digit required | 6 6th digit required | 7 7th digit required | 7th digit placeholder | + Additional code | Laterality

SP 7 **S61.220- Laceration with foreign body of right index finger without damage to nail**

SP 7 **S61.221- Laceration with foreign body of left index finger without damage to nail**

SP 7 **S61.222- Laceration with foreign body of right middle finger without damage to nail**

SP 7 **S61.223- Laceration with foreign body of left middle finger without damage to nail**

SP 7 **S61.224- Laceration with foreign body of right ring finger without damage to nail**

SP 7 **S61.225- Laceration with foreign body of left ring finger without damage to nail**

SP 7 **S61.226- Laceration with foreign body of right little finger without damage to nail**

SP 7 **S61.227- Laceration with foreign body of left little finger without damage to nail**

SP 7 **S61.228- Laceration with foreign body of other finger without damage to nail**

Laceration with foreign body of specified finger with unspecified laterality without damage to nail

IQ 7 **S61.229- Laceration with foreign body of unspecified finger without damage to nail**

6 **S61.23 Puncture wound without foreign body of finger without damage to nail**

SP 7 **S61.230- Puncture wound without foreign body of right index finger without damage to nail**

SP 7 **S61.231- Puncture wound without foreign body of left index finger without damage to nail**

SP 7 **S61.232- Puncture wound without foreign body of right middle finger without damage to nail**

SP 7 **S61.233- Puncture wound without foreign body of left middle finger without damage to nail**

SP 7 **S61.234- Puncture wound without foreign body of right ring finger without damage to nail**

SP 7 **S61.235- Puncture wound without foreign body of left ring finger without damage to nail**

SP 7 **S61.236- Puncture wound without foreign body of right little finger without damage to nail**

SP 7 **S61.237- Puncture wound without foreign body of left little finger without damage to nail**

SP 7 **S61.238- Puncture wound without foreign body of other finger without damage to nail**

Puncture wound without foreign body of specified finger with unspecified laterality without damage to nail

IQ 7 **S61.239- Puncture wound without foreign body of unspecified finger without damage to nail**

6 **S61.24 Puncture wound with foreign body of finger without damage to nail**

SP 7 **S61.240- Puncture wound with foreign body of right index finger without damage to nail**

SP 7 **S61.241- Puncture wound with foreign body of left index finger without damage to nail**

SP 7 **S61.242- Puncture wound with foreign body of right middle finger without damage to nail**

SP 7 **S61.243- Puncture wound with foreign body of left middle finger without damage to nail**

SP 7 **S61.244- Puncture wound with foreign body of right ring finger without damage to nail**

SP 7 **S61.245- Puncture wound with foreign body of left ring finger without damage to nail**

SP 7 **S61.246- Puncture wound with foreign body of right little finger without damage to nail**

SP 7 **S61.247- Puncture wound with foreign body of left little finger without damage to nail**

SP 7 **S61.248- Puncture wound with foreign body of other finger without damage to nail**

Puncture wound with foreign body of specified finger with unspecified laterality without damage to nail

IQ 7 **S61.249- Puncture wound with foreign body of unspecified finger without damage to nail**

6 **S61.25 Open bite of finger without damage to nail**

Bite of finger without damage to nail NOS

EXCLUDES 1 superficial bite of finger (S60.46-, S60.47-)

SP 7 **S61.250- Open bite of right index finger without damage to nail**

SP 7 **S61.251- Open bite of left index finger without damage to nail**

SP 7 **S61.252- Open bite of right middle finger without damage to nail**

SP 7 **S61.253- Open bite of left middle finger without damage to nail**

SP 7 **S61.254- Open bite of right ring finger without damage to nail**

SP 7 **S61.255- Open bite of left ring finger without damage to nail**

SP 7 **S61.256- Open bite of right little finger without damage to nail**

SP 7 **S61.257- Open bite of left little finger without damage to nail**

SP 7 **S61.258- Open bite of other finger without damage to nail**

Open bite of specified finger with unspecified laterality without damage to nail

IQ 7 **S61.259- Open bite of unspecified finger without damage to nail**

Chapter 19

S00-T88

5 **S61.3 Open wound of other finger with damage to nail**

6 **S61.30 Unspecified open wound of finger with damage to nail**

Laterality SP 7 **S61.300- Unspecified open wound of right index finger with damage to nail**

Laterality SP 7 **S61.301- Unspecified open wound of left index finger with damage to nail**

Laterality SP 7 **S61.302- Unspecified open wound of right middle finger with damage to nail**

Laterality SP 7 **S61.303- Unspecified open wound of left middle finger with damage to nail**

Laterality SP 7 **S61.304- Unspecified open wound of right ring finger with damage to nail**

Laterality SP 7 **S61.305- Unspecified open wound of left ring finger with damage to nail**

Laterality SP 7 **S61.306- Unspecified open wound of right little finger with damage to nail**

Laterality SP 7 **S61.307- Unspecified open wound of left little finger with damage to nail**

Laterality SP 7 **S61.308- Unspecified open wound of other finger with damage to nail**

Unspecified open wound of specified finger with unspecified laterality with damage to nail

Laterality IQ 7 **S61.309- Unspecified open wound of unspecified finger with damage to nail**

6 **S61.31 Laceration without foreign body of finger with damage to nail**

Laterality SP 7 **S61.310- Laceration without foreign body of right index finger with damage to nail**

Laterality SP 7 **S61.311- Laceration without foreign body of left index finger with damage to nail**

Laterality SP 7 **S61.312- Laceration without foreign body of right middle finger with damage to nail**

Laterality SP 7 **S61.313- Laceration without foreign body of left middle finger with damage to nail**

Laterality SP 7 **S61.314- Laceration without foreign body of right ring finger with damage to nail**

Laterality SP 7 **S61.315- Laceration without foreign body of left ring finger with damage to nail**

Laterality SP 7 **S61.316- Laceration without foreign body of right little finger with damage to nail**

Laterality SP 7 **S61.317- Laceration without foreign body of left little finger with damage to nail**

Laterality SP 7 **S61.318- Laceration without foreign body of other finger with damage to nail**

Laceration without foreign body of specified finger with unspecified laterality with damage to nail

Laterality IQ 7 **S61.319- Laceration without foreign body of unspecified finger with damage to nail**

6 **S61.32 Laceration with foreign body of finger with damage to nail**

Laterality SP 7 **S61.320- Laceration with foreign body of right index finger with damage to nail**

Laterality SP 7 **S61.321- Laceration with foreign body of left index finger with damage to nail**

Laterality SP 7 **S61.322- Laceration with foreign body of right middle finger with damage to nail**

Laterality SP 7 **S61.323- Laceration with foreign body of left middle finger with damage to nail**

Laterality SP 7 **S61.324- Laceration with foreign body of right ring finger with damage to nail**

Laterality SP 7 **S61.325- Laceration with foreign body of left ring finger with damage to nail**

Laterality SP 7 **S61.326- Laceration with foreign body of right little finger with damage to nail**

Laterality SP 7 **S61.327- Laceration with foreign body of left little finger with damage to nail**

Laterality SP 7 **S61.328- Laceration with foreign body of other finger with damage to nail**

Laceration with foreign body of specified finger with unspecified laterality with damage to nail

Laterality IQ 7 **S61.329- Laceration with foreign body of unspecified finger with damage to nail**

6 **S61.33 Puncture wound without foreign body of finger with damage to nail**

Laterality SP 7 **S61.330- Puncture wound without foreign body of right index finger with damage to nail**

Laterality SP 7 **S61.331- Puncture wound without foreign body of left index finger with damage to nail**

Laterality SP 7 **S61.332- Puncture wound without foreign body of right middle finger with damage to nail**

Laterality SP 7 **S61.333- Puncture wound without foreign body of left middle finger with damage to nail**

Laterality SP 7 **S61.334- Puncture wound without foreign body of right ring finger with damage to nail**

Laterality SP 7 **S61.335- Puncture wound without foreign body of left ring finger with damage to nail**

Laterality SP 7 **S61.336- Puncture wound without foreign body of right little finger with damage to nail**

Laterality SP 7 **S61.337- Puncture wound without foreign body of left little finger with damage to nail**

Laterality SP 7 **S61.338- Puncture wound without foreign body of other finger with damage to nail**

Puncture wound without foreign body of specified finger with unspecified laterality with damage to nail

S61.339- Puncture wound without foreign body of unspecified finger with damage to nail

S61.34 Puncture wound with foreign body of finger with damage to nail

S61.340- Puncture wound with foreign body of right index finger with damage to nail

S61.341- Puncture wound with foreign body of left index finger with damage to nail

S61.342- Puncture wound with foreign body of right middle finger with damage to nail

S61.343- Puncture wound with foreign body of left middle finger with damage to nail

S61.344- Puncture wound with foreign body of right ring finger with damage to nail

S61.345- Puncture wound with foreign body of left ring finger with damage to nail

S61.346- Puncture wound with foreign body of right little finger with damage to nail

S61.347- Puncture wound with foreign body of left little finger with damage to nail

S61.348- Puncture wound with foreign body of other finger with damage to nail

Puncture wound with foreign body of specified finger with unspecified laterality with damage to nail

S61.349- Puncture wound with foreign body of unspecified finger with damage to nail

S61.35 Open bite of finger with damage to nail

Bite of finger with damage to nail NOS

EXCLUDES 1 superficial bite of finger (S60.46-, S60.47-)

S61.350- Open bite of right index finger with damage to nail

S61.351- Open bite of left index finger with damage to nail

S61.352- Open bite of right middle finger with damage to nail

S61.353- Open bite of left middle finger with damage to nail

S61.354- Open bite of right ring finger with damage to nail

S61.355- Open bite of left ring finger with damage to nail

S61.356- Open bite of right little finger with damage to nail

S61.357- Open bite of left little finger with damage to nail

S61.358- Open bite of other finger with damage to nail

Open bite of specified finger with unspecified laterality with damage to nail

S61.359- Open bite of unspecified finger with damage to nail

S61.4 Open wound of hand

S61.40 Unspecified open wound of hand

S61.401- Unspecified open wound of right hand

S61.402- Unspecified open wound of left hand

S61.409- Unspecified open wound of unspecified hand

S61.41 Laceration without foreign body of hand

S61.411- Laceration without foreign body of right hand

S61.412- Laceration without foreign body of left hand

S61.419- Laceration without foreign body of unspecified hand

S61.42 Laceration with foreign body of hand

S61.421- Laceration with foreign body of right hand

S61.422- Laceration with foreign body of left hand

S61.429- Laceration with foreign body of unspecified hand

S61.43 Puncture wound without foreign body of hand

S61.431- Puncture wound without foreign body of right hand

S61.432- Puncture wound without foreign body of left hand

S61.439- Puncture wound without foreign body of unspecified hand

S61.44 Puncture wound with foreign body of hand

S61.441- Puncture wound with foreign body of right hand

S61.442- Puncture wound with foreign body of left hand

S61.449- Puncture wound with foreign body of unspecified hand

S61.45 Open bite of hand

Bite of hand NOS

EXCLUDES 1 superficial bite of hand (S60.56-, S60.57-)

S61.451- Open bite of right hand

S61.452- Open bite of left hand

S61.459- Open bite of unspecified hand

S61.5 Open wound of wrist

S61.50 Unspecified open wound of wrist

S61.501- Unspecified open wound of right wrist

S61.502- Unspecified open wound of left wrist

S61.509- Unspecified open wound of unspecified wrist

S61.51 Laceration without foreign body of wrist

S61.511- Laceration without foreign body of right wrist

S61.512- Laceration without foreign body of left wrist

S61.519- Laceration without foreign body of unspecified wrist

S61.52 Laceration with foreign body of wrist

S61.521- Laceration with foreign body of right wrist

S61.522- Laceration with foreign body of left wrist

S61.529- Laceration with foreign body of unspecified wrist

S61.53 Puncture wound without foreign body of wrist

S61.531- Puncture wound without foreign body of right wrist

S61.532- Puncture wound without foreign body of left wrist

S61.539- Puncture wound without foreign body of unspecified wrist

S61.54 Puncture wound with foreign body of wrist

S61.541- Puncture wound with foreign body of right wrist

S61.542- Puncture wound with foreign body of left wrist

S61.549- Puncture wound with foreign body of unspecified wrist

S61.55 Open bite of wrist

Bite of wrist NOS

EXCLUDES 1 superficial bite of wrist (S60.86-, S60.87-)

S61.551- Open bite of right wrist

S61.552- Open bite of left wrist

S61.559- Open bite of unspecified wrist

S62 Fracture at wrist and hand level

Note:

A fracture not indicated as displaced or nondisplaced should be coded to displaced

A fracture not indicated as open or closed should be coded to closed

EXCLUDES 1 traumatic amputation of wrist and hand (S68.-)

EXCLUDES 2 fracture of distal parts of ulna and radius (S52.-)

The appropriate 7th character is to be added to each code from category S62

A	initial encounter for closed fracture
B	initial encounter for open fracture
D	subsequent encounter for fracture with routine healing
G	subsequent encounter for fracture with delayed healing
K	subsequent encounter for fracture with nonunion
P	subsequent encounter for fracture with malunion
S	sequela

CODING TIPS✓ Fractures repaired by joint replacements are NOT coded with Z47.1. Fractures repaired by any other orthopedic surgery are NOT coded with Z47.89. Z codes are not appropriate for fractures of any kind. Code the fracture with 7th character D for fractures undergoing surgical repair.

CODING TIPS✓ 'D' is the 7th character for home care and hospice unless the physician or NPP has documented delayed healing, nonunion or malunion. A sequela is a condition left after the fracture has healed. The Gustilo open fracture classification must be used for open fractures. The default 7th character for open fractures is E.

CODING TIPS✓ A fracture not indicated as displaced or nondisplaced should be coded to displaced. A fracture not indicated as open or closed should be coded to closed.

S62.0 Fracture of navicular [scaphoid] bone of wrist

S62.00 Unspecified fracture of navicular [scaphoid] bone of wrist

S62.001- Unspecified fracture of navicular [scaphoid] bone of right wrist

S62.002- Unspecified fracture of navicular [scaphoid] bone of left wrist

S62.009- Unspecified fracture of navicular [scaphoid] bone of unspecified wrist

S62.01 Fracture of distal pole of navicular [scaphoid] bone of wrist

Fracture of volar tuberosity of navicular [scaphoid] bone of wrist

S62.011- Displaced fracture of distal pole of navicular [scaphoid] bone of right wrist

S62.012- Displaced fracture of distal pole of navicular [scaphoid] bone of left wrist

S62.013- Displaced fracture of distal pole of navicular [scaphoid] bone of unspecified wrist

S62.014- Nondisplaced fracture of distal pole of navicular [scaphoid] bone of right wrist

S62.015- Nondisplaced fracture of distal pole of navicular [scaphoid] bone of left wrist

S62.016- Nondisplaced fracture of distal pole of navicular [scaphoid] bone of unspecified wrist

S62.02 Fracture of middle third of navicular [scaphoid] bone of wrist

S62.021- Displaced fracture of middle third of navicular [scaphoid] bone of right wrist

S62.022- Displaced fracture of middle third of navicular [scaphoid] bone of left wrist

S62.023- Displaced fracture of middle third of navicular [scaphoid] bone of unspecified wrist

Chapter 19

S00-T88

SP 7 S62.024- Nondisplaced fracture of middle third of navicular [scaphoid] bone of right wrist

SP 7 S62.025- Nondisplaced fracture of middle third of navicular [scaphoid] bone of left wrist

!Q 7 S62.026- Nondisplaced fracture of middle third of navicular [scaphoid] bone of unspecified wrist

6 S62.03 Fracture of proximal third of navicular [scaphoid] bone of wrist

SP 7 S62.031- Displaced fracture of proximal third of navicular [scaphoid] bone of right wrist

SP 7 S62.032- Displaced fracture of proximal third of navicular [scaphoid] bone of left wrist

!Q 7 S62.033- Displaced fracture of proximal third of navicular [scaphoid] bone of unspecified wrist

SP 7 S62.034- Nondisplaced fracture of proximal third of navicular [scaphoid] bone of right wrist

SP 7 S62.035- Nondisplaced fracture of proximal third of navicular [scaphoid] bone of left wrist

!Q 7 S62.036- Nondisplaced fracture of proximal third of navicular [scaphoid] bone of unspecified wrist

5 S62.1 Fracture of other and unspecified carpal bone(s)

EXCLUDES 2 fracture of scaphoid of wrist (S62.0-)

6 S62.10 Fracture of unspecified carpal bone

Fracture of wrist NOS

SP 7 S62.101- Fracture of unspecified carpal bone, right wrist

SP 7 S62.102- Fracture of unspecified carpal bone, left wrist

!Q 7 S62.109- Fracture of unspecified carpal bone, unspecified wrist

6 S62.11 Fracture of triquetrum [cuneiform] bone of wrist

SP 7 S62.111- Displaced fracture of triquetrum [cuneiform] bone, right wrist

SP 7 S62.112- Displaced fracture of triquetrum [cuneiform] bone, left wrist

!Q 7 S62.113- Displaced fracture of triquetrum [cuneiform] bone, unspecified wrist

SP 7 S62.114- Nondisplaced fracture of triquetrum [cuneiform] bone, right wrist

SP 7 S62.115- Nondisplaced fracture of triquetrum [cuneiform] bone, left wrist

!Q 7 S62.116- Nondisplaced fracture of triquetrum [cuneiform] bone, unspecified wrist

6 S62.12 Fracture of lunate [semilunar]

SP 7 S62.121- Displaced fracture of lunate [semilunar], right wrist

SP 7 S62.122- Displaced fracture of lunate [semilunar], left wrist

!Q 7 S62.123- Displaced fracture of lunate [semilunar], unspecified wrist

SP 7 S62.124- Nondisplaced fracture of lunate [semilunar], right wrist

SP 7 S62.125- Nondisplaced fracture of lunate [semilunar], left wrist

!Q 7 S62.126- Nondisplaced fracture of lunate [semilunar], unspecified wrist

6 S62.13 Fracture of capitate [os magnum] bone

SP 7 S62.131- Displaced fracture of capitate [os magnum] bone, right wrist

SP 7 S62.132- Displaced fracture of capitate [os magnum] bone, left wrist

!Q 7 S62.133- Displaced fracture of capitate [os magnum] bone, unspecified wrist

SP 7 S62.134- Nondisplaced fracture of capitate [os magnum] bone, right wrist

SP 7 S62.135- Nondisplaced fracture of capitate [os magnum] bone, left wrist

!Q 7 S62.136- Nondisplaced fracture of capitate [os magnum] bone, unspecified wrist

6 S62.14 Fracture of body of hamate [unciform] bone

Fracture of hamate [unciform] bone NOS

SP 7 S62.141- Displaced fracture of body of hamate [unciform] bone, right wrist

SP 7 S62.142- Displaced fracture of body of hamate [unciform] bone, left wrist

!Q 7 S62.143- Displaced fracture of body of hamate [unciform] bone, unspecified wrist

SP 7 S62.144- Nondisplaced fracture of body of hamate [unciform] bone, right wrist

SP 7 S62.145- Nondisplaced fracture of body of hamate [unciform] bone, left wrist

!Q 7 S62.146- Nondisplaced fracture of body of hamate [unciform] bone, unspecified wrist

6 S62.15 Fracture of hook process of hamate [unciform] bone

Fracture of unciform process of hamate [unciform] bone

SP 7 S62.151- Displaced fracture of hook process of hamate [unciform] bone, right wrist

SP 7 S62.152- Displaced fracture of hook process of hamate [unciform] bone, left wrist

!Q 7 S62.153- Displaced fracture of hook process of hamate [unciform] bone, unspecified wrist

SP 7 S62.154- Nondisplaced fracture of hook process of hamate [unciform] bone, right wrist

SP 7 S62.155- Nondisplaced fracture of hook process of hamate [unciform] bone, left wrist

Chapter 19

S00-T88

S62.156- Nondisplaced fracture of hook process of hamate [unciform] bone, unspecified wrist

S62.16 Fracture of pisiform

S62.161- Displaced fracture of pisiform, right wrist

S62.162- Displaced fracture of pisiform, left wrist

S62.163- Displaced fracture of pisiform, unspecified wrist

S62.164- Nondisplaced fracture of pisiform, right wrist

S62.165- Nondisplaced fracture of pisiform, left wrist

S62.166- Nondisplaced fracture of pisiform, unspecified wrist

S62.17 Fracture of trapezium [larger multangular]

S62.171- Displaced fracture of trapezium [larger multangular], right wrist

S62.172- Displaced fracture of trapezium [larger multangular], left wrist

S62.173- Displaced fracture of trapezium [larger multangular], unspecified wrist

S62.174- Nondisplaced fracture of trapezium [larger multangular], right wrist

S62.175- Nondisplaced fracture of trapezium [larger multangular], left wrist

S62.176- Nondisplaced fracture of trapezium [larger multangular], unspecified wrist

S62.18 Fracture of trapezoid [smaller multangular]

S62.181- Displaced fracture of trapezoid [smaller multangular], right wrist

S62.182- Displaced fracture of trapezoid [smaller multangular], left wrist

S62.183- Displaced fracture of trapezoid [smaller multangular], unspecified wrist

S62.184- Nondisplaced fracture of trapezoid [smaller multangular], right wrist

S62.185- Nondisplaced fracture of trapezoid [smaller multangular], left wrist

S62.186- Nondisplaced fracture of trapezoid [smaller multangular], unspecified wrist

S62.2 Fracture of first metacarpal bone

S62.20 Unspecified fracture of first metacarpal bone

S62.201- Unspecified fracture of first metacarpal bone, right hand

S62.202- Unspecified fracture of first metacarpal bone, left hand

S62.209- Unspecified fracture of first metacarpal bone, unspecified hand

S62.21 Bennett's fracture

DEFINITION An intra-articular fracture dislocation of the base of the first metacarpal bone (thumb) extending into the carpometacarpal joint.

S62.211- Bennett's fracture, right hand

S62.212- Bennett's fracture, left hand

S62.213- Bennett's fracture, unspecified hand

S62.22 Rolando's fracture

S62.221- Displaced Rolando's fracture, right hand

S62.222- Displaced Rolando's fracture, left hand

S62.223- Displaced Rolando's fracture, unspecified hand

S62.224- Nondisplaced Rolando's fracture, right hand

S62.225- Nondisplaced Rolando's fracture, left hand

S62.226- Nondisplaced Rolando's fracture, unspecified hand

S62.23 Other fracture of base of first metacarpal bone

S62.231- Other displaced fracture of base of first metacarpal bone, right hand

S62.232- Other displaced fracture of base of first metacarpal bone, left hand

S62.233- Other displaced fracture of base of first metacarpal bone, unspecified hand

S62.234- Other nondisplaced fracture of base of first metacarpal bone, right hand

S62.235- Other nondisplaced fracture of base of first metacarpal bone, left hand

S62.236- Other nondisplaced fracture of base of first metacarpal bone, unspecified hand

S62.24 Fracture of shaft of first metacarpal bone

S62.241- Displaced fracture of shaft of first metacarpal bone, right hand

S62.242- Displaced fracture of shaft of first metacarpal bone, left hand

S62.243- Displaced fracture of shaft of first metacarpal bone, unspecified hand

S62.244- Nondisplaced fracture of shaft of first metacarpal bone, right hand

S62.245- Nondisplaced fracture of shaft of first metacarpal bone, left hand

S62.246- Nondisplaced fracture of shaft of first metacarpal bone, unspecified hand

S62.25 Fracture of neck of first metacarpal bone

S62.251- Displaced fracture of neck of first metacarpal bone, right hand

S62.252- Displaced fracture of neck of first metacarpal bone, left hand

S62.253- Displaced fracture of neck of first metacarpal bone, unspecified hand

SP 7 **S62.254-** **Nondisplaced fracture of neck of first metacarpal bone, right hand**

SP 7 **S62.255-** **Nondisplaced fracture of neck of first metacarpal bone, left hand**

IQ 7 **S62.256-** **Nondisplaced fracture of neck of first metacarpal bone, unspecified hand**

6 **S62.29** **Other fracture of first metacarpal bone**

SP 7 **S62.291-** **Other fracture of first metacarpal bone, right hand**

SP 7 **S62.292-** **Other fracture of first metacarpal bone, left hand**

IQ 7 **S62.299-** **Other fracture of first metacarpal bone, unspecified hand**

5 **S62.3** **Fracture of other and unspecified metacarpal bone**

EXCLUDES 2 fracture of first metacarpal bone (S62.2-)

6 **S62.30** **Unspecified fracture of other metacarpal bone**

SP 7 **S62.300-** **Unspecified fracture of second metacarpal bone, right hand**

SP 7 **S62.301-** **Unspecified fracture of second metacarpal bone, left hand**

SP 7 **S62.302-** **Unspecified fracture of third metacarpal bone, right hand**

SP 7 **S62.303-** **Unspecified fracture of third metacarpal bone, left hand**

SP 7 **S62.304-** **Unspecified fracture of fourth metacarpal bone, right hand**

SP 7 **S62.305-** **Unspecified fracture of fourth metacarpal bone, left hand**

SP 7 **S62.306-** **Unspecified fracture of fifth metacarpal bone, right hand**

SP 7 **S62.307-** **Unspecified fracture of fifth metacarpal bone, left hand**

IQ 7 **S62.308-** **Unspecified fracture of other metacarpal bone**

Unspecified fracture of specified metacarpal bone with unspecified laterality

IQ 7 **S62.309-** **Unspecified fracture of unspecified metacarpal bone**

6 **S62.31** **Displaced fracture of base of other metacarpal bone**

SP 7 **S62.310-** **Displaced fracture of base of second metacarpal bone, right hand**

SP 7 **S62.311-** **Displaced fracture of base of second metacarpal bone, left hand**

SP 7 **S62.312-** **Displaced fracture of base of third metacarpal bone, right hand**

SP 7 **S62.313-** **Displaced fracture of base of third metacarpal bone, left hand**

SP 7 **S62.314-** **Displaced fracture of base of fourth metacarpal bone, right hand**

SP 7 **S62.315-** **Displaced fracture of base of fourth metacarpal bone, left hand**

SP 7 **S62.316-** **Displaced fracture of base of fifth metacarpal bone, right hand**

SP 7 **S62.317-** **Displaced fracture of base of fifth metacarpal bone, left hand**

SP 7 **S62.318-** **Displaced fracture of base of other metacarpal bone**

Displaced fracture of base of specified metacarpal bone with unspecified laterality

SP IQ 7 **S62.319-** **Displaced fracture of base of unspecified metacarpal bone**

6 **S62.32** **Displaced fracture of shaft of other metacarpal bone**

SP 7 **S62.320-** **Displaced fracture of shaft of second metacarpal bone, right hand**

SP 7 **S62.321-** **Displaced fracture of shaft of second metacarpal bone, left hand**

SP 7 **S62.322-** **Displaced fracture of shaft of third metacarpal bone, right hand**

SP 7 **S62.323-** **Displaced fracture of shaft of third metacarpal bone, left hand**

SP 7 **S62.324-** **Displaced fracture of shaft of fourth metacarpal bone, right hand**

SP 7 **S62.325-** **Displaced fracture of shaft of fourth metacarpal bone, left hand**

SP 7 **S62.326-** **Displaced fracture of shaft of fifth metacarpal bone, right hand**

SP 7 **S62.327-** **Displaced fracture of shaft of fifth metacarpal bone, left hand**

SP 7 **S62.328-** **Displaced fracture of shaft of other metacarpal bone**

Displaced fracture of shaft of specified metacarpal bone with unspecified laterality

IQ 7 **S62.329-** **Displaced fracture of shaft of unspecified metacarpal bone**

6 **S62.33** **Displaced fracture of neck of other metacarpal bone**

SP 7 **S62.330-** **Displaced fracture of neck of second metacarpal bone, right hand**

SP 7 **S62.331-** **Displaced fracture of neck of second metacarpal bone, left hand**

SP 7 **S62.332-** **Displaced fracture of neck of third metacarpal bone, right hand**

SP 7 **S62.333-** **Displaced fracture of neck of third metacarpal bone, left hand**

SP 7 **S62.334-** **Displaced fracture of neck of fourth metacarpal bone, right hand**

SP 7 **S62.335-** **Displaced fracture of neck of fourth metacarpal bone, left hand**

SP 7 **S62.336-** **Displaced fracture of neck of fifth metacarpal bone, right hand**

SP 7 **S62.337-** **Displaced fracture of neck of fifth metacarpal bone, left hand**

SP 7 **S62.338-** **Displaced fracture of neck of other metacarpal bone**

Displaced fracture of neck of specified metacarpal bone with unspecified laterality

S62.339- **Displaced fracture of neck of unspecified metacarpal bone**

S62.34 **Nondisplaced fracture of base of other metacarpal bone**

S62.340- **Nondisplaced fracture of base of second metacarpal bone, right hand**

S62.341- **Nondisplaced fracture of base of second metacarpal bone, left hand**

S62.342- **Nondisplaced fracture of base of third metacarpal bone, right hand**

S62.343- **Nondisplaced fracture of base of third metacarpal bone, left hand**

S62.344- **Nondisplaced fracture of base of fourth metacarpal bone, right hand**

S62.345- **Nondisplaced fracture of base of fourth metacarpal bone, left hand**

S62.346- **Nondisplaced fracture of base of fifth metacarpal bone, right hand**

S62.347- **Nondisplaced fracture of base of fifth metacarpal bone, left hand**

S62.348- **Nondisplaced fracture of base of other metacarpal bone**
Nondisplaced fracture of base of specified metacarpal bone with unspecified laterality

S62.349- **Nondisplaced fracture of base of unspecified metacarpal bone**

S62.35 **Nondisplaced fracture of shaft of other metacarpal bone**

S62.350- **Nondisplaced fracture of shaft of second metacarpal bone, right hand**

S62.351- **Nondisplaced fracture of shaft of second metacarpal bone, left hand**

S62.352- **Nondisplaced fracture of shaft of third metacarpal bone, right hand**

S62.353- **Nondisplaced fracture of shaft of third metacarpal bone, left hand**

S62.354- **Nondisplaced fracture of shaft of fourth metacarpal bone, right hand**

S62.355- **Nondisplaced fracture of shaft of fourth metacarpal bone, left hand**

S62.356- **Nondisplaced fracture of shaft of fifth metacarpal bone, right hand**

S62.357- **Nondisplaced fracture of shaft of fifth metacarpal bone, left hand**

S62.358- **Nondisplaced fracture of shaft of other metacarpal bone**
Nondisplaced fracture of shaft of specified metacarpal bone with unspecified laterality

S62.359- **Nondisplaced fracture of shaft of unspecified metacarpal bone**

S62.36 **Nondisplaced fracture of neck of other metacarpal bone**

S62.360- **Nondisplaced fracture of neck of second metacarpal bone, right hand**

S62.361- **Nondisplaced fracture of neck of second metacarpal bone, left hand**

S62.362- **Nondisplaced fracture of neck of third metacarpal bone, right hand**

S62.363- **Nondisplaced fracture of neck of third metacarpal bone, left hand**

S62.364- **Nondisplaced fracture of neck of fourth metacarpal bone, right hand**

S62.365- **Nondisplaced fracture of neck of fourth metacarpal bone, left hand**

S62.366- **Nondisplaced fracture of neck of fifth metacarpal bone, right hand**

S62.367- **Nondisplaced fracture of neck of fifth metacarpal bone, left hand**

S62.368- **Nondisplaced fracture of neck of other metacarpal bone**
Nondisplaced fracture of neck of specified metacarpal bone with unspecified laterality

S62.369- **Nondisplaced fracture of neck of unspecified metacarpal bone**

S62.39 **Other fracture of other metacarpal bone**

S62.390- **Other fracture of second metacarpal bone, right hand**

S62.391- **Other fracture of second metacarpal bone, left hand**

S62.392- **Other fracture of third metacarpal bone, right hand**

S62.393- **Other fracture of third metacarpal bone, left hand**

S62.394- **Other fracture of fourth metacarpal bone, right hand**

S62.395- **Other fracture of fourth metacarpal bone, left hand**

S62.396- **Other fracture of fifth metacarpal bone, right hand**

S62.397- **Other fracture of fifth metacarpal bone, left hand**

S62.398- **Other fracture of other metacarpal bone**
Other fracture of specified metacarpal bone with unspecified laterality

S62.399- **Other fracture of unspecified metacarpal bone**

S62.5 **Fracture of thumb**

S62.50 **Fracture of unspecified phalanx of thumb**

S62.501- **Fracture of unspecified phalanx of right thumb**

S62.502- **Fracture of unspecified phalanx of left thumb**

S62.509- **Fracture of unspecified phalanx of unspecified thumb**

S62.51 **Fracture of proximal phalanx of thumb**

S62.511- **Displaced fracture of proximal phalanx of right thumb**

S62.512- **Displaced fracture of proximal phalanx of left thumb**

S62.513- **Displaced fracture of proximal phalanx of unspecified thumb**

Chapter 19

S00-T88

4th digit required 5th digit required 6th digit required 7th digit required 7th digit placeholder +Additional code Laterality

S62.514- Nondisplaced fracture of proximal phalanx of right thumb
S62.515- Nondisplaced fracture of proximal phalanx of left thumb
S62.516- Nondisplaced fracture of proximal phalanx of unspecified thumb

S62.52 Fracture of distal phalanx of thumb
S62.521- Displaced fracture of distal phalanx of right thumb
S62.522- Displaced fracture of distal phalanx of left thumb
S62.523- Displaced fracture of distal phalanx of unspecified thumb
S62.524- Nondisplaced fracture of distal phalanx of right thumb
S62.525- Nondisplaced fracture of distal phalanx of left thumb
S62.526- Nondisplaced fracture of distal phalanx of unspecified thumb

S62.6 Fracture of other and unspecified finger(s)
EXCLUDES 2 fracture of thumb (S62.5-)

S62.60 Fracture of unspecified phalanx of finger
S62.600- Fracture of unspecified phalanx of right index finger
S62.601- Fracture of unspecified phalanx of left index finger
S62.602- Fracture of unspecified phalanx of right middle finger
S62.603- Fracture of unspecified phalanx of left middle finger
S62.604- Fracture of unspecified phalanx of right ring finger
S62.605- Fracture of unspecified phalanx of left ring finger
S62.606- Fracture of unspecified phalanx of right little finger
S62.607- Fracture of unspecified phalanx of left little finger
S62.608- Fracture of unspecified phalanx of other finger
Fracture of unspecified phalanx of specified finger with unspecified laterality
S62.609- Fracture of unspecified phalanx of unspecified finger

S62.61 Displaced fracture of proximal phalanx of finger
S62.610- Displaced fracture of proximal phalanx of right index finger
S62.611- Displaced fracture of proximal phalanx of left index finger
S62.612- Displaced fracture of proximal phalanx of right middle finger
S62.613- Displaced fracture of proximal phalanx of left middle finger
S62.614- Displaced fracture of proximal phalanx of right ring finger
S62.615- Displaced fracture of proximal phalanx of left ring finger
S62.616- Displaced fracture of proximal phalanx of right little finger
S62.617- Displaced fracture of proximal phalanx of left little finger
S62.618- Displaced fracture of proximal phalanx of other finger
Displaced fracture of proximal phalanx of specified finger with unspecified laterality
S62.619- Displaced fracture of proximal phalanx of unspecified finger

S62.62 Displaced fracture of middle phalanx of finger
S62.620- Displaced fracture of middle phalanx of right index finger
S62.621- Displaced fracture of middle phalanx of left index finger
S62.622- Displaced fracture of middle phalanx of right middle finger
S62.623- Displaced fracture of middle phalanx of left middle finger
S62.624- Displaced fracture of middle phalanx of right ring finger
S62.625- Displaced fracture of middle phalanx of left ring finger
S62.626- Displaced fracture of middle phalanx of right little finger
S62.627- Displaced fracture of middle phalanx of left little finger
S62.628- Displaced fracture of middle phalanx of other finger
Displaced fracture of middle phalanx of specified finger with unspecified laterality
S62.629- Displaced fracture of middle phalanx of unspecified finger

S62.63 Displaced fracture of distal phalanx of finger
S62.630- Displaced fracture of distal phalanx of right index finger
S62.631- Displaced fracture of distal phalanx of left index finger
S62.632- Displaced fracture of distal phalanx of right middle finger
S62.633- Displaced fracture of distal phalanx of left middle finger
S62.634- Displaced fracture of distal phalanx of right ring finger
S62.635- Displaced fracture of distal phalanx of left ring finger
S62.636- Displaced fracture of distal phalanx of right little finger
S62.637- Displaced fracture of distal phalanx of left little finger
S62.638- Displaced fracture of distal phalanx of other finger
Displaced fracture of distal phalanx of specified finger with unspecified laterality
S62.639- Displaced fracture of distal phalanx of unspecified finger

S62.64 Nondisplaced fracture of proximal phalanx of finger
S62.640- Nondisplaced fracture of proximal phalanx of right index finger
S62.641- Nondisplaced fracture of proximal phalanx of left index finger

S62.642- Nondisplaced fracture of proximal phalanx of right middle finger

S62.643- Nondisplaced fracture of proximal phalanx of left middle finger

S62.644- Nondisplaced fracture of proximal phalanx of right ring finger

S62.645- Nondisplaced fracture of proximal phalanx of left ring finger

S62.646- Nondisplaced fracture of proximal phalanx of right little finger

S62.647- Nondisplaced fracture of proximal phalanx of left little finger

S62.648- Nondisplaced fracture of proximal phalanx of other finger

Nondisplaced fracture of proximal phalanx of specified finger with unspecified laterality

S62.649- Nondisplaced fracture of proximal phalanx of unspecified finger

S62.65 Nondisplaced fracture of middle phalanx of finger

S62.650- Nondisplaced fracture of middle phalanx of right index finger

S62.651- Nondisplaced fracture of middle phalanx of left index finger

S62.652- Nondisplaced fracture of middle phalanx of right middle finger

S62.653- Nondisplaced fracture of middle phalanx of left middle finger

S62.654- Nondisplaced fracture of middle phalanx of right ring finger

S62.655- Nondisplaced fracture of middle phalanx of left ring finger

S62.656- Nondisplaced fracture of middle phalanx of right little finger

S62.657- Nondisplaced fracture of middle phalanx of left little finger

S62.658- Nondisplaced fracture of middle phalanx of other finger

Nondisplaced fracture of middle phalanx of specified finger with unspecified laterality

S62.659- Nondisplaced fracture of middle phalanx of unspecified finger

S62.66 Nondisplaced fracture of distal phalanx of finger

S62.660- Nondisplaced fracture of distal phalanx of right index finger

S62.661- Nondisplaced fracture of distal phalanx of left index finger

S62.662- Nondisplaced fracture of distal phalanx of right middle finger

S62.663- Nondisplaced fracture of distal phalanx of left middle finger

S62.664- Nondisplaced fracture of distal phalanx of right ring finger

S62.665- Nondisplaced fracture of distal phalanx of left ring finger

S62.666- Nondisplaced fracture of distal phalanx of right little finger

S62.667- Nondisplaced fracture of distal phalanx of left little finger

S62.668- Nondisplaced fracture of distal phalanx of other finger

Nondisplaced fracture of distal phalanx of specified finger with unspecified laterality

S62.669- Nondisplaced fracture of distal phalanx of unspecified finger

S62.9 Unspecified fracture of wrist and hand

S62.90X- Unspecified fracture of unspecified wrist and hand

S62.91X- Unspecified fracture of right wrist and hand

S62.92X- Unspecified fracture of left wrist and hand

S63 Dislocation and sprain of joints and ligaments at wrist and hand level

INCLUDES
- avulsion of joint or ligament at wrist and hand level
- laceration of cartilage, joint or ligament at wrist and hand level
- sprain of cartilage, joint or ligament at wrist and hand level
- traumatic hemarthrosis of joint or ligament at wrist and hand level
- traumatic rupture of joint or ligament at wrist and hand level
- traumatic subluxation of joint or ligament at wrist and hand level
- traumatic tear of joint or ligament at wrist and hand level

Code also:
any associated open wound

EXCLUDES 2 strain of muscle, fascia and tendon of wrist and hand (S66.-)

The appropriate 7th character is to be added to each code from category S63
- A initial encounter
- D subsequent encounter
- S sequela

S63.0 Subluxation and dislocation of wrist and hand joints

S63.00 Unspecified subluxation and dislocation of wrist and hand

Dislocation of carpal bone NOS
Dislocation of distal end of radius NOS
Subluxation of carpal bone NOS
Subluxation of distal end of radius NOS

S63.001- Unspecified subluxation of right wrist and hand

S63.002- Unspecified subluxation of left wrist and hand

S63.003- Unspecified subluxation of unspecified wrist and hand

S63.004- Unspecified dislocation of right wrist and hand

Chapter 19
S00-T88

SP 7 S63.005- Unspecified dislocation of left wrist and hand
IQ 7 S63.006- Unspecified dislocation of unspecified wrist and hand

6 **S63.01 Subluxation and dislocation of distal radioulnar joint**
SP 7 S63.011- Subluxation of distal radioulnar joint of right wrist
SP 7 S63.012- Subluxation of distal radioulnar joint of left wrist
IQ 7 S63.013- Subluxation of distal radioulnar joint of unspecified wrist
SP 7 S63.014- Dislocation of distal radioulnar joint of right wrist
SP 7 S63.015- Dislocation of distal radioulnar joint of left wrist
IQ 7 S63.016- Dislocation of distal radioulnar joint of unspecified wrist

6 **S63.02 Subluxation and dislocation of radiocarpal joint**
SP 7 S63.021- Subluxation of radiocarpal joint of right wrist
SP 7 S63.022- Subluxation of radiocarpal joint of left wrist
IQ 7 S63.023- Subluxation of radiocarpal joint of unspecified wrist
SP 7 S63.024- Dislocation of radiocarpal joint of right wrist
SP 7 S63.025- Dislocation of radiocarpal joint of left wrist
IQ 7 S63.026- Dislocation of radiocarpal joint of unspecified wrist

6 **S63.03 Subluxation and dislocation of midcarpal joint**
SP 7 S63.031- Subluxation of midcarpal joint of right wrist
SP 7 S63.032- Subluxation of midcarpal joint of left wrist
IQ 7 S63.033- Subluxation of midcarpal joint of unspecified wrist
SP 7 S63.034- Dislocation of midcarpal joint of right wrist
SP 7 S63.035- Dislocation of midcarpal joint of left wrist
IQ 7 S63.036- Dislocation of midcarpal joint of unspecified wrist

6 **S63.04 Subluxation and dislocation of carpometacarpal joint of thumb**
EXCLUDES 2 interphalangeal subluxation and dislocation of thumb (S63.1-)
SP 7 S63.041- Subluxation of carpometacarpal joint of right thumb
SP 7 S63.042- Subluxation of carpometacarpal joint of left thumb
IQ 7 S63.043- Subluxation of carpometacarpal joint of unspecified thumb
SP 7 S63.044- Dislocation of carpometacarpal joint of right thumb
SP 7 S63.045- Dislocation of carpometacarpal joint of left thumb
IQ 7 S63.046- Dislocation of carpometacarpal joint of unspecified thumb

6 **S63.05 Subluxation and dislocation of other carpometacarpal joint**
EXCLUDES 2 subluxation and dislocation of carpometacarpal joint of thumb (S63.04-)
SP 7 S63.051- Subluxation of other carpometacarpal joint of right hand
SP 7 S63.052- Subluxation of other carpometacarpal joint of left hand
IQ 7 S63.053- Subluxation of other carpometacarpal joint of unspecified hand
SP 7 S63.054- Dislocation of other carpometacarpal joint of right hand
SP 7 S63.055- Dislocation of other carpometacarpal joint of left hand
IQ 7 S63.056- Dislocation of other carpometacarpal joint of unspecified hand

6 **S63.06 Subluxation and dislocation of metacarpal (bone), proximal end**
SP 7 S63.061- Subluxation of metacarpal (bone), proximal end of right hand
SP 7 S63.062- Subluxation of metacarpal (bone), proximal end of left hand
IQ 7 S63.063- Subluxation of metacarpal (bone), proximal end of unspecified hand
SP 7 S63.064- Dislocation of metacarpal (bone), proximal end of right hand
SP 7 S63.065- Dislocation of metacarpal (bone), proximal end of left hand
IQ 7 S63.066- Dislocation of metacarpal (bone), proximal end of unspecified hand

6 **S63.07 Subluxation and dislocation of distal end of ulna**
SP 7 S63.071- Subluxation of distal end of right ulna
SP 7 S63.072- Subluxation of distal end of left ulna
IQ 7 S63.073- Subluxation of distal end of unspecified ulna
SP 7 S63.074- Dislocation of distal end of right ulna
SP 7 S63.075- Dislocation of distal end of left ulna
IQ 7 S63.076- Dislocation of distal end of unspecified ulna

6 **S63.09 Other subluxation and dislocation of wrist and hand**
SP 7 S63.091- Other subluxation of right wrist and hand
SP 7 S63.092- Other subluxation of left wrist and hand
IQ 7 S63.093- Other subluxation of unspecified wrist and hand
SP 7 S63.094- Other dislocation of right wrist and hand
SP 7 S63.095- Other dislocation of left wrist and hand
IQ 7 S63.096- Other dislocation of unspecified wrist and hand

5 S63.1 Subluxation and dislocation of thumb

6 S63.10 Unspecified subluxation and dislocation of thumb

SP 7 S63.101- Unspecified subluxation of right thumb

SP 7 S63.102- Unspecified subluxation of left thumb

IQ 7 S63.103- Unspecified subluxation of unspecified thumb

SP 7 S63.104- Unspecified dislocation of right thumb

SP 7 S63.105- Unspecified dislocation of left thumb

IQ 7 S63.106- Unspecified dislocation of unspecified thumb

6 S63.11 Subluxation and dislocation of metacarpophalangeal joint of thumb

SP 7 S63.111- Subluxation of metacarpophalangeal joint of right thumb

SP 7 S63.112- Subluxation of metacarpophalangeal joint of left thumb

IQ 7 S63.113- Subluxation of metacarpophalangeal joint of unspecified thumb

SP 7 S63.114- Dislocation of metacarpophalangeal joint of right thumb

SP 7 S63.115- Dislocation of metacarpophalangeal joint of left thumb

IQ 7 S63.116- Dislocation of metacarpophalangeal joint of unspecified thumb

6 S63.12 Subluxation and dislocation of interphalangeal joint of thumb

IQ 7 S63.121- Subluxation of interphalangeal joint of right thumb

IQ 7 S63.122- Subluxation of interphalangeal joint of left thumb

IQ 7 S63.123- Subluxation of interphalangeal joint of unspecified thumb

IQ 7 S63.124- Dislocation of interphalangeal joint of right thumb

IQ 7 S63.125- Dislocation of interphalangeal joint of left thumb

IQ 7 S63.126- Dislocation of interphalangeal joint of unspecified thumb

5 S63.2 Subluxation and dislocation of other finger(s)

EXCLUDES 2 subluxation and dislocation of thumb (S63.1-)

6 S63.20 Unspecified subluxation of other finger

SP 7 S63.200- Unspecified subluxation of right index finger

SP 7 S63.201- Unspecified subluxation of left index finger

SP 7 S63.202- Unspecified subluxation of right middle finger

SP 7 S63.203- Unspecified subluxation of left middle finger

SP 7 S63.204- Unspecified subluxation of right ring finger

SP 7 S63.205- Unspecified subluxation of left ring finger

SP 7 S63.206- Unspecified subluxation of right little finger

SP 7 S63.207- Unspecified subluxation of left little finger

SP 7 S63.208- Unspecified subluxation of other finger

Unspecified subluxation of specified finger with unspecified laterality

IQ 7 S63.209- Unspecified subluxation of unspecified finger

6 S63.21 Subluxation of metacarpophalangeal joint of finger

SP 7 S63.210- Subluxation of metacarpophalangeal joint of right index finger

SP 7 S63.211- Subluxation of metacarpophalangeal joint of left index finger

SP 7 S63.212- Subluxation of metacarpophalangeal joint of right middle finger

SP 7 S63.213- Subluxation of metacarpophalangeal joint of left middle finger

SP 7 S63.214- Subluxation of metacarpophalangeal joint of right ring finger

SP 7 S63.215- Subluxation of metacarpophalangeal joint of left ring finger

SP 7 S63.216- Subluxation of metacarpophalangeal joint of right little finger

SP 7 S63.217- Subluxation of metacarpophalangeal joint of left little finger

SP IQ 7 S63.218- Subluxation of metacarpophalangeal joint of other finger

Subluxation of metacarpophalangeal joint of specified finger with unspecified laterality

IQ 7 S63.219- Subluxation of metacarpophalangeal joint of unspecified finger

6 S63.22 Subluxation of unspecified interphalangeal joint of finger

IQ 7 S63.220- Subluxation of unspecified interphalangeal joint of right index finger

IQ 7 S63.221- Subluxation of unspecified interphalangeal joint of left index finger

IQ 7 S63.222- Subluxation of unspecified interphalangeal joint of right middle finger

IQ 7 S63.223- Subluxation of unspecified interphalangeal joint of left middle finger

IQ 7 S63.224- Subluxation of unspecified interphalangeal joint of right ring finger

Chapter 19

S00-T88

IQ 7 S63.225- **Subluxation of unspecified interphalangeal joint of left ring finger**

IQ 7 S63.226- **Subluxation of unspecified interphalangeal joint of right little finger**

IQ 7 S63.227- **Subluxation of unspecified interphalangeal joint of left little finger**

IQ 7 S63.228- **Subluxation of unspecified interphalangeal joint of other finger**
Subluxation of unspecified interphalangeal joint of specified finger with unspecified laterality

IQ 7 S63.229- **Subluxation of unspecified interphalangeal joint of unspecified finger**

6 **S63.23 Subluxation of proximal interphalangeal joint of finger**

SP 7 S63.230- **Subluxation of proximal interphalangeal joint of right index finger**

SP 7 S63.231- **Subluxation of proximal interphalangeal joint of left index finger**

SP 7 S63.232- **Subluxation of proximal interphalangeal joint of right middle finger**

SP 7 S63.233- **Subluxation of proximal interphalangeal joint of left middle finger**

SP 7 S63.234- **Subluxation of proximal interphalangeal joint of right ring finger**

SP 7 S63.235- **Subluxation of proximal interphalangeal joint of left ring finger**

SP 7 S63.236- **Subluxation of proximal interphalangeal joint of right little finger**

SP 7 S63.237- **Subluxation of proximal interphalangeal joint of left little finger**

SP 7 S63.238- **Subluxation of proximal interphalangeal joint of other finger**
Subluxation of proximal interphalangeal joint of specified finger with unspecified laterality

IQ 7 S63.239- **Subluxation of proximal interphalangeal joint of unspecified finger**

6 **S63.24 Subluxation of distal interphalangeal joint of finger**

SP 7 S63.240- **Subluxation of distal interphalangeal joint of right index finger**

SP 7 S63.241- **Subluxation of distal interphalangeal joint of left index finger**

SP 7 S63.242- **Subluxation of distal interphalangeal joint of right middle finger**

SP 7 S63.243- **Subluxation of distal interphalangeal joint of left middle finger**

SP 7 S63.244- **Subluxation of distal interphalangeal joint of right ring finger**

SP 7 S63.245- **Subluxation of distal interphalangeal joint of left ring finger**

SP 7 S63.246- **Subluxation of distal interphalangeal joint of right little finger**

SP 7 S63.247- **Subluxation of distal interphalangeal joint of left little finger**

SP 7 S63.248- **Subluxation of distal interphalangeal joint of other finger**
Subluxation of distal interphalangeal joint of specified finger with unspecified laterality

IQ 7 S63.249- **Subluxation of distal interphalangeal joint of unspecified finger**

6 **S63.25 Unspecified dislocation of other finger**

SP 7 S63.250- **Unspecified dislocation of right index finger**

SP 7 S63.251- **Unspecified dislocation of left index finger**

SP 7 S63.252- **Unspecified dislocation of right middle finger**

SP 7 S63.253- **Unspecified dislocation of left middle finger**

SP 7 S63.254- **Unspecified dislocation of right ring finger**

SP 7 S63.255- **Unspecified dislocation of left ring finger**

SP 7 S63.256- **Unspecified dislocation of right little finger**

SP 7 S63.257- **Unspecified dislocation of left little finger**

SP 7 S63.258- **Unspecified dislocation of other finger**
Unspecified dislocation of specified finger with unspecified laterality

IQ 7 S63.259- **Unspecified dislocation of unspecified finger**
Unspecified dislocation of unspecified finger with unspecified laterality

6 **S63.26 Dislocation of metacarpophalangeal joint of finger**

SP 7 S63.260- **Dislocation of metacarpophalangeal joint of right index finger**

SP 7 S63.261- **Dislocation of metacarpophalangeal joint of left index finger**

SP 7 S63.262- **Dislocation of metacarpophalangeal joint of right middle finger**

SP 7 S63.263- **Dislocation of metacarpophalangeal joint of left middle finger**

SP 7 S63.264- **Dislocation of metacarpophalangeal joint of right ring finger**

S63.265- Dislocation of metacarpophalangeal joint of left ring finger

S63.266- Dislocation of metacarpophalangeal joint of right little finger

S63.267- Dislocation of metacarpophalangeal joint of left little finger

S63.268- Dislocation of metacarpophalangeal joint of other finger
Dislocation of metacarpophalangeal joint of specified finger with unspecified laterality

S63.269- Dislocation of metacarpophalangeal joint of unspecified finger

S63.27 Dislocation of unspecified interphalangeal joint of finger

S63.270- Dislocation of unspecified interphalangeal joint of right index finger

S63.271- Dislocation of unspecified interphalangeal joint of left index finger

S63.272- Dislocation of unspecified interphalangeal joint of right middle finger

S63.273- Dislocation of unspecified interphalangeal joint of left middle finger

S63.274- Dislocation of unspecified interphalangeal joint of right ring finger

S63.275- Dislocation of unspecified interphalangeal joint of left ring finger

S63.276- Dislocation of unspecified interphalangeal joint of right little finger

S63.277- Dislocation of unspecified interphalangeal joint of left little finger

S63.278- Dislocation of unspecified interphalangeal joint of other finger
Dislocation of unspecified interphalangeal joint of specified finger with unspecified laterality

S63.279- Dislocation of unspecified interphalangeal joint of unspecified finger
Dislocation of unspecified interphalangeal joint of unspecified finger without specified laterality

S63.28 Dislocation of proximal interphalangeal joint of finger

S63.280- Dislocation of proximal interphalangeal joint of right index finger

S63.281- Dislocation of proximal interphalangeal joint of left index finger

S63.282- Dislocation of proximal interphalangeal joint of right middle finger

S63.283- Dislocation of proximal interphalangeal joint of left middle finger

S63.284- Dislocation of proximal interphalangeal joint of right ring finger

S63.285- Dislocation of proximal interphalangeal joint of left ring finger

S63.286- Dislocation of proximal interphalangeal joint of right little finger

S63.287- Dislocation of proximal interphalangeal joint of left little finger

S63.288- Dislocation of proximal interphalangeal joint of other finger
Dislocation of proximal interphalangeal joint of specified finger with unspecified laterality

S63.289- Dislocation of proximal interphalangeal joint of unspecified finger

S63.29 Dislocation of distal interphalangeal joint of finger

S63.290- Dislocation of distal interphalangeal joint of right index finger

S63.291- Dislocation of distal interphalangeal joint of left index finger

S63.292- Dislocation of distal interphalangeal joint of right middle finger

S63.293- Dislocation of distal interphalangeal joint of left middle finger

S63.294- Dislocation of distal interphalangeal joint of right ring finger

S63.295- Dislocation of distal interphalangeal joint of left ring finger

S63.296- Dislocation of distal interphalangeal joint of right little finger

S63.297- Dislocation of distal interphalangeal joint of left little finger

S63.298- Dislocation of distal interphalangeal joint of other finger
Dislocation of distal interphalangeal joint of specified finger with unspecified laterality

S63.299- Dislocation of distal interphalangeal joint of unspecified finger

S63.3 Traumatic rupture of ligament of wrist

S63.30 Traumatic rupture of unspecified ligament of wrist

S63.301- Traumatic rupture of unspecified ligament of right wrist

SP 7 **S63.302- Traumatic rupture of unspecified ligament of left wrist**

IQ 7 **S63.309- Traumatic rupture of unspecified ligament of unspecified wrist**

6 **S63.31 Traumatic rupture of collateral ligament of wrist**

SP 7 **S63.311- Traumatic rupture of collateral ligament of right wrist**

SP 7 **S63.312- Traumatic rupture of collateral ligament of left wrist**

IQ 7 **S63.319- Traumatic rupture of collateral ligament of unspecified wrist**

6 **S63.32 Traumatic rupture of radiocarpal ligament**

SP 7 **S63.321- Traumatic rupture of right radiocarpal ligament**

SP 7 **S63.322- Traumatic rupture of left radiocarpal ligament**

IQ 7 **S63.329- Traumatic rupture of unspecified radiocarpal ligament**

6 **S63.33 Traumatic rupture of ulnocarpal (palmar) ligament**

SP 7 **S63.331- Traumatic rupture of right ulnocarpal (palmar) ligament**

SP 7 **S63.332- Traumatic rupture of left ulnocarpal (palmar) ligament**

IQ 7 **S63.339- Traumatic rupture of unspecified ulnocarpal (palmar) ligament**

6 **S63.39 Traumatic rupture of other ligament of wrist**

SP 7 **S63.391- Traumatic rupture of other ligament of right wrist**

SP 7 **S63.392- Traumatic rupture of other ligament of left wrist**

IQ 7 **S63.399- Traumatic rupture of other ligament of unspecified wrist**

5 **S63.4 Traumatic rupture of ligament of finger at metacarpophalangeal and interphalangeal joint(s)**

6 **S63.40 Traumatic rupture of unspecified ligament of finger at metacarpophalangeal and interphalangeal joint**

SP 7 **S63.400- Traumatic rupture of unspecified ligament of right index finger at metacarpophalangeal and interphalangeal joint**

SP 7 **S63.401- Traumatic rupture of unspecified ligament of left index finger at metacarpophalangeal and interphalangeal joint**

SP 7 **S63.402- Traumatic rupture of unspecified ligament of right middle finger at metacarpophalangeal and interphalangeal joint**

SP 7 **S63.403- Traumatic rupture of unspecified ligament of left middle finger at metacarpophalangeal and interphalangeal joint**

SP 7 **S63.404- Traumatic rupture of unspecified ligament of right ring finger at metacarpophalangeal and interphalangeal joint**

SP 7 **S63.405- Traumatic rupture of unspecified ligament of left ring finger at metacarpophalangeal and interphalangeal joint**

SP 7 **S63.406- Traumatic rupture of unspecified ligament of right little finger at metacarpophalangeal and interphalangeal joint**

SP 7 **S63.407- Traumatic rupture of unspecified ligament of left little finger at metacarpophalangeal and interphalangeal joint**

SP 7 **S63.408- Traumatic rupture of unspecified ligament of other finger at metacarpophalangeal and interphalangeal joint**

Traumatic rupture of unspecified ligament of specified finger with unspecified laterality at metacarpophalangeal and interphalangeal joint

IQ 7 **S63.409- Traumatic rupture of unspecified ligament of unspecified finger at metacarpophalangeal and interphalangeal joint**

6 **S63.41 Traumatic rupture of collateral ligament of finger at metacarpophalangeal and interphalangeal joint**

SP 7 **S63.410- Traumatic rupture of collateral ligament of right index finger at metacarpophalangeal and interphalangeal joint**

SP 7 **S63.411- Traumatic rupture of collateral ligament of left index finger at metacarpophalangeal and interphalangeal joint**

SP 7 **S63.412- Traumatic rupture of collateral ligament of right middle finger at metacarpophalangeal and interphalangeal joint**

SP 7 **S63.413- Traumatic rupture of collateral ligament of left middle finger at metacarpophalangeal and interphalangeal joint**

SP 7 **S63.414- Traumatic rupture of collateral ligament of right ring finger at metacarpophalangeal and interphalangeal joint**

SP 7 **S63.415- Traumatic rupture of collateral ligament of left ring finger at metacarpophalangeal and interphalangeal joint**

SP 7 **S63.416- Traumatic rupture of collateral ligament of right little finger at metacarpophalangeal and interphalangeal joint**

SP 7 **S63.417- Traumatic rupture of collateral ligament of left little finger at metacarpophalangeal and interphalangeal joint**

S63.418- Traumatic rupture of collateral ligament of other finger at metacarpophalangeal and interphalangeal joint

Traumatic rupture of collateral ligament of specified finger with unspecified laterality at metacarpophalangeal and interphalangeal joint

S63.419- Traumatic rupture of collateral ligament of unspecified finger at metacarpophalangeal and interphalangeal joint

S63.42 Traumatic rupture of palmar ligament of finger at metacarpophalangeal and interphalangeal joint

S63.420- Traumatic rupture of palmar ligament of right index finger at metacarpophalangeal and interphalangeal joint

S63.421- Traumatic rupture of palmar ligament of left index finger at metacarpophalangeal and interphalangeal joint

S63.422- Traumatic rupture of palmar ligament of right middle finger at metacarpophalangeal and interphalangeal joint

S63.423- Traumatic rupture of palmar ligament of left middle finger at metacarpophalangeal and interphalangeal joint

S63.424- Traumatic rupture of palmar ligament of right ring finger at metacarpophalangeal and interphalangeal joint

S63.425- Traumatic rupture of palmar ligament of left ring finger at metacarpophalangeal and interphalangeal joint

S63.426- Traumatic rupture of palmar ligament of right little finger at metacarpophalangeal and interphalangeal joint

S63.427- Traumatic rupture of palmar ligament of left little finger at metacarpophalangeal and interphalangeal joint

S63.428- Traumatic rupture of palmar ligament of other finger at metacarpophalangeal and interphalangeal joint

Traumatic rupture of palmar ligament of specified finger with unspecified laterality at metacarpophalangeal and interphalangeal joint

S63.429- Traumatic rupture of palmar ligament of unspecified finger at metacarpophalangeal and interphalangeal joint

S63.43 Traumatic rupture of volar plate of finger at metacarpophalangeal and interphalangeal joint

S63.430- Traumatic rupture of volar plate of right index finger at metacarpophalangeal and interphalangeal joint

S63.431- Traumatic rupture of volar plate of left index finger at metacarpophalangeal and interphalangeal joint

S63.432- Traumatic rupture of volar plate of right middle finger at metacarpophalangeal and interphalangeal joint

S63.433- Traumatic rupture of volar plate of left middle finger at metacarpophalangeal and interphalangeal joint

S63.434- Traumatic rupture of volar plate of right ring finger at metacarpophalangeal and interphalangeal joint

S63.435- Traumatic rupture of volar plate of left ring finger at metacarpophalangeal and interphalangeal joint

S63.436- Traumatic rupture of volar plate of right little finger at metacarpophalangeal and interphalangeal joint

S63.437- Traumatic rupture of volar plate of left little finger at metacarpophalangeal and interphalangeal joint

S63.438- Traumatic rupture of volar plate of other finger at metacarpophalangeal and interphalangeal joint

Traumatic rupture of volar plate of specified finger with unspecified laterality at metacarpophalangeal and interphalangeal joint

S63.439- Traumatic rupture of volar plate of unspecified finger at metacarpophalangeal and interphalangeal joint

S63.49 Traumatic rupture of other ligament of finger at metacarpophalangeal and interphalangeal joint

S63.490- Traumatic rupture of other ligament of right index finger at metacarpophalangeal and interphalangeal joint

S63.491- Traumatic rupture of other ligament of left index finger at metacarpophalangeal and interphalangeal joint

S63.492- Traumatic rupture of other ligament of right middle finger at metacarpophalangeal and interphalangeal joint

S63.493- Traumatic rupture of other ligament of left middle finger at metacarpophalangeal and interphalangeal joint

S63.494- Traumatic rupture of other ligament of right ring finger at metacarpophalangeal and interphalangeal joint

S63.495- Traumatic rupture of other ligament of left ring finger at metacarpophalangeal and interphalangeal joint

SP 7 **S63.496- Traumatic rupture of other ligament of right little finger at metacarpophalangeal and interphalangeal joint**

SP 7 **S63.497- Traumatic rupture of other ligament of left little finger at metacarpophalangeal and interphalangeal joint**

SP 7 **S63.498- Traumatic rupture of other ligament of other finger at metacarpophalangeal and interphalangeal joint**
Traumatic rupture of ligament of specified finger with unspecified laterality at metacarpophalangeal and interphalangeal joint

!Q 7 **S63.499- Traumatic rupture of other ligament of unspecified finger at metacarpophalangeal and interphalangeal joint**

5 **S63.5 Other and unspecified sprain of wrist**

6 **S63.50 Unspecified sprain of wrist**

SP 7 **S63.501- Unspecified sprain of right wrist**

SP 7 **S63.502- Unspecified sprain of left wrist**

!Q 7 **S63.509- Unspecified sprain of unspecified wrist**

6 **S63.51 Sprain of carpal (joint)**

SP 7 **S63.511- Sprain of carpal joint of right wrist**

SP 7 **S63.512- Sprain of carpal joint of left wrist**

!Q 7 **S63.519- Sprain of carpal joint of unspecified wrist**

6 **S63.52 Sprain of radiocarpal joint**
EXCLUDES 1 traumatic rupture of radiocarpal ligament (S63.32-)

SP 7 **S63.521- Sprain of radiocarpal joint of right wrist**

SP 7 **S63.522- Sprain of radiocarpal joint of left wrist**

!Q 7 **S63.529- Sprain of radiocarpal joint of unspecified wrist**

6 **S63.59 Other specified sprain of wrist**

SP 7 **S63.591- Other specified sprain of right wrist**

SP 7 **S63.592- Other specified sprain of left wrist**

!Q 7 **S63.599- Other specified sprain of unspecified wrist**

5 **S63.6 Other and unspecified sprain of finger(s)**
EXCLUDES 1 traumatic rupture of ligament of finger at metacarpophalangeal and interphalangeal joint (s) (S63.4-)

6 **S63.60 Unspecified sprain of thumb**

SP 7 **S63.601- Unspecified sprain of right thumb**

SP 7 **S63.602- Unspecified sprain of left thumb**

!Q 7 **S63.609- Unspecified sprain of unspecified thumb**

6 **S63.61 Unspecified sprain of other and unspecified finger(s)**

SP 7 **S63.610- Unspecified sprain of right index finger**

SP 7 **S63.611- Unspecified sprain of left index finger**

SP 7 **S63.612- Unspecified sprain of right middle finger**

SP 7 **S63.613- Unspecified sprain of left middle finger**

SP 7 **S63.614- Unspecified sprain of right ring finger**

SP 7 **S63.615- Unspecified sprain of left ring finger**

SP 7 **S63.616- Unspecified sprain of right little finger**

SP 7 **S63.617- Unspecified sprain of left little finger**

SP 7 **S63.618- Unspecified sprain of other finger**
Unspecified sprain of specified finger with unspecified laterality

!Q 7 **S63.619- Unspecified sprain of unspecified finger**

6 **S63.62 Sprain of interphalangeal joint of thumb**

SP 7 **S63.621- Sprain of interphalangeal joint of right thumb**

SP 7 **S63.622- Sprain of interphalangeal joint of left thumb**

!Q 7 **S63.629- Sprain of interphalangeal joint of unspecified thumb**

6 **S63.63 Sprain of interphalangeal joint of other and unspecified finger(s)**

SP 7 **S63.630- Sprain of interphalangeal joint of right index finger**

SP 7 **S63.631- Sprain of interphalangeal joint of left index finger**

SP 7 **S63.632- Sprain of interphalangeal joint of right middle finger**

SP 7 **S63.633- Sprain of interphalangeal joint of left middle finger**

SP 7 **S63.634- Sprain of interphalangeal joint of right ring finger**

SP 7 **S63.635- Sprain of interphalangeal joint of left ring finger**

SP 7 **S63.636- Sprain of interphalangeal joint of right little finger**

SP 7 **S63.637- Sprain of interphalangeal joint of left little finger**

SP 7 **S63.638- Sprain of interphalangeal joint of other finger**

!Q 7 **S63.639- Sprain of interphalangeal joint of unspecified finger**

6 **S63.64 Sprain of metacarpophalangeal joint of thumb**

SP 7 **S63.641- Sprain of metacarpophalangeal joint of right thumb**

SP 7 **S63.642- Sprain of metacarpophalangeal joint of left thumb**

!Q 7 **S63.649- Sprain of metacarpophalangeal joint of unspecified thumb**

6 **S63.65 Sprain of metacarpophalangeal joint of other and unspecified finger(s)**

SP 7 **S63.650- Sprain of metacarpophalangeal joint of right index finger**

Chapter 19

S00-T88

☐ SP 7 **S63.651-** Sprain of metacarpophalangeal joint of left index finger

☐ SP 7 **S63.652-** Sprain of metacarpophalangeal joint of right middle finger

☐ SP 7 **S63.653-** Sprain of metacarpophalangeal joint of left middle finger

☐ SP 7 **S63.654-** Sprain of metacarpophalangeal joint of right ring finger

☐ SP 7 **S63.655-** Sprain of metacarpophalangeal joint of left ring finger

☐ SP 7 **S63.656-** Sprain of metacarpophalangeal joint of right little finger

☐ SP 7 **S63.657-** Sprain of metacarpophalangeal joint of left little finger

☐ SP 7 **S63.658-** Sprain of metacarpophalangeal joint of other finger
Sprain of metacarpophalangeal joint of specified finger with unspecified laterality

☐ !Q 7 **S63.659-** Sprain of metacarpophalangeal joint of unspecified finger

6 **S63.68** Other sprain of thumb

☐ SP 7 **S63.681-** Other sprain of right thumb

☐ SP 7 **S63.682-** Other sprain of left thumb

☐ !Q 7 **S63.689-** Other sprain of unspecified thumb

6 **S63.69** Other sprain of other and unspecified finger(s)

☐ SP 7 **S63.690-** Other sprain of right index finger

☐ SP 7 **S63.691-** Other sprain of left index finger

☐ SP 7 **S63.692-** Other sprain of right middle finger

☐ SP 7 **S63.693-** Other sprain of left middle finger

☐ SP 7 **S63.694-** Other sprain of right ring finger

☐ SP 7 **S63.695-** Other sprain of left ring finger

☐ SP 7 **S63.696-** Other sprain of right little finger

☐ SP 7 **S63.697-** Other sprain of left little finger

☐ SP 7 **S63.698-** Other sprain of other finger
Other sprain of specified finger with unspecified laterality

☐ !Q 7 **S63.699-** Other sprain of unspecified finger

5 **S63.8** Sprain of other part of wrist and hand

6 **S63.8X** Sprain of other part of wrist and hand

☐ SP 7 **S63.8X1-** Sprain of other part of right wrist and hand

☐ SP 7 **S63.8X2-** Sprain of other part of left wrist and hand

☐ !Q 7 **S63.8X9-** Sprain of other part of unspecified wrist and hand

5 **S63.9** Sprain of unspecified part of wrist and hand

☐ !Q ☑ **S63.90X-** Sprain of unspecified part of unspecified wrist and hand

☐ SP ☑ **S63.91X-** Sprain of unspecified part of right wrist and hand

☐ SP ☑ **S63.92X-** Sprain of unspecified part of left wrist and hand

4 **S64** Injury of nerves at wrist and hand level
Code also:
any associated open wound (S61.-)

The appropriate 7th character is to be added to each code from category S64
A   initial encounter
D   subsequent encounter
S   sequela

5 **S64.0** Injury of ulnar nerve at wrist and hand level

☐ !Q ☑ **S64.00X-** Injury of ulnar nerve at wrist and hand level of unspecified arm

☐ SP ☑ **S64.01X-** Injury of ulnar nerve at wrist and hand level of right arm

☐ SP ☑ **S64.02X-** Injury of ulnar nerve at wrist and hand level of left arm

5 **S64.1** Injury of median nerve at wrist and hand level

☐ !Q ☑ **S64.10X-** Injury of median nerve at wrist and hand level of unspecified arm

☐ SP ☑ **S64.11X-** Injury of median nerve at wrist and hand level of right arm

☐ SP ☑ **S64.12X-** Injury of median nerve at wrist and hand level of left arm

5 **S64.2** Injury of radial nerve at wrist and hand level

☐ !Q ☑ **S64.20X-** Injury of radial nerve at wrist and hand level of unspecified arm

☐ SP ☑ **S64.21X-** Injury of radial nerve at wrist and hand level of right arm

☐ SP ☑ **S64.22X-** Injury of radial nerve at wrist and hand level of left arm

5 **S64.3** Injury of digital nerve of thumb

☐ !Q ☑ **S64.30X-** Injury of digital nerve of unspecified thumb

☐ SP ☑ **S64.31X-** Injury of digital nerve of right thumb

☐ SP ☑ **S64.32X-** Injury of digital nerve of left thumb

5 **S64.4** Injury of digital nerve of other and unspecified finger

!Q ☑ **S64.40X-** Injury of digital nerve of unspecified finger

6 **S64.49** Injury of digital nerve of other finger

☐ SP 7 **S64.490-** Injury of digital nerve of right index finger

☐ SP 7 **S64.491-** Injury of digital nerve of left index finger

☐ SP 7 **S64.492-** Injury of digital nerve of right middle finger

☐ SP 7 **S64.493-** Injury of digital nerve of left middle finger

☐ SP 7 **S64.494-** Injury of digital nerve of right ring finger

☐ SP 7 **S64.495-** Injury of digital nerve of left ring finger

☐ SP 7 **S64.496-** Injury of digital nerve of right little finger

☐ SP 7 **S64.497-** Injury of digital nerve of left little finger

☐ SP 7 **S64.498-** Injury of digital nerve of other finger
Injury of digital nerve of specified finger with unspecified laterality

5 **S64.8** Injury of other nerves at wrist and hand level

6 **S64.8X** Injury of other nerves at wrist and hand level

---

4 4th digit required   5 5th digit required   6 6th digit required   7 7th digit required   ☑ 7th digit placeholder   + Additional code   ☐ Laterality

SP 7 **S64.8X1-** Injury of other nerves at wrist and hand level of right arm

SP 7 **S64.8X2-** Injury of other nerves at wrist and hand level of left arm

!Q 7 **S64.8X9-** Injury of other nerves at wrist and hand level of unspecified arm

5 **S64.9** Injury of unspecified nerve at wrist and hand level

!Q 7 **S64.90X-** Injury of unspecified nerve at wrist and hand level of unspecified arm

!Q 7 **S64.91X-** Injury of unspecified nerve at wrist and hand level of right arm

!Q 7 **S64.92X-** Injury of unspecified nerve at wrist and hand level of left arm

4 **S65** **Injury of blood vessels at wrist and hand level**

Code also:

any associated open wound (S61.-)

The appropriate 7th character is to be added to each code from category S65

A initial encounter

D subsequent encounter

S sequela

5 **S65.0** Injury of ulnar artery at wrist and hand level

6 **S65.00** Unspecified injury of ulnar artery at wrist and hand level

SP 7 **S65.001-** Unspecified injury of ulnar artery at wrist and hand level of right arm

SP 7 **S65.002-** Unspecified injury of ulnar artery at wrist and hand level of left arm

!Q 7 **S65.009-** Unspecified injury of ulnar artery at wrist and hand level of unspecified arm

6 **S65.01** Laceration of ulnar artery at wrist and hand level

SP 7 **S65.011-** Laceration of ulnar artery at wrist and hand level of right arm

SP 7 **S65.012-** Laceration of ulnar artery at wrist and hand level of left arm

!Q 7 **S65.019-** Laceration of ulnar artery at wrist and hand level of unspecified arm

6 **S65.09** Other specified injury of ulnar artery at wrist and hand level

SP 7 **S65.091-** Other specified injury of ulnar artery at wrist and hand level of right arm

SP 7 **S65.092-** Other specified injury of ulnar artery at wrist and hand level of left arm

!Q 7 **S65.099-** Other specified injury of ulnar artery at wrist and hand level of unspecified arm

5 **S65.1** Injury of radial artery at wrist and hand level

6 **S65.10** Unspecified injury of radial artery at wrist and hand level

!Q 7 **S65.101-** Unspecified injury of radial artery at wrist and hand level of right arm

!Q 7 **S65.102-** Unspecified injury of radial artery at wrist and hand level of left arm

!Q 7 **S65.109-** Unspecified injury of radial artery at wrist and hand level of unspecified arm

6 **S65.11** Laceration of radial artery at wrist and hand level

SP 7 **S65.111-** Laceration of radial artery at wrist and hand level of right arm

SP 7 **S65.112-** Laceration of radial artery at wrist and hand level of left arm

!Q 7 **S65.119-** Laceration of radial artery at wrist and hand level of unspecified arm

6 **S65.19** Other specified injury of radial artery at wrist and hand level

SP 7 **S65.191-** Other specified injury of radial artery at wrist and hand level of right arm

SP 7 **S65.192-** Other specified injury of radial artery at wrist and hand level of left arm

!Q 7 **S65.199-** Other specified injury of radial artery at wrist and hand level of unspecified arm

5 **S65.2** Injury of superficial palmar arch

6 **S65.20** Unspecified injury of superficial palmar arch

!Q 7 **S65.201-** Unspecified injury of superficial palmar arch of right hand

!Q 7 **S65.202-** Unspecified injury of superficial palmar arch of left hand

!Q 7 **S65.209-** Unspecified injury of superficial palmar arch of unspecified hand

6 **S65.21** Laceration of superficial palmar arch

SP 7 **S65.211-** Laceration of superficial palmar arch of right hand

SP 7 **S65.212-** Laceration of superficial palmar arch of left hand

!Q 7 **S65.219-** Laceration of superficial palmar arch of unspecified hand

6 **S65.29** Other specified injury of superficial palmar arch

SP 7 **S65.291-** Other specified injury of superficial palmar arch of right hand

SP 7 **S65.292-** Other specified injury of superficial palmar arch of left hand

!Q 7 **S65.299-** Other specified injury of superficial palmar arch of unspecified hand

5 **S65.3** Injury of deep palmar arch

6 **S65.30** Unspecified injury of deep palmar arch

!Q 7 **S65.301-** Unspecified injury of deep palmar arch of right hand

!Q 7 **S65.302-** Unspecified injury of deep palmar arch of left hand

!Q 7 **S65.309-** Unspecified injury of deep palmar arch of unspecified hand

6 **S65.31** Laceration of deep palmar arch

Chapter 19

S00-T88

S65.311- Laceration of deep palmar arch of right hand
S65.312- Laceration of deep palmar arch of left hand
S65.319- Laceration of deep palmar arch of unspecified hand
S65.39 Other specified injury of deep palmar arch
S65.391- Other specified injury of deep palmar arch of right hand
S65.392- Other specified injury of deep palmar arch of left hand
S65.399- Other specified injury of deep palmar arch of unspecified hand
S65.4 Injury of blood vessel of thumb
S65.40 Unspecified injury of blood vessel of thumb
S65.401- Unspecified injury of blood vessel of right thumb
S65.402- Unspecified injury of blood vessel of left thumb
S65.409- Unspecified injury of blood vessel of unspecified thumb
S65.41 Laceration of blood vessel of thumb
S65.411- Laceration of blood vessel of right thumb
S65.412- Laceration of blood vessel of left thumb
S65.419- Laceration of blood vessel of unspecified thumb
S65.49 Other specified injury of blood vessel of thumb
S65.491- Other specified injury of blood vessel of right thumb
S65.492- Other specified injury of blood vessel of left thumb
S65.499- Other specified injury of blood vessel of unspecified thumb
S65.5 Injury of blood vessel of other and unspecified finger
S65.50 Unspecified injury of blood vessel of other and unspecified finger
S65.500- Unspecified injury of blood vessel of right index finger
S65.501- Unspecified injury of blood vessel of left index finger
S65.502- Unspecified injury of blood vessel of right middle finger
S65.503- Unspecified injury of blood vessel of left middle finger
S65.504- Unspecified injury of blood vessel of right ring finger
S65.505- Unspecified injury of blood vessel of left ring finger
S65.506- Unspecified injury of blood vessel of right little finger
S65.507- Unspecified injury of blood vessel of left little finger
S65.508- Unspecified injury of blood vessel of other finger
Unspecified injury of blood vessel of specified finger with unspecified laterality
S65.509- Unspecified injury of blood vessel of unspecified finger
S65.51 Laceration of blood vessel of other and unspecified finger
S65.510- Laceration of blood vessel of right index finger
S65.511- Laceration of blood vessel of left index finger
S65.512- Laceration of blood vessel of right middle finger
S65.513- Laceration of blood vessel of left middle finger
S65.514- Laceration of blood vessel of right ring finger
S65.515- Laceration of blood vessel of left ring finger
S65.516- Laceration of blood vessel of right little finger
S65.517- Laceration of blood vessel of left little finger
S65.518- Laceration of blood vessel of other finger
Laceration of blood vessel of specified finger with unspecified laterality
S65.519- Laceration of blood vessel of unspecified finger
S65.59 Other specified injury of blood vessel of other and unspecified finger
S65.590- Other specified injury of blood vessel of right index finger
S65.591- Other specified injury of blood vessel of left index finger
S65.592- Other specified injury of blood vessel of right middle finger
S65.593- Other specified injury of blood vessel of left middle finger
S65.594- Other specified injury of blood vessel of right ring finger
S65.595- Other specified injury of blood vessel of left ring finger
S65.596- Other specified injury of blood vessel of right little finger
S65.597- Other specified injury of blood vessel of left little finger
S65.598- Other specified injury of blood vessel of other finger
Other specified injury of blood vessel of specified finger with unspecified laterality
S65.599- Other specified injury of blood vessel of unspecified finger
S65.8 Injury of other blood vessels at wrist and hand level
S65.80 Unspecified injury of other blood vessels at wrist and hand level
S65.801- Unspecified injury of other blood vessels at wrist and hand level of right arm
S65.802- Unspecified injury of other blood vessels at wrist and hand level of left arm
S65.809- Unspecified injury of other blood vessels at wrist and hand level of unspecified arm

Chapter 19
S00-T88

6 **S65.81 Laceration of other blood vessels at wrist and hand level**
SP 7 **S65.811- Laceration of other blood vessels at wrist and hand level of right arm**
SP 7 **S65.812- Laceration of other blood vessels at wrist and hand level of left arm**
IQ 7 **S65.819- Laceration of other blood vessels at wrist and hand level of unspecified arm**
6 **S65.89 Other specified injury of other blood vessels at wrist and hand level**
SP 7 **S65.891- Other specified injury of other blood vessels at wrist and hand level of right arm**
SP 7 **S65.892- Other specified injury of other blood vessels at wrist and hand level of left arm**
IQ 7 **S65.899- Other specified injury of other blood vessels at wrist and hand level of unspecified arm**
5 **S65.9 Injury of unspecified blood vessel at wrist and hand level**
6 **S65.90 Unspecified injury of unspecified blood vessel at wrist and hand level**
IQ 7 **S65.901- Unspecified injury of unspecified blood vessel at wrist and hand level of right arm**
IQ 7 **S65.902- Unspecified injury of unspecified blood vessel at wrist and hand level of left arm**
IQ 7 **S65.909- Unspecified injury of unspecified blood vessel at wrist and hand level of unspecified arm**
6 **S65.91 Laceration of unspecified blood vessel at wrist and hand level**
SP 7 **S65.911- Laceration of unspecified blood vessel at wrist and hand level of right arm**
SP 7 **S65.912- Laceration of unspecified blood vessel at wrist and hand level of left arm**
IQ 7 **S65.919- Laceration of unspecified blood vessel at wrist and hand level of unspecified arm**
6 **S65.99 Other specified injury of unspecified blood vessel at wrist and hand level**
IQ 7 **S65.991- Other specified injury of unspecified blood vessel at wrist and hand of right arm**
IQ 7 **S65.992- Other specified injury of unspecified blood vessel at wrist and hand of left arm**
IQ 7 **S65.999- Other specified injury of unspecified blood vessel at wrist and hand of unspecified arm**
4 **S66 Injury of muscle, fascia and tendon at wrist and hand level**
Code also:
any associated open wound (S61.-)
EXCLUDES 2 sprain of joints and ligaments of wrist and hand (S63.-)

The appropriate 7th character is to be added to each code from category S66
A initial encounter
D subsequent encounter
S sequela

5 **S66.0 Injury of long flexor muscle, fascia and tendon of thumb at wrist and hand level**
6 **S66.00 Unspecified injury of long flexor muscle, fascia and tendon of thumb at wrist and hand level**
IQ 7 **S66.001- Unspecified injury of long flexor muscle, fascia and tendon of right thumb at wrist and hand level**
IQ 7 **S66.002- Unspecified injury of long flexor muscle, fascia and tendon of left thumb at wrist and hand level**
IQ 7 **S66.009- Unspecified injury of long flexor muscle, fascia and tendon of unspecified thumb at wrist and hand level**
6 **S66.01 Strain of long flexor muscle, fascia and tendon of thumb at wrist and hand level**
SP 7 **S66.011- Strain of long flexor muscle, fascia and tendon of right thumb at wrist and hand level**
SP 7 **S66.012- Strain of long flexor muscle, fascia and tendon of left thumb at wrist and hand level**
IQ 7 **S66.019- Strain of long flexor muscle, fascia and tendon of unspecified thumb at wrist and hand level**
6 **S66.02 Laceration of long flexor muscle, fascia and tendon of thumb at wrist and hand level**
SP 7 **S66.021- Laceration of long flexor muscle, fascia and tendon of right thumb at wrist and hand level**
SP 7 **S66.022- Laceration of long flexor muscle, fascia and tendon of left thumb at wrist and hand level**
IQ 7 **S66.029- Laceration of long flexor muscle, fascia and tendon of unspecified thumb at wrist and hand level**
6 **S66.09 Other specified injury of long flexor muscle, fascia and tendon of thumb at wrist and hand level**
SP 7 **S66.091- Other specified injury of long flexor muscle, fascia and tendon of right thumb at wrist and hand level**
SP 7 **S66.092- Other specified injury of long flexor muscle, fascia and tendon of left thumb at wrist and hand level**
IQ 7 **S66.099- Other specified injury of long flexor muscle, fascia and tendon of unspecified thumb at wrist and hand level**
5 **S66.1 Injury of flexor muscle, fascia and tendon of other and unspecified finger at wrist and hand level**

Chapter 19 S00-T88

EXCLUDES 2 Injury of long flexor muscle, fascia and tendon of thumb at wrist and hand level (S66.0-)

6 S66.10 **Unspecified injury of flexor muscle, fascia and tendon of other and unspecified finger at wrist and hand level**

⊟ !Q 7 S66.100- **Unspecified injury of flexor muscle, fascia and tendon of right index finger at wrist and hand level**

⊟ !Q 7 S66.101- **Unspecified injury of flexor muscle, fascia and tendon of left index finger at wrist and hand level**

⊟ !Q 7 S66.102- **Unspecified injury of flexor muscle, fascia and tendon of right middle finger at wrist and hand level**

⊟ !Q 7 S66.103- **Unspecified injury of flexor muscle, fascia and tendon of left middle finger at wrist and hand level**

⊟ !Q 7 S66.104- **Unspecified injury of flexor muscle, fascia and tendon of right ring finger at wrist and hand level**

⊟ !Q 7 S66.105- **Unspecified injury of flexor muscle, fascia and tendon of left ring finger at wrist and hand level**

⊟ !Q 7 S66.106- **Unspecified injury of flexor muscle, fascia and tendon of right little finger at wrist and hand level**

⊟ !Q 7 S66.107- **Unspecified injury of flexor muscle, fascia and tendon of left little finger at wrist and hand level**

⊟ !Q 7 S66.108- **Unspecified injury of flexor muscle, fascia and tendon of other finger at wrist and hand level**

Unspecified injury of flexor muscle, fascia and tendon of specified finger with unspecified laterality at wrist and hand level

⊟ !Q 7 S66.109- **Unspecified injury of flexor muscle, fascia and tendon of unspecified finger at wrist and hand level**

6 S66.11 **Strain of flexor muscle, fascia and tendon of other and unspecified finger at wrist and hand level**

⊟ SP 7 S66.110- **Strain of flexor muscle, fascia and tendon of right index finger at wrist and hand level**

⊟ SP 7 S66.111- **Strain of flexor muscle, fascia and tendon of left index finger at wrist and hand level**

⊟ SP 7 S66.112- **Strain of flexor muscle, fascia and tendon of right middle finger at wrist and hand level**

⊟ SP 7 S66.113- **Strain of flexor muscle, fascia and tendon of left middle finger at wrist and hand level**

⊟ SP 7 S66.114- **Strain of flexor muscle, fascia and tendon of right ring finger at wrist and hand level**

⊟ SP 7 S66.115- **Strain of flexor muscle, fascia and tendon of left ring finger at wrist and hand level**

⊟ SP 7 S66.116- **Strain of flexor muscle, fascia and tendon of right little finger at wrist and hand level**

⊟ SP 7 S66.117- **Strain of flexor muscle, fascia and tendon of left little finger at wrist and hand level**

⊟ SP 7 S66.118- **Strain of flexor muscle, fascia and tendon of other finger at wrist and hand level**

Strain of flexor muscle, fascia and tendon of specified finger with unspecified laterality at wrist and hand level

⊟ !Q 7 S66.119- **Strain of flexor muscle, fascia and tendon of unspecified finger at wrist and hand level**

6 S66.12 **Laceration of flexor muscle, fascia and tendon of other and unspecified finger at wrist and hand level**

⊟ SP 7 S66.120- **Laceration of flexor muscle, fascia and tendon of right index finger at wrist and hand level**

⊟ SP 7 S66.121- **Laceration of flexor muscle, fascia and tendon of left index finger at wrist and hand level**

⊟ SP 7 S66.122- **Laceration of flexor muscle, fascia and tendon of right middle finger at wrist and hand level**

⊟ SP 7 S66.123- **Laceration of flexor muscle, fascia and tendon of left middle finger at wrist and hand level**

⊟ SP 7 S66.124- **Laceration of flexor muscle, fascia and tendon of right ring finger at wrist and hand level**

⊟ SP 7 S66.125- **Laceration of flexor muscle, fascia and tendon of left ring finger at wrist and hand level**

⊟ SP 7 S66.126- **Laceration of flexor muscle, fascia and tendon of right little finger at wrist and hand level**

⊟ SP 7 S66.127- **Laceration of flexor muscle, fascia and tendon of left little finger at wrist and hand level**

⊟ SP 7 S66.128- **Laceration of flexor muscle, fascia and tendon of other finger at wrist and hand level**

Laceration of flexor muscle, fascia and tendon of specified finger with unspecified laterality at wrist and hand level

⊟ !Q 7 S66.129- **Laceration of flexor muscle, fascia and tendon of unspecified finger at wrist and hand level**

6 S66.19 **Other injury of flexor muscle, fascia and tendon of other and unspecified finger at wrist and hand level**

⊟ SP 7 S66.190- **Other injury of flexor muscle, fascia and tendon of right index finger at wrist and hand level**

⊟ SP 7 S66.191- **Other injury of flexor muscle, fascia and tendon of left index finger at wrist and hand level**

S66.192- **Other injury of flexor muscle, fascia and tendon of right middle finger at wrist and hand level**

S66.193- **Other injury of flexor muscle, fascia and tendon of left middle finger at wrist and hand level**

S66.194- **Other injury of flexor muscle, fascia and tendon of right ring finger at wrist and hand level**

S66.195- **Other injury of flexor muscle, fascia and tendon of left ring finger at wrist and hand level**

S66.196- **Other injury of flexor muscle, fascia and tendon of right little finger at wrist and hand level**

S66.197- **Other injury of flexor muscle, fascia and tendon of left little finger at wrist and hand level**

S66.198- **Other injury of flexor muscle, fascia and tendon of other finger at wrist and hand level**
Other injury of flexor muscle, fascia and tendon of specified finger with unspecified laterality at wrist and hand level

S66.199- **Other injury of flexor muscle, fascia and tendon of unspecified finger at wrist and hand level**

S66.2 **Injury of extensor muscle, fascia and tendon of thumb at wrist and hand level**

S66.20 **Unspecified injury of extensor muscle, fascia and tendon of thumb at wrist and hand level**

S66.201- **Unspecified injury of extensor muscle, fascia and tendon of right thumb at wrist and hand level**

S66.202- **Unspecified injury of extensor muscle, fascia and tendon of left thumb at wrist and hand level**

S66.209- **Unspecified injury of extensor muscle, fascia and tendon of unspecified thumb at wrist and hand level**

S66.21 **Strain of extensor muscle, fascia and tendon of thumb at wrist and hand level**

S66.211- **Strain of extensor muscle, fascia and tendon of right thumb at wrist and hand level**

S66.212- **Strain of extensor muscle, fascia and tendon of left thumb at wrist and hand level**

S66.219- **Strain of extensor muscle, fascia and tendon of unspecified thumb at wrist and hand level**

S66.22 **Laceration of extensor muscle, fascia and tendon of thumb at wrist and hand level**

S66.221- **Laceration of extensor muscle, fascia and tendon of right thumb at wrist and hand level**

S66.222- **Laceration of extensor muscle, fascia and tendon of left thumb at wrist and hand level**

S66.229- **Laceration of extensor muscle, fascia and tendon of unspecified thumb at wrist and hand level**

S66.29 **Other specified injury of extensor muscle, fascia and tendon of thumb at wrist and hand level**

S66.291- **Other specified injury of extensor muscle, fascia and tendon of right thumb at wrist and hand level**

S66.292- **Other specified injury of extensor muscle, fascia and tendon of left thumb at wrist and hand level**

S66.299- **Other specified injury of extensor muscle, fascia and tendon of unspecified thumb at wrist and hand level**

S66.3 **Injury of extensor muscle, fascia and tendon of other and unspecified finger at wrist and hand level**

EXCLUDES 2 Injury of extensor muscle, fascia and tendon of thumb at wrist and hand level (S66.2-)

S66.30 **Unspecified injury of extensor muscle, fascia and tendon of other and unspecified finger at wrist and hand level**

S66.300- **Unspecified injury of extensor muscle, fascia and tendon of right index finger at wrist and hand level**

S66.301- **Unspecified injury of extensor muscle, fascia and tendon of left index finger at wrist and hand level**

S66.302- **Unspecified injury of extensor muscle, fascia and tendon of right middle finger at wrist and hand level**

S66.303- **Unspecified injury of extensor muscle, fascia and tendon of left middle finger at wrist and hand level**

S66.304- **Unspecified injury of extensor muscle, fascia and tendon of right ring finger at wrist and hand level**

S66.305- **Unspecified injury of extensor muscle, fascia and tendon of left ring finger at wrist and hand level**

S66.306- **Unspecified injury of extensor muscle, fascia and tendon of right little finger at wrist and hand level**

S66.307- **Unspecified injury of extensor muscle, fascia and tendon of left little finger at wrist and hand level**

S66.308- **Unspecified injury of extensor muscle, fascia and tendon of other finger at wrist and hand level**
Unspecified injury of extensor muscle, fascia and tendon of specified finger with unspecified laterality at wrist and hand level

Chapter 19 S00-T88

S66.309- Unspecified injury of extensor muscle, fascia and tendon of unspecified finger at wrist and hand level

S66.31 Strain of extensor muscle, fascia and tendon of other and unspecified finger at wrist and hand level

S66.310- Strain of extensor muscle, fascia and tendon of right index finger at wrist and hand level

S66.311- Strain of extensor muscle, fascia and tendon of left index finger at wrist and hand level

S66.312- Strain of extensor muscle, fascia and tendon of right middle finger at wrist and hand level

S66.313- Strain of extensor muscle, fascia and tendon of left middle finger at wrist and hand level

S66.314- Strain of extensor muscle, fascia and tendon of right ring finger at wrist and hand level

S66.315- Strain of extensor muscle, fascia and tendon of left ring finger at wrist and hand level

S66.316- Strain of extensor muscle, fascia and tendon of right little finger at wrist and hand level

S66.317- Strain of extensor muscle, fascia and tendon of left little finger at wrist and hand level

S66.318- Strain of extensor muscle, fascia and tendon of other finger at wrist and hand level
Strain of extensor muscle, fascia and tendon of specified finger with unspecified laterality at wrist and hand level

S66.319- Strain of extensor muscle, fascia and tendon of unspecified finger at wrist and hand level

S66.32 Laceration of extensor muscle, fascia and tendon of other and unspecified finger at wrist and hand level

S66.320- Laceration of extensor muscle, fascia and tendon of right index finger at wrist and hand level

S66.321- Laceration of extensor muscle, fascia and tendon of left index finger at wrist and hand level

S66.322- Laceration of extensor muscle, fascia and tendon of right middle finger at wrist and hand level

S66.323- Laceration of extensor muscle, fascia and tendon of left middle finger at wrist and hand level

S66.324- Laceration of extensor muscle, fascia and tendon of right ring finger at wrist and hand level

S66.325- Laceration of extensor muscle, fascia and tendon of left ring finger at wrist and hand level

S66.326- Laceration of extensor muscle, fascia and tendon of right little finger at wrist and hand level

S66.327- Laceration of extensor muscle, fascia and tendon of left little finger at wrist and hand level

S66.328- Laceration of extensor muscle, fascia and tendon of other finger at wrist and hand level
Laceration of extensor muscle, fascia and tendon of specified finger with unspecified laterality at wrist and hand level

S66.329- Laceration of extensor muscle, fascia and tendon of unspecified finger at wrist and hand level

S66.39 Other injury of extensor muscle, fascia and tendon of other and unspecified finger at wrist and hand level

S66.390- Other injury of extensor muscle, fascia and tendon of right index finger at wrist and hand level

S66.391- Other injury of extensor muscle, fascia and tendon of left index finger at wrist and hand level

S66.392- Other injury of extensor muscle, fascia and tendon of right middle finger at wrist and hand level

S66.393- Other injury of extensor muscle, fascia and tendon of left middle finger at wrist and hand level

S66.394- Other injury of extensor muscle, fascia and tendon of right ring finger at wrist and hand level

S66.395- Other injury of extensor muscle, fascia and tendon of left ring finger at wrist and hand level

S66.396- Other injury of extensor muscle, fascia and tendon of right little finger at wrist and hand level

S66.397- Other injury of extensor muscle, fascia and tendon of left little finger at wrist and hand level

S66.398- Other injury of extensor muscle, fascia and tendon of other finger at wrist and hand level
Other injury of extensor muscle, fascia and tendon of specified finger with unspecified laterality at wrist and hand level

S66.399- Other injury of extensor muscle, fascia and tendon of unspecified finger at wrist and hand level

S66.4 Injury of intrinsic muscle, fascia and tendon of thumb at wrist and hand level

S66.40 Unspecified injury of intrinsic muscle, fascia and tendon of thumb at wrist and hand level

S66.401- Unspecified injury of intrinsic muscle, fascia and tendon of right thumb at wrist and hand level

S66.402- Unspecified injury of intrinsic muscle, fascia and tendon of left thumb at wrist and hand level

S66.409- Unspecified injury of intrinsic muscle, fascia and tendon of unspecified thumb at wrist and hand level

4th digit required | 5th digit required | 6th digit required | 7th digit required | 7th digit placeholder | + Additional code | Laterality

6 **S66.41 Strain of intrinsic muscle, fascia and tendon of thumb at wrist and hand level**

SP 7 **S66.411- Strain of intrinsic muscle, fascia and tendon of right thumb at wrist and hand level**

SP 7 **S66.412- Strain of intrinsic muscle, fascia and tendon of left thumb at wrist and hand level**

IQ 7 **S66.419- Strain of intrinsic muscle, fascia and tendon of unspecified thumb at wrist and hand level**

6 **S66.42 Laceration of intrinsic muscle, fascia and tendon of thumb at wrist and hand level**

SP 7 **S66.421- Laceration of intrinsic muscle, fascia and tendon of right thumb at wrist and hand level**

SP 7 **S66.422- Laceration of intrinsic muscle, fascia and tendon of left thumb at wrist and hand level**

IQ 7 **S66.429- Laceration of intrinsic muscle, fascia and tendon of unspecified thumb at wrist and hand level**

6 **S66.49 Other specified injury of intrinsic muscle, fascia and tendon of thumb at wrist and hand level**

SP 7 **S66.491- Other specified injury of intrinsic muscle, fascia and tendon of right thumb at wrist and hand level**

SP 7 **S66.492- Other specified injury of intrinsic muscle, fascia and tendon of left thumb at wrist and hand level**

IQ 7 **S66.499- Other specified injury of intrinsic muscle, fascia and tendon of unspecified thumb at wrist and hand level**

5 **S66.5 Injury of intrinsic muscle, fascia and tendon of other and unspecified finger at wrist and hand level**

EXCLUDES 2 injury of intrinsic muscle, fascia and tendon of thumb at wrist and hand level (S66.4-)

6 **S66.50 Unspecified injury of intrinsic muscle, fascia and tendon of other and unspecified finger at wrist and hand level**

IQ 7 **S66.500- Unspecified injury of intrinsic muscle, fascia and tendon of right index finger at wrist and hand level**

IQ 7 **S66.501- Unspecified injury of intrinsic muscle, fascia and tendon of left index finger at wrist and hand level**

IQ 7 **S66.502- Unspecified injury of intrinsic muscle, fascia and tendon of right middle finger at wrist and hand level**

IQ 7 **S66.503- Unspecified injury of intrinsic muscle, fascia and tendon of left middle finger at wrist and hand level**

IQ 7 **S66.504- Unspecified injury of intrinsic muscle, fascia and tendon of right ring finger at wrist and hand level**

IQ 7 **S66.505- Unspecified injury of intrinsic muscle, fascia and tendon of left ring finger at wrist and hand level**

IQ 7 **S66.506- Unspecified injury of intrinsic muscle, fascia and tendon of right little finger at wrist and hand level**

IQ 7 **S66.507- Unspecified injury of intrinsic muscle, fascia and tendon of left little finger at wrist and hand level**

IQ 7 **S66.508- Unspecified injury of intrinsic muscle, fascia and tendon of other finger at wrist and hand level**

Unspecified injury of intrinsic muscle, fascia and tendon of specified finger with unspecified laterality at wrist and hand level

IQ 7 **S66.509- Unspecified injury of intrinsic muscle, fascia and tendon of unspecified finger at wrist and hand level**

6 **S66.51 Strain of intrinsic muscle, fascia and tendon of other and unspecified finger at wrist and hand level**

SP 7 **S66.510- Strain of intrinsic muscle, fascia and tendon of right index finger at wrist and hand level**

SP 7 **S66.511- Strain of intrinsic muscle, fascia and tendon of left index finger at wrist and hand level**

SP 7 **S66.512- Strain of intrinsic muscle, fascia and tendon of right middle finger at wrist and hand level**

SP 7 **S66.513- Strain of intrinsic muscle, fascia and tendon of left middle finger at wrist and hand level**

SP 7 **S66.514- Strain of intrinsic muscle, fascia and tendon of right ring finger at wrist and hand level**

SP 7 **S66.515- Strain of intrinsic muscle, fascia and tendon of left ring finger at wrist and hand level**

SP 7 **S66.516- Strain of intrinsic muscle, fascia and tendon of right little finger at wrist and hand level**

SP 7 **S66.517- Strain of intrinsic muscle, fascia and tendon of left little finger at wrist and hand level**

SP 7 **S66.518- Strain of intrinsic muscle, fascia and tendon of other finger at wrist and hand level**

Strain of intrinsic muscle, fascia and tendon of specified finger with unspecified laterality at wrist and hand level

IQ 7 **S66.519- Strain of intrinsic muscle, fascia and tendon of unspecified finger at wrist and hand level**

6 **S66.52 Laceration of intrinsic muscle, fascia and tendon of other and unspecified finger at wrist and hand level**

Laterality SP 7 **S66.520- Laceration of intrinsic muscle, fascia and tendon of right index finger at wrist and hand level**

Laterality SP 7 **S66.521- Laceration of intrinsic muscle, fascia and tendon of left index finger at wrist and hand level**

Laterality SP 7 **S66.522- Laceration of intrinsic muscle, fascia and tendon of right middle finger at wrist and hand level**

Laterality SP 7 **S66.523- Laceration of intrinsic muscle, fascia and tendon of left middle finger at wrist and hand level**

Laterality SP 7 **S66.524- Laceration of intrinsic muscle, fascia and tendon of right ring finger at wrist and hand level**

Laterality SP 7 **S66.525- Laceration of intrinsic muscle, fascia and tendon of left ring finger at wrist and hand level**

Laterality SP 7 **S66.526- Laceration of intrinsic muscle, fascia and tendon of right little finger at wrist and hand level**

Laterality SP 7 **S66.527- Laceration of intrinsic muscle, fascia and tendon of left little finger at wrist and hand level**

Laterality SP 7 **S66.528- Laceration of intrinsic muscle, fascia and tendon of other finger at wrist and hand level**

Laceration of intrinsic muscle, fascia and tendon of specified finger with unspecified laterality at wrist and hand level

Laterality IQ 7 **S66.529- Laceration of intrinsic muscle, fascia and tendon of unspecified finger at wrist and hand level**

6 **S66.59 Other injury of intrinsic muscle, fascia and tendon of other and unspecified finger at wrist and hand level**

Laterality SP 7 **S66.590- Other injury of intrinsic muscle, fascia and tendon of right index finger at wrist and hand level**

Laterality SP 7 **S66.591- Other injury of intrinsic muscle, fascia and tendon of left index finger at wrist and hand level**

Laterality SP 7 **S66.592- Other injury of intrinsic muscle, fascia and tendon of right middle finger at wrist and hand level**

Laterality SP 7 **S66.593- Other injury of intrinsic muscle, fascia and tendon of left middle finger at wrist and hand level**

Laterality SP 7 **S66.594- Other injury of intrinsic muscle, fascia and tendon of right ring finger at wrist and hand level**

Laterality SP 7 **S66.595- Other injury of intrinsic muscle, fascia and tendon of left ring finger at wrist and hand level**

Laterality SP 7 **S66.596- Other injury of intrinsic muscle, fascia and tendon of right little finger at wrist and hand level**

Laterality SP 7 **S66.597- Other injury of intrinsic muscle, fascia and tendon of left little finger at wrist and hand level**

Laterality SP 7 **S66.598- Other injury of intrinsic muscle, fascia and tendon of other finger at wrist and hand level**

Other injury of intrinsic muscle, fascia and tendon of specified finger with unspecified laterality at wrist and hand level

Laterality IQ 7 **S66.599- Other injury of intrinsic muscle, fascia and tendon of unspecified finger at wrist and hand level**

5 **S66.8 Injury of other specified muscles, fascia and tendons at wrist and hand level**

6 **S66.80 Unspecified injury of other specified muscles, fascia and tendons at wrist and hand level**

Laterality IQ 7 **S66.801- Unspecified injury of other specified muscles, fascia and tendons at wrist and hand level, right hand**

Laterality IQ 7 **S66.802- Unspecified injury of other specified muscles, fascia and tendons at wrist and hand level, left hand**

Laterality IQ 7 **S66.809- Unspecified injury of other specified muscles, fascia and tendons at wrist and hand level, unspecified hand**

6 **S66.81 Strain of other specified muscles, fascia and tendons at wrist and hand level**

Laterality SP 7 **S66.811- Strain of other specified muscles, fascia and tendons at wrist and hand level, right hand**

Laterality SP 7 **S66.812- Strain of other specified muscles, fascia and tendons at wrist and hand level, left hand**

Laterality IQ 7 **S66.819- Strain of other specified muscles, fascia and tendons at wrist and hand level, unspecified hand**

6 **S66.82 Laceration of other specified muscles, fascia and tendons at wrist and hand level**

Laterality SP 7 **S66.821- Laceration of other specified muscles, fascia and tendons at wrist and hand level, right hand**

Laterality SP 7 **S66.822- Laceration of other specified muscles, fascia and tendons at wrist and hand level, left hand**

Laterality IQ 7 **S66.829- Laceration of other specified muscles, fascia and tendons at wrist and hand level, unspecified hand**

6 **S66.89 Other injury of other specified muscles, fascia and tendons at wrist and hand level**

Laterality SP 7 **S66.891- Other injury of other specified muscles, fascia and tendons at wrist and hand level, right hand**

Laterality SP 7 **S66.892- Other injury of other specified muscles, fascia and tendons at wrist and hand level, left hand**

Laterality IQ 7 **S66.899- Other injury of other specified muscles, fascia and tendons at wrist and hand level, unspecified hand**

S66.9 Injury of unspecified muscle, fascia and tendon at wrist and hand level

S66.90 Unspecified injury of unspecified muscle, fascia and tendon at wrist and hand level

S66.901- Unspecified injury of unspecified muscle, fascia and tendon at wrist and hand level, right hand

S66.902- Unspecified injury of unspecified muscle, fascia and tendon at wrist and hand level, left hand

S66.909- Unspecified injury of unspecified muscle, fascia and tendon at wrist and hand level, unspecified hand

S66.91 Strain of unspecified muscle, fascia and tendon at wrist and hand level

S66.911- Strain of unspecified muscle, fascia and tendon at wrist and hand level, right hand

S66.912- Strain of unspecified muscle, fascia and tendon at wrist and hand level, left hand

S66.919- Strain of unspecified muscle, fascia and tendon at wrist and hand level, unspecified hand

S66.92 Laceration of unspecified muscle, fascia and tendon at wrist and hand level

S66.921- Laceration of unspecified muscle, fascia and tendon at wrist and hand level, right hand

S66.922- Laceration of unspecified muscle, fascia and tendon at wrist and hand level, left hand

S66.929- Laceration of unspecified muscle, fascia and tendon at wrist and hand level, unspecified hand

S66.99 Other injury of unspecified muscle, fascia and tendon at wrist and hand level

S66.991- Other injury of unspecified muscle, fascia and tendon at wrist and hand level, right hand

S66.992- Other injury of unspecified muscle, fascia and tendon at wrist and hand level, left hand

S66.999- Other injury of unspecified muscle, fascia and tendon at wrist and hand level, unspecified hand

+ S67 Crushing injury of wrist, hand and fingers

Use additional code for all associated injuries, such as:
fracture of wrist and hand (S62.-)
open wound of wrist and hand (S61.-)

The appropriate 7th character is to be added to each code from category S67
A initial encounter
D subsequent encounter
S sequela

+ S67.0 Crushing injury of thumb

+ S67.00X- Crushing injury of unspecified thumb

+ S67.01X- Crushing injury of right thumb

+ S67.02X- Crushing injury of left thumb

+ S67.1 Crushing injury of other and unspecified finger(s)

EXCLUDES 2 crushing injury of thumb (S67.0-)

+ S67.10X- Crushing injury of unspecified finger(s)

+ S67.19 Crushing injury of other finger(s)

+ S67.190- Crushing injury of right index finger

+ S67.191- Crushing injury of left index finger

+ S67.192- Crushing injury of right middle finger

+ S67.193- Crushing injury of left middle finger

+ S67.194- Crushing injury of right ring finger

+ S67.195- Crushing injury of left ring finger

+ S67.196- Crushing injury of right little finger

+ S67.197- Crushing injury of left little finger

+ S67.198- Crushing injury of other finger

Crushing injury of specified finger with unspecified laterality

+ S67.2 Crushing injury of hand

EXCLUDES 2 crushing injury of fingers (S67.1-)
crushing injury of thumb (S67.0-)

+ S67.20X- Crushing injury of unspecified hand

+ S67.21X- Crushing injury of right hand

+ S67.22X- Crushing injury of left hand

+ S67.3 Crushing injury of wrist

+ S67.30X- Crushing injury of unspecified wrist

+ S67.31X- Crushing injury of right wrist

+ S67.32X- Crushing injury of left wrist

+ S67.4 Crushing injury of wrist and hand

EXCLUDES 1 crushing injury of hand alone (S67.2-)
crushing injury of wrist alone (S67.3-)

EXCLUDES 2 crushing injury of fingers (S67.1-)
crushing injury of thumb (S67.0-)

+ S67.40X- Crushing injury of unspecified wrist and hand

+ S67.41X- Crushing injury of right wrist and hand

+ S67.42X- Crushing injury of left wrist and hand

+ S67.9 Crushing injury of unspecified part(s) of wrist, hand and fingers

+ S67.90X- Crushing injury of unspecified part(s) of unspecified wrist, hand and fingers

⊟ SP + 7 S67.91X- **Crushing injury of unspecified part(s) of right wrist, hand and fingers**

⊟ SP + 7 S67.92X- **Crushing injury of unspecified part(s) of left wrist, hand and fingers**

4 **S68 Traumatic amputation of wrist, hand and fingers**

An amputation not identified as partial or complete should be coded to complete

The appropriate 7th character is to be added to each code from category S68
A initial encounter
D subsequent encounter
S sequela

CODING TIPS ✓ Use these codes only when the amputation was due to trauma. There is no need for adding Z89 with traumatic amputations. See Z47.81 for care of amputations not due to trauma.

5 **S68.0 Traumatic metacarpophalangeal amputation of thumb**

Traumatic amputation of thumb NOS

6 **S68.01 Complete traumatic metacarpophalangeal amputation of thumb**

⊟ SP 7 S68.011- **Complete traumatic metacarpophalangeal amputation of right thumb**

⊟ SP 7 S68.012- **Complete traumatic metacarpophalangeal amputation of left thumb**

⊟ IQ 7 S68.019- **Complete traumatic metacarpophalangeal amputation of unspecified thumb**

6 **S68.02 Partial traumatic metacarpophalangeal amputation of thumb**

⊟ SP 7 S68.021- **Partial traumatic metacarpophalangeal amputation of right thumb**

⊟ SP 7 S68.022- **Partial traumatic metacarpophalangeal amputation of left thumb**

⊟ IQ 7 S68.029- **Partial traumatic metacarpophalangeal amputation of unspecified thumb**

5 **S68.1 Traumatic metacarpophalangeal amputation of other and unspecified finger**

Traumatic amputation of finger NOS

EXCLUDES 2 traumatic metacarpophalangeal amputation of thumb (S68.0-)

6 **S68.11 Complete traumatic metacarpophalangeal amputation of other and unspecified finger**

⊟ SP 7 S68.110- **Complete traumatic metacarpophalangeal amputation of right index finger**

⊟ SP 7 S68.111- **Complete traumatic metacarpophalangeal amputation of left index finger**

⊟ SP 7 S68.112- **Complete traumatic metacarpophalangeal amputation of right middle finger**

⊟ SP 7 S68.113- **Complete traumatic metacarpophalangeal amputation of left middle finger**

⊟ SP 7 S68.114- **Complete traumatic metacarpophalangeal amputation of right ring finger**

⊟ SP 7 S68.115- **Complete traumatic metacarpophalangeal amputation of left ring finger**

⊟ SP 7 S68.116- **Complete traumatic metacarpophalangeal amputation of right little finger**

⊟ SP 7 S68.117- **Complete traumatic metacarpophalangeal amputation of left little finger**

⊟ SP 7 S68.118- **Complete traumatic metacarpophalangeal amputation of other finger**

Complete traumatic metacarpophalangeal amputation of specified finger with unspecified laterality

⊟ IQ 7 S68.119- **Complete traumatic metacarpophalangeal amputation of unspecified finger**

6 **S68.12 Partial traumatic metacarpophalangeal amputation of other and unspecified finger**

⊟ SP 7 S68.120- **Partial traumatic metacarpophalangeal amputation of right index finger**

⊟ SP 7 S68.121- **Partial traumatic metacarpophalangeal amputation of left index finger**

⊟ SP 7 S68.122- **Partial traumatic metacarpophalangeal amputation of right middle finger**

⊟ SP 7 S68.123- **Partial traumatic metacarpophalangeal amputation of left middle finger**

⊟ SP 7 S68.124- **Partial traumatic metacarpophalangeal amputation of right ring finger**

⊟ SP 7 S68.125- **Partial traumatic metacarpophalangeal amputation of left ring finger**

⊟ SP 7 S68.126- **Partial traumatic metacarpophalangeal amputation of right little finger**

⊟ SP 7 S68.127- **Partial traumatic metacarpophalangeal amputation of left little finger**

⊟ SP 7 S68.128- **Partial traumatic metacarpophalangeal amputation of other finger**

Partial traumatic metacarpophalangeal amputation of specified finger with unspecified laterality

S68.129- Partial traumatic metacarpophalangeal amputation of unspecified finger

S68.4 Traumatic amputation of hand at wrist level
Traumatic amputation of hand NOS
Traumatic amputation of wrist

S68.41 Complete traumatic amputation of hand at wrist level

S68.411- Complete traumatic amputation of right hand at wrist level
S68.412- Complete traumatic amputation of left hand at wrist level
S68.419- Complete traumatic amputation of unspecified hand at wrist level

S68.42 Partial traumatic amputation of hand at wrist level

S68.421- Partial traumatic amputation of right hand at wrist level
S68.422- Partial traumatic amputation of left hand at wrist level
S68.429- Partial traumatic amputation of unspecified hand at wrist level

S68.5 Traumatic transphalangeal amputation of thumb
Traumatic interphalangeal joint amputation of thumb

S68.51 Complete traumatic transphalangeal amputation of thumb

S68.511- Complete traumatic transphalangeal amputation of right thumb
S68.512- Complete traumatic transphalangeal amputation of left thumb
S68.519- Complete traumatic transphalangeal amputation of unspecified thumb

S68.52 Partial traumatic transphalangeal amputation of thumb

S68.521- Partial traumatic transphalangeal amputation of right thumb
S68.522- Partial traumatic transphalangeal amputation of left thumb
S68.529- Partial traumatic transphalangeal amputation of unspecified thumb

S68.6 Traumatic transphalangeal amputation of other and unspecified finger

S68.61 Complete traumatic transphalangeal amputation of other and unspecified finger(s)

S68.610- Complete traumatic transphalangeal amputation of right index finger
S68.611- Complete traumatic transphalangeal amputation of left index finger
S68.612- Complete traumatic transphalangeal amputation of right middle finger
S68.613- Complete traumatic transphalangeal amputation of left middle finger
S68.614- Complete traumatic transphalangeal amputation of right ring finger
S68.615- Complete traumatic transphalangeal amputation of left ring finger
S68.616- Complete traumatic transphalangeal amputation of right little finger
S68.617- Complete traumatic transphalangeal amputation of left little finger
S68.618- Complete traumatic transphalangeal amputation of other finger
Complete traumatic transphalangeal amputation of specified finger with unspecified laterality
S68.619- Complete traumatic transphalangeal amputation of unspecified finger

S68.62 Partial traumatic transphalangeal amputation of other and unspecified finger

S68.620- Partial traumatic transphalangeal amputation of right index finger
S68.621- Partial traumatic transphalangeal amputation of left index finger
S68.622- Partial traumatic transphalangeal amputation of right middle finger
S68.623- Partial traumatic transphalangeal amputation of left middle finger
S68.624- Partial traumatic transphalangeal amputation of right ring finger
S68.625- Partial traumatic transphalangeal amputation of left ring finger
S68.626- Partial traumatic transphalangeal amputation of right little finger
S68.627- Partial traumatic transphalangeal amputation of left little finger
S68.628- Partial traumatic transphalangeal amputation of other finger
Partial traumatic transphalangeal amputation of specified finger with unspecified laterality
S68.629- Partial traumatic transphalangeal amputation of unspecified finger

S68.7 Traumatic transmetacarpal amputation of hand

S68.71 Complete traumatic transmetacarpal amputation of hand

S68.711- Complete traumatic transmetacarpal amputation of right hand

Chapter 19 S00-T88

SP 7 **S68.712- Complete traumatic transmetacarpal amputation of left hand**

IQ 7 **S68.719- Complete traumatic transmetacarpal amputation of unspecified hand**

6 **S68.72 Partial traumatic transmetacarpal amputation of hand**

SP 7 **S68.721- Partial traumatic transmetacarpal amputation of right hand**

SP 7 **S68.722- Partial traumatic transmetacarpal amputation of left hand**

IQ 7 **S68.729- Partial traumatic transmetacarpal amputation of unspecified hand**

4 **S69 Other and unspecified injuries of wrist, hand and finger(s)**

The appropriate 7th character is to be added to each code from category S69

A initial encounter
D subsequent encounter
S sequela

5 **S69.8 Other specified injuries of wrist, hand and finger(s)**

IQ 7 **S69.80X- Other specified injuries of unspecified wrist, hand and finger(s)**

SP 7 **S69.81X- Other specified injuries of right wrist, hand and finger(s)**

SP IQ 7 **S69.82X- Other specified injuries of left wrist, hand and finger(s)**

5 **S69.9 Unspecified injury of wrist, hand and finger(s)**

IQ 7 **S69.90X- Unspecified injury of unspecified wrist, hand and finger(s)**

IQ 7 **S69.91X- Unspecified injury of right wrist, hand and finger(s)**

IQ 7 **S69.92X- Unspecified injury of left wrist, hand and finger(s)**

Injuries to the hip and thigh (S70-S79)

EXCLUDES 2 burns and corrosions (T20-T32)
frostbite (T33-T34)
snake bite (T63.0-)
venomous insect bite or sting (T63.4-)

GUIDELINES **Section I.C.19.c.2)**

Multiple fractures are sequenced in accordance with the severity of the fracture.

GUIDELINES **Section I.C.19.b.1)-2)**

When coding injuries, assign separate codes for each injury unless a combination code is provided, in which case the combination code is assigned ... Traumatic injury codes (S00-T14.9) are not to be used for normal, healing surgical wounds or to identify complications of surgical wounds. The code for the most serious injury, as determined by the provider and the focus of treatment, is sequenced first.

1) Superficial injuries such as abrasions or contusions are not coded when associated with more severe injuries of the same site.

2) When a primary injury results in minor damage to peripheral nerves or blood vessels, the primary injury is sequenced first with additional code(s) for injuries to nerves and spinal cord (such as category S04), and/or injury to blood vessels (such as category S15). When the primary injury is to the blood vessels or nerves, that injury should be sequenced first.

GUIDELINES **Section I.C.19.c**

Coding of Traumatic Fractures: The principles of multiple coding of injuries should be followed in coding fractures. Fractures of specified sites are coded individually by site in accordance with both the provisions within categories S02, S12, S22, S32, S42, S49, S52, S59, S62, S72, S79, S82, S89, S92 and the level of detail furnished by medical record content. A fracture not indicated as open or closed should be coded to closed. A fracture not indicated whether displaced or not displaced should be coded to displaced.

CODING TIPS ✓ 7th character A is acceptable in home health and hospice when active treatment is provided, such as antibiotics for an infected wound or a wound vac for a dehisced wound. D is used when the complication or injury is now healing. Think of D as aftercare. S is used for sequela of the injury or complication. Sequela is a residual deficit or condition produced as a result of the injury or complication after the original injury or complication has healed.

4 **S70 Superficial injury of hip and thigh**

The appropriate 7th character is to be added to each code from category S70

A initial encounter
D subsequent encounter
S sequela

5 **S70.0 Contusion of hip**

IQ 7 **S70.00X- Contusion of unspecified hip**

IQ 7 **S70.01X- Contusion of right hip**

IQ 7 **S70.02X- Contusion of left hip**

5 **S70.1 Contusion of thigh**

IQ 7 **S70.10X- Contusion of unspecified thigh**

IQ 7 **S70.11X- Contusion of right thigh**

IQ 7 **S70.12X- Contusion of left thigh**

5 **S70.2 Other superficial injuries of hip**

6 **S70.21 Abrasion of hip**

IQ 7 **S70.211- Abrasion, right hip**

IQ 7 **S70.212- Abrasion, left hip**

IQ 7 **S70.219- Abrasion, unspecified hip**

6 **S70.22 Blister (nonthermal) of hip**

IQ 7 **S70.221- Blister (nonthermal), right hip**

IQ 7 **S70.222- Blister (nonthermal), left hip**

S70.229- Blister (nonthermal), unspecified hip

S70.24 External constriction of hip

S70.241- External constriction, right hip

S70.242- External constriction, left hip

S70.249- External constriction, unspecified hip

S70.25 Superficial foreign body of hip
Splinter in the hip

S70.251- Superficial foreign body, right hip

S70.252- Superficial foreign body, left hip

S70.259- Superficial foreign body, unspecified hip

S70.26 Insect bite (nonvenomous) of hip

S70.261- Insect bite (nonvenomous), right hip

S70.262- Insect bite (nonvenomous), left hip

S70.269- Insect bite (nonvenomous), unspecified hip

S70.27 Other superficial bite of hip
EXCLUDES 1 open bite of hip (S71.05-)

S70.271- Other superficial bite of hip, right hip

S70.272- Other superficial bite of hip, left hip

S70.279- Other superficial bite of hip, unspecified hip

S70.3 Other superficial injuries of thigh

S70.31 Abrasion of thigh

S70.311- Abrasion, right thigh

S70.312- Abrasion, left thigh

S70.319- Abrasion, unspecified thigh

S70.32 Blister (nonthermal) of thigh

S70.321- Blister (nonthermal), right thigh

S70.322- Blister (nonthermal), left thigh

S70.329- Blister (nonthermal), unspecified thigh

S70.34 External constriction of thigh

S70.341- External constriction, right thigh

S70.342- External constriction, left thigh

S70.349- External constriction, unspecified thigh

S70.35 Superficial foreign body of thigh
Splinter in the thigh

S70.351- Superficial foreign body, right thigh

S70.352- Superficial foreign body, left thigh

S70.359- Superficial foreign body, unspecified thigh

S70.36 Insect bite (nonvenomous) of thigh

S70.361- Insect bite (nonvenomous), right thigh

S70.362- Insect bite (nonvenomous), left thigh

S70.369- Insect bite (nonvenomous), unspecified thigh

S70.37 Other superficial bite of thigh
EXCLUDES 1 open bite of thigh (S71.15)

S70.371- Other superficial bite of right thigh

S70.372- Other superficial bite of left thigh

S70.379- Other superficial bite of unspecified thigh

S70.9 Unspecified superficial injury of hip and thigh

S70.91 Unspecified superficial injury of hip

S70.911- Unspecified superficial injury of right hip

S70.912- Unspecified superficial injury of left hip

S70.919- Unspecified superficial injury of unspecified hip

S70.92 Unspecified superficial injury of thigh

S70.921- Unspecified superficial injury of right thigh

S70.922- Unspecified superficial injury of left thigh

S70.929- Unspecified superficial injury of unspecified thigh

S71 Open wound of hip and thigh
Code also:
any associated wound infection
EXCLUDES 1 open fracture of hip and thigh (S72.-)
traumatic amputation of hip and thigh (S78.-)
EXCLUDES 2 bite of venomous animal (T63.-)
open wound of ankle, foot and toes (S91.-)
open wound of knee and lower leg (S81.-)

The appropriate 7th character is to be added to each code from category S71
A initial encounter
D subsequent encounter
S sequela

CODING TIPS ✓ No aftercare code applies, including those indicating dressing changes, drain care, or suture removal. 7th character 'D' is the default for home care and hospice when providing aftercare for a healing or resolving condition; 'A' is used for active treatment such as antibiotics or more than routine wound care; 'S' may be used to indicate a residual condition after the original injury has healed.

CODING TIPS ✓ Open wound codes indicate a wound resulting from a traumatic origin. Do not assign a code for "open wound" unless the etiology of the wound is related to trauma.

S71.0 Open wound of hip

S71.00 Unspecified open wound of hip

S71.001- Unspecified open wound, right hip

S71.002- Unspecified open wound, left hip

S71.009- Unspecified open wound, unspecified hip

Chapter 19 S00-T88

6 **S71.01 Laceration without foreign body of hip**

Laterality SP 7 **S71.011- Laceration without foreign body, right hip**

Laterality SP 7 **S71.012- Laceration without foreign body, left hip**

Laterality !Q 7 **S71.019- Laceration without foreign body, unspecified hip**

6 **S71.02 Laceration with foreign body of hip**

Laterality SP 7 **S71.021- Laceration with foreign body, right hip**

Laterality SP 7 **S71.022- Laceration with foreign body, left hip**

Laterality !Q 7 **S71.029- Laceration with foreign body, unspecified hip**

6 **S71.03 Puncture wound without foreign body of hip**

Laterality SP 7 **S71.031- Puncture wound without foreign body, right hip**

Laterality SP 7 **S71.032- Puncture wound without foreign body, left hip**

Laterality !Q 7 **S71.039- Puncture wound without foreign body, unspecified hip**

6 **S71.04 Puncture wound with foreign body of hip**

Laterality SP 7 **S71.041- Puncture wound with foreign body, right hip**

Laterality SP 7 **S71.042- Puncture wound with foreign body, left hip**

Laterality !Q 7 **S71.049- Puncture wound with foreign body, unspecified hip**

6 **S71.05 Open bite of hip**

Bite of hip NOS

EXCLUDES 1 superficial bite of hip (S70.26, S70.27)

Laterality SP 7 **S71.051- Open bite, right hip**

Laterality SP 7 **S71.052- Open bite, left hip**

Laterality !Q 7 **S71.059- Open bite, unspecified hip**

5 **S71.1 Open wound of thigh**

6 **S71.10 Unspecified open wound of thigh**

Laterality SP 7 **S71.101- Unspecified open wound, right thigh**

Laterality SP 7 **S71.102- Unspecified open wound, left thigh**

Laterality !Q 7 **S71.109- Unspecified open wound, unspecified thigh**

6 **S71.11 Laceration without foreign body of thigh**

Laterality SP 7 **S71.111- Laceration without foreign body, right thigh**

Laterality SP 7 **S71.112- Laceration without foreign body, left thigh**

Laterality !Q 7 **S71.119- Laceration without foreign body, unspecified thigh**

6 **S71.12 Laceration with foreign body of thigh**

Laterality SP 7 **S71.121- Laceration with foreign body, right thigh**

Laterality SP 7 **S71.122- Laceration with foreign body, left thigh**

Laterality !Q 7 **S71.129- Laceration with foreign body, unspecified thigh**

6 **S71.13 Puncture wound without foreign body of thigh**

Laterality SP 7 **S71.131- Puncture wound without foreign body, right thigh**

Laterality SP 7 **S71.132- Puncture wound without foreign body, left thigh**

Laterality !Q 7 **S71.139- Puncture wound without foreign body, unspecified thigh**

6 **S71.14 Puncture wound with foreign body of thigh**

Laterality SP 7 **S71.141- Puncture wound with foreign body, right thigh**

Laterality SP 7 **S71.142- Puncture wound with foreign body, left thigh**

Laterality !Q 7 **S71.149- Puncture wound with foreign body, unspecified thigh**

6 **S71.15 Open bite of thigh**

Bite of thigh NOS

EXCLUDES 1 superficial bite of thigh (S70.37-)

Laterality SP 7 **S71.151- Open bite, right thigh**

Laterality SP 7 **S71.152- Open bite, left thigh**

Laterality !Q 7 **S71.159- Open bite, unspecified thigh**

Gustilo open fracture classification

Gustilo Grade	Definition
I	Open fracture, clean wound, wound <1 cm in length
II	Open fracture, wound > 1 cm but < 10 cm in length without extensive soft-tissue damage, flaps, avulsions
III	Open fracture with extensive soft-tissue laceration (>10 cm), damage, or loss or an open segmental fracture. This type also includes open fractures caused by farm injuries, fractures requiring vascular repair, or fractures that have been open for 8 hr prior to treatment
IIIA	Type III fracture with adequate periosteal coverage of the fracture bone despite the extensive soft-tissue laceration or damage
IIIB	Type III fracture with extensive soft-tissue loss and periosteal stripping and bone damage. Usually associated with massive contamination. Will often need further soft-tissue coverage procedure (i.e. free or rotational flap)
IIIC	Type III fracture associated with an arterial injury requiring repair, irrespective of degree of soft-tissue injury.
http://en.wikipedia.org/wiki/Gustilo_open_fracture_classification	

4 **S72 Fracture of femur**

Note:

A fracture not indicated as displaced or nondisplaced should be coded to displaced

A fracture not indicated as open or closed should be coded to closed

The open fracture designations are based on the Gustilo open fracture classification

EXCLUDES 1 traumatic amputation of hip and thigh (S78.-)

EXCLUDES 2 fracture of lower leg and ankle (S82.-)

fracture of foot (S92.-)

periprosthetic fracture of prosthetic implant of hip (M97.0-)

Chapter 19

S00-T88

4 4th digit required 5 5th digit required 6 6th digit required 7 7th digit required 7 7th digit placeholder + Additional code Laterality

The appropriate 7th character is to be added to all codes from category S72

- A initial encounter for closed fracture
- B initial encounter for open fracture type I or II
- C initial encounter for open fracture type IIIA, IIIB, or IIIC
- D subsequent encounter for closed fracture with routine healing
- E subsequent encounter for open fracture type I or II with routine healing
- F subsequent encounter for open fracture type IIIA, IIIB, or IIIC with routine healing
- G subsequent encounter for closed fracture with delayed healing
- H subsequent encounter for open fracture type I or II with delayed healing
- J subsequent encounter for open fracture type IIIA, IIIB, or IIIC with delayed healing
- K subsequent encounter for closed fracture with nonunion
- M subsequent encounter for open fracture type I or II with nonunion
- N subsequent encounter for open fracture type IIIA, IIIB, or IIIC with nonunion
- P subsequent encounter for closed fracture with malunion
- Q subsequent encounter for open fracture type I or II with malunion
- R subsequent encounter for open fracture type IIIA, IIIB, or IIIC with malunion
- S sequela

CODING TIPS✓ Fractures repaired by joint replacements are NOT coded with Z47.1. Fractures repaired by any other orthopedic surgery are NOT coded with Z47.89. Z codes are not appropriate for fractures of any kind. Code the fracture with 7th character D for fractures undergoing surgical repair.

CODING TIPS✓ A fracture not indicated as displaced or nondisplaced should be coded to displaced. A fracture not indicated as open or closed should be coded to closed. The open fracture designations are based on the Gustilo open fracture classification. The 7th characters E, H, M and Q are the default for the Gustilo classification when no information is available. Always query the physician or NPP.

CODING TIPS✓ "D" is the 7th character for home care and hospice unless the physician or NPP has documented delayed healing, nonunion or malunion. A sequela is a condition left after the fracture has healed.

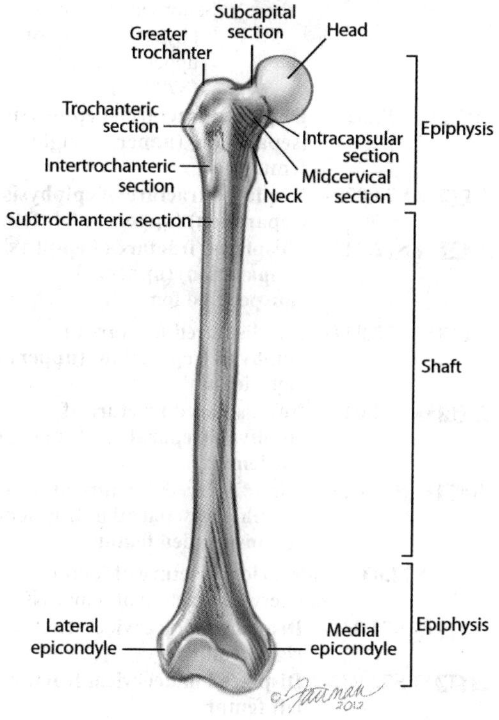

5 S72.0 Fracture of head and neck of femur

EXCLUDES 2 physeal fracture of upper end of femur (S79.0-)

6 S72.00 Fracture of unspecified part of neck of femur

Fracture of hip NOS

Fracture of neck of femur NOS

CODING TIPS✓ A fracture that is only reported as a "hip fracture" should be coded to S72.00- with the appropriate 6th character to indicate laterality, and a 7th character to indicate healing status and episode of care.

⊟ SP 7 S72.001- Fracture of unspecified part of neck of right femur

⊟ SP 7 S72.002- Fracture of unspecified part of neck of left femur

⊟ IQ 7 S72.009- Fracture of unspecified part of neck of unspecified femur

6 S72.01 Unspecified intracapsular fracture of femur

Subcapital fracture of femur

⊟ SP 7 S72.011- Unspecified intracapsular fracture of right femur

⊟ SP 7 S72.012- Unspecified intracapsular fracture of left femur

⊟ IQ 7 S72.019- Unspecified intracapsular fracture of unspecified femur

6 S72.02 Fracture of epiphysis (separation) (upper) of femur

Transepiphyseal fracture of femur

EXCLUDES 1 capital femoral epiphyseal fracture (pediatric) of femur (S79.01-)
Salter-Harris Type I physeal fracture of upper end of femur (S79.01-)

S72.021- **Displaced fracture of epiphysis (separation) (upper) of right femur**
S72.022- **Displaced fracture of epiphysis (separation) (upper) of left femur**
S72.023- **Displaced fracture of epiphysis (separation) (upper) of unspecified femur**
S72.024- **Nondisplaced fracture of epiphysis (separation) (upper) of right femur**
S72.025- **Nondisplaced fracture of epiphysis (separation) (upper) of left femur**
S72.026- **Nondisplaced fracture of epiphysis (separation) (upper) of unspecified femur**

6 **S72.03 Midcervical fracture of femur**
Transcervical fracture of femur NOS

S72.031- **Displaced midcervical fracture of right femur**
S72.032- **Displaced midcervical fracture of left femur**
S72.033- **Displaced midcervical fracture of unspecified femur**
S72.034- **Nondisplaced midcervical fracture of right femur**
S72.035- **Nondisplaced midcervical fracture of left femur**
S72.036- **Nondisplaced midcervical fracture of unspecified femur**

6 **S72.04 Fracture of base of neck of femur**
Cervicotrochanteric fracture of femur

S72.041- **Displaced fracture of base of neck of right femur**
S72.042- **Displaced fracture of base of neck of left femur**
S72.043- **Displaced fracture of base of neck of unspecified femur**
S72.044- **Nondisplaced fracture of base of neck of right femur**
S72.045- **Nondisplaced fracture of base of neck of left femur**
S72.046- **Nondisplaced fracture of base of neck of unspecified femur**

6 **S72.05 Unspecified fracture of head of femur**
Fracture of head of femur NOS

S72.051- **Unspecified fracture of head of right femur**
S72.052- **Unspecified fracture of head of left femur**
S72.059- **Unspecified fracture of head of unspecified femur**

6 **S72.06 Articular fracture of head of femur**

S72.061- **Displaced articular fracture of head of right femur**
S72.062- **Displaced articular fracture of head of left femur**
S72.063- **Displaced articular fracture of head of unspecified femur**
S72.064- **Nondisplaced articular fracture of head of right femur**
S72.065- **Nondisplaced articular fracture of head of left femur**
S72.066- **Nondisplaced articular fracture of head of unspecified femur**

6 **S72.09 Other fracture of head and neck of femur**

S72.091- **Other fracture of head and neck of right femur**
S72.092- **Other fracture of head and neck of left femur**
S72.099- **Other fracture of head and neck of unspecified femur**

5 **S72.1 Pertrochanteric fracture**

6 **S72.10 Unspecified trochanteric fracture of femur**
Fracture of trochanter NOS

S72.101- **Unspecified trochanteric fracture of right femur**
S72.102- **Unspecified trochanteric fracture of left femur**
S72.109- **Unspecified trochanteric fracture of unspecified femur**

6 **S72.11 Fracture of greater trochanter of femur**

S72.111- **Displaced fracture of greater trochanter of right femur**
S72.112- **Displaced fracture of greater trochanter of left femur**
S72.113- **Displaced fracture of greater trochanter of unspecified femur**
S72.114- **Nondisplaced fracture of greater trochanter of right femur**
S72.115- **Nondisplaced fracture of greater trochanter of left femur**
S72.116- **Nondisplaced fracture of greater trochanter of unspecified femur**

6 **S72.12 Fracture of lesser trochanter of femur**

S72.121- **Displaced fracture of lesser trochanter of right femur**
S72.122- **Displaced fracture of lesser trochanter of left femur**
S72.123- **Displaced fracture of lesser trochanter of unspecified femur**
S72.124- **Nondisplaced fracture of lesser trochanter of right femur**
S72.125- **Nondisplaced fracture of lesser trochanter of left femur**
S72.126- **Nondisplaced fracture of lesser trochanter of unspecified femur**

6 **S72.13 Apophyseal fracture of femur**
EXCLUDES 1 chronic (nontraumatic) slipped upper femoral epiphysis (M93.0-)

S72.131- **Displaced apophyseal fracture of right femur**
S72.132- **Displaced apophyseal fracture of left femur**

Chapter 19
S00-T88

4 4th digit required 5 5th digit required 6 6th digit required 7 7th digit required 7 7th digit placeholder + Additional code Laterality

S72.133- Displaced apophyseal fracture of unspecified femur
S72.134- Nondisplaced apophyseal fracture of right femur
S72.135- Nondisplaced apophyseal fracture of left femur
S72.136- Nondisplaced apophyseal fracture of unspecified femur

S72.14 Intertrochanteric fracture of femur
S72.141- Displaced intertrochanteric fracture of right femur
S72.142- Displaced intertrochanteric fracture of left femur
S72.143- Displaced intertrochanteric fracture of unspecified femur
S72.144- Nondisplaced intertrochanteric fracture of right femur
S72.145- Nondisplaced intertrochanteric fracture of left femur
S72.146- Nondisplaced intertrochanteric fracture of unspecified femur

S72.2 Subtrochanteric fracture of femur
S72.21X- Displaced subtrochanteric fracture of right femur
S72.22X- Displaced subtrochanteric fracture of left femur
S72.23X- Displaced subtrochanteric fracture of unspecified femur
S72.24X- Nondisplaced subtrochanteric fracture of right femur
S72.25X- Nondisplaced subtrochanteric fracture of left femur
S72.26X- Nondisplaced subtrochanteric fracture of unspecified femur

S72.3 Fracture of shaft of femur

S72.30 Unspecified fracture of shaft of femur
S72.301- Unspecified fracture of shaft of right femur
S72.302- Unspecified fracture of shaft of left femur
S72.309- Unspecified fracture of shaft of unspecified femur

S72.32 Transverse fracture of shaft of femur
S72.321- Displaced transverse fracture of shaft of right femur
S72.322- Displaced transverse fracture of shaft of left femur
S72.323- Displaced transverse fracture of shaft of unspecified femur
S72.324- Nondisplaced transverse fracture of shaft of right femur
S72.325- Nondisplaced transverse fracture of shaft of left femur
S72.326- Nondisplaced transverse fracture of shaft of unspecified femur

S72.33 Oblique fracture of shaft of femur
S72.331- Displaced oblique fracture of shaft of right femur
S72.332- Displaced oblique fracture of shaft of left femur
S72.333- Displaced oblique fracture of shaft of unspecified femur
S72.334- Nondisplaced oblique fracture of shaft of right femur
S72.335- Nondisplaced oblique fracture of shaft of left femur
S72.336- Nondisplaced oblique fracture of shaft of unspecified femur

S72.34 Spiral fracture of shaft of femur
S72.341- Displaced spiral fracture of shaft of right femur
S72.342- Displaced spiral fracture of shaft of left femur
S72.343- Displaced spiral fracture of shaft of unspecified femur
S72.344- Nondisplaced spiral fracture of shaft of right femur
S72.345- Nondisplaced spiral fracture of shaft of left femur
S72.346- Nondisplaced spiral fracture of shaft of unspecified femur

S72.35 Comminuted fracture of shaft of femur
S72.351- Displaced comminuted fracture of shaft of right femur
S72.352- Displaced comminuted fracture of shaft of left femur
S72.353- Displaced comminuted fracture of shaft of unspecified femur
S72.354- Nondisplaced comminuted fracture of shaft of right femur
S72.355- Nondisplaced comminuted fracture of shaft of left femur
S72.356- Nondisplaced comminuted fracture of shaft of unspecified femur

S72.36 Segmental fracture of shaft of femur
S72.361- Displaced segmental fracture of shaft of right femur
S72.362- Displaced segmental fracture of shaft of left femur
S72.363- Displaced segmental fracture of shaft of unspecified femur
S72.364- Nondisplaced segmental fracture of shaft of right femur
S72.365- Nondisplaced segmental fracture of shaft of left femur
S72.366- Nondisplaced segmental fracture of shaft of unspecified femur

S72.39 Other fracture of shaft of femur
S72.391- Other fracture of shaft of right femur
S72.392- Other fracture of shaft of left femur
S72.399- Other fracture of shaft of unspecified femur

S72.4 Fracture of lower end of femur
Fracture of distal end of femur
EXCLUDES 2 fracture of shaft of femur (S72.3-)
physeal fracture of lower end of femur (S79.1-)

S72.40 Unspecified fracture of lower end of femur
S72.401- Unspecified fracture of lower end of right femur

Chapter 19
S00-T88

S72.402- Unspecified fracture of lower end of left femur

S72.409- Unspecified fracture of lower end of unspecified femur

S72.41 Unspecified condyle fracture of lower end of femur

Condyle fracture of femur NOS

S72.411- Displaced unspecified condyle fracture of lower end of right femur

S72.412- Displaced unspecified condyle fracture of lower end of left femur

S72.413- Displaced unspecified condyle fracture of lower end of unspecified femur

S72.414- Nondisplaced unspecified condyle fracture of lower end of right femur

S72.415- Nondisplaced unspecified condyle fracture of lower end of left femur

S72.416- Nondisplaced unspecified condyle fracture of lower end of unspecified femur

S72.42 Fracture of lateral condyle of femur

S72.421- Displaced fracture of lateral condyle of right femur

S72.422- Displaced fracture of lateral condyle of left femur

S72.423- Displaced fracture of lateral condyle of unspecified femur

S72.424- Nondisplaced fracture of lateral condyle of right femur

S72.425- Nondisplaced fracture of lateral condyle of left femur

S72.426- Nondisplaced fracture of lateral condyle of unspecified femur

S72.43 Fracture of medial condyle of femur

S72.431- Displaced fracture of medial condyle of right femur

S72.432- Displaced fracture of medial condyle of left femur

S72.433- Displaced fracture of medial condyle of unspecified femur

S72.434- Nondisplaced fracture of medial condyle of right femur

S72.435- Nondisplaced fracture of medial condyle of left femur

S72.436- Nondisplaced fracture of medial condyle of unspecified femur

S72.44 Fracture of lower epiphysis (separation) of femur

EXCLUDES 1 Salter-Harris Type I physeal fracture of lower end of femur (S79.11-)

S72.441- Displaced fracture of lower epiphysis (separation) of right femur

S72.442- Displaced fracture of lower epiphysis (separation) of left femur

S72.443- Displaced fracture of lower epiphysis (separation) of unspecified femur

S72.444- Nondisplaced fracture of lower epiphysis (separation) of right femur

S72.445- Nondisplaced fracture of lower epiphysis (separation) of left femur

S72.446- Nondisplaced fracture of lower epiphysis (separation) of unspecified femur

S72.45 Supracondylar fracture without intracondylar extension of lower end of femur

Supracondylar fracture of lower end of femur NOS

EXCLUDES 1 supracondylar fracture with intracondylar extension of lower end of femur (S72.46-)

S72.451- Displaced supracondylar fracture without intracondylar extension of lower end of right femur

S72.452- Displaced supracondylar fracture without intracondylar extension of lower end of left femur

S72.453- Displaced supracondylar fracture without intracondylar extension of lower end of unspecified femur

S72.454- Nondisplaced supracondylar fracture without intracondylar extension of lower end of right femur

S72.455- Nondisplaced supracondylar fracture without intracondylar extension of lower end of left femur

S72.456- Nondisplaced supracondylar fracture without intracondylar extension of lower end of unspecified femur

S72.46 Supracondylar fracture with intracondylar extension of lower end of femur

EXCLUDES 1 supracondylar fracture without intracondylar extension of lower end of femur (S72.45-)

S72.461- Displaced supracondylar fracture with intracondylar extension of lower end of right femur

S72.462- Displaced supracondylar fracture with intracondylar extension of lower end of left femur

S72.463- Displaced supracondylar fracture with intracondylar extension of lower end of unspecified femur

S72.464- Nondisplaced supracondylar fracture with intracondylar extension of lower end of right femur

Chapter 19

S00-T88

SP 7 **S72.465- Nondisplaced supracondylar fracture with intracondylar extension of lower end of left femur**

IQ 7 **S72.466- Nondisplaced supracondylar fracture with intracondylar extension of lower end of unspecified femur**

6 **S72.47 Torus fracture of lower end of femur**

The appropriate 7th character is to be added to all codes in subcategory S72.47

A	initial encounter for closed fracture
D	subsequent encounter for fracture with routine healing
G	subsequent encounter for fracture with delayed healing
K	subsequent encounter for fracture with nonunion
P	subsequent encounter for fracture with malunion
S	sequela

CODING TIPS✓ Open fractures do not occur with torus fractures and greenstick fractures, therefore the 7th characters for open fractures are not available.

SP 7 **S72.471- Torus fracture of lower end of right femur**

SP 7 **S72.472- Torus fracture of lower end of left femur**

IQ 7 **S72.479- Torus fracture of lower end of unspecified femur**

6 **S72.49 Other fracture of lower end of femur**

SP 7 **S72.491- Other fracture of lower end of right femur**

SP 7 **S72.492- Other fracture of lower end of left femur**

IQ 7 **S72.499- Other fracture of lower end of unspecified femur**

5 **S72.8 Other fracture of femur**

6 **S72.8X Other fracture of femur**

SP 7 **S72.8X1- Other fracture of right femur**

SP 7 **S72.8X2- Other fracture of left femur**

IQ 7 **S72.8X9- Other fracture of unspecified femur**

5 **S72.9 Unspecified fracture of femur**

Fracture of thigh NOS
Fracture of upper leg NOS

EXCLUDES 1 fracture of hip NOS (S72.00-, S72.01-)

IQ 7 **S72.90X- Unspecified fracture of unspecified femur**

SP 7 **S72.91X- Unspecified fracture of right femur**

SP 7 **S72.92X- Unspecified fracture of left femur**

4 **S73 Dislocation and sprain of joint and ligaments of hip**

INCLUDES avulsion of joint or ligament of hip
laceration of cartilage, joint or ligament of hip
sprain of cartilage, joint or ligament of hip
traumatic hemarthrosis of joint or ligament of hip
traumatic rupture of joint or ligament of hip
traumatic subluxation of joint or ligament of hip
traumatic tear of joint or ligament of hip

Code also:
any associated open wound

EXCLUDES 2 strain of muscle, fascia and tendon of hip and thigh (S76.-)

The appropriate 7th character is to be added to each code from category S73

A	initial encounter
D	subsequent encounter
S	sequela

5 **S73.0 Subluxation and dislocation of hip**

EXCLUDES 2 dislocation and subluxation of hip prosthesis (T84.020, T84.021)

6 **S73.00 Unspecified subluxation and dislocation of hip**

Dislocation of hip NOS
Subluxation of hip NOS

IQ 7 **S73.001- Unspecified subluxation of right hip**

IQ 7 **S73.002- Unspecified subluxation of left hip**

IQ 7 **S73.003- Unspecified subluxation of unspecified hip**

IQ 7 **S73.004- Unspecified dislocation of right hip**

IQ 7 **S73.005- Unspecified dislocation of left hip**

IQ 7 **S73.006- Unspecified dislocation of unspecified hip**

6 **S73.01 Posterior subluxation and dislocation of hip**

SP 7 **S73.011- Posterior subluxation of right hip**

SP 7 **S73.012- Posterior subluxation of left hip**

IQ 7 **S73.013- Posterior subluxation of unspecified hip**

SP 7 **S73.014- Posterior dislocation of right hip**

SP 7 **S73.015- Posterior dislocation of left hip**

IQ 7 **S73.016- Posterior dislocation of unspecified hip**

6 **S73.02 Obturator subluxation and dislocation of hip**

SP 7 **S73.021- Obturator subluxation of right hip**

SP 7 **S73.022- Obturator subluxation of left hip**

IQ 7 **S73.023- Obturator subluxation of unspecified hip**

SP 7 **S73.024- Obturator dislocation of right hip**

SP 7 **S73.025- Obturator dislocation of left hip**

IQ 7 **S73.026- Obturator dislocation of unspecified hip**

6 **S73.03 Other anterior subluxation and dislocation of hip**

Chapter 19 S00-T88

S73.031- Other anterior subluxation of right hip
S73.032- Other anterior subluxation of left hip
S73.033- Other anterior subluxation of unspecified hip
S73.034- Other anterior dislocation of right hip
S73.035- Other anterior dislocation of left hip
S73.036- Other anterior dislocation of unspecified hip

S73.04 Central subluxation and dislocation of hip

S73.041- Central subluxation of right hip
S73.042- Central subluxation of left hip
S73.043- Central subluxation of unspecified hip
S73.044- Central dislocation of right hip
S73.045- Central dislocation of left hip
S73.046- Central dislocation of unspecified hip

S73.1 Sprain of hip

S73.10 Unspecified sprain of hip

S73.101- Unspecified sprain of right hip
S73.102- Unspecified sprain of left hip
S73.109- Unspecified sprain of unspecified hip

S73.11 Iliofemoral ligament sprain of hip

S73.111- Iliofemoral ligament sprain of right hip
S73.112- Iliofemoral ligament sprain of left hip
S73.119- Iliofemoral ligament sprain of unspecified hip

S73.12 Ischiocapsular (ligament) sprain of hip

S73.121- Ischiocapsular ligament sprain of right hip
S73.122- Ischiocapsular ligament sprain of left hip
S73.129- Ischiocapsular ligament sprain of unspecified hip

S73.19 Other sprain of hip

S73.191- Other sprain of right hip
S73.192- Other sprain of left hip
S73.199- Other sprain of unspecified hip

S74 Injury of nerves at hip and thigh level

Code also:
any associated open wound (S71.-)

EXCLUDES 2 injury of nerves at ankle and foot level (S94.-)
injury of nerves at lower leg level (S84.-)

The appropriate 7th character is to be added to each code from category S74
A initial encounter
D subsequent encounter
S sequela

S74.0 Injury of sciatic nerve at hip and thigh level

S74.00X- Injury of sciatic nerve at hip and thigh level, unspecified leg
S74.01X- Injury of sciatic nerve at hip and thigh level, right leg
S74.02X- Injury of sciatic nerve at hip and thigh level, left leg

S74.1 Injury of femoral nerve at hip and thigh level

S74.10X- Injury of femoral nerve at hip and thigh level, unspecified leg
S74.11X- Injury of femoral nerve at hip and thigh level, right leg
S74.12X- Injury of femoral nerve at hip and thigh level, left leg

S74.2 Injury of cutaneous sensory nerve at hip and thigh level

S74.20X- Injury of cutaneous sensory nerve at hip and thigh level, unspecified leg
S74.21X- Injury of cutaneous sensory nerve at hip and high level, right leg
S74.22X- Injury of cutaneous sensory nerve at hip and thigh level, left leg

S74.8 Injury of other nerves at hip and thigh level

S74.8X Injury of other nerves at hip and thigh level

S74.8X1- Injury of other nerves at hip and thigh level, right leg
S74.8X2- Injury of other nerves at hip and thigh level, left leg
S74.8X9- Injury of other nerves at hip and thigh level, unspecified leg

S74.9 Injury of unspecified nerve at hip and thigh level

S74.90X- Injury of unspecified nerve at hip and thigh level, unspecified leg
S74.91X- Injury of unspecified nerve at hip and thigh level, right leg
S74.92X- Injury of unspecified nerve at hip and thigh level, left leg

S75 Injury of blood vessels at hip and thigh level

Code also:
any associated open wound (S71.-)

EXCLUDES 2 injury of blood vessels at lower leg level (S85.-)
injury of popliteal artery (S85.0)

The appropriate 7th character is to be added to each code from category S75
A initial encounter
D subsequent encounter
S sequela

S75.0 Injury of femoral artery

S75.00 Unspecified injury of femoral artery

S75.001- Unspecified injury of femoral artery, right leg
S75.002- Unspecified injury of femoral artery, left leg
S75.009- Unspecified injury of femoral artery, unspecified leg

S75.01 Minor laceration of femoral artery

Incomplete transection of femoral artery
Laceration of femoral artery NOS
Superficial laceration of femoral artery

Chapter 19
S00-T88

4th digit required 5th digit required 6th digit required 7th digit required 7th digit placeholder + Additional code Laterality

SP 7 **S75.011- Minor laceration of femoral artery, right leg**

SP 7 **S75.012- Minor laceration of femoral artery, left leg**

!Q 7 **S75.019- Minor laceration of femoral artery, unspecified leg**

6 **S75.02 Major laceration of femoral artery**
Complete transection of femoral artery
Traumatic rupture of femoral artery

SP 7 **S75.021- Major laceration of femoral artery, right leg**

SP 7 **S75.022- Major laceration of femoral artery, left leg**

!Q 7 **S75.029- Major laceration of femoral artery, unspecified leg**

6 **S75.09 Other specified injury of femoral artery**

SP 7 **S75.091- Other specified injury of femoral artery, right leg**

SP 7 **S75.092- Other specified injury of femoral artery, left leg**

!Q 7 **S75.099- Other specified injury of femoral artery, unspecified leg**

5 **S75.1 Injury of femoral vein at hip and thigh level**

6 **S75.10 Unspecified injury of femoral vein at hip and thigh level**

!Q 7 **S75.101- Unspecified injury of femoral vein at hip and thigh level, right leg**

!Q 7 **S75.102- Unspecified injury of femoral vein at hip and thigh level, left leg**

!Q 7 **S75.109- Unspecified injury of femoral vein at hip and thigh level, unspecified leg**

6 **S75.11 Minor laceration of femoral vein at hip and thigh level**
Incomplete transection of femoral vein at hip and thigh level
Laceration of femoral vein at hip and thigh level NOS
Superficial laceration of femoral vein at hip and thigh level

SP 7 **S75.111- Minor laceration of femoral vein at hip and thigh level, right leg**

SP 7 **S75.112- Minor laceration of femoral vein at hip and thigh level, left leg**

!Q 7 **S75.119- Minor laceration of femoral vein at hip and thigh level, unspecified leg**

6 **S75.12 Major laceration of femoral vein at hip and thigh level**
Complete transection of femoral vein at hip and thigh level
Traumatic rupture of femoral vein at hip and thigh level

SP 7 **S75.121- Major laceration of femoral vein at hip and thigh level, right leg**

SP 7 **S75.122- Major laceration of femoral vein at hip and thigh level, left leg**

!Q 7 **S75.129- Major laceration of femoral vein at hip and thigh level, unspecified leg**

6 **S75.19 Other specified injury of femoral vein at hip and thigh level**

SP 7 **S75.191- Other specified injury of femoral vein at hip and thigh level, right leg**

SP 7 **S75.192- Other specified injury of femoral vein at hip and thigh level, left leg**

!Q 7 **S75.199- Other specified injury of femoral vein at hip and thigh level, unspecified leg**

5 **S75.2 Injury of greater saphenous vein at hip and thigh level**
EXCLUDES 1 greater saphenous vein NOS (S85.3)

6 **S75.20 Unspecified injury of greater saphenous vein at hip and thigh level**

!Q 7 **S75.201- Unspecified injury of greater saphenous vein at hip and thigh level, right leg**

!Q 7 **S75.202- Unspecified injury of greater saphenous vein at hip and thigh level, left leg**

!Q 7 **S75.209- Unspecified injury of greater saphenous vein at hip and thigh level, unspecified leg**

6 **S75.21 Minor laceration of greater saphenous vein at hip and thigh level**
Incomplete transection of greater saphenous vein at hip and thigh level
Laceration of greater saphenous vein at hip and thigh level NOS
Superficial laceration of greater saphenous vein at hip and thigh level

SP 7 **S75.211- Minor laceration of greater saphenous vein at hip and thigh level, right leg**

SP 7 **S75.212- Minor laceration of greater saphenous vein at hip and thigh level, left leg**

!Q 7 **S75.219- Minor laceration of greater saphenous vein at hip and thigh level, unspecified leg**

6 **S75.22 Major laceration of greater saphenous vein at hip and thigh level**
Complete transection of greater saphenous vein at hip and thigh level
Traumatic rupture of greater saphenous vein at hip and thigh level

SP 7 **S75.221- Major laceration of greater saphenous vein at hip and thigh level, right leg**

SP 7 **S75.222- Major laceration of greater saphenous vein at hip and thigh level, left leg**

!Q 7 **S75.229- Major laceration of greater saphenous vein at hip and thigh level, unspecified leg**

6 **S75.29 Other specified injury of greater saphenous vein at hip and thigh level**

SP 7 **S75.291- Other specified injury of greater saphenous vein at hip and thigh level, right leg**

SP 7 **S75.292- Other specified injury of greater saphenous vein at hip and thigh level, left leg**

Chapter 19

S00-T88

S75.299- Other specified injury of greater saphenous vein at hip and thigh level, unspecified leg

S75.8 Injury of other blood vessels at hip and thigh level

S75.80 Unspecified injury of other blood vessels at hip and thigh level

S75.801- Unspecified injury of other blood vessels at hip and thigh level, right leg

S75.802- Unspecified injury of other blood vessels at hip and thigh level, left leg

S75.809- Unspecified injury of other blood vessels at hip and thigh level, unspecified leg

S75.81 Laceration of other blood vessels at hip and thigh level

S75.811- Laceration of other blood vessels at hip and thigh level, right leg

S75.812- Laceration of other blood vessels at hip and thigh level, left leg

S75.819- Laceration of other blood vessels at hip and thigh level, unspecified leg

S75.89 Other specified injury of other blood vessels at hip and thigh level

S75.891- Other specified injury of other blood vessels at hip and thigh level, right leg

S75.892- Other specified injury of other blood vessels at hip and thigh level, left leg

S75.899- Other specified injury of other blood vessels at hip and thigh level, unspecified leg

S75.9 Injury of unspecified blood vessel at hip and thigh level

S75.90 Unspecified injury of unspecified blood vessel at hip and thigh level

S75.901- Unspecified injury of unspecified blood vessel at hip and thigh level, right leg

S75.902- Unspecified injury of unspecified blood vessel at hip and thigh level, left leg

S75.909- Unspecified injury of unspecified blood vessel at hip and thigh level, unspecified leg

S75.91 Laceration of unspecified blood vessel at hip and thigh level

S75.911- Laceration of unspecified blood vessel at hip and thigh level, right leg

S75.912- Laceration of unspecified blood vessel at hip and thigh level, left leg

S75.919- Laceration of unspecified blood vessel at hip and thigh level, unspecified leg

S75.99 Other specified injury of unspecified blood vessel at hip and thigh level

S75.991- Other specified injury of unspecified blood vessel at hip and thigh level, right leg

S75.992- Other specified injury of unspecified blood vessel at hip and thigh level, left leg

S75.999- Other specified injury of unspecified blood vessel at hip and thigh level, unspecified leg

S76 Injury of muscle, fascia and tendon at hip and thigh level

Code also:

any associated open wound (S71.-)

EXCLUDES 2 injury of muscle, fascia and tendon at lower leg level (S86)

sprain of joint and ligament of hip (S73.1)

The appropriate 7th character is to be added to each code from category S76

A initial encounter

D subsequent encounter

S sequela

S76.0 Injury of muscle, fascia and tendon of hip

S76.00 Unspecified injury of muscle, fascia and tendon of hip

S76.001- Unspecified injury of muscle, fascia and tendon of right hip

S76.002- Unspecified injury of muscle, fascia and tendon of left hip

S76.009- Unspecified injury of muscle, fascia and tendon of unspecified hip

S76.01 Strain of muscle, fascia and tendon of hip

S76.011- Strain of muscle, fascia and tendon of right hip

S76.012- Strain of muscle, fascia and tendon of left hip

S76.019- Strain of muscle, fascia and tendon of unspecified hip

S76.02 Laceration of muscle, fascia and tendon of hip

S76.021- Laceration of muscle, fascia and tendon of right hip

S76.022- Laceration of muscle, fascia and tendon of left hip

S76.029- Laceration of muscle, fascia and tendon of unspecified hip

S76.09 Other specified injury of muscle, fascia and tendon of hip

S76.091- Other specified injury of muscle, fascia and tendon of right hip

S76.092- Other specified injury of muscle, fascia and tendon of left hip

S76.099- Other specified injury of muscle, fascia and tendon of unspecified hip

S76.1 Injury of quadriceps muscle, fascia and tendon

Injury of patellar ligament (tendon)

S76.10 Unspecified injury of quadriceps muscle, fascia and tendon

Chapter 19 S00-T88

4th digit required 5th digit required 6th digit required 7th digit required 7th digit placeholder + Additional code Laterality

S76.101- Unspecified injury of right quadriceps muscle, fascia and tendon
S76.102- Unspecified injury of left quadriceps muscle, fascia and tendon
S76.109- Unspecified injury of unspecified quadriceps muscle, fascia and tendon
S76.11 Strain of quadriceps muscle, fascia and tendon
S76.111- Strain of right quadriceps muscle, fascia and tendon
S76.112- Strain of left quadriceps muscle, fascia and tendon
S76.119- Strain of unspecified quadriceps muscle, fascia and tendon
S76.12 Laceration of quadriceps muscle, fascia and tendon
S76.121- Laceration of right quadriceps muscle, fascia and tendon
S76.122- Laceration of left quadriceps muscle, fascia and tendon
S76.129- Laceration of unspecified quadriceps muscle, fascia and tendon
S76.19 Other specified injury of quadriceps muscle, fascia and tendon
S76.191- Other specified injury of right quadriceps muscle, fascia and tendon
S76.192- Other specified injury of left quadriceps muscle, fascia and tendon
S76.199- Other specified injury of unspecified quadriceps muscle, fascia and tendon
S76.2 Injury of adductor muscle, fascia and tendon of thigh
S76.20 Unspecified injury of adductor muscle, fascia and tendon of thigh
S76.201- Unspecified injury of adductor muscle, fascia and tendon of right thigh
S76.202- Unspecified injury of adductor muscle, fascia and tendon of left thigh
S76.209- Unspecified injury of adductor muscle, fascia and tendon of unspecified thigh
S76.21 Strain of adductor muscle, fascia and tendon of thigh
S76.211- Strain of adductor muscle, fascia and tendon of right thigh
S76.212- Strain of adductor muscle, fascia and tendon of left thigh
S76.219- Strain of adductor muscle, fascia and tendon of unspecified thigh
S76.22 Laceration of adductor muscle, fascia and tendon of thigh
S76.221- Laceration of adductor muscle, fascia and tendon of right thigh
S76.222- Laceration of adductor muscle, fascia and tendon of left thigh
S76.229- Laceration of adductor muscle, fascia and tendon of unspecified thigh
S76.29 Other injury of adductor muscle, fascia and tendon of thigh
S76.291- Other injury of adductor muscle, fascia and tendon of right thigh
S76.292- Other injury of adductor muscle, fascia and tendon of left thigh
S76.299- Other injury of adductor muscle, fascia and tendon of unspecified thigh
S76.3 Injury of muscle, fascia and tendon of the posterior muscle group at thigh level
S76.30 Unspecified injury of muscle, fascia and tendon of the posterior muscle group at thigh level
S76.301- Unspecified injury of muscle, fascia and tendon of the posterior muscle group at thigh level, right thigh
S76.302- Unspecified injury of muscle, fascia and tendon of the posterior muscle group at thigh level, left thigh
S76.309- Unspecified injury of muscle, fascia and tendon of the posterior muscle group at thigh level, unspecified thigh
S76.31 Strain of muscle, fascia and tendon of the posterior muscle group at thigh level
S76.311- Strain of muscle, fascia and tendon of the posterior muscle group at thigh level, right thigh
S76.312- Strain of muscle, fascia and tendon of the posterior muscle group at thigh level, left thigh
S76.319- Strain of muscle, fascia and tendon of the posterior muscle group at thigh level, unspecified thigh
S76.32 Laceration of muscle, fascia and tendon of the posterior muscle group at thigh level
S76.321- Laceration of muscle, fascia and tendon of the posterior muscle group at thigh level, right thigh
S76.322- Laceration of muscle, fascia and tendon of the posterior muscle group at thigh level, left thigh
S76.329- Laceration of muscle, fascia and tendon of the posterior muscle group at thigh level, unspecified thigh
S76.39 Other specified injury of muscle, fascia and tendon of the posterior muscle group at thigh level
S76.391- Other specified injury of muscle, fascia and tendon of the posterior muscle group at thigh level, right thigh
S76.392- Other specified injury of muscle, fascia and tendon of the posterior muscle group at thigh level, left thigh

S76.399- Other specified injury of muscle, fascia and tendon of the posterior muscle group at thigh level, unspecified thigh

S76.8 Injury of other specified muscles, fascia and tendons at thigh level

S76.80 Unspecified injury of other specified muscles, fascia and tendons at thigh level

S76.801- Unspecified injury of other specified muscles, fascia and tendons at thigh level, right thigh

S76.802- Unspecified injury of other specified muscles, fascia and tendons at thigh level, left thigh

S76.809- Unspecified injury of other specified muscles, fascia and tendons at thigh level, unspecified thigh

S76.81 Strain of other specified muscles, fascia and tendons at thigh level

S76.811- Strain of other specified muscles, fascia and tendons at thigh level, right thigh

S76.812- Strain of other specified muscles, fascia and tendons at thigh level, left thigh

S76.819- Strain of other specified muscles, fascia and tendons at thigh level, unspecified thigh

S76.82 Laceration of other specified muscles, fascia and tendons at thigh level

S76.821- Laceration of other specified muscles, fascia and tendons at thigh level, right thigh

S76.822- Laceration of other specified muscles, fascia and tendons at thigh level, left thigh

S76.829- Laceration of other specified muscles, fascia and tendons at thigh level, unspecified thigh

S76.89 Other injury of other specified muscles, fascia and tendons at thigh level

S76.891- Other injury of other specified muscles, fascia and tendons at thigh level, right thigh

S76.892- Other injury of other specified muscles, fascia and tendons at thigh level, left thigh

S76.899- Other injury of other specified muscles, fascia and tendons at thigh level, unspecified thigh

S76.9 Injury of unspecified muscles, fascia and tendons at thigh level

S76.90 Unspecified injury of unspecified muscles, fascia and tendons at thigh level

S76.901- Unspecified injury of unspecified muscles, fascia and tendons at thigh level, right thigh

S76.902- Unspecified injury of unspecified muscles, fascia and tendons at thigh level, left thigh

S76.909- Unspecified injury of unspecified muscles, fascia and tendons at thigh level, unspecified thigh

S76.91 Strain of unspecified muscles, fascia and tendons at thigh level

S76.911- Strain of unspecified muscles, fascia and tendons at thigh level, right thigh

S76.912- Strain of unspecified muscles, fascia and tendons at thigh level, left thigh

S76.919- Strain of unspecified muscles, fascia and tendons at thigh level, unspecified thigh

S76.92 Laceration of unspecified muscles, fascia and tendons at thigh level

S76.921- Laceration of unspecified muscles, fascia and tendons at thigh level, right thigh

S76.922- Laceration of unspecified muscles, fascia and tendons at thigh level, left thigh

S76.929- Laceration of unspecified muscles, fascia and tendons at thigh level, unspecified thigh

S76.99 Other specified injury of unspecified muscles, fascia and tendons at thigh level

S76.991- Other specified injury of unspecified muscles, fascia and tendons at thigh level, right thigh

S76.992- Other specified injury of unspecified muscles, fascia and tendons at thigh level, left thigh

S76.999- Other specified injury of unspecified muscles, fascia and tendons at thigh level, unspecified thigh

S77 Crushing injury of hip and thigh

Use additional code(s) for all associated injuries

EXCLUDES 2 crushing injury of ankle and foot (S97.-)
crushing injury of lower leg (S87.-)

The appropriate 7th character is to be added to each code from category S77
A initial encounter
D subsequent encounter
S sequela

S77.0 Crushing injury of hip

S77.00X- Crushing injury of unspecified hip

S77.01X- Crushing injury of right hip

S77.02X- Crushing injury of left hip

S77.1 Crushing injury of thigh

S77.10X- Crushing injury of unspecified thigh

S77.11X- Crushing injury of right thigh

S77.12X- Crushing injury of left thigh

S77.2 Crushing injury of hip with thigh

Chapter 19 S00-T88

4th digit required 5th digit required 6th digit required 7th digit required 7th digit placeholder +Additional code Laterality

IQ + 7 S77.20X- **Crushing injury of unspecified hip with thigh**

SP + 7 S77.21X- **Crushing injury of right hip with thigh**

SP + 7 S77.22X- **Crushing injury of left hip with thigh**

4 S78 **Traumatic amputation of hip and thigh**

An amputation not identified as partial or complete should be coded to complete

EXCLUDES 1 traumatic amputation of knee (S88.0-)

The appropriate 7th character is to be added to each code from category S78

A initial encounter
D subsequent encounter
S sequela

CODING TIPS ✓ Use these codes only when the amputation was due to trauma. There is no need for adding Z89 with traumatic amputations. See Z47.81 for care of amputations not due to trauma.

5 S78.0 **Traumatic amputation at hip joint**

6 S78.01 **Complete traumatic amputation at hip joint**

SP 7 S78.011- **Complete traumatic amputation at right hip joint**

SP 7 S78.012- **Complete traumatic amputation at left hip joint**

IQ 7 S78.019- **Complete traumatic amputation at unspecified hip joint**

6 S78.02 **Partial traumatic amputation at hip joint**

SP 7 S78.021- **Partial traumatic amputation at right hip joint**

SP 7 S78.022- **Partial traumatic amputation at left hip joint**

IQ 7 S78.029- **Partial traumatic amputation at unspecified hip joint**

5 S78.1 **Traumatic amputation at level between hip and knee**

EXCLUDES 1 traumatic amputation of knee (S88.0-)

6 S78.11 **Complete traumatic amputation at level between hip and knee**

SP 7 S78.111- **Complete traumatic amputation at level between right hip and knee**

SP 7 S78.112- **Complete traumatic amputation at level between left hip and knee**

IQ 7 S78.119- **Complete traumatic amputation at level between unspecified hip and knee**

6 S78.12 **Partial traumatic amputation at level between hip and knee**

SP 7 S78.121- **Partial traumatic amputation at level between right hip and knee**

SP 7 S78.122- **Partial traumatic amputation at level between left hip and knee**

IQ 7 S78.129- **Partial traumatic amputation at level between unspecified hip and knee**

5 S78.9 **Traumatic amputation of hip and thigh, level unspecified**

6 S78.91 **Complete traumatic amputation of hip and thigh, level unspecified**

SP 7 S78.911- **Complete traumatic amputation of right hip and thigh, level unspecified**

SP 7 S78.912- **Complete traumatic amputation of left hip and thigh, level unspecified**

IQ 7 S78.919- **Complete traumatic amputation of unspecified hip and thigh, level unspecified**

6 S78.92 **Partial traumatic amputation of hip and thigh, level unspecified**

SP 7 S78.921- **Partial traumatic amputation of right hip and thigh, level unspecified**

SP 7 S78.922- **Partial traumatic amputation of left hip and thigh, level unspecified**

IQ 7 S78.929- **Partial traumatic amputation of unspecified hip and thigh, level unspecified**

4 S79 **Other and unspecified injuries of hip and thigh**

Note:
A fracture not indicated as open or closed should be coded to closed

The appropriate 7th character is to be added to each code from subcategories S79.0 and S79.1

A initial encounter for closed fracture
D subsequent encounter for fracture with routine healing
G subsequent encounter for fracture with delayed healing
K subsequent encounter for fracture with nonunion
P subsequent encounter for fracture with malunion
S sequela

5 S79.0 **Physeal fracture of upper end of femur**

EXCLUDES 1 apophyseal fracture of upper end of femur (S72.13-)
nontraumatic slipped upper femoral epiphysis (M93.0-)

6 S79.00 **Unspecified physeal fracture of upper end of femur**

SP 7 S79.001- **Unspecified physeal fracture of upper end of right femur**

SP 7 S79.002- **Unspecified physeal fracture of upper end of left femur**

IQ 7 S79.009- **Unspecified physeal fracture of upper end of unspecified femur**

6 S79.01 **Salter-Harris Type I physeal fracture of upper end of femur**

Acute on chronic slipped capital femoral epiphysis (traumatic)
Acute slipped capital femoral epiphysis (traumatic)
Capital femoral epiphyseal fracture

EXCLUDES 1 chronic slipped upper femoral epiphysis (nontraumatic) (M93.02-)

Chapter 19 S00-T88

S79.011- Salter-Harris Type I physeal fracture of upper end of right femur

S79.012- Salter-Harris Type I physeal fracture of upper end of left femur

S79.019- Salter-Harris Type I physeal fracture of upper end of unspecified femur

S79.09 Other physeal fracture of upper end of femur

S79.091- Other physeal fracture of upper end of right femur

S79.092- Other physeal fracture of upper end of left femur

S79.099- Other physeal fracture of upper end of unspecified femur

S79.1 Physeal fracture of lower end of femur

S79.10 Unspecified physeal fracture of lower end of femur

S79.101- Unspecified physeal fracture of lower end of right femur

S79.102- Unspecified physeal fracture of lower end of left femur

S79.109- Unspecified physeal fracture of lower end of unspecified femur

S79.11 Salter-Harris Type I physeal fracture of lower end of femur

S79.111- Salter-Harris Type I physeal fracture of lower end of right femur

S79.112- Salter-Harris Type I physeal fracture of lower end of left femur

S79.119- Salter-Harris Type I physeal fracture of lower end of unspecified femur

S79.12 Salter-Harris Type II physeal fracture of lower end of femur

S79.121- Salter-Harris Type II physeal fracture of lower end of right femur

S79.122- Salter-Harris Type II physeal fracture of lower end of left femur

S79.129- Salter-Harris Type II physeal fracture of lower end of unspecified femur

S79.13 Salter-Harris Type III physeal fracture of lower end of femur

S79.131- Salter-Harris Type III physeal fracture of lower end of right femur

S79.132- Salter-Harris Type III physeal fracture of lower end of left femur

S79.139- Salter-Harris Type III physeal fracture of lower end of unspecified femur

S79.14 Salter-Harris Type IV physeal fracture of lower end of femur

S79.141- Salter-Harris Type IV physeal fracture of lower end of right femur

S79.142- Salter-Harris Type IV physeal fracture of lower end of left femur

S79.149- Salter-Harris Type IV physeal fracture of lower end of unspecified femur

S79.19 Other physeal fracture of lower end of femur

S79.191- Other physeal fracture of lower end of right femur

S79.192- Other physeal fracture of lower end of left femur

S79.199- Other physeal fracture of lower end of unspecified femur

S79.8 Other specified injuries of hip and thigh

The appropriate 7th character is to be added to each code in subcategory S79.8

A	initial encounter
D	subsequent encounter
S	sequela

S79.81 Other specified injuries of hip

S79.811- Other specified injuries of right hip

S79.812- Other specified injuries of left hip

S79.819- Other specified injuries of unspecified hip

S79.82 Other specified injuries of thigh

S79.821- Other specified injuries of right thigh

S79.822- Other specified injuries of left thigh

S79.829- Other specified injuries of unspecified thigh

S79.9 Unspecified injury of hip and thigh

The appropriate 7th character is to be added to each code in subcategory S79.9

A	initial encounter
D	subsequent encounter
S	sequela

S79.91 Unspecified injury of hip

S79.911- Unspecified injury of right hip

S79.912- Unspecified injury of left hip

S79.919- Unspecified injury of unspecified hip

S79.92 Unspecified injury of thigh

S79.921- Unspecified injury of right thigh

S79.922- Unspecified injury of left thigh

S79.929- Unspecified injury of unspecified thigh

Injuries to the knee and lower leg (S80-S89)

EXCLUDES 2 burns and corrosions (T20-T32)
frostbite (T33-T34)
injuries of ankle and foot, except fracture of ankle and malleolus (S90-S99)
insect bite or sting, venomous (T63.4)

GUIDELINES **Section I.C.19.c.2)**

Multiple fractures are sequenced in accordance with the severity of the fracture.

Chapter 19

S00-T88

4th digit required 5th digit required 6th digit required 7th digit required 7th digit placeholder + Additional code Laterality

GUIDELINES **Section I.C.19.b.1)-2)**

When coding injuries, assign separate codes for each injury unless a combination code is provided, in which case the combination code is assigned ... Traumatic injury codes (S00-T14.9) are not to be used for normal, healing surgical wounds or to identify complications of surgical wounds. The code for the most serious injury, as determined by the provider and the focus of treatment, is sequenced first.

1) Superficial injuries such as abrasions or contusions are not coded when associated with more severe injuries of the same site.

2) When a primary injury results in minor damage to peripheral nerves or blood vessels, the primary injury is sequenced first with additional code(s) for injuries to nerves and spinal cord (such as category S04), and/or injury to blood vessels (such as category S15). When the primary injury is to the blood vessels or nerves, that injury should be sequenced first.

GUIDELINES **Section I.C.19.c**

Coding of Traumatic Fractures: The principles of multiple coding of injuries should be followed in coding fractures. Fractures of specified sites are coded individually by site in accordance with both the provisions within categories S02, S12, S22, S32, S42, S49, S52, S59, S62, S72, S79, S82, S89, S92 and the level of detail furnished by medical record content. A fracture not indicated as open or closed should be coded to closed. A fracture not indicated whether displaced or not displaced should be coded to displaced.

CODING TIPS ✓ 7th character A is acceptable in home health and hospice when active treatment is provided, such as antibiotics for an infected wound or a wound vac for a dehisced wound. D is used when the complication or injury is now healing. Think of D as aftercare. S is used for sequela of the injury or complication. Sequela is a residual deficit or condition produced as a result of the injury or complication after the original injury or complication has healed.

4 S80 Superficial injury of knee and lower leg

EXCLUDES 2 superficial injury of ankle and foot (S90.-)

The appropriate 7th character is to be added to each code from category S80
A initial encounter
D subsequent encounter
S sequela

5 S80.0 Contusion of knee

H IQ 7 S80.00X- Contusion of unspecified knee
H IQ 7 S80.01X- Contusion of right knee
H IQ 7 S80.02X- Contusion of left knee

5 S80.1 Contusion of lower leg

H IQ 7 S80.10X- Contusion of unspecified lower leg
H IQ 7 S80.11X- Contusion of right lower leg
H IQ 7 S80.12X- Contusion of left lower leg

5 S80.2 Other superficial injuries of knee

6 S80.21 Abrasion of knee

H IQ 7 S80.211- Abrasion, right knee
H IQ 7 S80.212- Abrasion, left knee
H IQ 7 S80.219- Abrasion, unspecified knee

6 S80.22 Blister (nonthermal) of knee

H IQ 7 S80.221- Blister (nonthermal), right knee
H IQ 7 S80.222- Blister (nonthermal), left knee
H IQ 7 S80.229- Blister (nonthermal), unspecified knee

6 S80.24 External constriction of knee

H IQ 7 S80.241- External constriction, right knee
H IQ 7 S80.242- External constriction, left knee
H IQ 7 S80.249- External constriction, unspecified knee

6 S80.25 Superficial foreign body of knee
Splinter in the knee

H IQ 7 S80.251- Superficial foreign body, right knee
H IQ 7 S80.252- Superficial foreign body, left knee
H IQ 7 S80.259- Superficial foreign body, unspecified knee

6 S80.26 Insect bite (nonvenomous) of knee

H IQ 7 S80.261- Insect bite (nonvenomous), right knee
H IQ 7 S80.262- Insect bite (nonvenomous), left knee
H IQ 7 S80.269- Insect bite (nonvenomous), unspecified knee

6 S80.27 Other superficial bite of knee

EXCLUDES 1 open bite of knee (S81.05-)

H IQ 7 S80.271- Other superficial bite of right knee
H IQ 7 S80.272- Other superficial bite of left knee
H IQ 7 S80.279- Other superficial bite of unspecified knee

5 S80.8 Other superficial injuries of lower leg

6 S80.81 Abrasion of lower leg

H IQ 7 S80.811- Abrasion, right lower leg
H IQ 7 S80.812- Abrasion, left lower leg
H IQ 7 S80.819- Abrasion, unspecified lower leg

6 S80.82 Blister (nonthermal) of lower leg

H IQ 7 S80.821- Blister (nonthermal), right lower leg
H IQ 7 S80.822- Blister (nonthermal), left lower leg
H IQ 7 S80.829- Blister (nonthermal), unspecified lower leg

6 S80.84 External constriction of lower leg

H IQ 7 S80.841- External constriction, right lower leg
H IQ 7 S80.842- External constriction, left lower leg
H IQ 7 S80.849- External constriction, unspecified lower leg

6 S80.85 Superficial foreign body of lower leg
Splinter in the lower leg

H IQ 7 S80.851- Superficial foreign body, right lower leg
H IQ 7 S80.852- Superficial foreign body, left lower leg
H IQ 7 S80.859- Superficial foreign body, unspecified lower leg

6 S80.86 Insect bite (nonvenomous) of lower leg

H IQ 7 S80.861- Insect bite (nonvenomous), right lower leg
H IQ 7 S80.862- Insect bite (nonvenomous), left lower leg

Chapter 19 S00-T88

S80.869- Insect bite (nonvenomous), unspecified lower leg

S80.87 Other superficial bite of lower leg

EXCLUDES 1 open bite of lower leg (S81.85-)

S80.871- Other superficial bite, right lower leg

S80.872- Other superficial bite, left lower leg

S80.879- Other superficial bite, unspecified lower leg

S80.9 Unspecified superficial injury of knee and lower leg

S80.91 Unspecified superficial injury of knee

S80.911- Unspecified superficial injury of right knee

S80.912- Unspecified superficial injury of left knee

S80.919- Unspecified superficial injury of unspecified knee

S80.92 Unspecified superficial injury of lower leg

S80.921- Unspecified superficial injury of right lower leg

S80.922- Unspecified superficial injury of left lower leg

S80.929- Unspecified superficial injury of unspecified lower leg

S81 Open wound of knee and lower leg

Code also:

any associated wound infection

EXCLUDES 1 open fracture of knee and lower leg (S82.-)

traumatic amputation of lower leg (S88.-)

EXCLUDES 2 open wound of ankle and foot (S91.-)

The appropriate 7th character is to be added to each code from category S81

A	initial encounter
D	subsequent encounter
S	sequela

CODING TIPS✓ Open wound codes indicate a wound resulting from a traumatic origin. Do not assign a code for "open wound" unless the etiology of the wound is related to trauma.

CODING TIPS✓ No aftercare code applies, including those indicating dressing changes, drain care, or suture removal. 7th character 'D' is the default for home care and hospice when providing aftercare for a healing or resolving condition; 'A' is used for active treatment such as antibiotics or more than routine wound care; 'S' may be used to indicate a residual condition after the original injury has healed.

S81.0 Open wound of knee

S81.00 Unspecified open wound of knee

S81.001- Unspecified open wound, right knee

S81.002- Unspecified open wound, left knee

S81.009- Unspecified open wound, unspecified knee

S81.01 Laceration without foreign body of knee

S81.011- Laceration without foreign body, right knee

S81.012- Laceration without foreign body, left knee

S81.019- Laceration without foreign body, unspecified knee

S81.02 Laceration with foreign body of knee

S81.021- Laceration with foreign body, right knee

S81.022- Laceration with foreign body, left knee

S81.029- Laceration with foreign body, unspecified knee

S81.03 Puncture wound without foreign body of knee

S81.031- Puncture wound without foreign body, right knee

S81.032- Puncture wound without foreign body, left knee

S81.039- Puncture wound without foreign body, unspecified knee

S81.04 Puncture wound with foreign body of knee

S81.041- Puncture wound with foreign body, right knee

S81.042- Puncture wound with foreign body, left knee

S81.049- Puncture wound with foreign body, unspecified knee

S81.05 Open bite of knee

Bite of knee NOS

EXCLUDES 1 superficial bite of knee (S80.27-)

S81.051- Open bite, right knee

S81.052- Open bite, left knee

S81.059- Open bite, unspecified knee

S81.8 Open wound of lower leg

S81.80 Unspecified open wound of lower leg

S81.801- Unspecified open wound, right lower leg

S81.802- Unspecified open wound, left lower leg

S81.809- Unspecified open wound, unspecified lower leg

S81.81 Laceration without foreign body of lower leg

S81.811- Laceration without foreign body, right lower leg

S81.812- Laceration without foreign body, left lower leg

S81.819- Laceration without foreign body, unspecified lower leg

S81.82 Laceration with foreign body of lower leg

S81.821- Laceration with foreign body, right lower leg

S81.822- Laceration with foreign body, left lower leg

S81.829- Laceration with foreign body, unspecified lower leg

S81.83 Puncture wound without foreign body of lower leg

Chapter 19

S00-T88

SP 7 **S81.831- Puncture wound without foreign body, right lower leg**

SP 7 **S81.832- Puncture wound without foreign body, left lower leg**

IQ 7 **S81.839- Puncture wound without foreign body, unspecified lower leg**

6 **S81.84 Puncture wound with foreign body of lower leg**

SP 7 **S81.841- Puncture wound with foreign body, right lower leg**

SP 7 **S81.842- Puncture wound with foreign body, left lower leg**

IQ 7 **S81.849- Puncture wound with foreign body, unspecified lower leg**

6 **S81.85 Open bite of lower leg**

Bite of lower leg NOS

EXCLUDES 1 superficial bite of lower leg (S80.86-, S80.87-)

SP 7 **S81.851- Open bite, right lower leg**

SP 7 **S81.852- Open bite, left lower leg**

IQ 7 **S81.859- Open bite, unspecified lower leg**

▲ 4 **S82 Fracture of lower leg, including ankle**

Note:

A fracture not indicated as displaced or nondisplaced should be coded to displaced

A fracture not indicated as open or closed should be coded to closed

The open fracture designations are based on the Gustilo open fracture classification

INCLUDES fracture of malleolus

EXCLUDES 1 traumatic amputation of lower leg (S88.-)

EXCLUDES 2 fracture of foot, except ankle (S92.-)

periprosthetic fracture around internal prosthetic implant of knee joint (M97.1-)

The appropriate 7th character is to be added to all codes from category S82

A	initial encounter for closed fracture
B	initial encounter for open fracture type I or II
C	initial encounter for open fracture type IIIA, IIIB, or IIIC
D	subsequent encounter for closed fracture with routine healing
E	subsequent encounter for open fracture type I or II with routine healing
F	subsequent encounter for open fracture type IIIA, IIIB, or IIIC with routine healing
G	subsequent encounter for closed fracture with delayed healing
H	subsequent encounter for open fracture type I or II with delayed healing
J	subsequent encounter for open fracture type IIIA, IIIB, or IIIC with delayed healing
K	subsequent encounter for closed fracture with nonunion
M	subsequent encounter for open fracture type I or II with nonunion
N	subsequent encounter for open fracture type IIIA, IIIB, or IIIC with nonunion
P	subsequent encounter for closed fracture with malunion
Q	subsequent encounter for open fracture type I or II with malunion
R	subsequent encounter for open fracture type IIIA, IIIB, or IIIC with malunion
S	sequela

CODING TIPS ✓ Fractures repaired by joint replacements are NOT coded with Z47.1. Fractures repaired by any other orthopedic surgery are NOT coded with Z47.89. Z codes are not appropriate for fractures of any kind. Code the fracture with 7th character D for fractures undergoing surgical repair.

CODING TIPS ✓ "D" is the 7th character for home care and hospice unless the physician or NPP has documented delayed healing, nonunion or malunion. A sequela is a condition left after the fracture has healed.

CODING TIPS ✓ A fracture not indicated as displaced or nondisplaced should be coded to displaced. A fracture not indicated as open or closed should be coded to closed. The open fracture designations are based on the Gustilo open fracture classification. The 7th characters E, H, M and Q are the default for the Gustilo classification when no information is available. Always query the physician or NPP.

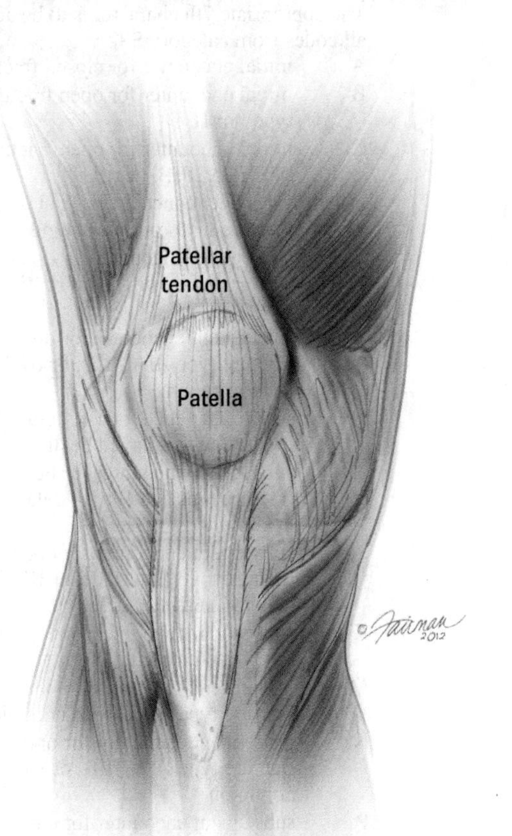

S82.0 Fracture of patella
Knee cap

S82.00 Unspecified fracture of patella

- **S82.001- Unspecified fracture of right patella**
- **S82.002- Unspecified fracture of left patella**
- **S82.009- Unspecified fracture of unspecified patella**

S82.01 Osteochondral fracture of patella

- **S82.011- Displaced osteochondral fracture of right patella**
- **S82.012- Displaced osteochondral fracture of left patella**
- **S82.013- Displaced osteochondral fracture of unspecified patella**
- **S82.014- Nondisplaced osteochondral fracture of right patella**
- **S82.015- Nondisplaced osteochondral fracture of left patella**
- **S82.016- Nondisplaced osteochondral fracture of unspecified patella**

S82.02 Longitudinal fracture of patella

- **S82.021- Displaced longitudinal fracture of right patella**
- **S82.022- Displaced longitudinal fracture of left patella**
- **S82.023- Displaced longitudinal fracture of unspecified patella**
- **S82.024- Nondisplaced longitudinal fracture of right patella**
- **S82.025- Nondisplaced longitudinal fracture of left patella**
- **S82.026- Nondisplaced longitudinal fracture of unspecified patella**

S82.03 Transverse fracture of patella

- **S82.031- Displaced transverse fracture of right patella**
- **S82.032- Displaced transverse fracture of left patella**
- **S82.033- Displaced transverse fracture of unspecified patella**
- **S82.034- Nondisplaced transverse fracture of right patella**
- **S82.035- Nondisplaced transverse fracture of left patella**
- **S82.036- Nondisplaced transverse fracture of unspecified patella**

S82.04 Comminuted fracture of patella

- **S82.041- Displaced comminuted fracture of right patella**
- **S82.042- Displaced comminuted fracture of left patella**
- **S82.043- Displaced comminuted fracture of unspecified patella**
- **S82.044- Nondisplaced comminuted fracture of right patella**
- **S82.045- Nondisplaced comminuted fracture of left patella**
- **S82.046- Nondisplaced comminuted fracture of unspecified patella**

S82.09 Other fracture of patella

- **S82.091- Other fracture of right patella**
- **S82.092- Other fracture of left patella**
- **S82.099- Other fracture of unspecified patella**

S82.1 Fracture of upper end of tibia
Fracture of proximal end of tibia

EXCLUDES 2 fracture of shaft of tibia (S82.2-)
physeal fracture of upper end of tibia (S89.0-)

S82.10 Unspecified fracture of upper end of tibia

- **S82.101- Unspecified fracture of upper end of right tibia**
- **S82.102- Unspecified fracture of upper end of left tibia**
- **S82.109- Unspecified fracture of upper end of unspecified tibia**

S82.11 Fracture of tibial spine

- **S82.111- Displaced fracture of right tibial spine**
- **S82.112- Displaced fracture of left tibial spine**
- **S82.113- Displaced fracture of unspecified tibial spine**
- **S82.114- Nondisplaced fracture of right tibial spine**
- **S82.115- Nondisplaced fracture of left tibial spine**
- **S82.116- Nondisplaced fracture of unspecified tibial spine**

Chapter 19
S00-T88

6 **S82.12 Fracture of lateral condyle of tibia**

- SP 7 **S82.121- Displaced fracture of lateral condyle of right tibia**
- SP 7 **S82.122- Displaced fracture of lateral condyle of left tibia**
- IQ 7 **S82.123- Displaced fracture of lateral condyle of unspecified tibia**
- SP 7 **S82.124- Nondisplaced fracture of lateral condyle of right tibia**
- SP 7 **S82.125- Nondisplaced fracture of lateral condyle of left tibia**
- IQ 7 **S82.126- Nondisplaced fracture of lateral condyle of unspecified tibia**

6 **S82.13 Fracture of medial condyle of tibia**

- SP 7 **S82.131- Displaced fracture of medial condyle of right tibia**
- SP 7 **S82.132- Displaced fracture of medial condyle of left tibia**
- IQ 7 **S82.133- Displaced fracture of medial condyle of unspecified tibia**
- SP 7 **S82.134- Nondisplaced fracture of medial condyle of right tibia**
- SP 7 **S82.135- Nondisplaced fracture of medial condyle of left tibia**
- IQ 7 **S82.136- Nondisplaced fracture of medial condyle of unspecified tibia**

6 **S82.14 Bicondylar fracture of tibia**

Fracture of tibial plateau NOS

- SP 7 **S82.141- Displaced bicondylar fracture of right tibia**
- SP 7 **S82.142- Displaced bicondylar fracture of left tibia**
- IQ 7 **S82.143- Displaced bicondylar fracture of unspecified tibia**
- SP 7 **S82.144- Nondisplaced bicondylar fracture of right tibia**
- SP 7 **S82.145- Nondisplaced bicondylar fracture of left tibia**
- IQ 7 **S82.146- Nondisplaced bicondylar fracture of unspecified tibia**

6 **S82.15 Fracture of tibial tuberosity**

- SP 7 **S82.151- Displaced fracture of right tibial tuberosity**
- SP 7 **S82.152- Displaced fracture of left tibial tuberosity**
- IQ 7 **S82.153- Displaced fracture of unspecified tibial tuberosity**
- SP 7 **S82.154- Nondisplaced fracture of right tibial tuberosity**
- SP 7 **S82.155- Nondisplaced fracture of left tibial tuberosity**
- IQ 7 **S82.156- Nondisplaced fracture of unspecified tibial tuberosity**

6 **S82.16 Torus fracture of upper end of tibia**

The appropriate 7th character is to be added to all codes in subcategory S82.16

A	initial encounter for closed fracture
D	subsequent encounter for fracture with routine healing
G	subsequent encounter for fracture with delayed healing
K	subsequent encounter for fracture with nonunion
P	subsequent encounter for fracture with malunion
S	sequela

CODING TIPS✓ Open fractures do not occur with torus fractures and greenstick fractures, therefore the 7th characters for open fractures are not available.

- SP 7 **S82.161- Torus fracture of upper end of right tibia**
- SP 7 **S82.162- Torus fracture of upper end of left tibia**
- IQ 7 **S82.169- Torus fracture of upper end of unspecified tibia**

6 **S82.19 Other fracture of upper end of tibia**

- SP 7 **S82.191- Other fracture of upper end of right tibia**
- SP 7 **S82.192- Other fracture of upper end of left tibia**
- IQ 7 **S82.199- Other fracture of upper end of unspecified tibia**

5 **S82.2 Fracture of shaft of tibia**

6 **S82.20 Unspecified fracture of shaft of tibia**

Fracture of tibia NOS

- SP 7 **S82.201- Unspecified fracture of shaft of right tibia**
- SP 7 **S82.202- Unspecified fracture of shaft of left tibia**
- IQ 7 **S82.209- Unspecified fracture of shaft of unspecified tibia**

6 **S82.22 Transverse fracture of shaft of tibia**

- SP 7 **S82.221- Displaced transverse fracture of shaft of right tibia**
- SP 7 **S82.222- Displaced transverse fracture of shaft of left tibia**
- IQ 7 **S82.223- Displaced transverse fracture of shaft of unspecified tibia**
- SP 7 **S82.224- Nondisplaced transverse fracture of shaft of right tibia**
- SP 7 **S82.225- Nondisplaced transverse fracture of shaft of left tibia**
- IQ 7 **S82.226- Nondisplaced transverse fracture of shaft of unspecified tibia**

6 **S82.23 Oblique fracture of shaft of tibia**

- SP 7 **S82.231- Displaced oblique fracture of shaft of right tibia**
- SP 7 **S82.232- Displaced oblique fracture of shaft of left tibia**
- IQ 7 **S82.233- Displaced oblique fracture of shaft of unspecified tibia**
- SP 7 **S82.234- Nondisplaced oblique fracture of shaft of right tibia**

Chapter 19

S00-T88

⊟ SP 7 S82.235- **Nondisplaced oblique fracture of shaft of left tibia**

⊟ !Q 7 S82.236- **Nondisplaced oblique fracture of shaft of unspecified tibia**

6 S82.24 **Spiral fracture of shaft of tibia**
Toddler fracture

⊟ SP 7 S82.241- **Displaced spiral fracture of shaft of right tibia**

⊟ SP 7 S82.242- **Displaced spiral fracture of shaft of left tibia**

⊟ !Q 7 S82.243- **Displaced spiral fracture of shaft of unspecified tibia**

⊟ SP 7 S82.244- **Nondisplaced spiral fracture of shaft of right tibia**

⊟ SP 7 S82.245- **Nondisplaced spiral fracture of shaft of left tibia**

⊟ !Q 7 S82.246- **Nondisplaced spiral fracture of shaft of unspecified tibia**

6 S82.25 **Comminuted fracture of shaft of tibia**

⊟ SP 7 S82.251- **Displaced comminuted fracture of shaft of right tibia**

⊟ SP 7 S82.252- **Displaced comminuted fracture of shaft of left tibia**

⊟ !Q 7 S82.253- **Displaced comminuted fracture of shaft of unspecified tibia**

⊟ SP 7 S82.254- **Nondisplaced comminuted fracture of shaft of right tibia**

⊟ SP 7 S82.255- **Nondisplaced comminuted fracture of shaft of left tibia**

⊟ !Q 7 S82.256- **Nondisplaced comminuted fracture of shaft of unspecified tibia**

6 S82.26 **Segmental fracture of shaft of tibia**

⊟ SP 7 S82.261- **Displaced segmental fracture of shaft of right tibia**

⊟ SP 7 S82.262- **Displaced segmental fracture of shaft of left tibia**

⊟ !Q 7 S82.263- **Displaced segmental fracture of shaft of unspecified tibia**

⊟ SP 7 S82.264- **Nondisplaced segmental fracture of shaft of right tibia**

⊟ SP 7 S82.265- **Nondisplaced segmental fracture of shaft of left tibia**

⊟ !Q 7 S82.266- **Nondisplaced segmental fracture of shaft of unspecified tibia**

6 S82.29 **Other fracture of shaft of tibia**

⊟ SP 7 S82.291- **Other fracture of shaft of right tibia**

⊟ SP 7 S82.292- **Other fracture of shaft of left tibia**

⊟ !Q 7 S82.299- **Other fracture of shaft of unspecified tibia**

5 S82.3 **Fracture of lower end of tibia**

EXCLUDES 1 bimalleolar fracture of lower leg (S82.84-)
fracture of medial malleolus alone (S82.5-)
Maisonneuve's fracture (S82.86-)
pilon fracture of distal tibia (S82.87-)
trimalleolar fractures of lower leg (S82.85-)

6 S82.30 **Unspecified fracture of lower end of tibia**

⊟ SP 7 S82.301- **Unspecified fracture of lower end of right tibia**

⊟ SP 7 S82.302- **Unspecified fracture of lower end of left tibia**

⊟ !Q 7 S82.309- **Unspecified fracture of lower end of unspecified tibia**

6 S82.31 **Torus fracture of lower end of tibia**

The appropriate 7th character is to be added to all codes in subcategory S82.31

A	initial encounter for closed fracture
D	subsequent encounter for fracture with routine healing
G	subsequent encounter for fracture with delayed healing
K	subsequent encounter for fracture with nonunion
P	subsequent encounter for fracture with malunion
S	sequela

CODING TIPS ✓ Open fractures do not occur with torus fractures and greenstick fractures, therefore the 7th characters for open fractures are not available.

⊟ SP 7 S82.311- **Torus fracture of lower end of right tibia**

⊟ SP 7 S82.312- **Torus fracture of lower end of left tibia**

⊟ !Q 7 S82.319- **Torus fracture of lower end of unspecified tibia**

6 S82.39 **Other fracture of lower end of tibia**

⊟ SP 7 S82.391- **Other fracture of lower end of right tibia**

⊟ SP 7 S82.392- **Other fracture of lower end of left tibia**

⊟ !Q 7 S82.399- **Other fracture of lower end of unspecified tibia**

5 S82.4 **Fracture of shaft of fibula**

EXCLUDES 2 fracture of lateral malleolus alone (S82.6-)

6 S82.40 **Unspecified fracture of shaft of fibula**

⊟ SP 7 S82.401- **Unspecified fracture of shaft of right fibula**

⊟ SP 7 S82.402- **Unspecified fracture of shaft of left fibula**

⊟ !Q 7 S82.409- **Unspecified fracture of shaft of unspecified fibula**

6 S82.42 **Transverse fracture of shaft of fibula**

⊟ SP 7 S82.421- **Displaced transverse fracture of shaft of right fibula**

⊟ SP 7 S82.422- **Displaced transverse fracture of shaft of left fibula**

⊟ !Q 7 S82.423- **Displaced transverse fracture of shaft of unspecified fibula**

⊟ SP 7 S82.424- **Nondisplaced transverse fracture of shaft of right fibula**

⊟ SP 7 S82.425- **Nondisplaced transverse fracture of shaft of left fibula**

Chapter 19
S00-T88

IQ 7 S82.426- Nondisplaced transverse fracture of shaft of unspecified fibula

6 S82.43 Oblique fracture of shaft of fibula

SP 7 S82.431- Displaced oblique fracture of shaft of right fibula

SP 7 S82.432- Displaced oblique fracture of shaft of left fibula

IQ 7 S82.433- Displaced oblique fracture of shaft of unspecified fibula

SP 7 S82.434- Nondisplaced oblique fracture of shaft of right fibula

SP 7 S82.435- Nondisplaced oblique fracture of shaft of left fibula

IQ 7 S82.436- Nondisplaced oblique fracture of shaft of unspecified fibula

6 S82.44 Spiral fracture of shaft of fibula

SP 7 S82.441- Displaced spiral fracture of shaft of right fibula

SP IQ 7 S82.442- Displaced spiral fracture of shaft of left fibula

IQ 7 S82.443- Displaced spiral fracture of shaft of unspecified fibula

SP 7 S82.444- Nondisplaced spiral fracture of shaft of right fibula

SP 7 S82.445- Nondisplaced spiral fracture of shaft of left fibula

SP IQ 7 S82.446- Nondisplaced spiral fracture of shaft of unspecified fibula

6 S82.45 Comminuted fracture of shaft of fibula

SP 7 S82.451- Displaced comminuted fracture of shaft of right fibula

SP 7 S82.452- Displaced comminuted fracture of shaft of left fibula

IQ 7 S82.453- Displaced comminuted fracture of shaft of unspecified fibula

SP 7 S82.454- Nondisplaced comminuted fracture of shaft of right fibula

SP 7 S82.455- Nondisplaced comminuted fracture of shaft of left fibula

IQ 7 S82.456- Nondisplaced comminuted fracture of shaft of unspecified fibula

6 S82.46 Segmental fracture of shaft of fibula

SP 7 S82.461- Displaced segmental fracture of shaft of right fibula

SP 7 S82.462- Displaced segmental fracture of shaft of left fibula

IQ 7 S82.463- Displaced segmental fracture of shaft of unspecified fibula

SP 7 S82.464- Nondisplaced segmental fracture of shaft of right fibula

SP 7 S82.465- Nondisplaced segmental fracture of shaft of left fibula

IQ 7 S82.466- Nondisplaced segmental fracture of shaft of unspecified fibula

6 S82.49 Other fracture of shaft of fibula

SP 7 S82.491- Other fracture of shaft of right fibula

SP 7 S82.492- Other fracture of shaft of left fibula

IQ 7 S82.499- Other fracture of shaft of unspecified fibula

5 S82.5 Fracture of medial malleolus

EXCLUDES 1 pilon fracture of distal tibia (S82.87-)
Salter-Harris type III of lower end of tibia (S89.13-)
Salter-Harris type IV of lower end of tibia (S89.14-)

SP 7 S82.51X- Displaced fracture of medial malleolus of right tibia

SP 7 S82.52X- Displaced fracture of medial malleolus of left tibia

IQ 7 S82.53X- Displaced fracture of medial malleolus of unspecified tibia

SP 7 S82.54X- Nondisplaced fracture of medial malleolus of right tibia

SP 7 S82.55X- Nondisplaced fracture of medial malleolus of left tibia

IQ 7 S82.56X- Nondisplaced fracture of medial malleolus of unspecified tibia

5 S82.6 Fracture of lateral malleolus

EXCLUDES 1 pilon fracture of distal tibia (S82.87-)

SP 7 S82.61X- Displaced fracture of lateral malleolus of right fibula

SP 7 S82.62X- Displaced fracture of lateral malleolus of left fibula

IQ 7 S82.63X- Displaced fracture of lateral malleolus of unspecified fibula

SP 7 S82.64X- Nondisplaced fracture of lateral malleolus of right fibula

SP 7 S82.65X- Nondisplaced fracture of lateral malleolus of left fibula

IQ 7 S82.66X- Nondisplaced fracture of lateral malleolus of unspecified fibula

5 S82.8 Other fractures of lower leg

6 S82.81 Torus fracture of upper end of fibula

The appropriate 7th character is to be added to all codes in subcategory S82.81

A	initial encounter for closed fracture
D	subsequent encounter for fracture with routine healing
G	subsequent encounter for fracture with delayed healing
K	subsequent encounter for fracture with nonunion
P	subsequent encounter for fracture with malunion
S	sequela

CODING TIPS ✓ Open fractures do not occur with torus fractures and greenstick fractures, therefore the 7th characters for open fractures are not available.

SP 7 S82.811- Torus fracture of upper end of right fibula

SP 7 S82.812- Torus fracture of upper end of left fibula

IQ 7 S82.819- Torus fracture of upper end of unspecified fibula

6 S82.82 Torus fracture of lower end of fibula

Chapter 19

S00-T88

The appropriate 7th character is to be added to all codes in subcategory S82.82

A initial encounter for closed fracture
D subsequent encounter for fracture with routine healing
G subsequent encounter for fracture with delayed healing
K subsequent encounter for fracture with nonunion
P subsequent encounter for fracture with malunion
S sequela

CODING TIPS✓ Open fractures do not occur with torus fractures and greenstick fractures, therefore the 7th characters for open fractures are not available.

S82.821- Torus fracture of lower end of right fibula
S82.822- Torus fracture of lower end of left fibula
S82.829- Torus fracture of lower end of unspecified fibula

S82.83 Other fracture of upper and lower end of fibula
S82.831- Other fracture of upper and lower end of right fibula
S82.832- Other fracture of upper and lower end of left fibula
S82.839- Other fracture of upper and lower end of unspecified fibula

S82.84 Bimalleolar fracture of lower leg
S82.841- Displaced bimalleolar fracture of right lower leg
S82.842- Displaced bimalleolar fracture of left lower leg
S82.843- Displaced bimalleolar fracture of unspecified lower leg
S82.844- Nondisplaced bimalleolar fracture of right lower leg
S82.845- Nondisplaced bimalleolar fracture of left lower leg
S82.846- Nondisplaced bimalleolar fracture of unspecified lower leg

S82.85 Trimalleolar fracture of lower leg
S82.851- Displaced trimalleolar fracture of right lower leg
S82.852- Displaced trimalleolar fracture of left lower leg
S82.853- Displaced trimalleolar fracture of unspecified lower leg
S82.854- Nondisplaced trimalleolar fracture of right lower leg
S82.855- Nondisplaced trimalleolar fracture of left lower leg
S82.856- Nondisplaced trimalleolar fracture of unspecified lower leg

S82.86 Maisonneuve's fracture
S82.861- Displaced Maisonneuve's fracture of right leg
S82.862- Displaced Maisonneuve's fracture of left leg
S82.863- Displaced Maisonneuve's fracture of unspecified leg
S82.864- Nondisplaced Maisonneuve's fracture of right leg
S82.865- Nondisplaced Maisonneuve's fracture of left leg
S82.866- Nondisplaced Maisonneuve's fracture of unspecified leg

S82.87 Pilon fracture of tibia
S82.871- Displaced pilon fracture of right tibia
S82.872- Displaced pilon fracture of left tibia
S82.873- Displaced pilon fracture of unspecified tibia
S82.874- Nondisplaced pilon fracture of right tibia
S82.875- Nondisplaced pilon fracture of left tibia
S82.876- Nondisplaced pilon fracture of unspecified tibia

S82.89 Other fractures of lower leg
Fracture of ankle NOS
S82.891- Other fracture of right lower leg
S82.892- Other fracture of left lower leg
S82.899- Other fracture of unspecified lower leg

S82.9 Unspecified fracture of lower leg
S82.90X- Unspecified fracture of unspecified lower leg
S82.91X- Unspecified fracture of right lower leg
S82.92X- Unspecified fracture of left lower leg

S83 Dislocation and sprain of joints and ligaments of knee

INCLUDES
- avulsion of joint or ligament of knee
- laceration of cartilage, joint or ligament of knee
- sprain of cartilage, joint or ligament of knee
- traumatic hemarthrosis of joint or ligament of knee
- traumatic rupture of joint or ligament of knee
- traumatic subluxation of joint or ligament of knee
- traumatic tear of joint or ligament of knee

Code also:
any associated open wound

EXCLUDES 2
- derangement of patella (M22.0-M22.3)
- injury of patellar ligament (tendon) (S76.1-)
- internal derangement of knee (M23.-)
- old dislocation of knee (M24.36)
- pathological dislocation of knee (M24.36)
- recurrent dislocation of knee (M22.0)
- strain of muscle, fascia and tendon of lower leg (S86.-)

Chapter 19 S00-T88

4th digit required 5th digit required 6th digit required 7th digit required 7th digit placeholder +Additional code Laterality

The appropriate 7th character is to be added to each code from category S83
A initial encounter
D subsequent encounter
S sequela

5 **S83.0 Subluxation and dislocation of patella**

6 **S83.00 Unspecified subluxation and dislocation of patella**

- H IQ 7 **S83.001- Unspecified subluxation of right patella**
- H IQ 7 **S83.002- Unspecified subluxation of left patella**
- H IQ 7 **S83.003- Unspecified subluxation of unspecified patella**
- H IQ 7 **S83.004- Unspecified dislocation of right patella**
- H IQ 7 **S83.005- Unspecified dislocation of left patella**
- H IQ 7 **S83.006- Unspecified dislocation of unspecified patella**

6 **S83.01 Lateral subluxation and dislocation of patella**

- H SP 7 **S83.011- Lateral subluxation of right patella**
- H SP 7 **S83.012- Lateral subluxation of left patella**
- H IQ 7 **S83.013- Lateral subluxation of unspecified patella**
- H SP 7 **S83.014- Lateral dislocation of right patella**
- H SP 7 **S83.015- Lateral dislocation of left patella**
- H IQ 7 **S83.016- Lateral dislocation of unspecified patella**

6 **S83.09 Other subluxation and dislocation of patella**

- H SP 7 **S83.091- Other subluxation of right patella**
- H SP 7 **S83.092- Other subluxation of left patella**
- H IQ 7 **S83.093- Other subluxation of unspecified patella**
- H SP 7 **S83.094- Other dislocation of right patella**
- H SP 7 **S83.095- Other dislocation of left patella**
- H IQ 7 **S83.096- Other dislocation of unspecified patella**

5 **S83.1 Subluxation and dislocation of knee**

EXCLUDES 2 instability of knee prosthesis (T84.022, T84.023)

6 **S83.10 Unspecified subluxation and dislocation of knee**

- H IQ 7 **S83.101- Unspecified subluxation of right knee**
- H IQ 7 **S83.102- Unspecified subluxation of left knee**
- H IQ 7 **S83.103- Unspecified subluxation of unspecified knee**
- H IQ 7 **S83.104- Unspecified dislocation of right knee**
- H IQ 7 **S83.105- Unspecified dislocation of left knee**
- H IQ 7 **S83.106- Unspecified dislocation of unspecified knee**

6 **S83.11 Anterior subluxation and dislocation of proximal end of tibia**

Posterior subluxation and dislocation of distal end of femur

- H SP 7 **S83.111- Anterior subluxation of proximal end of tibia, right knee**
- H SP 7 **S83.112- Anterior subluxation of proximal end of tibia, left knee**
- H IQ 7 **S83.113- Anterior subluxation of proximal end of tibia, unspecified knee**
- H SP 7 **S83.114- Anterior dislocation of proximal end of tibia, right knee**
- H SP 7 **S83.115- Anterior dislocation of proximal end of tibia, left knee**
- H IQ 7 **S83.116- Anterior dislocation of proximal end of tibia, unspecified knee**

6 **S83.12 Posterior subluxation and dislocation of proximal end of tibia**

Anterior dislocation of distal end of femur

- H SP 7 **S83.121- Posterior subluxation of proximal end of tibia, right knee**
- H SP 7 **S83.122- Posterior subluxation of proximal end of tibia, left knee**
- H IQ 7 **S83.123- Posterior subluxation of proximal end of tibia, unspecified knee**
- H SP 7 **S83.124- Posterior dislocation of proximal end of tibia, right knee**
- H SP 7 **S83.125- Posterior dislocation of proximal end of tibia, left knee**
- H IQ 7 **S83.126- Posterior dislocation of proximal end of tibia, unspecified knee**

6 **S83.13 Medial subluxation and dislocation of proximal end of tibia**

- H SP 7 **S83.131- Medial subluxation of proximal end of tibia, right knee**
- H SP 7 **S83.132- Medial subluxation of proximal end of tibia, left knee**
- H IQ 7 **S83.133- Medial subluxation of proximal end of tibia, unspecified knee**
- H SP 7 **S83.134- Medial dislocation of proximal end of tibia, right knee**
- H SP 7 **S83.135- Medial dislocation of proximal end of tibia, left knee**
- H IQ 7 **S83.136- Medial dislocation of proximal end of tibia, unspecified knee**

6 **S83.14 Lateral subluxation and dislocation of proximal end of tibia**

- H SP 7 **S83.141- Lateral subluxation of proximal end of tibia, right knee**
- H SP 7 **S83.142- Lateral subluxation of proximal end of tibia, left knee**
- H IQ 7 **S83.143- Lateral subluxation of proximal end of tibia, unspecified knee**
- H SP 7 **S83.144- Lateral dislocation of proximal end of tibia, right knee**
- H SP 7 **S83.145- Lateral dislocation of proximal end of tibia, left knee**
- H IQ 7 **S83.146- Lateral dislocation of proximal end of tibia, unspecified knee**

6 **S83.19 Other subluxation and dislocation of knee**

- H SP 7 **S83.191- Other subluxation of right knee**
- H SP 7 **S83.192- Other subluxation of left knee**

Chapter 19

S00-T88

S83.193- Other subluxation of unspecified knee
S83.194- Other dislocation of right knee
S83.195- Other dislocation of left knee
S83.196- Other dislocation of unspecified knee

S83.2 Tear of meniscus, current injury
EXCLUDES 1 old bucket-handle tear (M23.2)

S83.20 Tear of unspecified meniscus, current injury
Tear of meniscus of knee NOS
S83.200- Bucket-handle tear of unspecified meniscus, current injury, right knee
S83.201- Bucket-handle tear of unspecified meniscus, current injury, left knee
S83.202- Bucket-handle tear of unspecified meniscus, current injury, unspecified knee
S83.203- Other tear of unspecified meniscus, current injury, right knee
S83.204- Other tear of unspecified meniscus, current injury, left knee
S83.205- Other tear of unspecified meniscus, current injury, unspecified knee
S83.206- Unspecified tear of unspecified meniscus, current injury, right knee
S83.207- Unspecified tear of unspecified meniscus, current injury, left knee
S83.209- Unspecified tear of unspecified meniscus, current injury, unspecified knee

S83.21 Bucket-handle tear of medial meniscus, current injury
S83.211- Bucket-handle tear of medial meniscus, current injury, right knee
S83.212- Bucket-handle tear of medial meniscus, current injury, left knee
S83.219- Bucket-handle tear of medial meniscus, current injury, unspecified knee

S83.22 Peripheral tear of medial meniscus, current injury
S83.221- Peripheral tear of medial meniscus, current injury, right knee
S83.222- Peripheral tear of medial meniscus, current injury, left knee
S83.229- Peripheral tear of medial meniscus, current injury, unspecified knee

S83.23 Complex tear of medial meniscus, current injury
S83.231- Complex tear of medial meniscus, current injury, right knee
S83.232- Complex tear of medial meniscus, current injury, left knee
S83.239- Complex tear of medial meniscus, current injury, unspecified knee

S83.24 Other tear of medial meniscus, current injury
S83.241- Other tear of medial meniscus, current injury, right knee
S83.242- Other tear of medial meniscus, current injury, left knee
S83.249- Other tear of medial meniscus, current injury, unspecified knee

S83.25 Bucket-handle tear of lateral meniscus, current injury
S83.251- Bucket-handle tear of lateral meniscus, current injury, right knee
S83.252- Bucket-handle tear of lateral meniscus, current injury, left knee
S83.259- Bucket-handle tear of lateral meniscus, current injury, unspecified knee

S83.26 Peripheral tear of lateral meniscus, current injury
S83.261- Peripheral tear of lateral meniscus, current injury, right knee
S83.262- Peripheral tear of lateral meniscus, current injury, left knee
S83.269- Peripheral tear of lateral meniscus, current injury, unspecified knee

S83.27 Complex tear of lateral meniscus, current injury
S83.271- Complex tear of lateral meniscus, current injury, right knee
S83.272- Complex tear of lateral meniscus, current injury, left knee
S83.279- Complex tear of lateral meniscus, current injury, unspecified knee

S83.28 Other tear of lateral meniscus, current injury
S83.281- Other tear of lateral meniscus, current injury, right knee
S83.282- Other tear of lateral meniscus, current injury, left knee
S83.289- Other tear of lateral meniscus, current injury, unspecified knee

S83.3 Tear of articular cartilage of knee, current
S83.30X- Tear of articular cartilage of unspecified knee, current
S83.31X- Tear of articular cartilage of right knee, current
S83.32X- Tear of articular cartilage of left knee, current

S83.4 Sprain of collateral ligament of knee
S83.40 Sprain of unspecified collateral ligament of knee

Chapter 19
S00-T88

4th digit required | 5th digit required | 6th digit required | 7th digit required | 7th digit placeholder | + Additional code | Laterality

SP 7 **S83.401- Sprain of unspecified collateral ligament of right knee**

SP 7 **S83.402- Sprain of unspecified collateral ligament of left knee**

IQ 7 **S83.409- Sprain of unspecified collateral ligament of unspecified knee**

6 **S83.41 Sprain of medial collateral ligament of knee**
Sprain of tibial collateral ligament

SP 7 **S83.411- Sprain of medial collateral ligament of right knee**

SP 7 **S83.412- Sprain of medial collateral ligament of left knee**

IQ 7 **S83.419- Sprain of medial collateral ligament of unspecified knee**

6 **S83.42 Sprain of lateral collateral ligament of knee**
Sprain of fibular collateral ligament

SP 7 **S83.421- Sprain of lateral collateral ligament of right knee**

SP 7 **S83.422- Sprain of lateral collateral ligament of left knee**

IQ 7 **S83.429- Sprain of lateral collateral ligament of unspecified knee**

5 **S83.5 Sprain of cruciate ligament of knee**

6 **S83.50 Sprain of unspecified cruciate ligament of knee**

SP 7 **S83.501- Sprain of unspecified cruciate ligament of right knee**

SP 7 **S83.502- Sprain of unspecified cruciate ligament of left knee**

IQ 7 **S83.509- Sprain of unspecified cruciate ligament of unspecified knee**

6 **S83.51 Sprain of anterior cruciate ligament of knee**

SP 7 **S83.511- Sprain of anterior cruciate ligament of right knee**

SP 7 **S83.512- Sprain of anterior cruciate ligament of left knee**

IQ 7 **S83.519- Sprain of anterior cruciate ligament of unspecified knee**

6 **S83.52 Sprain of posterior cruciate ligament of knee**

SP 7 **S83.521- Sprain of posterior cruciate ligament of right knee**

SP 7 **S83.522- Sprain of posterior cruciate ligament of left knee**

IQ 7 **S83.529- Sprain of posterior cruciate ligament of unspecified knee**

5 **S83.6 Sprain of the superior tibiofibular joint and ligament**

IQ 7 **S83.60X- Sprain of the superior tibiofibular joint and ligament, unspecified knee**

SP 7 **S83.61X- Sprain of the superior tibiofibular joint and ligament, right knee**

SP 7 **S83.62X- Sprain of the superior tibiofibular joint and ligament, left knee**

5 **S83.8 Sprain of other specified parts of knee**

6 **S83.8X Sprain of other specified parts of knee**

SP 7 **S83.8X1- Sprain of other specified parts of right knee**

SP 7 **S83.8X2- Sprain of other specified parts of left knee**

IQ 7 **S83.8X9- Sprain of other specified parts of unspecified knee**

5 **S83.9 Sprain of unspecified site of knee**

IQ 7 **S83.90X- Sprain of unspecified site of unspecified knee**

SP 7 **S83.91X- Sprain of unspecified site of right knee**

SP 7 **S83.92X- Sprain of unspecified site of left knee**

4 **S84 Injury of nerves at lower leg level**
Code also:
any associated open wound (S81.-)
EXCLUDES 2 injury of nerves at ankle and foot level (S94.-)

The appropriate 7th character is to be added to each code from category S84
A initial encounter
D subsequent encounter
S sequela

5 **S84.0 Injury of tibial nerve at lower leg level**

IQ 7 **S84.00X- Injury of tibial nerve at lower leg level, unspecified leg**

SP 7 **S84.01X- Injury of tibial nerve at lower leg level, right leg**

SP 7 **S84.02X- Injury of tibial nerve at lower leg level, left leg**

5 **S84.1 Injury of peroneal nerve at lower leg level**

IQ 7 **S84.10X- Injury of peroneal nerve at lower leg level, unspecified leg**

SP 7 **S84.11X- Injury of peroneal nerve at lower leg level, right leg**

SP 7 **S84.12X- Injury of peroneal nerve at lower leg level, left leg**

5 **S84.2 Injury of cutaneous sensory nerve at lower leg level**

IQ 7 **S84.20X- Injury of cutaneous sensory nerve at lower leg level, unspecified leg**

SP 7 **S84.21X- Injury of cutaneous sensory nerve at lower leg level, right leg**

SP 7 **S84.22X- Injury of cutaneous sensory nerve at lower leg level, left leg**

5 **S84.8 Injury of other nerves at lower leg level**

6 **S84.80 Injury of other nerves at lower leg level**

SP 7 **S84.801- Injury of other nerves at lower leg level, right leg**

SP 7 **S84.802- Injury of other nerves at lower leg level, left leg**

IQ 7 **S84.809- Injury of other nerves at lower leg level, unspecified leg**

5 **S84.9 Injury of unspecified nerve at lower leg level**

IQ 7 **S84.90X- Injury of unspecified nerve at lower leg level, unspecified leg**

IQ 7 **S84.91X- Injury of unspecified nerve at lower leg level, right leg**

IQ 7 **S84.92X- Injury of unspecified nerve at lower leg level, left leg**

4 **S85 Injury of blood vessels at lower leg level**
Code also:
any associated open wound (S81.-)
EXCLUDES 2 injury of blood vessels at ankle and foot level (S95.-)

Chapter 19 S00-T88

The appropriate 7th character is to be added to each code from category S85
A initial encounter
D subsequent encounter
S sequela

S85.0 Injury of popliteal artery
S85.00 Unspecified injury of popliteal artery
IQ S85.001- Unspecified injury of popliteal artery, right leg
IQ S85.002- Unspecified injury of popliteal artery, left leg
IQ S85.009- Unspecified injury of popliteal artery, unspecified leg
S85.01 Laceration of popliteal artery
SP S85.011- Laceration of popliteal artery, right leg
SP S85.012- Laceration of popliteal artery, left leg
IQ S85.019- Laceration of popliteal artery, unspecified leg
S85.09 Other specified injury of popliteal artery
SP S85.091- Other specified injury of popliteal artery, right leg
SP S85.092- Other specified injury of popliteal artery, left leg
IQ S85.099- Other specified injury of popliteal artery, unspecified leg
S85.1 Injury of tibial artery
S85.10 Unspecified injury of unspecified tibial artery
Injury of tibial artery NOS
IQ S85.101- Unspecified injury of unspecified tibial artery, right leg
IQ S85.102- Unspecified injury of unspecified tibial artery, left leg
IQ S85.109- Unspecified injury of unspecified tibial artery, unspecified leg
S85.11 Laceration of unspecified tibial artery
SP S85.111- Laceration of unspecified tibial artery, right leg
SP S85.112- Laceration of unspecified tibial artery, left leg
IQ S85.119- Laceration of unspecified tibial artery, unspecified leg
S85.12 Other specified injury of unspecified tibial artery
SP S85.121- Other specified injury of unspecified tibial artery, right leg
SP S85.122- Other specified injury of unspecified tibial artery, left leg
IQ S85.129- Other specified injury of unspecified tibial artery, unspecified leg
S85.13 Unspecified injury of anterior tibial artery
IQ S85.131- Unspecified injury of anterior tibial artery, right leg
IQ S85.132- Unspecified injury of anterior tibial artery, left leg
SP IQ S85.139- Unspecified injury of anterior tibial artery, unspecified leg
S85.14 Laceration of anterior tibial artery
SP S85.141- Laceration of anterior tibial artery, right leg
SP S85.142- Laceration of anterior tibial artery, left leg
IQ S85.149- Laceration of anterior tibial artery, unspecified leg
S85.15 Other specified injury of anterior tibial artery
SP S85.151- Other specified injury of anterior tibial artery, right leg
SP S85.152- Other specified injury of anterior tibial artery, left leg
IQ S85.159- Other specified injury of anterior tibial artery, unspecified leg
S85.16 Unspecified injury of posterior tibial artery
IQ S85.161- Unspecified injury of posterior tibial artery, right leg
IQ S85.162- Unspecified injury of posterior tibial artery, left leg
IQ S85.169- Unspecified injury of posterior tibial artery, unspecified leg
S85.17 Laceration of posterior tibial artery
SP S85.171- Laceration of posterior tibial artery, right leg
SP S85.172- Laceration of posterior tibial artery, left leg
IQ S85.179- Laceration of posterior tibial artery, unspecified leg
S85.18 Other specified injury of posterior tibial artery
SP S85.181- Other specified injury of posterior tibial artery, right leg
SP S85.182- Other specified injury of posterior tibial artery, left leg
IQ S85.189- Other specified injury of posterior tibial artery, unspecified leg
S85.2 Injury of peroneal artery
S85.20 Unspecified injury of peroneal artery
IQ S85.201- Unspecified injury of peroneal artery, right leg
IQ S85.202- Unspecified injury of peroneal artery, left leg
IQ S85.209- Unspecified injury of peroneal artery, unspecified leg
S85.21 Laceration of peroneal artery
SP S85.211- Laceration of peroneal artery, right leg
SP S85.212- Laceration of peroneal artery, left leg
IQ S85.219- Laceration of peroneal artery, unspecified leg
S85.29 Other specified injury of peroneal artery
SP S85.291- Other specified injury of peroneal artery, right leg

Chapter 19
S00-T88

SP 7 S85.292- Other specified injury of peroneal artery, left leg

IQ 7 S85.299- Other specified injury of peroneal artery, unspecified leg

5 S85.3 Injury of greater saphenous vein at lower leg level
Injury of greater saphenous vein NOS
Injury of saphenous vein NOS

6 S85.30 Unspecified injury of greater saphenous vein at lower leg level

IQ 7 S85.301- Unspecified injury of greater saphenous vein at lower leg level, right leg

IQ 7 S85.302- Unspecified injury of greater saphenous vein at lower leg level, left leg

IQ 7 S85.309- Unspecified injury of greater saphenous vein at lower leg level, unspecified leg

6 S85.31 Laceration of greater saphenous vein at lower leg level

SP 7 S85.311- Laceration of greater saphenous vein at lower leg level, right leg

SP 7 S85.312- Laceration of greater saphenous vein at lower leg level, left leg

IQ 7 S85.319- Laceration of greater saphenous vein at lower leg level, unspecified leg

6 S85.39 Other specified injury of greater saphenous vein at lower leg level

SP 7 S85.391- Other specified injury of greater saphenous vein at lower leg level, right leg

SP 7 S85.392- Other specified injury of greater saphenous vein at lower leg level, left leg

IQ 7 S85.399- Other specified injury of greater saphenous vein at lower leg level, unspecified leg

5 S85.4 Injury of lesser saphenous vein at lower leg level

6 S85.40 Unspecified injury of lesser saphenous vein at lower leg level

IQ 7 S85.401- Unspecified injury of lesser saphenous vein at lower leg level, right leg

IQ 7 S85.402- Unspecified injury of lesser saphenous vein at lower leg level, left leg

IQ 7 S85.409- Unspecified injury of lesser saphenous vein at lower leg level, unspecified leg

6 S85.41 Laceration of lesser saphenous vein at lower leg level

SP 7 S85.411- Laceration of lesser saphenous vein at lower leg level, right leg

SP 7 S85.412- Laceration of lesser saphenous vein at lower leg level, left leg

IQ 7 S85.419- Laceration of lesser saphenous vein at lower leg level, unspecified leg

6 S85.49 Other specified injury of lesser saphenous vein at lower leg level

SP 7 S85.491- Other specified injury of lesser saphenous vein at lower leg level, right leg

SP 7 S85.492- Other specified injury of lesser saphenous vein at lower leg level, left leg

IQ 7 S85.499- Other specified injury of lesser saphenous vein at lower leg level, unspecified leg

5 S85.5 Injury of popliteal vein

6 S85.50 Unspecified injury of popliteal vein

IQ 7 S85.501- Unspecified injury of popliteal vein, right leg

IQ 7 S85.502- Unspecified injury of popliteal vein, left leg

IQ 7 S85.509- Unspecified injury of popliteal vein, unspecified leg

6 S85.51 Laceration of popliteal vein

SP 7 S85.511- Laceration of popliteal vein, right leg

SP 7 S85.512- Laceration of popliteal vein, left leg

SP IQ 7 S85.519- Laceration of popliteal vein, unspecified leg

6 S85.59 Other specified injury of popliteal vein

SP 7 S85.591- Other specified injury of popliteal vein, right leg

SP 7 S85.592- Other specified injury of popliteal vein, left leg

IQ 7 S85.599- Other specified injury of popliteal vein, unspecified leg

5 S85.8 Injury of other blood vessels at lower leg level

6 S85.80 Unspecified injury of other blood vessels at lower leg level

IQ 7 S85.801- Unspecified injury of other blood vessels at lower leg level, right leg

IQ 7 S85.802- Unspecified injury of other blood vessels at lower leg level, left leg

IQ 7 S85.809- Unspecified injury of other blood vessels at lower leg level, unspecified leg

6 S85.81 Laceration of other blood vessels at lower leg level

SP 7 S85.811- Laceration of other blood vessels at lower leg level, right leg

SP 7 S85.812- Laceration of other blood vessels at lower leg level, left leg

IQ 7 S85.819- Laceration of other blood vessels at lower leg level, unspecified leg

6 S85.89 Other specified injury of other blood vessels at lower leg level

SP 7 S85.891- Other specified injury of other blood vessels at lower leg level, right leg

SP 7 S85.892- Other specified injury of other blood vessels at lower leg level, left leg

IQ 7 S85.899- Other specified injury of other blood vessels at lower leg level, unspecified leg

5 S85.9 Injury of unspecified blood vessel at lower leg level

Chapter 19

S00-T88

6 **S85.90 Unspecified injury of unspecified blood vessel at lower leg level**

Laterality IQ 7 **S85.901- Unspecified injury of unspecified blood vessel at lower leg level, right leg**

Laterality IQ 7 **S85.902- Unspecified injury of unspecified blood vessel at lower leg level, left leg**

Laterality IQ 7 **S85.909- Unspecified injury of unspecified blood vessel at lower leg level, unspecified leg**

6 **S85.91 Laceration of unspecified blood vessel at lower leg level**

Laterality SP 7 **S85.911- Laceration of unspecified blood vessel at lower leg level, right leg**

Laterality SP 7 **S85.912- Laceration of unspecified blood vessel at lower leg level, left leg**

Laterality IQ 7 **S85.919- Laceration of unspecified blood vessel at lower leg level, unspecified leg**

6 **S85.99 Other specified injury of unspecified blood vessel at lower leg level**

Laterality IQ 7 **S85.991- Other specified injury of unspecified blood vessel at lower leg level, right leg**

Laterality IQ 7 **S85.992- Other specified injury of unspecified blood vessel at lower leg level, left leg**

Laterality IQ 7 **S85.999- Other specified injury of unspecified blood vessel at lower leg level, unspecified leg**

4 **S86 Injury of muscle, fascia and tendon at lower leg level**

Code also:
any associated open wound (S81.-)

EXCLUDES 2 injury of muscle, fascia and tendon at ankle (S96.-)
injury of patellar ligament (tendon) (S76.1-)
sprain of joints and ligaments of knee (S83.-)

The appropriate 7th character is to be added to each code from category S86
A initial encounter
D subsequent encounter
S sequela

5 **S86.0 Injury of Achilles tendon**

6 **S86.00 Unspecified injury of Achilles tendon**

Laterality IQ 7 **S86.001- Unspecified injury of right Achilles tendon**

Laterality IQ 7 **S86.002- Unspecified injury of left Achilles tendon**

Laterality IQ 7 **S86.009- Unspecified injury of unspecified Achilles tendon**

6 **S86.01 Strain of Achilles tendon**

Laterality SP 7 **S86.011- Strain of right Achilles tendon**

Laterality SP 7 **S86.012- Strain of left Achilles tendon**

Laterality IQ 7 **S86.019- Strain of unspecified Achilles tendon**

6 **S86.02 Laceration of Achilles tendon**

Laterality SP 7 **S86.021- Laceration of right Achilles tendon**

Laterality SP 7 **S86.022- Laceration of left Achilles tendon**

Laterality IQ 7 **S86.029- Laceration of unspecified Achilles tendon**

6 **S86.09 Other specified injury of Achilles tendon**

Laterality SP 7 **S86.091- Other specified injury of right Achilles tendon**

Laterality SP 7 **S86.092- Other specified injury of left Achilles tendon**

Laterality IQ 7 **S86.099- Other specified injury of unspecified Achilles tendon**

5 **S86.1 Injury of other muscle(s) and tendon(s) of posterior muscle group at lower leg level**

6 **S86.10 Unspecified injury of other muscle(s) and tendon(s) of posterior muscle group at lower leg level**

Laterality IQ 7 **S86.101- Unspecified injury of other muscle(s) and tendon(s) of posterior muscle group at lower leg level, right leg**

Laterality IQ 7 **S86.102- Unspecified injury of other muscle(s) and tendon(s) of posterior muscle group at lower leg level, left leg**

Laterality IQ 7 **S86.109- Unspecified injury of other muscle(s) and tendon(s) of posterior muscle group at lower leg level, unspecified leg**

6 **S86.11 Strain of other muscle(s) and tendon(s) of posterior muscle group at lower leg level**

Laterality SP 7 **S86.111- Strain of other muscle(s) and tendon(s) of posterior muscle group at lower leg level, right leg**

Laterality SP 7 **S86.112- Strain of other muscle(s) and tendon(s) of posterior muscle group at lower leg level, left leg**

Laterality IQ 7 **S86.119- Strain of other muscle(s) and tendon(s) of posterior muscle group at lower leg level, unspecified leg**

6 **S86.12 Laceration of other muscle(s) and tendon(s) of posterior muscle group at lower leg level**

Laterality SP 7 **S86.121- Laceration of other muscle(s) and tendon(s) of posterior muscle group at lower leg level, right leg**

Laterality SP 7 **S86.122- Laceration of other muscle(s) and tendon(s) of posterior muscle group at lower leg level, left leg**

Laterality IQ 7 **S86.129- Laceration of other muscle(s) and tendon(s) of posterior muscle group at lower leg level, unspecified leg**

6 **S86.19 Other injury of other muscle(s) and tendon(s) of posterior muscle group at lower leg level**

Laterality SP 7 **S86.191- Other injury of other muscle(s) and tendon(s) of posterior muscle group at lower leg level, right leg**

Laterality SP 7 **S86.192- Other injury of other muscle(s) and tendon(s) of posterior muscle group at lower leg level, left leg**

IQ 7 S86.199- Other injury of other muscle(s) and tendon(s) of posterior muscle group at lower leg level, unspecified leg

5 S86.2 Injury of muscle(s) and tendon(s) of anterior muscle group at lower leg level

6 S86.20 Unspecified injury of muscle(s) and tendon(s) of anterior muscle group at lower leg level

IQ 7 S86.201- Unspecified injury of muscle(s) and tendon(s) of anterior muscle group at lower leg level, right leg

IQ 7 S86.202- Unspecified injury of muscle(s) and tendon(s) of anterior muscle group at lower leg level, left leg

IQ 7 S86.209- Unspecified injury of muscle(s) and tendon(s) of anterior muscle group at lower leg level, unspecified leg

6 S86.21 Strain of muscle(s) and tendon(s) of anterior muscle group at lower leg level

SP 7 S86.211- Strain of muscle(s) and tendon(s) of anterior muscle group at lower leg level, right leg

SP 7 S86.212- Strain of muscle(s) and tendon(s) of anterior muscle group at lower leg level, left leg

IQ 7 S86.219- Strain of muscle(s) and tendon(s) of anterior muscle group at lower leg level, unspecified leg

6 S86.22 Laceration of muscle(s) and tendon(s) of anterior muscle group at lower leg level

SP 7 S86.221- Laceration of muscle(s) and tendon(s) of anterior muscle group at lower leg level, right leg

SP 7 S86.222- Laceration of muscle(s) and tendon(s) of anterior muscle group at lower leg level, left leg

IQ 7 S86.229- Laceration of muscle(s) and tendon(s) of anterior muscle group at lower leg level, unspecified leg

6 S86.29 Other injury of muscle(s) and tendon(s) of anterior muscle group at lower leg level

SP 7 S86.291- Other injury of muscle(s) and tendon(s) of anterior muscle group at lower leg level, right leg

SP 7 S86.292- Other injury of muscle(s) and tendon(s) of anterior muscle group at lower leg level, left leg

IQ 7 S86.299- Other injury of muscle(s) and tendon(s) of anterior muscle group at lower leg level, unspecified leg

5 S86.3 Injury of muscle(s) and tendon(s) of peroneal muscle group at lower leg level

6 S86.30 Unspecified injury of muscle(s) and tendon(s) of peroneal muscle group at lower leg level

IQ 7 S86.301- Unspecified injury of muscle(s) and tendon(s) of peroneal muscle group at lower leg level, right leg

IQ 7 S86.302- Unspecified injury of muscle(s) and tendon(s) of peroneal muscle group at lower leg level, left leg

IQ 7 S86.309- Unspecified injury of muscle(s) and tendon(s) of peroneal muscle group at lower leg level, unspecified leg

6 S86.31 Strain of muscle(s) and tendon(s) of peroneal muscle group at lower leg level

SP 7 S86.311- Strain of muscle(s) and tendon(s) of peroneal muscle group at lower leg level, right leg

SP 7 S86.312- Strain of muscle(s) and tendon(s) of peroneal muscle group at lower leg level, left leg

IQ 7 S86.319- Strain of muscle(s) and tendon(s) of peroneal muscle group at lower leg level, unspecified leg

6 S86.32 Laceration of muscle(s) and tendon(s) of peroneal muscle group at lower leg level

SP 7 S86.321- Laceration of muscle(s) and tendon(s) of peroneal muscle group at lower leg level, right leg

SP 7 S86.322- Laceration of muscle(s) and tendon(s) of peroneal muscle group at lower leg level, left leg

IQ 7 S86.329- Laceration of muscle(s) and tendon(s) of peroneal muscle group at lower leg level, unspecified leg

6 S86.39 Other injury of muscle(s) and tendon(s) of peroneal muscle group at lower leg level

SP 7 S86.391- Other injury of muscle(s) and tendon(s) of peroneal muscle group at lower leg level, right leg

SP 7 S86.392- Other injury of muscle(s) and tendon(s) of peroneal muscle group at lower leg level, left leg

IQ 7 S86.399- Other injury of muscle(s) and tendon(s) of peroneal muscle group at lower leg level, unspecified leg

5 S86.8 Injury of other muscles and tendons at lower leg level

6 S86.80 Unspecified injury of other muscles and tendons at lower leg level

IQ 7 S86.801- Unspecified injury of other muscle(s) and tendon(s) at lower leg level, right leg

IQ 7 S86.802- Unspecified injury of other muscle(s) and tendon(s) at lower leg level, left leg

IQ 7 S86.809- Unspecified injury of other muscle(s) and tendon(s) at lower leg level, unspecified leg

6 S86.81 Strain of other muscles and tendons at lower leg level

Chapter 19

S00-T88

S86.811- Strain of other muscle(s) and tendon(s) at lower leg level, right leg

S86.812- Strain of other muscle(s) and tendon(s) at lower leg level, left leg

S86.819- Strain of other muscle(s) and tendon(s) at lower leg level, unspecified leg

S86.82 Laceration of other muscles and tendons at lower leg level

S86.821- Laceration of other muscle(s) and tendon(s) at lower leg level, right leg

S86.822- Laceration of other muscle(s) and tendon(s) at lower leg level, left leg

S86.829- Laceration of other muscle(s) and tendon(s) at lower leg level, unspecified leg

S86.89 Other injury of other muscles and tendons at lower leg level

S86.891- Other injury of other muscle(s) and tendon(s) at lower leg level, right leg

S86.892- Other injury of other muscle(s) and tendon(s) at lower leg level, left leg

S86.899- Other injury of other muscle(s) and tendon(s) at lower leg level, unspecified leg

S86.9 Injury of unspecified muscle and tendon at lower leg level

S86.90 Unspecified injury of unspecified muscle and tendon at lower leg level

S86.901- Unspecified injury of unspecified muscle(s) and tendon(s) at lower leg level, right leg

S86.902- Unspecified injury of unspecified muscle(s) and tendon(s) at lower leg level, left leg

S86.909- Unspecified injury of unspecified muscle(s) and tendon(s) at lower leg level, unspecified leg

S86.91 Strain of unspecified muscle and tendon at lower leg level

S86.911- Strain of unspecified muscle(s) and tendon(s) at lower leg level, right leg

S86.912- Strain of unspecified muscle(s) and tendon(s) at lower leg level, left leg

S86.919- Strain of unspecified muscle(s) and tendon(s) at lower leg level, unspecified leg

S86.92 Laceration of unspecified muscle and tendon at lower leg level

S86.921- Laceration of unspecified muscle(s) and tendon(s) at lower leg level, right leg

S86.922- Laceration of unspecified muscle(s) and tendon(s) at lower leg level, left leg

S86.929- Laceration of unspecified muscle(s) and tendon(s) at lower leg level, unspecified leg

S86.99 Other injury of unspecified muscle and tendon at lower leg level

S86.991- Other injury of unspecified muscle(s) and tendon(s) at lower leg level, right leg

S86.992- Other injury of unspecified muscle(s) and tendon(s) at lower leg level, left leg

S86.999- Other injury of unspecified muscle(s) and tendon(s) at lower leg level, unspecified leg

+ S87 Crushing injury of lower leg

Use additional code(s) for all associated injuries

EXCLUDES 2 crushing injury of ankle and foot (S97.-)

The appropriate 7th character is to be added to each code from category S87

A initial encounter
D subsequent encounter
S sequela

+ S87.0 Crushing injury of knee

+ S87.00X- Crushing injury of unspecified knee

+ S87.01X- Crushing injury of right knee

+ S87.02X- Crushing injury of left knee

+ S87.8 Crushing injury of lower leg

+ S87.80X- Crushing injury of unspecified lower leg

+ S87.81X- Crushing injury of right lower leg

+ S87.82X- Crushing injury of left lower leg

S88 Traumatic amputation of lower leg

An amputation not identified as partial or complete should be coded to complete

EXCLUDES 1 traumatic amputation of ankle and foot (S98.-)

The appropriate 7th character is to be added to each code from category S88

A initial encounter
D subsequent encounter
S sequela

CODING TIPS ✓ Use these codes only when the amputation was due to trauma. There is no need for adding Z89 with traumatic amputations. See Z47.81 for care of amputations not due to trauma.

S88.0 Traumatic amputation at knee level

S88.01 Complete traumatic amputation at knee level

S88.011- Complete traumatic amputation at knee level, right lower leg

S88.012- Complete traumatic amputation at knee level, left lower leg

S88.019- Complete traumatic amputation at knee level, unspecified lower leg

S88.02 Partial traumatic amputation at knee level

S88.021- Partial traumatic amputation at knee level, right lower leg

Chapter 19

S00-T88

SP 7 S88.022- Partial traumatic amputation at knee level, left lower leg

IQ 7 S88.029- Partial traumatic amputation at knee level, unspecified lower leg

5 S88.1 Traumatic amputation at level between knee and ankle

6 S88.11 Complete traumatic amputation at level between knee and ankle

SP 7 S88.111- Complete traumatic amputation at level between knee and ankle, right lower leg

SP 7 S88.112- Complete traumatic amputation at level between knee and ankle, left lower leg

IQ 7 S88.119- Complete traumatic amputation at level between knee and ankle, unspecified lower leg

6 S88.12 Partial traumatic amputation at level between knee and ankle

SP 7 S88.121- Partial traumatic amputation at level between knee and ankle, right lower leg

SP 7 S88.122- Partial traumatic amputation at level between knee and ankle, left lower leg

IQ 7 S88.129- Partial traumatic amputation at level between knee and ankle, unspecified lower leg

5 S88.9 Traumatic amputation of lower leg, level unspecified

6 S88.91 Complete traumatic amputation of lower leg, level unspecified

SP 7 S88.911- Complete traumatic amputation of right lower leg, level unspecified

SP 7 S88.912- Complete traumatic amputation of left lower leg, level unspecified

IQ 7 S88.919- Complete traumatic amputation of unspecified lower leg, level unspecified

6 S88.92 Partial traumatic amputation of lower leg, level unspecified

SP 7 S88.921- Partial traumatic amputation of right lower leg, level unspecified

SP 7 S88.922- Partial traumatic amputation of left lower leg, level unspecified

IQ 7 S88.929- Partial traumatic amputation of unspecified lower leg, level unspecified

4 S89 Other and unspecified injuries of lower leg

Note:
A fracture not indicated as open or closed should be coded to closed

EXCLUDES 2 other and unspecified injuries of ankle and foot (S99.-)

The appropriate 7th character is to be added to each code from subcategories S89.0, S89.1, S89.2, and S89.3

- A initial encounter for closed fracture
- D subsequent encounter for fracture with routine healing
- G subsequent encounter for fracture with delayed healing
- K subsequent encounter for fracture with nonunion
- P subsequent encounter for fracture with malunion
- S sequela

CODING TIPS ✓ A fracture not indicated as open or closed should be coded to closed.

5 S89.0 Physeal fracture of upper end of tibia

6 S89.00 Unspecified physeal fracture of upper end of tibia

SP 7 S89.001- Unspecified physeal fracture of upper end of right tibia

SP 7 S89.002- Unspecified physeal fracture of upper end of left tibia

IQ 7 S89.009- Unspecified physeal fracture of upper end of unspecified tibia

6 S89.01 Salter-Harris Type I physeal fracture of upper end of tibia

SP 7 S89.011- Salter-Harris Type I physeal fracture of upper end of right tibia

SP 7 S89.012- Salter-Harris Type I physeal fracture of upper end of left tibia

IQ 7 S89.019- Salter-Harris Type I physeal fracture of upper end of unspecified tibia

6 S89.02 Salter-Harris Type II physeal fracture of upper end of tibia

SP 7 S89.021- Salter-Harris Type II physeal fracture of upper end of right tibia

SP 7 S89.022- Salter-Harris Type II physeal fracture of upper end of left tibia

IQ 7 S89.029- Salter-Harris Type II physeal fracture of upper end of unspecified tibia

6 S89.03 Salter-Harris Type III physeal fracture of upper end of tibia

SP 7 S89.031- Salter-Harris Type III physeal fracture of upper end of right tibia

SP 7 S89.032- Salter-Harris Type III physeal fracture of upper end of left tibia

IQ 7 S89.039- Salter-Harris Type III physeal fracture of upper end of unspecified tibia

6 S89.04 Salter-Harris Type IV physeal fracture of upper end of tibia

SP 7 S89.041- Salter-Harris Type IV physeal fracture of upper end of right tibia

SP 7 S89.042- Salter-Harris Type IV physeal fracture of upper end of left tibia

IQ 7 S89.049- Salter-Harris Type IV physeal fracture of upper end of unspecified tibia

6 S89.09 Other physeal fracture of upper end of tibia
SP 7 S89.091- Other physeal fracture of upper end of right tibia
SP 7 S89.092- Other physeal fracture of upper end of left tibia
IQ 7 S89.099- Other physeal fracture of upper end of unspecified tibia

5 S89.1 Physeal fracture of lower end of tibia
6 S89.10 Unspecified physeal fracture of lower end of tibia
SP 7 S89.101- Unspecified physeal fracture of lower end of right tibia
SP 7 S89.102- Unspecified physeal fracture of lower end of left tibia
IQ 7 S89.109- Unspecified physeal fracture of lower end of unspecified tibia
6 S89.11 Salter-Harris Type I physeal fracture of lower end of tibia
SP 7 S89.111- Salter-Harris Type I physeal fracture of lower end of right tibia
SP 7 S89.112- Salter-Harris Type I physeal fracture of lower end of left tibia
IQ 7 S89.119- Salter-Harris Type I physeal fracture of lower end of unspecified tibia
6 S89.12 Salter-Harris Type II physeal fracture of lower end of tibia
SP 7 S89.121- Salter-Harris Type II physeal fracture of lower end of right tibia
SP 7 S89.122- Salter-Harris Type II physeal fracture of lower end of left tibia
IQ 7 S89.129- Salter-Harris Type II physeal fracture of lower end of unspecified tibia
6 S89.13 Salter-Harris Type III physeal fracture of lower end of tibia
EXCLUDES 1 fracture of medial malleolus (adult) (S82.5-)
SP 7 S89.131- Salter-Harris Type III physeal fracture of lower end of right tibia
SP 7 S89.132- Salter-Harris Type III physeal fracture of lower end of left tibia
IQ 7 S89.139- Salter-Harris Type III physeal fracture of lower end of unspecified tibia
6 S89.14 Salter-Harris Type IV physeal fracture of lower end of tibia
EXCLUDES 1 fracture of medial malleolus (adult) (S82.5-)
SP 7 S89.141- Salter-Harris Type IV physeal fracture of lower end of right tibia
SP 7 S89.142- Salter-Harris Type IV physeal fracture of lower end of left tibia
IQ 7 S89.149- Salter-Harris Type IV physeal fracture of lower end of unspecified tibia
6 S89.19 Other physeal fracture of lower end of tibia
SP 7 S89.191- Other physeal fracture of lower end of right tibia
SP 7 S89.192- Other physeal fracture of lower end of left tibia
IQ 7 S89.199- Other physeal fracture of lower end of unspecified tibia

5 S89.2 Physeal fracture of upper end of fibula
6 S89.20 Unspecified physeal fracture of upper end of fibula
SP 7 S89.201- Unspecified physeal fracture of upper end of right fibula
SP 7 S89.202- Unspecified physeal fracture of upper end of left fibula
IQ 7 S89.209- Unspecified physeal fracture of upper end of unspecified fibula
6 S89.21 Salter-Harris Type I physeal fracture of upper end of fibula
SP 7 S89.211- Salter-Harris Type I physeal fracture of upper end of right fibula
SP 7 S89.212- Salter-Harris Type I physeal fracture of upper end of left fibula
IQ 7 S89.219- Salter-Harris Type I physeal fracture of upper end of unspecified fibula
6 S89.22 Salter-Harris Type II physeal fracture of upper end of fibula
SP 7 S89.221- Salter-Harris Type II physeal fracture of upper end of right fibula
SP 7 S89.222- Salter-Harris Type II physeal fracture of upper end of left fibula
IQ 7 S89.229- Salter-Harris Type II physeal fracture of upper end of unspecified fibula
6 S89.29 Other physeal fracture of upper end of fibula
SP 7 S89.291- Other physeal fracture of upper end of right fibula
SP 7 S89.292- Other physeal fracture of upper end of left fibula
IQ 7 S89.299- Other physeal fracture of upper end of unspecified fibula

5 S89.3 Physeal fracture of lower end of fibula
6 S89.30 Unspecified physeal fracture of lower end of fibula
SP 7 S89.301- Unspecified physeal fracture of lower end of right fibula
SP 7 S89.302- Unspecified physeal fracture of lower end of left fibula
IQ 7 S89.309- Unspecified physeal fracture of lower end of unspecified fibula
6 S89.31 Salter-Harris Type I physeal fracture of lower end of fibula
SP 7 S89.311- Salter-Harris Type I physeal fracture of lower end of right fibula
SP 7 S89.312- Salter-Harris Type I physeal fracture of lower end of left fibula
IQ 7 S89.319- Salter-Harris Type I physeal fracture of lower end of unspecified fibula
6 S89.32 Salter-Harris Type II physeal fracture of lower end of fibula

SP 7 **S89.321- Salter-Harris Type II physeal fracture of lower end of right fibula**

SP 7 **S89.322- Salter-Harris Type II physeal fracture of lower end of left fibula**

IQ 7 **S89.329- Salter-Harris Type II physeal fracture of lower end of unspecified fibula**

6 **S89.39 Other physeal fracture of lower end of fibula**

SP 7 **S89.391- Other physeal fracture of lower end of right fibula**

SP 7 **S89.392- Other physeal fracture of lower end of left fibula**

IQ 7 **S89.399- Other physeal fracture of lower end of unspecified fibula**

5 **S89.8 Other specified injuries of lower leg**

The appropriate 7th character is to be added to each code in subcategory S89.8
A initial encounter
D subsequent encounter
S sequela

IQ 7 **S89.80X- Other specified injuries of unspecified lower leg**

SP 7 **S89.81X- Other specified injuries of right lower leg**

SP 7 **S89.82X- Other specified injuries of left lower leg**

5 **S89.9 Unspecified injury of lower leg**

The appropriate 7th character is to be added to each code in subcategory S89.9
A initial encounter
D subsequent encounter
S sequela

IQ 7 **S89.90X- Unspecified injury of unspecified lower leg**

IQ 7 **S89.91X- Unspecified injury of right lower leg**

IQ 7 **S89.92X- Unspecified injury of left lower leg**

Injuries to the ankle and foot (S90-S99)

EXCLUDES 2 burns and corrosions (T20-T32)
fracture of ankle and malleolus (S82.-)
frostbite (T33-T34)
insect bite or sting, venomous (T63.4)

GUIDELINES **Section I.C.19.c.2)**

Multiple fractures are sequenced in accordance with the severity of the fracture.

GUIDELINES **Section I.C.19.b.1)-2)**

When coding injuries, assign separate codes for each injury unless a combination code is provided, in which case the combination code is assigned ... Traumatic injury codes (S00-T14.9) are not to be used for normal, healing surgical wounds or to identify complications of surgical wounds. The code for the most serious injury, as determined by the provider and the focus of treatment, is sequenced first.

1) Superficial injuries such as abrasions or contusions are not coded when associated with more severe injuries of the same site.

2) When a primary injury results in minor damage to peripheral nerves or blood vessels, the primary injury is sequenced first with additional code(s) for injuries to nerves and spinal cord (such as category S04), and/or injury to blood vessels (such as category S15). When the primary injury is to the blood vessels or nerves, that injury should be sequenced first.

GUIDELINES **Section I.C.19.c**

Coding of Traumatic Fractures: The principles of multiple coding of injuries should be followed in coding fractures. Fractures of specified sites are coded individually by site in accordance with both the provisions within categories S02, S12, S22, S32, S42, S49, S52, S59, S62, S72, S79, S82, S89, S92 and the level of detail furnished by medical record content. A fracture not indicated as open or closed should be coded to closed. A fracture not indicated whether displaced or not displaced should be coded to displaced.

CODING TIPS✓ 7th character A is acceptable in home health and hospice when active treatment is provided, such as antibiotics for an infected wound or a wound vac for a dehisced wound. D is used when the complication or injury is now healing. Think of D as aftercare. S is used for sequela of the injury or complication. Sequela is a residual deficit or condition produced as a result of the injury or complication after the original injury or complication has healed.

4 **S90 Superficial injury of ankle, foot and toes**

The appropriate 7th character is to be added to each code from category S90
A initial encounter
D subsequent encounter
S sequela

5 **S90.0 Contusion of ankle**

IQ 7 **S90.00X- Contusion of unspecified ankle**

IQ 7 **S90.01X- Contusion of right ankle**

IQ 7 **S90.02X- Contusion of left ankle**

5 **S90.1 Contusion of toe without damage to nail**

6 **S90.11 Contusion of great toe without damage to nail**

IQ 7 **S90.111- Contusion of right great toe without damage to nail**

IQ 7 **S90.112- Contusion of left great toe without damage to nail**

IQ 7 **S90.119- Contusion of unspecified great toe without damage to nail**

6 **S90.12 Contusion of lesser toe without damage to nail**

IQ 7 **S90.121- Contusion of right lesser toe(s) without damage to nail**

IQ 7 **S90.122- Contusion of left lesser toe(s) without damage to nail**

Chapter 19

S00-T88

S90.129- **Contusion of unspecified lesser toe(s) without damage to nail**
Contusion of toe NOS

S90.2 **Contusion of toe with damage to nail**

S90.21 **Contusion of great toe with damage to nail**

S90.211- **Contusion of right great toe with damage to nail**

S90.212- **Contusion of left great toe with damage to nail**

S90.219- **Contusion of unspecified great toe with damage to nail**

S90.22 **Contusion of lesser toe with damage to nail**

S90.221- **Contusion of right lesser toe(s) with damage to nail**

S90.222- **Contusion of left lesser toe(s) with damage to nail**

S90.229- **Contusion of unspecified lesser toe(s) with damage to nail**

S90.3 **Contusion of foot**
EXCLUDES 2 contusion of toes (S90.1-, S90.2-)

S90.30X- **Contusion of unspecified foot**
Contusion of foot NOS

S90.31X- **Contusion of right foot**

S90.32X- **Contusion of left foot**

S90.4 **Other superficial injuries of toe**

S90.41 **Abrasion of toe**

S90.411- **Abrasion, right great toe**

S90.412- **Abrasion, left great toe**

S90.413- **Abrasion, unspecified great toe**

S90.414- **Abrasion, right lesser toe(s)**

S90.415- **Abrasion, left lesser toe(s)**

S90.416- **Abrasion, unspecified lesser toe(s)**

S90.42 **Blister (nonthermal) of toe**

S90.421- **Blister (nonthermal), right great toe**

S90.422- **Blister (nonthermal), left great toe**

S90.423- **Blister (nonthermal), unspecified great toe**

S90.424- **Blister (nonthermal), right lesser toe(s)**

S90.425- **Blister (nonthermal), left lesser toe(s)**

S90.426- **Blister (nonthermal), unspecified lesser toe(s)**

S90.44 **External constriction of toe**
Hair tourniquet syndrome of toe

S90.441- **External constriction, right great toe**

S90.442- **External constriction, left great toe**

S90.443- **External constriction, unspecified great toe**

S90.444- **External constriction, right lesser toe(s)**

S90.445- **External constriction, left lesser toe(s)**

S90.446- **External constriction, unspecified lesser toe(s)**

S90.45 **Superficial foreign body of toe**
Splinter in the toe

S90.451- **Superficial foreign body, right great toe**

S90.452- **Superficial foreign body, left great toe**

S90.453- **Superficial foreign body, unspecified great toe**

S90.454- **Superficial foreign body, right lesser toe(s)**

S90.455- **Superficial foreign body, left lesser toe(s)**

S90.456- **Superficial foreign body, unspecified lesser toe(s)**

S90.46 **Insect bite (nonvenomous) of toe**

S90.461- **Insect bite (nonvenomous), right great toe**

S90.462- **Insect bite (nonvenomous), left great toe**

S90.463- **Insect bite (nonvenomous), unspecified great toe**

S90.464- **Insect bite (nonvenomous), right lesser toe(s)**

S90.465- **Insect bite (nonvenomous), left lesser toe(s)**

S90.466- **Insect bite (nonvenomous), unspecified lesser toe(s)**

S90.47 **Other superficial bite of toe**
EXCLUDES 1 open bite of toe (S91.15-, S91.25-)

S90.471- **Other superficial bite of right great toe**

S90.472- **Other superficial bite of left great toe**

S90.473- **Other superficial bite of unspecified great toe**

S90.474- **Other superficial bite of right lesser toe(s)**

S90.475- **Other superficial bite of left lesser toe(s)**

S90.476- **Other superficial bite of unspecified lesser toe(s)**

S90.5 **Other superficial injuries of ankle**

S90.51 **Abrasion of ankle**

S90.511- **Abrasion, right ankle**

S90.512- **Abrasion, left ankle**

S90.519- **Abrasion, unspecified ankle**

S90.52 **Blister (nonthermal) of ankle**

S90.521- **Blister (nonthermal), right ankle**

S90.522- **Blister (nonthermal), left ankle**

S90.529- **Blister (nonthermal), unspecified ankle**

S90.54 **External constriction of ankle**

S90.541- **External constriction, right ankle**

S90.542- **External constriction, left ankle**

S90.549- **External constriction, unspecified ankle**

S90.55 **Superficial foreign body of ankle**
Splinter in the ankle

S90.551- **Superficial foreign body, right ankle**

S90.552- **Superficial foreign body, left ankle**

S90.559- **Superficial foreign body, unspecified ankle**

6 **S90.56 Insect bite (nonvenomous) of ankle**
⊟ IQ 7 **S90.561- Insect bite (nonvenomous), right ankle**
⊟ IQ 7 **S90.562- Insect bite (nonvenomous), left ankle**
⊟ IQ 7 **S90.569- Insect bite (nonvenomous), unspecified ankle**
6 **S90.57 Other superficial bite of ankle**
EXCLUDES 1 open bite of ankle (S91.05-)
⊟ IQ 7 **S90.571- Other superficial bite of ankle, right ankle**
⊟ IQ 7 **S90.572- Other superficial bite of ankle, left ankle**
⊟ IQ 7 **S90.579- Other superficial bite of ankle, unspecified ankle**
5 **S90.8 Other superficial injuries of foot**
6 **S90.81 Abrasion of foot**
⊟ IQ 7 **S90.811- Abrasion, right foot**
⊟ IQ 7 **S90.812- Abrasion, left foot**
⊟ IQ 7 **S90.819- Abrasion, unspecified foot**
6 **S90.82 Blister (nonthermal) of foot**
⊟ IQ 7 **S90.821- Blister (nonthermal), right foot**
⊟ IQ 7 **S90.822- Blister (nonthermal), left foot**
⊟ IQ 7 **S90.829- Blister (nonthermal), unspecified foot**
6 **S90.84 External constriction of foot**
⊟ IQ 7 **S90.841- External constriction, right foot**
⊟ IQ 7 **S90.842- External constriction, left foot**
⊟ IQ 7 **S90.849- External constriction, unspecified foot**
6 **S90.85 Superficial foreign body of foot**
Splinter in the foot
⊟ IQ 7 **S90.851- Superficial foreign body, right foot**
⊟ IQ 7 **S90.852- Superficial foreign body, left foot**
⊟ IQ 7 **S90.859- Superficial foreign body, unspecified foot**
6 **S90.86 Insect bite (nonvenomous) of foot**
⊟ IQ 7 **S90.861- Insect bite (nonvenomous), right foot**
⊟ IQ 7 **S90.862- Insect bite (nonvenomous), left foot**
⊟ IQ 7 **S90.869- Insect bite (nonvenomous), unspecified foot**
6 **S90.87 Other superficial bite of foot**
EXCLUDES 1 open bite of foot (S91.35-)
⊟ IQ 7 **S90.871- Other superficial bite of right foot**
⊟ IQ 7 **S90.872- Other superficial bite of left foot**
⊟ IQ 7 **S90.879- Other superficial bite of unspecified foot**
5 **S90.9 Unspecified superficial injury of ankle, foot and toe**
6 **S90.91 Unspecified superficial injury of ankle**
⊟ IQ 7 **S90.911- Unspecified superficial injury of right ankle**
⊟ IQ 7 **S90.912- Unspecified superficial injury of left ankle**
⊟ IQ 7 **S90.919- Unspecified superficial injury of unspecified ankle**
6 **S90.92 Unspecified superficial injury of foot**
⊟ IQ 7 **S90.921- Unspecified superficial injury of right foot**
⊟ IQ 7 **S90.922- Unspecified superficial injury of left foot**
⊟ IQ 7 **S90.929- Unspecified superficial injury of unspecified foot**
6 **S90.93 Unspecified superficial injury of toes**
⊟ IQ 7 **S90.931- Unspecified superficial injury of right great toe**
⊟ IQ 7 **S90.932- Unspecified superficial injury of left great toe**
⊟ IQ 7 **S90.933- Unspecified superficial injury of unspecified great toe**
⊟ IQ 7 **S90.934- Unspecified superficial injury of right lesser toe(s)**
⊟ IQ 7 **S90.935- Unspecified superficial injury of left lesser toe(s)**
⊟ IQ 7 **S90.936- Unspecified superficial injury of unspecified lesser toe(s)**

4 **S91 Open wound of ankle, foot and toes**
Code also:
any associated wound infection
EXCLUDES 1 open fracture of ankle, foot and toes (S92.-with 7th character B)
traumatic amputation of ankle and foot (S98.-)

The appropriate 7th character is to be added to each code from category S91
A initial encounter
D subsequent encounter
S sequela

CODING TIPS✓ No aftercare code applies, including those for dressing changes, drain care, or suture removal. 7th character 'D' is the default for home care and hospice when providing aftercare for a healing or resolving condition; 'A' is used for active treatment such as antibiotics or more than routine wound care; 'S' may be used to indicate a residual condition after the original injury has healed.

CODING TIPS✓ Open wound codes indicate a wound resulting from a traumatic origin. Do not assign a code for "open wound" unless the etiology of the wound is related to trauma.

5 **S91.0 Open wound of ankle**
6 **S91.00 Unspecified open wound of ankle**
⊟ SP 7 **S91.001- Unspecified open wound, right ankle**
⊟ SP 7 **S91.002- Unspecified open wound, left ankle**
⊟ SP IQ 7 **S91.009- Unspecified open wound, unspecified ankle**
6 **S91.01 Laceration without foreign body of ankle**
⊟ SP 7 **S91.011- Laceration without foreign body, right ankle**
⊟ SP 7 **S91.012- Laceration without foreign body, left ankle**

Chapter 19
S00-T88

S91.019- Laceration without foreign body, unspecified ankle
S91.02 Laceration with foreign body of ankle
S91.021- Laceration with foreign body, right ankle
S91.022- Laceration with foreign body, left ankle
S91.029- Laceration with foreign body, unspecified ankle
S91.03 Puncture wound without foreign body of ankle
S91.031- Puncture wound without foreign body, right ankle
S91.032- Puncture wound without foreign body, left ankle
S91.039- Puncture wound without foreign body, unspecified ankle
S91.04 Puncture wound with foreign body of ankle
S91.041- Puncture wound with foreign body, right ankle
S91.042- Puncture wound with foreign body, left ankle
S91.049- Puncture wound with foreign body, unspecified ankle
S91.05 Open bite of ankle
EXCLUDES 1 superficial bite of ankle (S90.56-, S90.57-)
S91.051- Open bite, right ankle
S91.052- Open bite, left ankle
S91.059- Open bite, unspecified ankle
S91.1 Open wound of toe without damage to nail
S91.10 Unspecified open wound of toe without damage to nail
S91.101- Unspecified open wound of right great toe without damage to nail
S91.102- Unspecified open wound of left great toe without damage to nail
S91.103- Unspecified open wound of unspecified great toe without damage to nail
S91.104- Unspecified open wound of right lesser toe(s) without damage to nail
S91.105- Unspecified open wound of left lesser toe(s) without damage to nail
S91.106- Unspecified open wound of unspecified lesser toe(s) without damage to nail
S91.109- Unspecified open wound of unspecified toe(s) without damage to nail
S91.11 Laceration without foreign body of toe without damage to nail
S91.111- Laceration without foreign body of right great toe without damage to nail
S91.112- Laceration without foreign body of left great toe without damage to nail
S91.113- Laceration without foreign body of unspecified great toe without damage to nail
S91.114- Laceration without foreign body of right lesser toe(s) without damage to nail
S91.115- Laceration without foreign body of left lesser toe(s) without damage to nail
S91.116- Laceration without foreign body of unspecified lesser toe(s) without damage to nail
S91.119- Laceration without foreign body of unspecified toe without damage to nail
S91.12 Laceration with foreign body of toe without damage to nail
S91.121- Laceration with foreign body of right great toe without damage to nail
S91.122- Laceration with foreign body of left great toe without damage to nail
S91.123- Laceration with foreign body of unspecified great toe without damage to nail
S91.124- Laceration with foreign body of right lesser toe(s) without damage to nail
S91.125- Laceration with foreign body of left lesser toe(s) without damage to nail
S91.126- Laceration with foreign body of unspecified lesser toe(s) without damage to nail
S91.129- Laceration with foreign body of unspecified toe(s) without damage to nail
S91.13 Puncture wound without foreign body of toe without damage to nail
S91.131- Puncture wound without foreign body of right great toe without damage to nail
S91.132- Puncture wound without foreign body of left great toe without damage to nail
S91.133- Puncture wound without foreign body of unspecified great toe without damage to nail
S91.134- Puncture wound without foreign body of right lesser toe(s) without damage to nail
S91.135- Puncture wound without foreign body of left lesser toe(s) without damage to nail
S91.136- Puncture wound without foreign body of unspecified lesser toe(s) without damage to nail
S91.139- Puncture wound without foreign body of unspecified toe(s) without damage to nail
S91.14 Puncture wound with foreign body of toe without damage to nail
S91.141- Puncture wound with foreign body of right great toe without damage to nail

SP 7 **S91.142-** **Puncture wound with foreign body of left great toe without damage to nail**

IQ 7 **S91.143-** **Puncture wound with foreign body of unspecified great toe without damage to nail**

SP 7 **S91.144-** **Puncture wound with foreign body of right lesser toe(s) without damage to nail**

SP 7 **S91.145-** **Puncture wound with foreign body of left lesser toe(s) without damage to nail**

IQ 7 **S91.146-** **Puncture wound with foreign body of unspecified lesser toe(s) without damage to nail**

IQ 7 **S91.149-** **Puncture wound with foreign body of unspecified toe(s) without damage to nail**

6 **S91.15** **Open bite of toe without damage to nail**

Bite of toe NOS

EXCLUDES 1 superficial bite of toe (S90.46-, S90.47-)

SP 7 **S91.151-** **Open bite of right great toe without damage to nail**

SP 7 **S91.152-** **Open bite of left great toe without damage to nail**

IQ 7 **S91.153-** **Open bite of unspecified great toe without damage to nail**

SP 7 **S91.154-** **Open bite of right lesser toe(s) without damage to nail**

SP 7 **S91.155-** **Open bite of left lesser toe(s) without damage to nail**

IQ 7 **S91.156-** **Open bite of unspecified lesser toe(s) without damage to nail**

IQ 7 **S91.159-** **Open bite of unspecified toe(s) without damage to nail**

5 **S91.2** **Open wound of toe with damage to nail**

6 **S91.20** **Unspecified open wound of toe with damage to nail**

SP 7 **S91.201-** **Unspecified open wound of right great toe with damage to nail**

SP 7 **S91.202-** **Unspecified open wound of left great toe with damage to nail**

IQ 7 **S91.203-** **Unspecified open wound of unspecified great toe with damage to nail**

SP 7 **S91.204-** **Unspecified open wound of right lesser toe(s) with damage to nail**

SP 7 **S91.205-** **Unspecified open wound of left lesser toe(s) with damage to nail**

IQ 7 **S91.206-** **Unspecified open wound of unspecified lesser toe(s) with damage to nail**

IQ 7 **S91.209-** **Unspecified open wound of unspecified toe(s) with damage to nail**

6 **S91.21** **Laceration without foreign body of toe with damage to nail**

SP 7 **S91.211-** **Laceration without foreign body of right great toe with damage to nail**

SP 7 **S91.212-** **Laceration without foreign body of left great toe with damage to nail**

IQ 7 **S91.213-** **Laceration without foreign body of unspecified great toe with damage to nail**

SP 7 **S91.214-** **Laceration without foreign body of right lesser toe(s) with damage to nail**

SP 7 **S91.215-** **Laceration without foreign body of left lesser toe(s) with damage to nail**

IQ 7 **S91.216-** **Laceration without foreign body of unspecified lesser toe(s) with damage to nail**

IQ 7 **S91.219-** **Laceration without foreign body of unspecified toe(s) with damage to nail**

6 **S91.22** **Laceration with foreign body of toe with damage to nail**

SP 7 **S91.221-** **Laceration with foreign body of right great toe with damage to nail**

SP 7 **S91.222-** **Laceration with foreign body of left great toe with damage to nail**

IQ 7 **S91.223-** **Laceration with foreign body of unspecified great toe with damage to nail**

SP 7 **S91.224-** **Laceration with foreign body of right lesser toe(s) with damage to nail**

SP 7 **S91.225-** **Laceration with foreign body of left lesser toe(s) with damage to nail**

IQ 7 **S91.226-** **Laceration with foreign body of unspecified lesser toe(s) with damage to nail**

IQ 7 **S91.229-** **Laceration with foreign body of unspecified toe(s) with damage to nail**

6 **S91.23** **Puncture wound without foreign body of toe with damage to nail**

SP 7 **S91.231-** **Puncture wound without foreign body of right great toe with damage to nail**

SP 7 **S91.232-** **Puncture wound without foreign body of left great toe with damage to nail**

IQ 7 **S91.233-** **Puncture wound without foreign body of unspecified great toe with damage to nail**

SP 7 **S91.234-** **Puncture wound without foreign body of right lesser toe(s) with damage to nail**

SP 7 **S91.235-** **Puncture wound without foreign body of left lesser toe(s) with damage to nail**

IQ 7 **S91.236-** **Puncture wound without foreign body of unspecified lesser toe(s) with damage to nail**

IQ 7 **S91.239-** **Puncture wound without foreign body of unspecified toe(s) with damage to nail**

6 **S91.24** **Puncture wound with foreign body of toe with damage to nail**

S91.241- Puncture wound with foreign body of right great toe with damage to nail

S91.242- Puncture wound with foreign body of left great toe with damage to nail

S91.243- Puncture wound with foreign body of unspecified great toe with damage to nail

S91.244- Puncture wound with foreign body of right lesser toe(s) with damage to nail

S91.245- Puncture wound with foreign body of left lesser toe(s) with damage to nail

S91.246- Puncture wound with foreign body of unspecified lesser toe(s) with damage to nail

S91.249- Puncture wound with foreign body of unspecified toe(s) with damage to nail

S91.25 Open bite of toe with damage to nail

Bite of toe with damage to nail NOS

EXCLUDES 1 superficial bite of toe (S90.46-, S90.47-)

S91.251- Open bite of right great toe with damage to nail

S91.252- Open bite of left great toe with damage to nail

S91.253- Open bite of unspecified great toe with damage to nail

S91.254- Open bite of right lesser toe(s) with damage to nail

S91.255- Open bite of left lesser toe(s) with damage to nail

S91.256- Open bite of unspecified lesser toe(s) with damage to nail

S91.259- Open bite of unspecified toe(s) with damage to nail

S91.3 Open wound of foot

S91.30 Unspecified open wound of foot

S91.301- Unspecified open wound, right foot

S91.302- Unspecified open wound, left foot

S91.309- Unspecified open wound, unspecified foot

S91.31 Laceration without foreign body of foot

S91.311- Laceration without foreign body, right foot

S91.312- Laceration without foreign body, left foot

S91.319- Laceration without foreign body, unspecified foot

S91.32 Laceration with foreign body of foot

S91.321- Laceration with foreign body, right foot

S91.322- Laceration with foreign body, left foot

S91.329- Laceration with foreign body, unspecified foot

S91.33 Puncture wound without foreign body of foot

S91.331- Puncture wound without foreign body, right foot

S91.332- Puncture wound without foreign body, left foot

S91.339- Puncture wound without foreign body, unspecified foot

S91.34 Puncture wound with foreign body of foot

S91.341- Puncture wound with foreign body, right foot

S91.342- Puncture wound with foreign body, left foot

S91.349- Puncture wound with foreign body, unspecified foot

S91.35 Open bite of foot

EXCLUDES 1 superficial bite of foot (S90.86-, S90.87-)

S91.351- Open bite, right foot

S91.352- Open bite, left foot

S91.359- Open bite, unspecified foot

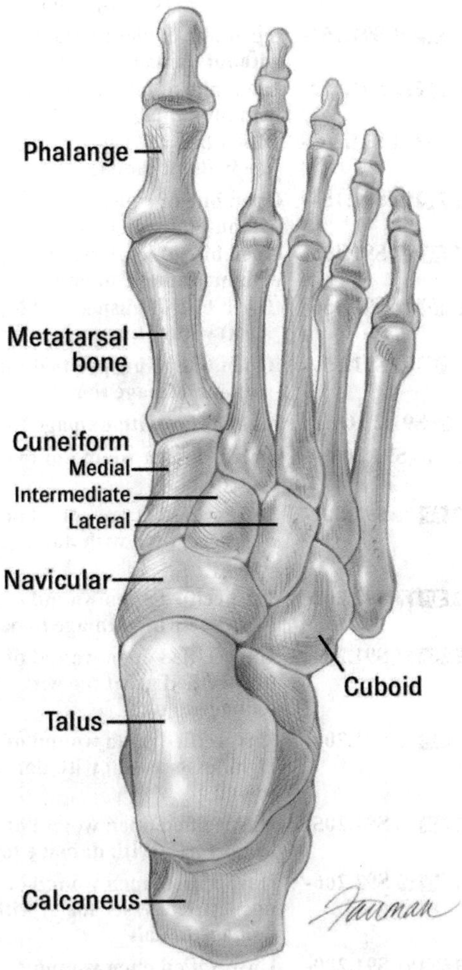

▲ S92 Fracture of foot and toe, except ankle

Note:

A fracture not indicated as displaced or nondisplaced should be coded to displaced

A fracture not indicated as open or closed should be coded to closed

4th digit required 5th digit required 6th digit required 7th digit required 7th digit placeholder +Additional code Laterality

Chapter 19 S00-T88

EXCLUDES 2 fracture of ankle (S82.-)
fracture of malleolus (S82.-)
traumatic amputation of ankle and foot (S98.-)

The appropriate 7th character is to be added to each code from category S92
A initial encounter for closed fracture
B initial encounter for open fracture
D subsequent encounter for fracture with routine healing
G subsequent encounter for fracture with delayed healing
K subsequent encounter for fracture with nonunion
P subsequent encounter for fracture with malunion
S sequela

CODING TIPS ✓ Fractures are not coded with aftercare. "D" is the 7th character for home care and hospice unless the physician or NPP has documented delayed healing, nonunion or malunion. A sequela is a condition left after the fracture has healed. The Gustilo open fracture classification must be used for open fractures.

CODING TIPS ✓ A fracture not indicated as displaced or nondisplaced should be coded to displaced. A fracture not indicated as open or closed should be coded to closed.

5 **S92.0 Fracture of calcaneus**
Heel bone
Os calcis
EXCLUDES 2 Physeal fracture of calcaneus (S99.0-)

6 **S92.00 Unspecified fracture of calcaneus**
SP 7 **S92.001- Unspecified fracture of right calcaneus**
SP 7 **S92.002- Unspecified fracture of left calcaneus**
!Q 7 **S92.009- Unspecified fracture of unspecified calcaneus**

6 **S92.01 Fracture of body of calcaneus**
SP 7 **S92.011- Displaced fracture of body of right calcaneus**
SP 7 **S92.012- Displaced fracture of body of left calcaneus**
!Q 7 **S92.013- Displaced fracture of body of unspecified calcaneus**
SP 7 **S92.014- Nondisplaced fracture of body of right calcaneus**
SP 7 **S92.015- Nondisplaced fracture of body of left calcaneus**
!Q 7 **S92.016- Nondisplaced fracture of body of unspecified calcaneus**

6 **S92.02 Fracture of anterior process of calcaneus**
SP 7 **S92.021- Displaced fracture of anterior process of right calcaneus**
SP 7 **S92.022- Displaced fracture of anterior process of left calcaneus**
!Q 7 **S92.023- Displaced fracture of anterior process of unspecified calcaneus**
SP 7 **S92.024- Nondisplaced fracture of anterior process of right calcaneus**
SP 7 **S92.025- Nondisplaced fracture of anterior process of left calcaneus**
!Q 7 **S92.026- Nondisplaced fracture of anterior process of unspecified calcaneus**

6 **S92.03 Avulsion fracture of tuberosity of calcaneus**
SP 7 **S92.031- Displaced avulsion fracture of tuberosity of right calcaneus**
SP 7 **S92.032- Displaced avulsion fracture of tuberosity of left calcaneus**
!Q 7 **S92.033- Displaced avulsion fracture of tuberosity of unspecified calcaneus**
SP 7 **S92.034- Nondisplaced avulsion fracture of tuberosity of right calcaneus**
SP 7 **S92.035- Nondisplaced avulsion fracture of tuberosity of left calcaneus**
!Q 7 **S92.036- Nondisplaced avulsion fracture of tuberosity of unspecified calcaneus**

6 **S92.04 Other fracture of tuberosity of calcaneus**
SP 7 **S92.041- Displaced other fracture of tuberosity of right calcaneus**
SP 7 **S92.042- Displaced other fracture of tuberosity of left calcaneus**
!Q 7 **S92.043- Displaced other fracture of tuberosity of unspecified calcaneus**
SP 7 **S92.044- Nondisplaced other fracture of tuberosity of right calcaneus**
SP 7 **S92.045- Nondisplaced other fracture of tuberosity of left calcaneus**
!Q 7 **S92.046- Nondisplaced other fracture of tuberosity of unspecified calcaneus**

6 **S92.05 Other extraarticular fracture of calcaneus**
SP 7 **S92.051- Displaced other extraarticular fracture of right calcaneus**
SP 7 **S92.052- Displaced other extraarticular fracture of left calcaneus**
!Q 7 **S92.053- Displaced other extraarticular fracture of unspecified calcaneus**
SP 7 **S92.054- Nondisplaced other extraarticular fracture of right calcaneus**
SP 7 **S92.055- Nondisplaced other extraarticular fracture of left calcaneus**
!Q 7 **S92.056- Nondisplaced other extraarticular fracture of unspecified calcaneus**

6 **S92.06 Intraarticular fracture of calcaneus**
SP 7 **S92.061- Displaced intraarticular fracture of right calcaneus**
SP 7 **S92.062- Displaced intraarticular fracture of left calcaneus**
!Q 7 **S92.063- Displaced intraarticular fracture of unspecified calcaneus**
SP 7 **S92.064- Nondisplaced intraarticular fracture of right calcaneus**
SP 7 **S92.065- Nondisplaced intraarticular fracture of left calcaneus**

⊟ !Q 7 S92.066- Nondisplaced intraarticular fracture of unspecified calcaneus

5 S92.1 Fracture of talus
Astragalus

6 S92.10 Unspecified fracture of talus

⊟ SP 7 S92.101- Unspecified fracture of right talus
⊟ SP 7 S92.102- Unspecified fracture of left talus
⊟ !Q 7 S92.109- Unspecified fracture of unspecified talus

6 S92.11 Fracture of neck of talus

⊟ SP 7 S92.111- Displaced fracture of neck of right talus
⊟ SP 7 S92.112- Displaced fracture of neck of left talus
⊟ !Q 7 S92.113- Displaced fracture of neck of unspecified talus
⊟ SP 7 S92.114- Nondisplaced fracture of neck of right talus
⊟ SP 7 S92.115- Nondisplaced fracture of neck of left talus
⊟ !Q 7 S92.116- Nondisplaced fracture of neck of unspecified talus

6 S92.12 Fracture of body of talus

⊟ SP 7 S92.121- Displaced fracture of body of right talus
⊟ SP 7 S92.122- Displaced fracture of body of left talus
⊟ !Q 7 S92.123- Displaced fracture of body of unspecified talus
⊟ SP 7 S92.124- Nondisplaced fracture of body of right talus
⊟ SP 7 S92.125- Nondisplaced fracture of body of left talus
⊟ !Q 7 S92.126- Nondisplaced fracture of body of unspecified talus

6 S92.13 Fracture of posterior process of talus

⊟ SP 7 S92.131- Displaced fracture of posterior process of right talus
⊟ SP 7 S92.132- Displaced fracture of posterior process of left talus
⊟ !Q 7 S92.133- Displaced fracture of posterior process of unspecified talus
⊟ SP 7 S92.134- Nondisplaced fracture of posterior process of right talus
⊟ SP 7 S92.135- Nondisplaced fracture of posterior process of left talus
⊟ !Q 7 S92.136- Nondisplaced fracture of posterior process of unspecified talus

6 S92.14 Dome fracture of talus
EXCLUDES 1 osteochondritis dissecans (M93.2)

⊟ SP 7 S92.141- Displaced dome fracture of right talus
⊟ SP 7 S92.142- Displaced dome fracture of left talus
⊟ !Q 7 S92.143- Displaced dome fracture of unspecified talus
⊟ SP 7 S92.144- Nondisplaced dome fracture of right talus
⊟ SP 7 S92.145- Nondisplaced dome fracture of left talus
⊟ !Q 7 S92.146- Nondisplaced dome fracture of unspecified talus

6 S92.15 Avulsion fracture (chip fracture) of talus

⊟ SP 7 S92.151- Displaced avulsion fracture (chip fracture) of right talus
⊟ SP 7 S92.152- Displaced avulsion fracture (chip fracture) of left talus
⊟ !Q 7 S92.153- Displaced avulsion fracture (chip fracture) of unspecified talus
⊟ SP 7 S92.154- Nondisplaced avulsion fracture (chip fracture) of right talus
⊟ SP 7 S92.155- Nondisplaced avulsion fracture (chip fracture) of left talus
⊟ !Q 7 S92.156- Nondisplaced avulsion fracture (chip fracture) of unspecified talus

6 S92.19 Other fracture of talus

⊟ SP 7 S92.191- Other fracture of right talus
⊟ SP 7 S92.192- Other fracture of left talus
⊟ !Q 7 S92.199- Other fracture of unspecified talus

5 S92.2 Fracture of other and unspecified tarsal bone(s)

6 S92.20 Fracture of unspecified tarsal bone(s)

⊟ !Q 7 S92.201- Fracture of unspecified tarsal bone(s) of right foot
⊟ !Q 7 S92.202- Fracture of unspecified tarsal bone(s) of left foot
⊟ !Q 7 S92.209- Fracture of unspecified tarsal bone(s) of unspecified foot

6 S92.21 Fracture of cuboid bone

⊟ SP 7 S92.211- Displaced fracture of cuboid bone of right foot
⊟ SP 7 S92.212- Displaced fracture of cuboid bone of left foot
⊟ !Q 7 S92.213- Displaced fracture of cuboid bone of unspecified foot
⊟ SP 7 S92.214- Nondisplaced fracture of cuboid bone of right foot
⊟ SP 7 S92.215- Nondisplaced fracture of cuboid bone of left foot
⊟ !Q 7 S92.216- Nondisplaced fracture of cuboid bone of unspecified foot

6 S92.22 Fracture of lateral cuneiform

⊟ SP 7 S92.221- Displaced fracture of lateral cuneiform of right foot
⊟ SP 7 S92.222- Displaced fracture of lateral cuneiform of left foot
⊟ !Q 7 S92.223- Displaced fracture of lateral cuneiform of unspecified foot
⊟ SP 7 S92.224- Nondisplaced fracture of lateral cuneiform of right foot
⊟ SP 7 S92.225- Nondisplaced fracture of lateral cuneiform of left foot
⊟ !Q 7 S92.226- Nondisplaced fracture of lateral cuneiform of unspecified foot

6 S92.23 Fracture of intermediate cuneiform

⊟ SP 7 S92.231- Displaced fracture of intermediate cuneiform of right foot

Chapter 19

S00-T88

SP 7 S92.232- Displaced fracture of intermediate cuneiform of left foot

!Q 7 S92.233- Displaced fracture of intermediate cuneiform of unspecified foot

SP 7 S92.234- Nondisplaced fracture of intermediate cuneiform of right foot

SP 7 S92.235- Nondisplaced fracture of intermediate cuneiform of left foot

!Q 7 S92.236- Nondisplaced fracture of intermediate cuneiform of unspecified foot

6 S92.24 Fracture of medial cuneiform

SP 7 S92.241- Displaced fracture of medial cuneiform of right foot

SP 7 S92.242- Displaced fracture of medial cuneiform of left foot

!Q 7 S92.243- Displaced fracture of medial cuneiform of unspecified foot

SP 7 S92.244- Nondisplaced fracture of medial cuneiform of right foot

SP 7 S92.245- Nondisplaced fracture of medial cuneiform of left foot

!Q 7 S92.246- Nondisplaced fracture of medial cuneiform of unspecified foot

6 S92.25 Fracture of navicular [scaphoid] of foot

SP 7 S92.251- Displaced fracture of navicular [scaphoid] of right foot

SP 7 S92.252- Displaced fracture of navicular [scaphoid] of left foot

!Q 7 S92.253- Displaced fracture of navicular [scaphoid] of unspecified foot

SP 7 S92.254- Nondisplaced fracture of navicular [scaphoid] of right foot

SP 7 S92.255- Nondisplaced fracture of navicular [scaphoid] of left foot

!Q 7 S92.256- Nondisplaced fracture of navicular [scaphoid] of unspecified foot

5 S92.3 Fracture of metatarsal bone(s)

EXCLUDES 2 Physeal fracture of metatarsal (S99.1-)

6 S92.30 Fracture of unspecified metatarsal bone(s)

SP !Q 7 S92.301- Fracture of unspecified metatarsal bone(s), right foot

SP !Q 7 S92.302- Fracture of unspecified metatarsal bone(s), left foot

!Q 7 S92.309- Fracture of unspecified metatarsal bone(s), unspecified foot

6 S92.31 Fracture of first metatarsal bone

SP 7 S92.311- Displaced fracture of first metatarsal bone, right foot

SP 7 S92.312- Displaced fracture of first metatarsal bone, left foot

!Q 7 S92.313- Displaced fracture of first metatarsal bone, unspecified foot

SP 7 S92.314- Nondisplaced fracture of first metatarsal bone, right foot

SP 7 S92.315- Nondisplaced fracture of first metatarsal bone, left foot

!Q 7 S92.316- Nondisplaced fracture of first metatarsal bone, unspecified foot

6 S92.32 Fracture of second metatarsal bone

SP 7 S92.321- Displaced fracture of second metatarsal bone, right foot

SP 7 S92.322- Displaced fracture of second metatarsal bone, left foot

!Q 7 S92.323- Displaced fracture of second metatarsal bone, unspecified foot

SP 7 S92.324- Nondisplaced fracture of second metatarsal bone, right foot

SP 7 S92.325- Nondisplaced fracture of second metatarsal bone, left foot

!Q 7 S92.326- Nondisplaced fracture of second metatarsal bone, unspecified foot

6 S92.33 Fracture of third metatarsal bone

SP 7 S92.331- Displaced fracture of third metatarsal bone, right foot

SP 7 S92.332- Displaced fracture of third metatarsal bone, left foot

!Q 7 S92.333- Displaced fracture of third metatarsal bone, unspecified foot

SP 7 S92.334- Nondisplaced fracture of third metatarsal bone, right foot

SP 7 S92.335- Nondisplaced fracture of third metatarsal bone, left foot

!Q 7 S92.336- Nondisplaced fracture of third metatarsal bone, unspecified foot

6 S92.34 Fracture of fourth metatarsal bone

SP 7 S92.341- Displaced fracture of fourth metatarsal bone, right foot

SP 7 S92.342- Displaced fracture of fourth metatarsal bone, left foot

!Q 7 S92.343- Displaced fracture of fourth metatarsal bone, unspecified foot

SP 7 S92.344- Nondisplaced fracture of fourth metatarsal bone, right foot

SP 7 S92.345- Nondisplaced fracture of fourth metatarsal bone, left foot

!Q 7 S92.346- Nondisplaced fracture of fourth metatarsal bone, unspecified foot

6 S92.35 Fracture of fifth metatarsal bone

SP 7 S92.351- Displaced fracture of fifth metatarsal bone, right foot

SP 7 S92.352- Displaced fracture of fifth metatarsal bone, left foot

!Q 7 S92.353- Displaced fracture of fifth metatarsal bone, unspecified foot

SP 7 S92.354- Nondisplaced fracture of fifth metatarsal bone, right foot

SP 7 S92.355- Nondisplaced fracture of fifth metatarsal bone, left foot

!Q 7 S92.356- Nondisplaced fracture of fifth metatarsal bone, unspecified foot

5 S92.4 Fracture of great toe

EXCLUDES 2 Physeal fracture of phalanx of toe (S99.2-)

6 **S92.40 Unspecified fracture of great toe**

Laterality SP 7 **S92.401- Displaced unspecified fracture of right great toe**

Laterality SP 7 **S92.402- Displaced unspecified fracture of left great toe**

Laterality IQ 7 **S92.403- Displaced unspecified fracture of unspecified great toe**

Laterality SP 7 **S92.404- Nondisplaced unspecified fracture of right great toe**

Laterality SP 7 **S92.405- Nondisplaced unspecified fracture of left great toe**

Laterality IQ 7 **S92.406- Nondisplaced unspecified fracture of unspecified great toe**

6 **S92.41 Fracture of proximal phalanx of great toe**

Laterality SP 7 **S92.411- Displaced fracture of proximal phalanx of right great toe**

Laterality SP 7 **S92.412- Displaced fracture of proximal phalanx of left great toe**

Laterality IQ 7 **S92.413- Displaced fracture of proximal phalanx of unspecified great toe**

Laterality SP 7 **S92.414- Nondisplaced fracture of proximal phalanx of right great toe**

Laterality SP 7 **S92.415- Nondisplaced fracture of proximal phalanx of left great toe**

Laterality IQ 7 **S92.416- Nondisplaced fracture of proximal phalanx of unspecified great toe**

6 **S92.42 Fracture of distal phalanx of great toe**

Laterality SP 7 **S92.421- Displaced fracture of distal phalanx of right great toe**

Laterality SP 7 **S92.422- Displaced fracture of distal phalanx of left great toe**

Laterality IQ 7 **S92.423- Displaced fracture of distal phalanx of unspecified great toe**

Laterality SP 7 **S92.424- Nondisplaced fracture of distal phalanx of right great toe**

Laterality SP 7 **S92.425- Nondisplaced fracture of distal phalanx of left great toe**

Laterality IQ 7 **S92.426- Nondisplaced fracture of distal phalanx of unspecified great toe**

6 **S92.49 Other fracture of great toe**

Laterality SP 7 **S92.491- Other fracture of right great toe**

Laterality SP 7 **S92.492- Other fracture of left great toe**

Laterality IQ 7 **S92.499- Other fracture of unspecified great toe**

5 **S92.5 Fracture of lesser toe(s)**

EXCLUDES 2 Physeal fracture of phalanx of toe (S99.2-)

6 **S92.50 Unspecified fracture of lesser toe(s)**

Laterality SP IQ 7 **S92.501- Displaced unspecified fracture of right lesser toe(s)**

Laterality SP IQ 7 **S92.502- Displaced unspecified fracture of left lesser toe(s)**

Laterality IQ 7 **S92.503- Displaced unspecified fracture of unspecified lesser toe(s)**

Laterality IQ 7 **S92.504- Nondisplaced unspecified fracture of right lesser toe(s)**

Laterality SP IQ 7 **S92.505- Nondisplaced unspecified fracture of left lesser toe(s)**

Laterality IQ 7 **S92.506- Nondisplaced unspecified fracture of unspecified lesser toe(s)**

6 **S92.51 Fracture of proximal phalanx of lesser toe(s)**

Laterality SP 7 **S92.511- Displaced fracture of proximal phalanx of right lesser toe(s)**

Laterality SP 7 **S92.512- Displaced fracture of proximal phalanx of left lesser toe(s)**

Laterality IQ 7 **S92.513- Displaced fracture of proximal phalanx of unspecified lesser toe(s)**

Laterality SP 7 **S92.514- Nondisplaced fracture of proximal phalanx of right lesser toe(s)**

Laterality SP 7 **S92.515- Nondisplaced fracture of proximal phalanx of left lesser toe(s)**

Laterality IQ 7 **S92.516- Nondisplaced fracture of proximal phalanx of unspecified lesser toe(s)**

6 **S92.52 Fracture of middle phalanx of lesser toe(s)**

Laterality SP 7 **S92.521- Displaced fracture of middle phalanx of right lesser toe(s)**

Laterality SP 7 **S92.522- Displaced fracture of middle phalanx of left lesser toe(s)**

Laterality IQ 7 **S92.523- Displaced fracture of middle phalanx of unspecified lesser toe(s)**

Laterality SP 7 **S92.524- Nondisplaced fracture of middle phalanx of right lesser toe(s)**

Laterality SP 7 **S92.525- Nondisplaced fracture of middle phalanx of left lesser toe(s)**

Laterality IQ 7 **S92.526- Nondisplaced fracture of middle phalanx of unspecified lesser toe(s)**

6 **S92.53 Fracture of distal phalanx of lesser toe(s)**

Laterality SP 7 **S92.531- Displaced fracture of distal phalanx of right lesser toe(s)**

Laterality SP 7 **S92.532- Displaced fracture of distal phalanx of left lesser toe(s)**

Laterality IQ 7 **S92.533- Displaced fracture of distal phalanx of unspecified lesser toe(s)**

Laterality SP 7 **S92.534- Nondisplaced fracture of distal phalanx of right lesser toe(s)**

Laterality SP 7 **S92.535- Nondisplaced fracture of distal phalanx of left lesser toe(s)**

Laterality IQ 7 **S92.536- Nondisplaced fracture of distal phalanx of unspecified lesser toe(s)**

6 **S92.59 Other fracture of lesser toe(s)**

Laterality SP 7 **S92.591- Other fracture of right lesser toe(s)**

Laterality SP 7 **S92.592- Other fracture of left lesser toe(s)**

Laterality IQ 7 **S92.599- Other fracture of unspecified lesser toe(s)**

5 **S92.8 Other fracture of foot, except ankle**

6 **S92.81 Other fracture of foot**

Sesamoid fracture of foot

Chapter 19

S00-T88

CODING TIPS✓ The sesamoid bones are a pair of small bones located on the bottom surface of the first metatarsal phalangeal joint within the tendons. Sesamoid fractures can be the result of a fall from a height, sports injury or overuse.

SP 7 **S92.811- Other fracture of right foot**
SP 7 **S92.812- Other fracture of left foot**
!Q 7 **S92.819- Other fracture of unspecified foot**

5 **S92.9 Unspecified fracture of foot and toe**

6 **S92.90 Unspecified fracture of foot**

SP 7 **S92.901- Unspecified fracture of right foot**
SP 7 **S92.902- Unspecified fracture of left foot**
!Q 7 **S92.909- Unspecified fracture of unspecified foot**

6 **S92.91 Unspecified fracture of toe**

SP 7 **S92.911- Unspecified fracture of right toe(s)**
SP 7 **S92.912- Unspecified fracture of left toe(s)**
!Q 7 **S92.919- Unspecified fracture of unspecified toe(s)**

4 **S93 Dislocation and sprain of joints and ligaments at ankle, foot and toe level**

INCLUDES avulsion of joint or ligament of ankle, foot and toe
laceration of cartilage, joint or ligament of ankle, foot and toe
sprain of cartilage, joint or ligament of ankle, foot and toe
traumatic hemarthrosis of joint or ligament of ankle, foot and toe
traumatic rupture of joint or ligament of ankle, foot and toe
traumatic subluxation of joint or ligament of ankle, foot and toe
traumatic tear of joint or ligament of ankle, foot and toe

Code also:
any associated open wound

EXCLUDES 2 strain of muscle and tendon of ankle and foot (S96.-)

The appropriate 7th character is to be added to each code from category S93
A initial encounter
D subsequent encounter
S sequela

5 **S93.0 Subluxation and dislocation of ankle joint**
Subluxation and dislocation of astragalus
Subluxation and dislocation of fibula, lower end
Subluxation and dislocation of talus
Subluxation and dislocation of tibia, lower end

SP 7 **S93.01X- Subluxation of right ankle joint**
SP 7 **S93.02X- Subluxation of left ankle joint**
!Q 7 **S93.03X- Subluxation of unspecified ankle joint**
SP 7 **S93.04X- Dislocation of right ankle joint**
SP 7 **S93.05X- Dislocation of left ankle joint**
!Q 7 **S93.06X- Dislocation of unspecified ankle joint**

5 **S93.1 Subluxation and dislocation of toe**

6 **S93.10 Unspecified subluxation and dislocation of toe**
Dislocation of toe NOS
Subluxation of toe NOS

!Q 7 **S93.101- Unspecified subluxation of right toe(s)**
!Q 7 **S93.102- Unspecified subluxation of left toe(s)**
!Q 7 **S93.103- Unspecified subluxation of unspecified toe(s)**
!Q 7 **S93.104- Unspecified dislocation of right toe(s)**
!Q 7 **S93.105- Unspecified dislocation of left toe(s)**
!Q 7 **S93.106- Unspecified dislocation of unspecified toe(s)**

6 **S93.11 Dislocation of interphalangeal joint**

SP 7 **S93.111- Dislocation of interphalangeal joint of right great toe**
SP 7 **S93.112- Dislocation of interphalangeal joint of left great toe**
!Q 7 **S93.113- Dislocation of interphalangeal joint of unspecified great toe**
SP 7 **S93.114- Dislocation of interphalangeal joint of right lesser toe(s)**
SP 7 **S93.115- Dislocation of interphalangeal joint of left lesser toe(s)**
!Q 7 **S93.116- Dislocation of interphalangeal joint of unspecified lesser toe(s)**
!Q 7 **S93.119- Dislocation of interphalangeal joint of unspecified toe(s)**

6 **S93.12 Dislocation of metatarsophalangeal joint**

SP 7 **S93.121- Dislocation of metatarsophalangeal joint of right great toe**
SP 7 **S93.122- Dislocation of metatarsophalangeal joint of left great toe**
!Q 7 **S93.123- Dislocation of metatarsophalangeal joint of unspecified great toe**
SP 7 **S93.124- Dislocation of metatarsophalangeal joint of right lesser toe(s)**
SP 7 **S93.125- Dislocation of metatarsophalangeal joint of left lesser toe(s)**
!Q 7 **S93.126- Dislocation of metatarsophalangeal joint of unspecified lesser toe(s)**
!Q 7 **S93.129- Dislocation of metatarsophalangeal joint of unspecified toe(s)**

6 **S93.13 Subluxation of interphalangeal joint**

Chapter 19

S00-T88

⊟ SP 7 S93.131- Subluxation of interphalangeal joint of right great toe

⊟ SP 7 S93.132- Subluxation of interphalangeal joint of left great toe

⊟ !Q 7 S93.133- Subluxation of interphalangeal joint of unspecified great toe

⊟ SP 7 S93.134- Subluxation of interphalangeal joint of right lesser toe(s)

⊟ SP 7 S93.135- Subluxation of interphalangeal joint of left lesser toe(s)

⊟ !Q 7 S93.136- Subluxation of interphalangeal joint of unspecified lesser toe(s)

⊟ !Q 7 S93.139- Subluxation of interphalangeal joint of unspecified toe(s)

6 S93.14 Subluxation of metatarsophalangeal joint

⊟ SP 7 S93.141- Subluxation of metatarsophalangeal joint of right great toe

⊟ SP 7 S93.142- Subluxation of metatarsophalangeal joint of left great toe

⊟ !Q 7 S93.143- Subluxation of metatarsophalangeal joint of unspecified great toe

⊟ SP 7 S93.144- Subluxation of metatarsophalangeal joint of right lesser toe(s)

⊟ SP 7 S93.145- Subluxation of metatarsophalangeal joint of left lesser toe(s)

⊟ !Q 7 S93.146- Subluxation of metatarsophalangeal joint of unspecified lesser toe(s)

⊟ !Q 7 S93.149- Subluxation of metatarsophalangeal joint of unspecified toe(s)

5 S93.3 Subluxation and dislocation of foot
EXCLUDES 2 dislocation of toe (S93.1-)

6 S93.30 Unspecified subluxation and dislocation of foot
Dislocation of foot NOS
Subluxation of foot NOS

⊟ !Q 7 S93.301- Unspecified subluxation of right foot

⊟ !Q 7 S93.302- Unspecified subluxation of left foot

⊟ !Q 7 S93.303- Unspecified subluxation of unspecified foot

⊟ !Q 7 S93.304- Unspecified dislocation of right foot

⊟ !Q 7 S93.305- Unspecified dislocation of left foot

⊟ !Q 7 S93.306- Unspecified dislocation of unspecified foot

6 S93.31 Subluxation and dislocation of tarsal joint

⊟ SP 7 S93.311- Subluxation of tarsal joint of right foot

⊟ SP 7 S93.312- Subluxation of tarsal joint of left foot

⊟ !Q 7 S93.313- Subluxation of tarsal joint of unspecified foot

⊟ SP 7 S93.314- Dislocation of tarsal joint of right foot

⊟ SP 7 S93.315- Dislocation of tarsal joint of left foot

⊟ !Q 7 S93.316- Dislocation of tarsal joint of unspecified foot

6 S93.32 Subluxation and dislocation of tarsometatarsal joint

⊟ SP 7 S93.321- Subluxation of tarsometatarsal joint of right foot

⊟ SP 7 S93.322- Subluxation of tarsometatarsal joint of left foot

⊟ !Q 7 S93.323- Subluxation of tarsometatarsal joint of unspecified foot

⊟ SP 7 S93.324- Dislocation of tarsometatarsal joint of right foot

⊟ SP 7 S93.325- Dislocation of tarsometatarsal joint of left foot

⊟ !Q 7 S93.326- Dislocation of tarsometatarsal joint of unspecified foot

6 S93.33 Other subluxation and dislocation of foot

⊟ SP 7 S93.331- Other subluxation of right foot

⊟ SP 7 S93.332- Other subluxation of left foot

⊟ !Q 7 S93.333- Other subluxation of unspecified foot

⊟ SP 7 S93.334- Other dislocation of right foot

⊟ SP 7 S93.335- Other dislocation of left foot

⊟ !Q 7 S93.336- Other dislocation of unspecified foot

5 S93.4 Sprain of ankle
EXCLUDES 2 injury of Achilles tendon (S86.0-)

6 S93.40 Sprain of unspecified ligament of ankle
Sprain of ankle NOS
Sprained ankle NOS

⊟ SP 7 S93.401- Sprain of unspecified ligament of right ankle

⊟ SP 7 S93.402- Sprain of unspecified ligament of left ankle

⊟ !Q 7 S93.409- Sprain of unspecified ligament of unspecified ankle

6 S93.41 Sprain of calcaneofibular ligament

⊟ SP 7 S93.411- Sprain of calcaneofibular ligament of right ankle

⊟ SP 7 S93.412- Sprain of calcaneofibular ligament of left ankle

⊟ !Q 7 S93.419- Sprain of calcaneofibular ligament of unspecified ankle

6 S93.42 Sprain of deltoid ligament

⊟ SP 7 S93.421- Sprain of deltoid ligament of right ankle

⊟ SP 7 S93.422- Sprain of deltoid ligament of left ankle

⊟ !Q 7 S93.429- Sprain of deltoid ligament of unspecified ankle

6 S93.43 Sprain of tibiofibular ligament

⊟ SP 7 S93.431- Sprain of tibiofibular ligament of right ankle

⊟ SP 7 S93.432- Sprain of tibiofibular ligament of left ankle

⊟ !Q 7 S93.439- Sprain of tibiofibular ligament of unspecified ankle

6 S93.49 Sprain of other ligament of ankle
Sprain of internal collateral ligament

4 4th digit required 5 5th digit required 6 6th digit required 7 7th digit required ⑦ 7th digit placeholder ✚ Additional code ⊟ Laterality

Chapter 19

S00-T88

Sprain of talofibular ligament

SP 7 **S93.491- Sprain of other ligament of right ankle**

SP 7 **S93.492- Sprain of other ligament of left ankle**

!Q 7 **S93.499- Sprain of other ligament of unspecified ankle**

5 **S93.5 Sprain of toe**

6 **S93.50 Unspecified sprain of toe**

SP 7 **S93.501- Unspecified sprain of right great toe**

SP 7 **S93.502- Unspecified sprain of left great toe**

!Q 7 **S93.503- Unspecified sprain of unspecified great toe**

SP 7 **S93.504- Unspecified sprain of right lesser toe(s)**

SP 7 **S93.505- Unspecified sprain of left lesser toe(s)**

!Q 7 **S93.506- Unspecified sprain of unspecified lesser toe(s)**

!Q 7 **S93.509- Unspecified sprain of unspecified toe(s)**

6 **S93.51 Sprain of interphalangeal joint of toe**

SP 7 **S93.511- Sprain of interphalangeal joint of right great toe**

SP 7 **S93.512- Sprain of interphalangeal joint of left great toe**

!Q 7 **S93.513- Sprain of interphalangeal joint of unspecified great toe**

SP 7 **S93.514- Sprain of interphalangeal joint of right lesser toe(s)**

SP 7 **S93.515- Sprain of interphalangeal joint of left lesser toe(s)**

!Q 7 **S93.516- Sprain of interphalangeal joint of unspecified lesser toe(s)**

!Q 7 **S93.519- Sprain of interphalangeal joint of unspecified toe(s)**

6 **S93.52 Sprain of metatarsophalangeal joint of toe**

SP 7 **S93.521- Sprain of metatarsophalangeal joint of right great toe**

SP 7 **S93.522- Sprain of metatarsophalangeal joint of left great toe**

!Q 7 **S93.523- Sprain of metatarsophalangeal joint of unspecified great toe**

SP 7 **S93.524- Sprain of metatarsophalangeal joint of right lesser toe(s)**

SP 7 **S93.525- Sprain of metatarsophalangeal joint of left lesser toe(s)**

!Q 7 **S93.526- Sprain of metatarsophalangeal joint of unspecified lesser toe(s)**

!Q 7 **S93.529- Sprain of metatarsophalangeal joint of unspecified toe(s)**

5 **S93.6 Sprain of foot**

EXCLUDES 2 sprain of metatarsophalangeal joint of toe (S93.52-)
sprain of toe (S93.5-)

6 **S93.60 Unspecified sprain of foot**

SP 7 **S93.601- Unspecified sprain of right foot**

SP 7 **S93.602- Unspecified sprain of left foot**

!Q 7 **S93.609- Unspecified sprain of unspecified foot**

6 **S93.61 Sprain of tarsal ligament of foot**

SP 7 **S93.611- Sprain of tarsal ligament of right foot**

SP 7 **S93.612- Sprain of tarsal ligament of left foot**

!Q 7 **S93.619- Sprain of tarsal ligament of unspecified foot**

6 **S93.62 Sprain of tarsometatarsal ligament of foot**

SP 7 **S93.621- Sprain of tarsometatarsal ligament of right foot**

SP 7 **S93.622- Sprain of tarsometatarsal ligament of left foot**

!Q 7 **S93.629- Sprain of tarsometatarsal ligament of unspecified foot**

6 **S93.69 Other sprain of foot**

SP 7 **S93.691- Other sprain of right foot**

SP 7 **S93.692- Other sprain of left foot**

!Q 7 **S93.699- Other sprain of unspecified foot**

4 **S94 Injury of nerves at ankle and foot level**

Code also:
any associated open wound (S91.-)

The appropriate 7th character is to be added to each code from category S94
A initial encounter
D subsequent encounter
S sequela

5 **S94.0 Injury of lateral plantar nerve**

!Q 7 **S94.00X- Injury of lateral plantar nerve, unspecified leg**

SP 7 **S94.01X- Injury of lateral plantar nerve, right leg**

SP 7 **S94.02X- Injury of lateral plantar nerve, left leg**

5 **S94.1 Injury of medial plantar nerve**

!Q 7 **S94.10X- Injury of medial plantar nerve, unspecified leg**

SP 7 **S94.11X- Injury of medial plantar nerve, right leg**

SP 7 **S94.12X- Injury of medial plantar nerve, left leg**

5 **S94.2 Injury of deep peroneal nerve at ankle and foot level**

Injury of terminal, lateral branch of deep peroneal nerve

!Q 7 **S94.20X- Injury of deep peroneal nerve at ankle and foot level, unspecified leg**

SP 7 **S94.21X- Injury of deep peroneal nerve at ankle and foot level, right leg**

SP 7 **S94.22X- Injury of deep peroneal nerve at ankle and foot level, left leg**

5 **S94.3 Injury of cutaneous sensory nerve at ankle and foot level**

!Q 7 **S94.30X- Injury of cutaneous sensory nerve at ankle and foot level, unspecified leg**

SP 7 **S94.31X- Injury of cutaneous sensory nerve at ankle and foot level, right leg**

SP 7 **S94.32X- Injury of cutaneous sensory nerve at ankle and foot level, left leg**

5 **S94.8 Injury of other nerves at ankle and foot level**

6 **S94.8X Injury of other nerves at ankle and foot level**

S94.8X1- Injury of other nerves at ankle and foot level, right leg

S94.8X2- Injury of other nerves at ankle and foot level, left leg

S94.8X9- Injury of other nerves at ankle and foot level, unspecified leg

S94.9 Injury of unspecified nerve at ankle and foot level

S94.90X- Injury of unspecified nerve at ankle and foot level, unspecified leg

S94.91X- Injury of unspecified nerve at ankle and foot level, right leg

S94.92X- Injury of unspecified nerve at ankle and foot level, left leg

S95 Injury of blood vessels at ankle and foot level

Code also:

any associated open wound (S91.-)

EXCLUDES 2 injury of posterior tibial artery and vein (S85.1-, S85.8-)

The appropriate 7th character is to be added to each code from category S95

A initial encounter

D subsequent encounter

S sequela

S95.0 Injury of dorsal artery of foot

S95.00 Unspecified injury of dorsal artery of foot

S95.001- Unspecified injury of dorsal artery of right foot

S95.002- Unspecified injury of dorsal artery of left foot

S95.009- Unspecified injury of dorsal artery of unspecified foot

S95.01 Laceration of dorsal artery of foot

S95.011- Laceration of dorsal artery of right foot

S95.012- Laceration of dorsal artery of left foot

S95.019- Laceration of dorsal artery of unspecified foot

S95.09 Other specified injury of dorsal artery of foot

S95.091- Other specified injury of dorsal artery of right foot

S95.092- Other specified injury of dorsal artery of left foot

S95.099- Other specified injury of dorsal artery of unspecified foot

S95.1 Injury of plantar artery of foot

S95.10 Unspecified injury of plantar artery of foot

S95.101- Unspecified injury of plantar artery of right foot

S95.102- Unspecified injury of plantar artery of left foot

S95.109- Unspecified injury of plantar artery of unspecified foot

S95.11 Laceration of plantar artery of foot

S95.111- Laceration of plantar artery of right foot

S95.112- Laceration of plantar artery of left foot

S95.119- Laceration of plantar artery of unspecified foot

S95.19 Other specified injury of plantar artery of foot

S95.191- Other specified injury of plantar artery of right foot

S95.192- Other specified injury of plantar artery of left foot

S95.199- Other specified injury of plantar artery of unspecified foot

S95.2 Injury of dorsal vein of foot

S95.20 Unspecified injury of dorsal vein of foot

S95.201- Unspecified injury of dorsal vein of right foot

S95.202- Unspecified injury of dorsal vein of left foot

S95.209- Unspecified injury of dorsal vein of unspecified foot

S95.21 Laceration of dorsal vein of foot

S95.211- Laceration of dorsal vein of right foot

S95.212- Laceration of dorsal vein of left foot

S95.219- Laceration of dorsal vein of unspecified foot

S95.29 Other specified injury of dorsal vein of foot

S95.291- Other specified injury of dorsal vein of right foot

S95.292- Other specified injury of dorsal vein of left foot

S95.299- Other specified injury of dorsal vein of unspecified foot

S95.8 Injury of other blood vessels at ankle and foot level

S95.80 Unspecified injury of other blood vessels at ankle and foot level

S95.801- Unspecified injury of other blood vessels at ankle and foot level, right leg

S95.802- Unspecified injury of other blood vessels at ankle and foot level, left leg

S95.809- Unspecified injury of other blood vessels at ankle and foot level, unspecified leg

S95.81 Laceration of other blood vessels at ankle and foot level

S95.811- Laceration of other blood vessels at ankle and foot level, right leg

S95.812- Laceration of other blood vessels at ankle and foot level, left leg

S95.819- Laceration of other blood vessels at ankle and foot level, unspecified leg

S95.89 Other specified injury of other blood vessels at ankle and foot level

S95.891- Other specified injury of other blood vessels at ankle and foot level, right leg

S95.892- Other specified injury of other blood vessels at ankle and foot level, left leg

S95.899- Other specified injury of other blood vessels at ankle and foot level, unspecified leg

S95.9 Injury of unspecified blood vessel at ankle and foot level

S95.90 Unspecified injury of unspecified blood vessel at ankle and foot level

S95.901- Unspecified injury of unspecified blood vessel at ankle and foot level, right leg

S95.902- Unspecified injury of unspecified blood vessel at ankle and foot level, left leg

S95.909- Unspecified injury of unspecified blood vessel at ankle and foot level, unspecified leg

S95.91 Laceration of unspecified blood vessel at ankle and foot level

S95.911- Laceration of unspecified blood vessel at ankle and foot level, right leg

S95.912- Laceration of unspecified blood vessel at ankle and foot level, left leg

S95.919- Laceration of unspecified blood vessel at ankle and foot level, unspecified leg

S95.99 Other specified injury of unspecified blood vessel at ankle and foot level

S95.991- Other specified injury of unspecified blood vessel at ankle and foot level, right leg

S95.992- Other specified injury of unspecified blood vessel at ankle and foot level, left leg

S95.999- Other specified injury of unspecified blood vessel at ankle and foot level, unspecified leg

S96 Injury of muscle and tendon at ankle and foot level

Code also:

any associated open wound (S91.-)

EXCLUDES 2 injury of Achilles tendon (S86.0-)

sprain of joints and ligaments of ankle and foot (S93.-)

The appropriate 7th character is to be added to each code from category S96

A	initial encounter
D	subsequent encounter
S	sequela

S96.0 Injury of muscle and tendon of long flexor muscle of toe at ankle and foot level

S96.00 Unspecified injury of muscle and tendon of long flexor muscle of toe at ankle and foot level

S96.001- Unspecified injury of muscle and tendon of long flexor muscle of toe at ankle and foot level, right foot

S96.002- Unspecified injury of muscle and tendon of long flexor muscle of toe at ankle and foot level, left foot

S96.009- Unspecified injury of muscle and tendon of long flexor muscle of toe at ankle and foot level, unspecified foot

S96.01 Strain of muscle and tendon of long flexor muscle of toe at ankle and foot level

S96.011- Strain of muscle and tendon of long flexor muscle of toe at ankle and foot level, right foot

S96.012- Strain of muscle and tendon of long flexor muscle of toe at ankle and foot level, left foot

S96.019- Strain of muscle and tendon of long flexor muscle of toe at ankle and foot level, unspecified foot

S96.02 Laceration of muscle and tendon of long flexor muscle of toe at ankle and foot level

S96.021- Laceration of muscle and tendon of long flexor muscle of toe at ankle and foot level, right foot

S96.022- Laceration of muscle and tendon of long flexor muscle of toe at ankle and foot level, left foot

S96.029- Laceration of muscle and tendon of long flexor muscle of toe at ankle and foot level, unspecified foot

S96.09 Other injury of muscle and tendon of long flexor muscle of toe at ankle and foot level

S96.091- Other injury of muscle and tendon of long flexor muscle of toe at ankle and foot level, right foot

S96.092- Other injury of muscle and tendon of long flexor muscle of toe at ankle and foot level, left foot

S96.099- Other injury of muscle and tendon of long flexor muscle of toe at ankle and foot level, unspecified foot

S96.1 Injury of muscle and tendon of long extensor muscle of toe at ankle and foot level

S96.10 Unspecified injury of muscle and tendon of long extensor muscle of toe at ankle and foot level

S96.101- Unspecified injury of muscle and tendon of long extensor muscle of toe at ankle and foot level, right foot

S96.102- Unspecified injury of muscle and tendon of long extensor muscle of toe at ankle and foot level, left foot

S96.109- Unspecified injury of muscle and tendon of long extensor muscle of toe at ankle and foot level, unspecified foot

6 S96.11 Strain of muscle and tendon of long extensor muscle of toe at ankle and foot level

SP 7 S96.111- Strain of muscle and tendon of long extensor muscle of toe at ankle and foot level, right foot

SP 7 S96.112- Strain of muscle and tendon of long extensor muscle of toe at ankle and foot level, left foot

!Q 7 S96.119- Strain of muscle and tendon of long extensor muscle of toe at ankle and foot level, unspecified foot

6 S96.12 Laceration of muscle and tendon of long extensor muscle of toe at ankle and foot level

SP 7 S96.121- Laceration of muscle and tendon of long extensor muscle of toe at ankle and foot level, right foot

SP 7 S96.122- Laceration of muscle and tendon of long extensor muscle of toe at ankle and foot level, left foot

!Q 7 S96.129- Laceration of muscle and tendon of long extensor muscle of toe at ankle and foot level, unspecified foot

6 S96.19 Other specified injury of muscle and tendon of long extensor muscle of toe at ankle and foot level

SP 7 S96.191- Other specified injury of muscle and tendon of long extensor muscle of toe at ankle and foot level, right foot

SP 7 S96.192- Other specified injury of muscle and tendon of long extensor muscle of toe at ankle and foot level, left foot

!Q 7 S96.199- Other specified injury of muscle and tendon of long extensor muscle of toe at ankle and foot level, unspecified foot

5 S96.2 Injury of intrinsic muscle and tendon at ankle and foot level

6 S96.20 Unspecified injury of intrinsic muscle and tendon at ankle and foot level

!Q 7 S96.201- Unspecified injury of intrinsic muscle and tendon at ankle and foot level, right foot

!Q 7 S96.202- Unspecified injury of intrinsic muscle and tendon at ankle and foot level, left foot

!Q 7 S96.209- Unspecified injury of intrinsic muscle and tendon at ankle and foot level, unspecified foot

6 S96.21 Strain of intrinsic muscle and tendon at ankle and foot level

SP 7 S96.211- Strain of intrinsic muscle and tendon at ankle and foot level, right foot

SP 7 S96.212- Strain of intrinsic muscle and tendon at ankle and foot level, left foot

!Q 7 S96.219- Strain of intrinsic muscle and tendon at ankle and foot level, unspecified foot

6 S96.22 Laceration of intrinsic muscle and tendon at ankle and foot level

SP 7 S96.221- Laceration of intrinsic muscle and tendon at ankle and foot level, right foot

SP 7 S96.222- Laceration of intrinsic muscle and tendon at ankle and foot level, left foot

!Q 7 S96.229- Laceration of intrinsic muscle and tendon at ankle and foot level, unspecified foot

6 S96.29 Other specified injury of intrinsic muscle and tendon at ankle and foot level

SP 7 S96.291- Other specified injury of intrinsic muscle and tendon at ankle and foot level, right foot

SP 7 S96.292- Other specified injury of intrinsic muscle and tendon at ankle and foot level, left foot

!Q 7 S96.299- Other specified injury of intrinsic muscle and tendon at ankle and foot level, unspecified foot

5 S96.8 Injury of other specified muscles and tendons at ankle and foot level

6 S96.80 Unspecified injury of other specified muscles and tendons at ankle and foot level

!Q 7 S96.801- Unspecified injury of other specified muscles and tendons at ankle and foot level, right foot

!Q 7 S96.802- Unspecified injury of other specified muscles and tendons at ankle and foot level, left foot

!Q 7 S96.809- Unspecified injury of other specified muscles and tendons at ankle and foot level, unspecified foot

6 S96.81 Strain of other specified muscles and tendons at ankle and foot level

SP 7 S96.811- Strain of other specified muscles and tendons at ankle and foot level, right foot

SP 7 S96.812- Strain of other specified muscles and tendons at ankle and foot level, left foot

!Q 7 S96.819- Strain of other specified muscles and tendons at ankle and foot level, unspecified foot

6 S96.82 Laceration of other specified muscles and tendons at ankle and foot level

SP 7 S96.821- Laceration of other specified muscles and tendons at ankle and foot level, right foot

SP 7 S96.822- Laceration of other specified muscles and tendons at ankle and foot level, left foot

!Q 7 S96.829- Laceration of other specified muscles and tendons at ankle and foot level, unspecified foot

6 S96.89 Other specified injury of other specified muscles and tendons at ankle and foot level

SP 7 S96.891- Other specified injury of other specified muscles and tendons at ankle and foot level, right foot

SP 7 **S96.892- Other specified injury of other specified muscles and tendons at ankle and foot level, left foot**

IQ 7 **S96.899- Other specified injury of other specified muscles and tendons at ankle and foot level, unspecified foot**

5 **S96.9 Injury of unspecified muscle and tendon at ankle and foot level**

6 **S96.90 Unspecified injury of unspecified muscle and tendon at ankle and foot level**

IQ 7 **S96.901- Unspecified injury of unspecified muscle and tendon at ankle and foot level, right foot**

IQ 7 **S96.902- Unspecified injury of unspecified muscle and tendon at ankle and foot level, left foot**

IQ 7 **S96.909- Unspecified injury of unspecified muscle and tendon at ankle and foot level, unspecified foot**

6 **S96.91 Strain of unspecified muscle and tendon at ankle and foot level**

SP 7 **S96.911- Strain of unspecified muscle and tendon at ankle and foot level, right foot**

SP 7 **S96.912- Strain of unspecified muscle and tendon at ankle and foot level, left foot**

IQ 7 **S96.919- Strain of unspecified muscle and tendon at ankle and foot level, unspecified foot**

6 **S96.92 Laceration of unspecified muscle and tendon at ankle and foot level**

SP 7 **S96.921- Laceration of unspecified muscle and tendon at ankle and foot level, right foot**

SP 7 **S96.922- Laceration of unspecified muscle and tendon at ankle and foot level, left foot**

IQ 7 **S96.929- Laceration of unspecified muscle and tendon at ankle and foot level, unspecified foot**

6 **S96.99 Other specified injury of unspecified muscle and tendon at ankle and foot level**

IQ 7 **S96.991- Other specified injury of unspecified muscle and tendon at ankle and foot level, right foot**

IQ 7 **S96.992- Other specified injury of unspecified muscle and tendon at ankle and foot level, left foot**

IQ 7 **S96.999- Other specified injury of unspecified muscle and tendon at ankle and foot level, unspecified foot**

+ 4 **S97 Crushing injury of ankle and foot**

Use additional code(s) for all associated injuries

The appropriate 7th character is to be added to each code from category S97

A	initial encounter
D	subsequent encounter
S	sequela

+ 5 **S97.0 Crushing injury of ankle**

IQ + 7 **S97.00X- Crushing injury of unspecified ankle**

SP + 7 **S97.01X- Crushing injury of right ankle**

SP + 7 **S97.02X- Crushing injury of left ankle**

+ 5 **S97.1 Crushing injury of toe**

+ 6 **S97.10 Crushing injury of unspecified toe(s)**

IQ + 7 **S97.101- Crushing injury of unspecified right toe(s)**

IQ + 7 **S97.102- Crushing injury of unspecified left toe(s)**

IQ + 7 **S97.109- Crushing injury of unspecified toe(s)**

Crushing injury of toe NOS

+ 6 **S97.11 Crushing injury of great toe**

SP + 7 **S97.111- Crushing injury of right great toe**

SP + 7 **S97.112- Crushing injury of left great toe**

IQ + 7 **S97.119- Crushing injury of unspecified great toe**

+ 6 **S97.12 Crushing injury of lesser toe(s)**

SP + 7 **S97.121- Crushing injury of right lesser toe(s)**

SP + 7 **S97.122- Crushing injury of left lesser toe(s)**

IQ + 7 **S97.129- Crushing injury of unspecified lesser toe(s)**

+ 5 **S97.8 Crushing injury of foot**

IQ + 7 **S97.80X- Crushing injury of unspecified foot**

Crushing injury of foot NOS

SP + 7 **S97.81X- Crushing injury of right foot**

SP + 7 **S97.82X- Crushing injury of left foot**

4 **S98 Traumatic amputation of ankle and foot**

An amputation not identified as partial or complete should be coded to complete

The appropriate 7th character is to be added to each code from category S98

A	initial encounter
D	subsequent encounter
S	sequela

CODING TIPS ✓ Use these codes only when the amputation was due to trauma. There is no need for adding Z89 with traumatic amputations. See Z47.81 for care of amputations not due to trauma.

5 **S98.0 Traumatic amputation of foot at ankle level**

6 **S98.01 Complete traumatic amputation of foot at ankle level**

SP 7 **S98.011- Complete traumatic amputation of right foot at ankle level**

SP 7 **S98.012- Complete traumatic amputation of left foot at ankle level**

IQ 7 **S98.019- Complete traumatic amputation of unspecified foot at ankle level**

6 **S98.02 Partial traumatic amputation of foot at ankle level**

SP 7 **S98.021- Partial traumatic amputation of right foot at ankle level**

SP 7 **S98.022- Partial traumatic amputation of left foot at ankle level**

IQ 7 **S98.029- Partial traumatic amputation of unspecified foot at ankle level**

5 **S98.1 Traumatic amputation of one toe**

6 **S98.11 Complete traumatic amputation of great toe**

SP 7 **S98.111- Complete traumatic amputation of right great toe**

SP 7 **S98.112- Complete traumatic amputation of left great toe**

IQ 7 **S98.119- Complete traumatic amputation of unspecified great toe**

6 **S98.12 Partial traumatic amputation of great toe**

SP 7 **S98.121- Partial traumatic amputation of right great toe**

SP 7 **S98.122- Partial traumatic amputation of left great toe**

IQ 7 **S98.129- Partial traumatic amputation of unspecified great toe**

6 **S98.13 Complete traumatic amputation of one lesser toe**

Traumatic amputation of toe NOS

SP 7 **S98.131- Complete traumatic amputation of one right lesser toe**

SP 7 **S98.132- Complete traumatic amputation of one left lesser toe**

IQ 7 **S98.139- Complete traumatic amputation of one unspecified lesser toe**

6 **S98.14 Partial traumatic amputation of one lesser toe**

SP 7 **S98.141- Partial traumatic amputation of one right lesser toe**

SP 7 **S98.142- Partial traumatic amputation of one left lesser toe**

IQ 7 **S98.149- Partial traumatic amputation of one unspecified lesser toe**

5 **S98.2 Traumatic amputation of two or more lesser toes**

6 **S98.21 Complete traumatic amputation of two or more lesser toes**

SP 7 **S98.211- Complete traumatic amputation of two or more right lesser toes**

SP 7 **S98.212- Complete traumatic amputation of two or more left lesser toes**

IQ 7 **S98.219- Complete traumatic amputation of two or more unspecified lesser toes**

6 **S98.22 Partial traumatic amputation of two or more lesser toes**

SP 7 **S98.221- Partial traumatic amputation of two or more right lesser toes**

SP 7 **S98.222- Partial traumatic amputation of two or more left lesser toes**

IQ 7 **S98.229- Partial traumatic amputation of two or more unspecified lesser toes**

5 **S98.3 Traumatic amputation of midfoot**

6 **S98.31 Complete traumatic amputation of midfoot**

SP 7 **S98.311- Complete traumatic amputation of right midfoot**

SP 7 **S98.312- Complete traumatic amputation of left midfoot**

IQ 7 **S98.319- Complete traumatic amputation of unspecified midfoot**

6 **S98.32 Partial traumatic amputation of midfoot**

SP 7 **S98.321- Partial traumatic amputation of right midfoot**

SP 7 **S98.322- Partial traumatic amputation of left midfoot**

IQ 7 **S98.329- Partial traumatic amputation of unspecified midfoot**

5 **S98.9 Traumatic amputation of foot, level unspecified**

6 **S98.91 Complete traumatic amputation of foot, level unspecified**

SP 7 **S98.911- Complete traumatic amputation of right foot, level unspecified**

SP 7 **S98.912- Complete traumatic amputation of left foot, level unspecified**

IQ 7 **S98.919- Complete traumatic amputation of unspecified foot, level unspecified**

6 **S98.92 Partial traumatic amputation of foot, level unspecified**

SP 7 **S98.921- Partial traumatic amputation of right foot, level unspecified**

SP 7 **S98.922- Partial traumatic amputation of left foot, level unspecified**

IQ 7 **S98.929- Partial traumatic amputation of unspecified foot, level unspecified**

4 **S99 Other and unspecified injuries of ankle and foot**

5 **S99.0 Physeal fracture of calcaneus**

The appropriate 7th character is to be added to each code from subcategories S99.0

A	initial encounter for closed fracture
B	initial encounter for open fracture
D	subsequent encounter for fracture with routine healing
G	subsequent encounter for fracture with delayed healing
K	subsequent encounter for fracture with nonunion
P	subsequent encounter for fracture with malunion
S	sequela

6 **S99.00 Unspecified physeal fracture of calcaneus**

SP 7 **S99.001- Unspecified physeal fracture of right calcaneus**

SP 7 **S99.002- Unspecified physeal fracture of left calcaneus**

IQ 7 **S99.009- Unspecified physeal fracture of unspecified calcaneus**

6 **S99.01 Salter-Harris Type I physeal fracture of calcaneus**

SP 7 **S99.011- Salter-Harris Type I physeal fracture of right calcaneus**

SP 7 S99.012- Salter-Harris Type I physeal fracture of left calcaneus

IQ 7 S99.019- Salter-Harris Type I physeal fracture of unspecified calcaneus

6 S99.02 Salter-Harris Type II physeal fracture of calcaneus

SP 7 S99.021- Salter-Harris Type II physeal fracture of right calcaneus

SP 7 S99.022- Salter-Harris Type II physeal fracture of left calcaneus

IQ 7 S99.029- Salter-Harris Type II physeal fracture of unspecified calcaneus

6 S99.03 Salter-Harris Type III physeal fracture of calcaneus

SP 7 S99.031- Salter-Harris Type III physeal fracture of right calcaneus

SP 7 S99.032- Salter-Harris Type III physeal fracture of left calcaneus

IQ 7 S99.039- Salter-Harris Type III physeal fracture of unspecified calcaneus

6 S99.04 Salter-Harris Type IV physeal fracture of calcaneus

SP 7 S99.041- Salter-Harris Type IV physeal fracture of right calcaneus

SP 7 S99.042- Salter-Harris Type IV physeal fracture of left calcaneus

IQ 7 S99.049- Salter-Harris Type IV physeal fracture of unspecified calcaneus

6 S99.09 Other physeal fracture of calcaneus

SP 7 S99.091- Other physeal fracture of right calcaneus

SP 7 S99.092- Other physeal fracture of left calcaneus

IQ 7 S99.099- Other physeal fracture of unspecified calcaneus

5 S99.1 Physeal fracture of metatarsal

The appropriate 7th character is to be added to each code from subcategories S99.1

A	initial encounter for closed fracture
B	initial encounter for open fracture
D	subsequent encounter for fracture with routine healing
G	subsequent encounter for fracture with delayed healing
K	subsequent encounter for fracture with nonunion
P	subsequent encounter for fracture with malunion
S	sequela

6 S99.10 Unspecified physeal fracture of metatarsal

SP 7 S99.101- Unspecified physeal fracture of right metatarsal

SP 7 S99.102- Unspecified physeal fracture of left metatarsal

IQ 7 S99.109- Unspecified physeal fracture of unspecified metatarsal

6 S99.11 Salter-Harris Type I physeal fracture of metatarsal

SP 7 S99.111- Salter-Harris Type I physeal fracture of right metatarsal

SP 7 S99.112- Salter-Harris Type I physeal fracture of left metatarsal

IQ 7 S99.119- Salter-Harris Type I physeal fracture of unspecified metatarsal

6 S99.12 Salter-Harris Type II physeal fracture of metatarsal

SP 7 S99.121- Salter-Harris Type II physeal fracture of right metatarsal

SP 7 S99.122- Salter-Harris Type II physeal fracture of left metatarsal

IQ 7 S99.129- Salter-Harris Type II physeal fracture of unspecified metatarsal

6 S99.13 Salter-Harris Type III physeal fracture of metatarsal

SP 7 S99.131- Salter-Harris Type III physeal fracture of right metatarsal

SP 7 S99.132- Salter-Harris Type III physeal fracture of left metatarsal

IQ 7 S99.139- Salter-Harris Type III physeal fracture of unspecified metatarsal

6 S99.14 Salter-Harris Type IV physeal fracture of metatarsal

SP 7 S99.141- Salter-Harris Type IV physeal fracture of right metatarsal

SP 7 S99.142- Salter-Harris Type IV physeal fracture of left metatarsal

IQ 7 S99.149- Salter-Harris Type IV physeal fracture of unspecified metatarsal

6 S99.19 Other physeal fracture of metatarsal

SP 7 S99.191- Other physeal fracture of right metatarsal

SP 7 S99.192- Other physeal fracture of left metatarsal

IQ 7 S99.199- Other physeal fracture of unspecified metatarsal

5 S99.2 Physeal fracture of phalanx of toe

The appropriate 7th character is to be added to each code from subcategories S99.2

A	initial encounter for closed fracture
B	initial encounter for open fracture
D	subsequent encounter for fracture with routine healing
G	subsequent encounter for fracture with delayed healing
K	subsequent encounter for fracture with nonunion
P	subsequent encounter for fracture with malunion
S	sequela

6 S99.20 Unspecified physeal fracture of phalanx of toe

SP 7 S99.201- Unspecified physeal fracture of phalanx of right toe

SP 7 S99.202- Unspecified physeal fracture of phalanx of left toe

IQ 7 S99.209- Unspecified physeal fracture of phalanx of unspecified toe

6 **S99.21 Salter-Harris Type I physeal fracture of phalanx of toe**

Laterality SP 7 **S99.211- Salter-Harris Type I physeal fracture of phalanx of right toe**

Laterality SP 7 **S99.212- Salter-Harris Type I physeal fracture of phalanx of left toe**

Laterality !Q 7 **S99.219- Salter-Harris Type I physeal fracture of phalanx of unspecified toe**

6 **S99.22 Salter-Harris Type II physeal fracture of phalanx of toe**

Laterality SP 7 **S99.221- Salter-Harris Type II physeal fracture of phalanx of right toe**

Laterality SP 7 **S99.222- Salter-Harris Type II physeal fracture of phalanx of left toe**

Laterality !Q 7 **S99.229- Salter-Harris Type II physeal fracture of phalanx of unspecified toe**

6 **S99.23 Salter-Harris Type III physeal fracture of phalanx of toe**

Laterality SP 7 **S99.231- Salter-Harris Type III physeal fracture of phalanx of right toe**

Laterality SP 7 **S99.232- Salter-Harris Type III physeal fracture of phalanx of left toe**

Laterality !Q 7 **S99.239- Salter-Harris Type III physeal fracture of phalanx of unspecified toe**

6 **S99.24 Salter-Harris Type IV physeal fracture of phalanx of toe**

Laterality SP 7 **S99.241- Salter-Harris Type IV physeal fracture of phalanx of right toe**

Laterality SP 7 **S99.242- Salter-Harris Type IV physeal fracture of phalanx of left toe**

Laterality !Q 7 **S99.249- Salter-Harris Type IV physeal fracture of phalanx of unspecified toe**

6 **S99.29 Other physeal fracture of phalanx of toe**

Laterality SP 7 **S99.291- Other physeal fracture of phalanx of right toe**

Laterality SP 7 **S99.292- Other physeal fracture of phalanx of left toe**

Laterality !Q 7 **S99.299- Other physeal fracture of phalanx of unspecified toe**

5 **S99.8 Other specified injuries of ankle and foot**

The appropriate 7th character is to be added to each code from subcategory S99.8
- A initial encounter
- D subsequent encounter
- S sequela

6 **S99.81 Other specified injuries of ankle**

Laterality SP 7 **S99.811- Other specified injuries of right ankle**

Laterality SP 7 **S99.812- Other specified injuries of left ankle**

Laterality !Q 7 **S99.819- Other specified injuries of unspecified ankle**

6 **S99.82 Other specified injuries of foot**

Laterality SP 7 **S99.821- Other specified injuries of right foot**

Laterality SP 7 **S99.822- Other specified injuries of left foot**

Laterality !Q 7 **S99.829- Other specified injuries of unspecified foot**

5 **S99.9 Unspecified injury of ankle and foot**

The appropriate 7th character is to be added to each code from subcategory S99.9
- A initial encounter
- D subsequent encounter
- S sequela

6 **S99.91 Unspecified injury of ankle**

Laterality !Q 7 **S99.911- Unspecified injury of right ankle**

Laterality !Q 7 **S99.912- Unspecified injury of left ankle**

Laterality !Q 7 **S99.919- Unspecified injury of unspecified ankle**

6 **S99.92 Unspecified injury of foot**

Laterality !Q 7 **S99.921- Unspecified injury of right foot**

Laterality !Q 7 **S99.922- Unspecified injury of left foot**

Laterality !Q 7 **S99.929- Unspecified injury of unspecified foot**

Injury, poisoning and certain other consequences of external causes (T07-T88)

Injuries involving multiple body regions (T07)

EXCLUDES 1 burns and corrosions (T20-T32)
frostbite (T33-T34)
insect bite or sting, venomous (T63.4)
sunburn (L55.-)

!Q 7th digit placeholder **T07.XXX- Unspecified multiple injuries**

EXCLUDES 1 injury NOS (T14.90)

The appropriate 7th character is to be added to code T07
- A initial encounter
- D subsequent encounter
- S sequela

Injury of unspecified body region (T14)

4 **T14 Injury of unspecified body region**

EXCLUDES 1 multiple unspecified injuries (T07)

The appropriate 7th character is to be added to each code from category T14
- A initial encounter
- D subsequent encounter
- S sequela

!Q 7th digit placeholder **T14.8XX- Other injury of unspecified body region**

Abrasion NOS
Contusion NOS
Crush injury NOS
Fracture NOS
Skin injury NOS
Vascular injury NOS
Wound NOS

5 **T14.9 Unspecified injury**

!Q 7th digit placeholder **T14.90X- Injury, unspecified**

Injury NOS

SP 7th digit placeholder **T14.91X- Suicide attempt**

Attempted suicide NOS

Chapter 19 S00-T88

4 4th digit required 5 5th digit required 6 6th digit required 7 7th digit required 7th digit placeholder + Additional code Laterality

Effects of foreign body entering through natural orifice (T15-T19)

EXCLUDES 2 foreign body accidentally left in operation wound (T81.5-)
foreign body in penetrating wound - See open wound by body region
residual foreign body in soft tissue (M79.5)
splinter, without open wound - See superficial injury by body region

4 T15 Foreign body on external eye

EXCLUDES 2 foreign body in penetrating wound of orbit and eye ball (S05.4-, S05.5-)
open wound of eyelid and periocular area (S01.1-)
retained foreign body in eyelid (H02.8-)
retained (old) foreign body in penetrating wound of orbit and eye ball (H05.5-, H44.6-, H44.7-)
superficial foreign body of eyelid and periocular area (S00.25-)

The appropriate 7th character is to be added to each code from category T15
A initial encounter
D subsequent encounter
S sequela

5 T15.0 Foreign body in cornea

H IQ 7 T15.00X- Foreign body in cornea, unspecified eye

H SP 7 T15.01X- Foreign body in cornea, right eye

H SP 7 T15.02X- Foreign body in cornea, left eye

5 T15.1 Foreign body in conjunctival sac

H IQ 7 T15.10X- Foreign body in conjunctival sac, unspecified eye

H SP 7 T15.11X- Foreign body in conjunctival sac, right eye

H SP 7 T15.12X- Foreign body in conjunctival sac, left eye

5 T15.8 Foreign body in other and multiple parts of external eye
Foreign body in lacrimal punctum

H IQ 7 T15.80X- Foreign body in other and multiple parts of external eye, unspecified eye

H SP 7 T15.81X- Foreign body in other and multiple parts of external eye, right eye

H SP 7 T15.82X- Foreign body in other and multiple parts of external eye, left eye

5 T15.9 Foreign body on external eye, part unspecified

H IQ 7 T15.90X- Foreign body on external eye, part unspecified, unspecified eye

H SP 7 T15.91X- Foreign body on external eye, part unspecified, right eye

H SP 7 T15.92X- Foreign body on external eye, part unspecified, left eye

4 T16 Foreign body in ear

INCLUDES foreign body in auditory canal

The appropriate 7th character is to be added to each code from category T16
A initial encounter
D subsequent encounter
S sequela

H SP 7 T16.1XX- Foreign body in right ear

H SP 7 T16.2XX- Foreign body in left ear

H IQ 7 T16.9XX- Foreign body in ear, unspecified ear

4 T17 Foreign body in respiratory tract

The appropriate 7th character is to be added to each code from category T17
A initial encounter
D subsequent encounter
S sequela

SP 7 T17.0XX- Foreign body in nasal sinus

SP 7 T17.1XX- Foreign body in nostril
Foreign body in nose NOS

5 T17.2 Foreign body in pharynx
Foreign body in nasopharynx
Foreign body in throat NOS

6 T17.20 Unspecified foreign body in pharynx

SP 7 T17.200- Unspecified foreign body in pharynx causing asphyxiation

SP 7 T17.208- Unspecified foreign body in pharynx causing other injury

6 T17.21 Gastric contents in pharynx
Aspiration of gastric contents into pharynx
Vomitus in pharynx

SP 7 T17.210- Gastric contents in pharynx causing asphyxiation

SP 7 T17.218- Gastric contents in pharynx causing other injury

6 T17.22 Food in pharynx
Bones in pharynx
Seeds in pharynx

SP 7 T17.220- Food in pharynx causing asphyxiation

SP 7 T17.228- Food in pharynx causing other injury

6 T17.29 Other foreign object in pharynx

SP 7 T17.290- Other foreign object in pharynx causing asphyxiation

SP 7 T17.298- Other foreign object in pharynx causing other injury

5 T17.3 Foreign body in larynx

6 T17.30 Unspecified foreign body in larynx

SP 7 T17.300- Unspecified foreign body in larynx causing asphyxiation

SP 7 T17.308- Unspecified foreign body in larynx causing other injury

6 T17.31 Gastric contents in larynx
Aspiration of gastric contents into larynx
Vomitus in larynx

SP 7 T17.310- Gastric contents in larynx causing asphyxiation

SP 7 T17.318- Gastric contents in larynx causing other injury

6 T17.32 Food in larynx
Bones in larynx
Seeds in larynx

SP 7 **T17.320- Food in larynx causing asphyxiation**
SP 7 **T17.328- Food in larynx causing other injury**
6 **T17.39 Other foreign object in larynx**
SP 7 **T17.390- Other foreign object in larynx causing asphyxiation**
SP 7 **T17.398- Other foreign object in larynx causing other injury**
5 **T17.4 Foreign body in trachea**
6 **T17.40 Unspecified foreign body in trachea**
SP 7 **T17.400- Unspecified foreign body in trachea causing asphyxiation**
SP 7 **T17.408- Unspecified foreign body in trachea causing other injury**
6 **T17.41 Gastric contents in trachea**
Aspiration of gastric contents into trachea
Vomitus in trachea
SP 7 **T17.410- Gastric contents in trachea causing asphyxiation**
SP 7 **T17.418- Gastric contents in trachea causing other injury**
6 **T17.42 Food in trachea**
Bones in trachea
Seeds in trachea
SP 7 **T17.420- Food in trachea causing asphyxiation**
SP 7 **T17.428- Food in trachea causing other injury**
6 **T17.49 Other foreign object in trachea**
SP 7 **T17.490- Other foreign object in trachea causing asphyxiation**
SP 7 **T17.498- Other foreign object in trachea causing other injury**
5 **T17.5 Foreign body in bronchus**
6 **T17.50 Unspecified foreign body in bronchus**
SP 7 **T17.500- Unspecified foreign body in bronchus causing asphyxiation**
SP 7 **T17.508- Unspecified foreign body in bronchus causing other injury**
6 **T17.51 Gastric contents in bronchus**
Aspiration of gastric contents into bronchus
Vomitus in bronchus
SP 7 **T17.510- Gastric contents in bronchus causing asphyxiation**
SP 7 **T17.518- Gastric contents in bronchus causing other injury**
6 **T17.52 Food in bronchus**
Bones in bronchus
Seeds in bronchus
SP 7 **T17.520- Food in bronchus causing asphyxiation**
SP 7 **T17.528- Food in bronchus causing other injury**
6 **T17.59 Other foreign object in bronchus**
SP 7 **T17.590- Other foreign object in bronchus causing asphyxiation**
SP 7 **T17.598- Other foreign object in bronchus causing other injury**
5 **T17.8 Foreign body in other parts of respiratory tract**
Foreign body in bronchioles
Foreign body in lung
6 **T17.80 Unspecified foreign body in other parts of respiratory tract**
SP 7 **T17.800- Unspecified foreign body in other parts of respiratory tract causing asphyxiation**
SP 7 **T17.808- Unspecified foreign body in other parts of respiratory tract causing other injury**
6 **T17.81 Gastric contents in other parts of respiratory tract**
Aspiration of gastric contents into other parts of respiratory tract
Vomitus in other parts of respiratory tract
SP 7 **T17.810- Gastric contents in other parts of respiratory tract causing asphyxiation**
SP 7 **T17.818- Gastric contents in other parts of respiratory tract causing other injury**
6 **T17.82 Food in other parts of respiratory tract**
Bones in other parts of respiratory tract
Seeds in other parts of respiratory tract
SP 7 **T17.820- Food in other parts of respiratory tract causing asphyxiation**
SP 7 **T17.828- Food in other parts of respiratory tract causing other injury**
6 **T17.89 Other foreign object in other parts of respiratory tract**
SP 7 **T17.890- Other foreign object in other parts of respiratory tract causing asphyxiation**
SP 7 **T17.898- Other foreign object in other parts of respiratory tract causing other injury**
5 **T17.9 Foreign body in respiratory tract, part unspecified**
6 **T17.90 Unspecified foreign body in respiratory tract, part unspecified**
SP 7 **T17.900- Unspecified foreign body in respiratory tract, part unspecified causing asphyxiation**
SP 7 **T17.908- Unspecified foreign body in respiratory tract, part unspecified causing other injury**
6 **T17.91 Gastric contents in respiratory tract, part unspecified**
Aspiration of gastric contents into respiratory tract, part unspecified
Vomitus in trachea respiratory tract, part unspecified
SP 7 **T17.910- Gastric contents in respiratory tract, part unspecified causing asphyxiation**
SP 7 **T17.918- Gastric contents in respiratory tract, part unspecified causing other injury**
6 **T17.92 Food in respiratory tract, part unspecified**
Bones in respiratory tract, part unspecified
Seeds in respiratory tract, part unspecified

SP 7 **T17.920- Food in respiratory tract, part unspecified causing asphyxiation**

SP 7 **T17.928- Food in respiratory tract, part unspecified causing other injury**

6 **T17.99 Other foreign object in respiratory tract, part unspecified**

SP 7 **T17.990- Other foreign object in respiratory tract, part unspecified in causing asphyxiation**

SP 7 **T17.998- Other foreign object in respiratory tract, part unspecified causing other injury**

4 **T18 Foreign body in alimentary tract**

EXCLUDES 2 foreign body in pharynx (T17.2-)

The appropriate 7th character is to be added to each code from category T18
A initial encounter
D subsequent encounter
S sequela

SP 7 **T18.0XX- Foreign body in mouth**

5 **T18.1 Foreign body in esophagus**

EXCLUDES 2 foreign body in respiratory tract (T17.-)

6 **T18.10 Unspecified foreign body in esophagus**

SP 7 **T18.100- Unspecified foreign body in esophagus causing compression of trachea**

Unspecified foreign body in esophagus causing obstruction of respiration

SP 7 **T18.108- Unspecified foreign body in esophagus causing other injury**

6 **T18.11 Gastric contents in esophagus**

Vomitus in esophagus

SP 7 **T18.110- Gastric contents in esophagus causing compression of trachea**

Gastric contents in esophagus causing obstruction of respiration

SP 7 **T18.118- Gastric contents in esophagus causing other injury**

6 **T18.12 Food in esophagus**

Bones in esophagus
Seeds in esophagus

SP 7 **T18.120- Food in esophagus causing compression of trachea**

Food in esophagus causing obstruction of respiration

SP 7 **T18.128- Food in esophagus causing other injury**

6 **T18.19 Other foreign object in esophagus**

SP 7 **T18.190- Other foreign object in esophagus causing compression of trachea**

Other foreign body in esophagus causing obstruction of respiration

SP 7 **T18.198- Other foreign object in esophagus causing other injury**

SP 7 **T18.2XX- Foreign body in stomach**

SP 7 **T18.3XX- Foreign body in small intestine**

SP 7 **T18.4XX- Foreign body in colon**

SP 7 **T18.5XX- Foreign body in anus and rectum**

Foreign body in rectosigmoid (junction)

SP 7 **T18.8XX- Foreign body in other parts of alimentary tract**

SP 7 **T18.9XX- Foreign body of alimentary tract, part unspecified**

Foreign body in digestive system NOS
Swallowed foreign body NOS

4 **T19 Foreign body in genitourinary tract**

EXCLUDES 2 complications due to implanted mesh (T83.7-)
mechanical complications of contraceptive device (intrauterine) (vaginal) (T83.3-)
presence of contraceptive device (intrauterine) (vaginal) (Z97.5)

The appropriate 7th character is to be added to each code from category T19
A initial encounter
D subsequent encounter
S sequela

SP 7 **T19.0XX- Foreign body in urethra**

SP 7 **T19.1XX- Foreign body in bladder**

SP 7 **T19.2XX- Foreign body in vulva and vagina**

SP 7 **T19.3XX- Foreign body in uterus**

SP 7 **T19.4XX- Foreign body in penis**

SP 7 **T19.8XX- Foreign body in other parts of genitourinary tract**

SP 7 **T19.9XX- Foreign body in genitourinary tract, part unspecified**

Burns and corrosions (T20-T32)

INCLUDES burns (thermal) from electrical heating appliances
burns (thermal) from electricity
burns (thermal) from flame
burns (thermal) from friction
burns (thermal) from hot air and hot gases
burns (thermal) from hot objects
burns (thermal) from lightning
burns (thermal) from radiation
chemical burn [corrosion] (external) (internal)
scalds

EXCLUDES 2 erythema [dermatitis] ab igne (L59.0)
radiation-related disorders of the skin and subcutaneous tissue (L55-L59)
sunburn (L55.-)

GUIDELINES **Section I.C.19.d.1)-5)**
Sequence first the code that reflects the highest degree of burn when more than one burn is present.
a. When the reason for the admission or encounter is for treatment of external multiple burns, sequence first the code that reflects the burn of the highest degree.
b. When a patient has both internal and external burns, the circumstances of admission govern the selection of the principal diagnosis or first-listed diagnosis.
c. When a patient is admitted for burn injuries and other related conditions such as smoke inhalation and/or respiratory failure, the circumstances of admission govern the selection of the principal or first-listed diagnosis.

Classify burns of the same anatomic site and on the same side but of different degrees to the subcategory identifying the highest degree recorded in the diagnosis (e.g., for second and third degree burns of right thigh, assign only code T24.311-).

Non-healing burns are coded as acute burns. Necrosis of burned skin should be coded as a non-healed burn.

For any documented infected burn site, use an additional code for the infection.

When coding burns, assign separate codes for each burn site. Codes for burns of "multiple sites" should only be assigned when the medical record documentation does not specify the individual sites.

GUIDELINES **Section I.C.19.d**
The ICD-10-CM makes a distinction between burns and corrosions. The burn codes are for thermal burns, except sunburns, that come from a heat source, such as a fire or hot appliance. The burn codes are also for burns resulting from electricity and radiation. Corrosions are burns due to chemicals. The guidelines are the same for burns and corrosions.

CODING TIPS✓ When a patient presents with a burn (other than sunburn), an additional code from Chapter 20 (External causes) should be added to indicate the cause (intent) of the burn.

CODING TIPS✓ A burn that is referred to as "not healing" should be coded as an acute burn using 7th character "A" or "D". Sequelae of a burn, such as contracture or keloid scarring, should be coded by first assigning the code for the residual condition, followed by the appropriate code to identify the burn with the 7th character "S" to indicate sequelae.

Burns and corrosions of external body surface, specified by site (T20-T25)

INCLUDES burns and corrosions of first degree [erythema]
burns and corrosions of second degree [blisters][epidermal loss]
burns and corrosions of third degree [deep necrosis of underlying tissue] [full- thickness skin loss]

Use additional code from category T31 or T32 to identify extent of body surface involved

GUIDELINES **Section I.C.19.d**
Current burns (T20-T25) are classified by depth, extent and by agent (X code). Burns are classified by depth as first degree (erythema), second degree (blistering), and third degree (full-thickness involvement). Burns of the eye and internal organs (T26-T28) are classified by site, but not by degree.

4 T20 Burn and corrosion of head, face, and neck
EXCLUDES 2 burn and corrosion of ear drum (T28.41, T28.91)
burn and corrosion of eye and adnexa (T26.-)
burn and corrosion of mouth and pharynx (T28.0)

The appropriate 7th character is to be added to each code from category T20
A initial encounter
D subsequent encounter
S sequela

CODING TIPS✓ Burns are classified according to degree. When there are multiple burns of different degrees to the same body part, code the burn at its highest degree. Remember, there is a convention requiring the external cause code at burns. Aftercare codes are not used for burns, including those for dressing changes, drain care, suture removal, or skin grafts. 7th character 'D' is the default for home care and hospice when providing aftercare for a healing or resolving condition; 'A' is used for active treatment such as antibiotics or more than routine wound care; 'S' is used to identify residual conditions when the burn has healed. Different burns heal at differing rates, so a current burn (with an A or D) can be coded at the same time as a sequela of a burn. A non-healing burn is still coded as a burn no matter how long it has been present.

+5 **T20.0 Burn of unspecified degree of head, face, and neck**
Use additional external cause code to identify the source, place and intent of the burn (X00-X19, X75-X77, X96-X98, Y92)

IQ +7 **T20.00X- Burn of unspecified degree of head, face, and neck, unspecified site**

+6 **T20.01 Burn of unspecified degree of ear [any part, except ear drum]**
EXCLUDES 2 burn of ear drum (T28.41-)

L IQ +7 **T20.011- Burn of unspecified degree of right ear [any part, except ear drum]**

L IQ +7 **T20.012- Burn of unspecified degree of left ear [any part, except ear drum]**

L IQ +7 **T20.019- Burn of unspecified degree of unspecified ear [any part, except ear drum]**

SP IQ +7 **T20.02X- Burn of unspecified degree of lip(s)**

IQ +7 **T20.03X- Burn of unspecified degree of chin**

IQ +7 **T20.04X- Burn of unspecified degree of nose (septum)**

IQ +7 **T20.05X- Burn of unspecified degree of scalp [any part]**

IQ +7 **T20.06X- Burn of unspecified degree of forehead and cheek**

IQ +7 **T20.07X- Burn of unspecified degree of neck**

IQ +7 **T20.09X- Burn of unspecified degree of multiple sites of head, face, and neck**

Chapter 19 S00-T88

+ 5 **T20.1 Burn of first degree of head, face, and neck**
Use additional external cause code to identify the source, place and intent of the burn (X00-X19, X75-X77, X96-X98, Y92)

IQ + 7 **T20.10X- Burn of first degree of head, face, and neck, unspecified site**

+ 6 **T20.11 Burn of first degree of ear [any part, except ear drum]**
EXCLUDES 2 burn of ear drum (T28.41-)

SP + 7 **T20.111- Burn of first degree of right ear [any part, except ear drum]**

SP + 7 **T20.112- Burn of first degree of left ear [any part, except ear drum]**

IQ + 7 **T20.119- Burn of first degree of unspecified ear [any part, except ear drum]**

SP + 7 **T20.12X- Burn of first degree of lip(s)**

SP + 7 **T20.13X- Burn of first degree of chin**

SP + 7 **T20.14X- Burn of first degree of nose (septum)**

SP + 7 **T20.15X- Burn of first degree of scalp [any part]**

SP + 7 **T20.16X- Burn of first degree of forehead and cheek**

SP + 7 **T20.17X- Burn of first degree of neck**

SP + 7 **T20.19X- Burn of first degree of multiple sites of head, face, and neck**

+ 5 **T20.2 Burn of second degree of head, face, and neck**
Use additional external cause code to identify the source, place and intent of the burn (X00-X19, X75-X77, X96-X98, Y92)

IQ + 7 **T20.20X- Burn of second degree of head, face, and neck, unspecified site**

+ 6 **T20.21 Burn of second degree of ear [any part, except ear drum]**
EXCLUDES 2 burn of ear drum (T28.41-)

SP + 7 **T20.211- Burn of second degree of right ear [any part, except ear drum]**

SP + 7 **T20.212- Burn of second degree of left ear [any part, except ear drum]**

IQ + 7 **T20.219- Burn of second degree of unspecified ear [any part, except ear drum]**

SP + 7 **T20.22X- Burn of second degree of lip(s)**

SP + 7 **T20.23X- Burn of second degree of chin**

SP + 7 **T20.24X- Burn of second degree of nose (septum)**

SP + 7 **T20.25X- Burn of second degree of scalp [any part]**

SP + 7 **T20.26X- Burn of second degree of forehead and cheek**

SP + 7 **T20.27X- Burn of second degree of neck**

SP + 7 **T20.29X- Burn of second degree of multiple sites of head, face, and neck**

+ 5 **T20.3 Burn of third degree of head, face, and neck**
Use additional external cause code to identify the source, place and intent of the burn (X00-X19, X75-X77, X96-X98, Y92)

IQ + 7 **T20.30X- Burn of third degree of head, face, and neck, unspecified site**

+ 6 **T20.31 Burn of third degree of ear [any part, except ear drum]**
EXCLUDES 2 burn of ear drum (T28.41-)

SP + 7 **T20.311- Burn of third degree of right ear [any part, except ear drum]**

SP + 7 **T20.312- Burn of third degree of left ear [any part, except ear drum]**

IQ + 7 **T20.319- Burn of third degree of unspecified ear [any part, except ear drum]**

SP + 7 **T20.32X- Burn of third degree of lip(s)**

SP + 7 **T20.33X- Burn of third degree of chin**

SP + 7 **T20.34X- Burn of third degree of nose (septum)**

SP + 7 **T20.35X- Burn of third degree of scalp [any part]**

SP + 7 **T20.36X- Burn of third degree of forehead and cheek**

SP + 7 **T20.37X- Burn of third degree of neck**

SP + 7 **T20.39X- Burn of third degree of multiple sites of head, face, and neck**

+ 5 **T20.4 Corrosion of unspecified degree of head, face, and neck**
Code first:
(T51-T65) to identify chemical and intent
Use additional external cause code to identify place (Y92)

IQ + 7 **T20.40X- Corrosion of unspecified degree of head, face, and neck, unspecified site**

+ 6 **T20.41 Corrosion of unspecified degree of ear [any part, except ear drum]**
EXCLUDES 2 corrosion of ear drum (T28.91-)

IQ + 7 **T20.411- Corrosion of unspecified degree of right ear [any part, except ear drum]**

IQ + 7 **T20.412- Corrosion of unspecified degree of left ear [any part, except ear drum]**

IQ + 7 **T20.419- Corrosion of unspecified degree of unspecified ear [any part, except ear drum]**

IQ + 7 **T20.42X- Corrosion of unspecified degree of lip(s)**

IQ + 7 **T20.43X- Corrosion of unspecified degree of chin**

IQ + 7 **T20.44X- Corrosion of unspecified degree of nose (septum)**

IQ + 7 **T20.45X- Corrosion of unspecified degree of scalp [any part]**

IQ + 7 **T20.46X- Corrosion of unspecified degree of forehead and cheek**

IQ + 7 **T20.47X- Corrosion of unspecified degree of neck**

IQ + 7 **T20.49X- Corrosion of unspecified degree of multiple sites of head, face, and neck**

Chapter 19 S00-T88

+ 5 **T20.5 Corrosion of first degree of head, face, and neck**
Code first:
(T51-T65) to identify chemical and intent
Use additional external cause code to identify place (Y92)

IQ + 7 **T20.50X- Corrosion of first degree of head, face, and neck, unspecified site**

+ 6 **T20.51 Corrosion of first degree of ear [any part, except ear drum]**
EXCLUDES 2 corrosion of ear drum (T28.91-)

⊟ IQ + 7 **T20.511- Corrosion of first degree of right ear [any part, except ear drum]**

⊟ IQ + 7 **T20.512- Corrosion of first degree of left ear [any part, except ear drum]**

⊟ IQ + 7 **T20.519- Corrosion of first degree of unspecified ear [any part, except ear drum]**

IQ + 7 **T20.52X- Corrosion of first degree of lip(s)**

IQ + 7 **T20.53X- Corrosion of first degree of chin**

IQ + 7 **T20.54X- Corrosion of first degree of nose (septum)**

IQ + 7 **T20.55X- Corrosion of first degree of scalp [any part]**

IQ + 7 **T20.56X- Corrosion of first degree of forehead and cheek**

IQ + 7 **T20.57X- Corrosion of first degree of neck**

IQ + 7 **T20.59X- Corrosion of first degree of multiple sites of head, face, and neck**

+ 5 **T20.6 Corrosion of second degree of head, face, and neck**
Code first:
(T51-T65) to identify chemical and intent
Use additional external cause code to identify place (Y92)

IQ + 7 **T20.60X- Corrosion of second degree of head, face, and neck, unspecified site**

+ 6 **T20.61 Corrosion of second degree of ear [any part, except ear drum]**
EXCLUDES 2 corrosion of ear drum (T28.91-)

⊟ SP + 7 **T20.611- Corrosion of second degree of right ear [any part, except ear drum]**

⊟ SP + 7 **T20.612- Corrosion of second degree of left ear [any part, except ear drum]**

⊟ IQ + 7 **T20.619- Corrosion of second degree of unspecified ear [any part, except ear drum]**

SP + 7 **T20.62X- Corrosion of second degree of lip(s)**

SP + 7 **T20.63X- Corrosion of second degree of chin**

SP + 7 **T20.64X- Corrosion of second degree of nose (septum)**

SP + 7 **T20.65X- Corrosion of second degree of scalp [any part]**

SP + 7 **T20.66X- Corrosion of second degree of forehead and cheek**

SP + 7 **T20.67X- Corrosion of second degree of neck**

SP + 7 **T20.69X- Corrosion of second degree of multiple sites of head, face, and neck**

+ 5 **T20.7 Corrosion of third degree of head, face, and neck**
Code first:
(T51-T65) to identify chemical and intent
Use additional external cause code to identify place (Y92)

IQ + 7 **T20.70X- Corrosion of third degree of head, face, and neck, unspecified site**

+ 6 **T20.71 Corrosion of third degree of ear [any part, except ear drum]**
EXCLUDES 2 corrosion of ear drum (T28.91-)

⊟ SP + 7 **T20.711- Corrosion of third degree of right ear [any part, except ear drum]**

⊟ SP + 7 **T20.712- Corrosion of third degree of left ear [any part, except ear drum]**

⊟ IQ + 7 **T20.719- Corrosion of third degree of unspecified ear [any part, except ear drum]**

SP + 7 **T20.72X- Corrosion of third degree of lip(s)**

SP + 7 **T20.73X- Corrosion of third degree of chin**

SP + 7 **T20.74X- Corrosion of third degree of nose (septum)**

SP + 7 **T20.75X- Corrosion of third degree of scalp [any part]**

SP + 7 **T20.76X- Corrosion of third degree of forehead and cheek**

SP + 7 **T20.77X- Corrosion of third degree of neck**

SP + 7 **T20.79X- Corrosion of third degree of multiple sites of head, face, and neck**

4 **T21 Burn and corrosion of trunk**
INCLUDES burns and corrosion of hip region
EXCLUDES 2 burns and corrosion of axilla (T22.- with fifth character 4)
burns and corrosion of scapular region (T22.- with fifth character 6)
burns and corrosion of shoulder (T22.- with fifth character 5)

The appropriate 7th character is to be added to each code from category T21
A initial encounter
D subsequent encounter
S sequela

CODING TIPS ✓ Do not use Z codes for skin grafts, dressing changes, drains, etc., for trauma wounds of any type, including burns. Continue to code the burn with the appropriate 7th character.

Chapter 19 S00-T88

CODING TIPS✓ Burns are classified according to degree. When there are multiple burns of different degrees to the same body part, code the burn at its highest degree. Remember, there is a convention requiring the external cause code at burns. Aftercare codes are not used for burns, including those for dressing changes, drain care, suture removal, or skin grafts. 7th character 'D' is the default for home care and hospice when providing aftercare for a healing or resolving condition; 'A' is used for active treatment such as antibiotics or more than routine wound care; 'S' is used to identify residual conditions when the burn has healed. Different burns heal at differing rates, so a current burn (with an A or D) can be coded at the same time as a sequela of a burn. A non-healing burn is still coded as a burn no matter how long it has been present.

+ 5 **T21.0 Burn of unspecified degree of trunk**
Use additional external cause code to identify the source, place and intent of the burn (X00-X19, X75-X77, X96-X98, Y92)

IQ + 7 **T21.00X- Burn of unspecified degree of trunk, unspecified site**

IQ + 7 **T21.01X- Burn of unspecified degree of chest wall**
Burn of unspecified degree of breast

IQ + 7 **T21.02X- Burn of unspecified degree of abdominal wall**
Burn of unspecified degree of flank
Burn of unspecified degree of groin

IQ + 7 **T21.03X- Burn of unspecified degree of upper back**
Burn of unspecified degree of interscapular region

IQ + 7 **T21.04X- Burn of unspecified degree of lower back**

IQ + 7 **T21.05X- Burn of unspecified degree of buttock**
Burn of unspecified degree of anus

IQ + 7 **T21.06X- Burn of unspecified degree of male genital region**
Burn of unspecified degree of penis
Burn of unspecified degree of scrotum
Burn of unspecified degree of testis

IQ + 7 **T21.07X- Burn of unspecified degree of female genital region**
Burn of unspecified degree of labium (majus) (minus)
Burn of unspecified degree of perineum
Burn of unspecified degree of vulva
EXCLUDES 2 burn of vagina (T28.3)

IQ + 7 **T21.09X- Burn of unspecified degree of other site of trunk**

+ 5 **T21.1 Burn of first degree of trunk**
Use additional external cause code to identify the source, place and intent of the burn (X00-X19, X75-X77, X96-X98, Y92)

IQ + 7 **T21.10X- Burn of first degree of trunk, unspecified site**

SP + 7 **T21.11X- Burn of first degree of chest wall**
Burn of first degree of breast

SP + 7 **T21.12X- Burn of first degree of abdominal wall**
Burn of first degree of flank
Burn of first degree of groin

SP + 7 **T21.13X- Burn of first degree of upper back**
Burn of first degree of interscapular region

SP + 7 **T21.14X- Burn of first degree of lower back**

SP + 7 **T21.15X- Burn of first degree of buttock**
Burn of first degree of anus

SP + 7 **T21.16X- Burn of first degree of male genital region**
Burn of first degree of penis
Burn of first degree of scrotum
Burn of first degree of testis

SP + 7 **T21.17X- Burn of first degree of female genital region**
Burn of first degree of labium (majus) (minus)
Burn of first degree of perineum
Burn of first degree of vulva
EXCLUDES 2 burn of vagina (T28.3)

SP + 7 **T21.19X- Burn of first degree of other site of trunk**

+ 5 **T21.2 Burn of second degree of trunk**
Use additional external cause code to identify the source, place and intent of the burn (X00-X19, X75-X77, X96-X98, Y92)

IQ + 7 **T21.20X- Burn of second degree of trunk, unspecified site**

SP + 7 **T21.21X- Burn of second degree of chest wall**
Burn of second degree of breast

SP + 7 **T21.22X- Burn of second degree of abdominal wall**
Burn of second degree of flank
Burn of second degree of groin

SP + 7 **T21.23X- Burn of second degree of upper back**
Burn of second degree of interscapular region

SP + 7 **T21.24X- Burn of second degree of lower back**

SP + 7 **T21.25X- Burn of second degree of buttock**
Burn of second degree of anus

SP + 7 **T21.26X- Burn of second degree of male genital region**
Burn of second degree of penis
Burn of second degree of scrotum
Burn of second degree of testis

SP + 7 **T21.27X- Burn of second degree of female genital region**
Burn of second degree of labium (majus) (minus)
Burn of second degree of perineum
Burn of second degree of vulva
EXCLUDES 2 burn of vagina (T28.3)

SP + 7 **T21.29X- Burn of second degree of other site of trunk**

+ 5 **T21.3 Burn of third degree of trunk**

Use additional external cause code to identify the source, place and intent of the burn (X00-X19, X75-X77, X96-X98, Y92)

IQ + T21.30X- **Burn of third degree of trunk, unspecified site**

SP + T21.31X- **Burn of third degree of chest wall**
Burn of third degree of breast

SP + T21.32X- **Burn of third degree of abdominal wall**
Burn of third degree of flank
Burn of third degree of groin

SP + T21.33X- **Burn of third degree of upper back**
Burn of third degree of interscapular region

SP + T21.34X- **Burn of third degree of lower back**

SP + T21.35X- **Burn of third degree of buttock**
Burn of third degree of anus

SP + T21.36X- **Burn of third degree of male genital region**
Burn of third degree of penis
Burn of third degree of scrotum
Burn of third degree of testis

SP + T21.37X- **Burn of third degree of female genital region**
Burn of third degree of labium (majus) (minus)
Burn of third degree of perineum
Burn of third degree of vulva
EXCLUDES 2 burn of vagina (T28.3)

SP + T21.39X- **Burn of third degree of other site of trunk**

+ T21.4 **Corrosion of unspecified degree of trunk**
Code first:
(T51-T65) to identify chemical and intent
Use additional external cause code to identify place (Y92)

IQ + T21.40X- **Corrosion of unspecified degree of trunk, unspecified site**

IQ + T21.41X- **Corrosion of unspecified degree of chest wall**
Corrosion of unspecified degree of breast

IQ + T21.42X- **Corrosion of unspecified degree of abdominal wall**
Corrosion of unspecified degree of flank
Corrosion of unspecified degree of groin

IQ + T21.43X- **Corrosion of unspecified degree of upper back**
Corrosion of unspecified degree of interscapular region

IQ + T21.44X- **Corrosion of unspecified degree of lower back**

IQ + T21.45X- **Corrosion of unspecified degree of buttock**
Corrosion of unspecified degree of anus

IQ + T21.46X- **Corrosion of unspecified degree of male genital region**
Corrosion of unspecified degree of penis
Corrosion of unspecified degree of scrotum
Corrosion of unspecified degree of testis

IQ + T21.47X- **Corrosion of unspecified degree of female genital region**
Corrosion of unspecified degree of labium (majus) (minus)
Corrosion of unspecified degree of perineum
Corrosion of unspecified degree of vulva
EXCLUDES 2 corrosion of vagina (T28.8)

IQ + T21.49X- **Corrosion of unspecified degree of other site of trunk**

+ T21.5 **Corrosion of first degree of trunk**
Code first:
(T51-T65) to identify chemical and intent
Use additional external cause code to identify place (Y92)

IQ + T21.50X- **Corrosion of first degree of trunk, unspecified site**

SP + T21.51X- **Corrosion of first degree of chest wall**
Corrosion of first degree of breast

SP + T21.52X- **Corrosion of first degree of abdominal wall**
Corrosion of first degree of flank
Corrosion of first degree of groin

SP + T21.53X- **Corrosion of first degree of upper back**
Corrosion of first degree of interscapular region

SP + T21.54X- **Corrosion of first degree of lower back**

SP + T21.55X- **Corrosion of first degree of buttock**
Corrosion of first degree of anus

SP + T21.56X- **Corrosion of first degree of male genital region**
Corrosion of first degree of penis
Corrosion of first degree of scrotum
Corrosion of first degree of testis

SP + T21.57X- **Corrosion of first degree of female genital region**
Corrosion of first degree of labium (majus) (minus)
Corrosion of first degree of perineum
Corrosion of first degree of vulva
EXCLUDES 2 corrosion of vagina (T28.8)

IQ + T21.59X- **Corrosion of first degree of other site of trunk**

+ T21.6 **Corrosion of second degree of trunk**
Code first:
(T51-T65) to identify chemical and intent
Use additional external cause code to identify place (Y92)

IQ + T21.60X- **Corrosion of second degree of trunk, unspecified site**

SP + T21.61X- **Corrosion of second degree of chest wall**
Corrosion of second degree of breast

Chapter 19

S00-T88

SP + 7 **T21.62X- Corrosion of second degree of abdominal wall**
Corrosion of second degree of flank
Corrosion of second degree of groin

SP + 7 **T21.63X- Corrosion of second degree of upper back**
Corrosion of second degree of interscapular region

SP + 7 **T21.64X- Corrosion of second degree of lower back**

SP + 7 **T21.65X- Corrosion of second degree of buttock**
Corrosion of second degree of anus

SP + 7 **T21.66X- Corrosion of second degree of male genital region**
Corrosion of second degree of penis
Corrosion of second degree of scrotum
Corrosion of second degree of testis

SP + 7 **T21.67X- Corrosion of second degree of female genital region**
Corrosion of second degree of labium (majus) (minus)
Corrosion of second degree of perineum
Corrosion of second degree of vulva
EXCLUDES 2 corrosion of vagina (T28.8)

!Q + 7 **T21.69X- Corrosion of second degree of other site of trunk**

+ 5 **T21.7 Corrosion of third degree of trunk**
Code first:
(T51-T65) to identify chemical and intent
Use additional external cause code to identify place (Y92)

!Q + 7 **T21.70X- Corrosion of third degree of trunk, unspecified site**

SP + 7 **T21.71X- Corrosion of third degree of chest wall**
Corrosion of third degree of breast

SP + 7 **T21.72X- Corrosion of third degree of abdominal wall**
Corrosion of third degree of flank
Corrosion of third degree of groin

SP + 7 **T21.73X- Corrosion of third degree of upper back**
Corrosion of third degree of interscapular region

SP + 7 **T21.74X- Corrosion of third degree of lower back**

SP + 7 **T21.75X- Corrosion of third degree of buttock**
Corrosion of third degree of anus

SP + 7 **T21.76X- Corrosion of third degree of male genital region**
Corrosion of third degree of penis
Corrosion of third degree of scrotum
Corrosion of third degree of testis

SP + 7 **T21.77X- Corrosion of third degree of female genital region**
Corrosion of third degree of labium (majus) (minus)
Corrosion of third degree of perineum
Corrosion of third degree of vulva
EXCLUDES 2 corrosion of vagina (T28.8)

!Q + 7 **T21.79X- Corrosion of third degree of other site of trunk**

4 **T22 Burn and corrosion of shoulder and upper limb, except wrist and hand**
EXCLUDES 2 burn and corrosion of interscapular region (T21.-)
burn and corrosion of wrist and hand (T23.-)

The appropriate 7th character is to be added to each code from category T22

A	initial encounter
D	subsequent encounter
S	sequela

CODING TIPS✓ Do not use Z codes for skin grafts, dressing changes, drains, etc., for trauma wounds of any type, including burns. Continue to code the burn with the appropriate 7th character.

CODING TIPS✓ Burns are classified according to degree. When there are multiple burns of different degrees to the same body part, code the burn at its highest degree. Remember, there is a convention requiring the external cause code at burns. Aftercare codes are not used for burns, including those for dressing changes, drain care, suture removal, or skin grafts. 7th character 'D' is the default for home care and hospice when providing aftercare for a healing or resolving condition; 'A' is used for active treatment such as antibiotics or more than routine wound care; 'S' is used to identify residual conditions when the burn has healed. Different burns heal at differing rates, so a current burn (with an A or D) can be coded at the same time as a sequela of a burn. A non-healing burn is still coded as a burn no matter how long it has been present.

+ 5 **T22.0 Burn of unspecified degree of shoulder and upper limb, except wrist and hand**
Use additional external cause code to identify the source, place and intent of the burn (X00-X19, X75-X77, X96-X98, Y92)

!Q + 7 **T22.00X- Burn of unspecified degree of shoulder and upper limb, except wrist and hand, unspecified site**

+ 6 **T22.01 Burn of unspecified degree of forearm**

H !Q + 7 **T22.011- Burn of unspecified degree of right forearm**

H !Q + 7 **T22.012- Burn of unspecified degree of left forearm**

H !Q + 7 **T22.019- Burn of unspecified degree of unspecified forearm**

+ 6 **T22.02 Burn of unspecified degree of elbow**

H !Q + 7 **T22.021- Burn of unspecified degree of right elbow**

H !Q + 7 **T22.022- Burn of unspecified degree of left elbow**

H !Q + 7 **T22.029- Burn of unspecified degree of unspecified elbow**

+ 6 **T22.03 Burn of unspecified degree of upper arm**

H !Q + 7 **T22.031- Burn of unspecified degree of right upper arm**

Chapter 19 S00-T88

[L] [IQ] + [7] T22.032- Burn of unspecified degree of left upper arm

[L] [IQ] + [7] T22.039- Burn of unspecified degree of unspecified upper arm

+ [6] T22.04 Burn of unspecified degree of axilla

[L] [IQ] + [7] T22.041- Burn of unspecified degree of right axilla

[L] [IQ] + [7] T22.042- Burn of unspecified degree of left axilla

[L] [IQ] + [7] T22.049- Burn of unspecified degree of unspecified axilla

+ [6] T22.05 Burn of unspecified degree of shoulder

[L] [IQ] + [7] T22.051- Burn of unspecified degree of right shoulder

[L] [IQ] + [7] T22.052- Burn of unspecified degree of left shoulder

[L] [IQ] + [7] T22.059- Burn of unspecified degree of unspecified shoulder

+ [6] T22.06 Burn of unspecified degree of scapular region

[L] [IQ] + [7] T22.061- Burn of unspecified degree of right scapular region

[L] [IQ] + [7] T22.062- Burn of unspecified degree of left scapular region

[L] [IQ] + [7] T22.069- Burn of unspecified degree of unspecified scapular region

+ [6] T22.09 Burn of unspecified degree of multiple sites of shoulder and upper limb, except wrist and hand

[L] [IQ] + [7] T22.091- Burn of unspecified degree of multiple sites of right shoulder and upper limb, except wrist and hand

[L] [IQ] + [7] T22.092- Burn of unspecified degree of multiple sites of left shoulder and upper limb, except wrist and hand

[L] [IQ] + [7] T22.099- Burn of unspecified degree of multiple sites of unspecified shoulder and upper limb, except wrist and hand

+ [5] T22.1 Burn of first degree of shoulder and upper limb, except wrist and hand

Use additional external cause code to identify the source, place and intent of the burn (X00-X19, X75-X77, X96-X98, Y92)

[IQ] + [7 placeholder] T22.10X- Burn of first degree of shoulder and upper limb, except wrist and hand, unspecified site

+ [6] T22.11 Burn of first degree of forearm

[L] [SP] + [7] T22.111- Burn of first degree of right forearm

[L] [SP] + [7] T22.112- Burn of first degree of left forearm

[L] [IQ] + [7] T22.119- Burn of first degree of unspecified forearm

+ [6] T22.12 Burn of first degree of elbow

[L] [SP] + [7] T22.121- Burn of first degree of right elbow

[L] [SP] + [7] T22.122- Burn of first degree of left elbow

[L] [IQ] + [7] T22.129- Burn of first degree of unspecified elbow

+ [6] T22.13 Burn of first degree of upper arm

[L] [SP] + [7] T22.131- Burn of first degree of right upper arm

[L] [SP] [IQ] + [7] T22.132- Burn of first degree of left upper arm

[L] [IQ] + [7] T22.139- Burn of first degree of unspecified upper arm

+ [6] T22.14 Burn of first degree of axilla

[L] [SP] + [7] T22.141- Burn of first degree of right axilla

[L] [SP] + [7] T22.142- Burn of first degree of left axilla

[L] [IQ] + [7] T22.149- Burn of first degree of unspecified axilla

+ [6] T22.15 Burn of first degree of shoulder

[L] [SP] + [7] T22.151- Burn of first degree of right shoulder

[L] [SP] + [7] T22.152- Burn of first degree of left shoulder

[L] [IQ] + [7] T22.159- Burn of first degree of unspecified shoulder

+ [6] T22.16 Burn of first degree of scapular region

[L] [SP] + [7] T22.161- Burn of first degree of right scapular region

[L] [SP] + [7] T22.162- Burn of first degree of left scapular region

[L] [IQ] + [7] T22.169- Burn of first degree of unspecified scapular region

+ [6] T22.19 Burn of first degree of multiple sites of shoulder and upper limb, except wrist and hand

[L] [SP] + [7] T22.191- Burn of first degree of multiple sites of right shoulder and upper limb, except wrist and hand

[L] [SP] + [7] T22.192- Burn of first degree of multiple sites of left shoulder and upper limb, except wrist and hand

[L] [SP] + [7] T22.199- Burn of first degree of multiple sites of unspecified shoulder and upper limb, except wrist and hand

+ [5] T22.2 Burn of second degree of shoulder and upper limb, except wrist and hand

Use additional external cause code to identify the source, place and intent of the burn (X00-X19, X75-X77, X96-X98, Y92)

[IQ] + [7 placeholder] T22.20X- Burn of second degree of shoulder and upper limb, except wrist and hand, unspecified site

+ [6] T22.21 Burn of second degree of forearm

[L] [SP] + [7] T22.211- Burn of second degree of right forearm

[L] [SP] + [7] T22.212- Burn of second degree of left forearm

[L] [IQ] + [7] T22.219- Burn of second degree of unspecified forearm

+ [6] T22.22 Burn of second degree of elbow

[L] [SP] + [7] T22.221- Burn of second degree of right elbow

[L] [SP] + [7] T22.222- Burn of second degree of left elbow

[L] [IQ] + [7] T22.229- Burn of second degree of unspecified elbow

+ [6] T22.23 Burn of second degree of upper arm

[4] 4th digit required [5] 5th digit required [6] 6th digit required [7] 7th digit required [7 placeholder] 7th digit placeholder + Additional code [L] Laterality

SP + 7 T22.231- Burn of second degree of right upper arm

SP + 7 T22.232- Burn of second degree of left upper arm

IQ + 7 T22.239- Burn of second degree of unspecified upper arm

+ 6 T22.24 Burn of second degree of axilla

SP + 7 T22.241- Burn of second degree of right axilla

SP + 7 T22.242- Burn of second degree of left axilla

IQ + 7 T22.249- Burn of second degree of unspecified axilla

+ 6 T22.25 Burn of second degree of shoulder

SP + 7 T22.251- Burn of second degree of right shoulder

SP + 7 T22.252- Burn of second degree of left shoulder

IQ + 7 T22.259- Burn of second degree of unspecified shoulder

+ 6 T22.26 Burn of second degree of scapular region

SP + 7 T22.261- Burn of second degree of right scapular region

SP + 7 T22.262- Burn of second degree of left scapular region

IQ + 7 T22.269- Burn of second degree of unspecified scapular region

+ 6 T22.29 Burn of second degree of multiple sites of shoulder and upper limb, except wrist and hand

SP + 7 T22.291- Burn of second degree of multiple sites of right shoulder and upper limb, except wrist and hand

SP + 7 T22.292- Burn of second degree of multiple sites of left shoulder and upper limb, except wrist and hand

SP + 7 T22.299- Burn of second degree of multiple sites of unspecified shoulder and upper limb, except wrist and hand

+ 5 T22.3 Burn of third degree of shoulder and upper limb, except wrist and hand

Use additional external cause code to identify the source, place and intent of the burn (X00-X19, X75-X77, X96-X98, Y92)

IQ + 7 T22.30X- Burn of third degree of shoulder and upper limb, except wrist and hand, unspecified site

+ 6 T22.31 Burn of third degree of forearm

SP + 7 T22.311- Burn of third degree of right forearm

SP + 7 T22.312- Burn of third degree of left forearm

IQ + 7 T22.319- Burn of third degree of unspecified forearm

+ 6 T22.32 Burn of third degree of elbow

SP + 7 T22.321- Burn of third degree of right elbow

SP + 7 T22.322- Burn of third degree of left elbow

IQ + 7 T22.329- Burn of third degree of unspecified elbow

+ 6 T22.33 Burn of third degree of upper arm

SP + 7 T22.331- Burn of third degree of right upper arm

SP + 7 T22.332- Burn of third degree of left upper arm

IQ + 7 T22.339- Burn of third degree of unspecified upper arm

+ 6 T22.34 Burn of third degree of axilla

SP + 7 T22.341- Burn of third degree of right axilla

SP + 7 T22.342- Burn of third degree of left axilla

IQ + 7 T22.349- Burn of third degree of unspecified axilla

+ 6 T22.35 Burn of third degree of shoulder

SP + 7 T22.351- Burn of third degree of right shoulder

SP + 7 T22.352- Burn of third degree of left shoulder

IQ + 7 T22.359- Burn of third degree of unspecified shoulder

+ 6 T22.36 Burn of third degree of scapular region

SP + 7 T22.361- Burn of third degree of right scapular region

SP + 7 T22.362- Burn of third degree of left scapular region

IQ + 7 T22.369- Burn of third degree of unspecified scapular region

+ 6 T22.39 Burn of third degree of multiple sites of shoulder and upper limb, except wrist and hand

SP + 7 T22.391- Burn of third degree of multiple sites of right shoulder and upper limb, except wrist and hand

SP + 7 T22.392- Burn of third degree of multiple sites of left shoulder and upper limb, except wrist and hand

SP + 7 T22.399- Burn of third degree of multiple sites of unspecified shoulder and upper limb, except wrist and hand

+ 5 T22.4 Corrosion of unspecified degree of shoulder and upper limb, except wrist and hand

Code first:
(T51-T65) to identify chemical and intent

Use additional external cause code to identify place (Y92)

IQ + 7 T22.40X- Corrosion of unspecified degree of shoulder and upper limb, except wrist and hand, unspecified site

+ 6 T22.41 Corrosion of unspecified degree of forearm

IQ + 7 T22.411- Corrosion of unspecified degree of right forearm

IQ + 7 T22.412- Corrosion of unspecified degree of left forearm

IQ + 7 T22.419- Corrosion of unspecified degree of unspecified forearm

+ 6 T22.42 Corrosion of unspecified degree of elbow

IQ + 7 T22.421- Corrosion of unspecified degree of right elbow

Chapter 19

S00-T88

T22.422- Corrosion of unspecified degree of left elbow
T22.429- Corrosion of unspecified degree of unspecified elbow
T22.43 Corrosion of unspecified degree of upper arm
T22.431- Corrosion of unspecified degree of right upper arm
T22.432- Corrosion of unspecified degree of left upper arm
T22.439- Corrosion of unspecified degree of unspecified upper arm
T22.44 Corrosion of unspecified degree of axilla
T22.441- Corrosion of unspecified degree of right axilla
T22.442- Corrosion of unspecified degree of left axilla
T22.449- Corrosion of unspecified degree of unspecified axilla
T22.45 Corrosion of unspecified degree of shoulder
T22.451- Corrosion of unspecified degree of right shoulder
T22.452- Corrosion of unspecified degree of left shoulder
T22.459- Corrosion of unspecified degree of unspecified shoulder
T22.46 Corrosion of unspecified degree of scapular region
T22.461- Corrosion of unspecified degree of right scapular region
T22.462- Corrosion of unspecified degree of left scapular region
T22.469- Corrosion of unspecified degree of unspecified scapular region
T22.49 Corrosion of unspecified degree of multiple sites of shoulder and upper limb, except wrist and hand
T22.491- Corrosion of unspecified degree of multiple sites of right shoulder and upper limb, except wrist and hand
T22.492- Corrosion of unspecified degree of multiple sites of left shoulder and upper limb, except wrist and hand
T22.499- Corrosion of unspecified degree of multiple sites of unspecified shoulder and upper limb, except wrist and hand

T22.5 Corrosion of first degree of shoulder and upper limb, except wrist and hand

Code first:
(T51-T65) to identify chemical and intent
Use additional external cause code to identify place (Y92)

T22.50X- Corrosion of first degree of shoulder and upper limb, except wrist and hand unspecified site
T22.51 Corrosion of first degree of forearm
T22.511- Corrosion of first degree of right forearm
T22.512- Corrosion of first degree of left forearm
T22.519- Corrosion of first degree of unspecified forearm
T22.52 Corrosion of first degree of elbow
T22.521- Corrosion of first degree of right elbow
T22.522- Corrosion of first degree of left elbow
T22.529- Corrosion of first degree of unspecified elbow
T22.53 Corrosion of first degree of upper arm
T22.531- Corrosion of first degree of right upper arm
T22.532- Corrosion of first degree of left upper arm
T22.539- Corrosion of first degree of unspecified upper arm
T22.54 Corrosion of first degree of axilla
T22.541- Corrosion of first degree of right axilla
T22.542- Corrosion of first degree of left axilla
T22.549- Corrosion of first degree of unspecified axilla
T22.55 Corrosion of first degree of shoulder
T22.551- Corrosion of first degree of right shoulder
T22.552- Corrosion of first degree of left shoulder
T22.559- Corrosion of first degree of unspecified shoulder
T22.56 Corrosion of first degree of scapular region
T22.561- Corrosion of first degree of right scapular region
T22.562- Corrosion of first degree of left scapular region
T22.569- Corrosion of first degree of unspecified scapular region
T22.59 Corrosion of first degree of multiple sites of shoulder and upper limb, except wrist and hand
T22.591- Corrosion of first degree of multiple sites of right shoulder and upper limb, except wrist and hand
T22.592- Corrosion of first degree of multiple sites of left shoulder and upper limb, except wrist and hand
T22.599- Corrosion of first degree of multiple sites of unspecified shoulder and upper limb, except wrist and hand

T22.6 Corrosion of second degree of shoulder and upper limb, except wrist and hand

Code first:
(T51-T65) to identify chemical and intent
Use additional external cause code to identify place (Y92)

T22.60X- Corrosion of second degree of shoulder and upper limb, except wrist and hand, unspecified site

Chapter 19 S00-T88

+ 6 T22.61 **Corrosion of second degree of forearm**

IQ + 7 T22.611- **Corrosion of second degree of right forearm**

IQ + 7 T22.612- **Corrosion of second degree of left forearm**

IQ + 7 T22.619- **Corrosion of second degree of unspecified forearm**

+ 6 T22.62 **Corrosion of second degree of elbow**

IQ + 7 T22.621- **Corrosion of second degree of right elbow**

IQ + 7 T22.622- **Corrosion of second degree of left elbow**

IQ + 7 T22.629- **Corrosion of second degree of unspecified elbow**

+ 6 T22.63 **Corrosion of second degree of upper arm**

IQ + 7 T22.631- **Corrosion of second degree of right upper arm**

IQ + 7 T22.632- **Corrosion of second degree of left upper arm**

IQ + 7 T22.639- **Corrosion of second degree of unspecified upper arm**

+ 6 T22.64 **Corrosion of second degree of axilla**

IQ + 7 T22.641- **Corrosion of second degree of right axilla**

IQ + 7 T22.642- **Corrosion of second degree of left axilla**

IQ + 7 T22.649- **Corrosion of second degree of unspecified axilla**

+ 6 T22.65 **Corrosion of second degree of shoulder**

IQ + 7 T22.651- **Corrosion of second degree of right shoulder**

IQ + 7 T22.652- **Corrosion of second degree of left shoulder**

IQ + 7 T22.659- **Corrosion of second degree of unspecified shoulder**

+ 6 T22.66 **Corrosion of second degree of scapular region**

IQ + 7 T22.661- **Corrosion of second degree of right scapular region**

IQ + 7 T22.662- **Corrosion of second degree of left scapular region**

IQ + 7 T22.669- **Corrosion of second degree of unspecified scapular region**

+ 6 T22.69 **Corrosion of second degree of multiple sites of shoulder and upper limb, except wrist and hand**

IQ + 7 T22.691- **Corrosion of second degree of multiple sites of right shoulder and upper limb, except wrist and hand**

IQ + 7 T22.692- **Corrosion of second degree of multiple sites of left shoulder and upper limb, except wrist and hand**

IQ + 7 T22.699- **Corrosion of second degree of multiple sites of unspecified shoulder and upper limb, except wrist and hand**

+ 5 T22.7 **Corrosion of third degree of shoulder and upper limb, except wrist and hand**

Code first:

(T51-T65) to identify chemical and intent

Use additional external cause code to identify place (Y92)

IQ + 7 T22.70X- **Corrosion of third degree of shoulder and upper limb, except wrist and hand, unspecified site**

+ 6 T22.71 **Corrosion of third degree of forearm**

IQ + 7 T22.711- **Corrosion of third degree of right forearm**

IQ + 7 T22.712- **Corrosion of third degree of left forearm**

IQ + 7 T22.719- **Corrosion of third degree of unspecified forearm**

+ 6 T22.72 **Corrosion of third degree of elbow**

IQ + 7 T22.721- **Corrosion of third degree of right elbow**

IQ + 7 T22.722- **Corrosion of third degree of left elbow**

IQ + 7 T22.729- **Corrosion of third degree of unspecified elbow**

+ 6 T22.73 **Corrosion of third degree of upper arm**

IQ + 7 T22.731- **Corrosion of third degree of right upper arm**

IQ + 7 T22.732- **Corrosion of third degree of left upper arm**

IQ + 7 T22.739- **Corrosion of third degree of unspecified upper arm**

+ 6 T22.74 **Corrosion of third degree of axilla**

IQ + 7 T22.741- **Corrosion of third degree of right axilla**

IQ + 7 T22.742- **Corrosion of third degree of left axilla**

IQ + 7 T22.749- **Corrosion of third degree of unspecified axilla**

+ 6 T22.75 **Corrosion of third degree of shoulder**

IQ + 7 T22.751- **Corrosion of third degree of right shoulder**

IQ + 7 T22.752- **Corrosion of third degree of left shoulder**

IQ + 7 T22.759- **Corrosion of third degree of unspecified shoulder**

+ 6 T22.76 **Corrosion of third degree of scapular region**

IQ + 7 T22.761- **Corrosion of third degree of right scapular region**

IQ + 7 T22.762- **Corrosion of third degree of left scapular region**

IQ + 7 T22.769- **Corrosion of third degree of unspecified scapular region**

+ 6 T22.79 **Corrosion of third degree of multiple sites of shoulder and upper limb, except wrist and hand**

IQ + 7 T22.791- **Corrosion of third degree of multiple sites of right shoulder and upper limb, except wrist and hand**

IQ + 7 T22.792- **Corrosion of third degree of multiple sites of left shoulder and upper limb, except wrist and hand**

IQ + 7 T22.799- **Corrosion of third degree of multiple sites of unspecified shoulder and upper limb, except wrist and hand**

4 T23 **Burn and corrosion of wrist and hand**

Chapter 19 S00-T88

The appropriate 7th character is to be added to each code from category T23
A initial encounter
D subsequent encounter
S sequela

CODING TIPS✓ Do not use Z codes for skin grafts, dressing changes, drains, etc., for trauma wounds of any type, including burns. Continue to code the burn with the appropriate 7th character.

CODING TIPS✓ Burns are classified according to degree. When there are multiple burns of different degrees to the same body part, code the burn at its highest degree. Remember, there is a convention requiring the external cause code at burns. Aftercare codes are not used for burns, including those for dressing changes, drain care, suture removal, or skin grafts. 7th character 'D' is the default for home care and hospice when providing aftercare for a healing or resolving condition; 'A' is used for active treatment such as antibiotics or more than routine wound care; 'S' is used to identify residual conditions when the burn has healed. Different burns heal at differing rates, so a current burn (with an A or D) can be coded at the same time as a sequela of a burn. A non-healing burn is still coded as a burn no matter how long it has been present.

+5 T23.0 **Burn of unspecified degree of wrist and hand**
Use additional external cause code to identify the source, place and intent of the burn (X00-X19, X75-X77, X96-X98, Y92)

+6 T23.00 **Burn of unspecified degree of hand, unspecified site**
L IQ +7 T23.001- **Burn of unspecified degree of right hand, unspecified site**
L IQ +7 T23.002- **Burn of unspecified degree of left hand, unspecified site**
L IQ +7 T23.009- **Burn of unspecified degree of unspecified hand, unspecified site**

+6 T23.01 **Burn of unspecified degree of thumb (nail)**
L IQ +7 T23.011- **Burn of unspecified degree of right thumb (nail)**
L IQ +7 T23.012- **Burn of unspecified degree of left thumb (nail)**
L IQ +7 T23.019- **Burn of unspecified degree of unspecified thumb (nail)**

+6 T23.02 **Burn of unspecified degree of single finger (nail) except thumb**
L IQ +7 T23.021- **Burn of unspecified degree of single right finger (nail) except thumb**
L IQ +7 T23.022- **Burn of unspecified degree of single left finger (nail) except thumb**
L IQ +7 T23.029- **Burn of unspecified degree of unspecified single finger (nail) except thumb**

+6 T23.03 **Burn of unspecified degree of multiple fingers (nail), not including thumb**
L IQ +7 T23.031- **Burn of unspecified degree of multiple right fingers (nail), not including thumb**
L IQ +7 T23.032- **Burn of unspecified degree of multiple left fingers (nail), not including thumb**
L IQ +7 T23.039- **Burn of unspecified degree of unspecified multiple fingers (nail), not including thumb**

+6 T23.04 **Burn of unspecified degree of multiple fingers (nail), including thumb**
L IQ +7 T23.041- **Burn of unspecified degree of multiple right fingers (nail), including thumb**
L IQ +7 T23.042- **Burn of unspecified degree of multiple left fingers (nail), including thumb**
L IQ +7 T23.049- **Burn of unspecified degree of unspecified multiple fingers (nail), including thumb**

+6 T23.05 **Burn of unspecified degree of palm**
L IQ +7 T23.051- **Burn of unspecified degree of right palm**
L IQ +7 T23.052- **Burn of unspecified degree of left palm**
L IQ +7 T23.059- **Burn of unspecified degree of unspecified palm**

+6 T23.06 **Burn of unspecified degree of back of hand**
L IQ +7 T23.061- **Burn of unspecified degree of back of right hand**
L IQ +7 T23.062- **Burn of unspecified degree of back of left hand**
L IQ +7 T23.069- **Burn of unspecified degree of back of unspecified hand**

+6 T23.07 **Burn of unspecified degree of wrist**
L IQ +7 T23.071- **Burn of unspecified degree of right wrist**
L IQ +7 T23.072- **Burn of unspecified degree of left wrist**
L IQ +7 T23.079- **Burn of unspecified degree of unspecified wrist**

+6 T23.09 **Burn of unspecified degree of multiple sites of wrist and hand**
L IQ +7 T23.091- **Burn of unspecified degree of multlple sites of right wrist and hand**
L IQ +7 T23.092- **Burn of unspecified degree of multiple sites of left wrist and hand**
L IQ +7 T23.099- **Burn of unspecified degree of multiple sites of unspecified wrist and hand**

+5 T23.1 **Burn of first degree of wrist and hand**
Use additional external cause code to identify the source, place and intent of the burn (X00-X19, X75-X77, X96-X98, Y92)

+6 T23.10 **Burn of first degree of hand, unspecified site**

Chapter 19

S00-T88

4 4th digit required 5 5th digit required 6 6th digit required 7 7th digit required X 7th digit placeholder + Additional code L Laterality

T23.101- Burn of first degree of right hand, unspecified site
T23.102- Burn of first degree of left hand, unspecified site
T23.109- Burn of first degree of unspecified hand, unspecified site
T23.11 Burn of first degree of thumb (nail)
T23.111- Burn of first degree of right thumb (nail)
T23.112- Burn of first degree of left thumb (nail)
T23.119- Burn of first degree of unspecified thumb (nail)
T23.12 Burn of first degree of single finger (nail) except thumb
T23.121- Burn of first degree of single right finger (nail) except thumb
T23.122- Burn of first degree of single left finger (nail) except thumb
T23.129- Burn of first degree of unspecified single finger (nail) except thumb
T23.13 Burn of first degree of multiple fingers (nail), not including thumb
T23.131- Burn of first degree of multiple right fingers (nail), not including thumb
T23.132- Burn of first degree of multiple left fingers (nail), not including thumb
T23.139- Burn of first degree of unspecified multiple fingers (nail), not including thumb
T23.14 Burn of first degree of multiple fingers (nail), including thumb
T23.141- Burn of first degree of multiple right fingers (nail), including thumb
T23.142- Burn of first degree of multiple left fingers (nail), including thumb
T23.149- Burn of first degree of unspecified multiple fingers (nail), including thumb
T23.15 Burn of first degree of palm
T23.151- Burn of first degree of right palm
T23.152- Burn of first degree of left palm
T23.159- Burn of first degree of unspecified palm
T23.16 Burn of first degree of back of hand
T23.161- Burn of first degree of back of right hand
T23.162- Burn of first degree of back of left hand
T23.169- Burn of first degree of back of unspecified hand
T23.17 Burn of first degree of wrist
T23.171- Burn of first degree of right wrist
T23.172- Burn of first degree of left wrist
T23.179- Burn of first degree of unspecified wrist
T23.19 Burn of first degree of multiple sites of wrist and hand
T23.191- Burn of first degree of multiple sites of right wrist and hand
T23.192- Burn of first degree of multiple sites of left wrist and hand
T23.199- Burn of first degree of multiple sites of unspecified wrist and hand
T23.2 Burn of second degree of wrist and hand
Use additional external cause code to identify the source, place and intent of the burn (X00-X19, X75-X77, X96-X98, Y92)
T23.20 Burn of second degree of hand, unspecified site
T23.201- Burn of second degree of right hand, unspecified site
T23.202- Burn of second degree of left hand, unspecified site
T23.209- Burn of second degree of unspecified hand, unspecified site
T23.21 Burn of second degree of thumb (nail)
T23.211- Burn of second degree of right thumb (nail)
T23.212- Burn of second degree of left thumb (nail)
T23.219- Burn of second degree of unspecified thumb (nail)
T23.22 Burn of second degree of single finger (nail) except thumb
T23.221- Burn of second degree of single right finger (nail) except thumb
T23.222- Burn of second degree of single left finger (nail) except thumb
T23.229- Burn of second degree of unspecified single finger (nail) except thumb
T23.23 Burn of second degree of multiple fingers (nail), not including thumb
T23.231- Burn of second degree of multiple right fingers (nail), not including thumb
T23.232- Burn of second degree of multiple left fingers (nail), not including thumb
T23.239- Burn of second degree of unspecified multiple fingers (nail), not including thumb
T23.24 Burn of second degree of multiple fingers (nail), including thumb
T23.241- Burn of second degree of multiple right fingers (nail), including thumb
T23.242- Burn of second degree of multiple left fingers (nail), including thumb
T23.249- Burn of second degree of unspecified multiple fingers (nail), including thumb
T23.25 Burn of second degree of palm
T23.251- Burn of second degree of right palm
T23.252- Burn of second degree of left palm

Chapter 19 S00-T88

T23.259- Burn of second degree of unspecified palm

T23.26 Burn of second degree of back of hand

T23.261- Burn of second degree of back of right hand

T23.262- Burn of second degree of back of left hand

T23.269- Burn of second degree of back of unspecified hand

T23.27 Burn of second degree of wrist

T23.271- Burn of second degree of right wrist

T23.272- Burn of second degree of left wrist

T23.279- Burn of second degree of unspecified wrist

T23.29 Burn of second degree of multiple sites of wrist and hand

T23.291- Burn of second degree of multiple sites of right wrist and hand

T23.292- Burn of second degree of multiple sites of left wrist and hand

T23.299- Burn of second degree of multiple sites of unspecified wrist and hand

T23.3 Burn of third degree of wrist and hand

Use additional external cause code to identify the source, place and intent of the burn (X00-X19, X75-X77, X96-X98, Y92)

T23.30 Burn of third degree of hand, unspecified site

T23.301- Burn of third degree of right hand, unspecified site

T23.302- Burn of third degree of left hand, unspecified site

T23.309- Burn of third degree of unspecified hand, unspecified site

T23.31 Burn of third degree of thumb (nail)

T23.311- Burn of third degree of right thumb (nail)

T23.312- Burn of third degree of left thumb (nail)

T23.319- Burn of third degree of unspecified thumb (nail)

T23.32 Burn of third degree of single finger (nail) except thumb

T23.321- Burn of third degree of single right finger (nail) except thumb

T23.322- Burn of third degree of single left finger (nail) except thumb

T23.329- Burn of third degree of unspecified single finger (nail) except thumb

T23.33 Burn of third degree of multiple fingers (nail), not including thumb

T23.331- Burn of third degree of multiple right fingers (nail), not including thumb

T23.332- Burn of third degree of multiple left fingers (nail), not including thumb

T23.339- Burn of third degree of unspecified multiple fingers (nail), not including thumb

T23.34 Burn of third degree of multiple fingers (nail), including thumb

T23.341- Burn of third degree of multiple right fingers (nail), including thumb

T23.342- Burn of third degree of multiple left fingers (nail), including thumb

T23.349- Burn of third degree of unspecified multiple fingers (nail), including thumb

T23.35 Burn of third degree of palm

T23.351- Burn of third degree of right palm

T23.352- Burn of third degree of left palm

T23.359- Burn of third degree of unspecified palm

T23.36 Burn of third degree of back of hand

T23.361- Burn of third degree of back of right hand

T23.362- Burn of third degree of back of left hand

T23.369- Burn of third degree of back of unspecified hand

T23.37 Burn of third degree of wrist

T23.371- Burn of third degree of right wrist

T23.372- Burn of third degree of left wrist

T23.379- Burn of third degree of unspecified wrist

T23.39 Burn of third degree of multiple sites of wrist and hand

T23.391- Burn of third degree of multiple sites of right wrist and hand

T23.392- Burn of third degree of multiple sites of left wrist and hand

T23.399- Burn of third degree of multiple sites of unspecified wrist and hand

T23.4 Corrosion of unspecified degree of wrist and hand

Code first:
(T51-T65) to identify chemical and intent

Use additional external cause code to identify place (Y92)

T23.40 Corrosion of unspecified degree of hand, unspecified site

T23.401- Corrosion of unspecified degree of right hand, unspecified site

T23.402- Corrosion of unspecified degree of left hand, unspecified site

T23.409- Corrosion of unspecified degree of unspecified hand, unspecified site

T23.41 Corrosion of unspecified degree of thumb (nail)

T23.411- Corrosion of unspecified degree of right thumb (nail)

T23.412- Corrosion of unspecified degree of left thumb (nail)

T23.419- Corrosion of unspecified degree of unspecified thumb (nail)

T23.42 Corrosion of unspecified degree of single finger (nail) except thumb

T23.421- Corrosion of unspecified degree of single right finger (nail) except thumb

T23.422- Corrosion of unspecified degree of single left finger (nail) except thumb

T23.429- Corrosion of unspecified degree of unspecified single finger (nail) except thumb

T23.43 Corrosion of unspecified degree of multiple fingers (nail), not including thumb

T23.431- Corrosion of unspecified degree of multiple right fingers (nail), not including thumb

T23.432- Corrosion of unspecified degree of multiple left fingers (nail), not including thumb

T23.439- Corrosion of unspecified degree of unspecified multiple fingers (nail), not including thumb

T23.44 Corrosion of unspecified degree of multiple fingers (nail), including thumb

T23.441- Corrosion of unspecified degree of multiple right fingers (nail), including thumb

T23.442- Corrosion of unspecified degree of multiple left fingers (nail), including thumb

T23.449- Corrosion of unspecified degree of unspecified multiple fingers (nail), including thumb

T23.45 Corrosion of unspecified degree of palm

T23.451- Corrosion of unspecified degree of right palm

T23.452- Corrosion of unspecified degree of left palm

T23.459- Corrosion of unspecified degree of unspecified palm

T23.46 Corrosion of unspecified degree of back of hand

T23.461- Corrosion of unspecified degree of back of right hand

T23.462- Corrosion of unspecified degree of back of left hand

T23.469- Corrosion of unspecified degree of back of unspecified hand

T23.47 Corrosion of unspecified degree of wrist

T23.471- Corrosion of unspecified degree of right wrist

T23.472- Corrosion of unspecified degree of left wrist

T23.479- Corrosion of unspecified degree of unspecified wrist

T23.49 Corrosion of unspecified degree of multiple sites of wrist and hand

T23.491- Corrosion of unspecified degree of multiple sites of right wrist and hand

T23.492- Corrosion of unspecified degree of multiple sites of left wrist and hand

T23.499- Corrosion of unspecified degree of multiple sites of unspecified wrist and hand

T23.5 Corrosion of first degree of wrist and hand

Code first:
(T51-T65) to identify chemical and intent
Use additional external cause code to identify place (Y92)

T23.50 Corrosion of first degree of hand, unspecified site

T23.501- Corrosion of first degree of right hand, unspecified site

T23.502- Corrosion of first degree of left hand, unspecified site

T23.509- Corrosion of first degree of unspecified hand, unspecified site

T23.51 Corrosion of first degree of thumb (nail)

T23.511- Corrosion of first degree of right thumb (nail)

T23.512- Corrosion of first degree of left thumb (nail)

T23.519- Corrosion of first degree of unspecified thumb (nail)

T23.52 Corrosion of first degree of single finger (nail) except thumb

T23.521- Corrosion of first degree of single right finger (nail) except thumb

T23.522- Corrosion of first degree of single left finger (nail) except thumb

T23.529- Corrosion of first degree of unspecified single finger (nail) except thumb

T23.53 Corrosion of first degree of multiple fingers (nail), not including thumb

T23.531- Corrosion of first degree of multiple right fingers (nail), not including thumb

T23.532- Corrosion of first degree of multiple left fingers (nail), not including thumb

T23.539- Corrosion of first degree of unspecified multiple fingers (nail), not including thumb

T23.54 Corrosion of first degree of multiple fingers (nail), including thumb

T23.541- Corrosion of first degree of multiple right fingers (nail), including thumb

T23.542- Corrosion of first degree of multiple left fingers (nail), including thumb

T23.549- Corrosion of first degree of unspecified multiple fingers (nail), including thumb

T23.55 Corrosion of first degree of palm

T23.551- Corrosion of first degree of right palm
T23.552- Corrosion of first degree of left palm
T23.559- Corrosion of first degree of unspecified palm
T23.56 Corrosion of first degree of back of hand
T23.561- Corrosion of first degree of back of right hand
T23.562- Corrosion of first degree of back of left hand
T23.569- Corrosion of first degree of back of unspecified hand
T23.57 Corrosion of first degree of wrist
T23.571- Corrosion of first degree of right wrist
T23.572- Corrosion of first degree of left wrist
T23.579- Corrosion of first degree of unspecified wrist
T23.59 Corrosion of first degree of multiple sites of wrist and hand
T23.591- Corrosion of first degree of multiple sites of right wrist and hand
T23.592- Corrosion of first degree of multiple sites of left wrist and hand
T23.599- Corrosion of first degree of multiple sites of unspecified wrist and hand
T23.6 Corrosion of second degree of wrist and hand
Code first:
(T51-T65) to identify chemical and intent
Use additional external cause code to identify place (Y92)
T23.60 Corrosion of second degree of hand, unspecified site
T23.601- Corrosion of second degree of right hand, unspecified site
T23.602- Corrosion of second degree of left hand, unspecified site
T23.609- Corrosion of second degree of unspecified hand, unspecified site
T23.61 Corrosion of second degree of thumb (nail)
T23.611- Corrosion of second degree of right thumb (nail)
T23.612- Corrosion of second degree of left thumb (nail)
T23.619- Corrosion of second degree of unspecified thumb (nail)
T23.62 Corrosion of second degree of single finger (nail) except thumb
T23.621- Corrosion of second degree of single right finger (nail) except thumb
T23.622- Corrosion of second degree of single left finger (nail) except thumb
T23.629- Corrosion of second degree of unspecified single finger (nail) except thumb
T23.63 Corrosion of second degree of multiple fingers (nail), not including thumb
T23.631- Corrosion of second degree of multiple right fingers (nail), not including thumb
T23.632- Corrosion of second degree of multiple left fingers (nail), not including thumb
T23.639- Corrosion of second degree of unspecified multiple fingers (nail), not including thumb
T23.64 Corrosion of second degree of multiple fingers (nail), including thumb
T23.641- Corrosion of second degree of multiple right fingers (nail), including thumb
T23.642- Corrosion of second degree of multiple left fingers (nail), including thumb
T23.649- Corrosion of second degree of unspecified multiple fingers (nail), including thumb
T23.65 Corrosion of second degree of palm
T23.651- Corrosion of second degree of right palm
T23.652- Corrosion of second degree of left palm
T23.659- Corrosion of second degree of unspecified palm
T23.66 Corrosion of second degree of back of hand
T23.661- Corrosion of second degree back of right hand
T23.662- Corrosion of second degree back of left hand
T23.669- Corrosion of second degree back of unspecified hand
T23.67 Corrosion of second degree of wrist
T23.671- Corrosion of second degree of right wrist
T23.672- Corrosion of second degree of left wrist
T23.679- Corrosion of second degree of unspecified wrist
T23.69 Corrosion of second degree of multiple sites of wrist and hand
T23.691- Corrosion of second degree of multiple sites of right wrist and hand
T23.692- Corrosion of second degree of multiple sites of left wrist and hand
T23.699- Corrosion of second degree of multiple sites of unspecified wrist and hand
T23.7 Corrosion of third degree of wrist and hand
Code first:
(T51-T65) to identify chemical and intent
Use additional external cause code to identify place (Y92)

Chapter 19 S00-T88

+6 **T23.70** Corrosion of third degree of hand, unspecified site

IQ +7 **T23.701-** Corrosion of third degree of right hand, unspecified site

IQ +7 **T23.702-** Corrosion of third degree of left hand, unspecified site

IQ +7 **T23.709-** Corrosion of third degree of unspecified hand, unspecified site

+6 **T23.71** Corrosion of third degree of thumb (nail)

IQ +7 **T23.711-** Corrosion of third degree of right thumb (nail)

IQ +7 **T23.712-** Corrosion of third degree of left thumb (nail)

IQ +7 **T23.719-** Corrosion of third degree of unspecified thumb (nail)

+6 **T23.72** Corrosion of third degree of single finger (nail) except thumb

IQ +7 **T23.721-** Corrosion of third degree of single right finger (nail) except thumb

IQ +7 **T23.722-** Corrosion of third degree of single left finger (nail) except thumb

IQ +7 **T23.729-** Corrosion of third degree of unspecified single finger (nail) except thumb

+6 **T23.73** Corrosion of third degree of multiple fingers (nail), not including thumb

IQ +7 **T23.731-** Corrosion of third degree of multiple right fingers (nail), not including thumb

IQ +7 **T23.732-** Corrosion of third degree of multiple left fingers (nail), not including thumb

IQ +7 **T23.739-** Corrosion of third degree of unspecified multiple fingers (nail), not including thumb

+6 **T23.74** Corrosion of third degree of multiple fingers (nail), including thumb

IQ +7 **T23.741-** Corrosion of third degree of multiple right fingers (nail), including thumb

IQ +7 **T23.742-** Corrosion of third degree of multiple left fingers (nail), including thumb

IQ +7 **T23.749-** Corrosion of third degree of unspecified multiple fingers (nail), including thumb

+6 **T23.75** Corrosion of third degree of palm

IQ +7 **T23.751-** Corrosion of third degree of right palm

IQ +7 **T23.752-** Corrosion of third degree of left palm

IQ +7 **T23.759-** Corrosion of third degree of unspecified palm

+6 **T23.76** Corrosion of third degree of back of hand

IQ +7 **T23.761-** Corrosion of third degree of back of right hand

IQ +7 **T23.762-** Corrosion of third degree of back of left hand

IQ +7 **T23.769-** Corrosion of third degree back of unspecified hand

+6 **T23.77** Corrosion of third degree of wrist

IQ +7 **T23.771-** Corrosion of third degree of right wrist

IQ +7 **T23.772-** Corrosion of third degree of left wrist

IQ +7 **T23.779-** Corrosion of third degree of unspecified wrist

+6 **T23.79** Corrosion of third degree of multiple sites of wrist and hand

IQ +7 **T23.791-** Corrosion of third degree of multiple sites of right wrist and hand

IQ +7 **T23.792-** Corrosion of third degree of multiple sites of left wrist and hand

IQ +7 **T23.799-** Corrosion of third degree of multiple sites of unspecified wrist and hand

4 **T24 Burn and corrosion of lower limb, except ankle and foot**

EXCLUDES 2 burn and corrosion of ankle and foot (T25.-)
burn and corrosion of hip region (T21.-)

The appropriate 7th character is to be added to each code from category T24
A initial encounter
D subsequent encounter
S sequela

CODING TIPS ✓ Do not use Z codes for skin grafts, dressing changes, drains, etc., for trauma wounds of any type, including burns. Continue to code the burn with the appropriate 7th character.

CODING TIPS ✓ Burns are classified according to degree. When there are multiple burns of different degrees to the same body part, code the burn at its highest degree. Remember, there is a convention requiring the external cause code at burns. Aftercare codes are not used for burns, including those for dressing changes, drain care, suture removal, or skin grafts. 7th character 'D' is the default for home care and hospice when providing aftercare for a healing or resolving condition; 'A' is used for active treatment such as antibiotics or more than routine wound care; 'S' is used to identify residual conditions when the burn has healed. Different burns heal at differing rates, so a current burn (with an A or D) can be coded at the same time as a sequela of a burn. A non-healing burn is still coded as a burn no matter how long it has been present.

+5 **T24.0** Burn of unspecified degree of lower limb, except ankle and foot

Use additional external cause code to identify the source, place and intent of the burn (X00-X19, X75-X77, X96-X98, Y92)

+6 **T24.00** Burn of unspecified degree of unspecified site of lower limb, except ankle and foot

IQ +7 **T24.001-** Burn of unspecified degree of unspecified site of right lower limb, except ankle and foot

Chapter 19 S00-T88

▤ **IQ** ✚ ⑦ **T24.002-** Burn of unspecified degree of unspecified site of left lower limb, except ankle and foot

▤ **IQ** ✚ ⑦ **T24.009-** Burn of unspecified degree of unspecified site of unspecified lower limb, except ankle and foot

✚ ⑥ **T24.01** Burn of unspecified degree of thigh

▤ **IQ** ✚ ⑦ **T24.011-** Burn of unspecified degree of right thigh

▤ **IQ** ✚ ⑦ **T24.012-** Burn of unspecified degree of left thigh

▤ **IQ** ✚ ⑦ **T24.019-** Burn of unspecified degree of unspecified thigh

✚ ⑥ **T24.02** Burn of unspecified degree of knee

▤ **IQ** ✚ ⑦ **T24.021-** Burn of unspecified degree of right knee

▤ **IQ** ✚ ⑦ **T24.022-** Burn of unspecified degree of left knee

▤ **IQ** ✚ ⑦ **T24.029-** Burn of unspecified degree of unspecified knee

✚ ⑥ **T24.03** Burn of unspecified degree of lower leg

▤ **IQ** ✚ ⑦ **T24.031-** Burn of unspecified degree of right lower leg

▤ **IQ** ✚ ⑦ **T24.032-** Burn of unspecified degree of left lower leg

▤ **IQ** ✚ ⑦ **T24.039-** Burn of unspecified degree of unspecified lower leg

✚ ⑥ **T24.09** Burn of unspecified degree of multiple sites of lower limb, except ankle and foot

▤ **IQ** ✚ ⑦ **T24.091-** Burn of unspecified degree of multiple sites of right lower limb, except ankle and foot

▤ **IQ** ✚ ⑦ **T24.092-** Burn of unspecified degree of multiple sites of left lower limb, except ankle and foot

▤ **IQ** ✚ ⑦ **T24.099-** Burn of unspecified degree of multiple sites of unspecified lower limb, except ankle and foot

✚ ⑤ **T24.1** Burn of first degree of lower limb, except ankle and foot
Use additional external cause code to identify the source, place and intent of the burn (X00-X19, X75-X77, X96-X98, Y92)

✚ ⑥ **T24.10** Burn of first degree of unspecified site of lower limb, except ankle and foot

▤ **IQ** ✚ ⑦ **T24.101-** Burn of first degree of unspecified site of right lower limb, except ankle and foot

▤ **IQ** ✚ ⑦ **T24.102-** Burn of first degree of unspecified site of left lower limb, except ankle and foot

▤ **IQ** ✚ ⑦ **T24.109-** Burn of first degree of unspecified site of unspecified lower limb, except ankle and foot

✚ ⑥ **T24.11** Burn of first degree of thigh

▤ **SP** ✚ ⑦ **T24.111-** Burn of first degree of right thigh

▤ **SP** ✚ ⑦ **T24.112-** Burn of first degree of left thigh

▤ **IQ** ✚ ⑦ **T24.119-** Burn of first degree of unspecified thigh

✚ ⑥ **T24.12** Burn of first degree of knee

▤ **SP** ✚ ⑦ **T24.121-** Burn of first degree of right knee

▤ **SP** ✚ ⑦ **T24.122-** Burn of first degree of left knee

▤ **IQ** ✚ ⑦ **T24.129-** Burn of first degree of unspecified knee

✚ ⑥ **T24.13** Burn of first degree of lower leg

▤ **SP** ✚ ⑦ **T24.131-** Burn of first degree of right lower leg

▤ **SP** ✚ ⑦ **T24.132-** Burn of first degree of left lower leg

▤ **IQ** ✚ ⑦ **T24.139-** Burn of first degree of unspecified lower leg

✚ ⑥ **T24.19** Burn of first degree of multiple sites of lower limb, except ankle and foot

▤ **SP** ✚ ⑦ **T24.191-** Burn of first degree of multiple sites of right lower limb, except ankle and foot

▤ **SP** ✚ ⑦ **T24.192-** Burn of first degree of multiple sites of left lower limb, except ankle and foot

▤ **IQ** ✚ ⑦ **T24.199-** Burn of first degree of multiple sites of unspecified lower limb, except ankle and foot

✚ ⑤ **T24.2** Burn of second degree of lower limb, except ankle and foot
Use additional external cause code to identify the source, place and intent of the burn (X00-X19, X75-X77, X96-X98, Y92)

✚ ⑥ **T24.20** Burn of second degree of unspecified site of lower limb, except ankle and foot

▤ **IQ** ✚ ⑦ **T24.201-** Burn of second degree of unspecified site of right lower limb, except ankle and foot

▤ **IQ** ✚ ⑦ **T24.202-** Burn of second degree of unspecified site of left lower limb, except ankle and foot

▤ **IQ** ✚ ⑦ **T24.209-** Burn of second degree of unspecified site of unspecified lower limb, except ankle and foot

✚ ⑥ **T24.21** Burn of second degree of thigh

▤ **SP** ✚ ⑦ **T24.211-** Burn of second degree of right thigh

▤ **SP** ✚ ⑦ **T24.212-** Burn of second degree of left thigh

▤ **IQ** ✚ ⑦ **T24.219-** Burn of second degree of unspecified thigh

✚ ⑥ **T24.22** Burn of second degree of knee

▤ **SP** ✚ ⑦ **T24.221-** Burn of second degree of right knee

▤ **SP** ✚ ⑦ **T24.222-** Burn of second degree of left knee

▤ **IQ** ✚ ⑦ **T24.229-** Burn of second degree of unspecified knee

✚ ⑥ **T24.23** Burn of second degree of lower leg

▤ **SP** ✚ ⑦ **T24.231-** Burn of second degree of right lower leg

▤ **SP** ✚ ⑦ **T24.232-** Burn of second degree of left lower leg

IQ 7 T24.239- Burn of second degree of unspecified lower leg

6 T24.29 **Burn of second degree of multiple sites of lower limb, except ankle and foot**

SP 7 T24.291- **Burn of second degree of multiple sites of right lower limb, except ankle and foot**

SP 7 T24.292- **Burn of second degree of multiple sites of left lower limb, except ankle and foot**

IQ 7 T24.299- Burn of second degree of multiple sites of unspecified lower limb, except ankle and foot

5 T24.3 **Burn of third degree of lower limb, except ankle and foot**

Use additional external cause code to identify the source, place and intent of the burn (X00-X19, X75-X77, X96-X98, Y92)

6 T24.30 Burn of third degree of unspecified site of lower limb, except ankle and foot

IQ 7 T24.301- Burn of third degree of unspecified site of right lower limb, except ankle and foot

IQ 7 T24.302- Burn of third degree of unspecified site of left lower limb, except ankle and foot

IQ 7 T24.309- Burn of third degree of unspecified site of unspecified lower limb, except ankle and foot

6 T24.31 **Burn of third degree of thigh**

SP 7 T24.311- **Burn of third degree of right thigh**

SP 7 T24.312- **Burn of third degree of left thigh**

IQ 7 T24.319- Burn of third degree of unspecified thigh

6 T24.32 **Burn of third degree of knee**

SP 7 T24.321- **Burn of third degree of right knee**

SP 7 T24.322- **Burn of third degree of left knee**

IQ 7 T24.329- Burn of third degree of unspecified knee

6 T24.33 **Burn of third degree of lower leg**

SP 7 T24.331- **Burn of third degree of right lower leg**

SP 7 T24.332- **Burn of third degree of left lower leg**

IQ 7 T24.339- Burn of third degree of unspecified lower leg

6 T24.39 **Burn of third degree of multiple sites of lower limb, except ankle and foot**

SP 7 T24.391- **Burn of third degree of multiple sites of right lower limb, except ankle and foot**

SP 7 T24.392- **Burn of third degree of multiple sites of left lower limb, except ankle and foot**

IQ 7 T24.399- Burn of third degree of multiple sites of unspecified lower limb, except ankle and foot

5 T24.4 Corrosion of unspecified degree of lower limb, except ankle and foot

Code first:

(T51-T65) to identify chemical and intent

Use additional external cause code to identify place (Y92)

6 T24.40 Corrosion of unspecified degree of unspecified site of lower limb, except ankle and foot

IQ 7 T24.401- Corrosion of unspecified degree of unspecified site of right lower limb, except ankle and foot

IQ 7 T24.402- Corrosion of unspecified degree of unspecified site of left lower limb, except ankle and foot

IQ 7 T24.409- Corrosion of unspecified degree of unspecified site of unspecified lower limb, except ankle and foot

6 T24.41 Corrosion of unspecified degree of thigh

IQ 7 T24.411- Corrosion of unspecified degree of right thigh

IQ 7 T24.412- Corrosion of unspecified degree of left thigh

IQ 7 T24.419- Corrosion of unspecified degree of unspecified thigh

6 T24.42 Corrosion of unspecified degree of knee

IQ 7 T24.421- Corrosion of unspecified degree of right knee

IQ 7 T24.422- Corrosion of unspecified degree of left knee

IQ 7 T24.429- Corrosion of unspecified degree of unspecified knee

6 T24.43 Corrosion of unspecified degree of lower leg

IQ 7 T24.431- Corrosion of unspecified degree of right lower leg

IQ 7 T24.432- Corrosion of unspecified degree of left lower leg

IQ 7 T24.439- Corrosion of unspecified degree of unspecified lower leg

6 T24.49 Corrosion of unspecified degree of multiple sites of lower limb, except ankle and foot

IQ 7 T24.491- Corrosion of unspecified degree of multiple sites of right lower limb, except ankle and foot

IQ 7 T24.492- Corrosion of unspecified degree of multiple sites of left lower limb, except ankle and foot

IQ 7 T24.499- Corrosion of unspecified degree of multiple sites of unspecified lower limb, except ankle and foot

5 T24.5 **Corrosion of first degree of lower limb, except ankle and foot**

Code first:

(T51-T65) to identify chemical and intent

Use additional external cause code to identify place (Y92)

Chapter 19

S00-T88

+ 6 T24.50 Corrosion of first degree of unspecified site of lower limb, except ankle and foot
L IQ + 7 T24.501- Corrosion of first degree of unspecified site of right lower limb, except ankle and foot
L IQ + 7 T24.502- Corrosion of first degree of unspecified site of left lower limb, except ankle and foot
L IQ + 7 T24.509- Corrosion of first degree of unspecified site of unspecified lower limb, except ankle and foot
+ 6 T24.51 Corrosion of first degree of thigh
L IQ + 7 T24.511- Corrosion of first degree of right thigh
L IQ + 7 T24.512- Corrosion of first degree of left thigh
L IQ + 7 T24.519- Corrosion of first degree of unspecified thigh
+ 6 T24.52 Corrosion of first degree of knee
L IQ + 7 T24.521- Corrosion of first degree of right knee
L IQ + 7 T24.522- Corrosion of first degree of left knee
L IQ + 7 T24.529- Corrosion of first degree of unspecified knee
+ 6 T24.53 Corrosion of first degree of lower leg
L IQ + 7 T24.531- Corrosion of first degree of right lower leg
L IQ + 7 T24.532- Corrosion of first degree of left lower leg
L IQ + 7 T24.539- Corrosion of first degree of unspecified lower leg
+ 6 T24.59 Corrosion of first degree of multiple sites of lower limb, except ankle and foot
L IQ + 7 T24.591- Corrosion of first degree of multiple sites of right lower limb, except ankle and foot
L IQ + 7 T24.592- Corrosion of first degree of multiple sites of left lower limb, except ankle and foot
L IQ + 7 T24.599- Corrosion of first degree of multiple sites of unspecified lower limb, except ankle and foot
+ 5 T24.6 Corrosion of second degree of lower limb, except ankle and foot
Code first:
(T51-T65) to identify chemical and intent
Use additional external cause code to identify place (Y92)
+ 6 T24.60 Corrosion of second degree of unspecified site of lower limb, except ankle and foot
L IQ + 7 T24.601- Corrosion of second degree of unspecified site of right lower limb, except ankle and foot
L IQ + 7 T24.602- Corrosion of second degree of unspecified site of left lower limb, except ankle and foot
L IQ + 7 T24.609- Corrosion of second degree of unspecified site of unspecified lower limb, except ankle and foot
+ 6 T24.61 Corrosion of second degree of thigh
L IQ + 7 T24.611- Corrosion of second degree of right thigh
L IQ + 7 T24.612- Corrosion of second degree of left thigh
L IQ + 7 T24.619- Corrosion of second degree of unspecified thigh
+ 6 T24.62 Corrosion of second degree of knee
L IQ + 7 T24.621- Corrosion of second degree of right knee
L IQ + 7 T24.622- Corrosion of second degree of left knee
L IQ + 7 T24.629- Corrosion of second degree of unspecified knee
+ 6 T24.63 Corrosion of second degree of lower leg
L IQ + 7 T24.631- Corrosion of second degree of right lower leg
L IQ + 7 T24.632- Corrosion of second degree of left lower leg
L IQ + 7 T24.639- Corrosion of second degree of unspecified lower leg
+ 6 T24.69 Corrosion of second degree of multiple sites of lower limb, except ankle and foot
L IQ + 7 T24.691- Corrosion of second degree of multiple sites of right lower limb, except ankle and foot
L IQ + 7 T24.692- Corrosion of second degree of multiple sites of left lower limb, except ankle and foot
L IQ + 7 T24.699- Corrosion of second degree of multiple sites of unspecified lower limb, except ankle and foot
+ 5 T24.7 Corrosion of third degree of lower limb, except ankle and foot
Code first:
(T51-T65) to identify chemical and intent
Use additional external cause code to identify place (Y92)
+ 6 T24.70 Corrosion of third degree of unspecified site of lower limb, except ankle and foot
L IQ + 7 T24.701- Corrosion of third degree of unspecified site of right lower limb, except ankle and foot
L IQ + 7 T24.702- Corrosion of third degree of unspecified site of left lower limb, except ankle and foot
L IQ + 7 T24.709- Corrosion of third degree of unspecified site of unspecified lower limb, except ankle and foot
+ 6 T24.71 Corrosion of third degree of thigh
L IQ + 7 T24.711- Corrosion of third degree of right thigh
L IQ + 7 T24.712- Corrosion of third degree of left thigh
L IQ + 7 T24.719- Corrosion of third degree of unspecified thigh

4 4th digit required 5 5th digit required 6 6th digit required 7 7th digit required 7 7th digit placeholder + Additional code L Laterality

+ 6 T24.72 Corrosion of third degree of knee

IQ + 7 T24.721- Corrosion of third degree of right knee

IQ + 7 T24.722- Corrosion of third degree of left knee

IQ + 7 T24.729- Corrosion of third degree of unspecified knee

+ 6 T24.73 Corrosion of third degree of lower leg

IQ + 7 T24.731- Corrosion of third degree of right lower leg

IQ + 7 T24.732- Corrosion of third degree of left lower leg

IQ + 7 T24.739- Corrosion of third degree of unspecified lower leg

+ 6 T24.79 Corrosion of third degree of multiple sites of lower limb, except ankle and foot

IQ + 7 T24.791- Corrosion of third degree of multiple sites of right lower limb, except ankle and foot

IQ + 7 T24.792- Corrosion of third degree of multiple sites of left lower limb, except ankle and foot

IQ + 7 T24.799- Corrosion of third degree of multiple sites of unspecified lower limb, except ankle and foot

4 T25 Burn and corrosion of ankle and foot

The appropriate 7th character is to be added to each code from category T25

A	initial encounter
D	subsequent encounter
S	sequela

CODING TIPS ✓ Do not use Z codes for skin grafts, dressing changes, drains, etc., for trauma wounds of any type, including burns. Continue to code the burn with the appropriate 7th character.

CODING TIPS ✓ Burns are classified according to degree. When there are multiple burns of different degrees to the same body part, code the burn at its highest degree. Remember, there is a convention requiring the external cause code at burns. Aftercare codes are not used for burns, including those for dressing changes, drain care, suture removal, or skin grafts. 7th character 'D' is the default for home care and hospice when providing aftercare for a healing or resolving condition; 'A' is used for active treatment such as antibiotics or more than routine wound care; 'S' is used to identify residual conditions when the burn has healed. Different burns heal at differing rates, so a current burn (with an A or D) can be coded at the same time as a sequela of a burn. A non-healing burn is still coded as a burn no matter how long it has been present.

+ 5 T25.0 Burn of unspecified degree of ankle and foot

Use additional external cause code to identify the source, place and intent of the burn (X00-X19, X75-X77, X96-X98, Y92)

+ 6 T25.01 Burn of unspecified degree of ankle

IQ + 7 T25.011- Burn of unspecified degree of right ankle

IQ + 7 T25.012- Burn of unspecified degree of left ankle

IQ + 7 T25.019- Burn of unspecified degree of unspecified ankle

+ 6 T25.02 Burn of unspecified degree of foot

EXCLUDES 2 burn of unspecified degree of toe (s) (nail) (T25.03-)

IQ + 7 T25.021- Burn of unspecified degree of right foot

IQ + 7 T25.022- Burn of unspecified degree of left foot

IQ + 7 T25.029- Burn of unspecified degree of unspecified foot

+ 6 T25.03 Burn of unspecified degree of toe(s) (nail)

IQ + 7 T25.031- Burn of unspecified degree of right toe(s) (nail)

IQ + 7 T25.032- Burn of unspecified degree of left toe(s) (nail)

IQ + 7 T25.039- Burn of unspecified degree of unspecified toe(s) (nail)

+ 6 T25.09 Burn of unspecified degree of multiple sites of ankle and foot

IQ + 7 T25.091- Burn of unspecified degree of multiple sites of right ankle and foot

IQ + 7 T25.092- Burn of unspecified degree of multiple sites of left ankle and foot

IQ + 7 T25.099- Burn of unspecified degree of multiple sites of unspecified ankle and foot

+ 5 T25.1 Burn of first degree of ankle and foot

Use additional external cause code to identify the source, place and intent of the burn (X00-X19, X75-X77, X96-X98, Y92)

+ 6 T25.11 Burn of first degree of ankle

SP + 7 T25.111- Burn of first degree of right ankle

SP + 7 T25.112- Burn of first degree of left ankle

IQ + 7 T25.119- Burn of first degree of unspecified ankle

+ 6 T25.12 Burn of first degree of foot

EXCLUDES 2 burn of first degree of toe (s) (nail) (T25.13-)

SP + 7 T25.121- Burn of first degree of right foot

SP + 7 T25.122- Burn of first degree of left foot

IQ + 7 T25.129- Burn of first degree of unspecified foot

+ 6 T25.13 Burn of first degree of toe(s) (nail)

SP + 7 T25.131- Burn of first degree of right toe(s) (nail)

SP + 7 T25.132- Burn of first degree of left toe(s) (nail)

IQ + 7 T25.139- Burn of first degree of unspecified toe(s) (nail)

+ 6 T25.19 Burn of first degree of multiple sites of ankle and foot

SP + 7 T25.191- Burn of first degree of multiple sites of right ankle and foot

Chapter 19

S00-T88

T25.192- Burn of first degree of multiple sites of left ankle and foot

T25.199- Burn of first degree of multiple sites of unspecified ankle and foot

T25.2 Burn of second degree of ankle and foot

Use additional external cause code to identify the source, place and intent of the burn (X00-X19, X75-X77, X96-X98, Y92)

T25.21 Burn of second degree of ankle

T25.211- Burn of second degree of right ankle

T25.212- Burn of second degree of left ankle

T25.219- Burn of second degree of unspecified ankle

T25.22 Burn of second degree of foot

EXCLUDES 2 burn of second degree of toe (s) (nail) (T25.23-)

T25.221- Burn of second degree of right foot

T25.222- Burn of second degree of left foot

T25.229- Burn of second degree of unspecified foot

T25.23 Burn of second degree of toe(s) (nail)

T25.231- Burn of second degree of right toe(s) (nail)

T25.232- Burn of second degree of left toe(s) (nail)

T25.239- Burn of second degree of unspecified toe(s) (nail)

T25.29 Burn of second degree of multiple sites of ankle and foot

T25.291- Burn of second degree of multiple sites of right ankle and foot

T25.292- Burn of second degree of multiple sites of left ankle and foot

T25.299- Burn of second degree of multiple sites of unspecified ankle and foot

T25.3 Burn of third degree of ankle and foot

Use additional external cause code to identify the source, place and intent of the burn (X00-X19, X75-X77, X96-X98, Y92)

T25.31 Burn of third degree of ankle

T25.311- Burn of third degree of right ankle

T25.312- Burn of third degree of left ankle

T25.319- Burn of third degree of unspecified ankle

T25.32 Burn of third degree of foot

EXCLUDES 2 burn of third degree of toe (s) (nail) (T25.33-)

T25.321- Burn of third degree of right foot

T25.322- Burn of third degree of left foot

T25.329- Burn of third degree of unspecified foot

T25.33 Burn of third degree of toe(s) (nail)

T25.331- Burn of third degree of right toe(s) (nail)

T25.332- Burn of third degree of left toe(s) (nail)

T25.339- Burn of third degree of unspecified toe(s) (nail)

T25.39 Burn of third degree of multiple sites of ankle and foot

T25.391- Burn of third degree of multiple sites of right ankle and foot

T25.392- Burn of third degree of multiple sites of left ankle and foot

T25.399- Burn of third degree of multiple sites of unspecified ankle and foot

T25.4 Corrosion of unspecified degree of ankle and foot

Code first:
(T51-T65) to identify chemical and intent

Use additional external cause code to identify place (Y92)

T25.41 Corrosion of unspecified degree of ankle

T25.411- Corrosion of unspecified degree of right ankle

T25.412- Corrosion of unspecified degree of left ankle

T25.419- Corrosion of unspecified degree of unspecified ankle

T25.42 Corrosion of unspecified degree of foot

EXCLUDES 2 corrosion of unspecified degree of toe (s) (nail) (T25.43-)

T25.421- Corrosion of unspecified degree of right foot

T25.422- Corrosion of unspecified degree of left foot

T25.429- Corrosion of unspecified degree of unspecified foot

T25.43 Corrosion of unspecified degree of toe(s) (nail)

T25.431- Corrosion of unspecified degree of right toe(s) (nail)

T25.432- Corrosion of unspecified degree of left toe(s) (nail)

T25.439- Corrosion of unspecified degree of unspecified toe(s) (nail)

T25.49 Corrosion of unspecified degree of multiple sites of ankle and foot

T25.491- Corrosion of unspecified degree of multiple sites of right ankle and foot

T25.492- Corrosion of unspecified degree of multiple sites of left ankle and foot

T25.499- Corrosion of unspecified degree of multiple sites of unspecified ankle and foot

T25.5 Corrosion of first degree of ankle and foot

Code first:
(T51-T65) to identify chemical and intent

Use additional external cause code to identify place (Y92)

+ 6 T25.51 Corrosion of first degree of ankle

IQ + 7 T25.511- Corrosion of first degree of right ankle

IQ + 7 T25.512- Corrosion of first degree of left ankle

IQ + 7 T25.519- Corrosion of first degree of unspecified ankle

+ 6 T25.52 Corrosion of first degree of foot

EXCLUDES 2 corrosion of first degree of toe (s) (nail) (T25.53-)

IQ + 7 T25.521- Corrosion of first degree of right foot

IQ + 7 T25.522- Corrosion of first degree of left foot

IQ + 7 T25.529- Corrosion of first degree of unspecified foot

+ 6 T25.53 Corrosion of first degree of toe(s) (nail)

IQ + 7 T25.531- Corrosion of first degree of right toe(s) (nail)

IQ + 7 T25.532- Corrosion of first degree of left toe(s) (nail)

IQ + 7 T25.539- Corrosion of first degree of unspecified toe(s) (nail)

+ 6 T25.59 Corrosion of first degree of multiple sites of ankle and foot

IQ + 7 T25.591- Corrosion of first degree of multiple sites of right ankle and foot

IQ + 7 T25.592- Corrosion of first degree of multiple sites of left ankle and foot

IQ + 7 T25.599- Corrosion of first degree of multiple sites of unspecified ankle and foot

+ 5 T25.6 Corrosion of second degree of ankle and foot

Code first:
(T51-T65) to identify chemical and intent

Use additional external cause code to identify place (Y92)

+ 6 T25.61 Corrosion of second degree of ankle

IQ + 7 T25.611- Corrosion of second degree of right ankle

IQ + 7 T25.612- Corrosion of second degree of left ankle

IQ + 7 T25.619- Corrosion of second degree of unspecified ankle

+ 6 T25.62 Corrosion of second degree of foot

EXCLUDES 2 corrosion of second degree of toe (s) (nail) (T25.63-)

IQ + 7 T25.621- Corrosion of second degree of right foot

IQ + 7 T25.622- Corrosion of second degree of left foot

IQ + 7 T25.629- Corrosion of second degree of unspecified foot

+ 6 T25.63 Corrosion of second degree of toe(s) (nail)

IQ + 7 T25.631- Corrosion of second degree of right toe(s) (nail)

IQ + 7 T25.632- Corrosion of second degree of left toe(s) (nail)

IQ + 7 T25.639- Corrosion of second degree of unspecified toe(s) (nail)

+ 6 T25.69 Corrosion of second degree of multiple sites of ankle and foot

IQ + 7 T25.691- Corrosion of second degree of right ankle and foot

IQ + 7 T25.692- Corrosion of second degree of left ankle and foot

IQ + 7 T25.699- Corrosion of second degree of unspecified ankle and foot

+ 5 T25.7 Corrosion of third degree of ankle and foot

Code first:
(T51-T65) to identify chemical and intent

Use additional external cause code to identify place (Y92)

+ 6 T25.71 Corrosion of third degree of ankle

IQ + 7 T25.711- Corrosion of third degree of right ankle

IQ + 7 T25.712- Corrosion of third degree of left ankle

IQ + 7 T25.719- Corrosion of third degree of unspecified ankle

+ 6 T25.72 Corrosion of third degree of foot

EXCLUDES 2 corrosion of third degree of toe (s) (nail) (T25.73-)

IQ + 7 T25.721- Corrosion of third degree of right foot

IQ + 7 T25.722- Corrosion of third degree of left foot

IQ + 7 T25.729- Corrosion of third degree of unspecified foot

+ 6 T25.73 Corrosion of third degree of toe(s) (nail)

IQ + 7 T25.731- Corrosion of third degree of right toe(s) (nail)

IQ + 7 T25.732- Corrosion of third degree of left toe(s) (nail)

IQ + 7 T25.739- Corrosion of third degree of unspecified toe(s) (nail)

+ 6 T25.79 Corrosion of third degree of multiple sites of ankle and foot

IQ + 7 T25.791- Corrosion of third degree of multiple sites of right ankle and foot

IQ + 7 T25.792- Corrosion of third degree of multiple sites of left ankle and foot

IQ + 7 T25.799- Corrosion of third degree of multiple sites of unspecified ankle and foot

Burns and corrosions confined to eye and internal organs (T26-T28)

CODING TIPS ✓ Burns to the eyes and internal organs are not coded to degree.

4 T26 Burn and corrosion confined to eye and adnexa

The appropriate 7th character is to be added to each code from category T26

A initial encounter
D subsequent encounter
S sequela

+ 5 T26.0 Burn of eyelid and periocular area
Use additional external cause code to identify the source, place and intent of the burn (X00-X19, X75-X77, X96-X98, Y92)

▣ **IQ** **+** ☑ **T26.00X-** Burn of unspecified eyelid and periocular area

▣ **SP** **+** ☑ **T26.01X-** Burn of right eyelid and periocular area

▣ **SP** **+** ☑ **T26.02X-** Burn of left eyelid and periocular area

+ 5 T26.1 Burn of cornea and conjunctival sac
Use additional external cause code to identify the source, place and intent of the burn (X00-X19, X75-X77, X96-X98, Y92)

▣ **IQ** **+** ☑ **T26.10X-** Burn of cornea and conjunctival sac, unspecified eye

▣ **SP** **+** ☑ **T26.11X-** Burn of cornea and conjunctival sac, right eye

▣ **SP** **+** ☑ **T26.12X-** Burn of cornea and conjunctival sac, left eye

+ 5 T26.2 Burn with resulting rupture and destruction of eyeball
Use additional external cause code to identify the source, place and intent of the burn (X00-X19, X75-X77, X96-X98, Y92)

▣ **IQ** **+** ☑ **T26.20X-** Burn with resulting rupture and destruction of unspecified eyeball

▣ **SP** **+** ☑ **T26.21X-** Burn with resulting rupture and destruction of right eyeball

▣ **SP** **+** ☑ **T26.22X-** Burn with resulting rupture and destruction of left eyeball

+ 5 T26.3 Burns of other specified parts of eye and adnexa
Use additional external cause code to identify the source, place and intent of the burn (X00-X19, X75-X77, X96-X98, Y92)

▣ **IQ** **+** ☑ **T26.30X-** Burns of other specified parts of unspecified eye and adnexa

▣ **SP** **+** ☑ **T26.31X-** Burns of other specified parts of right eye and adnexa

▣ **SP** **+** ☑ **T26.32X-** Burns of other specified parts of left eye and adnexa

+ 5 T26.4 Burn of eye and adnexa, part unspecified
Use additional external cause code to identify the source, place and intent of the burn (X00-X19, X75-X77, X96-X98, Y92)

▣ **IQ** **+** ☑ **T26.40X-** Burn of unspecified eye and adnexa, part unspecified

▣ **IQ** **+** ☑ **T26.41X-** Burn of right eye and adnexa, part unspecified

▣ **IQ** **+** ☑ **T26.42X-** Burn of left eye and adnexa, part unspecified

+ 5 T26.5 Corrosion of eyelid and periocular area
Code first:
(T51-T65) to identify chemical and intent
Use additional external cause code to identify place (Y92)

▣ **IQ** **+** ☑ **T26.50X-** Corrosion of unspecified eyelid and periocular area

▣ **IQ** **+** ☑ **T26.51X-** Corrosion of right eyelid and periocular area

▣ **IQ** **+** ☑ **T26.52X-** Corrosion of left eyelid and periocular area

+ 5 T26.6 Corrosion of cornea and conjunctival sac
Code first:
(T51-T65) to identify chemical and intent
Use additional external cause code to identify place (Y92)

▣ **IQ** **+** ☑ **T26.60X-** Corrosion of cornea and conjunctival sac, unspecified eye

▣ **IQ** **+** ☑ **T26.61X-** Corrosion of cornea and conjunctival sac, right eye

▣ **IQ** **+** ☑ **T26.62X-** Corrosion of cornea and conjunctival sac, left eye

+ 5 T26.7 Corrosion with resulting rupture and destruction of eyeball
Code first:
(T51-T65) to identify chemical and intent
Use additional external cause code to identify place (Y92)

▣ **IQ** **+** ☑ **T26.70X-** Corrosion with resulting rupture and destruction of unspecified eyeball

▣ **IQ** **+** ☑ **T26.71X-** Corrosion with resulting rupture and destruction of right eyeball

▣ **IQ** **+** ☑ **T26.72X-** Corrosion with resulting rupture and destruction of left eyeball

+ 5 T26.8 Corrosions of other specified parts of eye and adnexa
Code first:
(T51-T65) to identify chemical and intent
Use additional external cause code to identify place (Y92)

▣ **IQ** **+** ☑ **T26.80X-** Corrosions of other specified parts of unspecified eye and adnexa

▣ **IQ** **+** ☑ **T26.81X-** Corrosions of other specified parts of right eye and adnexa

▣ **IQ** **+** ☑ **T26.82X-** Corrosions of other specified parts of left eye and adnexa

+ 5 T26.9 Corrosion of eye and adnexa, part unspecified
Code first:
(T51-T65) to identify chemical and intent
Use additional external cause code to identify place (Y92)

▣ **IQ** **+** ☑ **T26.90X-** Corrosion of unspecified eye and adnexa, part unspecified

▣ **IQ** **+** ☑ **T26.91X-** Corrosion of right eye and adnexa, part unspecified

▣ **IQ** **+** ☑ **T26.92X-** Corrosion of left eye and adnexa, part unspecified

+ 4 T27 Burn and corrosion of respiratory tract
Use additional external cause code to identify the source and intent of the burn (X00-X19, X75-X77, X96-X98)
Use additional external cause code to identify place (Y92)

---

4 4th digit required   5 5th digit required   6 6th digit required   7 7th digit required   ☑ 7th digit placeholder   + Additional code   ▣ Laterality

The appropriate 7th character is to be added to each code from category T27
A initial encounter
D subsequent encounter
S sequela

SP + 7 **T27.0XX- Burn of larynx and trachea**

SP + 7 **T27.1XX- Burn involving larynx and trachea with lung**

SP + 7 **T27.2XX- Burn of other parts of respiratory tract**
Burn of thoracic cavity

!Q + 7 **T27.3XX- Burn of respiratory tract, part unspecified**

!Q + 7 **T27.4XX- Corrosion of larynx and trachea**
Code first:
(T51-T65) to identify chemical and intent

!Q + 7 **T27.5XX- Corrosion involving larynx and trachea with lung**
Code first:
(T51-T65) to identify chemical and intent

!Q + 7 **T27.6XX- Corrosion of other parts of respiratory tract**
Code first:
(T51-T65) to identify chemical and intent

!Q + 7 **T27.7XX- Corrosion of respiratory tract, part unspecified**
Code first:
(T51-T65) to identify chemical and intent

+ 4 **T28 Burn and corrosion of other internal organs**
Use additional external cause code to identify the source and intent of the burn (X00-X19, X75-X77, X96-X98)
Use additional external cause code to identify place (Y92)

The appropriate 7th character is to be added to each code from category T28
A initial encounter
D subsequent encounter
S sequela

SP + 7 **T28.0XX- Burn of mouth and pharynx**

SP + 7 **T28.1XX- Burn of esophagus**

SP + 7 **T28.2XX- Burn of other parts of alimentary tract**

SP + 7 **T28.3XX- Burn of internal genitourinary organs**

+ 5 **T28.4 Burns of other and unspecified internal organs**

!Q + 7 **T28.40X- Burn of unspecified internal organ**

+ 6 **T28.41 Burn of ear drum**

H SP + 7 **T28.411- Burn of right ear drum**

H SP + 7 **T28.412- Burn of left ear drum**

H !Q + 7 **T28.419- Burn of unspecified ear drum**

SP + 7 **T28.49X- Burn of other internal organ**

!Q + 7 **T28.5XX- Corrosion of mouth and pharynx**
Code first:
(T51-T65) to identify chemical and intent

!Q + 7 **T28.6XX- Corrosion of esophagus**
Code first:
(T51-T65) to identify chemical and intent

!Q + 7 **T28.7XX- Corrosion of other parts of alimentary tract**
Code first:
(T51-T65) to identify chemical and intent

!Q + 7 **T28.8XX- Corrosion of internal genitourinary organs**
Code first:
(T51-T65) to identify chemical and intent

+ 5 **T28.9 Corrosions of other and unspecified internal organs**
Code first:
(T51-T65) to identify chemical and intent

!Q + 7 **T28.90X- Corrosions of unspecified internal organs**

+ 6 **T28.91 Corrosions of ear drum**

H !Q + 7 **T28.911- Corrosions of right ear drum**

H !Q + 7 **T28.912- Corrosions of left ear drum**

H !Q + 7 **T28.919- Corrosions of unspecified ear drum**

!Q + 7 **T28.99X- Corrosions of other internal organs**

Burns and corrosions of multiple and unspecified body regions (T30-T32)

GUIDELINES Section I.C.19.d.6)-9)
Categories T31 and T32 are based on the classic "rule of nines" in estimating body surface involved: head and neck are assigned nine percent, each arm nine percent, each leg 18 percent, the anterior trunk 18 percent, posterior trunk 18 percent, and genitalia one percent. Providers may change these percentage assignments where necessary to accommodate infants and children who have proportionately larger heads than adults, and patients who have large buttocks, thighs, or abdomen that involve burns.

Encounters for the treatment of the late effects of burns or corrosions (i.e., scars or joint contractures) should be coded with a burn or corrosion code with the 7th character "S" for sequela.

When appropriate, both a code for a current burn or corrosion with 7th character "A" or "D" and a burn or corrosion code with 7th character "S" may be assigned on the same record (when both a current burn and sequelae of an old burn exist). Burns and corrosions do not heal at the same rate and a current healing wound may still exist with sequela of a healed burn or corrosion.

An external cause code should be used with burns and corrosions to identify the source and intent of the burn, as well as the place where it occurred.

4 **T30 Burn and corrosion, body region unspecified**

GUIDELINES Section I.C.19.d.5)
Category T30, Burn and corrosion, body region unspecified is extremely vague and should rarely be used.

CODING TIPS✓ This code should not be assigned in home health or hospice. The location of the burn should be identifiable by clinical assessment and supported by clinical record documentation. Code the burn to location/site and severity, specifically.

!Q **T30.0 Burn of unspecified body region, unspecified degree**

This code is not for inpatient use. Code to specified site and degree of burns
Burn NOS
Multiple burns NOS

!Q **T30.4 Corrosion of unspecified body region, unspecified degree**

This code is not for inpatient use. Code to specified site and degree of corrosion
Corrosion NOS
Multiple corrosion NOS

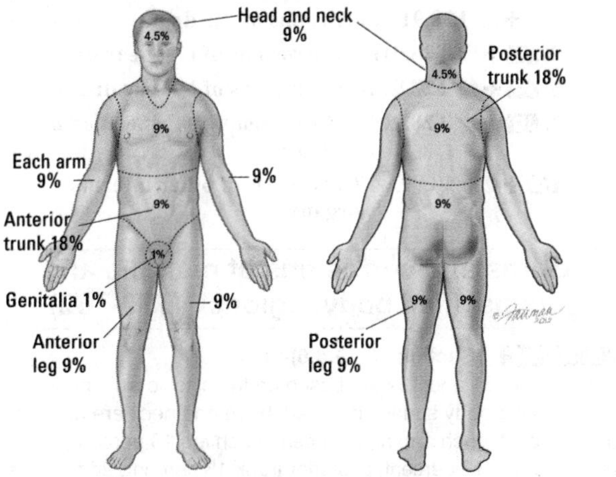

4 **T31 Burns classified according to extent of body surface involved**

Note:
This category is to be used as the primary code only when the site of the burn is unspecified. It should be used as a supplementary code with categories T20-T25 when the site is specified.

CODING TIPS✓ Do not use this code as primary in home care or hospice. T31 is used to identify the extent of a burn estimating body surface affected using the Rule of Nines and is only necessary in home care and hospice for patients who have 3rd degree burns over 20% or more of their bodies.

!Q **T31.0 Burns involving less than 10% of body surface**

5 **T31.1 Burns involving 10-19% of body surface**

!Q **T31.10 Burns involving 10-19% of body surface with 0% to 9% third degree burns**
Burns involving 10-19% of body surface NOS

!Q **T31.11 Burns involving 10-19% of body surface with 10-19% third degree burns**

5 **T31.2 Burns involving 20-29% of body surface**

!Q **T31.20 Burns involving 20-29% of body surface with 0% to 9% third degree burns**
Burns involving 20-29% of body surface NOS

!Q **T31.21 Burns involving 20-29% of body surface with 10-19% third degree burns**

!Q **T31.22 Burns involving 20-29% of body surface with 20-29% third degree burns**

5 **T31.3 Burns involving 30-39% of body surface**

!Q **T31.30 Burns involving 30-39% of body surface with 0% to 9% third degree burns**
Burns involving 30-39% of body surface NOS

!Q **T31.31 Burns involving 30-39% of body surface with 10-19% third degree burns**

!Q **T31.32 Burns involving 30-39% of body surface with 20-29% third degree burns**

!Q **T31.33 Burns involving 30-39% of body surface with 30-39% third degree burns**

5 **T31.4 Burns involving 40-49% of body surface**

!Q **T31.40 Burns involving 40-49% of body surface with 0% to 9% third degree burns**
Burns involving 40-49% of body surface NOS

!Q **T31.41 Burns involving 40-49% of body surface with 10-19% third degree burns**

!Q **T31.42 Burns involving 40-49% of body surface with 20-29% third degree burns**

!Q **T31.43 Burns involving 40-49% of body surface with 30-39% third degree burns**

!Q **T31.44 Burns involving 40-49% of body surface with 40-49% third degree burns**

5 **T31.5 Burns involving 50-59% of body surface**

!Q **T31.50 Burns involving 50-59% of body surface with 0% to 9% third degree burns**
Burns involving 50-59% of body surface NOS

!Q **T31.51 Burns involving 50-59% of body surface with 10-19% third degree burns**

!Q **T31.52 Burns involving 50-59% of body surface with 20-29% third degree burns**

!Q **T31.53 Burns involving 50-59% of body surface with 30-39% third degree burns**

!Q **T31.54 Burns involving 50-59% of body surface with 40-49% third degree burns**

!Q **T31.55 Burns involving 50-59% of body surface with 50-59% third degree burns**

5 **T31.6 Burns involving 60-69% of body surface**

IQ **T31.60 Burns involving 60-69% of body surface with 0% to 9% third degree burns**
Burns involving 60-69% of body surface NOS

IQ **T31.61 Burns involving 60-69% of body surface with 10-19% third degree burns**

IQ **T31.62 Burns involving 60-69% of body surface with 20-29% third degree burns**

IQ **T31.63 Burns involving 60-69% of body surface with 30-39% third degree burns**

IQ **T31.64 Burns involving 60-69% of body surface with 40-49% third degree burns**

IQ **T31.65 Burns involving 60-69% of body surface with 50-59% third degree burns**

IQ **T31.66 Burns involving 60-69% of body surface with 60-69% third degree burns**

5 **T31.7 Burns involving 70-79% of body surface**

IQ **T31.70 Burns involving 70-79% of body surface with 0% to 9% third degree burns**
Burns involving 70-79% of body surface NOS

IQ **T31.71 Burns involving 70-79% of body surface with 10-19% third degree burns**

IQ **T31.72 Burns involving 70-79% of body surface with 20-29% third degree burns**

IQ **T31.73 Burns involving 70-79% of body surface with 30-39% third degree burns**

IQ **T31.74 Burns involving 70-79% of body surface with 40-49% third degree burns**

IQ **T31.75 Burns involving 70-79% of body surface with 50-59% third degree burns**

IQ **T31.76 Burns involving 70-79% of body surface with 60-69% third degree burns**

IQ **T31.77 Burns involving 70-79% of body surface with 70-79% third degree burns**

5 **T31.8 Burns involving 80-89% of body surface**

IQ **T31.80 Burns involving 80-89% of body surface with 0% to 9% third degree burns**
Burns involving 80-89% of body surface NOS

IQ **T31.81 Burns involving 80-89% of body surface with 10-19% third degree burns**

IQ **T31.82 Burns involving 80-89% of body surface with 20-29% third degree burns**

IQ **T31.83 Burns involving 80-89% of body surface with 30-39% third degree burns**

IQ **T31.84 Burns involving 80-89% of body surface with 40-49% third degree burns**

IQ **T31.85 Burns involving 80-89% of body surface with 50-59% third degree burns**

IQ **T31.86 Burns involving 80-89% of body surface with 60-69% third degree burns**

IQ **T31.87 Burns involving 80-89% of body surface with 70-79% third degree burns**

IQ **T31.88 Burns involving 80-89% of body surface with 80-89% third degree burns**

5 **T31.9 Burns involving 90% or more of body surface**

IQ **T31.90 Burns involving 90% or more of body surface with 0% to 9% third degree burns**
Burns involving 90% or more of body surface NOS

IQ **T31.91 Burns involving 90% or more of body surface with 10-19% third degree burns**

IQ **T31.92 Burns involving 90% or more of body surface with 20-29% third degree burns**

IQ **T31.93 Burns involving 90% or more of body surface with 30-39% third degree burns**

IQ **T31.94 Burns involving 90% or more of body surface with 40-49% third degree burns**

IQ **T31.95 Burns involving 90% or more of body surface with 50-59% third degree burns**

IQ **T31.96 Burns involving 90% or more of body surface with 60-69% third degree burns**

IQ **T31.97 Burns involving 90% or more of body surface with 70-79% third degree burns**

IQ **T31.98 Burns involving 90% or more of body surface with 80-89% third degree burns**

IQ **T31.99 Burns involving 90% or more of body surface with 90% or more third degree burns**

4 **T32 Corrosions classified according to extent of body surface involved**
Note:
This category is to be used as the primary code only when the site of the corrosion is unspecified. It may be used as a supplementary code with categories T20-T25 when the site is specified.

IQ **T32.0 Corrosions involving less than 10% of body surface**

5 **T32.1 Corrosions involving 10-19% of body surface**

IQ **T32.10 Corrosions involving 10-19% of body surface with 0% to 9% third degree corrosion**
Corrosions involving 10-19% of body surface NOS

IQ **T32.11 Corrosions involving 10-19% of body surface with 10-19% third degree corrosion**

5 **T32.2 Corrosions involving 20-29% of body surface**

Chapter 19

S00-T88

IQ **T32.20** Corrosions involving 20-29% of body surface with 0% to 9% third degree corrosion

IQ **T32.21** Corrosions involving 20-29% of body surface with 10-19% third degree corrosion

IQ **T32.22** Corrosions involving 20-29% of body surface with 20-29% third degree corrosion

5 **T32.3** Corrosions involving 30-39% of body surface

IQ **T32.30** Corrosions involving 30-39% of body surface with 0% to 9% third degree corrosion

IQ **T32.31** Corrosions involving 30-39% of body surface with 10-19% third degree corrosion

IQ **T32.32** Corrosions involving 30-39% of body surface with 20-29% third degree corrosion

IQ **T32.33** Corrosions involving 30-39% of body surface with 30-39% third degree corrosion

5 **T32.4** Corrosions involving 40-49% of body surface

IQ **T32.40** Corrosions involving 40-49% of body surface with 0% to 9% third degree corrosion

IQ **T32.41** Corrosions involving 40-49% of body surface with 10-19% third degree corrosion

IQ **T32.42** Corrosions involving 40-49% of body surface with 20-29% third degree corrosion

IQ **T32.43** Corrosions involving 40-49% of body surface with 30-39% third degree corrosion

IQ **T32.44** Corrosions involving 40-49% of body surface with 40-49% third degree corrosion

5 **T32.5** Corrosions involving 50-59% of body surface

IQ **T32.50** Corrosions involving 50-59% of body surface with 0% to 9% third degree corrosion

IQ **T32.51** Corrosions involving 50-59% of body surface with 10-19% third degree corrosion

IQ **T32.52** Corrosions involving 50-59% of body surface with 20-29% third degree corrosion

IQ **T32.53** Corrosions involving 50-59% of body surface with 30-39% third degree corrosion

IQ **T32.54** Corrosions involving 50-59% of body surface with 40-49% third degree corrosion

IQ **T32.55** Corrosions involving 50-59% of body surface with 50-59% third degree corrosion

5 **T32.6** Corrosions involving 60-69% of body surface

IQ **T32.60** Corrosions involving 60-69% of body surface with 0% to 9% third degree corrosion

IQ **T32.61** Corrosions involving 60-69% of body surface with 10-19% third degree corrosion

IQ **T32.62** Corrosions involving 60-69% of body surface with 20-29% third degree corrosion

IQ **T32.63** Corrosions involving 60-69% of body surface with 30-39% third degree corrosion

IQ **T32.64** Corrosions involving 60-69% of body surface with 40-49% third degree corrosion

IQ **T32.65** Corrosions involving 60-69% of body surface with 50-59% third degree corrosion

IQ **T32.66** Corrosions involving 60-69% of body surface with 60-69% third degree corrosion

5 **T32.7** Corrosions involving 70-79% of body surface

IQ **T32.70** Corrosions involving 70-79% of body surface with 0% to 9% third degree corrosion

IQ **T32.71** Corrosions involving 70-79% of body surface with 10-19% third degree corrosion

IQ **T32.72** Corrosions involving 70-79% of body surface with 20-29% third degree corrosion

IQ **T32.73** Corrosions involving 70-79% of body surface with 30-39% third degree corrosion

IQ **T32.74** Corrosions involving 70-79% of body surface with 40-49% third degree corrosion

IQ **T32.75** Corrosions involving 70-79% of body surface with 50-59% third degree corrosion

IQ **T32.76** Corrosions involving 70-79% of body surface with 60-69% third degree corrosion

IQ **T32.77** Corrosions involving 70-79% of body surface with 70-79% third degree corrosion

5 **T32.8** Corrosions involving 80-89% of body surface

IQ **T32.80** Corrosions involving 80-89% of body surface with 0% to 9% third degree corrosion

IQ **T32.81** Corrosions involving 80-89% of body surface with 10-19% third degree corrosion

IQ **T32.82** Corrosions involving 80-89% of body surface with 20-29% third degree corrosion

IQ **T32.83** Corrosions involving 80-89% of body surface with 30-39% third degree corrosion

IQ **T32.84** Corrosions involving 80-89% of body surface with 40-49% third degree corrosion

IQ **T32.85** Corrosions involving 80-89% of body surface with 50-59% third degree corrosion

IQ **T32.86** Corrosions involving 80-89% of body surface with 60-69% third degree corrosion

IQ **T32.87** Corrosions involving 80-89% of body surface with 70-79% third degree corrosion

IQ T32.88 Corrosions involving 80-89% of body surface with 80-89% third degree corrosion

5 T32.9 Corrosions involving 90% or more of body surface

IQ T32.90 Corrosions involving 90% or more of body surface with 0% to 9% third degree corrosion

IQ T32.91 Corrosions involving 90% or more of body surface with 10-19% third degree corrosion

IQ T32.92 Corrosions involving 90% or more of body surface with 20-29% third degree corrosion

IQ T32.93 Corrosions involving 90% or more of body surface with 30-39% third degree corrosion

IQ T32.94 Corrosions involving 90% or more of body surface with 40-49% third degree corrosion

IQ T32.95 Corrosions involving 90% or more of body surface with 50-59% third degree corrosion

IQ T32.96 Corrosions involving 90% or more of body surface with 60-69% third degree corrosion

IQ T32.97 Corrosions involving 90% or more of body surface with 70-79% third degree corrosion

IQ T32.98 Corrosions involving 90% or more of body surface with 80-89% third degree corrosion

IQ T32.99 Corrosions involving 90% or more of body surface with 90% or more third degree corrosion

Frostbite (T33-T34)

EXCLUDES 2 hypothermia and other effects of reduced temperature (T68, T69.-)

4 T33 Superficial frostbite

INCLUDES frostbite with partial thickness skin loss

The appropriate 7th character is to be added to each code from category T33

- A initial encounter
- D subsequent encounter
- S sequela

5 T33.0 Superficial frostbite of head

6 T33.01 Superficial frostbite of ear

SP 7 T33.011- Superficial frostbite of right ear

SP 7 T33.012- Superficial frostbite of left ear

IQ 7 T33.019- Superficial frostbite of unspecified ear

SP 7 T33.02X- Superficial frostbite of nose

SP 7 T33.09X- Superficial frostbite of other part of head

SP 7 T33.1XX- Superficial frostbite of neck

SP 7 T33.2XX- Superficial frostbite of thorax

SP 7 T33.3XX- Superficial frostbite of abdominal wall, lower back and pelvis

5 T33.4 Superficial frostbite of arm

EXCLUDES 2 superficial frostbite of wrist and hand (T33.5-)

IQ 7 T33.40X- Superficial frostbite of unspecified arm

SP 7 T33.41X- Superficial frostbite of right arm

SP 7 T33.42X- Superficial frostbite of left arm

5 T33.5 Superficial frostbite of wrist, hand, and fingers

6 T33.51 Superficial frostbite of wrist

SP 7 T33.511- Superficial frostbite of right wrist

SP 7 T33.512- Superficial frostbite of left wrist

IQ 7 T33.519- Superficial frostbite of unspecified wrist

6 T33.52 Superficial frostbite of hand

EXCLUDES 2 superficial frostbite of fingers (T33.53-)

SP 7 T33.521- Superficial frostbite of right hand

SP 7 T33.522- Superficial frostbite of left hand

IQ 7 T33.529- Superficial frostbite of unspecified hand

6 T33.53 Superficial frostbite of finger(s)

SP 7 T33.531- Superficial frostbite of right finger(s)

SP 7 T33.532- Superficial frostbite of left finger(s)

IQ 7 T33.539- Superficial frostbite of unspecified finger(s)

5 T33.6 Superficial frostbite of hip and thigh

IQ 7 T33.60X- Superficial frostbite of unspecified hip and thigh

SP 7 T33.61X- Superficial frostbite of right hip and thigh

SP 7 T33.62X- Superficial frostbite of left hip and thigh

5 T33.7 Superficial frostbite of knee and lower leg

EXCLUDES 2 superficial frostbite of ankle and foot (T33.8-)

IQ 7 T33.70X- Superficial frostbite of unspecified knee and lower leg

SP 7 T33.71X- Superficial frostbite of right knee and lower leg

SP 7 T33.72X- Superficial frostbite of left knee and lower leg

5 T33.8 Superficial frostbite of ankle, foot, and toe(s)

6 T33.81 Superficial frostbite of ankle

SP 7 T33.811- Superficial frostbite of right ankle

SP 7 T33.812- Superficial frostbite of left ankle

IQ 7 T33.819- Superficial frostbite of unspecified ankle

6 T33.82 Superficial frostbite of foot

SP 7 T33.821- Superficial frostbite of right foot

SP 7 T33.822- Superficial frostbite of left foot

IQ 7 T33.829- Superficial frostbite of unspecified foot

6 T33.83 Superficial frostbite of toe(s)

SP 7 T33.831- Superficial frostbite of right toe(s)

SP 7 T33.832- Superficial frostbite of left toe(s)

IQ 7 T33.839- Superficial frostbite of unspecified toe(s)

5 T33.9 Superficial frostbite of other and unspecified sites

IQ ☑ T33.90X- **Superficial frostbite of unspecified sites**
Superficial frostbite NOS

SP ☑ T33.99X- **Superficial frostbite of other sites**
Superficial frostbite of leg NOS
Superficial frostbite of trunk NOS

4 T34 **Frostbite with tissue necrosis**

> The appropriate 7th character is to be added to each code from category T34
> A   initial encounter
> D   subsequent encounter
> S   sequela

5 T34.0 **Frostbite with tissue necrosis of head**

6 T34.01 **Frostbite with tissue necrosis of ear**

SP 7 T34.011- **Frostbite with tissue necrosis of right ear**

SP 7 T34.012- **Frostbite with tissue necrosis of left ear**

IQ 7 T34.019- **Frostbite with tissue necrosis of unspecified ear**

SP ☑ T34.02X- **Frostbite with tissue necrosis of nose**

SP ☑ T34.09X- **Frostbite with tissue necrosis of other part of head**

SP ☑ T34.1XX- **Frostbite with tissue necrosis of neck**

SP ☑ T34.2XX- **Frostbite with tissue necrosis of thorax**

SP ☑ T34.3XX- **Frostbite with tissue necrosis of abdominal wall, lower back and pelvis**

5 T34.4 **Frostbite with tissue necrosis of arm**
> **EXCLUDES 2** frostbite with tissue necrosis of wrist and hand (T34.5-)

IQ ☑ T34.40X- **Frostbite with tissue necrosis of unspecified arm**

SP ☑ T34.41X- **Frostbite with tissue necrosis of right arm**

SP ☑ T34.42X- **Frostbite with tissue necrosis of left arm**

5 T34.5 **Frostbite with tissue necrosis of wrist, hand, and finger(s)**

6 T34.51 **Frostbite with tissue necrosis of wrist**

SP 7 T34.511- **Frostbite with tissue necrosis of right wrist**

SP 7 T34.512- **Frostbite with tissue necrosis of left wrist**

IQ 7 T34.519- **Frostbite with tissue necrosis of unspecified wrist**

6 T34.52 **Frostbite with tissue necrosis of hand**
> **EXCLUDES 2** frostbite with tissue necrosis of finger (s) (T34.53-)

SP 7 T34.521- **Frostbite with tissue necrosis of right hand**

SP 7 T34.522- **Frostbite with tissue necrosis of left hand**

IQ 7 T34.529- **Frostbite with tissue necrosis of unspecified hand**

6 T34.53 **Frostbite with tissue necrosis of finger(s)**

SP 7 T34.531- **Frostbite with tissue necrosis of right finger(s)**

SP 7 T34.532- **Frostbite with tissue necrosis of left finger(s)**

IQ 7 T34.539- **Frostbite with tissue necrosis of unspecified finger(s)**

5 T34.6 **Frostbite with tissue necrosis of hip and thigh**

IQ ☑ T34.60X- **Frostbite with tissue necrosis of unspecified hip and thigh**

SP ☑ T34.61X- **Frostbite with tissue necrosis of right hip and thigh**

SP ☑ T34.62X- **Frostbite with tissue necrosis of left hip and thigh**

5 T34.7 **Frostbite with tissue necrosis of knee and lower leg**
> **EXCLUDES 2** frostbite with tissue necrosis of ankle and foot (T34.8-)

IQ ☑ T34.70X- **Frostbite with tissue necrosis of unspecified knee and lower leg**

SP ☑ T34.71X- **Frostbite with tissue necrosis of right knee and lower leg**

SP ☑ T34.72X- **Frostbite with tissue necrosis of left knee and lower leg**

5 T34.8 **Frostbite with tissue necrosis of ankle, foot, and toe(s)**

6 T34.81 **Frostbite with tissue necrosis of ankle**

SP 7 T34.811- **Frostbite with tissue necrosis of right ankle**

SP 7 T34.812- **Frostbite with tissue necrosis of left ankle**

IQ 7 T34.819- **Frostbite with tissue necrosis of unspecified ankle**

6 T34.82 **Frostbite with tissue necrosis of foot**

SP 7 T34.821- **Frostbite with tissue necrosis of right foot**

SP 7 T34.822- **Frostbite with tissue necrosis of left foot**

IQ 7 T34.829- **Frostbite with tissue necrosis of unspecified foot**

6 T34.83 **Frostbite with tissue necrosis of toe(s)**

SP 7 T34.831- **Frostbite with tissue necrosis of right toe(s)**

SP 7 T34.832- **Frostbite with tissue necrosis of left toe(s)**

IQ 7 T34.839- **Frostbite with tissue necrosis of unspecified toe(s)**

5 T34.9 **Frostbite with tissue necrosis of other and unspecified sites**

IQ ☑ T34.90X- **Frostbite with tissue necrosis of unspecified sites**
Frostbite with tissue necrosis NOS

SP ☑ T34.99X- **Frostbite with tissue necrosis of other sites**
Frostbite with tissue necrosis of leg NOS
Frostbite with tissue necrosis of trunk NOS

Poisoning by, adverse effects of and underdosing of drugs, medicaments and biological substances (T36-T50)

Note:
The drug giving rise to the adverse effect should be identified by use of codes from categories T36-T50 with fifth or sixth character 5.

---

4 4th digit required **5** 5th digit required **6** 6th digit required **7** 7th digit required **☑** 7th digit placeholder **+** Additional code **⊟** Laterality

INCLUDES adverse effect of correct substance properly administered
poisoning by overdose of substance
poisoning by wrong substance given or taken in error
underdosing by (inadvertently) (deliberately) taking less substance than prescribed or instructed

Code first, for adverse effects, the nature of the adverse effect, such as:
adverse effect NOS (T88.7)
aspirin gastritis (K29.-)
blood disorders (D56-D76)
contact dermatitis (L23-L25)
dermatitis due to substances taken internally (L27.-)
nephropathy (N14.0-N14.2)

Use additional code(s) to specify:
manifestations of poisoning
underdosing or failure in dosage during medical and surgical care (Y63.6, Y63.8-Y63.9)
underdosing of medication regimen (Z91.12-, Z91.13-)

EXCLUDES 1 toxic reaction to local anesthesia in pregnancy (O29.3-)

EXCLUDES 2 abuse and dependence of psychoactive substances (F10-F19)
abuse of non-dependence-producing substances (F55.-)
immunodeficiency due to drugs (D84.821)
drug reaction and poisoning affecting newborn (P00-P96)
pathological drug intoxication (inebriation) (F10-F19)

GUIDELINES **Section I.C.19.e.5)(c)**

Underdosing refers to taking less of a medication than is prescribed by a provider or a manufacturer's instruction. Discontinuing the use of a prescribed medication on the patient's own initiative (not directed by the patient's provider) is also classified as an underdosing. For underdosing, assign the code from categories T36-T50 (fifth or sixth character "6").

Codes for underdosing should never be assigned as principal or first-listed codes. If a patient has a relapse or exacerbation of the medical condition for which the drug is prescribed because of the reduction in dose, then the medical condition itself should be coded.

Noncompliance (Z91.12-, Z91.13- and Z91.14-) or complication of care (Y63.6-Y63.9) codes are to be used with an underdosing code to indicate intent, if known.

GUIDELINES **Section I.C.19.e.1)-4)**

Codes in categories T36-T65 are combination codes that include the substance that was taken as well as the intent. No additional external cause code is required for poisonings, toxic effects, adverse effects and underdosing codes.

Do not code directly from the Table of Drugs and Chemicals. Always refer back to the Tabular List. Use as many codes as necessary to describe completely all drugs, medicinal or biological substances. If the same code would describe the causative agent for more than one adverse reaction, poisoning, toxic effect or underdosing, assign the code only once. If two or more drugs, medicinal or biological substances are reported, code each individually unless a combination code is listed in the Table of Drugs and Chemicals.

GUIDELINES **Section I.C.19.e.5)(a)**

When coding an adverse effect of a drug that has been correctly prescribed and properly administered, assign the appropriate code for the nature of the adverse effect followed by the appropriate code for the adverse effect of the drug (T36-T50). The code for the drug should have a 5th or 6th character "5" (for example T36.0X5-). Examples of the nature of an adverse effect are tachycardia, delirium, gastrointestinal hemorrhaging, vomiting, hypokalemia, hepatitis, renal failure, or respiratory failure.

CODING TIPS ✓ Poisonings are coded as accidental unless there is provider documentation to indicate otherwise. 7th character 'A' means the effect of the drug/chemical requires active treatment. 'D' should be the 7th character if the effect is healing/resolving. 'S' should be used as the 7th character if the condition resulting is still a factor after the medication has long cleared from the body, i.e., glucocorticoids were taken last year resulting in diabetes.

4 **T36 Poisoning by, adverse effect of and underdosing of systemic antibiotics**

EXCLUDES 1 antineoplastic antibiotics (T45.1-)
locally applied antibiotic NEC (T49.0)
topically used antibiotic for ear, nose and throat (T49.6)
topically used antibiotic for eye (T49.5)

The appropriate 7th character is to be added to each code from category T36

A	initial encounter
D	subsequent encounter
S	sequela

GUIDELINES **Section I.C.19.e.5)(b)**

When coding a poisoning or reaction to the improper use of a medication (e.g., overdose, wrong substance given or taken in error, wrong route of administration), first assign the appropriate code from categories T36-T50. The poisoning codes have an associated intent as their 5th or 6th character (accidental, intentional self harm, assault and undetermined. If the intent of the poisoning is unknown or unspecified, code the intent as accidental intent. The undetermined intent is only for use if the documentation in the record specifies that the intent cannot be determined.

Use additional code(s) for all manifestations of poisonings. If there is also a diagnosis of abuse or dependence of the substance, the abuse or dependence is assigned as an additional code. *See Section I.C.4. if poisoning is the result of insulin pump malfunctions.*

5 **T36.0 Poisoning by, adverse effect of and underdosing of penicillins**

6 **T36.0X Poisoning by, adverse effect of and underdosing of penicillins**

SP IQ 7 **T36.0X1- Poisoning by penicillins, accidental (unintentional)**
Poisoning by penicillins NOS

SP 7 **T36.0X2- Poisoning by penicillins, intentional self-harm**

SP 7 **T36.0X3- Poisoning by penicillins, assault**

SP 7 **T36.0X4- Poisoning by penicillins, undetermined**

Chapter 19 S00-T88

!Q 7 **T36.0X5- Adverse effect of penicillins**

7 **T36.0X6- Underdosing of penicillins**

5 **T36.1 Poisoning by, adverse effect of and underdosing of cephalosporins and other beta-lactam antibiotics**

6 **T36.1X Poisoning by, adverse effect of and underdosing of cephalosporins and other beta-lactam antibiotics**

SP 7 **T36.1X1- Poisoning by cephalosporins and other beta-lactam antibiotics, accidental (unintentional)**
Poisoning by cephalosporins and other beta-lactam antibiotics NOS

SP 7 **T36.1X2- Poisoning by cephalosporins and other beta-lactam antibiotics, intentional self-harm**

SP 7 **T36.1X3- Poisoning by cephalosporins and other beta-lactam antibiotics, assault**

SP 7 **T36.1X4- Poisoning by cephalosporins and other beta-lactam antibiotics, undetermined**

!Q 7 **T36.1X5- Adverse effect of cephalosporins and other beta-lactam antibiotics**

7 **T36.1X6- Underdosing of cephalosporins and other beta-lactam antibiotics**

5 **T36.2 Poisoning by, adverse effect of and underdosing of chloramphenicol group**

6 **T36.2X Poisoning by, adverse effect of and underdosing of chloramphenicol group**

SP 7 **T36.2X1- Poisoning by chloramphenicol group, accidental (unintentional)**
Poisoning by chloramphenicol group NOS

SP 7 **T36.2X2- Poisoning by chloramphenicol group, intentional self-harm**

SP 7 **T36.2X3- Poisoning by chloramphenicol group, assault**

SP 7 **T36.2X4- Poisoning by chloramphenicol group, undetermined**

!Q 7 **T36.2X5- Adverse effect of chloramphenicol group**

7 **T36.2X6- Underdosing of chloramphenicol group**

5 **T36.3 Poisoning by, adverse effect of and underdosing of macrolides**

6 **T36.3X Poisoning by, adverse effect of and underdosing of macrolides**

SP 7 **T36.3X1- Poisoning by macrolides, accidental (unintentional)**
Poisoning by macrolides NOS

SP 7 **T36.3X2- Poisoning by macrolides, intentional self-harm**

SP 7 **T36.3X3- Poisoning by macrolides, assault**

SP 7 **T36.3X4- Poisoning by macrolides, undetermined**

!Q 7 **T36.3X5- Adverse effect of macrolides**

7 **T36.3X6- Underdosing of macrolides**

5 **T36.4 Poisoning by, adverse effect of and underdosing of tetracyclines**

6 **T36.4X Poisoning by, adverse effect of and underdosing of tetracyclines**

SP 7 **T36.4X1- Poisoning by tetracyclines, accidental (unintentional)**
Poisoning by tetracyclines NOS

SP 7 **T36.4X2- Poisoning by tetracyclines, intentional self-harm**

SP 7 **T36.4X3- Poisoning by tetracyclines, assault**

SP 7 **T36.4X4- Poisoning by tetracyclines, undetermined**

!Q 7 **T36.4X5- Adverse effect of tetracyclines**

7 **T36.4X6- Underdosing of tetracyclines**

5 **T36.5 Poisoning by, adverse effect of and underdosing of aminoglycosides**
Poisoning by, adverse effect of and underdosing of streptomycin

6 **T36.5X Poisoning by, adverse effect of and underdosing of aminoglycosides**

SP 7 **T36.5X1- Poisoning by aminoglycosides, accidental (unintentional)**
Poisoning by aminoglycosides NOS

SP 7 **T36.5X2- Poisoning by aminoglycosides, intentional self-harm**

SP 7 **T36.5X3- Poisoning by aminoglycosides, assault**

SP 7 **T36.5X4- Poisoning by aminoglycosides, undetermined**

!Q 7 **T36.5X5- Adverse effect of aminoglycosides**

7 **T36.5X6- Underdosing of aminoglycosides**

5 **T36.6 Poisoning by, adverse effect of and underdosing of rifampicins**

6 **T36.6X Poisoning by, adverse effect of and underdosing of rifampicins**

SP 7 **T36.6X1- Poisoning by rifampicins, accidental (unintentional)**
Poisoning by rifampicins NOS

SP 7 **T36.6X2- Poisoning by rifampicins, intentional self-harm**

SP 7 **T36.6X3- Poisoning by rifampicins, assault**

SP 7 **T36.6X4- Poisoning by rifampicins, undetermined**

!Q 7 **T36.6X5- Adverse effect of rifampicins**

7 **T36.6X6- Underdosing of rifampicins**

5 **T36.7 Poisoning by, adverse effect of and underdosing of antifungal antibiotics, systemically used**

6 **T36.7X Poisoning by, adverse effect of and underdosing of antifungal antibiotics, systemically used**

SP 7 **T36.7X1- Poisoning by antifungal antibiotics, systemically used, accidental (unintentional)**
Poisoning by antifungal antibiotics, systemically used NOS

SP 7 **T36.7X2- Poisoning by antifungal antibiotics, systemically used, intentional self-harm**

SP 7 **T36.7X3- Poisoning by antifungal antibiotics, systemically used, assault**

SP 7 **T36.7X4- Poisoning by antifungal antibiotics, systemically used, undetermined**

!Q 7 **T36.7X5- Adverse effect of antifungal antibiotics, systemically used**

7 **T36.7X6- Underdosing of antifungal antibiotics, systemically used**

5 **T36.8 Poisoning by, adverse effect of and underdosing of other systemic antibiotics**

6 **T36.8X Poisoning by, adverse effect of and underdosing of other systemic antibiotics**

SP 7 **T36.8X1- Poisoning by other systemic antibiotics, accidental (unintentional)**
Poisoning by other systemic antibiotics NOS

SP 7 **T36.8X2- Poisoning by other systemic antibiotics, intentional self-harm**

SP 7 **T36.8X3- Poisoning by other systemic antibiotics, assault**

SP 7 **T36.8X4- Poisoning by other systemic antibiotics, undetermined**

!Q 7 **T36.8X5- Adverse effect of other systemic antibiotics**

7 **T36.8X6- Underdosing of other systemic antibiotics**

5 **T36.9 Poisoning by, adverse effect of and underdosing of unspecified systemic antibiotic**

SP 7 **T36.91X- Poisoning by unspecified systemic antibiotic, accidental (unintentional)**
Poisoning by systemic antibiotic NOS

SP 7 **T36.92X- Poisoning by unspecified systemic antibiotic, intentional self-harm**

SP 7 **T36.93X- Poisoning by unspecified systemic antibiotic, assault**

SP 7 **T36.94X- Poisoning by unspecified systemic antibiotic, undetermined**

!Q 7 **T36.95X- Adverse effect of unspecified systemic antibiotic**

7 **T36.96X- Underdosing of unspecified systemic antibiotic**

4 **T37 Poisoning by, adverse effect of and underdosing of other systemic anti-infectives and antiparasitics**

EXCLUDES 1 anti-infectives topically used for ear, nose and throat (T49.6-)
anti-infectives topically used for eye (T49.5-)
locally applied anti-infectives NEC (T49.0-)

The appropriate 7th character is to be added to each code from category T37
A initial encounter
D subsequent encounter
S sequela

5 **T37.0 Poisoning by, adverse effect of and underdosing of sulfonamides**

6 **T37.0X Poisoning by, adverse effect of and underdosing of sulfonamides**

SP 7 **T37.0X1- Poisoning by sulfonamides, accidental (unintentional)**
Poisoning by sulfonamides NOS

SP 7 **T37.0X2- Poisoning by sulfonamides, intentional self-harm**

SP 7 **T37.0X3- Poisoning by sulfonamides, assault**

SP 7 **T37.0X4- Poisoning by sulfonamides, undetermined**

!Q 7 **T37.0X5- Adverse effect of sulfonamides**

7 **T37.0X6- Underdosing of sulfonamides**

5 **T37.1 Poisoning by, adverse effect of and underdosing of antimycobacterial drugs**

EXCLUDES 1 rifampicins (T36.6-)
streptomycin (T36.5-)

6 **T37.1X Poisoning by, adverse effect of and underdosing of antimycobacterial drugs**

SP 7 **T37.1X1- Poisoning by antimycobacterial drugs, accidental (unintentional)**
Poisoning by antimycobacterial drugs NOS

SP 7 **T37.1X2- Poisoning by antimycobacterial drugs, intentional self-harm**

SP 7 **T37.1X3- Poisoning by antimycobacterial drugs, assault**

SP 7 **T37.1X4- Poisoning by antimycobacterial drugs, undetermined**

!Q 7 **T37.1X5- Adverse effect of antimycobacterial drugs**

7 **T37.1X6- Underdosing of antimycobacterial drugs**

5 **T37.2 Poisoning by, adverse effect of and underdosing of antimalarials and drugs acting on other blood protozoa**

EXCLUDES 1 hydroxyquinoline derivatives (T37.8-)

6 **T37.2X Poisoning by, adverse effect of and underdosing of antimalarials and drugs acting on other blood protozoa**

SP 7 **T37.2X1- Poisoning by antimalarials and drugs acting on other blood protozoa, accidental (unintentional)**
Poisoning by antimalarials and drugs acting on other blood protozoa NOS

SP 7 **T37.2X2- Poisoning by antimalarials and drugs acting on other blood protozoa, intentional self-harm**

SP 7 **T37.2X3- Poisoning by antimalarials and drugs acting on other blood protozoa, assault**

SP 7 **T37.2X4- Poisoning by antimalarials and drugs acting on other blood protozoa, undetermined**

!Q 7 **T37.2X5- Adverse effect of antimalarials and drugs acting on other blood protozoa**

7 **T37.2X6- Underdosing of antimalarials and drugs acting on other blood protozoa**

5 **T37.3 Poisoning by, adverse effect of and underdosing of other antiprotozoal drugs**

6 **T37.3X Poisoning by, adverse effect of and underdosing of other antiprotozoal drugs**

SP 7 **T37.3X1- Poisoning by other antiprotozoal drugs, accidental (unintentional)**
Poisoning by other antiprotozoal drugs NOS

SP 7 **T37.3X2- Poisoning by other antiprotozoal drugs, intentional self-harm**

SP 7 **T37.3X3- Poisoning by other antiprotozoal drugs, assault**

SP 7 **T37.3X4- Poisoning by other antiprotozoal drugs, undetermined**

!Q 7 **T37.3X5- Adverse effect of other antiprotozoal drugs**

7 **T37.3X6- Underdosing of other antiprotozoal drugs**

5 **T37.4 Poisoning by, adverse effect of and underdosing of anthelminthics**

6 **T37.4X Poisoning by, adverse effect of and underdosing of anthelminthics**

SP 7 **T37.4X1- Poisoning by anthelminthics, accidental (unintentional)**
Poisoning by anthelminthics NOS

SP 7 **T37.4X2- Poisoning by anthelminthics, intentional self-harm**

SP 7 **T37.4X3- Poisoning by anthelminthics, assault**

SP 7 **T37.4X4- Poisoning by anthelminthics, undetermined**

!Q 7 **T37.4X5- Adverse effect of anthelminthics**

7 **T37.4X6- Underdosing of anthelminthics**

5 **T37.5 Poisoning by, adverse effect of and underdosing of antiviral drugs**

EXCLUDES 1 amantadine (T42.8-)
cytarabine (T45.1-)

6 **T37.5X Poisoning by, adverse effect of and underdosing of antiviral drugs**

SP 7 **T37.5X1- Poisoning by antiviral drugs, accidental (unintentional)**
Poisoning by antiviral drugs NOS

SP 7 **T37.5X2- Poisoning by antiviral drugs, intentional self-harm**

SP 7 **T37.5X3- Poisoning by antiviral drugs, assault**

SP 7 **T37.5X4- Poisoning by antiviral drugs, undetermined**

!Q 7 **T37.5X5- Adverse effect of antiviral drugs**

7 **T37.5X6- Underdosing of antiviral drugs**

5 **T37.8 Poisoning by, adverse effect of and underdosing of other specified systemic anti-infectives and antiparasitics**
Poisoning by, adverse effect of and underdosing of hydroxyquinoline derivatives

EXCLUDES 1 antimalarial drugs (T37.2-)

6 **T37.8X Poisoning by, adverse effect of and underdosing of other specified systemic anti-infectives and antiparasitics**

SP 7 **T37.8X1- Poisoning by other specified systemic anti-infectives and antiparasitics, accidental (unintentional)**
Poisoning by other specified systemic anti-infectives and antiparasitics NOS

SP 7 **T37.8X2- Poisoning by other specified systemic anti-infectives and antiparasitics, intentional self-harm**

SP 7 **T37.8X3- Poisoning by other specified systemic anti-infectives and antiparasitics, assault**

SP 7 **T37.8X4- Poisoning by other specified systemic anti-infectives and antiparasitics, undetermined**

!Q 7 **T37.8X5- Adverse effect of other specified systemic anti-infectives and antiparasitics**

7 **T37.8X6- Underdosing of other specified systemic anti-infectives and antiparasitics**

5 **T37.9 Poisoning by, adverse effect of and underdosing of unspecified systemic anti-infective and antiparasitics**

SP 7 **T37.91X- Poisoning by unspecified systemic anti-infective and antiparasitics, accidental (unintentional)**
Poisoning by, adverse effect of and underdosing of systemic anti-infective and antiparasitics NOS

SP 7 **T37.92X- Poisoning by unspecified systemic anti-infective and antiparasitics, intentional self-harm**

SP 7 **T37.93X- Poisoning by unspecified systemic anti-infective and antiparasitics, assault**

SP 7 **T37.94X- Poisoning by unspecified systemic anti-infective and antiparasitics, undetermined**

!Q 7 **T37.95X- Adverse effect of unspecified systemic anti-infective and antiparasitic**

7 **T37.96X- Underdosing of unspecified systemic anti-infectives and antiparasitics**

4 **T38 Poisoning by, adverse effect of and underdosing of hormones and their synthetic substitutes and antagonists, not elsewhere classified**

EXCLUDES 1 mineralocorticoids and their antagonists (T50.0-)
oxytocic hormones (T48.0-)
parathyroid hormones and derivatives (T50.9-)

The appropriate 7th character is to be added to each code from category T38

A	initial encounter
D	subsequent encounter
S	sequela

5 **T38.0 Poisoning by, adverse effect of and underdosing of glucocorticoids and synthetic analogues**

EXCLUDES 1 glucocorticoids, topically used (T49.-)

6 **T38.0X Poisoning by, adverse effect of and underdosing of glucocorticoids and synthetic analogues**

SP 7 **T38.0X1- Poisoning by glucocorticoids and synthetic analogues, accidental (unintentional)**
Poisoning by glucocorticoids and synthetic analogues NOS

SP 7 **T38.0X2- Poisoning by glucocorticoids and synthetic analogues, intentional self-harm**

SP 7 **T38.0X3- Poisoning by glucocorticoids and synthetic analogues, assault**

SP 7 **T38.0X4- Poisoning by glucocorticoids and synthetic analogues, undetermined**

!Q 7 **T38.0X5- Adverse effect of glucocorticoids and synthetic analogues**

7 **T38.0X6- Underdosing of glucocorticoids and synthetic analogues**

5 **T38.1 Poisoning by, adverse effect of and underdosing of thyroid hormones and substitutes**

6 **T38.1X Poisoning by, adverse effect of and underdosing of thyroid hormones and substitutes**

SP 7 **T38.1X1- Poisoning by thyroid hormones and substitutes, accidental (unintentional)**
Poisoning by thyroid hormones and substitutes NOS

SP 7 **T38.1X2- Poisoning by thyroid hormones and substitutes, intentional self-harm**

SP 7 **T38.1X3- Poisoning by thyroid hormones and substitutes, assault**

SP 7 **T38.1X4- Poisoning by thyroid hormones and substitutes, undetermined**

!Q 7 **T38.1X5- Adverse effect of thyroid hormones and substitutes**

7 **T38.1X6- Underdosing of thyroid hormones and substitutes**

5 **T38.2 Poisoning by, adverse effect of and underdosing of antithyroid drugs**

6 **T38.2X Poisoning by, adverse effect of and underdosing of antithyroid drugs**

SP 7 **T38.2X1- Poisoning by antithyroid drugs, accidental (unintentional)**
Poisoning by antithyroid drugs NOS

SP 7 **T38.2X2- Poisoning by antithyroid drugs, intentional self-harm**

SP 7 **T38.2X3- Poisoning by antithyroid drugs, assault**

SP 7 **T38.2X4- Poisoning by antithyroid drugs, undetermined**

!Q 7 **T38.2X5- Adverse effect of antithyroid drugs**

7 **T38.2X6- Underdosing of antithyroid drugs**

5 **T38.3 Poisoning by, adverse effect of and underdosing of insulin and oral hypoglycemic [antidiabetic] drugs**

6 **T38.3X Poisoning by, adverse effect of and underdosing of insulin and oral hypoglycemic [antidiabetic] drugs**

SP 7 **T38.3X1- Poisoning by insulin and oral hypoglycemic [antidiabetic] drugs, accidental (unintentional)**
Poisoning by insulin and oral hypoglycemic [antidiabetic] drugs NOS

GUIDELINES **Section I.C.4.a.5)(b)**
The principal or first-listed code for an encounter due to an insulin pump malfunction resulting in an overdose of insulin, should also be T85.6-, Mechanical complication of other specified internal and external prosthetic devices, implants and grafts, followed by code T38.3x1-.

SP 7 **T38.3X2- Poisoning by insulin and oral hypoglycemic [antidiabetic] drugs, intentional self-harm**

SP 7 **T38.3X3- Poisoning by insulin and oral hypoglycemic [antidiabetic] drugs, assault**

SP 7 **T38.3X4- Poisoning by insulin and oral hypoglycemic [antidiabetic] drugs, undetermined**

!Q 7 **T38.3X5- Adverse effect of insulin and oral hypoglycemic [antidiabetic] drugs**

7 **T38.3X6- Underdosing of insulin and oral hypoglycemic [antidiabetic] drugs**

GUIDELINES **Section I.C.4.a.5)(a)**
An underdose of insulin due to an insulin pump failure should be assigned to a code from subcategory T85.6, Mechanical complication of other specified internal and external prosthetic devices, implants and grafts, followed by code T38.3x6-. Additional codes for the type of diabetes mellitus and any associated complications due to the underdosing should also be assigned.

5 **T38.4 Poisoning by, adverse effect of and underdosing of oral contraceptives**
Poisoning by, adverse effect of and underdosing of multiple- and single-ingredient oral contraceptive preparations

6 **T38.4X Poisoning by, adverse effect of and underdosing of oral contraceptives**

SP 7 **T38.4X1- Poisoning by oral contraceptives, accidental (unintentional)**
Poisoning by oral contraceptives NOS

SP 7 **T38.4X2- Poisoning by oral contraceptives, intentional self-harm**

SP 7 **T38.4X3- Poisoning by oral contraceptives, assault**

SP 7 **T38.4X4- Poisoning by oral contraceptives, undetermined**

!Q 7 **T38.4X5- Adverse effect of oral contraceptives**

7 **T38.4X6- Underdosing of oral contraceptives**

5 **T38.5 Poisoning by, adverse effect of and underdosing of other estrogens and progestogens**
Poisoning by, adverse effect of and underdosing of estrogens and progestogens mixtures and substitutes

6 **T38.5X Poisoning by, adverse effect of and underdosing of other estrogens and progestogens**

SP 7 **T38.5X1- Poisoning by other estrogens and progestogens, accidental (unintentional)**
Poisoning by other estrogens and progestogens NOS

SP 7 **T38.5X2- Poisoning by other estrogens and progestogens, intentional self-harm**

SP 7 **T38.5X3- Poisoning by other estrogens and progestogens, assault**

SP 7 **T38.5X4- Poisoning by other estrogens and progestogens, undetermined**

!Q 7 **T38.5X5- Adverse effect of other estrogens and progestogens**

7 **T38.5X6- Underdosing of other estrogens and progestogens**

5 **T38.6 Poisoning by, adverse effect of and underdosing of antigonadotrophins, antiestrogens, antiandrogens, not elsewhere classified**

Poisoning by, adverse effect of and underdosing of tamoxifen

6 **T38.6X Poisoning by, adverse effect of and underdosing of antigonadotrophins, antiestrogens, antiandrogens, not elsewhere classified**

SP 7 **T38.6X1- Poisoning by antigonadotrophins, antiestrogens, antiandrogens, not elsewhere classified, accidental (unintentional)**

Poisoning by antigonadotrophins, antiestrogens, antiandrogens, not elsewhere classified NOS

SP 7 **T38.6X2- Poisoning by antigonadotrophins, antiestrogens, antiandrogens, not elsewhere classified, intentional self-harm**

SP 7 **T38.6X3- Poisoning by antigonadotrophins, antiestrogens, antiandrogens, not elsewhere classified, assault**

SP 7 **T38.6X4- Poisoning by antigonadotrophins, antiestrogens, antiandrogens, not elsewhere classified, undetermined**

!Q 7 **T38.6X5- Adverse effect of antigonadotrophins, antiestrogens, antiandrogens, not elsewhere classified**

7 **T38.6X6- Underdosing of antigonadotrophins, antiestrogens, antiandrogens, not elsewhere classified**

5 **T38.7 Poisoning by, adverse effect of and underdosing of androgens and anabolic congeners**

6 **T38.7X Poisoning by, adverse effect of and underdosing of androgens and anabolic congeners**

SP 7 **T38.7X1- Poisoning by androgens and anabolic congeners, accidental (unintentional)**

Poisoning by androgens and anabolic congeners NOS

SP 7 **T38.7X2- Poisoning by androgens and anabolic congeners, intentional self-harm**

SP 7 **T38.7X3- Poisoning by androgens and anabolic congeners, assault**

SP 7 **T38.7X4- Poisoning by androgens and anabolic congeners, undetermined**

!Q 7 **T38.7X5- Adverse effect of androgens and anabolic congeners**

7 **T38.7X6- Underdosing of androgens and anabolic congeners**

5 **T38.8 Poisoning by, adverse effect of and underdosing of other and unspecified hormones and synthetic substitutes**

6 **T38.80 Poisoning by, adverse effect of and underdosing of unspecified hormones and synthetic substitutes**

SP 7 **T38.801- Poisoning by unspecified hormones and synthetic substitutes, accidental (unintentional)**

Poisoning by unspecified hormones and synthetic substitutes NOS

SP 7 **T38.802- Poisoning by unspecified hormones and synthetic substitutes, intentional self-harm**

SP 7 **T38.803- Poisoning by unspecified hormones and synthetic substitutes, assault**

SP 7 **T38.804- Poisoning by unspecified hormones and synthetic substitutes, undetermined**

!Q 7 **T38.805- Adverse effect of unspecified hormones and synthetic substitutes**

7 **T38.806- Underdosing of unspecified hormones and synthetic substitutes**

6 **T38.81 Poisoning by, adverse effect of and underdosing of anterior pituitary [adenohypophyseal] hormones**

SP 7 **T38.811- Poisoning by anterior pituitary [adenohypophyseal] hormones, accidental (unintentional)**

Poisoning by anterior pituitary [adenohypophyseal] hormones NOS

SP 7 **T38.812- Poisoning by anterior pituitary [adenohypophyseal] hormones, intentional self-harm**

SP 7 **T38.813- Poisoning by anterior pituitary [adenohypophyseal] hormones, assault**

SP 7 **T38.814- Poisoning by anterior pituitary [adenohypophyseal] hormones, undetermined**

!Q 7 **T38.815- Adverse effect of anterior pituitary [adenohypophyseal] hormones**

7 **T38.816- Underdosing of anterior pituitary [adenohypophyseal] hormones**

6 **T38.89 Poisoning by, adverse effect of and underdosing of other hormones and synthetic substitutes**

SP 7 **T38.891- Poisoning by other hormones and synthetic substitutes, accidental (unintentional)**

Poisoning by other hormones and synthetic substitutes NOS

SP 7 **T38.892- Poisoning by other hormones and synthetic substitutes, intentional self-harm**

SP 7 **T38.893- Poisoning by other hormones and synthetic substitutes, assault**

SP 7 **T38.894- Poisoning by other hormones and synthetic substitutes, undetermined**

!Q 7 **T38.895- Adverse effect of other hormones and synthetic substitutes**

7 **T38.896- Underdosing of other hormones and synthetic substitutes**

5 **T38.9 Poisoning by, adverse effect of and underdosing of other and unspecified hormone antagonists**

6 **T38.90 Poisoning by, adverse effect of and underdosing of unspecified hormone antagonists**

SP 7 **T38.901- Poisoning by unspecified hormone antagonists, accidental (unintentional)**
Poisoning by unspecified hormone antagonists NOS

SP 7 **T38.902- Poisoning by unspecified hormone antagonists, intentional self-harm**

SP 7 **T38.903- Poisoning by unspecified hormone antagonists, assault**

SP 7 **T38.904- Poisoning by unspecified hormone antagonists, undetermined**

!Q 7 **T38.905- Adverse effect of unspecified hormone antagonists**

7 **T38.906- Underdosing of unspecified hormone antagonists**

6 **T38.99 Poisoning by, adverse effect of and underdosing of other hormone antagonists**

SP 7 **T38.991- Poisoning by other hormone antagonists, accidental (unintentional)**
Poisoning by other hormone antagonists NOS

SP 7 **T38.992- Poisoning by other hormone antagonists, intentional self-harm**

SP 7 **T38.993- Poisoning by other hormone antagonists, assault**

SP 7 **T38.994- Poisoning by other hormone antagonists, undetermined**

!Q 7 **T38.995- Adverse effect of other hormone antagonists**

7 **T38.996- Underdosing of other hormone antagonists**

4 **T39 Poisoning by, adverse effect of and underdosing of nonopioid analgesics, antipyretics and antirheumatics**

The appropriate 7th character is to be added to each code from category T39
A initial encounter
D subsequent encounter
S sequela

5 **T39.0 Poisoning by, adverse effect of and underdosing of salicylates**

6 **T39.01 Poisoning by, adverse effect of and underdosing of aspirin**
Poisoning by, adverse effect of and underdosing of acetylsalicylic acid

SP 7 **T39.011- Poisoning by aspirin, accidental (unintentional)**

SP 7 **T39.012- Poisoning by aspirin, intentional self-harm**

SP 7 **T39.013- Poisoning by aspirin, assault**

SP 7 **T39.014- Poisoning by aspirin, undetermined**

!Q 7 **T39.015- Adverse effect of aspirin**

7 **T39.016- Underdosing of aspirin**

6 **T39.09 Poisoning by, adverse effect of and underdosing of other salicylates**

SP 7 **T39.091- Poisoning by salicylates, accidental (unintentional)**
Poisoning by salicylates NOS

SP 7 **T39.092- Poisoning by salicylates, intentional self-harm**

SP 7 **T39.093- Poisoning by salicylates, assault**

SP 7 **T39.094- Poisoning by salicylates, undetermined**

!Q 7 **T39.095- Adverse effect of salicylates**

7 **T39.096- Underdosing of salicylates**

5 **T39.1 Poisoning by, adverse effect of and underdosing of 4-Aminophenol derivatives**

6 **T39.1X Poisoning by, adverse effect of and underdosing of 4-Aminophenol derivatives**

SP 7 **T39.1X1- Poisoning by 4-Aminophenol derivatives, accidental (unintentional)**
Poisoning by 4-Aminophenol derivatives NOS

SP 7 **T39.1X2- Poisoning by 4-Aminophenol derivatives, intentional self-harm**

SP 7 **T39.1X3- Poisoning by 4-Aminophenol derivatives, assault**

SP 7 **T39.1X4- Poisoning by 4-Aminophenol derivatives, undetermined**

!Q 7 **T39.1X5- Adverse effect of 4-Aminophenol derivatives**

7 **T39.1X6- Underdosing of 4-Aminophenol derivatives**

5 **T39.2 Poisoning by, adverse effect of and underdosing of pyrazolone derivatives**

6 **T39.2X Poisoning by, adverse effect of and underdosing of pyrazolone derivatives**

SP 7 **T39.2X1- Poisoning by pyrazolone derivatives, accidental (unintentional)**
Poisoning by pyrazolone derivatives NOS

SP 7 **T39.2X2- Poisoning by pyrazolone derivatives, intentional self-harm**

SP 7 **T39.2X3- Poisoning by pyrazolone derivatives, assault**

SP 7 **T39.2X4- Poisoning by pyrazolone derivatives, undetermined**

!Q 7 **T39.2X5- Adverse effect of pyrazolone derivatives**

7 **T39.2X6- Underdosing of pyrazolone derivatives**

5 **T39.3 Poisoning by, adverse effect of and underdosing of other nonsteroidal anti-inflammatory drugs [NSAID]**

6 **T39.31 Poisoning by, adverse effect of and underdosing of propionic acid derivatives**

Poisoning by, adverse effect of and underdosing of fenoprofen
Poisoning by, adverse effect of and underdosing of flurbiprofen
Poisoning by, adverse effect of and underdosing of ibuprofen
Poisoning by, adverse effect of and underdosing of ketoprofen
Poisoning by, adverse effect of and underdosing of naproxen
Poisoning by, adverse effect of and underdosing of oxaprozin

SP 7 **T39.311- Poisoning by propionic acid derivatives, accidental (unintentional)**
SP 7 **T39.312- Poisoning by propionic acid derivatives, intentional self-harm**
SP 7 **T39.313- Poisoning by propionic acid derivatives, assault**
SP 7 **T39.314- Poisoning by propionic acid derivatives, undetermined**
!Q 7 **T39.315- Adverse effect of propionic acid derivatives**
7 **T39.316- Underdosing of propionic acid derivatives**

6 **T39.39 Poisoning by, adverse effect of and underdosing of other nonsteroidal anti-inflammatory drugs [NSAID]**

SP 7 **T39.391- Poisoning by other nonsteroidal anti-inflammatory drugs [NSAID], accidental (unintentional)**
Poisoning by other nonsteroidal anti-inflammatory drugs NOS
SP 7 **T39.392- Poisoning by other nonsteroidal anti-inflammatory drugs [NSAID], intentional self-harm**
SP 7 **T39.393- Poisoning by other nonsteroidal anti-inflammatory drugs [NSAID], assault**
SP 7 **T39.394- Poisoning by other nonsteroidal anti-inflammatory drugs [NSAID], undetermined**
!Q 7 **T39.395- Adverse effect of other nonsteroidal anti-inflammatory drugs [NSAID]**
7 **T39.396- Underdosing of other nonsteroidal anti-inflammatory drugs [NSAID]**

5 **T39.4 Poisoning by, adverse effect of and underdosing of antirheumatics, not elsewhere classified**

EXCLUDES 1 poisoning by, adverse effect of and underdosing of glucocorticoids (T38.0-)
poisoning by, adverse effect of and underdosing of salicylates (T39.0-)

6 **T39.4X Poisoning by, adverse effect of and underdosing of antirheumatics, not elsewhere classified**

SP 7 **T39.4X1- Poisoning by antirheumatics, not elsewhere classified, accidental (unintentional)**
Poisoning by antirheumatics, not elsewhere classified NOS
SP 7 **T39.4X2- Poisoning by antirheumatics, not elsewhere classified, intentional self-harm**
SP 7 **T39.4X3- Poisoning by antirheumatics, not elsewhere classified, assault**
SP 7 **T39.4X4- Poisoning by antirheumatics, not elsewhere classified, undetermined**
!Q 7 **T39.4X5- Adverse effect of antirheumatics, not elsewhere classified**
7 **T39.4X6- Underdosing of antirheumatics, not elsewhere classified**

5 **T39.8 Poisoning by, adverse effect of and underdosing of other nonopioid analgesics and antipyretics, not elsewhere classified**

6 **T39.8X Poisoning by, adverse effect of and underdosing of other nonopioid analgesics and antipyretics, not elsewhere classified**

SP 7 **T39.8X1- Poisoning by other nonopioid analgesics and antipyretics, not elsewhere classified, accidental (unintentional)**
Poisoning by other nonopioid analgesics and antipyretics, not elsewhere classified NOS
SP 7 **T39.8X2- Poisoning by other nonopioid analgesics and antipyretics, not elsewhere classified, intentional self-harm**
SP 7 **T39.8X3- Poisoning by other nonopioid analgesics and antipyretics, not elsewhere classified, assault**
SP 7 **T39.8X4- Poisoning by other nonopioid analgesics and antipyretics, not elsewhere classified, undetermined**
!Q 7 **T39.8X5- Adverse effect of other nonopioid analgesics and antipyretics, not elsewhere classified**
7 **T39.8X6- Underdosing of other nonopioid analgesics and antipyretics, not elsewhere classified**

5 **T39.9 Poisoning by, adverse effect of and underdosing of unspecified nonopioid analgesic, antipyretic and antirheumatic**

SP X **T39.91X- Poisoning by unspecified nonopioid analgesic, antipyretic and antirheumatic, accidental (unintentional)**
Poisoning by nonopioid analgesic, antipyretic and antirheumatic NOS
SP X **T39.92X- Poisoning by unspecified nonopioid analgesic, antipyretic and antirheumatic, intentional self-harm**
SP X **T39.93X- Poisoning by unspecified nonopioid analgesic, antipyretic and antirheumatic, assault**
SP X **T39.94X- Poisoning by unspecified nonopioid analgesic, antipyretic and antirheumatic, undetermined**
!Q X **T39.95X- Adverse effect of unspecified nonopioid analgesic, antipyretic and antirheumatic**
X **T39.96X- Underdosing of unspecified nonopioid analgesic, antipyretic and antirheumatic**

Chapter 19
S00-T88

4 4th digit required 5 5th digit required 6 6th digit required 7 7th digit required X 7th digit placeholder + Additional code ⊟ Laterality

4 **T40 Poisoning by, adverse effect of and underdosing of narcotics and psychodysleptics [hallucinogens]**

EXCLUDES 2 drug dependence and related mental and behavioral disorders due to psychoactive substance use (F10.-F19.-)

The appropriate 7th character is to be added to each code from category T40
A initial encounter
D subsequent encounter
S sequela

5 **T40.0 Poisoning by, adverse effect of and underdosing of opium**
6 **T40.0X Poisoning by, adverse effect of and underdosing of opium**
SP 7 **T40.0X1- Poisoning by opium, accidental (unintentional)**
Poisoning by opium NOS
SP 7 **T40.0X2- Poisoning by opium, intentional self-harm**
SP 7 **T40.0X3- Poisoning by opium, assault**
SP 7 **T40.0X4- Poisoning by opium, undetermined**
!Q 7 **T40.0X5- Adverse effect of opium**
7 **T40.0X6- Underdosing of opium**
5 **T40.1 Poisoning by and adverse effect of heroin**
6 **T40.1X Poisoning by and adverse effect of heroin**
SP 7 **T40.1X1- Poisoning by heroin, accidental (unintentional)**
Poisoning by heroin NOS
SP 7 **T40.1X2- Poisoning by heroin, intentional self-harm**
SP 7 **T40.1X3- Poisoning by heroin, assault**
SP 7 **T40.1X4- Poisoning by heroin, undetermined**
5 **T40.2 Poisoning by, adverse effect of and underdosing of other opioids**
6 **T40.2X Poisoning by, adverse effect of and underdosing of other opioids**
SP 7 **T40.2X1- Poisoning by other opioids, accidental (unintentional)**
Poisoning by other opioids NOS
SP 7 **T40.2X2- Poisoning by other opioids, intentional self-harm**
SP 7 **T40.2X3- Poisoning by other opioids, assault**
SP 7 **T40.2X4- Poisoning by other opioids, undetermined**
!Q 7 **T40.2X5- Adverse effect of other opioids**
7 **T40.2X6- Underdosing of other opioids**
5 **T40.3 Poisoning by, adverse effect of and underdosing of methadone**
6 **T40.3X Poisoning by, adverse effect of and underdosing of methadone**
SP 7 **T40.3X1- Poisoning by methadone, accidental (unintentional)**
Poisoning by methadone NOS
SP 7 **T40.3X2- Poisoning by methadone, intentional self-harm**
SP 7 **T40.3X3- Poisoning by methadone, assault**
SP 7 **T40.3X4- Poisoning by methadone, undetermined**
!Q 7 **T40.3X5- Adverse effect of methadone**
7 **T40.3X6- Underdosing of methadone**
5 **T40.4 Poisoning by, adverse effect of and underdosing of other synthetic narcotics**
6 **T40.41 Poisoning by, adverse effect of and underdosing of fentanyl or fentanyl analogs**
SP 7 **T40.411- Poisoning by fentanyl or fentanyl analogs, accidental (unintentional)**
SP 7 **T40.412- Poisoning by fentanyl or fentanyl analogs, intentional self-harm**
SP 7 **T40.413- Poisoning by fentanyl or fentanyl analogs, assault**
SP 7 **T40.414- Poisoning by fentanyl or fentanyl analogs, undetermined**
7 **T40.415- Adverse effect of fentanyl or fentanyl analogs**
7 **T40.416- Underdosing of fentanyl or fentanyl analogs**
6 **T40.42 Poisoning by, adverse effect of and underdosing of tramadol**
SP 7 **T40.421- Poisoning by tramadol, accidental (unintentional)**
SP 7 **T40.422- Poisoning by tramadol, intentional self-harm**
SP 7 **T40.423- Poisoning by tramadol, assault**
SP 7 **T40.424- Poisoning by tramadol, undetermined**
7 **T40.425- Adverse effect of tramadol**
7 **T40.426- Underdosing of tramadol**
6 **T40.49 Poisoning by, adverse effect of and underdosing of other synthetic narcotics**
SP 7 **T40.491- Poisoning by other synthetic narcotics, accidental (unintentional)**
Poisoning by other synthetic narcotics NOS
SP 7 **T40.492- Poisoning by other synthetic narcotics, intentional self-harm**
SP 7 **T40.493- Poisoning by other synthetic narcotics, assault**
SP 7 **T40.494- Poisoning by other synthetic narcotics, undetermined**
7 **T40.495- Adverse effect of other synthetic narcotics**
7 **T40.496- Underdosing of other synthetic narcotics**
5 **T40.5 Poisoning by, adverse effect of and underdosing of cocaine**
6 **T40.5X Poisoning by, adverse effect of and underdosing of cocaine**
SP 7 **T40.5X1- Poisoning by cocaine, accidental (unintentional)**
Poisoning by cocaine NOS
SP 7 **T40.5X2- Poisoning by cocaine, intentional self-harm**
SP 7 **T40.5X3- Poisoning by cocaine, assault**
SP 7 **T40.5X4- Poisoning by cocaine, undetermined**
!Q 7 **T40.5X5- Adverse effect of cocaine**
7 **T40.5X6- Underdosing of cocaine**
5 **T40.6 Poisoning by, adverse effect of and underdosing of other and unspecified narcotics**

Chapter 19

S00-T88

6 T40.60 **Poisoning by, adverse effect of and underdosing of unspecified narcotics**

SP 7 T40.601- **Poisoning by unspecified narcotics, accidental (unintentional)**
Poisoning by narcotics NOS

SP 7 T40.602- **Poisoning by unspecified narcotics, intentional self-harm**

SP 7 T40.603- **Poisoning by unspecified narcotics, assault**

SP 7 T40.604- **Poisoning by unspecified narcotics, undetermined**

!Q 7 T40.605- **Adverse effect of unspecified narcotics**

7 T40.606- **Underdosing of unspecified narcotics**

6 T40.69 **Poisoning by, adverse effect of and underdosing of other narcotics**

SP 7 T40.691- **Poisoning by other narcotics, accidental (unintentional)**
Poisoning by other narcotics NOS

SP 7 T40.692- **Poisoning by other narcotics, intentional self-harm**

SP 7 T40.693- **Poisoning by other narcotics, assault**

SP 7 T40.694- **Poisoning by other narcotics, undetermined**

!Q 7 T40.695- **Adverse effect of other narcotics**

7 T40.696- **Underdosing of other narcotics**

5 T40.7 **Poisoning by, adverse effect of and underdosing of cannabis (derivatives)**

★ 6 T40.71 **Poisoning by, adverse effect of and underdosing of cannabis (derivatives)**

★ 7 T40.711- **Poisoning by cannabis, accidental (unintentional)**

★ 7 T40.712- **Poisoning by cannabis, intentional self-harm**

★ 7 T40.713- **Poisoning by cannabis, assault**

★ 7 T40.714- **Poisoning by cannabis, undetermined**

★ 7 T40.715- **Adverse effect of cannabis**

★ 7 T40.716- **Underdosing of cannabis**

★ 6 T40.72 **Poisoning by, adverse effect of and underdosing of synthetic cannabinoids**

★ 7 T40.721- **Poisoning by synthetic cannabinoids, accidental (unintentional)**

★ 7 T40.722- **Poisoning by synthetic cannabinoids, intentional self-harm**

★ 7 T40.723- **Poisoning by synthetic cannabinoids, assault**

★ 7 T40.724- **Poisoning by synthetic cannabinoids, undetermined**

★ 7 T40.725- **Adverse effect of synthetic cannabinoids**

★ 7 T40.726- **Underdosing of synthetic cannabinoids**

5 T40.8 **Poisoning by and adverse effect of lysergide [LSD]**

6 T40.8X **Poisoning by and adverse effect of lysergide [LSD]**

SP 7 T40.8X1- **Poisoning by lysergide [LSD], accidental (unintentional)**
Poisoning by lysergide [LSD] NOS

SP 7 T40.8X2- **Poisoning by lysergide [LSD], intentional self-harm**

SP 7 T40.8X3- **Poisoning by lysergide [LSD], assault**

SP 7 T40.8X4- **Poisoning by lysergide [LSD], undetermined**

5 T40.9 **Poisoning by, adverse effect of and underdosing of other and unspecified psychodysleptics [hallucinogens]**

6 T40.90 **Poisoning by, adverse effect of and underdosing of unspecified psychodysleptics [hallucinogens]**

SP 7 T40.901- **Poisoning by unspecified psychodysleptics [hallucinogens], accidental (unintentional)**

SP 7 T40.902- **Poisoning by unspecified psychodysleptics [hallucinogens], intentional self-harm**

SP 7 T40.903- **Poisoning by unspecified psychodysleptics [hallucinogens], assault**

SP 7 T40.904- **Poisoning by unspecified psychodysleptics [hallucinogens], undetermined**

!Q 7 T40.905- **Adverse effect of unspecified psychodysleptics [hallucinogens]**

7 T40.906- **Underdosing of unspecified psychodysleptics [hallucinogens]**

6 T40.99 **Poisoning by, adverse effect of and underdosing of other psychodysleptics [hallucinogens]**

SP 7 T40.991- **Poisoning by other psychodysleptics [hallucinogens], accidental (unintentional)**
Poisoning by other psychodysleptics [hallucinogens] NOS

SP 7 T40.992- **Poisoning by other psychodysleptics [hallucinogens], intentional self-harm**

SP 7 T40.993- **Poisoning by other psychodysleptics [hallucinogens], assault**

SP 7 T40.994- **Poisoning by other psychodysleptics [hallucinogens], undetermined**

!Q 7 T40.995- **Adverse effect of other psychodysleptics [hallucinogens]**

7 T40.996- **Underdosing of other psychodysleptics [hallucinogens]**

4 T41 **Poisoning by, adverse effect of and underdosing of anesthetics and therapeutic gases**

EXCLUDES 1 benzodiazepines (T42.4-)
cocaine (T40.5-)
complications of anesthesia during pregnancy (O29.-)
complications of anesthesia during labor and delivery (O74.-)

complications of anesthesia during the puerperium (O89.-)
opioids (T40.0-T40.2-)

The appropriate 7th character is to be added to each code from category T41
A initial encounter
D subsequent encounter
S sequela

5 **T41.0 Poisoning by, adverse effect of and underdosing of inhaled anesthetics**
EXCLUDES 1 oxygen (T41.5-)

6 **T41.0X Poisoning by, adverse effect of and underdosing of inhaled anesthetics**

SP 7 **T41.0X1- Poisoning by inhaled anesthetics, accidental (unintentional)**
Poisoning by inhaled anesthetics NOS

SP 7 **T41.0X2- Poisoning by inhaled anesthetics, intentional self-harm**

SP 7 **T41.0X3- Poisoning by inhaled anesthetics, assault**

SP 7 **T41.0X4- Poisoning by inhaled anesthetics, undetermined**

IQ 7 **T41.0X5- Adverse effect of inhaled anesthetics**

7 **T41.0X6- Underdosing of inhaled anesthetics**

5 **T41.1 Poisoning by, adverse effect of and underdosing of intravenous anesthetics**
Poisoning by, adverse effect of and underdosing of thiobarbiturates

6 **T41.1X Poisoning by, adverse effect of and underdosing of intravenous anesthetics**

SP 7 **T41.1X1- Poisoning by intravenous anesthetics, accidental (unintentional)**
Poisoning by intravenous anesthetics NOS

SP 7 **T41.1X2- Poisoning by intravenous anesthetics, intentional self-harm**

SP 7 **T41.1X3- Poisoning by intravenous anesthetics, assault**

SP 7 **T41.1X4- Poisoning by intravenous anesthetics, undetermined**

IQ 7 **T41.1X5- Adverse effect of intravenous anesthetics**

7 **T41.1X6- Underdosing of intravenous anesthetics**

5 **T41.2 Poisoning by, adverse effect of and underdosing of other and unspecified general anesthetics**

6 **T41.20 Poisoning by, adverse effect of and underdosing of unspecified general anesthetics**

SP 7 **T41.201- Poisoning by unspecified general anesthetics, accidental (unintentional)**
Poisoning by general anesthetics NOS

SP 7 **T41.202- Poisoning by unspecified general anesthetics, intentional self-harm**

SP 7 **T41.203- Poisoning by unspecified general anesthetics, assault**

SP 7 **T41.204- Poisoning by unspecified general anesthetics, undetermined**

IQ 7 **T41.205- Adverse effect of unspecified general anesthetics**

7 **T41.206- Underdosing of unspecified general anesthetics**

6 **T41.29 Poisoning by, adverse effect of and underdosing of other general anesthetics**

SP 7 **T41.291- Poisoning by other general anesthetics, accidental (unintentional)**
Poisoning by other general anesthetics NOS

SP 7 **T41.292- Poisoning by other general anesthetics, intentional self-harm**

SP 7 **T41.293- Poisoning by other general anesthetics, assault**

SP 7 **T41.294- Poisoning by other general anesthetics, undetermined**

IQ 7 **T41.295- Adverse effect of other general anesthetics**

7 **T41.296- Underdosing of other general anesthetics**

5 **T41.3 Poisoning by, adverse effect of and underdosing of local anesthetics**
Cocaine (topical)
EXCLUDES 2 poisoning by cocaine used as a central nervous system stimulant (T40.5X1-T40.5X4)

6 **T41.3X Poisoning by, adverse effect of and underdosing of local anesthetics**

SP 7 **T41.3X1- Poisoning by local anesthetics, accidental (unintentional)**
Poisoning by local anesthetics NOS

SP 7 **T41.3X2- Poisoning by local anesthetics, intentional self-harm**

SP 7 **T41.3X3- Poisoning by local anesthetics, assault**

SP 7 **T41.3X4- Poisoning by local anesthetics, undetermined**

IQ 7 **T41.3X5- Adverse effect of local anesthetics**

7 **T41.3X6- Underdosing of local anesthetics**

5 **T41.4 Poisoning by, adverse effect of and underdosing of unspecified anesthetic**

SP 7 **T41.41X- Poisoning by unspecified anesthetic, accidental (unintentional)**
Poisoning by anesthetic NOS

SP 7 **T41.42X- Poisoning by unspecified anesthetic, intentional self-harm**

SP 7 **T41.43X- Poisoning by unspecified anesthetic, assault**

SP 7 **T41.44X- Poisoning by unspecified anesthetic, undetermined**

IQ 7 **T41.45X- Adverse effect of unspecified anesthetic**

7 **T41.46X- Underdosing of unspecified anesthetics**

5 **T41.5 Poisoning by, adverse effect of and underdosing of therapeutic gases**

Chapter 19
S00-T88

6 **T41.5X Poisoning by, adverse effect of and underdosing of therapeutic gases**

SP 7 **T41.5X1- Poisoning by therapeutic gases, accidental (unintentional)**
Poisoning by therapeutic gases NOS

SP 7 **T41.5X2- Poisoning by therapeutic gases, intentional self-harm**

SP 7 **T41.5X3- Poisoning by therapeutic gases, assault**

SP 7 **T41.5X4- Poisoning by therapeutic gases, undetermined**

IQ 7 **T41.5X5- Adverse effect of therapeutic gases**

7 **T41.5X6- Underdosing of therapeutic gases**

4 **T42 Poisoning by, adverse effect of and underdosing of antiepileptic, sedative-hypnotic and antiparkinsonism drugs**

EXCLUDES 2 drug dependence and related mental and behavioral disorders due to psychoactive substance use (F10.--F19.-)

The appropriate 7th character is to be added to each code from category T42
A initial encounter
D subsequent encounter
S sequela

5 **T42.0 Poisoning by, adverse effect of and underdosing of hydantoin derivatives**

6 **T42.0X Poisoning by, adverse effect of and underdosing of hydantoin derivatives**

SP 7 **T42.0X1- Poisoning by hydantoin derivatives, accidental (unintentional)**
Poisoning by hydantoin derivatives NOS

SP 7 **T42.0X2- Poisoning by hydantoin derivatives, intentional self-harm**

SP 7 **T42.0X3- Poisoning by hydantoin derivatives, assault**

SP 7 **T42.0X4- Poisoning by hydantoin derivatives, undetermined**

IQ 7 **T42.0X5- Adverse effect of hydantoin derivatives**

7 **T42.0X6- Underdosing of hydantoin derivatives**

5 **T42.1 Poisoning by, adverse effect of and underdosing of iminostilbenes**
Poisoning by, adverse effect of and underdosing of carbamazepine

6 **T42.1X Poisoning by, adverse effect of and underdosing of iminostilbenes**

SP 7 **T42.1X1- Poisoning by iminostilbenes, accidental (unintentional)**
Poisoning by iminostilbenes NOS

SP 7 **T42.1X2- Poisoning by iminostilbenes, intentional self-harm**

SP 7 **T42.1X3- Poisoning by iminostilbenes, assault**

SP 7 **T42.1X4- Poisoning by iminostilbenes, undetermined**

IQ 7 **T42.1X5- Adverse effect of iminostilbenes**

7 **T42.1X6- Underdosing of iminostilbenes**

5 **T42.2 Poisoning by, adverse effect of and underdosing of succinimides and oxazolidinediones**

6 **T42.2X Poisoning by, adverse effect of and underdosing of succinimides and oxazolidinediones**

SP 7 **T42.2X1- Poisoning by succinimides and oxazolidinediones, accidental (unintentional)**
Poisoning by succinimides and oxazolidinediones NOS

SP 7 **T42.2X2- Poisoning by succinimides and oxazolidinediones, intentional self-harm**

SP 7 **T42.2X3- Poisoning by succinimides and oxazolidinediones, assault**

SP 7 **T42.2X4- Poisoning by succinimides and oxazolidinediones, undetermined**

IQ 7 **T42.2X5- Adverse effect of succinimides and oxazolidinediones**

7 **T42.2X6- Underdosing of succinimides and oxazolidinediones**

5 **T42.3 Poisoning by, adverse effect of and underdosing of barbiturates**

EXCLUDES 1 poisoning by, adverse effect of and underdosing of thiobarbiturates (T41.1-)

6 **T42.3X Poisoning by, adverse effect of and underdosing of barbiturates**

SP 7 **T42.3X1- Poisoning by barbiturates, accidental (unintentional)**
Poisoning by barbiturates NOS

SP 7 **T42.3X2- Poisoning by barbiturates, intentional self-harm**

SP 7 **T42.3X3- Poisoning by barbiturates, assault**

SP 7 **T42.3X4- Poisoning by barbiturates, undetermined**

IQ 7 **T42.3X5- Adverse effect of barbiturates**

7 **T42.3X6- Underdosing of barbiturates**

5 **T42.4 Poisoning by, adverse effect of and underdosing of benzodiazepines**

6 **T42.4X Poisoning by, adverse effect of and underdosing of benzodiazepines**

SP 7 **T42.4X1- Poisoning by benzodiazepines, accidental (unintentional)**
Poisoning by benzodiazepines NOS

SP 7 **T42.4X2- Poisoning by benzodiazepines, intentional self-harm**

SP 7 **T42.4X3- Poisoning by benzodiazepines, assault**

SP 7 **T42.4X4- Poisoning by benzodiazepines, undetermined**

IQ 7 **T42.4X5- Adverse effect of benzodiazepines**

7 **T42.4X6- Underdosing of benzodiazepines**

5 **T42.5 Poisoning by, adverse effect of and underdosing of mixed antiepileptics**

6 **T42.5X Poisoning by, adverse effect of and underdosing of antiepileptics**

SP 7 **T42.5X1- Poisoning by mixed antiepileptics, accidental (unintentional)**
Poisoning by mixed antiepileptics NOS

SP 7 **T42.5X2- Poisoning by mixed antiepileptics, intentional self-harm**

SP 7 **T42.5X3- Poisoning by mixed antiepileptics, assault**

Chapter 19

S00-T88

SP 7 **T42.5X4- Poisoning by mixed antiepileptics, undetermined**

IQ 7 **T42.5X5- Adverse effect of mixed antiepileptics**

7 **T42.5X6- Underdosing of mixed antiepileptics**

5 **T42.6 Poisoning by, adverse effect of and underdosing of other antiepileptic and sedative-hypnotic drugs**

Poisoning by, adverse effect of and underdosing of methaqualone

Poisoning by, adverse effect of and underdosing of valproic acid

EXCLUDES 1 poisoning by, adverse effect of and underdosing of carbamazepine (T42.1-)

6 **T42.6X Poisoning by, adverse effect of and underdosing of other antiepileptic and sedative-hypnotic drugs**

SP 7 **T42.6X1- Poisoning by other antiepileptic and sedative-hypnotic drugs, accidental (unintentional)**

Poisoning by other antiepileptic and sedative-hypnotic drugs NOS

SP 7 **T42.6X2- Poisoning by other antiepileptic and sedative-hypnotic drugs, intentional self-harm**

SP 7 **T42.6X3- Poisoning by other antiepileptic and sedative-hypnotic drugs, assault**

SP 7 **T42.6X4- Poisoning by other antiepileptic and sedative-hypnotic drugs, undetermined**

IQ 7 **T42.6X5- Adverse effect of other antiepileptic and sedative-hypnotic drugs**

7 **T42.6X6- Underdosing of other antiepileptic and sedative-hypnotic drugs**

5 **T42.7 Poisoning by, adverse effect of and underdosing of unspecified antiepileptic and sedative-hypnotic drugs**

SP 7 **T42.71X- Poisoning by unspecified antiepileptic and sedative-hypnotic drugs, accidental (unintentional)**

Poisoning by antiepileptic and sedative-hypnotic drugs NOS

SP 7 **T42.72X- Poisoning by unspecified antiepileptic and sedative-hypnotic drugs, intentional self-harm**

SP 7 **T42.73X- Poisoning by unspecified antiepileptic and sedative-hypnotic drugs, assault**

SP 7 **T42.74X- Poisoning by unspecified antiepileptic and sedative-hypnotic drugs, undetermined**

IQ 7 **T42.75X- Adverse effect of unspecified antiepileptic and sedative-hypnotic drugs**

7 **T42.76X- Underdosing of unspecified antiepileptic and sedative-hypnotic drugs**

5 **T42.8 Poisoning by, adverse effect of and underdosing of antiparkinsonism drugs and other central muscle-tone depressants**

Poisoning by, adverse effect of and underdosing of amantadine

6 **T42.8X Poisoning by, adverse effect of and underdosing of antiparkinsonism drugs and other central muscle-tone depressants**

SP 7 **T42.8X1- Poisoning by antiparkinsonism drugs and other central muscle-tone depressants, accidental (unintentional)**

Poisoning by antiparkinsonism drugs and other central muscle-tone depressants NOS

SP 7 **T42.8X2- Poisoning by antiparkinsonism drugs and other central muscle-tone depressants, intentional self-harm**

SP 7 **T42.8X3- Poisoning by antiparkinsonism drugs and other central muscle-tone depressants, assault**

SP 7 **T42.8X4- Poisoning by antiparkinsonism drugs and other central muscle-tone depressants, undetermined**

IQ 7 **T42.8X5- Adverse effect of antiparkinsonism drugs and other central muscle-tone depressants**

7 **T42.8X6- Underdosing of antiparkinsonism drugs and other central muscle-tone depressants**

4 **T43 Poisoning by, adverse effect of and underdosing of psychotropic drugs, not elsewhere classified**

EXCLUDES 1 appetite depressants (T50.5-)
barbiturates (T42.3-)
benzodiazepines (T42.4-)
methaqualone (T42.6-)
psychodysleptics [hallucinogens] (T40.7-T40.9-)

EXCLUDES 2 drug dependence and related mental and behavioral disorders due to psychoactive substance use (F10.- -F19.-)

The appropriate 7th character is to be added to each code from category T43
A initial encounter
D subsequent encounter
S sequela

5 **T43.0 Poisoning by, adverse effect of and underdosing of tricyclic and tetracyclic antidepressants**

6 **T43.01 Poisoning by, adverse effect of and underdosing of tricyclic antidepressants**

SP 7 **T43.011- Poisoning by tricyclic antidepressants, accidental (unintentional)**

Poisoning by tricyclic antidepressants NOS

SP 7 **T43.012- Poisoning by tricyclic antidepressants, intentional self-harm**

Chapter 19 S00-T88

SP 7 **T43.013- Poisoning by tricyclic antidepressants, assault**

SP 7 **T43.014- Poisoning by tricyclic antidepressants, undetermined**

!Q 7 **T43.015- Adverse effect of tricyclic antidepressants**

7 **T43.016- Underdosing of tricyclic antidepressants**

6 **T43.02 Poisoning by, adverse effect of and underdosing of tetracyclic antidepressants**

SP 7 **T43.021- Poisoning by tetracyclic antidepressants, accidental (unintentional)**
Poisoning by tetracyclic antidepressants NOS

SP 7 **T43.022- Poisoning by tetracyclic antidepressants, intentional self-harm**

SP 7 **T43.023- Poisoning by tetracyclic antidepressants, assault**

SP 7 **T43.024- Poisoning by tetracyclic antidepressants, undetermined**

!Q 7 **T43.025- Adverse effect of tetracyclic antidepressants**

7 **T43.026- Underdosing of tetracyclic antidepressants**

5 **T43.1 Poisoning by, adverse effect of and underdosing of monoamine-oxidase-inhibitor antidepressants**

6 **T43.1X Poisoning by, adverse effect of and underdosing of monoamine-oxidase-inhibitor antidepressants**

SP 7 **T43.1X1- Poisoning by monoamine-oxidase-inhibitor antidepressants, accidental (unintentional)**
Poisoning by monoamine-oxidase-inhibitor antidepressants NOS

SP 7 **T43.1X2- Poisoning by monoamine-oxidase-inhibitor antidepressants, intentional self-harm**

SP 7 **T43.1X3- Poisoning by monoamine-oxidase-inhibitor antidepressants, assault**

SP 7 **T43.1X4- Poisoning by monoamine-oxidase-inhibitor antidepressants, undetermined**

!Q 7 **T43.1X5- Adverse effect of monoamine-oxidase-inhibitor antidepressants**

7 **T43.1X6- Underdosing of monoamine-oxidase-inhibitor antidepressants**

5 **T43.2 Poisoning by, adverse effect of and underdosing of other and unspecified antidepressants**

6 **T43.20 Poisoning by, adverse effect of and underdosing of unspecified antidepressants**

SP 7 **T43.201- Poisoning by unspecified antidepressants, accidental (unintentional)**
Poisoning by antidepressants NOS

SP 7 **T43.202- Poisoning by unspecified antidepressants, intentional self-harm**

SP 7 **T43.203- Poisoning by unspecified antidepressants, assault**

SP 7 **T43.204- Poisoning by unspecified antidepressants, undetermined**

!Q 7 **T43.205- Adverse effect of unspecified antidepressants**
Antidepressant discontinuation syndrome

7 **T43.206- Underdosing of unspecified antidepressants**

6 **T43.21 Poisoning by, adverse effect of and underdosing of selective serotonin and norepinephrine reuptake inhibitors**
Poisoning by, adverse effect of and underdosing of SSNRI antidepressants

SP 7 **T43.211- Poisoning by selective serotonin and norepinephrine reuptake inhibitors, accidental (unintentional)**

SP 7 **T43.212- Poisoning by selective serotonin and norepinephrine reuptake inhibitors, intentional self-harm**

SP 7 **T43.213- Poisoning by selective serotonin and norepinephrine reuptake inhibitors, assault**

SP 7 **T43.214- Poisoning by selective serotonin and norepinephrine reuptake inhibitors, undetermined**

!Q 7 **T43.215- Adverse effect of selective serotonin and norepinephrine reuptake inhibitors**

7 **T43.216- Underdosing of selective serotonin and norepinephrine reuptake inhibitors**

6 **T43.22 Poisoning by, adverse effect of and underdosing of selective serotonin reuptake inhibitors**
Poisoning by, adverse effect of and underdosing of SSRI antidepressants

SP 7 **T43.221- Poisoning by selective serotonin reuptake inhibitors, accidental (unintentional)**

SP 7 **T43.222- Poisoning by selective serotonin reuptake inhibitors, intentional self-harm**

SP 7 **T43.223- Poisoning by selective serotonin reuptake inhibitors, assault**

SP 7 **T43.224- Poisoning by selective serotonin reuptake inhibitors, undetermined**

!Q 7 **T43.225- Adverse effect of selective serotonin reuptake inhibitors**

7 **T43.226- Underdosing of selective serotonin reuptake inhibitors**

6 **T43.29 Poisoning by, adverse effect of and underdosing of other antidepressants**

SP 7 **T43.291- Poisoning by other antidepressants, accidental (unintentional)**
Poisoning by other antidepressants NOS

SP 7 **T43.292- Poisoning by other antidepressants, intentional self-harm**

SP 7 **T43.293- Poisoning by other antidepressants, assault**

SP 7 **T43.294- Poisoning by other antidepressants, undetermined**

IQ 7 **T43.295- Adverse effect of other antidepressants**

7 **T43.296- Underdosing of other antidepressants**

5 **T43.3 Poisoning by, adverse effect of and underdosing of phenothiazine antipsychotics and neuroleptics**

6 **T43.3X Poisoning by, adverse effect of and underdosing of phenothiazine antipsychotics and neuroleptics**

SP 7 **T43.3X1- Poisoning by phenothiazine antipsychotics and neuroleptics, accidental (unintentional)**
Poisoning by phenothiazine antipsychotics and neuroleptics NOS

SP 7 **T43.3X2- Poisoning by phenothiazine antipsychotics and neuroleptics, intentional self-harm**

SP 7 **T43.3X3- Poisoning by phenothiazine antipsychotics and neuroleptics, assault**

SP 7 **T43.3X4- Poisoning by phenothiazine antipsychotics and neuroleptics, undetermined**

IQ 7 **T43.3X5- Adverse effect of phenothiazine antipsychotics and neuroleptics**

7 **T43.3X6- Underdosing of phenothiazine antipsychotics and neuroleptics**

5 **T43.4 Poisoning by, adverse effect of and underdosing of butyrophenone and thiothixene neuroleptics**

6 **T43.4X Poisoning by, adverse effect of and underdosing of butyrophenone and thiothixene neuroleptics**

SP 7 **T43.4X1- Poisoning by butyrophenone and thiothixene neuroleptics, accidental (unintentional)**
Poisoning by butyrophenone and thiothixene neuroleptics NOS

SP 7 **T43.4X2- Poisoning by butyrophenone and thiothixene neuroleptics, intentional self-harm**

SP 7 **T43.4X3- Poisoning by butyrophenone and thiothixene neuroleptics, assault**

SP 7 **T43.4X4- Poisoning by butyrophenone and thiothixene neuroleptics, undetermined**

IQ 7 **T43.4X5- Adverse effect of butyrophenone and thiothixene neuroleptics**

7 **T43.4X6- Underdosing of butyrophenone and thiothixene neuroleptics**

5 **T43.5 Poisoning by, adverse effect of and underdosing of other and unspecified antipsychotics and neuroleptics**

EXCLUDES 1 poisoning by, adverse effect of and underdosing of rauwolfia (T46.5-)

6 **T43.50 Poisoning by, adverse effect of and underdosing of unspecified antipsychotics and neuroleptics**

SP 7 **T43.501- Poisoning by unspecified antipsychotics and neuroleptics, accidental (unintentional)**
Poisoning by antipsychotics and neuroleptics NOS

SP 7 **T43.502- Poisoning by unspecified antipsychotics and neuroleptics, intentional self-harm**

SP 7 **T43.503- Poisoning by unspecified antipsychotics and neuroleptics, assault**

SP 7 **T43.504- Poisoning by unspecified antipsychotics and neuroleptics, undetermined**

IQ 7 **T43.505- Adverse effect of unspecified antipsychotics and neuroleptics**

7 **T43.506- Underdosing of unspecified antipsychotics and neuroleptics**

6 **T43.59 Poisoning by, adverse effect of and underdosing of other antipsychotics and neuroleptics**

SP 7 **T43.591- Poisoning by other antipsychotics and neuroleptics, accidental (unintentional)**
Poisoning by other antipsychotics and neuroleptics NOS

SP 7 **T43.592- Poisoning by other antipsychotics and neuroleptics, intentional self-harm**

SP 7 **T43.593- Poisoning by other antipsychotics and neuroleptics, assault**

SP 7 **T43.594- Poisoning by other antipsychotics and neuroleptics, undetermined**

IQ 7 **T43.595- Adverse effect of other antipsychotics and neuroleptics**

7 **T43.596- Underdosing of other antipsychotics and neuroleptics**

5 **T43.6 Poisoning by, adverse effect of and underdosing of psychostimulants**

EXCLUDES 1 poisoning by, adverse effect of and underdosing of cocaine (T40.5-)

6 **T43.60 Poisoning by, adverse effect of and underdosing of unspecified psychostimulant**

SP 7 **T43.601- Poisoning by unspecified psychostimulants, accidental (unintentional)**
Poisoning by psychostimulants NOS

SP 7 **T43.602- Poisoning by unspecified psychostimulants, intentional self-harm**

SP 7 **T43.603- Poisoning by unspecified psychostimulants, assault**

SP 7 **T43.604- Poisoning by unspecified psychostimulants, undetermined**

IQ 7 **T43.605- Adverse effect of unspecified psychostimulants**

7 **T43.606- Underdosing of unspecified psychostimulants**

6 **T43.61 Poisoning by, adverse effect of and underdosing of caffeine**

SP 7 **T43.611- Poisoning by caffeine, accidental (unintentional)**
Poisoning by caffeine NOS

SP 7 **T43.612- Poisoning by caffeine, intentional self-harm**

SP 7 **T43.613- Poisoning by caffeine, assault**

SP 7 **T43.614- Poisoning by caffeine, undetermined**

!Q 7 **T43.615- Adverse effect of caffeine**

7 **T43.616- Underdosing of caffeine**

6 **T43.62 Poisoning by, adverse effect of and underdosing of amphetamines**
Poisoning by, adverse effect of and underdosing of methamphetamines

SP 7 **T43.621- Poisoning by amphetamines, accidental (unintentional)**
Poisoning by amphetamines NOS

SP 7 **T43.622- Poisoning by amphetamines, intentional self-harm**

SP 7 **T43.623- Poisoning by amphetamines, assault**

SP 7 **T43.624- Poisoning by amphetamines, undetermined**

!Q 7 **T43.625- Adverse effect of amphetamines**

7 **T43.626- Underdosing of amphetamines**

6 **T43.63 Poisoning by, adverse effect of and underdosing of methylphenidate**

SP 7 **T43.631- Poisoning by methylphenidate, accidental (unintentional)**
Poisoning by methylphenidate NOS

SP 7 **T43.632- Poisoning by methylphenidate, intentional self-harm**

SP 7 **T43.633- Poisoning by methylphenidate, assault**

SP 7 **T43.634- Poisoning by methylphenidate, undetermined**

!Q 7 **T43.635- Adverse effect of methylphenidate**

7 **T43.636- Underdosing of methylphenidate**

6 **T43.64 Poisoning by ecstasy**
Poisoning by MDMA
Poisoning by 3,4-methylenedioxymethamphetamine

SP 7 **T43.641- Poisoning by ecstasy, accidental (unintentional)**
Poisoning by ecstasy NOS

SP 7 **T43.642- Poisoning by ecstasy, intentional self-harm**

SP 7 **T43.643- Poisoning by ecstasy, assault**

SP 7 **T43.644- Poisoning by ecstasy, undetermined**

6 **T43.69 Poisoning by, adverse effect of and underdosing of other psychostimulants**

SP 7 **T43.691- Poisoning by other psychostimulants, accidental (unintentional)**
Poisoning by other psychostimulants NOS

SP 7 **T43.692- Poisoning by other psychostimulants, intentional self-harm**

SP 7 **T43.693- Poisoning by other psychostimulants, assault**

SP 7 **T43.694- Poisoning by other psychostimulants, undetermined**

!Q 7 **T43.695- Adverse effect of other psychostimulants**

7 **T43.696- Underdosing of other psychostimulants**

5 **T43.8 Poisoning by, adverse effect of and underdosing of other psychotropic drugs**

6 **T43.8X Poisoning by, adverse effect of and underdosing of other psychotropic drugs**

SP 7 **T43.8X1- Poisoning by other psychotropic drugs, accidental (unintentional)**
Poisoning by other psychotropic drugs NOS

SP 7 **T43.8X2- Poisoning by other psychotropic drugs, intentional self-harm**

SP 7 **T43.8X3- Poisoning by other psychotropic drugs, assault**

SP 7 **T43.8X4- Poisoning by other psychotropic drugs, undetermined**

!Q 7 **T43.8X5- Adverse effect of other psychotropic drugs**

7 **T43.8X6- Underdosing of other psychotropic drugs**

5 **T43.9 Poisoning by, adverse effect of and underdosing of unspecified psychotropic drug**

SP 7 **T43.91X- Poisoning by unspecified psychotropic drug, accidental (unintentional)**
Poisoning by psychotropic drug NOS

SP 7 **T43.92X- Poisoning by unspecified psychotropic drug, intentional self-harm**

SP 7 **T43.93X- Poisoning by unspecified psychotropic drug, assault**

SP 7 **T43.94X- Poisoning by unspecified psychotropic drug, undetermined**

!Q 7 **T43.95X- Adverse effect of unspecified psychotropic drug**

7 **T43.96X- Underdosing of unspecified psychotropic drug**

4 **T44 Poisoning by, adverse effect of and underdosing of drugs primarily affecting the autonomic nervous system**

The appropriate 7th character is to be added to each code from category T44
- A initial encounter
- D subsequent encounter
- S sequela

5 **T44.0 Poisoning by, adverse effect of and underdosing of anticholinesterase agents**

6 **T44.0X Poisoning by, adverse effect of and underdosing of anticholinesterase agents**

SP 7 **T44.0X1- Poisoning by anticholinesterase agents, accidental (unintentional)**
Poisoning by anticholinesterase agents NOS

SP 7 **T44.0X2- Poisoning by anticholinesterase agents, intentional self-harm**

SP 7 **T44.0X3- Poisoning by anticholinesterase agents, assault**

SP 7 **T44.0X4- Poisoning by anticholinesterase agents, undetermined**

!Q 7 **T44.0X5- Adverse effect of anticholinesterase agents**

7 **T44.0X6- Underdosing of anticholinesterase agents**

5 **T44.1 Poisoning by, adverse effect of and underdosing of other parasympathomimetics [cholinergics]**

6 **T44.1X Poisoning by, adverse effect of and underdosing of other parasympathomimetics [cholinergics]**

SP 7 **T44.1X1- Poisoning by other parasympathomimetics [cholinergics], accidental (unintentional)**
Poisoning by other parasympathomimetics [cholinergics] NOS

SP 7 **T44.1X2- Poisoning by other parasympathomimetics [cholinergics], intentional self-harm**

SP 7 **T44.1X3- Poisoning by other parasympathomimetics [cholinergics], assault**

SP 7 **T44.1X4- Poisoning by other parasympathomimetics [cholinergics], undetermined**

!Q 7 **T44.1X5- Adverse effect of other parasympathomimetics [cholinergics]**

7 **T44.1X6- Underdosing of other parasympathomimetics [cholinergics]**

5 **T44.2 Poisoning by, adverse effect of and underdosing of ganglionic blocking drugs**

6 **T44.2X Poisoning by, adverse effect of and underdosing of ganglionic blocking drugs**

SP 7 **T44.2X1- Poisoning by ganglionic blocking drugs, accidental (unintentional)**
Poisoning by ganglionic blocking drugs NOS

SP 7 **T44.2X2- Poisoning by ganglionic blocking drugs, intentional self-harm**

SP 7 **T44.2X3- Poisoning by ganglionic blocking drugs, assault**

SP 7 **T44.2X4- Poisoning by ganglionic blocking drugs, undetermined**

!Q 7 **T44.2X5- Adverse effect of ganglionic blocking drugs**

7 **T44.2X6- Underdosing of ganglionic blocking drugs**

5 **T44.3 Poisoning by, adverse effect of and underdosing of other parasympatholytics [anticholinergics and antimuscarinics] and spasmolytics**
Poisoning by, adverse effect of and underdosing of papaverine

6 **T44.3X Poisoning by, adverse effect of and underdosing of other parasympatholytics [anticholinergics and antimuscarinics] and spasmolytics**

SP 7 **T44.3X1- Poisoning by other parasympatholytics [anticholinergics and antimuscarinics] and spasmolytics, accidental (unintentional)**
Poisoning by other parasympatholytics [anticholinergics and antimuscarinics] and spasmolytics NOS

SP 7 **T44.3X2- Poisoning by other parasympatholytics [anticholinergics and antimuscarinics] and spasmolytics, intentional self-harm**

SP 7 **T44.3X3- Poisoning by other parasympatholytics [anticholinergics and antimuscarinics] and spasmolytics, assault**

SP 7 **T44.3X4- Poisoning by other parasympatholytics [anticholinergics and antimuscarinics] and spasmolytics, undetermined**

!Q 7 **T44.3X5- Adverse effect of other parasympatholytics [anticholinergics and antimuscarinics] and spasmolytics**

7 **T44.3X6- Underdosing of other parasympatholytics [anticholinergics and antimuscarinics] and spasmolytics**

5 **T44.4 Poisoning by, adverse effect of and underdosing of predominantly alpha-adrenoreceptor agonists**
Poisoning by, adverse effect of and underdosing of metaraminol

6 **T44.4X Poisoning by, adverse effect of and underdosing of predominantly alpha-adrenoreceptor agonists**

SP 7 **T44.4X1- Poisoning by predominantly alpha-adrenoreceptor agonists, accidental (unintentional)**
Poisoning by predominantly alpha-adrenoreceptor agonists NOS

SP 7 **T44.4X2- Poisoning by predominantly alpha-adrenoreceptor agonists, intentional self-harm**

SP 7 **T44.4X3- Poisoning by predominantly alpha-adrenoreceptor agonists, assault**

SP 7 **T44.4X4- Poisoning by predominantly alpha-adrenoreceptor agonists, undetermined**

!Q 7 **T44.4X5- Adverse effect of predominantly alpha-adrenoreceptor agonists**

7 **T44.4X6- Underdosing of predominantly alpha-adrenoreceptor agonists**

5 **T44.5 Poisoning by, adverse effect of and underdosing of predominantly beta-adrenoreceptor agonists**
EXCLUDES 1 poisoning by, adverse effect of and underdosing of beta-adrenoreceptor agonists used in asthma therapy (T48.6-)

6 **T44.5X Poisoning by, adverse effect of and underdosing of predominantly beta-adrenoreceptor agonists**

Chapter 19
S00-T88

SP 7 **T44.5X1- Poisoning by predominantly beta-adrenoreceptor agonists, accidental (unintentional)**
Poisoning by predominantly beta-adrenoreceptor agonists NOS

SP 7 **T44.5X2- Poisoning by predominantly beta-adrenoreceptor agonists, intentional self-harm**

SP 7 **T44.5X3- Poisoning by predominantly beta-adrenoreceptor agonists, assault**

SP 7 **T44.5X4- Poisoning by predominantly beta-adrenoreceptor agonists, undetermined**

IQ 7 **T44.5X5- Adverse effect of predominantly beta-adrenoreceptor agonists**

7 **T44.5X6- Underdosing of predominantly beta-adrenoreceptor agonists**

5 **T44.6 Poisoning by, adverse effect of and underdosing of alpha-adrenoreceptor antagonists**
EXCLUDES 1 poisoning by, adverse effect of and underdosing of ergot alkaloids (T48.0)

6 **T44.6X Poisoning by, adverse effect of and underdosing of alpha-adrenoreceptor antagonists**

SP 7 **T44.6X1- Poisoning by alpha-adrenoreceptor antagonists, accidental (unintentional)**
Poisoning by alpha-adrenoreceptor antagonists NOS

SP 7 **T44.6X2- Poisoning by alpha-adrenoreceptor antagonists, intentional self-harm**

SP 7 **T44.6X3- Poisoning by alpha-adrenoreceptor antagonists, assault**

SP 7 **T44.6X4- Poisoning by alpha-adrenoreceptor antagonists, undetermined**

IQ 7 **T44.6X5- Adverse effect of alpha-adrenoreceptor antagonists**

7 **T44.6X6- Underdosing of alpha-adrenoreceptor antagonists**

5 **T44.7 Poisoning by, adverse effect of and underdosing of beta-adrenoreceptor antagonists**

6 **T44.7X Poisoning by, adverse effect of and underdosing of beta-adrenoreceptor antagonists**

SP 7 **T44.7X1- Poisoning by beta-adrenoreceptor antagonists, accidental (unintentional)**
Poisoning by beta-adrenoreceptor antagonists NOS

SP 7 **T44.7X2- Poisoning by beta-adrenoreceptor antagonists, intentional self-harm**

SP 7 **T44.7X3- Poisoning by beta-adrenoreceptor antagonists, assault**

SP 7 **T44.7X4- Poisoning by beta-adrenoreceptor antagonists, undetermined**

IQ 7 **T44.7X5- Adverse effect of beta-adrenoreceptor antagonists**

7 **T44.7X6- Underdosing of beta-adrenoreceptor antagonists**

▲ 5 **T44.8 Poisoning by, adverse effect of and underdosing of centrally-acting and adrenergic-neuron- blocking agents**
EXCLUDES 2 poisoning by, adverse effect of and underdosing of clonidine (T46.5)
poisoning by, adverse effect of and underdosing of guanethidine (T46.5)

6 **T44.8X Poisoning by, adverse effect of and underdosing of centrally-acting and adrenergic- neuron-blocking agents**

SP 7 **T44.8X1- Poisoning by centrally-acting and adrenergic-neuron-blocking agents, accidental (unintentional)**
Poisoning by centrally-acting and adrenergic-neuron-blocking agents NOS

SP 7 **T44.8X2- Poisoning by centrally-acting and adrenergic-neuron-blocking agents, intentional self-harm**

SP 7 **T44.8X3- Poisoning by centrally-acting and adrenergic-neuron-blocking agents, assault**

SP 7 **T44.8X4- Poisoning by centrally-acting and adrenergic-neuron-blocking agents, undetermined**

IQ 7 **T44.8X5- Adverse effect of centrally-acting and adrenergic-neuron-blocking agents**

7 **T44.8X6- Underdosing of centrally-acting and adrenergic-neuron-blocking agents**

5 **T44.9 Poisoning by, adverse effect of and underdosing of other and unspecified drugs primarily affecting the autonomic nervous system**
Poisoning by, adverse effect of and underdosing of drug stimulating both alpha and beta-adrenoreceptors

6 **T44.90 Poisoning by, adverse effect of and underdosing of unspecified drugs primarily affecting the autonomic nervous system**

SP 7 **T44.901- Poisoning by unspecified drugs primarily affecting the autonomic nervous system, accidental (unintentional)**
Poisoning by unspecified drugs primarily affecting the autonomic nervous system NOS

SP 7 **T44.902- Poisoning by unspecified drugs primarily affecting the autonomic nervous system, intentional self-harm**

SP 7 **T44.903- Poisoning by unspecified drugs primarily affecting the autonomic nervous system, assault**

SP 7 **T44.904- Poisoning by unspecified drugs primarily affecting the autonomic nervous system, undetermined**

IQ 7 **T44.905- Adverse effect of unspecified drugs primarily affecting the autonomic nervous system**

7 T44.906- **Underdosing of unspecified drugs primarily affecting the autonomic nervous system**

6 T44.99 **Poisoning by, adverse effect of and underdosing of other drugs primarily affecting the autonomic nervous system**

SP 7 T44.991- **Poisoning by other drug primarily affecting the autonomic nervous system, accidental (unintentional)**
Poisoning by other drugs primarily affecting the autonomic nervous system NOS

SP 7 T44.992- **Poisoning by other drug primarily affecting the autonomic nervous system, intentional self-harm**

SP 7 T44.993- **Poisoning by other drug primarily affecting the autonomic nervous system, assault**

SP 7 T44.994- **Poisoning by other drug primarily affecting the autonomic nervous system, undetermined**

!Q 7 T44.995- **Adverse effect of other drug primarily affecting the autonomic nervous system**

7 T44.996- **Underdosing of other drug primarily affecting the autonomic nervous system**

4 T45 **Poisoning by, adverse effect of and underdosing of primarily systemic and hematological agents, not elsewhere classified**

The appropriate 7th character is to be added to each code from category T45
A initial encounter
D subsequent encounter
S sequela

5 T45.0 **Poisoning by, adverse effect of and underdosing of antiallergic and antiemetic drugs**
EXCLUDES 1 poisoning by, adverse effect of and underdosing of phenothiazine-based neuroleptics (T43.3)

6 T45.0X **Poisoning by, adverse effect of and underdosing of antiallergic and antiemetic drugs**

SP 7 T45.0X1- **Poisoning by antiallergic and antiemetic drugs, accidental (unintentional)**
Poisoning by antiallergic and antiemetic drugs NOS

SP 7 T45.0X2- **Poisoning by antiallergic and antiemetic drugs, intentional self-harm**

SP 7 T45.0X3- **Poisoning by antiallergic and antiemetic drugs, assault**

SP 7 T45.0X4- **Poisoning by antiallergic and antiemetic drugs, undetermined**

!Q 7 T45.0X5- **Adverse effect of antiallergic and antiemetic drugs**

7 T45.0X6- **Underdosing of antiallergic and antiemetic drugs**

5 T45.1 **Poisoning by, adverse effect of and underdosing of antineoplastic and immunosuppressive drugs**
EXCLUDES 1 poisoning by, adverse effect of and underdosing of tamoxifen (T38.6)

6 T45.1X **Poisoning by, adverse effect of and underdosing of antineoplastic and immunosuppressive drugs**

SP 7 T45.1X1- **Poisoning by antineoplastic and immunosuppressive drugs, accidental (unintentional)**
Poisoning by antineoplastic and immunosuppressive drugs NOS

SP 7 T45.1X2- **Poisoning by antineoplastic and immunosuppressive drugs, intentional self-harm**

SP 7 T45.1X3- **Poisoning by antineoplastic and immunosuppressive drugs, assault**

SP 7 T45.1X4- **Poisoning by antineoplastic and immunosuppressive drugs, undetermined**

!Q 7 T45.1X5- **Adverse effect of antineoplastic and immunosuppressive drugs**

7 T45.1X6- **Underdosing of antineoplastic and immunosuppressive drugs**

5 T45.2 **Poisoning by, adverse effect of and underdosing of vitamins**
EXCLUDES 2 poisoning by, adverse effect of and underdosing of nicotinic acid (derivatives) (T46.7)
poisoning by, adverse effect of and underdosing of iron (T45.4)
poisoning by, adverse effect of and underdosing of vitamin K (T45.7)

6 T45.2X **Poisoning by, adverse effect of and underdosing of vitamins**

SP 7 T45.2X1- **Poisoning by vitamins, accidental (unintentional)**
Poisoning by vitamins NOS

SP 7 T45.2X2- **Poisoning by vitamins, intentional self-harm**

SP 7 T45.2X3- **Poisoning by vitamins, assault**

SP 7 T45.2X4- **Poisoning by vitamins, undetermined**

!Q 7 T45.2X5- **Adverse effect of vitamins**

7 T45.2X6- **Underdosing of vitamins**
EXCLUDES 1 vitamin deficiencies (E50-E56)

5 T45.3 **Poisoning by, adverse effect of and underdosing of enzymes**

6 T45.3X **Poisoning by, adverse effect of and underdosing of enzymes**

SP 7 T45.3X1- **Poisoning by enzymes, accidental (unintentional)**
Poisoning by enzymes NOS

SP 7 T45.3X2- **Poisoning by enzymes, intentional self-harm**

SP 7 T45.3X3- **Poisoning by enzymes, assault**

SP 7 T45.3X4- **Poisoning by enzymes, undetermined**

!Q 7 T45.3X5- **Adverse effect of enzymes**

7 T45.3X6- **Underdosing of enzymes**

Chapter 19 S00-T88

5 T45.4 Poisoning by, adverse effect of and underdosing of iron and its compounds

6 T45.4X Poisoning by, adverse effect of and underdosing of iron and its compounds

SP 7 T45.4X1- Poisoning by iron and its compounds, accidental (unintentional)
Poisoning by iron and its compounds NOS

SP 7 T45.4X2- Poisoning by iron and its compounds, intentional self-harm

SP 7 T45.4X3- Poisoning by iron and its compounds, assault

SP 7 T45.4X4- Poisoning by iron and its compounds, undetermined

!Q 7 T45.4X5- Adverse effect of iron and its compounds

7 T45.4X6- Underdosing of iron and its compounds
EXCLUDES 1 iron deficiency (E61.1)

5 T45.5 Poisoning by, adverse effect of and underdosing of anticoagulants and antithrombotic drugs

6 T45.51 Poisoning by, adverse effect of and underdosing of anticoagulants

SP 7 T45.511- Poisoning by anticoagulants, accidental (unintentional)
Poisoning by anticoagulants NOS

SP 7 T45.512- Poisoning by anticoagulants, intentional self-harm

SP 7 T45.513- Poisoning by anticoagulants, assault

SP 7 T45.514- Poisoning by anticoagulants, undetermined

!Q 7 T45.515- Adverse effect of anticoagulants

7 T45.516- Underdosing of anticoagulants

6 T45.52 Poisoning by, adverse effect of and underdosing of antithrombotic drugs
Poisoning by, adverse effect of and underdosing of antiplatelet drugs
EXCLUDES 2 poisoning by, adverse effect of and underdosing of aspirin (T39.01-)
poisoning by, adverse effect of and underdosing of acetylsalicylic acid (T39.01-)

SP 7 T45.521- Poisoning by antithrombotic drugs, accidental (unintentional)
Poisoning by antithrombotic drug NOS

SP 7 T45.522- Poisoning by antithrombotic drugs, intentional self-harm

SP 7 T45.523- Poisoning by antithrombotic drugs, assault

SP 7 T45.524- Poisoning by antithrombotic drugs, undetermined

!Q 7 T45.525- Adverse effect of antithrombotic drugs

7 T45.526- Underdosing of antithrombotic drugs

5 T45.6 Poisoning by, adverse effect of and underdosing of fibrinolysis-affecting drugs

6 T45.60 Poisoning by, adverse effect of and underdosing of unspecified fibrinolysis-affecting drugs

SP 7 T45.601- Poisoning by unspecified fibrinolysis-affecting drugs, accidental (unintentional)
Poisoning by fibrinolysis-affecting drug NOS

SP 7 T45.602- Poisoning by unspecified fibrinolysis-affecting drugs, intentional self-harm

SP 7 T45.603- Poisoning by unspecified fibrinolysis-affecting drugs, assault

SP 7 T45.604- Poisoning by unspecified fibrinolysis-affecting drugs, undetermined

!Q 7 T45.605- Adverse effect of unspecified fibrinolysis-affecting drugs

7 T45.606- Underdosing of unspecified fibrinolysis-affecting drugs

6 T45.61 Poisoning by, adverse effect of and underdosing of thrombolytic drugs

SP 7 T45.611- Poisoning by thrombolytic drug, accidental (unintentional)
Poisoning by thrombolytic drug NOS

SP 7 T45.612- Poisoning by thrombolytic drug, intentional self-harm

SP 7 T45.613- Poisoning by thrombolytic drug, assault

SP 7 T45.614- Poisoning by thrombolytic drug, undetermined

!Q 7 T45.615- Adverse effect of thrombolytic drugs

7 T45.616- Underdosing of thrombolytic drugs

6 T45.62 Poisoning by, adverse effect of and underdosing of hemostatic drugs

SP 7 T45.621- Poisoning by hemostatic drug, accidental (unintentional)
Poisoning by hemostatic drug NOS

SP 7 T45.622- Poisoning by hemostatic drug, intentional self-harm

SP 7 T45.623- Poisoning by hemostatic drug, assault

SP 7 T45.624- Poisoning by hemostatic drug, undetermined

!Q 7 T45.625- Adverse effect of hemostatic drug

7 T45.626- Underdosing of hemostatic drugs

6 T45.69 Poisoning by, adverse effect of and underdosing of other fibrinolysis-affecting drugs

SP 7 T45.691- Poisoning by other fibrinolysis-affecting drugs, accidental (unintentional)
Poisoning by other fibrinolysis-affecting drug NOS

SP 7 T45.692- Poisoning by other fibrinolysis-affecting drugs, intentional self-harm

SP 7 T45.693- Poisoning by other fibrinolysis-affecting drugs, assault

SP 7 **T45.694- Poisoning by other fibrinolysis-affecting drugs, undetermined**

IQ 7 **T45.695- Adverse effect of other fibrinolysis-affecting drugs**

7 **T45.696- Underdosing of other fibrinolysis-affecting drugs**

5 **T45.7 Poisoning by, adverse effect of and underdosing of anticoagulant antagonists, vitamin K and other coagulants**

6 **T45.7X Poisoning by, adverse effect of and underdosing of anticoagulant antagonists, vitamin K and other coagulants**

SP 7 **T45.7X1- Poisoning by anticoagulant antagonists, vitamin K and other coagulants, accidental (unintentional)**

Poisoning by anticoagulant antagonists, vitamin K and other coagulants NOS

SP 7 **T45.7X2- Poisoning by anticoagulant antagonists, vitamin K and other coagulants, intentional self-harm**

SP 7 **T45.7X3- Poisoning by anticoagulant antagonists, vitamin K and other coagulants, assault**

SP 7 **T45.7X4- Poisoning by anticoagulant antagonists, vitamin K and other coagulants, undetermined**

IQ 7 **T45.7X5- Adverse effect of anticoagulant antagonists, vitamin K and other coagulants**

7 **T45.7X6- Underdosing of anticoagulant antagonist, vitamin K and other coagulants**

EXCLUDES 1 vitamin K deficiency (E56.1)

5 **T45.8 Poisoning by, adverse effect of and underdosing of other primarily systemic and hematological agents**

Poisoning by, adverse effect of and underdosing of liver preparations and other antianemic agents

Poisoning by, adverse effect of and underdosing of natural blood and blood products

Poisoning by, adverse effect of and underdosing of plasma substitute

EXCLUDES 2 poisoning by, adverse effect of and underdosing of immunoglobulin (T50.Z1)
poisoning by, adverse effect of and underdosing of iron (T45.4)
transfusion reactions (T80.-)

6 **T45.8X Poisoning by, adverse effect of and underdosing of other primarily systemic and hematological agents**

SP 7 **T45.8X1- Poisoning by other primarily systemic and hematological agents, accidental (unintentional)**

Poisoning by other primarily systemic and hematological agents NOS

SP 7 **T45.8X2- Poisoning by other primarily systemic and hematological agents, intentional self-harm**

SP 7 **T45.8X3- Poisoning by other primarily systemic and hematological agents, assault**

SP 7 **T45.8X4- Poisoning by other primarily systemic and hematological agents, undetermined**

IQ 7 **T45.8X5- Adverse effect of other primarily systemic and hematological agents**

7 **T45.8X6- Underdosing of other primarily systemic and hematological agents**

5 **T45.9 Poisoning by, adverse effect of and underdosing of unspecified primarily systemic and hematological agent**

SP 7 **T45.91X- Poisoning by unspecified primarily systemic and hematological agent, accidental (unintentional)**

Poisoning by primarily systemic and hematological agent NOS

SP 7 **T45.92X- Poisoning by unspecified primarily systemic and hematological agent, intentional self-harm**

SP 7 **T45.93X- Poisoning by unspecified primarily systemic and hematological agent, assault**

SP 7 **T45.94X- Poisoning by unspecified primarily systemic and hematological agent, undetermined**

IQ 7 **T45.95X- Adverse effect of unspecified primarily systemic and hematological agent**

7 **T45.96X- Underdosing of unspecified primarily systemic and hematological agent**

4 **T46 Poisoning by, adverse effect of and underdosing of agents primarily affecting the cardiovascular system**

EXCLUDES 1 poisoning by, adverse effect of and underdosing of metaraminol (T44.4)

The appropriate 7th character is to be added to each code from category T46

A	initial encounter
D	subsequent encounter
S	sequela

5 **T46.0 Poisoning by, adverse effect of and underdosing of cardiac-stimulant glycosides and drugs of similar action**

6 **T46.0X Poisoning by, adverse effect of and underdosing of cardiac-stimulant glycosides and drugs of similar action**

SP 7 **T46.0X1- Poisoning by cardiac-stimulant glycosides and drugs of similar action, accidental (unintentional)**

Poisoning by cardiac-stimulant glycosides and drugs of similar action NOS

SP 7 **T46.0X2- Poisoning by cardiac-stimulant glycosides and drugs of similar action, intentional self-harm**

SP 7 **T46.0X3- Poisoning by cardiac-stimulant glycosides and drugs of similar action, assault**

SP 7 **T46.0X4- Poisoning by cardiac-stimulant glycosides and drugs of similar action, undetermined**

!Q 7 **T46.0X5- Adverse effect of cardiac-stimulant glycosides and drugs of similar action**

7 **T46.0X6- Underdosing of cardiac-stimulant glycosides and drugs of similar action**

5 **T46.1 Poisoning by, adverse effect of and underdosing of calcium-channel blockers**

6 **T46.1X Poisoning by, adverse effect of and underdosing of calcium-channel blockers**

SP 7 **T46.1X1- Poisoning by calcium-channel blockers, accidental (unintentional)**
Poisoning by calcium-channel blockers NOS

SP 7 **T46.1X2- Poisoning by calcium-channel blockers, intentional self-harm**

SP 7 **T46.1X3- Poisoning by calcium-channel blockers, assault**

SP 7 **T46.1X4- Poisoning by calcium-channel blockers, undetermined**

!Q 7 **T46.1X5- Adverse effect of calcium-channel blockers**

7 **T46.1X6- Underdosing of calcium-channel blockers**

5 **T46.2 Poisoning by, adverse effect of and underdosing of other antidysrhythmic drugs, not elsewhere classified**

EXCLUDES 1 poisoning by, adverse effect of and underdosing of beta-adrenoreceptor antagonists (T44.7-)

6 **T46.2X Poisoning by, adverse effect of and underdosing of other antidysrhythmic drugs**

SP 7 **T46.2X1- Poisoning by other antidysrhythmic drugs, accidental (unintentional)**
Poisoning by other antidysrhythmic drugs NOS

SP 7 **T46.2X2- Poisoning by other antidysrhythmic drugs, intentional self-harm**

SP 7 **T46.2X3- Poisoning by other antidysrhythmic drugs, assault**

SP 7 **T46.2X4- Poisoning by other antidysrhythmic drugs, undetermined**

!Q 7 **T46.2X5- Adverse effect of other antidysrhythmic drugs**

7 **T46.2X6- Underdosing of other antidysrhythmic drugs**

5 **T46.3 Poisoning by, adverse effect of and underdosing of coronary vasodilators**
Poisoning by, adverse effect of and underdosing of dipyridamole

EXCLUDES 1 poisoning by, adverse effect of and underdosing of calcium-channel blockers (T46.1)

6 **T46.3X Poisoning by, adverse effect of and underdosing of coronary vasodilators**

SP 7 **T46.3X1- Poisoning by coronary vasodilators, accidental (unintentional)**
Poisoning by coronary vasodilators NOS

SP 7 **T46.3X2- Poisoning by coronary vasodilators, intentional self-harm**

SP 7 **T46.3X3- Poisoning by coronary vasodilators, assault**

SP 7 **T46.3X4- Poisoning by coronary vasodilators, undetermined**

!Q 7 **T46.3X5- Adverse effect of coronary vasodilators**

7 **T46.3X6- Underdosing of coronary vasodilators**

5 **T46.4 Poisoning by, adverse effect of and underdosing of angiotensin-converting-enzyme inhibitors**

6 **T46.4X Poisoning by, adverse effect of and underdosing of angiotensin-converting-enzyme inhibitors**

SP 7 **T46.4X1- Poisoning by angiotensin-converting-enzyme inhibitors, accidental (unintentional)**
Poisoning by angiotensin-converting-enzyme inhibitors NOS

SP 7 **T46.4X2- Poisoning by angiotensin-converting-enzyme inhibitors, intentional self-harm**

SP 7 **T46.4X3- Poisoning by angiotensin-converting-enzyme inhibitors, assault**

SP 7 **T46.4X4- Poisoning by angiotensin-converting-enzyme inhibitors, undetermined**

!Q 7 **T46.4X5- Adverse effect of angiotensin-converting-enzyme inhibitors**

7 **T46.4X6- Underdosing of angiotensin-converting-enzyme inhibitors**

5 **T46.5 Poisoning by, adverse effect of and underdosing of other antihypertensive drugs**

EXCLUDES 2 poisoning by, adverse effect of and underdosing of beta-adrenoreceptor antagonists (T44.7)
poisoning by, adverse effect of and underdosing of calcium-channel blockers (T46.1)
poisoning by, adverse effect of and underdosing of diuretics (T50.0-T50.2)

6 **T46.5X Poisoning by, adverse effect of and underdosing of other antihypertensive drugs**

SP 7 **T46.5X1- Poisoning by other antihypertensive drugs, accidental (unintentional)**
Poisoning by other antihypertensive drugs NOS

SP 7 **T46.5X2- Poisoning by other antihypertensive drugs, intentional self-harm**

SP 7 **T46.5X3- Poisoning by other antihypertensive drugs, assault**

SP 7 **T46.5X4- Poisoning by other antihypertensive drugs, undetermined**

!Q 7 **T46.5X5- Adverse effect of other antihypertensive drugs**

7 **T46.5X6- Underdosing of other antihypertensive drugs**

5 **T46.6 Poisoning by, adverse effect of and underdosing of antihyperlipidemic and antiarteriosclerotic drugs**

6 **T46.6X Poisoning by, adverse effect of and underdosing of antihyperlipidemic and antiarteriosclerotic drugs**

SP 7 **T46.6X1- Poisoning by antihyperlipidemic and antiarteriosclerotic drugs, accidental (unintentional)**

Poisoning by antihyperlipidemic and antiarteriosclerotic drugs NOS

SP 7 **T46.6X2- Poisoning by antihyperlipidemic and antiarteriosclerotic drugs, intentional self-harm**

SP 7 **T46.6X3- Poisoning by antihyperlipidemic and antiarteriosclerotic drugs, assault**

SP 7 **T46.6X4- Poisoning by antihyperlipidemic and antiarteriosclerotic drugs, undetermined**

!Q 7 **T46.6X5- Adverse effect of antihyperlipidemic and antiarteriosclerotic drugs**

7 **T46.6X6- Underdosing of antihyperlipidemic and antiarteriosclerotic drugs**

5 **T46.7 Poisoning by, adverse effect of and underdosing of peripheral vasodilators**

Poisoning by, adverse effect of and underdosing of nicotinic acid (derivatives)

EXCLUDES 1 poisoning by, adverse effect of and underdosing of papaverine (T44.3)

6 **T46.7X Poisoning by, adverse effect of and underdosing of peripheral vasodilators**

SP 7 **T46.7X1- Poisoning by peripheral vasodilators, accidental (unintentional)**

Poisoning by peripheral vasodilators NOS

SP 7 **T46.7X2- Poisoning by peripheral vasodilators, intentional self-harm**

SP 7 **T46.7X3- Poisoning by peripheral vasodilators, assault**

SP 7 **T46.7X4- Poisoning by peripheral vasodilators, undetermined**

!Q 7 **T46.7X5- Adverse effect of peripheral vasodilators**

7 **T46.7X6- Underdosing of peripheral vasodilators**

5 **T46.8 Poisoning by, adverse effect of and underdosing of antivaricose drugs, including sclerosing agents**

6 **T46.8X Poisoning by, adverse effect of and underdosing of antivaricose drugs, including sclerosing agents**

SP 7 **T46.8X1- Poisoning by antivaricose drugs, including sclerosing agents, accidental (unintentional)**

Poisoning by antivaricose drugs, including sclerosing agents NOS

SP 7 **T46.8X2- Poisoning by antivaricose drugs, including sclerosing agents, intentional self-harm**

SP 7 **T46.8X3- Poisoning by antivaricose drugs, including sclerosing agents, assault**

SP 7 **T46.8X4- Poisoning by antivaricose drugs, including sclerosing agents, undetermined**

!Q 7 **T46.8X5- Adverse effect of antivaricose drugs, including sclerosing agents**

7 **T46.8X6- Underdosing of antivaricose drugs, including sclerosing agents**

5 **T46.9 Poisoning by, adverse effect of and underdosing of other and unspecified agents primarily affecting the cardiovascular system**

6 **T46.90 Poisoning by, adverse effect of and underdosing of unspecified agents primarily affecting the cardiovascular system**

SP 7 **T46.901- Poisoning by unspecified agents primarily affecting the cardiovascular system, accidental (unintentional)**

SP 7 **T46.902- Poisoning by unspecified agents primarily affecting the cardiovascular system, intentional self-harm**

SP 7 **T46.903- Poisoning by unspecified agents primarily affecting the cardiovascular system, assault**

SP 7 **T46.904- Poisoning by unspecified agents primarily affecting the cardiovascular system, undetermined**

!Q 7 **T46.905- Adverse effect of unspecified agents primarily affecting the cardiovascular system**

7 **T46.906- Underdosing of unspecified agents primarily affecting the cardiovascular system**

6 **T46.99 Poisoning by, adverse effect of and underdosing of other agents primarily affecting the cardiovascular system**

SP 7 **T46.991- Poisoning by other agents primarily affecting the cardiovascular system, accidental (unintentional)**

SP 7 **T46.992- Poisoning by other agents primarily affecting the cardiovascular system, intentional self-harm**

SP 7 **T46.993- Poisoning by other agents primarily affecting the cardiovascular system, assault**

SP 7 **T46.994- Poisoning by other agents primarily affecting the cardiovascular system, undetermined**

IQ 7 **T46.995- Adverse effect of other agents primarily affecting the cardiovascular system**

7 **T46.996- Underdosing of other agents primarily affecting the cardiovascular system**

4 **T47 Poisoning by, adverse effect of and underdosing of agents primarily affecting the gastrointestinal system**

The appropriate 7th character is to be added to each code from category T47
A initial encounter
D subsequent encounter
S sequela

5 **T47.0 Poisoning by, adverse effect of and underdosing of histamine H2-receptor blockers**

6 **T47.0X Poisoning by, adverse effect of and underdosing of histamine H2-receptor blockers**

SP 7 **T47.0X1- Poisoning by histamine H2-receptor blockers, accidental (unintentional)**
Poisoning by histamine H2-receptor blockers NOS

SP 7 **T47.0X2- Poisoning by histamine H2-receptor blockers, intentional self-harm**

SP 7 **T47.0X3- Poisoning by histamine H2-receptor blockers, assault**

SP 7 **T47.0X4- Poisoning by histamine H2-receptor blockers, undetermined**

IQ 7 **T47.0X5- Adverse effect of histamine H2-receptor blockers**

7 **T47.0X6- Underdosing of histamine H2-receptor blockers**

5 **T47.1 Poisoning by, adverse effect of and underdosing of other antacids and anti-gastric-secretion drugs**

6 **T47.1X Poisoning by, adverse effect of and underdosing of other antacids and anti-gastric-secretion drugs**

SP 7 **T47.1X1- Poisoning by other antacids and anti-gastric-secretion drugs, accidental (unintentional)**
Poisoning by other antacids and anti-gastric-secretion drugs NOS

SP 7 **T47.1X2- Poisoning by other antacids and anti-gastric-secretion drugs, intentional self-harm**

SP 7 **T47.1X3- Poisoning by other antacids and anti-gastric-secretion drugs, assault**

SP 7 **T47.1X4- Poisoning by other antacids and anti-gastric-secretion drugs, undetermined**

IQ 7 **T47.1X5- Adverse effect of other antacids and anti-gastric-secretion drugs**

7 **T47.1X6- Underdosing of other antacids and anti-gastric-secretion drugs**

5 **T47.2 Poisoning by, adverse effect of and underdosing of stimulant laxatives**

6 **T47.2X Poisoning by, adverse effect of and underdosing of stimulant laxatives**

SP 7 **T47.2X1- Poisoning by stimulant laxatives, accidental (unintentional)**
Poisoning by stimulant laxatives NOS

SP 7 **T47.2X2- Poisoning by stimulant laxatives, intentional self-harm**

SP 7 **T47.2X3- Poisoning by stimulant laxatives, assault**

SP 7 **T47.2X4- Poisoning by stimulant laxatives, undetermined**

IQ 7 **T47.2X5- Adverse effect of stimulant laxatives**

7 **T47.2X6- Underdosing of stimulant laxatives**

5 **T47.3 Poisoning by, adverse effect of and underdosing of saline and osmotic laxatives**

6 **T47.3X Poisoning by and adverse effect of saline and osmotic laxatives**

SP 7 **T47.3X1- Poisoning by saline and osmotic laxatives, accidental (unintentional)**
Poisoning by saline and osmotic laxatives NOS

SP 7 **T47.3X2- Poisoning by saline and osmotic laxatives, intentional self-harm**

SP 7 **T47.3X3- Poisoning by saline and osmotic laxatives, assault**

SP 7 **T47.3X4- Poisoning by saline and osmotic laxatives, undetermined**

IQ 7 **T47.3X5- Adverse effect of saline and osmotic laxatives**

7 **T47.3X6- Underdosing of saline and osmotic laxatives**

5 **T47.4 Poisoning by, adverse effect of and underdosing of other laxatives**

6 **T47.4X Poisoning by, adverse effect of and underdosing of other laxatives**

SP 7 **T47.4X1- Poisoning by other laxatives, accidental (unintentional)**
Poisoning by other laxatives NOS

SP 7 **T47.4X2- Poisoning by other laxatives, intentional self-harm**

SP 7 **T47.4X3- Poisoning by other laxatives, assault**

SP 7 **T47.4X4- Poisoning by other laxatives, undetermined**

IQ 7 **T47.4X5- Adverse effect of other laxatives**

7 **T47.4X6- Underdosing of other laxatives**

5 **T47.5 Poisoning by, adverse effect of and underdosing of digestants**

6 **T47.5X Poisoning by, adverse effect of and underdosing of digestants**

SP 7 **T47.5X1- Poisoning by digestants, accidental (unintentional)**
Poisoning by digestants NOS

SP 7 **T47.5X2- Poisoning by digestants, intentional self-harm**

SP 7 **T47.5X3- Poisoning by digestants, assault**

SP 7 **T47.5X4- Poisoning by digestants, undetermined**

IQ 7 **T47.5X5- Adverse effect of digestants**

7 **T47.5X6- Underdosing of digestants**

5 **T47.6 Poisoning by, adverse effect of and underdosing of antidiarrheal drugs**

EXCLUDES 2 poisoning by, adverse effect of and underdosing of systemic antibiotics and other anti-infectives (T36-T37)

Chapter 19 S00-T88

4 4th digit required 5 5th digit required 6 6th digit required 7 7th digit required 7 7th digit placeholder + Additional code Laterality

6 T47.6X Poisoning by, adverse effect of and underdosing of antidiarrheal drugs

SP 7 T47.6X1- **Poisoning by antidiarrheal drugs, accidental (unintentional)**
Poisoning by antidiarrheal drugs NOS

SP 7 T47.6X2- **Poisoning by antidiarrheal drugs, intentional self-harm**

SP 7 T47.6X3- **Poisoning by antidiarrheal drugs, assault**

SP 7 T47.6X4- **Poisoning by antidiarrheal drugs, undetermined**

!Q 7 T47.6X5- **Adverse effect of antidiarrheal drugs**

7 T47.6X6- **Underdosing of antidiarrheal drugs**

5 T47.7 **Poisoning by, adverse effect of and underdosing of emetics**

6 T47.7X **Poisoning by, adverse effect of and underdosing of emetics**

SP 7 T47.7X1- **Poisoning by emetics, accidental (unintentional)**
Poisoning by emetics NOS

SP 7 T47.7X2- **Poisoning by emetics, intentional self-harm**

SP 7 T47.7X3- **Poisoning by emetics, assault**

SP 7 T47.7X4- **Poisoning by emetics, undetermined**

!Q 7 T47.7X5- **Adverse effect of emetics**

7 T47.7X6- **Underdosing of emetics**

5 T47.8 **Poisoning by, adverse effect of and underdosing of other agents primarily affecting gastrointestinal system**

6 T47.8X **Poisoning by, adverse effect of and underdosing of other agents primarily affecting gastrointestinal system**

SP 7 T47.8X1- **Poisoning by other agents primarily affecting gastrointestinal system, accidental (unintentional)**
Poisoning by other agents primarily affecting gastrointestinal system NOS

SP 7 T47.8X2- **Poisoning by other agents primarily affecting gastrointestinal system, intentional self-harm**

SP 7 T47.8X3- **Poisoning by other agents primarily affecting gastrointestinal system, assault**

SP 7 T47.8X4- **Poisoning by other agents primarily affecting gastrointestinal system, undetermined**

!Q 7 T47.8X5- **Adverse effect of other agents primarily affecting gastrointestinal system**

7 T47.8X6- **Underdosing of other agents primarily affecting gastrointestinal system**

5 T47.9 **Poisoning by, adverse effect of and underdosing of unspecified agents primarily affecting the gastrointestinal system**

SP 7 T47.91X- **Poisoning by unspecified agents primarily affecting the gastrointestinal system, accidental (unintentional)**
Poisoning by agents primarily affecting the gastrointestinal system NOS

SP 7 T47.92X- **Poisoning by unspecified agents primarily affecting the gastrointestinal system, intentional self-harm**

SP 7 T47.93X- **Poisoning by unspecified agents primarily affecting the gastrointestinal system, assault**

SP 7 T47.94X- **Poisoning by unspecified agents primarily affecting the gastrointestinal system, undetermined**

!Q 7 T47.95X- **Adverse effect of unspecified agents primarily affecting the gastrointestinal system**

7 T47.96X- **Underdosing of unspecified agents primarily affecting the gastrointestinal system**

4 T48 **Poisoning by, adverse effect of and underdosing of agents primarily acting on smooth and skeletal muscles and the respiratory system**

The appropriate 7th character is to be added to each code from category T48
A initial encounter
D subsequent encounter
S sequela

5 T48.0 **Poisoning by, adverse effect of and underdosing of oxytocic drugs**
EXCLUDES 1 poisoning by, adverse effect of and underdosing of estrogens, progestogens and antagonists (T38.4-T38.6)

6 T48.0X **Poisoning by, adverse effect of and underdosing of oxytocic drugs**

SP 7 T48.0X1- **Poisoning by oxytocic drugs, accidental (unintentional)**
Poisoning by oxytocic drugs NOS

SP 7 T48.0X2- **Poisoning by oxytocic drugs, intentional self-harm**

SP 7 T48.0X3- **Poisoning by oxytocic drugs, assault**

SP 7 T48.0X4- **Poisoning by oxytocic drugs, undetermined**

!Q 7 T48.0X5- **Adverse effect of oxytocic drugs**

7 T48.0X6- **Underdosing of oxytocic drugs**

5 T48.1 **Poisoning by, adverse effect of and underdosing of skeletal muscle relaxants [neuromuscular blocking agents]**

6 T48.1X **Poisoning by, adverse effect of and underdosing of skeletal muscle relaxants [neuromuscular blocking agents]**

SP 7 T48.1X1- **Poisoning by skeletal muscle relaxants [neuromuscular blocking agents], accidental (unintentional)**

Chapter 19 S00-T88

Poisoning by skeletal muscle relaxants [neuromuscular blocking agents] NOS

SP 7 **T48.1X2- Poisoning by skeletal muscle relaxants [neuromuscular blocking agents], intentional self-harm**

SP 7 **T48.1X3- Poisoning by skeletal muscle relaxants [neuromuscular blocking agents], assault**

SP 7 **T48.1X4- Poisoning by skeletal muscle relaxants [neuromuscular blocking agents], undetermined**

IQ 7 **T48.1X5- Adverse effect of skeletal muscle relaxants [neuromuscular blocking agents]**

7 **T48.1X6- Underdosing of skeletal muscle relaxants [neuromuscular blocking agents]**

5 **T48.2 Poisoning by, adverse effect of and underdosing of other and unspecified drugs acting on muscles**

6 **T48.20 Poisoning by, adverse effect of and underdosing of unspecified drugs acting on muscles**

SP 7 **T48.201- Poisoning by unspecified drugs acting on muscles, accidental (unintentional)**

Poisoning by unspecified drugs acting on muscles NOS

SP 7 **T48.202- Poisoning by unspecified drugs acting on muscles, intentional self-harm**

SP 7 **T48.203- Poisoning by unspecified drugs acting on muscles, assault**

SP 7 **T48.204- Poisoning by unspecified drugs acting on muscles, undetermined**

IQ 7 **T48.205- Adverse effect of unspecified drugs acting on muscles**

7 **T48.206- Underdosing of unspecified drugs acting on muscles**

6 **T48.29 Poisoning by, adverse effect of and underdosing of other drugs acting on muscles**

SP 7 **T48.291- Poisoning by other drugs acting on muscles, accidental (unintentional)**

Poisoning by other drugs acting on muscles NOS

SP 7 **T48.292- Poisoning by other drugs acting on muscles, intentional self-harm**

SP 7 **T48.293- Poisoning by other drugs acting on muscles, assault**

SP 7 **T48.294- Poisoning by other drugs acting on muscles, undetermined**

IQ 7 **T48.295- Adverse effect of other drugs acting on muscles**

7 **T48.296- Underdosing of other drugs acting on muscles**

5 **T48.3 Poisoning by, adverse effect of and underdosing of antitussives**

6 **T48.3X Poisoning by, adverse effect of and underdosing of antitussives**

SP 7 **T48.3X1- Poisoning by antitussives, accidental (unintentional)**

Poisoning by antitussives NOS

SP 7 **T48.3X2- Poisoning by antitussives, intentional self-harm**

SP 7 **T48.3X3- Poisoning by antitussives, assault**

SP 7 **T48.3X4- Poisoning by antitussives, undetermined**

IQ 7 **T48.3X5- Adverse effect of antitussives**

7 **T48.3X6- Underdosing of antitussives**

5 **T48.4 Poisoning by, adverse effect of and underdosing of expectorants**

6 **T48.4X Poisoning by, adverse effect of and underdosing of expectorants**

SP 7 **T48.4X1- Poisoning by expectorants, accidental (unintentional)**

Poisoning by expectorants NOS

SP 7 **T48.4X2- Poisoning by expectorants, intentional self-harm**

SP 7 **T48.4X3- Poisoning by expectorants, assault**

SP 7 **T48.4X4- Poisoning by expectorants, undetermined**

IQ 7 **T48.4X5- Adverse effect of expectorants**

7 **T48.4X6- Underdosing of expectorants**

5 **T48.5 Poisoning by, adverse effect of and underdosing of other anti-common-cold drugs**

Poisoning by, adverse effect of and underdosing of decongestants

EXCLUDES 2 poisoning by, adverse effect of and underdosing of antipyretics, NEC (T39.9-)
poisoning by, adverse effect of and underdosing of non-steroidal antiinflammatory drugs (T39.3-)
poisoning by, adverse effect of and underdosing of salicylates (T39.0-)

6 **T48.5X Poisoning by, adverse effect of and underdosing of other anti-common-cold drugs**

SP 7 **T48.5X1- Poisoning by other anti-common-cold drugs, accidental (unintentional)**

Poisoning by other anti-common-cold drugs NOS

SP 7 **T48.5X2- Poisoning by other anti-common-cold drugs, intentional self-harm**

SP 7 **T48.5X3- Poisoning by other anti-common-cold drugs, assault**

SP 7 **T48.5X4- Poisoning by other anti-common-cold drugs, undetermined**

IQ 7 **T48.5X5- Adverse effect of other anti-common-cold drugs**

7 **T48.5X6- Underdosing of other anti-common-cold drugs**

5 **T48.6 Poisoning by, adverse effect of and underdosing of antiasthmatics, not elsewhere classified**

Poisoning by, adverse effect of and underdosing of beta-adrenoreceptor agonists used in asthma therapy

EXCLUDES 1 poisoning by, adverse effect of and underdosing of beta-adrenoreceptor agonists not used in asthma therapy (T44.5)

Chapter 19

S00-T88

4 4th digit required 5 5th digit required 6 6th digit required 7 7th digit required 7 7th digit placeholder + Additional code Laterality

poisoning by, adverse effect of and underdosing of anterior pituitary [adenohypophyseal] hormones (T38.8)

6 **T48.6X Poisoning by, adverse effect of and underdosing of antiasthmatics**

SP 7 **T48.6X1- Poisoning by antiasthmatics, accidental (unintentional)**
Poisoning by antiasthmatics NOS

SP 7 **T48.6X2- Poisoning by antiasthmatics, intentional self-harm**

SP 7 **T48.6X3- Poisoning by antiasthmatics, assault**

SP 7 **T48.6X4- Poisoning by antiasthmatics, undetermined**

IQ 7 **T48.6X5- Adverse effect of antiasthmatics**

7 **T48.6X6- Underdosing of antiasthmatics**

5 **T48.9 Poisoning by, adverse effect of and underdosing of other and unspecified agents primarily acting on the respiratory system**

6 **T48.90 Poisoning by, adverse effect of and underdosing of unspecified agents primarily acting on the respiratory system**

SP 7 **T48.901- Poisoning by unspecified agents primarily acting on the respiratory system, accidental (unintentional)**

SP 7 **T48.902- Poisoning by unspecified agents primarily acting on the respiratory system, intentional self-harm**

SP 7 **T48.903- Poisoning by unspecified agents primarily acting on the respiratory system, assault**

SP 7 **T48.904- Poisoning by unspecified agents primarily acting on the respiratory system, undetermined**

IQ 7 **T48.905- Adverse effect of unspecified agents primarily acting on the respiratory system**

7 **T48.906- Underdosing of unspecified agents primarily acting on the respiratory system**

6 **T48.99 Poisoning by, adverse effect of and underdosing of other agents primarily acting on the respiratory system**

SP 7 **T48.991- Poisoning by other agents primarily acting on the respiratory system, accidental (unintentional)**

SP 7 **T48.992- Poisoning by other agents primarily acting on the respiratory system, intentional self-harm**

SP 7 **T48.993- Poisoning by other agents primarily acting on the respiratory system, assault**

SP 7 **T48.994- Poisoning by other agents primarily acting on the respiratory system, undetermined**

IQ 7 **T48.995- Adverse effect of other agents primarily acting on the respiratory system**

7 **T48.996- Underdosing of other agents primarily acting on the respiratory system**

4 **T49 Poisoning by, adverse effect of and underdosing of topical agents primarily affecting skin and mucous membrane and by ophthalmological, otorhinorlaryngological and dental drugs**

INCLUDES poisoning by, adverse effect of and underdosing of glucocorticoids, topically used

The appropriate 7th character is to be added to each code from category T49
A initial encounter
D subsequent encounter
S sequela

5 **T49.0 Poisoning by, adverse effect of and underdosing of local antifungal, anti-infective and anti-inflammatory drugs**

6 **T49.0X Poisoning by, adverse effect of and underdosing of local antifungal, anti-infective and anti-inflammatory drugs**

SP 7 **T49.0X1- Poisoning by local antifungal, anti-infective and anti-inflammatory drugs, accidental (unintentional)**
Poisoning by local antifungal, anti-infective and anti-inflammatory drugs NOS

SP 7 **T49.0X2- Poisoning by local antifungal, anti-infective and anti-inflammatory drugs, intentional self-harm**

SP 7 **T49.0X3- Poisoning by local antifungal, anti-infective and anti-inflammatory drugs, assault**

SP 7 **T49.0X4- Poisoning by local antifungal, anti-infective and anti-inflammatory drugs, undetermined**

IQ 7 **T49.0X5- Adverse effect of local antifungal, anti-infective and anti-inflammatory drugs**

7 **T49.0X6- Underdosing of local antifungal, anti-infective and anti-inflammatory drugs**

5 **T49.1 Poisoning by, adverse effect of and underdosing of antipruritics**

6 **T49.1X Poisoning by, adverse effect of and underdosing of antipruritics**

SP 7 **T49.1X1- Poisoning by antipruritics, accidental (unintentional)**
Poisoning by antipruritics NOS

SP 7 **T49.1X2- Poisoning by antipruritics, intentional self-harm**

SP 7 **T49.1X3- Poisoning by antipruritics, assault**

SP 7 **T49.1X4- Poisoning by antipruritics, undetermined**

IQ 7 **T49.1X5- Adverse effect of antipruritics**

7 **T49.1X6- Underdosing of antipruritics**

5 **T49.2 Poisoning by, adverse effect of and underdosing of local astringents and local detergents**

6 **T49.2X Poisoning by, adverse effect of and underdosing of local astringents and local detergents**

SP 7 **T49.2X1- Poisoning by local astringents and local detergents, accidental (unintentional)**
Poisoning by local astringents and local detergents NOS

SP 7 **T49.2X2- Poisoning by local astringents and local detergents, intentional self-harm**

SP 7 **T49.2X3- Poisoning by local astringents and local detergents, assault**

SP 7 **T49.2X4- Poisoning by local astringents and local detergents, undetermined**

!Q 7 **T49.2X5- Adverse effect of local astringents and local detergents**

7 **T49.2X6- Underdosing of local astringents and local detergents**

5 **T49.3 Poisoning by, adverse effect of and underdosing of emollients, demulcents and protectants**

6 **T49.3X Poisoning by, adverse effect of and underdosing of emollients, demulcents and protectants**

SP 7 **T49.3X1- Poisoning by emollients, demulcents and protectants, accidental (unintentional)**
Poisoning by emollients, demulcents and protectants NOS

SP 7 **T49.3X2- Poisoning by emollients, demulcents and protectants, intentional self-harm**

SP 7 **T49.3X3- Poisoning by emollients, demulcents and protectants, assault**

SP 7 **T49.3X4- Poisoning by emollients, demulcents and protectants, undetermined**

!Q 7 **T49.3X5- Adverse effect of emollients, demulcents and protectants**

7 **T49.3X6- Underdosing of emollients, demulcents and protectants**

5 **T49.4 Poisoning by, adverse effect of and underdosing of keratolytics, keratoplastics, and other hair treatment drugs and preparations**

6 **T49.4X Poisoning by, adverse effect of and underdosing of keratolytics, keratoplastics, and other hair treatment drugs and preparations**

SP 7 **T49.4X1- Poisoning by keratolytics, keratoplastics, and other hair treatment drugs and preparations, accidental (unintentional)**
Poisoning by keratolytics, keratoplastics, and other hair treatment drugs and preparations NOS

SP 7 **T49.4X2- Poisoning by keratolytics, keratoplastics, and other hair treatment drugs and preparations, intentional self-harm**

SP 7 **T49.4X3- Poisoning by keratolytics, keratoplastics, and other hair treatment drugs and preparations, assault**

SP 7 **T49.4X4- Poisoning by keratolytics, keratoplastics, and other hair treatment drugs and preparations, undetermined**

!Q 7 **T49.4X5- Adverse effect of keratolytics, keratoplastics, and other hair treatment drugs and preparations**

7 **T49.4X6- Underdosing of keratolytics, keratoplastics, and other hair treatment drugs and preparations**

5 **T49.5 Poisoning by, adverse effect of and underdosing of ophthalmological drugs and preparations**

6 **T49.5X Poisoning by, adverse effect of and underdosing of ophthalmological drugs and preparations**

SP 7 **T49.5X1- Poisoning by ophthalmological drugs and preparations, accidental (unintentional)**
Poisoning by ophthalmological drugs and preparations NOS

SP 7 **T49.5X2- Poisoning by ophthalmological drugs and preparations, intentional self-harm**

SP 7 **T49.5X3- Poisoning by ophthalmological drugs and preparations, assault**

SP 7 **T49.5X4- Poisoning by ophthalmological drugs and preparations, undetermined**

!Q 7 **T49.5X5- Adverse effect of ophthalmological drugs and preparations**

7 **T49.5X6- Underdosing of ophthalmological drugs and preparations**

5 **T49.6 Poisoning by, adverse effect of and underdosing of otorhinolaryngological drugs and preparations**

6 **T49.6X Poisoning by, adverse effect of and underdosing of otorhinolaryngological drugs and preparations**

SP 7 **T49.6X1- Poisoning by otorhinolaryngological drugs and preparations, accidental (unintentional)**
Poisoning by otorhinolaryngological drugs and preparations NOS

SP 7 **T49.6X2- Poisoning by otorhinolaryngological drugs and preparations, intentional self-harm**

SP 7 **T49.6X3- Poisoning by otorhinolaryngological drugs and preparations, assault**

SP 7 **T49.6X4- Poisoning by otorhinolaryngological drugs and preparations, undetermined**

!Q 7 **T49.6X5- Adverse effect of otorhinolaryngological drugs and preparations**

IQ 7 **T49.6X6- Underdosing of otorhinolaryngological drugs and preparations**

5 **T49.7 Poisoning by, adverse effect of and underdosing of dental drugs, topically applied**

6 **T49.7X Poisoning by, adverse effect of and underdosing of dental drugs, topically applied**

SP 7 **T49.7X1- Poisoning by dental drugs, topically applied, accidental (unintentional)**
Poisoning by dental drugs, topically applied NOS

SP 7 **T49.7X2- Poisoning by dental drugs, topically applied, intentional self-harm**

SP 7 **T49.7X3- Poisoning by dental drugs, topically applied, assault**

SP 7 **T49.7X4- Poisoning by dental drugs, topically applied, undetermined**

IQ 7 **T49.7X5- Adverse effect of dental drugs, topically applied**

7 **T49.7X6- Underdosing of dental drugs, topically applied**

5 **T49.8 Poisoning by, adverse effect of and underdosing of other topical agents**
Poisoning by, adverse effect of and underdosing of spermicides

6 **T49.8X Poisoning by, adverse effect of and underdosing of other topical agents**

SP 7 **T49.8X1- Poisoning by other topical agents, accidental (unintentional)**
Poisoning by other topical agents NOS

SP 7 **T49.8X2- Poisoning by other topical agents, intentional self-harm**

SP 7 **T49.8X3- Poisoning by other topical agents, assault**

SP 7 **T49.8X4- Poisoning by other topical agents, undetermined**

IQ 7 **T49.8X5- Adverse effect of other topical agents**

7 **T49.8X6- Underdosing of other topical agents**

5 **T49.9 Poisoning by, adverse effect of and underdosing of unspecified topical agent**

SP 7 **T49.91X- Poisoning by unspecified topical agent, accidental (unintentional)**

SP 7 **T49.92X- Poisoning by unspecified topical agent, intentional self-harm**

SP 7 **T49.93X- Poisoning by unspecified topical agent, assault**

SP 7 **T49.94X- Poisoning by unspecified topical agent, undetermined**

IQ 7 **T49.95X- Adverse effect of unspecified topical agent**

7 **T49.96X- Underdosing of unspecified topical agent**

4 **T50 Poisoning by, adverse effect of and underdosing of diuretics and other and unspecified drugs, medicaments and biological substances**

The appropriate 7th character is to be added to each code from category T50
A initial encounter
D subsequent encounter
S sequela

5 **T50.0 Poisoning by, adverse effect of and underdosing of mineralocorticoids and their antagonists**

6 **T50.0X Poisoning by, adverse effect of and underdosing of mineralocorticoids and their antagonists**

SP 7 **T50.0X1- Poisoning by mineralocorticoids and their antagonists, accidental (unintentional)**
Poisoning by mineralocorticoids and their antagonists NOS

SP 7 **T50.0X2- Poisoning by mineralocorticoids and their antagonists, intentional self-harm**

SP 7 **T50.0X3- Poisoning by mineralocorticoids and their antagonists, assault**

SP 7 **T50.0X4- Poisoning by mineralocorticoids and their antagonists, undetermined**

IQ 7 **T50.0X5- Adverse effect of mineralocorticoids and their antagonists**

7 **T50.0X6- Underdosing of mineralocorticoids and their antagonists**

5 **T50.1 Poisoning by, adverse effect of and underdosing of loop [high-ceiling] diuretics**

6 **T50.1X Poisoning by, adverse effect of and underdosing of loop [high-ceiling] diuretics**

SP 7 **T50.1X1- Poisoning by loop [high-ceiling] diuretics, accidental (unintentional)**
Poisoning by loop [high-ceiling] diuretics NOS

SP 7 **T50.1X2- Poisoning by loop [high-ceiling] diuretics, intentional self-harm**

SP 7 **T50.1X3- Poisoning by loop [high-ceiling] diuretics, assault**

SP 7 **T50.1X4- Poisoning by loop [high-ceiling] diuretics, undetermined**

IQ 7 **T50.1X5- Adverse effect of loop [high-ceiling] diuretics**

7 **T50.1X6- Underdosing of loop [high-ceiling] diuretics**

5 **T50.2 Poisoning by, adverse effect of and underdosing of carbonic-anhydrase inhibitors, benzothiadiazides and other diuretics**
Poisoning by, adverse effect of and underdosing of acetazolamide

6 **T50.2X Poisoning by, adverse effect of and underdosing of carbonic-anhydrase inhibitors, benzothiadiazides and other diuretics**

SP 7 **T50.2X1- Poisoning by carbonic-anhydrase inhibitors, benzothiadiazides and other diuretics, accidental (unintentional)**
Poisoning by carbonic-anhydrase inhibitors, benzothiadiazides and other diuretics NOS

Chapter 19 S00-T88

SP 7 **T50.2X2- Poisoning by carbonic-anhydrase inhibitors, benzothiadiazides and other diuretics, intentional self-harm**

SP 7 **T50.2X3- Poisoning by carbonic-anhydrase inhibitors, benzothiadiazides and other diuretics, assault**

SP 7 **T50.2X4- Poisoning by carbonic-anhydrase inhibitors, benzothiadiazides and other diuretics, undetermined**

IQ 7 **T50.2X5- Adverse effect of carbonic-anhydrase inhibitors, benzothiadiazides and other diuretics**

7 **T50.2X6- Underdosing of carbonic-anhydrase inhibitors, benzothiadiazides and other diuretics**

5 **T50.3 Poisoning by, adverse effect of and underdosing of electrolytic, caloric and water-balance agents**
Poisoning by, adverse effect of and underdosing of oral rehydration salts

6 **T50.3X Poisoning by, adverse effect of and underdosing of electrolytic, caloric and water-balance agents**

SP 7 **T50.3X1- Poisoning by electrolytic, caloric and water-balance agents, accidental (unintentional)**
Poisoning by electrolytic, caloric and water-balance agents NOS

SP 7 **T50.3X2- Poisoning by electrolytic, caloric and water-balance agents, intentional self-harm**

SP 7 **T50.3X3- Poisoning by electrolytic, caloric and water-balance agents, assault**

SP 7 **T50.3X4- Poisoning by electrolytic, caloric and water-balance agents, undetermined**

!Q 7 **T50.3X5- Adverse effect of electrolytic, caloric and water-balance agents**

7 **T50.3X6- Underdosing of electrolytic, caloric and water-balance agents**

5 **T50.4 Poisoning by, adverse effect of and underdosing of drugs affecting uric acid metabolism**

6 **T50.4X Poisoning by, adverse effect of and underdosing of drugs affecting uric acid metabolism**

SP 7 **T50.4X1- Poisoning by drugs affecting uric acid metabolism, accidental (unintentional)**
Poisoning by drugs affecting uric acid metabolism NOS

SP 7 **T50.4X2- Poisoning by drugs affecting uric acid metabolism, intentional self-harm**

SP 7 **T50.4X3- Poisoning by drugs affecting uric acid metabolism, assault**

SP 7 **T50.4X4- Poisoning by drugs affecting uric acid metabolism, undetermined**

IQ 7 **T50.4X5- Adverse effect of drugs affecting uric acid metabolism**

7 **T50.4X6- Underdosing of drugs affecting uric acid metabolism**

5 **T50.5 Poisoning by, adverse effect of and underdosing of appetite depressants**

6 **T50.5X Poisoning by, adverse effect of and underdosing of appetite depressants**

SP 7 **T50.5X1- Poisoning by appetite depressants, accidental (unintentional)**
Poisoning by appetite depressants NOS

SP 7 **T50.5X2- Poisoning by appetite depressants, intentional self-harm**

SP 7 **T50.5X3- Poisoning by appetite depressants, assault**

SP 7 **T50.5X4- Poisoning by appetite depressants, undetermined**

IQ 7 **T50.5X5- Adverse effect of appetite depressants**

7 **T50.5X6- Underdosing of appetite depressants**

5 **T50.6 Poisoning by, adverse effect of and underdosing of antidotes and chelating agents**
Poisoning by, adverse effect of and underdosing of alcohol deterrents

6 **T50.6X Poisoning by, adverse effect of and underdosing of antidotes and chelating agents**

SP 7 **T50.6X1- Poisoning by antidotes and chelating agents, accidental (unintentional)**
Poisoning by antidotes and chelating agents NOS

SP 7 **T50.6X2- Poisoning by antidotes and chelating agents, intentional self-harm**

SP 7 **T50.6X3- Poisoning by antidotes and chelating agents, assault**

SP 7 **T50.6X4- Poisoning by antidotes and chelating agents, undetermined**

IQ 7 **T50.6X5- Adverse effect of antidotes and chelating agents**

7 **T50.6X6- Underdosing of antidotes and chelating agents**

5 **T50.7 Poisoning by, adverse effect of and underdosing of analeptics and opioid receptor antagonists**

6 **T50.7X Poisoning by, adverse effect of and underdosing of analeptics and opioid receptor antagonists**

SP 7 **T50.7X1- Poisoning by analeptics and opioid receptor antagonists, accidental (unintentional)**
Poisoning by analeptics and opioid receptor antagonists NOS

SP 7 **T50.7X2- Poisoning by analeptics and opioid receptor antagonists, intentional self-harm**

SP 7 **T50.7X3- Poisoning by analeptics and opioid receptor antagonists, assault**

SP 7 **T50.7X4- Poisoning by analeptics and opioid receptor antagonists, undetermined**

IQ 7 **T50.7X5- Adverse effect of analeptics and opioid receptor antagonists**

7 **T50.7X6- Underdosing of analeptics and opioid receptor antagonists**

5 **T50.8 Poisoning by, adverse effect of and underdosing of diagnostic agents**

6 T50.8X Poisoning by, adverse effect of and underdosing of diagnostic agents

SP 7 T50.8X1- Poisoning by diagnostic agents, accidental (unintentional)
Poisoning by diagnostic agents NOS

SP 7 T50.8X2- Poisoning by diagnostic agents, intentional self-harm

SP 7 T50.8X3- Poisoning by diagnostic agents, assault

SP 7 T50.8X4- Poisoning by diagnostic agents, undetermined

!Q 7 T50.8X5- Adverse effect of diagnostic agents

7 T50.8X6- Underdosing of diagnostic agents

5 T50.A Poisoning by, adverse effect of and underdosing of bacterial vaccines

6 T50.A1 Poisoning by, adverse effect of and underdosing of pertussis vaccine, including combinations with a pertussis component

SP 7 T50.A11- Poisoning by pertussis vaccine, including combinations with a pertussis component, accidental (unintentional)

SP 7 T50.A12- Poisoning by pertussis vaccine, including combinations with a pertussis component, intentional self-harm

SP 7 T50.A13- Poisoning by pertussis vaccine, including combinations with a pertussis component, assault

SP 7 T50.A14- Poisoning by pertussis vaccine, including combinations with a pertussis component, undetermined

!Q 7 T50.A15- Adverse effect of pertussis vaccine, including combinations with a pertussis component

7 T50.A16- Underdosing of pertussis vaccine, including combinations with a pertussis component

6 T50.A2 Poisoning by, adverse effect of and underdosing of mixed bacterial vaccines without a pertussis component

SP 7 T50.A21- Poisoning by mixed bacterial vaccines without a pertussis component, accidental (unintentional)

SP 7 T50.A22- Poisoning by mixed bacterial vaccines without a pertussis component, intentional self-harm

SP 7 T50.A23- Poisoning by mixed bacterial vaccines without a pertussis component, assault

SP 7 T50.A24- Poisoning by mixed bacterial vaccines without a pertussis component, undetermined

!Q 7 T50.A25- Adverse effect of mixed bacterial vaccines without a pertussis component

7 T50.A26- Underdosing of mixed bacterial vaccines without a pertussis component

6 T50.A9 Poisoning by, adverse effect of and underdosing of other bacterial vaccines

SP 7 T50.A91- Poisoning by other bacterial vaccines, accidental (unintentional)

SP 7 T50.A92- Poisoning by other bacterial vaccines, intentional self-harm

SP 7 T50.A93- Poisoning by other bacterial vaccines, assault

SP 7 T50.A94- Poisoning by other bacterial vaccines, undetermined

!Q 7 T50.A95- Adverse effect of other bacterial vaccines

7 T50.A96- Underdosing of other bacterial vaccines

5 T50.B Poisoning by, adverse effect of and underdosing of viral vaccines

6 T50.B1 Poisoning by, adverse effect of and underdosing of smallpox vaccines

SP 7 T50.B11- Poisoning by smallpox vaccines, accidental (unintentional)

SP 7 T50.B12- Poisoning by smallpox vaccines, intentional self-harm

SP 7 T50.B13- Poisoning by smallpox vaccines, assault

SP 7 T50.B14- Poisoning by smallpox vaccines, undetermined

!Q 7 T50.B15- Adverse effect of smallpox vaccines

7 T50.B16- Underdosing of smallpox vaccines

6 T50.B9 Poisoning by, adverse effect of and underdosing of other viral vaccines

SP 7 T50.B91- Poisoning by other viral vaccines, accidental (unintentional)

SP 7 T50.B92- Poisoning by other viral vaccines, intentional self-harm

SP 7 T50.B93- Poisoning by other viral vaccines, assault

SP 7 T50.B94- Poisoning by other viral vaccines, undetermined

!Q 7 T50.B95- Adverse effect of other viral vaccines

7 T50.B96- Underdosing of other viral vaccines

5 T50.Z Poisoning by, adverse effect of and underdosing of other vaccines and biological substances

6 T50.Z1 Poisoning by, adverse effect of and underdosing of immunoglobulin

SP 7 T50.Z11- Poisoning by immunoglobulin, accidental (unintentional)

SP 7 T50.Z12- Poisoning by immunoglobulin, intentional self-harm

SP 7 T50.Z13- Poisoning by immunoglobulin, assault

SP 7 T50.Z14- Poisoning by immunoglobulin, undetermined

!Q 7 T50.Z15- Adverse effect of immunoglobulin

7 T50.Z16- Underdosing of immunoglobulin

6 T50.Z9 Poisoning by, adverse effect of and underdosing of other vaccines and biological substances

SP 7 T50.Z91- Poisoning by other vaccines and biological substances, accidental (unintentional)

SP 7 **T50.Z92- Poisoning by other vaccines and biological substances, intentional self-harm**

SP 7 **T50.Z93- Poisoning by other vaccines and biological substances, assault**

SP 7 **T50.Z94- Poisoning by other vaccines and biological substances, undetermined**

IQ 7 **T50.Z95- Adverse effect of other vaccines and biological substances**

7 **T50.Z96- Underdosing of other vaccines and biological substances**

5 **T50.9 Poisoning by, adverse effect of and underdosing of other and unspecified drugs, medicaments and biological substances**

6 **T50.90 Poisoning by, adverse effect of and underdosing of unspecified drugs, medicaments and biological substances**

SP 7 **T50.901- Poisoning by unspecified drugs, medicaments and biological substances, accidental (unintentional)**

SP 7 **T50.902- Poisoning by unspecified drugs, medicaments and biological substances, intentional self-harm**

SP 7 **T50.903- Poisoning by unspecified drugs, medicaments and biological substances, assault**

SP 7 **T50.904- Poisoning by unspecified drugs, medicaments and biological substances, undetermined**

IQ 7 **T50.905- Adverse effect of unspecified drugs, medicaments and biological substances**

SP 7 **T50.906- Underdosing of unspecified drugs, medicaments and biological substances**

6 **T50.91 Poisoning by, adverse effect of and underdosing of multiple unspecified drugs, medicaments and biological substances**

Multiple drug ingestion NOS

Code also:

any specific drugs, medicaments and biological substances

SP 7 **T50.911- Poisoning by multiple unspecified drugs, medicaments and biological substances, accidental (unintentional)**

SP 7 **T50.912- Poisoning by multiple unspecified drugs, medicaments and biological substances, intentional self-harm**

SP 7 **T50.913- Poisoning by multiple unspecified drugs, medicaments and biological substances, assault**

SP 7 **T50.914- Poisoning by multiple unspecified drugs, medicaments and biological substances, undetermined**

7 **T50.915- Adverse effect of multiple unspecified drugs, medicaments and biological substances**

7 **T50.916- Underdosing of multiple unspecified drugs, medicaments and biological substances**

6 **T50.99 Poisoning by, adverse effect of and underdosing of other drugs, medicaments and biological substances**

SP 7 **T50.991- Poisoning by other drugs, medicaments and biological substances, accidental (unintentional)**

SP 7 **T50.992- Poisoning by other drugs, medicaments and biological substances, intentional self-harm**

SP 7 **T50.993- Poisoning by other drugs, medicaments and biological substances, assault**

SP 7 **T50.994- Poisoning by other drugs, medicaments and biological substances, undetermined**

IQ 7 **T50.995- Adverse effect of other drugs, medicaments and biological substances**

SP 7 **T50.996- Underdosing of other drugs, medicaments and biological substances**

Toxic effects of substances chiefly nonmedicinal as to source (T51-T65)

Note:

When no intent is indicated code to accidental. Undetermined intent is only for use when there is specific documentation in the record that the intent of the toxic effect cannot be determined.

Use additional code(s):

for all associated manifestations of toxic effect, such as:

respiratory conditions due to external agents (J60-J70)

personal history of foreign body fully removed (Z87.821)

to identify any retained foreign body, if applicable (Z18.-)

EXCLUDES 1 contact with and (suspected) exposure to toxic substances (Z77.-)

GUIDELINES **Section I.C.19.e.1)-4)**

Codes in categories T36-T65 are combination codes that include the substance that was taken as well as the intent. No additional external cause code is required for poisonings, toxic effects, adverse effects and underdosing codes.

Do not code directly from the Table of Drugs and Chemicals. Always refer back to the Tabular List. Use as many codes as necessary to describe completely all drugs, medicinal or biological substances. If the same code would describe the causative agent for more than one adverse reaction, poisoning, toxic effect or underdosing, assign the code only once. If two or more drugs, medicinal or biological substances are reported, code each individually unless a combination code is listed in the Table of Drugs and Chemicals.

GUIDELINES **Section I.C.19.e.5)(d)**

When a harmful substance is ingested or comes in contact with a person, this is classified as a toxic effect. The toxic effect codes are in categories T51-T65. Toxic effect codes have an associated intent: accidental, intentional self-harm, assault and undetermined.

CODING TIPS✓ When coding toxic effects, first assign the code from T51-T65 to identify the substance and intent, followed by an additional code to identify the manifestations of the toxic substance that resulted in the effect(s). If the intent is not documented, accidental intent should be coded. Undetermined intent should only be coded when documentation specifically indicates that the intent cannot be determined.

CODING TIPS✓ Note there are only codes for poisonings or toxic effects. There are no therapeutic uses for the following substances, therefore there are no codes for adverse effects or underdosing.

4 **T51 Toxic effect of alcohol**

The appropriate 7th character is to be added to each code from category T51
A initial encounter
D subsequent encounter
S sequela

5 **T51.0 Toxic effect of ethanol**
Toxic effect of ethyl alcohol
EXCLUDES 2 acute alcohol intoxication or 'hangover' effects (F10.129, F10.229, F10.929)
drunkenness (F10.129, F10.229, F10.929)
pathological alcohol intoxication (F10.129, F10.229, F10.929)

6 **T51.0X Toxic effect of ethanol**

SP 7 **T51.0X1- Toxic effect of ethanol, accidental (unintentional)**
Toxic effect of ethanol NOS

SP 7 **T51.0X2- Toxic effect of ethanol, intentional self-harm**

SP 7 **T51.0X3- Toxic effect of ethanol, assault**

SP 7 **T51.0X4- Toxic effect of ethanol, undetermined**

5 **T51.1 Toxic effect of methanol**
Toxic effect of methyl alcohol

6 **T51.1X Toxic effect of methanol**

SP 7 **T51.1X1- Toxic effect of methanol, accidental (unintentional)**
Toxic effect of methanol NOS

SP 7 **T51.1X2- Toxic effect of methanol, intentional self-harm**

SP 7 **T51.1X3- Toxic effect of methanol, assault**

SP 7 **T51.1X4- Toxic effect of methanol, undetermined**

5 **T51.2 Toxic effect of 2-Propanol**
Toxic effect of isopropyl alcohol

6 **T51.2X Toxic effect of 2-Propanol**

SP 7 **T51.2X1- Toxic effect of 2-Propanol, accidental (unintentional)**
Toxic effect of 2-Propanol NOS

SP 7 **T51.2X2- Toxic effect of 2-Propanol, intentional self-harm**

SP 7 **T51.2X3- Toxic effect of 2-Propanol, assault**

SP 7 **T51.2X4- Toxic effect of 2-Propanol, undetermined**

5 **T51.3 Toxic effect of fusel oil**
Toxic effect of amyl alcohol
Toxic effect of butyl [1-butanol] alcohol
Toxic effect of propyl [1-propanol] alcohol

6 **T51.3X Toxic effect of fusel oil**

SP 7 **T51.3X1- Toxic effect of fusel oil, accidental (unintentional)**
Toxic effect of fusel oil NOS

SP 7 **T51.3X2- Toxic effect of fusel oil, intentional self-harm**

SP 7 **T51.3X3- Toxic effect of fusel oil, assault**

SP 7 **T51.3X4- Toxic effect of fusel oil, undetermined**

5 **T51.8 Toxic effect of other alcohols**

6 **T51.8X Toxic effect of other alcohols**

SP 7 **T51.8X1- Toxic effect of other alcohols, accidental (unintentional)**
Toxic effect of other alcohols NOS

SP 7 **T51.8X2- Toxic effect of other alcohols, intentional self-harm**

SP 7 **T51.8X3- Toxic effect of other alcohols, assault**

SP 7 **T51.8X4- Toxic effect of other alcohols, undetermined**

5 **T51.9 Toxic effect of unspecified alcohol**

SP X **T51.91X- Toxic effect of unspecified alcohol, accidental (unintentional)**

SP X **T51.92X- Toxic effect of unspecified alcohol, intentional self-harm**

SP X **T51.93X- Toxic effect of unspecified alcohol, assault**

SP X **T51.94X- Toxic effect of unspecified alcohol, undetermined**

4 **T52 Toxic effect of organic solvents**
EXCLUDES 1 halogen derivatives of aliphatic and aromatic hydrocarbons (T53.-)

The appropriate 7th character is to be added to each code from category T52
A initial encounter
D subsequent encounter
S sequela

5 **T52.0 Toxic effects of petroleum products**
Toxic effects of gasoline [petrol]
Toxic effects of kerosene [paraffin oil]
Toxic effects of paraffin wax
Toxic effects of ether petroleum
Toxic effects of naphtha petroleum
Toxic effects of spirit petroleum

6 **T52.0X Toxic effects of petroleum products**

SP 7 **T52.0X1- Toxic effect of petroleum products, accidental (unintentional)**
Toxic effects of petroleum products NOS

SP 7 **T52.0X2- Toxic effect of petroleum products, intentional self-harm**

SP 7 **T52.0X3- Toxic effect of petroleum products, assault**

SP 7 **T52.0X4- Toxic effect of petroleum products, undetermined**

5 **T52.1 Toxic effects of benzene**
EXCLUDES 1 homologues of benzene (T52.2)
nitroderivatives and aminoderivatives of benzene and its homologues (T65.3)

6 **T52.1X Toxic effects of benzene**

Chapter 19 S00-T88

SP 7 **T52.1X1- Toxic effect of benzene, accidental (unintentional)**
Toxic effects of benzene NOS

SP 7 **T52.1X2- Toxic effect of benzene, intentional self-harm**

SP 7 **T52.1X3- Toxic effect of benzene, assault**

SP 7 **T52.1X4- Toxic effect of benzene, undetermined**

5 **T52.2 Toxic effects of homologues of benzene**
Toxic effects of toluene [methylbenzene]
Toxic effects of xylene [dimethylbenzene]

6 **T52.2X Toxic effects of homologues of benzene**

SP 7 **T52.2X1- Toxic effect of homologues of benzene, accidental (unintentional)**
Toxic effects of homologues of benzene NOS

SP 7 **T52.2X2- Toxic effect of homologues of benzene, intentional self-harm**

SP 7 **T52.2X3- Toxic effect of homologues of benzene, assault**

SP 7 **T52.2X4- Toxic effect of homologues of benzene, undetermined**

5 **T52.3 Toxic effects of glycols**

6 **T52.3X Toxic effects of glycols**

SP 7 **T52.3X1- Toxic effect of glycols, accidental (unintentional)**
Toxic effects of glycols NOS

SP 7 **T52.3X2- Toxic effect of glycols, intentional self-harm**

SP 7 **T52.3X3- Toxic effect of glycols, assault**

SP 7 **T52.3X4- Toxic effect of glycols, undetermined**

5 **T52.4 Toxic effects of ketones**

6 **T52.4X Toxic effects of ketones**

SP 7 **T52.4X1- Toxic effect of ketones, accidental (unintentional)**
Toxic effects of ketones NOS

SP 7 **T52.4X2- Toxic effect of ketones, intentional self-harm**

SP 7 **T52.4X3- Toxic effect of ketones, assault**

SP 7 **T52.4X4- Toxic effect of ketones, undetermined**

5 **T52.8 Toxic effects of other organic solvents**

6 **T52.8X Toxic effects of other organic solvents**

SP 7 **T52.8X1- Toxic effect of other organic solvents, accidental (unintentional)**
Toxic effects of other organic solvents NOS

SP 7 **T52.8X2- Toxic effect of other organic solvents, intentional self-harm**

SP 7 **T52.8X3- Toxic effect of other organic solvents, assault**

SP 7 **T52.8X4- Toxic effect of other organic solvents, undetermined**

5 **T52.9 Toxic effects of unspecified organic solvent**

SP 7 **T52.91X- Toxic effect of unspecified organic solvent, accidental (unintentional)**

SP 7 **T52.92X- Toxic effect of unspecified organic solvent, intentional self-harm**

SP 7 **T52.93X- Toxic effect of unspecified organic solvent, assault**

SP 7 **T52.94X- Toxic effect of unspecified organic solvent, undetermined**

4 **T53 Toxic effect of halogen derivatives of aliphatic and aromatic hydrocarbons**

The appropriate 7th character is to be added to each code from category T53
A initial encounter
D subsequent encounter
S sequela

5 **T53.0 Toxic effects of carbon tetrachloride**
Toxic effects of tetrachloromethane

6 **T53.0X Toxic effects of carbon tetrachloride**

SP 7 **T53.0X1- Toxic effect of carbon tetrachloride, accidental (unintentional)**
Toxic effects of carbon tetrachloride NOS

SP 7 **T53.0X2- Toxic effect of carbon tetrachloride, intentional self-harm**

SP 7 **T53.0X3- Toxic effect of carbon tetrachloride, assault**

SP 7 **T53.0X4- Toxic effect of carbon tetrachloride, undetermined**

5 **T53.1 Toxic effects of chloroform**
Toxic effects of trichloromethane

6 **T53.1X Toxic effects of chloroform**

SP 7 **T53.1X1- Toxic effect of chloroform, accidental (unintentional)**
Toxic effects of chloroform NOS

SP 7 **T53.1X2- Toxic effect of chloroform, intentional self-harm**

SP 7 **T53.1X3- Toxic effect of chloroform, assault**

SP 7 **T53.1X4- Toxic effect of chloroform, undetermined**

5 **T53.2 Toxic effects of trichloroethylene**
Toxic effects of trichloroethene

6 **T53.2X Toxic effects of trichloroethylene**

SP 7 **T53.2X1- Toxic effect of trichloroethylene, accidental (unintentional)**
Toxic effects of trichloroethylene NOS

SP 7 **T53.2X2- Toxic effect of trichloroethylene, intentional self-harm**

SP 7 **T53.2X3- Toxic effect of trichloroethylene, assault**

SP 7 **T53.2X4- Toxic effect of trichloroethylene, undetermined**

5 **T53.3 Toxic effects of tetrachloroethylene**
Toxic effects of perchloroethylene
Toxic effect of tetrachloroethene

6 **T53.3X Toxic effects of tetrachloroethylene**

SP 7 **T53.3X1- Toxic effect of tetrachloroethylene, accidental (unintentional)**
Toxic effects of tetrachloroethylene NOS

SP 7 **T53.3X2- Toxic effect of tetrachloroethylene, intentional self-harm**

SP 7 **T53.3X3- Toxic effect of tetrachloroethylene, assault**

SP 7 **T53.3X4- Toxic effect of tetrachloroethylene, undetermined**

Chapter 19

S00-T88

4 4th digit required 5 5th digit required 6 6th digit required 7 7th digit required 7 7th digit placeholder + Additional code Laterality

5 **T53.4 Toxic effects of dichloromethane**
Toxic effects of methylene chloride
6 **T53.4X Toxic effects of dichloromethane**
SP 7 **T53.4X1- Toxic effect of dichloromethane, accidental (unintentional)**
Toxic effects of dichloromethane NOS
SP 7 **T53.4X2- Toxic effect of dichloromethane, intentional self-harm**
SP 7 **T53.4X3- Toxic effect of dichloromethane, assault**
SP 7 **T53.4X4- Toxic effect of dichloromethane, undetermined**
5 **T53.5 Toxic effects of chlorofluorocarbons**
6 **T53.5X Toxic effects of chlorofluorocarbons**
SP 7 **T53.5X1- Toxic effect of chlorofluorocarbons, accidental (unintentional)**
Toxic effects of chlorofluorocarbons NOS
SP 7 **T53.5X2- Toxic effect of chlorofluorocarbons, intentional self-harm**
SP 7 **T53.5X3- Toxic effect of chlorofluorocarbons, assault**
SP 7 **T53.5X4- Toxic effect of chlorofluorocarbons, undetermined**
5 **T53.6 Toxic effects of other halogen derivatives of aliphatic hydrocarbons**
6 **T53.6X Toxic effects of other halogen derivatives of aliphatic hydrocarbons**
SP 7 **T53.6X1- Toxic effect of other halogen derivatives of aliphatic hydrocarbons, accidental (unintentional)**
Toxic effects of other halogen derivatives of aliphatic hydrocarbons NOS
SP 7 **T53.6X2- Toxic effect of other halogen derivatives of aliphatic hydrocarbons, intentional self-harm**
SP 7 **T53.6X3- Toxic effect of other halogen derivatives of aliphatic hydrocarbons, assault**
SP 7 **T53.6X4- Toxic effect of other halogen derivatives of aliphatic hydrocarbons, undetermined**
5 **T53.7 Toxic effects of other halogen derivatives of aromatic hydrocarbons**
6 **T53.7X Toxic effects of other halogen derivatives of aromatic hydrocarbons**
SP 7 **T53.7X1- Toxic effect of other halogen derivatives of aromatic hydrocarbons, accidental (unintentional)**
Toxic effects of other halogen derivatives of aromatic hydrocarbons NOS
SP 7 **T53.7X2- Toxic effect of other halogen derivatives of aromatic hydrocarbons, intentional self-harm**
SP 7 **T53.7X3- Toxic effect of other halogen derivatives of aromatic hydrocarbons, assault**
SP 7 **T53.7X4- Toxic effect of other halogen derivatives of aromatic hydrocarbons, undetermined**
5 **T53.9 Toxic effects of unspecified halogen derivatives of aliphatic and aromatic hydrocarbons**
SP 7 **T53.91X- Toxic effect of unspecified halogen derivatives of aliphatic and aromatic hydrocarbons, accidental (unintentional)**
SP 7 **T53.92X- Toxic effect of unspecified halogen derivatives of aliphatic and aromatic hydrocarbons, intentional self-harm**
SP 7 **T53.93X- Toxic effect of unspecified halogen derivatives of aliphatic and aromatic hydrocarbons, assault**
SP 7 **T53.94X- Toxic effect of unspecified halogen derivatives of aliphatic and aromatic hydrocarbons, undetermined**
4 **T54 Toxic effect of corrosive substances**

The appropriate 7th character is to be added to each code from category T54
A initial encounter
D subsequent encounter
S sequela

5 **T54.0 Toxic effects of phenol and phenol homologues**
6 **T54.0X Toxic effects of phenol and phenol homologues**
SP 7 **T54.0X1- Toxic effect of phenol and phenol homologues, accidental (unintentional)**
Toxic effects of phenol and phenol homologues NOS
SP 7 **T54.0X2- Toxic effect of phenol and phenol homologues, intentional self-harm**
SP 7 **T54.0X3- Toxic effect of phenol and phenol homologues, assault**
SP 7 **T54.0X4- Toxic effect of phenol and phenol homologues, undetermined**
5 **T54.1 Toxic effects of other corrosive organic compounds**
6 **T54.1X Toxic effects of other corrosive organic compounds**
SP 7 **T54.1X1- Toxic effect of other corrosive organic compounds, accidental (unintentional)**
Toxic effects of other corrosive organic compounds NOS
SP 7 **T54.1X2- Toxic effect of other corrosive organic compounds, intentional self-harm**
SP 7 **T54.1X3- Toxic effect of other corrosive organic compounds, assault**
SP 7 **T54.1X4- Toxic effect of other corrosive organic compounds, undetermined**
5 **T54.2 Toxic effects of corrosive acids and acid-like substances**
Toxic effects of hydrochloric acid
Toxic effects of sulfuric acid
6 **T54.2X Toxic effects of corrosive acids and acid-like substances**

SP 7 **T54.2X1- Toxic effect of corrosive acids and acid-like substances, accidental (unintentional)**
Toxic effects of corrosive acids and acid-like substances NOS

SP 7 **T54.2X2- Toxic effect of corrosive acids and acid-like substances, intentional self-harm**

SP 7 **T54.2X3- Toxic effect of corrosive acids and acid-like substances, assault**

SP 7 **T54.2X4- Toxic effect of corrosive acids and acid-like substances, undetermined**

5 **T54.3 Toxic effects of corrosive alkalis and alkali-like substances**
Toxic effects of potassium hydroxide
Toxic effects of sodium hydroxide

6 **T54.3X Toxic effects of corrosive alkalis and alkali-like substances**

SP 7 **T54.3X1- Toxic effect of corrosive alkalis and alkali-like substances, accidental (unintentional)**
Toxic effects of corrosive alkalis and alkali-like substances NOS

SP 7 **T54.3X2- Toxic effect of corrosive alkalis and alkali-like substances, intentional self-harm**

SP 7 **T54.3X3- Toxic effect of corrosive alkalis and alkali-like substances, assault**

SP 7 **T54.3X4- Toxic effect of corrosive alkalis and alkali-like substances, undetermined**

5 **T54.9 Toxic effects of unspecified corrosive substance**

SP X **T54.91X- Toxic effect of unspecified corrosive substance, accidental (unintentional)**

SP X **T54.92X- Toxic effect of unspecified corrosive substance, intentional self-harm**

SP X **T54.93X- Toxic effect of unspecified corrosive substance, assault**

SP X **T54.94X- Toxic effect of unspecified corrosive substance, undetermined**

4 **T55 Toxic effect of soaps and detergents**

The appropriate 7th character is to be added to each code from category T55
A initial encounter
D subsequent encounter
S sequela

5 **T55.0 Toxic effect of soaps**

6 **T55.0X Toxic effect of soaps**

SP 7 **T55.0X1- Toxic effect of soaps, accidental (unintentional)**
Toxic effect of soaps NOS

SP 7 **T55.0X2- Toxic effect of soaps, intentional self-harm**

SP 7 **T55.0X3- Toxic effect of soaps, assault**

SP 7 **T55.0X4- Toxic effect of soaps, undetermined**

5 **T55.1 Toxic effect of detergents**

6 **T55.1X Toxic effect of detergents**

SP 7 **T55.1X1- Toxic effect of detergents, accidental (unintentional)**
Toxic effect of detergents NOS

SP 7 **T55.1X2- Toxic effect of detergents, intentional self-harm**

SP 7 **T55.1X3- Toxic effect of detergents, assault**

SP 7 **T55.1X4- Toxic effect of detergents, undetermined**

+ 4 **T56 Toxic effect of metals**

INCLUDES toxic effects of fumes and vapors of metals
toxic effects of metals from all sources, except medicinal substances

Use additional code to identify any retained metal foreign body, if applicable (Z18.0-, T18.1-)

EXCLUDES 1 arsenic and its compounds (T57.0)
manganese and its compounds (T57.2)

The appropriate 7th character is to be added to each code from category T56
A initial encounter
D subsequent encounter
S sequela

+ 5 **T56.0 Toxic effects of lead and its compounds**

+ 6 **T56.0X Toxic effects of lead and its compounds**

SP + 7 **T56.0X1- Toxic effect of lead and its compounds, accidental (unintentional)**
Toxic effects of lead and its compounds NOS

SP + 7 **T56.0X2- Toxic effect of lead and its compounds, intentional self-harm**

SP + 7 **T56.0X3- Toxic effect of lead and its compounds, assault**

SP + 7 **T56.0X4- Toxic effect of lead and its compounds, undetermined**

+ 5 **T56.1 Toxic effects of mercury and its compounds**

+ 6 **T56.1X Toxic effects of mercury and its compounds**

SP + 7 **T56.1X1- Toxic effect of mercury and its compounds, accidental (unintentional)**
Toxic effects of mercury and its compounds NOS

SP + 7 **T56.1X2- Toxic effect of mercury and its compounds, intentional self-harm**

SP + 7 **T56.1X3- Toxic effect of mercury and its compounds, assault**

SP + 7 **T56.1X4- Toxic effect of mercury and its compounds, undetermined**

+ 5 **T56.2 Toxic effects of chromium and its compounds**

+ 6 **T56.2X Toxic effects of chromium and its compounds**

SP + 7 **T56.2X1- Toxic effect of chromium and its compounds, accidental (unintentional)**
Toxic effects of chromium and its compounds NOS

SP + 7 **T56.2X2- Toxic effect of chromium and its compounds, intentional self-harm**

SP + 7 **T56.2X3- Toxic effect of chromium and its compounds, assault**

SP + 7 **T56.2X4- Toxic effect of chromium and its compounds, undetermined**

\+ 5 **T56.3 Toxic effects of cadmium and its compounds**

\+ 6 **T56.3X Toxic effects of cadmium and its compounds**

SP + 7 **T56.3X1- Toxic effect of cadmium and its compounds, accidental (unintentional)**
Toxic effects of cadmium and its compounds NOS

SP + 7 **T56.3X2- Toxic effect of cadmium and its compounds, intentional self-harm**

SP + 7 **T56.3X3- Toxic effect of cadmium and its compounds, assault**

SP + 7 **T56.3X4- Toxic effect of cadmium and its compounds, undetermined**

\+ 5 **T56.4 Toxic effects of copper and its compounds**

\+ 6 **T56.4X Toxic effects of copper and its compounds**

SP + 7 **T56.4X1- Toxic effect of copper and its compounds, accidental (unintentional)**
Toxic effects of copper and its compounds NOS

SP + 7 **T56.4X2- Toxic effect of copper and its compounds, intentional self-harm**

SP + 7 **T56.4X3- Toxic effect of copper and its compounds, assault**

SP + 7 **T56.4X4- Toxic effect of copper and its compounds, undetermined**

\+ 5 **T56.5 Toxic effects of zinc and its compounds**

\+ 6 **T56.5X Toxic effects of zinc and its compounds**

SP + 7 **T56.5X1- Toxic effect of zinc and its compounds, accidental (unintentional)**
Toxic effects of zinc and its compounds NOS

SP + 7 **T56.5X2- Toxic effect of zinc and its compounds, intentional self-harm**

SP + 7 **T56.5X3- Toxic effect of zinc and its compounds, assault**

SP + 7 **T56.5X4- Toxic effect of zinc and its compounds, undetermined**

\+ 5 **T56.6 Toxic effects of tin and its compounds**

\+ 6 **T56.6X Toxic effects of tin and its compounds**

SP + 7 **T56.6X1- Toxic effect of tin and its compounds, accidental (unintentional)**
Toxic effects of tin and its compounds NOS

SP + 7 **T56.6X2- Toxic effect of tin and its compounds, intentional self-harm**

SP + 7 **T56.6X3- Toxic effect of tin and its compounds, assault**

SP + 7 **T56.6X4- Toxic effect of tin and its compounds, undetermined**

\+ 5 **T56.7 Toxic effects of beryllium and its compounds**

\+ 6 **T56.7X Toxic effects of beryllium and its compounds**

SP + 7 **T56.7X1- Toxic effect of beryllium and its compounds, accidental (unintentional)**
Toxic effects of beryllium and its compounds NOS

SP + 7 **T56.7X2- Toxic effect of beryllium and its compounds, intentional self-harm**

SP + 7 **T56.7X3- Toxic effect of beryllium and its compounds, assault**

SP + 7 **T56.7X4- Toxic effect of beryllium and its compounds, undetermined**

\+ 5 **T56.8 Toxic effects of other metals**

\+ 6 **T56.81 Toxic effect of thallium**

SP + 7 **T56.811- Toxic effect of thallium, accidental (unintentional)**
Toxic effect of thallium NOS

SP + 7 **T56.812- Toxic effect of thallium, intentional self-harm**

SP + 7 **T56.813- Toxic effect of thallium, assault**

SP + 7 **T56.814- Toxic effect of thallium, undetermined**

\+ 6 **T56.89 Toxic effects of other metals**

SP + 7 **T56.891- Toxic effect of other metals, accidental (unintentional)**
Toxic effects of other metals NOS

SP + 7 **T56.892- Toxic effect of other metals, intentional self-harm**

SP + 7 **T56.893- Toxic effect of other metals, assault**

SP + 7 **T56.894- Toxic effect of other metals, undetermined**

\+ 5 **T56.9 Toxic effects of unspecified metal**

SP + 7 **T56.91X- Toxic effect of unspecified metal, accidental (unintentional)**

SP + 7 **T56.92X- Toxic effect of unspecified metal, intentional self-harm**

SP + 7 **T56.93X- Toxic effect of unspecified metal, assault**

SP + 7 **T56.94X- Toxic effect of unspecified metal, undetermined**

4 **T57 Toxic effect of other inorganic substances**

The appropriate 7th character is to be added to each code from category T57
A initial encounter
D subsequent encounter
S sequela

5 **T57.0 Toxic effect of arsenic and its compounds**

6 **T57.0X Toxic effect of arsenic and its compounds**

SP 7 **T57.0X1- Toxic effect of arsenic and its compounds, accidental (unintentional)**
Toxic effect of arsenic and its compounds NOS

SP 7 **T57.0X2- Toxic effect of arsenic and its compounds, intentional self-harm**

SP 7 **T57.0X3- Toxic effect of arsenic and its compounds, assault**

SP 7 **T57.0X4- Toxic effect of arsenic and its compounds, undetermined**

Chapter 19 S00-T88

5 **T57.1 Toxic effect of phosphorus and its compounds**

EXCLUDES 1 organophosphate insecticides (T60.0)

6 **T57.1X Toxic effect of phosphorus and its compounds**

SP 7 **T57.1X1- Toxic effect of phosphorus and its compounds, accidental (unintentional)**

Toxic effect of phosphorus and its compounds NOS

SP 7 **T57.1X2- Toxic effect of phosphorus and its compounds, intentional self-harm**

SP 7 **T57.1X3- Toxic effect of phosphorus and its compounds, assault**

SP 7 **T57.1X4- Toxic effect of phosphorus and its compounds, undetermined**

5 **T57.2 Toxic effect of manganese and its compounds**

6 **T57.2X Toxic effect of manganese and its compounds**

SP 7 **T57.2X1- Toxic effect of manganese and its compounds, accidental (unintentional)**

Toxic effect of manganese and its compounds NOS

SP 7 **T57.2X2- Toxic effect of manganese and its compounds, intentional self-harm**

SP 7 **T57.2X3- Toxic effect of manganese and its compounds, assault**

SP 7 **T57.2X4- Toxic effect of manganese and its compounds, undetermined**

5 **T57.3 Toxic effect of hydrogen cyanide**

6 **T57.3X Toxic effect of hydrogen cyanide**

SP 7 **T57.3X1- Toxic effect of hydrogen cyanide, accidental (unintentional)**

Toxic effect of hydrogen cyanide NOS

SP 7 **T57.3X2- Toxic effect of hydrogen cyanide, intentional self-harm**

SP 7 **T57.3X3- Toxic effect of hydrogen cyanide, assault**

SP 7 **T57.3X4- Toxic effect of hydrogen cyanide, undetermined**

5 **T57.8 Toxic effect of other specified inorganic substances**

6 **T57.8X Toxic effect of other specified inorganic substances**

SP 7 **T57.8X1- Toxic effect of other specified inorganic substances, accidental (unintentional)**

Toxic effect of other specified inorganic substances NOS

SP 7 **T57.8X2- Toxic effect of other specified inorganic substances, intentional self-harm**

SP 7 **T57.8X3- Toxic effect of other specified inorganic substances, assault**

SP 7 **T57.8X4- Toxic effect of other specified inorganic substances, undetermined**

5 **T57.9 Toxic effect of unspecified inorganic substance**

SP 7 **T57.91X- Toxic effect of unspecified inorganic substance, accidental (unintentional)**

SP 7 **T57.92X- Toxic effect of unspecified inorganic substance, intentional self-harm**

SP 7 **T57.93X- Toxic effect of unspecified inorganic substance, assault**

SP 7 **T57.94X- Toxic effect of unspecified inorganic substance, undetermined**

4 **T58 Toxic effect of carbon monoxide**

INCLUDES asphyxiation from carbon monoxide
toxic effect of carbon monoxide from all sources

The appropriate 7th character is to be added to each code from category T58

A initial encounter
D subsequent encounter
S sequela

5 **T58.0 Toxic effect of carbon monoxide from motor vehicle exhaust**

Toxic effect of exhaust gas from gas engine

Toxic effect of exhaust gas from motor pump

SP 7 **T58.01X- Toxic effect of carbon monoxide from motor vehicle exhaust, accidental (unintentional)**

SP 7 **T58.02X- Toxic effect of carbon monoxide from motor vehicle exhaust, intentional self-harm**

SP 7 **T58.03X- Toxic effect of carbon monoxide from motor vehicle exhaust, assault**

SP 7 **T58.04X- Toxic effect of carbon monoxide from motor vehicle exhaust, undetermined**

5 **T58.1 Toxic effect of carbon monoxide from utility gas**

Toxic effect of acetylene

Toxic effect of gas NOS used for lighting, heating, cooking

Toxic effect of water gas

SP 7 **T58.11X- Toxic effect of carbon monoxide from utility gas, accidental (unintentional)**

SP 7 **T58.12X- Toxic effect of carbon monoxide from utility gas, intentional self-harm**

SP 7 **T58.13X- Toxic effect of carbon monoxide from utility gas, assault**

SP 7 **T58.14X- Toxic effect of carbon monoxide from utility gas, undetermined**

5 **T58.2 Toxic effect of carbon monoxide from incomplete combustion of other domestic fuels**

Toxic effect of carbon monoxide from incomplete combustion of coal, coke, kerosene, wood

6 **T58.2X Toxic effect of carbon monoxide from incomplete combustion of other domestic fuels**

SP 7 **T58.2X1- Toxic effect of carbon monoxide from incomplete combustion of other domestic fuels, accidental (unintentional)**

Chapter 19 S00-T88

4 4th digit required 5 5th digit required 6 6th digit required 7 7th digit required 7 7th digit placeholder + Additional code Laterality

SP 7 **T58.2X2- Toxic effect of carbon monoxide from incomplete combustion of other domestic fuels, intentional self-harm**

SP 7 **T58.2X3- Toxic effect of carbon monoxide from incomplete combustion of other domestic fuels, assault**

SP 7 **T58.2X4- Toxic effect of carbon monoxide from incomplete combustion of other domestic fuels, undetermined**

5 **T58.8 Toxic effect of carbon monoxide from other source**

Toxic effect of carbon monoxide from blast furnace gas

Toxic effect of carbon monoxide from fuels in industrial use

Toxic effect of carbon monoxide from kiln vapor

6 **T58.8X Toxic effect of carbon monoxide from other source**

SP 7 **T58.8X1- Toxic effect of carbon monoxide from other source, accidental (unintentional)**

SP 7 **T58.8X2- Toxic effect of carbon monoxide from other source, intentional self-harm**

SP 7 **T58.8X3- Toxic effect of carbon monoxide from other source, assault**

SP 7 **T58.8X4- Toxic effect of carbon monoxide from other source, undetermined**

5 **T58.9 Toxic effect of carbon monoxide from unspecified source**

SP 7 **T58.91X- Toxic effect of carbon monoxide from unspecified source, accidental (unintentional)**

SP 7 **T58.92X- Toxic effect of carbon monoxide from unspecified source, intentional self-harm**

SP 7 **T58.93X- Toxic effect of carbon monoxide from unspecified source, assault**

SP 7 **T58.94X- Toxic effect of carbon monoxide from unspecified source, undetermined**

4 **T59 Toxic effect of other gases, fumes and vapors**

INCLUDES aerosol propellants

EXCLUDES 1 chlorofluorocarbons (T53.5)

The appropriate 7th character is to be added to each code from category T59

A initial encounter

D subsequent encounter

S sequela

5 **T59.0 Toxic effect of nitrogen oxides**

6 **T59.0X Toxic effect of nitrogen oxides**

SP 7 **T59.0X1- Toxic effect of nitrogen oxides, accidental (unintentional)**

Toxic effect of nitrogen oxides NOS

SP 7 **T59.0X2- Toxic effect of nitrogen oxides, intentional self-harm**

SP 7 **T59.0X3- Toxic effect of nitrogen oxides, assault**

SP 7 **T59.0X4- Toxic effect of nitrogen oxides, undetermined**

5 **T59.1 Toxic effect of sulfur dioxide**

6 **T59.1X Toxic effect of sulfur dioxide**

SP 7 **T59.1X1- Toxic effect of sulfur dioxide, accidental (unintentional)**

Toxic effect of sulfur dioxide NOS

SP 7 **T59.1X2- Toxic effect of sulfur dioxide, intentional self-harm**

SP 7 **T59.1X3- Toxic effect of sulfur dioxide, assault**

SP 7 **T59.1X4- Toxic effect of sulfur dioxide, undetermined**

5 **T59.2 Toxic effect of formaldehyde**

6 **T59.2X Toxic effect of formaldehyde**

SP 7 **T59.2X1- Toxic effect of formaldehyde, accidental (unintentional)**

Toxic effect of formaldehyde NOS

SP 7 **T59.2X2- Toxic effect of formaldehyde, intentional self-harm**

SP 7 **T59.2X3- Toxic effect of formaldehyde, assault**

SP 7 **T59.2X4- Toxic effect of formaldehyde, undetermined**

5 **T59.3 Toxic effect of lacrimogenic gas**

Toxic effect of tear gas

6 **T59.3X Toxic effect of lacrimogenic gas**

SP 7 **T59.3X1- Toxic effect of lacrimogenic gas, accidental (unintentional)**

Toxic effect of lacrimogenic gas NOS

SP 7 **T59.3X2- Toxic effect of lacrimogenic gas, intentional self-harm**

SP 7 **T59.3X3- Toxic effect of lacrimogenic gas, assault**

SP 7 **T59.3X4- Toxic effect of lacrimogenic gas, undetermined**

5 **T59.4 Toxic effect of chlorine gas**

6 **T59.4X Toxic effect of chlorine gas**

SP 7 **T59.4X1- Toxic effect of chlorine gas, accidental (unintentional)**

Toxic effect of chlorine gas NOS

SP 7 **T59.4X2- Toxic effect of chlorine gas, intentional self-harm**

SP 7 **T59.4X3- Toxic effect of chlorine gas, assault**

SP 7 **T59.4X4- Toxic effect of chlorine gas, undetermined**

5 **T59.5 Toxic effect of fluorine gas and hydrogen fluoride**

6 **T59.5X Toxic effect of fluorine gas and hydrogen fluoride**

SP 7 **T59.5X1- Toxic effect of fluorine gas and hydrogen fluoride, accidental (unintentional)**

Toxic effect of fluorine gas and hydrogen fluoride NOS

SP 7 **T59.5X2- Toxic effect of fluorine gas and hydrogen fluoride, intentional self-harm**

SP 7 **T59.5X3- Toxic effect of fluorine gas and hydrogen fluoride, assault**

SP 7 **T59.5X4- Toxic effect of fluorine gas and hydrogen fluoride, undetermined**

5 **T59.6 Toxic effect of hydrogen sulfide**

6 **T59.6X Toxic effect of hydrogen sulfide**

SP 7 **T59.6X1- Toxic effect of hydrogen sulfide, accidental (unintentional)**

Toxic effect of hydrogen sulfide NOS

SP 7 **T59.6X2- Toxic effect of hydrogen sulfide, intentional self-harm**

SP 7 **T59.6X3- Toxic effect of hydrogen sulfide, assault**

SP 7 **T59.6X4- Toxic effect of hydrogen sulfide, undetermined**

5 **T59.7 Toxic effect of carbon dioxide**

6 **T59.7X Toxic effect of carbon dioxide**

SP 7 **T59.7X1- Toxic effect of carbon dioxide, accidental (unintentional)**

Toxic effect of carbon dioxide NOS

SP 7 **T59.7X2- Toxic effect of carbon dioxide, intentional self-harm**

SP 7 **T59.7X3- Toxic effect of carbon dioxide, assault**

SP 7 **T59.7X4- Toxic effect of carbon dioxide, undetermined**

5 **T59.8 Toxic effect of other specified gases, fumes and vapors**

6 **T59.81 Toxic effect of smoke**

Smoke inhalation

EXCLUDES 2 toxic effect of cigarette (tobacco) smoke (T65.22-)

SP 7 **T59.811- Toxic effect of smoke, accidental (unintentional)**

Toxic effect of smoke NOS

SP 7 **T59.812- Toxic effect of smoke, intentional self-harm**

SP 7 **T59.813- Toxic effect of smoke, assault**

SP 7 **T59.814- Toxic effect of smoke, undetermined**

6 **T59.89 Toxic effect of other specified gases, fumes and vapors**

SP 7 **T59.891- Toxic effect of other specified gases, fumes and vapors, accidental (unintentional)**

SP 7 **T59.892- Toxic effect of other specified gases, fumes and vapors, intentional self-harm**

SP 7 **T59.893- Toxic effect of other specified gases, fumes and vapors, assault**

SP 7 **T59.894- Toxic effect of other specified gases, fumes and vapors, undetermined**

5 **T59.9 Toxic effect of unspecified gases, fumes and vapors**

SP 7 **T59.91X- Toxic effect of unspecified gases, fumes and vapors, accidental (unintentional)**

SP 7 **T59.92X- Toxic effect of unspecified gases, fumes and vapors, intentional self-harm**

SP 7 **T59.93X- Toxic effect of unspecified gases, fumes and vapors, assault**

SP 7 **T59.94X- Toxic effect of unspecified gases, fumes and vapors, undetermined**

4 **T60 Toxic effect of pesticides**

INCLUDES toxic effect of wood preservatives

The appropriate 7th character is to be added to each code from category T60

A	initial encounter
D	subsequent encounter
S	sequela

5 **T60.0 Toxic effect of organophosphate and carbamate insecticides**

6 **T60.0X Toxic effect of organophosphate and carbamate insecticides**

SP 7 **T60.0X1- Toxic effect of organophosphate and carbamate insecticides, accidental (unintentional)**

Toxic effect of organophosphate and carbamate insecticides NOS

SP 7 **T60.0X2- Toxic effect of organophosphate and carbamate insecticides, intentional self-harm**

SP 7 **T60.0X3- Toxic effect of organophosphate and carbamate insecticides, assault**

SP 7 **T60.0X4- Toxic effect of organophosphate and carbamate insecticides, undetermined**

5 **T60.1 Toxic effect of halogenated insecticides**

EXCLUDES 1 chlorinated hydrocarbon (T53.-)

6 **T60.1X Toxic effect of halogenated insecticides**

SP 7 **T60.1X1- Toxic effect of halogenated insecticides, accidental (unintentional)**

Toxic effect of halogenated insecticides NOS

SP 7 **T60.1X2- Toxic effect of halogenated insecticides, intentional self-harm**

SP 7 **T60.1X3- Toxic effect of halogenated insecticides, assault**

SP 7 **T60.1X4- Toxic effect of halogenated insecticides, undetermined**

5 **T60.2 Toxic effect of other insecticides**

6 **T60.2X Toxic effect of other insecticides**

SP 7 **T60.2X1- Toxic effect of other insecticides, accidental (unintentional)**

Toxic effect of other insecticides NOS

SP 7 **T60.2X2- Toxic effect of other insecticides, intentional self-harm**

SP 7 **T60.2X3- Toxic effect of other insecticides, assault**

SP 7 **T60.2X4- Toxic effect of other insecticides, undetermined**

5 **T60.3 Toxic effect of herbicides and fungicides**

6 **T60.3X Toxic effect of herbicides and fungicides**

SP 7 **T60.3X1- Toxic effect of herbicides and fungicides, accidental (unintentional)**

Toxic effect of herbicides and fungicides NOS

SP 7 **T60.3X2- Toxic effect of herbicides and fungicides, intentional self-harm**

SP 7 **T60.3X3- Toxic effect of herbicides and fungicides, assault**

SP 7 **T60.3X4- Toxic effect of herbicides and fungicides, undetermined**

5 **T60.4 Toxic effect of rodenticides**

EXCLUDES 1 strychnine and its salts (T65.1)
thallium (T56.81-)

6 **T60.4X Toxic effect of rodenticides**

SP 7 **T60.4X1- Toxic effect of rodenticides, accidental (unintentional)**
Toxic effect of rodenticides NOS

SP 7 **T60.4X2- Toxic effect of rodenticides, intentional self-harm**

SP 7 **T60.4X3- Toxic effect of rodenticides, assault**

SP 7 **T60.4X4- Toxic effect of rodenticides, undetermined**

5 **T60.8 Toxic effect of other pesticides**

6 **T60.8X Toxic effect of other pesticides**

SP 7 **T60.8X1- Toxic effect of other pesticides, accidental (unintentional)**
Toxic effect of other pesticides NOS

SP 7 **T60.8X2- Toxic effect of other pesticides, intentional self-harm**

SP 7 **T60.8X3- Toxic effect of other pesticides, assault**

SP 7 **T60.8X4- Toxic effect of other pesticides, undetermined**

5 **T60.9 Toxic effect of unspecified pesticide**

SP 7 **T60.91X- Toxic effect of unspecified pesticide, accidental (unintentional)**

SP 7 **T60.92X- Toxic effect of unspecified pesticide, intentional self-harm**

SP 7 **T60.93X- Toxic effect of unspecified pesticide, assault**

SP 7 **T60.94X- Toxic effect of unspecified pesticide, undetermined**

4 **T61 Toxic effect of noxious substances eaten as seafood**

EXCLUDES 1 allergic reaction to food, such as:
anaphylactic reaction or shock due to adverse food reaction (T78.0-)
bacterial foodborne intoxications (A05.-)
dermatitis (L23.6, L25.4, L27.2)
food protein-induced enterocolitis syndrome (K52.21)
food protein-induced enteropathy (K52.22)
gastroenteritis (noninfective) (K52.29)
toxic effect of aflatoxin and other mycotoxins (T64)
toxic effect of cyanides (T65.0-)
toxic effect of harmful algae bloom (T65.82-)
toxic effect of hydrogen cyanide (T57.3-)
toxic effect of mercury (T56.1-)
toxic effect of red tide (T65.82-)

The appropriate 7th character is to be added to each code from category T61

A	initial encounter
D	subsequent encounter
S	sequela

5 **T61.0 Ciguatera fish poisoning**

SP 7 **T61.01X- Ciguatera fish poisoning, accidental (unintentional)**

SP 7 **T61.02X- Ciguatera fish poisoning, intentional self-harm**

SP 7 **T61.03X- Ciguatera fish poisoning, assault**

SP 7 **T61.04X- Ciguatera fish poisoning, undetermined**

5 **T61.1 Scombroid fish poisoning**
Histamine-like syndrome

SP 7 **T61.11X- Scombroid fish poisoning, accidental (unintentional)**

SP 7 **T61.12X- Scombroid fish poisoning, intentional self-harm**

SP 7 **T61.13X- Scombroid fish poisoning, assault**

SP 7 **T61.14X- Scombroid fish poisoning, undetermined**

5 **T61.7 Other fish and shellfish poisoning**

6 **T61.77 Other fish poisoning**

SP 7 **T61.771- Other fish poisoning, accidental (unintentional)**

SP 7 **T61.772- Other fish poisoning, intentional self-harm**

SP 7 **T61.773- Other fish poisoning, assault**

SP 7 **T61.774- Other fish poisoning, undetermined**

6 **T61.78 Other shellfish poisoning**

SP 7 **T61.781- Other shellfish poisoning, accidental (unintentional)**

SP 7 **T61.782- Other shellfish poisoning, intentional self-harm**

SP 7 **T61.783- Other shellfish poisoning, assault**

SP 7 **T61.784- Other shellfish poisoning, undetermined**

5 **T61.8 Toxic effect of other seafood**

6 **T61.8X Toxic effect of other seafood**

SP 7 **T61.8X1- Toxic effect of other seafood, accidental (unintentional)**

SP 7 **T61.8X2- Toxic effect of other seafood, intentional self-harm**

SP 7 **T61.8X3- Toxic effect of other seafood, assault**

SP 7 **T61.8X4- Toxic effect of other seafood, undetermined**

5 **T61.9 Toxic effect of unspecified seafood**

SP 7 **T61.91X- Toxic effect of unspecified seafood, accidental (unintentional)**

SP 7 **T61.92X- Toxic effect of unspecified seafood, intentional self-harm**

SP 7 **T61.93X- Toxic effect of unspecified seafood, assault**

SP 7 **T61.94X- Toxic effect of unspecified seafood, undetermined**

4 **T62 Toxic effect of other noxious substances eaten as food**

EXCLUDES 1 allergic reaction to food, such as:

Chapter 19 S00-T88

anaphylactic shock (reaction) due to adverse food reaction (T78.0-)
bacterial food borne intoxications (A05.-)
dermatitis (L23.6, L25.4, L27.2)
food protein-induced enterocolitis syndrome (K52.21)
food protein-induced enteropathy (K52.22)
gastroenteritis (noninfective) (K52.29)
toxic effect of aflatoxin and other mycotoxins (T64)
toxic effect of cyanides (T65.0-)
toxic effect of hydrogen cyanide (T57.3-)
toxic effect of mercury (T56.1-)

The appropriate 7th character is to be added to each code from category T62
A initial encounter
D subsequent encounter
S sequela

5 **T62.0 Toxic effect of ingested mushrooms**

6 **T62.0X Toxic effect of ingested mushrooms**

SP 7 **T62.0X1- Toxic effect of ingested mushrooms, accidental (unintentional)**
Toxic effect of ingested mushrooms NOS

SP 7 **T62.0X2- Toxic effect of ingested mushrooms, intentional self-harm**

SP 7 **T62.0X3- Toxic effect of ingested mushrooms, assault**

SP 7 **T62.0X4- Toxic effect of ingested mushrooms, undetermined**

5 **T62.1 Toxic effect of ingested berries**

6 **T62.1X Toxic effect of ingested berries**

SP 7 **T62.1X1- Toxic effect of ingested berries, accidental (unintentional)**
Toxic effect of ingested berries NOS

SP 7 **T62.1X2- Toxic effect of ingested berries, intentional self-harm**

SP 7 **T62.1X3- Toxic effect of ingested berries, assault**

SP 7 **T62.1X4- Toxic effect of ingested berries, undetermined**

5 **T62.2 Toxic effect of other ingested (parts of) plant(s)**

6 **T62.2X Toxic effect of other ingested (parts of) plant(s)**

SP 7 **T62.2X1- Toxic effect of other ingested (parts of) plant(s), accidental (unintentional)**
Toxic effect of other ingested (parts of) plant(s) NOS

SP 7 **T62.2X2- Toxic effect of other ingested (parts of) plant(s), intentional self-harm**

SP 7 **T62.2X3- Toxic effect of other ingested (parts of) plant(s), assault**

SP 7 **T62.2X4- Toxic effect of other ingested (parts of) plant(s), undetermined**

5 **T62.8 Toxic effect of other specified noxious substances eaten as food**

6 **T62.8X Toxic effect of other specified noxious substances eaten as food**

SP 7 **T62.8X1- Toxic effect of other specified noxious substances eaten as food, accidental (unintentional)**
Toxic effect of other specified noxious substances eaten as food NOS

SP 7 **T62.8X2- Toxic effect of other specified noxious substances eaten as food, intentional self-harm**

SP 7 **T62.8X3- Toxic effect of other specified noxious substances eaten as food, assault**

SP 7 **T62.8X4- Toxic effect of other specified noxious substances eaten as food, undetermined**

5 **T62.9 Toxic effect of unspecified noxious substance eaten as food**

SP 7 **T62.91X- Toxic effect of unspecified noxious substance eaten as food, accidental (unintentional)**
Toxic effect of unspecified noxious substance eaten as food NOS

SP 7 **T62.92X- Toxic effect of unspecified noxious substance eaten as food, intentional self-harm**

SP 7 **T62.93X- Toxic effect of unspecified noxious substance eaten as food, assault**

SP 7 **T62.94X- Toxic effect of unspecified noxious substance eaten as food, undetermined**

4 **T63 Toxic effect of contact with venomous animals and plants**

INCLUDES bite or touch of venomous animal
pricked or stuck by thorn or leaf

EXCLUDES 2 ingestion of toxic animal or plant (T61.-, T62.-)

The appropriate 7th character is to be added to each code from category T63
A initial encounter
D subsequent encounter
S sequela

5 **T63.0 Toxic effect of snake venom**

6 **T63.00 Toxic effect of unspecified snake venom**

SP 7 **T63.001- Toxic effect of unspecified snake venom, accidental (unintentional)**
Toxic effect of unspecified snake venom NOS

SP 7 **T63.002- Toxic effect of unspecified snake venom, intentional self-harm**

SP 7 **T63.003- Toxic effect of unspecified snake venom, assault**

SP 7 **T63.004- Toxic effect of unspecified snake venom, undetermined**

6 **T63.01 Toxic effect of rattlesnake venom**

SP 7 **T63.011- Toxic effect of rattlesnake venom, accidental (unintentional)**
Toxic effect of rattlesnake venom NOS

SP 7 **T63.012- Toxic effect of rattlesnake venom, intentional self-harm**

SP 7 **T63.013- Toxic effect of rattlesnake venom, assault**

SP 7 **T63.014- Toxic effect of rattlesnake venom, undetermined**

6 **T63.02 Toxic effect of coral snake venom**

SP 7 **T63.021- Toxic effect of coral snake venom, accidental (unintentional)**
Toxic effect of coral snake venom NOS

SP 7 **T63.022- Toxic effect of coral snake venom, intentional self-harm**

SP 7 **T63.023- Toxic effect of coral snake venom, assault**

SP 7 **T63.024- Toxic effect of coral snake venom, undetermined**

6 **T63.03 Toxic effect of taipan venom**

SP 7 **T63.031- Toxic effect of taipan venom, accidental (unintentional)**
Toxic effect of taipan venom NOS

SP 7 **T63.032- Toxic effect of taipan venom, intentional self-harm**

SP 7 **T63.033- Toxic effect of taipan venom, assault**

SP 7 **T63.034- Toxic effect of taipan venom, undetermined**

6 **T63.04 Toxic effect of cobra venom**

SP 7 **T63.041- Toxic effect of cobra venom, accidental (unintentional)**
Toxic effect of cobra venom NOS

SP 7 **T63.042- Toxic effect of cobra venom, intentional self-harm**

SP 7 **T63.043- Toxic effect of cobra venom, assault**

SP 7 **T63.044- Toxic effect of cobra venom, undetermined**

6 **T63.06 Toxic effect of venom of other North and South American snake**

SP 7 **T63.061- Toxic effect of venom of other North and South American snake, accidental (unintentional)**
Toxic effect of venom of other North and South American snake NOS

SP 7 **T63.062- Toxic effect of venom of other North and South American snake, intentional self-harm**

SP 7 **T63.063- Toxic effect of venom of other North and South American snake, assault**

SP 7 **T63.064- Toxic effect of venom of other North and South American snake, undetermined**

6 **T63.07 Toxic effect of venom of other Australian snake**

SP 7 **T63.071- Toxic effect of venom of other Australian snake, accidental (unintentional)**
Toxic effect of venom of other Australian snake NOS

SP 7 **T63.072- Toxic effect of venom of other Australian snake, intentional self-harm**

SP 7 **T63.073- Toxic effect of venom of other Australian snake, assault**

SP 7 **T63.074- Toxic effect of venom of other Australian snake, undetermined**

6 **T63.08 Toxic effect of venom of other African and Asian snake**

SP 7 **T63.081- Toxic effect of venom of other African and Asian snake, accidental (unintentional)**
Toxic effect of venom of other African and Asian snake NOS

SP 7 **T63.082- Toxic effect of venom of other African and Asian snake, intentional self-harm**

SP 7 **T63.083- Toxic effect of venom of other African and Asian snake, assault**

SP 7 **T63.084- Toxic effect of venom of other African and Asian snake, undetermined**

6 **T63.09 Toxic effect of venom of other snake**

SP 7 **T63.091- Toxic effect of venom of other snake, accidental (unintentional)**
Toxic effect of venom of other snake NOS

SP 7 **T63.092- Toxic effect of venom of other snake, intentional self-harm**

SP 7 **T63.093- Toxic effect of venom of other snake, assault**

SP 7 **T63.094- Toxic effect of venom of other snake, undetermined**

5 **T63.1 Toxic effect of venom of other reptiles**

6 **T63.11 Toxic effect of venom of gila monster**

SP 7 **T63.111- Toxic effect of venom of gila monster, accidental (unintentional)**
Toxic effect of venom of gila monster NOS

SP 7 **T63.112- Toxic effect of venom of gila monster, intentional self-harm**

SP 7 **T63.113- Toxic effect of venom of gila monster, assault**

SP 7 **T63.114- Toxic effect of venom of gila monster, undetermined**

6 **T63.12 Toxic effect of venom of other venomous lizard**

SP 7 **T63.121- Toxic effect of venom of other venomous lizard, accidental (unintentional)**
Toxic effect of venom of other venomous lizard NOS

SP 7 **T63.122- Toxic effect of venom of other venomous lizard, intentional self-harm**

SP 7 **T63.123- Toxic effect of venom of other venomous lizard, assault**

SP 7 **T63.124- Toxic effect of venom of other venomous lizard, undetermined**

6 **T63.19 Toxic effect of venom of other reptiles**

SP 7 **T63.191- Toxic effect of venom of other reptiles, accidental (unintentional)**
Toxic effect of venom of other reptiles NOS

Chapter 19

S00-T88

SP 7 **T63.192- Toxic effect of venom of other reptiles, intentional self-harm**
SP 7 **T63.193- Toxic effect of venom of other reptiles, assault**
SP 7 **T63.194- Toxic effect of venom of other reptiles, undetermined**
5 **T63.2 Toxic effect of venom of scorpion**
6 **T63.2X Toxic effect of venom of scorpion**
SP 7 **T63.2X1- Toxic effect of venom of scorpion, accidental (unintentional)**
Toxic effect of venom of scorpion NOS
SP 7 **T63.2X2- Toxic effect of venom of scorpion, intentional self-harm**
SP 7 **T63.2X3- Toxic effect of venom of scorpion, assault**
SP 7 **T63.2X4- Toxic effect of venom of scorpion, undetermined**
5 **T63.3 Toxic effect of venom of spider**
6 **T63.30 Toxic effect of unspecified spider venom**
SP 7 **T63.301- Toxic effect of unspecified spider venom, accidental (unintentional)**
SP 7 **T63.302- Toxic effect of unspecified spider venom, intentional self-harm**
SP 7 **T63.303- Toxic effect of unspecified spider venom, assault**
SP 7 **T63.304- Toxic effect of unspecified spider venom, undetermined**
6 **T63.31 Toxic effect of venom of black widow spider**
SP 7 **T63.311- Toxic effect of venom of black widow spider, accidental (unintentional)**
SP 7 **T63.312- Toxic effect of venom of black widow spider, intentional self-harm**
SP 7 **T63.313- Toxic effect of venom of black widow spider, assault**
SP 7 **T63.314- Toxic effect of venom of black widow spider, undetermined**
6 **T63.32 Toxic effect of venom of tarantula**
SP 7 **T63.321- Toxic effect of venom of tarantula, accidental (unintentional)**
SP 7 **T63.322- Toxic effect of venom of tarantula, intentional self-harm**
SP 7 **T63.323- Toxic effect of venom of tarantula, assault**
SP 7 **T63.324- Toxic effect of venom of tarantula, undetermined**
6 **T63.33 Toxic effect of venom of brown recluse spider**
SP 7 **T63.331- Toxic effect of venom of brown recluse spider, accidental (unintentional)**
SP 7 **T63.332- Toxic effect of venom of brown recluse spider, intentional self-harm**
SP 7 **T63.333- Toxic effect of venom of brown recluse spider, assault**
SP 7 **T63.334- Toxic effect of venom of brown recluse spider, undetermined**
6 **T63.39 Toxic effect of venom of other spider**
SP 7 **T63.391- Toxic effect of venom of other spider, accidental (unintentional)**
SP 7 **T63.392- Toxic effect of venom of other spider, intentional self-harm**
SP 7 **T63.393- Toxic effect of venom of other spider, assault**
SP 7 **T63.394- Toxic effect of venom of other spider, undetermined**
5 **T63.4 Toxic effect of venom of other arthropods**
6 **T63.41 Toxic effect of venom of centipedes and venomous millipedes**
SP 7 **T63.411- Toxic effect of venom of centipedes and venomous millipedes, accidental (unintentional)**
SP 7 **T63.412- Toxic effect of venom of centipedes and venomous millipedes, intentional self-harm**
SP 7 **T63.413- Toxic effect of venom of centipedes and venomous millipedes, assault**
SP 7 **T63.414- Toxic effect of venom of centipedes and venomous millipedes, undetermined**
6 **T63.42 Toxic effect of venom of ants**
SP 7 **T63.421- Toxic effect of venom of ants, accidental (unintentional)**
SP 7 **T63.422- Toxic effect of venom of ants, intentional self-harm**
SP 7 **T63.423- Toxic effect of venom of ants, assault**
SP 7 **T63.424- Toxic effect of venom of ants, undetermined**
6 **T63.43 Toxic effect of venom of caterpillars**
SP 7 **T63.431- Toxic effect of venom of caterpillars, accidental (unintentional)**
SP 7 **T63.432- Toxic effect of venom of caterpillars, intentional self-harm**
SP 7 **T63.433- Toxic effect of venom of caterpillars, assault**
SP 7 **T63.434- Toxic effect of venom of caterpillars, undetermined**
6 **T63.44 Toxic effect of venom of bees**
SP 7 **T63.441- Toxic effect of venom of bees, accidental (unintentional)**
SP 7 **T63.442- Toxic effect of venom of bees, intentional self-harm**
SP 7 **T63.443- Toxic effect of venom of bees, assault**
SP 7 **T63.444- Toxic effect of venom of bees, undetermined**
6 **T63.45 Toxic effect of venom of hornets**
SP 7 **T63.451- Toxic effect of venom of hornets, accidental (unintentional)**
SP 7 **T63.452- Toxic effect of venom of hornets, intentional self-harm**
SP 7 **T63.453- Toxic effect of venom of hornets, assault**
SP 7 **T63.454- Toxic effect of venom of hornets, undetermined**
6 **T63.46 Toxic effect of venom of wasps**
Toxic effect of yellow jacket

SP 7 T63.461- Toxic effect of venom of wasps, accidental (unintentional)
SP 7 T63.462- Toxic effect of venom of wasps, intentional self-harm
SP 7 T63.463- Toxic effect of venom of wasps, assault
SP 7 T63.464- Toxic effect of venom of wasps, undetermined
6 T63.48 Toxic effect of venom of other arthropod
SP 7 T63.481- Toxic effect of venom of other arthropod, accidental (unintentional)
SP 7 T63.482- Toxic effect of venom of other arthropod, intentional self-harm
SP 7 T63.483- Toxic effect of venom of other arthropod, assault
SP 7 T63.484- Toxic effect of venom of other arthropod, undetermined
5 T63.5 Toxic effect of contact with venomous fish
EXCLUDES 2 poisoning by ingestion of fish (T61.-)
6 T63.51 Toxic effect of contact with stingray
SP 7 T63.511- Toxic effect of contact with stingray, accidental (unintentional)
SP 7 T63.512- Toxic effect of contact with stingray, intentional self-harm
SP 7 T63.513- Toxic effect of contact with stingray, assault
SP 7 T63.514- Toxic effect of contact with stingray, undetermined
6 T63.59 Toxic effect of contact with other venomous fish
SP 7 T63.591- Toxic effect of contact with other venomous fish, accidental (unintentional)
SP 7 T63.592- Toxic effect of contact with other venomous fish, intentional self-harm
SP 7 T63.593- Toxic effect of contact with other venomous fish, assault
SP 7 T63.594- Toxic effect of contact with other venomous fish, undetermined
5 T63.6 Toxic effect of contact with other venomous marine animals
EXCLUDES 1 sea-snake venom (T63.09)
EXCLUDES 2 poisoning by ingestion of shellfish (T61.78-)
▲ 6 T63.61 Toxic effect of contact with Portuguese Man-o-war
Toxic effect of contact with bluebottle
▲ SP 7 T63.611- Toxic effect of contact with Portuguese Man-o-war, accidental (unintentional)
▲ SP 7 T63.612- Toxic effect of contact with Portuguese Man-o-war, intentional self-harm
▲ SP 7 T63.613- Toxic effect of contact with Portuguese Man-o-war, assault
▲ SP 7 T63.614- Toxic effect of contact with Portuguese Man-o-war, undetermined
6 T63.62 Toxic effect of contact with other jellyfish
SP 7 T63.621- Toxic effect of contact with other jellyfish, accidental (unintentional)
SP 7 T63.622- Toxic effect of contact with other jellyfish, intentional self-harm
SP 7 T63.623- Toxic effect of contact with other jellyfish, assault
SP 7 T63.624- Toxic effect of contact with other jellyfish, undetermined
6 T63.63 Toxic effect of contact with sea anemone
SP 7 T63.631- Toxic effect of contact with sea anemone, accidental (unintentional)
SP 7 T63.632- Toxic effect of contact with sea anemone, intentional self-harm
SP 7 T63.633- Toxic effect of contact with sea anemone, assault
SP 7 T63.634- Toxic effect of contact with sea anemone, undetermined
6 T63.69 Toxic effect of contact with other venomous marine animals
SP 7 T63.691- Toxic effect of contact with other venomous marine animals, accidental (unintentional)
SP 7 T63.692- Toxic effect of contact with other venomous marine animals, intentional self-harm
SP 7 T63.693- Toxic effect of contact with other venomous marine animals, assault
SP 7 T63.694- Toxic effect of contact with other venomous marine animals, undetermined
5 T63.7 Toxic effect of contact with venomous plant
6 T63.71 Toxic effect of contact with venomous marine plant
SP 7 T63.711- Toxic effect of contact with venomous marine plant, accidental (unintentional)
SP 7 T63.712- Toxic effect of contact with venomous marine plant, intentional self-harm
SP 7 T63.713- Toxic effect of contact with venomous marine plant, assault
SP 7 T63.714- Toxic effect of contact with venomous marine plant, undetermined
6 T63.79 Toxic effect of contact with other venomous plant
SP 7 T63.791- Toxic effect of contact with other venomous plant, accidental (unintentional)
SP 7 T63.792- Toxic effect of contact with other venomous plant, intentional self-harm
SP 7 T63.793- Toxic effect of contact with other venomous plant, assault
SP 7 T63.794- Toxic effect of contact with other venomous plant, undetermined
5 T63.8 Toxic effect of contact with other venomous animals
6 T63.81 Toxic effect of contact with venomous frog
EXCLUDES 1 contact with nonvenomous frog (W62.0)

SP 7 **T63.811- Toxic effect of contact with venomous frog, accidental (unintentional)**

SP 7 **T63.812- Toxic effect of contact with venomous frog, intentional self-harm**

SP 7 **T63.813- Toxic effect of contact with venomous frog, assault**

SP 7 **T63.814- Toxic effect of contact with venomous frog, undetermined**

6 **T63.82 Toxic effect of contact with venomous toad**

EXCLUDES 1 contact with nonvenomous toad (W62.1)

SP 7 **T63.821- Toxic effect of contact with venomous toad, accidental (unintentional)**

SP 7 **T63.822- Toxic effect of contact with venomous toad, intentional self-harm**

SP 7 **T63.823- Toxic effect of contact with venomous toad, assault**

SP 7 **T63.824- Toxic effect of contact with venomous toad, undetermined**

6 **T63.83 Toxic effect of contact with other venomous amphibian**

EXCLUDES 1 contact with nonvenomous amphibian (W62.9)

SP 7 **T63.831- Toxic effect of contact with other venomous amphibian, accidental (unintentional)**

SP 7 **T63.832- Toxic effect of contact with other venomous amphibian, intentional self-harm**

SP 7 **T63.833- Toxic effect of contact with other venomous amphibian, assault**

SP 7 **T63.834- Toxic effect of contact with other venomous amphibian, undetermined**

6 **T63.89 Toxic effect of contact with other venomous animals**

SP 7 **T63.891- Toxic effect of contact with other venomous animals, accidental (unintentional)**

SP 7 **T63.892- Toxic effect of contact with other venomous animals, intentional self-harm**

SP 7 **T63.893- Toxic effect of contact with other venomous animals, assault**

SP 7 **T63.894- Toxic effect of contact with other venomous animals, undetermined**

5 **T63.9 Toxic effect of contact with unspecified venomous animal**

SP X **T63.91X- Toxic effect of contact with unspecified venomous animal, accidental (unintentional)**

SP X **T63.92X- Toxic effect of contact with unspecified venomous animal, intentional self-harm**

SP X **T63.93X- Toxic effect of contact with unspecified venomous animal, assault**

SP X **T63.94X- Toxic effect of contact with unspecified venomous animal, undetermined**

4 **T64 Toxic effect of aflatoxin and other mycotoxin food contaminants**

The appropriate 7th character is to be added to each code from category T64
A initial encounter
D subsequent encounter
S sequela

5 **T64.0 Toxic effect of aflatoxin**

SP X **T64.01X- Toxic effect of aflatoxin, accidental (unintentional)**

SP X **T64.02X- Toxic effect of aflatoxin, intentional self-harm**

SP X **T64.03X- Toxic effect of aflatoxin, assault**

SP X **T64.04X- Toxic effect of aflatoxin, undetermined**

5 **T64.8 Toxic effect of other mycotoxin food contaminants**

SP X **T64.81X- Toxic effect of other mycotoxin food contaminants, accidental (unintentional)**

SP X **T64.82X- Toxic effect of other mycotoxin food contaminants, intentional self-harm**

SP X **T64.83X- Toxic effect of other mycotoxin food contaminants, assault**

SP X **T64.84X- Toxic effect of other mycotoxin food contaminants, undetermined**

4 **T65 Toxic effect of other and unspecified substances**

The appropriate 7th character is to be added to each code from category T65
A initial encounter
D subsequent encounter
S sequela

5 **T65.0 Toxic effect of cyanides**

EXCLUDES 1 hydrogen cyanide (T57.3-)

6 **T65.0X Toxic effect of cyanides**

SP 7 **T65.0X1- Toxic effect of cyanides, accidental (unintentional)**
Toxic effect of cyanides NOS

SP 7 **T65.0X2- Toxic effect of cyanides, intentional self-harm**

SP 7 **T65.0X3- Toxic effect of cyanides, assault**

SP 7 **T65.0X4- Toxic effect of cyanides, undetermined**

5 **T65.1 Toxic effect of strychnine and its salts**

6 **T65.1X Toxic effect of strychnine and its salts**

SP 7 **T65.1X1- Toxic effect of strychnine and its salts, accidental (unintentional)**
Toxic effect of strychnine and its salts NOS

SP 7 **T65.1X2- Toxic effect of strychnine and its salts, intentional self-harm**

SP 7 **T65.1X3- Toxic effect of strychnine and its salts, assault**

SP 7 **T65.1X4- Toxic effect of strychnine and its salts, undetermined**

5 **T65.2 Toxic effect of tobacco and nicotine**

EXCLUDES 2 nicotine dependence (F17.-)

6 **T65.21 Toxic effect of chewing tobacco**

SP 7 **T65.211- Toxic effect of chewing tobacco, accidental (unintentional)**

Chapter 19

S00-T88

4 4th digit required 5 5th digit required 6 6th digit required 7 7th digit required X 7th digit placeholder + Additional code ⊟ Laterality

Toxic effect of chewing tobacco NOS

SP 7 **T65.212- Toxic effect of chewing tobacco, intentional self-harm**

SP 7 **T65.213- Toxic effect of chewing tobacco, assault**

SP 7 **T65.214- Toxic effect of chewing tobacco, undetermined**

+ 6 **T65.22 Toxic effect of tobacco cigarettes**

Toxic effect of tobacco smoke

Use additional code for exposure to second hand tobacco smoke (Z57.31, Z77.22)

SP + 7 **T65.221- Toxic effect of tobacco cigarettes, accidental (unintentional)**

Toxic effect of tobacco cigarettes NOS

SP + 7 **T65.222- Toxic effect of tobacco cigarettes, intentional self-harm**

SP + 7 **T65.223- Toxic effect of tobacco cigarettes, assault**

SP + 7 **T65.224- Toxic effect of tobacco cigarettes, undetermined**

6 **T65.29 Toxic effect of other tobacco and nicotine**

SP 7 **T65.291- Toxic effect of other tobacco and nicotine, accidental (unintentional)**

Toxic effect of other tobacco and nicotine NOS

SP 7 **T65.292- Toxic effect of other tobacco and nicotine, intentional self-harm**

SP 7 **T65.293- Toxic effect of other tobacco and nicotine, assault**

SP 7 **T65.294- Toxic effect of other tobacco and nicotine, undetermined**

5 **T65.3 Toxic effect of nitroderivatives and aminoderivatives of benzene and its homologues**

Toxic effect of anilin [benzenamine]

Toxic effect of nitrobenzene

Toxic effect of trinitrotoluene

6 **T65.3X Toxic effect of nitroderivatives and aminoderivatives of benzene and its homologues**

SP 7 **T65.3X1- Toxic effect of nitroderivatives and aminoderivatives of benzene and its homologues, accidental (unintentional)**

Toxic effect of nitroderivatives and aminoderivatives of benzene and its homologues NOS

SP 7 **T65.3X2- Toxic effect of nitroderivatives and aminoderivatives of benzene and its homologues, intentional self-harm**

SP 7 **T65.3X3- Toxic effect of nitroderivatives and aminoderivatives of benzene and its homologues, assault**

SP 7 **T65.3X4- Toxic effect of nitroderivatives and aminoderivatives of benzene and its homologues, undetermined**

5 **T65.4 Toxic effect of carbon disulfide**

6 **T65.4X Toxic effect of carbon disulfide**

SP 7 **T65.4X1- Toxic effect of carbon disulfide, accidental (unintentional)**

Toxic effect of carbon disulfide NOS

SP 7 **T65.4X2- Toxic effect of carbon disulfide, intentional self-harm**

SP 7 **T65.4X3- Toxic effect of carbon disulfide, assault**

SP 7 **T65.4X4- Toxic effect of carbon disulfide, undetermined**

5 **T65.5 Toxic effect of nitroglycerin and other nitric acids and esters**

Toxic effect of 1,2,3-Propanetriol trinitrate

6 **T65.5X Toxic effect of nitroglycerin and other nitric acids and esters**

SP 7 **T65.5X1- Toxic effect of nitroglycerin and other nitric acids and esters, accidental (unintentional)**

Toxic effect of nitroglycerin and other nitric acids and esters NOS

SP 7 **T65.5X2- Toxic effect of nitroglycerin and other nitric acids and esters, intentional self-harm**

SP 7 **T65.5X3- Toxic effect of nitroglycerin and other nitric acids and esters, assault**

SP 7 **T65.5X4- Toxic effect of nitroglycerin and other nitric acids and esters, undetermined**

5 **T65.6 Toxic effect of paints and dyes, not elsewhere classified**

6 **T65.6X Toxic effect of paints and dyes, not elsewhere classified**

SP 7 **T65.6X1- Toxic effect of paints and dyes, not elsewhere classified, accidental (unintentional)**

Toxic effect of paints and dyes NOS

SP 7 **T65.6X2- Toxic effect of paints and dyes, not elsewhere classified, intentional self-harm**

SP 7 **T65.6X3- Toxic effect of paints and dyes, not elsewhere classified, assault**

SP 7 **T65.6X4- Toxic effect of paints and dyes, not elsewhere classified, undetermined**

5 **T65.8 Toxic effect of other specified substances**

6 **T65.81 Toxic effect of latex**

SP 7 **T65.811- Toxic effect of latex, accidental (unintentional)**

Toxic effect of latex NOS

SP 7 **T65.812- Toxic effect of latex, intentional self-harm**

SP 7 **T65.813- Toxic effect of latex, assault**

SP 7 **T65.814- Toxic effect of latex, undetermined**

6 **T65.82 Toxic effect of harmful algae and algae toxins**

Toxic effect of (harmful) algae bloom NOS

Toxic effect of blue-green algae bloom

Toxic effect of brown tide

Toxic effect of cyanobacteria bloom

Toxic effect of Florida red tide

Toxic effect of pfiesteria piscicida

Toxic effect of red tide

SP 7 **T65.821- Toxic effect of harmful algae and algae toxins, accidental (unintentional)**

Toxic effect of harmful algae and algae toxins NOS

SP 7 **T65.822- Toxic effect of harmful algae and algae toxins, intentional self-harm**

SP 7 **T65.823- Toxic effect of harmful algae and algae toxins, assault**

SP 7 **T65.824- Toxic effect of harmful algae and algae toxins, undetermined**

6 **T65.83 Toxic effect of fiberglass**

SP 7 **T65.831- Toxic effect of fiberglass, accidental (unintentional)**

Toxic effect of fiberglass NOS

SP 7 **T65.832- Toxic effect of fiberglass, intentional self-harm**

SP 7 **T65.833- Toxic effect of fiberglass, assault**

SP 7 **T65.834- Toxic effect of fiberglass, undetermined**

6 **T65.89 Toxic effect of other specified substances**

SP 7 **T65.891- Toxic effect of other specified substances, accidental (unintentional)**

Toxic effect of other specified substances NOS

SP 7 **T65.892- Toxic effect of other specified substances, intentional self-harm**

SP 7 **T65.893- Toxic effect of other specified substances, assault**

SP 7 **T65.894- Toxic effect of other specified substances, undetermined**

5 **T65.9 Toxic effect of unspecified substance**

SP 7 **T65.91X- Toxic effect of unspecified substance, accidental (unintentional)**

Poisoning NOS

SP 7 **T65.92X- Toxic effect of unspecified substance, intentional self-harm**

SP 7 **T65.93X- Toxic effect of unspecified substance, assault**

SP 7 **T65.94X- Toxic effect of unspecified substance, undetermined**

Other and unspecified effects of external causes (T66-T78)

SP 7 **T66.XXX- Radiation sickness, unspecified**

EXCLUDES 1 specified adverse effects of radiation, such as:
- burns (T20-T31)
- leukemia (C91-C95)
- radiation gastroenteritis and colitis (K52.0)
- radiation pneumonitis (J70.0)
- radiation related disorders of the skin and subcutaneous tissue (L55-L59)
- sunburn (L55.-)

The appropriate 7th character is to be added to code T66
- A initial encounter
- D subsequent encounter
- S sequela

CODING TIPS ✓ To code a burn or other effect of radiation, other than radiation sickness, code the burn and then the external cause code to indicate the cause, such as Y84.2.

4 **T67 Effects of heat and light**

EXCLUDES 1 erythema [dermatitis] ab igne (L59.0)
- malignant hyperpyrexia due to anesthesia (T88.3)
- radiation-related disorders of the skin and subcutaneous tissue (L55-L59)

EXCLUDES 2 burns (T20-T31)
- sunburn (L55.-)
- sweat disorder due to heat (L74-L75)

The appropriate 7th character is to be added to each code from category T67
- A initial encounter
- D subsequent encounter
- S sequela

+ 5 **T67.0 Heatstroke and sunstroke**

Use additional code(s) to identify any associated complications of heatstroke, such as:
- coma and stupor (R40.-)
- rhabdomyolysis (M62.82)
- systemic inflammatory response syndrome (R65.1-)

SP + 7 **T67.01X- Heatstroke and sunstroke**

Heat apoplexy
Heat pyrexia
Siriasis
Thermoplegia

SP + 7 **T67.02X- Exertional heatstroke**

SP + 7 **T67.09X- Other heatstroke and sunstroke**

SP 7 **T67.1XX- Heat syncope**

Heat collapse

SP 7 **T67.2XX- Heat cramp**

SP 7 **T67.3XX- Heat exhaustion, anhydrotic**

Heat prostration due to water depletion

EXCLUDES 1 heat exhaustion due to salt depletion (T67.4)

SP 7 **T67.4XX- Heat exhaustion due to salt depletion**

Heat prostration due to salt (and water) depletion

SP 7 **T67.5XX- Heat exhaustion, unspecified**

Heat prostration NOS

SP 7 **T67.6XX- Heat fatigue, transient**

SP 7 **T67.7XX- Heat edema**

SP 7 **T67.8XX- Other effects of heat and light**

SP 7 **T67.9XX- Effect of heat and light, unspecified**

SP + 7 **T68.XXX- Hypothermia**

Accidental hypothermia
Hypothermia NOS

Use additional code to identify source of exposure:
- Exposure to excessive cold of man-made origin (W93)
- Exposure to excessive cold of natural origin (X31)

EXCLUDES 1 hypothermia following anesthesia (T88.51)
hypothermia not associated with low environmental temperature (R68.0)
hypothermia of newborn (P80.-)

EXCLUDES 2 frostbite (T33-T34)

The appropriate 7th character is to be added to code T68
A initial encounter
D subsequent encounter
S sequela

+ 4 **T69 Other effects of reduced temperature**
Use additional code to identify source of exposure:
Exposure to excessive cold of man-made origin (W93)
Exposure to excessive cold of natural origin (X31)

EXCLUDES 2 frostbite (T33-T34)

The appropriate 7th character is to be added to each code from category T69
A initial encounter
D subsequent encounter
S sequela

+ 5 **T69.0 Immersion hand and foot**
+ 6 **T69.01 Immersion hand**
SP + 7 **T69.011- Immersion hand, right hand**
SP + 7 **T69.012- Immersion hand, left hand**
SP + 7 **T69.019- Immersion hand, unspecified hand**
+ 6 **T69.02 Immersion foot**
Trench foot
SP + 7 **T69.021- Immersion foot, right foot**
SP + 7 **T69.022- Immersion foot, left foot**
SP + 7 **T69.029- Immersion foot, unspecified foot**
SP + 7 **T69.1XX- Chilblains**
SP + 7 **T69.8XX- Other specified effects of reduced temperature**
SP + 7 **T69.9XX- Effect of reduced temperature, unspecified**

4 **T70 Effects of air pressure and water pressure**

The appropriate 7th character is to be added to each code from category T70
A initial encounter
D subsequent encounter
S sequela

SP 7 **T70.0XX- Otitic barotrauma**
Aero-otitis media
Effects of change in ambient atmospheric pressure or water pressure on ears
SP 7 **T70.1XX- Sinus barotrauma**
Aerosinusitis
Effects of change in ambient atmospheric pressure on sinuses
5 **T70.2 Other and unspecified effects of high altitude**
EXCLUDES 2 polycythemia due to high altitude (D75.1)
SP 7 **T70.20X- Unspecified effects of high altitude**
SP 7 **T70.29X- Other effects of high altitude**
Alpine sickness
Anoxia due to high altitude
Barotrauma NOS
Hypobaropathy
Mountain sickness
SP 7 **T70.3XX- Caisson disease [decompression sickness]**
Compressed-air disease
Diver's palsy or paralysis
SP 7 **T70.4XX- Effects of high-pressure fluids**
Hydraulic jet injection (industrial)
Pneumatic jet injection (industrial)
Traumatic jet injection (industrial)
SP 7 **T70.8XX- Other effects of air pressure and water pressure**
SP 7 **T70.9XX- Effect of air pressure and water pressure, unspecified**

4 **T71 Asphyxiation**
Mechanical suffocation
Traumatic suffocation

EXCLUDES 1 acute respiratory distress (syndrome) (J80)
anoxia due to high altitude (T70.2)
asphyxia NOS (R09.01)
asphyxia from carbon monoxide (T58.-)
asphyxia from inhalation of food or foreign body (T17.-)
asphyxia from other gases, fumes and vapors (T59.-)
respiratory distress (syndrome) in newborn (P22.-)

The appropriate 7th character is to be added to each code from category T71
A initial encounter
D subsequent encounter
S sequela

5 **T71.1 Asphyxiation due to mechanical threat to breathing**
Suffocation due to mechanical threat to breathing
6 **T71.11 Asphyxiation due to smothering under pillow**
SP 7 **T71.111- Asphyxiation due to smothering under pillow, accidental**
Asphyxiation due to smothering under pillow NOS
SP 7 **T71.112- Asphyxiation due to smothering under pillow, intentional self-harm**
SP 7 **T71.113- Asphyxiation due to smothering under pillow, assault**
SP 7 **T71.114- Asphyxiation due to smothering under pillow, undetermined**
6 **T71.12 Asphyxiation due to plastic bag**
SP 7 **T71.121- Asphyxiation due to plastic bag, accidental**
Asphyxiation due to plastic bag NOS
SP 7 **T71.122- Asphyxiation due to plastic bag, intentional self-harm**
SP 7 **T71.123- Asphyxiation due to plastic bag, assault**

SP 7 **T71.124- Asphyxiation due to plastic bag, undetermined**

6 **T71.13 Asphyxiation due to being trapped in bed linens**

SP 7 **T71.131- Asphyxiation due to being trapped in bed linens, accidental**
Asphyxiation due to being trapped in bed linens NOS

SP 7 **T71.132- Asphyxiation due to being trapped in bed linens, intentional self-harm**

SP 7 **T71.133- Asphyxiation due to being trapped in bed linens, assault**

SP 7 **T71.134- Asphyxiation due to being trapped in bed linens, undetermined**

6 **T71.14 Asphyxiation due to smothering under another person's body (in bed)**

SP 7 **T71.141- Asphyxiation due to smothering under another person's body (in bed), accidental**
Asphyxiation due to smothering under another person's body (in bed) NOS

SP 7 **T71.143- Asphyxiation due to smothering under another person's body (in bed), assault**

SP 7 **T71.144- Asphyxiation due to smothering under another person's body (in bed), undetermined**

6 **T71.15 Asphyxiation due to smothering in furniture**

SP 7 **T71.151- Asphyxiation due to smothering in furniture, accidental**
Asphyxiation due to smothering in furniture NOS

SP 7 **T71.152- Asphyxiation due to smothering in furniture, intentional self-harm**

SP 7 **T71.153- Asphyxiation due to smothering in furniture, assault**

SP 7 **T71.154- Asphyxiation due to smothering in furniture, undetermined**

+ 6 **T71.16 Asphyxiation due to hanging**
Hanging by window shade cord
Use additional code for any associated injuries, such as:
crushing injury of neck (S17.-)
fracture of cervical vertebrae (S12.0-S12.2-)
open wound of neck (S11.-)

SP + 7 **T71.161- Asphyxiation due to hanging, accidental**
Asphyxiation due to hanging NOS
Hanging NOS

SP + 7 **T71.162- Asphyxiation due to hanging, intentional self-harm**

SP + 7 **T71.163- Asphyxiation due to hanging, assault**

SP + 7 **T71.164- Asphyxiation due to hanging, undetermined**

6 **T71.19 Asphyxiation due to mechanical threat to breathing due to other causes**

SP 7 **T71.191- Asphyxiation due to mechanical threat to breathing due to other causes, accidental**
Asphyxiation due to other causes NOS

SP 7 **T71.192- Asphyxiation due to mechanical threat to breathing due to other causes, intentional self-harm**

SP 7 **T71.193- Asphyxiation due to mechanical threat to breathing due to other causes, assault**

SP 7 **T71.194- Asphyxiation due to mechanical threat to breathing due to other causes, undetermined**

5 **T71.2 Asphyxiation due to systemic oxygen deficiency due to low oxygen content in ambient air**
Suffocation due to systemic oxygen deficiency due to low oxygen content in ambient air

SP X **T71.20X- Asphyxiation due to systemic oxygen deficiency due to low oxygen content in ambient air due to unspecified cause**

SP + X **T71.21X- Asphyxiation due to cave-in or falling earth**
Use additional code for any associated cataclysm (X34-X38)

6 **T71.22 Asphyxiation due to being trapped in a car trunk**

SP 7 **T71.221- Asphyxiation due to being trapped in a car trunk, accidental**

SP 7 **T71.222- Asphyxiation due to being trapped in a car trunk, intentional self-harm**

SP 7 **T71.223- Asphyxiation due to being trapped in a car trunk, assault**

SP 7 **T71.224- Asphyxiation due to being trapped in a car trunk, undetermined**

6 **T71.23 Asphyxiation due to being trapped in a (discarded) refrigerator**

SP 7 **T71.231- Asphyxiation due to being trapped in a (discarded) refrigerator, accidental**

SP 7 **T71.232- Asphyxiation due to being trapped in a (discarded) refrigerator, intentional self-harm**

SP 7 **T71.233- Asphyxiation due to being trapped in a (discarded) refrigerator, assault**

SP 7 **T71.234- Asphyxiation due to being trapped in a (discarded) refrigerator, undetermined**

SP X **T71.29X- Asphyxiation due to being trapped in other low oxygen environment**

SP X **T71.9XX- Asphyxiation due to unspecified cause**
Suffocation (by strangulation) due to unspecified cause
Suffocation NOS
Systemic oxygen deficiency due to low oxygen content in ambient air due to unspecified cause
Systemic oxygen deficiency due to mechanical threat to breathing due to unspecified cause
Traumatic asphyxia NOS

4 **T73 Effects of other deprivation**

The appropriate 7th character is to be added to each code from category T73
A initial encounter
D subsequent encounter
S sequela

SP 7 **T73.0XX- Starvation**
Deprivation of food

SP 7 **T73.1XX- Deprivation of water**

SP 7 **T73.2XX- Exhaustion due to exposure**

SP 7 **T73.3XX- Exhaustion due to excessive exertion**
Exhaustion due to overexertion

SP 7 **T73.8XX- Other effects of deprivation**

SP !Q 7 **T73.9XX- Effect of deprivation, unspecified**

+ 4 **T74 Adult and child abuse, neglect and other maltreatment, confirmed**
Use additional code, if applicable, to identify any associated current injury
Use additional external cause code to identify perpetrator, if known (Y07.-)
EXCLUDES 1 abuse and maltreatment in pregnancy (O9A.3-, O9A.4-, O9A.5-)
adult and child maltreatment, suspected (T76.-)

The appropriate 7th character is to be added to each code from category T74
A initial encounter
D subsequent encounter
S sequela

GUIDELINES **Section I.C.19.f**
Sequence first the appropriate code from categories T74.- (Adult and child abuse, neglect and other maltreatment, confirmed) or T76.- (Adult and child abuse, neglect and other maltreatment, suspected) for abuse, neglect and other maltreatment, followed by any accompanying mental health or injury code(s). If the documentation in the medical record states abuse or neglect it is coded as confirmed (T74.-). It is coded as suspected if it is documented as suspected (T76.-).

For cases of confirmed abuse or neglect an external cause code from the assault section (X92-Y09) should be added to identify the cause of any physical injuries. A perpetrator code (Y07) should be added when the perpetrator of the abuse is known. For suspected cases of abuse or neglect, do not report external cause or perpetrator code. If a suspected case of abuse, neglect or mistreatment is ruled out during an encounter code Z04.71, Encounter for examination and observation following alleged physical adult abuse, ruled out, or code Z04.72, Encounter for examination and observation following alleged child physical abuse, ruled out, should be used, not a code from T76.

+ 5 **T74.0 Neglect or abandonment, confirmed**

SP + 7 **T74.01X- Adult neglect or abandonment, confirmed**

SP + 7 **T74.02X- Child neglect or abandonment, confirmed**

+ 5 **T74.1 Physical abuse, confirmed**
EXCLUDES 2 sexual abuse (T74.2-)

SP + 7 **T74.11X- Adult physical abuse, confirmed**

SP + 7 **T74.12X- Child physical abuse, confirmed**
EXCLUDES 2 shaken infant syndrome (T74.4)

+ 5 **T74.2 Sexual abuse, confirmed**
Rape, confirmed
Sexual assault, confirmed

SP + 7 **T74.21X- Adult sexual abuse, confirmed**

SP + 7 **T74.22X- Child sexual abuse, confirmed**

+ 5 **T74.3 Psychological abuse, confirmed**
Bullying and intimidation, confirmed
Intimidation through social media, confirmed

SP + 7 **T74.31X- Adult psychological abuse, confirmed**

SP + 7 **T74.32X- Child psychological abuse, confirmed**

SP + 7 **T74.4XX- Shaken infant syndrome**

+ 5 **T74.5 Forced sexual exploitation, confirmed**

SP + 7 **T74.51X- Adult forced sexual exploitation, confirmed**

SP + 7 **T74.52X- Child sexual exploitation, confirmed**

+ 5 **T74.6 Forced labor exploitation, confirmed**

!Q + 7 **T74.61X- Adult forced labor exploitation, confirmed**

!Q + 7 **T74.62X- Child forced labor exploitation, confirmed**

+ 5 **T74.9 Unspecified maltreatment, confirmed**

!Q + 7 **T74.91X- Unspecified adult maltreatment, confirmed**

!Q + 7 **T74.92X- Unspecified child maltreatment, confirmed**

4 **T75 Other and unspecified effects of other external causes**
EXCLUDES 1 adverse effects NEC (T78.-)
EXCLUDES 2 burns (electric) (T20-T31)

The appropriate 7th character is to be added to each code from category T75
A initial encounter
D subsequent encounter
S sequela

5 **T75.0 Effects of lightning**
Struck by lightning

!Q 7 **T75.00X- Unspecified effects of lightning**
Struck by lightning NOS

SP 7 **T75.01X- Shock due to being struck by lightning**

SP + 7 **T75.09X- Other effects of lightning**
Use additional code for other effects of lightning

!Q 7 **T75.1XX- Unspecified effects of drowning and nonfatal submersion**
Immersion
EXCLUDES 1 specified effects of drowning- code to effects

5 **T75.2 Effects of vibration**

!Q 7 **T75.20X- Unspecified effects of vibration**

SP 7 **T75.21X- Pneumatic hammer syndrome**

SP 7 **T75.22X- Traumatic vasospastic syndrome**

SP 7 **T75.23X- Vertigo from infrasound**

Chapter 19 S00-T88

EXCLUDES 1 vertigo NOS (R42)

SP **T75.29X- Other effects of vibration**

SP + **T75.3XX- Motion sickness**
Airsickness
Seasickness
Travel sickness
Use additional external cause code to identify vehicle or type of motion (Y92.81-, Y93.5-)

SP **T75.4XX- Electrocution**
Shock from electric current
Shock from electroshock gun (taser)

5 **T75.8 Other specified effects of external causes**

SP **T75.81X- Effects of abnormal gravitation [G] forces**

SP **T75.82X- Effects of weightlessness**

SP **T75.89X- Other specified effects of external causes**

+ 4 **T76 Adult and child abuse, neglect and other maltreatment, suspected**
Use additional code, if applicable, to identify any associated current injury
EXCLUDES 1 adult and child maltreatment, confirmed (T74.-)
suspected abuse and maltreatment in pregnancy (O9A.3-, O9A.4-, O9A.5-)
suspected adult physical abuse, ruled out (Z04.71)
suspected adult sexual abuse, ruled out (Z04.41)
suspected child physical abuse, ruled out (Z04.72)
suspected child sexual abuse, ruled out (Z04.42)

The appropriate 7th character is to be added to each code from category T76

A	initial encounter
D	subsequent encounter
S	sequela

GUIDELINES **Section I.C.19.f**
Sequence first the appropriate code from categories T74.- (Adult and child abuse, neglect and other maltreatment, confirmed) or T76.- (Adult and child abuse, neglect and other maltreatment, suspected) for abuse, neglect and other maltreatment, followed by any accompanying mental health or injury code(s). If the documentation in the medical record states abuse or neglect it is coded as confirmed (T74.-). It is coded as suspected if it is documented as suspected (T76.-).

For cases of confirmed abuse or neglect an external cause code from the assault section (X92-Y09) should be added to identify the cause of any physical injuries. A perpetrator code (Y07) should be added when the perpetrator of the abuse is known. For suspected cases of abuse or neglect, do not report external cause or perpetrator code. If a suspected case of abuse, neglect or mistreatment is ruled out during an encounter code Z04.71, Encounter for examination and observation following alleged physical adult abuse, ruled out, or code Z04.72, Encounter for examination and observation following alleged child physical abuse, ruled out, should be used, not a code from T76.

+ 5 **T76.0 Neglect or abandonment, suspected**

SP + **T76.01X- Adult neglect or abandonment, suspected**

SP + **T76.02X- Child neglect or abandonment, suspected**

+ 5 **T76.1 Physical abuse, suspected**

SP + **T76.11X- Adult physical abuse, suspected**

SP + **T76.12X- Child physical abuse, suspected**

+ 5 **T76.2 Sexual abuse, suspected**
Rape, suspected
EXCLUDES 1 alleged abuse, ruled out (Z04.7)

SP + **T76.21X- Adult sexual abuse, suspected**

SP + **T76.22X- Child sexual abuse, suspected**

+ 5 **T76.3 Psychological abuse, suspected**
Bullying and intimidation, suspected
Intimidation through social media, suspected

SP + **T76.31X- Adult psychological abuse, suspected**

SP + **T76.32X- Child psychological abuse, suspected**

+ 5 **T76.5 Forced sexual exploitation, suspected**

SP + **T76.51X- Adult forced sexual exploitation, suspected**

SP + **T76.52X- Child sexual exploitation, suspected**

+ 5 **T76.6 Forced labor exploitation, suspected**

IQ + **T76.61X- Adult forced labor exploitation, suspected**

IQ + **T76.62X- Child forced labor exploitation, suspected**

+ 5 **T76.9 Unspecified maltreatment, suspected**

IQ + **T76.91X- Unspecified adult maltreatment, suspected**

Chapter 19

S00-T88

4 4th digit required 5 5th digit required 6 6th digit required 7 7th digit required 7th digit placeholder + Additional code Laterality

IQ + 7 T76.92X- **Unspecified child maltreatment, suspected**

4 **T78 Adverse effects, not elsewhere classified**

EXCLUDES 2 complications of surgical and medical care NEC (T80-T88)

The appropriate 7th character is to be added to each code from category T78

A initial encounter
D subsequent encounter
S sequela

5 **T78.0 Anaphylactic reaction due to food**

Anaphylactic reaction due to adverse food reaction
Anaphylactic shock or reaction due to nonpoisonous foods
Anaphylactoid reaction due to food

IQ 7 T78.00X- **Anaphylactic reaction due to unspecified food**

SP 7 T78.01X- **Anaphylactic reaction due to peanuts**

SP 7 T78.02X- **Anaphylactic reaction due to shellfish (crustaceans)**

SP 7 T78.03X- **Anaphylactic reaction due to other fish**

SP 7 T78.04X- **Anaphylactic reaction due to fruits and vegetables**

SP 7 T78.05X- **Anaphylactic reaction due to tree nuts and seeds**

EXCLUDES 2 anaphylactic reaction due to peanuts (T78.01)

SP 7 T78.06X- **Anaphylactic reaction due to food additives**

SP 7 T78.07X- **Anaphylactic reaction due to milk and dairy products**

SP 7 T78.08X- **Anaphylactic reaction due to eggs**

SP 7 T78.09X- **Anaphylactic reaction due to other food products**

SP + 7 T78.1XX- **Other adverse food reactions, not elsewhere classified**

Use additional code to identify the type of reaction, if applicable

EXCLUDES 1 anaphylactic reaction or shock due to adverse food reaction (T78.0-)
anaphylactic reaction due to food (T78.0-)
bacterial food borne intoxications (A05.-)

EXCLUDES 2 allergic and dietetic gastroenteritis and colitis (K52.29)
allergic rhinitis due to food (J30.5)
dermatitis due to food in contact with skin (L23.6, L24.6, L25.4)
dermatitis due to ingested food (L27.2)
food protein-induced enterocolitis syndrome (K52.21)
food protein-induced enteropathy (K52.22)

SP 7 T78.2XX- **Anaphylactic shock, unspecified**

Allergic shock
Anaphylactic reaction
Anaphylaxis

EXCLUDES 1 anaphylactic reaction or shock due to adverse effect of correct medicinal substance properly administered (T88.6)
anaphylactic reaction or shock due to adverse food reaction (T78.0-)
anaphylactic reaction or shock due to serum (T80.5-)

SP 7 T78.3XX- **Angioneurotic edema**

Allergic angioedema
Giant urticaria
Quincke's edema

EXCLUDES 1 serum urticaria (T80.6-)
urticaria (L50.-)

5 **T78.4 Other and unspecified allergy**

EXCLUDES 1 specified types of allergic reaction such as:
allergic diarrhea (K52.29)
allergic gastroenteritis and colitis (K52.29)
dermatitis (L23-L25, L27.-)
food protein-induced enterocolitis syndrome (K52.21)
food protein-induced enteropathy (K52.22)
hay fever (J30.1)

SP 7 T78.40X- **Allergy, unspecified**

Allergic reaction NOS
Hypersensitivity NOS

SP 7 T78.41X- **Arthus phenomenon**

Arthus reaction

SP 7 T78.49X- **Other allergy**

SP 7 T78.8XX- **Other adverse effects, not elsewhere classified**

Certain early complications of trauma (T79)

4 **T79 Certain early complications of trauma, not elsewhere classified**

EXCLUDES 2 acute respiratory distress syndrome (J80)
complications occurring during or following medical procedures (T80-T88)
complications of surgical and medical care NEC (T80-T88)
newborn respiratory distress syndrome (P22.0)

The appropriate 7th character is to be added to each code from category T79

A initial encounter
D subsequent encounter
S sequela

SP 7 T79.0XX- **Air embolism (traumatic)**

Chapter 19

S00-T88

EXCLUDES 1 air embolism complicating abortion or ectopic or molar pregnancy (O00-O07, O08.2)
air embolism complicating pregnancy, childbirth and the puerperium (O88.0)
air embolism following infusion, transfusion, and therapeutic injection (T80.0)
air embolism following procedure NEC (T81.7-)

CODING TIPS ✓ Code T79.0- should not be assigned for an air embolus that is not specified as due to a traumatic cause.

SP 7 **T79.1XX- Fat embolism (traumatic)**

EXCLUDES 1 fat embolism complicating:
abortion or ectopic or molar pregnancy (O00-O07, O08.2)
pregnancy, childbirth and the puerperium (O88.8)

SP 7 **T79.2XX- Traumatic secondary and recurrent hemorrhage and seroma**

▲ SP 7 **T79.4XX- Traumatic shock**

Shock (immediate) (delayed) following injury

EXCLUDES 1 anaphylactic shock due to adverse food reaction (T78.0-)
anaphylactic shock due to correct medicinal substance properly administered (T88.6)
anaphylactic shock due to serum (T80.5-)
anaphylactic shock NOS (T78.2)
electric shock (T75.4)
nontraumatic shock NEC (R57.-)
obstetric shock (O75.1)
postprocedural shock (T81.1-)
septic shock (R65.21)
shock complicating abortion or ectopic or molar pregnancy (O00-O07, O08.3)
shock due to anesthesia (T88.2)
shock due to lightning (T75.01)
shock NOS (R57.9)

SP 7 **T79.5XX- Traumatic anuria**

Crush syndrome
Renal failure following crushing

SP 7 **T79.6XX- Traumatic ischemia of muscle**

Traumatic rhabdomyolysis
Volkmann's ischemic contracture

EXCLUDES 2 anterior tibial syndrome (M76.8)
compartment syndrome (traumatic) (T79.A-)
nontraumatic ischemia of muscle (M62.2-)

SP 7 **T79.7XX- Traumatic subcutaneous emphysema**

EXCLUDES 2 emphysema NOS (J43)
emphysema (subcutaneous) resulting from a procedure (T81.82)

5 **T79.A Traumatic compartment syndrome**

EXCLUDES 1 fibromyalgia (M79.7)
nontraumatic compartment syndrome (M79.A-)

EXCLUDES 2 traumatic ischemic infarction of muscle (T79.6)

CODING TIPS ✓ Do not assign any code from subcategory T79.A- to indicate compartment syndrome that is not specifically stated as due to a traumatic cause. Non-traumatic compartment syndrome is coded to M79.A-.

IQ 7 **T79.A0X- Compartment syndrome, unspecified**

Compartment syndrome NOS

6 **T79.A1 Traumatic compartment syndrome of upper extremity**

Traumatic compartment syndrome of shoulder, arm, forearm, wrist, hand, and fingers

Laterality SP 7 **T79.A11- Traumatic compartment syndrome of right upper extremity**

Laterality SP 7 **T79.A12- Traumatic compartment syndrome of left upper extremity**

Laterality IQ 7 **T79.A19- Traumatic compartment syndrome of unspecified upper extremity**

6 **T79.A2 Traumatic compartment syndrome of lower extremity**

Traumatic compartment syndrome of hip, buttock, thigh, leg, foot, and toes

Laterality SP 7 **T79.A21- Traumatic compartment syndrome of right lower extremity**

Laterality SP 7 **T79.A22- Traumatic compartment syndrome of left lower extremity**

Laterality IQ 7 **T79.A29- Traumatic compartment syndrome of unspecified lower extremity**

SP 7 **T79.A3X- Traumatic compartment syndrome of abdomen**

SP 7 **T79.A9X- Traumatic compartment syndrome of other sites**

SP 7 **T79.8XX- Other early complications of trauma**

IQ 7 **T79.9XX- Unspecified early complication of trauma**

Complications of surgical and medical care, not elsewhere classified (T80-T88)

Use additional code for adverse effect, if applicable, to identify drug (T36-T50 with fifth or sixth character 5)

Use additional code(s) to identify the specified condition resulting from the complication

Use additional code to identify devices involved and details of circumstances (Y62-Y82)

EXCLUDES 2 any encounters with medical care for postprocedural conditions in which no complications are present, such as:
- artificial opening status (Z93.-)
- closure of external stoma (Z43.-)
- fitting and adjustment of external prosthetic device (Z44.-)

burns and corrosions from local applications and irradiation (T20-T32)
complications of surgical procedures during pregnancy, childbirth and the puerperium (O00-O9A)
mechanical complication of respirator [ventilator] (J95.850)
poisoning and toxic effects of drugs and chemicals (T36-T65 with fifth or sixth character 1-4 or 6)
postprocedural fever (R50.82)
specified complications classified elsewhere, such as:
- cerebrospinal fluid leak from spinal puncture (G97.0)
- colostomy malfunction (K94.0-)
- disorders of fluid and electrolyte imbalance (E86-E87)
- functional disturbances following cardiac surgery (I97.0-I97.1)
- intraoperative and postprocedural complications of specified body systems (D78.-, E36.-, E89.-, G97.3-, G97.4, H59.3-, H59.-, H95.2-, H95.3, I97.4-, I97.5, J95.6-, J95.7, K91.6-, L76.-, M96.-, N99.-)
- ostomy complications (J95.0-, K94.-, N99.5-)
- postgastric surgery syndromes (K91.1)
- postlaminectomy syndrome NEC (M96.1)
- postmastectomy lymphedema syndrome (I97.2)
- postsurgical blind-loop syndrome (K91.2)
- ventilator associated pneumonia (J95.851)

GUIDELINES **Section I.B.16**

Documentation of Complication of Care: Code assignment is based on the provider's documentation of the relationship between the condition and the care or procedure. The guideline extends to any complications of care, regardless of the chapter the code is located in. It is important to note that not all conditions that occur during or following medical care or surgery are classified as complications. There must be a cause-and-effect relationship between the care provided and the condition, and an indication in the documentation that it is a complication. Query the provider for clarification, if the complication is not clearly documented.

GUIDELINES **Section I.C.19.g.5)**

Intraoperative and postprocedural complication codes are found within the body system chapters with codes specific to the organs and structures of that body system. These codes should be sequenced first, followed by a code(s) for the specific complication, if applicable.

CODING TIPS✓ Conditions classifiable to T80-T88 are classifiable as complications of surgical and medical care. These conditions should only be assigned when diagnostic statements clearly indicate that the condition is a complication. Additional codes may be assigned to fully describe the complication.

4 T80 Complications following infusion, transfusion and therapeutic injection

INCLUDES complications following perfusion

EXCLUDES 2 bone marrow transplant rejection (T86.01)
febrile nonhemolytic transfusion reaction (R50.84)
fluid overload due to transfusion (E87.71)
posttransfusion purpura (D69.51)
transfusion associated circulatory overload (TACO) (E87.71)
transfusion (red blood cell) associated hemochromatosis (E83.111)
transfusion related acute lung injury (TRALI) (J95.84)

The appropriate 7th character is to be added to each code from category T80
- A initial encounter
- D subsequent encounter
- S sequela

CODING TIPS✓ No aftercare code applies, including dressing changes, drain care, and suture removal. 7th character 'D' is the default for home care and hospice when providing aftercare for a healing or resolving condition; 'A' is used for active treatment such as antibiotics or more than routine wound care; 'S' may be used to indicate a residual condition after the original injury has healed. Once complication is repaired in the acute setting, continue to code the complication in home care and hospice with 7th character D if healing/resolving.

SP 7 **T80.0XX- Air embolism following infusion, transfusion and therapeutic injection**

SP + 7 **T80.1XX- Vascular complications following infusion, transfusion and therapeutic injection**

Use additional code to identify the vascular complication

EXCLUDES 2 extravasation of vesicant agent (T80.81-)
infiltration of vesicant agent (T80.81-)
vascular complications specified as due to prosthetic devices, implants and grafts (T82.8-, T83.8-, T84.8-, T85.8-)
postprocedural vascular complications (T81.7-)

+ 5 **T80.2 Infections following infusion, transfusion and therapeutic injection**

Use additional code to identify the specific infection, such as:
sepsis (A41.9)

Use additional code (R65.2-) to identify severe sepsis, if applicable

Chapter 19

S00-T88

EXCLUDES 2 infections specified as due to prosthetic devices, implants and grafts (T82.6-T82.7, T83.5-T83.6, T84.5-T84.7, T85.7)
postprocedural infections (T81.4-)

CODING TIPS ✓ These codes indicate complications of central lines, including, but not limited to, Hickman catheters, PICC lines, port-a-caths, Swan-Ganz and triple lumen catheters. Do not use Z45.2 for routine care of the venous catheter when it is documented as infected.

+ 6 **T80.21 Infection due to central venous catheter**
Infection due to pulmonary artery catheter (Swan-Ganz catheter)

SP + 7 **T80.211- Bloodstream infection due to central venous catheter**
Catheter-related bloodstream infection (CRBSI) NOS
Central line-associated bloodstream infection (CLABSI)
Bloodstream infection due to Hickman catheter
Bloodstream infection due to peripherally inserted central catheter (PICC)
Bloodstream infection due to portacath (port-a-cath)
Bloodstream infection due to pulmonary artery catheter
Bloodstream infection due to triple lumen catheter
Bloodstream infection due to umbilical venous catheter

SP + 7 **T80.212- Local infection due to central venous catheter**
Exit or insertion site infection
Local infection due to Hickman catheter
Local infection due to peripherally inserted central catheter (PICC)
Local infection due to portacath (port-a-cath)
Local infection due to pulmonary artery catheter
Local infection due to triple lumen catheter
Local infection due to umbilical venous catheter
Port or reservoir infection
Tunnel infection

SP + 7 **T80.218- Other infection due to central venous catheter**
Other central line-associated infection
Other infection due to Hickman catheter
Other infection due to peripherally inserted central catheter (PICC)
Other infection due to portacath (port-a-cath)
Other infection due to pulmonary artery catheter
Other infection due to triple lumen catheter
Other infection due to umbilical venous catheter

IQ + 7 **T80.219- Unspecified infection due to central venous catheter**
Central line-associated infection NOS
Unspecified infection due to Hickman catheter
Unspecified infection due to peripherally inserted central catheter (PICC)
Unspecified infection due to portacath (port-a-cath)
Unspecified infection due to pulmonary artery catheter
Unspecified infection due to triple lumen catheter
Unspecified infection due to umbilical venous catheter

SP + 7 **T80.22X- Acute infection following transfusion, infusion, or injection of blood and blood products**

SP + 7 **T80.29X- Infection following other infusion, transfusion and therapeutic injection**

5 **T80.3 ABO incompatibility reaction due to transfusion of blood or blood products**
EXCLUDES 1 minor blood group antigens reactions (Duffy) (E) (K) (Kell) (Kidd) (Lewis) (M) (N) (P) (S) (T80.A-)

SP 7 **T80.30X- ABO incompatibility reaction due to transfusion of blood or blood products, unspecified**
ABO incompatibility blood transfusion NOS
Reaction to ABO incompatibility from transfusion NOS

6 **T80.31 ABO incompatibility with hemolytic transfusion reaction**

SP 7 **T80.310- ABO incompatibility with acute hemolytic transfusion reaction**
ABO incompatibility with hemolytic transfusion reaction less than 24 hours after transfusion
Acute hemolytic transfusion reaction (AHTR) due to ABO incompatibility

SP 7 **T80.311- ABO incompatibility with delayed hemolytic transfusion reaction**
ABO incompatibility with hemolytic transfusion reaction 24 hours or more after transfusion
Delayed hemolytic transfusion reaction (DHTR) due to ABO incompatibility

SP 7 **T80.319- ABO incompatibility with hemolytic transfusion reaction, unspecified**
ABO incompatibility with hemolytic transfusion reaction at unspecified time after transfusion
Hemolytic transfusion reaction (HTR) due to ABO incompatibility NOS

Chapter 19
S00-T88

SP 7 **T80.39X- Other ABO incompatibility reaction due to transfusion of blood or blood products**
Delayed serologic transfusion reaction (DSTR) from ABO incompatibility
Other ABO incompatible blood transfusion
Other reaction to ABO incompatible blood transfusion

5 **T80.4 Rh incompatibility reaction due to transfusion of blood or blood products**
Reaction due to incompatibility of Rh antigens (C) (c) (D) (E) (e)

SP 7 **T80.40X- Rh incompatibility reaction due to transfusion of blood or blood products, unspecified**
Reaction due to Rh factor in transfusion NOS
Rh incompatible blood transfusion NOS

6 **T80.41 Rh incompatibility with hemolytic transfusion reaction**

SP 7 **T80.410- Rh incompatibility with acute hemolytic transfusion reaction**
Acute hemolytic transfusion reaction (AHTR) due to Rh incompatibility
Rh incompatibility with hemolytic transfusion reaction less than 24 hours after transfusion

SP 7 **T80.411- Rh incompatibility with delayed hemolytic transfusion reaction**
Delayed hemolytic transfusion reaction (DHTR) due to Rh incompatibility
Rh incompatibility with hemolytic transfusion reaction 24 hours or more after transfusion

SP 7 **T80.419- Rh incompatibility with hemolytic transfusion reaction, unspecified**
Rh incompatibility with hemolytic transfusion reaction at unspecified time after transfusion
Hemolytic transfusion reaction (HTR) due to Rh incompatibility NOS

SP 7 **T80.49X- Other Rh incompatibility reaction due to transfusion of blood or blood products**
Delayed serologic transfusion reaction (DSTR) from Rh incompatibility
Other reaction to Rh incompatible blood transfusion

5 **T80.A Non-ABO incompatibility reaction due to transfusion of blood or blood products**
Reaction due to incompatibility of minor antigens (Duffy) (Kell) (Kidd) (Lewis) (M) (N) (P) (S)

SP 7 **T80.A0X- Non-ABO incompatibility reaction due to transfusion of blood or blood products, unspecified**
Non-ABO antigen incompatibility reaction from transfusion NOS

6 **T80.A1 Non-ABO incompatibility with hemolytic transfusion reaction**

SP 7 **T80.A10- Non-ABO incompatibility with acute hemolytic transfusion reaction**
Acute hemolytic transfusion reaction (AHTR) due to non-ABO incompatibility
Non-ABO incompatibility with hemolytic transfusion reaction less than 24 hours after transfusion

SP 7 **T80.A11- Non-ABO incompatibility with delayed hemolytic transfusion reaction**
Delayed hemolytic transfusion reaction (DHTR) due to non-ABO incompatibility
Non-ABO incompatibility with hemolytic transfusion reaction 24 or more hours after transfusion

SP 7 **T80.A19- Non-ABO incompatibility with hemolytic transfusion reaction, unspecified**
Hemolytic transfusion reaction (HTR) due to non-ABO incompatibility NOS
Non-ABO incompatibility with hemolytic transfusion reaction at unspecified time after transfusion

SP 7 **T80.A9X- Other non-ABO incompatibility reaction due to transfusion of blood or blood products**
Delayed serologic transfusion reaction (DSTR) from non-ABO incompatibility
Other reaction to non-ABO incompatible blood transfusion

5 **T80.5 Anaphylactic reaction due to serum**
Allergic shock due to serum
Anaphylactic shock due to serum
Anaphylactoid reaction due to serum
Anaphylaxis due to serum
EXCLUDES 1 ABO incompatibility reaction due to transfusion of blood or blood products (T80.3-)
allergic reaction or shock NOS (T78.2)
anaphylactic reaction or shock NOS (T78.2)
anaphylactic reaction or shock due to adverse effect of correct medicinal substance properly administered (T88.6)
other serum reaction (T80.6-)

SP 7 **T80.51X- Anaphylactic reaction due to administration of blood and blood products**

SP 7 **T80.52X- Anaphylactic reaction due to vaccination**

SP 7 **T80.59X- Anaphylactic reaction due to other serum**

5 **T80.6 Other serum reactions**
Intoxication by serum
Protein sickness
Serum rash

Chapter 19

S00-T88

Serum sickness
Serum urticaria
EXCLUDES 2 serum hepatitis (B16-B19)

SP T80.61X- **Other serum reaction due to administration of blood and blood products**

SP T80.62X- **Other serum reaction due to vaccination**

SP T80.69X- **Other serum reaction due to other serum**
Code also:
, if applicable, arthropathy in hypersensitivity reactions classified elsewhere (M36.4)

5 T80.8 **Other complications following infusion, transfusion and therapeutic injection**

6 T80.81 **Extravasation of vesicant agent**
Infiltration of vesicant agent

SP 7 T80.810- **Extravasation of vesicant antineoplastic chemotherapy**
Infiltration of vesicant antineoplastic chemotherapy

SP 7 T80.818- **Extravasation of other vesicant agent**
Infiltration of other vesicant agent

★ + T80.82X- **Complication of immune effector cellular therapy**
Complication of chimeric antigen receptor (CAR-T) cell therapy
Complication of IEC therapy
Use additional code to identify the specific complication, such as:
cytokine release syndrome (D89.83-)
immune effector cell-associated neurotoxicity syndrome (G92.0-)
EXCLUDES 2 complication of bone marrow transplant (T86.0)
complication of stem cell transplant (T86.5)

SP + T80.89X- **Other complications following infusion, transfusion and therapeutic injection**
Delayed serologic transfusion reaction (DSTR), unspecified incompatibility
Use additional code to identify graft-versus-host reaction, if applicable, (D89.81-)

5 T80.9 **Unspecified complication following infusion, transfusion and therapeutic injection**

SP T80.90X- **Unspecified complication following infusion and therapeutic injection**

6 T80.91 **Hemolytic transfusion reaction, unspecified incompatibility**
EXCLUDES 1 ABO incompatibility with hemolytic transfusion reaction (T80.31-)
Non-ABO incompatibility with hemolytic transfusion reaction (T80.A1-)
Rh incompatibility with hemolytic transfusion reaction (T80.41-)

SP 7 T80.910- **Acute hemolytic transfusion reaction, unspecified incompatibility**

SP 7 T80.911- **Delayed hemolytic transfusion reaction, unspecified incompatibility**

SP 7 T80.919- **Hemolytic transfusion reaction, unspecified incompatibility, unspecified as acute or delayed**
Hemolytic transfusion reaction NOS

SP T80.92X- **Unspecified transfusion reaction**
Transfusion reaction NOS

+ 4 T81 **Complications of procedures, not elsewhere classified**
Use additional code for adverse effect, if applicable, to identify drug (T36-T50 with fifth or sixth character 5)
EXCLUDES 2 complications following immunization (T88.0-T88.1)
complications following infusion, transfusion and therapeutic injection (T80.-)
complications of transplanted organs and tissue (T86.-)
specified complications classified elsewhere, such as:
complication of prosthetic devices, implants and grafts (T82-T85)
dermatitis due to drugs and medicaments (L23.3, L24.4, L25.1, L27.0-L27.1)
endosseous dental implant failure (M27.6-)
floppy iris syndrome (IFIS) (intraoperative) H21.81
intraoperative and postprocedural complications of specific body system (D78.-, E36.-, E89.-, G97.3-, G97.4, H59.3-, H59.-, H95.2-, H95.3, I97.4-, I97.5, J95, K91.-, L76.-, M96.-, N99.-)
ostomy complications (J95.0-, K94.-, N99.5-)
plateau iris syndrome (post-iridectomy) (postprocedural) H21.82
poisoning and toxic effects of drugs and chemicals (T36-T65 with fifth or sixth character 1-4 or 6)

The appropriate 7th character is to be added to each code from category T81
A initial encounter
D subsequent encounter
S sequela

CODING TIPS✓ No aftercare code applies, including dressing changes, drain care, and suture removal. 7th character 'D' is the default for home care and hospice when providing aftercare for a healing or resolving condition; 'A' is used for active treatment such as antibiotics or more than routine wound care; 'S' may be used to indicate a residual condition after the original injury has healed. Once complication is repaired in the acute setting, continue to code the complication in home care and hospice with 7th character D if healing/resolving.

▲ + 5 **T81.1 Postprocedural shock**

Shock during or resulting from a procedure, not elsewhere classified

EXCLUDES 1 anaphylactic shock NOS (T78.2)
anaphylactic shock due to correct substance properly administered (T88.6)
anaphylactic shock due to serum (T80.5-)
electric shock (T75.4)
obstetric shock (O75.1)
septic shock (R65.21)
shock due to anesthesia (T88.2)
shock following abortion or ectopic or molar pregnancy (O00-O07, O08.3)
traumatic shock (T79.4)

SP + 7 **T81.10X- Postprocedural shock unspecified**

Collapse NOS during or resulting from a procedure, not elsewhere classified
Postprocedural failure of peripheral circulation
Postprocedural shock NOS

SP + 7 **T81.11X- Postprocedural cardiogenic shock**

IQ + 7 **T81.12X- Postprocedural septic shock**

Postprocedural endotoxic shock resulting from a procedure, not elsewhere classified
Postprocedural gram-negative shock resulting from a procedure, not elsewhere classified
Code first:
underlying infection
Use additional code, to identify any associated acute organ dysfunction, if applicable

GUIDELINES **Section I.C.1.d.5)(b-c)**
For infections following a procedure, a code from T81.40, to T81.43 Infection following a procedure, or a code from O86.00 to O86.03, Infection of obstetric surgical wound, that identifies the site of the infection should be coded first, if known. Assign an additional code for sepsis following a procedure (T81.44) or sepsis following an obstetrical procedure (O86.04). Use an additional code to identify the infectious agent. If the patient has severe sepsis, the appropriate code from subcategory R65.2 should also be assigned with the additional code(s) for any acute organ dysfunction.

If a postprocedural infection has resulted in postprocedural septic shock, assign the codes indicated above for sepsis due to a postprocedural infection, followed by code T81.12-, Postprocedural septic shock. Do not assign code R65.21, Severe sepsis with septic shock. Additional code(s) should be assigned for any acute organ dysfunction.

CODING TIPS✓ **Documentation:** Only assign T81.12- when the provider diagnostic statements clearly indicate septic shock as a postprocedural complication.

SP + 7 **T81.19X- Other postprocedural shock**

Postprocedural hypovolemic shock

+ 5 **T81.3 Disruption of wound, not elsewhere classified**

Disruption of any suture materials or other closure methods

EXCLUDES 1 breakdown (mechanical) of permanent sutures (T85.612)
displacement of permanent sutures (T85.622)
disruption of cesarean delivery wound (O90.0)
disruption of perineal obstetric wound (O90.1)
mechanical complication of permanent sutures NEC (T85.692)

CODING TIPS✓ No aftercare code applies including dressing changes, drain care, and suture removal. The 7th character "D" is the default for home care and hospice when providing aftercare for a healing or resolving condition; "A" is used for active treatment such as antibiotics or more than routine wound care; "S" may be used to indicate a residual condition after the original injury has healed.

SP + 7 **T81.30X- Disruption of wound, unspecified**

Disruption of wound NOS

Chapter 19 S00-T88

CODING TIPS ✓ Code T81.30x- should not be used as it indicates unspecified wound, not unspecified surgical wound.

SP + 7 T81.31X- Disruption of external operation (surgical) wound, not elsewhere classified

Dehiscence of operation wound NOS
Disruption of operation wound NOS
Disruption or dehiscence of closure of cornea
Disruption or dehiscence of closure of mucosa
Disruption or dehiscence of closure of skin and subcutaneous tissue
Full-thickness skin disruption or dehiscence
Superficial disruption or dehiscence of operation wound

EXCLUDES 1 dehiscence of amputation stump (T87.81)

CODING TIPS ✓ These codes may be assigned for dehisced surgical wounds. If assigned as primary, the payment is based on the wound grouper. Do not use Z48.01 codes with these codes. Once the surgical wound is not healing due to dehiscence, do not change the code to T81.89.

CODING TIPS ✓ T81.31x- indicates external dehiscence of a surgical wound, as well as dehiscence of a surgical wound unspecified, whether external or internal. Reference the inclusion note for examples of external dehiscence. This code is a NEC code and there may be another more specific code for dehiscence that should be used instead.

SP + 7 T81.32X- Disruption of internal operation (surgical) wound, not elsewhere classified

Deep disruption or dehiscence of operation wound NOS
Disruption or dehiscence of closure of internal organ or other internal tissue
Disruption or dehiscence of closure of muscle or muscle flap
Disruption or dehiscence of closure of ribs or rib cage
Disruption or dehiscence of closure of skull or craniotomy
Disruption or dehiscence of closure of sternum or sternotomy
Disruption or dehiscence of closure of tendon or ligament
Disruption or dehiscence of closure of superficial or muscular fascia

CODING TIPS ✓ These codes may be assigned for dehisced surgical wounds. If assigned as primary, the payment is based on the wound grouper. Do not use Z48.01 codes with these codes. Once the surgical wound is not healing due to dehiscence, do not change the code to T81.89.

CODING TIPS ✓ T81.32x- indicates internal dehiscence of a surgical wound. Reference the inclusion note for examples of internal dehiscence.This code is a NEC code and there may be another more specific code for dehiscence that should be used instead. Note the inclusion note at this code.

SP + 7 T81.33X- Disruption of traumatic injury wound repair

Disruption or dehiscence of closure of traumatic laceration (external) (internal)

CODING TIPS ✓ These codes may be assigned for dehisced surgical wounds. If assigned as primary, the payment is based on the wound grouper. Do not use Z48.01 codes with these codes. Once the surgical wound is not healing due to dehiscence, do not change the code to T81.89.

CODING TIPS ✓ Assign code T81.33- for a repaired (sutured) traumatic laceration, which has dehisced. Also code the traumatic wound.

+ 5 T81.4 Infection following a procedure

Wound abscess following a procedure
Use additional code to identify infection
Use additional code (R65.2-) to identify severe sepsis, if applicable

EXCLUDES 2 bleb associated endophthalmitis (H59.4-)
infection due to infusion, transfusion and therapeutic injection (T80.2-)
infection due to prosthetic devices, implants and grafts (T82.6-T82.7, T83.5-T83.6, T84.5-T84.7, T85.7)
obstetric surgical wound infection (O86.0-)
postprocedural fever NOS (R50.82)
postprocedural retroperitoneal abscess (K68.11)

GUIDELINES **Section I.C.1.d.5)(b-c)**
For infections following a procedure, a code from T81.40, to T81.43 Infection following a procedure, or a code from O86.00 to O86.03, Infection of obstetric surgical wound, that identifies the site of the infection should be coded first, if known. Assign an additional code for sepsis following a procedure (T81.44) or sepsis following an obstetrical procedure (O86.04). Use an additional code to identify the infectious agent. If the patient has severe sepsis, the appropriate code from subcategory R65.2 should also be assigned with the additional code(s) for any acute organ dysfunction.

If a postprocedural infection has resulted in postprocedural septic shock, assign the codes indicated above for sepsis due to a postprocedural infection, followed by code T81.12-, Postprocedural septic shock. Do not assign code R65.21, Severe sepsis with septic shock. Additional code(s) should be assigned for any acute organ dysfunction.

CODING TIPS✓ Assign a specific code from the T81.4- category to indicate post-operative infections such as postprocedural sepsis, postoperative wound infections, and intra-abdominal abscess following a procedure. Surgical site infections are commonly classified according to their depth: superficial incisional, deep incisional, and organ/space infection.

CODING TIPS✓ No aftercare code applies including dressing changes, drain care, and suture removal. The 7th character "D" is the default for home care and hospice when providing aftercare for a healing or resolving condition; "A" is used for active treatment such as antibiotics or more than routine wound care; "S" may be used to indicate a residual condition after the original injury has healed.

IQ + 7 **T81.40X- Infection following a procedure, unspecified**
CODING TIPS✓ Avoid using this code for an infected surgical wound. The default code is T81.49-.

SP + 7 **T81.41X- Infection following a procedure, superficial incisional surgical site**
Subcutaneous abscess following a procedure
Stitch abscess following a procedure
CODING TIPS✓ These codes may be assigned for infected surgical wounds. If assigned as primary, the payment is based on the wound grouper. Do not use Z48.01 codes with these codes. Once the surgical wound is not healing due to infection, do not change the code to T81.89.

CODING TIPS✓ A superficial incisional infection involves only the skin and subcutaneous tissue and may be indicated by localized signs such as redness, pain, heat or swelling at the site of the incision or by the drainage of pus.

SP + 7 **T81.42X- Infection following a procedure, deep incisional surgical site**
Intra-muscular abscess following a procedure
CODING TIPS✓ These codes may be assigned for infected surgical wounds. If assigned as primary, the payment is based on the wound grouper. Do not use Z48.01 codes with these codes. Once the surgical wound is not healing due to infection, do not change the code to T81.89.
CODING TIPS✓ A deep incisional infection involves deep tissues, such as fascial and muscle layers, and may be indicated by the presence of pus or an abscess, fever with tenderness of the wound, or separation of incision edges exposing deeper tissues.

SP + 7 **T81.43X- Infection following a procedure, organ and space surgical site**
Intra-abdominal abscess following a procedure
Subphrenic abscess following a procedure
CODING TIPS✓ These codes may be assigned for infected surgical wounds. If assigned as primary, the payment is based on the wound grouper. Do not use Z48.01 codes with these codes. Once the surgical wound is not healing due to infection, do not change the code to T81.89.
CODING TIPS✓ An organ and space infection involves any part of the anatomy in organs and spaces other than the incision, which was opened or manipulated during operation, such as the joint or the peritoneum, and may be indicated by the drainage of pus or the formation of an abscess detected by histopathological or radiological examination or during re-operation; does not include organ infection.

SP + 7 **T81.44X- Sepsis following a procedure**
Use additional code to identify the sepsis
CODING TIPS✓ This code is used for postprocedural sepsis. Code the specified infection first, then T81.44-, then the A code for the sepsis.

SP + 7 **T81.49X- Infection following a procedure, other surgical site**

Chapter 19

S00-T88

CODING TIPS✓ These codes may be assigned for infected surgical wounds. If assigned as primary, the payment is based on the wound grouper. Do not use Z48.01 codes with these codes. Once the surgical wound is not healing due to infection, do not change the code to T81.89.

CODING TIPS✓ T81.49 is the default code for infected surgical wound when the depth of the wound/infection is not indicated by the physician or NPP.

+ 5 T81.5 Complications of foreign body accidentally left in body following procedure

+ 6 T81.50 Unspecified complication of foreign body accidentally left in body following procedure

L IQ + 7 T81.500- Unspecified complication of foreign body accidentally left in body following surgical operation

L IQ + 7 T81.501- Unspecified complication of foreign body accidentally left in body following infusion or transfusion

L IQ + 7 T81.502- Unspecified complication of foreign body accidentally left in body following kidney dialysis

L IQ + 7 T81.503- Unspecified complication of foreign body accidentally left in body following injection or immunization

L IQ + 7 T81.504- Unspecified complication of foreign body accidentally left in body following endoscopic examination

L IQ + 7 T81.505- Unspecified complication of foreign body accidentally left in body following heart catheterization

L IQ + 7 T81.506- Unspecified complication of foreign body accidentally left in body following aspiration, puncture or other catheterization

L IQ + 7 T81.507- Unspecified complication of foreign body accidentally left in body following removal of catheter or packing

L IQ + 7 T81.508- Unspecified complication of foreign body accidentally left in body following other procedure

L IQ + 7 T81.509- Unspecified complication of foreign body accidentally left in body following unspecified procedure

+ 6 T81.51 Adhesions due to foreign body accidentally left in body following procedure

L SP + 7 T81.510- Adhesions due to foreign body accidentally left in body following surgical operation

L SP + 7 T81.511- Adhesions due to foreign body accidentally left in body following infusion or transfusion

L SP + 7 T81.512- Adhesions due to foreign body accidentally left in body following kidney dialysis

L SP + 7 T81.513- Adhesions due to foreign body accidentally left in body following injection or immunization

L SP + 7 T81.514- Adhesions due to foreign body accidentally left in body following endoscopic examination

L SP + 7 T81.515- Adhesions due to foreign body accidentally left in body following heart catheterization

L SP + 7 T81.516- Adhesions due to foreign body accidentally left in body following aspiration, puncture or other catheterization

L SP + 7 T81.517- Adhesions due to foreign body accidentally left in body following removal of catheter or packing

L SP + 7 T81.518- Adhesions due to foreign body accidentally left in body following other procedure

L IQ + 7 T81.519- Adhesions due to foreign body accidentally left in body following unspecified procedure

+ 6 T81.52 Obstruction due to foreign body accidentally left in body following procedure

L SP + 7 T81.520- Obstruction due to foreign body accidentally left in body following surgical operation

L SP + 7 T81.521- Obstruction due to foreign body accidentally left in body following infusion or transfusion

L SP + 7 T81.522- Obstruction due to foreign body accidentally left in body following kidney dialysis

L SP + 7 T81.523- Obstruction due to foreign body accidentally left in body following injection or immunization

L SP + 7 T81.524- Obstruction due to foreign body accidentally left in body following endoscopic examination

L SP + 7 T81.525- Obstruction due to foreign body accidentally left in body following heart catheterization

L SP + 7 T81.526- Obstruction due to foreign body accidentally left in body following aspiration, puncture or other catheterization

L SP + 7 T81.527- Obstruction due to foreign body accidentally left in body following removal of catheter or packing

L SP + 7 T81.528- Obstruction due to foreign body accidentally left in body following other procedure

L SP + 7 T81.529- Obstruction due to foreign body accidentally left in body following unspecified procedure

Chapter 19

S00-T88

+ 6 T81.53 **Perforation due to foreign body accidentally left in body following procedure**

SP + 7 T81.530- **Perforation due to foreign body accidentally left in body following surgical operation**

SP + 7 T81.531- **Perforation due to foreign body accidentally left in body following infusion or transfusion**

SP + 7 T81.532- **Perforation due to foreign body accidentally left in body following kidney dialysis**

SP + 7 T81.533- **Perforation due to foreign body accidentally left in body following injection or immunization**

SP + 7 T81.534- **Perforation due to foreign body accidentally left in body following endoscopic examination**

SP + 7 T81.535- **Perforation due to foreign body accidentally left in body following heart catheterization**

SP + 7 T81.536- **Perforation due to foreign body accidentally left in body following aspiration, puncture or other catheterization**

SP + 7 T81.537- **Perforation due to foreign body accidentally left in body following removal of catheter or packing**

SP + 7 T81.538- **Perforation due to foreign body accidentally left in body following other procedure**

SP + 7 T81.539- **Perforation due to foreign body accidentally left in body following unspecified procedure**

+ 6 T81.59 **Other complications of foreign body accidentally left in body following procedure**

EXCLUDES 2 obstruction or perforation due to prosthetic devices and implants intentionally left in body (T82.0-T82.5, T83.0-T83.4, T83.7, T84.0-T84.4, T85.0-T85.6)

SP + 7 T81.590- **Other complications of foreign body accidentally left in body following surgical operation**

SP + 7 T81.591- **Other complications of foreign body accidentally left in body following infusion or transfusion**

SP + 7 T81.592- **Other complications of foreign body accidentally left in body following kidney dialysis**

SP + 7 T81.593- **Other complications of foreign body accidentally left in body following injection or immunization**

SP + 7 T81.594- **Other complications of foreign body accidentally left in body following endoscopic examination**

SP + 7 T81.595- **Other complications of foreign body accidentally left in body following heart catheterization**

SP + 7 T81.596- **Other complications of foreign body accidentally left in body following aspiration, puncture or other catheterization**

SP + 7 T81.597- **Other complications of foreign body accidentally left in body following removal of catheter or packing**

SP + 7 T81.598- **Other complications of foreign body accidentally left in body following other procedure**

IQ + 7 T81.599- **Other complications of foreign body accidentally left in body following unspecified procedure**

+ 5 T81.6 **Acute reaction to foreign substance accidentally left during a procedure**

EXCLUDES 2 complications of foreign body accidentally left in body cavity or operation wound following procedure (T81.5-)

IQ + 7 T81.60X- **Unspecified acute reaction to foreign substance accidentally left during a procedure**

SP + 7 T81.61X- **Aseptic peritonitis due to foreign substance accidentally left during a procedure**
Chemical peritonitis

SP + 7 T81.69X- **Other acute reaction to foreign substance accidentally left during a procedure**

+ 5 T81.7 **Vascular complications following a procedure, not elsewhere classified**
Air embolism following procedure NEC
Phlebitis or thrombophlebitis resulting from a procedure

EXCLUDES 1 embolism complicating abortion or ectopic or molar pregnancy (O00-O07, O08.2)
embolism complicating pregnancy, childbirth and the puerperium (O88.-)
traumatic embolism (T79.0)

EXCLUDES 2 embolism due to prosthetic devices, implants and grafts (T82.8-, T83.81, T84.8-, T85.81-)
embolism following infusion, transfusion and therapeutic injection (T80.0)

+ 6 T81.71 **Complication of artery following a procedure, not elsewhere classified**

SP + 7 T81.710- **Complication of mesenteric artery following a procedure, not elsewhere classified**

SP + 7 T81.711- **Complication of renal artery following a procedure, not elsewhere classified**

SP + 7 T81.718- **Complication of other artery following a procedure, not elsewhere classified**

SP + 7 T81.719- **Complication of unspecified artery following a procedure, not elsewhere classified**

Chapter 19
S00-T88

SP + 7 **T81.72X- Complication of vein following a procedure, not elsewhere classified**

+ 5 **T81.8 Other complications of procedures, not elsewhere classified**

EXCLUDES 2 hypothermia following anesthesia (T88.51)
malignant hyperpyrexia due to anesthesia (T88.3)

SP + 7 **T81.81X- Complication of inhalation therapy**

SP + 7 **T81.82X- Emphysema (subcutaneous) resulting from a procedure**

SP + 7 **T81.83X- Persistent postprocedural fistula**

SP + 7 **T81.89X- Other complications of procedures, not elsewhere classified**

Use additional code to specify complication, such as:
postprocedural delirium (F05)

CODING TIPS✓ If assigned as primary, the payment is based on the wound grouper. Do not use Z48.01 codes with this code.

CODING TIPS✓ This code is used for non-healing surgical wounds when no other code applies. It is a NEC code so ensure that another complication code is not more appropriate. For example, do not switch from the infected surgical wound or dehisced surgical wound to T81.89x- just because the wound remains open. The 'use additional code' note does not apply when using the code for non-healing surgical wounds.

L IQ + 7 **T81.9XX- Unspecified complication of procedure**

4 **T82 Complications of cardiac and vascular prosthetic devices, implants and grafts**

EXCLUDES 2 failure and rejection of transplanted organs and tissue (T86.-)

The appropriate 7th character is to be added to each code from category T82

A	initial encounter
D	subsequent encounter
S	sequela

CODING TIPS✓ No aftercare code applies, including dressing changes, drain care, and suture removal. 7th character 'D' is the default for home care and hospice when providing aftercare for a healing or resolving condition; 'A' is used for active treatment such as antibiotics or more than routine wound care; 'S' may be used to indicate a residual condition after the original injury has healed. Once complication is repaired in the acute setting, continue to code the complication in home care and hospice with 7th character D if healing/resolving.

5 **T82.0 Mechanical complication of heart valve prosthesis**

Mechanical complication of artificial heart valve

EXCLUDES 1 mechanical complication of biological heart valve graft (T82.22-)

CODING TIPS✓ Do not use Z95.2 to indicate presence of a heart valve prosthesis when there is a complication of the prosthesis.

SP 7 **T82.01X- Breakdown (mechanical) of heart valve prosthesis**

SP 7 **T82.02X- Displacement of heart valve prosthesis**

Malposition of heart valve prosthesis

SP 7 **T82.03X- Leakage of heart valve prosthesis**

SP 7 **T82.09X- Other mechanical complication of heart valve prosthesis**

Obstruction (mechanical) of heart valve prosthesis
Perforation of heart valve prosthesis
Protrusion of heart valve prosthesis

5 **T82.1 Mechanical complication of cardiac electronic device**

6 **T82.11 Breakdown (mechanical) of cardiac electronic device**

SP 7 **T82.110- Breakdown (mechanical) of cardiac electrode**

SP 7 **T82.111- Breakdown (mechanical) of cardiac pulse generator (battery)**

SP 7 **T82.118- Breakdown (mechanical) of other cardiac electronic device**

IQ 7 **T82.119- Breakdown (mechanical) of unspecified cardiac electronic device**

6 **T82.12 Displacement of cardiac electronic device**

Malposition of cardiac electronic device

SP 7 **T82.120- Displacement of cardiac electrode**

SP 7 **T82.121- Displacement of cardiac pulse generator (battery)**

SP 7 **T82.128- Displacement of other cardiac electronic device**

IQ 7 **T82.129- Displacement of unspecified cardiac electronic device**

6 **T82.19 Other mechanical complication of cardiac electronic device**

Leakage of cardiac electronic device
Obstruction of cardiac electronic device
Perforation of cardiac electronic device
Protrusion of cardiac electronic device

SP 7 **T82.190- Other mechanical complication of cardiac electrode**

SP 7 **T82.191- Other mechanical complication of cardiac pulse generator (battery)**

SP 7 **T82.198- Other mechanical complication of other cardiac electronic device**

IQ 7 **T82.199- Other mechanical complication of unspecified cardiac device**

5 **T82.2 Mechanical complication of coronary artery bypass graft and biological heart valve graft**

EXCLUDES 1 mechanical complication of artificial heart valve prosthesis (T82.0-)

CODING TIPS✓ Do not use Z95.5 to indicate presence of a coronary bypass graft when there is a complication of the graft.

6 **T82.21 Mechanical complication of coronary artery bypass graft**

SP 7 **T82.211- Breakdown (mechanical) of coronary artery bypass graft**

SP 7 **T82.212- Displacement of coronary artery bypass graft**
Malposition of coronary artery bypass graft

SP 7 **T82.213- Leakage of coronary artery bypass graft**

SP 7 **T82.218- Other mechanical complication of coronary artery bypass graft**
Obstruction, mechanical of coronary artery bypass graft
Perforation of coronary artery bypass graft
Protrusion of coronary artery bypass graft

6 **T82.22 Mechanical complication of biological heart valve graft**

SP 7 **T82.221- Breakdown (mechanical) of biological heart valve graft**

SP 7 **T82.222- Displacement of biological heart valve graft**
Malposition of biological heart valve graft

SP 7 **T82.223- Leakage of biological heart valve graft**

SP 7 **T82.228- Other mechanical complication of biological heart valve graft**
Obstruction of biological heart valve graft
Perforation of biological heart valve graft
Protrusion of biological heart valve graft

5 **T82.3 Mechanical complication of other vascular grafts**

6 **T82.31 Breakdown (mechanical) of other vascular grafts**

SP 7 **T82.310- Breakdown (mechanical) of aortic (bifurcation) graft (replacement)**

SP 7 **T82.311- Breakdown (mechanical) of carotid arterial graft (bypass)**

SP 7 **T82.312- Breakdown (mechanical) of femoral arterial graft (bypass)**

SP 7 **T82.318- Breakdown (mechanical) of other vascular grafts**

IQ 7 **T82.319- Breakdown (mechanical) of unspecified vascular grafts**

6 **T82.32 Displacement of other vascular grafts**
Malposition of other vascular grafts

SP 7 **T82.320- Displacement of aortic (bifurcation) graft (replacement)**

SP 7 **T82.321- Displacement of carotid arterial graft (bypass)**

SP 7 **T82.322- Displacement of femoral arterial graft (bypass)**

SP 7 **T82.328- Displacement of other vascular grafts**

IQ 7 **T82.329- Displacement of unspecified vascular grafts**

6 **T82.33 Leakage of other vascular grafts**

SP 7 **T82.330- Leakage of aortic (bifurcation) graft (replacement)**

SP 7 **T82.331- Leakage of carotid arterial graft (bypass)**

SP 7 **T82.332- Leakage of femoral arterial graft (bypass)**

SP 7 **T82.338- Leakage of other vascular grafts**

IQ 7 **T82.339- Leakage of unspecified vascular graft**

6 **T82.39 Other mechanical complication of other vascular grafts**
Obstruction (mechanical) of other vascular grafts
Perforation of other vascular grafts
Protrusion of other vascular grafts

SP 7 **T82.390- Other mechanical complication of aortic (bifurcation) graft (replacement)**

SP 7 **T82.391- Other mechanical complication of carotid arterial graft (bypass)**

SP 7 **T82.392- Other mechanical complication of femoral arterial graft (bypass)**

SP 7 **T82.398- Other mechanical complication of other vascular grafts**

IQ 7 **T82.399- Other mechanical complication of unspecified vascular grafts**

5 **T82.4 Mechanical complication of vascular dialysis catheter**
Mechanical complication of hemodialysis catheter

EXCLUDES 1 mechanical complication of intraperitoneal dialysis catheter (T85.62)

CODING TIPS✓ Care for dialysis catheters under the home health benefit is limited to abandoned dialysis catheters. Code the reason that the dialysis catheter cannot be used.

IQ 7 **T82.41X- Breakdown (mechanical) of vascular dialysis catheter**

IQ 7 **T82.42X- Displacement of vascular dialysis catheter**
Malposition of vascular dialysis catheter

IQ 7 **T82.43X- Leakage of vascular dialysis catheter**

IQ 7 **T82.49X- Other complication of vascular dialysis catheter**
Obstruction (mechanical) of vascular dialysis catheter
Perforation of vascular dialysis catheter
Protrusion of vascular dialysis catheter

5 **T82.5 Mechanical complication of other cardiac and vascular devices and implants**

EXCLUDES 2 mechanical complication of epidural and subdural infusion catheter (T85.61)

6 **T82.51 Breakdown (mechanical) of other cardiac and vascular devices and implants**

IQ 7 **T82.510- Breakdown (mechanical) of surgically created arteriovenous fistula**

IQ 7 **T82.511- Breakdown (mechanical) of surgically created arteriovenous shunt**

SP 7 **T82.512- Breakdown (mechanical) of artificial heart**

SP 7 **T82.513- Breakdown (mechanical) of balloon (counterpulsation) device**

SP 7 **T82.514- Breakdown (mechanical) of infusion catheter**

SP 7 **T82.515- Breakdown (mechanical) of umbrella device**

SP 7 **T82.518- Breakdown (mechanical) of other cardiac and vascular devices and implants**

IQ 7 **T82.519- Breakdown (mechanical) of unspecified cardiac and vascular devices and implants**

6 **T82.52 Displacement of other cardiac and vascular devices and implants**

Malposition of other cardiac and vascular devices and implants

IQ 7 **T82.520- Displacement of surgically created arteriovenous fistula**

IQ 7 **T82.521- Displacement of surgically created arteriovenous shunt**

SP 7 **T82.522- Displacement of artificial heart**

SP 7 **T82.523- Displacement of balloon (counterpulsation) device**

SP 7 **T82.524- Displacement of infusion catheter**

SP 7 **T82.525- Displacement of umbrella device**

SP 7 **T82.528- Displacement of other cardiac and vascular devices and implants**

IQ 7 **T82.529- Displacement of unspecified cardiac and vascular devices and implants**

6 **T82.53 Leakage of other cardiac and vascular devices and implants**

IQ 7 **T82.530- Leakage of surgically created arteriovenous fistula**

IQ 7 **T82.531- Leakage of surgically created arteriovenous shunt**

SP 7 **T82.532- Leakage of artificial heart**

SP 7 **T82.533- Leakage of balloon (counterpulsation) device**

SP 7 **T82.534- Leakage of infusion catheter**

SP 7 **T82.535- Leakage of umbrella device**

SP 7 **T82.538- Leakage of other cardiac and vascular devices and implants**

IQ 7 **T82.539- Leakage of unspecified cardiac and vascular devices and implants**

6 **T82.59 Other mechanical complication of other cardiac and vascular devices and implants**

Obstruction (mechanical) of other cardiac and vascular devices and implants

Perforation of other cardiac and vascular devices and implants

Protrusion of other cardiac and vascular devices and implants

IQ 7 **T82.590- Other mechanical complication of surgically created arteriovenous fistula**

IQ 7 **T82.591- Other mechanical complication of surgically created arteriovenous shunt**

SP 7 **T82.592- Other mechanical complication of artificial heart**

SP 7 **T82.593- Other mechanical complication of balloon (counterpulsation) device**

SP 7 **T82.594- Other mechanical complication of infusion catheter**

SP 7 **T82.595- Other mechanical complication of umbrella device**

SP 7 **T82.598- Other mechanical complication of other cardiac and vascular devices and implants**

IQ 7 **T82.599- Other mechanical complication of unspecified cardiac and vascular devices and implants**

SP + 7 **T82.6XX- Infection and inflammatory reaction due to cardiac valve prosthesis**

Use additional code to identify infection

SP + 7 **T82.7XX- Infection and inflammatory reaction due to other cardiac and vascular devices, implants and grafts**

Use additional code to identify infection

5 **T82.8 Other specified complications of cardiac and vascular prosthetic devices, implants and grafts**

6 **T82.81 Embolism due to cardiac and vascular prosthetic devices, implants and grafts**

SP 7 **T82.817- Embolism due to cardiac prosthetic devices, implants and grafts**

SP 7 **T82.818- Embolism due to vascular prosthetic devices, implants and grafts**

6 **T82.82 Fibrosis due to cardiac and vascular prosthetic devices, implants and grafts**

SP 7 **T82.827- Fibrosis due to cardiac prosthetic devices, implants and grafts**

SP 7 **T82.828- Fibrosis due to vascular prosthetic devices, implants and grafts**

6 **T82.83 Hemorrhage due to cardiac and vascular prosthetic devices, implants and grafts**

SP 7 **T82.837- Hemorrhage due to cardiac prosthetic devices, implants and grafts**

SP 7 **T82.838- Hemorrhage due to vascular prosthetic devices, implants and grafts**

6 **T82.84 Pain due to cardiac and vascular prosthetic devices, implants and grafts**

SP 7 **T82.847- Pain due to cardiac prosthetic devices, implants and grafts**

SP 7 **T82.848- Pain due to vascular prosthetic devices, implants and grafts**

6 **T82.85 Stenosis due to cardiac and vascular prosthetic devices, implants and grafts**

Chapter 19

S00-T88

CODING TIPS✓ Approximately 30% of peripheral and bare metal coronary stents will restenose within a year of placement. This condition is variously called restenosis of stent, in-stent stenosis or in-stent restenosis (ISR). The area of in-stent stenosis has a different makeup than is seen in native areas of atherosclerotic plaque and vessel stenosis.

SP 7 **T82.855- Stenosis of coronary artery stent**
In-stent stenosis (restenosis) of coronary artery stent
Restenosis of coronary artery stent

SP 7 **T82.856- Stenosis of peripheral vascular stent**
In-stent stenosis (restenosis) of peripheral vascular stent
Restenosis of peripheral vascular stent

SP 7 **T82.857- Stenosis of other cardiac prosthetic devices, implants and grafts**

SP 7 **T82.858- Stenosis of other vascular prosthetic devices, implants and grafts**

6 **T82.86 Thrombosis of cardiac and vascular prosthetic devices, implants and grafts**

SP 7 **T82.867- Thrombosis due to cardiac prosthetic devices, implants and grafts**

SP 7 **T82.868- Thrombosis due to vascular prosthetic devices, implants and grafts**

6 **T82.89 Other specified complication of cardiac and vascular prosthetic devices, implants and grafts**

SP 7 **T82.897- Other specified complication of cardiac prosthetic devices, implants and grafts**

SP 7 **T82.898- Other specified complication of vascular prosthetic devices, implants and grafts**

IQ 7 **T82.9XX- Unspecified complication of cardiac and vascular prosthetic device, implant and graft**

4 **T83 Complications of genitourinary prosthetic devices, implants and grafts**

EXCLUDES 2 failure and rejection of transplanted organs and tissue (T86.-)

The appropriate 7th character is to be added to each code from category T83
A initial encounter
D subsequent encounter
S sequela

CODING TIPS✓ No aftercare code applies, including dressing changes, drain care, and suture removal. 7th character 'D' is the default for home care and hospice when providing aftercare for a healing or resolving condition; 'A' is used for active treatment such as antibiotics or more than routine wound care; 'S' may be used to indicate a residual condition after the original injury has healed. Once complication is repaired in the acute setting, continue to code the complication in home care and hospice with 7th character D if healing/resolving.

5 **T83.0 Mechanical complication of urinary catheter**

EXCLUDES 2 complications of stoma of urinary tract (N99.5-)

CODING TIPS✓ These codes are for mechanical complications of urinary catheters of all kinds. They may be coded with the complication of stoma code, as applicable (N99.5-). Do not use Z46.6 when a complication of the urinary catheter is documented.

6 **T83.01 Breakdown (mechanical) of urinary catheter**

SP 7 **T83.010- Breakdown (mechanical) of cystostomy catheter**

SP 7 **T83.011- Breakdown (mechanical) of indwelling urethral catheter**

SP 7 **T83.012- Breakdown (mechanical) of nephrostomy catheter**

SP 7 **T83.018- Breakdown (mechanical) of other urinary catheter**
Breakdown (mechanical) of Hopkins catheter
Breakdown (mechanical) of ileostomy catheter
Breakdown (mechanical) urostomy catheter

6 **T83.02 Displacement of urinary catheter**
Malposition of urinary catheter

SP 7 **T83.020- Displacement of cystostomy catheter**

SP 7 **T83.021- Displacement of indwelling urethral catheter**

SP 7 **T83.022- Displacement of nephrostomy catheter**

SP 7 **T83.028- Displacement of other urinary catheter**
Displacement of Hopkins catheter
Displacement of ileostomy catheter
Displacement of urostomy catheter

6 **T83.03 Leakage of urinary catheter**

SP 7 **T83.030- Leakage of cystostomy catheter**

SP 7 **T83.031- Leakage of indwelling urethral catheter**

SP 7 **T83.032- Leakage of nephrostomy catheter**

SP 7 **T83.038- Leakage of other urinary catheter**
Leakage of Hopkins catheter
Leakage of ileostomy catheter
Leakage of urostomy catheter

6 **T83.09 Other mechanical complication of urinary catheter**

Chapter 19

S00-T88

Obstruction (mechanical) of urinary catheter
Perforation of urinary catheter
Protrusion of urinary catheter

SP 7 **T83.090- Other mechanical complication of cystostomy catheter**

SP 7 **T83.091- Other mechanical complication of indwelling urethral catheter**

SP 7 **T83.092- Other mechanical complication of nephrostomy catheter**

SP 7 **T83.098- Other mechanical complication of other urinary catheter**
Other mechanical complication of Hopkins catheter
Other mechanical complication of ileostomy catheter
Other mechanical complication of urostomy catheter

5 **T83.1 Mechanical complication of other urinary devices and implants**

6 **T83.11 Breakdown (mechanical) of other urinary devices and implants**

SP 7 **T83.110- Breakdown (mechanical) of urinary electronic stimulator device**
EXCLUDES 2 Breakdown (mechanical) of electrode (lead) for sacral nerve neurostimulator (T85.111)
Breakdown (mechanical) of implanted electronic sacral neurostimulator, pulse generator or receiver (T85.113)

SP 7 **T83.111- Breakdown (mechanical) of implanted urinary sphincter**

SP 7 **T83.112- Breakdown (mechanical) of indwelling ureteral stent**

SP 7 **T83.113- Breakdown (mechanical) of other urinary stents**
Breakdown (mechanical) of ileal conduit stent
Breakdown (mechanical) of nephroureteral stent

SP 7 **T83.118- Breakdown (mechanical) of other urinary devices and implants**

6 **T83.12 Displacement of other urinary devices and implants**
Malposition of other urinary devices and implants

SP 7 **T83.120- Displacement of urinary electronic stimulator device**
EXCLUDES 2 Displacement of electrode (lead) for sacral nerve neurostimulator (T85.121)
Displacement of implanted electronic sacral neurostimulator, pulse generator or receiver (T85.123)

SP 7 **T83.121- Displacement of implanted urinary sphincter**

SP 7 **T83.122- Displacement of indwelling ureteral stent**

SP 7 **T83.123- Displacement of other urinary stents**
Displacement of ileal conduit stent
Displacement of nephroureteral stent

SP 7 **T83.128- Displacement of other urinary devices and implants**

6 **T83.19 Other mechanical complication of other urinary devices and implants**
Leakage of other urinary devices and implants
Obstruction (mechanical) of other urinary devices and implants
Perforation of other urinary devices and implants
Protrusion of other urinary devices and implants

SP 7 **T83.190- Other mechanical complication of urinary electronic stimulator device**
EXCLUDES 2 Other mechanical complication of electrode (lead) for sacral nerve neurostimulator (T85.191)
Other mechanical complication of implanted electronic sacral neurostimulator, pulse generator or receiver (T85.193)

SP 7 **T83.191- Other mechanical complication of implanted urinary sphincter**

SP 7 **T83.192- Other mechanical complication of indwelling ureteral stent**

SP 7 **T83.193- Other mechanical complication of other urinary stent**
Other mechanical complication of ileal conduit stent
Other mechanical complication of nephroureteral stent

SP 7 **T83.198- Other mechanical complication of other urinary devices and implants**

5 **T83.2 Mechanical complication of graft of urinary organ**

SP 7 **T83.21X- Breakdown (mechanical) of graft of urinary organ**

SP 7 **T83.22X- Displacement of graft of urinary organ**
Malposition of graft of urinary organ

SP 7 **T83.23X- Leakage of graft of urinary organ**

SP 7 **T83.24X- Erosion of graft of urinary organ**

SP 7 **T83.25X- Exposure of graft of urinary organ**

SP 7 **T83.29X- Other mechanical complication of graft of urinary organ**
Obstruction (mechanical) of graft of urinary organ
Perforation of graft of urinary organ
Protrusion of graft of urinary organ

5 **T83.3 Mechanical complication of intrauterine contraceptive device**

SP 7 **T83.31X- Breakdown (mechanical) of intrauterine contraceptive device**

SP 7 **T83.32X- Displacement of intrauterine contraceptive device**
Malposition of intrauterine contraceptive device
Missing string of intrauterine contraceptive device

SP 7 **T83.39X- Other mechanical complication of intrauterine contraceptive device**
Leakage of intrauterine contraceptive device
Obstruction (mechanical) of intrauterine contraceptive device
Perforation of intrauterine contraceptive device
Protrusion of intrauterine contraceptive device

5 **T83.4 Mechanical complication of other prosthetic devices, implants and grafts of genital tract**

6 **T83.41 Breakdown (mechanical) of other prosthetic devices, implants and grafts of genital tract**

SP 7 **T83.410- Breakdown (mechanical) of implanted penile prosthesis**
Breakdown (mechanical) of penile prosthesis cylinder
Breakdown (mechanical) of penile prosthesis pump
Breakdown (mechanical) of penile prosthesis reservoir

SP 7 **T83.411- Breakdown (mechanical) of implanted testicular prosthesis**

SP 7 **T83.418- Breakdown (mechanical) of other prosthetic devices, implants and grafts of genital tract**

6 **T83.42 Displacement of other prosthetic devices, implants and grafts of genital tract**
Malposition of other prosthetic devices, implants and grafts of genital tract

SP 7 **T83.420- Displacement of implanted penile prosthesis**
Displacement of penile prosthesis cylinder
Displacement of penile prosthesis pump
Displacement of penile prosthesis reservoir

SP 7 **T83.421- Displacement of implanted testicular prosthesis**

SP 7 **T83.428- Displacement of other prosthetic devices, implants and grafts of genital tract**

6 **T83.49 Other mechanical complication of other prosthetic devices, implants and grafts of genital tract**
Leakage of other prosthetic devices, implants and grafts of genital tract
Obstruction, mechanical of other prosthetic devices, implants and grafts of genital tract
Perforation of other prosthetic devices, implants and grafts of genital tract
Protrusion of other prosthetic devices, implants and grafts of genital tract

SP 7 **T83.490- Other mechanical complication of implanted penile prosthesis**
Other mechanical complication of penile prosthesis cylinder
Other mechanical complication of penile prosthesis pump
Other mechanical complication of penile prosthesis reservoir

SP 7 **T83.491- Other mechanical complication of implanted testicular prosthesis**

SP 7 **T83.498- Other mechanical complication of other prosthetic devices, implants and grafts of genital tract**

+ 5 **T83.5 Infection and inflammatory reaction due to prosthetic device, implant and graft in urinary system**
Use additional code to identify infection

CODING TIPS ✓ Do not use Z43 or Z93 codes for routine care when a complication is documented.

+ 6 **T83.51 Infection and inflammatory reaction due to urinary catheter**
EXCLUDES 2 complications of stoma of urinary tract (N99.5-)

SP + 7 **T83.510- Infection and inflammatory reaction due to cystostomy catheter**

SP + 7 **T83.511- Infection and inflammatory reaction due to indwelling urethral catheter**

SP + 7 **T83.512- Infection and inflammatory reaction due to nephrostomy catheter**

SP + 7 **T83.518- Infection and inflammatory reaction due to other urinary catheter**
Infection and inflammatory reaction due to Hopkins catheter
Infection and inflammatory reaction due to ileostomy catheter
Infection and inflammatory reaction due to urostomy catheter

+ 6 **T83.59 Infection and inflammatory reaction due to prosthetic device, implant and graft in urinary system**

SP + 7 **T83.590- Infection and inflammatory reaction due to implanted urinary neurostimulation device**
EXCLUDES 2 Infection and inflammatory reaction due to electrode lead of sacral nerve neurostimulator (T85.732)
Infection and inflammatory reaction due to pulse generator or receiver of sacral nerve neurostimulator (T85.734)

SP + 7 **T83.591- Infection and inflammatory reaction due to implanted urinary sphincter**

Chapter 19 S00-T88

SP + 7 **T83.592- Infection and inflammatory reaction due to indwelling ureteral stent**

SP + 7 **T83.593- Infection and inflammatory reaction due to other urinary stents**
Infection and inflammatory reaction due to ileal conduit stents
Infection and inflammatory reaction due to nephroureteral stent

SP + 7 **T83.598- Infection and inflammatory reaction due to other prosthetic device, implant and graft in urinary system**

+ 5 **T83.6 Infection and inflammatory reaction due to prosthetic device, implant and graft in genital tract**
Use additional code to identify infection

SP + 7 **T83.61X- Infection and inflammatory reaction due to implanted penile prosthesis**
Infection and inflammatory reaction due to penile prosthesis cylinder
Infection and inflammatory reaction due to penile prosthesis pump
Infection and inflammatory reaction due to penile prosthesis reservoir

SP + 7 **T83.62X- Infection and inflammatory reaction due to implanted testicular prosthesis**

SP + 7 **T83.69X- Infection and inflammatory reaction due to other prosthetic device, implant and graft in genital tract**

5 **T83.7 Complications due to implanted mesh and other prosthetic materials**

6 **T83.71 Erosion of implanted mesh and other prosthetic materials to surrounding organ or tissue**

SP 7 **T83.711- Erosion of implanted vaginal mesh to surrounding organ or tissue**
Erosion of implanted vaginal mesh into pelvic floor muscles

SP 7 **T83.712- Erosion of implanted urethral mesh to surrounding organ or tissue**
Erosion of implanted female urethral sling
Erosion of implanted male urethral sling
Erosion of implanted urethral mesh into pelvic floor muscles

SP 7 **T83.713- Erosion of implanted urethral bulking agent to surrounding organ or tissue**

SP 7 **T83.714- Erosion of implanted ureteral bulking agent to surrounding organ or tissue**

SP 7 **T83.718- Erosion of other implanted mesh to organ or tissue**

SP 7 **T83.719- Erosion of other prosthetic materials to surrounding organ or tissue**

6 **T83.72 Exposure of implanted mesh and other prosthetic materials into surrounding organ or tissue**
Extrusion of implanted mesh

SP 7 **T83.721- Exposure of implanted vaginal mesh into vagina**
Exposure of implanted vaginal mesh through vaginal wall

SP 7 **T83.722- Exposure of implanted urethral mesh into urethra**
Exposure of implanted female urethral sling
Exposure of implanted male urethral sling
Exposure of implanted urethral mesh through urethral wall

SP 7 **T83.723- Exposure of implanted urethral bulking agent into urethra**

SP 7 **T83.724- Exposure of implanted ureteral bulking agent into ureter**

SP 7 **T83.728- Exposure of other implanted mesh into organ or tissue**

SP 7 **T83.729- Exposure of other prosthetic materials into organ or tissue**

SP 7 **T83.79X- Other specified complications due to other genitourinary prosthetic materials**

5 **T83.8 Other specified complications of genitourinary prosthetic devices, implants and grafts**

SP 7 **T83.81X- Embolism due to genitourinary prosthetic devices, implants and grafts**

SP 7 **T83.82X- Fibrosis due to genitourinary prosthetic devices, implants and grafts**

SP 7 **T83.83X- Hemorrhage due to genitourinary prosthetic devices, implants and grafts**

SP 7 **T83.84X- Pain due to genitourinary prosthetic devices, implants and grafts**

SP 7 **T83.85X- Stenosis due to genitourinary prosthetic devices, implants and grafts**

SP 7 **T83.86X- Thrombosis due to genitourinary prosthetic devices, implants and grafts**

SP 7 **T83.89X- Other specified complication of genitourinary prosthetic devices, implants and grafts**

IQ 7 **T83.9XX- Unspecified complication of genitourinary prosthetic device, implant and graft**

4 **T84 Complications of internal orthopedic prosthetic devices, implants and grafts**
EXCLUDES 2 failure and rejection of transplanted organs and tissues (T86.-)
fracture of bone following insertion of orthopedic implant, joint prosthesis or bone plate (M96.6)

The appropriate 7th character is to be added to each code from category T84
A initial encounter
D subsequent encounter
S sequela

Chapter 19

S00-T88

CODING TIPS ✓ Code T84 includes all of the complications of orthopedic prostheses, implants and grafts. Most of these codes indicate the joint affected so there is no need to add the Z96.6- code to indicate the prosthesis. Periprosthetic fractures are no longer considered complications and can be found in M97.

CODING TIPS ✓ No aftercare code applies, including dressing changes, drain care, and suture removal. 7th character 'D' is the default for home care and hospice when providing aftercare for a healing or resolving condition; 'A' is used for active treatment such as antibiotics or more than routine wound care; 'S' may be used to indicate a residual condition after the original injury has healed. Once complication is repaired in the acute setting, continue to code the complication in home care and hospice with 7th character D if healing/resolving.

5 T84.0 Mechanical complication of internal joint prosthesis

CODING TIPS ✓ This subcategory includes complications of internal prosthetic joints. Most include the joint affected, so there is no need to add Z96.6 for the joint unless the complication code does not indicate the joint.

6 T84.01 Broken internal joint prosthesis
Breakage (fracture) of prosthetic joint
Broken prosthetic joint implant
EXCLUDES 1 periprosthetic joint implant fracture (M97.-)

H SP 7 **T84.010- Broken internal right hip prosthesis**

H SP 7 **T84.011- Broken internal left hip prosthesis**

H SP 7 **T84.012- Broken internal right knee prosthesis**

H SP 7 **T84.013- Broken internal left knee prosthesis**

H SP + 7 **T84.018- Broken internal joint prosthesis, other site**
Use additional code to identify the joint (Z96.6-)

H IQ 7 **T84.019- Broken internal joint prosthesis, unspecified site**

6 T84.02 Dislocation of internal joint prosthesis
Instability of internal joint prosthesis
Subluxation of internal joint prosthesis

H SP 7 **T84.020- Dislocation of internal right hip prosthesis**

H SP 7 **T84.021- Dislocation of internal left hip prosthesis**

H SP 7 **T84.022- Instability of internal right knee prosthesis**

H SP 7 **T84.023- Instability of internal left knee prosthesis**

H SP + 7 **T84.028- Dislocation of other internal joint prosthesis**
Use additional code to identify the joint (Z96.6-)

H IQ 7 **T84.029- Dislocation of unspecified internal joint prosthesis**

6 T84.03 Mechanical loosening of internal prosthetic joint
Aseptic loosening of prosthetic joint

H SP 7 **T84.030- Mechanical loosening of internal right hip prosthetic joint**

H SP 7 **T84.031- Mechanical loosening of internal left hip prosthetic joint**

H SP 7 **T84.032- Mechanical loosening of internal right knee prosthetic joint**

H SP 7 **T84.033- Mechanical loosening of internal left knee prosthetic joint**

H SP + 7 **T84.038- Mechanical loosening of other internal prosthetic joint**
Use additional code to identify the joint (Z96.6-)

H IQ 7 **T84.039- Mechanical loosening of unspecified internal prosthetic joint**

+ **6 T84.05 Periprosthetic osteolysis of internal prosthetic joint**
Use additional code to identify major osseous defect, if applicable (M89.7-)

H SP + 7 **T84.050- Periprosthetic osteolysis of internal prosthetic right hip joint**

H SP + 7 **T84.051- Periprosthetic osteolysis of internal prosthetic left hip joint**

H SP + 7 **T84.052- Periprosthetic osteolysis of internal prosthetic right knee joint**

H SP + 7 **T84.053- Periprosthetic osteolysis of internal prosthetic left knee joint**

H SP + 7 **T84.058- Periprosthetic osteolysis of other internal prosthetic joint**
Use additional code to identify the joint (Z96.6-)

H IQ + 7 **T84.059- Periprosthetic osteolysis of unspecified internal prosthetic joint**

6 T84.06 Wear of articular bearing surface of internal prosthetic joint

H SP 7 **T84.060- Wear of articular bearing surface of internal prosthetic right hip joint**

H SP 7 **T84.061- Wear of articular bearing surface of internal prosthetic left hip joint**

H SP 7 **T84.062- Wear of articular bearing surface of internal prosthetic right knee joint**

H SP 7 **T84.063- Wear of articular bearing surface of internal prosthetic left knee joint**

H SP + 7 **T84.068- Wear of articular bearing surface of other internal prosthetic joint**
Use additional code to identify the joint (Z96.6-)

H IQ 7 **T84.069- Wear of articular bearing surface of unspecified internal prosthetic joint**

6 T84.09 Other mechanical complication of internal joint prosthesis
Prosthetic joint implant failure NOS

H SP 7 **T84.090- Other mechanical complication of internal right hip prosthesis**

H SP 7 **T84.091- Other mechanical complication of internal left hip prosthesis**

Chapter 19 S00-T88

T84.092- Other mechanical complication of internal right knee prosthesis
T84.093- Other mechanical complication of internal left knee prosthesis
T84.098- Other mechanical complication of other internal joint prosthesis
Use additional code to identify the joint (Z96.6-)
T84.099- Other mechanical complication of unspecified internal joint prosthesis

T84.1 Mechanical complication of internal fixation device of bones of limb
EXCLUDES 2 mechanical complication of internal fixation device of bones of feet (T84.2-)
mechanical complication of internal fixation device of bones of fingers (T84.2-)
mechanical complication of internal fixation device of bones of hands (T84.2-)
mechanical complication of internal fixation device of bones of toes (T84.2-)

T84.11 Breakdown (mechanical) of internal fixation device of bones of limb
T84.110- Breakdown (mechanical) of internal fixation device of right humerus
T84.111- Breakdown (mechanical) of internal fixation device of left humerus
T84.112- Breakdown (mechanical) of internal fixation device of bone of right forearm
T84.113- Breakdown (mechanical) of internal fixation device of bone of left forearm
T84.114- Breakdown (mechanical) of internal fixation device of right femur
T84.115- Breakdown (mechanical) of internal fixation device of left femur
T84.116- Breakdown (mechanical) of internal fixation device of bone of right lower leg
T84.117- Breakdown (mechanical) of internal fixation device of bone of left lower leg
T84.119- Breakdown (mechanical) of internal fixation device of unspecified bone of limb

T84.12 Displacement of internal fixation device of bones of limb
Malposition of internal fixation device of bones of limb
T84.120- Displacement of internal fixation device of right humerus
T84.121- Displacement of internal fixation device of left humerus
T84.122- Displacement of internal fixation device of bone of right forearm
T84.123- Displacement of internal fixation device of bone of left forearm
T84.124- Displacement of internal fixation device of right femur
T84.125- Displacement of internal fixation device of left femur
T84.126- Displacement of internal fixation device of bone of right lower leg
T84.127- Displacement of internal fixation device of bone of left lower leg
T84.129- Displacement of internal fixation device of unspecified bone of limb

T84.19 Other mechanical complication of internal fixation device of bones of limb
Obstruction (mechanical) of internal fixation device of bones of limb
Perforation of internal fixation device of bones of limb
Protrusion of internal fixation device of bones of limb
T84.190- Other mechanical complication of internal fixation device of right humerus
T84.191- Other mechanical complication of internal fixation device of left humerus
T84.192- Other mechanical complication of internal fixation device of bone of right forearm
T84.193- Other mechanical complication of internal fixation device of bone of left forearm
T84.194- Other mechanical complication of internal fixation device of right femur
T84.195- Other mechanical complication of internal fixation device of left femur
T84.196- Other mechanical complication of internal fixation device of bone of right lower leg
T84.197- Other mechanical complication of internal fixation device of bone of left lower leg
T84.199- Other mechanical complication of internal fixation device of unspecified bone of limb

T84.2 Mechanical complication of internal fixation device of other bones
T84.21 Breakdown (mechanical) of internal fixation device of other bones
T84.210- Breakdown (mechanical) of internal fixation device of bones of hand and fingers
T84.213- Breakdown (mechanical) of internal fixation device of bones of foot and toes
T84.216- Breakdown (mechanical) of internal fixation device of vertebrae
T84.218- Breakdown (mechanical) of internal fixation device of other bones
T84.22 Displacement of internal fixation device of other bones
Malposition of internal fixation device of other bones
T84.220- Displacement of internal fixation device of bones of hand and fingers

Chapter 19 S00-T88

4 4th digit required 5 5th digit required 6 6th digit required 7 7th digit required 7 7th digit placeholder + Additional code Laterality

SP 7 **T84.223- Displacement of internal fixation device of bones of foot and toes**

SP 7 **T84.226- Displacement of internal fixation device of vertebrae**

SP 7 **T84.228- Displacement of internal fixation device of other bones**

6 **T84.29 Other mechanical complication of internal fixation device of other bones**
Obstruction (mechanical) of internal fixation device of other bones
Perforation of internal fixation device of other bones
Protrusion of internal fixation device of other bones

SP 7 **T84.290- Other mechanical complication of internal fixation device of bones of hand and fingers**

SP 7 **T84.293- Other mechanical complication of internal fixation device of bones of foot and toes**

SP 7 **T84.296- Other mechanical complication of internal fixation device of vertebrae**

SP 7 **T84.298- Other mechanical complication of internal fixation device of other bones**

5 **T84.3 Mechanical complication of other bone devices, implants and grafts**
EXCLUDES 2 other complications of bone graft (T86.83-)

6 **T84.31 Breakdown (mechanical) of other bone devices, implants and grafts**

SP 7 **T84.310- Breakdown (mechanical) of electronic bone stimulator**

SP 7 **T84.318- Breakdown (mechanical) of other bone devices, implants and grafts**

6 **T84.32 Displacement of other bone devices, implants and grafts**
Malposition of other bone devices, implants and grafts

SP 7 **T84.320- Displacement of electronic bone stimulator**

SP 7 **T84.328- Displacement of other bone devices, implants and grafts**

6 **T84.39 Other mechanical complication of other bone devices, implants and grafts**
Obstruction (mechanical) of other bone devices, implants and grafts
Perforation of other bone devices, implants and grafts
Protrusion of other bone devices, implants and grafts

SP 7 **T84.390- Other mechanical complication of electronic bone stimulator**

SP 7 **T84.398- Other mechanical complication of other bone devices, implants and grafts**

5 **T84.4 Mechanical complication of other internal orthopedic devices, implants and grafts**

6 **T84.41 Breakdown (mechanical) of other internal orthopedic devices, implants and grafts**

SP 7 **T84.410- Breakdown (mechanical) of muscle and tendon graft**

SP 7 **T84.418- Breakdown (mechanical) of other internal orthopedic devices, implants and grafts**

6 **T84.42 Displacement of other internal orthopedic devices, implants and grafts**
Malposition of other internal orthopedic devices, implants and grafts

SP 7 **T84.420- Displacement of muscle and tendon graft**

SP 7 **T84.428- Displacement of other internal orthopedic devices, implants and grafts**

6 **T84.49 Other mechanical complication of other internal orthopedic devices, implants and grafts**
Mechanical complication of other internal orthopedic devices, implants and grafts NOS
Obstruction (mechanical) of other internal orthopedic devices, implants and grafts
Perforation of other internal orthopedic devices, implants and grafts
Protrusion of other internal orthopedic devices, implants and grafts

SP 7 **T84.490- Other mechanical complication of muscle and tendon graft**

SP 7 **T84.498- Other mechanical complication of other internal orthopedic devices, implants and grafts**

+ 5 **T84.5 Infection and inflammatory reaction due to internal joint prosthesis**
Use additional code to identify infection

CODING TIPS ✓ If wound care is the focus of care for infection complications of prostheses, devices, implants and grafts, assign T84.89 first.

CODING TIPS ✓ If septic joint or septic arthritis is documented, use an additional code from M00.- to identify the organism.

IQ + 7 **T84.50X- Infection and inflammatory reaction due to unspecified internal joint prosthesis**

SP + 7 **T84.51X- Infection and inflammatory reaction due to internal right hip prosthesis**

SP + 7 **T84.52X- Infection and inflammatory reaction due to internal left hip prosthesis**

SP + 7 **T84.53X- Infection and inflammatory reaction due to internal right knee prosthesis**

SP + 7 **T84.54X- Infection and inflammatory reaction due to internal left knee prosthesis**

SP + 7 **T84.59X- Infection and inflammatory reaction due to other internal joint prosthesis**

+ 5 **T84.6 Infection and inflammatory reaction due to internal fixation device**
Use additional code to identify infection

CODING TIPS ✓ If wound care is the focus of care for infection complications of prostheses, devices, implants and grafts, assign T84.89 first.

Chapter 19 S00-T88

IQ + 7 **T84.60X- Infection and inflammatory reaction due to internal fixation device of unspecified site**

+ 6 **T84.61 Infection and inflammatory reaction due to internal fixation device of arm**

L SP + 7 **T84.610- Infection and inflammatory reaction due to internal fixation device of right humerus**

L SP + 7 **T84.611- Infection and inflammatory reaction due to internal fixation device of left humerus**

L SP + 7 **T84.612- Infection and inflammatory reaction due to internal fixation device of right radius**

L SP + 7 **T84.613- Infection and inflammatory reaction due to internal fixation device of left radius**

L SP + 7 **T84.614- Infection and inflammatory reaction due to internal fixation device of right ulna**

L SP + 7 **T84.615- Infection and inflammatory reaction due to internal fixation device of left ulna**

L IQ + 7 **T84.619- Infection and inflammatory reaction due to internal fixation device of unspecified bone of arm**

+ 6 **T84.62 Infection and inflammatory reaction due to internal fixation device of leg**

L SP + 7 **T84.620- Infection and inflammatory reaction due to internal fixation device of right femur**

L SP + 7 **T84.621- Infection and inflammatory reaction due to internal fixation device of left femur**

L SP + 7 **T84.622- Infection and inflammatory reaction due to internal fixation device of right tibia**

L SP + 7 **T84.623- Infection and inflammatory reaction due to internal fixation device of left tibia**

L SP + 7 **T84.624- Infection and inflammatory reaction due to internal fixation device of right fibula**

L SP IQ + 7 **T84.625- Infection and inflammatory reaction due to internal fixation device of left fibula**

L IQ + 7 **T84.629- Infection and inflammatory reaction due to internal fixation device of unspecified bone of leg**

SP + 7 **T84.63X- Infection and inflammatory reaction due to internal fixation device of spine**

SP + 7 **T84.69X- Infection and inflammatory reaction due to internal fixation device of other site**

SP + 7 **T84.7XX- Infection and inflammatory reaction due to other internal orthopedic prosthetic devices, implants and grafts**

Use additional code to identify infection

CODING TIPS✓ If wound care is the focus of care for infection complications of prostheses, devices, implants and grafts, assign T84.89 first.

5 **T84.8 Other specified complications of internal orthopedic prosthetic devices, implants and grafts**

SP 7 **T84.81X- Embolism due to internal orthopedic prosthetic devices, implants and grafts**

SP 7 **T84.82X- Fibrosis due to internal orthopedic prosthetic devices, implants and grafts**

SP 7 **T84.83X- Hemorrhage due to internal orthopedic prosthetic devices, implants and grafts**

SP 7 **T84.84X- Pain due to internal orthopedic prosthetic devices, implants and grafts**

CODING TIPS✓ A G89.- code may be added to indicate the nature of the pain, e.g. post surgical vs traumatic, and acute vs chronic.

SP 7 **T84.85X- Stenosis due to internal orthopedic prosthetic devices, implants and grafts**

SP 7 **T84.86X- Thrombosis due to internal orthopedic prosthetic devices, implants and grafts**

SP 7 **T84.89X- Other specified complication of internal orthopedic prosthetic devices, implants and grafts**

IQ 7 **T84.9XX- Unspecified complication of internal orthopedic prosthetic device, implant and graft**

4 **T85 Complications of other internal prosthetic devices, implants and grafts**

EXCLUDES 2 failure and rejection of transplanted organs and tissue (T86.-)

The appropriate 7th character is to be added to each code from category T85

A	initial encounter
D	subsequent encounter
S	sequela

CODING TIPS✓ No aftercare code applies, including dressing changes, drain care, and suture removal. 7th character 'D' is the default for home care and hospice when providing aftercare for a healing or resolving condition; 'A' is used for active treatment such as antibiotics or more than routine wound care; 'S' may be used to indicate a residual condition after the original injury has healed. Once complication is repaired in the acute setting, continue to code the complication in home care and hospice with 7th character D if healing/resolving.

5 **T85.0 Mechanical complication of ventricular intracranial (communicating) shunt**

CODING TIPS✓ Do not use Z98.2 to indicate presence of a ventricular shunt when there is a complication of the shunt.

SP 7 **T85.01X- Breakdown (mechanical) of ventricular intracranial (communicating) shunt**

SP 7 **T85.02X- Displacement of ventricular intracranial (communicating) shunt**

Malposition of ventricular intracranial (communicating) shunt

Chapter 19 S00-T88

4 4th digit required 5 5th digit required 6 6th digit required 7 7th digit required 7 7th digit placeholder + Additional code L Laterality

SP 7 **T85.03X- Leakage of ventricular intracranial (communicating) shunt**

SP 7 **T85.09X- Other mechanical complication of ventricular intracranial (communicating) shunt**
Obstruction (mechanical) of ventricular intracranial (communicating) shunt
Perforation of ventricular intracranial (communicating) shunt
Protrusion of ventricular intracranial (communicating) shunt

5 **T85.1 Mechanical complication of implanted electronic stimulator of nervous system**

6 **T85.11 Breakdown (mechanical) of implanted electronic stimulator of nervous system**

SP 7 **T85.110- Breakdown (mechanical) of implanted electronic neurostimulator of brain electrode (lead)**

SP 7 **T85.111- Breakdown (mechanical) of implanted electronic neurostimulator of peripheral nerve electrode (lead)**
Breakdown of electrode (lead) for cranial nerve neurostimulators
Breakdown of electrode (lead) for gastric neurostimulator
Breakdown of electrode (lead) for sacral nerve neurostimulator
Breakdown of electrode (lead) for vagal nerve neurostimulators

SP 7 **T85.112- Breakdown (mechanical) of implanted electronic neurostimulator of spinal cord electrode (lead)**

SP 7 **T85.113- Breakdown (mechanical) of implanted electronic neurostimulator, generator**
Breakdown (mechanical) of implanted electronic neurostimulator generator, brain, peripheral, gastric, spinal
Breakdown (mechanical) of implanted electronic sacral neurostimulator, pulse generator or receiver

SP 7 **T85.118- Breakdown (mechanical) of other implanted electronic stimulator of nervous system**

6 **T85.12 Displacement of implanted electronic stimulator of nervous system**
Malposition of implanted electronic stimulator of nervous system

SP 7 **T85.120- Displacement of implanted electronic neurostimulator of brain electrode (lead)**

SP 7 **T85.121- Displacement of implanted electronic neurostimulator of peripheral nerve electrode (lead)**
Displacement of electrode (lead) for cranial nerve neurostimulators
Displacement of electrode (lead) for gastric neurostimulator
Displacement of electrode (lead) for sacral nerve neurostimulator
Displacement of electrode (lead) for vagal nerve neurostimulators

SP 7 **T85.122- Displacement of implanted electronic neurostimulator of spinal cord electrode (lead)**

SP 7 **T85.123- Displacement of implanted electronic neurostimulator, generator**
Displacement of implanted electronic neurostimulator generator, brain, peripheral, gastric, spinal
Displacement of implanted electronic sacral neurostimulator, pulse generator or receiver

SP 7 **T85.128- Displacement of other implanted electronic stimulator of nervous system**

6 **T85.19 Other mechanical complication of implanted electronic stimulator of nervous system**
Leakage of implanted electronic stimulator of nervous system
Obstruction (mechanical) of implanted electronic stimulator of nervous system
Perforation of implanted electronic stimulator of nervous system
Protrusion of implanted electronic stimulator of nervous system

SP 7 **T85.190- Other mechanical complication of implanted electronic neurostimulator of brain electrode (lead)**

SP 7 **T85.191- Other mechanical complication of implanted electronic neurostimulator of peripheral nerve electrode (lead)**
Other mechanical complication of electrode (lead) for cranial nerve neurostimulators
Other mechanical complication of electrode (lead) for gastric neurostimulator
Other mechanical complication of electrode (lead) for sacral nerve neurostimulator
Other mechanical complication of electrode (lead) for vagal nerve neurostimulators

SP 7 **T85.192- Other mechanical complication of implanted electronic neurostimulator of spinal cord electrode (lead)**

SP 7 **T85.193- Other mechanical complication of implanted electronic neurostimulator, generator**
Other mechanical complication of implanted electronic neurostimulator generator, brain, peripheral, gastric, spinal
Other mechanical complication of implanted electronic sacral neurostimulator, pulse generator or receiver

SP 7 **T85.199- Other mechanical complication of other implanted electronic stimulator of nervous system**

Chapter 19 S00-T88

5 **T85.2 Mechanical complication of intraocular lens**

SP 7 **T85.21X- Breakdown (mechanical) of intraocular lens**

SP 7 **T85.22X- Displacement of intraocular lens**
Malposition of intraocular lens

SP 7 **T85.29X- Other mechanical complication of intraocular lens**
Obstruction (mechanical) of intraocular lens
Perforation of intraocular lens
Protrusion of intraocular lens

5 **T85.3 Mechanical complication of other ocular prosthetic devices, implants and grafts**
EXCLUDES 2 other complications of corneal graft (T86.84-)

6 **T85.31 Breakdown (mechanical) of other ocular prosthetic devices, implants and grafts**

Laterality SP 7 **T85.310- Breakdown (mechanical) of prosthetic orbit of right eye**

Laterality SP 7 **T85.311- Breakdown (mechanical) of prosthetic orbit of left eye**

Laterality SP 7 **T85.318- Breakdown (mechanical) of other ocular prosthetic devices, implants and grafts**

6 **T85.32 Displacement of other ocular prosthetic devices, implants and grafts**
Malposition of other ocular prosthetic devices, implants and grafts

Laterality SP 7 **T85.320- Displacement of prosthetic orbit of right eye**

Laterality SP 7 **T85.321- Displacement of prosthetic orbit of left eye**

Laterality SP 7 **T85.328- Displacement of other ocular prosthetic devices, implants and grafts**

6 **T85.39 Other mechanical complication of other ocular prosthetic devices, implants and grafts**
Obstruction (mechanical) of other ocular prosthetic devices, implants and grafts
Perforation of other ocular prosthetic devices, implants and grafts
Protrusion of other ocular prosthetic devices, implants and grafts

Laterality SP 7 **T85.390- Other mechanical complication of prosthetic orbit of right eye**

Laterality SP 7 **T85.391- Other mechanical complication of prosthetic orbit of left eye**

Laterality SP 7 **T85.398- Other mechanical complication of other ocular prosthetic devices, implants and grafts**

5 **T85.4 Mechanical complication of breast prosthesis and implant**

SP 7 **T85.41X- Breakdown (mechanical) of breast prosthesis and implant**

SP 7 **T85.42X- Displacement of breast prosthesis and implant**
Malposition of breast prosthesis and implant

SP 7 **T85.43X- Leakage of breast prosthesis and implant**

SP 7 **T85.44X- Capsular contracture of breast implant**

SP 7 **T85.49X- Other mechanical complication of breast prosthesis and implant**
Obstruction (mechanical) of breast prosthesis and implant
Perforation of breast prosthesis and implant
Protrusion of breast prosthesis and implant

5 **T85.5 Mechanical complication of gastrointestinal prosthetic devices, implants and grafts**

6 **T85.51 Breakdown (mechanical) of gastrointestinal prosthetic devices, implants and grafts**

SP 7 **T85.510- Breakdown (mechanical) of bile duct prosthesis**

SP 7 **T85.511- Breakdown (mechanical) of esophageal anti-reflux device**

SP 7 **T85.518- Breakdown (mechanical) of other gastrointestinal prosthetic devices, implants and grafts**

6 **T85.52 Displacement of gastrointestinal prosthetic devices, implants and grafts**
Malposition of gastrointestinal prosthetic devices, implants and grafts

SP 7 **T85.520- Displacement of bile duct prosthesis**

SP 7 **T85.521- Displacement of esophageal anti-reflux device**

SP 7 **T85.528- Displacement of other gastrointestinal prosthetic devices, implants and grafts**

6 **T85.59 Other mechanical complication of gastrointestinal prosthetic devices, implants and**
Obstruction, mechanical of gastrointestinal prosthetic devices, implants and grafts
Perforation of gastrointestinal prosthetic devices, implants and grafts
Protrusion of gastrointestinal prosthetic devices, implants and grafts

SP 7 **T85.590- Other mechanical complication of bile duct prosthesis**

SP 7 **T85.591- Other mechanical complication of esophageal anti-reflux device**

SP 7 **T85.598- Other mechanical complication of other gastrointestinal prosthetic devices, implants and grafts**

5 **T85.6 Mechanical complication of other specified internal and external prosthetic devices, implants and grafts**

Chapter 19

S00-T88

GUIDELINES Section I.C.4.a.5)(a)-(b)
An underdose of insulin due to an insulin pump failure should be assigned to a code from subcategory T85.6 followed by code T38.3x6-, Underdosing of insulin and oral hypoglycemic [antidiabetic] drugs. Additional codes for the type of diabetes mellitus and any associated complications due to the underdosing should also be assigned.

The principal or first-listed code for an encounter due to an insulin pump malfunction resulting in an overdose of insulin, should also be T85.6- followed by code T38.3x1-, Poisoning by insulin and oral hypoglycemic [antidiabetic] drugs, accidental (unintentional).

6 **T85.61 Breakdown (mechanical) of other specified internal prosthetic devices, implants and grafts**

SP 7 **T85.610- Breakdown (mechanical) of cranial or spinal infusion catheter**
Breakdown (mechanical) of epidural infusion catheter
Breakdown (mechanical) of intrathecal infusion catheter
Breakdown (mechanical) of subarachnoid infusion catheter
Breakdown (mechanical) of subdural infusion catheter

SP 7 **T85.611- Breakdown (mechanical) of intraperitoneal dialysis catheter**
EXCLUDES 1 mechanical complication of vascular dialysis catheter (T82.4-)

SP 7 **T85.612- Breakdown (mechanical) of permanent sutures**
EXCLUDES 1 mechanical complication of permanent (wire) suture used in bone repair (T84.1-T84.2)

SP 7 **T85.613- Breakdown (mechanical) of artificial skin graft and decellularized allodermis**
Failure of artificial skin graft and decellularized allodermis
Non-adherence of artificial skin graft and decellularized allodermis
Poor incorporation of artificial skin graft and decellularized allodermis
Shearing of artificial skin graft and decellularized allodermis

SP 7 **T85.614- Breakdown (mechanical) of insulin pump**

SP 7 **T85.615- Breakdown (mechanical) of other nervous system device, implant or graft**
Breakdown (mechanical) of intrathecal infusion pump

SP 7 **T85.618- Breakdown (mechanical) of other specified internal prosthetic devices, implants and grafts**

6 **T85.62 Displacement of other specified internal prosthetic devices, implants and grafts**
Malposition of other specified internal prosthetic devices, implants and grafts

SP 7 **T85.620- Displacement of cranial or spinal infusion catheter**
Displacement of epidural infusion catheter
Displacement of intrathecal infusion catheter
Displacement of subarachnoid infusion catheter
Displacement of subdural infusion catheter

SP 7 **T85.621- Displacement of intraperitoneal dialysis catheter**
EXCLUDES 1 mechanical complication of vascular dialysis catheter (T82.4-)

SP 7 **T85.622- Displacement of permanent sutures**
EXCLUDES 1 mechanical complication of permanent (wire) suture used in bone repair (T84.1-T84.2)

SP 7 **T85.623- Displacement of artificial skin graft and decellularized allodermis**
Dislodgement of artificial skin graft and decellularized allodermis

SP 7 **T85.624- Displacement of insulin pump**

SP 7 **T85.625- Displacement of other nervous system device, implant or graft**
Displacement of intrathecal infusion pump

SP 7 **T85.628- Displacement of other specified internal prosthetic devices, implants and grafts**

6 **T85.63 Leakage of other specified internal prosthetic devices, implants and grafts**

SP 7 **T85.630- Leakage of cranial or spinal infusion catheter**
Leakage of epidural infusion catheter
Leakage of intrathecal infusion catheter infusion catheter
Leakage of subdural infusion catheter
Leakage of subarachnoid infusion catheter

SP IQ 7 **T85.631- Leakage of intraperitoneal dialysis catheter**
EXCLUDES 1 mechanical complication of vascular dialysis catheter (T82.4)

SP IQ 7 **T85.633- Leakage of insulin pump**

Chapter 19

S00-T88

SP 7 **T85.635- Leakage of other nervous system device, implant or graft**
Leakage of intrathecal infusion pump

SP 7 **T85.638- Leakage of other specified internal prosthetic devices, implants and grafts**

6 **T85.69 Other mechanical complication of other specified internal prosthetic devices, implants and grafts**
Obstruction, mechanical of other specified internal prosthetic devices, implants and grafts
Perforation of other specified internal prosthetic devices, implants and grafts
Protrusion of other specified internal prosthetic devices, implants and grafts

SP 7 **T85.690- Other mechanical complication of cranial or spinal infusion catheter**
Other mechanical complication of epidural infusion catheter
Other mechanical complication of intrathecal infusion catheter
Other mechanical complication of subarachnoid infusion catheter
Other mechanical complication of subdural infusion catheter

SP 7 **T85.691- Other mechanical complication of intraperitoneal dialysis catheter**
EXCLUDES 1 mechanical complication of vascular dialysis catheter (T82.4)

SP 7 **T85.692- Other mechanical complication of permanent sutures**
EXCLUDES 1 mechanical complication of permanent (wire) suture used in bone repair (T84.1-T84.2)

SP 7 **T85.693- Other mechanical complication of artificial skin graft and decellularized allodermis**

SP 7 **T85.694- Other mechanical complication of insulin pump**

SP 7 **T85.695- Other mechanical complication of other nervous system device, implant or graft**
Other mechanical complication of intrathecal infusion pump

SP 7 **T85.698- Other mechanical complication of other specified internal prosthetic devices, implants and grafts**
Mechanical complication of nonabsorbable surgical material NOS

+ 5 **T85.7 Infection and inflammatory reaction due to other internal prosthetic devices, implants and grafts**
Use additional code to identify infection

SP + 7 **T85.71X- Infection and inflammatory reaction due to peritoneal dialysis catheter**

SP + 7 **T85.72X- Infection and inflammatory reaction due to insulin pump**

+ 6 **T85.73 Infection and inflammatory reaction due to nervous system devices, implants and graft**

SP + 7 **T85.730- Infection and inflammatory reaction due to ventricular intracranial (communicating) shunt**

SP + 7 **T85.731- Infection and inflammatory reaction due to implanted electronic neurostimulator of brain, electrode (lead)**

SP + 7 **T85.732- Infection and inflammatory reaction due to implanted electronic neurostimulator of peripheral nerve, electrode (lead)**
Infection and inflammatory reaction due to electrode (lead) for cranial nerve neurostimulators
Infection and inflammatory reaction due to electrode (lead) for gastric neurostimulator
Infection and inflammatory reaction due to electrode (lead) for sacral nerve neurostimulator
Infection and inflammatory reaction due to electrode (lead) for vagal nerve neurostimulators

SP + 7 **T85.733- Infection and inflammatory reaction due to implanted electronic neurostimulator of spinal cord, electrode (lead)**

SP + 7 **T85.734- Infection and inflammatory reaction due to implanted electronic neurostimulator, generator**
Generator pocket infection

SP + 7 **T85.735- Infection and inflammatory reaction due to cranial or spinal infusion catheter**
Infection and inflammatory reaction due to epidural catheter
Infection and inflammatory reaction due to intrathecal infusion catheter
Infection and inflammatory reaction due to subarachnoid catheter
Infection and inflammatory reaction due to subdural catheter

SP + 7 **T85.738- Infection and inflammatory reaction due to other nervous system device, implant or graft**
Infection and inflammatory reaction due to intrathecal infusion pump

SP + 7 **T85.79X- Infection and inflammatory reaction due to other internal prosthetic devices, implants and grafts**

5 **T85.8 Other specified complications of internal prosthetic devices, implants and grafts, not elsewhere classified**

6 **T85.81 Embolism due to internal prosthetic devices, implants and grafts, not elsewhere classified**

Chapter 19
S00-T88

SP 7 **T85.810- Embolism due to nervous system prosthetic devices, implants and grafts**

SP 7 **T85.818- Embolism due to other internal prosthetic devices, implants and grafts**

6 **T85.82 Fibrosis due to internal prosthetic devices, implants and grafts, not elsewhere classified**

SP 7 **T85.820- Fibrosis due to nervous system prosthetic devices, implants and grafts**

SP 7 **T85.828- Fibrosis due to other internal prosthetic devices, implants and grafts**

6 **T85.83 Hemorrhage due to internal prosthetic devices, implants and grafts, not elsewhere classified**

SP 7 **T85.830- Hemorrhage due to nervous system prosthetic devices, implants and grafts**

SP 7 **T85.838- Hemorrhage due to other internal prosthetic devices, implants and grafts**

6 **T85.84 Pain due to internal prosthetic devices, implants and grafts, not elsewhere classified**

SP 7 **T85.840- Pain due to nervous system prosthetic devices, implants and grafts**

SP 7 **T85.848- Pain due to other internal prosthetic devices, implants and grafts**

6 **T85.85 Stenosis due to internal prosthetic devices, implants and grafts, not elsewhere classified**

SP 7 **T85.850- Stenosis due to nervous system prosthetic devices, implants and grafts**

SP 7 **T85.858- Stenosis due to other internal prosthetic devices, implants and grafts**

6 **T85.86 Thrombosis due to internal prosthetic devices, implants and grafts, not elsewhere classified**

SP 7 **T85.860- Thrombosis due to nervous system prosthetic devices, implants and grafts**

SP 7 **T85.868- Thrombosis due to other internal prosthetic devices, implants and grafts**

6 **T85.89 Other specified complication of internal prosthetic devices, implants and grafts, not elsewhere classified**

Erosion or breakdown of subcutaneous device pocket

SP 7 **T85.890- Other specified complication of nervous system prosthetic devices, implants and grafts**

SP 7 **T85.898- Other specified complication of other internal prosthetic devices, implants and grafts**

IQ 7 **T85.9XX- Unspecified complication of internal prosthetic device, implant and graft**

Complication of internal prosthetic device, implant and graft NOS

+ 4 **T86 Complications of transplanted organs and tissue**

Use additional code to identify other transplant complications, such as:
graft-versus-host disease (D89.81-)
malignancy associated with organ transplant (C80.2)
post-transplant lymphoproliferative disorders (PTLD) (D47.Z1)

GUIDELINES **Section I.C.19.g.3)(a)**

Codes under category T86, Complications of transplanted organs and tissues, are for use for both complications and rejection of transplanted organs. A transplant complication code is only assigned if the complication affects the function of the transplanted organ. Two codes are required to fully describe a transplant complication: the appropriate code from category T86 and a secondary code that identifies the complication.

Pre-existing conditions or conditions that develop after the transplant are not coded as complications unless they affect the function of the transplanted organs.

GUIDELINES **Section I.C.2.r**

A malignant neoplasm of a transplanted organ should be coded as a transplant complication. Assign first the appropriate code from category T86.-, Complications of transplanted organs and tissue, followed by code C80.2. Use an additional code for the specific malignancy.

CODING TIPS✓ If the organ must be removed due to failure or rejection, use Z98.85 for removal status.

CODING TIPS✓ Do not assume dysfunction in a transplanted organ to be a complication of a transplanted organ unless specifically stated by a provider diagnostic statement. The only exception to this is a malignant neoplasm of a transplanted organ. A neoplasm associated with a transplant is coded as an "other complication of transplant" unless specified by the physician as a failure or rejection.

CODING TIPS✓ This category includes complications for organ transplants, including skin grafts. Note that these complication codes do not require a 7th character.

+ 5 **T86.0 Complications of bone marrow transplant**

IQ + **T86.00 Unspecified complication of bone marrow transplant**

SP + **T86.01 Bone marrow transplant rejection**

SP + **T86.02 Bone marrow transplant failure**

SP + **T86.03 Bone marrow transplant infection**

SP + **T86.09 Other complications of bone marrow transplant**

+ 5 **T86.1 Complications of kidney transplant**

Chapter 19 S00-T88

GUIDELINES Section I.C.19.g.3)(b)
Patients who have undergone kidney transplant may still have some form of chronic kidney disease (CKD) because the kidney transplant may not fully restore kidney function ... Code T86.1- should not be assigned for post kidney transplant patients who have CKD unless a transplant complication such as transplant failure or rejection is documented. If the documentation is unclear as to whether the patient has a complication of the transplant, query the provider.

Conditions that affect the function of the transplanted kidney, other than CKD, should be assigned a code from subcategory T86.1 and a secondary code that identifies the complication. For patients with CKD following a kidney transplant, but who do not have a complication such as failure or rejection, *see section I.C.14. Chronic kidney disease and kidney transplant status.*

!Q + **T86.10 Unspecified complication of kidney transplant**

SP + **T86.11 Kidney transplant rejection**

SP + **T86.12 Kidney transplant failure**

SP + **T86.13 Kidney transplant infection**
Use additional code to specify infection

SP + **T86.19 Other complication of kidney transplant**

▲ + 5 **T86.2 Complications of heart transplant**
EXCLUDES 1 complication of:
artificial heart device (T82.5-)
heart-lung transplant (T86.3-)

!Q + **T86.20 Unspecified complication of heart transplant**

SP + **T86.21 Heart transplant rejection**

SP + **T86.22 Heart transplant failure**

SP + **T86.23 Heart transplant infection**
Use additional code to specify infection

+ 6 **T86.29 Other complications of heart transplant**

SP + **T86.290 Cardiac allograft vasculopathy**
EXCLUDES 1 atherosclerosis of coronary arteries (I25.75-, I25.76-, I25.81-)

SP + **T86.298 Other complications of heart transplant**

+ 5 **T86.3 Complications of heart-lung transplant**

!Q + **T86.30 Unspecified complication of heart-lung transplant**

SP + **T86.31 Heart-lung transplant rejection**

SP + **T86.32 Heart-lung transplant failure**

SP + **T86.33 Heart-lung transplant infection**
Use additional code to specify infection

SP + **T86.39 Other complications of heart-lung transplant**

+ 5 **T86.4 Complications of liver transplant**

!Q + **T86.40 Unspecified complication of liver transplant**

SP + **T86.41 Liver transplant rejection**

SP + **T86.42 Liver transplant failure**

SP + **T86.43 Liver transplant infection**
Use additional code to identify infection, such as:
Cytomegalovirus (CMV) infection (B25.-)

SP + **T86.49 Other complications of liver transplant**

SP + **T86.5 Complications of stem cell transplant**
Complications from stem cells from peripheral blood
Complications from stem cells from umbilical cord

+ 5 **T86.8 Complications of other transplanted organs and tissues**

+ 6 **T86.81 Complications of lung transplant**
EXCLUDES 1 complication of heart-lung transplant (T86.3-)

SP + **T86.810 Lung transplant rejection**

SP + **T86.811 Lung transplant failure**

SP + **T86.812 Lung transplant infection**
Use additional code to specify infection

SP + **T86.818 Other complications of lung transplant**

!Q + **T86.819 Unspecified complication of lung transplant**

+ 6 **T86.82 Complications of skin graft (allograft) (autograft)**
EXCLUDES 2 complication of artificial skin graft (T85.693)

SP + **T86.820 Skin graft (allograft) rejection**

SP + **T86.821 Skin graft (allograft) (autograft) failure**

SP + **T86.822 Skin graft (allograft) (autograft) infection**
Use additional code to specify infection

SP + **T86.828 Other complications of skin graft (allograft) (autograft)**

!Q + **T86.829 Unspecified complication of skin graft (allograft) (autograft)**

+ 6 **T86.83 Complications of bone graft**
EXCLUDES 2 mechanical complications of bone graft (T84.3-)

SP + **T86.830 Bone graft rejection**

SP + **T86.831 Bone graft failure**

SP + **T86.832 Bone graft infection**
Use additional code to specify infection

SP + **T86.838 Other complications of bone graft**

!Q + **T86.839 Unspecified complication of bone graft**

+ 6 **T86.84 Complications of corneal transplant**
EXCLUDES 2 mechanical complications of corneal graft (T85.3-)

⊟ SP + 7 **T86.840 Corneal transplant rejection**

CODING TIPS✓ For codes T86.840 - T86.842, T86.848-T86.849, assign a 7th character to indicate laterality, such as right (1), left (2), bilateral (3), or unspecified (9).

Chapter 19
S00-T88

SP + 7 T86.841 Corneal transplant failure

SP + 7 T86.842 Corneal transplant infection
Use additional code to specify infection

SP + 7 T86.848 Other complications of corneal transplant

IQ + 7 T86.849 Unspecified complication of corneal transplant

+ 6 T86.85 Complication of intestine transplant

SP + T86.850 Intestine transplant rejection

SP + T86.851 Intestine transplant failure

SP + T86.852 Intestine transplant infection
Use additional code to specify infection

SP + T86.858 Other complications of intestine transplant

IQ + T86.859 Unspecified complication of intestine transplant

+ 6 T86.89 Complications of other transplanted tissue
Transplant failure or rejection of pancreas

SP + T86.890 Other transplanted tissue rejection

SP + T86.891 Other transplanted tissue failure

SP + T86.892 Other transplanted tissue infection
Use additional code to specify infection

SP + T86.898 Other complications of other transplanted tissue

IQ + T86.899 Unspecified complication of other transplanted tissue

+ 5 T86.9 Complication of unspecified transplanted organ and tissue

IQ + T86.90 Unspecified complication of unspecified transplanted organ and tissue

IQ + T86.91 Unspecified transplanted organ and tissue rejection

IQ + T86.92 Unspecified transplanted organ and tissue failure

IQ + T86.93 Unspecified transplanted organ and tissue infection
Use additional code to specify infection

IQ + T86.99 Other complications of unspecified transplanted organ and tissue

4 T87 Complications peculiar to reattachment and amputation

CODING TIPS✓ Complications of amputations include both traumatic amputations with complications as well as surgical amputations with complications. Note that most, but not all, of the complication codes include the extremity affected. These codes are more specific than the T81 codes and should be used for any amputation complications. These complications do not require 7th characters.

CODING TIPS✓ A pressure injury on the stump related to a prosthesis is considered a Medical Device Related Pressure Injury (MDRPI). This describes an etiology. Use the L89 codes for pressure ulcer/injury and the staging system to stage. A Y79.- code may be added to indicate the cause as a medical device.

5 T87.0 Complications of reattached (part of) upper extremity

6 T87.0X Complications of reattached (part of) upper extremity

SP T87.0X1 Complications of reattached (part of) right upper extremity

SP T87.0X2 Complications of reattached (part of) left upper extremity

IQ T87.0X9 Complications of reattached (part of) unspecified upper extremity

5 T87.1 Complications of reattached (part of) lower extremity

6 T87.1X Complications of reattached (part of) lower extremity

SP T87.1X1 Complications of reattached (part of) right lower extremity

SP T87.1X2 Complications of reattached (part of) left lower extremity

IQ T87.1X9 Complications of reattached (part of) unspecified lower extremity

SP T87.2 Complications of other reattached body part

5 T87.3 Neuroma of amputation stump

IQ T87.30 Neuroma of amputation stump, unspecified extremity

SP T87.31 Neuroma of amputation stump, right upper extremity

SP T87.32 Neuroma of amputation stump, left upper extremity

SP T87.33 Neuroma of amputation stump, right lower extremity

SP T87.34 Neuroma of amputation stump, left lower extremity

5 T87.4 Infection of amputation stump

CODING TIPS✓ If the focus of care is wound care for an infected amputation stump, sequence T87.89 as primary, followed by the appropriate T87.4 code.

CODING TIPS✓ When a patient presents with an infected amputation stump wound, assign the appropriate code from T87.4-. When both dehiscence and infection are present, code the dehiscence first (T87.81), followed by infection. The T87.81 sequenced first will result in the wound grouper. Use an additional code to specify the infection.

IQ T87.40 Infection of amputation stump, unspecified extremity

SP T87.41 Infection of amputation stump, right upper extremity

SP T87.42 Infection of amputation stump, left upper extremity

SP T87.43 Infection of amputation stump, right lower extremity

SP T87.44 Infection of amputation stump, left lower extremity

5 T87.5 Necrosis of amputation stump

L IQ T87.50 Necrosis of amputation stump, unspecified extremity

L SP T87.51 Necrosis of amputation stump, right upper extremity

L SP T87.52 Necrosis of amputation stump, left upper extremity

L SP T87.53 Necrosis of amputation stump, right lower extremity

L SP T87.54 Necrosis of amputation stump, left lower extremity

5 T87.8 Other complications of amputation stump

SP T87.81 Dehiscence of amputation stump

CODING TIPS ✓ When a patient presents with a dehiscence of an amputation stump wound, assign code T87.81. When both dehiscence and infection are present, code the dehiscence first (T87.81), followed by infection. Use an additional code to specify the infection.

SP T87.89 Other complications of amputation stump

Amputation stump contracture
Amputation stump contracture of next proximal joint
Amputation stump flexion
Amputation stump edema
Amputation stump hematoma

EXCLUDES 2 phantom limb syndrome (G54.6-G54.7)

CODING TIPS ✓ If the focus of care is wound care for an infected amputation stump, sequence T87.89 as primary, followed by the appropriate T87.4 code.

CODING TIPS ✓ Do not assign a code for complication of an amputation stump for an ulcer (due to pressure, diabetic ulcer, arterial, trauma, stasis, or other) of the amputation stump. Ulcers of the amputation stump are not considered amputation stump complications. A pressure injury on the stump related to a prosthesis is considered a Medical Device Related Pressure Injury (MDRPI). This describes an etiology. Use the L89 codes for pressure ulcer/injury and the staging system to stage. A Y79.- code may be added to indicate the cause as a medical device.

IQ T87.9 Unspecified complications of amputation stump

4 T88 Other complications of surgical and medical care, not elsewhere classified

EXCLUDES 2
complication following infusion, transfusion and therapeutic injection (T80.-)
complication following procedure NEC (T81.-)
complications of anesthesia in labor and delivery (O74.-)
complications of anesthesia in pregnancy (O29.-)
complications of anesthesia in puerperium (O89.-)
complications of devices, implants and grafts (T82-T85)
complications of obstetric surgery and procedure (O75.4)
dermatitis due to drugs and medicaments (L23.3, L24.4, L25.1, L27.0-L27.1)
poisoning and toxic effects of drugs and chemicals (T36-T65 with fifth or sixth character 1-4 or 6)
specified complications classified elsewhere

The appropriate 7th character is to be added to each code from category T88

A	initial encounter
D	subsequent encounter
S	sequela

CODING TIPS ✓ No aftercare code applies, including dressing changes, drain care, and suture removal. 7th character 'D' is the default for home care and hospice when providing aftercare for a healing or resolving condition; 'A' is used for active treatment such as antibiotics or more than routine wound care; 'S' may be used to indicate a residual condition after the original injury has healed. Once complication is repaired in the acute setting, continue to code the complication in home care and hospice with 7th character D if healing/resolving.

SP 7 T88.0XX- Infection following immunization

Sepsis following immunization

SP 7 T88.1XX- Other complications following immunization, not elsewhere classified

Generalized vaccinia
Rash following immunization

EXCLUDES 1 vaccinia not from vaccine (B08.011)

EXCLUDES 2
anaphylactic shock due to serum (T80.5-)
other serum reactions (T80.6-)
postimmunization arthropathy (M02.2)
postimmunization encephalitis (G04.02)
postimmunization fever (R50.83)

SP + 7 T88.2XX- Shock due to anesthesia

Use additional code for adverse effect, if applicable, to identify drug (T41.- with fifth or sixth character 5)

EXCLUDES 1 complications of anesthesia (in) :
labor and delivery (O74.-)
pregnancy (O29.-)
puerperium (O89.-)
postprocedural shock NOS (T81.1-)

SP + 7 T88.3XX- Malignant hyperthermia due to anesthesia

4 4th digit required 5 5th digit required 6 6th digit required 7 7th digit required 7 7th digit placeholder + Additional code L Laterality

Use additional code for adverse effect, if applicable, to identify drug (T41.- with fifth or sixth character 5)

SP 7 **T88.4XX- Failed or difficult intubation**

+ 5 **T88.5 Other complications of anesthesia**

Use additional code for adverse effect, if applicable, to identify drug (T41.- with fifth or sixth character 5)

SP + 7 **T88.51X- Hypothermia following anesthesia**

SP + 7 **T88.52X- Failed moderate sedation during procedure**

Failed conscious sedation during procedure

EXCLUDES 2 personal history of failed moderate sedation (Z92.83)

SP + 7 **T88.53X- Unintended awareness under general anesthesia during procedure**

EXCLUDES 2 personal history of unintended awareness under general anesthesia (Z92.84)

SP + 7 **T88.59X- Other complications of anesthesia**

SP + 7 **T88.6XX- Anaphylactic reaction due to adverse effect of correct drug or medicament properly administered**

Anaphylactic shock due to adverse effect of correct drug or medicament properly administered

Anaphylactoid reaction NOS

Use additional code for adverse effect, if applicable, to identify drug (T36-T50 with fifth or sixth character 5)

EXCLUDES 1 anaphylactic reaction due to serum (T80.5-)

anaphylactic shock or reaction due to adverse food reaction (T78.0-)

IQ + 7 **T88.7XX- Unspecified adverse effect of drug or medicament**

Drug hypersensitivity NOS

Drug reaction NOS

Use additional code for adverse effect, if applicable, to identify drug (T36-T50 with fifth or sixth character 5)

EXCLUDES 1 specified adverse effects of drugs and medicaments (A00-R94 and T80-T88.6, T88.8)

SP + 7 **T88.8XX- Other specified complications of surgical and medical care, not elsewhere classified**

Use additional code to identify the complication

IQ 7 **T88.9XX- Complication of surgical and medical care, unspecified**

Chapter 19

S00-T88

Chapter 19 Scenarios: Injury, poisoning and certain other consequences of external causes (S00-T88)

Sepsis due to midline catheter infection

A 66-year-old woman is admitted to home health for treatment with IV antibiotics, of gram-negative sepsis caused by a midline catheter infection. She is morbidly obese and has insulin-dependent diabetes and hypertension. The focus of care is the systemic infection itself and teaching hygiene and care of the IV catheter. The patient's family will be instructed in antibiotic administration and will provide some doses, if safe and able.

Description	Code
Primary: Infection and inflammatory reaction due to other cardiac and vascular devices, implants and grafts, initial encounter	T82.7XXA
Secondary: Gram-negative sepsis, unspecified	A41.50
Secondary: Type 2 diabetes mellitus without complications	E11.9
Secondary: Essential (primary) hypertension	I10
Secondary: Morbid (severe) obesity due to excess calories	E66.01
Secondary: Encounter for adjustment and management of vascular access device	Z45.2
Secondary: Long term (current) use of antibiotics	Z79.2
Secondary: Long term (current) use of insulin	Z79.4

Sepsis due to a midline catheter infection should be coded first with T82.7- followed by the code for the sepsis as the code choice should be driven by the location of the catheter, not its use, according to Q1 2019 Coding Clinic guidance. A seventh character "A" is assigned as the condition is receiving active treatment. Diabetes and hypertension are relevant comorbidities that will impact her care and are thus coded. Morbid obesity is always clinically relevant and should be assigned whether it's the focus of home health treatment, per Q4 2018 Coding Clinic guidance. The administration of IV antibiotics and the dependence on insulin, as a non-type 1 diabetic, are captured with Z45.2, Z79.2 and Z79.4. If the IV is not the primary reason the patient requires home health care, but where there may be some sort of intervention noted on the home health plan of care, then it would be appropriate to report Z45.2 (but not as the principal or first secondary diagnosis), according to CMS.

Skin graft care, burn

A 62-year-old woman is admitted to home care after having a skin graft onto her right thigh following a third-degree burn that occurred when she accidentally spilled hot oil on herself while cooking. Her doctor has ordered daily dressing changes. The skin donor site has healed and does not require care

Description	Code
Primary: Burn of third degree of right thigh, subsequent encounter	T24.311D
Secondary: Contact with fats and cooking oils, subsequent encounter	X10.2xxD

A burn that is covered with a graft is still considered a burn. Because aftercare codes for injury and trauma do not exist in ICD-10, the acute burn is coded with the appropriate seventh character, "D" to indicate that it is a subsequent encounter. The T24.- category has a "use additional code" note to include the external cause code. That code is included to specify that the burn occurred from contact with hot cooking oil.

Hip fracture

A 72-year-old man was admitted to the hospital following a surgical repair of a left hip fracture. Home physical therapy was initiated for continued aftercare. The referral indicated no other pertinent medical history except for the fall that caused the fracture.

Description	Code
Primary: Fracture of unspecified part of neck of left femur, subsequent encounter for closed fracture with routine healing	S72.002D
Secondary: Unspecified fall, subsequent encounter	W19.xxxD

Even though the fracture was treated surgically, it is still coded with the active fracture code, with a "D" to indicate the subsequent nature of the encounter, per coding guidelines. Code Z91.81 (History of falling) is not included here as there was no indication of any past history or further risks for falls. Without other documentation, a fracture not indicated as open or closed should be coded as closed. A fracture not indicated whether displaced or not displaced should be coded as displaced. Note that it's important to code whether the fracture affects the left or right hip. Unspecified hip fracture is an unacceptable primary diagnosis in PDGM.

Aftercare, amputation

A patient was trimming hedges and dropped the electric trimmer on his right foot, almost severing his foot at the ankle. The patient has a long history of diabetic PVD, hypertension, and stage 4 chronic kidney disease. The surgeon completed the amputation as a Syme amputation of the foot and ankle, and home health was ordered for amputation aftercare, including dressing changes.

Description	Code
Primary: Traumatic amputation partial of right foot at ankle level, subsequent encounter	S98.021D
Secondary: Diabetes with peripheral angiopathy without gangrene	E11.51
Secondary: Type 2 diabetes mellitus with diabetic chronic kidney disease	E11.22
Secondary: Hypertensive chronic kidney disease with stage 1 through stage 4 chronic kidney disease, or unspecified chronic kidney disease	I12.9
Secondary: Chronic kidney disease, stage 4 (severe)	N18.4
Secondary: Contact with powered garden and outdoor hand tools and machinery, subsequent encounter	W29.3xxD

Aftercare codes for traumatic injuries do not exist in ICD-10. Instead 7th characters are used to indicate the nature of the care provided following an injury. When a 7th character is required and the code has fewer than six characters, a placeholder "x" must be used, according to coding guidelines. The external cause code for how the injury occurred is recommended to further paint the clinical picture *[I.A.4]*. Additional codes for diabetes with PVD (angiopathy), as well as diabetes with chronic kidney disease, hypertension, and chronic kidney disease stage 4 are assigned as these conditions have an impact on the patient's prognosis and care plan, as well as may provide important comorbidity adjustment.

Infected wound

A patient's initial injury was a cat bite on her left hand. When her wound became infected, she was referred to home health for wound care and IV antibiotics. The PICC line also became infected. MRSA has grown out of the PICC line. Other diagnoses include diabetes and hypertension. The focus of care is the wound.

Description	Code
Primary: Open bite of left hand, initial encounter	S61.452A
Secondary: Other infection due to central venous catheter, initial encounter	T80.218A
Secondary: MRSA	B95.62
Secondary: Diabetes mellitus without mention of complication	E11.9
Secondary: Essential hypertension, unspecified	I10
Secondary: Long term (current) use of antibiotics	Z79.2
Secondary: Encounter for adjustment and management of vascular access device	Z45.2
Secondary: Bitten by cat, initial encounter	W55.01XA

Open wound codes are divided into groups of lacerations, puncture wounds, bites and other wounds. If the skin is unbroken, the bite is coded as a superficial injury. There is no different code to indicate complicated. The MRSA code is included because the open bite code and the catheter infection code both have a "use additional code" note to specify the infection, if known. The seventh character "A" is used for both the injury and infected catheter codes because the patient is still receiving active treatment, via the IV antibiotics. Codes Z45.2 and Z79.2 are additionally assigned to capture the administration of IV antibiotics. If the IV is not the primary reason the patient requires home health care, but where there may be some sort of intervention noted on the home health plan of care, then it would be appropriate to report Z45.2 (but not as the principal or first secondary diagnosis), according to CMS. An external cause code (W55.01xA) is assigned to capture how the patient sustained the bite and carries the same seventh character as the wound, in accordance with coding guidelines. *[I.C.20.a.2]*

Underdosing

A patient with diagnosis of hypertension continued to experience elevated blood pressure while taking blood pressure meds. Upon patient interview, it was found the patient was taking medication once daily instead of twice daily because of the cost of the drug. The face-to-face encounter notes provided with the home health referral also indicate the patient has recently diagnosed Parkinson's disease.

Description	Code
Primary: Essential (primary) hypertension	I10
Secondary: Underdosing of other antihypertensive drugs, subsequent encounter	T46.5x6D
Secondary: Parkinson's disease	G20
Secondary: Patient's intentional underdosing of medication regimen due to financial hardship	Z91.120

Codes for underdosing should never be assigned as principal or first-listed codes, according to coding guidelines. If a patient has a relapse or exacerbation of the medical condition for which the drug is prescribed because of the reduction in dose, then the medical condition itself should be coded, according to coding guidelines. Report underdosing with codes from T36-T50 with sixth character of "6" to delineate that the adverse effect was due to "underdosing." Finally, report the appropriate Z code for the underdosing reason *[I.C.19.e.5.c]*. An additional code for the patient's recently-diagnosed Parkinson's disease is assigned due to the impact of this condition on the patient's prognosis and care plan.

Lasix poisoning

A patient has taken his Lasix 40mg every morning and night for congestive heart failure (CHF). The prescription bottle reads 40mg daily. Patient is dehydrated and hypokalemic.

Description	Code
Primary: Poisoning by diuretics	T50.1x1D
Secondary: Dehydration	E86.0
Secondary: Hypokalemia	E87.6
Secondary: Heart failure, unspecified	I50.9

This is a poisoning because the patient took an incorrect amount of the drug, from what was prescribed. When coding a poisoning or improper use of a medication first assign the appropriate code from categories T36-T50, according to coding guidelines. Use additional code(s) for manifestations of poisonings. The reason for the patient taking the Lasix in the first place, CHF, is also coded, following the manifestations of the poisoning, the dehydration and hypokalemia. *[I.C.19.e.5.b]*

Digoxin adverse effect

A patient has been taking the prescribed amount of Digoxin to treat paroxysmal atrial fibrillation. However, he's began to experience serious side effects, including visual disturbance, a pulse of 42, and bradycardia has been diagnosed. He is toxic according to lab values. Skilled nursing is ordered for observation and assessment, teaching and venipuncture for monitoring levels.

Description	Code
Primary: Other visual disturbances	H53.8
Secondary: Bradycardia	R00.1
Secondary: Adverse effect of cardiac-stimulant glycosides and drugs of similar action, subsequent encounter	T46.0x5D
Secondary: Paroxysmal atrial fibrillation	I48.0
Secondary: Encounter for therapeutic drug level monitoring	Z51.81
Secondary: Other long term (current) drug therapy	Z79.899

When coding an adverse effect of a drug that has been correctly prescribed and properly administered, assign the appropriate code for the nature of the adverse effects (the visual disturbance and bradycardia in this case) followed by the appropriate code for the adverse effect of the drug (T46.0x5D), according to coding guidelines. Do not code bradycardia as the primary diagnosis as it is not an acceptable primary reason for a home health admission. The reason the Digoxin was prescribed in the first place, paroxysmal atrial fibrillation, is also coded following the adverse effect. Codes Z51.81 and Z79.899 capture the venipuncture and drug monitoring. An adverse effect is defined as "hypersensitivity," "reaction," etc. of correct substance properly administered. *[I.C.19.e.5.a]*

Dehisced laceration, diabetic PVD

A 57-year-old woman suffered a deep laceration to her right thigh when she accidentally dropped a large kitchen knife. The wound was surgically repaired in the hospital, but later dehisced. She was admitted to home health for wound care, and also has diabetic peripheral neuropathy. She is insulin dependent.

Description	Code
Primary: Disruption of traumatic injury wound repair, initial encounter	T81.33XA
Secondary: Laceration without foreign body, right thigh, initial encounter	S71.111A
Secondary: Type 2 diabetes mellitus with diabetic polyneuropathy	E11.42
Secondary: Long term (current) use of insulin	Z79.4
Secondary: Contact with knife, initial encounter	W26.0XXA

The patient's dehisced wound is a traumatic wound that was repaired surgically and later reopened. Therefore, it codes to T81.33-. The seventh character "A" is used because there has been dehiscence, which constitutes active treatment according to the Coding Clinic. An additional code for the laceration to her thigh provides the necessary information about the type, location and laterality of the wound. Diabetic peripheral neuropathy is captured with the combination code E11.42. An additional code for insulin use is required because the patient is dependent on insulin but not said to be a Type 1 diabetic. An external cause code is used to help explain how she got the laceration.

Muscle flap failure, wheelchair confinement, obesity

An 80-year-old man underwent surgery to repair a stage 4 pressure ulcer/injury on his left buttocks with a muscle flap, which failed but is still covering the original pressure ulcer/injury. He is now in home health for wound care. He is also obese and confined to his wheelchair and has chronic obstructive bronchitis. His BMI is calculated at 42.

Description	Code
Primary: Other transplanted tissue failure	T86.891
Secondary: Pressure ulcer of left buttock, unstageable	L89.320
Secondary: Chronic obstructive pulmonary disease, unspecified	J44.9
Secondary: Obesity, unspecified	E66.9
Secondary: Body mass index (BMI) 40.0-44.9, adult	Z68.41
Secondary: Dependence on wheelchair	Z99.3

Because the stage 4 pressure ulcer/injury was treated with muscle flap that failed, it should be captured with a complication code that specifies the failure of transplanted tissue. There isn't a specific listing for this type of complication in the index. Thus, the appropriate code choice is found in the "specified tissue NEC" option, which is T86.891 (Other transplanted tissue failure). The pressure ulcer/injury is also coded as unstageable due to the fact that the flap is obscuring the wound bed, according to coding guidelines.

The patient has a diagnosis of chronic obstructive bronchitis, which is included in category J44., chronic obstructive bronchitis. The patient is diagnosed as obese, and the tabular instruction at E66.9 says to use an additional code for BMI, which can easily be calculated by the assessing clinician. Obesity should always be coded when it's documented, according to Q4 2018 Coding Clinic guidance. Therefore, Z68.41 is coded directly following E66.9. His wheelchair confinement is captured with Z99.3.

Dehiscence following appendectomy, obesity, diabetic kidney disease

A 67-year-old woman is admitted to home health with an abdominal wound resulting from an appendectomy. The wound has dehisced through the skin closures. She is also obese, with a BMI of 37, and has hypertension and stage 3 unspecified chronic kidney disease resulting from her Type 1 diabetes.

Description	Code
Primary: Disruption of external operation (surgical) wound, not elsewhere classified, initial encounter	T81.31XA
Secondary: Type 1 diabetes mellitus with diabetic chronic kidney disease	E10.22
Secondary: Hypertensive chronic kidney disease with stage 1 through stage 4 chronic kidney disease, or unspecified chronic kidney disease	I12.9
Secondary: Chronic kidney disease, stage 3 unspecified	N18.30
Secondary: Obesity, unspecified	E66.9
Secondary: Body mass index (BMI) 37.0-37.9, adult	Z68.37

The surgical wound has dehisced, and because it is described as through the skin, it can be coded as an externally dehisced wound, with T81.31XA. The seventh character "A" is used because the wound has dehisced, according to Coding Clinic guidance. Though the diabetic chronic kidney disease can be captured with the combination code E10.22, an additional code, N18.3-, is required to specify the stage. The ICD-10-CM classification assumes a classification between hypertension and chronic kidney disease and a combination code for hypertensive chronic kidney disease is assigned. As a type 1 diabetic, insulin dependence is assumed and does not have to be stated with a Z code. Obesity should be coded when it's documented, according to Q4 2018 Coding Clinic guidance.

Burn from battery acid

A 59-year-old man was working in his machine shop when he accidentally spilled battery acid on his right thigh, causing a third degree burn over 15 percent of his body area. He was admitted to home health for daily wound care to his thigh.

Description	Code
Primary: Toxic effect of corrosive acids and acid-like substances, accidental (unintentional), subsequent encounter	T54.2x1D
Secondary: Corrosion of third degree of right thigh, subsequent encounter	T24.711D

The burn was caused by a corrosive chemical and should therefore be coded as a corrosion burn. The code identifying the chemical that caused the burn, T54.2x1D, must be coded first, according to tabular instruction. Because the third degree burns have not affected 20 percent or more of the patient's body, a code from the T32.- category isn't necessary.

Puncture wound

A 69-year-old woman slipped and fell while looking in boxes in her basement, suffering a puncture wound when she impaled her left calf on a sharp piece of wood that was sticking out from behind the stairway. She received nine stiches in the emergency room and was discharged to home health for wound care. Skilled nursing will be providing wound care and closely monitoring her recovery as she has diabetic peripheral angiopathy and her doctor is concerned about slow wound healing.

Description	Code
Primary: Puncture wound without foreign body, left lower leg, subsequent encounter	S81.832D
Secondary: Type 2 diabetes mellitus with diabetic peripheral angiopathy without gangrene	E11.51
Secondary: Fall on same level from slipping, tripping and stumbling with subsequent striking against other sharp object, subsequent encounter	W01.118D

The puncture wound is the focus of care and is coded primary. Her diabetes is coded as it will impact her recovery and wound healing. The external cause code is added to help explain the nature of the injury. The external cause code carries the same seventh character as the injury code, in accordance with coding guidelines.

Laceration from hedge trimmer

A 67-year-old man cut his left lower leg while trimming the bushes in front of his home with a powered hedge trimmer, resulting in a deep laceration that required surgery. Following his surgery he was admitted to home health for continue his recovery and for wound care with wet-to-dry dressings. His wound is progressing normally and the care provided is routine. He is also type 1 diabetic with diabetic stage 2 chronic kidney disease, and has comorbid diastolic congestive heart failure that is not currently exacerbated.

Description	Code
Primary: Laceration without foreign body, left lower leg, subsequent encounter	S81.812D
Secondary: Type 1 diabetes mellitus with diabetic chronic kidney disease	E10.22
Secondary: Chronic kidney disease, stage 2 (mild)	N18.2
Secondary: Chronic diastolic (congestive) heart failure	I50.32
Secondary: Contact with powered garden and outdoor hand tools and machinery, subsequent encounter	W29.3xxD

Even though the patient underwent surgery to treat the wound, it is still coded as a trauma wound, in accordance with official coding guidelines. His diabetes and diabetic chronic kidney disease have the potential to impact his recovery and ability to fully heal from this trauma wound and therefore they are coded as well. As a type 1 diabetic, insulin dependence is assumed and the code for insulin use is therefore not required. A code for the chronic diastolic heart failure is also assigned even though the condition is not exacerbated because the condition has a significant impact on the care plan and prognosis for the patient. The external cause code to capture how the wound occurred carries the same seventh character as the other codes in the scenario, in accordance with official coding guidelines.
[I.C.21.c.7] [I.C.20.a.2]

Traumatic periprosthetic fracture

A 74-year-old man was walking down the stairs in his home when he accidentally missed a step and fell the rest of the way down. He was sent to the emergency room and was later admitted to the hospital after undergoing surgery to repair a traumatic periprosthetic fracture of the upper end of his left femur, near his left prosthetic hip joint. The prosthetic hip joint was placed two years ago. Following his hospitalization, he was admitted to home health care for skilled nursing and physical and occupational therapy. He has comorbidities of hypertension and stage 4 CKD. The fracture is the focus of care.

Description	Code
Primary: Fracture of unspecified part of neck of left femur, subsequent encounter for closed fracture with routine healing	S72.002D
Secondary: Periprosthetic fracture around internal prosthetic left hip joint, subsequent encounter	M97.02xD
Secondary: Hypertensive chronic kidney disease with stage 1 through stage 4 chronic kidney disease, or unspecified chronic kidney disease	I12.9
Secondary: Chronic kidney disease, stage 4 (severe)	N18.4
Secondary: Fall (on) (from) unspecified stairs and steps, subsequent encounter	W10.9xxD

As the focus of care, the fracture is coded first, with the code for the traumatic fracture sequenced ahead of the periprosthetic fracture, in accordance with Q4 2016 Coding Clinic guidance. The etiology of the fracture is traumatic and is thus coded as a traumatic fracture with S72.002D. Note that coding the specific location of the fracture (left or right side) is critical as a code for a fracture of an unspecified hip is not an acceptable primary diagnosis code in PDGM.The patient's comorbidities of hypertension and stage 4 CKD have the potential to impact his recovery and thus should be coded. The ICD-10-CM classification assumes a relationship between these conditions, so a combination code is assigned for the hypertension. An external cause code, W10.9xxD, is used to describe how the patient suffered the traumatic fracture, in a fall down the stairs.

Shoulder fracture, joint replacement

A 70-year-old man underwent surgery to replace his right shoulder after slipping on an ice-covered walkway and sustaining a fracture of the upper end of his right humerus. He also has comorbid diagnoses of diet-controlled type 2 diabetes and hypertension.

Description	Code
Primary: Unspecified fracture of upper end of right humerus, subsequent encounter for fracture with routine healing	S42.201D
Secondary: Type 2 diabetes mellitus without complications	E11.9
Secondary: Essential (primary) hypertension	I10
Secondary: Presence of right artificial shoulder joint	Z96.611
Secondary: Fall on same level due to ice and snow, subsequent encounter	W00.0xxD

The impetus for the patient's shoulder replacement surgery was a fracture. Because an injury necessitated surgery, a surgical aftercare code is not appropriate. Instead, the fracture itself is coded with the seventh character "D" to denote the subsequent nature of the home health encounter. Diabetes and hypertension are coded as relevant comorbidities that will impact his recovery. A status code to capture the site of the implanted joint is assigned. An external cause code is assigned to help explain how the patient sustained the fracture.

Fibula fracture, infected wound, stitch abscess

A 79-year-old man fractured the shaft of his left fibula and underwent an ORIF procedure to repair it. His fracture is healing normally but the surgical incision site developed a stitch abscess. He arrives in home health with orders for wound care and is still taking oral antibiotics to treat the infection. He will also receive physical and occupational therapy. He also has type 2 diabetes, which is currently stable.

Description	Code
Primary: Infection following a procedure, superficial incisional surgical site, initial encounter	T81.41xA
Secondary: Unspecified fracture of shaft of left fibula, subsequent encounter for closed fracture with routine healing	S82.402D
Secondary: Type 2 diabetes mellitus without complications	E11.9
Secondary: Long term (current) use of antibiotics	Z79.2

The incision site is still requiring active treatment for the infection, which was described as a stitch abscess and thus is coded with T81.41-. The seventh character "A" is assigned because the infection is still being actively treated with antibiotics. The fracture is healing normally and is thus coded with "D." Diabetes is coded as a relevant comorbidity that will require monitoring. The patient continues to take antibiotics and thus Z79.2 is coded to capture this.

Healing infected surgical wound

A 67-year-old man is being recerted for another episode of home health to continue wound care to a surgical wound. He underwent coronary artery bypass graft (CABG) surgery to treat coronary artery disease and the surgical wound became infected at the superficial incisional surgical site. The infection has now resolved but wound care is still required.

Description	Code
Primary: Infection following a procedure, superficial incisional surgical site, subsequent encounter	T81.41xD
Secondary: Atherosclerotic heart disease of native coronary artery without angina pectoris	I25.10
Secondary: Presence of aortocoronary bypass graft	Z95.1

The infection has resolved and so an infecting organism is not coded. But the wound was previously complicated and thus should still be coded with a complication code, T81.41-. The seventh character "D" signifies that the wound has progressed into the healing phase and is no longer being actively treated. Though the patient had the CABG surgery to treat his coronary artery disease, the operation does not cure the condition; it only treats it. Thus, coronary artery disease is still coded with I25.10. The status of his CABG is captured with Z95.1.

Broken internal hip joint

A 68-year-old woman who has had an internal right hip joint prosthesis for more than three years, was experiencing severe pain in that hip for two days. A trip to the ER revealed a break in her prosthetic hip joint. She recalled falling on some ice on the sidewalk in front of her home several months prior but did not recall any specific injuries from that fall and could not think of any more recent trauma. She was admitted to home health for physical therapy for strengthening until she undergoes surgery to replace the broken prosthetic.

Description	Code
Primary: Broken internal right hip prosthesis, subsequent encounter	T84.010D
Secondary: Fall on same level due to ice and snow, subsequent encounter	W00.0xxD

The internal joint prosthetic itself is broken, necessitating a code from T84.01-. The right hip is affected, making the proper primary diagnosis code T84.010D, with a seventh character "D" for the subsequent nature of the home health encounter. A status code for the replaced joint is not assigned in this scenario as the complication code captures it.

Brown recluse spider bite

A 67-year-old man sustained a bite on the left ankle from a brown recluse spider. The area ulcerated, developing cellulitis due to the venom and now requires wound care, including dressing changes three times a week to be done by home health nursing. Provider documentation indicates that the ulceration has penetrated the muscle but no necrosis is present. The focus of care is managing the wound and specifically the healing of the ulcer due to the bite. He also has diabetes, which is stable and diet-controlled.

Description	Code
Primary: Toxic effect of venom of brown recluse spider, accidental (unintentional), subsequent encounter	T63.331D
Secondary: Non-pressure chronic ulcer of left ankle with muscle involvement without evidence of necrosis	L97.325
Secondary: Cellulitis of left lower limb	L03.116
Secondary: Type 2 diabetes mellitus without complications	E11.9

A venomous spider bite is coded as a poisoning with a code from the Table of Drugs and Chemicals, according to the alphabetic index. The code for toxic effect should always be listed first, followed by the manifestations of the toxic effect. Diabetes is a relevant comorbidity that could impact his recovery and is thus coded.

Dog bite

A 70-year-old man was mowing his lawn when a dog attacked him and bit his left ankle. The wound is clean without evidence of infection. He also has diagnoses of diabetes and PVD, which could complicate his wound healing. He will receive skilled nursing for wound care.

Description	Code
Primary: Open bite, left ankle, subsequent encounter	S91.052D
Secondary: Type 2 diabetes mellitus with diabetic peripheral angiopathy without gangrene	E11.51
Secondary: Bitten by dog, subsequent encounter	W54.0xxD

The patient has a wound resulting from the dog bite that is the focus of care; thus it is coded as primary. Diabetes and PVD can be assumed to be connected in the absence of another stated etiology. Thus, E11.51 is assigned. While there is no requirement to assign external cause codes, it paints the picture of the patient and his injuries and will help support the care provided.

Revision of right hip prosthesis

A 68-year-old man comes to home health for skilled nursing and physical therapy after undergoing revision surgery to his right prosthetic hip after part of it became dislocated. He has an underlying diagnosis of rheumatoid arthritis.

Description	Code
Primary: Dislocation of internal right hip prosthesis, subsequent encounter	T84.020D
Secondary: Rheumatoid arthritis, unspecified	M06.9

The patient underwent a joint prosthesis revision and thus the complication that necessitated the revision should be coded, not surgical aftercare. In this case, it was a dislocation and thus T84.020D is assigned to capture the dislocation of a right hip prosthesis. His rheumatoid arthritis will impact his recovery and will be a factor in his physical therapy. Therefore it is coded as a relevant comorbidity. No status code is assigned because the complication code identifies the joint.

Mechanical loosening of joint prosthesis

An 82-year-old man comes to home health for surgical aftercare following a revision to his right prosthetic hip joint after a part of it had loosened. He also has right heart failure, which will require monitoring and for which he just started new medications. He will receive skilled nursing and physical therapy.

Description	Code
Primary: Mechanical loosening of internal right hip prosthetic joint, subsequent encounter	T84.030D
Secondary: Right heart failure, unspecified	I50.810

While the patient will be receiving aftercare, the patient underwent a joint prosthetic revision due to a mechanical loosening, which is a complication. Therefore, an aftercare code from Z47.3- (Aftercare following explantation of joint prosthesis) is not appropriate in this scenario. The complication itself is coded instead. The patient's right heart failure is coded because he is starting new medications and the condition will require monitoring. No status code is required because the complication code identifies the replaced joint.

Traumatic subdural hemorrhage

A 74-year-old patient was diagnosed with Alzheimer's dementia with behavioral problems, dysphagia and hypertension two years ago. Two months ago she suffered a domestic violence assault in which her former husband hit her in the head with a shoe causing her to lose consciousness for about 20 minutes. The patient had a burr hole evacuation procedure to evacuate a hematoma that had increased in size. The surgeon diagnosed a chronic subdural hemorrhage and noted that re-accumulation of blood was likely which would lead to additional hematomas and neurological deficits. Her family opted for no further imaging and has elected the hospice benefit. She requires total care.

Description	Code
Primary: Traumatic subdural hemorrhage with loss of consciousness of 30 minutes or less, subsequent encounter	S06.5x1D
Secondary: Alzheimer's disease, unspecified	G30.9
Secondary: Dementia in other diseases classified elsewhere with behavioral disturbance	F02.81
Secondary: Essential (primary) hypertension	I10
Secondary: Dysphagia, unspecified	R13.10
Secondary: Assault by blunt object, subsequent encounter	Y00.xxxD

The patient's head injury was treated but is not resolved and the patient's family is opting to forgo further investigation. Thus, the head injury is coded in the primary position with the seventh character "D." The Alzheimer's disease with behaviors, dysphagia and hypertension are coded as relevant comorbidities that will impact her care. The external cause code Y00.xxxD is assigned to explain how the patient became injured; in this case, it was an assault.

Infected wound, knee replacement, lupus

A 72-year-old woman recently underwent a right knee replacement to treat osteoarthritis that affects both knees. Her surgical wound incision is documented as infected by the documentation states that the infection is superficial and only affecting the incision itself. The prosthesis is uncomplicated. She was prescribed oral antibiotics for several weeks for the incisional infection. Skilled nursing will provide and teach wound care and dressing changes, medication management, and monitoring PT/INRs. She'll also receive physical and occupational therapy. Other diagnoses include hypertension and systemic lupus erythematosus. She is on an anticoagulant and long-term prednisone due to her lupus.

Description	Code
Primary: Infection following a procedure, superficial incisional surgical site, initial encounter	T81.41xA
Secondary: Unilateral primary osteoarthritis, left knee	M17.12
Secondary: Systemic lupus erythematosus, unspecified	M32.9
Secondary: Essential (primary) hypertension	I10
Secondary: Presence of right artificial knee joint	Z96.651
Secondary: Encounter for therapeutic drug level monitoring	Z51.81
Secondary: Long term (current) use of antibiotics	Z79.2
Secondary: Long term (current) use of anticoagulants	Z79.01
Secondary: Long term (current) use of systemic steroids	Z79.52

Though the surgical wound is infected, it is only affecting the incision and the joint prosthetic is healing normally. Therefore, T81.41- is the appropriate code choice. The seventh character "A" is used because the infection is being actively treated with antibiotics. The patient's comordidities of lupus and hypertension are coded as secondary diagnoses that will require monitoring. A status code is assigned to denote the replaced knee joint, because the joint prosthetic itself is not complicated. PT/INR monitoring and her use of antibiotics, systemic steroids and anticoagulants are coded as well.

Chapter 20: External Causes of Morbidity (V00-Y99)

Chapter 20 encompasses codes with alpha characters V, W, X and Y, and contains a massive expansion from ICD-9-CM. This chapter permits the classification of environmental events and circumstances as the cause of injury and other adverse effects. Where a code from this section is applicable, it is intended that it shall be used secondary to a code from another ICD-10 chapter indicating the nature of the condition. Most often the condition will be classifiable to Chapter 19, Injury, poisoning and certain other consequences of external causes (S00-T88). Other conditions that may be stated to be due to external causes are classified in Chapters 1 through 18. For these conditions, codes from Chapter 20 may be used to provide additional information as to the cause of the condition.

External cause codes are intended to provide data for injury research and evaluation of injury prevention strategies. However, an external cause code(s) may be used with any code in the range of A00.0-T88.9, Z00-Z99, indicating a health condition due to an external cause such as infections, a disease due to an external source, or another health condition such as a heart attack that occurs during strenuous physical activity.

The codes capture how the injury or health condition happened (cause); the intent (unintentional or accidental; or intentional, such as suicide or assault); the place where the event occurred; the activity of the patient at the time of the event; and the person's status (e.g., civilian, military). The acronym IPAS can be used to remember the sequence of external cause codes – Intent/injury, Place, Activity and Status.

There is no national requirement for mandatory ICD-10-CM external cause code reporting. Unless a provider is subject to a state-based external cause code reporting mandate or these codes are required by a particular payer, reporting of ICD-10-CM codes found in Chapter 20, External Causes of Morbidity, is not required. In the absence of a mandatory reporting requirement, providers are encouraged to voluntarily report external cause codes, as they provide valuable data for injury research and evaluation of injury prevention strategies. (*Source: ICD-10-CM Official Guidelines for Coding and Reporting, 2014*)

Reminder: Within the Official Coding Guidelines, the term provider is used throughout the guidelines to mean physician or any qualified health care practitioner who is legally accountable for establishing the patient's diagnosis.

If an agency chooses to voluntarily report external cause codes, only the code for the intent/cause should be reported. External cause codes for place of encounter, activity and status codes are **used only once at the initial encounter for treatment.** Home health or hospice is never the initial encounter site for treatment (e.g., the patient was seen by a physician in the ER or urgent-care center to diagnose and order treatment first).

External Cause Coding Guidelines

- External cause codes utilize a 7th character to designate the initial encounter, subsequent encounter or sequela for the entire length of treatment for which the injury or condition is being treated.
- The full range of external cause codes is used to completely describe the cause, intent, place of occurrence, and if applicable, the activity of the patient **at the time of the event.**
- No external cause code from Chapter 20 is needed if the external cause and intent are included in the code from another chapter (e.g., T36.0X1, poisoning by penicillins, accidental (unintentional).

Place of Occurrence Guidelines

- Codes from category Y92, Place of occurrence of the external cause, are secondary codes for use after other external cause codes to identify the location of the patient at the time of injury or other condition.
- **A place of occurrence code is used only once, at the initial encounter for treatment.** No 7th characters are used for Y92 and only one Y92 code should be recorded on a medical record. A place of occurrence should be used in conjunction with an activity code, Y93.
- **Do not use** Y92.9, unknown location, if the place of occurrence is not stated or is not applicable.

Activity Code

- Assign a code from category Y93 to describe the activity of the patient at the time the injury or when another health condition occurred, such as a heart attack (I21.3) while shoveling snow (Y93.H1) where the MI resulted from the activity or was contributed to by the activity.
- Activity codes are appropriate for use for both acute injuries, such as those from Chapter 19, and conditions that are due to the long-term, cumulative effects of an activity, such as those from Chapter 13. They are also appropriate for use

with external cause and intent codes if identifying the activity provides additional information about the event.

- **An activity code is used only once, at the initial encounter for treatment** and only one code from Y93 should be recorded on a medical record. An activity code should be used in conjunction with codes for external cause status (Y99) and place of occurrence code, Y92.
- The activity codes are not applicable to poisonings, adverse effects, misadventures or sequela.
- **Do not assign** Y93.9, Unspecified activity, if the activity is not stated.

External Cause Status

A code from category Y99, External cause status, should be assigned in all cases when any other external cause code is assigned for an encounter, including an activity code, except for the specific events noted below. Assign a code from category Y99, External cause status, to indicate the work status of the person at the time the event occurred. The status code indicates whether the event occurred during military activity, whether a non-military person was at work, or whether an individual including a student or volunteer was involved in a non-work activity at the time of the causal event.

- A code from Y99, External cause status, should be assigned, when applicable, with other external cause codes, such as transport accidents and falls. The external cause status codes are ***not applicable*** to poisonings, adverse effects, misadventures or late effects. Do not assign a code from category Y99 if no other external cause codes (cause, activity) are applicable for the encounter.
- ***An external cause status code is only used once, at the initial encounter for treatment.*** Only one code from Y99 should be reported on a medical record.
- Do not assign code Y99.9, Unspecified external cause status, if the status is not stated.

When applicable, place of occurrence, activity and external cause status codes are sequenced after the main external cause code(s). Regardless of the number of external cause codes assigned, there should be only one place of occurrence code, one activity code, and one external cause status code assigned to an encounter.

Multiple External Cause Coding Guidelines

- If the reporting format permits the capture of additional external cause codes, the cause /intent, including medical misadventures, of the additional events should be reported rather than the codes for place, activity or external status.
- When two or more events cause separate injuries, an external cause code should be assigned for each cause. The assignment of the external cause codes should be sequenced in the following priority:
  - The first-listed external cause code(s) for child and adult abuse takes priority over all other external cause codes.
  - External cause codes for terrorism events take priority over all other external cause codes except child and adult abuse.
  - External cause codes for cataclysmic events take priority over all other external cause codes except child and adult abuse, and terrorism.
  - Activity and external cause status codes are assigned following all causal (intent) external cause codes.
  - The first-listed external cause code should correspond to the cause of the most serious diagnosis due to an assault, accident, or self-harm, following the order of hierarchy listed above.

Adult and child abuse, neglect and maltreatment are classified as assault. Any of the assault codes may be used to indicate the external cause of an injury resulting from confirmed abuse. For confirmed cases of abuse, neglect and maltreatment, when the perpetrator is known, a code from Y07, Perpetrator of maltreatment and neglect, should accompany any other assault codes.

Unknown intent: If the intent (accident, self-harm, assault) of the cause of an injury or other condition is unknown or unspecified, code the intent as accidental intent. All transport accident categories assume accidental intent. External cause codes for events of undetermined intent are only for use if the documentation in the record specifies that the intent cannot be determined.

Sequelae (Late Effects) of External Cause

- Sequelae are reported using the external cause code with the 7th character "S" for sequela. These codes should be used with any report of a late effect or sequela resulting from a previous injury.
- A sequela external cause code should never be used with a related current nature of injury code.
- Use a late effect external cause code for subsequent visits when a late effect of the initial injury is being treated. **Do not use** a late effect external cause code for subsequent visits for

follow-up care (e.g., to assess healing, to receive rehabilitative therapy) of the injury when no late effect of the injury has been documented.

Terrorism Guidelines

- When the cause of an injury is ***defined by the Federal Government (FBI)*** as terrorism, the first-listed external cause code should be a code from category Y38, Terrorism. The definition of terrorism used by the FBI is found at the inclusion note at the beginning of category Y38. An additional code for place of occurrence (Y92.-) also is used. More than one Y38 code may be assigned if the injury is the result of more than one mechanism of terrorism.
- When the cause of the injury is ***suspected*** to be the result of terrorism, a code from category Y38 should ***not*** be assigned. Suspected cases should be classified as assault.
- Assign code Y38.9, Terrorism, secondary effects, for conditions occurring subsequent to the terrorist event. This code should not be assigned for conditions that are due to the initial terrorist act.
- It is acceptable to assign code Y38.9 with another code from Y38 if there is an injury due to the initial terrorist event and an injury that is a subsequent result of the terrorist event.

Major Categories in Chapter 20

Transport Accidents (V00-V99) involve a variety of types of injuries that are associated with the various types of transport vehicles, including:

- Pedestrians injured in transport accident (V00-V09)
- Pedal cycle rider injured in transport accidents (V10-V19)
- Motorcycle rider injured in transport accident (V20-V29)
- Occupant of three-wheeled motor vehicle injured in transport accident (V30-V39)
- Car occupant injured in transport accident (V40-V49)
- Occupant of pick-up truck or van injured in transport accident (V50-V59)
- Occupant of heavy transport vehicle injured in transport accident (V60-V69)
- Bus occupant injured in transport accident (V70-V79)
- Other land transport accidents (V80-V89)
- Water transport accidents (V90-V94)
- Air and space transport accidents (V95-V97)
- Other and unspecified transport accidents (V98-V99)

Other external causes of accidental injury (W00-X58)

- Slipping, tripping, stumbling and falls (W00-W19): includes falls from stairs or steps, ladders or scaffolding, out of building or other structures, down manholes or wells, into water, and other tripping, slipping and stumbling.
- Exposure to inanimate mechanical forces (W20-W49)
- Exposure to animate mechanical forces (W50-W64): involves injury by person, rodent, dog, cat, other mammals, nonvenomous marine animal, nonvenomous insect or arthropod, crocodile or alligator, nonvenomous plant thorns, spines or sharp leaves, birds, and nonvenomous amphibians
- Accidental non-transport drowning and submersion (W65-74)
- Exposure to electric current, radiation and extreme ambient temperature and pressure (W85-W99)
- Exposure to smoke, fire and flames (X00-X08)
- Contact with heat and hot substances (X10-X19)
- Exposure to forces of nature (X30-X39)
- Accidental exposure to other specified factors (X52-X58)
- Intentional self-harm (X71-X83)
- Assault (X92-Y09)
- Event of undetermined intent (Y21-Y33)
- Legal intervention, operations of war, military operations, and terrorism (Y35-Y38)

Complications of medical and surgical care (Y62-Y84)

- Misadventures to patients during surgical and medical care (Y62-Y69)
- Medical devices associated with adverse incidents in diagnostic and therapeutic use (Y70-Y82)
- Surgical and other medical procedures as the cause of abnormal reaction of the patient, or later complication, without mention of misadventure at the time of the procedure (Y83-Y84)
- Supplementary factors related to causes of morbidity classified elsewhere (Y90-Y99); physician must determine if this occurred.

CHAPTER 20: EXTERNAL CAUSES OF MORBIDITY (V00-Y99)

Note:
This chapter permits the classification of environmental events and circumstances as the cause of injury, and other adverse effects. Where a code from this section is applicable, it is intended that it shall be used secondary to a code from another chapter of the Classification indicating the nature of the condition. Most often, the condition will be classifiable to Chapter 19, Injury, poisoning and certain other consequences of external causes (S00-T88). Other conditions that may be stated to be due to external causes are classified in Chapters I to XVIII. For these conditions, codes from Chapter 20 should be used to provide additional information as to the cause of the condition.

GUIDELINES **Section I.C.20**
The external causes of morbidity codes should never be sequenced as the first-listed or principal diagnosis. External cause codes are intended to provide data for injury research and evaluation of injury prevention strategies. These codes capture how the injury or health condition happened (cause), the intent (unintentional or accidental; or intentional, such as suicide or assault), the place where the event occurred the activity of the patient at the time of the event, and the person's status (e.g., civilian, military).

There is no national requirement for mandatory ICD-10-CM external cause code reporting. Unless a provider is subject to a state-based external cause code reporting mandate or these codes are required by a particular payer, reporting of ICD-10-CM codes in Chapter 20, External Causes of Morbidity, is not required. In the absence of a mandatory reporting requirement, providers are encouraged to voluntarily report external cause codes, as they provide valuable data for injury research and evaluation of injury prevention strategies.

GUIDELINES **Section I.C.20.a.2)**
Most categories in chapter 20 have a 7th character requirement for each applicable code. ... While the patient may be seen by a new or different provider over the course of treatment for an injury or condition, assignment of the 7th character for external cause should match the 7th character of the code assigned for the associated injury or condition for the encounter.

CODING TIPS✓ These codes are used to explain injuries. External cause codes for accidents should not be assigned if there is no injury coded on the claim.

CODING TIPS✓ These codes can never be placed as primary. Guidelines indicate that they are encouraged, but not required, for home care and hospice. However, if a convention (tabular instruction) indicates to use an additional code, the coder should query for more information and use the code (i.e. for L57 and burns).

CODING TIPS✓ External cause codes may be coded based on documentation other than the physician or NPP's.

This chapter contains the following blocks:

V00-X58	Accidents
V00-V99	Transport accidents
V00-V09	Pedestrian injured in transport accident
V10-V19	Pedal cycle rider injured in transport accident
V20-V29	Motorcycle rider injured in transport accident
V30-V39	Occupant of three-wheeled motor vehicle injured in transport accident
V40-V49	Car occupant injured in transport accident
V50-V59	Occupant of pick-up truck or van injured in transport accident
V60-V69	Occupant of heavy transport vehicle injured in transport accident
V70-V79	Bus occupant injured in transport accident
V80-V89	Other land transport accidents
V90-V94	Water transport accidents
V95-V97	Air and space transport accidents
V98-V99	Other and unspecified transport accidents
W00-X58	Other external causes of accidental injury
W00-W19	Slipping, tripping, stumbling and falls
W20-W49	Exposure to inanimate mechanical forces
W50-W64	Exposure to animate mechanical forces
W65-W74	Accidental non-transport drowning and submersion
W85-W99	Exposure to electric current, radiation and extreme ambient air temperature and pressure
X00-X08	Exposure to smoke, fire and flames
X10-X19	Contact with heat and hot substances
X30-X39	Exposure to forces of nature
X50	Overexertion and strenuous or repetitive movements
X52-X58	Accidental exposure to other specified factors
X71-X83	Intentional self-harm
X92-Y09	Assault
Y21-Y33	Event of undetermined intent
Y35-Y38	Legal intervention, operations of war, military operations, and terrorism
Y62-Y84	Complications of medical and surgical care
Y62-Y69	Misadventures to patients during surgical and medical care
Y70-Y82	Medical devices associated with adverse incidents in diagnostic and therapeutic use
Y83-Y84	Surgical and other medical procedures as the cause of abnormal reaction of the patient, or of later complication, without mention of misadventure at the time of the procedure
Y90-Y99	Supplementary factors related to causes of morbidity classified elsewhere

Accidents (V00-X58)

Transport accidents (V00-V99)

Note:
This section is structured in 12 groups. Those relating to land transport accidents (V00-V89) reflect the victim's mode of transport and are subdivided to identify the victim's 'counterpart' or the type of event. The vehicle of which the injured person is an occupant is identified in the first two characters since it is seen as the most important factor to identify for prevention purposes. A transport accident is one in which the vehicle involved must be moving or running or in use for transport purposes at the time of the accident.
Definitions related to transport accidents:
(a) A transport accident (V00-V99) is any accident involving a device designed primarily for, or used at the time primarily for, conveying persons or good from one place to another.
(b) A public highway [trafficway] or street is the entire width between property lines (or other boundary lines) of land open to the public as a matter of right or custom for purposes of moving persons or property from one place to another. A roadway is that part of the public highway designed, improved and customarily used for vehicular traffic.
(c) A traffic accident is any vehicle accident occurring on the public highway [i.e. originating on, terminating on, or involving a vehicle partially on the highway]. A vehicle accident is assumed to have occurred on the public highway unless another place is specified, except in the case of accidents involving only off-road motor vehicles, which are classified as nontraffic accidents unless the contrary is stated.

4th digit required | 5th digit required | 6th digit required | 7th digit required | 7th digit placeholder | +Additional code | Laterality

(d) A nontraffic accident is any vehicle accident that occurs entirely in any place other than a public highway.

(e) A pedestrian is any person involved in an accident who was not at the time of the accident riding in or on a motor vehicle, railway train, streetcar or animal-drawn or other vehicle, or on a pedal cycle or animal. This includes, a person changing a tire, working on a parked car, or a person on foot. It also includes the user of a pedestrian conveyance such as a baby stroller, ice-skates, skis, sled, roller skates, a skateboard, nonmotorized or motorized wheelchair, motorized mobility scooter, or nonmotorized scooter.

(f) A driver is an occupant of a transport vehicle who is operating or intending to operate it.

(g) A passenger is any occupant of a transport vehicle other than the driver, except a person traveling on the outside of the vehicle.

(h) A person on the outside of a vehicle is any person being transported by a vehicle but not occupying the space normally reserved for the driver or passengers, or the space intended for the transport of property. This includes a person travelling on the bodywork, bumper, fender, roof, running board or step of a vehicle, as well as, hanging on the outside of the vehicle.

(i) A pedal cycle is any land transport vehicle operated solely by nonmotorized pedals including a bicycle or tricycle.

(j) A pedal cyclist is any person riding a pedal cycle or in a sidecar or trailer attached to a pedal cycle.

(k) A motorcycle is a two-wheeled motor vehicle with one or two riding saddles and sometimes with a third wheel for the support of a sidecar. The sidecar is considered part of the motorcycle. This includes a moped, motor scooter, or motorized bicycle.

(l) A motorcycle rider is any person riding a motorcycle or in a sidecar or trailer attached to the motorcycle.

(m) A three-wheeled motor vehicle is a motorized tricycle designed primarily for on-road use. This includes a motor-driven tricycle, a motorized rickshaw, or a three-wheeled motor car.

(n) A car [automobile] is a four-wheeled motor vehicle designed primarily for carrying up to 7 persons. A trailer being towed by the car is considered part of the car. It does not include a van or minivan - see definition (o)

(o) A pick-up truck or van is a four or six-wheeled motor vehicle designed for carrying passengers as well as property or cargo weighing less than the local limit for classification as a heavy goods vehicle, and not requiring a special driver's license. This includes a minivan and a sport-utility vehicle (SUV).

(p) A heavy transport vehicle is a motor vehicle designed primarily for carrying property, meeting local criteria for classification as a heavy goods vehicle in terms of weight and requiring a special driver's license.

(q) A bus (coach) is a motor vehicle designed or adapted primarily for carrying more than 10 passengers, and requiring a special driver's license.

(r) A railway train or railway vehicle is any device, with or without freight or passenger cars couple to it, designed for traffic on a railway track. This includes subterranean (subways) or elevated trains.

(s) A streetcar, is a device designed and used primarily for transporting passengers within a municipality, running on rails, usually subject to normal traffic control signals, and operated principally on a right-of-way that forms part of the roadway. This includes a tram or trolley that runs on rails. A trailer being towed by a streetcar is considered part of the streetcar.

(t) A special vehicle mainly used on industrial premises is a motor vehicle designed primarily for use within the buildings and premises of industrial or commercial establishments. This includes battery-powered airport passenger vehicles or baggage/mail trucks, forklifts, coal-cars in a coal mine, logging cars and trucks used in mines or quarries.

(u) A special vehicle mainly used in agriculture is a motor vehicle designed specifically for use in farming and agriculture (horticulture), to work the land, tend and harvest crops and transport materials on the farm. This includes harvesters, farm machinery and tractor and trailers.

(v) A special construction vehicle is a motor vehicle designed specifically for use on construction and demolition sites. This includes bulldozers, diggers, earth levellers, dump trucks. backhoes, front-end loaders, pavers, and mechanical shovels.

(w) A special all-terrain vehicle is a motor vehicle of special design to enable it to negotiate over rough or soft terrain, snow or sand. Examples of special design are high construction, special wheels and tires, tracks, and support on a cushion of air. This includes snow mobiles, All-terrain vehicles (ATV), and dune buggies. It does not include passenger vehicle designated as Sport Utility Vehicles. (SUV)

(x) A watercraft is any device designed for transporting passengers or goods on water. This includes motor or sail boats, ships, and hovercraft.

(y) An aircraft is any device for transporting passengers or goods in the air. This includes hot-air balloons, gliders, helicopters and airplanes.

(z) A military vehicle is any motorized vehicle operating on a public roadway owned by the military and being operated by a member of the military.

Use additional code to identify:
- Airbag injury (W22.1)
- Type of street or road (Y92.4-)
- Use of cellular telephone and other electronic equipment at the time of the transport accident (Y93.C-)

EXCLUDES 1 agricultural vehicles in stationary use or maintenance (W31.-)
assault by crashing of motor vehicle (Y03.-)
automobile or motor cycle in stationary use or maintenance- code to type of accident
crashing of motor vehicle, undetermined intent (Y32)
intentional self-harm by crashing of motor vehicle (X82)

EXCLUDES 2 transport accidents due to cataclysm (X34-X38)

Pedestrian injured in transport accident (V00-V09)

INCLUDES person changing tire on transport vehicle
person examining engine of vehicle broken down in (on side of) road

EXCLUDES 1 fall due to non-transport collision with other person (W03)
pedestrian on foot falling (slipping) on ice and snow (W00.-)
struck or bumped by another person (W51)

+ 4 **V00 Pedestrian conveyance accident**

Use additional place of occurrence and activity external cause codes, if known (Y92.-, Y93.-)

EXCLUDES 1 collision with another person without fall (W51)
fall due to person on foot colliding with another person on foot (W03)

fall from non-moving wheelchair, nonmotorized scooter and motorized mobility scooter without collision (W05.-)
pedestrian (conveyance) collision with other land transport vehicle (V01-V09)
pedestrian on foot falling (slipping) on ice and snow (W00.-)

The appropriate 7th character is to be added to each code from category V00
A initial encounter
D subsequent encounter
S sequela

+ 5 **V00.0 Pedestrian on foot injured in collision with pedestrian conveyance**

IQ + 7 **V00.01X- Pedestrian on foot injured in collision with roller-skater**

IQ + 7 **V00.02X- Pedestrian on foot injured in collision with skateboarder**

+ 6 **V00.03 Pedestrian on foot injured in collision with standing micro-mobility pedestrian conveyance**

+ 7 **V00.031- Pedestrian on foot injured in collision with rider of standing electric scooter**

+ 7 **V00.038- Pedestrian on foot injured in collision with rider of other standing micro-mobility pedestrian conveyance**
Pedestrian on foot injured in collision with rider of hoverboard
Pedestrian on foot injured in collision with rider of segway

IQ + 7 **V00.09X- Pedestrian on foot injured in collision with other pedestrian conveyance**

+ 5 **V00.1 Rolling-type pedestrian conveyance accident**
EXCLUDES 1 accident with baby stroller (V00.82-)
accident with wheelchair (powered) (V00.81-)
accident with motorized mobility scooter (V00.83-)

+ 6 **V00.11 In-line roller-skate accident**

IQ + 7 **V00.111- Fall from in-line roller-skates**

IQ + 7 **V00.112- In-line roller-skater colliding with stationary object**

IQ + 7 **V00.118- Other in-line roller-skate accident**
EXCLUDES 1 roller-skater collision with other land transport vehicle (V01-V09 with 5th character 1)

+ 6 **V00.12 Non-in- line roller-skate accident**

IQ + 7 **V00.121- Fall from non-in-line roller-skates**

IQ + 7 **V00.122- Non-in-line roller-skater colliding with stationary object**

IQ + 7 **V00.128- Other non-in-line roller-skating accident**
EXCLUDES 1 roller-skater collision with other land transport vehicle (V01-V09 with 5th character 1)

+ 6 **V00.13 Skateboard accident**

IQ + 7 **V00.131- Fall from skateboard**

IQ + 7 **V00.132- Skateboarder colliding with stationary object**

IQ + 7 **V00.138- Other skateboard accident**
EXCLUDES 1 skateboarder collision with other land transport vehicle (V01-V09 with 5th character 2)

+ 6 **V00.14 Scooter (nonmotorized) accident**
EXCLUDES 1 motor scooter accident (V20-V29)

IQ + 7 **V00.141- Fall from scooter (nonmotorized)**

IQ + 7 **V00.142- Scooter (nonmotorized) colliding with stationary object**

IQ + 7 **V00.148- Other scooter (nonmotorized) accident**
EXCLUDES 1 scooter (nonmotorized) collision with other land transport vehicle (V01-V09 with fifth character 9)

+ 6 **V00.15 Heelies accident**
Rolling shoe
Wheeled shoe
Wheelies accident

IQ + 7 **V00.151- Fall from heelies**

IQ + 7 **V00.152- Heelies colliding with stationary object**

IQ + 7 **V00.158- Other heelies accident**

+ 6 **V00.18 Accident on other rolling-type pedestrian conveyance**

IQ + 7 **V00.181- Fall from other rolling-type pedestrian conveyance**

IQ + 7 **V00.182- Pedestrian on other rolling-type pedestrian conveyance colliding with stationary object**

IQ + 7 **V00.188- Other accident on other rolling-type pedestrian conveyance**

+ 5 **V00.2 Gliding-type pedestrian conveyance accident**

+ 6 **V00.21 Ice-skates accident**

IQ + 7 **V00.211- Fall from ice-skates**

IQ + 7 **V00.212- Ice-skater colliding with stationary object**

IQ + 7 **V00.218- Other ice-skates accident**
EXCLUDES 1 ice-skater collision with other land transport vehicle (V01-V09 with 5th character 9)

+ 6 **V00.22 Sled accident**

IQ + 7 **V00.221- Fall from sled**

IQ + 7 **V00.222- Sledder colliding with stationary object**

IQ + 7 **V00.228- Other sled accident**

Chapter 20
V00-Y99

EXCLUDES 1 sled collision with other land transport vehicle (V01-V09 with 5th character 9)

+ 6 **V00.28 Other gliding-type pedestrian conveyance accident**

!Q + 7 **V00.281- Fall from other gliding-type pedestrian conveyance**

!Q + 7 **V00.282- Pedestrian on other gliding-type pedestrian conveyance colliding with stationary object**

!Q + 7 **V00.288- Other accident on other gliding-type pedestrian conveyance**

EXCLUDES 1 gliding-type pedestrian conveyance collision with other land transport vehicle (V01-V09 with 5th character 9)

+ 5 **V00.3 Flat-bottomed pedestrian conveyance accident**

+ 6 **V00.31 Snowboard accident**

!Q + 7 **V00.311- Fall from snowboard**

!Q + 7 **V00.312- Snowboarder colliding with stationary object**

!Q + 7 **V00.318- Other snowboard accident**

EXCLUDES 1 snowboarder collision with other land transport vehicle (V01-V09 with 5th character 9)

+ 6 **V00.32 Snow-ski accident**

!Q + 7 **V00.321- Fall from snow-skis**

!Q + 7 **V00.322- Snow-skier colliding with stationary object**

!Q + 7 **V00.328- Other snow-ski accident**

EXCLUDES 1 snow-skier collision with other land transport vehicle (V01-V09 with 5th character 9)

+ 6 **V00.38 Other flat-bottomed pedestrian conveyance accident**

!Q + 7 **V00.381- Fall from other flat-bottomed pedestrian conveyance**

!Q + 7 **V00.382- Pedestrian on other flat-bottomed pedestrian conveyance colliding with stationary object**

!Q + 7 **V00.388- Other accident on other flat-bottomed pedestrian conveyance**

+ 5 **V00.8 Accident on other pedestrian conveyance**

+ 6 **V00.81 Accident with wheelchair (powered)**

!Q + 7 **V00.811- Fall from moving wheelchair (powered)**

EXCLUDES 1 fall from non-moving wheelchair (W05.0)

!Q + 7 **V00.812- Wheelchair (powered) colliding with stationary object**

!Q + 7 **V00.818- Other accident with wheelchair (powered)**

+ 6 **V00.82 Accident with baby stroller**

!Q + 7 **V00.821- Fall from baby stroller**

!Q + 7 **V00.822- Baby stroller colliding with stationary object**

!Q + 7 **V00.828- Other accident with baby stroller**

+ 6 **V00.83 Accident with motorized mobility scooter**

!Q + 7 **V00.831- Fall from motorized mobility scooter**

EXCLUDES 1 fall from non-moving motorized mobility scooter (W05.2)

!Q + 7 **V00.832- Motorized mobility scooter colliding with stationary object**

!Q + 7 **V00.838- Other accident with motorized mobility scooter**

+ 6 **V00.84 Accident with standing micro-mobility pedestrian conveyance**

+ 7 **V00.841- Fall from standing electric scooter**

+ 7 **V00.842- Pedestrian on standing electric scooter colliding with stationary object**

+ 7 **V00.848- Other accident with standing micro-mobility pedestrian conveyance**

Accident with hoverboard

Accident with segway

+ 6 **V00.89 Accident on other pedestrian conveyance**

!Q + 7 **V00.891- Fall from other pedestrian conveyance**

!Q + 7 **V00.892- Pedestrian on other pedestrian conveyance colliding with stationary object**

!Q + 7 **V00.898- Other accident on other pedestrian conveyance**

EXCLUDES 1 other pedestrian (conveyance) collision with other land transport vehicle (V01-V09 with 5th character 9)

4 **V01 Pedestrian injured in collision with pedal cycle**

The appropriate 7th character is to be added to each code from category V01

A	initial encounter
D	subsequent encounter
S	sequela

5 **V01.0 Pedestrian injured in collision with pedal cycle in nontraffic accident**

!Q 7 **V01.00X- Pedestrian on foot injured in collision with pedal cycle in nontraffic accident**

Pedestrian NOS injured in collision with pedal cycle in nontraffic accident

!Q 7 **V01.01X- Pedestrian on roller-skates injured in collision with pedal cycle in nontraffic accident**

!Q 7 **V01.02X- Pedestrian on skateboard injured in collision with pedal cycle in nontraffic accident**

Chapter 20 V00-Y99

6 **V01.03 Pedestrian on standing micro-mobility pedestrian conveyance injured in collision with pedal cycle in nontraffic accident**

7 **V01.031- Pedestrian on standing electric scooter injured in collision with pedal cycle in nontraffic accident**

7 **V01.038- Pedestrian on other standing micro-mobility pedestrian conveyance injured in collision with pedal cycle in nontraffic accident**
Pedestrian on hoverboard injured in collision with pedal cycle in nontraffic accident
Pedestrian on segway injured in collision with pedal cycle in nontraffic accident

IQ 7 **V01.09X- Pedestrian with other conveyance injured in collision with pedal cycle in nontraffic accident**
Pedestrian with baby stroller injured in collision with pedal cycle in nontraffic accident
Pedestrian on ice-skates injured in collision with pedal cycle in nontraffic accident
Pedestrian on nonmotorized scooter injured in collision with pedal cycle in nontraffic accident
Pedestrian on sled injured in collision with pedal cycle in nontraffic accident
Pedestrian on snowboard injured in collision with pedal cycle in nontraffic accident
Pedestrian on snow-skis injured in collision with pedal cycle in nontraffic accident
Pedestrian in wheelchair (powered) injured in collision with pedal cycle in nontraffic accident
Pedestrian in motorized mobility scooter injured in collision with pedal cycle in nontraffic accident

5 **V01.1 Pedestrian injured in collision with pedal cycle in traffic accident**

IQ 7 **V01.10X- Pedestrian on foot injured in collision with pedal cycle in traffic accident**
Pedestrian NOS injured in collision with pedal cycle in traffic accident

IQ 7 **V01.11X- Pedestrian on roller-skates injured in collision with pedal cycle in traffic accident**

IQ 7 **V01.12X- Pedestrian on skateboard injured in collision with pedal cycle in traffic accident**

6 **V01.13 Pedestrian on standing micro-mobility pedestrian conveyance injured in collision with pedal cycle in traffic accident**

7 **V01.131- Pedestrian on standing electric scooter injured in collision with pedal cycle in traffic accident**

7 **V01.138- Pedestrian on other standing micro-mobility pedestrian conveyance injured in collision with pedal cycle in traffic accident**
Pedestrian on hoverboard injured in collision with pedal cycle in traffic accident
Pedestrian on segway injured in collision with pedal cycle in traffic accident

IQ 7 **V01.19X- Pedestrian with other conveyance injured in collision with pedal cycle in traffic accident**
Pedestrian with baby stroller injured in collision with pedal cycle in traffic accident
Pedestrian on ice-skates injured in collision with pedal cycle in traffic accident
Pedestrian on nonmotorized scooter injured in collision with pedal cycle in traffic accident
Pedestrian on sled injured in collision with pedal cycle in traffic accident
Pedestrian on snowboard injured in collision with pedal cycle in traffic accident
Pedestrian on snow-skis injured in collision with pedal cycle in traffic accident
Pedestrian in wheelchair (powered) injured in collision with pedal cycle in traffic accident
Pedestrian in motorized mobility scooter injured in collision with pedal cycle in traffic accident

5 **V01.9 Pedestrian injured in collision with pedal cycle, unspecified whether traffic or nontraffic accident**

IQ 7 **V01.90X- Pedestrian on foot injured in collision with pedal cycle, unspecified whether traffic or nontraffic accident**
Pedestrian NOS injured in collision with pedal cycle, unspecified whether traffic or nontraffic accident

IQ 7 **V01.91X- Pedestrian on roller-skates injured in collision with pedal cycle, unspecified whether traffic or nontraffic accident**

IQ 7 **V01.92X- Pedestrian on skateboard injured in collision with pedal cycle, unspecified whether traffic or nontraffic accident**

6 **V01.93 Pedestrian on standing micro-mobility pedestrian conveyance injured in collision with pedal cycle, unspecified whether traffic or nontraffic accident**

7 **V01.931- Pedestrian on standing electric scooter injured in collision with pedal cycle, unspecified whether traffic or nontraffic accident**

7 **V01.938- Pedestrian on other standing micro-mobility pedestrian conveyance injured in collision with pedal cycle, unspecified whether traffic or nontraffic accident**

Pedestrian on hoverboard injured in collision with pedal cycle, unspecified whether traffic or nontraffic accident

Pedestrian on segway injured in collision with pedal cycle, unspecified whether traffic or nontraffic accident

IQ 7 **V01.99X- Pedestrian with other conveyance injured in collision with pedal cycle, unspecified whether traffic or nontraffic accident**

Pedestrian with baby stroller injured in collision with pedal cycle, unspecified whether traffic or nontraffic accident

Pedestrian on ice-skates injured in collision with pedal cycle unspecified, whether traffic or nontraffic accident

Pedestrian on nonmotorized scooter injured in collision with pedal cycle, unspecified whether traffic or nontraffic accident

Pedestrian on sled injured in collision with pedal cycle unspecified, whether traffic or nontraffic accident

Pedestrian on snowboard injured in collision with pedal cycle, unspecified whether traffic or nontraffic accident

Pedestrian on snow-skis injured in collision with pedal cycle, unspecified whether traffic or nontraffic accident

Pedestrian in wheelchair (powered) injured in collision with pedal cycle, unspecified whether traffic or nontraffic accident

Pedestrian in motorized mobility scooter injured in collision with pedal cycle, unspecified whether traffic or nontraffic accident

4 **V02 Pedestrian injured in collision with two- or three-wheeled motor vehicle**

The appropriate 7th character is to be added to each code from category V02

A	initial encounter
D	subsequent encounter
S	sequela

5 **V02.0 Pedestrian injured in collision with two- or three-wheeled motor vehicle in nontraffic accident**

IQ 7 **V02.00X- Pedestrian on foot injured in collision with two- or three-wheeled motor vehicle in nontraffic accident**

Pedestrian NOS injured in collision with two- or three-wheeled motor vehicle in nontraffic accident

IQ 7 **V02.01X- Pedestrian on roller-skates injured in collision with two- or three-wheeled motor vehicle in nontraffic accident**

IQ 7 **V02.02X- Pedestrian on skateboard injured in collision with two- or three-wheeled motor vehicle in nontraffic accident**

6 **V02.03 Pedestrian on standing micro-mobility pedestrian conveyance injured in collision with two- or three-wheeled motor vehicle in nontraffic accident**

7 **V02.031- Pedestrian on standing electric scooter injured in collision with two- or three-wheeled motor vehicle in nontraffic accident**

7 **V02.038- Pedestrian on other standing micro-mobility pedestrian conveyance injured in collision with two- or three-wheeled motor vehicle in nontraffic accident**

Pedestrian on hoverboard injured in collision with two-or three wheeled motor vehicle in nontraffic accident

Pedestrian on segway injured in collision with two- or three-wheeled motor vehicle in nontraffic accident

IQ 7 **V02.09X- Pedestrian with other conveyance injured in collision with two- or three-wheeled motor vehicle in nontraffic accident**

Pedestrian with baby stroller injured in collision with two- or three-wheeled motor vehicle in nontraffic accident

Pedestrian on ice-skates injured in collision with two- or three-wheeled motor vehicle in nontraffic accident

Pedestrian on nonmotorized scooter injured in collision with two- or three-wheeled motor vehicle in nontraffic accident

Pedestrian on sled injured in collision with two- or three-wheeled motor vehicle in nontraffic accident

Pedestrian on snowboard injured in collision with two- or three-wheeled motor vehicle in nontraffic accident

Pedestrian on snow-skis injured in collision with two- or three-wheeled motor vehicle in nontraffic accident

Pedestrian in wheelchair (powered) injured in collision with two- or three-wheeled motor vehicle in nontraffic accident

Pedestrian in motorized mobility scooter injured in collision with two- or three-wheeled motor vehicle in nontraffic accident

V02.1 Pedestrian injured in collision with two- or three-wheeled motor vehicle in traffic accident

V02.10X- Pedestrian on foot injured in collision with two- or three-wheeled motor vehicle in traffic accident

Pedestrian NOS injured in collision with two- or three-wheeled motor vehicle in traffic accident

V02.11X- Pedestrian on roller-skates injured in collision with two- or three-wheeled motor vehicle in traffic accident

V02.12X- Pedestrian on skateboard injured in collision with two- or three-wheeled motor vehicle in traffic accident

V02.13 Pedestrian on standing micro-mobility pedestrian conveyance injured in collision with two- or three-wheeled motor vehicle in traffic accident

V02.131- Pedestrian on standing electric scooter injured in collision with two- or three-wheeled motor vehicle in traffic accident

V02.138- Pedestrian on other standing micro-mobility pedestrian conveyance injured in collision with two- or three-wheeled motor vehicle in traffic accident

Pedestrian on hoverboard injured in collision with two-or three wheeled motor vehicle in traffic accident

Pedestrian on segway injured in collision with two- or three-wheeled motor vehicle in traffic accident

V02.19X- Pedestrian with other conveyance injured in collision with two- or three-wheeled motor vehicle in traffic accident

Pedestrian with baby stroller injured in collision with two- or three-wheeled motor vehicle in traffic accident

Pedestrian on ice-skates injured in collision with two- or three-wheeled motor vehicle in traffic accident

Pedestrian on nonmotorized scooter injured in collision with two- or three-wheeled motor vehicle in traffic accident

Pedestrian on sled injured in collision with two- or three-wheeled motor vehicle in traffic accident

Pedestrian on snowboard injured in collision with two- or three-wheeled motor vehicle in traffic accident

Pedestrian on snow-skis injured in collision with two- or three-wheeled motor vehicle in traffic accident

Pedestrian in wheelchair (powered) injured in collision with two- or three-wheeled motor vehicle in traffic accident

Pedestrian in motorized mobility scooter injured in collision with two- or three-wheeled motor vehicle in traffic accident

V02.9 Pedestrian injured in collision with two- or three-wheeled motor vehicle, unspecified whether traffic or nontraffic accident

V02.90X- Pedestrian on foot injured in collision with two- or three-wheeled motor vehicle, unspecified whether traffic or nontraffic accident

Pedestrian NOS injured in collision with two- or three-wheeled motor vehicle, unspecified whether traffic or nontraffic accident

V02.91X- Pedestrian on roller-skates injured in collision with two- or three-wheeled motor vehicle, unspecified whether traffic or nontraffic accident

V02.92X- Pedestrian on skateboard injured in collision with two- or three-wheeled motor vehicle, unspecified whether traffic or nontraffic accident

V02.93 Pedestrian on standing micro-mobility pedestrian conveyance injured in collision with two- or three-wheeled motor vehicle, unspecified whether traffic or nontraffic accident

V02.931- Pedestrian on standing electric scooter injured in collision with two- or three wheeled motor vehicle, unspecified whether traffic or nontraffic accident

V02.938- Pedestrian on other standing micro-mobility pedestrian conveyance injured in collision with two- or three wheeled motor vehicle, unspecified whether traffic or nontraffic accident

Pedestrian on hoverboard injured in collision with two-three-wheeled motor vehicle, unspecified whether traffic or nontraffic accident

Pedestrian on segway injured in collision with two- or three wheeled motor vehicle, unspecified whether traffic or nontraffic accident

V02.99X- Pedestrian with other conveyance injured in collision with two- or three-wheeled motor vehicle, unspecified whether traffic or nontraffic accident

Pedestrian with baby stroller injured in collision with two- or three-wheeled motor vehicle, unspecified whether traffic or nontraffic accident
Pedestrian on ice-skates injured in collision with two- or three-wheeled motor vehicle, unspecified whether traffic or nontraffic accident
Pedestrian on nonmotorized scooter injured in collision with two- or three-wheeled motor vehicle, unspecified whether traffic or nontraffic accident
Pedestrian on sled injured in collision with two- or three-wheeled motor vehicle, unspecified whether traffic or nontraffic accident
Pedestrian on snowboard injured in collision with two- or three-wheeled motor vehicle, unspecified whether traffic or nontraffic accident
Pedestrian on snow-skis injured in collision with two- or three-wheeled motor vehicle, unspecified whether traffic or nontraffic accident
Pedestrian in wheelchair (powered) injured in collision with two- or three-wheeled motor vehicle, unspecified whether traffic or nontraffic accident
Pedestrian in motorized mobility scooter injured in collision with two- or three-wheeled motor vehicle, unspecified whether traffic or nontraffic accident

4 **V03 Pedestrian injured in collision with car, pick-up truck or van**

The appropriate 7th character is to be added to each code from category V03
A initial encounter
D subsequent encounter
S sequela

5 **V03.0 Pedestrian injured in collision with car, pick-up truck or van in nontraffic accident**

IQ 7 **V03.00X- Pedestrian on foot injured in collision with car, pick-up truck or van in nontraffic accident**
Pedestrian NOS injured in collision with car, pick-up truck or van in nontraffic accident

IQ 7 **V03.01X- Pedestrian on roller-skates injured in collision with car, pick-up truck or van in nontraffic accident**

IQ 7 **V03.02X- Pedestrian on skateboard injured in collision with car, pick-up truck or van in nontraffic accident**

6 **V03.03 Pedestrian on standing micro-mobility pedestrian conveyance injured in collision with car, pick-up or van in nontraffic accident**

7 **V03.031- Pedestrian on standing electric scooter injured in collision with car, pick-up or van in nontraffic accident**

7 **V03.038- Pedestrian on other standing micro-mobility pedestrian conveyance injured in collision with car, pick-up or van in nontraffic accident**
Pedestrian on hoverboard injured in collision with car, pick-up or van in nontraffic accident
Pedestrian on segway injured in collision with car, pick-up or van in nontraffic accident

IQ 7 **V03.09X- Pedestrian with other conveyance injured in collision with car, pick-up truck or van in nontraffic accident**
Pedestrian with baby stroller injured in collision with car, pick-up truck or van in nontraffic accident
Pedestrian on ice-skates injured in collision with car, pick-up truck or van in nontraffic accident
Pedestrian on nonmotorized scooter injured in collision with car, pick-up truck or van in nontraffic accident
Pedestrian on sled injured in collision with car, pick-up truck or van in nontraffic accident
Pedestrian on snowboard injured in collision with car, pick-up truck or van in nontraffic accident
Pedestrian on snow-skis injured in collision with car, pick-up truck or van in nontraffic accident
Pedestrian in wheelchair (powered) injured in collision with car, pick-up truck or van in nontraffic accident
Pedestrian in motorized mobility scooter injured in collision with car, pick-up truck or van in nontraffic accident

5 **V03.1 Pedestrian injured in collision with car, pick-up truck or van in traffic accident**

IQ 7 **V03.10X- Pedestrian on foot injured in collision with car, pick-up truck or van in traffic accident**
Pedestrian NOS injured in collision with car, pick-up truck or van in traffic accident

IQ 7 **V03.11X- Pedestrian on roller-skates injured in collision with car, pick-up truck or van in traffic accident**

IQ 7 **V03.12X- Pedestrian on skateboard injured in collision with car, pick-up truck or van in traffic accident**

6 **V03.13 Pedestrian on standing micro-mobility pedestrian conveyance injured in collision with car, pick-up or van in traffic accident**

7 **V03.131- Pedestrian on standing electric scooter injured in collision with car, pick-up or van in traffic accident**

7 **V03.138- Pedestrian on other standing micro-mobility pedestrian conveyance injured in collision with car, pick-up or van in traffic accident**
Pedestrian on hoverboard injured in collision with car, pick-up or van in traffic accident
Pedestrian on segway injured in collision with car, pick-up or van in traffic accident

IQ 7 **V03.19X- Pedestrian with other conveyance injured in collision with car, pick-up truck or van in traffic accident**
Pedestrian with baby stroller injured in collision with car, pick-up truck or van in traffic accident
Pedestrian on ice-skates injured in collision with car, pick-up truck or van in traffic accident
Pedestrian on nonmotorized scooter injured in collision with car, pick-up truck or van in traffic accident
Pedestrian on sled injured in collision with car, pick-up truck or van in traffic accident
Pedestrian on snowboard injured in collision with car, pick-up truck or van in traffic accident
Pedestrian on snow-skis injured in collision with car, pick-up truck or van in traffic accident
Pedestrian in wheelchair (powered) injured in collision with car, pick-up truck or van in traffic accident
Pedestrian in motorized mobility scooter injured in collision with car, pick-up truck or van in traffic accident

5 **V03.9 Pedestrian injured in collision with car, pick-up truck or van, unspecified whether traffic or nontraffic accident**

IQ 7 **V03.90X- Pedestrian on foot injured in collision with car, pick-up truck or van, unspecified whether traffic or nontraffic accident**
Pedestrian NOS injured in collision with car, pick-up truck or van, unspecified whether traffic or nontraffic accident

IQ 7 **V03.91X- Pedestrian on roller-skates injured in collision with car, pick-up truck or van, unspecified whether traffic or nontraffic accident**

IQ 7 **V03.92X- Pedestrian on skateboard injured in collision with car, pick-up truck or van, unspecified whether traffic or nontraffic accident**

6 **V03.93 Pedestrian on standing micro-mobility pedestrian conveyance injured in collision with car, pick-up or van, unspecified whether traffic or nontraffic accident**

7 **V03.931- Pedestrian on standing electric scooter injured in collision with car, pick-up or van, unspecified whether traffic or nontraffic accident**

7 **V03.938- Pedestrian on other standing micro-mobility pedestrian conveyance injured in collision with car, pick-up or van, unspecified whether traffic or nontraffic accident**
Pedestrian on hoverboard injured in collision with car, pick-up or van, unspecified whether traffic or nontraffic accident
Pedestrian on segway injured in collision with car, pick-up or van, unspecified whether traffic or nontraffic accident

IQ 7 **V03.99X- Pedestrian with other conveyance injured in collision with car, pick-up truck or van, unspecified whether traffic or nontraffic accident**
Pedestrian with baby stroller injured in collision with car, pick-up truck or van, unspecified whether traffic or nontraffic accident
Pedestrian on ice-skates injured in collision with car, pick-up truck or van, unspecified whether traffic or nontraffic accident
Pedestrian on nonmotorized scooter injured in collision with car, pick-up truck or van, unspecified whether traffic or nontraffic accident
Pedestrian on sled injured in collision with car, pick-up truck or van in nontraffic accident
Pedestrian on snowboard injured in collision with car, pick-up truck or van, unspecified whether traffic or nontraffic accident
Pedestrian on snow-skis injured in collision with car, pick-up truck or van, unspecified whether traffic or nontraffic accident
Pedestrian in wheelchair (powered) injured in collision with car, pick-up truck or van, unspecified whether traffic or nontraffic accident
Pedestrian in motorized mobility scooter injured in collision with car, pick-up truck or van, unspecified whether traffic or nontraffic accident

4 **V04 Pedestrian injured in collision with heavy transport vehicle or bus**
EXCLUDES 1 pedestrian injured in collision with military vehicle (V09.01, V09.21)

The appropriate 7th character is to be added to each code from category V04
A initial encounter
D subsequent encounter
S sequela

Chapter 20

V00-Y99

5 **V04.0 Pedestrian injured in collision with heavy transport vehicle or bus in nontraffic accident**

IQ 7 **V04.00X- Pedestrian on foot injured in collision with heavy transport vehicle or bus in nontraffic accident**

Pedestrian NOS injured in collision with heavy transport vehicle or bus in nontraffic accident

IQ 7 **V04.01X- Pedestrian on roller-skates injured in collision with heavy transport vehicle or bus in nontraffic accident**

IQ 7 **V04.02X- Pedestrian on skateboard injured in collision with heavy transport vehicle or bus in nontraffic accident**

6 **V04.03 Pedestrian on standing micro-mobility pedestrian conveyance injured in collision with heavy transport vehicle or bus in nontraffic accident**

7 **V04.031- Pedestrian on standing electric scooter injured in collision with heavy transport vehicle or bus in nontraffic accident**

7 **V04.038- Pedestrian on other standing micro-mobility pedestrian conveyance injured in collision with heavy transport vehicle or bus in nontraffic accident**

Pedestrian on hoverboard injured in collision with heavy transport vehicle or bus in nontraffic accident

Pedestrian on segway injured in collision with heavy transport vehicle or bus in nontraffic accident

IQ 7 **V04.09X- Pedestrian with other conveyance injured in collision with heavy transport vehicle or bus in nontraffic accident**

Pedestrian with baby stroller injured in collision with heavy transport vehicle or bus in nontraffic accident

Pedestrian on ice-skates injured in collision with heavy transport vehicle or bus in nontraffic accident

Pedestrian on nonmotorized scooter injured in collision with heavy transport vehicle or bus in nontraffic accident

Pedestrian on sled injured in collision with heavy transport vehicle or bus in nontraffic accident

Pedestrian on snowboard injured in collision with heavy transport vehicle or bus in nontraffic accident

Pedestrian on snow-skis injured in collision with heavy transport vehicle or bus in nontraffic accident

Pedestrian in wheelchair (powered) injured in collision with heavy transport vehicle or bus in nontraffic accident

Pedestrian in motorized mobility scooter injured in collision with heavy transport vehicle or bus in nontraffic accident

5 **V04.1 Pedestrian injured in collision with heavy transport vehicle or bus in traffic accident**

IQ 7 **V04.10X- Pedestrian on foot injured in collision with heavy transport vehicle or bus in traffic accident**

Pedestrian NOS injured in collision with heavy transport vehicle or bus in traffic accident

IQ 7 **V04.11X- Pedestrian on roller-skates injured in collision with heavy transport vehicle or bus in traffic accident**

IQ 7 **V04.12X- Pedestrian on skateboard injured in collision with heavy transport vehicle or bus in traffic accident**

6 **V04.13 Pedestrian on standing micro-mobility pedestrian conveyance injured in collision with heavy transport vehicle or bus in traffic accident**

7 **V04.131- Pedestrian on standing electric scooter injured in collision with heavy transport vehicle or bus in traffic accident**

7 **V04.138- Pedestrian on other standing micro-mobility pedestrian conveyance injured in collision with heavy transport vehicle or bus in traffic accident**

Pedestrian on hoverboard injured in collision with heavy transport vehicle or bus in traffic accident

Pedestrian on segway injured in collision with heavy transport vehicle or bus in traffic accident

IQ 7 **V04.19X- Pedestrian with other conveyance injured in collision with heavy transport vehicle or bus in traffic accident**

Pedestrian with baby stroller injured in collision with heavy transport vehicle or bus in traffic accident

Pedestrian on ice-skates injured in collision with heavy transport vehicle or bus in traffic accident

Pedestrian on nonmotorized scooter injured in collision with heavy transport vehicle or bus in traffic accident

Pedestrian on sled injured in collision with heavy transport vehicle or bus in traffic accident

Pedestrian on snowboard injured in collision with heavy transport vehicle or bus in traffic accident

Pedestrian on snow-skis injured in collision with heavy transport vehicle or bus in traffic accident

Pedestrian in wheelchair (powered) injured in collision with heavy transport vehicle or bus in traffic accident

Pedestrian in motorized mobility scooter injured in collision with heavy transport vehicle or bus in traffic accident

⑤ V04.9 Pedestrian injured in collision with heavy transport vehicle or bus, unspecified whether traffic or nontraffic accident

!Q ☑ V04.90X- Pedestrian on foot injured in collision with heavy transport vehicle or bus, unspecified whether traffic or nontraffic accident

Pedestrian NOS injured in collision with heavy transport vehicle or bus, unspecified whether traffic or nontraffic accident

!Q ☑ V04.91X- Pedestrian on roller-skates injured in collision with heavy transport vehicle or bus, unspecified whether traffic or nontraffic accident

!Q ☑ V04.92X- Pedestrian on skateboard injured in collision with heavy transport vehicle or bus, unspecified whether traffic or nontraffic accident

⑥ V04.93 Pedestrian on standing micro-mobility pedestrian conveyance injured in collision with heavy transport vehicle or bus, unspecified whether traffic or nontraffic accident

⑦ V04.931- Pedestrian on standing electric scooter injured in collision with heavy transport vehicle or bus, unspecified whether traffic or nontraffic accident

⑦ V04.938- Pedestrian on other standing micro-mobility pedestrian conveyance injured in collision with heavy transport vehicle or bus, unspecified whether traffic or nontraffic accident

Pedestrian on hoverboard injured in collision with heavy transport vehicle or bus, unspecified whether traffic or nontraffic accident

Pedestrian on segway injured in collision with heavy transport vehicle or bus, unspecified whether traffic or nontraffic accident

!Q ☑ V04.99X- Pedestrian with other conveyance injured in collision with heavy transport vehicle or bus, unspecified whether traffic or nontraffic accident

Pedestrian with baby stroller injured in collision with heavy transport vehicle or bus, unspecified whether traffic or nontraffic accident

Pedestrian on ice-skates injured in collision with heavy transport vehicle or bus, unspecified whether traffic or nontraffic accident

Pedestrian on nonmotorized scooter injured in collision with heavy transport vehicle or bus, unspecified whether traffic or nontraffic accident

Pedestrian on sled injured in collision with heavy transport vehicle or bus, unspecified whether traffic or nontraffic accident

Pedestrian on snowboard injured in collision with heavy transport vehicle or bus, unspecified whether traffic or nontraffic accident

Pedestrian on snow-skis injured in collision with heavy transport vehicle or bus, unspecified whether traffic or nontraffic accident

Pedestrian in wheelchair (powered) injured in collision with heavy transport vehicle or bus, unspecified whether traffic or nontraffic accident

Pedestrian in motorized mobility scooter injured in collision with heavy transport vehicle or bus, unspecified whether traffic or nontraffic accident

④ V05 Pedestrian injured in collision with railway train or railway vehicle

The appropriate 7th character is to be added to each code from category V05
A   initial encounter
D   subsequent encounter
S   sequela

⑤ V05.0 Pedestrian injured in collision with railway train or railway vehicle in nontraffic accident

!Q ☑ V05.00X- Pedestrian on foot injured in collision with railway train or railway vehicle in nontraffic accident
Pedestrian NOS injured in collision with railway train or railway vehicle in nontraffic accident

!Q ☑ V05.01X- Pedestrian on roller-skates injured in collision with railway train or railway vehicle in nontraffic accident

!Q ☑ V05.02X- Pedestrian on skateboard injured in collision with railway train or railway vehicle in nontraffic accident

⑥ V05.03 Pedestrian on standing micro-mobility pedestrian conveyance injured in collision with railway train or railway vehicle in nontraffic accident

④ 4th digit required   ⑤ 5th digit required   ⑥ 6th digit required   ⑦ 7th digit required   ☑ 7th digit placeholder   ✚ Additional code   ▤ Laterality

7 **V05.031- Pedestrian on standing electric scooter injured in collision with railway train or railway vehicle in nontraffic accident**

7 **V05.038- Pedestrian on other standing micro-mobility pedestrian conveyance injured in collision with railway train or railway vehicle in nontraffic accident**
Pedestrian on hoverboard injured in collision with railway train or railway vehicle in nontraffic accident
Pedestrian on segway injured in collision with railway train or railway vehicle in nontraffic accident

IQ 7 **V05.09X- Pedestrian with other conveyance injured in collision with railway train or railway vehicle in nontraffic accident**
Pedestrian with baby stroller injured in collision with railway train or railway vehicle in nontraffic accident
Pedestrian on ice-skates injured in collision with railway train or railway vehicle in nontraffic accident
Pedestrian on nonmotorized scooter injured in collision with railway train or railway vehicle in nontraffic accident
Pedestrian on sled injured in collision with railway train or railway vehicle in nontraffic accident
Pedestrian on snowboard injured in collision with railway train or railway vehicle in nontraffic accident
Pedestrian on snow-skis injured in collision with railway train or railway vehicle in nontraffic accident
Pedestrian in wheelchair (powered) injured in collision with railway train or railway vehicle in nontraffic accident
Pedestrian in motorized mobility scooter injured in collision with railway train or railway vehicle in nontraffic accident

5 **V05.1 Pedestrian injured in collision with railway train or railway vehicle in traffic accident**

IQ 7 **V05.10X- Pedestrian on foot injured in collision with railway train or railway vehicle in traffic accident**
Pedestrian NOS injured in collision with railway train or railway vehicle in traffic accident

IQ 7 **V05.11X- Pedestrian on roller-skates injured in collision with railway train or railway vehicle in traffic accident**

IQ 7 **V05.12X- Pedestrian on skateboard injured in collision with railway train or railway vehicle in traffic accident**

6 **V05.13 Pedestrian on standing micro-mobility pedestrian conveyance injured in collision with railway train or railway vehicle in traffic accident**

7 **V05.131- Pedestrian on standing electric scooter injured in collision with railway train or railway vehicle in traffic accident**

7 **V05.138- Pedestrian on other standing micro-mobility pedestrian conveyance injured in collision with railway train or railway vehicle in traffic accident**
Pedestrian on hoverboard injured in collision with railway train or railway vehicle in traffic accident
Pedestrian on segway injured in collision with railway train or railway vehicle in traffic accident

IQ 7 **V05.19X- Pedestrian with other conveyance injured in collision with railway train or railway vehicle in traffic accident**
Pedestrian with baby stroller injured in collision with railway train or railway vehicle in traffic accident
Pedestrian on ice-skates injured in collision with railway train or railway vehicle in traffic accident
Pedestrian on nonmotorized scooter injured in collision with railway train or railway vehicle in traffic accident
Pedestrian on sled injured in collision with railway train or railway vehicle in traffic accident
Pedestrian on snowboard injured in collision with railway train or railway vehicle in traffic accident
Pedestrian on snow-skis injured in collision with railway train or railway vehicle in traffic accident
Pedestrian in wheelchair (powered) injured in collision with railway train or railway vehicle in traffic accident
Pedestrian in motorized mobility scooter injured in collision with railway train or railway vehicle in traffic accident

5 **V05.9 Pedestrian injured in collision with railway train or railway vehicle, unspecified whether traffic or nontraffic accident**

IQ 7 **V05.90X- Pedestrian on foot injured in collision with railway train or railway vehicle, unspecified whether traffic or nontraffic accident**
Pedestrian NOS injured in collision with railway train or railway vehicle, unspecified whether traffic or nontraffic accident

IQ 7 **V05.91X- Pedestrian on roller-skates injured in collision with railway train or railway vehicle, unspecified whether traffic or nontraffic accident**

!Q ⁷ **V05.92X- Pedestrian on skateboard injured in collision with railway train or railway vehicle, unspecified whether traffic or nontraffic accident**

⁶ **V05.93 Pedestrian on standing micro-mobility pedestrian conveyance injured in collision with railway train or railway vehicle, unspecified whether traffic or nontraffic accident**

⁷ **V05.931- Pedestrian on standing electric scooter injured in collision with railway train or railway vehicle, unspecified whether traffic or nontraffic accident**

⁷ **V05.938- Pedestrian on other standing micro-mobility pedestrian conveyance injured in collision with railway train or railway vehicle, unspecified whether traffic or nontraffic accident**

Pedestrian on hoverboard injured in collision with railway train or railway vehicle, unspecified whether traffic or nontraffic accident

Pedestrian on segway injured in collision with railway train or railway vehicle, unspecified whether traffic or nontraffic accident

!Q ⁷ **V05.99X- Pedestrian with other conveyance injured in collision with railway train or railway vehicle, unspecified whether traffic or nontraffic accident**

Pedestrian with baby stroller injured in collision with railway train or railway vehicle, unspecified whether traffic or nontraffic

Pedestrian on ice-skates injured in collision with railway train or railway vehicle, unspecified whether traffic or nontraffic

Pedestrian on nonmotorized scooter injured in collision with railway train or railway vehicle, unspecified whether traffic or nontraffic

Pedestrian on sled injured in collision with railway train or railway vehicle, unspecified whether traffic or nontraffic

Pedestrian on snowboard injured in collision with railway train or railway vehicle, unspecified whether traffic or nontraffic

Pedestrian on snow-skis injured in collision with railway train or railway vehicle, unspecified whether traffic or nontraffic

Pedestrian in wheelchair (powered) injured in collision with railway train or railway vehicle, unspecified whether traffic or nontraffic

Pedestrian in motorized mobility scooter injured in collision with railway train or railway vehicle, unspecified whether traffic or nontraffic

⁴ **V06 Pedestrian injured in collision with other nonmotor vehicle**

INCLUDES collision with animal-drawn vehicle, animal being ridden, nonpowered streetcar

EXCLUDES 1 pedestrian injured in collision with pedestrian conveyance (V00.0-)

The appropriate 7th character is to be added to each code from category V06

A initial encounter
D subsequent encounter
S sequela

⁵ **V06.0 Pedestrian injured in collision with other nonmotor vehicle in nontraffic accident**

!Q ⁷ **V06.00X- Pedestrian on foot injured in collision with other nonmotor vehicle in nontraffic accident**

Pedestrian NOS injured in collision with other nonmotor vehicle in nontraffic accident

!Q ⁷ **V06.01X- Pedestrian on roller-skates injured in collision with other nonmotor vehicle in nontraffic accident**

!Q ⁷ **V06.02X- Pedestrian on skateboard injured in collision with other nonmotor vehicle in nontraffic accident**

⁶ **V06.03 Pedestrian on standing micro-mobility pedestrian conveyance injured in collision with other nonmotor vehicle in nontraffic accident**

⁷ **V06.031- Pedestrian on standing electric scooter injured in collision with other nonmotor vehicle in nontraffic accident**

⁷ **V06.038- Pedestrian on other standing micro-mobility pedestrian conveyance injured in collision with other nonmotor vehicle in nontraffic accident**

Pedestrian on hoverboard injured in collision with other nonmotor vehicle in nontraffic accident

Pedestrian on segway injured in collision with other nonmotor vehicle in nontraffic accident

!Q ⁷ **V06.09X- Pedestrian with other conveyance injured in collision with other nonmotor vehicle in nontraffic accident**

Pedestrian with baby stroller injured in collision with other nonmotor vehicle in nontraffic accident

Pedestrian on ice-skates injured in collision with other nonmotor vehicle in nontraffic accident

Pedestrian on nonmotorized scooter injured in collision with other nonmotor vehicle in nontraffic accident

Pedestrian on sled injured in collision with other nonmotor vehicle in nontraffic accident
Pedestrian on snowboard injured in collision with other nonmotor vehicle in nontraffic accident
Pedestrian on snow-skis injured in collision with other nonmotor vehicle in nontraffic accident
Pedestrian in wheelchair (powered) injured in collision with other nonmotor vehicle in nontraffic accident
Pedestrian in motorized mobility scooter injured in collision with other nonmotor vehicle in nontraffic accident

5 **V06.1 Pedestrian injured in collision with other nonmotor vehicle in traffic accident**

IQ 7 **V06.10X- Pedestrian on foot injured in collision with other nonmotor vehicle in traffic accident**
Pedestrian NOS injured in collision with other nonmotor vehicle in traffic accident

IQ 7 **V06.11X- Pedestrian on roller-skates injured in collision with other nonmotor vehicle in traffic accident**

IQ 7 **V06.12X- Pedestrian on skateboard injured in collision with other nonmotor vehicle in traffic accident**

6 **V06.13 Pedestrian on standing micro-mobility pedestrian conveyance injured in collision with other nonmotor vehicle in traffic accident**

7 **V06.131- Pedestrian on standing electric scooter injured in collision with other nonmotor vehicle in traffic accident**

7 **V06.138- Pedestrian on other standing micro-mobility pedestrian conveyance injured in collision with other nonmotor vehicle in traffic accident**
Pedestrian on hoverboard injured in collision with other nonmotor vehicle in traffic accident
Pedestrian on segway injured in collision with other nonmotor vehicle in traffic accident

IQ 7 **V06.19X- Pedestrian with other conveyance injured in collision with other nonmotor vehicle in traffic accident**
Pedestrian with baby stroller injured in collision with other nonmotor vehicle in nontraffic accident
Pedestrian on ice-skates injured in collision with other nonmotor vehicle in traffic accident
Pedestrian on nonmotorized scooter injured in collision with other nonmotor vehicle in traffic accident
Pedestrian on sled injured in collision with other nonmotor vehicle in traffic accident
Pedestrian on snowboard injured in collision with other nonmotor vehicle in traffic accident
Pedestrian on snow-skis injured in collision with other nonmotor vehicle in traffic accident
Pedestrian in wheelchair (powered) injured in collision with other nonmotor vehicle in traffic accident
Pedestrian in motorized mobility scooter injured in collision with other nonmotor vehicle in traffic accident

5 **V06.9 Pedestrian injured in collision with other nonmotor vehicle, unspecified whether traffic or nontraffic accident**

IQ 7 **V06.90X- Pedestrian on foot injured in collision with other nonmotor vehicle, unspecified whether traffic or nontraffic accident**
Pedestrian NOS injured in collision with other nonmotor vehicle, unspecified whether traffic or nontraffic accident

IQ 7 **V06.91X- Pedestrian on roller-skates injured in collision with other nonmotor vehicle, unspecified whether traffic or nontraffic accident**

IQ 7 **V06.92X- Pedestrian on skateboard injured in collision with other nonmotor vehicle, unspecified whether traffic or nontraffic accident**

6 **V06.93 Pedestrian on standing micro-mobility pedestrian conveyance injured in collision with other nonmotor vehicle, unspecified whether traffic or nontraffic accident**

7 **V06.931- Pedestrian on standing electric scooter injured in collision with other nonmotor vehicle, unspecified whether traffic or nontraffic accident**

7 **V06.938- Pedestrian on other standing micro-mobility pedestrian conveyance injured in collision with other nonmotor vehicle, unspecified whether traffic or nontraffic accident**
Pedestrian on hoverboard injured in collision with other nonmotor, unspecified whether traffic or nontraffic accident
Pedestrian on segway injured in collision with other nonmotor vehicle, unspecified whether traffic or nontraffic accident

IQ 7 **V06.99X- Pedestrian with other conveyance injured in collision with other nonmotor vehicle, unspecified whether traffic or nontraffic accident**
Pedestrian with baby stroller injured in collision with other nonmotor vehicle, unspecified whether traffic or nontraffic accident

Pedestrian on ice-skates injured in collision with other nonmotor vehicle, unspecified whether traffic or nontraffic accident
Pedestrian on nonmotorized scooter injured in collision with other nonmotor vehicle, unspecified whether traffic or nontraffic accident
Pedestrian on sled injured in collision with other nonmotor vehicle, unspecified whether traffic or nontraffic accident
Pedestrian on snowboard injured in collision with other nonmotor vehicle, unspecified whether traffic or nontraffic accident
Pedestrian on snow-skis injured in collision with other nonmotor vehicle, unspecified whether traffic or nontraffic accident
Pedestrian in wheelchair (powered) injured in collision with other nonmotor vehicle, unspecified whether traffic or nontraffic accident
Pedestrian in motorized mobility scooter injured in collision with other nonmotor vehicle, unspecified whether traffic or nontraffic accident

4 **V09 Pedestrian injured in other and unspecified transport accidents**

The appropriate 7th character is to be added to each code from category V09
A initial encounter
D subsequent encounter
S sequela

5 **V09.0 Pedestrian injured in nontraffic accident involving other and unspecified motor vehicles**

IQ X **V09.00X- Pedestrian injured in nontraffic accident involving unspecified motor vehicles**

IQ X **V09.01X- Pedestrian injured in nontraffic accident involving military vehicle**

IQ X **V09.09X- Pedestrian injured in nontraffic accident involving other motor vehicles**
Pedestrian injured in nontraffic accident by special vehicle

IQ X **V09.1XX- Pedestrian injured in unspecified nontraffic accident**

5 **V09.2 Pedestrian injured in traffic accident involving other and unspecified motor vehicles**

IQ X **V09.20X- Pedestrian injured in traffic accident involving unspecified motor vehicles**

IQ X **V09.21X- Pedestrian injured in traffic accident involving military vehicle**

IQ X **V09.29X- Pedestrian injured in traffic accident involving other motor vehicles**

IQ X **V09.3XX- Pedestrian injured in unspecified traffic accident**

IQ X **V09.9XX- Pedestrian injured in unspecified transport accident**

Pedal cycle rider injured in transport accident (V10-V19)

INCLUDES any non-motorized vehicle, excluding an animal-drawn vehicle, or a sidecar or trailer attached to the pedal cycle

EXCLUDES 2 rupture of pedal cycle tire (W37.0)

4 **V10 Pedal cycle rider injured in collision with pedestrian or animal**

EXCLUDES 1 pedal cycle rider collision with animal-drawn vehicle or animal being ridden (V16.-)

The appropriate 7th character is to be added to each code from category V10
A initial encounter
D subsequent encounter
S sequela

IQ X **V10.0XX- Pedal cycle driver injured in collision with pedestrian or animal in nontraffic accident**

IQ X **V10.1XX- Pedal cycle passenger injured in collision with pedestrian or animal in nontraffic accident**

IQ X **V10.2XX- Unspecified pedal cyclist injured in collision with pedestrian or animal in nontraffic accident**

IQ X **V10.3XX- Person boarding or alighting a pedal cycle injured in collision with pedestrian or animal**

IQ X **V10.4XX- Pedal cycle driver injured in collision with pedestrian or animal in traffic accident**

IQ X **V10.5XX- Pedal cycle passenger injured in collision with pedestrian or animal in traffic accident**

IQ X **V10.9XX- Unspecified pedal cyclist injured in collision with pedestrian or animal in traffic accident**

4 **V11 Pedal cycle rider injured in collision with other pedal cycle**

The appropriate 7th character is to be added to each code from category V11
A initial encounter
D subsequent encounter
S sequela

IQ X **V11.0XX- Pedal cycle driver injured in collision with other pedal cycle in nontraffic accident**

IQ X **V11.1XX- Pedal cycle passenger injured in collision with other pedal cycle in nontraffic accident**

IQ X **V11.2XX- Unspecified pedal cyclist injured in collision with other pedal cycle in nontraffic accident**

IQ X **V11.3XX- Person boarding or alighting a pedal cycle injured in collision with other pedal cycle**

IQ X **V11.4XX- Pedal cycle driver injured in collision with other pedal cycle in traffic accident**

IQ X **V11.5XX- Pedal cycle passenger injured in collision with other pedal cycle in traffic accident**

IQ 7 V11.9XX- Unspecified pedal cyclist injured in collision with other pedal cycle in traffic accident

4 **V12 Pedal cycle rider injured in collision with two- or three-wheeled motor vehicle**

The appropriate 7th character is to be added to each code from category V12
A initial encounter
D subsequent encounter
S sequela

IQ 7 **V12.0XX- Pedal cycle driver injured in collision with two- or three-wheeled motor vehicle in nontraffic accident**

IQ 7 **V12.1XX- Pedal cycle passenger injured in collision with two- or three-wheeled motor vehicle in nontraffic accident**

IQ 7 **V12.2XX- Unspecified pedal cyclist injured in collision with two- or three-wheeled motor vehicle in nontraffic accident**

IQ 7 **V12.3XX- Person boarding or alighting a pedal cycle injured in collision with two- or three-wheeled motor vehicle**

IQ 7 **V12.4XX- Pedal cycle driver injured in collision with two- or three-wheeled motor vehicle in traffic accident**

IQ 7 **V12.5XX- Pedal cycle passenger injured in collision with two- or three-wheeled motor vehicle in traffic accident**

IQ 7 **V12.9XX- Unspecified pedal cyclist injured in collision with two- or three-wheeled motor vehicle in traffic accident**

4 **V13 Pedal cycle rider injured in collision with car, pick-up truck or van**

The appropriate 7th character is to be added to each code from category V13
A initial encounter
D subsequent encounter
S sequela

IQ 7 **V13.0XX- Pedal cycle driver injured in collision with car, pick-up truck or van in nontraffic accident**

IQ 7 **V13.1XX- Pedal cycle passenger injured in collision with car, pick-up truck or van in nontraffic accident**

IQ 7 **V13.2XX- Unspecified pedal cyclist injured in collision with car, pick-up truck or van in nontraffic accident**

IQ 7 **V13.3XX- Person boarding or alighting a pedal cycle injured in collision with car, pick-up truck or van**

IQ 7 **V13.4XX- Pedal cycle driver injured in collision with car, pick-up truck or van in traffic accident**

IQ 7 **V13.5XX- Pedal cycle passenger injured in collision with car, pick-up truck or van in traffic accident**

IQ 7 **V13.9XX- Unspecified pedal cyclist injured in collision with car, pick-up truck or van in traffic accident**

4 **V14 Pedal cycle rider injured in collision with heavy transport vehicle or bus**

EXCLUDES 1 pedal cycle rider injured in collision with military vehicle (V19.81)

The appropriate 7th character is to be added to each code from category V14
A initial encounter
D subsequent encounter
S sequela

IQ 7 **V14.0XX- Pedal cycle driver injured in collision with heavy transport vehicle or bus in nontraffic accident**

IQ 7 **V14.1XX- Pedal cycle passenger injured in collision with heavy transport vehicle or bus in nontraffic accident**

IQ 7 **V14.2XX- Unspecified pedal cyclist injured in collision with heavy transport vehicle or bus in nontraffic accident**

IQ 7 **V14.3XX- Person boarding or alighting a pedal cycle injured in collision with heavy transport vehicle or bus**

IQ 7 **V14.4XX- Pedal cycle driver injured in collision with heavy transport vehicle or bus in traffic accident**

IQ 7 **V14.5XX- Pedal cycle passenger injured in collision with heavy transport vehicle or bus in traffic accident**

IQ 7 **V14.9XX- Unspecified pedal cyclist injured in collision with heavy transport vehicle or bus in traffic accident**

4 **V15 Pedal cycle rider injured in collision with railway train or railway vehicle**

The appropriate 7th character is to be added to each code from category V15
A initial encounter
D subsequent encounter
S sequela

IQ 7 **V15.0XX- Pedal cycle driver injured in collision with railway train or railway vehicle in nontraffic accident**

IQ 7 **V15.1XX- Pedal cycle passenger injured in collision with railway train or railway vehicle in nontraffic accident**

IQ 7 **V15.2XX- Unspecified pedal cyclist injured in collision with railway train or railway vehicle in nontraffic accident**

IQ 7 **V15.3XX- Person boarding or alighting a pedal cycle injured in collision with railway train or railway vehicle**

IQ 7 **V15.4XX- Pedal cycle driver injured in collision with railway train or railway vehicle in traffic accident**

IQ 7 **V15.5XX- Pedal cycle passenger injured in collision with railway train or railway vehicle in traffic accident**

IQ 7 **V15.9XX- Unspecified pedal cyclist injured in collision with railway train or railway vehicle in traffic accident**

4 **V16 Pedal cycle rider injured in collision with other nonmotor vehicle**

INCLUDES collision with animal-drawn vehicle, animal being ridden, streetcar

Chapter 20 V00-Y99

The appropriate 7th character is to be added to each code from category V16
A   initial encounter
D   subsequent encounter
S   sequela

!Q ☑ V16.0XX- Pedal cycle driver injured in collision with other nonmotor vehicle in nontraffic accident

!Q ☑ V16.1XX- Pedal cycle passenger injured in collision with other nonmotor vehicle in nontraffic accident

!Q ☑ V16.2XX- Unspecified pedal cyclist injured in collision with other nonmotor vehicle in nontraffic accident

!Q ☑ V16.3XX- Person boarding or alighting a pedal cycle injured in collision with other nonmotor vehicle in nontraffic accident

!Q ☑ V16.4XX- Pedal cycle driver injured in collision with other nonmotor vehicle in traffic accident

!Q ☑ V16.5XX- Pedal cycle passenger injured in collision with other nonmotor vehicle in traffic accident

!Q ☑ V16.9XX- Unspecified pedal cyclist injured in collision with other nonmotor vehicle in traffic accident

4 V17 Pedal cycle rider injured in collision with fixed or stationary object

The appropriate 7th character is to be added to each code from category V17
A   initial encounter
D   subsequent encounter
S   sequela

!Q ☑ V17.0XX- Pedal cycle driver injured in collision with fixed or stationary object in nontraffic accident

!Q ☑ V17.1XX- Pedal cycle passenger injured in collision with fixed or stationary object in nontraffic accident

!Q ☑ V17.2XX- Unspecified pedal cyclist injured in collision with fixed or stationary object in nontraffic accident

!Q ☑ V17.3XX- Person boarding or alighting a pedal cycle injured in collision with fixed or stationary object

!Q ☑ V17.4XX- Pedal cycle driver injured in collision with fixed or stationary object in traffic accident

!Q ☑ V17.5XX- Pedal cycle passenger injured in collision with fixed or stationary object in traffic accident

!Q ☑ V17.9XX- Unspecified pedal cyclist injured in collision with fixed or stationary object in traffic accident

4 V18 Pedal cycle rider injured in noncollision transport accident

INCLUDES   fall or thrown from pedal cycle (without antecedent collision) overturning pedal cycle NOS overturning pedal cycle without collision

The appropriate 7th character is to be added to each code from category V18
A   initial encounter
D   subsequent encounter
S   sequela

!Q ☑ V18.0XX- Pedal cycle driver injured in noncollision transport accident in nontraffic accident

!Q ☑ V18.1XX- Pedal cycle passenger injured in noncollision transport accident in nontraffic accident

!Q ☑ V18.2XX- Unspecified pedal cyclist injured in noncollision transport accident in nontraffic accident

!Q ☑ V18.3XX- Person boarding or alighting a pedal cycle injured in noncollision transport accident

!Q ☑ V18.4XX- Pedal cycle driver injured in noncollision transport accident in traffic accident

!Q ☑ V18.5XX- Pedal cycle passenger injured in noncollision transport accident in traffic accident

!Q ☑ V18.9XX- Unspecified pedal cyclist injured in noncollision transport accident in traffic accident

4 V19 Pedal cycle rider injured in other and unspecified transport accidents

The appropriate 7th character is to be added to each code from category V19
A   initial encounter
D   subsequent encounter
S   sequela

5 V19.0 Pedal cycle driver injured in collision with other and unspecified motor vehicles in nontraffic accident

!Q ☑ V19.00X- Pedal cycle driver injured in collision with unspecified motor vehicles in nontraffic accident

!Q ☑ V19.09X- Pedal cycle driver injured in collision with other motor vehicles in nontraffic accident

5 V19.1 Pedal cycle passenger injured in collision with other and unspecified motor vehicles in nontraffic accident

!Q ☑ V19.10X- Pedal cycle passenger injured in collision with unspecified motor vehicles in nontraffic accident

!Q ☑ V19.19X- Pedal cycle passenger injured in collision with other motor vehicles in nontraffic accident

5 V19.2 Unspecified pedal cyclist injured in collision with other and unspecified motor vehicles in nontraffic accident

!Q ☑ V19.20X- Unspecified pedal cyclist injured in collision with unspecified motor vehicles in nontraffic accident

Pedal cycle collision NOS, nontraffic

!Q ☑ V19.29X- Unspecified pedal cyclist injured in collision with other motor vehicles in nontraffic accident

!Q ☑ V19.3XX- Pedal cyclist (driver) (passenger) injured in unspecified nontraffic accident

4 4th digit required   **5** 5th digit required   **6** 6th digit required   **7** 7th digit required   **☑** 7th digit placeholder   **+** Additional code   **⊟** Laterality

1810   *DecisionHealth's* FY 2022 Complete Home Health ICD-10-CM Diagnosis Coding Manual

Chapter 20

V00-Y99

Pedal cycle accident NOS, nontraffic
Pedal cyclist injured in nontraffic accident NOS

5 **V19.4 Pedal cycle driver injured in collision with other and unspecified motor vehicles in traffic accident**

IQ 7 **V19.40X- Pedal cycle driver injured in collision with unspecified motor vehicles in traffic accident**

IQ 7 **V19.49X- Pedal cycle driver injured in collision with other motor vehicles in traffic accident**

5 **V19.5 Pedal cycle passenger injured in collision with other and unspecified motor vehicles in traffic accident**

IQ 7 **V19.50X- Pedal cycle passenger injured in collision with unspecified motor vehicles in traffic accident**

IQ 7 **V19.59X- Pedal cycle passenger injured in collision with other motor vehicles in traffic accident**

5 **V19.6 Unspecified pedal cyclist injured in collision with other and unspecified motor vehicles in traffic accident**

IQ 7 **V19.60X- Unspecified pedal cyclist injured in collision with unspecified motor vehicles in traffic accident**

Pedal cycle collision NOS (traffic)

IQ 7 **V19.69X- Unspecified pedal cyclist injured in collision with other motor vehicles in traffic accident**

5 **V19.8 Pedal cyclist (driver) (passenger) injured in other specified transport accidents**

IQ 7 **V19.81X- Pedal cyclist (driver) (passenger) injured in transport accident with military vehicle**

IQ 7 **V19.88X- Pedal cyclist (driver) (passenger) injured in other specified transport accidents**

IQ 7 **V19.9XX- Pedal cyclist (driver) (passenger) injured in unspecified traffic accident**

Pedal cycle accident NOS

Motorcycle rider injured in transport accident (V20-V29)

INCLUDES moped
motorcycle with sidecar
motorized bicycle
motor scooter

EXCLUDES 1 three-wheeled motor vehicle (V30-V39)

4 **V20 Motorcycle rider injured in collision with pedestrian or animal**

EXCLUDES 1 motorcycle rider collision with animal-drawn vehicle or animal being ridden (V26.-)

The appropriate 7th character is to be added to each code from category V20
A initial encounter
D subsequent encounter
S sequela

IQ 7 **V20.0XX- Motorcycle driver injured in collision with pedestrian or animal in nontraffic accident**

IQ 7 **V20.1XX- Motorcycle passenger injured in collision with pedestrian or animal in nontraffic accident**

IQ 7 **V20.2XX- Unspecified motorcycle rider injured in collision with pedestrian or animal in nontraffic accident**

IQ 7 **V20.3XX- Person boarding or alighting a motorcycle injured in collision with pedestrian or animal**

IQ 7 **V20.4XX- Motorcycle driver injured in collision with pedestrian or animal in traffic accident**

IQ 7 **V20.5XX- Motorcycle passenger injured in collision with pedestrian or animal in traffic accident**

IQ 7 **V20.9XX- Unspecified motorcycle rider injured in collision with pedestrian or animal in traffic accident**

4 **V21 Motorcycle rider injured in collision with pedal cycle**

The appropriate 7th character is to be added to each code from category V21
A initial encounter
D subsequent encounter
S sequela

IQ 7 **V21.0XX- Motorcycle driver injured in collision with pedal cycle in nontraffic accident**

IQ 7 **V21.1XX- Motorcycle passenger injured in collision with pedal cycle in nontraffic accident**

IQ 7 **V21.2XX- Unspecified motorcycle rider injured in collision with pedal cycle in nontraffic accident**

IQ 7 **V21.3XX- Person boarding or alighting a motorcycle injured in collision with pedal cycle**

IQ 7 **V21.4XX- Motorcycle driver injured in collision with pedal cycle in traffic accident**

IQ 7 **V21.5XX- Motorcycle passenger injured in collision with pedal cycle in traffic accident**

IQ 7 **V21.9XX- Unspecified motorcycle rider injured in collision with pedal cycle in traffic accident**

4 **V22 Motorcycle rider injured in collision with two- or three-wheeled motor vehicle**

The appropriate 7th character is to be added to each code from category V22
A initial encounter
D subsequent encounter
S sequela

IQ 7 **V22.0XX- Motorcycle driver injured in collision with two- or three-wheeled motor vehicle in nontraffic accident**

IQ 7 **V22.1XX- Motorcycle passenger injured in collision with two- or three-wheeled motor vehicle in nontraffic accident**

IQ 7 **V22.2XX- Unspecified motorcycle rider injured in collision with two- or three-wheeled motor vehicle in nontraffic accident**

IQ 7 **V22.3XX- Person boarding or alighting a motorcycle injured in collision with two- or three-wheeled motor vehicle**

!Q x V22.4XX- **Motorcycle driver injured in collision with two- or three-wheeled motor vehicle in traffic accident**

!Q x V22.5XX- **Motorcycle passenger injured in collision with two- or three-wheeled motor vehicle in traffic accident**

!Q x V22.9XX- **Unspecified motorcycle rider injured in collision with two- or three-wheeled motor vehicle in traffic accident**

4 **V23 Motorcycle rider injured in collision with car, pick-up truck or van**

The appropriate 7th character is to be added to each code from category V23
A initial encounter
D subsequent encounter
S sequela

!Q x V23.0XX- **Motorcycle driver injured in collision with car, pick-up truck or van in nontraffic accident**

!Q x V23.1XX- **Motorcycle passenger injured in collision with car, pick-up truck or van in nontraffic accident**

!Q x V23.2XX- **Unspecified motorcycle rider injured in collision with car, pick-up truck or van in nontraffic accident**

!Q x V23.3XX- **Person boarding or alighting a motorcycle injured in collision with car, pick-up truck or van**

!Q x V23.4XX- **Motorcycle driver injured in collision with car, pick-up truck or van in traffic accident**

!Q x V23.5XX- **Motorcycle passenger injured in collision with car, pick-up truck or van in traffic accident**

!Q x V23.9XX- **Unspecified motorcycle rider injured in collision with car, pick-up truck or van in traffic accident**

4 **V24 Motorcycle rider injured in collision with heavy transport vehicle or bus**

EXCLUDES 1 motorcycle rider injured in collision with military vehicle (V29.81)

The appropriate 7th character is to be added to each code from category V24
A initial encounter
D subsequent encounter
S sequela

!Q x V24.0XX- **Motorcycle driver injured in collision with heavy transport vehicle or bus in nontraffic accident**

!Q x V24.1XX- **Motorcycle passenger injured in collision with heavy transport vehicle or bus in nontraffic accident**

!Q x V24.2XX- **Unspecified motorcycle rider injured in collision with heavy transport vehicle or bus in nontraffic accident**

!Q x V24.3XX- **Person boarding or alighting a motorcycle injured in collision with heavy transport vehicle or bus**

!Q x V24.4XX- **Motorcycle driver injured in collision with heavy transport vehicle or bus in traffic accident**

!Q x V24.5XX- **Motorcycle passenger injured in collision with heavy transport vehicle or bus in traffic accident**

!Q x V24.9XX- **Unspecified motorcycle rider injured in collision with heavy transport vehicle or bus in traffic accident**

4 **V25 Motorcycle rider injured in collision with railway train or railway vehicle**

The appropriate 7th character is to be added to each code from category V25
A initial encounter
D subsequent encounter
S sequela

!Q x V25.0XX- **Motorcycle driver injured in collision with railway train or railway vehicle in nontraffic accident**

!Q x V25.1XX- **Motorcycle passenger injured in collision with railway train or railway vehicle in nontraffic accident**

!Q x V25.2XX- **Unspecified motorcycle rider injured in collision with railway train or railway vehicle in nontraffic accident**

!Q x V25.3XX- **Person boarding or alighting a motorcycle injured in collision with railway train or railway vehicle**

!Q x V25.4XX- **Motorcycle driver injured in collision with railway train or railway vehicle in traffic accident**

!Q x V25.5XX- **Motorcycle passenger injured in collision with railway train or railway vehicle in traffic accident**

!Q x V25.9XX- **Unspecified motorcycle rider injured in collision with railway train or railway vehicle in traffic accident**

4 **V26 Motorcycle rider injured in collision with other nonmotor vehicle**

INCLUDES collision with animal-drawn vehicle, animal being ridden, streetcar

The appropriate 7th character is to be added to each code from category V26
A initial encounter
D subsequent encounter
S sequela

!Q x V26.0XX- **Motorcycle driver injured in collision with other nonmotor vehicle in nontraffic accident**

!Q x V26.1XX- **Motorcycle passenger injured in collision with other nonmotor vehicle in nontraffic accident**

!Q x V26.2XX- **Unspecified motorcycle rider injured in collision with other nonmotor vehicle in nontraffic accident**

!Q x V26.3XX- **Person boarding or alighting a motorcycle injured in collision with other nonmotor vehicle**

!Q x V26.4XX- **Motorcycle driver injured in collision with other nonmotor vehicle in traffic accident**

IQ 7 V26.5XX- **Motorcycle passenger injured in collision with other nonmotor vehicle in traffic accident**

IQ 7 V26.9XX- **Unspecified motorcycle rider injured in collision with other nonmotor vehicle in traffic accident**

4 V27 **Motorcycle rider injured in collision with fixed or stationary object**

The appropriate 7th character is to be added to each code from category V27
A initial encounter
D subsequent encounter
S sequela

IQ 7 V27.0XX- **Motorcycle driver injured in collision with fixed or stationary object in nontraffic accident**

IQ 7 V27.1XX- **Motorcycle passenger injured in collision with fixed or stationary object in nontraffic accident**

IQ 7 V27.2XX- **Unspecified motorcycle rider injured in collision with fixed or stationary object in nontraffic accident**

IQ 7 V27.3XX- **Person boarding or alighting a motorcycle injured in collision with fixed or stationary object**

IQ 7 V27.4XX- **Motorcycle driver injured in collision with fixed or stationary object in traffic accident**

IQ 7 V27.5XX- **Motorcycle passenger injured in collision with fixed or stationary object in traffic accident**

IQ 7 V27.9XX- **Unspecified motorcycle rider injured in collision with fixed or stationary object in traffic accident**

4 V28 **Motorcycle rider injured in noncollision transport accident**

INCLUDES fall or thrown from motorcycle (without antecedent collision)
overturning motorcycle NOS
overturning motorcycle without collision

The appropriate 7th character is to be added to each code from category V28
A initial encounter
D subsequent encounter
S sequela

IQ 7 V28.0XX- **Motorcycle driver injured in noncollision transport accident in nontraffic accident**

IQ 7 V28.1XX- **Motorcycle passenger injured in noncollision transport accident in nontraffic accident**

IQ 7 V28.2XX- **Unspecified motorcycle rider injured in noncollision transport accident in nontraffic accident**

IQ 7 V28.3XX- **Person boarding or alighting a motorcycle injured in noncollision transport accident**

IQ 7 V28.4XX- **Motorcycle driver injured in noncollision transport accident in traffic accident**

IQ 7 V28.5XX- **Motorcycle passenger injured in noncollision transport accident in traffic accident**

IQ 7 V28.9XX- **Unspecified motorcycle rider injured in noncollision transport accident in traffic accident**

4 V29 **Motorcycle rider injured in other and unspecified transport accidents**

The appropriate 7th character is to be added to each code from category V29
A initial encounter
D subsequent encounter
S sequela

5 V29.0 **Motorcycle driver injured in collision with other and unspecified motor vehicles in nontraffic accident**

IQ 7 V29.00X- **Motorcycle driver injured in collision with unspecified motor vehicles in nontraffic accident**

IQ 7 V29.09X- **Motorcycle driver injured in collision with other motor vehicles in nontraffic accident**

5 V29.1 **Motorcycle passenger injured in collision with other and unspecified motor vehicles in nontraffic accident**

IQ 7 V29.10X- **Motorcycle passenger injured in collision with unspecified motor vehicles in nontraffic accident**

IQ 7 V29.19X- **Motorcycle passenger injured in collision with other motor vehicles in nontraffic accident**

5 V29.2 **Unspecified motorcycle rider injured in collision with other and unspecified motor vehicles in nontraffic accident**

IQ 7 V29.20X- **Unspecified motorcycle rider injured in collision with unspecified motor vehicles in nontraffic accident**
Motorcycle collision NOS, nontraffic

IQ 7 V29.29X- **Unspecified motorcycle rider injured in collision with other motor vehicles in nontraffic accident**

IQ 7 V29.3XX- **Motorcycle rider (driver) (passenger) injured in unspecified nontraffic accident**
Motorcycle accident NOS, nontraffic
Motorcycle rider injured in nontraffic accident NOS

5 V29.4 **Motorcycle driver injured in collision with other and unspecified motor vehicles in traffic accident**

IQ 7 V29.40X- **Motorcycle driver injured in collision with unspecified motor vehicles in traffic accident**

IQ 7 V29.49X- **Motorcycle driver injured in collision with other motor vehicles in traffic accident**

5 V29.5 **Motorcycle passenger injured in collision with other and unspecified motor vehicles in traffic accident**

IQ 7 V29.50X- **Motorcycle passenger injured in collision with unspecified motor vehicles in traffic accident**

Chapter 20

V00-Y99

!Q ☑ V29.59X- Motorcycle passenger injured in collision with other motor vehicles in traffic accident

⑤ V29.6 Unspecified motorcycle rider injured in collision with other and unspecified motor vehicles in traffic accident

!Q ☑ V29.60X- Unspecified motorcycle rider injured in collision with unspecified motor vehicles in traffic accident

Motorcycle collision NOS (traffic)

!Q ☑ V29.69X- Unspecified motorcycle rider injured in collision with other motor vehicles in traffic accident

⑤ V29.8 Motorcycle rider (driver) (passenger) injured in other specified transport accidents

!Q ☑ V29.81X- Motorcycle rider (driver) (passenger) injured in transport accident with military vehicle

!Q ☑ V29.88X- Motorcycle rider (driver) (passenger) injured in other specified transport accidents

!Q ☑ V29.9XX- Motorcycle rider (driver) (passenger) injured in unspecified traffic accident

Motorcycle accident NOS

Occupant of three-wheeled motor vehicle injured in transport accident   (V30-V39)

INCLUDES   motorized tricycle
motorized rickshaw
three-wheeled motor car
EXCLUDES 1   all-terrain vehicles (V86.-)
motorcycle with sidecar (V20-V29)
vehicle designed primarily for off-road use (V86.-)

④ V30 Occupant of three-wheeled motor vehicle injured in collision with pedestrian or animal

EXCLUDES 1   three-wheeled motor vehicle collision with animal-drawn vehicle or animal being ridden (V36.-)

The appropriate 7th character is to be added to each code from category V30
A   initial encounter
D   subsequent encounter
S   sequela

!Q ☑ V30.0XX- Driver of three-wheeled motor vehicle injured in collision with pedestrian or animal in nontraffic accident

!Q ☑ V30.1XX- Passenger in three-wheeled motor vehicle injured in collision with pedestrian or animal in nontraffic accident

!Q ☑ V30.2XX- Person on outside of three-wheeled motor vehicle injured in collision with pedestrian or animal in nontraffic accident

!Q ☑ V30.3XX- Unspecified occupant of three-wheeled motor vehicle injured in collision with pedestrian or animal in nontraffic accident

!Q ☑ V30.4XX- Person boarding or alighting a three-wheeled motor vehicle injured in collision with pedestrian or animal

!Q ☑ V30.5XX- Driver of three-wheeled motor vehicle injured in collision with pedestrian or animal in traffic accident

!Q ☑ V30.6XX- Passenger in three-wheeled motor vehicle injured in collision with pedestrian or animal in traffic accident

!Q ☑ V30.7XX- Person on outside of three-wheeled motor vehicle injured in collision with pedestrian or animal in traffic accident

!Q ☑ V30.9XX- Unspecified occupant of three-wheeled motor vehicle injured in collision with pedestrian or animal in traffic accident

④ V31 Occupant of three-wheeled motor vehicle injured in collision with pedal cycle

The appropriate 7th character is to be added to each code from category V31
A   initial encounter
D   subsequent encounter
S   sequela

!Q ☑ V31.0XX- Driver of three-wheeled motor vehicle injured in collision with pedal cycle in nontraffic accident

!Q ☑ V31.1XX- Passenger in three-wheeled motor vehicle injured in collision with pedal cycle in nontraffic accident

!Q ☑ V31.2XX- Person on outside of three-wheeled motor vehicle injured in collision with pedal cycle in nontraffic accident

!Q ☑ V31.3XX- Unspecified occupant of three-wheeled motor vehicle injured in collision with pedal cycle in nontraffic accident

!Q ☑ V31.4XX- Person boarding or alighting a three-wheeled motor vehicle injured in collision with pedal cycle

!Q ☑ V31.5XX- Driver of three-wheeled motor vehicle injured in collision with pedal cycle in traffic accident

!Q ☑ V31.6XX- Passenger in three-wheeled motor vehicle injured in collision with pedal cycle in traffic accident

!Q ☑ V31.7XX- Person on outside of three-wheeled motor vehicle injured in collision with pedal cycle in traffic accident

!Q ☑ V31.9XX- Unspecified occupant of three-wheeled motor vehicle injured in collision with pedal cycle in traffic accident

④ V32 Occupant of three-wheeled motor vehicle injured in collision with two- or three-wheeled motor vehicle

The appropriate 7th character is to be added to each code from category V32
A   initial encounter
D   subsequent encounter
S   sequela

---

④ 4th digit required   ⑤ 5th digit required   ⑥ 6th digit required   ☑ 7th digit required   ☑ 7th digit placeholder   ✚ Additional code   ⊟ Laterality

IQ 7 V32.0XX- **Driver of three-wheeled motor vehicle injured in collision with two- or three-wheeled motor vehicle in nontraffic accident**

IQ 7 V32.1XX- **Passenger in three-wheeled motor vehicle injured in collision with two- or three-wheeled motor vehicle in nontraffic accident**

IQ 7 V32.2XX- **Person on outside of three-wheeled motor vehicle injured in collision with two- or three-wheeled motor vehicle in nontraffic accident**

IQ 7 V32.3XX- **Unspecified occupant of three-wheeled motor vehicle injured in collision with two- or three-wheeled motor vehicle in nontraffic accident**

IQ 7 V32.4XX- **Person boarding or alighting a three-wheeled motor vehicle injured in collision with two- or three-wheeled motor vehicle**

IQ 7 V32.5XX- **Driver of three-wheeled motor vehicle injured in collision with two- or three-wheeled motor vehicle in traffic accident**

IQ 7 V32.6XX- **Passenger in three-wheeled motor vehicle injured in collision with two- or three-wheeled motor vehicle in traffic accident**

IQ 7 V32.7XX- **Person on outside of three-wheeled motor vehicle injured in collision with two- or three-wheeled motor vehicle in traffic accident**

IQ 7 V32.9XX- **Unspecified occupant of three-wheeled motor vehicle injured in collision with two- or three-wheeled motor vehicle in traffic accident**

4 V33 **Occupant of three-wheeled motor vehicle injured in collision with car, pick-up truck or van**

The appropriate 7th character is to be added to each code from category V33
A initial encounter
D subsequent encounter
S sequela

IQ 7 V33.0XX- **Driver of three-wheeled motor vehicle injured in collision with car, pick-up truck or van in nontraffic accident**

IQ 7 V33.1XX- **Passenger in three-wheeled motor vehicle injured in collision with car, pick-up truck or van in nontraffic accident**

IQ 7 V33.2XX- **Person on outside of three-wheeled motor vehicle injured in collision with car, pick-up truck or van in nontraffic accident**

IQ 7 V33.3XX- **Unspecified occupant of three-wheeled motor vehicle injured in collision with car, pick-up truck or van in nontraffic accident**

IQ 7 V33.4XX- **Person boarding or alighting a three-wheeled motor vehicle injured in collision with car, pick-up truck or van**

IQ 7 V33.5XX- **Driver of three-wheeled motor vehicle injured in collision with car, pick-up truck or van in traffic accident**

IQ 7 V33.6XX- **Passenger in three-wheeled motor vehicle injured in collision with car, pick-up truck or van in traffic accident**

IQ 7 V33.7XX- **Person on outside of three-wheeled motor vehicle injured in collision with car, pick-up truck or van in traffic accident**

IQ 7 V33.9XX- **Unspecified occupant of three-wheeled motor vehicle injured in collision with car, pick-up truck or van in traffic accident**

4 V34 **Occupant of three-wheeled motor vehicle injured in collision with heavy transport vehicle or bus**

EXCLUDES 1 occupant of three-wheeled motor vehicle injured in collision with military vehicle (V39.81)

The appropriate 7th character is to be added to each code from category V34
A initial encounter
D subsequent encounter
S sequela

IQ 7 V34.0XX- **Driver of three-wheeled motor vehicle injured in collision with heavy transport vehicle or bus in nontraffic accident**

IQ 7 V34.1XX- **Passenger in three-wheeled motor vehicle injured in collision with heavy transport vehicle or bus in nontraffic accident**

IQ 7 V34.2XX- **Person on outside of three-wheeled motor vehicle injured in collision with heavy transport vehicle or bus in nontraffic accident**

IQ 7 V34.3XX- **Unspecified occupant of three-wheeled motor vehicle injured in collision with heavy transport vehicle or bus in nontraffic accident**

IQ 7 V34.4XX- **Person boarding or alighting a three-wheeled motor vehicle injured in collision with heavy transport vehicle or bus**

IQ 7 V34.5XX- **Driver of three-wheeled motor vehicle injured in collision with heavy transport vehicle or bus in traffic accident**

IQ 7 V34.6XX- **Passenger in three-wheeled motor vehicle injured in collision with heavy transport vehicle or bus in traffic accident**

IQ 7 V34.7XX- **Person on outside of three-wheeled motor vehicle injured in collision with heavy transport vehicle or bus in traffic accident**

IQ 7 V34.9XX- **Unspecified occupant of three-wheeled motor vehicle injured in collision with heavy transport vehicle or bus in traffic accident**

4 V35 **Occupant of three-wheeled motor vehicle injured in collision with railway train or railway vehicle**

The appropriate 7th character is to be added to each code from category V35
A initial encounter
D subsequent encounter
S sequela

V35.0XX- Driver of three-wheeled motor vehicle injured in collision with railway train or railway vehicle in nontraffic accident

V35.1XX- Passenger in three-wheeled motor vehicle injured in collision with railway train or railway vehicle in nontraffic accident

V35.2XX- Person on outside of three-wheeled motor vehicle injured in collision with railway train or railway vehicle in nontraffic accident

V35.3XX- Unspecified occupant of three-wheeled motor vehicle injured in collision with railway train or railway vehicle in nontraffic accident

V35.4XX- Person boarding or alighting a three-wheeled motor vehicle injured in collision with railway train or railway vehicle

V35.5XX- Driver of three-wheeled motor vehicle injured in collision with railway train or railway vehicle in traffic accident

V35.6XX- Passenger in three-wheeled motor vehicle injured in collision with railway train or railway vehicle in traffic accident

V35.7XX- Person on outside of three-wheeled motor vehicle injured in collision with railway train or railway vehicle in traffic accident

V35.9XX- Unspecified occupant of three-wheeled motor vehicle injured in collision with railway train or railway vehicle in traffic accident

V36 Occupant of three-wheeled motor vehicle injured in collision with other nonmotor vehicle

INCLUDES collision with animal-drawn vehicle, animal being ridden, streetcar

The appropriate 7th character is to be added to each code from category V36
A initial encounter
D subsequent encounter
S sequela

V36.0XX- Driver of three-wheeled motor vehicle injured in collision with other nonmotor vehicle in nontraffic accident

V36.1XX- Passenger in three-wheeled motor vehicle injured in collision with other nonmotor vehicle in nontraffic accident

V36.2XX- Person on outside of three-wheeled motor vehicle injured in collision with other nonmotor vehicle in nontraffic accident

V36.3XX- Unspecified occupant of three-wheeled motor vehicle injured in collision with other nonmotor vehicle in nontraffic accident

V36.4XX- Person boarding or alighting a three-wheeled motor vehicle injured in collision with other nonmotor vehicle

V36.5XX- Driver of three-wheeled motor vehicle injured in collision with other nonmotor vehicle in traffic accident

V36.6XX- Passenger in three-wheeled motor vehicle injured in collision with other nonmotor vehicle in traffic accident

V36.7XX- Person on outside of three-wheeled motor vehicle injured in collision with other nonmotor vehicle in traffic accident

V36.9XX- Unspecified occupant of three-wheeled motor vehicle injured in collision with other nonmotor vehicle in traffic accident

V37 Occupant of three-wheeled motor vehicle injured in collision with fixed or stationary object

The appropriate 7th character is to be added to each code from category V37
A initial encounter
D subsequent encounter
S sequela

V37.0XX- Driver of three-wheeled motor vehicle injured in collision with fixed or stationary object in nontraffic accident

V37.1XX- Passenger in three-wheeled motor vehicle injured in collision with fixed or stationary object in nontraffic accident

V37.2XX- Person on outside of three-wheeled motor vehicle injured in collision with fixed or stationary object in nontraffic accident

V37.3XX- Unspecified occupant of three-wheeled motor vehicle injured in collision with fixed or stationary object in nontraffic accident

V37.4XX- Person boarding or alighting a three-wheeled motor vehicle injured in collision with fixed or stationary object

V37.5XX- Driver of three-wheeled motor vehicle injured in collision with fixed or stationary object in traffic accident

V37.6XX- Passenger in three-wheeled motor vehicle injured in collision with fixed or stationary object in traffic accident

V37.7XX- Person on outside of three-wheeled motor vehicle injured in collision with fixed or stationary object in traffic accident

V37.9XX- Unspecified occupant of three-wheeled motor vehicle injured in collision with fixed or stationary object in traffic accident

Chapter 20
V00-Y99

4 **V38 Occupant of three-wheeled motor vehicle injured in noncollision transport accident**

INCLUDES fall or thrown from three-wheeled motor vehicle
overturning of three-wheeled motor vehicle NOS
overturning of three-wheeled motor vehicle without collision

The appropriate 7th character is to be added to each code from category V38
A initial encounter
D subsequent encounter
S sequela

IQ 7 **V38.0XX- Driver of three-wheeled motor vehicle injured in noncollision transport accident in nontraffic accident**

IQ 7 **V38.1XX- Passenger in three-wheeled motor vehicle injured in noncollision transport accident in nontraffic accident**

IQ 7 **V38.2XX- Person on outside of three-wheeled motor vehicle injured in noncollision transport accident in nontraffic accident**

IQ 7 **V38.3XX- Unspecified occupant of three-wheeled motor vehicle injured in noncollision transport accident in nontraffic accident**

IQ 7 **V38.4XX- Person boarding or alighting a three-wheeled motor vehicle injured in noncollision transport accident**

IQ 7 **V38.5XX- Driver of three-wheeled motor vehicle injured in noncollision transport accident in traffic accident**

IQ 7 **V38.6XX- Passenger in three-wheeled motor vehicle injured in noncollision transport accident in traffic accident**

IQ 7 **V38.7XX- Person on outside of three-wheeled motor vehicle injured in noncollision transport accident in traffic accident**

IQ 7 **V38.9XX- Unspecified occupant of three-wheeled motor vehicle injured in noncollision transport accident in traffic accident**

4 **V39 Occupant of three-wheeled motor vehicle injured in other and unspecified transport accidents**

The appropriate 7th character is to be added to each code from category V39
A initial encounter
D subsequent encounter
S sequela

5 **V39.0 Driver of three-wheeled motor vehicle injured in collision with other and unspecified motor vehicles in nontraffic accident**

IQ 7 **V39.00X- Driver of three-wheeled motor vehicle injured in collision with unspecified motor vehicles in nontraffic accident**

IQ 7 **V39.09X- Driver of three-wheeled motor vehicle injured in collision with other motor vehicles in nontraffic accident**

5 **V39.1 Passenger in three-wheeled motor vehicle injured in collision with other and unspecified motor vehicles in nontraffic accident**

IQ 7 **V39.10X- Passenger in three-wheeled motor vehicle injured in collision with unspecified motor vehicles in nontraffic accident**

IQ 7 **V39.19X- Passenger in three-wheeled motor vehicle injured in collision with other motor vehicles in nontraffic accident**

5 **V39.2 Unspecified occupant of three-wheeled motor vehicle injured in collision with other and unspecified motor vehicles in nontraffic accident**

IQ 7 **V39.20X- Unspecified occupant of three-wheeled motor vehicle injured in collision with unspecified motor vehicles in nontraffic accident**
Collision NOS involving three-wheeled motor vehicle, nontraffic

IQ 7 **V39.29X- Unspecified occupant of three-wheeled motor vehicle injured in collision with other motor vehicles in nontraffic accident**

IQ 7 **V39.3XX- Occupant (driver) (passenger) of three-wheeled motor vehicle injured in unspecified nontraffic accident**
Accident NOS involving three-wheeled motor vehicle, nontraffic
Occupant of three-wheeled motor vehicle injured in nontraffic accident NOS

5 **V39.4 Driver of three-wheeled motor vehicle injured in collision with other and unspecified motor vehicles in traffic accident**

IQ 7 **V39.40X- Driver of three-wheeled motor vehicle injured in collision with unspecified motor vehicles in traffic accident**

IQ 7 **V39.49X- Driver of three-wheeled motor vehicle injured in collision with other motor vehicles in traffic accident**

5 **V39.5 Passenger in three-wheeled motor vehicle injured in collision with other and unspecified motor vehicles in traffic accident**

IQ 7 **V39.50X- Passenger in three-wheeled motor vehicle injured in collision with unspecified motor vehicles in traffic accident**

IQ 7 **V39.59X- Passenger in three-wheeled motor vehicle injured in collision with other motor vehicles in traffic accident**

5 **V39.6 Unspecified occupant of three-wheeled motor vehicle injured in collision with other and unspecified motor vehicles in traffic accident**

IQ 7 V39.60X- **Unspecified occupant of three-wheeled motor vehicle injured in collision with unspecified motor vehicles in traffic accident**

Collision NOS involving three-wheeled motor vehicle (traffic)

IQ 7 V39.69X- **Unspecified occupant of three-wheeled motor vehicle injured in collision with other motor vehicles in traffic accident**

5 V39.8 **Occupant (driver) (passenger) of three-wheeled motor vehicle injured in other specified transport accidents**

IQ 7 V39.81X- **Occupant (driver) (passenger) of three-wheeled motor vehicle injured in transport accident with military vehicle**

IQ 7 V39.89X- **Occupant (driver) (passenger) of three-wheeled motor vehicle injured in other specified transport accidents**

IQ 7 V39.9XX- **Occupant (driver) (passenger) of three-wheeled motor vehicle injured in unspecified traffic accident**

Accident NOS involving three-wheeled motor vehicle

Car occupant injured in transport accident (V40-V49)

INCLUDES a four-wheeled motor vehicle designed primarily for carrying passengers
automobile (pulling a trailer or camper)

EXCLUDES 1 bus (V50-V59)
minibus (V50-V59)
minivan (V50-V59)
motorcoach (V70-V79)
pick-up truck (V50-V59)
sport utility vehicle (SUV) (V50-V59)

4 V40 **Car occupant injured in collision with pedestrian or animal**

EXCLUDES 1 car collision with animal-drawn vehicle or animal being ridden (V46.-)

The appropriate 7th character is to be added to each code from category V40
A initial encounter
D subsequent encounter
S sequela

IQ 7 V40.0XX- **Car driver injured in collision with pedestrian or animal in nontraffic accident**

IQ 7 V40.1XX- **Car passenger injured in collision with pedestrian or animal in nontraffic accident**

IQ 7 V40.2XX- **Person on outside of car injured in collision with pedestrian or animal in nontraffic accident**

IQ 7 V40.3XX- **Unspecified car occupant injured in collision with pedestrian or animal in nontraffic accident**

IQ 7 V40.4XX- **Person boarding or alighting a car injured in collision with pedestrian or animal**

IQ 7 V40.5XX- **Car driver injured in collision with pedestrian or animal in traffic accident**

IQ 7 V40.6XX- **Car passenger injured in collision with pedestrian or animal in traffic accident**

IQ 7 V40.7XX- **Person on outside of car injured in collision with pedestrian or animal in traffic accident**

IQ 7 V40.9XX- **Unspecified car occupant injured in collision with pedestrian or animal in traffic accident**

4 V41 **Car occupant injured in collision with pedal cycle**

The appropriate 7th character is to be added to each code from category V41
A initial encounter
D subsequent encounter
S sequela

IQ 7 V41.0XX- **Car driver injured in collision with pedal cycle in nontraffic accident**

IQ 7 V41.1XX- **Car passenger injured in collision with pedal cycle in nontraffic accident**

IQ 7 V41.2XX- **Person on outside of car injured in collision with pedal cycle in nontraffic accident**

IQ 7 V41.3XX- **Unspecified car occupant injured in collision with pedal cycle in nontraffic accident**

IQ 7 V41.4XX- **Person boarding or alighting a car injured in collision with pedal cycle**

IQ 7 V41.5XX- **Car driver injured in collision with pedal cycle in traffic accident**

IQ 7 V41.6XX- **Car passenger injured in collision with pedal cycle in traffic accident**

IQ 7 V41.7XX- **Person on outside of car injured in collision with pedal cycle in traffic accident**

IQ 7 V41.9XX- **Unspecified car occupant injured in collision with pedal cycle in traffic accident**

4 V42 **Car occupant injured in collision with two- or three-wheeled motor vehicle**

The appropriate 7th character is to be added to each code from category V42
A initial encounter
D subsequent encounter
S sequela

IQ 7 V42.0XX- **Car driver injured in collision with two- or three-wheeled motor vehicle in nontraffic accident**

IQ 7 V42.1XX- **Car passenger injured in collision with two- or three-wheeled motor vehicle in nontraffic accident**

IQ 7 V42.2XX- **Person on outside of car injured in collision with two- or three-wheeled motor vehicle in nontraffic accident**

IQ 7 V42.3XX- **Unspecified car occupant injured in collision with two- or three-wheeled motor vehicle in nontraffic accident**

IQ 7 V42.4XX- **Person boarding or alighting a car injured in collision with two- or three-wheeled motor vehicle**

IQ 7 V42.5XX- Car driver injured in collision with two- or three-wheeled motor vehicle in traffic accident

IQ 7 V42.6XX- Car passenger injured in collision with two- or three-wheeled motor vehicle in traffic accident

IQ 7 V42.7XX- Person on outside of car injured in collision with two- or three-wheeled motor vehicle in traffic accident

IQ 7 V42.9XX- Unspecified car occupant injured in collision with two- or three-wheeled motor vehicle in traffic accident

4 V43 Car occupant injured in collision with car, pick-up truck or van

The appropriate 7th character is to be added to each code from category V43
A initial encounter
D subsequent encounter
S sequela

5 V43.0 Car driver injured in collision with car, pick-up truck or van in nontraffic accident

IQ 7 V43.01X- Car driver injured in collision with sport utility vehicle in nontraffic accident

IQ 7 V43.02X- Car driver injured in collision with other type car in nontraffic accident

IQ 7 V43.03X- Car driver injured in collision with pick-up truck in nontraffic accident

IQ 7 V43.04X- Car driver injured in collision with van in nontraffic accident

5 V43.1 Car passenger injured in collision with car, pick-up truck or van in nontraffic accident

IQ 7 V43.11X- Car passenger injured in collision with sport utility vehicle in nontraffic accident

IQ 7 V43.12X- Car passenger injured in collision with other type car in nontraffic accident

IQ 7 V43.13X- Car passenger injured in collision with pick-up truck in nontraffic accident

IQ 7 V43.14X- Car passenger injured in collision with van in nontraffic accident

5 V43.2 Person on outside of car injured in collision with car, pick-up truck or van in nontraffic accident

IQ 7 V43.21X- Person on outside of car injured in collision with sport utility vehicle in nontraffic accident

IQ 7 V43.22X- Person on outside of car injured in collision with other type car in nontraffic accident

IQ 7 V43.23X- Person on outside of car injured in collision with pick-up truck in nontraffic accident

IQ 7 V43.24X- Person on outside of car injured in collision with van in nontraffic accident

5 V43.3 Unspecified car occupant injured in collision with car, pick-up truck or van in nontraffic accident

IQ 7 V43.31X- Unspecified car occupant injured in collision with sport utility vehicle in nontraffic accident

IQ 7 V43.32X- Unspecified car occupant injured in collision with other type car in nontraffic accident

IQ 7 V43.33X- Unspecified car occupant injured in collision with pick-up truck in nontraffic accident

IQ 7 V43.34X- Unspecified car occupant injured in collision with van in nontraffic accident

5 V43.4 Person boarding or alighting a car injured in collision with car, pick-up truck or van

IQ 7 V43.41X- Person boarding or alighting a car injured in collision with sport utility vehicle

IQ 7 V43.42X- Person boarding or alighting a car injured in collision with other type car

IQ 7 V43.43X- Person boarding or alighting a car injured in collision with pick-up truck

IQ 7 V43.44X- Person boarding or alighting a car injured in collision with van

5 V43.5 Car driver injured in collision with car, pick-up truck or van in traffic accident

IQ 7 V43.51X- Car driver injured in collision with sport utility vehicle in traffic accident

IQ 7 V43.52X- Car driver injured in collision with other type car in traffic accident

IQ 7 V43.53X- Car driver injured in collision with pick-up truck in traffic accident

IQ 7 V43.54X- Car driver injured in collision with van in traffic accident

5 V43.6 Car passenger injured in collision with car, pick-up truck or van in traffic accident

IQ 7 V43.61X- Car passenger injured in collision with sport utility vehicle in traffic accident

IQ 7 V43.62X- Car passenger injured in collision with other type car in traffic accident

IQ 7 V43.63X- Car passenger injured in collision with pick-up truck in traffic accident

IQ 7 V43.64X- Car passenger injured in collision with van in traffic accident

5 V43.7 Person on outside of car injured in collision with car, pick-up truck or van in traffic accident

IQ 7 V43.71X- Person on outside of car injured in collision with sport utility vehicle in traffic accident

IQ 7 V43.72X- Person on outside of car injured in collision with other type car in traffic accident

IQ 7 V43.73X- Person on outside of car injured in collision with pick-up truck in traffic accident

IQ 7 V43.74X- Person on outside of car injured in collision with van in traffic accident

⑤ V43.9 Unspecified car occupant injured in collision with car, pick-up truck or van in traffic accident

!Q ☑ **V43.91X-** Unspecified car occupant injured in collision with sport utility vehicle in traffic accident

!Q ☑ **V43.92X-** Unspecified car occupant injured in collision with other type car in traffic accident

!Q ☑ **V43.93X-** Unspecified car occupant injured in collision with pick-up truck in traffic accident

!Q ☑ **V43.94X-** Unspecified car occupant injured in collision with van in traffic accident

④ V44 Car occupant injured in collision with heavy transport vehicle or bus

> **EXCLUDES 1**   car occupant injured in collision with military vehicle (V49.81)

The appropriate 7th character is to be added to each code from category V44
A   initial encounter
D   subsequent encounter
S   sequela

!Q ☑ **V44.0XX-** Car driver injured in collision with heavy transport vehicle or bus in nontraffic accident

!Q ☑ **V44.1XX-** Car passenger injured in collision with heavy transport vehicle or bus in nontraffic accident

!Q ☑ **V44.2XX-** Person on outside of car injured in collision with heavy transport vehicle or bus in nontraffic accident

!Q ☑ **V44.3XX-** Unspecified car occupant injured in collision with heavy transport vehicle or bus in nontraffic accident

!Q ☑ **V44.4XX-** Person boarding or alighting a car injured in collision with heavy transport vehicle or bus

!Q ☑ **V44.5XX-** Car driver injured in collision with heavy transport vehicle or bus in traffic accident

!Q ☑ **V44.6XX-** Car passenger injured in collision with heavy transport vehicle or bus in traffic accident

!Q ☑ **V44.7XX-** Person on outside of car injured in collision with heavy transport vehicle or bus in traffic accident

!Q ☑ **V44.9XX-** Unspecified car occupant injured in collision with heavy transport vehicle or bus in traffic accident

④ V45 Car occupant injured in collision with railway train or railway vehicle

The appropriate 7th character is to be added to each code from category V45
A   initial encounter
D   subsequent encounter
S   sequela

!Q ☑ **V45.0XX-** Car driver injured in collision with railway train or railway vehicle in nontraffic accident

!Q ☑ **V45.1XX-** Car passenger injured in collision with railway train or railway vehicle in nontraffic accident

!Q ☑ **V45.2XX-** Person on outside of car injured in collision with railway train or railway vehicle in nontraffic accident

!Q ☑ **V45.3XX-** Unspecified car occupant injured in collision with railway train or railway vehicle in nontraffic accident

!Q ☑ **V45.4XX-** Person boarding or alighting a car injured in collision with railway train or railway vehicle

!Q ☑ **V45.5XX-** Car driver injured in collision with railway train or railway vehicle in traffic accident

!Q ☑ **V45.6XX-** Car passenger injured in collision with railway train or railway vehicle in traffic accident

!Q ☑ **V45.7XX-** Person on outside of car injured in collision with railway train or railway vehicle in traffic accident

!Q ☑ **V45.9XX-** Unspecified car occupant injured in collision with railway train or railway vehicle in traffic accident

④ V46 Car occupant injured in collision with other nonmotor vehicle

> **INCLUDES**   collision with animal-drawn vehicle, animal being ridden, streetcar

The appropriate 7th character is to be added to each code from category V46
A   initial encounter
D   subsequent encounter
S   sequela

!Q ☑ **V46.0XX-** Car driver injured in collision with other nonmotor vehicle in nontraffic accident

!Q ☑ **V46.1XX-** Car passenger injured in collision with other nonmotor vehicle in nontraffic accident

!Q ☑ **V46.2XX-** Person on outside of car injured in collision with other nonmotor vehicle in nontraffic accident

!Q ☑ **V46.3XX-** Unspecified car occupant injured in collision with other nonmotor vehicle in nontraffic accident

!Q ☑ **V46.4XX-** Person boarding or alighting a car injured in collision with other nonmotor vehicle

!Q ☑ **V46.5XX-** Car driver injured in collision with other nonmotor vehicle in traffic accident

!Q ☑ **V46.6XX-** Car passenger injured in collision with other nonmotor vehicle in traffic accident

!Q ☑ **V46.7XX-** Person on outside of car injured in collision with other nonmotor vehicle in traffic accident

!Q ☑ **V46.9XX-** Unspecified car occupant injured in collision with other nonmotor vehicle in traffic accident

④ V47 Car occupant injured in collision with fixed or stationary object

---

④ 4th digit required   ⑤ 5th digit required   ⑥ 6th digit required   ⑦ 7th digit required   ☑ 7th digit placeholder   ✚ Additional code   ⊟ Laterality

The appropriate 7th character is to be added to each code from category V47
A initial encounter
D subsequent encounter
S sequela

IQ 7 **V47.0XX- Car driver injured in collision with fixed or stationary object in nontraffic accident**

IQ 7 **V47.1XX- Car passenger injured in collision with fixed or stationary object in nontraffic accident**

IQ 7 **V47.2XX- Person on outside of car injured in collision with fixed or stationary object in nontraffic accident**

IQ 7 **V47.3XX- Unspecified car occupant injured in collision with fixed or stationary object in nontraffic accident**

IQ 7 **V47.4XX- Person boarding or alighting a car injured in collision with fixed or stationary object**

IQ 7 **V47.5XX- Car driver injured in collision with fixed or stationary object in traffic accident**

IQ 7 **V47.6XX- Car passenger injured in collision with fixed or stationary object in traffic accident**

IQ 7 **V47.7XX- Person on outside of car injured in collision with fixed or stationary object in traffic accident**

IQ 7 **V47.9XX- Unspecified car occupant injured in collision with fixed or stationary object in traffic accident**

4 **V48 Car occupant injured in noncollision transport accident**

INCLUDES overturning car NOS
overturning car without collision

The appropriate 7th character is to be added to each code from category V48
A initial encounter
D subsequent encounter
S sequela

IQ 7 **V48.0XX- Car driver injured in noncollision transport accident in nontraffic accident**

IQ 7 **V48.1XX- Car passenger injured in noncollision transport accident in nontraffic accident**

IQ 7 **V48.2XX- Person on outside of car injured in noncollision transport accident in nontraffic accident**

IQ 7 **V48.3XX- Unspecified car occupant injured in noncollision transport accident in nontraffic accident**

IQ 7 **V48.4XX- Person boarding or alighting a car injured in noncollision transport accident**

IQ 7 **V48.5XX- Car driver injured in noncollision transport accident in traffic accident**

IQ 7 **V48.6XX- Car passenger injured in noncollision transport accident in traffic accident**

IQ 7 **V48.7XX- Person on outside of car injured in noncollision transport accident in traffic accident**

IQ 7 **V48.9XX- Unspecified car occupant injured in noncollision transport accident in traffic accident**

4 **V49 Car occupant injured in other and unspecified transport accidents**

The appropriate 7th character is to be added to each code from category V49
A initial encounter
D subsequent encounter
S sequela

5 **V49.0 Driver injured in collision with other and unspecified motor vehicles in nontraffic accident**

IQ 7 **V49.00X- Driver injured in collision with unspecified motor vehicles in nontraffic accident**

IQ 7 **V49.09X- Driver injured in collision with other motor vehicles in nontraffic accident**

5 **V49.1 Passenger injured in collision with other and unspecified motor vehicles in nontraffic accident**

IQ 7 **V49.10X- Passenger injured in collision with unspecified motor vehicles in nontraffic accident**

IQ 7 **V49.19X- Passenger injured in collision with other motor vehicles in nontraffic accident**

5 **V49.2 Unspecified car occupant injured in collision with other and unspecified motor vehicles in nontraffic accident**

IQ 7 **V49.20X- Unspecified car occupant injured in collision with unspecified motor vehicles in nontraffic accident**

Car collision NOS, nontraffic

IQ 7 **V49.29X- Unspecified car occupant injured in collision with other motor vehicles in nontraffic accident**

IQ 7 **V49.3XX- Car occupant (driver) (passenger) injured in unspecified nontraffic accident**

Car accident NOS, nontraffic
Car occupant injured in nontraffic accident NOS

5 **V49.4 Driver injured in collision with other and unspecified motor vehicles in traffic accident**

IQ 7 **V49.40X- Driver injured in collision with unspecified motor vehicles in traffic accident**

IQ 7 **V49.49X- Driver injured in collision with other motor vehicles in traffic accident**

5 **V49.5 Passenger injured in collision with other and unspecified motor vehicles in traffic accident**

IQ 7 **V49.50X- Passenger injured in collision with unspecified motor vehicles in traffic accident**

IQ 7 **V49.59X- Passenger injured in collision with other motor vehicles in traffic accident**

Chapter 20 V00-Y99

5 V49.6 Unspecified car occupant injured in collision with other and unspecified motor vehicles in traffic accident

!Q ☑ V49.60X- Unspecified car occupant injured in collision with unspecified motor vehicles in traffic accident

Car collision NOS (traffic)

!Q ☑ V49.69X- Unspecified car occupant injured in collision with other motor vehicles in traffic accident

5 V49.8 Car occupant (driver) (passenger) injured in other specified transport accidents

!Q ☑ V49.81X- Car occupant (driver) (passenger) injured in transport accident with military vehicle

!Q ☑ V49.88X- Car occupant (driver) (passenger) injured in other specified transport accidents

!Q ☑ V49.9XX- Car occupant (driver) (passenger) injured in unspecified traffic accident

Car accident NOS

Occupant of pick-up truck or van injured in transport accident   (V50-V59)

INCLUDES a four or six wheel motor vehicle designed primarily for carrying passengers and property but weighing less than the local limit for classification as a heavy goods vehicle
minibus
minivan
sport utility vehicle (SUV)
truck
van

EXCLUDES 1 heavy transport vehicle (V60-V69)

4 V50 Occupant of pick-up truck or van injured in collision with pedestrian or animal

EXCLUDES 1 pick-up truck or van collision with animal-drawn vehicle or animal being ridden (V56.-)

The appropriate 7th character is to be added to each code from category V50
A   initial encounter
D   subsequent encounter
S   sequela

!Q ☑ V50.0XX- Driver of pick-up truck or van injured in collision with pedestrian or animal in nontraffic accident

!Q ☑ V50.1XX- Passenger in pick-up truck or van injured in collision with pedestrian or animal in nontraffic accident

!Q ☑ V50.2XX- Person on outside of pick-up truck or van injured in collision with pedestrian or animal in nontraffic accident

!Q ☑ V50.3XX- Unspecified occupant of pick-up truck or van injured in collision with pedestrian or animal in nontraffic accident

!Q ☑ V50.4XX- Person boarding or alighting a pick-up truck or van injured in collision with pedestrian or animal

!Q ☑ V50.5XX- Driver of pick-up truck or van injured in collision with pedestrian or animal in traffic accident

!Q ☑ V50.6XX- Passenger in pick-up truck or van injured in collision with pedestrian or animal in traffic accident

!Q ☑ V50.7XX- Person on outside of pick-up truck or van injured in collision with pedestrian or animal in traffic accident

!Q ☑ V50.9XX- Unspecified occupant of pick-up truck or van injured in collision with pedestrian or animal in traffic accident

4 V51 Occupant of pick-up truck or van injured in collision with pedal cycle

The appropriate 7th character is to be added to each code from category V51
A   initial encounter
D   subsequent encounter
S   sequela

!Q ☑ V51.0XX- Driver of pick-up truck or van injured in collision with pedal cycle in nontraffic accident

!Q ☑ V51.1XX- Passenger in pick-up truck or van injured in collision with pedal cycle in nontraffic accident

!Q ☑ V51.2XX- Person on outside of pick-up truck or van injured in collision with pedal cycle in nontraffic accident

!Q ☑ V51.3XX- Unspecified occupant of pick-up truck or van injured in collision with pedal cycle in nontraffic accident

!Q ☑ V51.4XX- Person boarding or alighting a pick-up truck or van injured in collision with pedal cycle

!Q ☑ V51.5XX- Driver of pick-up truck or van injured in collision with pedal cycle in traffic accident

!Q ☑ V51.6XX- Passenger in pick-up truck or van injured in collision with pedal cycle in traffic accident

!Q ☑ V51.7XX- Person on outside of pick-up truck or van injured in collision with pedal cycle in traffic accident

!Q ☑ V51.9XX- Unspecified occupant of pick-up truck or van injured in collision with pedal cycle in traffic accident

4 V52 Occupant of pick-up truck or van injured in collision with two- or three-wheeled motor vehicle

The appropriate 7th character is to be added to each code from category V52
A   initial encounter
D   subsequent encounter
S   sequela

!Q ☑ V52.0XX- Driver of pick-up truck or van injured in collision with two- or three-wheeled motor vehicle in nontraffic accident

!Q ☑ V52.1XX- Passenger in pick-up truck or van injured in collision with two- or three-wheeled motor vehicle in nontraffic accident

!Q ☑ V52.2XX- Person on outside of pick-up truck or van injured in collision with two- or three-wheeled motor vehicle in nontraffic accident

4 4th digit required   5 5th digit required   6 6th digit required   7 7th digit required   ☑ 7th digit placeholder   ✚ Additional code   ▤ Laterality

V52.3XX- **Unspecified occupant of pick-up truck or van injured in collision with two- or three-wheeled motor vehicle in nontraffic accident**

V52.4XX- **Person boarding or alighting a pick-up truck or van injured in collision with two- or three-wheeled motor vehicle**

V52.5XX- **Driver of pick-up truck or van injured in collision with two- or three-wheeled motor vehicle in traffic accident**

V52.6XX- **Passenger in pick-up truck or van injured in collision with two- or three-wheeled motor vehicle in traffic accident**

V52.7XX- **Person on outside of pick-up truck or van injured in collision with two- or three-wheeled motor vehicle in traffic accident**

V52.9XX- **Unspecified occupant of pick-up truck or van injured in collision with two- or three-wheeled motor vehicle in traffic accident**

V53 **Occupant of pick-up truck or van injured in collision with car, pick-up truck or van**

The appropriate 7th character is to be added to each code from category V53
A initial encounter
D subsequent encounter
S sequela

V53.0XX- **Driver of pick-up truck or van injured in collision with car, pick-up truck or van in nontraffic accident**

V53.1XX- **Passenger in pick-up truck or van injured in collision with car, pick-up truck or van in nontraffic accident**

V53.2XX- **Person on outside of pick-up truck or van injured in collision with car, pick-up truck or van in nontraffic accident**

V53.3XX- **Unspecified occupant of pick-up truck or van injured in collision with car, pick-up truck or van in nontraffic accident**

V53.4XX- **Person boarding or alighting a pick-up truck or van injured in collision with car, pick-up truck or van**

V53.5XX- **Driver of pick-up truck or van injured in collision with car, pick-up truck or van in traffic accident**

V53.6XX- **Passenger in pick-up truck or van injured in collision with car, pick-up truck or van in traffic accident**

V53.7XX- **Person on outside of pick-up truck or van injured in collision with car, pick-up truck or van in traffic accident**

V53.9XX- **Unspecified occupant of pick-up truck or van injured in collision with car, pick-up truck or van in traffic accident**

V54 **Occupant of pick-up truck or van injured in collision with heavy transport vehicle or bus**

EXCLUDES 1 occupant of pick-up truck or van injured in collision with military vehicle (V59.81)

The appropriate 7th character is to be added to each code from category V54
A initial encounter
D subsequent encounter
S sequela

V54.0XX- **Driver of pick-up truck or van injured in collision with heavy transport vehicle or bus in nontraffic accident**

V54.1XX- **Passenger in pick-up truck or van injured in collision with heavy transport vehicle or bus in nontraffic accident**

V54.2XX- **Person on outside of pick-up truck or van injured in collision with heavy transport vehicle or bus in nontraffic accident**

V54.3XX- **Unspecified occupant of pick-up truck or van injured in collision with heavy transport vehicle or bus in nontraffic accident**

V54.4XX- **Person boarding or alighting a pick-up truck or van injured in collision with heavy transport vehicle or bus**

V54.5XX- **Driver of pick-up truck or van injured in collision with heavy transport vehicle or bus in traffic accident**

V54.6XX- **Passenger in pick-up truck or van injured in collision with heavy transport vehicle or bus in traffic accident**

V54.7XX- **Person on outside of pick-up truck or van injured in collision with heavy transport vehicle or bus in traffic accident**

V54.9XX- **Unspecified occupant of pick-up truck or van injured in collision with heavy transport vehicle or bus in traffic accident**

V55 **Occupant of pick-up truck or van injured in collision with railway train or railway vehicle**

The appropriate 7th character is to be added to each code from category V55
A initial encounter
D subsequent encounter
S sequela

V55.0XX- **Driver of pick-up truck or van injured in collision with railway train or railway vehicle in nontraffic accident**

V55.1XX- **Passenger in pick-up truck or van injured in collision with railway train or railway vehicle in nontraffic accident**

V55.2XX- **Person on outside of pick-up truck or van injured in collision with railway train or railway vehicle in nontraffic accident**

IQ 7 **V55.3XX-** **Unspecified occupant of pick-up truck or van injured in collision with railway train or railway vehicle in nontraffic accident**

IQ 7 **V55.4XX-** **Person boarding or alighting a pick-up truck or van injured in collision with railway train or railway vehicle**

IQ 7 **V55.5XX-** **Driver of pick-up truck or van injured in collision with railway train or railway vehicle in traffic accident**

IQ 7 **V55.6XX-** **Passenger in pick-up truck or van injured in collision with railway train or railway vehicle in traffic accident**

IQ 7 **V55.7XX-** **Person on outside of pick-up truck or van injured in collision with railway train or railway vehicle in traffic accident**

IQ 7 **V55.9XX-** **Unspecified occupant of pick-up truck or van injured in collision with railway train or railway vehicle in traffic accident**

4 **V56** **Occupant of pick-up truck or van injured in collision with other nonmotor vehicle**

INCLUDES collision with animal-drawn vehicle, animal being ridden, streetcar

The appropriate 7th character is to be added to each code from category V56
A initial encounter
D subsequent encounter
S sequela

IQ 7 **V56.0XX-** **Driver of pick-up truck or van injured in collision with other nonmotor vehicle in nontraffic accident**

IQ 7 **V56.1XX-** **Passenger in pick-up truck or van injured in collision with other nonmotor vehicle in nontraffic accident**

IQ 7 **V56.2XX-** **Person on outside of pick-up truck or van injured in collision with other nonmotor vehicle in nontraffic accident**

IQ 7 **V56.3XX-** **Unspecified occupant of pick-up truck or van injured in collision with other nonmotor vehicle in nontraffic accident**

IQ 7 **V56.4XX-** **Person boarding or alighting a pick-up truck or van injured in collision with other nonmotor vehicle**

IQ 7 **V56.5XX-** **Driver of pick-up truck or van injured in collision with other nonmotor vehicle in traffic accident**

IQ 7 **V56.6XX-** **Passenger in pick-up truck or van injured in collision with other nonmotor vehicle in traffic accident**

IQ 7 **V56.7XX-** **Person on outside of pick-up truck or van injured in collision with other nonmotor vehicle in traffic accident**

IQ 7 **V56.9XX-** **Unspecified occupant of pick-up truck or van injured in collision with other nonmotor vehicle in traffic accident**

4 **V57** **Occupant of pick-up truck or van injured in collision with fixed or stationary object**

The appropriate 7th character is to be added to each code from category V57
A initial encounter
D subsequent encounter
S sequela

IQ 7 **V57.0XX-** **Driver of pick-up truck or van injured in collision with fixed or stationary object in nontraffic accident**

IQ 7 **V57.1XX-** **Passenger in pick-up truck or van injured in collision with fixed or stationary object in nontraffic accident**

IQ 7 **V57.2XX-** **Person on outside of pick-up truck or van injured in collision with fixed or stationary object in nontraffic accident**

IQ 7 **V57.3XX-** **Unspecified occupant of pick-up truck or van injured in collision with fixed or stationary object in nontraffic accident**

IQ 7 **V57.4XX-** **Person boarding or alighting a pick-up truck or van injured in collision with fixed or stationary object**

IQ 7 **V57.5XX-** **Driver of pick-up truck or van injured in collision with fixed or stationary object in traffic accident**

IQ 7 **V57.6XX-** **Passenger in pick-up truck or van injured in collision with fixed or stationary object in traffic accident**

IQ 7 **V57.7XX-** **Person on outside of pick-up truck or van injured in collision with fixed or stationary object in traffic accident**

IQ 7 **V57.9XX-** **Unspecified occupant of pick-up truck or van injured in collision with fixed or stationary object in traffic accident**

4 **V58** **Occupant of pick-up truck or van injured in noncollision transport accident**

INCLUDES overturning pick-up truck or van NOS
overturning pick-up truck or van without collision

The appropriate 7th character is to be added to each code from category V58
A initial encounter
D subsequent encounter
S sequela

IQ 7 **V58.0XX-** **Driver of pick-up truck or van injured in noncollision transport accident in nontraffic accident**

IQ 7 **V58.1XX-** **Passenger in pick-up truck or van injured in noncollision transport accident in nontraffic accident**

IQ 7 **V58.2XX-** **Person on outside of pick-up truck or van injured in noncollision transport accident in nontraffic accident**

IQ 7 **V58.3XX-** **Unspecified occupant of pick-up truck or van injured in noncollision transport accident in nontraffic accident**

Chapter 20

V00-Y99

IQ 7 **V58.4XX- Person boarding or alighting a pick-up truck or van injured in noncollision transport accident**

IQ 7 **V58.5XX- Driver of pick-up truck or van injured in noncollision transport accident in traffic accident**

IQ 7 **V58.6XX- Passenger in pick-up truck or van injured in noncollision transport accident in traffic accident**

IQ 7 **V58.7XX- Person on outside of pick-up truck or van injured in noncollision transport accident in traffic accident**

IQ 7 **V58.9XX- Unspecified occupant of pick-up truck or van injured in noncollision transport accident in traffic accident**

4 **V59 Occupant of pick-up truck or van injured in other and unspecified transport accidents**

The appropriate 7th character is to be added to each code from category V59
A initial encounter
D subsequent encounter
S sequela

5 **V59.0 Driver of pick-up truck or van injured in collision with other and unspecified motor vehicles in nontraffic accident**

IQ 7 **V59.00X- Driver of pick-up truck or van injured in collision with unspecified motor vehicles in nontraffic accident**

IQ 7 **V59.09X- Driver of pick-up truck or van injured in collision with other motor vehicles in nontraffic accident**

5 **V59.1 Passenger in pick-up truck or van injured in collision with other and unspecified motor vehicles in nontraffic accident**

IQ 7 **V59.10X- Passenger in pick-up truck or van injured in collision with unspecified motor vehicles in nontraffic accident**

IQ 7 **V59.19X- Passenger in pick-up truck or van injured in collision with other motor vehicles in nontraffic accident**

5 **V59.2 Unspecified occupant of pick-up truck or van injured in collision with other and unspecified motor vehicles in nontraffic accident**

IQ 7 **V59.20X- Unspecified occupant of pick-up truck or van injured in collision with unspecified motor vehicles in nontraffic accident**

Collision NOS involving pick-up truck or van, nontraffic

IQ 7 **V59.29X- Unspecified occupant of pick-up truck or van injured in collision with other motor vehicles in nontraffic accident**

IQ 7 **V59.3XX- Occupant (driver) (passenger) of pick-up truck or van injured in unspecified nontraffic accident**

Accident NOS involving pick-up truck or van, nontraffic
Occupant of pick-up truck or van injured in nontraffic accident NOS

5 **V59.4 Driver of pick-up truck or van injured in collision with other and unspecified motor vehicles in traffic accident**

IQ 7 **V59.40X- Driver of pick-up truck or van injured in collision with unspecified motor vehicles in traffic accident**

IQ 7 **V59.49X- Driver of pick-up truck or van injured in collision with other motor vehicles in traffic accident**

5 **V59.5 Passenger in pick-up truck or van injured in collision with other and unspecified motor vehicles in traffic accident**

IQ 7 **V59.50X- Passenger in pick-up truck or van injured in collision with unspecified motor vehicles in traffic accident**

IQ 7 **V59.59X- Passenger in pick-up truck or van injured in collision with other motor vehicles in traffic accident**

5 **V59.6 Unspecified occupant of pick-up truck or van injured in collision with other and unspecified motor vehicles in traffic accident**

IQ 7 **V59.60X- Unspecified occupant of pick-up truck or van injured in collision with unspecified motor vehicles in traffic accident**

Collision NOS involving pick-up truck or van (traffic)

IQ 7 **V59.69X- Unspecified occupant of pick-up truck or van injured in collision with other motor vehicles in traffic accident**

5 **V59.8 Occupant (driver) (passenger) of pick-up truck or van injured in other specified transport accidents**

IQ 7 **V59.81X- Occupant (driver) (passenger) of pick-up truck or van injured in transport accident with military vehicle**

IQ 7 **V59.88X- Occupant (driver) (passenger) of pick-up truck or van injured in other specified transport accidents**

IQ 7 **V59.9XX- Occupant (driver) (passenger) of pick-up truck or van injured in unspecified traffic accident**

Accident NOS involving pick-up truck or van

Occupant of heavy transport vehicle injured in transport accident (V60-V69)

INCLUDES 18 wheeler
armored car
panel truck

EXCLUDES 1 bus
motorcoach

4 **V60 Occupant of heavy transport vehicle injured in collision with pedestrian or animal**

EXCLUDES 1 heavy transport vehicle collision with animal-drawn vehicle or animal being ridden (V66.-)

The appropriate 7th character is to be added to each code from category V60
A   initial encounter
D   subsequent encounter
S   sequela

IQ ☑ V60.0XX- Driver of heavy transport vehicle injured in collision with pedestrian or animal in nontraffic accident

IQ ☑ V60.1XX- Passenger in heavy transport vehicle injured in collision with pedestrian or animal in nontraffic accident

IQ ☑ V60.2XX- Person on outside of heavy transport vehicle injured in collision with pedestrian or animal in nontraffic accident

IQ ☑ V60.3XX- Unspecified occupant of heavy transport vehicle injured in collision with pedestrian or animal in nontraffic accident

IQ ☑ V60.4XX- Person boarding or alighting a heavy transport vehicle injured in collision with pedestrian or animal

IQ ☑ V60.5XX- Driver of heavy transport vehicle injured in collision with pedestrian or animal in traffic accident

IQ ☑ V60.6XX- Passenger in heavy transport vehicle injured in collision with pedestrian or animal in traffic accident

IQ ☑ V60.7XX- Person on outside of heavy transport vehicle injured in collision with pedestrian or animal in traffic accident

IQ ☑ V60.9XX- Unspecified occupant of heavy transport vehicle injured in collision with pedestrian or animal in traffic accident

④ V61 Occupant of heavy transport vehicle injured in collision with pedal cycle

The appropriate 7th character is to be added to each code from category V61
A   initial encounter
D   subsequent encounter
S   sequela

IQ ☑ V61.0XX- Driver of heavy transport vehicle injured in collision with pedal cycle in nontraffic accident

IQ ☑ V61.1XX- Passenger in heavy transport vehicle injured in collision with pedal cycle in nontraffic accident

IQ ☑ V61.2XX- Person on outside of heavy transport vehicle injured in collision with pedal cycle in nontraffic accident

IQ ☑ V61.3XX- Unspecified occupant of heavy transport vehicle injured in collision with pedal cycle in nontraffic accident

IQ ☑ V61.4XX- Person boarding or alighting a heavy transport vehicle injured in collision with pedal cycle while boarding or alighting

IQ ☑ V61.5XX- Driver of heavy transport vehicle injured in collision with pedal cycle in traffic accident

IQ ☑ V61.6XX- Passenger in heavy transport vehicle injured in collision with pedal cycle in traffic accident

IQ ☑ V61.7XX- Person on outside of heavy transport vehicle injured in collision with pedal cycle in traffic accident

IQ ☑ V61.9XX- Unspecified occupant of heavy transport vehicle injured in collision with pedal cycle in traffic accident

④ V62 Occupant of heavy transport vehicle injured in collision with two- or three-wheeled motor vehicle

The appropriate 7th character is to be added to each code from category V62
A   initial encounter
D   subsequent encounter
S   sequela

IQ ☑ V62.0XX- Driver of heavy transport vehicle injured in collision with two- or three-wheeled motor vehicle in nontraffic accident

IQ ☑ V62.1XX- Passenger in heavy transport vehicle injured in collision with two- or three-wheeled motor vehicle in nontraffic accident

IQ ☑ V62.2XX- Person on outside of heavy transport vehicle injured in collision with two- or three-wheeled motor vehicle in nontraffic accident

IQ ☑ V62.3XX- Unspecified occupant of heavy transport vehicle injured in collision with two- or three-wheeled motor vehicle in nontraffic accident

IQ ☑ V62.4XX- Person boarding or alighting a heavy transport vehicle injured in collision with two- or three-wheeled motor vehicle

IQ ☑ V62.5XX- Driver of heavy transport vehicle injured in collision with two- or three-wheeled motor vehicle in traffic accident

IQ ☑ V62.6XX- Passenger in heavy transport vehicle injured in collision with two- or three-wheeled motor vehicle in traffic accident

IQ ☑ V62.7XX- Person on outside of heavy transport vehicle injured in collision with two- or three-wheeled motor vehicle in traffic accident

IQ ☑ V62.9XX- Unspecified occupant of heavy transport vehicle injured in collision with two- or three-wheeled motor vehicle in traffic accident

④ V63 Occupant of heavy transport vehicle injured in collision with car, pick-up truck or van

④ 4th digit required   ⑤ 5th digit required   ⑥ 6th digit required   ⑦ 7th digit required   ☑ 7th digit placeholder   ✚ Additional code   ▤ Laterality

1826   DecisionHealth's FY 2022 Complete Home Health ICD-10-CM Diagnosis Coding Manual

Chapter 20

V00-Y99

The appropriate 7th character is to be added to each code from category V63
A   initial encounter
D   subsequent encounter
S   sequela

!Q ✓ V63.0XX- **Driver of heavy transport vehicle injured in collision with car, pick-up truck or van in nontraffic accident**

!Q ✓ V63.1XX- **Passenger in heavy transport vehicle injured in collision with car, pick-up truck or van in nontraffic accident**

!Q ✓ V63.2XX- **Person on outside of heavy transport vehicle injured in collision with car, pick-up truck or van in nontraffic accident**

!Q ✓ V63.3XX- **Unspecified occupant of heavy transport vehicle injured in collision with car, pick-up truck or van in nontraffic accident**

!Q ✓ V63.4XX- **Person boarding or alighting a heavy transport vehicle injured in collision with car, pick-up truck or van**

!Q ✓ V63.5XX- **Driver of heavy transport vehicle injured in collision with car, pick-up truck or van in traffic accident**

!Q ✓ V63.6XX- **Passenger in heavy transport vehicle injured in collision with car, pick-up truck or van in traffic accident**

!Q ✓ V63.7XX- **Person on outside of heavy transport vehicle injured in collision with car, pick-up truck or van in traffic accident**

!Q ✓ V63.9XX- **Unspecified occupant of heavy transport vehicle injured in collision with car, pick-up truck or van in traffic accident**

4 V64 **Occupant of heavy transport vehicle injured in collision with heavy transport vehicle or bus**

> **EXCLUDES 1** occupant of heavy transport vehicle injured in collision with military vehicle (V69.81)

The appropriate 7th character is to be added to each code from category V64
A   initial encounter
D   subsequent encounter
S   sequela

!Q ✓ V64.0XX- **Driver of heavy transport vehicle injured in collision with heavy transport vehicle or bus in nontraffic accident**

!Q ✓ V64.1XX- **Passenger in heavy transport vehicle injured in collision with heavy transport vehicle or bus in nontraffic accident**

!Q ✓ V64.2XX- **Person on outside of heavy transport vehicle injured in collision with heavy transport vehicle or bus in nontraffic accident**

!Q ✓ V64.3XX- **Unspecified occupant of heavy transport vehicle injured in collision with heavy transport vehicle or bus in nontraffic accident**

!Q ✓ V64.4XX- **Person boarding or alighting a heavy transport vehicle injured in collision with heavy transport vehicle or bus while boarding or alighting**

!Q ✓ V64.5XX- **Driver of heavy transport vehicle injured in collision with heavy transport vehicle or bus in traffic accident**

!Q ✓ V64.6XX- **Passenger in heavy transport vehicle injured in collision with heavy transport vehicle or bus in traffic accident**

!Q ✓ V64.7XX- **Person on outside of heavy transport vehicle injured in collision with heavy transport vehicle or bus in traffic accident**

!Q ✓ V64.9XX- **Unspecified occupant of heavy transport vehicle injured in collision with heavy transport vehicle or bus in traffic accident**

4 V65 **Occupant of heavy transport vehicle injured in collision with railway train or railway vehicle**

The appropriate 7th character is to be added to each code from category V65
A   initial encounter
D   subsequent encounter
S   sequela

!Q ✓ V65.0XX- **Driver of heavy transport vehicle injured in collision with railway train or railway vehicle in nontraffic accident**

!Q ✓ V65.1XX- **Passenger in heavy transport vehicle injured in collision with railway train or railway vehicle in nontraffic accident**

!Q ✓ V65.2XX- **Person on outside of heavy transport vehicle injured in collision with railway train or railway vehicle in nontraffic accident**

!Q ✓ V65.3XX- **Unspecified occupant of heavy transport vehicle injured in collision with railway train or railway vehicle in nontraffic accident**

!Q ✓ V65.4XX- **Person boarding or alighting a heavy transport vehicle injured in collision with railway train or railway vehicle**

!Q ✓ V65.5XX- **Driver of heavy transport vehicle injured in collision with railway train or railway vehicle in traffic accident**

!Q ✓ V65.6XX- **Passenger in heavy transport vehicle injured in collision with railway train or railway vehicle in traffic accident**

!Q ✓ V65.7XX- **Person on outside of heavy transport vehicle injured in collision with railway train or railway vehicle in traffic accident**

Chapter 20

V00-Y99

★ New ▲ Revised Px Primary SP PDGM Px SL Low CoM SH High CoM !Q Quest. Encounter H Hospice non-cancer Dx Unspecified M *Manifestation*

[IQ] [✓] V65.9XX- **Unspecified occupant of heavy transport vehicle injured in collision with railway train or railway vehicle in traffic accident**

[4] V66 **Occupant of heavy transport vehicle injured in collision with other nonmotor vehicle**

> **INCLUDES** collision with animal-drawn vehicle, animal being ridden, streetcar

> The appropriate 7th character is to be added to each code from category V66
> A   initial encounter
> D   subsequent encounter
> S   sequela

[IQ] [✓] V66.0XX- **Driver of heavy transport vehicle injured in collision with other nonmotor vehicle in nontraffic accident**

[IQ] [✓] V66.1XX- **Passenger in heavy transport vehicle injured in collision with other nonmotor vehicle in nontraffic accident**

[IQ] [✓] V66.2XX- **Person on outside of heavy transport vehicle injured in collision with other nonmotor vehicle in nontraffic accident**

[IQ] [✓] V66.3XX- **Unspecified occupant of heavy transport vehicle injured in collision with other nonmotor vehicle in nontraffic accident**

[IQ] [✓] V66.4XX- **Person boarding or alighting a heavy transport vehicle injured in collision with other nonmotor vehicle**

[IQ] [✓] V66.5XX- **Driver of heavy transport vehicle injured in collision with other nonmotor vehicle in traffic accident**

[IQ] [✓] V66.6XX- **Passenger in heavy transport vehicle injured in collision with other nonmotor vehicle in traffic accident**

[IQ] [✓] V66.7XX- **Person on outside of heavy transport vehicle injured in collision with other nonmotor vehicle in traffic accident**

[IQ] [✓] V66.9XX- **Unspecified occupant of heavy transport vehicle injured in collision with other nonmotor vehicle in traffic accident**

[4] V67 **Occupant of heavy transport vehicle injured in collision with fixed or stationary object**

> The appropriate 7th character is to be added to each code from category V67
> A   initial encounter
> D   subsequent encounter
> S   sequela

[IQ] [✓] V67.0XX- **Driver of heavy transport vehicle injured in collision with fixed or stationary object in nontraffic accident**

[IQ] [✓] V67.1XX- **Passenger in heavy transport vehicle injured in collision with fixed or stationary object in nontraffic accident**

[IQ] [✓] V67.2XX- **Person on outside of heavy transport vehicle injured in collision with fixed or stationary object in nontraffic accident**

[IQ] [✓] V67.3XX- **Unspecified occupant of heavy transport vehicle injured in collision with fixed or stationary object in nontraffic accident**

[IQ] [✓] V67.4XX- **Person boarding or alighting a heavy transport vehicle injured in collision with fixed or stationary object**

[IQ] [✓] V67.5XX- **Driver of heavy transport vehicle injured in collision with fixed or stationary object in traffic accident**

[IQ] [✓] V67.6XX- **Passenger in heavy transport vehicle injured in collision with fixed or stationary object in traffic accident**

[IQ] [✓] V67.7XX- **Person on outside of heavy transport vehicle injured in collision with fixed or stationary object in traffic accident**

[IQ] [✓] V67.9XX- **Unspecified occupant of heavy transport vehicle injured in collision with fixed or stationary object in traffic accident**

[4] V68 **Occupant of heavy transport vehicle injured in noncollision transport accident**
> **INCLUDES** overturning heavy transport vehicle NOS
> overturning heavy transport vehicle without collision

> The appropriate 7th character is to be added to each code from category V68
> A   initial encounter
> D   subsequent encounter
> S   sequela

[IQ] [✓] V68.0XX- **Driver of heavy transport vehicle injured in noncollision transport accident in nontraffic accident**

[IQ] [✓] V68.1XX- **Passenger in heavy transport vehicle injured in noncollision transport accident in nontraffic accident**

[IQ] [✓] V68.2XX- **Person on outside of heavy transport vehicle injured in noncollision transport accident in nontraffic accident**

[IQ] [✓] V68.3XX- **Unspecified occupant of heavy transport vehicle injured in noncollision transport accident in nontraffic accident**

[IQ] [✓] V68.4XX- **Person boarding or alighting a heavy transport vehicle injured in noncollision transport accident**

[IQ] [✓] V68.5XX- **Driver of heavy transport vehicle injured in noncollision transport accident in traffic accident**

[IQ] [✓] V68.6XX- **Passenger in heavy transport vehicle injured in noncollision transport accident in traffic accident**

[IQ] [✓] V68.7XX- **Person on outside of heavy transport vehicle injured in noncollision transport accident in traffic accident**

---

[4] 4th digit required   [5] 5th digit required   [6] 6th digit required   [7] 7th digit required   [✓] 7th digit placeholder   **+** Additional code   [⊟] Laterality

IQ 7 **V68.9XX- Unspecified occupant of heavy transport vehicle injured in noncollision transport accident in traffic accident**

4 **V69 Occupant of heavy transport vehicle injured in other and unspecified transport accidents**

The appropriate 7th character is to be added to each code from category V69
A initial encounter
D subsequent encounter
S sequela

5 **V69.0 Driver of heavy transport vehicle injured in collision with other and unspecified motor vehicles in nontraffic accident**

IQ 7 **V69.00X- Driver of heavy transport vehicle injured in collision with unspecified motor vehicles in nontraffic accident**

IQ 7 **V69.09X- Driver of heavy transport vehicle injured in collision with other motor vehicles in nontraffic accident**

5 **V69.1 Passenger in heavy transport vehicle injured in collision with other and unspecified motor vehicles in nontraffic accident**

IQ 7 **V69.10X- Passenger in heavy transport vehicle injured in collision with unspecified motor vehicles in nontraffic accident**

IQ 7 **V69.19X- Passenger in heavy transport vehicle injured in collision with other motor vehicles in nontraffic accident**

5 **V69.2 Unspecified occupant of heavy transport vehicle injured in collision with other and unspecified motor vehicles in nontraffic accident**

IQ 7 **V69.20X- Unspecified occupant of heavy transport vehicle injured in collision with unspecified motor vehicles in nontraffic accident**

Collision NOS involving heavy transport vehicle, nontraffic

IQ 7 **V69.29X- Unspecified occupant of heavy transport vehicle injured in collision with other motor vehicles in nontraffic accident**

IQ 7 **V69.3XX- Occupant (driver) (passenger) of heavy transport vehicle injured in unspecified nontraffic accident**

Accident NOS involving heavy transport vehicle, nontraffic
Occupant of heavy transport vehicle injured in nontraffic accident NOS

5 **V69.4 Driver of heavy transport vehicle injured in collision with other and unspecified motor vehicles in traffic accident**

IQ 7 **V69.40X- Driver of heavy transport vehicle injured in collision with unspecified motor vehicles in traffic accident**

IQ 7 **V69.49X- Driver of heavy transport vehicle injured in collision with other motor vehicles in traffic accident**

5 **V69.5 Passenger in heavy transport vehicle injured in collision with other and unspecified motor vehicles in traffic accident**

IQ 7 **V69.50X- Passenger in heavy transport vehicle injured in collision with unspecified motor vehicles in traffic accident**

IQ 7 **V69.59X- Passenger in heavy transport vehicle injured in collision with other motor vehicles in traffic accident**

5 **V69.6 Unspecified occupant of heavy transport vehicle injured in collision with other and unspecified motor vehicles in traffic accident**

IQ 7 **V69.60X- Unspecified occupant of heavy transport vehicle injured in collision with unspecified motor vehicles in traffic accident**

Collision NOS involving heavy transport vehicle (traffic)

IQ 7 **V69.69X- Unspecified occupant of heavy transport vehicle injured in collision with other motor vehicles in traffic accident**

5 **V69.8 Occupant (driver) (passenger) of heavy transport vehicle injured in other specified transport accidents**

IQ 7 **V69.81X- Occupant (driver) (passenger) of heavy transport vehicle injured in transport accidents with military vehicle**

IQ 7 **V69.88X- Occupant (driver) (passenger) of heavy transport vehicle injured in other specified transport accidents**

IQ 7 **V69.9XX- Occupant (driver) (passenger) of heavy transport vehicle injured in unspecified traffic accident**

Accident NOS involving heavy transport vehicle

Bus occupant injured in transport accident (V70-V79)

INCLUDES motorcoach
EXCLUDES 1 minibus (V50-V59)

4 **V70 Bus occupant injured in collision with pedestrian or animal**

EXCLUDES 1 bus collision with animal-drawn vehicle or animal being ridden (V76.-)

The appropriate 7th character is to be added to each code from category V70
A initial encounter
D subsequent encounter
S sequela

IQ 7 **V70.0XX- Driver of bus injured in collision with pedestrian or animal in nontraffic accident**

IQ 7 **V70.1XX- Passenger on bus injured in collision with pedestrian or animal in nontraffic accident**

Chapter 20 V00-Y99

!Q V70.2XX- Person on outside of bus injured in collision with pedestrian or animal in nontraffic accident

!Q V70.3XX- Unspecified occupant of bus injured in collision with pedestrian or animal in nontraffic accident

!Q V70.4XX- Person boarding or alighting from bus injured in collision with pedestrian or animal

!Q V70.5XX- Driver of bus injured in collision with pedestrian or animal in traffic accident

!Q V70.6XX- Passenger on bus injured in collision with pedestrian or animal in traffic accident

!Q V70.7XX- Person on outside of bus injured in collision with pedestrian or animal in traffic accident

!Q V70.9XX- Unspecified occupant of bus injured in collision with pedestrian or animal in traffic accident

V71 Bus occupant injured in collision with pedal cycle

The appropriate 7th character is to be added to each code from category V71
A initial encounter
D subsequent encounter
S sequela

!Q V71.0XX- Driver of bus injured in collision with pedal cycle in nontraffic accident

!Q V71.1XX- Passenger on bus injured in collision with pedal cycle in nontraffic accident

!Q V71.2XX- Person on outside of bus injured in collision with pedal cycle in nontraffic accident

!Q V71.3XX- Unspecified occupant of bus injured in collision with pedal cycle in nontraffic accident

!Q V71.4XX- Person boarding or alighting from bus injured in collision with pedal cycle

!Q V71.5XX- Driver of bus injured in collision with pedal cycle in traffic accident

!Q V71.6XX- Passenger on bus injured in collision with pedal cycle in traffic accident

!Q V71.7XX- Person on outside of bus injured in collision with pedal cycle in traffic accident

!Q V71.9XX- Unspecified occupant of bus injured in collision with pedal cycle in traffic accident

V72 Bus occupant injured in collision with two- or three-wheeled motor vehicle

The appropriate 7th character is to be added to each code from category V72
A initial encounter
D subsequent encounter
S sequela

!Q V72.0XX- Driver of bus injured in collision with two- or three-wheeled motor vehicle in nontraffic accident

!Q V72.1XX- Passenger on bus injured in collision with two- or three-wheeled motor vehicle in nontraffic accident

!Q V72.2XX- Person on outside of bus injured in collision with two- or three-wheeled motor vehicle in nontraffic accident

!Q V72.3XX- Unspecified occupant of bus injured in collision with two- or three-wheeled motor vehicle in nontraffic accident

!Q V72.4XX- Person boarding or alighting from bus injured in collision with two- or three-wheeled motor vehicle

!Q V72.5XX- Driver of bus injured in collision with two- or three-wheeled motor vehicle in traffic accident

!Q V72.6XX- Passenger on bus injured in collision with two- or three-wheeled motor vehicle in traffic accident

!Q V72.7XX- Person on outside of bus injured in collision with two- or three-wheeled motor vehicle in traffic accident

!Q V72.9XX- Unspecified occupant of bus injured in collision with two- or three-wheeled motor vehicle in traffic accident

V73 Bus occupant injured in collision with car, pick-up truck or van

The appropriate 7th character is to be added to each code from category V73
A initial encounter
D subsequent encounter
S sequela

!Q V73.0XX- Driver of bus injured in collision with car, pick-up truck or van in nontraffic accident

!Q V73.1XX- Passenger on bus injured in collision with car, pick-up truck or van in nontraffic accident

!Q V73.2XX- Person on outside of bus injured in collision with car, pick-up truck or van in nontraffic accident

!Q V73.3XX- Unspecified occupant of bus injured in collision with car, pick-up truck or van in nontraffic accident

!Q V73.4XX- Person boarding or alighting from bus injured in collision with car, pick-up truck or van

!Q V73.5XX- Driver of bus injured in collision with car, pick-up truck or van in traffic accident

!Q V73.6XX- Passenger on bus injured in collision with car, pick-up truck or van in traffic accident

!Q V73.7XX- Person on outside of bus injured in collision with car, pick-up truck or van in traffic accident

!Q V73.9XX- Unspecified occupant of bus injured in collision with car, pick-up truck or van in traffic accident

V74 Bus occupant injured in collision with heavy transport vehicle or bus

EXCLUDES 1 bus occupant injured in collision with military vehicle (V79.81)

Chapter 20

V00-Y99

The appropriate 7th character is to be added to each code from category V74
A initial encounter
D subsequent encounter
S sequela

IQ 7 **V74.0XX- Driver of bus injured in collision with heavy transport vehicle or bus in nontraffic accident**
IQ 7 **V74.1XX- Passenger on bus injured in collision with heavy transport vehicle or bus in nontraffic accident**
IQ 7 **V74.2XX- Person on outside of bus injured in collision with heavy transport vehicle or bus in nontraffic accident**
IQ 7 **V74.3XX- Unspecified occupant of bus injured in collision with heavy transport vehicle or bus in nontraffic accident**
IQ 7 **V74.4XX- Person boarding or alighting from bus injured in collision with heavy transport vehicle or bus**
IQ 7 **V74.5XX- Driver of bus injured in collision with heavy transport vehicle or bus in traffic accident**
IQ 7 **V74.6XX- Passenger on bus injured in collision with heavy transport vehicle or bus in traffic accident**
IQ 7 **V74.7XX- Person on outside of bus injured in collision with heavy transport vehicle or bus in traffic accident**
IQ 7 **V74.9XX- Unspecified occupant of bus injured in collision with heavy transport vehicle or bus in traffic accident**

4 **V75 Bus occupant injured in collision with railway train or railway vehicle**

The appropriate 7th character is to be added to each code from category V75
A initial encounter
D subsequent encounter
S sequela

IQ 7 **V75.0XX- Driver of bus injured in collision with railway train or railway vehicle in nontraffic accident**
IQ 7 **V75.1XX- Passenger on bus injured in collision with railway train or railway vehicle in nontraffic accident**
IQ 7 **V75.2XX- Person on outside of bus injured in collision with railway train or railway vehicle in nontraffic accident**
IQ 7 **V75.3XX- Unspecified occupant of bus injured in collision with railway train or railway vehicle in nontraffic accident**
IQ 7 **V75.4XX- Person boarding or alighting from bus injured in collision with railway train or railway vehicle**
IQ 7 **V75.5XX- Driver of bus injured in collision with railway train or railway vehicle in traffic accident**
IQ 7 **V75.6XX- Passenger on bus injured in collision with railway train or railway vehicle in traffic accident**
IQ 7 **V75.7XX- Person on outside of bus injured in collision with railway train or railway vehicle in traffic accident**
IQ 7 **V75.9XX- Unspecified occupant of bus injured in collision with railway train or railway vehicle in traffic accident**

4 **V76 Bus occupant injured in collision with other nonmotor vehicle**

INCLUDES collision with animal-drawn vehicle, animal being ridden, streetcar

The appropriate 7th character is to be added to each code from category V76
A initial encounter
D subsequent encounter
S sequela

IQ 7 **V76.0XX- Driver of bus injured in collision with other nonmotor vehicle in nontraffic accident**
IQ 7 **V76.1XX- Passenger on bus injured in collision with other nonmotor vehicle in nontraffic accident**
IQ 7 **V76.2XX- Person on outside of bus injured in collision with other nonmotor vehicle in nontraffic accident**
IQ 7 **V76.3XX- Unspecified occupant of bus injured in collision with other nonmotor vehicle in nontraffic accident**
IQ 7 **V76.4XX- Person boarding or alighting from bus injured in collision with other nonmotor vehicle**
IQ 7 **V76.5XX- Driver of bus injured in collision with other nonmotor vehicle in traffic accident**
IQ 7 **V76.6XX- Passenger on bus injured in collision with other nonmotor vehicle in traffic accident**
IQ 7 **V76.7XX- Person on outside of bus injured in collision with other nonmotor vehicle in traffic accident**
IQ 7 **V76.9XX- Unspecified occupant of bus injured in collision with other nonmotor vehicle in traffic accident**

4 **V77 Bus occupant injured in collision with fixed or stationary object**

The appropriate 7th character is to be added to each code from category V77
A initial encounter
D subsequent encounter
S sequela

IQ 7 **V77.0XX- Driver of bus injured in collision with fixed or stationary object in nontraffic accident**
IQ 7 **V77.1XX- Passenger on bus injured in collision with fixed or stationary object in nontraffic accident**
IQ 7 **V77.2XX- Person on outside of bus injured in collision with fixed or stationary object in nontraffic accident**
IQ 7 **V77.3XX- Unspecified occupant of bus injured in collision with fixed or stationary object in nontraffic accident**

V77.4XX- Person boarding or alighting from bus injured in collision with fixed or stationary object

V77.5XX- Driver of bus injured in collision with fixed or stationary object in traffic accident

V77.6XX- Passenger on bus injured in collision with fixed or stationary object in traffic accident

V77.7XX- Person on outside of bus injured in collision with fixed or stationary object in traffic accident

V77.9XX- Unspecified occupant of bus injured in collision with fixed or stationary object in traffic accident

V78 Bus occupant injured in noncollision transport accident

INCLUDES overturning bus NOS
overturning bus without collision

The appropriate 7th character is to be added to each code from category V78
A initial encounter
D subsequent encounter
S sequela

V78.0XX- Driver of bus injured in noncollision transport accident in nontraffic accident

V78.1XX- Passenger on bus injured in noncollision transport accident in nontraffic accident

V78.2XX- Person on outside of bus injured in noncollision transport accident in nontraffic accident

V78.3XX- Unspecified occupant of bus injured in noncollision transport accident in nontraffic accident

V78.4XX- Person boarding or alighting from bus injured in noncollision transport accident

V78.5XX- Driver of bus injured in noncollision transport accident in traffic accident

V78.6XX- Passenger on bus injured in noncollision transport accident in traffic accident

V78.7XX- Person on outside of bus injured in noncollision transport accident in traffic accident

V78.9XX- Unspecified occupant of bus injured in noncollision transport accident in traffic accident

V79 Bus occupant injured in other and unspecified transport accidents

The appropriate 7th character is to be added to each code from category V79
A initial encounter
D subsequent encounter
S sequela

V79.0 Driver of bus injured in collision with other and unspecified motor vehicles in nontraffic accident

V79.00X- Driver of bus injured in collision with unspecified motor vehicles in nontraffic accident

V79.09X- Driver of bus injured in collision with other motor vehicles in nontraffic accident

V79.1 Passenger on bus injured in collision with other and unspecified motor vehicles in nontraffic accident

V79.10X- Passenger on bus injured in collision with unspecified motor vehicles in nontraffic accident

V79.19X- Passenger on bus injured in collision with other motor vehicles in nontraffic accident

V79.2 Unspecified bus occupant injured in collision with other and unspecified motor vehicles in nontraffic accident

V79.20X- Unspecified bus occupant injured in collision with unspecified motor vehicles in nontraffic accident
Bus collision NOS, nontraffic

V79.29X- Unspecified bus occupant injured in collision with other motor vehicles in nontraffic accident

V79.3XX- Bus occupant (driver) (passenger) injured in unspecified nontraffic accident
Bus accident NOS, nontraffic
Bus occupant injured in nontraffic accident NOS

V79.4 Driver of bus injured in collision with other and unspecified motor vehicles in traffic accident

V79.40X- Driver of bus injured in collision with unspecified motor vehicles in traffic accident

V79.49X- Driver of bus injured in collision with other motor vehicles in traffic accident

V79.5 Passenger on bus injured in collision with other and unspecified motor vehicles in traffic accident

V79.50X- Passenger on bus injured in collision with unspecified motor vehicles in traffic accident

V79.59X- Passenger on bus injured in collision with other motor vehicles in traffic accident

V79.6 Unspecified bus occupant injured in collision with other and unspecified motor vehicles in traffic accident

V79.60X- Unspecified bus occupant injured in collision with unspecified motor vehicles in traffic accident
Bus collision NOS (traffic)

V79.69X- Unspecified bus occupant injured in collision with other motor vehicles in traffic accident

V79.8 Bus occupant (driver) (passenger) injured in other specified transport accidents

V79.81X- Bus occupant (driver) (passenger) injured in transport accidents with military vehicle

V79.88X- Bus occupant (driver) (passenger) injured in other specified transport accidents

IQ 7 **V79.9XX- Bus occupant (driver) (passenger) injured in unspecified traffic accident**
Bus accident NOS

Other land transport accidents (V80-V89)

4 **V80 Animal-rider or occupant of animal-drawn vehicle injured in transport accident**

The appropriate 7th character is to be added to each code from category V80
A initial encounter
D subsequent encounter
S sequela

5 **V80.0 Animal-rider or occupant of animal drawn vehicle injured by fall from or being thrown from animal or animal-drawn vehicle in noncollision accident**

6 **V80.01 Animal-rider injured by fall from or being thrown from animal in noncollision accident**

IQ 7 **V80.010- Animal-rider injured by fall from or being thrown from horse in noncollision accident**

IQ 7 **V80.018- Animal-rider injured by fall from or being thrown from other animal in noncollision accident**

IQ 7 **V80.02X- Occupant of animal-drawn vehicle injured by fall from or being thrown from animal-drawn vehicle in noncollision accident**
Overturning animal-drawn vehicle NOS
Overturning animal-drawn vehicle without collision

5 **V80.1 Animal-rider or occupant of animal-drawn vehicle injured in collision with pedestrian or animal**
EXCLUDES 1 animal-rider or animal-drawn vehicle collision with animal-drawn vehicle or animal being ridden (V80.7)

IQ 7 **V80.11X- Animal-rider injured in collision with pedestrian or animal**

IQ 7 **V80.12X- Occupant of animal-drawn vehicle injured in collision with pedestrian or animal**

5 **V80.2 Animal-rider or occupant of animal-drawn vehicle injured in collision with pedal cycle**

IQ 7 **V80.21X- Animal-rider injured in collision with pedal cycle**

IQ 7 **V80.22X- Occupant of animal-drawn vehicle injured in collision with pedal cycle**

5 **V80.3 Animal-rider or occupant of animal-drawn vehicle injured in collision with two- or three-wheeled motor vehicle**

IQ 7 **V80.31X- Animal-rider injured in collision with two- or three-wheeled motor vehicle**

IQ 7 **V80.32X- Occupant of animal-drawn vehicle injured in collision with two- or three-wheeled motor vehicle**

5 **V80.4 Animal-rider or occupant of animal-drawn vehicle injured in collision with car, pick-up truck, van, heavy transport vehicle or bus**
EXCLUDES 1 animal-rider injured in collision with military vehicle (V80.910)
occupant of animal-drawn vehicle injured in collision with military vehicle (V80.920)

IQ 7 **V80.41X- Animal-rider injured in collision with car, pick-up truck, van, heavy transport vehicle or bus**

IQ 7 **V80.42X- Occupant of animal-drawn vehicle injured in collision with car, pick-up truck, van, heavy transport vehicle or bus**

5 **V80.5 Animal-rider or occupant of animal-drawn vehicle injured in collision with other specified motor vehicle**

IQ 7 **V80.51X- Animal-rider injured in collision with other specified motor vehicle**

IQ 7 **V80.52X- Occupant of animal-drawn vehicle injured in collision with other specified motor vehicle**

5 **V80.6 Animal-rider or occupant of animal-drawn vehicle injured in collision with railway train or railway vehicle**

IQ 7 **V80.61X- Animal-rider injured in collision with railway train or railway vehicle**

IQ 7 **V80.62X- Occupant of animal-drawn vehicle injured in collision with railway train or railway vehicle**

5 **V80.7 Animal-rider or occupant of animal-drawn vehicle injured in collision with other nonmotor vehicles**

6 **V80.71 Animal-rider or occupant of animal-drawn vehicle injured in collision with animal being ridden**

IQ 7 **V80.710- Animal-rider injured in collision with other animal being ridden**

IQ 7 **V80.711- Occupant of animal-drawn vehicle injured in collision with animal being ridden**

6 **V80.72 Animal-rider or occupant of animal-drawn vehicle injured in collision with other animal-drawn vehicle**

IQ 7 **V80.720- Animal-rider injured in collision with animal-drawn vehicle**

IQ 7 **V80.721- Occupant of animal-drawn vehicle injured in collision with other animal-drawn vehicle**

6 **V80.73 Animal-rider or occupant of animal-drawn vehicle injured in collision with streetcar**

IQ 7 **V80.730- Animal-rider injured in collision with streetcar**

IQ 7 **V80.731- Occupant of animal-drawn vehicle injured in collision with streetcar**

6 **V80.79 Animal-rider or occupant of animal-drawn vehicle injured in collision with other nonmotor vehicles**

IQ 7 **V80.790- Animal-rider injured in collision with other nonmotor vehicles**

Chapter 20

V00-Y99

!Q 7 V80.791- Occupant of animal-drawn vehicle injured in collision with other nonmotor vehicles

5 V80.8 Animal-rider or occupant of animal-drawn vehicle injured in collision with fixed or stationary object

!Q ✓ V80.81X- Animal-rider injured in collision with fixed or stationary object

!Q ✓ V80.82X- Occupant of animal-drawn vehicle injured in collision with fixed or stationary object

5 V80.9 Animal-rider or occupant of animal-drawn vehicle injured in other and unspecified transport accidents

6 V80.91 Animal-rider injured in other and unspecified transport accidents

!Q 7 V80.910- Animal-rider injured in transport accident with military vehicle

!Q 7 V80.918- Animal-rider injured in other transport accident

!Q 7 V80.919- Animal-rider injured in unspecified transport accident

Animal rider accident NOS

6 V80.92 Occupant of animal-drawn vehicle injured in other and unspecified transport accidents

!Q 7 V80.920- Occupant of animal-drawn vehicle injured in transport accident with military vehicle

!Q 7 V80.928- Occupant of animal-drawn vehicle injured in other transport accident

!Q 7 V80.929- Occupant of animal-drawn vehicle injured in unspecified transport accident

Animal-drawn vehicle accident NOS

4 V81 Occupant of railway train or railway vehicle injured in transport accident

INCLUDES derailment of railway train or railway vehicle
person on outside of train

EXCLUDES 1 streetcar (V82.-)

The appropriate 7th character is to be added to each code from category V81
A   initial encounter
D   subsequent encounter
S   sequela

!Q ✓ V81.0XX- Occupant of railway train or railway vehicle injured in collision with motor vehicle in nontraffic accident

EXCLUDES 1 Occupant of railway train or railway vehicle injured due to collision with military vehicle (V81.83)

!Q ✓ V81.1XX- Occupant of railway train or railway vehicle injured in collision with motor vehicle in traffic accident

EXCLUDES 1 Occupant of railway train or railway vehicle injured due to collision with military vehicle (V81.83)

!Q ✓ V81.2XX- Occupant of railway train or railway vehicle injured in collision with or hit by rolling stock

!Q ✓ V81.3XX- Occupant of railway train or railway vehicle injured in collision with other object

Railway collision NOS

!Q ✓ V81.4XX- Person injured while boarding or alighting from railway train or railway vehicle

!Q ✓ V81.5XX- Occupant of railway train or railway vehicle injured by fall in railway train or railway vehicle

!Q ✓ V81.6XX- Occupant of railway train or railway vehicle injured by fall from railway train or railway vehicle

!Q ✓ V81.7XX- Occupant of railway train or railway vehicle injured in derailment without antecedent collision

5 V81.8 Occupant of railway train or railway vehicle injured in other specified railway accidents

!Q ✓ V81.81X- Occupant of railway train or railway vehicle injured due to explosion or fire on train

!Q ✓ V81.82X- Occupant of railway train or railway vehicle injured due to object falling onto train

Occupant of railway train or railway vehicle injured due to falling earth onto train

Occupant of railway train or railway vehicle injured due to falling rocks onto train

Occupant of railway train or railway vehicle injured due to falling snow onto train

Occupant of railway train or railway vehicle injured due to falling trees onto train

!Q ✓ V81.83X- Occupant of railway train or railway vehicle injured due to collision with military vehicle

!Q ✓ V81.89X- Occupant of railway train or railway vehicle injured due to other specified railway accident

!Q ✓ V81.9XX- Occupant of railway train or railway vehicle injured in unspecified railway accident

Railway accident NOS

4 V82 Occupant of powered streetcar injured in transport accident

INCLUDES interurban electric car
person on outside of streetcar
tram (car)
trolley (car)

EXCLUDES 1 bus (V70-V79)
motorcoach (V70-V79)
nonpowered streetcar (V76.-)
train (V81.-)

The appropriate 7th character is to be added to each code from category V82
A   initial encounter
D   subsequent encounter
S   sequela

4 4th digit required   5 5th digit required   6 6th digit required   7 7th digit required   ✓ 7th digit placeholder   + Additional code   Laterality

!Q 7 **V82.0XX- Occupant of streetcar injured in collision with motor vehicle in nontraffic accident**

!Q 7 **V82.1XX- Occupant of streetcar injured in collision with motor vehicle in traffic accident**

!Q 7 **V82.2XX- Occupant of streetcar injured in collision with or hit by rolling stock**

!Q 7 **V82.3XX- Occupant of streetcar injured in collision with other object**

EXCLUDES 1 collision with animal-drawn vehicle or animal being ridden (V82.8)

!Q 7 **V82.4XX- Person injured while boarding or alighting from streetcar**

!Q 7 **V82.5XX- Occupant of streetcar injured by fall in streetcar**

EXCLUDES 1 fall in streetcar:
while boarding or alighting (V82.4)
with antecedent collision (V82.0-V82.3)

!Q 7 **V82.6XX- Occupant of streetcar injured by fall from streetcar**

EXCLUDES 1 fall from streetcar:
while boarding or alighting (V82.4)
with antecedent collision (V82.0-V82.3)

!Q 7 **V82.7XX- Occupant of streetcar injured in derailment without antecedent collision**

EXCLUDES 1 occupant of streetcar injured in derailment with antecedent collision (V82.0-V82.3)

!Q 7 **V82.8XX- Occupant of streetcar injured in other specified transport accidents**

Streetcar collision with military vehicle
Streetcar collision with train or nonmotor vehicles

!Q 7 **V82.9XX- Occupant of streetcar injured in unspecified traffic accident**

Streetcar accident NOS

4 **V83 Occupant of special vehicle mainly used on industrial premises injured in transport accident**

INCLUDES battery-powered airport passenger vehicle
battery-powered truck (baggage) (mail)
coal-car in mine
forklift (truck)
logging car
self-propelled industrial truck
station baggage truck (powered)
tram, truck, or tub (powered) in mine or quarry

EXCLUDES 1 special construction vehicles (V85.-)
special industrial vehicle in stationary use or maintenance (W31.-)

The appropriate 7th character is to be added to each code from category V83
A initial encounter
D subsequent encounter
S sequela

!Q 7 **V83.0XX- Driver of special industrial vehicle injured in traffic accident**

!Q 7 **V83.1XX- Passenger of special industrial vehicle injured in traffic accident**

!Q 7 **V83.2XX- Person on outside of special industrial vehicle injured in traffic accident**

!Q 7 **V83.3XX- Unspecified occupant of special industrial vehicle injured in traffic accident**

!Q 7 **V83.4XX- Person injured while boarding or alighting from special industrial vehicle**

!Q 7 **V83.5XX- Driver of special industrial vehicle injured in nontraffic accident**

!Q 7 **V83.6XX- Passenger of special industrial vehicle injured in nontraffic accident**

!Q 7 **V83.7XX- Person on outside of special industrial vehicle injured in nontraffic accident**

!Q 7 **V83.9XX- Unspecified occupant of special industrial vehicle injured in nontraffic accident**

Special-industrial-vehicle accident NOS

4 **V84 Occupant of special vehicle mainly used in agriculture injured in transport accident**

INCLUDES self-propelled farm machinery
tractor (and trailer)

EXCLUDES 1 animal-powered farm machinery accident (W30.8-)
contact with combine harvester (W30.0)
special agricultural vehicle in stationary use or maintenance (W30.-)

The appropriate 7th character is to be added to each code from category V84
A initial encounter
D subsequent encounter
S sequela

!Q 7 **V84.0XX- Driver of special agricultural vehicle injured in traffic accident**

!Q 7 **V84.1XX- Passenger of special agricultural vehicle injured in traffic accident**

!Q 7 **V84.2XX- Person on outside of special agricultural vehicle injured in traffic accident**

!Q 7 **V84.3XX- Unspecified occupant of special agricultural vehicle injured in traffic accident**

!Q 7 **V84.4XX- Person injured while boarding or alighting from special agricultural vehicle**

!Q 7 **V84.5XX- Driver of special agricultural vehicle injured in nontraffic accident**

!Q 7 **V84.6XX- Passenger of special agricultural vehicle injured in nontraffic accident**

🆀 ☑ V84.7XX- Person on outside of special agricultural vehicle injured in nontraffic accident

🆀 ☑ V84.9XX- Unspecified occupant of special agricultural vehicle injured in nontraffic accident

Special-agricultural vehicle accident NOS

④ V85 Occupant of special construction vehicle injured in transport accident

> INCLUDES
> bulldozer
> digger
> dump truck
> earth-leveller
> mechanical shovel
> road-roller
>
> EXCLUDES 1
> special industrial vehicle (V83.-)
> special construction vehicle in stationary use or maintenance (W31.-)

The appropriate 7th character is to be added to each code from category V85
A   initial encounter
D   subsequent encounter
S   sequela

🆀 ☑ V85.0XX- Driver of special construction vehicle injured in traffic accident

🆀 ☑ V85.1XX- Passenger of special construction vehicle injured in traffic accident

🆀 ☑ V85.2XX- Person on outside of special construction vehicle injured in traffic accident

🆀 ☑ V85.3XX- Unspecified occupant of special construction vehicle injured in traffic accident

🆀 ☑ V85.4XX- Person injured while boarding or alighting from special construction vehicle

🆀 ☑ V85.5XX- Driver of special construction vehicle injured in nontraffic accident

🆀 ☑ V85.6XX- Passenger of special construction vehicle injured in nontraffic accident

🆀 ☑ V85.7XX- Person on outside of special construction vehicle injured in nontraffic accident

🆀 ☑ V85.9XX- Unspecified occupant of special construction vehicle injured in nontraffic accident

Special-construction-vehicle accident NOS

④ V86 Occupant of special all-terrain or other off-road motor vehicle, injured in transport accident

> EXCLUDES 1
> special all-terrain vehicle in stationary use or maintenance (W31.-)
> sport-utility vehicle (V50-V59)
> three-wheeled motor vehicle designed for on-road use (V30-V39)

The appropriate 7th character is to be added to each code from category V86
A   initial encounter
D   subsequent encounter
S   sequela

⑤ V86.0 Driver of special all-terrain or other off-road motor vehicle injured in traffic accident

🆀 ☑ V86.01X- Driver of ambulance or fire engine injured in traffic accident

🆀 ☑ V86.02X- Driver of snowmobile injured in traffic accident

🆀 ☑ V86.03X- Driver of dune buggy injured in traffic accident

🆀 ☑ V86.04X- Driver of military vehicle injured in traffic accident

🆀 ☑ V86.05X- Driver of 3- or 4- wheeled all-terrain vehicle (ATV) injured in traffic accident

🆀 ☑ V86.06X- Driver of dirt bike or motor/cross bike injured in traffic accident

🆀 ☑ V86.09X- Driver of other special all-terrain or other off-road motor vehicle injured in traffic accident

Driver of go cart injured in traffic accident

Driver of golf cart injured in traffic accident

⑤ V86.1 Passenger of special all-terrain or other off-road motor vehicle injured in traffic accident

🆀 ☑ V86.11X- Passenger of ambulance or fire engine injured in traffic accident

🆀 ☑ V86.12X- Passenger of snowmobile injured in traffic accident

🆀 ☑ V86.13X- Passenger of dune buggy injured in traffic accident

🆀 ☑ V86.14X- Passenger of military vehicle injured in traffic accident

🆀 ☑ V86.15X- Passenger of 3- or 4- wheeled all-terrain vehicle (ATV) injured in traffic accident

🆀 ☑ V86.16X- Passenger of dirt bike or motor/cross bike injured in traffic accident

🆀 ☑ V86.19X- Passenger of other special all-terrain or other off-road motor vehicle injured in traffic accident

Passenger of go cart injured in traffic accident

Passenger of golf cart injured in traffic accident

⑤ V86.2 Person on outside of special all-terrain or other off-road motor vehicle injured in traffic accident

🆀 ☑ V86.21X- Person on outside of ambulance or fire engine injured in traffic accident

🆀 ☑ V86.22X- Person on outside of snowmobile injured in traffic accident

🆀 ☑ V86.23X- Person on outside of dune buggy injured in traffic accident

🆀 ☑ V86.24X- Person on outside of military vehicle injured in traffic accident

🆀 ☑ V86.25X- Person on outside of 3- or 4- wheeled all-terrain vehicle (ATV) injured in traffic accident

Chapter 20

V00-Y99

④ 4th digit required   ⑤ 5th digit required   ⑥ 6th digit required   ⑦ 7th digit required   ☑ 7th digit placeholder   ✚ Additional code   ⊟ Laterality

IQ ☑ **V86.26X-** Person on outside of dirt bike or motor/cross bike injured in traffic accident

IQ ☑ **V86.29X-** Person on outside of other special all-terrain or other off-road motor vehicle injured in traffic accident

Person on outside of go cart in traffic accident

Person on outside of golf cart injured in traffic accident

☐ **V86.3** Unspecified occupant of special all-terrain or other off-road motor vehicle injured in traffic accident

IQ ☑ **V86.31X-** Unspecified occupant of ambulance or fire engine injured in traffic accident

IQ ☑ **V86.32X-** Unspecified occupant of snowmobile injured in traffic accident

IQ ☑ **V86.33X-** Unspecified occupant of dune buggy injured in traffic accident

IQ ☑ **V86.34X-** Unspecified occupant of military vehicle injured in traffic accident

IQ ☑ **V86.35X-** Unspecified occupant of 3- or 4- wheeled all-terrain vehicle (ATV) injured in traffic accident

IQ ☑ **V86.36X-** Unspecified occupant of dirt bike or motor/cross bike injured in traffic accident

IQ ☑ **V86.39X-** Unspecified occupant of other special all-terrain or other off-road motor vehicle injured in traffic accident

Unspecified occupant of go cart injured in traffic accident

Unspecified occupant of golf cart injured in traffic accident

☐ **V86.4** Person injured while boarding or alighting from special all-terrain or other off-road motor vehicle

IQ ☑ **V86.41X-** Person injured while boarding or alighting from ambulance or fire engine

IQ ☑ **V86.42X-** Person injured while boarding or alighting from snowmobile

IQ ☑ **V86.43X-** Person injured while boarding or alighting from dune buggy

IQ ☑ **V86.44X-** Person injured while boarding or alighting from military vehicle

IQ ☑ **V86.45X-** Person injured while boarding or alighting from a 3- or 4- wheeled all-terrain vehicle (ATV)

IQ ☑ **V86.46X-** Person injured while boarding or alighting from a dirt bike or motor/cross bike

IQ ☑ **V86.49X-** Person injured while boarding or alighting from other special all-terrain or other off-road motor vehicle

Person injured while boarding or alighting from go cart

Person injured while boarding or alighting from golf cart

☐ **V86.5** Driver of special all-terrain or other off-road motor vehicle injured in nontraffic accident

IQ ☑ **V86.51X-** Driver of ambulance or fire engine injured in nontraffic accident

IQ ☑ **V86.52X-** Driver of snowmobile injured in nontraffic accident

IQ ☑ **V86.53X-** Driver of dune buggy injured in nontraffic accident

IQ ☑ **V86.54X-** Driver of military vehicle injured in nontraffic accident

IQ ☑ **V86.55X-** Driver of 3- or 4- wheeled all-terrain vehicle (ATV) injured in nontraffic accident

IQ ☑ **V86.56X-** Driver of dirt bike or motor/cross bike injured in nontraffic accident

IQ ☑ **V86.59X-** Driver of other special all-terrain or other off-road motor vehicle injured in nontraffic accident

Driver of go cart injured in nontraffic accident

Driver of golf cart injured in nontraffic accident

☐ **V86.6** Passenger of special all-terrain or other off-road motor vehicle injured in nontraffic accident

IQ ☑ **V86.61X-** Passenger of ambulance or fire engine injured in nontraffic accident

IQ ☑ **V86.62X-** Passenger of snowmobile injured in nontraffic accident

IQ ☑ **V86.63X-** Passenger of dune buggy injured in nontraffic accident

IQ ☑ **V86.64X-** Passenger of military vehicle injured in nontraffic accident

IQ ☑ **V86.65X-** Passenger of 3- or 4- wheeled all-terrain vehicle (ATV) injured in nontraffic accident

IQ ☑ **V86.66X-** Passenger of dirt bike or motor/cross bike injured in nontraffic accident

IQ ☑ **V86.69X-** Passenger of other special all-terrain or other off-road motor vehicle injured in nontraffic accident

Passenger of go cart injured in nontraffic accident

Passenger of golf cart injured in nontraffic accident

☐ **V86.7** Person on outside of special all-terrain or other off-road motor vehicle injured in nontraffic accident

IQ ☑ **V86.71X-** Person on outside of ambulance or fire engine injured in nontraffic accident

IQ ☑ **V86.72X-** Person on outside of snowmobile injured in nontraffic accident

IQ ☑ **V86.73X-** Person on outside of dune buggy injured in nontraffic accident

IQ ☑ **V86.74X-** Person on outside of military vehicle injured in nontraffic accident

IQ ☑ **V86.75X-** Person on outside of 3- or 4- wheeled all-terrain vehicle (ATV) injured in nontraffic accident

IQ ☑ **V86.76X-** Person on outside of dirt bike or motor/cross bike injured in nontraffic accident

IQ ☑ **V86.79X-** Person on outside of other special all-terrain or other off-road motor vehicles injured in nontraffic accident

Chapter 20

V00-Y99

★ New ▲ Revised Px Primary **SP** PDGM Px **SL** Low CoM **SH** High CoM **IQ** Quest. Encounter ⊞ Hospice non-cancer Dx Unspecified **M** *Manifestation*

Person on outside of go cart injured in nontraffic accident
Person on outside of golf cart injured in nontraffic accident

5 **V86.9 Unspecified occupant of special all-terrain or other off-road motor vehicle injured in nontraffic accident**

!Q 7 **V86.91X- Unspecified occupant of ambulance or fire engine injured in nontraffic accident**

!Q 7 **V86.92X- Unspecified occupant of snowmobile injured in nontraffic accident**

!Q 7 **V86.93X- Unspecified occupant of dune buggy injured in nontraffic accident**

!Q 7 **V86.94X- Unspecified occupant of military vehicle injured in nontraffic accident**

!Q 7 **V86.95X- Unspecified occupant of 3- or 4-wheeled all-terrain vehicle (ATV) injured in nontraffic accident**

!Q 7 **V86.96X- Unspecified occupant of dirt bike or motor/cross bike injured in nontraffic accident**

!Q 7 **V86.99X- Unspecified occupant of other special all-terrain or other off-road motor vehicle injured in nontraffic accident**

Off-road motor-vehicle accident NOS
Other motor-vehicle accident NOS
Unspecified occupant of go cart injured in nontraffic accident
Unspecified occupant of golf cart injured in nontraffic accident

4 **V87 Traffic accident of specified type but victim's mode of transport unknown**

EXCLUDES 1 collision involving:
pedal cycle (V10-V19)
pedestrian (V01-V09)

The appropriate 7th character is to be added to each code from category V87
A initial encounter
D subsequent encounter
S sequela

!Q 7 **V87.0XX- Person injured in collision between car and two- or three-wheeled powered vehicle (traffic)**

!Q 7 **V87.1XX- Person injured in collision between other motor vehicle and two- or three-wheeled motor vehicle (traffic)**

!Q 7 **V87.2XX- Person injured in collision between car and pick-up truck or van (traffic)**

!Q 7 **V87.3XX- Person injured in collision between car and bus (traffic)**

!Q 7 **V87.4XX- Person injured in collision between car and heavy transport vehicle (traffic)**

!Q 7 **V87.5XX- Person injured in collision between heavy transport vehicle and bus (traffic)**

!Q 7 **V87.6XX- Person injured in collision between railway train or railway vehicle and car (traffic)**

!Q 7 **V87.7XX- Person injured in collision between other specified motor vehicles (traffic)**

!Q 7 **V87.8XX- Person injured in other specified noncollision transport accidents involving motor vehicle (traffic)**

!Q 7 **V87.9XX- Person injured in other specified (collision)(noncollision) transport accidents involving nonmotor vehicle (traffic)**

4 **V88 Nontraffic accident of specified type but victim's mode of transport unknown**

EXCLUDES 1 collision involving:
pedal cycle (V10-V19)
pedestrian (V01-V09)

The appropriate 7th character is to be added to each code from category V88
A initial encounter
D subsequent encounter
S sequela

!Q 7 **V88.0XX- Person injured in collision between car and two- or three-wheeled motor vehicle, nontraffic**

!Q 7 **V88.1XX- Person injured in collision between other motor vehicle and two- or three-wheeled motor vehicle, nontraffic**

!Q 7 **V88.2XX- Person injured in collision between car and pick-up truck or van, nontraffic**

!Q 7 **V88.3XX- Person injured in collision between car and bus, nontraffic**

!Q 7 **V88.4XX- Person injured in collision between car and heavy transport vehicle, nontraffic**

!Q 7 **V88.5XX- Person injured in collision between heavy transport vehicle and bus, nontraffic**

!Q 7 **V88.6XX- Person injured in collision between railway train or railway vehicle and car, nontraffic**

!Q 7 **V88.7XX- Person injured in collision between other specified motor vehicle, nontraffic**

!Q 7 **V88.8XX- Person injured in other specified noncollision transport accidents involving motor vehicle, nontraffic**

!Q 7 **V88.9XX- Person injured in other specified (collision)(noncollision) transport accidents involving nonmotor vehicle, nontraffic**

4 **V89 Motor- or nonmotor-vehicle accident, type of vehicle unspecified**

The appropriate 7th character is to be added to each code from category V89
A initial encounter
D subsequent encounter
S sequela

!Q 7 **V89.0XX- Person injured in unspecified motor-vehicle accident, nontraffic**

Motor-vehicle accident NOS, nontraffic

Chapter 20
V00-Y99

!Q ✓ **V89.1XX-** **Person injured in unspecified nonmotor-vehicle accident, nontraffic**

Nonmotor-vehicle accident NOS (nontraffic)

!Q ✓ **V89.2XX-** **Person injured in unspecified motor-vehicle accident, traffic**

Motor-vehicle accident [MVA] NOS
Road (traffic) accident [RTA] NOS

!Q ✓ **V89.3XX-** **Person injured in unspecified nonmotor-vehicle accident, traffic**

Nonmotor-vehicle traffic accident NOS

!Q ✓ **V89.9XX-** **Person injured in unspecified vehicle accident**

Collision NOS

Water transport accidents (V90-V94)

④ **V90** **Drowning and submersion due to accident to watercraft**

EXCLUDES 1 civilian water transport accident involving military watercraft (V94.81-)
fall into water not from watercraft (W16.-)
military watercraft accident in military or war operations (Y36.0-, Y37.0-)
water-transport-related drowning or submersion without accident to watercraft (V92.-)

The appropriate 7th character is to be added to each code from category V90
A   initial encounter
D   subsequent encounter
S   sequela

⑤ **V90.0** **Drowning and submersion due to watercraft overturning**

!Q ✓ **V90.00X-** **Drowning and submersion due to merchant ship overturning**

!Q ✓ **V90.01X-** **Drowning and submersion due to passenger ship overturning**

Drowning and submersion due to Ferry-boat overturning
Drowning and submersion due to Liner overturning

!Q ✓ **V90.02X-** **Drowning and submersion due to fishing boat overturning**

!Q ✓ **V90.03X-** **Drowning and submersion due to other powered watercraft overturning**

Drowning and submersion due to Hovercraft (on open water) overturning
Drowning and submersion due to Jet ski overturning

!Q ✓ **V90.04X-** **Drowning and submersion due to sailboat overturning**

!Q ✓ **V90.05X-** **Drowning and submersion due to canoe or kayak overturning**

!Q ✓ **V90.06X-** **Drowning and submersion due to (nonpowered) inflatable craft overturning**

!Q ✓ **V90.08X-** **Drowning and submersion due to other unpowered watercraft overturning**

Drowning and submersion due to windsurfer overturning

!Q ✓ **V90.09X-** **Drowning and submersion due to unspecified watercraft overturning**

Drowning and submersion due to boat NOS overturning
Drowning and submersion due to ship NOS overturning
Drowning and submersion due to watercraft NOS overturning

⑤ **V90.1** **Drowning and submersion due to watercraft sinking**

!Q ✓ **V90.10X-** **Drowning and submersion due to merchant ship sinking**

!Q ✓ **V90.11X-** **Drowning and submersion due to passenger ship sinking**

Drowning and submersion due to Ferry-boat sinking
Drowning and submersion due to Liner sinking

!Q ✓ **V90.12X-** **Drowning and submersion due to fishing boat sinking**

!Q ✓ **V90.13X-** **Drowning and submersion due to other powered watercraft sinking**

Drowning and submersion due to Hovercraft (on open water) sinking
Drowning and submersion due to Jet ski sinking

!Q ✓ **V90.14X-** **Drowning and submersion due to sailboat sinking**

!Q ✓ **V90.15X-** **Drowning and submersion due to canoe or kayak sinking**

!Q ✓ **V90.16X-** **Drowning and submersion due to (nonpowered) inflatable craft sinking**

!Q ✓ **V90.18X-** **Drowning and submersion due to other unpowered watercraft sinking**

!Q ✓ **V90.19X-** **Drowning and submersion due to unspecified watercraft sinking**

Drowning and submersion due to boat NOS sinking
Drowning and submersion due to ship NOS sinking
Drowning and submersion due to watercraft NOS sinking

⑤ **V90.2** **Drowning and submersion due to falling or jumping from burning watercraft**

!Q ✓ **V90.20X-** **Drowning and submersion due to falling or jumping from burning merchant ship**

!Q ✓ **V90.21X-** **Drowning and submersion due to falling or jumping from burning passenger ship**

Drowning and submersion due to falling or jumping from burning Ferry-boat
Drowning and submersion due to falling or jumping from burning Liner

!Q ✓ **V90.22X-** **Drowning and submersion due to falling or jumping from burning fishing boat**

★ New ▲ Revised Px Primary SP PDGM Px SL Low CoM SH High CoM !Q Quest. Encounter H Hospice non-cancer Dx Unspecified M *Manifestation*

IQ 7 **V90.23X- Drowning and submersion due to falling or jumping from other burning powered watercraft**
Drowning and submersion due to falling and jumping from burning Hovercraft (on open water)
Drowning and submersion due to falling and jumping from burning Jet ski

IQ 7 **V90.24X- Drowning and submersion due to falling or jumping from burning sailboat**

IQ 7 **V90.25X- Drowning and submersion due to falling or jumping from burning canoe or kayak**

IQ 7 **V90.26X- Drowning and submersion due to falling or jumping from burning (nonpowered) inflatable craft**

IQ 7 **V90.27X- Drowning and submersion due to falling or jumping from burning water-skis**

IQ 7 **V90.28X- Drowning and submersion due to falling or jumping from other burning unpowered watercraft**
Drowning and submersion due to falling and jumping from burning surf-board
Drowning and submersion due to falling and jumping from burning windsurfer

IQ 7 **V90.29X- Drowning and submersion due to falling or jumping from unspecified burning watercraft**
Drowning and submersion due to falling or jumping from burning boat NOS
Drowning and submersion due to falling or jumping from burning ship NOS
Drowning and submersion due to falling or jumping from burning watercraft NOS

5 **V90.3 Drowning and submersion due to falling or jumping from crushed watercraft**

IQ 7 **V90.30X- Drowning and submersion due to falling or jumping from crushed merchant ship**

IQ 7 **V90.31X- Drowning and submersion due to falling or jumping from crushed passenger ship**
Drowning and submersion due to falling and jumping from crushed Ferry boat
Drowning and submersion due to falling and jumping from crushed Liner

IQ 7 **V90.32X- Drowning and submersion due to falling or jumping from crushed fishing boat**

IQ 7 **V90.33X- Drowning and submersion due to falling or jumping from other crushed powered watercraft**
Drowning and submersion due to falling and jumping from crushed Hovercraft
Drowning and submersion due to falling and jumping from crushed Jet ski

IQ 7 **V90.34X- Drowning and submersion due to falling or jumping from crushed sailboat**

IQ 7 **V90.35X- Drowning and submersion due to falling or jumping from crushed canoe or kayak**

IQ 7 **V90.36X- Drowning and submersion due to falling or jumping from crushed (nonpowered) inflatable craft**

IQ 7 **V90.37X- Drowning and submersion due to falling or jumping from crushed water-skis**

IQ 7 **V90.38X- Drowning and submersion due to falling or jumping from other crushed unpowered watercraft**
Drowning and submersion due to falling and jumping from crushed surf-board
Drowning and submersion due to falling and jumping from crushed windsurfer

IQ 7 **V90.39X- Drowning and submersion due to falling or jumping from crushed unspecified watercraft**
Drowning and submersion due to falling and jumping from crushed boat NOS
Drowning and submersion due to falling and jumping from crushed ship NOS
Drowning and submersion due to falling and jumping from crushed watercraft NOS

5 **V90.8 Drowning and submersion due to other accident to watercraft**

IQ 7 **V90.80X- Drowning and submersion due to other accident to merchant ship**

IQ 7 **V90.81X- Drowning and submersion due to other accident to passenger ship**
Drowning and submersion due to other accident to Ferry-boat
Drowning and submersion due to other accident to Liner

IQ 7 **V90.82X- Drowning and submersion due to other accident to fishing boat**

IQ 7 **V90.83X- Drowning and submersion due to other accident to other powered watercraft**
Drowning and submersion due to other accident to Hovercraft (on open water)
Drowning and submersion due to other accident to Jet ski

IQ 7 **V90.84X- Drowning and submersion due to other accident to sailboat**

IQ 7 **V90.85X- Drowning and submersion due to other accident to canoe or kayak**

IQ 7 **V90.86X- Drowning and submersion due to other accident to (nonpowered) inflatable craft**

IQ 7 **V90.87X- Drowning and submersion due to other accident to water-skis**

IQ 7 **V90.88X- Drowning and submersion due to other accident to other unpowered watercraft**
Drowning and submersion due to other accident to surf-board
Drowning and submersion due to other accident to windsurfer

IQ 7 V90.89X- **Drowning and submersion due to other accident to unspecified watercraft**
Drowning and submersion due to other accident to boat NOS
Drowning and submersion due to other accident to ship NOS
Drowning and submersion due to other accident to watercraft NOS

4 V91 **Other injury due to accident to watercraft**
INCLUDES any injury except drowning and submersion as a result of an accident to watercraft
EXCLUDES 1 civilian water transport accident involving military watercraft (V94.81-)
military watercraft accident in military or war operations (Y36, Y37.-)
EXCLUDES 2 drowning and submersion due to accident to watercraft (V90.-)

The appropriate 7th character is to be added to each code from category V91
A initial encounter
D subsequent encounter
S sequela

5 V91.0 **Burn due to watercraft on fire**
EXCLUDES 1 burn from localized fire or explosion on board ship without accident to watercraft (V93.-)

IQ 7 V91.00X- **Burn due to merchant ship on fire**

IQ 7 V91.01X- **Burn due to passenger ship on fire**
Burn due to Ferry-boat on fire
Burn due to Liner on fire

IQ 7 V91.02X- **Burn due to fishing boat on fire**

IQ 7 V91.03X- **Burn due to other powered watercraft on fire**
Burn due to Hovercraft (on open water) on fire
Burn due to Jet ski on fire

IQ 7 V91.04X- **Burn due to sailboat on fire**

IQ 7 V91.05X- **Burn due to canoe or kayak on fire**

IQ 7 V91.06X- **Burn due to (nonpowered) inflatable craft on fire**

IQ 7 V91.07X- **Burn due to water-skis on fire**

IQ 7 V91.08X- **Burn due to other unpowered watercraft on fire**

IQ 7 V91.09X- **Burn due to unspecified watercraft on fire**
Burn due to boat NOS on fire
Burn due to ship NOS on fire
Burn due to watercraft NOS on fire

5 V91.1 **Crushed between watercraft and other watercraft or other object due to collision**
Crushed by lifeboat after abandoning ship in a collision
Note:
select the specified type of watercraft that the victim was on at the time of the collision

IQ 7 V91.10X- **Crushed between merchant ship and other watercraft or other object due to collision**

IQ 7 V91.11X- **Crushed between passenger ship and other watercraft or other object due to collision**
Crushed between Ferry-boat and other watercraft or other object due to collision
Crushed between Liner and other watercraft or other object due to collision

IQ 7 V91.12X- **Crushed between fishing boat and other watercraft or other object due to collision**

IQ 7 V91.13X- **Crushed between other powered watercraft and other watercraft or other object due to collision**
Crushed between Hovercraft (on open water) and other watercraft or other object due to collision
Crushed between Jet ski and other watercraft or other object due to collision

IQ 7 V91.14X- **Crushed between sailboat and other watercraft or other object due to collision**

IQ 7 V91.15X- **Crushed between canoe or kayak and other watercraft or other object due to collision**

IQ 7 V91.16X- **Crushed between (nonpowered) inflatable craft and other watercraft or other object due to collision**

IQ 7 V91.18X- **Crushed between other unpowered watercraft and other watercraft or other object due to collision**
Crushed between surfboard and other watercraft or other object due to collision
Crushed between windsurfer and other watercraft or other object due to collision

IQ 7 V91.19X- **Crushed between unspecified watercraft and other watercraft or other object due to collision**
Crushed between boat NOS and other watercraft or other object due to collision
Crushed between ship NOS and other watercraft or other object due to collision
Crushed between watercraft NOS and other watercraft or other object due to collision

5 V91.2 **Fall due to collision between watercraft and other watercraft or other object**
Fall while remaining on watercraft after collision
Note:
select the specified type of watercraft that the victim was on at the time of the collision
EXCLUDES 1 crushed between watercraft and other watercraft and other object due to collision (V91.1-)
drowning and submersion due to falling from crushed watercraft (V90.3-)

Chapter 20
V00-Y99

IQ 7 **V91.20X- Fall due to collision between merchant ship and other watercraft or other object**

IQ 7 **V91.21X- Fall due to collision between passenger ship and other watercraft or other object**
Fall due to collision between Ferry-boat and other watercraft or other object
Fall due to collision between Liner and other watercraft or other object

IQ 7 **V91.22X- Fall due to collision between fishing boat and other watercraft or other object**

IQ 7 **V91.23X- Fall due to collision between other powered watercraft and other watercraft or other object**
Fall due to collision between Hovercraft (on open water) and other watercraft or other object
Fall due to collision between Jet ski and other watercraft or other object

IQ 7 **V91.24X- Fall due to collision between sailboat and other watercraft or other object**

IQ 7 **V91.25X- Fall due to collision between canoe or kayak and other watercraft or other object**

IQ 7 **V91.26X- Fall due to collision between (nonpowered) inflatable craft and other watercraft or other object**

IQ 7 **V91.29X- Fall due to collision between unspecified watercraft and other watercraft or other object**
Fall due to collision between boat NOS and other watercraft or other object
Fall due to collision between ship NOS and other watercraft or other object
Fall due to collision between watercraft NOS and other watercraft or other object

5 **V91.3 Hit or struck by falling object due to accident to watercraft**
Hit or struck by falling object (part of damaged watercraft or other object) after falling or jumping from damaged watercraft
EXCLUDES 2 drowning or submersion due to fall or jumping from damaged watercraft (V90.2-, V90.3-)

IQ 7 **V91.30X- Hit or struck by falling object due to accident to merchant ship**

IQ 7 **V91.31X- Hit or struck by falling object due to accident to passenger ship**
Hit or struck by falling object due to accident to Ferry-boat
Hit or struck by falling object due to accident to Liner

IQ 7 **V91.32X- Hit or struck by falling object due to accident to fishing boat**

IQ 7 **V91.33X- Hit or struck by falling object due to accident to other powered watercraft**
Hit or struck by falling object due to accident to Hovercraft (on open water)
Hit or struck by falling object due to accident to Jet ski

IQ 7 **V91.34X- Hit or struck by falling object due to accident to sailboat**

IQ 7 **V91.35X- Hit or struck by falling object due to accident to canoe or kayak**

IQ 7 **V91.36X- Hit or struck by falling object due to accident to (nonpowered) inflatable craft**

IQ 7 **V91.37X- Hit or struck by falling object due to accident to water-skis**
Hit by water-skis after jumping off of waterskis

IQ 7 **V91.38X- Hit or struck by falling object due to accident to other unpowered watercraft**
Hit or struck by surf-board after falling off damaged surf-board
Hit or struck by object after falling off damaged windsurfer

IQ 7 **V91.39X- Hit or struck by falling object due to accident to unspecified watercraft**
Hit or struck by falling object due to accident to boat NOS
Hit or struck by falling object due to accident to ship NOS
Hit or struck by falling object due to accident to watercraft NOS

5 **V91.8 Other injury due to other accident to watercraft**

IQ 7 **V91.80X- Other injury due to other accident to merchant ship**

IQ 7 **V91.81X- Other injury due to other accident to passenger ship**
Other injury due to other accident to Ferry-boat
Other injury due to other accident to Liner

IQ 7 **V91.82X- Other injury due to other accident to fishing boat**

IQ 7 **V91.83X- Other injury due to other accident to other powered watercraft**
Other injury due to other accident to Hovercraft (on open water)
Other injury due to other accident to Jet ski

IQ 7 **V91.84X- Other injury due to other accident to sailboat**

IQ 7 **V91.85X- Other injury due to other accident to canoe or kayak**

IQ 7 **V91.86X- Other injury due to other accident to (nonpowered) inflatable craft**

IQ 7 **V91.87X- Other injury due to other accident to water-skis**

IQ 7 **V91.88X- Other injury due to other accident to other unpowered watercraft**
Other injury due to other accident to surf-board
Other injury due to other accident to windsurfer

IQ 7 **V91.89X- Other injury due to other accident to unspecified watercraft**
Other injury due to other accident to boat NOS
Other injury due to other accident to ship NOS

Other injury due to other accident to watercraft NOS

4 V92 Drowning and submersion due to accident on board watercraft, without accident to watercraft

EXCLUDES 1 civilian water transport accident involving military watercraft (V94.81-)
drowning or submersion due to accident to watercraft (V90-V91)
drowning or submersion of diver who voluntarily jumps from boat not involved in an accident (W16.711, W16.721)
fall into water without watercraft (W16.-)
military watercraft accident in military or war operations (Y36, Y37)

The appropriate 7th character is to be added to each code from category V92
A initial encounter
D subsequent encounter
S sequela

5 V92.0 Drowning and submersion due to fall off watercraft
Drowning and submersion due to fall from gangplank of watercraft
Drowning and submersion due to fall overboard watercraft
EXCLUDES 2 hitting head on object or bottom of body of water due to fall from watercraft (V94.0-)

IQ 7 V92.00X- Drowning and submersion due to fall off merchant ship

IQ 7 V92.01X- Drowning and submersion due to fall off passenger ship
Drowning and submersion due to fall off Ferry-boat
Drowning and submersion due to fall off Liner

IQ 7 V92.02X- Drowning and submersion due to fall off fishing boat

IQ 7 V92.03X- Drowning and submersion due to fall off other powered watercraft
Drowning and submersion due to fall off Hovercraft (on open water)
Drowning and submersion due to fall off Jet ski

IQ 7 V92.04X- Drowning and submersion due to fall off sailboat

IQ 7 V92.05X- Drowning and submersion due to fall off canoe or kayak

IQ 7 V92.06X- Drowning and submersion due to fall off (nonpowered) inflatable craft

IQ 7 V92.07X- Drowning and submersion due to fall off water-skis
EXCLUDES 1 drowning and submersion due to falling off burning water-skis (V90.27)
drowning and submersion due to falling off crushed water-skis (V90.37)
hit by boat while water-skiing NOS (V94.X)

IQ 7 V92.08X- Drowning and submersion due to fall off other unpowered watercraft
Drowning and submersion due to fall off surf-board
Drowning and submersion due to fall off windsurfer
EXCLUDES 1 drowning and submersion due to fall off burning unpowered watercraft (V90.28)
drowning and submersion due to fall off crushed unpowered watercraft (V90.38)
drowning and submersion due to fall off damaged unpowered watercraft (V90.88)
drowning and submersion due to rider of nonpowered watercraft being hit by other watercraft (V94.-)
other injury due to rider of nonpowered watercraft being hit by other watercraft (V94.-)

IQ 7 V92.09X- Drowning and submersion due to fall off unspecified watercraft
Drowning and submersion due to fall off boat NOS
Drowning and submersion due to fall off ship
Drowning and submersion due to fall off watercraft NOS

5 V92.1 Drowning and submersion due to being thrown overboard by motion of watercraft
EXCLUDES 1 drowning and submersion due to fall off surf-board (V92.08)
drowning and submersion due to fall off water-skis (V92.07)
drowning and submersion due to fall off windsurfer (V92.08)

IQ 7 V92.10X- Drowning and submersion due to being thrown overboard by motion of merchant ship

IQ 7 V92.11X- Drowning and submersion due to being thrown overboard by motion of passenger ship
Drowning and submersion due to being thrown overboard by motion of Ferry-boat

Drowning and submersion due to being thrown overboard by motion of Liner

IQ 7 **V92.12X- Drowning and submersion due to being thrown overboard by motion of fishing boat**

IQ 7 **V92.13X- Drowning and submersion due to being thrown overboard by motion of other powered watercraft**
Drowning and submersion due to being thrown overboard by motion of Hovercraft

IQ 7 **V92.14X- Drowning and submersion due to being thrown overboard by motion of sailboat**

IQ 7 **V92.15X- Drowning and submersion due to being thrown overboard by motion of canoe or kayak**

IQ 7 **V92.16X- Drowning and submersion due to being thrown overboard by motion of (nonpowered) inflatable craft**

IQ 7 **V92.19X- Drowning and submersion due to being thrown overboard by motion of unspecified watercraft**
Drowning and submersion due to being thrown overboard by motion of boat NOS
Drowning and submersion due to being thrown overboard by motion of ship NOS
Drowning and submersion due to being thrown overboard by motion of watercraft NOS

5 **V92.2 Drowning and submersion due to being washed overboard from watercraft**
Code first:
any associated cataclysm (X37.0-)

IQ 7 **V92.20X- Drowning and submersion due to being washed overboard from merchant ship**

IQ 7 **V92.21X- Drowning and submersion due to being washed overboard from passenger ship**
Drowning and submersion due to being washed overboard from Ferry-boat
Drowning and submersion due to being washed overboard from Liner

IQ 7 **V92.22X- Drowning and submersion due to being washed overboard from fishing boat**

IQ 7 **V92.23X- Drowning and submersion due to being washed overboard from other powered watercraft**
Drowning and submersion due to being washed overboard from Hovercraft (on open water)
Drowning and submersion due to being washed overboard from Jet ski

IQ 7 **V92.24X- Drowning and submersion due to being washed overboard from sailboat**

IQ 7 **V92.25X- Drowning and submersion due to being washed overboard from canoe or kayak**

IQ 7 **V92.26X- Drowning and submersion due to being washed overboard from (nonpowered) inflatable craft**

IQ 7 **V92.27X- Drowning and submersion due to being washed overboard from water-skis**
EXCLUDES 1 drowning and submersion due to fall off water-skis (V92.07)

IQ 7 **V92.28X- Drowning and submersion due to being washed overboard from other unpowered watercraft**
Drowning and submersion due to being washed overboard from surf-board
Drowning and submersion due to being washed overboard from windsurfer

IQ 7 **V92.29X- Drowning and submersion due to being washed overboard from unspecified watercraft**
Drowning and submersion due to being washed overboard from boat NOS
Drowning and submersion due to being washed overboard from ship NOS
Drowning and submersion due to being washed overboard from watercraft NOS

4 **V93 Other injury due to accident on board watercraft, without accident to watercraft**
EXCLUDES 1 civilian water transport accident involving military watercraft (V94.81-)
other injury due to accident to watercraft (V91.-)
military watercraft accident in military or war operations (Y36, Y37.-)
EXCLUDES 2 drowning and submersion due to accident on board watercraft, without accident to watercraft (V92.-)

The appropriate 7th character is to be added to each code from category V93
A initial encounter
D subsequent encounter
S sequela

5 **V93.0 Burn due to localized fire on board watercraft**
EXCLUDES 1 burn due to watercraft on fire (V91.0-)

IQ 7 **V93.00X- Burn due to localized fire on board merchant vessel**

IQ 7 **V93.01X- Burn due to localized fire on board passenger vessel**
Burn due to localized fire on board Ferry-boat
Burn due to localized fire on board Liner

IQ 7 **V93.02X- Burn due to localized fire on board fishing boat**

IQ 7 **V93.03X- Burn due to localized fire on board other powered watercraft**
Burn due to localized fire on board Hovercraft

Chapter 20
V00-Y99

4 4th digit required 5 5th digit required 6 6th digit required 7 7th digit required 7 7th digit placeholder + Additional code Laterality

Burn due to localized fire on board Jet ski

IQ ☑ **V93.04X- Burn due to localized fire on board sailboat**

IQ ☑ **V93.09X- Burn due to localized fire on board unspecified watercraft**

Burn due to localized fire on board boat NOS
Burn due to localized fire on board ship NOS
Burn due to localized fire on board watercraft NOS

5 **V93.1 Other burn on board watercraft**

Burn due to source other than fire on board watercraft

EXCLUDES 1 burn due to watercraft on fire (V91.0-)

IQ ☑ **V93.10X- Other burn on board merchant vessel**

IQ ☑ **V93.11X- Other burn on board passenger vessel**

Other burn on board Ferry-boat
Other burn on board Liner

IQ ☑ **V93.12X- Other burn on board fishing boat**

IQ ☑ **V93.13X- Other burn on board other powered watercraft**

Other burn on board Hovercraft
Other burn on board Jet ski

IQ ☑ **V93.14X- Other burn on board sailboat**

IQ ☑ **V93.19X- Other burn on board unspecified watercraft**

Other burn on board boat NOS
Other burn on board ship NOS
Other burn on board watercraft NOS

5 **V93.2 Heat exposure on board watercraft**

EXCLUDES 1 exposure to man-made heat not aboard watercraft (W92)
exposure to natural heat while on board watercraft (X30)
exposure to sunlight while on board watercraft (X32)

EXCLUDES 2 burn due to fire on board watercraft (V93.0-)

IQ ☑ **V93.20X- Heat exposure on board merchant ship**

IQ ☑ **V93.21X- Heat exposure on board passenger ship**

Heat exposure on board Ferry-boat
Heat exposure on board Liner

IQ ☑ **V93.22X- Heat exposure on board fishing boat**

IQ ☑ **V93.23X- Heat exposure on board other powered watercraft**

Heat exposure on board hovercraft

IQ ☑ **V93.24X- Heat exposure on board sailboat**

IQ ☑ **V93.29X- Heat exposure on board unspecified watercraft**

Heat exposure on board boat NOS
Heat exposure on board ship NOS
Heat exposure on board watercraft NOS

5 **V93.3 Fall on board watercraft**

EXCLUDES 1 fall due to collision of watercraft (V91.2-)

IQ ☑ **V93.30X- Fall on board merchant ship**

IQ ☑ **V93.31X- Fall on board passenger ship**

Fall on board Ferry-boat
Fall on board Liner

IQ ☑ **V93.32X- Fall on board fishing boat**

IQ ☑ **V93.33X- Fall on board other powered watercraft**

Fall on board Hovercraft (on open water)
Fall on board Jet ski

IQ ☑ **V93.34X- Fall on board sailboat**

IQ ☑ **V93.35X- Fall on board canoe or kayak**

IQ ☑ **V93.36X- Fall on board (nonpowered) inflatable craft**

IQ ☑ **V93.38X- Fall on board other unpowered watercraft**

IQ ☑ **V93.39X- Fall on board unspecified watercraft**

Fall on board boat NOS
Fall on board ship NOS
Fall on board watercraft NOS

5 **V93.4 Struck by falling object on board watercraft**

Hit by falling object on board watercraft

EXCLUDES 1 struck by falling object due to accident to watercraft (V91.3)

IQ ☑ **V93.40X- Struck by falling object on merchant ship**

IQ ☑ **V93.41X- Struck by falling object on passenger ship**

Struck by falling object on Ferry-boat
Struck by falling object on Liner

IQ ☑ **V93.42X- Struck by falling object on fishing boat**

IQ ☑ **V93.43X- Struck by falling object on other powered watercraft**

Struck by falling object on Hovercraft

IQ ☑ **V93.44X- Struck by falling object on sailboat**

IQ ☑ **V93.48X- Struck by falling object on other unpowered watercraft**

IQ ☑ **V93.49X- Struck by falling object on unspecified watercraft**

5 **V93.5 Explosion on board watercraft**

Boiler explosion on steamship

EXCLUDES 2 fire on board watercraft (V93.0-)

IQ ☑ **V93.50X- Explosion on board merchant ship**

IQ ☑ **V93.51X- Explosion on board passenger ship**

Explosion on board Ferry-boat
Explosion on board Liner

IQ ☑ **V93.52X- Explosion on board fishing boat**

IQ ☑ **V93.53X- Explosion on board other powered watercraft**

Explosion on board Hovercraft
Explosion on board Jet ski

IQ ☑ **V93.54X- Explosion on board sailboat**

IQ ☑ **V93.59X- Explosion on board unspecified watercraft**

Explosion on board boat NOS
Explosion on board ship NOS
Explosion on board watercraft NOS

5 **V93.6 Machinery accident on board watercraft**

EXCLUDES 1 machinery explosion on board watercraft (V93.4-)

machinery fire on board
watercraft (V93.0-)

!Q ☑ V93.60X- **Machinery accident on board merchant ship**

!Q ☑ V93.61X- **Machinery accident on board passenger ship**
Machinery accident on board Ferry-boat
Machinery accident on board Liner

!Q ☑ V93.62X- **Machinery accident on board fishing boat**

!Q ☑ V93.63X- **Machinery accident on board other powered watercraft**
Machinery accident on board Hovercraft

!Q ☑ V93.64X- **Machinery accident on board sailboat**

!Q ☑ V93.69X- **Machinery accident on board unspecified watercraft**
Machinery accident on board boat NOS
Machinery accident on board ship NOS
Machinery accident on board watercraft NOS

⑤ V93.8 Other injury due to other accident on board watercraft
Accidental poisoning by gases or fumes on watercraft

!Q ☑ V93.80X- **Other injury due to other accident on board merchant ship**

!Q ☑ V93.81X- **Other injury due to other accident on board passenger ship**
Other injury due to other accident on board Ferry-boat
Other injury due to other accident on board Liner

!Q ☑ V93.82X- **Other injury due to other accident on board fishing boat**

!Q ☑ V93.83X- **Other injury due to other accident on board other powered watercraft**
Other injury due to other accident on board Hovercraft
Other injury due to other accident on board Jet ski

!Q ☑ V93.84X- **Other injury due to other accident on board sailboat**

!Q ☑ V93.85X- **Other injury due to other accident on board canoe or kayak**

!Q ☑ V93.86X- **Other injury due to other accident on board (nonpowered) inflatable craft**

!Q ☑ V93.87X- **Other injury due to other accident on board water-skis**
Hit or struck by object while waterskiing

!Q ☑ V93.88X- **Other injury due to other accident on board other unpowered watercraft**
Hit or struck by object while surfing
Hit or struck by object while on board windsurfer

!Q ☑ V93.89X- **Other injury due to other accident on board unspecified watercraft**
Other injury due to other accident on board boat NOS

Other injury due to other accident on board ship NOS
Other injury due to other accident on board watercraft NOS

④ V94 **Other and unspecified water transport accidents**

> **EXCLUDES 1** military watercraft accidents in military or war operations (Y36, Y37)

The appropriate 7th character is to be added to each code from category V94
A   initial encounter
D   subsequent encounter
S   sequela

!Q ☑ V94.0XX- **Hitting object or bottom of body of water due to fall from watercraft**
> **EXCLUDES 2** drowning and submersion due to fall from watercraft (V92.0-)

⑤ V94.1 Bather struck by watercraft
Swimmer hit by watercraft

!Q ☑ V94.11X- **Bather struck by powered watercraft**

!Q ☑ V94.12X- **Bather struck by nonpowered watercraft**

⑤ V94.2 Rider of nonpowered watercraft struck by other watercraft

!Q ☑ V94.21X- **Rider of nonpowered watercraft struck by other nonpowered watercraft**
Canoer hit by other nonpowered watercraft
Surfer hit by other nonpowered watercraft
Windsurfer hit by other nonpowered watercraft

!Q ☑ V94.22X- **Rider of nonpowered watercraft struck by powered watercraft**
Canoer hit by motorboat
Surfer hit by motorboat
Windsurfer hit by motorboat

⑤ V94.3 Injury to rider of (inflatable) watercraft being pulled behind other watercraft

!Q ☑ V94.31X- **Injury to rider of (inflatable) recreational watercraft being pulled behind other watercraft**
Injury to rider of inner-tube pulled behind motor boat

!Q ☑ V94.32X- **Injury to rider of non-recreational watercraft being pulled behind other watercraft**
Injury to occupant of dingy being pulled behind boat or ship
Injury to occupant of life-raft being pulled behind boat or ship

!Q ☑ V94.4XX- **Injury to barefoot water-skier**
Injury to person being pulled behind boat or ship

⑤ V94.8 Other water transport accident

⑥ V94.81 Water transport accident involving military watercraft

!Q ☑ V94.810- **Civilian watercraft involved in water transport accident with military watercraft**

---

④ 4th digit required   ⑤ 5th digit required   ⑥ 6th digit required   ☑ 7th digit required   ☑ 7th digit placeholder   ✚ Additional code   ▣ Laterality

Passenger on civilian watercraft injured due to accident with military watercraft

IQ 7 **V94.811- Civilian in water injured by military watercraft**

IQ 7 **V94.818- Other water transport accident involving military watercraft**

IQ 7 **V94.89X- Other water transport accident**

IQ 7 **V94.9XX- Unspecified water transport accident**

Water transport accident NOS

Air and space transport accidents (V95-V97)

EXCLUDES 1 military aircraft accidents in military or war operations (Y36, Y37)

4 **V95 Accident to powered aircraft causing injury to occupant**

The appropriate 7th character is to be added to each code from category V95
A initial encounter
D subsequent encounter
S sequela

5 **V95.0 Helicopter accident injuring occupant**

IQ 7 **V95.00X- Unspecified helicopter accident injuring occupant**

IQ 7 **V95.01X- Helicopter crash injuring occupant**

IQ 7 **V95.02X- Forced landing of helicopter injuring occupant**

IQ 7 **V95.03X- Helicopter collision injuring occupant**

Helicopter collision with any object, fixed, movable or moving

IQ 7 **V95.04X- Helicopter fire injuring occupant**

IQ 7 **V95.05X- Helicopter explosion injuring occupant**

IQ 7 **V95.09X- Other helicopter accident injuring occupant**

5 **V95.1 Ultralight, microlight or powered-glider accident injuring occupant**

IQ 7 **V95.10X- Unspecified ultralight, microlight or powered-glider accident injuring occupant**

IQ 7 **V95.11X- Ultralight, microlight or powered-glider crash injuring occupant**

IQ 7 **V95.12X- Forced landing of ultralight, microlight or powered-glider injuring occupant**

IQ 7 **V95.13X- Ultralight, microlight or powered-glider collision injuring occupant**

Ultralight, microlight or powered-glider collision with any object, fixed, movable or moving

IQ 7 **V95.14X- Ultralight, microlight or powered-glider fire injuring occupant**

IQ 7 **V95.15X- Ultralight, microlight or powered-glider explosion injuring occupant**

IQ 7 **V95.19X- Other ultralight, microlight or powered-glider accident injuring occupant**

5 **V95.2 Other private fixed-wing aircraft accident injuring occupant**

IQ 7 **V95.20X- Unspecified accident to other private fixed-wing aircraft, injuring occupant**

IQ 7 **V95.21X- Other private fixed-wing aircraft crash injuring occupant**

IQ 7 **V95.22X- Forced landing of other private fixed-wing aircraft injuring occupant**

IQ 7 **V95.23X- Other private fixed-wing aircraft collision injuring occupant**

Other private fixed-wing aircraft collision with any object, fixed, movable or moving

IQ 7 **V95.24X- Other private fixed-wing aircraft fire injuring occupant**

IQ 7 **V95.25X- Other private fixed-wing aircraft explosion injuring occupant**

IQ 7 **V95.29X- Other accident to other private fixed-wing aircraft injuring occupant**

5 **V95.3 Commercial fixed-wing aircraft accident injuring occupant**

IQ 7 **V95.30X- Unspecified accident to commercial fixed-wing aircraft injuring occupant**

IQ 7 **V95.31X- Commercial fixed-wing aircraft crash injuring occupant**

IQ 7 **V95.32X- Forced landing of commercial fixed-wing aircraft injuring occupant**

IQ 7 **V95.33X- Commercial fixed-wing aircraft collision injuring occupant**

Commercial fixed-wing aircraft collision with any object, fixed, movable or moving

IQ 7 **V95.34X- Commercial fixed-wing aircraft fire injuring occupant**

IQ 7 **V95.35X- Commercial fixed-wing aircraft explosion injuring occupant**

IQ 7 **V95.39X- Other accident to commercial fixed-wing aircraft injuring occupant**

5 **V95.4 Spacecraft accident injuring occupant**

IQ 7 **V95.40X- Unspecified spacecraft accident injuring occupant**

IQ 7 **V95.41X- Spacecraft crash injuring occupant**

IQ 7 **V95.42X- Forced landing of spacecraft injuring occupant**

IQ 7 **V95.43X- Spacecraft collision injuring occupant**

Spacecraft collision with any object, fixed, moveable or moving

IQ 7 **V95.44X- Spacecraft fire injuring occupant**

IQ 7 **V95.45X- Spacecraft explosion injuring occupant**

IQ 7 **V95.49X- Other spacecraft accident injuring occupant**

IQ 7 **V95.8XX- Other powered aircraft accidents injuring occupant**

IQ 7 **V95.9XX- Unspecified aircraft accident injuring occupant**

Aircraft accident NOS
Air transport accident NOS

4 **V96 Accident to nonpowered aircraft causing injury to occupant**

The appropriate 7th character is to be added to each code from category V96
A   initial encounter
D   subsequent encounter
S   sequela

⑤ V96.0 Balloon accident injuring occupant

!Q ☑ V96.00X-   Unspecified balloon accident injuring occupant

!Q ☑ V96.01X- Balloon crash injuring occupant

!Q ☑ V96.02X- Forced landing of balloon injuring occupant

!Q ☑ V96.03X- Balloon collision injuring occupant
Balloon collision with any object, fixed, moveable or moving

!Q ☑ V96.04X- Balloon fire injuring occupant

!Q ☑ V96.05X- Balloon explosion injuring occupant

!Q ☑ V96.09X- Other balloon accident injuring occupant

⑤ V96.1 Hang-glider accident injuring occupant

!Q ☑ V96.10X-   Unspecified hang-glider accident injuring occupant

!Q ☑ V96.11X- Hang-glider crash injuring occupant

!Q ☑ V96.12X- Forced landing of hang-glider injuring occupant

!Q ☑ V96.13X- Hang-glider collision injuring occupant
Hang-glider collision with any object, fixed, moveable or moving

!Q ☑ V96.14X- Hang-glider fire injuring occupant

!Q ☑ V96.15X- Hang-glider explosion injuring occupant

!Q ☑ V96.19X- Other hang-glider accident injuring occupant

⑤ V96.2 Glider (nonpowered) accident injuring occupant

!Q ☑ V96.20X-   Unspecified glider (nonpowered) accident injuring occupant

!Q ☑ V96.21X- Glider (nonpowered) crash injuring occupant

!Q ☑ V96.22X- Forced landing of glider (nonpowered) injuring occupant

!Q ☑ V96.23X- Glider (nonpowered) collision injuring occupant
Glider (nonpowered) collision with any object, fixed, moveable or moving

!Q ☑ V96.24X- Glider (nonpowered) fire injuring occupant

!Q ☑ V96.25X- Glider (nonpowered) explosion injuring occupant

!Q ☑ V96.29X- Other glider (nonpowered) accident injuring occupant

!Q ☑ V96.8XX- Other nonpowered-aircraft accidents injuring occupant
Kite carrying a person accident injuring occupant

!Q ☑ V96.9XX-   Unspecified nonpowered-aircraft accident injuring occupant
Nonpowered-aircraft accident NOS

④ V97   Other specified air transport accidents

The appropriate 7th character is to be added to each code from category V97
A   initial encounter
D   subsequent encounter
S   sequela

!Q ☑ V97.0XX- Occupant of aircraft injured in other specified air transport accidents
Fall in, on or from aircraft in air transport accident
> EXCLUDES 1   accident while boarding or alighting aircraft (V97.1)

!Q ☑ V97.1XX- Person injured while boarding or alighting from aircraft

⑤ V97.2 Parachutist accident

!Q ☑ V97.21X- Parachutist entangled in object
Parachutist landing in tree

!Q ☑ V97.22X- Parachutist injured on landing

!Q ☑ V97.29X- Other parachutist accident

⑤ V97.3 Person on ground injured in air transport accident

!Q ☑ V97.31X- Hit by object falling from aircraft
Hit by crashing aircraft
Injured by aircraft hitting house
Injured by aircraft hitting car

!Q ☑ V97.32X- Injured by rotating propeller

!Q ☑ V97.33X- Sucked into jet engine

!Q ☑ V97.39X- Other injury to person on ground due to air transport accident

⑤ V97.8 Other air transport accidents, not elsewhere classified
> EXCLUDES 1   aircraft accident NOS (V95.9)
> exposure to changes in air pressure during ascent or descent (W94.-)

⑥ V97.81 Air transport accident involving military aircraft

!Q ☑ V97.810- Civilian aircraft involved in air transport accident with military aircraft
Passenger in civilian aircraft injured due to accident with military aircraft

!Q ☑ V97.811- Civilian injured by military aircraft

!Q ☑ V97.818- Other air transport accident involving military aircraft

!Q ☑ V97.89X- Other air transport accidents, not elsewhere classified
Injury from machinery on aircraft

Other and unspecified transport accidents (V98-V99)

> EXCLUDES 1   vehicle accident, type of vehicle unspecified (V89.-)

④ V98   Other specified transport accidents

The appropriate 7th character is to be added to each code from category V98
A   initial encounter
D   subsequent encounter
S   sequela

④ 4th digit required   ⑤ 5th digit required   ⑥ 6th digit required   ⑦ 7th digit required   ☑ 7th digit placeholder   ➕ Additional code   ⊟ Laterality

IQ 7 V98.0XX- **Accident to, on or involving cable-car, not on rails**
Caught or dragged by cable-car, not on rails
Fall or jump from cable-car, not on rails
Object thrown from or in cable-car, not on rails

IQ 7 V98.1XX- **Accident to, on or involving land-yacht**

IQ 7 V98.2XX- **Accident to, on or involving ice yacht**

IQ 7 V98.3XX- **Accident to, on or involving ski lift**
Accident to, on or involving ski chair-lift
Accident to, on or involving ski-lift with gondola

IQ 7 V98.8XX- **Other specified transport accidents**

IQ 7 V99.XXX- **Unspecified transport accident**

The appropriate 7th character is to be added to code V99
A initial encounter
D subsequent encounter
S sequela

Other external causes of accidental injury (W00-X58)

CODING TIPS ✓ Do not assign a code for other external causes of accidental injury as an external cause of morbidity when there is no injury coded on the claim.

Slipping, tripping, stumbling and falls (W00-W19)

EXCLUDES 1 assault involving a fall (Y01-Y02)
fall from animal (V80.-)
fall (in) (from) machinery (in operation) (W28-W31)
fall (in) (from) transport vehicle (V01-V99)
intentional self-harm involving a fall (X80-X81)

EXCLUDES 2 at risk for fall (history of fall) Z91.81
fall (in) (from) burning building (X00.-)
fall into fire (X00-X04, X08)

4 W00 **Fall due to ice and snow**

INCLUDES pedestrian on foot falling (slipping) on ice and snow

EXCLUDES 1 fall on (from) ice and snow involving pedestrian conveyance (V00.-)
fall from stairs and steps not due to ice and snow (W10.-)

The appropriate 7th character is to be added to each code from category W00
A initial encounter
D subsequent encounter
S sequela

IQ 7 W00.0XX- **Fall on same level due to ice and snow**

IQ 7 W00.1XX- **Fall from stairs and steps due to ice and snow**

IQ 7 W00.2XX- **Other fall from one level to another due to ice and snow**

IQ 7 W00.9XX- **Unspecified fall due to ice and snow**

4 W01 **Fall on same level from slipping, tripping and stumbling**

INCLUDES fall on moving sidewalk

EXCLUDES 1 fall due to bumping (striking) against object (W18.0-)
fall in shower or bathtub (W18.2-)
fall on same level NOS (W18.30)
fall on same level from slipping, tripping and stumbling due to ice or snow (W00.0)
fall off or from toilet (W18.1-)
slipping, tripping and stumbling NOS (W18.40)
slipping, tripping and stumbling without falling (W18.4-)

The appropriate 7th character is to be added to each code from category W01
A initial encounter
D subsequent encounter
S sequela

IQ 7 W01.0XX- **Fall on same level from slipping, tripping and stumbling without subsequent striking against object**
Falling over animal

5 W01.1 **Fall on same level from slipping, tripping and stumbling with subsequent striking against object**

IQ 7 W01.10X- **Fall on same level from slipping, tripping and stumbling with subsequent striking against unspecified object**

6 W01.11 **Fall on same level from slipping, tripping and stumbling with subsequent striking against sharp object**

IQ 7 W01.110- **Fall on same level from slipping, tripping and stumbling with subsequent striking against sharp glass**

IQ 7 W01.111- **Fall on same level from slipping, tripping and stumbling with subsequent striking against power tool or machine**

IQ 7 W01.118- **Fall on same level from slipping, tripping and stumbling with subsequent striking against other sharp object**

IQ 7 W01.119- **Fall on same level from slipping, tripping and stumbling with subsequent striking against unspecified sharp object**

6 W01.19 **Fall on same level from slipping, tripping and stumbling with subsequent striking against other object**

IQ 7 W01.190- **Fall on same level from slipping, tripping and stumbling with subsequent striking against furniture**

IQ 7 W01.198- **Fall on same level from slipping, tripping and stumbling with subsequent striking against other object**

IQ 7 W03.XXX- **Other fall on same level due to collision with another person**

Chapter 20 V00-Y99

Fall due to non-transport collision with other person

EXCLUDES 1 collision with another person without fall (W51)
crushed or pushed by a crowd or human stampede (W52)
fall involving pedestrian conveyance (V00-V09)
fall due to ice or snow (W00)
fall on same level NOS (W18.30)

The appropriate 7th character is to be added to code W03
A initial encounter
D subsequent encounter
S sequela

IQ 7 **W04.XXX- Fall while being carried or supported by other persons**
Accidentally dropped while being carried

The appropriate 7th character is to be added to code W04
A initial encounter
D subsequent encounter
S sequela

4 **W05 Fall from non-moving wheelchair, nonmotorized scooter and motorized mobility scooter**

EXCLUDES 1 fall from moving wheelchair (powered) (V00.811)
fall from moving motorized mobility scooter (V00.831)
fall from nonmotorized scooter (V00.141)

The appropriate 7th character is to be added to each code from category W05
A initial encounter
D subsequent encounter
S sequela

IQ 7 **W05.0XX- Fall from non-moving wheelchair**
IQ 7 **W05.1XX- Fall from non-moving nonmotorized scooter**
IQ 7 **W05.2XX- Fall from non-moving motorized mobility scooter**
IQ 7 **W06.XXX- Fall from bed**

The appropriate 7th character is to be added to code W06
A initial encounter
D subsequent encounter
S sequela

IQ 7 **W07.XXX- Fall from chair**

The appropriate 7th character is to be added to code W07
A initial encounter
D subsequent encounter
S sequela

IQ 7 **W08.XXX- Fall from other furniture**

The appropriate 7th character is to be added to code W08
A initial encounter
D subsequent encounter
S sequela

4 **W09 Fall on and from playground equipment**

EXCLUDES 1 fall involving recreational machinery (W31)

The appropriate 7th character is to be added to each code from category W09
A initial encounter
D subsequent encounter
S sequela

IQ 7 **W09.0XX- Fall on or from playground slide**
IQ 7 **W09.1XX- Fall from playground swing**
IQ 7 **W09.2XX- Fall on or from jungle gym**
IQ 7 **W09.8XX- Fall on or from other playground equipment**

4 **W10 Fall on and from stairs and steps**

EXCLUDES 1 Fall from stairs and steps due to ice and snow (W00.1)

The appropriate 7th character is to be added to each code from category W10
A initial encounter
D subsequent encounter
S sequela

IQ 7 **W10.0XX- Fall (on)(from) escalator**
IQ 7 **W10.1XX- Fall (on)(from) sidewalk curb**
IQ 7 **W10.2XX- Fall (on)(from) incline**
Fall (on) (from) ramp
IQ 7 **W10.8XX- Fall (on) (from) other stairs and steps**
IQ 7 **W10.9XX- Fall (on) (from) unspecified stairs and steps**
IQ 7 **W11.XXX- Fall on and from ladder**

The appropriate 7th character is to be added to code W11
A initial encounter
D subsequent encounter
S sequela

IQ 7 **W12.XXX- Fall on and from scaffolding**

The appropriate 7th character is to be added to code W12
A initial encounter
D subsequent encounter
S sequela

4 **W13 Fall from, out of or through building or structure**

The appropriate 7th character is to be added to each code from category W13
A initial encounter
D subsequent encounter
S sequela

IQ 7 **W13.0XX- Fall from, out of or through balcony**
Fall from, out of or through railing
IQ 7 **W13.1XX- Fall from, out of or through bridge**
IQ 7 **W13.2XX- Fall from, out of or through roof**
IQ 7 **W13.3XX- Fall through floor**
▲ IQ 7 **W13.4XX- Fall from, out of or through window**

Chapter 20

V00-Y99

EXCLUDES 2 fall with subsequent striking against sharp glass (W01.110-)

IQ 7 **W13.8XX- Fall from, out of or through other building or structure**
Fall from, out of or through viaduct
Fall from, out of or through wall
Fall from, out of or through flag-pole

IQ 7 **W13.9XX- Fall from, out of or through building, not otherwise specified**
EXCLUDES 1 collapse of a building or structure (W20.-)
fall or jump from burning building or structure (X00.-)

IQ 7 **W14.XXX- Fall from tree**

The appropriate 7th character is to be added to code W14
A initial encounter
D subsequent encounter
S sequela

IQ 7 **W15.XXX- Fall from cliff**

The appropriate 7th character is to be added to code W15
A initial encounter
D subsequent encounter
S sequela

4 **W16 Fall, jump or diving into water**
EXCLUDES 1 accidental non-watercraft drowning and submersion not involving fall (W65-W74)
effects of air pressure from diving (W94.-)
fall into water from watercraft (V90-V94)
hitting an object or against bottom when falling from watercraft (V94.0)
EXCLUDES 2 striking or hitting diving board (W21.4)

The appropriate 7th character is to be added to each code from category W16
A initial encounter
D subsequent encounter
S sequela

5 **W16.0 Fall into swimming pool**
Fall into swimming pool NOS
EXCLUDES 1 fall into empty swimming pool (W17.3)

6 **W16.01 Fall into swimming pool striking water surface**

IQ 7 **W16.011- Fall into swimming pool striking water surface causing drowning and submersion**
EXCLUDES 1 drowning and submersion while in swimming pool without fall (W67)

IQ 7 **W16.012- Fall into swimming pool striking water surface causing other injury**

6 **W16.02 Fall into swimming pool striking bottom**

IQ 7 **W16.021- Fall into swimming pool striking bottom causing drowning and submersion**
EXCLUDES 1 drowning and submersion while in swimming pool without fall (W67)

IQ 7 **W16.022- Fall into swimming pool striking bottom causing other injury**

6 **W16.03 Fall into swimming pool striking wall**

IQ 7 **W16.031- Fall into swimming pool striking wall causing drowning and submersion**
EXCLUDES 1 drowning and submersion while in swimming pool without fall (W67)

IQ 7 **W16.032- Fall into swimming pool striking wall causing other injury**

5 **W16.1 Fall into natural body of water**
Fall into lake
Fall into open sea
Fall into river
Fall into stream

6 **W16.11 Fall into natural body of water striking water surface**

IQ 7 **W16.111- Fall into natural body of water striking water surface causing drowning and submersion**
EXCLUDES 1 drowning and submersion while in natural body of water without fall (W69)

IQ 7 **W16.112- Fall into natural body of water striking water surface causing other injury**

6 **W16.12 Fall into natural body of water striking bottom**

IQ 7 **W16.121- Fall into natural body of water striking bottom causing drowning and submersion**
EXCLUDES 1 drowning and submersion while in natural body of water without fall (W69)

IQ 7 **W16.122- Fall into natural body of water striking bottom causing other injury**

6 **W16.13 Fall into natural body of water striking side**

IQ 7 **W16.131- Fall into natural body of water striking side causing drowning and submersion**
EXCLUDES 1 drowning and submersion while in natural body of water without fall (W69)

IQ 7 **W16.132- Fall into natural body of water striking side causing other injury**

5 **W16.2 Fall in (into) filled bathtub or bucket of water**

6 **W16.21 Fall in (into) filled bathtub**
EXCLUDES 1 fall into empty bathtub (W18.2)

IQ 7 **W16.211- Fall in (into) filled bathtub causing drowning and submersion**

EXCLUDES 1 drowning and submersion while in filled bathtub without fall (W65)

!Q 7 **W16.212- Fall in (into) filled bathtub causing other injury**

6 **W16.22 Fall in (into) bucket of water**

!Q 7 **W16.221- Fall in (into) bucket of water causing drowning and submersion**

!Q 7 **W16.222- Fall in (into) bucket of water causing other injury**

5 **W16.3 Fall into other water**

Fall into fountain

Fall into reservoir

6 **W16.31 Fall into other water striking water surface**

!Q 7 **W16.311- Fall into other water striking water surface causing drowning and submersion**

EXCLUDES 1 drowning and submersion while in other water without fall (W73)

!Q 7 **W16.312- Fall into other water striking water surface causing other injury**

6 **W16.32 Fall into other water striking bottom**

!Q 7 **W16.321- Fall into other water striking bottom causing drowning and submersion**

EXCLUDES 1 drowning and submersion while in other water without fall (W73)

!Q 7 **W16.322- Fall into other water striking bottom causing other injury**

6 **W16.33 Fall into other water striking wall**

!Q 7 **W16.331- Fall into other water striking wall causing drowning and submersion**

EXCLUDES 1 drowning and submersion while in other water without fall (W73)

!Q 7 **W16.332- Fall into other water striking wall causing other injury**

5 **W16.4 Fall into unspecified water**

!Q 7 **W16.41X- Fall into unspecified water causing drowning and submersion**

!Q 7 **W16.42X- Fall into unspecified water causing other injury**

5 **W16.5 Jumping or diving into swimming pool**

6 **W16.51 Jumping or diving into swimming pool striking water surface**

!Q 7 **W16.511- Jumping or diving into swimming pool striking water surface causing drowning and submersion**

EXCLUDES 1 drowning and submersion while in swimming pool without jumping or diving (W67)

!Q 7 **W16.512- Jumping or diving into swimming pool striking water surface causing other injury**

6 **W16.52 Jumping or diving into swimming pool striking bottom**

!Q 7 **W16.521- Jumping or diving into swimming pool striking bottom causing drowning and submersion**

EXCLUDES 1 drowning and submersion while in swimming pool without jumping or diving (W67)

!Q 7 **W16.522- Jumping or diving into swimming pool striking bottom causing other injury**

6 **W16.53 Jumping or diving into swimming pool striking wall**

!Q 7 **W16.531- Jumping or diving into swimming pool striking wall causing drowning and submersion**

EXCLUDES 1 drowning and submersion while in swimming pool without jumping or diving (W67)

!Q 7 **W16.532- Jumping or diving into swimming pool striking wall causing other injury**

5 **W16.6 Jumping or diving into natural body of water**

Jumping or diving into lake

Jumping or diving into open sea

Jumping or diving into river

Jumping or diving into stream

6 **W16.61 Jumping or diving into natural body of water striking water surface**

!Q 7 **W16.611- Jumping or diving into natural body of water striking water surface causing drowning and submersion**

EXCLUDES 1 drowning and submersion while in natural body of water without jumping or diving (W69)

!Q 7 **W16.612- Jumping or diving into natural body of water striking water surface causing other injury**

6 **W16.62 Jumping or diving into natural body of water striking bottom**

!Q 7 **W16.621- Jumping or diving into natural body of water striking bottom causing drowning and submersion**

EXCLUDES 1 drowning and submersion while in natural body of water without jumping or diving (W69)

!Q 7 **W16.622- Jumping or diving into natural body of water striking bottom causing other injury**

5 **W16.7 Jumping or diving from boat**

EXCLUDES 1 Fall from boat into water -see watercraft accident (V90-V94)

6 **W16.71 Jumping or diving from boat striking water surface**

IQ 7 **W16.711- Jumping or diving from boat striking water surface causing drowning and submersion**

IQ 7 **W16.712- Jumping or diving from boat striking water surface causing other injury**

6 **W16.72 Jumping or diving from boat striking bottom**

IQ 7 **W16.721- Jumping or diving from boat striking bottom causing drowning and submersion**

IQ 7 **W16.722- Jumping or diving from boat striking bottom causing other injury**

5 **W16.8 Jumping or diving into other water**

Jumping or diving into fountain

Jumping or diving into reservoir

6 **W16.81 Jumping or diving into other water striking water surface**

IQ 7 **W16.811- Jumping or diving into other water striking water surface causing drowning and submersion**

EXCLUDES 1 drowning and submersion while in other water without jumping or diving (W73)

IQ 7 **W16.812- Jumping or diving into other water striking water surface causing other injury**

6 **W16.82 Jumping or diving into other water striking bottom**

IQ 7 **W16.821- Jumping or diving into other water striking bottom causing drowning and submersion**

EXCLUDES 1 drowning and submersion while in other water without jumping or diving (W73)

IQ 7 **W16.822- Jumping or diving into other water striking bottom causing other injury**

6 **W16.83 Jumping or diving into other water striking wall**

IQ 7 **W16.831- Jumping or diving into other water striking wall causing drowning and submersion**

EXCLUDES 1 drowning and submersion while in other water without jumping or diving (W73)

IQ 7 **W16.832- Jumping or diving into other water striking wall causing other injury**

5 **W16.9 Jumping or diving into unspecified water**

IQ 7 **W16.91X- Jumping or diving into unspecified water causing drowning and submersion**

IQ 7 **W16.92X- Jumping or diving into unspecified water causing other injury**

4 **W17 Other fall from one level to another**

The appropriate 7th character is to be added to each code from category W17

A initial encounter

D subsequent encounter

S sequela

IQ 7 **W17.0XX- Fall into well**

IQ 7 **W17.1XX- Fall into storm drain or manhole**

IQ 7 **W17.2XX- Fall into hole**

Fall into pit

IQ 7 **W17.3XX- Fall into empty swimming pool**

EXCLUDES 1 fall into filled swimming pool (W16.0-)

IQ 7 **W17.4XX- Fall from dock**

5 **W17.8 Other fall from one level to another**

IQ 7 **W17.81X- Fall down embankment (hill)**

IQ 7 **W17.82X- Fall from (out of) grocery cart**

Fall due to grocery cart tipping over

IQ 7 **W17.89X- Other fall from one level to another**

Fall from cherry picker

Fall from lifting device

Fall from mobile elevated work platform [MEWP]

Fall from sky lift

4 **W18 Other slipping, tripping and stumbling and falls**

The appropriate 7th character is to be added to each code from category W18

A initial encounter

D subsequent encounter

S sequela

5 **W18.0 Fall due to bumping against object**

Striking against object with subsequent fall

EXCLUDES 1 fall on same level due to slipping, tripping, or stumbling with subsequent striking against object (W01.1-)

IQ 7 **W18.00X- Striking against unspecified object with subsequent fall**

IQ 7 **W18.01X- Striking against sports equipment with subsequent fall**

IQ 7 **W18.02X- Striking against glass with subsequent fall**

IQ 7 **W18.09X- Striking against other object with subsequent fall**

5 **W18.1 Fall from or off toilet**

IQ 7 **W18.11X- Fall from or off toilet without subsequent striking against object**

Fall from (off) toilet NOS

IQ 7 **W18.12X- Fall from or off toilet with subsequent striking against object**

IQ 7 **W18.2XX- Fall in (into) shower or empty bathtub**

EXCLUDES 1 fall in full bathtub causing drowning or submersion (W16.21-)

5 **W18.3 Other and unspecified fall on same level**

IQ ☒ **W18.30X- Fall on same level, unspecified**

IQ ☒ **W18.31X- Fall on same level due to stepping on an object**
Fall on same level due to stepping on an animal
EXCLUDES 1 slipping, tripping and stumbling without fall due to stepping on animal (W18.41)

IQ ☒ **W18.39X- Other fall on same level**

5 **W18.4 Slipping, tripping and stumbling without falling**
EXCLUDES 1 collision with another person without fall (W51)

IQ ☒ **W18.40X- Slipping, tripping and stumbling without falling, unspecified**

IQ ☒ **W18.41X- Slipping, tripping and stumbling without falling due to stepping on object**
Slipping, tripping and stumbling without falling due to stepping on animal
EXCLUDES 1 slipping, tripping and stumbling with fall due to stepping on animal (W18.31)

IQ ☒ **W18.42X- Slipping, tripping and stumbling without falling due to stepping into hole or opening**

IQ ☒ **W18.43X- Slipping, tripping and stumbling without falling due to stepping from one level to another**

IQ ☒ **W18.49X- Other slipping, tripping and stumbling without falling**

IQ ☒ **W19.XXX- Unspecified fall**
Accidental fall NOS

The appropriate 7th character is to be added to code W19
A initial encounter
D subsequent encounter
S sequela

Exposure to inanimate mechanical forces (W20-W49)

EXCLUDES 1 assault (X92-Y09)
contact or collision with animals or persons (W50-W64)
exposure to inanimate mechanical forces involving military or war operations (Y36.-, Y37.-)
intentional self-harm (X71-X83)

4 **W20 Struck by thrown, projected or falling object**
Code first any associated:
cataclysm (X34-X39)
lightning strike (T75.00)
EXCLUDES 1 falling object in machinery accident (W24, W28-W31)
falling object in transport accident (V01-V99)
object set in motion by explosion (W35-W40)
object set in motion by firearm (W32-W34)
struck by thrown sports equipment (W21.-)

The appropriate 7th character is to be added to each code from category W20
A initial encounter
D subsequent encounter
S sequela

IQ ☒ **W20.0XX- Struck by falling object in cave-in**
EXCLUDES 2 asphyxiation due to cave-in (T71.21)

IQ ☒ **W20.1XX- Struck by object due to collapse of building**
EXCLUDES 1 struck by object due to collapse of burning building (X00.2, X02.2)

IQ ☒ **W20.8XX- Other cause of strike by thrown, projected or falling object**
EXCLUDES 1 struck by thrown sports equipment (W21.-)

4 **W21 Striking against or struck by sports equipment**
EXCLUDES 1 assault with sports equipment (Y08.0-)
striking against or struck by sports equipment with subsequent fall (W18.01)

The appropriate 7th character is to be added to each code from category W21
A initial encounter
D subsequent encounter
S sequela

5 **W21.0 Struck by hit or thrown ball**

IQ ☒ **W21.00X- Struck by hit or thrown ball, unspecified type**

IQ ☒ **W21.01X- Struck by football**

IQ ☒ **W21.02X- Struck by soccer ball**

IQ ☒ **W21.03X- Struck by baseball**

IQ ☒ **W21.04X- Struck by golf ball**

IQ ☒ **W21.05X- Struck by basketball**

IQ ☒ **W21.06X- Struck by volleyball**

IQ ☒ **W21.07X- Struck by softball**

IQ ☒ **W21.09X- Struck by other hit or thrown ball**

5 **W21.1 Struck by bat, racquet or club**

IQ ☒ **W21.11X- Struck by baseball bat**

IQ ☒ **W21.12X- Struck by tennis racquet**

IQ ☒ **W21.13X- Struck by golf club**

IQ ☒ **W21.19X- Struck by other bat, racquet or club**

5 **W21.2 Struck by hockey stick or puck**

6 **W21.21 Struck by hockey stick**

IQ 7 **W21.210- Struck by ice hockey stick**

IQ 7 **W21.211- Struck by field hockey stick**

6 **W21.22 Struck by hockey puck**

IQ 7 **W21.220- Struck by ice hockey puck**

IQ 7 **W21.221- Struck by field hockey puck**

5 **W21.3 Struck by sports foot wear**

IQ ☒ **W21.31X- Struck by shoe cleats**
Stepped on by shoe cleats

IQ ☒ **W21.32X- Struck by skate blades**
Skated over by skate blades

IQ ☒ **W21.39X- Struck by other sports foot wear**

IQ + ☒ **W21.4XX- Striking against diving board**

Use additional code for subsequent falling into water, if applicable (W16.-)

5 **W21.8 Striking against or struck by other sports equipment**

IQ 7 **W21.81X- Striking against or struck by football helmet**

IQ 7 **W21.89X- Striking against or struck by other sports equipment**

IQ 7 **W21.9XX- Striking against or struck by unspecified sports equipment**

4 **W22 Striking against or struck by other objects**

EXCLUDES 1 striking against or struck by object with subsequent fall (W18.09)

The appropriate 7th character is to be added to each code from category W22
A initial encounter
D subsequent encounter
S sequela

5 **W22.0 Striking against stationary object**

EXCLUDES 1 striking against stationary sports equipment (W21.8)

IQ 7 **W22.01X- Walked into wall**

IQ 7 **W22.02X- Walked into lamppost**

IQ 7 **W22.03X- Walked into furniture**

6 **W22.04 Striking against wall of swimming pool**

IQ 7 **W22.041- Striking against wall of swimming pool causing drowning and submersion**

EXCLUDES 1 drowning and submersion while swimming without striking against wall (W67)

IQ 7 **W22.042- Striking against wall of swimming pool causing other injury**

IQ 7 **W22.09X- Striking against other stationary object**

5 **W22.1 Striking against or struck by automobile airbag**

IQ 7 **W22.10X- Striking against or struck by unspecified automobile airbag**

IQ 7 **W22.11X- Striking against or struck by driver side automobile airbag**

IQ 7 **W22.12X- Striking against or struck by front passenger side automobile airbag**

IQ 7 **W22.19X- Striking against or struck by other automobile airbag**

IQ 7 **W22.8XX- Striking against or struck by other objects**

Striking against or struck by object NOS

EXCLUDES 1 struck by thrown, projected or falling object (W20.-)

4 **W23 Caught, crushed, jammed or pinched in or between objects**

EXCLUDES 1 injury caused by cutting or piercing instruments (W25-W27)
injury caused by firearms malfunction (W32.1, W33.1-, W34.1-)
injury caused by lifting and transmission devices (W24.-)
injury caused by machinery (W28-W31)
injury caused by nonpowered hand tools (W27.-)
injury caused by transport vehicle being used as a means of transportation (V01-V99)
injury caused by struck by thrown, projected or falling object (W20.-)

The appropriate 7th character is to be added to each code from category W23
A initial encounter
D subsequent encounter
S sequela

IQ 7 **W23.0XX- Caught, crushed, jammed, or pinched between moving objects**

IQ 7 **W23.1XX- Caught, crushed, jammed, or pinched between stationary objects**

4 **W24 Contact with lifting and transmission devices, not elsewhere classified**

EXCLUDES 1 transport accidents (V01-V99)

The appropriate 7th character is to be added to each code from category W24
A initial encounter
D subsequent encounter
S sequela

IQ 7 **W24.0XX- Contact with lifting devices, not elsewhere classified**

Contact with chain hoist
Contact with drive belt
Contact with pulley (block)

IQ 7 **W24.1XX- Contact with transmission devices, not elsewhere classified**

Contact with transmission belt or cable

▲ IQ 7 **W25.XXX- Contact with sharp glass**

Code first any associated:
injury due to flying glass from explosion or firearm discharge (W32-W40)
transport accident (V00-V99)

EXCLUDES 1 fall on same level due to slipping, tripping and stumbling with subsequent striking against sharp glass (W01.110-)
striking against sharp glass with subsequent fall (W18.02-)

EXCLUDES 2 glass embedded in skin (W45.-)

The appropriate 7th character is to be added to code W25
A initial encounter
D subsequent encounter
S sequela

▲ 4 **W26 Contact with other sharp objects**

EXCLUDES 2 sharp object (s) embedded in skin (W45.-)

Chapter 20 V00-Y99

> The appropriate 7th character is to be added to each code from category W26
> A initial encounter
> D subsequent encounter
> S sequela

IQ ☑ **W26.0XX- Contact with knife**
EXCLUDES 1 contact with electric knife (W29.1)

IQ ☑ **W26.1XX- Contact with sword or dagger**

IQ ☑ **W26.2XX- Contact with edge of stiff paper**
Paper cut

IQ ☑ **W26.8XX- Contact with other sharp object(s), not elsewhere classified**
Contact with tin can lid

IQ ☑ **W26.9XX- Contact with unspecified sharp object(s)**

[4] **W27 Contact with nonpowered hand tool**

> The appropriate 7th character is to be added to each code from category W27
> A initial encounter
> D subsequent encounter
> S sequela

IQ ☑ **W27.0XX- Contact with workbench tool**
Contact with auger
Contact with axe
Contact with chisel
Contact with handsaw
Contact with screwdriver

IQ ☑ **W27.1XX- Contact with garden tool**
Contact with hoe
Contact with nonpowered lawn mower
Contact with pitchfork
Contact with rake

IQ ☑ **W27.2XX- Contact with scissors**

IQ ☑ **W27.3XX- Contact with needle (sewing)**
EXCLUDES 1 contact with hypodermic needle (W46.-)

IQ ☑ **W27.4XX- Contact with kitchen utensil**
Contact with fork
Contact with ice-pick
Contact with can-opener NOS

IQ ☑ **W27.5XX- Contact with paper-cutter**

IQ ☑ **W27.8XX- Contact with other nonpowered hand tool**
Contact with nonpowered sewing machine
Contact with shovel

IQ ☑ **W28.XXX- Contact with powered lawn mower**
Powered lawn mower (commercial) (residential)
EXCLUDES 1 contact with nonpowered lawn mower (W27.1)
EXCLUDES 2 exposure to electric current (W86.-)

> The appropriate 7th character is to be added to code W28
> A initial encounter
> D subsequent encounter
> S sequela

[4] **W29 Contact with other powered hand tools and household machinery**
EXCLUDES 1 contact with commercial machinery (W31.82)
contact with hot household appliance (X15)
contact with nonpowered hand tool (W27.-)
exposure to electric current (W86)

> The appropriate 7th character is to be added to each code from category W29
> A initial encounter
> D subsequent encounter
> S sequela

IQ ☑ **W29.0XX- Contact with powered kitchen appliance**
Contact with blender
Contact with can-opener
Contact with garbage disposal
Contact with mixer

IQ ☑ **W29.1XX- Contact with electric knife**

IQ ☑ **W29.2XX- Contact with other powered household machinery**
Contact with electric fan
Contact with powered dryer (clothes) (powered) (spin)
Contact with washing-machine
Contact with sewing machine

IQ ☑ **W29.3XX- Contact with powered garden and outdoor hand tools and machinery**
Contact with chainsaw
Contact with edger
Contact with garden cultivator (tiller)
Contact with hedge trimmer
Contact with other powered garden tool
EXCLUDES 1 contact with powered lawn mower (W28)

IQ ☑ **W29.4XX- Contact with nail gun**

IQ ☑ **W29.8XX- Contact with other powered hand tools and household machinery**
Contact with do-it-yourself tool NOS

[4] **W30 Contact with agricultural machinery**
INCLUDES animal-powered farm machine
EXCLUDES 1 agricultural transport vehicle accident (V01-V99)
explosion of grain store (W40.8)
exposure to electric current (W86.-)

> The appropriate 7th character is to be added to each code from category W30
> A initial encounter
> D subsequent encounter
> S sequela

IQ ☑ **W30.0XX- Contact with combine harvester**
Contact with reaper
Contact with thresher

IQ ☑ **W30.1XX- Contact with power take-off devices (PTO)**

IQ ☑ **W30.2XX- Contact with hay derrick**

IQ ☑ **W30.3XX- Contact with grain storage elevator**
EXCLUDES 1 explosion of grain store (W40.8)

[5] **W30.8 Contact with other specified agricultural machinery**

IQ ☑ **W30.81X- Contact with agricultural transport vehicle in stationary use**

Contact with agricultural transport vehicle under repair, not on public roadway

EXCLUDES 1 agricultural transport vehicle accident (V01-V99)

IQ 7 **W30.89X- Contact with other specified agricultural machinery**

IQ 7 **W30.9XX- Contact with unspecified agricultural machinery**

Contact with farm machinery NOS

4 **W31 Contact with other and unspecified machinery**

EXCLUDES 1 contact with agricultural machinery (W30.-)
contact with machinery in transport under own power or being towed by a vehicle (V01-V99)
exposure to electric current (W86)

The appropriate 7th character is to be added to each code from category W31
A initial encounter
D subsequent encounter
S sequela

IQ 7 **W31.0XX- Contact with mining and earth-drilling machinery**

Contact with bore or drill (land) (seabed)
Contact with shaft hoist
Contact with shaft lift
Contact with undercutter

IQ 7 **W31.1XX- Contact with metalworking machines**

Contact with abrasive wheel
Contact with forging machine
Contact with lathe
Contact with mechanical shears
Contact with metal drilling machine
Contact with milling machine
Contact with power press
Contact with rolling-mill
Contact with metal sawing machine

IQ 7 **W31.2XX- Contact with powered woodworking and forming machines**

Contact with band saw
Contact with bench saw
Contact with circular saw
Contact with molding machine
Contact with overhead plane
Contact with powered saw
Contact with radial saw
Contact with sander

EXCLUDES 1 nonpowered woodworking tools (W27.0)

IQ 7 **W31.3XX- Contact with prime movers**

Contact with gas turbine
Contact with internal combustion engine
Contact with steam engine
Contact with water driven turbine

5 **W31.8 Contact with other specified machinery**

IQ 7 **W31.81X- Contact with recreational machinery**

Contact with roller coaster

IQ 7 **W31.82X- Contact with other commercial machinery**

Contact with commercial electric fan
Contact with commercial kitchen appliances
Contact with commercial powered dryer (clothes) (powered) (spin)
Contact with commercial washing-machine
Contact with commercial sewing machine

EXCLUDES 1 contact with household machinery (W29.-)
contact with powered lawn mower (W28)

IQ 7 **W31.83X- Contact with special construction vehicle in stationary use**

Contact with special construction vehicle under repair, not on public roadway

EXCLUDES 1 special construction vehicle accident (V01-V99)

IQ 7 **W31.89X- Contact with other specified machinery**

IQ 7 **W31.9XX- Contact with unspecified machinery**

Contact with machinery NOS

4 **W32 Accidental handgun discharge and malfunction**

INCLUDES accidental discharge and malfunction of gun for single hand use
accidental discharge and malfunction of pistol
accidental discharge and malfunction of revolver
Handgun discharge and malfunction NOS

EXCLUDES 1 accidental airgun discharge and malfunction (W34.010, W34.110)
accidental BB gun discharge and malfunction (W34.010, W34.110)
accidental pellet gun discharge and malfunction (W34.010, W34.110)
accidental shotgun discharge and malfunction (W33.01, W33.11)
assault by handgun discharge (X93)
handgun discharge involving legal intervention (Y35.0-)
handgun discharge involving military or war operations (Y36.4-)
intentional self-harm by handgun discharge (X72)
Very pistol discharge and malfunction (W34.09, W34.19)

The appropriate 7th character is to be added to each code from category W32
A initial encounter
D subsequent encounter
S sequela

W32.0XX- Accidental handgun discharge

W32.1XX- Accidental handgun malfunction
Injury due to explosion of handgun (parts)
Injury due to malfunction of mechanism or component of handgun
Injury due to recoil of handgun
Powder burn from handgun

W33 Accidental rifle, shotgun and larger firearm discharge and malfunction

INCLUDES rifle, shotgun and larger firearm discharge and malfunction NOS

EXCLUDES 1 accidental airgun discharge and malfunction (W34.010, W34.110)
accidental BB gun discharge and malfunction (W34.010, W34.110)
accidental handgun discharge and malfunction (W32.-)
accidental pellet gun discharge and malfunction (W34.010, W34.110)
assault by rifle, shotgun and larger firearm discharge (X94)
firearm discharge involving legal intervention (Y35.0-)
firearm discharge involving military or war operations (Y36.4-)
intentional self-harm by rifle, shotgun and larger firearm discharge (X73)

The appropriate 7th character is to be added to each code from category W33
A initial encounter
D subsequent encounter
S sequela

W33.0 Accidental rifle, shotgun and larger firearm discharge

W33.00X- Accidental discharge of unspecified larger firearm
Discharge of unspecified larger firearm NOS

W33.01X- Accidental discharge of shotgun
Discharge of shotgun NOS

W33.02X- Accidental discharge of hunting rifle
Discharge of hunting rifle NOS

W33.03X- Accidental discharge of machine gun
Discharge of machine gun NOS

W33.09X- Accidental discharge of other larger firearm
Discharge of other larger firearm NOS

W33.1 Accidental rifle, shotgun and larger firearm malfunction
Injury due to explosion of rifle, shotgun and larger firearm (parts)
Injury due to malfunction of mechanism or component of rifle, shotgun and larger firearm
Injury due to piercing, cutting, crushing or pinching due to (by) slide trigger mechanism, scope or other gun part
Injury due to recoil of rifle, shotgun and larger firearm
Powder burn from rifle, shotgun and larger firearm

W33.10X- Accidental malfunction of unspecified larger firearm
Malfunction of unspecified larger firearm NOS

W33.11X- Accidental malfunction of shotgun
Malfunction of shotgun NOS

W33.12X- Accidental malfunction of hunting rifle
Malfunction of hunting rifle NOS

W33.13X- Accidental malfunction of machine gun
Malfunction of machine gun NOS

W33.19X- Accidental malfunction of other larger firearm
Malfunction of other larger firearm NOS

W34 Accidental discharge and malfunction from other and unspecified firearms and guns

The appropriate 7th character is to be added to each code from category W34
A initial encounter
D subsequent encounter
S sequela

W34.0 Accidental discharge from other and unspecified firearms and guns

W34.00X- Accidental discharge from unspecified firearms or gun
Discharge from firearm NOS
Gunshot wound NOS
Shot NOS

W34.01 Accidental discharge of gas, air or spring-operated guns

W34.010- Accidental discharge of airgun
Accidental discharge of BB gun
Accidental discharge of pellet gun

W34.011- Accidental discharge of paintball gun
Accidental injury due to paintball discharge

W34.018- Accidental discharge of other gas, air or spring-operated gun

W34.09X- Accidental discharge from other specified firearms
Accidental discharge from Very pistol [flare]

W34.1 Accidental malfunction from other and unspecified firearms and guns

W34.10X- Accidental malfunction from unspecified firearms or gun
Firearm malfunction NOS

W34.11 Accidental malfunction of gas, air or spring-operated guns

W34.110- Accidental malfunction of airgun
Accidental malfunction of BB gun

Accidental malfunction of pellet gun

IQ 7 **W34.111- Accidental malfunction of paintball gun**
Accidental injury due to paintball gun malfunction

IQ 7 **W34.118- Accidental malfunction of other gas, air or spring-operated gun**

IQ 7 **W34.19X- Accidental malfunction from other specified firearms**
Accidental malfunction from Very pistol [flare]

IQ 7 **W35.XXX- Explosion and rupture of boiler**
EXCLUDES 1 explosion and rupture of boiler on watercraft (V93.4)

The appropriate 7th character is to be added to code W35
A initial encounter
D subsequent encounter
S sequela

4 **W36 Explosion and rupture of gas cylinder**

The appropriate 7th character is to be added to each code from category W36
A initial encounter
D subsequent encounter
S sequela

IQ 7 **W36.1XX- Explosion and rupture of aerosol can**

IQ 7 **W36.2XX- Explosion and rupture of air tank**

IQ 7 **W36.3XX- Explosion and rupture of pressurized-gas tank**

IQ 7 **W36.8XX- Explosion and rupture of other gas cylinder**

IQ 7 **W36.9XX- Explosion and rupture of unspecified gas cylinder**

4 **W37 Explosion and rupture of pressurized tire, pipe or hose**

The appropriate 7th character is to be added to each code from category W37
A initial encounter
D subsequent encounter
S sequela

IQ 7 **W37.0XX- Explosion of bicycle tire**

IQ 7 **W37.8XX- Explosion and rupture of other pressurized tire, pipe or hose**

IQ 7 **W38.XXX- Explosion and rupture of other specified pressurized devices**

The appropriate 7th character is to be added to code W38
A initial encounter
D subsequent encounter
S sequela

IQ 7 **W39.XXX- Discharge of firework**

The appropriate 7th character is to be added to code W39
A initial encounter
D subsequent encounter
S sequela

4 **W40 Explosion of other materials**
EXCLUDES 1 assault by explosive material (X96)
explosion involving legal intervention (Y35.1-)
explosion involving military or war operations (Y36.0-, Y36.2-)
intentional self-harm by explosive material (X75)

The appropriate 7th character is to be added to each code from category W40
A initial encounter
D subsequent encounter
S sequela

IQ 7 **W40.0XX- Explosion of blasting material**
Explosion of blasting cap
Explosion of detonator
Explosion of dynamite
Explosion of explosive (any) used in blasting operations

IQ 7 **W40.1XX- Explosion of explosive gases**
Explosion of acetylene
Explosion of butane
Explosion of coal gas
Explosion in mine NOS
Explosion of explosive gas
Explosion of fire damp
Explosion of gasoline fumes
Explosion of methane
Explosion of propane

IQ 7 **W40.8XX- Explosion of other specified explosive materials**
Explosion in dump NOS
Explosion in factory NOS
Explosion in grain store
Explosion in munitions
EXCLUDES 1 explosion involving legal intervention (Y35.1-)
explosion involving military or war operations (Y36.0-, Y36.2-)

IQ 7 **W40.9XX- Explosion of unspecified explosive materials**
Explosion NOS

4 **W42 Exposure to noise**

The appropriate 7th character is to be added to each code from category W42
A initial encounter
D subsequent encounter
S sequela

IQ 7 **W42.0XX- Exposure to supersonic waves**

IQ 7 **W42.9XX- Exposure to other noise**
Exposure to sound waves NOS

4 **W45 Foreign body or object entering through skin**
INCLUDES foreign body or object embedded in skin
nail embedded in skin
EXCLUDES 2 contact with hand tools (nonpowered) (powered) (W27-W29)
contact with other sharp object(s) (W26.-)
contact with sharp glass (W25.-)
struck by objects (W20-W22)

Chapter 20 V00-Y99

The appropriate 7th character is to be added to each code from category W45
A   initial encounter
D   subsequent encounter
S   sequela

IQ ☑ W45.0XX- Nail entering through skin

IQ ☑ W45.8XX- Other foreign body or object entering through skin
Splinter in skin NOS

4 W46 Contact with hypodermic needle

The appropriate 7th character is to be added to each code from category W46
A   initial encounter
D   subsequent encounter
S   sequela

IQ ☑ W46.0XX- Contact with hypodermic needle
Hypodermic needle stick NOS

IQ ☑ W46.1XX- Contact with contaminated hypodermic needle

4 W49 Exposure to other inanimate mechanical forces

> INCLUDES   exposure to abnormal gravitational [G] forces
> exposure to inanimate mechanical forces NEC

> EXCLUDES 1   exposure to inanimate mechanical forces involving military or war operations (Y36.-, Y37.-)

The appropriate 7th character is to be added to each code from category W49
A   initial encounter
D   subsequent encounter
S   sequela

5 W49.0 Item causing external constriction

IQ ☑ W49.01X- Hair causing external constriction

IQ ☑ W49.02X- String or thread causing external constriction

IQ ☑ W49.03X- Rubber band causing external constriction

IQ ☑ W49.04X- Ring or other jewelry causing external constriction

IQ ☑ W49.09X- Other specified item causing external constriction

IQ ☑ W49.9XX- Exposure to other inanimate mechanical forces

Exposure to animate mechanical forces (W50-W64)

> EXCLUDES 1   Toxic effect of contact with venomous animals and plants (T63.-)

4 W50 Accidental hit, strike, kick, twist, bite or scratch by another person

> INCLUDES   hit, strike, kick, twist, bite, or scratch by another person NOS

> EXCLUDES 1   assault by bodily force (Y04)
> struck by objects (W20-W22)

The appropriate 7th character is to be added to each code from category W50
A   initial encounter
D   subsequent encounter
S   sequela

IQ ☑ W50.0XX- Accidental hit or strike by another person
Hit or strike by another person NOS

IQ ☑ W50.1XX- Accidental kick by another person
Kick by another person NOS

IQ ☑ W50.2XX- Accidental twist by another person
Twist by another person NOS

IQ ☑ W50.3XX- Accidental bite by another person
Human bite
Bite by another person NOS

IQ ☑ W50.4XX- Accidental scratch by another person
Scratch by another person NOS

IQ ☑ W51.XXX- Accidental striking against or bumped into by another person

> EXCLUDES 1   assault by striking against or bumping into by another person (Y04.2)
> fall due to collision with another person (W03)

The appropriate 7th character is to be added to code W51
A   initial encounter
D   subsequent encounter
S   sequela

IQ ☑ W52.XXX- Crushed, pushed or stepped on by crowd or human stampede
Crushed, pushed or stepped on by crowd or human stampede with or without fall

The appropriate 7th character is to be added to code W52
A   initial encounter
D   subsequent encounter
S   sequela

4 W53 Contact with rodent

> INCLUDES   contact with saliva, feces or urine of rodent

The appropriate 7th character is to be added to each code from category W53
A   initial encounter
D   subsequent encounter
S   sequela

5 W53.0 Contact with mouse

IQ ☑ W53.01X- Bitten by mouse

IQ ☑ W53.09X- Other contact with mouse

5 W53.1 Contact with rat

IQ ☑ W53.11X- Bitten by rat

IQ ☑ W53.19X- Other contact with rat

5 W53.2 Contact with squirrel

IQ ☑ W53.21X- Bitten by squirrel

IQ ☑ W53.29X- Other contact with squirrel

5 W53.8 Contact with other rodent

IQ ☑ W53.81X- Bitten by other rodent

IQ ☑ W53.89X- Other contact with other rodent

4 W54 Contact with dog

> INCLUDES   contact with saliva, feces or urine of dog

---

4 4th digit required   **5** 5th digit required   **6** 6th digit required   **7** 7th digit required   **☑** 7th digit placeholder   **+** Additional code   **⊟** Laterality

Chapter 20

V00-Y99

The appropriate 7th character is to be added to each code from category W54
A initial encounter
D subsequent encounter
S sequela

IQ 7 **W54.0XX- Bitten by dog**

IQ 7 **W54.1XX- Struck by dog**
Knocked over by dog

IQ 7 **W54.8XX- Other contact with dog**

4 **W55 Contact with other mammals**

INCLUDES contact with saliva, feces or urine of mammal

EXCLUDES 1 animal being ridden- see transport accidents
bitten or struck by dog (W54)
bitten or struck by rodent (W53.-)
contact with marine mammals (W56.-)

The appropriate 7th character is to be added to each code from category W55
A initial encounter
D subsequent encounter
S sequela

5 **W55.0 Contact with cat**

IQ 7 **W55.01X- Bitten by cat**

IQ 7 **W55.03X- Scratched by cat**

IQ 7 **W55.09X- Other contact with cat**

5 **W55.1 Contact with horse**

IQ 7 **W55.11X- Bitten by horse**

IQ 7 **W55.12X- Struck by horse**

IQ 7 **W55.19X- Other contact with horse**

5 **W55.2 Contact with cow**
Contact with bull

IQ 7 **W55.21X- Bitten by cow**

IQ 7 **W55.22X- Struck by cow**
Gored by bull

IQ 7 **W55.29X- Other contact with cow**

5 **W55.3 Contact with other hoof stock**
Contact with goats
Contact with sheep

IQ 7 **W55.31X- Bitten by other hoof stock**

IQ 7 **W55.32X- Struck by other hoof stock**
Gored by goat
Gored by ram

IQ 7 **W55.39X- Other contact with other hoof stock**

5 **W55.4 Contact with pig**

IQ 7 **W55.41X- Bitten by pig**

IQ 7 **W55.42X- Struck by pig**

IQ 7 **W55.49X- Other contact with pig**

5 **W55.5 Contact with raccoon**

IQ 7 **W55.51X- Bitten by raccoon**

IQ 7 **W55.52X- Struck by raccoon**

IQ 7 **W55.59X- Other contact with raccoon**

5 **W55.8 Contact with other mammals**

IQ 7 **W55.81X- Bitten by other mammals**

IQ 7 **W55.82X- Struck by other mammals**

IQ 7 **W55.89X- Other contact with other mammals**

4 **W56 Contact with nonvenomous marine animal**

EXCLUDES 1 contact with venomous marine animal (T63.-)

The appropriate 7th character is to be added to each code from category W56
A initial encounter
D subsequent encounter
S sequela

5 **W56.0 Contact with dolphin**

IQ 7 **W56.01X- Bitten by dolphin**

IQ 7 **W56.02X- Struck by dolphin**

IQ 7 **W56.09X- Other contact with dolphin**

5 **W56.1 Contact with sea lion**

IQ 7 **W56.11X- Bitten by sea lion**

IQ 7 **W56.12X- Struck by sea lion**

IQ 7 **W56.19X- Other contact with sea lion**

5 **W56.2 Contact with orca**
Contact with killer whale

IQ 7 **W56.21X- Bitten by orca**

IQ 7 **W56.22X- Struck by orca**

IQ 7 **W56.29X- Other contact with orca**

5 **W56.3 Contact with other marine mammals**

IQ 7 **W56.31X- Bitten by other marine mammals**

IQ 7 **W56.32X- Struck by other marine mammals**

IQ 7 **W56.39X- Other contact with other marine mammals**

5 **W56.4 Contact with shark**

IQ 7 **W56.41X- Bitten by shark**

IQ 7 **W56.42X- Struck by shark**

IQ 7 **W56.49X- Other contact with shark**

5 **W56.5 Contact with other fish**

IQ 7 **W56.51X- Bitten by other fish**

IQ 7 **W56.52X- Struck by other fish**

IQ 7 **W56.59X- Other contact with other fish**

5 **W56.8 Contact with other nonvenomous marine animals**

IQ 7 **W56.81X- Bitten by other nonvenomous marine animals**

IQ 7 **W56.82X- Struck by other nonvenomous marine animals**

IQ 7 **W56.89X- Other contact with other nonvenomous marine animals**

IQ 7 **W57.XXX- Bitten or stung by nonvenomous insect and other nonvenomous arthropods**

EXCLUDES 1 contact with venomous insects and arthropods (T63.2-, T63.3-, T63.4-)

The appropriate 7th character is to be added to code W57
A initial encounter
D subsequent encounter
S sequela

4 **W58 Contact with crocodile or alligator**

The appropriate 7th character is to be added to each code from category W58
A initial encounter
D subsequent encounter
S sequela

5 **W58.0 Contact with alligator**

W58.01X- Bitten by alligator
W58.02X- Struck by alligator
W58.03X- Crushed by alligator
W58.09X- Other contact with alligator
W58.1 Contact with crocodile
W58.11X- Bitten by crocodile
W58.12X- Struck by crocodile
W58.13X- Crushed by crocodile
W58.19X- Other contact with crocodile

W59 Contact with other nonvenomous reptiles
EXCLUDES 1 contact with venomous reptile (T63.0-, T63.1-)

The appropriate 7th character is to be added to each code from category W59
A initial encounter
D subsequent encounter
S sequela

W59.0 Contact with nonvenomous lizards
W59.01X- Bitten by nonvenomous lizards
W59.02X- Struck by nonvenomous lizards
W59.09X- Other contact with nonvenomous lizards
Exposure to nonvenomous lizards
W59.1 Contact with nonvenomous snakes
W59.11X- Bitten by nonvenomous snake
W59.12X- Struck by nonvenomous snake
W59.13X- Crushed by nonvenomous snake
W59.19X- Other contact with nonvenomous snake
W59.2 Contact with turtles
EXCLUDES 1 contact with tortoises (W59.8-)
W59.21X- Bitten by turtle
W59.22X- Struck by turtle
W59.29X- Other contact with turtle
Exposure to turtles
W59.8 Contact with other nonvenomous reptiles
W59.81X- Bitten by other nonvenomous reptiles
W59.82X- Struck by other nonvenomous reptiles
W59.83X- Crushed by other nonvenomous reptiles
W59.89X- Other contact with other nonvenomous reptiles

W60.XXX- Contact with nonvenomous plant thorns and spines and sharp leaves
EXCLUDES 1 Contact with venomous plants (T63.7-)

The appropriate 7th character is to be added to code W60
A initial encounter
D subsequent encounter
S sequela

W61 Contact with birds (domestic) (wild)
INCLUDES contact with excreta of birds

The appropriate 7th character is to be added to each code from category W61
A initial encounter
D subsequent encounter
S sequela

W61.0 Contact with parrot
W61.01X- Bitten by parrot
W61.02X- Struck by parrot
W61.09X- Other contact with parrot
Exposure to parrots
W61.1 Contact with macaw
W61.11X- Bitten by macaw
W61.12X- Struck by macaw
W61.19X- Other contact with macaw
Exposure to macaws
W61.2 Contact with other psittacines
W61.21X- Bitten by other psittacines
W61.22X- Struck by other psittacines
W61.29X- Other contact with other psittacines
Exposure to other psittacines
W61.3 Contact with chicken
W61.32X- Struck by chicken
W61.33X- Pecked by chicken
W61.39X- Other contact with chicken
Exposure to chickens
W61.4 Contact with turkey
W61.42X- Struck by turkey
W61.43X- Pecked by turkey
W61.49X- Other contact with turkey
W61.5 Contact with goose
W61.51X- Bitten by goose
W61.52X- Struck by goose
W61.59X- Other contact with goose
W61.6 Contact with duck
W61.61X- Bitten by duck
W61.62X- Struck by duck
W61.69X- Other contact with duck
W61.9 Contact with other birds
W61.91X- Bitten by other birds
W61.92X- Struck by other birds
W61.99X- Other contact with other birds
Contact with bird NOS

W62 Contact with nonvenomous amphibians
EXCLUDES 1 contact with venomous amphibians (T63.81-R63.83)

The appropriate 7th character is to be added to each code from category W62
A initial encounter
D subsequent encounter
S sequela

W62.0XX- Contact with nonvenomous frogs
W62.1XX- Contact with nonvenomous toads
W62.9XX- Contact with other nonvenomous amphibians

W64.XXX- Exposure to other animate mechanical forces
INCLUDES exposure to nonvenomous animal NOS

EXCLUDES 1 contact with venomous animal (T63.-)

The appropriate 7th character is to be added to code W64
A initial encounter
D subsequent encounter
S sequela

Accidental non-transport drowning and submersion (W65-W74)

EXCLUDES 1 accidental drowning and submersion due to fall into water (W16.-)
accidental drowning and submersion due to water transport accident (V90.-, V92.-)

EXCLUDES 2 accidental drowning and submersion due to cataclysm (X34-X39)

IQ 7 **W65.XXX- Accidental drowning and submersion while in bath-tub**

EXCLUDES 1 accidental drowning and submersion due to fall in (into) bathtub (W16.211)

The appropriate 7th character is to be added to code W65
A initial encounter
D subsequent encounter
S sequela

IQ 7 **W67.XXX- Accidental drowning and submersion while in swimming-pool**

EXCLUDES 1 accidental drowning and submersion due to fall into swimming pool (W16.011, W16.021, W16.031)
accidental drowning and submersion due to striking into wall of swimming pool (W22.041)

The appropriate 7th character is to be added to code W67
A initial encounter
D subsequent encounter
S sequela

IQ 7 **W69.XXX- Accidental drowning and submersion while in natural water**

Accidental drowning and submersion while in lake
Accidental drowning and submersion while in open sea
Accidental drowning and submersion while in river
Accidental drowning and submersion while in stream

EXCLUDES 1 accidental drowning and submersion due to fall into natural body of water (W16.111, W16.121, W16.131)

The appropriate 7th character is to be added to code W69
A initial encounter
D subsequent encounter
S sequela

IQ 7 **W73.XXX- Other specified cause of accidental non-transport drowning and submersion**

Accidental drowning and submersion while in quenching tank
Accidental drowning and submersion while in reservoir

EXCLUDES 1 accidental drowning and submersion due to fall into other water (W16.311, W16.321, W16.331)

The appropriate 7th character is to be added to code W73
A initial encounter
D subsequent encounter
S sequela

IQ 7 **W74.XXX- Unspecified cause of accidental drowning and submersion**

Drowning NOS

The appropriate 7th character is to be added to code W74
A initial encounter
D subsequent encounter
S sequela

Exposure to electric current, radiation and extreme ambient air temperature and pressure (W85-W99)

EXCLUDES 1 exposure to:
failure in dosage of radiation or temperature during surgical and medical care (Y63.2-Y63.5)
lightning (T75.0-)
natural cold (X31)
natural heat (X30)
natural radiation NOS (X39)
radiological procedure and radiotherapy (Y84.2)
sunlight (X32)

IQ 7 **W85.XXX- Exposure to electric transmission lines**

Broken power line

The appropriate 7th character is to be added to code W85
A initial encounter
D subsequent encounter
S sequela

4 **W86 Exposure to other specified electric current**

The appropriate 7th character is to be added to each code from category W86
A initial encounter
D subsequent encounter
S sequela

IQ 7 **W86.0XX- Exposure to domestic wiring and appliances**

IQ 7 **W86.1XX- Exposure to industrial wiring, appliances and electrical machinery**

Exposure to conductors

Chapter 20

V00-Y99

Exposure to control apparatus
Exposure to electrical equipment and
machinery
Exposure to transformers

!Q ☑ W86.8XX- Exposure to other electric current
Exposure to wiring and appliances in
or on farm (not farmhouse)
Exposure to wiring and appliances
outdoors
Exposure to wiring and appliances in
or on public building
Exposure to wiring and appliances in
or on residential institutions
Exposure to wiring and appliances in
or on schools

4 W88   Exposure to ionizing radiation
EXCLUDES 1   exposure to sunlight (X32)

The appropriate 7th character is to be added to
each code from category W88
A   initial encounter
D   subsequent encounter
S   sequela

!Q ☑ W88.0XX- Exposure to X-rays

!Q ☑ W88.1XX- Exposure to radioactive isotopes

**!Q ☑ W88.8XX- Exposure to other ionizing
radiation**

**4 W89   Exposure to man-made visible and
ultraviolet light**
INCLUDES   exposure to welding light (arc)
EXCLUDES 2   exposure to sunlight (X32)

The appropriate 7th character is to be added to
each code from category W89
A   initial encounter
D   subsequent encounter
S   sequela

!Q ☑ W89.0XX- Exposure to welding light (arc)

!Q ☑ W89.1XX- Exposure to tanning bed

**!Q ☑ W89.8XX- Exposure to other man-made
visible and ultraviolet light**

**!Q ☑ W89.9XX- Exposure to unspecified man-
made visible and ultraviolet light**

4 W90   Exposure to other nonionizing radiation
EXCLUDES 2   exposure to sunlight (X32)

The appropriate 7th character is to be added to
each code from category W90
A   initial encounter
D   subsequent encounter
S   sequela

!Q ☑ W90.0XX- Exposure to radiofrequency

!Q ☑ W90.1XX- Exposure to infrared radiation

!Q ☑ W90.2XX- Exposure to laser radiation

**!Q ☑ W90.8XX- Exposure to other nonionizing
radiation**

**!Q ☑ W92.XXX- Exposure to excessive heat of man-
made origin**

The appropriate 7th character is to be
added to code W92
A   initial encounter
D   subsequent encounter
S   sequela

**4 W93   Exposure to excessive cold of man-made
origin**

The appropriate 7th character is to be added to
each code from category W93
A   initial encounter
D   subsequent encounter
S   sequela

5 W93.0 Contact with or inhalation of dry ice

!Q ☑ W93.01X- Contact with dry ice

!Q ☑ W93.02X- Inhalation of dry ice

5 W93.1 Contact with or inhalation of liquid air

!Q ☑ W93.11X- Contact with liquid air
Contact with liquid hydrogen
Contact with liquid nitrogen

!Q ☑ W93.12X- Inhalation of liquid air
Inhalation of liquid hydrogen
Inhalation of liquid nitrogen

**!Q ☑ W93.2XX- Prolonged exposure in deep freeze
unit or refrigerator**

**!Q ☑ W93.8XX- Exposure to other excessive cold of
man-made origin**

**4 W94   Exposure to high and low air pressure and
changes in air pressure**

The appropriate 7th character is to be added to
each code from category W94
A   initial encounter
D   subsequent encounter
S   sequela

**!Q ☑ W94.0XX- Exposure to prolonged high air
pressure**

5 W94.1 Exposure to prolonged low air pressure

**!Q ☑ W94.11X- Exposure to residence or
prolonged visit at high altitude**

**!Q ☑ W94.12X- Exposure to other prolonged low
air pressure**

**5 W94.2 Exposure to rapid changes in air
pressure during ascent**

**!Q ☑ W94.21X- Exposure to reduction in
atmospheric pressure while
surfacing from deep-water diving**

**!Q ☑ W94.22X- Exposure to reduction in
atmospheric pressure while
surfacing from underground**

**!Q ☑ W94.23X- Exposure to sudden change in air
pressure in aircraft during ascent**

**!Q ☑ W94.29X- Exposure to other rapid changes
in air pressure during ascent**

**5 W94.3 Exposure to rapid changes in air
pressure during descent**

**!Q ☑ W94.31X- Exposure to sudden change in air
pressure in aircraft during descent**

**!Q ☑ W94.32X- Exposure to high air pressure
from rapid descent in water**

**!Q ☑ W94.39X- Exposure to other rapid changes
in air pressure during descent**

**!Q ☑ W99.XXX- Exposure to other man-made
environmental factors**

The appropriate 7th character is to be
added to code W99
A   initial encounter
D   subsequent encounter
S   sequela

4 4th digit required   5 5th digit required   6 6th digit required   7 7th digit required   ☑ 7th digit placeholder   ✚ Additional code   ⊟ Laterality

Exposure to smoke, fire and flames (X00-X08)

EXCLUDES 1 arson (X97)

EXCLUDES 2 explosions (W35-W40)
lightning (T75.0-)
transport accident (V01-V99)

4 X00 **Exposure to uncontrolled fire in building or structure**

INCLUDES conflagration in building or structure

Code first:
any associated cataclysm

EXCLUDES 2 Exposure to ignition or melting of nightwear (X05)
Exposure to ignition or melting of other clothing and apparel (X06.-)
Exposure to other specified smoke, fire and flames (X08.-)

The appropriate 7th character is to be added to each code from category X00
A   initial encounter
D   subsequent encounter
S   sequela

!Q ☑ X00.0XX- **Exposure to flames in uncontrolled fire in building or structure**

!Q ☑ X00.1XX- **Exposure to smoke in uncontrolled fire in building or structure**

!Q ☑ X00.2XX- **Injury due to collapse of burning building or structure in uncontrolled fire**

EXCLUDES 1 injury due to collapse of building not on fire (W20.1)

!Q ☑ X00.3XX- **Fall from burning building or structure in uncontrolled fire**

!Q ☑ X00.4XX- **Hit by object from burning building or structure in uncontrolled fire**

!Q ☑ X00.5XX- **Jump from burning building or structure in uncontrolled fire**

!Q ☑ X00.8XX- **Other exposure to uncontrolled fire in building or structure**

4 X01 **Exposure to uncontrolled fire, not in building or structure**

INCLUDES exposure to forest fire

The appropriate 7th character is to be added to each code from category X01
A   initial encounter
D   subsequent encounter
S   sequela

!Q ☑ X01.0XX- **Exposure to flames in uncontrolled fire, not in building or structure**

!Q ☑ X01.1XX- **Exposure to smoke in uncontrolled fire, not in building or structure**

!Q ☑ X01.3XX- **Fall due to uncontrolled fire, not in building or structure**

!Q ☑ X01.4XX- **Hit by object due to uncontrolled fire, not in building or structure**

!Q ☑ X01.8XX- **Other exposure to uncontrolled fire, not in building or structure**

4 X02 **Exposure to controlled fire in building or structure**

INCLUDES exposure to fire in fireplace
exposure to fire in stove

The appropriate 7th character is to be added to each code from category X02
A   initial encounter
D   subsequent encounter
S   sequela

!Q ☑ X02.0XX- **Exposure to flames in controlled fire in building or structure**

!Q ☑ X02.1XX- **Exposure to smoke in controlled fire in building or structure**

!Q ☑ X02.2XX- **Injury due to collapse of burning building or structure in controlled fire**

EXCLUDES 1 injury due to collapse of building not on fire (W20.1)

!Q ☑ X02.3XX- **Fall from burning building or structure in controlled fire**

!Q ☑ X02.4XX- **Hit by object from burning building or structure in controlled fire**

!Q ☑ X02.5XX- **Jump from burning building or structure in controlled fire**

!Q ☑ X02.8XX- **Other exposure to controlled fire in building or structure**

4 X03 **Exposure to controlled fire, not in building or structure**

INCLUDES exposure to bon fire
exposure to camp-fire
exposure to trash fire

The appropriate 7th character is to be added to each code from category X03
A   initial encounter
D   subsequent encounter
S   sequela

!Q ☑ X03.0XX- **Exposure to flames in controlled fire, not in building or structure**

!Q ☑ X03.1XX- **Exposure to smoke in controlled fire, not in building or structure**

!Q ☑ X03.3XX- **Fall due to controlled fire, not in building or structure**

!Q ☑ X03.4XX- **Hit by object due to controlled fire, not in building or structure**

!Q ☑ X03.8XX- **Other exposure to controlled fire, not in building or structure**

!Q ☑ X04.XXX- **Exposure to ignition of highly flammable material**
Exposure to ignition of gasoline
Exposure to ignition of kerosene
Exposure to ignition of petrol

EXCLUDES 2 exposure to ignition or melting of nightwear (X05)
exposure to ignition or melting of other clothing and apparel (X06)

The appropriate 7th character is to be added to code X04
A   initial encounter
D   subsequent encounter
S   sequela

!Q ☑ X05.XXX- **Exposure to ignition or melting of nightwear**

★ New ▲ Revised Px Primary SP PDGM Px SL Low CoM SH High CoM !Q Quest. Encounter H Hospice non-cancer Dx Unspecified M *Manifestation*

EXCLUDES 2 exposure to uncontrolled fire in building or structure (X00.-)
exposure to uncontrolled fire, not in building or structure (X01.-)
exposure to controlled fire in building or structure (X02.-)
exposure to controlled fire, not in building or structure (X03.-)
exposure to ignition of highly flammable materials (X04.-)

The appropriate 7th character is to be added to code X05
A initial encounter
D subsequent encounter
S sequela

4 **X06 Exposure to ignition or melting of other clothing and apparel**

EXCLUDES 2 exposure to uncontrolled fire in building or structure (X00.-)
exposure to uncontrolled fire, not in building or structure (X01.-)
exposure to controlled fire in building or structure (X02.-)
exposure to controlled fire, not in building or structure (X03.-)
exposure to ignition of highly flammable materials (X04.-)

The appropriate 7th character is to be added to each code from category X06
A initial encounter
D subsequent encounter
S sequela

IQ 7 **X06.0XX- Exposure to ignition of plastic jewelry**
IQ 7 **X06.1XX- Exposure to melting of plastic jewelry**
IQ 7 **X06.2XX- Exposure to ignition of other clothing and apparel**
IQ 7 **X06.3XX- Exposure to melting of other clothing and apparel**

4 **X08 Exposure to other specified smoke, fire and flames**

The appropriate 7th character is to be added to each code from category X08
A initial encounter
D subsequent encounter
S sequela

5 **X08.0 Exposure to bed fire**
Exposure to mattress fire

IQ 7 **X08.00X- Exposure to bed fire due to unspecified burning material**
IQ 7 **X08.01X- Exposure to bed fire due to burning cigarette**
IQ 7 **X08.09X- Exposure to bed fire due to other burning material**

5 **X08.1 Exposure to sofa fire**

IQ 7 **X08.10X- Exposure to sofa fire due to unspecified burning material**
IQ 7 **X08.11X- Exposure to sofa fire due to burning cigarette**
IQ 7 **X08.19X- Exposure to sofa fire due to other burning material**

5 **X08.2 Exposure to other furniture fire**

IQ 7 **X08.20X- Exposure to other furniture fire due to unspecified burning material**
IQ 7 **X08.21X- Exposure to other furniture fire due to burning cigarette**
IQ 7 **X08.29X- Exposure to other furniture fire due to other burning material**

IQ 7 **X08.8XX- Exposure to other specified smoke, fire and flames**

Contact with heat and hot substances (X10-X19)

EXCLUDES 1 exposure to excessive natural heat (X30)
exposure to fire and flames (X00-X08)

4 **X10 Contact with hot drinks, food, fats and cooking oils**

The appropriate 7th character is to be added to each code from category X10
A initial encounter
D subsequent encounter
S sequela

IQ 7 **X10.0XX- Contact with hot drinks**
IQ 7 **X10.1XX- Contact with hot food**
IQ 7 **X10.2XX- Contact with fats and cooking oils**

4 **X11 Contact with hot tap-water**

INCLUDES contact with boiling tap-water
contact with boiling water NOS

EXCLUDES 1 contact with water heated on stove (X12)

The appropriate 7th character is to be added to each code from category X11
A initial encounter
D subsequent encounter
S sequela

IQ 7 **X11.0XX- Contact with hot water in bath or tub**
EXCLUDES 1 contact with running hot water in bath or tub (X11.1)

IQ 7 **X11.1XX- Contact with running hot water**
Contact with hot water running out of hose
Contact with hot water running out of tap

IQ 7 **X11.8XX- Contact with other hot tap-water**
Contact with hot water in bucket
Contact with hot tap-water NOS

IQ 7 **X12.XXX- Contact with other hot fluids**
Contact with water heated on stove
EXCLUDES 1 hot (liquid) metals (X18)

The appropriate 7th character is to be added to code X12
A initial encounter
D subsequent encounter
S sequela

4 **X13 Contact with steam and other hot vapors**

Chapter 20

V00-Y99

The appropriate 7th character is to be added to each code from category X13
A   initial encounter
D   subsequent encounter
S   sequela

IQ ☑ X13.0XX- **Inhalation of steam and other hot vapors**

IQ ☑ X13.1XX- **Other contact with steam and other hot vapors**

④ X14 **Contact with hot air and other hot gases**

The appropriate 7th character is to be added to each code from category X14
A   initial encounter
D   subsequent encounter
S   sequela

IQ ☑ X14.0XX- **Inhalation of hot air and gases**

IQ ☑ X14.1XX- **Other contact with hot air and other hot gases**

④ X15 **Contact with hot household appliances**
EXCLUDES 1   contact with heating appliances (X16)
contact with powered household appliances (W29.-)
exposure to controlled fire in building or structure due to household appliance (X02.8)
exposure to household appliances electrical current (W86.0)

The appropriate 7th character is to be added to each code from category X15
A   initial encounter
D   subsequent encounter
S   sequela

IQ ☑ X15.0XX- **Contact with hot stove (kitchen)**

IQ ☑ X15.1XX- **Contact with hot toaster**

IQ ☑ X15.2XX- **Contact with hotplate**

IQ ☑ X15.3XX- **Contact with hot saucepan or skillet**

IQ ☑ X15.8XX- **Contact with other hot household appliances**
Contact with cooker
Contact with kettle
Contact with light bulbs

IQ ☑ X16.XXX- **Contact with hot heating appliances, radiators and pipes**
EXCLUDES 1   contact with powered appliances (W29.-)
exposure to controlled fire in building or structure due to appliance (X02.8)
exposure to industrial appliances electrical current (W86.1)

The appropriate 7th character is to be added to code X16
A   initial encounter
D   subsequent encounter
S   sequela

IQ ☑ X17.XXX- **Contact with hot engines, machinery and tools**
EXCLUDES 1   contact with hot heating appliances, radiators and pipes (X16)

contact with hot household appliances (X15)

The appropriate 7th character is to be added to code X17
A   initial encounter
D   subsequent encounter
S   sequela

IQ ☑ X18.XXX- **Contact with other hot metals**
Contact with liquid metal

The appropriate 7th character is to be added to code X18
A   initial encounter
D   subsequent encounter
S   sequela

IQ ☑ X19.XXX- **Contact with other heat and hot substances**
EXCLUDES 1   objects that are not normally hot, e.g., an object made hot by a house fire (X00-X08)

The appropriate 7th character is to be added to code X19
A   initial encounter
D   subsequent encounter
S   sequela

Exposure to forces of nature (X30-X39)

IQ ☑ X30.XXX- **Exposure to excessive natural heat**
Exposure to excessive heat as the cause of sunstroke
Exposure to heat NOS
EXCLUDES 1   excessive heat of man-made origin (W92)
exposure to man-made radiation (W89)
exposure to sunlight (X32)
exposure to tanning bed (W89)

The appropriate 7th character is to be added to code X30
A   initial encounter
D   subsequent encounter
S   sequela

IQ ☑ X31.XXX- **Exposure to excessive natural cold**
Excessive cold as the cause of chilblains NOS
Excessive cold as the cause of immersion foot or hand
Exposure to cold NOS
Exposure to weather conditions
EXCLUDES 1   cold of man-made origin (W93.-)
contact with or inhalation of dry ice (W93.-)
contact with or inhalation of liquefied gas (W93.-)

Chapter 20

V00-Y99

★ New ▲ Revised Px Primary SP PDGM Px SL Low CoM SH High CoM IQ Quest. Encounter H Hospice non-cancer Dx Unspecified M Manifestation

The appropriate 7th character is to be added to code X31
A initial encounter
D subsequent encounter
S sequela

X32.XXX- Exposure to sunlight
EXCLUDES 1 man-made radiation (tanning bed) (W89)
EXCLUDES 2 radiation-related disorders of the skin and subcutaneous tissue (L55-L59)

The appropriate 7th character is to be added to code X32
A initial encounter
D subsequent encounter
S sequela

X34.XXX- Earthquake
EXCLUDES 2 tidal wave (tsunami) due to earthquake (X37.41)

The appropriate 7th character is to be added to code X34
A initial encounter
D subsequent encounter
S sequela

X35.XXX- Volcanic eruption
EXCLUDES 2 tidal wave (tsunami) due to volcanic eruption (X37.41)

The appropriate 7th character is to be added to code X35
A initial encounter
D subsequent encounter
S sequela

X36 Avalanche, landslide and other earth movements
INCLUDES victim of mudslide of cataclysmic nature
EXCLUDES 1 earthquake (X34)
EXCLUDES 2 transport accident involving collision with avalanche or landslide not in motion (V01-V99)

The appropriate 7th character is to be added to each code from category X36
A initial encounter
D subsequent encounter
S sequela

X36.0XX- Collapse of dam or man-made structure causing earth movement
X36.1XX- Avalanche, landslide, or mudslide
X37 Cataclysmic storm

The appropriate 7th character is to be added to each code from category X37
A initial encounter
D subsequent encounter
S sequela

X37.0XX- Hurricane
Storm surge
Typhoon
X37.1XX- Tornado
Cyclone
Twister
X37.2XX- Blizzard (snow)(ice)
X37.3XX- Dust storm
X37.4 Tidalwave
X37.41X- Tidal wave due to earthquake or volcanic eruption
Tidal wave NOS
Tsunami
X37.42X- Tidal wave due to storm
X37.43X- Tidal wave due to landslide
X37.8XX- Other cataclysmic storms
Cloudburst
Torrential rain
EXCLUDES 2 flood (X38)
X37.9XX- Unspecified cataclysmic storm
Storm NOS
EXCLUDES 1 collapse of dam or man-made structure causing earth movement (X36.0)
X38.XXX- Flood
Flood arising from remote storm
Flood of cataclysmic nature arising from melting snow
Flood resulting directly from storm
EXCLUDES 1 collapse of dam or man-made structure causing earth movement (X36.0)
tidal wave NOS (X37.41)
tidal wave caused by storm (X37.42)

The appropriate 7th character is to be added to code X38
A initial encounter
D subsequent encounter
S sequela

X39 Exposure to other forces of nature

The appropriate 7th character is to be added to each code from category X39
A initial encounter
D subsequent encounter
S sequela

X39.0 Exposure to natural radiation
EXCLUDES 1 contact with and (suspected) exposure to radon and other naturally occurring radiation (Z77.123)
exposure to man-made radiation (W88-W90)
exposure to sunlight (X32)
X39.01X- Exposure to radon
X39.08X- Exposure to other natural radiation
X39.8XX- Other exposure to forces of nature

Overexertion and strenuous or repetitive movements (X50)

X50 Overexertion and strenuous or repetitive movements

Chapter 20
V00-Y99

4th digit required 5th digit required 6th digit required 7th digit required 7th digit placeholder +Additional code Laterality

The appropriate 7th character is to be added to each code from category X50
A initial encounter
D subsequent encounter
S sequela

IQ X50.0XX- **Overexertion from strenuous movement or load**
Lifting heavy objects
Lifting weights

IQ X50.1XX- **Overexertion from prolonged static or awkward postures**
Prolonged bending
Prolonged kneeling
Prolonged reaching
Prolonged sitting
Prolonged standing
Prolonged twisting
Static bending
Static kneeling
Static reaching
Static sitting
Static standing
Static twisting

IQ X50.3XX- **Overexertion from repetitive movements**
Use of hand as hammer
EXCLUDES 2 Overuse from prolonged static or awkward postures (X50.1)

IQ X50.9XX- **Other and unspecified overexertion or strenuous movements or postures**
Contact pressure
Contact stress

Accidental exposure to other specified factors (X52-X58)

IQ X52.XXX- **Prolonged stay in weightless environment**
Weightlessness in spacecraft (simulator)

The appropriate 7th character is to be added to code X52
A initial encounter
D subsequent encounter
S sequela

IQ X58.XXX- **Exposure to other specified factors**
Accident NOS
Exposure NOS

The appropriate 7th character is to be added to code X58
A initial encounter
D subsequent encounter
S sequela

Intentional self-harm (X71-X83)

Purposely self-inflicted injury
Suicide (attempted)

CODING TIPS Do not assign a code for intentional self harm as an external cause of morbidity when there is no injury coded on the claim.

4 X71 **Intentional self-harm by drowning and submersion**

The appropriate 7th character is to be added to each code from category X71
A initial encounter
D subsequent encounter
S sequela

IQ X71.0XX- **Intentional self-harm by drowning and submersion while in bathtub**

IQ X71.1XX- **Intentional self-harm by drowning and submersion while in swimming pool**

IQ X71.2XX- **Intentional self-harm by drowning and submersion after jump into swimming pool**

IQ X71.3XX- **Intentional self-harm by drowning and submersion in natural water**

IQ X71.8XX- **Other intentional self-harm by drowning and submersion**

IQ X71.9XX- **Intentional self-harm by drowning and submersion, unspecified**

IQ X72.XXX- **Intentional self-harm by handgun discharge**
Intentional self-harm by gun for single hand use
Intentional self-harm by pistol
Intentional self-harm by revolver
EXCLUDES 1 Very pistol (X74.8)

The appropriate 7th character is to be added to code X72
A initial encounter
D subsequent encounter
S sequela

4 X73 **Intentional self-harm by rifle, shotgun and larger firearm discharge**
EXCLUDES 1 airgun (X74.01)

The appropriate 7th character is to be added to each code from category X73
A initial encounter
D subsequent encounter
S sequela

IQ X73.0XX- **Intentional self-harm by shotgun discharge**

IQ X73.1XX- **Intentional self-harm by hunting rifle discharge**

IQ X73.2XX- **Intentional self-harm by machine gun discharge**

IQ X73.8XX- **Intentional self-harm by other larger firearm discharge**

IQ X73.9XX- **Intentional self-harm by unspecified larger firearm discharge**

4 X74 **Intentional self-harm by other and unspecified firearm and gun discharge**

The appropriate 7th character is to be added to each code from category X74
A initial encounter
D subsequent encounter
S sequela

5 X74.0 **Intentional self-harm by gas, air or spring-operated guns**

IQ X74.01X- **Intentional self-harm by airgun**
Intentional self-harm by BB gun discharge
Intentional self-harm by pellet gun discharge

Chapter 20 V00-Y99

X74.02X- Intentional self-harm by paintball gun

X74.09X- Intentional self-harm by other gas, air or spring-operated gun

X74.8XX- Intentional self-harm by other firearm discharge
Intentional self-harm by Very pistol [flare] discharge

X74.9XX- Intentional self-harm by unspecified firearm discharge

X75.XXX- Intentional self-harm by explosive material

The appropriate 7th character is to be added to code X75
A initial encounter
D subsequent encounter
S sequela

X76.XXX- Intentional self-harm by smoke, fire and flames

The appropriate 7th character is to be added to code X76
A initial encounter
D subsequent encounter
S sequela

X77 Intentional self-harm by steam, hot vapors and hot objects

The appropriate 7th character is to be added to each code from category X77
A initial encounter
D subsequent encounter
S sequela

X77.0XX- Intentional self-harm by steam or hot vapors

X77.1XX- Intentional self-harm by hot tap water

X77.2XX- Intentional self-harm by other hot fluids

X77.3XX- Intentional self-harm by hot household appliances

X77.8XX- Intentional self-harm by other hot objects

X77.9XX- Intentional self-harm by unspecified hot objects

X78 Intentional self-harm by sharp object

The appropriate 7th character is to be added to each code from category X78
A initial encounter
D subsequent encounter
S sequela

X78.0XX- Intentional self-harm by sharp glass

X78.1XX- Intentional self-harm by knife

X78.2XX- Intentional self-harm by sword or dagger

X78.8XX- Intentional self-harm by other sharp object

X78.9XX- Intentional self-harm by unspecified sharp object

X79.XXX- Intentional self-harm by blunt object

The appropriate 7th character is to be added to code X79
A initial encounter
D subsequent encounter
S sequela

X80.XXX- Intentional self-harm by jumping from a high place
Intentional fall from one level to another

The appropriate 7th character is to be added to code X80
A initial encounter
D subsequent encounter
S sequela

X81 Intentional self-harm by jumping or lying in front of moving object

The appropriate 7th character is to be added to each code from category X81
A initial encounter
D subsequent encounter
S sequela

X81.0XX- Intentional self-harm by jumping or lying in front of motor vehicle

X81.1XX- Intentional self-harm by jumping or lying in front of (subway) train

X81.8XX- Intentional self-harm by jumping or lying in front of other moving object

X82 Intentional self-harm by crashing of motor vehicle

The appropriate 7th character is to be added to each code from category X82
A initial encounter
D subsequent encounter
S sequela

X82.0XX- Intentional collision of motor vehicle with other motor vehicle

X82.1XX- Intentional collision of motor vehicle with train

X82.2XX- Intentional collision of motor vehicle with tree

X82.8XX- Other intentional self-harm by crashing of motor vehicle

X83 Intentional self-harm by other specified means

EXCLUDES 1 intentional self-harm by poisoning or contact with toxic substance- See Table of Drugs and Chemicals

The appropriate 7th character is to be added to each code from category X83
A initial encounter
D subsequent encounter
S sequela

X83.0XX- Intentional self-harm by crashing of aircraft

X83.1XX- Intentional self-harm by electrocution

X83.2XX- Intentional self-harm by exposure to extremes of cold

X83.8XX- Intentional self-harm by other specified means

Assault (X92-Y09)

INCLUDES homicide
injuries inflicted by another person with intent to injure or kill, by any means

EXCLUDES 1 injuries due to legal intervention (Y35.-)
injuries due to operations of war (Y36.-)
injuries due to terrorism (Y38.-)

CODING TIPS✓ Do not assign a code for assault as an external cause of morbidity when there is no injury coded on the claim.

4 **X92 Assault by drowning and submersion**

The appropriate 7th character is to be added to each code from category X92
A initial encounter
D subsequent encounter
S sequela

IQ 7 **X92.0XX- Assault by drowning and submersion while in bathtub**
IQ 7 **X92.1XX- Assault by drowning and submersion while in swimming pool**
IQ 7 **X92.2XX- Assault by drowning and submersion after push into swimming pool**
IQ 7 **X92.3XX- Assault by drowning and submersion in natural water**
IQ 7 **X92.8XX- Other assault by drowning and submersion**
IQ 7 **X92.9XX- Assault by drowning and submersion, unspecified**

IQ 7 **X93.XXX- Assault by handgun discharge**
Assault by discharge of gun for single hand use
Assault by discharge of pistol
Assault by discharge of revolver
EXCLUDES 1 Very pistol (X95.8)

The appropriate 7th character is to be added to code X93
A initial encounter
D subsequent encounter
S sequela

4 **X94 Assault by rifle, shotgun and larger firearm discharge**
EXCLUDES 1 airgun (X95.01)

The appropriate 7th character is to be added to each code from category X94
A initial encounter
D subsequent encounter
S sequela

IQ 7 **X94.0XX- Assault by shotgun**
IQ 7 **X94.1XX- Assault by hunting rifle**
IQ 7 **X94.2XX- Assault by machine gun**
IQ 7 **X94.8XX- Assault by other larger firearm discharge**
IQ 7 **X94.9XX- Assault by unspecified larger firearm discharge**

4 **X95 Assault by other and unspecified firearm and gun discharge**

The appropriate 7th character is to be added to each code from category X95
A initial encounter
D subsequent encounter
S sequela

5 **X95.0 Assault by gas, air or spring-operated guns**
IQ 7 **X95.01X- Assault by airgun discharge**
Assault by BB gun discharge
Assault by pellet gun discharge
IQ 7 **X95.02X- Assault by paintball gun discharge**
IQ 7 **X95.09X- Assault by other gas, air or spring-operated gun**
IQ 7 **X95.8XX- Assault by other firearm discharge**
Assault by very pistol [flare] discharge
IQ 7 **X95.9XX- Assault by unspecified firearm discharge**

4 **X96 Assault by explosive material**
EXCLUDES 1 incendiary device (X97)
terrorism involving explosive material (Y38.2-)

The appropriate 7th character is to be added to each code from category X96
A initial encounter
D subsequent encounter
S sequela

IQ 7 **X96.0XX- Assault by antipersonnel bomb**
EXCLUDES 1 antipersonnel bomb use in military or war (Y36.2-)
IQ 7 **X96.1XX- Assault by gasoline bomb**
IQ 7 **X96.2XX- Assault by letter bomb**
IQ 7 **X96.3XX- Assault by fertilizer bomb**
IQ 7 **X96.4XX- Assault by pipe bomb**
IQ 7 **X96.8XX- Assault by other specified explosive**
IQ 7 **X96.9XX- Assault by unspecified explosive**

IQ 7 **X97.XXX- Assault by smoke, fire and flames**
Assault by arson
Assault by cigarettes
Assault by incendiary device

The appropriate 7th character is to be added to code X97
A initial encounter
D subsequent encounter
S sequela

4 **X98 Assault by steam, hot vapors and hot objects**

The appropriate 7th character is to be added to each code from category X98
A initial encounter
D subsequent encounter
S sequela

IQ 7 **X98.0XX- Assault by steam or hot vapors**
IQ 7 **X98.1XX- Assault by hot tap water**
IQ 7 **X98.2XX- Assault by hot fluids**
IQ 7 **X98.3XX- Assault by hot household appliances**
IQ 7 **X98.8XX- Assault by other hot objects**
IQ 7 **X98.9XX- Assault by unspecified hot objects**

4 **X99 Assault by sharp object**
EXCLUDES 1 assault by strike by sports equipment (Y08.0-)

The appropriate 7th character is to be added to each code from category X99
A initial encounter
D subsequent encounter
S sequela

!Q ☑ **X99.0XX- Assault by sharp glass**

!Q ☑ **X99.1XX- Assault by knife**

!Q ☑ **X99.2XX- Assault by sword or dagger**

!Q ☑ **X99.8XX- Assault by other sharp object**

!Q ☑ **X99.9XX- Assault by unspecified sharp object**
Assault by stabbing NOS

!Q ☑ **Y00.XXX- Assault by blunt object**
EXCLUDES 1 assault by strike by sports equipment (Y08.0-)

The appropriate 7th character is to be added to code Y00
A initial encounter
D subsequent encounter
S sequela

!Q ☑ **Y01.XXX- Assault by pushing from high place**

The appropriate 7th character is to be added to code Y01
A initial encounter
D subsequent encounter
S sequela

4 **Y02 Assault by pushing or placing victim in front of moving object**

The appropriate 7th character is to be added to each code from category Y02
A initial encounter
D subsequent encounter
S sequela

!Q ☑ **Y02.0XX- Assault by pushing or placing victim in front of motor vehicle**

!Q ☑ **Y02.1XX- Assault by pushing or placing victim in front of (subway) train**

!Q ☑ **Y02.8XX- Assault by pushing or placing victim in front of other moving object**

4 **Y03 Assault by crashing of motor vehicle**

The appropriate 7th character is to be added to each code from category Y03
A initial encounter
D subsequent encounter
S sequela

!Q ☑ **Y03.0XX- Assault by being hit or run over by motor vehicle**

!Q ☑ **Y03.8XX- Other assault by crashing of motor vehicle**

4 **Y04 Assault by bodily force**
EXCLUDES 1 assault by:
submersion (X92.-)
use of weapon (X93-X95, X99, Y00)

The appropriate 7th character is to be added to each code from category Y04
A initial encounter
D subsequent encounter
S sequela

!Q ☑ **Y04.0XX- Assault by unarmed brawl or fight**

!Q ☑ **Y04.1XX- Assault by human bite**

!Q ☑ **Y04.2XX- Assault by strike against or bumped into by another person**

!Q ☑ **Y04.8XX- Assault by other bodily force**
Assault by bodily force NOS

4 **Y07 Perpetrator of assault, maltreatment and neglect**
Note:
Codes from this category are for use only in cases of confirmed abuse (T74.-)
Selection of the correct perpetrator code is based on the relationship between the perpetrator and the victim
INCLUDES perpetrator of abandonment
perpetrator of emotional neglect
perpetrator of mental cruelty
perpetrator of physical abuse
perpetrator of physical neglect
perpetrator of sexual abuse
perpetrator of torture

5 **Y07.0 Spouse or partner, perpetrator of maltreatment and neglect**
Spouse or partner, perpetrator of maltreatment and neglect against spouse or partner

!Q **Y07.01 Husband, perpetrator of maltreatment and neglect**

!Q **Y07.02 Wife, perpetrator of maltreatment and neglect**

!Q **Y07.03 Male partner, perpetrator of maltreatment and neglect**

!Q **Y07.04 Female partner, perpetrator of maltreatment and neglect**

5 **Y07.1 Parent (adoptive) (biological), perpetrator of maltreatment and neglect**

!Q **Y07.11 Biological father, perpetrator of maltreatment and neglect**

!Q **Y07.12 Biological mother, perpetrator of maltreatment and neglect**

!Q **Y07.13 Adoptive father, perpetrator of maltreatment and neglect**

!Q **Y07.14 Adoptive mother, perpetrator of maltreatment and neglect**

5 **Y07.4 Other family member, perpetrator of maltreatment and neglect**

6 **Y07.41 Sibling, perpetrator of maltreatment and neglect**
EXCLUDES 1 stepsibling, perpetrator of maltreatment and neglect (Y07.435, Y07.436)

!Q **Y07.410 Brother, perpetrator of maltreatment and neglect**

!Q **Y07.411 Sister, perpetrator of maltreatment and neglect**

6 **Y07.42 Foster parent, perpetrator of maltreatment and neglect**

!Q **Y07.420 Foster father, perpetrator of maltreatment and neglect**

!Q **Y07.421 Foster mother, perpetrator of maltreatment and neglect**

6 **Y07.43 Stepparent or stepsibling, perpetrator of maltreatment and neglect**

!Q **Y07.430 Stepfather, perpetrator of maltreatment and neglect**

Chapter 20 V00-Y99

IQ Y07.432 Male friend of parent (co-residing in household), perpetrator of maltreatment and neglect
IQ Y07.433 Stepmother, perpetrator of maltreatment and neglect
IQ Y07.434 Female friend of parent (co-residing in household), perpetrator of maltreatment and neglect
IQ Y07.435 Stepbrother, perpetrator or maltreatment and neglect
IQ Y07.436 Stepsister, perpetrator of maltreatment and neglect
6 Y07.49 Other family member, perpetrator of maltreatment and neglect
IQ Y07.490 Male cousin, perpetrator of maltreatment and neglect
IQ Y07.491 Female cousin, perpetrator of maltreatment and neglect
IQ Y07.499 Other family member, perpetrator of maltreatment and neglect
5 Y07.5 Non-family member, perpetrator of maltreatment and neglect
IQ Y07.50 Unspecified non-family member, perpetrator of maltreatment and neglect
6 Y07.51 Daycare provider, perpetrator of maltreatment and neglect
IQ Y07.510 At-home childcare provider, perpetrator of maltreatment and neglect
IQ Y07.511 Daycare center childcare provider, perpetrator of maltreatment and neglect
IQ Y07.512 At-home adultcare provider, perpetrator of maltreatment and neglect
IQ Y07.513 Adultcare center provider, perpetrator of maltreatment and neglect
IQ Y07.519 Unspecified daycare provider, perpetrator of maltreatment and neglect
6 Y07.52 Healthcare provider, perpetrator of maltreatment and neglect
IQ Y07.521 Mental health provider, perpetrator of maltreatment and neglect
IQ Y07.528 Other therapist or healthcare provider, perpetrator of maltreatment and neglect
Nurse perpetrator of maltreatment and neglect
Occupational therapist perpetrator of maltreatment and neglect
Physical therapist perpetrator of maltreatment and neglect
Speech therapist perpetrator of maltreatment and neglect
IQ Y07.529 Unspecified healthcare provider, perpetrator of maltreatment and neglect
IQ Y07.53 Teacher or instructor, perpetrator of maltreatment and neglect
Coach, perpetrator of maltreatment and neglect
IQ Y07.59 Other non-family member, perpetrator of maltreatment and neglect
IQ Y07.6 Multiple perpetrators of maltreatment and neglect
IQ Y07.9 Unspecified perpetrator of maltreatment and neglect
4 Y08 Assault by other specified means

The appropriate 7th character is to be added to each code from category Y08
A initial encounter
D subsequent encounter
S sequela

5 Y08.0 Assault by strike by sport equipment
IQ 7 Y08.01X- Assault by strike by hockey stick
IQ 7 Y08.02X- Assault by strike by baseball bat
IQ 7 Y08.09X- Assault by strike by other specified type of sport equipment
5 Y08.8 Assault by other specified means
IQ 7 Y08.81X- Assault by crashing of aircraft
IQ 7 Y08.89X- Assault by other specified means
IQ Y09 Assault by unspecified means
Assassination (attempted) NOS
Homicide (attempted) NOS
Manslaughter (attempted) NOS
Murder (attempted) NOS

Event of undetermined intent (Y21-Y33)

Undetermined intent is only for use when there is specific documentation in the record that the intent of the injury cannot be determined. If no such documentation is present, code to accidental (unintentional)

CODING TIPS✓ Do not assign a code for event of undetermined intent as an external cause of morbidity when there is no injury coded on the claim.

4 Y21 Drowning and submersion, undetermined intent

The appropriate 7th character is to be added to each code from category Y21
A initial encounter
D subsequent encounter
S sequela

IQ 7 Y21.0XX- Drowning and submersion while in bathtub, undetermined intent
IQ 7 Y21.1XX- Drowning and submersion after fall into bathtub, undetermined intent
IQ 7 Y21.2XX- Drowning and submersion while in swimming pool, undetermined intent
IQ 7 Y21.3XX- Drowning and submersion after fall into swimming pool, undetermined intent
IQ 7 Y21.4XX- Drowning and submersion in natural water, undetermined intent
IQ 7 Y21.8XX- Other drowning and submersion, undetermined intent
IQ 7 Y21.9XX- Unspecified drowning and submersion, undetermined intent
IQ 7 Y22.XXX- Handgun discharge, undetermined intent
Discharge of gun for single hand use, undetermined intent
Discharge of pistol, undetermined intent

Chapter 20 V00-Y99

Discharge of revolver, undetermined intent

EXCLUDES 2 very pistol (Y24.8)

The appropriate 7th character is to be added to code Y22
A initial encounter
D subsequent encounter
S sequela

4 Y23 Rifle, shotgun and larger firearm discharge, undetermined intent

EXCLUDES 2 airgun (Y24.0)

The appropriate 7th character is to be added to each code from category Y23
A initial encounter
D subsequent encounter
S sequela

IQ 7 Y23.0XX- Shotgun discharge, undetermined intent

IQ 7 Y23.1XX- Hunting rifle discharge, undetermined intent

IQ 7 Y23.2XX- Military firearm discharge, undetermined intent

IQ 7 Y23.3XX- Machine gun discharge, undetermined intent

IQ 7 Y23.8XX- Other larger firearm discharge, undetermined intent

IQ 7 Y23.9XX- Unspecified larger firearm discharge, undetermined intent

4 Y24 Other and unspecified firearm discharge, undetermined intent

The appropriate 7th character is to be added to each code from category Y24
A initial encounter
D subsequent encounter
S sequela

IQ 7 Y24.0XX- Airgun discharge, undetermined intent

BB gun discharge, undetermined intent

Pellet gun discharge, undetermined intent

IQ 7 Y24.8XX- Other firearm discharge, undetermined intent

Paintball gun discharge, undetermined intent

Very pistol [flare] discharge, undetermined intent

IQ 7 Y24.9XX- Unspecified firearm discharge, undetermined intent

IQ 7 Y25.XXX- Contact with explosive material, undetermined intent

The appropriate 7th character is to be added to code Y25
A initial encounter
D subsequent encounter
S sequela

IQ 7 Y26.XXX- Exposure to smoke, fire and flames, undetermined intent

The appropriate 7th character is to be added to code Y26
A initial encounter
D subsequent encounter
S sequela

4 Y27 Contact with steam, hot vapors and hot objects, undetermined intent

The appropriate 7th character is to be added to each code from category Y27
A initial encounter
D subsequent encounter
S sequela

IQ 7 Y27.0XX- Contact with steam and hot vapors, undetermined intent

IQ 7 Y27.1XX- Contact with hot tap water, undetermined intent

IQ 7 Y27.2XX- Contact with hot fluids, undetermined intent

IQ 7 Y27.3XX- Contact with hot household appliance, undetermined intent

IQ 7 Y27.8XX- Contact with other hot objects, undetermined intent

IQ 7 Y27.9XX- Contact with unspecified hot objects, undetermined intent

4 Y28 Contact with sharp object, undetermined intent

The appropriate 7th character is to be added to each code from category Y28
A initial encounter
D subsequent encounter
S sequela

IQ 7 Y28.0XX- Contact with sharp glass, undetermined intent

IQ 7 Y28.1XX- Contact with knife, undetermined intent

IQ 7 Y28.2XX- Contact with sword or dagger, undetermined intent

IQ 7 Y28.8XX- Contact with other sharp object, undetermined intent

IQ 7 Y28.9XX- Contact with unspecified sharp object, undetermined intent

IQ 7 Y29.XXX- Contact with blunt object, undetermined intent

The appropriate 7th character is to be added to code Y29
A initial encounter
D subsequent encounter
S sequela

IQ 7 Y30.XXX- Falling, jumping or pushed from a high place, undetermined intent

Victim falling from one level to another, undetermined intent

The appropriate 7th character is to be added to code Y30
A initial encounter
D subsequent encounter
S sequela

IQ 7 Y31.XXX- Falling, lying or running before or into moving object, undetermined intent

The appropriate 7th character is to be added to code Y31
A initial encounter
D subsequent encounter
S sequela

IQ 7 Y32.XXX- Crashing of motor vehicle, undetermined intent

The appropriate 7th character is to be added to code Y32
A initial encounter
D subsequent encounter
S sequela

IQ 7 **Y33.XXX- Other specified events, undetermined intent**

The appropriate 7th character is to be added to code Y33
A initial encounter
D subsequent encounter
S sequela

Legal intervention, operations of war, military operations, and terrorism (Y35-Y38)

4 **Y35 Legal intervention**

INCLUDES any injury sustained as a result of an encounter with any law enforcement official, serving in any capacity at the time of the encounter, whether on-duty or off-duty. Includes: injury to law enforcement official, suspect and bystander

The appropriate 7th character is to be added to each code from category Y35
A initial encounter
D subsequent encounter
S sequela

5 **Y35.0 Legal intervention involving firearm discharge**

6 **Y35.00 Legal intervention involving unspecified firearm discharge**

Legal intervention involving gunshot wound
Legal intervention involving shot NOS

IQ 7 **Y35.001- Legal intervention involving unspecified firearm discharge, law enforcement official injured**

IQ 7 **Y35.002- Legal intervention involving unspecified firearm discharge, bystander injured**

IQ 7 **Y35.003- Legal intervention involving unspecified firearm discharge, suspect injured**

7 **Y35.009- Legal intervention involving unspecified firearm discharge, unspecified person injured**

6 **Y35.01 Legal intervention involving injury by machine gun**

IQ 7 **Y35.011- Legal intervention involving injury by machine gun, law enforcement official injured**

IQ 7 **Y35.012- Legal intervention involving injury by machine gun, bystander injured**

IQ 7 **Y35.013- Legal intervention involving injury by machine gun, suspect injured**

7 **Y35.019- Legal intervention involving injury by machine gun, unspecified person injured**

6 **Y35.02 Legal intervention involving injury by handgun**

IQ 7 **Y35.021- Legal intervention involving injury by handgun, law enforcement official injured**

IQ 7 **Y35.022- Legal intervention involving injury by handgun, bystander injured**

IQ 7 **Y35.023- Legal intervention involving injury by handgun, suspect injured**

7 **Y35.029- Legal intervention involving injury by handgun, unspecified person injured**

6 **Y35.03 Legal intervention involving injury by rifle pellet**

IQ 7 **Y35.031- Legal intervention involving injury by rifle pellet, law enforcement official injured**

IQ 7 **Y35.032- Legal intervention involving injury by rifle pellet, bystander injured**

IQ 7 **Y35.033- Legal intervention involving injury by rifle pellet, suspect injured**

7 **Y35.039- Legal intervention involving injury by rifle pellet, unspecified person injured**

6 **Y35.04 Legal intervention involving injury by rubber bullet**

IQ 7 **Y35.041- Legal intervention involving injury by rubber bullet, law enforcement official injured**

IQ 7 **Y35.042- Legal intervention involving injury by rubber bullet, bystander injured**

IQ 7 **Y35.043- Legal intervention involving injury by rubber bullet, suspect injured**

7 **Y35.049- Legal intervention involving injury by rubber bullet, unspecified person injured**

6 **Y35.09 Legal intervention involving other firearm discharge**

IQ 7 **Y35.091- Legal intervention involving other firearm discharge, law enforcement official injured**

IQ 7 **Y35.092- Legal intervention involving other firearm discharge, bystander injured**

IQ 7 **Y35.093- Legal intervention involving other firearm discharge, suspect injured**

7 **Y35.099- Legal intervention involving other firearm discharge, unspecified person injured**

5 **Y35.1 Legal intervention involving explosives**

6 **Y35.10 Legal intervention involving unspecified explosives**

IQ 7 **Y35.101- Legal intervention involving unspecified explosives, law enforcement official injured**

IQ 7 **Y35.102- Legal intervention involving unspecified explosives, bystander injured**

IQ 7 Y35.103- Legal intervention involving unspecified explosives, suspect injured

7 Y35.109- Legal intervention involving unspecified explosives, unspecified person injured

6 Y35.11 Legal intervention involving injury by dynamite

IQ 7 Y35.111- Legal intervention involving injury by dynamite, law enforcement official injured

IQ 7 Y35.112- Legal intervention involving injury by dynamite, bystander injured

IQ 7 Y35.113- Legal intervention involving injury by dynamite, suspect injured

7 Y35.119- Legal intervention involving injury by dynamite, unspecified person injured

6 Y35.12 Legal intervention involving injury by explosive shell

IQ 7 Y35.121- Legal intervention involving injury by explosive shell, law enforcement official injured

IQ 7 Y35.122- Legal intervention involving injury by explosive shell, bystander injured

IQ 7 Y35.123- Legal intervention involving injury by explosive shell, suspect injured

7 Y35.129- Legal intervention involving injury by explosive shell, unspecified person injured

6 Y35.19 Legal intervention involving other explosives

Legal intervention involving injury by grenade

Legal intervention involving injury by mortar bomb

IQ 7 Y35.191- Legal intervention involving other explosives, law enforcement official injured

IQ 7 Y35.192- Legal intervention involving other explosives, bystander injured

IQ 7 Y35.193- Legal intervention involving other explosives, suspect injured

7 Y35.199- Legal intervention involving other explosives, unspecified person injured

5 Y35.2 Legal intervention involving gas

Legal intervention involving asphyxiation by gas

Legal intervention involving poisoning by gas

6 Y35.20 Legal intervention involving unspecified gas

IQ 7 Y35.201- Legal intervention involving unspecified gas, law enforcement official injured

IQ 7 Y35.202- Legal intervention involving unspecified gas, bystander injured

IQ 7 Y35.203- Legal intervention involving unspecified gas, suspect injured

7 Y35.209- Legal intervention involving unspecified gas, unspecified person injured

6 Y35.21 Legal intervention involving injury by tear gas

IQ 7 Y35.211- Legal intervention involving injury by tear gas, law enforcement official injured

IQ 7 Y35.212- Legal intervention involving injury by tear gas, bystander injured

IQ 7 Y35.213- Legal intervention involving injury by tear gas, suspect injured

7 Y35.219- Legal intervention involving injury by tear gas, unspecified person injured

6 Y35.29 Legal intervention involving other gas

IQ 7 Y35.291- Legal intervention involving other gas, law enforcement official injured

IQ 7 Y35.292- Legal intervention involving other gas, bystander injured

IQ 7 Y35.293- Legal intervention involving other gas, suspect injured

7 Y35.299- Legal intervention involving other gas, unspecified person injured

5 Y35.3 Legal intervention involving blunt objects

Legal intervention involving being hit or struck by blunt object

6 Y35.30 Legal intervention involving unspecified blunt objects

IQ 7 Y35.301- Legal intervention involving unspecified blunt objects, law enforcement official injured

IQ 7 Y35.302- Legal intervention involving unspecified blunt objects, bystander injured

IQ 7 Y35.303- Legal intervention involving unspecified blunt objects, suspect injured

7 Y35.309- Legal intervention involving unspecified blunt objects, unspecified person injured

6 Y35.31 Legal intervention involving baton

IQ 7 Y35.311- Legal intervention involving baton, law enforcement official injured

IQ 7 Y35.312- Legal intervention involving baton, bystander injured

IQ 7 Y35.313- Legal intervention involving baton, suspect injured

7 Y35.319- Legal intervention involving baton, unspecified person injured

6 Y35.39 Legal intervention involving other blunt objects

IQ 7 Y35.391- Legal intervention involving other blunt objects, law enforcement official injured

IQ 7 Y35.392- Legal intervention involving other blunt objects, bystander injured

IQ 7 Y35.393- **Legal intervention involving other blunt objects, suspect injured**

7 Y35.399- **Legal intervention involving other blunt objects, unspecified person injured**

5 Y35.4 **Legal intervention involving sharp objects**
Legal intervention involving being cut by sharp objects
Legal intervention involving being stabbed by sharp objects

6 Y35.40 **Legal intervention involving unspecified sharp objects**

IQ 7 Y35.401- **Legal intervention involving unspecified sharp objects, law enforcement official injured**

IQ 7 Y35.402- **Legal intervention involving unspecified sharp objects, bystander injured**

IQ 7 Y35.403- **Legal intervention involving unspecified sharp objects, suspect injured**

7 Y35.409- **Legal intervention involving unspecified sharp objects, unspecified person injured**

6 Y35.41 **Legal intervention involving bayonet**

IQ 7 Y35.411- **Legal intervention involving bayonet, law enforcement official injured**

IQ 7 Y35.412- **Legal intervention involving bayonet, bystander injured**

IQ 7 Y35.413- **Legal intervention involving bayonet, suspect injured**

7 Y35.419- **Legal intervention involving bayonet, unspecified person injured**

6 Y35.49 **Legal intervention involving other sharp objects**

IQ 7 Y35.491- **Legal intervention involving other sharp objects, law enforcement official injured**

IQ 7 Y35.492- **Legal intervention involving other sharp objects, bystander injured**

IQ 7 Y35.493- **Legal intervention involving other sharp objects, suspect injured**

7 Y35.499- **Legal intervention involving other sharp objects, unspecified person injured**

5 Y35.8 **Legal intervention involving other specified means**

6 Y35.81 **Legal intervention involving manhandling**

IQ 7 Y35.811- **Legal intervention involving manhandling, law enforcement official injured**

IQ 7 Y35.812- **Legal intervention involving manhandling, bystander injured**

IQ 7 Y35.813- **Legal intervention involving manhandling, suspect injured**

7 Y35.819- **Legal intervention involving manhandling, unspecified person injured**

6 Y35.83 **Legal intervention involving a conducted energy device**
Electroshock device (taser)
Stun gun

7 Y35.831- **Legal intervention involving a conducted energy device, law enforcement official injured**

7 Y35.832- **Legal intervention involving a conducted energy device, bystander injured**

7 Y35.833- **Legal intervention involving a conducted energy device, suspect injured**

7 Y35.839- **Legal intervention involving a conducted energy device, unspecified person injured**

6 Y35.89 **Legal intervention involving other specified means**

IQ 7 Y35.891- **Legal intervention involving other specified means, law enforcement official injured**

IQ 7 Y35.892- **Legal intervention involving other specified means, bystander injured**

IQ 7 Y35.893- **Legal intervention involving other specified means, suspect injured**

★ 7 Y35.899- **Legal intervention involving other specified means, unspecified person injured**

5 Y35.9 **Legal intervention, means unspecified**

IQ 7 Y35.91X- **Legal intervention, means unspecified, law enforcement official injured**

IQ 7 Y35.92X- **Legal intervention, means unspecified, bystander injured**

IQ 7 Y35.93X- **Legal intervention, means unspecified, suspect injured**

7 Y35.99X- **Legal intervention, means unspecified, unspecified person injured**

4 Y36 **Operations of war**

INCLUDES injuries to military personnel and civilians caused by war, civil insurrection, and peacekeeping missions

EXCLUDES 1 injury to military personnel occurring during peacetime military operations (Y37.-)
military vehicles involved in transport accidents with non-military vehicle during peacetime (V09.01, V09.21, V19.81, V29.81, V39.81, V49.81, V59.81, V69.81, V79.81)

The appropriate 7th character is to be added to each code from category Y36
A initial encounter
D subsequent encounter
S sequela

5 Y36.0 **War operations involving explosion of marine weapons**

6 Y36.00 **War operations involving explosion of unspecified marine weapon**
War operations involving underwater blast NOS

Chapter 20

V00-Y99

IQ 7 Y36.000- **War operations involving explosion of unspecified marine weapon, military personnel**

IQ 7 Y36.001- **War operations involving explosion of unspecified marine weapon, civilian**

6 Y36.01 **War operations involving explosion of depth-charge**

IQ 7 Y36.010- **War operations involving explosion of depth-charge, military personnel**

IQ 7 Y36.011- **War operations involving explosion of depth-charge, civilian**

6 Y36.02 **War operations involving explosion of marine mine**

War operations involving explosion of marine mine, at sea or in harbor

IQ 7 Y36.020- **War operations involving explosion of marine mine, military personnel**

IQ 7 Y36.021- **War operations involving explosion of marine mine, civilian**

6 Y36.03 **War operations involving explosion of sea-based artillery shell**

IQ 7 Y36.030- **War operations involving explosion of sea-based artillery shell, military personnel**

IQ 7 Y36.031- **War operations involving explosion of sea-based artillery shell, civilian**

6 Y36.04 **War operations involving explosion of torpedo**

IQ 7 Y36.040- **War operations involving explosion of torpedo, military personnel**

IQ 7 Y36.041- **War operations involving explosion of torpedo, civilian**

6 Y36.05 **War operations involving accidental detonation of onboard marine weapons**

IQ 7 Y36.050- **War operations involving accidental detonation of onboard marine weapons, military personnel**

IQ 7 Y36.051- **War operations involving accidental detonation of onboard marine weapons, civilian**

6 Y36.09 **War operations involving explosion of other marine weapons**

IQ 7 Y36.090- **War operations involving explosion of other marine weapons, military personnel**

IQ 7 Y36.091- **War operations involving explosion of other marine weapons, civilian**

5 Y36.1 **War operations involving destruction of aircraft**

6 Y36.10 **War operations involving unspecified destruction of aircraft**

IQ 7 Y36.100- **War operations involving unspecified destruction of aircraft, military personnel**

IQ 7 Y36.101- **War operations involving unspecified destruction of aircraft, civilian**

6 Y36.11 **War operations involving destruction of aircraft due to enemy fire or explosives**

War operations involving destruction of aircraft due to air to air missile

War operations involving destruction of aircraft due to explosive placed on aircraft

War operations involving destruction of aircraft due to rocket propelled grenade [RPG]

War operations involving destruction of aircraft due to small arms fire

War operations involving destruction of aircraft due to surface to air missile

IQ 7 Y36.110- **War operations involving destruction of aircraft due to enemy fire or explosives, military personnel**

IQ 7 Y36.111- **War operations involving destruction of aircraft due to enemy fire or explosives, civilian**

6 Y36.12 **War operations involving destruction of aircraft due to collision with other aircraft**

IQ 7 Y36.120- **War operations involving destruction of aircraft due to collision with other aircraft, military personnel**

IQ 7 Y36.121- **War operations involving destruction of aircraft due to collision with other aircraft, civilian**

6 Y36.13 **War operations involving destruction of aircraft due to onboard fire**

IQ 7 Y36.130- **War operations involving destruction of aircraft due to onboard fire, military personnel**

IQ 7 Y36.131- **War operations involving destruction of aircraft due to onboard fire, civilian**

6 Y36.14 **War operations involving destruction of aircraft due to accidental detonation of onboard munitions and explosives**

IQ 7 Y36.140- **War operations involving destruction of aircraft due to accidental detonation of onboard munitions and explosives, military personnel**

IQ 7 Y36.141- **War operations involving destruction of aircraft due to accidental detonation of onboard munitions and explosives, civilian**

6 Y36.19 **War operations involving other destruction of aircraft**

IQ 7 Y36.190- **War operations involving other destruction of aircraft, military personnel**

IQ 7 Y36.191- **War operations involving other destruction of aircraft, civilian**

5 Y36.2 **War operations involving other explosions and fragments**

EXCLUDES 1 war operations involving explosion of aircraft (Y36.1-)

Chapter 20

V00-Y99

war operations involving explosion of marine weapons (Y36.0-)
war operations involving explosion of nuclear weapons (Y36.5-)
war operations involving explosion occurring after cessation of hostilities (Y36.8-)

6 **Y36.20 War operations involving unspecified explosion and fragments**
War operations involving air blast NOS
War operations involving blast NOS
War operations involving blast fragments NOS
War operations involving blast wave NOS
War operations involving blast wind NOS
War operations involving explosion NOS
War operations involving explosion of bomb NOS

!Q 7 **Y36.200- War operations involving unspecified explosion and fragments, military personnel**

!Q 7 **Y36.201- War operations involving unspecified explosion and fragments, civilian**

6 **Y36.21 War operations involving explosion of aerial bomb**

!Q 7 **Y36.210- War operations involving explosion of aerial bomb, military personnel**

!Q 7 **Y36.211- War operations involving explosion of aerial bomb, civilian**

6 **Y36.22 War operations involving explosion of guided missile**

!Q 7 **Y36.220- War operations involving explosion of guided missile, military personnel**

!Q 7 **Y36.221- War operations involving explosion of guided missile, civilian**

6 **Y36.23 War operations involving explosion of improvised explosive device [IED]**
War operations involving explosion of person-borne improvised explosive device [IED]
War operations involving explosion of vehicle-borne improvised explosive device [IED]
War operations involving explosion of roadside improvised explosive device [IED]

!Q 7 **Y36.230- War operations involving explosion of improvised explosive device [IED], military personnel**

!Q 7 **Y36.231- War operations involving explosion of improvised explosive device [IED], civilian**

6 **Y36.24 War operations involving explosion due to accidental detonation and discharge of own munitions or munitions launch device**

!Q 7 **Y36.240- War operations involving explosion due to accidental detonation and discharge of own munitions or munitions launch device, military personnel**

!Q 7 **Y36.241- War operations involving explosion due to accidental detonation and discharge of own munitions or munitions launch device, civilian**

6 **Y36.25 War operations involving fragments from munitions**

!Q 7 **Y36.250- War operations involving fragments from munitions, military personnel**

!Q 7 **Y36.251- War operations involving fragments from munitions, civilian**

6 **Y36.26 War operations involving fragments of improvised explosive device [IED]**
War operations involving fragments of person-borne improvised explosive device [IED]
War operations involving fragments of vehicle-borne improvised explosive device [IED]
War operations involving fragments of roadside improvised explosive device [IED]

!Q 7 **Y36.260- War operations involving fragments of improvised explosive device [IED], military personnel**

!Q 7 **Y36.261- War operations involving fragments of improvised explosive device [IED], civilian**

6 **Y36.27 War operations involving fragments from weapons**

!Q 7 **Y36.270- War operations involving fragments from weapons, military personnel**

!Q 7 **Y36.271- War operations involving fragments from weapons, civilian**

6 **Y36.29 War operations involving other explosions and fragments**
War operations involving explosion of grenade
War operations involving explosions of land mine
War operations involving shrapnel NOS

!Q 7 **Y36.290- War operations involving other explosions and fragments, military personnel**

!Q 7 **Y36.291- War operations involving other explosions and fragments, civilian**

5 **Y36.3 War operations involving fires, conflagrations and hot substances**
War operations involving smoke, fumes, and heat from fires, conflagrations and hot substances
EXCLUDES 1 war operations involving fires and conflagrations aboard military aircraft (Y36.1-)

Chapter 20
V00-Y99

war operations involving fires and conflagrations aboard military watercraft (Y36.0-)
war operations involving fires and conflagrations caused indirectly by conventional weapons (Y36.2-)
war operations involving fires and thermal effects of nuclear weapons (Y36.53-)

6 **Y36.30 War operations involving unspecified fire, conflagration and hot substance**

!Q 7 **Y36.300- War operations involving unspecified fire, conflagration and hot substance, military personnel**

!Q 7 **Y36.301- War operations involving unspecified fire, conflagration and hot substance, civilian**

6 **Y36.31 War operations involving gasoline bomb**
War operations involving incendiary bomb
War operations involving petrol bomb

!Q 7 **Y36.310- War operations involving gasoline bomb, military personnel**

!Q 7 **Y36.311- War operations involving gasoline bomb, civilian**

6 **Y36.32 War operations involving incendiary bullet**

!Q 7 **Y36.320- War operations involving incendiary bullet, military personnel**

!Q 7 **Y36.321- War operations involving incendiary bullet, civilian**

6 **Y36.33 War operations involving flamethrower**

!Q 7 **Y36.330- War operations involving flamethrower, military personnel**

!Q 7 **Y36.331- War operations involving flamethrower, civilian**

6 **Y36.39 War operations involving other fires, conflagrations and hot substances**

!Q 7 **Y36.390- War operations involving other fires, conflagrations and hot substances, military personnel**

!Q 7 **Y36.391- War operations involving other fires, conflagrations and hot substances, civilian**

5 **Y36.4 War operations involving firearm discharge and other forms of conventional warfare**

6 **Y36.41 War operations involving rubber bullets**

!Q 7 **Y36.410- War operations involving rubber bullets, military personnel**

!Q 7 **Y36.411- War operations involving rubber bullets, civilian**

6 **Y36.42 War operations involving firearms pellets**

!Q 7 **Y36.420- War operations involving firearms pellets, military personnel**

!Q 7 **Y36.421- War operations involving firearms pellets, civilian**

6 **Y36.43 War operations involving other firearms discharge**
War operations involving bullets NOS
EXCLUDES 1 war operations involving munitions fragments (Y36.25-)
war operations involving incendiary bullets (Y36.32-)

!Q 7 **Y36.430- War operations involving other firearms discharge, military personnel**

!Q 7 **Y36.431- War operations involving other firearms discharge, civilian**

6 **Y36.44 War operations involving unarmed hand to hand combat**
EXCLUDES 1 war operations involving combat using blunt or piercing object (Y36.45-)
war operations involving intentional restriction of air and airway (Y36.46-)
war operations involving unintentional restriction of air and airway (Y36.47-)

!Q 7 **Y36.440- War operations involving unarmed hand to hand combat, military personnel**

!Q 7 **Y36.441- War operations involving unarmed hand to hand combat, civilian**

6 **Y36.45 War operations involving combat using blunt or piercing object**

!Q 7 **Y36.450- War operations involving combat using blunt or piercing object, military personnel**

!Q 7 **Y36.451- War operations involving combat using blunt or piercing object, civilian**

6 **Y36.46 War operations involving intentional restriction of air and airway**

!Q 7 **Y36.460- War operations involving intentional restriction of air and airway, military personnel**

!Q 7 **Y36.461- War operations involving intentional restriction of air and airway, civilian**

6 **Y36.47 War operations involving unintentional restriction of air and airway**

!Q 7 **Y36.470- War operations involving unintentional restriction of air and airway, military personnel**

!Q 7 **Y36.471- War operations involving unintentional restriction of air and airway, civilian**

6 **Y36.49 War operations involving other forms of conventional warfare**

!Q 7 **Y36.490- War operations involving other forms of conventional warfare, military personnel**

!Q 7 **Y36.491- War operations involving other forms of conventional warfare, civilian**

5 Y36.5 War operations involving nuclear weapons
War operations involving dirty bomb NOS

6 Y36.50 War operations involving unspecified effect of nuclear weapon

IQ 7 Y36.500- War operations involving unspecified effect of nuclear weapon, military personnel

IQ 7 Y36.501- War operations involving unspecified effect of nuclear weapon, civilian

6 Y36.51 War operations involving direct blast effect of nuclear weapon
War operations involving blast pressure of nuclear weapon

IQ 7 Y36.510- War operations involving direct blast effect of nuclear weapon, military personnel

IQ 7 Y36.511- War operations involving direct blast effect of nuclear weapon, civilian

6 Y36.52 War operations involving indirect blast effect of nuclear weapon
War operations involving being thrown by blast of nuclear weapon
War operations involving being struck or crushed by blast debris of nuclear weapon

IQ 7 Y36.520- War operations involving indirect blast effect of nuclear weapon, military personnel

IQ 7 Y36.521- War operations involving indirect blast effect of nuclear weapon, civilian

6 Y36.53 War operations involving thermal radiation effect of nuclear weapon
War operations involving direct heat from nuclear weapon
War operation involving fireball effects from nuclear weapon

IQ 7 Y36.530- War operations involving thermal radiation effect of nuclear weapon, military personnel

IQ 7 Y36.531- War operations involving thermal radiation effect of nuclear weapon, civilian

6 Y36.54 War operation involving nuclear radiation effects of nuclear weapon
War operation involving acute radiation exposure from nuclear weapon
War operation involving exposure to immediate ionizing radiation from nuclear weapon
War operation involving fallout exposure from nuclear weapon
War operation involving secondary effects of nuclear weapons

IQ 7 Y36.540- War operation involving nuclear radiation effects of nuclear weapon, military personnel

IQ 7 Y36.541- War operation involving nuclear radiation effects of nuclear weapon, civilian

6 Y36.59 War operation involving other effects of nuclear weapons

IQ 7 Y36.590- War operation involving other effects of nuclear weapons, military personnel

IQ 7 Y36.591- War operation involving other effects of nuclear weapons, civilian

5 Y36.6 War operations involving biological weapons

6 Y36.6X War operations involving biological weapons

IQ 7 Y36.6X0- War operations involving biological weapons, military personnel

IQ 7 Y36.6X1- War operations involving biological weapons, civilian

5 Y36.7 War operations involving chemical weapons and other forms of unconventional warfare
EXCLUDES 1 war operations involving incendiary devices (Y36.3-, Y36.5-)

6 Y36.7X War operations involving chemical weapons and other forms of unconventional warfare

IQ 7 Y36.7X0- War operations involving chemical weapons and other forms of unconventional warfare, military personnel

IQ 7 Y36.7X1- War operations involving chemical weapons and other forms of unconventional warfare, civilian

5 Y36.8 War operations occurring after cessation of hostilities
War operations classifiable to categories Y36.0-Y36.8 but occurring after cessation of hostilities

6 Y36.81 Explosion of mine placed during war operations but exploding after cessation of hostilities

IQ 7 Y36.810- Explosion of mine placed during war operations but exploding after cessation of hostilities, military personnel

IQ 7 Y36.811- Explosion of mine placed during war operations but exploding after cessation of hostilities, civilian

6 Y36.82 Explosion of bomb placed during war operations but exploding after cessation of hostilities

IQ 7 Y36.820- Explosion of bomb placed during war operations but exploding after cessation of hostilities, military personnel

IQ 7 Y36.821- Explosion of bomb placed during war operations but exploding after cessation of hostilities, civilian

6 Y36.88 Other war operations occurring after cessation of hostilities

IQ 7 Y36.880- Other war operations occurring after cessation of hostilities, military personnel

IQ 7 Y36.881- Other war operations occurring after cessation of hostilities, civilian

6 **Y36.89 Unspecified war operations occurring after cessation of hostilities**

!Q 7 **Y36.890- Unspecified war operations occurring after cessation of hostilities, military personnel**

!Q 7 **Y36.891- Unspecified war operations occurring after cessation of hostilities, civilian**

5 **Y36.9 Other and unspecified war operations**

!Q 7 **Y36.90X- War operations, unspecified**

!Q 7 **Y36.91X- War operations involving unspecified weapon of mass destruction [WMD]**

!Q 7 **Y36.92X- War operations involving friendly fire**

4 **Y37 Military operations**

INCLUDES injuries to military personnel and civilians occurring during peacetime on military property and during routine military exercises and operations

EXCLUDES 1 military aircraft involved in aircraft accident with civilian aircraft (V97.81-)
military vehicles involved in transport accident with civilian vehicle (V09.01, V09.21, V19.81, V29.81, V39.81, V49.81, V59.81, V69.81, V79.81)
military watercraft involved in water transport accident with civilian watercraft (V94.81-)
war operations (Y36.-)

The appropriate 7th character is to be added to each code from category Y37
A initial encounter
D subsequent encounter
S sequela

5 **Y37.0 Military operations involving explosion of marine weapons**

6 **Y37.00 Military operations involving explosion of unspecified marine weapon**

Military operations involving underwater blast NOS

!Q 7 **Y37.000- Military operations involving explosion of unspecified marine weapon, military personnel**

!Q 7 **Y37.001- Military operations involving explosion of unspecified marine weapon, civilian**

6 **Y37.01 Military operations involving explosion of depth-charge**

!Q 7 **Y37.010- Military operations involving explosion of depth-charge, military personnel**

!Q 7 **Y37.011- Military operations involving explosion of depth-charge, civilian**

6 **Y37.02 Military operations involving explosion of marine mine**

Military operations involving explosion of marine mine, at sea or in harbor

!Q 7 **Y37.020- Military operations involving explosion of marine mine, military personnel**

!Q 7 **Y37.021- Military operations involving explosion of marine mine, civilian**

6 **Y37.03 Military operations involving explosion of sea-based artillery shell**

!Q 7 **Y37.030- Military operations involving explosion of sea-based artillery shell, military personnel**

!Q 7 **Y37.031- Military operations involving explosion of sea-based artillery shell, civilian**

6 **Y37.04 Military operations involving explosion of torpedo**

!Q 7 **Y37.040- Military operations involving explosion of torpedo, military personnel**

!Q 7 **Y37.041- Military operations involving explosion of torpedo, civilian**

6 **Y37.05 Military operations involving accidental detonation of onboard marine weapons**

!Q 7 **Y37.050- Military operations involving accidental detonation of onboard marine weapons, military personnel**

!Q 7 **Y37.051- Military operations involving accidental detonation of onboard marine weapons, civilian**

6 **Y37.09 Military operations involving explosion of other marine weapons**

!Q 7 **Y37.090- Military operations involving explosion of other marine weapons, military personnel**

!Q 7 **Y37.091- Military operations involving explosion of other marine weapons, civilian**

5 **Y37.1 Military operations involving destruction of aircraft**

6 **Y37.10 Military operations involving unspecified destruction of aircraft**

!Q 7 **Y37.100- Military operations involving unspecified destruction of aircraft, military personnel**

!Q 7 **Y37.101- Military operations involving unspecified destruction of aircraft, civilian**

6 **Y37.11 Military operations involving destruction of aircraft due to enemy fire or explosives**

Military operations involving destruction of aircraft due to air to air missile
Military operations involving destruction of aircraft due to explosive placed on aircraft
Military operations involving destruction of aircraft due to rocket propelled grenade [RPG]
Military operations involving destruction of aircraft due to small arms fire

Chapter 20 V00-Y99

Military operations involving destruction of aircraft due to surface to air missile

IQ 7 **Y37.110- Military operations involving destruction of aircraft due to enemy fire or explosives, military personnel**

IQ 7 **Y37.111- Military operations involving destruction of aircraft due to enemy fire or explosives, civilian**

6 **Y37.12 Military operations involving destruction of aircraft due to collision with other aircraft**

IQ 7 **Y37.120- Military operations involving destruction of aircraft due to collision with other aircraft, military personnel**

IQ 7 **Y37.121- Military operations involving destruction of aircraft due to collision with other aircraft, civilian**

6 **Y37.13 Military operations involving destruction of aircraft due to onboard fire**

IQ 7 **Y37.130- Military operations involving destruction of aircraft due to onboard fire, military personnel**

IQ 7 **Y37.131- Military operations involving destruction of aircraft due to onboard fire, civilian**

6 **Y37.14 Military operations involving destruction of aircraft due to accidental detonation of onboard munitions and explosives**

IQ 7 **Y37.140- Military operations involving destruction of aircraft due to accidental detonation of onboard munitions and explosives, military personnel**

IQ 7 **Y37.141- Military operations involving destruction of aircraft due to accidental detonation of onboard munitions and explosives, civilian**

6 **Y37.19 Military operations involving other destruction of aircraft**

IQ 7 **Y37.190- Military operations involving other destruction of aircraft, military personnel**

IQ 7 **Y37.191- Military operations involving other destruction of aircraft, civilian**

5 **Y37.2 Military operations involving other explosions and fragments**

EXCLUDES 1 military operations involving explosion of aircraft (Y37.1-)
military operations involving explosion of marine weapons (Y37.0-)
military operations involving explosion of nuclear weapons (Y37.5-)

6 **Y37.20 Military operations involving unspecified explosion and fragments**

Military operations involving air blast NOS
Military operations involving blast NOS
Military operations involving blast fragments NOS
Military operations involving blast wave NOS
Military operations involving blast wind NOS
Military operations involving explosion NOS
Military operations involving explosion of bomb NOS

IQ 7 **Y37.200- Military operations involving unspecified explosion and fragments, military personnel**

IQ 7 **Y37.201- Military operations involving unspecified explosion and fragments, civilian**

6 **Y37.21 Military operations involving explosion of aerial bomb**

IQ 7 **Y37.210- Military operations involving explosion of aerial bomb, military personnel**

IQ 7 **Y37.211- Military operations involving explosion of aerial bomb, civilian**

6 **Y37.22 Military operations involving explosion of guided missile**

IQ 7 **Y37.220- Military operations involving explosion of guided missile, military personnel**

IQ 7 **Y37.221- Military operations involving explosion of guided missile, civilian**

6 **Y37.23 Military operations involving explosion of improvised explosive device [IED]**

Military operations involving explosion of person-borne improvised explosive device [IED]
Military operations involving explosion of vehicle-borne improvised explosive device [IED]
Military operations involving explosion of roadside improvised explosive device [IED]

IQ 7 **Y37.230- Military operations involving explosion of improvised explosive device [IED], military personnel**

IQ 7 **Y37.231- Military operations involving explosion of improvised explosive device [IED], civilian**

6 **Y37.24 Military operations involving explosion due to accidental detonation and discharge of own munitions or munitions launch device**

IQ 7 **Y37.240- Military operations involving explosion due to accidental detonation and discharge of own munitions or munitions launch device, military personnel**

IQ 7 **Y37.241- Military operations involving explosion due to accidental detonation and discharge of own munitions or munitions launch device, civilian**

6 **Y37.25 Military operations involving fragments from munitions**

IQ 7 Y37.250- Military operations involving fragments from munitions, military personnel

IQ 7 Y37.251- Military operations involving fragments from munitions, civilian

6 Y37.26 Military operations involving fragments of improvised explosive device [IED]

Military operations involving fragments of person-borne improvised explosive device [IED]

Military operations involving fragments of vehicle-borne improvised explosive device [IED]

Military operations involving fragments of roadside improvised explosive device [IED]

IQ 7 Y37.260- Military operations involving fragments of improvised explosive device [IED], military personnel

IQ 7 Y37.261- Military operations involving fragments of improvised explosive device [IED], civilian

6 Y37.27 Military operations involving fragments from weapons

IQ 7 Y37.270- Military operations involving fragments from weapons, military personnel

IQ 7 Y37.271- Military operations involving fragments from weapons, civilian

6 Y37.29 Military operations involving other explosions and fragments

Military operations involving explosion of grenade

Military operations involving explosions of land mine

Military operations involving shrapnel NOS

IQ 7 Y37.290- Military operations involving other explosions and fragments, military personnel

IQ 7 Y37.291- Military operations involving other explosions and fragments, civilian

5 Y37.3 Military operations involving fires, conflagrations and hot substances

Military operations involving smoke, fumes, and heat from fires, conflagrations and hot substances

EXCLUDES 1 military operations involving fires and conflagrations aboard military aircraft (Y37.1-)

military operations involving fires and conflagrations aboard military watercraft (Y37.0-)

military operations involving fires and conflagrations caused indirectly by conventional weapons (Y37.2-)

military operations involving fires and thermal effects of nuclear weapons (Y36.53-)

6 Y37.30 Military operations involving unspecified fire, conflagration and hot substance

IQ 7 Y37.300- Military operations involving unspecified fire, conflagration and hot substance, military personnel

IQ 7 Y37.301- Military operations involving unspecified fire, conflagration and hot substance, civilian

6 Y37.31 Military operations involving gasoline bomb

Military operations involving incendiary bomb

Military operations involving petrol bomb

IQ 7 Y37.310- Military operations involving gasoline bomb, military personnel

IQ 7 Y37.311- Military operations involving gasoline bomb, civilian

6 Y37.32 Military operations involving incendiary bullet

IQ 7 Y37.320- Military operations involving incendiary bullet, military personnel

IQ 7 Y37.321- Military operations involving incendiary bullet, civilian

6 Y37.33 Military operations involving flamethrower

IQ 7 Y37.330- Military operations involving flamethrower, military personnel

IQ 7 Y37.331- Military operations involving flamethrower, civilian

6 Y37.39 Military operations involving other fires, conflagrations and hot substances

IQ 7 Y37.390- Military operations involving other fires, conflagrations and hot substances, military personnel

IQ 7 Y37.391- Military operations involving other fires, conflagrations and hot substances, civilian

5 Y37.4 Military operations involving firearm discharge and other forms of conventional warfare

6 Y37.41 Military operations involving rubber bullets

IQ 7 Y37.410- Military operations involving rubber bullets, military personnel

IQ 7 Y37.411- Military operations involving rubber bullets, civilian

6 Y37.42 Military operations involving firearms pellets

IQ 7 Y37.420- Military operations involving firearms pellets, military personnel

IQ 7 Y37.421- Military operations involving firearms pellets, civilian

6 Y37.43 Military operations involving other firearms discharge

Military operations involving bullets NOS

EXCLUDES 1 military operations involving munitions fragments (Y37.25-)

Chapter 20 V00-Y99

military operations involving incendiary bullets (Y37.32-)

!Q 7 **Y37.430- Military operations involving other firearms discharge, military personnel**

!Q 7 **Y37.431- Military operations involving other firearms discharge, civilian**

6 **Y37.44 Military operations involving unarmed hand to hand combat**

EXCLUDES 1 military operations involving combat using blunt or piercing object (Y37.45-)
military operations involving intentional restriction of air and airway (Y37.46-)
military operations involving unintentional restriction of air and airway (Y37.47-)

!Q 7 **Y37.440- Military operations involving unarmed hand to hand combat, military personnel**

!Q 7 **Y37.441- Military operations involving unarmed hand to hand combat, civilian**

6 **Y37.45 Military operations involving combat using blunt or piercing object**

!Q 7 **Y37.450- Military operations involving combat using blunt or piercing object, military personnel**

!Q 7 **Y37.451- Military operations involving combat using blunt or piercing object, civilian**

6 **Y37.46 Military operations involving intentional restriction of air and airway**

!Q 7 **Y37.460- Military operations involving intentional restriction of air and airway, military personnel**

!Q 7 **Y37.461- Military operations involving intentional restriction of air and airway, civilian**

6 **Y37.47 Military operations involving unintentional restriction of air and airway**

!Q 7 **Y37.470- Military operations involving unintentional restriction of air and airway, military personnel**

!Q 7 **Y37.471- Military operations involving unintentional restriction of air and airway, civilian**

6 **Y37.49 Military operations involving other forms of conventional warfare**

!Q 7 **Y37.490- Military operations involving other forms of conventional warfare, military personnel**

!Q 7 **Y37.491- Military operations involving other forms of conventional warfare, civilian**

5 **Y37.5 Military operations involving nuclear weapons**

Military operation involving dirty bomb NOS

6 **Y37.50 Military operations involving unspecified effect of nuclear weapon**

!Q 7 **Y37.500- Military operations involving unspecified effect of nuclear weapon, military personnel**

!Q 7 **Y37.501- Military operations involving unspecified effect of nuclear weapon, civilian**

6 **Y37.51 Military operations involving direct blast effect of nuclear weapon**

Military operations involving blast pressure of nuclear weapon

!Q 7 **Y37.510- Military operations involving direct blast effect of nuclear weapon, military personnel**

!Q 7 **Y37.511- Military operations involving direct blast effect of nuclear weapon, civilian**

6 **Y37.52 Military operations involving indirect blast effect of nuclear weapon**

Military operations involving being thrown by blast of nuclear weapon
Military operations involving being struck or crushed by blast debris of nuclear weapon

!Q 7 **Y37.520- Military operations involving indirect blast effect of nuclear weapon, military personnel**

!Q 7 **Y37.521- Military operations involving indirect blast effect of nuclear weapon, civilian**

6 **Y37.53 Military operations involving thermal radiation effect of nuclear weapon**

Military operations involving direct heat from nuclear weapon
Military operation involving fireball effects from nuclear weapon

!Q 7 **Y37.530- Military operations involving thermal radiation effect of nuclear weapon, military personnel**

!Q 7 **Y37.531- Military operations involving thermal radiation effect of nuclear weapon, civilian**

6 **Y37.54 Military operation involving nuclear radiation effects of nuclear weapon**

Military operation involving acute radiation exposure from nuclear weapon
Military operation involving exposure to immediate ionizing radiation from nuclear weapon
Military operation involving fallout exposure from nuclear weapon
Military operation involving secondary effects of nuclear weapons

!Q 7 **Y37.540- Military operation involving nuclear radiation effects of nuclear weapon, military personnel**

!Q 7 **Y37.541- Military operation involving nuclear radiation effects of nuclear weapon, civilian**

6 **Y37.59 Military operation involving other effects of nuclear weapons**

!Q 7 **Y37.590- Military operation involving other effects of nuclear weapons, military personnel**

IQ 7 **Y37.591- Military operation involving other effects of nuclear weapons, civilian**

5 **Y37.6 Military operations involving biological weapons**

6 **Y37.6X Military operations involving biological weapons**

IQ 7 **Y37.6X0- Military operations involving biological weapons, military personnel**

IQ 7 **Y37.6X1- Military operations involving biological weapons, civilian**

5 **Y37.7 Military operations involving chemical weapons and other forms of unconventional warfare**

EXCLUDES 1 military operations involving incendiary devices (Y36.3-, Y36.5-)

6 **Y37.7X Military operations involving chemical weapons and other forms of unconventional warfare**

IQ 7 **Y37.7X0- Military operations involving chemical weapons and other forms of unconventional warfare, military personnel**

IQ 7 **Y37.7X1- Military operations involving chemical weapons and other forms of unconventional warfare, civilian**

5 **Y37.9 Other and unspecified military operations**

IQ 7 **Y37.90X- Military operations, unspecified**

IQ 7 **Y37.91X- Military operations involving unspecified weapon of mass destruction [WMD]**

IQ 7 **Y37.92X- Military operations involving friendly fire**

+ 4 **Y38 Terrorism**

These codes are for use to identify injuries resulting from the unlawful use of force or violence against persons or property to intimidate or coerce a Government, the civilian population, or any segment thereof, in furtherance of political or social objective

Use additional code for place of occurrence (Y92.-)

The appropriate 7th character is to be added to each code from category Y38

A	initial encounter
D	subsequent encounter
S	sequela

+ 5 **Y38.0 Terrorism involving explosion of marine weapons**

Terrorism involving depth-charge
Terrorism involving marine mine
Terrorism involving mine NOS, at sea or in harbor
Terrorism involving sea-based artillery shell
Terrorism involving torpedo
Terrorism involving underwater blast

+ 6 **Y38.0X Terrorism involving explosion of marine weapons**

IQ + 7 **Y38.0X1- Terrorism involving explosion of marine weapons, public safety official injured**

IQ + 7 **Y38.0X2- Terrorism involving explosion of marine weapons, civilian injured**

IQ + 7 **Y38.0X3- Terrorism involving explosion of marine weapons, terrorist injured**

+ 5 **Y38.1 Terrorism involving destruction of aircraft**

Terrorism involving aircraft burned
Terrorism involving aircraft exploded
Terrorism involving aircraft being shot down
Terrorism involving aircraft used as a weapon

+ 6 **Y38.1X Terrorism involving destruction of aircraft**

IQ + 7 **Y38.1X1- Terrorism involving destruction of aircraft, public safety official injured**

IQ + 7 **Y38.1X2- Terrorism involving destruction of aircraft, civilian injured**

IQ + 7 **Y38.1X3- Terrorism involving destruction of aircraft, terrorist injured**

+ 5 **Y38.2 Terrorism involving other explosions and fragments**

Terrorism involving antipersonnel (fragments) bomb
Terrorism involving blast NOS
Terrorism involving explosion NOS
Terrorism involving explosion of breech block
Terrorism involving explosion of cannon block
Terrorism involving explosion (fragments) of artillery shell
Terrorism involving explosion (fragments) of bomb
Terrorism involving explosion (fragments) of grenade
Terrorism involving explosion (fragments) of guided missile
Terrorism involving explosion (fragments) of land mine
Terrorism involving explosion of mortar bomb
Terrorism involving explosion of munitions
Terrorism involving explosion (fragments) of rocket
Terrorism involving explosion (fragments) of shell
Terrorism involving shrapnel
Terrorism involving mine NOS, on land

EXCLUDES 1 terrorism involving explosion of nuclear weapon (Y38.5)
terrorism involving suicide bomber (Y38.81)

+ 6 **Y38.2X Terrorism involving other explosions and fragments**

IQ + 7 **Y38.2X1- Terrorism involving other explosions and fragments, public safety official injured**

IQ + 7 **Y38.2X2- Terrorism involving other explosions and fragments, civilian injured**

IQ + 7 **Y38.2X3- Terrorism involving other explosions and fragments, terrorist injured**

Chapter 20

V00-Y99

4 4th digit required 5 5th digit required 6 6th digit required 7 7th digit required 7 7th digit placeholder + Additional code Laterality

+ 5 **Y38.3 Terrorism involving fires, conflagration and hot substances**
Terrorism involving conflagration NOS
Terrorism involving fire NOS
Terrorism involving petrol bomb
EXCLUDES 1 terrorism involving fire or heat of nuclear weapon (Y38.5)

+ 6 **Y38.3X Terrorism involving fires, conflagration and hot substances**

IQ + 7 **Y38.3X1- Terrorism involving fires, conflagration and hot substances, public safety official injured**

IQ + 7 **Y38.3X2- Terrorism involving fires, conflagration and hot substances, civilian injured**

IQ + 7 **Y38.3X3- Terrorism involving fires, conflagration and hot substances, terrorist injured**

+ 5 **Y38.4 Terrorism involving firearms**
Terrorism involving carbine bullet
Terrorism involving machine gun bullet
Terrorism involving pellets (shotgun)
Terrorism involving pistol bullet
Terrorism involving rifle bullet
Terrorism involving rubber (rifle) bullet

+ 6 **Y38.4X Terrorism involving firearms**

IQ + 7 **Y38.4X1- Terrorism involving firearms, public safety official injured**

IQ + 7 **Y38.4X2- Terrorism involving firearms, civilian injured**

IQ + 7 **Y38.4X3- Terrorism involving firearms, terrorist injured**

+ 5 **Y38.5 Terrorism involving nuclear weapons**
Terrorism involving blast effects of nuclear weapon
Terrorism involving exposure to ionizing radiation from nuclear weapon
Terrorism involving fireball effect of nuclear weapon
Terrorism involving heat from nuclear weapon

+ 6 **Y38.5X Terrorism involving nuclear weapons**

IQ + 7 **Y38.5X1- Terrorism involving nuclear weapons, public safety official injured**

IQ + 7 **Y38.5X2- Terrorism involving nuclear weapons, civilian injured**

IQ + 7 **Y38.5X3- Terrorism involving nuclear weapons, terrorist injured**

+ 5 **Y38.6 Terrorism involving biological weapons**
Terrorism involving anthrax
Terrorism involving cholera
Terrorism involving smallpox

+ 6 **Y38.6X Terrorism involving biological weapons**

IQ + 7 **Y38.6X1- Terrorism involving biological weapons, public safety official injured**

IQ + 7 **Y38.6X2- Terrorism involving biological weapons, civilian injured**

IQ + 7 **Y38.6X3- Terrorism involving biological weapons, terrorist injured**

+ 5 **Y38.7 Terrorism involving chemical weapons**
Terrorism involving gases, fumes, chemicals
Terrorism involving hydrogen cyanide
Terrorism involving phosgene
Terrorism involving sarin

+ 6 **Y38.7X Terrorism involving chemical weapons**

IQ + 7 **Y38.7X1- Terrorism involving chemical weapons, public safety official injured**

IQ + 7 **Y38.7X2- Terrorism involving chemical weapons, civilian injured**

IQ + 7 **Y38.7X3- Terrorism involving chemical weapons, terrorist injured**

+ 5 **Y38.8 Terrorism involving other and unspecified means**

IQ + 7 **Y38.80X- Terrorism involving unspecified means**
Terrorism NOS

+ 6 **Y38.81 Terrorism involving suicide bomber**

IQ + 7 **Y38.811- Terrorism involving suicide bomber, public safety official injured**

IQ + 7 **Y38.812- Terrorism involving suicide bomber, civilian injured**

+ 6 **Y38.89 Terrorism involving other means**
Terrorism involving drowning and submersion
Terrorism involving lasers
Terrorism involving piercing or stabbing instruments

IQ + 7 **Y38.891- Terrorism involving other means, public safety official injured**

IQ + 7 **Y38.892- Terrorism involving other means, civilian injured**

IQ + 7 **Y38.893- Terrorism involving other means, terrorist injured**

+ 5 **Y38.9 Terrorism, secondary effects**
Note:
This code is for use to identify conditions occurring subsequent to a terrorist attack not those that are due to the initial terrorist attack

+ 6 **Y38.9X Terrorism, secondary effects**

IQ + 7 **Y38.9X1- Terrorism, secondary effects, public safety official injured**

IQ + 7 **Y38.9X2- Terrorism, secondary effects, civilian injured**

Complications of medical and surgical care (Y62-Y84)

INCLUDES complications of medical devices
surgical and medical procedures as the cause of abnormal reaction of the patient, or of later complication, without mention of misadventure at the time of the procedure

Misadventures to patients during surgical and medical care (Y62-Y69)

EXCLUDES 1 surgical and medical procedures as the cause of abnormal reaction of the patient, without mention of misadventure at the time of the procedure (Y83-Y84)

EXCLUDES 2 breakdown or malfunctioning of medical device (during procedure) (after implantation) (ongoing use) (Y70-Y82)

4 **Y62 Failure of sterile precautions during surgical and medical care**

!Q Y62.0 Failure of sterile precautions during surgical operation

!Q Y62.1 Failure of sterile precautions during infusion or transfusion

!Q Y62.2 Failure of sterile precautions during kidney dialysis and other perfusion

!Q Y62.3 Failure of sterile precautions during injection or immunization

!Q Y62.4 Failure of sterile precautions during endoscopic examination

!Q Y62.5 Failure of sterile precautions during heart catheterization

!Q Y62.6 Failure of sterile precautions during aspiration, puncture and other catheterization

!Q Y62.8 Failure of sterile precautions during other surgical and medical care

!Q Y62.9 Failure of sterile precautions during unspecified surgical and medical care

4 Y63 Failure in dosage during surgical and medical care

EXCLUDES 2 accidental overdose of drug or wrong drug given in error (T36-T50)

!Q Y63.0 Excessive amount of blood or other fluid given during transfusion or infusion

!Q Y63.1 Incorrect dilution of fluid used during infusion

!Q Y63.2 Overdose of radiation given during therapy

!Q Y63.3 Inadvertent exposure of patient to radiation during medical care

!Q Y63.4 Failure in dosage in electroshock or insulin-shock therapy

!Q Y63.5 Inappropriate temperature in local application and packing

!Q Y63.6 Underdosing and nonadministration of necessary drug, medicament or biological substance

GUIDELINES **Section I.C.19.e.5)(c)**
Noncompliance (Z91.12-, Z91.13- and Z91.14-) or complication of care (Y63.6-Y63.9) codes are to be used with an underdosing code to indicate intent, if known.

!Q Y63.8 Failure in dosage during other surgical and medical care

GUIDELINES **Section I.C.19.e.5)(c)**
Noncompliance (Z91.12-, Z91.13- and Z91.14-) or complication of care (Y63.6-Y63.9) codes are to be used with an underdosing code to indicate intent, if known.

!Q Y63.9 Failure in dosage during unspecified surgical and medical care

GUIDELINES **Section I.C.19.e.5)(c)**
Noncompliance (Z91.12-, Z91.13- and Z91.14-) or complication of care (Y63.6-Y63.9) codes are to be used with an underdosing code to indicate intent, if known.

4 Y64 Contaminated medical or biological substances

!Q Y64.0 Contaminated medical or biological substance, transfused or infused

!Q Y64.1 Contaminated medical or biological substance, injected or used for immunization

!Q Y64.8 Contaminated medical or biological substance administered by other means

!Q Y64.9 Contaminated medical or biological substance administered by unspecified means

Administered contaminated medical or biological substance NOS

4 Y65 Other misadventures during surgical and medical care

!Q Y65.0 Mismatched blood in transfusion

!Q Y65.1 Wrong fluid used in infusion

!Q Y65.2 Failure in suture or ligature during surgical operation

!Q Y65.3 Endotracheal tube wrongly placed during anesthetic procedure

!Q Y65.4 Failure to introduce or to remove other tube or instrument

5 Y65.5 Performance of wrong procedure (operation)

!Q Y65.51 Performance of wrong procedure (operation) on correct patient

Wrong device implanted into correct surgical site

EXCLUDES 1 performance of correct procedure (operation) on wrong side or body part (Y65.53)

!Q Y65.52 Performance of procedure (operation) on patient not scheduled for surgery

Performance of procedure (operation) intended for another patient

Performance of procedure (operation) on wrong patient

!Q Y65.53 Performance of correct procedure (operation) on wrong side or body part

Performance of correct procedure (operation) on wrong side

Performance of correct procedure (operation) on wrong site

!Q Y65.8 Other specified misadventures during surgical and medical care

!Q Y66 Nonadministration of surgical and medical care

Premature cessation of surgical and medical care

EXCLUDES 1 DNR status (Z66)
palliative care (Z51.5)

!Q Y69 Unspecified misadventure during surgical and medical care

Medical devices associated with adverse incidents in diagnostic and therapeutic use (Y70-Y82)

INCLUDES breakdown or malfunction of medical devices (during use) (after implantation) (ongoing use)

EXCLUDES 2 later complications following use of medical devices without breakdown or malfunctioning of device (Y83-Y84)
misadventure to patients during surgical and medical care, classifiable to (Y62-Y69)

surgical and other medical procedures as the cause of abnormal reaction of the patient, or of later complication, without mention of misadventure at the time of the procedure (Y83-Y84)

4 **Y70 Anesthesiology devices associated with adverse incidents**

IQ **Y70.0 Diagnostic and monitoring anesthesiology devices associated with adverse incidents**

IQ **Y70.1 Therapeutic (nonsurgical) and rehabilitative anesthesiology devices associated with adverse incidents**

IQ **Y70.2 Prosthetic and other implants, materials and accessory anesthesiology devices associated with adverse incidents**

IQ **Y70.3 Surgical instruments, materials and anesthesiology devices (including sutures) associated with adverse incidents**

IQ **Y70.8 Miscellaneous anesthesiology devices associated with adverse incidents, not elsewhere classified**

4 **Y71 Cardiovascular devices associated with adverse incidents**

IQ **Y71.0 Diagnostic and monitoring cardiovascular devices associated with adverse incidents**

IQ **Y71.1 Therapeutic (nonsurgical) and rehabilitative cardiovascular devices associated with adverse incidents**

IQ **Y71.2 Prosthetic and other implants, materials and accessory cardiovascular devices associated with adverse incidents**

IQ **Y71.3 Surgical instruments, materials and cardiovascular devices (including sutures) associated with adverse incidents**

IQ **Y71.8 Miscellaneous cardiovascular devices associated with adverse incidents, not elsewhere classified**

4 **Y72 Otorhinolaryngological devices associated with adverse incidents**

IQ **Y72.0 Diagnostic and monitoring otorhinolaryngological devices associated with adverse incidents**

IQ **Y72.1 Therapeutic (nonsurgical) and rehabilitative otorhinolaryngological devices associated with adverse incidents**

IQ **Y72.2 Prosthetic and other implants, materials and accessory otorhinolaryngological devices associated with adverse incidents**

IQ **Y72.3 Surgical instruments, materials and otorhinolaryngological devices (including sutures) associated with adverse incidents**

IQ **Y72.8 Miscellaneous otorhinolaryngological devices associated with adverse incidents, not elsewhere classified**

4 **Y73 Gastroenterology and urology devices associated with adverse incidents**

IQ **Y73.0 Diagnostic and monitoring gastroenterology and urology devices associated with adverse incidents**

IQ **Y73.1 Therapeutic (nonsurgical) and rehabilitative gastroenterology and urology devices associated with adverse incidents**

IQ **Y73.2 Prosthetic and other implants, materials and accessory gastroenterology and urology devices associated with adverse incidents**

IQ **Y73.3 Surgical instruments, materials and gastroenterology and urology devices (including sutures) associated with adverse incidents**

IQ **Y73.8 Miscellaneous gastroenterology and urology devices associated with adverse incidents, not elsewhere classified**

4 **Y74 General hospital and personal-use devices associated with adverse incidents**

IQ **Y74.0 Diagnostic and monitoring general hospital and personal-use devices associated with adverse incidents**

IQ **Y74.1 Therapeutic (nonsurgical) and rehabilitative general hospital and personal-use devices associated with adverse incidents**

IQ **Y74.2 Prosthetic and other implants, materials and accessory general hospital and personal-use devices associated with adverse incidents**

IQ **Y74.3 Surgical instruments, materials and general hospital and personal-use devices (including sutures) associated with adverse incidents**

IQ **Y74.8 Miscellaneous general hospital and personal-use devices associated with adverse incidents, not elsewhere classified**

4 **Y75 Neurological devices associated with adverse incidents**

IQ **Y75.0 Diagnostic and monitoring neurological devices associated with adverse incidents**

IQ **Y75.1 Therapeutic (nonsurgical) and rehabilitative neurological devices associated with adverse incidents**

IQ **Y75.2 Prosthetic and other implants, materials and neurological devices associated with adverse incidents**

IQ **Y75.3 Surgical instruments, materials and neurological devices (including sutures) associated with adverse incidents**

IQ **Y75.8 Miscellaneous neurological devices associated with adverse incidents, not elsewhere classified**

4 **Y76 Obstetric and gynecological devices associated with adverse incidents**

IQ **Y76.0 Diagnostic and monitoring obstetric and gynecological devices associated with adverse incidents**

IQ **Y76.1 Therapeutic (nonsurgical) and rehabilitative obstetric and gynecological devices associated with adverse incidents**

IQ **Y76.2 Prosthetic and other implants, materials and accessory obstetric and gynecological devices associated with adverse incidents**

!Q Y76.3 Surgical instruments, materials and obstetric and gynecological devices (including sutures) associated with adverse incidents

!Q Y76.8 Miscellaneous obstetric and gynecological devices associated with adverse incidents, not elsewhere classified

4 Y77 Ophthalmic devices associated with adverse incidents

!Q Y77.0 Diagnostic and monitoring ophthalmic devices associated with adverse incidents

5 Y77.1 Therapeutic (nonsurgical) and rehabilitative ophthalmic devices associated with adverse incidents

!Q Y77.11 Contact lens associated with adverse incidents
Rigid gas permeable contact lens associated with adverse incidents
Soft (hydrophilic) contact lens associated with adverse incidents

!Q Y77.19 Other therapeutic (nonsurgical) and rehabilitative ophthalmic devices associated with adverse incidents

!Q Y77.2 Prosthetic and other implants, materials and accessory ophthalmic devices associated with adverse incidents

!Q Y77.3 Surgical instruments, materials and ophthalmic devices (including sutures) associated with adverse incidents

!Q Y77.8 Miscellaneous ophthalmic devices associated with adverse incidents, not elsewhere classified

4 Y78 Radiological devices associated with adverse incidents

!Q Y78.0 Diagnostic and monitoring radiological devices associated with adverse incidents

!Q Y78.1 Therapeutic (nonsurgical) and rehabilitative radiological devices associated with adverse incidents

!Q Y78.2 Prosthetic and other implants, materials and accessory radiological devices associated with adverse incidents

!Q Y78.3 Surgical instruments, materials and radiological devices (including sutures) associated with adverse incidents

!Q Y78.8 Miscellaneous radiological devices associated with adverse incidents, not elsewhere classified

4 Y79 Orthopedic devices associated with adverse incidents

!Q Y79.0 Diagnostic and monitoring orthopedic devices associated with adverse incidents

!Q Y79.1 Therapeutic (nonsurgical) and rehabilitative orthopedic devices associated with adverse incidents

CODING TIPS✓ This code may be used to indicate the cause of a pressure injury from a prosthetic limb or other therapeutic orthopedic device.

!Q Y79.2 Prosthetic and other implants, materials and accessory orthopedic devices associated with adverse incidents

!Q Y79.3 Surgical instruments, materials and orthopedic devices (including sutures) associated with adverse incidents

!Q Y79.8 Miscellaneous orthopedic devices associated with adverse incidents, not elsewhere classified

4 Y80 Physical medicine devices associated with adverse incidents

!Q Y80.0 Diagnostic and monitoring physical medicine devices associated with adverse incidents

!Q Y80.1 Therapeutic (nonsurgical) and rehabilitative physical medicine devices associated with adverse incidents

!Q Y80.2 Prosthetic and other implants, materials and accessory physical medicine devices associated with adverse incidents

!Q Y80.3 Surgical instruments, materials and physical medicine devices (including sutures) associated with adverse incidents

!Q Y80.8 Miscellaneous physical medicine devices associated with adverse incidents, not elsewhere classified

4 Y81 General- and plastic-surgery devices associated with adverse incidents

!Q Y81.0 Diagnostic and monitoring general- and plastic-surgery devices associated with adverse incidents

!Q Y81.1 Therapeutic (nonsurgical) and rehabilitative general- and plastic-surgery devices associated with adverse incidents

!Q Y81.2 Prosthetic and other implants, materials and accessory general- and plastic-surgery devices associated with adverse incidents

!Q Y81.3 Surgical instruments, materials and general- and plastic-surgery devices (including sutures) associated with adverse incidents

!Q Y81.8 Miscellaneous general- and plastic-surgery devices associated with adverse incidents, not elsewhere classified

4 Y82 Other and unspecified medical devices associated with adverse incidents

!Q Y82.8 Other medical devices associated with adverse incidents

!Q Y82.9 Unspecified medical devices associated with adverse incidents

Surgical and other medical procedures as the cause of abnormal reaction of the patient, or of later complication, without mention of misadventure at the time of the procedure (Y83-Y84)

EXCLUDES 1 misadventures to patients during surgical and medical care, classifiable to (Y62-Y69)

EXCLUDES 2 breakdown or malfunctioning of medical device (after implantation) (during procedure) (ongoing use) (Y70-Y82)

4 Y83 Surgical operation and other surgical procedures as the cause of abnormal reaction of the patient, or of later complication, without mention of misadventure at the time of the procedure

IQ **Y83.0 Surgical operation with transplant of whole organ as the cause of abnormal reaction of the patient, or of later complication, without mention of misadventure at the time of the procedure**

IQ **Y83.1 Surgical operation with implant of artificial internal device as the cause of abnormal reaction of the patient, or of later complication, without mention of misadventure at the time of the procedure**

IQ **Y83.2 Surgical operation with anastomosis, bypass or graft as the cause of abnormal reaction of the patient, or of later complication, without mention of misadventure at the time of the procedure**

IQ **Y83.3 Surgical operation with formation of external stoma as the cause of abnormal reaction of the patient, or of later complication, without mention of misadventure at the time of the procedure**

IQ **Y83.4 Other reconstructive surgery as the cause of abnormal reaction of the patient, or of later complication, without mention of misadventure at the time of the procedure**

IQ **Y83.5 Amputation of limb(s) as the cause of abnormal reaction of the patient, or of later complication, without mention of misadventure at the time of the procedure**

IQ **Y83.6 Removal of other organ (partial) (total) as the cause of abnormal reaction of the patient, or of later complication, without mention of misadventure at the time of the procedure**

IQ **Y83.8 Other surgical procedures as the cause of abnormal reaction of the patient, or of later complication, without mention of misadventure at the time of the procedure**

IQ **Y83.9 Surgical procedure, unspecified as the cause of abnormal reaction of the patient, or of later complication, without mention of misadventure at the time of the procedure**

4 **Y84 Other medical procedures as the cause of abnormal reaction of the patient, or of later complication, without mention of misadventure at the time of the procedure**

IQ **Y84.0 Cardiac catheterization as the cause of abnormal reaction of the patient, or of later complication, without mention of misadventure at the time of the procedure**

IQ **Y84.1 Kidney dialysis as the cause of abnormal reaction of the patient, or of later complication, without mention of misadventure at the time of the procedure**

IQ **Y84.2 Radiological procedure and radiotherapy as the cause of abnormal reaction of the patient, or of later complication, without mention of misadventure at the time of the procedure**

CODING TIPS✓ This indicates an adverse effect of radiation, such as radiation burns or radiodermatitis from therapeutic use of radiation, e.g. for the treatment of cancer.

IQ **Y84.3 Shock therapy as the cause of abnormal reaction of the patient, or of later complication, without mention of misadventure at the time of the procedure**

IQ **Y84.4 Aspiration of fluid as the cause of abnormal reaction of the patient, or of later complication, without mention of misadventure at the time of the procedure**

IQ **Y84.5 Insertion of gastric or duodenal sound as the cause of abnormal reaction of the patient, or of later complication, without mention of misadventure at the time of the procedure**

IQ **Y84.6 Urinary catheterization as the cause of abnormal reaction of the patient, or of later complication, without mention of misadventure at the time of the procedure**

IQ **Y84.7 Blood-sampling as the cause of abnormal reaction of the patient, or of later complication, without mention of misadventure at the time of the procedure**

IQ **Y84.8 Other medical procedures as the cause of abnormal reaction of the patient, or of later complication, without mention of misadventure at the time of the procedure**

IQ **Y84.9 Medical procedure, unspecified as the cause of abnormal reaction of the patient, or of later complication, without mention of misadventure at the time of the procedure**

Supplementary factors related to causes of morbidity classified elsewhere (Y90-Y99)

Note:
These categories may be used to provide supplementary information concerning causes of morbidity. They are not to be used for single-condition coding.

4 **Y90 Evidence of alcohol involvement determined by blood alcohol level**
Code first:
any associated alcohol related disorders (F10)

IQ **Y90.0 Blood alcohol level of less than 20 mg/100 ml**

IQ **Y90.1 Blood alcohol level of 20-39 mg/100 ml**

IQ **Y90.2 Blood alcohol level of 40-59 mg/100 ml**

IQ **Y90.3 Blood alcohol level of 60-79 mg/100 ml**

IQ **Y90.4 Blood alcohol level of 80-99 mg/100 ml**

IQ **Y90.5 Blood alcohol level of 100-119 mg/100 ml**

IQ **Y90.6 Blood alcohol level of 120-199 mg/100 ml**

IQ **Y90.7 Blood alcohol level of 200-239 mg/100 ml**

IQ **Y90.8 Blood alcohol level of 240 mg/100 ml or more**

IQ **Y90.9 Presence of alcohol in blood, level not specified**

4 **Y92 Place of occurrence of the external cause**
The following category is for use, when relevant, to identify the place of occurrence of the external cause. Use in conjunction with an activity code.
Place of occurrence should be recorded only at the initial encounter for treatment

5 **Y92.0 Non-institutional (private) residence as the place of occurrence of the external cause**
EXCLUDES 1 abandoned or derelict house (Y92.89)
home under construction but not yet occupied (Y92.6-)
institutional place of residence (Y92.1-)

6 **Y92.00 Unspecified non-institutional (private) residence as the place of occurrence of the external cause**

IQ **Y92.000 Kitchen of unspecified non-institutional (private) residence as the place of occurrence of the external cause**

IQ **Y92.001 Dining room of unspecified non-institutional (private) residence as the place of occurrence of the external cause**

IQ **Y92.002 Bathroom of unspecified non-institutional (private) residence as the place of occurrence of the external cause**

IQ **Y92.003 Bedroom of unspecified non-institutional (private) residence as the place of occurrence of the external cause**

IQ **Y92.007 Garden or yard of unspecified non-institutional (private) residence as the place of occurrence of the external cause**

IQ **Y92.008 Other place in unspecified non-institutional (private) residence as the place of occurrence of the external cause**

IQ **Y92.009 Unspecified place in unspecified non-institutional (private) residence as the place of occurrence of the external cause**
Home (NOS) as the place of occurrence of the external cause

6 **Y92.01 Single-family non-institutional (private) house as the place of occurrence of the external cause**
Farmhouse as the place of occurrence of the external cause
EXCLUDES 1 barn (Y92.71)
chicken coop or hen house (Y92.72)
farm field (Y92.73)
orchard (Y92.74)
single family mobile home or trailer (Y92.02-)
slaughter house (Y92.86)

IQ **Y92.010 Kitchen of single-family (private) house as the place of occurrence of the external cause**

IQ **Y92.011 Dining room of single-family (private) house as the place of occurrence of the external cause**

IQ **Y92.012 Bathroom of single-family (private) house as the place of occurrence of the external cause**

IQ **Y92.013 Bedroom of single-family (private) house as the place of occurrence of the external cause**

IQ **Y92.014 Private driveway to single-family (private) house as the place of occurrence of the external cause**

IQ **Y92.015 Private garage of single-family (private) house as the place of occurrence of the external cause**

IQ **Y92.016 Swimming-pool in single-family (private) house or garden as the place of occurrence of the external cause**

IQ **Y92.017 Garden or yard in single-family (private) house as the place of occurrence of the external cause**

IQ **Y92.018 Other place in single-family (private) house as the place of occurrence of the external cause**

IQ **Y92.019 Unspecified place in single-family (private) house as the place of occurrence of the external cause**

6 **Y92.02 Mobile home as the place of occurrence of the external cause**

IQ **Y92.020 Kitchen in mobile home as the place of occurrence of the external cause**

IQ **Y92.021 Dining room in mobile home as the place of occurrence of the external cause**

IQ **Y92.022 Bathroom in mobile home as the place of occurrence of the external cause**

IQ **Y92.023 Bedroom in mobile home as the place of occurrence of the external cause**

IQ **Y92.024 Driveway of mobile home as the place of occurrence of the external cause**

IQ **Y92.025 Garage of mobile home as the place of occurrence of the external cause**

IQ **Y92.026 Swimming-pool of mobile home as the place of occurrence of the external cause**

IQ **Y92.027 Garden or yard of mobile home as the place of occurrence of the external cause**

IQ **Y92.028 Other place in mobile home as the place of occurrence of the external cause**

IQ **Y92.029 Unspecified place in mobile home as the place of occurrence of the external cause**

6 **Y92.03 Apartment as the place of occurrence of the external cause**
Condominium as the place of occurrence of the external cause
Co-op apartment as the place of occurrence of the external cause

IQ **Y92.030 Kitchen in apartment as the place of occurrence of the external cause**

IQ **Y92.031 Bathroom in apartment as the place of occurrence of the external cause**

IQ **Y92.032 Bedroom in apartment as the place of occurrence of the external cause**

IQ **Y92.038 Other place in apartment as the place of occurrence of the external cause**

IQ **Y92.039 Unspecified place in apartment as the place of occurrence of the external cause**

6 **Y92.04 Boarding-house as the place of occurrence of the external cause**

IQ **Y92.040 Kitchen in boarding-house as the place of occurrence of the external cause**

IQ **Y92.041 Bathroom in boarding-house as the place of occurrence of the external cause**

IQ **Y92.042 Bedroom in boarding-house as the place of occurrence of the external cause**

IQ **Y92.043 Driveway of boarding-house as the place of occurrence of the external cause**

IQ **Y92.044 Garage of boarding-house as the place of occurrence of the external cause**

IQ **Y92.045 Swimming-pool of boarding-house as the place of occurrence of the external cause**

IQ **Y92.046 Garden or yard of boarding-house as the place of occurrence of the external cause**

IQ **Y92.048 Other place in boarding-house as the place of occurrence of the external cause**

IQ **Y92.049 Unspecified place in boarding-house as the place of occurrence of the external cause**

6 **Y92.09 Other non-institutional residence as the place of occurrence of the external cause**

IQ **Y92.090 Kitchen in other non-institutional residence as the place of occurrence of the external cause**

IQ **Y92.091 Bathroom in other non-institutional residence as the place of occurrence of the external cause**

IQ **Y92.092 Bedroom in other non-institutional residence as the place of occurrence of the external cause**

IQ **Y92.093 Driveway of other non-institutional residence as the place of occurrence of the external cause**

IQ **Y92.094 Garage of other non-institutional residence as the place of occurrence of the external cause**

IQ **Y92.095 Swimming-pool of other non-institutional residence as the place of occurrence of the external cause**

IQ **Y92.096 Garden or yard of other non-institutional residence as the place of occurrence of the external cause**

IQ **Y92.098 Other place in other non-institutional residence as the place of occurrence of the external cause**

CODING TIPS ✓ Assign Y92.098, Other place in other noninstitutional residence, as the place of occurrence of the external cause, for an assisted living facility.

IQ **Y92.099 Unspecified place in other non-institutional residence as the place of occurrence of the external cause**

5 **Y92.1 Institutional (nonprivate) residence as the place of occurrence of the external cause**

IQ **Y92.10 Unspecified residential institution as the place of occurrence of the external cause**

6 **Y92.11 Children's home and orphanage as the place of occurrence of the external cause**

IQ **Y92.110 Kitchen in children's home and orphanage as the place of occurrence of the external cause**

IQ **Y92.111 Bathroom in children's home and orphanage as the place of occurrence of the external cause**

IQ **Y92.112 Bedroom in children's home and orphanage as the place of occurrence of the external cause**

IQ **Y92.113 Driveway of children's home and orphanage as the place of occurrence of the external cause**

IQ **Y92.114 Garage of children's home and orphanage as the place of occurrence of the external cause**

IQ **Y92.115 Swimming-pool of children's home and orphanage as the place of occurrence of the external cause**

IQ **Y92.116 Garden or yard of children's home and orphanage as the place of occurrence of the external cause**

IQ **Y92.118 Other place in children's home and orphanage as the place of occurrence of the external cause**

IQ **Y92.119 Unspecified place in children's home and orphanage as the place of occurrence of the external cause**

6 **Y92.12 Nursing home as the place of occurrence of the external cause**
Home for the sick as the place of occurrence of the external cause
Hospice as the place of occurrence of the external cause

IQ **Y92.120 Kitchen in nursing home as the place of occurrence of the external cause**

IQ **Y92.121 Bathroom in nursing home as the place of occurrence of the external cause**

IQ **Y92.122 Bedroom in nursing home as the place of occurrence of the external cause**
IQ **Y92.123 Driveway of nursing home as the place of occurrence of the external cause**
IQ **Y92.124 Garage of nursing home as the place of occurrence of the external cause**
IQ **Y92.125 Swimming-pool of nursing home as the place of occurrence of the external cause**
IQ **Y92.126 Garden or yard of nursing home as the place of occurrence of the external cause**
IQ **Y92.128 Other place in nursing home as the place of occurrence of the external cause**
IQ **Y92.129 Unspecified place in nursing home as the place of occurrence of the external cause**

6 **Y92.13 Military base as the place of occurrence of the external cause**
EXCLUDES 1 military training grounds (Y92.83)

IQ **Y92.130 Kitchen on military base as the place of occurrence of the external cause**
IQ **Y92.131 Mess hall on military base as the place of occurrence of the external cause**
IQ **Y92.133 Barracks on military base as the place of occurrence of the external cause**
IQ **Y92.135 Garage on military base as the place of occurrence of the external cause**
IQ **Y92.136 Swimming-pool on military base as the place of occurrence of the external cause**
IQ **Y92.137 Garden or yard on military base as the place of occurrence of the external cause**
IQ **Y92.138 Other place on military base as the place of occurrence of the external cause**
IQ **Y92.139 Unspecified place military base as the place of occurrence of the external cause**

6 **Y92.14 Prison as the place of occurrence of the external cause**

IQ **Y92.140 Kitchen in prison as the place of occurrence of the external cause**
IQ **Y92.141 Dining room in prison as the place of occurrence of the external cause**
IQ **Y92.142 Bathroom in prison as the place of occurrence of the external cause**
IQ **Y92.143 Cell of prison as the place of occurrence of the external cause**
IQ **Y92.146 Swimming-pool of prison as the place of occurrence of the external cause**
IQ **Y92.147 Courtyard of prison as the place of occurrence of the external cause**
IQ **Y92.148 Other place in prison as the place of occurrence of the external cause**
IQ **Y92.149 Unspecified place in prison as the place of occurrence of the external cause**

6 **Y92.15 Reform school as the place of occurrence of the external cause**

IQ **Y92.150 Kitchen in reform school as the place of occurrence of the external cause**
IQ **Y92.151 Dining room in reform school as the place of occurrence of the external cause**
IQ **Y92.152 Bathroom in reform school as the place of occurrence of the external cause**
IQ **Y92.153 Bedroom in reform school as the place of occurrence of the external cause**
IQ **Y92.154 Driveway of reform school as the place of occurrence of the external cause**
IQ **Y92.155 Garage of reform school as the place of occurrence of the external cause**
IQ **Y92.156 Swimming-pool of reform school as the place of occurrence of the external cause**
IQ **Y92.157 Garden or yard of reform school as the place of occurrence of the external cause**
IQ **Y92.158 Other place in reform school as the place of occurrence of the external cause**
IQ **Y92.159 Unspecified place in reform school as the place of occurrence of the external cause**

6 **Y92.16 School dormitory as the place of occurrence of the external cause**
EXCLUDES 1 reform school as the place of occurrence of the external cause (Y92.15-)
school buildings and grounds as the place of occurrence of the external cause (Y92.2-)
school sports and athletic areas as the place of occurrence of the external cause (Y92.3-)

IQ **Y92.160 Kitchen in school dormitory as the place of occurrence of the external cause**
IQ **Y92.161 Dining room in school dormitory as the place of occurrence of the external cause**
IQ **Y92.162 Bathroom in school dormitory as the place of occurrence of the external cause**
IQ **Y92.163 Bedroom in school dormitory as the place of occurrence of the external cause**
IQ **Y92.168 Other place in school dormitory as the place of occurrence of the external cause**

Chapter 20 V00-Y99

IQ **Y92.169 Unspecified place in school dormitory as the place of occurrence of the external cause**

6 **Y92.19 Other specified residential institution as the place of occurrence of the external cause**

IQ **Y92.190 Kitchen in other specified residential institution as the place of occurrence of the external cause**

IQ **Y92.191 Dining room in other specified residential institution as the place of occurrence of the external cause**

IQ **Y92.192 Bathroom in other specified residential institution as the place of occurrence of the external cause**

IQ **Y92.193 Bedroom in other specified residential institution as the place of occurrence of the external cause**

IQ **Y92.194 Driveway of other specified residential institution as the place of occurrence of the external cause**

IQ **Y92.195 Garage of other specified residential institution as the place of occurrence of the external cause**

IQ **Y92.196 Pool of other specified residential institution as the place of occurrence of the external cause**

IQ **Y92.197 Garden or yard of other specified residential institution as the place of occurrence of the external cause**

IQ **Y92.198 Other place in other specified residential institution as the place of occurrence of the external cause**

IQ **Y92.199 Unspecified place in other specified residential institution as the place of occurrence of the external cause**

5 **Y92.2 School, other institution and public administrative area as the place of occurrence of the external cause**

Building and adjacent grounds used by the general public or by a particular group of the public

EXCLUDES 1 building under construction as the place of occurrence of the external cause (Y92.6)
residential institution as the place of occurrence of the external cause (Y92.1)
school dormitory as the place of occurrence of the external cause (Y92.16-)
sports and athletics area of schools as the place of occurrence of the external cause (Y92.3-)

6 **Y92.21 School (private) (public) (state) as the place of occurrence of the external cause**

IQ **Y92.210 Daycare center as the place of occurrence of the external cause**

IQ **Y92.211 Elementary school as the place of occurrence of the external cause**

Kindergarten as the place of occurrence of the external cause

IQ **Y92.212 Middle school as the place of occurrence of the external cause**

IQ **Y92.213 High school as the place of occurrence of the external cause**

IQ **Y92.214 College as the place of occurrence of the external cause**

University as the place of occurrence of the external cause

IQ **Y92.215 Trade school as the place of occurrence of the external cause**

IQ **Y92.218 Other school as the place of occurrence of the external cause**

IQ **Y92.219 Unspecified school as the place of occurrence of the external cause**

IQ **Y92.22 Religious institution as the place of occurrence of the external cause**

Church as the place of occurrence of the external cause

Mosque as the place of occurrence of the external cause

Synagogue as the place of occurrence of the external cause

6 **Y92.23 Hospital as the place of occurrence of the external cause**

EXCLUDES 1 ambulatory (outpatient) health services establishments (Y92.53-)
home for the sick as the place of occurrence of the external cause (Y92.12-)
hospice as the place of occurrence of the external cause (Y92.12-)
nursing home as the place of occurrence of the external cause (Y92.12-)

IQ **Y92.230 Patient room in hospital as the place of occurrence of the external cause**

IQ **Y92.231 Patient bathroom in hospital as the place of occurrence of the external cause**

IQ **Y92.232 Corridor of hospital as the place of occurrence of the external cause**

IQ **Y92.233 Cafeteria of hospital as the place of occurrence of the external cause**

IQ **Y92.234 Operating room of hospital as the place of occurrence of the external cause**

IQ **Y92.238 Other place in hospital as the place of occurrence of the external cause**

IQ **Y92.239 Unspecified place in hospital as the place of occurrence of the external cause**

6 **Y92.24 Public administrative building as the place of occurrence of the external cause**

IQ **Y92.240 Courthouse as the place of occurrence of the external cause**

IQ **Y92.241 Library as the place of occurrence of the external cause**

IQ **Y92.242 Post office as the place of occurrence of the external cause**

IQ **Y92.243 City hall as the place of occurrence of the external cause**

IQ **Y92.248 Other public administrative building as the place of occurrence of the external cause**

6 **Y92.25 Cultural building as the place of occurrence of the external cause**

IQ **Y92.250 Art Gallery as the place of occurrence of the external cause**

IQ **Y92.251 Museum as the place of occurrence of the external cause**

IQ **Y92.252 Music hall as the place of occurrence of the external cause**

IQ **Y92.253 Opera house as the place of occurrence of the external cause**

IQ **Y92.254 Theater (live) as the place of occurrence of the external cause**

IQ **Y92.258 Other cultural public building as the place of occurrence of the external cause**

IQ **Y92.26 Movie house or cinema as the place of occurrence of the external cause**

IQ **Y92.29 Other specified public building as the place of occurrence of the external cause**

Assembly hall as the place of occurrence of the external cause

Clubhouse as the place of occurrence of the external cause

5 **Y92.3 Sports and athletics area as the place of occurrence of the external cause**

6 **Y92.31 Athletic court as the place of occurrence of the external cause**

EXCLUDES 1 tennis court in private home or garden (Y92.09)

IQ **Y92.310 Basketball court as the place of occurrence of the external cause**

IQ **Y92.311 Squash court as the place of occurrence of the external cause**

IQ **Y92.312 Tennis court as the place of occurrence of the external cause**

IQ **Y92.318 Other athletic court as the place of occurrence of the external cause**

6 **Y92.32 Athletic field as the place of occurrence of the external cause**

IQ **Y92.320 Baseball field as the place of occurrence of the external cause**

IQ **Y92.321 Football field as the place of occurrence of the external cause**

IQ **Y92.322 Soccer field as the place of occurrence of the external cause**

IQ **Y92.328 Other athletic field as the place of occurrence of the external cause**

Cricket field as the place of occurrence of the external cause

Hockey field as the place of occurrence of the external cause

6 **Y92.33 Skating rink as the place of occurrence of the external cause**

IQ **Y92.330 Ice skating rink (indoor) (outdoor) as the place of occurrence of the external cause**

IQ **Y92.331 Roller skating rink as the place of occurrence of the external cause**

IQ **Y92.34 Swimming pool (public) as the place of occurrence of the external cause**

EXCLUDES 1 swimming pool in private home or garden (Y92.016)

IQ **Y92.39 Other specified sports and athletic area as the place of occurrence of the external cause**

Golf-course as the place of occurrence of the external cause

Gymnasium as the place of occurrence of the external cause

Riding-school as the place of occurrence of the external cause

Stadium as the place of occurrence of the external cause

5 **Y92.4 Street, highway and other paved roadways as the place of occurrence of the external cause**

EXCLUDES 1 private driveway of residence (Y92.014, Y92.024, Y92.043, Y92.093, Y92.113, Y92.123, Y92.154, Y92.194)

6 **Y92.41 Street and highway as the place of occurrence of the external cause**

IQ **Y92.410 Unspecified street and highway as the place of occurrence of the external cause**

Road NOS as the place of occurrence of the external cause

IQ **Y92.411 Interstate highway as the place of occurrence of the external cause**

Freeway as the place of occurrence of the external cause

Motorway as the place of occurrence of the external cause

IQ **Y92.412 Parkway as the place of occurrence of the external cause**

IQ **Y92.413 State road as the place of occurrence of the external cause**

IQ **Y92.414 Local residential or business street as the place of occurrence of the external cause**

IQ **Y92.415 Exit ramp or entrance ramp of street or highway as the place of occurrence of the external cause**

6 **Y92.48 Other paved roadways as the place of occurrence of the external cause**

IQ **Y92.480 Sidewalk as the place of occurrence of the external cause**

IQ **Y92.481 Parking lot as the place of occurrence of the external cause**

IQ **Y92.482 Bike path as the place of occurrence of the external cause**

IQ **Y92.488 Other paved roadways as the place of occurrence of the external cause**

5 **Y92.5 Trade and service area as the place of occurrence of the external cause**

EXCLUDES 1 garage in private home (Y92.015)
schools and other public administration buildings (Y92.2-)

6 **Y92.51 Private commercial establishments as the place of occurrence of the external cause**

!Q **Y92.510 Bank as the place of occurrence of the external cause**

!Q **Y92.511 Restaurant or café as the place of occurrence of the external cause**

!Q **Y92.512 Supermarket, store or market as the place of occurrence of the external cause**

!Q **Y92.513 Shop (commercial) as the place of occurrence of the external cause**

6 **Y92.52 Service areas as the place of occurrence of the external cause**

!Q **Y92.520 Airport as the place of occurrence of the external cause**

!Q **Y92.521 Bus station as the place of occurrence of the external cause**

!Q **Y92.522 Railway station as the place of occurrence of the external cause**

!Q **Y92.523 Highway rest stop as the place of occurrence of the external cause**

!Q **Y92.524 Gas station as the place of occurrence of the external cause**
Petroleum station as the place of occurrence of the external cause
Service station as the place of occurrence of the external cause

6 **Y92.53 Ambulatory health services establishments as the place of occurrence of the external cause**

!Q **Y92.530 Ambulatory surgery center as the place of occurrence of the external cause**
Outpatient surgery center, including that connected with a hospital as the place of occurrence of the external cause
Same day surgery center, including that connected with a hospital as the place of occurrence of the external cause

!Q **Y92.531 Health care provider office as the place of occurrence of the external cause**
Physician office as the place of occurrence of the external cause

!Q **Y92.532 Urgent care center as the place of occurrence of the external cause**

!Q **Y92.538 Other ambulatory health services establishments as the place of occurrence of the external cause**

!Q **Y92.59 Other trade areas as the place of occurrence of the external cause**
Office building as the place of occurrence of the external cause
Casino as the place of occurrence of the external cause
Garage (commercial) as the place of occurrence of the external cause
Hotel as the place of occurrence of the external cause
Radio or television station as the place of occurrence of the external cause
Shopping mall as the place of occurrence of the external cause
Warehouse as the place of occurrence of the external cause

5 **Y92.6 Industrial and construction area as the place of occurrence of the external cause**

!Q **Y92.61 Building [any] under construction as the place of occurrence of the external cause**

!Q **Y92.62 Dock or shipyard as the place of occurrence of the external cause**
Dockyard as the place of occurrence of the external cause
Dry dock as the place of occurrence of the external cause
Shipyard as the place of occurrence of the external cause

!Q **Y92.63 Factory as the place of occurrence of the external cause**
Factory building as the place of occurrence of the external cause
Factory premises as the place of occurrence of the external cause
Industrial yard as the place of occurrence of the external cause

!Q **Y92.64 Mine or pit as the place of occurrence of the external cause**
Mine as the place of occurrence of the external cause

!Q **Y92.65 Oil rig as the place of occurrence of the external cause**
Pit (coal) (gravel) (sand) as the place of occurrence of the external cause

!Q **Y92.69 Other specified industrial and construction area as the place of occurrence of the external cause**
Gasworks as the place of occurrence of the external cause
Power-station (coal) (nuclear) (oil) as the place of occurrence of the external cause
Tunnel under construction as the place of occurrence of the external cause
Workshop as the place of occurrence of the external cause

5 **Y92.7 Farm as the place of occurrence of the external cause**
Ranch as the place of occurrence of the external cause
EXCLUDES 1 farmhouse and home premises of farm (Y92.01-)

!Q **Y92.71 Barn as the place of occurrence of the external cause**

!Q **Y92.72 Chicken coop as the place of occurrence of the external cause**
Hen house as the place of occurrence of the external cause

!Q **Y92.73 Farm field as the place of occurrence of the external cause**

!Q **Y92.74 Orchard as the place of occurrence of the external cause**

!Q **Y92.79 Other farm location as the place of occurrence of the external cause**

5 **Y92.8 Other places as the place of occurrence of the external cause**

6 **Y92.81 Transport vehicle as the place of occurrence of the external cause**

EXCLUDES 1 transport accidents (V00-V99)

IQ **Y92.810 Car as the place of occurrence of the external cause**

IQ **Y92.811 Bus as the place of occurrence of the external cause**

IQ **Y92.812 Truck as the place of occurrence of the external cause**

IQ **Y92.813 Airplane as the place of occurrence of the external cause**

IQ **Y92.814 Boat as the place of occurrence of the external cause**

IQ **Y92.815 Train as the place of occurrence of the external cause**

IQ **Y92.816 Subway car as the place of occurrence of the external cause**

IQ **Y92.818 Other transport vehicle as the place of occurrence of the external cause**

6 **Y92.82 Wilderness area**

IQ **Y92.820 Desert as the place of occurrence of the external cause**

IQ **Y92.821 Forest as the place of occurrence of the external cause**

IQ **Y92.828 Other wilderness area as the place of occurrence of the external cause**

Swamp as the place of occurrence of the external cause

Mountain as the place of occurrence of the external cause

Marsh as the place of occurrence of the external cause

Prairie as the place of occurrence of the external cause

6 **Y92.83 Recreation area as the place of occurrence of the external cause**

IQ **Y92.830 Public park as the place of occurrence of the external cause**

IQ **Y92.831 Amusement park as the place of occurrence of the external cause**

IQ **Y92.832 Beach as the place of occurrence of the external cause**

Seashore as the place of occurrence of the external cause

IQ **Y92.833 Campsite as the place of occurrence of the external cause**

IQ **Y92.834 Zoological garden (Zoo) as the place of occurrence of the external cause**

IQ **Y92.838 Other recreation area as the place of occurrence of the external cause**

IQ **Y92.84 Military training ground as the place of occurrence of the external cause**

IQ **Y92.85 Railroad track as the place of occurrence of the external cause**

IQ **Y92.86 Slaughter house as the place of occurrence of the external cause**

IQ **Y92.89 Other specified places as the place of occurrence of the external cause**

Derelict house as the place of occurrence of the external cause

IQ **Y92.9 Unspecified place or not applicable**

4 **Y93 Activity codes**

Note:
Category Y93 is provided for use to indicate the activity of the person seeking healthcare for an injury or health condition, such as a heart attack while shoveling snow, which resulted from, or was contributed to, by the activity. These codes are appropriate for use for both acute injuries, such as those from chapter 19, and conditions that are due to the long-term, cumulative effects of an activity, such as those from chapter 13. They are also appropriate for use with external cause codes for cause and intent if identifying the activity provides additional information on the event. These codes should be used in conjunction with codes for external cause status (Y99) and place of occurrence (Y92).

This section contains the following broad activity categories:

Y93.0 Activities involving walking and running
Y93.1 Activities involving water and water craft
Y93.2 Activities involving ice and snow
Y93.3 Activities involving climbing, rappelling, and jumping off
Y93.4 Activities involving dancing and other rhythmic movement
Y93.5 Activities involving other sports and athletics played individually
Y93.6 Activities involving other sports and athletics played as a team or group
Y93.7 Activities involving other specified sports and athletics
Y93.A Activities involving other cardiorespiratory exercise
Y93.B Activities involving other muscle strengthening exercises
Y93.C Activities involving computer technology and electronic devices
Y93.D Activities involving arts and handcrafts
Y93.E Activities involving personal hygiene and interior property and clothing maintenance
Y93.F Activities involving caregiving
Y93.G Activities involving food preparation, cooking and grilling
Y93.H Activities involving exterior property and land maintenance, building and construction
Y93.I Activities involving roller coasters and other types of external motion
Y93.J Activities involving playing musical instrument
Y93.K Activities involving animal care
Y93.8 Activities, other specified
Y93.9 Activity, unspecified

5 **Y93.0 Activities involving walking and running**

EXCLUDES 1 activity, walking an animal (Y93.K1)
activity, walking or running on a treadmill (Y93.A1)

IQ **Y93.01 Activity, walking, marching and hiking**

Activity, walking, marching and hiking on level or elevated terrain

Chapter 20 V00-Y99

EXCLUDES 1 activity, mountain climbing (Y93.31)

IQ **Y93.02 Activity, running**

5 **Y93.1 Activities involving water and water craft**

EXCLUDES 1 activities involving ice (Y93.2-)

IQ **Y93.11 Activity, swimming**

IQ **Y93.12 Activity, springboard and platform diving**

IQ **Y93.13 Activity, water polo**

IQ **Y93.14 Activity, water aerobics and water exercise**

IQ **Y93.15 Activity, underwater diving and snorkeling**

Activity, SCUBA diving

IQ **Y93.16 Activity, rowing, canoeing, kayaking, rafting and tubing**

Activity, canoeing, kayaking, rafting and tubing in calm and turbulent water

IQ **Y93.17 Activity, water skiing and wake boarding**

IQ **Y93.18 Activity, surfing, windsurfing and boogie boarding**

Activity, water sliding

IQ **Y93.19 Activity, other involving water and watercraft**

Activity involving water NOS

Activity, parasailing

Activity, water survival training and testing

5 **Y93.2 Activities involving ice and snow**

EXCLUDES 1 activity, shoveling ice and snow (Y93.H1)

IQ **Y93.21 Activity, ice skating**

Activity, figure skating (singles) (pairs)

Activity, ice dancing

EXCLUDES 1 activity, ice hockey (Y93.22)

IQ **Y93.22 Activity, ice hockey**

IQ **Y93.23 Activity, snow (alpine) (downhill) skiing, snowboarding, sledding, tobogganing and snow tubing**

EXCLUDES 1 activity, cross country skiing (Y93.24)

IQ **Y93.24 Activity, cross country skiing**

Activity, nordic skiing

IQ **Y93.29 Activity, other involving ice and snow**

Activity involving ice and snow NOS

5 **Y93.3 Activities involving climbing, rappelling and jumping off**

EXCLUDES 1 activity, hiking on level or elevated terrain (Y93.01)
activity, jumping rope (Y93.56)
activity, trampoline jumping (Y93.44)

IQ **Y93.31 Activity, mountain climbing, rock climbing and wall climbing**

IQ **Y93.32 Activity, rappelling**

IQ **Y93.33 Activity, BASE jumping**

Activity, Building, Antenna, Span, Earth jumping

IQ **Y93.34 Activity, bungee jumping**

IQ **Y93.35 Activity, hang gliding**

IQ **Y93.39 Activity, other involving climbing, rappelling and jumping off**

5 **Y93.4 Activities involving dancing and other rhythmic movement**

EXCLUDES 1 activity, martial arts (Y93.75)

IQ **Y93.41 Activity, dancing**

IQ **Y93.42 Activity, yoga**

IQ **Y93.43 Activity, gymnastics**

Activity, rhythmic gymnastics

EXCLUDES 1 activity, trampolining (Y93.44)

IQ **Y93.44 Activity, trampolining**

IQ **Y93.45 Activity, cheerleading**

IQ **Y93.49 Activity, other involving dancing and other rhythmic movements**

5 **Y93.5 Activities involving other sports and athletics played individually**

EXCLUDES 1 activity, dancing (Y93.41)
activity, gymnastic (Y93.43)
activity, trampolining (Y93.44)
activity, yoga (Y93.42)

IQ **Y93.51 Activity, roller skating (inline) and skateboarding**

IQ **Y93.52 Activity, horseback riding**

IQ **Y93.53 Activity, golf**

IQ **Y93.54 Activity, bowling**

IQ **Y93.55 Activity, bike riding**

IQ **Y93.56 Activity, jumping rope**

IQ **Y93.57 Activity, non-running track and field events**

EXCLUDES 1 activity, running (any form) (Y93.02)

IQ **Y93.59 Activity, other involving other sports and athletics played individually**

EXCLUDES 1 activities involving climbing, rappelling, and jumping (Y93.3-)
activities involving ice and snow (Y93.2-)
activities involving walking and running (Y93.0-)
activities involving water and watercraft (Y93.1-)

5 **Y93.6 Activities involving other sports and athletics played as a team or group**

EXCLUDES 1 activity, ice hockey (Y93.22)
activity, water polo (Y93.13)

IQ **Y93.61 Activity, american tackle football**

Activity, football NOS

IQ **Y93.62 Activity, american flag or touch football**

IQ **Y93.63 Activity, rugby**

IQ **Y93.64 Activity, baseball**

Activity, softball

IQ **Y93.65 Activity, lacrosse and field hockey**

IQ **Y93.66 Activity, soccer**

IQ **Y93.67 Activity, basketball**

IQ **Y93.68 Activity, volleyball (beach) (court)**

Chapter 20

V00-Y99

IQ **Y93.6A Activity, physical games generally associated with school recess, summer camp and children**
Activity, capture the flag
Activity, dodge ball
Activity, four square
Activity, kickball

IQ **Y93.69 Activity, other involving other sports and athletics played as a team or group**
Activity, cricket

5 **Y93.7 Activities involving other specified sports and athletics**

IQ **Y93.71 Activity, boxing**

IQ **Y93.72 Activity, wrestling**

IQ **Y93.73 Activity, racquet and hand sports**
Activity, handball
Activity, racquetball
Activity, squash
Activity, tennis

IQ **Y93.74 Activity, frisbee**
Activity, ultimate frisbee

IQ **Y93.75 Activity, martial arts**
Activity, combatives

IQ **Y93.79 Activity, other specified sports and athletics**
EXCLUDES 1 sports and athletics activities specified in categories Y93.0-Y93.6

5 **Y93.A Activities involving other cardiorespiratory exercise**
Activities involving physical training

IQ **Y93.A1 Activity, exercise machines primarily for cardiorespiratory conditioning**
Activity, elliptical and stepper machines
Activity, stationary bike
Activity, treadmill

IQ **Y93.A2 Activity, calisthenics**
Activity, jumping jacks
Activity, warm up and cool down

IQ **Y93.A3 Activity, aerobic and step exercise**

IQ **Y93.A4 Activity, circuit training**

IQ **Y93.A5 Activity, obstacle course**
Activity, challenge course
Activity, confidence course

IQ **Y93.A6 Activity, grass drills**
Activity, guerilla drills

IQ **Y93.A9 Activity, other involving cardiorespiratory exercise**
EXCLUDES 1 activities involving cardiorespiratory exercise specified in categories Y93.0-Y93.7

5 **Y93.B Activities involving other muscle strengthening exercises**

IQ **Y93.B1 Activity, exercise machines primarily for muscle strengthening**

IQ **Y93.B2 Activity, push-ups, pull-ups, sit-ups**

IQ **Y93.B3 Activity, free weights**
Activity, barbells
Activity, dumbbells

IQ **Y93.B4 Activity, pilates**

IQ **Y93.B9 Activity, other involving muscle strengthening exercises**
EXCLUDES 1 activities involving muscle strengthening specified in categories Y93.0-Y93.A

5 **Y93.C Activities involving computer technology and electronic devices**
EXCLUDES 1 activity, electronic musical keyboard or instruments (Y93.J-)

IQ **Y93.C1 Activity, computer keyboarding**
Activity, electronic game playing using keyboard or other stationary device

IQ **Y93.C2 Activity, hand held interactive electronic device**
Activity, cellular telephone and communication device
Activity, electronic game playing using interactive device
EXCLUDES 1 activity, electronic game playing using keyboard or other stationary device (Y93.C1)

IQ **Y93.C9 Activity, other involving computer technology and electronic devices**

5 **Y93.D Activities involving arts and handcrafts**
EXCLUDES 1 activities involving playing musical instrument (Y93.J-)

IQ **Y93.D1 Activity, knitting and crocheting**

IQ **Y93.D2 Activity, sewing**

IQ **Y93.D3 Activity, furniture building and finishing**
Activity, furniture repair

IQ **Y93.D9 Activity, other involving arts and handcrafts**

5 **Y93.E Activities involving personal hygiene and interior property and clothing maintenance**
EXCLUDES 1 activities involving cooking and grilling (Y93.G-)
activities involving exterior property and land maintenance, building and construction (Y93.H-)
activities involving caregiving (Y93.F-)
activity, dishwashing (Y93.G1)
activity, food preparation (Y93.G1)
activity, gardening (Y93.H2)

IQ **Y93.E1 Activity, personal bathing and showering**

IQ **Y93.E2 Activity, laundry**

IQ **Y93.E3 Activity, vacuuming**

IQ **Y93.E4 Activity, ironing**

IQ **Y93.E5 Activity, floor mopping and cleaning**

IQ **Y93.E6 Activity, residential relocation**
Activity, packing up and unpacking involved in moving to a new residence

IQ **Y93.E8 Activity, other personal hygiene**

IQ **Y93.E9 Activity, other interior property and clothing maintenance**

5 **Y93.F Activities involving caregiving**

Chapter 20
V00-Y99

Activity involving the provider of caregiving

IQ **Y93.F1 Activity, caregiving, bathing**

IQ **Y93.F2 Activity, caregiving, lifting**

IQ **Y93.F9 Activity, other caregiving**

5 **Y93.G Activities involving food preparation, cooking and grilling**

IQ **Y93.G1 Activity, food preparation and clean up**
Activity, dishwashing

IQ **Y93.G2 Activity, grilling and smoking food**

IQ **Y93.G3 Activity, cooking and baking**
Activity, use of stove, oven and microwave oven

IQ **Y93.G9 Activity, other involving cooking and grilling**

5 **Y93.H Activities involving exterior property and land maintenance, building and construction**

IQ **Y93.H1 Activity, digging, shoveling and raking**
Activity, dirt digging
Activity, raking leaves
Activity, snow shoveling

IQ **Y93.H2 Activity, gardening and landscaping**
Activity, pruning, trimming shrubs, weeding

IQ **Y93.H3 Activity, building and construction**

IQ **Y93.H9 Activity, other involving exterior property and land maintenance, building and construction**

5 **Y93.I Activities involving roller coasters and other types of external motion**

IQ **Y93.I1 Activity, roller coaster riding**

IQ **Y93.I9 Activity, other involving external motion**

5 **Y93.J Activities involving playing musical instrument**
Activity involving playing electric musical instrument

IQ **Y93.J1 Activity, piano playing**
Activity, musical keyboard (electronic) playing

IQ **Y93.J2 Activity, drum and other percussion instrument playing**

IQ **Y93.J3 Activity, string instrument playing**

IQ **Y93.J4 Activity, winds and brass instrument playing**

5 **Y93.K Activities involving animal care**
EXCLUDES 1 activity, horseback riding (Y93.52)

IQ **Y93.K1 Activity, walking an animal**

IQ **Y93.K2 Activity, milking an animal**

IQ **Y93.K3 Activity, grooming and shearing an animal**

IQ **Y93.K9 Activity, other involving animal care**

5 **Y93.8 Activities, other specified**

IQ **Y93.81 Activity, refereeing a sports activity**

IQ **Y93.82 Activity, spectator at an event**

IQ **Y93.83 Activity, rough housing and horseplay**

IQ **Y93.84 Activity, sleeping**

IQ **Y93.85 Activity, choking game**
Activity, blackout game
Activity, fainting game
Activity, pass out game

IQ **Y93.89 Activity, other specified**

IQ **Y93.9 Activity, unspecified**

IQ **Y95 Nosocomial condition**

4 **Y99 External cause status**
Note:
A single code from category Y99 should be used in conjunction with the external cause code(s) assigned to a record to indicate the status of the person at the time the event occurred.

IQ **Y99.0 Civilian activity done for income or pay**
Civilian activity done for financial or other compensation
EXCLUDES 1 military activity (Y99.1)
volunteer activity (Y99.2)

IQ **Y99.1 Military activity**
EXCLUDES 1 activity of off duty military personnel (Y99.8)

IQ **Y99.2 Volunteer activity**
EXCLUDES 1 activity of child or other family member assisting in compensated work of other family member (Y99.8)

IQ **Y99.8 Other external cause status**
Activity NEC
Activity of child or other family member assisting in compensated work of other family member
Hobby not done for income
Leisure activity
Off-duty activity of military personnel
Recreation or sport not for income or while a student
Student activity
EXCLUDES 1 civilian activity done for income or compensation (Y99.0)
military activity (Y99.1)

IQ **Y99.9 Unspecified external cause status**

Chapter 20 Scenarios: External causes of morbidity (V00-Y99)

Leukemia due to radiation exposure

A 42-year-old male is admitted to home health for observation and assessment of dehydration, fever and shortness of breath, which are stated to be side effects of experimental chemotherapy taken to treat chronic lymphocytic leukemia. The medical record states that the leukemia resulted from occupational exposure to radiation due to his job as a registered nurse in an emergency room setting.

Description	Code
Primary: Dehydration	E86.0
Secondary: Fever, unspecified	R50.9
Secondary: Shortness of breath	R06.02
Secondary: Adverse effect of antineoplastic and immunosuppressive drugs, subsequent encounter	T45.1X5D
Secondary: Chronic lymphocytic leukemia of B-cell type not having achieved remission	C91.10
Secondary: Exposure to X-rays, sequela	W88.0XXS

Because the dehydration, fever and shortness of breath resulted from the proper use of the experimental drug, they're coded as adverse effects. The dehydration, fever and shortness of breath are coded first, followed by the code for the drug that caused it. The patient's leukemia is still an active condition and so it is included as well. Because it was said to be caused by radiation exposure, an external cause code is assigned to indicate that. The seventh character "S" is assigned to the external cause code to indicate that the leukemia occurred from past radiation exposure.

Radiation burn to chest wall

A 69-year-old woman comes to home health for active treatment to a third degree burn on her chest wall caused by radiation for cancer in the lower inner quadrant of her left breast.

Description	Code
Primary: Burn of third degree of chest wall, initial encounter	T21.31XA
Secondary: Radiological procedure and radiotherapy as the cause of abnormal reaction of the patient, or of later complication, without mention of misadventure at the time of the procedure	Y84.2
Secondary: Malignant neoplasm of lower-inner quadrant of left female breast	C50.312

A radiation burn is treated as a burn, according to the alphabetic index. The seventh character "A" is used because the home health agency will be providing active treatment to the burn. An external cause code, Y84.2, is assigned to indicate that radiation is the source of the burn. Since the cancer is an active diagnosis, it is also coded.

Burn of palm on hot pan

A 68-year-old man sustained a second degree burn to his left palm after accidently pressing his hand down on a hot skillet on the stove. He was admitted to home health to continue wound care to the site. He is a type 1 diabetic and has mild polyneuropathy and newly diagnosed dementia.

Description	Code
Primary: Burn of second degree of left palm, subsequent encounter	T23.252D
Secondary: Type 1 diabetes mellitus with diabetic polyneuropathy	E10.42
Secondary: Unspecified dementia without behavioral disturbance	F03.90
Secondary: Contact with hot saucepan or skillet, subsequent encounter	X15.3xxD

The appropriate seventh character "D" is used on the burn code, in accordance with coding conventions, to denote the subsequent nature of the care being given. The external cause code indicating how the wound was sustained carries the same seventh character as the injury code, "D," in accordance with coding guidelines. Two placeholder x's are used here because the external cause code, X15.3-, has only four characters but requires a seventh character. Thus, the two empty places are filled with placeholder x. The patient's type 1 diabetes with polyneuropathy has the potential to impact his ability to heal from the burn, so it is included as well. The patient's dementia may also impact the patient's care planning and this is also coded. An additional code for insulin use is not required because it is assumed in type 1 diabetes.

Gunshot wound, child abuse

A 13-year-old male patient underwent surgery in the hospital for a gunshot wound to the right lower quadrant of his abdomen; the bullet fragment was removed. In a recent domestic violence incident, his father shot and killed his mother with a shotgun, then shot the patient and finally committed suicide. The medical record also documents that prior to the shooting, the patient had suffered severe abuse at the hands of his father which left him underweight with a body mass index (BMI) that is less than the fifth percentile for his age. The patient was admitted to home health for continued wound care and physical therapy to regain strength.

Description	Code
Primary: Child physical abuse, confirmed, subsequent encounter	T74.12xD
Secondary: Puncture wound of abdominal wall with foreign body, right lower quadrant without penetration into peritoneal cavity, subsequent encounter	S31.143D
Secondary: Biological father, perpetrator of maltreatment and neglect	Y07.11
Secondary: Assault by shotgun, subsequent encounter	X94.0xxD
Secondary: Underweight	R63.6
Secondary: Body mass index (BMI) pediatric, less than 5th percentile for age	Z68.51

Because this is a documented case of child abuse, the child abuse code is assigned first, in accordance with coding guidelines. There is a "use additional code" note which gives instructions to code any associated current injury as well as an external cause code to identify the perpetrator. In this case, the injury is a gunshot wound from the shotgun and the perpetrator is the patient's biological father. The patient is coming to home health to continue healing, versus to receive active treatment. Thus, the seventh character "D" is used. The gunshot wound is coded as a puncture wound, according to Q3 2016 Coding Clinic guidance. Since the wound was brought about with a bullet, the code for "with foreign body" is used. The seventh character "D" captures that initial treatment, including removing the bullet fragment, is completed and the patient is now in the healing and recovery phase. An additional code, Y07.11, is assigned the show that the patient's abuse was perpetrated by his father, in accordance with tabular instruction. An external cause code is also assigned to indicate that a shotgun was used to perpetrate the assault/abuse and led to the injuries now needing treatment. The patient was diagnosed as underweight, and thus R63.6 is assigned to capture this. An additional code, Z68.51, is used to show his BMI, which is less than the fifth percentile for his age, in accordance with tabular instruction. Because the patient is between 2-19 years of age, pediatric BMI codes are used.

Chapter 21: Factors Influencing Health Status and Contact with Health Services (Z00-Z99)

Categories Z00-Z99 are provided for occasions when circumstances other than a disease, injury or external cause classifiable to categories A00-Y89, are recorded as 'diagnoses' or problems. This can arise in two main ways:

a. When a person who may or may not be sick encounters the health services for some specific purpose, such as to receive limited care or service for a current condition, to donate an organ or tissue, to receive prophylactic vaccination (immunization), or to discuss a problem which in itself is not a disease or injury.

b. When some circumstance or problem is present which influences the person's health status but is not in itself a current illness or injury.

Z codes are for use in any healthcare setting and may be used as either a first-listed (principal diagnosis code) or a secondary code, depending on the circumstances of the encounter. Certain Z codes may only be used as first-listed or principal diagnosis.

Chapter 21 has significant changes from ICD-9-CM, including expansions of some categories, especially the history codes, while eliminating other codes such as encounter for rehabilitation, aftercare codes for healing fractures, and aftercare for injury codes. Injuries, including traumatic and pathological fractures, require assignment of the acute injury or fracture code with use of the appropriate 7th character extension (for subsequent care).

Don't look for a so-called "rehab code" to capture a therapy-only case. Instead, capture the therapy a patient is receiving with ICD-10 codes that describe the reason for the therapy, such as I50.31 (Acute diastolic (congestive) heart failure).

As with all coding, it is important to search for codes first in the Alphabetical Index and confirm the code and read all of the notes in the Tabular List (code definitions, Excludes 1 and 2 notes, code first and add an additional code).

Z codes are organized by categories. The most important categories to home health are Status, History and Aftercare. Here is a look at all of the blocks within chapter 21:

Persons encountering health services for examinations (Z00-Z13)

These codes are primarily used in clinic and physician offices for examinations and disease and disorder screenings.

Genetic carrier and genetic susceptibility to disease (Z14-Z15)

These are status codes indicating the person carries a gene associated with a particular disease, which may be passed to offspring who may develop that disease. Genetic carrier codes (Z14.-) indicate the person does not have the disease and is not at risk of developing the disease. Z15, Genetic susceptibility to disease, indicates that a person has a gene that increases the risk of that person developing the disease. Examples include: Genetic susceptibility to malignant neoplasm of: breast (Z15.01), ovary, prostate (Z15.03), endometrium (Z15.04), and other malignant neoplasm (Z15.09). Codes from Z15 should not be used as first-listed codes. If the patient has the condition to which he is susceptible, and that condition is the reason for the encounter, the code for the current condition should be sequenced first. If the patient is being seen for follow-up after completed treatment for the disease, and the condition no longer exists, a follow-up code should be sequenced first, followed by the appropriate personal history and genetic susceptibility codes.

Resistance to antimicrobial drugs (Z16)

This code indicates that a patient has a condition that is resistant to antimicrobial drug treatment. Z16 includes a 'code first' note for the infection and a second note that codes in this category are provided for use as additional codes to identify the resistance and non-responsiveness of a condition to antimicrobial drugs. Z16.1- refers to resistance to beta lactam antibiotics including resistance to penicillin/amoxicillin/ampicillin (Z16.11). Z16.2- refers to resistance to other antibiotics such as vancomycin (Z16.21), resistance to multiple antibiotics (Z16.24), and other single antibiotics (Z16.29). Z16.3- covers other antimicrobial drugs such as resistance to antiparasitic, antifungal, antiviral or antimycobacterial drugs; multiple and other antimicrobial drugs.

Estrogen receptor status (Z17)

These codes are consolidated to indicate status codes for **estrogen receptor positive (Z17.0) and estrogen receptor negative (Z17.1)** with a note to code first malignant neoplasm of the breast (C50.-).

Retained foreign body fragments (Z18)

A series of 5-character codes describe the nature of the foreign body fragments as radioactive (Z18.0-), metal (Z18.1-), plastic (Z18.2), organic such as animal quills or spines, tooth or wood (Z18.3-), other specified retained foreign body (Z18.8-), and retained foreign body fragments of unspecified material (Z18.9).

Hormone sensitivity malignancy status (Z19)

This category was added in FY2017, and contains codes Z19.1 (Hormone sensitive malignancy status) and Z19.2 (Hormone resistant malignancy status). This category of codes has a note to code first malignant neoplasm (see Table of Neoplasms).

Persons with potential health hazards related to communicable diseases (Z20-Z29)

These codes indicate contact with, and suspected exposure to, communicable diseases. They are reported for patients who do not show any signs or symptoms of a disease, but are suspected to have been exposed to it by close personal contact with an infected individual or are in an area where the disease is epidemic. These codes may be assigned as principal diagnoses to explain an encounter for testing, or as an additional diagnosis to identify a potential risk.

Codes include contact with and (suspected) exposure to communicable diseases such as intestinal infectious diseases, **contact with/exposure to TB (Z20.1),** sexually transmitted diseases, rabies (Z20.3), rubella (Z20.4), **viral hepatitis (Z20.5), HIV (Z20.6)**, pediculosis, acariasis and other infestations (Z20.7), and a number of other bacterial and viral communicable diseases (V20.8-).

Other potential health hazards include HIV status **(Z21) that indicates that a patient has tested positive for HIV, but has not manifested any signs or symptoms of the disease.** Z22.- are carrier status codes indicating that a person harbors the specific organisms of a disease without manifesting symptoms, but is capable of transmitting the infection.

Code Z23 is for encounters for inoculations and vaccinations. It indicates the patient is being seen to receive prophylactic inoculation against a disease. Procedure codes are required to identify the actual administration of the injection and the type(s) of immunizations given.

Codes for immunization not carried out (with reasons) include Z28.0-, Z28.2-, Z28.8-, Z28.9, and **under- immunization status (Z28.3).**

Persons encountering health services in circumstances related to reproduction (Z30-Z39)

This category is used primarily for:

- Counseling on contraceptive management, supervision of normal pregnancy, etc.
- Pregnancy state incidental (Z33.1) is a status code
- Weeks of gestation (Z3A.-) for use only on maternal record to show weeks of gestation of the pregnancy with a note to code first obstetric condition or encounter for delivery (O09-O60, O80-O82).
- Outcome of delivery on the mother's record (Z37.-)
- Encounter and care for postpartum care and follow-up (Z39.-).

Encounters for other specific health care (Z40-Z53)

These categories are intended for use to indicate a reason for care. They may be used for patients who already have been treated for a disease or injury, but who are receiving aftercare or prophylactic care, or care to consolidate the treatment, or to deal with a residual state. These categories have an Excludes 2 note for follow-up examination for medical surveillance after treatment (Z08-Z09). More specifically, they include:

- Z40 Encounter for prophylactic surgery such as **prophylactic removal of breast (Z40.01)** and other organs.
- Z41 Encounter for procedures for purposes other than remedying health state such as cosmetic surgery (Z41.1)
- Z42 Encounter for plastic and reconstructive surgery following medical procedure or healed injury such as **breast reconstruction following mastectomy (Z42.1)** or encounter for other plastic and reconstructive surgery following medical procedure or healed injury (Z42.8).
- Z43 Encounter for attention to artificial openings includes passage of sounds, reforming the artificial opening, removal of catheter and toileting or cleansing. Examples include: **attention to tracheostomy (Z43.0), colostomy (Z43.3), other artificial opening of urinary tract (Z43.6), other artificial opening (Z43.8).** Note, that once the artificial opening has been closed, codes from category Z43.- are no longer applicable since the patient no longer has the ostomy. If the patient is seen for wound care following closure of the site, assign a code from category Z48.- (Encounter for other postprocedural aftercare).
- Z44 Encounter for fitting and adjustment of external prosthetic device including artificial arm (Z44.0-) or leg (Z44.1-). Fitting and adjustment examples include: Fitting and adjustment complete left artificial arm (Z44.012) or partial artificial right arm (Z44.021), external breast prosthesis (Z44.3-), Fitting and adjustment other external prosthetic device (Z44.8),
- Z45 Encounter for **checking and testing cardiac pacemaker pulse generator (Z45.010), or adjustment and management of automated implantable defibrillator (Z45.02) ; encounter for adjustment and management of vascular access device (Z45.2); encounter for adjustment and management of implanted hearing device (Z45.32); adjustment and management of cerebrospinal fluid drainage device (Z45.41).**
- Z46 Fitting and adjustment of other devices such as **encounter for fitting and adjustment of gastric lap band (Z46.51), fitting and adjustment of urinary device (intermittent or indwelling**

catheter) (Z46.6), fitting and adjustment of insulin pump, encounter for insulin pump titration **or encounter for insulin pump instruction and training (Z46.81).**

- Z47 Orthopedic aftercare including **aftercare following joint prosthesis (Z47.1); aftercare following explantation of joint prosthesis (Z47.3-); encounter for orthopedic aftercare following surgical amputation (Z47.81) encounter for orthopedic aftercare following scoliosis surgery (Z47.82).** Assign an aftercare code if the condition for which a patient is receiving rehab services is no longer present unless the patient sustained an injury. In these scenarios, assign the injury code with the appropriate 7th character. For example: A hip replacement that was done to treat a right intertrochanteric femur fracture, would be coded with S72.141D (Displaced intertrochanteric fracture of right femur, subsequent encounter for closed fracture with routine healing), not Z47.1 (Aftercare following joint replacement surgery), according to coding guidelines.
- Z48 Encounter for other post-procedural aftercare such as **change/removal nonsurgical wound dressing (Z48.00) or change/removal of surgical wound dressings (Z48.01);** Encounter for aftercare following organ transplant (Z48.2-); **Aftercare following surgery for a neoplasm (Z48.3)**; or Aftercare for surgical aftercare following surgery on specific body systems (Z48.81-).
- Z49 Encounter for care involving renal dialysis codes have a note to code also end stage renal disease (N18.6)
- Z51 Encounter for other aftercare and medical care such as: **Z51.11, encounter for antineoplastic chemotherapy or Z51.12, encounter for antineoplastic immunotherapy; and encounter for therapeutic drug level monitoring (Z51.81).**
- Z52 Donors of organs and tissues
- Z53 Persons encountering health services for specific procedures and treatment, not carried out due to specific reasons such as contraindications, patient smoking, reasons of belief and group pressure, and patient's decision.

Persons with potential health hazards related to socioeconomic and psychosocial circumstances (Z55-Z65)

Codes in categories Z55-Z65 (Persons with potential hazards related to socioeconomic and psychosocial circumstances) capture social information, rather than medical diagnoses, and can thus be reported based on information documented by other clinicians, not just the physician, who are involved in the care of the patient, according to Q1 2018 Coding Clinic guidance.

- Z55 includes codes for problems related to education and literacy, while Z56 contains codes related to problems related to employment and unemployment.
- Z57 includes codes for occupational exposure to risk factors such as noise, radiation, dust, tobacco smoke, other air contaminants, toxic agents in agriculture and other industries, extreme temperature, and exposure to other & unspecified risk factors.
- Z59 includes codes for problems related to housing and economic circumstances such as homelessness, inadequate housing, discord with neighbors, lodgers & landlord, problems related to living in residential institution, lack of adequate food & safe drinking water, extreme poverty & low income, and other problems related to housing and economic circumstances.
- Z60 codes describe problems related to social environment such as problems of life style adjustment, living alone, acculturation, social exclusion & rejection and adverse discrimination & persecution.
- Z62, problems relate to upbringing includes inadequate parental supervision & control, parental overprotection, hostility toward & scapegoating of child, personal history of abuse in childhood, and parent-child conflict.
- Z63, Other problems related to primary support group and family circumstances including a variety of stressful life events affecting family and household.
- Z64 and Z65, Problems related to psychosocial circumstances such as unwanted pregnancy, multiparity, conviction without imprisonment, imprisonment & other legal circumstances, etc.

Do not resuscitate status (Z66), Blood Type (Z67) and Body mass Index (Z68)

Code Z66, Do not resuscitate, may only be used when the provider documents that a patient is a "do not resuscitate" at any time during the patient's stay. BMI codes (Z68) should only be assigned when there is an associated, reportable diagnosis (such as obesity), according to coding guidelines. Do not assign BMI codes during pregnancy.

Persons encountering health services in other circumstances (Z69-Z76)

- Z69, Encounter for mental health services for victim and perpetrator of abuse
- Z71, Other counseling and medical advice, not elsewhere classified such as counseling and surveillance for dietary, alcohol abuse, drug abuse,

tobacco abuse, HIV, and spiritual or religious counseling.

- Z72, Problems related to lifestyle such as tobacco use, lack of physical exercise, inappropriate diet and eating habits, high risk sexual & antisocial behavior, and sleep problems (deprivation, inadequate sleep hygiene).
- Z73, Problems related to life management difficulty such as burn out, Type A behavior pattern, lack of relaxation and leisure, stress NOS, inadequate social skills or social role conflict, limitation of activities due to disability, and other problems relate to life management difficulty.
- Z74, Problems related to care provider dependency such as **bed confinement status (Z74.01)**, need for assistance with personal care, assistance at home and no other household member able to render care, and need for continuous supervision.
- Z75, Problems related to medical facilities and other health care such as person awaiting admission to adequate facility elsewhere, unavailability and inaccessibility of other helping agencies, and holiday relief care.
- Z76, Personal encountering health services in other circumstances such as issue of repeat prescription medications, malingerer, **awaiting organ transplant status (Z76.82).**

Persons with potential health hazards related to family and personal history and certain conditions influencing health status (Z77-Z99)

- Z77, Other contact with and (suspected) exposures hazardous to health such as chiefly nonmedicinal metals & chemicals (e.g., **exposure to lead Z77.011)**, environmental pollution & hazards in the physical environment e.g., **(mold Z77.120)**, and other hazardous substances **(e.g., environmental tobacco smoke, Z77.22).** These codes may be used as first-listed to explain an encounter for testing, or more commonly, as a secondary code to identify a potential risk.
- Z78, Other specified health status, including **physical restraint status (Z78.1).**
- Z79, Long term (current) drug therapy includes **long term use of anticoagulants (Z79.01), antithrombotics/antiplatelets (Z79.02), NSAID (Z79.1), antibiotics Z79.2),** hormonal contraceptives (Z79.3), **insulin (Z79.4),** inhaled steroids (Z79.51), system steroids (Z79.52), aspirin (Z79.82), bisphosphonates (Z79.83); **oral hypoglycemic drugs (Z79.84);** opiate analgesic (Z79.891); use of agents affecting estrogen receptors and estrogen levels – includes both code first and use additional codes notes and six character codes for an expanded list of SERMS, aromatase inhibitors & other agents (Z79.81); and other such as hormone replacement therapy (Z79.890).

  Codes from this category indicate a patient's continuous use of a prescription drug (including aspirin therapy) for the long-term treatment of a condition or for prophylactic use. A code from Z79 is assigned for a patient who is receiving medication for an extended period as a prophylactic measure (such as for the prevention of deep vein thrombosis) or as treatment of a chronic condition (such as arthritis) or a disease requiring a lengthy course of treatment (such as cancer). A code from Z79 is ***not assigned for medication being administered for a brief period to treat an acute illness or injury*** (such as a course of antibiotics to treat acute bronchitis).

  The Z79 codes are ***not*** for use for patients who have addictions to drugs, or medications for detoxification, or maintenance programs to prevent withdrawal symptoms in patients with drug dependence (e.g., methadone maintenance for opiate dependence). Instead assign the appropriate drug dependence code for those patients.

- Z80, Family history of primary malignant neoplasm by body site. Example: **family history of leukemia (Z80.6)** or **family history of other malignant neoplasms of lymphoid, hematopoietic and related tissue (Z80.7).**
- Z81 – Z84 are all family history codes and are broken into categories as follows: Family history of mental and behavioral disorders (Z81.-), Family history of certain disabilities and chronic diseases (leading to disablement) (Z82.-), Family history of other specific disorders (Z83.-), and Family history of other conditions (Z84.-).
- Z85, Personal history of malignant neoplasm by body system and identification of conditions classifiable to categories in Chapter 2. Be aware of the code first note and use additional codes listed at the top of the category. Examples include: **Z85.110, personal history of malignant carcinoid tumor of bronchus and lung or Z85.820, Personal history of malignant melanoma of skin.**
- Z86, Personal history of certain other diseases includes codes for Personal history of in-situ and benign neoplasm and neoplasms of uncertain behavior (Z86.0-); Personal history of infectious and parasitic diseases (Z86.1-) such as **Personal history of polio (Z86.12) or TB (Z86.11)**; Personal history of endocrine, nutritional and metabolic diseases (Z86.3-) such as **Personal history of diabetic foot ulcer (Z86.31)**; plus Personal history of combat and operational stress reaction (Z86.51) and other mental and behavioral disorder (Z86.59); Personal history of infections of the CNS

(Z86.61) or nervous system and sense organs (Z86.69); and Personal history of diseases of the circulatory system (Z86.7-) such as **Personal history of pulmonary embolism (Z86.711) or Personal history of TIA and cerebral infarction without residual deficits (Z86.73).**

- Z87 Personal history of other diseases and conditions may be used in conjunction with follow-up codes. These codes explain a patient's past medical condition that no longer exists and is not receiving any current treatment, but has a potential for recurrence, and therefore may require continued monitoring and may also alter the type of treatment ordered. Examples include: **Personal history of pneumonia (Z87.01), personal history** of other diseases of the respiratory system (Z87.09); **Personal history of peptic ulcer disease (Z87.11)** or Personal history of other diseases of the digestive system (Z87.19); Personal history off diseases of the skin and subcutaneous tissue (Z87.2); Personal history of diseases of the musculoskeletal system and connective tissue (Z87.3-) such **as Personal history of (healed) osteoporosis fracture (Z87.310), or Personal history of other pathological fracture (Z87.311), or Personal history of stress fracture (Z87.312);** Personal history of diseases of genitourinary system (Z87.4-) such as **Personal history of urinary tract infection (Z87.440);** Personal history of other complications of pregnancy, childbirth and the puerperium (Z87.59) or Personal history of pre-term labor (Z87.51); Personal history of other specified conditions (Z87.8-) such as **personal history of (healed) traumatic fracture (Z87.81)** or Personal history of traumatic brain injury (Z87.820) or Personal history of nicotine dependence (Z87.891).
- Z88, Allergy status to drugs, medicaments, and biological substances, such as **Allergy status to penicillin (Z88.0), Allergy status to analgesic agent (Z88.6) or Allergy status to other anti-infective agents (Z88.3).**
- Z89, Acquired absence of a limb (amputation status, post-procedural loss of limb, or post-traumatic loss of limb) are status codes that include codes for acquired absence of a thumb, fingers, hand, wrist, upper limb above wrist, upper limb below or above elbow, shoulder, toes, foot, ankle, leg above or below knee, knee, and hip with specific codes for laterality. These codes can ***only be used*** if there are no complications of the amputation site. For example, **acquired absence of right shoulder (Z89.231) or acquired absence of left great toe (Z89.412) or disarticulation of a right ankle (Z89.441) or acquired absence of left hip joint following explantation of hip joint prosthesis with or without presence of an antibiotic-impregnated spacer (Z89.622).**
- Z90, Acquired absence of organs, not elsewhere classified, are also status codes that can only be used when there are no complications present. Examples include acquired absence of larynx (Z90.02), or **acquired absence of bilateral breasts and nipples (Z90.13) or acquired absence of uterus with remaining cervical stump (Z90.711).**
- Z91, Personal risk factors, not elsewhere classified, includes status codes for allergy status, other than to drugs and biological substances such as **latex allergy (Z91.040).** Z91.1- codes relate to patient's noncompliance with medical treatment and regimen such as **noncompliance with dietary regimen (Z91.11), or patient's noncompliance with renal dialysis (Z91.15).** Other codes in this category include: **Personal history of falling (Z91.81)**, and **Personal history of wandering in diseases classified elsewhere (Z91.83).**
- Z92, Personal history of medical treatment includes the following: **Z92.21, Personal history of antineoplastic chemotherapy; Z92.240, Personal history of inhaled steroid therapy.**
- Z93, Artificial opening status codes ***exclude*** artificial openings requiring attention or management which are coded to Z43.- and complications of external stoma (J95.0, K94.-, N99.5). These status codes indicate the patient or family caregiver is providing the care for the stoma, not the home health personnel. Some examples of these status codes are: **Z93.3, Colostomy status or Z93.51, Cutaneous-vesicostomy** status.
- Z94, Transplanted organ and tissue status codes indicate an organ or tissue replaced by heterogenous or homogenous transplant. These codes are not to be used in the presence of complications of the transplant organ or tissue. Examples include: **Z94.1, Heart transplant status** that excludes an artificial heart status (Z95.811) or heart-valve replacement status (Z95.2-X95.4); and **Bone marrow transplant status (Z94.81).**
- Z95, Presence of cardiac and vascular implants and grafts includes status codes such as: **Presence of cardiac pacemaker (Z95.0), aortocoronary bypass graft (Z95.1), presence of automatic (implanted) defibrillator (Z95.810).**
- Z96, Presence of orthopedic joint implants are status codes and exclude complications of internal prosthetic devices, implants or grafts, but these codes may be coded in addition to the codes from Z96.6-. Examples include **presence of right artificial hip joint (Z96.641), presence of left artificial knee joint (Z96.652), and presence of right artificial shoulder (Z96.611).** Other functional implants coded at Z96 include: presence of an artificial larynx (Z96.3) or presence of artificial skin (Z96.81).

- Z97, Presence of other devices includes codes for **presence of artificial right arm (complete) or (partial) (Z97.11), presence of bilateral artificial legs, bilateral (complete) (partial) (Z97.16),** and presence of external hearing aid (Z97.4)
- Z98, Other post procedural states has an Excludes 2 note for aftercare (Z43-Z49, Z51), follow-up medical care (Z08-Z09), and post procedural complications. Examples of codes from this category include: **coronary angioplasty status (Z98.61)**, excluding coronary angioplasty status with implant and graft (Z95.5); **breast implant status (Z98.82),** excluding breast implant removal status (Z98.86)**; bariatric surgery status (Z98.84)**; and **transplant organ removal status (Z98.85)** that is used to indicate a transplanted organ has been previously removed due to complication, failure, rejection or infection.
- Z99, Dependence on enabling machines and devices, not elsewhere classified, includes codes such as **Dependence on respirator/ ventilator (Z99.1-),** Dependence on renal dialysis (Z99.2), Dependence on wheelchair (Z99.3), and **Dependence on supplemental oxygen** (Z99.81).

Special Instructions related to Z code use

Note: Categories Z89-Z90 and Z93-Z99 can only be used when there are no complications, malfunctions of the organ or tissue replaced, the amputation site or the equipment on which the patient is dependent.

Aftercare codes (Z42-Z49, Z51) are heavily used in home health care for situations when the initial treatment of a disease has been performed and the patient requires continued care during the healing or recovery phase, or for the long-term consequences of the disease. The aftercare Z code should not be used if treatment is directed at a current, acute disease. The diagnosis code is to be used in these cases.

Additional guidance on aftercare codes includes:

- Exceptions to these rules are Z51.0, Encounter for antineoplastic radiation therapy, and Z51.1, Encounter for antineoplastic chemotherapy and immunotherapy. These codes are the first-listed, followed by the diagnosis code when a patient's encounter is solely to receive radiation therapy, chemotherapy or immunotherapy for the treatment of a neoplasm.
- The aftercare Z codes should **not** be used for aftercare for injuries including traumatic fractures. Instead, assign the original (acute) injury code with the appropriate 7th character (for subsequent care).
- The aftercare codes are generally first-listed to explain the specific reason for the encounter. An aftercare code may be used as an additional code when some type of aftercare is provided in addition to the reason for admission and no diagnosis code is applicable. An example of this would be the closure of a colostomy during an encounter for treatment of another condition.
- Aftercare codes should be used in conjunction with other aftercare codes or diagnosis codes to provide better detail on the specifics of an aftercare encounter visit, unless otherwise directed by the classification.
- Certain aftercare Z code categories need a secondary diagnosis code to describe the resolving condition or sequelae. For others, the condition is included in the code title.
- Status Z codes may be used with aftercare Z codes to indicate the nature of the aftercare. For example, Z95.1, Presence of aortocoronary bypass graft, may be used with code Z48.812, Encounter for surgical aftercare following surgery on the circulatory system, to indicate surgery for which the aftercare is being performed. A status code should not be used when the aftercare code indicates the type of status, such as using Z43.0, Encounter for attention to tracheostomy, with Z93.0, Tracheostomy status.

Follow-up codes (Z08-Z09, Z39, follow up-examination after completed treatment for malignant neoplasm, for conditions other than neoplasms and maternal postpartum care) are used to explain continuing surveillance following completed treatment of a disease, condition or injury. They imply that the condition has been fully treated and no longer exists. They should not be confused with aftercare codes, or injury codes with a 7th character for subsequent encounter, that explain ongoing care of a healing condition or its sequelae.

Prophylactic Organ Removal

For encounters specifically for prophylactic removal of an organ, the principal or first-listed code should be a code from category Z40, Encounter for prophylactic surgery.

Note, you would assign code Z48.3 (Aftercare following surgery for neoplasm) if your agency is providing care during the healing and recovery phase, following the initial treatment (surgery) for removal of the breast. You can also assign an additional code from subcategory Z90.1- (Acquired absence of breast and nipple) to provide additional information, according to the Coding Clinic (in a letter dated Aug. 17, 2016).

You would not assign code Z40.01 (Encounter for prophylactic removal of breast) since the home health visit is not the encounter where the breast is actually removed. Also you would not assign an aftercare visit code, such as Z42.1 (Encounter for breast reconstruction following mastectomy) since the breast is not reconstructed during the home health visit, according to Coding Clinic.

CHAPTER 21: FACTORS INFLUENCING HEALTH STATUS AND CONTACT WITH HEALTH SERVICES (Z00-Z99)

Note:
Z codes represent reasons for encounters. A corresponding procedure code must accompany a Z code if a procedure is performed. Categories Z00-Z99 are provided for occasions when circumstances other than a disease, injury or external cause classifiable to categories A00-Y89 are recorded as 'diagnoses' or 'problems'. This can arise in two main ways:
(a) When a person who may or may not be sick encounters the health services for some specific purpose, such as to receive limited care or service for a current condition, to donate an organ or tissue, to receive prophylactic vaccination (immunization), or to discuss a problem which is in itself not a disease or injury.
(b) When some circumstance or problem is present which influences the person's health status but is not in itself a current illness or injury.

ALERT Sometimes payer policy conflicts with official guidelines, rules and conventions, and other official guidance. When a payer refuses to pay based on code(s) used in compliance with that guidance, take the following steps: 1) Determine whether the denial or rejection is truly a coding dispute and not a different coverage or payment issue; 2) Remind the payer that following official guidelines and conventions is required by HIPAA code set standards and provide the official guidance in question. If a payer does have a policy that clearly conflicts with official coding rules or guidelines, every effort should be made to resolve the issue with the payer; 3) If the payer refuses to change its policy, obtain the payer requirements in writing. If the payer refuses to provide their policy in writing, document all discussions, including dates and names of individuals involved; 4) Conform to the payer's policy if the payer continues to deny or reject the claim; 5) Keep a permanent file of the documentation obtained regarding payer coding policies. It may be come in handy in the event of an audit.

GUIDELINES **Section I.C.21.a**
Z codes are for use in any healthcare setting. Z codes may be used as either a first-listed (principal diagnosis code in the inpatient setting) or secondary code, depending on the circumstances of the encounter. Certain Z codes may only be used as first-listed or principal diagnosis.

CODING TIPS✓ Aftercare Z codes should not be used for aftercare of injuries. For aftercare of an injury, assign the injury code with the appropriate 7th character, usually "D" if the condition meets the definition of aftercare (patient requires continued care during the healing or recovery phase or long term consequences of the disease/Injury). Do not use aftercare Z codes for complications. Continue to code the complication with a D to indicate aftercare.

This chapter contains the following blocks:

Z00-Z13	Persons encountering health services for examinations
Z14-Z15	Genetic carrier and genetic susceptibility to disease
Z16	Resistance to antimicrobial drugs
Z17	Estrogen receptor status
Z18	Retained foreign body fragments
Z19	Hormone sensitivity malignancy status
Z20-Z29	Persons with potential health hazards related to communicable diseases
Z30-Z39	Persons encountering health services in circumstances related to reproduction
Z40-Z53	Encounters for other specific health care
Z55-Z65	Persons with potential health hazards related to socioeconomic and psychosocial circumstances
Z66	Do not resuscitate status
Z67	Blood type
Z68	Body mass index (BMI)
Z69-Z76	Persons encountering health services in other circumstances
Z77-Z99	Persons with potential health hazards related to family and personal history and certain conditions influencing health status

Persons encountering health services for examinations (Z00-Z13)

Note:
Nonspecific abnormal findings disclosed at the time of these examinations are classified to categories R70-R94.

EXCLUDES 1 examinations related to pregnancy and reproduction (Z30-Z36, Z39.-)

CODING TIPS✓ These codes are generally for physician and NPP use with the exception of Z03.818, Z09 and Z11.59.

4 **Z00 Encounter for general examination without complaint, suspected or reported diagnosis**
EXCLUDES 1 encounter for examination for administrative purposes (Z02.-)
EXCLUDES 2 encounter for pre-procedural examinations (Z01.81-)
special screening examinations (Z11-Z13)

5 **Z00.0 Encounter for general adult medical examination**
Encounter for adult periodic examination (annual) (physical) and any associated laboratory and radiologic examinations
EXCLUDES 1 encounter for examination of sign or symptom- code to sign or symptom
general health check-up of infant or child (Z00.12.-)

Px IQ **Z00.00 Encounter for general adult medical examination without abnormal findings**
Encounter for adult health check-up NOS

Px IQ + **Z00.01 Encounter for general adult medical examination with abnormal findings**
Use additional code to identify abnormal findings

5 **Z00.1 Encounter for newborn, infant and child health examinations**

+ 6 **Z00.11 Newborn health examination**
Health check for child under 29 days old
Use additional code to identify any abnormal findings
EXCLUDES 1 health check for child over 28 days old (Z00.12-)

Px IQ + **Z00.110 Health examination for newborn under 8 days old**
Health check for newborn under 8 days old

Px IQ + **Z00.111 Health examination for newborn 8 to 28 days old**
Health check for newborn 8 to 28 days old
Newborn weight check

6 **Z00.12 Encounter for routine child health examination**
Health check (routine) for child over 28 days old
Immunizations appropriate for age
Routine developmental screening of infant or child
Routine vision and hearing testing
EXCLUDES 1 health check for child under 29 days old (Z00.11-)
health supervision of foundling or other healthy infant or child (Z76.1-Z76.2)
newborn health examination (Z00.11-)

Px IQ + **Z00.121 Encounter for routine child health examination with abnormal findings**
Use additional code to identify abnormal findings

Px IQ **Z00.129 Encounter for routine child health examination without abnormal findings**
Encounter for routine child health examination NOS

Px IQ **Z00.2 Encounter for examination for period of rapid growth in childhood**

Px IQ **Z00.3 Encounter for examination for adolescent development state**
Encounter for puberty development state

Px IQ **Z00.5 Encounter for examination of potential donor of organ and tissue**

IQ **Z00.6 Encounter for examination for normal comparison and control in clinical research program**
Examination of participant or control in clinical research program

5 **Z00.7 Encounter for examination for period of delayed growth in childhood**

Px IQ **Z00.70 Encounter for examination for period of delayed growth in childhood without abnormal findings**

Px IQ + **Z00.71 Encounter for examination for period of delayed growth in childhood with abnormal findings**
Use additional code to identify abnormal findings

Px IQ **Z00.8 Encounter for other general examination**
Encounter for health examination in population surveys

4 **Z01 Encounter for other special examination without complaint, suspected or reported diagnosis**
Note:
Codes from category Z01 represent the reason for the encounter. A separate procedure code is required to identify any examinations or procedures performed
INCLUDES routine examination of specific system
EXCLUDES 1 encounter for examination for administrative purposes (Z02.-)
encounter for examination for suspected conditions, proven not to exist (Z03.-)
encounter for laboratory and radiologic examinations as a component of general medical examinations (Z00.0-)
encounter for laboratory, radiologic and imaging examinations for sign (s) and symptom(s) - code to the sign(s) or symptom(s)
EXCLUDES 2 screening examinations (Z11-Z13)

5 **Z01.0 Encounter for examination of eyes and vision**
EXCLUDES 1 examination for driving license (Z02.4)

Px IQ **Z01.00 Encounter for examination of eyes and vision without abnormal findings**
Encounter for examination of eyes and vision NOS

Px IQ + **Z01.01 Encounter for examination of eyes and vision with abnormal findings**
Use additional code to identify abnormal findings

▲ 6 **Z01.02 Encounter for examination of eyes and vision following failed vision screening**
EXCLUDES 1 encounter for examination of eyes and vision with abnormal findings (Z01.01)
encounter for examination of eyes and vision without abnormal findings (Z01.00)

Px **Z01.020 Encounter for examination of eyes and vision following failed vision screening without abnormal findings**

Px + **Z01.021 Encounter for examination of eyes and vision following failed vision screening with abnormal findings**
Use additional code to identify abnormal findings

5 **Z01.1 Encounter for examination of ears and hearing**

Px IQ **Z01.10 Encounter for examination of ears and hearing without abnormal findings**
Encounter for examination of ears and hearing NOS

6 **Z01.11 Encounter for examination of ears and hearing with abnormal findings**

Px IQ **Z01.110 Encounter for hearing examination following failed hearing screening**

Px IQ + **Z01.118 Encounter for examination of ears and hearing with other abnormal findings**
Use additional code to identify abnormal findings

Px IQ **Z01.12 Encounter for hearing conservation and treatment**

5 **Z01.2 Encounter for dental examination and cleaning**

4 4th digit required 5 5th digit required 6 6th digit required 7 7th digit required X 7th digit placeholder + Additional code L Laterality

Px IQ **Z01.20 Encounter for dental examination and cleaning without abnormal findings**
Encounter for dental examination and cleaning NOS

Px IQ + **Z01.21 Encounter for dental examination and cleaning with abnormal findings**
Use additional code to identify abnormal findings

5 **Z01.3 Encounter for examination of blood pressure**

Px IQ **Z01.30 Encounter for examination of blood pressure without abnormal findings**
Encounter for examination of blood pressure NOS

Px IQ + **Z01.31 Encounter for examination of blood pressure with abnormal findings**
Use additional code to identify abnormal findings

5 **Z01.4 Encounter for gynecological examination**
EXCLUDES 2 pregnancy examination or test (Z32.0-)
routine examination for contraceptive maintenance (Z30.4-)

+ 6 **Z01.41 Encounter for routine gynecological examination**
Encounter for general gynecological examination with or without cervical smear
Encounter for gynecological examination (general) (routine) NOS
Encounter for pelvic examination (annual) (periodic)
Use additional code:
for screening for human papillomavirus, if applicable, (Z11.51)
for screening vaginal pap smear, if applicable (Z12.72)
to identify acquired absence of uterus, if applicable (Z90.71-)
EXCLUDES 1 gynecologic examination status-post hysterectomy for malignant condition (Z08)
screening cervical pap smear not a part of a routine gynecological examination (Z12.4)

Px IQ + **Z01.411 Encounter for gynecological examination (general) (routine) with abnormal findings**
Use additional code to identify abnormal findings

Px IQ + **Z01.419 Encounter for gynecological examination (general) (routine) without abnormal findings**

Px IQ **Z01.42 Encounter for cervical smear to confirm findings of recent normal smear following initial abnormal smear**

5 **Z01.8 Encounter for other specified special examinations**

6 **Z01.81 Encounter for preprocedural examinations**
Encounter for preoperative examinations
Encounter for radiological and imaging examinations as part of preprocedural examination

Px IQ **Z01.810 Encounter for preprocedural cardiovascular examination**

Px IQ **Z01.811 Encounter for preprocedural respiratory examination**

Px IQ **Z01.812 Encounter for preprocedural laboratory examination**
Blood and urine tests prior to treatment or procedure

Px IQ **Z01.818 Encounter for other preprocedural examination**
Encounter for preprocedural examination NOS
Encounter for examinations prior to antineoplastic chemotherapy

Px IQ **Z01.82 Encounter for allergy testing**
EXCLUDES 1 encounter for antibody response examination (Z01.84)

Px IQ **Z01.83 Encounter for blood typing**
Encounter for Rh typing

Px IQ **Z01.84 Encounter for antibody response examination**
Encounter for immunity status testing
EXCLUDES 1 encounter for allergy testing (Z01.82)

Px IQ **Z01.89 Encounter for other specified special examinations**

4 **Z02 Encounter for administrative examination**

Px IQ **Z02.0 Encounter for examination for admission to educational institution**
Encounter for examination for admission to preschool (education)
Encounter for examination for re-admission to school following illness or medical treatment

Px IQ **Z02.1 Encounter for pre-employment examination**

Px IQ **Z02.2 Encounter for examination for admission to residential institution**
EXCLUDES 1 examination for admission to prison (Z02.89)

Px IQ **Z02.3 Encounter for examination for recruitment to armed forces**

Px IQ **Z02.4 Encounter for examination for driving license**

Px IQ **Z02.5 Encounter for examination for participation in sport**
EXCLUDES 1 blood-alcohol and blood-drug test (Z02.83)

Px IQ **Z02.6 Encounter for examination for insurance purposes**

5 **Z02.7 Encounter for issue of medical certificate**
EXCLUDES 1 encounter for general medical examination (Z00-Z01, Z02.0-Z02.6, Z02.8-Z02.9)

Px IQ **Z02.71 Encounter for disability determination**
Encounter for issue of medical certificate of incapacity
Encounter for issue of medical certificate of invalidity

Chapter 21

Z00-Z99

Px IQ **Z02.79 Encounter for issue of other medical certificate**

5 **Z02.8 Encounter for other administrative examinations**

Px IQ **Z02.81 Encounter for paternity testing**

Px IQ **Z02.82 Encounter for adoption services**

Px IQ + **Z02.83 Encounter for blood-alcohol and blood-drug test**
Use additional code for findings of alcohol or drugs in blood (R78.-)

Px IQ **Z02.89 Encounter for other administrative examinations**
Encounter for examination for admission to prison
Encounter for examination for admission to summer camp
Encounter for immigration examination
Encounter for naturalization examination
Encounter for premarital examination
EXCLUDES 1 health supervision of foundling or other healthy infant or child (Z76.1-Z76.2)

Px IQ **Z02.9 Encounter for administrative examinations, unspecified**

4 **Z03 Encounter for medical observation for suspected diseases and conditions ruled out**
This category is to be used when a person without a diagnosis is suspected of having an abnormal condition, without signs or symptoms, which requires study, but after examination and observation, is ruled out. This category is also for use for administrative and legal observation status.
EXCLUDES 1 contact with and (suspected) exposures hazardous to health (Z77.-)
encounter for observation and evaluation of newborn for suspected diseases and conditions ruled out (Z05.-)
person with feared complaint in whom no diagnosis is made (Z71.1)
signs or symptoms under study-code to signs or symptoms

CODING TIPS✓ Observation codes are typically primary only codes and as such are not appropriate for home care or hospice. Observation codes may be assigned as a secondary diagnosis code when the patient is being observed for a condition that is ruled out and is unrelated to the principal/first-listed diagnosis (e.g., patient presents for treatment following injuries sustained in a motor vehicle accident and is also observed for suspected COVID-19 infection that is subsequently ruled out).

IQ **Z03.6 Encounter for observation for suspected toxic effect from ingested substance ruled out**
Encounter for observation for suspected adverse effect from drug
Encounter for observation for suspected poisoning

5 **Z03.7 Encounter for suspected maternal and fetal conditions ruled out**
Encounter for suspected maternal and fetal conditions not found
EXCLUDES 1 known or suspected fetal anomalies affecting management of mother, not ruled out (O26.-, O35.-, O36.-, O40.-, O41.-)

IQ **Z03.71 Encounter for suspected problem with amniotic cavity and membrane ruled out**
Encounter for suspected oligohydramnios ruled out
Encounter for suspected polyhydramnios ruled out

IQ **Z03.72 Encounter for suspected placental problem ruled out**

IQ **Z03.73 Encounter for suspected fetal anomaly ruled out**

IQ **Z03.74 Encounter for suspected problem with fetal growth ruled out**

IQ **Z03.75 Encounter for suspected cervical shortening ruled out**

IQ **Z03.79 Encounter for other suspected maternal and fetal conditions ruled out**

5 **Z03.8 Encounter for observation for other suspected diseases and conditions ruled out**

6 **Z03.81 Encounter for observation for suspected exposure to biological agents ruled out**

IQ **Z03.810 Encounter for observation for suspected exposure to anthrax ruled out**

IQ **Z03.818 Encounter for observation for suspected exposure to other biological agents ruled out**

6 **Z03.82 Encounter for observation for suspected foreign body ruled out**
EXCLUDES 1 retained foreign body (Z18.-)
retained foreign body in eyelid (H02.81)
residual foreign body in soft tissue (M79.5)
EXCLUDES 2 confirmed foreign body ingestion or aspiration including:
foreign body in alimentary tract (T18)
foreign body in ear (T16)
foreign body on external eye (T15)
foreign body in respiratory tract (T17)

IQ **Z03.821 Encounter for observation for suspected ingested foreign body ruled out**

IQ **Z03.822 Encounter for observation for suspected aspirated (inhaled) foreign body ruled out**

IQ **Z03.823 Encounter for observation for suspected inserted (injected) foreign body ruled out**
Encounter for observation for suspected inserted (injected) foreign body in eye ruled out

4 4th digit required 5 5th digit required 6 6th digit required 7 7th digit required 7 7th digit placeholder + Additional code Laterality

Encounter for observation for suspected inserted (injected) foreign body in orifice ruled out
Encounter for observation for suspected inserted (injected) foreign body in skin ruled out

IQ **Z03.89 Encounter for observation for other suspected diseases and conditions ruled out**

4 **Z04 Encounter for examination and observation for other reasons**

INCLUDES encounter for examination for medicolegal reasons

This category is to be used when a person without a diagnosis is suspected of having an abnormal condition, without signs or symptoms, which requires study, but after examination and observation, is ruled-out. This category is also for use for administrative and legal observation status.

CODING TIPS✓ Observation codes are typically primary only codes and as such are not appropriate for home care or hospice. Observation codes may be assigned as a secondary diagnosis code when the patient is being observed for a condition that is ruled out and is unrelated to the principal/first-listed diagnosis (e.g., patient presents for treatment following injuries sustained in a motor vehicle accident and is also observed for suspected COVID-19 infection that is subsequently ruled out).

Px IQ **Z04.1 Encounter for examination and observation following transport accident**

EXCLUDES 1 encounter for examination and observation following work accident (Z04.2)

Px IQ **Z04.2 Encounter for examination and observation following work accident**

Px IQ **Z04.3 Encounter for examination and observation following other accident**

5 **Z04.4 Encounter for examination and observation following alleged rape**

Encounter for examination and observation of victim following alleged rape
Encounter for examination and observation of victim following alleged sexual abuse

Px IQ **Z04.41 Encounter for examination and observation following alleged adult rape**

Suspected adult rape, ruled out
Suspected adult sexual abuse, ruled out

Px IQ **Z04.42 Encounter for examination and observation following alleged child rape**

Suspected child rape, ruled out
Suspected child sexual abuse, ruled out

Px IQ **Z04.6 Encounter for general psychiatric examination, requested by authority**

5 **Z04.7 Encounter for examination and observation following alleged physical abuse**

Px IQ **Z04.71 Encounter for examination and observation following alleged adult physical abuse**

Suspected adult physical abuse, ruled out

EXCLUDES 1 confirmed case of adult physical abuse (T74.-)
encounter for examination and observation following alleged adult sexual abuse (Z04.41)
suspected case of adult physical abuse, not ruled out (T76.-)

Px IQ **Z04.72 Encounter for examination and observation following alleged child physical abuse**

Suspected child physical abuse, ruled out

EXCLUDES 1 confirmed case of child physical abuse (T74.-)
encounter for examination and observation following alleged child sexual abuse (Z04.42)
suspected case of child physical abuse, not ruled out (T76.-)

5 **Z04.8 Encounter for examination and observation for other specified reasons**

Encounter for examination and observation for request for expert evidence

Px IQ **Z04.81 Encounter for examination and observation of victim following forced sexual exploitation**

Px IQ **Z04.82 Encounter for examination and observation of victim following forced labor exploitation**

Px IQ **Z04.89 Encounter for examination and observation for other specified reasons**

Px IQ **Z04.9 Encounter for examination and observation for unspecified reason**

Encounter for observation NOS

4 **Z05 Encounter for observation and evaluation of newborn for suspected diseases and conditions ruled out**

This category is to be used for newborns, within the neonatal period (the first 28 days of life), who are suspected of having an abnormal condition, but without signs or symptoms, and which, after examination and observation, is ruled out.

CODING TIPS✓ Observation codes are typically primary only codes and as such are not appropriate for home care or hospice. Observation codes may be assigned as a secondary diagnosis code when the patient is being observed for a condition that is ruled out and is unrelated to the principal/first-listed diagnosis (e.g., patient presents for treatment following injuries sustained in a motor vehicle accident and is also observed for suspected COVID-19 infection that is subsequently ruled out).

IQ **Z05.0 Observation and evaluation of newborn for suspected cardiac condition ruled out**

Chapter 21

Z00-Z99

IQ **Z05.1 Observation and evaluation of newborn for suspected infectious condition ruled out**

IQ **Z05.2 Observation and evaluation of newborn for suspected neurological condition ruled out**

IQ **Z05.3 Observation and evaluation of newborn for suspected respiratory condition ruled out**

5 **Z05.4 Observation and evaluation of newborn for suspected genetic, metabolic or immunologic condition ruled out**

IQ **Z05.41 Observation and evaluation of newborn for suspected genetic condition ruled out**

IQ **Z05.42 Observation and evaluation of newborn for suspected metabolic condition ruled out**

IQ **Z05.43 Observation and evaluation of newborn for suspected immunologic condition ruled out**

IQ **Z05.5 Observation and evaluation of newborn for suspected gastrointestinal condition ruled out**

IQ **Z05.6 Observation and evaluation of newborn for suspected genitourinary condition ruled out**

5 **Z05.7 Observation and evaluation of newborn for suspected skin, subcutaneous, musculoskeletal and connective tissue condition ruled out**

IQ **Z05.71 Observation and evaluation of newborn for suspected skin and subcutaneous tissue condition ruled out**

IQ **Z05.72 Observation and evaluation of newborn for suspected musculoskeletal condition ruled out**

IQ **Z05.73 Observation and evaluation of newborn for suspected connective tissue condition ruled out**

IQ **Z05.8 Observation and evaluation of newborn for other specified suspected condition ruled out**

IQ **Z05.9 Observation and evaluation of newborn for unspecified suspected condition ruled out**

IQ + **Z08 Encounter for follow-up examination after completed treatment for malignant neoplasm**

Medical surveillance following completed treatment

Use additional code to identify any acquired absence of organs (Z90.-)

Use additional code to identify the personal history of malignant neoplasm (Z85.-)

EXCLUDES 1 aftercare following medical care (Z43-Z49, Z51)

IQ + **Z09 Encounter for follow-up examination after completed treatment for conditions other than malignant neoplasm**

Medical surveillance following completed treatment

Use additional code to identify any applicable history of disease code (Z86.-, Z87.-)

EXCLUDES 1 aftercare following medical care (Z43-Z49, Z51)

surveillance of contraception (Z30.4-)

surveillance of prosthetic and other medical devices (Z44-Z46)

GUIDELINES **Section I.C.1.g.1)(j)**

For individuals who previously had COVID-19 and are being seen for follow-up evaluation, and COVID-19 test results are negative, assign codes Z09, Encounter for follow-up examination after completed treatment for conditions other than malignant neoplasm, and Z86.16, Personal history of COVID-19.

CODING TIPS✓ Official guidance indicates this is the correct code for follow-up after the former COVID-19 patient no longer has symptoms. It is to be used along with Z86.16.

4 **Z11 Encounter for screening for infectious and parasitic diseases**

Screening is the testing for disease or disease precursors in asymptomatic individuals so that early detection and treatment can be provided for those who test positive for the disease.

EXCLUDES 1 encounter for diagnostic examination-code to sign or symptom

IQ **Z11.0 Encounter for screening for intestinal infectious diseases**

IQ **Z11.1 Encounter for screening for respiratory tuberculosis**

Encounter for screening for active tuberculosis disease

IQ **Z11.2 Encounter for screening for other bacterial diseases**

IQ **Z11.3 Encounter for screening for infections with a predominantly sexual mode of transmission**

EXCLUDES 2 encounter for screening for human immunodeficiency virus [HIV] (Z11.4)

encounter for screening for human papillomavirus (Z11.51)

IQ **Z11.4 Encounter for screening for human immunodeficiency virus [HIV]**

5 **Z11.5 Encounter for screening for other viral diseases**

EXCLUDES 2 encounter for screening for viral intestinal disease (Z11.0)

IQ **Z11.51 Encounter for screening for human papillomavirus (HPV)**

SP **Z11.52 Encounter for screening for COVID-19**

CODING TIPS✓ During the COVID-19 pandemic, a screening code is generally not appropriate. Do not assign code Z11.52, Encounter for screening for COVID-19. Assign Z20.822 instead.

IQ **Z11.59 Encounter for screening for other viral diseases**

IQ **Z11.6 Encounter for screening for other protozoal diseases and helminthiases**

EXCLUDES 2 encounter for screening for protozoal intestinal disease (Z11.0)

Z11.7 Encounter for testing for latent tuberculosis infection

IQ **Z11.8 Encounter for screening for other infectious and parasitic diseases**
Encounter for screening for chlamydia
Encounter for screening for rickettsial
Encounter for screening for spirochetal
Encounter for screening for mycoses

IQ **Z11.9 Encounter for screening for infectious and parasitic diseases, unspecified**

+ 4 **Z12 Encounter for screening for malignant neoplasms**
Screening is the testing for disease or disease precursors in asymptomatic individuals so that early detection and treatment can be provided for those who test positive for the disease.
Use additional code to identify any family history of malignant neoplasm (Z80.-)
EXCLUDES 1 encounter for diagnostic examination-code to sign or symptom

IQ + **Z12.0 Encounter for screening for malignant neoplasm of stomach**

+ 5 **Z12.1 Encounter for screening for malignant neoplasm of intestinal tract**

IQ + **Z12.10 Encounter for screening for malignant neoplasm of intestinal tract, unspecified**

IQ + **Z12.11 Encounter for screening for malignant neoplasm of colon**
Encounter for screening colonoscopy NOS

IQ + **Z12.12 Encounter for screening for malignant neoplasm of rectum**

IQ + **Z12.13 Encounter for screening for malignant neoplasm of small intestine**

IQ + **Z12.2 Encounter for screening for malignant neoplasm of respiratory organs**

+ 5 **Z12.3 Encounter for screening for malignant neoplasm of breast**

IQ + **Z12.31 Encounter for screening mammogram for malignant neoplasm of breast**
EXCLUDES 1 inconclusive mammogram (R92.2)

IQ + **Z12.39 Encounter for other screening for malignant neoplasm of breast**

IQ + **Z12.4 Encounter for screening for malignant neoplasm of cervix**
Encounter for screening pap smear for malignant neoplasm of cervix
EXCLUDES 1 when screening is part of general gynecological examination (Z01.4-)
EXCLUDES 2 encounter for screening for human papillomavirus (Z11.51)

IQ + **Z12.5 Encounter for screening for malignant neoplasm of prostate**

IQ + **Z12.6 Encounter for screening for malignant neoplasm of bladder**

+ 5 **Z12.7 Encounter for screening for malignant neoplasm of other genitourinary organs**

IQ + **Z12.71 Encounter for screening for malignant neoplasm of testis**

IQ + **Z12.72 Encounter for screening for malignant neoplasm of vagina**
Vaginal pap smear status-post hysterectomy for non-malignant condition
Use additional code to identify acquired absence of uterus (Z90.71-)
EXCLUDES 1 vaginal pap smear status-post hysterectomy for malignant conditions (Z08)

IQ + **Z12.73 Encounter for screening for malignant neoplasm of ovary**

IQ + **Z12.79 Encounter for screening for malignant neoplasm of other genitourinary organs**

+ 5 **Z12.8 Encounter for screening for malignant neoplasm of other sites**

IQ + **Z12.81 Encounter for screening for malignant neoplasm of oral cavity**

IQ + **Z12.82 Encounter for screening for malignant neoplasm of nervous system**

IQ + **Z12.83 Encounter for screening for malignant neoplasm of skin**

IQ + **Z12.89 Encounter for screening for malignant neoplasm of other sites**

IQ + **Z12.9 Encounter for screening for malignant neoplasm, site unspecified**

4 **Z13 Encounter for screening for other diseases and disorders**
Screening is the testing for disease or disease precursors in asymptomatic individuals so that early detection and treatment can be provided for those who test positive for the disease.
EXCLUDES 1 encounter for diagnostic examination-code to sign or symptom

IQ **Z13.0 Encounter for screening for diseases of the blood and blood-forming organs and certain disorders involving the immune mechanism**

IQ **Z13.1 Encounter for screening for diabetes mellitus**

5 **Z13.2 Encounter for screening for nutritional, metabolic and other endocrine disorders**

IQ **Z13.21 Encounter for screening for nutritional disorder**

6 **Z13.22 Encounter for screening for metabolic disorder**

IQ **Z13.220 Encounter for screening for lipoid disorders**
Encounter for screening for cholesterol level
Encounter for screening for hypercholesterolemia
Encounter for screening for hyperlipidemia

IQ **Z13.228 Encounter for screening for other metabolic disorders**

▲ IQ **Z13.29 Encounter for screening for other suspected endocrine disorder**
EXCLUDES 2 encounter for screening for diabetes mellitus (Z13.1)

5 **Z13.3 Encounter for screening examination for mental health and behavioral disorders**

IQ **Z13.30 Encounter for screening examination for mental health and behavioral disorders, unspecified**

IQ **Z13.31 Encounter for screening for depression**
Encounter for screening for depression, adult
Encounter for screening for depression for child or adolescent

IQ **Z13.32 Encounter for screening for maternal depression**
Encounter for screening for perinatal depression

IQ **Z13.39 Encounter for screening examination for other mental health and behavioral disorders**
Encounter for screening for alcoholism
Encounter for screening for intellectual disabilities

5 **Z13.4 Encounter for screening for certain developmental disorders in childhood**
Encounter for development testing of infant or child
Encounter for screening for developmental handicaps in early childhood
EXCLUDES 2 encounter for routine child health examination (Z00.12-)

IQ **Z13.40 Encounter for screening for unspecified developmental delays**

IQ **Z13.41 Encounter for autism screening**

IQ **Z13.42 Encounter for screening for global developmental delays (milestones)**
Encounter for screening for developmental handicaps in early childhood

IQ **Z13.49 Encounter for screening for other developmental delays**

IQ **Z13.5 Encounter for screening for eye and ear disorders**
EXCLUDES 2 encounter for general hearing examination (Z01.1-)
encounter for general vision examination (Z01.0-)

IQ **Z13.6 Encounter for screening for cardiovascular disorders**

5 **Z13.7 Encounter for screening for genetic and chromosomal anomalies**
EXCLUDES 1 genetic testing for procreative management (Z31.4-)

IQ **Z13.71 Encounter for nonprocreative screening for genetic disease carrier status**

IQ **Z13.79 Encounter for other screening for genetic and chromosomal anomalies**

5 **Z13.8 Encounter for screening for other specified diseases and disorders**
EXCLUDES 2 screening for malignant neoplasms (Z12.-)

6 **Z13.81 Encounter for screening for digestive system disorders**

IQ **Z13.810 Encounter for screening for upper gastrointestinal disorder**

IQ **Z13.811 Encounter for screening for lower gastrointestinal disorder**
EXCLUDES 1 encounter for screening for intestinal infectious disease (Z11.0)

IQ **Z13.818 Encounter for screening for other digestive system disorders**

6 **Z13.82 Encounter for screening for musculoskeletal disorder**

IQ **Z13.820 Encounter for screening for osteoporosis**

IQ **Z13.828 Encounter for screening for other musculoskeletal disorder**

IQ **Z13.83 Encounter for screening for respiratory disorder NEC**
EXCLUDES 1 encounter for screening for respiratory tuberculosis (Z11.1)

IQ **Z13.84 Encounter for screening for dental disorders**

6 **Z13.85 Encounter for screening for nervous system disorders**

IQ **Z13.850 Encounter for screening for traumatic brain injury**

IQ **Z13.858 Encounter for screening for other nervous system disorders**

IQ **Z13.88 Encounter for screening for disorder due to exposure to contaminants**
EXCLUDES 1 those exposed to contaminants without suspected disorders (Z57.-, Z77.-)

IQ **Z13.89 Encounter for screening for other disorder**
Encounter for screening for genitourinary disorders

IQ **Z13.9 Encounter for screening, unspecified**

Genetic carrier and genetic susceptibility to disease (Z14-Z15)

4 **Z14 Genetic carrier**

5 **Z14.0 Hemophilia A carrier**

IQ **Z14.01 Asymptomatic hemophilia A carrier**

IQ **Z14.02 Symptomatic hemophilia A carrier**

IQ **Z14.1 Cystic fibrosis carrier**

IQ **Z14.8 Genetic carrier of other disease**

+ 4 **Z15 Genetic susceptibility to disease**
INCLUDES confirmed abnormal gene
Use additional code, if applicable, for any associated family history of the disease (Z80-Z84)
EXCLUDES 1 chromosomal anomalies (Q90-Q99)
GUIDELINES **Section I.C.21.c.3)**
Codes from category Z15 should not be used as principal or first-listed codes. If the patient has the condition to which he/she is susceptible, and that condition is the reason for the encounter, the code for the current condition should be sequenced first.

+ 5 **Z15.0 Genetic susceptibility to malignant neoplasm**
Code first:
, if applicable, any current malignant neoplasm (C00-C75, C81-C96)

Use additional code, if applicable, for any personal history of malignant neoplasm (Z85.-)

CODING TIPS✓ These codes should always be used with prophylactic removal of the particular organ, when documented.

IQ + **Z15.01 Genetic susceptibility to malignant neoplasm of breast**

CODING TIPS✓ Assign Z15.01 for a patient who has prophylactic breast removal due to genetic susceptibility to breast cancer.

IQ + **Z15.02 Genetic susceptibility to malignant neoplasm of ovary**

IQ + **Z15.03 Genetic susceptibility to malignant neoplasm of prostate**

IQ + **Z15.04 Genetic susceptibility to malignant neoplasm of endometrium**

IQ + **Z15.09 Genetic susceptibility to other malignant neoplasm**

+ 5 **Z15.8 Genetic susceptibility to other disease**

IQ + **Z15.81 Genetic susceptibility to multiple endocrine neoplasia [MEN]**

EXCLUDES 1 multiple endocrine neoplasia [MEN] syndromes (E31.2-)

IQ + **Z15.89 Genetic susceptibility to other disease**

Resistance to antimicrobial drugs (Z16)

CODING TIPS✓ Assign as many codes from Z16 as necessary to identify all antimicrobial resistance documented.

CODING TIPS✓ When resistance to antibiotics is documented, add the Z16 codes after the codes that indicate the bacteria causing the sepsis (A40-A41), or other bacterial infections (B95-B96), or the combination codes when the bacteria is included in the code (J15.211). Do not use Z16.11 for MRSA because the resistance to penicillins is already included in the MRSA codes. If the MRSA is also documented as resistant to another antibiotic, such as Vancomycin, a Z16 code is added for the other antibiotic.

4 **Z16 Resistance to antimicrobial drugs**

Note:

The codes in this category are provided for use as additional codes to identify the resistance and non-responsiveness of a condition to antimicrobial drugs.

Code first:

the infection

EXCLUDES 1 Methicillin resistant Staphylococcus aureus infection (A49.02)
Methicillin resistant Staphylococcus aureus pneumonia (J15.212)
Sepsis due to Methicillin resistant Staphylococcus aureus (A41.02)

GUIDELINES **Section I.C.1.c**

Many bacterial infections are resistant to current antibiotics. It is necessary to identify all infections documented as antibiotic resistant. Assign a code from category Z16, Resistance to antimicrobial drugs, following the infection code only if the infection code does not identify drug resistance.

5 **Z16.1 Resistance to beta lactam antibiotics**

IQ **Z16.10 Resistance to unspecified beta lactam antibiotics**

IQ **Z16.11 Resistance to penicillins**

Resistance to amoxicillin
Resistance to ampicillin

GUIDELINES **Section I.C.e.1)(a)**

When a patient is diagnosed with an infection that is due to methicillin resistant Staphylococcus aureus (MRSA), and that infection has a combination code that includes the causal organism (e.g., sepsis, pneumonia) assign the appropriate combination code for the condition.

Do not assign code B95.62, MRSA infection as the cause of diseases classified elsewhere, as an additional code, because the combination code includes the type of infection and the MRSA organism. Do not assign a code from subcategory Z16.11, Resistance to penicillins, as an additional diagnosis.

IQ **Z16.12 Extended spectrum beta lactamase (ESBL) resistance**

EXCLUDES 2 Methicillin resistant Staphylococcus aureus infection in diseases classified elsewhere (B95.62)

IQ **Z16.19 Resistance to other specified beta lactam antibiotics**

Resistance to cephalosporins

5 **Z16.2 Resistance to other antibiotics**

IQ **Z16.20 Resistance to unspecified antibiotic**

Resistance to antibiotics NOS

IQ **Z16.21 Resistance to vancomycin**

IQ **Z16.22 Resistance to vancomycin related antibiotics**

IQ **Z16.23 Resistance to quinolones and fluoroquinolones**

IQ **Z16.24 Resistance to multiple antibiotics**

IQ **Z16.29 Resistance to other single specified antibiotic**

Resistance to aminoglycosides
Resistance to macrolides
Resistance to sulfonamides
Resistance to tetracyclines

5 **Z16.3 Resistance to other antimicrobial drugs**

EXCLUDES 1 resistance to antibiotics (Z16.1-, Z16.2-)

IQ **Z16.30 Resistance to unspecified antimicrobial drugs**

Drug resistance NOS

IQ **Z16.31 Resistance to antiparasitic drug(s)**

Resistance to quinine and related compounds

IQ **Z16.32 Resistance to antifungal drug(s)**

IQ **Z16.33 Resistance to antiviral drug(s)**

6 **Z16.34 Resistance to antimycobacterial drug(s)**

Resistance to tuberculostatics

IQ **Z16.341 Resistance to single antimycobacterial drug**

Resistance to antimycobacterial drug NOS

IQ **Z16.342 Resistance to multiple antimycobacterial drugs**

IQ **Z16.35 Resistance to multiple antimicrobial drugs**

EXCLUDES 1 Resistance to multiple antibiotics only (Z16.24)

IQ **Z16.39 Resistance to other specified antimicrobial drug**

Estrogen receptor status (Z17)

CODING TIPS✓ When a patient has breast cancer and the estrogen receptor status is specified, the appropriate code from category Z17 should be assigned to indicate the ER positive or negative status. Breast cancers that are ER+ may be treated with selective estrogen receptor modulators (SERMs). When SERM therapy is also present in an ER+ breast cancer patient, an additional Z code may be assigned to identify SERM therapy (Z79.81-).

4 **Z17 Estrogen receptor status**

Code first:

malignant neoplasm of breast (C50.-)

IQ **Z17.0 Estrogen receptor positive status [ER+]**

IQ **Z17.1 Estrogen receptor negative status [ER-]**

Retained foreign body fragments (Z18)

4 **Z18 Retained foreign body fragments**

INCLUDES embedded fragment (status)
embedded splinter (status)
retained foreign body status

EXCLUDES 1 artificial joint prosthesis status (Z96.6-)
foreign body accidentally left during a procedure (T81.5-)
foreign body entering through orifice (T15-T19)
in situ cardiac device (Z95.-)
organ or tissue replaced by means other than transplant (Z96.-, Z97.-)
organ or tissue replaced by transplant (Z94.-)
personal history of retained foreign body fully removed Z87.821
superficial foreign body (non-embedded splinter) - code to superficial foreign body, by site

5 **Z18.0 Retained radioactive fragments**

IQ **Z18.01 Retained depleted uranium fragments**

IQ **Z18.09 Other retained radioactive fragments**

Other retained depleted isotope fragments
Retained nontherapeutic radioactive fragments

5 **Z18.1 Retained metal fragments**

EXCLUDES 1 retained radioactive metal fragments (Z18.01-Z18.09)

IQ **Z18.10 Retained metal fragments, unspecified**

Retained metal fragment NOS

IQ **Z18.11 Retained magnetic metal fragments**

IQ **Z18.12 Retained nonmagnetic metal fragments**

IQ **Z18.2 Retained plastic fragments**

Acrylics fragments
Diethylhexyl phthalates fragments
Isocyanate fragments

5 **Z18.3 Retained organic fragments**

IQ **Z18.31 Retained animal quills or spines**

IQ **Z18.32 Retained tooth**

IQ **Z18.33 Retained wood fragments**

IQ **Z18.39 Other retained organic fragments**

5 **Z18.8 Other specified retained foreign body**

IQ **Z18.81 Retained glass fragments**

IQ **Z18.83 Retained stone or crystalline fragments**

Retained concrete or cement fragments

IQ **Z18.89 Other specified retained foreign body fragments**

IQ **Z18.9 Retained foreign body fragments, unspecified material**

Hormone sensitivity malignancy status (Z19)

4 **Z19 Hormone sensitivity malignancy status**

Code first:

malignant neoplasm - see Table of Neoplasms, by site, malignant

IQ **Z19.1 Hormone sensitive malignancy status**

DEFINITION Identifies cancers that are known to be hormone dependent and for which the use of hormone therapy drugs in treatment is effective.

IQ **Z19.2 Hormone resistant malignancy status**

Castrate resistant prostate malignancy status

Persons with potential health hazards related to communicable diseases (Z20-Z29)

4 **Z20 Contact with and (suspected) exposure to communicable diseases**

EXCLUDES 1 carrier of infectious disease (Z22.-)
diagnosed current infectious or parasitic disease -see Alphabetic Index

EXCLUDES 2 personal history of infectious and parasitic diseases (Z86.1-)

GUIDELINES **Section I.C.21.c.1)**
Category Z20 indicates contact with, and suspected exposure to, communicable diseases. These codes are for patients who do not show any sign or symptom of a disease but are suspected to have been exposed to it by close personal contact with an infected individual or are in an area where a disease is epidemic. Category Z77 indicates contact with and suspected exposures hazardous to health.

Contact/exposure codes may be used as a first-listed code to explain an encounter for testing, or, more commonly, as a secondary code to identify a potential risk.

5 **Z20.0 Contact with and (suspected) exposure to intestinal infectious diseases**

IQ **Z20.01 Contact with and (suspected) exposure to intestinal infectious diseases due to Escherichia coli (E. coli)**

IQ **Z20.09 Contact with and (suspected) exposure to other intestinal infectious diseases**

IQ **Z20.1 Contact with and (suspected) exposure to tuberculosis**

IQ **Z20.2 Contact with and (suspected) exposure to infections with a predominantly sexual mode of transmission**

IQ **Z20.3 Contact with and (suspected) exposure to rabies**

IQ **Z20.4 Contact with and (suspected) exposure to rubella**

IQ **Z20.5 Contact with and (suspected) exposure to viral hepatitis**

IQ **Z20.6 Contact with and (suspected) exposure to human immunodeficiency virus [HIV]**

EXCLUDES 1 asymptomatic human immunodeficiency virus [HIV] HIV infection status (Z21)

IQ **Z20.7 Contact with and (suspected) exposure to pediculosis, acariasis and other infestations**

5 **Z20.8 Contact with and (suspected) exposure to other communicable diseases**

6 **Z20.81 Contact with and (suspected) exposure to other bacterial communicable diseases**

IQ **Z20.810 Contact with and (suspected) exposure to anthrax**

IQ **Z20.811 Contact with and (suspected) exposure to meningococcus**

IQ **Z20.818 Contact with and (suspected) exposure to other bacterial communicable diseases**

6 **Z20.82 Contact with and (suspected) exposure to other viral communicable diseases**

IQ **Z20.820 Contact with and (suspected) exposure to varicella**

IQ **Z20.821 Contact with and (suspected) exposure to Zika virus**

SP **Z20.822 Contact with and (suspected) exposure to COVID-19**

Contact with and (suspected) exposure to SARS-CoV-2

GUIDELINES **Section I.C.1.g.1)(l)**
If an individual with a known or suspected exposure to COVID-19, and no current COVID-19 infection or history of COVID-19, develops MIS, assign codes M35.81, Multisystem inflammatory syndrome, and Z20.822, Contact with and (suspected) exposure to COVID-19.

GUIDELINES **Section I.C.1.g.1)(e)**
For asymptomatic individuals with actual or suspected exposure to COVID-19, assign code Z20.822, Contact with and (suspected) exposure to COVID-19.
For symptomatic individuals with actual or suspected exposure to COVID-19 and the infection has been ruled out, or test results are inconclusive or unknown, assign code Z20.822, Contact with and (suspected) exposure to COVID-19.

GUIDELINES **Section I.C.1.g.1)(g)**
For patients presenting with any signs/symptoms associated with COVID-19 (such as fever, etc.) but a definitive diagnosis has not been established, assign the appropriate code(s) for each of the presenting signs and symptoms such as: R05 (Cough), R06.02 (Shortness of breath), R50.9 (Fever, unspecified).

If a patient with signs/symptoms associated with COVID-19 also has an actual or suspected contact with or exposure to someone who has COVID-19, assign Z20.822, Contact with and (suspected) exposure to COVID-19, as an additional code.

IQ **Z20.828 Contact with and (suspected) exposure to other viral communicable diseases**

CODING TIPS✓ Do not use this code for actual or suspected exposure to COVID-19. Use Z20.822.

IQ **Z20.89 Contact with and (suspected) exposure to other communicable diseases**

IQ **Z20.9 Contact with and (suspected) exposure to unspecified communicable disease**

IQ **Z21 Asymptomatic human immunodeficiency virus [HIV] infection status**

HIV positive NOS

Code first:

Human immunodeficiency virus [HIV] disease complicating pregnancy, childbirth and the puerperium, if applicable (O98.7-)

EXCLUDES 1 acquired immunodeficiency syndrome (B20)
contact with human immunodeficiency virus [HIV] (Z20.6)
exposure to human immunodeficiency virus [HIV] (Z20.6)

Chapter 21

Z00-Z99

human immunodeficiency virus [HIV] disease (B20)
inconclusive laboratory evidence of human immunodeficiency virus [HIV] (R75)

GUIDELINES Patients with asymptomatic HIV infection status admitted (or presenting for a health care encounter) during pregnancy, childbirth, or the puerperium should receive codes of O98.7- and Z21.

GUIDELINES **Section I.C.1.a.2)(f)**
Patients with any known prior diagnosis of an HIV-related illness should be coded to B20. Once a patient has developed an HIV-related illness, the patient should always be assigned code B20 on every subsequent admission/ encounter. Patients previously diagnosed with any HIV illness (B20) should never be assigned to R75 or Z21, Asymptomatic human immunodeficiency virus [HIV] infection status.

GUIDELINES **Section I.C.1.a.2)(d)**
Z21, Asymptomatic human immunodeficiency virus [HIV] infection status, is to be applied when the patient without any documentation of symptoms is listed as being "HIV positive," "known HIV," "HIV test positive," or similar terminology. Do not use this code if the term "AIDS" is used or if the patient is treated for any HIV-related illness or is described as having any condition(s) resulting from his/her HIV positive status; use B20 in these cases.

4 **Z22 Carrier of infectious disease**
INCLUDES colonization status
suspected carrier
EXCLUDES 2 carrier of viral hepatitis (B18.-)

IQ **Z22.0 Carrier of typhoid**

IQ **Z22.1 Carrier of other intestinal infectious diseases**

IQ **Z22.2 Carrier of diphtheria**

5 **Z22.3 Carrier of other specified bacterial diseases**

IQ **Z22.31 Carrier of bacterial disease due to meningococci**

6 **Z22.32 Carrier of bacterial disease due to staphylococci**

GUIDELINES **Section I.C.1.e.1)(c)**
Assign code Z22.322 for patients documented as having MRSA colonization. Assign code Z22.321 for patient documented as having MSSA colonization. Colonization is not necessarily indicative of a disease process or as the cause of a specific condition the patient may have unless documented as such by the provider.

IQ **Z22.321 Carrier or suspected carrier of Methicillin susceptible Staphylococcus aureus**
MSSA colonization

IQ **Z22.322 Carrier or suspected carrier of Methicillin resistant Staphylococcus aureus**
MRSA colonization

GUIDELINES **Section I.C.1.e.1)(d)**
If a patient is documented as having both MRSA colonization and infection during a hospital admission, code Z22.322 and a code for the MRSA infection may both be assigned.

CODING TIPS✓ This code should be used when "MRSA screen positive" or "nasal swab positive" is documented. Colonization by MRSA makes teaching a patient/caregiver how to do their own wound dressings more difficult and sometimes impractical.

6 **Z22.33 Carrier of bacterial disease due to streptococci**

IQ **Z22.330 Carrier of Group B streptococcus**
EXCLUDES 1 Carrier of streptococcus group B (GBS) complicating pregnancy, childbirth and the puerperium (O99.82-)

IQ **Z22.338 Carrier of other streptococcus**

IQ **Z22.39 Carrier of other specified bacterial diseases**

IQ **Z22.4 Carrier of infections with a predominantly sexual mode of transmission**

IQ **Z22.6 Carrier of human T-lymphotropic virus type-1 [HTLV-1] infection**

Z22.7 Latent tuberculosis
Latent tuberculosis infection (LTBI)
EXCLUDES 1 nonspecific reaction to cell mediated immunity measurement of gamma interferon antigen response without active tuberculosis (R76.12)
nonspecific reaction to tuberculin skin test without active tuberculosis (R76.11)

DEFINITION Latent tuberculosis infection (LTBI) occurs when a person is infected with the bacteria Mycobacterium tuberculosis, but does not have active tuberculosis (TB) disease. The only sign of a tuberculosis infection is a positive reaction to the tuberculin skin test or tuberculosis blood test. Compared to active tuberculosis, persons with latent tuberculosis infection are not infectious, cannot spread TB and normally do not develop TB disease. But in persons who have a weak immune system, the bacteria can become active, multiply and cause tuberculosis disease.

IQ **Z22.8 Carrier of other infectious diseases**

IQ **Z22.9 Carrier of infectious disease, unspecified**

▲ IQ **Z23 Encounter for immunization**

Note:
procedure codes are required to identify the types of immunizations given
Code first:
any routine childhood examination
Code also:
, if applicable, encounter for immunization safety counseling (Z71.85)

GUIDELINES **Section I.C.21.c.2)**
Code Z23 is for encounters for inoculations and vaccinations. It indicates that a patient is being seen to receive a prophylactic inoculation against a disease. Procedure codes are required to identify the actual administration of the injection and the type(s) of immunizations given. Code Z23 may be used as a secondary code if the inoculation is given as a routine part of preventive health care, such as a well-baby visit.

▲4 **Z28 Immunization not carried out and underimmunization status**
INCLUDES vaccination not carried out
Code also:
, if applicable, encounter for immunization safety counseling (Z71.85)

5 **Z28.0 Immunization not carried out because of contraindication**

IQ **Z28.01 Immunization not carried out because of acute illness of patient**

IQ **Z28.02 Immunization not carried out because of chronic illness or condition of patient**

IQ **Z28.03 Immunization not carried out because of immune compromised state of patient**

IQ **Z28.04 Immunization not carried out because of patient allergy to vaccine or component**

IQ **Z28.09 Immunization not carried out because of other contraindication**

IQ **Z28.1 Immunization not carried out because of patient decision for reasons of belief or group pressure**
Immunization not carried out because of religious belief

5 **Z28.2 Immunization not carried out because of patient decision for other and unspecified reason**

IQ **Z28.20 Immunization not carried out because of patient decision for unspecified reason**

IQ **Z28.21 Immunization not carried out because of patient refusal**

IQ **Z28.29 Immunization not carried out because of patient decision for other reason**

IQ **Z28.3 Underimmunization status**
Delinquent immunization status
Lapsed immunization schedule status

5 **Z28.8 Immunization not carried out for other reason**

IQ **Z28.81 Immunization not carried out due to patient having had the disease**

IQ **Z28.82 Immunization not carried out because of caregiver refusal**
Immunization not carried out because of guardian refusal
Immunization not carried out because of parent refusal
EXCLUDES 1 immunization not carried out because of caregiver refusal because of religious belief (Z28.1)

IQ **Z28.83 Immunization not carried out due to unavailability of vaccine**
Delay in delivery of vaccine
Lack of availability of vaccine
Manufacturer delay of vaccine

IQ **Z28.89 Immunization not carried out for other reason**

IQ **Z28.9 Immunization not carried out for unspecified reason**

4 **Z29 Encounter for other prophylactic measures**
EXCLUDES 1 desensitization to allergens (Z51.6)
prophylactic surgery (Z40.-)

5 **Z29.1 Encounter for prophylactic immunotherapy**
Encounter for administration of immunoglobulin

IQ **Z29.11 Encounter for prophylactic immunotherapy for respiratory syncytial virus (RSV)**

IQ **Z29.12 Encounter for prophylactic antivenin**

IQ **Z29.13 Encounter for prophylactic Rho(D) immune globulin**

IQ **Z29.14 Encounter for prophylactic rabies immune globin**

IQ **Z29.3 Encounter for prophylactic fluoride administration**

IQ **Z29.8 Encounter for other specified prophylactic measures**

IQ **Z29.9 Encounter for prophylactic measures, unspecified**

Persons encountering health services in circumstances related to reproduction (Z30-Z39)

4 **Z30 Encounter for contraceptive management**

5 **Z30.0 Encounter for general counseling and advice on contraception**

6 **Z30.01 Encounter for initial prescription of contraceptives**
EXCLUDES 1 encounter for surveillance of contraceptives (Z30.4-)

IQ **Z30.011 Encounter for initial prescription of contraceptive pills**

IQ **Z30.012 Encounter for prescription of emergency contraception**
Encounter for postcoital contraception

IQ **Z30.013 Encounter for initial prescription of injectable contraceptive**

IQ **Z30.014 Encounter for initial prescription of intrauterine contraceptive device**
EXCLUDES 1 encounter for insertion of intrauterine contraceptive device (Z30.430, Z30.432)

IQ **Z30.015 Encounter for initial prescription of vaginal ring hormonal contraceptive**

IQ **Z30.016 Encounter for initial prescription of transdermal patch hormonal contraceptive device**

IQ **Z30.017 Encounter for initial prescription of implantable subdermal contraceptive**

IQ **Z30.018 Encounter for initial prescription of other contraceptives**
Encounter for initial prescription of barrier contraception
Encounter for initial prescription of diaphragm

IQ **Z30.019 Encounter for initial prescription of contraceptives, unspecified**

IQ **Z30.02 Counseling and instruction in natural family planning to avoid pregnancy**

IQ **Z30.09 Encounter for other general counseling and advice on contraception**
Encounter for family planning advice NOS

IQ **Z30.2 Encounter for sterilization**

5 **Z30.4 Encounter for surveillance of contraceptives**

IQ **Z30.40 Encounter for surveillance of contraceptives, unspecified**

IQ **Z30.41 Encounter for surveillance of contraceptive pills**
Encounter for repeat prescription for contraceptive pill

IQ **Z30.42 Encounter for surveillance of injectable contraceptive**

6 **Z30.43 Encounter for surveillance of intrauterine contraceptive device**

IQ **Z30.430 Encounter for insertion of intrauterine contraceptive device**

IQ **Z30.431 Encounter for routine checking of intrauterine contraceptive device**

IQ **Z30.432 Encounter for removal of intrauterine contraceptive device**

IQ **Z30.433 Encounter for removal and reinsertion of intrauterine contraceptive device**
Encounter for replacement of intrauterine contraceptive device

IQ **Z30.44 Encounter for surveillance of vaginal ring hormonal contraceptive device**

IQ **Z30.45 Encounter for surveillance of transdermal patch hormonal contraceptive device**

IQ **Z30.46 Encounter for surveillance of implantable subdermal contraceptive**
Encounter for checking, reinsertion or removal of implantable subdermal contraceptive

IQ **Z30.49 Encounter for surveillance of other contraceptives**
Encounter for surveillance of barrier contraception
Encounter for surveillance of diaphragm

IQ **Z30.8 Encounter for other contraceptive management**
Encounter for postvasectomy sperm count
Encounter for routine examination for contraceptive maintenance
EXCLUDES 1 sperm count following sterilization reversal (Z31.42)
sperm count for fertility testing (Z31.41)

IQ **Z30.9 Encounter for contraceptive management, unspecified**

▲ 4 **Z31 Encounter for procreative management**
EXCLUDES 2 complications associated with artificial fertilization (N98.-)
female infertility (N97.-)
male infertility (N46.-)

IQ **Z31.0 Encounter for reversal of previous sterilization**

5 **Z31.4 Encounter for procreative investigation and testing**
EXCLUDES 1 postvasectomy sperm count (Z30.8)

IQ **Z31.41 Encounter for fertility testing**
Encounter for fallopian tube patency testing
Encounter for sperm count for fertility testing

IQ **Z31.42 Aftercare following sterilization reversal**
Sperm count following sterilization reversal

+ 6 **Z31.43 Encounter for genetic testing of female for procreative management**
Use additional code for recurrent pregnancy loss, if applicable (N96, O26.2-)
EXCLUDES 1 nonprocreative genetic testing (Z13.7-)

IQ + **Z31.430 Encounter of female for testing for genetic disease carrier status for procreative management**

IQ + **Z31.438 Encounter for other genetic testing of female for procreative management**

6 **Z31.44 Encounter for genetic testing of male for procreative management**
EXCLUDES 1 nonprocreative genetic testing (Z13.7-)

IQ **Z31.440 Encounter of male for testing for genetic disease carrier status for procreative management**

IQ **Z31.441 Encounter for testing of male partner of patient with recurrent pregnancy loss**

IQ **Z31.448 Encounter for other genetic testing of male for procreative management**

IQ **Z31.49 Encounter for other procreative investigation and testing**

IQ **Z31.5 Encounter for procreative genetic counseling**

5 **Z31.6 Encounter for general counseling and advice on procreation**

IQ **Z31.61 Procreative counseling and advice using natural family planning**

IQ **Z31.62 Encounter for fertility preservation counseling**
Encounter for fertility preservation counseling prior to cancer therapy

Encounter for fertility preservation counseling prior to surgical removal of gonads

IQ **Z31.69 Encounter for other general counseling and advice on procreation**

IQ **Z31.7 Encounter for procreative management and counseling for gestational carrier**

EXCLUDES 1 pregnant state, gestational carrier (Z33.3)

5 **Z31.8 Encounter for other procreative management**

Px IQ **Z31.81 Encounter for male factor infertility in female patient**

IQ **Z31.82 Encounter for Rh incompatibility status**

Px IQ + **Z31.83 Encounter for assisted reproductive fertility procedure cycle**

Patient undergoing in vitro fertilization cycle

Use additional code to identify the type of infertility

EXCLUDES 1 pre-cycle diagnosis and testing - code to reason for encounter

Px IQ **Z31.84 Encounter for fertility preservation procedure**

Encounter for fertility preservation procedure prior to cancer therapy

Encounter for fertility preservation procedure prior to surgical removal of gonads

IQ **Z31.89 Encounter for other procreative management**

IQ **Z31.9 Encounter for procreative management, unspecified**

4 **Z32 Encounter for pregnancy test and childbirth and childcare instruction**

5 **Z32.0 Encounter for pregnancy test**

IQ **Z32.00 Encounter for pregnancy test, result unknown**

Encounter for pregnancy test NOS

IQ **Z32.01 Encounter for pregnancy test, result positive**

IQ **Z32.02 Encounter for pregnancy test, result negative**

IQ **Z32.2 Encounter for childbirth instruction**

IQ **Z32.3 Encounter for childcare instruction**

Encounter for prenatal or postpartum childcare instruction

4 **Z33 Pregnant state**

IQ **Z33.1 Pregnant state, incidental**

Pregnancy NOS

Pregnant state NOS

EXCLUDES 1 complications of pregnancy (O00-O9A)
pregnant state, gestational carrier (Z33.3)

GUIDELINES **Section I.C.15.a.1)**

Should the provider document that the pregnancy is incidental to the encounter, then code Z33.1 should be used in place of any chapter 15 codes. It is the provider's responsibility to state that the condition being treated is not affecting the pregnancy.

Px IQ **Z33.2 Encounter for elective termination of pregnancy**

EXCLUDES 1 early fetal death with retention of dead fetus (O02.1)
late fetal death (O36.4)
spontaneous abortion (O03)

IQ **Z33.3 Pregnant state, gestational carrier**

EXCLUDES 1 encounter for procreative management and counseling for gestational carrier (Z31.7)

4 **Z34 Encounter for supervision of normal pregnancy**

EXCLUDES 1 any complication of pregnancy (O00-O9A)
encounter for pregnancy test (Z32.0-)
encounter for supervision of high risk pregnancy (O09.-)

5 **Z34.0 Encounter for supervision of normal first pregnancy**

Px IQ **Z34.00 Encounter for supervision of normal first pregnancy, unspecified trimester**

Px IQ **Z34.01 Encounter for supervision of normal first pregnancy, first trimester**

Px IQ **Z34.02 Encounter for supervision of normal first pregnancy, second trimester**

Px IQ **Z34.03 Encounter for supervision of normal first pregnancy, third trimester**

5 **Z34.8 Encounter for supervision of other normal pregnancy**

Px IQ **Z34.80 Encounter for supervision of other normal pregnancy, unspecified trimester**

Px IQ **Z34.81 Encounter for supervision of other normal pregnancy, first trimester**

Px IQ **Z34.82 Encounter for supervision of other normal pregnancy, second trimester**

Px IQ **Z34.83 Encounter for supervision of other normal pregnancy, third trimester**

5 **Z34.9 Encounter for supervision of normal pregnancy, unspecified**

Px IQ **Z34.90 Encounter for supervision of normal pregnancy, unspecified, unspecified trimester**

Px IQ **Z34.91 Encounter for supervision of normal pregnancy, unspecified, first trimester**

Px IQ **Z34.92 Encounter for supervision of normal pregnancy, unspecified, second trimester**

Px IQ **Z34.93 Encounter for supervision of normal pregnancy, unspecified, third trimester**

4 **Z36 Encounter for antenatal screening of mother**

INCLUDES Encounter for placental sample (taken vaginally)
Screening is the testing for disease or disease precursors in asymptomatic individuals so that early detection and treatment can be provided for those who test positive for the disease.

EXCLUDES 1 diagnostic examination- code to sign or symptom

Chapter 21

Z00-Z99

encounter for suspected maternal and fetal conditions ruled out (Z03.7-)
suspected fetal condition affecting management of pregnancy - code to condition in Chapter 15

EXCLUDES 2 abnormal findings on antenatal screening of mother (O28.-)
genetic counseling and testing (Z31.43-, Z31.5)
routine prenatal care (Z34)

IQ **Z36.0 Encounter for antenatal screening for chromosomal anomalies**

IQ **Z36.1 Encounter for antenatal screening for raised alphafetoprotein level**
Encounter for antenatal screening for elevated maternal serum alphafetoprotein level

IQ **Z36.2 Encounter for other antenatal screening follow-up**
Non-visualized anatomy on a previous scan

IQ **Z36.3 Encounter for antenatal screening for malformations**
Screening for a suspected anomaly

IQ **Z36.4 Encounter for antenatal screening for fetal growth retardation**
Intrauterine growth restriction (IUGR)/small-for-dates

IQ **Z36.5 Encounter for antenatal screening for isoimmunization**

5 **Z36.8 Encounter for other antenatal screening**

IQ **Z36.81 Encounter for antenatal screening for hydrops fetalis**

IQ **Z36.82 Encounter for antenatal screening for nuchal translucency**

IQ **Z36.83 Encounter for fetal screening for congenital cardiac abnormalities**

IQ **Z36.84 Encounter for antenatal screening for fetal lung maturity**

IQ **Z36.85 Encounter for antenatal screening for Streptococcus B**

IQ **Z36.86 Encounter for antenatal screening for cervical length**
Screening for risk of pre-term labor

IQ **Z36.87 Encounter for antenatal screening for uncertain dates**

IQ **Z36.88 Encounter for antenatal screening for fetal macrosomia**
Screening for large-for-dates

IQ **Z36.89 Encounter for other specified antenatal screening**

IQ **Z36.8A Encounter for antenatal screening for other genetic defects**

IQ **Z36.9 Encounter for antenatal screening, unspecified**

▲ 4 **Z3A Weeks of gestation**
Note:
Codes from category Z3A are for use, only on the maternal record, to indicate the weeks of gestation of the pregnancy, if known.
Code first:
obstetric condition or encounter for delivery (O09-O60, O80-O82)

5 **Z3A.0 Weeks of gestation of pregnancy, unspecified or less than 10 weeks**

IQ **Z3A.00 Weeks of gestation of pregnancy not specified**

IQ **Z3A.01 Less than 8 weeks gestation of pregnancy**

IQ **Z3A.08 8 weeks gestation of pregnancy**

IQ **Z3A.09 9 weeks gestation of pregnancy**

5 **Z3A.1 Weeks of gestation of pregnancy, weeks 10-19**

IQ **Z3A.10 10 weeks gestation of pregnancy**

IQ **Z3A.11 11 weeks gestation of pregnancy**

IQ **Z3A.12 12 weeks gestation of pregnancy**

IQ **Z3A.13 13 weeks gestation of pregnancy**

IQ **Z3A.14 14 weeks gestation of pregnancy**

IQ **Z3A.15 15 weeks gestation of pregnancy**

IQ **Z3A.16 16 weeks gestation of pregnancy**

IQ **Z3A.17 17 weeks gestation of pregnancy**

IQ **Z3A.18 18 weeks gestation of pregnancy**

IQ **Z3A.19 19 weeks gestation of pregnancy**

5 **Z3A.2 Weeks of gestation of pregnancy, weeks 20-29**

IQ **Z3A.20 20 weeks gestation of pregnancy**

IQ **Z3A.21 21 weeks gestation of pregnancy**

IQ **Z3A.22 22 weeks gestation of pregnancy**

IQ **Z3A.23 23 weeks gestation of pregnancy**

IQ **Z3A.24 24 weeks gestation of pregnancy**

IQ **Z3A.25 25 weeks gestation of pregnancy**

IQ **Z3A.26 26 weeks gestation of pregnancy**

IQ **Z3A.27 27 weeks gestation of pregnancy**

IQ **Z3A.28 28 weeks gestation of pregnancy**

IQ **Z3A.29 29 weeks gestation of pregnancy**

5 **Z3A.3 Weeks of gestation of pregnancy, weeks 30-39**

IQ **Z3A.30 30 weeks gestation of pregnancy**

IQ **Z3A.31 31 weeks gestation of pregnancy**

IQ **Z3A.32 32 weeks gestation of pregnancy**

IQ **Z3A.33 33 weeks gestation of pregnancy**

IQ **Z3A.34 34 weeks gestation of pregnancy**

IQ **Z3A.35 35 weeks gestation of pregnancy**

IQ **Z3A.36 36 weeks gestation of pregnancy**

IQ **Z3A.37 37 weeks gestation of pregnancy**

IQ **Z3A.38 38 weeks gestation of pregnancy**

IQ **Z3A.39 39 weeks gestation of pregnancy**

5 **Z3A.4 Weeks of gestation of pregnancy, weeks 40 or greater**

IQ **Z3A.40 40 weeks gestation of pregnancy**

IQ **Z3A.41 41 weeks gestation of pregnancy**

IQ **Z3A.42 42 weeks gestation of pregnancy**

IQ **Z3A.49 Greater than 42 weeks gestation of pregnancy**

4 **Z37 Outcome of delivery**
This category is intended for use as an additional code to identify the outcome of delivery on the mother's record. It is not for use on the newborn record.

EXCLUDES 1 stillbirth (P95)

IQ **Z37.0 Single live birth**

IQ **Z37.1 Single stillbirth**

IQ **Z37.2 Twins, both liveborn**

IQ **Z37.3 Twins, one liveborn and one stillborn**

4 4th digit required 5 5th digit required 6 6th digit required 7 7th digit required 7 7th digit placeholder + Additional code Laterality

IQ Z37.4 **Twins, both stillborn**

5 Z37.5 **Other multiple births, all liveborn**

IQ Z37.50 **Multiple births, unspecified, all liveborn**

IQ Z37.51 **Triplets, all liveborn**

IQ Z37.52 **Quadruplets, all liveborn**

IQ Z37.53 **Quintuplets, all liveborn**

IQ Z37.54 **Sextuplets, all liveborn**

IQ Z37.59 **Other multiple births, all liveborn**

5 Z37.6 **Other multiple births, some liveborn**

IQ Z37.60 **Multiple births, unspecified, some liveborn**

IQ Z37.61 **Triplets, some liveborn**

IQ Z37.62 **Quadruplets, some liveborn**

IQ Z37.63 **Quintuplets, some liveborn**

IQ Z37.64 **Sextuplets, some liveborn**

IQ Z37.69 **Other multiple births, some liveborn**

IQ Z37.7 **Other multiple births, all stillborn**

IQ Z37.9 **Outcome of delivery, unspecified**

Multiple birth NOS
Single birth NOS

4 Z38 **Liveborn infants according to place of birth and type of delivery**

This category is for use as the principal code on the initial record of a newborn baby. It is to be used for the initial birth record only. It is not to be used on the mother's record.

5 Z38.0 **Single liveborn infant, born in hospital**

Single liveborn infant, born in birthing center or other health care facility

Px IQ Z38.00 **Single liveborn infant, delivered vaginally**

Px IQ Z38.01 **Single liveborn infant, delivered by cesarean**

Px IQ Z38.1 **Single liveborn infant, born outside hospital**

Px IQ Z38.2 **Single liveborn infant, unspecified as to place of birth**

Single liveborn infant NOS

5 Z38.3 **Twin liveborn infant, born in hospital**

Px IQ Z38.30 **Twin liveborn infant, delivered vaginally**

Px IQ Z38.31 **Twin liveborn infant, delivered by cesarean**

Px IQ Z38.4 **Twin liveborn infant, born outside hospital**

Px IQ Z38.5 **Twin liveborn infant, unspecified as to place of birth**

5 Z38.6 **Other multiple liveborn infant, born in hospital**

Px IQ Z38.61 **Triplet liveborn infant, delivered vaginally**

Px IQ Z38.62 **Triplet liveborn infant, delivered by cesarean**

Px IQ Z38.63 **Quadruplet liveborn infant, delivered vaginally**

Px IQ Z38.64 **Quadruplet liveborn infant, delivered by cesarean**

Px IQ Z38.65 **Quintuplet liveborn infant, delivered vaginally**

Px IQ Z38.66 **Quintuplet liveborn infant, delivered by cesarean**

Px IQ Z38.68 **Other multiple liveborn infant, delivered vaginally**

Px IQ Z38.69 **Other multiple liveborn infant, delivered by cesarean**

Px IQ Z38.7 **Other multiple liveborn infant, born outside hospital**

Px IQ Z38.8 **Other multiple liveborn infant, unspecified as to place of birth**

4 Z39 **Encounter for maternal postpartum care and examination**

Px IQ Z39.0 **Encounter for care and examination of mother immediately after delivery**

Care and observation in uncomplicated cases when the delivery occurs outside a healthcare facility

EXCLUDES 1 care for postpartum complication- see Alphabetic index

Px IQ Z39.1 **Encounter for care and examination of lactating mother**

Encounter for supervision of lactation

EXCLUDES 1 disorders of lactation (O92.-)

Px IQ Z39.2 **Encounter for routine postpartum follow-up**

Encounters for other specific health care (Z40-Z53)

Categories Z40-Z53 are intended for use to indicate a reason for care. They may be used for patients who have already been treated for a disease or injury, but who are receiving aftercare or prophylactic care, or care to consolidate the treatment, or to deal with a residual state

EXCLUDES 2 follow-up examination for medical surveillance after treatment (Z08-Z09)

4 Z40 **Encounter for prophylactic surgery**

EXCLUDES 1 organ donations (Z52.-)
therapeutic organ removal-code to condition

CODING TIPS ✓ Official guidance indicates the Z40 category is for use for physician encounters only. Z48.816 should be used as the aftercare code for prophylactic removal of breasts, ovaries, and other genitourinary organs.

+ 5 Z40.0 **Encounter for prophylactic surgery for risk factors related to malignant neoplasms**

Admission for prophylactic organ removal
Use additional code to identify risk factor

Px IQ + Z40.00 **Encounter for prophylactic removal of unspecified organ**

Px IQ + Z40.01 **Encounter for prophylactic removal of breast**

Px IQ + Z40.02 **Encounter for prophylactic removal of ovary(s)**

Encounter for prophylactic removal of ovary(s) and fallopian tube(s)

IQ + Z40.03 **Encounter for prophylactic removal of fallopian tube(s)**

Px IQ + Z40.09 **Encounter for prophylactic removal of other organ**

Px IQ Z40.8 **Encounter for other prophylactic surgery**

Px IQ Z40.9 **Encounter for prophylactic surgery, unspecified**

4 Z41 **Encounter for procedures for purposes other than remedying health state**

IQ **Z41.1 Encounter for cosmetic surgery**
Encounter for cosmetic breast implant
Encounter for cosmetic procedure
EXCLUDES 1 encounter for plastic and reconstructive surgery following medical procedure or healed injury (Z42.-)
encounter for post-mastectomy breast implantation (Z42.1)

IQ **Z41.2 Encounter for routine and ritual male circumcision**

IQ **Z41.3 Encounter for ear piercing**

IQ **Z41.8 Encounter for other procedures for purposes other than remedying health state**

IQ **Z41.9 Encounter for procedure for purposes other than remedying health state, unspecified**

4 **Z42 Encounter for plastic and reconstructive surgery following medical procedure or healed injury**
EXCLUDES 1 encounter for cosmetic plastic surgery (Z41.1)
encounter for plastic surgery for treatment of current injury - code to relevent injury

Px IQ **Z42.1 Encounter for breast reconstruction following mastectomy**
EXCLUDES 1 deformity and disproportion of reconstructed breast (N65.1-)

CODING TIPS ✓ Official guidance indicates the Z42.1 code is for use for physician encounters only. For home care, either the Z48.816 or the Z48.3 code is recommended for aftercare following reconstruction following mastectomy depending on the circumstances of the mastectomy, i.e. prophylactic removal or cancer.

Px IQ **Z42.8 Encounter for other plastic and reconstructive surgery following medical procedure or healed injury**

4 **Z43 Encounter for attention to artificial openings**
INCLUDES closure of artificial openings
passage of sounds or bougies through artificial openings
reforming artificial openings
removal of catheter from artificial openings
toilet or cleansing of artificial openings
EXCLUDES 1 complications of external stoma (J95.0-, K94.-, N99.5-)
EXCLUDES 2 fitting and adjustment of prosthetic and other devices (Z44-Z46)

CODING TIPS ✓ Z43 codes are in the complex nursing grouper. Assign Z43 codes as primary only if the ostomy is the focus of care and the agency is providing active care/intervention to the artificial opening. If the opening has been reversed, codes from category Z43 are no longer applicable since the patient no longer has the ostomy. If the patient is seen for wound care following closure, assign a code from category Z48. If the ostomy is allowed to close on its own, the Z43 codes are appropriate for any care provided.
Do not use codes in the Z43 category with status ostomy codes (Z93) for the same ostomy or when the ostomy is complicated.

CODING TIPS ✓ When assigning a code from Z43 for an encounter for attention to artificial openings, such as a tracheostomy or cystostomy, the plan of care should include interventions for the treatment of the artificial opening.

SP **Z43.0 Encounter for attention to tracheostomy**

SP **Z43.1 Encounter for attention to gastrostomy**
EXCLUDES 2 artificial opening status only, without need for care (Z93.-)

SP **Z43.2 Encounter for attention to ileostomy**

SP **Z43.3 Encounter for attention to colostomy**

SP **Z43.4 Encounter for attention to other artificial openings of digestive tract**

SP **Z43.5 Encounter for attention to cystostomy**
CODING TIPS ✓ This code may be assigned for the attention to the cystostomy in addition to Z46.6 if the catheter is also being changed.

SP **Z43.6 Encounter for attention to other artificial openings of urinary tract**
Encounter for attention to nephrostomy
Encounter for attention to ureterostomy
Encounter for attention to urethrostomy

SP **Z43.7 Encounter for attention to artificial vagina**

SP **Z43.8 Encounter for attention to other artificial openings**

IQ **Z43.9 Encounter for attention to unspecified artificial opening**

4 **Z44 Encounter for fitting and adjustment of external prosthetic device**
INCLUDES removal or replacement of external prosthetic device
EXCLUDES 1 malfunction or other complications of device - see Alphabetical Index
presence of prosthetic device (Z97.-)

5 **Z44.0 Encounter for fitting and adjustment of artificial arm**

6 **Z44.00 Encounter for fitting and adjustment of unspecified artificial arm**

Laterality IQ **Z44.001 Encounter for fitting and adjustment of unspecified right artificial arm**

Laterality IQ **Z44.002 Encounter for fitting and adjustment of unspecified left artificial arm**

Z44.009 Encounter for fitting and adjustment of unspecified artificial arm, unspecified arm

Z44.01 Encounter for fitting and adjustment of complete artificial arm

Z44.011 Encounter for fitting and adjustment of complete right artificial arm

Z44.012 Encounter for fitting and adjustment of complete left artificial arm

Z44.019 Encounter for fitting and adjustment of complete artificial arm, unspecified arm

Z44.02 Encounter for fitting and adjustment of partial artificial arm

Z44.021 Encounter for fitting and adjustment of partial artificial right arm

Z44.022 Encounter for fitting and adjustment of partial artificial left arm

Z44.029 Encounter for fitting and adjustment of partial artificial arm, unspecified arm

Z44.1 Encounter for fitting and adjustment of artificial leg

Z44.10 Encounter for fitting and adjustment of unspecified artificial leg

Z44.101 Encounter for fitting and adjustment of unspecified right artificial leg

Z44.102 Encounter for fitting and adjustment of unspecified left artificial leg

Z44.109 Encounter for fitting and adjustment of unspecified artificial leg, unspecified leg

Z44.11 Encounter for fitting and adjustment of complete artificial leg

Z44.111 Encounter for fitting and adjustment of complete right artificial leg

Z44.112 Encounter for fitting and adjustment of complete left artificial leg

Z44.119 Encounter for fitting and adjustment of complete artificial leg, unspecified leg

Z44.12 Encounter for fitting and adjustment of partial artificial leg

Z44.121 Encounter for fitting and adjustment of partial artificial right leg

Z44.122 Encounter for fitting and adjustment of partial artificial left leg

Z44.129 Encounter for fitting and adjustment of partial artificial leg, unspecified leg

Z44.2 Encounter for fitting and adjustment of artificial eye

EXCLUDES 1 mechanical complication of ocular prosthesis (T85.3)

Z44.20 Encounter for fitting and adjustment of artificial eye, unspecified

Z44.21 Encounter for fitting and adjustment of artificial right eye

Z44.22 Encounter for fitting and adjustment of artificial left eye

Z44.3 Encounter for fitting and adjustment of external breast prosthesis

EXCLUDES 1 complications of breast implant (T85.4-)
encounter for adjustment or removal of breast implant (Z45.81-)
encounter for initial breast implant insertion for cosmetic breast augmentation (Z41.1)
encounter for breast reconstruction following mastectomy (Z42.1)

Z44.30 Encounter for fitting and adjustment of external breast prosthesis, unspecified breast

Z44.31 Encounter for fitting and adjustment of external right breast prosthesis

Z44.32 Encounter for fitting and adjustment of external left breast prosthesis

Z44.8 Encounter for fitting and adjustment of other external prosthetic devices

Z44.9 Encounter for fitting and adjustment of unspecified external prosthetic device

Z45 Encounter for adjustment and management of implanted device

INCLUDES removal or replacement of implanted device

EXCLUDES 1 malfunction or other complications of device - see Alphabetical Index

EXCLUDES 2 encounter for fitting and adjustment of non-implanted device (Z46.-)

Z45.0 Encounter for adjustment and management of cardiac device

Z45.01 Encounter for adjustment and management of cardiac pacemaker

Encounter for adjustment and management of cardiac resynchronization therapy pacemaker (CRT-P)

EXCLUDES 1 encounter for adjustment and management of automatic implantable cardiac defibrillator with synchronous cardiac pacemaker (Z45.02)

CODING TIPS ✓ See Z95.0 for presence of cardiac pacemaker.

Z45.010 Encounter for checking and testing of cardiac pacemaker pulse generator [battery]

Encounter for replacing cardiac pacemaker pulse generator [battery]

Z45.018 Encounter for adjustment and management of other part of cardiac pacemaker

EXCLUDES 1 presence of other part of cardiac pacemaker (Z95.0)

EXCLUDES 2 presence of prosthetic and other devices (Z95.1-Z95.5, Z95.811-Z97)

IQ **Z45.02 Encounter for adjustment and management of automatic implantable cardiac defibrillator**

Encounter for adjustment and management of automatic implantable cardiac defibrillator with synchronous cardiac pacemaker

Encounter for adjustment and management of cardiac resynchronization therapy defibrillator (CRT-D)

IQ **Z45.09 Encounter for adjustment and management of other cardiac device**

IQ **Z45.1 Encounter for adjustment and management of infusion pump**

CODING TIPS✓ See also Z46.81, which may be more appropriate to the care being provided.

SP **Z45.2 Encounter for adjustment and management of vascular access device**

Encounter for adjustment and management of vascular catheters

EXCLUDES 1 encounter for adjustment and management of renal dialysis catheter (Z49.01)

CODING TIPS✓ This code as primary or first secondary places the patient into the complex nursing primary grouper. Use the code as primary only if the care of the infusion line is the only care provided and the underlying condition is not being treated. This code may be placed as a secondary for Medicare data purposes.

CODING TIPS✓ This code is used for routine care of vascular access devices, including peripheral, PICC and central lines. Do not use this code if the line is complicated. See T80 for complications.

5 **Z45.3 Encounter for adjustment and management of implanted devices of the special senses**

IQ **Z45.31 Encounter for adjustment and management of implanted visual substitution device**

6 **Z45.32 Encounter for adjustment and management of implanted hearing device**

EXCLUDES 1 Encounter for fitting and adjustment of hearing aide (Z46.1)

IQ **Z45.320 Encounter for adjustment and management of bone conduction device**

IQ **Z45.321 Encounter for adjustment and management of cochlear device**

IQ **Z45.328 Encounter for adjustment and management of other implanted hearing device**

5 **Z45.4 Encounter for adjustment and management of implanted nervous system device**

IQ **Z45.41 Encounter for adjustment and management of cerebrospinal fluid drainage device**

Encounter for adjustment and management of cerebral ventricular (communicating) shunt

IQ **Z45.42 Encounter for adjustment and management of neurostimulator**

Encounter for adjustment and management of brain neurostimulator

Encounter for adjustment and management of gastric neurostimulator

Encounter for adjustment and management of peripheral nerve neurostimulator

Encounter for adjustment and management of sacral nerve neurostimulator

Encounter for adjustment and management of spinal cord neurostimulator

Encounter for adjustment and management of vagus nerve neurostimulator

IQ **Z45.49 Encounter for adjustment and management of other implanted nervous system device**

5 **Z45.8 Encounter for adjustment and management of other implanted devices**

▲6 **Z45.81 Encounter for adjustment or removal of breast implant**

Encounter for elective implant exchange (different material) (different size)

Encounter for removal of tissue expander with or without synchronous insertion of permanent implant

EXCLUDES 1 complications of breast implant (T85.4-)
encounter for initial breast implant insertion for cosmetic breast augmentation (Z41.1)
encounter for breast reconstruction following mastectomy (Z42.1)

⊟ IQ **Z45.811 Encounter for adjustment or removal of right breast implant**

⊟ IQ **Z45.812 Encounter for adjustment or removal of left breast implant**

⊟ IQ **Z45.819 Encounter for adjustment or removal of unspecified breast implant**

IQ **Z45.82 Encounter for adjustment or removal of myringotomy device (stent) (tube)**

IQ **Z45.89 Encounter for adjustment and management of other implanted devices**

IQ **Z45.9 Encounter for adjustment and management of unspecified implanted device**

4 **Z46 Encounter for fitting and adjustment of other devices**

INCLUDES removal or replacement of other device

EXCLUDES 1 malfunction or other complications of device - see Alphabetical Index

EXCLUDES 2 encounter for fitting and management of implanted devices (Z45.-)
issue of repeat prescription only (Z76.0)
presence of prosthetic and other devices (Z95-Z97)

IQ **Z46.0 Encounter for fitting and adjustment of spectacles and contact lenses**

IQ **Z46.1 Encounter for fitting and adjustment of hearing aid**

EXCLUDES 1 encounter for adjustment and management of implanted hearing device (Z45.32-)

IQ **Z46.2 Encounter for fitting and adjustment of other devices related to nervous system and special senses**

EXCLUDES 2 encounter for adjustment and management of implanted nervous system device (Z45.4-)
encounter for adjustment and management of implanted visual substitution device (Z45.31)

IQ **Z46.3 Encounter for fitting and adjustment of dental prosthetic device**

Encounter for fitting and adjustment of dentures

IQ **Z46.4 Encounter for fitting and adjustment of orthodontic device**

5 **Z46.5 Encounter for fitting and adjustment of other gastrointestinal appliance and device**

EXCLUDES 1 encounter for attention to artificial openings of digestive tract (Z43.1-Z43.4)

IQ **Z46.51 Encounter for fitting and adjustment of gastric lap band**

IQ **Z46.59 Encounter for fitting and adjustment of other gastrointestinal appliance and device**

SP **Z46.6 Encounter for fitting and adjustment of urinary device**

EXCLUDES 2 attention to artificial openings of urinary tract (Z43.5, Z43.6)

CODING TIPS✓ This code may be assigned for the changing of cystostomy catheters in addition to attention to the cystomy (Z43.5).

CODING TIPS✓ Complications of urinary catheters should be coded to complications, such as T83.0.

CODING TIPS✓ Code Z46.6 includes removal and intermittent catheterization as well as indwelling catheter care.

5 **Z46.8 Encounter for fitting and adjustment of other specified devices**

IQ **Z46.81 Encounter for fitting and adjustment of insulin pump**

Encounter for insulin pump instruction and training
Encounter for insulin pump titration

IQ **Z46.82 Encounter for fitting and adjustment of non-vascular catheter**

CODING TIPS✓ Non-vascular catheters include subcutaneous infusions, intrathecal infusions, epidural infusions and even NG tubes. Urinary catheters are not included.

IQ **Z46.89 Encounter for fitting and adjustment of other specified devices**

Encounter for fitting and adjustment of wheelchair

IQ **Z46.9 Encounter for fitting and adjustment of unspecified device**

4 **Z47 Orthopedic aftercare**

EXCLUDES 1 aftercare for healing fracture-code to fracture with 7th character D

CODING TIPS✓ Do not use Z47 codes for surgery for injuries, including surgery for trauma or pathologic fractures. Use the injury (fracture) code instead with D as the 7th character.

SP + **Z47.1 Aftercare following joint replacement surgery**

Use additional code to identify the joint (Z96.6-)

CODING TIPS✓ These aftercare codes place the patient in the MS Rehab grouper. Wound care is not usually the focus of care for these patients, but if wound care is the focus of care, consider Z48.01 as primary instead.

CODING TIPS✓ Do NOT use Z47.1 for fractures, even if the fracture was treated with a joint replacement. Code the fracture with 7th character D and the appropriate Z96.6- code to indicate the presence of the joint prosthesis.

IQ **Z47.2 Encounter for removal of internal fixation device**

EXCLUDES 1 encounter for adjustment of internal fixation device for fracture treatment- code to fracture with appropriate 7th character
encounter for removal of external fixation device-code to fracture with 7th character D
infection or inflammatory reaction to internal fixation device (T84.6-)
mechanical complication of internal fixation device (T84.1-)

CODING TIPS✓ These aftercare codes place the patient in the MS Rehab grouper. Wound care is not usually the focus of care for these patients, but if wound care is the focus of care, consider Z48.01 as primary instead.

CODING TIPS✓ Pay close attention to the Excludes 1 note. Most instances for removal of an internal fixation device are for complications or actual treatment, like an infection. Z47.2 will most often be used for the physician encounter.

5 Z47.3 Aftercare following explantation of joint prosthesis

Aftercare following explantation of joint prosthesis, staged procedure

Encounter for joint prosthesis insertion following prior explantation of joint prosthesis

CODING TIPS ✓ These aftercare codes place the patient in the MS Rehab grouper. Wound care is not usually the focus of care for these patients, but if wound care is the focus of care, consider Z48.01 as primary instead.

CODING TIPS ✓ Pay close attention to the Excludes 1 note. Most instances for removal of an internal prosthesis are for complications or actual treatment of the fracture. If a mechanical complication has been repaired, continue to code the complication with a D until healed. This code is meant for a staged procedure and is appropriate for a new prosthesis once an infection has resolved.

CODING TIPS ✓ If the joint prosthesis was removed and not replaced, code M96.89 provides additional information regarding instability of the joint, if documented.

SP Z47.31 Aftercare following explantation of shoulder joint prosthesis

EXCLUDES 1 acquired absence of shoulder joint following prior explantation of shoulder joint prosthesis (Z89.23-)
shoulder joint prosthesis explantation status (Z89.23-)

SP Z47.32 Aftercare following explantation of hip joint prosthesis

EXCLUDES 1 acquired absence of hip joint following prior explantation of hip joint prosthesis (Z89.62-)
hip joint prosthesis explantation status (Z89.62-)

SP Z47.33 Aftercare following explantation of knee joint prosthesis

EXCLUDES 1 acquired absence of knee joint following prior explantation of knee prosthesis ()
knee joint prosthesis explantation status (Z89.52-)

5 Z47.8 Encounter for other orthopedic aftercare

SP + Z47.81 Encounter for orthopedic aftercare following surgical amputation

Use additional code to identify the limb amputated (Z89.-)

CODING TIPS ✓ These aftercare codes place the patient in the MS Rehab grouper. Wound care is not usually the focus of care for these patients, but if wound care is the focus of care, consider Z48.01 as primary instead.

CODING TIPS ✓ If amputation was performed because of a diabetic foot ulcer, use an additional code to indicate the history of diabetic ulcer (Z86.31).

CODING TIPS ✓ This code is only used for planned amputations. Do not assign Z47.81 for care following a traumatic amputation or when a surgical amputation is complicated by infection, dehiscence, or other complication.

SP Z47.82 Encounter for orthopedic aftercare following scoliosis surgery

CODING TIPS ✓ If the condition treated by surgery is coded with a M41 code, this aftercare code is correct.

SP Z47.89 Encounter for other orthopedic aftercare

CODING TIPS ✓ These aftercare codes place the patient in the MS Rehab grouper. Wound care is not usually the focus of care for these patients, but if wound care is the focus of care, consider Z48.01 as primary instead.

CODING TIPS ✓ Do not use this code for fracture repair. Code the fracture with 7th character D. Do not use this code for trauma to the musculoskeletal system. Use the appropriate trauma code with 7th character D.

CODING TIPS ✓ This code is the best choice for aftercare following musculoskeletal surgery that does not fit into any of the other Z47 codes, such as lumbar fusion or rotator cuff repair resulting from disuse. It is not to be used for aftercare for musculoskeletal injuries. Injuries should continue to be coded with the injury with 7th character D to indicate a healing/resolving injury.

4 Z48 Encounter for other postprocedural aftercare

EXCLUDES 1 encounter for follow-up examination after completed treatment (Z08-Z09)
encounter for aftercare following injury - code to Injury, by site, with appropriate 7th character for subsequent encounter

EXCLUDES 2 encounter for attention to artificial openings (Z43.-)
encounter for fitting and adjustment of prosthetic and other devices (Z44-Z46)

CODING TIPS ✓ Do not use Z48 codes for surgery for injuries. Use the injury code with D as the 7th character.

5 Z48.0 Encounter for attention to dressings, sutures and drains

EXCLUDES 1 encounter for planned postprocedural wound closure (Z48.1)

CODING TIPS ✓ Do not use dressing change codes for complicated wounds. The dressing change code may be placed as primary in home health to indicate the wound care is the primary focus of care. If the wound care is not the focus of care for a surgical wound, consider the aftercare following surgery code as the first code. The dressing change code should not be primary in hospice.

SP **Z48.00 Encounter for change or removal of nonsurgical wound dressing**

Encounter for change or removal of wound dressing NOS

CODING TIPS ✓ Z48.00 is an acceptable primary code to indicate that wound care is the focus of care for non-surgical wounds.

SP **Z48.01 Encounter for change or removal of surgical wound dressing**

CODING TIPS ✓ Z48.01 is an acceptable primary code to indicate the routine wound care of a surgical wound. Do not use this code for complicated surgical wounds. Z48.01 may be placed prior to the aftercare following surgery code to indicate that the wound care is the focus of care.

SP **Z48.02 Encounter for removal of sutures**

Encounter for removal of staples

SP **Z48.03 Encounter for change or removal of drains**

CODING TIPS ✓ This code may be used for care of drains of all kinds. The appropriate aftercare code for the reason for the drain may be coded first. Z48.03 should not be coded if the condition is complicated.

IQ **Z48.1 Encounter for planned postprocedural wound closure**

EXCLUDES 1 encounter for attention to dressings and sutures (Z48.0-)

5 **Z48.2 Encounter for aftercare following organ transplant**

CODING TIPS ✓ These aftercare following organ transplant codes do not require a second status code for the organ transplanted. If wound care is the focus of care, assign Z48.01 as primary. To indicate the status of a transplanted organ, see Z94. If the transplant is documented as complicated (failure, rejection, etc.) then use T86 codes instead.

SP **Z48.21 Encounter for aftercare following heart transplant**

SP **Z48.22 Encounter for aftercare following kidney transplant**

SP **Z48.23 Encounter for aftercare following liver transplant**

SP **Z48.24 Encounter for aftercare following lung transplant**

6 **Z48.28 Encounter for aftercare following multiple organ transplant**

SP **Z48.280 Encounter for aftercare following heart-lung transplant**

SP **Z48.288 Encounter for aftercare following multiple organ transplant**

6 **Z48.29 Encounter for aftercare following other organ transplant**

SP **Z48.290 Encounter for aftercare following bone marrow transplant**

SP **Z48.298 Encounter for aftercare following other organ transplant**

SP + **Z48.3 Aftercare following surgery for neoplasm**

Use additional code to identify the neoplasm

CODING TIPS ✓ When coding Z48.3, an additional code should be assigned to identify the neoplasm. If it is unclear if the neoplasm has been eradicated or if there are plans to continue treatment for the neoplastic disease, assign the appropriate code from Chapter 2 to indicate the neoplasm. If documentation clearly indicates that the neoplasm has been eradicated, assign the appropriate Z85 or Z86 code to report personal history of neoplasm. If wound care is the focus of care, assign Z48.01 as the primary code.

5 **Z48.8 Encounter for other specified postprocedural aftercare**

6 **Z48.81 Encounter for surgical aftercare following surgery on specified body systems**

These codes identify the body system requiring aftercare. They are for use in conjunction with other aftercare codes to fully explain the aftercare encounter. The condition treated should also be coded if still present.

EXCLUDES 1 aftercare for injury- code the injury with 7th character D

aftercare following surgery for neoplasm (Z48.3)

EXCLUDES 2 aftercare following organ transplant (Z48.2-)

orthopedic aftercare (Z47.-)

CODING TIPS ✓ If a dressing change is part of the aftercare, the dressing change code can precede the Z48.81- code. The dressing change is NOT part of the aftercare following surgery code. Status codes may be useful to indicate more fully the post-operative status. Also consider the use of Z90 codes to indicate acquired absence of a body part or organ. Do not use aftercare codes for complications that have been repaired or are resolving. Use the complication code with 7th character D. These codes are used to indicate care after procedures. Do not confuse what OASIS considers a surgical wound.

SP **Z48.810 Encounter for surgical aftercare following surgery on the sense organs**

CODING TIPS✓ Use this aftercare code for pre-operative conditions coded with H codes.

SP **Z48.811 Encounter for surgical aftercare following surgery on the nervous system**

EXCLUDES 2 encounter for surgical aftercare following surgery on the sense organs (Z48.810)

CODING TIPS✓ Use this aftercare code for pre-operative conditions coded with G codes.

SP **Z48.812 Encounter for surgical aftercare following surgery on the circulatory system**

CODING TIPS✓ Use this aftercare code for pre-operative conditions coded with I codes.

SP **Z48.813 Encounter for surgical aftercare following surgery on the respiratory system**

CODING TIPS✓ Use this aftercare code for pre-operative conditions coded with J codes.

SP **Z48.814 Encounter for surgical aftercare following surgery on the teeth or oral cavity**

SP **Z48.815 Encounter for surgical aftercare following surgery on the digestive system**

CODING TIPS✓ Use this aftercare code for pre-operative conditions coded with K codes.

SP **Z48.816 Encounter for surgical aftercare following surgery on the genitourinary system**

EXCLUDES 1 encounter for aftercare following sterilization reversal (Z31.42)

CODING TIPS✓ Use this aftercare code for pre-operative conditions coded with N codes.

SP **Z48.817 Encounter for surgical aftercare following surgery on the skin and subcutaneous tissue**

CODING TIPS✓ Use this aftercare code for pre-operative conditions coded with L codes.

SP **Z48.89 Encounter for other specified surgical aftercare**

4 **Z49 Encounter for care involving renal dialysis**

Code also:

associated end stage renal disease (N18.6)

CODING TIPS✓ These codes are not appropriate for home care or hospice. This care would be considered duplication of services in home health.

5 **Z49.0 Preparatory care for renal dialysis**

Encounter for dialysis instruction and training

IQ **Z49.01 Encounter for fitting and adjustment of extracorporeal dialysis catheter**

Removal or replacement of renal dialysis catheter

Toilet or cleansing of renal dialysis catheter

IQ **Z49.02 Encounter for fitting and adjustment of peritoneal dialysis catheter**

5 **Z49.3 Encounter for adequacy testing for dialysis**

IQ **Z49.31 Encounter for adequacy testing for hemodialysis**

IQ **Z49.32 Encounter for adequacy testing for peritoneal dialysis**

Encounter for peritoneal equilibration test

4 **Z51 Encounter for other aftercare and medical care**

Code also:

condition requiring care

EXCLUDES 1 follow-up examination after treatment (Z08-Z09)

GUIDELINES **Section I.C.2.e.2)**

If a patient admission/encounter is solely for the administration of chemotherapy, immunotherapy or external beam radiation therapy, assign code Z51.0, Encounter for antineoplastic radiation therapy, or Z51.11, Encounter for antineoplastic chemotherapy, or Z51.12, Encounter for antineoplastic immunotherapy as the first-listed or principal diagnosis.

The malignancy for which the therapy is being administered should be assigned as a secondary diagnosis.

If a patient admission/encounter is for the insertion or implantation of radioactive elements (e.g., brachytherapy) the appropriate code for the malignancy is sequenced as the principal or first-listed diagnosis. Code Z51.0 should not be assigned.

CODING TIPS✓ Only the provider administering the radiation, chemotherapy or immunotherapy may assign a code from category Z51 to report encounter for radiation, chemotherapy, or immunotherapy.

Px IQ **Z51.0 Encounter for antineoplastic radiation therapy**

GUIDELINES **Section I.C.2.e.3)**

When a patient is admitted for the purpose of external beam radiotherapy, immunotherapy or chemotherapy and develops complications such as uncontrolled nausea and vomiting or dehydration, the principal or first-listed diagnosis is Z51.0 or Z51.11 or Z51.12, followed by any codes for the complications.

CODING TIPS✓ This code is primary only and should only be used if home care is actually administering the therapy. Z codes are not appropriate as primary in hospice.

5 **Z51.1 Encounter for antineoplastic chemotherapy and immunotherapy**

EXCLUDES 2 encounter for chemotherapy and immunotherapy for nonneoplastic condition - code to condition

Px SP **Z51.11 Encounter for antineoplastic chemotherapy**

CODING TIPS✓ This code is primary only and should only be used if home care is actually administering the therapy. Z codes are not appropriate as primary in hospice.

Px SP **Z51.12 Encounter for antineoplastic immunotherapy**

CODING TIPS✓ This code is primary only and should only be used if home care is actually administering the therapy. Z codes are not appropriate as primary in hospice.

SP **Z51.5 Encounter for palliative care**

CODING TIPS✓ Z51.5 may be assigned as a primary diagnosis to indicate palliative care in home health. The condition(s) requiring palliative care may be coded as primary or secondary in home health. This code is appropriate for hospice, end of life care and palliative care as a secondary code. But note hospice claims do not allow Z codes as primary.

IQ **Z51.6 Encounter for desensitization to allergens**

5 **Z51.8 Encounter for other specified aftercare**

EXCLUDES 1 holiday relief care (Z75.5)

IQ **Z51.81 Encounter for therapeutic drug level monitoring**

Code also:

any long-term (current) drug therapy (Z79.-)

EXCLUDES 1 encounter for blood-drug test for administrative or medicolegal reasons (Z02.83)

CODING TIPS✓ This code is usually associated with venipuncture and should only be used if monitoring drug levels. Use a code from Z79 to indicate the drug monitored.

IQ **Z51.89 Encounter for other specified aftercare**

CODING TIPS✓ If the myocardial infarction patient still requires care related to the MI after 4 weeks, assign Z51.89 followed by I25.2. Neither one of these codes may be primary under PDGM.

CODING TIPS✓ This is not the code for admission for therapy. Assign the appropriate code for the condition for which rehabilitation services are being provided.

4 **Z52 Donors of organs and tissues**

INCLUDES autologous and other living donors

EXCLUDES 1 cadaveric donor - omit code examination of potential donor (Z00.5)

5 **Z52.0 Blood donor**

6 **Z52.00 Unspecified blood donor**

Px IQ **Z52.000 Unspecified donor, whole blood**

Px IQ **Z52.001 Unspecified donor, stem cells**

Px IQ **Z52.008 Unspecified donor, other blood**

6 **Z52.01 Autologous blood donor**

Px IQ **Z52.010 Autologous donor, whole blood**

Px IQ **Z52.011 Autologous donor, stem cells**

Px IQ **Z52.018 Autologous donor, other blood**

6 **Z52.09 Other blood donor**

Volunteer donor

Px IQ **Z52.090 Other blood donor, whole blood**

Px IQ **Z52.091 Other blood donor, stem cells**

Px IQ **Z52.098 Other blood donor, other blood**

5 **Z52.1 Skin donor**

Px IQ **Z52.10 Skin donor, unspecified**

Px IQ **Z52.11 Skin donor, autologous**

Px IQ **Z52.19 Skin donor, other**

5 **Z52.2 Bone donor**

Px IQ **Z52.20 Bone donor, unspecified**

Px IQ **Z52.21 Bone donor, autologous**

Px IQ **Z52.29 Bone donor, other**

Px IQ **Z52.3 Bone marrow donor**

Px IQ **Z52.4 Kidney donor**

Px IQ **Z52.5 Cornea donor**

Px IQ **Z52.6 Liver donor**

5 **Z52.8 Donor of other specified organs or tissues**

6 **Z52.81 Egg (Oocyte) donor**

Px IQ **Z52.810 Egg (Oocyte) donor under age 35, anonymous recipient**

Egg donor under age 35 NOS

Px IQ **Z52.811 Egg (Oocyte) donor under age 35, designated recipient**

Px IQ **Z52.812 Egg (Oocyte) donor age 35 and over, anonymous recipient**

Egg donor age 35 and over NOS

Px IQ **Z52.813 Egg (Oocyte) donor age 35 and over, designated recipient**

Px IQ **Z52.819 Egg (Oocyte) donor, unspecified**

Px IQ **Z52.89 Donor of other specified organs or tissues**

IQ **Z52.9 Donor of unspecified organ or tissue**

Donor NOS

4 **Z53 Persons encountering health services for specific procedures and treatment, not carried out**

5 **Z53.0 Procedure and treatment not carried out because of contraindication**

IQ **Z53.01 Procedure and treatment not carried out due to patient smoking**

IQ **Z53.09 Procedure and treatment not carried out because of other contraindication**

IQ **Z53.1 Procedure and treatment not carried out because of patient's decision for reasons of belief and group pressure**

5 **Z53.2 Procedure and treatment not carried out because of patient's decision for other and unspecified reasons**

IQ **Z53.20 Procedure and treatment not carried out because of patient's decision for unspecified reasons**

IQ **Z53.21 Procedure and treatment not carried out due to patient leaving prior to being seen by health care provider**

Chapter 21

Z00-Z99

IQ **Z53.29 Procedure and treatment not carried out because of patient's decision for other reasons**

5 **Z53.3 Procedure converted to open procedure**

IQ **Z53.31 Laparoscopic surgical procedure converted to open procedure**

IQ **Z53.32 Thoracoscopic surgical procedure converted to open procedure**

IQ **Z53.33 Arthroscopic surgical procedure converted to open procedure**

IQ **Z53.39 Other specified procedure converted to open procedure**

IQ **Z53.8 Procedure and treatment not carried out for other reasons**

IQ **Z53.9 Procedure and treatment not carried out, unspecified reason**

Persons with potential health hazards related to socioeconomic and psychosocial circumstances (Z55-Z65)

CODING TIPS✓ Social determinants of health may be coded based on the clinician's documentation and patient report.

4 **Z55 Problems related to education and literacy**

EXCLUDES 1 disorders of psychological development (F80-F89)

IQ **Z55.0 Illiteracy and low-level literacy**

IQ **Z55.1 Schooling unavailable and unattainable**

IQ **Z55.2 Failed school examinations**

IQ **Z55.3 Underachievement in school**

IQ **Z55.4 Educational maladjustment and discord with teachers and classmates**

★ **Z55.5 Less than a high school diploma**

No general equivalence degree (GED)

IQ **Z55.8 Other problems related to education and literacy**

Problems related to inadequate teaching

IQ **Z55.9 Problems related to education and literacy, unspecified**

Academic problems NOS

4 **Z56 Problems related to employment and unemployment**

EXCLUDES 2 occupational exposure to risk factors (Z57.-)
problems related to housing and economic circumstances (Z59.-)

IQ **Z56.0 Unemployment, unspecified**

IQ **Z56.1 Change of job**

IQ **Z56.2 Threat of job loss**

IQ **Z56.3 Stressful work schedule**

IQ **Z56.4 Discord with boss and workmates**

IQ **Z56.5 Uncongenial work environment**

Difficult conditions at work

IQ **Z56.6 Other physical and mental strain related to work**

5 **Z56.8 Other problems related to employment**

IQ **Z56.81 Sexual harassment on the job**

IQ **Z56.82 Military deployment status**

Individual (civilian or military) currently deployed in theater or in support of military war, peacekeeping and humanitarian operations

IQ **Z56.89 Other problems related to employment**

IQ **Z56.9 Unspecified problems related to employment**

Occupational problems NOS

4 **Z57 Occupational exposure to risk factors**

IQ **Z57.0 Occupational exposure to noise**

IQ **Z57.1 Occupational exposure to radiation**

IQ **Z57.2 Occupational exposure to dust**

5 **Z57.3 Occupational exposure to other air contaminants**

IQ **Z57.31 Occupational exposure to environmental tobacco smoke**

EXCLUDES 2 exposure to environmental tobacco smoke (Z77.22)

IQ **Z57.39 Occupational exposure to other air contaminants**

IQ **Z57.4 Occupational exposure to toxic agents in agriculture**

Occupational exposure to solids, liquids, gases or vapors in agriculture

IQ **Z57.5 Occupational exposure to toxic agents in other industries**

Occupational exposure to solids, liquids, gases or vapors in other industries

IQ **Z57.6 Occupational exposure to extreme temperature**

IQ **Z57.7 Occupational exposure to vibration**

IQ **Z57.8 Occupational exposure to other risk factors**

IQ **Z57.9 Occupational exposure to unspecified risk factor**

★ 4 **Z58 Problems related to physical environment**

Excludes:2: occupational exposure (Z57.-)

★ **Z58.6 Inadequate drinking-water supply**

Lack of safe drinking water

EXCLUDES 2 deprivation of water (T73.1)

4 **Z59 Problems related to housing and economic circumstances**

EXCLUDES 2 problems related to upbringing (Z62.-)

▲ 5 **Z59.0 Homelessness**

★ **Z59.00 Homelessness unspecified**

★ **Z59.01 Sheltered homelessness**

Doubled up

Living in a shelter such as: motel, scattered site housing, temporary or transitional living situation

★ **Z59.02 Unsheltered homelessness**

Residing in place not meant for human habitation such as: abandoned buildings, cars, parks, sidewalk

Residing on the street

IQ **Z59.1 Inadequate housing**

Lack of heating

Restriction of space

Technical defects in home preventing adequate care

Unsatisfactory surroundings

EXCLUDES 1 problems related to the natural and physical environment (Z77.1-)

IQ **Z59.2 Discord with neighbors, lodgers and landlord**

IQ **Z59.3 Problems related to living in residential institution**
Boarding-school resident
EXCLUDES 1 institutional upbringing (Z62.2)

▲ 5 **Z59.4 Lack of adequate food**
EXCLUDES 2 deprivation of food (T73.0)
effects of hunger (T73.0)
inappropriate diet or eating habits (Z72.4)
malnutrition (E40-E46)

★ **Z59.41 Food insecurity**

★ **Z59.48 Other specified lack of adequate food**
Inadequate food
Lack of food

IQ **Z59.5 Extreme poverty**

IQ **Z59.6 Low income**

IQ **Z59.7 Insufficient social insurance and welfare support**

▲ 5 **Z59.8 Other problems related to housing and economic circumstances**

★ 6 **Z59.81 Housing instability, housed**
Foreclosure on home loan
Past due on rent or mortgage
Unwanted multiple moves in the last 12 months

★ **Z59.811 Housing instability, housed, with risk of homelessness**
Imminent risk of homelessness

★ **Z59.812 Housing instability, housed, homelessness in past 12 months**

★ **Z59.819 Housing instability, housed unspecified**

★ **Z59.89 Other problems related to housing and economic circumstances**
Foreclosure on loan
Isolated dwelling
Problems with creditors

IQ **Z59.9 Problem related to housing and economic circumstances, unspecified**

4 **Z60 Problems related to social environment**

IQ **Z60.0 Problems of adjustment to life-cycle transitions**
Empty nest syndrome
Phase of life problem
Problem with adjustment to retirement [pension]

IQ **Z60.2 Problems related to living alone**

IQ **Z60.3 Acculturation difficulty**
Problem with migration
Problem with social transplantation

IQ **Z60.4 Social exclusion and rejection**
Exclusion and rejection on the basis of personal characteristics, such as unusual physical appearance, illness or behavior.
EXCLUDES 1 target of adverse discrimination such as for racial or religious reasons (Z60.5)

IQ **Z60.5 Target of (perceived) adverse discrimination and persecution**
EXCLUDES 1 social exclusion and rejection (Z60.4)

IQ **Z60.8 Other problems related to social environment**

IQ **Z60.9 Problem related to social environment, unspecified**

4 **Z62 Problems related to upbringing**
INCLUDES current and past negative life events in childhood
current and past problems of a child related to upbringing
EXCLUDES 2 maltreatment syndrome (T74.-)
problems related to housing and economic circumstances (Z59.-)

IQ **Z62.0 Inadequate parental supervision and control**

IQ **Z62.1 Parental overprotection**

5 **Z62.2 Upbringing away from parents**
EXCLUDES 1 problems with boarding school (Z59.3)

IQ **Z62.21 Child in welfare custody**
Child in care of non-parental family member
Child in foster care
EXCLUDES 2 problem for parent due to child in welfare custody (Z63.5)

IQ **Z62.22 Institutional upbringing**
Child living in orphanage or group home

IQ **Z62.29 Other upbringing away from parents**

IQ **Z62.3 Hostility towards and scapegoating of child**

IQ **Z62.6 Inappropriate (excessive) parental pressure**

5 **Z62.8 Other specified problems related to upbringing**

6 **Z62.81 Personal history of abuse in childhood**

IQ **Z62.810 Personal history of physical and sexual abuse in childhood**
EXCLUDES 1 current child physical abuse (T74.12, T76.12)
current child sexual abuse (T74.22, T76.22)

IQ **Z62.811 Personal history of psychological abuse in childhood**
EXCLUDES 1 current child psychological abuse (T74.32, T76.32)

IQ **Z62.812 Personal history of neglect in childhood**
EXCLUDES 1 current child neglect (T74.02, T76.02)

IQ **Z62.813 Personal history of forced labor or sexual exploitation in childhood**

IQ **Z62.819 Personal history of unspecified abuse in childhood**
EXCLUDES 1 current child abuse NOS (T74.92, T76.92)

6 **Z62.82 Parent-child conflict**

IQ **Z62.820 Parent-biological child conflict**
Parent-child problem NOS

IQ **Z62.821 Parent-adopted child conflict**

IQ **Z62.822 Parent-foster child conflict**

6 **Z62.89 Other specified problems related to upbringing**

Chapter 21

Z00-Z99

IQ **Z62.890 Parent-child estrangement NEC**

IQ **Z62.891 Sibling rivalry**

IQ **Z62.898 Other specified problems related to upbringing**

IQ **Z62.9 Problem related to upbringing, unspecified**

4 **Z63 Other problems related to primary support group, including family circumstances**

EXCLUDES 2 maltreatment syndrome (T74.-, T76)
parent-child problems (Z62.-)
problems related to negative life events in childhood (Z62.-)
problems related to upbringing (Z62.-)

IQ **Z63.0 Problems in relationship with spouse or partner**

Relationship distress with spouse or intimate partner

EXCLUDES 1 counseling for spousal or partner abuse problems (Z69.1)
counseling related to sexual attitude, behavior, and orientation (Z70.-)

IQ **Z63.1 Problems in relationship with in-laws**

5 **Z63.3 Absence of family member**

EXCLUDES 1 absence of family member due to disappearance and death (Z63.4)
absence of family member due to separation and divorce (Z63.5)

IQ **Z63.31 Absence of family member due to military deployment**

Individual or family affected by other family member being on military deployment

EXCLUDES 1 family disruption due to return of family member from military deployment (Z63.71)

IQ **Z63.32 Other absence of family member**

IQ **Z63.4 Disappearance and death of family member**

Assumed death of family member
Bereavement

IQ **Z63.5 Disruption of family by separation and divorce**

Marital estrangement

IQ **Z63.6 Dependent relative needing care at home**

5 **Z63.7 Other stressful life events affecting family and household**

IQ **Z63.71 Stress on family due to return of family member from military deployment**

Individual or family affected by family member having returned from military deployment (current or past conflict)

IQ **Z63.72 Alcoholism and drug addiction in family**

IQ **Z63.79 Other stressful life events affecting family and household**

Anxiety (normal) about sick person in family
Health problems within family
Ill or disturbed family member
Isolated family

IQ **Z63.8 Other specified problems related to primary support group**

Family discord NOS
Family estrangement NOS
High expressed emotional level within family
Inadequate family support NOS
Inadequate or distorted communication within family

IQ **Z63.9 Problem related to primary support group, unspecified**

Relationship disorder NOS

4 **Z64 Problems related to certain psychosocial circumstances**

IQ **Z64.0 Problems related to unwanted pregnancy**

IQ **Z64.1 Problems related to multiparity**

IQ **Z64.4 Discord with counselors**

Discord with probation officer
Discord with social worker

4 **Z65 Problems related to other psychosocial circumstances**

IQ **Z65.0 Conviction in civil and criminal proceedings without imprisonment**

IQ **Z65.1 Imprisonment and other incarceration**

IQ **Z65.2 Problems related to release from prison**

IQ **Z65.3 Problems related to other legal circumstances**

Arrest
Child custody or support proceedings
Litigation
Prosecution

IQ **Z65.4 Victim of crime and terrorism**

Victim of torture

IQ **Z65.5 Exposure to disaster, war and other hostilities**

EXCLUDES 1 target of perceived discrimination or persecution (Z60.5)

IQ **Z65.8 Other specified problems related to psychosocial circumstances**

Religious or spiritual problem

IQ **Z65.9 Problem related to unspecified psychosocial circumstances**

Do not resuscitate status (Z66)

IQ **Z66 Do not resuscitate**

DNR status

CODING TIPS ✓ The use of this code requires a physician's order for Do Not Resuscitate (DNR). Check state law to learn if NPPs are allowed to write DNR orders in your state.

Blood type (Z67)

4 **Z67 Blood type**

5 **Z67.1 Type A blood**

IQ **Z67.10 Type A blood, Rh positive**

IQ **Z67.11 Type A blood, Rh negative**

5 **Z67.2 Type B blood**

IQ **Z67.20 Type B blood, Rh positive**

IQ **Z67.21 Type B blood, Rh negative**

5 **Z67.3 Type AB blood**

IQ **Z67.30 Type AB blood, Rh positive**

IQ **Z67.31 Type AB blood, Rh negative**

5 **Z67.4 Type O blood**

IQ **Z67.40 Type O blood, Rh positive**

IQ **Z67.41 Type O blood, Rh negative**

5 **Z67.9 Unspecified blood type**

IQ **Z67.90 Unspecified blood type, Rh positive**

IQ **Z67.91 Unspecified blood type, Rh negative**

Body mass index [BMI] (Z68)

CODING TIPS✓ BMI may not be coded without an associated diagnosis from the physician or NPP, e.g., overweight, obesity, morbid obesity, or low weight diagnoses. Provider documentation indicating that condition as a diagnosis is required. If suspected, but not present, the coder may query the provider to obtain confirmation of the condition, but may not code obesity without confirmation from the provider. BMI may be calculated and documented based upon nursing documentation (height and weight used to calculate), however the BMI may only be coded if a physician-provided diagnosis, such as overweight, obesity, underweight is coded.

4 **Z68 Body mass index [BMI]**

Kilograms per meters squared

Note:

BMI adult codes are for use for persons 20 years of age or older

BMI pediatric codes are for use for persons 2-19 years of age.

These percentiles are based on the growth charts published by the Centers for Disease Control and Prevention (CDC)

CODING TIPS✓ BMI adult codes are for use in persons 20 years of age or older. Pediatric BMI codes (Z68.5-) are for use in persons aged 2-19 years of age. Percentiles are based on growth charts published by the CDC.

IQ **Z68.1 Body mass index [BMI] 19.9 or less, adult**

5 **Z68.2 Body mass index [BMI] 20-29, adult**

IQ **Z68.20 Body mass index [BMI] 20.0-20.9, adult**

IQ **Z68.21 Body mass index [BMI] 21.0-21.9, adult**

IQ **Z68.22 Body mass index [BMI] 22.0-22.9, adult**

IQ **Z68.23 Body mass index [BMI] 23.0-23.9, adult**

IQ **Z68.24 Body mass index [BMI] 24.0-24.9, adult**

IQ **Z68.25 Body mass index [BMI] 25.0-25.9, adult**

IQ **Z68.26 Body mass index [BMI] 26.0-26.9, adult**

IQ **Z68.27 Body mass index [BMI] 27.0-27.9, adult**

IQ **Z68.28 Body mass index [BMI] 28.0-28.9, adult**

IQ **Z68.29 Body mass index [BMI] 29.0-29.9, adult**

5 **Z68.3 Body mass index [BMI] 30-39, adult**

IQ **Z68.30 Body mass index [BMI] 30.0-30.9, adult**

IQ **Z68.31 Body mass index [BMI] 31.0-31.9, adult**

IQ **Z68.32 Body mass index [BMI] 32.0-32.9, adult**

IQ **Z68.33 Body mass index [BMI] 33.0-33.9, adult**

IQ **Z68.34 Body mass index [BMI] 34.0-34.9, adult**

IQ **Z68.35 Body mass index [BMI] 35.0-35.9, adult**

IQ **Z68.36 Body mass index [BMI] 36.0-36.9, adult**

IQ **Z68.37 Body mass index [BMI] 37.0-37.9, adult**

IQ **Z68.38 Body mass index [BMI] 38.0-38.9, adult**

IQ **Z68.39 Body mass index [BMI] 39.0-39.9, adult**

5 **Z68.4 Body mass index [BMI] 40 or greater, adult**

IQ **Z68.41 Body mass index [BMI] 40.0-44.9, adult**

IQ **Z68.42 Body mass index [BMI] 45.0-49.9, adult**

IQ **Z68.43 Body mass index [BMI] 50.0-59.9, adult**

IQ **Z68.44 Body mass index [BMI] 60.0-69.9, adult**

IQ **Z68.45 Body mass index [BMI] 70 or greater, adult**

5 **Z68.5 Body mass index [BMI] pediatric**

IQ **Z68.51 Body mass index [BMI] pediatric, less than 5th percentile for age**

IQ **Z68.52 Body mass index [BMI] pediatric, 5th percentile to less than 85th percentile for age**

IQ **Z68.53 Body mass index [BMI] pediatric, 85th percentile to less than 95th percentile for age**

IQ **Z68.54 Body mass index [BMI] pediatric, greater than or equal to 95th percentile for age**

Persons encountering health services in other circumstances (Z69-Z76)

4 **Z69 Encounter for mental health services for victim and perpetrator of abuse**

INCLUDES counseling for victims and perpetrators of abuse

5 **Z69.0 Encounter for mental health services for child abuse problems**

6 **Z69.01 Encounter for mental health services for parental child abuse**

IQ **Z69.010 Encounter for mental health services for victim of parental child abuse**

Encounter for mental health services for victim of child abuse by parent

Encounter for mental health services for victim of child neglect by parent

Encounter for mental health services for victim of child psychological abuse by parent

Encounter for mental health services for victim of child sexual abuse by parent

IQ **Z69.011 Encounter for mental health services for perpetrator of parental child abuse**
Encounter for mental health services for perpetrator of parental child neglect
Encounter for mental health services for perpetrator of parental child psychological abuse
Encounter for mental health services for perpetrator of parental child sexual abuse
EXCLUDES 1 encounter for mental health services for non-parental child abuse (Z69.02-)

6 **Z69.02 Encounter for mental health services for non-parental child abuse**

IQ **Z69.020 Encounter for mental health services for victim of non-parental child abuse**
Encounter for mental health services for victim of non-parental child neglect
Encounter for mental health services for victim of non-parental child psychological abuse
Encounter for mental health services for victim of non-parental child sexual abuse

IQ **Z69.021 Encounter for mental health services for perpetrator of non-parental child abuse**
Encounter for mental health services for perpetrator of non-parental child neglect
Encounter for mental health services for perpetrator of non-parental child psychological abuse
Encounter for mental health services for perpetrator of non-parental child sexual abuse

5 **Z69.1 Encounter for mental health services for spousal or partner abuse problems**

IQ **Z69.11 Encounter for mental health services for victim of spousal or partner abuse**
Encounter for mental health services for victim of spouse or partner neglect
Encounter for mental health services for victim of spouse or partner psychological abuse
Encounter for mental health services for victim of spouse or partner violence, physical

IQ **Z69.12 Encounter for mental health services for perpetrator of spousal or partner abuse**
Encounter for mental health services for perpetrator of spouse or partner neglect
Encounter for mental health services for perpetrator of spouse or partner psychological abuse
Encounter for mental health services for perpetrator of spouse or partner violence, physical
Encounter for mental health services for perpetrator of spouse or partner violence, sexual

5 **Z69.8 Encounter for mental health services for victim or perpetrator of other abuse**

IQ **Z69.81 Encounter for mental health services for victim of other abuse**
Encounter for mental health services for victim of non-spousal adult abuse
Encounter for mental health services for victim of spouse or partner violence, sexual
Encounter for rape victim counseling

IQ **Z69.82 Encounter for mental health services for perpetrator of other abuse**
Encounter for mental health services for perpetrator of non-spousal adult abuse

4 **Z70 Counseling related to sexual attitude, behavior and orientation**
INCLUDES encounter for mental health services for sexual attitude, behavior and orientation
EXCLUDES 2 contraceptive or procreative counseling (Z30-Z31)

IQ **Z70.0 Counseling related to sexual attitude**

IQ **Z70.1 Counseling related to patient's sexual behavior and orientation**
Patient concerned regarding impotence
Patient concerned regarding non-responsiveness
Patient concerned regarding promiscuity
Patient concerned regarding sexual orientation

IQ **Z70.2 Counseling related to sexual behavior and orientation of third party**
Advice sought regarding sexual behavior and orientation of child
Advice sought regarding sexual behavior and orientation of partner
Advice sought regarding sexual behavior and orientation of spouse

IQ **Z70.3 Counseling related to combined concerns regarding sexual attitude, behavior and orientation**

IQ **Z70.8 Other sex counseling**
Encounter for sex education

IQ **Z70.9 Sex counseling, unspecified**

4 **Z71 Persons encountering health services for other counseling and medical advice, not elsewhere classified**
EXCLUDES 2 contraceptive or procreation counseling (Z30-Z31)
sex counseling (Z70.-)

IQ **Z71.0 Person encountering health services to consult on behalf of another person**
Person encountering health services to seek advice or treatment for non-attending third party
EXCLUDES 2 anxiety (normal) about sick person in family (Z63.7)
expectant (adoptive) parent(s) pre-birth pediatrician visit (Z76.81)

IQ **Z71.1 Person with feared health complaint in whom no diagnosis is made**

Person encountering health services with feared condition which was not demonstrated
Person encountering health services in which problem was normal state
'Worried well'
EXCLUDES 1 medical observation for suspected diseases and conditions proven not to exist (Z03.-)

IQ **Z71.2 Person consulting for explanation of examination or test findings**

IQ + **Z71.3 Dietary counseling and surveillance**
Use additional code for any associated underlying medical condition
Use additional code to identify body mass index (BMI), if known (Z68.-)

+ 5 **Z71.4 Alcohol abuse counseling and surveillance**
Use additional code for alcohol abuse or dependence (F10.-)

IQ + **Z71.41 Alcohol abuse counseling and surveillance of alcoholic**

IQ + **Z71.42 Counseling for family member of alcoholic**
Counseling for significant other, partner, or friend of alcoholic

+ 5 **Z71.5 Drug abuse counseling and surveillance**
Use additional code for drug abuse or dependence (F11-F16, F18-F19)

IQ + **Z71.51 Drug abuse counseling and surveillance of drug abuser**

IQ + **Z71.52 Counseling for family member of drug abuser**
Counseling for significant other, partner, or friend of drug abuser

IQ + **Z71.6 Tobacco abuse counseling**
Use additional code for nicotine dependence (F17.-)

IQ **Z71.7 Human immunodeficiency virus [HIV] counseling**

5 **Z71.8 Other specified counseling**
EXCLUDES 2 counseling for contraception (Z30.0-)

IQ **Z71.81 Spiritual or religious counseling**

IQ **Z71.82 Exercise counseling**

IQ **Z71.83 Encounter for nonprocreative genetic counseling**
EXCLUDES 1 counseling for procreative genetics (Z31.5)
counseling for procreative management (Z31.6)

Z71.84 Encounter for health counseling related to travel
Encounter for health risk and safety counseling for (international) travel
Code also:
, if applicable, encounter for immunization (Z23)
EXCLUDES 2 encounter for administrative examination (Z02.-)
encounter for other special examination without complaint, suspected or reported diagnosis (Z01.-)

★ **Z71.85 Encounter for immunization safety counseling**
Encounter for vaccine product safety counseling
Code also:
, if applicable, encounter for immunization (Z23)
, if applicable, immunization not carried out (Z28.-)
EXCLUDES 1 encounter for health counseling related to travel (Z71.84)

IQ **Z71.89 Other specified counseling**

IQ **Z71.9 Counseling, unspecified**
Encounter for medical advice NOS

4 **Z72 Problems related to lifestyle**
EXCLUDES 2 problems related to life-management difficulty (Z73.-)
problems related to socioeconomic and psychosocial circumstances (Z55-Z65)

CODING TIPS ✓ These codes should be assigned only when the documentation specifies that the patient has an associated problem.

IQ **Z72.0 Tobacco use**
Tobacco use NOS
EXCLUDES 1 history of tobacco dependence (Z87.891)
nicotine dependence (F17.2-)
tobacco dependence (F17.2-)
tobacco use during pregnancy (O99.33-)

CODING TIPS ✓ If the physician or NPP documents "smoker," use code F17.2- instead.

IQ **Z72.3 Lack of physical exercise**

▲ IQ **Z72.4 Inappropriate diet and eating habits**
EXCLUDES 1 behavioral eating disorders of infancy or childhood (F98.2.-F98.3)
eating disorders (F50.-)
lack of adequate food (Z59.48)
malnutrition and other nutritional deficiencies (E40-E64)

5 **Z72.5 High risk sexual behavior**
Promiscuity
EXCLUDES 1 paraphilias (F65)

IQ **Z72.51 High risk heterosexual behavior**

IQ **Z72.52 High risk homosexual behavior**

IQ **Z72.53 High risk bisexual behavior**

IQ **Z72.6 Gambling and betting**
EXCLUDES 1 compulsive or pathological gambling (F63.0)

5 **Z72.8 Other problems related to lifestyle**

6 **Z72.81 Antisocial behavior**
EXCLUDES 1 conduct disorders (F91.-)

IQ **Z72.810 Child and adolescent antisocial behavior**
Antisocial behavior (child) (adolescent) without manifest psychiatric disorder
Delinquency NOS
Group delinquency
Offenses in the context of gang membership
Stealing in company with others
Truancy from school

IQ **Z72.811 Adult antisocial behavior**
Adult antisocial behavior without manifest psychiatric disorder

6 **Z72.82 Problems related to sleep**

IQ **Z72.820 Sleep deprivation**
Lack of adequate sleep
EXCLUDES 1 insomnia (G47.0-)

IQ **Z72.821 Inadequate sleep hygiene**
Bad sleep habits
Irregular sleep habits
Unhealthy sleep wake schedule
EXCLUDES 1 insomnia (F51.0-, G47.0-)

IQ **Z72.89 Other problems related to lifestyle**
Self-damaging behavior

IQ **Z72.9 Problem related to lifestyle, unspecified**

4 **Z73 Problems related to life management difficulty**
EXCLUDES 2 problems related to socioeconomic and psychosocial circumstances (Z55-Z65)

IQ **Z73.0 Burn-out**

IQ **Z73.1 Type A behavior pattern**

IQ **Z73.2 Lack of relaxation and leisure**

IQ **Z73.3 Stress, not elsewhere classified**
Physical and mental strain NOS
EXCLUDES 1 stress related to employment or unemployment (Z56.-)

IQ **Z73.4 Inadequate social skills, not elsewhere classified**

IQ **Z73.5 Social role conflict, not elsewhere classified**

IQ **Z73.6 Limitation of activities due to disability**
EXCLUDES 1 care-provider dependency (Z74.-)

5 **Z73.8 Other problems related to life management difficulty**

6 **Z73.81 Behavioral insomnia of childhood**

IQ **Z73.810 Behavioral insomnia of childhood, sleep-onset association type**

IQ **Z73.811 Behavioral insomnia of childhood, limit setting type**

IQ **Z73.812 Behavioral insomnia of childhood, combined type**

IQ **Z73.819 Behavioral insomnia of childhood, unspecified type**

IQ **Z73.82 Dual sensory impairment**

IQ **Z73.89 Other problems related to life management difficulty**

IQ **Z73.9 Problem related to life management difficulty, unspecified**

4 **Z74 Problems related to care provider dependency**
EXCLUDES 2 dependence on enabling machines or devices NEC (Z99.-)

CODING TIPS✓ These codes are useful to explain the circumstances of the patient and/or the caregiver to assist in explanation of the need for skilled care.

5 **Z74.0 Reduced mobility**
CODING TIPS✓ These codes are useful to explain reduced mobility for hospice prognosis purposes as well as homebound for home health patients.

IQ **Z74.01 Bed confinement status**
Bedridden

IQ **Z74.09 Other reduced mobility**
Chairridden
Reduced mobility NOS
EXCLUDES 2 wheelchair dependence (Z99.3)

IQ **Z74.1 Need for assistance with personal care**

IQ **Z74.2 Need for assistance at home and no other household member able to render care**

IQ **Z74.3 Need for continuous supervision**

IQ **Z74.8 Other problems related to care provider dependency**

IQ **Z74.9 Problem related to care provider dependency, unspecified**

4 **Z75 Problems related to medical facilities and other health care**

IQ **Z75.0 Medical services not available in home**
EXCLUDES 1 no other household member able to render care (Z74.2)

IQ **Z75.1 Person awaiting admission to adequate facility elsewhere**

IQ **Z75.2 Other waiting period for investigation and treatment**

IQ **Z75.3 Unavailability and inaccessibility of health-care facilities**
EXCLUDES 1 bed unavailable (Z75.1)

IQ **Z75.4 Unavailability and inaccessibility of other helping agencies**

IQ **Z75.5 Holiday relief care**

IQ **Z75.8 Other problems related to medical facilities and other health care**

IQ **Z75.9 Unspecified problem related to medical facilities and other health care**

4 **Z76 Persons encountering health services in other circumstances**

IQ **Z76.0 Encounter for issue of repeat prescription**
Encounter for issue of repeat prescription for appliance
Encounter for issue of repeat prescription for medicaments
Encounter for issue of repeat prescription for spectacles
EXCLUDES 2 issue of medical certificate (Z02.7)
repeat prescription for contraceptive (Z30.4-)

Px IQ **Z76.1 Encounter for health supervision and care of foundling**

Px IQ **Z76.2 Encounter for health supervision and care of other healthy infant and child**
Encounter for medical or nursing care or supervision of healthy infant under circumstances such as adverse socioeconomic conditions at home
Encounter for medical or nursing care or supervision of healthy infant under circumstances such as awaiting foster or adoptive placement
Encounter for medical or nursing care or supervision of healthy infant under circumstances such as maternal illness
Encounter for medical or nursing care or supervision of healthy infant under circumstances such as number of children at home preventing or interfering with normal care

IQ **Z76.3 Healthy person accompanying sick person**

▲ IQ **Z76.4 Other boarder to healthcare facility**
EXCLUDES 1 homelessness (Z59.0-)

IQ **Z76.5 Malingerer [conscious simulation]**
Person feigning illness (with obvious motivation)
EXCLUDES 1 factitious disorder (F68.1-, F68.A)
peregrinating patient (F68.1-)

5 **Z76.8 Persons encountering health services in other specified circumstances**

IQ **Z76.81 Expectant parent(s) prebirth pediatrician visit**
Pre-adoption pediatrician visit for adoptive parent(s)

IQ **Z76.82 Awaiting organ transplant status**
Patient waiting for organ availability

IQ **Z76.89 Persons encountering health services in other specified circumstances**
Persons encountering health services NOS

Persons with potential health hazards related to family and personal history and certain conditions influencing health status (Z77-Z99)

Code also:
any follow-up examination (Z08-Z09)

4 **Z77 Other contact with and (suspected) exposures hazardous to health**
INCLUDES contact with and (suspected) exposures to potential hazards to health
EXCLUDES 2 contact with and (suspected) exposure to communicable diseases (Z20.-)
exposure to (parental) (environmental) tobacco smoke in the perinatal period (P96.81)
newborn affected by noxious substances transmitted via placenta or breast milk (P04.-)
occupational exposure to risk factors (Z57.-)
retained foreign body (Z18.-)
retained foreign body fully removed (Z87.821)
toxic effects of substances chiefly nonmedicinal as to source (T51-T65)

GUIDELINES **Section I.C.21.c.1)**
Category Z20 indicates contact with, and suspected exposure to, communicable diseases. These codes are for patients who do not show any sign or symptom of a disease but are suspected to have been exposed to it by close personal contact with an infected individual or are in an area where a disease is epidemic. Category Z77 indicates contact with and suspected exposures hazardous to health.

Contact/exposure codes may be used as a first-listed code to explain an encounter for testing, or, more commonly, as a secondary code to identify a potential risk.

5 **Z77.0 Contact with and (suspected) exposure to hazardous, chiefly nonmedicinal, chemicals**

6 **Z77.01 Contact with and (suspected) exposure to hazardous metals**

IQ **Z77.010 Contact with and (suspected) exposure to arsenic**

IQ **Z77.011 Contact with and (suspected) exposure to lead**

IQ **Z77.012 Contact with and (suspected) exposure to uranium**
EXCLUDES 1 retained depleted uranium fragments (Z18.01)

IQ **Z77.018 Contact with and (suspected) exposure to other hazardous metals**
Contact with and (suspected) exposure to chromium compounds
Contact with and (suspected) exposure to nickel dust

6 **Z77.02 Contact with and (suspected) exposure to hazardous aromatic compounds**

IQ **Z77.020 Contact with and (suspected) exposure to aromatic amines**

IQ **Z77.021 Contact with and (suspected) exposure to benzene**

IQ **Z77.028 Contact with and (suspected) exposure to other hazardous aromatic compounds**
Aromatic dyes NOS
Polycyclic aromatic hydrocarbons

6 **Z77.09 Contact with and (suspected) exposure to other hazardous, chiefly nonmedicinal, chemicals**

IQ **Z77.090 Contact with and (suspected) exposure to asbestos**

IQ **Z77.098 Contact with and (suspected) exposure to other hazardous, chiefly nonmedicinal, chemicals**
Dyes NOS

5 **Z77.1 Contact with and (suspected) exposure to environmental pollution and hazards in the physical environment**

6 **Z77.11 Contact with and (suspected) exposure to environmental pollution**

Chapter 21
Z00-Z99

IQ **Z77.110 Contact with and (suspected) exposure to air pollution**

IQ **Z77.111 Contact with and (suspected) exposure to water pollution**

IQ **Z77.112 Contact with and (suspected) exposure to soil pollution**

IQ **Z77.118 Contact with and (suspected) exposure to other environmental pollution**

6 **Z77.12 Contact with and (suspected) exposure to hazards in the physical environment**

IQ **Z77.120 Contact with and (suspected) exposure to mold (toxic)**

IQ **Z77.121 Contact with and (suspected) exposure to harmful algae and algae toxins**

Contact with and (suspected) exposure to (harmful) algae bloom NOS

Contact with and (suspected) exposure to blue-green algae bloom

Contact with and (suspected) exposure to brown tide

Contact with and (suspected) exposure to cyanobacteria bloom

Contact with and (suspected) exposure to Florida red tide

Contact with and (suspected) exposure to pfiesteria piscicida

Contact with and (suspected) exposure to red tide

IQ **Z77.122 Contact with and (suspected) exposure to noise**

IQ **Z77.123 Contact with and (suspected) exposure to radon and other naturally occurring radiation**

EXCLUDES 2 radiation exposure as the cause of a confirmed condition (W88-W90, X39.0-)

radiation sickness NOS (T66)

IQ **Z77.128 Contact with and (suspected) exposure to other hazards in the physical environment**

5 **Z77.2 Contact with and (suspected) exposure to other hazardous substances**

IQ **Z77.21 Contact with and (suspected) exposure to potentially hazardous body fluids**

IQ **Z77.22 Contact with and (suspected) exposure to environmental tobacco smoke (acute) (chronic)**

Exposure to second hand tobacco smoke (acute) (chronic)

Passive smoking (acute) (chronic)

EXCLUDES 1 nicotine dependence (F17.-)

tobacco use (Z72.0)

EXCLUDES 2 occupational exposure to environmental tobacco smoke (Z57.31)

IQ **Z77.29 Contact with and (suspected) exposure to other hazardous substances**

CODING TIPS✓ This code may be used to indicate passive exposure to e-cigarettes or vaping.

IQ **Z77.9 Other contact with and (suspected) exposures hazardous to health**

4 **Z78 Other specified health status**

EXCLUDES 2 asymptomatic human immunodeficiency virus [HIV] infection status (Z21)

postprocedural status (Z93-Z99)

sex reassignment status (Z87.890)

IQ **Z78.0 Asymptomatic menopausal state**

Menopausal state NOS

Postmenopausal status NOS

EXCLUDES 2 symptomatic menopausal state (N95.1)

IQ **Z78.1 Physical restraint status**

EXCLUDES 1 physical restraint due to a procedure - omit code

IQ **Z78.9 Other specified health status**

4 **Z79 Long term (current) drug therapy**

INCLUDES long term (current) drug use for prophylactic purposes

Code also:

any therapeutic drug level monitoring (Z51.81)

EXCLUDES 2 drug abuse and dependence (F11-F19)

drug use complicating pregnancy, childbirth, and the puerperium (O99.32-)

GUIDELINES **Section I.C.21.c.3)**

Codes from this category [Z79] indicate a patient's continuous use of a prescribed drug (including such things as aspirin therapy) for the long-term treatment of a condition or for prophylactic use. It is not for use for patients who have addictions to drugs. This subcategory is not for use of medications for detoxification or maintenance programs to prevent withdrawal symptoms in patients with drug dependence (e.g., methadone maintenance for opiate dependence). Assign the appropriate code for the drug dependence instead.

Assign a code from Z79 if the patient is receiving a medication for an extended period as a prophylactic measure (such as for the prevention of deep vein thrombosis) or as treatment of a chronic condition (such as arthritis) or a disease requiring a lengthy course of treatment (such as cancer). Do not assign a code from category Z79 for medication being administered for a brief period of time to treat an acute illness or injury (such as a course of antibiotics to treat acute bronchitis).

CODING TIPS✓ Medications prescribed on an as needed basis (PRN), e.g. rescue medications for asthma, are not assigned Z79 codes. [AHA: 1Q 2021]

CODING TIPS ✓ "Long-term use" refers to multiple refills, long term prophylaxis, etc. Use the code if the medication is pertinent to the plan of care.

CODING TIPS ✓ Codes classifiable to category Z79 should not be assigned as primary diagnoses. When the management of any of these medications is integral to the plan of care, consider the confirmed diagnosis for which the patient is under treatment with the medication. This diagnosis should be coded, with a code from Z79 as an additional diagnosis.

5 **Z79.0 Long term (current) use of anticoagulants and antithrombotics/antiplatelets**

EXCLUDES 2 long term (current) use of aspirin (Z79.82)

IQ **Z79.01 Long term (current) use of anticoagulants**

IQ **Z79.02 Long term (current) use of antithrombotics/antiplatelets**

IQ **Z79.1 Long term (current) use of non-steroidal anti-inflammatories (NSAID)**

EXCLUDES 2 long term (current) use of aspirin (Z79.82)

IQ **Z79.2 Long term (current) use of antibiotics**

CODING TIPS ✓ Do not use this code for routine 7-10 days of oral antibiotics.

IQ **Z79.3 Long term (current) use of hormonal contraceptives**

Long term (current) use of birth control pill or patch

▲ IQ **Z79.4 Long term (current) use of insulin**

EXCLUDES 2 long term (current) use of oral hypoglycemic drugs (Z79.84)
long term (current) use of oral antidiabetic drugs (Z79.84)

GUIDELINES **Section I.C.4.a.6)(a)**
For patients with secondary diabetes mellitus who routinely use insulin or oral hypoglycemic drugs, an additional code from category Z79 should be assigned to identify the long-term (current) use of insulin or oral hypoglycemic drugs. If the patient is treated with both oral medications and insulin, only the code for long-term (current) use of insulin should be assigned. If the patient is treated with both insulin and an injectable non-insulin antidiabetic drug, assign codes Z79.4, Long-term (current) use of insulin, and Z79.899, Other long term (current) drug therapy. If the patient is treated with both oral hypoglycemic drugs and an injectable non-insulin antidiabetic drug, assign codes Z79.84, Long-term (current) use of oral hypoglycemic drugs, and Z79.899, Other long-term (current) drug therapy. Code Z79.4 should not be assigned if insulin is given temporarily to bring a secondary diabetic patient's blood sugar under control during an encounter.

GUIDELINES **Section I.C.4.a.3)**
If the documentation in a medical record does not indicate the type of diabetes but does indicate that the patient uses insulin, code E11, Type 2 diabetes mellitus, should be assigned. An additional code should be assigned from category Z79 to identify the long-term (current) use of insulin or oral hypoglycemic drugs. If the patient is treated with both oral medications and insulin, only the code for long-term (current) use of insulin should be assigned.

GUIDELINES **Section I.C.15.i**
Code Z79.4, Long-term (current) use of insulin or code Z79.84, Long-term (current) use of oral hypoglycemic drugs, should not be assigned with codes from subcategory O24.4.

5 **Z79.5 Long term (current) use of steroids**

IQ **Z79.51 Long term (current) use of inhaled steroids**

CODING TIPS ✓ Flonase is not classified as an inhaled steroid nor a systemic steroid. Use Z79.899 for Flonase.

IQ **Z79.52 Long term (current) use of systemic steroids**

5 **Z79.8 Other long term (current) drug therapy**

+ 6 **Z79.81 Long term (current) use of agents affecting estrogen receptors and estrogen levels**

Code first, if applicable:
malignant neoplasm of breast (C50.-)
malignant neoplasm of prostate (C61)
Use additional code, if applicable, to identify:
estrogen receptor positive status (Z17.0)
family history of breast cancer (Z80.3)
genetic susceptibility to malignant neoplasm (cancer) (Z15.0-)
personal history of breast cancer (Z85.3)
personal history of prostate cancer (Z85.46)
postmenopausal status (Z78.0)

EXCLUDES 1 hormone replacement therapy (Z79.890)

CODING TIPS ✓ These types of agents are used for both active treatment of malignancies (see the "code first" note) and for prevention of recurring malignancies (see the "use additional code" for history and susceptibility). The clinician/coder should query the physician or NPP for further information when the patient is taking one of these drugs to determine whether to code the malignancy, the history of malignant neoplasm or other condition.

IQ + **Z79.810 Long term (current) use of selective estrogen receptor modulators (SERMs)**

Long term (current) use of raloxifene (Evista)

Long term (current) use of tamoxifen (Nolvadex)
Long term (current) use of toremifene (Fareston)

IQ + **Z79.811 Long term (current) use of aromatase inhibitors**
Long term (current) use of anastrozole (Arimidex)
Long term (current) use of exemestane (Aromasin)
Long term (current) use of letrozole (Femara)

IQ + **Z79.818 Long term (current) use of other agents affecting estrogen receptors and estrogen levels**
Long term (current) use of estrogen receptor downregulators
Long term (current) use of fulvestrant (Faslodex)
Long term (current) use of gonadotropin-releasing hormone (GnRH) agonist
Long term (current) use of goserelin acetate (Zoladex)
Long term (current) use of leuprolide acetate (leuprorelin) (Lupron)
Long term (current) use of megestrol acetate (Megace)

IQ **Z79.82 Long term (current) use of aspirin**

IQ **Z79.83 Long term (current) use of bisphosphonates**

IQ **Z79.84 Long term (current) use of oral hypoglycemic drugs**
Long term (current) use of oral antidiabetic drugs
EXCLUDES 2 long term (current) use of insulin (Z79.4)

6 **Z79.89 Other long term (current) drug therapy**

IQ **Z79.890 Hormone replacement therapy**

IQ **Z79.891 Long term (current) use of opiate analgesic**
Long term (current) use of methadone for pain management
EXCLUDES 1 methodone use NOS (F11.9-)
use of methodone for treatment of heroin addiction (F11.2-)

IQ **Z79.899 Other long term (current) drug therapy**

4 **Z80 Family history of primary malignant neoplasm**

GUIDELINES **Section I.C.21.c.4)**
There are two types of history Z codes, personal and family. Personal history codes explain a patient's past medical condition that no longer exists and is not receiving any treatment, but that has the potential for recurrence, and therefore may require continued monitoring.

Family history codes are for use when a patient has a family member(s) who has had a particular disease that causes the patient to be at higher risk of also contracting the disease. Personal history codes may be used in conjunction with follow-up codes and family history codes may be used in conjunction with screening codes to explain the need for a test or procedure. History codes are also acceptable on any medical record regardless of the reason for visit. A history of an illness, even if no longer present, is important information that may alter the type of treatment ordered.

IQ **Z80.0 Family history of malignant neoplasm of digestive organs**
Conditions classifiable to C15-C26

IQ **Z80.1 Family history of malignant neoplasm of trachea, bronchus and lung**
Conditions classifiable to C33-C34

IQ **Z80.2 Family history of malignant neoplasm of other respiratory and intrathoracic organs**
Conditions classifiable to C30-C32, C37-C39

IQ **Z80.3 Family history of malignant neoplasm of breast**
Conditions classifiable to C50.-

5 **Z80.4 Family history of malignant neoplasm of genital organs**
Conditions classifiable to C51-C63

IQ **Z80.41 Family history of malignant neoplasm of ovary**

IQ **Z80.42 Family history of malignant neoplasm of prostate**

IQ **Z80.43 Family history of malignant neoplasm of testis**

IQ **Z80.49 Family history of malignant neoplasm of other genital organs**

5 **Z80.5 Family history of malignant neoplasm of urinary tract**
Conditions classifiable to C64-C68

IQ **Z80.51 Family history of malignant neoplasm of kidney**

IQ **Z80.52 Family history of malignant neoplasm of bladder**

IQ **Z80.59 Family history of malignant neoplasm of other urinary tract organ**

IQ **Z80.6 Family history of leukemia**
Conditions classifiable to C91-C95

IQ **Z80.7 Family history of other malignant neoplasms of lymphoid, hematopoietic and related tissues**
Conditions classifiable to C81-C90, C96.-

IQ **Z80.8 Family history of malignant neoplasm of other organs or systems**
Conditions classifiable to C00-C14, C40-C49, C69-C79

IQ **Z80.9 Family history of malignant neoplasm, unspecified**
Conditions classifiable to C80.1

4 **Z81 Family history of mental and behavioral disorders**

GUIDELINES **Section I.C.21.c.4)**
There are two types of history Z codes, personal and family. Personal history codes explain a patient's past medical condition that no longer exists and is not receiving any treatment, but that has the potential for recurrence, and therefore may require continued monitoring.

Family history codes are for use when a patient has a family member(s) who has had a particular disease that causes the patient to be at higher risk of also contracting the disease. Personal history codes may be used in conjunction with follow-up codes and family history codes may be used in conjunction with screening codes to explain the need for a test or procedure. History codes are also acceptable on any medical record regardless of the reason for visit. A history of an illness, even if no longer present, is important information that may alter the type of treatment ordered.

IQ **Z81.0 Family history of intellectual disabilities**
Conditions classifiable to F70-F79

IQ **Z81.1 Family history of alcohol abuse and dependence**
Conditions classifiable to F10.-

IQ **Z81.2 Family history of tobacco abuse and dependence**
Conditions classifiable to F17.-

IQ **Z81.3 Family history of other psychoactive substance abuse and dependence**
Conditions classifiable to F11-F16, F18-F19

IQ **Z81.4 Family history of other substance abuse and dependence**
Conditions classifiable to F55

IQ **Z81.8 Family history of other mental and behavioral disorders**
Conditions classifiable elsewhere in F01-F99

4 **Z82 Family history of certain disabilities and chronic diseases (leading to disablement)**

GUIDELINES **Section I.C.21.c.4)**
There are two types of history Z codes, personal and family. Personal history codes explain a patient's past medical condition that no longer exists and is not receiving any treatment, but that has the potential for recurrence, and therefore may require continued monitoring.

Family history codes are for use when a patient has a family member(s) who has had a particular disease that causes the patient to be at higher risk of also contracting the disease. Personal history codes may be used in conjunction with follow-up codes and family history codes may be used in conjunction with screening codes to explain the need for a test or procedure. History codes are also acceptable on any medical record regardless of the reason for visit. A history of an illness, even if no longer present, is important information that may alter the type of treatment ordered.

IQ **Z82.0 Family history of epilepsy and other diseases of the nervous system**
Conditions classifiable to G00-G99

IQ **Z82.1 Family history of blindness and visual loss**
Conditions classifiable to H54.-

IQ **Z82.2 Family history of deafness and hearing loss**
Conditions classifiable to H90-H91

IQ **Z82.3 Family history of stroke**
Conditions classifiable to I60-I64

▲ 5 **Z82.4 Family history of ischemic heart disease and other diseases of the circulatory system**
Conditions classifiable to I00-I5A, I65-I99

IQ **Z82.41 Family history of sudden cardiac death**

IQ **Z82.49 Family history of ischemic heart disease and other diseases of the circulatory system**

IQ **Z82.5 Family history of asthma and other chronic lower respiratory diseases**
Conditions classifiable to J40-J47

EXCLUDES 2 family history of other diseases of the respiratory system (Z83.6)

5 **Z82.6 Family history of arthritis and other diseases of the musculoskeletal system and connective tissue**
Conditions classifiable to M00-M99

IQ **Z82.61 Family history of arthritis**

IQ **Z82.62 Family history of osteoporosis**

IQ **Z82.69 Family history of other diseases of the musculoskeletal system and connective tissue**

5 **Z82.7 Family history of congenital malformations, deformations and chromosomal abnormalities**
Conditions classifiable to Q00-Q99

IQ **Z82.71 Family history of polycystic kidney**

IQ **Z82.79 Family history of other congenital malformations, deformations and chromosomal abnormalities**

IQ **Z82.8 Family history of other disabilities and chronic diseases leading to disablement, not elsewhere classified**

4 **Z83 Family history of other specific disorders**

EXCLUDES 2 contact with and (suspected) exposure to communicable disease in the family (Z20.-)

GUIDELINES **Section I.C.21.c.4)**

There are two types of history Z codes, personal and family. Personal history codes explain a patient's past medical condition that no longer exists and is not receiving any treatment, but that has the potential for recurrence, and therefore may require continued monitoring.

Family history codes are for use when a patient has a family member(s) who has had a particular disease that causes the patient to be at higher risk of also contracting the disease. Personal history codes may be used in conjunction with follow-up codes and family history codes may be used in conjunction with screening codes to explain the need for a test or procedure. History codes are also acceptable on any medical record regardless of the reason for visit. A history of an illness, even if no longer present, is important information that may alter the type of treatment ordered.

IQ **Z83.0 Family history of human immunodeficiency virus [HIV] disease**

Conditions classifiable to B20

IQ **Z83.1 Family history of other infectious and parasitic diseases**

Conditions classifiable to A00-B19, B25-B94, B99

IQ **Z83.2 Family history of diseases of the blood and blood-forming organs and certain disorders involving the immune mechanism**

Conditions classifiable to D50-D89

IQ **Z83.3 Family history of diabetes mellitus**

Conditions classifiable to E08-E13

5 **Z83.4 Family history of other endocrine, nutritional and metabolic diseases**

Conditions classifiable to E00-E07, E15-E88

IQ **Z83.41 Family history of multiple endocrine neoplasia [MEN] syndrome**

IQ **Z83.42 Family history of familial hypercholesterolemia**

6 **Z83.43 Family history of other disorder of lipoprotein metabolism and other lipidemias**

IQ **Z83.430 Family history of elevated lipoprotein(a)**

Family history of elevated Lp(a)

IQ **Z83.438 Family history of other disorder of lipoprotein metabolism and other lipidemia**

Family history of familial combined hyperlipidemia

IQ **Z83.49 Family history of other endocrine, nutritional and metabolic diseases**

5 **Z83.5 Family history of eye and ear disorders**

6 **Z83.51 Family history of eye disorders**

Conditions classifiable to H00-H53, H55-H59

EXCLUDES 2 family history of blindness and visual loss (Z82.1)

IQ **Z83.511 Family history of glaucoma**

IQ **Z83.518 Family history of other specified eye disorder**

IQ **Z83.52 Family history of ear disorders**

Conditions classifiable to H60-H83, H92-H95

EXCLUDES 2 family history of deafness and hearing loss (Z82.2)

IQ **Z83.6 Family history of other diseases of the respiratory system**

Conditions classifiable to J00-J39, J60-J99

EXCLUDES 2 family history of asthma and other chronic lower respiratory diseases (Z82.5)

5 **Z83.7 Family history of diseases of the digestive system**

Conditions classifiable to K00-K93

IQ **Z83.71 Family history of colonic polyps**

EXCLUDES 2 family history of malignant neoplasm of digestive organs (Z80.0)

IQ **Z83.79 Family history of other diseases of the digestive system**

4 **Z84 Family history of other conditions**

GUIDELINES **Section I.C.21.c.4)**

There are two types of history Z codes, personal and family. Personal history codes explain a patient's past medical condition that no longer exists and is not receiving any treatment, but that has the potential for recurrence, and therefore may require continued monitoring.

Family history codes are for use when a patient has a family member(s) who has had a particular disease that causes the patient to be at higher risk of also contracting the disease. Personal history codes may be used in conjunction with follow-up codes and family history codes may be used in conjunction with screening codes to explain the need for a test or procedure. History codes are also acceptable on any medical record regardless of the reason for visit. A history of an illness, even if no longer present, is important information that may alter the type of treatment ordered.

IQ **Z84.0 Family history of diseases of the skin and subcutaneous tissue**

Conditions classifiable to L00-L99

IQ **Z84.1 Family history of disorders of kidney and ureter**

Conditions classifiable to N00-N29

IQ **Z84.2 Family history of other diseases of the genitourinary system**

Conditions classifiable to N30-N99

IQ **Z84.3 Family history of consanguinity**

5 **Z84.8 Family history of other specified conditions**

IQ **Z84.81 Family history of carrier of genetic disease**

IQ **Z84.82 Family history of sudden infant death syndrome**
Family history of SIDS

IQ **Z84.89 Family history of other specified conditions**

+ 4 **Z85 Personal history of malignant neoplasm**
Code first:
any follow-up examination after treatment of malignant neoplasm (Z08)
Use additional code to identify:
alcohol use and dependence (F10.-)
exposure to environmental tobacco smoke (Z77.22)
history of tobacco dependence (Z87.891)
occupational exposure to environmental tobacco smoke (Z57.31)
tobacco dependence (F17.-)
tobacco use (Z72.0)

EXCLUDES 2 personal history of benign neoplasm (Z86.01-)
personal history of carcinoma-in-situ (Z86.00-)

GUIDELINES **Section I.C.2.m**

When a primary malignancy has been excised but further treatment, such as an additional surgery for the malignancy, radiation therapy or chemotherapy is directed to that site, the primary malignancy code should be used until treatment is completed.

When a primary malignancy has been previously excised or eradicated from its site, there is no further treatment (of the malignancy) directed at that site, and there is no evidence of any existing primary malignancy, a code from category Z85 should be used to indicate the former site of the malignancy.

Subcategories Z85.0 – Z85.7 should only be assigned for the former site of a primary malignancy, not the site of a secondary malignancy. Codes from subcategory Z85.8-, may be assigned for the former site(s) of either a primary or secondary malignancy included in this subcategory.

GUIDELINES **Section I.C.21.c.4)**

There are two types of history Z codes, personal and family. Personal history codes explain a patient's past medical condition that no longer exists and is not receiving any treatment, but that has the potential for recurrence, and therefore may require continued monitoring.

Family history codes are for use when a patient has a family member(s) who has had a particular disease that causes the patient to be at higher risk of also contracting the disease. Personal history codes may be used in conjunction with follow-up codes and family history codes may be used in conjunction with screening codes to explain the need for a test or procedure. History codes are also acceptable on any medical record regardless of the reason for visit. A history of an illness, even if no longer present, is important information that may alter the type of treatment ordered.

CODING TIPS✓ The codes in this section are commonly referred to as the "history of cancer" codes. "History" in this case means the cancer has been eradicated from its primary site. Because the cancer may have already metastasized to other sites, it does not necessarily mean the patient no longer has cancer.

+ 5 **Z85.0 Personal history of malignant neoplasm of digestive organs**

IQ + **Z85.00 Personal history of malignant neoplasm of unspecified digestive organ**

IQ + **Z85.01 Personal history of malignant neoplasm of esophagus**
Conditions classifiable to C15

+ 6 **Z85.02 Personal history of malignant neoplasm of stomach**

IQ + **Z85.020 Personal history of malignant carcinoid tumor of stomach**
Conditions classifiable to C7A.092

IQ + **Z85.028 Personal history of other malignant neoplasm of stomach**
Conditions classifiable to C16

+ 6 **Z85.03 Personal history of malignant neoplasm of large intestine**

IQ + **Z85.030 Personal history of malignant carcinoid tumor of large intestine**
Conditions classifiable to C7A.022-C7A.025, C7A.029

IQ + **Z85.038 Personal history of other malignant neoplasm of large intestine**
Conditions classifiable to C18

+ 6 **Z85.04 Personal history of malignant neoplasm of rectum, rectosigmoid junction, and anus**

IQ + **Z85.040 Personal history of malignant carcinoid tumor of rectum**
Conditions classifiable to C7A.026

IQ + **Z85.048 Personal history of other malignant neoplasm of rectum, rectosigmoid junction, and anus**
Conditions classifiable to C19-C21

IQ + Z85.05 **Personal history of malignant neoplasm of liver**
Conditions classifiable to C22

+ 6 Z85.06 **Personal history of malignant neoplasm of small intestine**

IQ + Z85.060 **Personal history of malignant carcinoid tumor of small intestine**
Conditions classifiable to C7A.01-

IQ + Z85.068 **Personal history of other malignant neoplasm of small intestine**
Conditions classifiable to C17

IQ + Z85.07 **Personal history of malignant neoplasm of pancreas**
Conditions classifiable to C25

IQ + Z85.09 **Personal history of malignant neoplasm of other digestive organs**

+ 5 Z85.1 **Personal history of malignant neoplasm of trachea, bronchus and lung**

+ 6 Z85.11 **Personal history of malignant neoplasm of bronchus and lung**

IQ + Z85.110 **Personal history of malignant carcinoid tumor of bronchus and lung**
Conditions classifiable to C7A.090

IQ + Z85.118 **Personal history of other malignant neoplasm of bronchus and lung**
Conditions classifiable to C34

IQ + Z85.12 **Personal history of malignant neoplasm of trachea**
Conditions classifiable to C33

+ 5 Z85.2 **Personal history of malignant neoplasm of other respiratory and intrathoracic organs**

IQ + Z85.20 **Personal history of malignant neoplasm of unspecified respiratory organ**

IQ + Z85.21 **Personal history of malignant neoplasm of larynx**
Conditions classifiable to C32

IQ + Z85.22 **Personal history of malignant neoplasm of nasal cavities, middle ear, and accessory sinuses**
Conditions classifiable to C30-C31

+ 6 Z85.23 **Personal history of malignant neoplasm of thymus**

IQ + Z85.230 **Personal history of malignant carcinoid tumor of thymus**
Conditions classifiable to C7A.091

IQ + Z85.238 **Personal history of other malignant neoplasm of thymus**
Conditions classifiable to C37

IQ + Z85.29 **Personal history of malignant neoplasm of other respiratory and intrathoracic organs**

IQ + Z85.3 **Personal history of malignant neoplasm of breast**
Conditions classifiable to C50.-

+ 5 Z85.4 **Personal history of malignant neoplasm of genital organs**
Conditions classifiable to C51-C63

IQ + Z85.40 **Personal history of malignant neoplasm of unspecified female genital organ**

IQ + Z85.41 **Personal history of malignant neoplasm of cervix uteri**

IQ + Z85.42 **Personal history of malignant neoplasm of other parts of uterus**

IQ + Z85.43 **Personal history of malignant neoplasm of ovary**

IQ + Z85.44 **Personal history of malignant neoplasm of other female genital organs**

IQ + Z85.45 **Personal history of malignant neoplasm of unspecified male genital organ**

IQ + Z85.46 **Personal history of malignant neoplasm of prostate**

IQ + Z85.47 **Personal history of malignant neoplasm of testis**

IQ + Z85.48 **Personal history of malignant neoplasm of epididymis**

IQ + Z85.49 **Personal history of malignant neoplasm of other male genital organs**

+ 5 Z85.5 **Personal history of malignant neoplasm of urinary tract**
Conditions classifiable to C64-C68

IQ + Z85.50 **Personal history of malignant neoplasm of unspecified urinary tract organ**

IQ + Z85.51 **Personal history of malignant neoplasm of bladder**

+ 6 Z85.52 **Personal history of malignant neoplasm of kidney**
EXCLUDES 1 personal history of malignant neoplasm of renal pelvis (Z85.53)

IQ + Z85.520 **Personal history of malignant carcinoid tumor of kidney**
Conditions classifiable to C7A.093

IQ + Z85.528 **Personal history of other malignant neoplasm of kidney**
Conditions classifiable to C64

IQ + Z85.53 **Personal history of malignant neoplasm of renal pelvis**

IQ + Z85.54 **Personal history of malignant neoplasm of ureter**

IQ + Z85.59 **Personal history of malignant neoplasm of other urinary tract organ**

IQ + Z85.6 **Personal history of leukemia**
Conditions classifiable to C91-C95
EXCLUDES 1 leukemia in remission C91.0-C95.9 with 5th character 1

+ 5 Z85.7 **Personal history of other malignant neoplasms of lymphoid, hematopoietic and related tissues**

IQ + Z85.71 **Personal history of Hodgkin lymphoma**
Conditions classifiable to C81

IQ + Z85.72 **Personal history of non-Hodgkin lymphomas**
Conditions classifiable to C82-C85

IQ + Z85.79 **Personal history of other malignant neoplasms of lymphoid, hematopoietic and related tissues**
Conditions classifiable to C88-C90, C96
EXCLUDES 1 multiple myeloma in remission (C90.01)
plasma cell leukemia in remission (C90.11)

plasmacytoma in remission (C90.21)

GUIDELINES **Section I.C.2.n**

The categories for leukemia, and category C90, Multiple myeloma and malignant plasma cell neoplasms, have codes indicating whether or not the leukemia has achieved remission. There are also codes Z85.6, Personal history of leukemia, and Z85.79, Personal history of other malignant neoplasms of lymphoid, hematopoietic and related tissues. If the documentation is unclear, as to whether the leukemia has achieved remission, the provider should be queried.

+ 5 **Z85.8 Personal history of malignant neoplasms of other organs and systems**
Conditions classifiable to C00-C14, C40-C49, C69-C75, C7A.098, C76-C79

+ 6 **Z85.81 Personal history of malignant neoplasm of lip, oral cavity, and pharynx**
Conditions classifiable to C00-C14

IQ + **Z85.810 Personal history of malignant neoplasm of tongue**

IQ + **Z85.818 Personal history of malignant neoplasm of other sites of lip, oral cavity, and pharynx**

IQ + **Z85.819 Personal history of malignant neoplasm of unspecified site of lip, oral cavity, and pharynx**

+ 6 **Z85.82 Personal history of malignant neoplasm of skin**

IQ + **Z85.820 Personal history of malignant melanoma of skin**
Conditions classifiable to C43

IQ + **Z85.821 Personal history of Merkel cell carcinoma**
Conditions classifiable to C4A

IQ + **Z85.828 Personal history of other malignant neoplasm of skin**
Conditions classifiable to C44

+ 6 **Z85.83 Personal history of malignant neoplasm of bone and soft tissue**
Conditions classifiable to C40-C41; C45-C49

IQ + **Z85.830 Personal history of malignant neoplasm of bone**

IQ + **Z85.831 Personal history of malignant neoplasm of soft tissue**
EXCLUDES 2 personal history of malignant neoplasm of skin (Z85.82-)

+ 6 **Z85.84 Personal history of malignant neoplasm of eye and nervous tissue**
Conditions classifiable to C69-C72

IQ + **Z85.840 Personal history of malignant neoplasm of eye**

IQ + **Z85.841 Personal history of malignant neoplasm of brain**

IQ + **Z85.848 Personal history of malignant neoplasm of other parts of nervous tissue**

+ 6 **Z85.85 Personal history of malignant neoplasm of endocrine glands**
Conditions classifiable to C73-C75

IQ + **Z85.850 Personal history of malignant neoplasm of thyroid**

IQ + **Z85.858 Personal history of malignant neoplasm of other endocrine glands**

IQ + **Z85.89 Personal history of malignant neoplasm of other organs and systems**
Conditions classifiable to C7A.098, C76, C77-C79

IQ + **Z85.9 Personal history of malignant neoplasm, unspecified**
Conditions classifiable to C7A.00, C80.1

4 **Z86 Personal history of certain other diseases**
Code first:
any follow-up examination after treatment (Z09)

GUIDELINES **Section I.C.21.c.4)**

There are two types of history Z codes, personal and family. Personal history codes explain a patient's past medical condition that no longer exists and is not receiving any treatment, but that has the potential for recurrence, and therefore may require continued monitoring.

Family history codes are for use when a patient has a family member(s) who has had a particular disease that causes the patient to be at higher risk of also contracting the disease. Personal history codes may be used in conjunction with follow-up codes and family history codes may be used in conjunction with screening codes to explain the need for a test or procedure. History codes are also acceptable on any medical record regardless of the reason for visit. A history of an illness, even if no longer present, is important information that may alter the type of treatment ordered.

5 **Z86.0 Personal history of in-situ and benign neoplasms and neoplasms of uncertain behavior**
EXCLUDES 2 personal history of malignant neoplasms (Z85.-)

6 **Z86.00 Personal history of in-situ neoplasm**
Conditions classifiable to D00-D09

IQ **Z86.000 Personal history of in-situ neoplasm of breast**
Conditions classifiable to D05

IQ **Z86.001 Personal history of in-situ neoplasm of cervix uteri**
Conditions classifiable to D06
Personal history of cervical intraepithelial neoplasia III [CIN III]

Z86.002 Personal history of in-situ neoplasm of other and unspecified genital organs
Conditions classifiable to D07
Personal history of high-grade prostatic intraepithelial neoplasia III [HGPIN III]
Personal history of vaginal intraepithelial neoplasia III [VAIN III]

Personal history of vulvar intraepithelial neoplasia III [VIN III]

Z86.003 Personal history of in-situ neoplasm of oral cavity, esophagus and stomach
Conditions classifiable to D00

Z86.004 Personal history of in-situ neoplasm of other and unspecified digestive organs
Conditions classifiable to D01
Personal history of anal intraepithelial neoplasia (AIN III)

Z86.005 Personal history of in-situ neoplasm of middle ear and respiratory system
Conditions classifiable to D02

Z86.006 Personal history of melanoma in-situ
Conditions classifiable to D03
EXCLUDES 2 sites other than skin - code to personal history of in-situ neoplasm of the site

Z86.007 Personal history of in-situ neoplasm of skin
Conditions classifiable to D04
Personal history of carcinoma in situ of skin

IQ **Z86.008 Personal history of in-situ neoplasm of other site**
Conditions classifiable to D09

6 **Z86.01 Personal history of benign neoplasm**

IQ **Z86.010 Personal history of colonic polyps**

IQ **Z86.011 Personal history of benign neoplasm of the brain**

IQ **Z86.012 Personal history of benign carcinoid tumor**

IQ **Z86.018 Personal history of other benign neoplasm**

IQ **Z86.03 Personal history of neoplasm of uncertain behavior**

5 **Z86.1 Personal history of infectious and parasitic diseases**
Conditions classifiable to A00-B89, B99
EXCLUDES 1 personal history of infectious diseases specific to a body system
sequelae of infectious and parasitic discascs (B90-B94)

IQ **Z86.11 Personal history of tuberculosis**
CODING TIPS✓ This code is for the patient who has had TB in the past and currently has no residual effects from the TB.

IQ **Z86.12 Personal history of poliomyelitis**
CODING TIPS✓ This code is for the patient who has had polio in the past and currently has no residual effects from the polio.

IQ **Z86.13 Personal history of malaria**

IQ **Z86.14 Personal history of Methicillin resistant Staphylococcus aureus infection**
Personal history of MRSA infection
CODING TIPS✓ This code is for the patient who has had a MRSA infection in the past that is resolved and currently is not nasal swab positive. If nasal swab positive, use Z22.322.

Z86.15 Personal history of latent tuberculosis infection

▲ IQ **Z86.16 Personal history of COVID-19**
EXCLUDES 1 post COVID-19 condition (U09.9)
GUIDELINES **Section I.C.1.g.1)(i)**
For patients with a history of COVID-19, assign code Z86.16, Personal history of COVID-19.
GUIDELINES **Section I.C.1.g.1)(l)**
If an individual with a history of COVID-19 develops MIS and the provider does not indicate the MIS is due to the previous COVID-19 infection, assign codes M35.81, Multisystem inflammatory syndrome, and Z86.16, Personal history of COVID-19.
CODING TIPS✓ Use this code for patients who no longer have COVID-19 or any residual conditions of the COVID-19. If the patient still has residuals, code the residuals and U09.9.

IQ **Z86.19 Personal history of other infectious and parasitic diseases**
CODING TIPS✓ Do not use this code for history of COVID-19. Use Z86.16 instead.

IQ **Z86.2 Personal history of diseases of the blood and blood-forming organs and certain disorders involving the immune mechanism**
Conditions classifiable to D50-D89

5 **Z86.3 Personal history of endocrine, nutritional and metabolic diseases**
Conditions classifiable to E00-E88

IQ **Z86.31 Personal history of diabetic foot ulcer**
EXCLUDES 2 current diabetic foot ulcer (E08.621, E09.621, E10.621, E11.621, E13.621)

IQ **Z86.32 Personal history of gestational diabetes**
Personal history of conditions classifiable to O24.4-
EXCLUDES 1 gestational diabetes mellitus in current pregnancy (O24.4-)

IQ **Z86.39 Personal history of other endocrine, nutritional and metabolic disease**
CODING TIPS✓ Assign code Z86.39 when the physician has documented the diabetes as resolved by bariatric surgery or pancreatic transplant.

5 **Z86.5 Personal history of mental and behavioral disorders**
Conditions classifiable to F40-F59

IQ **Z86.51 Personal history of combat and operational stress reaction**

IQ **Z86.59 Personal history of other mental and behavioral disorders**

5 Z86.6 Personal history of diseases of the nervous system and sense organs
Conditions classifiable to G00-G99, H00-H95

IQ Z86.61 Personal history of infections of the central nervous system
Personal history of encephalitis
Personal history of meningitis

IQ Z86.69 Personal history of other diseases of the nervous system and sense organs

5 Z86.7 Personal history of diseases of the circulatory system
Conditions classifiable to I00-I99
EXCLUDES 2 old myocardial infarction (I25.2)
personal history of anaphylactic shock (Z87.892)
postmyocardial infarction syndrome (I24.1)

6 Z86.71 Personal history of venous thrombosis and embolism
CODING TIPS✓ Prior to assigning these codes, ensure that the clot is dissolved. It can take 3-6 months for the clot to dissipate and in the meantime, the acute condition should be coded.

IQ Z86.711 Personal history of pulmonary embolism

IQ Z86.718 Personal history of other venous thrombosis and embolism

IQ Z86.72 Personal history of thrombophlebitis

IQ Z86.73 Personal history of transient ischemic attack (TIA), and cerebral infarction without residual deficits
Personal history of prolonged reversible ischemic neurological deficit (PRIND)
Personal history of stroke NOS without residual deficits
EXCLUDES 1 personal history of traumatic brain injury (Z87.820)
sequelae of cerebrovascular disease (I69.-)

GUIDELINES **Section I.C.9.d.3)**
Codes from category I69, Sequela of cerebrovascular disease, should not be assigned if the patient does not have neurologic deficits. Assign Z86.73, Personal history of transient ischemic attack (TIA) and cerebral infarction

IQ Z86.74 Personal history of sudden cardiac arrest
Personal history of sudden cardiac death successfully resuscitated

IQ Z86.79 Personal history of other diseases of the circulatory system

4 Z87 Personal history of other diseases and conditions
Code first:
any follow-up examination after treatment (Z09)

GUIDELINES **Section I.C.21.c.4)**
There are two types of history Z codes, personal and family. Personal history codes explain a patient's past medical condition that no longer exists and is not receiving any treatment, but that has the potential for recurrence, and therefore may require continued monitoring.

Family history codes are for use when a patient has a family member(s) who has had a particular disease that causes the patient to be at higher risk of also contracting the disease. Personal history codes may be used in conjunction with follow-up codes and family history codes may be used in conjunction with screening codes to explain the need for a test or procedure. History codes are also acceptable on any medical record regardless of the reason for visit. A history of an illness, even if no longer present, is important information that may alter the type of treatment ordered.

5 Z87.0 Personal history of diseases of the respiratory system
Conditions classifiable to J00-J99

IQ Z87.01 Personal history of pneumonia (recurrent)

IQ Z87.09 Personal history of other diseases of the respiratory system

5 Z87.1 Personal history of diseases of the digestive system
Conditions classifiable to K00-K93

IQ Z87.11 Personal history of peptic ulcer disease

IQ Z87.19 Personal history of other diseases of the digestive system

IQ Z87.2 Personal history of diseases of the skin and subcutaneous tissue
Conditions classifiable to L00-L99
EXCLUDES 2 personal history of diabetic foot ulcer (Z86.31)

5 Z87.3 Personal history of diseases of the musculoskeletal system and connective tissue
Conditions classifiable to M00-M99
EXCLUDES 2 personal history of (healed) traumatic fracture (Z87.81)

6 Z87.31 Personal history of (healed) nontraumatic fracture
CODING TIPS✓ The patient can have a current fracture and a history of healed fracture at the same time. History of healed osteoporosis fracture qualifies the patient for Calcimar injections. See Z87.81 for history of healed traumatic fracture.

IQ Z87.310 Personal history of (healed) osteoporosis fracture
Personal history of (healed) fragility fracture
Personal history of (healed) collapsed vertebra due to osteoporosis

GUIDELINES **Section I.C.13.d.1)**
Category M81, Osteoporosis without current pathological fracture, is for use for patients with osteoporosis who do not currently have a pathologic fracture due to the osteoporosis, even if they have had a fracture in the past. For patients with a history of osteoporosis fractures, status code Z87.310, Personal history of (healed) osteoporosis fracture, should follow the code from M81.

IQ **Z87.311 Personal history of (healed) other pathological fracture**
Personal history of (healed) collapsed vertebra NOS
EXCLUDES 2 personal history of osteoporosis fracture (Z87.310)

IQ **Z87.312 Personal history of (healed) stress fracture**
Personal history of (healed) fatigue fracture

IQ **Z87.39 Personal history of other diseases of the musculoskeletal system and connective tissue**

5 **Z87.4 Personal history of diseases of genitourinary system**
Conditions classifiable to N00-N99

6 **Z87.41 Personal history of dysplasia of the female genital tract**
EXCLUDES 1 personal history of intraepithelial neoplasia III of female genital tract (Z86.001, Z86.008)
personal history of malignant neoplasm of female genital tract (Z85.40-Z85.44)

IQ **Z87.410 Personal history of cervical dysplasia**

IQ **Z87.411 Personal history of vaginal dysplasia**

IQ **Z87.412 Personal history of vulvar dysplasia**

IQ **Z87.42 Personal history of other diseases of the female genital tract**

6 **Z87.43 Personal history of diseases of male genital organs**

IQ **Z87.430 Personal history of prostatic dysplasia**
EXCLUDES 1 personal history of malignant neoplasm of prostate (Z85.46)

IQ **Z87.438 Personal history of other diseases of male genital organs**

6 **Z87.44 Personal history of diseases of urinary system**
EXCLUDES 1 personal history of malignant neoplasm of cervix uteri (Z85.41)

IQ **Z87.440 Personal history of urinary (tract) infections**

IQ **Z87.441 Personal history of nephrotic syndrome**

IQ **Z87.442 Personal history of urinary calculi**
Personal history of kidney stones

IQ **Z87.448 Personal history of other diseases of urinary system**

5 **Z87.5 Personal history of complications of pregnancy, childbirth and the puerperium**
Conditions classifiable to O00-O9A
EXCLUDES 2 recurrent pregnancy loss (N96)

IQ **Z87.51 Personal history of pre-term labor**
EXCLUDES 1 current pregnancy with history of pre-term labor (O09.21-)

IQ **Z87.59 Personal history of other complications of pregnancy, childbirth and the puerperium**
Personal history of trophoblastic disease

5 **Z87.7 Personal history of (corrected) congenital malformations**
Conditions classifiable to Q00-Q89 that have been repaired or corrected
EXCLUDES 1 congenital malformations that have been partially corrected or repair but which still require medical treatment - code to condition
EXCLUDES 2 other postprocedural states (Z98.-)
personal history of medical treatment (Z92.-)
presence of cardiac and vascular implants and grafts (Z95.-)
presence of other devices (Z97.-)
presence of other functional implants (Z96.-)
transplanted organ and tissue status (Z94.-)

6 **Z87.71 Personal history of (corrected) congenital malformations of genitourinary system**

IQ **Z87.710 Personal history of (corrected) hypospadias**

IQ **Z87.718 Personal history of other specified (corrected) congenital malformations of genitourinary system**

6 **Z87.72 Personal history of (corrected) congenital malformations of nervous system and sense organs**

IQ **Z87.720 Personal history of (corrected) congenital malformations of eye**

IQ **Z87.721 Personal history of (corrected) congenital malformations of ear**

IQ **Z87.728 Personal history of other specified (corrected) congenital malformations of nervous system and sense organs**

6 **Z87.73 Personal history of (corrected) congenital malformations of digestive system**

IQ **Z87.730 Personal history of (corrected) cleft lip and palate**

IQ **Z87.738 Personal history of other specified (corrected) congenital malformations of digestive system**

IQ **Z87.74 Personal history of (corrected) congenital malformations of heart and circulatory system**

IQ **Z87.75 Personal history of (corrected) congenital malformations of respiratory system**

IQ **Z87.76 Personal history of (corrected) congenital malformations of integument, limbs and musculoskeletal system**

6 **Z87.79 Personal history of other (corrected) congenital malformations**

IQ **Z87.790 Personal history of (corrected) congenital malformations of face and neck**

IQ **Z87.798 Personal history of other (corrected) congenital malformations**

▲ 5 **Z87.8 Personal history of other specified conditions**

EXCLUDES 2 personal history of self harm (Z91.5-)

IQ **Z87.81 Personal history of (healed) traumatic fracture**

EXCLUDES 2 personal history of (healed) nontraumatic fracture (Z87.31-)

CODING TIPS✓ The patient can have a current fracture and a history of healed fracture at the same time. See Z87.31 for history of healed pathologic fractures.

6 **Z87.82 Personal history of other (healed) physical injury and trauma**

Conditions classifiable to S00-T88, except traumatic fractures

IQ **Z87.820 Personal history of traumatic brain injury**

EXCLUDES 1 personal history of transient ischemic attack (TIA), and cerebral infarction without residual deficits (Z86.73)

IQ **Z87.821 Personal history of retained foreign body fully removed**

IQ **Z87.828 Personal history of other (healed) physical injury and trauma**

6 **Z87.89 Personal history of other specified conditions**

IQ **Z87.890 Personal history of sex reassignment**

IQ **Z87.891 Personal history of nicotine dependence**

EXCLUDES 1 current nicotine dependence (F17.2-)

CODING TIPS✓ Code history of tobacco dependence (Z87.891) for someone who was a smoker but who isn't now. Use this code if the physician or NPP uses the term "history." Remission is coded to F17.2 codes.

IQ **Z87.892 Personal history of anaphylaxis**

Code also allergy status such as:
- allergy status to drugs, medicaments and biological substances (Z88.-)
- allergy status, other than to drugs and biological substances (Z91.0-)

IQ **Z87.898 Personal history of other specified conditions**

4 **Z88 Allergy status to drugs, medicaments and biological substances**

EXCLUDES 2 Allergy status, other than to drugs and biological substances (Z91.0-)

IQ **Z88.0 Allergy status to penicillin**

IQ **Z88.1 Allergy status to other antibiotic agents**

IQ **Z88.2 Allergy status to sulfonamides**

IQ **Z88.3 Allergy status to other anti-infective agents**

IQ **Z88.4 Allergy status to anesthetic agent**

IQ **Z88.5 Allergy status to narcotic agent**

IQ **Z88.6 Allergy status to analgesic agent**

IQ **Z88.7 Allergy status to serum and vaccine**

IQ **Z88.8 Allergy status to other drugs, medicaments and biological substances**

IQ **Z88.9 Allergy status to unspecified drugs, medicaments and biological substances**

4 **Z89 Acquired absence of limb**

INCLUDES amputation status
- postprocedural loss of limb
- post-traumatic loss of limb

EXCLUDES 1 acquired deformities of limbs (M20-M21)
- congenital absence of limbs (Q71-Q73)

CODING TIPS✓ These codes are used to indicate the absence of the limb after surgical amputation, as well as healed traumatic amputations that no longer require care.

5 **Z89.0 Acquired absence of thumb and other finger(s)**

6 **Z89.01 Acquired absence of thumb**

⊟ IQ **Z89.011 Acquired absence of right thumb**

⊟ IQ **Z89.012 Acquired absence of left thumb**

⊟ IQ **Z89.019 Acquired absence of unspecified thumb**

6 **Z89.02 Acquired absence of other finger(s)**

EXCLUDES 2 acquired absence of thumb (Z89.01-)

⊟ IQ **Z89.021 Acquired absence of right finger(s)**

⊟ IQ **Z89.022 Acquired absence of left finger(s)**

⊟ IQ **Z89.029 Acquired absence of unspecified finger(s)**

5 **Z89.1 Acquired absence of hand and wrist**

6 **Z89.11 Acquired absence of hand**

⊟ IQ **Z89.111 Acquired absence of right hand**

⊟ IQ **Z89.112 Acquired absence of left hand**

⊟ IQ **Z89.119 Acquired absence of unspecified hand**

6 **Z89.12 Acquired absence of wrist**

Disarticulation at wrist

⊟ IQ **Z89.121 Acquired absence of right wrist**

Z89.122 Acquired absence of left wrist
Z89.129 Acquired absence of unspecified wrist
Z89.2 Acquired absence of upper limb above wrist
Z89.20 Acquired absence of upper limb, unspecified level
Z89.201 Acquired absence of right upper limb, unspecified level
Z89.202 Acquired absence of left upper limb, unspecified level
Z89.209 Acquired absence of unspecified upper limb, unspecified level
Acquired absence of arm NOS
Z89.21 Acquired absence of upper limb below elbow
Z89.211 Acquired absence of right upper limb below elbow
Z89.212 Acquired absence of left upper limb below elbow
Z89.219 Acquired absence of unspecified upper limb below elbow
Z89.22 Acquired absence of upper limb above elbow
Disarticulation at elbow
Z89.221 Acquired absence of right upper limb above elbow
Z89.222 Acquired absence of left upper limb above elbow
Z89.229 Acquired absence of unspecified upper limb above elbow
Z89.23 Acquired absence of shoulder
Acquired absence of shoulder joint following explantation of shoulder joint prosthesis, with or without presence of antibiotic-impregnated cement spacer
Z89.231 Acquired absence of right shoulder
Z89.232 Acquired absence of left shoulder
Z89.239 Acquired absence of unspecified shoulder
Z89.4 Acquired absence of toe(s), foot, and ankle
Z89.41 Acquired absence of great toe
Z89.411 Acquired absence of right great toe
Z89.412 Acquired absence of left great toe
Z89.419 Acquired absence of unspecified great toe
Z89.42 Acquired absence of other toe(s)
EXCLUDES 2 acquired absence of great toe (Z89.41-)
Z89.421 Acquired absence of other right toe(s)
Z89.422 Acquired absence of other left toe(s)
Z89.429 Acquired absence of other toe(s), unspecified side
Z89.43 Acquired absence of foot
CODING TIPS Because "absence of" codes indicate partial or total absence, unless otherwise noted, a transmetatarsal amputation is coded as absence of foot.
Z89.431 Acquired absence of right foot
Z89.432 Acquired absence of left foot
Z89.439 Acquired absence of unspecified foot
Z89.44 Acquired absence of ankle
Disarticulation of ankle
Z89.441 Acquired absence of right ankle
Z89.442 Acquired absence of left ankle
Z89.449 Acquired absence of unspecified ankle
Z89.5 Acquired absence of leg below knee
Z89.51 Acquired absence of leg below knee
Z89.511 Acquired absence of right leg below knee
Z89.512 Acquired absence of left leg below knee
Z89.519 Acquired absence of unspecified leg below knee
Z89.52 Acquired absence of knee
Acquired absence of knee joint following explantation of knee joint prosthesis, with or without presence of antibiotic-impregnated cement spacer
Z89.521 Acquired absence of right knee
Z89.522 Acquired absence of left knee
Z89.529 Acquired absence of unspecified knee
Z89.6 Acquired absence of leg above knee
Z89.61 Acquired absence of leg above knee
Acquired absence of leg NOS
Disarticulation at knee
Z89.611 Acquired absence of right leg above knee
Z89.612 Acquired absence of left leg above knee
Z89.619 Acquired absence of unspecified leg above knee
Z89.62 Acquired absence of hip
Acquired absence of hip joint following explantation of hip joint prosthesis, with or without presence of antibiotic-impregnated cement spacer
Disarticulation at hip
Z89.621 Acquired absence of right hip joint
Z89.622 Acquired absence of left hip joint
Z89.629 Acquired absence of unspecified hip joint
Z89.9 Acquired absence of limb, unspecified
Z90 Acquired absence of organs, not elsewhere classified
INCLUDES postprocedural or post-traumatic loss of body part NEC
EXCLUDES 1 congenital absence - see Alphabetical Index
EXCLUDES 2 postprocedural absence of endocrine glands (E89.-)
CODING TIPS These codes are used to indicate a new or old surgical removal of that particular body part. They are not used for congenital absence.

Z90.0 Acquired absence of part of head and neck

Z90.01 Acquired absence of eye

Z90.02 Acquired absence of larynx

Z90.09 Acquired absence of other part of head and neck
Acquired absence of nose
EXCLUDES 2 teeth (K08.1)

Z90.1 Acquired absence of breast and nipple

Z90.10 Acquired absence of unspecified breast and nipple

Z90.11 Acquired absence of right breast and nipple

Z90.12 Acquired absence of left breast and nipple

Z90.13 Acquired absence of bilateral breasts and nipples

Z90.2 Acquired absence of lung [part of]

Z90.3 Acquired absence of stomach [part of]

Z90.4 Acquired absence of other specified parts of digestive tract

+ Z90.41 Acquired absence of pancreas
Code also:
exocrine pancreatic insufficiency (K86.81)
Use additional code to identify any associated:
diabetes mellitus, postpancreatectomy (E13.-)
insulin use (Z79.4)

GUIDELINES **Section I.C.4.a.6)(b)(i)**
For postpancreatectomy diabetes mellitus (lack of insulin due to the surgical removal of all or part of the pancreas), assign code E89.1, Postprocedural hypoinsulinemia. Assign a code from category E13 and a code from subcategory Z90.41-, Acquired absence of pancreas, as additional codes.

+ Z90.410 Acquired total absence of pancreas
Acquired absence of pancreas NOS

+ Z90.411 Acquired partial absence of pancreas

Z90.49 Acquired absence of other specified parts of digestive tract

Z90.5 Acquired absence of kidney

Z90.6 Acquired absence of other parts of urinary tract
Acquired absence of bladder

Z90.7 Acquired absence of genital organ(s)
EXCLUDES 1 personal history of sex reassignment (Z87.890)
EXCLUDES 2 female genital mutilation status (N90.81-)

Z90.71 Acquired absence of cervix and uterus

Z90.710 Acquired absence of both cervix and uterus
Acquired absence of uterus NOS
Status post total hysterectomy

Z90.711 Acquired absence of uterus with remaining cervical stump
Status post partial hysterectomy with remaining cervical stump

Z90.712 Acquired absence of cervix with remaining uterus

Z90.72 Acquired absence of ovaries

Z90.721 Acquired absence of ovaries, unilateral

Z90.722 Acquired absence of ovaries, bilateral

Z90.79 Acquired absence of other genital organ(s)

Z90.8 Acquired absence of other organs

Z90.81 Acquired absence of spleen

Z90.89 Acquired absence of other organs

Z91 Personal risk factors, not elsewhere classified
EXCLUDES 2 contact with and (suspected) exposures hazardous to health (Z77.-)
exposure to pollution and other problems related to physical environment (Z77.1-)
female genital mutilation status (N90.81-)
personal history of physical injury and trauma (Z87.81, Z87.82-)
occupational exposure to risk factors (Z57.-)

Z91.0 Allergy status, other than to drugs and biological substances
EXCLUDES 2 Allergy status to drugs, medicaments, and biological substances (Z88.-)

Z91.01 Food allergy status
EXCLUDES 2 food additives allergy status (Z91.02)

Z91.010 Allergy to peanuts

Z91.011 Allergy to milk products
EXCLUDES 1 lactose intolerance (E73.-)

Z91.012 Allergy to eggs

Z91.013 Allergy to seafood
Allergy to shellfish
Allergy to octopus or squid ink

Z91.014 Allergy to mammalian meats
Allergy to beef
Allergy to lamb
Allergy to pork
Allergy to red meats

Z91.018 Allergy to other foods
Allergy to nuts other than peanuts

Z91.02 Food additives allergy status

Z91.03 Insect allergy status

Z91.030 Bee allergy status

Z91.038 Other insect allergy status

Z91.04 Nonmedicinal substance allergy status

Z91.040 Latex allergy status
Latex sensitivity status

Z91.041 Radiographic dye allergy status
Allergy status to contrast media used for diagnostic X-ray procedure

Z91.048 Other nonmedicinal substance allergy status

IQ **Z91.09 Other allergy status, other than to drugs and biological substances**

5 **Z91.1 Patient's noncompliance with medical treatment and regimen**

CODING TIPS✓ Be careful regarding use of noncompliance codes. Noncompliance may be a reason for initiating care, but continued noncompliance after teaching interventions have been completed usually indicates a lack of medical necessity. The exception is intentional or unintentional underdosing of medications. Underdosing codes are sequenced after the condition not being adequately treated and the T36-T50 code for underdosing, to explain the reason for underdosing.

IQ **Z91.11 Patient's noncompliance with dietary regimen**

6 **Z91.12 Patient's intentional underdosing of medication regimen**

Code first:
underdosing of medication (T36-T50) with fifth or sixth character 6

EXCLUDES 1 adverse effect of prescribed drug taken as directed- code to adverse effect
poisoning (overdose) -code to poisoning

GUIDELINES **Section I.C.19.e.5)(c)**
Noncompliance (Z91.12-, Z91.13- and Z91.14-) or complication of care (Y63.6-Y63.9) codes are to be used with an underdosing code to indicate intent, if known.

CODING TIPS✓ A code from Z91.12-, Z91.13- or Z91.14- should be assigned when underdosing has been identified and coded in the plan of care/medical record.

IQ **Z91.120 Patient's intentional underdosing of medication regimen due to financial hardship**

IQ **Z91.128 Patient's intentional underdosing of medication regimen for other reason**

6 **Z91.13 Patient's unintentional underdosing of medication regimen**

Code first:
underdosing of medication (T36-T50) with fifth or sixth character 6

EXCLUDES 1 adverse effect of prescribed drug taken as directed- code to adverse effect
poisoning (overdose) -code to poisoning

GUIDELINES **Section I.C.19.e.5)(c)**
Noncompliance (Z91.12-, Z91.13- and Z91.14-) or complication of care (Y63.6-Y63.9) codes are to be used with an underdosing code to indicate intent, if known.

CODING TIPS✓ A code from Z91.12-, Z91.13- or Z91.14- should be assigned when underdosing has been identified and coded in the plan of care/medical record.

IQ **Z91.130 Patient's unintentional underdosing of medication regimen due to age-related debility**

IQ **Z91.138 Patient's unintentional underdosing of medication regimen for other reason**

IQ **Z91.14 Patient's other noncompliance with medication regimen**

Patient's underdosing of medication NOS

GUIDELINES **Section I.C.19.e.5)(c)**
Noncompliance (Z91.12-, Z91.13- and Z91.14-) or complication of care (Y63.6-Y63.9) codes are to be used with an underdosing code to indicate intent, if known.

CODING TIPS✓ A code from Z91.12-, Z91.13- or Z91.14- should be assigned when underdosing has been identified and coded in the plan of care/medical record.

IQ **Z91.15 Patient's noncompliance with renal dialysis**

IQ **Z91.19 Patient's noncompliance with other medical treatment and regimen**

Nonadherence to medical treatment

5 **Z91.4 Personal history of psychological trauma, not elsewhere classified**

GUIDELINES **Section I.C.21.c.4)**
There are two types of history Z codes, personal and family. Personal history codes explain a patient's past medical condition that no longer exists and is not receiving any treatment, but that has the potential for recurrence, and therefore may require continued monitoring.

Family history codes are for use when a patient has a family member(s) who has had a particular disease that causes the patient to be at higher risk of also contracting the disease. Personal history codes may be used in conjunction with follow-up codes and family history codes may be used in conjunction with screening codes to explain the need for a test or procedure. History codes are also acceptable on any medical record regardless of the reason for visit. A history of an illness, even if no longer present, is important information that may alter the type of treatment ordered.

6 **Z91.41 Personal history of adult abuse**

EXCLUDES 2 personal history of abuse in childhood (Z62.81-)

IQ **Z91.410 Personal history of adult physical and sexual abuse**

EXCLUDES 1 current adult physical abuse (T74.11, T76.11)

current adult sexual abuse (T74.21, T76.11)

IQ **Z91.411 Personal history of adult psychological abuse**

IQ **Z91.412 Personal history of adult neglect**

EXCLUDES 1 current adult neglect (T74.01, T76.01)

IQ **Z91.419 Personal history of unspecified adult abuse**

IQ **Z91.42 Personal history of forced labor or sexual exploitation**

IQ **Z91.49 Other personal history of psychological trauma, not elsewhere classified**

▲ 5 **Z91.5 Personal history of self-harm**

Code also:
mental health disorder, if known

★ **Z91.51 Personal history of suicidal behavior**

Personal history of parasuicide
Personal history of self-poisoning
Personal history of suicide attempt

★ **Z91.52 Personal history of nonsuicidal self-harm**

Personal history of nonsuicidal self-injury
Personal history of self-inflicted injury without suicidal intent
Personal history of self-mutilation

5 **Z91.8 Other specified personal risk factors, not elsewhere classified**

IQ **Z91.81 History of falling**

At risk for falling

GUIDELINES **Section I.C.21.c.4)**
There are two types of history Z codes, personal and family. Personal history codes explain a patient's past medical condition that no longer exists and is not receiving any treatment, but that has the potential for recurrence, and therefore may require continued monitoring.

Family history codes are for use when a patient has a family member(s) who has had a particular disease that causes the patient to be at higher risk of also contracting the disease. Personal history codes may be used in conjunction with follow-up codes and family history codes may be used in conjunction with screening codes to explain the need for a test or procedure. History codes are also acceptable on any medical record regardless of the reason for visit. A history of an illness, even if no longer present, is important information that may alter the type of treatment ordered.

GUIDELINES **Section I.C.18.d**
Code R29.6, Repeated falls, is for use for encounters when a patient has recently fallen and the reason for the fall is being investigated. Code Z91.81, History of falling, is for use when a patient has fallen in the past and is at risk for future falls. When appropriate, both codes R29.6 and Z91.81 may be assigned together.

CODING TIPS✓ Use this code when a patient has fallen in the past and is at risk for future falls.

IQ **Z91.82 Personal history of military deployment**

Individual (civilian or military) with past history of military war, peacekeeping and humanitarian deployment (current or past conflict)
Returned from military deployment

IQ **Z91.83 Wandering in diseases classified elsewhere**

Code first underlying disorder such as:
Alzheimer's disease (G30.-)
autism or pervasive developmental disorder (F84.-)
intellectual disabilities (F70-F79)
unspecified dementia with behavioral disturbance (F03.9-)

CODING TIPS✓ Wandering is considered a behavior when coding dementia.

6 **Z91.84 Oral health risk factors**

IQ **Z91.841 Risk for dental caries, low**

IQ **Z91.842 Risk for dental caries, moderate**

IQ **Z91.843 Risk for dental caries, high**

IQ **Z91.849 Unspecified risk for dental caries**

IQ **Z91.89 Other specified personal risk factors, not elsewhere classified**

CODING TIPS✓ Stage A of the ABCD Classification of the American College of Cardiology (ACC)/American Heart Association (AHA) is the presence of heart failure risk factors but no heart disease and no symptoms. This should not be coded to the regular heart failure codes, but rather to code Z91.89, Other specified personal risk factors, not elsewhere classified.

4 **Z92 Personal history of medical treatment**

EXCLUDES 2 postprocedural states (Z98.-)

IQ **Z92.0 Personal history of contraception**

EXCLUDES 1 counseling or management of current contraceptive practices (Z30.-)
long term (current) use of contraception (Z79.3)
presence of (intrauterine) contraceptive device (Z97.5)

5 **Z92.2 Personal history of drug therapy**

EXCLUDES 2 long term (current) drug therapy (Z79.-)

IQ **Z92.21 Personal history of antineoplastic chemotherapy**

IQ **Z92.22 Personal history of monoclonal drug therapy**

IQ **Z92.23 Personal history of estrogen therapy**

6 **Z92.24 Personal history of steroid therapy**

IQ **Z92.240 Personal history of inhaled steroid therapy**

IQ **Z92.241 Personal history of systemic steroid therapy**

Personal history of steroid therapy NOS

▲ IQ **Z92.25 Personal history of immunosuppression therapy**

EXCLUDES 2 personal history of steroid therapy (Z92.24)

IQ **Z92.29 Personal history of other drug therapy**

IQ **Z92.3 Personal history of irradiation**

Personal history of exposure to therapeutic radiation

EXCLUDES 1 exposure to radiation in the physical environment (Z77.12)
occupational exposure to radiation (Z57.1)

5 **Z92.8 Personal history of other medical treatment**

IQ **Z92.81 Personal history of extracorporeal membrane oxygenation (ECMO)**

IQ **Z92.82 Status post administration of tPA (rtPA) in a different facility within the last 24 hours prior to admission to current facility**

Code first condition requiring tPA administration, such as:
acute cerebral infarction (I63.-)
acute myocardial infarction (I21.-, I22.-)

IQ **Z92.83 Personal history of failed moderate sedation**

Personal history of failed conscious sedation

EXCLUDES 2 failed moderate sedation during procedure (T88.52)

IQ **Z92.84 Personal history of unintended awareness under general anesthesia**

EXCLUDES 2 unintended awareness under general anesthesia during procedure (T88.53)

★ 6 **Z92.85 Personal history of cellular therapy**

★ **Z92.850 Personal history of Chimeric Antigen Receptor T-cell therapy**

Personal history of CAR T-cell therapy

★ **Z92.858 Personal history of other cellular therapy**

★ **Z92.859 Personal history of cellular therapy, unspecified**

★ **Z92.86 Personal history of gene therapy**

IQ **Z92.89 Personal history of other medical treatment**

4 **Z93 Artificial opening status**

EXCLUDES 1 artificial openings requiring attention or management (Z43.-)
complications of external stoma (J95.0-, K94.-, N99.5-)

CODING TIPS ✓ Assign codes from category Z93 to indicate artificial openings which are present but do not require intervention or management by the agency. Do not use codes in the Z93 category with attention to artificial opening codes (Z43) codes for the same ostomy or when the ostomy is complicated.

IQ **Z93.0 Tracheostomy status**

IQ **Z93.1 Gastrostomy status**

IQ **Z93.2 Ileostomy status**

IQ **Z93.3 Colostomy status**

IQ **Z93.4 Other artificial openings of gastrointestinal tract status**

5 **Z93.5 Cystostomy status**

IQ **Z93.50 Unspecified cystostomy status**

IQ **Z93.51 Cutaneous-vesicostomy status**

IQ **Z93.52 Appendico-vesicostomy status**

IQ **Z93.59 Other cystostomy status**

IQ **Z93.6 Other artificial openings of urinary tract status**

Nephrostomy status
Ureterostomy status
Urethrostomy status

IQ **Z93.8 Other artificial opening status**

IQ **Z93.9 Artificial opening status, unspecified**

4 **Z94 Transplanted organ and tissue status**

INCLUDES organ or tissue replaced by heterogenous or homogenous transplant

EXCLUDES 1 complications of transplanted organ or tissue - see Alphabetical Index

EXCLUDES 2 presence of vascular grafts (Z95.-)

CODING TIPS ✓ These are status codes and are used to 1) indicate that a transplant has occurred in the past; and 2) to provide more information as to type of transplant, **if needed**, in the case of aftercare (Z48.2) or transplant complications (T86).

IQ **Z94.0 Kidney transplant status**

IQ **Z94.1 Heart transplant status**

EXCLUDES 1 artificial heart status (Z95.812)
heart-valve replacement status (Z95.2-Z95.4)

IQ **Z94.2 Lung transplant status**

IQ **Z94.3 Heart and lungs transplant status**

IQ **Z94.4 Liver transplant status**

IQ **Z94.5 Skin transplant status**

Autogenous skin transplant status

IQ **Z94.6 Bone transplant status**

IQ **Z94.7 Corneal transplant status**

5 **Z94.8 Other transplanted organ and tissue status**

IQ **Z94.81 Bone marrow transplant status**

IQ **Z94.82 Intestine transplant status**

IQ **Z94.83 Pancreas transplant status**

IQ **Z94.84 Stem cells transplant status**

IQ **Z94.89 Other transplanted organ and tissue status**

IQ **Z94.9 Transplanted organ and tissue status, unspecified**

4 Z95 Presence of cardiac and vascular implants and grafts

EXCLUDES 2 complications of cardiac and vascular devices, implants and grafts (T82.-)

CODING TIPS✓ Assign codes from this category with the aftercare code Z48.812 to provide more information on the aftercare, or alone when aftercare is no longer required. Do not use these codes if there is a complication. If there has been an angioplasty without a stent or implant, see Z98.6.

IQ Z95.0 Presence of cardiac pacemaker

Presence of cardiac resynchronization therapy (CRT-P) pacemaker

EXCLUDES 1 adjustment or management of cardiac device (Z45.0-)
adjustment or management of cardiac pacemaker (Z45.0)
presence of automatic (implantable) cardiac defibrillator with synchronous cardiac pacemaker (Z95.810)

IQ Z95.1 Presence of aortocoronary bypass graft

Presence of coronary artery bypass graft

CODING TIPS✓ Z95.1 and Z95.5 are used to indicate the presence of a coronary bypass grafts and implants without complications. If complications are documented, see T82.2-.

IQ Z95.2 Presence of prosthetic heart valve

Presence of heart valve NOS

CODING TIPS✓ Code Z95.2 is used to indicate the presence of a heart valve prosthesis without complications. If complications are documented, see T82.0-.

IQ Z95.3 Presence of xenogenic heart valve

IQ Z95.4 Presence of other heart-valve replacement

IQ Z95.5 Presence of coronary angioplasty implant and graft

EXCLUDES 1 coronary angioplasty status without implant and graft (Z98.61)

CODING TIPS✓ Z95.1 and Z95.5 are used to indicate the presence of a coronary bypass grafts and implants without complications. If complications are documented, see T82.2-.

5 Z95.8 Presence of other cardiac and vascular implants and grafts

6 Z95.81 Presence of other cardiac implants and grafts

CODING TIPS✓ Do not use these codes if the condition is complicated, unless the status code provides information about the specific type of device. See T82 for complications.

IQ Z95.810 Presence of automatic (implantable) cardiac defibrillator

Presence of automatic (implantable) cardiac defibrillator with synchronous cardiac pacemaker

Presence of cardiac resynchronization therapy defibrillator (CRT-D)

Presence of cardioverter-defibrillator (ICD)

CODING TIPS✓ This code is generally accepted for the coding of the presence of a "vest."

IQ Z95.811 Presence of heart assist device

CODING TIPS✓ This code is generally accepted for the coding of the presence of a LVAD.

IQ Z95.812 Presence of fully implantable artificial heart

IQ Z95.818 Presence of other cardiac implants and grafts

CODING TIPS✓ This code is generally accepted for the coding of the presence of a loop recorder.

6 Z95.82 Presence of other vascular implants and grafts

IQ Z95.820 Peripheral vascular angioplasty status with implants and grafts

EXCLUDES 1 peripheral vascular angioplasty without implant and graft (Z98.62)

IQ Z95.828 Presence of other vascular implants and grafts

Presence of intravascular prosthesis NEC

IQ Z95.9 Presence of cardiac and vascular implant and graft, unspecified

4 Z96 Presence of other functional implants

EXCLUDES 2 complications of internal prosthetic devices, implants and grafts (T82-T85)
fitting and adjustment of prosthetic and other devices (Z44-Z46)

IQ Z96.0 Presence of urogenital implants

IQ Z96.1 Presence of intraocular lens

Presence of pseudophakia

5 Z96.2 Presence of otological and audiological implants

IQ Z96.20 Presence of otological and audiological implant, unspecified

IQ Z96.21 Cochlear implant status

IQ Z96.22 Myringotomy tube(s) status

IQ Z96.29 Presence of other otological and audiological implants

Presence of bone-conduction hearing device

Presence of eustachian tube stent

Stapes replacement

IQ Z96.3 Presence of artificial larynx

5 Z96.4 Presence of endocrine implants

IQ Z96.41 Presence of insulin pump (external) (internal)

CODING TIPS✓ If the patient uses an insulin pump, use Z96.41 as an secondary code. If there is a complication involving the insulin pump, use a code from T85.6- or T85.7- instead of the Z code.

IQ Z96.49 Presence of other endocrine implants

IQ Z96.5 Presence of tooth-root and mandibular implants

5 Z96.6 Presence of orthopedic joint implants

CODING TIPS ✓ Codes from Z96.6- should be assigned with aftercare code Z47.1. They also may be assigned to indicate the presence of a prosthetic joint even after no care is needed. When a joint replacement is performed to repair a fracture, code the fracture with a 7th character D and use the Z96.6 code to indicate the presence of the joint prosthesis. When a complication is present to a joint prosthesis, assign a complication code from category T84.-, which will identify the joint replaced, as well as the complication. No Z96.6- code is required when a complication is present if the joint is identified in the complication code. If the patient has bilateral joint replacements of the same joint, the coder may assign the bilateral code, or separate codes if the joints were replaced in different encounters.

IQ Z96.60 Presence of unspecified orthopedic joint implant

6 Z96.61 Presence of artificial shoulder joint

⊟ IQ Z96.611 Presence of right artificial shoulder joint

⊟ IQ Z96.612 Presence of left artificial shoulder joint

⊟ IQ Z96.619 Presence of unspecified artificial shoulder joint

6 Z96.62 Presence of artificial elbow joint

⊟ IQ Z96.621 Presence of right artificial elbow joint

⊟ IQ Z96.622 Presence of left artificial elbow joint

⊟ IQ Z96.629 Presence of unspecified artificial elbow joint

6 Z96.63 Presence of artificial wrist joint

⊟ IQ Z96.631 Presence of right artificial wrist joint

⊟ IQ Z96.632 Presence of left artificial wrist joint

⊟ IQ Z96.639 Presence of unspecified artificial wrist joint

6 Z96.64 Presence of artificial hip joint

Hip-joint replacement (partial) (total)

⊟ IQ Z96.641 Presence of right artificial hip joint

⊟ IQ Z96.642 Presence of left artificial hip joint

⊟ IQ Z96.643 Presence of artificial hip joint, bilateral

⊟ IQ Z96.649 Presence of unspecified artificial hip joint

6 Z96.65 Presence of artificial knee joint

⊟ IQ Z96.651 Presence of right artificial knee joint

⊟ IQ Z96.652 Presence of left artificial knee joint

⊟ IQ Z96.653 Presence of artificial knee joint, bilateral

⊟ IQ Z96.659 Presence of unspecified artificial knee joint

6 Z96.66 Presence of artificial ankle joint

⊟ IQ Z96.661 Presence of right artificial ankle joint

⊟ IQ Z96.662 Presence of left artificial ankle joint

⊟ IQ Z96.669 Presence of unspecified artificial ankle joint

6 Z96.69 Presence of other orthopedic joint implants

⊟ IQ Z96.691 Finger-joint replacement of right hand

⊟ IQ Z96.692 Finger-joint replacement of left hand

⊟ IQ Z96.693 Finger-joint replacement, bilateral

⊟ IQ Z96.698 Presence of other orthopedic joint implants

IQ Z96.7 Presence of other bone and tendon implants

Presence of skull plate

5 Z96.8 Presence of other specified functional implants

IQ Z96.81 Presence of artificial skin

Z96.82 Presence of neurostimulator

Presence of brain neurostimulator
Presence of gastric neurostimulator
Presence of peripheral nerve neurostimulator
Presence of sacral nerve neurostimulator
Presence of spinal cord neurostimulator
Presence of vagus nerve neurostimulator

IQ Z96.89 Presence of other specified functional implants

IQ Z96.9 Presence of functional implant, unspecified

4 Z97 Presence of other devices

EXCLUDES 1 complications of internal prosthetic devices, implants and grafts (T82-T85)

EXCLUDES 2 fitting and adjustment of prosthetic and other devices (Z44-Z46)
presence of cerebrospinal fluid drainage device (Z98.2)

IQ Z97.0 Presence of artificial eye

5 Z97.1 Presence of artificial limb (complete) (partial)

⊟ IQ Z97.10 Presence of artificial limb (complete) (partial), unspecified

⊟ IQ Z97.11 Presence of artificial right arm (complete) (partial)

⊟ IQ Z97.12 Presence of artificial left arm (complete) (partial)

⊟ IQ Z97.13 Presence of artificial right leg (complete) (partial)

⊟ IQ Z97.14 Presence of artificial left leg (complete) (partial)

⊟ IQ Z97.15 Presence of artificial arms, bilateral (complete) (partial)

⊟ IQ Z97.16 Presence of artificial legs, bilateral (complete) (partial)

IQ Z97.2 Presence of dental prosthetic device (complete) (partial)

Presence of dentures (complete) (partial)

IQ Z97.3 Presence of spectacles and contact lenses

IQ Z97.4 Presence of external hearing-aid

IQ Z97.5 Presence of (intrauterine) contraceptive device

EXCLUDES 1 checking, reinsertion or removal of implantable subdermal contraceptive (Z30.46)
checking, reinsertion or removal of intrauterine contraceptive device (Z30.43-)

IQ **Z97.8 Presence of other specified devices**

4 **Z98 Other postprocedural states**

EXCLUDES 2 aftercare (Z43-Z49, Z51)
follow-up medical care (Z08-Z09)
postprocedural complication - see Alphabetical Index

IQ **Z98.0 Intestinal bypass and anastomosis status**

EXCLUDES 2 bariatric surgery status (Z98.84)
gastric bypass status (Z98.84)
obesity surgery status (Z98.84)

IQ **Z98.1 Arthrodesis status**

CODING TIPS✓ Ankylosis of the joint is caused by arthritis, traumatic injury or infection. The joint will assume the least painful position and become permanently fixed. A surgical fusion is coded Z98.1. Surgical fusions are never coded with M43.

CODING TIPS✓ If spinal fusion has taken place, also use a code from M43.2-.

IQ **Z98.2 Presence of cerebrospinal fluid drainage device**

Presence of CSF shunt

CODING TIPS✓ Do not use this code if the condition is complicated. See T85.0-.

IQ **Z98.3 Post therapeutic collapse of lung status**

Code first:
underlying disease

+ 5 **Z98.4 Cataract extraction status**

Use additional code to identify intraocular lens implant status (Z96.1)

EXCLUDES 1 aphakia (H27.0)

H IQ + **Z98.41 Cataract extraction status, right eye**

H IQ + **Z98.42 Cataract extraction status, left eye**

H IQ + **Z98.49 Cataract extraction status, unspecified eye**

5 **Z98.5 Sterilization status**

EXCLUDES 1 female infertility (N97.-)
male infertility (N46.-)

IQ **Z98.51 Tubal ligation status**

IQ **Z98.52 Vasectomy status**

5 **Z98.6 Angioplasty status**

CODING TIPS✓ Assign codes from this category with the aftercare code Z48.812 to provide more information on the aftercare, or alone when aftercare is no longer required. Do not use these codes if there is a complication.

IQ **Z98.61 Coronary angioplasty status**

EXCLUDES 1 coronary angioplasty status with implant and graft (Z95.5)

IQ **Z98.62 Peripheral vascular angioplasty status**

EXCLUDES 1 peripheral vascular angioplasty status with implant and graft (Z95.820)

5 **Z98.8 Other specified postprocedural states**

6 **Z98.81 Dental procedure status**

IQ **Z98.810 Dental sealant status**

IQ **Z98.811 Dental restoration status**

Dental crown status
Dental fillings status

IQ **Z98.818 Other dental procedure status**

IQ **Z98.82 Breast implant status**

EXCLUDES 1 breast implant removal status (Z98.86)

IQ **Z98.83 Filtering (vitreous) bleb after glaucoma surgery status**

EXCLUDES 1 Inflammation (infection) of postprocedural bleb (H59.4-)

IQ **Z98.84 Bariatric surgery status**

Gastric banding status
Gastric bypass status for obesity
Obesity surgery status

EXCLUDES 1 bariatric surgery status complicating pregnancy, childbirth, or the puerperium (O99.84)

EXCLUDES 2 intestinal bypass and anastomosis status (Z98.0)

CODING TIPS✓ Code Z98.84 is not appropriate if there is a complication. Use a code from K95 instead.

IQ **Z98.85 Transplanted organ removal status**

Transplanted organ previously removed due to complication, failure, rejection or infection

EXCLUDES 1 encounter for removal of transplanted organ -code to complication of transplanted organ (T86.-)

GUIDELINES **Section I.C.21.c.3)**
Assign code Z98.85, Transplanted organ removal status, to indicate that a transplanted organ has been previously removed. This code should not be assigned for the encounter in which the transplanted organ is removed. The complication necessitating removal of the transplant organ should be assigned for that encounter.

IQ **Z98.86 Personal history of breast implant removal**

6 **Z98.87 Personal history of in utero procedure**

IQ **Z98.870 Personal history of in utero procedure during pregnancy**

EXCLUDES 2 complications from in utero procedure for current pregnancy (O35.7)

supervision of current pregnancy with history of in utero procedure during previous pregnancy (O09.82-)

IQ **Z98.871 Personal history of in utero procedure while a fetus**

6 **Z98.89 Other specified postprocedural states**

IQ **Z98.890 Other specified postprocedural states**
Personal history of surgery, not elsewhere classified

IQ **Z98.891 History of uterine scar from previous surgery**
EXCLUDES 1 Maternal care due to uterine scar from previous surgery (O34.2-)

▲ 4 **Z99 Dependence on enabling machines and devices, not elsewhere classified**

SP **Z99.0 Dependence on aspirator**
CODING TIPS✓ Even though this code is acceptable as a primary diagnosis under PDGM, it is a status code and is usually not an acceptable primary diagnosis. Choose the condition requiring the dependence on the respiratory treatment as the primary instead.

5 **Z99.1 Dependence on respirator**
Dependence on ventilator

SP **Z99.11 Dependence on respirator [ventilator] status**
CODING TIPS✓ Even though this code is acceptable as a primary diagnosis under PDGM, it is a status code and is usually not an acceptable primary diagnosis. Choose the condition requiring the dependence on the respiratory treatment as the primary instead.

Px IQ **Z99.12 Encounter for respirator [ventilator] dependence during power failure**
EXCLUDES 1 mechanical complication of respirator [ventilator] (J95.850)

IQ **Z99.2 Dependence on renal dialysis**
Hemodialysis status
Peritoneal dialysis status
Presence of arteriovenous shunt for dialysis
Renal dialysis status NOS
EXCLUDES 1 encounter for fitting and adjustment of dialysis catheter (Z49.0-)
EXCLUDES 2 noncompliance with renal dialysis (Z91.15)

IQ **Z99.3 Dependence on wheelchair**
Wheelchair confinement status
Code first cause of dependence, such as:
muscular dystrophy (G71.0-)
obesity (E66.-)
CODING TIPS✓ Code Z74.09 may be used in conjunction with this code.

5 **Z99.8 Dependence on other enabling machines and devices**

IQ **Z99.81 Dependence on supplemental oxygen**
Dependence on long-term oxygen

IQ **Z99.89 Dependence on other enabling machines and devices**
Dependence on machine or device NOS

Chapter 21 Scenarios: Factors influencing health status and contact with health services (Z00-Z99)

Exacerbated heart failure, history of tuberculosis

An 83-year-old man is admitted to home health following hospitalization with acutely exacerbated chronic systolic congestive heart failure. He also has hypertension, chronic obstructive asthma and a history of resolved tuberculosis.

Description	Code
Primary: Hypertensive heart disease with heart failure	I11.0
Secondary: Acute on chronic combined systolic (congestive) and diastolic (congestive) heart failure	I50.43
Secondary: Chronic obstructive pulmonary disease, unspecified	J44.9
Secondary: Personal history of tuberculosis	Z86.11

The ICD-10 classification assumes a relationship between hypertension and heart failure. Thus, the patient's heart failure is coded as hypertensive heart disease, which requires first coding I11.0 followed by I50.43. Chronic obstructive asthma is coded with J44.9, according to the alphabetic index. Finally, Z86.11 is assigned to capture the patient's history of resolved tuberculosis.

Joint replacement

A 70-year-old male patient is admitted to home health for physical therapy following a second right knee replacement for bilateral primary osteoarthritis. The patient had previously had a knee replacement but the prosthetic joint became infected and had to be removed. He was treated with antibiotics and the infection completely resolved prior to the placement of the new right knee prosthesis. He still suffers from osteoarthritis in his left knee and will undergo a left knee replacement in the near future. His discharge summary encounter notes report comorbid hypertension and heart failure, currently under control.

Description	Code
Primary: Aftercare following explantation of knee joint prosthesis	Z47.33
Secondary: Unilateral primary osteoarthritis, left knee	M17.12
Secondary: Hypertensive heart disease with heart failure	I11.0
Secondary: Heart failure, unspecified	I50.9
Secondary: Presence of right artificial knee joint	Z96.651

Because the complication (the infection) resolved completely prior to the placement of the second right knee prosthesis and thus the patient's care is routine, Z47.33 is the appropriate primary code choice. The right knee replacement resolved the primary osteoarthritis in his right knee, but it is still in his left knee and will impact his care. Therefore it is coded as a secondary diagnosis. Hypertension and heart failure have an assumed relationship in the ICD-10-CM classification and a combination code is assigned for hypertensive heart disease, followed by the appropriate heart failure code. The Z96.651 code is assigned to capture the presence of the right prosthetic knee joint.

Post pulmonary embolectomy

The patient developed chest pain, severe shortness of breath, and was hospitalized. Pulmonary scans and arteriograms revealed that more than half of the major pulmonary arteries were occluded; smaller vessels also were obstructed. Pulmonary embolectomy was performed on major vessels. The patient was sent home on Coumadin. The patient has a history of chronic emphysematous bronchitis and hypertension. Home health orders are for wound care, teaching of the disease process, meds and lab draws for PT/INR.

Description	Code
Primary: Aftercare following surgery of circulatory system	Z48.812
Secondary: Other pulmonary embolism without acute cor pulmonale	I26.99
Secondary: Chronic obstructive pulmonary disease, unspecified	J44.9
Secondary: Essential primary hypertension	I10
Secondary: Therapeutic drug monitoring	Z51.81
Secondary: Long term use of anticoagulants	Z79.01

Although the embolectomy removed occlusions of the major vessels, this patient continues to have occlusions of the small vessels and is undergoing treatment. Thus, I26.99 is still coded. Do not use the history code (Z86.711) in the presence of the acute diagnosis. The chronic emphysematous bronchitis and hypertension are coded as relevant comorbidities. Monitoring of PT/INR and use of anticoagulants are also captured with Z51.81 and Z79.01.

Surgical aftercare, hip replacement

A patient is admitted for surgical aftercare following right hip joint replacement due to primary generalized osteoarthritis.

Description	Code
Primary: Aftercare following joint replacement surgery	Z47.1
Secondary: Primary generalized (osteo)arthritis	M15.0
Secondary: Presence of right artificial hip joint	Z96.641

Code Z47.1 (Aftercare following joint replacement surgery) does not specify the joint replaced. So it does require the use of an additional code to identify the joint (Z96.641). The code title includes laterality. Primary generalized arthritis continues to be assigned even after the joint replacement because it is generalized and therefore occurs in more than just the joint that was just replaced. Thus it is still an active diagnosis.

Surgical aftercare, shoulder replacement

A patient had a right shoulder joint replacement due to localized degenerative joint disease (DJD) in that shoulder. Nursing and therapy are ordered for aftercare.

Description	Code
Primary: Aftercare following joint replacement surgery	Z47.1
Secondary: Presence of right artificial shoulder joint	Z96.611

Aftercare following replacement of a joint (Z47.- category) should be listed as the primary diagnosis. Tabular instructions note this code identifies that a joint has been replaced but a second code needs to be added to identify which joint was replaced. Even though the Z96.611 code is a status code, it is categorized in the Alphabetic Index under the main term "presence." The condition treated also should be coded if still present. In this example, the condition (localized DJD) resolved with the surgery and would not be listed.

Amputation due to PVD

A 70-year-old patient is admitted with a below the knee right leg amputation due to peripheral vascular disease (PVD).

Description	Code
Primary: Encounter for orthopedic aftercare following surgical amputation	Z47.81
Secondary: Peripheral vascular disease, unspecified	I73.9
Secondary: Acquired absence of right leg below knee	Z89.511

The amputation is done because of the PVD but it does not resolve the condition. Therefore, it should still be coded. A code from Z89.- is assigned to identify the amputated limb, according to tabular instruction.

Infected left hip replacement

A 68-year-old female patient was admitted to home care with an infected left hip prosthesis. Home health orders include IV antibiotics, and peak and trough in addition to the wound care.

Description	Code
Primary: Infection and inflammatory reaction due to internal left hip prosthesis, initial encounter	T84.52xA
Secondary: Encounter for adjustment and management of vascular access device	Z45.2
Secondary: Encounter for therapeutic drug level monitoring	Z51.81
Secondary: Long term (current) use of antibiotics	Z79.2

The hip replacement is complicated and therefore an aftercare code is not appropriate. The patient continues to receive active treatment for the complication, necessitating the use of an initial encounter seventh encounter. Codes Z45.2, Z51.81 and Z79.2 are included to capture the antibiotics and peak and trough measuring. Because the patient requires IV antibiotic administration and this is the primary skilled need, Z45.2 is appropriate to assign in the first secondary position according to CMS. It should be noted that the assignment of Z45.2 as primary or first secondary diagnosis classifies any PDGM episode to the Complex Nursing Interventions primary diagnosis clinical group.

New ileostomy, diabetes

A patient is admitted to home health with a newly created ileostomy and is currently unable to independently care for the ostomy. He has a history of prostate cancer, now resolved, and is being treated for diabetes, which is diet-controlled.

Description	Code
Primary: Encounter for attention to ileostomy	Z43.2
Secondary: Type 2 diabetes mellitus without complications	E11.9
Secondary: Personal history of malignant neoplasm of prostate	Z85.46

In this scenario, a code from “encounter for attention to” (Z43.2) is used because the agency will be providing hands-on care and teaching for this patient who needs assistance with his new ileostomy.

HOME HEALTH CODING SCENARIOS

Mitral valve replacement

A 72-year-old man complained of increasing shortness of breath during a routine doctor's appointment. A cardiovascular workup revealed severe mitral valve stenosis that a cardiologist determined needed immediate treatment. Shortly thereafter, he underwent surgery to replace the damaged valve with a prosthetic one, which resolved the mitral valve disease. He also has hypertension and is on Coumadin.

Description	Code
Primary: Encounter for surgical aftercare following surgery on the circulatory system	Z48.812
Secondary: Essential (primary) hypertension	I10
Secondary: Presence of prosthetic heart valve	Z95.2
Secondary: Long term (current) use of anticoagulants	Z79.01

The patient underwent heart valve replacement surgery. The condition that necessitated the procedure, mitral valve stenosis, affects the circulatory system. Therefore, the correct surgical aftercare code is Z48.812. As the focus of the home health admission Z48.812 is coded in the primary position. The heart valve replacement surgery resolved the heart valve disease and thus that condition is not coded as an active condition. The status code Z95.2 is assigned to indicate the presence of the patient's prosthetic valve. The fact that the patient is taking Coumadin needs to be captured with Z79.01.

Hip replacement, history of breast cancer, use of Tamoxifen

A 68-year-old woman comes to home health for surgical aftercare following a right hip replacement to treat localized traumatic arthritis. Her medical record states that she has a history of breast cancer in her right breast from five years ago. She underwent a bilateral mastectomy and additional treatment with chemotherapy and radiation. Her treatment was completed four years ago. She continues to take tamoxifen but her history and physical states that it is prescribed prophylactically and she is receiving no active treatment for the cancer.

Description	Code
Primary: Aftercare following joint replacement surgery	Z47.1
Secondary: Presence of right artificial hip joint	Z96.641
Secondary: Personal history of malignant neoplasm of breast	Z85.3
Secondary: Long term (current) use of selective estrogen receptor modulators (SERMs)	Z79.810
Secondary: Acquired absence of bilateral breasts and nipples	Z90.13

As the focus of care the surgical aftercare is coded primary and an additional code to capture the replaced joint is assigned in accordance with tabular instruction. Traumatic arthritis is not coded as it was said to be localized and was thus resolved by the joint replacement procedure. The patient is no longer undergoing treatment for breast cancer and is taking tamoxifen prophylactically, thus making the use of the history code for breast cancer appropriate, versus a code for active cancer. Her long-term use of tamoxifen is captured with Z79.810. Finally, Z90.13 is assigned to capture the absence of her breasts due to bilateral mastectomy.

Out of control diabetes

A 57-year-old man comes to home health with diabetes that is out of control. His history and physician states that the patient admitted to being unable to read and as a result, wasn't able to read his glipizide medication instructions, which led to his dangerously high blood sugar levels because he was taking far less than the prescribed daily dosage. He will receive skilled nursing and medical social work services.

Description	Code
Primary: Type 2 diabetes mellitus with hyperglycemia	E11.65
Secondary: Underdosing of insulin and oral hypoglycemic [antidiabetic] drugs, subsequent encounter	T38.3x6D
Secondary: Patient's unintentional underdosing of medication regimen for other reason	Z91.138
Secondary: Illiteracy and low-level literacy	Z55.0
Secondary: Long term (current) use of oral hypoglycemic drugs	Z79.84

The patient unintentionally underdosed his diabetes medications because he couldn't read the instructions, leading to his diabetes becoming out of control. Out of control diabetes codes to diabetes with hyperglycemia, according to the alphabetic index. The code for underdosing of the drug is coded next, in accordance with coding guidelines. Code Z91.138 helps explain why the patient experienced an underdosing and Z55.0 is assigned to capture that the patient struggles with literacy. Codes in categories Z55 to Z65 can be assigned based on clinician, versus physician, documentation, according to Q1 2018 Coding Clinic guidance. The patient's use of oral hypoglycemic medication is captured with Z79.84.

Old MI with symptoms

An 81-year-old man with a history of late-onset Alzheimer's dementia, suffered an ST-elevation MI five weeks ago and is returning home, with home health support, after being in rehab following his hospitalization. He continues to suffer from symptoms related to the MI, including chest pain and dyspnea. His record does not indicate anywhere that he's been diagnosed with coronary artery disease (CAD) or any other form of heart disease. His physician did not return repeated calls for further information on the chest pain and dyspnea symptoms. His panic disorder, newly diagnosed after the heart attack, will be the focus of care.

Description	Code
Primary: Panic disorder [episodic paroxysmal anxiety]	F41.0
Secondary: Chest pain, unspecified	R07.9
Secondary: Dyspnea, unspecified	R06.00
Secondary: Encounter for other specified aftercare	Z51.89
Secondary: Alzheimer's disease with late onset	G30.1
Secondary: Dementia in other diseases classified elsewhere without behavioral disturbance	F02.80

His newly-diagnosed panic disorder is the focus of care and is coded first. He is still receiving care following the MI, though is it no longer considered an acute condition being more than four weeks old, so Z51.89 is coded to indicate that he's still experiencing symptoms related to the MI, in accordance with official coding guidelines and Coding Clinic guidance. Though a diagnosis of CAD is a possibility, it is not coded because the record didn't indicate it and the physician could not be reached to confirm it. Note that symptom codes for chest pain and dyspnea are unacceptable as primary diagnoses under PDGM. Late onset Alzheimer's dementia is also coded due to the impact this condition has on the management of the new anxiety disorder and the overall plan of care and prognosis.

Stage A heart failure

A 77-year-old woman is admitted to home health following hospitalization for exacerbated emphysema and COPD. Her record states she has also been diagnosed with Stage A heart failure. The emphysema is the focus of care. She is dependent on oxygen and was a smoker for 22 years but quit three years ago.

Description	Code
Primary: Emphysema, unspecified	J43.9
Secondary: Dependence on supplemental oxygen	Z99.81
Secondary: Personal history of nicotine dependence	Z87.891
Secondary: Other specified personal risk factors, not elsewhere classified	Z91.89

A diagnosed specified as "emphysema and COPD" codes to J43.9, according to the alphabetic index. Even though the diagnosis is exacerbated, J43.9 is still the appropriate code, according to Q4 2017 and Q1 2019 Coding Clinic guidance. The fact that the patient used to smoke must be captured with Z87.891, according to tabular instruction. Her use of oxygen is captured with Z99.81. The patient has been diagnosed with Stage A heart failure, which indicates the presence of heart failure risk factors but is not a diagnosis of heart failure. Thus, Z91.89 (Other specified personal risk factors not elsewhere classified) is the correct code for this diagnosis.

Chapter 22: Codes for Special Purposes (U00-U85)

This chapter is for the provisional assignment of new diseases of uncertain etiology or emergency use. Specifically, codes U00-U49 are to be used by WHO for the provisional assignment of new diseases of uncertain etiology or emergency use. Included in Chapter 22 are three codes:

- U07.0, Vaping-related disorder
- U07.1, COVID-19
- U09.9, Post COVID-19 condition, unspecified

U07.0 Vaping-Related Disorder

The purpose of U07.0 is for coding encounters related to E-cigarette, or Vaping, Product Use.

Code U07.0, Vaping-related disorder, has been implemented in response to the recent occurrences of vaping-related disorders. The incorporation of this diagnosis code is consistent with certain provisions of the Health Insurance Portability and Accountability Act of 1996 (HIPAA) for diagnosis coding, including the *Official ICD-10-CM Guidelines for Coding and Reporting*, as maintained and distributed by the U.S. Department of Health and Human Services.

The code is consistent with the emergency code established by the World Health Organization (WHO). The code resulted from a meeting of the WHO Framework Convention on Tobacco Control and the WHO Family of International Classifications (WHOFIC) Network Classification and Statistics Advisory Committee (CSAC).

According to the U.S. Centers for Disease Control and Prevention (CDC), using an electronic cigarette (e-cigarette) is commonly called vaping. E-cigarettes are also called vapes, e-hookahs, vape pens, tank systems, mods, and electronic nicotine delivery systems (ENDS). E-cigarettes work by heating a liquid to produce an aerosol that users inhale into their lungs. The liquid can contain nicotine, tetrahydrocannabinol (THC) and cannabinoid (CBD) oils, and other substances, flavorings, and additives. THC is the psychoactive mind-altering compound of marijuana that produces the "high." The U.S. Food and Drug Administration (FDA) and the U.S. Centers for Disease Control and Prevention (CDC) continue to investigate the incidents of severe respiratory illness associated with use of vaping products.

General guidance for assigning U07.0

Per tabular instructions, when assigning U07.0, use additional code to identify manifestations, such as:

- abdominal pain (R10.84)
- acute respiratory distress syndrome (J80)
- diarrhea (R19.7)
- drug-induced interstitial lung disorder (J70.4)
- lipoid pneumonia (J69.1)
- weight loss (R63.4)

Coding guidance for vaping-related disorders

The guidance in this section is from the FY2021 coding guidelines, effective Jan. 1, 2021, unless otherwise noted. The guidelines for proper assignment of U07.0 can be found in Chapter 10 of the official coding guidelines.

For patients presenting with condition(s) related to vaping, assign code U07.0, Vaping-related disorder, as the principal diagnosis. For lung injury due to vaping, assign only code U07.0. Assign additional codes for other manifestations, such as acute respiratory failure (subcategory J96.0-) or pneumonitis (code J68.0).

Associated respiratory signs and symptoms due to vaping, such as cough, shortness of breath, etc., are not coded separately, when a definitive diagnosis has been established. However, it would be appropriate to code separately any gastrointestinal symptoms, such as diarrhea and abdominal pain.

Poisoning and toxicity

Acute nicotine exposure can be toxic. Children and adults have been poisoned by swallowing, breathing, or absorbing e-cigarette liquid through their skin or eyes. For these patients assign code:

- T65.291-, Toxic effect of other nicotine and tobacco, accidental (unintentional); includes Toxic effect of other tobacco and nicotine NOS.

Substance use, abuse and dependence

For patients with documented substance use/abuse/dependence, additional codes identifying the substance(s) used should be assigned.

When the provider documentation refers to use, abuse and dependence of the same substance (e.g. nicotine, cannabis, etc.), only one code should be assigned to identify the pattern of use based on the following hierarchy:

- If both use and abuse are documented, assign only the code for abuse
- If both abuse and dependence are documented, assign only the code for dependence
- If use, abuse and dependence are all documented, assign only the code for dependence
- If both use and dependence are documented, assign only the code for dependence.

Assign as many codes, as appropriate. Examples:

- Cannabis related disorders: F12.---
- Nicotine related disorders: F17.----

Specifically, for vaping of nicotine, assign code F17.29-, Nicotine dependence, other tobacco products. Electronic nicotine delivery systems (ENDS) are non-combustible tobacco products.

Signs and symptoms

For patients presenting with any signs/symptoms (such as fever, etc.) and where a definitive diagnosis has **not** been established, assign the appropriate code(s) for each of the presenting signs and symptoms such as:

- M79.10, Myalgia, unspecified site
- R06.00, Dyspnea, unspecified
- R06.02, Shortness of breath
- R06.2, Wheezing
- R06.82, Tachypnea, not elsewhere classified
- R07.9, Chest pain, unspecified
- R09.02, Hypoxemia
- R09.89, Other specified symptoms and signs involving the circulatory and respiratory systems (includes chest congestion)
- R10.84, Generalized abdominal pain
- R10.9, Unspecified abdominal pain
- R11.10, Vomiting, unspecified
- R11.11, Vomiting without nausea
- R11.2, Nausea with vomiting, unspecified
- R19.7, Diarrhea, unspecified
- R50.-, Fever of other and unknown origin
- R53.83, Other fatigue
- R61, Generalized hyperhidrosis (night sweats)
- R63.4, Abnormal weight loss
- R68.83, Chills (without fever)

This coding guidance has been approved by the four organizations that make up the Cooperating Parties: The National Center for Health Statistics, the American Health Information Management Association, the American Hospital Association, and the Centers for Medicare & Medicaid Services.

U07.1 COVID-19 Infections (Infections due to SARS-CoV-2)

The purpose of U07.1 is for coding encounters related to infections due to SARS-CoV-2.

Code U07.1, COVID-19, has been implemented in response to the recent pandemic. A national emergency has been declared in the United States concerning the COVID-19 Outbreak. Given these developments, and the critical need to report COVID-19 in claims and surveillance data, the Centers for Disease Control (CDC), under the National Emergencies Act Section 201 and 301, announced a change in the effective date of new diagnosis code U07.1, COVID-19, as April 1, 2020. This off-cycle update was unprecedented and is an exception to the code set updating process established under HIPAA. Code U07.1 was also included in the FY2021 code update, effective Jan. 1, 2021. The guidance in this section is from the FY2021 coding guidelines, effective Jan. 1, 2021, unless otherwise noted. The guidelines for proper assignment of U07.1 can be found in Chapter 1 of the official coding guidelines.

General Guidance

Per tabular instruction, when assigning U07.1, use additional code to identify pneumonia or other manifestations.

Code only a confirmed diagnosis of the 2019 novel coronavirus disease (COVID-19) as documented by the provider or documentation of a positive COVID-19 test result. For a confirmed diagnosis, assign code U07.1, COVID-19. This is an exception to the hospital inpatient guideline Section II, H. In this context, "confirmation" does not require documentation of a positive test result for COVID-19; the provider's documentation that the individual has COVID-19 is sufficient.

If the provider documents "suspected," "possible," "probable," or "inconclusive" COVID-19, do not assign code U07.1. Instead, code the signs and symptoms reported.

Sequencing of codes

When COVID-19 meets the definition of principal diagnosis, code U07.1, COVID-19, should be sequenced first, followed by the appropriate codes for associated manifestations, except when another guideline requires that certain codes be sequenced first, such as obstetrics, sepsis, or transplant complications.

Acute respiratory illnesses due to COVID-19

When the reason for the encounter/admission is a respiratory manifestation of COVID-19, assign U07.1 as the principal/first-listed diagnosis and assign code(s) for the respiratory manifestation(s) as additional diagnoses.

The following conditions are examples of common respiratory manifestations confirmed as due to COVID-19.

- **Pneumonia:** Assign codes U07.1 (COVID-19) and J12.82 (Pneumonia due to coronavirus disease 2019).
- **Acute bronchitis:** Assign U07.1 and J20.8 (Acute bronchitis due to other specified organisms). Note: Bronchitis not otherwise specified (NOS) due to COVID-19 should be coded using code U07.1 and J40 (Bronchitis, not specified as acute or chronic).
- **Lower respiratory infection:** If the COVID-19 is documented as being associated with a lower respiratory infection, not otherwise specified (NOS), or an acute respiratory infection, NOS, assign U07.1 and J22 (Unspecified acute lower respiratory infection). If the COVID-19 is documented as being associated with a respiratory infection, NOS, assign U07.1 and J98.8 (Other specified respiratory disorders).
- **Acute respiratory distress syndrome:** Assign U07.1 and J80 (Acute respiratory distress syndrome).
- **Acute respiratory failure:** Assign U07.1 and J96.0- (Acute respiratory failure).

When the reason for the encounter/admission is a non-respiratory manifestation (e.g., viral enteritis) of COVID-19, assign code U07.1, COVID-19, as the principal/first-listed diagnosis and assign code(s) for the manifestation(s) as additional diagnoses.

Additional COVID-19 guidance

- **Exposure:** For asymptomatic individuals with actual or suspected exposure to COVID-19, assign code Z20.822 (Contact with and (suspected) exposure to COVID-19). For symptomatic individuals with actual or suspected exposure to COVID-19 and the infection has been ruled out, or test results are inconclusive or unknown, assign code Z20.822.
- **Screening:** During the COVID-19 pandemic, a screening code is generally not appropriate. Do not assign code Z11.52 (Encounter for screening for COVID-19). For encounters for COVID-19 testing, including preoperative testing, code as exposure to COVID-19.
- **Signs and symptoms without definitive diagnosis of COVID-19:** For patients who have any symptoms that are associated with COVID-19, but a definitive diagnosis has not be confirmed, assign the appropriate codes for each of the symptoms such as R05.- (Cough), R06.02 (Shortness or breath) or R50.9 (Fever, unspecified). If a patient with signs/symptoms associated with COVID-19 also has an actual or suspected contact with or exposure to COVID-19, assign Z20.822 as an additional code.
- **Asymptomatic individuals who test positive for COVID-19:** See guideline I.C.1.g.1.a. Although the individual is asymptomatic, the individual has tested positive and is considered to have the COVID-19 infection.
- **Personal history of COVID-19:** For patients with a history of COVID-19, assign code Z86.16 (Personal history of COVID-19).

  Important: Coding experts warn that a subsequent negative test does NOT automatically mean you report Z86.16 instead of U07.1, especially when a patient is still experiencing active sequela of COVID. Before assigning Z86.16 ensure you have clear provider documentation that states "resolved" or "history". There's no guideline that says you can code history from a negative test.
- **Follow-up visits after COVID-19 infection has resolved:** For individuals who previously had COVID-19 and are being seen for follow-up evaluation, and COVID-19 test results are negative, assign codes Z09, Encounter for follow-up examination after completed treatment for conditions other than malignant neoplasm, and Z86.16, Personal history of COVID-19.
- **Encounter for antibody testing:** For an encounter for antibody testing that is not being performed to confirm a current COVID-19 infection, nor is a follow-up test after resolution of COVID-19, assign Z01.84, Encounter for antibody response examination.

  Follow the applicable guidelines above if the individual is being tested to confirm a current COVID-19 infection.

  For follow-up testing after a COVID-19 infection, see guideline I.C.1.g.1.j.
- **Multisystem Inflammatory Syndrome:** For individuals with multisystem inflammatory syndrome (MIS) and COVID-19, assign code U07.1, COVID-19, as the principal/first-listed diagnosis and assign code M35.81, Multisystem inflammatory syndrome, as an additional diagnosis.

If MIS develops as a result of a previous COVID-19 infection, assign codes M35.81, Multisystem inflammatory syndrome, and U09.9 (Post COVID-19 condition, unspecified).

If an individual with a history of COVID-19 develops MIS and the provider does not indicate the MIS is due to the previous COVID-19 infection, assign codes M35.81, Multisystem inflammatory syndrome, and Z86.16, Personal history of COVID-19.

If an individual with a known or suspected exposure to COVID-19, and no current COVID-19 infection or history of COVID-19, develops MIS, assign codes M35.81, Multisystem inflammatory syndrome, and Z20.822, Contact with and (suspected) exposure to COVID-19.

Additional codes should be assigned for any associated complications of MIS.

COVID-19 infection in pregnancy, childbirth, and the puerperium

During pregnancy, childbirth or the puerperium, when COVID-19 is the reason for admission/encounter, code O98.5-, Other viral diseases complicating pregnancy, childbirth and the puerperium, should be sequenced as the principal/first-listed diagnosis, and code U07.1, COVID-19, and the appropriate codes for associated manifestation(s) should be assigned as additional diagnoses. Codes from Chapter 15 always take sequencing priority.

If the reason for admission/encounter is unrelated to COVID-19 but the patient tests positive for COVID-19 during the admission/encounter, the appropriate code for the reason for admission/encounter should be sequenced as the principal/first- listed diagnosis, and codes O98.5- and U07.1, as well as the appropriate codes for associated COVID-19 manifestations, should be assigned as additional diagnoses.

Post COVID-19 condition, unspecified (U09.9)

This code is not to be used in cases that are still presenting with active COVID-19. However, an exception is made in cases of re-infection with COVID-19, occurring with a condition related to prior COVID-19, according to Tabular instruction. When assigning code U09.9, you must code first the specific condition related to COVID-19 if known.

CHAPTER 22: CODES FOR SPECIAL PURPOSES (U00-U85)

This chapter contains the following blocks:
U00-U49 Provisional assignment of new diseases of uncertain etiology or emergency use

Provisional assignment of new diseases of uncertain etiology or emergency use (U00-U49)

4 U07 Emergency use of U07

SP + U07.0 Vaping-related disorder
Dabbing related lung damage
Dabbing related lung injury
E-cigarette, or vaping, product use associated lung injury [EVALI]
Electronic cigarette related lung damage
Electronic cigarette related lung injury
Use additional code to identify manifestations, such as:
abdominal pain (R10.84)
acute respiratory distress syndrome (J80)
diarrhea (R19.7)
drug-induced interstitial lung disorder (J70.4)
lipoid pneumonia (J69.1)
weight loss (R63.4)

GUIDELINES **Section I.C.10.e.**
For patients presenting with condition(s) related to vaping, assign code U07.0, Vaping-related disorder, as the principal diagnosis. For lung injury due to vaping, assign only code U07.0. Assign additional codes for other manifestations, such as acute respiratory failure (subcategory J96.0-) or pneumonitis (code J68.0).

Associated respiratory signs and symptoms due to vaping, such as cough, shortness of breath, etc., are not coded separately, when a definitive diagnosis has been established. However, it would be appropriate to code separately any gastrointestinal symptoms, such as diarrhea and abdominal pain.

DEFINITION E-cigarette or vaping product use associated lung injury (EVALI) is the lung disease linked to vaping. Symptoms include cough, shortness of breath, acute respiratory distress, chest pain, fever, stomach pain, diarrhea, nausea, vomiting and weight loss. Damaging lung effects can be so severe as to stop the lungs from functioning. It is thought that vitamin E acetate or other harmful chemical byproduct produced by the heated liquid disrupt the lung's surfactant lining or otherwise interferes with the lung's ability to expand. Treatment includes the use of a ventilator or supplemental oxygen depending on illness severity; corticosteroids to reduce inflammation; and antibiotics or antivirals until test results for EVALI are finalized.

SP SL + U07.1 COVID-19
Use additional code to identify pneumonia or other manifestations, such as:
pneumonia due to COVID-19 (J12.82)

EXCLUDES 2 coronavirus as the cause of diseases classified elsewhere (B97.2-)
coronavirus infection, unspecified (B34.2)
pneumonia due to SARS-associated coronavirus (J12.81)

GUIDELINES **Section I.C.1.g.1)(c)(i)**
For a patient with pneumonia confirmed as due to COVID-19, assign codes U07.1, COVID-19, and J12.82, Pneumonia due to coronavirus disease 2019.

GUIDELINES **Section I.C.1.g.1)(c)(v)**
For acute respiratory failure due to COVID-19, assign code U07.1, and code J96.0-, Acute respiratory failure.

GUIDELINES **Section I.C.1.g.1)(d)**
When the reason for the encounter/admission is a non-respiratory manifestation (e.g., viral enteritis) of COVID-19, assign code U07.1, COVID-19, as the principal/first-listed diagnosis and assign code(s) for the manifestation(s) as additional diagnoses.

GUIDELINES **Section I.C.1.g.1)(l)**
For individuals with multisystem inflammatory syndrome (MIS) and COVID-19, assign code U07.1, COVID-19, as the principal/first-listed diagnosis and assign code M35.81, Multisystem inflammatory syndrome, as an additional diagnosis.

GUIDELINES **Section I.C.1.g.1)(g)**
For patients presenting with any signs/symptoms associated with COVID-19 (such as fever, etc.) but a definitive diagnosis has not been established, assign the appropriate code(s) for each of the presenting signs and symptoms such as: R05 (Cough), R06.02 (Shortness of breath), R50.9 (Fever, unspecified).

If a patient with signs/symptoms associated with COVID-19 also has an actual or suspected contact with or exposure to someone who has COVID-19, assign Z20.822, Contact with and (suspected) exposure to COVID-19, as an additional code.

Chapter 22
U00-U85

GUIDELINES **Section I.C.1.g.1)(a)**
Code only a confirmed diagnosis of the 2019 novel coronavirus disease (COVID-19) as documented by the provider or documentation of a positive COVID-19 test result. For a confirmed diagnosis, assign code U07.1, COVID-19. This is an exception to the hospital inpatient guideline Section II, H. In this context, "confirmation" does not require documentation of a positive test result for COVID-19; the provider's documentation that the individual has COVID-19 is sufficient.

If the provider documents "suspected," "possible," "probable," or "inconclusive" COVID-19, do not assign code U07.1. Instead, code the signs and symptoms reported.

GUIDELINES **Section I.C.1.g.1)(b)**
When COVID-19 meets the definition of principal diagnosis, code U07.1, COVID-19, should be sequenced first, followed by the appropriate codes for associated manifestations, except when another guideline requires that certain codes be sequenced first, such as obstetrics, sepsis, or transplant complications.

Section I.C.1.g.1)(c)
Acute respiratory manifestations of COVID-19 When the reason for the encounter/admission is a respiratory manifestation of COVID-19, assign code U07.1, COVID-19, as the principal/first-listed diagnosis and assign code(s) for the respiratory manifestation(s) as additional diagnoses.

CODING TIPS✓ Possible manifestations of COVID-19 are not assumed related. They must be linked to the COVID-19 by the physician or NPP.

CODING TIPS✓ If the provider documents suspected, possible or probable COVID-19, do not assign U07.1. U07.1 is assigned when the test results are positive, or documented by the provider. If test results are returned and are negative, the provider should be queried.

CODING TIPS✓ U07.1 is assigned as a primary code when the COVID-19 infection is the primary focus of care. Follow with the specified manifestations of the COVID-19, i.e., pneumonia. If COVID-19 does not meet the definition of primary, use U07.1 as a secondary diagnosis.

DEFINITION COVID-19, caused by the 2019 novel coronavirus, causes respiratory illness with flu-like symptoms that range from mild to severe illness and death. Symptoms may appear 2-14 days after exposure and include cough, fever, shortness of breath, or difficulty breathing in serious cases. Emergency warning signs for COVID-19 infection that require immediate medical attention include trouble breathing; continual pain or pressure in the chest; a newly altered mental state such as confusion or the inability to be aroused; and a bluish tint to the lips or face. The virus is spread primarily through contact with an infected person by saliva droplets or nasal discharge whenever the person coughs or sneezes.

★ 4 **U09 Post COVID-19 condition**

★ **U09.9 Post COVID-19 condition, unspecified**

Note:
This code enables establishment of a link with COVID-19.
This code is not to be used in cases that are still presenting with active COVID-19. However, an exception is made in cases of re-infection with COVID-19, occurring with a condition related to prior COVID-19.
Post-acute sequela of COVID-19
Code first the specific condition related to COVID-19 if known, such as:
- chronic respiratory failure (J96.1-)
- loss of smell (R43.8)
- loss of taste (R43.8)
- multisystem inflammatory syndrome (M35.81)
- pulmonary embolism (I26.-)
- pulmonary fibrosis (J84.10)

DEFINITION Any long-term physical, cognitive or psychological symptom or illness experienced as a post-acute sequela of a COVID-19 (SARS-CoV-2 virus) infection, generally persisting more than a month after the initial, active COVID-19 diagnosis.

Chapter 22 Scenarios: Codes for special purposes (U00-U85)

Positive COVID-19

A 68-year old female has been referred for home health therapy following hospitalization due to severe weakness with diarrhea and hypertensive urgency, which have now resolved. The discharge summary lists positive test for COVID-19 upon admission and NSTEMI occurring upon admission (now 16 days ago). The patient has a pre-existing diagnosis of hypertension.

Description	Code
Primary: COVID-19	U07.1
Secondary: Non-ST elevation (NSTEMI) myocardial infarction	I21.4
Secondary: Essential (primary) hypertension	I10

Coding guidelines require that when COVID-19 meets the definition of principal diagnosis, U07.1 should be sequenced first, followed by the appropriate codes for associated manifestations. This patient did test positive for COVID-19 and should be coded using U07.1 for this reason. If the documentation is unclear as to whether the COVID-19 is active or resolved, query the physician. This patient experienced weakness, diarrhea, and hypertensive urgency, which are all stated as resolved, so no manifestations remain. The NSTEMI that the patient experienced is within the past 4 weeks and can still be coded as an acute MI. Hypertension should additionally be coded due to its relevance to the current plan of care and impact on the overall prognosis.

Down syndrome, COVID-19, E. coli pneumonia

A 52-year-old man was admitted to home health 3 weeks ago with a diagnosis of COVID-19 positive with associated viral pneumonia, then re-hospitalized when his respiratory condition declined. He is now being resumed at home for care to continue recovery from a new diagnosis of E. coli pneumonia that developed from his already compromised respiratory condition. He continues to take oral antibiotics and will for several weeks. Inpatient medical records from this recent hospitalization report that the patient was re-tested for COVID-19 and was still positive at admission, but negative when re-tested at discharge. He has Down syndrome with severe intellectual disabilities.

Description	Code
Primary: COVID-19	U07.1
Secondary: Pneumonia due to coronavirus disease 2019	J12.82
Secondary: Pneumonia due to Escherichia coli	J15.5
Secondary: Down syndrome, unspecified	Q90.9
Secondary: Severe intellectual disabilities	F72
Secondary: Long term (current) use of antibiotics	Z79.2

This patient tested positive for COVID-19 and was diagnosed with associated viral pneumonia. While he was re-hospitalized and did have one negative test, the patient has been diagnosed with a subsequent bacterial pneumonia due to his respiratory compromise and his diagnosis of COVID-19 is not yet resolved based upon the available medical records and treatment plan. Per updated coding guidelines that took effect 1/1/21, for a pneumonia case confirmed as due to the 2019 novel coronavirus (COVID-19), assign U07.1 and J12.82. Because the COVID-19 and associated pneumonia has caused the patient's overall respiratory decline, it is coded first, followed by the E. Coli pneumonia.

His Down syndrome will impact his plan of care and is also coded. His severe intellectual disabilities are coded following the Down syndrome code, in accordance with tabular instruction. Since he will be taking antibiotics for several more weeks, the code for long-term antibiotic use is assigned.

COVID-19, Gastroenteritis, PE

A 58-year-old male patient with right upper lobe lung cancer was diagnosed with COVID-19 one month ago. He was sent home, developed shortness of breath and was re-hospitalized due to pulmonary embolism and viral gastroenteritis secondary to the COVID-19 infection. Home health services have been ordered for skilled nursing and physical therapy due to severe debility, new oxygen dependence, and infection.

Description	Code
Primary: COVID-19	U07.1
Secondary: Other viral enteritis	A08.39
Secondary: Other pulmonary embolism without acute cor pulmonale	I26.99
Secondary: Malignant neoplasm of upper lobe, right bronchus or lung	C34.11
Secondary: Dependence on supplemental oxygen	Z99.81

While this patient was first diagnosed with COVID-19 one month prior, the infection cannot be presumed to be resolved and the condition would be coded as current. Conditions should not be coded as sequela(e) of COVID-19 unless it is specified that the virus itself has been resolved and other conditions resulting from the infection remain. Q1 2021 Coding Clinic guidance specifies that non respiratory and other conditions related to a current COVID-19 infection should be sequenced after U07.1, so this is listed first, followed by the gastroenteritis and pulmonary embolism. The current lung neoplasm and new dependence on oxygen should also be coded.

Post COVID-19 Condition, Chronic Respiratory Failure

A 68-year-old female is referred for home health. Her records indicate she was previously diagnosed with severe COVID-19 in January 2020, hospitalized for 3 months, and while the infection resolved, she developed chronic hypoxic respiratory failure. She now presents after an extended inpatient stay for COVID-19 reinfection. Her physician has noted that she has "post-COVID post-inflammatory pulmonary fibrosis" as result of the reinfection but is no longer COVID-19 positive and will now need continuous oxygen due to the severity of her pulmonary conditions. She also has a history of hypertension and chronic diastolic heart failure.

Description	Code
Primary: Pulmonary fibrosis, unspecified	J84.10
Secondary: Chronic respiratory failure with hypoxia	J96.11
Secondary: Post COVID-19 condition, unspecified	U09.9
Secondary: Hypertensive heart disease with heart failure	I11.0
Secondary: Chronic diastolic (congestive) heart failure	I50.32
Secondary: Dependence on supplemental oxygen	Z99.81

This patient was infected with COVID-19 previously and developed a sequela - chronic hypoxic respiratory failure. She later was reinfected and suffered an additional residual effect of the second infection. A residual condition that persists after the causative condition resolves is coded as a sequela(e). Unless otherwise directed by specific code notes, the residual condition(s) are assigned first, followed by the sequela code. Sequela(e) of a COVID-19 infection that has resolved are coded by the assignment of U09.9, Post COVID-19 condition, unspecified, which notes to "code first" the specified residual condition related to the COVID-19 infection. While this patient experience two separate periods of infection, both are resolved, and she has sequela(e) conditions specified due to infection(s) that are resolved. Both residual conditions must be sequenced prior to U09.9, which may only be listed once. **Also note** that while U07.1, COVID-19 (active infection) is an excludes 1 condition to U09.9, there is a note indicating an exception to this at U09.9 if the patient has a clearly documented, specified, separate re-infection with the virus that is current following an initial infection that resulted in a sequela(e). However, in this case, the patient's reinfection is noted to be resolved, not active, so both infection periods are considered resolved infections with residual conditions, requiring the assignment of only U09.9 to identify the COVID-19 as the cause.

Hospice coding primer: Learn to code hospice claims accurately

Code ***all*** unresolved diagnoses on a hospice patient's claim, not just those that are related to the terminal diagnosis.

Hospices must report all diagnoses of the beneficiary on the hospice claim as a part of the ongoing data collection efforts for possible future hospice payment refinements. Reporting of all diagnoses on the hospice claim aligns with current coding guidelines as well as admission requirements for hospice certifications, CMS stated in its FY2016 Hospice Wage Index rule, and then reiterated in its FY2017 payment hospice rule.

The confusion over how to decide which diagnoses were related or unrelated, and therefore which diagnoses to include on the claim, was resolved in the FY2016 Hospice Wage Index when the rule instructed hospices to include every diagnosis.

The rule cited the importance of a comprehensive approach to hospice patients' care, the fact that a large majority of hospice claims still include only one diagnosis and the confusion about "related" versus "unrelated" diagnoses as reasoning for the rule change.

Data reported in the FY2019 proposed hospice payment rule indicates that hospices are acting in compliance with CMS's repeated request that they code every unresolved diagnosis a hospice patient has regardless of its relation to the terminal one.

In fact, analysis of FY2018 hospice claims show that 100% of claims included at least one diagnosis, 90% included at least two diagnoses, and 82% included at least three diagnoses, according to CMS.

The focus on and changes in hospice coding began with the forbidding of assigning debility (R53.81) and adult failure to thrive (R62.7), as well as unspecified dementia (F03.9-) and dementia manifestation codes (F02.8-) as ***primary terminal*** diagnoses starting Oct. 1, 2014.

Recall that if this directive is not heeded, hospice claims will be returned to provider (RTP'd) for correction.

As a result of this policy, there has been a shift in coding patterns on hospice claims. The top five most commonly reported principal diagnoses in FY2019 were G30.9 (Alzheimer's disease, unspecified), G31.1 (Senile degeneration of brain, not elsewhere classified), J44.9 (Chronic obstructive pulmonary disease, unspecified), I50.9 (Heart failure, unspecified), and C34.90 (Malignant neoplasm of unspecified part of unspecified bronchus or lung), according to the FY2022 proposed hospice rule. "Our ongoing analysis of diagnosis reporting finds that neurological and organ-based failure conditions remain the top-reported principal diagnoses," CMS stated in the FY2022 proposed rule.

Determine the primary diagnosis

Sometimes the primary hospice diagnosis as well as the documentation necessary to support it, is readily apparent. The patient may have terminal cancer, decompensated COPD, end-stage renal disease or Alzheimer's disease.

But other times it isn't so easy. For some patients, there is no one single diagnosis that is the primary reason for his or her terminal condition.

The patient may have several chronic diagnoses or symptomatic conditions that, when combined, are leading to the patient having a life expectancy of six months or less.

In these cases, it becomes a clinical decision, made by the hospice's interdisciplinary group (IDG), as to which of the diagnoses is the ***most contributory*** to the terminal prognosis.

Get back to the basics

Adhere to the ICD-10-CM official coding guidelines when coding hospice claims, or risk getting claims denials or additional documentation requests (ADRs).

Although some mistakenly believe that hospice coders don't have to follow these guidelines, they ***do*** apply to hospice as much as they apply to home health, and closely adhering to them is the best way to steer clear of trouble.

Here are examples of official coding guidelines to which hospice coders must pay particular attention:

- Do ***not*** report a Z code, such as Z51.5 (Encounter for palliative care) or Z48.812 (Encounter for surgical aftercare following surgery on the circulatory system), as a primary diagnosis, according to Chapter 11 of the Medicare Claims Processing Manual.
- Do ***not*** report diagnosis codes that cannot be used as the principal diagnosis, such as F02.80 (Dementia in other diseases classified elsewhere without behavioral disturbance). Note that F02.80 is a manifestation code that ***can only be sequenced after*** its corresponding etiology. *[I.A.13]*

- Follow sequencing instruction provided in the tabular. For example, you must assign E10.22 (Type 1 diabetes mellitus with diabetic chronic kidney disease) ahead of N18.6 (End stage renal disease) when diabetes is the cause of the end-stage renal disease, even if N18.6 is the terminal diagnosis, according to tabular instruction.
- Ensure that the documentation supports the appropriateness for coverage under the hospice benefit.
- Report any mental health disorders or conditions that would affect the patient's plan of care.

Scenario: Metastatic bone cancer

The patient is an 88-year-old female with a history of breast cancer that was treated 20 years ago with bilateral mastectomies, chemotherapy and radiation therapy and the cancer was thought to be resolved. She was recently hospitalized for a fracture of the shaft of her right femur that was determined to be the result of metastatic bone cancer consistent with breast cancer primary. She also has COPD, insulin-dependent diabetes and hypertension. She has a history of smoking two packs of cigarettes a day for 30 years, quitting approximately three years ago and has elected to go home with hospice care. Metastatic bone cancer is the primary terminal diagnosis.

Code the scenario:

Primary and Secondary Diagnoses		
Primary	Secondary malignant neoplasm of bone	C79.51
Secondary	Pathological fracture in neoplastic disease, left femur, subsequent encounter for fracture with routine healing	M84.552D
Secondary	Personal history of malignant neoplasm of breast	Z85.3
Secondary	Chronic obstructive pulmonary disease, unspecified	J44.9
Secondary	Essential (primary) hypertension	I10
Secondary	Type 2 diabetes mellitus without complications	E11.9

Additional diagnoses: *Z79.4 (Long term (current) use of insulin), Z87.891 (Personal history of nicotine dependence), Z51.5 (Encounter for palliative care)*

Rationale:

- ICD-10 guidelines state that when the cancer is the primary focus of care, it is sequenced first followed by the code for the neoplastic fracture.
- Because the primary breast cancer (Z85.3) was stated to be resolved, the code for personal history is assigned.
- Additional codes are assigned to capture all of the patient's current diagnoses, including her insulin-dependent diabetes, hypertension, COPD and smoking history.
- ***Tip:*** Include a code for a patient's current or past nicotine use when assigning certain respiratory and cardiac codes in ICD-10, including J44.9.

Scenario: End-stage renal disease

A male patient is referred to hospice for end stage renal disease. He has refused dialysis and wishes comfort care only. He also has hypertension, type 2 diabetes, PVD, COPD, coronary artery disease and angina. He is tobacco dependent, having smoked one pack of cigarettes per day for 40 years and continues to smoke.

Code the scenario:

Primary and Secondary Diagnoses		
Primary	Hypertensive chronic kidney disease with stage 5 chronic kidney disease or end stage renal disease	I12.0
Secondary	Type 2 diabetes mellitus with diabetic chronic kidney disease	E11.22
Secondary	End stage renal disease	N18.6
Secondary	Type 2 diabetes mellitus with diabetic peripheral angiopathy without gangrene	E11.51
Secondary	Chronic obstructive pulmonary disease, unspecified	J44.9
Secondary	Atherosclerotic heart disease of native coronary artery with unspecified angina pectoris	I25.119
Secondary	Nicotine dependence, cigarettes, uncomplicated	F17.210

Additional diagnoses: *Z51.5 (Encounter for palliative care)*

Rationale:

- Although the physician states the patient is terminal due to their end stage renal disease, the ICD-10 classification assumes a relationship between the hypertension, diabetes and end-stage renal disease. Hypertension and diabetes must be coded before N18.6, according to coding guidelines.
- The classification also assumes a relationship between diabetes and PVD in the absence of another stated etiology, and thus the diagnosis is coded with E11.51.
- ***Tip:*** Remember that in ICD-10 there is an assumed relationship between the coronary artery disease and angina and is captured by a combination code, I25.119.

Scenario: End-stage vascular dementia

A female patient comes to hospice care for end stage vascular dementia due to multiple CVAs. She also has oropharyngeal dysphagia and left-side dominant hemiplegia from the CVAs. She also has a history of chronic diastolic heart failure, COPD with chronic hypoxic respiratory failure, is on 4L/min of oxygen via nasal cannula, has a stage three sacral pressure ulcer and an unstageable pressure ulcer on her left heel.

Code the scenario:

Primary and Secondary Diagnoses		
Primary	Other symptoms and signs involving cognitive functions following cerebral infarction	I69.318
Secondary	Vascular dementia without behavioral disturbance	F01.50
Secondary	Hemiplegia and hemiparesis following cerebral infarction affecting left dominant side	I69.352
Secondary	Dysphagia following cerebral infarction	I69.391
Secondary	Dysphagia, oropharyngeal phase	R13.12
Secondary	Chronic obstructive pulmonary disease, unspecified	J44.9

Additional diagnoses: J96.11 (Chronic respiratory failure with hypoxia), L89.153 (Pressure ulcer of sacral region, stage 3), L89.620 (Pressure ulcer of left heel, unstageable), Z99.81 (Dependence on supplemental oxygen), Z51.5 (Encounter for palliative care)

Rationale:

- Coding guidelines require that the cause of the vascular dementia, CVAs in this case, be coded first. Therefore, this patient's terminal condition is coded first with I69.318 and then with F01.50. – *This article was written by guest editor Maurice Frear, HCS-D and is current as of the Manual's publication date.*

Code only confirmed diagnoses on hospice claims, stay in compliance

Hospice coders should not code "probable," "suspected," "likely" or "possible" diagnoses as if they were confirmed diagnoses, according to Q1 2016 Coding Clinic guidance.

This means that hospices may not code lung cancer, for example, in a patient who is suspected of having the disease but either refuses to or cannot undergo further diagnostic testing to confirm it.

Hospice coders are required to following the official coding guidelines. The exception mentioned in Section III, C that allows the coding of unconfirmed diagnosis does not apply to them, according to the Coding Clinic.

That exception is only for inpatient admissions to short-term, acute, long-term care and psychiatric hospitals, the Coding Clinic said.

This guidance aligns with the opinion of CMS's ICD-10 ombudsman Dr. William Rogers, M.D., who previously said that coding unconfirmed diagnoses in hospice is hard to justify and that signs, symptoms and other conditions should be coded in these scenarios to help support the patient's medical necessity for the hospice benefit.

This can be an issue for hospice coders in situations involving patients who elect hospice care due to suspected metastatic cancer, for example. But, the patient is either too frail to undergo further diagnostic testing or refuses it, says Brandi Whitemyer, HCS-D, independent home health & hospice consultant in Canton, Ohio.

Hospice coders have been left wondering how to appropriately capture why the patient is terminally ill, having to choose between an unconfirmed diagnosis and one, such as "lung mass," that is unacceptably vague, Whitemyer says.

Documentation is key to compliance

Ensure that detailed clinical documentation about the patient's health status and his or her appropriateness for hospice care accompanies a hospice record in which a vague diagnosis like "mass" is coded in the primary position due to a lack of diagnostic confirmation.

"Documentation is very critical in the situations when there is no specific diagnosis that can be reported in the principal spot. Therefore, the coder and clinician must be sure any other diagnoses, symptoms, clinical findings, diagnostic studies, etc. that support the patient's eligibility for the hospice benefit are included in the clinical record," says Judy Adams, HCS-D, president of Adams Home Care Consulting in Chapel Hill, N.C.

When hospice coder Maurice Frear comes across records where a patient is either too frail to undergo further diagnostic testing or refuses it, he assigns the diagnosis that is available, such as a "mass" and is sure to include any other diagnoses that are contributing to the patient's decline in six months or less.

These include conditions like malnutrition, anorexia and weight loss. It's also wise to include a code for the patient's BMI (body mass index) along with codes for weight loss, says Frear, HCS-D, coder for Bon Secours Home Health and Hospice in Virginia Beach.

To his knowledge, Frear has never suffered negative consequences, such as claims denials, for taking this approach.

6 more hospice coding tips

Tip: Make sure there's adequate documentation explaining why the patient or the patient's family has refused diagnostic testing or why the patient cannot undergo further testing to determine the etiology of the mass, for example.

Tip: Include a code for a history of cancer, such as Z85.3 (Personal history of malignant neoplasm of breast), if the patient has suspected metastasized cancer resulting from cancer previously thought to be eradicated. This will work together with documentation describing a mass that is suspected but unconfirmed cancer, for example, to further explain the patient's condition.

Tip: Don't assign a code from the F50.0- category (Anorexia nervosa) without a documented diagnosis. These codes refer to a psychiatric disorder, which requires a physician's diagnosis. The loss of appetite experienced by hospice patients, also referred to as anorexia, is a symptom code and is captured with R63.0 (Anorexia/Loss of appetite), according to the alphabetic index.

Tip: Avoid, if possible, coding unspecified diagnoses in the primary position on hospice claims. However, if you cannot get further detail about a diagnosis, make sure the medical record includes supporting information to show why the unspecified diagnosis is the best alternative to use as a principal diagnosis and how the patient qualifies for the hospice benefit.

Tip: Be aware of unspecified diagnoses, such as F03.90 (Unspecified dementia without behavioral disturbance), that CMS has already deemed unacceptable for use as primary hospice diagnoses. For a full list of unallowable terminal diagnosis codes, refer to CMS Transmittal 8877, which you can view at *https://go.cms.gov/1Vh1SBs*.

Tip: Attempt to get an attending physician and/or the medical director of the hospice to make that commitment to the cancer based on what else is going on, e.g. tumor markers, progression of debility.

Scenario: Probable metastatic cancer, anorexia

A 96-year-old woman elected hospice care after her doctor found a large mass on her lung that he believes is metastasized cancer resulting from breast cancer previously treated and believed eradicated 30 years ago. She has refused all further diagnostic testing and wants only comfort care. She has very little appetite, refuses to eat most days and has lost a significant amount of weight. Her BMI is now 16.

Code the scenario:

Primary and Secondary Diagnoses	
Primary diagnosis: Lung mass NOS found on diagnostic imaging of lung	R91.8
Additional diagnosis: Anorexia/Loss of appetite	R63.0
Additional diagnosis: Abnormal weight loss	R63.4
Additional diagnosis: Body mass index (BMI) 19 or less, adult	Z68.1
Additional diagnosis: Personal history of malignant neoplasm of breast	Z85.3

Rationale:

- While the patient's physician suspects metastatic lung cancer, the diagnosis hasn't and won't be confirmed with diagnostic testing, because the patient refused. Therefore, the primary diagnosis is the lung mass.
- Additional diagnoses that are contributing to her terminal status, such as her loss of appetite, weight loss and low BMI, are also coded to further support the admission.
- She has a history of breast cancer that her physician believes is the source of her lung mass. Because it was believed to be eradicated, the history code Z85.3 is assigned.

Do not assign fractures as primary hospice diagnosis, or risk auditor scrutiny

Avoid assigning a fracture code, such as S72.031D (Displaced midcervical fracture of right femur, subsequent encounter for closed fracture with routine healing) as the primary diagnosis on a hospice claim or you could risk a review.

This issue was non-existent in ICD-9 when fractures could only be captured with aftercare V codes (such as with V54.1x, Aftercare for healing traumatic fracture) and V codes weren't eligible to be primary hospice diagnoses.

But now that fracture codes can be assigned, some hospice coders are wondering whether a fracture could ever be appropriate as a primary hospice diagnosis. But it's not a wise choice, experts say.

It's unlikely that a fracture would ever be the main reason for a patient being in hospice care, says Brandi Whitemyer, HCS-D, independent home health & hospice consultant in Canton, Ohio..

Rather, consider what medical issues have resulted from or have been exacerbated by the patient's condition with the fracture and how these may have resulted in a terminal prognosis, says Whitemyer.

For example, a patient with a terminal diagnosis of metastatic bone cancer may have suffered a pathologic hip fracture due to bones that are weakened by the advancing disease, she says.

Scenario: Alzheimer's disease, fracture

A patient with Alzheimer's dementia fractured his hip after falling at home. He is now admitted to hospice as the patient's physician determined that the patient is not appropriate for surgery and the patient is no longer ambulating and his nutritional status has now significantly declined. He is no longer taking in any food by mouth. His terminal diagnosis is reported as Alzheimer's, with related diagnoses of left hip fracture and anorexia/loss of appetite. He is bedfast.

Code the scenario:

Primary and Secondary Diagnoses		
Primary:	Alzheimer's disease, unspecified	G30.9
Secondary:	Dementia in other diseases classified elsewhere without behavioral disturbance	F02.80
Secondary:	Fracture of unspecified part of neck of left femur, subsequent encounter for closed fracture with routine healing	S72.002D
Secondary:	Loss of appetite	R63.0
Secondary:	Bed confinement status	Z74.01
Secondary:	Unspecified fall, subsequent encounter	W19.xxxD

Rationale:

- The primary terminal diagnosis is Alzheimer's diagnosis, which should be reported as G30.9, Alzheimer's disease.
- It should be followed by the manifestation code for dementia in diseases classified elsewhere, F02.80. Note that when coding Alzheimer's, the manifestation code for dementia in diseases classified elsewhere, F02.8-, must always be additionally assigned, according to Coding Clinic.
- The fracture should be listed as well, due to the related nature of the fracture to the terminal condition.
- Also code the anorexia (R63.0) and a Z code for bed confinement status (Z74.01).Do not assign the 7th character "A" when reporting a fracture on a hospice claim.
- An external cause code, W19.xxxD, is also assigned to explain how the patient sustained the fall. It carries the same seventh character as the fracture code, in accordance with coding guidelines.

Use caution when assigning malnutrition as primary hospice diagnosis

Ensure there's adequate documentation explaining how malnutrition is causing a hospice patient's death, or prepare to see those records returned, or even denied.

For example, E46 (Malnutrition NOS) is not specific enough to communicate why a patient's life span is limited to six months or less, which is the requirement for the hospice benefit.

There have been reports of hospices getting denials for using malnutrition codes as a primary hospice diagnoses, says Judy Adams, HCS-D, president of Adams Home Care Consulting in Chapel Hill, N.C., who speculates that it likely began as a reaction from Medicare Administrative Contractors (MACs) to all of the sudden seeing a rash of claims with primary terminal diagnosis codes it hadn't previously seen before.

However, the issue has now become one of inadequate documentation, as the MACs are beginning to deny hospice claims that don't support why malnutrition is causing a patient's death, she says.

Part of the problem is that the hospice industry is not used to documenting at the level that Medicare wants to see to support these diagnoses, Adams says. In the past, their documentation has focused simply on how the patient is doing at each visit.

But what needs to be in the record, if the primary terminal diagnosis is something like severe protein-calorie malnutrition, is measurements of the patient's weight, his or her arm circumference, documentation about how the patient is eating, that his or her muscles are wasting away and skin is hanging, she says.

Additionally, do not assign E41 (Nutritional marasmus) for a patient who is diagnosed with "emaciation" or documented as "emaciated," according to Q3 2017 Coding Clinic guidance. Instead, you should assign R64 (Cachexia).

This is true even though the alphabetic index leads to E41 when searching under "emaciation." The reason for this is that the diagnosis captured by E41 refers to a type of malnutrition that occurs in infants and young children. If that's not applicable to the scenario you're coding, E41 is not the right code, the Coding Clinic said.

Tip: Don't assign a code, even if the alphabetic index leads you there, if it doesn't fit the particulars of the scenario you're working on, according to Coding Clinic guidance.

Hospice FAQ: What you need to know to avoid claim denials

Q: Can I assign "suspected" or "probable" diagnoses on a hospice claim?

A: No. If a hospice has a patient with a suspected or probable diagnosis but no other clinical information to support that diagnosis, the hospice medical director should query the provider who documented the suspected diagnosis for additional clinical information. Hospice coders should not code "probable," "suspected," "likely" or "possible" diagnoses as if they were confirmed diagnoses, according to Q1 2016 Coding Clinic guidance.

If no definitive information can be obtained, the hospice should assign appropriate codes for signs, symptoms and other conditions which lend support for the patient's terminal status and need for hospice care.

Q: Can I code debility or adult failure to thrive as a primary diagnosis on the hospice claim?

A: No, effective Oct. 1, 2014, CMS started to return to provider (RTP) all hospice claims that list in the primary position the vague diagnoses debility (R53.81), adult failure to thrive (R62.7), or an unspecified dementia code (such as F03.90, Unspecified dementia). These diagnoses can still be listed as secondary diagnoses however.

Also claims were returned starting on Oct. 1, 2014, for incorrect assignment of a manifestation code without an appropriate preceding etiology code, such as F02.80 (Dementia in conditions classified elsewhere without behavioral disturbance). CMS added edits to the Medicare Code Editor (MCE) to detect claims that reflect inappropriate assignment of primary and secondary diagnoses and incorrect sequencing of etiology/manifestation pairs.

Keep in mind that coding conventions and guidelines, to which hospices must adhere, require the assignment of an etiology code before its manifestation, such as assigning G30.9 (Alzheimer's disease, unspecified) before F02.80.

Q: What is the etiology-manifestation convention?

A: An etiology is an underlying condition that can cause other diseases, or manifestations. Diabetic chronic kidney disease is an example of an etiology-manifestation pair. Diabetes is the etiology, or underlying cause, of the chronic kidney disease, the manifestation. The etiology-manifestation convention requires you to sequence the code for the etiology (for example, E11.22 for Type 2 diabetes mellitus with diabetic chronic kidney disease) ***immediately before*** you assign the code for the manifestation (such as N18.6 for end-stage renal disease).

Q: What do I do if a hospice patient has multiple diagnoses but none of them is singularly responsible for the patient's life expectancy being six months or less, and the physician says the terminal diagnosis is "debility"?

A: Go back to the hospice interdisciplinary group (IDG), which should include the physician, and explain that CMS will send back the claim if it has a primary diagnosis of debility. Then, have the group list all of the conditions and symptoms that are contributing to the patient's terminal prognosis and decide which of those is the ***most contributory*** toward the patient's terminal state.

For example, a patient may be severely debilitated by end-stage liver disease, congestive heart failure (CHF) and chronic obstructive pulmonary disease (COPD). Though none of the conditions by itself may cause death, together they are leading to her severe debility. In cases like these, if the IDG determines that the CHF is the condition most responsible for exacerbating the other two and therefore causing death, code the CHF in the primary position and include the other diagnoses, including debility if desired, as secondary conditions.

Q: How do I determine whether a condition is "related" to a patient's terminal diagnosis?

A: You don't need to spend time trying to figure this out. In its FY2016 hospice wage index, CMS said to code every unresolved condition a hospice patient has whether it's related or unrelated to the terminal diagnosis. CMS then reiterated this directive in its FY2017 hospice rule. This directive clarifies previous guidance to include comorbid diagnoses that are related to the terminal condition on hospice claims.

Q: Many times hospice patients have a lot of trouble with eating — they either cannot eat or have simply stopped eating. How do I code this? Does R63.0 (Loss of appetite) cover it or is there something else?

A: Search for the most specific diagnosis to capture a hospice patient's eating difficulties. Consider the malnutrition codes available in the code set's nutritional deficiencies section; for example code E43 (Other severe protein calorie malnutrition). Symptom codes, such as R63.0 (Loss of appetite) may be assigned if a definitive diagnosis cannot be reached. You may also want to include codes for weight loss (R63.4) and a low BMI (Z68.-) if these apply.

While the symptom codes mentioned above can be assigned as the primary diagnosis on hospice claims without the risk of being returned to provider, the reason for the loss of appetite, for example, should be determined and coded when known. Be sure to verify all diagnoses with the physician before coding them.

Q: What if the hospice patient's chart indicates that the terminal diagnosis is a fracture; what should I code?

A: Look for another reason, such as a bone cancer, as it's highly unusual that a fracture would be a terminal diagnosis.

Discuss with the physician and the IDG whether there's another condition more appropriate for selection as the terminal diagnosis that may have put the patient at a risk for falls wherein a fracture would be sustained. Investigate what's happened to the patient within the past three to six months that has led to his terminal status.

Q: What if the patient's terminal diagnosis is listed simply as "dementia" with no stated etiology?

A: Seek to change the patient's terminal diagnosis through discussion with the interdisciplinary group.

Look for an underlying condition that may be responsible for the dementia, such as Alzheimer's disease or Parkinson's disease. If there's no known underlying disease, code the dementia as F03.90 or F03.91 depending on whether the patient has behavioral disturbance. Then, look at other conditions the patient may have that are contributing to his or her terminal status, and choose one of those conditions that is most contributory to the terminal status to list as the principal diagnosis making the unspecified dementia a secondary code.

And, remember that patients with unspecified dementia, adult failure to thrive, debility and other vague diagnoses don't have just one condition that is responsible for their terminal status, but rather a combination of conditions and factors that has led to their being terminal. It's the job of the hospice to identify and code every condition and diagnosis that's contributing to the patient's terminal prognosis.

Source: FY2014, 2015, 2016, 2017, 2018, 2019, 2020, 2021 and 2022 Hospice Wage Index rules; coding experts Brandi Whitemyer, HCS-D, independent home health & hospice consultant, and Judy Adams, HCS-D, president of Adams Home Care Consulting in Asheville, N.C.